D1187603

Companion to

Clinical Neurology

Companion to

Clinical Neurology

Third Edition

William Pryse-Phillips, MD, FRCP (Lond.), FRCP (C), DPM

Professor of Medicine (emeritus)
Memorial University
St. John's, Newfoundland, Canada

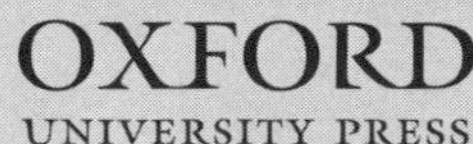

2009

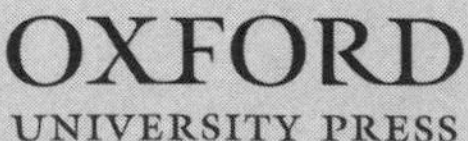

Oxford University Press, Inc., publishes works that further
Oxford University's objective of excellence
in research, scholarship, and education.

Oxford New York
Auckland Cape Town Dar es Salaam Hong Kong Karachi
Kuala Lumpur Madrid Melbourne Mexico City Nairobi
New Delhi Shanghai Taipei Toronto

With offices in
Argentina Austria Brazil Chile Czech Republic France Greece
Guatemala Hungary Italy Japan Poland Portugal Singapore
South Korea Switzerland Thailand Turkey Ukraine Vietnam

Published by Oxford University Press, Inc.
198 Madison Avenue, New York, New York 10016
http://www.oup.com

Library of Congress Cataloging-in-Publication Data

Pryse-Phillips, William.
Companion to clinical neurology/William Pryse-Phillips. — 3rd ed.
p. ; cm.
Includes bibliographical references.
ISBN 978-0-19-536772-0 (alk.paper)
Neurology—Dictionaries. I. Title.
[DNLM: 1. Neurology—Dictionary—English. 2. Nervous System Diseases—Dictionary—English.
WL 13 P973c 2009]
RC334.P79 2009
616.8003—dc22
2008043010

1 3 5 7 9 8 6 4 2

Printed in the United States of America
on acid-free paper

Foreword
to the First Edition

In these days of publish-or-perish, novelty seldom rises above the flat sea of new reviews and books that simply confirm what's already well known. Dr. Pryse-Phillips, however, has chosen a new tack and, in the process, brought us an astonishingly large, clinically oriented compendium of things neurological. In form, *Companion to Clinical Neurology* takes its place alongside such source references as the renowned and informative *Oxford Companions*. Its contents describe at varying length but with great clarity the phenomenological world of clinical neurology from its hesitant beginning over a century ago to its current vigorous strength. Ranging between brief, identifying sentences defining minor neurological facts to longer descriptions about diseases and their classifications, Pryse-Phillips depicts or explains neurology's bygone leaders as well as its symptoms, signs, syndromes, diseases, eponyms, operative procedures, and diagnostic tests. In the breadth of its topics the book has a gently nostalgic, British-Continental flavor of a more relaxed scientific day. Nevertheless, it by no means ignores American sources or recent contributions, including genetic classifications.

Certain features stand out. The *Companion* gives special attention to the clinical expressions and electrophysiological mechanisms of the epilepsies. The text also interestingly and informatively reflects Pryse-Phillips' longstanding interest in neurology's cognitive and behavioral aspects. But these are just a few of its extraordinary riches. Did you, the reader, know that although Munchausen's syndrome was named by Asher in 1951, the disorder's content had been described by Meige in his graduation thesis (Paris) in 1893? Or that the condition has three synonyms and three subsets? I didn't. Would you be surprised to find that ataxia has been defined in 41 different forms, or that it is included in 40 different identified syndromes? I was. These historic pearls and many others await the reader's eye, whether to entertain as nightly pre-sleep browsing or to act as a sourcebook from which to identify past foundations of tomorrow's neuroscience.

Companion to Clinical Neurology provides a remarkably thorough, pithy view of the world of clinical neurology and its close co-disciplines. With well over 15,000 entries and 5,000 references, it successfully reflects the prodigious (and nowadays rare) scholarship of its author. Within these pages the novitiate will discover the past richness of clinical neurology, and experienced neurologists will find informative explanations about all kinds of common and arcane aspects of their discipline's heritage.

In short, *Companion to Clinical Neurology* provides the best compact source I know in which one can quickly refresh one's memory about a fact well known or dig out a hitherto unknown item about the most philosophically and biologically interesting of all the medical specialties.

Fred Plum, M.D.

Preface
to the Third Edition

Impatient to recall where I had put the reprints of published diagnostic criteria that I had occasionally culled from the literature for, e.g., Parkinson disease, motor neuron disease and a host of other conditions in order to reassure myself of the validity of my clinical diagnoses, I conceived 20 years ago a plan to incorporate all of them in a booklet that might eventually be published. But then I felt it would be of interest to add some background; to define also the terms that we clinical neurologists use, or at least meet in our daily practice; to reinforce understanding with a little history; and to indicate resources that a clinical neurologist might now and then need to consult. What started as a 75,000 word work has turned into this, because neurology is expanding explosively; and because it was such an interesting task to try to define the whole vocabulary of our trade.

In choosing entries, I have had to be selective. This book contains what I think that I should know (and certainly want to know) or a least be able to access quickly. Readers will identify omissions, obviously; the whole field of neurology is beyond the compass of one individual. I must have missed or rejected some potentially valuable entries, but this is a very personal book, without the benefit of co-authors or editors as to fact. I apologize for any perceived errors of omission or commission and again I offer it with the hope that it will inform and occasionally divert my colleagues and that it will assist them in the care of their patients.

William Pryse-Phillips

St. John's, Newfoundland, Canada
January 2009

Preface
to the Second Edition

The kind comments of those who wrote reviews of the first edition of my *Companion* delighted me. I am particularly pleased that what was written originally for my own use as a practicing clinical neurologist was also found appropriate by so many of my colleagues and I was further honored when Japanese colleagues called for an edition in their own language.

The format of the book has not changed in this second edition. I have continued to list certain items twice if either of their two names seems likely to be the word or phrase that requires authentication, and have selected from some thousands of journal articles scanned only those definitions, criteria, or comments that were most meaningful to me. I have made comments that may not amuse the General Staff, but they come from where the action is: in the trenches.

Advances in neurology are occurring at least as fast as in any other area of medicine and I recognize that in the year between the delivery of my manuscript and its publication, new information will have been presented that will make some of my definitions passé. I ask the reader's forbearance. I also must restate the comment that I made in preparing the first edition of my *Companion*: "I have aimed [only] for reasonable completeness," suitable for almost all (but of course not quite all) the situations that the clinical neurologist is likely to meet in which an authoritative definition is required. The decisions on what to include and to exclude were mine, based on my experience and my enthusiasms, so this is a very personal compilation, stemming from my insights (and sometimes probably the lack of them) into the neurology of today that rides upon yesterday's shoulders. I offer it with the hope that it will inform and occasionally divert my colleagues and that it will benefit their patients.

W.P-P.

Preface
to the First Edition

A confused and equivocal terminology is the fruitful parent of confused and equivocal thinking.
—*Sir Francis Walshe*, 1947

One of the most difficult tasks for the beginning neurologist is that of understanding the jargon of the subject. It has been estimated that over 20,000 new words are learned or at least interpreted by a mature physician; a high percentage of them must be used in neurology. Not only derivations from Latin and Greek, but also eponymous disorders, names of chemicals, acronyms, neologisms, and pet-names spill repeatedly from neurologists' lips. Because they are not all widely known they often cloud meaning and impair communication, even though their original intent was to define, to categorize, or to distinguish concepts, clinical experience, or scientific truths.

Who were all these people whose names are attached to syndromes or diseases or tests? How do dysphagia and dysphasia differ? Why isn't Bell's phenomenon the same as Bell's palsy and why doesn't it involve the long thoracic nerve of Bell? Is there common ground in the definition of criteria for this or that condition? Such questions are naïve to an experienced neurologist, but need an answer when asked by students or by physicians who are not so trained, or by professional workers in allied disciplines.

Companion to Clinical Neurology is a personal endeavour to provide answers to questions like these. I have tried to incorporate within it some science, some art, some history, some practical experience. It is also a hive in which there nest numerous bees formerly resident in my bonnet and which needed more *lebensraum*. It is designed for the bedside and, I hope, for a reasonably low shelf in a room where a physician does his or her work. At least one reference is included for most of the entries delineating diseases, usually representing that publication on the subject which brought the material first to attention or one to which the interested reader may turn in order to receive more precise directions along the road to further knowledge; but in some instances it is to that paper on the subject which I most enjoyed reading.

The *Companion* is designed as a guide wherein the menu of neurological practice is laid out and from which suggestions for further reading may be obtained. I have assembled what I believe to be the best published definitions of neurological phenomena, and where none is available, have provided a brief description of my own. This is not a treatise on differential diagnosis; only, when a word or a phrase is encountered which is not fully understood, I trust that it will have been given a definition here, and in certain cases, some background to assist memorization.

My selection of items or names for inclusion has been on the basis of what problems I think a neurologist might expect to meet over the years of clinical practice. The major entry is in each case that name which I believe to be the one most commonly used, and therefore the most recognizable. Bracketed thereafter are synonyms also in recent use. Where words other than major entries are printed in boldface, this indicates that the item is itself a separate entry; italics indicate foreign words, emphasis, journals, or variants not entered elsewhere. Where two or more authors have given their names to a condition, the reference given is to that paper first appearing, or occasionally to that which corrected the errors of the first with such dexterity that the alternate eponym is preferable—as with Jakob and Creutzfeldt. However, where usage of the two (or three or, God help us, more) names has led to numerous variations depending on the order in which those names are placed, only that combination which seemed to me to be the most familiar has been included. The same restriction applies to the seemingly endless permutations of derived Latinisms, only a few of which appear. To save the bother of incessant turning of pages, brief summaries of some conditions are also included under their alternative names.

In this *Companion* I have aimed for reasonable completeness, but realize that neurology is too large a subject for one head to contain. Among the readers of this book there will be many with special knowledge which could lead to improvements upon some of the definitions that I have attempted here; their offers of contributions would be accepted with delight and acknowledged with gratitude.

W.P-P.

Acknowledgments

Over the years that I wrote the first edition of this book, many people gave me help and advice. In particular I was fortunate in being able to access the private collection of medical biographies compiled by the late Mr. Austin Seckersen, formerly of the Bodleian Library at the University of Oxford. His generosity greatly speeded the completion of the work. The initial writing was done during a sabbatical year from Memorial University. I thank Lord Walton, then Warden of Green College, and the late Professor John Newsom-Davis of the University of Oxford for providing me with a visiting scholarship at Green College and with membership of the Oxford Department of Neurology.

Substantial assistance in the writing of the first edition was provided by Drs. Milton Alter, Peter Dunne, Roger Duvoisin, Joseph Foley, Andrew Kertesz, Wayne Massey, David Neary, Charles Poser, R. Mark Sadler, Patrick Sweeney, the late Professors P.K. Thomas and Anita Harding, and Mr. James Woodrow. Mr. Theo Dunnett of the Bodleian Library provided skilled help without limit in the location and selection of sources, particularly in the production of the illustrations in the second edition. Many corrections and additions were suggested by Dr. Homer J. Moore. To all I repeat my hearty thanks.

In some instances an original reference was not available to me; I acknowledge again with pleasure (and with admiration) the work of Dr. Michael Baraitser and Dr. Robin Winter and their colleagues which led to the publication of the London Neurogenetic Database; this and the encyclopedic works of Dr. Victor McKusick and (through his superb Web site) Dr. Alan Pestronk provided me with data on, and analyses of, many disorders that I would otherwise failed to catalogue.

The transformation of the second to the third edition has required over a year of full-time effort, aided by the Internet and the assistance of scholarly peers. I wish to record again my debt to Dr. Alan Pestronk of Washington University, St. Louis, United States, for his generous permission to access and use the comprehensive material on his Internet site, mentioned throughout the text; to Dr. Chrysostom Panayiotopoulos of the University of London, UK for his similar permission to abstract entries from his masterly book *Epileptic Syndromes and their Treatment*; and to Professor George Ebers of the University of Oxford for his kindness in allowing me access to his personal library. I am also grateful to the reviewers of the two preceding editions, to many colleagues for their kind comments and suggestions and to Dr. Chern Lim, currently (2009) a senior resident in our neurology program, who assisted me greatly in the discovery and analysis of many of the Web sites listed here.

I am most grateful to Dr. John Noseworthy, the American Academy of Neurology and Lippincott Williams and Wilkins for their generous permission to use material from *Neurology*; and to the American Academy of Sleep Medicine, the American Medical Association, the British Medical Association, the Canadian Journal of Neurological Sciences, Elsevier Science, the International Headache Society and Wiley-Blackwell Publications, the International League Against Epilepsy, the United States Government, and the World Health Organization for their generosity in the matter of fees for reproducing much or all of their copyrighted material. The entries here taken from the American Association of Neuromuscular and Electrodiagnostic Medicine's Glossary of Terms in Electrodiagnostic Medicine © 2001 are reproduced by their generous permission. Without all of this gracious support, another edition of the *Companion* would have been impossible to produce. Again, I offer my sincere thanks.

I gladly acknowledge my debt to Oxford University Press (a not-or-profit publisher) and to my editors Craig Panner and David D'Addona for their confidence in the book and for enhancing it through their advice, their skills, and their gentle criticisms.

And I thank my family, Gwyneth, Amy, and Sam, for their continual support and for understanding the realities even of a retired academic life.

William Pryse-Phillips

St. John's, Newfoundland, Canada
January 2009

Abbreviations

used in this book

AAN	American Academy of Neurology
AANEM	American Academy of Neuromuscular and Electrodiagnostic Medicine
AASM	American Academy of Sleep Medicine
ADEM	Acute disseminated encephalomyelitis
AIDS	acquired immunodeficiency disease
AIP	Acute inflammatory polyneuropathy
AK	Dr. Andrew Kertesz
ASDA	American Sleep Disorders Association
AVM	arteriovenous malformation
BPPV	benign positional paroxysmal vertigo
CDH	Chronic daily headache
Chr	chromosome
CIDP	Chronic inflammatory demyelinating polyneiropathy
CK	creatine kinase
CNS	central nervous system
CMAP	compound muscle action potential
CMD	Congenital muscular dystrophies
CP	cerebral palsy
CPTase	carnitine palmitoyl transferase
CT	computed (axial) tomography
CSF	cerebrospinal fluid
DLB	Dementia with Lewy bodies
DSM	*Diagnostic and Statistical Manual of the American Psychiatry Association*
EEG	electroencephalogram
EDX	Electrodiagnosis
EMG	electromyo(gram)graph
EWM	Dr. E Wayne Massey
FIRDA	Frontal intermittent rhythmic delta activity
g	gram
GAD	Glutamic acid dehydrogenase
GTCS	generalized tonic clonic seizures
HWM	Dr. Homer Moore
h.	hour
Hz	Hertz (cycles/second)
ICD-10	International classification of disease, version 10
IASP	International Association for the Study of Pain
ICHD	International Classification of Headache Disorders
IFCN	International Federation of Clinical Neurophysiology
ILAE	International League Against Epilepsy
JF	(The late) Dr. Joseph Foley
LGMD	Limb Girdle Muscular Dystrophy
MAG	myelin-associated glycoprotein
mg	milligram
mm	millimeter
MOH	Medication overuse headache
MAOIs	monoamine oxidase inhibitors
MNCV	motor nerve conduction velocity
MRI	magnetic resonance imaging
NBIA	neurodegeneration with brain iron accumulation

NIH	National Institutes of Health
NINCDS	National Institute of Communicative and Neurological Diseases and Stroke
OCD	Obsessive-Compulsive Disorder
OED	Oxford English dictionary
PBI	Protein boung iodine
PDD	Parkinson disease with dementia
PME	Progressive Myoclonic Epilepsy
PNS	peripheral nervous system
QST	Quantitative sensory testing
RCD	Dr. RC Duvoisin
RMS	Dr. R. Mark Sadler
sec.	seconds
SNAP	sensory nerve action potential
SPECT	Single Photon Emission Computed Tomography
SSEP	short-latency somatosensory evoked potential
SSRI	selective serotonin reuptake inhibitor
VaD	Vascular dementia
VEP	Visual Evoked Potential
WAIS	Wechsler Adult Intelligence scale
WHO	World Health Organization
WISC	Wechsler Intelligence scale for Children

Companion to

Clinical Neurology

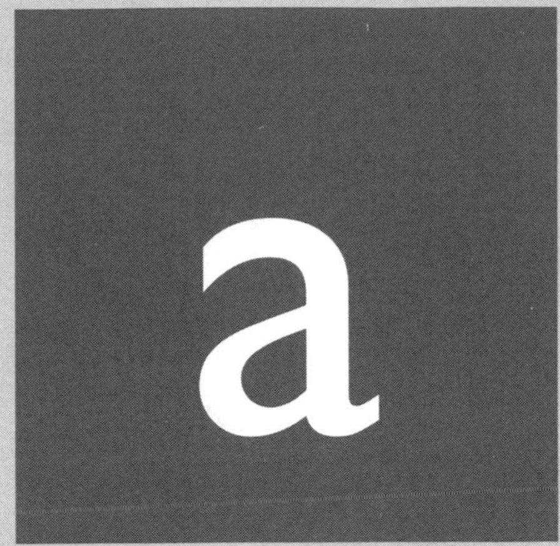

AAAA syndrome See **Allgrove syndrome**.

A band Dark, anisotropic, thick filaments in muscle which with the I bands make up a myofibril. Upon them is a dark transverse M-line surrounded by a lighter H-zone.

A pattern deviation A nonparalytic form of horizontal strabismus or **tropia** in which the visual axes are directed to closer objects (**esotropia**) as the subject looks up or separate (**exotropia**) as the subject looks down. Thus the horizontal deviation of the visual axes varies with the vertical position of the eyes. See also **V pattern deviation**, which is the reverse of this.

A test (Random Letter test) A simple test of **vigilance** in which the examiner reads out a random series of letters, and the patient is required to tap on the table with a pencil whenever a specific letter such as "A" is spoken.

A wave A compound muscle action potential that follows the M wave, evoked consistently from a muscle by submaximal electric stimuli and frequently abolished by supramaximal stimuli. Its amplitude is similar to that of an F wave, but the latency is more constant. Usually occurs before the F wave but may also occur afterwards. It is thought to be due to extra discharges in the nerve, ephapses, or axonal branching. This term is preferred over axon reflex, axon wave, or axon response. Cf. **F wave**.[19] (From the 2001 Report of the Nomenclature Committee of the American Academy of Neuromuscular and Electrodiagnostic Medicine and reproduced by kind permission of the Academy.)

A_1, A_2 electrodes The conventional terms in electroencephalography for recording electrodes placed respectively on the left and right ears.

A_c electrode The conventional term in electroencephalography for a recording electrode placed on the contralateral ear with respect to any other electrode.

Aase–Smith syndrome
A congenital dysmorphic syndrome characterized by cardiac and skeletal abnormalities, adrenal tumors, **holoprosencephaly**, **Dandy–Walker malformation** and hydrocephalus.[25]

AB variant A form of gangliosidosis characterized by deficiency of GM_2 activator factor, leading to the accumulation of GM_2 ganglioside. See **GM_2 gangliosidosis**.

Aβ-related angiitis (isolated or primary angiitis of the nervous system, ABRA, granulomatous angiitis) An idiopathic relapsing, focal, necrotizing, giant-cell angiitis of young or middle-aged adults, characterized by sterile inflammation of the small- and medium-sized intracranial, intraspinal, or intraocular vessels, exclusively.

Clinically, severe headache, lethargy and malaise, confusion with hallucinations, nausea, vomiting, seizures, or myelopathic signs appear first, followed by multifocal neurological symptoms and signs. Fever, myalgia, and arthralgia are uncommon presentations, as is that with subarachnoid hemorrhage. Abnormal cell and protein levels in the (sterile) CSF, the arteriographic finding of alternating areas of dilatation or constriction in any of the cerebral arteries, white matter hyperintensities on MRI, and the proliferation of mesenchymal cells in the intima and adventitia or in all layers of the vessel wall, with giant cells seen on leptomeningeal and cortical biopsy specimens, allow the diagnosis.[980, 5876]

The disorder is unlikely to be homogeneous; numerous etiologies may be responsible[1314, 2728] and it has been reported in association with sporadic, amyloid ß peptide (Aß)-related cerebral amyloid angiopathy.[5684] The following diagnostic criteria have been suggested:[123]

1. A clinical presentation with multifocal strokes or encephalopathy, with headache
2. Cerebral angiography shows changes consistent with vasculitis such as segmental stenosis, irregularity of small- or medium-sized vessels' lumina, beading, and an aneurysmal appearance, as above
3. Systemic infection, neoplasm, and toxic exposure can be excluded
4. Leptomeningeal or cortical biopsy demonstrates vascular inflammation and excludes other (such as infectious or malignant) causes of vascular inflammation

Reproduced by kind permission of the American Academy of Neurology and Lippincott Williams and Wilkins.

In *variant forms*, the spinal cord is involved rather than the brain; or children are affected;[3696] or uveitis, optic neuritis, or retinal vasculitis accompany the disease.

See also **isolated benign cerebral vasculitis**, **microangiopathic encephalopathy** (so-called; probably the same as **Susac syndrome**), **RED-M syndrome**.

Abadie, Charles A. (1842–1932) French ophthalmologist who practiced in Paris. He described alcohol injection of the Gasserian ganglion for **trigeminal neuralgia** as well as the **Abadie sign** (Dalrymple sign), retraction of the upper lid as a result of contraction of the levator palpebrae muscles in hyperthyroidism.[27]

Abadie, Jean-Louis-Irenée-Jean (1873–1946) French neurologist and psychiatrist who graduated with a thesis on the internal capsule and who became professor of nervous and mental diseases in Bordeaux. He described the Abadie sign in 1905; his other publications dealt with such topics as hysterical polyuria, epilepsy, **tabes**, and diabetes insipidus.

Abadie sign Loss of deep pain sensation, shown by insensibility to hard pressure upon the Achilles' tendon in patients with **tabes dorsalis**; it was said to have been the third most common sign in that condition. See also **Biernacki sign** and **Pitres sign**, both of which are also typically positive in tabes.

abasia An inability to maintain an upright posture, as described with **astasia** by **Blocq** in patients with hysterical disorders.[684]

abasic gait apraxia A syndrome resulting from small hemorrhages into the posterior internal capsule and/or putamen bilaterally, manifesting clinically as an inability to maintain the upright stance or to walk, although the muscle actions underlying these activities are unaffected when the subject makes the same movements while lying down.[5782]

Abbreviated Injury Scale An anatomic scale grading the severity of injury, developed by the Association for the Advancement of Automotive Medicine.[2293]

ABC syndrome (angry backfiring C-nociceptor syndrome) A fanciful term for what is likely to be the **complex regional pain syndrome**.

Abdallat neurocutaneous syndrome A congenital dysmorphic syndrome characterized by patchy depigmentation of skin and hair, spasticity, and sensorimotor peripheral neuropathy.[381]

abdominal epilepsy A nonconvulsive seizure manifesting as abdominal pain, vomiting, pallor or flushing of the face, and perspiration as the major manifestation(s) of a partial seizure in children.[1699] It is frequently associated with altered consciousness and brief and simple automatisms. Coexisting EEG abnormalities include bilateral spike-and-wave, polyspike-and-wave, low-voltage fast, and 10-Hz fast activity.[72]

abdominal migraine Recurrent attacks of abdominal pain, vomiting, pallor, and sometimes fever in school-age children who have a family history of migraine and who, in many cases, later go on to develop more typical migrainous features.[406] The pain is usually a diffuse burning or aching in periumbilical or epigastric regions and may have been preceded by well-recognized prodromal symptoms of migraine. The following diagnostic criteria have been defined:

A. At least five attacks fulfilling criteria B–D
B. Attacks of abdominal pain lasting 1–72 h (untreated or unsuccessfully treated)
C. Abdominal pain has all of the following characteristics:
   1. Midline location, periumbilical, or poorly localized
   2. Dull or "just sore" quality
   3. Moderate or severe intensity
D. During abdominal pain at least 2 of the following will be present:
   1. Anorexia
   2. Nausea
   3. Vomiting
   4. Pallor
E. Not attributed to another disorder

From the International Classification of Headache Disorders (Headache Classification Committee of the International Headache Society. *Cephalalgia* 2004;**24**[Suppl 1]) by kind permission of Dr. Jes Olesen, the International Headache Society and Wiley-Blackwell Publications.

abdominal neuroblastoma See **neuroblastoma**.

abdominal pain–nerve entrapment syndrome Unilateral segmental pain felt in the abdominal wall and due to entrapment of cutaneous nerves as they pass through its muscular layer, usually at the outer border of the rectus sheath. The origin of the pain is localized to a point below the examining finger, and it is worsened by tensing the abdominal muscles, as with trunk flexion in the supine position.

abdominal paradox Inward movement of the abdominal wall during inspiration, as seen in some cases of neuromuscular disease leading to ventilatory failure.

abdominal (muscle) reflex Contraction of the rectus abdominis and other muscles of the abdominal wall in response to a tap on the muscle itself at its upper or lower end. The reflex is not always found in the normal subject but may be increased in patients with pyramidal lesions above T6.

Numerous sites for the elicitation of the reflex have been described, including the rectus abdominis lateral to the umbilicus, the nipple, the symphysis pubis, the anterior superior iliac spine, the costal margin, or the thoracic wall. Another method described is to insert the finger into the umbilicus and to tap it.

abdominal (skin) reflex Contraction of the muscles of the abdominal wall such that the umbilicus is drawn slightly toward the site of a gentle scratch of the overlying skin in any of the four quadrants. It was first described by Rosenbach in 1876.

This represents a spinal polysynaptic reflex that is normally present, but it may be absent in pyramidal lesions at sites above T6, and in multiple sclerosis, because of diminished excitability of the spinal reflex center. It is seldom present after pregnancies, in the very obese, and in those who have had numerous abdominal operations. When the cord lesion is at T10, the reflex will only be present over the upper half of the abdomen. Further localization of a spinal cord lesion according to the presence of the reflex in upper, middle, and lower abdominal regions is of more theoretical than practical value.

abdominal reflex dissociation Augmentation of the **abdominal muscle reflex** with disappearance of the **abdominal skin reflex**; a sign of an upper motor neuron lesion above T6.

abducens (Lat, to lead away from) The sixth cranial nerve, described by Eustachius in 1564 and so called because it supplies the lateral rectus muscle which draws the eye to the side, away from the midline.

abduction The movement by which part of the body is drawn away from the sagittal line or a digit is drawn aside from the medial line of the hand. See also (ocular) **duction**.

abduction nystagmus (ataxic nystagmus, internuclear ophthalmoplegia) A form of dissociated nystagmus in which the abnormal movement is seen in the abducting eye either exclusively or else far more obviously than in the other eye, which may fail to adduct normally. See **internuclear ophthalmoplegia**.

abductor digiti quinti sign Slight abduction of the fifth finger on one side when patient with mild hemiparesis extend the arms out in front of them. When this is seen bilaterally, however, the sign has no significance.

The phenomenon was noted by **Wartenberg**, but he ascribed it to cerebellar disease. The **Souques sign**, in which all the fingers are separated, is similar, as is the **pinky finger sign**.

abductor laryngeal paralysis A dominantly inherited congenital syndrome manifesting as hoarse voice and dysphagia.

abductor sign A modification of the **Hoover sign** in which the patient is asked to abduct the legs at the hips rather than to flex them, in order to detect nonorganic paresis of the leg by the presence of contralateral synergic movements.[5953]

Abercrombie, John (1781–1844) Scottish physician who published the first book devoted to the neuropathology of both the central and the peripheral nervous systems, in which he classified three types of apoplexy (1828). He was also the first to describe **subdural empyema**.

Aberfeld syndrome A recessively inherited syndrome of myotonia, dwarfism, multiple joint contractures, facial dysmorphism, blepharophimosis, poor muscle development, and bone disease resembling **Morquio–Brailsford disease**.

aberrant regeneration The inappropriate redirection of fibers sprouting from a site of injury. This has been described most typically in compression of the third cranial nerve by an intracavernous meningioma. In this situation, retraction of the upper eyelid on downward gaze or adduction of the eye, restricted upward movement of the globe, and impairment of the pupillary light response are found.

abetalipoproteinemia (Bassen–Kornzweig syndrome) A recessively inherited, progressive ataxic syndrome of childhood or youth due to a deficiency of apoprotein B, which is an important factor in transporting lipids from the intestine to the plasma. The responsible gene is located at 4q24. The accompanying neuropathy is probably due to vitamin E deficiency.

Clinically, the disease resembles **Friedreich ataxia**, with cerebellar signs, ptosis, ophthalmoplegia, and sensorimotor neuropathy, but in addition pigmentary retinopathy and steatorrhea are found, low-density lipoproteins are absent from the plasma, triglyceride and cholesterol levels and chylomicron counts are low, and acanthocytes are found in fresh smears.[2754] See also **cerebellar ataxias** (*variants*), **hypobetalipoproteinemia**.

abiotrophic dementia See **Creutzfeldt–Jakob disease**.

abiotrophy (Gr, lack of + organism + turn) A derivation of Sir William **Gowers**, this term signifies the cessation of growth of an organ. It is used to label a process whereby the previously normal metabolism of certain cell lines ceases, frequently as an age-related process. The word was first used by Gowers in his discussion of the spinocerebellar degenerations. Garrod AE. In *The Inborn Factors in Disease* (Oxford, Oxford University Press, 1931) described them as "maladies, inherited and obviously inborn, in which there are no obvious tissue defects at birth nor in early childhood, but in which there appear, at some period in early life, signs of a progressive disease." Many hereditary cerebellar diseases, inborn errors of metabolism, neuropathies, and muscular dystrophies are included in this category and they form the basis of what Galton described as "the steady and pitiless march of the hidden weaknesses in our constitutions through illness to death."

Diseases labeled abiotrophic include **Huntington chorea**, adult-onset acid maltase deficiency, **Parkinson** disease, **amyotrophic lateral sclerosis**, and many more; but as the infective, genetic, or other etiologies of neurological diseases are progressively discovered, the blanket term seems to have less and less utility. Probably the last condition to warrant the name of abiotrophy will be such age-related changes as cortical cell loss resulting in memory impairment.

able autism See **Asperger syndrome**.

ablepharon Absence of the eyelids. In the most severe form, the skin of the forehead and the skin of the face are fused, but the condition may be incomplete or unilateral. Autosomal recessive inheritance has been shown in many cases.

abluminal Outside the lumen of a vessel, such as a blood vessel.

abnormal illness behavior See **hysteria**.

abnormal involuntary movement scale A five-point scale for the evaluation of abnormal involuntary movements affecting the face and mouth, the extremities, and the trunk, with an added global judgment of severity.

The assessment is based upon a formal examination in which subjects remove their shoes and socks and sit with their legs apart, their feet flat on the floor, and their hands on their knees or hanging unsupported. Opening of the mouth, protrusion of the tongue, tapping the thumb with each finger as fast as possible, standing, extending both arms in front, walking, and alternate flexion and extension of the arms are then observed and the abnormalities rated between 0 (none, normal) and 4 (severe impairment). The muscles of facial expression, lips and perioral regions, jaw, tongue, upper and lower limbs, and trunk are examined separately, and a global assessment is made of the severity of any abnormal movements and of the incapacity which they induce.[5136]

abnormal swallowing syndrome

Brief awakenings from normal sleep as a result of aspiration of normal secretions that have not been swallowed efficiently, leading to choking and coughing.[2628, 1629] See also **sleep disorders**.

abortive disseminated encephalitis

(Redlich encephalitis) See **encephalitis lethargica**.

About BFS

A Web site providing information on **benign fasciculation syndrome**. Web site: http://www.nextination.com/aboutbfs/.

abscess, cerebral

A circumscribed collection of pus within the brain. The first accurate account of the phenomenon was that of Hermann Lebert (1813–1878), a French physician, in 1856, although Sauveur Morand (1697–1773), a French surgeon, is credited with a successful drainage procedure for temporosphenoidal abscess in 1752.[5619] MacEwen performed the first modern procedure.[3996] An historical review was published by Garfield.[2284] See also **epidural abscess, spinal subdural abscess**.

absence epilepsy

(petit mal epilepsy, centrencephalic epilepsy, minor motor seizures, myoclonicastatic seizures, myokinetic epilepsy, typical absence attacks, pyknolepsy)

A seizure disorder in which the seizures consist typically of frequent brief (2–15 s) alterations in consciousness without motor accompaniments apart from fluttering of the eyelids, automatisms, or association with myoclonic or atonic seizures (*complex absences*). In all cases there is an immediate return to normal activity and mentation at the end of the attack. In *simple absence attacks*, there is only impairment of consciousness, although simple and limited motor activity such as eyelid fluttering may occur. An hereditary tendency is notable in some families.[3959, 1903]

The original diagnostic criteria of the ILAE have been reviewed:[767]

1. A form of epilepsy with onset before puberty (childhood AE), or before age 17 years (juvenile AE)
2. Occurring in previously mentally and neurologically normal children
3. Absences are the initial type of seizures
4. Very frequent absence seizures of any kind, except myoclonic absences
5. Absence seizures are associated on the EEG with bilateral, symmetric, and synchronous discharge of regular 3/s spike-and-wave complexes with normal background activity. Less regular spike-wave activity is possible, when compatible with a diagnosis of typical absences.

Typical and atypical forms are recognized. In the *typical form*, the clinical manifestations are as above, and the EEG shows generalized, synchronous, symmetrical 2.5-Hz (or more) spike-and-wave or multiple spike-and-wave activity. In the *atypical form* (see **atypical absences**) such activity is at <2.5 Hz or is >2.5 Hz but with irregular frequency or asymmetrical voltage; clinically the duration is greater and abnormal interictal records, multiple seizure types including myoclonus and loss of postural tone, mental retardation, and developmental delay are all more common, while automatisms are less so. Atypical absences may also be associated with other EEG patterns including small-amplitude fast activity or rhythmic, high-voltage 10-Hz activity. Substantial overlap occurs between the two varieties. *Myoclonic absences* are seizures with myoclonic components that are rhythmic (2.5–4.5 Hz) clonic rather than truly myoclonic, and that have a tonic component. *Absence status epilepticus* occurs in elderly patients without a prior history of epilepsy. See also **absence status**.

Distinctions have been made between **childhood absence epilepsy** and **juvenile absence epilepsy**. In the *childhood* form, the onset of brief spells occurring many times each day is before the age of 10 years, often remitting in young adult life. The EEG features are as above. In the *juvenile* form the onset is before the age of 16 and brief spells occur infrequently, but tonic-clonic seizures are commonly associated. The EEG shows generalized polyspike-and-wave activity triggered by hyperventilation and remission of seizures is uncommon.[4039]

In further *variant forms*, myoclonic jerks, versive movements, or atonic periods are associated, in which case the tendency for the typical or complex absence attacks to cease at puberty is not manifest. Generalized tonic-clonic seizures may also occur in patients with typical absence attacks,[2968, 2968] as may myoclonus.

The term was first employed to describe temporary mental confusion by Louis-Florentin Calmeil (1798–1895), a French physician, in his graduate thesis on epilepsy. See also **childhood absence epilepsy, Dravet syndrome, epilepsy with continuous spikes and waves during slow-wave sleep, epilepsy with myoclonic astatic seizures, frontal lobe epilepsies, generalized epilepsies with febrile seizures plus, epilepsy with myoclonic absences, perioral myoclonia with absences, idiopathic generalized epilepsy with phantom absences, idiopathic photosensitive occipital lobe epilepsy, idiopathic reading epilepsy, juvenile absence epilepsy, juvenile myoclonic epilepsy, Jeavons syndrome, Lennox-Gastaut syndrome, Landau-Kleffner syndrome, myoclonic status in nonprogressive encephalopathies, photosensitive epilepsy, reflex seizures and related epileptic syndromes, self-induced seizures, television epilepsy**.

absence status

(petit mal status, spike-wave stupor, nonconvulsive status, minor status) An epileptic syndrome characterized by clouding of consciousness, apathy or stupor with fluctuating confusion, interspersed with atonic or myoclonic head nods, fluttering of the eyelids or slight erratic myoclonus of the face or segments of the limbs, lasting from hours to days. These behavioral changes are accompanied by generalized continuous or near-continuous EEG abnormalities, usually comprising complexes of spikes and slow waves occurring at 3 Hz (2.5–6 Hz) and representing a change from the usual interictal EEG pattern. Incoordination resembling that of cerebellar ataxia may also occur. The condition is usually found in subjects with pre-existing generalized epileptic syndromes, such as the **Lennox–Gastaut syndrome**. See also **twilight states, status epilepticus, complex partial status.**

In a *variant form*, similar features appear in adults without any pre-existing seizure disorder, and they show rhythmic irregular spike-wave discharges on the EEG.[6279]

absent muscles The congenital absence of certain muscles such as the pectoralis, serratus anterior, latissimus dorsi, trapezius, supraspinatus, or thenar muscles. The more usual deficiency of the right rather than of the left pectoralis is unexplained. See **Souques syndrome**.

absolute refractory period That interval following depolarization of a nerve or muscle during which it cannot be excited by further stimuli.

abstraction ability The ability to discern the meaning or signification of ideas. The ability to think in nonrepresentative rather than in concrete terms, to form concepts, use categories, generalize from a single instance, apply procedural rules, and distinguish the properties of a part from the mass of the whole.

Abul Quasim Arabian physician of the tenth century whose writings contained the first known account of **experiential hallucinations** in epilepsy.

abulia (Gr, without + will) A state in which the patient manifests lack of initiative and spontaneity in normal consciousness. An apathetic blunting of feeling, drive, mentation, and behavior exists such that all actions are performed only slowly and after a delay.

Clinically, it is a sign of lesions such as a tumor affecting the under side of the frontal lobes, bilateral lacunar strokes, or **normal pressure hydrocephalus**.[4333]

Academy of Neurological and Orthopedic Medicine and Surgery A professional society. Address: 522 Rossmore Drive, Las Vegas, NV 89110. Tel: 702-452-9538.

acalculia Difficulties in reading, writing, and comprehending numbers and in calculating, usually accompanied by an inability to copy (**acopia**). The condition was described and named by Henschen in 1919. Lesions of the dominant frontal or parieto-occipital lobes are responsible. Hécaen[2825] defined three forms:

Aphasic acalculia. Impaired comprehension and writing of numbers, due to a lesion of the dominant hemisphere.

Visuospatial acalculia. Defective alignment of numbers and of arithmetic grammar, with retained comprehension of the numbers themselves.

Anarithmic acalculia. An inability to comprehend numeration and the principles of mathematics, often accompanied by other evidence of dominant hemisphere lesions. See also **anarithmia**.

acanthamoebocytosis Infection with *acanthamoeba polyphaga*, usually acquired from swimming in infected pools. The neurological complications include meningoencephalitis.

acanthocytes (Gr, thorn + cells) Red cells with a spiky outline, seen only in fresh blood smear preparations.

acanthocytosis The presence of **acanthocytes** (spiky red cells) in the blood; a finding in **abetalipoproteinemia, familial hypobetalipoproteinemia, amyotrophic chorea with acanthocytosis, HARP syndrome, Hallervorden–Spatz disease, mitochondrial cytopathies, Wolman disease**, and the **McLeod phenotype**.[2750, 6054] See **neuroacanthocytosis**.

acatalasemia A peroxisomal disorder without neurological features.

acataposis (Gr, not + to swallow) Dysphagia.

acceleration injury (cervical acceleration injury) A complicated pain syndrome resulting from sudden movement of the head and neck in relation to the rest of the body. The older term, ***whiplash injury,*** though more evocative, has now been superseded in the scientific literature (as has **railway spine**), but not here.

acceleration injury syndrome A post-traumatic syndrome of persistent neck pain, headache, dizziness and disequilibration, impaired concentration, irritability, and emotional lability following such an injury, usually caused by a motor vehicle accident. The underlying pathology, if any, is not determined.

accelerator nerves The sympathetic nerves to the heart.

accessory nerve The eleventh cranial nerve, so named by Thomas **Willis** in his *Cerebri Anatome* (1664) because he realized that it receives additional fibers from the C2–3 spinal roots.

accessory nerve palsy A focal motor neuropathy causing weakness and wasting of the sternomastoid and/or trapezius muscles. The most common cause is surgical trauma at the time of lymph node biopsy; blunt trauma is etiologically less common.[588]

accident neurosis See **disability neurosis**.

accommodation 1. In neuronal physiology, a rise in the threshold transmembrane depolarization required to initiate a spike, when depolarization is slow or a subthreshold depolarization is maintained. In the older literature, the observation that the final intensity of current applied in a slowly rising fashion to stimulate a nerve was greater than the intensity of a pulse of current required to stimulate the same nerve. The latter may largely be an artifact of the nerve sheath and bears little relation to true accommodation as measured intracellularly. (From the 2001 Report of the Nomenclature Committee of the American Association of Electromyography and Electrodiagnosis.[19] Reproduced by kind permission of the AANEM.)

2. In the older literature, *accommodation* was used to describe the observation that the final intensity of current applied in a slowly rising fashion to stimulate a nerve was greater than the intensity of a pulse of current required to stimulate the same nerve. The latter may largely be an artifact of the nerve sheath and bears little relation to true accommodation as measured intracellularly.

3. (ocular) The process whereby the lens changes its shape to refract more, and the pupil constricts as the eyes converge in order to improve the focusing of objects at a short range. Retinal blur is diminished and (as in the case of cameras) the smaller aperture improves the depth of focus. The power of accommodation decreases with age because of decreased power of the ciliary muscle and

decreased elasticity of the lens. The phenomenon was first described by Thomas Young (1773–1829), an English physician, at the age of 20 years.

accommodation curve See **strength-duration curve**.

accommodative effort syndrome Blurring of images with persisting near fixation, due to impaired ocular divergence with a normal near point for accommodation and convergence, and with an **esophoria** during near vision which is relieved by plus lenses.[5205]

accommodative insufficiency Impairment of accommodation for near vision, as a result of congenital or acquired causes; the latter include disorders both of the eye and of the central and the peripheral nervous systems and muscles.

acephalgic migraine (migraine equivalent) The occurrence of a migraine aura without the succeeding headache, more commonly seen in patients of advanced age. Symptoms of cortical or brainstem dysfunction occur, with gradual onset and are less than an hour in duration. In childhood, occipital seizures may cause the same symptoms. See also **aura, migraine without aura**. A familial form has been described.[5793]

aceruloplasminemia A recessively inherited syndrome affecting iron metabolism manifesting as cerebellar ataxia, early dementia, involuntary movements, retinal dystrophy, and diabetes, with absence of ceruloplasmin in the plasma.[3896] As a result of such Cp ferroxidase deficiency the subject is unable to oxidate the ferrous to the ferric form of iron.[6193]

acervuli See **psammoma bodies**.

acesis (from Gr, to heal) A cure.

acetylcholine Acetyl trimethyl-β-acetyl-ethylammonium hydroxide, a transmitter substance liberated from terminals of the vagus nerve (Otto Loewi, 1921), from parasympathetic synapses, and from motor nerve endings (Sir Henry Dale, 1933, 1936).

acetylcholine deficiency A variant syndrome of childhood **myasthenia gravis**, in which a deficiency of acetylcholine at the nerve terminals is due to a defect in resynthesis at that site.[2787]

acetylcholine receptor deficiency A recessively inherited myasthenia-like syndrome characterized by a marked deficiency of acetylcholine receptors and presenting clinically as bulbar, limb, and ocular muscle weakness from infancy and electrically marked by small miniature end-plate potentials.[1361]

acetylcholinesterase deficiency A rare variant syndrome of infantile **myasthenia gravis** in which the acetylcholine is not hydrolyzed after its release at the end plate, leading to prolonged depolarization and repetitive potentials following a single stimulus.[1876]

The clinical features resemble those of other forms of myasthenia with weakness and fatigability of the bulbar, extraocular, and spinal musculature, but EMG studies reveal repetitive muscle action potentials in response to single nerve stimulation as well as the usual decrementing response to repetitive stimuli.

achalasia Failure of relaxation of any kind of hollow tube, as in the case of degeneration of Auerbach's plexus in the esophagus, which leads to impaired esophageal contractions presenting clinically as dysphagia or vomiting. The condition usually occurs in infancy.[4397]

achalasia and microcephaly A congenital syndrome characterized by this disorder of esophageal motility, with accompanying microcephaly and mental and developmental delay.[381]

Achard–Foix–Mouzon syndrome Reduction of the number of lumbar or sacrococcygeal vertebrae usually associated with a **conus medullaris syndrome** and sometimes causing leg weakness as well.[43]

achee See **akee**.

Achilles reflex (triceps surae reflex) The ankle jerk.

Achilles tendon The gastrocnemius tendon inserting into the calcaneum, so named because of the association with Achilles' heel.

The fable underlying the nomenclature is that the mother of this Greek hero held him by the heel when dipping him into the river Styx, a procedure conferring invulnerability to all those parts touched by the water. The heel was not protected and it was a wound to this region delivered by his enemy Paris that killed him. In these days of flourishing neuromythology, it is unwise to scoff at this kind of story.

Achillodynia (Albert disease, Swediaur disease) Pain in the heel due to Achilles' tendonitis. This was first described in 1893 by Edward Albert (1841–1900), an Austrian surgeon.[5619]

achondroplasia A craniofacial dysplasia in which the formation of enchondral bone is also deficient. The condition is dominantly inherited in 20% of cases. The major clinical features are facial dysmorphism, dwarfism, tripod hands, and lumbar lordosis. See also **Jeune syndrome** and **Ellis–van Creveld syndrome**, which are similar.

The condition was described by Parrot in 1878, but in greater detail by Pierre **Marie** in 1880.

ACHOO See **photic sneeze reflex**. Unlike most others, this acronym should have won a prize.

Achor–Smith syndrome A syndrome of acute skeletal muscle degeneration with profound weakness in the setting of prolonged nutritional deficiency manifesting features of pernicious anemia, sprue, and pellagra, complicated by acute diarrhea resulting in hypokalemia and severe renal insufficiency.

achromasia (Gr,. lack of + color) The impaired uptake of chemical stains by cells undergoing chromatolysis.

achromatic Having or producing no color; a term applied to those lenses which cause no color dispersion.

achromatopsia (Gr, lack of + color + eyesight) (color blindness, cortical or central achromatopsia) An acquired disorder of color perception involving all or part of the visual field, with preservation of vision for form. The retinal color receptors are not affected. The condition is frequently associated with visual agnosia and with a field defect. It is caused by focal damage to the visual association cortex or its subjacent white matter.[1430] See also **dyschromatopsia, cone dystrophy**.

In a *variant form*, the same problem is inherited as an X-linked deficit.

acid albumen turbidity test A screening test for the detection of mucopolysaccharides in blood or urine.

acid maltase (δ 1,4- and δ 1,6-glucosidase) A lysosomal enzyme which hydrolyzes glycogen, maltose, and other oligosaccharides to yield free glucose, deficient in **glycogen storage disease** type II due to a defective GAA gene.

acid maltase deficiency A syndrome of muscle weakness with respiratory difficulty due to lymphocyte α-glucosidase deficiency. See **glycogen storage diseases**.

acid phosphatase deficiency A recessively inherited syndrome of intermittent vomiting, hypotonia, lethargy, and opisthotonus, with death in early infancy, due to deficiency of lysosomal acid phosphatase.[4570]

acidemia See **organic acidemia**.

Ackerman's angle A measurement at the skull base, considered characteristic in encephalocele and hydrocephalus but not now in use. It was described in 1882 by Konrad Ackerman (1825–1896), a German pathologist who was a professor at Rostock.

acne fulminans with inflammatory myopathy A syndrome characterized by the sudden onset of severe ulcerative acne on the chest, back, and face, associated with fever and leukocytosis and accompanied by pain in the pelvic girdle muscles with wasting, myalgia, and arthralgia but with normal serum creatine kinase levels.[4711]

acopia Difficulty in making a copy on paper from a printed or written text, regardless of whether reading is affected or not.

acoria (aplestia) Inability to attain satiety after eating.

Acosta disease See **acute mountain sickness**.

acoustic EMG (AMG; acoustic myography) A record of the sounds emitted by muscles during their contraction as a result of mechanical vibrations set up within the muscle. The mean frequency of the sounds increases in parallel with the contractile force derived. The technique is used in monitoring fatigue and force of contraction and in the control of prosthetic devices.[422, 19]

acoustic myography See **acoustic EMG**.

acoustic neuroma A benign tumor of the vestibular portion of the eighth cranial nerve, and actually a Schwannoma. It was first described by **Cushing** in 1917,[1390] and it accounts for 5–10% of all intracranial tumors.

Clinically, hearing loss, tinnitus, and dysequilibrium lead on to headache, incoordination, and imbalance, involvement of the adjacent cranial nerves, and eventually symptoms of increased intracranial pressure and bulbar symptoms. The use of **computerized axial tomography, magnetic resonance imaging** and **brainstem auditory-evoked responses** in the diagnosis of the condition has been reviewed.[2785]

Relevant Web sites are http://www.ucsf.edu/nreview/06.4-Oncology-Histological Type/AcousticNeuroma.html, which details the epidemiology, pathology, and clinical features of this condition, the Australian **Acoustic Neuroma Association NSW Inc.** http://www.acousticneuroma.com.au/. See also **Acoustic Neuroma Association** and **Acoustic Neuroma Association of Canada**.

Acoustic Neuroma Association A charitable organization in this field. Address: 600 Peachtree Parkway, Suite 108, Cumming, GA 30041. E-mail: anusa@aol.com. Web site: http://www.anausa.org.

Acoustic Neuroma Association of Canada A charitable organization. Address: P.O. Box 369, Edmonton, Alberta, Canada T5J 2J6. Tel: 403-428-3384. Web site: http://www.anac.ca.

acoustic reflex Contraction of the stapedius muscles bilaterally in response to a loud sound, recorded by measuring the acoustic impedance in the ear. The quietest sound producing such a contraction is known as the *acoustic threshold*; it is elevated in lesions of the cochlear nerve, but also with VII cranial nerve or middle ear disease.

acoustic startle reflex Violent muscle jerks (e.g., in the biceps muscle) following an unexpected sound stimulus, as in **stiff person syndrome** and **hyperekplexia**, and also in some patients with stroke or spinal cord injury.

acoustic threshold See **acoustic reflex**.

acousticomotor seizures See **startle epilepsy**.

acousticopalpebral reflex See **palpebral reflex**.

acquired central alveolar hypoventilation A syndrome of hypoventilation occurring during sleep, typically related to bilateral posterolateral medullary lesions, which are most often vascular occlusions.[1616]

acquired epileptic aphasia See **Landau–Kleffner syndrome**.

acquired fixation nystagmus See **acquired nystagmus, fixation nystagmus**.

acquired generalized repetitive myoclonus An atypical generalized whole-body tremor syndrome actually due to repetitive low-amplitude myoclonus (polymyoclonus) as shown by the absence of true periodicity on surface electromyography. Clinically, the onset of tremor or gait disturbance is usually subacute, in middle life. Surface EMG shows nonperiodic muscle bursts lasting less than 50 ms as is typical of myoclonus. Causes include autoimmunity and drug-induced toxicity.[4240]

acquired hepatocerebral encephalopathy (portosystemic shunt encephalopathy, non-Wilsonian hepatocerebral degeneration) A cerebral degenerative disease complicating chronic liver failure and producing a syndrome of drowsiness, impaired memory, ataxia, dysarthria, asterixis, choreoathetosis, and progressive dementia. The pathological hallmarks of the disorder are the presence of plump (Alzheimer Type II) astrocytes in the striatum, cortex, and dentate nucleus and of spongy changes in the third cerebral cortical layer in laminar distribution. The condition was described by Victor and Adams in 1965, although F. Morel had noted a similar condition in 1939.[4471]

A *variant condition* is *early childhood hepatocerebral degeneration*, in which progressive liver disease (the Huttenlocher variant of **Alpers disease**) and brain disease are manifest by recurrent partial, secondarily generalized seizures followed by mental and motor regression. The liver disease is exacerbated by valproic acid administration.[617]

In another *variant form*, the clinical appearances are those of **Wilson disease**, but the metabolic disorder affecting copper is distinct.[2421] See also **non-Wilsonian extrapyramidal disease**.

acquired horizontal jerk nystagmus

acquired horizontal jerk nystagmus The most common form of acquired nystagmus, subdivided between **vestibular** and **gaze-evoked** or **gaze-paretic** forms.

acquired immunodeficiency syndrome (AIDS)

acquired immunodeficiency syndrome (AIDS) Infection with the human immunodeficiency virus (HIV), a lentivirus which causes systemic and neurological disease, the latter by primary infection, malignancy, or through opportunistic infection. The various neurological syndromes produced have been classified as in Chart A–1 below:[6416, 4200]

Chart A–1. Neurological Complications of Acquired Immunodeficiency Syndrome

Opportunistic infection

CNS toxoplasmosis
Cryptococcal meningitis
Progressive multifocal leukoencephalopathy
Herpesvirus infections

Malignancy

Primary CNS lymphoma
Systemic lymphoma

Primary Infection

AIDS-related dementia (See **HIV encephalopathy**)
HIV encephalopathy
HIV myelopathy
Acute atypical meningitis
Acute sensory neuropathy
AIDS radiculopathy

See also **HIV-associated** conditions.

acquired inflammatory demyelinating polyneuropathies

acquired inflammatory demyelinating polyneuropathies Inflammatory demyelinating diseases of the peripheral nerves and nerve roots, often with extensive secondary axonal degeneration and resulting from immunological disturbances. Acute (**acute inflammatory demyelinating polyneuropathy**), chronic (**chronic inflammatory demyelinating polyneuropathy**), and dysproteinemic or paraneoplastic (**gammopathic neuropathy**) forms are described.[101]

acquired mutism

acquired mutism A condition of complete absence of speech that is not associated with other aphasic symptomatology or alteration of consciousness. See **mutism, cerebellar mutism**.

acquired myotonia

acquired myotonia See **idiopathic neuromyotonia**.

acquired pendular nystagmus

acquired pendular nystagmus A rare form of horizontal, vertical, or rotatory nystagmus in any plane with a quasi-sinusoidal form. It can be monocular or asymmetric. The phases are similar in duration in each direction, as a result of which there is no "jerk" component. It leads to complaints of blurred vision with **oscillopsia** and is often associated with a head tremor. The usual causes are cerebellar or brainstem disease, most likely due to vascular or demyelinating pathologies.[2574] It is also a feature of the syndromes of **oculopalatal myoclonus**,[308] **Whipple disease**, and drug toxicity.[26]

acquired slow-channel syndrome

acquired slow-channel syndrome See **myasthenia gravis**.

acquired verbal auditory agnosia with convulsive disorder

acquired verbal auditory agnosia with convulsive disorder See **Landau–Kleffner syndrome**.

acrocallosal syndrome

acrocallosal syndrome (Nelson syndrome, Schinzel syndrome) A dysmorphic syndrome characterized by unusual facial appearance, mental retardation, absent corpus callosum, duplication of the halluces, and mental retardation.[4624] Macrocephaly and clinodactyly are also common, and hyperreflexia with hypotonia is usual.[5609]

acrocephalopolysyndactyly

acrocephalopolysyndactyly The combination of cranial vault abnormality with polysyndactyly. At least four forms are differentiated[379]

Type I (**Noack syndrome, Pfeiffer syndrome**) A (dominantly inherited?) syndrome of acrocephaly, large toes with syndactyly, and brachydactyly of the toes and sometimes of the fingers.

Type II (**Carpenter syndrome**) The combination of acrocephaly, polysyndactyly, short stature, obesity, mental retardation (usually), and congenital cardiac defects.[5341]

Type III The combination of acrocephaly, syndactyly of fingers and toes, and other skeletal abnormalities.[5507]

Type IV A congenital dysmorphic syndrome characterized by acrocephalopolysyndactyly and craniosynostosis.[379]

Hootnick–Holmes syndrome is a further *variant form* characterized by webbed fingers, polysyndactyly, and craniostenosis.[2979]

See also **acrocephalosyndactyly**, **Apert syndrome**.

acrocephalosyndactyly

acrocephalosyndactyly Dominantly inherited syndromes characterized by the occurrence of both tower skull and fusion of digits. The distinction between some of the syndromes that follow may be artificial.[379]

Type I See **Apert syndrome**.

Type II Probably the same as **Apert syndrome**.

Type III (Saethre–Chozen syndrome) A congenital dysmorphic syndrome characterized also by low frontal hairline, ptosis, facial asymmetry, and soft-tissue syndactyly of the hands.[612]

Type IV (Waardenburg syndrome) A rare congenital dysmorphic syndrome characterized by genital, digital, and cardiac anomalies; acrocephaly; and craniosynostosis.[6251]

Type V (Pfeiffer syndrome) A rare congenital dysmorphic syndrome characterized by acrocephaly, hypertelorism with normal intelligence, and soft tissue syndactyly of the hands.[4127] See **Pfeiffer syndrome**.

Other *variants* without CNS findings are recorded.[379] See also **Carpenter syndrome**.

acrocephaly (Gr,. pointed + head) A developmental defect in skull shape such that the anteroposterior diameter is reduced, the occiput is flattened, and the forehead is high, as with fusion of both of the coronal or of all the cranial sutures. See also **Crouzon syndrome**.

acrodermatitis chronica atrophicans (Hopf syndrome) A chronically progressive dermatological disease in young adults, probably of tick-borne spirochetal origin and leading to widespread livid blue-red discoloration of the skin and later dermal atrophy.[2983] It is often complicated by an asymmetric sensory polyneuropathy.[4711]

acrodermatitis enteropathica See **subacute myelo-optico-neuropathy**.

acrodynia (Gr, the extremities + pain) 1. See **Pink disease**. 2. The distal limb pain felt in nutritional neuropathies and in ergotism. The term is now seldom used.

acrodysostosis A congenital dysmorphic syndrome characterized by short stature, psychomotor retardation, brachycephaly, thick calvarium, and hydrocephalus.[5869]

acrodystrophic neuropathy A sensory neuropathy causing painless plantar ulcers or trophic changes, often with destruction of the bones of the hands and feet.

In this group are the **hereditary sensory and autonomic neuropathies** and some acquired neuropathies such as those due to **leprosy**, **diabetes**, and alcoholism.[5502]

acrofacial dysostosis See **orofaciodigital syndrome II**.

acrofacial syndrome See **fetal hydantoin syndrome**.

acromegalic myopathy A syndrome of mild proximal muscle weakness with elevated levels of serum creatine kinase and associated with hypertrophy of both type I and type II muscle fibers in patchy distribution,[4155] sometimes seen in this condition of excess growth hormone production.

In a *variant form*, muscle hypertrophy is the only abnormality.

acromegalic neuropathy An uncommon, severe, debilitating, progressive peripheral neuropathy complicating hypothyroidism, with marked enlargement of the peripheral nerves and characterized by endoneurial hypertrophy and axonal degeneration.[6055] Features of the **carpal tunnel syndrome** may be the earliest presentation.

acromial reflex Flexion of the elbow in response to a tap on the coracoid or the acromion, present in upper motor neuron lesions affecting that limb[5333] and probably resulting from transmitted vibrations rather than from direct stretch of any tendon.

acromicria A skeletal deformity appearing in many congenital syndromes, characterized by smallness of the extremities.

acro-osteolysis with osteoporosis See **osteopetrosis**.

acroparesthesias Tingling sensations in the distal parts of the limbs, the classic complaint of people with **carpal tunnel syndrome** but also voiced by some with sensory polyneuropathies.

acroparesthesia syndrome See **carpal tunnel syndrome**.

acropathy Disfiguring damage sustained by the most distal parts of the body—the digits, ears, and nose, for example. This is seen in many mutilating sensory neuropathies,[6269] such as **hereditary sensory and autonomic neuropathies** and **leprosy**, as well as with cord lesions interrupting pain pathways, such as **syringomyelia**.

acrus The term of Hippocrates for the state of the body when it is at the height of its well-being.

acrylamide An industrial polymer used to form slurries. It is toxic to axons since it impairs the process of fast (bidirectional) axonal transport, leading to **dying-back neuropathies**.[175]

Acta Neurochiurgica A neurosurgical journal. Web site: http://link.springer.de/link/service/journals/00701/about.htm.

Acta Neurologica Belgica (*Acta Neurol Belg*) A neurological journal. Address: Association des Sociétés Scientifiques Medicales Belgiques, 43 rue des Champs Elyssées, B-1050 Brussels, Belgium. Web site: http://www.ulb.ac.be/medecine/loce/Acta_Medica_Belgica/journal/Acta_Neurologica_Belgica.htm.

Acta Neurologica Scandinavica (*Acta Neurol Scand*) A neurological journal. Web site: http://www.blackwellpublishing.com/journal.asp?ref=0001-6314&site=1.

Acta Neuropathologica A neuropathological journal. Web site: http://link.springer.de/link/service/journals/00401/index.htm.

actin A structural protein in vertebrate muscles.

actin-related myopathy An unique limb girdle–type myopathy marked by F-actin and thin filament–containing plaques within muscle fibers.

action myoclonus (intention myoclonus) Brief, sudden, arrhythmic, fine or coarse myoclonic jerks followed by a period of inhibition, excited by willed movements and startle, affecting variable muscle groups but usually those activated voluntarily and leading to fragmentation of contraction. It is the characteristic finding in the **Lance-Adams syndrome**.[3660] See also **myoclonus**.

action myoclonus–renal failure syndrome A recessively inherited syndrome in which patients present in the second or third decades of life with renal failure and/or neurological features. It is characterized by severe progressive action myoclonus on voluntary movement, a fine finger tremor (likely a **cortical tremor**), ataxia, dysarthria, infrequent generalized seizures, and renal impairment presenting with as proteinuria and progressing to renal failure due to a glomerulopathy and requiring transplantation by the third decade. There is no mental involvement.[188, 329] The EEG shows spike and spike–wave complexes syndrome indicating cortical hyperexcitability as in cortical myoclonus.

Effective treatment of the renal failure extends the lifespan but does not improve the neurological signs. See also **uremic encephalopathy**.

action myotonia Delayed muscle relaxation following voluntary contraction of the muscle.

action potential (AP) The brief regenerative electric potential that propagates along a single axon or muscle fiber membrane. An all-or-none phenomenon; whenever the stimulus is at or above threshold, the action potential generated has a constant size and configuration. See also **compound action potential, motor unit action potential**. (From the 2001 Report of the Nomenclature Committee of the American Association of Electromyography and Electrodiagnosis.[19] Reproduced by kind permission of the AANEM.)

action tremor 1. Physiological tremor accentuated by muscle contraction, as is seen both in normal subjects and in those with **Parkinson disease**. 2. Any tremor on voluntary contraction of muscles, including postural, kinetic, and isometric tremors.[1615] See also **cerebellar tremors**.

activated protein C resistance factor (Leiden) A dominantly inherited disorder due to a mutation at 1q23, resulting in an increased liability to stroke.

activation 1. In physiology, a general term for the initiation of a process. 2. The process of motor unit action potential firing. The force of muscle contraction is determined by the number of motor units and their firing rate. (From the 2001 Report of the Nomenclature Committee of the American Association of Electromyography and Electrodiagnosis.[19] Reproduced by kind permission of the AANEM.)

activation procedure A technique used to detect defects of neuromuscular transmission during repetitive nerve stimulation testing. Most commonly a sustained voluntary contraction is performed to elicit facilitation or postactivation depression. (From the 2001 Report of the Nomenclature Committee of the American Association of Electromyography and Electrodiagnosis.[19] Reproduced by kind permission of the AANEM.)

activator mutant A form of **gangliosidosis** with two *variants*:

Infantile (AB variant) A disorder presenting similarly to Tay–Sachs disease (**GM_2 gangliosidosis**) with the infantile onset of myoclonus, seizures, hypotonia and, later, spasticity, dementia, and death. A cherry-red retinal spot is present.[5537]

Adult (AB variant) A syndrome of adult-onset normal pressure hydrocephalus, seizures, and dementia with increased hexosaminidase A and B activity.[379]

active continence The maintenance of bladder outlet closure at rest through increased reflex activity in the pudendal nerve, which causes increased activity in the striated muscle around the urethra and thus increases the resistance to fluid flow.

active electrode (exploring electrode, input terminal 1, grid 1, G1) The recording electrode close to the source of the activity to be recorded. In EEG, the first of two inputs to a differential amplifier. [RMS] See also **recording electrode**.

active sleep A sleep stage in newborn children, similar to **REM Sleep**.

activities of daily living (ADL) The range of those behaviors which are normally required for personal self-maintenance and independent life within a community. These activities are usually divided into two categories:

Physical ADL represents the most basic personal care tasks such as feeding, excretion (bowels, bladder), toileting, dressing, cleanliness (grooming, bathing), and motility (transfers, wheelchair, walking, stairs).

Instrumental ADL embodies more complex activities including handling of personal finances, preparing meals, shopping, using the telephone, traveling, and housework.

Items included within *extended ADL* include the following:[393]

Getting about	*Household activities*	*Other activities*
Carrying a hot drink	Washing up	Gardening
Working outside	Washing clothes	Managing money
Crossing roads	Housework	Going out socially
Getting in/out of a car	Shopping	Employment/Work
Using public transport	Making hot drinks/snack	Hobbies/leisure
Driving a car	Reading	
	Telephoning	
	Writing	

Scores on ADL scales correlate well with scores on psychometric test batteries.[2] See also **Katz Activities of Daily Living Scale, Physical Self-Maintenance Scale, Instrumental Activities of Daily Living Scale**, and **Functional Assessment Staging**.

acuity A term expressing the efficiency of a sensory pathway. It is most often employed in the realm of vision, with normal acuity being the ability to resolve an image at a distance similar to that required by a normal population. Thus a visual acuity of 20/40 implies that the subject is only capable of resolving an image 20 feet away while the normal is to do so when it is 40 feet away. Auditory acuity is also measureable, but measurements of tactile acuity are complex and unresolved.

acupressure (Gr, needle + to press) Formerly a method of arresting hemorrhage; currently the term is used for a system of pain relief by digital or other pressure on certain sites on a patient's body, known only to practitioners of the mystery.

acupuncture An Oriental system of treatment of disease by the insertion and subsequent rotation of long needles through the tautened skin; the insertions are made along certain charted meridians. Acupuncture was introduced into England in 1683 by a Dr. Rhyne but was not accepted until espoused by Berlioz in 1816. Since it is a method of alternative medicine, scientific evaluation is often rejected.

acusia (acousis) The faculty of hearing.

acute Sudden, urgent, short-term, or fast-appearing.

acute abstinence encephalopathy An acute confusional state occurring on withdrawal from a cerebral depressant agent which had been chronically ingested. **Delirium tremens** is an example.

acute acquired postconvulsive hemiplegia See HHE syndrome.

acute active multiple sclerosis (Marburg variant) That form of **multiple sclerosis** characterized by extensive areas of confluent demyelination within the brainstem or spinal cord and leading to death within months of the clinical onset of the disease.

acute alcoholic myopathy An acute syndrome of muscle pain, tenderness, swelling, weakness, and wasting of proximal muscles with myoglobinuria and consequent renal failure,[1831, 2829] following another bout of excessive ingestion of alcohol by chronic alcoholics.

Pathologically the condition is marked by myofibrillar degeneration especially of type 1 fibers. See also **alcoholic myopathy, acute hypokalemic myopathy of alcoholism**.

acute amnestic syndromes See **Wernicke–Korsakoff syndrome**.

acute anterior poliomyelitis See **poliomyelitis**.

acute areflexic paralysis A syndrome occurring in malnourished patients who become acutely hypophosphatemic as a result of being fed with nutrients which do not contain phosphate.

Clinically, initial paresthesias lead on to acute muscular weakness affecting the ocular and bulbar as well as the truncal and limb muscles; areflexia; sensory neuropathy; and ageusia. Central signs include somnolence or coma, confusional states, seizures and pyramidal signs. The serum phosphorus level is always below 1 mg/dl and the signs remit when the levels are raised.[5841]

acute ascending polyneuropathy See **acute inflammatory demyelinating polyneuropathy**.

acute ataxia See **acute cerebellar ataxia**.

acute atrophic paralysis A defunct name for **poliomyelitis**.

acute atypical meningitis A manifestation of the initial direct infection of the meninges or brain with HIV and presenting a self-limited syndrome of meningitis, headache, long tract signs, and cranial nerve deficits.[2951]

acute autonomic neuropathy An uncommon syndrome, usually affecting healthy young people. Presentation is often dramatic with gastrointestinal involvement heralding widespread dysautonomia. Acute autonomic neuropathy can be primarily cholinergic without orthostatic hypotension (26%) or pandysautonomic (74%) involving sympathetic adrenergic functions. Onset has been temporally related to viral syndromes in 20% of cases, with autonomic deficits usually evolving over 1–3 weeks. Gastroparesis (69%) and syncope (12%) are frequent presenting complaints. Spinal fluid protein levels are often (75%) elevated in pandysautonomic subtypes. Prolonged and incomplete recovery is the rule (60%), with persistent gastroparesis and orthostatic hypotension.

Other specific diseases that occasionally mimic acute autonomic neuropathy include botulism, porphyria, amyloidosis, and paraneoplastic neuropathies. Acute autonomic neuropathy shares several clinical features with and is likely to be a variant of **acute inflammatory demyelinating polyneuropathy**, suggesting an immune-mediated pathogenesis.[2786] See also **autonomic neuropathy**.

acute axonal motor neuropathy See **Chinese paralytic syndrome**.

acute axonal motor neuropathy with anti-GM$_1$ antibodies and *Campylobacter* infection See **immune-mediated neuropathies**.

acute benign hydrocephalus (Marie–See syndrome) **Idiopathic intracranial hypertension** occurring in children as a result of the excessive ingestion of vitamin A.

acute brachial neuropathy See **neuralgic amyotrophy**.

acute brachial plexitis See **neuralgic amyotrophy**.

acute brachial plexopathy See **neuralgic amyotrophy**.

acute brain stem (Bickerstaff) encephalitis See **disseminated vasculomyelinopathy**.

acute brain swelling See **parainfectious noninflammatory encephalomyelitis, cerebral edema**.

acute central cervical spinal cord injury Acute hyperextension injury to the cervical spine producing hemorrhagic necrosis of the central cord. See **central cord syndrome**. The resulting clinical syndrome is comprised of weakness (greater in the arms than in the legs), variable impairment of sensation below the level of the lesion, and urinary incontinence.[5626] See also **hematomyelia, Minor disease**.

acute cerebellar ataxia 1. (Zappert syndrome, acute cerebellitis) An acute reversible cerebellitis following viral infections such as varicella or after immunization and presenting with truncal, gait, and limb ataxia and **opsoclonus**.[2453] The prognosis for full recovery is good.[1270] 2. (Westphal–Leyden syndrome) An acute ataxic syndrome described in an adult by Leyden in 1891 and having both cerebral (cerebellar) and peripheral (sensory) forms.[3824] The condition was thought not to be a toxic manifestation and may have represented a postinfectious or demyelinating disorder. It is not clearly distinguished from Zappert syndrome.

acute cerebellar degeneration A pan-cerebellar syndrome manifesting as ataxia and dysarthria in which there are no antibodies to Yo antigen nor to Purkinje cells and which is unassociated with underlying carcinoma or other structural disease.[5382]

acute cerebellitis See **acute cerebellar ataxia**.

acute cerebral schistosomiasis An acute encephalitis or encephalomyelitis presenting with personality change, angioneurotic edema, and pyramidal signs but progressing to coma with seizures. Marked peripheral eosinophilia is detected. The condition may be a form of allergic encephalopathy.[6858] See also **chronic cerebral schistosomiasis**.

acute compartment syndrome of the thigh A potentially devastating disorder due to damage to neural and vascular structures as a result of acute swelling of the thigh muscles following severe (or sometimes not severe) trauma.[5676]

Compartment syndromes may occur wherever muscles are overlaid by fascial coverings. The **anterior tibial syndrome** is the best known, but other sites include the supraspinatus, anconeus and forearm muscles, the abdomen, and the posterior thigh and foot.

acute confusional migraine

(dysphrenic migraine) An agitated and confused state lasting minutes to hours and occurring occasionally in children (and even less commonly in adults) with a personal or family history of migraine. The confusional episode is not itself accompanied by headache, however.[2295]

acute corticosteroid myopathy

An acute necrotizing myopathy associated with the use of corticosteroids with or without neuromuscular junction blocking agents, occasionally seen in patients in intensive care. See **acute quadriplegic myopathy**.

acute delayed measles encephalitis

A chronic progressive encephalopathy occurring 3 months after an attack of measles and characterized by high antimeasles antibody levels, the presence of intranuclear inclusions in glial and neuronal nuclei, destruction of the ependyma, hydrocephalus, and clinically intractable **epilepsia partialis continua** and coma.[3978] See also **subacute sclerosing panencephalitis**.

acute dialysis encephalopathy

See **dialysis encephalopathy**.

acute dialysis neuropathy

An asymmetrical sensorimotor neuropathy (an acute **multiple mononeuropathy**) considered to be caused by ischemia due to vasoconstriction, occurring in patients with chronic renal failure undergoing dialysis.[4346]

acute disseminated (demyelinating) encephalomyelitis

(ADEM, post- or parainfectious encephalomyelitis, acute perivascular myelinoclasia) A monophasic immune-mediated demyelinating disease of the CNS that typically follows a febrile infection or a vaccination. Children are predominantly affected. This monophasic, postinfectious or postvaccinial autoallergic, inflammatory, and demyelinating encephalopathy has major effects upon the white matter of the cerebral hemispheres, cerebellum, optic nerves, and spinal cord in response to antigenic challenge. It is characterized pathologically by the presence of perivascular mononuclear cell infiltration in the brain and spinal cord, edema of the white matter, and variable perivenous and confluent demyelination with relative preservation of axons.[6253] The name was first applied by C.F. **Westphal** in 1872, but the condition was defined pathologically by Hurst only in 1941.[3059]

Clinically it is manifested by the acute onset of fever, seizures and altered consciousness, meningismus, headache, nausea, and vomiting, with developing evidence of widespread CNS damage such as bilateral optic neuritis and other cranial nerve palsies, visual field defects, aphasia, hemiparesis, seizures, and cerebellar ataxia, all developing days or weeks after a viral or streptococcal infection or other immunologic challenge.[108] MRI studies reveal multifocal areas of increased signal intensity on T2 weighted sequences, enhancing with contrast, in both white and gray matter. In most cases the course is monophasic and recovery occurs with steroid therapy, but recurrences occur in a third of patients[5682] and the only way to make the differentiation is long-term follow-up. The cerebrospinal fluid may disclose a mild lymphocytic pleocytosis and elevated albumin levels. Oligoclonal bands are not always present in ADEM and if so, may be transient.[4310]

Vaccination-associated ADEM is most frequently observed after measles, mumps, or rubella vaccinations. However, it has also been reported after poliomyelitis and European tick-borne encephalitis vaccinations. Consensus definitions proposed for monophasic ADEM in pediatric populations[3574] indicate that there should be an acute or subacute onset of a first clinical event with a presumed inflammatory or demyelinating cause affecting many brain areas, and thus polysymptomatic. The encephalopathy will be manifest by alterations in consciousness and behavioral changes such as confusion and irritability but improvement should follow, though clinical and MRI deficits may persist. There should have been no previous history of a similar event and there should nto be any other likely cause. It is recognized that the clinical and MRI findings may fluctuate over the course of the next 3 months.

In such cases, focal or multifocal white matter lesions are shown on MRI scans, without evidence of previous destructive brain disease. The T2 weighted or FLAIR images show large (1–2 cm) and multifocal lesions that are hyperintense; rarely a single white matter lesion and/or added intramedullary cord lesions may be acceptable for the diagnosis.

The same authors define *recurrent* and *multphasic ADEM* as follows:

Recurrent New event of ADEM with a recurrence of the initial symptoms and signs, in 3 or more months after the first ADEM event, without involvement of new clinical areas by history, examination, or neuroimaging. Event does not occur while on steroids and occurs at least 1 month after completing therapy. MRI shows no new lesions; original lesions may have enlarged. No better explanation exists.

Multiphasic ADEM followed by a new clinical event also meeting criteria for ADEM, but involving new anatomic areas of the CNS as confirmed by history, neurologic examination, and neuroimaging.

The subsequent event must occur at least 3 months after the onset of the initial ADEM event and at least 1 month after completing steroid therapy. The subsequent event must include a polysymptomatic presentation including encephalopathy, with neurologic symptoms or signs that differ from the initial event (mental status changes may not differ from the initial event).

The brain MRI must show new areas of involvement but also demonstrate complete or partial resolution of those lesions associated with the first ADEM event.

When acute and fulminating with multiple intracerebral hemorrhages, the condition is known as *acute hemorrhagic leukoencephalitis*, Hurst disease, or Strumpell–Leichtenstern syndrome.[6101]

Hymenoptera (bee) stings can produce demyelinating complications in the central and/or peripheral nervous system resembling ADEM, presumably related to the autoimmune system. See also **disseminated vasculomyelinopathy, brainstem encephalitis, Miller Fisher syndrome, multiphasic disseminated encephalomyelitis**.

acute disseminated perivenous encephalomyelitis

See **acute disseminated encephalomyelitis**.

acute dystonia of thalamic origin

A lacunar syndrome.[2092]

acute encephalopathy of infancy (fatal infantile mitochondrial disease) A fatal mitochondrial disease with Complex IV or cytochrome-c oxidase deficiency, presenting in neonates with hypotonia, vomiting, weakness, ptosis and areflexia with renal tubular acidosis and sometimes cardiomyopathy and lactic acidosis.[379, 1653]

acute facial diplegia and hyperreflexia See **acute inflammatiory polyneuropathy**.

acute flexion-extension injury See **whiplash; acceleration injury syndrome**.

acute fulminant myoglobinuric polymyositis A form of **polymyositis** distinguished from other forms by its extreme severity and by the presence of picornavirus-like particles in the muscles.[2236]

acute headache attributed to other head and/or neck trauma See **post-traumatic headaches**.

acute headache attributed to whiplash injury See **post-traumatic headaches**.

acute hemiconcern A transient behavioral syndrome rarely following stroke involving the territory of the right anterior parietal artery, in which patients with profound left hemisensory loss persistently examine and manipulate the left side of their bodies with their intact right arm.[707]

acute hemiplegia of childhood Hemiplegia occurring in early childhood due to occlusive vascular disease or from unknown causes, as opposed to those cases in which trauma, heart disease, infection, sickle-cell disease, or other pathologies can be incriminated.[5945] See also **moya-moya disease**.

acute hemorrhagic leukoencephalitis (acute necrotizing hemorrhagic encephalopathy, Hurst syndrome, Strumpell–Leichtenstern syndrome) A form of autoallergic encephalitis following a viral illness in young adults, representing the most severe form of **acute disseminated encephalomyelitis**, in which there is inflammation within and around vessels with petechial hemorrhages, maximal in white matter. All of these features, excepting the petechiae, resemble those of **experimental allergic encephalomyelitis**. See **disseminated vasculomyelinopathy**. The condition may be dominantly inherited.[4612]

The condition is usually acute and fatal, but patients with slow progression and even with recovery have been described.[3017] It was first described by Hurst in 1941 from Australia.

acute hypokalemic myopathy of alcoholism An acute myopathy without muscle pain, tenderness or swelling, associated with severe hypokalemia within the context of alcoholism.[5460]

acute illness myopathy See **Hopkins syndrome, critical care myopathy**.

acute infantile hemiplegia The abrupt occurrence of a brain infarct (usually thrombotic in nature) in a previously healthy infant or child who lacks any predisposing condition. Coma, seizures and fever often result from the localized defect. The causes of the condition have been reviewed by Golden.[2444]

acute infantile spinal muscular atrophy type I See **hereditary motor neuropathy**.

acute infectious torticollis An epidemic syndrome reported from China, characterized by the occurrence of nonspecific prodromal symptoms suggesting viral infection, followed by painful spasm of the neck muscles with head tilt, torticollis, tongue stiffness and spasm of other muscles including the oculomotor, lingual and oral muscles, and distant dystonia.[4627]

acute inflammatory demyelinating polyneuropathy (acute ascending polyneuropathy, Landry–Guillain–Barré [–Strohl] syndrome, acute postinfective polyradiculoneuropathy, acute plexitis, etc.; Jablonski[3113] lists 21 synonyms)

Forms of peripheral neuropathy of uncertain cause but with an immune-mediated pathology, characterized by lymphocytic infiltration of the peripheral nerves and by destruction of myelin. The basis of the condition is the occurrence of aberrant immune responses directed against components of peripheral nerve, likely following cytomegalovirus, Epstein–Barr virus, HIV, or vaccinia virus infection.

Clinically this presents typically as an acute or subacute polyneuropathy with progressive motor weakness, areflexia, minor sensory changes and almost invariably some autonomic instability.[2621, 3678] The face is often involved, and the eyes rarely so (except in the **Miller Fisher** variant). Antecedent events are often detected, these events typically including virus infections, surgery, trauma, malignancy, injection of sera and vaccines, or the presence of lymphoma or other malignancies, although in many cases there are no known preceding events. Symptoms reach their nadir in less than 3 weeks, but 80% of patients improve to some degree by 6 weeks.

The CSF protein is frequently raised but the cell count is not (**albumino-cytologic dissociation**). The disease presents one of the classic "catch-22" dilemmas; those who respond best to **plasmapheresis** are also those whose signs have progressed rapidly over the first week, but the best response is obtained when this treatment is given in the first 7 days. Antibodies to GM1, GD1a, LM1, sulfatide and other glycolipids are variously detectable.[6807]

Descriptive clinical[258] and electrodiagnostic[101] criteria have been defined (but criticized by Poser[5095]) and some are reproduced in Chart A–2.

The condition was first reported by Wardrop and Ollivier in 1834–1837 and then by Jean-Baptiste-Octave **Landry** (1826–1865), a French physician, who correctly concluded in 1859 that it is a disease of the peripheral nerves. **Guillain** and **Barré** added the CSF findings ("dissociation albumino-cytologique" or Sicard–Foix syndrome) in 1891.

Organizations devoted to this condition include the following:

American Autoimmune Related Diseases Association A charitable organization in this field. Address: 22100 Gratiot Ave. Eastpointe, East Detroit, MI 48201-2227. Tel: 586-776-3900; 800-598-4668. E-mail: aarda@aol.com. Web site: http://www.aarda.org/.

Guillain–Barre Foundation International P.O. Box 262. Wynnewood, PA 19096. E-mail: gbint@netcom.com. Tel: 610-667-0131. Web site: http://www.webmast.com/gbs.

Proposed electrodiagnostic criteria for demyelination of peripheral nerve are included with the above, but are somewhat complex. A more recent and much simpler set[88] is given in Chart A–3:

Chart A–2. Diagnostic Criteria for Guillain–Barre Syndrome (Acute Infectious Polyneuropathy)

I. *Features required for diagnosis*

A. Progressive motor weakness of more than one limb. The degree ranges from minimal weakness of the legs, with or without mild areflexia, to total paralysis of the muscles of all four extremities and the trunk, bulbar and facial paralysis, and external ophthalmoplegia.
B. Areflexia (loss of tendon jerks). Universal areflexia is the rule, although distal areflexia with definite hyporeflexia of the biceps and knee jerks will suffice if other features are consistent.

II. *Features strongly suggestive of the diagnosis*

A. Clinical features (ranked in order of importance)

1. Progression. Symptoms and signs of motor weakness develop rapidly but cease to progress by 4 weeks into the illness. Approximately 50% will reach the nadir by 2 weeks, 80% by 3 weeks, and more than 90% by 4 weeks.
2. Relative symmetry. Symmetry is seldom absolute, but usually, if one limb is affected, the opposite is as well.
3. Mild sensory symptoms or signs.
4. Cranial nerve involvement. Facial weakness occurs in approximately 50% and is frequently bilateral. Other cranial nerves may be involved, particularly those innervating the tongue and muscles of deglutition, and sometimes the extraocular motor nerves. On occasion (less than 50%) the neuropathy may begin in the nerves to the extraocular muscles or other cranial nerves.
5. Recovery. It usually begins 2–4 weeks after progression stops. Recovery may be delayed for months. Most patients recover functionally.
6. Autonomic dysfunction. Tachycardia and other arrhythmias, postural hypotension, hypertension, and vasomotor symptoms, when present, support the diagnosis. These findings may fluctuate. Care must be exercised to exclude other bases for these symptoms, such as pulmonary embolism.
7. Absence of fever at the onset of neuritic symptoms.
8. Absence of manifestations of systemic illness or constitutional symptoms or both, either preceding or coinciding with onset of neuropathy.

Variants (not ranked). The presence of one of these need not rule out the diagnosis if other features are strongly supportive, but the presence of two of them makes the diagnosis unlikely.

1. Fever at onset of neuritic symptoms.
2. Severe sensory loss with pain.
3. Progression beyond 4 weeks. Occasionally, a patient's disease will continue to progress for much longer than 4 weeks or the patient will have a minor relapse.
4. Cessation of progression without recovery or with major permanent residual deficit remaining.
5. Sphincter function. Usually the sphincters are not affected, but transient bladder paralysis may occur during the evolution of symptoms.
6. CNS involvement. Ordinarily, Guillain–Barré syndrome is thought of as a disease of the peripheral nervous system. Evidence of CNS involvement is controversial. In occasional patients, such findings as severe ataxia interpretable as cerebellar in origin, dysarthria, extensor plantar responses, and ill-defined sensory levels are demonstrable, and these need not exclude the diagnosis if other features are typical.

B. CSF features strongly supportive of the diagnosis.

1. CSF protein. After the first week of symptoms CSF protein is elevated or has been shown to rise on serial lumbar punctures.
2. CSF cells. Counts of 10 or fewer mononuclear leukocytes/mm^3 in the CSF.

Variants include the following:

1. No CSF protein rise in the period of 1–10 weeks after the onset of symptoms (rare).
2. Counts of 10–50 mononuclear leukocytes per cubic millimeter in CSF (common in patients seropositive for HIV, however).

C. Electrodiagnostic features strongly supportive of the diagnosis (see below). Approximately 80% will have evidence of nerve conduction slowing or block at some point during the illness. Conduction velocity is usually less than 60% of normal, but the process is patchy and not all nerves are affected. Distal latencies may be increased to as much as three times the normal value. Use of F-wave responses often gives good indication of slowing over proximal portions of nerve trunks and roots. Up to 20% of patients will have normal conduction studies. Conduction studies may not become abnormal until several weeks into the illness.

III. *Features Casting Doubt on the Diagnosis*

A. Marked, persistent asymmetry of weakness
B. Persistent bladder or bowel dysfunction
C. Bladder or bowel dysfunction at onset
D. More than 50 mononuclear leukocytes/mm^3 in CSF
E. Presence of polymorphonuclear leukocytes in CSF
F. Sharp sensory level

IV. *Features that rule out the diagnosis*

A. Current history of hexacarbon abuse (volatile solvents; n-hexane; and methyl n-butyl ketone). This includes huffing of paint lacquer vapors or addictive glue sniffing.

B. Abnormal porphyrin metabolism indicating a diagnosis of acute intermittent porphyria. This would manifest as increased excretion of porphobilinogen and d-aminolevulinic acid in the urine.
C. A history or finding of recent diphtheritic infection, either faucial or wound, with or without myocarditis.
D. Features clinically consistent with lead neuropathy (upper limb weakness with prominent wrist drop; may be asymmetrical) and evidence of lead intoxication.
E. Occurrence of a purely sensory syndrome.
F. A definite diagnosis of a condition such as poliomyelitis, botulism, hysterical paralysis, or toxic neuropathy (e.g., from nitrofurantoin, dapsone, or organo-phosphorus compounds), which occasionally may be confused with Guillain–Barré syndrome

The criteria have been established by an ad hoc committee of the NINCDS, Dr. A.K. Asbury, Chairman and are reproduced by kind permission.[258]

Chart A–3. Criteria for Electrophysiological Classification

Normal	Normal nerve conduction studies
Nondiagnostic	Nonspecific or nonlocalizing abnormalities, including an isolated absent H reflex without definite demyelination
Suggested	Sural sparing pattern, or two or more nerves with absent or prolonged minimum F wave latency (with relatively normal distal seat and a peak amplitudes) and absent H-reflex
Highly suggestive	Sural sparing pattern and two or more nerves with absent or prolonged minimum F wave latency (with relatively normal distal CMAP amplitudes) and absent H reflex
Definite	Both signs of demyelination to be present in two motor nerves: 1. Focal slowing, temporal dispersion, and/or conduction blocks 2. Absent or prolonged minimum F-wave latency (with relatively normal distal CMAP amplitude) and with absent H reflex.

The sural sparing pattern is defined as a normal or relatively preserved sural SNAPs compared with at least two abnormal SNAPs in the upper limb (median, ulnar, and radial SNAPs)

About 5% of patients with this condition will show evidence of axonal damage.[258,259] See also **demyelination**.

Variants of the usual clinical syndrome include

Ataxia, areflexia, and facial diplegia
acute facial diplegia and hyperreflexia
Acute motor axonal neuropathy (AMAN) (An acute axonal form with a poor prognosis for recovery, often due to *Campylobacter infection*.)[1979]
Acute motor and sensory neuropathy (AMSN)
Acute multiple cranial neuropathy
Acute pandysautonomia
Acute sensory neuronopathy
Acute small fiber sensory neuropathy
Distal acquired demyelinating sensory and motor neuropathy (DADS)
Miller Fisher syndrome
Multifocal motor neuropathy
Polyneuritis cranialis
AIDP occurring in the setting of Hodgkin disease.

A *pharyngeal-cervical-brachial variant* has the following diagnostic criteria suggested by Ropper et al.[5387] and reproduced here by kind permission of Oxford University Press.

Clinical Features

1. Paresthesias in the feet and hands
2. No weakness or respiratory failure
3. Areflexia or hyporeflexia in all limbs by 1 week
4. Distally diminished sensation involving mainly vibration and joint position
5. Proximal progression of numbness and sensory loss on the limbs over several days to 1 month
6. Improvement in paresthesias and sensory loss by 2–4 months from onset

Laboratory Abnormalities That Confirm the Diagnosis

7. Elevated CSF protein concentration (>45 mg/dl) within 3 weeks of onset
8. Severe sensory nerve conduction abnormalities
9. Minimal motor conduction and late response abnormalities

Anti-GD1a and anti-GT1a antibodies have been detected in some cases of this condition.

A *pure motor variant* has the following diagnostic criteria suggested by Ropper et al.[5387] Reproduced by kind permission of Oxford University Press.

Simpler clinical criteria for the typical syndrome (and variants) have been suggested by Ropper et al.[5387] and are reproduced here by kind permission of Oxford University Press.

Clinical Features

1. Weakness that is approximately symmetric in all the limbs
2. Paresthesias in the feet and hands
3. Areflexia or hyporeflexia in all limbs by 1 week
4. Progression of the above three features over several days to 1 month

Laboratory Abnormalities That Confirm the Diagnosis:

5. Elevated CSF protein concentration (>45 mg/dl) within 3 weeks from onset
6. Abnormalities of F waves in at least two limbs, or motor nerve conduction block, or slowing (motor nerve conduction velocity below 80% of normal)

Clinical Features

1. Progressive, relatively symmetric weakness in all limbs
1. No paresthesias or sensory loss
3. Areflexia or hyporeflexia in all limbs by 1 week
4. Progression of weakness over 1 day to 3 weeks

Laboratory Abnormalities That Confirm the Diagnosis

5. Elevated CSF protein concentration (>45 mg/dl) within 3 weeks of onset
6. Abnormalities of F waves in at least two limbs or motor nerve conduction block, or slowing
7. Normal sensory nerve potentials

A *paraparetic variant* has the following diagnostic criteria suggested by Ropper et al.[5387] Reproduced by kind permission of Oxford University Press.

Clinical Features

1. Progressive leg weakness over 1–3 weeks
2. Areflexia or hyporeflexia in the legs by 1 week of illness
3. Normal (or virtually normal) power and reflexes in the arms and cranial nerve innervated muscles
4. Minimal or no paresthesias or sensory loss

Laboratory Abnormalities That Confirm the Diagnosis

5. Variable, usually slight, elevation of CSF protein concentration
6. Abnormal motor nerve conduction and late responses in the legs

Acute facial diplegia and hyperreflexia[6139]

Acute motor conduction block neuropathy A form of pure motor neuropathy with conduction blocks, normal or brisk muscle stretch reflexes, and relatively fast recovery.[1002]

Acute ophthalmoparesis without ataxia A rare form presenting with relatively symmetric ophthalmoparesis progressing over 4 weeks, unaccompanied by ataxia or limb weakness. The condition usually follows an infectious illness. The CSF shows albuminocytological dissociation and anti-GQ1b IgG antibodies are detectable in the serum.[4751]

Acute small fiber sensory neuropathy. 1. A pure sensory variant presenting with acute numbness and burning dysesthesias in a symmetric glove-and-stocking distribution in the limbs, with areflexia, normal muscle strength, and electrophysiological evidence of demyelinating neuropathy. The CSF protein levels may be raised. The condition increases for up to a month and then slowly remits. (Oh et al. *Neurology* 2001;56:82–6) 2. A similar syndrome in which, however, there is evidence only of thin sensory fiber involvement, the electrodiagnostic studies being normal, and the muscle stretch reflexes retained.[5727]

AIP associated with mycoplasma pneumoniae infection Also manifesting bilateral optic neuritis and extensive CNS white matter lesions on MRI.[4569]

Facial diplegia Presents with ataxia and areflexia but with minimal limb weakness or sensory deficit.[1114]

acute intermittent porphyria

A dominantly inherited disorder characterized by deficiency of hydroxymethylbilane synthase (porphobilinogen deaminase) and manifesting episodes of acute abdominal pain, vomiting, and porphyrinuria, sometimes with acute distal motor axonopathy. Exacerbations are triggered in most instances by exposure to environmental triggers (barbiturates, dilantin, griseofulvin, sulfonamides, and estrogens; alcohol; infections; or starvation).[5370] The responsible gene maps to 11q23.2-qter.

Neurological features complicate a third of attacks and include the acute or subacute occurrence of proximal motor neuropathy affecting the arms more than the legs (often asymmetrically) as well as the face and autonomic system in the setting of other features of the disease including dermal photosensitivity, limb, chest, and abdominal pain, vomiting, tachycardia, hypertension, and often seizures. Delirium, psychosis, and neurotic behavior patterns are the abnormal mental features described, as in the case of King George III of England. Sensory loss may be detected in the **bathing suit area**. The ankle jerks are preserved but all other muscle stretch reflexes are diminished.

Widespread central, peripheral, and autonomic system lesions have been found.[6115]

acute intrinsic myelopathy

(acute transverse myelitis, acute necrotic myelopathy) An acutely developing spinal cord lesion, involving both sides of the cord at one or more adjacent levels, ascending or static, occurring at any age without prior neurological features and neither due to compression nor surgery. The condition may remain at one level or may ascend through new levels of the cord. Onset in less than 3 weeks of symmetrical motor and sensory dysfunction referable to a distinct spinal cord level, with sphincter dysfunction, are typical features.

Typically, this occurs as a postinfectious autoimmune demyelinating condition, but ischemic infarction, bleeding from arteriovenous malformations, demyelinating disease, viral infections, and paraneoplastic syndromes are also possible causes.[6754] See also **acute necrotic myelopathy**, **acute toxic myelopathy**.

acute lethal catatonia

Muscle rigidity with an increase in creatine kinase (CK) levels without involuntary movements or autonomic signs in subjects exposed to neuroleptic drugs. The condition represents a rare variant of the **neuroleptic malignant syndrome**, from which it cannot be distinguished clinically.[54]

acute midbrain syndrome

See **diencephalic autonomic seizures**.

acute motor axonal neuropathy

(AMAN) An axonal form of acute inflammatory polyneuropathy characterized clinically by rapid onset of weakness, an early nadir, distal weakness initially, relative sparing of cranial nerves, and occurrence mainly in summer. Many cases are associated with *C. jejuni* infection and the presence of IgG anti-GM1 antibodies, some of which may be cross-reactive with lipopolysaccharides. AMAN may also occur following infusion of parenteral gangliosides, composed primarily of GM1. These disorders have been further subdivided on the basis of electrophysiology and pathology into acute motor axonal neuropathy (AMAN) and acute motor-sensory axonal neuropathy (AMSAN).

Pathologic findings in AMAN and AMSAN include axonal degeneration of the affected nerves and the presence of periaxonal macrophages (in motor roots in AMAN and in motor and sensory roots in AMSAN). The cause is unknown. Campylobacter infections, present in many patients with AMAN and in other forms of Guillain-Barre Syndrome, may play a role in triggering such a process possibly by "molecular mimicry."[1979, 4241]

acute mountain sickness

(Acosta syndrome) A clinical syndrome comprising of headache, insomnia, anorexia, nausea, dizziness, dyspnea, peripheral edema, vomiting, and incoordination, occurring between 6 and 24 h after attainment of high elevations, peaking on the second or third day and resolving after about a week.

While it is usually self-limiting, the syndrome can progress to pulmonary and cerebral edema. It is hypothesized that the pathogenesis is increased cerebral blood flow causing cerebral edema as a result of hypoxia, which itself is due to improper or too rapid acclimatization.[2666] See also **altitude insomnia.**

acute multifocal placoid pigment epitheliopathy (AMPPE) A rare, probably postviral condition that can be associated with neurologic problems, including headache, CNS arteritis, and sagittal sinus thrombosis.[4734]

acute multiple cranial neuropathy A syndrome of complete or partial ophthalmoplegia with bilateral facial and bulbar dysfunction, possibly a regional (cranial) form of **acute inflammatory polyneuropathy.**[3982]

acute myelitis See **acute intrinsic myelopathy.**

acute necrotic myelopathy (myelomalacia) A form of **acute intrinsic myelopathy** presenting with flaccid paralysis and total sensory loss ascending over a few days from the legs to the thoracic regions or higher with loss of sphincter control and without recovery. Pathologically, the condition is characterized by extensive necrosis of the white, more than of the gray, matter of a large part of the cord, without vascular disease or neoplasia but sometimes with evidence of inflammation.[6754] Changes in the CSF are inconstant but may include an abnormally high protein content, either with few cells or with pleocytosis.

The condition is thought to be a form of **acute disseminated encephalomyelitis** or of **Devic disease** but a similar syndrome may be associated with carcinoma or tuberculosis and with some toxic or infectious agents. It may also represent a postinfectious phenomenon.[5099] See also **subacute necrotic myelopathy.**

acute (necroticizing) myopathy A myopathy complicating infection with influenza A or B virus, coxsackie virus B5, echovirus 9, adenovirus 21, Epstein–Barr virus, or herpes simplex virus and presenting with lymphadenopathy, proximal myopathic weakness, muscle pain and cramp and myoglobinuria due to rhabdomyolysis. Biopsy shows phagocytosis and fiber necrosis.

A similar myopathy may complicate carcinoma or alcoholism. See also **acute fulminant myoglobinuric polymyositis, acute quadriplegic myopathy, myoglobinuria, Hopkins syndrome.**

acute necrotizing encephalopathy A complication of infection with certain strains of influenza and other viruses presenting with high fever, seizures and alterations in mental status that rapidly progress to coma. Brain imaging may demonstrate symmetric white matter, thalamic, basal ganglia, and/or pontine involvement in which there is necrosis associated with punctate hemorrhages. Permanent and severe disability or death often result.[4067]

acute necrotizing encephalopathy of childhood A syndrome of coma, seizures, vomiting, hyperpyrexia, and hepatomegaly reported in Japanese children following acute respiratory infections. The presence of diarrhea and of raised CSF protein and the absence of hyperammonemia or hypoglycemia are considered to differentiate the condition from **Reye syndrome.**[4417]

acute necrotizing hemorrhagic encephalopathy See **acute hemorrhagic leukoencephalitis.**

acute necrotizing myopathy of intensive care See **quadriplegic myopathy.**

acute nonsuppurative encephalitis See **parainfectious noninflammatory encephalomyelits.**

acute ocular oscillations See **opsoclonus.**

acute-onset lethargia and prolonged abulia A syndrome resulting from infarction of the genu of the left internal capsule. See **strategic-infarct dementia, capsular genu syndrome, multi-infarct dementia.**

acute ophthalmoparesis without ataxia See **acute inflammatory demyelinating neuropathy** (*variants*).

acute (and recurrent) optic neuritis See **disseminated vasculomyelinopathy.**

acute painful ophthalmoplegia A syndrome closely resembling **superior orbital fissure syndrome** but with frequent involvement of the optic nerve, reported from the Far East.[6228]

acute pandysautonomia See **autonomic neuropathy (I).**

acute peripheral vestibulopathy (vestibular neuronitis, labyrinthitis, neurolabyrinthitis) A clinical syndrome of vertigo and vomiting, falls, past-pointing toward the affected side, horizontal or rotatory direction-fixed spontaneous nystagmus toward the affected side and unilateral canal paresis with normal hearing. While it is usually supposed to have a viral origin affecting the eighth nerve and/or the labyrinth, pontine lesions can produce an identical syndrome.[6295, 68]

acute persistent akathisia A variety of chronic **akathisia** in which the abnormal movements appear shortly after institution of therapy with a neuroleptic agent, and which persist.[945]

acute phase shift of sleep See **rapid time zone change syndrome.**

acute plexitis See **acute inflammatory demyelinating polyneuropathy.**

acute polioclastic encephalitis A form of encephalitis in which the gray matter of the cerebral cortex bears the brunt of the damage caused by the inflammatory process.

acute polymyopathy A rapidly progressive syndrome of proximal weakness, muscle pain, tenderness, and swelling with elevated creatine kinase levels. It is considered to be due to deficiency of essential fatty acids during prolonged total peripheral nutrition.[6060] See also **acute (necrotic) myopathy, polymyositis.**

acute polyneuropathy with edema. Beriberi in modern form.[1465]

acute polyradiculitis See **acute inflammatory demyelinating polyneuropathy**.

acute posterior multifocal placoid pigment epitheliopathy A syndrome characterized by sudden, usually binocular, blurring of vision, in which multifocal yellowish-white lesions are seen in the pigment epithelium of the retina. The disease, considered to be a manifestation of diffuse cerebral vasculitis, is usually self-limiting and visual function returns eventually.[2301]

acute postasthmatic amyotrophy See **Hopkins syndrome**.

acute postinfectious encephalomyelitis See **acute disseminated encephalomyelitis**.

acute postinfective polyradiculoneuropathy See **acute inflammatory demyelinating polyneuropathy**.

acute post-traumatic headache attributed to moderate or severe head injury See **post-traumatic headaches**.

acute quadriplegic myopathy (acute necrotizing myopathy of intensive care, critical illness myopathy, thick filament myopathy, floppy person syndrome) A syndrome of severe, rapid-onset diffuse myopathic weakness and wasting, complicating urgent steroid therapy, as in the course of treatment of acute asthmatic attacks, with or without the addition of nondepolarizing blocking agents in patients with severe systemic illness.[2913, 6982] Typically, the clinical picture is of flaccid quadriparesis with ventilatory muscle involvement, marked wasting, and hyporeflexia. EMG findings are a mix of neuropathic, myopathic, and end-plate abnormalities. Muscle biopsy reveals severe atrophy of most muscle fibers, with disorganization and necrosis of myofibrils and selective loss of thick (myosin) filaments.[2913] See also **Hopkins syndrome** and **acute (necroticizing) myopathy**.

acute rhabdomyolysis An uncommon acute necrotic myopathy occurring during various viral infections and causing muscle destruction with myoglobinuria. Clinically, muscle pain, tenderness, weakness, and myoglobinuria occur, sometimes complicated by renal failure. See **acute (necrotic) myopathy**.

A similar but more limited syndrome occurs in association with unaccustomed heavy exercise. See **squat-jump myoglobinuria** and **rhabdomyolysis**.

acute sensory (ataxic) neuronopathy An acutely developing, monophasic, purely sensory neuropathy involving mainly large-fiber modalities in the limbs and trunk with sensory ataxia and areflexia, and in which the underlying lesions are thought to be of the dorsal root and Gasserian ganglion cells. The condition is probably immune-mediated or due to vascular causes in the absence of underlying carcinoma. The autonomic system may also be involved; occasionally, muscle stretch reflexes are preserved.[4768]

The syndrome has also been recorded following exposure to adriamycin, pyridoxine, mercury, and antibiotics and following infections with herpes zoster. The prognosis for recovery is poor.[6038]

acute serous encephalitis (Brown–Symmers disease) A rapidly progressive encephalopathy characterized by irritability, anorexia, vomiting, and evidence of raised intracranial pressure with bulbar signs in the form of respiratory irregularity. Ptosis, nystagmus, papilledema, convulsions, contraction of the angle of the mouth, muscle twitching, rigidity of the neck, hemiplegia, and coma lead on to death if affected children are not treated within 2 days.[887] See **parainfectious noninflammatory encephalomyelitis, acute disseminated encephalomyelitis**.

acute severe combined demyelination The concurrence of Guillain–Barré syndrome and acute disseminated encephalomyelitis in acute and fulminant form, presenting with acute onset of coma and flaccid, areflexic quadriparesis, elevated CSF protein levels, and delayed F waves, with MRI evidence of extensive multifocal demyelination. Prompt clinical response followed by recovery may be achieved by treatment with corticosteroids.[182]

acute sinus headache Headache and facial pain during an attack of acute sinusitis. See **sinus headache**.

acute small fiber sensory neuropathy See **acute inflammatory polyneuropathy**.

acute superior hemorrhagic polioencephalitis The term of **Gayet** for what is now known as **Wernicke–Korsakoff syndrome**.

acute suppurative myositis (pyomyositis) Direct bacterial (or syphilitic) infection of muscle, with staphylococci, clostridia, streptococci, and anaerobes being the organisms most commonly isolated. Clinical findings include localized pain, tenderness, and swelling with systemic evidence of infection. The condition is uncommon in temperate regions, especially since paraldehyde is now seldom administered intramuscularly.

acute symptomatic seizures See **situation-related seizures**.

acute syphilitic meningitis A benign meningitic illness occurring in the secondary stage of syphilis but without fever, but often complicated by hydrocephalus or cranial nerve involvement. The CSF almost always shows abnormality. The illness usually occurs same time as the rash occurs and within 2 years of infection. Cerebrovascular syphilitic syndromes follow within years at most.

acute thalamic esotropia Adduction of one eye, which remains immobile while the other eye responds normally to vestibuloocular stimulation, in the presence of altered consciousness, long tract signs, and impaired upward gaze. The condition results from lesions of the contralateral posterior thalamus.[2459]

acute thyrotoxic encephalomyelopathy (Waldenstrom syndrome) An acute complication of hyperthyroidism, usually seen in the elderly, who present with sixth, seventh, and bulbar cranial nerve palsies, an hallucinatory psychosis with lethargy and apathy or excitement, and a variety of signs of cortical dysfunction. Eventually they slip into coma.[6595] See also **thyrotoxic crises**.

acute thyrotoxic myopathy Rapidly progressive bulbar weakness complicating a thyroid storm (acute hyperthyroidism); a condition of uncertain nature, myasthenia, periodic paralysis, and encephalopathy also having been suggested variously as the underlying cause.

acute toxic encephalitis/ encephalopathy See **parainfectious noninflammatory encephalomyelitis, disseminated vasculomyelinopathy**.

acute toxic myelopathy An **acute intrinsic myelopathy** occasionally associated with intravenous illicit drug usage, spinal angiography, aortic angiography, intrathecal penicillin, or chemotherapeutic injections, or spinal anesthesia. See also **lathyrism**.

acute transverse myelitis (idiopathic acute transverse myelitis) Suggested diagnostic criteria for this and for recurrent transverse myelitis require bilateral sensory, motor, or autonomic dysfunction referable to the spinal cord, with a clearly defined sensory level progressing to a nadir at between 4 and 21 days from onset. MRI must eliminate structural causes and reveal evidence of an inflammatory etiology. Also, evidence of an inflammatory origin must be shown by enhanced MRI or by CSF findings of pleocytosis or increased IgG levels.[6264]

For diagnostic confidence, there should be evidence of spinal cord inflammation as shown by CSF pleocytosis or elevated CSF IgG index and gadolinium enhancement on a spinal MRI. In children particularly, MRI assists diagnosis by showing that the cord involvement extends over six segments or more.

In a *variant* form, unrelated to systemic disease, there is a relapsing course.[5710] See also **disseminated vasculomyelinopathy, acute intrinsic myelopathy**.

acute traumatic central cord syndrome A clinical presentation most commonly seen in older people with cervical spondylosis and canal stenosis as a consequence of direct compression of the spinal cord, which is trapped anteriorly by osteophytes and posteriorly by buckling of the hypertrophied ligamentum flavum. Clinically it presents with weakness in the arms but with preservation of strength in the legs. Patchy sensory loss and variable sphincter involvement are also described.[1916] See also **bodybuilder sign, Hirayama syndrome**.

acute vertical myoclonus Vertical, pendular, large-amplitude oscillations of the eyes, occurring in some patients with recent brainstem strokes.[3762]

acute viral encephalitis Infection of the substance of the brain by a virus (such as herpes simplex, Epstein–Barr, mumps, influenza, Coxsackie, or echo), leading to disease which may be mild and transient or fulminant and lethal.

Clinically, headache, hemiparesis, fever, nausea, drowsiness, coma, neck stiffness, papilledema, seizures, and various other neurological signs are the commonest findings. The CSF may be under increased pressure; it contains mononuclear cells (and typically red cells in herpes encephalitis) but the protein level may be normal. EEG abnormalities usually include generalized or focal slowing, or bursts of spike-and-wave activity.[3382]

Descriptions of more serious forms of the infection can be found at the Centers for Disease Control Web site: http://www.cdc.gov/ncphi/disss/nndss/casedef/encephalitiscurrent.htm/.

acute Werdnig–Hoffman disease See **hereditary motor neuropathy**.

acute-onset lethargia and prolonged abulia A syndrome resulting from infarction of the genu of the left internal capsule. See **strategic-infarct dementia, capsular genu syndrome, multi-infarct dementia**.

acyl coenzyme A dehydrogenase deficiency Recessively inherited mitochondrial diseases in childhood, characterized by disorders of the short-, medium-, or long-chain forms of the enzyme. *Medium-chain acyl coenzyme A* dehydrogenase deficiency is perhaps the commonest disorder of fatty acid oxidation.

Clinical features variously include vomiting, coma, muscle weakness (lipid myopathy with cardiomyopathy), and mental retardation. Hepatomegaly, nonketotic hypoglycemia, myoglobinuria resulting from rhabdomyolysis, and dicarboxylic aciduria are usual laboratory features of these conditions.[6015]

Multiple acyl coenzyme A dehydrogenase deficiency is listed under **glutaric aciduria type II**.

AD 8 A brief informant or patient interview used to detect early dementia, correlating well with the **MMSE** and the **Clinical Dementia Rating** Scale in differentiating nondemented from demented individuals.[2265] It is accessible at http://alzheimer.wustl.edu/About_Us/PDFs/AD8form2005.pdf/.

adacrya (Gr, without + to weep) Inability to form tears.

Adamantiades-Behçet syndrome See **Behçet syndrome**.

adamantinoma (Gr, hard mineral substance) See **craniopharyngioma**.

Adamkiewicz, Albert (1850–1921) Polish professor of pathology at Kraków. The artery of Adamkiewicz is a branch of the abdominal aorta, representing the major segmental arterial supply of the spinal cord at that level, which it approaches close to or at L1, usually from the left side. Adamkiewicz also described the demilunes found beneath the neurilemma of medullated nerves.

Adams, Robert (1771–1875) Dublin physician.

Adams-Stokes-Morgagni syndrome (Stokes–Adams syndrome) Syncope of cardiac origin, the usual cause being complete atrioventricular block, with bradycardia usually at a rate below 40 per min.[50] Morgagni's original (1761) note in his *De Sedibus et Causis Morborum* (Letter the Ninth, which treats of epilepsy) clearly describes seizures with cessation of the heart beat, but Adams' report was more precise in detail. Stokes published his observations in 1846.

Adams syndrome (tachycardia and hypertension) A congenital syndrome characterized by microphthalmia, cataract, ECG abnormality, aminoaciduria, renal stones, hypertension, and seizures.[381]

adaptation 1. A decline in the response to a repetitive stimulus. 2. A decline in the frequency of the spike discharge as typically recorded from sensory axons in response to a maintained stimulus.[19] 3. (Neuro-ophthalmology) Diminished responsiveness of central mechanisms in response to a persistent abnormality disturbing function. Adaptation modifies the direct effects of a neurological lesion; thus the nystagmus in **internuclear ophthalmoplegia** reflects the excessive innervation of the weak medial rectus with spill-over to the abducting eye. Saccadic dysmetria and macrosaccadic oscillations occur in **myasthenia gravis** and with cerebellar lesions as adaptive changes to weakness but become maladaptive when strength returns temporarily in the Tensilon test.

adaptation rate The rate at which a sensory receptor reduces its afferent discharge in response to a persisting adequate stimulus.

adaptive behavior The capacity of an individual to function with respect to the physical and the human environment. See also **Vineland Adaptive Behavior Scale, Woodcock-Johnson Scales of Independent Behavior, Minnesota Child Development Inventory, Adaptive Behavior Scale.**

Adaptive Behavior Scale A questionnaire used in the assessment of levels of functioning and maladaptive behavior in retarded people or those with acquired brain damage.[4673]

Addenbrooke's Cognitive Evaluation A short instrument for the early detection of dementia, usefully expanding the MMSE. It consists of six components evaluating orientation (10 points), attention (8), memory (35), verbal fluency (14), language (28), and visuospatial ability (5). The orientation and attention components are as in the MMSE. The memory component evaluates episodic memory (recall of three items from the MMSE plus a "name and address learning and delayed recall" test) and semantic memory. The language component requires naming 12 line drawings, repetition of words and sentences, reading regular and irregular words, and comprehension and writing tasks. The visuospatial test requires copying of overlapping pentagons (from the MMSE) and of a wire cube, and drawing a clock face. Verbal fluency examines letter fluency for words beginning with the letter "P" and category fluency (animals). Scores for each of the six domains can be calculated separately; their sum gives a composite score out of 100. The MMSE score can also be calculated. The instrument is published in 19 languages. It can be reviewed as an appendix on the *Neurology* Web site (www.neurology.org)[4168] but is also available at http://pn.bmj.com/supplemental/.

Addison, Thomas (1793–1860) English physician who trained in Edinburgh but spent almost all of his professional life as physician to Guy's Hospital in London, where he showed particular interest in the skin and described pernicious anemia, adrenal failure, xanthomas, vitiligo (Addison–Gull disease), morphea, and the use of electricity in "spasmodic diseases."

Addison disease The systemic disorder resulting from a deficiency of corticosteroid hormones as a result of adrenal disease. Neurological complications include a mild myopathy and a syndrome of idiopathic intracranial hypertension, with or without cerebral edema and encephalopathy.

Addison–Schilder disease See **adrenoleukodystrophy**.

adducted thumbs syndrome See **Christian syndrome, craniosynostosis**.

adduction (from Lat, to lead toward) The movement by which a body part is drawn toward the sagittal line or a finger moves toward the center line of the hand. See also (ocular) **duction**.

adduction lag A reduction in the amplitude and in the velocity of the (adducting) fast phase of jerk nystagmus induced in the eye on the same side as a lesion of the median longitudinal fasciculus (**internuclear ophthalmoplegia**).[5919]

adductor laryngeal breathing dystonia (Gerhardt syndrome) A rare task-specific dystonia in which the adductor spasm of the vocal cords occurs during inspiration but not while speaking (unlike spasmodic dysphonia in which the vocal cords adduct involuntarily during speech but function normally during breathing). Patients present with severe stridor with the risk of life-threatening respiratory obstruction. It can occur sporadically or as a manifestation of a drug-induced dystonia.

adductor reflex Adduction of the abducted leg in response to a tap on the medial epicondyle of the femur and, in cases of pyramidal disease, from many other sites on the pelvis, leg, and spine (*spinal adductor reflex*). It is a marker for lower motor neuron lesions at L2 and, like other muscle stretch reflexes, is increased in pyramidal tract disease.

adductor reflex of the foot (Hirschberg sign) Stroking the inner border of the foot from the hallux back toward the heel leads to adduction, inversion, and plantar flexion of the foot due to contraction of the tibialis posterior in patients with pyramidal tract disease.

adductor spread of knee jerk See **developmental reflexes**.

Adelaide craniosynostosis A rare, dominantly inherited syndrome linked to chromosome 4p (see also **craniosynostosis**).

adenoma sebaceum (Bourneville disease) A papular skin lesion in **tuberous sclerosis**, first described in 1826 by Pierre Rayer (1793–1867), a French dermatologist, although Pringle had already noted the facial lesions.

adenylate deaminase deficiency See **muscle adenylate deaminase deficiency**.

adenylosuccinate lysase deficiency A rare disorder of purine synthesis in infancy or childhood with multiple presentations including autism, hypotonia, psychomotor retardation, and seizures.[1181]

adermonervia (Gr, lack of + skin + nerves) Loss of skin sensation.

adhalin (from Arabic, muscle) A 50-kd dystrophin-associated glycoprotein (α-sarcoglycan); a component of the sarcoglycan complex of the muscle cell membrane. The disorders consequent upon deficiency of the protein were first detected in North Africa; hence the derivation of the term.

adhalinopathies (α-sarcoglycanopathies) Unusual, heterogeneous forms of muscular dystrophy characterized by deficiency of adhalin and presenting clinically as severe childhood autosomal recessive muscular dystrophy (SCARMD) resembling **Duchenne dystrophy** in its clinical features and course but without involvement of the cardiac, facial, ocular, or pharyngeal muscles. This form has been mapped to chromosome 17q21 and is due to a primary defect of adhalin. In another form presenting as a milder limb girdle muscular dystrophy, the absence of adhalin is secondary to a separate defect on chromosome 13q12 or 4q12.[92, 1940] See also **quadriceps myopathy, severe childhood autosomal recessive muscular dystrophy**.

Primary adhalinopathy may be a common cause of autosomal recessive muscular dystrophy of variable severity.[5018]

adhesive arachnoiditis (chronic idiopathic adhesive arachnoiditis) Chronic inflammation of the arachnoid membrane, usually in lumbar regions, constricting the spinal cord, the nerve roots, and the blood vessels and leading to a slowly progressive ascending myelopathy or to multiple painful radiculopathies.

This condition was a complication of myelography using oily contrast media, or the injection of any foreign substance into the subarachnoid space, and also of syphilis and chronic granulomatous diseases; but these causes are now rare and when the condition is detected, commonly no cause is found. See **spinal arachnoiditis**.

adhesive capsulitis of the shoulder See **Duplay syndrome**.

adiadochokinesis See **dysdiadochokinesis**.

adiaphoresis (Gr, lack of + to throw off by perspiration) Lack of sweating.

Adie, William John (1887–1935) An Australian neurologist who trained in Edinburgh and in Europe before being appointed to the staff of the **National Hospital**, Queen Square, and the Charing Cross Hospital. During World War I, he was mentioned in despatches for gallantry and for devising a temporary gas mask, consisting of clothing soaked in urine.[2066] (However, a more acceptable gas mask was invented by Dr. Cluny MacPherson, a Newfoundland physician.)

He wrote on a variety of subjects such as **narcolepsy** (in his M.D. thesis), **myotonic dystrophy**, pituitary tumors, forced grasping, and **multiple sclerosis** but is best remembered for his 1931 description[55] of the pupillary anomaly which bears his name, although he gave credit to colleagues for having described it in 1902. However, the first report was probably that of James Ware[5704] in a paper read to the Royal Society in 1812, and others since then had also briefly noted the phenomenon.

Adie–Critchley syndrome Forced grasping and groping in cases of tumor of the contralateral frontal lobe, described by these authors in 1927.[56]

Adie–Holmes syndrome See **Adie pupil, Holmes–Adie syndrome**.

Adie pupil (tonic pupil, pupillotonic pseudotabes, Markus syndrome, pseudo-Argyll Robertson pupil, myotonic pupillary reaction, Saenger syndrome, Kehrer–Adie syndrome, iridoplegia interna, pseudotonic pupillotonia) The condition in which one enlarged pupil (seldom both) reacts extremely slowly if at all to light but does constrict on prolonged accommodation and then remains persistently constricted after the stimulus is removed. It is usually seen in young women.

The lesion causing the partial denervation of the pupillary sphincter is in the ciliary ganglion; it is diagnosed definitively by the hypersensitivity of the pupil to 0.125% pilocarpine or 2.5% methacholine and is a benign condition which nevertheless disturbs the naïve who look into a mirror and notice a single dilated pupil. Scheie had previously introduced the methacholine test and Adie concluded that the lesion was in the postganglionic parasympathetic fibers as the pupils showed denervation hypersensitivity to that substance.

This pupillary phenomenon was reported by Piltz in 1899 and by at least three other authors before Holmes and Adie[55, 2960] each reported it in 1931. The pupillary changes are often combined with reduction or loss of the muscle stretch reflexes in the legs (**Holmes–Adie syndrome**), as reported by both authors[57, 4997] and occasionally with anhidrosis or generalized weakness.

Adie Syndrome A Web site providing data on this condition. http://www.ninds.nih.gov/disorders/holmes_adie/holmes_adie.htm/.

adiposis dolorosa See **Dercum disease**.

adiposogenital syndrome Arrest or delay in sexual development with obesity and due to destruction of the tuberal nuclei of the hypothalamus. The cause of most cases is not determined, but a craniopharyngioma is present in some cases.

adipsia A decreased sensation of thirst, usually due to damage to the osmoreceptors of the anterior hypothalamus, such that in the presence of a high plasma osmolality there is an inappropriate lack of thirst and water losses are not replenished by drinking.

The hypothalamic lesion may also cause a reduction in antidiuretic hormone secretion, so that the problem of thirst is complicated by excessive water loss.[192]

adjustment sleep disorder Sleep disturbances temporally related to acute stress, conflict, or environmental change causing persistent emotional arousal. The complaints of insomnia or excessive sleepiness are related in time to an identifiable stressor and remit when the stress is removed or if adaptation to it improves. Polysomnography reveals an increased sleep latency, reduced sleep efficiency, or increased number and duration of awakenings; a prolonged total sleep time; or reduced mean sleep latency on the **minimum sleep latency test**.[1629]

adolescent familial cramps A relatively benign X-linked recessively or dominantly inherited myopathic syndrome of adolescence, characterized by cramps following exercise, elevated serum creatine kinase levels, normal production of lactate by muscle under ischemic conditions, and minimal weakness or wasting.[2738] See **cramps**.

adolescent stretch syncope

The occurrence of syncope when the subject stretches the trunk with the neck hyperextended, resulting from compression of the craniocervical arteries.[6112]

ADR syndrome

(ataxia, deafness, mental retardation) See **cerebellar ataxias**, **Richards Rundle syndrome**.

adrenal hypoplasia with mental retardation and muscular dystrophy

See **Renier syndrome**.

adrenergic receptors

(adrenoceptors) Sites of the action of noradrenaline in the CNS. There are three types of receptor: alpha-1 (found in the cerebral cortex and thalamus), alpha-2, and beta.

adrenocorticotrophic hormone

A peptide secreted by the hypothalamus, possessed also of functions within the CNS to do with task discrimination, approach–avoidance behavior, and memory.

adrenoleukodystrophy

(Addison–Schilder disease, Siemerling–Creutzfeldt disease, sudanophilic leukodystrophy, melanodermic leukodystrophy, adrenoleukomyeloneuropathy, adrenomyelodystrophy; OMIM 300100) A group of progressive, X-linked recessive peroxisomal degenerative disorders of myelin (leukodystrophies), the responsible gene mapping to Xq28. They are characterized by a deficiency of lignoceroyl coenzyme A synthetase.

The diagnosis is established by finding abnormal levels of very long chain (C_{26}) fatty acids (VLCFAs) in the plasma, cultured fibroblasts, and brain,[4514, 4513] for which a single peroxisomal deficiency is responsible. The abnormal VLCFA levels are considered responsible for interference with myelin formation, shown by the presence of severe myelinoclastic diffuse sclerosis not sparing the U fibers, especially in parieto-occipital regions. Axonal loss also occurs. Increased CSF protein levels, abnormal EEGs and nucleide scans, and the biochemical consequences of primary adrenal failure are also found.

The condition was first reported by Creutzfeldt in 1923, although Schilder had published reports of patients with various other white matter diseases (some accompanying adrenal insufficiency) in 1911. The status of **Schilder disease** as a separate entity is uncertain; it may not exist.

In the classical *X-linked juvenile variety* of adrenoleukodystrophy, the onset of symptoms is in childhood or youth, with progressive spastic gait disturbance due to myelopathy, often with neuropathy and hypoadrenalism, sometimes with extrapyramidal or cerebellar signs, demyelinating sensorimotor peripheral neuropathy, and unmyelinated fiber loss.[2578] Intellectual functions are usually intact. This form may also present as **hereditary spastic paraparesis**.

In younger children with the X-linked form, progressive encephalopathy with cortical blindness, dementia, deafness, optic atrophy, and seizures are described; the same features may appear only later in life in males and are sometimes manifested in female carriers. Isolated myelopathy and isolated hypoadrenalism are other rare phenotypes.

At least six different phenotypes are recognized:

Childhood cerebral ALD A variant characterized by rapidly progressive cerebral demyelination

Adolescent cerebral ALD A phenotype which is similar but with slightly later onset age

Adult cerebral ALD (OMIM 169500) A rare, dominantly inherited variant, sometimes presenting with psychosis

Adrenomyeloneuropathy An X-linked metabolic defect in which deficiency of peroxisomal oxidation of VLCFAs leads to accumulation of these acids, especially hexocosanoate (C26:0) with a high C26/C22 ratio in plasma and fibroblasts. The gene locus has been mapped to Xq28. The condition is a clinically and genetically distinct variant of childhood **adrenoleukodystrophy**.[2578] It presents as a syndrome of adrenal insufficiency beginning in youth or early adult life, with the later development of progressive spastic paraparesis in the third decade, hypogonadism, and distal, axonal, dying-back, symmetrical polyneuropathy with autonomic involvement (causing impotence and sphincter disturbances) beginning in early adult life. Cerebellar dysfunction, dementia, and hemiparesis are also described.

X-linked Addison disease A phenotype without neurological involvement

Adult-onset forms Including adrenomyeloneuroathy as above and other forms with purely tract or lobar affection or with generalized cerebral involvement[3595]

Asymptomatic forms[6494]

The correct classification of the following three conditions is uncertain:

Naidu variant A disorder characterized by neonatal seizures, hypotonia, hepatomegaly, hypsarrhythmia, and developmental delay, with elevated VLCFA levels but normal liver peroxisomes[4578]

Infantile sudanophilic leukodystrophy A disorder resembling typical adrenoleukodystrophy beginning in infancy and characterized by severe seizures and psychomotor retardation.[636] It resembles (and may be the same as) **Zellweger syndrome**, another peroxisomal disorder

Neonatal adrenoleukodystrophy (recessive type) A congenital **peroxisomal disorder** in which multiple peroxisomal functions are deficient, inherited in a recessive manner, and characterized by frontal bossing, cataract, optic atrophy, pigmentary retinal degeneration, enlarged liver, adrenal hypoplasia, dementia, seizures, nystagmus, cerebral atrophy, diffusely increased skin pigmentation, and hyperpipecolic acidemia.[3372, 3371] Clinically, the features are almost identical with those of **Zellweger syndrome**, differing only in the milder involvement and longer survival of the affected infant (death ensuing at ages up to 10 years).[5389] See also **female adrenoleukodystrophy**, **Pelizaeus-Merzbacher disease**.

adrenoleukomyeloneuropathy

See **adrenoleukodystrophy**.

adrenomyelodystrophy

See **adrenoleukodystrophy**.

adrenomyeloneuropathy

See **adrenoleukodystrophy**.

Adrian, Edgar Douglas, Lord

(1889–1977) English physiologist who was educated at Cambridge, where his neurophysiological studies included important research leading to the elucidation of the **"all-or-nothing" response**. He trained in neurology at the **National Hospital** and served in military hospitals during World War I, returning thereafter to Cambridge, where he devoted the rest of his life to studies of the electrical reactions of muscle and nerve, the physiology of the retinal receptors, the all-or-nothing response,[62] receptor adaptation to stimuli (1926), the EEG, and the general principles of neural transmission, introducing many new investigative techniques including coaxial needles for electromyography. For these studies, he shared the Nobel Prize in 1932 with C.S. **Sherrington**. He was the first scientist to acknowledge and understand the significance of Hans **Berger**'s EEG work, which had been ridiculed as artifact by others, but which he confirmed and elaborated.

He was made professor of physiology at Cambridge in 1937 and later became master of Trinity College, after that vice-chancellor, and then chancellor of the university. He was the president of the Royal Society from 1951 to 1955 and was raised to the peerage on relinquishing that position.

Adson, Alfred Washington (1887–1951) American surgeon at the Mayo Clinic.

Adson syndrome (Naffziger syndrome) See **thoracic outlet syndrome**.

Adson test A maneuver for the diagnosis of vasogenic **thoracic outlet syndrome**. The subject leans forward with the neck extended and turned to one or the other side, and then inhales deeply. Elevation of the rib cage puts further pressure on the subclavian artery and thus reduces the radial pulse on the side to which the head is turned. However, the same occurs in many asymptomatic people, so the value of the test is unproven. Even the existence of the syndrome is disputed.[64] The performance of a Valsalva maneuver during hyperextension of the neck is an alternative method of doing this test.

adult acid maltase deficiency See **glycogen storage disease**.

adult amaurotic idiocy See **neurodegeneration with brain iron accumulation**.

adult amylopectinosis See **glycogen storage diseases**.

adult cretinism (Gull syndrome) See **myxedema**.[2635]

adult familial myoclonic epilepsy See **benign adult familial myoclonic epilepsy**.

adult myoclonic epilepsy A syndrome of idiopathic generalized epilepsy in which myoclonic seizures beginning in adult life accompany absence or generalized tonic-clonic seizures. The family history is usually positive for seizures. The clinical examination and imaging studies are normal. The EEG shows generalized epileptiform abnormalities.[2383]

adult occult hydrocephalus See **normal pressure hydrocephalus**.

adult-onset absence epilepsy A syndrome of absence (and occasional tonic-clonic) seizures with onset in adult life, in which the EEG shows 3–4 Hz spike-and-wave discharges.[4083]

adult-onset cerebellar ataxia and sensory deafness (of Schimke) See **cerebellar ataxias** (*variants*).

adult-onset dementia with argyrophilic grains A progressive dementing disorder with clinical features indistinguishable from **Alzheimer disease** but in which no tangles are found in the cerebral cortex and with argyrophilic grains staining positive with Alz-50 monoclonal antibody.[3107]

adult-onset foot dystonia A rare form of localized **dystonia**, sometimes occurring as a presenting feature of Parkinson disease.[3518]

adult-onset leukodystrophies See **18q syndrome, adrenoleukodystrophy, Alexander disease, Canavan disease, Cockayne syndrome, Krabbe disease, metachromatic leukodystrophy, multiple sulfatase deficiency, Pelizaeus-Merzbacher disease, childhood ataxia with CNS hypomyelination, sudanophilic leukodystrophies**.

Although most of these conditions more commonly start in childhood, all can occasionally appear first in adult life.[448]

adult-onset myoclonic epilepsy A syndrome of myoclonus and occasional tonic-clonic seizures, often precipitated by sleep deprivation and alcohol, with onset in adult life. The myoclonus affects only the arms, and occurs mainly in the morning. The EEG shows spike-and-wave or polyspike–and-wave discharges.[4083] See also **FAME**.

adult-onset primary lower limb dystonia The unusual occurrence of lower limb dystonia in adults (although childhood-onset dystonia typically begins in the foot). The most common patterns are plantar flexion of all of the toes and inversion of the foot, typically activated with standing or walking. Dystonia elsewhere is unusual. A family history of dystonia is unusual.[5629] See also **runners' dystonia**.

adult-onset tonic-clonic epilepsy A syndrome of tonic-clonic seizures occurring in adult life sometimes provoked by sleep deprivation or photic stimulation. Some attacks occur soon after waking. The EEG shows 4–5 Hz generalized spike-and-wave and polyspike-and-wave discharges, with bifrontal predominance.[4083]

adult polyglucosan body disease A rare neurological disorder of unknown cause characterized by diffuse central and peripheral nervous system dysfunction, manifesting clinically as progressive upper and lower motor neuron involvement of the limbs, disturbances of the sphincters, sensory loss, and cognitive impairment. Pathologically the condition is distinguished by the widespread accumulation of polyglucosan bodies throughout the nervous system. Assay of leucocyte glycogen brancher enzymes may assist in diagnosis.

The condition is considered to be inherited as an autosomal recessive trait in which abnormalities of branching enzyme activity in white cells are implicated[3917, 5343] but it is likely to be heterogeneous.

Adult Polyglucosan Body Disease (APBD) Research Foundation A charitable organization. Web site: www.apbdrf.org.

adult polysaccharidosis A rare syndrome characterized by the intracellular accumulation of abnormal polysaccharides resembling amylopectin in the form of cytoplasmic spheroids similar to those of **Lafora body disease** but presenting in adult life. Clinically the condition starts with paraparesis, progressing to quadriparesis, sensory loss in the legs, dementia, and death.[4983]

adult proximal spinal muscular atrophy See **hereditary motor neuropathy** (*variants*).

adult spinal muscular atrophy See **hereditary motor neuropathy, type IV**.

advanced sleep phase syndrome (phase lead, phase advance, evening somnolence, and early morning wakefulness) A syndrome of persistent and consistent expedition in the times of sleep onset and of waking compared to the times that were formerly normal for that patient, leading to complaints of excessive evening sleepiness and of early waking. Sleep architecture is normal.[4823] In this disorder the major sleep episode is advanced in relation to the desired clock-time, resulting in symptoms of compelling evening sleepiness and an awakening that is earlier than desired. Diagnostic criteria have been suggested:[1629]

A. Inability to stay awake until the desired bedtime or inability to remain asleep until the desired time of awakening
B. There is a phase advance of the major sleep episode in relation to the desired time for sleep
C. Symptoms are present for at least 3 months.
D. When not required to remain awake until the desired (later) bedtime, patients will
    1. have a habitual sleep period that is of normal quality and duration, with sleep onset earlier than desired;
    2. awaken spontaneously earlier than desired;
    3. maintain stable entrainment to a 24-h sleep–wake pattern.
E. Does not meet criteria for any other disorder causing inability to maintain sleep or excessive sleepiness.

From AASM Diagnostic Classification Steering Committee. *The International Classification of Sleep Disorders Diagnostic and Coding Manual*. Rochester, MN. American Academy of Sleep Disorders, 1991/2001. Reproduced by kind permission of the Academy.

See also http://www.sleepeducation.com/Disorders.aspx.

Advances in Applied Neurological Sciences (*Adv Appl Neurol Sci*) A neurological journal. Address: Springer-Verlag New York Inc., 175 Fifth Ave., New York, NY 10010.

Advances in Neurogerontology (*Adv Neurogerontol*) A neurological subspecialty journal. Address: Praeger Publishers, 1 Madison Ave., New York, NY 10010-3603.

Advances in Neurology (*Adv Neurol*) A neurological review book series. Address: Raven Press, 1185 Avenue of the Americas, Department 1B, New York, NY 10036.

Advances in Neuropsychology and Behavioral Neurology (*Adv Neuropsychol Behav Neurol*) A neurological journal. Address: Guilford Publications Inc., 72 Spring St., New York, NY 10012.

adversive seizure A variety of partial complex epilepsy in which there is tonic or clonic deviation of the head and eyes to one side with or without jerking of the arm on that side and the adoption of a raised, flexed posture of that arm. Though formerly regarded as indicating that the origin of the seizure is in the frontal lobe on the side from which the head turns away, the localizing value of the sign is now questioned.

adynamesthesia (Gr, lack of + power + feeling) Lack of appreciation of the force applied in a motor act, described with lesions in the contralateral pre-Rolandic cortex.[5358]

adynamia (Gr, lack of + power) Weakness.

adynamia episodica hereditaria, adynamia-hyperkalemia (Gamstorp syndrome) See **familial periodic paralysis**.[2267]

adynamia periodica hereditaria A dominantly inherited disorder of the muscle membrane with secondary effects on potassium metabolism in which attacks of muscle weakness with areflexia and percussion myotonia occur from childhood onwards, precipitated by rest after exercise, hunger, and cold. See **familial periodic paralysis** (*hyperkalemic form*).

aerocele See **pneumo(cephalo)cele**.

aerotitis syndrome Middle ear petechiae and inflammation following barotrauma, leading to complaints of fullness or pain in the ear, mild conduction deafness and vertigo.[1765]

aesthesiometer An instrument for measuring the sense of touch on the skin.

aesthesioneuroblastoma (olfactory neuroblastoma) See **neuroblastoma**.

afebrile occasional seizures Simple or complex motor seizures occurring as a symptom of underlying brain disease and not recurring after the underlying cause is no longer operating.

The list of causes includes intracranial infections or other encephalopathies, metabolic diseases, and head trauma.[72]

affect (feeling-tone) The range, depth, and appropriateness of a subject's emotional responsiveness.

affective aura An epileptic aura comprising symptoms such as fear, depression, joy, and (rarely) anger. See also **temporal lobe epilepsy**.

affective-psychic seizure (dreamy state, psychic variant, automatism, vertige épileptique, psychomotor seizure) A form of simple partial seizure (thus without alteration of consciousness) characterized by alterations in mood or cognitive function as a result of the epileptic discharge. The seizures resemble those of complex partial type inasmuch as they may also be components of such attacks, and they have similar pathologies.

afferent (Lat, carrying toward) Applied to neural impulses running into the CNS from the periphery, or to impulses running toward any identified structure.

Affiliated National Dystonia Association A charitable organization comprising **the Dystonia Medical Research Foundation** and the **National Spasmodic Dysphonia Association. WE MOVE** also participates. The association awards research grants to discover the cause and cure of dystonia, sponsors symposia for the medical profession and for patients, publishes educational materials and a newsletter, and builds chapters and patient support groups. Web site: http://www.dystonia-foundation.org.

affricate A consonant which is produced by first blocking the airflow, as for a stop, and then slowly releasing it, causing turbulence as in a fricative sound—for example, /c/ as in cheese.[3949]

African trypanosomiasis See **sleeping sickness**.

afterdischarge 1. The continuation of action potentials in a neuron, axon, or muscle fiber following the termination of an applied stimulus. 2. The continuation of firing of muscle action potentials after cessation of voluntary activation, for example, in myotonia. (From the 2001 Report of the Nomenclature Committee of the American Association of Electromyography and Electrodiagnosis.[19] Reproduced by kind permission of the AANEM.) 3. An EEG seizure pattern following repetitive electrical stimulation of a discrete area of the brain via cortical or intracerebral electrodes. 4. A burst of rhythmic activity following a transient such as an evoked potential or a spike. (Adapted from the 1974 Report of the Committee on Terminology, IFCN[1117] © 1974 with permission from Elsevier Science.)

afterimage The persistence of a visual image after extinction of the original stimulus as a result of retinal changes during exposure to it. The perception may be similar to that of a photographic negative.

afternoon ectropion Weakness of the periocular muscles increasing during the day, thus leading to ectropion in the evening in patients with **myasthenia gravis**.[6617]

after-nystagmus Transient **nystagmus** occurring after a period of rotation of the body (as in a **Barany chair**) has ceased, as a result of the continued movement of endolymph.

afterpotential The membrane potential between the end of the spike and the time when the membrane potential is restored to its resting value. The membrane during this period may be depolarized or hyperpolarized at different times. (From the 2001 Report of the Nomenclature Committee of the American Association of Electromyography and Electrodiagnosis.[19] Reproduced by kind permission of the AANEM.)

age Years of life, the groupings having been arbitrarily defined in 1879 as embryonic (9 months), infancy to 3 years, childhood to 12 years, adolescence to 25 years, maturity to 50 years and decline thereafter. "Boyhood" and "girlhood" are defined as the period from the second dentition to puberty.[5103]

age-associated memory impairment (age-associated cognitive decline, benign senescent forgetfulness) A state of minor cognitive impairment in the form of disturbances of memory function in people aged over 50 years.[1352] The following diagnostic criteria have been suggested (Adapted from Crook[1350] and McEntee[4220]):

I. Inclusion

A. Patient aged over 50 years
B. Complaints of gradually progressive memory loss reflected in everyday circumstances
C. Memory test performance at least 1 standard deviation below the mean established for young adults on a standardized test of recent memory (e.g., **Benton Visual Retention Test**, Logical Memory Scale, or Associate Learning subtests of the **Wechsler Memory Scale**)
D. Evidence of adequate intellectual function as determined by a scaled score of at least 9 on the Vocabulary subtest of the **Wechsler Adult Intelligence Scale**
E. Absence of dementia, as suggested by a score of 24 or higher on the **Mini-Mental State examination**

II. Exclusion

A. Evidence of delirium, confusion, or alteration in consciousness or of any general medical or neurological disorder which could cause cognitive deterioration
B. History of any infective or inflammatory brain disease
C. Evidence of significant cerebrovascular pathology; of repeated head injury; of depression, mania, or any other major psychiatric disorder
D. Current diagnosis or history of substance abuse or use of psychotropic drug in the previous month

Whether or not this condition blends over time into a true dementing illness remains to be seen, now as at the time of publication of the first edition of this book; the author prognosticates that it will eventually be shown to do so. See also **minimal cognitive impairment**.

agenesis The failure of the formation of a body part during embryological development. In the case of the corpus callosum, agenesis may occur alone or in association with other cerebral malformations or as part of a number of other syndromes such as alobar **holoprosencephaly**, and it may also be a marker for certain inherited metabolic diseases.[3521, 4316]

Agenesis of the cerebellar vermis may be asymptomatic or may be associated with impaired motor coordination.

agenesis of the cerebellar vermis See **Joubert syndrome**.

agenesis of the cerebellum An uncommon malformation characterized by improper development of the dentate nuclei, vermis, and cerebellar peduncles.[3489] Unilateral maldevelopment of the cerebellum is more common.

agenesis of the corpus callosum (callosal agenesis) A dysmorphic developmental syndrome presenting clinically with brachycephaly, hypertelorism, and hyperhidrosis in childhood with abnormality in consciousness, flushing, poor temperature control, and mental and developmental delay.[498] **Microcephaly** and **heterotopias** may be associated. Both recessive and X-linked transmission have been described.

The anatomical defect was described first by Reil in 1812. The same anomaly complicates a number of other congenital degenerative syndromes.[379]

Variants include the following:

Agenesis of the corpus callosum, X-linked A congenital syndrome comprising megacolon, adducted thumbs, and mental and developmental delay in addition to the dysmorphogenesis.[3295]

Agenesis of the corpus callosum with hypothermia A syndrome which has been reported in childhood and adult life. Some cases show spongy white matter disease.[5034]

Agenesis of the corpus callosum with anterior horn cell disease (Charlevoix County disease) A dysmorphic condition described in Quebec in which the agenesis is complicated by lower motor neuron lesions causing flaccid quadriparesis, areflexia, sensory neuropathy, and mental retardation.[185] See also **acrocallosal syndrome**.

agenesis of the septum pellucidum with porencephaly A congenital dysmorphic syndrome characterized by heterotopias within the cerebrum, microcephaly, hydranencephaly, or porencephaly; polymicrogyria; and absence of the septum pellucidum. Clinically it manifests with mental and developmental delay, pyramidal signs, and dystonia.[381]

ageotropic nystagmus (apogeotropic nystagmus) See **vestibular nystagmus**.

age-related cognitive decline See **age-associated memory impairment**.

age-related white matter changes Deep cerebral signals on CT or MRI seen increasingly as age advances, especially in those with a history of hypertension and/or stroke, and associated with impaired results on testing speed, attention, and executive function.

ageusia (Gr, lack of + the sensation of taste) Loss of taste sensation, usually resulting from lesions of the chorda tympani, and less commonly resulting from disorders of the brainstem or of the temporal lobes.

aggressive myoclonic epilepsies Syndromes characterized by myoclonic jerks, fragmental and usually erratic. See **progressive myoclonic epilepsy**.

agnathia-holoprosencephaly A congenital dysmorphic syndrome characterized by an absent or small mandible and holoprosencephaly.[381]

agnosia Impairment of the ability to recognize stimuli which were formerly recognized—in the absence of disturbances of perception, intellect, or language—due to acquired lesions of the cerebral cortex. In Teuber's words, perceptions are stripped of meaning. Vision, hearing, gustatory, and tactile sensations may also be affected.

The term was coined by Sigmund Freud in 1891; but others, using the terms *visual perceptive centers*, *asymbolia*, and *imperceptions*, had clearly recognized the existence of the condition.[4339] The causal lesions are usually in the posterior part of the parietal lobe, but they can also be in the callosum or deeper white matter where they act to disconnect the speech area from the primary sensory cortex, indicating that, as Geschwind had originally proposed, most agnosias are modality-specific naming defects with a marked confabulatory response and represent disconnection syndromes.

Visual agnosia is "a disorder of higher behaviour confined to the visual realm in which an alert, attentive, intelligent and non-aphasic patient with normal visual perception gives evidence of not knowing the meaning of [or of not recognizing visual] stimuli."[1430]

Prosopagnosia (from Gr, a face + to know) is a form of visual agnosia characterized by an inability to recognize previously known faces or other complex visual stimuli and to learn new ones.

Generic recognition (a face) may remain but specific recognition (Uncle Fred) is lost, indicating a failure of visually triggered episodic memory. Bilateral lesions of the central visual system are responsible.

Visual object agnosia is often associated with prosopagnosia and with failures of generic recognition. The lesions are bilateral and extensive, affecting the ventral and mesial occipitotemporal visual cortex. Object agnosia without prosopagnosia is sometimes seen with a unilateral lesion of the left occipitotemporal region.

See also **apperceptive agnosia**, **associative agnosia**.

agnosopsia The ability to discriminate in the absence of awareness of what is being discriminated. See **Riddoch syndrome**.

agonist 1. (prime mover, protagonist) A muscle, the major action of which is to produce a particular movement in question. See **prime mover; antagonist**. 2. A chemical substance that binds to a receptor, thus exciting it.

agoraphobia (Gr, an assembly or marketplace + fear) Pathological fear of open spaces; the term was introduced by **Westphal** in 1871.[6739]

agrammatic aphasia See **Broca aphasia**.

agrammatism (telegraphic speech, nonfluent aphasia) An aphasic disorder which impairs syntax rather than vocabulary and which leads to effortful, dysprosodic speech, often with associated dysarthria and improper sentence construction. It results from an inability to organize words so that sentences follow grammatical rules, and from the improper use or nonuse of grammatical morphemes (e.g., conjunctions, prepositions, and bound inflectional affixes such as *-ed, -ment, or -ing*).[2473]

The substantive content of speech uttered is high but the supporting grammar distortion makes the speech sound like pidgin English or a telegram. The causal lesion is in the Sylvian cortex. The term was first used by **Pick** in 1913.

agranular cortex The motor strip, containing pyramidal rather than granular cells.

agraphesthesia Lack of the ability to perceive figures drawn on the skin, as with lesions of the contralateral parietal lobe, of subcortical structures, of the spinal cord, and of the peripheral nerves.

This is a sensitive and consistent indicator of defective perception of cutaneous sensory space but it is not of value in localizing the cause of sensory disturbance to the parietal lobe. The faculty had been identified by Hall and Donaldson in 1885, but the word was only introduced 40 years later.[509] See also **tactile agnosia**.

agraphia (Gr, lack of + writing) Difficulty experienced in self-expression by means of writing.[1337] The term is generally restricted to that inability to write due to a cerebral lesion but which is not traceable to a gross motor handicap. The first modern descriptions were those of Jean Pitres (1848–1928) in 1884, and of **Déjèrine**.[1538]

Various classifications exist:

Anterior agraphia Writing is characterized by large, crude, and scrawled letters, written usually with the left hand, as seen in dextrals who have suffered an anterior lesion of the dominant hemisphere.

Posterior agraphia Writing is characterized by well-formed letters composed into sentences but with omissions, misspellings, and incorrect word order, seen in dextrals who have suffered a posterior lesion of the dominant hemisphere.

Visuospatial agraphia Writing is characterized by inappropriate placement of normal words and letters on the page, as seen in patients who have suffered a nondominant hemisphere lesion.

An alternative descriptive classification[452] recognizes the following:

Aphasic agraphia The agraphia accompanies Broca, Wernicke, conduction, or transcortical sensory **dysphasia**.

Agraphia with **alexia** (parietal agraphia) A disorder which occurs with dominant parietal lobe lesions and leads to the poor formation of letters and to spelling errors.

Pure agraphia Writing is characterized by poor spelling, although the words are well formed; neither alexia nor aphasia is present.

Apraxic agraphia A dominant parietal lobe syndrome characterized by difficulty in forming letters and words when writing spontaneously or to dictation, often accompanied by errors in copying and in oral spelling.

Spatial agraphia Writing is distorted by abnormal placement of the letters on the page, often explicable by visual neglect, because a nondominant parietal lobe lesion is the usual cause.

To the above forms, these may yet be added:

Deep agraphia A disorder characterized by lexicalizations and semantic errors. [AK]

Surface agraphia A disorder in which irregular spelling is regularized. [AK]

Phonological agraphia A disorder in which there is specific impairment of the conversion from phoneme to grapheme and in which dictated nonwords cannot be transcribed. [AK]

agraphia with alexia See **agraphia**.

agrypnia (Gr, lack of + sleep) Total and prolonged absence of sleep. A condition characterized by total insomnia without tiredness.[2073]

It has been described in *agrypnia with fibrillary chorea of Morvan*[4506] as a syndrome of unknown cause characterized by complete absence of sleep and of sleepiness, evening hallucinations, generalized fasciculations and paresthesias, and abnormal movements as in **Morvan disease**. Some relief of the agrypnia has been obtained by oral 5-hydroxytryptophan ingestion. The cause is unknown; both viral infection and mercury poisoning have been incriminated.

Aguecheek disease A literary allusion to the Shakespearean character, Sir Andrew Aguecheek in *Twelfth Night* (1602), whose former intellect appears to have been commendable: "[he]. . . plays o'the viol de Gamboys, and speaks three or four languages word for word without the book and hath all the good gifts of Nature" (Act I, Scene 3) but, having been drunk nightly, lost important mental powers: "for many do call me a fool" (Act II, Scene 5). Moreover, his drinking companion Sir Toby Belch considered that " if you were to find so much blood in [Andrew's] liver as would clog the foot of a flea, I'll eat the rest of the anatomy."

Shakespeare gave Sir Andrew himself some insight: "Methinks I have no more wit than a Christian or an ordinary man has; but I am a great eater of beef, and I believe that does harm to my wit."

Summerskill[6126] has neatly suggested that this was the first account of **chronic porto-systemic encephalopathy**.

Aguilar syndrome A congenital dysmorphic syndrome characterized by conjunctival telangiectasias, immunoglobulin deficiency, seizures, and mental and developmental delay.[70] See **ataxia-telangiectasia-like syndrome**.

agyria Absence of gyri in the cerebral cortex. See **lissencephaly**.

ai An old Gascon word for tenosynovitis, evocative when spoken loudly.

Aicardi syndrome A rare syndrome in infant girls characterized by **infantile spasms, agenesis of the corpus callosum**, and chorioretinal lacunae. Other features of note are myoclonus, psychomotor deterioration, optic hypoplasia, microphthalmia, chorioretinopathy, vertebral and other dysplastic bony anomalies including microcephaly and atypical asynchronous burst–suppression EEG patterns in the two hemispheres. Axial hypotonia, bilateral pyramidal signs, and swallowing difficulties are always present; skeletal anomalies and facial dysmorphisms may also be found.

An unidentified intrauterine insult during the first trimester has been considered to be the cause,[593] but the condition may be X-linked dominant (at Xp22) with lethality in affected males.[379]

Aicardi Syndrome Foundation A charitable organization in this field. Address: 450 Winterwood Drive, Roselle, IL 60172. Tel: 800-374-8518. E-mail: aicardi@aol.com. Web site: http://www.aicardi.com.

Aicardi-Goutieres syndrome (microcephaly with basal ganglion calcification) A congenital autosomal recessive progressive leukodystrophic syndrome, characterized by microcephaly, seizures, basal ganglion calcification, hydrocephalus, CSF lymphocytosis, and mental and developmental delay.[77] Most patients present with severe developmental retardation, microcephaly, abnormal eye movements, pyramidal tract signs, and prominent dystonic movements. Although genetically heterogeneous, one locus has been identified at chromosome 3p21.[5522]

AIDS See HIV. Organizations offering information and support in this disease include the *Elizabeth Glaser Pediatric AIDS Foundation.* Address: 2950 31st St., Suite 125, Santa Monica, CA 90405. Tel: 310-314-1459; 888-499-4673. E-mail: info@pedAIDS.org/. Web site: http://www.pedAIDS.org/; the *American Foundation for AIDS Research*. Address: 120 Wall St. 13th Floor, New York, NY 10005-3902. Tel: 212-806-1600. E-mail: publications@amfar.org/. Web site: http://www.amfar.org/; the *National Association of People with AIDS.* Address: 1413 K Street, NW 7th Floor Washington, DC 20005-3442. Tel: 202-898-0414 ext. 124. E-mail: jmbrevelle@napwa.org. Web site: http://www.napwa.org/; the *National NeuroAIDS Tissue Consortium.* Address: 1050 Forest Hill Rd., Staten Island, NY 10314. Tel: 800-510-1678. E-mail: Joanna@hivbrainbanks.org/. Web site: http://www.hivbrainbanks.org/; and the *National Institute of Allergy and Infectious Diseases* (NIAID). Address: National Institutes of Health, 31 Center Drive, Rm. 7A50 MSC 2520, Bethesda, MD 20892-2520. Tel: 301-496-5717. Web site: http://www.niaid.nih.gov.

AIDS-dementia complex See **HIV encephalopathy**.

AIDS radiculopathy An inflammatory demyelinating polyneuropathy resembling **acute** or **chronic inflammatory demyelinating polyneuropathy**, considered to be immune-mediated and to reflect disordered immune regulation in patients infected with the human T-cell lymphotropic virus type III.

A predominantly sensory mixed axonal-demyelinating polyneuropathy is also found in patients with AIDS-related complex, and features of multiple mononeuropathy also occur in some of these patients. Another neuropathy with painful dysesthesias and symmetrical distal sensory loss has also been reported.[1288, 5931] See also **HIV-associated progressive polyneuropathy**.

AIDS-related dementia See HIV **encephalopathy**.

ainhum Spontaneous amputation of the smallest toes without anesthesia; a tropical disease seen in the Black races.

akataphasia (Gr, negative + to declare) See **Broca aphasia**.

akathisia (Gr, an inability to stay down) A feeling of restlessness or an irresistible urge to move, of which the patient is painfully aware. The urge is usually expressed as complex, stereotyped, and repetitive movements. The condition is most commonly induced by dopamine receptor–blocking drugs.[2358]

Complex stereotypies, accompanied by restlessness, are also common in patients with akathisia. Both early *acute persistent* and *chronic tardive* forms have been distinguished, the former when the dose of a neuroleptic drug is being increased and the latter at a late stage of therapy, during its reduction. See also **restless legs syndrome**, **Tourette syndrome**.

The following rating scale has been designed:[5488]

Subjective

1. Feeling of restlessness, especially in the legs
2. Inability to keep the legs still
3. Inability to remain still, standing or sitting

Objective (rate each item as 0 = absent, 1 = mild, 2 = moderate, 3 = severe)

1. Sitting:

   Semi-purposeful/purposeless leg/feet movements
   Semi-purposeful hand/arm movements
   Shifting body position in chair
   Inability to remain seated

2. Standing:

   Purposeless/semi-purposeful leg/feet movements
   Shifting weight from foot to foot or walking on the spot
   Inability to remain standing in one place (walking/pacing)

akee (achee) A West Indian fruit containing hypoglycin, an inhibitor of acyl coenzyme A dehydrogenases. Intoxication leads to a picture resembling **isovaleric acidemia**.[4313]

akinesia (akinesis) (Gr, lack of + set in motion) Defined by an international committee as a movement disorder "characterized by poverty and slowness of initiation and execution of willed and associated movements, and difficulty in changing one motor pattern to another in the absence of paralysis. This may include an inability to sustain repetitive movements and difficulty in performing repetitive motor acts and may vary in severity from slight (sometimes called hypokinesia) to severe and complete immobility."[6868]

akinesia algera (Möbius syndrome, atremia) The loss of voluntary motion as a result of pain produced by such motion. In the absence of any detectable physical disease likely to be responsible, the condition is considered to be functional or psychogenic.[5984]

akinesthesia Loss of directional sensitivity in the skin and joints.

akinetic freezing of gait A hypokinetic form of fluctuation in Parkinsonian patients on long-term levadopa therapy.

akinetic mutism (persistent vegetative state) The term introduced by Cairns[977] for the state in which patients appear awake and maintain a sleep–wake cycle but are unable to communicate in any way (i.e., not by speech, by gesture, nor by facial expression). The condition is characterized by continuous or prolonged deep NREM hypersomnia or coma with some retention of eye movements but with loss of REM sleep and of arousal mechanisms. The **Glasgow Coma Scale** score will be 4-1-1 or less. There is little evidence of damage to the descending corticospinal pathways.

Cairns' original patient had an epidermoid tumor of the third ventricle, but patients with lesions in the region of the thalamus, basal ganglia, anterior cingulate gyrus, or pons, or with obstructive hydrocephalus, and those with **Creutzfeldt–Jakob** disease may also enter this state. Those with lesions in the paramedian part of the posterior diencephalon, the anterior thalamic peduncle, or the midbrain are said to have "posterior" or "mesencephalic" akinetic mutism, and those with bifrontal lesions disconnecting the cingulate cortex to have the "anterior" or "frontal" form.

Since damage to both afferent and efferent pathways and to the rostral reticular activating system has caused the syndrome, it cannot be called homogeneous, although the clinical syndrome shows little variation. See **persistent vegetative state** (the preferred term) in which, however, spasticity is common, and also **de-efferented state**.

A *variant* is *akinetic mutism with blepharospasm, anomic aphasia, and delirium* which may complicate treatment with the immunosuppressive agent Muromonab-CD3 (OKT3). The MRI shows meningeal enhancement. Transient aseptic meningitis is a more usual complication.[5041]

akinetic-rigid syndrome Loss of the ability to initiate and to execute movements, associated with a loss of postural stability; negative symptoms, as typically seen in basal ganglion syndromes such as Parkinson disease but also as a result of heatstroke, as a toxic effect, and in numerous other neurological disorders. The subject was reviewed by Riley and Lang in 1996.[5305]

akinetic rigid syndromes Degenerative brain diseases producing these features.[6859]

They include **Wilson disease; dopa responsive dystonia; Juvenile Huntington disease; SCA3/MJD;DRPLA; Pelizaeus–Merzbacher disease; ataxia-telangectasia; Lesch–Nyhan syndrome; neurodegeneration with brain iron accumulation (NBIA); familial prion diseases**; autosomal dominant and autosomal recessive **juvenile Parkinson disease; X-linked dystonia parkinsonism (Lubag), and DDPAC**.

akinetic rigidity See **arteriosclerotic rigidity**.

akinetic seizures (centerencephalic myoclonic-astatic petit mal seizures) A syndrome in which seizures manifest by sudden and complete loss of muscle tone or absences are accompanied by severe mental retardation and often by major motor (grand mal) seizures.[3051] See also **Lennox–Gastaut syndrome**.

akinetic syndrome See **Parkinson disease**.

akinetopsia See **cerebral akinetopsia**.

akopia See **acopia**.

Akureyri disease See **von Economo disease**.

ALADIN See **Allgrove syndrome**.

Alajouanine, Theophile (1869–1959) French neurologist who was a pupil of the **Déjèrines** in Paris.

Alajouanine–Foix syndrome See **subacute necrotic myelopathy**.

Alajouanine syndrome Congenital bilateral paralysis of the sixth and seventh cranial nerves, with clubfoot.[91]

alalia (Gr, lack of + to talk) Speechlessness due to paralysis of the vocal apparatus.

Aland disease An X-linked disease reported (only) from the Aland Islands, characterized by deafness, seizures, mental retardation, latent nystagmus, and tapetoretinal degeneration.[2154]

alaninuria-microcephaly-dwarfism-diabetes syndrome See **Stimmler syndrome**.

alarm-clock headache A term reflecting the regularity of the attacks of head pain in **cluster headache**.

alarm reaction The first of the three stages of adaptive reaction to stressful situations defined by Hans **Selye**. It is marked by strong sympathetic activity, sufficient for the fight-or-flight response.

Albers–Schonberg disease (osteopetrosis, osteosclerosis fragilis, marble bone disease) A dominantly or recessively inherited syndrome characterized by increased density of the bones throughout the skeleton with unusual brittleness and associated with anemia and macrocephaly. The condition occasionally leads to cranial nerve (e.g., I, II, III, V, VII, VIII) palsies, nystagmus, or hydrocephalus.[3483, 6405]

The condition was described in 1904 by Heinreich Ernst Albers-Schonberg (1865–1921), a German radiologist and professor at Hamburg, who devoted his life to the study of X-rays and clinical radiology without being fully aware of their dangers.[102] See also **osteopetrosis**.

In a *variant form*, osteopetrosis is combined with syndactyly.[6405]

Albert disease See **achillodynia**.

Albert test A screening test for visual neglect in which the subject is required to cross out a series of lines ruled on a sheet of paper; the percentage of lines left uncrossed gives a score which in patients with acute stroke is related to cognitive outcome 6 months later.[104] See also **neglect**.

albinism Hereditary syndromes characterized by deficiency of melanin production in the eyes and/or skin. Most have no neurological complications other than congenital nystagmus.

The Rev. Mr. Spooner, a classicist don and warden of New College Oxford, was albino and it has been suggested that his verbal distortions ("Sir! You have hissed all my mystery lectures; you shall leave Oxford by the town drain") could be accounted for by his nystagmus which jumbled the words that he read; however, his abnormal speech was by all accounts spontaneous as much as read, so this explanation may be insufficient.

albinism with degenerative features A dominantly inherited syndrome of deaf–mutism with albinism.[6319]

Albright hereditary osteodystrophy (Fuller Albright syndrome, osteitis fibrosa disseminata, polyostotic fibrous dysplasia) A rare disorder with onset in childhood, characterized by replacement of bone by fibrous tissue, bony cysts, precocious puberty in female patients, areas of brown skin pigmentation, and, in some cases, papilledema and optic atrophy.[110]

Albright syndrome (pseudohypoparathyroidism and pseudopseudo hypoparathyroidism) A congenital dysmetabolic, dysmorphic **neurocutaneous syndrome** characterized by obesity; short stature; brachydactyly; dental anomalies; precocious puberty in females; hypocalcemia; intracranial, intramuscular, and subcutaneous calcification; skin hyperpigmentation; and mental and developmental delay.[3] Ocular symptoms reported include proptosis, visual field defects, optic atrophy, and papilledema.[110]

albumino-cytologic dissociation A marked increase in the level of protein in the cerebrospinal fluid without a similarly large increase in the cell count. See **Froin syndrome**.

alcohol A sedative drug that relaxes inhibitions first and provides transient emotional relief. Also, it is the cause of much social and medical misery. . King Darius of the Persians had inscribed on his tomb "I could drink much wine and bear it well" and William Pitt found that he could retire during a lively debate for a couple of bottles of port to refresh and enliven his faculties, but most heavy drinkers (i.e., more than three drinks per day for men or two for women) suffer some medical consequences. Some of the neurological problems associated with alcohol are listed in the following entries.

alcohol blackouts Temporary, complete inability to form long-term memories as the result of a high blood alcohol level. The inability may be partial or fragmentary with spotty losses of memory; or it could be complete, in which case memory is lost for the events that transpired during whole periods of time, including anything from general social to more intimate forms of intercourse. Their duration ranges between 6 h and 3 days. A rapidly rising blood alcohol level is a likely prerequisite.[6746]

Such periods of amnesia are primarily "anterograde," in that alcohol impairs the ability to form new memories while the person is intoxicated, rather than erasing memories formed before intoxication and are explained in part by the fact that alcohol impairs especially the transfer of information from short-term to long-term storage through the hippocampus.

alcohol-dependent sleep disorder A disorder characterized by persistent attempts to assist initiation of sleep by the ingestion of ethanol, used here for its sedative effect.[1629] Other alcoholic patients claim that they persistently wake up too early in the morning.

alcohol-induced headache The ICHD[2820] distinguishes two forms of headache related to alcohol ingestion:

Immediate alcohol-induced headache (cocktail headache) for which the diagnostic criteria are:

A. Headache with at least one of the following characteristics and fulfilling criteria C and D:
   1. Bilateral
   2. Frontotemporal location
   3. Pulsating quality
   4. Aggravated by physical activity
B. Ingestion of beverage containing alcohol
C. Headache develops within 3 h after ingestion of alcoholic beverage
D. Headache resolves within 72 h

Delayed alcohol-induced headache (hangover headache) for which the diagnostic criteria are:

A. Headache with at least one of the following characteristics and fulfilling criteria C and D:
   1. Bilateral
   2. Frontotemporal location
   3. Pulsating quality
   4. Aggravated by physical activity
B. Ingestion of a modest amount of alcoholic beverage by a migraine sufferer or an intoxicating amount by a nonmigraine sufferer
C. Headache develops after blood alcohol level declines or reduces to zero
D. Headache resolves within 72 h

From the International Classification of Headache Disorders (Headache Classification Committee of the International Headache Society. *Cephalalgia* 2004;**24**[Suppl 1]) by kind permission of Dr. Jes Olesen, the International Headache Society and Wiley-Blackwell Publications.

Alcohol-Use Disorders Identification Test (AUDIT) A screening test to evaluate problems with alcohol use.[5562]

alcohol withdrawal syndrome A clinical syndrome occurring in alcohol-dependent people within 1–2 days of the consumption of their last drink. Clinically, anxiety, tremor, headache, agitated delirium of any degree of severity (often with hallucinations), insomnia, and signs of excessive CNS and autonomic (sympathetic) activation are the prime features. The condition is particularly serious as it represents a possible precursor to **delirium tremens** and withdrawal seizures.[4242a]

alcoholic cerebellar degeneration A uniform syndrome in chronic alcoholics resulting from atrophy, especially of the cerebellar vermis. The clinical features include a broad-based, staggering gait, impaired heel–toe walking, slow leg tremor, and terminal oscillations in the finger–nose test with minimal involvement of the arms and without nystagmus or dysarthria.

The disorder is associated with destruction of all the neurocellular elements of the cerebellar cortex, and with damage to the anterior and superior aspects of the vermis and the olivary nuclei. Cerebral cortical atrophy is also likely to accompany this syndrome.[2902]

alcoholic dementia Widespread affections of intellectual function, subtle or severe, occurring in chronic alcoholics who have no evidence of Alzheimer disease, multi-infarct dementia, or **Wernicke–Korsakoff syndrome** (which is the diagnosis usually applied in the cases where the onset was not abrupt), and in whom there is a tendency for cortical shrinkage and ventricular dilatation on head CT scans.[3864] The absence of any typical pathology makes the existence of the entity as a primary condition suspect, however.[6542] See also **Marchiafava–Bignami disease, pellagrous encephalopathy, acquired hepatocerebral degeneration**.

alcoholic encephalopathy Alcohol-engendered **pellagra** affecting the brain, leading to central chromatolysis, especially marked in the brainstem pontine nuclei and cerebellar dentate nuclei, and in the nuclei of the third, sixth, seventh, and eighth cranial nerves.[2799]

alcoholic myopathy A syndrome of acute or chronic weakness due to the toxic effects of alcohol.

The *acute form* (**acute alcoholic myopathy**) is a necrotizing myopathy presenting with muscle pain, tenderness, swelling, and weakness which begins during a period of heavy alcohol intake. Myoglobinuria is commonly detectable, as are other manifestations of acute alcohol toxicity or withdrawal, many of which lead to excessive muscular activity.[1831]

The *chronic form* is a slowly progressive, painless proximal myopathy with retained reflexes, affecting the legs more than the arms. It improves with cessation of alcohol ingestion and improved nutrition.[1831]

A form associated with *hypokalemia* (**acute hypokalemic myopathy of alcoholism**) is also described.[3025]

alcoholic neuropathy (athrodynia a potu) A painful, centripetal, sensorimotor axonal neuropathy due at least in part to nutritional deficiencies in alcoholics. The condition was first described in 1779 by Lettsom (1744–1815), a physician in the Virgin Islands, and later in 1822 by James Jackson Sr. (1777–1867).

Clinically, insidiously progressive, distal weakness, paresthesias, and burning pain are the usual symptoms, felt in the legs much more than in the arms; hyperesthesias and hyperpathias are also common complaints. Symmetrical hyporeflexia, distal weakness, and the usual features of sensorimotor and autonomic neuropathy, with trophic changes, are typical signs.

A *variant* is *acute alcoholic axonal polyneuropathy*, presenting with flaccid tetraplegia and areflexia in subjects with malnutrition related to heavy alcohol consumption.[6841] See also **Wernicke–Korsakoff syndrome, Strachan syndrome, beriberi**.

alcoholic paraplegia Weakness of the legs associated with excessive alcohol abuse, described first in 1868 by Samuel Wilks (1824–1911), physician to Guy's Hospital, London.[6787] The condition is likely to represent either a severe motor neuropathy or a proximal myopathy, as described in the preceding entries.

Alcoholics Anonymous General services office. Address: P.O. Box 459, Grand Central Station, New York, NY 10017.

aldolase A deficiency A congenital dysmorphic syndrome characterized also by dwarfism; strabismus; ptosis; dental, dermal, skeletal, and cardiac anomalies; enlarged liver; microcephaly; and mental and developmental delay.[381]

alertness A phasic, graded state of arousal in which the subject is awake and responsive to environmental stimuli.

Alexander Graham Bell Association for the Deaf A charitable organization. Address: 3417 Volta Pl., NW, Washington, DC 20007-2778.

Alexander disease (fibrinoid degeneration of astrocytes, dysmyelinogenic leukodystrophy; OMIM 203450) A rare, fatal, sporadic leukodystrophy, usually occurring in infants and characterized by fibrinoid degeneration of astrocytes surrounding blood vessels, especially under the ependyma in frontal and parietal regions, which contain deposits resembling **Rosenthal fibers**, with widespread demyelination but preservation of neurons. The major component of Rosenthal fibers is glial fibrillary acidic protein resulting from GFAP mutations. Its biochemical basis is undefined. Linkage to 11q13 has been established. The many pathogenic mutations are listed at http://www.waisman.wisc.edu/alexander.

The major clinical features include psychomotor retardation, growth delay, seizures, spastic quadriparesis, and megalencephaly; death ensues within a few years.[6485] The condition was described by W.S. Alexander in 1949.[119]

MRI criteria have been suggested and include the presence of extensive symmetrical white matter lesions, especially frontally; a periventricular rim of low signal on T2 weighted images; swelling or atrophy of basal ganglia and thalamus; brain stem lesions; and contrast enhancement in the ventricular lining, periventricular rim, frontal white matter, optic chiasm, fornix, basal ganglia, thalamus, dentate, cerebellar cortex, or brainstem. The presence of four of these suggests the diagnosis. (For reference, see van der Knaap, 2006.)[6485]

Variants include the following:

A *localized form* in infants, characterized by spastic dysarthria, dysphagia, and fasciculations.[381]

A *juvenile type*, characterized by self-mutilation, seizures, bulbar weakness, nystagmus, ataxia, and pyramidal signs.[752]

Even rarer *adult forms* are characterized by dominantly inherited manifest nystagmus, dysarthria, palatal myoclonus, ataxia, intracranial calcification, cerebral gliosis, and diffuse demyelination[5477, 5670] with medullary atrophy and, in some cases, dementia.

Alexander's laws 1. The amplitude of the nystagmus caused by central lesions changes with the direction of gaze, being greater when gaze is directed in the direction of the fast phase.[5338, 5731] 2. Nystagmus of vestibular origin is separable into three degrees. First degree; present only when gaze is in the direction of the fast phase of the nystagmus; second degree; present also in the primary position; third degree; present when gaze is in any direction. Thus, in sum, nystagmus of vestibular origin is of greatest amplitude when the subject looks in the direction of its fast component. This last series of statements was enunciated by Dr. Gustav Alexander, an Austrian otolaryngologist, in 1912.

alexia (Gr, lack of + lexicon) Inability to comprehend the meaning of written or printed language symbols.[1330] Auditory comprehension is retained and spontaneous speech is normal in the pure form, which is rare and is marked by the subjects' ability to read letter by letter with errors, but not to manage whole words.

The condition was separated from other varieties of language impairment in 1885 by Lichtheim. **Déjèrine** described the two major varieties (***with agraphia*** and ***without agraphia***) in 1891–1892 and determined that the left angular gyrus is the center for the interpretation of the visual images which constitute written language.

A third form (*anterior or frontal alexia*; preangular, literal alexia, letter blindness) also exists, in association with **Broca aphasia** caused by a lesion in the posterior part of the dominant frontal lobe. It may represent inability to read out loud while internal comprehension is retained (in which case it is not really an alexia at all) or the exposure of a lifelong reading problem, but is most often a feature of the primary lesion.

Its features include **syntactic alexia**, anomia for letters though there is some success with comprehension of spelled words. Spelling aloud is poor. There is severe agraphia, poor ability to comprehend spelled words and to spell aloud, nonfluent aphasia, poor, clumsy copying with omissions, and accompanying right hemiparesis, motor apraxia, and mild sensory loss.[526, 522]

A fourth form, *deep dyslexia*, is a condition of total alexia and agraphia with an added lack of comprehension of words spelled out and is due to a lesion of the posterior parts of the cortical language areas. It occurs usually in the context of recovery from total alexia. In this condition, a patient can read only by lexical–semantic association, which leads to speech containing a number of synonyms which are spoken in place of the words read.

With *surface alexia*, words with irregular spelling are not read.

Finally, *neglect alexia*, seen in subjects with right pariental lesions, is characterized by their neglect of the first few letters of a word; thus "barnyard" might be read as "yard." See also **deep dyslexia**.

alexia with agraphia (central alexia; associative, verbal, literal, semantic, subangular, aphasic, total, parietal-temporal, letter, or cortical alexia; angular gyrus syndrome; word and letter blindness; word blindness; acquired illiteracy)A symptom complex identified by Déjèrine in 1891, comprising impairment of reading and naming, especially of letters but also of words (literal and verbal alexia); severe impairment of both spontaneous writing and writing to dictation, with retention of only a slavish ability to copy (agraphia); and an inability to comprehend spelled words and to spell aloud.[2905] Fluent aphasia, anomia, right hemisensory deficits with hemianopia, and the features of Gerstmann syndrome are occasionally found. The causal lesion is in the dominant parietotemporal region.[1538]

alexia without agraphia (posterior, occipital, sensory, verbal, agnosic, optic, associative, splenio-occipital, postangular, visual or pure alexia; pure word blindness) A disconnection syndrome described by **Déjèrine** (1892) and the first for which clear anatomical evidence was forthcoming. The major feature is an inability to read letters, words, or musical notation, in association with a right hemianopia and difficulties with color naming. Copying, writing spontaneously and to dictation, and the interpretation of pictures and letter naming are preserved, however, and verbal output is fluent and appropriate. Comprehension of spelled words and spelling aloud are retained.

A patient with the syndrome was recorded by Johann Schmidt in 1673 as follows: "He could not read written characters, much less combine them in any way. He did not know a single letter nor could he distinguish one from one another. But it is remarkable that, if some name were given to him to be written, he could write it readily, spelling it correctly. However, he could not read what he had written even though it was in his own hand."

The causal lesions are of the left occipital lobe and of the splenium of the corpus callosum, disconnecting the intact right visual cortex (area 18) from the left angular gyrus.[2338]

alexithymia An alteration in the regulation of affect such that subjects cannot identify nor describe feelings and have difficulty distinguishing feelings from bodily sensations of emotional arousal, impaired symbolization, and an externally oriented cognitive style, occurring usually in the context of clinical depression. Alexithymia may contribute to the development and severity of somatic and psychopathological disorders.

algesthesis (Gr, pain + perception) An antique term for any painful condition.

algetic (Gr, pain) Producing pain.

algodystrophy (Sudeck atrophy) See **complex regional pain syndrome**.

algoneurodystrophy See **reflex sympathetic dystrophy**.

Alice-in-Wonderland syndrome (depersonalization syndrome, Lilliputian syndrome) A syndrome of bizarre disturbances of the body image, feelings of levitation, alteration of the sense of the passage of time, depersonalization, **metamorphopsia**, and doubting of personality that may occur in the setting of migraine, epilepsy, parietal lobe disease, hypnagogic states, schizophrenia, delirious states, or the ingestion of hallucinogens. In migraine at least, the patient retains insight into the unreality of the experiences. The syndrome is also well described in children.[3004]

The same feelings of detachment, unreal changes in the outside world, fantastic distortions of the sizes and shapes of people and things, and the bewilderment that plagued Alice also affect the victims of this syndrome, as was noted by J.W. Todd in 1955.[6336] The fact that Lewis Carroll suffered from migraine may also have led to the appellation,[4294] and as Alice drank several mysterious vials of liquid before her strange experiences, so also have a number of victims of this syndrome ingested drugs such as LSD and hashish.[5704]

alien hand (limb) syndromes (la main étrangère; anarchic hand) Failure to recognize ownership of a limb in the absence of visual cues, associated with autonomous activity of that limb, which are perceived by the subject as outside his control; thus a circumstance in which one of the patient's hands behaves idiosyncratically and automatically in a way which the patient finds foreign, or at least uncooperative. It usually complicates a callosal lesion and may be accompanied by grasp reflexes, cortical myoclonus, involuntary groping toward (or manipulation of) objects perceived, intermanual conflict, mirror movements, and motor perseveration.[373] In many cases **apraxias** are also present. The patients frequently express astonishment and frustration at the errant limb (*autocriticism*). They experience it as being controlled by an external agent and often refer to it in the third person.

Alien hand syndrome most commonly follows lesions in the medial frontal lobes and corpus callosum. It is also encountered with more posterior strokes (posterior alien hand syndrome) and in patients with corticobasal ganglionic degeneration.[651] Various forms are recognized:

The *callosal form* is characterized by intermanual conflict (in which the hands act at cross-purposes with each other) and the *frontal type* by reflex grasping. The former usually occurs in the nondominant hand and is temporary, while the latter is due to left medial frontal lesions with callosal involvement and is persistent; the alien phenomena are seen in the contralateral dominant hand.[5608] A major recent review of that of Fisher.[2103] A *sensory alien hand syndrome* is also described, involuntary movements of choking and attack on the left side of the body by the right arm following a stroke in right posterior cerebral artery territory. Multiple disorders of primary sensation, sensory processing, hemispatial attention and visual association, and severe left arm ataxia are also present.[312] A posterior form with sensory ataxia and hemineglect due to a thalamic lesion has also been described.

The term *diagonistic dyspraxia* indicates a conflict between the desired act and that which is performed; *agonistic dyspraxia* is the compulsive automatic execution of orders by one hand when the patient is asked to perform that movement with the other one. *Magnetic apraxia/repellent apraxia* refers to instinctive grasping or avoiding with an abnormal posture.

In a *variant form* which may be ictal, the phenomenon occurs paroxysmally. The cortical lesions described were frontomedial or posteroparietal.[3763]

alien tissue lesions Hamartomatous masses commonly found in the temporal lobes of patients operated on for complex partial seizures. They are of three main types: *glial forms* may be astroglial or oligodendroglial; *mixed neuroglial forms* include gangliogliomas and cortical dysplasias, neither of which acts like a tumor. The *vascular lesions* occurring in this context represent angiomatous malformations.[6]

aliquorrhea A syndrome of low intracranial pressure following lumbar puncture or traumatic meningeal tears, occasionally seen with subdural hematomas or occurring spontaneously. The leading clinical symptom is headache occurring in the upright position, which fades quickly when the recumbent position is attained. See also **spontaneous intracranial hypotension**.

allachesthesia See **alloesthesia**.

Allan-Herndon-Dudley syndrome A rare X-linked variant of **hereditary spastic paraparesis** characterized by neonatal hypotonia, markedly delayed motor milestones, decreased muscle bulk, contractures at large and small joints, spastic paraplegia, extrapyramidal signs (variable), mental retardation (usually severe), dysarthria, ataxia, abnormal faces (elongated face with normal head circumference, bitemporal narrowing, and large ears), scoliosis, and broad, shallow pectus excavatum, and sometimes by mental retardation. Neck drop ("limber neck") is a characteristic finding. Linkage to chromosome Xq213 has been reported.[717]

allele (allelic) diseases Conditions in which the same genetic abnormality leads to differing clinical manifestations.

Allen–Dent syndrome See **argininosuccinase deficiency**, **citrullinemia**.

Allen diagnostic scale A scoring system devised to aid in the clinical diagnosis of the pathology underlying acute stroke.[130]

Allen reflex 1. (Gonda reflex) A variant of the **Babinski reflex** in which dorsiflexion of the hallux is sought in response to downward stretching and sudden release of the second toe. See also **Stransky reflex**.

2. (Cleckley reflex) A variant of the **Babinski reflex** in which dorsiflexion of the hallux is sought in response to upward flicking and sudden release of the second toe.

Allen score A scale with prognostic value in patients with stroke. The features recorded are:

Age in years
Loss of consciousness at onset of stroke
Drowsy or comatose 24 h after onset (or later)
Complete limb paralysis (no movement better than palpable contraction, MRC 1)
Higher cerebral dysfunction (HCD)

Aphasia and/or Parietal deficit:

Sensory or visual inattention or
Visuospatial neglect or
Loss of joint position sense

Homonymous visual field deficit to confrontation (HHA)

Patients with a score of <0 are likely to die or to have severe impairments if they live. Those with a score >0 will probably survive and will walk again.[129]

From Allen CMC. Clinical diagnosis of the acute stroke syndrome. *Quart J Med* 1983;52:515–23, reprinted by kind permission.

Calculation of Score	
Constant (start with)	+40
Complete limb paralysis	−12
HCD with HHA and hemiplegia	−11
Drowsy/comatose at 24 h	−10
Age in years	− (age × 0.4)
Initial loss of consciousness	− 9
Uncomplicated hemiparesis	+8

Allen diagnostic scale

Variable	*Clinical Feature*	*Score*
Apoplectic onset with two or more of the following:	None or one Two or more	0
loss of consciousness, headache within 2 h, vomiting, or neck stiffness		21.9
Level of consciousness 24 h after admission	Alert	0
	Drowsy	7.3
	Coma	14.6
Plantar responses	Both down or one upgoing	0
	Bilaterally upgoing	7.1
Diastolic blood pressure 24 h after admission		× 0.17
History of angina, claudication, or diabetes	None	0
	1 or more	−3.7
History of hypertension	Not present	0
	Present	−3.7
Previous transient ischemic attack or stroke	None	0
	Any previous event	−6.7
Heart disease	None	0
	Aortic or mitral murmur	−4.3
	Cardiac failure	−4.3
	Cardiomyopathy	−4.3
	Atrial fibrillation	−4/3
	Cardiomegaly on chest X-ray	−4.3
	Myocardial infarct in past 6/12 months	−4.3
Constant heart disease		−12

A score of <4 suggests ischemic stroke and a score of >24 suggests intracranial hemorrhage with fair reliability.[1066] See also **Siriraj score, NIH Stroke Scale, Canadian Neurological Scale.**

allergic angiitis and granulomatosis (Churg–Strauss syndrome) Vasculitic syndromes characterized by fibrinoid necrosis with eosinophilic and granulomatous tissue reactivity in capillaries, venules, and the small- and medium-sized muscular arteries.[6087] See **Churg–Strauss syndrome**. The clinical presentations resemble those of **polyarteritis nodosa**.[2728]

In a *variant form, necrotizing granulomatous angiitis with a predilection for the CNS* (Feisen–Cravioto syndrome) the effects are confined to the brain and spinal cord.

allergic polyneuritis A subacute motor neuropathy following prophylactic immunization against **Rabies**.[3724]

allesthesia See **alloesthesia**.

Allgrove syndrome (ALADIN, AAA or AAAA syndrome; OMIM 231550) A rare, recessively inherited multisystem peroxisomal disease of childhood, linked to a mutation at 12q13 and characterized by alacrima, achalasia, autonomic and sensorimotor polyneuropathy, and insensitivity to ACTH, largely as a result of cholinergic nerve dysfunction.[136] The condition usually presents in infancy with dysphagia, hypoglycaemia, and hypotension, which progresses to polyneuropathy and dementia, although survival to adult life has been reported.[3433] Many other neurological disorders have been reported in association.

The words ALacrima, achalasia, ADrenal Insufficiency and Neurological disorder have been manipulated into *aladin*, the name bestowed upon the faulty gene product.

Alliance of Genetic Support Groups A charitable organization. Address: 4301 Connecticut Ave. NW, Suite 404 Washington, DC 20008-2369. Tel: 202-966-5557; fax: 202-966-8553. E-mail: info@geneticalliance.org.

Allison leg jitters See **restless legs syndrome**.

all-median hand The anomalous condition in which all of the intrinsic hand muscles are supplied by the median nerve, which normally supplies only the opponens and abductor pollicis brevis, the lateral two lumbricals and half of the flexor pollicis brevis. The clinical significance is slight unless the patient happens to sustain an ulnar nerve lesion (in which case the hand continues to function normally) or a median nerve lesion (in which case the hand does not function at all).[4080]

all-or-nothing (none) response (of sensory nerve fibers) A phenomenon described first by Keith Lucas but further analyzed by **Adrian** in 1918 and then more fully 4 years later.[62] Adrian stated the All-or-Nothing principle as follows: "In a normal nerve fibre, where the impulse is not conducted with a decrement, the intensity of the impulse at any point depends only on the local condition of the fiber at that point [but neither] on the strength of the stimulus which set the impulse in motion nor on the amount of reduction which the impulse may have suffered in regions of decrement as it passed down the nerve."

all-ulnar hand Anomalous motor innervation of all of the intrinsic hand muscles by the ulnar nerve, the sensory innervation pattern being normal. The anatomical basis is the Riche–Cannieu anastomosis, through which the motor fibers from the median nerve transfer to the ulnar nerve in the palm.[5490]

allo- Greek prefix, signifying "other."

allocheiria (allochiria) Faulty localization of a stimulus, such that e.g., a subject touched on the left hand claims to having been touched on the right; a sign of right (nondominant) parietal lobe disease, described by **Bamberger** and by Obersteiner in 1881.

allochiria See **allocheiria**.

allocortex (rhinencephalon) The four-layered, differentiated paleocortex including the hippocampal formation and the pyriform cortex. With the **corticoid areas**, it constitutes the cortical expression of the **limbic system**.

allodynia (Gr, other + pain) (hyperpathia, hyperalgesia) Pain felt following a stimulus that is not usually noxious or painful. This frequently occurs in association with **causalgia** following prior axonal injury and indicates the presence of hyperexcitable axonal sprouts able to generate electrical impulses ab initio or else to encourage **ephaptic transmission**. **Sensitization** of peripheral nociceptors and disinhibition within the trigeminocaudal system are other postulated mechanisms,[2258] as are development of spontaneous activity in afferent inputs, sprouting of large primary efferents and of sympathetic efferents into neuromas and dorsal root and ganglion cells, the elimination of intrinsic modulatory systems, and up-regulation of receptors in the dorsal horn which mediate excitatory processes.See also **hyperalgesia**.

At the bedside, *brush allodynia* (provoked by stroking the skin with an artist's paintbrush) is most easily tested and will be found present over the face and scalp in a range of primary headache disorders.

Although its pathophysiological significance has only been appreciated recently, Dr. William Salmon wrote on this matter in his *Theory and Practice of Physick* (3rd edition, London, 1695) as follows: "if the film that covereth the skull be affected, the Pain is so vehement that the Sick cannot suffer the skin thereof to be touched by ones Hand."

alloesthesia (allesthesia)
1. Displacement of a sensation—usually tactile or visual—away from the true position of the stimulating object. Thus, a patient with a right parietal lesion touched on the left hand which is resting on a table may claim that it was actually the table that was touched. 2. Displacement of a perception (in any modality) from the correct to another side or site, seen with lesions of the right parietal lobe or spinal cord. Thus with visual alloesthesia, the percept may be displaced from an intact to a blind half-field.

Obersteiner described the sign first in 1880 in a patient with a spinal cord lesion and others have noted it in patients with hysteria or parietal lobe lesions. It is thought that damage to the crossing fibers causes sensory inputs to be channeled through uncrossed fibers on the opposite side.[3346]

allokinesis 1. Perception of an ordinary nonpruritic stimulus as itchy (HJM).[5853] 2. The performance of movements requested of the patient by the wrong limb. Thus a paralyzed left arm will not obey a request to touch an object, but the left leg will do so involuntarily.[2097]

allophones Minor variations in a phoneme.

allotriogeusia (Gr, another + taste) Perversion of taste. See **ageusia**.

alogia Poverty of speech production and content.

alopecia-mental retardation-seizures syndrome A congenital dysmorphic syndrome in which alopecia, fine, brittle hair, dental caries, seizures, and mental and developmental delay are associated. See **dermotrichic syndrome**.

alopecia, neurological defects, and endocrinopathy syndrome A recessively inherited syndrome (7q31.32, *RBM28*) described in an Arab Moslem kindred and characterized by loss of hair and subcutaneous fat, mental retardation, hypogonadotropic hypogonadism, central adrenal insufficiency, gynecomastia, short stature, microcephaly, and kyphoscoliosis.[4992]

Alpers, Bernard Jacob (1900–1981) American neurologist who trained at Harvard and studied as a postgraduate in Madrid with **Rio-Hortega**. He was professor and chairman of neurology at Jefferson Medical College, Philadelphia, for 27 years. He described the infantile gray matter degenerative disease, **Alpers disease**, named for him in 1931.

His comment on differential diagnosis: "based on collective data, clinical problems deal entirely with pertinent possibilities and not with a long list of all possibilities" represents a message which, in the context of Grand Rounds, has still not been widely understood.

Alpers disease (progressive neuronal degeneration of childhood with liver disease, progressive cerebral poliodystrophy; spongy glioneuronal dystrophy; diffuse cerebral degeneration in infancy; diffuse progressive cerebral cortical atrophy; progressive neuronal degeneration of childhood; Christensen–Krabbé syndrome; OMIM 203700)

A rare, sporadic or recessively inherited mitochondrial disease of unknown cause in which there is degeneration of the gray matter and glial tissue (infantile poliodystrophy) and a subacute hepatitis beginning early in life, often after a transiently normal infancy. It is the result of mutations in a mitochondrial DNA (mtDNA) polymerase gene (*POLG1*),

Clinically, the disease is characterized by progressive mental deterioration, developmental delay, spasticity, myoclonus and intractable generalized convulsions, choreoathetosis, ataxia, optic atrophy with blindness, deafness, vomiting, and early death from liver failure in association with abnormal lactate and pyruvate metabolism.[142] Adolescent onset has also been recorded.The differences between this condition and **Leigh disease** are questionable. See also **familial poliodystrophy**, **MNGIE and** the Web site: http://www.ninds.nih.gov/disorders/alpersdisease/alpersdisease.htm/.

alpha-aminoadipic aciduria A rare diffuse encephalopathy, probably recessively inherited and a possible cause of mental retardation, characterized by this urinary finding.[2070]

alpha coma (alpha pattern coma) The presence of an EEG pattern predominantly within the alpha frequency band, paradoxically resembling waking EEG patterns but unreactive to touch, sound, or pain and often widely distributed over the head, seen in apparently comatose patients. See **persistent vegetative state** (the preferred term).

This is most commonly seen in hypoxic patients following cardiac arrest, those with localized brainstem lesions at or just caudal to the pontomesencephalic junction, or those with drug intoxication or concussion.[6545, 300]

Its outcome may be predicted by the reactivity of the EEG to noxious stimuli but the finding carries a poor prognosis; the few survivors seldom have meaningful recovery.[3296]

alpha-fetoprotein A protein. Its levels are elevated in the amniotic fluid of fetuses that have neural tube deficits. Acetylcholinesterase levels, however, have more specificity.

alpha galactosidase The enzyme deficient in **Fabry disease**.

alpha-glycerophosphate dehydrogenase deficiency See **glycerophosphate dehydrogenase deficiency**.

alpha ketoadipic aciduria A rare diffuse encephalopathy of infants due to an error in lysine metabolism (failure of conversion of α-ketoadipic acid to glutaryl coenzyme A) and characterized by impairment of mental and physical development, metabolic acidosis, skin rash, hypotonia, and seizures.[6719]

alpha-mannosidosis deficiency (OMIM248500) A recessively inherited lysosomal storage disease associated with decreased activity of α-mannosidase, an enzyme that degrades oligosaccharides and glycoproteins in neural and visceral tissues. Two disease phenotypes are described: type I, the severe infantile phenotype, and type II, which progresses more slowly and allows survival to a state of adult leukoencephalopathy.[1056]

alpha-methyl-aceto-acetyl-coenzyme (Aß-ketothiolase deficiency) A hyperammonemic syndrome causing accumulation of acetoacetic and other organic acids, and clinically characterized by episodic vomiting, impairment of consciousness, seizures, hyperglycemia, and ketoacidosis.[1471]

alpha-methyl-ß-hydroxybutyric aciduria A diffuse encephalopathy due to deficiency in thiolase activity, characterized by mental retardation, metabolic acidosis, and altered consciousness.[1471]

alpha rhythm Regular, rhythmic activity on the EEG at 8–13 Hz occurring during wakefulness over the posterior regions of the head, generally with higher voltage over the occipital area. Its amplitude is variable but is mostly below 50 uV in the adult and it is best seen with the eyes closed and under conditions of physical relaxation and relative mental inactivity. The rhythm is blocked or attenuated by attention (especially visual), mental effort, and drowsiness.

The use of the term must be restricted to those rhythms that fulfil all these criteria. Activities in the alpha band which differ from the alpha rhythm as regards their topography and/or reactivity either have specific appellations (e.g., the mu rhythm) or should be referred to as rhythms of alpha frequency. (Adapted from the 1974 Report of the Committee on Terminology, IFCN[1117] and reproduced by kind permission of Elsevier science.)

alpha-sarcoglycan deficiency A muscular dystrophy presenting in childhood with easy fatigue, hyperCKemia, and mild scapular winging with the later development of exercise intolerance and myoglobinuria. Muscle biopsy demonstrates slight fiber size variability but dystrophin is normally distributed; carnitine palmitoyl transferase and glycolytic enzyme levels are normal. Immunohistochemistry shows marked reduction of α-sarcoglycan. Genetically, there is compound heterozygosity with Arg284Cys and Glu137Lys substitutions, corresponding to nucleotide changes C850 T and G409 A in the gene.[4446]

alpha variant rhythms Certain characteristic EEG rhythms which are recorded most prominently over the posterior regions of the head and differ in frequency but resemble in reactivity the alpha rhythm. Cf. **fast alpha variant rhythm** and **slow alpha variant rhythms**. (Adapted from the 1974 Report of the Committee on Terminology, IFCN[1117] and reproduced by kind permission of Elsevier science.) This rhythm tends to have a frequency that is harmonic of the fundamental EEG rhythm.

alpine sickness See **altitude insomnia**.

Alport, A. Cecil (1890–1959) American physician.

Alport syndrome (dominant nephritis and hearing loss) A dominantly or incomplete sex-linked recessively inherited disease of childhood, characterized by progressive renal impairment with interstitial foamy cells in the kidneys; neural deafness; abnormalities of the lens including spherophakia and caaracts; macular degeneration; and optic nerve **drusen**.[147, 2201]

ALS See **amyotrophic lateral sclerosis**. Charitable organizations in this field include: The *Family Caregiver Alliance*. Address: 690 Market St., Suite 600, San Francisco, CA 94104. Tel: 415-434-3388; 800-445-8106. E-mail: info@caregiver.org. Web site: http://www.caregiver.org; the **ALS Association**; the **ALS Society of Canada**; the Forbes Norris ALS Research Center. Address: California Pacific Medical Center, 2324 Sacramento St., San Francisco, CA 94115. Tel: 415-923-3604; the *Les Turner ALS Foundation*. Address: 8142 North Lawndale Ave., Skokie, IL 60076. Tel: 888-ALS-1107. Web site: info@lesturnerals.org; and the **International Alliance of ALS/MND Associations**, a coordinating body for national organizations supporting people living with ALS Web site: http://www.alsmndalliance.org/.

ALS and Associated Web Sites A patient-based site providing links to other sites related to ALS, including chat rooms and message boards.

ALS and Neuromuscular Research Foundation A charitable organization. Address: California Pacific Medical Center, 3698 California St. Room 545, San Francisco, CA 94118. Tel: 415-923-3604.

ALS Association A charitable organization dedicated to finding the cause and cure of this disease. It provides funding for research, conducts scientific symposia, and provides both public and professional education programs and patient counseling. Address: 21021 Ventura Blvd., Suite 321, Woodland Hills, CA 91364-2206. Tel: 818-340-7500; Fax: 1-800-782-4747.

ALS Forums An online support group, moderated by people with that condition and intended for others affected.

ALS Foundation for Life A nonprofit organization dedicated to increasing public awareness of Amyotrophic Lateral Sclerosis. Web site: http://www.alsfoundation.org/.

ALS mimic syndromes See **multifocal motor neuropathy, Kennedy syndrome, motor neuropathy, noncompressive myelopathy, spinal muscular atrophy, cervical spondylitic myelopathy, hereditary spastic paraparesis, postpolio syndrome, hyperthyroidism,** and **Pancoast syndrome.**

ALS Network A resource and support for people with ALS, their families, and caregivers and helps unite with other PALS to educate the public about the condition.

ALS-Parkinson-dementia syndromes See **amyotrophic lateral sclerosis** (*variants*).

ALS Ride for Life An ALS site with charitable functions.

ALS Society of Canada A charitable organization dedicated to providing care and finding the cure for ALS. Web site: http://www.als.ca.

ALSSQOL A tool for assessing the quality of life in patients with **amyotrophic lateral** sclerosis and surveying negative emotions, interaction with people and the environment, intimacy, religiosity (sic), physical symptoms, and bulbar functions.[5845] See also **Sickness Impact Profile, McGill Quality of Life Inventory.**

Alstrom–Hallgren syndrome (recessive retinal degeneration, diabetes, obesity, and hearing loss) A rare, recessively transmitted syndrome of infancy or childhood characterized by loss of central vision because of pigmentary retinal degeneration (cone-rod dystrophy), diabetes mellitus, progressive neural deafness, hypogonadism, interstitial nephropathy, and, sometimes, acanthosis nigricans, mental retardation, or obesity.[149] See also **Bardet–Biedl syndrome, Usher syndrome.**

alternans nystagmus See **periodic nystagmus.**

alternate brachial diplegia See **cruciate paralysis.**

alternate cover test See **cover test.**

alternate fixation The ability of a subject to fixate with either eye with equal facility.

alternate inferior paralysis See **Millard–Gubler syndrome.**

alternate paralysis A condition described in the nineteenth century, in which there is paralysis of movement on one side of the body and of sensation on the other.[5103] A low brainstem lesion could account for this rare occurrence.

alternating abducent hemiplegia See **Raymond syndrome.**

alternating contraction anisocoria A rare consequence of damage to the pathway from the pretectal area to the Edinger–Westphal nucleus. There is increased reactivity of the affected eye to light, but the size of the pupils is equal in darkness.

alternating current nystagmus See **vestibular nystagmus.**

alternating eye deviation sign Consistent deviation of the eyes in parallel away from the side on which the examiner is standing, occurring when the examiner attempts to open the subject's eyes. The condition is considered to be a conversion reaction.[246]

alternating hemiplegia Paresis of cranial nerves on one side of the body and of the trunk and limbs on the other, constituting clear evidence of a lesion of the brainstem. The term was introduced by Gubler. See also the **Weber, Benedikt, Foville, Millard–Gubler, Jackson** and **Villaret syndromes,** and the **alternating hypoglossal hemiplegia syndrome.** *Alternating Hemiplegia* is a Web-based information sheet compiled by the National Institute of Neurological Disorders and Stroke.

alternating hemiplegia of childhood A rare, progressive disease with onset before the age of 18 months, characterized by sudden and repeated attacks of hemiplegia lasting hours to days, involving each side alternately, relieved by sleep, associated with other paroxysmal phenomena (tonic attacks, posturing, nystagmus, chorea or athetosis) or with autonomic disturbances, and with progressive mental and neurological deterioration.[73] Ocular palsies and fixed motor deficits are additional features described. In infancy, screaming attacks may precede the motor manifestations.[1047] The condition may reflect mitochondrial dysfunction.

In *variant forms,* the condition is dominantly inherited,[4355] affects all four limbs, or is a benign syndrome occurring repetitively during sleep. See also **periodic syndromes.**

The syndrome also appears in *infantile hypotonia and paroxysmal dystonia, paroxysmal symptomatic alternating dystonia with hemiparesis,* **migraine coma,** *alternating diplegia with livedo reticularis,* and **pyruvate dehydrogenase deficiency.**[184]

alternating Horner syndrome The apparent alternation with time of the side on which there is a **Horner syndrome.** This represents a *variant* in which the miosis, ptosis, and facial flushing in patients with lower cervical cord disease alternate from side to side over days, presumably as a result of a lesion of the ciliospinal centers of Budge.[2251]

Another explanation would be that one side is normal but that on the other, the manifestations of the Horner syndrome alternate with those of a **Pourfour du Petit syndrome**.

alternating hypoglossal hemiplegia syndrome (anterior bulbar syndrome, Déjèrine syndrome) A vascular medial brainstem syndrome in which damage to the pyramid and twelfth cranial nerve nucleus on one side causes wasting and weakness of the tongue with anesthesia of the soft palate and posterior pharyngeal wall on the same side as the infarct; and a contralateral hemiparesis.

In a *variant form (alternating hypoglossal hemiplegia-hemianesthesia syndrome)*, contralateral numbness also occurs, due to involvement of the medial lemniscus. See also **Déjèrine syndromes**.

alternating nystagmus See **periodic nystagmus**.

alternating oculomotor paralysis See **Weber syndrome**.

alternating parallel syndrome The association of spastic hemiparesis, cerebellar ataxia, and trigeminal analgesia on the side of a brainstem lesion, with analgesia of the trunk and limbs on the contralateral side, due to an adjacent or extending lesion affecting the cervical cord.[6340]

alternating sensory loss Impairment of certain modalities of sensation on different sides of the head and of the trunk and limbs. Thus, in the **lateral medullary syndrome,** damage to the descending spinal nucleus and tract and to the ascending spinothalamic pathway leads to loss of pain and temperature sensation over the face on the same side and of the trunk and limbs on the other side. See **alternating thermoanalgesia, alternating hemiplegia**.

alternating sequences test A test of concentration, planning, and resistance to interference, in which the subject is required to write some lines of alternating letters or shapes.[3965]

alternating thermoanalgesia A subjective diminution of the sense of sharp pain and of temperature on one side of the face and the opposite side of the trunk and limbs. This combination of signs signifies the presence of a lateral brainstem lesion, as in the **Wallenberg syndrome** or the **anterior inferior cerebellar artery syndrome**. See **alternating sensory loss**.

alternating windmill nystagmus See **circular nystagmus**.

alternobaric vertigo An acute form of vestibular vertigo occurring in pilots during marked change in altitude, usually following straining movements (Valsalva) designed to "clear the ears" and always due to obstruction of the Eustachian tubes. Nystagmus and oscillopsia are the usual accompaniments.

altitude insomnia (acute mountain sickness, Acosta disease, Andes disease, Alpine sickness, hypobaropathy) An acute insomnia usually accompanied by headaches, loss of appetite, and fatigue following ascent to high altitudes. Diagnostic criteria include the following:[1629]

A. A complaint of insomnia
B. A temporally related ascent to a high altitude (typically above 4000 m)
C. Polysomnographic monitoring that demonstrates:
    1. Reduced total sleep duration, decreased sleep efficiency with an increased sleep latency, and increased arousals and awake time
    2. A pattern of periodic breathing during sleep
    3. Oxygen desaturation during sleep
D. Other medical or psychiatric disorders can be present but are not the cause of the primary complaint
E. The complaint is not caused by other sleep disorders, such as obstructive sleep apnea syndrome, central sleep apnea syndrome, or other causes of insomnia.

From AASM Diagnostic Classification Steering Committee. *The International Classification of Sleep Disorders Diagnostic and Coding Manual*. Rochester, MN. American Academy of Sleep Medicine 1991/2001. Reproduced by kind permission of the Academy. See also http://www.sleepeducation.com/Disorders.aspx/.

altitudinal defects Visual field defects which do not cross the equator of vision (but may cross the vertical meridian) and which indicate the presence of an acquired lesion of the retina or choroid, or of the more proximal portion of the visual pathway. They also occur with congenital hypoplasia of the optic nerve.

altitudinal headache See **high-altitude headache**.

altitudinal hemianopia Loss of half of the visual field above or below the (horizontal) equator. This is usually evidence of retinal vascular insufficiency or of anterior ischemic optic neuropathy. See also **hemianopia**, **altitudinal defects**.

altitudinal neglect Neglect of half of the visual field above or below the equator. This is usually evidence of bilateral parietal lobe lesions.[5197]

alveolar hypoventilation DIMS (disorders of initiating and maintaining sleep) syndrome A syndrome of insomnia due to the disruption of sleep occasioned by central apnea superimposed upon hypopnea with alveolar hypoventilation, associated with daytime unresponsiveness to chemical regulators of ventilation (see also **sleep disorders** and **Ondine's curse**).

alveolar hypoventilation DOES (disorders of excessive sleep) syndrome The appearance or worsening during sleep of conditions characterized by impaired ventilation (reduced tidal volume or respiratory rate) but without prolonged apneic spells. See **sleep disorders**.

alveolar sarcoma A rare malignant primary tumor of muscle occurring in children and young adults, in which muscle cell differentiation can be differentiated microscopically.

Alzheimer, Alois (1864–1915) German neuropsychiatrist and pathologist, professor of psychiatry in Munich and then Breslau. He first described the disease named for him, differentiating it from "arteriosclerotic dementia" on the basis of the presence of neurofibrillary tangles and refractive plaques in the presence of only minimal vascular changes in a lecture given in Tubingen in 1906, publishing this a year later. **Kraepelin**, with whom he was working, recognized the description as definitive and named the disease for Alzheimer in 1910.

Alzheimer also made important contributions in the areas of syphilis, Huntington, and Parkinson diseases and vascular dementias[5704] although these contributions are less well remembered.

Alzheimer Association An American charitable organization with 217 chapters nationwide. Research, education, chapter formation, advocacy, and patient and family services are its goals. Funding is available for pilot and multiyear research proposals in the basic, clinical and social sciences with relevance to Alzheimer disease. Address: 919 N. Michigan Ave., Suite 1000, Chicago, IL 60611-1696. Tel: 312-335-8700. E-mail: info@alz.org. Web site: http://www.alz.org. Also Alzheimer's Association Home Page.

Alzheimer disease The proper name for what was formerly known by the pejorative term *senile dementia* (introduced by **Binswanger** in 1898). At last it has become a respectable subject for research, in part because of the economic threat that it poses to Western civilization as the population ages and the prevalence increases. Order has been brought to the clinical diagnostic process by the acceptance of diagnostic guidelines (see Chart A–4). Progressive memory loss, aphasia, apraxias, and visuospatial abnormalities are the most important features.

The most common genetic flaws appear to be in *PS-1* (presenilin 1) on chromosome 14. Less often, *PS-2*, on chromosome 1, is implicated, and still more rarely, a third gene, *amyloid precursor protein* (*APP*) on chromosome 21. In all three cases, the mutations are autosomal dominant. Among them, *APP* encodes the polypeptide amyloid precursor protein, of which a fragment is toxic to the brain. The tangles consist mainly of *tau*, a microtubule-associated protein. Rare kindreds have been identified carrying tau mutations associated with a familial form of frontotemporal dementia. On the basis of the known cleavage sites in the A-beta precursor protein, a set of proteolytic enzymes had been predicted, the so-called alpha, beta, and gamma secretases. Among them, the beta and gamma enzymes liberate A-beta, while the alpha enzyme cleaves within the A-beta sequence, precluding A-beta production. A-beta secretase has now been identified and named beta-site APP cleaving enzyme (BACE).

Criteria for pathological diagnosis have also been defined: cortical atrophy, neuronal loss, "senile" plaques, vacuoles, neurofibrillary tangles (the earliest change observed), and meningeal fibrosis are characteristic; all were described by Alzheimer verbally in 1906 or in subsequent publications in 1907[155] and 1911.[3336]

Internet sites of interest include: www.alz.org, www.alzforum.org, www.alzheimer.ca, and www.alzheimer's.org; See also the Alzheimer's Disease Fact Sheet at http://www.ninds.nih.gov/disorders/alzheimersdisease/alzheimersdisease.htm (providing information compiled by the National Institute of Neurological Disorders and Stroke) and the Alzheimer's Information Site at http://www.alzinfo.org/ (offering information on the disease, current research, and resources).

See also **dementia** and **frontotemporal dementia** (from which the differentiation may be difficult).[4304]

Chart A–4. NINCDS Criteria for the Clinical Diagnosis of Alzheimer disease[4600]

I. The criteria for the clinical diagnosis of PROBABLE Alzheimer disease include

A. Dementia, established by clinical examination and documented by the **Mini-Mental State examination**, the **Blessed Dementia Scale**, or some similar examination, and confirmed by neuropsychological tests
B. Deficits in two or more areas of cognition
C. Progressive worsening of memory and other cognitive functions
D. No disturbance of consciousness
E. Onset between ages 40 and 90, most often after age 65 years
F. Absence of systemic disorders or other brain diseases that in and of themselves could account for the progressive deficits in memory and cognition

II. The diagnosis of PROBABLE Alzheimer disease is supported by

A. Progressive deterioration of specific cognitive functions such as language (aphasia), motor skills (apraxia), and perception (agnosia)
B. Impaired activities of daily living and altered patterns of behavior
C. Family history of similar disorders, particularly if confirmed neuropathologically
D. Laboratory results: Normal lumbar puncture as evaluated by standard techniques; normal pattern or nonspecific changes in EEG, such as increased slow-wave activity; and evidence of cerebral atrophy on CT scanning with progression documented by serial observation

III. *Features that make the diagnosis of PROBABLE Alzheimer disease uncertain or unlikely*

A. Sudden, apoplectic onset
B. Focal neurological findings such as hemiparesis, sensory loss, visual field deficits, and incoordination early in the course of the illness
C. Seizures or gait disturbances at the onset or very early in the course of the illness

IV. *Clinical diagnosis of POSSIBLE Alzheimer disease*

A. May be made on the basis of the dementia syndrome; in the absence of other neurological, psychiatric, or systemic disorders sufficient to cause dementia; and in the presence of variations in the onset, in the presentation, or in the clinical course
B. May be made in the presence of a second systemic or brain disorder sufficient to produce dementia, which is not considered to be the cause of the dementia
C. Should be used in research studies when a single, gradually progressive severe cognitive deficit is identified in the absence of other identifiable cause

Alternative Research Diagnostic Criteria have been formulated, e.g., by Berg.[549] The American Psychiatric Association *DSM IV-TR diagnostic guidelines*.[172] differ slightly; they can be found at http://www.behavenet.com/capsules/disorders/dsm4TRclassification.htm/.

Variants include the following:

Alzheimer disease with spongy changes and myoclonus A syndrome in which the onset of dementia is between the ages of 20 and 50 years, with added myoclonic seizures. Pathologically, cerebral atrophy, neurofibrillary tangles, senile plaques, and spongy changes are found in the brain.[381]

Familial Alzheimer disease Relatively uncommon dominantly inherited types of the disease.[379] Early-onset forms are associated with the gene presenilin 1 on chromosome 14 (14q24), amyloid precursor protein on chromosome 21 (21q11.2–21q21) or presenilin 2 on chromosome 2. A later-onset form maps to chromosome l9 (19q13). In each case, the clinical picture is much the same as that in patients with the sporadic form.

A dominantly inherited form associated with spastic paraparesis and non-neuritic "cotton wool" plaques, with a deletion of exon 9 of the presenilin-1 (PS-1) gene.[879]

Early-onset autosomal dominant dementia with ataxia, extrapyramidal features, and epilepsy.[2049]

Visual variant of Alzheimer disease A form characterized by early visual agnosia and abnormal contrast sensitivity without defects of acuity or color vision, slowly progressing over years to a demented state with the pathological features of Alzheimer disease.[3808]

Alzheimer disease with cerebrovascular disease A category of dementia reserved for patients fulfilling the clinical criteria for possible **Alzheimer disease** who also present clinical or brain-imaging evidence of relevant cerebrovascular disease.

Early-onset Alzheimer disease A dominantly inherited variant mapping to chromosome 14q 23.

Dominantly inherited Alzheimer disease with spastic paraparesis and non-neuritic "cotton wool" plaques, associated with a deletion of exon 9 of the *presenilin-1* gene. Clinically, individuals with paraparesis at presentation have a later than average age at onset of dementia symptoms.[879]

Alzheimer disease with spastic paraparesis See **familial British dementia**.

A *psychotic phenotype* characterized by a rapid decline in cognitive and functional capacities and a tendency toward aggressive behavior with a suggestive familial basis.[6165]

Alzheimer Disease and Associated Disorders

Alzheimer Disease and Associated Disorders (*Alzheimer Dis Assoc Disord*) A subspecialty neurological journal. Web site: http://www.alzheimerjournal.com/.

Alzheimer Disease Assessment Battery

Alzheimer Disease Assessment Battery A computer-based behavioral assessment package designed to detect deterioration of cognitive functioning in **Alzheimer disease**.[809]

The battery examines intellectual deterioration, pathological memory loss, word-finding disturbance, and spatial disorientation. A selective reminding task is incorporated and word fluency, spatial disorientation, and remote memory are also assessed.

Alzheimer Disease Assessment Scale

Alzheimer Disease Assessment Scale A 21-item scale designed to assess the severity of cognitive and noncognitive behavioral impairments in a patient with dementia due to **Alzheimer disease**.

The scale includes short neuropsychological tests and items rated by the clinical examiner on the basis of observation of the patient's behavior and after an interview with the caregiver. It is divided into two sections, the first employing short tests of memory, language, and praxis to give a *cognitive sub-scale*, and the second rating mood, distractibility, vegetative functions, agitation, delusions, hallucinations, and concentration to give a 10-item *noncognitive subscale*.[5396]

Alzheimer's Disease Fact Sheet

An information sheet compiled by the National Institute of Neurological Disorders and Stroke. Web site: http://www.ninds.nih.gov/disorders/alzheimersdisease/alzheimersdisease.htm/.

Alzheimer Disease Society

A British charitable organization. Address: 3rd floor, Bank Buildings, Fulham Broadway, London SW6 1EP, UK.

Alzheimer Foundation

Alzheimer Foundation An organization devoted to facilitating clinical and basic research in Alzheimer disease. The official journal of the foundation is the *Journal of Geriatric Psychiatry and Neurology*. Address: 8177 South Harvard M/C-114. Tulsa, OK 74137. A Web site allowing access to many related sites is at http://www.alz.org/

Alzheimer Society of Canada—Société Alzheimer du Canada

A charitable organization providing information on Alzheimer Disease, related dementias, caregiving, support, research, treatment, and programs and services. Address: 1320 Yonge St., Suite 201, Toronto, ON M4T 1X2. Tel: 416-925-3552.

Alzheimer type I astrocyte

Alzheimer type I astrocyte An astrocyte with a large lobulated vesicular nucleus and abundant vacuolated cytoplasm, resulting from aberrant cell division and described in the striatum of patients with **Wilson disease** and with other chronic liver diseases.

Alzheimer type II astrocyte

Alzheimer type II astrocyte An astrocyte with a large, irregularly shaped, and lobulated nucleus encompassed by a narrow rim of poorly staining cytoplasm. It is characteristically found in patients with ammonia toxicity, as in hepatic failure.

Alzheimer's Association

A charitable organization in this field. Address: 919 North Michigan Ave., Suite 1100, Chicago, IL 60611-1676. Tel: 312-335-8700; 800-272-3900. E-mail: info@alz.org. Web site: http://www.alz.org/.

Alzheimer's Center

Alzheimer's Center A Mayo Clinic site offering information, explanations, and advice about treatment and care for patients with Alzheimer disease. Web site: http://www.mayoclinic.com/health/alzheimers/AZ99999.

Alzheimer's Disease Education and Referral Center (ADEAR)

A site providing data on current research and clinical trials and with links to other Federal resources, a service of the National Institutes of Health. Address: P.O. Box 8250, Silver Spring, MD 20907-8250. Tel: 301-495-3311; 800-438-4380. E-mail: adear@alzheimers.org. Web site: http://www.nia.nih.gov/alzheimers.

Amalric syndrome

Amalric syndrome (macular dystrophy–deaf–muteness syndrome) A recessively inherited syndrome of congenital partial deafness and atypical pigmentary retinopathy without impaired night vision.[156] Its similarities to **Alport**, **Cockayne**, **Laurence-Moon-Biedl**, and **Hallgren syndromes** are notable.

amaurosis (from Gr, darkness) The term used by Hippocrates for "a becoming dull of sight" in seventeenth-century England for the condition "when the sight is gone and no fault is to be seen."[5886] It is now used almost exclusively for **transient monocular blindness** of vascular origin.

amaurosis congenita See **Leber disease**.

amaurosis fugax A term signifying **transient monocular blindness** (TMB), the latter being a more precise and contemporary label. It is usually due to platelet–cholesterol emboli, but in about 20% of cases is migrainous. Since the etiological diagnosis is almost impossible to make clinically, the precision of studies of the various treatments for amaurosis is questionable.

Wray has discerned four types, differentiated by their underlying pathologies and reproduced by kind permission.[6875]

Type I (transient retinal ischemia— embolic) is characterized by the abrupt loss of all or a part of the vision in one eye, lasting seconds to minutes, with total recovery. The partial visual impairment may be described as a curtain, ascending, descending, or moving sideways, and producing a uniocular altitudinal or hemianopic defect. Patients may experience a central scotoma, a paracentral scotoma or an area of segmental visual loss. In addition, they may complain of vertical or horizontal stationary scintillating scotomas, which may be associated with (a) vague, irregular, background shadows that rapidly move to the periphery and (b) vague, irregular shadows suddenly appearing paracentrally and moving toward the periphery in seconds. Intensely bright, tiny scintillating lights suddenly appear paracentrally and move peripherally (seconds) in a straight horizontal line, leaving behind a faint glowing line for 2 or 3 s.

Most commonly, the visual loss is complete, the patient stating that "everything is completely black." Vision recovers in seconds to minutes, with recovery taking longer than loss. *Variants* include graying, dimming, or blurring of vision.

The pathophysiological mechanism is thought to be arterial occlusion due to emboli to the ophthalmic artery or to the retinal artery.

Type II (retinal vascular insufficiency— hypoperfusion) is characterized by a less rapid onset of visual loss. In general, it is of longer duration, lasting minutes to hours (thus temporary rather than transient). Many of these patients complain of peculiar visual aberrations such as loss of or excessive contrast vision, dazzle, photographic negative imagery, flickering lights, photopsias, and dyschromatopsias. In addition, many experience a blurring or total loss of vision when they go out into (or come in from) bright light, or upon assuming a sitting or an upright position. The visual loss is often described as a concentric contraction of the visual field ("iris diaphragm effect"), especially when it is bilateral. Rarely, a patient will report blindness after eating. Often, while reading, the subject will complain that the page becomes excessively bright. Complaints of chronic ocular or retro-ocular pain of an insidious and aching nature are also recorded.

In all of these cases there is severe carotid stenosis, either ipsilaterally or bilaterally, marked by low perfusion pressures on ophthalmodynamometric testing.

Type III (angiospastic form) is characterized by the sudden onset of total visual loss or progressive contraction of the visual field sparing fixation. These attacks are usually short lived in terms of minutes, but may be prolonged. Direct observations of the fundus during such attacks have revealed:
(a) narrowing of the retinal arteries and veins, cessation of blood flow, segmentation of the blood columns, and optic disc pallor; and (b) narrowing of the retinal veins.

Fluorescein angiography reveals early filling of the optic disc capillaries with late filling (30 s) of the retinal arterioles in the former case (a), and a delay in filling of the central retinal artery in the latter (b). Many of these patients have a known migraine diathesis.

Type IV (idiopathic forms) is a "wastebasket" category in which the signs and symptoms defy classification. The type of visual disturbance in this group of patients closely resembles that of Type I, except for the duration of the attack, which may be very short (like a transient obscuration of vision) or very long (thus resembling a type III attack). In general, the patients suffer from multiple attacks, some occurring as frequently as one or two times per day. No identifiable pathophysiological mechanism can be determined,[939] but anticardiolipid antibodies may be tarred with guilt by association.

amaurosis-hemiplegia syndrome (Espildora–Luque syndrome) Blindness in one eye with contralateral hemiparesis, due to reflex spasm of the homolateral middle cerebral artery (as originally described), to separate emboli to that artery, or to occlusion of the internal carotid at the takeoff of the ophthalmic artery.[1657] See **Espildora-Luque syndrome**.

amaurotic familial idiocy (Tay–Sachs disease) The original term for the **gangliosidoses**, applied by Bernard Sachs (1858–1954), an American neurologist. The term is now defunct, having been replaced by the names of the two broad categories of disease which the condition represents, namely the **gangliosidoses** and the **neuronal ceroid lipofuscinoses**.

amaurotic pupil A pupil that does not constrict despite maximal light stimulation of the eye, because of damage to the afferent pathway.

ambient echolalia The use of words suggested by irrelevant local visual or auditory stimuli rather than by the context of the conversation. This occurs as a manifestation of delirious states and some dementias.[2097]

ambiguo-hypoglossal paralysis See **Tapia syndrome**.

ambiguo-spinothalamic syndrome See **Avellis syndrome**.

ambiopia See **diplopia**.

amblyaphia (Gr, dulled + the sense of touch) Numbness.

amblyopia (Gr, dulled or blunted + eye) Impairment or loss of vision in a healthy eye which is not due to an error in refraction nor to other disease of the eye itself.

Squint and **anisometropia** are the commoner causes, although Hippocrates used the word for dimness of vision in old age, which indicates that the use of the word has been modified substantially.

Amblyopia ex anopsia is diminished vision due to suppression of images from a ("lazy") strabismic eye.

ambulation index A simple scale of some value in assessing the stage of disease in multiple sclerosis.[2477]

AMC See **arthrogryposis multiplex congenita**.

AMC ([Dutch] Academic Medical Centre) Linear Disability score A scale for measuring disability in patients with **Parkinson disease**.[6708]

amebiasis Infection with *Naegleria* or with *Entamoeba histolytica*; in each case, a potential cause of meningoencephalitis or of cerebral abscess.[1045]

ameloblastoma See **craniopharyngioma**.

amenorrhea-galactorrhea syndrome The occurrence of these problems due to the excessive secretion of prolactin by a pituitary basophilic adenoma.

American Academy of Cerebral Developmental Medicine A professional organization. Address: 2315 Westwood Ave., P.O. Box 11086, Richmond, VA 23230.

American Academy of Clinical Neurophysiology A professional organization. Address: 5700 Old Orchard Rd., First floor, Skokie, IL 60077-1057. Tel: 708-966-0050. Web site: www.pressenter.com/-dtjorneh/.

American Academy of Neurological and Orthopedic Medicine and Surgery A professional organization. Address: 320 Ranchero Drive, Suite 108, Las Vegas, NV 89102.

American Academy of Neurological Surgery A professional organization. Address: Massachussetts General Hospital, Department of Neurosurgery, Fruit Street, Boston, MA 02114. Tel: 617-726-2000.

American Academy of Neurology (AAN) A leading professional organization founded in 1948 against the strident opposition of some members of the **American Neurological Association** (ANA), in order to cater to the educational and scientific needs of all neurologists and to be a forum for the younger members of the discipline. Unlike the ANA, the AAN offers ordinary membership to any individual with Board qualifications and associate and junior membership categories are also available. Fellows are elected from the ranks of those clinical neurologist members who have attended sufficient annual meetings.

Dr. A.B. **Baker** was the prime mover in the founding of the academy in March 1948; he and Drs. Forster, Aird, and **Wartenberg** were the first directors. The house journal is *Neurology*. The early history of the academy was recounted by Brown.[892] Address: 2221 University Ave. SE, Suite 335, Minneapolis, MN 55414. Tel: 612-623-8115; Fax: 612-623-3504. Web site: http://www.aan.com/. The Web site for the practice guidelines of AAN is at www.aan.com/professionals/practice/guidelines.cfm/.

American Academy of Neuromuscular and Electrodiagnostic Medicine (AANEM) (formerly the American Association of Electromyography and Electrodiagnosis) A professional society concerned with education, practice standards, and research into neuromuscular disease, founded in 1953 by Dr. James G. Golseth, an American neurologist. *Muscle and Nerve* is the official publication of the association. Tel: 507-288-0100. Web site: http://www.aanem.org/.

American Academy of Pain Management A professional specialist organization in this field. Web site: http://www.aapainmanage.org/.

American Academy of Sleep Medicine (formerly American Sleep Disorders Association) A professional society in the medical subspecialty of sleep medicine. Its mission is to set clinical standards for the field of sleep medicine, advocate for recognition, diagnosis, and treatment of sleep disorders, educate professionals dedicated to providing optimal sleep health care, and foster the development and application of scientific knowledge in this field. Fax: 708-492-0943. Web site: http://www.aasmnet.org/.

American Association for the Study of Headache See **American Headache Society**.

American Association of Acoustic Neuroma A professional organization. Address: P.O. Box 398, Carlisle, PA 17013. Tel: 717-249-4783; Fax: 717-249-0353.

American Association of Electrodiagnostic Technologists A professional organization. Address: Box 40, Davey, NE 68336.

American Association of Neurological Surgeons A professional society. Address: 625 N. Michigan Ave., Suite 1519, Chicago, IL 60611. Tel: 312-993-0043. Web site: http://www.aans.org/.

American Association of Neuropathologists (AANP) A professional society of neuropathologists seeking to advance research and training. The official forum of the AANP is the *Journal of Neuropathology and Experimental Neurology*, Web site: http://www.neuropath.org/pt/re/aanp/home.htm.

American Association of Neuroscience A professional organization. Address: 224 N. Des Plaines, Suite 601, Chicago, IL 60661. Tel: 312-993-0043.

American Association of Neuroscience Nurses A professional organization. Web site: http://www.aann.org.

American Association of Physical Medicine and Rehabilitation A professional organization. Address: One IBM Plaza, Suite 2500, Chicago, IL 60611-3604. Tel: 312 464-9700. E-mail: info@aapmr.org. Web site: http://www.aapmr.org.

American Autoimmune Related Diseases Association A charitable organization in this field. Address: 22100 Gratiot Ave., Eastpointe, East Detroit, MI 48201-2227. Tel: 586-776-3900; 800-598-4668. E-mail: aarda@aol.com. Web site: http://www.aarda.org.

American Behcet's Disease Association A charitable organization in this field. Address: P.O. Box 15247, Chattanooga, TN 37415. Tel: 800-723-4238. E-mail: mharting@ix.netcom.com. Web site: http://www.behcets.com.

American Board of Clinical Neurophysiology A professional organization. Address: 1111 Lac de Ville Blvd., Rochester, NY 14618. Tel: 804-627-0713.

American Board of Electrodiagnostic Medicine A body established in 1988 to control the process of specialization in this field and to oversee the recognition of those considered to be qualified in electromyography and related disciplines. Address: 21 Second St., Suite 306, Rochester, MN 55902. See also **American Academy of Neuromuscular and Electrodiagnostic Medicine**.

American Board of Electroencephalography and Neurophysiology A body established to control the process of specialization and to oversee the recognition of those considered to be qualified in electroencephalography and related disciplines. Address: 850 Elm Grove Rd., Elm Grove, WI 53122.

American Board of Neurological Surgery An American regulatory body. Address: School of Medicine, LSU Medical Center, 1542 Tulane Ave., New Orleans, LA 70112. Tel: 504-568-5036.

American Board of Psychiatry and Neurology A body established in 1934 to control the process of specialization and to oversee the recognition of those considered to be qualified in these disciplines.

American Brain Tumor Association A charitable association in this field. Address: 2720 River Rd., Suite 146, Des Plaines, IL 60018. Tel: 708-827-9910. Web site: http://www.abta.org.

American Brain Tumor Association's Primer A patient manual providing information about brain tumors and their treatments.

American Chronic Pain Association A charitable organization providing support and information on this condition. Address: P.O. Box 850, Rocklin, CA 95677. Tel: 916-632-0922. Web site: http://www.theacpa.org.

American Clinical Neurophysiology Society A specialist professional organization. Web site: www.acns.org.

American College of Neuropsychopharmacology A professional association. Address: 134 Wesley Hall, Vanderbilt University, Nashville, TN 37240. Tel: 615-322-7417.

American Council for Headache Education (ACHE) A charitable organization concerned with public education about the nature and management of headache. Address: 19 Mantua Rd., Mt. Royal, NJ 08061. Tel: 856-423-0258; 800-255-2243. E-mail: achehq@talley.com. Web site: http://www.achenet.org.

American Electroencephalographic Society A professional organization for physicians and others with interests in basic systems neurobiology, neuroimaging, and neurobehavior. Address: 1 Regency Dr., P.O. Box 30, Bloomfield, CT 06002. Tel: 203-243-3977.

American Epilepsy Society A professional society promoting interdisciplinary communication and the exchange of basic and clinical information about epilepsy. Address: 638 Prospect Ave., Hartford, CT 06105. Tel: 203-232-4825. Web site: http://www.aesnet.org/.

American Foundation for the Blind A charitable organization. Address: 15 W. 16th St., New York, NY 10011. Tel: 212-620-2000.

American Headache Society A professional organization for physicians and others interested in the study and management of headache and facial pain, founded in 1959. Its objectives are to promote the exchange of ideas concerning the cause and treatment of headache and related painful disorders, the education of physicians and other health professionals, and the encouragement of scientific research. Address: 19 Mantua Rd., Mt. Royal, NJ 08061. Tel: 856-423-0043. Web site: http://www.americanheadachesociety.org/.

American Heart Association A charitable organization providing support and information on vascular disease including stroke. Address: 7272 Greenville Ave., Dallas, TX 7523I. Tel: 214-373-6300. Web site: www.americanheart.org/.

American Insomnia Association A patient-based organization dedicated to assisting and providing resources to insomniacs. Web site: http://www.americaninsomniaassociation.org/.

American Journal of EEG Technology (*Am J EEG Technol*) A subspecialty EEG journal. Address: ASET Executive Office, 204 West 7th St., Carroll, IA 51401.

American Journal of Neuroradiology (*Am J Neuroradiol*) A neuro-radiological journal. Address: Waverly Press Inc., 428 E. Preston St., Baltimore, MD 21202. Web site: http://www.ajnr.org/.

American Lyme Disease Foundation, Inc. A charitable association in this field. Address: Royal Executive Park, 3. International Dr., Rye Brook, NY 10573. Tel: 914-277-6970.

American Medical Electroencephalographic Association A professional organization. Address: 850 Elm Grove Rd., Elm Grove, WI 53122. Tel: 414-796-1149.

American Narcolepsy Association A charitable organization providing support and information on this condition. P.O. Box 26230, San Francisco, CA 94126-6230. Tel: 415-788-4793.

American Neurological Association (ANA) A leading professional society devoted to the cultivation of neurological science in its normal and pathological relations, founded by William **Hammond**, J.J. Putnam, and others in 1875. The ANA was the first of the national neurological associations to be formed, the British one coming into existence in 1886, the French one in 1899, and the German one in 1907.

The neurological trauma cases produced by the Civil War led to a great increase in interest in neurology in the latter half of the nineteenth century in the United States and the ANA flourished, with **Ramsay Hunt**, **C.L. Dana**, **Bernard Sachs**, Pearce Bailey, Charles K. Mills, **Silas Weir Mitchell**, George Beard, and James Jewell among its members.

The association's journal was the *Archives of Neurology* until 1975, when it sponsored the **Annals of Neurology** under the editorship of Dr. Fred Plum. A retrospective anniversary volume was published in 1975.[1596] Membership today is by election and requires evidence of significant scientific contributions on the part of the candidate. Address: 2221 University Ave. SE, Suite 350, Minneapolis, MN 55414. Tel: 612-623-2401. Web site: http://www.aneuroa.org/.

American Nystagmus Network A nonprofit organization serving the needs and interests of those affected by nystagmus. Web site: http://www.nystagmus.org/.

American Pain Society A charitable association in this field. Address: 5700 Old Orchard Rd., Skokie, IL 60077. Tel: 708-966-5595. Web site: http://www.ampainsoc.org/.

American Paralysis Association A charitable organization concerned with research, care, and treatment of spinal cord injury and other paralyzing or disabling conditions. Address: 500 Morris Ave., Springfield, NJ 07081. Tel: 201-379-2690; 1-800-225-0292. A related Web site is at: http://www.familyvillage.wisc.edu/lib_sci.htm.

American Paraplegia Society A charitable organization providing support and information on this condition. Address: 75-20 Astoria Blvd Jackson Heights, NY 11370. Tel: 718-303-3782. Web site: http://www.apssci.org.

American Parkinson Disease Association A charitable organization that provides an educational, referral, and support programme to medical professionals, patients and their families, and the public at large through regional symposia and educational literature and videotapes. The association has 48 information and referral centers, 90 chapters, and more than 350 support groups. It also sponsors research on Parkinson disease by funding Advanced Centers for Research, fellowships, and research grants. Web site: http://www.apdaparkinson.org/.

American Psychiatric Association *Diagnostic and Statistical Manual* A compilation, revised periodically of all psychiatric and many neurological disorders, with diagnostic criteria. The *Diagnostic and Statistical Manual, IV Edition (Text Revision)* is the current volume.[172]

American Sleep Apnea Association A charitable organization in this field. Address: 1424 K St. NW. Suite 302, Washington, DC 20005. Tel: 202-293-3650. E-mail: asaa@sleepapnea.org. Web site: http://www.sleepapnea.org.

American Sleep Disorders Association See the American Academy of Sleep Medicine.

American Sleep Disorders Association Diagnostic Classification of Sleep Disorders See sleep disorders.

American Sleep Medicine Foundation A not-for-profit charitable and scientific organization established by the American Academy of Sleep Medicine. Address: One Wesbrook Corporate Center, Suite 920, Westchester, IL 60154. Tel: 708-492-0930; Fax: 708-492-0943. E-mail: info@discoversleep.org.

American Society for Clinical Evoked Potentials A professional organization. Address: 41 East Point Rd., White Plains, NY 10601.

American Society for Experimental Neurotherapeutics A professional organization. Web site: www.asent.org.

American Society for Neuroradiology A professional organization. Web site: www.asnr.org/.

American Society for Neurorehabilitation A professional organization. Web site: www.asnr.com.

American Society for Stereotactic and Functional Neurosurgery A professional organization. Address: Division of Neurosurgery, 636431 Fannen, University of Texas Medical School, Houston, TX 77030. Tel: 713-792-2121.

American Society of Electroneurodiagnostic Technologists The national professional organization for EEG/EP/PSG/NCV technologists, physicians, managers, institutions, and students. It provides education, employment services, a newsletter, insurance services, and an annual scientific forum and publishes the *American Journal of EEG Technology*. Address: 204 W. 7th St., Carroll, IA 51401-2317. Tel: 712-792-2978.

American Society of Neuroimaging A professional scientific organization dedicated to the advancement of all types of neuroimaging through literature and the promotion of scientific and educational programs. Address: 2221 University Ave. SE, Suite 340, Minneapolis, MN 55414. Tel: 612-623-2404. Web site: http://www.asnweb.org/.

American Society of Neuroradiology A professional association. Address: Rush Presbyterian Medical Center, 1753 West Congress Parkway, Chicago, IL 60612. Tel: 312-942-5000.

American Society of Neurorehabilitation A professional organization dedicated to improving patient care and fostering and encouraging research, teaching, and training in all areas of neurorehabilitation. Address: 2221

University Ave. SE, Suite 360, Minneapolis, MN 55414. Tel: 612-623-2405. Web site: http://www.asnr.com/.

American Speech Language Hearing Association (ASHA) A charitable organization in this field. Address; 10801 Rockville Pike, Rockville, MD 20852-3279. Tel: 301-897-5700; 800-638-8255. E-mail: actioncenter@asha.org. Web site: http://www.asha.org/.

American Stroke Association A division of the American Heart Association. Address: 7272 Greenville Ave., Dallas, TX 75231-4596. Tel: 1-888-478-7653. E-mail: strokeassociation@heart.org. Web site: http://www.strokeassociation.org.

American Syringomyelia Alliance Project A charitable organization providing support and information on this condition. Address: P.O. Box 1586, Longview, TX 75606-1586. Tel: 903-236-7079; 1-800-ASAP-282. Web site: http://www.asap4sm.com/.

American Tinnitus Association A charitable organization providing support and information on this condition. Address: P.O. Box 5, Portland, OR 97207. Tel: 503-248-0024; 503-248-9985.

American Tourette Syndrome Association A charitable organization providing support and information on this condition. Address: 42-40 Bell Blvd Bayside, New York, NY 11361-2861. Tel: 718-224-299; 1-800-237-0717. Web site: http://www.nlm.nih.gov./medlineplus/tourettesyndrome.html/.

amimia Loss of the power to copy gestures.

Amin-Amat syndrome (inverse Marcus Gunn phenomenon, inverse jaw-winking) A rare condition in which the homolateral eye closes as the external pterygoid muscle moves the jaw to the opposite side. It is due to inhibition of the levator palpebrae during the activation of the fifth nerve; in some cases this occurs as a congenital anomaly.[3943]

aminoacidopathies Inborn errors of metabolism presenting usually in the neonatal period with depression of neurological function and increase or decrease in muscle tone. See **hyperglycinemia, homocystinuria, hypervalinemia, phenylketonuria, maple syrup urine disease.**

aminoaciduria-retardation-dwarfism and muscular dystrophy syndrome See Stransky **syndrome.**

aminoacylase 1 deficiency A recessively inherited organic aciduria manifesting as developmental delay with seizures in childhood, caused due to various ACY1 mutations.[5553]

Ammon, Friedrich Augustus von (1799–1861) German physician who studied medicine in Leipzig and Gottingen, specialized in ophthalmology in Dresden, and was then professor of pathology and materia medica at that university.

Ammon's horn The hippocampus. The god Jupiter was considered capable of assuming the form of a ram, in which guise his name was Ammon. The name refers to the shape of a ram's horn.

Ammon's horn sclerosis Gliosis of the hippocampus, the most common single lesion found in the temporal lobectomy specimens of patients with **complex partial seizures**. It was first described by Sommer in 1880.

amnemonic (Gr, lack of + memory) Diseases characterized by loss of memory.

amnesia (Gr, lack of + memory) Forgetfulness, or inability to learn new material currently perceived unless repeatedly rehearsed. Amnesia exists both for events and for facts. Broca's use of the word in the phrase *verbal amnesia*, meaning "impaired word-finding", is no longer current. See also **hysterical amnesia, post-traumatic amnesia, primary amnesia, retrograde amnesia, topographic amnesia,** and **transient global amnesia**.

Amnesia Association A charitable organization. Address: 25 Prebend Gardens, London, W4 1TN, United Kingdom.

amnesic aphasia Originally, a fluent aphasia (see **anomic aphasia**).

amnesic automatisms An occasional feature of the narcolepsy complex, in which the subject acts automatically (but usually appropriately) without subsequent recall. See also **transient global amnesia.**

amnesic shellfish poisoning See **shellfish poisoning**.

amnesic stroke Persistent or transient amnesic syndromes resulting from infarction in the territory of the posterior cerebral arteries, usually accompanied by visual field deficits. Rarely, unilateral (usually left-sided) infarctions in the territories of the posterior cerebral, anterior choroidal, or thalamic penetrating arteries affecting the hippocampus or thalamus may cause a similar pure amnesic state.[4831]

amnestic A term for diseases causing loss of memory.

amnestic aphasia A form of aphasia in which there is a failure to recall the names of people or of other nouns in conversation when they are presented visually or verbally.

amnestic color anomia An inability to recall the names of colors but with retention of the ability to distinguish them.

amnestic-confabulatory syndrome See **Korsakoff syndrome**.

amnestic disorder A disorder of memory due to bilateral lesions of the hippocampal–limbic circuit in which the subject is unable to store new memories ("loss of recent memory") and to some extent fails to recall previously learned data. It causes significant impairment in social and occupational functioning. Classic causes are **Wernicke–Korsakoff encephalopathy** and **herpes simplex encephalitis**. Craniocerebral trauma is also one of the many other causes.

The diagnostic guidelines provided by American Psychiatric Association *DSM IV-TR*[172] can be found at http://www.behavenet.com/capsules/disorders/dsm4TRclassification.htm/.

An amnestic syndrome with anterograde, retrograde, and postevent amnesia and relative preservation of recognition memory[2228] can also occur after basal forebrain infarction.

amniotic bands A congenital dysmorphic syndrome caused by compression of the fetus by fibrous bands of amniotic origin *in utero*.

The clinical results of this include omphalocele; constriction rings of the arms, legs, or digits; and syndactyly. **Craniosynostosis, hydrocephalus, holoprosencephaly, encephalocele,** and **cranial meningocele** have all been described in association.[3024]

amoeboid movements Variable distortions of a dilated pupil, considered to reflect excessive activity in the ciliary ganglion or of the long ciliary nerve.[6617]

amok A self-limited syndrome of spontaneous, wild, and murderous agitation, the word coming from Malaya, where this behavior is described with greater frequency than elsewhere, mainly in young men. Whether the cause is toxic or psychological is not determined.

amorphin A structural protein in the Z-lines of muscle.

amorphosynthesis 1. A *variant* term for **constructional apraxia** as a result of parietal lobe dysfunction. 2. Inability to comprehend or be aware of parts or functions of the body. Tactile extinction would be a minor form of this condition, hemiasomatagnosia a maximal form.[1593]

amphigory Fluent, grammatical, but nonsensical or irrelevant speech in demented patients who do not have dysphasia.[2087] Central and medial temporal lobe lesions are usually responsible.

amphiphilic drug myopathy Form of myopathy associated with the ingestion of large, cationic amphiphilic molecules (i.e., with both hydrophilic and hydrophobic sites). Such agents include imipramine, amiodarone, chloroquine, and colchicine.[3600]

amphiphysin autoimmunity The production of IgG antibodies to the synaptic vesicle protein amphiphysin in association with underlying malignancy; clinically presenting with neuropathy, encephalopathy, myelopathy, **stiff-person**, or cerebellar syndromes.[5043]

amphoamphoterodiplopia (Gr, both + both of two + double sight) Diplopia which is both uni- and binocular. The length of the word is inversely proportional to the importance of the condition.

amplitude With reference to an action potential, the maximum voltage difference between two points, usually baseline-to-peak or peak-to-peak. By convention, the amplitude of potentials that have an initial negative deflection from the baseline, such as the compound muscle action potential and the antidromic sensory nerve action potential are measured from baseline to the most negative peak. In contrast, the amplitude of a compound sensory nerve action potential, motor unit potential, fibrillation potential, positive sharp wave, fasciculation potential, and most other action potentials is measured from the most positive peak to the most negative peak.[19] (From the 2001 Report of the Nomenclature Committee of the American Association of Electromyography and Electrodiagnosis.[19] Reproduced by kind permission of the AANEM.)

amplitude decay The percent change in the amplitude of the M wave or the compound sensory nerve action potential between two different stimulation points along the nerve.
Decay = 100 × ($amplitude_{distal}$ – $amplitude_{proximal}$ / $amplitude_{distal}$.). It is said to be useful in the evaluation of conduction block. Abnormal decay without increased temporal dispersion may indicate a conduction block.

Ampole syndrome A congenital dysmorphic syndrome characterized also by short stature, strabismus, double ureters, arachnodactyly, skeletal deformities, dry skin, seizures, and mental and developmental delay.[381]

amputation illusion A sensation that may occur after spinal cord injury in which the subject feels that an anesthetic part is no longer present at all.[5827]

amputation neuroma A swelling at the distal end of the proximal segment of a cut nerve, composed of bundles of randomly oriented axons (**neurites**), Schwann cells, and connective tissue.

Amsterdam dwarfism See **De Lange syndrome**.

Amsterdam Short Term Memory (ASTM) test A test of memory and concentration, reported to be of value in detecting malingering in subjects after whiplash injury and leading to the suggestion that the cognitive complaints of nonmalingering postwhiplash patients are likely to result from chronic pain, chronic fatigue, or depression.[5613]

amusement park stroke Stroke, usually due to dissection of a vertebral artery, as a result of hyperextension of the neck during a roller-coaster ride.[946] Headache, subdural hematoma, acute anxiety, vertigo, and vomiting are other complications of this leisure activity.

amusia (Gr, lack of + to do with the Muses—in this case those concerned with melodies) Inability to discern the elements of music such as rhythm, pitch, melody, modulation, intonation, and accentuation of musical sounds. Like aphasia, this has both expressive and receptive forms, both of which seem to be unusually common among people who otherwise appear healthy and many of whom today are in the forefront of composition.

The faculty of musical expression is probably dependent on the normal function of the anterior parts of the right or left temporal and posterior inferior frontal convolutions. On the sensory side, *tone deafness* and *note blindness* were the other terms suggested by Knoblauch (1888) for those disorders of communication involving music which correspond to aphasia in the realm of language. The **Luria–Nebraska Battery** examines some such functions.

Numerous other disorders have also been identified in the musical field[4339] including motor and sensory amusia, *paramusia*, *musical agraphia*, *amnestic amusia*, *musical alexia*, *instrumental apraxia*, and **amimia**.

amyelotrophy (Gr, lack of + marrow + nourishment) Atrophy of the spinal cord.

amygdala (Gr, almond) A nucleus, part of the limbic system, situated deep in the inferomesial aspect of the temporal lobe at the tail of the caudate. Its major roles are in motivation, affect, and emotional display.

amygdalar sclerosis Severe neuronal loss and sclerosis in the amygdala without accompanying hippocampal pathology, associated with seizures and described in subjects who have had temporal lobe surgery for that indication.[4369]

amygdalo-hippocampal seizures (mesiobasal limbic or rhinencephalic seizures) Hippocampal seizures are the most common form; the symptoms are those described under **temporal lobe syndromes** except that auditory symptoms may not occur. The interictal scalp EEG may be normal, or may show interictal uni- or bilateral temporal sharp or slow waves, which may be synchronous or asynchronous. The intracranial interictal EEG may show mesial anterior temporal spikes or sharp waves.

Clinically, the seizures are characterized by rising epigastric discomfort, nausea, marked autonomic signs, and other symptoms including borborygmi, belching, pallor, fullness of the face, flushing of the face, arrest of respiration, pupillary dilatation, fear, panic, and olfactory–gustatory hallucinations,[1264] and the seizures tend to increase during REM sleep.

amyloid (β-amyloid protein) (from Lat, starch) An insoluble fibrous membrane protein, part of the β-amyloid precursor protein, which exhibits green birefringence in polarized light after staining with Congo red. It is encoded by a gene on chromosome 21. The β-protein form is found in the CNS in neurofibrillary tangles, in plaques, and in the walls of cerebral vessels, typically in **congophilic angiopathy**, **Alzheimer disease**, and **Down syndrome**. The prion protein form is also found in scrapie and in **Jakob–Creutzfeldt disease**.

Primary amyloidosis is that form associated with the AL amyloid protein, an immunoglobulin light-chain fragment produced by plasma cells. The same amyloid protein is also found with **multiple myeloma**, Waldenstrom **macroglobulinemia**, and agammaglobulinemia. The main findings are cardiac and renal, but painful sensorimotor and autonomic peripheral axonal neuropathy and amyloid myopathy are neurological complications, mainly in elderly men. Genetic forms are also recognized; see **familial amyloid neuropathy** and below.

In *secondary amyloidosis* (as with various chronic diseases, Hodgkin disease, and familial Mediterranean fever) the protein is of the AA type, derived from a plasma protein precursor in patients with chronic inflammatory disease or with malignancy such as renal cell carcinoma and Hodgkin disease. Yet other forms of amyloid protein are expressed in dialysis patients and those with different mitotic lesions or **Alzheimer disease**.

In a *variant* form, *AA amyloidosis* may be associated with autonomic neuropathy, vestibulocochlear dysfunction, and lattice corneal dystrophy.[6413]

Variant forms of amyloidosis are described at http://neuromuscular.wustl.edu/nother/amyloid.htm/.

amyloid angiopathy See **congophilic angiopathy**.

amyloid-associated muscle pseudohypertrophy General hypertrophy of muscles attributed to the deposition of extracellular amyloid within skeletal muscles, producing proximal limb stiffness, aching, and weakness.[5310]

amyloid myopathy An occasional manifestation of primary systemic amyloidosis in which there is infiltration of muscles with amyloid material, forming nodules and compressing muscle fibers, leading to atrophy or pseudohypertrophy, weakness, hardness of muscles, macroglossia, and hoarseness. It is seen mainly in older males. The EMG findings are of chronic myositis.[3202, 2336]

amyloid neuropathy Forms of neuropathy characterized by the deposition of amyloid (fragments of an immunoglobulin light chain) within tissues in cases of sporadic **amyloidosis**. *Primary amyloid neuropathy* presents with sensorimotor polyneuropathy, **carpal tunnel syndrome,** and **autonomic neuropathy,** complicating renal and cardiac failure.[49] *Secondary amyloidosis* leads only to entrapment neuropathies. See also **familial amyloid neuropathy**.

amyloidoma Large deposits of amyloid material within the parenchyma of the nervous system and choroid plexus where they may give rise to clinical features resembling those of a tumor.[1232]

amyloidopathies Neurodegenerative disorders characterized by the production/deposition of normal or abnormal amyloid material within cells of the nervous system. Examples are **Alzheimer disease,** some forms of **primary systemic amyloidosis,** and **familial British** (or Danish) **dementia**.

amyloidosis Deposition of **amyloid** within tissues, as occurs in familial, primary, or secondary amyloidosis. See **familial amyloid neuropathy, myeloma, gammopathic neuropathy**.

amylo-transglucosidase deficiency See **glycogen storage diseases**.

amylo-1,6-glucosidase debrancher deficiency See **glycogen storage diseases**.

amyoplasia congenita See **arthrogryposis multiplex congenita**.

amyostatic syndrome (Gr, lack of + muscle + standing still) An old term for tremor in **Parkinson disease**.

amyosthenia (Gr, lack of + muscle + force) Weakness.

amyotonia congenita (Oppenheim disease) A sporadic congenital disorder characterized by muscular weakness and hypotonia at birth without local muscle wasting, mainly peripherally, and with no tendency to spread to muscles previously unaffected. The usual course is for progressive improvement, even with a return of muscle stretch reflexes.

Despite these guidelines to the clinical features, so many exceptions to the original rules governing the diagnosis have been recorded that it is more likely that this is not a disease *sui generis* but represents either a nonprogressive myopathy or a form of **hereditary motor neuropathy**.[6424]

The term replaced Oppenheim's *myatonia congenita* because the latter was too similar to **myotonia congenita** but was itself later replaced at the suggestion of Walton by **benign congenital hypotonia**[7] and then by the vernacular **floppy baby syndrome**.

See also **benign congenital hypotonia, Oppenheim disease, hereditary motor neuropathy type I**.

amyotrophic cervical myelopathy

A sporadic syndrome of asymmetric muscular atrophy of the distal upper limbs seen predominantly in young males and reported mainly from Japan.[6344]

amyotrophic choreoacanthocytosis

(amyotrophic choreoathetosis) A rare, dominantly or recessively inherited disease with adult onset, characterized by orofacial dyskinesias, chorea, lip or tongue biting, and neurogenic muscular atrophy accompanied by atrophy of the caudate nuclei and acanthocytosis but without abnormalities in plasma lipoproteins.[2591, 5732] See also **neuroacanthocytosis**.

Criteria for the diagnosis have been suggested;[3809] these include extrapyramidal movement disorders, generalized muscle weakness, acanthocytosis (1–50%), normal intelligence, and, in some cases, ataxia, epilepsy, or schizophrenia.

amyotrophic choreo-athetosis

See **amyotrophic chorea-acanthocytosis**.

amyotrophic dystonic paraplegia

A syndrome of slowly progressive dystonia, spasticity, weakness, and muscle wasting, dominantly inherited with variable expression. The dystonia affects the bulbar, trunk, and limb muscles and is accompanied over time by spastic paraparesis and later by neurogenic muscle atrophy.[2385]

amyotrophic lateral sclerosis

(ALS; Charcot syndrome; Aran syndrome; motor neuron disease; progressive muscular atrophy; Aran–Duchenne disease; progressive bulbar palsy; progressive muscular atrophy; primary lateral sclerosis; Mills disease, Lou Gehrig disease) A sporadic, fatal, degenerative disease of unknown cause occurring in adult life, in which pure involvement of the cranial and spinal upper and lower motor neuron systems is manifested by rapid, inexorably progressive and ultimately generalized muscle weakness and wasting and by pyramidal signs.

Clinically, older adults are affected with any combination of upper and lower motor signs such as weakness, wasting, fasciculations, and hyperreflexia, witnessing damage to the bulbar and spinal motor nuclei and pyramidal tracts, although the ocular muscles are spared. The course is usually fatal within 5 years of onset. Stages of involvement based on single-fiber EMG data (early reinnervation; well-compensated reinnervation; early decompensation—late reinnervation; and late decompensation—reinnervation failure) have been defined.[6159] Cognitive impairment is increasingly recognized in this condition.[5318]

This group includes sporadic cases with atypical features: e.g., ophthalmoplegia; nystagmus; sporadic multisystem disorders with amyotrophy, cerebellar disorder, and ophthalmoplegia; **monomelic**; and other restricted forms. See also **motor neuronal diseases, lower motor neuron disease**.

Pathologically, there is loss of the large motor neurons in the cerebral cortex, brainstem, and spinal cord, leading to a combination of upper and lower motor neuron lesions. Subclinical involvement of other neuronal systems also occurs.[6203] Ubiquitin-containing intraneuronal inclusions are found in the nuclei or upper and lower motor neurons.

This invariably fatal disease is survived only by medical students and impressionable neurologists who notice the extent of their (normal) fasciculations for the first time. Although it is subsumed under the category of **abiotrophy**, studies of the Chamorro and other Guamian peoples indicate that toxicity from ingestion of the cycad root may be the cause of the **ALS–Parkinson–dementia syndromes** prevalent there, and by extension it is supposed that toxic causes may in fact be important in ALS as well.

More information is available at Web sites including ALS http://www.wfnals.org/links/index.html/ **ALS Association** http://www.alsa.org/ (a nonprofit health organization); the Muscular Dystrophy Association (**MDA**) http://www.als-mda.org/disease/als.html; the **Amyotrophic Lateral Sclerosis Information Page** http://www.ninds.nih.gov/disorders/amyotrophiclateralsclerosis/amyotrophiclateralsclerosis.htm (provides information compiled by the National Institute of Neurological Disorders and Stroke); the **International Alliance of ALS/MND Associations** http://www.alsmndalliance.org/ (the central coordinating body for national organizations supporting people living with ALS); the **ALS Foundation for Life** http://www.alsfoundation.org/ (a nonprofit organization dedicated to increasing public awareness of ALS); and **ALS Society of Canada** http://www.als.ca/ (a Canadian organization providing ALS information).

It is likely that the first description was given by Sir Charles **Bell** in 1830, but Duchenne[1736], Aran,[229], Cruveilhier in 1852, and Charcot[1101] in 1881 further defined the condition, and it was Charcot who introduced the term *amyotrophic lateral sclerosis*. Marie reviewed the validity of the syndrome in 1897,[4071] and Poser the diagnostic criteria for the disease.[5092] Charcot also distinguished true (progressive)

Chart A–5. Stage of Involvement of Individual Muscles in Amyotrophic Lateral Sclerosis

Stage	*Strength*	*Wasting*	*Fiber Density*	*Jitter*
1	Normal	None	Normal/slightly increased <2.5	None/slightly increased
2	Normal	None	Increased >2.5	Increased
3	Weak and easily fatigable	Often present	Markedly increased	Markedly increased
4	Very weak	Prominent	Slightly increased may be unrecordable	Prominent if recordable

Criteria for the diagnosis of ALS were defined at a workshop held under the auspices of the World Federation of Neurology in 1989[6867] and have been further revised (Subcommittee on Motor Neuron Diseases of World Federation of Neurology Research Group on Neuromuscular Diseases, El Escorial "Revisited: Revised (1998) Criteria for the Diagnosis of Amyotrophic Lateral Sclerosis.

Chart A–6. Revised Criteria for the Diagnosis of Amyotrophic Lateral Sclerosis

The diagnosis of Amyotrophic Lateral Sclerosis [ALS] requires:

A – the presence of:

(A:1) Evidence of *lower motor neuron (LMN) degeneration* by clinical, electrophysiological or neuropathologic examination,
(A:2) Evidence of *upper motor neuron (UMN) degeneration* by clinical examination, and
(A:3) *Progressive spread of symptoms or signs* within a region or to other regions, as determined by history or examination, together with

B – the absence of:

(B:1) *Electrophysiological and pathological evidence of other disease processes* that might explain the signs of LMN and/or UMN degeneration, and
(B:2) *Neuroimaging evidence of other disease processes* that might explain the observed clinical and electrophysiological signs.

It is generally held that the presence of any of the following excludes the diagnosis:
Sensory signs (except those attributable to aging)
Neurogenic sphincter abnormalities
Clinical evidence of CNS disease with a natural history of progression (e.g., Parkinson disease, dementia) other than ALS
Clinically evident peripheral nervous system disease with a natural history of progression (e.g., diabetic polyneuropathy, hereditary polyneuropathy)

From http://www.wfnals.org/guidelines/1998elescorial/elescorial1998.htm.

and pseudobulbar palsy. His "spastic spinal paralysis" was probably what we call primary lateral sclerosis—a variant of ALS. Familial ALS (<10% of all ALS cases) has both recessive and dominant inheritance patterns with variable penetrance. About 20% of familial cases are associated with mutations in the superoxide dismutase gene (dominant forms) or of the alsin, senataxin dynactin or *VAPB* (recessive forms). A recent review is that of Rowland and Shneider.[5447]
Chart A–5 lists the stages of involvement of individual muscles in ALS.

Clinical Studies in the Diagnosis of Amyotrophic Lateral Sclerosis **(http:// www.wfnals.org/guidelines/ 1998elescorial/elescorial1998.htm)**
Newer criteria[876] indicate that the diagnosis of *definite ALS* requires the presence of each of the following:

A progressive course and upper motor neuron (UPN) and lower motor neuron (LPN) signs in three of the following sites: brainstem, cervical, thoracic, or lumbar spinal cord.
The diagnosis of *probable ALS* requires the same, but affecting two regions only.
The diagnosis of *clinically probable ALS with laboratory support* requires: upper and lower motor neuron signs in only one region, upper motor neuron signs in one region, and lower motor neuron signs in at least two limbs, with proper application of neuroimaging and clinical laboratory protocols allowing exclusion of other causes.
The diagnosis of *clinically possible ALS* requires:
upper and lower motor neuron signs in only one region,
upper motor neuron signs alone in two or more regions, and
lower motor neuron signs found rostral to upper motor neuron signs.

A careful history and physical and neurological examination are essential to search for clinical evidence of UMN and LMN signs in four regions of the CNS—brainstem, and cervical, thoracic, or lumbosacral spinal cord. Ancillary tests should be reasonably applied, as clinically indicated, to exclude other disease processes. These should include electrodiagnostic, neurophysiological, neuroimaging, and clinical laboratory studies.

Clinical evidence of LMN and UMN degeneration is required for the diagnosis of ALS. The clinical diagnosis of ALS without pathological confirmation may be categorized into various levels of certainty by clinical assessment alone depending on the presence of both UMN and LMN signs in the same topographical anatomic region in the brainstem (bulbar cranial motor neurons), cervical, thoracic, or lumbosacral spinal cord (anterior horn motor neurons). The terms *clinically definite ALS* and *clinically probable ALS* are used to describe these categories of clinical diagnostic certainty on clinical criteria alone, as follows:

Clinically Definite ALS There is clinical evidence alone of the presence of UMN, as well as LMN signs, in three regions.
Clinically Probable ALS There is clinical evidence alone of UMN and LMN signs in at least two regions with some UMN signs necessarily rostral to (above) the LMN signs. The terms *clinically probable ALS–Laboratory-supported* and *clinically possible ALS* are used to describe these categories of clinical certainty on clinical and criteria, or only clinical criteria:
Clinically Probable–Laboratory-supported ALS Clinical signs of UMN and LMN dysfunction are in only one region, or when UMN signs alone are present in one region and LMN signs defined by EMG criteria are present in at least two limbs, with proper application of neuroimaging and clinical laboratory protocols to exclude other causes.
Clinically Possible ALS Clinical signs of UMN and LMN dysfunction are found together in only one region or UMN signs are found alone in two or more regions, or LMN signs are found rostral to UMN signs and the diagnosis of clinically probable–laboratory-supported ALS cannot be proven by evidence on clinical grounds in conjunction with electrodiagnostic, neurophysiologic, neuroimaging, or clinical laboratory studies. Other diagnoses must have been excluded to accept a diagnosis of clinically possible ALS.

Clinically suspected ALS is a pure LMN syndrome in which the diagnosis of ALS cannot be regarded as sufficiently certain to include the patient in a research study. Hence, this category was deleted from the revised El Escorial Criteria for the Diagnosis of ALS.

***Clinical Types and Patterns of Amyotrophic Lateral Sclerosis* (http://www.wfnals.org/guidelines/1998elescorial/elescorial1998.htm)**

Sporadic ALS—ALS occurs alone or is present incidentally with other preexisting disease processes.

Genetically determined (familial, hereditary) ALS—ALS present in one or more generations is associated with different modes of inheritance and defined pathogenic mutations such as superoxide dismutase-1 (SOD-1) mutations or hexosaminidase A/B deficiency. ALS may occur as a genetically determined disease and, in some cases, the pathogenic mutation has been determined, e.g., mutations of the SOD-1 gene. When there is a family history of such a defined pathogenic mutation, the diagnosis may be upgraded to *Clinically Definite Familial–Laboratory-supported ALS* or ALS presenting with progressive upper and/or lower motor neuron signs in at least a single region (in the absence of another cause for the abnormal neurological signs). However, in genetically determined cases where the gene has not been identified (even if linkage is established), the criteria for the diagnosis of sporadic ALS apply.

ALS plus syndromes ALS is present in association with clinical features of other neurological diseases which develop in addition to the phenotype of ALS or develop in parallel with the ALS, e.g., extra-pyramidal features or dementia.

ALS with laboratory abnormalities of uncertain significance. ALS is present in association with laboratory-defined abnormalities that are of uncertain significance to the pathogenesis of ALS.

ALS-mimic syndromes These syndromes occur as a consequence of other, non-ALS pathogenic processes and do not represent other forms of ALS. ALS-mimic syndromes include the postpoliomyelitis syndrome, multifocal motor neuropathy with or without conduction block, endocrinopathies, especially hyperparathyroid or hyperthyroid states; lead intoxication; infections; and paraneoplastic syndromes.

***Electrophysiological Studies in the Diagnosis of Amyotrophic Lateral Sclerosis* (http://www.wfnals.org/guidelines/1998elescorial/elescorial1998.htm)**

Patients in whom the diagnosis of ALS is considered on clinical grounds should have electrophysiological studies performed to confirm LMN dysfunction in clinically affected regions, detect electrophysiological evidence of LMN dysfunction in clinically uninvolved regions, and exclude other pathophysiological processes.

These electrophysiological studies should be performed by qualified physicians according to established standards. It is essential to interpret the electrophysiological results in conjunction with the clinical and other ancillary findings. The El Escorial criteria for electrophysiological studies are given below:

Electrophysiological features required to identify definite primary LMN degeneration include all of the following:

- Reduced interference pattern with firing rates higher than 10 Hz
- Large motor unit potential (large amplitude, long duration)
- Fibrillation potentials

Electrophyiological features that support the identification of probable primary LMN degeneration include one or both of the following:

- Reduced recruitment or large motor unit potential (MUP) and fibrillation potentials and unstable MUP
- Reduced motor unit estimates and increased macro-EMG MUP

Electrophysiological features that support the identification of possible primary LMN degeneration include one or more of the following:

- Reduced recruitment, large MUP, fibrillation potentials, or unstable MUP alone
- Polyphasic MUP or increased single fiber density alone
- Low-amplitude MUP if the disease has lasted more than 5 years or if there is associated atrophy
- Low-amplitude compound motor unit potential (CMAP)
- CMAP change between proximal and distal sites of stimulation is uniform along the length of the nerve
- Up to 30% decrement in motor conduction velocity established normal values if a low-amplitude CMAP is above 10% of normal is present
- Up to 50% decrement in motor conduction velocity established normal values if the CMAP is less than 10% of normal
- Up to 20% decrement of the CMAP on 2-Hz repetitive stimulation
- Up to 10% decrement in sensory nerve conduction velocity and action potential amplitude from established normal values
- Complex repetitive discharges
- Presence (*originally published as "absence"*) of fasciculations

These criteria, however, have been persuasively criticized by Wilbourn.[6776]

Neuroimaging Studies in the Diagnosis of Amyotrophic Lateral Sclerosis

Neuroimaging studies should be selected in order to exclude other conditions which may cause UMN and/or LMN signs that may stimulate sporadic ALS. There are no neuroimaging tests which provide positive support for the diagnosis of ALS, although there are neuroimaging methods (e.g., nuclear magnetic resonance spectroscopy) that may in the future support the diagnosis of UMN involvement. Rarely, brain T2-weighted MRI may show increased signal in the corticospinal tracts.

Clinical Laboratory Studies in the Diagnosis of Amyotrophic Lateral Sclerosis.

The diagnostic process employed to confirm the diagnosis of sporadic ALS when the diagnosis is uncertain includes repeated clinical examinations to document progression, repeated electrophysiological and/or neuroimaging examinations to exclude structural disorders, and laboratory examinations to exclude other disorders or support the diagnosis of ALS-plus syndromes, ALS-mimic syndromes, or ALS with laboratory abnormalities of uncertain significance.

Neuropathological Studies in the Diagnosis of Amyotrophic Lateral Sclerosis

The diagnosis of sporadic ALS may be supported or excluded by muscle and/or biopsy studies in the living patient. The diagnosis of sporadic ALS may be proven or excluded by autopsy examination.

****

Amyotrophic lateral sclerosis variants comprise clinical syndromes in which the predominant presentation is that seen in sporadic ALS, but which includes one or more additional features. These features are outlined below.

1. *Forms with documented genetic transmission*

   A. *Familial ALS* (Hirano–Lewy body disease). In uncommon instances the condition is a familial trait, usually compatible with an autosomal dominant mode of transmission.[4538] The responsible gene maps to chromosome 21.q22.1–q22.2.

Familial ALS and Related Disorders: Known Inheritance Patterns

Inheritance Pattern	*Chromosomal Linkage*	*Notable Features*
Autosomal Dominant		
ALS	1p36	
ALS 1	21q22.1	Cu/Zn superoxide dismutase (SOD) mutations
ALS X	Xpll–q12	Adult onset
ALS 3	18q21	Adult onset; absence of linkage to Cu/Zn superoxide dismutase
ALS 4	9q34	A *senataxin* mutation; juvenile onset; complete penetrance; very slow progression of distal limb amyotrophy; pyramidal signs[5163]
ALS6	16q.12	Classic ALS
ALS8	20q13	
ALS9	14q11	*Angiogenin* mutation.
ALS-FTD	9q21–q22	(*motor neuron disease with presenile dementia*) onset in mature adult life; frontal-lobe form of dementia, ophthalmoplegias, and cerebral atrophy; with usual features of ALS[760]
ALS-FTD2	9p13	ALS with bulbar onset; Japanese family; juvenile presentation, prominent early onset bulbar dysfunction; slow progression with dementia.
Distal **hereditary motor neuropathy**	7B 2p13	*Dynactin* mutation; facial and vocal cord pareses; later distal limb weakness
NFH	22q12.1–q22	Mutations in neurofilament heavy chain; (not observed in familial, only in sporadic ALS)
Linkages of pure ALS to loci on 12.12, 16q21, 14q11.2, and 20p13 have also been detected.		
Autosomal Recessive		
ALS 2	2q33–q35	*Alsin* mutation; causing a pseudobulbar syndrome with spastic paraplegia; childhood-onset; with slow progression
ALS 5	15q15.1–q21.1	Onset in adolescence; with atrophy of arm muscles and spasticity in all limbs; long-term survival; no pseudobulbar signs
Brown-Vialetto-Van Laere syndrome	Sporadic, or dominant or recessive inheritance; progressive bulbar paralysis, progressive sensorineural deafness, and pyramidal signs; childhood-onset	
AAA syndrome 12q13; Fazio-Londe (can also be dominant)	*Aladin* mutation Bulbar ALS	
X-linked		
Bulbospinal muscular atrophy Xq12	(Kennedy) Progressive muscle atrophy; gynecomastia; reduced fertility. Androgen receptor gene mutation (trinucleotide [CAG] repeat)	
Worster–Drought syndrome:	(congenital suprabulbar paralysis) It may also be dominantly inherited.	
Miscellaneous		
Hexosaminidase	A, B 15q23–q24	A late-onset GM2 gangliosidosis
Disinhibition-dementia Chr.17	Allelic with frontotemporal dementia and Parkinsonism-amyotrophy syndrome	
Western Pacific form	?	
Foix–Chavany–Marie syndrome	Faciopharyngoglossomasticatory diplegia	

Synthesized from Strong[6095] and from the WUSTL neuromuscular Web site at http://neuromuscular.wustl.edu/synmot.html#sma5q/ by kind permission of Dr. Alan Pestronk.

Recessive transmission of the pure syndrome has also been described. In most cases, pyramidal and posterior column signs are present; in some cases, dementia and/or extrapyramidal signs (Parkinsonism) are found as well.[151, 6187, 2911]

B. **Adult polyglycosan body disease**.

C. *Amyotrophic lateral sclerosis with autosomal dominant familial* ***Parkinsonism***.[6006]

D. *Familial juvenile motor neuron disease* (juvenile bulbar palsy) A slowly progressive dominant or recessive *variant* characterized by the onset in childhood of bulbar and spinal muscle atrophy with pyramidal signs.[2715] See **Fazio-Londe syndrome**. The gene maps to 2q 33–35.

In another form of juvenile ALS, dementia is associated.

E. *Progressive muscular atrophy with microcephaly and mental retardation*.[5993]

F. *Corticospinal tract deficit and axonal motor polyneuropathy*, in which weakness, intermittent dysphagia, weight loss, atrophy and fasciculations of the distal muscles, pseudobulbar dysarthria, hyperactive reflexes, and upgoing plantar responses are found without sensory loss in patients with hyperparathyroidism.[2108]

G. *Juvenile spinal muscular atrophy of the distal upper extremity* A syndrome in which the features of ALS are accompanied by minipolymyoclonus of the fingers and worsening of symptoms with cold. It has been described in young male Japanese and is caused by a structural abnormality of the cervical cord. **X-linked bulbospinal muscular atrophy** (Kennedy disease), adult **GM2 gangliosidosis, Machado-Joseph disease, multiple system atrophy**, and **hexosaminidase A deficiency** are phenotypically similar.

H. Respiratory chain defects can also mimic ALS and should be considered in the differential diagnosis.[2912]

2. *Forms with unusual age at presentation or unusual course:*

A. *Sporadic juvenile ALS*. A variant in which neuronal inclusions derived from the Nissl substance are formed, and with neurofibrillary degeneration in the motor cortex.[4280] A form with a spastin gene mutation and prolonged survival has been described. See ALS4 above.

B. *Progressive muscular atrophy with malignant course*. A form which is fatal within 1 year but which is not clearly different from autosomal dominant ALS.

C. *Slow motor neuron disease*. A variant in which survival extends well beyond 5 years, and in which the etiology may differ from that of the more usual forms.

D. *Subacute reversible motor neuron disease*. A syndrome of weakness and wasting with fasciculations and some upper motor neuron signs occurring in adults with spontaneous resolution of the signs over a year, in the absence of any other demonstrable pathology.[6417]

E. *Brachial amyotrophic diplegia* A sporadic form in which weakness and muscle atrophy without pyramidal signs affects only the upper limbs and is slowly progressive over years. A **man-in-the-barrel** syndrome results.[3331]

3. *Geographic location (Western Pacific, Guam, Kii, etc.)*

A. *ALS-Parkinson-dementia syndrome of Guam*. (**Lytico–Bodig**, Hirano parkinsonism/dementia, Western Pacific ALS). A disease of the Chamorro race of the Western Pacific island of Guam in the Mariana Island group, first described by Hirano and others in 1961, at which time it accounted for 10% of adult deaths. The condition also occurs in clusters in Japan and Western New Guinea. Insidious but severe progressive dementia, parkinsonism, and motor neuron involvement occur in any combination in adult patients, especially males, all show the reptilian stare, akinesia, and stooped posture of typical Parkinson disease, but tremor is slight or absent and rigidity is often absent too. Ophthalmoplegia, cerebellar and pyramidal signs, and evidence of dementia may be found, but typical signs of ALS are found in only about one-third of the cases. Death occurs within 3–5 years of the onset of symptoms.[2910] Pathologically, the brain and spinal cord are found to contain an excess of neurofibrillary tangles without amyloid plaques.

Intensive study of the Chamorros has shown this to be a toxic disease as a result of eating flour made of the seeds of the False Sago palm *Cycas circinalis* which contains an excitatory nonprotein aminoacid neurotoxin;[5970] the disease is manifested in those who are genetically susceptible.

A similar condition is recognized among the Japanese people on the Kii peninsula and among the Akai and Ayau people of Western New Guinea.

B. **Madras type**. A sporadic or recessive form characterized by the onset in youth of bulbar palsy, hearing loss, and minipolymyoclonus of the fingers, recorded in southern India.

4. *Forms with concurrent dementia*

A. ALS phenotypes with the pathological features of nbia (*Martha-Alma* or *Hallervorden-Spatz disease*)[760] or with *aphasic dementia*[1053] have been described.

B. *Amyotrophic Lateral Sclerosis-Parkinson-dementia syndrome* The association of these three entities occurs as a sporadic or familial disease, most commonly seen in Guam (see III-A, above) but also in Europeans, in whom it may be inherited as a recessive trait.[2910] The pathological features of typical ALS are occasionally accompanied by mild dementia, language disturbance or parkinsonism but this is more common in subjects with the familial form of the disease.[5622]

5. *Forms with extrapyramidal signs* (may be recessively inherited):

A. **Amyotrophic dystonic paraplegia**.

6. *Forms with objective sensory, autonomic or cerebellar abnormalities:*

A. *Amyotrophic lateral sclerosis with posterior column involvement*. A variant which is dominantly inherited with clinical and pathological features of degeneration of upper and lower motor neurons and with posterior column demyelination.[1890]

B. *Spinal muscular atrophy with amyotrophic lateral sclerosis, spinocerebellar ataxia and deafness*.

C. *Motor neuron disease (amyotrophic lateral sclerosis) with sensory involvement* A variant characterized by the onset in mature adult life of loss of pain and temperature sensation along with the usual features of ALS.

D. **Progressive muscular atrophy with ALS** An entity of uncertain validity, presenting as a combination of **hereditary motor and sensory neuropathy** and pyramidal features.

E. *Spastic paraplegia with amyotrophy of hands*.

F. *Focal motor neuron disease*. See **monomelic spinal muscular atrophy**.

G. *ALS with ophthalmoplegia*. A rare variant in which there is extensive neuronal loss and gliosis in the nuclei of the third, fourth, and sixth cranial nerves.[2791]

H. Forms with associated evidence of degeneration of the posterior columns or other tracts in the spinal cord, of **tics**, or of **Luysopallidalnigral atrophy**.

7. *Forms with involvement of other body systems or with other identified disease*

A. *Amyotrophic lateral sclerosis with hyperparathyroidism*. A syndrome of corticospinal tract deficit and axonal motor polyneuropathy, in which weakness, intermittent dysphagia, weight loss, atrophy and fasciculations of the distal muscles, pseudobulbar dysarthria, hyperactive reflexes and up-going plantar responses are found without sensory loss in patients with hyperparathyroidism.[2108]

B. *Paraneoplastic amyotrophic lateral sclerosis.* Here, the typical findings of ALS are associated with underlying bronchial carcinoma, and remit when the tumor is resected.[4399] Carcinomatous motor neuron disease is only possibly a specific syndrome but amyotrophy may be seen in paraneoplastic encephalomyelopathy and may improve after removal of the tumor.

C. *Amyotrophic lateral sclerosis with plasma cell dyscrasia and monoclonal paraproteinemia* such as Waldenstrom macroglobulinemia, multiple myeloma or chronic lymphatic leukemia. Both monoclonal and polyclonal gammopathies involving either IgM or IgG have been detected.[4254] See **gammopathic neuropathy**.

D. ALS associated with adrenocorticotrophic hormone deficiency.[3075]

E. *ALS-like syndromes* resemble but are not ALS and include; spondylotic myelopathy, vascular, lymphoma, nontumor endocrine abnormalities, hyperthyroidism, hyperparathyroidism, prior irradiation of the spinal cord, acute infection, postinfectious, monoclonal gammopathy, dysimmune states such as multifocal motor neuropathy with conduction block, exogenous toxins such as lead,[990] and genetic/acquired enzyme defects such as hexosaminidase A deficiency in younger patients (Adapted from the Scottish MND Register.)[5694]

Amyotrophic Lateral Sclerosis and Other Motor Neuron Disorders The official publication of the World Federation of Neurology Research Group on Motor Neuron Disease, published by Martin Dunitz. Web site: http://www.tandf.co.uk/journals/alphalist.html.

Amyotrophic Lateral Sclerosis Information Page ALS information sheet compiled bythe National Institute of Neurological Disorders and Stroke (NINDS). Web site: http://www.ninds.nih.gov/disorders/amyotrophiclateralsclerosis/amyotrophiclateralsclerosis.htm/.

Amyotrophic Lateral Sclerosis Association See ALS Association.

Amyotrophic Lateral Sclerosis Functional Rating Scale A validated rating instrument for monitoring the progression of disability in patients with ALS[1064] under the following criteria:

Bulbar (swallowing, speech, salivation)
Respiratory (based upon ventilatory capacity)
Muscle strength in the upper and lower extremities, grip, and lateral pinch

Leg muscle function (standing from a chair, standing from the supine position, walking 20 feet, the need for assistive devices, climbing and descending four standard steps, and functions of hips and legs)

Arm muscle function (dressing and feeding, propelling a wheelchair for 20 feet, arm and shoulder power, and the ability to cut, to perform a pegboard test, or to handle a block test).

A revised version incorporates additional assessments of dyspnea, orthopnea, and the need for ventilatory support. The revision is provided at Chahin et al. (2008).[1079]

Amyotrophic Lateral Sclerosis score A standardized method of assessment of motor functions in patients with ALS, which are rated as 3 (normal), 2 (impaired), 1 (trace), or 0.

Items assessed include holding up the head, chewing food, swallowing, speaking, turning in bed, sitting up, emptying the bowel and bladder, breathing and coughing. The subject is also scored on writing his name, fastening buttons or zippers, feeding himself, gripping objects, lifting himself, lifting a book or a tray, lifting a fork or a pencil, changing arm position, climbing one flight of stairs, walking one block, walking across a room, walking with assistance, standing up, and changing position. Stretch reflexes in the arms and legs, the jaw jerk, and the plantar responses bilaterally are also assessed, as are fasciculations and wasting in the face, tongue, arms, shoulders, legs, and hips. Emotional lability, fatigability, and leg rigidity are other factors examined. The theoretical maximum score is 100.[4705]

Amyotrophic Lateral Sclerosis Society of Canada A charitable organization. Address: 90 Adelaide St. E. Suite B-101, Toronto, ON, Canada M5C 2R4. Tel: 416-362-0269.

amyotrophic syphilitic myelopathy See **syphilitic amyotrophy**.

amyotrophy (from Lat, lack of + muscle + growth) Muscle atrophy. The word is used in the context of acute shoulder girdle pain and weakness (**neuralgic amyotrophy**), **syphilitic amyotrophy**, **diabetic amyotrophy**, and various genetically determined malformations; but as it is descriptive rather than definitive, its employment is properly limited. There is a convention, however, that it is used when the seat of the pathology is in the anterior horn cells.

The word is an unfortunate neologism; while lack of muscle growth is indeed present in patients with amyotrophy, the word *atrophy* is better known to us, and *myoatrophy* would have been a better construction. But since *amyotrophy* has been around for twice as long as this author, he will not tilt at windmills.

anabolic GM$_3$ gangliosidosis See **hematosidosis**.

anaerobic threshold The level of muscular activity at which respiratory rate, plasma lactate levels, and other signs of anaerobic metabolic activity first appear.

anal reflex The *superficial* anal reflex is a (polysynaptic) reflex contraction of the anal sphincter in response to stimulation of the perianal skin, mediated by the somatic fibers at S4–S5, described by Rossimolo in 1891. It is lost in tabes dorsalis and with local lesions at these levels.

The *deep (internal)* reflex consists of the contraction of the internal anal sphincter muscle in response to muscle stretch, as by the gloved finger introduced, and is mediated by sympathetic fibers from L1–L2, and by coughing or sneezing.

anal triangle An anatomical region, the two sides of which are formed by the gluteus maximus and the base by the superficial transverse perineal muscles. The anus, along with the surrounding external anal sphincter, is in the middle. The entire area is covered by the levator ani.

anal wink Transitory contraction of the anal sphincter upon coughing.

analgagnosia Unawareness of the unpleasant qualities of painful stimuli, as shown by the subject's lack of reactivity to them.

analgesia (Gr, lack of + pain) 1. Reduction or loss of sensitivity to a stimulus which would normally be painful. This meaning, however, is often included in the nonspecific term **anesthesia**. 2. Insensibility to pain, or lack of pain sensation, without effects on consciousness.

analgesia panaris See **hereditary sensory and autonomic neuropathy type II**.

analgesic headache See **analgesic-overuse headache**.

analgesic-overuse headache (analgesic rebound headache; analgesic headache; rebound headache; medication-induced headache) A headache syndrome with the clinical characteristics of both **migraine** and of **tension-type headaches**, occurring in chronic migraine or tension-type headache sufferers who have taken to consuming acetylsalicylic acid, acetaminophen, nonsteroidal anti-inflammatory agents, benzodiazepines, ergot compounds, caffeine, narcotics, barbiturates, or combinations of these agents in increasing doses and on a regular basis, usually daily.[5195] A headache with characteristics of **hemicrania continua** has also been reported as a *variant*.

The mechanism is unknown, but the morning accentuation of the symptom would support chemical dependence such that the headaches are triggered by falling analgesic levels. This perpetuates and worsens instead of alleviating the headaches. Diagnostic criteria have been defined:

A. Headache present on >15 days/month with at least one of the following characteristics and fulfilling criteria C and D:
   1. Bilateral
   2. Pressing/tightening (nonpulsating) quality
   3. Mild or moderate intensity
B. Intake of simple analgesics on ≥15 days/month for >3 months
C. Headache has developed or markedly worsened during analgesic overuse
D. Headache resolves or reverts to its previous pattern within 2 months after discontinuation of analgesics

From the International Classification of Headache Disorders (Headache Classification Committee of the International Headache Society. *Cephalalgia* 2004;**24**[Suppl 1]) by kind permission of Dr. Jes Olesen, the International Headache Society and Wiley-Blackwell Publications.

See also **ergotamine-**, **opioid-**, and **triptan overuse headaches**.

analgesic rebound headache See **analgesic-overuse headache**.

analphalipoproteinemia See **Tangier disease**.

anamnesia (Gr, anew + memory) Recollection of phenomena prior to a given period in the disease.

anamnestic Recalling to memory. Thus as *anamnesis*, the history of the disease.

anamnestic color blindness Difficulty in finding the correct word for a colored object, errors being made in which the patient may perseverate. This is probably a combination of a mild disorder of visual perception and minimal dysphasia.

anapeiratic (Gr, to do again, to repeat exercises) The term applied by **Hammond** to those pareses brought on by excessive use of a body part. See **occupational cramps**.

anaplastic meningioma See **meningioma**.

anarchic hand See **alien hand (limb) syndromes**.

anarithmetrica See **anarithmia**.

anarithmia (anarithmetrica) Inability to comprehend numeration and the principles of mathematics, as presumably is the case in **Gerstmann syndrome**. See also **acalculia**.

anarthria Complete inability to articulate speech sounds, due to local causes or lesions of the medulla, pons, or bulbar cranial nerves. The original Greek derivation actually indicates a defect or absence of the limbs. See also **logopenia**.

anastic aphasia See **anomia**.

anastomosis (Gr, to bring to a mouth) The communication of the branches of vessels with one another, as if one mouth (or open end of a vessel) were joined to another.

anaudia (Gr, negative + speech) See **aphonia**. The term has also been employed for **catalepsy**.

ancient change The presence of large, pleomorphic, scattered, hyperchromatic nuclei within **Schwannomas**, and particularly in long-standing acoustic neuromas.[6]

Ander disease See **Dercum disease**.

Andermann syndrome 1. See **Landau–Kleffner syndrome**. 2. (**agenesis of the corpus callosum**) A recessively inherited dysmorphic syndrome characterized by agenesis of the corpus callosum and progressive sensorimotor neuropathy, presenting in infancy with delayed motor milestones, hypotonia, areflexia, and mainly distal muscular weakness. Patients start to walk with support and braces between 4 years and 8 years, but some never achieve independent gait. Progressive motor deterioration ensues with increased weakness, amyotrophy, and contractures of the distal musculature and progressive scoliosis. Most patients are confined to a wheelchair by early adolescence. The condition was first described in a French–Canadian population living in the Saguenay-Lac St-Jean region in the Province of Québec, Canada.

Mental and developmental delay, mild distal sensory loss, progressive flaccid and distal amyotrophy with hypotonia and areflexia, nonprogressive bilateral ptosis, slight limitation of upward gaze, dysarthria, and intention tremor of the arms are other features. The progressive motor deterioration is due to increasing weakness, amyotrophy, and contractures of the distal musculature. Scoliosis occurs at the end of the first decade.[1757]

Dysmorphisms include elongated and asymmetrical facies, hypertelorism, high-arched palate, hypoplastic maxilla, large angle of the mandible, protruding ears, short neck and low hairline, pigeon-chest deformities, long tapering fingers with digitalization of the thumbs, partial syndactyly, scoliosis, pes cavus, and overriding of the toes. Few subjects survive beyond the mid-twenties.[3699]

Andersen brown forehead ring (linea fusca) A brown pigmentation on the forehead, found in some patients with chronic CNS diseases, especially postencephalitic Parkinsonism and syphilis. The cause is unknown.[4348]

Andersen–Tawil syndrome (glycogen storage disease type IV; D-1, 4 glucan 6-glucosyltransferase brancher enzyme deficiency) A rare, dominantly inherited multisystem channelopathy characterized by periodic paralyses (all types), long QT (LQT) with ventricular arrhythmias, skeletal developmental abnormalities and dysmorphisms, caused by mutations in *KCNJ2*, which encodes the inward rectifier K^+ channel Kir2.1 on chromosome 17q23. The major features are hepatic cirrhosis, splenomegaly, hypotonia with muscle atrophy (especially in the legs), and delay in acquisition of motor skills.[191] Multiple phenotypic variants, some with cognitive deficits, have also been recorded.[6389] See also **glycogen storage diseases**.

Andersen, Dorothy (1901–1963) American pediatrician and pathologist.

Andersen syndrome (Klein-Lisak syndrome) A rare potassium channelopathy comprising potassium-sensitive periodic paralysis without myotonia, ventricular arrhythmias leading potentially to syncope or sudden death and dysmorphisms (clinodactyly, syndactyly, hypoplastic mandible, hypertelorism, low-set ears). A prolonged QTc interval is detected in many cases; other cardiac manifestations include a LQT syndrome, premature ventricular contractions, complex ventricular ectopy, or polymorphic or bidirectional ventricular tachycardias.[5102] Tubular aggregates may be found on muscle biopsy. The deficit is linked to mutations in *KCNJ2*.[6389] A dominant *variant* has also been reported.[6226]

Anderson, W. (1842–1900) English surgeon and anatomist at St. Thomas Hospital, where he was also a dermatologist.

Anderson–Fabry disease A rare X-linked lysosomal storage disorder due to deficiency of; α-galactosidase A, which results in the deposition of neutral glycosphingolipids (mainly trihexosyl ceramide) in endothelial and smooth muscle cells.

The clinical features include a skin rash (**angiokeratoma**); pain and paresthesias in the extremities; abnormalities of cutaneous thermal sensation; episodic painful crises, sometimes precipitated by exercise or other stress; acroparesthesias; and a tendency toward acute ischemic hemorrhagic brain lesions. Death is due to renal failure and cerebrovascular accidents.[1945, 660, 194]

Andes disease See **altitude insomnia**.

Andrade neuropathy (familial amyloid neuropathy, Portuguese neuropathy) A dominantly inherited acropathic sensorimotor and autonomic neuropathy with adult onset, complicating primary amyloidosis, in which gastrointestinal complaints (cyclic diarrhea and constipation) are common.[196]

André-Thomas (1867–1961) French neurologist, born in Paris, where he trained in medicine, serving under **Raymond**, Bouchard, and **Déjèrine**. After graduation he worked as chef de laboratoire for Déjèrine, remaining at the **Salpêtrière** until 1917, but was not accepted onto the staff. From 1911 until his death he was attached to the Hôpital Saint-Joseph. He assumed the hyphen between his Christian name and surname in order to distinguish himself from André Thomas, the contemporary physiologist.

His contributions to neurology extend over about 70 years, the greater part concerned with clinical and anatomical studies of the cerebellum and spinal cord, psychotherapy, and neurophysiology. He commenced his studies of the development of the newborn at the age of 78; these culminated in his landmark book *The Neurological Examination of the Infant* (1954, in collaboration).

André-Thomas sign (springlike phenomenon) This is essentially the same as **rebound**.[5333]

anemic headache A frontal or generalized headache, once considered to be associated with increased blood flow in patients with severe anemia.

anencephaly (Gr, lack of + brain) (acrania, exencephaly, craniorachischisis) A lethal defect due to failure in the formation of the cephalad part of the neural tube, resulting in the complete absence of development of the cerebral hemispheres[1549] and of the vault of the skull. This developmental aberration is commonly accompanied by failure of closure of the neural tube, presenting as **myelocele** or **meningomyelocele**.

It is suggested that anencephalics are capable of performing certain of those intellectual functions commonly considered to require the presence of cerebral cortex, but they seldom live long enough for evidence of this to be detected.

anerethisia (Gr, lack of + to excite) Lack of incentive or motivation.

anergy (Gr, lack of + energy) (anergia, anenergia) Lack of strength, vigor, or energy.

anesthesia (Gr, lack of + sensation) Lack of feeling, though not necessarily of pain. The term was suggested by Oliver Wendell Holmes (1804–1894), the American physician and author, in a letter to Dr. William Morton, an American dentist who pioneered the use of pain-relieving agents in his practice. Holmes used the diphthong.

anesthesia dolorosa 1. Persistent and painful anesthesia or hypesthesia in the distribution of the trigeminal nerve or one of its divisions or of the occipital nerves, occurring most often after rhizotomy or thermocoagulation performed for treatment of classical trigeminal neuralgia. Diagnostic criteria have been defined:

A. Persistent pain and dysesthesia within the area of distribution of one or more divisions of the trigeminal nerve or of the occipital nerves
B. Diminished sensation to pin-prick and sometimes other sensory loss over the affected area
C. Presence of a lesion of the relevant nerve or its central connections

From the International Classification of Headache Disorders (Headache Classification Committee of the International Headache Society. *Cephalalgia* 2004;**24**[Suppl 1]) by kind permission of Dr. Jes Olesen, the International Headache Society and Wiley-Blackwell Publications.

2. Painful insensitivity of a body part, occurring as a result of incomplete nerve injury, usually traumatic or postherpetic.

anesthetic leprosy (Danielsson–Boeck disease) A form of **leprosy** in which hyperesthesia gives way to anesthesia with mutilation.[1443] See **leprosy**.

aneurysm (Gr, a widening) An expansion of the diameter of a blood vessel, usually an artery, due to disease of its wall. Various forms occur:

Berry ("saccular") aneurysms (naturalistic, not eponymic) are focal "blowouts" at points where arteries bifurcate, at which sites there is attenuation of the medial muscular and of the elastic layers of the arterial wall. They are found on the vessels of the anterior circulation in 85% of cases; in 25% of cases, more than one aneurysm is present.

Cirsoid (Gr, enlargement of a vein + likeness) or racemose (Lat, clusters) aneurysms are irregular dilatations of arteries, leading to many sinuous bulges.

Dissecting aneurysms are those occurring in both intracranial and extracranial arteries in which there is a tear in the media, the blood under pressure rupturing and splitting the media before tracking back into the true lumen of the vessel at a higher level.

Fusiform aneurysms (dolichoectasia, atherosclerotic aneurysm) are dilatations of the whole circumference over a length of the vessel, mainly caused by atheroma. They are found most commonly in the vertebrobasilar and internal carotid arteries in elderly people, and they produce symptoms mainly by compression of adjacent structures.[2051]

Mycotic aneurysms are focal dilations of cerebral arteries resulting from inflammation of the walls of the vessels, tending distally and usually occurring as a complication of bacteremia.

aneurysm of the great vein of Galen Aneurysmal dilation of this vein as a result of the shunting of excessive amounts of arterial blood into it, seen in infants with developmental cerebrovascular anomalies such as **arteriovenous malformations**.

In early infancy, the usual presentation is with high-output cardiac failure, accompanied by a cranial bruit,[5875] while in later months the aneurysm may act as a mass lesion causing aqueductal compression and resulting hydrocephalus; seizures and dilated scalp veins are other features of note. When the presentation is not until later childhood, seizures, the effects of intracranial bleeding, and both brainstem and cerebellar findings are commonly noted, but usually no bruit is audible.

anfracta cerebri The cerebral fissures.

anfractuosity (Lat, a turning or bending around) Applied to the sulci between the cerebral convolutions.

Angelman syndrome (happy puppet syndrome (OMIM 105830) A congenital neurobehavioral disorder characterized by brachycephaly, microcephaly, and a horizontal depression in the occipital bone; cerebral atrophy and primary optic atrophy; multifocal seizures with **hypsarrhythmia**; ataxic, jerky (puppet-like) limb movements (hence the alternative name); prognathism; unusually protrusive tongue; easily provoked and prolonged paroxysms of laughter but no speech; hypopigmentation; and mental and developmental delay.[204] A microdeletion at chromosome 15q11–q13 is present, almost always of maternal inheritance.

See also **Prader–Willi syndrome**, in which the same deletion is of paternal inheritance, and http://www.ninds.nih.gov/disorders/angelman/angelman.htm/.

Angelucci syndrome (allergic conjunctivitis syndrome) A syndrome of recurrent conjunctivitis, often associated with dermal and mucosal pruritic lesions and occasionally with signs of proximal myopathy.[205] The cause is unknown.

angiectasia (Gr, a blood vessel + dilation) Pathological widening of the blood vessels, usually applied to dilatation of the capillaries (telangiectasis).

angiitis See **primary angiitis of the nervous system** and **Aβ related-angüitis.**

angioblastic meningioma See **meningioma.**

angiodysgenetic myelomalacia See **subacute necrotizing myelopathy** (Foix–Alajouanine syndrome).

angioendotheliomatosis Invasion of cerebral and other blood vessels by anaplastic malignant cells.

angiographically occult CNS vascular malformation Slow-flow vascular lesions within the brain which appear avascular on angiography. They include venous angioma, telangiectasis, thrombosed arteriovenous angioma, and cavernous angioma.

angiography A series of techniques for visualizing the anatomy and pathology of the arterial system by means of the injection of radio-opaque dyes with X-ray imaging, ultrasound (**Doppler** studies), or **magnetic resonance imaging**.

The first of these was introduced by the Portuguese surgeon Egaz Moniz in 1936, providing the first opportunity for physicians to obtain even an indirect representation of the intracranial structures. A history of angiography has been written by Gurdjian.[2642]

angioid streaks (Knapp syndrome) Brown or gray lines visible on the retinae. They represent defects in Brusch's membrane or other retinal degenerative changes and resemble blood vessels, except that they are not usually directed radially.

Angioid streaks are typically seen in **pseudoxanthoma elasticum** but also occur in other diseases of the retinal vessels[3493] and are occasionally found in normal subjects.

angiokeratoma Warty growths in the skin with telangiectasia, the skin lesion clustered in the swimming trunk area, characteristic of **Anderson–Fabry disease** and in Mibelli disease, described first in 1877 by Dr. E.W. Cottle (d. 1919), an English physician.[5619]

angiokeratoma corporis diffusum (universale) (Fabry disease) See **Anderson–Fabry disease**.

angiolipoma A rare benign tumor composed of adipose tissue and abnormal vascular elements, usually in the posterior epidural space of the spinal canal and sometimes infiltrating local bone.[2163]

angioma A common vascular malformation (rather than a true neoplasm), comprising four types:

Arteriovenous malformations

Capillary telangiectases

Cavernous angiomas (cavernomas) Compact aggregations of sinusoidal blood vessels with minimal or no neural tissue between the vessels, most common within the brainstem and in Sylvian regions and sometimes multiple. Calcification may occur. Clinically, bleeding is uncommon, but seizures may occur.

Venous angiomas (developmental venous anomalies) Common malformations consisting of loose collections of venous channels with intervening neural tissue, situated anywhere in the nervous system and often multiple. They are seldom symptomatic.

Angioma Alliance Web site A resource for cavernous angioma information and support.

angioma capillare et venosum calcificans See **Sturge–Weber syndrome**.

angiomatosis meningo-oculofacialis See **Sturge–Weber syndrome**.

angiomatosis retinae (cystica) See **von Hippel–Lindau disease**.

angiomatosis retino-cerebellaris See **von Hippel–Lindau disease**.

angiomatous malformation See **arteriovenous malformation**.

angiomatous meningioma See **meningioma**.

angioparalytic hemicrania See **hemiplegic migraine**.

angiopathia retinae juvenalis See **Eales disease**.

angiopathic myopathy An ischemic myopathy complicating polyarteritis nodosa or giant-cell arteritis.[3724]

angiopathic neuropathy Typically, a **multiple mononeuropathy** causing pain, weakness, and sensory loss in the distribution of a number of nerves as a result of numerous nerve microinfarcts in small-vessel occlusive diseases, causing both axonal damage and demyelination. Diabetes and polyarteritis are the more common causes.[1775]

angiophrasia The repetitive insertion of a meaningless sound into otherwise normal speech, as in "hemming and hawing."

angiosarcoma A vascular sarcoma.

angiosclerotic paroxysmal myasthenia (Determan) See **Charcot**.

angiostrongyliasis An infestion by *Angiostrongylus cantonensis*, acquired through the ingestion of inadequately cooked snails, prawns, or frogs, or the vegetable matter upon which they have resided. Both sensory radiculopathies and CNS infestation are the main complications.

Anglade, Dominique (b. 1867) French neurologist who first demonstrated the value of Victoria Blue as a staining technique for neuroglia, according to Lasègue.[3708]

angle tumors Conventionally synonymous with cerebellopontine angle tumors. The typical syndrome was first described in accurate detail by **Cushing**,[1390] who noted that there had been reports as far back as 1830 but based his account on a personal series of 30 such cases. Tinnitus; deafness; vertigo; suboccipital discomfort; frank cerebellar signs; involvement of the fifth, sixth, seventh, and bulbar cranial nerves; features of raised intracranial pressure; and "cerebellar crises" (extreme suboccipital pain with neck retraction and reduction in consciousness, angor animi, bradycardia, and apnea, indicating intermittent increases in intracranial pressure) occurred, generally in that order.

angular gyrus syndrome The clinical effects of damage to the heteromodal cortex adjacent to Wernicke area, including any combination of anomia, alexia, acalculia, constructional deficits, dysgraphia, defects in finger identification, and left/right naming difficulties. See also Gerstmann syndromes, alexia.

anhedonia A term used mainly in psychiatry, signifying the inability to experience pleasure and loss of the power of enjoyment. By extension, it represents a telling symptom of depressed affect.

anhidrosis (Gr, lack of + sweat) Absence of sweating; a local phenomenon with damage to postganglionic sympathetic cholinergic pathways, or a generalized problem as a result of degenerative or chemically induced sympathetic failure. *Generalized anhidrosis* is a rare congenital or acquired disease with heat intolerance and lack of sweating with or without autonomic neuropathy.

The condition may occur congenitally as a recessively inherited trait in which there is a failure of differentiation of sweat glands.[4019] See also **Riley–Day syndrome, multiple system atrophy, familial amyloid neuropathy**.

anhidrotic ectodermal dysplasia (Christ-Siemens-Touraine syndrome) An X-linked recessive syndrome comprising anhidrosis, hypotrichosis, saddle nose, dental anomalies, periorbital pigmentation, and sometimes mental delay.[6450]

anhydromyelia (Gr, lack of + water + marrow) Deficiency of CSF.

anima (derivative of Lat, soul or spirit) The soul or vital life-force, applied also to the intellectual principle of humans.

aniridia A dominantly inherited congenital malformation characterized by absence of the iris, usually bilaterally associated with photophobia, amblyopia, nystagmus, and sometimes ataxia.[5772] Other anomalies are also described in a few of the patients.

In a *variant form* (*aniridia, mental retardation, genital abnormalities*), these features and nystagmus, cataract, and glaucoma are found in association with abnormalities of chromosome 11p13.[4674] See also **Gillespie syndrome**.

aniseikonia Perception of one object viewed by the two eyes as having two different sizes or shapes.

anismus Constipation due to functional obstruction of the pelvic outlet by paradoxical contraction of the striated sphincter muscles during defecation straining. This may represent a focal dystonia.[4163]

anisocoria (Gr, negative + equal + pupil) Inequality of the diameter of the pupils of 0.4 mm or more, suggesting the presence of a lesion of the sympathetic pathway to the eye on one side or of the parasympathetic pathway on the other if any disease is present at all.

In this form, *simple, essential, or central anisocoria*, the pupils react to light and accommodation, the difference in their size is maintained under different conditions of illumination, and pharmacological responses are normal. The condition is regarded as a normal variant.

anisometropia (Gr, negative + equal + measure + eye) A difference in the refraction of the two eyes, or a difference in the anteroposterior diameter of the two eyes. In each case, it is a common cause of **amblyopia**.

anisomorphic gliosis The irregular orientation of the glial fibers in severely damaged neural tissues.

anisosthenic (Gr, negative + the same + strength) Inequality in the force of contraction of different muscles.

ankyloblepharon The presence of a variable degree of fusion of the lid margins, a malformation that may be dominantly or recessively inherited.

ankylosis (from Gr, the bend of the arm) A stiffening of a joint by disease.

Annals of Neurology The journal of the American Neurological Association (Web site: http://www.aneuroa.org/) and of the Child Neurology Society (Web site: http://www.childneurologysociety.org/), publishing articles on all aspects of the human nervous system, both normal and abnormal, published by Wiley-Blackwell Publications. *Wiley InterScience* (Web site: http://www3.interscience.wiley.com/journal/76507645/home)

annectant gyri The convolutions passing from the parietal to the occipital lobes.[2531]

Annual Review of Neuroscience (*Annu Rev Neurosci*) A neurological/neuroscience review book series published by Annuals Reviews Inc. Address: Annual Reviews Inc., 4139 El Camino Way, Palo Alto, CA 94303-0897. Web site: http://neuro.annualreviews.org/.

anodal block A local block of nerve conduction caused by membrane hyperpolarization under a stimulating anode.

anode The positive terminal of an electric current source. Cf. **cathode**.

anodyne (Gr, lack of + pain) An analgesic medicine; until the earliest part of this century the word was applied to drugs such as opium, chloroform, and hemp, only the last of which is easily obtainable today.

anoetic Capable of thought.

anomalous reflex A reflex with no known survival value, e.g., vomiting with vertigo.

anomia (from Lat, deprivative + a name) The inability to generate and utter names; a facility impaired in all forms of aphasia but also in many cerebral diseases not causing aphasia. Four forms are distinguished:[527]

Word-production anomia The patient knows the required name but is unable to produce it correctly without some form of cuing, because of difficulty in initiating articulation, or in evoking the word, or as a result of **paraphasia**.

Word-selection anomia A pure word-finding problem in which the patient can recognize and describe the function of the object presented, but cannot evoke its name.

Semantic anomia A failure of both the comprehension and the use of the name of an object; a situation in which the word has lost its semantic meaning for the patient.

Disconnection anomia Inability to evoke the name of an object presented in one modality while the word is recalled when it is presented in another (*modality specific anomia*); a naming failure in a single category only, such as color (*category-specific anomia*); and inability to name an object recognized after placement in the left hand, as after callosal section (*callosal anomia*).

See also **progressive pure anomia**.

anomic aphasia The most common form of aphasia, characterized by fluency, retention of repetition, and fair or good comprehension but poor naming ability. The anomia is a defect of naming, not of recognition. Semantic errors and the use of circumlocutions and general words ("thing," "whatsit," "you know") for specific nouns are characteristic. The lesion is of the low angular gyrus and posterior middle temporal gyrus but the phenomenon is also a socially pervasive form of communication (?) in modern teenagers.

anophthalmia (Gr, lack or + eye) A rare, usually recessively inherited **craniofacial malformation** characterized by a lack of traces even of ocular development as the result of failure of formation of the primary optic vesicle.[3087] See also the syndromes of **Goldenhar**, **Wildervanck**, **Franceschetti**, and **Hallermann and Streiff**.

Another *variant* is *anophthalmia with intracranial germinoma*, a congenital syndrome in which the anophthalmia is complicated by polyuria, hypopituitarism, hydrocephalus, cerebral teratoma, and mental and developmental delay.[381]

anopsia (Gr, lack of + vision) Loss of sight.

anorexia hysterica See **anorexia nervosa**.

anorexia nervosa (Gr, lack of + appetite) (apepsia hysterica; anorexia hysterica) An eating disorder (psychogenic food refusal) characterized by an exaggerated fear of obesity, a desire for thinness, and a distorted body image. Refusal of food leads to drastic weight loss, often accompanied by overexercising and the abuse of laxatives. With this, there is a disturbance in perception of body image such that the subject claims to feel fat even when emaciated or believes that one area of the body is "too fat" even when this is obviously not the case. Total body weight is at least 15% below the expected weight, and in females, thre will be absence of at least three consecutive menstrual cycles when otherwise expected to occur (primary or secondary amenorrhea). The APA diagnostic guidelines may be found at: http://www.psychiatryonline.com/content.aspx?aID=3617.

The condition was first described by Richard Morton in 1689, but there is some evidence that Mary, Queen of Scots, had suffered from this disorder in the previous century. The name was coined by Sir William **Gull** in 1874 but is not fully accurate, as many patients retain a feeling of hunger at least until well into the illness.[995, 2285] It was also described by **William Hammond** (*Fasting Girls*, 1879, New York, Putnam's Sons), who, however, showed that in some cases their allegations that they had not eaten for weeks or months were fraudulent.

anorgasmia Inability to experience orgasm, due to psychological reasons, medications, local genital causes, or lesions of the anterolateral spinal cord or of the nervi erigentes.[566]

anosmia (Gr, lack of + smell) Loss of the sense of smell. When unilateral, it suggests the presence of local nasal disease or of a mass lesion such as a meningioma, glioma, or abscess in the anterior cranial fossa; when bilateral, its localizing value is diluted and either local nasal or intracranial disorders may be responsible. The condition may be inherited as an autosomal dominant trait.[5866] See also **Kallmann syndrome**.

anosognosia (from Gr, nosos [illness] and gnosis [knowledge/awareness] [denial syndrome]) A term introduced by Josef **Babinski** for the unawareness or denial of physical deficits.[325] This is seen most often with lesions of the right parietal lobe, in which case the unawareness is of the deficits on the left side of the body. This may actually lead to denial of ownership of a (paretic) limb, usually the left, in patients with infarct of the right supramarginal cortex or the thalamocortical radiations projecting to it. In a minor key, the phenomenon consists merely of unconcern about an admitted deficit. Denial of numerous other kinds of deficit such as those of memory, sight, praxis, or speech also occurs. Anosognosia may also be a feature of **Alzheimer disease**. See also **simultagnosia**.

anosognosic graphopmimia See **hypergraphia**.

anoxic myelopathy The occurrence of symmetrical gray matter lesions in the spinal cords of patients who had suffered systemic anoxic episodes or circulatory arrest. These changes, though generalized, are most marked in lumbosacral regions.[315]

anoxic seizures A heterogeneous group of paroxysmal events that include some degree of abrogation of consciousness and various motor and sensory phenomena occurring as a result of cortical anoxia and representing a type of **nonepileptic seizure**.

ansa (Lat, a handle) A curved structure.

ansa hypoglossi A looped branch running between the twelfth cranial nerve and the cervical plexus.

ansa lenticularis A fiber tract carrying impulses from the globus pallidus to the thalamus.

ansa subclavia The left recurrent laryngeal nerve.

antagonist 1. A muscle, the main action of which opposes the function of another (**agonist**) muscle. See also **synergist**.
2. A chemical substance that binds to a receptor and inhibits its activity.

antagonistic anterior tibial reflex (Piotrowski reflex) Plantar flexion at the ankle in response to a tap on the tibialis anterior muscle belly. The reflex is sometimes elicited in patients with pyramidal lesions. See **Piotrowski sign**.

antagonistic reflexes Occasional variant forms of the usual muscle stretch reflexes, modified in certain conditions by the underlying pathology and by the method of elicitation.[6656]

antalgic (Gr, against + pain) Analgesic.

antalgic gait Limping as a result of pain felt (from any cause, such as arthropathy) during walking.

antebrachium (Lat, before + arm) The forearm.

antecollis (Lat, before + neck) A focal dystonia characterized by sustained involuntary contractions of the neck muscles, which result in abnormal flexion of the head on the neck. See **cervical dystonia**.

anterior (rostral) In front.

anterior agraphia See **agraphia**.

anterior alexia See **alexia**.

anterior apraxia See **apraxia**.

anterior bulbar syndrome Anterior spinal artery occlusion causing ischemic infarction of the pyramid, the twelfth cranial nerve, and possibly the medial lemniscus, thus producing a homolateral hypoglossal paralysis and contralateral hemiparesis (and hemianesthesia). It was first described by Déjèrine.[3113] See also **alternating hypoglossal hemiplegia syndrome**, **Déjèrine syndromes**.

anterior cavernous syndrome A syndrome of painful ophthalmoplegia with **Horner syndrome** and trigeminal anesthesia due to a lesion in this situation. It was first described in detail by **Jefferson**[3113] and later by Foix in 1925. See **Tolosa–Hunt syndrome**.

anterior cerebral artery syndromes Occlusion of the main trunk proximal to Heubner's artery leading to severe contralateral hemiplegia with sensory loss in the leg, urinary incontinence, emotional and intellectual changes, and left-sided apraxia with a right-side occlusion, or transcortical aphasia if it is on the left. Sensory neglect and micrographia have also been described in this circumstance. Abulia is associated with frontal pole, corpus callosum, and cingulate gyrus infarcts. Callosal infarcts often induce a grasp reflex.

Occlusion distal to Heubner's artery leads to hemiplegia with crural predominance, indefinite sensory impairment, left-sided ideomotor apraxia, forced grasping and groping in the left arm, dysphasia with a left-sided occlusion, and emotional and intellectual changes. Main stem occlusions distal to this point lead to crural paresis and mental changes only. Occlusion of Heubner's artery alone leads to hemiparesis affecting the arm more than the face or leg, and occlusions of other arterial branches cause varying degrees of crural weakness only.[1324] The most severe motor dysfunction occurs with involvement of the supplementary motor area/paracentral lobule.

anterior choroidal artery A branch of the internal carotid artery supplying part of the posterior limb of the internal capsule, the lateral geniculate body, the globus pallidus, part of the optic radiation, and the middle third of the crus cerebri. Occlusion leads to a constant clinical picture. See **anterior choroidal artery syndrome**.

anterior choroidal artery syndrome (von Monakow syndrome) The occurrence of contralateral hemiplegia, hemianesthesia, and homonymous hemianopia without cognitive deficit, due to occlusion or hemorrhage of the artery with infarction of the posterior limb of the internal capsule or the medial globus pallidus, the ventral posterolateral thalamus, and the lateral geniculate body.[6027]

Left-sided spatial neglect and minor speech disturbances may also occur according to the side of the infarction.[1529] Despite the eponymous attribution, Foix and Chavanay gave a complete description in 1925.[2140]

anterior cingulate gyrus epilepsy A variety of frontal focal cortical epilepsy involving the pericallosal gyrus. It has variable clinical manifestations including head turning, head dropping, apparent absences, and psychotic behavior and there is no typical EEG pattern.[5523]

anterior cingulate syndrome Apathy, akinesia, drowsiness, and mutism, said to be fatal in weeks, in which case the causative lesion is more likely to be of the thalamus with secondary expansion effects on the corpus callosum, since surgical removal of the anterior cingulate gyri causes no such signs.

anterior cornual syndrome (Schantz syndrome) Damage to the anterior horn cells in a segment of the spinal cord, resulting from any one of the various possible pathologies.

anterior crural syndrome See **anterior tibial syndrome**.

anterior encephalocele The congenital appearance of a frontal cranial meningocele. See **dysraphism**.

anterior ethmoidal nerve syndrome Bilateral recurrent nasal pain or severe headache with neck stiffness lasting a day or more at a time.[948] The nature of this condition requires further study.

anterior frontopolar region seizures A form of epilepsy. The patterns of which include forced thinking or initial loss of contact and adversive movements of head and eyes, with possible evolution including contraversive movements and axial clonic jerks and falls and autonomic signs. (From the revised ILAE Classification,[1264] reproduced by kind permission from Wiley-Blackwell Publications.)

anterior horn cell disease with cerebellar hypoplasia in infants See **hereditary motor neuropathy** (*variants*).

anterior horn cell disease with pontocerebellar hypoplasia See **hereditary motor neuropathy** (*variants*).

anterior inferior cerebellar artery syndrome The constellation of signs following infarction of the territory supplied by this artery.

The signs include vertigo and nystagmus; tinnitus and homolateral deafness; gait and homolateral limb ataxia; homolateral facial palsy; **alternating thermoanalgesia** (homolateral face and contralateral trunk and limb involvement); and homolateral **Horner syndrome**.

anterior internuclear ophthalmoplegia See **internuclear ophthalmoplegia**. It is not certain that Lutz and Lhermitte's differentiation between the so-called anterior and posterior forms of the syndrome is appropriate.

anterior interosseous nerve syndrome (Kiloh–Nevin syndrome) Weakness and wasting of flexor pollicis longus, of that part of the flexor digitorum profundus innervated by the median nerve, and of pronator quadratus as a result of proximal compression of the anterior interosseous branch of the median nerve between the two heads of pronator teres, usually by a fibrous band or as a result of local trauma.[4728]

Clincally, there is weakness in flexion of the terminal phalanges of digits I–III, through its innervation of the flexor digitorum profundus I and II, flexor pollicis longus (FPL), and pronator quadratus. Sensation is preserved.

The flexor carpi radialis and flexor digitorum sublimis are spared, being supplied by the main trunk of the median nerve. The pronator teres is seldom affected. See also **pinch sign**.

anterior ischemic optic neuropathy Infarction of the laminar and retrolaminar parts of the optic nerve due to small-vessel disease of the choroidal or posterior ciliary branches of the ophthalmic arteries. The condition is most commonly associated with hypertension or **giant cell arteritis** (when it is frequently bilateral), other collagen–vascular diseases, **drusen**, diabetes, and such vascular disorders as hypotension resulting from blood loss; nevertheless, over a quarter of the patients have no detectable underlying disease.

Clinically, the major features are abrupt painless visual field loss, with an **altitudinal defect** and pallor and swelling of all or only a sector of the optic nerve head, later leading on to **optic atrophy**. Peripapillary hemorrhages are commonly seen in the acute stages.[703]

anterior midline structure syndrome See **Zeman–King syndrome**.

anterior opercular syndrome (Foix-Chavanay-Marie syndrome, facio-linguo-pharyngo-masticatory diplegia) Loss of voluntary control of facial, pharyngeal, lingual, masticatory, and sometimes ocular muscle activity due to bilateral anterior perisylvian lesions involving the primary motor cortex within the frontal and parietal opercula. Bilateral opercular polymicrogyria or infarction is the usual cause.[4053]

Clinically, the *acquired form* of the condition is characterized by acute onset, inability to perform voluntary movements with the bulbar muscles, decreased gag reflex, and absence of **emotionalism**. In the *developmental form*, inability to protrude or wiggle the tongue, seizures, mild mental retardation, and brisk reflexes with normal Babinski responses are typical features.[2139] Bilateral infarcts or herpes encephalitis are usually responsible. See also **bilateral central macrogyria: epilepsy, pseudobulbar palsy, and mental retardation**.

anterior sacral meningiocele Herniation of the dural sac that contains cerebrospinal fluid and sometimes neural elements through a defect in the anterior surface of the sacrum. Constipation and urinary incontinence with evidence of a pelvic mass are the usual presenting features.

anterior slow alpha of drowsiness An EEG pattern recorded in drowsiness from midline frontocentral regions; also distinct from true alpha activity by virtue of being slightly slower.[884]

anterior spinal artery syndrome (Beck syndrome) Infarction of the anterior portion of the spinal cord due to occlusion of the anterior spinal artery, leading abruptly to pain, pyramidal and spinothalamic deficits, and loss of sphincter control below the level of the lesion and to pain, hyperalgesia, and evidence of a lower motor neuron lesion at its site. The senses of vibration and of joint position are spared.

Such infarcts are most usual in thoracic regions, the clinical picture varying with the level of cord involvement. Aortic dissection, syphilis, and aortic surgery are the most common causes of the condition which was first described by Preobrashenski in 1904,[5113] although a fuller account was later provided by Beck.[468]

anterior spinal hernia Thoracic myelopathy due to anterior spinal artery segmental branch ischemia in a cord chronically trapped in a congenital anterior meningocele.[6747]

anterior-superior cerebellar artery syndrome The clinical picture resulting from infarcts in the territory of this artery.[5081] The typical clinical presentation includes dysarthria, unsteadiness and/or vertigo, homolateral limb ataxia, and dysmetria with axial lateropulsion, but it may also mimic the lacunar **dysarthria-clumsy hand syndrome**. Coma at onset (or delayed) and tetraplegia are also described. Cardiogenic embolism is the commonest single cause.

anterior tarsal tunnel syndrome Entrapment of the terminal parts of the mixed deep peroneal nerve below the inferior extensor retinaculum, presenting clinically with numbness and tingling over the first web space of the foot and frequently with a **Tinel sign** over the sensory branch of the deep peroneal nerve on the anterior aspect of the ankle.[5088]

anterior tibial sign Involuntary extension of the hallux with forcible flexion of the hip; seen in pyramidal lesions.[5333]

anterior tibial syndrome (anterior crural syndrome; march syndrome) Pain in the anterior tibial compartment with weakness of the muscles and sensory loss in the distribution of the anterior tibial nerve, due to swelling of the muscles with a resultant increase in local pressure below the fascial covering of the compartment, and with subsequent ischemic necrosis of all the soft tissues within it.[4529]

The condition was first described by Karl Beck, and later by **Vogt** in 1943.

anterocollis A form of sporadic focal **dystonia**.

anterograde Forward.

anterograde amnesia 1. (anterograde memory deficits) Loss of the capacity for learning new material which may lead to decreased attention and inaccurate perception. This term corresponds to memory difficulties as they are usually understood. Cf. **retrograde amnesia**. 2. Loss of recall for events following a neurological insult. Anterograde memory is commonly the last function to return after recovery from loss of consciousness.

anthrax meningoencephalitis The major neurologic complication of infection by *Bacillus anthracis* through the skin or by inhalation; a fulminant and rapidly fatal hemorrhagic meningoencephalitis with dark necrotic pustules forming in the skin of the extremities, fever, malaise, meningism, delirium, stupor, or coma. Gram-positive rods are found in the CSF and there are multifocal areas of unexplained intracerebral hemorrhage on CT scans.[3691, 4343]

anthropology The study of the characteristics of past and present human populations. Subdivisions of anthropology include the sociocultural, archeological, biological, and linguistic branches.

anthropomorphism The ascription of human characteristics to animals.

anti- (Lat, against) A prefix signifying "in opposition to."

antiamphiphysin antibodies Antibodies detected rarely in patients with breast cancer who manifest paraneoplastic encephalomyelitis or **stiff-person syndromes.**[1422]

antibasal ganglion antibodies Markers of the presence of a postinfectious autoimmune inflammatory disorder, usually following a streptococcal infection. The syndromes include **Sydenham chorea, PANDAs**, and **acute disseminated encephalomyelitis**.

anti-CAR antibody An antibody used as a marker for (small-cell lung cancer) **cancer-associated retinopathy**. Such antibodies may be detected in some patients with small-cell lung cancer who manifest photoreceptor degeneration.[1422]

anticardiolipin antibodies Circulating immunoglobulin A, G, and M antibodies associated with a tendency toward arterial or venous thrombosis and thrombocytopenia, in part as a result of inhibition of prostacycline release from the endothelial walls.

Associations with ischemic (multiple) cerebral infarction, **Sneddon syndrome**, **chorea**, seizures, **optic neuritis**, **acute inflammatory demyelinating polyneuropathy**, and **migraine** have been shown.[618]

anticholinergic syndrome The association of fever, flushing, dilated pupils, and drowsiness, delirium or coma, sometimes with extrapyramidal signs, as a result of a toxic reaction to anticholinergic drugs.[2001]

anticipation The presentation of a genetic disease earlier and more severely in succeeding generations. It is seen mainly in dominantly inherited diseases such as **myotonic dystrophy**, **hereditary spastic paraplegia**, and **Huntington disease**.

anticipatory nystagmus Predictive, slow eye movements that occur prior to ramp or step target movements of the eyes, interspersed with saccades in the opposite direction.[1561] See **induced nystagmus**.

anticipatory postural reflexes Alterations of the position of the trunk and limbs prior to the performance of a movement of the whole body. An example is the truncal and leg flexion which precedes the rising from a chair.[4723] (Reproduced by kind permission of the American Academy of Neurology and Lippincott Williams and Wilkins.)

anticonvulsant A drug that inhibits epileptic seizures. As many such agents have other effects (such as inhibition of activity in pain pathways), use of the term is only appropriate in the context of epilepsy.

anti-CV2 antibodies Antibodies detected in some patients with small-cell lung cancer who manifest encephalomyelitis or cerebellar degeneration syndromes.[1422]

antidepressant A drug that elevates depressed mood. As many such agents have other effects (such as the prophylaxis of migraine), use of the term is only appropriate in the context of depression.

antidromic Propagation of a nerve impulse in the direction opposite to physiologic conduction—e.g., conduction along motor nerve fibers away from the muscle and conduction along sensory fibers away from the spinal cord. Cf. **orthodromic**. (From the 2001 Report of the Nomenclature Committee of the American Association of Electromyography and Electrodiagnosis. Reproduced by kind permission of the AANEM.)[19]

anti-GD1b antibody syndrome An ataxic form of Guillain-Barré syndrome with profound loss of proprioception and generalized areflexia, sometimes with mild external ophthalmoplegia, associated with high titers of monospecific anti-GD1b IgG antibodies during the acute phase.[4878]

anti-GM1 antibodies Antibodies directed at ganglioside epitopes, capable of inducing conduction block and associated with the clinical conditions such as **multifocal neuropathy with conduction block**, a motor variant of **chronic inflammatory demyelinating ganglioradiculopathy, amyotrophic lateral sclerosis** (seldom), and other motor neuropathies.

anti-GQ1b antibody syndrome The common autoimmune mechanism in **Miller Fisher syndrome, acute inflammatory demyelinating polyneuropathy, Bickerstaff brainstem encephalitis,** and **acute ophthalmoparesis without ataxia**.[4751]

anti-Hu antibodies Antibodies directed at neuronal nuclei in the central and peripheral nervous systems, characteristically found in paraneoplastic encephalomyelitis affecting the cerebellum and limbic system and with sensory and autonomic neuropathies. Small-cell lung cancer and neuroblastoma are the more common underlying tumors.[4437, 1421]

anti-Jo-1 antibodies Antibodies present in some syndromes characterized by muscle weakness and pain, the Raynaud phenomenon, interstitial lung disease, arthritis, and skin rashes.[4528]

anti-Ma antibodies Antibodies detected to Ma1 and Ma2 proteins in patients with various cancers who manifest paraneoplastic limbic, cerebellar, and brainstem syndromes.[1422]

anti-Ma2-associated encephalitis A variant of paraneoplastic encephalitis, usually presenting with isolated or combined limbic, diencephalic, or brainstem dysfunction and excessive daytime sleepiness due to diencephalic–hypothalamic involvement. Vertical gaze paresis, external ophthalmoplegia, and atypical Parkinsonism or a severe hypokinetic syndrome are the described features. In young male patients the primary tumor is usually in the testis, in others the commonest neoplasm is lung cancer.[1420]

anti-MAG-associated neuropathy See **immune-mediated neuropathies**.

anti-MysB antibodies Antibodies detected rarely in patients with small-cell lung cancer who manifest a myasthenic syndrome.[1422]

antineuronal antibodies Autoantibodies occasionally identified in the serum of patients with a paraneoplastic disorder of the nervous system. The *antinucleoprotein antibody* (Hu) is mainly associated with small-cell carcinoma of the lung, while the *antiPurkinje* antibody is usually found in patients with breast or ovarian cancer.[4438] Anti-Ro/SS-A and anti-La/SSB antibodies occur in some patients with **Sjögren syndrome**. Anti-Yo antibodies are found in paraneoplastric cerebellar degeneration. Other neuronal antigens include myelin-associated glycoprotein; GM1, GQ1b, and other gangliosides; and sulfatide and chondroitin sulfate.[5151]

antiphospholipid antibodies A family of immunoglobulin antibodies to phospholipids, including the lupus anticoagulant and anticardiolipin antibodies (IgG, IgM, and IgA isotypes). They are most commonly found in women, in people aged less than 50 years, and in those with cerebral, optic, and other ischemic syndromes, headaches, thrombotic events, biologically false-positive reactions to syphilis, or thrombocytopenia. They also occur in 1–2% of the general population and in up to 50% of patients with **systemic lupus erythematosus**.

These antibodies may be considered markers of stroke risk, but their precise relationship to the event is uncertain.[3811]

antiphospholipid antibody syndrome An autoimmune thrombophilic disorder defined by the presence in the blood of the lupus anticoagulant or anticardiolipin antibodies, usually in high titer, and clinically by recurrent fetal losses, recurrent arterial or venous thromboses, or thrombocytopenia.[3811]

Patients who are antiphospholipid-antibody positive and who present with recurrent fetal loss, venous or arterial occlusion, or thrombocytopenia but without clinical evidence of systemic lupus erythematosus are said to have the primary syndrome. The cerebral syndromes may involve the small or the larger arteries, presenting a **stroke, transient ischemic attacks**, or **multi-infarct dementia**.[835] Occasional neurological presentations include transverse myelitis, chorea, and a syndrome resembling **acute inflammatory demyelinating polyneuropathy**. Classification criteria have been suggested[6821] and require one or more episodes of vascular thrombosis, pregnancy morbidity (deaths of a neonate, or three or more spontaneous abortions before 10 weeks). Laboratory criteria include the detection of anticardiolipin antibodies or lupus anticoagulant according to listed guidelines. See also **Sneddon syndrome**.[2887]

anti-Ri antibodies Antibodies detected rarely in patients with breast cancer who manifest opsoclonuis, nystagmus, dysarthria, and ataxia.[1421, 4437]

antisaccades Deviations of the eyes from a central fixation point not *toward* a new visual stimulus but *away from* it. Failure to make such movements in the test situation is evidence of frontal lobe dysfunction.[3460]

anti-Ta antibodies Antibodies detected rarely in some patients with testicular cancer who manifest a paraneoplastic syndrome of limbic and brainstem encephalitis.[1422]

antithrombin III deficiency A dominantly inherited disorder of hemaglobin predisposing patients to stroke and due to a mutation in the antithrombin III gene at 1q23–25.

anti-Tr antibodies Antibodies detected rarely in patients with Hodgkin lymphoma who manifest a paraneoplastic syndrome of cerebellar degeneration.[1422]

anti-VGCC antibodies Antibodies detected in some patients with small-cell lung cancer who manifest a paraneoplastic myasthenic (Lambert–Eaton) syndrome.[1422]

anti-Yo antibodies Antibodies detected rarely in patients with breast or ovarian cancer who manifest a paraneoplastic subacute cerebellar syndrome with nystagmus and dysarthria.[4437, 1421]

Anton, Gabriel (1858–1933) Austrian neurologist who worked with **Pick** and **Meynert** before holding appointments successively in Innsbruck, Graz, and Halle (where he succeeded **Wernicke** as professor in 1905). In 1899, he described a loss of awareness of focal cerebral somatosensory defects in patients suffering from visual agnosia or word deafness (*anosognosia* in **Babinski**'s terminology).

Anton syndrome Anosognosia for blindness, with denial of that blindness. Such usage actually extends the definition of the syndrome described by Anton in 1899.

Although overtly unable to see, often because of bilateral occipital lobe ischemic damage, the patients deny that this is so and may resort to confabulation about things "seen."[211, 5228] **Allocheiria** is another inconstant accompaniment.

Anton–Babinski syndrome A rare neuropsychiatric syndrome featuring bilateral cortical blindness, visual anosognosia, and denial of the blindness and usually of an accompanying left hemiparesis, as it is classically a result of a right parietal lesion. The patient is commonly unaware of the paralysis or, if aware, remains indifferent.

The names of Redlich and Bonvicini are also sometimes attached to this condition, but their reports were up to 20 years later than those of Anton and Babinski.

Antonini type A areas Regions within **Schwannomas** characterized by sheaths of spindle cells with long nuclei and fine intercellular cytoplasmic processes.[6]

Antonini type B areas Regions within **Schwannomas** characterized by populations of cells with small round nuclei and fine cytoplasmic processes intermixed with mast cells.[6]

anxietas tibiarum See **restless legs syndrome**.

Anyane Yeboa syndrome (clefting-corneal opacity-retardation) A congenital dysmorphic syndrome characterized by short stature, cloudy corneas, cleft upper lip and palate, urinary system anomalies, hydrocephalus, and mental and developmental delay.[381]

aortic arch arteritis See **aortic arch disease**.

aortic arch disease (Takayasu disease, pulseless disease, aortic arch arteritis) An obliterative panarteritis affecting the major branches of the arch of the aorta, usually in young women, leading to cerebral and systemic ischemic symptoms and loss of pulses at the appropriate sites. Evidence of the formation of a collateral circulation, cardiac enlargement, systemic hypertension in the legs, and an elevated erythrocyte sedimentation rate are also characteristic.[6191]

The condition was described by Broadbent in 1875 (as "subclavian stenosis") and by Takayasu in 1908. Sixteen synonyms are listed by Jablonski.[3113, 3114]

In a *variant* of the syndrome (*aortic arch syndrome*), similar features occur, mainly in young males in the Far East, in the absence of such arteritic pathology and without evidence of fibromuscular hyperplasia or atheroma. There is, however, intense collagen proliferation at the origins of the great vessels leaving the aorta.[1415]

APACHE score A severity-of-disease classification system deriving a point score based upon the initial values of 12 routine physiological measurements, age, and previous health status. Increasing scores are closely correlated with the risk of subsequent hospital death.[3495]

apallic syndrome The original term of Kretschmer[3562] for the **persistent vegetative state**.

apathetic thyrotoxicosis A variant form of acute hyperthyroidism in the elderly, characterized by lethargy, depression, abdominal pain, nausea, and vomiting.

apathy (Gr, without + feeling) A pathological behavioral state characterized by a reduction in spontaneous action and speech, with delayed, short, slow, or absent responses to stimuli and a flat affect.[1027, 6025a]

Apathy, abulia from frontal lobe disorders, psychomotor retardation in depression, and bradykinesia with "bradyphrenia" from extrapyramidal disorders can be difficult to tell apart clinically.[3816] Apathy does not correlate well with depression but does correlate with lowered cognitive function. See also **athymhormia**, **Lille Apathy Rating Scale**.[5940]

ape hand (simian hand) Generalized atrophy and weakness of the intrinsic muscles of the hand, leading to a decline of the position of the thumb into the plane of the palm, as in severe motor neuropathies with predominant effects on the median nerve.[645]

Apelt-Gerkin-Lenz syndrome See **cleft lip-palate and tetraphocomelia**.

apepsia hysterica See **anorexia nervosa**.

aperiodic 1. EEG waves or complexes occurring in a sequence but at an irregular rate. 2. EEG waves or complexes occurring intermittently at irregular intervals. (Adapted from the 1974 Report of the Committee on Terminology, IFCN[1117] and reproduced by kind permission of Elsevier Science.)

aperiodic alternating nystagmus See **periodic alternating nystagmus**.

Apert, Eugene (1868–1940) French pediatrician practicing in Paris, with a major interest in developmental abnormalities.

Apert syndrome (Type I acrocephalosyndactyly; Apert-Park-Powers syndrome; syndrome of Lobstein, van der Hoeve, Spurway, Henzschell, von Ammon, Looser, or Eddowes) A rare, sporadic (rarely autosomal dominant) craniofacial malformation stemming from abnormal bony fusion (craniostenosis) affecting the skull (**acrocephaly, turricephaly, brachycephaly**), facial bones, hands, and feet (**syndactyly**). In some cases, the inability of the skull to expand leads to increased intracranial pressure as the brain grows, leading to ophthalmoplegia, optic atrophy with visual failure, and mental retardation. Shallow orbits are responsible for the slight exophthalmos. Agenesis of the corpus callosum or of limbic structures, blue sclerae, deafness, bilateral fourth cranial nerve palsy, and bony fragility are also reported.[216] Linkage to chromosome 10q has been achieved.

It was first described by Oribasius (325–403 AD) and may have been recognized by Homer, whose hero Thersites was described as if being so afflicted. It was reviewed and fully described in 1906 by Apert after a preceding description by Troquart in 1886.

The skull shape of Louis-Philippe of France ("tête en poire") may have been due to such brachycephaly. The conditions of acrocephaly and acrocephalosyndactyly have been reviewed by Ferriman[2032] and by Baraitser.[379] See also **Crouzon syndrome, acrocephalosyndactyly**.

Apert-Park-Powers syndrome See **Apert syndrome**.

Apgar scores A practical, semiquantitative method of evaluation of the newborn infant, the observations being made 1 min after birth and sometimes repeated at 10 min.

In the scale, up to 2 points may be given each for respiratory effort, reflex irritability, muscle tone, heart rate, and color.[217] The scale has predictive value in terms of future motor and mental development.

Apgar scores

Score	*Heart Rate*	*Respiratory Effort*	*Reflex Irritability*	*Muscle Tone*	*Color*
2	100–140	Normal cry	Normal	Good	Pink
1	100	Irregular and shallow	Depressed	Fair	Fair
0	>60	Apnea	Absent	Flaccid	Cyanotic

aphagia algera The loss of the ability to eat as a result of pain produced by eating, leading to emaciation. In the absence of any detectable physical disease likely to be responsible, the condition is considered to be functional or psychogenic.[5984] See also **akinesia algera**.

aphakia (Gr, negative + a lentil) The condition of absence of the lens of the eye.

aphasia (Gr, lack of + speech) (dysphasia) A disturbance of word choice and/or grammar or of comprehension in communicating through language due to brain disease; a disturbance in communication using language, not primarily due to motor or sensory deficits. Or, in the terms of Sir Henry **Head**, a disorder of symbolic formulation and expression.

The first modern report of motor aphasia was by **Broca**, who demonstrated a case (of "aphemie") in 1861 associated with a lesion of the left second and third frontal convolutions. Broca later correctly narrowed the site of the lesion to the posterior part of the left inferior frontal convolution, although Pierre **Marie** sectioned that patient's brain in 1906 and found that the lesion was much more extensive.[4072]

The condition had been described by Hippocrates and by Schmidt in 1679 and was recognized by Carl von Linne (Linnaeus) in 1745. In 1683, Peter Rommeliu (1643–1708) described what he called a "rare form of aphonia." His lucid description, the embodiment of the modern aphasia examination, identifies the syndrome as Broca aphasia. **Alexia, paraphasia**, unawareness of defects, amnesic aphasia, jargon aphasia, and agraphia had also been mentioned variously by others before the nineteenth century.[4339] In 1825, Bouillard noted that the faculty for forming words could be lost even though the muscles of articulation were intact; in 1836, Marc Dax stated that the site of speech memories was the left hemisphere; and in 1864, **Trousseau** suggested the use of the word *aphasia* rather than *aphemie*. A survey of the earliest accounts of aphasia from those of Hippocrates on was provided by Benton and Joynt, who noted that most of the forms of aphasia had been described piecemeal before Broca's contribution.[534] The early history has also been reviewed.[5298]

The sensory type of aphasia was first described as such by **Wernicke** in 1874, although others had written of the deficits before him. The most important summations of knowledge have been those of Henry **Head**, whose two-volume work *Aphasia and Kindred Disorders of Speech* was published in 1926, and more recently that of Critchley.[2911]

See also **Broca aphasia, Wernicke aphasia, conduction aphasia, transcortical aphasia, global aphasia, nonoptic aphasia, amnestic aphasia, alexia**.

Aphasia, Apraxia, Agnosia A subspecialty neurological journal. Address: Biolinguistics, P.O. Box 11356, Chicago, IL 60611.

aphasia–agnosia–apraxia syndrome (Pick syndrome, Bianchi syndrome) The combination of dementia, apperceptive blindness, and loss of reflex gaze.[5228] See **posterior cortical dementia**.

aphasia batteries Standardized schemes for the diagnosis and assessment of aphasic disorders, for use informally at the bedside or in the neuropsychology laboratory.

Batteries in common clinical use include the **Western Aphasia battery**,[3401] the **Aphasia Language Performance Scales**, the **Boston Diagnostic Aphasia Examination**,[2474] the Eisenson Examination for Aphasia,[1826] the **Minnesota Test for the Differential Diagnosis of Aphasia**, and the **Porch Index of Communicative Ability**.[5080]

Screening tests include the **Aphasia Screening Test**, the **Frenchay Aphasia Screening Test**, the **Sheffield screening test for Acquired Language Disorders**, and the **Token Test**. The use of these (and other) tools is reviewed by Lezak.[3825]

Aphasia Language Performance Scale A formalized, portable interview technique for assessing a patient's skills in listening, talking, reading, and writing.

aphasia quotient The relationship of fluency, information, comprehension, repetition, and naming scores on the **Western Aphasia Battery** to the hypothetical normal score of 100, as a measure of the severity of language impairment.[3407]

Aphasia Screening Test A popular instrument for the assessment, classification, and grading of language dysfunction and some nonlanguage communications skills.[2711] The test is included within the **Halstead-Reitan Test Battery**.

The following truncated version is suggested as a tool for distinguishing between right and left hemisphere damage.[2843]

1. Copy a square, a Greek cross, and a triangle without lifting the pencil from the paper.
2. Name each copied figure.
3. Spell each name.
4. Repeat "He shouted the warning" and then explain and write it down.

Patients with left hemisphere lesions may be able to copy the designs but not to write, but those with right hemisphere lesions will be able to write but may not manage to reproduce the designs.[3825] The test differentiates between patients with right and with left hemisphere lesions, but it should not be relied upon to do more than that.

aphasic acalculia See **acalculia**.

aphasic agraphia See **agraphia**.

aphasic perseveration therapy A method of reducing aphasic errors by encouraging speech free from that **perseveration** which is considered to be an integral component of aphasic symptoms.[2848]

aphasic seizures Those focal seizures that impair speech production or comprehension when the dominant hemisphere is involved.

aphasiology A study of the phenomena of central disorders of language.[1336]

Aphasiology A specialist professional journal. Web site: http://www.tandf.co.uk/journals/pp/02687038.html.

aphemia 1. (pure word dumbness; cortical dumbness; cortical anarthria; simple aphasia; subcortical motor aphasia; ataxic aphasia; severe apraxia of speech) A nonfluent aphasia characterized by a disturbance of oral verbal output, in which spoken language is poorly articulated, slow, and effortful, and repetition is impaired. Comprehension, word choice, grammar, syntax, and writing are not affected. See **logopenia**.

The syndrome commonly evolves from an initial state of right hemiparesis and mutism. The underlying lesion interrupts the path from Broca's area to the motor area.[521]

The word was originally selected by **Broca** to indicate loss of articulate speech due to a cerebral lesion, the motor and sensory functions remaining unaffected, but it was rejected by **Trousseau** in 1864 because a literal translation from modern Greek is *infamy*, which seems inappropriate.

Bastian thought that, in aphasia, the area for kinesthetic images for words was destroyed and thinking was thus disturbed; in aphemia, he considered the lesion to be of the motor paths linking this area with the muscles of articulation so that intellectual functions remained. The lesion is now considered to be restricted within Broca's area or in the subjacent cortex.[4431] See also **aphasia**, **foreign accent syndrome**, **diplegia with dissociation**, **oralbuccal apraxia**.

2. Selective loss of volitional (as opposed to emotional) movements, as in the case of the facial muscles in the **anterior opercular syndrome**.[5598]

apheresis (Gr, to take away) (plasmapheresis) The term used for the separation of the constituents of blood by centrifugation, after which the protein fractions containing the antibodies responsible for the pathology can be removed and the remainder of the blood, with added albumin, replaced.

aphonia (Gr, negative + the voice) 1. The inability to produce vocal sounds or phonate. 2. Loss of the power of intonation, although articulation is preserved (obsolete).

aphonia clericorum Loss of speech due to laryngitis, from excessive use of the voice.

aphrasia (Gr, negative + to speak) Broca's term for **aphasia**.

aphthongia (Gr, negative + a clear sound) A peculiar affection described by Fleury, allied to stuttering, in which an attempt to speak brings on spasm of the tongue and of the muscles attached to the hyoid bone[2531] and representing dysarthria due to orofacial dystonia with spasm of the hypoglossus. The condition has certain similarities to **writer's cramp**.

aplestia (acoria) Inability to attain satiety after eating.

apnea (Gr, negative + to breathe) Cessation of the ventilatory airflow for at least 10 s.

apnea index The number of periods of apnea occurring in the course of 1 h of sleep, recorded by **polysomnography**. The normal number is 5 or less.

apnea test A necessary test in **brain death** protocols. The comatose patient is ventilated with pure oxygen (or oxygen with CO_2) for 10 min. After which, ventilation is terminated but a passive flow of oxygen is maintained for 10 min. Spontaneous ventilatory efforts stimulated by a rise in $PaCO_2$ over 60 mmHg indicate retention of some brainstem function.

apneic spells Cessation of airflow at the nose and mouth lasting longer than 10 s. See **sleep apnea**.

apneic threshold The partial pressure of arterial CO_2 below which respiratory motor output is so inhibited that the normal breathing rhythm is significantly disrupted; a pathophysiological mechanism involved in sleep apnea.[1574]

apneusis See **apneustic breathing**.

apneustic breathing (Gr, lack of + to breathe) A respiratory pattern in which the usual pause taken at the end of expiration is replaced by one at the end of inspiration. Pauses at the end of inspiration lasting 2 or 3 s may alternate with pauses at the end of expiration and reflect damage to the respiratory control mechanisms in the mid- or caudal pons. Apneustic breathing is therefore a late sign of rostrocaudal deterioration. In comatose patients, this pattern of respiration has serious significance because the probable cause is a lesion low in the pons.

apneustic center A site in the caudal pons adjacent to the trigeminal motor nucleus, damage to which may lead to apneustic breathing.

apoceruloplasmin deficiency A recessively inherited syndrome characterized by adult-onset blepharospasm with facial dystonia, high-density basal ganglion lesions on CT scans, low serum copper and ceruloplasmin levels (but no **Kayser–Fleischer rings**), low serum apoceruloplasmin and intestinal copper absorption, but increased liver uptake of copper.[4413]

apo-E A plasma glycoprotein involved in lipid metabolism, with three variants (apo-E2, E3, and E4). The E4 allele is associated with decreased longevity, raised plasma cholesterol, and **Alzheimer disease** with β-amyloid and tangle pathology.

apogeotropic nystagmus See **vestibular nystagmus**.

apomorphine test The assessment of motor functions such as tapping and walking before and repetitively after a subcutaneous injection of apomorphine, a dopamine receptor. Doses are increased from 1 up to 10 mg until either a positive response occurs or intolerance develops. The test is considered to predict responsiveness to levadopa administration in Parkinsonian syndromes and may differentiate idiopathic Lewy body **Parkinson disease** from **parkinsonism-plus** syndromes such as multisystem atrophy and cerebellar atrophy.[1407]

aponeurotic ptosis Drooping of the upper lid in association with lengthening or disease of the aponeurosis. The muscle function is normal but the upper lid is seen to be thinned above the tarsal plate.[1524]

apoplexy (Gr, a violent striking down) A sudden, sometimes catastrophic event such as a stroke, or hemorrhage into an organ, usually the brain. In Hippocratic writings, the word was also used for paralysis of part of the body occurring as a result of a stroke.[1191] The term was also used by Areteus and Galen and can be found in Chaucer's work; the meaning was a paralysis of *all* the body with loss of sensation, motion, and understanding ("a total deprivation of sense and motion, excepting that of respiration, which is performed with difficulty, and snoring.") while for partial paralyses the term *palsy* was used. Johann **Wepfer** (1620–1695) demonstrated in 1658 that hemorrhage into the brain was the cause[5619] and Marshall **Hall** agreed. **Abercrombie** differentiated three forms, corresponding to subarachnoid hemorrhage, left middle cerebral artery occlusion, and intracerebral bleeding. The term *pontine apoplexy* was used from 1845 for primary intrapontine hemorrhage and *cerebellar apoplexy*, similarly.

The word is also used today for acute events affecting the labyrinth or the pituitary. The former is typically due to occlusion of the artery of the internal auditory meatus, the latter is a life-threatening condition in which pituitary infarction leads to the acute onset of ophthalmoplegia with bilateral amaurosis, drowsiness, or coma; subarachnoid hemorrhage, CSF pleocytosis, and increased protein are also usually associated.

apoptosis A gene-directed process of programmed cell death characterized by raised levels of cytosolic calcium in the dying cells, triggering digesting endonuclease activity without inflammatory changes. The process is normal in the embryo and in healthy adult tissues, and in the latter case, it leads to the disposal of neutrophils and the elimination of self-reactive T-cell clones.[125, 5266] Prevention of apoptosis is a therapeutic option in ischemic and traumatic brain disease.[11]

apparent/real nystagmus see **stepping-around nystagmus**.

apperception Sensation accompanied by comprehension of what is perceived.

apperceptive agnosia An inability to recognize objects in the absence of a primary visual sensory deficit seen in patients with lesions of the right hemisphere. Lissauer considered that visual perception began with a stage of conscious awareness of a sensory impression (apperception) followed by a stage in which associating semantic ideas added meaning.[3868]

appetite An emotion requiring the satisfaction of a perceived need.

applause sign See **three clap test**.

approach–avoidance equilibrium A state of immobility in which a stimulus to act is balanced by a countervailing disincentive.

apractagnosia (minor hemisphere syndrome) Unawareness of the significance of painful sensations, disturbances of the body schema, denial of contralateral hemiparesis, lack of spontaneous movement of the contralateral side, dressing apraxia, **asymbolia for pain**, and loss of visuospatial functions and orientation due to lesions of the minor (effectively, the right) hemisphere.[2826] The term is not specific, since it encompasses too many separate symptoms, and is thus seldom employed now. See also **anosognosia, constructional apraxia**.

apractagnosia for spatial orientation See **visuospatial agnosia**.

aprataxin (*APTX*) A nuclear protein with a potential role in DNA repair; the causative protein for EAOH.

apraxia 1. An inability to use body parts successfully. 2. An inability to carry out learned skilled, purposeful movements to command or in imitation, despite intact motor and sensory systems, good comprehension, normal volition and cognition, and full cooperation. The subject thus cannot produce the correct movement in response to a verbal command, nor imitate correctly a movement performed by the examiner, nor perform a movement correctly in response to a scene or object, nor handle an object correctly. 3. The loss of those mental faculties required to guide or execute purposeful movements, not explained by elementary motor or sensory deficits, impairment of perception or comprehension, or severe mental deterioration.

The first definition (of Nathan) is appropriate when apraxias occur as a result of a lesion of the motor system, as in the case of apraxic dysarthria in the **anterior opercular syndrome**. Geschwind suggested[2338] that apraxias result from disconnections of the posterior speech area from the association areas lying anterior to the primary motor cortex, and from disconnections of the visual association areas from these "motor association areas." Sparing of whole-body movements is not uncommon in such cases, perhaps because of preservation of the **Bundle of Turck**.

The definition of apraxia specifies that the disturbance of performed skilled movements cannot be explained by the motor impairments experienced by patients with movement disorders. Bradykinesia and dystonia compromise the ability to establish the presence of loss of dexterity and deftness that constitutes limb-kinetic apraxia.[6943]

Standard tests for apraxia include the imitation of gestures, with or without meaning; pantomime of the use of imagined objects; tests of orobuccal movements; and a sequencing task such as the **fist-palm-side test**.[3449]

The recognition of apraxia and its first classification were the work of Hugo Carl Liepmann (1863–1925), a German neurologist, in 1900; he described three varieties[3845] but further subgroups are defined today:

1. *Ideomotor apraxia* (motor apraxia) The inability to perform a motor act on command which can be performed spontaneously, so that the implementation of the gesture in a precise motor program is disrupted. In right-handed subjects, it is associated with lesions of the left hemisphere and thus is a common finding in patients with aphasia. Further subcategories include *sympathetic dyspraxia*; the failure of a patient with Broca's aphasia to perform actions to command with the left hand; *parietal apraxia* resulting from damage to the arcuate fasciculus; *callosal apraxia*, an inability of the patient to perform an action with one hand while he can do so with the other, as in cases of anterior lesions of the corpus callosum; and *anterior* or *frontal apraxia*, in which the subject fails in the performance of tasks requiring bimanual interaction, because of a lesion of the left supplementary motor area.[842]
2. *Ideational apraxia* (conceptual apraxia) The inability to perform the coordinated sequence of actions that constitute a goal-directed activity despite the patient's ability to perform the individual components of the actions in isolation; or the inability to select and use objects as a result of disruption of the normal integration of systems subserving the functional knowledge of actions and those involved in object knowledge.[3764]
3. *Limb-kinetic apraxia* Limb apraxia has been divided between forms because of a failure of a conceptual system (ideational apraxia, above) and impairment of the production of the movement—ideomotor or limb-kinetic apraxia—which is an entity of doubtful validity, the clumsiness that forms the basis for the condition probably being due to paresis.

Specific forms of apraxia (slightly modified here) have been defined by Koski et al. (2002)[3540]

Buccofacial apraxia Impairment in performing mouth or face actions on verbal command or imitation (see also **orofacial apraxia**).

Conceptual apraxia A form in which the concept of the action is lost; characterized by an impaired ability to solve tool/mechanical problems and also to understand meaningful gestures. The distinguishing feature of the deficit is the loss of tool–object associations, actions associated with tools, and the mechanical advantage of using tools. This deficit is more representative of a loss of knowledge of proper performance than loss of motor function.

Constructional apraxia Inability to assemble component parts into a coherent whole.

Ideational apraxia Impairment in the sequential use of multiple objects. Traditionally, the term has also been used to refer to impairment in conceptualizing an action. The term **conceptual apraxia** (see above) was coined to distinguish between these two dissociable impairments which are easily confused. Ideational apraxia is characterized as a failure to sequence task elements correctly—conceptual problems are not the main issue. The distinguishing factor is that patients can convey knowledge of how to perform a sequence task (e.g., making a ham sandwich), but they fail to order the elements of the task properly and so omit steps or do them out of order.

Ideomotor apraxia A disorder commonly seen in patients with stroke involving the left hemisphere. It is characterized by deficits in properly performing tool-use pantomimes (e.g., pretending to use a hammer) and communicative gestures (e.g., waving goodbye). These deficits are typically identified with movements made to verbal command or imitation. It is also present in conditions such as **corticobasal degeneration** (CBD), **Parkinson disease, Alzheimer disease, progressive supranuclear palsy**, and **Huntington disease**.[6742]

Limb apraxia The term used to refer to ideomotor apraxia of the limbs. It frequently includes impaired performance of actions that also depend on the hands and fingers.

Limb-kinetic apraxia Slowness and stiffness of movements with a loss of fine and precise movements. Limb-kinetic apraxia involves deficits mainly in fine and precise finger movements, such as those used in picking up a small coin or paper clip. Grasping with the full hand may also be affected. It is a basic motor coordination deficit, not explainable by more elemental deficits implicating areas such as the cerebellum or corticospinal tract.[6742]

Optical apraxia Impairment in performing saccadic eye movements on command.

Orofacial apraxia Impairment in performing mouth or face actions on verbal command or imitation (see also *buccofacial apraxia*).

Speech apraxia A selective impairment in the ability to produce speech sounds.

Tactile apraxia Impairment of hand movements for the use of, and interaction with, an object; a selective disturbance of active touch. Hand skills not related to object exploration and manipulation remain intact. The disturbance is not specific for tool use, but affects any use of the hand as a sense organ.

Unimodal apraxia Any form of apraxia that is specific to actions demonstrated in a single modality, e.g., visual but not auditory.

Verbal–motor dissociation apraxia (disassociation apraxia) A condition in which, patients fail to respond to verbal commands to make movements. This disorder may be more involved with speech processing than motor performance.

Based upon Wheaton[6742] and Koski L, et al. Deconstructing stroke: understanding disorders of intentional movement after stroke. *Curr Opin Neurol Neurosurg* 2002;15:71.

The term *apraxia* has also been applied to other motor disturbances, such as gait apraxia and apraxia of eyelid opening but probably incorrectly. See **Bruns gait apraxia, lid apraxia, apraxia of eyelid opening, dressing apraxia, Luria-Nebraska battery** and also the following entries.

apraxia for dressing See **dressing apraxia**.

apraxia of eyelid closure

(compulsive lid opening) The inability of awake patients to initiate or sustain lid closure voluntarily in the presence of intact reflex lid closure due to bilateral hemispheric damage.[3353]

apraxia of eyelid opening

(blepharocolysis, eyelid apraxia, focal eyelid dystonia, eyelid freezing, involuntary levator inhibition) A supranuclear disorder manifested by an inability of the alert subject to open the closed lids at will, in the absence of **ptosis** from any cause, of failed language comprehension, and of **blepharospasm**.

The responsible lesion may be in the right hemisphere, in both, or in the basal ganglia; and is due to inhibition of normal tonic activity in the levator muscle.[3240, 3359] It may be an accompaniment of such basal ganglion syndromes as **Parkinson** or **Wilson disease**,[1620, 228] sometimes with sustained contraction of the orbicularis oculi with or without failure of levator palpebrae inhibition.

apraxia of gait See **apraxic gait**, **Bruns gait apraxia**.

apraxia of gaze A supranuclear disorder characterized by a transient, atonic inability to move the eyes in the direction desired, or to scan a picture for features surrounding the central point, in the absence of evidence of a lower motor neuron lesion of the III, IV, or VI cranial nerves.

The condition is a feature of **progressive supranuclear palsy** and of various pyramidal syndromes of hemispheric origin and may occur in the **Balint syndrome**.

apraxia of speech Impairment of purposive speech with word-finding errors and paraphasias, while emotional or automatic speech is unaffected; as occurs with inferior frontal lesions in the dominant hemisphere.[1454]

apraxic agraphia An agraphic syndrome characterized by a selective disturbance of writing in the absence of any abnormality in letter or name selection, so that in the pure variety, spelling and reading are intact and there are no other disturbances of language function.[452] The causal lesion may be frontal, parietal, or thalamic.

apraxic dysarthria Inability to make purposeful speech sounds in the absence of **dysphasia**, as occurs in the **anterior opercular syndrome**.[4053]

apraxic gait (apractic gait, magnetic gait, Bruns gait apraxia) Inability to initiate the process of forward motion by alternating steps, although the power and coordination of the legs are normal in the lying and sitting positions. The maintenance of the feet on the floor, removed only with great effort, has led to the alternative name *magnetic gait*.

aprosencephaly See **cerebellar syndromes** (congenital ataxias).

aproscencephaly with Rieger-type eye anomalies A congenital syndrome characterized by anterior chamber abnormalities, adrenal hypoplasia, and aproscencephaly.[381]

aprosexia An abnormal inability to pay attention, often with a lack of interest in anything; similar to accedia, one of the seven deadly sins.

aprosodia (aprosody) Lack of **prosody** in speech, which thus loses the inflections that add meaning and emotional content so that patients talk as though the language used were foreign to them.

Prosody is an affective component of language, as is emotional gesturing, and is organized within the right hemisphere in a manner similar to left hemispheric language functions so that motor, sensory, global, transcortical, and conduction forms of aprosodia may be differentiated.[5418]

In *motor aprosodia* the lesion affects the right frontal and anterior parietal opercula and produces speech that is flat, devoid of emotional tone and unaccompanied by gestures. Repetition of affective prosody is impaired but its comprehension and the interpretation of emotional gesturing remain.

In *sensory aprosodia* emotional prosody in speech and active gesturing are normal but their visual and auditory comprehension is impaired, as is their repetition. The lesion is of the right posterior temporal and parietal opercula.

In *global aprosodia*, due to a large right perisylvian lesion, affect can neither be displayed nor comprehended. A left hemiparesis is also likely to be present.

Transcortical aprosodias resemble the motor, sensory, and global forms, except that repetition is preserved.

Impairment of both the production and comprehension of language components such as stress, pauses, cadences, accent, melody, and intonation that allow the translation of internal states is termed *affective aprosodia*.[1027]

aqueduct of Sylvius (cerebral aqueduct) The narrow passage between the third and fourth ventricles described by Franciscus de la Boe (**Sylvius**) in about 1650.

aqueduct syndrome See **syndrome of the mesencephalic gray matter**, **Sylvian aqueduct syndrome**.

aqueductal forking A developmental error in which representation of the aqueduct for part of its course is by two distinct channels in the sagittal plane, separated from each other by normal nervous tissue.[1708]

aqueductal stenosis Narrowing of the aqueduct of Sylvius in the absence of branching of the channel, gliosis, inflammation, or tumor; a cause of **noncommunicating hydrocephalus**.[1708] Acquired causes or congenital narrowing, forking or gliosis of the aqueduct, or the presence of a septum may be responsible.

arachnoid (Gr, resembling a spider's web) The word was used by Herophilus and later by Galen for any thin membrane. In neurology, it refers to the gossamer thin middle (but watertight) layer of the three meninges enclosing, with the pia mater, the CSF. Its anatomy was described in 1800 by Bichat.[5886]

arachnoid cysts (leptomeningeal cysts) A developmental abnormality consisting of benign, extra-parenchymal, nongenetic, slowly growing cysts composed of a thickened and fibrotic arachnoid membrane, usually situated over the lateral aspects of the hemispheres or within the spinal canal containing CSF. They are considered to represent splitting or duplication of the arachnoid membrane.

They usually arise within and expand the margins of CSF cisterns such as those of the Sylvian fissures and suprasellar and cerebellopontine regions. They have been blamed for cognitive impairment, seizures, developmental delay, headache, hydrocephalus, focal signs and raised intracranial pressure, but are most often asymptomatic. See also **porencephalic cyst**.[6736]

The Arachnoid Cyst Foundation An organization offering guides, support, therapies, diet, and personal stories about arachnoid cyst.

arachnoid diverticula (spinal arachnoid cyst; leptomeningeal cyst; intradural meningeal cyst; circumscribed serous spinal meningitis; localized adhesive spinal arachnoiditis; meningeal hydrops) Small diverticula in free communication with the subarachnoid space, arising from the septum posticum of Schwalbe (a sagittal membrane dividing the posterior spinal subarachnoid space) and occasionally causing pain, percussion tenderness, and myelopathic signs in erect adult subjects.[3427]

arachnoid granulations Normally, small outpouchings of arachnoid projecting into the dural venous sinuses to allow the transfer of CSF and some of its contents. *Giant arachnoid granulations* may cause a syndrome mimicking dural **sinus thrombosis**.

Aran disease See **amyotrophic lateral sclerosis**.

Aran, Francois-Amilcar (1817–1861) French physician who was born in Bordeaux but who was trained and worked in Paris. He was mainly interested in cardiology but described progressive muscular atrophy (**amyotrophic lateral sclerosis**) in 1850, a year after **Duchenne** (whose work he acknowledged) but 3 years before Cruveilhier (whose name is also sometimes attached to the syndrome).

Aran–Duchenne disease See **amyotrophic lateral sclerosis**.

arbovirus encephalitis Direct viral infections of the brain due to RNA viruses of the togavirus, bunyaviruses, or reoviruses class. Most are zoonoses of birds or lower vertebrates and are transmitted through an arthropod vector, such as mosquitoes or ticks. The *togavirus* diseases include Eastern, Western, Venezuelan, and Semlicki forest encephalitis. St. Louis, Japanese, Murray Valley, West Nile, Ilheus, Russian, Spring Summer, Central European encephalitis, and Louping ill and Powassan encephalitis are also produced by *flaviviruses* of the togavirus group. *Bunyavirus*-caused encephalitides are those of the California encephalitis group. *Reoviruses* include Colorado tick-borne encephalitis and Bhanja.[6858] See also the CDC Web site: http://www.cdc.gov/DiseasesConditions/az/E.html.

arcade of Frohse A fibrous tunnel at the origin of the supinator muscle, under which runs the posterior interosseous nerve as it enters the forearm. Hence, this is a place where that nerve may be entrapped.

arceau rhythm See **mu rhythm**.

archenteric cyst See **neurenteric cyst**.

Archimedes spiral Fine motor coordination may be assessed by getting the subject to draw a two-dimensional spiral figure from the center outwards. Tremor, athetosis, and other involuntary movement disorders and also pyramidal lesions may disturb the smooth execution of the drawing.

architectonics The microscopical study of the appearances of cells and fibers in the cerebral cortex, leading to the definition of morphologically distinct areas. The major work was done by **Korbimian Brodmann**, **von Economo**, and the **Vogts**.

Archives de Neurologie A neurological journal founded by **Charcot** in 1880 and edited by him until his death in 1893.

Archives of Neurology (*Arch Neurol*) An American neurological journal founded in 1959 with Harold **Wolff** as the first chief editor. It was sponsored by the American Neurological Association and published by the American Medical Association, taking over from the **Archives of Neurology and Psychiatry**. The American Neurological Association later adopted the newly formed **Annals of Neurology** as its official organ. Web sites: http://archneur.amaassn.org/. Archives of Neurology Homepage.

Archives of Neurology and Psychiatry A professional journal founded in 1918 with Weisenburg as editor, to provide a vehicle for neurological papers that were not then finding adequate space in the *Journal of Nervous and Mental Diseases*.

ARCO A childhood mitochondriopathy manifesting sensory neuropathy, dysarthria, and ophthalmoparesis.

arctic hysteria (Myriatchit) See **Latah**.

arcuate fasciculus (Lat, bowed + a bundle) A cerebral fiber pathway originating in the cortex of the supratemporal plane, arching posteriorly around the Sylvian fissure, and running in the superior longitudinal fasciculus across the insula to the lower frontal region. This and the local auditory cortex, insula, and supramarginal gyrus are the structures damaged in patients with **conduction aphasia**, in which the faculty of word repetition is especially affected.[1435]

arcuate scotoma A visual field defect described first by **Bjerrum**.[663] It has a curved shape, skirting the central fixation spot, and is due to segmental (compressive) lesions of the optic nerve fibers running from the temporal retina both above and below the maculopapillar bundle.

area postrema A region in the floor of the fourth ventricle where the blood-brain barrier is deficient.

areflexia without pupillary changes A benign and nonprogressive anomaly of unknown cause.[6466] See also **Holmes–Adie syndrome**.

areflexic syncope (syndrome) See **paralytic postural syncope**.

Aretaeus of Cappadocia (81–138 AD) Arabian physician who described complex partial seizures (in a patient with a depressed skull fracture) and gave a full account of the different forms of **aura**. Noting the contralateral signs, he postulated decussation of the motor pathways in the brain. He also introduced the terms ***paraplegia*** (localized loss of touch and movement), ***paresis*** (loss of motor power only), and ***apoplexy*** (a generalized loss of movement, sensation, and understanding).

arginase deficiency (argininemia) A very rare, recessively inherited hyperammonemic syndrome presenting as a diffuse encephalopathy in infancy or childhood, with the added features of microcephaly, developmental delay, seizures, spasticity, ataxia, chorea, athetosis, opisthotonos, persistent vomiting, and intolerance of protein feeds.[5936] Argininemia, arginemia, and aminoaciduria are other characteristic laboratory findings.[2754]

argininemia See **arginase deficiency**.

argininosuccinase deficiency (Allen-Dent syndrome; citrullinemia) A rare, usually recessively inherited hyperammonemic disorder presenting in childhood with toe-walking, vomiting, lethargy, and failure to thrive, usually followed in 6–12 months by progressive developmental delay, seizures, abnormal involuntary movements, ataxia, paraparesis, friability of the hair, attention-deficit/hyperactivity disorder, hepatomegaly, and persistent vomiting. A few patients with nearly normal development have been reported.[127] Plasma citrulline levels are markedly raised.

argininosuccinic aciduria A rare, recessive hyperammonemic syndrome due to deficiency of arginosuccinate lysase. The abnormal gene is located on chromosome 7 (7cen–q11.2).

The condition presents clinically with lethargy, seizures, and coma in newborn children who have sparse, brittle, and coarse hair. Failure to thrive, seizures, hepatosplenomegaly, jaundice, and mental retardation are the usual presenting features in infancy; and seizures, ataxia and psychomotor retardation, often with episodic vomiting and hypotonia, in childhood. Aminoacidemia, moderate citrullinemia, and hyperammonemia are noted at all ages.[1065]

Argyll Robertson, Douglas Moray Cooper Lamb (1837–1909) Scottish ophthalmologist who was trained in Edinburgh, St. Andrews, and Berlin. After his studies abroad, he returned to Edinburgh and eventually became president of the Royal College of Surgeons in that city. He gave credit to the German neurologist **Remak** for first showing him the pupillary abnormality which now bears his own name.

Argyll Robertson pupils Pupils that are small, irregular, unequal, and hardly reactive to light, though quite reactive to accommodation.

Described in 1869, the lesion is of the pathways between the pretectal region of the midbrain and the Edinger–Westphal nucleus. Syphilis is the classic etiology, but other mesencephalic lesions and diabetes may also be responsible. The inequality and irregularity of the spastic pupils are not explained by the known neurological defects;[5329] possibly syphilitic iritis producing local scarring is the immediate cause.[239]

argyrophilic grain disease A sporadic neurodegenerative disease of old age (a tauopathy) in which silver-staining fibrils derived from dendrites are detected throughout the cortex, rather than the usual plaques and tangles of **Alzheimer disease**, which this condition otherwise resembles closely.[3107] It accounts for about 5% of all cases of dementia. Clinical symptoms largely depend on the extension of the grains together with the very common associated tauopathies, such as **Alzheimer disease, progressive supranuclear palsy, corticobasal degeneration**, and the **synucleinopathies**.[2030]

arhinencephaly A congenital malformation in which the olfactory pathway is absent. It is neither a morphological nor a single etiological entity, since numerous associated malformations of the eyes, pyramidal pathways, cerebellum and dentato-olivary complex, craniofacial dysmorphisms, and cardiac, renal, and endocrine disorders are variously described in association.[3508] See also **olfactory dysgenesis, holoprosencephaly**.

Arieti-Gray syndrome See **Sturge–Weber syndrome**.

arm-diaphragm synkinesis Arm movements occurring in time with respiratory movements, as a result of aberrant regeneration of phrenic nerve fibers following brachial plexus or cervical root lesions.[6166]

arm drop A test for functional weakness, only occasionally of value, in which the supine patient's arm is raised above the face and then let go; in functional disorders the arm is likely to fall away from the face but with *complete* "organic" weakness, it should drop right onto the face.

arm-dropping test See **Bekhterev signs**, No. 9.

arm recoil The arms of the supine infant are first flexed maximally and then extended; in the normal mature infant the arms return to the fully flexed position.

Armendares syndrome An X-linked recessive or autosomal recessive syndrome characterized by microcephaly with cranial asymmetry, craniosynostosis, small face, microcephaly, high-arched palate, ptosis, pigmentary retinopathy, short stature, delayed skeletal maturation, short fifth fingers, and simian creases of the hand.[245] See also **craniosynostosis**.

Arnold, Friedrich (1803–1890) German anatomist who in 1838 made precise differentiation between the frontal, parietal, occipital, and temporosphenoidal lobes. He also described the frontopontine tract, the arcuate nuclei, the otic ganglion, and the auricular branch of the vagus nerve and its canal.

Arnold, Julius (1835–1915) Heidelberg physician (the son of Friedrich) who described **superior laryngeal neuralgia**[3113] and the **Chiari malformation** (in 1894, 3 years after Chiari).

Arnold–Chiari malformation See **Chiari malformation**.

Arnold syndrome See **superior laryngeal neuralgia**.

Arnold's nerve cough Coughing with stabbing pain felt in the suboccipital region, thought to be due to irritation of the auricular branch of the vagus nerve.[96]

aromatic L-amino acid decarboxylase deficiency A rare recessively inherited inborn error of metabolism in which absence of this enzyme prevents the synthesis of normal amounts of catecholamines and of serotonin.

Clinically, the disorder is characterized by oculogyric crises and extreme axial hypotonia, with hypokinesia and athetosis. Ptosis, sweating, lability of blood pressure and temperature, and nasal congestion witness the catecholamine deficiency. Abnormal sleep, feeding difficulties, and esophageal reflux are other features. A response to monoamine oxidase A inhibitors and to dopamine agonists is reported.[3067]

arousal 1. An abrupt change from a deeper to a lighter stage of nonrapid eye movement sleep or from rapid eye movement sleep to the awake state.[280] 2. A period of at least 1.5 s in which there is increased EMG activity in association with a return of desynchronization of the EEG during sleep.

arousal disorders Parasomnias occurring in the first third of nocturnal sleep during stages 3 or 4 of NREM sleep, when the subject is unrousable. A spectrum of behaviors is identified, increasing in severity from face rubbing, chewing and mumbling through sleeptalking, sitting up in bed, sleepwalking, thrashing about in bed, night terrors, and panic attacks. See **parasomnias, confusional arousals, sleepwalking, sleep terrors**.

array A regular arrangement of electrodes over the scalp or brain or within the brain substance.

arrhythmic activity A sequence of waves of inconstant period. Cf. **rhythm**.

arrhythmokinesis Disturbances in rapid alternating ballistic movements in patients with cerebellar dysfunction.[6733]

arrow sign A finding on CT scans due to blood in the Sylvian fissure, typically as a result of seepage between the insula and the frontal and temporal opercula of the sylvian cistern near the MCA trifurcation.[4055]

Arroyo sign Sluggishness of the pupillary light reaction in hypoadrenalism.[5333]

arsenic neuropathy The neurological features of arsenic poisoning resemble those of lead neuropathy but with added cramps and muscle tenderness.

arterial gas embolism Air embolism occurring typically when a diver ascends (decompresses) without exhaling, as a result of which the expanding air in the respiratory passages expands and causes alveolar rupture, the air entering the systemic circulation.

Pain, respiratory distress, and cerebral and brainstem signs are the usual sequelae.[2571]

arterial stationary wave An angiographic appearance resembling ringed constrictions, described in the distal part of the internal carotid artery in Tolosa–Hunt syndrome (**superior orbital fissure syndrome**).

arteriography The depiction of the lumen of the larger arteries by X-rays, the artery having been injected with a radio-opaque medium. The technique was introduced by Egas Moniz (1874–1955).[1815]

arteriosclerotic Parkinsonism See **frontal gait disorder, isolated gait ignition failure**.

arteriosclerotic rigidity (akinetic rigidity; hypertonia of opposition; paratonia) The expression employed by Macdonald Critchley for increased muscular resistance to passive stretch, made worse by instructions given to the patient to relax. It thus resembles **paratonia**.

arteriovenous fistula Any connection between an artery and a vein allowing arterial blood to flow into the venous system directly without interposed capillaries. See **spinal dural arteriovenous fistula**.

arteriovenous malformation (AVM) (tumor circoidius; racemose aneurysm; racemose angioma; angiomatous malformation) An uncommon congenital vascular malformation (**angioma**) in which gliotic neural tissue is present between the vascular elements. It is due to an arrest in development that results in the formation of direct artery-to-vein communications of any size from cryptic to tumorous, without an intervening capillary bed. The condition is usually sporadic but may be familial.

The lesion evolves during life with increased blood flow and attenuation of distended venous channels, leading to clinical manifestations usually after the second decade. Hemorrhage, ischemia resulting from steal of arterial blood, irritation of the underlying brain, and local brain atrophy may be responsible for the clinical manifestations which include intracerebral or subarachnoid bleeding, seizures, focal signs, headache, bruits, and even cardiac failure in patients with large-volume shunts through the malformation.[4989, 6030, 3561]

See also **angioma, cerebral blood vessel hamartoma, aneurysm of the vein of Galen, capillary telangiectasia, cavernous angioma, venous malformations**. A grading system for all forms of AVM has been suggested.[5974]

A *variant* is *spinal avm, epidermal nevus, and rhabdomyosarcoma*.[5661]

Arteriovenous Malformation Grading Scale A prognostic tool based on the size of the AVM, the eloquence of the adjacent brain, and the pattern of venous drainage.[4120]

arteriovenous malformations with cavernous hemangiomas A dominantly inherited syndrome of **cerebral blood vessel hamartoma** in which both of these abnormalities occur, without skin or retinal lesions.[3585]

arteritis Inflammatory disease of the arterial walls. See **giant-cell arteritis**.

artery of migraine The posterior cerebral artery,[2096] so called because of the close association between migraine and visual disturbances.

artery of Percheron A perforating artery branching from the precommunal part of the posterior cerebral artery and supplying the upper paramedian midbrain and thalamus.

arthrogryposis (Gr, joint + to become bent) Congenital ankylosis of more than one joint. A condition of fixation of joints due to contractures in local tissues, occurring either in isolation or in association with neural or muscular diseases in childhood (see **arthrogryposis multiplex congenita**).

Arthrogryposis Association A charitable organization. Address: 106 Herkheimer St., Northville, NY 11710.

arthrogryposis multiplex congenita (AMC) (multiple congenital articular rigidities; amyoplasia congenita; Guerin–Stern disease; myodystrophia fetalis deformans) A group of disorders of infants and children characterized by multiple fibrotic joint contractures appearing at or just after birth, leading to immobility of the limbs with fixation in certain postures due to contracture of the muscles.[2610] The spine and temporomandibular joints, however, are never affected.

Most cases are sporadic, and are neither neural nor myopathic in origin; presumably this form is not heritable and represents an intrauterine or developmental disorder of joints. However, AMC may be associated with either neuropathic or myopathic disease[372, 1703] and may be inherited either as a dominant or as a recessive characteristic. The syndrome was first described by Otto in 1841.

Congenital cerebral maldevelopments such as micropolygyria, heterotopias, dilated ventricles, absent corticospinal tracts, anterior cell degeneration, and facial nerve nuclear degeneration may accompany the joint disorder.[2978] Absence of abdominal muscles, myelocele, club feet, dislocation of hips and knees, congenital heart disease, and hernias are also described in association.

Major forms of AMC include:

Distal arthrogryposis (DA1) is a genetically heterogeneous but usually dominantly inherited syndrome characterized by clenched fists at birth, overlapping fingers, ulnar deviation and **camptodactyly**, foot deformities, and variable contractures of major joints.[3432]

Freeman–Sheldon syndrome (DA2A) presents with facial anomalies (e.g., small mouth, deep set eyes, micrognathia) and distal joint contractures. A milder form is known as DA2B. The abnormality is on chromosome 11.

Variant forms include the following:

1. *Arthrogryposis is dominantly inherited* but neither atrophy nor weakness is apparent.[1408]
2. The anterior horn cells of the spinal cord are affected, and there is liver disease with pigment overload and renal dysfunction. Death ensues within weeks or months.[4656]
3. Multiple articular rigidities and nodular protuberances of the anterior vertebral columns are present with an almost total absence of myelin and Schwann cells.[4972]
4. *Dominantly inherited lower motor neuron disorder with arthrogryposis* is a nonprogressive, congenital disorder restricted to the lower part of the body, with atrophy of spinal motor neurons and absence of muscle spindles.[3569] Expression of the gene is variable.[2128]
5. The *myopathic type* is characterized by the occurrence of arthrogryposis with a primary myopathic disorder, such as **congenital muscular dystrophy**.
6. *AMC* associated with pulmonary hypoplasia
7. Distal X-linked *AMC* also manifesting anterior horn cell disease
8. AMC accompanying a congenital neuropathy[2978]

See also **Kuskowim disease**.

arthrokinetic-induced nystagmus (Stransky nystagmus; somatosensory nystagmus) That form of nystagmus induced in darkness by passive movement of the arm or, if the subject sits inside a rotating drum, by feeling its inner surface with the hands. Build-up and decay are slow and the fast phase beats away from the arm that is moved.

articulated labials Those consonants (*B*, *P*, *M*, *W*) which depend for their utterance upon intact lip function. See also **modified labials**, **dentolabials**.

articulation The distinct utterance of vocal speech sounds.

artifact (artefact) 1. Any potential difference due to an extracerebral source recorded in EEG tracings. 2. Any modification of the EEG caused by extracerebral factors such as alterations of the media surrounding the brain, instrumental distortion or malfunction, and operational errors. (Adapted from the 1974 Report of the Committee on Terminology, IFCN[1117] with permission from Elsevier Science.) 3. Any symptom or physical sign which is unrelated to the pathology which induced the present consultation. 4. A voltage change generated by a biologic or nonbiologic source other than the ones of interest. The stimulus artifact (or shock artifact) represents cutaneous spread of stimulating current to the recording electrode and the delay in return to baseline which is dependent on the ability of filters to respond to high voltage. Stimulus artifacts may precede or overlap the activity of interest.

Movement artifact refers to a distortion in the trace due to movement of the recording electrodes.

artistic agnosia Inability to comprehend the nuances of an artistic production; an uncommon sign of right hemisphere disease. In a diluted but much more common form, this incapacity affects many otherwise normal people, both in the visual and auditory spheres.

ARX (Aristaless-related homebox gene) A developmental gene located at Xp22 which is associated with infantile spasms and such developmental problems as mental retardation, ambiguous genitalia, neonatal poikilothermia, callosal agenesis, dystonias, dysarthria, autism, and gait disturbance. See **Partington syndrome, West syndrome, X-linked mental retardation, X-linked infantile spasms, X-linked myoclonic epilepsy with generalized spasticity and intellectual disability,** and **X-linked lissencephaly** *with abnormal genitalia.*

arylsulfatase A family of enzymes coded on chromosome 22 responsible for cleaving the sulfatase ester from the galactose portion of the sulfatide molecule. Sulfatase A is deficient in **metachromatic leukodystrophy**. The B and C forms are also missing in the condition of **multiple sulfatase deficiency**.

ascending neuritis An inflammatory reaction in the peripheral nerves capable of progressing proximally and thereby leading to dysfunction of the CNS as hypothesized by **Charcot**. In the absence of supportive evidence, the hypothesis generates intestinal rather than cerebral sympathy.

Aschner cardiac phenomenon See **oculocardiac reflex**.

Aschner sign See **oculocardiac reflex**.

asemasia (Gr, lack of + to show by signs) Loss of the power of communication by language or by signs.

aseptic lymphocytic meningoencephalitis See **disseminated vasculomyelinopathy**.

aseptic meningitis (lymphocytic choriomeningitis) 1. A disease with acute onset characterized by meningeal signs, pleocytosis in the CSF (mainly mononuclear cells), and sterile CSF culture. 2. A benign lymphocytic meningitis due to an RNA virus, usually transmitted by mice, in which the cellular response is monocytic (lymphocytic) rather than granulocytic.

Clinically, a typical meningitic illness with headache, fever, photophobia, and nuchal rigidity follows a prodromal febrile, influenza-like illness after 4–7 days, and lasts for up to 4 weeks, with minor residua such as arthralgias and drowsiness being common over the next few months. In the acute stage, the CSF shows monocytic pleocytosis but glucose levels are normal and cultures are negative. Enteroviruses account for most viral causes. Herpes simplex, adenovirus, mumps, etc. may also be responsible.The term was first applied in 1920 by James Bourne Ayer (b. 1882), a Boston neurologist.[3373] A **chronic benign**

lymphocytic form of meningitis also occurs.[2986]

Diagnostic criteria for *headache attributed to lymphocytic meningitis* have been defined:

A. Diffuse headache fulfilling criterion D
B. Examination of CSF shows lymphocytic pleocytosis, mildly elevated protein and normal glucose in the absence of infectious organisms
C. Use of one of the following: ibuprofen, immunoglobulins, penicillin or trimethoprim, intrathecal injections, or insufflations
D. Headache resolves within 3 months after withdrawal of the offending substance

From the International Classification of Headache Disorders (Headache Classification Committee of the International Headache Society. *Cephalalgia* 2004;**24**[Suppl 1]) by kind permission of Dr. Jes Olesen, the International Headache Society and Wiley-Blackwell Publications.

ash leaf spots Hypomelanotic macules seen in the skin in over 80% of patients with tuberous sclerosis.

Ashworth scale A validated scale for assessing the severity of spasticity, initially designed for children with cerebral palsy when such an assessment is important.[274]

0. No increase in muscle tone
1. Slight increase in tone, giving a catch when the affected part is moved in flexion or extension, followed by minimal resistance throughout the remainder of the range of movement
2. More marked increase in tone through most of the range of movement, but the affected parts are easily moved
3. Considerable increase in tone, making passive movement difficult
4. Affected part rigid in flexion or extension.[720]

See also **Spasm score**.

asimultagnosia (extinction, sensory competition) Difficulty in perceiving the whole of the visual field at one time, or in appreciating the occurrence of simultaneously presented tactile or auditory stimuli on each side of the body. Those affected with the visual form see their field piecemeal and identify objects in parts of it only, thus failing to enumerate the number of objects (crosses, letters, etc.) written on a card, although those that they *do* perceive, they perceive normally. The condition is a feature of **Balint syndrome**.

asomatognosia 1. Lack of awareness of the deep sensations (joint position sense, deep pain, muscle sense) from part of the body, usually due to posterior column or peripheral nerve (thick-fiber) disease.
2. Inability to recognize a paretic limb as one's own. See **anosognosia**.

asomnia Pathologically persistent wakefulness. See **agrypnia**.

aspartate A dicarboxylic acid excitatory neurotransmitter.

aspartylglycosaminuria A rare, recessively inherited lysosomal storage disease producing diffuse encephalopathy and presenting as intellectual retardation from infancy, accompanied by skin photosensitivity; short neck and short stature; brachycephaly; facial dysmorphism; joint laxity; macroglossia; behavioral disturbances; pyramidal, retinal, and corneal abnormalities; glycoasparginuria; and aminoaciduria.

The biopsy of almost any tissue shows the presence of vacuoles in the cytoplasm. The responsible gene has been located at 4q24-qter.[5069, 6720]

Asperger syndrome (able autism) A minor form of autism first described in 1944 by Hans Asperger, an Austrian pediatrician, in which there are few if any problems with language and learning but many in the realm of social interaction. This pervasive developmental disorder is characterized by social impairments, restricted interests, and repetitive behaviors, though not associated with delay in language development. Subjects lack empathy, appear self-centered, and are only comfortable in predictable situations. They may not use appropriate loudness levels, may make socially unacceptable statements about the appearance of others (see **verbal dysdecorum**) or yawn widely as one talks to them, and may miss the nonliteral meaning of language and/or the suprasegmental intent of language communicated through prosodic rhythm and melody as opposed to the words said, as well as the nonverbal message. Many also demonstrate a kind of rigidity in thought and action, which presents as stereotyped, manneristic, or obsessional behavior. Other common features include pedantic styles of communication, gross motor clumsiness, poor motor skills, sensory oversensitivity, seizures, and sleep disturbance. Depression and anxiety are also common.

The overwhelming prevalence of both autism and Asperger syndrome in males suggests X-linked influences, but specific markers have not been identified, although it has been mapped to chromosome 3p21.

The American Psychiatric Association *DSM IV-TR* diagnostic guidelines[172] are similar to those for autistic disorder. They can be found at http://www.behavenet.com/capsules/disorders/dsm4TRclassification.htm/ See also **fragile-X syndrome** and the Web site http://www.ummed.edu/pub/o/ozbayrak/asperger.html/.

Asperger Syndrome Coalition of the U.S. A charitable organization in this field. Address: P.O. Box 351268, Jacksonville, FL 32235-1268. Tel: 866-427-7747. E-mail: info@asc-us.org. Web site: http://www.asc-us.org.

aspergillosis Infection with *Aspergillus fumigatus*, seldom affecting the nervous system, but occasionally causing cerebral abscess or basal meningitis. Hematogenous spread from pulmonary aspergillosis commonly causes an infectious cerebral vasculitis, especially involving the thalamoperforating and lenticulostriate arteries and leading to thalamic or basal nuclei lesions, or septic infarction of the brain. Non-neurologic features helpful in diagnosis are the presence of risk factors (major or prolonged neutropenia, hematologic malignancies, prolonged corticosteroid treatment, bone marrow or solid organ transplant, AIDS); persistent fever not responding to antibacterials; and respiratory signs.[6223]

Assessment of Quality of Movement for Unilateral Arm Function An arm assessment test for children with cerebral palsy.[3229]

associated movements 1. Tonic or postural reflex reactions (i.e., variations in muscle tone or attitude), typically appearing in hemiparetic limbs and characterized by long latency, constant form and slow development, and decline. Their adequate stimulus is the tonically maintained voluntary contraction of some other part of the skeletal musculature.[6622] 2. An involuntary association between the movements of paralyzed limbs and other parts of the body, thus a paralyzed arm may be adducted strongly during a yawn.[6300]

associated nystagmus See **induced nystagmus**.

Association Canadienne de l' Ataxie de Friedreich A Canadian charitable organization. Address: 5620 rue CA Jobin St., Montreal, PQ H1P 1H8, Canada.
Tel: 514-321-8684.

association cortex 1. Those parts of the cerebral cortex not recognized as having specific motor or sensory functions, although lesions of these regions lead to deficits in attention, sensation, language, and other higher cerebral functions.[1742]
2. Homotypical six-layered isocortex, some of which is modality-specific (*unimodal*) and some *heteromodal* (polymodal, multimodal, supramodal, polysensory, or high-order association cortex) in its response to differing kinds of stimulation.

The unimodal areas act as obligatory relays for the intracortical transfer of sensory information from the primary receptive areas to other parts of the cortex. The heteromodal areas allow intermodal association and have close relationships with limbic and paralimbic function. Lesions here give rise to complex, multimodality disorders such as **Gerstmann syndrome**, confusional states, or **Balint syndrome**.[4332]

Association for Alzheimer's Disease and Related Disorders A charitable organization. Address: 70 East Lake St., Chicago, IL 60601. Tel: 312-853-3060. Web site: http://www.alzhi.org/.

Association for Brain Tumor Research A national charitable organization providing free written information about brain tumors and treatment options, including facts about medical specialists, facilities, and support groups. The organization also funds medical research. Address: 208 South LaSalle St., Suite 1426, Chicago, IL 60604. Tel: 312-782-4311. Web site: http://www.abta.org/.

Association for Children and Adults with Learning Disabilities A charitable organization. Address: 4156 Library Rd., Pittsburgh, PA 15234. Tel: 412-881-2253.

Association for Neuro-Metabolic Disorders A charitable organization in this field. Address: c/o Cheryl Volk, 5223 Brookfield Lane, Sylvania, OH 43560. Tel: 419-885-1497. E-mail: VOLK4OLKS@aol.com.

Association for Persons with Severe Handicaps A charitable organization. Address: 7010 Roosevelt Way, NE, Seattle, WA 98115. Tel: 206-361-8870.

Association for Research in Nervous and Mental Disease A professional organization. Address: 1. Gustave Levy Pl., P.O. Box 1052, New York, NY 10029.

Association Française contre les Myopathies A charitable organization. Address. 13 Place de Rungis, 75013 Paris, France. Tel: 1-4565-1300.

Association of British Neurologists A professional society that represents clinical and academic neurologists in the United Kingdom. Address: Ormond House, 27. Boswell St., London WC1N 3JZ, UK. Web site: http://www.theabn.org/.

Association of Professional Sleep Disorders Clinics A grouping of the three major U.S. societies involved with clinical and research studies on sleep. Address: 604 Second St. SW, Rochester, MN 55902. Tel: 507-287-6006.

Association of Rehabilitation Nurses A professional organization. Address: 2506 Gross Point Rd., Evanston, IL 60201. Tel: 708-966-3433.

Association of Sleep Disorders Centers See **American Academy of Sleep Medicine**. Web site: http://www.aasmnet.org/.

Association of University Professors of Neurology A professional organization. Web site: www.aupn.org.

associative agnosia One of the two forms of agnosia differentiated by Lissauer (1891), the other being **apperceptive agnosia** (in which the perceptual mechanism is thought to be disturbed). Associative agnosia is a true defect of recognition caused by an impairment of the normal processing mechanisms of the associative cortex by which perceived stimuli are matched with previously encoded information to allow recognition. As a result, the perception is normal but it is stripped of its meaning; thus there is a loss of the ability to identify objects seen,[1105] so that while an object seen may be drawn accurately, the subject nevertheless does not recognize what it is.

associative visual agnosia without alexia A rare syndrome in which the subject is unable to appreciate the meaning of visually presented, nonverbal but meaningful stimuli, while perception of such stimuli through other channels is retained. A right hemianopia is usually present.

The condition represents the effect of both an interhemispheric visual–verbal disconnection and a specific categorization defect for visual, nonverbal meaningful stimuli.[107]

astasia–abasia The inability to maintain an upright posture, despite normal function of the legs in bed; usually a manifestation of hysteria. The opposite condition (legs paralyzed in bed but able to sustain gait) is also recognized.[684] The words mean "inability to stand and walk." It may be better to use the term *hysterical dysbasia* for the difficulty with gait and the term *stasibasiphobia* for the fear of standing or walking. In hysterical dysbasia there is often marked swaying from side to side, with superfluous movements; the patient may fall far to the side or to the front or back when walking but is usually able to regain balance without falling to the floor. If a fall does occur, it is in a theatrical manner but usually without injury. It can frequently be demonstrated in hysterical dysbasia that, although unable to walk forwards, the patient may be able to walk backwards or to one side or even to run without difficulty.

Charcot, in describing this as "a special variety of motor feebleness of the legs from want of coordination in relation to position in rest and progression," indicated that he regarded the condition as an ability to move the legs in the recumbent but not in the upright position. See also **Blocq syndrome**, **frontal disequilibrium**, and **subcortical disequilibrium**.

astasia trepidante (astasia trepidans) A peculiar fear of walking, occurring rarely in elderly people in whom no specific abnormalities can be found to explain their apprehension. Occasionally, they may be so fearful of walking that they will not take a step at all and "freeze"; when encouraged to step out, they may clutch onto things or drop to their knees. In many cases, **normal pressure hydrocephalus** is considered to be the cause, and in some cases it is.

The **Petren gait** is a dilute version of the same condition.

astatesthesia Inability to recognize the position of a limb in space.

astatic seizure (drop attack) A motor seizure causing loss of the erect posture that results from an atonic, myoclonic, or tonic mechanism.

astereognosis A failure of judgement regarding the spatial characteristics of a tactile stimulus, due to a lesion of the contralateral parietal cortex.

asterixis (negative myoclonus) Brief, irregular, and jerky movements resulting from the temporary loss of muscle stimulation during which muscle tone is lost from an extended limb. This leads to momentary dropping of all or part of it (lapses in posture),[6931] or to a tremor when the interruptions in innervation last <200 ms. When bilateral, asterixis is the result of metabolic or toxic diseases, such as renal or hepatic failure; when unilateral, lesions of the opposite hemisphere or of the midbrain or brainstem on either side are responsible.[5246] Truncal asterixis is also described.

asteroid hyalitis Deposition of calcium compounds in the vitreous humor as a result of trauma or in the elderly.

asthenia (Gr, lack of + strength) 1. A languid, fragile, and vulnerable constitutional tendency, leaving the subject prone to complaints but without diagnosable disease. 2. Generalized weakness or disinclination to attempt muscular activity. 3. Early subjective fatigue preventing the continuation of motor activity without clinical or laboratory-demonstrated weakness.[2692] See also **fatigue**.

asthenia crurum dolorosa (paresthetica) See **Ekbom syndrome**.

asthenia of upward gaze Progressive ptosis with descent of the globe after the maintenance of upward gaze for a minute or so; a sign of end-plate fatigue in **myasthenia gravis**.

asthenic bulbar paralysis See **myasthenia gravis**.

asthenic ophthalmoplegia Ocular **myasthenia gravis**.

asthenopia (Gr, lack of + strength + eye) 1. (accomodative asthenopia) Frontal headache, fatigue, and failure of continued accommodation (leading to complaints of blurred or indistinct vision) and of concentration, occurring in some subjects after prolonged close work. 2. A similar phenomenon occurs during the later stages of recovery from cortical blindness.

asthmatic amyotrophy See **Hopkins syndrome**.

astigmatism (Gr, lack of + a point) A defect of the refractive media of the eye in which parallel rays of light arising from a single source are not brought to a common point on the retina, usually due to differences in the curvature of the cornea at different places.[2636]

astonagaza See **dancing mania**.

astroblastoma See **astrocytoma**.

astrocyte (Gr, star + cell) A glial cell in the CNS. *Gemistocyctic* astrocytes (goose-fat cells), plump reactive astrocytes found abundantly in areas of demyelination, and *protoplasmic* astrocytes (now type I) found largely in gray matter, were the two forms differentiated by Ramon y **Cajal** in 1881. *Fibrous* astrocytes (spider cells) are abundant in white matter and in the optic nerve.

astrocytoma A slowly growing primary neuroectodermal tumor of the cerebrum, cerebellum, or spinal cord composed of astrocytic cells with fine fibrillary processes and indistinct cell borders in well-differentiated types and lacking both collagen and reticulin fibers. Glial fibrillary acidic protein is present in most astrocytoma cells.

On the basis of their distribution, histology, and predominant cell type, the following forms are recognized:

- *Fibrillary* (diffuse) The commonest (90%) form of astrocytoma, occurring particularly in the cerebral hemispheres of adults or in the pons in children. The tumor is graded[5315] between astrocytoma, malignant (anaplastic) astrocytoma, and glioblastoma multiforme (in which malignant change is seen in discrete areas of previously well-differentiated astrocytomas arising in the cerebral hemispheres of adults).[6]
- *Pilocytic* Relatively slowly growing fibrillary astrocytic tumors occurring particularly in the cerebellum, hypothalamus, optic nerve and chiasm, and the brainstem in children. The tumors are characterized by the elongation of some of their constituent cells lying in parallel rows and by the presence of **Rosenthal fibers**.

Less common forms include the following:

- *Subependymal giant-cell astrocytomas* Calcified astrocytomas found in the thalamus and periventricular regions in some patients with **tuberous sclerosis**
- *Protoplasmic astrocytomas* Tumors containing stellate cells with fine processes and minimal neuroglial fibers
- *Gemistocytic astrocytomas* Tumors containing plump cells with eosinophilic cytoplasm displacing the nucleus peripherally
- *Pleomorphic xanthoastrocytomas* More malignant tumors with exceptionally large cells, occasionally found in the superficial cortex of the hemispheres in young people
- *Astroblastomas* Poorly differentiated astrocytomas with pleomorphism, mitoses, and perivascular rosette formation

These histological differences do not correlate well with prognosis, however, and an alternative method of classification defines the astrocytoma as a mildly hypercellular tumor with pleomorphism but without vascular proliferation or necrosis; the anaplastic astrocytoma as a tumor with vascular proliferation, moderate pleomorphism and hypercellularity; and the glioblastoma multiforme as the same with added necrosis.[940]

In yet another system, nuclear atypia, mitoses, endothelial proliferation, and necrosis are used as the criteria for grading.[1474]

In a *variant* familial syndrome, cutaneous malignant melanomas are associated.[3338]

Two relevant Web sites are http://www.cancer.gov/cancertopics/pdq/treatment/adultbrain/HealthProfessional/page8/ from the National Cancer Institute, which describes treatment options available, and http://www.cancerbackup.org.uk/Cancertype/Brain/Typesofbraintumour/Astrocytictumours/.

astrocytosis See **gliosis**.

astroglia Astrocytes of all kinds.

astroglial neoplasms An encompassing term for all tumors arising from astrocytes.

astrogliosis Proliferation of astrocytes (mainly type I) in response to local injury. See **gliosis**.

asymbolia (e) (Gr, lack of + a sign) Loss of the power of forming or comprehending a symbol of thought, in any medium. The term was suggested by Finkelberg as more encompassing than **aphasia**.[5103]

asymbolia for pain Unawareness of the unpleasant qualities of painful sensations, first described by Schilder and Stengel in 1938. A patient can distinguish between some sensations, e.g., sharp from dull, but shows no response either to pain or to threatening gestures while such a response is seen to verbal threats. The syndrome is strongly associated with lesions of the dominant parietal lobe and may be accompanied by the features of **Gerstmann syndrome**. Other areas of the brain considered to subserve the processing of painful stimuli include the parietal lobes and/or the anterior cingulate or insular cortices.

asymmetric cortical degenerative syndromes Dementing disorders with features suggesting only localized cortical involvement, at least in the early stages.[1052] See **primary progressive aphasia**, **frontal lobe dementia**, and **parietal degeneration**.

asymmetric crying facies See **cardio-facial syndrome**.

asymmetric limb weakness with motor conduction block An acquired syndrome of slowly progressive, asymmetric, multifocal limb weakness with regions of profound, circumscribed motor conduction block in proximal or intermediate limb regions, sparing the extremities, the cranial nerves, and sensory fibers.[3557] See **multifocal motor neuropathy with conduction block**.

asymmetry 1. The unequal amplitude, form, or frequency of EEG activity over homologous areas on opposite sides of the head. 2. The unequal development of EEG waves about the baseline.

asymptomatic carotid bruit The presence of an audible bruit over a carotid artery in the absence of a history of neurological deficit. The finding suggests that the subject has generalized arteriosclerosis and has a 1% annual risk of stroke (but is at considerably greater risk of myocardial infarction). Detection of such a bruit was once regarded as an indication for carotid endarterectomy rather than cardiac evaluation (a decision analogous to repairing the stable door after the horse has been sold), but conservative management is now more widely advocated unless the carotid stenosis is extreme.[6909]

asymptomatic neurosyphilis A mild spirochetal meningitis without clinical effect but due to active treponemal invasion, commonly within months of infection and accompanied by an inflammatory reaction and positive reagin tests in the CSF. Untreated, progression to a symptomatic form of neurosyphilis is likely.

asymptomatic polysomographic finding Features that are recorded during polysomnography but are not the basis of any subjective complaints.[280]

asynchrony The nonsimultaneous occurrence of EEG activities over regions on the same side or on opposite sides of the head.

asynergia (asynergy) 1. A disturbance in the normal cooperation of agonists and antagonists, as is supposed to occur with disease of the cerebellum. 2. The inability to perform the various components of a movement at the right time and in the appropriate order or place. See **dyssynergia**.

asynkinesia A consistent pattern of impairment in the ability to perform two tasks simultaneously with the two hands (e.g., drawing a triangle while squeezing a bulb). The deficit is described in **Parkinson disease**.[900]

atavism Some strange recurrence to a primitive past; with more resemblance to remote ancestors than to parents (OED). A number of pathological states, e.g., **Down syndrome** and recidivism, were ascribed to atavism until genetic research determined the nature of the former and sociology demonstrated that the latter was explicable without reference to genetics at all. However, as Medawar points out, reappearance of a recessive trait in remote descendants as a manifestation of a recessive gene could be regarded as atavism too.

atavistic speech See **Worster-Drought-Allen syndrome**.

ataxia (Gr, without + order; disarranged) (ataxy) A term of Hippocrates, still in general use to characterize incoordination or awkwardness in the performance of a motor task. This may be due to lesions of the motor (including cerebellar) or sensory pathways or to local factors such as arthritis.

When due to impairment of cerebellar function, it is known as *cerebellar ataxia* and when due to loss of proprioceptive information, as *sensory*, *special sensory*, *or posterior column ataxia*.

In *frontal ataxia* the disorder of movements results from a lesion of the contralateral frontocorticopontine pathway. *Parietal ataxia* is better regarded as a form of **apraxia**. *Truncal ataxia* is that form in which sitting and standing stance are mainly affected, due to a lesion of the (midline) archicerebellum. *Gait ataxia* is wide based and staggering; it is due to lesions of the paleocerebellum (vermis and anterior lobe).

See also **cerebellar ataxia, episodic ataxia, posterior column ataxia, retinitis pigmentosa**. For quantitation of ataxia, see **Nobile-Orazio Ataxia Scale, Ataxia Assessment and Rating Scale**[5623] and the Web site: http://www.ataxia.org.

ataxia-analgia hysterica (Briquet ataxia) Inability to maintain the upright posture with anesthesia of the skin; a psychogenic disorder described by **Briquet** in 1859.

ataxia and adult-onset dementia An X-linked syndrome of

early-onset ataxia, tremor, and pyramidal signs and slowly progressive dementia with onset in adult life. Optic atrophy and extrapyramidal findings are not part of this syndrome.[1968]

ataxia and albinism See **cerebellar ataxias** (*variants*).

ataxia and cirrhosis See **cerebellar ataxias** (*variants*).

ataxia and dementia See **cerebellar syndromes** (congenital ataxias).

ataxia and epilepsy See **cerebellar syndromes** (congenital ataxias).

ataxia and hypergonadotrophic hypogonadism (of Skre) See **cerebellar ataxias** (*variants*).

ataxia and mental retardation See **cerebellar syndromes** (congenital ataxias).

ataxia and other neurological deficits with hyperuricemia See **cerebellar ataxias** (*variants*).

ataxia and sideroblastic anemia See **cerebellar syndromes** (congenital ataxias).

ataxia, aniridia, and mental retardation (Gillespie syndrome) See **cerebellar ataxias** (*variants*).

ataxia, areflexia, and facial diplegia A variant of **acute inflammatory demyelinating polyneuropathy** in which the seventh cranial nerves are affected bilaterally, the CSF protein is elevated and ataxia and areflexia are typically found in the virtual absence of limb weakness or significant sensory disturbances. The prognosis for recovery is excellent.[1114]

ataxia, areflexia, and ophthalmoplegia A variant presentation of **acute inflammatory demyelinating polyneuropathy**. See **Miller Fisher syndrome**.

Ataxia Assessment and Rating Scale A checklist evaluating gait, stance, sitting, speech disturbance, finger chase score, finger–nose test, fast alternating hand movements, and heel-shin slide.[5623]

ataxia, cataracts, hemiballismus, and dementia See **cerebellar ataxias** (*variants*).

ataxia, deaf-mutism, and muscular wasting 1, early onset See **cerebellar ataxias** (*variants*).

ataxia, deaf-mutism, and muscular wasting 2, late onset See **cerebellar ataxias** (*variants*).

ataxia, deafness, and leukodystrophy A progressive familial disorder of early onset with unknown cause.[3797]

ataxia hereditaria See **Friedreich ataxia**.

ataxia, ichthyosis, and hepatosplenomegly (of Harper) See **cerebellar ataxias** (*variants*).

ataxia, juvenile cataract, myopathy, and mental retardation See **cerebellar ataxias** (*variants*).

ataxia muscularis See **Thomsen disease**.

ataxia-oculomotor apraxia A recessively inherited ataxia associated with an elevation in α-fetoprotein as in **ataxia-telangiectasia** and, in one *variant*, with mutations in senataxin.[4576] See **cerebellar ataxias** (*variants*).

ataxia oligophrenia myocardial sclerosis, sensory deafness See **cerebellar ataxias** (*variants*).

ataxia, photomyoclonus, skeletal deformities See **cerebellar ataxias** (*variants*).

ataxia-plus See **Machado–Joseph disease**.

ataxia, sensory deafness, and optic atrophy See **cerebellar ataxias** (*variants*).

ataxia-telangiectasia (Louis-Bar syndrome) A rare, recessively inherited syndrome of neurological deterioration and failure of DNA repair in which there are breaks at 11q22–q23 (ATM gene). The condition is named for Mme. Louis-Bar, who gave the first complete description.[3922]

The main clinical features are the onset in infancy of progressive cerebellar ataxia (mainly truncal) with dysarthria; telangiectasia of the bulbar conjunctiva and malar areas of the face; progeric changes in the skin and hair; chorea and athetosis; apraxia of eye movements with impaired pursuit, gaze-holding, and convergence; mental retardation; demyelinating sensorimotor neuropathy with hyporeflexia; predisposition to malignancies; recurrent sinopulmonary infections; and hypersensitivity to ionising radiation.

Increased serum α-fetoprotein, deficiency of immunoglobulins, absent or hypoplastic thymus and T-cell deficiency with impairment of the synthesis of antibodies, and degeneration of the cerebellar cortex, dentate nucleus, inferior olives, and cranial nerve nuclei are other notable characteristics.[4224, 1752, 3997] *Variants* include the following:

1. *Ataxia without telangiectasia*. An inherited ataxic syndrome with onset in infancy or childhood and also characterized by dysarthria, immunoglobulin deficiency, dementia, dystonia, ophthalmoplegia, athetosis, and neurogenic muscle atrophy.[381]
2. A syndrome of ataxia, choreoathetosis, and horizontal and vertical ocular motor apraxia.[76]

See also the **Ataxia Telangiectasia Society** Web site: http://www.atsociety.org.uk/.

ataxia-telangiectasia-like syndrome (epilepsy-telangiectasia syndrome) A recessively inherited dysmorphic syndrome (11q21) characterized by conjunctival telangiectasias, brachydactyly, seizures, and mental retardation.

Ataxia Telangiectasia Children's Project A charitable organization in this field acting as a clearinghouse for ataxia-telangiectasia information. Address: 668 South Military Trail, Deerfield Beach, FL 33442-3023. Tel: 954-481-6611; 800-543-5728. E-mail: Info@atcp.org. Web site: http://www.atcp.org.

Ataxia Telangiectasia Medical Research Foundation A charitable organization in this field. Address: 5241 Round Meadow Rd., Hidden Hills, CA 91302. Tel: 818-704-8146. E-mail: becca4435@aol.com.

Ataxia Telangiectasia Society A British organization committed to helping, supporting, and advising families affected by ataxia telangiectasia and other cerebellar ataxias. Web site: http://www.atsociety.org.uk/.

ataxia with downbeat nystagmus See **cerebellar ataxias** (*variants*).

ataxia with hypogonadism and retinopathy See **cerebellar ataxias** (*variants*).

ataxia with motor neuron disease See **cerebellar ataxias** (*variants*).

ataxia with paroxysmal dystonia See **cerebellar ataxias** (*variants*).

ataxia with sensory neuropathy A syndrome characterized by the onset in childhood of speech defect/dysarthria, cerebellar signs, and demyelinating sensorimotor neuropathy. Developmental deformities of the cerebellum, pons, and basal ganglia are also found.[381]

ataxia with severe mental retardation See **cerebellar syndromes** (congenital ataxias).

ataxia without telangiectasia See **ataxia-telangiectasia**.

ataxic aphasia The term of **Lichtheim** for the disconnection syndrome in which the pathway from Broca's area to the motor areas is interrupted, producing nonfluent speech with poor repetition but with preservation of both writing and comprehension. See **Broca aphasia** and **aphemia**.

ataxic breathing See **Biot breathing**.

ataxic cerebral palsy See **congenital cerebellar hypoplasia**.

ataxic cerebral palsy See **cerebellar syndromes** (congenital ataxias).

ataxic conjugate movements See **opsoclonus**.

ataxic diplegia A congenital syndrome characterized by T-cell deficiency, absence or hypoplasia of the thymus, spasticity, and ataxia.[381]

ataxic gait A disorder in which the gait is irregular, lurching, and wide-based; the steps taken are irregular and of unequal length and falling to the side is common. It is due to the impairment of the righting reflexes. This form of gait disturbance is accentuated when the subject attempts to walk on a narrow base, as with heel–toe walking.

ataxic hemiparesis (dysarthria—clumsy hand syndrome, homolateral ataxia, and crural paresis) A **lacunar syndrome** in which weakness and cerebellar ataxia occur on the same side of the body, the leg being most affected.

The lesion is in the posterior limb of the internal capsule or in the basis pontis on the side opposite to the signs in most cases.[2105, 2474]

ataxic neuropathy Any form of neuropathy in which the thick fibers subserving proprioception are particularly affected. See **sensory ataxia** and **chronic sensory gangliopathies**.

ataxic nystagmus (abduction nystagmus, internuclear ophthalmoplegia) A form of dissociated nystagmus seen in the abducting eye either exclusively or far more than in the other eye, which may fail to adduct normally. See **abduction nystagmus**, **internuclear ophthalmoplegia**, and **saccadic pulses**.

ataxic paramyotonia (Gr, beside + a muscle + a stretching) (paramyotonia) An acquired nervous disease characterized by tonic spasms in certain muscle groups associated with ataxia and both sensory and motor deficits, described by **Gowers**.

ataxic syndromes Inherited or acquired conditions characterized by the appearance of limb or truncal ataxia, nystagmus, and other signs of cerebellar and other neurological impairment at varying stages of life. The biochemical causes of the several conditions are not completely known and the group may be regarded as a set of variants on the forms of inherited **cerebellar ataxias** listed elsewhere, to which group some of these possibly belong.

ataxic tremor See **cerebellar tremors**.

ataxic tropical neuropathy A diffuse affection of the CNS producing optic atrophy and sensory ataxia as a result of chronic cyanide poisoning from the excessive consumption of cassava root, seen in Central and West African countries. See **Nigerian neuropathy**.[2668]

ataxy See **ataxia**, **cerebellar ataxia**.

atelencephaly A congenital dysmorphic syndrome characterized by microcephaly, hydranencephaly or porencephaly, hydrocephalus, and cerebral atrophy.[381]

ateliosis (from Gr, incompleteness + a state) Dwarfism with incomplete development of all body organs (as in the Lorain-Levi syndrome); a term introduced by Gilford in 1902 but which has not been much employed.

atelo- (Gr, imperfect development of) Prefix denoting maldevelopment; thus *ateloencephalia*, *atelomyelia*, and *atelostomia* indicate imperfect development of the brain, the spine, and the mouth, respectively.

atherothrombotic brain infarction Cerebral infarction due to occlusion of a supplying vessel which is the site of atherosclerosis. Diagnostic criteria include the following:

1. The rapid onset and persistence for over 24 h of focal neurological symptoms or signs such as uni- or binocular visual loss; dysphasia or dysarthria; symptoms of bulbar paresis; uni- or bilateral paresis; uni- or bilateral sensory impairment; disturbance in the level of consciousness, *and*
2. Stenosis or obstruction of a carotid or vertebral artery or a major branch thereof shown by some form of angiography; *or* abnormal uptake of tracer elements consistent with infarction on radionucleide brain scan or SPECT scan; *or* focal abnormality consistent with infarction on CT or MRI scan.

athetoid cerebral palsy See **athetoid syndrome**.

athetoid syndrome (double athetosis, infantile partial striatal sclerosis, Little disease with involuntary movements, distal dystonia) A nonprogressive but evolving form of **cerebral palsy** caused by damage to the basal ganglia of the full-term brain and characterized by impairment of postural reflexes, arrhythmic involuntary movements, and dysarthria, with sparing of sensation, ocular movements, and often of intelligence.

Affected children thus cannot sit, cannot move at will, and cannot talk, but yet take everything in.[2142] Intranatal asphyxia or neonatal jaundice are the usual etiologies, and marbling of the basal ganglia (**état marbré**) is the typical pathology.

A *variant* is *BD MCA* (athetoid cerebral palsy), a congenital dysmorphic syndrome characterized by microphthalmia, colobomas of the iris, blue sclera, breast and skeletal anomalies, microcephaly, pyramidal and extrapyramidal signs, and mental and developmental delay.[381]

athétose double (Fr, bilateral athetosis) A severe form of cerebral palsy manifesting with bilateral athetosis and profound mental delay, described by Paul Oulmont.[7]

athetosis (Gr, lack of + a fixed place; thus, without a fixed position) (Hammond disease) An involuntary movement disorder characterized by irregular, forceful, slow, writhing movements generally of the extremities, very often with finger movements and with co-contraction of agonists and antagonists. Primary and secondary causes are recognized.[6868, 2720]

Both negative and positive phenomena have been described as constituting the clinical features. The *negative phenomena* include impairment of postural reactions, dysarthria, and early paresis of upward gaze. The *positive phenomena* comprise athetotic involuntary movements (a release of anticipatory postural reactions) and the athetoid "dance on hot bricks," dysphagia, and snorting, which witness athetosis of the bulbar muscles.

In certain syndromes in which athetosis is the dominant feature, other phenomena such as **intention tremors** and signs witnessing the release of brainstem and other primitive reflexes (an overactive bite reflex and **Moro response**, extension spasms, asymmetrical **tonic neck reflexes**, eye-avoiding and face-avoiding reactions) also may emerge.[2142]

The condition was described and named by William **Hammond** in 1871[2720] but had previously been known (as *"morbus sacer"*). Hammond was incorrect in maintaining that the movements persist in sleep as they do not. Sir Victor **Horsley** showed in 1909 that excision of the precentral cortex relieved or abolished the movements.[2998] In 1911, the Vogts defined *double athetosis* (bilateral athetosis) as a pure striatal syndrome, the clinical correlate of the **état marbré**, which they also distinguished. See also **athetoid syndrome, spinal pseudoathetosis**.

athrodynia à potu See **alcoholic neuropathy**.

athymhormia Loss of self-psychic activation—a lack of motivation, with apathy, aspontaneity, and loss of motor and affective drive but without suffering or cognitive impairment. The cause is usually bilateral infarcts in the region of the centrum semiovale.[1027]

Atkin oculo-cerebro-acral syndrome An X-linked congenital dysmorphic syndrome characterized also by seizures, skeletal, ocular, cardiac, and renal malformations, delayed closure of fontanelles, and cerebellar atrophy with the Dandy–Walker malformation with macrocephaly and mental and developmental delay.[286]

atlantoaxial dislocation Abnormal congenital or acquired mobility between **atlas** and **axis** as a result of absence or nonfusion of the odontoid peg, or of abnormal laxity of the ligament binding the odontoid to the anterior arch of the atlas.[5980]

Such forward displacement of the atlas may occur as a result of trauma or as a congenital anomaly (as in **Down syndrome**). The narrowing of the spinal canal may lead to chronic compressive or ischemic myelopathy affecting the posterior columns and pyramidal tracts most severely and leading to extensive degeneration of anterior horn cells throughout the cervical cord.

Clinically, affected people complain of neck pain, stiffness, and both static and progressive symptoms which mainly indicate damage to the upper motor neuron in the spinal cord, with less evidence of lower motor neuron or posterior column involvement. Cranial nerve palsies are not a feature. The dislocation may be congenital in Asian people.[6584] Three forms are defined:

1. Occipitalization of the atlas with fusion of the second and third cervical vertebrae, posterior dislocation of the odontoid, and cord compression as a result of maldevelopment of the transverse ligament
2. Maldevelopment of the odontoid process only
3. Dislocation of the odontoid only during flexion of the neck

atlanto-dens interval The separation of the first and second cervical vertebrae, normally less than 5 mm. A greater separation suggests the presence of atlantoaxial dislocation.

atlas The first cervical vertebra, carrying the weight of the head. It is named for the Greek mythological figure who was changed by Perseus into stone—the Atlas mountain that was so lofty that it was considered to hold up the sky. A variation of the myth, more relevant to the function of the vertebra under discussion, has Atlas supporting variously the pillars of heaven or the earth upon his shoulders (hence the name for a book of maps), which led Vesalius to name the vertebra so.

atonia-astasia See **Foerster atonic diplegia**.[3113]

atonic absences Atypical absences accompanied by loss of postural tone. See **atonic seizures**.

atonic cerebral diplegia A congenital "cerebral palsy" syndrome comprising flaccid weakness with marked delay in the attainment of motor milestones, severe mental defect, and absent or rudimentary speech. Microcephaly, seizures, and congenital heart disease may also be associated.[1715]

atonic motor seizure An **atonic seizure** in which there is a sudden loss or diminution of muscle tone without apparent preceding myoclonic or tonic event lasting 1–2 s or more and involving head, trunk, jaw, or limb musculature.

atonic-sclerotic muscular dystrophy See **congenital muscular dystrophy**.

atonic seizures (atonic absences) Epileptic syndromes characterized by the sudden loss of motor power, sometimes with an initial tonic or myoclonic component, leading to sudden falls or slumping of all or part of the body and accompanied on EEG by slow spike-waves, 3 Hz-spike waves, polyspike-and-waves or fast recruiting rhythms, and on EMG by suppression of normal tonic activity in the involved muscles.[72]

If they are very brief, they are known as **negative myoclonus**.

atremia See **akinesia algera**.

atrophia myotonica See **myotonic dystrophy**.

atrophy (Gr, Negative + to nourish) Emaciation or wasting, usually of muscles, and most often accompanied by loss of strength.

Progressive muscular atrophy is a term for **amyotrophic lateral sclerosis**.

attack (of multiple sclerosis) The occurrence of a symptom or symptoms of neurological dysfunction in the setting of multiple sclerosis, with or without objective confirmation, and lasting more than 24 h.[5094]

attention The complex capacity for focusing upon one of a number of competing sensory stimuli or for maintaining readiness to record specific stimuli, without being distracted by others that are extraneous. "When any object of external sense, or of thought, occupies the mind in such a degree that a person does not receive a clear perception from any other one, he is said to attend to it."

Orientation, exploration, concentration, motivation, and vigilance are prerequisites for, or aspects of, this capacity, while attention itself is the major prerequisite for intellectual, reflective, and meaningful motor activity. The faculty is particularly likely to be disturbed when a lesion affects the frontal lobe.[4332] Useful tests include the Trailmaking test and tests of cancellation, reversal of digits, and serial-seven subtractions.

The processes underlying attention include *tonic attention*, which requires mechanisms regulating the span or efficiency of vigilance, and *selective attention*, which determines its object.

Standard methods of testing include **digit** span, reciting the months of the year, or spelling a word (e.g., "world") backwards.

attention deficit/hyperactivity disorder (ADHD) A condition predominantly seen in childhood, in which the patient manifests stimulus-oriented behavior, distractibility, shortened attention span, lack of tolerance of frustration, and lack of fear.[1747] The cause is unknown.

Lack of investment of organization and maintenance of attention and effort in completing tasks; inability to inhibit impulsive responses; lack of modulation of arousal levels to meet the demands of the situation; and unusually strong inclination to seek immediate gratification are considered the primary deficits.[1700, 3]

The principal characteristics of ADHD are **inattention**, **hyperactivity**, and **impulsivity** appearing gradually early in life. Impulsiveness and hyperactivity precede inattention, which may not emerge for a year or more. The impulsive child who acts before thinking may be considered just a "discipline problem," while the child who is passive or sluggish may be viewed as merely unmotivated. Yet, both may have different types of ADHD. All children are sometimes restless, sometimes act without thinking, and sometimes daydream the time away. When the child's hyperactivity, distractibility, poor concentration, or impulsivity begin to affect performance in school, social relationships with other children, or behavior at home, ADHD may be suspected. But because the symptoms vary so much across settings, ADHD is not easy to diagnose. This is especially true when inattentiveness is the primary symptom.

Three patterns of behavior are differentiated: the **predominantly hyperactive-impulsive type** (without marked inattention); the **predominantly inattentive type** (without marked hyperactive-impulsive behavior); and a **combined type** in which both inattentive and hyperactive-impulsive symptoms occur.

Hyperactive children always seem to be "on the go" or constantly in motion. *Impulsive* children do not curb their immediate reactions and do not think enough before they act. They will often blurt out inappropriate comments, display their emotions without restraint, and act without regard for the consequences. Signs of hyperactivity-impulsivity include feelings of restlessness, fidgeting with the hands or feet, or squirming while seated; inappropriate behavior in situations where sitting or quiet behavior is expected; blurting out answers before hearing the whole question; and having difficulty waiting in line or taking turns.

Children who are inattentive have a hard time keeping their minds on any one thing and may get bored with a task quickly unless they thoroughly enjoy doing it. Homework is particularly hard for these children. The *DSM-IV-TR* gives these signs of *inattention*: often becoming easily distracted by irrelevant sights and sounds, failing to pay attention to details, and making careless mistakes; rarely following instructions carefully and completely losing or forgetting things like toys, pencils, or books, and tools needed for a task; and skipping from one uncompleted activity to another. (Abstracted from the NIMH Web site: http://www.nimh.nih.gov/health/publications/adhd/symptoms.shtml/.)

The diagnostic criteria defined by the American Psychiatric Association in *DSM IV-TR*[172] can be found at: http://www.behavenet.com/capsules/disorders/dsm4TRclassification.htm/.

attenuation 1. Reduction in amplitude of EEG activity. This may occur transiently in response to physiological or other stimuli, such as electrical stimulation of the brain, or can result from pathological conditions. Cf. **blocking**. 2. Reduction of sensitivity of an EEG channel, i.e., decrease in output pen deflection by operation of the sensitivity or filter controls. It is customarily expressed as relative reduction of sensitivity at certain stated frequencies. (Adapted from the 1974 Report of the Committee on Terminology, IFCN[1117] © 1974 with kind permission from Elsevier Science.) 3. Decrease in any neurological phenomenon induced by some extrinsic factor.

attitude en chien de fusil The French term for that posture of rigid trunk extension and maximal flexion of the hips and knees (resembling that of a gundog keeping down) adopted by patients with severe meningeal irritation.

atypical absences Absence seizures unassociated with the typical 3-Hz spike-wave pattern and marked clinically by a brief period of immobility with staring, decreased responsiveness, and, on the EEG, bursts of diffuse and often asymmetrically slow spike-waves at rates of up to 2.5 Hz or the various EEG patterns associated with tonic seizures.[72] The attacks have slower onset and termination and tend to occur more often and for longer than typical absence attacks. In some cases, motor activity is retained during the seizure.[1291]

In some cases, the condition presents as atonic or tonic seizures lasting 5–20 s with a frequency of a few per day to nearly continuous; it is often associated with changes in postural tone which may cause the patient to fall. Eyelid clonus, mild tonic, or autonomic features and automatisms may also be observed. Association with tonic seizures and slow spikes and waves would classify this as the **Lennox-Gastaut syndrome** while when combined with generalized tonic-clonic and myoclonic seizures, the diagnosis would be **myoclonic-astatic epilepsy**. See **continuous spike waves in slow sleep**.

atypical Alzheimer disease See **congophilic angiopathy**.

atypical benign partial epilepsy An epileptic encephalopathy of childhood characterized by atypical absence, atonic, myoclonic, partial, or secondarily generalized motor seizures and with Rolandic sharp waves and electrical status epilepticus in sleep.[6833]

atypical bobbing See **reverse ocular bobbing**.

atypical cluster headache A dubious entity, in which otherwise typical cluster headaches are accompanied by interparoxysmal changes in the EEG and by episodes of retrobulbar neuritis.

atypical facial pain See **persistent idiopathic facial pain**. See also **atypical trigeminal neuralgia**.

atypical myopathy with myofibrillar aggregates See **myofibrillar myopathy**.

atypical neurologic disease syndrome (ANDS) Assorted symptom complexes experienced initially by women after the surgical insertion of bags containing silicone in sub-mammary regions, but more recently following other traumatic life events, such as participation in military conflict; and characterized by multiple apparent rheumatological or neurological complaints without accompanying clinical or laboratory abnormalities. Fatigue, myalgias, memory problems, blurred vision, numbness, impaired balance etc. are the usual presentations. See also **silicone encephalopathy**.

A learned judgement delivered in an Alabama (U.S.) court appears to have taken responsibility for defining medical criteria for nonmedical (or at least nonorganic) disorders; these are reproduced here with some editing but without critical comment, in order to save this author from having to invoke the First Amendment.

1. A diagnosis of atypical neurological disease syndrome (ANDS) shall be based on the clinical findings and laboratory tests set forth below. The clinical and laboratory presentation of these neurologic syndromes will have an atypical presentation from the natural disease and will also have additional neuromuscular, rheumatic, or nonspecific autoimmune signs and symptoms.
2. Eligibility for ANDS requires both:
   Satisfying the requirements for one of the four neurologic disease types set forth in paragraph 5 below, and
   Any three additional (nonduplicative) neuromuscular, rheumatic, or nonspecific symptoms or findings set forth in the definition for atypical connective tissue disease (ACTD).
3. An individual will fit into this category if her primary symptoms are characteristic of a neurologic disease as diagnosed by a Board-certified neurologist or by a physician Board certified in internal medicine.
4. If the individual's qualified medical doctor determines that a symptom is clearly and specifically caused by a source other than breast implants, that symptom will not be utilized in the diagnosis of ANDS unless the Claims Office determines that other submissions indicate that the symptom should be utilized. A symptom that may be caused only in part by a source other than breast implants is not excluded from such utilization.
5. Neurological disease types:

   Polyneuropathies. This disease category requires a diagnosis of polyneuropathy that is confirmed by one or more of the following:

   - Objectively demonstrated loss of sensation to pinprick, vibration, touch, or position
   - Proximal or distal muscle weakness
   - Tingling and/or burning pain in the extremities
   - Signs of dysesthesia
   - Loss of tendon reflex

Plus one or more of the following laboratory findings:

- Abnormal levels of anti-mag or anti-sulfatide or anti-GM1 antibodies
- Abnormal sural nerve biopsy
- Abnormal electrodiagnostic testing (EMG or nerve conduction studies, etc.)

Multiple sclerosis-like syndrome. This disease category requires definite evidence of CNS disease, with a history and physical findings compatible with multiple sclerosis or multiple sclerosis-like syndrome, involving one or more of the following signs and symptoms:

- Weakness in the pyramidal distribution
- Evidence of optic neuritis documented by an ophthalmologist
- Increased deep tendon reflexes
- Absent superficial abdominal reflexes
- Ataxia or dysdiadochokinesia as the sign of cerebellar involvement
- Neurologically induced tremors
- Internuclear ophthalmoplegia and/or bladder or speech involvement secondary to CNS disease

Plus one or more of the following:

- Abnormal brain MRI with foci of increased signal abnormality suggestive of demyelinating lesions
- Delayed visual-evoked responses or abnormal-evoked potentials
- Abnormal CSF with oligoclonal bands

Amyotrophic lateral sclerosis-like syndrome. This disease category requires documented evidence of progressive upper and widespread lower motor neuron involvement, plus one or more of the following:

- Neurologic autoantibodies such as anti-mag, anti-sulfatide, and anti-GM1
- Abnormal sural nerve biopsy
- Chronic inflammation on muscle or nerve biopsies
- Abnormal EMG

- Documentation on neurologic examination of both upper and lower motor neuron disease and/or bulbar involvement

Disease of neuromuscular junction. This disease category requires a diagnosis of myasthenia gravis or myasthenia gravis–like syndrome or disorders of the neuromuscular junction made by a Board-certified neurologist and confirmed by abnormal EMG showing typical findings of decrement on repetitive stimulation testing and/or elevated acetylcholine receptor antibodies.

atypical ocular bobbing See **reverse ocular bobbing**.

atypical parkinsonism Syndromes resembling **Parkinson disease** in which there occur early involvement of speech, gait, or balance; relative paucity of tremor; symmetrical involvement; increased axial rather than limb tone; and poor response to levadopa treatment. MRI scans may show increased T2 signal intensities in the putamen and caudate, perhaps reflecting the accumulation of iron in those sites. Two major groups are defined; **progressive supranuclear palsy** and **multiple system degeneration**, the latter encompassing **striatonigral degeneration**, **Shy-Drager syndrome**, and **olivopontocerebellar atrophy**. See also **corticobasal degeneration**.

atypical partial benign epilepsy of childhood An epileptic syndrome in which the onset is between 2 and 6 years of age in children with previously normal development and examination. They display at least two different seizure types including partial nocturnal seizures, generalized atonic-clonic seizures, brief absences, massive myoclonic jerks, and atonic seizures occurring in clusters lasting up to a month and separated by free intervals of several months' duration. The EEG shows intense diffuse slow spike-wave activity during slow-wave sleep in these periods. Focal spikes and central regions are recorded in the awake state. Atonic seizures and mental deterioration do not occur and the disease appears to remit before the age of 9 years.[72]

atypical rapid spike-wave activity See **irregular generalized spike-wave activity**.

atypical repetitive spike-and-slow-waves A term referring to paroxysms consisting of a sequence of spike-and-slow-wave complexes which occur bilaterally and synchronously but do not meet one or more of the criteria of 3-Hz spike-and-slow-waves. (Adapted from the 1974 Report of the Committee on Terminology, IFCN[1117]. © 1974 with kind permission from Elsevier Science.)

atypical sensory syndrome A pattern of sensory loss involving all sensations, but only in isolated parts of the body, and occurring with variously sited infarcts of a parietal lobe.[434] See also **parietal stroke**.

atypical teratoma See **dysgerminoma, germinoma**.

atypical trigeminal neuralgia The occurrence of pain persisting between acute attacks in patients with trigeminal neuralgia, who exhibit both episodic, lancinating unilateral facial pains with shock-free intervals and variable-intensity but constant unilateral facial pain, thus combining features of both classical trigeminal neuralgia and trigeminal neuropathy. See also **atypical facial pain**.

atz See **wolfing reflex**.

audiogenic epilepsy See **musciogenic epilepsy**.

audiokinetic nystagmus A form of jerk nystagmus induced in darkness by a loud noise that rotates around the subject.

audiometry Techniques for the quantitative measurement of auditory acuity. See also **Bekesy audiometry**.

audiospinal reaction Brief (startle-like) muscle contraction of the trunk and limbs in response to an unexpected, loud auditory stimulus. The response can be quantitated by examining the facilitation of the **H reflex** that it induces.[1567]

audiovestibular syndrome A dominantly inherited, late-onset, progressive disorder manifesting bilateral sensorineural hearing loss, intermittent brief attacks of vertigo.and increasing permanent disequilibrium.[3102]

audiovestibular Web sites http://www.dizziness-and-balance.com/, a privately produced site with data for patients and physicians; http://www.ghr.lmnihgov/ghr/page/home/, a listing of genetic disorders; http://www.emedicine.com/ent/topic 479.htm/, a site addressing auditory rehabilitation.

auditory affective agnosia Impairment in the comprehension of affective speech, as opposed to propositional speech; this may occur in subjects with right hemisphere dysfunction and a neglect syndrome.[2840]

auditory agnosia A disorder of recognition of sounds in a subject with normal hearing, alertness, and intelligence. Both *verbal* (inability to interpret spoken language) and *nonverbal types* (inability to interpret nonverbal sounds) occur; the former is due to bilateral lesions of the auditory cortex, the latter to a similar lesion on the right side.[2840] See also **cortical deafness**.

auditory-evoked potential Electric waveforms of biologic origin elicited in response to sound stimuli. Classified by their latency as short-latency brainstem auditory evoked potential (BAEP) with a latency of up to 10 ms, middle-latency with a latency of 10–50 ms, and long-latency with a latency of over 50 ms. See **brainstem auditory evoked potential**. (From the 2001 Report of the Nomenclature Committee of the American Association of Electromyography and Electrodiagnosis.[19] Reproduced by kind permission of the AANEM.)

auditory imperception (word deafness) Failure of a patient to comprehend the meaning of what he hears although he knows well that the sounds represent speech.[929, 4694] See **word deafness**.

auditory neuropathy An acquired or hereditary condition still under study, characterized by hearing deficits (especially for speech); normal cochlear function; and abnormal brainstem auditory evoked potentials.[6023]

auditory-oculogyric reflex Immediate turning of the head and eyes in the direction of an unexpected, sudden, and loud noise. A cochlear reflex, once invoked as a test for hysterical deafness.[5333]

auditory-palpebral reflex (cochleopalpebral reflex) Immediate blinking in response to a sudden, loud, and unexpected sound.[5333] See **palpebral reflex**.

auditory receptive dysphasia See **Wernicke aphasia**.

Auditory Verbal Learning Test A memory test, requiring the subject to learn 15 nouns in five trials, recalling them 20 min later, after which a recognition test is given.[6480]

auditory vertigo Illusory physiological sensations of movement of the self (with audiokinetic nystagmus) induced by moving sound fields.[819]

Auerbach, Leopold (1828–1897) German anatomist and neuropathologist of Breslau.

Auerbach's plexus (myenteric plexus) The autonomic plexus between the circular and the longitudinal coats of the intestinal wall described by Auerbach in 1862.[3373]

augmentation An increase in the amplitude of recorded electrical activity.

Aujesky, Aladar (1869–1933) Hungarian pathologist, working in Budapest, who described the "scratching pest."

aura (Gr, a soft breath of wind) 1. The events comprising that part of an epileptic seizure which a subject can recall afterwards. The classical form, known to Aretaeus of Cappadocia and to Galen, was the **epigastric aura** "as if a blast of cold air ascended from the lowest parts toward the heart and head."[5886] 2. Reversible neurological symptoms that may precede, accompany, or follow the pain phase of a migraine.

Typical aura with migraine headache It may consist of visual and/or sensory and/or speech symptoms with gradual development, duration of less than 1 h, a mix of positive and negative features, and complete reversibility characterize the aura which precedes (usually) a headache fulfilling the criteria for **migraine without aura**. Diagnostic criteria have been defined:

A. At least 2 attacks fulfilling criteria B–D
B. Aura consisting of at least one of the following, but no motor weakness:
   1. Fully reversible visual symptoms including positive features (e.g., flickering lights, spots, or lines) and/or negative features (i.e., loss of vision)
   2. Fully reversible sensory symptoms including positive features (i.e., pins and needles) and/or negative features (i.e., numbness)
   3. Fully reversible dysphasic speech disturbance
C. At least two of the following:
   1. Homonymous visual symptoms and/or unilateral sensory symptoms
   2. At least one aura symptom develops gradually over ≥5 min and/or different aura symptoms occur in succession over ≥5 min
   3. Each symptom lasts ≥5 and <60 min
D. Headache fulfilling criteria B–D for migraine without aura begins during the aura or follows aura within 60 min
E. Not attributed to another disorder

From the International Classification of Headache Disorders (Headache Classification Committee of the International Headache Society. *Cephalalgia* 2004;**24**[Suppl 1]) by kind permission of Dr. Jes Olesen, the International Headache Society and Wiley-Blackwell Publications.

A related disorder is *typical aura with nonmigraine headache* which is a typical aura consisting of visual and/or sensory and/or speech symptoms developing gradually over less than 1 h with a mixture of positive and negative features and complete reversibility. These IHS criteria are exactly the same as for **aura** (typical aura with migraine headache) except that under "D" the entry is "Headache that does not fulfill criteria B–D" for **migraine without aura**.

aura continua Prolonged episodes of sensory symptoms similar or identical to a seizure aura lasting hours to days, representing a subtype of status epilepticus. This rare manifestation of focal epilepsy usually occurs with retained consciousness. The variable dysesthesias, painful sensations, and visual disturbances experienced may be associated with a motor component. Aura continua involving the limbic system is the most common clinical pattern, typically presenting as fear or as a rising epigastric sensation and recurring every few minutes for hours without progressive to an observable seizure with impairment of awareness.[5740, 4882]

aural vertigo See **Ménière syndrome**.

auricular myoclonus Repetitive, intermittent, or constant clonic movements of the antitragicus muscle at rates of up to 70 Hz, suppressed only by strong contraction of the limbs, as a result of excessive irritability of the facial nerve of unknown cause.[3452]

auriculotemporal neuralgia See **superior laryngeal neuralgia**.

auriculotemporal syndrome (Gustatory sweating, chorda tympani syndrome) Flushing and sweating of one side of the face during mastication, particularly when eating highly spiced foods, as a result of abnormal regeneration of the terminal axons of parasympathetic fibers following damage to the auriculotemporal nerve, a branch of the mandibular.[2199] See **Frey syndrome**.

auscultatory percussion A technique designed to detect intracranial mass lesions. The examiner percusses the frontal bone in the midline while listening with a stethoscope applied successively to different parts of the scalp; reduction in perceived sound intensity is claimed to indicate the presence of an intracranial mass between the site of tapping and the area of reduced sound transmission.[2602]

Austin disease See **multiple sulfatase deficiency**

Austin fluff test A screening test for the detection of metachromatic lipids.[301]

Austin variant See **metachromatic leukodystrophy**.

Australian X disease See **Murray valley encephalitis**.

Austregesilo, Antonio (1876–1956?) Brazilian neurologist and psychiatrist, who was professor of clinical medicine and then of neurology in Rio de Janeiro. He described epidemic neuromyelitis following an epidemic in 1931 and wrote particularly on tropical neurology, extrapyramidal disorders, and Schilder disease, and in addition the elicitation of the Babinski response by stimulation of the thigh, recognizing this as being due to spread of the receptive area for the reflex.

autism A polygenetic developmental neurobiologic disorder with multiorgan system involvement, though it predominantly involves the association cortices of the brain. The term was introduced by Bleuler for that form of psychosis in which the individual is "divorced from reality." The word is used now, after Kanner, for a life-long, static developmental disorder with a genetic basis, comprising a spectrum of biological or organic childhood psychoses (infantile autism or autistic disorder) which may be postencephalitic (*autism with polioencephalopathy*), schizophrenic or, probably very commonly, due to a disorder of the association cortex, impairing intrahemispheric connectivity. The multiorgan system involvement and diversity of central nervous system findings suggest an epigenetic mechanism.[4395]

Clinical manifestations include profound impairment in social relationships, severe developmental disturbances of verbal and nonverbal communication, ritualistic and compulsive behavior, and disturbances of motility and of attention. Perseveration, concreteness of thought, affective blunting, and lack of insight into the thinking of others (lack of empathy) are usual features. There is also delay of, or abnormal functioning in, social interaction, language (e.g., in social conversation) and/or symbolic and imaginative play. Seizures and cognitive disturbances may also be present,[1566, 1429] as may any of a range of defined neurological conditions such as chromosomal abnormalities, **Rett syndrome**, **phenylketonuria**, etc.[74] See also **Asperger syndrome**.

Autism is characterized by impaired social interaction, problems with verbal and nonverbal communication, and unusual, repetitive, or severely limited activities and interests. Males are four times more likely to have autism than females. Three distinctive behaviors ranging in impact from mild to disabling are:

1. *Difficulties with social interaction (the hallmark feature)* Even in infancy, a baby with autism may be unresponsive to people or focus intently on one item to the exclusion of others for long periods of time. A child with autism may appear to develop normally and then withdraw and become indifferent to social engagement.
2. *Problems with verbal and nonverbal communication* Children with autism lack empathy. They may fail to respond to their name and often avoid eye contact with other people. They have difficulty interpreting what others are thinking or feeling because they cannot understand social cues, such as tone of voice or facial expressions.
3. *Repetitive behaviors or narrow, obsessive interests* Performance of repetitive movements such as rocking and twirling, or in self-abusive behavior such as biting or head-banging, is common. Autistic children start speaking later than other children and may refer to themselves by name instead of "I" or "me." Autistic children seldom play interactively.

Core behaviors suggesting autism include:

- An impaired ability to make friends or to initiate or sustain conversations
- The absence or impairment of imaginative and social play
- Stereotyped, repetitive, or unusual use of language
- Restricted patterns of interest that are abnormal in intensity or focus, often with a preoccupation with certain objects or subjects
- Inflexible adherence to specific routines or rituals.

Children with autism have an unusually high risk for **fragile X syndrome**, **tuberous sclerosis**, seizures, **Tourette syndrome**, learning disabilities, and **attention deficit hyperactivity disorder**. (After data on the NIMH Web site: http://www.nimh.nih.gov/health/publications/adhd/symptoms.shtml/.)

A practice guideline for screening and diagnosis has been developed by the American Academy of Neurology.[2047]

Autism Network International A charitable organization in this field. Address: P.O. Box 35448, Syracuse, NY 13235-5448. E-mail: jisincla@mailbox.syr.edu. Web site: http://www.ani.ac.

Autism Society of America A charitable organization in this field. Address: 7910 Woodmont Ave., Suite 300, Bethesda, MD 20814-3067. Tel: 301-657-0881; 800-328-8476. E-mail: info@autism-society.org. Web site: http://www.autism-society.org.

Autism Society of Canada 129 Yorkville Ave., Suite 202, Toronto, ON, Canada M5R 1C4. Tel: 416-922-0302; fax: 416-922-1032.

autism with polioencephalopathy See **autism**.

autochthonous Proceeding from within the self, as opposed to being triggered by external stimuli. The term is usually used in the descriptions of forms of delusional activity.

autoecholalia See **palilalia**.

autoimmune polyglandular syndrome A rare combination of chronic polyendocrinopathy, candidiasis of the skin and mucosae, alopecia, and ectodermal dystrophy, recessively inherited. Neurological associations reported include autoimmune polyneuropathy, CNS demyelination resembling multiple sclerosis with cerebellar and pyramidal signs, extrapyramidal manifestations, proximal muscle weakness, Tolosa-Hunt syndrome, and complications secondary to the various endocrine failures.[556]

autolysis Enzymatic autodigestion of cells in which there is initially clumping of the chromatin, swelling of mitochondria, and dispersion of ribosomes. The process is typified by the changes occurring in the brain when it remains warm and unfixed after death.

automatic behavior syndrome The frequent occurrence of complex automatisms lasting seconds to hours and involving activities not requiring great learned skill, during a state of altered consciousness due to repetitive microsleeps, a state that is facilitated by performing repetitive or boring tasks such as long drives inducing drowsiness. There is amnesia for events occurring during the episode, which occurs in patients with **narcolepsy** and other causes of **excessive daytime sleepiness**.[2626]

automatic bladder Reflex contraction of the bladder wall with relaxation of its sphincter, in response to increased distension pressure, occurring when the bladder has lost its upper motor neuron or lower motor neuron innervation. As a result, normal cortical inhibition is impossible and the bladder discharges, usually with low volumes of urine contained therein, as a result of its own inherent response to stretch of the detrusor. Such automatic expulsion of the contents of the bladder occurs some 25 days after complete division of the spinal cord, when the bladder contents reach a certain amount. At this time, the sphincter relaxes and urine is passed involuntarily.

Automatic micturition may be facilitated by any afferent stimulus passing into the lower part of the cord, especially if it evokes a flexor spasm, or by deep breathing. Generalized sweating due to activity of the nervous system below the level of the lesion may accompany the bladder contraction.

In a different form in which there is a lower motor neuron lesion as a result of damage to the cauda equina or conus medullaris, contractions occur initially but later distension or infection leads to damage to the stretch receptors in the bladder wall, and overdistension occurs with dribbling incontinence. In a third form, following complete division of the spinal cord above L5, the reflex is intact but detrusor contraction occurs in response to stretch without inhibition from higher levels.[2817]

automatic decomposition EMG (ADEMG) A computerized method for extracting individual motor unit action potentials from an interference pattern. (From the 2001 Report of the Nomenclature Committee of the American Association of Electromyography and Electrodiagnosis.[19] Reproduced by kind permission of the AANEM.)

automatic language Overlearned sequences of speech (such as numbers or the alphabet) and emotional speech such as expletives.

automatism 1. More-or-less coordinated and adapted involuntary activity that would be purposeful if the subject were aware of it, occurring during a state of clouding of consciousness, either in the course of or after an epileptic seizure and usually followed by amnesia for the event.[3126, 1912] 2. Behavioral sequences that unfold without voluntary control and usually with loss or impairment of awareness, as components of **complex partial**, prolonged absence, or other types of seizures, or postictally. In a few cases, consciousness is retained during the performance of the automatic movement.[4289] They often resemble voluntary movements and may consist of inappropriate continuation of ongoing preictal motor activity. See also **affective-psychic seizures**.

autonomic (Gr, self + law; hence self-governing or automatic) The term **autonomic nervous system** was suggested by **Langley** for the sympathetic and parasympathetic systems in about 1898.

autonomic aura In the context of epilepsy, the experience of sensations consistent with involvement of the autonomic nervous system, including cardiovascular, gastrointestinal, sudomotor, vasomotor, and thermoregulatory symptoms.

autonomic diencephalic epilepsy Unusual seizures, manifestations of which include apnea, stridor, laryngospasm, chest pain, and cardiac arrhythmias. See **Penfield syndrome**.

Autonomic Disorders Association A charitable organization. Address: Sarah Matheson Trust, Pickering Unit, St. Mary's Hospital, Praed St., London W2 1 UK. Tel: 0171-886-1520. Web site: http://www.msaweb.co.uk/professionals.htm.

autonomic dysfunction syndrome See **diencephalic autonomic seizures**.

autonomic dysreflexia (autonomic hyperreflexia) The occurrence of paroxysmal hypertensive episodes, headache, malaise, nausea, sweating above the level of the lesion, and bradycardia, due to increased sympathetic output in response to such triggers as somatic pain, fecal impaction, and bladder distension. The causative spinal lesion is at or above T6 and the condition is triggered by sensory inputs below that level. Intracerebral hemorrhage, hypertension, seizures, and pulmonary edema are complications.[671] The mechanism is considered to be disconnection of spinal sympathetic centers from supraspinal control. See also **Head-Riddoch syndrome**.

Autonomic Dysreflexia A Web-based fact sheet addressing this condition and spinal cord injury. http://www.sci-info-pages.com/ad.html.

autonomic function tests Measurements of end-organ responsiveness to the activation of neural reflex arcs, reflecting autonomic function. The noninvasive tests in more general use[5211] include the following:

Sympathetic Division:

1. One drop of 4–10% cocaine dilates the pupil if the postganglionic sympathetic activity is intact but will not have this effect if there is a lesion of the sympathetic pathway at any site. Cocaine blocks the re-uptake of adrenaline from the synaptic cleft.
2. One drop of 0.1% (1 in 1000) adrenaline has no effect on a normal pupil but causes dilatation when there is postganglionic failure due to denervation supersensitivity.
3. One drop of 1% hydroxyamphetamine (Paredrine®) dilates the normal pupil by releasing noradrenaline from the nerve ending into the synaptic cleft; absence of dilation signifies a lesion of the third neuron. Dilation lag occurs when the active dilation of the pupil is absent because of lack of sympathetic activity.
4. Postural hypotension. A fall in blood pressure of more than 30 mmHg systolic and more than 20 mmHg. diastolic on standing for 2 min is abnormal, although if the heart rate increases this may be evidence of reduced blood volume. The arm must be extended horizontally during the test. Orthostatic stress tests may accentuate abnormalities; have the patient do 12 squats (or take sublingual glyceryl trinitrite) and then repeat the blood pressure recording.
5. Isometric exercise (sustained handgrip) should increase systolic and diastolic blood pressures by 15 mmHg; heart rate and cardiac output should also increase.[1937]
6. **Cold pressor test**. The hand is immersed in ice water for 1 min, as a result of which the blood pressure should rise by 20/15 mmHg.
7. **Thermoregulatory sweat test**. The naked patient is heated by more than 1°C, and that area of the skin painted with alizarin-red which has changed color is measured. This test assesses the postganglionic sympathetic (cholinergic) activity.[3929] Quinizarin[1650, 2648] was formerly used.
8. Supine noradrenaline and vanillylmandelic acid levels provide information about net postganglionic adrenergic activity. With preganglionic lesions, supine noradrenaline levels are normal but there will be no response to standing.
9. **Psychogalvanic response**. This test assesses a polysynaptic, postganglionic,

somatosympathetic reflex pathway, skin voltage changing in response to emotion, an electrical shock, or an inspiratory gasp.[3930]

10. **Quantitative sudomotor axon reflex test** (Q-SART). A 10% solution of acetylcholine is iontophoresed into the skin of the proximal foot and medial forearm for 10 mA-min. This will produce sweating within 1–2 min in preganglionic but not in postganglionic sympathetic disorders.
11. Intradermal acetylcholine injection leads normally to a sweating response. This test and the preceding test assess postganglionic sympathetic sudomotor function.[169, 1906]
12. Silastic imprint. Pilocarpine is iontophoresed over skin covered with silastic, which is marked by each sweat droplet.[3386]
13. Skin vasomotor reflexes. In this test, the skin blood flow is measured by a laser Doppler flowmeter in the toe or finger pads. The stimulus employed may be an inspiratory gasp, contralateral cold stimulation, the response to standing, or the Valsalva maneuver.[3928]
14. **Venoarteriolar reflex**. A local axon reflex, relying on postganglionic sympathetic C fiber activity which normally increases total peripheral resistance. Reflex arteriolar constriction should reduce the blood flow by half in response to a rise in venous transmural pressure of more than 25 mmHg, as by lowering the leg 40 cm.
15. Baroreflex activity. The alteration in heart rate with sudden or sustained changes in blood pressure is assessed.[3929]

Parasympathetic Division

1. One drop of 2.5% methacholine or 0.125% pilocarpine has no effect on a normal pupil but constricts one with pre- or postganglionic parasympathetic denervation (supersensitivity again).
2. **Sinus arrhythmia**. Beat-to-beat variation during respiration depends on cardiac parasympathetic activity. Normally, the heart beats faster (so the R-R interval shortens) toward the end of inspiration and beats slower (the R-R interval lengthens) toward the end of expiration. With normal vagal activity, the ECG recorded at six respirations per minute should demonstrate differences of 15 beats per minute (bpm) between inspiration and expiration. A change of less than 10 bpm suggests abnormal vagal activity.
3. **E:I ratio**. The mean of the longest R-R interval during expiration divided by the mean of the shortest R-R intervals during inspiration should be more than 1.2 in patients aged less than 40 years. The test is a modified way of expressing the beat-to-beat variation in heart rate with simple breathing.
4. **30:15 ratio**. The ratio of the R-R intervals at the 30th and the 15th beats after standing position following a period lyingdown. A ratio of greater than 1.03 is abnormal, and it suggests a lesion of the vagal pathway. The supine-to-erect heart rate normally increases by 11–29 bpm, the maximum usually occurring at the 15th beat and the heart slowing to a stable rate by the 30th beat. See also **pNN50**.
5. Carotid sinus massage should cause bradycardia.
6. Atropine, 1 mg IV, should increase heart rate by 30–40 bpm.
7. **Valsalva ratio**. This is an expression of the maximum heart rate generated by a Valsalva maneuver (blowing against 40 mmHg for 15 s) divided by the minimum rate occurring within 30 s of the maximum rate. The ratio of the longest to the shortest R-R interval should be 1.45 in young people. This is more accurately measured invasively.
8. The bulbocavernosus reflex and anal sphincter tone can be assessed with specialized instrumentation.

Invasive tests including measurements of skin blood flow during mental arithmetic or with an inspiratory gasp, hot/cold stimulation, or radiant heating need a well-tuned autonomic laboratory. The tests currently most favored have been reviewed.[8]

autonomic ganglionopathy

See **autonomic neuropathy**.

autonomic hyperreflexia

See **autonomic dysreflexia, Head-Riddoch syndrome**.

autonomic nervous system

(vegetative nervous system) A division of the nervous system responsible for the automatic regulation of all the other systems of the body. Its existence was known to Galen, who regarded the sympathetic chain and the ninth, tenth, and eleventh nerve complex as forming the sixth nerve in his classification. He was also aware of the superior cervical ganglion and the rami communicantes.

It was Eustachius (1524–1574) who differentiated the vagus from the sympathetic, but the relative functions of the two systems were not considered until **Pourfour Du Petit** (1644–1741) sectioned the sympathetic chain in a dog and observed the resulting features of Horner syndrome. **Remak** first described unmyelinated nerve fibers in 1838 and believed that they arose from the sympathetic chain. Kolliker, Claude **Bernard**, and **Brown-Séquard** each demonstrated sympathetic vasoconstrictor effects, while E.F. and E.H. Weber slowed the heart by vagal stimulation and introduced the concept of inhibition in the nervous system. Hering and Breuer discovered the pulmonary reflex resulting from inflation of the lung in 1868.

W.H. Gaskell (1874–1914) and John Newport Langley (1852–1925), working in Cambridge, described pre- and postganglionic neurons, noted the antagonistic functions of the sympathetic and parasympathetic systems (respectively exciting and inhibiting glandular and smooth muscle activity), and divided the autonomic system between the cranial (bulbar) and sacral parasympathetic and thoracolumbar sympathetic outflows. It was Langley who suggested the name *autonomic nervous system*.[45]

autonomic neuropathy

(acute autonomic neuropathy, acute pandysautonomia, autoimmune autonomic ganglionopathy, idiopathic autonomic neuropathy) The acute or subacute onset of pandysautonomia occurring usually over several weeks, often followed by recovery and usually unaccompanied by evidence of involvement of the central or peripheral nervous systems, preceding infection and other systemic disease. The condition is an immune-mediated disorder, possibly considered as a *variant form* of **acute inflammatory demyelinating polyneuropathy**. Antibodies to the nicotinic ganglionic acetylcholine receptor are frequently detectable and are responsible for the attack upon autonomic ganglia.[6534]

Clinically, lethargy, tiredness, orthostatic hypotension, blurred vision with pupillary paresis, anhidrosis, dry mouth, abdominal pain, constipation, urinary retention, and impotence are the usual features.[6294, 6638] *Pure cholinergic dysautonomia* has also been described.[4251]

Ropper et al.[5387] have defined diagnostic criteria for the *pure autonomic variant* of **acute inflammatory demyelinating polyneuropathy**, suggesting that progressive sympathetic and parasympathetic dysfunction over a period of up to 3 weeks in the absence of limb weakness, ophthalmoplegia, and ataxia with areflexia (or at least hyporeflexia) within the first week are required and that some improvement of some autonomic dysfunction should occur within 4 months. The laboratory abnormalities that confirm the diagnosis would be an elevated CSF protein concentration, normal (or virtually normal) motor nerve conduction studies, and abnormal sensory nerve conduction studies.

Generalized autonomic failure without evidence of sensory neuropathy may also be due to autoimmune autonomic ganglionopathy, as in **Sjögren syndrome**.[5506]

Neuropathies affecting the autonomic nervous system also occur as part of a more generalized affection as with diabetes, amyloidosis, porphyria, and the **hereditary sensory and autonomic neuropathies**, etc.[4251] and as a **paraneoplastic syndrome**.[5232] The National Dysautonomia Research Foundation http://www.ndrf.org/ is a site providing information on autonomic nervous system disorders.

Autonomic Neuroscience: Basic and Clinical (formerly the *Journal of the Autonomic Nervous System*) The official publication of the International Society for Autonomic Neuroscience. Web site: http://www.isanweb.org.

autonomic seizure An objectively documented and distinct alteration of autonomic nervous system function involving cardiovascular, pupillary, gastrointestinal, sudomotor, vasomotor, and thermoregulatory functions.

autonomic storm See **episodic autonomic dysreflexia**; **diencephalic autonomic seizures**.

Autonomic Symptom Profile A question bank assessing secretomotor function, male sexual dysfunction, urinary, gastrointestinal, pupillomotor, vasomotor and sleep functions, and reflex syncope.[6114]

autonomous bladder 1. (reflex neurogenic bladder) The state of the bladder following loss of all supraspinal inhibitory influences; the volume tolerated is reduced and reflex emptying occurs through a contracted sphincter. 2. (autonomous or paralytic neurogenic bladder) The state of the bladder deprived of lower motor neuron innervation or in the early stages of spinal shock; the bladder is flaccid and dilated, with dribbling incontinence through a lax sphincter and loss of voluntary control of the initiation or termination of voiding.

autophagy The localization of intracellular debris and organelles within membranes of the endoplasmic reticulum.

autoregulation The ability of the brain to maintain a constant cerebral blood flow despite changes in perfusion pressure by variation in size of precapillary resistance vessels (arterioles). A metabolic mechanism is likely, perhaps based on the release of adenosine or other vasodilator metabolites with incipient hypoxia. With fully relaxed smooth muscle, increases in transmural pressure cause passive widening of the lumen. If the smooth muscle is normally responsive, increased transmural pressure causes constriction and decreased pressure, dilatation. Maximum dilatation occurs below 60 and above 160 mmHg. (Below or above those levels, the perfusion rate follows the perfusion pressure; in other words, autoregulation is lost.)

With severe hypertension, the arterioles dilate maximally and the **blood-brain barrier** breaks down. Substances such as protein cross as a result of increased vesicular transport and endothelial disruption, not by opening of the tight junctions. The result is edema.

autoscopy The vision of oneself at a distance, most often occurring during REM sleep with lucid dreams and in association with sleep paralysis. The experience can also be produced experimentally by stimulation of the nondominant angular gyrus.

autosomal dominant acute necrotizing encephalopathy (ADANE) An incompletely penetrant genetic disorder mapped to chromosome 2, primarily affecting children who experience a sudden-onset encephalopathy 2 or 3 days after the onset of a febrile illness. Coma, seizures, and other neurological deficits comprise the initial presenting signs. The disorder is fatal in some patients; most recover from the coma but may experience mild to severe developmental regression, spastic quadriplegia, and mental retardation but half of the survivors experience a recurrent encephalopathy with a worse outcome. During the acute episode FLAIR-MRI shows T2-weighted hyperintensities primarily in the thalamus and brainstem.[4611]

autosomal dominant cerebellar ataxia (ADCA, olivopontocerebellar atrophy) A group of spinocerebellar degenerations including what were once known as **Sanger-Brown** and **Marie ataxias** and **olivopontocerebellar**, **"primary" parenchymatous cerebellar cortical**, and **cerebellopontine atrophies**, with onset in young adult life. In these conditions, cerebellar and corticospinal features coexist variously with optic atrophy, involuntary movements (chorea, dystonia, or Parkinsonian features), lower motor neuron lesions, ptosis, myoclonus, bulbar palsy, pigmentary retinal degeneration, and/or ophthalmoplegia; sensory loss is not found.

Harding[2753] classified them as follows:

ADCA I Cerebellar ataxia associated with supranuclear ophthalmoplegia, optic atrophy, dementia, lower motor neuron lesions, and/or extrapyramidal features. Pathologically there is degeneration of the spinal cord, brainstem nuclei, and cerebellar afferent pathways. This class is genetically heterogeneous.

ADCA II Cerebellar ataxia, visual failure due to pigmentary retinal degeneration and sometimes dementia, and both pyramidal and extrapyramidal features

ADCA III A rare pure cerebellar ataxia with onset over the age of 50 years

ADCA IV Cerebellar ataxia with photosensitive myoclonus and deafness

A few rare, dominantly inherited forms remain: one with *periodic ataxic manifestations*, another *associated with essential tremor*, and others still whose various manifestations demonstrate that these disorders are essentially **multiple system degenerations**, potentially involving almost any part of the nervous system.

Yet other *variant forms* are autosomal or X-linked recessively inherited or occur sporadically.

autosomal dominant cerebellar atrophy with optic atrophy, progressive external ophthalmoplegia, dementia, extra-pyramidal signs, and lower motor neuron lesions See **Joseph disease**.

autosomal dominant chin tremor See hereditary quivering of the chin.

autosomal dominant cortical myoclonus and epilepsy See benign adult familial myoclonic epilepsy.

autosomal dominant episodic ataxia A heterogenous condition characterized by episodic ataxia and a clinical response to acetazolamide. In many cases nystagmus is also found. In various other kindreds, paroxysmal ataxia, paroxysmal choreoathetosis, and myotonia have been found.[2269]

autosomal dominant juvenile amyotrophic lateral sclerosis See amyotrophic lateral sclerosis.

autosomal dominant muscular dystrophy with humeropelvic distribution and cardiomyopathy See myopathies.

autosomal dominant myopathy with myofibrillar inclusions See myofibrillar myopathy.

autosomal dominant myopathy with proximal weakness and early respiratory muscle involvement A titinopathy with these clinical features.[4676]

autosomal dominant nocturnal frontal lobe epilepsy A dominantly inherited syndrome characterized by brief clusters of nocturnal seizures preceded by an aura lasting less than a minute, with onset in childhood or youth. Patients often present with a personal or familial history of parasomnia. Tonic spasms or hyperkinetic motor seizures occurring frequently at night are the usual phenotypes. Partial awareness may be maintained. Years of seizures are likely in most of these patients, at least until later adult life. Linkage to both 20q (OMIM 600513) and 15q (OMIM 603204) has been established. In the latter case, the syndrome presents with tonic hyperkinetic movements. The EEG is usually normal but frontal lobe epileptiform abnormalities may be seen, especially during sleep. The diagnosis of **parasomnia** or of **paroxysmal nocturnal dystonia** is often made if sleep EEGs are not performed.[5585, 4882, 5484]

All affected family members have nocturnal frontal lobe seizures. In some families, mutations in neuronal nicotinic acetylcholine receptor genes are found, but in many families the genetic etiology is unknown.[1861]

autosomal dominant "partial" epilepsy with auditory features See **familial temporal lobe epilepsies**.

autosomal dominant "partial" epilepsy with variable foci A syndrome with onset in childhood in which heterogeneous complex partial or secondarily generalized seizures occur in members of the same family, by day or night. Interictal EEGs are abnormal in the patients and in some asymptomatic relatives.[5585]

autosomal dominant rolandic epilepsy with speech dyspraxia A syndrome with the onset in early childhood of typical nocturnal rolandic seizures, centrotemporal spikes in the interictal EEG with the addition of speech dyspraxia and cognitive deterioration becoming more severe in subsequent generations as a result of anticipation.[5585]

autosomal dominant torsion dystonia See dopa-responsive dystonia.

autosomal recessive mitochondrial ataxic syndrome A progressive recessively inherited disorder due to mutations in *POLG*, starting with episodic symptoms including migraine-like headache or seizures, with the later development of ataxia and ophthalmoplegia. The seizures are usually focal with an occipital lobe origin; myoclonus and status epilepticus may occur.[6831]

autosomal recessive muscular dystrophy A severe and progressive recessively inherited muscular dystrophy characterized by the onset in childhood of proximal muscle weakness and atrophy affecting the girdle and truncal muscles predominantly. Joint contractures, pseudohypertrophy, scoliosis, cardiomyopathy, calf hypertrophy, and markedly increased serum creatine kinase levels are other features.

The best-recognized form, also known as **adhalinopathy**, is characterized by at least near-complete absence of this muscle membrane protein with normal staining for dystrophin. The gene responsible is located on chromosome 17q. The clinical disorders reported range from severe childhood muscular dystrophy resembling **Duchenne dystrophy** (but seldom with cardiomyopathy and with a more benign course) to a late-onset syndrome of mild myopathic muscle weakness.[5018] Another form is due to a mutation at 13q, and is hardly distinguishable from **Duchenne dystrophy** except for the absence here of mental retardation and the occurrence of the disorder mainly (so far) in Tunisian patients.[502] See also **severe childhood autosomal recessive muscular dystrophy**.

There is marked variability in the intensity of symptoms and severity of the course of the disease between siblings.[2714] See also **limb-girdle muscular dystrophy**, **myopathies**.

autosomal recessive sensory neuropathy. See hereditary sensory neuropathy.

autotopagnosia Impairment in the localization and naming of one's own body parts, described by **Pick** in 1908.

Avellis, Georg (1864–1916) German laryngologist.

Avellis syndrome (ambiguospinothalamic syndrome) Paralysis of one vocal cord and the pharynx and soft palate on the same side (tenth cranial nerve) with contralateral hemianesthesia. This is due to a lesion of the medullary tegmentum affecting the vagal nuclei and the spinothalamic tract, or from a lesion at the jugular foramen. A **Horner** syndrome or contralateral spinothalamic tract deficits may be associated.[305]

In the original cases, only the IX and X cranial nerves were affected, and the lesion was most likely at the jugular foramen; but the more generalized effects of a medullary lesion are now regarded as appropriately included with this condition.

average potential reference (Goldman-Offner reference) An average of the potentials of all or of many EEG electrodes, used as a reference.

averaging A method for extracting time-locked potentials from random background noise by sequentially adding traces and dividing by the total number of traces.

aviation neurology The branch of neurology concerning fitness to fly in an airplane as aircrew or passenger. Guidelines for fitness status were compiled by a committee of the American Medical Association and published in 1979.

Avicenna (980–1036) Persian physician and Islamic philosopher. His book on the laws of medicine was published in Arabic and, when translated into Latin, served as a basic textbook for medicine in Europe until the eighteenth century. In it he described facial palsy, trigeminal neuralgia, and perhaps hemifacial spasm and also introduced the word *epilepsy*.[161]

AVM Support Group An academically based site providing information on such conditions. Web-site: http://neurosurgery.mgh.harvard.edu/Interventional/AVMspt.htm.

awakening The return to the polysomnographically defined awake state from any nonrapid eye movement stage or from rapid eye movement sleep, characterized by the appearance of α and β waves on the EEG, tonic EMG activity, voluntary eye movements, and eye blinking.[280] See also **arousal**.

awakening grand mal An epileptic syndrome, representing a form of primary generalized epilepsy of adolescence, characterized by the onset, after the age of 8 years (usually in the mid-teen years) of primary generalized seizures, occurring mainly in the half hour following awakening but sometimes also during sleep. Seizures are easily provoked by deprivation of sleep and by photic stimulation. See also **juvenile myoclonic epilepsy**.

Axelrod sensory neuropathy with skeletal dysplasia A congenital dysmorphic syndrome characterized by skeletal deformities, absent or sparse tears, seizures, sensory and autonomic neuropathy, and craniorachischisis.[381]

Axenfeld, Karl Theodor Paul Polycarpus (1867–1930) German ophthalmologist.

Axenfeld-Rieger anomaly A dominantly inherited syndrome characterized by hypoplasia of the anterior iris, partial absence of the eye muscles, proptosis, mild sensorineural deafness, short stature, hypertelorism, communicating hydrocephalus, and psychomotor retardation.[4992]

Axenfeld-Schurenberg syndrome (cyclic oculomotor paralysis) A congenital unilateral third cranial nerve palsy with mydriasis alternating with phases of pupillary constriction and contraction of muscles supplied by the third nerve, and thus leading to elevation of the upper lid and nasal deviation of the eye (although lateral deviation is also described).[311] See also **cyclic oculomotor palsy**.

axial dystonia Dystonia affecting the back and trunk, causing scoliosis, lordosis, tortipelvis, etc.

axial hyperkinesia Rocking at the hips in a to-and-fro movement, often with an element of pelvic thrusting. It is seen in some patients with dystonic states such as **tardive dyskinesia**.

axial myopia Congenital increase in the anteroposterior diameter of the eye, leading to the appearance of unilateral proptosis of up to 4 mm.[4822]

axial skeletal–neural dysraphic disorders Complex developmental malformations due to original paraxial mesodermal insufficiency affecting the formation of the axial basicranium and the elevation of the neural folds interfering with their closure. Three types are recognized, in which the skeletal, neural, and oropharyngeal elements are partially or totally unclosed (e.g., **anencephaly** and **occipital encephalocele**) or are closed but abnormal (e.g., **Chiari malformation**).[4078]

axial tonic seizures Seizures in which stiffening of the posterior neck muscles produces an erect posture of the head. Opening of the eyes and mouth, rigidity of the paraspinal and abdominal muscles, and apnea are other common characteristics.[2312]

axilemma (axolemma, Mauthner's sheath) The axon sheath. Ludwig Mauthner (1840–1894), a Bohemian ophthalmologist, described and so named it in 1882.

axilla (Gr, the point on which a wheel revolves + arm) The armpit.

axillary nerve palsy (circumflex nerve palsy) A mononeuropathy occurring particularly as a result of dislocation of the shoulder, leading to weakness and wasting of the deltoid and teres minor muscles and to a patch of numbness over the lateral aspect of the shoulder and upper arm.

axis The second cervical vertebra.

axis cylinder (axon, Remak's band) The core and conducting element of the nerve fiber; the long extension of a neuronal cell body containing **microtubules**, **neurofilaments**, and **smooth endoplasmic reticulum**.

Robert Remak (1815–1865), a German physiologist and neurologist, described and named it in 1838.[5619]

axon The conducting element of the nerve trunk. See **axis cylinder**.

axon reaction See **chromatolysis**.

axon reflex (axon response, axon wave) A late response recorded from nerves after peripheral stimulation and disappearing when the stimulus is supramaximal. It may witness **ephaptic transmission** and is detected in neuropathies or after nerve injury.[2240] See also **A wave**.

axon reflex test Local vasodilation with the production of a flare normally follows a prick delivered through one drop of 1% histamine solution placed on the skin, indicating that the axons in that region are intact. See also **autonomic function tests**.

axon response A triple response in the skin, consisting of local vasodilatation, formation of a wheal, and further surrounding vasodilatation (the flare) occurring after the intradermal injection of 1% histamine acid phosphate or a strong local tactile stimulus. See also **axon reflex**.

It is present normally and in areas in which denervation has occurred as a result of preganglionic nerve lesions. With postganglionic nerve lesions, the response is not present in anesthetic regions, when it thus represents a hopeful prognostic sign.[742]

axon stains Histological enhancement methods used to demonstrate axons preferentially. These include the Bodian and Bielschowsky methods employing silver salts and a reducing agent. See also **myelin stains**.

axon wave See **axon reflex**.

axonal cross-talk See **ephaptic transmission**.

axonal degenerations Forms of neuropathy in which the basic fault is disruption of neuronal metabolism to the extent that axonal transport mechanisms fail. See also **Wallerian degeneration**.

axonal sensory neuropathy with antineurofilament (200 kDa) antibodies An acquired neuropathy of later adult life characterized by sensory loss in all modalities in the presence of monoclonal IgM antibodies targeting the neurofilament heavy chain.[4992] See also **opsoclonus-myoclonus.**

axonal sensory neuropathy with IgM binding to trisulfated heparin disaccharide A rare acquired axonal neuropathy of later adult life characterized by painful, distal, symmetrical sensory loss in most modalities, and areflexia, all in the presence of antibodies to trisulfated heparin disaccharide (TS-HDS).[4992]

axonal sheath Three concentric layers of tissue about the axon. From within outwards, these comprise the Schwann cells and two connective-tissue membranes, the neurilemma and the endoneurium. In some nerves, a layer of myelin is interposed between the Schwann cell layer and the axon.

axonal transport (axoplasmic transport) The process whereby constituents of the axoplasm pass both centrifugally from and centripetally toward the perikaryon. Two systems exist: the slow transport system is that process whereby the constituents of axoplasm such as **neurofilaments** and **microtubules** are delivered from the cell body down the axon to its terminal at rates of up to 3 mm/day; the fast system is bidirectional and carries substances of high molecular weight (small vesicles, mitochondria, and membrane-bound tubules) at speeds of up to 400 mm/day both toward and away from the cell body.

The existence of such a system was correctly surmised by Descartes, although he was unaware of the electrical properties of nerves.

axonopathy Disease of the axon, as opposed to disease primarily affecting the neuronal cell body (which is called **neuronopathy**). In the dying-back form, there is initial degeneration of the longer fibers with progression of the lesion from distal to proximal.

axonotmesis A lesion of a peripheral nerve producing discontinuity of axons, while the supporting structures of the nerve (Schwann tubes, endoneurium and perineurium) are more or less preserved. There is nevertheless such disturbance of the nerve fibers that true Wallerian degeneration occurs peripherally.

The condition represents one of the three types of nerve injury described by Seddon,[5705] the others being **neurapraxia** and **neurotmesis**.

axoplasm The circulating cytoplasm contained within the axonal tubes.

axorhizomelic tonic seizures A type of tonic seizure which begins in the same way as axial tonic seizures but which continues with tonic contraction of the proximal part of the contralateral arm, causing abduction and elevation of the semiflexed arm and shoulder.

axotomy, axonotomy See **axonotmesis**.

Ayala quotient (index) A formula for measuring the effect on the intraspinal pressure of removing a volume of CSF. Its value may correlate with the size of the cerebrospinal fluid reservoir but it finds little use today.

Ayer, James Bourne (1882–1963) Boston neurologist who described cisternal puncture and suggested the name **aseptic meningitis**.[3373]

Azorean disease (Azorean ataxia, Joseph disease). A dominantly inherited syndrome with **cerebellar ataxia**. See **Joseph disease**.

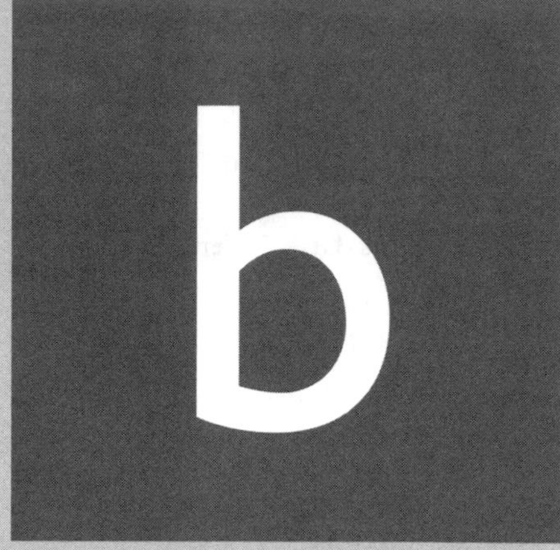

B cells Type B lymphocytes, the precursors of immunoglobulin-producing cells.

B waves Spontaneous oscillations of intracranial pressure of between 10 and 50 mmHg, occurring at 0.5–2 min intervals during sleep and in patients with periodic (**Cheyne–Stokes**) respirations. Their physiological mechanisms are not known.

Baastrup disease The presence of lumbar pain due to soft tissue disease affecting the interspinous ligaments and adjacent soft tissues.[318]

Babcock sentence "One thing that a nation must have to become rich and great is a large, secure supply of wood."

The inability to repeat exactly this rather pedestrian economic statement after three presentations was once considered a strong indication of impaired short-term memory, but three-item recall sequences are now preferred.

Babes nodules Collections of microglia in the nervous system, found in **rabies**.

Babiński, Josef-Francois-Felix (1857–1932) French neurologist of Polish descent who became *chef de clinique* under **Charcot**, following Pierre **Marie** and preceding Gilles de la **Tourette**. He did not succeed **Charcot** as professor at the Salpêtrière for internal political reasons, but instead led the neurology service at the Pitié, an adjacent Paris hospital, from 1895. He remained a bachelor, living with his older brother Henri, a gourmet of distinction.

Babiński regarded his work on spinal cord compression to be his best, but today his most lasting legacy is considered to be the sign bearing his name, which he described in 1896 (in 28 lines). He is also remembered for his definition of many cerebellar signs and for the introduction of the terms **dysdiadochokinesis** and **asynergia**; for the platysma, reinforcement, trunk-thigh, and **pronator signs**; and for the **Babiński–Frölich (adiposo-genital) syndrome** which he described in 1900, a year before Fröhlich. The **Babiński–Nageotte** and **Anton–Babiński** (anosognosia) **syndromes** also bear witness to his astonishing clinical perspicacity. It is also remembered that he pointed out that the hysterical symptoms of many patients at the Salpêtrière died with Charcot. He was an early proponent of the use of the reflex hammer.

Babiński attracted many important neurologists from abroad to his service, but his failure to gain appointment at the **Salpêtrière** reduced his influence within France, although he was a founder of the Société de Neurologie, edited the *Revue Neurologique*, and was elected to the Parisian Academy of Medicine in 1914. In the end, dispassionately, from abroad, he was properly regarded as the most outstanding of all the pupils of Charcot.[3097] Like Henry **Head**, he died from complications of **Parkinson disease**.

Babiński signs 1. Described by Babiński as "the phenomenon of the toes," the sign consists of the upward (dorsiflexion or extension) movement of the hallux with uncomfortable or painful stimulation of the sole of the foot, while the normal response would be for the toes to move downward. As he noted in his original[321] or in later papers published between 1896 and 1903, flexion at the hip and knee, ankle dorsiflexion, and fanning of the toes ("signe de l'éventail") may also occur.

The (upgoing toe) sign is present in the presence of a disturbance in the pyramidal system, regardless of its duration, intensity, or extent. It represents a part of the flexor reflex in humans.

Marshall **Hall, Vulpian,** and **Strumpell** had previously noted this phenomenon and

Remak had described extension of the hallux on plantar stimulation in transverse myelitis 3 years before, but Babiński investigated the phenomenon in depth, principally in an attempt to distinguish organic from hysterical weakness, and deserves the eponym. Some reports show him using a feather, but his words indicate that he elicited the sign by pricking the skin of the sole.[321]

Numerous other methods of eliciting the sign (**Chaddock, Bing, Oppenheim, Gordon, Thomas, Stransky**, etc.) have also been described and are complementary but rather less useful.[6496]

2. Diminution or absence of the Achilles' reflex in sciatica. Babiński introduced the preferred method of examining the reflex, the patient kneeling on a chair.

3. Fanning of the toes on the side on which there is clinical evidence of a pyramidal lesion, when the supine patient attempts to sit up.

4. Greater contraction of the platysma on the healthy than on the affected side in hemiparesis, tested by getting the patient to open the mouth wide or to try to whistle.

5. (**pronator sign**) Increased pronation of the paretic arm in hemiparetic states, such that when the examiner places the patient's hands in a position of supination, only the hand on the side affected returns to the pronated position.

6. Pupillary changes with aortic aneurysms.[322] See **Horner syndrome**.

7. Paradoxical raising of the eyebrow on the side of hemifacial spasm as a result of contraction of the frontalis muscle as well as the orbicularis oculi.[324] Possibly this is better recalled as the brow-lift sign.[6014]

Babiński trunk-thigh test (combined flexion phenomenon) If the recumbent patient with leg weakness is asked to sit up with his arms flexed his chest, the legs may move as follows:

- Involuntary flexion of the paretic limb occurs in organic hemiplegia; the heel may lift off the examining table.
- Involuntary flexion of both limbs occurs in organic paraplegia.
- Only the normal leg is flexed in hysterical hemiparesis.
- Neither leg is flexed in hysterical paraparesis.

Thus an unusual situation obtains, namely that the retention of some movement denotes the presence of organic disease.

Babiński–Fröhlich syndrome (pituitary tumor without acromegaly but with arrest of genital development) See **Fröhlich syndrome**.

Babiński–Froment syndrome Post-traumatic paralysis with hypotonia and hyporeflexia but also with excessive mechanical excitability. A syndrome of wartime, with an uncertain basis.[326]

Babiński–Nageotte syndrome (medullary tegmental paralysis, combined lateral and medial medullary syndrome) A paramedian pontomedullary lesion causing homolateral **Horner syndrome**; ipsilateral weakness of the soft palate, pharynx, larynx, and tongue; loss of taste of the posterior third of the tongue; cerebellar ataxia with nystagmus; and contralateral hemiparesis and hemianesthesia.[327] The **Cestan–Chenais syndrome** is almost identical.

Babiński–Weil Test The blindfolded patient with a unilateral vestibular disorder, when asked to take 10 steps forward and 10 backward, deviates to the right while walking forward and to the left going backward, or vice versa. This gait pattern has been termed *star walking*.

Babkin reflex (hand–mouth reflex) Opening of the mouth and flexion of the forearm and the neck when the palm of a normal infant is pressed. The reflex is normally present until the fourth month of life.

backaveraging Averaging a signal which occurs in a time epoch preceding a triggering event; often used to extract a time-locked EEG signal preceding voluntary or involuntary movement, usually triggered by the onset of the EMG activity of the movement. An example is the **Bereitschaftspotential**. (From the 2001 Report of the Nomenclature Committee of the American Association of Electromyography and Electrodiagnosis.[19] Reproduced by kind permission of the AANEM.)

backfiring The discharge of an antidromically activated motor neuron.

background activity 1. Any EEG activity representing the setting in which a given normal or abnormal pattern appears and from which such pattern is distinguished. This is not, however, a synonym for any individual rhythm such as the alpha rhythm. (Adapted from the 1974 Report of the Committee on Terminology, IFCN.[1117] Copyright 1974, with the kind permission of Elsevier Science.)

2. In electromyography, no background activity is normally recorded unless the needle tip is close to a motor end plate. See **end-plate noise**.

back-handing The process of arising from the squatting position with the aid of the hands placed on the floor beside and behind the feet to give a push upward; a sign of mild pelvic girdle weakness. See also **Gowers signs**.

back-kneeing Locking of the knee in hyperextension, a posture adopted by patients with quadriceps weakness in order to prevent sudden flexion at the joint while walking or standing.

back-up saccades See **catch-up saccades**.

Badal, Jules (1840–1929) French neuro-ophthalmologist, the first holder of a chair in that subject in France (at Bordeaux). He was at first a soldier, being decorated in the field during the Franco-Prussian war, but left the army for medicine. He published in 1888 a description of his patient Valerie, who developed a posteclamptic state of visual disorientation with features of what is now known as **Gerstmann syndrome**.

Badal–Gerstmann syndrome See **Gerstmann syndromes**.

BADS syndrome The association of a loss of the **Bell phenomenon** with **corneal anesthesia** and a dry eye in a patient with VII cranial nerve palsy, leading to traumatic corneal damage.

Baer nystagmus See **reflex sensory nystagmus**.

Baetz–Greenwalt syndrome A congenital dysmorphic syndrome characterized also by microcephaly, holoprosencephaly, or arhinencephaly and by congenital cardiac anomalies.[381]

bag fibers Intrafusal muscle fibers of two types, one reacting to the velocity and acceleration of stretch and the other to the acceleration of the stretching force.

Bailey, Pearce (1902–1976) American neurologist, who trained in medicine at Princeton and Columbia, receiving also a Ph.D. in psychology from the Sorbonne, before training in neurology at Bellevue Hospital in New York. His later clinical post was as professor at Georgetown University. He was the first director of the National Institute of Neurological and Communicative Disorders and Stroke, where he organized an intensive program of research into seizure disorders, multiple sclerosis, muscular disease, perinatal disease, and diseases of the eye and ear, training and assisting the careers of many now-prominent scholar-neurologists. With **Cushing** he classified malignant cerebral tumors in 1926.

Bailey was a founder of the World Federation of Neurology and both nationally and internationally was prominent in the organization of associations dedicated to the furtherance of social, research, or clinical goals within the neurological sciences. The Pearce Bailey medal and prize of the Epilepsy Foundation of America were created in his honor.

Bailey, Perceval (1892–1973) American neurosurgeon, anatomist, and scholar who trained in medicine at Chicago and Northwestern Universities and then studied with **Cushing** at Harvard, in Chicago and in Paris. Returning to Harvard, he embarked upon a study of cerebral tumors, which culminated in his classification of gliomas, completed while working under Cushing, who, in the tradition of nineteenth-century European schools, published it himself in 1926. Bailey continued to collaborate with Cushing on tumor classification but returned to the University of Chicago in 1928 where he became head of the Department of Neurology and Neurosurgery. His major work was *Intracranial Tumors of Infancy and Childhood* (1939), published in collaboration. He transferred to the University of Illinois in 1940, where he continued his work until retirement.[7]

Bailey–Cushing tumor See **medulloblastoma**.

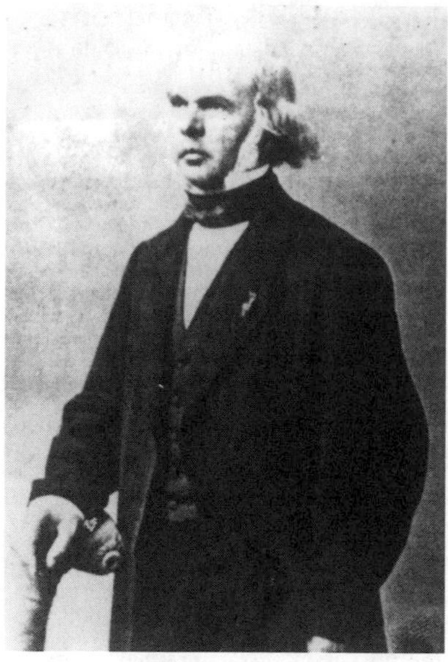

Figure B–1 Jules-Gabriel-Francois Baillarger.

Baillarger, Jean-Gabriel-Francois (1809–1890) An outstanding figure in French neurology and psychiatry in the nineteenth century. He worked at the Salpêtrière from 1840, whence he described the cycles of manic-depressive illness and melancholic stupor and wrote extensively on hallucinations, syphilis; brain anatomy, etc., until his retirement in 1870.[337, 338]

Baillarger lines The bands of fibers visible to the naked eye in sections of the occipital cortex. The striae Gennarii are such laminations. Six layers were described by Baillarger, a finding later confirmed histologically by **Remak**.

Baillarger sign Unilateral dilatation of the pupil in tertiary syphilis, for which neither Baillarger nor anyone else has adduced a satisfactory explanation.[337]

Baillarger syndrome See **Frey syndrome**.

Baillarger–Jackson principle The ability of aphasic patients to enunciate words involuntarily which they cannot utter at will.[92] The phenomenon puts one in mind of the words of Dr. Samuel Johnson: "Things too silly to be said may yet be sung."

Baillie, Matthew (1761–1823) Scottish morbid anatomist who gave the first accounts of cerebral pathology.

Bainbridge, Francis Arthur (1874–1921) English physiologist who was professor of physiology successively at Durham and at St. Bartholemew's hospital in London.[1972] His best-remembered work was that showing that cardiac acceleration occurs as a result of inhibition of vagal tone, as by an increase in blood pressure or distension of the right atrium.

Bainbridge reflex Increased sympathetic activity with tachycardia in response to an increase in venous and in right atrial pressure, due to vagal inhibition.

Bajonet posture Hyperpronation and hyperflexion of the hands and feet with permanent dorsiflexion of the hallux (**pseudo-Babiński sign**), seen in some basal ganglion disorders such as the later stages of Parkinsonism and **pallidal atrophies**.

balance The maintenance of the upright posture during sitting, standing, and locomotion through the detection and correction of displacement of the individual's line of gravity beyond the base of support.

balanced amplifier An amplifier which consists of two identical single-ended amplifiers operated as a pair but in opposite phases.

Balci oculo-cerebral syndrome A congenital dysmorphic syndrome characterized by cloudy corneae or sclerocornea, microphthalmia, mental and developmental delay, seizures, microcephaly, and spasticity with aminoaciduria.[381]

balderdash syndrome A colloquial term for **Ganser syndrome**.

Balduzzi reflex Adduction and inward rotation of the contralateral leg in response to the vibration set up by a tap on the sole of the foot, present in normal subjects but increased in patients with pyramidal tract disease.

The sign was described in 1926 by Ottorino Balduzzi, an Italian neurologist at the University of Rome.[347]

Balint, Rudolf (1874–1929) Hungarian neurologist, professor at Budapest.

Balint syndrome 1. (Balint–Holmes syndrome, psychic paralysis of visual fixation, cortical paralysis of visual fixation) A rare syndrome resulting from bilateral parieto-occipital disease and characterized by inability to direct the eyes to a certain point in the visual field despite the retention of intact eye movements (ocular apraxia, psychic paralysis of gaze); **optic ataxia**, a disorder of visual reaching; inability to read; impaired depth perception and fluctuating visual inattention for any stimulus not exciting the macula (visual disorientation or **simultagnosia**).[3389]

Balint's patient had left-sided visual inattention but inability to perform directed movements with the right hand (his left-handed movements were faultless), suggesting a **disconnection syndrome**. Fragments of receptive aphasia, agraphia, and ideomotor apraxia may coexist.[350, 6426] See also **posterior cortical atrophy**.

2. Loss of all voluntary extra-ocular movements and pupillary paralysis with retention of reflex eye movements, seen in hyperthyroidism.[5704]

Balint–Holmes syndrome See **Balint syndrome**.

balking The increasingly angry refusal of demented patients to cooperate in the routine procedures of daily care.

Baller–Gerold syndrome (craniosynostosis and radial aplasia) A recessively inherited congenital syndrome characterized by craniosynostosis affecting the coronal suture, short stature, radial aplasia, and absent fingers.[351]

ballet dancer's foot A focal occupational dystonia affecting the foot muscles.[6035]

Ballet, Gilbert (1853–1916) French neurologist and psychiatrist who trained in Limoges and Paris, became Chef de Clinique to **Charcot**, rising through the ranks to professor of the history of medicine and then of mental diseases in 1908.

Ballet sign Retention of the pupillary reflexes despite external ophthalmoplegia in **dysthyroid ophthalmopathy**.

Ballet syndrome External ophthalmoplegia with paresis in the muscles supplied by the V, VII, and XII cranial nerves and by the vagus in patients with hyperthyroidism.[352]

ballism (ballismus) (from Gr, to dance) Extensive, vigorous, fast, poorly patterned, nonadaptive movements of the facial, limb, or truncal muscles. These violent, flinging, involuntary movements are due to lesions of the subthalamic nucleus of Luys, most often following a **lacunar stroke**.

Hemiballism is the term applied when the movements are unilateral, as is more common. *Paraballism* denotes bilateral ballism.

ballismic cerebral palsy An ill-defined form of cerebral palsy characterized by uni- or bilateral ballism affecting the arms or legs.

ballismus See **ballism**.

ballistic Not subject to modification after initiation.

ballistic movement overflow myoclonus A form of **essential myoclonus**, characterized by involuntary movements occurring in 50–100 min bursts of activity in the agonist muscle, accelerating a limb, followed by the same in the antagonist muscles (slowing it down) and then by further brief contraction in the agonist. The phenomenon has been described in patients with **familial essential myoclonus**.

This pattern differs from that occurring in *reticular* and in *cortical loop myoclonus*, in which the duration of the burst is only 10–30 min.[2698]

balloon cells Grossly distended neurons with displacement of the nucleus and Nissl substance to the periphery, as in the **gangliosidoses**, in which the undegraded gangliosides distend neuronal cell bodies.

balloon sickness A syndrome of limb and truncal paralysis, blindness, and subsequent loss of consciousness as a result of severe decompression. The first account was written in 1862, describing such symptoms in the context of a hot-air balloon ascent to 37 000 feet over central England. See **altitude insomnia**.

Baló, József Matayas (1895–1979) Hungarian pathologist who trained and worked in Budapest where he became chairman of the department of pathology and, for a period, dean of the medical school. He reported his case of concentric sclerosis in 1926.

Baló concentric sclerosis (encephalitis periaxialis concentrica) A rare subacute, progressive dysmyelinating disease, perhaps a variant of **multiple sclerosis**, described by Baló in Hungary in 1927. Bands of intact myelin alternating with zones of demyelination are found in the white matter especially of the frontal lobes, varying in size from 1 to 3 cm and arranged in irregular concentric rings, witnessing the patchy destruction of myelin with reformation at the edge of each large plaque and thus explaining the laminated appearance. The axons are intact within these foci.[353]

The clinical features include progressive spastic paralysis and other widely varying evidence of diffuse cerebral disease, with childhood onset.

Baltic myoclonus (Nordic myoclonus, Unverricht–Lundborg–Lafora syndrome) A recessively inherited form of **progressive myoclonic epilepsy**. The onset of the myoclonus and tonic-clonic seizures is between 8 and 13 years. Neurological signs such as gradual intellectual failure, dysarthria, ataxia, and intention tremor appear later. Absence and drop attacks sometimes occur. The myoclonus may be precipitated by movement, stress and sensory stimuli, and repetitive morning myoclonus is common. Survival into adult life is usual. The gene locus has been mapped to chromosome 21. The diagnostic feature of Lafora body disease is the PAS-positive inclusion body found in neurons throughout the gray matter of the brain including the dentate nucleus of the cerebellum and on biopsy of axillary skin, liver, or skeletal muscle.

The syndrome was first reported by Unverricht in 1891 and appears to occur mainly in the populations of eastern Sweden and Finland, determining the name.[6449] There is suggestive evidence that **dyssynergia cerebellaris myoclonica** is the same condition as this disease. See also **Unverricht–Lundborg-Lafora syndrome** (which differs only in a slightly older onset age and earlier onset of intellectual impairment).

Bamberger, H. von (1822–1888) German physician who trained in Prague and Vienna and later became professor of pathology first at Wurzburg and then at Vienna. In 1872 he described the findings now regarded as typical of **Pick disease**, as well as the disease next entered.

Bamberger disease (palmus) The sudden onset of clonic spasms of the legs, producing a jumping or springing motion. It was sometimes a manifestation of hysteria, sometimes of psychosis. Guttmann (1867), Frey (1875), and **Gowers**[2531] also wrote on the same condition, which they thought in at least some cases was organic. Bamberger also described **allocheiria**.

The author has seen one possible case but knows of no other report in the last century.[2529] See **saltatory spasm**.

band A portion of the frequency spectrum of the EEG, including the delta, theta, alpha, and beta bands.

band heterotopia A form of gray matter heterotopia in which there is premature arrest of gray matter migration, resulting in a symmetric band of subcortical gray matter, referred to as the "double cortex sign." There may be some associated cortical pachygyria. Clinically, patients manifest an age-related epileptogenic encephalopathy with multiple types of generalized seizures and progressive cognitive decline. Association with the *Lennox–Gastaut syndrome* has been reported.[398] See **diffuse cortical dysplasia**.

band keratopathy Horizontal ribbons of calcium deposition in the cornea and conjunctiva, occurring in hypercalcemic states.

bands of Büngner Chains of multiplying Schwann cells which act as templates for the regenerating axons following **Wallerian degeneration**.

bandwidth (EEG channel) The range of frequencies between which the response of an EEG channel is within stated limits. This is determined by the frequency response of the amplifier–writer combination and the frequency filters used. However, the manner in which the EEG channel bandwidth is specified by different manufacturers is not standardized.

Bannayan–Zonana syndrome A congenital dysmorphic syndrome characterized by mental and developmental delay, macrocephaly, an unusual frequency of brain tumors such as capillary or cavernous hemangiomas, subcutaneous lipomas, and musculoskeletal maldevelopment.[4356]

Bannwarth syndrome (lymphocytic meningo-radiculitis) Subacute or chronic lymphocytic meningitis due to tick-borne infection with *Borrelia burgdorferi* and presenting with severe radicular pain and sensory and motor signs associated with cranial nerve palsies, especially facial paralysis.[375] See **Lyme disease** (of which this is the European version).

Baraitser syndrome A craniofacial malformation syndrome characterized by cleft lip or palate, choroidal **colobomas**, seizures, mental retardation, short broad digits, and renal dysplasia.[382]

Bárány, Robert (1876–1936) Hungarian otologist, born in Vienna who studied medicine, psychiatry, and neurology in Austria and Germany. He was awarded the Nobel Prize in 1914 for his work on otovestibular physiology and medicine. Although working in Vienna as a physician, he was captured by the Russian forces in the Austro-Hungarian army during World War I (although he was himself a pacifist) and was interned as a prisoner, being released by the Czar to work in Uppsala at the behest of Prince Carl of Sweden.

His publications on the genesis of vertigo and on caloric testing have been disputed because he failed to give any credit to the contributions of his colleague Gustav Alexander.[359] He claimed to have been the first to note that nystagmus followed aural lavage and that the direction of the fast component was away from the cooled side, leading him to propose that the caloric response occurred as a result of the movement of fluid in the semicircular canals. His invention of the rotating chair was based upon his reasoning that gravitational forces would have the same effect.

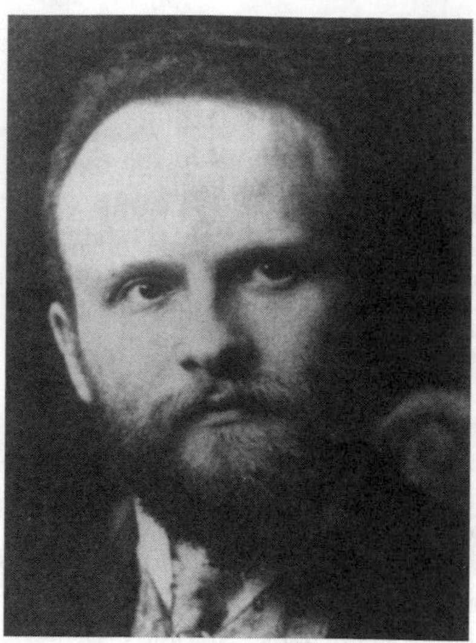

Figure B–2 Robert Bárány.

Bárány positional vertigo See **benign positional vertigo**.

Bárány sign Complete or partial reduction of the response of the labyrinth to caloric stimulation.

Bárány syndrome Unilateral posterior headache, periodic ipsilateral deafness, vertigo, tinnitus, and imperfect pointing.[384] See also **Ménière disease**.

Bárány Test 1. (*caloric test*) Production of nystagmus by irrigation of the external auditory meatus first with hot and then with cold water. Hot water irrigation leads to nystagmus with its fast component to the same side; with cold water irrigation, the fast component is to the opposite side. Reduction in the amplitude and duration of the nystagmus indicates the presence of labyrinthine disease. The test was introduced by Bárány in 1906.

2. (*pointing test*) The subject points to a stationary object first with the eyes open and then with them closed; deviation of the arm(s) only with the eyes closed suggests a posterior column lesion, while deviation both with the eyes open and with them closed suggests ipsilateral cerebellar or vestibular disease. In such conditions, the deviation of the arm is in the same direction as the slow component of any accompanying nystagmus.

3. (*chair test*) Rotation of a subject who is sitting on a chair wearing opaque lenses and with the head inclined 30° forward (in order to bring the horizontal semicircular canals into the true horizontal plane). With normal

labyrinthine function, horizontal nystagmus is produced in the direction opposite to the direction of rotation and lasts about 10–30 s.

Barbeau, André (1931–1986) Quebec neurologist, professor at the Université de Montreal, who trained in Chicago and Montreal and became a leading figure in Canadian Neurology as a result of his dynamic interest in neurogenetic diseases and movement disorders.

barber's chair sign See **Lhermitte sign**.

Barber syndrome A congenital dysmorphic syndrome characterized also by skeletal maldevelopment, mental and developmental delay, microcephaly, microphthalmia, ptosis and blepharophimosis, and spina bifida occulta.[381]

Bard sign Nystagmus due to an organic lesion increases in amplitude with fixation of a moving object, but with congenital nystagmus, this may cause the abnormal movements to cease.

Bardet, Georges (b. 1885) Parisian physician.

Bardet–Biedl Syndrome A recessively inherited syndrome manifesting obesity, severe pigmentary retinal dystrophy, renal failure, syndactyly, brachydactyly, and (less often) polydactyly.[390, 631]

It represents a variant form of **Laurence–Moon–Biedl syndrome**, from which it differs through the absence of spastic paraparesis. However, mental retardation, diabetes, congenital cardiac anomalies, multiple renal cysts, hydronephrosis, and hypogenitalism (males) or hypogonadism (females) are other features described.[2559, 2774]

baresthesia The sense of weight or graded pressure.

barkers See **dancing mania**.

Barkhof criteria A system used in the diagnosis of multiple sclerosis using MRI. One or more juxtacortical lesions, one or more enhancing lesions, one or more infraentorial lesions, and three or more periventricular lesions provide evidence for the diagnosis. A threshold of at least three positive criteria and substitution of the need for a gadolinium-enhanced lesion with the presence of nine or more T2 lesions has been proposed by Tintoré and is generally accepted.[397] See also **McDonald criteria**.

Barlow, Sir Thomas (1845–1945) London physician, who described **acute disseminated encephalomyelitis** following measles, in 1887.

Barnard–Scholz syndrome A syndrome of retinal degeneration and ophthalmoplegia of unknown cause; one of the original patients at least had syphilis, another had cerebellar signs.[408]

Reports that the condition resembles **Kjellin syndrome** appear mistaken, as spastic paraplegia was not a feature of the cases reported by Barnard and Scholz.

Barnes myopathy See **limb-girdle muscular dystrophy**.

barognosis The ability to discriminate between weights using the cutaneous, muscle, tendon, and joint senses. Disturbance of the faculty was investigated by Gordon **Holmes** after 1910, who determined that subjects with unilateral cerebellar disease tend to overestimate weights placed in the ataxic hand. Parietal lesions may also be responsible.

baroreceptors Specialized detectors of pressure change situated in the carotid sinus and aortic arch and relaying information to the nucleus tractus solitarius along the IX cranial nerve. Increase in blood pressure leads to reflex bradycardia and decrease in both peripheral resistance and myocardial contractility.

baroreflex The arterial baroreflex maintains ongoing control over arterial blood pressure, sensing and buffering its acute increases or decreases. It is mediated by the IX and X cranial nerves through their influences upon peripheral arterial resistance (sympathetic) and cardiac rate (vagal parasympathetic). Failure of the baroreflex can lead to hypertensive crises, **malignant vagotonia** and (less often) orthostatic tachycardia or episodic labile hypertension. Disorders of the carotid sinus in the neck or of the tractus solitarius in the brainstem are the more likely causes. (For a full review, see Benarroch, EE. The arterial baroreflex. *Neurology* 2008;71;1733–1738).

baroreflexes Alterations in blood pressure as a result of stimulation of the baroreceptors in the great vessels of the neck, buffering changes in arterial blood pressure in order to avoid excessive fluctuations; thus they mediate the blood pressure response to standing, carotid sinus compression, etc.[2576]

baroreflex failure syndrome A syndrome of labile or sustained hypertension alternating with hypotension, and tachycardia resulting from lesions of the carotid sinus, of its afferent pathways, or of the brainstem. Sweating, flushing, headache, and emotional lability are other symptoms recorded.

Tachycardia occurs with such stresses as the ice-water immersion test and bradycardia with sedation; but hypotension resulting from nitroprusside infusion does not cause tachycardia, nor does phenylephrine-induced hypertension lead to bradycardia. Generalized autonomic failure is seldom an accompaniment.[5330]

barotrauma The effects on the body of alterations in atmospheric pressure, as with deep-water diving or ascent to high altitudes. The sinuses, middle ears, nervous system, and skin are especially affected in the various syndromes.[1611]

Barré, J.A. (1880–1967) French physician who interned with **Babiński** in Paris and worked with **Guillain** during World War I. He became professor of neurology in Strasbourg in 1919, working largely on vestibular functions.

Barré signs 1. The patient, lying prone with the knees flexed, is unable to keep the lower leg vertical on the side of a pyramidal lesion. 2. Downward drift of the outstretched arm when affected by a pyramidal lesion. 3. (straight arm raising) When the patient extends his arms parallel to the floor with the forearm pronated, the wrist dorsiflexed, and the fingers extended and abducted, failure to maintain that position for 1 min suggests the presence of a pyramidal lesion. Although attributed to Barré, Mingazzini actually described it first.

Barré syndrome (Barré–Lieou syndrome, posterior cervical sympathetic syndrome) Occipital headache, corneal ulceration with pain in the eyes and also in the ears, vertigo, tinnitus, vasomotor disorders, and facial spasm, thought to be due to irritation of the sympathetic plexus on the vertebral artery in patients with rheumatism of the cervical spine.

The condition was first described in 1928 in the thesis of Dr. Y.C. Lieou, a student of Barré in Strasbourg. Also see **acceleration injury syndrome**,[419] **whiplash**, and **cervical migraine**.

Barré–Lieou syndrome See Barré syndrome.

Barrow Neurological Institute A nonprofit neurological research institution. Address: 305 W. Thomas Rd., Phoenix, AZ 85013, USA. Tel: 602-285-3186.

Barry–Albright Dystonia Scale An instrument assessing spasticity in children with cerebral palsy.[423]

Bartel nystagmus See induced nystagmus.

bartender's sign Extension of the shoulder so that the elbow is pulled backward—a trick used by patients with weakness of the biceps to resist the examiner's attempt to extend the elbow.

The name derives from the pulling movement made by bartenders who draw beer from a barrel in the old-fashioned way (by suction rather than with the benefit of compressed air).

Barth syndrome An X-linked dilated cardiomyopathy linked to chromosome Xp28 (allelic with X-linked fatal infantile cardiomyopathy) and due to a mutation on the Tafazzin protein. The clinical features include onset in infancy with mild and nonprogressive hypotonia, learning disability, and lethal dilated cardiomyopathy.

A variant is Barth-like syndrome with mtRNA Leu mutations, which may be either progressive or self-limiting. See http://www.neuro.wustl.edu/.

Barthel Index of Activities of Daily Living A reliable 10-item instrument for the assessment by an observer of a patient's actual abilities in self- care and ambulation, of particular use in assessing the degree of dependence in the elderly.[3894, 4024] A score of greater than 60 correlates with eventual return to home and of greater than 95 indicates independent self-care. The drawback to the Barthel Index is its lack of inclusion of cognitive and language function. A five-item short form (rating transfers, bathing, use of the toilet, stair climbing, and mobility) has also been validated.[2926] The scale can be viewed online at http://www.dundee.ac.uk/medther/Stroke/Scales/barthel.htm. See Chart B–1.

Chart B–1. Barthel Index of Activities of Daily Living

Self-care Index

1. Drinking from a cup
2. Eating
3. Dressing upper body
4. Dressing lower body
5. Putting on brace or artificial limb
6. Grooming
7. Washing or bathing
8. Urinary incontinence
9. Bowel incontinence

Mobility Index

10. Getting into and out of chair
11. Getting onto and off the toilet
12. Getting into and out of a bathtub or shower
13. Walking 50 yards on level surface
14. Walking up/down one flight of stairs
15. Propelling or pushing wheelchair (if unable to walk)

In using the scale, one should aim to record what the patient actually DOES do in daily life, not what he/she can do. The score reflects the degree of INDEPENDENCE from help provided by another person: if supervision is required, the patient is NOT independent, if aids and devices are used but no help is required, the patient IS independent. Use the best available evidence, asking the patient or relatives, carers, nurses, and therapists and using common sense. Observing the patient is helpful, but direct testing is NOT necessary. Middle categories imply that the patient supplies over 50% of the effort. Ask about abilities before admission or acute illness, and enter in *the column marked "Estimate of previous score."*

Bowels

2 Continent (for preceding week).
1 Occasional accident (once a week or less).
0 Any worse grade of incontinence (or needs enemas for continence).

Bladder

2 Continent (for preceding week) or able to manage any device (e.g., catheter, bag) without help.
1 Occasional accident (once a day or less), or catheterized and needs help with device.
0 Any worse grade of incontinence.

Feeding, food placed within reach by others

2 Able to cut up food, spread butter, etc., without help
1 Needs some help cutting or spreading
0 Needs to be fed.

Grooming

1 Independent washing face, combing hair, shaving, and cleaning teeth (when implements are provided).
0 Needs help.

Dressing

2 Independent putting on all clothes, including fastening buttons, zips, etc. (Clothes may be adapted).
1 Needs some help, but can do at least half.
0 Needs more help than this.

Transfer, bed to chair and back

3 Needs no help.
2 Needs minor help, verbal or physical: can transfer with one person easily, or needs supervision.
1 Needs major help: two people or one strong/trained person, but can sit unaided.
0 Cannot sit; needs skilled lift by two people (or hoist).

Toilet use

2 Able to get on and off toilet or commode, undress and dress sufficiently, and wipe self without physical or verbal help.
1 Needs some help, can wipe self, and do some of the rest with minimal help only.
0 Needs more help than this.

Mobility around house or ward, indoors

3 May use aid (stick or frame, etc., but not wheelchair).
2 Needs help of one person, verbal or physical, including help standing up.
1 Independent in wheelchair, including able to negotiate doors and corners unaided.
0 Needs more help than this.

Stairs

2 Independent up and down, and can carry any necessary walking aid.
1 Needs help, verbal or physical or help carrying aid.
0 Unable.

Bathing

1 Able to get in and out of bath or shower, wash self without help (may use any aids).
0 Unable.

From Mahoney FI, Barthel D. Functional Evaluation: The Barthel Index. Maryland State Med J *1965;14:56–61. Reproduced with permission.*

Modifications to this part of the instrument (mainly as regards scoring) have been suggested. See also **Functional Impairment measure, Functional Independence measure, stroke scales, disability scales, Katz activities of daily living index, Nottingham 10-point Activities of Daily Living index, Rivermead Activities of Daily Living Scale.**

Bartschi-Rochaix syndrome See **cervical migraine**.

basal cell nevus syndrome A chromosomal disorder characterized by mental retardation, frontal and biparietal bossing, hypertelorism, basal cell nevi, and an increased frequency of **medulloblastomas** or **astrocytomas**.[2507]

basal electrode An electrode placed close to the base of the skull, such as nasopharyngeal and sphenoidal electrodes.

basal ganglia The term of Gowers (1885) for the deep cerebral nuclei concerned with the elaboration of motor activity and including the caudate, putamen and globus pallidus, substantia nigra, subthalamic nucleus, and amygdala. These he referred to as the "dark basement of the brain."

basal ganglion calcification with mental retardation and steatorrhea A rare syndrome with these features. See also **striato-pallidal calcification, bilateral occipital calcification, epilepsy**, and **celiac disease**.

basal ganglion disorders A popular inclusive term for those syndromes which manifest, *inter alia*, athetosis, ballism, chorea, dystonia, or Parkinsonism.

basal ganglion "epilepsy" Paroxysmal **dystonias** lasting a few seconds or minutes only. Despite the (old) name, the movements do not represent epilepsy nor seizures at all.

basal vein of Rosenthal A neuroradiological landmark, the basal cerebral vein is a tributary of the internal cerebral vein. It was described by Friedrich Rosenthal (1780–1829), a German anatomist.

basal-frontal syndrome See **Foster Kennedy syndrome**.

Basedow, Karl Adolph von (1799–1854) German physician.

Basedow disease Exophthalmic goiter, described by Basedow in Germany in 1840, but in England by **Graves** 5 years and by **Parry** 15 years previously.

Basedow paraplegia A subacute areflexic motor polyneuropathy affecting the legs in patients with hyperthyroidism, with sparing of sphincter functions.[1162] The attribution to Basedow was made by Charcot.[1986]

That this entity and **acute inflammatory demyelinating polyneuropathy** are different conditions remains uncertain. Proximal myopathy is another complication with a similar presentation. See **hyperthyroidism**.

baseline (isoelectric line) 1. (EEG) Strictly, a line obtained when an identical voltage is applied to the two input terminals of an EEG amplifier or when the instrument is in the calibrate position, but no calibration signal is applied. 2. Colloquially, an imaginary line corresponding to the approximate mean value of all the EEG activity assessed visually in an EEG derivation over a period of time. (Adapted from the 1974 report of the Committee on Terminology, IFCN. In: Chatrian GE, Bergamini L, Dondey M, et al. A glossary of terms most commonly used by clinical electroencephalographers. *EEG Clin Neurophysiol* 1974;**37**:538–48. Reproduced by kind permission of the IFCN and Elsevier Science.) 3. A potential recorded from a biologic system while it is at rest. 4. A flat trace on the recording instrument. (From the 2001 Report of the Nomenclature Committee of the American Association of Electromyography and Electrodiagnosis.[19] Reproduced by kind permission of the AANEM.)

basilar (Gr, arising from the base of a thing) Term denoting its Greek derivation.

basilar artery migraine See **basilar migraine**.

basilar impression (basilar invagination) A deformity of the base of the skull, consisting of an elevation into the cranial cavity of a variable part of the bony rim of the foramen magnum, not always associated with an increase in the basal angle of the skull and thus not quite the same as **platybasia**.[5980] The condition was first described by Ackerman in 1790, but this term was first used by Berg and Retzius in 1855. A violation by at least 6.6 mm of the **Chamberlain line** by the odontoid process of the axis process defines basilar invagination.

The upward movement of the rim of the foramen magnum causes the floor of the posterior fossa to rise up so that the upper cervical spine invaginates the posterior fossa, thus diminishing its volume. The basal angle of the skull (Weckler's angle, normally 132–145°) is increased to over 150°. The importance of measuring this angle is now rather less since diagnosis is more readily made with MRI scanning.

Invagination is common in conditions marked by softening of the bones, such as Paget disease, osteomalacia, and rickets; is associated with shortness of the neck; and may lead to local pain, raised intracranial pressure, bilateral cerebellar disturbance, interference of the function of the lower cranial nerves, or high spinal cord compression.[4731] See also **platybasia**.

basilar insufficiency See **vertebrobasilar insufficiency**.

basilar invagination See **basilar impression**.

basilar-type migraine (basilar artery migraine, Bickerstaff migraine, syncopal migraine, vertebrobasilar migraine). Migraine with typical aura symptoms clearly originating from the brainstem or cerebellum or from both hemispheres but without motor weakness. The headache is preceded by symptoms of dysfunction in vertebro-basilar territory, including alteration of consciousness in the form of stupor or coma. See also **migraine-coma**. Diagnostic criteria have been defined:

A. At least two attacks fulfilling criteria B–D
B. Aura consisting of at least two of the following fully reversible symptoms but no motor weakness:
   1. Dysarthria
   2. Tinnitus
   3. Hypacusis
   4. Diplopia
   5. Visual symptoms simultaneously in both temporal and nasal fields of both eyes
   6. Ataxia
   7. Decreased level of consciousness
   8. Simultaneously bilateral paresthesias
C. At least one of the following:
   1. At least one aura symptom develops gradually over ≥5 min and/or different aura symptoms occur in succession over ≥5 min
   2. Each aura symptom lasts ≥5 and <60 min
D. Headache fulfilling criteria B–D for **migraine without aura** begins during the aura or follows aura within 60 min
E. Not attributed to another disorder

Adapted from the International Classification of Headache Disorders (Headache Classification Committee of the International Headache Society. *Cephalalgia* 2004;**24[Suppl** 1]) by kind permission of Dr. Jes Olesen, the International Headache Society and Wiley-Blackwell Publications.

The condition is characterized by signs compatible with ischemia in the territory of the posterior circulation, presumably on the basis of migrainous vasospasm, occurring typically in adolescent and preadolescent females. The attacks usually last less than 1 h and usually precede a severe migrainous headache. Common symptoms include bilateral scintillating visual scotomata, ataxia, nausea, and vomiting. Rarer symptoms are nystagmus and decreased hearing. Bickerstaff's description,[620] published in 1961, has not been equalled.

A *variant* is the combination of *basilar migraine*, *seizures*, and *severe epileptiform EEG abnormalities*. This is a benign syndrome in adolescents characterized by the occurrence of rare focal or generalized seizures and rhythmic temporo-occipital spike wave complexes in association with the clinical features of basilar migraine as detailed above.[987] Whether this is the same condition as **benign occipital epilepsy of childhood** or is different remains undetermined.

basket brain A developmental abnormality characterized by the presence of bilateral fluid-filled cysts in the cerebral hemispheres. The condition represents a milder degree of damage than **hydranencephaly**.

Bassen, F.A. (b. 1903) Canadian born internist and hematologist, who practiced at the Mount Sinai Hospital in New York.

Bassen–Kornzweig syndrome See **abetalipoproteinemia**.[432]

Bassoe syndrome A congenital dysmorphic syndrome characterized by distal myopathic weakness, cataract, ptosis, kyphosis, hypogonadotrophic hypogonadism, gonadal dysgenesis, and osteoporosis.[381]

Bastian, Henry Charlton (1837–1915) English neurologist, professor of medicine at University College Hospital, London, and on the staff of the **National Hospital**, Queen Square. His publications include excellent descriptions of spinal shock, pareses, word deafness, word blindness, and other aphasias,[439] and a successful book, *The Brain as the Organ of Mind* (1880). Nevertheless, he appears to have been outshone by contemporary luminaries of greater incandescence. His dictum "We think in words," the basis of the **phonological system** of speech, will not, however, be eclipsed, although his beliefs in the essential unity of living and nonliving matter and in spontaneous generation have not been popularly accepted.

Bastian aphasia See **Wernicke aphasia**. Nevertheless, Bastian described it 5 years before Wernicke did.

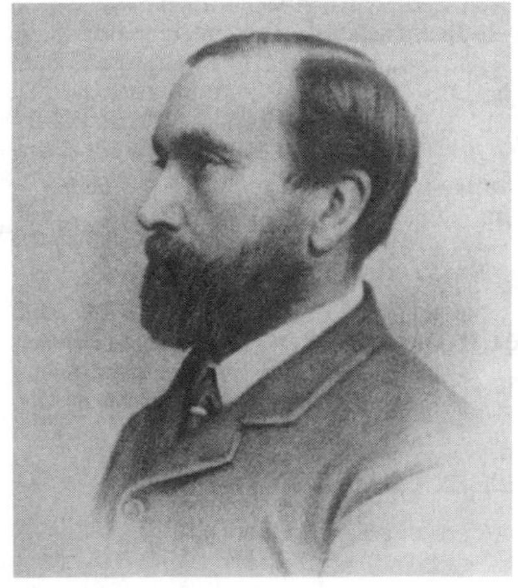

Figure B–3 Henry Charlton Bastian.

Bastian's law Transverse lesions of the spinal cord above the lumbar enlargement result in the abolition of the muscle stretch reflexes in the legs.[440] This is true enough in the early stages during the period of spinal shock but not later on.

Batelle developmental inventory A developmental screening test assessing gross and fine motor development, academic, social and cognitive skills, receptive and expressive language activity, and self-help skills. The inventory is suitable for children up to 8 years of age. It relies upon a questionnaire, observation of the child and specific testing.

bathing headache (bath headache) A form of **thunderclap headache**[3835] affecting mainly middle-aged Oriental women in contact with cold water. See also **cold stimulus headache**.

bathing suit area The shoulder and pelvic girdle regions of the trunk, distinguished only because sensory losses may occasionally be found in such areas in, for example, **acute intermittent porphyria** or **leprosy**. Changes in fashion have made this appellation seriously outdated.

bathmocephaly (from Gr, threshold + head) A developmental malformation characterized by parieto-occipital overdevelopment with marked prominence of the occiput.

bathyesthesia Deep sensibility—awareness of sensations emanating from muscles, tendons, joints, etc., and including the senses of position, movement, and deep pressure, as well as vibration.

Batson's plexus The prevertebral venous plexus, a valveless system extending from the dural venous sinuses and thought to act as a potential path for the distribution of infection or tumor cells.

Batten, Frederic Eustace (1865–1918) English neurologist who trained at Cambridge and St. Bartholemew's Hospital and whose clinical career was based at the **National Hospital** and the Hospital for Sick Children, where he concentrated mainly upon the pathology of diseases of the nervous system in children. He described cerebellar diplegia (**ataxic cerebral palsy**) in 1908 and noted that both congenital and acquired causes were relevant, and progressive muscular atrophy a year after the report by Werdnig in Germany. His first work on cerebroretinal degeneration was published in 1903.

Batten disease (Batten–Vogt disease) See **neuronal ceroid lipofuscinosis**. Apposite Web sites are **Batten Disease Information Page** http://www.ninds.nih.gov/disorders/batten/batten.htm and the site listed next.

Batten Disease Support and Research Association A charitable association in this field. Address: 2660 Parsons Ave., Columbus, OH 43207. Tel: 800-614-448-4570. Web site: http://www.bdsra.org/.

Batten–Gibb disease See **myotonic dystrophy**.

Batten–Mayou disease See **neuronal ceroid lipofuscinosis**, **gangliosidoses**.

Batten–Russell–Collier disease See **diencephalic syndrome**.

Batten–Steinert–Curschmann disease See **myotonic dystrophy**.

Batten–Turner syndrome See **congenital muscular dystrophy**.[6175]

Batten–Vogt disease See **neuronal ceroid lipofuscinosis**.

battered baby syndrome The effect of nonaccidental trauma to infants, resulting in skeletal and soft-tissue injury. Neurological lesions include concussion, subdural hematomas, skull fractures, cerebral contusions, and **diffuse axonal injury**.[6575]

Battle, W.H. (1855–1936) English surgeon, practicing at St. Thomas' and the Royal Free Hospitals in London.

Battle sign Bruising and swelling of the skin behind the ear and over the mastoid, as occurs with local skull fractures and with dural sinus thrombosis.[2066]

Bayle, Antoine-Laurent-Jesse (1799–1858) French psychiatrist and pathologist, whose thesis after internship gave the first definitive account of **general paralysis of the insane** (although this condition had been recorded by Esquirol) in which he described the delusions of grandeur, delirium, dementia, paresis, tremor, ataxia, gait disturbance, sensory loss and deafness, and chronic adhesive arachnoiditis. Unfortunately, his thesis was received with antagonism by the medical establishment and Bayle drifted away from neurology to general medicine and bibliography. He did, however, summarize the features of general paralysis superbly, as follows in translation:[455]

> The symptoms of chronic arachnoiditis can all be included in the condition of general incomplete paralysis and derangement of the intellectual functions . . . First, enunciation is noticeably impeded, the gait is unsteady, the disorder of the patients' understanding is manifested by a weakening of his intelligence and a monomaniacal dementia that more or less dominates the sick man, who is often considerably elated.
>
> In the second stage, speech disturbance and partial paralysis of the arms may [remain the same or] become worse. The dementia remains maniacal and general, often accompanied by dominant ideas; the patient may become agitated, a condition varying with his volubility and mobility; this causes him to become restless. . .and occasionally his furor is completely violent and uncontrollable.
>
> Finally, the third period is usually characterized by a state of dementia and a partial paralysis which may be partial or complete. The patient's speech is faltering, tremulous, and sometimes unintelligible. The gait is vacillating, staggering, or even impossible . . . Understanding is extremely weakened; he retains only a few ideas that are incoherent and fixed and at this stage he becomes calm and immobile, though at times he may have periods of severe agitation. This stage . . . ends in paralysis and complete idiocy [with] tremors and convulsive movements.

The correctness of his original conclusions that the mental symptoms and paralysis were the consequence of the changes he recorded in the brain and meninges was only confirmed 2 years after Bayle's death by **Baillarger**.

Bayle disease See **general paralysis of the insane**.

Bayle, Francois (1622–1709) French physician who first noted calcification and plaques in the arterial walls and related these appearances of arterial atherosclerosis to apoplexy.

Bayley scales of infant development A measure of sensorimotor development in infants up to the age of 30 months.[3]

BBB syndrome See **Opitz syndrome**.

BD MCA See **athetoid syndrome**.

Beals syndrome A dominantly inherited disorder in which the appearance of **Marfan syndrome** is complicated by the presence of multiple contractures, dysmorphic ears, and congenital cardiac defects.[5178]

(BEAM-D) Scale See **Behavioral and Emotional Activities Manifested in Dementia Scale**

Bean syndrome See **blue rubber bleb nevus syndrome**.

Beard, George Miller (1839–1883) American physician who after training at Yale and in New York, interrupted by a period in Lincoln's navy, practiced neuropsychiatry at the New York Hospital and introduced the concept of **neurasthenia**,[459] devoting most of his energy to that dubious entity which he treated with vigor, electrotherapy, and some success. His book *American Nervousness* (Boston, 1881) inspired many to believe in the organicity of their symptoms.

Beard–Valleix points See **Valleix points**.

Beare syndrome A congenital dysmorphic syndrome characterized by short stature, sensorineural deafness, ichthyosis, erythema, abnormal nails, sensorimotor neuropathy, and mental and developmental delay.[381]

Beck depression inventory A self-report questionnaire devised by Dr. Aaron Beck, with 21 groups of statements to do with both psychological and somatic symptoms, designed to determine the level of depression but frequently used as a screening test.[467] In disabled people, the scale may measure distress rather than depression.[6581] See also **Hamilton Rating Scale, Zung Self-rating Depression Scale**.

Beck, Karl German neurologist at Heidelberg who described the white rami in 1846.

Beck syndrome See **anterior spinal artery syndrome**.

Becker, P.E. German geneticist whose work was done mainly at the Universities of Freyburg and of Göttingen, where he was professor of human genetics. His publications concentrated upon the myotonic and other muscular dystrophies.[2066] See also the next entry.

Becker muscle dystrophy An X-linked recessive muscular dystrophy with the gene locus in the Xp21 band (on the short arm of the X chromosome). Clinically, the disease is allelic with, and resembles, **Duchenne dystrophy** in every clinical feature excepting its later onset, facial sparing, lesser severity of somatic, cardiac and enzymatic manifestations; slower rate of progression and resultant longer survival.[472]

Becker myotonia The autosomal recessive form of **myotonia congenita**.

Beckwith–Wiedemann syndrome A chromosomal anomaly (duplication of the terminal segment of 11p) characterized clinically by high birth weight and rapid postnatal growth, neonatal leucine-induced hypoglycemia with seizures, macrosomia with macroglossia and muscular hypertrophy, microcephaly, umbilical hernia, and renal hyperplasia. Additional features may include facial nevus flammeus.[6678, 1260]

Beemer syndrome A congenital dysmorphic syndrome characterized by delayed closure of the fontanelles, wide cranial sutures, hydrocephalus, Fallot tetralogy, ambiguous genitalia, and osteopetrosis.[381]

beer potomania See **beer-drinkers hyponatremia**

beer-drinkers hyponatremia (beer-drinkers potomania) A hypo-osmolar state with low serum sodium and potassium levels, resulting from the intake of large quantities of low-electrolyte fluid. Fatigue, confusion, and seizures are the common clinical results.

The mechanism is considered to be a combination of primary polydipsia and impaired water excretion in subjects with an excessive water load (e.g., 5 liters of beer daily) and with a low intake of solutes and protein. As a result, urea formation is reduced too, so that there is insufficient solute available to allow excretion of the water.[2900]

Beevor, Charles Edward (1854–1908) British neurologist who trained at University College Hospital and in Europe before joining the staff of the **National Hospital**, Queen Square. There he worked closely with Sir Victor **Horsley** on cerebral localization. Such work established him as one of the leading British neurologists, a reputation further solidified by his complete description of the arterial supply to the brain.[479]

Beevor signs 1. In the supine patient with a cord lesion at T9–T10, attempted flexion of the neck and upper trunk leads to upward movement of the umbilicus, due to weakness of the lower half of the rectus abdominis. It may also be present in many patients with **facioscapulohumeral muscular dystrophy**.

2. Contraction of both agonists and antagonists during attempted muscle contraction in hysterical states, described by Beevor in 1904.

BEHAVE AD See **Behavioral Pathology in Alzheimer Disease**.

Behavioral and Emotional Activities Manifested in Dementia (BEAM-D) A validated rating scale of behaviors which are directly observable (such as wandering and aggression) and of those signs which must be inferred from the subject's behaviors (such as delusions and hallucinations). It is used mainly to assess the effects of treatment in dementing conditions.[5870]

Behavioral Assessment of Dysexecutive syndrome A validated schedule for assessing executive deficits in schizophrenia and dementing disorders.[6811]

Behavioral Dyscontrol Scale (BDS) A measure of frontal lobe impairment designed to predict the capacity for independent regulation of purposeful behavior. It has been shown to predict functional autonomy and both impulsivity and apathy among geriatric patients. The scale appears to assess a different functional domain than do the **Mini-Mental State Examination** (MMSE) and similar measures, which rely heavily on the evaluation of orientation and gross cognitive status.[3350, 5452]

Behavioral Inattention Test A battery of tests for the assessment of visuospatial neglect, including pointing to objects and reading a menu and a newspaper, sensitive for detecting lesions of both the right and left hemispheres.[6071] The battery employs six conventional tests: line crossing (**Albert Test**), letter cancellation, star cancellation, figure and shape copying, and line bisection and representational drawing; and 9 behavioral tests: picture scanning, telephone dialling, menu reading, article reading, telling and setting the time (digital clock), coin sorting, address and sentence copying, map navigation, and card sorting.[6813]

Behavioural Neurology A journal publishing mainly on the relationship between disordered human behavior and its underlying biological mechanisms. Web site: http://www.iospress.nl/site/html/09534180.html.

Behavioral Neurology assessment A validated mental status examination for use in the ambulatory or in-patient setting that is reasonably brief to administer, covers all major cognitive domains, and provides qualitative as well as quantitative information, requiring only pencil and paper.[1463]

The long form consists of 24 subtests divided into the cognitive domains of attention, memory, language, visuospatial function, executive function, and praxis, and allows a maximum total score of 250. Its positive predictive value is equivalent to that of the MMSE, but it provides superior negative predictive value. A short form is also available.

Behavioral Pathology in Alzheimer Disease (BEHAVE-AD) A 25-item scale designed to chart behavioral symptoms related to Alzheimer disease and to measure treatment outcomes, the ratings made by clinicians who interview the patient and also by a caregiver. Such items as delusional ideation, hallucinations, disturbances in activity, aggression, sleep disturbances, affective symptoms, and anxiety symptoms are examined.[5251]

Behavioral Problem Checklist An instrument designed to assess the range of behavioral problems that dementia patients may exhibit when living at home, and the upset caused to family members or other caregivers. The instrument is an expansion and modification of the memory and behavioral problems checklist of Zarit and incorporates additional items. The frequency, duration, and reaction to 52 separate activities or normal behaviors are scored.

Behavioral Rating Scale for Dementia A 51-item scale rating the signs and symptoms of psychopathology in patients with dementing diseases and completed by a caregiver.[6212]

Behavioral Rating Scale for Geriatric Patients An instrument for measuring global change in the status of patients with dementia.

Behavioral Rating Scales See **Geriatric Rating Scale**; **Sandoz Clinical Assessment-Geriatric**; **Dementia Rating Scale**; **Vineland Social Maturity Scale**; **Adaptive Behavior Scale**; **Glasgow Coma Scale**; **Galveston Orientation and Amnesia Test**; **Glasgow Outcome Scale**; **Rappaport Disability Rating Scale**; **Quality of Life**.

behaviorism A psychological paradigm, the theory underlying it being that all overt human behavior is the result of the building up of a series of conditioned reflexes throughout life.

Behçet, Halushi (1889–1948) Turkish dermatologist.

Behçet syndrome (Adamantiades–Behcet syndrome, triple symptom complex, oculo-bucco-genital syndrome) A chronic recurrent systemic vasculitic syndrome of unknown etiology, thought originally[482] to comprise the triad of recurrent oral and genital aphthous ulcers and hypopyon iritis. In some cases, synovitis, cutaneous pustules, erythema nodosum, meningoencephalitis, systemic and pulmonary arterial aneurysms, phlebitis, and intestinal ulcers are added features and subclinical involvement of the CNS is also common,[597] occurring in about a third of sufferers who are usually young males. Diagnostic criteria suggested by International Study Group for Behçet disease (1990) included recurrent oral aphthous ulcers occurring at least 3 times a year, plus any two of the following:

- Genital ulcerations
- Skin lesions such as erythema nodosum folliculitis or ulcers
- Anterior or posterior uveitis or retinal vasculitis
- Hyperreactivity of the skin to pinprick, a sterile pustule being formed in <48 h.

The diverse neurological features include headache and less commonly meningoencephalitis involving the optic nerves; brainstem, cerebellar and vestibular syndromes; myelopathy; seizures; benign intracranial hypertension (probably following cerebral venous thrombosis), Parkinsonism, and dementia.[4733] Peripheral nerve involvement also occurs but rarely. The CSF contains excess cells and protein and brain MRI shows scattered T2-hyperintense lesions in the white matter of the brainstem, cerebellum, basal ganglia, or thalamus.

The first description of the disease was that of Hippocrates in his third *Book of Endemic Diseases*, the next by another Athenian, Benediktos Adamantiades, in 1930–1931. At least 18 synonyms for the condition are recorded.[3113, 3419]

Behr, Carl Julius Peter (b. 1876) German ophthalmologist who studied in Freyburg, Kiel, Munich, and Berlin, actually graduating from Kiel. After holding various positions he became professor of ophthalmology at Hamburg.

Behr disease 1. (Behr syndrome, complicated hereditary infantile optic atrophy, optic atrophy-ataxia syndrome) A recessively inherited combination of degeneration of the maculae with chorioretinitis, optic atrophy and pigmentary retinopathy, cerebellar and pyramidal signs, peripheral sensory axonal neuropathy, and mental retardation, with onset in early childhood.[483] See **cerebellar syndromes**. 2. (Central tapetoretinal degeneration) A foveal dystrophy of adults.[484] 3. Calcification in the basal ganglia in hyperparathyroidism.[6289]

Behr pupil Dilation of the pupil opposite to the side of damage to the optic tract. The sign is inconsistent and of no utility.

Behr syndrome See **Behr disease**.

Békésy audiometry An audiometric test measuring the increments in volume which are required for a patient to hear continuous rather than interrupted tones at low levels of stimulation. Five categories of abnormality have been differentiated and the test can distinguish between cochlear and retro-cochlear lesions.

Bekhterev, Vladimir Mikhailovich von (1857–1927) Russian neuropathologist and psychiatrist at Kazan and later in Leningrad. He trained with Fleschig, **Meynert**, **Westphal**, and **Charcot** and authored over 500 papers on anatomy, the vestibular system, cortical localization, and psychology. He described spondylitis deformans (Bekhterev–Marie–Strumpell disease) as well as the conditions defined in the following entries. He maintained poor relations with Pavlov, his colleague at Leningrad, who did not consider his work to be of much merit.[2066]

Bekhterev layer A plane of the cerebral cortex between the Baillarger lines and the tangential fibers.

Bekhterev nucleus The superior vestibular nucleus in the brainstem.

Bekhterev nystagmus (Bekhterev phenomenon, compensatory nystagmus) Reversal of the direction of the eye and head nystagmus and body turning induced by unilateral labyrinthectomy when the second labyrinth is also removed. See **vestibular nystagmus**.

Bekhterev phenomenon See **Bekhterev nystagmus**.

Bekhterev signs A number of clinical signs described by Bekhterev, of greater or less clinical utility. 1. The Russian alternative to the **Babiński sign**, described independently but in a language less conducive to international understanding. 2. Paradoxical dilation of a pupil with light stimulation in syphilis. 3. Plantar flexion of the foot when the dorsum is tapped with a percussion hammer, seen in pyramidal tract disease. 4. In pyramidal disease of the cord and in hemiplegia: "where the foot is passively bent in a plantar direction, when released, dorsal flexion of the foot occurs with flexion of the knee and the hip on the opposite side."[5333] 5. (*hypogastric reflex*) Normal contraction of the muscles of the lower part of the abdominal wall when the thigh is scratched. 6. Lack of pain when the peroneal nerve is compressed, seen in tertiary neurosyphilis. This is the same as the **Biernacki sign** but in a different nerve. It also resembles the **Abadie sign**. 7. (*nasal reflex*) Contraction of the facial muscles on the same side when the nose is tickled (a normal phenomenon). 8. When the patient with severe sciatic nerve irritation extends the sound leg, the affected leg cannot be extended at all. 9. (*arm dropping test*) When the arms are supported with the shoulders and elbows flexed and the support is suddenly removed, they will fall to the side after a momentary delay in normal subjects, but will "hang" in the air for a second or so in patients with pyramidal disease. 10. Extension and adduction of the thumb in response to a gentle pressure sliding down the border of the radius; a sign of pyramidal tract disease.[1500]

Bekhterev–Brissaud syndrome Spasmodic laughter and weeping in patients with hemiplegia; probably the first account of **pathological emotionality** since involvement of the brain stem was suggested by the original papers of Brissaud.[490, 852]

Bekhterev–Mendel reflex Elicitation of the **plantar muscle reflex** by tapping on the dorsum of the foot, thus depressing it, lengthening the arch, and stretching the plantar muscles, thus leading to plantar flexion of the toes; dorsiflexion being the normal response.

Belgian Society of Clinical Neurophysiology A professional organization. Web site: http://www.neuro.be/bscn/page.asp?lang=en&mod=home&page=index.

Bell, Sir Charles (1774–1842) Scottish anatomist, surgeon, and artist who went to London in 1804, returning as professor of surgery at Edinburgh in 1835. Many of his discoveries were enabled in part by his attendance on the wounded after the battles of Corunna and Waterloo. He was a man of great good humor, acknowledged as the leading anatomist of his day. He described facial palsy in 1821, and later reported **myotonia** and pseudohypertrophic muscular dystrophy. He determined that muscles only twitched when the anterior spinal roots were sectioned, but thought that these roots carried both motor and sensory impulses. He was aware that posterior root section produced loss of pain, but thought that the pathway for unconscious impressions (position sense) was through the posterior roots to the cerebellum; it was **Magendie** who showed their general sensory function, in 1822—a view that Bell accepted fully.

Bell also noted that the trigeminal nerve has both motor and sensory functions. He identified the long thoracic nerve,[493] and was the first to postulate the existence of a "sixth" sense, that of movement in muscles or joints; this and many other of his anatomical findings were published in his books *The Anatomy of the Body* (1802) or *The Nervous System of the Human Body* (London, Longman, Reed, 1830). He also described **jelly nystagmus** and **amyotrophic lateral sclerosis** and noted that **hemifacial spasm** was mediated by the VII nerve.

His engaging personality prompted the text of his epitaph in Hallow Churchyard, Worcestershire:

Sacred to the Memory
of
Sir Charles Bell
Who after Unfolding with
Unrivalled Sagacity, Patience and Success
the Wonderful Structure of our Mortal
Bodies, Esteemed Lightly of his Greatest
Discoveries
Except only as they Tended to Impress
Himself and Others with a Deeper Sense
of
The Infinite Wisdom and Ineffable Goodness
of the
Almighty Creator.

Bell palsy (facial palsy, refrigeration palsy, rheumatic palsy) Facial paralysis due to a lesion of the seventh cranial nerve peripheral to the brain stem and commonly high in the facial canal, where viral infection (HSV) is considered the most common cause.

Pain in the mastoid region may be the first symptom, after which the face is weak as shown by inability to wrinkle the forehead or to close the eye on that side; tearing; dysarthria due to drooping of the corner of the mouth; and loss of the nasolabial fold. As Bell noticed, the nostril on the affected side collapses with inspiration. The sense of taste may be lost over the anterior two-thirds of the tongue. Recovery occurs within 6 months in over 80% of patients.[493] The site of the pathology is usually in the suprageniculate segment of the nerve.

The alternative name reflects the long-held but unproven belief that cooling of the face may precipitate the palsy, as Bell himself noted in one case. Melotte[4299] indicates that an account of the palsy was given by Richard Powell 8 years before Bell's classic description. Recurrent facial palsy may in some instances be familial when it carries a worse prognosis for recovery.[115] Uncommonly associated involvement of the greater petrosal nerve leads to some numbness of the face or tongue.

A *variant form* is *familial recurrent Bell palsy with ocular motor palsies*, a dominantly inherited syndrome with the first episode of facial weakness occurring at any age and the first episode of oculomotor paresis (with pupillary sparing) occurring in mature adult life. The pathogenesis is unknown.[115]

Bell phenomenon (palpebro-oculogyric reflex) The normal tendency of the eyes to roll upward when a person tries to close them. In the presence of facial palsy, with resulting paralysis of the orbicularis oculi, this deviation, normally hidden, is visible since the eye is no longer covered by the eyelid. Bell described it in 1826.[494] The elevation of the globe occurs through the action of the inferior oblique muscle.

Bell–Magendie law The anterior spinal roots are motor, the posterior roots sensory. The name of Sir Charles **Bell** should not really join that of **Magendie** here, because no such conclusion was drawn by him until after Magendie had published.

Bell, Luther Nineteenth-century American psychiatrist and superintendent of an asylum in Somerville, Massachusetts.

Bell mania Acute delirium.

Bell Test A cancellation test that allows for a quantitative and qualitative assessment of visual neglect in near-extrapersonal space.

belly-dancer's dystonia (dyskinesia) Focal dyskinetic movements affecting the abdominal wall muscles, most often as an unwanted effect of metoclopramide. Forward thrusting of the pelvis is another such movement similarly occasioned.[3078] The condition is usually described following laparotomy.[3754] Rhythmic long-lasting (0.8–1 s) low-frequency EMG discharges lasting 30–40/min can be recorded.

belly dancer's spinal myoclonus A form of **propriospinal myoclonus** involving abdominal, thoracic, and lumbar paraspinal muscles with EMG evidence of focal neurogenic damage, suggesting anterior horn/root involvement, as with thoracic disk herniation with mild compressive effects on ventral roots and ventral columns.

Bender, Morris B. (d. 1983) American neurologist at Mount Sinai Hospital, New York. His major area of interest was neuro-ophthalmology and the higher functions associated with vision. A superb intuitive clinician and teacher, he was rewarded with a personal Chair in Clinical Neurology and was at one time president of the **American Neurological Association**.

Bender Gestalt Test A test of visuospatial praxis in which the subject is required to copy designs shown for a brief period.[505] The results allow comment upon right hemisphere and frontal lobe functions.

Bender-type myopathy See **congenital myopathy**.

bending reflex Flexion of the elbow and shoulder when the wrist is forcibly passively flexed; it is present in normal subjects but is markedly increased with bifrontal lesions, especially those affecting the parasagittal, precentral regions. In severe cases, the elbow flexion can be elicited by gentle radial deviation of the patient's wrist (radial bending reflex). The reflexes of **Leri** and of **Mayer** are related.[5746]

bending-over vertigo The physiological occurrence of vertigo or postural imbalance induced when a subject bends maximally at the waist, caused by the same mechanism as **head-extension vertigo** with the addition of increased intracranial pressure.[819]

bends See **decompression sickness**.

Benedek, Laszlo (b. 1887) Hungarian. Professor of Neuropsychiatry at Debrecen University and later at Budapest.

Benedek klazomania (Gr, klazo, I howl) Compulsive palilalic shouting in postencephalitic patients, differentiated by Benedek from the encephalitic complications of rage attacks, somnambulism, delirium, chorea, and Parkinsonism, the latter having been present in all of his postencephalitic patients.[511]

benediction hand The appearance of the hand when trying to make a fist when there is a high lesion of the median nerve preventing flexion of the index and middle fingers because of paresis of the flexor digitorum sublimis and of the median half of the flexor digitorum profundus. The postures with Dupuytren's contracture and ischemic contracture of the hand look much the same. See also **claw hand**.

Benedikt, Moritz (1835–1920) An Austrian physician who practiced in Vienna. His interest in cerebral localization led him to embrace phrenology, in the course of which studies he was one of the first physicians to X-ray the skull. His description of the syndrome now known by his name (1889) was brief and somewhat distorted by the facts that his 4-year-old patient also had a left cerebellar and many frontal tuberculomas, a right cingulate gyrus lesion and another in the cerebral peduncle, and syphilis; but his intuitive localization of the responsible lesion to the midbrain was nevertheless correct.[513] He was also a pioneer in electrotherapy and in the study of the occupational neuroses.

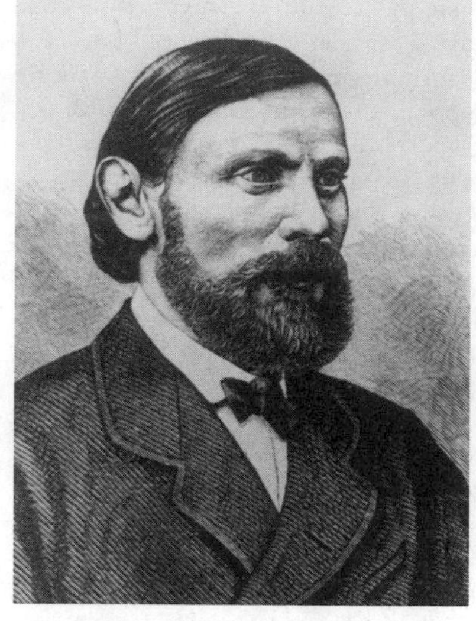

Figure B–4 Moritz Benedikt.

Benedikt inferior syndrome A pontine lesion, usually vascular, causing contralateral hemiplegia, hemiataxia, and sensory change.[5333]

Benedikt syndrome (tegmental syndrome) The association of a III cranial nerve palsy with ipsilateral cerebellar tremor and contralateral **rubral tremor**, involuntary movements resembling Parkinsonian tremor, and hemiparesis, usually as a result of a small infarct or tumor in the region of the red nucleus which damages both this and the adjacent corticospinal fibers in the cerebral peduncle.[513] Benedikt actually described it in a patient with a tuberculoma at that site.

Motor fibers have crossed to the red nucleus from the contralateral dentate nucleus and will cross back to influence the performance of motor actions on the other side of the body, whereas the corticospinal fibers are also uncrossed at this level—so there appears the unusual association of both cerebellar-like and pyramidal findings on the same side.[513]

benign abducens nerve palsy of childhood A rare, self-limiting condition seen in infancy and childhood. The diagnosis is essentially one of exclusion;[1238] its pathophysiology is ill-defined.

benign acute childhood myositis (myalgia cruris epidemica) An acute infectious syndrome of children causing muscle inflammation, after which myalgia involves the calves and thighs more frequently than other muscles; mild weakness and local tenderness are present and serum creatine kinase levels are markedly increased.[209] Recovery usually occurs within a week.

Influenza A and B, parainfluenza virus and adenovirus 2 are the commoner causal agents. See also **postinfluenzal myositis**.

benign adult familial myoclonic epilepsy A dominantly inherited nonprogressive syndrome characterized by adult-onset cortical tremor and generalized seizures. It is mapped variously to chromosomes 8q24 and 2p11.[1493] See also **familial cortical myoclonic tremor with epilepsy**.

benign age and localization-related idiopathic epilepsy See **benign childhood epilepsy with centrotemporal spikes, benign childhood epilepsy with occipital paroxysms**.

benign angiopathy of the central nervous system See **benign cerebral vasculitis**.

benign cerebral vasculitis (benign angiopathy of the central nervous system) An inflammatory disorder of the intracranial arteries (**Aβ angiitis**) associated with segmental narrowing seen on angiography. The condition may be asymptomatic or it may cause seizures and focal neurological signs. The reversibility of the arteriographic findings and the absence of biopsy reports allow speculation that vasospasm (rather than vasculitis) is the cause in at least some cases.[5728] Despite this alternative name, the condition is not usually very benign. See also **Call–Fleming syndrome**.

benign childhood epilepsy with affective symptoms A disputed epileptic syndrome, in which frequent brief periods of extreme fear occur in young children without alteration in consciousness but with the usual autonomic symptoms of extreme anxiety. No consistent EEG abnormality is associated. The condition appears to be self-limiting within a year or two, clearing without residua.[4880, 1419]

benign childhood epilepsy with centrotemporal spikes (Rolandic seizures, Sylvian epilepsy, benign epilepsy, benign Sylvian seizures with midtemporal spike foci, benign childhood epilepsy with Rolandic paroxysmal discharges, lingual syndrome, centrotemporal epilepsy; OMIM 117100) A common form of "benign age and localization-related idiopathic epilepsy" characterized by brief, simple, partial, hemifacial motor seizures, frequently having associated somatosensory symptoms which have a tendency to evolve into generalized tonic-clonic seizures. Both seizure types are often related to sleep. The onset of these attacks is between the ages of 3 and 13 years (peak: 9–10 years) and recovery occurs spontaneously before the age of 16 years. Genetic predisposition is frequent (linked to chr. 15q14) and there is male predominance.[3904]

Clinically, there are infrequent focal unilateral facial sensory-motor symptoms, oro-pharyngo-laryngeal manifestations such as unilateral numbness and dysaesthesias inside the mouth, cheek, teeth, and tongue alone or with motor phenomena producing strange sounds such as death rattle, gargling, guttural sounds or speech arrest, with hypersalivation. Hemifacial seizures consist of clonic contractions of the lower lip, sometimes spreading to the arm.

The EEG shows blunt high-voltage centrotemporal spikes, often followed by slow waves that are activated by sleep and tend to spread or shift from side to side (From Dreifuss FE, et al. Commission for classification and terminology, ILAE. Proposal for Revised Classifications of Epilepsies and Epileptic syndromes. *Epilepsia* 1989;30:389–99, by kind permission of Wiley-Blackwell Publications) and Panayioutopoulos.[4882]

In brief, it is a rare example of a distinct syndrome of epilepsy, occurring mainly during sleep in prepubertal children who are without neurological or intellectual abnormalities. The seizures are usually brief and infrequent, and the whole disorder only occupies a few years of the child's life.[72] The seizures tend to be controllable without great difficulty and after their termination, the child is left without physical or psychological handicap.[3786]

Despite the usual eponym, given above, the syndrome was actually first described by Martinus Rulando in 1597.[6500]

Variant forms include the following:

One in which the condition is dominantly inherited and complicated by speech dyspraxia.[5584]

The presence of atypical clinical manifestations including hemifacial seizures, dysarthria or anarthria, and persistent drooling.[5437]

Malignant Rolandic–Sylvian epilepsy, a form characterized by refractory sensorimotor seizures, cognitive disturbances, normal MRI findings, perisylvian spikes on magnetoencephalography, and frontotemporal spikes on the EEG.[4830]

Thus this condition also is not always benign, although forms that are not occur in only a small percentage of patients and may represent related conditions.

benign childhood epilepsy with frontal or with midline spikes

A syndrome with clinical features resembling those of **benign childhood epilepsy with centrotemporal spikes** in which, however, the spikes are recorded from these differing locations.

benign childhood epilepsy with occipital paroxysms

A form of "benign age and localization-related idiopathic epilepsy" occurring before the age of 13 years and characterized by unequivocal clinical evidence of epileptic seizures (mainly tonic deviation of the eyes and vomiting, often with evolution to generalized tonic-clonic or to simple motor seizures) and with paroxysms maximal in the occipital areas on at least one EEG, and neither clinical nor EEG manifestations of primary generalized epilepsy or of any other distinctive syndrome; no evidence of neurological or intellectual deficit; and a normal appearance of the CT brain scan.[4879, 2310]

benign childhood epilepsy with Rolandic paroxysmal discharges

See **benign childhood epilepsy with centrotemporal spikes**.

benign childhood epilepsy with somatosensory-evoked spikes

An epileptic syndrome of children in the first decade, characterized clinically by daytime versive seizures affecting the head and body, not always with alteration in consciousness; and electrically by sharp- and slow-wave complexes recorded in parietal or parasagittal regions, elicited by somatosensory stimulation, such as tapping the limbs. The attacks tend to remit after a year or so.[4880]

benign childhood focal seizures

Nonfebrile, usually nocturnal and infrequent, seizures that remit within 1–3 years from onset. Brief or prolonged seizures, even status epilepticus, may be the only clinical event of the patient's lifetime. Ictal autonomic manifestations are frequent and may occasionally appear in isolation as in pure autonomic seizures. Febrile seizures are common. Neurological examination and intellect are normal, but some children may experience mild and reversible neuropsychological problems during the active stage of the disorder. Brain imaging is normal. The severe high-amplitude focal spikes on the EEG are disproportionate to the frequency of seizures.[4882]

benign childhood partial epilepsies

A group of syndromes characterized by the occurrence of partial epileptic seizures in young children, occurring over the space of a few years only, usually at night, and often accompanied by hypersalivation, vomiting, headache, pallor, and sweating. Abundant high-amplitude focal sharp- and slow-wave discharges are recorded interictally on the EEG from various cephalic regions, especially during sleep, but all other tests give normal results. Febrile convulsions are common in these children.

The syndromes delineated to date include **benign childhood epilepsy with affective seizures; benign childhood epilepsy with centrotemporal spikes; Panayiotopoulos syndrome; benign childhood epilepsy with occipital paroxysms; benign childhood epilepsy with somatosensory-evoked spikes**; and **benign childhood epilepsy with frontal** or with **midline spikes**.[4880] See also **Landau–Kleffner syndrome**.

benign congenital hypotonia

A syndrome diagnosed on the basis of a clinical impression that an infant shows more hypotonia than weakness. This is unlikely to be a single entity and some of the conditions are probably not even myopathic. See **benign congenital myopathy**.

benign congenital myopathy

(Oppenheim disease, myotonia, amyotonia congenita, benign congenital hypotonia, minimal change myopathy, floppy infant syndrome) A heterogeneous group of conditions affecting infants in which hypotonia, muscle weakness, and lax (hypermobile) joints, but normal muscle biopsy, serum enzymes, and EMG findings are the major features.[1966]

The subjects correctly diagnosed in retrospect are those that recover after the first year of life. Others (obviously not suffering from a benign disease) die of respiratory complications of their weakness[4802, 6631, 6424] and should be classified as having some other condition.

When combined with hyperexcitability of the CNS, the condition has been known as *Ullrich syndrome*.[3113, 6632]

benign congenital myotonia See **benign hereditary myopathy**.

benign cough headache A brief, bilateral headache precipitated by coughing in the absence of any intracranial disorder such as a posterior fossa mass lesion.

benign distal cranial arteritis See **isolated benign cerebral vasculitis**.

benign dystonia A congenital dystonic syndrome characterized by dystonias without accompanying features.[381]

benign early-onset Parkinson disease A Parkinsonian syndrome characterized by unilateral tremor and rigidity of long duration and minimal progression with onset usually in the fourth decade, sometimes following a severe febrile illness.[5691]

benign encephalomyelitis See **postinfection fatigue syndrome**.

benign epilepsy of children with Rolandic spikes See **benign childhood epilepsy with centrotemporal spikes**.

benign epilepsy syndrome One characterized by epileptic seizures that are easily treated or require no treatment and which remit without sequelae.[1861]

benign epilepsy with occipital paroxysms See **benign occipital epilepsy of childhood**.

benign epileptic aphasia One of the benign focal (partial) epilepsies of childhood manifesting with pure intermittent speech disturbances. See **benign occipital epilepsy of childhood, occipital lobar epilepsy**, and **intercalated migraine**.

benign epileptiform discharges of childhood Regional or multiregional sharp waves, which are normally followed by a negative slow wave with lower amplitude than the negative peak of the sharp wave and which typically show a bipolar distribution with a positive sink in the midfrontal region. These sharp waves often have a multiregional distribution and are easy to recognize by their typical morphology. If they occur in the centrotemporal region, they are also called Rolandic spikes. They typically increase during sleep and tend to appear in series. (From Noachtar S, Binnie C, Ebersole J, et al. A glossary of terms most commonly used by clinical electroencephalographers and proposal for the report form for the EEG findings. The International Federation of Clinical Neurophysiology. EEG Clin Neurophysiol Suppl 1999;52:21–41. Reproduced by kind permission of Elsevier Science and the IFCN.)

benign epileptiform transients of sleep (small/big/large sharp spikes) The appearance of spike activity between 5 and 135 mV recorded on the EEG uni- or bilaterally over the anterior and middle temporal lobe regions of young people during nonrapid eye movement sleep stages 1 and 2, especially after a period of sleep deprivation, first described by Grey–Walter. They are considered to have no pathological significance, but their differentiation from similar spikes associated with partial epilepsy of temporal lobe origin may cause confusion.[6751] See also **small sharp spikes**.

benign episodic mydriasis Intermittent unilateral pupillary dilation, of unknown cause.[2699, 1806]

benign essential blepharospasm See **blepharospasm.** A Google search retrieves over 32 000 entries for this condition.

Benign Essential Blepharospasm/Meige Research Foundation Inc. A nonprofit organization dedicated to finding the cause of and cure for blepharospasm, Meige disease, and related disorders. The foundation has support groups nationwide in the United States, promotes awareness and research, distributes educational materials to patients and physicians, and serves as a referral clearing house. Web site: http://www.healthfinder.gov/orgs/HR2032.htm/; also see www.blepharospasm.org/.

benign essential chorea See **hereditary nonprogressive chorea**.

benign essential tremor See **essential tremor**.[1437]

benign exertional headache A bilateral, throbbing headache lasting for minutes to hours and precipitated by any form of exercise. It may develop migrainous features in patients already subject to migraine headaches. Subvarieties such as *weight-lifters headache* and *effort headache in runners*[4144] are also recognized.

benign familial chorea See **hereditary nonprogressive chorea**.

benign familial (and nonfamilial) infantile seizures (Watanabe–Vigevano syndrome, benign epilepsy, Fukuyama disease; OMIM 601764)A rare syndrome (probably a channelopathy) with onset between 3 and 20 months in otherwise normal children The familial form is autosomal dominantly inherited with genetic heterogeneity (chromosomes 19q, 16, or 2). Clinically, there are diurnal brief (<3 min) focal seizures with arrest of movement, decreased responsiveness, staring, eye and head deviation, simple automatisms, and mild clonic movements, frequently alternating between sides. They occur in clusters of up to 8–10 per day for 1–3 days and may recur after 1–3 months. They sometimes progress to generalized convulsions. The Ictal EEG shows focal parieto-occipital discharges. Subsequent development is normal and seizures do not persist.[4882]

Paroxysmal choreoathetosis may be associated at a later age.[571] The locus on chromosome 16 is also associated with paroxysmal choreoathetosis (*infantile convulsions and choreoathetosis*).[6544]

Despite the eponyms given, the condition was first described by Dr. Andreas Rett in 1964.

benign familial macrocephaly A syndrome with the following diagnostic criteria suggested by De Myer, adapted here.[1513] (See Chart B–2.)

benign familial myoclonic epilepsy See **Rabot epilepsy**.

benign familial neonatal convulsions (OMIM 121200) A dominantly inherited epileptic syndrome in which multiple generalized tonic-clonic

Chart B–2. Criteria for the Diagnosis of Benign Familial Macrocephaly

Occipito-frontal diameter >2 standard deviations above the mean or >98th percentile.
No increase in intracranial pressure (as would be shown by bulging fontanelle, palpably split sutures, or persistent vomiting).
Normal neurological and developmental examinations.
Absence of neurocutaneous stigmata and other somatic anomalies.
A family history of megalencephaly.
Follow-up visits establish the normality of the patient's developmental course, and the occipito-frontal circumference curve levels off and, although it remains high, begins to parallel the normal curve. Radiographic demonstration of normal or only slightly enlarged ventricles in one of the family members with an enlarged occipito-frontal circumference, establishing that the condition is megalencephaly, not arrested hydrocephalus or another lesion.
Negative chemical screening tests for metabolic disorders or lysosomal enzyme deficits in those patients lacking some of the other criteria.

Adapted from De Myer W. Megalencephaly: Types, Clinical Syndromes and Management. Pediatr Neurol *1986;***2***:321–27 © 1986 by permission from Elsevier Science.*

seizures occur daily, starting on or after the second day of life (but always in the first month) and disappearing spontaneously within weeks, although occasional seizures may occur thereafter[3297] in a variant form. The physical examination findings and the children's subsequent neurodevelopmental progress are normal. The responsible genes have been mapped to chromosomes 20q13.3 and 8q24.

Ocular, autonomic, tonic, and respiratory seizure manifestations and automatisms are also recorded.[5374]

benign fasciculation potential A fasciculation potential occurring (in retrospect) in the context of a nonprogressive neuromuscular disorder. Unfortunately, its electrical characteristics do not allow confident distinction from fasciculations occurring in progressive neuromuscular disorders, so the value of the term is questionable. They have a high firing rate and normal EMG morphologic parameters.

benign fasciculations and cramps (Denny–Brown and Foley syndrome) The occurrence of fasciculations in healthy people who do not have other features suggesting **amyotrophic lateral sclerosis** nor of other lower motor neuron disorders such as weakness, wasting; and neither EMG nor biopsy evidence of denervation.[5229, 1595] The fasciculations are most commonly in the leg muscles but can affect any region and tend to recur in the same point of a muscle on any particular occasion.

The cramps are usually felt in the calves. The origin of the disorder is not known, but progression to **amyotrophic lateral sclerosis** is seldom seen. Only about 6% of subjects aged 45 years and older with fasciculations as their only complaint go on to develop this disorder. A relevant Web site is About BFS at http://www.nextination.com/aboutbfs/.

benign febrile myoclonus A rare, benign presentation in which frequent myoclonic jerks resolve when the fever abates in children who were otherwise healthy.[1691]

benign focal amyotrophy A sporadic, clinically heterogeneous syndrome of nonprogressive asymmetrical uni- or bilateral segmental muscle weakness and atrophy localized to one limb or both homologous limbs markedly, occurring in young males. Sensory loss and CNS involvement do not occur. The electrophysiological, radiological and muscle histopathological findings suggest chronic focal anterior horn cell disease.[3429] It is distinguished from other more common forms of motor neuron disease by the restricted limb involvement, absence of upper motor neuron signs, and slow progression for months to years followed by disease stabilization.[2006] Benign calf amyotrophy is an example. See **monomelic amyotrophy** and **hereditary motor neuropathy**, of which this could be a *variant*.

benign focal atrophy (amyotrophy) See **monomelic amyotrophy**.

benign focal epilepsy See **benign childhood epilepsy with centrotemporal spikes**.

benign focal epilepsy with centrotemporal spikes See **benign childhood epilepsy with centrotemporal spikes**.

benign focal epilepsy with occipital lobe spike waves See **occipital lobe epilepsy and intercalated migraine**.

benign hereditary chorea (OMIM 118700) A rare, dominantly inherited but heterogeneous syndrome characterized by chorea affecting all body parts, clumsy gait, sometimes with dystonia and with onset in infancy, childhood, or youth,[5342, 5159] improving with the years. The condition is mapped to 14q (mutations in the *TITF-1* gene)[1619] and to chromosome 8q21.3–q23.3 (*BHC2*).

This is surely no more than a variety of **hereditary nonprogressive chorea**. However, *variant* forms are described in which there are also manifest axial or limb dystonia, myoclonic jerks, dysarthria, and/or gait disturbance.

benign hereditary myopathy See **benign congenital myopathy**.

benign idiopathic dystonia Dystonia occurring in the first year of life, ceasing by 18 months of age.[6792] See **dystonia**.

benign infantile mitochondrial myopathy (mitochondria-lipid-glycogen disease of muscle) A reversible expression of inherited deficiency in cytochrome *c* oxidase (complex IV), leading clinically to hypotonia, weakness, macroglossia, and lactic acidosis after birth, which, however, abates over months and leads only to residual mild proximal weakness.[1645]

benign influenzal myopathy A transient painful affection of the legs, with elevated serum creatine kinase levels, seen occasionally in children recovering from acute influenzal infections.[4352]

benign intracranial hypertension One of two acceptable alternative terms for the syndrome of increased intracranial pressure in the absence of a causative mass lesion, documented elsewhere in this book under **idiopathic intracranial hypertension**.

benign juvenile focal muscular atrophy of upper extremities See **monomelic amyotrophy.**

benign masturbatory cephalalgia An acute **benign exertional headache**, usually experienced in private.[6551] See **headache associated with sexual activity**.

benign monoclonal gammopathy See **paraproteinemic neuropathy**.

benign monomelic amyotrophy See **monomelic amyotrophy**.

benign motor neuron disorder See **cramp fasciculation syndrome**.

benign multiple sclerosis That form of multiple sclerosis which, having been present with a relapsing and remitting course, has left the patient with little functional disability (rating 2 or less on the **Kurtzke Scale**) after 15 years. This form is more commonly seen in younger women who presented with sensory symptoms and/or optic neuritis. However, some of these patients do go on to develop the chronic progressive form eventually.

benign muscular dystrophy with contractures A variant of **Emery–Dreifuss syndrome** with likely autosomal dominant inheritance (though Y-to-Y transmission is also possible),[335] characterized by proximal myopathy, contractures and rigidity of paraspinal muscles without cardiomyopathy.[335]

benign myalgic encephalomyelitis See **chronic fatigue syndrome**.

benign myoclonic epilepsy in childhood See **benign myoclonic epilepsy in infancy**.

benign myoclonic epilepsy in infancy 1. A syndrome characterized by jerks that occur in clusters of four or five at about 1/s and involve mainly the limbs, occasionally affecting distal muscle roots most obviously. The onset is usually in the first week of life. The disorder is self-limited and benign, lasting at most a few months. There is often a family history of convulsions or epilepsy. The physical examination is normal.

They are not accompanied by any other type of seizure, although generalized tonic-clonic seizures may occur during adolescence, when they are easily controlled. The epileptic syndrome may be accompanied by a relative delay of intellectual development and minor personality disorders. The EEG shows generalized 3 Hz spike-waves occurring in brief bursts during the early stages of sleep. (From Dreifuss FE, et al. Commission for classification and terminology, ILAE. Proposal for Revised Classifications of Epilepsies and Epileptic syndromes. *Epilepsia* 1989;**30**:389–99 by kind permission of Wiley Blackwell.)

2. (benign neonatal sleep myoclonus, benign myoclonic epilepsy in childhood) A rare idiopathic generalized epilepsy syndrome characterized by a partial arousal response manifesting as bilateral, synchronous and repetitive rhythmic jerking of the limbs and occasional jerks of the trunk, fingers, wrists, elbows, and ankles, occurring without other clinical abnormality during any phase of sleep in otherwise-normal neonates up to the age of 2 years.[1298] The usual onset is between 6 months and 3 years in otherwise normal children. Its genetic basis is not established. Consciousness is retained but mild clouding may occur during the clusters of jerks. No other types of seizure occur apart from simple febrile seizures in a small number of cases. Photosensitivity and unexpected acoustic or tactile stimuli may precipitate attacks but these usually occur on awakening or during the first hours of sleep. The interictal EEG is normal but the ictal EEG shows generalized polyspike or spike and slow wave discharges. Remission usually occurs within 1 year (6 months to 6 years), but a minority of children develop infrequent generalized tonic-clonic seizures in their early teens and a very few develop mild cognitive, behavioral, or motor deficits if untreated.[4882] Thus the term "benign" may be incorrect here, according to the most recent definitions of the International League Against Epilepsy.

benign myoclonus of early infancy A clinical syndrome of repetitive jerking movements resembling **West syndrome** but self-limiting by the age of 2 years and lacking the neurological and developmental arrest, the **hypsarrhythmic** EEG pattern, and the fatal prognosis of that condition.[3905] It may actually be a form of **tic disorder**.

benign myopathy A dominantly inherited syndrome with onset in childhood after normal infantile motor development and characterized by weakness of the neck flexors, girdle muscles and limb extensors, and, in some cases, by flexion contracture of the elbows and by hyporeflexia. Muscle biopsy findings are nonspecific but suggest myopathy.[3223]

benign neonatal convulsions (fifth-day fits) Frequently repeated clonic or apneic seizures occurring at about the fifth day of life, without known etiology or concomitant metabolic disturbance. The interictal EEG often shows alternating sharp theta waves. There is no recurrence of seizures and psychomotor development is not affected. (Adapted from Dreifuss FE, et al. Commission for classification and terminology, ILAE. Proposal for Revised Classifications of Epilepsies and Epileptic syndromes. *Epilepsia* 1989;**30**:389–99 by kind permission of Wiley-Blackwell Publications.) Such self-limited events without sequelae do not require the diagnosis of epilepsy.[1861]

benign neonatal familial convulsions Rare, dominantly inherited disorders manifesting most commonly on the second and third days of life, with frequently repeated clonic or apneic seizures lasting for a few days or weeks, without specific EEG criteria. The history and investigations reveal no etiologic factors. About 14% of these patients later develop epilepsy, commonly in adult life. (Adapted from Dreifuss FE, et al. Commission for classification and terminology, ILAE. Proposal for Revised Classifications of Epilepsies and Epileptic syndromes. *Epilepsia* 1989;**30**:389–99 by kind permission of the

IFCN and Wiley-Blackwell Publications.) One responsible gene lies at chromosome 20q13.3.

benign neonatal sleep myoclonus See **benign myoclonic epilepsy in infancy**.

benign (nonfamilial) neonatal seizures (fifth-day fits) Repetitive, unilateral clonic convulsions affecting the face and limbs, lasting 1–3 min and occurring between the fourth and sixth days of life in otherwise normal infants. The manifestations may change sides and are occasionally bilateral. A spell of apnea is common. The whole event lasts from 2 h to 3 days, with a median of ~20 h and does not recur. The interictal EEG may show a "theta pointu alternant" pattern or focal or multifocal, nonspecific abnormalities or a discontinuous pattern or it may be normal. The ictal paroxysms may be unilateral, generalized, or first localized, then generalizing. Subsequent development is normal and there is no recurrence of seizures.[4882] See (the identical?) **benign neonatal convulsions**.

benign occipital epilepsy of childhood (benign epilepsy with occipital paroxysms, BEOPS) One of the benign focal (partial) epilepsies of childhood, thus related to **benign childhood epilepsy with centrotemporal spikes** and **benign epileptic aphasia**. Clinically, the condition presents in the middle of the first decade with infrequent and easily controlled seizures comprising positive or negative visual phenomena, without focal neurological or ocular signs or mental disturbance but with striking irregular occipital spike-wave discharges on the EEG.[2310] In a number of cases these are followed by hemisensory, motor, or psychomotor seizures and by migraine-like headaches.[2307] See also **Panayiotopoulos syndrome**.

benign occipital spikes The appearance of uniform diphasic or triphasic sharp waves over one or both occipital regions, attenuated by eye opening but activated by sleep. The electrographic finding is most commonly associated with migraine; seizures, if they occur at all, usually remit after puberty.[2307]

benign paroxysmal cranial neuralgia (cephalgia fugax) A benign syndrome of unknown cause, characterized by the occurrence of frequent, repetitive (120 per day), sharp, neuralgia-like head pains occurring in bouts, with long remissions between them.[4950]

benign paroxysmal positional vertigo See **benign positional vertigo**.

benign paroxysmal torticollis in infancy A self-limited disorder with onset during the first month of life, recurring at varying intervals until the ages of 1–5 years and characterized by periods of torticollic posturing of the head.[1239]

benign paroxysmal vertigo of childhood (paroxysmal torticollis in infancy) Multiple, brief, sporadic episodes of severe vertigo occurring in otherwise healthy children aged between 1 and 5 years who stop all activities, appear frightened, refuse to move or stand and may be nauseated or vomit. The attacks last between minutes and hours. The condition may be a migraine equivalent of childhood or adolescence. It remits spontaneously after some years. Diagnostic criteria have been defined:

A. At least 5 attacks fulfilling criterion B
B. Multiple episodes of severe vertigo, occurring without warning and resolving spontaneously after minutes to hours
C. Normal neurological examination and audiometric and vestibular functions between attacks
D. Normal electroencephalogram

From the International Classification of Headache Disorders (Headache Classification Committee of the International Headache Society; *Cephalalgia* 2004;**24**[Suppl 1]) by kind permission of Dr. Jes Olesen, the International Headache Society and Wiley-Blackwell Publications.

The criteria require a normal neurological examination and a normal EEG, since recurrent vertigo can be a symptom of epilepsy (**tornado epilepsy**).[1598] See also **periodic syndromes**.

benign partial epilepsy of childhood A syndrome of benign seizures occurring only during sleep, involving mainly the mouth and face, disappearing by puberty and accompanied by marked Rolandic spike discharges during rapid eye movement sleep periods, but the EEG is normal interictally.[4757] The neurological examination is normal. See **benign childhood epilepsy with centrotemporal spikes**—which is surely the same thing.

benign partial epilepsy of childhood with occipital paroxysms A syndrome characterized by interictal paroxysms of high-amplitude spike waves or sharp waves, recurring more or less rhythmically on the occipital and postero-temporal areas of one or both hemispheres and occurring only when the eyes are closed. Ictally, the initial visual symptoms such as amaurosis, phosphenes, visual illusions or hallucinations are often followed by a hemiclonic seizure or by automatisms when the occipital discharge spreads to central or temporal regions. A migraine-like headache ensues in a quarter of the cases.

benign partial epilepsy with affective symptoms during the attacks The ictal symptomatology is mainly constituted by a terror feeling and autonomic signs without evident loss of consciousness. EEG abnormalities are variable and situated in frontal and mid-temporal areas.

benign partial epilepsy with centrotemporal spikes (atypical benign partial epilepsy of childhood) A rare condition, not recognized as an epileptic syndrome by the ILAE. Its manifestations include male predominance; the onset before the age of 6 years, often with recovery before 16 years of brief, usually nocturnal, hemifacial Rolandic-like focal motor seizures or atonic seizures,[4882] with frequent associated somatosensory symptoms, sometimes generalizing. The EEG shows blunt, high-voltage centrotemporal spikes, often followed by slow waves, activated by sleep and tending to spread and/or to shift from side to side.

benign partial epilepsy with extreme somatosensory-evoked potentials A form of **benign partial epilepsy of childhood**, affected children having large somatosensory-evoked potentials evoked by heel-tapping. Later, spontaneous EEG abnormalities in the parietal area and partial motor seizures with adversion appear.

benign partial epilepsy with occipital sharp waves See **benign childhood epilepsy with occipital paroxysms.**

benign pontine hypertrophy Although the condition is neither benign nor truly hypertrophic, the name was once applied to slowly growing pontine gliomas.

benign positional nystagmus A subtype of **benign positional vertigo** affecting one or more of the semicircular canals.

benign positional vertigo (BPPV; benign peripheral/paroxysmal positional vertigo, paroxysmal positional nystagmus) A common syndrome characterized by acute, transient, episodic, rotational vertigo, precipitated (after a few seconds latency) by rapid changes in the position of the head, characteristically declining after seconds or minutes and fatiguing with repeated postural changes. Nausea, vomiting, and peripheral nystagmus are typically associated,[362, 3692] but auditory symptoms are not.

The condition is most commonly seen in adult females. The cause is uncertain but may be the dislocation and random movement of the canaliths (otoconia) that stimulate the hair cells in the posterior (less commonly the horizontal) semicircular canal of the undermost ear. The condition was first described by Bárány in 1921.[384] It is frequently relieved by **canalith repositioning** or by the **Semont** or the **Epley liberatory maneuvers** which are supposed to move the otoliths from the affected canal to the vestibule.

Diagnostic criteria have been suggested[6566] and are reproduced by kind permission.

Vestibular vertigo (one criterion has to be fulfilled)

1. Spontaneous rotational vertigo
2. Positional vertigo
3. Recurrent dizziness with nausea and oscillopsia or imbalance

Benign paroxysmal positional vertigo (A–D must be fulfilled)

A. Recurrent vestibular vertigo
B. Duration of an attack always <1 min
C. Symptoms are invariably provoked by the changes of head position (lying down or turning in the supine position) or by at least two of the following maneuvers:
   reclining the head
   rising up from a supine position
   bending forward
D. Not attributable to another disorder.

Variants include the following:

A disabling form.[3165]
A form in which a horizontal semicircular canal is implicated; in this type the nystagmus is direction-changing, horizontal, and nonfatiguing.
A form in which the nystagmus is direction-changing, probably due to pathology affecting the horizontal semicircular canal.[357]

See also **Dix-Hallpike maneuver**. Other diagnostic tests such as the Pagnini-McClure and the Lempert roll maneuvers are described by Fife et al. (2008).[2045]

benign positional vertigo of childhood A migraine precursor, in many cases presenting in childhood and lasting between seconds and days. Central or peripheral forms of nystagmus may accompany the symptom.[4632]

benign postural myoclonus A rare syndrome manifesting position-dependent myoclonus, responsive to clonazepam and valproic acid.

benign recurrent vertigo (vestibular migraine) A benign, recurrent, episodic syndrome of vertigo, nausea, vomiting, and hyperhidrosis without evidence of vestibulopathy, occurring mainly on waking and seen in women with a personal (or at least a family) history of recurrent headaches at the time of their menstrual periods.[4473]

benign Rolandic epilepsy (benign focal epilepsy linked to 15q) See **benign childhood epilepsy with centrotemporal spikes.**

benign senescent forgetfulness A nonprogressive, fluctuating amnestic syndrome in elderly people, whose recollection of remote names and dates, but not of events, is impaired on certain occasions, the data bubbling up later.[3552] See **minimal cognitive impairment (age-associated memory impairment).**

benign sensorimotor epilepsy with parietal spikes See **extreme somatosensory-evoked potential.**

benign sex headache See **headache associated with sexual activity.**

benign VI nerve palsy Isolated, painless, and self-limited paresis of one of the sixth nerves in children, occurring 10–20 days after an upper respiratory infection.[3503]

benign spinal muscular atrophy with calf hypertrophy See **hereditary motor neuropathy.**

benign sporadic sleep spikes See **small sharp spikes.**

benign sylvian seizures with midtemporal spike foci See **benign childhood epilepsy with centrotemporal spikes.**

benign symmetric lipomatosis See **familial multiple symmetrical lipomatosis with peripheral neuropathy.**

benign torticollis of infancy Recurrent attacks in which the head tilts, occurring during the first year of life and persisting for a few months to several years. The attacks occur predominantly in the morning and last between 2 and 24 h. Associated symptoms include irritability, drowsiness, pallor or flushing, and dysequilibrium.[1598] The etiology is not determined.

benign tremulous Parkinsonism A syndrome of isolated tremor without other signs of **Parkinson disease**, occurring in a single limb, in elderly patients, and without progression over the course of years of observation.

benign tumors Tumors which are slowly growing and noninvasive and which show no vascular proliferation, few mitoses, and minimal necrosis histologically.

benign X-linked muscular dystrophy (Waida dystrophy) A variant form of muscular dystrophy characterized by the onset in youth of proximal and distal muscle atrophy and weakness, pseudohypertrophy, and cardiomyopathy.[381] See **Becker muscle dystrophy**.

bent knee pulling A variation of the **femoral stretch** maneuver in which the examiner passively extends the patient's hip by pulling backward on the foot with the knee flexed and exerting forward pressure on the buttock, with the patient in the semiprone position. The action stretches the femoral nerve. Pain felt as a result is a useful sign of root irritation at L3.[3117]

bent spine syndrome (camptocormia; from Greek bent + tree trunk) A focal axial myopathy seen mainly in elderly people and causing progressive paravertebral muscle weakness, leading to a posture of anterior flexion of the trunk, with bent spine on standing but normal supine posture. Weakness of the neck extensors may lead to dropping of the head. Serum creatine kinase is normal or moderately increased, paraspinal EMG nonspecific and biopsy myopathic. The syndrome may be caused by a late-onset paraspinal muscle dystrophy but is heterogeneous in origin.[5735] See also **camptocormia**.

Benton facial recognition test An instrument used to assess facial recognition abilities, commercially available.

Benton Visual Retention Test A test of visuospatial praxis and nonverbal memory in which the subject sees and is required to memorize and later to reproduce a series of simple but progressively more complex line drawings.

It is said to be able to distinguish between the normal elderly and those with **Alzheimer disease**.[531]

Benton–van Allen Test of facial discrimination A pictorial test for visual agnosia.

Berant syndrome A dominantly inherited congenital syndrome characterized by acrocephaly, elbow joint and radio-ulnar synostosis, and craniosynostosis affecting the sagittal suture.[539]

Berdon syndrome See **megacystis-microcolon-intestinal hypoperistalsis syndrome**.

bereitschraft potential (readiness potential) An EEG potential recorded maximally at the vertex, probably emanating from the supplementary motor area and preceding a self-paced voluntary movement.[1634] It is a component of the movement-related cortical potential. See also **backaveraging**.

Berg Balance Scale A measure of balance in older adults, available at the Web site http://www.strokecenter.org/trials/scales/berg.html/.

Bergara–Wartenberg sign Loss of those fine vibrations which are palpable when the examiner places his finger on the closed eyelids of a normal patient. The sign is positive in patients with facial palsy.[551]

Berger, E. (1855–1926) Austrian ophthalmologist who studied in Vienna, Berlin, and Paris where he later set up in practice, becoming professor of ophthalmology at the École de Médicine. He was a voluminous writer on many aspects of ophthalmology.

Berger sign Irregularity of the pupil, which may be elliptical in the early stages of tertiary syphilis.[552]

Berger, Johannes (Hans) (1873–1941) German physiologist who trained at Jena, where he became professor of psychiatry, succeeding **Bingswanger**. He was the first to record cortical electrical potentials in humans (1924), describing the alpha and the beta rhythms.[553] In 1932, he established the association in humans between unilateral spike discharges on the EEG and contralateral clonic jerks. He died by his own hand in 1941; he was an outspoken anti-Nazi and the régime had closed his clinic for that reason, at which he became despondent.

Berger rhythm The alpha rhythm of the EEG.

Berger, Oskar (1844–1885) German neurologist and neuropathologist who studied in Breslau, Berlin, and Vienna, graduating from Berlin and eventually becoming professor at Breslau where his main interests were hypnotism, neuropathology, neuralgias, and electrotherapy.

Berger paresthesia Distal paresthesias in young subjects. Berger's paper was published in a Breslau journal in 1879, but no pathology was reported, and it is likely that the condition represents benign nerve compression, as in **carpal tunnel syndrome**.

Bergeron, Etienne-Jules (1817–1900) French pediatrician who trained in Paris and worked in the French military and at the Hôpital Trousseau, as well as being prominent in the field of public health.

Bergeron disease (electric chorea) A disease of childhood characterized by violent rhythmical spasms ceasing in sleep and with a short and benign course. In this the condition differs from Dubini disease, which was frequently fatal.

The first description was attributed to Dr. E.J. Bergeron in 1880 by his pupil René Berland in his graduation thesis (University of Paris), but the condition had been previously noted by James Begbie in 1847.[480, 5704] Its nature remains unexplained. See also **Dubini disease**.

Bergmann glial cells A layer of astrocytes within the Purkinje layer of the cerebellar cortex which hypertrophy in those conditions in which the Purkinje cells atrophy. They were described by Gottlieb Bergmann (1781–1861), a German physician.

Bergmeister papilla An ocular remnant of the anterior hyaloid artery producing a preretinal fibrous veil. Another remnant, placed further anteriorly, is known as a *Mittendorf dot*.

beriberi (probably derived from a Sinhalese word signifying weakness, the repetition adding emphasis) A syndrome of cardiomyopathy and sensorimotor peripheral neuropathy resulting from dietary deficiency of vitamin B_1 (thiamine).

The condition was first described in the East Indies in 1642 by Jacob Bontius, a Dutch physician. In 1889, another Dutch physician, Christiaan Eijkman, demonstrated that the dietary deficiency was due to a lack of thiamine because of the polishing of rice, thus removing the husks, which is where the thiamine is. More recently, the name has been used in remote areas to refer to any form of severe neuropathy. It is still seen in third-world countries in starvation areas, in severely dietarily deprived alcoholics, and occasionally in people on severely restricted "fad" diets.

The chronic, dry, *atrophic form* represents a mainly motor neuropathy and occurs in alcoholics. The *subacute form* is a centripetal symmetrical sensorimotor neuropathy affecting especially those limbs most utilized in the individual's activities of daily living, with the later addition of cardiac failure.

Acute beriberi is a syndrome of chest pain with cardiac failure and leads rapidly to death.[5047]

Berlin syndrome A recessively inherited dysmorphic syndrome of physical and mental retardation with generalized mottling of the skin, hyperkeratosis, reduced sweating, and impaired eruption of the teeth.[573]

Berman disease See **mucolipidosis**.

Berman syndrome A familial, perhaps recessive disorder characterized by progressive ataxia, deafness, mental retardation, and signs of both upper and lower motor neuron lesions.

The condition resembles the **Richards–Rundle syndrome** except that it lacks the endocrinopathy and aminoaciduria.[579]

Bernard, Claude (1813–1878) An outstanding French physician and physiologist who was first apprenticed to an apothecary and embarked upon a career as a playwright (with very modest success) before he became a medical student graduating in 1839, and eventually a pupil of **Magendie** in Paris, from whom he learned much of the experimental method. He described the ocular changes which are now known as **Horner syndrome** in 1862, 7 years before Horner did,[582] and also discovered the existence of vasomotor nerves.[581]

His early work was on the chorda tympani, gastric digestion, and the role of pancreatic juices. He later studied the metabolism of glycogen and discovered the role of the sympathetic nerves in vasomotor regulation. His successes led to his appointment in 1847 as deputy to Magendie at the College de France (and later as his successor) and to a personal chair in experimental physiology and appointment to the Academie Francaise. Bernard was also the first to describe the action of curare in producing neuromuscular blockade although the muscle remained susceptible to direct stimulation, and he first identified the *milieu intérieur*, gluconeogenesis, the functions of gastric secretions and lipolysis by pancreatic secretions. His book *An Introduction to the Study of Experimental Medicine* (1865) laid the foundations for the scientific study of the human body.

Among the honors accorded him was the issue of a French stamp bearing his portrait and carrying a surcharge to be used for the support of unemployed intellectuals.

Bernard–Horner syndrome See **Horner syndrome**.

Bernhardt, Martin (1844–1915) German neurologist who graduated from Berlin and later worked with Leyden and Westphal. He himself was eventually professor at Berlin. He described **meralgia paresthetica** in 1878 and a form of progressive spinal muscular atrophy in 1893, as well as publishing good descriptions of cerebral tumors, syphilitic apoplexy, and diseases of the spinal cord.

Bernhardt–Roth (Rot) paresthesia See **meralgia paresthetica**.

Berry aneurysm See **aneurysm**.

Berry pins A set of three 8 cm pins with white, green, or red spots of different sizes painted upon their globular heads, used for the assessment of the central visual fields by confrontation at the bedside.[587] Dr. Henry Berry is a Canadian neurologist.

Berry spot test A test for detecting mucopolysaccharides, used in the diagnosis of Hurler syndrome, one of the **mucopolysaccharidoses**.

Bertolotti syndrome Numbness, pain, and/or hypersensitivity in the distribution of the sciatic nerve associated with sacralization of the fifth lumbar vertebra.[591]

Bertoletti–Garcin syndrome See **Garcin syndrome**.

Besnier–Boeck–Schaumann disease See **sarcoidosis**.

Bessman–Baldwin syndrome A recessively inherited syndrome characterized by blindness due to pigmentary macular degeneration, seizures, and mental and motor retardation. Excessive urinary excretion of carnitine and of various amino acids is another feature of the syndrome.[598]

beta band EEG activity in the frequency band over 13 Hz. Practically, most EEG machines using pen writers appreciably attenuate all frequencies higher than 75 Hz, and the customary use of relatively slow paper speeds further limits the interpreter's ability to resolve visually waves of frequencies over 35 Hz. However, this does not justify limiting unduly the high frequency response of the EEG channels, for EEG waves include transients such as spikes and sharp waves with components at frequencies above 50 Hz. (Adapted from the 1974 Report of the Committee on Terminology, IFCN. In: Chatrian, GE, Bergamini L, Dondey M, et al. A glossary of terms most commonly used by clinical electroencephalographers. *EEG Clin Neurophysiol* 1974;37:538–48. Reproduced by kind permission of Elsevier Science and the IFCN.)

beta rhythm In general, any EEG rhythm faster than 13 Hz, but more characteristically used to describe a rhythm from 13 to 35 Hz recorded over the frontocentral regions of the head during wakefulness. The amplitude of such beta rhythm is variable but is mostly below 30 μV. Other beta rhythms are most prominent in other locations or are diffuse. (Adapted from the 1974 report of the Committee on Terminology, IFCN. In: Chatrian GE, Bergamini L, Dondey M, et al. A glossary of terms most commonly used by clinical electroencephalographers. *EEG ClinNeurophysiol* 1974;37:538–48. Reproduced by kind permission of Elsevier Science and the IFCN.)

This rhythm is especially susceptible to enhancement by medications such as benzodiazepines and barbiturates.

beta-enolase deficiency A defect of distal glycolysis that may present as a metabolic myopathy and manifesting myalgias and exercise intolerance during adult life.[1261] See also **phosphoglycerate kinase, phosphoglycerate mutase, lactate dehydrogenase**, and **aldolase A deficiencies**.

beta-galactosidase-neuraminidase deficiency See **galactosialidosis**.

beta-glucuronidase deficiency See **mucopolysaccharidoses**.

beta-hydroxyisovaleric aciduria A syndrome of hereditary motor neuropathy resembling type 1 **hereditary motor neuropathy**, with associated abnormal aminoaciduria, and leading to early death. The condition is considered to be due to a failure of the enzymes in the leucine degradation pathway.[1835]

beta-interferon The first therapy for remitting-relapsing **multiple sclerosis** shown to be capable of reducing the number of exacerbations of the disease, at least during the first 3 years in which it is taken.

beta-ketothiolase deficiency (short chain 3-ketothiolase deficiency) An inborn error of metabolism presenting in infancy with intermittent acidosis, hyperammonemia, lethargy, vomiting, feeding difficulty, hyponatremia, hyperkalemia, and alteration in consciousness down to coma. Aminoaciduria is not a feature of the syndrome.[1472]

beta-methylcrotonylglycinuria A rare **organic acidemia** presenting in infancy with **infantile spasms**, lethargy, irritability, tachypnea, feeding difficulties, and failure to thrive.[379]

Beth Israel dystonia screen A short standardized telephone interview for use as a diagnostic instrument for dystonia. The interview questions whether subjects had noticed head turning, tilting, or shifting in any direction, whether the head shakes or jerks, or whether they had ever seen a doctor about such problems; whether others had remarked that their head pulls to either side, forward or backward, or that there was a head tremor; whether the shoulders lift or pull up or down involuntarily; and whether there is pain or stiffness in the neck most of the time and whether there is a head position that they can assume in order to stop the movement or the pain.[5564] (Reproduced by kind permission of the American Academy of Neurology and Lippincott Williams and Wilkins.)

Bethlem myopathy (early-onset benign autosomal dominant limb-girdle myopathy with contractures; OMIM 158810) (21q22.3; 2q37) A dominantly inherited, slowly progressive muscle disease with onset of limb-girdle weakness, hyotonia, and mild atrophy in infancy or childhood, without facial or cardiac involvement. Contractures of the long finger flexors and of the elbows and ankles are common. The first evidence may be reduction in fetal movements in the last trimester, hypotonia in the neonatal period, or weakness and contractures presenting in early childhood, but the onset can also be in late adult life with mild diffuse proximal > distal weakness, occasional respiratory muscle weakness, cramps, and falls. The condition may arrest at any time and it is compatible with a normal life span,[3223] although some disability is usual after the age of 50 years. Ten gene mutations, mainly affecting subunits of collagen type VI (*COL6A1,2,3*) are known to be responsible. See also **Ullrich congenital muscular dystrophy**.

Serum CK levels are normal or slightly elevated, the EMG is myopathic, and muscle biopsy indicates nonspecific myopathy. The condition has been mapped variously to chromosomes 21q22.3 and 2q37.

Better Hearing Institute A charitable organization. Address: Box 1840, Washington, DC 20013.

Betz, Vladimir Aleksandrovich (1834–1894) Russian professor of anatomy at Kiev (1868–1889).[1670] He described the giant pyramidal cells in 1874.

Betz cells The largest motor pyramidal cells of the fifth cerebral cortical layer.[602]

Beveridge syndrome A congenital dysmorphic syndrome characterized by macrocephaly, delayed closure of the fontanelles and cranial sutures, skeletal maldevelopments, visceromegaly, rhizomelia of the upper limbs, and patchy depigmentation of the skin.[381]

Bezold-Jarisch reflex Reflex cardiovascular depression with vasodilation and bradycardia (vasovagal syncope). The circulatory response changes from the normal maintenance of arterial pressure, to parasympathetic activation and sympathetic inhibition, causing hypotension. This change is triggered by reduced cardiac venous return leading to mechanical or chemical stimulation in the heart's left ventricle, where the afferent limb of the reflex evidently arises (HJM) as well as through affective mechanisms such as pain or fear. It is probably mediated in part via afferent nerves from the heart, but also by various noncardiac baroreceptors which may become paradoxically active. This response may occur during regional anesthesia, hemorrhage, or supine inferior vena cava compression in pregnancy; these factors are additive when combined. In these circumstances hypotension may be more severe than that caused by bradycardia alone, because of unappreciated vasodilation.[1403, 3447] See also **neurocardiogenic syncope**.

Bianchi syndrome The occurrence of sensory aphasia, apraxia, and alexia occurring in patients with left-sided lesions involving the parietal lobe, with transient hemiplegia and hemianesthesia, and described by Leonardo Bianchi (1848–1927),[613] an Italian psychiatrist. See **aphasia–agnosia–apraxia syndrome**.

bias 1. People who survive a disease for some time (prevalent cases) may differ from new (incident) cases by virtue of a confounding factor which is actually enhancing survival rather than acting as an etiologic factor.[4655] 2. Prejudgement.

biceps femoris reflex Contraction of this muscle in response to a tap over its tendon just above the fibular head. This is one of the few reflexes allowing assessment of the L5 reflex arc. See also **external hamstring reflex**.

biceps reflex Contraction of the biceps in response to a tap on its tendon, usually elicited by placing the examiner's index finger over the biceps tendon and tapping the finger, thus both palpating and visualizing the resultant muscle contraction. The reflex is increased in pyramidal disease affecting that limb and diminished with C5,6 lesions.

Bichat, Marie-François-Xavier (1771–1802) Anatomist, histologist, and physician at the Hotel-Dieu in Paris from the unusually early age of 28. Among his many contributions were his descriptions of the arachnoid membrane and of the subarachnoid space.[616]

Bickerstaff brainstem "encephalitis" A syndrome of ophthalmoplegia, ataxia, and normal or decreased muscle stretch reflexes, preceded by a febrile illness and leading on to gradual paralysis of cranial nerve function, descending from the oculomotor muscles to the whole brainstem, with slow subsequent recovery, during which a Parkinsonian picture may develop transiently. During the acute illness, drowsiness or a moribund state may occur, although with supportive care patients slowly return to normal, without sequelae. However, presentation with flaccid quadripatesis and coma has been described.[2161] Pupillary abnormalities, deafness bulbar palsy, ataxia, extensor plantar responses, and upper motor neurone features or hemisensory loss are also described as are cortical EEG abnormalities and areflexia. The disease runs a monophasic remitting course, usually with a good outcome.[4752]

As in Miller Fisher syndrome, IgG anti-GQ1b antibodies are frequently present. MRI scans, brainstem-evoked responses, and more recently autopsies have indicated the presence of a brainstem lesion and there is pleocytosis in the CSF.[83, 621] The condition tends to occur in small groups in geographically related areas.
Dr. E.R. Bickerstaff was an English neurologist practicing in the West Midlands.

The relationship of this condition to the **Miller Fisher syndrome** (a variant of **acute inflammatory demyelinating polyneuropathy**) is likely to be intimate; indeed they may be identical,[6823] since anti-GQ1b antibodies are not limited by the blood–brain barrier in the sites of their attack. The anti-GQ1b antibodies found in both conditions are considered to be pathogenic.[4839] The increased cells in the CSF, normal peripheral nerve conduction studies, and localized abnormality of evoked potentials in typical cases of "brainstem encephalitis" suggest that the condition involves the brainstem with or without peripheral nerve involvement,[6902] but the simultaneous involvement of both sites is common (brainstem encephalitis with an added (axonal subtype of) Guillain–Barré syndrome) and central and peripheral demyelination can occur together. See also **basilar migraine, disseminated vasculomyelinopathy**.

Bickerstaff migraine See **basilar migraine**.

bicuculline A potent epileptogenic agent which acts by blockade of gamma-aminohydroxybutyric acid, the inhibitory neurotransmitter.

Biedel, Arthur (1869–1933) Polish endocrinologist.

Bielschowsky, Alfred (1871–1940) German ophthalmologist practicing in Berlin, who gave the first account of **internuclear ophthalmoplegia**.[628] See also **Roth–Bielschowsky syndrome**.

Bielschowsky–Lutz–Cogan syndrome See **internuclear ophthalmoplegia**.

Bielschowsky head tilt test Patients with diplopia due to a IV cranial nerve palsy will note that the images fuse if they tilt the head toward the opposite shoulder but separate further when they tilt the head toward the side of the IV nerve palsy. As an example, with a left IV nerve palsy, the vertical deviation is more marked when the head is tilted down toward the left shoulder, and less marked when the head is tilted the other way.

Bielschowsky, Max (1869–1940) German neurobiologist, a student under Edinger and Nissl, who graduated from Munich and worked with Weigl and Edinger before moving to the Neurobiological Institute in Berlin. There his work was mainly on cytoarchitecture (**Vogt** was the director of the institute). He sought asylum from the Nazis in Spain and then in Holland in 1936, but was brought back by threat; he fled to England just before the start of World War II.

He introduced the technique for the silver staining of neurons which is still the basis of that now used and investigated the pathology of numerous brain diseases, such as that next following.[7]

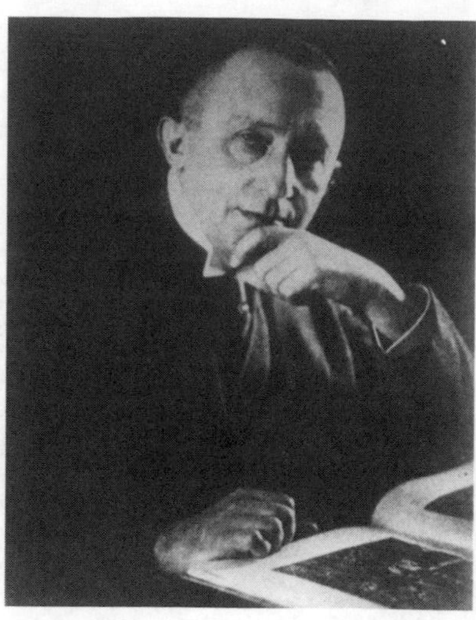

Figure B–5 Max Bielschowsky.

Bielschowsky bodies Intraneuronal inclusion bodies restricted to neurons in the external pallidum in cases of choreoathetosis and cerebral palsy.[3900] See also **corpora amylacea, Lafora bodies**.

Bielschowsky–(Dollinger)–Jansky disease (late infantile amaurotic familial idiocy) A rare, recessively inherited lipid storage disease characterized by seizures in early childhood, mental and motor impairment, cerebellar atrophy, and retinal degeneration (without the **cherry-red spot**), described by Bielschowsky in 1914.[629] See **neuronal ceroid lipidosis**.

Biemond, Arie (b. 1902) Dutch neurologist who trained in Amsterdam where he later became professor of neurology. His book *Brain Diseases* was published in 1970.

Biemond ataxia (OMIM 176250) A rare, dominantly inherited spinocerebellar degeneration resembling SCA4 with onset in youth or young adult life, and in which there is loss of posterior root ganglion cells with posterior column demyelination and of cerebellar Purkinje cells. Loss of vibration and postural sensation, areflexia, and scoliosis are the usual clinical manifestations.[632, 379] The condition has been mapped to the short arm of chromosome 16.

There is uncertainty as to whether this is a specific disorder, even though it is often referred to as a syndrome of pure posterior column ataxia (sensory ataxia). Primary degeneration of the large dorsal root ganglion cells would cause exactly the same symptoms (loss of thick-fiber sensory functions and hypo- or areflexia).[2754] The condition was first described by Mollaret in 1929.

Variants are: A recessively inherited form with *added pigmentary retinopathy*.[2895]

Sensory neuropathy with scoliosis A dominantly inherited or sporadic syndrome with onset at any time of a sensory neuropathy with ataxia and positive Romberg sign and with areflexia due to the peripheral loss of myelinated axons, and scoliosis. Nerve conductions show a loss of SNAPs.

Sensory ataxic neuropathy A dominantly inherited or sporadic syndrome with onset in adult life, characterized by loss of thick-fiber functions such as position and vibration sense, giving rise to sensory ataxia with hyporeflexia. Minor small-fiber loss accounts for some reduction in pain perception. The primary pathology is a loss of peripheral myelinated fibers.

See also **familial posterior column ataxia**, **cerebellar ataxias**.

Biemond syndrome 1. (brachydactyly-ataxia) A congenital dominantly inherited dysmorphic syndrome characterized by brachydactyly, abnormal metatarsals, and cerebellar signs.[630]

2. (obesity-polydactyly-iris coloboma) A congenital, recessive, dysmorphic syndrome characterized by obesity, iris coloboma, pigmentary retinal degeneration, hypogonadotrophic hypogonadism, polydactyly, hydrocephalus, and mental and developmental delay.[631] See **hydrocephalus with polydactyly**.

Biernacki sign Anesthesia in ulnar distribution or absence of pain when the ulnar nerve is pinched, described in tertiary neurosyphilis.[5333]

big blind spot syndrome The occurrence of an enlarged blind spot in the absence of any optic disk edema, the increased size of the blind spot being due to focal peripapillary retinopathy. Central acuity and color vision are unaffected, but a sharply defined scotoma is present, corresponding to the blind spot. The syndrome appears to be evanescent.[2126] See also **multiple evanescent white dot syndrome**, **papillophlebitis**.

big Broca aphasia See **Broca aphasia**.

big/large Spikes See **benign epileptiform transients of sleep**.

Bignami, Amico (1862–1929) Italian pathologist who graduated from the University of Rome where he became professor of general pathology in 1902. Most of his important communications were made in conjunction with **Marchiafava**.

Bijlsma syndrome A congenital dysmorphic syndrome characterized by aqueduct stenosis with hydrocephalus and gaze palsies, spasticity, and mental and developmental delay.[381]

Bikele sign 1. Resistance to extension of the elbow when the arm is elevated at the shoulder in patients with **neuralgic amyotrophy**, probably due to traction upon the irritated nerve roots.[6675] 2. Pain felt in the shoulder with contraction of the biceps, when the abducted, externally rotated arm is extended. The sign is described in patients with cerebral tumor[5704] or meningism.

bilateral (Gr, double + the side) On both sides.

bilateral biparietal atrophy See **posterior cortical atrophy**

bilateral central macrogyria (epilepsy, pseudobulbar palsy, and mental retardation, developmental Foix–Chavany–Marie syndrome) A neuronal migration disorder manifesting pseudobulbar palsy, mild pyramidal signs, mild mental retardation, and intractable secondary or multifocal epileptic syndromes (such as **infantile spasms**, generalized tonic-clonic or partial complex seizures, atonic attacks, head-dropping spells). The bilateral cerebral macrogyria is demonstrable on MRI scans.[3619]

bilateral distal vertebral artery occlusion A rare syndrome with a grave prognosis seen in patients with marked vasculopathy and characterized by the slow progression of signs of cerebellar and lateral medullary ischemia due to chronically reduced perfusion in vertebrobasilar territory, with a tendency to sudden death.[1008]

bilateral facial agenesis See **mandibulofacial dysostosis**.

bilateral facial spasm See **blepharospasm**.

bilateral frontal polymicrogyria See **polymicrogyria**.

bilateral generalized polymicrogyria A group of syndromes including *bilateral frontal polymicrogyria*, *bilateral parasagittal parieto-occipital polymicrogyria*, *bilateral perisylvian polymicrogyria*, and *bilateral frontoparietal polymicrogyria*. See **polymicrogyria**.

bilateral occipital calcification, epilepsy, and celiac disease An uncommon epileptic syndrome resembling **Sturge–Weber disease** and characterized by malabsorption; bilateral cortical and subcortical calcifications, mainly posteriorly but sometimes extending into frontal regions; and partial epilepsy. The latter may consist either of occipital seizures with a benign course and without mental deterioration or neurological signs or of drug-resistant occipital seizures with mental deterioration. No cutaneous abnormalities are described; there is no lobar atrophy, and MRI scans are normal.[4016]

bilateral paraspasm See **dystonia**.

bilateral periventricular nodular heterotopia (OMIM 300049) A malformation of neuronal migration or proliferation in which nodular masses of gray matter line the lateral ventricles and protrude into its lumen. Most cases have been in females, who present with various types of seizure, but who are otherwise normal. The condition is dominant and mapped to chromosome Xq28.

In a *variant* form in boys, mental retardation and frontonasal malformations also occur.[1673, 2614] See also **X-linked lissencephaly**, **congenital bilateral perisylvian syndrome**, and **subcortical band heterotopia**.

bilateral simultaneous optic neuropathy See **optic neuropathy**.

bilateral striatal necrosis, dystonia, and optic atrophy A rare syndrome, probably recessively inherited, characterized by dystonic movements and postures, generalized hypokinesia, subacute visual loss, and bilateral selective striatal necrotic lesions visualized by CT and MRI scans. Cognitive functions are unimpaired.[3796] See also **Leigh disease**, **infantile bilateral striatal necrosis**, and **Leber optic atrophy**.

bilateral vestibular paresis Loss of vestibular function following local infection, leading to **sensory ataxia** when the eyes can no longer compensate for the loss of vestibular input. Rotation and caloric stimulation tests do not induce vertigo for the same reason.[1177]

bilirubin encephalopathy See **kernicterus**.

bimodal extinction The failure to perceive and to report sensory signals from one side in more than one mode, for example, tactile and visual.

binasal hemianopia Isolated loss of both of the nasal fields of vision due to bilateral involvement of the uncrossed fibers at the optic chiasm, typically as a result of displacement of these fibers by a local mass lesion or increased intracranial pressure, or due to their compression by masses such as aneurysms of the internal carotid artery or meningiomas which are often (but not always) bilateral.[4730]

binaural (Lat, twice + ear) Relating to both ears.

Binet, Alfred (1856–1911) French psychologist, who with Theodor Simon devised the first validated test of intelligence at the request of the French government. The early tests gave a "mental age," and allowed classifications of intellectually impaired people as *idiots* (mental age 1–2 years), *imbeciles* (3–7 years), and *morons* (8–12 years). Above that age, people were classified as backward, normal, or advanced.

Later, an intelligence quotient was calculated as the mental age divided by the chronological age and expressed as a percentage. The Binet–Simon tests led on to refinements such as the Stanford–Binet and Herring–Binet tests, derivatives of which are still in use.

Bing, Robert Paul (1878–1956) Swiss neurologist and neuropathologist, who studied under **Horsley**, His, **Edinger**, **Oppenheim**, and **Déjèrine**, eventually becoming professor of neurology at Basel. His *Kompendium* (1909) was a manual of localization in clinical neurology based upon a superb exposition of clinical neuroanatomy; it was translated into three languages and most recently revised in English by Webb **Haymaker** (1969). The book remains, however, an essential introduction to the subject for aspiring neurologists. It was followed by his *Lehrbuch der Nerven-Krankenheiten* (1913), the fifth edition of which was also translated by Haymaker in 1939.

Bing headache (syndrome) See **cluster headache**.

Bing reflex 1. Watering of the eyes when eating food with a strong taste. 2. A variant method of eliciting the Babiński response, whereby the dorsum of the foot is pricked with a pin.[645]

Bing–Neel syndrome A syndrome of encephalomyelopathy and polyradiculopathy in association with macroglobulinemia. Systemic clinical features include fever, emaciation, anorexia, weight loss, and lymphadenopathy; common neurological findings are personality change, delusions, dementia, and variously pyramidal, cerebellar, and unclear sensory findings. The erythrocyte sedimentation rate is elevated, and IgM hyperglobulinemia, resembling **Waldenstrom macroglobulinemia**, is usual.[644]

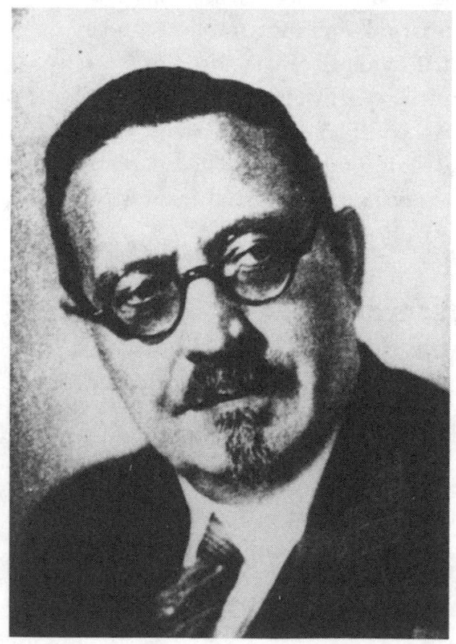

Figure B–6 Robert Paul Bing.

Dr. Bing is an American and Dr. A.V. Neel a Scandinavian physician.

binge eating The continuing ingestion of food despite reported satiety, sometimes associated with damage to a right-sided orbito-frontal-insular-striatal circuit in humans.[6864]

binocular (Lat, twice + eyes) Relating to both eyes.

binocular diplopia See **diplopia**.

Binswanger, Otto Ludwig (1852–1929) Swiss physician who qualified in Medicine at Zurich and who later studied psychiatry under Meynert in Vienna. He became professor of psychiatry at Jena and directed a military hospital during World War I. He is best remembered for his paper "The Differentiation of Progressive General Paralysis" published in 1894,[648] in which he suggested a vascular rather than a syphilitic cause for the dementing syndrome now named for him, but he also wrote extensively on epilepsy, hysteria, and delirium. He retired, following a severe attack of "Spanish" influenza (**encephalitis lethargica**) in 1919.

Binswanger disease (Binswanger encephalitis, subacute arteriosclerotic encephalopathy, progressive subcortical arteriosclerotic encephalopathy, encephalitis subcorticalis chronica progressiva, lacunar dementia, subcortical vascular dementia)

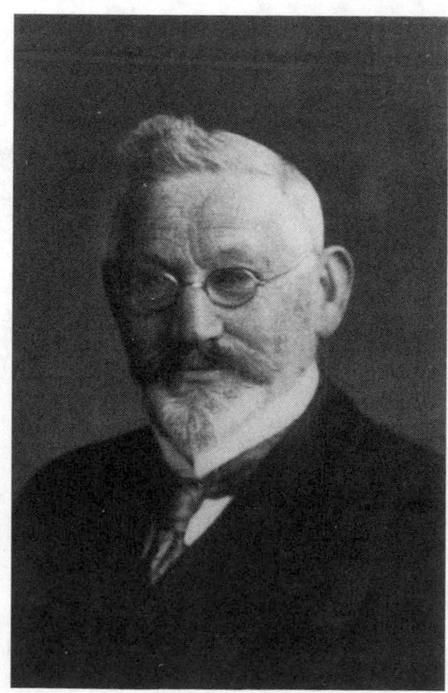

Figure B–7 Otto Ludwig Bingswanger.

An entity characterized by an ischemic periventricular leukoencephalopathy typically sparing the arcuate subcortical U fibers and manifested clinically by subcortical frontal executive dysfunction, Parkinsonian gait disturbances, urinary incontinence, mood changes, and pseudobulbar palsy. It is one of the most common forms of vascular dementia in the elderly. Clinically, it may be suspected in middle-aged hypertensive patients with evidence of systemic vascular disease who develop insidious, fluctuating **subcortical dementia** with especial involvement of memory, mood, and cognition, seizures as well as evidence of pyramidal, extrapyramidal, and cerebellar[515] dysfunction presenting as mild strokes.

This leukoencephalopathy is likely caused by hypoxia-ischemia of distal watershed periventricular territories, the combined effects of arteriolosclerosis and elongation of medullary arterioles, dilatation of the perivascular spaces (état criblé), and decreased brain perfusion from hypotension or low cardiac output. Lacunes may be markers of Binswanger-type lesions in these patients. Increased fibrinogen levels and hyperviscosity may be found.[2107, 1012]

Binswanger did not provide a full account of the neuropathology of the condition (this was remedied by **Nissl** and by **Alzheimer**, who also named the disease), and his patients were not notably hypertensive. One assumes with slight justification that the condition defined as follows is that which Binswanger actually described. Criteria for the diagnosis of Binswanger disease have been suggested.[518] (See Chart B–3.)

This condition Binswanger differentiated from syphilis (although in retrospect it is likely that his patients did have syphilis), and his pathological examination showed the presence of arteriolosclerosis, hemorrhages and infarcts deep in the cerebral hemispheres, extensive white matter atrophy mainly in the periventricular and occipitotemporal distribution, and only slight atrophy of the cortex.[648] The pathological features of note are **lacunes**, subcortical white matter demyelination, the **état criblé**, neuronal loss, gliosis, ventricular dilatation, and atheroma of the larger cerebral vessels. CT scans show enlarged ventricles, symmetrical periventricular lucencies, and lacunar and sometimes cortical infarcts.

Olszewski emphasized the presence of the lacunes in 1962 and suggested the term *subcortical arteriosclerotic encephalopathy*, but the eponym presumes less and is preferred for its brevity. The definitive major review is that of Babikian and Ropper.[320]

A familial form of Binswanger disease presenting in younger patients in the absence of vascular risk factors should raise the possibility of **cerebral autosomal dominant arteriopathy with subcortical infarcts and leukoencephalopathy**.

Symptoms are related to the disruption of subcortical neural circuits that control *executive cognitive functioning* which includes short-term memory, organization, mood, the regulation of attention, the ability to act or make decisions, and appropriate behavior. The most characteristic feature is psychomotor slowness; other symptoms include forgetfulness (but not as severe as the forgetfulness of Alzheimer disease), changes in speech, an unsteady gait, clumsiness or frequent falls, changes in personality or mood (most likely apathy, irritability, and depression), and urinary symptoms. See the NIMH Web site: http://www.nimh.nih.gov/health/publications/adhd/symptoms.shtml/.

Binswanger encephalitis See **Binswanger disease**.

biological clocks Pacemaking mechanisms in the brain controlling circadian rhythms, likely situated within the suprachiasmatic nuclei in the anterior hypothalamus.

Bio-Med Central Neurology A professional electronic-only journal. Web site: www.biomedcentral.com/bmcneurol.

biopsy The surgical removal of tissue (such as muscle, nerve, or brain) for microscopic or bacteriological study.

biopterin deficiency See **phenylketonuria**.

Biot breathing (ataxic breathing) A pattern of respiration marked by irregular grouping of the breaths which vary in depth and between which there are apneic pauses of different lengths. These occur in patients with dorsolateral medullary lesions and in such diffuse diseases as meningitis and uremia. The pattern is not (as has sometimes been suggested) regular, rapid, or rhythmical.

Dr. C. Biot (1848–1918) was a French physician who published his description in 1876 while an intern in Lyon.[649] See also **Cheyne–Stokes respiration** and **apneustic breathing**.

Chart B–3. Criteria for the Diagnosis of Binswanger Disease

1. Dementia must be established by clinical examination and confirmed by neuropsychological tests.
2. One finding from two of the following three groups must be present:
   The presence of a vascular risk factor or evidence of systemic vascular disease (e.g., hypertension, diabetes, a history of myocardial infarction, cardiac arrhythmia, or congestive heart failure)
   Evidence of focal cerebrovascular disease (e.g., a history of stroke or demonstration of focal pyramidal or sensory signs).
   Evidence of "subcortical" cerebral dysfunction (e.g., Parkinsonian, magnetic, or "senile" gait, Parkinsonian or gegenhalten rigidity, or a history of incontinence secondary to a spastic bladder).
3. The radiological criteria requires bilateral **leukoaraiosis** on computed tomography (CT), or bilateral and multiple or diffuse subcortical high signal T2-weighted lesions greater than 2 × 2 mm on MRI scans.

The proposed criteria lose their validity in the presence
1. of multiple or bilateral cortical lesions on CT or MRI scans; or
2. of severe dementia (e.g., **Mini-Mental state** score of less than 10).

Adapted from Bennett DA, Wilson RS, Gilley, et al. *Clinical diagnosis of Binswanger's disease.* J Neurol Neurosurg Psychiatr *1990;53:961–65. Reproduced by kind permission of BMJ Publications.*

biotin-responsive encephalopathy (OMIM 252260) A recessively inherited progressive neurological syndrome of early childhood due to deficiency of biotinidase.[6850] It is mapped to 3p25.

Clinically, the disease is phenotypically diverse and may be characterized by alopecia, skin rash, encephalopathy, ataxia, hypotonia, hearing loss, myoclonus, neonatal seizures, developmental delay, lactic acidosis, and/or aminoaciduria.[5510] The condition is one cause of the **Ramsay–Hunt syndrome** of seizures, myoclonus, and ataxia. See **multiple carboxylase deficiency**.

biotin-responsive multiple carboxylase deficiency See **holo-carboxylase deficiency**.

biphasic action potential An action potential that crosses the baseline only once, producing two phases (one above and the other below the baseline).

biphasic end-plate activity See **end-plate activity**.

biphasic motor reaction The occurrence of a **flexor reflex** followed by extension of the legs in patients with incomplete spinal cord lesions, after any form of stimulation given to sites below the level of the lesion.

biphasic wave See **diphasic wave**.

bipolar With two opposite poles or states. Hence *bipolar depression*, *bipolar cells* (neurons with two axons), and the following entries.

bipolar derivation A recording from a pair of exploring electrodes. See also **exploring electrode** and **bipolar montage**.

bipolar montage Multiple bipolar derivations in which no electrode is common to all derivations. In most cases, bipolar derivations are linked, that is, adjacent derivations from electrodes along the same array have one electrode in common, connected to the input terminal 2 of one amplifier and to the input terminal 1 of the following amplifier. See also **referential montage**. (Adapted from the 1974 Report of the Committee on Terminology, IFCN. In: Chatrian GE, Bergamini L, Dondey M, et al. A glossary of terms most commonly used by clinical electroencephalographers. *EEG Clin Neurophysiol* 1974;37:538–48. Reproduced by kind permission of Elsevier Science and the IFCN.)

bipolar needle electrode A recording electrode that measures the voltage between two insulated wires cemented side by side in a steel cannula. The bare tips of the electrodes are flush with the level of the cannula which may serve as a ground. (From the 2001 Report of the Nomenclature Committee of the American Association of Electromyography and Electrodiagnosis.[19] Reproduced by kind permission of the AANEM.)

bird-like face syndrome See **Seckel bird-headed dwarfism**.

Birnbaum syndrome A syndrome of chronic progressive chorea with cerebellar atrophy, described in 1941.[659]

bisynchronous An tautologous contraction of the equally tautologous "bilaterally synchronous."

bitemporal hemianopia Loss or reduction in efficacy of the visual field on the temporal side in each eye. The first complete analytic description was in 1915 by Cushing and Walker,[1394] who pointed out that the usual cause was a hypophyseal tumor and that the defects were rarely symmetrical.

They divided such visual defects between eight stages according to their severity, among which stage 1 represented a slant in the upper boundary of the temporal field and a corresponding quadrantic defect in the color peripheries; stage 4 represented hemianopsia, often with macular sparing; while stage 8 indicated complete blindness.

The development of the deficit was charted by Traquair, who showed that it characteristically begins in the upper outer quadrant, proceeding clockwise in the right and anticlockwise in the left field, so that the upper nasal quadrant remains longest. The central defect behaves in the same way.[6372] See also **hemianopia**, **Traquair scotoma**.

bizarre high-frequency discharge See **complex repetitive discharge**.

bizarre repetitive discharge See **complex repetitive discharge**.

bizarre repetitive potential See **complex repetitive discharge**.

Bjerrum, Jamik Peterson (1851–1926) Danish professor of ophthalmology in Copenhagen, who described **arcuate scotomas** in patients with glaucoma in 1890. He also developed the tangent screen, still in general use, employing a cloth pinned to the door of his office.[2066]

Bjerrum screen (tangent screen) A dark felt cloth 1 m^2 marked with a central point, radii, and concentric rings, set vertically in a darkened room, upon which the subject gazes while a lighted object is brought into his field of vision from the periphery as a test of the peripheral visual fields and the extent of the blind spot.

Björnstadt syndrome See **pili torti**.

black widow spider An arachnid, the venom of which induces the rapid release of transmitter from nerve terminals, causing initial muscular contractions followed by paralysis. This may be fatal in young children and the frail elderly. The spider (so called because she eats her mate) is recognized by the characteristic red "hourglass" pattern on her belly by those prepared to turn her over.

bladder disorders See **automatic bladder**, **deafferented bladder**, **hypertonic bladder**, **incontinence**, and **motor paralytic bladder**.

Blanchet syndrome Unilateral lumbar meningopolyradiculoneuritis associated with inflammation of the lumbar sympathetic chain.[673] Further reports of this syndrome are not available and the nature of the condition is unknown.

blast (Gr, bud) A suffix denoting development.

blennophobia An exaggerated fear of slime or mucus.

blepharismus (from Gr, the eyelid) Winking.

blepharoclonus Repetitive blinking, sometimes amounting to forced eye closure, heralding the later development of **blepharospasm**. See **spasmus nictitans**.

blepharocolysis (Gr, an eyelid + inhibition) (lid opening apraxia) A supranuclear movement disorder with involuntary closure of the eyelids and an inability to open the eyes, due to an involuntary over-inhibition of the levator palpebrae muscles without ongoing activity in the orbicularis oculi. It occurs in idiopathic dystonias and less often with rostral brainstem lesions.[1919] The transient atonic inability to initiate eyelid opening occurs in the absence of a definable lesion of the supranuclear or infranuclear oculomotor pathways. Despite the alternative name, the condition is not really an apraxia at all. See also **blepharospasm**, **apraxia of lid opening**.

blepharonasofacial syndrome A dominantly inherited dysmorphic syndrome characterized by stenosis of the lacrimal puncta, syndactyly, pyramidal and cerebellar signs, dystonia, and mental retardation.[4921]

blepharophimosis A dominantly inherited condition characterized by shortness and narrowing of the palpebral fissures, shortening of the upper eyelid (with deficiency of the levator palpebrae superioris also contributing to ptosis), hypoplasia of the orbicularis oculi and flattening of the root of the nose.[4]

blepharophimosis syndrome A heterogeneous, dominantly inherited congenital dysmorphic syndrome characterized by blepharophimosis and, variously, ptosis, telecanthus, nystagmus, strabismus, reversible joint contractures, cleft palate, dolichocephaly, arachnodactyly, skeletal and cerebellar dysgeneses, hypotonia, and mandibular hypoplasia.[2117] Type 1 is dominantly inherited (3q23, *FOXL2*) and presents with ptosis and epicanthus inversus (a small skin-fold arising from the lower lid and running in and up toward the nose) with or without ovarian failure. *Variants* are as follows:

Congenital blepharophimosis, characterized by general diminution of the palpebral fissure in all its dimensions but with the eyelids normally differentiated. Associated eye defects include nystagmus, microphthalmos, anophthalmos, ptosis, epicanthus inversus, and hypermetropia. Facial dysmorphisms are also frequently associated. The condition may be dominantly inherited as uncomplicated blepharophimosis; associated with micropthalmos and anophthalmos; with rigidity and dysfunction of the extra-ocular muscles; or as part of the **Waardenburg syndrome**.

Criteria for the diagnosis of congenital blepharophimosis have been suggested[6153] and are adapted here:

1. Diminution of the palpebral fissure by 2–4 mm width over a length of 10–15 mm on opening the lids. These measurements remain constant throughout life.
2. The distance between the internal canthi is often double the length of the palpebral fissure.
3. The nasal bridge is flattened.
4. The aplasia of the palpebral levators and the tautness of the skin cause stiffness of the lids and obliteration of the tarsal folds.
5. The eyelid covers the pupil; for improvement the head is usually tilted back and there is continued overaction of the occipitofrontalis muscle.
6. The eyelids are defectively developed with thin, smooth atrophic skin, and rudimentary tarsal plates.
7. The eyelashes are underdeveloped and grow irregularly.
8. There is lateral displacement of the lachrymal puncta.
9. The lack of contact within the bulb and the lids, especially nasally, results in epiphora.

Variants include the following:

Saethre-Chotzen Syndrome (SCS; blepharophimosis 2) (7p21, *TWIST*)

Blepharophimosis with short stature An autosomal recessive syndrome of blepharophimosis, ptosis, ophthalmoplegia and prognathism, synophrys, short stature and syndactyly of the toes, borderline mental retardation, and anosmia.[4992]

Ohdo syndrome of mental retardation, congenital heart disease, blepharophimosis and blepharoptosis with hypoplastic teeth.[4992]

Dubowitz syndrome (ptosis, blepharophimosis, lateral telecanthus, microcephaly, short stature, and mental retardation).

See also **Marden–Walker syndrome**, **Schwartz–Jampel syndrome**.

blepharoplegia (Gr, eyelid + weakness) Ptosis due to paresis of the levator palpebrae.

blepharoptosis (Gr, eyelid + a fall) Drooping of the upper eyelid. See **ptosis**.

blepharoschisis A malformation affecting the eyelids which may be a simple cleft up to complete absence (*ablepharon*).[4] See also **coloboma**.

blepharospasm (facial paraspasm, bilateral facial spasm, benign essential blepharospasm) Symmetrical, repetitive, involuntary, sustained, tight closure of the eyes as a result of involuntary contractions of the orbiculari oculi, in the absence of ocular pathology,[2549, 3160] although the R2 component of the **blink reflex** is abnormally prolonged. The involuntary overactivity of the orbicularis oculi with co-contraction of the levator palpebrae manifests as frequent and prolonged blinks, clonic bursts, prolonged tonic contractions, or a blend of all of these. It occurs in idiopathic dystonias and less often with rostral brainstem lesions and represents a focal dystonic syndrome, most common in adult women. The muscular contractions are often increased by bright light and reduced by other voluntary activity, despite which they may be so intractable as to produce functional blindness.[1853, 1919, 3163] See also **Meige syndrome**.

Rating scales for blepharospasm have been constructed.[1947]

In *variant* forms, patients with **Parkinson disease** or **progressive supranuclear palsy** are unable to initiate or sustain eye opening in the absence of overt spasm of the orbicularis muscles;[1852] or the condition occurs as a familial disorder (but with great phenotypic variability). See also **apraxia of lid opening**.

blepharospasm-oromandibular dystonia See **Breughel syndrome**.

Blessed-Roth dementia instruments (Newcastle dementia scale, information-memory-concentration test) A two-part measure designed to quantify the cognitive and behavioral symptoms of dementia, comparing these manifestations with measures of underlying brain neuropathology. Some of the elements have been included in the **CAMDEX**[5429] and in the CERAD Instrument.[4498]

The *Blessed Dementia Scale* is a behavioral rating scale evaluating functional and emotional impairment and consisting of 22 items measuring changes in the performance of everyday activities, in self-care habits and in personality interests and drives. The Blessed Information-Memory-Concentration test[681] is a well-validated measure of cognitive impairment. Dr. G. Blessed is a neuro-psychologist in Newcastle, UK. See **information-memory-concentration test**.

blind headache A once-popular term for **migraine**.

blind spot A physiological defect in the visual fields due to the absence of rod and cone receptors on the head of the optic nerve. Its presence was first remarked in 1688 by E. Mariotte (1620–1684), a French physicist, who also described the **red reflex**.

blindisms (digito-ocular maneuver) The repetitive rubbing of the eyes, an action performed frequently by some people with congenital pigmentary retinal degenerations.

blindsight The capacity to detect (or at least make saccadic movements in the direction of) visual stimuli presented within the area of a field defect in the absence of acknowledged awareness. This may occur when the blindness results from damage to the striate cortex.[6703]

blink rate The frequency of involuntary repetitive blinking. In the normal subject this is 24 ± 15 per min. The rate is decreased in depressive illnesses, **Parkinson disease**, and **progressive supranuclear palsy**.[5470]

blink reflex 1. Clinically, closure of the eyes with sudden visual stimulation or with tactile stimulation of the upper part of the face. The reflex was known to Descartes and to Jean Fernel (1506–1588). See also **palpebral reflex** and **orbicularis oculi reflex**. 2. In electromyography, **compound muscle action potentials** evoked from orbicularis oculi muscles as a result of brief electric or mechanical stimuli applied to the cutaneous area innervated by the supraorbital (or less commonly, the infraorbital) branch of the trigeminal nerve. Typically, there is an early compound muscle action potential (RJ wave) ipsilateral to the stimulation site with a latency of about 10 msec and a bilateral late compound muscle action potential (R2 wave) with a latency of approximately 30 msec. Generally, only the R2 wave is associated with a visible contraction of the muscle. The configuration, amplitude, duration, and latency of the two components, along with the sites of recording and stimulation, should be specified. The Rl and R2 waves are oligosynaptic and polysynaptic brainstem reflexes, respectively. Together they are called the blink reflex. The afferent arc is provided by the sensory branches of the trigeminal nerve and the efferent arc is provided by facial nerve motor fibers. (From the 2001 Report of the Nomenclature Committee of the American Association of Electromyography and Electrodiagnosis.[19] Reproduced by kind permission of the AANEM.)

The reflex is considered abnormal when there is unilateral loss of R1; unilateral delay by 1.4 ms or more; or uni- or bilateral delay above the age-related mean + 2.5 SEM.[2982]

blink response See **blink reflex**.

blink-saccade synkinesis The tendency for blink and saccadic movements to occur together. This is both normal and efficient, although normally either movement may be made alone. Inability to make saccades without blinking has been described as a sign of posterior fossa disease.[6957]

blip syndrome Irregularly recurrent, momentary sensations in the head suggesting impending loss of consciousness, felt in the relaxed state by subjects without evidence of neurological disease. It has a benign prognosis.[3659]

See also **exploding head syndrome**.

blips Torsional eye deviations during and after saccadic eye movements.[2849]

Bliss symbols A pictographic, ideographic writing system of about 100 symbols developed by Charles K. Bliss that can be decoded in all languages and is intended to function as an auxiliary language for international communication. It has been adapted as a communication medium for prereading, severely communicatively impaired children.

The symbols express both items and ideas and are laid out on large cards, enabling the subject to point to them successively in order to convey information or requests.[4264] However, newer language systems such as *Rebus* and *Picsyms* have been adopted more widely because many people find them easier to learn.

blitz-nick-salaam krampfe See **West syndrome**.

Bloch, Bruno (1878–1933) Swiss physician.

Bloch–Sulzberger syndrome See **incontinentia pigmenti**.

Block Design Test A constructional task, a subtest of the **Wechsler Adult Intelligence Scale**, wherein the subject is required to manipulate multiple-patterned blocks in order to match a composite pattern presented on a card. It is a measure of right hemispheric spatial functioning (constructional praxis).[6688]

block vertebral anomaly A rare spinal column and cord anomaly with scoliosis, abnormal rib cage, and local myelopathy resulting from a failure of segmentation at the affected level.[5611]

blocking 1.The apparent temporary obliteration of EEG rhythms in response to physiological or other stimuli such as electrical stimulation of the brain. See **attenuation**. 2. A condition of temporary unresponsiveness of the EEG amplifier caused by major overload and manifested initially by extreme flat-topped pen excursion(s) lasting up to a few seconds. See also **clipping**. (Adapted from the 1974 Report of the Committee on Terminology, IFCN. In: Chatrian GE, Bergamini L, Dondey M, et al. A glossary of terms most commonly used by clinical electroencephalographers. *EEG Clin Neurophysiol* 1974;37:538–48.) 3. A brief interruption of a train of thought with a temporary difficulty in logical verbal expression. Although this is a common occurrence in the normal, fatigued person and increases with age, repetitive brief periods of complete inhibition of thought is a symptom of schizophrenia of the first rank, and can occur in depressive illness. 4. A term used in **single fiber electromyography** to describe dropout of one or more components of the potential during sequential firings. If more than one component drop out simultaneously, this is described as concomitant blocking and is usually seen when jitter values exceed 80–100 μs. Blocking is a sign of abnormal neuromuscular transmission, which may be due to primary neuromuscular transmission disorders, such as **myasthenia gravis** and other myasthenic syndromes. It is also seen as a result of degeneration and reinnervation in neuropathies or myopathies. Concomitant blocking may be generated by a split muscle fiber or failure of conduction at an axon branch serving several muscle fibers. (Adapted from the 2001 Report of the Nomenclature Committee of the American Association of Electromyography and Electrodiagnosis.[19] Reproduced by kind permission of the AANEM.)

blocking reaction The abrupt inhibition or cessation of a voluntary movement.

Blocq, Paul-Oscar (1860–1896) French neuropsychiatrist, born and trained in Paris, where he worked at the Salpêtrière before his premature death. He published his own textbook in 1894, contributed chapters on chorea and syphilis to Charcot's "Traité de Médicine" and described the syndrome of **astasia-abasia** in 1888.[684]

Blocq syndrome (astasia-abasia) Hysterical inability to walk or even stand, although all movements are normal in the lying position. Jacoud, Charcot, and Weir Mitchell had touched upon the subject, but Blocq's 1888 monograph was the definitive text.[684] As he put it, the patient "can even jump in some cases or walk on all fours, but has lost the memory of the specialized movements necessary to hold himself upright (astasia) and to walk (abasia)."

All but one of Blocq's patients were under 28 years old. By his description there appears to be some resemblance to Bamberger's saltatory spasms, but Blocq denied this. In fact, both were manifestations of hysteria. However, with vermis lesions (e.g., due to medulloblastoma in children), leg movements may be unimpaired in recumbency even though the gait is very ataxic. [JF]

blood–brain barrier A physico-chemical mechanism whereby solutes and materials in suspension in the blood are held back from entering the internal environment of the brain.

The search for the nature of this barrier was initiated by Ehrlich in 1886 as a result of his work on aniline dyes as staining reagents, during which he noticed that the vital acid dyes such as trypan blue stained everything in the body except the brain, which *was* however stained by the basic dyes. In 1913, Goldman injected acid dyes into the ventricles and showed that they did then stain the brain tissue, indicating the presence of a selectively permeable barrier between blood and brain, considered to be at the level of the endothelial cell.[6355]

Within the brain, only the area postrema, median eminence, pineal gland, neurohypophysis, pineal crest, and a few other areas are not shielded by this barrier. Clinically, it is highly effective in preventing entry into the CNS of various medications, including some antibiotics. The barrier may, however, be lowered by inflammation, as in meningitis, and by certain other toxins. The barrier is crossed more easily by nonionized, low molecular weight, lipid-soluble molecules.

Bloom syndrome A congenital dysmorphic syndrome characterized also by microcephaly, short stature, hirsutism, facial telangiectasias, vitiligo, café-au-lait spots, and photosensitivity of the skin.[5749]

blowout fracture A fracture of the floor of the orbit as a result of blunt trauma to the globe or to the inferior orbital rim. Multiple ocular motor palsies may result, and entrapment of the inferior rectus muscle within the fracture may lead to restriction of upward gaze.[3762]

blue diaper syndrome (Drummond syndrome) A recessively inherited diffuse encephalopathy characterized by hypercalcemia, nephrocalcinosis, and indicanuria. Craniostenosis, mental retardation, and dwarfism are less constant features. It is due to the slow absorption of tryptophan from the bowel, followed by its conversion to indoles which are absorbed and excreted in the urine to produce the bluish staining.[1716]

blue edema See **Charcot edema**.

blue jeans syndrome Compression of the sciatic nerve by shrinking wet jeans.[4167]

blue rubber bleb nevus syndrome An uncommon congenital neurocutaneous disorder manifesting blue hemangiomas of the skin and vascular malformations of internal organs, sometimes including the brain and its venous sinuses but more commonly the gastrointestinal tract. Seizures may be a complication. It was first described by William Bean in 1958.[5561] Most cases are sporadic but linkage to chromosome 9p has been reported.

b-mode ultrasonography A technique whereby high-frequency sound waves are transmitted through tissues, the returning echoes providing an image of the area evaluated. It allows identification of the arterial wall and lumen of vessels to the extent that even minor disease of the internal carotid can be detected, but it does not readily distinguish flowing blood from clot.

bobbing See **ocular bobbing**.

bobble-headed doll syndrome A congenital syndrome characterized by intermittent, arrhythmic, to-and-fro (flexion-extension) bobbing or nodding movements of the head at 2–3 Hz associated with rhythmic flexion and extension of the arms and legs in the presence of severe, slowly progressive hydrocephalus. It is usually caused by a tumor of the third ventricle, but tumors of the corpus callosum, frontal lobe, or basal ganglia may also be responsible.[536, 6770]

Generalized obesity, optic atrophy, behavioral problems, emotional lability, sensory deficits, choroid plexus tumors, and arachnoid cysts are other reported features.[3754]

Bode-Heinemann Measure of Post-Traumatic Confusion and Amnesia An adaptation of the **Galveston Orientation and Amnesia Test** from the Kessler Medical Rehabilitation Research and Education Corporation 1199 Pleasant Valley Way, West Orange, NJ 07052.

The items are administered starting with the easiest first, progressing through more difficult ones and include the following:

What is your name? Where do you live? When were you born?

If less than 2 are correct the test is aborted and a severe confusional state (aka PTA) is diagnosed. If 2 or more are correct, the test continues with the following questions:

Where are you now (city)? Where are you now (hospital)? What year is it? What month is it? What day of the week is it? What time is it? What day of the month is it?

If less than 6 answers are correct the test is halted and a moderate confusional state (aka disorientation/PTA) is diagnosed. If 6 or more are correct, the test continues with the final questions:

What is your last memory before your injury? What is your first memory after your injury? (With details of the subject's last memory.)

Details of first memory are then requested, and the questions "How did you get here?"

and

"When did you get here?" are put.

10 or less correct answers indicates the diagnosis of a confusional state. A recheck on the second day is advised.

Boder–Sedgwick syndrome See **ataxia-telangiectasia**.

Bodian, David (b. 1910) American anatomist.

Bodian stain A method for staining nerve fibers and nerve endings, using colloidal silver, invented by Bodian in 1936.[696]

bodybuilder sign A posture of abduction of the arms at the shoulders with full flexion at the elbows and wrists, resembling the pose of a bodybuilder and occurring as a result of acute traumatic central cervical cord injury, usually in the elderly.[1916] A partial illustration of this was given in C.A. Elsberg's book *Diseases of the Spinal Cord and Membranes* (Saunders, Philadelphia, 1926, pp. 212–13).

body clock That mechanism within the brain which regulates cycles of human activity as a pacemaker. It is considered to exist within the suprachiasmatic nucleus.

body image agnosia See **topographical agnosia, finger agnosia**.

body righting reflex See **righting reflexes**.

body schema See **body scheme**.

body scheme (body schema) The term of **Head, Holmes**, and **Brain** for an individual's conception of his body's size, shape and position, the body parts, right and left sides, etc. The mechanism is directly involved when a person cannot recognize parts of his own body—**asomatagnosia**.

Boe, Franciscus de la (1614–1672) Dutch physiologist and professor of the practice of medicine at Leyden; also known as **Sylvius**. He described the lateral (Sylvian) fissure in 1637 and named the aqueduct, although he was not the first to describe it. He also made the first differentiation between static, postural and action tremors.

Bogorad, F.A. (fl. 1928) Russian neurologist.

Bogorad syndrome See **crocodile tears**, the syndrome aptly named by Bogorad in 1928,[704] but previously described by **Oppenheim** in 1913.

bombesin A peptide found in the brain and in the gastrointestinal tract that causes a feeling of satiety.

bonbon sign Movement of the tongue inside the mouth, producing a bulge in the cheek, as though the subject has a candy in his mouth. It is seen in dystonic or choreic states.

Bondin–Barbizet syndrome See **epileptic-endocrine syndrome**.

Bonhoeffer, Karl Ludwig (1868–1948) German psychiatrist who studied in Tubingen and Munich. After psychiatric training in France and Germany, he became an assistant to **Wernicke** and later succeeded Kraepelin at Heidelberg before moving on, eventually to Berlin as professor of psychiatry. He authored nearly 100 publications on various topics in neurology, psychiatry, pathology, and alcoholism. He died 3 years after his son, a Lutheran pastor, was hanged for outspoken criticism of the Nazi régime.

Bonhoeffer symptom Chorea, which he considered to be caused by a lesion in a region posterior to the optic thalamus, presumably the caudate, in which case he was right.[734]

Bonhoeffer syndrome (exogenous psychosis) See **delirium**.

Bonnet, Amedée (1809–1858) French surgeon who trained in Lyon and Paris and after internship there returned to Lyon where he became professor of clinical surgery in due course.

Bonnet sign Pain in the back occurring with adduction of the thigh, but not when flexion is passively performed without adduction; it is positive in lumbosacral root irritation. The sign was described incidentally, in Bonnet's two-volume book on joint disease (1845).

Bonnet, Charles (1720–1793) Swiss lawyer, naturalist, and philosopher. A wealthy man, he never practiced law (which he disliked) but rather studied natural history. He wrote on sensation and discernment in plants and anticipated Darwin's theory of evolution, by implication. His studies of respiratory pores in *Lepidoptera* led to his election as a fellow of the Royal Society, although he never left Switzerland.[5704] After his sight failed, he turned from biology to philosophy. He described the **Bonnet syndrome** in his grandfather.

Bonnet syndrome (syndrome of Charles Bonnet) The occurrence in elderly people with normal mental faculties of monosymptomatic and recurrent, vivid, dynamic, neutral, or pleasant visual pseudo-hallucinations. The original description was of this problem and autoscopy occurring in Charles Bonnet's grandfather who had had an operation for cataract 11 years before. "His double, the smoker, appeared regularly each evening the moment he lit his pipe. Immediately after he would describe another

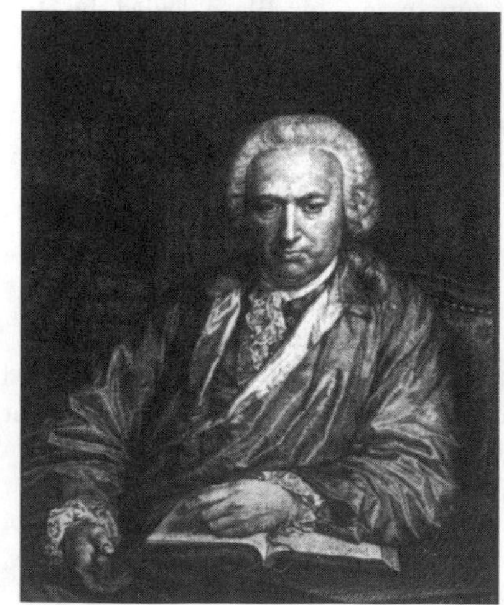

Figure B–8 Charles Bonnet.

decoration or some other vision; and having jested over these fictions of the brain, he would calmly resume his discourse."[737] Strangely, when Charles Bonnet went blind at the end of his life, he also experienced visual hallucinations.[1428]

The hallucinations usually lack any personal meaning and are easily dismissed as unreal by the patient, unlike the hallucinations in Parkinson disease which may be dismissed as unreal, but often are loaded with personal meaning—such as visions of dead relatives; they may be associated with other psychotic symptoms such as paranoid delusions.

It has been suggested that four criteria allow the diagnosis. These are the sudden, unexpected onset of visual hallucinations which are complex, repetitive, and stereotyped; insight is fully or partially retained; there is an absence of delusions and no other types of hallucinations occur.[2437]

The condition is not all that rare if elderly people are asked directly about such experiences, but they seldom volunteer the information.[JF] Although originally described in people with eye disease, it may also occur as a cortical dissociation syndrome and may be the result of deafferentation in the occipital cortex.

Bonnet, Paul Contemporary French ophthalmologist in Lyon.

Bonnet syndrome
1. (trigeminosympathetic neuralgia) **trigeminal neuralgia** with **Horner syndrome** and with vasomotor disturbance in the area supplied by the trigeminal nerve.[738, 5704] The condition may be a form of **Raeder syndrome**. 2. (Bonnet–Dechaume–Blanc syndrome, neuroretinoangiomatosis.) Unilateral tortuosity of the retinal vessels (cirsoid aneurysms) with vascular malformations of the orbit or midbrain and of the face, described by Bonnet and his colleagues in 1937.[739, 740]

Miscellaneous other lesions of the orbits, central or peripheral nervous systems, or skin are also described. See also **Wyburn–Mason syndrome**—which may be the same thing.

Bonnet–Collet syndrome See **Collet–Sicard syndrome**.

Bonnet–Dechaume–Blanc syndrome See **Bonnet syndrome** (#2).

Bonnevie, Kristine (1872–1950) Norwegian zoologist.

Bonnevie–Ullrich syndrome A sporadic congenital syndrome characterized by ptosis, ophthalmopareses, cataracts, hyperelastic skin, hypertrichosis, muscular hypotrophy, and lymphangiectatic edema of the extremities. The condition may be a variant of Turner syndrome.[3365]

Bonnier, Paul (1861–1918) French physician.

Bonnier syndrome (Deiter's nucleus syndrome) Vertigo, pallor, tachycardia, somnolence, trigeminal pain, weakness, and marked apprehension; contralateral hemiplegia may be a feature. The syndrome is due to a vascular or neoplastic lesion of Deiter's nucleus.[743]

Bontius, Jacobus (1592–1631) Dutch physician who gave the first account of **beriberi** and of **nutritional amblyopia** in his book *De Medicina Indorum* after working for the Dutch East India Company.

Boorgard angle (foraminobasilar angle) The angle defined by the intersection of the plane of the clivus and the plane of the foramen magnum, normally 126–136°. The value changes with age and increase is not always associated with genuine basilar invagination, so this measurement is now little employed.[5980]

borderland of epilepsy The term of Sir William **Gowers** for a group of disorders including fainting, vagal and vaso-vagal attacks, vertigo, migraine, and sleep disorders which by their abrupt onset, repetitive nature, and brief duration resemble seizure disorders. The clinical characteristics of these conditions, with speculations on their underlying pathophysiology, were published by Gowers in a book of the same name in 1907.[2528]

borderzone infarction Infarctions along the boundaries of recognized vascular territories, most commonly following an episode of profound reduction in global cerebral perfusion.

Bordier–Fränkel sign Upward and outward deviation of the eye on the side of a peripheral facial nerve lesion.[5333]

Börjeson–Forssman–Lehmann syndrome A rare X-linked recessive dysmorphic syndrome (or at least expressed fully only in males) consisting of severe obesity, genital infantilism, hypogonadism, seizures, mental retardation, hypothyroidism, narrow palpebral fissures, and acromegaloid facial appearance. Short stature, nystagmus, strabismus, ptosis, blepharophimosis, microcephaly, seizures, and hypogonadotrophic hypogonadism are also described.[750, 5704]

Borna virus A recently detected virus capable of causing damage to the central nervous system (especially to the hippocampus) without evidence of inflammation.[5458]

Bornholm Disease See **epidemic pleurodynia**.

borreliosis (relapsing fever) Infection with *Borrelia recurrentis*, a spirochete transmitted to humans by lice or ticks. The disease is characterized by malaise, high fever, headache, vomiting, and myalgias followed by hepatosplenomegaly with jaundice, bronchitis, a petechial skin rash, and meningoencephalopathy causing confusion, drowsiness up to coma, seizures, and focal neurological signs. The CSF often shows a lymphocytic pleocytosis. Further but milder relapses of the initial illness occur over the next few weeks.[927] Acrodermatitis chronica atrophicans is a late manifestation and is associated with a distal sensory polyneuropathy.[3437] See also **Lyme disease**.

Borries syndrome Headache, fever, increased cells and protein in the CSF, and focal signs suggesting brain abscess but in fact due to localized nonsuppurative encephalitis.[753]

The condition was described in 1921 by GVT Borries, a Danish physician in Copenhagen.

Bors–Comarr classification A system for grading the degree of bladder involvement, introduced for the management of patients following spinal shock.[754] See Chart B–4.

Boston craniosynostosis A dominantly inherited form of craniosynostosis mapped to chromosome 5q.

Chart B–4. Bors-Comarr Classification of Bladder Disorders

Complete Lesions Above Conus (S2–4); Somatic Upper Motor Neuron Lesion	
Balanced: (Automatic or neurogenic reflex bladder)	Small capacity, increased residual urine; reflex, spontaneous or conditioned initiation; no inhibition; no desire to void
Imbalanced:	Initially flaccid-atonic with large capacity, 400 ml or more; later autonomous with capacity 150–250 ml; finally spastic, with capacity less than 150 ml.
Incomplete Lesions Above Conus (S2–4); Somatic Upper Motor Neuron Lesion	
Balanced:(Uninhibited neurogenic bladder)	Residual 10–20%, capacity 200–300 ml; desire to micturate present; initiation precipitate; inhibition inadequate.
Imbalanced:	Residual 10% or more; capacity 200–1000 ml or more.
Complete Lesions at or Below Conus (S2–4); Somatic Lower Motor Neuron Lesion	
Balanced: (Autonomous/Automatic bladder)	Residual 0–10%, capacity 400 ml or more; desire to micturate absent; initiation with straining; Inhibition passive.
Imbalanced:	Residual 10% or more; capacity 400 ml or more.
Incomplete Lesions at or Below Conus (S2–4); Somatic Lower Motor Neuron Lesion	
Balanced:	Residual 0–10%, capacity 300–400 ml; desire to micturate present; initiation with straining or normal; inhibition active but inadequate;
Imbalanced: (tabetic bladder)	Residual 10% or more; capacity 600 ml or more; sensation absent.

The term "balanced" here refers to coordination of the forces of expulsion and relaxation. The amount of residual urine is considered to be in proportion to the imbalance between these functions. From Bors E. Urological aspects of rehabilitation in spinal cord injuries. JAMA *1951;*146*:225–9. © 1951. American Medical Association. Reproduced by kind permission of the AMA.*

Boston Diagnostic Aphasia examination A comprehensive instrument for assessing language, in particular spontaneous speech, naming, repetition, comprehension of oral language, reading and writing, used for classifying as well as detecting aphasias.[2475] The examination may be prolonged and requires expertise on the part of the interviewer.

Boston Naming Test A sensitive test of visual confrontation naming ability, wherein the subject is required to name a series of 60 objects presented as line drawings, standardized verbal or phonemic clues being provided when initial recognition fails.[3292] A shorter version is also available for use with demented patients.[3998]

Boston Society of Psychiatry and Neurology One of the oldest medical societies in the United States, it was founded in 1880, largely with the inspiration of Walter Channing, for the informal and social discussion of medical subjects. Its proceedings were reported in the *Boston Medical and Surgical Reporter* (the forerunner of the *New England Journal of Medicine*). Members have continued to present and discuss topics in both psychiatry and neurology at monthly meetings held continuously since its foundation.[1895]

Boston sign Intermittent descent of the globe on downward gaze, seen in **dysthyroid orbitopathy**.[5333]

bottoms-up dissection Dissection of the extracranial carotid artery considered to have been produced by repetitive neck extension during the act of throwing back the head in order to drain the contents of drinking glasses.[6397]

botulinus toxin A group of seven serologically distinct neuroparalytic toxins produced by *Clostridium botulinum*, all of which block the release of acetylcholine by the nerve terminal and cause slowly reversible effects indistinguishable from typical denervation. The type A toxin is used therapeutically to produce local suppression of muscle contraction in certain **dystonias** and in **hemifacial spasm**. Guidelines for its use were suggested by the American Academy of Neurology in 1990.[22]

The use of the agent in the management of headaches and of the facial evidences of aging is less well substantiated.

botulism (from Lat, a sausage) Poisoning with the exotoxin of *Clostridium botulinus* (commonly of types A, B, and E), initially described after poisoning by infected sausages.

The toxin binds to cholinergic nerve terminals, inhibiting acetylcholine release and clinically leading to weakness especially of the ocular and bulbar muscles, acute autonomic dysfunction (pupillary dilatation occurs in half the cases), and gastrointestinal symptoms. The electrical signs resemble those of the **Lambert–Eaton myasthenic syndrome**, but nerve conduction velocities are normal.

Infantile botulism results from botulinal neurotoxin produced *in vivo* following colonization of the gastrointestinal tract in children aged 1–9 months. The disease spectrum varies from "failure to thrive" to "the floppy baby syndrome" (the most common form) and sudden infant death syndrome or "crib death." Typical symptoms in the floppy baby syndrome include lethargy, diminished sucking, constipation, weakness, feeble cry, and diminished spontaneous activity with loss of head control, followed by extensive flaccid paralysis.[1133, 1134]

Adult botulism is usually caused by ingestion of preformed toxin and less often from wound infection. Progressive descending paralysis develops involving extraocular, bilbar, respiratory, and proximal more than distal limb muscle weakness with autonomic dysfunction. A useful, if anxiety-provoking Web site is **Botulism Emergency Preparedness and Response**, which examines botulism when used as a biological weapon at http://www.bt.cdc.gov/agent/botulism/.

Bouchard, Charles (1837–1909) French neurologist who trained in Lyon and Paris; he studied under **Charcot** at the

Salpêtrière for some of this time and coauthored a number of papers with him, particularly on the relationship of miliary aneurysms to cerebral hemorrhage, the subject of his doctoral thesis. Bouchard rose quickly in the hierarchy and was appointed professor of general pathology in the University of Paris in 1879. After this, however, he distanced himself from Charcot and strove for the advancement of his own students against Charcot's; thus he prevented the appointment of **Babiński** to the position of *professeur agrégé*.[3097]

In his book *Pathology of Cerebral Haemorrhage* (trans. MacLagan TJ. London, MacLachan and Stewart, 1872), he described "a sclerous condition of the small arteries with atrophy of the middle coat and the secondary production of aneurysms, whose rupture is the proximate cause of the [hemorrhage]." Bouchard found these on the surfaces of the convolutions but more numerously in the deep gray matter.

bouche de Tapir (Fr, mouth of a Tapir) Involuntary protrusion of the upper lip, a sign of bilateral facial weakness as in some cases of facial myopathy, described by Karl **Westphal** in 1886. Pouting of the mouth, as seen in facioscapulohumeral muscular dystrophy.

Bouillard, Jean-Baptiste (1796–1881) French physician, professor of medicine at the Charité in Paris. He differentiated between expressive and receptive dysphasias and was the first to localize the lesion to the frontal lobes.

boundary infarct See **watershed infarct.**

Bourdon test A test of attention in which the subject is required to strike out all the examples of a given letter in a line of printed random letters.

Bourneville, Desiré-Magloire (1840–1909) French physician who trained under **Charcot** and became a pediatric neurologist and psychiatrist at the Bicêtre hospital in Paris where he was in charge of care of the mentally retarded patients. Apart from his description of **tuberous sclerosis**, he also demonstrated the virtual identity of cretinism and myxedema (1880), wrote on multiple sclerosis, hysteria, medical photography, and thermometry, and was a founder both of the French *Archives de Neurologie* in 1880 and of the *La Presse Medicale*. Bourneville was an important figure in arranging the publication of Charcot's lectures.

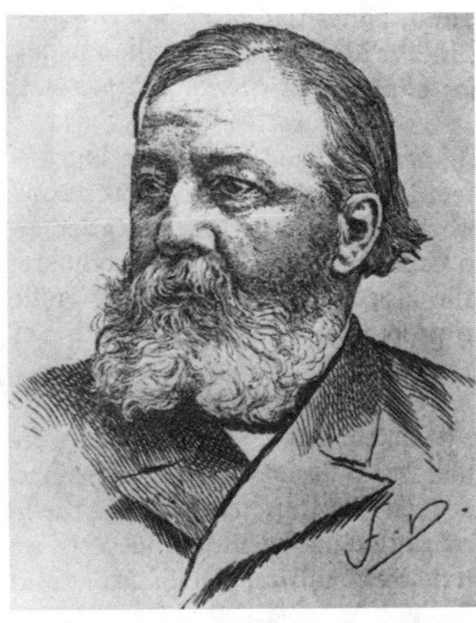

Figure B–9 Desiré-Magloire Bourneville.

He described tuberous sclerosis in 1880,[770, 771] the same year as Hartdegen in Germany reported the condition independently (but von Recklinghausen[1339] had already noted the same features in 1863). Outside medicine, he was elected to the Chambre des Deputés in Paris in 1873, and introduced legislation to improve hospital conditions and medical practice in obstetrics.[7]

Bourneville disease See **tuberous sclerosis.**

Bourneville–Brissaud disease See **tuberous sclerosis.**

Bourneville–Pellizzi disease See **tuberous sclerosis.**

Bourneville–Pringle disease See **tuberous sclerosis.**

bovine spongiform encephalopathy ("mad cow disease") A neurological disease of cattle transmitted by an unconventional, resistant agent (an aberrant isoform of **prion** protein), with a latency of some 18 months; a "slow virus" disease, equivalent to the disease **scrapie** in sheep.[6718]

The possibility that this condition might be responsible for a future outbreak of **Creutzfeldt–Jakob disease** has recently caused concern in Europe and North America.

Bowditch law Peripheral nerve fibers do not fatigue with repetitive stimulation; a truth enunciated by Henry Pickering Bowditch (1840–1911), an American physiologist, in 1890 (and 6 years previously by Nikolai Wedensky in Russia).[5619]

bowed-head sign (Gould sign) Forward flexion of the head on the neck in an effort to compensate for an inferior hemianopia.

bowel-bladder functional scale A sensitive questionnaire developed to assess the nature and severity of sphincter dysfunction, mainly in patients with **multiple sclerosis.**[6423]

Bowen–Conradi syndrome A lethal, congenital, recessively inherited dysmorphic syndrome characterized also by dolicho- or scaphocephaly, microcephaly, dwarfism, and other musculoskeletal maldevelopments. The condition has been reported to occur among the Hutterite people of North America.[779]

bow hunters syndrome See **rotational vertebral artery occlusion.**

bowing reflex If an infant with anencephaly is placed in the supine position and the thigh is extended at the hip joints, the head then lifts itself slowly in flexion and the trunk does the same, so that the infant achieves the sitting position. The reflex is seen only in anencephalic children or in normal premature infants of 7 months gestation.[4939]

bow-leggedness See **genu varum.**

bowlers' cramp An occupational dystonic syndrome described in cricketers, whose attempts to put spin on the ball being bowled lead instead to involuntary gripping of it and a delayed or inaccurate delivery.[5131]

Bowman, Sir William (1816–1892) English ophthalmic surgeon and anatomist, professor of anatomy and physiology at King's College, London.[1670]

Bowman membrane The anterior elastic membrane of the cornea.

bowstring sign (Cram test) A sign of lumbar root irritation elicited by flexing the hip with the knee flexed 30°, the heel resting on the examiner's shoulder; the examiner presses upon the posterior tibial nerve in the popliteal fossa with his thumb and then depresses the knee into extension. Pain felt in the leg or in the low back suggests root irritation.[1310]

bow-tie atrophy The pattern of retinal atrophy secondary to the presence of a lesion at the junction of the optic tract and chiasm, damaging there the fibers from the homolateral temporal and contralateral nasal retinas; relative superior and inferior temporal atrophy of the homolateral disk and nasal and temporal atrophy of the contralateral disk occurs, the abnormal region being defined by the normal arcuate fibers above and below.[4646]

bow-tie nystagmus A drug-induced oscillation of the eyes consisting of upbeat nystagmus coupled with alternating horizontal saccades synchronized with the vertical fast phases; thus the movement of the eyes traces the outline of a bow tie (diabolo, butterfly, etc.).[1561] See also **induced nystagmus, anticipatory nystagmus.**

Box and Block test A manipulation task, assessing dexterity in the arms and hands.[2477]

boxing An organized attempt of two people to inflict head injuries upon one another for the pleasure of the spectators and (if the latter pay to witness the event) for the profit of the promoter.

While acutely inflicted injuries such as concussion are deemed especially praiseworthy, the causation of post-concussion syndrome, intracranial hemorrhage, and cerebral contusion does not detract from the victor's kudos, whereas chronic traumatic encephalopathy in boxers is only taken into account outside public scrutiny. The neurological aspects of this "sport" have been reviewed.[3247]

Boyle, Robert Seventeenth-century English chemist and member of the Royal Society who gave an account of a diurnal variety of **essential tremor**, relieved by drinking a (alcoholic) chocolate liqueur.

Braak stages A six-stage system relating the progression of **Parkinson disease** to the underlying neuropathology.[788] The first stage denotes degeneration of the olfactory bulb and the anterior olfactory nucleus, whereas the second characterizes progression of the process to the lower brainstem. Stages 3 and 4 indicate involvement of the substantia nigra and other deep nuclei of the midbrain and of the forebrain, and are accompanied clinically by tremor, rigidity, and bradykinesia. Stages 5 and 6 correlate with the presence of Lewy bodies in limbic structures and the neocortex. At this point, neuropsychiatric symptoms are likely to be present.

brachial (from Lat, arm) Of or pertaining to the arm.

brachial amyotrophic diplegia (flail arm) A slowly progressive variety of **amyotrophic lateral sclerosis** in which a lower motor neuron syndrome is confined to the arms and shoulder girdle, often for some years.[3331] Pyramidal signs are not found and survival is prolonged. See also **man-in-a-barrel syndrome.**

brachial neuritis See **neuralgic amyotrophy.**

brachial neuropathy Any neuropathic disorder affecting the brachial plexus or its branches peripherally in the arms.[3866]

brachial plexopathy (traumatic) Damage to the brachial plexus, usually a closed injury resulting from severe distraction of the shoulder from the neck and in Western society usually seen in young males as a result of motor cycle accidents. Supraclavicular injuries are more common, more severe, and more likely to require surgery, and are associated with a worse prognosis compared with infraclavicular injuries.[5187] See also **neuralgic amyotrophy, hypertrophic brachial plexus neuropathy.**

brachial plexus neuropathy See **neuralgic amyotrophy, hypertrophic brachial plexus neuropathy.**

brachial-basilar insufficiency syndrome See **subclavian steal syndrome.**

brachialgia statica progressiva Nocturnal arm paresthesiae. See **sensory perineuritis.** In fact, this is probably **carpal tunnel syndrome.**

brachioradial pruritus An itching sensation on the dorsolateral aspect of the upper arm relieved by a local cooling and occurring after an injury producing neuropathy at the C5-6 level.[1320]

brachioradialis reflex (supinator, radial, forearm, or styloradial reflex) Contraction of this muscle in response to a sudden stretch caused by a tap on the radius. It is increased as a result of an upper motor neuron lesion sited above C6.

Brachmann-de Lange syndrome See **de Lange syndrome.**

brachy- (Gr, short) Prefix denoting its etymological meaning.

brachycephaly (Gr, short + head) A craniofacial dysmorphism characterized by premature bilateral fusion of the coronal sutures which leads to a relative increase in the transverse compared with the longitudinal diameter of the skull (usually quoted as being above 80% or in a ratio of 4:5).[4]

The appearance is of recession of the supraorbital rim and of the forehead (which bulges out above the root of the nose) while the temporal fossa bulges laterally in compensation. One or both orbits show an elliptic "Harlequin" or "devil-like" appearance. Upward growth of the skull leads to **turricephaly** and if the anterior fontanelle is slow to close, the top of the head has a pointed appearance (**acrocephaly**).

Clinically, cleft palate and syndactyly occur often, and raised intracranial pressure, blindness, and mental retardation are sometimes associated.

brachydactyly-ataxia See **Biemond syndrome.**

brachydactyly-spheroplakia See **Weill–Marchesani syndrome.**

brachytherapy The implantation of radioactive materials by catheter directly into a tumor.

Bradborn sign (Thorburn phenomenon) Adoption of a posture of flexion of the wrist and fingers when the arm is adducted at the shoulder and flexed at the elbow, seen in patients with bilateral C7 lesions. When unilateral, this is also known as the *Jolly sign*.

Bradbury–Eggleston triad Orthostatic hypotension, impotence, and anhidrosis, as components of the **Shy–Drager syndrome** or of **progressive autonomic failure**.

bradycoria Slowing of the pupillary reaction to light or accommodation.

bradykinesia (Gr, slow + movement) Abnormal slowness in the execution of motor tasks, as in depressive illness, hypothyroidism, Parkinsonism, and disinclination to undertake the task in hand.

bradykinin A neuropeptide vasodilator.

bradylalia (Gr, slow + babbling) Slowness and monotony in speech with pauses between syllables, as in **Parkinsonism** and with **pseudobulbar palsy**.

bradyphrasia Slowness of speech due to slowness of the underlying mental operations.[5103]

bradyphrenia Slowness in thinking, as suggested by delay in responding to questions. See also **abulia**.

Bragard sign Aggravation of the back pain induced during straight leg raising as a result of passive dorsiflexion of the ankle.[421] The **Sicard sign** is the same except that in this case only the hallux is dorsiflexed.

Braid, James (1795–1860) English surgeon in Manchester who attended a series of popular demonstrations of hypnotism in 1841. He was converted into believing that it was "a simple, speedy, and certain method for throwing the nervous system into a new condition, which may be rendered eminently available in the cure of certain disorders" and in 1843 published a book (*Neurypnology*) on the subject, advocating its use for the treatment of hysterical paralysis, tic douloureux, headache, epilepsy, palpitations, etc.

In this and other publications, however, he did explode the fancies of the Mesmerists and showed that the basis of the state was suggestion. He also introduced the term *hypnotism*.

Braid strabismus Accommodation for close vision of an object held above the line of sight, reputedly useful in the attainment of the hypnotic state.

Braidism Hypnosis or Mesmerism.

Braille A system for the reading of words adapted in 1830 by Louis Braille (1809–1852), a blind French teacher of the blind, from a prototype designed by Charles Barbier 10 years before.[797] It uses 63 groups of raised points 2.5 or 3 mm apart to represent each letter or punctuation mark, and can be read fluently by a blind person using one finger (the *reading finger*) of each hand, but less well or not at all when using other fingers. Although complex, the system remains that most often used today, despite the introduction of other systems, such as the English method of Dr. William Moon (1845).

Alexia for reading Braille has been reported and considered to be an apperceptive tactile agnosia.

brain What this is all about. The word is a generic term for that part of the CNS within the cranium subserving (as Sherrington regarded it in essence) the management of the muscles but also the regulation of the bodily functions of the animal, its will and the apparatus required for perception of the internal and external environment. The word is derived from the Anglo-Saxon word braegen, which could have a common root with the Greek **bregma**.

Brain A professional journal of neurology, published continuously since April 1878. Bucknill, Crighton-Brown, Ferrier, and Hughlings-**Jackson** were the first editors, but Dr. A. de Watteville took over the editorship in 1886 with committee assistance until 1900 and Henry **Head** occupied the editor's chair from shortly thereafter. The publication was adopted by the Neurological Society of London as its organ in 1887, 2 years after its foundation. It is currently published by the Oxford University Press, Walton St., Oxford oX2 6DP UK. Web site: http://brain.oupjournals.org/.

The BrainWeb A site offering information about depression, injury, aging, learning, addiction, and diseases, all in relation to the brain.

Brain, W. Russell (Lord Brain, 1895–1966) Pre-eminent English neurologist who trained at Oxford and at the London Hospital before entering neurology as a junior staff member at the Maida Vale Hospital for Nervous Diseases. He was elected to a consultant appointment at both hospitals and practiced from them for all of his professional life. His honors included the presidency of the Royal College of Physicians of London and of the Association of British Neurologists, Fellowship of the Royal Society, a peerage, and honors bestowed by other Universities, Royal Societies, and Foreign Institutions. He was the editor of **Brain** from 1954 until his death.

Lord Brain's research contributions were essentially clinical, leading him to define first or to describe best such conditions as the carpal tunnel syndrome, dysthyroid ophthalmopathy, some paraneoplastic syndromes, the dysphasias, and the complications of cervical spondylosis. His textbooks *Diseases of the Nervous System* and the shorter *Clinical Neurology* were each a model of clarity, selectiveness and accuracy, and both went into several editions during his lifetime and thereafter. His literary output turned to the poetical and philosophical later in his life (*Some Reflections on Genius and Other Essays* in 1960 and *Tea with Walter de la Mare* in 1957). In addition, he was well placed to guide public and political opinion in matters relating to humanitarian care of the sick and numerous aspects of public health policy, responsibilities which he fulfilled completely. He was acknowledged at his death to be the foremost neurologist in England by virtue of his abilities in every field of endeavor to which he turned his hand or his heart.

Brain and Development. The official journal of the Japanese Society for Child Neurology, published by Elsevier. Web site: http://www.elsevier.nl/locate/braindev.

Brain and Language (*Brain Lang*) A neurological journal. Address: Academic Press Inc., 1250 6th Ave., San Diego, CA 92101. Editors: Drs. Harry A. Whitaker and Andre Roch Lecours.

Brain and Mind An electronic (Web-based) neuroscience magazine. Web site: http://www.epub.org.br/cm/.

Brain and Nerve (No To Shinkei) A neurological journal. Address: Igaku Shoin Ltd., 5-24-3 Hongo Bunkyo-ku, Tokyo 113-91, Japan.

Brain and Spine Foundation A British charitable organization. Web site: www.brainandspine.org.uk.

brain attack A term introduced to remind all those who treat stroke lightly that this condition requires and is benefited by emergency management in the same way as is heart attack.

Brain Attack Coalition A professional group dedicated to improving stroke care and comprising the **American Academy of Neurology, American Association of Neurological Surgeons, American College of Emergency Physicians,** American Heart Association Stroke Council, **American Society of Neuroradiology, National Institute of Neurological Disease and Stroke,** and the **National Stroke Association**. Web site: www.stroke-site.org.

brain autolysis Enzymatic autodigestion of the brain, following prolonged circulatory stoppage and death.

brain death (cerebral death) Loss of the clinical function of the brain, including the brainstem when the proximate cause is known and demonstrably irreversible. The three cardinal findings upon which the clinical diagnosis is based are coma or unresponsiveness, absence of brainstem reflexes and apnea. The concept of brain death was created out of advances in therapeutic technology. The criteria for determining of brain death in adults and in children suggested by the President's Commission are reproduced in Charts B–5 and B–6. Competing but not necessarily conflicting alternatives have also been published.[6263] (Reproduced by kind permission of the American Academy of Neurology and Lippincott Williams and Wilkins.) Six other original sets of criteria can be found at http://www.medal.org/visitor/www/active/ch17/ch17.aspx. See also **persistent vegetative state**.

Chart B–5. Criteria for the Determination of Brain Death

An individual presenting the findings in either section A (cardiopulmonary) or section B (neurological) is dead. In either section a diagnosis of death requires that both *cessation of functions*, as set forth in subsection 1, and *irreversibility*, as set forth in subsection 2, be demonstrated.

A. An individual with irreversible cessation of circulatory and respiratory functions is dead.

1. Cessation is recognized by an appropriate clinical examination. Clinical examination will disclose absence of responsiveness, heartbeat, and respiratory effort. Medical circumstances may require the use of confirmatory tests, such as an ECG.
2. Irreversibility is recognized by persistent cessation of functions during an appropriate period of observation and/or trial of therapy.

In clinical situations where death is expected, where the course has been gradual, and where irregular agonal respiration or heartbeat finally ceases, the period of observation following the cessation may be only the few minutes required to complete the examination. Similarly, if resuscitation is not undertaken and ventricular fibrillation and standstill develop in a monitored patient, the required period of observation thereafter may be as short as a few minutes. When a possible death is unobserved, unexpected, or sudden, the examination may need to be more detailed and repeated over a longer period, while appropriate resuscitative effort is maintained as a test of cardiovascular responsiveness. Diagnosis in individuals who are first observed with rigor mortis or putrefaction may require only the observation period necessary to establish that fact.

B. An individual with irreversible cessation of all functions of the entire brain, including the brainstem, is dead. The "functions of the entire brain" that are relevant to the diagnosis are those that are clinically ascertainable. Where indicated, the clinical diagnosis is subject to confirmation by laboratory tests, as described in the following portions of the text. Consultation with a physician experienced in this diagnosis is advisable.

1. Cessation is recognized when evaluation discloses findings of a and b:
   a. Cerebral functions are absent, and there must be deep coma, that is, cerebral unreceptivity and unresponsivity. Medical circumstances may require the use of confirmatory studies such as an EEG or blood-flow study.
   b. Brainstem functions are absent.

Reliable testing of brainstem reflexes requires a perceptive and experienced physician using adequate stimuli. Pupillary light, corneal, oculocephalic, oculovestibular, oropharyngeal, and respiratory (apnea) reflexes should be tested. When these reflexes cannot be adequately assessed, confirmatory tests are recommended.

Adequate testing for apnea is very important. An accepted method is ventilation with pure oxygen or an oxygen and carbon dioxide mixture for 10 min before withdrawal of the ventilator, followed by passive flow of oxygen. (This procedure allows $PaCO_2$ to rise without hazardous hypoxia.) Hypercarbia adequately stimulates respiratory effort within 30 s when $PaCO_2$ is greater than 60 mmHg. A 10 min period of apnea is usually sufficient to attain this level of hypercarbia. Testing of arterial blood gases can be used to confirm this level. Spontaneous breathing efforts indicate that part of the brainstem is functioning.

Peripheral nervous system activity and spinal cord reflexes may persist after death. True decerebrate or decorticate posturing or seizures are inconsistent with the diagnosis of death.

2. Irreversibility is recognized when evaluation discloses findings of a, b, and c:
   a. The cause of coma is established and is sufficient to account for the loss of brain functions and so on.
   Most difficulties with the determination of death on the basis of neurological criteria have resulted from inadequate attention to this basic diagnostic prerequisite. In addition to a careful clinical examination and investigation of history, relevant knowledge of causation may be acquired by CT scan, measurement of core temperature, drug screening, EEG, angiography, or other procedures.

b. The possibility of recovery of any brain functions is excluded, and the most important reversible conditions are sedation, hypothermia, neuromuscular blockade, and shock. In the unusual circumstance where a sufficient cause cannot be established, irreversibility can be reliably inferred only after extensive evaluation for drug intoxication, extended observation, and other testing. A determination that blood flow to the brain is absent can be used to demonstrate a sufficient and irreversible condition.
c. The cessation of all brain functions persists for an appropriate period of observation and/or trial of therapy.

Even when coma is known to have started at an earlier time, the absence of all brain functions must be established by an experienced physician at the initiation of the observation period. The duration of observation periods is a matter of clinical judgment, and some physicians recommend shorter or longer periods than those given here.

Except for patients with drug intoxication, hypothermia, young age, or shock, medical centers with substantial experience in diagnosing death neurologically report no cases of brain functions returning following a 6 h cessation, documented by clinical examination and confirmatory EEG. In the absence of confirmatory tests, a period of observation of at least 12 h is recommended when an irreversible condition is well established. For anoxic brain damage where the extent of damage is more difficult to ascertain, observation for 24 h is generally desirable. In anoxic injury, the observation period may be reduced if a test shows cessation of cerebral blood flow or if an EEG shows electrocerebral silence in an adult patient without drug intoxication, hypothermia, or shock.

Confirmation of clinical findings by EEG is desirable when objective documentation is needed to substantiate the clinical findings. Electrocerebral silence verifies irreversible loss of cortical function except in patients with drug intoxication or hypothermia. (Important technical details are provided in "Minimal Technical Standards for EEG Recording in Suspected Cerebral Death" [Guidelines in EEG 1980, Atlanta, *American Electroencephalographic Society*, 1980, section 4, pp. 19–24].) When joined with the clinical findings of absent brainstem functions, electrocerebral silence confirms the diagnosis.

Complete cessation of circulation to the normothermic adult brain for more than 10 min is incompatible with survival of brain tissue. Documentation of this circulatory failure is therefore evidence of death of the entire brain. Four-vessel intracranial angiography is definitive for diagnosing cessation of circulation to the entire brain (both cerebrum and posterior fossa) but entails substantial practical difficulties and risks. Tests are available that assess circulation only in the cerebral hemispheres, namely radioisotope bolus cerebral angiography and gamma camera imaging with radioisotope cerebral angiography. Without complicating conditions, absent cerebral blood flow as measured by these tests, in conjunction with the clinical determination of cessation of all brain functions for at least 6 h, is diagnostic of death.

Complicating Conditions

A. Drug and Metabolic Intoxication. Drug intoxication is the most serious problem in the determination of death, especially when multiple drugs are used. Cessation of brain functions caused by the sedative and anesthetic drugs, such as barbiturates, benzodiazepines, meprobamate, methaqualone, and trichloroethylene, may be completely reversible even though they produce clinical cessation of brain functions and electrocerebral silence. In cases where there is any likelihood of sedative presence, toxicology screening for all likely drugs is required. If exogenous intoxication is found, death may not be declared until the intoxicant is metabolized or intracranial circulation is tested and found to have ceased.

Total paralysis may cause unresponsiveness, areflexia, and apnea that closely simulates death. Exposure to drugs such as neuromuscular blocking agents or aminoglycoside antibiotics and diseases like myasthenia gravis are usually apparent by careful review of the history. Prolonged paralysis after use of succinylcholine chloride and related drugs requires evaluation for pseudocholinesterase deficiency. If there is any question, low-dose atropine stimulation, electromyogram, peripheral nerve stimulation, EEG, tests of intracranial circulation, or extended observation, as indicated, will make the diagnosis clear.

In drug-induced coma, EEG activity may return or persist while the patient remains unresponsive, and therefore the EEG may be an important evaluation along with extended observation. If the EEG shows electrocerebral silence, short latency auditory or somatosensory-evoked potentials may be used to test brainstem functions, since these potentials are unlikely to be affected by drugs.

Some severe illnesses (e.g., hepatic encephalopathy, hyperosmolar coma, and preterminal uremia) can cause deep coma. Before irreversible cessation of brain functions can be determined, metabolic abnormalities should be considered and, if possible, corrected. Confirmatory tests of circulation or EEG may be necessary.

B. *Hypothermia.* Criteria for reliable recognition of death are not available in the presence of hypothermia (below 32.2°C core temperature). The variables of cerebral circulation in hypothermic patients are not sufficiently well studied to know whether tests of absent or diminished circulation are confirmatory. Hypothermia can mimic brain death by ordinary clinical criteria and can protect against neurological damage due to hypoxia. Further complications arise since hypothermia also usually precedes and follows death. If these complicating factors make it unclear whether an individual is alive, the only available measure to resolve the issue is to restore normothermia. Hypothermia is not a common cause of difficulty in the determination of death.

C. *Children.* The brains of infants and young children have increased resistance to damage and may recover substantial functions even after exhibiting unresponsiveness on neurological examination for longer periods compared with adults. Physicians should be particularly cautious in applying neurological criteria to determine death in children younger than 5 years.

D. *Shock.* Physicians should also be particularly cautious in applying neurological criteria to determine death in patients in shock because the reduction in cerebral circulation can render clinical examination and laboratory tests unreliable.

From President's commission. Guidelines for the determination of death. JAMA *1981;*246:*2184–6.*

Chart B–6. Guidelines for the Determination of Brain Death in Children

History

The critical initial assessment is the clinical history and examination. The most important factor is determination of the proximate cause of coma to ensure absence of remediable or reversible conditions. Most difficulties with the determination of death on the basis of neurological criteria have resulted from overlooking this basic fact. Especially important are detection of toxic and metabolic disorders, sedative-hypnotic drugs, paralytic agents, hypothermia, hypotension, and surgically remediable conditions. The physical examination is necessary to determine the failure of brain function.

Physical Examination Criteria

1. Coma and apnea must coexist. The patient must exhibit complete loss of consciousness, vocalization, and volitional activity.
2. Absence of brainstem function as defined by:
   a. Midposition or fully dilated pupils which do not respond to light. Drugs may influence and invalidate pupillary assessment.
   b. Absence of spontaneous eye movements and those induced by oculocephalic and caloric (oculovestibular) testing.
   c. Absence of movement of bulbar musculature including facial and oropharyngeal muscles. The corneal, gag, cough, sucking, and rooting reflexes are absent.
   d. Respiratory movements are absent with the patient off the respirator. Apnea testing using standardized methods can be performed, but this is done after other criteria are met.
3. The patient must not be significantly hypothermic or hypotensive for age.
4. Flaccid tone and absence of spontaneous or induced movements, excluding spinal cord events such as reflex withdrawal or spinal myoclonus, should exist.
5. The examination should remain consistent with brain death throughout the observation and testing period.

Observation Periods According to Age

The recommended observation period depends on the age of the patient and the laboratory test utilized.

7 days to 2 months: The Task Force recommends two examinations and electro-encephalograms (EEGs) separated by at least 48 h.

2 months to 1 year: The Task Force recommends two examinations and EEGs separated by at least 24 h. A repeat examination and EEG are not necessary if a concomitant radionuclide angiographic (CRAG) study demonstrates no visualization of cerebral arteries.

Over 1 year: When an irreversible cause exists, laboratory testing is not required and the Task Force recommends an observation period of at least 12 h. There are conditions, particularly hypoxic–ischemic encephalopathy, in which it is difficult to assess the extent and reversibility of brain damage. This is particularly true if the first examination is performed soon after the acute event. Therefore, in this situation, the Task Force recommends a more prolonged period of at least 24 h of observation. The observation period may be reduced if the EEG demonstrates electrocerebral silence or the CRAG does not visualize cerebral arteries.

Laboratory Testing

Electroencephalography Electroencephalography to document electrocerebral silence should, if performed, be done over a 30 min period using standardized techniques for brain death determinations. In small children it may not be possible to meet the standard requirement for 10 cm electrode separation. The interelectrode distance should be decreased proportional to the patient's head size. Drug concentrations should be insufficient to suppress EEG activity.

Angiography CRAG confirms cerebral death by demonstrating the lack of visualization of the cerebral circulation. A technically satisfactory CRAG that demonstrates arrest of carotid circulation at the base of the skull and absence of intracranial arterial circulation can be considered confirmatory of brain death, even though there may be some visualization of the intracranial venous sinuses (8–10). The value of this study in infants under 2 months is under investigation. Contrast angiography can document lack of effective blood flow to the brain.

RAG = cerebral radionuclide angiogram

From American Neurological Association Task Force: Guidelines for the determination of brain death in children. Ann Neurol *1987;***21***:616–7. Reproduced by permission.*

brain distension See **normal pressure hydrocephalus**.

brain electrical activity mapping (BEAM) A computer-controlled method for collecting and displaying spatiotemporal information about brain electrical activity contained in recordings from multiple scalp electrodes, whereby colored topographic maps of regional electrical activity (EEG or evoked potential) are displayed.[1744] The place of this technique vis-à-vis other methods for the diagnostic localization of cerebral lesions is still undetermined.

brain ferrocalcinosis See **striopallidal calcification**.

brain fever See **chronic fatigue syndrome**.

brain herniation Displacement of brain structures as a result of pressure from an expanding mass lesion elsewhere in the cranium. Examples are a cerebellar pressure cone at the foramen magnum, uncal herniation down through the tentorium, transtentorial herniation of the brainstem, subfalcial herniation of the cinguate gyrus, and upward cerebellar herniation through the tentorium. The relevance of these tissue shifts has been questioned, the suggestion being made that the only really important event is midbrain compression as a result of lateral shift at the level of the tentorium.[2102]

Brain Information Service Address: Health Science Room 43–67, University of California, Los Angeles, CA 90024.

Brain Injury A specialist neurological journal. Web site: http://www.tandf.co.uk/journals/titles/02699052.asp.

Brain Injury Association of America A charitable organization. Tel.: 703-761-0750; fax: 703-761-0755. Web site: http://www.biausa.org/.

Brain Injury Research Center A research database with educational materials for people with traumatic brain injury, their families, and professionals. Web site: http://www.tbicommunity.org/

brain mapping A digital technique whereby the EEG tracing from 16 to 32 electrodes arranged in a grid pattern is analyzed to create an isoelectric display of the electrical field over the head, usually in color. It can be used to study the topography of any feature at a point in time, or to average recurring events, as with evoked potentials. Its usefulness stems from the ease with which such abnormalities may be seen or localized, rather than from its ability to show features invisible to trained electroencephalographers. The technique is not a substitute for neuroimaging in any form.[646]

brain reflex (quadripedal reflex) The flexed arm of a hemiparetic patient extends when the patient assumes the quadripedal position.[5333]

Brain Research A neurological journal. Web site: http://www.elsevier.com/wps/find/journaldescription.cws_home/622287/description#description.

Brain Research Bulletin The official journal of the International Behavioral Neuroscience Society. Web site: http://www.brb.cf.ac.uk/.

Brain Research Fund Foundation of London A charitable association in this field. Address: 111 Waterloo St., Suite 600, London, Ontario N6B 2M4, Canada. Tel.: 519-642-7755.

brain sand Gritty particles (**psammoma bodies**) found in certain cerebral tumors, such as meningiomas, but also in many normal people.

brain shift The movement of parts of the brain across the midline or downward in response to the effects of an intracranial mass lesion. Such displacements include those of the cingulate gyrus herniating beneath the falx; of the uncus or cerebellar tonsils which descend through the tentorial aperture or the foramen magnum, respectively; and of the brain stem which moves across the midline and also downward. In the case of masses within the posterior fossa, upward herniation of the cerebellum may also occur.

brain stones See **cerebral calculi**.

Brain Talk communities A resource center. Web site: www.braintalk.org.

Brain Tissue Resource Center An association promoting research through the collection and banking of human postmortem brain tissue. Tel.: 1-800 Brain Bank. Web site: http://www.brainbank.mclean.org/.

brain tumor Benign or malignant neoplasms of the brain. These have been classified by the World Health Organization as follows, but most of the entries are cataloged in this book under their individual names. The method of grading is available at http://neurosurgery.mgh.harvard.edu/newwhobt.htm.

Neuroepithelial Tumors of the Central Nervous System and other CNS Neoplasms

1. *Astrocytic tumors* (glial tumors—categories I–V, below. [See Grading of Astrocytic Tumors] They may also be subclassified as invasive or noninvasive, although this is not formally part of the WHO system. The noninvasive tumor types are indicated below. Categories in italics are also not recognized by the new WHO classification system, but are in common use.)
   1. Astrocytoma [WHO grade II]
      Variants: protoplasmic, gemistocytic, fibrillary, mixed
   2. Anaplastic (malignant) astrocytoma [WHO grade III]
      Hemispheric, diencephalic. optic, brain stem, and cerebellar sites
   3. Glioblastoma multiforme [WHO grade IV]
      Variants: giant cell glioblastoma, gliosarcoma
   4. Pilocytic astrocytoma [noninvasive, WHO grade I]
      Hemispheric, diencephalic. optic, brain stem, and cerebellar sites
   5. Subependymal giant cell astrocytoma [noninvasive, WHO grade I]
   6. Pleomorphic xanthroastrocytoma [noninvasive, WHO grade I]
2. *Oligodendroglial tumors*
   1. Oligodendroglioma [WHO grade II]
   2. Anaplastic oligodendroglioma [WHO grade III]
3. *Ependymal cell tumors*
   1. Ependymoma [WHO grade II]
      Variants are cellular, papillary, epithelial, clear cell, and mixed
   2. Anaplastic ependymoma [WHO grade III]
   3. Myxopapillary ependymoma
   4. Subependymoma [WHO grade I]
4. *Mixed gliomas*
   1. Mixed oligoastrocytoma [WHO grade II]
   2. Anaplastic (malignant) oligodastrocytoma [WHO grade III]
   3. Other (e.g., ependymo-astrocytoma)
5. *Neuroepithelial tumors of uncertain origin*
   1. Polar spongioblastoma [WHO grade IV]
   2. Astroblastoma [WHO grade IV]
   3. Gliomatosis cerebri [WHO grade IV]
6. *Tumors of the choroids plexus*
   1. Choroid plexus papilloma
   2. Choroid plexus carcinoma (anaplastic choroids plexus papilloma)
7. *Neuronal and mixed neuronal-glial tumors*
   1. Gangliocytoma
   2. Dysplastic gangliocytoma of the cerebellum (Lhermitte–Duclos)
   3. Ganglioglioma
   4. Anaplastic (malignant) ganglioglioma
   5. Desmoplastic infantile ganglioglioma (*desmoplastic infantile astrocytoma*)
   6. Central neurocytoma
   7. Dysembryoplastic neuroepithelial tumor
   8. Olfactory neuroblastoma (esthesioneuroblastoma) (variant: olfactory neuroepithelioma)
8. *Pineal parenchyma tumors*
   1. Pineocytoma
   2. Pineoblastoma
   3. Mixed pineocytoma/pineoblastoma
9. *Tumors with neuroblastic or glioblastic elements (embryonal tumors)*
   1. Medulloepithelioma
   2. Primitive neuroectodermal tumors with multipotent differentiation
      i. medulloblastoma (variants: medullomyoblastoma, melanocytic medulloblastoma, desmoplastic medulloblastoma)
      ii. cerebral primitive neuroectodermal tumor
   3. Neuroblastoma (variant: ganglioneuroblastoma)
   4. Retinoblastoma
   5. Ependymoblastoma.

Other CNS Neoplasms

1. Tumors of the sellar region; pituitary adenoma, pituitary carcinoma, craniopharyngioma
2. Hematopoietic tumors; primary malignant lymphomas, plasmacytoma, granulocytic sarcoma, and others
3. Germ cell tumors; germinoma, embryonal carcinoma, yolk sac tumor (endodermal sinus tumor), choriocarcinoma, teratoma, mixed germ cell tumors
4. Tumors of the meninges:
   1. Meningioma (variants: meningothelial, fibrous (fibroblastic), transitional (mixed), psammomatous, angiomatous, microcystic, secretory, clear cell, chordoid, lymphoplasmacyte-rich, and metaplastic subtypes)
   2. Atypical meningioma
   3. Anaplastic (malignant) meningioma
5. Nonmeningothelial tumors of the meninges
   1. Benign mesenchymal (osteocartilaginous tumors, lipoma, fibrous histiocytoma, and others)
   2. Malignant mesenchymal (chondrosarcoma, hemangiopericytoma, rhabdomyosarcoma, meningeal sarcomatosis, and others)
   3. Primary melanocytic lesions (diffuse melanosis, melanocytoma, malignant melanoma, and the variant meningeal melanomatosis)
   4. Hemopoietic neoplasms (malignant lymphoma, plasmactoma, granulocytic sarcoma)
   5. Tumors of uncertain histogenesis Hemangioblastoma (capillary hemangioblastoma)
6. Tumors of cranial and spinal nerves
   1. Schwannoma (neurinoma, neurilemoma); cellular, plexiform, and melanotic subtypes
   2. Neurofibroma (circumscribed (solitary) neurofibroma; plexiform neurofibroma)
   3. Malignant peripheral nerve sheath tumor (malignant schwannoma); epithelioid, divergent mesenchymal, or epithelial differentiation; melanotic
7. Local Extensions from Regional Tumors; paraganglioma (chemodectoma); chordoma; chondroma; chondrosarcoma; carcinoma
8. Metastatic tumors
9. Unclassified tumors
10. Cysts and tumor-like lesions; Rathke cleft cyst, epidermoid, dermoid, colloid cyst of the third ventricle, enterogenous cyst, neuroglial cyst, granular cell tumor (choristoma, pituicytoma), hypothalamic neuronal hamartoma, nasal glial heterotopia, plasma cell granuloma.

A number of grading systems are in common use for tumors of astrocytic lineage (i.e., astrocytomas, anaplastic astrocytomas, and glioblastomas). Grades are assigned solely based on the microsopic appearance of the tumor. The numerical grade assigned for a given tumor, however, can vary depending on which grading system (Kernohan, Mayo) is used. Thus, it is important to specify the grading system referred to when a grade is specified. The St. Anne/Mayo grade has proven to correlate better with survival than the previously favored Kernohan grading system. It can only be applied to invasive tumors of astrocytic lineage; it is otherwise similar to the WHO grading system.

Brain Tumor Foundation for Children Inc. A charitable organization. Address: 2231 Perimeter Park Drive, Suite 9, Atlanta, GA 30341, USA. Tel: 404-458-5564.

Brain Tumor Society A charitable organization. Address: 258 Harvard Street, Suite 308, Brookline, MA 02146, USA. Tel: 617-433-7033. Web site: http://www.tbts.org/.

brainstem attack See **diencephalic autonomic seizures**.

brainstem auditory evoked potentials (BAEPs, AEPs, BAERs) Electric waveforms of biologic origin elicited in response to sound stimuli. Normally consists of a sequence of up to seven waves, designated I–VII, which occur during the first 10 msec after the onset of the stimulus and have positive polarity at the vertex of the head. (From the 2001 Report of the Nomenclature Committee of the American Association of Electromyography and Electrodiagnosis.[19] Reproduced by kind permission of the AANEM.)

The normal BAEP consists of a sequence of up to seven waves, named I–VII, which occurs during the first 10 min after the onset of the stimulus and have positive polarity at the vertex of the head.[162] The generators for waves I–V are respectively the acoustic nerve, cochlear nuclei, superior olivary nuclei, lateral lemniscus, and inferior colliculi. The generators for waves VI and VII are uncertain.

Recording of BAEPs may be of value in the assessment of brainstem function in a variety of disorders, including multiple sclerosis, central pontine myelinolysis, and brain death.[1144]

brainstem encephalitis 1. See **basilar migraine** (Bickerstaff brainstem encephalitis).[83] 2. A paraneoplastic syndrome characterized by cranial nerve palsies, cerebellar ataxia, and long tract signs. Myoclonus, movement disorders, and neurogenic hypoventilation are less common.[5232]

brainstem gliomas Malignant tumors of the brainstem, usually arising in childhood, adolescence, or early adult life with death supervening usually within a year. Diffuse intrinsic pontine, tectal, and cervicomedullary locations are most common, but tectal and cervicomedullary sites are also described.[2624] See also **gliomas**.

brainstem hallucinations Pure visual hallucinations resulting from lesions of the midbrain, pons, or thalamus.[2101] See **peduncular hallucinosis**.

brainstem malformations Congenital anomalies of the pons, midbrain, or medulla or of more than one region, and including malformations with abnormal brainstem segmentation; those with segmental hypoplasia or postsegmentation malformations or associated with abnormal cortical organization.[405] See also **oculocerebrocutaneous syndromes**.

brainstem ptosis Bilateral ptosis in alert patients without pupillary changes in the setting of brainstem infarctions. The cause is not known.[2086]

brainstem reflexes Colloquially, the **corneal**, **gag**, **oculocephalic**, **oculovestibular**, and **cough reflexes**. The **carotid sinus**, **cardio-respiratory**, and other vegetative reflexes are not usually included under this heading.

BrainWeb A site that provides information and links to validated sites suitable for lay readers about some common brain diseases and disorders. These include outside resources reviewed by scientific advisors, as well as articles in Dana publications. Web site: http://www.dana.org/resources/brainweb/default.aspx/.

braking saccades Saccades which stop the movement of the quick phase of jerk nystagmus, preceding the ensuing slow drift of the eyes which comprises the next part of the cycle.

Bramwell, Byrom (1847–1931) Scottish physician, who contributed substantially to the understanding of the principles of localization within the spinal cord,[806] and of tumors of the nervous system. His book *The Diseases of the Spinal Cord* (Edinburgh, Maclachan, and Stewart, 1882) dealt with the anatomy, pathology, and clinical aspects of the cord and was the most complete account then published. It was profusely and superbly illustrated, mainly by himself.

branch atheromatous disease Narrowing or occlusion of the mouth of a branching artery by an atheromatous process different from lipohyalinosis, considered to be a potential cause of **lacunar syndromes**.[1010]

branched-chain ketoaciduria (maple syrup urine disease) A congenital dysmetabolic syndrome characterized by neonatal seizures and feeding problems, hypotonia alternating with dystonia, and aminoaciduria. The condition progresses to seizures, coma, and death. Classic, intermediate, intermittent, and thiamine-responsive types have been differentiated.[379]

Another *variant* is *maple syrup urine disease, variant form*, a congenital syndrome characterized by neonatal feeding problems, seizures and disturbed consciousness, hypotonia, ophthalmoplegia, XII cranial nerve palsy, and aminoaciduria.

brancher enzyme deficiency A rare recessively inherited and fatal form of glycogen storage disease characterized by the accumulation of polysaccharides in the liver, brain, and both cardiac and skeletal muscles.

The condition presents in infancy with hypotonia and weakness and is fatal within 2 years.[4257] See also **glycogen storage diseases**.

branchial muscle hypertrophy See **branchial myopathy**.

branchial myoclonus Rhythmical myoclonus-like movements of the palate, pharynx, larynx, tongue, and face (the branchial musculature) occurring as a hereditary disease or as a result of disease affecting the dentatorubroolivary pathways in the brainstem (the **Guillain–Mollaret triangle**).

branchial myopathy (hypertrophic branchial myopathy, branchial muscle hypertrophy) A rare syndrome of unknown cause, characterized by tender hypertrophy of the temporalis and masseter muscles.[3650, 4037]

brass arm (telegraphist's cramp) A repetitive strain injury. See **occupational cramp**.

brassfounders ague Sweating, nervousness, and paresthesias, possibly as a result of zinc oxide poisoning.

Brauch–Romberg sign See **Romberg sign**.

Bravais, Louis French physician who gave an account of focal (hemiplegic) seizures in his thesis on graduation from the University of Paris in 1827, thus antedating even Richard **Bright**. Bravais was actually the first to describe **Jacksonian epilepsy** (1827) but did so in an incomplete manner.

brawny induration (old Fr, slice of flesh + from Lat, to make hard) Discoloration and abnormal firmness developing in soft tissues, as in cellulitis.

breach rhythm Nonepileptogenic mu-like EEG activity with enhanced amplitude, recorded in the vicinity of a skull defect.[3469] See also **wicket rhythm**.

breadcrumbing tremor An alternative and rather better name for the (inaccurately titled) **pill-rolling tremor** of Parkinsonism.

breath-holding spells Forms of **reflex syncope** in children. Episodes of altered consciousness occurring in children under the age of 5 years. Two forms are defined: *Cyanotic* spells result from performing a Valsalva maneuvre and are characterized by emotional provocation, apnea in expiration, cyanosis, brief stiffening of the body, and loss of consciousness, in that order, before the infant breathes again and regains awareness. See also **sobbing spasms**. *Pallid breath-holding spells* (**reflex anoxic seizures**) are provoked by minor head trauma and are characterized by pallor, accelerated loss of consciousness, stiffening of the trunk and limbs with myoclonus and downbeating of the eyes, and result from asystole due to vagal cardiac standstill. Crying is seldom a feature.[3906]

breathing arm Co-contraction of the diaphragm and proximal arm muscles as a result of aberrant regeneration of injured phrenic nerves or of the C.3,4,5 roots as a result of obstetric brachial plexopathy.

breathing hand Co-contraction of the diaphragm and distal upper limb muscles as a result of aberrant regeneration of injured upper thorax roots or intercostal nerves as a result of obstetric brachial plexopathy.[2200]

breathlessness with effort intolerance See **chronic fatigue syndrome**.

Breathnach syndrome (premature aging with telangiectasias) A congenital dysmorphic syndrome characterized by pigmentary retinopathy, chorioretinitis, and intracranial calcification with seizures. Multiple fractures, skin telangiectasia, and angiokeratomas are other manifestations.[381]

Bregeat syndrome An embryologic malformation comprising angiomatosis of the oculo-orbital vessels, homolateral thalamencephalic angioma of the choroidal plexus, and contralateral cutaneous angioma on the forehead. The condition is thus very similar to the **Wyburn–Mason syndrome**.[826]

bregma (Gr, to moisten) The forepart of the head, the anterior fontanelle at the junction of the coronal, and sagittal sutures of the skull, which is soft and moist in the newborn. The word was used by Aristotle and Galen to apply to the **vertex**, but **Broca** applied it as we use it now.

bregmo-cardiac reflex Bradycardia occurring as a result of compression of the anterior fontanelle in infants.

Bremer, Friedreich Wilhelm (fl. 1926) German neurologist at Munich whose major work on dysraphism was published in 1926.[827] He was also the first to show changes in the EEG during different sleep stages and used the **cerveau isolé** preparation (in which the transection is performed behind the III nerve nucleus) in the cat to show that coma can occur with the EEG appearance of nonrapid eye movement sleep; contrasting this with the findings in the **encephale isolé** preparation (in which a cut is made at the level of the cervicomedullary junction) when normal sleep–wake cycles are retained.

Bremer syndrome See **dysraphism**.

Breughel syndrome (blepharospasm-oromandibular dystonia, Meige syndrome) A **cranial dystonia** marked by combinations of prolonged involuntary spasmodic contractions of the muscles of the face, mouth, tongue, and jaw, due to a disorder of the basal ganglia in the elderly, the blepharospasm often making the patients functionally blind.

The condition is named after the contorted facial expressions of the individuals depicted in some of the paintings of Peter Breughel the elder, a Flemish artist (1712–1765).[4099, 4290] Unlike those of Breughel, the equally graphic depictions of dystonia by William Blake do not include representations of oromandibular dystonia.

Brickner, Richard Max (1896–1959) American neurologist in New York, who studied extensively the effects of temperature on function in **multiple sclerosis**.

Brickner phenomenon The **oscillopsia** originally described in multiple sclerosis.[837]

Brief Cognitive Rating Scale (BCRS) An instrument designed to assess the severity of cognitive decline and sometimes employed in the investigation of pharmacological agents used to treat dementia in the elderly. The test excludes measures of mood change but provides ratings in 5 other areas, although scoring is somewhat subjective. See Chart B-7. In a modification (BCRS part 2), speech and

Chart B–7. Brief Cognitive Rating Scale (Reisberg, 1988)[5255]

1. *Concentration*

1. No objective or subjective evidence of deficit in concentration.
2. Subjective decrement in concentration ability.
3. Minor objective signs of poor concentration (e.g., serial 7s).
4. Definite concentration deficit for background (e.g., marked deficit on serial 7s; frequent deficit in subtraction of serial 4s from 40).
5. Marked concentration deficit (e.g., gives months backward or problem with serial 2s from 20)
6. Forgets the concentration task. Frequently begins to count forward when asked to count backward from 10 by 1s.
7. Marked difficulty counting forward to 10 by 1s.

2. *Recent Memory*

1. No objective or subjective evidence of deficit.
2. Subjective impairment only (forgetting names more than before).
3. Deficit in recall of specific events evident on detailed questioning. No deficit in the recall of major recent events.
4. Cannot recall major events of previous weekend or week. Scanty knowledge (not detailed) of current events, favorite TV shows, etc.
5. Unsure of weather, current President, or current address.
6. Occasional knowledge of some recent events. Little or no idea of current address, weather, etc.
7. No knowledge of any recent events.

3. *Past Memory*

1. No subjective or objective impairment in present memory.
2. Subjective impairment only. Can recall 2 or more school teachers.
3. Some gaps in past memory upon detailed questioning. Able to recall at least one childhood teacher and/or one childhood friend.
4. Clear-cut deficit. The spouse recalls more of the patient's past than the patient. Cannot recall childhood friends and/or teachers but knows the names of most schools attended. Confuses chronology in reciting personal history.
5. Major past events sometimes not recalled (e.g., names of schools attended).
6. Some residual memory of past (e.g., may recall country of birth or former occupation).
7. No memory of the past.

4. *Orientation*

1. No deficit in memory for time, place, identity of self or others.
2. Subjective impairment only. Knows time to nearest hour, location.
3. Any mistake in time >2 h; day of week >1 day; date >3 days.
4. Mistakes in month >10 days, or year >1 month.
5. Unsure of month and/or year and/or season; unsure of locale.
6. No idea of date. Identifies spouse but may not recall name. Knows own name.
7. Cannot identify spouse. May be unsure of personal identity.

5. *Functioning and Self-care*

1. No difficulty, either subjectively or objectively.
2. Complains of forgetting location of objects. Subjective work difficulties.
3. Decreased job functioning evident to co-workers. Difficulty in traveling to new locations.
4. Decreased ability to perform complex tasks (e.g., planning dinner for guests, handling finances, marketing, etc.).
5. Needs help in choosing proper clothing
6. Needs help in feeding, toileting, bathing, and/or ambulating.
7. Requires constant assistance in all activities of daily life.

From Reisberg B, Ferris SH. *Psychopharmacol Bull* 1988;24:629. Permission sought from MedWorks Media LLC. With thanks to the (US) National Institute for Mental Health.

language capacity, psychomotor function, mood and behavior, praxis and calculation ability are also assessed.[5255, 5252]

Brief Psychiatric Rating Scale A relatively short observer-rated scale assessing 18 items including depressive symptoms with the object of assessing changes after treatment.[4837] The scale concentrates on psychopathology with less emphasis on the manifestations of dementia such as somatic and self-care factors.

A similar scale for the assessment of geriatric patients has also been constructed.[4935]

Brief Repeatable Battery of Neuropsychological Tests A sensitive measure of cognitive impairment in multiple sclerosis, using five validated measures of spatial memory, verbal memory, short- and long-term recall, attention, and verbal fluency.[749]

brief small abundant motor-unit action potentials A pattern of voluntary EMG activity which suggests, but is by no means diagnostic of, primary myopathy.[1884] See **BSAPPs**.

brief symptom inventory A self-report questionnaire used for individual screening of depressive symptoms.[1607]

Bright, Richard (1789–1858) English physician and pathologist born in Bristol. After training in Edinburgh, at Guy's Hospital, and in Europe, he practiced in London where he was appointed physician to Guy's Hospital in 1824. He is best remembered for his descriptions of chronic renal disease and of various neurological conditions, collected in the two volumes of his *Reports of Medical Cases* (1827–1831), in which *inter alia* he described the features of certain seizure types, recognizing the sensory march,[838] painful lateralized seizures, secondary generalization of focal seizures, ictal amaurosis, and olfactory auras.

His account of postictal paralysis preceded that of **R.B. Todd**. He described absence attacks as follows: "Often it is the momentary absence of mind, the eye fixed in thought, yet gazing vacantly, no convulsion, no sound, the occupation of the hand ceases while the mind for the moment is annihilated; the cloud passes off, the intellect returns and often unconscious that its operation has been suspended, the patient resumes the occupation in which he was engaged."

He obtained and himself performed autopsies whenever possible, leading both to a superb pathological collection (still retained at Guy's) and to contemporary recognition of the value of understanding the pathology of disease. Thus he was able to show that focal epilepsy was as likely to originate from brain disease as was the generalized variety, at a time when **Brown-Séquard**, for example, was advocating amputations for the control of focal seizures.[6926]

He was also a noted geologist; his collection, expanded by the purchase of the fossil section of that amassed by James **Parkinson**, passed eventually to the Institute of Geological Sciences.

Briquet, Paul (1796–1881) French physician whose two theses were on varicose veins and artificial illumination, respectively, but who also published on tuberculosis, cholera, and hysteria.

Briquet syndrome 1. Aphonia and dyspnea, considered by Briquet (1859) to be due to hysterical paralysis of the diaphragm; this is almost certainly the **hyperventilation syndrome**. 2. Hysteria, specifically hysterical anesthesia of the skin with consequent imprecision of movements ("ataxia") Briquet regarded this as a "neurosis of the brain" in which unpleasant environmental events acted upon the "affective part" of the brain in a susceptible and predisposed person. His book[844] finally disposed of the old concept that hysteria was in some way associated with wanderings of the uterus. 3. A chronic illness characterized by the occurrence of multiple symptoms affecting multiple organ systems, resulting from **conversion disorder**.

His work and concepts of hysteria have been reviewed.[4028]

Brissaud, Edouard (1852–1909) French neuropsychiatrist. As a student he trained under **Charcot**, Millard, and **Lasègue** and after graduation became chef de clinique at the Pitié. He later deputized for Charcot in his absences, filling the Chair at the Salpêtrière temporarily after Charcot's death.

He was elected professor of the history of medicine in the Faculté de médicine in Paris and later was professor of pathology. With Pierre **Marie** he founded the *Revue Neurologique* in 1893. Brissaud wrote extensively on such subjects as neuroanatomy, hysteria, asthma,

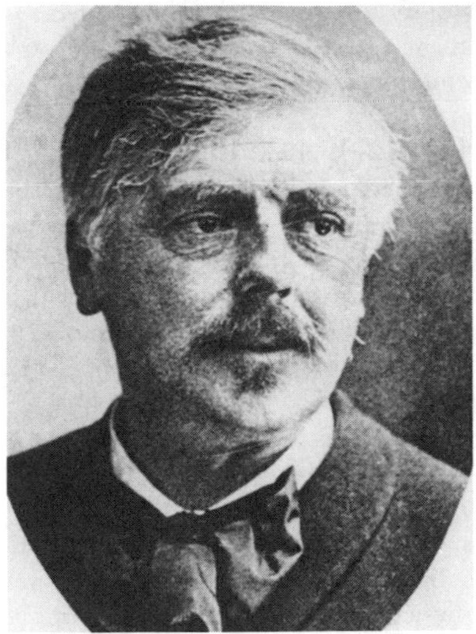

Figure B–10 Edouard Brissaud.

acromegaly, Parkinsonism, syphilis, involuntary movements, hypnosis, and medical history. He also gave a good account of **tuberous sclerosis**, but after Bourneville. **Horsley** operated on his brain tumor in Paris, but this did not prolong his life.

Brissaud convolution The gyrus parietalis transversus.

Brissaud disease (chorea variabilis) See **Tourette syndrome** (which was in fact what he was describing).[845]

Brissaud infantilism A syndrome of the persistence of infantile characteristics beyond the age of puberty, with retarded growth and delayed mental development. Round, chubby face, underdeveloped genitalia, dwarfism, lack of body hair, and delayed epiphyseal ossification are characteristics. The condition probably represents infantile myxedema.[846]

Brissaud reflex Contraction of the tensor fascia lata in response to scratching the sole of the foot; seen in pyramidal disease.

Brissaud syndrome 1. See **Brissaud infantilism**. 2. Sinistrosis ("shell-shock") but the term was used by him to describe the features of traumatic or **compensation neurosis**; "It is a pathological attitude in an injured person who refuses to recognise that he is cured as he genuinely believes that he has not obtained just legal compensation for the injury received. He is basically a claimant who over-estimated his right to be indemnified."[847]

Brissaud–Lereboullet syndrome (hemicraniosis) Hemifacial and hemicranial hyperostosis associated with underlying meningiomas or sarcomas, raised intracranial pressure, visual disturbances, exophthalmos, and seizures.

The condition probably represents sarcomatous change in a long-standing meningioma.[848]

Brissaud–Marie syndrome Hysterical glossolabial paralysis in which the deviation of the face and of the tongue are unphysiological with respect to the limb weakness.[849, 851, 5333]

Brissaud–Meige syndrome See **hemifacial spasm**.

Brissaud–Sicard syndrome Facial hemispasm associated with contralateral hemiparesis due to a caudal-ventral pontine lesion, described in 1908.[850]

Bristowe, John Syer (fl. 1885) English neurologist and Fellow of the Royal Society who described the effects of callosal tumors in ***Brain*** in 1885.

Bristowe syndrome (callosal syndrome) The pattern of symptoms associated with tumors of the corpus callosum, comprising negativism, disturbances of memory, concentration and personality, and hemiparesis.[143] Tumors affecting the anterior part of the corpus callosum may lead to apraxias of the left hand as well.

British Journal of Neurosurgery A neurosurgical journal. Address: Carfax Publishing Company, P.O. Box 25, Abingdon, Oxfordshire OX14 3UE, England. Web site: http://www.tandf.co.uk/journals/titles/02688697.html.

British Medical Journal A leading general medical journal, publishing also neurological papers. Web site: http://www.bmj.com.

British Neuropsychiatry Association (BNPA) An academic and professional body for medical practitioners and professionals allied to medicine working at the interface of the clinical and cognitive neurosciences and psychiatry.

British Neuroscience Association (formerly The Brain Research Association) was relaunched in 1997 to represent all aspects of neuroscience while continuing many of the traditions of the BRA with a new style.

British Paediatric Neurology Association A professional organization. Web site: www.bpna.org.uk.

British Society for Clinical Neurophysiology A professional organization. Web site: www.bscn.org.uk.

British Society of Neuroradiologists A professional organization.Web site: www.bsnr.co.uk.

Brixa–Koppens sign See **Gowers signs**.

broad A band disease A rare, benign congenital myopathy characterized clinically by neonatal hypotonia, with or without congenital blindness due to retinal dystrophy, and delay in speech and development. Ultrastructural abnormalities include disorganization of myosin thick filaments leading to a loss of A band/I band demarcation and an impression of broadening of the A band. See also **Leber congenital amaurosis**.[4530]

Broadbent, Sir William Henry (1835–1907) English neurologist and cardiologist who trained in Manchester and London, studying further under Trousseau in Paris after graduation. He practiced largely from St. Mary's Hospital, London, and was elected a fellow of the Royal Society in 1896. He was created a baronet as a result of his services as physician to Queen Victoria and King Edward VII.

His neurological publications concerned hemiplegia, aphasia, and the following.

Broadbent apoplexy Intracerebral hemorrhage which penetrates into the ventricles.[857]

Broadbent Law With a lesion of the upper motor neuron above the facial colliculus in the pons, the hand and arm are the most affected, the leg next so, and the lower face and tongue only slightly.

Broca, Pierre-Paul (1824–1880) French anthropologist, anatomist, and professor of clinical surgery at the Bicêtre in Paris, later a politician. He described hemispheric dominance and determined that right-handedness was associated with the representation of speech in the left hemisphere, thus defining the anatomical correlate of nonfluent aphasia (1861).[858] He also described the major features of motor or expressive aphasia in his patient "Tan" and was the first to trephine for a cerebral abscess which he had localized correctly by clinical means (the only means available).

He reported in 1865 the cases of 8 aphasic ("aphemic") right-handers with left hemisphere lesions and stated that the left inferior frontal convolution was the center for articulate speech.[859, 2856] He also described muscular dystrophy before **Duchenne**, rickets, the treatment of cerebral aneurysms, clubfeet, fractures, and the use of hypnotism in surgery.

As an anthropologist he was interested in craniology (naming the inion, bregma, dacryon, lambda, metopion, obelion, and opisthion) and he was involved in the discovery and reports on Neanderthal man. He founded the French school of Anthropology.

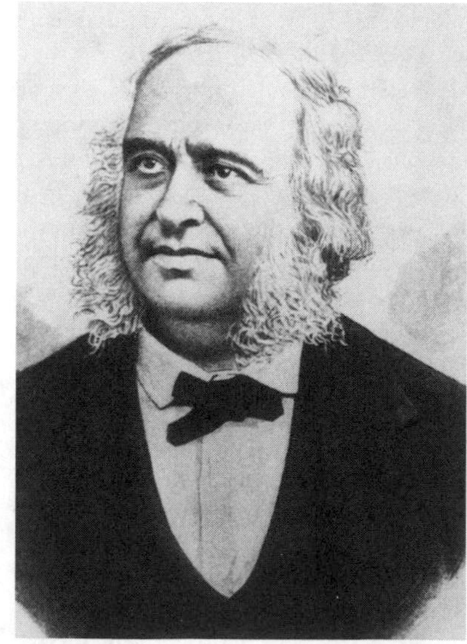

Figure B–11 Pierre-Paul Broca.

Broca aphasia (Broca dysphasia, nonfluent aphasia, agrammatic aphasia) A classic nonfluent dysphasia characterized by awkward slow and effortful articulation, loss of **prosody**, impairment of repetition and naming, and restriction to simple grammatical forms in speech and writing (**agrammatism**) so that spontaneous speech is of a "telegraphic" type.

Agrammatism leads to the use of single words, words with a high substantive content (nouns and verbs) but few articles, pronouns, prepositions, or conjunctions. The normal syntactic relations are lost. Repetition and confrontation naming are also much affected but there is relative preservation of comprehension. Phonetic disintegration (mainly shown as trouble in initiating speech and in selecting and blending words) and mispronunciation of phonemes (such as B for P) also occurs.

The causative lesion involves the posterior part of the inferior frontal gyrus of the dominant hemisphere, the anterior parietal region, the insula, and both banks of the Rolandic fissure with deep extension.[858]

The condition has been separated into two types:

Persisting Broca aphasia (big or true Broca aphasia) which usually begins with a global aphasia and right-sided paresis with evolution to a state in which spoken language is comprehended but nonfluent and agrammatical speech with poor repetition remains, due to extensive damage affecting not only the inferior left frontal gyrus but also the surrounding cortex and the underlying white matter and basal ganglia, as above.

Broca area infarction syndrome (little, mild, or acute Broca aphasia) A nonfluent agrammatic output is present at the beginning of the disorder, comprehension is preserved, and the speech disturbance improves to a state of near normality except for some impairment in prosody. Any initial **mutism** is replaced by rapidly abating dyspraxic and effortful articulation and there is significant permanent disturbance in language function. The lesion responsible is a restricted infarction of the posterior portion of the dominant inferior frontal gyrus.[4431]

Broca dysphasia See **Broca aphasia**.

Broca's area (Broca's convolution) The motor speech area; the posterior part of the inferior (third) frontal convolution, on the left side in a large majority of people.

Broca's area infarction syndrome See **Broca aphasia**.

Broca's convolution See **Broca area**.

Brodmann, Korbinian (1868–1918) German physician who initially trained in psychiatry in Jena, Frankfurt, and Berlin but who was later appointed professor of anatomy successively in Tubingen, Halle, and Munich, where he pioneered the study of **cytoarchitectonics**.

Brodmann areas Fifty-two cortical areas, containing 11 regions distinguished by the structure and disposition of their cellular layers (**cytoarchitectonics**) defined by Brodmann in 1903–1908.[1670]

Brody syndrome (Lambert–Brody syndrome) A slowly progressive, recessive muscle disease of childhood mapped to chromosome 16p12; and due to functional deficiency of Ca^{2+} ATPase in the sarcoplasmic reticulum of fast-twitch skeletal muscle. The onset is in childhood with impaired muscle relaxation after voluntary contraction, in the limbs and face, stiffness, cramping and myalgias, worsened by exercise and cold. Strength is normal between episodes. Serum CK levels may be mildly elevated, but rhabdomyolysis is rare. The EMG shows that the cramps are electrically silent. Muscle biopsy reveals only type II fiber atrophy.[862, 293, 540] Dominant inheritance has also been reported.

bromide A halogen introduced by Locock for the treatment of "hysterical" epilepsy in 1857[3890] on the bases that epilepsy was (at least in some cases) a manifestation of abnormal sexual tendencies and that bromides had been found to cause impotence. As a result of Locock's paper, Drs. C.B. Radcliffe and Sir Samuel Wilks both generalized the indications for its use to organic epilepsy.

bromide partition test A chemical test performed on CSF samples providing evidence for or against a diagnosis of tuberculous meningitis.[4043]

Bronx cheer A derogatory expression, a compound of eructation and retching. When involuntary, it is classified as a complex vocal tic, a manifestation of **Tourette syndrome**; when voluntary, it is classified merely as an expression of opinion.

Brossard, Jules (1855–1911) French physician.

Brossard scapulo-distal syndrome A **scapulo-peroneal syndrome**, probably recessively inherited.[880]

Brown, Charles Leonard (b. 1899) American pathologist, practicing in Boston and New York.

Brown–Peterson paradigm A test used for the assessment of short-term memory. It typically consists of the presentation of a set of three items, after which the patient is asked to engage in some distracting activity such as counting backward from a three-digit number for between 2 and 30 s. Reproduction of the originally presented material is then requested. Between 10 and 20 trials are usually administered.[5003]

Brown–Symmers disease (acute serous encephalitis) See **acute disseminated encephalomyelitis**.[887]

Brown, Jason W. American neurologist in Los Angeles.

Brown syndrome ("A syndrome of the neural crest") 1. Loss of deep pain sensitivity, retention of superficial pain, autonomic dysfunction, hypoplasia of dental enamel, meningeal thickening and cystic change, hyporeflexia, mild mental retardation, and blond hair, blue-green eyes, and a fair complexion.[893]

The authors suggested that this association of signs indicated that there was a failure of differentiation of the neural crest as the underlying embryonic abnormality. 2. See **superior orbital fissure syndrome**.

Brown syndrome See **superior oblique tendon syndrome**. The condition was described by Dr. H.W. Brown in 1950.

Brown, Sanger (1852–1928) Canadian-born neurologist who trained in medicine at Bellevue. He introduced a new

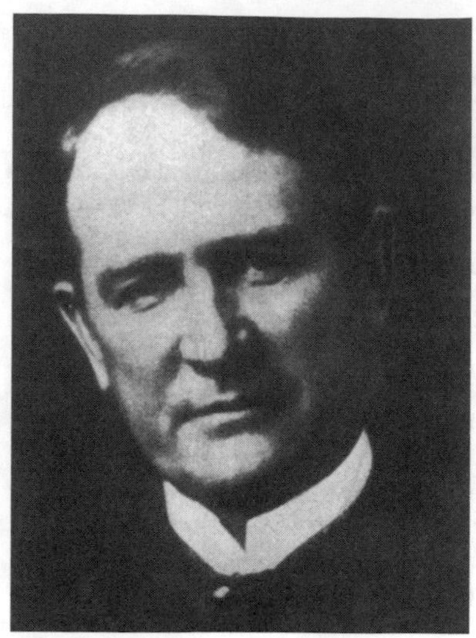

Figure B–12 Sanger Brown.

system of classification of patients at the mental hospital where he was first appointed which led to the discharge of a number of them; and he achieved prominence in psychiatry, going on to be medical superintendent in other hospitals in the northeastern United States.

In 1886 he studied neurology with Sharpey-Shafer in London and established the role of the occipital lobe in vision. He settled in Chicago in 1890, becoming professor of forensic medicine and hygiene at Rush and of clinical neurology at the University of Illinois.

Brown ataxia See **Sanger Brown ataxia**.

Brown-Séquard, Charles-Edouard (1817–1894) A neurologist of Eurasian and Irish-American parentage who was born in Mauritius (and was thus a British citizen) but who trained in Paris, first for a literary and later for a medical career. Trousseau was one of his teachers, and after graduation he worked with Baron Larrey. His thesis on the physiology of the spinal cord was accepted in Paris in 1846; in it, he described the sensory decussation within the cord. Constrained by the Second Empire and short of money, he left France on a slow ship (chosen so that he would have time to learn the English language) and visited New York, returning later to Mauritius (where a gold medal was struck to commemorate his handling of a cholera epidemic) before settling to practice in Richmond, Virginia in 1855, from which city he felt it proper to withdraw following a tactless remark of his about slavery and the resulting remarks of others upon his own mixed blood.

He returned to Paris in that year and published his findings on the functions of the adrenal glands. In 1858 he lectured in London, Glasgow, and Dublin, after which he was held in the highest esteem and was elected Fellow of the Royal Society and also Fellow of the Royal College of Physicians in 1860. At this time he was appointed as the first physician to the **National Hospital**, Queen Square, a position which he held until 1863 when he accepted the Chair of Nervous Pathology at Harvard. There he remained until the death of his wife in 1868, when he returned to Paris and accepted the Chair of Experimental Physiology at the Faculté de Médicine. In 1872 he returned to New York and remarried, but he went again to Paris on the death of his second wife 2 years later. He crossed the Atlantic over 60 times.

In 1877 he accepted the post of professor of physiology at Geneva, married for the third time, and remained in Geneva for a year before succeeding Claude **Bernard** as professor of experimental medicine at the Collège de France in Paris, a post that he retained until his death.

Although noted for many physiological observations, including that of caloric testing (45 years before **Bárány**), of the effects of removal of the suprarenal glands and of the vasomotor functions of sympathetic nerves, his name is chiefly remembered for his descriptions in 1850 and 1851 of the syndrome resulting from lateral hemisection of the spinal cord, popularly (but probably incorrectly) thought to have been brought to his attention by the activities of the Parisian mafioso who settled their scores with stilettos so thin as to be able to penetrate into the spinal canal[903] and for his demonstration that excision of the adrenal glands was followed by features of Addison disease. He also reported (1856) spontaneous "convulsions" with limited generalization resulting from disease of the spinal cord and also resembling the pains of trigeminal neuralgia (see next entry).

His medical interests exceeded neurology,[6427] and he reported, late in life on the effects he experienced from the self-injection of an extract of guinea pig testicles, which he regarded as entirely satisfactory.

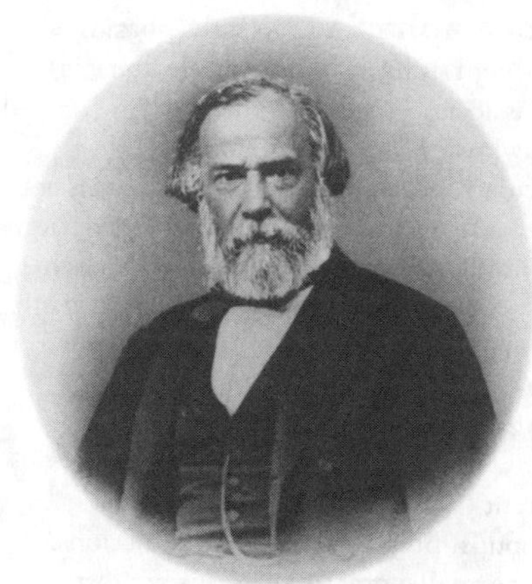

Figure B–13 Charles-Edouard Brown-Séquard.

Brown-Séquard spinal epilepsy
Muscle spasms resulting from the presence of an irritative lesion affecting the motor fibers in the spinal cord. Despite the name, the condition is not truly epileptic but rather a form of segmental myoclonus.[645]

Brown-Séquard syndrome
Damage to the lateral half of the spinal cord, leading to ipsilateral loss of pyramidal and posterior column function and contralateral spino-thalamic loss, with evidence of a root lesion at the site of the cord injury. Direct trauma was once, an extrinsic compressive lesion is now, the commonest cause.[903]

Brown–Vialetto–Van Laere syndrome See **pontobulbar palsy with deafness**.

Bruch membrane The structure supporting the pigmented epithelial layer overlying the rods and cones in the retina.

Bruck–de Lange syndrome A fatal infantile syndrome of psychomotor delay, extrapyramidal rigidity, movement disorder, and local or generalized muscular hypertrophy.[1504] See **De Lange syndrome**.

Brudzinski, Josef (1874–1917) Polish physician who graduated from Moscow and specialized in pediatrics. After a tour of European schools he returned to Warsaw and then was appointed head of a children's hospital in Lodz, transferring to Warsaw again as Rector of the University. The sign for which he is best remembered (entry following) was described in 1909.[908]

Brudzinski signs 1. *Neck phenomenon* Flexion of the hips and knees (sometimes with extension of the hallux and fanning of the toes) in response to passive neck flexion.

2. *Contralateral leg sign* The involuntary flexion or extension of one leg in response to forceful passive flexion of the other leg at the hip (straight leg raising).[908] In each case it is a sign of meningeal irritation or inflammation. *The reciprocal contralateral leg sign* is seen when one leg is flexed at the hip and knee and the other is extended. When the flexed limb is lowered to the bed, the other leg flexes.

3. (*Cheek sign*) Flexion of the elbows with upward jerking of both arms in response to pressure on the cheeks.[909]

4. (*Symphysis sign*) Flexion of the legs in response to suprapubic pressure.[421]
Most of these signs were described in patients with tuberculous meningitis.[5333, 5704]

Brueghel syndrome See **orofaciomandibular dystonia**.

Brugada syndrome Right bundle branch block with ST segment elevation of the caved in type in EKG leads V1–V5, predisposing to ventricular arrhythmias or sudden death in up to 8% in 2 years.

bruit (Fr, noise) An abnormal sound generated as a result of the turbulent flow of blood within arteries and heard through a stethoscope.

bruit de pôt fêlé See **cracked-pot note**.

Brumback syndrome A congenital dysmorphic syndrome characterized by microcephaly, cerebral atrophy, agenesis of the corpus callosum, and **Brushfield spots** on the iris.

Brunauer syndrome A dominantly inherited syndrome of mental retardation, defective enamel formation, and hyperhidrosis with hyperkeratosis of the palms and soles.[2506]

Bruns, Ludwig (1858–1916) German neurologist who studied at Munich and Göttingen and trained in neurology with Hitzig and later in Paris. After some time in

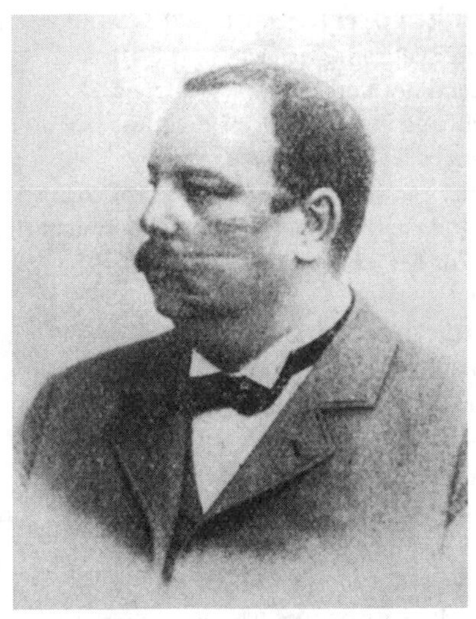

Figure B–14 Ludwig Bruns.

Berlin with **Westphal** and **Oppenheim**, he left to direct the department of internal medicine in Hanover where he was later appointed professor.

In 1892 he described the gait disorder named for him[917] and wrote on hysteria, callosal tumors, goiter, tetanus, Parkinsonism, the optic nerve, birth injuries, and diabetes. He was also the author (in collaboration) of a large and influential *Textbook of Pediatric Neurology*.[919]

Bruns ataxia See **Bruns gait apraxia**.

Bruns gait apraxia (Bruns ataxia, apractic, or magnetic gait) Inability to initiate the process of forward motion by alternating steps, although the power and coordination of the legs is normal in the lying or sitting positions. The maintenance of the feet on the floor, removed only with great effort, has led to the alternative name *magnetic gait*.

This static ataxia in the presence of frontal lobe disorders is due to involvement of the descending efferent frontocerebellar fibers and was originally described in the setting of frontal lobe tumors but is now more commonly seen in frontal ischemic disease. The constellation of abulia, psychomotor retardation, primitive reflexes, and ideomotor apraxia with cerebellar findings is suggestive.[917]

The entity is of uncertain validity and has been considered to have cerebellar, apraxic, agnosic, and labyrinthine components.[919] See **frontal dysequilibrium**.

Bruns nystagmus The combination of small-amplitude, rapid jerk nystagmus in the primary position, beating away from the side of an extra-axial mass lesion compressing the vestibular nerve and the brainstem, in association with slow, large-amplitude gaze-evoked or gaze-paretic nystagmus toward the side of the lesion.[6910]

The syndrome occurs typically with cerebello-pontine angle tumors characterized by **gaze paretic nystagmus** evoked by gaze to the side of the tumor and by **vestibular nystagmus** evoked by gaze to the opposite side.

Bruns syndrome Vertigo, vomiting, headache, and visual disturbance during change in head posture; a sign of cerebral tumors, usually in the posterior fossa but also occurring with, for example, bilateral subdural hematomas.[918] The original description was of a man with cysticercosis, who had no symptoms unless he moved his head quickly.[144]

brush allodynia The perception of pain in response to a non-noxious cutaneous stimulus, such as stroking the skin with an artist's paintbrush or a piece of gauze. See **allodynia.**

Brushfield, Thomas (1856–1933) English psychiatrist working in mental deficiency.

Brushfield spots Mottled or speckled, white or light yellow pinpoints regularly placed in a ring near the outer margin of the iris, found in 90% of people with **Down syndrome** and in about a quarter of normal subjects when they are known as **Wolfflin nodules**.

Brushfield could not find the spots in patients with brown irides.[920]

Brushfield syndrome See **Sturge–Weber syndrome**.

Brushfield–Wyatt syndrome Generalized and trigeminal port-wine stains with a calcified angioma in the underlying cerebral hemisphere producing hemianopia and hemiparesis, and mental defect.[921] The similarity to **Sturge–Weber syndrome** is obvious.

The term has also been used for **tuberous sclerosis**.

bruxism (nocturnal tooth-grinding) A stereotyped movement disorder occurring during partial arousal from sleep (and thus a **parasomnia**), characterized by unconscious tight jaw closure with stereotyped rhythmic grinding of the teeth occurring especially during nonrapid eye movement stage 2 sleep, unassociated with EEG abnormalities.[5555] See also **sleep disorders**.[1629] Damage to the teeth and to the temporomandibular joints may result. The condition also occurs during periods of rapid eye movement sleep.

bruxomania Persistent, conscious tooth-grinding.

BSA(P)Ps (Brief, Small, Abundant Polyphasic Potentials) A recruitment pattern of motor unit action potentials recorded during electromyography, usually during minimal contraction and usually suggesting the presence of primary muscle disease. Although the term is discouraged by the AANEM nomenclature subcommittee,[19] the pattern is quite distinctive and the acronym quite satisfactory to most electromyographers.

buccal apraxia (oral apraxia) Impairment in performing mouth or face actions on verbal command or imitation (see also **orofacial apraxia**) or to perform learned, skilled movements with the facial and bulbar muscles—for example, inability to protrude the tongue to command. With this is associated difficulty in imitating meaningless movements made by the examiner. The responsible lesion is of the opercula or the anterior perisylvian regions.[41, 3540] See also **apraxia**.

buccal reflex (snouting; Toulouse, Vurpas, oral, nasomental reflex) Approximation of the lips when the upper lip is tapped; a sign of pseudobulbar palsy. See also **orbicularis oris reflex**.

For a sign of relatively slight importance, this number of alternative names is peculiar.

Buchem syndrome See **hyperostosis corticalis generalisata familiaris**.

buckling sign Involuntary flexion of the extended knee when the hip is flexed during straight leg raising. This is evidence of irritation of the sciatic spinal nerve roots.

buckthorn neuropathy (tullidora) A toxic syndrome characterized by flaccid ascending motor weakness and ataxia, resulting from the ingestion of the berries of *Karwinskia humboldtiana*, a Central American shrub. The pathological changes include both segmental demyelination of the motor nerves and neuronopathy.[4398]

buckthorn plant Ingestion of the berries of this plant may cause an ascending Guillain–Barré-like paralysis.

Budge, Julius Ludwig (1811–1884) Professor of anatomy and physiology in Bonn and later in Pomerania.[1670]

Budge centers The spinal cord at C7–T6, from which fibers pass out to the sympathetic chain, named the *cilio-spinal center* by Budge and Waller; they also identified the *genito-spinal center* in the sacral cord.

buffer amplifier An amplifier generally with a voltage gain of l, a high-input impedance and a low-output impedance, and used to isolate the input signal from the loading effects of an immediately following circuit. In some EEG machines, each input is connected to a buffer amplifier located in the jack box to reduce cable artifact and interference. (Adapted from the 1974 report of the Committee on Terminology, IFCN. In: Chatrian, GE, Bergamini L, Dondey M, et al. A glossary of terms most commonly used by clinical electroencephalographers. *EEG Clin Neurophysiol* 1974; 37:538–48 and reproduced by kind permission of Elsevier Science and the IFCN.)

bulbar (from Gr, a bulb or any rounded structure) Of or pertaining to the medulla oblongata.

bulbar encephalitis See **Bickerstaff brainstem encephalitis**.

bulbar myoclonus See **palatal myoclonus**.

bulbar palsy Lower motor neuron weakness of those muscles supplied by the VII through XII cranial nerves as a result usually of pontomedullary lesions, motor neuropathies, nerve compression at the skull base or **myasthenia gravis**; and leading thus to weakness of the face and tongue, dysphagia, dysarthria, and dysphonia.

The first description was that of John Bunyan in 1680.

bulbar palsy with deafness See **Vialetto–van Laere syndrome**

bulbar palsy with deafness and pigmentary retinopathy See **hereditary motor neuropathy** (*variants*).

bulbar palsy with olivopontocerebellar atrophy See **cerebellar ataxias**.

bulbar spinal muscular atrophy of childhood See **Fazio–Londe disease**.

bulbar spinal muscular atrophy with deafness See **Vialetto–van Laere syndrome**.

bulbocavernosus reflex (virile reflex) Sudden contraction of the bulbocavernosus and ischiocavernosus muscles and of the anal sphincter with squeezing or irritation of the glans penis or clitoris. The same reflex can be elicited with electrical stimulation of the dorsal nerve of the penis, with recording by a single-fiber needle in the bulbocavernosus muscle.[6557]

The reflex was described as a normal phenomenon in 1890 by Jacques **Onanoff**, but he noted that it is absent with advancing age and regarded it more useful as evidence of retained virility than of neurological disease, considering that when it was present in impotent or in neurasthenic patients it signified that the condition did not have an organic basis. Absence of the reflex suggests a neurogenic cause for bladder dysfunction, indicating neural integrity of L5–S5, but mainly of the S2,3,4 segments. The response is increased in patients with pyramidal tract lesions.[1909]

bulbomimic reflex (Mondonesi reflex) In metabolic coma, eyeball pressure leads to bilateral facial grimacing; with coma due to a focal brain lesion, the grimace is seen on one side only.

bulbospinal neuronopathy (spinal and bulbar muscular atrophy, Kennedy syndrome) A heterogeneous group of disorders of unknown cause affecting infants or young adults who present with distal weakness, fasciculations, and postural tremor. Twitching of the chin is a typical finding. Dysarthria and dysphagia follow later. The depression of muscle stretch reflexes and the detection of mild sensory disturbances differentiate the condition from motor neuron disease and from hereditary motor neuropathies.

Inheritance by all modes has been described and the course of the disease shows extreme variability. *Variant forms* include:

1. *Kennedy syndrome* (Kennedy–Alter–Sung syndrome) A relatively benign X-linked bulbospinal neuronopathy due to a triplet repeat (CAG) mapping to Xq21.3–q12, also with onset in adult life, in which gynecomastia, bulbar and facial weakness, perioral fasciculations, hypertrophy and cramping of the calves, and postural tremor are the most prominent features.[3385, 288] **Progressive proximal spinal and bulbar atrophy of late onset** is probably the same condition.
2. The juvenile form of X-linked proximal spinal muscular atrophy, with calf enlargement.
3. A rare phenotype of **GM_2 gangliosidosis.**[6290]
4. *Familial bulbospinal neuronopathy with optic atrophy.*[4891]

See also **lower motor neuron disease.**

bulbospinal system Pathways which originate in the brainstem, descend to spinal levels and are concerned in the control of movement and of posture.

bulimia (Gr, a particle + hunger) Morbid hunger; excessive appetite with decreased satiety after eating.

bulimia nervosa (Gr, a particle + hunger) (Binge eating) 1. Morbid hunger; excessive appetite with decreased satiety after eating. 2. A chronic but self-limiting eating disorder characterized by an episodic desire to eat large amounts of food, accompanied by a sense of loss of control and often of depression; each episode being followed by purging, starvation, and fasting.

As with **anorexia**, the patients manifest a fear of fatness, a desire for thinness, a distorted body image, and a denial of illness.[5475] The American Psychiatric Association criteria (*DSM-IV-TR*)[171] amplify this description. Web site: http://www.psychiatryonline.com/content.aspx?aID=3610.

Bull angle The angle between the plane of the hard palate and the plane of the atlas vertebra on a true lateral skull X-Ray film. The normal angle is less than 5°, while patients with basilar impression often have an angle measuring over 13°.[934]

Although a popular measure, it has been criticized because the first reference point is not part of the base of the skull, and is therefore unsuitable when defining the relationship of different parts thereof, such as the rim of the foramen magnum.

bulldog reflex Involuntary clenching of the teeth in response to the sensation of any object placed between them; shown by some patients with frontal lobe tumors.[645]

Bumke, Oswald Conrad Edward (1877–1950) German neurologist and psychiatrist who studied medicine in various German universities, graduating from Kiel. He rose through the ranks in Freyberg, Halle, Rostock, Breslau, Leipzig, and Munich, succeeding Kraepelin in Munich. He is best remembered for describing the pupillary sign, but he also published extensively on various psychiatric topics.[5704]

He collaborated with **Foerster** in the production of the *Handbuch der Neurologie* (1935–1937), which became the most influential book (in 17 volumes) on the subject in European neurology. He attended Lenin in his last illness (a stroke).

Bumke (anxiety) pupils Dilatation of the normal pupil in response to a stressful psychic stimulus, with an impaired light response. The sign was described by Bumke in his book *Die Pupillenstorungen* (Jena, 1903) and is said to be absent in schizophrenia, presumably because of lack of affect.

bundle of Turck A fiber pathway running from the posterior temporal region to the pontine nuclei and thence to the cerebellar vermis, probably responsible for the retention of whole-body movements in cases of apraxia.

bungarotoxin (a-BTX) The lethal factor in the venom of the banded krait, which binds so completely and specifically to acetylcholine receptor sites that it supplies a method for their quantification.

Büngner bands Basal laminae which assist in the orientation of sprouting axons.

Bunina bodies Eosinophilic, rounded or elongated intra-cytoplasmic inclusion bodies with clear haloes found in the motor neurons of the spinal cord, brainstem, and motor cortex in **amyotrophic lateral sclerosis**.

Burdach, Karl Friedrich (1776–1847) German physician, anatomist, and physiologist; professor in these disciplines in Dorpat and then in Königsberg. He was a member of the "Naturphilosophen" group, concerned with speculative generalizations on brain functions.

He introduced the terms *biology* and *morphology* to medicine and named the globus pallidus (1819), internal capsule, putamen, lenticular nucleus, red nucleus, cingulum, cuneus, and amygdaloid nucleus and classified the thalamic nuclei, as well as writing widely in other areas of pathology and physiology.[4338] He named the fasciculus cuneatus and discovered the red nucleus before Stilling. He was also a neuro-anatomical historian; in his *Vom Baue und Leben des Gehirns* (1819–1826) he attributed to **Willis** the first description of the corpus striatum, pyramids, olives, and the anterior commissure, and the description of the anatomy of the connections of the cerebellar peduncles, the stria medullaris, and of the XI cranial nerve.

Burdach column (fasciculus cuneatus) The lateral part of the posterior (dorsal) columns of the spinal cord, named by Burdach in 1819. The medial part (fasciculus gracilis) is named for **Goll**. The Burdach nucleus is the cuneate nucleus. See also **cuneate fasciculus** and **nucleus**.

Burkitt lymphoma A multicentric tumor composed of poorly differentiated lymphoid cells, common in East Africa and described by Sir Denis Burkitt from Uganda in 1958. Clinically, swellings of the jaw, orbit, and face and ovarian infiltration are the usual features.

Neurological complications include direct or ischemic myelopathy, multiple cranial neuropathies affecting especially the oculomotor and VII cranial nerves, malignant meningitis, seizures, and delirium.

burn encephalopathy The acute onset of reduction in the level of consciousness, often with confusion, seizures, or neurological signs, or any of these in combination, in patients (especially children) suffering from severe burns. The syndrome is not homogeneous. It affects some 5% of children at risk (usually with over 30% of the body surface burned) within a few days of the injury, but is usually reversible. Multiple metabolic problems are considered to be responsible.[4426] The syndrome was first noted by Dupuytren in 1832.

burn neuropathy Multiple mononeuropathies occurring in severely burned patients, often with associated complications of sepsis. Vascular occlusion of the vasa nervorum, direct thermal injury, and a disseminated neurotoxin are suggested as mechanisms.[4097]

burner–stinger syndrome Stretch injury of the upper fibres of the brachial plexus, not causing nerve root avulsion but sufficient to rupture some axons. It is usually seen following an athletic injury in which the head was forcibly distracted away from the side of the plexus injury. Clinically, there is immediate, severe burning pain in the shoulder region and distally, with paresthesias, dysesthesias, and sometimes arm weakness, lasting minutes. The prognosis for recovery is good.

Burnett syndrome (milk–alkali syndrome) The occurrence of weakness, depression, nausea, headache, and mental confusion in patients with hypercalcemia and alkalosis, due to excessive intake of milk and soluble alkalis.[947]

Burnier, Louis-Rene (1880–1952) French dermatologist, practicing in Paris.

Burnier syndrome (hypophysial nanism) A syndrome of short stature, optic atrophy, and adiposogenital dystrophy, with or without obesity, due to a pituitary tumor destroying the anterior lobe in childhood.[949]

burning feet syndrome (Gopalan syndrome, hot feet, happy feet, painful feet, jittery legs) A sensory neuropathy causing aching, burning, numbness, tingling, and aching in the legs with vasodilation of the feet, worse with heat and better with cold. It is generally due to deficiency in B-complex vitamins, as occurs in malnutrition states and uremia[2485] but a dominantly inherited form has been reported.[6067]

burning hands syndrome A *forme fruste* of the **central cord syndrome** in which limited injury has spared many of the fibers usually affected in that condition but has led to reduced input into the spino-thalamic tract from the cervical segments.[4093]

burning mouth syndrome (glossodynia, glossopyrosis, oral dysesthesias) A syndrome of persistent awareness of a painful, burning sensation in the mouth and/or tongue seen mainly in mature adult women, for which no medical or dental cause can be found. The causes are multifactorial; ill-fitting dentures, vitamin B deficiency, anxiety, depression, and cancerphobia are all cited as etiological factors.[3652] Diagnostic criteria have been defined:

A. Pain in the mouth present daily and persisting for most of the day
B. Oral mucosa is of normal appearance
C. Local and systemic diseases have been excluded

From the International Classification of Headache Disorders (Headache Classification Committee of the International Headache Society; *Cephalalgia* 2004;**24** [Suppl 1]) by kind permission of Dr. Jes Olesen, the International Headache Society and Wiley-Blackwell Publications.

Burns syndrome See **oculoauriculocutaneous syndrome**.

burst A group of waves which appear and disappear abruptly and are distinguished from background activity by differences in frequency and/or amplitude. The term does not imply abnormality and is not a synonym for **paroxysm**. (Adapted from the 1974 Report of the Committee on Terminology, IFCN. In: Chatrian GE, Bergamini L, Dondey M, et al. A glossary of terms most commonly used by clinical electroencephalographers. *EEG Clin Neurophysiol* 1974;**37**:538–48. Reproduced by kind permission of Elsevier Science and the IFCN.)

burst lobe The occurrence of an intracerebral or intracerebellar hematoma in continuity with a subdural hematoma, following cerebral trauma.

burst neurons Neurons which, with pause neurons, are found in the paramedian pontine reticular formation (PPRF) and which generate the high-frequency burst discharges that act as the command for saccades to occur.

burst suppression An EEG pattern characterized by bursts of theta and/or delta waves, at times intermixed with faster waves and with intervening periods of relative quiescence.

The term should be used to describe the EEG effects of some anesthetic drugs at certain levels of anesthesia. (Adapted from the 1974 Report of the Committee on Terminology, IFCN. In: Chatrian GE, Bergamini L, Dondey M, et al. A glossary of terms most commonly used by clinical electroencephalographers. *EEG Clin Neurophysiol* 1974;**37**:538–48. Reproduced by kind permission of Elsevier Science and the IFCN.)

The pattern is typically seen in hypoxic brain damage and in prolonged status epilepticus, and it indicates significant compromise of the brain's metabolic integrity, with a poor prognosis.

Burton sign The blue line in the gums just below their junction with the teeth in chronic lead poisoning, described by Dr. H. Burton (1799–1849), a physician at St. Thomas Hospital in London.

Buschke Cued Recall (selective reminding) test A test of verbal learning and memory using confrontation naming, which coordinates the encoding and retrieval of new information for cued recall with an initial search strategy. The subject is required to name the objects shown in a series of pictures (e.g., "Which one is a piece of clothing?"), is prompted if he fails to name it, and finally is told the answer. Following a distracting task, he is required to recall as many of the 12 pictures shown as he can.[956,957]

Buschke–Fuld selective reminding procedure A test of recent memory wherein the subject learns 12 words over a dozen trials, being reminded only of those words which he failed to recall on the preceding trial. After 12 trials, he is required to note from a multiple choice list those words with which he had difficulty.[957] The test is very sensitive to the presence of cognitive change.

Busse–Buschke disease See **cryptococcal meningitis**.

butterfly area The nasal and adjacent malar regions of the face.

butterfly glioma A glioma which has spread from one hemisphere to the other directly through the corpus callosum. These lesions may have started within the corpus callosum and, by infiltrating both frontal lobes, lead either to increasing stupor or to emotional lability, irritability, or delusional states.[5648]

butterfly infarct The pattern of infarction with occlusion of the precommunal part of the posterior cerebral artery and thus of the penetrating arteries springing from it; and involving the medial part of the midbrain tegmentum and the medial part of the thalamus bilaterally.

Pupillary disorders and disturbances of eye movement result.

Buzzard, E.F. (1871–1945) English physician, Regius Professor of Medicine at Oxford.

Buzzard reflex A variant of the knee jerk, in this case obtained as the patient sits with his toes pressing on the floor as a facilitatory maneuver.[5333] See **nocioceptive reflex**.

Bywaters syndrome Traumatic/ischemic myositis with myoglobinemia and myoglobinuria and shock, sometimes leading to renal failure and usually described after extensive crush injuries.[969]

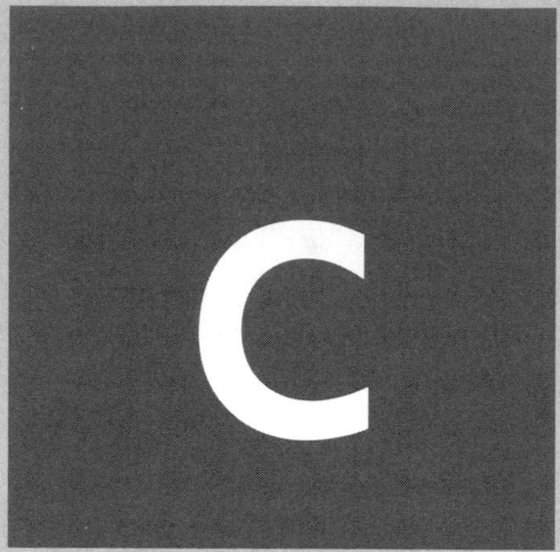

C fibers Unmyelinated sensory nerve fibers in the peripheral nervous system, feeding in from receptors which respond to temperature, chemical, and high-threshold mechanical stimulation.

C reflex An abnormal reflex response representing the electrophysiologic correlate of sensory-evoked myoclonus. The term "C" was chosen to indicate that the reflex might be mediated in the cerebral cortex, which is sometimes, but not always, true.[19]

This enhanced long-latency EMG response is found in a stimulated muscle (and sometimes in the homologous muscle on the opposite side), particularly in patients with myoclonic disorders, time-locked to a peripheral nerve electrical stimulus and equating a myoclonic jerk.

C syndrome (Opitz trigonocephaly syndrome) A recessively inherited craniofacial malformation syndrome characterized by trigonocephaly and microcephaly with ridging in the metopic region due to synostosis of the metopic suture, hypotelorism, Mongoloid slant to the eyes, epicanthic folds, strabismus, short neck, congenital cardiac malformations, and skeletal anomalies including syndactyly.[4799, 4808]

C waves (Traub–Hering waves) Low-amplitude fluctuations of the CSF pressure occurring at 4–8/min, normally present but enhanced in states of raised intracranial pressure. The waves correspond with changes in arterial blood pressure.

cacacusis Frightening echoes of mechanical sounds or of words heard or said, symptomatic of right hemisphere lesions.[5521] See also **palinacousis**.

CACH (vanishing white matter disease) A heterogeneous leukodystrophic condition of childhood with variable course resulting from maldevelopments of myelin formation (dys- or hypomyelination) rather than from demyelination.[5600, 6484] See **fatal infantile leukodystrophy**.

cachectic myopathy (neuromyopathy) A syndrome of proximal atrophy with relative retention of power. Both neuropathic and myopathic causes are suspected, whereas the underlying problem is considered to be nutritional.

cachexia (Gr, bad + a habit) Severe loss of subcutaneous tissue and muscle bulk, the latter without commensurate weakness; muscle biopsy shows the presence of scattered atrophic fibers. The condition is the result of severe malnutrition, malignancy, or other systemic illness. *Cachexia mercurialis* was the term applied to widespread ulceration occurring in syphilitic patients treated with mercury; *cachexia saturnia* is an old term for chronic lead poisoning.

cachodic (from Gr, a bad smell) Having a bad smell.

cacogenesis (Gr, bad + origin) A morbid malformation, such as a monster.

cacogeusia (Gr, bad + taste) The perception that all food in the mouth has a foul taste; a symptom of local disease, partial damage to the olfactory nerve, or depressive illness.

cacophonia (Gr, bad + lack of + voice) Hoarseness of the voice.

cacosmia (Gr, bad + smell) Perception of all food as having a foul smell. The causes are similar to those of **cacogeusia**.

CADASIL See **cerebral autosomal dominant arteripathy with subcortical infarcts and leukoencephalopathy**. See also **CARASIL**.

CADASIL coma An uncommon complication of the underlying arteriopathy, manifesting as an acute encephalopathy lasting a week or two after presenting with fever, acute confusion, coma, and seizures. There is eventual full recovery but the condition may recur.[5636]

cadet palsy See **rucksack palsy**.

cadiva insania (Lat, falling + senseless) An ancient term for epilepsy.

caducus (Lat, falling) Hence *caducus morbus*—another ancient term for epilepsy.

Cadwalader, Thomas (1708–1779) American physician who first described lead palsy and lead colic in his *Essay on the West Indian Dry-Gripes* published in Philadelphia by Benjamin Franklin in 1746.[5333]

caeruleus (ceruleus) (from Lat, dark blue) Blue, azure.

café-au-lait spots Brown skin macules, possessed by many healthy people but a diagnostic requirement for **von Recklinghausen** disease, in which condition there must be more than six present. At least one of these should measure over 5 mm in its longest axis in prepubertal people; after puberty, at least one should measure more than 15 mm.

Caffey–Silverman syndrome See **infantile cortical hyperostosis.**

cage paralysis Vitamin B_{12} deficiency in captive primates fed a fruit diet deficient in that vitamin.

caida de mollera See **fallen fontanelle**.

Cairns, Sir Hugh William Bell (1896–1952) Australian neurosurgeon, born and educated in Adelaide and seeing service in World War I before returning to Australia, graduating in 1917. He was later elected to a Rhodes scholarship at Balliol College, Oxford, and, following that, worked at the London Hospital. After studying with Harvey **Cushing** on a Rockefeller fellowship, he turned to neurosurgery and later joined the staff first of the London Hospital and the **National Hospitals** for Nervous Diseases in Queen Square and Maida Vale and subsequently of the Radcliffe Infirmary as the first Regius Professor of Surgery at the University of Oxford.

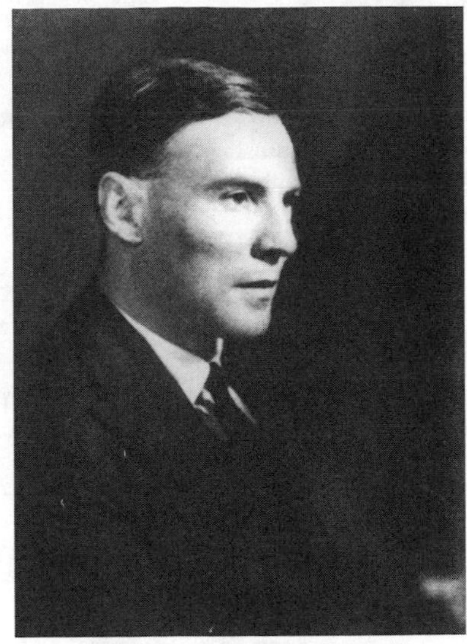

Figure C–1 Sir Hugh William Bell Cairns.

During World War II he established and ran a head injury base hospital in Oxford and organized mobile neurosurgical teams for the front. He designed a crash helmet and leg guard for motor cyclists which led to the saving of many lives and fractures. His numerous publications included studies of gliomas and subdural hematomas, the use of antibiotics, problems of consciousness, and neuro ophthalmology.[3181, 5666]

Cairns syndrome 1. **persistent vegetative state** with near complete loss of all but ocular movements and of emotional response. "Oft-repeated commands may be carried out in a feeble, slow, and incomplete manner but usually there are no movements of a voluntary character." Voluntary extraocular movements, chewing, swallowing, and breathing are maintained. There is incontinence, and in some cases, decorticate rigidity. Fluctuations may occur.

The condition is produced by lesions in and around the third ventricle. Cairns considered that this state was due to a disorder of cortical function secondary to a diencephalic lesion.[977] 2. Hydrocephalus due to blockage of the CSF pathways by meningitic exudate.[976]

caisson disease See **decompression sickness**.

Cajal, Santiago Ramon y (1852–1934) Spanish neurohistologist and anatomist who trained in Saragossa. He was appointed professor of anatomy at Valencia at the age of 29 but later transferred to Bologna and then returned to Spain as professor of histology and morbid anatomy in Madrid. His major work *Histologie du système nerveuse de l'homme and des vertèbres* (Paris, 1909–1911) established him as the father of neurohistology, although some of the credit belongs to Camillo **Golgi**, a modification of whose silver stain Cajal used and with whom he shared the Nobel Prize in 1906. His textbook of general pathology[5176] became a standard source. Cajal also introduced a silver nitrate stain to show the content of the neuronal cytoplasm; this stain was employed by **Alzheimer** to demonstrate neuro-fibrillary tangles. Among his students or collaborators were **Lorente de No**, **Lafora**, and Wilder **Penfield**.

Cajal enunciated his neuronal theory in three parts. First, nerve cells are independent elements which do not anastomose (as in a syncytium) but make contact only at specific points. Second, nervous impulses are always transmitted from the cell body out to the axon. Third, the axon conducts *away from* the cell body. His autobiography has recently been published.[5177]

Cajal cells Astrocytes.

Cajal stain A metallic impregnation method of staining astrocytes, using gold chloride sublimate.

calamus scriptorius (Lat, a quill or reed + of a writer) The inverted triangle, somewhat resembling the point of a pen, on the dorsum of the medulla in the floor of the fourth ventricle; so named by Herophilus, a Greek physician and anatomist in Athens (335–280 BC).

calcification of the basal ganglia 1. An asymptomatic condition discovered fortuitously on X-ray studies, CT scans, or MRI scans of the head. 2. Calcium deposition in the basal ganglia as occurs in numerous progressive white matter degenerations, true and pseudo-hypoparathyroidism, hyperparathyroidism, mitochondrial cytopathies, some infections including HIV infection and toxoplasmosis, tuberous sclerosis, Down syndrome and systemic lupus erythematosus, and also following many forms of toxic, radiation, or other damage to neural tissue. See **striato-pallidal calcification**. 3. A specific fatal syndrome in infants who present with microcephaly, bilateral spasticity, dystonia, and CSF lymphocytosis.[77] See also **choroido-cerebral calcification syndrome**.

calcinosis universalis See **Profichet syndrome**.

calcitonin myopathy A myopathic syndrome also characterized by medullary carcinoma of the thyroid, neuromas of the tongue and eyelid, prominence of the lips, and stigmata of **Marfan syndrome** and skin pigmentation.[1381]

calcium ATPase deficiency A rare disorder of muscle characterized by exertional muscle contractures with rhabdomyolysis and impaired muscle relaxation, due to a deficiency in sarcoplasmic reticulum-ATPase.[5060]

calcium gene-related peptide A neurotransmitter normally found at cholinergic sites in the motor system but also released in the walls of cranial vessels in migraine attacks, at which sites it has a local inflammatory action.

Calderon syndrome (kinky hair–photosensitivity–mental retardation) A congenital dysmorphic syndrome characterized by sparse, brittle, and kinky hair, absent eyebrows and eyelashes, skin photosensitivity, and mental and developmental delay.[381] See also **Menkes disease**.

calf head sign A suggested appearance of the dorsal muscles in **Miyoshi myopathy** seen when patients raise their arms with the shoulders abducted and the elbows flexed to 90°.[5106]

calibration The testing and recording of the responses of EEG channels to voltage differences applied to the input terminals of their respective amplifiers. DC (usually) or AC voltages of magnitude comparable to the amplitudes of EEG waves are used.

California encephalitis Direct viral infection of brain due to bunyavirus members of the arbovirus group. Clinically, the disease typically affects children in the central and eastern parts of the United States and southern Canada and occurs seasonally, mainly in early fall, presenting with typical features of encephalitis with focal neurological signs and stupor but with a low mortality and few residua.[3227] See also www.cdc.gov/ncidod/diseases/submenus/sub_encephalitis.htm.

California Verbal Learning Test A test of aural learning, recall, and recognition memory for a list of words over five trials and allowing assessment of different components of memory as well as of retrieval strategy and other executive functions.[1558]

Call–Fleming syndrome (benign angiopathy of the central nervous system, postpartum angiopathy, thunderclap headache with reversible vasospasm, migrainous vasospasm, migraine angiitis, drug-induced cerebral arteritis) The occurrence of vasospasm following subarachnoid hemorrhage, hemorrhagic stroke, or numerous other conditions including eclampsia, exposure to vasoactive and antidepressant drugs and to blood products, pheochromocytoma, unruptured cerebral aneurysm, head trauma, migraine, and exertion.[979]

The clinical presentation is most common in adult women who present with **thunderclap headache**, nausea, vomiting, photosensitivity, and various neurologic symptoms and signs occurring secondary to ischemia of brain regions now perfused by a very constricted artery. Seizures and transient hypertension are also described. The CSF is normal but angiography or MRA shows multifocal segmental areas of cerebral arterial vasoconstriction and interspersed dilatation ("beading"). These findings and the clinical deficits should return to normal within 3 months unless an infarct has occurred.

The condition is classified as a **reversible cerebral vasoconstriction syndrome**.[979] See also **posterior reversible leukoencephalopathy** and **primary angiitis of the central nervous system**.

callosal agenesis Failure of formation of the corpus callosum due to a developmental failure during embryogenesis. See **agenesis of the corpus callosum**.

callosal anomia See **anomia**.

callosal apraxia A disconnection syndrome manifesting apraxia of the left hand as a result of infarction of the anterior corpus callosum.[6671] See **apraxia**.

callosal disconnection The association of tactile anomia, agraphia, and apraxia affecting the left hand, described in **multiple sclerosis**.[5630] Left-ear suppression on dichotic listening tasks is another feature of the syndrome.

callosal fissure The space between the dorsum of the corpus callosum and the overlying hemisphere.

callosal syndrome See **Bristowe syndrome**.

callosotomy Section of the corpus callosum: a surgical therapy for intractable generalized and akinetic seizure disorders for half a century, now more widely accepted than heretofore on account of reduced morbidity from the use of microsurgical techniques.[4756]

Calmeil, Louis-Florentin (1798–1895) French physician, chief of the Charenton Hospital, who described **general paralysis** in a book in 1826, immediately after **Bayle**'s description of the same condition. He also introduced the term *absence* into medicine. His book *Malades Inflammatoires du Cerveau* (1859) included accurate descriptions of cerebral hemorrhages, syphilis and other acute and chronic infections, delirium, and meningitis.

calmodulin The main calcium-binding protein in cells. Ca^{2+} ATPase is the main enzyme responsible for removal. With depletion of high-energy phosphates resulting from ischemia, the Ca^{2+} ATPase system quits and Ca^{2+} levels increase within cells. High Ca^{2+} levels are cytotoxic, and cell death only occurs in the presence of Ca^{2+}.

caloric after-nystagmus See **vestibular nystagmus**.

caloric nystagmus Nystagmus of the type seen in peripheral vestibular lesions and induced by warm or cold stimulation of the labyrinths. Cold stimulation leads to nystagmus with its fast component away from the irrigated side, and warm stimulation produces nystagmus in the other direction. See **vestibular nystagmus**.

caloric paresis A relative decrease in the responsiveness of one side compared with the other on caloric testing. See **canal paresis**.

caloric tests (caloric irrigation tests) The introduction of hot or cold (44°C or 30°C) water or air into the external auditory meatus to test VIII (vestibular) cranial nerve function through stimulation of the receptors in the semicircular canals. The change in ambient temperature sets up convection currents in the endolymph of the horizontal semicircular canal when the subject lies supine with the head elevated 30° from the horizontal. These induce vertigo and nystagmus (with the fast component away from the canal when irrigated with cold, and toward the canal when irrigated with warm) in the normal subject, the maximal velocity of the slow component being recorded using electronystagmography. See also **canal paresis, directional preponderance**, and **Barany Test**.

calpainopathy Mutations of the calpain-3 gene, the most common cause of adult-onset, recessively inherited limb girdle muscular dystrophy with the usual onset in late childhood or adolescence of scapular–humeral–pelvic muscle weakness and atrophy and with the early development of severe contractures.[3454]

calsequestrin storage myopathy A mild "surplus protein" myopathy, sometimes only presenting as asymptomatic elevated serum CK levels, in which toluidine blue-stained semithin sections of muscle specimens reveal heteromorphic inclusions, likely to be constituted by an excess of proteins normally present in the terminal cisternae of sarcoplasmic reticulum.[6346]

calvaria, calvarium (from Lat, baldness) The vault of the cranium.

calvarial hyperostosis (Morgagni syndrome) See **hyperostosis frontalis interna**.

Cambridge Behavioral Inventory A reliable informant-based assessment of neuropsychiatric symptoms and everyday functioning of people with dementia. Cross-validation with the **Neuropsychiatric Inventory** shows good concurrent validity, which has been used to show that disinhibition, stereotypic behavior, elation, anxiety, poor self-care, and changes in eating habits occur more commonly in patients with frontotemporal lobar degeneration than in those with **Alzheimer disease**.[6690]

CAMDEX (Cambridge Diagnostic Examination) A highly reliable clinical instrument, of value in diagnosing dementia, in measuring cognitive impairment, and in assessing behavior and adaptation in everyday life. The measure includes a standardized, structured interview with a relative or other caregiver and incorporates data from other sources, including a patient interview, a cognitive examination, and interviewer observations. Three diagnostic scores (for organicity, multi-infarct dementia, and depression) can be derived. Items of the **Blessed Dementia Scale** are included within the CAMDEX as one of the measures of cognitive decline.[5429, 5429] See also the **CERAD** instrument.[4499]

camel sign The appearance of a sensory action potential with two peaks when recorded over the median nerve at the wrist with stimulation of the fourth finger.

The mechanism concerns the innervation of the fourth finger by both the ulnar and the median nerves; in **carpal tunnel syndrome** a small-amplitude ulnar sensory nerve action potential can be recorded from a point over the median nerve, as can the delayed median sensory nerve action potential, the two producing the "double-humped" appearance. The sign was originally noted by Dr. Charles Simpson of Victoria, British Columbia, who also pointed out that the normal response is a potential with a single peak (the dromedary response), the abnormal one having two, like a Bactrian camel.[5855]

Camera syndrome (neuralgic osteopathy) Lumbosacral inflammatory osteopathy of adults, causing radiculopathic pain which is worse at night, and weight loss.[590] The similarity to ankylosing spondylitis is great.

CAMFAK syndrome A recessively inherited syndrome of **CA**taracts, **M**icrocephaly, **F**ailure to thrive, **A**rthrogryposis, and **K**yphoscoliosis; also with decreased myelination in the CNS, cerebral calcifications, pyramidal signs, and peripheral neuropathy.

Whether this condition has its own identity or is merely a severe variant of **Cockayne syndrome** is not yet determined.[6197]

CAMOS See **cerebellar syndromes** (congenital ataxias).

campimetry The measurement or plotting of the visual fields.

campomelic dwarfism See **campomelic variant**.

campomelic syndrome See **campomelic variant**.

campomelic variant (campomelic syndrome, campomelic dwarfism) A congenital dysmorphic syndrome characterized by dwarfism, hypertelorism, nasal hemangiomas, micrognathia, cleft palate, platyspondyly, mesomelia of upper and lower limbs, and skeletal anomalies of the skull, long bones, and spine, with delayed closure of the fontanelles, wide cranial sutures, and hydrocephalus.[4094]

camptocormia (from Gr, kamptos [curved] + kormos [the trunk]; [functional bent back, Souques disease]) 1. In the elderly, an acquired kyphosis increasing during walking, totally reducible in the dorsal horizontal position, and sometimes accompanied by other neurological or systemic disorders.[2904] 2. A posture of severe maintained neck flexion resulting from, for example, **amyotrophic lateral sclerosis**; myopathy such as **inclusion body myositis, facio-scapulo-humeral dystrophy**, or **nemaline myopathy**; stroke; **dystonias**; or **Parkinson** disease or its variants.[6442] There are some even less common etiologies.[313] 3. A bizarre posture of maximal trunk flexion, adopted primarily while walking. In some cases, it represents a hysterical condition in which the spine is greatly flexed, even though it remains flexible and in which there is compensatory extension of the head on the neck. It was first described by Sir Benjamin **Brodie** in 1837 and has been known by his name; practically all the cases seen early in the last century were soldiers during the two world wars. **Hurst** regarded it as always hysterical in nature,[5963] but the first two categories above indicate that he was wrong. See also **Pisa syndrome**.

camptodactyly A dominantly inherited abnormality of the hands characterized by permanent flexion of one of more fingers, usually at the proximal interphalangeal joints.[3676] In *variant* forms, deafness and muscular hypoplasia are also described. The condition is also a feature of various other congenital malformation syndromes. See also **CAP disease**, **Pena–Shokeir phenotypes**, **Tel-Hashomer camptodactyly**, and **camptomelic variant**.

Camurati–Engelman syndrome A genetic craniotubular hyperostotic and osteosclerotic syndrome stemming from active overgrowth of bone, in which sclerosis and hyperostosis of the base of the skull and the long bones appear in the first year, associated with conductive deafness and proximal and distal myopathic weakness. The condition has been reviewed.[4045] See **progressive diaphyseal dysplasia**.

Canadian Association for Narcolepsy A Canadian charitable association. Web site: www.connexions.org/Groups/Subscribers/cxg10972.htm.

Canadian Association of Neurological Nurses A professional organization. Web site: www.cann.ca/.

Canadian Brain and Nerve Health Coalition An organization established as a coalition of various Canadian voluntary health organizations with an interest in neurological disorders, committed to improving quality of life by promoting access to cost-effective treatments, supporting research and education and promoting public and government awareness of the incidence and impact of nervous system disorders and injuries. Web site: www.cnsfederation.org/gen_info_CBANCH.html/.

A list of affiliated organizations follows. Those that are not listed separately in this book can be accessed through the Web site above.

Acoustic Neuroma Association of Canada
ALS Society of Canada
Alzheimer's Society of Canada
Autism Society of Canada
Brain Injury Association of Canada
Brain Injury Association of Alberta
Brain Tumour Foundation of Canada
Canadian Alliance of Brain Tumour Organizations
Canadian Association of Neuroscience (CAN)
Canadian Association of Neuroscience Nurses (CANN)
Canadian Brain Tissue Bank
Canadian Neurological Sciences Federation (CNSF)
Canadian Continence Foundation
Canadian Down Syndrome Society National Office
Canadian Institutes of Health Research
Canadian Paraplegic Association (CPA)
Canadian Psychiatric Research Foundation
Canadian Spinal Research Organization
Canadian Syringomyelia Network
Canadian VHL Family Alliance
Central Okanagan Brain Injury Society
Cerebral Palsy Association of British Columbia
Epilepsy Canada
Heart and Stroke Foundation of Canada
Heart and Stroke Foundation of Ontario
Huntington Society of Canada
Institute of Neurosciences, Mental Health and Addictions (INMHA)
Multiple Sclerosis Society of Canada
Muscular Dystrophy Association of Canada
Neuroscience Canada Foundation
Ontario Brain Injury Association
Parkinson Society Canada
Le Regroupment des associations de personnes tramatisées cranio-cérébrales du Québec
Spina Bifida and Hydrocephalus Association of Canada
Think First Foundation of Canada
Tourette Syndrome Foundation of Canada
Tuberous Sclerosis Canada

Canadian Brain Tissue Bank Address: Banting Institute, Room 128, 100 College St, Toronto, ON M5G 1L5, Canada. Web site: www.utoronto.ca/neuropathology/cbb.html.

Canadian Cerebral Palsy Association A charitable organization. Web site (based upon a medical malpractice site): www.lawmedmal.ca/cp_association.htm.

Canadian Congress of Neurological Sciences See **Canadian Neurological Sciences Federation.**

Canadian Down Syndrome Society A charitable organization. Web site: www.cdss.ca/.

Canadian Headache Society A professional society, now merged with the Headache Network Canada. Web site: www.headachenetwork.ca/.

Canadian Journal of Neurological Sciences (*Can J Neurol Sci*) The official organ of the Canadian Neurological, Neurosurgical, Child Neurology, and Clinical Neurophysiology Societies (Canadian Neurological Sciences Federation). Address: P.O. Box 4220, Station C, Calgary, AB T2T 5N1, Canada.Web site: www.canjneurolsci.org/.

Canadian Liver Foundation: Hepatic Encephalopathy A site providing an overview of this complication of liver disease.

Canadian Liver Foundation: Wilson Disease A site giving an overview of the condition that includes description, causes, symptoms, diagnosis, treatment, and precautions, at www.liver.ca/Home.aspx

Canadian Mental Health Association A charitable organization. Address: 180 Dundas St. W, Suite 2301, Toronto, ON M5G 1Z8, Canada. Tel: 416-977-5580. Web site: www.cmha.ca/bins/index.asp/.

Canadian Movement Disorder Group A professionally inspired informational source for patients with disorders of movement and their caregivers. Web site: www.cmdg.org/index.htm.

Canadian Neurological Coalition A group formed by the association of a number of Canadian Charitable Foundations concerned with various neurological disorders for the purposes of advocacy, information sharing, and the support of research. Web site: www.cnsfederation.org/gen_info_ CBANCH.html.

Canadian Neurological Scale A semiquantitative tool for the assessment of neurologic function. It was designed primarily for use in patients following cerebrovascular accident, in which situation it has been shown to be both valid and reliable. The scale rates mentation (level of consciousness, orientation, and speech); motor weakness (face and both proximal and distal arm and leg function); and motor responses, comparing the two sides with respect to the face, arms, and legs.[1295] (Reproduced by kind permission of the American Academy of Neurology and Lippincott Williams and Wilkins.) (See Chart C–1.)

Canadian Neurological Sciences Federation An umbrella organization representing four member societies—the Canadian Neurological Society, the Canadian Neurosurgical Society, the Canadian Society of Clinical Neurophysiologists, and the Canadian Association of Child Neurologists—and publishing the *Canadian Journal of Neurological Sciences*. Web site: www.cnsfederation.org/index.html.

Canadian Neuropathy Association A charitable organization that provides support for people with neuropathies by providing education, conducting research, and sharing information. Web site: www.canadianneuropathyassociation.org/.

Canadian Paraplegic Association A charitable organization providing support and information on this condition. Web site: www.canparaplegic.org/en/.

Canadian Porphyria Foundation Inc. A charitable organization providing support and information on this condition. Web site: www.cpf-inc.ca/.

Canadian (Ontario) Rett Syndrome Association A charitable organization providing support and information on this condition. Address: 555 Fairway Rd., Suite 301, Kitchener, ON N2C 1X4, Canada. Tel: 416-494-1954. Web site accessible through www.rettsyndrome.org.uk/RS_organisations.htm.

Canadian Stroke Strategy A public initiative of charitable and professional groups in Canada designed to improve Canadian stroke care. Web site: www.canadianstrokestrategy.ca/.

canal (Lat, a furrow) A groove in or a passage through bone or other tissues. Thus Arnold's canal for the lesser superficial petrosal nerve, Huguier's canal for the chorda tympani, and Jacobson's canal for the tympanic branch of the IX cranial nerve. The spinal canal was identified by **Etienne**.

canal paresis Decreased responsiveness of the vestibular apparatus as shown by reduced duration of nystagmus in response to caloric stimulation with water 7°C above or below body temperature. The lesion may lie anywhere between the vestibular nuclei in the brainstem and the semicircular canals, but when due to a central lesion, the nystagmus is not enhanced by preventing visual fixation.[2172] See also **directional preponderance**.

Chart C–1. The Canadian Neurological Scale

Level of consciousness

Alert: Normal consciousness
Drowsy: The patient when stimulated verbally, remains awake and alert for a short period of time but tends to doze even when examined
Stuporous: The patient responds to loud verbal stimuli and/or strong touch; and may vocalize but does not become alert nor completely wake up
Comatose: The patient responds to deep pain (i.e., sternal pressure)

1. Only by purposeful movement of limb toward noxious stimuli and/or grimacing and/or moaning (no verbal response)
2. By nonpurposeful movements, flexion of upper limbs (i.e., decortication) or extension of upper limbs (i.e., decerebration)
3. No response to noxious stimuli

Note: If the patient is alert or drowsy, monitor progress with Section A, but if stuporous or comatose, monitor with Section B.

Mentation

1. Orientation
   A. Oriented: Patient is oriented both to place (i.e., city or hospital) and to time (i.e., patient must give at least correct month and year). If early in month (i.e., first 3 days), previous month is acceptable. Speech can be dysarthric (mispronounced or slurred) but intelligible.
   B. Disoriented or nonapplicable: If for any reason patient cannot answer the preceding questions on orientation (i.e., does not know answer, gives wrong answer, answers only partially, cannot express himself either by lack of words or unintelligible speech or finally ignores questions).
2. Speech (language and pronunciation)
   A. Receptive language
      The patient is asked,
      a. "Close your eyes."
      b. "Does a stone sink in water?"
      c. "Point to the ceiling." Repeat twice if necessary.
         If the patient obeys all three commands, continue to (B) expressive language; but if he obeys only two commands or fewer, score the receptive defect in the Speech Scale, and then proceed directly to motor function testing.
   B. Expressive language
      In this section pay special attention to not only the answers but also the word pronunciation, for example, dysarthria or slurring.
      a. Ask the patient to name a pencil, key, and watch; make sure that he can see them. If he names only two or less of them, score "expressive defect" in Speech Scale but if all three objects are correctly named, proceed to (b).

continued

Chart C–1. *(continued)*

b. Ask the patient,
"What do you do with a pencil?"
"What do you do with a key?"
"What do you do with a watch?"
If all three questions are correctly answered, score "normal speech."

Note: (1) The above scoring system relates to language only. Problems with pronunciation of words (dysarthria or slurred speech) are graded directly on the Speech Scale. (2) The patient should always be scored according to worst speech deficit (i.e., language score or mispronunciation) (3) Do not mimic commands in Section A on receptive language.

Speech Scale

Normal speech: Answers all commands and questions in speech section; patient can have slurred speech (dysarthria) but has to be still intelligible.
Expressive defect: The patient obeys commands in receptive language section but makes one or more errors in the section on expressive language and/or mispronounces words (slurred speech), so that the speech is totally or partially unintelligible (severe dysarthria).
Receptive defect: The patient obeys only two or less commands in section on receptive language.

Motor function

When evaluating strength and range of motion in limbs, always submit both limbs to same testing (i.e., apply same resistance at same position bilaterally).

Section A1. For patients who do not have comprehension problems (i.e., normal speech or expressive defect only).

1. Face: Ask patient to show his teeth or gums.
   No weakness: symmetrical grin, no asymmetry in smile.
   Weakness: facial asymmetry; one corner of mouth lower than other, either at rest or while showing teeth.
2. Upper limb (proximal)
   The patient should be tested in sitting position if possible.
   Test: abduction arms (to 90°).
   If the patient is lying in bed: elevate arms to approximately 45°–90°. The strength in both arms is to be tested simultaneously; resistance must be applied at midpoint between shoulder and elbow at all times.
3. Upper limb (distal):
   The patient is tested in the sitting or the lying position with the arms elevated and is asked to make fists and to extend his wrists. Compare the range of movement in both wrists simultaneously.
   If there is a full range of extension in both wrists, proceed to test strength by applying resistance separately to both fists while stabilizing the patient's arms firmly.
4. Lower limb
   The patient lying in bed for testing should always be scored according to his worst deficit, either (a) or (b). Test:
   a. Hip flexion. Ask patient to flex thighs toward trunk with knees flexed to 90°. Movement in both thighs is tested separately.
   b. Dorsiflexion of foot. Ask patient to point toes and foot upward. Compare both feet simultaneously (i.e., complete and partial movement).

In both (a) and (b) apply resistance alternately to each thigh and foot after the full movement has been completed to test strength.

Gradation of Motor Deficit

No detectable weakness.
Mild weakness: normal range of motion against gravity, but succumbs to resistance by observer either partially or totally.
Significant weakness: cannot completely overcome gravity in range of motion (i.e., partial movement).
Total weakness: absence of motion in movement tested or only contraction of muscles without actual movement of limb.

Section A2. For patients with comprehension problems (i.e., receptive defect in Speech Scale). Motor function in this section can be monitored in one of two ways:

1. The ability of the patient to maintain a fixed posture in the upper or lower limbs for a few (3–5) seconds. The observer will alternately place the limbs in the desired position.
   a. Upper limbs: place arms outstretched at 90° in front of patient.
   b. Lower limbs: flex thighs with knees flexed at 90°.
   c. Facial power: have the patient mimic your own grin.
   If the patient does not cooperate, then proceed to:
2. Comparison of motor response to a noxious stimuli (i.e., pressure on the nail-bed of the fingers or toes with a pencil). Facial response (grimacing) to pain is tested by applying pressure on sternum.
   a. Face (grimacing)
      Symmetrical
      Asymmetrical (note side)
   b. Upper limbs:
      Equal motor response: patient can maintain the fixed posture equally in both upper limbs for a few seconds or withdraws equally on both sides to pain.
      Unequal motor response: patient cannot maintain the fixed posture equally on both sides; weakness is noted on one side or there is an unequal withdrawal to pain. Note the side on which the withdrawal is not as brisk.

c. Lower limbs:
Equal motor response: patient can maintain the fixed posture equally in both lower limbs for a few seconds or withdraws equally on both sides to pain.
Unequal motor response: patient cannot maintain the fixed posture equally on both sides; weakness is noted on one side or there is an unequal withdrawal to pain. Note the side where withdrawal is not as brisk.

Symptomatology

1. Presenting symptoms	*2. New Symptoms (recurrence)*
Type	Type
Localization	Localization
Duration	Duration
Frequency	Frequency

The above symptoms and any remarks should be noted in the progress notes. The side of the weakness should always be identified and the modalities graded numerically on the score sheet. If the patient is stuporous or comatose, monitor progress with the **Glasgow Coma Scale**.

Scoring

Mentation

Level of consciousness	Alert	30	Arm: proximal	None	15	Leg: distal	None	15
	Drowsy	15		Mild	10		Mild	10
Orientation	Oriented	10		Significant	05		Significant	05
	Disoriented or NA	00		Total	00		Total	00
Speech	Normal	10	Arm: distal	None	15	*With comprehension deficit motor response*		
	Expressive deficit	05		Mild	10			
				Significant	05	Face	Symmetrical	05
	Receptive deficit	00		Total	00		Asymmetrical	00
Motor functions: weakness (no comprehension deficit)			Leg: proximal	None	15	Arms	Equal	15
				Mild	10		Unequal	00
Face:	None	05		Significant	05	Legs	Equal	15
	Present	00		Total	00		Unequal	00

NA = not applicable. *Adapted from Coté R, Battista RN, Wolfson C, et al. The Canadian Neurological Scale: validation and reliability assessment. Neurology 1989; 39: 638–43 with kind permission of the American Academy of Neurology and Lippincott Williams and Wilkins.*

canalolithiasis A state in which the calcific particles normally present in the semicircular canals move abnormally in response to postural changes of the head, exciting the hair cell receptors of the canals and producing a hallucination of rotation. This is considered especially relevant in the genesis of posterior canal **benign positional vertigo**. See also **cupolithiasis**.

canalith repositioning A manuever employed in the treatment of patients with **benign paroxysmal positional vertigo**, whereby the Dix–Hallpike maneuver is performed and the supine subject's extended head is then rotated to the left or right, held in that position for half a minute, and then turned another 90° in the same direction, the trunk following, for another half minute, after which the subject is raised to the sitting position. The aim of the procedure is to reposition those otoliths floating aberrantly in the semicircular canal into the vestibule. This and other relevant procedures were redescribed by Fife et al. (2008).[2045]

Canavan, Myrtelle M. (1879–1953) American neuropathologist who trained at the Women's Medical College in Philadelphia and who became pathologist at the Boston State Hospital and later curator of the Warren Anatomical Museum at Harvard. Her paper on a form of spongy degeneration was published in 1931.

Canavan leukodystrophy (Canavan–van Bogaert–Bertrand disease; aspartoacyclase deficiency; spongy degeneration of infancy; infantile CNS spongy degeneration; cavitating leukodystrophy; OMIM 271900) A rare, recessively inherited leukodystrophy, considered to be due to asparto-acylase deficiency, in which spongy vacuolation of the brain and spinal cord and demyelination are the pathological hallmarks.[3] It is mapped to 17pter-p13, and experimental gene therapy has been reported.

The *neonatal form* presents with hypotonia and failure to thrive, and is lethal.

The *infantile form* is a recessively inherited syndrome occurring among Eastern European Jewish children, and is characterized pathologically by **lissencephaly**, spongy degeneration and vacuolation of the cerebral white matter, and loss of myelin with little glial reaction. Increased urinary excretion of *N*-acetyl aspartic acid is a characteristic finding. The main clinical features include the early onset of psychomotor arrest, **megalencephaly**, seizures, and drooping of the head due to particular weakness of the neck muscles. Myoclonus, spasticity, involuntary movements, optic atrophy, blindness, and deafness also occur before the final phase of decerebration and death before the age of 5 years.[996]

The *juvenile form* begins after the age of 5 years and is characterized by a progressive cerebellar syndrome, optic atrophy, pigmentary retinal degeneration, and dementia.

The condition was first differentiated by Van Bogaert and Bertrand in 1949. Canavan herself had considered the condition to be a form of **Schilder disease**.

A *variant* condition is *cavitating leukodystrophy with autonomic failure*, characterized by the onset in young adult life of ataxia, orthostatic hypotension, neurogenic bladder, spasticity, and constipation in presence of the same pathological findings.

Canavan–van Bogaert–Bertrand disease See **Canavan leukodystrophy**.

cancellation tests Tests of attention, specifically for visual neglect, wherein the subject is required to find and circle all instances of a specific letter in a field of printed letters or of a specific design in a printed field of designs.[4332]

cancer-associated retinopathy (CAR syndrome)[3481] See **visual paraneoplastic syndrome**.

candle drippings The irregular outgrowths of the ependyma into the ventricles, producing small tumor-like nodules containing excessive numbers of astrocytes, calcium, and groups of bizarre and vacuolated cells of large diameter as in **tuberous sclerosis**.

Cannon, Walter Bradford (1871–1945) American neurologist and professor of physiology at Harvard, who described stress reactions in the ANS and showed that sympathetic nerves liberate a substance ("sympathin") which has an adrenaline-like action—and is indeed adrenaline. He was also a pioneer in the physiology of the gastrointestinal tract, suffering excessive X-ray exposure as a result.

His emergency theory, summarized today by the phrase "fight or flight" in relation to the functions of the sympathetic nervous system, provided the basis for Hans **Selye**'s categorization of the body's reactions to chronic stress.

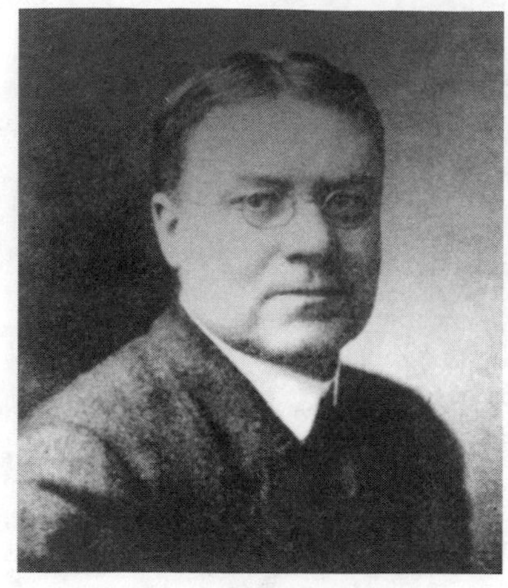

Figure C–2 Walter Bradford Cannon.

Cannon's law (law of denervation) Denervated end-organs become supersensitive to their physiological transmitters.

cannula plexopathy Injury to the upper or lower brachial plexus resulting from cannulation of the jugular vein, usually in the setting of cardiac surgery. Associated complications include damage to the vagus, accessory or hypoglossal nerves, Horner syndrome, and phrenic nerve palsy.

Cantelli sign (Widowitz sign, doll's-eye sign) Dissociated movements of the head and the eyes in diphtheria. When the head is raised, the eyes are lowered, and vice versa.[5333] This is not the same as the abnormalities of **doll's head eye movements** described in comatose patients with brainstem lesions.

Cao syndrome (agenesis of corpus callosum and microcephaly) A congenital dysmorphic syndrome characterized by optic atrophy, pigmented retinas, microcephaly, spasticity, aqueduct stenosis, and callosal agenesis with mental and developmental delay.[381]

CAP congenital myopathy See **CAP disease**. See also **congenital myopathy with caps**.

CAP disease (CAP congenital myopathy) A rare, nonprogressive congenital myopathy associated with Camptodactyly, Arthropathy, and Pericarditis. Neurological features are facial, proximal, and distal atrophy and weakness, short stature, high palate, kyphoscoliosis, pectus excavatum, and seizures. Pathologically the condition is distinguished by a lack of ATPase peripherally in many of the myofibrils, type I fiber predominance, a decrease of myosin, and an abnormal sarcomere pattern.[2041]

capillary hemangioma See **nevus flammeus**.

capillary leak syndrome A potentially fatal condition characterized by generalized increased permeability of capillaries and presenting with widespread edema, including cerebral edema and multiple microinfarctions.[5620]

capillary nevus See **nevus flammeus**.

capillary telangiectasia A small **vascular malformation** composed of multiple irregular clusters of dilated capillaries, usually separated by some neural parenchyma and found in the cerebral cortex, white matter, or brainstem (mainly in the pons). Occasionally, they bleed and lead to destruction of small regions locally, producing seizures or focal deficits such as hearing loss, ataxia, vertigo, diplopia, and limb weakness.[5572, 6] They are also found in association with Weber–Rendu–Osler disease but are usually of no clinical significance.[6030]

Capgras, J.M. (1873–1950) French psychiatrist.

Capgras syndrome (Fr, *l'illusion des sosies*—the illusion of doubles) A chronic delusional psychosis occurring in clear consciousness, in which patients make the remarkable complaint that certain people whom they see (usually family members) are only their own doubles, or that they have replaced another person of emotional importance to the patient, such as the spouse.[1004, 6382]

Cappeto syndrome A disease of unknown cause, possibly immune based and certainly resembling **systemic lupus erythematosus** in its usual occurrence in young women and its clinical features. These include multiple retinal branch occlusions with retinal hemorrhages, field defects, gaze palsies, and encephalopathy with confusion, psychosis, seizures, pyramidal signs, and almost any other neurological features.[1003]

capsaicin A neurotoxic agent derived from red peppers (paprika) which initially causes pain but later analgesia to chemical and heat stimuli (but not to mechanical touch) by first stimulating and then blocking unmyelinated sensory fibers. It can be used topically in the treatment of **post-herpetic neuralgia**.[6670]

capsular genu syndrome A facio-lingual stroke syndrome in which the infarct or hemorrhage is limited to the genu of the internal capsule, leading to contralateral facial and lingual hemiparesis with dysarthria but with only mild limb weakness.[711]

When the inferior part of the internal capsule is infarcted, fluctuating alertness, hypokinesia, memory disturbances, and **abulia** are typical clinical features; the whole may resemble **akinetic mutism**. The syndrome is considered to arise as a result of occlusion of the perforating vessels arising from the internal carotid, anterior cerebral, or anterior choroidal arteries supplying the thalamic peduncles. The condition was first described by **Déjèrine**.[1541]

capsular warning syndrome (crescendo TIAs) A distinct syndrome of repetitive motor and/or sensory transient ischemic attacks affecting the face, arm, and leg, considered to be related to the region of the internal capsule and frequently succeeded by evidence of capsular infarction, usually lacunar in nature.[1687] The ischemia is most often due to hemodynamic phenomena in diseased single, small penetrating vessels. When cerebral infarction develops it is usually lacunar and involves a single penetrating vessel, although occasionally striatocapsular or anterior choroidal artery territory infarction occurs.

capsulothalamic syndrome See **thalamic syndrome**.

CAR syndrome See **paraneoplastic syndromes**.

car toll neuropathy Compression of the sciatic nerve under the pirformis muscle, in this case by loose change carried in the hip pocket by the driver of the car.[576] See **piriformis syndrome, toilet seat neuropathy**, and **credit card wallet sciatica**.

CARASIL (cerebral autosomal recessive arteriopathy with subcortical infarcts and leukoencephalopathy) A condition similar to **CADASIL** but also associated with spinal deformities.

carbamoyl phosphate synthetase deficiency A rare congenital **hyperammonemic syndrome** leading to severe leukoencephalopathy with neonatal feeding problems, altered consciousness, cyclic vomiting, seizures, and secondary cerebrovascular disease, usually in infants with mental and developmental delay (but also described in an adult). The condition is due to deficiency of the enzyme essential in the early stages of the urea cycle.[6613] The responsible gene maps to chromosome 2q33.

A *variant* is an incomplete form that appears in later childhood.[116]

carbohydrate-deficient glycoprotein syndrome A group of recessively inherited metabolic disorders. Type I presents with early-onset psychomotor retardation and pigmentary retinopathy, usually combined with mild hepatic dysfunction, facial dysmorphisms, subcutaneous lipodystrophy, stroke-like episodes during childhood, and generalized seizures. Thoracic deformities are also described. The prognosis for life is good. Types II and III are associated with demyelination or hypomyelination and are less well recognized. Patients with type III manifest severe psychomotor retardation, tetrapareses, cerebral and optic atrophy, retinal pigmentary degeneration, and cerebellar hypoplasia.[6063] A raised serum level of carbohydrate-deficient transferrin is a marker for the condition.[6063] See **cerebellar syndromes** (congenital ataxias).

carbon dioxide narcosis A generalized encephalopathy with increased cerebral blood flow and cerebral edema, resulting from chronic ventilatory insufficiency and carbon dioxide retention.

carbon monoxide encephalopathy A severe encephalopathy resulting from the conversion of oxyhemoglobin to carboxyhemoglobin, a compound which does not liberate oxygen with the same facility as does oxyhemoglobin. The resulting histotoxic anoxia leads to reduction in consciousness in the early stages. In fatal cases, cerebral edema, petechial hemorrhages, degeneration of the globus pallidus, and eventually leukoencephalopathy occur.[768]

carbonic anhydrase II deficiency (marble brain disease) A congenital dysmorphic syndrome characterized by short stature, deafness, optic atrophy with blindness, abnormal dental development, renal tubular acidosis, proximal and distal myopathic weakness, myopathy, intracranial calcifications, multiple fractures, osteosclerosis or osteopetrosis, wide metaphyses, and mental and developmental delay.[381]

carcinoid myopathy An acquired proximal myopathy with advanced atrophy of type II muscle fibers, developing in subjects with carcinoid syndrome of long standing.[6156]

carcinomatous meningitis (meningeal carcinomatosis) A rare, usually fatal complication of solid tumors in which the leptomeninges are diffusely invaded by metastatic tumor cells, coating the surface of the brain and spinal cord and infiltrating the **Virchow–Robin spaces**. The most common primary sites are the breast and lung; melanomas can produce a similar picture.

Both clinically and pathologically, the condition resembles meningitis rather than tumor. Headache, visual failure, raised intracranial pressure, multiple cranial nerve palsies, areflexia, meningism, and a variable degree of dementia are the leading clinical features.[2074] Malignant cells are found in the cerebrospinal fluid and there is marked meningeal enhancement on brain CT scans. See also **cerebral metastases**.[6663]

carcinomatous myopathy A syndrome of monomyositis multiplex with the chief complaint of pain of sudden onset of a few days duration as a result of infarction, possibly from nonbacterial thrombotic endocarditis,[2834] or of direct carcinomatous emboli to the proximal muscles.[1696] Generalized muscle atrophy (**cachexia**) in association with systemic carcinoma and acute myonecrosis complicating distant carcinoma[6452] are further syndromes under this heading.

carcinomatous neuromyopathy Syndromes of proximal and axial weakness, usually neurogenic in origin. They are most often considered to be the result of an autoimmune attack but may also be associated with the treatment for an underlying carcinoma with, for example, steroids. See **paraneoplastic syndromes**.

carcinomatous neuropathy See **paraneoplastic syndromes**.

carcinomatous sensory neuropathy/radiculopathy A **paraneoplastic syndrome** of dorsal root ganglionitis and neuronal degeneration presenting subacutely with isolated sensory loss, usually in association with oat-cell carcinoma of the lung.[1585] See **paraneoplastic sensory neuropathy**.

cardiac cephalalgia Headache occurring in association with acute myocardial ischemia. Diagnostic criteria suggested in the ICHD[2820] require that the headache, which may be severe, occurs in the context of acute myocardial ischemia, is aggravated by exertion, and is accompanied by nausea; also that the headache resolves and does not recur after effective medical therapy for myocardial ischemia.

cardiac encephalopathy 1. Altered alertness with cognitive and behavioral changes seen particularly in patients in congestive heart failure. 2. Apathy and abulia with retained alertness resulting from fluid retention in the cranial cavity in patients with congestive heart failure or other conditions leading to substantial fluid retention.[1014]

cardiac syncope Syncope due to diminished cardiac output as a result of dysrhythmia or outflow obstruction.

cardinal points reflex Deviation of the lip and the tongue to the point where a baby's lip is touched by the examiner's finger. Further movements of the finger up toward the nose or down to the chin lead to extension and to flexion of the neck, respectively.

cardinal positions of gaze The nine classic points to which gaze may be directed. They are up-left, up-center, up-right; left, center, and right in the horizontal plane; and down-left, down-center, and down-right.

cardioembolic stroke See **cardiogenic embolism**.

cardio-facial syndrome (asymmetrical crying facies) A dominant congenital syndrome (22q11.2) of unilateral weakness of the depressor muscles of the lower lip with variable severity accompanied by atrial or ventricular septal defect, mild myopathy with raised serum CK, and variation in fiber size on muscle biopsy. Cervical vertebral fusion, adducted thumbs, facial dysmorphisms, microcephaly, thymic hypoplasia, and mental retardation are sometimes found in association. The asymmetry only appears in infants when they cry. The sign itself is of small import, except that it may be a marker for other congenital anomalies, usually cardiac.[2504]

Although this is usually considered to represent damage to fibers of the VII nerve, the facts that the weakness is only of the lower quadrant and appears only with emotional movements, and that any other deficits are on the same side of the body as the facial weakness, all suggest that the original lesion is cerebral.

cardiogenic dementia Impairment in cognitive function occurring in patients with cardiac dysrhythmia and resulting relative hypotension and impairment of cerebral perfusion.[3681]

cardiogenic embolism (cardioembolic stroke) Emboli arising from the heart and proceeding to the cerebral circulation. They are considered to account for cerebral ischemic infarction in 15% of cases of stroke.

The cardiac pathologies responsible and the therapeutic methods have been reviewed and the clinical features suggesting embolism listed[1069] Diagnostic criteria have also been suggested.[2329, 4381] (Reproduced by kind permission of the American Academy of Neurology and Lippincott Williams and Wilkins.) (See Charts C–2 to C–5.) A problem in diagnosis is that emboli are often dispatched when the heart rhythm reverts to normal after a period of fibrillation. [JF]

cardio-inhibitory syncope Fainting due to extreme bradycardia resulting from excessive vagal stimulation of the heart. The effect is clinically demonstrable by increasing vagal cardiac activity by placing pressure on the eyeball—the *oculo-cardiac reflex*. See **cardiac syncope**.

Chart C–2. Clinical Features of Cerebral Embolism

1. Abrupt onset of maximal deficit
2. Presence of a potentially embolic source
3. Multiple brain infarcts involving the cortex or cerebellum in multiple vascular territories
4. Hemorrhagic infarct shown by computed tomography
5. Absence of atherosclerotic arterial disease by angiography
6. Angiographic evidence of vanishing occlusions
7. Evidence of embolism to other organs
8. Cardiac thrombi demonstrated by various imaging techniques

Chart C–3. Diagnostic Criteria for Cardiogenic Cerebral Embolism

Definite Cardioembolic Stroke

All of the following;

1. No antecedent TIAs in the same vascular distribution within 2 weeks of stroke onset.
2. Maximal neurologic deficit at stroke onset.
3. CT or MRI evidence of lesion $\geq$2 cm or involving cortex or symptoms suggesting cortical involvement.
4. Arterial imaging showing no evidence of significant occlusive disease. (Greater than or equal to 50% linear stenosis in proximal large vessel supply.)

Probable Cardioembolic Stroke

One of the following;

1. At least two of 1, 2, 3, above, no lacunar syndrome present, *and* arterial imaging required with no evidence of significant occlusive disease.
2. Vertebrobasilar distribution *and* 1, 2, 3, above all true *and* no arterial imaging.

Adapted from Miller et al. (1993).[4381] Reproduced by kind permission of the American Academy of Neurology and Lippincott Williams and Wilkins.

cardioskeletal myopathy with intrasarcoplasmic-dense granulofilamentous material See **myofibrillar myopathy**.

cardiovascular autonomic reflex testing Studies of pulse rate or blood pressure with deep breathing, Valsalva maneuver or tilting. See **autonomic function tests**.

Chart C–4. Diagnostic Criteria for Cerebral Embolism (2)

***Criteria for the Diagnosis of Cardiac-Originating Embolism*:**

Presence of any *one* of the following:
1. Mitral stenosis
2. Prosthetic valve
3. Endocarditis
4. Myocardial infarction within 6 weeks of qualifying stroke
5. Myocardial aneurysm
6. Intracardiac clot or mass
7. Mitral valve prolapse, age under 45, in the absence of a reasonable alternative explanation for the qualifying stroke

Or, the presence of any *two* of the following:
1. Atrial fibrillation (chronic or paroxysmal)
2. Sick sinus syndrome
3. Recent involvement of more than one vascular territory
4. Seizure at onset
5. Hemorrhagic infarct
6. Cerebral artery branch occlusion(s) without overt evidence of extracranial or cavernous sinus carotid disease on arteriography.

Adapted from Gent M, Blakeley J, Easton JD, et al. Canadian–American Ticlopidine study; thromboembolic stroke. Stroke *1988;19:1203–10. Reproduced by permission.*

cardio-vocal syndrome See **Ortner syndrome**.

Care4Dystonia, Inc. A charitable organization. Web site: www.care4dystonia.org/.

CARE Acronym for the Comprehensive Assessment and Referral Evaluation, a long, semistructured instrument which covers psychiatric symptoms, physical symptoms, and performance in the activities of daily living, and requests information about nutrition and economic matters. A short form is available.[2644] The tool has been widely used in the assessment of elderly people who might need referral to health or social services.[2645]

Caregiver Questionnaire An instrument to measure the quality of life in children with cerebral palsy.[5625]

Carney complex (Swiss syndrome) A dominantly inherited disorder characterized by mesenchymal and peripheral nerve tumors, skin pigmentation, and endocrine overactivity.[1774] See **familial Cushing syndrome**.

Carey–Fineman–Ziter Syndrome A recessively inherited congenital syndrome characterized by nonprogressive myopathy with hypotonia and muscle hypoplasia, features of **Möbius syndrome**, facial weakness, dysphagia leading to feeding disorders, microcephaly, facial and skeletal dysmorphisms, and developmental delay. Muscle biopsy shows fiber size variation and type II fiber predominance.

carnitine A small water-soluble molecule, both synthesized in the liver and ingested, which is stored in skeletal and cardiac muscle, where it plays an important role in the transport of the coenzyme A–fatty acid complex across the mitochondrial membrane, and thus in energy availability. It is also concerned in the buffering of organic acids.

carnitine deficiency A diffuse disorder, of which two major forms have been defined: muscular and systemic.[1657]

Type I lipid storage myopathy (myopathic carnitine deficiency) A recessively inherited lipid storage vacuolar myopathy leading to fluctuating but progressive proximal muscle weakness and kyphoscoliosis. Lipid excess is confined to muscle and low levels of carnitine are found in type I muscle fibers[1371] but not in the serum. In some cases, oral L-carnitine ingestion reverses the signs of the disease,[1868] which has resulted from a deficit in the carnitine-acylcarnitine carrier system.

Type II lipid storage myopathy (systemic carnitine deficiency) A recessively inherited syndrome with onset in infancy or childhood, leading to episodic attacks of metabolic acidosis and hypoglycemia causing encephalopathy, and to slowly progressive proximal weakness with lipid storage in muscles, cardiomyopathy, and low carnitine levels in liver, heart, and muscle. The affected infants may present with features resembling **Reye syndrome** with nausea, vomiting, liver failure, encephalopathy, and lipid storage myopathy.[1657, 3312]

In a *variant form, dominant lipid myopathy with normal carnitine*, lifelong weakness, and fat intolerance are associated with lipid storage in type I muscle fibers and with type II muscle fiber atrophy.[275]

Low carnitine levels are found secondarily in patients with cirrhosis or schistosomiasis, in those on dialysis, and in those with chronic renal failure not on dialysis, as well as in people receiving total parenteral nutrition or suffering from Fanconi syndrome, **mitochondrial myopathies**, organic acidemias, or muscular dystrophy. The cardiomyopathy of dialysis is due to carnitine deficiency. See also **lipid myopathies**.

Carnitine Palmitoyltransferase Deficiency A newsletter for health care professionals and patients interested in CPT deficiency.

carnitine palmityl transferase deficiency An autosomal or X-linked recessively inherited lipid storage myopathy due to deficiency of this enzyme, which is normally involved in fatty acid metabolism in muscles.

Clinically, it presents in infancy as a generalized lethal disease with severe cardiomyopathy; or in childhood, youth, or adult life with exercise intolerance, muscle pain and cramp, recurrent myoglobinuria with nephropathy, and chronic myopathic girdle weakness[1648, 3032] following prolonged exertion, fasting, or cold.[907] Fat intolerance and raised serum triglyceride levels are usually detected.[1039] During fasting, serum creatine kinase levels remain low and ketogenesis is normal. Deficiency of the enzyme may be associated with susceptibility to **malignant hyperthermia**. The genetic mutation in CPT_2 is on chromosome 1. In *variant forms*:

- CPT_2 is deficient in skeletal muscle and leukocytes but the CPT_1 level is normal.[5633]
- A lipid myopathy is associated with reduced exercise capacity, intolerance to fasting, and reduced concentration of carnitine in muscle and serum, but with normal CPTase activity. The possibility of flavoprotein deficiency is adduced.[1040]
- Myoglobinuria and weakness occur, progressing even to acute respiratory failure following an infection (*adult* form).[595]
- Carnitine deficiency is induced by repeated *hemodialysis*.[446]
- Carnitine deficiency accompanies a riboflavine-responsive **lipid myopathy**.[1040]

carnosinase deficiency See **carnosinemia**.

carnosine A neuropeptide substance.

carnosinemia (carnosinase deficiency) A congenital, recessively inherited neurodegenerative syndrome characterized by kyphoscoliosis, aminoaciduria, arachnodactyly, and cerebral atrophy with myoclonic and generalized tonic-clonic seizures, pyramidal and extrapyramidal signs, and severe progressive psychomotor retardation[4991] in the presence of high plasma levels of carnosine.

carotico-cavernous fistula (Foix–Jefferson syndrome) Rupture of an aneurysm of the intracavernous internal carotid artery creating an arteriovenous anastomosis, arterial blood thus flowing into the sinus. Local pain, an ocular bruit (often audible to the patient), visual loss, and diplopia are the usual symptoms, and retinal congestion and pulsatile exophthalmos with variable lesions of the III, IV, ophthalmic V, and VI cranial nerves are characteristic signs.[40]

carotid (from Gr, to cast into a deep sleep, to throttle) The arteries of the neck were so called because it was known in ancient times that animals became sleepy when these vessels were compressed, a fact well known to professional wrestlers today.

carotid angioplasty headache Any new acute headache developing within a week after extra- or intracranial angioplasty has been performed and resolving in a month.[2820]

carotid artery syndrome 1. (ocular ischemic syndrome) Transient or permanent painless visual loss, lachrymation, visual field losses due to retinal ischemia, vascular retinopathy, and transient ischemic attacks, due to reduced flow within, or emboli from, the homolateral carotid artery. See **ocular ischemic syndrome**. 2. See **red-eyed shunt syndrome**.

carotid body A chromaffin-containing chemoreceptor situated at the bifurcation of the common carotid artery.

carotid body tumor (ganglion nodosum tumor) A chromaffinoma (chemodectoma) which infiltrates the region of the jugular foramen and leads to complaints of pulsatile tinnitus, hoarseness, and dysarthria due to dysfunction of cranial nerves VII, IX, and X and local pain. Compression of the carotid sinus may also occur, leading to bradycardia and syncope. The first pathological account was given in 1891 by Felix Marchand (1846–1928), a German pathologist.

carotid-cavernous fistula (dural carotid-cavernous fistula) A rare syndrome caused by abnormal communications between meningeal branches of the internal external carotid artery and the cavernous sinus. It is most commonly seen in post-menopausal women and may present with proptosis, ophthalmoplegia, visual impairment, or intracranial hemorrhage.[6265]

carotid compression test (Matas Test) Digital massage of the carotid sinuses, and then compression of the two carotid arteries in turn during electroencephalography, with the patient's head facing forward or turned to the left or right, in an attempt to assess the adequacy of blood flow in the carotid and vertebral systems as judged by the clinical or EEG changes induced.

The method is now seldom employed; hypotension, cardiac asystole, displacement of atheromatous debris, and ischemic stroke are potential hazards; a vague idea of arterial patency the questionable reward.

carotid hypoplasia See **familial hypoplasia of the carotid arteries**.

carotid sinus A dilation of the proximal portion of the internal carotid artery, containing baroreceptors which send information on blood pressure via the IX nerve to the medulla.

carotid sinus hypersensitivity (carotid sinus syncope/syndrome, CSS, Charcot–Weiss–Baker syndrome[1099]) Syncope, confusion, faintness, or seizures resulting from decreased cerebral perfusion due to extreme bradycardia or asystole in response to excessive afferent input from the carotid sinus, usually in older patients with atheroma, in whom it may lead to significant morbidity related to trauma suffered during falls. In the clinic, manual massage of the carotid sinus is the required diagnostic maneuver.

The *cardioinhibitory* form is diagnosed when stimulation of the carotid sinuses leads to 3 s of cardiac asystole or atrioventricular block; the less common *depressor* type is said to occur when a drop in blood pressure of 50 mmHg results. Slowing of the pulse by 30 bpm or a fall in blood pressure of 30 mmHg characterizes borderline states.[5592] The syndrome was first described in 1933 by Soma Weiss (1898–1942) and James P. Baker, two American physicians.[5619]

The central mechanisms involved in CSS may be similar to those that result in neurocardiogenic syncope. Tilt testing may be helpful in diagnosis and SSRIs in treatment.[1436]

carotid sinus reflex Bradycardia resulting from increased pressure within the carotid sinuses; a parasympathetic response on both the afferent and efferent sides.[6350] Either an increase in blood pressure or manipulation of the sinus by pressure from without will normally induce slowing of the heart rate.

The reflex is mediated by the IX and X cranial nerves; it was first described by Torald Sollamn (b. 1874), an American pharmacologist, but his description was elaborated upon by Heinrich Hering (1866–1948), a German physiologist, in 1923. See also **carotid sinus hypersensitivity**.

carotid sinus syncope/ syndrome See **carotid sinus hypersensitivity**.

carotid tubercle The mass on the anterior aspect of the transverse processes of the sixth cervical vertebra, in front of which lies the carotid artery.

carotidynia (facial migraine, atypical facial neuralgia, Hilger syndrome) A dull, intermittent, aching pain in the neck and in the lower half of the face, sometimes with a throbbing component, with tenderness of the carotid artery. The condition is thought to arise from the adventitial coat of the common carotid artery, either as a form of migraine or as a result of subclinical carotid artery dissection, but superior laryngeal neuralgia has been suggested as another possible cause,[4738] and the nonspecificity of the pathologies causing transient unilateral neck pain has led to a suggestion that the whole condition could be expunged from medical nosology.[650] The condition was initially described in 1927, but more fully by Dr. J.A. Hilger.[2901]

carpal tunnel syndrome A common entity in which affected subjects (who are usually female) complain of paresthesias, numbness, and pain in the hands, especially on waking and following repetitive manual tasks. The cause is compression of the median nerve beneath the transverse carpal ligament at the wrist, the cure surgical decompression. The original description by Putnam[5144] seems to have been ignored until the syndrome was rediscovered by **Phalen** at the Cleveland Clinic and by Lord **Brain** in London, UK, in 1946. See also **Phalen sign, Tinel sign** and **flick sign**.

Diagnostic guidelines have been suggested by the American Academy of Neurology.[21] (See Chart C–5.) These also list differential diagnostic possibilities, confirmatory studies, further diagnostic tests, and treatment.[21]

Familial carpal tunnel syndrome is an occasional *variant*, with its usual onset in adult life.[1447]

The median-thenar to ulnar thenar latency difference (TTLD) and the median-thenar to ulnar-hypothenar latency difference (THLD) may be the most sensitive electrodiagnostic tests in this condition. The abnormal cutoffs are TTLD, 0.8 ms; THLD, 1.2 ms.

In *severe carpal tunnel syndrome* the subject has evidence of denervation of the thenar muscles as well as the signs listed above.

Chart C–5. Diagnostic Guidelines for Carpal Tunnel Syndrome

1. *History:* The likelihood of CTS increases with the number of standard symptoms and provocative factors listed:
   - Dull aching discomfort in the hand, forearm, or upper arm
   - Paresthesias in the hand
   - Weakness or clumsiness of the hand
   - Dry skin, swelling, or color changes in the hand
   - Occurrence of any of these symptoms within the median distribution

   Provocative factors include sleep, sustained hand and/or arm positions, and repetitive actions of the hand or wrist.

   Mitigating factors include changes in hand posture and shaking the hand
2. *Physical examination*:
   - May be normal
   - Symptoms elicited by tapping or direct pressure over the median nerve at the wrist (**Tinel sign**) or with forced extension or flexion of the wrist (**Phalen sign**)
   - Sensory loss in the median nerve distribution
   - Weakness or atrophy of the thenar muscles
   - Dry skin on digits 1–3 (a rare complaint)

Adapted from the American Academy of Neurology Quality Standards Committee. Practice Parameters; Carpal Tunnel Syndrome *(1993) and reproduced by kind permission of the American Academy of Neurology and Lippincott Williams and Wilkins.*

Carpenter syndrome

(acrocephalopolysyndactyly) A rare recessively inherited disorder characterized by premature fusion of all the cranial sutures, which leads to **acrocephaly** and **brachycephaly**. Facial dysmorphism, corneal opacities, mental retardation, obesity, syndactyly, pes cavus, polydactyly, congenital cardiac anomalies, and aminoaciduria are also described.[1029] See also **acrocallosal syndrome** and **acrocephalosyndactyly**.

carphology (Gr, chaff + to collect) Picking at the bedclothes, once thought characteristic of typhoidal delirium but in fact a nonspecific sign both of delirium and dementia.

carpometacarpal reflex (carpophalangeal reflex, von Bechterew reflex) Flexion of the fingers in response to a tap on the back of the wrist when the arm is extended; a sign with the same significance as the **finger flexion reflex**, of which it is a *variant*.

carpopedal spasm Cupping of the palm of the hand with extension of the fingers and adduction of the thumb as a result of spasm of the intrinsic hand muscles in **tetany**. It is typically due to abnormal calcium control of sodium channels leading to axonal hyperexcitability, as in hypomagnesemia, hypoparathyroidism, and respiratory alkalosis normocalcemic tetany. All forms are worsened by alkalosis resulting from hyperventilation and by ischemia. A dominantly inherited form is described. Electromyographically, there are spontaneous repetitive discharges at up to 300 Hz arising in peripheral axons.

carpophalangeal reflex See **carpometacarpal reflex**.

carpus (Gr, the wrist) Pertaining to the wrist.

Carraro syndrome A recessively inherited syndrome characterized by the absence of the tibias and by nerve deafness.[1036]

Carrión disease See **Oroya fever**.

carus (Gr, heavy sleep) An ancient term for deep sleep or coma and also for loss of sensation and voluntary movement.

Casal, Gaspar (1679–1759) Spanish physician who wrote the first definitive account of the features of **pellagra**, including the pigmentation of the upper chest wall, sometimes known as the *Casal necklace*.

CASM See **cerebellar syndromes** (congenital ataxias).

Casserio, Giulio See **Gasser, Johann Lorenz**.

Castro-Gago syndrome

(microcephaly–albinism–limb defects) A congenital dysmorphic syndrome characterized by generalized depigmentation of the hair and skin, acral defects such as hypoplastic phalanges and absent or hypoplastic hallux, microcephaly, and mental and developmental delay.[381]

cat-box effect A familiar name applied by H.H. Jasper to the activation of the cat's EEG through increased activity of the reticular activating system, brought on by the desire of the cat to urinate.

cat cry syndrome See **cri-du-chat syndrome**.

cat eye syndrome (coloboma–anal atresia syndrome) A chromosomal disorder characterized by colobomas of the iris and choroid, facial dysmorphisms, urogenital anomalies, congenital cardiac defects, and mental and developmental delay. In many cases, trisomy 22 is present.[3279]

CAT scan See **computerized axial tomography**.

cat scratch encephalitis An acute nonfatal febrile illness with encephalopathy (or myelopathy or radiculopathy) due to *Bartonella henselae*, distinguished by normalcy of the CSF. Seizures and a variety of neurological signs occur with an acute febrile illness and meningism. It complicates *cat scratch disease*, a benign and self-limited disorder manifested usually in children by a skin rash, local lymphadenopathy, and fever.[3818, 3979, 5068, 5699]

CAT syndrome A congenital dysmorphic syndrome also characterized by skeletal anomalies affecting the skull, spine, facial and limb bones and teeth, sparse fine hair, muscle atrophy, metaphyseal dysplasia, ichthyosis, and mental and developmental delay.[381]

cataclysmic migraine An unusual vascular episode in the territory of the posterior cerebral artery, in which headache, visual symptoms, sensory and motor deficits, and signs of involvement of the III cranial nerve develop suddenly, clearing but leaving permanent neurological sequelae such as a hemianopias. The syndrome is commoner in females, especially those below the age of 40 years.[2094] See **posterior cerebral artery syndrome, Call-Fleming syndrome.**

catalentia Paracelsus' term for **epilepsy**.

catalepsy (from Gr, a seizure) Increase in muscle tone, leading to the assumption of fixed postures which can be held for long periods without fatigue or other voluntary movement. It is usually associated with psychiatric disease (including schizophrenia and hysteria) or epilepsy. The term has also been used in quite the opposite sense for the astatic, falling attacks in **narcolepsy**.

catalepsy of awakening See **sleep paralysis**.

cataleptic hallucinatory fear syndrome See **Rosenthal syndrome**.

catamenial seizures Those occurring principally or exclusively during any one phase of the menstrual cycle.

cataphasia (Gr, an affirmative proposition) Spontaneous or evoked repetition of the same word or phrase.

cataphora (Gr, to fall down) An ancient alternative term for deep sleep or coma.

cataplexy (Gr, to strike down) A rapid eye movement sleep disorder triggered by events which stir the emotions and consisting of the sudden, episodic, reversible, generalized, or localized loss of muscle power and areflexia, without any alteration of consciousness and with abrupt return to normalcy after a few seconds. It is considered to represent a dissociation of awareness and behavior.

The clinical manifestations range between a sagging of the jaw, with flexion of the neck and knees, up to sudden powerlessness of abrupt onset lasting between seconds and half an hour. If the attack lasts more than a minute, a dreamlike state supervenes.[2626] The sphincters are not affected but other features of the narcoleptic tetrad are often present. The episodes may occur unprovoked or as a reaction to an emotional stimulus, tiredness, or a heavy meal. Unilateral cataplexy is also described but is extremely rare.

The term was known to Hippocrates, to whom it denoted any sudden illness but in its modern form was first applied by Henneberg in 1916. See also **narcolepsy** and the AASM Diagnostic Classification.[1629]

In *status cataplecticus*, hundreds of partial cataplectic attacks each day, at a rate of one every few seconds, associated with a peculiar variation of posture and tone. The gait has been described as resembling a puppet on strings, with periods of sagging of the face, limp arms, and buckling knees (limp man syndrome). Various brainstem pathologies have been regarded as causal.[5848]

cataptosis (from Gr, to fall down) A term of Galen for epilepsy, apoplexy, or sudden paralysis.

cataract–sensorineural deafness syndrome A dominantly inherited syndrome in which the deafness is progressive.[4571]

cataract–spasticity–mental retardation syndrome (Martsolf syndrome) A recessively inherited congenital dysmorphic syndrome characterized by cataract, ataxia, spasticity, and mental and developmental delay.[4128]

cataracts–renal tubular necrosis–encephalopathy See **Crome syndrome**.

catastrophic migraine See **cataclysmic migraine, posterior cerebral artery syndrome.**[2096]

catastrophic reaction A brief emotional outburst, the behavioral response of a brain-injured or demented subject to frustration, sorrow, or anger because of inability to cope in the performance of a task. The reaction is characterized by acute anxiety, agitation, and tearfulness, cessation of meaningful or cooperative activity, and sometimes uncontrolled hostility. It is associated especially with nonfluent aphasias and with left opercular lesions, and likely results from disturbances in frontotemporal-limbic-basal ganglion circuitry.[1026]

Catastrophic Reaction Scale An 11-item instrument quantitating the severity of this reaction during the clinical interview.[6021]

cathernia (from Gr, like a groan) A parasomnia characterized by monotonous irregular groans occurring during both NREM and especially REM sleep, alternating with normal breathing. There appear to be no long-term clinical consequences. Patients are unaware, but typically bed-partners are alarmed by the frequent nocturnal noise.[6539] The patients have neither respiratory distress or an anguished expression during the groaning, nor are there any abnormal motor behaviors nor any recall of vivid dreams.

catatonia (from Gr, stretching tight, depressed)[5886] A psychiatric and motor disturbance characterized by the presence of at least one motor sign (catalepsy, posturing, or waxy flexibility of the limbs) in combination with at least one sign of psychosocial withdrawal or excitement and/or bizarre repetitive movements (mutism, negativism, grimacing, impulsiveness, stereotypes, mannerisms, command automatism, echopraxia/echolalia, or verbigeration). The EEG shows low-voltage fast activity.

Other definitions suggest unresponsiveness to the environment with the appearance of consciousness (eyes open but unblinking, oculocephalic responses impaired but caloric responses intact).

The condition was first described by **Kahlbaum** in 1868 and is most commonly associated with affective illnesses and schizophrenia but also occurs in a wide range of metabolic, systemic, toxic, and organic cerebral diseases.[1548]

catch-up saccades (back-up saccades) Brief, small corrective saccades which augment the velocity of pursuit movements in order that they shall match that of the moving visual target. When the velocity of the pursuit movements is too high, *back-up saccades* exert a braking function with the same purpose. See **gain of pursuit eye movements**.

category fluency test A test of language in which the subject is asked to generate the names of as many different kinds of fruit, vegetables, or animals as he can in 1 min. See also **letter fluency test**.

category test (of Halstead) A sensitive test of abstract reasoning, concept formation, and organizational ability wherein the subject is required to discern similarities and differences between, and to sort and classify, colored shapes on changing bases of reference.

category specific anomia See **anomia**.

category-specific dysphasia The selective preservation or impairment of specific semantic categories among patients with aphasia; these include specific deficits in comprehension of the names of body parts or of colors or inanimate objects.

cathode The negative pole of a galvanic battery.

cathodic (Gr, downward + a way) Proceeding downward, as in the case of the efferent nerve impulse.

cation An electrically charged body which seeks the negative pole in an electrical field.

Catlin mark (fenestra parietalia symmetricae, foramina parietalia permagna) A familial anomaly consisting of bilateral defects in the parietal bones, first described by Lancisi in 1707. Clinically, the subjects are themselves aware of the defects, but headaches and seizures have only been associated loosely.[3462]

catochus (Gr, from + to detain) An ancient term for **catalepsy** and for **persistent vegetative state**.

Caton, Richard (1842–1926) Scottish physician, whose physiological researches led to the first (1874) description of the electrical potential changes in the brain, described while he was a lecturer at Liverpool, where he later became professor of physiology.[5978] His work was not recognized until **Berger** referred to it in his seminal paper in 1929.

cattle-trucking Retinal arteriolar stasis; the breaking up of the columns of blood in the retinal arterioles, seen after death. The sign is sometimes dignified by the names of Salsbury and Melvin.

Caucasian A term first used in 1776 by Blumenbach to define the white-skinned races and currently still employed by those who do not know that the term *Europoid* is anthropologically more correct.

cauda equina (Lat, a tail + of a horse) The nerve roots of the lumbar and sacral segments which, on leaving the cord within the dural sac, stream downward with something like the appearance of a horse's tail.

cauda equina syndrome Weakness, reflex change, pain and sensory disturbances in the territory of any of the roots forming the cauda equina (L2, -3, -4, -5, and S1), but often sparing the conus medullaris and thus bladder and bowel sphincter function and the motor and sensory functions of S2, -3, -4 (**sacral sparing**).

Clinically, the motor weakness is variable and asymmetrical but typically there is weakness of external rotation and extension of the thigh at the hip, of knee flexion, and of all muscles below the knee. Erectile dysfunction may occur in males. The sensory losses are also variable, but assymmetric perineal and saddle sensory loss with loss of erotic genital sensation is typical. Distally referred pain or dysesthesia and radicular pain may be present (cf. **conus medullaris syndrome**). Urinary and rectal incontinence and retention are both described.

Compression by an intra- or extradural mass is the most common cause, but it may occur with any form of spinal injury below the terminus of the spinal cord at the L1–L2 disk space. So-called intermittent claudication of the cord[3344] is a *variant* due to **lumbar spinal stenosis**.

It must be noted that lesions seldom affect the nervous system in this nicely classified manner, so that the features of both of these syndromes often occur together.[5440] See also **conus medullaris syndrome**.

caudal Toward the tail; posterior.

caudal dysplasia syndrome See **caudal regression syndrome**.

caudal paramedian midbrain syndrome A rare brainstem syndrome manifesting bilateral cerebellar dysfunction with dysarthria, ataxia of the trunk and gait, and dysmetric movements of the limbs, worse on one side. Some ocular movement abnormalities may be seen. Although the MRI shows bilateral inferior olivary degeneration, palatal tremor is uncommon. The lesion presumably involves the decussation of the superior cerebellar peduncles.[4519]

caudal regression syndrome (caudal dysplasia syndrome, sacral agenesis, mermaid syndrome) A congenital developmental disorder characterized by spinal dysraphism, complete or partial absence (aplasia) of the bony structures of the lower spine (sacrum and coccyx), anal anomalies, aplasia of the lumber facets, and usually visceral anomalies, incontinence, and a neurogenic bladder depending on the extent of involvement of the lumbosacral cord and roots.[1746, 5551, 6712]

The cause of the syndrome is unknown but maternal diabetes is a common association, while in other cases autosomal dominant inheritance has been recorded.

caudate (Lat, equipped with a tail) A nucleus within the basal ganglion complex, its long "tail" curving around in a C-shape.

cauloplegia (Gr, stem + a stroke) Paralysis of the penis.[5103] Presumably this means impotence.

causalgia (Gr, burning heat) (reflex dystrophy, shoulder-hand syndrome, mimoausalgia, algodystrophy, neurodynia, traumatic neuralgia, post-traumatic pain syndrome, reflex sympathetic dystrophy, sympathalgia, Sudeck atrophy, minor causalgia, sympathalgia, deafferentation pain) A syndrome of severe, persistent burning pain, felt commonly in the distribution of a nerve at any time following partial damage to that nerve (especially the proximal median, ulnar or sciatic), but also felt in more distant regions, occurring in patients with nontraumatic nerve lesions or a phantom limb; and accompanied by sudomotor and vasomotor changes and eventually secondary atrophy of skin, joints, muscle, and bone in the affected region.[5643] Abnormal discharges in sympathetic efferents, sensitization of peripheral receptors, or ephaptic transmission between sympathetic and nociceptive afferent fibers has been incriminated in causation; sensitization of spinal cord nociceptive neurons is a likely central mechanism.

Typically, the subject cannot bear anything to touch the affected areas, and heat, movement, and emotion worsen it, although local cooling or block of the sympathetic fibers at a proximal level may provide relief. Tremor, dystonias, and chorea occur in a few cases. The syndrome also occurs sometimes with diseases of the CNS such as stroke, myelopathy, cervical osteoarthritis, and multiple sclerosis, with immobility after myocardial infarction, following frostbite and burns and with phenobarbital ingestion.

Stages have been defined: the acute stage of pain, hyperpathia, and allodynia last weeks after injury and is succeeded by the dystrophic stage after about 3 months. The pain now radiates more widely, joints swell, muscles atrophy, and osteoporosis can be shown. The atrophic stage is the end-stage of the condition, in which there are irreversible trophic changes in the skin and underlying structures, with joint contractures.

Weir **Mitchell**, as a result of his Civil War experiences, saw this condition frequently and applied the term to such a severe, persistent, and burning pain following nerve injury,[4402] although the first modern account of all was that of Denmark,[1579] whose patient had been injured in the Peninsular War. The term is probably best reserved for the combination of burning pain and autonomic disturbances occurring in the circumstances he described (nerve injury), the syndrome similar in whole or part (or when arising in other contexts) being termed **reflex sympathetic dystrophy**. See also **deafferentation pain** and **complex regional pain syndrome**.

causalgia–dystonia A psychogenic disorder characterized by fixed spasms resembling contractures, with rapid onset, severe pain and vasomotor, sudomotor, and trophic changes. There is no benefit from sleep, the *geste antagoniste* is not seen, and there is no response to botulinus toxin injections.[608]

cautious gait (elderly gait, senile gait) A gait disorder characterized by a normal to mildly widened base, short and slow stride, and *en bloc* turns. There are no shuffling, freezing nor hesitancies in initiating gait. Cadence and foot clearance of the support surface are normal. There is mild disequilibrium as judged by the response to a push and the difficulty in balancing on one foot.

Most patients with this gait pattern are aware of impaired balance and express the need for caution to avoid falls. Other neurological symptoms and signs are generally mild and do not form a consistent picture. The pattern is associated with musculoskeletal lesions in the peripheral or central nervous systems.[4723] (Reproduced [modified] by kind permission of the American Academy of Neurology and Lippincott Williams and Wilkins.)

cava septi pellucidi et vergae (fifth ventricle, ventricle of Arantius, pseudocele) Cavities within the septum pellucidum, developing at the site of fusion of the two cerebral hemispheres as a secondary cleavage with necrobiosis as the fibers of the corpus callosum cross the midline.

The cavities (vergae being the posterior of the two and closing first) are normally present during prenatal life but are obliterated in most people within weeks of birth. Although they may rarely enlarge to obliterate the foramina of Monro, thus producing hydrocephalus, in an overwhelming majority of cases they have no clinical effects at all.[5769] Their presence was first recorded by Julius Caesar Arantius (1530–1589), an Italian physician, in 1571.[5619]

Cavanagh variant See **hereditary spastic paraparesis**.

caveolin-3 A muscle-specific transmembrane protein, mutations of which are responsible for **rippling muscle disease**. Caveolin-3 protein deficiency is a sensitive and specific marker for primary caveolinopathy.

caveolinopathies Mutations in the caveolin-3 gene (*CAV-3*) causing **limb girdle muscular dystrophy** type IC and other muscle diseases. Caveolinopathies may represent 1% of both unclassified LGMD and other phenotypes or with asymptomatic elevation of blood levels of creatine kinase, myalgias, rippling muscle disease, or distal myopathy.[3454]

cavernoma See **cavernous angioma**.

cavernous angioma (hemangioma, cavernoma) Benign vascular malformations consisting of masses of abnormally dilated and undifferentiated sinusoidal vascular channels with no direct arteriovenous communication, lined by a single layer of endothelium and packed together with little or no neural tissue between.[6, 4467] They also occur in the skin and liver.

When dominantly inherited, cavernous angiomas are often multiple, occurring mainly in the cerebral hemispheres, less often in the pons and spinal cord. Seizures and the effects of hemorrhage are the usual neurological presentations. They are seldom visualized on arteriograms because of the slow flow of the blood within them, but they are well shown on CT and MRI scans. Clinically, they are characterized by either the lack of symptoms, or by seizures, headaches, or focal neurological signs, which may result from intracerebral hemorrhage. On T2-weighted MRI scans they show as tiny hypodense areas, or as larger areas of mixed signal intensity with a low intensity rim, due to the deposition of hemosiderin.[5270] A responsible gene (CCM1) has been mapped to chromosome 7q11–q22. See also **arteriovenous malformation** and **angioma**.

cavernous sinus A plexus of small veins within a split in the dural sac beside the pituitary, through which pass the internal carotid artery and cranial nerves III, IV, V (ophthalmic division), and VI.

cavernous sinus syndrome Painful dysfunction of cranial nerves III, IV, and VI, of the first (and occasionally second) division of the V nerve, and in some cases of the sympathetic fibers, due to a lesion within the cavernous sinus.

The syndrome was described by Foix in 1922[2136] and by Jefferson in 1938.[3180] See **superior orbital fissure syndrome**.

cavernous sinus–lateral wall syndrome See **superior orbital fissure syndrome**.

cavernous sinus–nasopharyngeal tumor syndrome See **Godtfredsen syndrome**.

cavernous sinus syndrome of Raeder See **superior orbital fissure syndrome**.

cavernous sinus thrombosis Occlusion of the venous channels comprising the cavernous sinus.[1663] It was most often seen secondary to sepsis, especially mastoiditis, in the preantibiotic era, but today it is usually a complication of marantic conditions such as severe dehydration and in cachectic states associated with cancer.

Diagnostic criteria were suggested by Eagleton prior to the introduction of modern investigative procedures;[1795] and comprise

1. a known site of infection, or septicemia;
2. early destructive signs (such as full retinal veins, proptosis, exophthalmos, collateral venous circulation);
3. oculomotor pareses and trigeminal nerve involvement
4. neighborhood abscesses from the thrombophlebitis situated in the orbit, nasopharynx, occiput or neck, and
5. symptoms of complicating disease such as headache, papilledema, and meningeal signs.

cavitating sudanophilic leukodystrophy A group of demyelinating diseases occurring at any time of life and characterized clinically by developmental delay or dementia, tonic or clonic seizures, cerebellar and pyramidal signs, and cavitating changes in the CNS.[215] See **Canavan leukodystrophy**.

cavum (from Lat, a hollow) A cavity or space.

cavum septi pellucidi (Lat, a compartment or hole + a fence + transparent) (the "fifth ventricle") A cystic structure within the septum pellucidum, occurring as a developmental variant and declining in prevalence with age.[4010] This is a common incidental finding in normal subjects, but may also be associated with **holoproscencephaly**, optic nerve hypoplasia, or the following syndrome, and may be acquired as a result of cranial trauma or hydrocephalus,[4370] or itself act as a cause of obstructive hydrocephalus.

cavum vergae A congenital syndrome characterized by macrocephaly, posteriorly sited cavum septi pellucidi, and mental/developmental delay.[4370]

Cawthorne–Cooksey exercises A regimen of physical therapy exercises for the eyes and body designed to diminish vertigo due to labyrinthine lesions. See also **Semont liberatory maneuver**.

cebocephaly (from Lat, a monkey + head) A form of frontal median clefting of the face, in which there is orbital hypotelorism with a single blind nostril, the nasal cavity correctly placed but with no septum nor columella.[379]

-cele (Gr, a tumor) Suffix denoting tumor.

celiac disease A malabsorption syndrome resulting from intolerance to dietary gluten. In around 10% of cases, neurological syndromes occur, such as peripheral neuropathy, progressive multifocal leukoencephalopathy, cerebellar ataxia, progressive myoclonic ataxia, myelopathy, dementia, or myopathy.[4968] Burning, tingling, and numbness in the hands and feet are typical presentations of cases with neuropathy. Nerve biopsy shows axonal loss.[1149] Antigliadin antibodies can be found in subjects with neurological dysfunction of unknown cause, particularly in sporadic cerebellar ataxia. See also **gluten ataxia**.

In a *variant form*, celiac disease is accompanied by migraine and cerebral calcifications in the occipital and parietal regions.[1405]

cellulalgia 1. Unusually severe pain felt with gentle compression (pinching) of the skin. This is a characteristic feature in patients with **myofascial pain syndromes** and with **cervicogenic headaches** and may represent referred hyperesthesia, although the underlying pathology is quite uncertain. 2. Thickened and tender skin in the territory of one dermatome, the root of which is irritated or compressed.[4029]

Celsus, Aurelius Cornelius (53 BC to AD 7) Roman gentleman and writer on medicine, probably not a doctor, even though occasionally described as physician to Caligula. He compiled Greek medical writings into a book *De Medicina* which flourished but was later lost, bursting forth again in 1478 as one of the first books to be made after the invention of printing and remaining a standard medical text for nearly 300 years at a time when "many men would not look at the new moon out of respect for the old." In it, Celsus described anesthetic leprosy, migraine, seizures, apoplexy, paralysis, hydrocephalus, spinal injury, and facial neuralgia. See also **Paracelsus**.

Center for Epidemiological Studies Depression Scale (CES-D) A self-report questionnaire found to be both reliable and valid as a screening tool to identify the presence of depressive symptoms. See Chart C–6. The interview is given by a nurse who shows the depression

Chart C–6. Center for Epidemiological Studies Depression Scale

Depression scale

0 Rarely or at no time (less than 1 day)
1 Some or a little of the time (1–2 days)
2 Occasionally or a moderate amount of time (3–4 days)
3 Most or all of the time (5–7 days)

Statements

1. I was bothered by things that usually don't bother me.
2. I did not feel like eating; my appetite was poor.
3. I felt that I could not shake off the blues even with help from my family or friends.
4. I felt that I was just as good as other people.
5. I had trouble keeping my mind on what I was doing.
6. I felt depressed (blue or down).
7. I felt that everything I did was an effort.
8. I felt hopeful about the future.
9. I thought my life had been a failure.
10. I felt fearful.
11. My sleep was restless.
12. I was happy.
13. I talked less than usual.
14. I felt lonely.
15. People were unfriendly.
16. I enjoyed life.
17. I had crying spells.
18. I felt sad.
19. I felt that people disliked me.
20. I could not get "going."

Adapted from Radloff LS. The CES-D scale. Appl Psychol Meas *1977;1:385–401 and reproduced by kind permission of Dr. David Weiss.*

scale response cards to the patient and asks him or her (for each item) to pick the card "which best describes how you felt or behaved this past week," recording the responses on a form.[5806, 5165]

Center for Inherited Disorders of Energy Metabolism (CIDEM)

A group of interdisciplinary, clinical diagnostic laboratories which focus on disorders of mitochondrial function, based at Case Western Reserve University.

Center for Narcolepsy

A university-based research institute. Web site: http://med.stanford.edu/school/Psychiatry/narcolepsy/index.html.

Centre for the Research and Rehabilitation of the Hereditary Ataxias www.ataxia.org/

The Web site of the National Ataxia Foundation, which is dedicated to improving the lives of persons affected by ataxia through support, education, and research.

central and peripheral demyelination

A syndrome comprising features of both **multiple sclerosis** and **chronic inflammatory demyelinating polyradiculoneuropathy.**[6288] See **chronic demyelinating neuropathy with multifocal CNS demyelination**.

central alveolar hypoventilation syndrome

A disorder characterized by ventilatory impairment resulting in arterial oxygen desaturation that is worsened by sleep, and occurring in patients with normal mechanical properties of the lung. Diagnostic criteria have been suggested:[1629] (See Chart C–7.)

See also www.sleepeducation.com/Disorders.aspx/ and congenital central hypoventilation syndrome.

Chart C–7. Central Alveolar Hypoventilation Syndrome

A. The patient can have a complaint of either insomnia or excessive sleepiness. The patient is usually unaware of the clinical features observed by others, such as hypoventilation during sleep.
B. Frequent episodes of shallow breathing during sleep.
C. The absence of primary lung disease, skeletal malformations, or peripheral neuromuscular disorder affecting ventilation.
D. Polysomnographic monitoring demonstrates:
   1. Episodes of shallow breathing greater than 10 s in duration associated with arterial oxygen desaturation, and one or more of the following:
   2. Frequent arousals from sleep associated with the breathing disturbances;
   3. Bradytachycardia; and
   4. A minimal sleep latency test that demonstrates mean sleep latency of less than 10 min.
E. The disorder can be associated with neurological disorders that affect the CNS control of breathing.
F. Other sleep disorders can be present, such as periodic limb moment disorder, central sleep apnea syndrome, or obstructive sleep apnea syndrome.

From AASM Diagnostic Classification Steering Committee. The International Classification of Sleep Disorders Diagnostic and Coding Manual. *Rochester, MN. American Academy of Sleep Medicine 1991/2001. Reproduced by kind permission of the AASM.*

central anisocoria

Variable inequality of the pupils with normal light reactions at all times and with normal dilation in response to psychosensory or pharmacological stimuli. A lesion of the brainstem, as in **multiple sclerosis**, has been considered to be causal.[6617]

central anticholinergic syndrome

Signs suggesting atropine poisoning (dry, flushed and warm skin, dilated pupils, decreased bowel sounds and urinary retention, and confusion) occurring as a result of exposure of the CNS to anticholinergic agents in toxic concentrations. See **anticholinergic syndrome**.

central aphasia

A form of aphasia described by Goldstein, now regarded as an incomplete form of **Wernicke (receptive) aphasia** resembling **conduction aphasia**.

central cervical cord syndrome

See **central cord syndrome**.

central conduction time

The latencies between stimulation of the cortical motor areas and the cervical cord, and the onset of the peripheral response. Either a magnetic stimulator or stimulation using a low-output impedance stimulator is employed. The technique allows assessment of conduction in the descending motor pathways between the cortex and the cord, and has been found useful in demonstrating lesions of this pathway in, e.g., multiple sclerosis.[4386] See also **central motor conduction**.

central congenital alveolar hypoventilation

See **central alveolar hypoventilation syndrome**.

central cord syndrome

The occurrence of signs of spinothalamic and pyramidal tract dysfunction below, and of areflexia and hyper- or hypoesthesia at the site of a lesion affecting the central regions of the spinal cord. This may follow hyperextension injuries and other causes of ischemia, or may be the manifestation of intrinsic cord tumors, infections, or syringomyelia.[5182]

The *central cervical cord syndrome* leads to complaints of severe pain in the shoulder girdle region and arms, with more weakness of the upper than of the lower limbs, retention of urine, and variable impairment of sensation below the level of the lesion. It results from central cord lesions following severe hyperextension injuries to the cervical spine[2985] or to midline cervical disk protrusion.

See also **burning hands syndrome**.

central core disease

(Shy–Magee disease; MIM 117000) An uncommon, relatively benign, dominantly or recessively inherited, usually nonprogressive myopathy in which frozen sections of muscle demonstrate single or multiple regions within type I myofibers which lack reactivity for oxidative enzymes, phosphorylase, and glycogen, and which have a smudgy appearance with the modified trichrome stain. Electron microscopy of the **cores** shows lack or absence of mitochondria, reduced glycogen content, and changes in the contractile apparatus. The gene responsible is located at 19q12–q13.1 and impairs function of the *ryanodine* receptor. Many mutations have been identified.

The clinical features include onset in infancy, proximal muscle weakness, and hypotonia with delayed motor development, and, in adults, mild proximal weakness affecting the pelvic girdle mainly, and the facial muscles in some cases. At any age, flat feet, kyphoscoliosis, pes cavus, congenital dislocation of the hips, joint contractures, poor temperature control, and stiffness of the muscles during exercise are often found. Eye movements are normal. The condition is a cause of "idiopathic" hyperCKemia.

Both dominant and recessive *RYR1* mutations have been reported. Such mutations lead to a broad spectrum and high prevalence of clinical phenotypes and are pathologically responsible for eccentric or peripheral cores, multiple minicores, uniformity of type I fibers with an absence of cores, unevenness of oxidative enzyme staining, marked muscle replacement by fatty tissue in association with cores, or an increase in internal nuclei. They are responsible for this condition as for **malignant hyperthermia** susceptibility.[4554, 5813]

Central cores may also be a nonspecific marker for a metabolic disorder. The condition was first recognized by Shy and Magee in 1956.[5823]

Variants include *multicore disease*, a syndrome of nonprogressive weakness in which small, short cores lie transversely across the muscle fiber;[1874] *minicore disease*, in which very small foci of Z-line streaming are seen within the muscle fibers;[1384] a recessive form resembling **multi-minicore disease**;[2029] and a form with *muscle diphosphatase deficiency* presenting as a nonfamilial congenital nonprogressive myopathy.[3301]

central dazzle See **central photophobia**.

central deafness See **word deafness**.

central-distal axonopathy Axonal damage in the peripheral extremities of axons within the CNS, one cause of which is prolonged low-level exposure to acrylamide, an industrial polymer, while the effects of MPTP, clioquinol, and lathyrism, and possibly the biochemical deficits underlying **Friedreich ataxia** and **hereditary spastic paraplegia** are others.

The clinical syndromes produced include the subacutely evolving onset and progression of a sensorimotor/autonomic peripheral neuropathy, spasticity, optic atrophy, and cerebellar ataxia.[6286] See also **subacute myelo-optico-neuropathy**.

central electromyography The electrodiagnostic study of reflexes and of the control of movement by the spinal cord and brain, using for example **transcranial magnetic stimulation**. See also **central motor conduction**.

Central European encephalitis A direct infection of brain by a flavivirus member of the togavirus group of arboviruses, characterized by an illness resembling **Russian spring–summer encephalitis** except that it is milder and usually resolves without sequelae.[6858]

central facial palsy Weakness of the lower quadrant of the face due to a lesion of the upper motor neuron pathway from the contralateral hemisphere. When isolated, this may be a **lacunar syndrome**.[3019] The upper quadrant (the forehead) is largely spared because the neurons innervating the frontalis muscles receive (supranuclear) input from the motor cortex of both hemispheres, but those innervating the muscles of the lower half do not. See also **volitional facial palsy**, **emotional facial palsy**, and **lacunes**.

central fatigue Failure to maintain sustained maximal force due to an unidentified, nonvolitional safety mechanism within the CNS which shuts off the neuromuscular unit when the latter seems to be at risk of damage from excessive contraction.[873] The organic nature of the problem was proved by the slowness of recovery times of motor-evoked potential amplitudes using transcranial magnetic stimulation.[3844]

central glare See **central photophobia**.

central hematomyelia Traumatic myelopathy, the clinical features resembling those of **syringomyelia** but in this case resulting from bleeding into the substance of the spinal cord.[4393] See **Minor disease**.

central herniation 1. The lateral and forward shift of the diencephalon and the downward thrusting of the centrum semiovale through the tentorium cerebelli consequent upon raised intracranial pressure (giving rise to the **central syndrome**). 2. Backward protrusion of a herniating intervertebral disk in the midline.

central midtemporal spikes (Rolandic or Sylvian spikes) Uniform diphasic or triphasic sharp waves occurring focally in the central and midtemporal regions in children between the ages of 4 and 13 years of age, unilaterally, bilaterally or shifting between the two sides. The number of sharp waves is markedly increased by sleep, and discharges may be absent during the waking state. The EEG finding is not necessarily associated with clinical seizure activity.[3787]

central motor conduction The speed of conduction in central motor pathways, estimated by measurement of the latency of response in a muscle with magnetic stimulation of the motor cortex and of the appropriate nerve roots.[3086]

central nervous deficiency syndrome Garland's term for the syndrome affecting starved prisoners of war who developed failing vision with optic atrophy, nerve deafness, and numbness and paresthesias of the legs, presumably due to nutritional deficiencies.[2288] See also **Strachan syndrome**.

central nervous system The brain, the I and II cranial nerves, and the spinal cord.

Central Nervous System and Brain Disorders Network An alliance of the National Foundation for Brain Research, the National Association for Clinical NeuroServices, and the National Coalition for Research in Neurological Disorders.

central neurofibromatosis See **neurofibromatosis** and **Gardner syndrome**.

central neurogenic hyperventilation Hyperventilation characterized by sustained tachypnea that persists despite an elevated arterial pO_2 and pH and a low arterial pCO_2. It occurs in the absence of a respiratory stimulant and persists during sleep. In most cases it is due to hepatic encephalopathy or brainstem tumors, or is a sign of rostral-caudal deterioration in patients with generalized brain swelling. The mechanism of its occurrence is uncertain.[5050]

central nystagmus A direction-changing nystagmus caused by a lesion of the CNS (as opposed to disease of the eyes or of the labyrinths), usually in the cerebellum or brainstem. Vertical, horizontal, or torsional forms occur; they may be uni- or bidirectional and are neither fatigable nor suppressed by fixation. Other signs of CNS dysfunction are commonly present. Any vertigo accompanying it is relatively mild. See **direction-changing nystagmus**.

central oscillopsia Subjective awareness of movement of visual images resulting from brainstem or temporal lobe disorders affecting the central vestibular apparatus.

central pain (funicular pain) Deeply felt, amorphous, indefinable, and severe pain arising from lesions (almost all of which are strokes) completely or mainly confined to the CNS, with a latent period between injury and onset and invariably associated with some sensory disturbance.This dynamic process is influenced by the effects of past pain and other experiences and is shown by the development of sensitization, wind-up, or expansion of receptive fields of CNS neurons, by the enhancement of flexion reflexes, and by the persistence of pain or hyperalgesia after inputs from injured tissues are blocked.

Such pain is felt in regions distant from, but related to, spinal cord or cerebral lesions. Diffuse paresthesias, **allodynia**, and **hyperpathia** are commonly associated. The mechanisms are unknown. Up- or downregulation of receptors for adrenergic transmitters; sensitization of C nociceptors with low thresholds, capable of prolonged discharges after sensitization; abnormal hypersensitivity of damaged fibers; the generation of new receptors; alteration in the central pattern of impulse conduction; alterations in inhibitory mechanisms; and activation of secondary polysynaptic pathways, all are possibilities, but in every case there appears to be some interruption of the spino-thalamo-cortical nociceptive pathways.[3081, 4300, 565] Both non-NMDA and NMDA glutamate receptor or NK1 substance P receptor antagonists prevent such central sensitization. See also **thalamic syndrome**.

central paroxysmal positional nystagmus A form of positional nystagmus in any direction, lasting 30 s or so, non-fatiguing, and accompanied by other features of brainstem disease.

central photophobia (central glare, central dazzle) A subjective complaint of excessive brightness in patients with a homonymous hemianopia, probably in association with a calcarine lesion and interpretable as the visual correlate of paresthesia.[1374, 2086] The same symptom may result from digitalis poisoning.

central pontine myelinolysis See **osmotic demyelination syndrome**.

central post-stroke pain Unilateral pain and dysesthesia associated with impaired sensation involving part or the whole of the face, not explicable by a lesion of the trigeminal nerve. It is attributed to a lesion of the quintothalamic (trigeminothalamic) pathway, thalamus, or thalamocortical projection. Symptoms may also involve the trunk and/or limbs of the affected *or contralateral* side. Diagnostic criteria have been defined:

A. Pain and dysesthesia in one half of the face, associated with loss of sensation to pin-prick, temperature, and/or touch, and fulfilling criteria C and D
B. One or both of the following:
   1. History of sudden onset suggesting a vascular lesion (stroke)
   2. Demonstration by CT or MRI of a vascular lesion in an appropriate site
C. Pain and dysesthesias develop within 6 months of stroke
D. Not explicable by a lesion of the trigeminal nerve

From the International Classification of Headache Disorders (Headache Classification Committee of the International Headache Society; *Cephalalgia* 2004;24[Suppl 1]) by kind permission of Dr. Jes Olesen, the International Headache Society and Wiley-Blackwell Publications.

central razzle Excessive discomfort from stimulation by loud sounds due to cortical lesions and thought to be due to loss of a centrifugal inhibitory pathway which may function to sharpen images.[292]

central retinal artery occlusion An ophthalmological emergency occurring mainly in the elderly, in which retinal ischemia and infarction cause acute and severe visual loss, with attenuation of the retinal vessels, retinal pallor, and edema, and a **cherry-red spot**. The usual causes are an arterial embolism, arteritis, or vasospasm; in the case of the first of these, massage of the eye and lowering of intraocular pressure may improve the chances of restoring some sight.[220]

central retinal vein occlusion An acquired disorder causing reduction in vision, swelling of the optic nerve head, dilation of the retinal veins, and hemorrhages in the retinal nerve fiber layer. The cause is usually not determined, but the condition may be associated with hypertension and other vascular diseases.[3363] One cause may be compression of the vein by a dilated, atheromatous central retinal artery. See also **venous stasis retinopathy**.

central scotoma 1. A defect in the field of vision corresponding to that part of the field subtended by the macula, due to a lesion of the papillomacular fibers. 2. A defect in the field of vision which is surrounded by an intact field. See **scotoma**.

central sensitization Propagation (and possibly augmentation) of impulses within the central nervous system relating to data about a pain stimulus that outlasts the original stimulus; "an activity-dependent change in the excitability and synaptic strength of neurons in the dorsal horn of the spinal cord . . . responsible for the generation of secondary hyperalgesia and allodynia in acute and chronic pain states."[3680]

Such changes are due to the altered behavior of neurons characterized by enlarged receptive fields, increased spontaneous firing or evoked firing rate, or firing to novel stimuli which did not previously cause such activation: The phenomenon is thought to underlie the increasing and persisting pain in such central syndromes as **migraine**, in which condition, for example, patients say that touching their head or combing their hair are painful during (and sometimes after) an attack.[2411]

central serous retinopathy (central angiospastic retinopathy) A syndrome of unknown cause occurring in young adult males, characterized by the accumulation of serous fluid at one macula, beneath the retina or the adjacent pigmented epithelium. Clinical features include complaints of metamorphopsia, positive scotomas, and micropsia. The prognosis for recovery is good but in about a quarter of all cases, the condition recurs.

central sleep apnea syndrome A disorder characterized by a cessation or

Chart C–8. Central Sleep Apnea Syndrome

A. The patient has a complaint of either insomnia or excessive sleepiness. Occasionally, the patient may be unaware of clinical features observed by others.
B. Frequent episodes of shallow or absent breathing during sleep.
C. Associated features include at least one of the following:
  1. Gasps, grunts, or choking during sleep;
  2. Frequent body movements;
  3. Cyanosis during sleep.
D. Polysomnographic monitoring demonstrates:
  1. Central apneic pauses greater than 10 s (20 s in infancy) in duration, and one or more of the following
  2. Frequent arousals from sleep associated with the apneas;
  3. Brady-tachycardia;
  4. Oxygen desaturation in association with the apneic episodes; with or without
  5. A **minimal sleep latency test** that demonstrates mean sleep latency of less than 10 min.
E. Other sleep disorders can be present, for example, periodic limb movement disorder, obstructive sleep apnea syndrome, or **central alveolar hypoventilation syndrome**.

From AASM Diagnostic Classification Steering Committee. The International Classification of Sleep Disorders Diagnostic and Coding Manual. Rochester, MN. *American Academy of Sleep Disorders, 1991/2001. Reproduced by kind permission of the AASM.*

decrease of ventilatory effort during rapid eye movement sleep, usually with associated oxygen desaturation and without any accompanying respiratory effort, as a result of an unusually high apneic threshold. The condition may occur as a complication of numerous CNS lesions, hypoxia, and metabolic diseases but is most commonly found in healthy people at high altitudes. Diagnostic criteria have been suggested.[1629] (See Chart C–8.)

See also the Web site: www.sleepeducation.com/Disorders.aspx.

central syndrome Downward displacement of the upper brainstem at the junction with the diencephalon through the tentorial opening, leading to an orderly sequence of events which witness the functional disturbance of progressively more caudal levels of the brainstem.[5053] These include reduction in conscious level and Cheyne–Stokes respirations (*diencephalic stage*); midposition fixed pupils, loss of oculocephalic reflexes, and central neurogenic hyperventilation (*pontine stage*); decorticate posturing, ataxic or no respirations, bradycardia, and hypertension (*medullary stage*); and ultimately death.

central tapetoretinal degeneration See **Behr disease**.

central tegmental tract Fibers which descend from the red nucleus and elsewhere in the lower diencephalon and mesencephalon, running to the ipsilateral olive. It was first described by von Bechterew in 1885. Bilateral lesions of the tract appear to induce the phenomenon of **palatal myoclonus**.

central vestibular nystagmus See **vestibular nystagmus**.

central vestibular vertigo The form of vertigo caused by lesions of the vestibular nuclei or of the vestibulocerebellum, and characterized by change in direction with gaze to either side. The nystagmus may be pendular and is usually purely horizontal, vertical, or rotatory.

centrencephalic epilepsy The term applied to the supposed site of origin of generalized tonic-clonic seizures, based on the fact that bilateral epileptic discharges can be set up in homologous areas of the two hemispheres following stimulation of subcortical structures such as the intralaminar thalamic nuclei of experimental animals. **Penfield** in 1938 considered that one area in the nervous system functions to integrate the electrical activity of the two hemispheres, probably the rostral brainstem and thalamus, and that this area also constituted the neural substratum of consciousness.

Abnormal discharges in this region would give rise to those seizures which Penfield labelled *centrencephalic*. However, it is notable that lesions of other parts of the brain may also induce seizures with exactly the same clinical and electrographic characteristics. See **absence seizures**.

centrencephalic myoclonic-astatic petit mal See **centrencephalic myoclonic-astatic epilepsy**.

centrencephalic myoclonic-astatic epilepsy (infantile myoclonic petit mal, centrencephalic myoclonic-astatic petit mal, true myoclonic epilepsy) An older term for forms of myoclonic-astatic epilepsy for which there is no detectable pathological basis. In such cases, there is frequently a positive family history of seizures.[1693] The patient may be mentally normal or retarded, and first exhibits symptoms usually in the second to fifth years of life. Myoclonic and atonic seizures, absences, petit mal status, tonic seizures, etc., are the usual phenotypes. See **akinetic seizures**, **juvenile myoclonic epilepsy of Janz**, and **centrencephalic epilepsy**.

centrifugal (Lat, center + fleeing from) Movement of a phenomenon (such as sensory loss in developing peripheral neuropathy) from proximal to distal parts of the body.

centrifugal nerve A motor nerve.

centripetal (Lat, center + seeking) Movement of a phenomenon (such as sensory loss in developing peripheral neuropathy) from distal to proximal parts of the body.

centripetal nystagmus A form of **gaze-evoked nystagmus** that increases with prolonged eccentric gaze, but may reverse in direction if the position of the eyes is maintained yet longer. It is most commonly seen in ocular **myasthenia gravis**[3751] or in diseases of the cerebellum.

See also **rebound nystagmus**, in which again nystagmus in the opposite direction occurs when the eyes are returned from the deviated to the primary position.

centrocecal scotoma A scotoma which involves the area of the visual field subtended by both the macula and the blind spot. It reflects pathology affecting the fibers running to the optic nerve head from the macula and from the retina between the macula and the optic disk.

centronuclear myopathies (myotubular myopathies) Sporadic or variously inherited **congenital myopathies** with occasional onset in childhood or adult life, characterized by the presence of structures resembling fetal myotubes and central nuclei in the extrafusal muscle fibers with predominance and hypotrophy of type I fibers.[1966, 5783] The commonest form maps to Xq27–q28, Both autosomal dominant (late) and recessive (early) forms are recorded.[3175] Clinically the appearances vary; facial, extraocular, and limb weakness with equinovarus deformity of the feet and, in adults, a syndrome of moderate limb-girdle weakness both having been associated with these biopsy appearances, although a syndrome of nonprogressive myopathy with weakness of the facial and extraocular muscles and hypotonia is a characteristic presentation. Muscle pain and stiffness after exertion, with relief by rest, are other common symptoms.

Muscle biopsy shows a high proportion of histochemical type II fibers commonly containing myotubes (with a peripheral ring of myofibrils and a central area in which myofibrillar components and nuclei are present). Type I fiber atrophy and the nonspecific features of myopathy are other common findings.[4485, 5992]

It is possible that **centronuclear** myopathies and **type I fiber atrophy with central nuclei** are forms of the same disease.[601]

Variant members of the class are

X-linked recessive centronuclear (myotubular) myopathy (OMIM 310400) A fatal congenital myopathy presenting with weak fetal movements, fetal distress, respiratory distress in the neonate, proximal myopathic weakness, hypotonia, and atrophy. Tubular aggregates are found in muscle biopsy specimens.[5836] The responsible gene maps to Xq28.[6508]

Centronuclear myopathy with type I fiber atrophy and myotubules A slowly progressive form of centronuclear myopathy with onset in childhood, affecting the muscles of the pelvic girdle and legs, in which the muscle biopsy reveals type I fiber atrophy, central nuclei, and fibers resembling myotubes.[601]

A form in which *type I fiber hypotrophy and fingerprint inclusions* are found in muscle biopsy specimens. The clinical syndrome includes slowly progressive muscular weakness and features of Malins syndrome.[4717]

A *dominantly inherited form* (12q21) presenting in youth or adult life with proximal muscle wasting, the facial, extraocular, and distal muscles sometimes being involved as well. The condition is slowly progressive and can be compatible with a normal life span. Muscle biopsy shows central nuclei with a clear surrounding zone in 60% of the fibers, both types I and II.[4249] Different missense mutations affecting the middle domain of the dynamin 2 (*DNM2*) have been shown to cause at least one autosomal dominant form.

In other *dominantly or recessively inherited forms* presenting in childhood or adult life, *variants* showing proximal muscle weakness and wasting with sparing of the cranial muscles; calf muscle hypertrophy;[637] cardiomyopathy; weakness beginning in adolescence or early adulthood with bilateral ptosis, more distal than proximal weakness and evidence of mild axonal peripheral nerve involvement as well as myopathic changes[2068] (*DNM2*-CNM; mapped to 19p13) have all been reported.

The British Web site http://tonilouise.tripod.com/ is an information point for those suffering from these and other muscle disorders.

centro-temporal epilepsy See **benign childhood epilepsy with centrotemporal spikes**.

centrum ovale infarcts Stroke from acute infarction in the centrum ovale which receives its blood supply from the superficial (pial) middle cerebral artery (MCA) system through perforating medullary branches which course toward the lateral ventricles.[712]

centrum semiovale The hemispheric mass of gray and white matter which remains at the top of the brainstem when the cerebrum is removed. It comprises the basal ganglia and internal capsules.

cephalaea An ancient term for a form of headache resembling migraine.

cephalalgia (Gr, the head + pain) Headache.

Cephalalgia The organ of the International Headache Society, devoted to the topic of headache and related pains. Web site: www.blackwellpublishing.com/journals/cha.

cephalgia fugax See **benign paroxysmal cranial neuralgia**.

cephalic (Gr, pertaining to the head) Sensations in the head such as light-headedness, tingling, or headache.

cephalic bellows sound A cranial bruit heard best over the anterior fontanelle of children with hydrocephalus and raised intracranial pressure. It was described first in 1833 by Dr. John Dix Fisher (1797–1850), a physician in Massachussetts,[2494] and was thought by him to indicate the presence of cerebral pathology, but it was dismissed by Osler as without pathological significance in 1880.

cephalic index A craniometric sign—the breadth of the head divided by the length and multiplied by 100, the product having no known significance.

cephalic tetanus (Rose tetanus, Rose-Villar syndrome) A form of **tetanus** affecting the facial or oculomotor muscles.

cephalitis An ancient term for inflammation of the brain and its membranes.

cephalocele Herniation of the intracranial contents through a defect in the skull. Such midline cranio-cerebral cystic defects result from failure in the normal development of the neural tube and consist of **meningoceles**, within which there is no neural tissue, and **encephaloceles** proper, in which some neural tissue is present.[4247] They are classified as *primary* (occipital, parietal, **sincipital**, and basal) and *secondary* (following surgery or trauma or with a craniofacial cleft).[1476]

Occipital cephaloceles have been reported as a dominantly inherited condition presenting with bulging of the scalp even at birth but without other abnormalities.[437]

cephalohematoma (Gr, head + blood + a mass) A blood clot lying beneath the scalp but outside the cranium, most often seen in infants as a complication of a traumatic delivery.

cephalo-oculo-cutaneous telangiectasia See **Louis-Bar syndrome**.

cephaloponia (Gr, head + pain) An ancient term for a severe or heavy pain in the head.

cephalosyndactyly See **Waardenbeng syndrome**.

CERAD The Consortium to Establish a Registry for Alzheimer Disease, a research group formed in the United States to standardize examination techniques, facilitate cooperative study, and perform annual assessments on a defined population.[4499]

CERAD Global Deterioration Scale (GDS) A rating instrument for staging the magnitude of cognitive and functional impairment in normal aging, age-associated memory impairment, and primary degenerative dementia, composed of a battery of tests designed to provide brief and accurate assessment of the presenting symptoms. The levels of cognitive functioning are rated from no cognitive decline to very mild, moderate, moderately severe, severe, and very severe decline, and for each of these, a full notation of definitions is given.[4499]

CERAD test battery A selection of tests designed to provide a brief and accurate assessment of the presenting manifestations and cognitive changes in patients with **Alzheimer disease** or other cognitive disorders in the elderly.

Aside from information on demographics, a drug inventory, and history, physical and general neurological examinations are performed and a diagnostic impression recorded. Tests of verbal fluency, the modified **Boston Naming Test**, the Mini-Mental State Examination, tests of constructional praxis, word lists to recall, and word list recognition tests are also administered.[4498]

ceramidase deficiency See **Farber disease**.

ceramide lactoside lipidosis (ceramidosis) See **Farber disease**.

cerebellar and pancreatic aplasia See **cerebellar ataxia**.

cerebellar abscess A purulent collection within the cerebellum, usually associated with pyogenic inflammation of the middle ear. Clinically, headache, vomiting, drowsiness, ataxia of gait and limb movements, nystagmus, meningism, and evidence of increased intracranial pressure are the leading features.

cerebellar ataxia (ataxy, Zappert syndrome, SCA) 1. An inclusive term for all the clinical motor manifestations of cerebellar disease, especially incoordination or awkwardness in the performance of a motor task due to disease of the cerebellum or its connections.

The term thus begs the question: "What are the signs of cerebellar disease?" Although an experienced clinician may have no doubt that certain mild abnormalities of voluntary movements are due to loss of cerebellar coordinating functions, no precise differentiation between these abnormalities and those caused by, e.g., proprioceptive disorders or subtle weakness in corticospinal lesions is possible, other than by the exclusion of such alternatives by determining that the other signs of such lesions are not to be found. All of the tests to elicit "cerebellar signs" (discoordination, dysmetria, dysdiadochokinesis, etc.) may in fact be abnormal on the basis of frontal lobe, internal capsule, or other pathway lesions.

Acquired cerebellar cortical degenerations may be caused by the production of anti-Yo antibodies cross-reacting against cerebellar Purkinje cells, most often in the context of carcinoma of the lung or ovary. However, the syndrome has also been associated with carcinoma in other organs and with malignant melanoma and lymphomas. The symptoms of cerebellar degeneration often precede the diagnosis of the responsible neoplasm.

2. (*cerebellar ataxias*, spino-cerebellar ataxias) Inherited diseases of the cerebellum or of its connections, presenting with typical signs of cerebellar dysfunction and frequently complicated damage to other parts of the nervous system. These are here distinguished from those conditions which have no known hereditary basis, which are listed here.

A comprehensive classification of the multitude of the inherited cerebellar ataxias was that of Harding,[2755] who defined five groups, to which the condition of **hereditary spastic paraparesis** may conveniently be added. Chart C–9 is based upon the classification on Dr. Alan Pestronk's Web site, http://neuromuscular.wustl.edu/ataxia/,[4992] with many thanks for his kind permission, but is adapted by the addition of syndromes taken from the extensive listing by Baraitser,[379] and from Schelhaas,[5591]Subramony,[6116] Hammans,[2719] and Dr. Will Garrett (personal communication). In all forms, clinical limb and gait ataxia, nystagmus, and dysarthria are present, to which many variable features are added in those cases not labeled as "pure" cerebellar ataxias.

Web sites of interest include: www.ataxiacubana.sld.cu/ataxia_en_index.htm, relating to a project developed by the Cuban Revolution to carry out research on ataxia and to help those affected.

www.fara.org.au/, which summarizes recent progress in ataxia research and treatment from the Friedreich Ataxia Research Association.

www.ninds.nih.gov/disorders/friedreichs_ataxia/detail_friedreichs_ataxia.htm, a resource guide and fact sheet

Chart C–9a. The Autosomal Dominant (Spino-)Cerebellar Ataxias (SCAs)

At least 28 genes have been linked with the dominantly inherited forms. They are due variously to CAG repeat expansions that encode a pure repeat of the amino acid glutamine in the disease protein, producing toxic proteins (SCA 1, 2, 3, 6, 7, and 17), as well as at least three other diseases that are not primarily ataxic syndromes such as **Huntington disease, spinobulbar muscular atrophy,** and **dentatorubropallidoluysian atrophy**; to noncoding repeats; or to conventional mutations in specific genes (SCA 5, 13, 14, and 27). The six polyglutamine repeat SCAs are the most common causes of dominantly inherited ataxia. A second category comprises the SCAs that are due to repeat expansions falling outside of the protein-coding region of the respective disease genes.

In the following, the chromosome location, the gene/locus and the forms of mutation will be given for each SCA subtype,

SCA 1 (6p22.3 ATXN1; CAG repeat) Clinically, gait disturbance and speech problems are the typical onset symptoms, usually in the twenties; ophthalmoplegia, optic atrophy, pyramidal and extrapyramidal signs, peripheral sensorimotor neuropathy, mild dementia, and amyotrophy follow. This is the most frequent single example of the SCAs reported to date.

SCA 2 (12q24.13; ATXN2, CAG repeat) Slow saccades, Parkinsonian features, motor neuropathy, and postural tremor. Clinically, it resembles SCA 1 but for the presence of hyporeflexia. Saccades are particularly slow and both myoclonus and cramps are reported.[492] In variant forms, there are added Parkinsonism[2654] (Pulst et al., 1996) or retinal degeneration.[520]

continued

Chart C–9a. *(continued)*

SCA 3 (14q32.12; ATXN3, CAG repeat) (Machado–Joseph disease) A syndrome with onset usually in mid-adult life, comprising progressive ataxia and supervening pyramidal signs, dysarthria, and vertical gaze pareses associated with cerebellar and brainstem atrophy with perioral fasciculations. Optic atrophy, chorea, Parkinsonism, dystonic or rigid dystonias, distal weakness and wasting, and retained reflexes are common additional findings; saccade velocities are not reduced. In some kinships the responsible gene maps to 6p24-p23.[2755, 5668] (Takiyama et al., 1993; Stevanin et al., 1994b). The condition was first described in detail by Menzel in 1891.[4317] See also **Joseph disease**.

SCA 4 (16q24-qter; SCA4) A form with prominent sensory axonal neuropathy and hyporeflexia but without eye movement disorders.

SCA 5 (11q13.2; SPTBN2) A slowly developing cerebellar and pyramidal syndrome with onset in the third decade, with global cerebellar atrophy. One *variant* is *cerebellar ataxia with spasmodic cough*, a pure late-onset dominantly inherited ataxia with a benign evolution in which attacks of spasmodic coughing precede ataxia for one to three decades. Clinically, it resembles SCAs 5 and 12.[14] Another is a pure cerebellar syndrome with downbeat nystagmus and slow progression.

SCA 6 (19p13.13; CACNA1A, CAG repeat) This pure cerebellar ataxia resembles SCA 5 but is manifested in older adults and posterior column function is impaired. Life span is normal. Downbeat nystagmus is an added feature but the brainstem is otherwise unaffected. The mutation is allelic with **episodic ataxia** type II.[6050, 2337] The condition is linked to **familial hemiplegic migraine** both clinically and through shared abnormalities of the CACNA1A P/Q-type calcium channel α_1 subunit.

SCA 7 (3p14.1 or 3p12-p21.1; ATXN7, CAG repeat) (formerly listed as OPCA II or III) Syndromes resembling SCA 1 with onset usually in childhood, comprising progressive visual failure (due to pigmentary maculopathy), ataxia, seizures, and supervening gaze pareses. Pyramidal signs including hyperreflexia, posterior column sensory loss, and dementia are found. The syndrome is associated with atrophic changes in the cerebellum, basal ganglia, and spinal cord.[6694, 2527] This must be the same condition as that formerly called *ADCA II: with pigmentary retinal degeneration/progressive macular degeneration.* Clinically, the cerebellar syndrome is accompanied by progressive visual loss and evidence of anterior horn cell degeneration. It is mapped to[1859]

SCA 8 (13q21; KLHL1AS, CTG repeat) A slowly progressive form with cerebellar, pyramidal, and cognitive signs and evidence of sensory neuropathy.[3264] It is associated with a large CTG repeat expansion that is not fully penetrant (i.e., not all individuals with the expansion develop disease).

SCA 9 Not yet reallocated

SCA 10 (22q13.31; ATXN10, ATTCT repeat) A pure cerebellar syndrome with seizures as an added feature, described from Brazil and Mexico.[5206, 6593] It is caused by an expansion in an intron of the *ATXN10* gene.

SCA 11 (15q14-q21.3; SCA11) A relatively benign form with normal life span.

SCA 12 (5q32; PPP2R2B, CAG repeat) Characterized clinically by action tremor in the head and arms with onset in the fourth decade of hyperreflexia and mild to moderate cerebellar signs such as ataxia, dysmetria, and dysarthria. Parkinsonism and dementia have been recorded later in life.[4735]

SCA 13 (19q13.33; KCNC3) A form manifest in childhood with added psychomotor failure. SCA 13 encodes a voltage-gated K^+ channel, mutations of which impair the electrophysiological properties of the multi-subunit K^+ channel, and lead to disease phenotypes with neurodevelopmental and neurodegenerative features.

SCA 14 (19q13.42; PRKCG) A form caused by various missense, deletion, and splice site mutations in the PRKCG gene encoding protein kinase C. Most affected patients display a late-onset uncomplicated form of ataxia with occasional mild extrapyramidal features such as dystonia or myoclonus.[1127]

SCA 15 (3p25.2-pter; ITRP1 I) A pure ataxic syndrome reported in a single Australian family.[6080]

SCA 16 (3p26.2) Head and hand tremors are reported in adults.

SCA 17 (OPCA 5?) (6q27; TBP TBP, CAG repeat) Chorea, seizures, psychiatric manifestations, dementia.[5360] Initiation of smooth pursuit eye movements is markedly impaired.

SCA 18 (7q22-q32) A form with added sensorimotor neuropathy

*SCA 19 (*1p21-q21)* A form with added myoclonus and cognitive impairment.

SCA 20 11 A dominantly inherited form with dentate nucleus calcification producing a low signal on MRI sequences. Dysarthria/spasmodic dysphonia are typically the initial manifestations. Mild pyramidal signs, palatal tremor, and hypermetric saccades are noted in most cases.[3497]

SCA 21 (7p21.3-p15.1) A slowly progressive form with added Parkinsonism, unresponsive to levadopa.[6577]

SCA 22 (1p21-q23) Pure ataxia.

SCA 23 (20p13-p12.2) A form with added pyramidal signs and sensory neuropathy.

SCA 24 (1p36) Genotype and phenotype unclear.

SCA 25 (2p21-p1) A form with added severe sensory neuropathy.[6049]

SCA 26 (19p13.3) Pure ataxia with adult onset.[6936]

SCA 27 (13q34; FGF14. AD) Characterized by impaired cognitive abilities and slowly progressive ataxia and caused by mutations in fibroblast growth factor 14.

SCA 28 (18p11.22-q11.2) A slowly progressive form with juvenile onset and with added ophthalmoplegia, nystagmus, ptosis, and hyperreflexia.[974]

DRPLA (12p13.31; ATN1 Atrophin 1, CAG repeat) See **dentato-rubro-pallido-Luysian atrophy.**

ADCA III: Unlinked Pure Ataxia

Unnumbered variants:

Autosomal dominant sensory ataxia A syndrome of gait difficulty associated with diminished sensation in the limbs and with areflexia due to a mutation on the *SNAX1* gene.[6459] This form closely resembles **Biemond ataxia**.

Branchial myoclonus with spastic paraparesis and ataxia.

CAPOS syndrome Episodic Cerebellar ataxia with fever, childhood onset, Areflexia without polyneuropathy, Pes cavus, Optic atrophy, and Sensorineural hearing loss.

Cerebellar ataxia with mental retardation
Cerebellar ataxia, deafness and narcolepsy
Cerebellar vermal aplasia
Cerebelloparenchymal degeneration A form with adult onset and added dysarthria and dementia.
Familial (British or Danish) dementia
Familial **essential tremor** (3q13).
Glucose transporter 1 deficiency syndrome (1p35)
Hereditary ataxia with thermoanalgesia and loss of fungiform papillae
Holmes ataxia is a pure ataxia, but a *variant* is *ataxia with hypogonadotrophic hypergondadism*, a recessively inherited syndrome of gait and limb ataxia, with onset in youth or early adult life. The condition is also characterized by pigmentary retinopathy, small penis and testes, pes cavus, dementia, hypotonia, dysarthria, choreoathetosis, distal weakness and wasting, loss of pain and joint position senses, short stature, and mental and developmental delay.[2956]
Multiple hamartoma syndrome See **Cowden disease** and **Lhermitte–Duclos syndrome.**
Myelocerebellar disorder A form with added pyramidal signs and a predisposition to leukemia.
Prion disease *(20p.12)* See **Gerstmann–Straussler–Scheinker disease** and **Creutzfeldt–Jakob disease.**
SCA with chronic cough A pure late-onset form with a benign course. Spasmodic coughing attacks precede ataxia for one to three decades. Clinically, it resembles SCAs 5 and 12.[1304]
Skeleton–skin–brain syndrome (4p16; FGFR-3)
Spinocerebellar ataxia with rigidity and neuropathy A late-onset form with added rigidity, bradykinesia, dysarthria, spasticity, muscle atrophy, and peripheral neuropathy.
Syndrome of vertical (downbeat) and horizontal nystagmus.
von Hippel–Lindau Syndrome.

Undefined forms
a. *(16q22.1; PLEKHG4)* A form with added sensory neuropathy; resembles SCA 4
b. *(16q21–q23)*
In yet other forms, ataxia is accompanied by generalized tonic-clonic epilepsy.[2575] Two rare forms of ataxia, one with epilepsy, sensory ataxic neuropathy, dysarthria, and ophthalmoparesis, and an infantile onset spinocerebellar ataxia, have been described and found to be caused by defective mitochondrial proteins. Children present with generalized tonic-clonic epilepsy, ataxia, and mental retardation, but have neither myoclonus nor mental deterioration. MRI and muscle biopsy of one patient revealed, respectively, posterior white matter hyperintensities and vacuolization of the sarcotubular system.

Episodic ataxias (periodic ataxias, hereditary paroxysmal cerebellar ataxia) are channelopathies, of which many dominantly inherited forms are decribed;
EA1 (12p13; KCNA 1) Brief attacks (lasting minutes) in childhood, precipitated by exercise and startle, and complicated by joint contractures and neuromyotonia/myokymia, due to a mutation of the potassium channel gene.
EA2 (19p13; α_{1A} Ca^{2+} *{CACNA1A} channel) (many mutations)* Paroxysmal attacks in childhood lasting minutes to days, precipitated by stress, exercise, and fatigue with a progressive cerebellar syndrome and permanent gaze-evoked nystagmus.
EA3 (1q42) Brief attacks with added vertigo and tinnitus
These three forms respond to acetazolamide.[2719]m1>*EA4 (PATX)* Adult onset, with added vertigo and diplopia

EA5 (2q22; ACNB4β4) Adult onset, with added seizures and vertigo
EA6 (5p13; SLC1A3) Childhood onset; added **migraine with prolonged aura.**
EA7 (19q13) Longer-lasting attacks with onset in youth.
Episodic ataxia with paroxysmal choreoathetosis and spasticity (dystonia-9; DYT9) 1p
Childhood onset of attacks lasting <20 min with the above features and headaches, also responsive to acetazolamide.
See also **pyruvate decarboxylase deficiency, pyruvate dehydrogenase deficiency, maple syrup urine disease, Hartnup disease,** and defects of ammonia metabolism.

Chart C–9b. The Recessive Ataxias

The knowledge base is ever expanding; this chart is largely derived from Dr. Alan Pestronk's Web site with many thanks for his kind permission to do so. For further updates the reader is referred http://neuromuscular.wustl.edu/ataxia/recatax.html#ataxmacdys/.
In all of the following variant syndromes, cerebellar signs such as limb and gait ataxia, nystagmus, and dysarthria are assumed. A further classification will in time be adopted, relying upon genetic data. In the following list, the abbreviation, locus, and gene mutation are shown after each entry, where they are known.

Adult-onset ataxia with thalamic lesions Clinically, in this form, dysarthria and dysphagia present in adult life and there are vacuolar changes in the thalamus.

continued

Chart C–9b. *(continued)*

ARCA1 (autosomal recessive cerebellar ataxia 1, SCAR8) *(16q25; SYNE)* A pure ataxia with adult onset.

ARCA2 (SCAR9) *(1q42; CABC1)* A form with childhood onset, and with added seizures and often intellectual; impairment and associated ubiquitone deficiency.

Ataxia telangectasia *(11q22; ATM)* and *ataxia telangectasia-like syndrome (11q21)*

Ataxia with axonal neuropathy (SCAN 1) *(14q31; TDP1)* Onset in youth with added sensorimotor neuropathy.

Ataxia with bulls-eye macular dystrophy A form with childhood onset of ataxia and impaired vision.

Ataxia with epilepsy and mental retardation (16q21–23) A Saudi Arabian kindred presenting with the onset in infancy of seizures and cognitive delay.

Ataxia with hypogonadotrophic hypergonadism (Holmes syndrome) A recessively inherited syndrome of gait and limb ataxia, with onset in youth or early adult life. The condition is also characterized by pigmentary retinopathy, small penis and testes, pes cavus, dementia, hypotonia, dysarthria, choreoathetosis, distal weakness and wasting, loss of pain and joint position senses, short stature, and mental and developmental delay.[2956]

Ataxia with muscle coenzyme Q10 deficiency (9p13; Aprataxin) Forms presenting with a fatal mitochondrial encephalomyopathy and renal impairment at birth, an ataxic syndrome in childhood and youth, or a myopathic syndrome with pyramidal signs and hypogonadism in adult life.[2392]

Ataxia-oculomotor apraxia AOA1 *(19p13; Aprataxin)* Childhood onset, with added sensorimotor neuropathy.[5542]

Ataxia with saccadic intrusions SCAR4 *(1p36)* The onset of this form is in adult life, with macrosaccadic oscillations, fasciculations, pyramidal signs, and evidence of an axonal sensorimotor neuropathy.

Ataxia with slow eye movements A single kinship with a progressive syndrome of slow or absent saccades, intellectual impairment, extrapyramidal features, and peripheral neuropathy.

Ataxia with upgaze palsy A slowly progressive form with onset in early childhood of added seizures, myoclonus, and sensory neuropathy.

Ataxia-oculomotor apraxia (SCAR1) *(29q34; Senataxin)* Onset in youth with extrapyramidal signs, sensory neuropathy, and impaired saccaders.

Baltic myoclonus (**Unverricht–Lundborg**) *(21q22; Cystatin B)*

Cayman ataxia (ATCAY) *(19p13)* A geographically restricted, nonprogressive form.

Cerebellar hypoplasia, mental retardation, and quadripedal locomotion (17p) A Turkish kinship manifesting an inability to walk on two legs, mental retardation with lack or speech, kyphosis, and short stature.

Cerebelloparenchymal disorders (CPD) II A pure ataxia with adult onset. V. See **dyssynergia cerebellaris myoclonica** (types I, III, and IV are also described).

Charlevoix–Saguenay spastic ataxia: *(13q12; Sacsin)*

Childhood onset ataxia (SCAR7) *(11p15)* A form with added upper and lower motor neuron signs and pontocerebellar atrophy.

Cockayne Syndrome A (ERCC8) *(5q12)*

Cockayne Syndrome B (ERCC6) *(10q11)*

Cytochrome c oxidase I deficiency A mitochondriopathy in which hearing loss, cataracts, myoclonic seizures, and myopathic signs appear in early childhood.

Dilated cardiomyopathy and ataxia (DNAJC) *(19 3q26)* An infantile form associated with a long QT syndrome and optic atrophy.

Early-onset cerebellar ataxia with retained reflexes (EOCA) *(13q12)* Onset in childhood or youth with added peripheral neuropathy (thus resembling **Friedreich ataxia**) but with retained reflexes and slow progression.

Friedreich ataxia: (FRDA) *(9q13; Frataxin)* and Friedreich ataxia 2 *(FRDA 2; 9p23)*

Hearing loss and optic atrophy (SCAR3; *6p21*) Cochlear degeneration and optic atrophy with onset in childhood.

Infantile onset spinocerebellar ataxia: *(10q24; Twinkle)* A form with athetosis, sensorimotor polyneuropathy, and hyporeflexia.

Karak syndrome (PLA2G6) *(22q13)* An early-onset form with spasticity, dystonia, and intellectual impairment. The **eye of the tiger** sign may be present due to iron deposition in the basal ganglia.

Laryngeal paralysis and motor neuronopathy A form that resembles **multiple system atrophy** with adult onset, presenting with laryngeal abductor paralysis and stridor and with motor neuropathy.

Marinesco–Sjögren syndrome (SIL1) *(5q31)*

Mitochondrial recessive ataxia syndrome (MIRAS) *(15q25; POLG1)* A form described in Finland, characterized by the childhood or adult onset of seizures, polyneuropathy, cramps, athetosis, and tremor.

Portneuf spastic ataxia (SPAX3) *(2q33–34)* Reported in a French-Canadian kindred with the onset in childhood or later of a spastic-ataxic syndrome with dystonias, scoliosis, and sometimes evidence of cortical atrophy.

Posterior column + retinitis pigmentosa (1q31) A form presenting in early childhood with visual failure, thick-fiber sensory neuropathy and areflexia, and achalasia.

Recessive ataxia of the Beauce (6q) A nearly pure form of ataxia described from Quebec with adult onset and slow progression, showing minimal pyramidal findings.

Recessive ataxia with upward gaze palsy and seizures (9q34) An early-onset form.[6088]

Salla syndrome (sialic acid storage disease) (SLC17A) *(6q14)*

Spastic ataxia with leukopencephalopathy

Vanishing white matter disease See **fatal infantile leukodystrophy.**

Vitamin E deficiency: α-tocopherol transfer protein: *(8q13)* An early-onset form resembling **Friedereich ataxia** but also manifesting thick-fiber sensory losses, skin xanthelasmas, and sometimes dystonias or titubation

Xeroderma pigmentosum.

Chart C–9c. The Congenital Ataxias

Aprosencephaly *with cerebellar dysgenesis*. A syndrome in which the optic chiasm and mesencephalon are absent, the metencephalon: poorly formed, and the cerebellum severely dysplastic.

Ataxia and pancreatic aplasia (PTF1A) *(10p13)*

Ataxia with photomyoclonus A dominantly inherited syndrome characterized by extreme sensitivity to light, with myoclonus, cerebellar ataxia, ataxic gait, pes cavus, kyphosis, and dementia.[1830] It may manifest later in life. This condition and **MERRF** (myoclonus epilepsy with ragged red fibers) are probably the same.

Ataxic **cerebral palsy** *(9p12–q12)* Described in one Asian family.

A type formerly called *ADCA type IV*. Cerebellar signs with myoclonus and deafness characterize this group, which may not be a distinct entity. See *May-White syndrome* and **MERRF**.

Behr syndrome The combination of bilateral optic atrophy, pyramidal and posterior column signs, mental retardation, and ataxia.

Carbohydrate deficient glycoprotein syndrome (PMM2) *(16p.13.2)* A recessively inherited syndrome of psychomotor retardation, hypotonia, truncal ataxia, and demyelinating polyneuropathy as well as systemic dysmorphisms.

Cerebellar hemisphere hypoplasia (congenital granular cell hypoplasia) A syndrome of ataxia and mental retardation, each of variable severity.[6766]

Cerebellar ataxia 1 (CLA1; Norman; CPD III; SCAR2) *(9q34-9qter)* A nonprogressive ataxic syndrome with cognitive failure and short stature, reported in a single Lebanese family.

CAMOS (SCAR5) *(15q24) A recessive form reported from the Lebanon, characterized by congenitalataxia, pyramidal signs, mental retardation, optic atrophy, and microcephaly.*

Cerebellar ataxia 3 (SCAR6) *(20q11)* A nonprogressive, recessive syndrome of motor and speech impairment with cerebellar ataxia, mild pyramidal signs, short stature, and pes planus, reported from Norway.

Cerebellar hypoplasia with cerebral gyral simplification (VLDLR) *(9p24)* Described in the Hutterite population, this nonprogressive syndrome comprises mental retardation, strabismus, pes planus, seizures, and short stature.

Cerebellotrigeminaldermal dysplasia (Gómez–López-Hernández syndrome) A recessive or sporadic syndrome manifesting craniosynostosis, short stature, corneal, opacities, facial dysmorphisms, trigeminal anesthesia, and mental retardation.

COACH syndrome A syndrome of early-onset ataxia, mental retardation, spasticity, and craniofacial dysmorphisms.

Congenital ataxia with choroidal colobomas (**Pfeiffer syndrome**)

Congenital cerebellar atrophy A dominantly inherited syndrome in which ataxia complicates early mild motor delay.[2244]

Congenital muscular dystrophies

Dandy–Walker syndrome

Dysequilibrium syndrome A rare congenital, nonprogressive autosomal recessively inherited ataxic syndrome characterized by ataxia, hypotonia, severe postural disturbance, strabismus, delay in achieving language, and often severe mental and motor retardation.[2677]

Fibroblast growth factor receptor-3 deficiency

Gillespie syndrome A congenital ataxia with partial aniridia, fixed dilated pupils, infantile spasms hypotonia, choreoathetosis, and mental and developmental delay. The inheritance pattern is undefined.[2382]

Joubert syndromes (recessively inherited congenital ataxia with episodic hyperpnea, abnormal eye movements, and mental retardation).

Lhermitte–Duclos disease (*granular cell hypertrophy*)

Lissencephaly

A. *With cleft palate and cerebellar hypoplasia* A syndrome lethal in the first week of life.

B. *With cerebellar hypoplasia (7q22)* Recessively inherited lissencephaly with added cognitive delay, seizures, nystagmus, myopia, hypotonia, and lymphedema.

NARP syndrome (**N**europathy, **A**taxia, and **R**etinitis **P**igmentosa).

Neonatal cerebellar atrophy with retinal dystrophy A fatal syndrome of neonatal ataxia with retinal dystrophy and limitation of joint movement complicated by diarrhea, vomiting, pericardial effusion, and hepatic fibrosis.

Olivopontocerebellar atrophy with hepatic cirrhosis and retinal dystrophy A congenitally inherited ataxic syndrome with cerebellar hemisphere hypoplasia, characterized by pericarditis, neonatal feeding problems, hypotonia, pigmentary retinopathy, abnormal enlarged liver, joint contractures, and mental and developmental delay.[381]

Paine syndrome

Pitt–Hopkins syndrome (TCF-4) *(18q21)* A syndrome of mental retardation with intermittent hyperventilation, severe psychomotor delay, facial dysmorphisms, and seizures.

Pontocerebellar hypoplasia

PCH1: An ataxic syndrome with added *spinal muscular atrophy*;

PCH2: With progressive cerebral atrophy, dyskinesias, microcephaly, and spasticity;

PCH3: With progressive microcephaly (CLAM) *(7q11)* described in Oman;

PCH4: A fatal infantile form with microcephaly, myoclonus, and hypertonia;

PCH5: With fetal onset, lethal *in utero*;

PCH6: Pontocerebellar hypoplasia;

RARS2; A syndrome of microcephaly, spasticity, and seizures. Almost all of these are recessively inherited.

Progressive ataxia, retinal degeneration, peripheral neuropathy, myopathy, and mental subnormality A rare congenital syndrome in which the above manifestations are accompanied by hypoparathyroidism.

There are also other forms associated with **congenital muscular dystrophies**, chromosomal abnormalities, etc.

Chart C–9d. X-Linked Cerebellar Ataxias

These are rare syndromes characterized by various combinations of visual loss, mild spastic paraparesis, mental slowing, myoclonic seizures, extrapyramidal deficits, posterior column demyelination, peripheral motor neuropathy, and pes cavus with onset in infancy.[254, 2755] They include the following:

Arts syndrome (PRPS1) *(Xq22.3)* A form presenting with early-onset hypotonia, leading on to flaccid tetraplegia with areflexia, and deafness.
Ataxia + epilepsy (OPHN1) *(Xq12)* A recessively inherited syndrome manifesting mental retardation, seizures, and myoclonus, hypotonia, squint, facial dysmorphisms, and hypogenitalism.
Ataxia and dementia (SCAX4) A syndrome of ataxia with dementia, described in one kinship, with delayed walking, tremor, pyramidal tract signs, and cognitive failure; the onset can be at any time from childhood to adult life.
Ataxia and sideroblastic anemia (ABC7) *(Xq13)* A nonprogressive ataxic syndrome also manifesting pyramidal signs, anemia, and the presence of ring sideroblasts in the bone marrow.
Ataxia with severe mental retardation (Xq24–q27) A recessively inherited syndrome with epilepsy, ophthalmoplegia, and craniofacial dysmorphisms.
CASM (Xpter-q13.1) The combination of cataracts, ataxia, short stature, and mental retardation added to the ataxia.
Congenital X-linked ataxia (SCAX1) *(Xp11)* This form manifests nonprogressive ataxia, hypotonia, and motor delay from birth.
Congenital X-linked ataxia (SCAX2) A single kindred reported, with spasticity, rigidity, and early death.
Congenital X-linked ataxia (ataxia-deafness syndrome) (SCAX3) A progressive and lethal syndrome, whose clinical features are onset in infancy with hypotonia, sensorineural deafness, optic atrophy, and developmental delay.
Congenital X-linked ataxia (SCAX5) *(Xq25)* A single kindred presenting with severe but nonprogressive neonatal hypotonia and motor developmental delay.
Congenital X-linked ataxia (Xq23) A form manifesting delay in walking and speaking, dysarthria, and external ophthalmoplegia which is nonprogressive after childhood.
Hoyeraal-Hreidarsson syndrome (Xq28; DKC1, dyskerin) A progressive syndrome, with onset in infancy manifesting pancytopenia, dyskeratosis, and growth retardation.
Mental retardation-epilepsy (Xq24; SLC9A6) A form resembling **Angelman syndrome**, characterized by the onset of seizures within the first 2 years of life with severe mental retardation, occasional pyramidal signs, and dysphagia.
Tremor and cognitive decline (FXTAS) *(Xq27; FMR1)* See **Fragile X syndrome.**
X-*linked mental retardation with short stature, small testes, muscle wasting and tremor (Xq23; Cullin 4B)* A recessive form characterized by low birth weight, mental and developmental delay, impaired or absent speech, seizures, short stature, increased head circumference, and hyperextensible joints.
See also **Pelizaeus–Merzbacher syndrome** (allelic variant), **adrenomyeloneuropathy**, and **Rett syndrome.**

Chart C–10. Cerebellar Ataxias (*variants* or Forms Not Classified Above)

I. Ataxias with Known Metabolic or Other Cause

A. Intermittent ataxic syndromes:
Hyperammonemias:
Citrullinemia (ornithine transcarbylamase deficiency)
Hyperornithinemia
Aminoacidurias
Hartnup disease
Pyruvate and lactic acid dysmetabolism
Episodic ataxias
Argininosuccinuria
Arginase deficiency
PDH deficiency

B. Other progressive ataxic syndromes:
Abetalipoproteinemia
Adrenoleukodystrophy
Celiac disease
Cerebrotendinous xanthomatosis
GDH deficiency
Hexosaminidase deficiency
(GM_2 gangliosidosis)
Hypobetalipoproteinemia
Hypoxanthine-guanine phosphoribotransferase deficiency.
Krabbe leukodystrophy
Metachromatic leukodystrophy
Mitochondrial encephalomyopathies
Neuronal ceroid lipofuscinosis

Sialidosis
Sphingomyelin storage disorders
Vitamin E deficiency
Wilson disease
X-linked ataxia, ichthyosis, and tapetoretinal dystrophy (arylsulfatase C deficiency)
See also **metachromatic leukodystrophy**.

C. Ataxic disorders associated with defective DNA repair
Ataxia-telangiectasia
Xeroderma pigmentosum
Cockayne syndrome

II. *Early-onset ataxias of unknown cause (onset usually before 20 years)*

Friedreich ataxia Among the spinocerebellar degenerations in this group, this is the form most commonly diagnosed, but such a statement (while true globally) is inappropriate in certain parts of the world, where variants may be far more frequent. Next most commonly reported is the syndrome of early-onset cerebellar ataxia with retained reflexes (see the following entry). Most of these syndromes are recessively inherited and differ from Friedreich ataxia in the absence (with certain exceptions as below) of optic atrophy, diabetes, cardiac involvement, and severe skeletal deformity.

A *variant* is *early onset cerebellar ataxia of unknown cause* (Friedreich ataxia with retained reflexes) A syndrome resembling **Friedreich ataxia** but with retention of the muscle stretch reflexes and with a better prospect of continuing function.[3488]

"Pure" cerebellar ataxias with late onset (formerly known as adult-onset cerebellar ataxia III: olivopontocerebellar atrophy, parenchymatous cerebellar cortical atrophy, cerebellopontine atrophy, late cortical cerebellar atrophy, Marie–Foix–Alajouanine syndrome, Thomas atrophy). This is a group of ataxic disorders of unknown etiology (often dominantly inherited) with onset usually after the age of 50 years,[2753] in which corticospinal, extrapyramidal, and ocular features are not prominent and sensory loss is absent. The chief pathological change is cerebellar cortical atrophy with loss of the Purkinje cell layer.[199, 2940] Some of the syndromes are complicated by **myoclonus** (see **Ramsay Hunt syndrome**) while occasional families have also been described in which the ataxia is associated with deafness, tapetoretinal or pigmentary retinal degeneration, optic atrophy, macular degeneration, dementia, extrapyramidal disorders, peripheral neuropathy, etc.:

Ataxia with ocular motor apraxia type I (AOA1) A recessively inherited ataxic syndrome of childhood associated with oculomotor apraxia, hypoalbuminemia, and hypercholesterolemia. Cerebellar ataxia with cerebellar atrophy on MRI and severe axonal sensorimotor neuropathy are invariable; oculomotor apraxia, hypoalbuminemia, hypercholesterolemia, and initial choreic movements are frequent. Missense or truncating mutations in the aprataxin gene (*APTX*) appear responsible.[3731] The disorder is mapped to 9q13 and is reported mainly from Japan and Portugal.

Ataxia-oculomotor apraxia 17 A recessively inherited ataxia associated with an elevation in α-fetoprotein as in ataxia-telangiectasia and, in one *variant*, with mutations in senataxin.[4576]

Ataxia with OLG mutations A syndrome of ataxia with various CNS features including epilepsy, myoclonus, cognitive decline, nystagmus, dysarthria, thalamic and cerebellar white matter lesions on MRI, and neuronal loss in discrete gray nuclei on autopsy. Gastrointestinal dysmotility, weight loss, cardiomyopathy, and valproate-induced hepatotoxicity occurr less frequently.

Hypo- or hypergonadism: ataxia with hypergonadotrophic hypogonadism (Skre syndrome) A recessively inherited syndrome of gait and limb ataxia, also characterized by cataract, primary amenorrhea, streak ovaries, small testes, ophthalmoplegias, loss of pain sensation, and mental and developmental delay.[4182]

Myoclonus

Ramsay Hunt syndrome This represents more than one condition, including **mitochondrial encephalomyopathy**, **sialidosis**, and **Baltic myoclonus**. See **progressive myoclonus epilepsy**.

Childhood ataxia with diffuse central nervous system demyelination A progressive neurological disorder, also classified as a leukodystrophy, characterized clinically by progressive ataxic diplegia with onset before the age of 5 and with MRI and pathological evidence of confluent white matter disease.[5599]

Forms with congenital or childhood-onset deafness

Ataxia with sensory deafness and optic atrophy A dominantly inherited ataxic syndrome with onset in childhood, characterized by sensorineural deafness, optic atrophy, and neurogenic muscle atrophy.[381]

Ataxia with deaf-mutism and muscular wasting 1. (early onset) A congenital inherited ataxic syndrome characterized by sensorineural deafness, pyramidal signs, neurogenic muscle atrophy with fasciculations, and thick-fiber sensory neuropathy.[1714, 2328] 2. (late onset) An inherited ataxic syndrome characterized by sensorineural deafness, endocrinopathy, spasticity, axonal motor neuropathy, and thick-fiber sensory neuropathy.

Forms with optic atrophy, pigmentary retinopathy, or cataract, with or without mental retardation

Richards–Rundle syndrome

Marinesco–Sjögren syndrome A recessively inherited ataxic syndrome with onset in childhood, also characterized by cataract, proximal and distal myopathy, and mental and developmental delay.[4082]

Ataxia with retinal degeneration A dominantly inherited ataxic syndrome characterized variously by such additional features as macular degeneration, optic atrophy, pigmentary retinopathy, nerve deafness, peripheral neuropathy, mental retardation, external ophthalmoplegia, pyramidal and extrapyramidal signs, myoclonus, myocardial sclerosis and skin lesions, and the presence of abnormal mitochondria.[2755, 3156] Kinships in which this syndrome is recessively inherited are also described.[2755] See also MERRF.

continued

Chart C–10. (*continued*)

Other variant early-onset ataxias of unknown etiology include the following:

Ataxia with albinism An inherited ataxic syndrome characterized by dysarthria, motor neuropathy, diffuse depigmentation of skin, and mental and developmental delay.[381]

Ataxia with ocular motor apraxia An inherited ataxic syndrome with onset in infancy or childhood also characterized by chorea and athetosis.[76] This and **ataxia-telangiectasia** are possibly the same condition.

Ataxia with pallido-nigro-luysian atrophy and Lewy bodies.[4490]

Ataxia with paroxysmal dystonia An inherited ataxic syndrome with onset in infancy or childhood, also characterized by dysarthria, paroxysmal dystonia, and pyramidal signs.[2542]

Ataxia with pupillary paralysis A static inherited ataxic syndrome with onset in early adult life in which these features accompany pes cavus, kyphoscoliosis, VI nerve palsy, cataract, kyphoscoliosis, and pes cavus.[6141]

Benign cerebellatr ataxia with extensive thermoanalgesia A dominantly inherited variant with associated demyelinating neuropathy affecting especially the smaller fibers. [5071]

Early onset ataxia with cardiomyopathy and retained reflexes A variant phenotype of **Friedreich ataxia,** also mapping to chromosome 9q.[4864]

Early-onset recessive cerebellar ataxia and progressive distal limb wasting without ocular or other telangiectasias, frequent infections or immunodeficiencies, also characterized by incapacitating myoclonus in childhood and youth, in which cytogenetic analysis isactually compatible with the diagnosis of ataxia-telagiectasia.[2537]

Familial intermittent ataxia An X-linked recessive, paroxysmal ataxic syndrome with onset in infancy or early childhood, also characterized by dysarthria, apraxias, neurodegenerative regression and abnormal lactate, and pyruvate metabolism.[3883]

Familial spinocerebellar degeneration with corneal dystrophy An inherited ataxic syndrome with congenital or infantile onset, also characterized by cloudy corneas.[381]

Jeune syndrome.

Myokymia and periodic ataxia An inherited ataxic syndrome with onset in infancy and also characterized by paroxysmal dystonia and myokymia.[5321]

Progressive visual and hearing loss, progressive spastic paraplegia, cerebellar ataxia, and dementia A syndrome with these findings may be dominantly or recessively inherited.

Spino-olivo-cerebellar degeneration with ophthalmoplegia A recessively inherited ataxic syndrome characterized by colobomas of the optic nerve, dementia, ophthalmoplegia, paraplegia, demyelination, and pancytopenia.[1448]

Wadia–Swami syndrome

In still other rare *variants* (summarized by Baraitser[379]) cerebellar ataxia is combined with brachydactyly and nystagmus, erythrokeratodermia, gutathione deficiency, or skin hyperpigmentation, and there remain others not easily classified:

Adult onset cerebellar ataxia and sensory deafness (of Schimke) An inherited ataxic syndrome with onset in adult life, also manifesting sensorineural deafness and high arches of the feet.[381]

Adult-onset autosomal recessive ataxia with thalamic lesions described once in a Finnish family.[5188]

Ataxia and other neurological deficits with hyperuricemia An inherited ataxic syndrome with onset in youth or adult life, characterized by ophthalmoplegia, facial palsy, sensorineural deafness, dysarthria, cardiomyopathy, nephropathy, and hyperuricemia.[381]

Ataxia with cataracts, hemiballismus, and dementia An inherited ataxic syndrome with onset in adult life, also characterized by cataract, tics, pyramidal and extrapyramidal signs, muscle cramp, and dementia.[381]

Ataxia with downbeat nystagmus A recessively inherited ataxic syndrome with onset in young adult life characterized also by dysarthria, dysphagia, vertical nystagmus, and pyramidal signs.[381]

Ataxia with fasciculations A dominantly inherited condition with onset in young adult life, described (once) in India.[5865]

Ataxia with ichthyosis and hepatosplenomegaly (of Harper) An inherited ataxic syndrome with onset in mature adult life, characterized by dysarthria, enlarged liver and spleen, dementia, ophthalmoplegia, hyperkeratosis, and ichthyosis.[381]

Ataxia with photomyoclonus and skeletal deformities An inherited ataxic syndrome with onset in adult life and characterized by dysarthria kyphosis, high arches of feet, dementia, and myoclonus.[381]

Ataxia with vitamin E deficiency[4832]

Ataxia-telangiectasia

Autosomal recessive late-onset ataxia A rare, recessively inherited syndrome with onset in adult life, characterized by ataxia, supranuclear ophthalmoplegias, facial impassivity, pseudobulbar and pyramidal signs, peripheral neuropathy, and pure cerebellar cortical atrophy.[2758] Thalamic lesions also may occur.[5188]

Benign hereditary cerebellar ataxia with extensive thermoanalgesia A dominantly inherited variant in which a length-dependent axonal neuropathy results from the loss of primary sensory afferents subserving pain and temperature sensation.[5070]

Cerebellar ataxia with myoclonus and deafness (May–White syndrome) A very slowly progressive, dominantly inherited syndrome characterized by onset in late childhood or adolescence of cerebellar ataxia and impaired vision due to pigmentary retinopathy. Spasticity occurs in some cases but mental deterioration is not found.[4187]

Familial cerebellar ataxia with cerebrovascular amyloid An inherited ataxic syndrome with onset in young adult life characterized by dementia, pyramidal signs, and cerebrovascular disease.[3925]

Familial periodic ataxia A syndrome characterized by the onset in childhood of attacks of ataxia, dysarthria, vertigo, and nystagmus lasting hours to days. Drowsiness, headache, fever, and vomiting may also occur. A response to acetazolamide is reported. The signs usually remit completely between attacks.[1685] Similarities to **basilar migraine** are notable.

Familial spastic ataxia A dominantly inherited ataxic syndrome with onset at any age, characterized by spastic-ataxic dysarthria, dementia, vertical nystagmus, optic atrophy, pyramidal signs, and variable sensory neuropathic signs.

Idiopathic late-onset cerebellar ataxia A heterogeneous group of familial or sporadic cerebellar syndromes without a known familial basis.[2751]

Late-onset hereditary ataxia with global thermoanalgesia and absence of fungiform papillae on the tongue An ataxic syndrome, probably dominantly inherited, with these features and sensorineural deafness, canal paresis, ageusia and numerous signs of autonomic disease, thus resembling **hereditary sensory and autonomic neuropathy** types II or III. The onset in the single Japanese report published was in mid-adult life.[2235]

Spinocerebellar degeneration with motor system involvement A rare variant with onset in adult life, characterized by ataxia, amyotrophy, and ophthalmoplegia, resembling spinocerebellar degenerative diseases.[2804] Pyramidal signs and generalized neuropathic muscle atrophy and weakness leading to respiratory difficulties have also been described in this cluster.

Spinopontine degeneration.

III. Late-onset recessive ataxias

These are very rare and no diagnostic criteria are available. See also **palatal tremor.**

Baraitser[379] summarized the reports of the adult-onset cerebellar ataxias above (cerebellar ataxia plus) and classified them as follows:

1. Syndromes with added ophthalmological signs and pyramidal or extrapyramidal signs
2. Syndromes with added retinitis pigmentosa
3. Syndromes with added peripheral neuropathy; in which features of **hereditary motor and sensory neuropathy** are found in association with cerebellar ataxia. One such is *Ziegler syndrome*, in which ataxia, rigidity, fasciculations, Parkinsonism, and signs of peripheral neuropathy are found.
4. Late-onset pure cerebellar ataxias without associated features. These comprise two groups of complicated and "pure" ataxic syndromes with onset in adult life.
   A. *Recessive inheritance* Those inherited recessively are rarer than other recessive ataxias. They may be variously associated with downbeat nystagmus, hypogonadism, deafness, pigmentary retinopathy, or optic atrophy.
   B. *Dominant inheritance* Rare syndromes in which affected family members also show other features apart from the ataxia and which thus are not completely "pure."[2751]

Cerebellar ataxia is also a feature of the following syndromes, noted elsewhere:

Ataxia-telangiectasia	**Chediak–Higashi syndrome**
Flynn–Aird syndrome	**Hartnup disease**
Ketotic hyperglycinemia	**Non-ketotic hyperglycinemia**
Pyruvate decarboxylase deficiency	**Richards–Rundle syndrome**
Intermittent branched-chain ketoaciduria	

See also **Biemond ataxia, Kuru, hypertrophia musculorum vera, periodic ataxias, idiopathic late-onset cerebellar ataxias, Joseph disease,** and **delayed-onset cerebellar syndrome.**

Hereditary spastic parapareses/paraplegias This final group again includes both pure and complicated forms. A historical review was provided by Konigsmark.[3527] See **hereditary spastic paraparesis.**

---

compiled by the National Institute of Neurological Disorders and Stroke.

www.ncbi.nlm.nih.gov/bookshelf/br.fcgi?book=gene&part=friedreich/, an informational site.

cerebellar ataxia with celiac disease

The concurrence of these conditions; the patients do not have specific or diagnostic neurological signs other than the ataxia.[4968]

cerebellar ataxia with crossed III nerve palsy

(Claude syndrome) A **lacunar syndrome** presenting with dysarthria, cerebellar ataxia, and facial numbness.[2092, 2106]

cerebellar ataxia with hypogonadotrophic hypogonadism

See **cerebellar ataxias.**

cerebellar ataxia with myoclonus and deafness

See **cerebellar ataxias.**

cerebellar ataxia with retained reflexes

See **cerebellar ataxias.**

cerebellar ataxia with retinal degeneration

See **cerebellar ataxias.**

cerebellar ataxia with torticollis

The combination of a slowly progressive ataxic syndrome and cervical dystonia. Onset is in childhood or adult life and transmission either autosomal dominant or mitochondrial.[6475]

cerebellar catalepsy sign

Oscillation of the trunk and legs of patients with cerebellar lesions when their legs, flexed at the hips and knees, are passively raised from the bed. The sign was described by **Babiński** in 1902, but has not found favor.[323]

cerebellar cataplexy

The ability of certain patients with cerebellar disease to hold a static posture of the legs with statuesque immobility while they cannot walk or move the legs through space without gross ataxia. The test serves when positive to differentiate between sensory ataxias and those of cerebellar origin.[1548] This sign was first described by Babiński in 1902.

cerebellar catatonia

The ability of certain patients with cerebellar disease to hold a posture of the legs with statuesque immobility while they cannot walk or move the legs through space without gross ataxia. When positive, the test serves to differentiate between sensory ataxias and those of cerebellar origin.[1548]

cerebellar cognitive affective syndrome Behavioral changes occurring in patients with lesions involving the posterior lobe of the cerebellum and the vermis, characterized by impairment of executive functions such as planning, set shifting, verbal fluency, abstract reasoning, and working memory; difficulties with spatial cognition including visual-spatial organization and memory; personality change with blunting of affect or disinhibited and inappropriate behavior; and language deficits including agrammatism and dysprosodia. Lesions of the anterior lobe of the cerebellum produce only minor changes in executive and visual-spatial functions.

The constellation of deficits is suggestive of disruption of the cerebellar modulation of neural circuits that link prefrontal, posterior parietal, superior temporal, and limbic cortices with the cerebellum.[5612]

cerebellar cortical degeneration An autoimmune nonmetastatic **paraneoplastic syndrome** of the CNS manifesting evidence of widespread cerebellar atrophy with loss of Purkinje cells, occurring in patients with carcinoma of the bronchus or ovary or with lymphoma, and in which an immunologic response induced by the tumor causes a secondary immune reaction in specific brain areas because of shared antigens.[803]

cerebellar diaschisis A reduction in blood flow and oxygen utilization in the cerebellar hemisphere contralateral to a supratentorial infarct[416, 417] due to an interruption of afferent input along the corticopontocerebellar pathway.

cerebellar diplegia The term applied by Frederick **Batten** in 1903 to what is now known as **ataxic cerebral palsy**.

cerebellar disorders Syndromes characterized by **ataxia**, **nystagmus**, alterations in muscle tone, and **gait disorder** resulting from disorders affecting the cerebellum or its connections.

These are classified in this book as **cerebellar ataxias**, where there is a known hereditary basis for the condition; as **ataxic syndromes**, where the ataxia is a major feature but no familial tendency is known; and randomly, where cerebellar signs occur as one feature of other syndromes.

cerebellar "fits" Tonic extensor spasms of the trunk and limbs resulting from tonsillar herniation or a **Chiari malformation**. Clinical evidence of raised intracranial pressure will be present. The EEG shows only slow activity with no suggestion of epilepsy.

cerebellar hemangioblastoma A malignant vascular tumor of the cerebellum, commonly occurring in patients with **von Hippel–Lindau** disease.

cerebellar hemisphere hypoplasia See **cerebellar ataxias.**

cerebellar hypoplasia with cerebral gyral simplification See **cerebellar ataxia.**

cerebellar imitation synkineses Similar movements occurring in the hand or foot 200 ms or so after the contralateral one is moved. This may occur in patients with cerebellar degenerative diseases.[3257]

cerebellar migraine A distinct form of late-onset autosomal dominant **cerebellar ataxia** in which the ataxia occurs during recovery from attacks of hemiplegic migraine, the patients ultimately suffering from persistent ataxia, with cerebellar atrophy shown radiologically.[5271] See also **familial hemiplegic migraine**.

cerebellar mutism (mutism and subsequent dysarthria) Loss of speech a day or two after an acute cerebellar event such as removal of a chronic mid-cerebellar tumor, or with stroke or encephalitis. Speech returns usually within 6 months, but there is severe ataxic dysarthria. Consciousness is retained and there are no accompanying deficits on examination of the lower cranial nerves but in children, neurobehavioral disorders and pyramidal signs may be manifest.

The mechanism is not determined but the condition is associated with hydrocephalus at presentation, localization of the tumor adjacent to the IV ventricle, and post-surgical edema of the pontine tegmentum.[1406, 6491]

cerebellar outflow tremor See **rubral or midbrain tremor**.

cerebellar posture A term introduced by **Batten** in 1903 for that position of the head in which "the occiput is turned to one side and the chin to the other and at the same time flexed to the side to which the occiput was directed." The same posture occurs after labyrinthine extirpation and "is the result of interference with a tonic reflex in which the extensor muscles of the neck, under the influence of impulses from the labyrinths, are maintained in a state of tonus adequate to resist the effect of gravity on the head."[798]

cerebellar seizures See **diencephalic autonomic seizures.**

cerebellar signs Postural **hypotonia**, **pendular reflexes**, **asthenia** and fatigability, **ataxia**, **decomposition of movement**, **asynergy**, **nystagmus**, **dysmetria**, **tremor**, loss of associated movements, drooping of the shoulder, and abnormalities in the rate, regularity, and force of voluntary movements occurring as a result of disease of the cerebellum or of its connections.[2962] See **cerebellar tremors**. In patients with cerebellar tumors, symptoms and signs have been defined as vertigo, deafness, tinnitus, weakness in homolateral conjugate gaze, VI nerve palsies, skew deviation, horizontal jerk nystagmus, involvement of the V and VII cranial nerves, homolateral limb weakness with asthenia, paresis of homolateral trunk muscles, hypotonia of the homolateral limbs, ataxia, with reeling gait, intention tremour, postural deficits, and variable muscle stretch reflex activity.[6062]

cerebellar tonic seizures See **diencephalic autonomic seizures**.

cerebellar tremors Various forms of involuntary alternating movement due to disease of the cerebellum or of its connections. Such tremors are proximal, occur with movement, displace the limb at right angles to the intended direction of movement, and increase in amplitude when they approach the target.[JF] The frequency is usually less than 5 Hz.

The various forms of cerebellar tremor have been classified by Sabra and Hallet [5486] (See Chart C–11.) See also **titubation**.

cerebello-olivary degeneration A dominantly inherited form of cerebellar ataxia[2956] with abnormal motor and sensory conduction in peripheral nerves. See **Holmes disease**.

Chart C–11. Varieties of Cerebellar Tremor

Action tremor: A tremor occurring with postural maintenance or goal-directed movement.
Cerebellar tremor at rest: A tremor seen when the body part appears to be completely relaxed, although there is actually some slight background muscular contraction.
Epipaxic postural tremor: A tremor occurring just after the performance of a goal-directed movement.
Intention tremor (kinetic cerebellar, ataxia or hyperkinetic tremor): A tremor appearing with goal-directed movements, often worse terminally.
Mild postural cerebellar tremor (postural, simple, static, propaxic postural, or epipaxic postural tremors): A mild tremor occurring early or late during sustained postural maintenance or just before (propaxic) or after (epipaxic) a goal-directed movement.
Propaxic postural tremor: Tremor occurring just before the performance of a goal-directed movement.
Severe postural cerebellar tremor (rubral, superior cerebellar peduncle, peduncular, or hyperkinetic tremor): A severe tremor at 2.5–4 Hz occurring with postural maintenance, present at rest, persisting during maintenance of a posture, and worsening with goal-directed movements. It is usually associated with **dysmetria**.

Adapted from Sabra AF, Hallett M. Action tremor with alternating activity in antagonist muscles. Neurology *1984;34:151–6. Reproduced by kind permission of the American Academy of Neurology and Lippincott Williams and Wilkins.)*

cerebellopontine angle tumor Any extra-axial mass situated beside the pontomedullary junction and abutting the internal auditory meatus. Pressure upon the roots of cranial nerves V, VII, and VIII and on the cerebellum are responsible for the usual clinical findings.[364] The most common form is the vestibular **schwannoma**.

cerebellotrigeminodermal dysplasia See **cerebellar ataxia**.

cerebellum (Lat, diminutive of brain) The hindbrain, situated in the posterior fossa and behind the pons. It was considered to be the seat of sexual appetite by Fraser (1880) but was shown to function in the coordination of voluntary movements by **Flourens** and regarded as the head ganglion of the proprioceptive system by **Sherrington**. The name was first applied by Erasistratus, a Greek physician and anatomist, around 300–250 BC.

cerebral (from Lat, cerebrum, the brain) Pertaining to the brain.

cerebral abscess An infective lesion of the brain substance. Though commonly bacterial, other organisms may produce focal encephalitis with liquefaction and the formation of a capsule, which are the hallmarks of an abscess. *Toxoplasma, Cryptococcus,* and *Mycobacterium tuberculosis* are all nonpyogenic causes of abscess, but pyogenic abscesses are more common. Infection may spread hematologically from a distant site, particularly in patients with congenital heart disease; or may spread directly from infected cranial structures such as the middle ear or the nasal sinuses. The clinical features are those of increased intracranial pressure, focal deficits and meningeal inflammation in any combination. The frequency of cerebral abscesses, particularly of those due to toxoplasmosis, is now increasing in the wake of the epidemic of HIV infections.

The first systematic account was published in 1856 by Hermann Lebert (1813–1878).

cerebral acanthocytosis An hereditary syndrome of tics, self-mutilation, dystonia, and personality change associated with the presence of acanthocytes in the fresh peripheral blood smear. See **neuroacanthocytosis**.

cerebral akinetopsia (cerebral motion blindness) A syndrome in which a patient loses specifically the ability to perceive visual motion, as a result of cortical lesions outside the striate area.[6963]

cerebral amyloid angiopathy (congophilic angiopathy, cerebral angiopathy, dyshoric angiopathy) An age-related condition characterized by deposition of amyloid protein (Aβ) fibrils outside the internal elastic lamina of the small- and medium-sized leptomeningeal vessels and the pial and cortical arterioles, with acellular thickening of their walls. The amorphous, eosinophilic amyloid material stains with Congo red and shows birefringence under polarized light. The peripheral vessels are unaffected.

The condition is progressively more common in older populations; it occurs sporadically, but dominantly inherited forms have been described in Iceland and the Netherlands.[3321] The vessels affected are those running from the leptomeninges to the cerebral cortex, leading to hypoperfusion and multiple small infarcts and hemorrhages into the cortex (lobar hemorrhages) and to demyelination of the underlying white matter. Systemic amyloidosis is not present.

Clinically the picture is that of multiple or recurrent lobar intracerebral hemorrhages (15% of all cases) with pyramidal signs, internal and external ophthalmoplegias, and dementia (if there are symptoms at all; the condition has been detected in healthy elderly people and in those with **Down syndrome, Alzheimer disease**, and other dementing illnesses of that type[913]). For further discussion of the dementing syndrome, see **congophilic angiopathy**. *Variants* are listed under **familial amyloid neuropathy**.

cerebral aneurysmal arteriopathy Diffuse dilation of the arteries arising from the circle of Willis, due to hypoperfusion and/or septic emboli and seen particularly in children with AIDS.[1734]

cerebral angiomas Arteriovenous communications which are established through the medium of a mass of abnormal cerebral vessels which take the place of the usual capillary bed. The usual clinical presentation is with focal seizures followed by **Todd paresis** in patients aged less than 30 years at the first presentation, and who develop a slowly progressive hemiparesis or sensory loss on the affected side. In some cases, headache, subarachnoid hemorrhage, or the presence of a bruit suggests the diagnosis.[4002]

cerebral angiopathy (dyshoric angiopathy) See **cerebral amyloid angiopathy**.

cerebral angiopathy of toxemia Multisegment narrowing of the cerebral arteries resulting from hypertension-induced vasoconstriction in women with toxemia of pregnancy. The syndrome presents with headache, focal neurological signs, seizures, and decreased consciousness; there may be lymphocytic pleocytosis in the CSF. The prognosis is generally favorable.[6394]

cerebral apophysis The pineal gland.

cerebral apoplexy Intracerebral hemorrhage.

cerebral atonic-astatic syndrome See **Forster syndrome**.

cerebral auscultation See **cephalic bellows sound**.

cerebral autosomal dominant arteriopathy with subcortical infarcts and leukoencephalopathy (CADASIL) A dominantly inherited systemic vascular disease and a cause of multiple lacunar infarcts in adults, mainly in the white matter and basal ganglia. The clinical presentation is usually with multiple episodes of migraine (usually associated with aura) in young adult life, later leading to recurrent subcortical infarcts with pseudobulbar palsy and vascular dementia. However, the infarcts that occur are often silent.

Other manifestations appearing within 20 years of onset include gait disturbance, pseudobulbar palsy, mood disturbances, neurosensory hearing loss, urinary incontinence, cognitive impairment, and seizures. The dementia has a subcortical and frontal presentation, with behavioral symptoms, amnesia, disturbed executive functions, bradyphrenia, slowing of information processing, and frontal symptoms without aphasia, apraxia, or agnosia.

The condition is due to a *NOTCH3* mutation on chromosome 19p13 (or 19p12). Histopathologically, an eosinophilic granular deposit is seen in the media of the small penetrating cerebral arteries causing vascular obliteration and multiple infarcts, mainly in the white matter, basal ganglia, and leptomeninges. Magnetic resonance imaging shows hyperintensities in the periventricular and deep white matter, basal ganglia, and brainstem, but the diagnosis is best made by skin biopsy, which shows granular, electron-dense osmophilic material.[1074, 1801, 5462] See also **CADASIL coma**.

cerebral beriberi See **Wernicke syndrome**.

cerebral blood flow The totality of the volume of blood delivered to the brain. This is usually constant at 55 ml/100 g/min if the pCO_2 is constant, depending on local activation. Measurement is with intracarotid or inhaled xenon,[133] a gamma emitter, using the Kety–Schmidt equation (the amount of a substance entering or leaving the brain in a given time is equal to the difference in its arteriovenous concentration times the blood flow; thus the cerebral metabolic rate of oxygen = $\{PaO_2 - PvO_2\} \times$ blood flow). Two clearance rates are normally measured, fast from gray matter and slow from white matter and scalp.

cerebral calcifications and cerebellar hypoplasia A congenital syndrome of optic nerve colobomas leading to blindness with hypotonia, myoclonic seizures, microcephaly, quadriplegia, and mental and developmental delay.

Cerebral and cerebellar atrophy with intracranial calcifications and the **Dandy–Walker malformation** are also found.[381]

cerebral calculi (brain stones) Large, solitary or multiple, well-circumscribed, bony hard areas of pathological cerebral calcification, within preexisting cerebral tumors, hemorrhage, inflammation, or degenerative pathology. Clinically, if symptomatic, they usually present with recurrent seizures.[6317]

cerebral cavernous malformations Thin-walled sinusoidal vascular malformations lined only by endothelium, without smooth muscle or elastin, and with little or no intercalated brain parenchyma. Four varieties are defined: **arteriovenous, venous**, and **cavernous** (angiomas) **malformations**, and **capillary telangiectasias**. They tend to be surrounded by deposits of hemosiderin from spilled blood and are surrounded by a gliotic rim.[5213]

cerebral cortex (Gr, brain + rind or bark) The outer surface of the brain, composed largely of neuronal cell bodies and glial tissue. The six-layered cortex was first described and illustrated by Berlin in his inaugural thesis of 1858; following this insight, he continued on to become a distinguished ophthalmologist. Three- and four-layered cortices are also found, the former as the olfactory cortex and the latter as the cerebral expression of the limbic system.

cerebral death See **brain death**.

cerebral diplegia See **Little disease**. The term applied by Sigmund **Freud** to cerebral palsies with bilateral involvement. The condition had, however, been recognized by Nicholas André in 1741.

cerebral diplopia (polyopia) A rare symptom of perception of more than one object as a result of a lesion of the occipital lobe. The underlying mechanism is not precisely determined.[510]

cerebral dominance Specialization of one hemisphere for the performance of a function in humans and animals, influenced by both genetic and nongenetic factors. Dominance varies according to the modality examined; thus, while almost all right-handers have left hemispheric dominance for speech, so do at least 60% of left-handers. Commonly, the left hemisphere is dominant for language and manual skills, while the right is more involved in certain spatial and musical abilities, attention, and many aspects of emotion.[2341]

Broca in 1863 and **Dax** in 1865 first stated that language functions resided in the left hemisphere in right-handed people.

cerebral dropsy See **hydrocephalus**.

cerebral dyschromatopsia Acquired defects in color perception resulting (rarely) from cerebral lesions, usually in the parietal or occipital regions.[4954]

cerebral dysgenesis Disorders of embryological development of the brain. These have been classified by Cochrane and colleagues. (See Chart C–12.)

cerebral edema An increase in the volume of the brain as a result of an increase in the water content of the brain itself. Three major forms are recognized:[2115]

Vasogenic edema, due to increased capillary permeability, as with tumors, abscess, or purulent meningitis resulting from damage to the vessel walls. The fluid, a protein-containing filtrate, collects mainly

Chart C–12. Types of Cerebral Dysgenesis

A. *Dysgenesis presenting because of or associated with ventriculomegaly*
   1. Hydrocephalus is usually present.
      Dandy–Walker syndrome.
      Aqueductal stenosis.
      Chiari type II malformation.
      Lhermitte–Duclos disease.
   2. Hydrocephalus may not be present.
      Lobar **holoprosencephaly**.
      Agenesis of the corpus callosum associated with a dorsal sac.
   3. Hydrocephalus is not usually present.
      Alobar **holoprosencephaly**.
      Megalencephaly.
      Periventricular **heterotopias**.

B. *Dysgenesis presenting because of craniofacial dysmorphism*
   1. **Encephalocele** (occipital/frontobasal/sphenoidal).
   2. **Amniotic band syndrome**.

C. *Dysgenesis presenting because of focal neurological dysfunction*
   1. Hypothalamic hamartomas.
   2. Cortical dysplasia.
   3. **Chiari malformation**.

From Cochrane DD, Poskitt KJ, Normal MG. Surgical implications of cerebral dysgenesis. Can J Neurol Sci *1991;18:181–95. Reproduced by kind permission.*

in the white matter, increasing the extracellular fluid volume.

Cytotoxic edema, in which cellular swelling affects the neurons and glia in both the gray and white matter, as with hypoxia or hypo-osmolality states. The extracelluar volume is here decreased.

Interstitial edema, in which there is increased brain fluid due to a reduction in absorption of CSF. This occurs initially in the periventricular white matter, as in obstructive hydrocephalus. The extracellular fluid volume is increased.

cerebral embolism Occlusion of a cerebral blood vessel by a clot of blood or a mass of other material (cholesterol, air, cardiac valve fragments, etc.). This may be symptomless or may lead to clinical evidence of a stroke syndrome.[1069] See **cardiogenic embolism**.

cerebral enlargement See **normal pressure hydrocephalus**.

cerebral equipotentiality The concept that all parts of the cortex are functionally equivalent. The concept was propounded by Golz in 1812 and grew during the eighteenth century, gaining further strength from **Flourens**' and from **Lashley's** demonstrations that intelligent behavior in rats (learning to run mazes after ablation of their cerebral cortex) was determined by the amount of tissue removed rather than by the actual site of its removal. This Lashley called the "law of mass action," but he himself modified this later by suggesting that *area* rather than *total* equipotentiality was more likely to be relevant.

cerebral gigantism (Sotos syndrome) A dominantly inherited or sporadic congenital dysmorphic syndrome characterized by increased birth weight and body length for the first 5 years or so of life, with the rapid development of acromegalic features, accelerated skeletal maturation, macrocrania, hypertelorism, dolichocephaly or scaphocephaly, renal tumors, seizures, strabismus, and mental and developmental delay. Prognathism, antimongolian slant, high-arched palate, mental retardation, and ataxia are other usual clinical signs.[5958]

cerebral granulomatous angiitis See **isolated angiitis of the nervous system**.

cerebral hemispheric attention vise The right hemisphere is considered to activate spacial representational mechanisms in both hemispheres, while the left can only activate its own. Damage to the right hemisphere then causes reduced arousal in both hemispheres, prevents left hemispheric symptoms from compensating for the deficit, and results in left sided neglect, whereas damage to the left hand side will still allow the right hemisphere to function in overcoming right-sided neglect.[3445]

cerebral hemorrhage Bleeding into the brain substance. Most commonly this occurs as a result of the rupture of small deep penetrating arterioles in the basal ganglia, deep cerebral white matter, pons, or cerebellum, typically in hypertensive patients, but trauma, hemostatic disorders, and vascular pathologies such as aneurysms and angiomas are other important, if less common, causes.

A *variant* is *lobar cerebral hemorrhage*, in which the bleeding is into the cortex or the subjacent white matter, usually as a result of local structural disease, trauma, or **cerebral amyloid angiopathy**.

cerebral hydatid disease The presence of intracerebral cysts as accidental parasites of *Echinococcus granularis*. The condition is usually seen in children who come into close contact with dogs in sheep-rearing areas. The symptoms are mainly of raised intracranial pressure, seizures, and focal signs with the Schroeder tetrad.[6858] Rupture of the cyst, most often due to puncture during surgery when the disease was neither anticipated nor diagnosed preoperatively, produces a chemical meningeal reaction which may be lethal.

Cranio-vertebral hydatid disease is a *variant* condition in which hydatid cysts are found mainly within the lower thoracic vertebrae or in extraspinal soft tissue masses which infiltrate or compress the spinal cord or, with high cervical lesions, cause cranial nerve pareses.[5654, 5655] See also **Schroeder tetrad**.

cerebral hyperperfusion syndrome The combination of ipsilateral throbbing headache and facial pain, vomiting, confusion, hypertension, and focal neurological deficits (including seizures) following carotid endarterectomy or other measures taken to improve cerebral blood flow. Ironically, the greater the increase in cerebral blood flow achieved, the more likely is the syndrome to occur. If ignored, cerebral edema and hemorrhage can result.[6502]

cerebral hypoperfusion Reduction in blood supply to the whole brain (or to a defined region of the brain) of such a degree as to induce symptoms.

cerebral hypoxia A reduction in the supply of oxygen to the brain of such a degree as to induce symptoms. This may reflect either **cerebral hypoperfusion** or a diminution of the arterial p_aO_2.

cerebral infantile paralysis Poliomyelitis extending from its usual major site of attack in the spinal cord, to cause encephalitis. See **Strumpell disease**.

cerebral infarction Irreversible ischemic damage to all cell types within a region of the brain, usually following incomplete ischemia.

cerebral ischemia That condition marked by inadequate blood supply to the brain, either locally or globally and with or without symptoms arising as a result.

cerebral lymphoma (microglioma) Primary malignant lymphomas of the CNS. Spinal (extradural) lymphomas also occur. See **primary CNS lymphoma** and **HIV**.

cerebral malaria A diffuse encephalopathy following infection with *Plasmodium falciparum*, transmitted by the bites of female anopheles mosquitoes. The condition is found in Central Africa, Southeast Asia, South America, India, and Central America, but cerebral complications ensue in only some 2% of cases of *P. falciparum* infection, mainly in infants and those who have had no previous exposure to such infection.

Such complications are due to occlusion of small cerebral vessels by clumps of cells and plasmodia, giving rise to a number of defined syndromes reflecting the numerous vessels which may be occluded. Clinically, chills, rigors and headache, followed by periods of high fever with delirium, more severe headache, and abdominal pain, occur at 48 h intervals. Neurologically, meningitic, mono- or hemiplegic, cerebellar, myelitic, aphasic, and comatose forms, and others manifesting various focal neurological syndromes resulting from spinal or peripheral nerve involvement, are reported.[1458, 6858] Criteria for the diagnosis in adults have been suggested.[4651, 4652]

cerebral metastases Secondary tumors of the brain or meninges, arising most commonly from the lung, breast, kidney, or thyroid gland. Choriocarcinomas, malignant melanoma, and leukemias are the other more common types of secondary malignancy directly affecting the nervous system.

cerebral microangiopathy See **idiopathic calcification of the basal ganglia**.

cerebral motion blindness See **cerebral akinetopsia**.

cerebral nerve See **cranial nerve**.

cerebral palsy (Little disease) A symptom complex comprising nonprogressive (but not unchanging) disorders of posture and movement, sometimes with epilepsy, visuomotor, or other learning difficulties or extrapyramidal syndromes, secondary to lesions or anomalies of the brain arising in the early stages of its development or (in a minority of cases) to post-neonatal events such as meningoencephalitis, vascular occlusion, or trauma.

The condition is classed as a **static encephalopathy** and is segregated according to the extremities involved—hence mono-, hemi-, di-, and quadriplegic forms. It is supposed to arise as a result of cerebral insults, either congenital or sustained during pregnancy (such as anoxia or infections), or in the perinatal period (such as intracerebral hemorrhage or anoxia), but major risk factors include maternal mental retardation, the presence of congenital malformations outside the CNS, birth weight below 2,000 g, and breech presentation (though not breech delivery). Most affected children do not show evidence of severe fetal distress during labor nor of depression of cerebral function in the neonatal period.[937, 4621] A discussion of causes and mechanisms has been published.[3580] Characteristic signs are spasticity, rigidity and other movement disorders, weakness, and ataxia.[3523] There may or may not be intellectual impairment. Named varieties are as follows:

ataxic cerebral palsy

ataxic diplegia A combination of **ataxic cerebral palsy** and signs of corticospinal tract dysfunction.

athetoid type A congenital syndrome manifesting cerebellar ataxia, with rigidity, athetosis, and often dystonia. See **athetoid syndrome**.

dyskinetic cerebral palsy

hemiparetic cerebral palsy

hypotonic cerebral palsy

spastic cerebral palsy (**Little disease**) A congenital syndrome manifesting microcephaly, pyramidal signs (hemiparesis, paraparesis, quadriparesis), spasticity, athetosis, myoclonus, and mental and developmental delay.

Historical reviews have been published.[3088, 3345] See also **Little WJ**, **Gowers W**, **Hammond W**, and **Foerster W**. A useful Web site is at www.ninds.nih.gov/disorders/cerebral_palsy/cerebral_palsy.htm.

Cerebral Palsy Bulletin See **Developmental Medicine and Child Neurology**.

cerebral peduncle syndrome (Leyden syndrome) See **Weber syndrome**.

cerebral perfusion pressure The difference between the mean arterial blood pressure and the intracranial pressure. Cerebral blood flow can usually be maintained by autoregulation until the perfusion pressure falls below 40 mmHg.

cerebral pseudosclerosis See **Wilson disease**.

cerebral ptosis Bilateral, often asymmetrical ptosis occurring in association with acute right hemisphere lesions and conjugate deviation of the eyes to the right.[1767, 3782]

cerebral radionecrosis Necrosis of brain tissue as a late complication of prior radiotherapy. Clinically, the damaged brain tissue acts as an expanding mass lesion, producing increased intracranial pressure, focal deficits, and seizures, or causes a milder syndrome of progressive intellectual deficits with seizures.

cerebral salt-wasting An electrolyte balance disorder that can complicate the course of acute neurologic disorders such as intracerebral hemorrhage and meningoencephalitis. It is characterized by a volume-depleted state secondary to primary natriuresis with hyponatremia, signs of hypovolemia ([reflex] tachycardia, postural hypotension, reduced skin turgor, and low central venous pressure), and diuresis (high urine volume, high renal sodium excretion, and normal or high urine osmolality). The natriuresis with losses of water and of sodium occurs despite hyponatremia and contraction of the extracellular volume. Treatment is by replacement of salt and water. Diagnosis is assisted by the finding of increased urinary volumes with high sodium content; increased packed cell volume; reduced central venous pressure; and normal or increased serum osmolality.[4999]

The syndrome must be distinguished from the **syndrome of inappropriate secretion of ADH** because it is the opposite of dilutional hyponatremia, with increased extracellular fluid caused by inappropriate ADH secretion. The underlying mechanism is not fully understood, but impaired sodium resorption of the proximal nephron has been suggested.

cerebral signs, nonspecific

Nonlocalizing but suggestive evidence of organic pathology in the brain. These include **perseveration**, **drowsiness**, irritability, inversion of sleep rhythms, **amnesia**, and personality changes.

cerebral thrombosis The occlusion of an artery supplying the brain as a result of disease of the arterial wall *in situ*, as opposed to embolism from a point in the vascular system closer to the heart. The result is commonly atherothrombotic brain infarction.

cerebral tumors Benign or malignant tumors of the brain. By popular extension, tumors of the meninges and blood vessels may also be included with them although properly these are intracranial/intraspinal but not necessarily cerebral. A listing is given in Chart C–13.

Web sites relevant to the subject of cerebral tumors include the following:

Childhood Brain Tumor Treatment
www.cancer.gov/cancertopics/pdq/treatment/childbrain/Patient/page2/ provides information about the types of childhood brain tumors and treatment options.

Childhood Brain Stem Glioma
www.meb.uni-bonn.de/cancer.gov/CDR0000062761.html is a German site providing an overview of the diagnosis, classification, treatment, and prognosis for childhood brainstem gliomas.

www.cancer.gov/cancertopics/pdq/treatment/child-brain-stem-glioma/Patient Features/ provides information about the treatment, diagnosis, stages, and recurrence of the disease.

Childhood Cerebellar Astrocytoma
www.cancer.gov/cancertopics/pdq/treatment/child-cerebellar-astrocytoma/patient/ providing a review of treatment options for childhood cerebellar astrocytoma and a disease description, causes, stages, and available resources.

Childhood Ependymoma Treatment
www.cancer.gov/cancertopics/pdq/treatment/childependymoma/ provides information about the treatment of childhood ependymoma.

Childhood Supratentorial PNET
www.cancer.gov/cancertopics/pdq/treatment/childSPNET/patient/ provides general information about the tumors, stages, and treatment options.

Childhood Visual Pathway Glioma
www.cancer.gov/cancertopics/pdq/treatment/ child-visual-pathway/Patient is an information summary about the treatment of childhood visual pathway and hypothalamic gliomas.

Classification of Spinal Cord Tumors
www.cancer.gov/cancertopics/pdq/treatment/childbrain/HealthProfessional/page4 reviews the types of spinal cord tumor found in children, with treatment options, links, and references.

CNS Pathology Index provides images of CNS hemorrhage, infarction, edema and herniation, infections, congenital malformations, acquired and congenital degenerative diseases, dementias, and neoplasms.

www.cancer.gov/cancertopics/pdq/treatment/adultbrain/patient/ provides patient and professional information about adult brain tumors, including treatment options, staging, grades, types, and prognosis.

www.cancer.gov/cancertopics/pdq/treatment/adultbrain/HealthProfessional/page14 provides information about **medulloblastoma**, treatment options, links, and references.

www.rare-cancer.org/desmoplastic-infantile-ganglioglioma/ provides information and support for desmoplastic infantile ganglioglioma of childhood.

www.cancerbackup.org.uk/Cancertype/Childrenscancers/Typesofchildrenscancers/Neuroblastoma provides information about specific cancers, including causes, definition, symptoms, diagnosis, staging, treatment, and resources concerning neuroblastoma.

www.cancer.gov/templates/doc.aspx?viewid=7c0524a3-4751-4a6e-b357-0ad39c16c0ba§ionid=126&version=1 is an information summary about **oligodendroglial tumors** with treatment options, links, and references.

www.cancer.gov/templates/doc.aspx?viewid=7c0524a3-4751-4a6e-b357-0ad39c16c0ba§ionid=170&version=1 provides information about Grade I meningioma and Grade II and III meningioma and hemangiopericytoma, including treatment options and references.

www.cancer.gov/templates/doc.aspx?viewid=7c0524a3-4751-4a6e b357-0ad39c16c0ba§ionid=139&version=1 provides information on mixed bliomas, summarizing treatment options, with links and references.

www.chordomafoundation.org/ is a Web site of a nonprofit organization dedicated to furthering the exploration of the treatment of chordomas.

www.cancer.gov/cancertopics/wyntk/brain ("What You Need To Know About Brain Tumors") provides information about the detection, symptoms, diagnosis, and treatment of brain tumors from the U.S. National Cancer Institute.

www.meb.uni-bonn.de/cancer.gov/CDR0000062775.html provides general information including cellular classifications, treatment options, stages, and recurrences of supratentorial primitive neuroectodermal tumors and pineoblastoma.

Chart C–13. Neuroectodermal Tumors

Astrocytoma
Brainstem glioma
Cerebellar astrocytoma
Ependymoma
Glioblastoma
Medulloblastoma
Oligodendroglioma

Other tumors

Chordoma
Craniopharyngioma
Hemangioma, hemangioblastoma
Lymphoproliferative diseases
Meningioma
Neurilemmoma
Neurofibromas
Pituitary adenoma
Reticulum cell sarcoma (microgliomatosis)
Secondary tumors

cerebral vasculitis Inflammatory disease of the arteries supplying the brain. See **giant cell arteritis** and **isolated benign cerebral vasculitis**.

cerebral venous sinus thrombosis Thrombotic occlusion of the great venous sinuses or of other cerebral veins; the superior sagittal sinus is that most often affected. Both septic and aseptic forms are recognized; the former are less common than in past years, while the latter have occurred, especially in young adults, with a wide range of associated diseases, most of which impact upon coagulation.[307, 6497]

Clinical syndromes resulting include the usual features of raised intracranial pressure; headache; reduced conscious level; seizures; and various focal deficits pointing to the hemispheric or posterior fossa lesion, which is usually a venous infarct.[307, 776] The causes have been reviewed.[773]

In children, presentations are with lethargy, anorexia, headache, vomiting, seizures, focal signs or coma, and with positive neuroimaging. Recent infections, anemias, and prothrombotic disorders may be causal. The superficial venous system is more commonly involved than the deep.[5702]

With lateral sinus thrombosis, headache (including **thunderclap headache**) may be the sole manifestation. See also **cord sign**, **empty delta sign**, and **dense triangle sign**.

cerebral ventricostium The spontaneous formation of a communication between the cerebral ventricles and the surface of the brain in patients with hydrocephalus.[3285]

cerebration The use of the brain; thinking (colloquial).

Cerebri Anatome The anatomical masterpiece of Thomas **Willis**, published in 1664.

cerebritis Inflammation of the substance of the brain. The term is most commonly employed to denote the earliest stages of pyogenic infection, which progress toward abscess formation.

cerebroarthrodigital syndrome A congenital dysmorphic syndrome characterized by absence of the sacrum, reduction deformity of the arms, absent fingers or oligodactyly, brachydactyly, joint contractures, hypoplasia of muscles, microcephaly, and hydrocephalus.[6000]

cerebrocardiac neurosis See **depersonalization**.

cerebrocerebellar lissencephaly A congenital malformation characterized by **lissencephaly** of the cerebrum, cerebellum, and corpus callosum, with mental and developmental delay.[4698] See **lissencephaly**.

cerebrocostomandibular syndrome A congenital, recessively inherited dysmorphic syndrome characterized by dwarfism, micrognathia, cleft palate, narrow thorax, tracheal anomalies, and mental and developmental delay.[5838]

cerebrofaciothoracic dysplasia See **Pascual-Castroviejo syndrome**.

cerebrohepatorenal syndrome See **Zellweger disease**.

cerebromacular degeneration (cerebromacular dystrophy, Stock–Spielmeyer–Vogt disease) See **gangliosidoses** and **neuronal ceroid lipofuscinosis**.

cerebromacular dystrophy See **cerebromacular degeneration**.

cerebromalacia (Lat and Gr, brain + softness) Local softening of the brain, usually as the result of ischemia.

cerebromedullary disconnection See **locked-in syndrome**.

cerebro-ocular dysgenesis See **Walker–Warburg syndrome**.

cerebro-ocular dysplasia with muscular dystrophy See **congenital muscular dystrophy** (*variants*) and **Walker–Warburg syndrome**.

cerebro-oculofacioskeletal syndrome A recessively inherited congenital dysmorphic syndrome characterized by microphthalmia, cataract, blepharophimosis, micrognathia, rocker-bottom feet, vertical talus bones, camptodactyly, intracranial calcifications, agenesis of the corpus callosum, microcephaly, and mental and developmental delay.[4973] See **Pena–Shokeir syndrome**.

cerebro-oculo-muscular syndrome (COMS) A congenital syndrome characterized by cloudy corneas, microphthalmia, colobomas of the iris, cataract, hypoplasia of the optic nerve or retina, optic atrophy, pigmentary retinopathy, and blindness, with adducted thumbs, joint contractures, macrocephaly, distal myopathic weakness, cerebral atrophy, aqueduct stenosis, hydrocephalus, lissencephaly, the **Dandy–Walker malformation**, and mental and developmental delay.[2836] See **congenital muscular dystrophy** and **Walker–Warburg syndrome**.

cerebro-osteo-nephrodysplasia A congenital dysmorphic syndrome, also characterized by dwarfism, large tongue, umbilical hernia, protuberant abdomen, enlarged liver and spleen, skeletal anomalies including clefts of the vertebrae, platyspondyly, brachycephaly, microcephaly, delayed closure of fontanelles, camptodactyly and rhizomelia of the limbs, nephropathy, seizures, spasticity, fasciculations, cerebral atrophy, hydrocephalus, and mental and developmental delay.[381]

cerebroretinal angiomatosis See **von Hippel–Lindau disease**.

cerebroretinal arteriovenous aneurysm See **Wyburn–Mason syndrome**.

cerebroretinal degeneration See **neuronal ceroid lipofuscinosis**.

cerebroretinal lipofuscinosis See **neuronal ceroid lipofuscinosis**.

cerebroretinal microangiopathy with calcifications and cysts A rare syndrome manifesting features of **Coats disease** and leukoencephalopathy with calcifications and cysts, likely due to an underlying obliterative cerebral angiopathy involving small vessels and leading to dystrophic calcification and secondary white matter abnormalities.[3861] Retinal vascular changes, skeletal abnormalities, and intestinal bleeding are other recorded features. See also **striatopallidal calcification**.

cerebroretinal vasculopathy (hereditary cerebroretinal vasculopathy) A rare dominantly inherited disorder presenting with progressive visual loss, dysarthria, intellectual decline, and gait disturbances starting after the age of 30 years and due to the presence of abnormalities of small blood vessels in the retina and brain and of cerebral pseudotumors. Periventricular leukoencephalopathy suggesting small vessel occlusions is evident on MRI scans.[2548]

cerebroside Phosphate-free nitrogenous lipids containing galactose and found in brain myelin.

cerebroside lipidosis See **glucosylceramide lipidosis**.

cerebrospinal Relating both to the brain and the spinal cord.

cerebrospinal block syndrome See **Zange–Kindler syndrome**.

cerebrospinal fever Meningococcal meningitis.

cerebrospinal fluid (CSF) A clear watery secretion of the choroid plexus and brain. The existence of the CSF was proved by **Domenic Cotugno** (1736–1822), an Italian anatomist, in 1764, but the term was not used until introduced by Magendie in 1827.[5886] The first analyses of the fluid were performed nearly a hundred years later (Corning, 1855), preceding the studies of **Quincke**.

The fluid is formed principally by the choroid plexus within the ventricles but also from brain extracellular fluid, enters the subarachnoid space through the foramina of Luschka and **Magendie**, and circulates (the third circulation of Harvey **Cushing**) down into the spinal canal before rising again and passing diffusely over the hemispheres to its final site of absorption by the pacchionian granulations in the dural venous sinuses, minimal amounts also being absorbed through the arachnoid root sleeves along the cranial and spinal nerve roots. It functions as a protective surround for the brain and cord, as a pathway for neurotransmitters, as a metabolic sink, and possibly as a coolant. The methods of secretion and absorption and the normal pressure, cytology, and biochemistry of the fluid have been reviewed.[1398, 2115, 3971]

cerebrospinal fluid fistula headache See **post-dural puncture headache**.

cerebrospinal fluid hypovolemia See **idiopathic intracranial hypotension**.

cerebrospinal fluid rhinorrhea Escape of CSF through the anterior cranial fossa to the nasal cavities. The causes are divided between those which are traumatic and those which are not, the latter group including cases of high- and normal pressure leaks.[4794]

cerebrotendinous xanthomatosis (cholestanolosis; OMIM 213700) A rare autosomal recessive lipid storage disease characterized by the deposition of cholestanol (a cholesterol metabolite) in the body tissues (replacing cholesterol in the myelin of the central and peripheral nervous systems) and by raised plasma levels of cholestanol; the result of a defect in the activity of sterol 27-hydroxylase, a mitochondrial enzyme responsible for the synthesis of bile acids.[6472] The genetic abnormality maps to 2q33-ter. *(cyp27a1)*

Clinically, the disease is manifest in early life with cataracts, xanthomatous swelling of tendons (particularly the Achilles tendons), mild mental slowing, ataxia and eventually cerebellar and pyramidal signs, and a sensorimotor peripheral neuropathy. Seizures, early atheroma, osteoporosis, bone fractures, pes cavus, hypercholestanolemia, and myopathic facies are other features. The condition progresses to a state of progressive myoclonus dementia with spastic, dysarthric helplessness, and death, usually before the age of 30 years.[561, 2754] The condition was first described by van Bogaert in 1937.

cerebrovascular disease See **strokes**.

Cerebrovascular Diseases A neurological subspecialty journal. Address: S. Karger AG, P.O. Box 10, Allschwilerstrasse, CH-4009 Basel, Switzerland. www.karger.ch/journals/ced/ced_jh.htm.

cerebrovascular insufficiency The term of **Denny-Brown** denoting episodes of focal reversible ischemia of the brain resulting from failure of the collateral blood supply, as occurs during systemic hypotension in people with severe but previously subclinical carotid or vertebro-basilar disease, leading to a reduction in perfusion pressure in defined brain regions.[6966]

Cardiac abnormalities or mere postural change may be responsible for the hypotensive episodes. The clinical effects include brief, repetitive episodes of transient neurological dysfunction (amaurosis, clumsiness, weakness, paresthesias, etc.), frequently with involuntary jerking of the affected limbs, accompanied by slow activity on the EEG.[2314] See also **limb shaking**.

cerebrovascular reserve 1. The capacity of the brain to withstand a limited period of ischemia without undergoing infarction. 2. The capacity of the cerebral circulation to protect the brain from the potentially damaging effects of ischemia by maintaining the delivery of glucose and oxygen despite reductions in local or global perfusion pressure.

cerebrovascular syphilis A form of tertiary syphilis in which arteritis leads to vascular occlusion, usually in the territory of the middle cerebral artery, after a prolonged prodrome of nonspecific headaches, malaise, vertigo, insomnia, etc. The CSF cell count, protein, and serology findings are always abnormal.

cerebrum (Lat, the brain) Originally the whole thing, but the cerebellum was differentiated by Erasistratus in the third century BC. The word appeared in English in 1565.[5886]

ceroid An acid-fast, sudanophilic fluorescent substance of unknown chemical composition which is found in human tissues such as liver, muscle, intestine, and nervous system, in association with several disease processes. See **lipofuscin**.

ceroid lipofuscinosis See **neuronal ceroid lipofuscinosis**.

ceroid storage disease A disease resulting from an inborn metabolic error and once known as *Landing–Oppenheim disease*,[3671] but now subdivided according to the chemical deficits obtaining. See **neuronal ceroid lipofuscinosis**.

ceruleum See **caeruleum**.

ceruloplasmin deficiency with hemosiderosis An hereditary syndrome of progressive dementia, extrapyramidal disorders, cerebellar ataxia, and diabetes mellitus with low serum cereloplasmin and raised ferritin levels, reported from Japan.[4491] Linkage to 3q23–q24 has been established.

cerveau isolé A physiological preparation, the brain (classically of a cat) being isolated from the remainder of the CNS by a cut made at the intercollicular level, just beneath the III nerve nucleus.[828]

Interruption of the activity of the ascending reticular activating system leads to permanent sleep, apart from the motor and sensory effects.

cervical (from Lat, the neck) Pertaining to the neck.

cervical acceleration injury See **whiplash**.

cervical band syndrome A form of **thoracic outlet syndrome**, supposed to be produced by pressure upon the lower fibers of the brachial plexus by a fibrous tissue remnant stretching from the transverse processes of the lowest cervical vertebra to the clavicle. The existence of such bands, which are visible only to surgeons and which cannot be imaged, must be extremely rare.

cervical dystonia (spasmodic torticollis, idiopathic cervical dystonia [ICD]) The commonest form of adult-onset focal **dystonia** characterized by sustained involuntary contractions of the neck muscles, which result in abnormal movements and postures of the head and neck. Tremor may be associated.[3162] Dystonia in other regions and concomitant head or hand tremor are also present in a minority of cases. When the onset is in adult life the symptoms do not generalize, but segmental spread may occur and pain can increase independent of the dystonia.

Because the movements are not always spasmodic and because torticollis is not the invariable clinical result of the muscle contractions (**laterocollis, retrocollis**, and **antecollis** also occur), the alternative term is now preferred to that used for over a century. The etiology is unknown; painful trauma may be involved in the pathogenesis of the condition but the underlying physiology is speculative. In inherited adult-onset cervical dystonia, linkage to chromosome 18p has been demonstrated.[1470]

cervical migraine (posterior cervical sympathetic syndrome of Barré, Bärtschi-Rochaix syndrome, cervical vertigo syndrome) A syndrome characterized by occipital headache, scotomas, vertigo, tinnitus, vasomotor disorders, paresthesiae, facial spasm, and neck stiffness, ascribed by M.J. Barré[420] to irritation of the sympathetic plexus around the vertebral artery in patients with cervical arthropathy.

Whether this represents **migraine** or **vertebrobasilar insufficiency** or arises as a result of structural pathology in the cervical spine, is not determined.[4702] See also **cervicogenic headache**.

cervical nystagmus (neck torsion nystagmus, vertebrobasilar insufficiency nystagmus) A form of jerk nystagmus with or without other vestibular signs, supposed to result from lesions of the proprioceptive mechanisms in the cervical cord, but which is commonly due either to toxicity or to positional changes.

cervical radiculopathy Compression or ischemia of the cervical nerve roots as a result of local degenerative or some other disease. The clinical features have been analyzed and comprise pain in the neck, shoulders, arm, or forearm, paresthesias, muscle weakness and atrophy, hyporeflexia, and objective disturbances of sensation in the appropriate dermatomal distributions.[6921] Diagnostic criteria have been suggested.

1. **Symptoms:**
   - A. Pain in the neck, the arm, or both
   - B. Paresthesias, dysesthesias, or hypesthesia in nerve root distribution
   - C. Muscle weakness

2. **Signs:**
   - A. Sensory changes in dermatomal distribution
   - B. Weakness, atrophy, or fasciculation in myotomal distribution
   - C. Unilaterally diminished muscle stretch reflexes

3. **Diagnostic procedures**:
   - A. EMG evidence of acute denervation in cervical paraspinal muscles or in a myotome
   - B. Demonstrable abnormality on myelography, CT-assisted myelography, or MRI, correlating with the clinical features
   - C. Identification of an affected cervical root at operation

The diagnosis of definite radiculopathy can be made in the presence of 3C; 3A; 2A, 2B, and 2C; or 3B and 1A and either 1B or 1C. The diagnosis of probable radiculopathy can be made in the presence of more than one of 1A, -B, and -C with any one of 2; or with any one of 1 with 3B; or 1A with any two of 2.

Cervical radiculopathy is deemed *not* present if only one of 1 is present, in the presence of an abnormal imaging test without evidence of a recent radiculopathy, or if the EMG changes suggest chronicity rather than a recent cervical root injury. (Amended from the criteria of Dr. William J. Litchy, Mayo Clinic, with many thanks.)

cervical rib A benign anomaly, first described by Naffziger[4573] and sometimes detected in patients who complain of neck or arm pain and who are then at risk of operation to remove the rib, which is thought to be causing a **thoracic outlet syndrome**.

cervical spinal muscular atrophy See **hereditary motor neuropathy, type I**.

cervical spondylosis Degenerative changes in the vertebrae and their joints and in the annulus fibrosus of the disks with or without accompanying arthritis of the synovial joints of the cervical spine (cervical osteoarthritis) leading to any combination of degeneration or prolapse of the intervertebral disks, thickening and buckling of the ligamentum flavum, and osteophyte formation.[4946] The local fibrosis, hypertrophy, and distortion lead sometimes to ischemic or compressive effects upon the spinal cord and nerve roots at the affected levels.

The condition was recognized as a cause of paraplegia by Strümpell in 1888, but only in 1926 was it shown (by Eliott) that spondylotic narrowing of the intervertebral foramina could lead to radicular symptoms.[802]

cervical spondylotic myelopathy Ischemic-compressive disease of the spinal cord resulting from degenerative arthropathy of the cervical spine, in particular affecting the intervertebral disks and the zygapophyseal joints and leading to hypertrophy of the ligamentum flavum. Disk protrusion compounds the clinical deficit.[6207] Clinically, compression leads to conduction block in the cord, especially between C3 and C5, producing pyramidal signs and evidence of root compression. Compression of the vertebral arteries augmenting cord ischemia is another complication.

The condition had attracted little attention until the papers of Brain and Wilkinson demonstrated the ability of such incursions upon the spinal canal to compromise the functions of the cord at this site. The further studies of Yoss et al.[6921] confirmed the clinical and radiological picture, which is composed of the triad of reduced mobility of the neck, long tract signs below (often far below) the level of the lesion(s), and local radiculopathic features. *Thoracic myelopathy* is far less common; local tumors or disk herniation are the commoner causes. See also **midcervical central cord syndrome**.

cervical sympathetic irritation syndrome See **Pourfour du Petit syndrome**.

cervical vertigo Subjective hallucinations of rotational acceleration thought likely to arise as a result of lesions of the cervical proprioceptive mechanisms. The existence of the phenomenon in humans is, however, controversial.[818]

cervical vertigo syndrome See **cervical migraine**.

cervicobrachial neuralgia Pain felt in the neck and referred to the regions of the arm supplied by the four lower cervical and the first thoracic roots.

cervicocollic reflex A muscle stretch reflex allowing compensatory adjustments to the position of the head in response to neck and truncal movements.

cervicogenic headache Recurrent, persistent, uni- or bilateral, moderate to severe pulsating head pain in any region, referred from a primary nociceptive source in the musculoskeletal tissues innervated by the cranial nerves, but usually associated with some disorder of the cervical spine, most commonly in women. It was first described by John Hilton, an English surgeon, in 1860.

Consistent reproduction of the pain by neck movement, painful limitation of neck movement, accentuation of pain with sudden head movement, abnormal postures of the head and neck, abnormal mobility of the craniocervical junction, and sensory abnormalities implicating the upper cervical cord or lower medulla are features characteristically associated.[1808] Dizziness, conjunctival injection, phonophobia, photophobia, nausea, and vomiting are also described—which have led to persistent concerns since Liveing's contention in 1873 that the differentiation of this condition from **migraine** is inappropriate.[1807] Convergence of afferents from the upper cervical roots upon the nucleus caudalis of the trigeminal tract is the most commonly accepted neurophysiological explanation.[212] See also **posterior cervical sympathetic syndrome** and **cervical migraine**.

cervicolinguomasticatory syndrome (Kulenkampff–Tarnow syndrome) Probably an earlier description of **Meige syndrome**. See **tardive dyskinesia**.

cervico-ocular reflex (neck–eye loop) A postural reflex elicited by angular motion of the trunk relative to the fixed head or *vice versa*, holding still the position of the eyes and head to ensure gaze stability during movement of the trunk.[867]

cervicooculoacoustic syndrome See **Wildervanck syndrome**.

cervicoosteofacial syndrome See **Wildervanck syndrome**.

CES-D Scale See Center for Epidemiologic Studies Depression Scale.

Céstan, Étienne Jacques-Marie-Raymond (1872–1933) French neurologist and psychiatrist who worked at the **Salpêtrière**, for some years as *chef de clinique* to **Raymond**, before returning to his native Toulouse, where he practiced as professor of mental and nervous diseases or clinical medicine. His publications spanned numerous areas of neuropathology and clinical neurology without a single focus.

Chart C–14. Diagnostic Criteria for Cervicogenic Headache

Here follows a variant form of the diagnostic criteria proposed by Sjaastad et al. (1990)[5880] and reviewed by Antonaci et al.[213]

1. Unilateral headache without side-shift
2. Symptoms and signs of neck involvement:
   a. Pain triggered by neck movement and/or sustained awkward position and/or external pressure over the ipsilateral upper, posterior neck, or occipital region
   b. Ipsilateral neck, shoulder, and arm pain of a rather vague, non-radicular nature;
   c. Reduced range of motion in the cervical spine
3. Pain episodes of varying duration or fluctuating, continuous pain
4. Moderate, non-excruciating pain, usually of a non-throbbing nature
5. Pain starting in the neck, eventually spreading to oculo-frontotemporal areas, where the maximum pain is often located
6. a. Anaesthetic blockades of the major occipital nerve and/or the C2 root or other appropriate blockades on the symptomatic side abolish the pain transiently, provided complete anaesthesia is obtained or
   b. Sustained a whiplash (neck trauma) a relatively short time prior to the onset
7. Various attack-related phenomena: autonomic symptoms and signs, nausea, vomiting (ipsilateral edema and flushing mostly in the periocular area; dizziness; photo- and phonophobia; blurred vision on the eye ipsilateral to the pain)

The International Classification of Headache Disorders[2820] includes similar (but not identical) criteria.

A *variant* is *constant pain caused by compression, irritation or distortion of cranial nerves or upper cervical roots by structural lesions* in which there is constant headache or facial pain caused by a lesion directly compromising afferent fibers in nerves mediating pain sensation from the head and/or neck. Sensory deficits may be detected within the appropriate distribution. Diagnostic criteria are:

A. Constant and/or jabbing pain in the territory supplied by a cranial sensory nerve, fulfilling criteria C and D
B. Evidence of compression, irritation, or distortion of the appropriate cranial nerve
C. Pain and compression, irritation, or distortion occur simultaneously and correspond in location
D. Pain is relieved by removal of the cause of compression, irritation, or distortion

Céstan syndrome (Céstan–Chenais syndrome) Unilateral paralysis of the soft palate and vocal cords with **Horner syndrome**, ataxia, alternating hemiplegia, and hemianesthesia for proprioception and discriminative touch (medial lemniscus); the spino-thalamic fibers, placed laterally, are spared. The syndrome is due to infarction of the medial part of the medullary tegmentum as a result of vertebral artery occlusion below the origin of the posterior inferior cerebellar artery.[1072]

Dr. L.J. Chenais (1872–1950) was also a French physician.

Céstan–Chenais syndrome See **Céstan syndrome**.

Céstan–LeJonne syndrome See **Emery-Dreifuss syndrome**.

cGy The unit of measurement of radiation.

Chaddock, Charles Gilbert (1861–1936) American neurologist and psychiatrist who trained in Michigan and later in Paris under **Babiński** at the Bicêtre. He became professor of neurological diseases at the St. Louis University School of Medicine. He is remembered for the sign described next and for having translated Kraft-Ebing's work *Psychopathia Sexualis* and some of **Babiński**'s papers into English.[1972]

Chaddock reflex 1. (*external malleolar sign*) A variant method of eliciting the **Babiński reflex** (plantar reflex) by scratching the skin below the lateral malleolus from behind forward, its advantage being the lesser amount of withdrawal excited. There is evidence that this is the only method with greater sensitivity than the original.[1076] The same method had been described by Kisaku Yoshimura, a Japanese physician, in 1906, 5 years before Chaddock's description. The reversed Chaddock sign[6216] is the same thing done (obviously) backward. 2. (*wrist sign*) Flexion of the wrist and abduction of the fingers when the ulnar side of the lower forearm is stimulated; seen in pyramidal tract disease.[5333]

chaeromania (from Gr, to rejoice + madness) Mania or euphoria—a psychotic state characterized by unwonted cheerfulness.

Chagas Disease An arthropod-borne zoonosis due to infection with *Trypanosoma cruzi*, first described by Chagas in 1907. The clinical features are of chronic meningitis with evidence of cortical inflammation and demyelination; late in the course of the disease there is evidence of autonomic neuropathy.[5986] See **South American trypanosomiasis**.

chair tests 1. The production of nystagmus in the direction opposite to rotation when the subject revolves on a chair with his head flexed 30° forward (in order to bring the horizontal semicircular canal truly into a horizontal position) and while wearing **Frenzel glasses**. The test was described by **Barany**.

The normal response after rotation of the chair to the right is for horizontal jerk nystagmus to the left to persist for 10–30 s. See **Barany Test**. 2. If the chair on which the normal subject sits is suddenly tilted backward, he reflexly sits forward. The subject with bilateral labyrinthine lesions or with **Parkinson disease** makes no such reaction.

chalasia (from Gr, chalasis; to relax or grow languid) 1. A term of Hippocrates for relaxation. 2. Failure of contraction of the cardiac sphincter of the stomach, leading to acid reflux.

chalastic fits (inhibitory epilepsy) Attacks of general limpness, resembling **cataplexy** but symptomatic of lesions affecting the medial aspects of both frontal lobes.[1921]

Chalfont Seizure Severity Scale A scale which assesses and scores the components of seizure attacks which cause patients the greatest disturbance. Factors such as the presence of falling, injuries, loss of awareness, and any warning of seizures; the occurrence of dropping objects, incontinence, automatisms, and convulsions; and duration of the seizures and the time taken to regain normal functioning are rated.[1750] See also the **National Hospital Seizure Severity Scale**, derived from the Chalfont Scale.

Chamberlain, W.E. (b. 1891) American radiologist in Philadelphia.

Chamberlain line A line drawn on a true lateral X-ray of the skull from the back of the hard palate to the posterior border of the foramen magnum. The line normally crosses above all parts of the atlas and axis; if basilar impression is present, part of the odontoid process and, in severe cases, other parts of the axis and of the atlas project above this line. However, the same is true in some normal subjects and a better measurement is that of the **Bull angle**.[934]

chameleon tongue Involuntary withdrawal of the tongue which is being protruded voluntarily; a sign commonly seen in patients with chorea.

champagne-cork papilledema Severe papilledema such that the optic nerve head bulges forward and extends outward in all directions into the vitreous humor, thus resembling a champagne cork (or a mushroom).

chancre An indolent, painless skin or mucosal ulcer at the site of a primary infection with *Treponema pallidum*, which can be isolated from it.

channel The complete system for the detection, amplification, and display of potential differences between a pair of electrodes.

channelopathies Genetically determined metabolic disturbances of the calcium, chloride, or potassium voltage-gated ion channels in the cell membrane, leading to disparate manifestations. In migraine, epilepsy, and cardiac arrhythmias, the electrical signals critical to the function of neurons, muscle cells, and heart cells are distorted by abnormalities in the proteins that regulate electrical signalling in these cells. Many of the disorders recognized are listed below, some with notes on the sites of the chromosomal anomaly. Acquired channelopathies are auto-antibody-mediated disorders that may follow an infection or occur in the presence of a neoplasm .[5137]

chanson de parler See **prosody**.

Chapple syndrome Unilateral facial weakness with contralateral laryngeal palsy occurring in the newborn. The latter problem is thought to be due to compression of the superior laryngeal nerve by the thyroid

Chart C–15a. Channelopathies

Disorder	Site of Chromosomal Anomaly
Acquired **autonomic neuropathies** (antibodies to an acetylcholine receptor type)	
Acquired neuromyotonia (voltage-gated K^+ channel antibodies)	
AD nocturnal frontal lobe epilepsy	20q13
Andersen syndrome (potassium) Anderson–Tawil syndrome	*KCNJ2*
Batten disease	16p 12.1
Benign familial infantile convulsions	18q?
Benign familial neonatal convulsions	29q 13. 8q24?
Central core disease	
Cherry red spot myoclonus syndrome	6p 21.3
Congenital myasthenic syndrome	*CHRNA/B/E*
Episodic ataxia with myokymia	CACNA1 12p13; *KCNA1*
Episodic ataxia with nystagmus*2*	*CACNIA*
Familial adult myoclonic epilepsy	8q 24
Familial hemiplegic migraine (episodic ataxia 2 is closely linked) voltage-gated potassium/calcium channels	*CACNIA; ATPIA2*
Familial hemiplegic migraine	CACNL4
Familial hyperkalemic periodic paralyses (skeletal muscle Na^+ channel)	SCN4A, 17q23–25b
Familial hypokalemic periodic paralyses (voltage-gated Ca^{++} or K^+ channels)	*CACNL3*
Febrile convulsions	8q
Generalized epilepsy with febrile seizures	19q13
Hereditary hyperekplexia	*GLRA1*
Juvenile **Gaucher disease** 1q 21	
Juvenile myoclonic epilepsy (Janz) 6p	
Lafora disease 6q 24	
Lambert–Eaton myasthenic syndrome	
Long QT syndrome (an episodic cardiac dysrhythmia) Types I, II, III, IV, V, VII; voltage-gated Na^+ or K^+ channels.	
Malignant hyperthermia (ryanodine)	
MERRF mt DNA	
Myasthenic syndrome phenotype	*CHRNA/B/E*
Myotonia congenita (Thomsen, Becker) (chloride)	CLCN1; 7q
Myotonia fluctuans (sodium)	
Myotonia permanens (sodium)	
Paramyotonia congenita (skeletal muscle Na channel)	SCN4A 17q 23–25
Partial epilepsy	10q22
Paraneoplastic **limbic encephalitis**	
Potassium aggravated myotonia	*SCN4A*
Rasmussen encephalitis (antibodies to a glutamate receptor)	
Spinocerebellar ataxia, type VI	*CACNIA*
Unverricht-Lundberg syndrome	21q22

cartilage *in utero* as a consequence of excessive lateral flexion of the neck.[1096] The syndrome was described by Dr. Charles Chapple of Philadelphia in 1956.

Charcot, Jean-Martin (1825–1893)

French neurologist, psychiatrist, and anatomist. After graduation from the University of Paris in 1853 he interned at the Salpêtrière, an asylum in Paris for the mentally ill and for those suffering from various chronic diseases, for 4 years from 1848, seeing there a huge variety of hitherto unclassified disease. He returned in 1862 as attending physician and over the next 30 years developed it into a school of neurology which became internationally famous. He was elected professor of pathological anatomy in 1872, succeeding **Vulpian**. Ten years after that, a special chair of nervous diseases was created for him, although his observations did not extend solely to neurology—as evident from his accounts of Charcot–Leyden crystals in the sputum of asthmatics, of intermittent claudication, and of biliary (Charcot) fever.

The starting point for this triumph was his meticulous recording of physical signs in all the 5000 patients housed in the hospital, signs which he later attributed to the specific neurological lesions found when the patients came to autopsy. This was the clinico-anatomic method which became the hallmark of the **Salpêtrière** and later of neurology in general. From 1866, Charcot offered lectures on neurological subjects which quickly became popular as a result of the inclusion of pathophysiology with the clinical demonstrations, of his own dominating and self-assured manner, and of the theatricality of the presentations. At these sessions (the Tuesday Lectures), symptoms, diagnoses, and pathology were discussed, focusing upon a number of patients brought in for demonstration. The extent to which he actually examined (as opposed to observed) the patients is unclear.

Charcot's private practice was large, his hospital practice even larger. Honored in his day, he may be considered in retrospect to be the father of modern neurology. It was Charcot who differentiated tics from chorea. His other studies encompassed rheumatism and changes in abdominal organs and lungs in old age, organic disease of the nervous system such as muscular atrophy, **poliomyelitis**, aneurysms, **multiple sclerosis** (differentiated for the first time in the Tuesday Lectures of 1868), motor neuron disease (**amyotrophic lateral sclerosis**), in which he demonstrated the involvement of the anterior roots as well as the lateral columns in 1869, stroke syndromes, **Ménière syndrome**, tabetic arthropathy and lightning pains, encephalitis, cord compression, cerebral hemorrhage, **hysteria** and hypnotism, the psychoneuroses, and art as applied to the nervous system. Charcot himself did not hypnotize his demonstrated subjects (that was done by his assistants), but he may have failed to realize the multiple other cues that were picked by the suggestible patients as to the responses expected of them. Shortly before his death, he determined that his former views on hysteria needed revision, but he did not live to complete that task (Guillain G. *J.-M. Charcot: His Life and Work*. Trans. Bailey P. New York: Hoeber, 1959).

His complete works were published in nine volumes. The *Tuesday Lectures* were translated into English after 1877 by George Sigerson (New Sydenham Society).[2430, 5704]

Charcot artery The lenticulo-striate branch of the middle cerebral artery, known as the "artery of cerebral hemorrhage."

Charcot–Bouchard aneurysm A defect in the muscular coat of an arteriole among the deep penetrating vessels of the brain affected by **lipohyalinosis** in chronically hypertensive people. These are most often in the basal ganglia, thalamus, pons, and cerebellum. The arteriolar wall is here comprised merely of the intimal layer and some surrounding gliosis. As a result, it is fragile and in the event of its rupture in association with increased blood pressure, bleeding will not be controllable by the usual mechanism of muscle spasm.

Charcot disease 1. See **amyotrophic lateral sclerosis**.[1108] 2. Chorea in the elderly, of which he gave the neat description: "the movements are gesticulatory; they cover a wide area, are irregular, unrhythmical, contradictory, and render the accomplishment of any definite act a difficult matter."[1102] The status of the disorder may be in some doubt.

Charcot edema (blue edema) Non-pitting stasis edema, coldness and peripheral cyanosis, usually with sensory loss and weakness and occurring as a result of disuse of a limb—a manifestation of hysterical paralyses in many of Charcot's patients but also sometimes seen following injury or stroke.[2618]

Charcot–Erb paresis (syphilitic myelitis) See **Erb–Charcot syndrome**.

Charcot-Joffroy syndrome See **hypertrophic spinal meningitis**.

Charcot joint Painless, often gross deformity and destruction of joints in tabes dorsalis and other conditions (e.g., syringomyelia, hereditary sensory neuropathy) in which the sensation of pain is lost.[1098] The absence of proprioceptive sense is also likely to be relevant by denying restraint to the muscular contractions and thus permitting abnormal joint positions to be assumed. [JF] See also **neurogenic arthropathy**.

Charcot–Marie–Tooth Association A charitable organization which provides education and support to the patient with Charcot–Marie–Tooth disease and his family as well as the medical/scientific community. The association's program is composed of a quarterly newsletter, regional conferences, a medical referral system, a videotape program, and area support groups. The association also maintains a registry of patients with the disease. Web site: www.charcot-marie-tooth.org/.

Charcot–Marie–Tooth disease See **hereditary motor and sensory neuropathies**. While Charcot and Marie[1109] had priority of publication, they considered the condition to be a myelopathy, an error corrected by Tooth (who noted that **Virchow** had already described the same condition).

Charcot–Marie–Tooth disease neuropathy score A standardized method of assessing the disability of patients with this disorder. It assesses sensory and motor symptoms, sensation to pinprick and vibration, strength in the arms and legs, and ulnar and median CMAPs and SNAPs, all on a scale of 0–4.[5824]

Charcot–Marie–Tooth disease with distal spinal muscular atrophy See **hereditary motor and sensory neuropathy, type II**.

Charcot–Marie–Tooth disease with progressive ataxia and tremor See **hereditary motor and sensory neuropathy, type I**.

Charcot sign Elevation of the eyebrow on the side of a peripheral facial palsy and its depression when the patient attempts to close the eye. The sign has also been interpreted as consisting of depression of the eyebrows when the eyes are closed, indicating blepharospasm; or their elevation, indicating apraxia of eye closure.

Charcot syndrome See **amyotrophic lateral sclerosis**.

Charcot triad The combination of nystagmus, intention tremor, and scanning speech, which he suggested was diagnostic of **multiple sclerosis**.[1103] This is no longer considered to be so.

Charcot vertigo (laryngeal vertigo, laryngeal epilepsy) The occurrence of syncope or vertigo caused by a severe bout of coughing, sometimes with laryngospasm.[1104] That this actually represents epilepsy is unproven, though it has been suggested to be so.[6760] **Cough syncope** is perhaps a more likely cause.

Charcot–Weiss–Baker syndrome See **carotid sinus hypersensitivity**.

Charcot–Wilbrand syndrome Visual agnosia with an inability to revisualize images formerly seen, due to an infarct in the territory of the posterior cerebral artery.[1106]

Dr. H. Wilbrand (1851–1935) was a German neuro-ophthalmologist and a professor in Hamburg.

CHARGE association syndrome A congenital dysmorphic syndrome characterized by Colobomas of iris and retina, congenital Heart disease, choanal Atresia, mental and developmental Retardation, Genital hypoplasia and cryptorchid testes, and Ear deformities and deafness. Four of these six manifestations are taken as sufficient for the diagnosis.

Facial palsy, cleft palate, hypopituitarism, esophageal and renal deformities, etc., also occur[2687] but could not be worked into the acronym.

Charles Bonnet syndrome See **Bonnet syndrome**.

Charlevoix–Saguenay spastic ataxic syndrome A recessive form of slowly progressive complicated hereditary spastic paraplegia with ataxia and with onset in childhood, first reported from Quebec and mapped to chromosome 13q11–12.[4532]

Clinically, the pyramidal syndrome is accompanied by dysarthria, ataxia, hypermyelinated retinal nerve fibers, and abnormal eye movements; mitral incompetence and a motor neuropathy may be associated.[762] See **hereditary spastic paraplegia**; but the condition could equally well be classified as an early-onset **cerebellar ataxia** with retained reflexes.

Charlie M syndrome A congenital syndrome characterized by ocular hyperteleorism, facial paralysis, cleft palate, and digital and dental abnormalities.[2498]

Charlin Correa, Carlos (1885–1945) A Chilean ophthalmologist.

Charlin syndrome Brief bouts of severe unilateral pain at the root and ala of the nose accompanied by catarrh, uveitis with photophobia, conjunctivitis, and lacrimation.[1111] See **ciliary neuralgia**. The problem has been considered to be a selective neuritis of the maxillary branch of the trigeminal nerve, but may equally well be a form of **cluster headache**.

Chaslin, Pierre French pathologist, who first described the appearances of gliosis.[1115]

Chaslin gliosis (marginal gliosis) A condensation of usually delicate horizontal glial fibers which are normally found in the cortex, immediately beneath the pial surface; thought to be the consequence of convulsions. The gliosis is ubiquitous but most noticeable in the hippocampal gyrus and the surface of Ammon's horn; in severe cases it may extend through the cortex down to the subependymal regions.

chasma See yawning.

Chassaignac disease Pain in the limbs caused by trauma in children aged between 2 and 5 years, leading to incomplete paralysis or pseudo-paralysis and with prompt and full recovery.[1116] It was described by Charles-Marie-Édouard Chassaignac (1805–1879), who was a French physician.

CHAT classification of stroke A brief method of classifying the Clinical, Historical, Arterial (anatomical), and Target (pathological) features that relate to the stroke process.[585]

chatterbox syndrome See **cocktail party syndrome**.

Chavany, J.-A. E. (1892–1959) French neurologist.

Chavany–Brunhes syndrome The occurrence of headaches and various other (probably psychogenic) complaints in patients who are found to have benign calcification of the falx. The original description[1122] suggested a causal association.

check reflex Involuntary inhibition of a muscular contraction with a degree of restitution. Thus, when a patient's arm is extended horizontally in front of him and downward pressure on the wrist applied by the examiner, when that pressure is suddenly released, the arm normally flies upward for a short distance, then stops and descends slightly. The latter movement is also known as *rebound* or *recoil*. Failure to inhibit the upward movement and loss of the downward restitution are together considered as signs of cerebellar disease on the same side and are due to abnormal slowing of the desired contraction or relaxation of muscles required to maintain the position of the limb when the resistance is removed.

"When a person attempts to execute movement against resistance with a normal limb, and the resistance is suddenly removed, the limb rapidly moves a short distance in the desired direction till abruptly checked, or it may recoil. In a spastic limb, the amount of recoil is excessive; in functional cases there may be neither primary movement, nor recoil. In homolateral cerebellar disease, the range of movement is excessive, generally continued till it is no longer mechanically possible, and there is little or no recoil."[6062]

checkerboard fields Alternating squares of different colors, conveniently represented upon a television monitor. Repeated reversals of the colors of the squares (e.g., black becomes white, white becomes black) is the most effective stimulus known for the formation of **visual-evoked responses**.

Chediak, Moises (b. 1903) Cuban physician, professor of clinical pathology in Havana.

Chediak–Higashi disease A rare congenital recessively inherited **neurocutaneous syndrome** manifesting partial oculocutaneous albinism in childhood with photophobia, decreased lacrimation, peripheral neuropathy, enlarged liver, spleen, and lymph glands, and signs of cerebellar and basal ganglion disease with intermittent febrile episodes.

Other neurological signs such as mental and developmental delay, seizures, papilledema, nystagmus, ataxia, and motor neuropathy have also been recorded. The diagnosis is confirmed by the finding of peroxidase-positive panleukocytic granules. Only a few patients live into their adult years, usually because of recurrent infections[687] or the development of lymphomas.

Dr. O. Higashi is a Japanese pediatrician.

Chedoke-McMaster Stroke Assessment Disability Inventory A two-part scale measuring the physical impairments and disabilities affecting patients after stroke and yielding scores on shoulder pain, postural control, the arm, the hand, the leg, and the foot.[2534] (See Chart C–15.) See also **stroke scales**.

Chart C–15. Chedoke-McMaster Stroke Assessment Disability Inventory

Gross motor function index

1. Supine to side lying on strong side.
2. Supine to side lying on weak side.
3. Side lying to long sitting through strong side.
4. Side lying to sitting on side of the bed through strong side.
5. Side lying to sitting on side of the bed through weak side.
6. Standing.
7. Transfer to and from bed toward strong side.
8. Transfer to and from bed toward weak side.
9. Transfer up and down from floor and chair.
10. Transfer up and down from floor and standing.

Walking index

11. Walking indoors.
12. Walking outdoors, over rough ground, ramps, and curbs.
13. Walking outdoors several blocks.
14. Stairs.
15. Age- and sex-appropriate walking distance (in meters) for 2 min (2-point bonus).

Scoring Key

Independence (no helper)
- 7. Complete independence (timely, safely)
- 6. Modified independence (device)

Modified dependence (helper)
- 5. Supervision
- 4. Minimal assist (subject = 75%)
- 3. Moderate assist (subject = 50%)

Complete dependence (helper)
- 2. Maximal assist (subject = 25%)
- 1. Total assist (subject = 0%)

Adapted from Gowland C., Stratford P., Ward M. et al. Measuring physical impairment and disability woth the Chedoke-McMaster stroke assessment. Stroke 1993;24:58–63.[2534] *Reproduced by permission of Wolters–Kluwer.*

cheek sign See **Brudzinski signs**.

cheilalgia (Gr, lip + pain) Pain in the lips.

cheiralgia paresthetica (Gr, the hand + pain) (cheiralgia, Wartenberg disease) Isolated painful neuropathy of the superficial branch of the radial nerve, described by Wartenberg in 1917.

cheiro-oral migraine Migraine headaches preceded by an aura comprising paresthesias of the hand and cheek on one side, sometimes combined with aphasia.

cheiro-oral syndrome The combination of a sensory defect around the corner of the mouth and on the homolateral palm of the hand or thumb, due to a small lesion in the contralateral parietal cortex, or less often in the contralateral corona radiata, or in the pons (where the medial lemniscus is involved).[4173, 4792]

A *variant* is *crossed cheiro-oral syndrome* Perioral and contralateral acral paresthesias resulting from dorsal or dorsolateral brainstem infarction and often progressing to a full-blown **lateral medullary syndrome**.

cheiro-oral-pedal syndrome A sensory disturbance at the corner of the mouth, in the hand, and in the foot on the same side, usually due to a lesion in the thalamocortical projections or in the thalamus or brainstem as a result of a lacunar infarct.[3070]

chemical meningitis A syndrome of meningism associated with the rupture of a dermoid cyst, or resulting from the presence of blood or chemicals in the CSF. The cells in the CSF are largely of mononuclear type. A similar syndrome occurs rarely as a complication of primary cerebral tumors.

chemical terrorism The use of nervous system agents such as saxin, saxitoxin, botulinus toxin, metabolic and cellular poisons (e.g., cyanide, arsine), pulmonary agents such as chlorine and phosgene, or substances affecting epidermal structures (e.g., sulfur and nitrogen mustards, lewisite) for political purposes.[3218]

chemoaffinity The hypothesis of Sperry that each developing neuron or group of neurons acquires a distinct chemical label which defines both its functional class and its position within the population of neurons of which it is a part, and to identify and form connections with their target cells such as receptor organs.

chemodactoma A benign, highly vascular, locally invasive paraganglioma of non-chromaffin cells, often arising in the glomus jugulare region and characterized by the presence of thin-walled vessels and clear cells with intervening reticulin.[4743] See **glomus jugulare tumor** and **carotid body tumor**.

chemonucleolysis An invasive therapeutic procedure involving the injection of digesting enzymes (chymopapain) into an intervertebral disk in order to cause it to shrink as the nucleus pulposus is digested, thus relieving symptoms of disk protrusion. The effectiveness of the procedure in patients with prolapsed intervertebral disks, neurological signs, and failed conservative therapy is not questioned, but the unwanted effects of the injection include anaphylaxis and transverse myelitis.

chemopallidectomy The production of destructive lesions in the globus pallidus by stereotaxic procaine or alcohol injection as a therapeutic measure to relieve rigidity and tremor in **Parkinson disease.** Both the newer operation of ventrolateral thalamotomy and the advent of useful oral medications led to the abandonment of this technique, popular in the 1950s; but should such a measure be required at this time to contain severe and resistant tremors, radiofrequency lesions would be used rather than chemicals.

chemoreceptors Carotid and aortic bodies sensitive to alterations in the tissue tensions of pH, oxygen, and carbon dioxide. Decreased arterial pO_2, increased pCO_2, or decreased pH of the blood lead to hyperpnea and redistribution of blood to cerebral and coronary beds, but induce vasoconstriction. Similar bodies in the floor of the medulla are sensitive to changes in the pH of the CSF, a fall leading to hyperpnea.

Chernogubov syndrome See **Ehlers–Danlos syndrome**.

cherry-red spot The appearance of the macula which remains red when surrounded by a pale retina, reflecting the storage of an opaque material in the perifoveal ganglion cells; a characteristic sign in Tay–Sachs disease (classic **GM_2 gangliosidosis**) and in numerous other neuronal storage diseases, in central retinal artery occlusion, and in macular trauma or hemorrhage. In patients with storage diseases, disappearance of the spot occurs when the retinal ganglion cells atrophy. Fourteen conditions in which the spot is seen have been listed.[3465]

cherry-red spot-myoclonus syndrome (type I juvenile sialidosis) A lysosomal storage disease in which sialoligosaccharides are accumulated, manifesting corneal clouding and the retinal spot in childhood with the later appearance of severe, progressive stimulus-sensitive myoclonus and generalized seizures, hypotonia, hyperreflexia, and dysarthria.[5193] See **sialidosis type I**.

The association of such abnormalities also occurs in Tay–Sachs disease, Niemann–Pick disease, **GM_1 and GM_2 gangliosidoses**, **metachromatic leukodystrophy**, and the **glycogenoses**.

cheshire cat sign 1. The inappropriate persistence of a smile on the face of a patient with myotonic dystrophy.[1811] 2. The situations described by Bywaters in which patients exhibit the typical features of a condition although the diagnosis cannot be confirmed by pathological examination; or in which patients have a disease without any clinical evidence thereof.[968]

cheval de frise A device made of a hexagonal beam to which were attached radial wooden stakes or iron spikes, placed atop a wall to repel invaders. The pattern resulting resembles, in the minds of some migraineurs, the visual auras of migraine attacks.[5044]

chewing oscillopsia See **oscillopsia**.

Cheyne, George (1671–1743) Scottish physician who studied in Edinburgh and Aberdeen, was elected to the Royal Society within a year of graduation, and entered practice in London. He enjoyed a somewhat intemperate way of life, became ill, renounced his former indulgencies and retired to Bath, where his publications advocated temperance and a strict regimen in daily life, suggested methods of treating gout, and advised on diet. Much of this material must have been written on the basis of personal experience.[5704] He is best remembered for his book *The English Malady*.

Cheyne disease (The English Malady) Morbid concern about health matters, considered by George Cheyne to be due to the moisture and variability of the climate in the British isles[1141] but not a significant problem today in Newfoundland, where the weather is even worse.

Cheyne, John (1777–1836) Scottish physician, though physician to the Dublin hospitals, and an early neuropathologist. He published accounts of acute hydrocephalus, probably due to tuberculous meningitis, ischemic stroke, and subarachnoid hemorrhage, drawn in part from the pathological specimens of his friend Sir **Charles Bell**. Although he presciently blamed stress, alcohol, and tobacco as causes of strokes, he is best remembered for his description of periodic (Cheyne–Stokes) respirations in 1818, 35 years before **Stokes** (who acknowledged this). Neither seems to have been aware that **Robert Whytt** had also remarked upon the phenomenon.

Cheyne–Stokes respiration The occurrence of a series of inspirations increasing to a maximum and then declining in force and length until a state of apparent apnea is established; when, after a more or less prolonged period, sometimes of apparent death, a low inspiration, followed by one more decided, marks the commencement of a new ascending and then descending series of inspirations. "For several days his breathing was irregular; it would cease entirely for a quarter of a minute, then it would become very perceptible, although very low, then by degrees it became heaving and quick, and then it would gradually cease again; this revolution in the state of his breathing occupied about a minute, during which there were about thirty acts of respiration."[1142]

The phenomenon was named for **John Cheyne** and **William Stokes** (1804–1878) an Irish physician, Regius professor of medicine at Dublin from 1845.

Chiari, Hans (1851–1916) Austrian pathologist who trained in Vienna and worked there with Heschl before moving to Prague and later to Strasbourg. He described the first three of the malformations bearing his name between 1891 and 1896. Other contributions included his description of choriocarcinoma and thrombosis of the hepatic vein (Budd–Chiari syndrome), and, in 1906, recognition of the association of

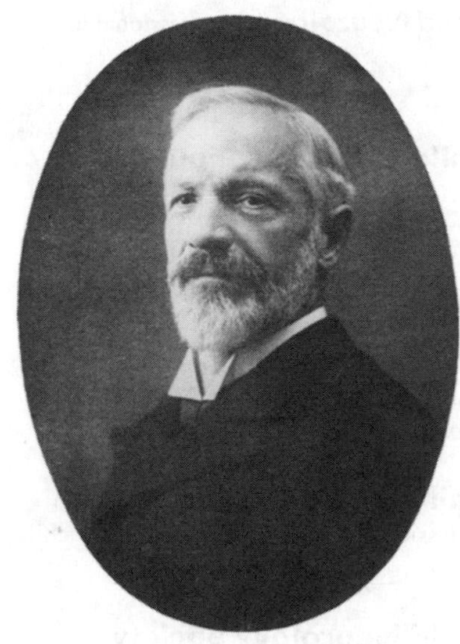

Figure C–3 Hans Chiari.

carotid artery plaques with thrombi in the intracranial portion of the carotid artery.[4233]

Chiari malformation (Arnold–Chiari malformation, List syndrome)[3869] Congenital caudal displacement of the brainstem, cerebellum, spinal cord, cervical spine, and posterior fossa, often manifesting only in adult life. A short neck, obstructive hydrocephalus, cerebellar signs, evidence of damage to the lower cranial nerves, and nystagmus are the principal manifestations when the disorder becomes symptomatic, but a syringomyelic syndrome (lumbosacral radiculopathy) may also occur and the condition may be complicated by meningomyelocele.[251]

In *type I* (adult type, familial occipital dysplasia, Arnold–Chiari–Schwalbe–Gredig–Penfield–Coburn syndrome), there is downward displacement of the pons, medulla, fourth ventricle, and cerebellar tonsils down to or through the foramen magnum, associated with spinal dysraphism and sometimes with hydrocephalus. This usually presents with pyramidal or cerebellar signs, downbeat nystagmus, hydrocephalus, and variable cranial nerve disturbances in adult life. Syringomyelia is also commonly present. The condition may be dominantly inherited.[4468]

In *type II* (infantile type, Chiari type), the fourth ventricle may descend far down into the cervical spine, and the hypoplastic cerebellar vermis and tonsils and possibly the elongated medulla all herniate down through, and may impact within, the foramen magnum. Meningomyelocele is associated.

This is the commonest form and presents in infancy or childhood. Spina bifida of any degree, platybasia, assimilation of the atlas with the occipital bones, **Klippel–Feil syndrome**, hydrocephalus, and other cerebral anomalies (microgyria, tectal anomalies) often coexist.

Type III (Chiari–Parker–McConnell–Aring) is characterized by downward displacement of the medulla and cerebellar tonsils, with an accompanying occipital encephalocele through which the cerebellum projects.

Type IV is cerebellar hypoplasia, the same condition as the **Dandy–Walker** cyst.

Despite the usual eponymous title, the first description was actually that of John Cleland (an English anatomist, surgeon, and poet) in 1883, but the report of Chiari in 1891 drew more attention.[1146] **Arnold** described one case in 1894.[7]

For the headache attributed to **Chiari malformation** type I, diagnostic criteria have been defined:

A. Headache characterized by at least one of the following and fulfilling criterion D:
   1. Precipitated by cough and/or Valsalva maneuver
   2. Protracted (hours to days) occipital and/or sub-occipital headache
   3. Associated with symptoms and/or signs of brainstem, cerebellar, and/or cervical cord dysfunction

B. Cerebellar tonsillar herniation as defined by one of the following on craniocervical MRI:
   1. ≥5 mm caudal descent of the cerebellar tonsils
   2. ≥3 mm caudal descent of the cerebellar tonsils plus at least one of the following indicators of crowding of the subarachnoid space in the area of the craniocervical junction:
      a. Compression of the CSF spaces posterior and lateral to the cerebellum
      b. Reduced height of the supraocciput
      c. Increased slope of the tentorium
      d. Kinking of the medulla oblongata

C. Evidence of posterior fossa dysfunction, based on at least two of the following:
   1. Otoneurological symptoms and/or signs (e.g., dizziness, disequilibrium, sensations of alteration in ear pressure, hypacusis or hyperacusis, vertigo, downbeat nystagmus, oscillopsia)

2. Transient visual symptoms (spark photopsias, visual blurring, diplopia or transient visual field deficits)
3. Demonstration of clinical signs relevant to cervical cord, brainstem, or lower cranial nerves or of ataxia or dysmetria

D. Headache resolves within 3 months after successful treatment of the Chiari malformation.

From the International Classification of Headache Disorders (Headache Classification Committee of the International Headache Society. *Cephalalgia* 2004;24[Suppl 1]) by kind permission of Dr. Jes Olesen, the International Headache Society and Wiley-Blackwell Publications.

chiasma (Gr, two lines crossing like an X) The decussation of the fibers of the optic nerve.

chiasmal apoplexy An acutely evolving syndrome of retro-orbital or frontal headache with abrupt visual loss due to hemorrhage into the optic chiasm. Young adults are most often affected. The underlying pathology is most commonly a small intrachiasmatic arteriovenous malformation.[4032]

chiasmal syndrome The clinical effects of compression of the chiasm in the presence of a normal-sized sella turcica by, for instance, a pituitary adenoma or a suprasellar meningioma. The clinical features include complaints of visual deterioration with dimming of vision, diplopia, headache, and vertigo, and on examination, a central scotoma, bitemporal field defects, and optic atrophy are found.[1392] See **Cushing syndrome**. See also **hemifield slide** and **postfixation blindness**.

CHILD Syndrome (Congenital Hemidysplasia, Ichthyosiform erythroderma and Limb Defects) An X-linked dominantly inherited malformation (Xq28) manifesting hypoplasia of the psoas muscle, the lung, thyroid, lower cranial nerves, and the pons, medulla, cerebellum, and spinal cord.

Child Behaviour Checklist A rating instrument for child behavior, used in the classification of pediatric neurobehavioral disorders.[44]

Child Neurology A professional journal. Web site: www.waisman.wisc.edu/child-neuro/.

Child Neurology Foundation A charitable organization. Web site: www.childneurologyfoundation.org.

Child Neurology Home Page A site coordinating the available internet resources in Child Neurology, both for professionals and patients. Web site: http://www-personal.umich.edu/~leber/c-n/.

Child Neurology in the UK A professional resource. Web site: www.child-neuro.org.uk.

Child Neurology Society A professional organization of child neurologists. Address: 475 Cleveland Ave. N. Suite, 220, St. Paul, MN 55104-5051. Tel: 612-641-1584.Web site: www.childneurologysociety.org/.

childhood absence epilepsy (pyknolepsy; OMIM 600131) A relatively common form of **idiopathic generalized epilepsy** occurring in children of school age (peak manifestations at age 6–7 years), with a strong genetic predisposition in otherwise normal children. It appears more frequently in girls than in boys and is characterized by very frequent absences (several to many hundreds per day), typically precipitated by hyperventilation and starting and ending abruptly in less than 20 s. Unresponsiveness, interruption of the ongoing voluntary activity, and transient eyelid or facial myoclonia are classic features. The neurological examination is normal and the condition usually remits in adolescence.[4882]

The suggested diagnostic criteria available on the ILAE Web site: (www.ilae-epilepsy.org/ctf/childhood_absence.html) are the following:

1. Age at onset between 4 and 10 years and a peak at 5–7 years.
2. Normal neurologic state and development.
3. Brief (4–20 s, exceptionally longer) and frequent (tens per day) absence seizures with abrupt and severe impairment (loss) of consciousness. Automatisms are frequent but have no significance in the diagnosis.
4. EEG ictal discharges of generalized high-amplitude spike and double (maximum of occasional three spikes are allowed) spike and slow-wave complexes. They are rhythmic at around 3 Hz with a gradual and regular slowdown from the initial to the terminal phase of the discharge. Their duration varies from 4 to 20 s.

Exclusion criteria

The following may be incompatible with childhood absence epilepsy:

1. Other than typical absence seizures such as GTCS, or myoclonic jerks prior to or during the active stage of absences. (However, some patients do develop GTC seizures in adolescence or early adult life.)
2. Eyelid myoclonia, perioral myoclonia, rhythmic massive limb jerking, and single or arrhythmic myoclonic jerks of the head, trunk, or limbs. However, mild myoclonic elements of the eyes, eyebrows, and eyelids may be featured, particularly in the first 3 s of the absence seizure.
3. Retention of consciousness during the 3–4 Hz discharges.
4. Brief EEG 3–4 Hz spike-wave paroxysms of less than 4 s, multiple spikes (more than 3) or ictal discharge fragmentations.
5. Visual (photic) and other sensory precipitation of clinical seizures.

Adapted from Dreifuss FE, et al. Commission for classification and terminology, ILAE. Proposal for revised classifications of epilepsies and epileptic syndromes. *Epilepsia* 1989;30:389–99 by kind permission of the IFCN and Wiley-Blackwell Publications.

childhood ataxia with diffuse CNS hypomyelination (fatal infantile leukodystrophy; CACH; vanishing white matter disease) A progressive heterogeneous leukodystrophic disorder of unknown etiology with onset in childhood, sometimes following cranial trauma or fever. It is characterized by normal head size, ataxic diplegia, lack of dementia, late optic atrophy, and a diffuse confluent CNS white matter abnormality on CT and MRI scans shown pathologically to be due to hypomyelination.[5599, 6484] The condition has also been reported to occur first in adult life.[448]

childhood dermatomyositis or polymyositis associated with vasculitis (juvenile dermatomyositis) An acquired, progressive, noninfectious, nongranulomatous proximal painful inflammatory myopathy of children or youth with a slow, relapsing, or monophasic course. Clinically, a skin rash and calcinosis are both common in association with the weakness. Pathologically, muscle fiber necrosis is rare and limited to lesions resembling infarcts; capillary necrosis at the periphery of muscle fascicles, the presence of undulating tubules in endothelial cells, lymphocytes, pericytes and pseudosatellite cells, and variable inflammatory infiltrates in connective tissue septa are the major features.[1030]

A strong association with HLA Class II DQa1*0501 antigen has been shown.

childhood epilepsy with centrotemporal spikes See **benign Rolandic epilepsy**.

childhood epilepsy with occipital paroxysms The syndrome is, in general, similar to that of benign childhood epilepsy with centrotemporal spikes. The seizures start with visual symptoms (amaurosis, phosphenes, illusions, or hallucinations) and are often followed by a hemiclonic seizure or automatisms. In 25% of cases, the seizures are immediately followed by migrainous headache. The EEG has paroxysms of high-amplitude spike-waves or sharp waves recurring rhythmically on the occipital and posterior temporal areas of one or both hemispheres, but only when the eyes are closed. During seizures, the occipital discharge may spread to the central or temporal region. At present, no definite statement on prognosis is possible. (Adaped from Dreifuss, F.E. et al. Commission for classification and terminology, ILAE. Proposal for revised classifications of epilepsies and epileptic syndromes. *Epilepsia* 1989;30:389–99. Reproduced by kind permission of Wiley-Blackwell Publications.)

Other criteria have been suggested as follows:[4879] 1. Unequivocal clinical evidence of epileptic seizures and paroxysms maximal in the occipital areas on at least one EEG, and no clinical nor EEG manifestations of primary generalized epilepsy or of another distinctive epileptic syndrome; 2. No evidence of neurological or intellectual deficit; and 3. Normal appearance of CT brain scan.

childhood muscular dystrophies See **limb girdle muscular dystrophies** (LGMD 2B); distal myopathy (**Miyoshi myopathy**) which are both deficient in this same gene product; and **Fukuyama** congenital muscular dystrophy.[6408]

childhood myoclonic epilepsies See **myoclonus**.

childhood polymyositis Inflammatory muscle disease occurring before the (arbitrary) age of 16 years. See **polymyositis**.

A *variant* form is *acquired infantile polymyositis*, which is a variant of **childhood polymyositis** presenting in infancy with hypotonia without CNS involvement and showing a good response to steroid therapy.[6299]

childhood schizophrenia See **Heller disease**.

childhood-onset DIMS Difficulties in the initiation and maintenance of sleep starting before puberty and persisting into adult life, resulting in complaints of insomnia. (See also ASDA diagnostic classification and **sleep disorders**.[1629])

childhood-onset idiopathic torsion dystonia A syndrome presenting first after the age of 6 years with arm dystonia but without rest tremor, bradykinesia, or rigidity. Any response to levadopa is but slight.[942]

childhood-onset Parkinsonism A Parkinsonian syndrome presenting first before the age of 12 years, with foot dystonia, rest tremor, bradykinesia, and rigidity. A response to levadopa is notable.[2333]

Children's Brain Tumor Foundation A charitable organization. Web site: http://cbtf.org/cms/.

Children's Coma Score A scale designed for use with infants and toddlers aged 0–3 years who have incurred head injury.[5170] (Chart C–16; see also **Glasgow Coma Scale**.)

Child's Brain See **Pediatric Neurosciences**.

chimera An organism created from the genetic material of two different species. The term is derived from the Greek word signifying a monster.

Chart C–16. Children's Coma Score

Score	Response
Ocular Responses	
4	Pursuit
3	Extra-ocular muscles intact and reactive pupils
2	Fixed pupils, *or* extraocular movements impaired
1	Fixed pupils *and* extraocular movements impaired
Verbal Responses	
3	Cries
2	Spontaneous respirations
1	Apneic
Motor Responses	
4	Flexes and extends
3	Withdraws from painful stimuli
2	Hypertonic
1	Flaccid

Chinese paralytic syndrome An acute axonal motor neuropathy occurring in the summer months and causing a rapidly progressive ascending tetraparesis in children or young adults, often with ventilatory failure but without sensory changes, fever, CSF pleocytosis or systemic illness. In some cases, anti-GM_1 antibodies suggesting recent *Campylobacter* infection are detectable. The prognosis is good if the severe complications are appropriately managed.

The name was applied as a result of the first reports of the disorder which had affected many children in northern China, but the infection is worldwide.[2364, 4241, 4242] See also **immune-mediated neuropathies**.

Chinese restaurant syndrome (Kwok's quease, post sino-cibal syndrome, Sin-Cib-Syn) Monosodium glutamate (MSG) poisoning, manifesting as tightness of the masseters, limb paresthesias, burning of the face, limbs, and chest and precordial discomfort occurring after ingestion of MSG (usually in a restaurant serving Chinese food) but self-limited over a few hours.[3622]

chiralgia See **cheiralgia paresthetica**.

chirismus An old term for spasm of the wrists, hands, or fingers during a convulsion.

chiromegaly Trophic changes leading to proliferation of the soft tissues of the hand, as in some cases of syringomyelia.

chiropodal paralysis Weakness and atrophy of the small muscles of the hands and feet, once thought typical of arsenical polyneuritis but in fact common in almost every form of motor neuropathy.

chloroma (Balfour disease) A rare condition in which hyperplasia of the leukocyte parent cells, usually myeloblasts, results in widespread tumor formation, frequently affecting the orbits and skull. The eponym follows the report of Dr. J.H. Balfour to the Medico-Chiurgical society in 1834 but the nature of the syndrome is uncertain.

chlorosis (from Gr, greening) Until the early twentieth century, this was considered a disease entity, affecting young women around puberty and manifest by a greenish pallor, oligomenorrhea, and numerous symptoms which would today be regarded as evidence of hypochondriasis. See **chronic fatigue syndrome**.

Chodzko reflex Contraction of several muscles of the arm on one or both sides when the manubrium is percussed,[1156] presumably witnessing hyperirritability of some kind.

Dr. W. Chodkzo was a Polish neurologist.

choked disk See **papilledema**.

cholecystokinin A complex of octapeptide neurotransmitter hormones found in the gut and in the brain with a role in feeding behavior.

cholestanol A biological substance closely resembling cholesterol, deposited in **cholestanolosis**.

cholestanolosis See **cerebrotendinous xanthomatosis**.

cholesteatoma Small tumors usually found on the base of the skull, for instance at the cerebellopontine angle, and composed of epithelial cells arranged in concentric layers.

cholesterol emboli syndrome (atheromatous embolization) A multisystem disorder caused by peripheral embolization of cholesterol crystals, for example, after angiography, aortic surgery, or other trauma. The findings may occur remotely, even months after the inciting event. The clinical features include blue toe syndrome, gangrene, livedo reticularis; pain in the legs, feet, toes, abdomen, flank or back; hematuria; accelerated hypertension; impaired renal function; and (less commonly) spinal cord, penile, splenic, or adrenal infarction.[499]

cholinergic crisis An acute exacerbation of myasthenia-like symptoms of weakness and fatigability (**cholinergic paralysis**) often with evidence of generalized parasympathetic overactivity, as a result of excessive ingestion of anticholinergic drugs, in a patient with **myasthenia gravis**.

The condition mimics, and is hardly differentiated clinically from, **myasthenic crisis**. The use of edrophonium for diagnosis in this situation is dangerous, but a régime comprising discontinuation of anticholinesterase drugs, ventilatory support, and time invariably provides the answer.

cholinergic paralysis Weakness as a result of excessive depolarization of the motor end plate. Poisoning with anti-cholinesterase compounds such as nerve gases, depolarizing drugs, or black widow spider venom are typical causes. See also **neuromuscular transmission defects**.

cholosis An extinct term for lameness.

chondrodystrophia calcificans punctata congenita See **Conradi–Hünerman syndrome**.

chondrodytrophic myotonia See **Schwartz–Jampel syndrome**.

chondroectodermal dysplasia See **Ellis–van Creveld syndrome**.

chondromas Benign cartilaginous tumors which occasionally arise from the synchrondroses at the base of the skull or from the vault.[3629]

chopper A device consisting of a mechanical or electronic switch used in some EEG amplifiers for interrupting (chopping) DC and low-frequency AC signals and converting them into square waves of relatively high frequency. The same device may provide synchronous rectification of these square waves after amplification to reconvert them to the form of the original signal at the output. (From the 1974 Report of the Committee on Terminology, IFCN. In: Chatrian GE, Bergamini L, Dondey M, et al. A glossary of terms most commonly used by clinical electroencephalographers. *EEG Clin Neurophysiol* 1974;37:538–48. Reproduced with kind permission from the IFCN and Elsevier Science.)

chopper amplifier A direct current amplifier in which a chopper interrupts DC and low-frequency AC signals and converts them into square waves of relatively high frequency. These are magnified by an AC amplifier and then reconverted by synchronous rectification to the form of the original signal at the output. (From the 1974 Report of the Committee on Terminology, IFCN. In: Chatrian GE, Bergamini L, Dondey M, et al. A glossary of terms most commonly used by clinical electroencephalographers. *EEG Clin Neurophysiol* 1974;37:538–48. Reproduced with kind permission from the IFCN and Elsevier Science.)

chorda (Lat, the string, as of a musical instrument) A tendon or fiber bundle.

chorda tympani (Gr, bowstring + drum) A branch of the VII cranial nerve, crossing through the middle ear applied to the eardrum and carrying afferent fibers subserving taste sensation from the anterior two-thirds of the tongue. It was first described by Bartolommeo Eustachius (1524–1574), an Italian anatomist, in 1563.[5619]

chordoma An uncommon tumor arising from the remnants of the primitive notochord, either in the clivus at the base of the cranium or at the level of the sacrum. It was first described and named by Moritz Ribbert (1855–1920), a Swiss pathologist.[5619]

Symptoms occur as a result of local compression of neurological and other structures. Histologically they are characterized by sheets of **physaliphorous cells** containing periodic acid-Schiff-positive material, bone fragments, keratin, S100 protein, and epithelial membrane antigen.[6]

chorea (Gr, dancing) (Fr, folie musculaire) Excessive spontaneous, random, brief, abrupt, non-repetitive irregular movements with distal predominance, flowing randomly from one body part to another. They result from numerous diseases of the basal ganglia, including the caudate nucleus. The severity of the movements varies from mild motor restlessness and fidgeting to constant, dance-like, or even violent and disabling instability of limbs, posture, and gait. The original description was by Thomas Sydenham (see *The Entire Works.* Trans. Swan D. London, Edward Cave, 1742). In this book of 623 pages only about 5 are devoted to disorders of the nervous system—chorea, apoplexy, and epilepsy. The most relevant entry follows

> *This disorder is a kind of convulsion which seizes children of both sexes, from the tenth to the fourteenth year: it manifests itself by a halting or unsteadiness of one of the legs which the patient draws after him like an idiot. If the hand of the same side be applied to the breast, or any other part of the body, the child can't keep it a moment in the same posture but it will be drawn into a different one by a convulsion, notwithstanding all his efforts to the contrary. Before a child who has this disorder can get a glass or a cup to his mouth, he uses abundance of odd gestures; for he does not bring it in a straight line thereto but his hand being drawn sideways by the spasm, he moves it backwards and forwards until at length, the glass accidently coming nearer his lips, he throws the liquor hastily into his mouth and swallows it greedily, as if he meant to divert the spectators.*

The names of four saints (Vitus [Guy], Valentine, Modesti, and John) have been associated with chorea over the ages. Power and Sedgwick (1882) identify 39 varieties of chorea; apart from the succeeding entries, these include diaphragmatic or laryngeal chorea (probably hiccoughs), chorea dimitiata (hemichorea), epidemic chorea, chorea magna and chorea germanorum (dancing mania, epidemic or hysterical chorea, or tarantulism), chorea nutans (head nodding), chorea festinans and saltatoria (forms in which the subject is compelled to run or jump), and chorea senilis, an inaccurate synonym for **Parkinson disease**.[5103]

For a historical review, see McHenry.[4233] See also the following entries and **dystonic choreoathetosis induced by exercise, familial inverted choreoathetosis** and **kinesigenic choreoathetosis, benign hereditary chorea, benign essential chorea, hereditary progressive chorea without dementia, Huntington disease**, and **Sydenham chorea**.

chorea-acanthocytosis (OMIM #200150) A recessively inherited disorder caused by deficiency in VPS13A on chr. 9q21, which encodes *chorein*. It is characterized by neuronal degeneration and acanthocytosis of red cells.The onset is in young adult life, with chorea and dystonia, occasionally Parkinsonism, and prominent orofacial and lingual dyskinesias that result in self-mutilating lip- and tongue-biting. Abnormal eye movements, bizarre gait, and peripheral neuropathy and myopathy with raised CK levels are usual. Neuropsychiatric, disinhibition, obsessive-compulsive disorder, self-neglect, tics, affective disturbances with agitation, and dementia are all frequently seen.

chorea anglorum See Sydenham chorea.

chorea electrica (Bergeron disease, electric chorea) See **Dubini disease**.

chorea fibrillaris See Morvan chorea.

chorea gravidarum Monosymptomatic chorea resembling that of **Sydenham chorea** but occurring during the earlier months of pregnancy.[545]

chorea lascivia The name applied by Paracelsus to **dancing mania**.

chorea major Originally dancing mania; now **Huntington chorea**, if employed at all.

chorea minor (chorea anglorum) See Sydenham chorea.

chorea progressive hereditaria See Huntington disease.

chorea St. Viti See Sydenham chorea.

chorea variabilis A term used both for **Tourette syndrome** and Brissaud disease.

chorea with curvilinear bodies A rare, possibly recessively inherited syndrome characterized by chorea, paroxysmal dystonia, intractable tonic-clonic seizures, pyramidal signs, and mental and developmental delay with onset in childhood. Curvilinear bodies are detected in brain neurons and in peripheral white cells.[1409]

chorea-amyotrophy with chronic hemolytic anemia A condition resembling **choreoacanthocytosis** except for the substitution of hemolytic anemia for the acanthocytosis. Clinically, the disorder appears in adult life and manifests facial and vocal tics, tongue-biting, pes cavus, hyporeflexia, neuropathy or myopathy, and increased serum CK levels.[5971] See also **Fotopoulos syndrome**.

choreic gait Unsteady progression with irregular lurches induced by involuntary choreic movements of the legs, giving an impression fancifully described as dance-like.

choreic hand Flexion of the wrist with overextension of the metacarpo-phalangeal joints when the arms are extended in front of the body.[6819]

choreiform syndrome The persistent movements and akathisiac restlessness in school-age boys with the **attentional defect hyperactivity syndrome**. The validity of the syndrome is uncertain.[5111]

choreoacanthocytosis The coexistence of these entities, sometimes with added Parkinsonian features. See **neuroacanthocytosis**.

choreoathetosis While **chorea** and **athetosis** are clinically different, and result from lesions in different areas of the basal ganglia, they often coexist; but more often this term reflects the uncertainty of the observer as to which condition is being viewed.

choreoathetosis/spasticity disease A syndrome with these features mapped to 1p, a region containing a cluster of potassium (K^+) channel genes.

choreoathetotic cerebral palsy See **cerebral palsy**. The original description of athetosis was by **Hammond** in 1867.

choreofacient An agent which produces limb tremor; the name was formerly applied to heavy metals such as mercury.

choreomania epidemic chorea. See **dancing mania**.

choresthesia (Gr, place + sensation) A term encompassing the somatic sense of space, and thus a synthesis of joint position sense, depth sense, and two-point discrimination.[5267, 5895]

choristoma A benign, microscopic granular cell tumor of the neurohypophysis, usually found accidentally in elderly people.

choroid (Gr, chorion + like) A vascular structure; thus the vascular layer of the eye or the secretory villi beneath the ependyma and within the cerebral ventricles.

choroid plexus papilloma An uncommon, benign, primary neuroectodermal vascular tumor arising from the choroid plexus in the lateral ventricles in children and the fourth ventricles in adults. Benign (well-differentiated) forms are characterized histologically by an uniform columnar epithelium with few mitoses, frequent calcification, and positive staining for carbonic anhydrase C, S100 protein, **glial acidic fibrillary protein**, and cytokeratins: malignant (poorly differentiated) forms show pleomorphism, irregularity of structure and local invasiveness, and stain only for cytokeratins.[6]

Clinically, it may lead to a syndrome of headache with raised intracranial pressure without localizing signs with seizures, but it may also remain asymptomatic.

choroideremia An X-linked recessive condition (Xq21.2) causing retinitis pigmentosa, choroidal degeneration, and visual loss.[1317]

choroiditis Inflammation of the choroid layer of the eye.

choroidocerebral calcification syndrome A rare syndrome of mental retardation, dense calcification of the lateral ventricular choroid plexus, and increased CSF protein, seen first in infancy.[5864]

Christensen–Krabbe syndrome See **Alpers disease**.

Christian syndrome 1. (adducted thumbs syndrome, Christian–Andrews–Conneally–Molar syndrome) A congenital recessively inherited dysmorphic syndrome characterized also by brachydactyly, hirsutism, micrognathia, cleft palate, pectus excavatum, adducted thumbs, club foot, ophthalmoplegia, muscle fasciculations, preaxial polysyndactyly, varus joint contractures, craniosynostosis with microcephaly and hypertelorism, and mental and developmental delay.[1170] See also **craniosynostosis**. 2. An X-linked syndrome characterized by dwarfism, ridging of the metopic sutures, cervical vertebral fusion, thoracic and sacral vertebral deformities, VI cranial nerve palsy, and imperforate anus.[1169]

Christian–Andrews–Conneally–Molar syndrome (adducted thumbs syndrome) See **Christian syndrome** (1).

chromatic sensitive epilepsy A seizure disorder in boys who convulse while watching cartoons on television. Like many others, they were not known to suffer from epilepsy, although some had a family history of epilepsy. The flickering blue and red background is considered to be the most important precipitating factor.

chromatin positive Turner syndrome See **Noonan syndrome**.

chromatolysis (axon reaction) Morphologic changes within neuronal cell bodies, including the disruption, dispersal, and eventual disappearance of the granular endoplasmic reticulum (Nissl substance) as a result of damage to its axon. Loss of stainable material from a damaged neuron.

Two forms are described. In *central chromatolysis*, the loss of basophilic Nissl substance leads to eosinophilic staining of the cytoplasm, initially close to the cell nucleus. When chromatolysis occurs as a response to *axonal injury*, the Nissl substance degenerates but the nucleus also moves to an eccentric position, the nucleolus enlarges, and swelling of the perikaryon and basophilia within the cytoplasm also occurs. The word was introduced by **Marinesco** in 1909.

chromatopsia The abnormal perception of colors investing objects seen or their backgrounds.

chromophobe adenoma A benign pituitary tumor, the cells of which take up little stain. The tumor provides evidence of its existence mainly through exerting local pressure on the surrounding structures (optic chiasm, hypothalamus, cavernous sinus), rather than through the effects of its hormonal secretions.

chromosome 4p partial deletion A dysmorphic syndrome characterized also by mental and physical delay, nystagmus, ptosis, and strabismus.[240] See **Wolf-Hirschorn syndrome**.

chromosome 5p deletion See **cri-du-chat syndrome**.

chromosome 13 trisomy syndrome (Patau syndrome) See **trisomy 13 syndrome**.

chromosome 18 partial deletion 1. (long arm; de Grouchy syndrome) A congenital dysmorphic syndrome manifesting midface dysplasia, short stature, mental and physical delay, nystagmus, seizures, hypotonia, optic atrophy, retinal degeneration, and congenital cardiac anomalies.[3719] 2. (short arm) A congenital dysmorphic syndrome with midface dysplasia, manifesting also mental and physical delay, hypertelorism, epicanthic folds, strabismus, and (later) aphasia. Arhinencephaly or microcephaly are also reported in some cases.[3135]

chromosome 21q deletion A congenital dysmorphic syndrome characterized by microcephaly, hypertonia, antimongoloid slant, mental delay, and pyloric stenosis.[5257]

chromotopia Loss of the perception of colors when there is no loss for white objects. Clinically, it is usually a hemichromatopia, due to a lesion of the contralateral pathways less severe than is required to produce hemianopia.

chronaxie (chronaxy) (Gr, time + value) The time for which a current twice as strong as the galvanic threshold must flow in order to excite the muscle stimulated. The concept was introduced by Louis Lapique (b. 1866), a French physiologist, in 1909. Both the term and the concept are obsolete. See **strength–duration curve**.

chronaxy See **chronaxie**.

chronic (Gr, concerning time) Long continued.

chronic acquired hepatocerebral degeneration A heterogeneous disorder affecting patients with porto-systemic collaterals or surgically created shunts. Clinical presentations can be neuropsychiatric (apathy, lethargy, dementia, excessive somnolence), a movement disorder (dysarthria, ataxia, tremor, choreoathetosis which affects the cranial musculature predominantly but also that of the trunk and extremities, Parkinsonism, myoclonus, pyramidal signs, and/or dystonia). Diffuse muscular rigidity, grasp reflexes, tremor at rest, nystagmus, action myoclonus, and persistent asterixis are less common signs. A coarse rhythmic tremor of the arms in certain sustained postures and diffuse slowing on the EEG complete the typical clinical picture. Elevation of the blood ammonia level or an abnormality of ammonia tolerance are typical findings.

At the cellular level, cortical laminar necrosis and polymicrocavitation in the cortex and basal ganglia are combined with cerebral and cerebellar atrophy. Microscopically, Alzheimer type II astrocytes and cytoplasmic glycogen granules are characteristic. Recent neuroradiological observations in patients with liver failure have shown a specific MRI imaging appearance with a hyperintense T1 signal in the pallidum, putamen, and, rarely, in the mesencephalon.[3225]

chronic AIDS encephalopathy See **HIV-associated cognitive/motor complex**.

chronic akathisia A form of drug-induced akathisia in which the abnormal movements occur either as the neuroleptic dose is being increased early in therapy (**acute persistent akathisia**) or coinciding with a reduction of the dose at the end of the course of treatment (**tardive akathisia**).[945]

chronic alcoholic myopathy See **alcoholic myopathy** and **Schultze Test**.

chronic anterior poliomyelitis (Cruveilhier atrophy) See **amyotrophic lateral sclerosis**.

chronic asymmetric spinal muscular atrophy A rare syndrome, commoner in males, with its onset in the first four decades of life and manifesting slowly progressive asymmetrical neurogenic muscular atrophy (usually of one arm) without bulbar or pyramidal involvement and with slight depression of the muscle stretch reflexes.[2757] Patients with this condition probably represent that small proportion of those diagnosed as having **amyotrophic lateral sclerosis** whose survival is prolonged. See also **hereditary motor neuropathy** (*variants*).

chronic ataxic neuropathy with ophthalmoplegia, IgM paraprotein, cold agglutinins, and anti-GG1b disialosylantibodies (CANOMAD) An acquired chronic ataxic neuropathy with features resembling a dorsal midbrain syndrome.[231]

chronic atrophic paralysis An old name for hereditary motor neuropathy.

chronic axon loss polyradiculoneuropathy See **chronic inflammatory demyelinating polyradiculoneuropathy**.

chronic benign lymphocytic meningitis (chronic lymphocytic meningitis) A benign and chronic syndrome of headache, depression, malaise, and subtle personality change in patients with persistent elevation of CSF cell counts following an episode of meningitis. The etiology is unknown[2986] but rarely conditions such as **Wegener granulomatosis** or **multiple sclerosis** are found. A subgroup of patients responds to corticosteroids.[1110]

chronic brain syndrome See **dementia**. The term is inappropriate, evasive, and redundant.

chronic brain syndrome of infantile hydrocephalus See **cocktail party syndrome**.

chronic cerebral schistosomiasis A granulomatous disease resulting from invasion of the brain, usually by *Schistosoma japonicum*. The granulomas may produce focal signs and frequently seizures.[6858]

chronic childhood spinal muscular atrophy (Werdnig–Hoffman, Oppenheimer, [Wohlfart–] Kugelberg–Welander disease, Krabbe universal muscular hypoplasia, amyotonia congenita, hereditary proximal SMA, infantile muscular atrophy) A recessively (seldom dominantly) inherited syndrome manifesting progressive disorder of anterior horn cells with initial proximal selectivity but without pyramidal tract involvement, which does not itself cause death in less than 18 months. Most cases have their onset before the age of 8 years.[4956] See **hereditary motor neuropathy**, types I, II, and III.

chronic chorea See **trigeminal neuralgia**.

chronic cluster headache (chronic migrainous neuralgia) Headaches in which the attacks occur for more than 1 year without remission or with remissions only lasting less than 14 days. They occur mainly in males and are related to smoking. This definition and the diagnostic criteria are suggested by the Headache Classification Committee of the International Headache Society. (See Chart C–17.)

Chart C–17. Chronic Cluster Headache

A. All letter headings of **cluster headache**.
B. Absence of remission phases for 1 year or more with remissions lasting less than 14 days.[2820]

Two subvarieties are defined:

Chronic cluster headache unremitting from onset (primary chronic cluster)

A. All letter headings of **chronic cluster headache**.
B. Absence of remission periods lasting 14 days or more from onset.

Chronic cluster headache evolved from episodic (secondary chronic cluster)

A. All letter headings of **chronic cluster headache**.
B. At least one interim remission period lasting 14 days or more within 1 year after onset, followed by unremitting course for at least 1 year.

These diagnostic criteria were suggested by the Headache Classification Committee of the International Headache Society (Classification of headache disorders, cranial neuralgias and facial pains; and diagnostic criteria for primary headache disorders. Cephalalgia *1988;***8***(Suppl):1–96) and are reproduced by kind permission. They do not, however, mention auras such as nasal and ocular congestion, changes in mood and bowel function, and more typical visual, paresthetic, or aphasic symptoms which can also occur.*

chronic congenital TORCH encephalopathies Polio-encephalopathies resulting from intrauterine infection with Toxoplasmosis, Other viruses, Rubella, Cytomegalovirus or Herpesvirus, or with *Treponema.*

Developmental delay, myoclonic seizures, retinopathy, hepatosplenomegaly, and hematological disorders are potential consequences common to all these infections.[2055]

chronic congenital toxoplasmosis with late degeneration A polioencephalopathy characterized by the development of chorioretinitis, intracranial calcification, cerebral cortical atrophy, microcephaly, and various neurological signs in infants after 3 months of age with congenital toxoplasmosis which had formerly been asymptomatic.[1791] See **congenital toxoplasmosis**.

chronic cytomegalovirus disease An encephalopathy resulting from prenatal or perinatal cytomegalovirus infection, the virus acting like a slow virus infection, and liable to cause mild hydrocephalus progressing to extensive loss of brain substance or polycystic encephalomalacia. The virus can be cultured in the urine or leukocytes, indicating that it is capable of causing both static and progressive encephalopathies. The static encephalopathy usually consists of microcephaly, spasticity, seizures, and retinal abnormalities besides hearing loss and mental retardation. In the progressive form, the virus has not been cultured from the brain.[822]

chronic dacryoadenitis See **orbital pseudotumor syndrome**.

chronic daily headache (CDH) A compound headache syndrome characterized by persistence, clinical features reminiscent of both migraine and tension-type headache and debilitation, all in the absence of evidence of organic disease. The diagnosis requires frequent headaches including those headaches associated with overuse of medications. So-called chronic tension-type headache is the leading cause of primary CDH. In clinic populations, this is the commonest causes of headaches and is usually complicated by persistent analgesic usage.

Primary CDH sufferers have headaches more than 15 days/month unrelated to a structural or systemic illness. In the United States, Europe, and the Orient, 4–5% of the general population can be so diagnosed. The disorders subsumed include chronic migraine, **chronic tension-type headache, new daily persistent headache,** and **hemicrania continua.** Headaches lasting less than 4 h per day in this category **include SUNCT, chronic paroxysmal hemicrania, hypnic headache,** and **chronic cluster headache.**

Secondary causes include post-traumatic headache, cervical spine disorders, and headache associated with vascular disease and nonvascular intracranial disorders. Most patients with chronic daily headache overuse symptomatic medication.[5832]

Analgesic overuse is a possible causal factor for CDH in individuals with episodic headaches who use caffeine-containing combination products, narcotics, benzodiazepines, triptans, etc., all which may trigger that form of CDH (whereas the use of aspirin alone may be protective). Patients with CDH also can have **idiopathic intracranial hypertension.**

chronic demyelinating neuropathy with multifocal CNS demyelination (central and peripheral demyelination) A syndrome combining the features of chronic demyelinating peripheral neuropathy with slow nerve conduction velocities, peripheral nerve hypertrophy, and elevation of the CSF protein levels. Its onset is insidious and there is continuous progression with evidence of multifocal lesions in the CNS, including optic neuritis, brainstem involvement, and cerebellar and pyramidal signs, with episodic expression.[6288] These findings actually fulfil the diagnostic criteria for clinically definite **multiple sclerosis**. They also suggest the co-incidence of a chronic inflammatory demyelinating polyneuropathy and multiple sclerosis, which might be supposed to represent central and peripheral responses to a common antigen at some time past.

chronic encephalitis of Rasmussen See **Rasmussen encephalitis**.

chronic encephalopathy with hepatic insufficiency See **acquired hepatocerebral degeneration**.

chronic encephalopathy with pulmonary insufficiency See **chronic pulmonary encephalopathy**.

chronic Epstein–Barr virus infection 1. A syndrome of recurrent fever, upper respiratory tract infections, lymphadenopathy, fatigue, malaise, uveitis, keratitis, conjunctivitis, and corneal edema due to persistent or reactivating EB virus infection.[6855]

2. See **chronic fatigue syndrome**.

chronic factitious disorder with physical symptoms See **Munchausen syndrome**.

chronic familial vascular encephalopathy See **familial subcortical dementia with arteriosclerotic leukoencephalopathy**.

chronic fatigue syndrome (Royal Free disease, Iceland disease) A combination of symptoms such as apparent weakness, lack of mental drive, listlessness, and fatigue (easy tiring after exertion) in the absence of demonstrable organic pathology, substantially reducing a patient's daily activities for over 6 months. Any pathophysiology remains unknown, although both a hyperserotonergic state or hypoactivity of the hypothalamic-pituitary-adrenal axis have been postulated.[1155]

Numerous other conditions can be subsumed under this heading with greater or lesser degrees of confidence; effort syndrome, Da Costa syndrome, benign myalgic encephalomyelitis, chronic Epstein–Barr virus infection, post-viral asthenia, post-infection fatigue syndrome, brain fever, breathlessness with effort intolerance, melancholy, the vapors, chlorosis, neurasthenia, repetitive strain injury, and other named conditions have been considered by many to have no organic cause, while just as many others claim (or once claimed, for there is a fashion to these things) that these are physical rather than mental illnesses.

The presence of the above-mentioned symptoms without appropriate physical signs and a tendency in some instances for the symptoms to spread in communities with epidemic speed are the only notable clinical features. Objective testing of patients with typical fatigue syndromes revealed normal muscle strength in one study,[3885] though this has been disputed. The demonstration of slowed reaction times, impaired performance on complex attentional and memory tasks, and slowness in acquiring and processing new information suggest that an organic cause may remain to be found.[4518] In some patients there is an abnormal lactate response to exercise, reflecting impaired muscle energy metabolism, in the presence of enterovirus sequences in muscles.

Fatigue can be of central or peripheral origin, and particularly in the former case may not yet be susceptible to etiologic diagnosis, in acknowledgment of which it may be best to keep an open mind with respect to the possible cause in any one case.[6153] Discussions on the very existence of this contentious syndrome as an organic entity have been emotional. Even though rapid event-related functional MRI suggests that CFS may be associated with dysfunctional motor planning, it also indicates the presence of some motivational disturbances.[1505] Various sets of criteria for the diagnosis have been suggested.[2969] Chart C–18 reproduces those of the U.S. Centers for Disease Control.[2230]

Chart C–18. Guidelines for the Diagnosis of Chronic Fatigue Syndrome

Clinically evaluated, medically unexplained fatigue of at least 6 months duration that is:

- Of new onset
- Not a result of ongoing exertion
- Not substantially alleviated by rest
- The cause of a substantial reduction in the patient's previous levels of activity.

Four or more of the following symptoms should be present:

- Subjective memory impairment; tender lymph nodes; muscle or joint pain; headaches; unrefreshing sleep; and postexertional malaise lasting >24 h.

Exclusion criteria include the presence of active unresolvable suspected disease that could be causal, depressive illness, psychotic disorders, dementia, anorexia or bulimia nervosa, alcohol or other substance misuse, and severe obesity.

chronic Guillain-Barré syndrome See **chronic inflammatory demyelinating polyradiculoneuropathy**.

chronic headache attributed to other head and/or neck trauma See **post-traumatic headaches**.

chronic headache attributed to whiplash injury See **post-traumatic headaches**.

chronic hepatic encephalopathy and Parkinsonism (acquired [non-Wilsonian] chronic hepatocerebral degeneration) A syndrome of variable dementia, a rather characteristic dysarthria, ataxia, intention tremor, and choreoathetosis which affects the cranial musculature predominantly but also that of the trunk and extremities; a coarse rhythmic tremor of the arms, maximized in certain sustained postures, pyramidal tract signs, and diffuse slowing on the EEG complete the typical clinical picture. Diffuse muscular rigidity, grasp reflexes, tremor at rest, nystagmus, and persistent asterixis are less common signs. Action myoclonus and combined system disease of the spinal cord have been found in isolated instances.

The condition may complicate any type of liver disease (postnecrotic, portal, and biliary cirrhosis). All patients have had portal-systemic collaterals or surgically created shunts and have either an elevation of blood ammonia levels or abnormal ammonia tolerance. The major neuropathologic changes consist of a diffuse but patchy cortical laminar or pseudo-laminar necrosis and polymicrocavitation at the corticomedullary junctions and in the striatum. In addition, there is a diffuse increase in the size and number of protoplasmic astrocytes as is so often encountered in other forms of liver failure.

chronic hereditary spinocerebellar degeneration See **cerebellar ataxias**.

chronic hexosaminidase A and B deficiency See **hexosaminidase deficiency**.

chronic hyperphosphatemia tarda See **hyperostosis corticalis generalisata**.

chronic idiopathic adhesive arachnoiditis Smoldering inflammation of the arachnoid membrane, seldom due to a cause which can be determined (although fungi may occasionally be responsible[1481]), leading to constriction and ischemia of the cord and the nerve roots at those levels. See **adhesive arachnoiditis**.

chronic idiopathic anhidrosis The condition of isolated local failure of sudomotor function in adult life, other evidence of autonomic failure being absent. Both pre- and postganglionic lesions may be responsible for the anhidrosis, which is not total, but which involves wide areas of the body, not always in contiguous sites. Clinically, the patients manifest heat intolerance, becoming flushed, dizzy, dyspneic, and weak in high ambient temperatures, in which they do not sweat.[3930]

chronic idiopathic ataxic neuropathy Sensory ataxia due to a chronic, large-fiber pure sensory neuronopathy, the principal lesion being of the dorsal root ganglia in the absence of cancer, nutritional deficiency, pyridoxine abuse, or previous acute infectious polyneuropathy. Sural nerve biopsy reveals severe destruction of myelinated axons.

The clinical features include paresthesias, profound disturbance of proprioception and kinesthetic sense, absent muscle stretch reflexes, and normal muscle strength.[1411, 5851] The EMG and motor conduction speeds are normal but sensory potentials cannot be recorded. See also **chronic inflammatory demyelinating polyradiculoneuropathy** and **progressive sensory radiculopathy**.

chronic idiopathic axonal polyneuropathy A heterogeneous condition of painful or painless sensory or sensorimotor neuropathy typically presenting with gradually progressive neuropathic features that cause mild to moderate disability and reduce the quality of life. Fasting insulin concentrations are significantly raised and familial causes, environmental toxin exposure, and hypertriglyceridemia may have etiological roles. See also **chronic inflammatory demyelinating polyradiculoneuropathy**.

chronic idiopathic headache See **chronic tension-type headache unassociated with disorder of pericranial muscles**.

chronic immune demyelinating polyneuropathy (CIDP) See **chronic inflammatory demyelinating polyradiculoneuropathy**.

chronic immune sensory polyneuropathy See **chronic inflammatory demyelinating polyradiculoneuropathy**.

chronic immune sensory polyradiculopathy A slowly progressive syndrome of gait ataxia, large-fiber sensory loss, paresthesias, and frequent falls but with retained sural sensory nerve action potentials, although SSEPs suggest sensory nerve root involvement. The CSF protein level is usually elevated. The condition appears to be a variant of **chronic inflammatory demyelinating polyradiculoneuropathy**.[5872] See **sensory ataxic neuropathy with anti-GD1b antibodies**.

chronic infantile spinal muscular atrophy See **hereditary motor neuropathy, type II**.

chronic inflammatory demyelinating polyradiculoneuropathy (CIDP, relapsing corticosteroid-dependent polyneuritis, steroid-responsive recurrent polyneuropathy, relapsing hypertrophic neuritis, subacute demyelinating proximal and distal polyneuropathy, chronic axon loss polyradiculoneuropathy, chronic idiopathic axonal polyneuropathy, chronic Guillain–Barré syndrome) A heterogeneous syndrome of acquired subacute or chronic, symmetrical, slowly progressive, or relapsing polyneuropathies with pathological or electrophysiological evidence of demyelination and inflammatory cell infiltration within nerves, occurring mainly in adult males in the absence of detectable underlying causal disease such as carcinoma and paraproteinemia (CIDP-1). In the presence of such pathologies, the appellation *CIDP-2* has been suggested.

The neuropathy is usually sensorimotor, but pure motor and pure sensory (**chronic sensory demyelinating neuropathy**) forms also occur. The interval between onset and nadir of this condition is greater than 4 weeks and the average duration from onset to peak deficit is between three and 15 years. Sensory and autonomic changes are more, and identifiable antecedent events less common than in the acute form. Clinically there is hypo- or areflexia with often asymmetrical distal > proximal weakness; pain, painful paresthesias or numbness, autonomic signs, and clinically evident nerve hypertrophy may be noted. Mild, symmetric facial, or bulbar weakness occasionally occurs. The course is chronic and progressive in most cases, taking up to 2 years to reach a plateau. About a third of cases have a relapsing course. Two-thirds of patients respond to steroid therapy, most of the remainder to other forms of immunosuppression.[4205, 413]

Pathologically, the spinal roots and peripheral nerves may show mild inflammation but demyelination and remyelination are more typical. Onion bulbs are seen in the peripheral nerves. The CSF protein is high and myelopathy can occur due to cord compression from the enlarged nerve roots.[4353] Electrophysiologic testing reveals conduction block, marked slowing of nerve conduction velocities, temporal dispersion of the CMAP, prolonged distal latencies, and impersistence of F-waves. Serum IgM and IgG autoantibodies against tubulin are characteristic. MRI may show hypertrophy of spinal roots and plexus, especially in cases of long duration. Anti-GM1 ganglioside antibodies are seldom found.

In a minority of cases, periventricular, subcortical, and brainstem white matter lesions indistinguishable from those seen in MS are also seen, supporting the existence of a central–peripheral inflammatory demyelinating syndrome.[4307, 4569]

See also **GALOP syndrome, GD1a antibody motor-sensory neuropathy, multifocal motor neuropathy, MAG antibody associated neuropathy, osteosclerotic myeloma, POEMS syndrome,** and **sulfatide antibody associated neuropathy**.

Many systemic disorders are associated with CIDP, including those associated with paraproteins, autoimmune disorders, HIV, infection, chronic active hepatitis, and more.[4838] Various sets of criteria for the diagnosis[413, 20] have been blended by Saperstein et al.[5549] and are reproduced here. (See Chart C–19.) Electrodiagnostic criteria for demyelination (from a different source) have also been suggested.

chronic insomnia Prolonged difficulty in sleeping; **primary chronic insomnia**, **chronic pseudo-insomnia**, insomnia due to other disease, and forms due to another sleep disorder are distinguished.[4904]

chronic juvenile amyotrophic lateral sclerosis See **hereditary motor system disease** and **hereditary motor neuropathy**, type III.

chronic limb-girdle myasthenia gravis See **myasthenia gravis**.

chronic lymphocytic leukemia A group of malignancies characterized by the proliferation of small, immunologically mature lymphoid cells in the peripheral blood, most of which as B-cell in origin. Neurological complications include herpes zoster and other opportunistic infections, and less commonly direct invasion or hemorrhage in the central nervous system.[782]

chronic lymphocytic meningitis See **chronic benign lymphocytic meningitis**.

chronic manganese encephalopathy A syndrome of involuntary movement disorders characterized by widespread cell loss in the caudate and putamen as a result of chronic manganese intoxication.[6894]

chronic meningitis That form of meningitis in which the clinical and CSF abnormalities persist for longer than 4 weeks.[1848] Tuberculosis, brucellosis, and spirochetal infections are the commonest infectious causes; granulomatous diseases and neoplastic meningeal disorders are others.

chronic migraine A complication of migraine in which migraine headaches occur on 15 or more days per month for more than 3 months in the absence of medication overuse. Diagnostic criteria have been defined and adapted.[2820, 4783]

A. Headache (tension-type and/or migraine) on $\geq$15 days per month for at least 3 months.
B. Occurring in a patient who has had at least five attacks fulfilling criteria for **migraine without aura**.
C. On $\geq$ 8 days per month for at least 3 months headache has fulfilled C1 and/or C2 below, that is, has fulfilled criteria for pain and associated symptoms of migraine without aura.
   1. Has at least two of a–d: (a) unilateral location, (b) pulsating quality, (c) moderate or severe pain intensity, and (d) aggravation by or causing avoidance of routine physical activity (e.g., walking or climbing stairs); and at least one of a or b: (a) nausea and/or vomiting and (b) photophobia and phonophobia.
   2. Treated and relieved by triptan(s) or ergot before the expected development of C1 above.
D. No medication overuse and not attributed to another causative disorder.

Chart C–19. Chronic Inflammatory Demyelinating Polyradiculoneuropathy

1. Clinical
Mandatory clinical features

Major; symmetric proximal and distal weakness
Minor; exclusively distal weakness or sensory loss
Hypo- or areflexia [This will usually involve all four limbs]
Duration 2 months or more

Laboratory features

Mandatory: CSF protein >45 mg/dl
Supportive: Cell count <10/cu. mm
Nerve biopsy shows predominant features of demyelination*
Electrodiagnostic studies (see below)

Requirements for diagnostic categories

Definite: Clinical major electrodiagnostic and CSF (biopsy not mandatory)
Probable: Clinical major electrodiagnostic or CSF and biopsy
Possible: Clinical major and 1 of 3 laboratory features

**Unequivocal nerve biopsy evidence of demyelination and remyelination includes demyelination shown by either electron microscopy (>5 fibers) or teased fiber studies (>12% of 50 teased fibers, minimum of four internodes each, demonstrating demyelination/remyelination); subperineurial or endoneurial edema; mononuclear cell infiltration; onion bulb formation; and prominent variation in the degree of demyelination between fascicles.*

Exclusion factors would be vasculitis, neurofilamentous swollen axons, amyloid deposits, or intracytoplasmic inclusions in Schwann cells or macrophages indicating adrenoleukodystrophy, metachromatic leukodystrophy, globoid cell leukodystrophy, or other evidence of specific pathology.

Clinical exclusions noted in the 1991 AAN ad hoc committee recommendations[20] were:

1. Mutilation of hands or feet, retinitis pigmentosa, ichthyosis, appropriate history of drug or toxic exposure known to cause a similar peripheral neuropathy, or family history of a genetically based peripheral neuropathy.
2. Sensory level.
3. Unequivocal sphincter disturbance.

(From Saperstein D.S., Katz J.S., Barohn R.J. Clinical spectrum of chronic acquired demyelinating polyneuropathies. Muscle Nerve 2001;**24**:311–24. *Reproduced by kind permission of John Wiley and Sons. Inc.)*

2. Physiological studies
Neurophysiological Criteria for Diagnosis of CIDP
These criteria require documentation of conduction block or temporal dispersion, F-waves, conduction velocity, and/or distal latency abnormalities in at least three nerves:

Any one of the following:

Conduction block (CB) or temporal dispersion (TD) must be present in at least three different nerves with abnormal conduction values suggestive of demyelination in at least one other nerve including one of the nerves with CB/TD

The CB/TD must be present in two different nerves and abnormal conduction values in at least one other nerve.

CB/ TD must be present in one nerve and abnormal conduction values in at least two other nerves

No CB/TD, but abnormal conduction values must be present in three different nerves.

Definitions:
Conduction block Amplitude drop of ≥30% between proximal and distal sites of stimulation except with Erb point.stimulation ≥50% amplitude drop. Tibial nerve excluded.
Temporal dispersion Increase in CMAP duration of >15% after proximal stimulation with regards to distal stimulation. Tibial nerve excluded.
Significantly reduced conduction velocity <80% of the lower limits of normal (LLN) or, if distal motor CMAP amplitude <80% of LLN, <70% of LLN.
Significantly prolonged distal motor latency >125% of upper limit of normal (ULN) or if amplitude <80% *of normal,* >150% of ULN.
Abnormal F-waves Absent F-waves or F-wave minimal latency >120% of ULN or if amplitude < 80% of normal, F-wave minimal latency >150% of ULN.

Bilateral testing of the median, ulnar, peroneal, and tibial nerves is required. At least 10 consecutive F-waves are to be recorded from each nerve and the minimal latency measured.

A simpler set of criteria is as follows:[5501]

1. Motor conduction velocity (MCV) less than 75% of the lower limit of normal.
2. Distal motor latencies greater than 140% of normal.
3. Conduction block and/or temporal dispersion of the motor unit action potentials.
4. F wave latency increased to greater than 120% of normal.

Laboratory studies.

Depending on the results of the laboratory tests, those patients meeting the criteria above will be classified into the groups listed below.

The following studies are suggested: Complete blood count, erythrocyte sedimentation rate, creatine kinase, antinuclear antibody, CK, ANA, routine biochemical screen, thyroid function tests, serum and urine immunoglobulin studies (to include either immunofixation electrophoresis or immunoelectrophoresis), and HIV and hepatitis serology. The list of laboratory studies is not comprehensive. For instance, in certain clinical circumstances other studies may be indicated, such as phytanic acid, long-chain fatty acids, porphyrins, urine heavy metals, α-lipoprotein, β-lipoprotein, glucose tolerance test, imaging studies of the CNS, and lymph node or bone marrow biopsy.

continued

Chart C–19. *(continued)*

Idiopathic CIDP is said to occur when there is no concurrent disease. The presence of such diseases (depending on laboratory studies or other clinical features) indicates that the patient has an *acquired demyelinating polyneuropathy*. The conditions so far described include systemic lupus erythematosus, hyperthyroidism, HIV infection,[166] monoclonal or biclonal gammopathy (macroglobulinemia, POEMS syndrome, osteosclerotic myeloma, Hodgkin disease, and monoclonal gammopathies of undetermined significance), hereditary motor and sensory neuropathy, chronic active hepatitis, inflammatory bowel disease, Castleman disease, diabetes mellitus, and CNS demyelination.

(Adapted from Hughes RAC et al. Randomized controlled trial of intravenous immunoglobulin versus oral prednisolone in chronic inflammatory demyelinating polyneuropathy. Ann Neurol *2001;***50***:195–201*[3040] *and from Nicholas G, et al. Proposed revised electrophysiological criteria for chronic inflammatory demyelinating polyradiculoneuropathy.* Muscle Nerve *2002;***25***:26–30.*[4660] *© 2002. Reproduced by kind permission of John Wiley and Sons. Inc.)*

Variant forms are as follows;

anti-MAG antibody syndrome

Focal and multifocal neuropathy and CIDP Chronic inflammatory demyelinating polyneuropathy (CIDP) presents in rare instances with numbness, paresthesias, weakness, and pain in focal or multifocal upper limb distribution. The criteria for conduction block are often not met; demyelination is sometimes restricted to proximal nerves and roots, so proximal nerve and nerve root stimulation may be necessary. In a study of proximal root stimulation, only 7 of 31 cases met published demyelinating criteria. Even totally normal conduction studies should not exclude the diagnosis of CIDP.[5501]

Chronic sensory demyelinating polyneuropathy A variant of CIDP presenting with isolated ataxia, pains, and paresthesias of legs, sometimes followed around 5 years later by motor signs. Both thick- and thin-fiber functions are impaired. In about half the patients the CSG protein levels are modestly raised. At least one motor conduction parameter (MCV, distal, and F-wave latency) suggests demyelination in almost all cases and that conduction blocks and temporal dispersion are present in a third.of the cases. Sensory conduction velocity was in the demyelinating range in 56% of the patients. Needle EMG shows subclinical motor involvement in all patients. In chronic sensory demyelinating polyneuropathy demyelination may also be restricted to sensory nerves or to dorsal root ganglia.[5501] This is strikingly similar to a *sensory form* with distal pansensory loss and pain and normal power or minimal distal weakness, in which electrophysiology shows evidence of motor and sensory demyelination, conduction block, slow NCV, and long distal latency in which the manifestations are more of a sensory than of a motor deficit.[4764]

A form with onset in childhood (when the disease may be monophasic with remission) and in which associations with diabetes and serum M-proteins are described. In a few cases, a multifocal presentation, perineuritis, sensory manifestations, and arm involvement have been noted. Pathologically there is patchy loss of myelinated axons with some axonal regeneration.

An adult form in which the pathology suggests mainly axonal involvement.[6445]

Miller Fisher syndrome

Multifocal neuropathy with persistent conduction block

Multifocal demyelinating CIDP (**Lewis–Sumner syndrome**) A slowly progressive, or relapsing–remitting disorder of adult life presenting with asymmetric, mainly distal weakness in arms > legs. Occasionally, a proximal syndrome involving the phrenic or suprascapular nerves occurs. Sensory loss is mainly distal but is rarely severe or disabling. Electrophysiology shows multifocal conduction blocks and variably slowed nerve conduction velocities with prolonged distal latencies. The CSF protein level is raised but is usually <100 mg/dl. IgM anti-GM1 antibodies are not present. MRI may show swollen nerves in brachial plexus. Pathologically, there is patchy demyelination and some axonal loss. This is probably the same as **multifocal acquired demyelinating sensory and motor neuropathy** (*MADSAM*).

Chronic demyelinating neuropathy with multifocal CNS demyelination. A central–peripheral inflammatory demyelinating syndrome in which periventricular, subcortical, and brainstem white matter lesions indistinguishable from those seen in MS are found in association with the peripheral neuropathy.[4307, 6288]

Childhood CIDP A variant often following infections or vaccinations and with a monophasic or chronic course, weakness, and disability persisting in some cases. The disease here may be monophasic with remission.

CIDP associated with IgG or IgA M-protein, which presents a similar clinical syndrome to typical CIDP with slowly progressive symmetric weakness.

CIDP + diabetes mellitus A condition similar to CIDP, but the subjects are older, gait imbalance is especially marked, and there is evidence of significant axonal loss.

Distal acquired demyelinating symmetric neuropathy (DADS)

Multifocal acquired sensory and motor neuropathy

An *infantile form*, which is a hypertrophic, demyelinating, sensorimotor peripheral neuropathy with muscle weakness and atrophy, accompanied by scoliosis, pes cavus, and raised CSF protein levels.

Pure motor chronic inflammatory demyelinating polyradiculoneuropathy A syndrome of symmetric or asymmetric proximal and distal weakness in all four limbs progressing over weeks to months. Clinically, proximal and distal weakness with preserved muscle bulk and areflexia are notable; there may also be minor, distal sensory loss. Nerve conduction studies show significantly slow NCS with relative preservation of CMAP, and SNCVs may also be slowed. Dispersion or multifocal conduction blocks are prominent. The CSF protein is significantly elevated (>100 mg/dl). In a few cases, a multifocal presentation, perineuritis, sensory manifestations, and arm involvement have been noted. See also **monoclonal gammopathy of uncertain significance**, the clinical features of which may be identical with those of CIDP. See also the Web site http://neuromuscular.wustl.edu/ for yet more detailed current information.

See also **migraine**.

More inclusive criteria for chronic migraine and medication overuse headache are included in the appendix of ICHD-2, primarily for further scientific evaluation. It is now recommended that the MOH diagnosis should no longer require improvement after discontinuation of medication overuse but should be assigned to patients if they have a primary headache *and* ongoing medication overuse (defined previously as 10 days or more of intake of triptans, ergot alkaloids, mixed analgesics, or opioids, or 15 days or more of analgesics/NSAIDs or the combined use of more than one substance). If these new criteria for CM and MOH prove useful in future testing they will be included in a future version of the ICHD.[4784]

chronic migrainous neuralgia See **chronic cluster headache**.

chronic motor axonal neuropathy A diffuse inflammatory motor polyradiculoneuropathy not associated with the presence of antiGM1 antibodies or paraproteinemia.[2513] See also

chronic inflammatory dysimmune polyneuropathy.

chronic motor tic disorder A syndrome of stereotyped, unifocal, and unvarying motor or vocal tics (not both), occurring for over a year and usually presenting in adult life. The condition probably falls within the spectrum of **Tourette syndrome.**[2443]

chronic muscle contraction headache See **chronic tension-type headache associated with disorder of pericranial muscles.**

chronic myelopathy (progressive myelopathy) An isolated, slowly progressive unifocal myelopathy with predominantly motor findings, considered to be due to a single site of involvement by **multiple sclerosis** in cases in whom **amyotrophic lateral sclerosis, structural lesions,** and **subacute combined degeneration of the cord** have been excluded.[4937]

chronic myopathy The rare production of a syndrome of muscle weakness and wasting in children as a result of persisting viral infection.[4157]

chronic neurogenic quadriceps amyotrophy A rare focal wasting disease of the thighs, with childhood onset. See **Furukawa syndrome**[2248] and **hereditary motor neuropathy** (*variants*).

Chronic Pain Outreach A charitable organization. Web site: www.chronicpain.org/.

chronic pain syndromes These are listed variously by name in this book. A taxonomy has been devised by the International Association for the Study of Pain.[3069]

chronic paroxysmal hemicrania (Sjaastad syndrome) Attacks with largely the same characteristics of pain and associated symptoms and signs as **cluster headache**, but shorter lasting, more frequent, and occurring mostly in females and with absolute effectiveness of indomethacin. This type of head pain almost exactly resembles **cluster headache**, the notable differences being the increased frequency (and reduced duration) of the pains, its predilection for women, precipitation often by neck movement, and the near-specific responsiveness to indomethacin.

This definition and the following diagnostic criteria are suggested by the Headache Classification Committee of the International Headache Society.[2820] (See Chart C–20.)

chronic paroxysmal hemicraniatic syndrome A rare **trigeminal-autonomic cephalalgia** in which these two syndromes occur together.[6984]

chronic polymyositis (acquired inflammatory polyneuropathy, late-life muscular dystrophy, menopausal muscular dystrophy) A very slowly progressive form of **idiopathic inflammatory polymyositis** occurring in adult life, affecting the arms and legs, often asymmetrically, without pain, muscle swelling, or associated skin changes.

In a *variant* form, intranuclear and intracytoplasmic aggregates with tubular structures are found on muscle biopsy.[1164]

chronic polyneuropathy of undetermined cause Sensory, motor, or mixed neuropathies usually with onset in mature adult life, symmetrical and present for more than 1 year. They are usually accompanied by mild slowing of motor conduction, an impairment of sensory conduction, and with chronic axonal degeneration shown on sural nerve biopsy. The condition is only slowly progressive; in some two-thirds of patients prolonged follow-up does not yield any clues as to the underlying etiology. The group has been thought to make up some 13% of an unselected series of patients with peripheral neuropathy referred to a neurological center.[4253]

chronic polyradiculoneuropathy of infancy A fatal syndrome of progressive muscular weakness and wasting with areflexia and elevation of the CSF protein levels occurring in infancy, and characterized pathologically by near-total deficiency of myelin in the cranial and spinal nerve roots.[3323]

chronic portosystemic encephalopathy See **acquired hepatocerebral encephalopathy.**

chronic post-craniotomy headache See **post-traumatic headaches.**

chronic post-traumatic headache attributed to moderate or severe head injury See **post-traumatic headaches.**

chronic post-traumatic headache A headache syndrome without special features that is indistinguishable from chronic tension-type headache and migraine without aura. It is associated with reduced regional cerebral blood flow and hemispheric asymmetries, which supports an organic basis.[2657] See also **post-traumatic headache.**

chronic progressive dementia See **Alzheimer disease.**

chronic progressive disseminated encephalomyelitis See **disseminated vasculomyelinopathy.**

Chart C–20. Chronic Paroxysmal Hemicrania: Diagnostic Criteria

A. At least 20 attacks fulfilling B–D
B. Severe unilateral orbital, supraorbital, or temporal pain lasting 2–3 min
C. Headache is accompanied by at least one of the following:
   1. Ipsilateral conjunctival injection and/or lacrimation
   2. Ipsilateral nasal congestion and/or rhinorrhea
   3. Forehead and facial sweating
   4. Ipsilateral eyelid edema
   5. Ipsilateral forehead and facial sweating
   6. Ipsilateral miosis and/or ptosis
D. Attacks have a frequency above five per day for more than half the time, although periods with lower frequency may occur
E. Attacks are prevented completely by therapeutic doses of indomethacin
F. *Not attributed to another disorder*

Episodic paroxysmal headache attacks occur in periods lasting 7 days to a year, separated by pain-free periods lasting a month or more. *Chronic paroxysmal headache* attacks occur for more than a year without remission or with remissions lasting less than a month.

chronic progressive encephalitis A slow-virus disease of the brain possibly associated with preceding infection with the virus of **Russian spring-summer encephalitis**, clinically manifesting as mental, visual, auditory, pyramidal, and cerebellar disorders.

chronic progressive external ophthalmoplegia (CPEO; von Graefe syndrome) Disorders of conjugate gaze, usually without diplopia but with marked ptosis. The syndrome may be accompanied by any of various other clinical features including dementia, mitochondrial myopathy, and encephalopathy (**Leigh disease**). It is often caused by deletions in mitochondrial DNA and is conveniently classified as an encephalomyeloneuromyopathy, thus ending the tedious disputes of the last 30 years as to whether the disorder is of central or peripheral origin.

The syndromes are usually dominantly inherited. Clinically, the ophthalmoplegia (a constant) may be associated with weakness of other muscle groups and/or with evidence of central or peripheral nervous system dysfunction. The course of the disorder with large-scale mitochondrial mtDNA deletions varies from a mild, slowly progressive myopathy to cardiac conduction defects and involvement of the brain, inner ear, or retina.[298] See **Kearns–Sayre syndrome**, **mitochondrial diseases**, and **progressive external ophthalmoplegia**.

chronic progressive myelopathy The clinical entity of a slowly progressive spastic paraparesis (with spastic gait, leg weakness, hyperreflexia, and variable degrees of sensory loss) without evidence of spinal cord compression, disseminated lesions, or disease of the lower motor neurons. Most of these patients are eventually determined to suffer from **multiple sclerosis**.[4937]

chronic progressive radiation myelopathy See **radiation myelopathy**.

chronic progressive spinobulbar spasticity A syndrome with onset in adult life characterized by spasticity, dysphasia, and XII cranial nerve abnormalities.[381]

chronic pseudoinsomnia The complaint of insomnia starting in adult life with daytime sleepiness and malaise but without demonstrable abnormality of the duration or structure of sleep on investigation in the sleep laboratory.

chronic psychogenic headache See **chronic tension-type headache unassociated with disorder of pericranial muscles**.

chronic pulmonary encephalopathy (chronic encephalopathy with pulmonary insufficiency) A progressive degenerative disease of premature infants with severe respiratory distress. Cerebral cortical and brainstem forms are differentiated, each with a fatal prognosis.[1847, 4313]

chronic relapsing polyneuropathy The term applied to those forms of chronic inflammatory demyelinating polyradiculoneuropathy in which remissions and recurrences occur.

chronic relapsing plexus neuropathy with persistent conduction block See **multifocal inflammatory CIDP variant** and **multifocal inflammatory demyelinating neuropathy**.

chronic segmental spinal muscular atrophy of the upper limbs A sporadic or familial disorder characterized by juvenile-onset, uni- or bilateral localization of muscle atrophy to the hands and forearms, and a benign course.[2916]

chronic sensory ataxic neuropathy See **chronic sensory demyelinating neuropathy**.

chronic sensory demyelinating neuropathy (chronic sensory ganglionopathy) A form of **chronic inflammatory demyelinating neuropathy** with its pathology localized mainly in the dorsal root ganglion cells, characterized by the subacute or chronic progression of a pure sensory neuropathy (though with electrical evidence that the demyelinating process affects motor as well as sensory fibers), loss of proprioceptive and kinaesthetic sensation, raised CSF protein, and a good response to immunosuppression.[4764] Malignancies, **Sjögren syndrome**, paraproteinemia and idiopathic causes are recognized.[3266]

chronic sensory ganglionopathy See **chronic sensory demyelinating neuropathy**.

chronic sensory neuropathy (chronic sensory ganglionopathy) An insidiously progressive large-fiber sensory neuronopathy with ataxia as its most prominent clinical feature.[5851] See **chronic idiopathic ataxic neuropathy**.

chronic sinus headache A dilute form of **migraine**, beloved of the purveyors of antihistamines, vasoconstrictors, and analgesics, many of which can transform the condition to **medication overuse headache**.

chronic spinal meningitis (radicular myelopathy associated with spinal neuronitis, meningitis circumscripta spinalis) A rapidly progressive radicular myelopathy due to extensive spinal meningitis, often occurring as a first expression of tuberculosis in the nervous system. Syphilis, pyogenic organisms, *Cryptococcus*, and chemicals may also be causal in a few cases. The condition was first described by Harley in 1909. See **spinal arachnoiditis**.

chronic spinal muscular atrophy with pallidal degeneration See **hereditary motor neuropathy** (*variants*).

chronic subdural hematoma (pachymeningitis hemorrhagica interna) Subdural hemorrhage present at 2 weeks or more after head trauma which has displaced the brain in an anterior–posterior direction, tearing the veins as they enter the superior longitudinal sinus and leading to blood loss into the subdural space, with the eventual formation of a membrane.

Clinical signs typically include headache, depression of consciousness, and fluctuating focal deficits; increased intracranial pressure and such transient neurological signs as weakness, dysarthria, dysphasia, and visual field deficits are also recorded as presenting signs. The condition is an important cause of reversible dementia. The latent interval between the trauma and the development of clinical signs may be months or years,[6399] so that the patient and his family and friends may be unaware of the occurrence of the preceding head trauma.

chronic tension-type headache (chronic daily headache) Headache present for at least 15 days a month during at least 6 months. The headache is usually pressing/tightening in quality, mild or moderate in severity, bilateral, and does not worsen with routine physical activity. Nausea, photophobia, or phonophobia may occur.

This definition and the diagnostic criteria are suggested by the Headache Classification Committee of the International Headache Society. (From Classification of headache disorders, cranial neuralgias and facial pains; and diagnostic criteria for primary headache disorders. *Cephalalgia* 1988;8[Suppl]:1–96 by kind permission of Dr. Jes Olesen, the International Headache Society and Wiley-Blackwell Publications.) (See Chart C–21.) The definition is valid but the diverse manifestations of this heterogeneous form of headache may not always comply.

chronic tension-type headache associated with disorder of pericranial muscles (chronic muscle contraction headache) A form of chronic tension-type headache recognized by the IHS. It meets the criteria for **chronic tension-type headache** but is also associated with tenderness of the pericranial muscles to palpation, or these may show increased EMG activity. The distinction between the two is, at best, fine.

chronic tension-type headache unassociated with disorder of pericranial muscles (chronic idiopathic headache, chronic psychogenic headache) An older name, essentially subsumed now under chronic tension-type headache.

chronic tetanus A rare *variant* occurring in patients partially immune to tetanus, and producing such symptoms as stiffness and muscle spasms, worsened by volitional movements and startle, and lasting months. Electrodiagnostic studies and muscle biopsy study show evidence of motor neuropathy.[5321]

chronic tetany (sporadic tetany) See **idiopathic neuromyotonia**.

chronic tic disorder See **Tourette syndrome**.

chronic TORCH encephalopathy with myoclonia A variant of chronic congenital TORCH encephalopathies with this added complication.

chronic traumatic edema See **reflex sympathetic dystrophy**.

chronic Werdnig–Hoffmann disease See **hereditary motor neuropathy, type II**.

Chart C–21. Chronic Tension-Type Headache: Diagnostic Criteria

A. Average headache frequency ≥15 days/month (180 days/year) for ≥6 months fulfilling criteria B–D, listed below:
B. At least two of the following pain characteristics:
   1. Pressing/tightening quality.
   2. Mild or moderate severity (may inhibit, but does not prohibit activities).
   3. Bilateral location.
   4. No aggravation by walking stairs or similar routine physical activity.
C. Both of the following:
   1. No vomiting.
   2. No more than one of nausea, photophobia, or phonophobia.
D. At least one of the following:
   1. History and physical and neurological examinations do not suggest one of the disorders listed in groups 5–11 (see **headache**).
   2. History and/or physical and/or neurological examinations do suggest such a disorder, but it is ruled out by appropriate investigations.
   3. Such disorder is present, but tension-type headache does not occur for the first time in close temporal relation to the disorder.

From the International Classification of Headache Disorders (Headache Classification Committee of the International Headache Society. Cephalalgia *2004;24(Suppl 1)) by kind permission of Dr. Jes Olesen, the International Headache Society and Wiley-Blackwell Publications.*

chronic whiplash See **whiplash-associated disorder**.

chronodispersion The difference between minimum and maximum latency values in a series of F-waves.

chronotaraxis A disturbance of temporal orientation, of time interval estimation, or of chronological order of events for symptoms that is peculiar to circumscribed lesions of the anterior ventral and medio-dorsal thalamic nuclei.[3598, 5975] It is well described after a thalamic stroke affecting the mediodorsal nucleus.

chronotherapy 1. A form of therapy for sleep disorders in which the times for waking and sleeping are rigidly prescribed. 2. Selective treatment of certain diseases with regard to the patient's diurnal rhythms. Thus, steroid treatment of multiple sclerosis relapses has been found to be more effective when given at night.[2406]

Churg–Strauss syndrome (leucocytoclastic angiitis, allergic granulomatosis, eosinophilic granulomatous vasculitis) An auto-allergic vasculopathy of unknown cause, affecting small- to medium-sized vessels, not certainly defined as a specific entity but characterized as part of the spectrum of **polyarteritis nodosa**. Adult males are more commonly affected.

Clinically, it is characterized by asthma, fever, hypereosinophilia with widespread necrotizing arteritis, erythema multiforme, allergic rhinitis, and extravascular granulomatosis. Neurological features occur in about 25% of cases and include deficits of cranial nerves II, III, VII, and VIII, headache, hemorrhagic stroke, myositis and polyneuropathy or multiple mononeuropathy,[5582, 6087] and other focal deficits such as the **Balint syndrome**. MR imaging reveals diffuse hypointense lesions on T2-weighted images in the frontal meninges and anterior falx cerebri with diffuse enhancement.[6338] See also **allergic angiitis** and **granulomatosis**. The typical pathology shows angiitis and extravascular granulomas with eosinophilic infiltrates. A prodromal period with rhinitis may last for years, followed then by the development of eosinophilia and later asthma which precedes the vasculitis. Peripheral nerve involvement is recognized in 65–75% of the patients.

Chvostek, Frantisek (1835–1884) Austrian physician who trained in Vienna and worked there for all of his life. He published an account of his sign in 1876. His other contributions were in various fields of internal medicine.

Chvostek sign Tapping over the facial nerve anterior to the ear leads to twitching of the homolateral facial muscles due to hyperexcitability of the nerve, as in hypocalcemic tetany.

The related **Chvostek phenomenon** consists of hyperexcitability of any of the peripheral nerves to percussion, as in cases of tetanus.[1180]

chymopapain A proteolytic digestive enzyme used for **chemonucleolysis**.

cicatrix A gliotic scar in the CNS, often leading to the local origination of epileptic discharges and detectable during life by **MRI**.

ciguatera A widespread ichthyosarcotoxaemia with dramatic and clinically important neurological features. The clinical syndrome results from the ingestion of ciguatera toxin, a substance found in various species of periequatorial reef fish as the result of their ingestion of algae containing the toxin that increases the permeability of nerve and muscle membranes to sodium. The condition is most common in Polynesian and Caribbean waters. Captain James Cook suffered from this in 1777, probably as a result of eating a large grouper. The neurotoxin is stored in the viscera of fish that have eaten the dinoflagellate and concentrated it upward throughout the food chain toward progressively larger species, including humans. Both Pacific (P-CTX-1) and Caribbean (C-CTX-1) ciguatoxins are potent, heat-stable lipophilic sodium channel activator toxins which bind to and maintain open the voltage-sensitive sodium channel on the cell membranes of all excitable tissues.

The clinical manifestations include oral and peripheral paresthesias, dysesthesias and allodynia, metallic taste, pruritis, nausea, vomiting, malaise, anorexia, burning joint pain, **cold reversal**, diarrhoea, vomiting, skin itching, cramps, and joint and muscle pains within 30 min to 2 days after ingestion. Temperature perception reversal has been described as "pathognomonic" for ciguatera poisoning. Cerebellar dysfunction, hyporeflexia, cranial nerve palsies, and (rarely) respiratory paralysis have also been recorded. Autonomic dysfunction leads to hypotension, bradycardia, dilated pupils, and hypersalivation in severe cases.[1167, 4955, 42, 2484]

The differential diagnosis includes organophosphate, botulinus, **tetrodotoxin**, and neurologic shellfish poisoning. See also **scombroid, paralytic shellfish poisoning,** and **domoic acid**.

ciliary (from Lat, the eyelid or eyelash) Pertinent to the eyelid.

ciliary arteries Anterior and posterior, long and short branches of the ophthalmic artery supplying the external ocular muscles, and the conjunctiva, sclera, ciliary apparatus, and choroid.

ciliary body The ciliary muscle and anterior part of the choroid (corona ciliaris), with specialized functions in secreting the aqueous fluid into the anterior chamber of the eye. It was known to **Herodotus** (ca. 290 BC), but the term was applied by **Fallopius** (ca. AD 1550) to the whole of the anterior part of the choroid, the more restrictive definition being that of Frederich Henle (1809–1885), a German anatomist.

ciliary ganglion A ganglion situated immediately behind the eye, in which relay parasympathetic fibers destined for the ciliary body, and sympathetic fibers with a similar destination pass through without synapsing. It was described by Anders Retzius (1796–1860), a Swedish anatomist (ca. 1840).[5619]

ciliary muscles Smooth muscles of the ciliary body, the circumferential fibers described in 1858 by Heinrich Müller (1820–1864) and the radial in 1847 by William Bowman (1816–1892).[5619] Together they control the aperture of the pupil and the degree of curvature of the lens.

ciliary neuralgia Intermittent bouts of severe pain in the cheek, temple, and eye. See **cluster headache** and **Charlin syndrome**.

ciliary reflex Touching the eyelashes causes blinking of the homolateral eyelid.[6898]

ciliospinal center of Budge The site of the cell bodies of the second neuron of the descending sympathetic pathway, situated at the C8–T2 cord levels. Their fibers are pupillo-dilator neurons.

ciliospinal reflex Dilation of the pupil homolateral to a painful stimulus such as pinching the neck. The presence of the sign indicates the integrity of the afferent pathway through the cervical nerves and of the efferent sympathetic pathway which traverses the whole of the brainstem.

cilosis (from Lat, an eyelash) Spasmodic trembling of the eyelid. A form of facial **myokymia**.

cinchona The extract of the bark of the Peruvian Oak, so named after the Countess of Cinchon, wife of the Spanish Governor of Peru, who was cured of a fever (presumably malaria) through its use. The active principle is quinine.

cinchonism Quinine toxicity, manifest by headache, tinnitus, tremor, pallor, and jaundice.

cinerea (Lat, ash-colored) Hence *tuber cinereum*—the "gray root" of the pituitary.

cinesialgia (Gr, movement + pain) An extinct term for painful muscle cramps or muscle pain during contraction.

cinetic (from Gr, with reference to motion) Now usually written as *kinetic.*

cingulate (from Lat, a belt or girdle) Encompassing.

cingulate gyrus The four-layered paleocortex representing the cortical expression of the **limbic system** and sited above the corpus callosum on the medial aspect of the frontal lobes.

cingulate gyrus syndrome See **Nielsen syndrome**.

cingulate seizures A seizure disorder in which the seizure patterns are complex partial with complex motor gestural automatisms at the onset. Autonomic signs are common, as are changes in mood and affect. (Adapted from Dreifuss, F.E. et al. Commission for Classification and

Terminology, ILAE. Proposal for revised classifications of epilepsies and epileptic syndromes. *Epilepsia* 1989;30:389–99, by kind permission of the ILAE and Wiley–Blackwell Publications.)

These complex partial seizures often end with a temper tantrum. They may be provoked by stress and are often accompanied by frequent absence attacks, autonomic disturbances, and motor signs.[4194]

cingulosynapsis A form of lobar **holoproscencephaly** in which the hemispheres are well developed but joined by a band of neocortex over the corpus callosum.[3508]

cinonosos (Gr, to move + disease) An obsolete term for any disease affecting muscular motion.

circadian rhythm Alternations of sleeping and waking and of activity, body temperature, and hormonal levels with a cycle of about a day, paced by a "clock" function within the suprachiasmatic nucleus.

Two circadian rhythms exist, each with a 25 h length: the sleep-wake/growth hormone/urinary electrolytes cycle and the rapid eye movement sleep, cortisol, and body temperature cycle.

circadian rhythm sleep disorders Varieties of **dyssomnia** reflecting disturbance of the timing of sleep rather than its nature. They are classified by the **American Academy of Sleep Disorders** as follows:[1629]

1. Time zone change (jet lag) syndrome
2. Shift work sleep disorder
3. Irregular sleep–wake pattern
4. Delayed sleep phase syndrome
5. Advanced sleep phase syndrome
6. Non-24-h sleep–wake disorder
7. Circadian rhythm sleep disorder not otherwise specified.See also **sleep disorders.**

   Useful Web sites are www.mentalhelp.net/poc/view_index.php?idx=26/, which describes the general symptoms of circadian rhythm sleep disorder, from Mental Health Net; and that of the Circadian Sleep Disorders Association, www.circadiandisorders.org/, providing information and support to those affected by circadian sleep disorders such as **delayed sleep phase syndrome**.

circle of Haller The network of blood vessels surrounding the optic nerves. Also the attachments of the mitral and tricuspid valves in the heart.

circle of Willis The anastomotic ring of arteries (two posterior cerebral, posterior communicating, internal carotid and anterior cerebral; one anterior communicating and the basilar) which encircles the pituitary stalk anterior and inferior to the base of the brain. It was first depicted in 1647 by Johann Vesling, but Thomas **Willis** further defined the structures in 1664 and his name is applied to the configuration.

circular nystagmus (diagonal, elliptic, oblique, alternating windmill, circumduction, gyratory, radiary nystagmus) Types of acquired pendular nystagmus in which the fine, fast, vertical, and horizontal oscillations are in opposite directions. In circular nystagmus, they have similar amplitudes; in elliptical nystagmus, they are different. The resulting ocular movements are as their names suggest. The retinal image and the perceived motion (**oscillopsia**) are in the same direction as the eye movement.[1561] Such disorders are most commonly due to brainstem disease but are sometimes congenital.

circumduction An abnormality of gait wherein the pelvis is elevated on the side of a hemiparesis when the weight is borne on the other leg, in order that the affected leg (longer now as a result of hip and knee extension and ankle plantar flexion) does not scrape upon the ground.

circumduction nystagmus See **circular nystagmus**.

circumferential bipolar montage A montage consisting of derivations from pairs of electrodes along circumferential arrays. (From the 1974 Report of the Committee on Terminology, IFCN. In: Chatrian GE, Bergamini L, Dondey M, et al. A glossary of terms most commonly used by clinical electroencephalographers. *EEG Clin Neurophysiol* 1974;37:538–48. Reproduced by kind permission of the IFCN and Elsevier Science.)

circumlocution Discursive wordiness, indirectly providing information rather than defining the objects to be communicated. Charles Dickens' Mr. Micawber is a well-drawn example, but he did not appear to suffer from that amnesic aphasia which is a typical pathology causing this form of speech disturbance.

circumscribed cortical atrophy See **Pick disease**.

circumscribed serous spinal meningitis See **arachnoid diverticula**.

circumscript meningitis See **subdural empyema**.

cisplatin An anti-neoplastic drug that can cause a length-dependent sensory neuronopathy in a stocking-glove distribution.[3558]

cirsoid aneurysm of the scalp A congenital syndrome characterized by paroxysmal vascular headaches and the presence of cirsoid aneurysms.[381] See also **aneurysm**.

cisterna chiasmatica The subarachnoid space between the optic chiasm and the rostral end of the corpus callosum.

cisterna interpeduncularis The subarachnoid space between the crura cerebri (cerebral peduncles).

cisterna magna (Lat, large reservoir) The subarachnoid space behind the transverse fissure of the cerebellum.

cisternal block syndrome See **Zange–Kindler syndrome**.

cisternal puncture Insertion of a needle through the atlanto-occipital membrane into the cisterna magna. This is done to collect a CSF sample when it cannot be obtained at the usual lumbar site, or to insert contrast medium above the level of a spinal block. Precise measurement of the depth of the puncture is required, since the next structure to be encountered after the cistern is the medulla oblongata.

The procedure was introduced by Obregia in 1908 and further refined by James B. Ayer (b. 1882), an American neurologist, in 1920.

cisternography An invasive test designed to assess the circulation of the CSF, performed by the injection of a radionuclide such as radio-iodinated albumin into the lumbar subarachnoid space, the passage of this marker indicating CSF flow patterns when the spine and later the head are scanned with a gamma camera at intervals over the following 72 h.

citrullinemia (Allen–Dent syndrome) A recessively inherited hyperammonemic syndrome of infants due to deficiency of argininosuccinate synthetase, an essential enzyme in the urea cycle. The responsible gene maps to 9q34. Three forms (neonatal/infantile types I and III and adult type II) are recognized. The genetic defect of the latter is in the "citrin" gene (SLC25A13) and the clinical manifestations are mainly those of hepatic encephalopathy with raised plasma levels of citrulline and ammonia.[3076]

Types I and III are characterized by attacks of ataxia, vomiting, irritability, seizures, involuntary movements, and confusion, which occur from early childhood, precipitated by dietary protein and fever in children who are mentally retarded.[4260] High plasma levels of argininosuccinic acid are found.[6489] Although the condition may be lethal due to brain edema, in some cases it is actually asymptomatic.

A *variant* is reported from the Orient, in which the disease presents only in adult life, with cyclical bizarre behavior patterns and recurrent coma. Dysarthria, motor weakness, dementia, and hepatomegaly follow. See also **argininosuccinase deficiency.**

Clarke, Jacob Augustus Lockhart (1817–1880) English anatomist and neurologist who trained first at Guy's Hospital in London and later at St. Andrews. After his initial anatomical publications, which started in 1851 when he described the nucleus dorsalis, he was elected a Fellow of the Royal Society (1854) and he received their gold medal 10 years later. Although initially a general practitioner, he was appointed to the staff of the Hospital for Epilepsy and Paralysis in Regent's Park, London (now the **National Hospital**, Queen Square), on the basis of his research output. Most of his other papers were on the subjects of diabetes, the muscular atrophies, paraplegias, and tetanus, but he collaborated with **Jackson** in describing **syringomyelia** and **syringobulbia**.

Clarke cells Pigmented cells in the nucleus dorsalis.

Clarke column The dorsal or posterior columns of the spinal cord,[1670] described by **Clarke** in 1851.

clasp-knife rigidity If the examiner attempts to extend the flexed limb of a patient with a pyramidal lesion, **Gowers** noted that "When near full extension the spasm [of the extensor muscles] suddenly comes on and completes the movement, as the blade of a pocket knife moves under the influence of a spring."[2531] Today it is considered that sudden inhibition of the resistive flexor force is a more likely explanation. This is presumably due to the activation of the Golgi tendon organs by the force of the stretch, leading to the usual generation of their impulses inhibiting activity in the reflex arc.

class hysteria Contagious behavioral excess. The **dancing mania** is a relatively benign example of such activity; teen behavior at rock concerts is another; and mob violence still another, but more malignant.

classical torsion dystonia See **dystonia.**

Classics in the History of Psychology A large compilation of psychology links containing full text versions of some of the most important papers in this subject and even some complete books from the last 150 years. Web site: www.vanguard.edu/faculty/ddegelman/amoebaweb.

classification of neurologic disease "It is impossible to base a classification on the pathological evidence alone; this is only part of the clinical picture. Any classification must be based on genealogic, clinical, and pathological manifestations" (Waggoner, 1938).

This excellent advice is not always heeded, and the common phenotypic variability of dominantly inherited diseases provides a rich mine, ripe for eponymous excavations.

Claude, Henri Charles Jules (1869–1945) French neurologist who graduated and then trained further in Paris, at one time assistant to Raymond and Bouchard. He was later appointed to the staff of the **Salpêtrière** in Paris.

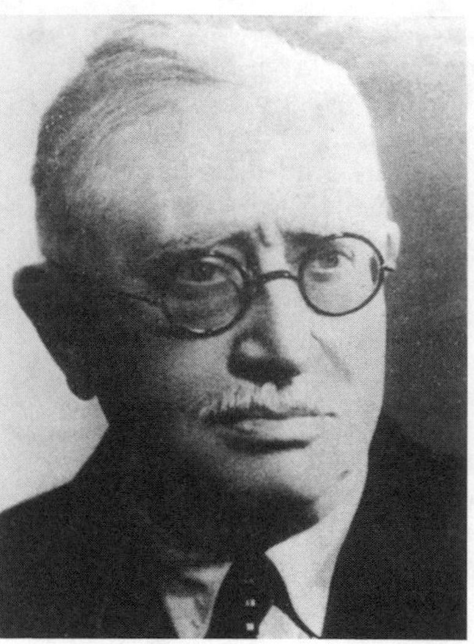

Figure C–4 Henri Charles Jules Claude.

His earliest contributions were studies in pathology, but he later turned to psychiatry and neurology and was concerned with movement disorders, hysteria, peripheral nerve lesions, epilepsy, and the physical treatment of the psychoses in particular.[1972]

Claude hyperkinesis Painful stimuli applied to paretic muscles excite reflex flexion or extension movements of those muscles; presented as evidence of organic weakness.

Claude syndrome The combination of III and IV cranial nerve palsies with contralateral cerebellar ataxia, rubral tremor, and hemianesthesia, resulting from a paramedian midbrain tegmental lesion involving the red nucleus and the superior cerebellar peduncle. The etiology is usually a stroke, tumor, or aneurysm.[1197] See **cerebellar ataxia with crossed III nerve palsy.**

Claude topoanesthesia See **Verger–Déjèrine syndrome.**

claudication (from Lat, to halt or be lame) Limping. The word is speculatively considered to have been introduced through the lameness of the Roman Emperor Claudius.

claudication of the cord Inability to continue the act of walking due to acutely progressive weakness of the legs. See **lumbar spinal stenosis.**

Clauss phenomenon The Toe phenomenon—see **Strümpell sign**—although it was described independently in 1926 by Clauss.

claustrophobia (from Lat, a bolt + Gr, fear) Mental anguish from being enclosed within a small confining space.

claustrum (Lat, a barrier or fence) A thin gray matter strip described by **Meynert**, lying lateral to the lenticular nucleus and beneath the insula.

clavus hystericus (Lat, a nail + hysterical) Sharp, sudden, stabbing, local head pain, as though a nail were being driven in.[2531] Despite the name, there is no suggestion that this is a psychiatric disorder. See **ice pick pains.**

claw foot ("le pied en griffe") The position taken up by the foot with paralysis of its intrinsic muscles. The mechanical effect of unopposed action of the long toe extensors is to cause raising of the arch with shortening of the foot, dorsiflexion of the proximal phalanges, and plantar flexion at the distal joints.

claw hand ("le main en griffe") The position taken up by the hand with paralysis of its small intrinsic muscles such as the interossei and lumbricals; the long finger flexors produce flexion at the proximal and distal interphalangeal joints while extension at the metacarpo-phalangeal joints is maintained by the long extensors.

CLEAT syndrome The acronym of Cerebral infarcts, Livedo reticularis, Endocardial lesions, Amaurosis fugax, and Thrombosis, these comprising selected but characteristic clinical manifestations of the **antiphospholipid antibody syndrome**.

Cleckley reflex See **Allen reflex**.

cleft lip-palate and tetraphocomelia (Appelt–Gerkin–Lenz syndrome) A recessively inherited syndrome characterized by bilateral cleft lip and palate, tetraphocomelia with a reduction in the number of digits, proptosis, hyperteleorism, and dwarfism. Hydrocephalus, encephalocele, spina bifida, and cardiac defects have also been described in association.[219] See **Roberts syndrome**.

clefting A craniofacial malformation in which there is persistence of epithelium between the borders of the facial bony processes which normally fuse during development. Clefts thus occur at the sites of normal fusion, as between the lateral or medial nasal and the maxillary processes (naso-ocular clefts and cleft lip); between the palatine processes of the maxillae (cleft palate); or between the maxillary and mandibular processes (macrostomia).[4]

clefting with skeletal anomalies See **Crane syndrome**.

clefting-corneal opacity-retardation syndrome See **Anyane Yeboa syndrome**.

Clifton Assessment Procedure for the Elderly (CAPE) A brief mental status examination assessing orientation, mental abilities, and psychomotor abilities in chronic psychiatric and geriatric patients and able to differentiate dementing from functional disorders. The scale has two parts: the first concerns information/orientation and is scored after interview with the subject, while the second is a behavior rating scale in which activities of daily living are also scored.[4935]

Clinical Autonomic Research A journal communicating data on research and treatment related to autonomic function and dysfunction. It is the official journal of the American Autonomic Society, the Clinical Autonomic Research Society, and the European Federation of Autonomic Societies. Web site: www.springerlink.com/content/108933/.

Clinical Dementia Rating Scale A composite instrument for the assessment of the severity of dementia on the basis of a semistructured interview procedure with the patient and an informed caregiver. Six areas of functioning (memory, judgment and problem solving, orientation, community affairs, home/hobbies, and personal care) are each rated on a 5-point scale (0 = None; 0.5 = Questionable; 1 = Mild impairment; 2 = Moderate impairment; and 3 = Severe impairment). Language and praxis are not assessed.[3036, 548]

Two additional categories have been suggested, to allow a rating of more severely impaired people:

CDR 4: Profound indicates severe impairment of language or comprehension, with inability to walk unaided, difficulty in feeding, in recognizing family or in controlling bladder or bowel function.

CDR 5: Terminal is applied to subjects who require total care and are completely uncommunicative, bedridden, vegetative, and incontinent.

Clinical EEG Electroencephalography (*Clin EEG Electroencephalogr*) A subspecialty medical journal. Web site: www.ecnsweb.com/ce_clinicaleeg.htm.

clinical electromyography (electroneuromyography) A term encompassing all electrodiagnostic studies of peripheral nerves and muscles. See also **electromyography** and **nerve conduction studies.**

Clinical Neurological Assessment tool A 21-item instrument assessing various parameters of activity in patients following head trauma. The scale is strengthened by the incorporation of items relating to brainstem function. (See Chart C–22.) The scores attained on this scale correlate well with those of the **Glasgow Coma Scale.** It is discussed online at www.baillement.com/index-neuro-crosby.html.

Clinical Neurology and Neurosurgery (*Clin Neurol Neurosurg*) A clinical neuroscience journal. Web site: www.sciencedirect.com/science/journal/03038467/.

Clinical Neurophysiology (formerly *EEG and Clinical Neurophysiology*) A professional journal. Web site: www.elsevier.nl/inca/publications/store/6/0/1/5/2/8/index.htt/.

Clinical Neurophysiology A Web-based resource describing the basics of the subject. Web site: www.clinicalneurophysiology.org.uk/.

Clinical Neurophysiology on the Internet A Web site providing data on basic neurophysiology and on the basis of EEG, EMG, and evoked potentials. Web site: www.neurophys.com.

Chart C–22. Clinical Neurological Assessment Tool

I. *Assessment of patient's response following verbal stimulation.*

1. *Response to verbal stimulation.* Assessor will say, "Hello [patient's nickname or first name]. This is [assessor's name]. How are you?"
   1. No response.
   2. Minimally aroused/slight movement.
   3. Becomes agitated/startles.
   4. Opens eyes, lids fluttering and blinking.
   5. Orients toward verbal stimulation/ demonstrates signs of recognition.
2. *Eye movement in response to verbal stimulation.*
   1. No response.
   2. Slight movement of eyelids/eyes.
   3. Opens eyes sluggishly.
   4. Opens eyes, lids fluttering and blinking.
   5. Opens eyes briskly, purposeful blinking.

II. *Assessment of patient's response to tactile stimulation. Firmly grasp left or right arm and shake it.*

3. *Body response to touch.*
   1. No response.
   2. Startles or becomes agitated/ demonstrates posturing.
   3. Slight movement.
   4. Movement away from source.
   5. Movement toward source.
   6. Movement toward source/attempts to grasp assessor.
   7. Able to discriminate areas of light touch.
4. *Eye movement in response to touch.*
   1. No response.
   2. Slight movement of eyelids.
   3. Opens eyes sluggishly.
   4. Opens eyes, lids fluttering and blinking.
   5. Opens eyes briskly, purposeful blinking.
5. *Response to painful stimulation.*
   1. No response.
   2. Startles or becomes agitated/ demonstrates posturing.
   3. Sluggish/delayed motor response.
   4. Moves away from source of pain.
   5. Localizes to pain source.
   6. Purposeful avoidance of pain/grimace.
   7. Able to discriminate sharp from dull stimulation.

III. *Assessment of patient's ability to follow commands.*

6. *Request patient to follow movement of finger with eyes*: "[Patient's name], follow my finger."
   1. No response.
   2. Opens eyes.
   3. Follows <30° arc.
   4. Follows >30° arc but <90° arc.
   5. Follows 90° arc.
7. *Response to command to squeeze and release assessor's hand.* Record best score, right hand versus left hand.
   1. No response.
   2. Delayed but slow squeeze.
   3. Slow squeeze.
   4. Brisk squeeze.
   5. Squeeze and release.
8. *Demonstrates subjective behavior.*
   1. None.
   2. Willful uncooperative activity.
   3. Willing but unable to cooperate.
   4. Willful cooperative activity.

IV. *Assessment of patient's muscle tone and resistance.*

9. *Muscle tone of biceps.* Record best score, right arm versus left arm.
   1. Flaccid.
   2. Rigid.
   3. Tense.
   4. Normal.
10. *Resistance associated with flexion/extension of arms.* Record best score, right versus left.
    1. Flaccid.
    2. Rigid.
    3. Tense.
    4. Normal.
11. *Muscle tone of quadriceps.* Record best score, right versus left leg.
    1. Flaccid.
    2. Rigid.
    3. Tense.
    4. Normal.
12. *Resistance associated with flexion/extension of legs.* Record best score, right versus left.
    1. Flaccid/no resistance.
    2. Inability to flex/fixed.
    3. Flexion/rigid (clasp-knife).
    4. Flexion/nonpurposeful resistance.
    5. Flexion normal.

V. *Assessment of patient's body and extremity position/movement.*

13. *Body position in bed.*
    1. Motionless/remains stationary.
    2. Position secondary to posturing.
    3. Skewed/nonaligned.
    4. Relaxed/purposeful/sleeplike.
14. *Arm activity.*
    1. Motionless/flaccid.
    2. Both extended and internally rotated (decerebrate).
    3. One arm extended and one arm flexed (decorticate/decerebrate).
    4. Both decorticate.
    5. Semiflexed/appears tense.
    6. Normal/flexed.
15. *Leg activity.*
    1. Motionless/flaccid.
    2. Both extended (decerebrate).
    3. Semiflexed/appears tense.
    4. Normal/flexed.
16. *General voluntary body movement.*
    1. No voluntary movement or posturing
    2. Slight movement.
    3. Restlessness, rolling, and turning.
    4. Aroused/nonpurposeful movement.
    5. Purposeful movement.
17. *Position of eyelids.* Record best score.
    1. Half open.
    2. Closed/no movement.
    3. Closed with oscillation of eyes.
    4. Closed with blinking/fluttering.
    5. Tightly closed/purposeful.
    6. Open and blinking/fluttering.

VI. *Assessment of patient's chewing, yawning, verbalization.*

18. *Chewing.*
    1. Absent.
    2. Nonpurposeful.
    3. Grinds teeth.
    4. Normal purposeful.
19. *Yawning.*
    1. Absent.
    2. Present.

    If chewing and yawning are not observed, consult with person caring for patient. If no one has observed chewing or yawning, mark absent.
20. *Verbalization.*
    1. Unconscious/no sound.
    2. Moaning and/or babbling.
    3. Conscious/no attempts at speech.
    4. Single-word answers/nodding or shaking head.
    5. Spontaneous communication to self or others.
    6. Meaningful communication yet word retrieval problems.
    7. Meaningful communication (written, verbal, and/or gestures).
21. *Orientation.*
    1. Unable to communicate (this does not mean because of tracheostomy).
    2. Disoriented.
    3. Oriented to time, place, person, situation (reason for hospitalization) (if incorrect responses, patient should be classified disoriented).

From Crosby L, Parsons LC. Clinical neurological assessment tool. Heart Lung 1989;**18:**121–9.[1353]

The Clinical Neuropsychologist The official journal of the American Academy of Clinical Neurophysiology.

clinically definite multiple sclerosis 1. That form of **multiple sclerosis** fulfilling all of the **Schumacher criteria.**[5663] 2. A diagnostic category of **multiple sclerosis** characterized by the occurrence of two preceding attacks, with evidence of involvement of two or more sites in the nervous system (clinically probable multiple sclerosis, CPMS) A1 or with two previous attacks, clinical evidence of one involved site in the nervous system, and paraclinical evidence of multiple sclerosis such as positive oligoclonal banding, positive MRI findings, or abnormal evoked responses. See **Poser criteria.** See also **McDonald–Halliday criteria.**[4217]

clinically isolated syndrome An acute or subacute episode of neurological disturbance due to a single lesion in the white matter, usually diagnosed in young adults. Optic neuritis, internuclear ophthalmopegia, and brainstem or partial spinal cord syndromes are examples. Between 30 and 70% of patients with this syndrome later develop **multiple sclerosis.** Both a new method of detecting oligoclonal bands[4141] and the MRI have been used as prognostic markers, with some success.[4363, 6330]

In children, this is defined as a first acute clinical episode of CNS symptoms with a presumed inflammatory demyelinating cause for which there is no prior history of a demyelinating event.[3574] This clinical event may be either monofocal or multifocal, but usually does not include encephalopathy, except in cases of brainstem syndromes. Examples include, but are not limited to, optic neuritis, transverse myelitis, and brainstem, cerebellar, and/or hemispheric dysfunction.

Because MS is diagnosed on the basis of two or more attacks separated in space and time, delay of a second attack after the appearance of symptoms of the first clinical event as a result of using immunomodulating agents somewhat delays the diagnosis of multiple sclerosis using current criteria. Clinically isolated syndromes also occur with **antiphospholipid syndrome, systemic lupus, Behcet disease,** and **Sjögren syndrome**.

clinically probable multiple sclerosis A diagnostic category of **multiple sclerosis** characterized by evidence of two preceding attacks with clinical evidence of one abnormal site in the nervous system (CPMS C1); of one prior attack and evidence of two involved sites in the nervous system (CPMS C2); or of evidence of one prior attack, clinical evidence of one site involved in the nervous system and the presence of paraclinical evidence of multiple sclerosis (CPMS C3). See **Poser criteria.** See also **McDonald–Halliday criteria.**[4217]

Clinician Interview-Based Impression of Change (CIBIC) An FDA-mandated attempt to assess a physician's gestalt in the context of clinical trials of medications for **Alzheimer disease.** Minimally or very much improved/worsened are the preferred ratings.[3499] Augmentation by garnering the opinion of a caregiver adds a "plus" to the title.

At least the vehicle underlines the fact that medicine is as much an art as a science.

clinocephaly (Gr, bed or inclination + head) A cranial developmental malformation in which there is depression of the cranial vault behind the bregma; the vertex is thus flattened into the shape of a couch.[4]

clinodactyly Incurving and shortening of the little finger; a common feature in developmental diseases such as **Down syndrome**.

clinoid (Gr, in the shape of a bed) Shaped like an antique bed.

clipping Distortion of EEG waves as a result of overload, which makes them appear flat-topped in the paper write-out.

clitoral crises Paroxysms of sexual excitement in females with **tabes dorsalis.**[2531] An unnecessary term for a rare manifestation of an unusual disease in a restricted population.

clivus That part of the sphenoid bone forming the central portion of the base of the skull.

clivus edge syndrome See **Kernohan notch syndrome** and **transtentorial herniation.** The term is not altogether appropriate since it is the tentorial free edge, not the clivus, that compresses the brainstem.

Clock Drawing Test A simple and reliable test of executive function in which the subject is asked to draw the face of a clock, putting in the numbers from 1 through 12 and indicating the position of the hands at some arbitrary chosen time. The test is sensitive in detecting early executive cognitive dysfunction which can precede memory disturbances in dementing illnesses. More than one scoring system has been devised but that of Sunderland et al. (*J Am Ger Soc* 1989)[6132] is relatively simple (© Wiley–Blackwell Publications; reproduced here by kind permission). The scores obtained correlate with global measures of dementia .

Another Clock Drawing Test is offered as a screening tool to evaluate global cognitive functioning as it reflects even subtle changes in cortical integration. Benefits are that it is easy to administer (though not always to score) and that it is not influenced by language, cultural, ethnic, or educational factors.[383]

Ability to Follow Instructions and Draw a Clock	Score
Either no attempt or an uninterpretable effort is made	1
Drawing reveals some evidence of instructions being received, but only a vague representation of a clock	2
Numbers and clock face no longer obviously connected in the drawing. Hands are not present	3
Distortion of number sequence. Integrity of clock face is now gone (numbers may be missing, placed outside of boundaries of clock face, etc.)	4
Crowding of numbers at one end of the clock, or a reversal of the numbers. Hands may be present in some fashion	5
Inappropriate use of clock hands (use a digital display, circle numbers despite repeated instructions)	6
Placement of hands is significantly off course	7
Noticeable errors in the placement of hours and minute hands	8
Slight errors in the placement of the hands	9
Hands are in correct position to indicate "2:45"	10

clonic absence attacks See **myoclonic absence attacks.**

clonic facial spasm See **hemifacial spasm.**

clonic seizures (rhythmic myoclonus) Those forms of seizure in which the repetitive muscular contractions are intermittent at a frequency of about 2–3 Hz. The repetitive discharges appear to be due primarily to rhythmic excitation. In the case of focal seizures, the jerks involve a part of the face or part or all of one limb. Consciousness is usually preserved.[4192, 1861]

clonic status epilepticus See **status epilepticus.**

clonic-tonic-clonic seizures Tonic-clonic seizures preceded by prominent myoclonic jerks.[1556]

clonus (from Gr, a commotion or tumult) Repetitive involuntary alternating contractions of agonist and antagonist muscle groups at about 5 Hz in response to a sudden maintained stretching force. It is due to disinhibition of a spinal generator within the reflex arc at that level, as in pyramidal tract lesions.[6614]

closing-in phenomenon The tendency to draw upon or close to the pattern to be copied in drawing tests, seen in patients with diffuse cortical disease.[4190]

clouding An alteration of consciousness such that perceptions are reduced in number, immediacy, and strength, the speed and clarity of thought are diminished, and, in many but not all cases, the patient is abnormally distractible. Clouding is a common sign in the early stages of delirium and in patients with severe dementia.

Clouston disease (hidrotic ectodermal dysplasia) A dominantly inherited syndrome characterized by nail dystrophy, telangiectasias, hair defects, hyperkeratosis of the palms and soles, cataract, and strabismus.[1205]

cloverleaf skull (Holtermüller–Weidemann syndrome) A deformity resulting from premature synostosis of the parieto-temporal sutures.[2970]

CLOX An executive clock drawing task that correlates closely with cognitive test scores and discriminates between healthy and demented elderly people. The test is divided into two parts. CLOX1 is an unprompted task that is sensitive to executive control, while CLOX2 is a copied version that is less dependent on executive skills. CLOX1 is more "executive" than several other comparable clock-drawing tasks. CLOX1, but not CLOX2, makes a significant independent contribution to the level of care received by elderly retirees.[5453]

club foot Shortening of the foot with elevation of the arch, usually a congenital deformity inherited as a recessive trait, although a majority of patients are male. The problem is usually bilateral.

The term was in use in England in the mid-sixteenth century. The earliest full description was made in 1794 by Antonius Scarpa (1747–1832), an Italian anatomist and surgeon who also described the (Scarpa's) canal in the inner ear, and the nerve, canal, fascia, and triangle to which his name is also given. He was also the first to identify disease of the medial wall of arteries as the basis of aneurysms.[5333]

cluneal nerve syndrome A myofascial pain syndrome presenting with paravertebral and gluteal pain and stiffness with palpable trigger zones in the affected areas.[6094] See also **piriformis syndrome.**

cluster headache (Bing headache [syndrome/erythroprosopalgia of/ciliary erythromelalgia of the head], periodic migrainous neuralgia of Wilfred Harris, hemicrania angioparalytica, histaminic cephalalgia, Horton headache, migrainous neuralgia, petrosal neuralgia [Gardner], Sluder neuralgia, spheno-palatine neuralgia, vidian neuralgia) A trigeminal autonomic cephalgia presenting with attacks of severe, strictly unilateral pain occurring in the orbital, supraorbital, and/or temporal regions lasting 15–180 min and occurring from once every other day to 8 times a day. The pain is associated with one or more of the following; conjunctival injection, lacrimation, nasal congestion, rhinorrhea, forehead and facial sweating, miosis, ptosis, and eyelid edema. The headaches are classically and almost uniquely associated with a sense of restlessness or agitation. The inferior posterior hypothalamic gray matter homolateral to the pain is activated during attacks of headache unresponsive to medication. The attacks occur in series lasting for weeks or months (so-called cluster periods) separated by remissions lasting months or years. About 10% of the patients have chronic symptoms (chronic cluster headache). Even fewer have a preceding aura.

The clinical features suggest excessive cranial parasympathetic discharge and abnormal activation of the suprachiasmatic nucleus has been postulated as a causal factor. Autosomal dominant transmission has been recorded. A polymorphism of the hypocretin receptor 2 gene may be associated. The first recorded descriptions were by Nicholas Tulp in1641 and Thomas Wllis in 1672.

The following diagnostic criteria are suggested by the Headache Classification Committee of the International Headache Society.[2820] (See Chart C–23.)

Episodic cluster headache occurs in periods lasting 7 days to 1 year separated by pain-free periods lasting 1 month or more fulfilling all the above criteria and with at least two cluster periods lasting from 7 to 365 days and separated by pain-free remissions of 1 month or more. *Chronic cluster headache* attacks occur for more than 1 year without remission or with remissions that last less than 1 month.

In *secondary cluster headache*, the clinical features are the same except for lack of the periodicity seen in the primary form, but follow injury or disease in the trigeminal distribution or vertebral artery dissection.[1316]

In another *variant* form, all the autonomic features are present but there is no headache.[1643]

See also **episodic cluster headache, chronic cluster headache,** and **chronic paroxysmal hemicrania**.

The tireless reader who has examined the contents of this book from A to C will have found already, and will still find, references to this condition from (in all) about 16 entries, so various are the names which have been given to it. The now-fashionable name **cluster headache** was the happy invention of Kunkle (1954), who remarked on the periodicity of the attacks 80 years after the condition was first described by Eulenberg.[3583] The most arresting descriptions, however, were those of Symonds[6175] and Horton.[3001]

cluster headache variant An alternative name for **chronic cluster headache**, in which atypical cluster

Chart C–23. Cluster Headache: Diagnostic Criteria

Cluster headache (ciliary neuralgia, erythromelalgia of the head, erythroprosopalgia of Bing, hemicrania angioparalytica, hemicrania neuralgiformis chronica, histaminic cephalalgia, Horton headache, Harris–Horton disease, migrainous neuralgia (of Harris), petrosal neuralgia of Gardner)

Attacks of severe, strictly unilateral pain which is orbital, supraorbital, temporal, or in any combination of these sites, lasting 15–180 min and occurring from once every other day to eight times a day. The attacks are associated with one or more of the following, all of which are ipsilateral: conjunctival injection, lacrimation, nasal congestion, rhinorrhoea, forehead and facial sweating, miosis, ptosis, and eyelid edema. Most patients are restless or agitated during an attack. Diagnostic criteria have been defined:

A. At least five attacks fulfilling criteria B–D
B. Severe/very severe unilateral orbital, supraorbital, and/or temporal pain lasting 15–180 min if untreated
C. Headache is accompanied by at least one of the following:
   1. Ipsilateral conjunctival injection and/or lacrimation
   2. Ipsilateral nasal congestion and/or rhinorrhea
   3. Ipsilateral eyelid edema
   4. Ipsilateral forehead and facial sweating
   5. Ipsilateral miosis and/or ptosis
   6. A sense of restlessness or agitation
D. Attacks have a frequency from one every other day to eight per day
E. Not attributed to another disorder

(From the International Classification of Headache Disorders (Headache Classification Committee of the International Headache Society. *Cephalalgia* 2004;24[Suppl 1]) by kind permission of Dr. Jes Olesen, the International Headache Society and Wiley-Blackwell Publications.)

The usual form is *episodic cluster headache*—attacks occurring in periods lasting 7 days to 1 year, separated by pain-free periods lasting a month or longer. The cluster periods usually last between 2 weeks and 3 months. Diagnostic criteria have been defined:

A. Attacks fulfilling criteria A–E **for cluster headache**
B. At least two cluster periods lasting 7–365 days and separated by pain-free remission periods of ≥1 month.

A *variant* is *chronic cluster headache*—cluster headache attacks occurring for more than 1 year without remission or with remissions lasting less than 1 month. Diagnostic criteria have been defined:

A. Attacks fulfilling criteria A–E for **cluster headache**
B. Attacks recur over >1 year without remission periods or with remission periods lasting <1 month

---

headache, multiple jabs of pain, and background vascular headache occur. The headache is atypical in that it occurs several times daily, shifts sides, is less severe and briefer than the typical cluster headache, does not recur in bouts, and is less constantly accompanied by signs of autonomic overactivity.[4277]

cluster headache-like disorder not fulfilling criteria Headache attacks diagnosable as cluster headache or chronic paroxysmal hemicrania which do not quite meet the IHS operational diagnostic criteria for cluster headache or chronic paroxysmal hemicrania, one item only being unfulfilled.

cluster-migraine A syndrome combining some of the components of cluster headache and of migraine headache, without abnormal findings on neurological examination. An example might be the occurrence of a typical (migrainous) visual aura preceding a cluster headache.[5947]

cluster minibouts Episodes of **cluster headache** lasting only 1–2 weeks.[5879]

cluster-tic syndrome A variant of **cluster headache** in which **trigeminal neuralgia** is associated. The pains respond somewhat to carbamazepine and baclofen but not to methysergide.[5947]

cluster vertigo The association of cluster headaches with episodic vertigo which occurs during the cluster headache periods.[2372]

cluttered speech (tachyphemia) A developmental articulatory disorder in which the speed of speech is increased beyond the patient's control, the patient varies the inflexions and division of syllables in a manner which is not euphonious, and speech is arrhythmic and repetitious.

These features may be accompanied by hyperactivity, impaired concentration, poor musical ability, and disturbances of reading and writing. The site and nature of the causal lesion are not known.[234]

Clutton joints Painful (sometimes painless) hydrarthrosis of the knees in children with congenital syphilis. This was first described by Dr. Henry Clutton (1850–1909) in 1886.

CMT International (Charcot-Marie-Tooth Disease International) A charitable organization based in the UK. Web site: www.cmt.org.uk/.

CNS germ cell tumors of childhood Uncommon childhood malignancies usually arising in the pineal and supra-sellar regions or elsewhere along the neuraxis. Pure germinoma, embryonal carcinoma, yolk sac tumor, choriocarcinoma, teratoma, and mixed germ cell tumors are differentiated.[1315]

CNS hypersomnia syndrome A chronic disorder of excessive daytime somnolence. The cause is not known, but prior infection with Epstein–Barr virus may play a part.

CNS Pathology Index A Web page with links to full-color images of the brain, found at http://library.med.utah.edu/WebPath/CNSHTML/CNSIDX.html/.

COACH syndrome A congenital syndrome manifesting Cerebellar vermis hypoplasia, Oligophrenia, Ataxia, Colobomata, and Hepatic fibrosis. See **cerebellar ataxia.**

coat-hanger headache Headache in the distribution of the neck and trapezius muscle, sometimes related to orthostatic hypotension.

coat-hanger sign One end of a coat hanger is placed on the patient's forehead and a "target", such as a piece of tape, is affixed to the other end, arranged so that it is directly in front of the patient. The patient's head is then passively moved while keeping the target directly in front of the patient's field of vision. A positive "coat-hanger sign" is the inability to maintain the eyes directed at the target during passive head movement (i.e., inability to suppress the **vestibular-ocular reflex**). This can be seen early in **progressive supranuclear palsy.**

Coats, G. (1876–1915) A Scottish ophthalmologist working in London.

Coats syndrome A syndrome consisting of unilateral telangiectasias of the retina with exudates; optic atrophy; and sensorineural deafness, sometimes associated with a port wine stain or with a **facioscapulohumeral muscular dystrophy**. It is most commonly seen in boys.[6233] See also **cerebroretinal microangiopathy with calcifications and cysts.**

coaxial needle electrode See **concentric needle electrode.**

cobalamin C disease An inborn error in cobalamin metabolism usually presenting in the first year of life with microcephaly, seizures, hypotonia, speech and developmental delay, failure to thrive due to poor feeding; vomiting; anemia and thrombocytopenia; low levels of vitamin B_{12}, and microthrombotic disease. The condition is associated with mutations in the *MMACHG* gene.

A rare *variant* adult-onset form is also described, with multiple neurologic presentations, some resulting from thromboembolic events.[6261]

Cobb, Stanley (1887–1968) American neurologist and psychiatrist who trained at Harvard and in British and European centers before returning to the United States and serving as chief of the neurology service at Boston City Hospital, from where he published widely on the cerebral circulation and demonstrated the reactivity of its arterial system to carbon dioxide rather than oxygen. He transferred to become head of psychiatry at the Massachusetts General Hospital in 1934, from which post he retired in 1954.

Cobb as much as anyone helped to reintegrate neurology and psychiatry, and demonstrated the utility and possibility of running a psychiatric service within a general hospital. His broad training in the basic neurosciences also allowed him an imaginative view of the nervous system which was perhaps unique for a psychiatrist who espoused the psychoanalytical school.[6748]

Cobb syndrome (cutaneo-meningo-spinal angiomatosis) A sporadic **neurocutaneous syndrome** characterized by the association of pial venous hemangiomas of the spinal cord behaving as extradural mass lesions with compression of the spinal cord or nerve roots; and by nevi in the overlying skin of the corresponding dermatomes.[1207] Those nevi in cervical regions may be associated with lesions of the lower cranial nerves. See **cutaneo-meningo-spinal angiomatosis** and **Klippel–Trenaunay–Weber Syndrome.**[4196]

cobblestone complex Forms of **lissencephaly** (malformations due to abnormal neuronal migration) in which the brain is not abnormally smooth. A version of Barkovich's classification[399] follows:

1. Cobblestone complex with congenital muscular dystrophy syndromes:
   a. Walker–Warburg syndrome (WWS)
   b. Muscle–eye–brain disease (MEB)
   c. Fukuyama **congenital muscular dystrophy** (FCMD) with or without retinal dystrophy

   In both the Walker–Warburg syndrome and muscle–eye–brain disease, various different mutations (e.g., of *POMT*, *FKRP*, *POMGnTl* or *LARGE*) have been identified.
2. Syndromes without involvement of muscle
   a. Cobblestone complex MEB pattern with normal eyes and muscle
   b. Cobblestone complex diffuse with normal eyes and muscle

(Based upon Barkovich AJ, Kuzniecky R, Jackson GG, et al. Classification system for malformations of cortical development. *Neurology* 2001;57:2168–78.)

Another *variant* is *cobblestone-like brain dysgenesis with cutis laxa* manifesting facial dysmorphisms, connective tissue disorders and neurologic impairment. (van Maldergem et al. *Neurology* 2008;71:1602–8)

cocaine test One drop of 10% cocaine solution is instilled into each eye, followed by another drop in each eye 1 min later. A normal pupil will dilate by the time the eyes are re-examined in 45 min, but a pupil with loss of its sympathetic innervation will not do so. The mechanism is the prevention by the cocaine of the reuptake of norepinephrine at the sympathetic junctions of the normal iris, leading to an excessive local adrenergic dilator effect; when there is a distal lesion of the sympathetic pathway, less norepinephrine than usual is available. See also **hydroxyamphetamine test.**

coccidioidomycosis An uncommon infection with the soil fungus *Coccidioides immitis*, capable of causing a chronic basal granulomatous leptomeningitis; which usually results from the spread of cranial osteomyelitis, and choroiditis, uveitis, optic nerve granuloma, papilledema, and VI cranial nerve palsy.[497]

coccydynia (coccygodynia) Persistent pain felt in the coccygeal area, especially on sitting and with local pressure, with no known cause.

coccygodynia See **coccydynia.**

coccyx (Gr, the cuckoo) The four lowest small, fused, triangular vertebrae.

cochlea (Lat, a snail; Gr, a winding staircase) A tapering coiled tube in the anterior part of the labyrinth within the petrous temporal bone; the auditory end-organ.

cochlear aplasia Developmental disorders of the inner ear and usually of the VII cranial nerve. See **Michel**, **Mondini**, and **Scheibe defects.**

cochlear deafness, myopia and oligophrenia syndrome See **Flynn–Aird syndrome.**

cochleoorbicularis reflex See **cochleopalpebral reflex.**

cochleopalpebral reflex (cochleoorbicularis reflex) Blinking of the eyes in response to a sudden loud noise.[6898] See also **palpebral reflex.**

cochleopupillary reflex Mydriasis in response to a sudden and unexpected loud noise; a normal phenomenon.

cochleovestibular atrophies A group of inherited disorders, often with congenital onset, manifesting nerve deafness and/or vestibular malfunction.

Cochrane Library A professional resource providing meta-analyses of clinical trials and recommendations as to therapies. Web site: www.update-software.com/cochrane.

Cockayne, Edward Alfred (1880–1956) English lepidopterist and physician or pediatrician, to the Middlesex and Great Ormond St. Children's Hospitals, respectively. His major interests were endocrinopathies and genetic diseases.[1972]

Cockayne syndrome (type VI sudanophilic leukodystrophy, dwarfism with retinal atrophy and deafness) A rare, recessively inherited hypomyelinating leukoencephalopathy (or possibly a leukodystrophy) in which there is failure of DNA repair.[1210]

Clinically, the children appear normal at birth but later develop mental retardation, prognathism, thickened microcephalic skull, an abnormally old facial appearance, anhidrosis, cachexia, skin photosensitivity, kyphosis, dwarfism with large hands and feet, and joint contractures. Neurological features include sensori-neural deafness, optic atrophy, cataracts, cerebellar ataxia, demyelinating sensorimotor peripheral neuropathy, and pigmentary retinal degeneration.[4463, 6414] Death occurs by the third decade, by which time marked spasticity and often tremor, nystagmus, ataxia, seizures, choreoathetosis, patchy CNS demyelination, and both basal ganglion and perivascular calcification are usually notable.[5941] See also **Neill–Dingwall syndrome** and the Web page "Cockayne syndrome" at www.ncbi.nlm.nih.gov/books/bv.fcgi?call=bv.View..ShowSection&rid=gnd.section.159.

cocktail party deafness Those forms of minor or moderate nerve deafness in which speech discrimination is markedly diminished as a result of background noise.

cocktail party syndrome (chatterbox syndrome, chronic brain syndrome of infantile hydrocephalus) A syndrome manifest in children with arrested hydrocephalus who appear bright and very talkative but in whom mental development is profoundly affected.[3089]

co-contraction The concurrent contraction of antagonist muscles when an agonist is activated. The phenomenon is regarded as evidence of a **functional disorder**.

codfish vertebrae Biconcavity of the posterior aspects of the vertebral bodies, seen in homocystinuria.[6291]

coenesthesis (Gr, common + sensation) Subjective awareness without precision as to the modes stimulated which produce that awareness; the total impression of internal bodily sensations. The reality of such a sensory mode, and the different interpretations placed upon the meaning of the word in the last 200 years, have made the word and possibly the concept obsolescent.[5604]

coenzyme Q deficiency A rare mitochondrial disorder manifesting focal seizures and hypotonia.

Coffin syndrome (lean spastic dwarfism) A familial dysmorphic syndrome, also characterized by spastic quadriparesis, seizures, predisposition to infections, congenital cardiac anomalies, and mental and motor delay.[1214]

Coffin–Lowry syndrome (fifth digit syndrome) A congenital X-linked dysmorphic syndrome mapping to Xp 22.2, characterized by mental and developmental delay, growth retardation, scoliosis, thickened calvarium, hypotonia, lax joints, ptosis, hypertrichosis, and abnormal development of the fifth digits and their nails, and sometimes of other digits as well. The **Dandy–Walker malformation** or other hindbrain abnormalities are associated with unusual frequency.[1526]

Coffin–Siris syndrome A congenital syndrome comprising mild microcephaly, coarse facial features, absent or hypoplastic fifth digits and their nails, hypotonia and psychomotor delay, accompanied by the **Dandy–Walker malformation**.[1526]

Cofs syndrome (cerebro-oculo-facio-skeletal syndrome) See **Pena-Shokeir phenotype**.

CogSport A computerized cognitive test battery consisting of eight tasks designed as card games examining simple reaction time, choice reaction time, complex reaction time, a monitoring task, and four others. It has been shown to be useful in the assessment of cerebral concussion and in monitoring recovery.[1252]

Cogan sign (lid twitch sign) The patient is asked to look down, then up, and down and up twice more. As a result of fatigue of the weaker levator muscle in **myasthenia gravis**, both lids go up, but the weaker one then slowly descends again, as if overshooting and then settling.[1220]

Cogan syndrome 1. (congenital oculomotor apraxia, Wieacker syndrome) An inability to perform voluntary saccadic horizontal eye movements, although spontaneous and reflex movements are possible, described by Cogan in 1953. Thus the child is unable to deviate his eyes when asked to examine an object set to one side, but rather turns his head, at which the eyes actually deviate the other way due to the integrity of the vestibulo-ocular reflex.[1216]

As a result of the abnormal movements of the head and eyes during attempted changes in the direction of gaze, only delayed and hypometric horizontal jerk saccades can be made when the head is immobilized; when it is not, the subject makes thrusting and overshooting head movements in order to compensate for the inability to move the eyes voluntarily. A history of prematurity, delayed psychomotor development, strabismus, and slight clumsiness are common accompaniments. The anatomical substrate for the condition is not certainly defined.[6960] See also **ocular apraxia.**

2. *Non-syphilitic interstitial keratitis* occurring in young adults, who present with photophobia, blurred vision, recurrent attacks of vertigo, vomiting, tinnitus, and deafness, resembling the symptoms of **Ménière disease** but due to diffuse vasculitis.[1215]

Other neurological and systemic manifestations are variably present.[627]

3. A congenital syndrome manifesting hemianopia, loss of optokinetic nystagmus, dyslexia, spasm of conjugate gaze, lateral disorientation, finger agnosia, dysgraphia, and dyscalculia.

Cogan twitch sign (eyelid twitch sign) Transient elevation or twitching of the upper eyelid when the subject returns gaze to the midposition after looking down. The sign is present in **myasthenia gravis.**[1220] See **Cogan sign.**

cognition (Lat, with + knowledge) A generic term for the quality of knowing, which in this context has been said to include abstraction ability, attention (the appropriate selection of a principal perception or task); conceiving; imagining; judgement; memory (the ability to store and retrieve percepts or concepts); perception; praxis (executive function); problem solving and reasoning; sensing (or the symbolic conception of sensory information); and use of language.

This motley collection of mental accomplishments constitutes a summation of adaptive behavior. Some also include emotion and the assignment of appropriate affective significance to a perception.

Cognitive Capacity Screening Examination A formalized, short, bedside screening test of cognitive function with adequate reliability but with a substantial false negative rate. It consists of 30 questions testing orientation to place and time, concentration, short-term memory, abstraction, digit recall, and arithmetic ability.[3132]

cognitive closure The mental completion of an incomplete stimulus; the ability to perceive a complete pattern where only an incomplete one is presented. Tests of such gestalt operations are considered to give information on right hemisphere functioning. See also **Gollin Incomplete Figures Test.**

cognitive dissonance The acceptance of both of two opposing viewpoints; a match/mismatch situation in which a subject wishing to believe in a pair of mutually exclusive ideas frequently experiences emotional distress.

cognitive domains The functions of orientation, attention, language, visuospatial functions, executive functions, motor control, and praxis.

Cognitive Failures Questionnaire A series of 25 questions to do with minor errors of memory or judgment which subjects may make ("Do you fail to listen to people's names when you are meeting them?") presented as a list for the patient to score between 0 (never) to 4 (very often). In a second part, a relative is asked to rate the patient on a different series with eight questions.[855]

cognitive fatigue A decline in cognitive performance during a single psychological testing session documented in multiple sclerosis,[3577] but likely to be a nonspecific finding.

cognitive processing epilepsy A composite of seizure types (generalized tonic-clonic, myoclonic, absence) sharing the common bond of precipitation by higher cortical processes such as performing mathematical problems, making decisions, playing board or card games, drawing, etc.[622] **Epilepsy arithmetices**, *decision-related epilepsy*, and *drawing-induced seizures* are named examples.

cognitive reserve A proposed mechanism accounting for the fact that some people show more and some show less cognitive impairment after similar brain injuries; and explaining nicely the protective effect of higher education in the prevention or delay of the symptoms of **Alzheimer disease**. Other contributing factors include genetics, head size, linguistic and reading abilities, lifestyle, and occupational attainment.[679]

cognitive screening tests Thirty-nine of these have been reviewed and assessed[1370] but no single instrument was judged superior to the others. Those judged most promising are italicized in the following compilation:

Modified Mini-Mental State Examination; Three Word Recall; 7-Minute Screen; AB Cognitive Screen; ***Addenbrooke's Cognitive Examination***; Abbreviated Mental Test; Brief Alzheimer Screen; Brief Cognitive Scale; *Cognitive Abilities Screening Instrument*; Cognitive Assessment Screening Test; Cognitive Capacity Screening Examination; **Clock Drawing Test;** Deterioration Cognitive Observé; DemTect; Dementia Questionnaire; General Practitioner Assessment of Cognition; Hopkins Verbal Learning Test; Informant Questionnaire on Cognitive Decline in the Elderly; Informant Questionnaire on Cognitive Decline in the Elderly-short form; Minnesota Cognitive Acuity Screen; Mini-Cog; Memory Impairment Screen; Montpellier Screen; Neurobehavioral Cognitive Status Examination (Cognistat); Rotterdam version of the Cambridge Cognitive Examination; Rapid Dementia Screening Test; *Short and Sweet Screening Instrument;* Symptoms of Dementia Screener; Six Item Screener; Short Memory Questionnaire; Short Orientation Memory Concentration Test (AKA 6-CIT, AKA Short **IMC** [Blessed] **Test**); Short Portable Mental Status Questionnaire; *Short Test of Mental Status*; Time and Change; Telephone Interview of Cognitive Status-Modified; Trail making Test; Verbal Fluency-Categories; Modified WORLD Test.

Yet others are the AD8, a brief informant interview sensitive to early signs of cognitive change,[2265] the Cognitive Abilities Screening Instrument, and the Rowland Universal Dementia Assessment Scale, both described by Galvin.

cogwheel phenomenon The arrhythmic, repetitive alteration of resistance to passive stretch occurring during passive movement of a joint; a palpable tremor. Such regular involuntary interruptions to the smooth flow of passive movements are a sign of disease of the basal ganglia, as in Parkinsonism.

cogwheel (saccadic) pursuit eye movement The occurrence of **catch-up saccades** during pursuit eye movement in an effort to compensate for a diminished velocity of those eye movements caused by, for example, reduced consciousness from any cause, or diffuse hemispheric or brainstem disease.[3761]

Coh syndrome A craniofacial malformation characterized by **cloverleaf skull** with fusion of all sutures, polymicrogyria, absent olfactory tracts and bulbs, duplication of the thumbs, micropenis, and bifid scrotum.[4]

Cohen hamartoma syndrome

A congenital dysmorphic syndrome characterized by asymmetrical eyes, heterochromia iridis, epibulbar dermoids, cataract, detached retina, malocclusion of teeth, asymmetrical leg hypertrophy with varicose veins, macrocephaly, hydrocephalus, and mental and developmental delay. Papules, capillary hemangiomas, lipomata, and other tumors of the skin are often present.[381]

Cohen-Mansfield Agitation Inventory A seven-item rating scale assessing the frequency of various agitated and related behaviors, completed by a caregiver usually in a nursing home setting.

Cohen syndrome A recessively inherited syndrome characterized by facial, oral, and ocular abnormalities, with microcephaly, microphthalmia, myopia, lax joints, brachydactyly, syndactyly, scoliosis, obesity, and hypotonia. The condition may be a manifestation of hyper-β-alaninemia.[1237, 3694, 2894]

coin-in-the-hand test A bedside or office test used to determine the organicity of claimed amnesia in which the subject is shown a coin in one of the examiner's hands and after 10 s of eye closure is asked to indicate the hand in which the coin was held, over 10 trials. Malingering patients perform at chance levels, but those with delayed memory failure, as after herpes encephalitis, usually attain a perfect score.[3299]

coital cephalgia See **headache associated with sexual activity.**

cold The sensation that an object contacted is at a lower temperature than the self. "In medicine, the sensation was formerly described as having three degrees of intensity; *algor*, when there was merely the feeling of cold; *horror*, when there was the creeping feeling of chilliness; and *rigor*, when there was actual shivering."[5103]

The phenomenon of cold is of interest in neurology because subjective descriptions of localized sensations of cold are occasionally heard in patients with myelopathy, particularly that due to **multiple sclerosis.** Cold itself may, however, have a beneficial effect in multiple sclerosis, while heat often induces an increase in symptoms, perhaps through alterations in the functioning of the neural potassium pump. With cerebral lesions, such as strokes, the affected limbs, especially the leg, may be several degrees cooler than the unaffected limbs.

cold face test The measurement of cardiac rate following the application of cold compresses to the face, which induce bradycardia, decreased cardiac output, selective vasoconstriction of the skin and viscera, and maintained blood pressure depending upon the function of the trigeminal–brainstem–vagal reflex pathway. The *diving reflex* and the *simulated diving reflex* (for which the stimuli are, respectively, immersion of the body and of the face in cold water) depend upon the same pathways.[3415] See also **cold pressor test.**

cold-induced sweating The occurrence of sweating over the head, trunk, and arms with a reduction in core body temperature, unassociated with any evidence of peripheral autonomic dysfunction. Facial and upper limb dysmorphisms may be present. The precise nature and site of the central sudomotor abnormality is undetermined. A defect in the *CRLF1* gene at 19p12 has been identified.

cold nerve injury Nerve damage as a result of nonfreezing cold injury following a period in which temperatures fluctuate, likely because of repeated reperfusion injury.[3221]

cold pain See **post-traumatic neuralgia.**

cold pressor test A measure of sympathetic efferent vasoconstrictor activity. When a patient's hand is placed in ice water for 1 min, or when ice is applied to the neck (**cold face test**), the forearm blood flow diminishes and the blood pressure should rise by 20/15 mmHg,[4252] but it does not do so in the presence of a central or an efferent sympathetic lesion.[3928] Bradycardia also occurs, in the absence of a parasympathetic lesion.

cold reversal (cold allodynia/hyperpathia) The sensation of heat and pain occurring with cold stimulation of the skin, as in **ciguatera** poisoning.

cold stimulus headache Generalized headache following exposure of the unprotected head to a low environmental temperature as in very cold weather or in diving into cold water Generalized headache following exposure of the unprotected head to a low environmental temperature as in subzero weather or when diving into cold water. The headache was first described by Robert **Whytt.** The ICHD criteria are the following:

A. Diffuse and/or non-pulsating headache fulfilling criteria C and D
B. Presence of external cold stimulus to the head
C. Headache developing during cold stimulus
D. Headache resolving after removal of cold stimulus

A *variant* is *headache attributed to ingestion or inhalation of a cold stimulus* (ice-cream headache) A short-lasting pain produced in susceptible individuals by the passage of cold material, solid or liquid, over the palate and posterior pharyngeal wall. Diagnostic criteria have been defined:

A. Acute frontal non-pulsatile headache fulfilling criteria C and D
B. Cold stimulus to palate and/or posterior pharyngeal wall due to ingestion of cold food or drink or to inhalation of cold air
C. Headache develops immediately, and only, after cold stimulus
D. Headache resolves within 5 min after removal of cold stimulus

From the International Classification of Headache Disorders (Headache Classification Committee of the International Headache Society. *Cephalalgia* 2004;24[Suppl 1]) by kind permission of Dr. Jes Olesen, the International Headache Society and Wiley-Blackwell Publications.

cold test Local cooling, which reduces myasthenic fatigability; this is well shown in the ptotic eyelids of the myasthenic patient which open after ice has been applied to them, until they warm again. The mechanism is not known.[748]

cold vasodilatation Capillary vasodilation of the skin causing transient rises in the skin temperature following immersion of the fingers in cold water. This is uninfluenced by sympathetic nerve integrity but is absent after section of the somatic nerves and so is likely to be due to a sensory nerve axon reflex.[2562]

Coleman syndrome (cervical spine trauma with injury of the head and shoulder girdle) A nonspecific cervical spine injury occurring in association with combined injuries to the head and the shoulder girdle. The lesion may include a fracture of the odontoid process, rotary dislocation of the atlas on the axis, fractured dislocation of the cervical vertebrae, and fracture of the transverse spinal processes. Cervical cord contusion is a possible reason for these features.[4320]

collagen VI An extracellular matrix protein that is widely expressed and is encoded by genes on 21q22.3 and 2q37. The typical phenotype occurring with mutations includes congenital kyphosis, torticollis, proximal contractures, and distal hyperlaxity, followed by delayed motor development and later respiratory compromise. Milder phenotypes also exist.[4555].

collapse (from Lat, to fall together) More or less sudden prostration as a result of severe physical or emotional illness such as fever, shock, seizure, or overwhelming affect.

Though formerly a respectable word in medicine, its clear meaning has endeared it to the laity; the profession therefore largely eschews it.

collapsing weakness The sudden "giving-way" of a limb from a normal position after minimal applied pressure. Thus the extended arms fall after only minimal downward pressure from the examiner. The phenomenon is regarded as evidence of a **functional disorder.**

collateral (Lat, with + the side) 1. That which accompanies or runs beside; an alternate pathway. Thus an auxiliary blood supply of a body part. 2. A branch of an axon.

collateral circulation The auxiliary pathways for blood supply to the brain, comprising extracranial arterial connections, the persistence of vessels running between the extracranial and intracranial circulations (middle-anterior meningeal, facial, anterior choroidal-posterior cerebral) and intracranial cerebral arterial anastomoses, such as the circle of Willis and superficial anastomoses between branches of the three major cerebral arteries.[3293]

collateral reinnervation The growth of nerve sprouts from a healthy axon's subterminal fiber to innervate a denervated motor end plate. An indicator of the presence of neurogenic disease.

Collet, Frederic Justin (b. 1870) French otolaryngologist; he described the following condition in 1915, 2 years before the account by J.A. Sicard, a French radiologist.

Collet–Sicard syndrome (posterior lacero-condylar syndrome, Bonnet–Collet syndrome, Weisenberg–Sicard–Robineau syndrome) Unilateral paresis of the bulbar nerves IX, X, XI, and XII, from which result loss of taste on the posterior third of the tongue, paralysis of the vocal cords and palate, weakness of the sternomastoid and trapezius muscles, and hemianesthesia of the palate, tongue, and pharyngeal walls. In contradistinction to the findings in **Villaret syndrome**, there is no **Horner syndrome.**[1251]

Although Collet's patient had a bullet lodged in his head, the syndrome is usually due to compression or infiltration by local infection such as tuberculosis or by tumors such as lymphomas, chromaffinomas, or parotid body tumors causing ischemia in the territory of the neuromeningeal trunk of the ascending pharyngeal artery. See also **Vernet syndrome.**

colliculus (Lat, a little hill) In the CNS, the anterior and posterior quadrigeminal bodies in the midbrain, parts of the optic and auditory reflex pathways, respectively.

Collier, James Stansfield (1870–1935) English neurologist and neuropathologist who trained at St. Mary's Hospital and who was later on the staffs of the **National Hospital**, and St. George's and the Bethlem Hospitals, where he was known as a dramatic and inspiring teacher and a superb diagnostic clinician.

Although he recognized that cerebral palsy was often the result of arrested development *in utero*, his best known works were his contribution to the study of **subacute combined degeneration of the cord** with **Russell** and **Batten**, and his description of cerebellar tonsillar herniation, **false localizing signs**, and the **superior orbital fissure syndrome** (which he considered to be a periostitis and was possibly right). It was he who first suggested that the dilated lateral ventricles in patients with **hydrocephalus** stretch and displace those descending motor fibers destined to control leg movements, thus explaining the relatively increased spasticity in the legs in that condition.

Collier sign (posterior fossa stare, tucked lid sign, lid retraction) Bilateral symmetrical lid retraction in the dorsal midbrain syndrome, resembling that of hyperthyroidism, but here accompanied by light-near dissociation and without lid lag on down-gaze.

Collins, Edward Treacher (1862–1932) English ophthalmologist who practiced at Moorfields and Charing Cross hospitals in London. He described what we call **Treacher Collins syndrome** in 1900, but there had been a prior report in 1846.

collision When used with reference to nerve conduction studies, the interaction of two action potentials propagated toward each other from opposite directions on the same nerve fiber so that the refractory periods of the two potentials prevent propagation past each other.

colloid cyst (Gr, glue-like + a bag) Benign thin-walled cysts, usually detected in the anterior end of the third ventricle, with a columnar or cuboidal epithelial wall and soft colloid contents. They are considered to arise from the embryonic remnant of the stomatodeum.

Their clinical effects result only when the cyst causes obstruction of CSF flow, when they may be manifest by intermittent paroxysms of acute headache with a notable postural factor, and by signs of raised intracranial pressure, coma, and profound mental changes, but usually eventual complete recovery. This classical picture is, however, uncommon, syndromes of raised intracranial pressure without any localizing signs, of sudden weakness of the legs with falling, or of progressive or fluctuating dementia being at least as common.[3376, 6, 1019]

In a *congenital* form, microphthalmia, seizures, cranial meningocele, hydranencephaly, porencephaly, or aqueduct stenosis may accompany these choroid plexus tumors.[381] See also **neuroepithelial cyst.**

colloidal gold test An indirect assessment of the amount and nature of γ-globulin present in a fluid specimen, relying on the tendency of colloidal gold to precipitate in the presence of slowly migrating γ-globulins. Quantitative tests have largely replaced this measure, which was at one time considered able to differentiate between paretic, luetic, and meningitic reactions in neurosyphilis according to the pattern of precipitation seen in the graded concentrations of colloidal gold test solutions—the early, middle, or late zone rises.[3687]

coloboma (Gr, the part taken away after mutilation) 1. A sporadic congenital malformation of the optic nerve head or of the iris resulting from developmental arrest (defective closure of the fetal fissure).

Clinically, the disk is usually enlarged, often with a deep cup, abnormally pigmented, and crossed by abnormal glial remnants and embryonic blood vessels. The condition leads to field defects in the region of the disk, and is commonly associated with basal encephalocele, midline facial dysmorphisms, and hypopituitarism.[2400] 2. A developmental defect of the eyelid, affecting primarily the upper or the lower lid margin. At its most severe, the eyelid is absent (*ablepharon*) while minimal degrees lead only to notching of the lid.[4]

coloboma-anal atresia syndrome See **cat eye syndrome**.

color agnosia Inability to name colors in the presence of normal color discrimination; impairment in relating a color to its name in the absence of deficits in color discrimination. This is revealed by normal performance on, for example, the ishihara charts, with difficulty in naming colors at sight and in matching dictated color names to color choices.

color anomia (color-naming disorder) Failure to name a color, or to indicate colors when given their names, in the absence of demonstrable defects in color perception or of aphasia,[1430] as shown by a retained ability to point to and to sort colors. The condition is usually associated with a right homonymous hemianopia and intact color perception in the left half-field; the lesion is subsplenial, lying between the occipital and temporal lobes in the left hemisphere.[4332]

Errors are made when naming colors or when the subject is asked to point to a named color, although color matching and interpretation of the ishihara pseudoisochromatic plates are normal. The syndrome is usually associated with a right-sided visual defect and with pure alexia caused by infarction in the territory of the left posterior cerebral artery. Two varieties are described—one a primary aphasic disorder, the other a disconnection syndrome separating the visual input and the cerebral structures subserving language function.[4842]

color association The ability to indicate the color of known common objects, impaired in patients with auditory–verbal deficits but intact in those with color anomia.

color blindness (deuteranopia) An X-linked recessive trait, wherein the subject cannot perceive certain colors. Red-green blindness is the usual form, blue-yellow blindness (**tritanopia**) being less common. It was first described in detail by the color-blind English chemist John Dalton (1766–1844) in 1794, although there is report of a letter to Joseph Priestly by Joseph Huddard in 1777 in which the phenomenon was reported. See also **achromatopsia.**

color desaturation Subjective reduction in the intensity of hue of a perceived object, usually as a result of disease of the optic nerve.

color duplex sonography A refinement of doppler sonography in which color-coding systems provide a real-time color image of blood flow in vessels, superimposed on the simultaneously generated b-mode image, so that areas of major blood flow disturbance are readily identified.[4678]

color flickerings Periodic visual phenomena at the margin of a field defect, as in the auras of migraine.

color naming disorder See **color anomia.**

color vision The theory of three types of retinal receptor, each responding maximally to one of three colors, was first suggested by Young and then developed by Helmholtz in 1852.

colorado tick fever A benign acute fever due to infection with a reovirus member of the arbovirus group, seen mainly in the western United States and Canada. It is a rare cause of encephalitis.[6002]

colpocephaly A dysmorphogenetic condition in which there is enlargement of the occipital horns of the ventricles in underdeveloped brains. The condition is associated with mental retardation and frequently with varied signs of neurological dysfunction, such as optic atrophy, seizures, and pyramidal signs.[2286]

Columbia Rating Scale A scale for assessment of change in patients with Parkinson disease.[1942] The scale rates *tremor* (in the arms, head, and legs); *rigidity* (in the arms, neck, and legs); *bradykinesia* (including gait disturbance, posture, postural stability, and rising from a chair); *functional performance* (finger dexterity, alternating movements, foot tapping, facial expression, seborrhea, and sialorrhea); and *speech disorder*. See also **Hoehn and Yahr Scale, Parkinson Disease Impairment Index**, and **Unified Rating Scale for Parkinsonism.**

coma (Gr, a deep sleep) The term used by Hippocrates to mean lethargy but now used to describe a state characterized by a reduction of conscious level to a point where the subject is unable to make meaningful responses to environmental stimuli due to either dysfunction of the reticular activating system or widespread depression of cerebral

Coma classification

Category	Subcategory
I Delta/theta > 50% of record	A. Reactivity B. No reactivity
II Triphasic waves	
III Burst suppression	A. With epileptiform activity B. Without epileptiform activity
IV Alpha/theta/spindle coma (unreactive)	
V Epileptiform activity (not in burst suppression pattern)	A. Generalized B. Focal or multifocal
VI Suppression	A. $<20\,\mu V$ but $>10\,\mu V$

cortical function. The score on the **Glasgow Coma Scale** will be 2-4-2 or less.

coma classification An electroencephalographic classification has been proposed and has been shown to have high intraobserver reliability.[6928]

Coma Outcome Scale A 5-point scale rating the functional outcome from coma, designed to allow comparisons between the results of different treatment plans:[3205]

1. No recovery; comatose until death
2. Persistent vegetative state
3. Severe disability; some cognitive function but dependent upon others for daily support
4. Moderate disability; independent in activities of daily life but unable to resume normal function
5. Good recovery; able to lead a normal life or to resume normal activity in the presence of a preexisting disability

(Adapted from Jennett B and Bond MR. Assessment of outcome after severe brain damage. *Lancet* 1975;1:480. Reproduced by kind permission.)

Coma Recovery Scale A wide-ranging assessment tool designed to predict the outcome in minimally responsive patients. Six items to do with *arousal and attention*, five with *auditory functions*, seven with *visual functions*, seven with *motor functions*, two with *oromotor functions*, six with *communication abilities*, and two concerned with *initiative* are rated. The possible scores range between 0 and 35.[2354] The scale scores correlate well with those of the **Glasgow Coma Scale.**

coma scales See **Glasgow Coma Scale, Reaction Level Scale, Innsbruck Coma Scale, Glasgow–Liege Scale, Coma Recovery Scale,** and **Comprehensive Level of Consciousness Scale.**

coma vigil 1. Originally, a lethargic delirious state described by French physicians in those moribund as a result of typhoid fever. It was **Osler** who recognized that it also occurred in typhus. 2. For present use, see **persistent vegetative state.**

Coma Waiting A Web site offering a glossary of terms used for brain injury, A–Z. Web site: www.waiting.com/

comatose In a state of coma.

comb rhythm See **mu rhythm.**

combined central and peripheral myelinopathy A syndrome characterized by the occurrence of both a primary demyelinating polyneuropathy and features of a **leukodystrophy** such as **adrenomyeloneuropathy, metachromatic leukodystrophy,** or **Krabbé disease.**[6288]

combined flexion phenomenon See **Babiński trunk-thigh test.**

combined lateral and medial medullary syndrome See **Babiński–Nageotte syndrome.**

combined plantar sign Described as "the simultaneous disappearance of the cortical and spinal plantar reflex met with in hysteria,"[5333] this sign probably requires further verification before it is generally adopted.

combined system diseases Disorders affecting both the lateral and posterior columns of the spinal cord. Although **subacute combined degeneration of the cord** is now regarded as the classic example, **Friedreich ataxia** was once so considered and other hereditary, nutritional, toxic, and other conditions may also be responsible.

comma-shaped degeneration The appearance of the short vertical fibers of the posterior columns in stained preparations of the cord taken from below a transection.[2531]

commissural myelotomy Sagittal incision of the spinal cord made in an attempt to divide the crossing fibers in the anterior commissure destined for the spino-thalamic tracts, and thus to relieve pain. This aim has often been achieved, while the absence of permanent alteration in thermal sensitivity remains unexplained.[1273]

The *Bischoff myelotomy* is performed to relieve spasticity; it incises the cord laterally at a number of levels in order to interrupt the fibers of the stretch reflex running from the dorsal root entry zone to the anterior horn cell pool.

commissure (Lat, a joining-together) Those fibers which join the two cerebral hemispheres—the corpus callosum, and the anterior, posterior, habenular, and hippocampal commissures.

commissure aphasia See **conduction aphasia.**

commissurotomy Incision of the anterior or posterior commissures, usually performed in an attempt to reduce the frequency of epileptic seizures.

common EEG input test A procedure in which the same pair of EEG electrodes is connected to the two input terminals of all the channels of an EEG machine as an adjunct to the calibration procedure. See also **calibration.**

common mode rejection A characteristic of differential amplifiers whereby they provide markedly reduced amplification of common mode signals compared to differential signals. It is expressed as the common mode rejection ratio, that is, the ratio of amplifications of differential and common mode signals. Thus:

$$\frac{\text{amplification; differential}}{1} = \frac{20,000}{\text{amplification}} = \frac{20,000:1}{\text{common mode}}.$$

common mode signal The common component of the two signals applied to the two respective input terminals of a differential EEG amplifier. In EEG recordings, external interference frequently occurs in this manner.

common peroneal nerve palsy A mononeuropathy affecting most often the deep branch of the nerve at the fibular head as the result of local compression, prolonged squatting, or direct injury, although more proximal lesions can occur. Clinically, the usual findings consist of weakness and wasting of the muscles of the anterior compartment (leading to weakness of ankle dorsiflexion and eversion, and of toe dorsiflexion) with altered sensation over the lateral aspect of the shin and the dorsum of the foot. A **Tinel sign** is often elicitable at the site of the nerve lesion.

The area of sensory disturbance cannot be differentiated from that associated with a lesion of the L5 root, but lumbar pain or any lower motor neuron signs in the glutei, tensor fascia lata, hamstrings, or tibialis posterior would indicate that it is the root rather than the nerve which is involved.

common reference electrode A reference electrode connected to the input terminal 2 of several or all EEG amplifiers.

common reference montage Several referential derivations sharing a single reference electrode. See also **referential derivation** and **reference electrode**.

commotio cerebri Originally, an intracranial hemorrhagic lesion resulting from a blow to the head, or brain injury in the absence of skull fracture as described by Ambrose Paré. Nowadays—see **concussion**.

communicating hydrocephalus That form of hydrocephalus in which there is obstruction to the circulation of CSF between the roof of the fourth ventricle and the superior sagittal sinus.

compartment syndromes 1. Disorders resulting from an increase in the interstitial pressure within a closed anatomical space, such as an osseofascial compartment, that leads to microvascular compromise. 2. Compressive ischemia of muscles and nerves lying within a compartment bounded on all sides by muscle, connective tissues, and/or bone, and occurring when there is pathological swelling of muscle or with any other cause of increased interstitial pressure within that compartment. Excessive pressure within such enclosed regions leads to pain, edema, muscle necrosis with myoglobinuria, and nerve ischemia, with the expected clinical deficits for each nerve affected.[4534]

In the leg, the *anterior tibial compartment* contains the tibialis anterior muscle, the long ankle and toe dorsiflexors, and the anterior tibial nerve (see **anterior tibial syndrome**); the *peroneal compartment* contains the peroneal muscles and the superficial peroneal nerve; the *deep posterior (tibial) compartment* contains the long plantar flexors of the ankle and toes and the posterior tibial nerve; and the *superficial posterior (triceps surae) compartment* contains the gastrocnemius-soleus muscles and the sural nerve.

In the forearm, the structures anterior to the radius and ulna are within the *volar compartment*, those posterior to the radius are within the *dorsal (extensor) compartment*. In the trunk, the *rectus abdominis* muscle may similarly compress the emerging spinal nerves.[769, 5676]

compass gait Rotation toward the side affected by a cerebellar lesion, best tested by having the patient walk a few steps forward and backward in an open area with the eyes closed. See also **star walking**.

compelled movements Involuntary movements arising due to abnormal excitation of some part of the CNS. The term has been supplanted by **dystonia**.

compensation neurosis Symptoms not of organic origin but produced without conscious intent, determined by an individual's quest for financial reward as a result of injury. Differentiation is made from **malingering**, in which the patient consciously fabricates symptoms and signs for the same purpose. See **disability neurosis**.

compensation syndrome See **nystagmus-blockage syndrome**.

compensatory nystagmus See **vestibular nystagmus**.

competency A legal term, signifying an individual's capacity to make rational medical (and other) decisions that are to be respected unless an opposing view is represented by a better lawyer.

complementary neuromotor examination A system of examination of neonates and infants in which the active participation of the alerted infant is obtained through close contact and by suppressing the intrusive **Moro reflex**, the latter achieved by fixing the infant's neck so that he reacts as if possessed of the amount of head control which normally appears only by the age of 3 months. Using this method, an 8-week-old infant can be brought actively to raise himself up into the sitting position.[176]

complete ophthalmoplegia Loss of all external eye movements, as may occur with **Miller–Fisher syndrome** or **acute inflammatory demyelinating polyneuropathy**, midbrain infarction, or **myasthenia gravis**; while skull base tumors, botulism, mucormycosis, phenytoin toxicity, and trauma are less common causes.

completed stroke 1. A stroke syndrome in which the progression of the deficit has stopped (**stable stroke**). 2. The attainment of maximal impairment such as complete hemiplegia or hemianesthesia, such that the symptoms could not get any worse.[4678]

completion phenomenon A variety of visual illusion in which there occurs the psychological "filling-in" of images of which part fall in a hemianopic field; this results in the patient reporting that he can perceive, for example, the whole face of the examiner when only half of it can actually be seen because of the hemianopic defect.[2303]

complex A sequence of two or more waves having a characteristic form or recurring with a fairly consistent form and distinguishable from background activity.

complex absence A form of generalized seizure disorder in which prolonged absences occur in conjunction with myoclonic activity or atonic attacks in children with preexisting brain damage.

complex I disease Rare recessively inherited mitochondrial respiratory chain diseases resulting from deficiency of *NADH coenzyme q-reductase.* Typically, they present in infancy or early childhood with features resembling **Leigh disease**, *fatal infantile lactic acidosis, cardiomyopathy and lactic acidosis with or without cataract, macrocephaly and leukodystrophy,* or *hepatopathy with tubulopathy*. See also **mitochondrial diseases**.[3893]

complex II disease A rare mitochondrial respiratory chain disease due to deficiency of succinate coenzyme *q*-reductase. See also **mitochondrial diseases**.

complex III disease A rare mitochondrial respiratory chain disease presenting with ptosis and fatigable weakness due to deficiency of coenzyme *q* cytochrome *c* reductase, a respiratory chain enzyme.[2806] Cardiomyopathy, Wolff–Parkinson–White syndrome, cerebellar atrophy, and myoglobinuria are also described features. See also **mitochondrial diseases** and **septo-optic dysplasia.**

complex IV disease A rare mitochondrial respiratory chain disease due to deficiency of cytochrome *c* oxidase. See also **mitochondrial diseases.**

complex figures test See Rey–Osterreith Test.

complex motor unit action potential A motor unit action potential that is polyphasic or serrated. See preferred terms, **polyphasic action potential**, or **serrated action potential**. (From the 2001 Report of the Nomenclature Committee of the American Association of Electromyography and Electrodiagnosis.[19] Reproduced by kind permission of the AANEM.)

More than five phases (crossings of the baseline) are required before a motor unit action potential is considered to be polyphasic. The normal proportion of such units recorded is <10%, but it may be higher in some muscles such as the deltoid.

complex partial seizures Forms of epilepsy originating locally in a limited area of one cerebral hemisphere, presenting most often in adolescence or adult life and manifesting simple or elaborate automatisms (especially of the trunk and limbs), impairment of awareness or responsiveness to externally applied stimuli (including absence attacks), and, in some cases, clonic movements, loss of body tone, and ictal or postictal speech disturbances.

They usually last for 1 min but occasionally for up to 15 min and are seldom preceded by an aura. No single typical EEG manifestation is described[6267] in brief, partial seizures with motor, sensory, and/or psychological manifestations in which there is always some impairment of consciousness.

In a *variant* form, complex partial seizures occur with generalized nocturnal seizures and MRI findings of hyperintensity in the temporal lobes on T2-weighted studies with a "fat" hippocampus.

complex partial status epilepticus The rare repetition of the manifestations of **complex partial seizures** leading to a confusional state, automatic behavior, and subsequent amnesia, usually seen in children and associated with a variety of cerebral lesions.[2462]

complex regional pain syndrome (reflex sympathetic dystrophy, RSD; Sudeck atrophy; major causalgia, minor causalgia, mimocausalgia, shoulder-hand syndrome, algoneurodystrophy, reflex neurovascular dystrophy, post-traumatic osteoporosis, pain syndrome, edema, or angiospasm; traumatic angiospasm; peripheral acute trophoneurosis; postinfarctional sclerodactly; Steinbrocker disease, chronic traumatic edema) A condition of painful swelling, dryness, **allodynia**, and warmth of the hand not limited to the distribution of a single peripheral nerve, with immobility enforced by the pain and with developing osteoporosis and atrophy of skin, underlying muscles and bones.[6117, 5644] The condition appears to be due to prolonged vasoconstriction, tissue hypoxia, and tissue metabolic acidosis.

Two varieties are distinguished, without (type I) and with (type II) a proximate cause in nerve injury. So-called *type I* has been defined by the International Association for the Study of Pain as a pain syndrome, occurring

- in the presence of an initiating noxious event or a cause of immobilization (however, this is not always accepted);
- if the subject manifests continuing pain, allodynia, or hyperalgesia, but the degree of pain experienced appears to be disproportional in severity and duration to the inciting event (if there is one);
- if there is evidence at some time of edema, changes in skin blood flow, color, and temperature, or other abnormal autonomic activity in the region of the body affected by the pain. This is usually the distal aspect of an affected extremity or it may have a distal-to-proximal gradient.
- if there is a reduction in the range of motion of the affected parts with stiffness, weakness, and tremor[6016]

  The diagnosis would be excluded, however, in the presence of other conditions that could otherwise account for the degree of pain and dysfunction experienced.

(From *Pain* 1995;**63**:127–33. Stanton-Hicks M et al. Reflex sympathetic dystrophy: changing concepts and taxonomy. © 1995 Elsevier Science. Reproduced by kind permission.)

Other criteria variously suggested have included the presence of pain, allodynia, or hyperalgesia, the pain being disproportional in severity and duration in relation to the inciting event (if there is one); and the presence of edema, changes in skin blood flow, color, and temperature, skin mottling, and abnormal sudomotor activity in the region of the pain (usually the distal aspect of an affected extremity or with a distal-to-proximal gradient). Reduction in the range of motion of the affected areas with stiffness, weakness, and tremor are further common clinical features.

Type II represents what was known formerly as **causalgia.** In this case, prior nerve injury shall have occurred.[6016] In association with the intractable pain and trophic changes described above, pareses, incoordination, tremor, myoclonus, and dystonia are also occasionally manifest. The condition is seen after myocardial infarction, injuries to the arm or shoulder, with cervical or shoulder joint disease and with numerous diseases of both the central and peripheral nervous systems, stroke in particular.[5683] It was once thought to signify damage to the sympathetic innervation of the affected limb but the pathogenesis remains uncertain although in patients with stroke, avoidance of traction damage to the shoulder may supply some protection.

Suggested criteria[4326] are as follows:

1. The presence of continuing pain, allodynia, or hypalgesia after a nerve injury, not necessarily limited to the distribution of the injured nerve
2. Evidence, at some time, of edema, changes in skin blood flow, or abnormal sudomotor activity in the region of the pain

The diagnosis would be excluded, however, by the existence of conditions that would otherwise account for the degree of pain and dysfunction.

Web sites devoted to this subject include www.ninds.nih.gov/disorders/reflex_sympathetic_dystrophy/reflex_sympathetic_dystrophy.htm (compiled by the National Institute of Neurological Disorders and Stroke); the Web site of the International Research Foundation for RSD/CRPS, http://rsdfoundation.org/, a multilingual site providing clinical guidelines for treatment of reflex sympathetic dystrophy, physician and patient resources, and scientific advice; and http://familydoctor.org/online/famdocen/home/common/pain/disorders/238.html, a site providing patient information from the American Academy of Family Physicians.

complex repetitive discharge A type of spontaneous activity consisting of a regularly repeating series of complex polyphasic or serrated potentials that begin abruptly after needle electrode movement or spontaneously. The potentials have a uniform shape, amplitude, and discharge frequency ranging from 5 to 100 Hz. The discharge typically terminates abruptly. May be seen in both myopathic and neurogenic disorders, usually chronic. They are thought to be due to ephaptic excitation of adjacent muscle fibers in a cyclic fashion. This term is preferred to **bizarre high-frequency discharge, bizarre repetitive discharge, bizarre repetitive potential, near-constant frequency trains, pseudomyotonic discharge,** and **synchronized fibrillation.** (From the 2001 Report of the Nomenclature Committee of the American Association of Electromyography and Electrodiagnosis.[19] Reproduced by kind permission of the AANEM.)

complex visual hallucinations

Abnormal visual perceptions that affect some normal individuals on going to sleep and are also seen in association with sleep disturbances. The content of the hallucinations is striking and relatively stereotyped, often involving animals and human figures in bright colors and dramatic settings. Causes include the narcolepsy-cataplexy syndrome, peduncular hallucinosis, treated idiopathic **Parkinson disease, Lewy body** disease, migraine coma, Charles **Bonnet syndrome**, schizophrenia, hallucinogen-induced states, and epilepsy.

Pathogeneses cited include epileptic hallucinations due to a direct irritative process acting on cortical centers integrating complex visual information; visual pathway lesions with defective visual processing or an abnormal cortical release phenomenon; or brainstem lesions affecting ascending cholinergic and serotonergic pathways are considered.[4040]

complicated acrocephalopolysyndactly

See **craniosynostosis.**

complicated amyotrophic lateral sclerosis

The association of dementia, posterior column degeneration, or Parkinsonism in patients with familial or classical amyotrophic lateral sclerosis. In sporadic amyotrophic lateral sclerosis, posterior column degeneration is uncommon. Familial amyotrophic lateral sclerosis in children is recessively inherited; that in adults is dominantly inherited. The association of these conditions has been reviewed.[3027] See **amyotrophic lateral sclerosis.**

complicated hemianopias

See **hemianopia.**

complicated hereditary infantile optic atrophy

See Behr **disease.**

compound action potential

A potential or waveform resulting from the summation of multiple individual axon or muscle fiber action potentials. See **compound mixed nerve action potential, compound motor nerve action potential, compound nerve action potential, compound sensory nerve action potential, and compound muscle action potential**. (From the 2001 Report of the Nomenclature Committee of the American Association of Electromyography and Electrodiagnosis.[19] Reproduced by kind permission of the AANEM.)

compound granular corpuscles

(gitterzellen) Microglial cells swollen with lipid droplets following local tissue injury and cell breakdown.

compound mixed nerve action potential

A compound nerve action potential recorded from a mixed nerve when an electric stimulus is applied to a segment of the nerve that contains both afferent and efferent fibers. The amplitude, latency, duration, and phases should be noted. (From the 2001 Report of the Nomenclature Committee of the American Association of Electromyography and Electrodiagnosis.[19] Reproduced by kind permission of the AANEM.)

compound motor nerve action potential

(compound motor NAP) A compound nerve action potential recorded from efferent fibers of a motor nerve or a motor branch of a mixed nerve. Elicited by stimulation of a motor nerve, a motor branch of a mixed nerve, or a ventral nerve root. The amplitude, latency, duration, and number of phases should be noted. Distinguished from compound muscle action potential. (From the 2001 Report of the Nomenclature Committee of the American Association of Electromyography and Electrodiagnosis.[19] Reproduced by kind permission of the AANEM.)

compound movements

Those movements which involve change of posture at two or more joints, as bringing a finger to the nose or a heel to the opposite knee.[2962]

compound muscle action potential (CMAP)

The summation of nearly synchronous muscle fiber action potentials recorded from a muscle, commonly produced by stimulation of the nerve supplying the muscle either directly or indirectly. Baseline-to-peak amplitude, duration, and latency of the negative phase should be noted, along with details of the method of stimulation and recording. Use of specific named potentials is recommended, e.g., **M-wave, F-wave, H-wave, T-wave, A-wave,** and **R1 wave** or **R2 wave** (see **blink responses**). (Adapted from the 2001 Report of the Nomenclature Committee of the American Association of Electromyography and Electrodiagnosis.[19] Reproduced by kind permission of the AANEM.)

compound nerve action potential

(compound NAP) The summation of nearly synchronous nerve fiber action potentials recorded from a nerve trunk, commonly produced by stimulation of the nerve directly or indirectly. Details of the method of stimulation and recording should be specified, together with the fiber type (sensory, motor, or mixed nerve). (From the 2001 Report of the Nomenclature Committee of the American Association of Electromyography and Electrodiagnosis.[19] Reproduced by kind permission of the AANEM.)

compound sensory nerve action potential

(compound SNAP) A compound nerve action potential recorded from the afferent fibers of a sensory nerve, a sensory branch of a mixed nerve, or in response to stimulation of a sensory nerve or a dorsal nerve root. May also be elicited when an adequate stimulus is applied synchronously to sensory receptors. The amplitude, latency, duration, and configuration should be noted. Generally, the amplitude is measured as the maximum peak-to-peak voltage when there is an initial positive deflection or from baseline to peak when there is an initial negative deflection. The latency is measured as either the time to the initial deflection or the negative peak, and the duration as the interval from the first deflection of the waveform from the baseline to its final return to the baseline. Also referred to by the less preferred terms *sensory response*, *sensory potential*, or *SNAP*.

(From the 2001 Report of the Nomenclature Committee of the American Association of Electromyography and Electrodiagnosis.[19] Reproduced by kind permission of the AANEM.)

Comprehensive Level of Consciousness Scale (CLOCS)

A system for assessing physical signs relating to consciousness.[6017] (See Chart C–24.) See also **coma scales.**

Comprehensive Psychopathology Rating Scale

A scale containing 66 items representing neuropsychological symptoms or signs detected in a clinical interview and rated between 0 and 3; the scale is highly sensitive and specific, particularly for the detection of depression in elderly patients.[256]

Chart C–24. Comprehensive Level of Consciousness Scale

1: Posture
4 Posture is under volitional control and is normally flexible.
0 No abnormal posture but muscle tonus is completely flaccid.

2: Eye position at rest
6 Midposition and conjugate.
0 Skew deviation.

3: Spontaneous eye opening
4 Volitional control of eye opening.
0 No spontaneous or elicited eye opening.

4: General motor functioning
6 Normal spontaneous movements within the limits of the patient's physical abilities.
0 No spontaneous motor movements.

5: Abnormal ocular movements
6 None.
0 Complete absence of ocular motility.

6: Pupillary light reflexes
7 Normal direct and consensual light reflexes.
0 Wide pupillary dilatation and fixed to all stimuli or bilaterally small (pinpoint) pupils which are fixed to all stimuli.

7: General responsiveness
8 The person is fully aroused and alert, or, if asleep, arouses and attends to the examiner after only mild or moderate stimulation. The arousal outlasts the duration of the stimulus.
0 Total absence of discernible motor activity even in response to noxious stimulation.

8: Best communicative effort
7 Normal communication is possible through speech, writing, gesturing, etc.
0 No elicited or spontaneous vocalizations, searching behaviors, or eye contact.

From Stanzak et al. (1984),[6017] reproduced from the J Neurosurg © *1984 by kind permission.)*

compressed spectral array

A mathematical method of displaying EEG signals depicting changes in the amplitude and frequency of brain activity.[623] The sequential spectra of the mean frequencies of EEG activity over a defined period are closely applied in the printout, creating a graphic pseudo-three-dimensional representation. Analysis of such recordings taken over a prolonged period may be of value in determining prognosis in comatose patients.

compression neuropathy Deficits within the territory of a nerve as a result of continued pressure causing ischemic conduction block within the nerve.

compression nystagmus See **vestibular nystagmus.**

compulsive tics See **Tourette syndrome.**

computerized axial tomography (CAT scan) A refinement of plain radiological tomography in which electronic detectors receive X-rays from a source rotating 180° on the opposite side of the subject, examining him thus from all angles to provide accurate cross sections in the axial plane. Computer analysis of the images allows for two-dimensional reconstruction of the structures irradiated at any number of transverse levels. Further computer analysis of the data to allow coronal or sagittal reconstructions is also possible.

Following the initial mathematical work by Allan Cormack up to 1963, and by Dr. W.H. **Oldendorf**, Dr. Godfrey Hounsfield developed the method for CT scanning in humans, for which he and Prof. Cormack were awarded the Nobel Prize in 1979.

Computerized Everyday Memory Battery An automated instrument in which the subject's abilities in such tasks as telephone dialing with or without interference, name/face association (with both immediate and delayed recall), recognition of faces with immediate and delayed signal detection, reaction times, selective reminding, tests of associative learning and memory, visual (nonlanguage) memory, and narrative recall. The battery is used to evaluate potential cognition-enhancing pharmaceutical compounds.[3701]

conation (Lat, to try) The products of thought, as opposed to the **cognitive** powers which allow such exertions to occur.

concentration The ability to maintain focused attention upon one item or activity over a period of time. This capacity tends to be lost early in the dementias and at the outset in delirious states.

Digit span and serial seven subtraction tests are those generally used at the bedside to assess concentration.

concentric lacunar leukoencephalopathy A subacutely progressive demyelinating disorder of the CNS, related to **neuromyelitis optica**, in which zones of cavitation alternate with glial septa devoid of axons and myelin sheaths. Clinically, the condition presents in adult life with cortical blindness, seizures, and focal deficits.[1385]

concentric macro EMG A technique for studying the concentric motor unit action potential alongside the macro-potential, using a needle electrode combining concentric and macro recording surfaces.[3116]

concentric needle electrode

Recording electrode that measures an electric potential difference between a centrally insulated wire and the cannula of the needle through which it runs. (From the 2001 Report of the Nomenclature Committee of the American Association of Electromyography and Electrodiagnosis.[19] Reproduced by kind permission of the AANEM.)

conceptual apraxia A form of apraxia in which the concept of the action is lost. It is characterized by impaired ability to use tools and to understand meaningful gestures.[3540] See **apraxia.**

concussion (From Lat, to shake violently) (*commotio cerebri, embranlement*) A clinical syndrome, traumatic in origin, characterized by immediate neurological dysfunction (usually involving at least transient impairment of consciousness and awareness) which is fully reversible and unassociated with demonstrable gross changes, though *microscopic* brainstem and cortical abnormalities may exist. Later, a **post-concussional syndrome** may occur manifesting headache, impaired memory and concentration, sleep disturbance, anxiety and depression, fatigue, irritability, and vertigo.

Concussions are considered to be "complex" if there are specific sequelae such as seizures; with loss of consciousness lasting more than a minute; in the presence of persistent symptoms or prolonged cognitive impairment; and with a prior history of concussions.

Concussion affects the cerebrum and the spinal cord similarly. The mechanism is considered to result from rotation of the cerebral hemispheres in the anterior–posterior plane around the fulcrum of the upper brainstem which is relatively fixed.[5385] Cranial impact is not a necessary factor in causation; acute acceleration injury affecting the cervical cord or brainstem has also been held responsible. The subject has recently received major reviews.[4209, 5385]

Two sets of decision rules for ordering a CT scan after a concussion have been framed (in New Orleans and Canada). The latter apply to subjects with Glasgow Coma Scale scores of 13–15 aged 16 years and older; and advise intervention if the GCS score is <15 within 2 h of injury, with a suspected depressed or open skull fracture or basal skull fracture, two or more episodes of vomiting, and age over 65 years. There is thought to be a moderate risk of brain injury detected by CT scans if there is retrograde amnesia for 30 min or more, and if the mechanism of the injury was "dangerous"—being struck by or ejected from a motor vehicle, or a fall from 3 feet or more, or over five stairs, for example.

Stages of recovery from cerebral concussion have been defined:[4905]

4 Respiratory arrest with somatic immobility
3 Shallow, irregular respirations with somatic immobility
2 Normal respiratory movements with inadequate, ineffective, and inappropriate somatic movements
1 Normal posture, gait speed, and attitude but impaired performance of complex tasks
0 Full recovery

Immediate features of concussion include headache, dizziness, vertigo, and nausea in the short term and headache, inattention, light-headedness, impaired memory, fatigability, irritability, light and noise intolerance, anxiety, and sleep disturbances days or weeks later.[3375] Guidelines for classification of concussion suffered during sports have been defined by a committee of the AAN[5150] as follows (Reproduced by kind permission of the American Academy of Neurology and Lippincott Williams and Wilkins.)

Grade 1
Transient confusion
No loss of consciousness
"Bell rung" or "dinged"
Concussion symptoms or mental status abnormalities on examination resolve in <15 min

Grade 2
Transient confusion
No loss of consciousness
Concussion symptoms or mental status abnormalities on examination resolve in >15 min

Grade 3
Any loss of consciousness, brief (seconds) or prolonged (minutes)

In brief, Grade 1 (mild) signifies no loss of consciousness and post-traumatic amnesia lasting less than 30 min. In Grade 2 (moderate) loss of consciousness lasted for less than 5 min or post-traumatic amnesia was for more than 30 min. In Grade 3 (severe) the loss of consciousness was for more than 5 min or the post-traumatic amnesia lasted more than 24 h.

Grade 0 of Nelson (*Phys Sports Medicine* 1984;12[3]:103–7; not a part of the AAN classification system above) may be assigned when the athlete's head is struck or moved rapidly, but the athlete is not stunned or dazed initially but subsequently complains of headache and difficulty in concentrating.

Suggested guidelines for the management of sport-related injuries (first or second concussion) may be found at the Web site: www.neurology.org/cgi/content/full/48/3/581.

The range of disabilities caused by minor head injuries has been reviewed[5307] and guidelines for the management of and the performance of CT scans after sports-related concussions have been created and were reviewed by Ropper and Gorson (2007).[5385] See also **second impact syndrome, chronic fatigue syndrome, ding, post-concussional syndrome**, and **whiplash concussion**.

conditionally responsive extrapyramidal syndrome

See **paroxysmal kinesigenic choreoathetosis**.

conditioned insomnia

The occurrence of chronic insomnia as a result of a learned negative emotional association between sleeping and a particular environment. (Adapted from the Association of Sleep Disorders Centers. Diagnostic classifications of sleep and arousal disorders. *Sleep* 1979;2:1–137.[280])

conditioned reflex

Reflex responses to stimuli which do not normally produce such responses, these responses being acquired as a result of training and repetition. The two stimuli must be related in time and the conditional stimulus must precede the unconditional. Such reflexes are in contradistinction to unconditional reflexes or instincts which are native to the organism. **Pavlov** introduced the concept and the term in 1898, following his research on food rewards and secretion in the canine stomach.

The theory underlying **behaviorism** is that overt human behavior is the result of the building up of series of conditioned reflexes throughout life.

conduction aphasia

(central aphasia, leitungaphasie, commissure aphasia) That form of dysphasia produced by lesions of the supramarginal gyrus and the subjacent arcuate fasciculus (which extends from the supramarginal gyrus anteriorly to the motor association and Broca areas) in which the auditory language comprehension center is separated from the verbal motor center. Repetition of spoken speech is seriously affected, word-finding and naming are impaired, and there are many circumlocutions and phonemic (literal) **paraphasias** with self-correction, but with retention of comprehension. Spontaneous speech and writing are usually fluent and copious. Facial apraxias are also commonly found.[4202]

Such fluent paraphasic speech with normal comprehension but severely impaired repetition was described by Wernicke (1874), who recognized that it was due to disconnection of the first temporal and third frontal gyri, and called it aphasia of the insular region, later, however, correctly incriminating lesions of the arcuate fasciculus. Goldstein regarded it as a disturbance of **inner speech.**

conduction apraxia

A syndrome resulting from damage to the left

hemisphere and characterized by good performance to pantomime on verbal command but impaired performance on attempted imitation in the presence of severe ideomotor apraxia to verbal command and naming. Reception of the gestures is spared.[4746]

conduction block Failure of an action potential to propagate past a particular point upon an intact axon in the nervous system as a result of failure of depolarization of the axonal membrane because of the increased capacitance induced by demyelination. Conduction nevertheless is possible below the point of the block. It is documented by demonstration of a reduction in the area of a compound muscle action potential greater than that normally seen with stimulation at two different points on a nerve trunk; anatomic variations of nerve pathways and technical factors related to nerve stimulation must be excluded as the cause of the reduction in area. (From the 2001 Report of the Nomenclature Committee of the American Association of Electromyography and Electrodiagnosis.[19] Reproduced by kind permission of the AANEM.)

The finding of a 50% reduction in such amplitudes with no more than a 15% increase in the duration of the CMAP is characteristic of demyelinating but not of axonal neuropathies. Conduction block is also documented by demonstration of a reduction in the area of an evoked potential greater than that normally seen with electrical stimulation at two different points on a nerve trunk; anatomical variations of nerve pathways and technical factors related to nerve stimulation must be excluded as the cause of the reduction in area. (From the American Association of Electromyography and Electrodiagnosis [AAEE]. Glossary of terms in clinical electromyography. *Muscle Nerve* 1987;10S:G5–G23. © 1987. Reproduced by permission of John Wiley and Sons Inc.)

conduction syndromes See **disconnection syndromes.**

conduction velocity (CV) Speed of propagation of an action potential along a nerve or muscle fiber. The nerve fibers studied (motor, sensory, autonomic, or mixed nerve) should be specified. For a nerve trunk, the maximum conduction velocity is calculated from the latency of the evoked potential (muscle or nerve) at maximal or supramaximal intensity of stimulation at two different points. The distance between the two points (conduction distance) is divided by the difference between the corresponding latencies (conduction time). The calculated result is the conduction velocity of the fastest fibers and is usually expressed in meters per second (m/s). As commonly used, CV refers to the maximum conduction velocity. By specialized techniques, the conduction velocity of other fibers can also be determined and should be specified, for example, minimum conduction velocity. (From the 2001 Report of the Nomenclature Committee of the American Association of Electromyography and Electrodiagnosis.[19] Reproduced by kind permission of the AANEM.)

conduit d'apprendre (Fr, literally, learning pathway) The struggle of paraphasic subjects to utter the correct word, achieved (or not) after many incorrect attempts.

cone dysfunction syndromes See **cone dystrophy.**

cone dystrophy (achromatopsia, cone dysfunction syndromes) Retinal degenerative syndromes characterized by selective loss of retinal cone function and presenting with bilateral diminution of visual acuity and of color vision, photophobia, dayblindness (**hemeralopia**), central visual field defects, and abnormal single-flash and flicker **electroretinogram** (ERG).

Most cases are dominantly inherited and occur in association with evidence of hereditary **cerebellar ataxias**, but all forms of inheritance have been described.[2479, 5319]

Variant forms are *rod monochromatism*, in which there is congenital absence of cones with marked impairment of visual acuity and color vision, nystagmus, and abnormal photopic (cone-mediated) but normal scotopic (rod-mediated) electroretinogram responses; and the *macular form of pigmentary retinopathy* (inversa form), which is a selective loss of cone function at the macula.

cone–rod dystrophy See **pigmentary retinal degeneration.**

confabulation The uttering of incorrect statements by a patient who believes them to be true; involving the fabrication of details in order to compensate for loss of memory.[525] Two forms have been differentiated: *spontaneous confabulation*, which may result from the superimposition of frontal lobe dysfunction on an organic amnesia, and in which the statements made represent inadvertent displacement of memories taken from the past to the present; and the *provoked form*, which is considered a reasonable response in the presence of a faulty memory.

It is necessary for one to be unaware of the memory deficits suffered in order to confabulate. As Miller Fisher pointed out: "The subject cannot say 'I don't know' if he is unaware of his deficit. His answer is whatever comes to mind. 'I don't know' represents a relatively preserved intellect." Thus Miller Fisher designated confabulation as "false recollections and delusions with anosognosia (various types)."[2099] See also **Wernicke–Korsakoff syndrome.**

Confabulation Questionnaire A scale useful in excluding confabulation, as would be common in the **Wernicke–Korsakoff syndrome** and in certain toxic dementias, but rare in **Alzheimer disease.**

confirmed epilepsy The occurrence of at least two unprovoked seizures separated by more than 24 h.[3901]

confrontation An insensitive technique for assessing visual fields in which the examiner stands immediately in front of the patient who is asked to fix his gaze on the examiner and to identify the side on which the latter moves his fingers, placed in various parts of the field, or to count the number of fingers raised.

Suprathreshold techniques involve the stationary presentation of fingers or targets well within the visual field; *threshold* techniques require the patient to identify the point of first awareness as the fingers are brought into the field from outside it. The sensitivity can be improved if colored targets are used.[6391]

confusion See **confusional state.**

confusional arousals (excessive sleep inertia, schlaftrunkenheit, l'ivresse du sommeil) Episodes of confusion occurring during and following arousals from sleep, usually from deep sleep in the first part of the night. See **sleep drunkenness**. Diagnostic criteria have been suggested:[1629]

A. A complaint by the patient or an observer of recurrent mental confusion upon arousal or awakening
B. Spontaneous confusional episodes can be induced by forced arousal

C. Absence of fear, walking behavior, or intense hallucinations in association with the episodes
D. Polysomnography demonstrates arousals from slow-wave sleep
E. Not associated with the medical disorders such as partial complex seizures
F. Does not meet the diagnostic criteria for other sleep disorders causing the complaint, such as sleep terrors and sleepwalking.

From AASM Diagnostic Classification Steering Committee. *The International Classification of Sleep Disorders Diagnostic and Coding Manual*. Rochester, MN. American Academy of Sleep Medicine 1991/2001. Reproduced by kind permission of the AASM.) See also the Web site: www.sleepeducation.com/Disorders.aspx/.

Confusional Assessment Method An instrument for the detection of delirium, based upon clinical observation, and using a diagnostic algorithm for confusion based on the *DSM IIIR* criteria. It depends on the presence of four features: acute onset, fluctuating course, inattention, and disorganized thinking *or* altered level of consciousness. This leads on to the assessment of orientation, memory, perception, psychomotor agitation, and retardation and disturbances of the sleep–wake cycle. The presence of such features reliably predicts delirium.[3092]

confusional migraine A migraine syndrome which occurs more commonly in boys, characterized by a typical aura, a headache (which may be insignificant), and confusion (inattention, distractibility, and difficulty maintaining speech and other motor activities) which may precede or follow the headache.

Agitation, memory disturbances, obscene utterances, and violent behavior are not uncommon. Single attacks are typical, multiple attacks rare. Both may be triggered by mild head trauma. If the level of consciousness is more profoundly disturbed, **migraine stupor** lasting 2–5 days can occur.[3004] See **dysphrenic migraine.**

confusional state (confusion, delirium) 1. An alteration in mental state characterized by some degree of reduction in consciousness, in which the most salient deficits are those of attention, leading in turn to impairments in clear thinking, perception, orientation, and memory. The **Glasgow Coma Scale** score will be 4-6-4. 2. An inability to think with one's customary clarity and coherence, reflecting an impairment in abstract thinking. In addition to impairment of consciousness, thinking, memory, psychomotor behavior, perception, and emotion are affected.

Clinically, fluctuating disturbances of vigilance and of attentiveness (i.e., distractibility); impairment of coherence in the stream of thought and of skilled, goal-directed movements; perceptual distortions; disorientation; impaired judgment, blunted insight, and labile affect; apathy or agitation; and anomia, dysgraphia, acalculia, and failure of constructional abilities are the more notable features.[4332] See also **Confusional Assessment Method, delirium,** and **Galveston Orientation** and **Amnesia Test.**

congenital absence of the pectoral muscles See **Souques syndrome.**

congenital amaurosis See **Leber congenital amaurosis.**

congenital analgesia See **congenital indifference to pain.**

congenital aphasia See **developmental dysphasia** and **congenital auditory imperception.**

congenital apnea A malformation syndrome in which medullary and olivary hypoplasia are associated with periods of apnea in infants.[3442]

congenital ataxia with aniridia See **cerebellar ataxias (*variants*).**

congenital ataxia with choroidal coloboma See **Pfeiffer syndrome.**

congenital atlanto-axial dislocation First observed in 1960 by the Mumbai neurologist N.H. Wadia,[6582] this condition is rare in the West but is well recognized in India. Symptoms are precipitated by neck movement and include cervical pain and stiffness, transitory attacks of paralysis, paresthesias, visual loss or loss of consciousness, and progressive pyramidal dysfunction. Young men with short necks are mainly affected. Occipitalization of the atlas, fusion of the second and third cervical vertebrae, and an abnormal odontoid process are the more common structural findings. The treatment is surgical.

congenital auditory imperception (congenital aphasia, developmental aphasia, congenital word deafness) Impaired discrimination of sounds, including speech sounds, leading to reliance on gesture, facial expression, and lip reading and to delayed attainment of speech expression and comprehension with **idioglossia.** The condition is considered to be a developmental speech disorder syndrome.[131] See **Worster-Drought–Allen syndrome.**

congenital bilateral perisylvian syndrome (Foix–Chavany–Marie syndrome) A familial (probably X-linked dominant) developmental syndrome characterized by the association of facio-pharyngo-glosso-masticatory diplegia and bilateral perisylvian polymicrogyria. The usual clinical features include pseudobulbar signs, cognitive deficits, epilepsy, and perisylvian abnormalities on imaging studies, but the presentations are variable.[2611] See also **bilateral periventricular nodular heterotopia** and **anterior operculum syndrome.**

congenital brachial palsy Intra-partum stretch injury of the (upper) brachial plexus, frequently bilateral though asymmetrical.[5573]

congenital brevicollis See **Klippel–Feil anomaly.**

congenital bulbar palsy See **Möbius syndrome.**

congenital cataracts, facial dysmorphism neuropathy syndrome A recessively inherited disorder of children, detected in Wallachian gypsies, characterized by microcornea and cataracts, a mainly motor neuropathy starting in the legs, mild nonprogressive cognitive impairment, and in some cases pyramidal signs and chorea. Short stature, facial dysmorphism, and hypogonadotrophic hypogonadism are other features of the syndrome.[6361]

congenital central apnea Failure to breathe from birth, associated in one case with medullary hypoplasia and malformations of the inferior olives.[3442]

congenital central hypoventilation syndrome

(central alveolar hypoventilation syndrome, primary alveolar hypoventilation syndrome) A syndrome occurring, usually within the first few days of life and characterized by episodes of apnea at sleep onset, due to a defect in the function of central chemoreceptor function.[467] See **Ondine's curse.**

Failure of the autonomic control of ventilation occurs due to a decrease in the density of neurons and myelinated fibers in the medullary respiratory centers, and may lead to a fatal outcome.[4286] The syndrome is characterized by hypoventilation, which is worse during sleep than wakefulness, and which is unexplained by primary pulmonary disease or ventilatory muscle weakness. In central alveolar hypoventilation, there is considered to be a failure of the automatic control of breathing.[4930]

Clinical diagnostic criteria have been suggested.[1629]

A. Shallow breathing, or cyanosis and apnea, worse during sleep than in wakefulness, which has a perinatal onset
B. Hypoventilation that is worse during sleep than in wakefulness
C. Absent or diminished ventilatory response to hypoxia and hypercapnia
D. Polysomnographic monitoring demonstrates hypercapnia and hypoxia during sleep, predominantly without apnea
E. The absence of primary lung disease or ventilatory muscle dysfunction that can explain the hypoventilation
F. Not due to any other sleep disorder, such as infant sleep apnea

From AASM Diagnostic Classification Steering Committee. *The International Classification of Sleep Disorders Diagnostic and Coding Manual*. Rochester, MN. American Academy of Sleep Medicine 1991/2001. Reproduced by kind permission of the AASM.) See also the Web site: www.sleepeducation.com/Disorders.aspx/.

congenital cerebellar ataxia

See **cerebellar ataxias.**

congenital cerebellar atrophy

See **cerebellar ataxias.**

congenital cerebellar hypoplasia

(ataxic cerebral palsy) A congenital developmental syndrome characterized by colobomas of the retina, strabismus, dysarthria, and cerebellar signs due to cerebellar hypoplasia, sometimes with mental delay. See **cerebral palsy.**

congenital cervical spinal muscular atrophy

A nonfamilial, neurogenic type of **arthrogryposis** limited to the upper limbs, characterized by severe symmetrical muscle wasting with areflexia and congenital contractures of the shoulders and arms. Sensory and bulbar symptoms, long tract signs, scoliosis, and leg involvement are absent.[2679]

congenital chiasmal dysplasia

Developmental anomalies usually associated with other midline malformations affecting, for example, the hypothalamus and the lateral or third ventricles. **Optic nerve hypoplasia** is a milder variant. See also **septo-optic dysplasia.**

congenital chorea

See **Vogt syndrome.**

congenital cranial osteoporosis

See **craniotabes.**

congenital cytomegalovirus infection

Infection by this double-stranded DNA herpes virus follows maternal viremia and affects up to some 2% of all live-born children, most, however, remaining asymptomatic.

Clinically, the disease is characterized by multiple organ system involvement, low birth weight, jaundice, a petechial skin rash, and chorioretinitis. Neurologically, microcephaly, ventricular enlargement, periventricular calcification, mental retardation, spasticity, and deafness are the commonest features in symptomatic infants.

Some infected children who are asymptomatic at birth develop neurological problems later, particularly behavioral disturbances and arrest of intellectual development, over the course of the next few years. Deafness is also a common complication.[822, 5281] The pathology is that of a chronic encephalitis with particular damage to the periventricular subependymal tissues.[6858]

congenital deafness and otitic meningitis

The combination of congenital unilateral deafness and nontraumatic otorrhea due to a malformation of the inner ear, this latter leading on to recurrent episodes of meningitis.[4635]

congenital demyelinating encephalopathy

A syndrome of mental retardation with epileptic seizures and spastic paresis of congenital onset, accompanied by particular damage to CNS myelin with destruction of axis cylinders and with reactive gliosis. The etiology is unknown; perinatal asphyxia may be responsible.[4000]

congenital demyelinating neuropathy with multifocal CNS demyelination

A syndrome combining the features of chronic demyelinating peripheral neuropathy (with slow nerve conduction velocities, peripheral nerve hypertrophy, elevation of CSF protein levels, insidious onset, and continuous progression) with evidence of multifocal lesions in the CNS, including optic neuritis, brainstem involvement, and cerebellar and pyramidal signs, with episodic expression.[6288] The latter fulfil diagnostic criteria for clinically definite **multiple sclerosis.**

The findings suggest the coincidence of a chronic inflammatory demyelinating polyneuropathy and multiple sclerosis, which might be supposed to represent central and peripheral responses to a common antigen at some time past.

congenital encephalo-ophthalmic dysplasia

See **Krause syndrome.**

congenital end-plate acetylcholine receptor deficiency

A rare variant of congenital myasthenia with electrical responses resembling those found in the adult disease.[1866] See also **myasthenia gravis.**

congenital end-plate acetylcholinesterase deficiency

A rare variant of congenital myasthenia manifesting severe weakness and fatigability of all muscles from birth, refractory to anti-cholinesterase drugs, and with a decrement at all rates of stimulation on electrical testing.[1876]

congenital facial-abducens paralysis See Möbius syndrome.

congenital facial diplegia and **congenital nuclear agenesis/aplasia** See Möbius syndrome.

congenital facial palsy A dominantly inherited facial palsy present (usually bilaterally) at birth and due to nuclear agenesis as in **Möbius syndrome** or as a result of more peripheral damage to the nerves, though not occasioned by trauma during birth.[4234] See also **Bell palsy.**

congenital familial fibrosis A rare form of restrictive ophthalmoplegia characterized by the replacement of the extraocular muscles by fibrous tissue.[2770]

congenital fiber type disproportion An idiopathic nonprogressive or slowly progressive **congenital myopathy** presenting with hypotonia and proximal and distal weakness in the neonatal period, and in which biopsy changes in muscle include uniform smallness and numerical predominance of type I muscle fibers and hypertrophy of type II fibers (particularly of subtype IIb). Although generally benign, it has a variable natural course.[5938] Ophthalmoplegia, arthrogryposis, and scoliosis are also described, with moderate to severe, mainly proximal, muscle weakness without loss of ambulation. Nerve conduction studies are normal; the EMG may be normal or myopathic.

The weakness often involves the respiratory muscles; in addition there are delay in achieving motor milestones, short stature, high palate, scoliosis, joint contractures, macrocephaly, and the later development of muscle and joint contractures and skeletal deformities such as congenital dislocation of the hips.[1888, 2408] The serum CK levels are only slightly, if at all, raised.

Subtypes are defined as follows: A *dominant form* (1q42, *α-actin*) with a phenotype of severe diffuse congenital weakness leading to early death. A *recessive form* with onset in youth or early adult life, mapped to 1p35-p36 and due to mutations in *selenoprotein-N*, 1 (*SEPN1*), with congenital truncal hypotonia causing neck weakness and respiratory impairment; *CFTD2* (Xq13.1), a recessive form with bilateral ptosis and facial weakness, generalized hypotonia, respiratory insufficiency, and early death;[7721] and a form with slowly progressive proximal weakness occurs in children in whom muscle biopsy specimens show the presence of a relative excess of type I fibers and minimally enlarged type II fibers,[1827] and in **Krabbe disease.**[1535]

Type I fiber predominance is a frequent finding in several types of congenital myopathy and may actually approach type I fiber uniformity in **central core disease.** Fiber-type disproportion (a morphological pattern in muscles in which predominance and smallness of type I fibers appear as pathological features when compared with type II fibers in the same muscles) may be a nonspecific variation of type I fiber predominance. In the soleus muscle, type I fiber predominance is physiological. The pattern of fiber-type predominance has been seen in a wide variety of neuromuscular disorders such as some congenital myopathies, infantile **myotonic dystrophy, Krabbe** and **metachromatic leukodystrophies,** and in adult myotonic dystrophy. The finding is also present in some patients as a manifestation of a CNS disorder.

congenital fibrosis of extraocular muscles (CFEOM) A set of hereditary disorders of ocular muscle development. Varieties include the following:

CFEOM1 (12p11.2–q12; *kinesin*) is dominant or sporadic and presents with bilateral ptosis, and restriction of eye movements, the eyes fixed in a position below the horizontal, compensated for by neck extension. Blepharophimosis is associated.

CFEOM2 (11q13.3, *ARIX*) is a recessive trait with limited extraocular movements, the eyes being fixed in abduction. The ptosis markedly reduces vision and there is also miosis. Central ocular motility reflexes (smooth pursuit, saccades, vestibulo-ocular reflex, and optokinetic reflex) are intact but convergence is lost. Light and near reflexes are absent.[755]

This is a primary neurogenic abnormality with secondary myopathic changes that results from mutations in the transcription factor associated with the anatomical absence of cranial nerves III and probably IV bilaterally.

CFEOM3 (16q24) is a dominant trait with the variable expression of asymmetric ptosis and limitation of extraocular movements, especially vertically.

CFEOM with ulnar hand anomalies (21qter) is a recessively inherited syndrome of ophthalmoplegia with limited upgaze or worse and oligodactyly or oligosyndactyly.[7720]

congenital hemihypertrophy (Curtius syndrome) A congenital syndrome manifesting an increase in the size of all or part of one side of the body, including the face and limbs, or of a single system (nervous, vascular, muscular) only, with dilated and tortuous veins, associated variously with hypogenitalism, mental delay, facial dysmorphisms, tumors of the kidney or adrenal glands, cataracts, and psychosis.[1388]

congenital hydrocephalus-hydranencephaly A syndrome of aqueduct atresia and arthrogryposis, complicated by hydramnios.[2167]

congenital hypomyelination polyneuropathy (congenital hypomyelination neuropathy) A group of rare, recessively inherited or sporadic neuropathies characterized by the presence in infancy of severe distal weakness and difficulties with feeding and respiration; motor development is retarded in surviving children. Motor nerve conduction speeds are extremely slow. Most of the few patients described in literature die within the first years of life.

The condition is probably a variant of Déjèrine–Sottas disease (HMSN type III, itself probably a form of HMSN type 1).[2653] Pathologically, there is evidence of a hypertrophic neuropathy with severe hypomyelination or even the complete absence of myelin in all the fibers of peripheral motor and sensory nerves. The condition resembles **hereditary motor and sensory neuropathy** (HMSN) type III, but has the atypical pathological features of absence of myelin breakdown products, **onion bulbs,** and inflammatory infiltrates.[349] The number of axons is markedly reduced.[2653] Mutations have been described in the following genes: MPZ, EGR2, PMP22, and MTMR2.[5897]

Variant forms include a form with **arthrogryposis multiplex congenita** in association,[786] as well as *late infantile* and *juvenile* (groups 2 and 3) onset forms. See also **hereditary motor and sensory neuropathy** type III.

congenital hypotonia-sclerotic muscular dystrophy A possible variant of **congenital muscular dystrophy** characterized by muscle dystrophy, unimpaired intelligence, and recurrent respiratory infections.[2250]

congenital hypotonia with small type II fibers A **congenital myopathy** distinguished by the presence in muscle biopsy specimens of hypotrophy of the type II fibers.

congenital hypotonia with type I fiber predominance A mild and nonprogressive or abating **congenital myopathy** with decreased reflexes and skeletal deformities, distinguished by the presence in muscle biopsy specimens of a relative excess of type I fibers.

congenital hypotonic-sclerotic muscular dystrophy See **congenital muscular dystrophy.**

congenital indifference to pain (congenital analgesia, congenital universal insensitivity to pain) A sporadic or dominantly or recessively inherited congenital syndrome in which pain is perceived as a sensation but one to which there is no emotional response, although subjects can differentiate between hot and cold and between sharp and dull. The sensation of "pain" does not lead to aversion nor to withdrawal from the causative stimuli. Touch sensation, muscle stretch reflexes, the histamine flare response, and light microscopy and EM findings in peripheral nerves are normal. The corneal responses are absent and itching is not perceived. Some affected subjects also manifest developmental delay and multiple fractures. A central origin of the syndrome is presumed.

One prominent patient reported in the nineteenth century styled himself "The Human Pincushion" and exhibited himself in the United States for a fee; his *pièce de (non-) résistance* was his crucifixion on stage, the performance of which, however, had to be terminated prematurely on account of the more acute sensibilities of some of the audience.[1525]

See also **hereditary sensory and autonomic neuropathy** and **pain asymbolia.**

congenital inflammatory myopathy A form of myositis with antenatal or neonatal presentation and clinically resembling **congenital muscular dystrophy**, but associated with microcephaly and intellectual impairment. The serum creatine kinase levels are raised. Muscle biopsy findings include inflammatory infiltrates, muscle fiber damage, and class 1 major histocompatibility complex products in the muscle sarcolemma.[5794]

congenital insensitivity to pain A recessively inherited condition present from birth in which patients have a markedly impaired ability to perceive the type, intensity, and quality of painful stimuli due to abnormal sensory nerve conduction in small-diameter C- and A-λ fibers. There is minimal or no impairment of other sensory modalities or of the muscle stretch reflexes.

Whether the lesion is in the peripheral nervous system (though undetected in some studies) or is a manifestation of a central disorder, remains undetermined; both forms probably occur. Those patients with various forms of **hereditary sensory and autonomic neuropathy** (e.g., types IV and V) also present with loss of pain awareness, but in such cases other modalities are clearly affected as well.[6307]

Variants are *congenital insensitivity to pain with anhidrosis* (see **hereditary sensory and autonomic neuropathy** type IV); and *congenital insensitivity to pain, dominant form,* which is a congenital neuropathic syndrome comprising sclerocornea, hyperactivity, self-mutilation, paroxysmal headache, loss of pain and temperature sensation, paresthesia or hyperesthesia, and flushing.[1263] See also **hereditary sensory and autonomic neuropathy** (recessive and *variant* forms) and **congenital indifference to pain.**

congenital lactic acidosis The result of an inborn error of pyruvate metabolism with numerous phenotypes.

congenital lower motor neuron disease with arthrogryposis See **hereditary motor neuropathy.**

congenital muscle fiber type disproportion An idiopathic neuromuscular disorder which may be the manifestation of a CNS or of a lower motor neuron disorder and which presents with polymorphic features including severe generalized weakness (often involving the respiratory muscles), hypertonia, and a variable outcome.[2408]

congenital muscular dystrophy 1. A heterogeneous group of genetically determined disorders characterized by severe muscle wasting from birth or shortly thereafter. 2. All congenital myopathies, not otherwise specified. 3. (Donner type) Congenital muscle disease manifest by hypotonia, facial and proximal weakness, and often contractures at birth, with biopsy evidence of primary muscle disease. An increased incidence of spinal tumors has been reported but otherwise CNS or retinal lesions are only occasionally associated.[4688, 5436] Diagnostic criteria have been suggested by Fenichel:[2008]

1. Hypotonia, weakness, or arthrogryposis is present at birth. Children who appear normal at birth and develop clinical features of muscle disease during infancy should not be considered to have congenital muscular dystrophy unless there is another family member with a similar disorder whose clinical symptoms *were* present at birth.
2. The muscle biopsy findings should be consistent with myopathy (i.e., spectrum of fiber sizes, degeneration of medium-sized fibers, and fat and collagen replacement of muscle fibers) and should specifically exclude denervation.
3. Other myopathies of the newborn with recognizable clinical or pathological features are excluded.

See also **cerebellar ataxia**

Brooke[869] distinguished five subcategories of congenital muscular dystrophy. The first two account for the large majority of cases:

1. *Undifferentiated type* (Batten–Turner syndrome) The classical (occidental) form is a relatively benign, probably autosomal recessive syndrome consisting of hypotonia, girdle weakness, and motor delay in young children whose muscle biopsy findings suggest a primary myopathy.[6425] No evidence of CNS involvement is apparent. Two subtypes are determined according to the presence or absence of merosin.
   a. *The merosin negative* type shows marked motor disability with normal mentation but white matter lucencies on MRI scans and is mapped to chromosome 6q22–23.
   b. *The merosin positive* type is characterized by reduced fetal

movements in the last trimester of pregnancy, poor sucking, hypotonia, and weakness in post-natal life; delayed developmental milestones with psychomotor impairment; and absence of CNS findings.[3507] Subtypes are described.

2. **Fukuyama type** (congenital muscular dystrophy with CNS involvement; **Walker–Warburg syndrome**) A recessively inherited congenital or infantile form (9q31–33; 9q3, variously ascribed) in which the features of severe muscle dystrophy with joint contractures in infancy and complex malformations of the brain and the eyes are accompanied by marked mental retardation, seizures, and skeletal deformities.[2237] Bulbar weakness, pyramidal signs, cerebral atrophy, hydrocephalus, lissencephaly, polymicrogyria, and heterotopias are also described. Vision is normal. See also **muscle–eye–brain disease.**
3. *Atonic-sclerotic type* (**Ullrich syndrome**) (21q2; 2q3; 3p23, variously ascribed) A congenital muscle dystrophy with proximal joint contractures but with hyperextensibility of the digits, kyphoscoliosis, dysmorphisms, hyperhidrosis, and a tendency to recurrent infections.[6440] Kyphoscoliosis, protruded calcanei, and follicular hyperkeratosis are also associated. There is no intellectual deficit. Complete deficiency of collagen VI has been reported. Three forms are currently recognized.
4. *stick-man type*: A delayed-onset form of congenital muscle dystrophy characterized by atrophy which is disproportionately severe in comparison to the extent of weakness, contractures, and nonrandom distribution of the small muscle fibers.[869, 2427]
5. **rigid spine syndrome**: Forms of muscular dystrophy with marked limitation of flexion of the spine along its length, in association with kyphosis, myopathic limb weakness and contractures, seizures, and mental and developmental delay.[1731] In *variant* forms, the onset is later in life and spinal extensor contractures are notable,[2123] or the syndrome is not linked to 1p.

Kirschner[3454] has provided a recent classification of the congenital muscular dystrophies:

1. CMDs with normal mental development
   A. Primary laminin-2 (*merosin*) deficiency due to mutations in the laminin-α_2 chain (MDC1A). Patients present at or soon after birth with muscular hypotonia, contractures, and respiratory and feeding problems. Facial weakness is often prominent and motor development is markedly delayed, precluding independent ambulation. Most patients develop respiratory insufficiency requiring ventilatory support during the first decade. T2-weighted MRI scans commonly show white matter abnormalities. Electrophysiologically most children show a demyelinating motor neuropathy. The condition maps to 6q2.
   B. Mutations in *FKRP* lead to deficiency of *laminin-2* and can cause an LGMD phenotype, often with pseudohypertrophy of leg and other muscles, evidence of left ventricular dilated cardiomyopathy and neuropathy. One variety is the relatively common *congenital muscular dystrophy 1C* with a wide spectrum of severity. The "typical" form presents with weakness and hypotonia from birth or soon after, with a marked delay of subsequent motor milestones but with normal brain imaging and intelligence and without arthrogryposis. Progressive respiratory muscle weakness leads to ventilatory insufficiency in the first or second decade of life.[4555]
   C. **Ullrich syndrome** (and as above).
   D. Autosomal dominant mutations of collagen VI cause both the milder phenotype of **Bethlem myopathy** and a severe phenotype of Ullrich CMD.[3454]
   E. *CMD with rigid spine* (selenoprotein N-related myopathy) is characterized by early rigidity of the spine and a restrictive respiratory syndrome, often preceded by hypotonia in the first months of life and predominantly axial muscle weakness. Independent ambulation is normally achieved before 18 months of age. It maps to 1p3 mutations of selenoprotein N have described, as also in patients with multiminicore disease.[3454]
2. CMD with abnormal brain development and mental retardation.

Fukuyama CMD, **muscle–eye–brain disease**, and **Walker–Warburg syndrome** are caused by mutations in genes encoding glycosyltransferases and related proteins involved in α-dystroglycan metabolism. Common characteristics include severe muscular dystrophy, neuronal migration defects including **lissencephaly** type II (**cobblestone complex**), **pachygyria**, cerebellar, and brainstem abnormalities, and variable ocular anomalies. Some forms map to 9q31-q33 and involve a mutation of the *fukutin* protein.

Fukuyama CMD is characterized by congenital weakness, profound delay of motor development mostly precluding independent ambulation, and severe mental retardation but the clinical phenotype is heterogeneous. Typical findings on cerebral imaging include abnormal gyral formation, a flattened brainstem, and cerebellar hypoplasia.[3454]

Other *variants* are the following:

Cerebro-ocular dysplasia with muscular dystrophy (**muscle–eye–brain disease**, Santavuori syndrome) A congenital form of muscular dystrophy complicated by glaucoma, optic atrophy, myopia, choroidal hypoplasia, ophthalmoplegia, seizures, mental and developmental delay, and hypodensities in the white matter on CT scans.[5544]

A *severe recessive form* linked to 4p16 with neonatal onset.

Congenital muscle disease with abnormal CT findings which is a congenital form of muscular dystrophy with pyramidal signs, hydrocephalus, and hypodensities in the white matter on CT scans, but normal intelligence.[4688]

Congenital muscular dystrophy with joint hyperlaxity[1758] linked to 3p23–21 and presenting with muscle weakness, proximal contractures, and distal joint hyperlaxity, reported in a French–Canadian kinship.

integrin α7 deficiency A recessive form mapping to 12q13 and characterized by proximal weakness and delayed motor milestones.

CMD with mental retardation and pachygyria mapping to 22q *CNS atrophy and absence of large myelinated peripheral nerve axons* A recessive variant with arthrogryposis, facial dysmorphisms, and psychomotor retardation.[4992]

Congenital muscular dystrophy, with muscle hypertrophy, microcephaly, and mental retardation A recessively inherited form reported from Italy, characterized by the neonatal onset of hypotonia, joint contractures, psychomotor retardation, and diffuse weakness with muscle hypertrophy in the tongue, quadriceps, and calves. Serum CK levels are very high. Muscle biopsy shows dystrophic changes and an enlarged cisterna magna and cerebellar vermis and hemisphere hypoplasia are seen on MRI.[4992]

Congenital muscular dystrophy with severe mental retardation and abnormal glycosylation A recessive syndrome (22q12.3) described once; and characterized by onset in infancy of the typical features of congenital muscular dystrophy, with slow improvement over the first decade, and by moderate muscle hypertrophy of the quadriceps; calves and arm muscles with mainly proximal weakness. Profound mental retardation, mirror movements, and a pyramidal syndrome are also found. Contractures at the ankle and elbow are mild. The serum CK is high and the EMG myopathic. Muscle biopsy shows reduced immunolabeling of *α-dystroglycan*.[4992]

Marinesco–Sjögren syndrome

Forms with desmin inclusions (1p36, SEPN1)[4992]

Congenital muscular dystrophy with familial junctional epidermolysis bullosa A slowly progressive recessive variant (8q24; *plectin*) with congenital onset of proximal, distal, facial, and ocular weakness, hypotonia with skin blistering with trauma and heat. A myasthenic syndrome is also described. Elbow contractures, alopecia, dental caries, laryngeal webs, and brain atrophy with large ventricles are additional features. The serum CK levels are high. Repetitive nerve stimulation shows a decrement and the EMG is myopathic. Muscle biopsy is myopathic, with absent or reduced plectin. Focal desmin deposits are widespread.

Congenital muscular dystrophy with muscle hypertrophy A recessively inherited syndrome (19q13.3, *fukutin-related protein FKRP*), allelic with **LGMD** 2i. The onset is in the first weeks of life with hypotonia, reduced activity, and diffuse weakness, eventually allowing unassisted sitting but preventing ambulation. The calves are hypertrophic but there is girdle wasting and occasionally contractures at the knees, ankles, elbows, and spine. Scoliosis is also described. The serum CK levels are very high and the EMG is myopathic. Muscle biopsy shows variable fiber size, increased connective tissue, and a marked reduction in staining for *α-dystroglycan*.[4992]

CMD variants without identified genetic defects include CMD with mental retardation and isolated cerebellar hypoplasia; CMD and mental retardation with cataracts; CMD and mental retardation with adducted thumbs and ophthalmoplegia; "*Italian muscle–eye–brain disease*" with cerebellar hypoplasia and large cisterna magna; CMD with limb-girdle muscular dystrophy and microcephaly; and CMD/mental retardation with peripheral neuropathy.[4992]

Congenital muscular dystrophy: genes and proteins identified

CMD	Gene location	Protein
CMD (M−)	6q2	Merosin (α2-laminin)
CMD (M−)	–	–
CMD (M+) RSS	1q	–
CMD (M−) RSS	–	–
CMD (M+)	12q13	Integrin
Fukuyama CMD	9q31–q33	Fukutin
Muscle–eye–brain	1q	–
Walker–Warburg	?	–

congenital muscular dystrophy with joint hyperlaxity[1758]

See **Ullrich syndrome** under **congenital muscular dystrophy**.

congenital muscular hypertrophy

Abnormal enlargement of skeletal muscles from birth, with development of normal strength. Hypertrophy is also seen in the **de Lange**, **Debré–Semelaigne**, and other syndromes reviewed by Zellweger.[6965] Such conditions were first described by Bruck in 1889. Linkages to chromosomes 1, 19q13.3, and 1d 22q12.3 have been established.

congenital myasthenia

Inherited disorders in which the safety margin of neuromuscular transmission is compromised by one or more defective proteins in the nerve terminal, the synaptic basal lamina, or in the postsynaptic region of the neuromuscular end-plate. This is a generally benign, heterogeneous group of genetically determined forms of myasthenia gravis, present at birth or during the first 2 years of life in children born to women without myasthenia and manifesting mainly ocular, but also some facial, bulbar, and limb involvement.[4862, 1867] Anti-acetycholine receptor (AchR) antibodies are typically detected. The fatigability results from defects in presynaptic, synaptic basal lamina, or postsynaptic proteins. The presynaptic varieties are due to impairment of the release of acetylcholine quanta or of ACh resynthesis resulting from mutations in choline acetyltransferase. For reviews, see Richman et al. (1994)[5286] and Engel (2003).[1863]

The oculomotor palsies are sometimes incomplete but tend to be symmetrical and they are permanent. While these clinical features are similar to those in the adult form, no anti-AchR antibodies and no evidence of an immunological defect are detected, and the usual therapies with immunosuppressants and plasma exchange are ineffective.[2007] The problem appears to be one of defective acetylcholine synthesis or mobilization[1877] as a result of presynaptic defects that reduce quantal size or alter quantal release or from postsynaptic defects that impair quantal efficiency. At least nine mutations have been shown to be responsible, but in the Western hemisphere it is RAPSN mutations that are found most often.

One *variant* is *congenital myasthenia with facial malformations*, a recessively inherited syndrome described in Iraqi and Iranian Jewish children, characterized by ptosis, face and jaw muscle weakness, and fatigability, responsive to cholinesterase inhibitors and due to a postsynaptic abnormality.[5492] Other *variant* forms include **familial infantile myasthenia, congenital end-plate acetylcholinesterase deficiency, congenital end-plate acetylcholine receptor deficiency**, and **refractory congenital myasthenia.** See **myasthenia gravis.**[1867]

Synaptic basal lamina-associated defects involve end-plate AChE deficiency, while *postsynaptic defects* involve kinetic abnormality of AChR with/without AChR deficiency (**slow- and fast-channel syndromes**), and AChR deficiency with/without minor kinetic abnormality and abnormalities of rapsyn or plectin.[1863]

Clinical syndromes due to *presynaptic* defects are

1. associated with episodic apnea (CMS-EA) caused by defects in choline acetyltransferase (ChAT) with sudden and unexpected episodes of severe dyspnea and bulbar weakness and apnea;
2. with paucity of synaptic vesicles and reduced quantal release;
3. resembling the Lambert–Eaton syndrome;
4. with reduced quantal release due to an undefined mechanism.

Other myasthenic symptoms spare the external ocular muscles but are accompanied by other neurological symptoms such as ataxia or nystagmus.[1863]

Another clinical syndrome associated with the *synaptic basal lamina* is *end-plate acetylcholinesterase deficiency,* caused by the absence of AChE from the synaptic space, usually with neonatal onset and disabling but sometimes presenting in childhood and only disabling in adolescence or later. Features helpful in diagnosis are as follows: 1. a decrementing EMG response; 2. a repetitive CMAP of smaller amplitude and decrements faster than the first CMAP; 3. ineffectiveness of AChE inhibitors for the decrementing response, the repetitive CMAP, or the clinical state; and 4. a slow pupillary light response in some patients. The diagnosis is confirmed by demonstrating the absence of AChE from the end-plate or the presence of pathogenic mutations in *COLQ*.

Clinical syndromes due to *postsynaptic defects* are as follows:

Slow-channel syndromes caused by dominant gain-of-function mutations. The clinical phenotypes vary, with onset at any age from childhood to adult life and any degree of severity, although selective severe involvement of cervical and of wrist and finger extensor muscles is a diagnostic pointer. The cranial muscles tend to be spared but progressive spinal deformities and respiratory embarrassment are common late complications.

Fast-channel mutations presenting with features resembling those of autoimmune myasthenia gravis, again with widely variable severity.

AChR deficiency caused by mutations in AChR subunit genes, AChR deficiency caused by mutations in rapsyn, and congenital myasthenic syndrome associated with plectin deficiency are also described.[1863]

congenital myopathies

Neuromuscular disorders, mostly of childhood but occasionally of adult onset, that occur chiefly in a familial but occasionally in a sporadic fashion. Often of slow progression but exceptionally having a more rapid course, they are marked by disease-specific structural abnormalities in muscle fibers. Their recognition and characterization are a product of modern myopathological techniques, enzyme histochemistry, and electron microscopy.[2424] Members of the group are distinguished by individually characteristic changes on muscle biopsy, although these may overlap.

Clinically, they are characterized by muscle hypotrophy; weakness of the ocular, bulbar, facial, truncal, or limb muscles; and hypotonia, with a resulting delay in motor milestones. The condition is often accompanied by skeletal deformities and contractures. The better-established varieties are listed in Chart C–25

Chart C–25. Varieties of Congenital Myopathy

Actin-related myopathy
Apoptotic changes
Bender-type myopathy
Broad a-band disease
Cardiofacial syndrome
Carey–Fineman–Ziter syndrome
Central core disease
Centronuclear myopathy
Congenital fiber type disproportion
Congenital hypotonia with small type II fibers
Congenital hypotonia with type I fiber predominance
Congenital myopathy with apoptotic changes
Congenital myopathy with caps
Congenital myopathy with intracytoplasmic inclusions
Congenital myopathy with caps
Congenital myopathy with cytoplasmic bodies See **congenital myopathies with intracytoplasmic inclusions**
Congenital myopathy with excess of thin filaments
Congenital myopathy with multifocal degeneration of muscle fibers See **multicore myopathy**
Congenital myopathy with muscle spindle excess
Congenital myopathy with trilaminar muscle fibers
Congenital neuromuscular disease with uniform type I fibers
Cylindrical spirals myopathy
Cytoplasmic body myopathy
Desminopathy (2q35; desmin)
Desmin-related myopathies (2q21, 10q22.3, 12, 15q22)
Distal myopathy with onset in infancy
Fatal infantile myopathy
Fingerprint body myopathy
Granulofilamentous myopathy
Hexagonal tubular arrays
Hyaline body myopathy
Mallory body-like myopathy
Minimal change myopathy See **benign congenital myopathy**[1966]
Multicore myopathy (congenital myopathy with multifocal degeneration of muscle fibers)
Multi-minicore disease
Muscle spindle excess
Myopathy with cylindrical spiral inclusions
Myopathy with focal loss of cross striations and multicores
Myopathy with lysis of myofibrils in type II fibers
Myopathy with tubulomembranous inclusions
Myosin-related myopathy
Myotubular myopathy
Nemaline (rod) myopathy
Neonatal perifascicular myopathy
Reducing body myopathy
Sarcoplasmic body myopathy
Sarcotubular myopathy
Spheroid body myopathy

Trilaminar myopathy A syndrome with neonatal onset characterized by hypertonia and contractures with high serum CK and with a trilaminar appearance in muscle fibers stained with NADH (showing dark inner and outer zones) and with ATPase (showing pale inner and outer zones), reported in one sporadic case.

Tubular aggregate myopathy
Tubulin-reactive crystalline inclusions 2
Tubulofilamentous tubular aggregates
X-linked myotubular myopathies
Zebra body myopathy

and at www.neuro.wustl.edu/neuromuscular/maltbrain.html.

congenital myopathy with apoptotic changes Congenital generalized hypotonia, atrophy, and delayed psychomotor development. Muscle biopsy shows small and Bax-positive (pro-apoptotic) muscle fibers.[4992]

congenital myopathy with caps (9p13, *β-tropomyosin 2* [*TPM2*]) A dominantly inherited congenital syndrome characterized by hypotonia, slowly progressive proximal, distal, facial, and respiratory weakness, and Marfanoid features, leading to death in youth. The EMG is myopathic and muscle biopsy shows caps on the ends of muscle fibers staining dark on Gomori trichrome. A *variant* recessive form is also described.[1073]

congenital myopathy with excess of thin filaments A sporadic congenital syndrome (1q42, α-actin; *ACTA1*) presenting with hypotonia, respiratory insufficiency, and cardiomyopathy, sometimes leading to early death. The serum CK levels are normal. Muscle biopsy shows masses of thin actin filaments. See also **congenital fiber type size disproportion** and **rod myopathy.**

congenital myopathy with fatal dilated cardiomyopathy A recessive form (2q24) due to *titin* mutations and characterized by early onset of hypotonia, proximal more than distal weakness and delayed motor milestones, cardiomyopathy supervening a few years later. It is allelic with *Finnish distal myopathy*, *dilated cardiomyopathy 1G*, and **limb girdle muscular dystrophy** 2J.[4992]

congenital myopathy with intracytoplasmic inclusions (congenital myopathy with cytoplasmic bodies) Rare syndromes conforming to the usually benign clinical features of the congenital myopathies, with facial, proximal, and distal myopathic weakness, dysphagia and feeding problems in infants, joint contractures and laxity, chorea, and athetosis, but in which electron microscopy demonstrates characteristic inclusions such as **zebra bodies**, **fingerprint bodies**, and cytoplasmic bodies. See **zebra body myopathy**, **fingerprint inclusion myopathy**, and **cytoplasmic body myopathy.**

The diagnosis of such conditions is solely within the purview of the electron microscopist; the functional and pathological significance of the findings are unknown.[1966] See also **neuromyopathy.**

congenital myopathy with multifocal degeneration of muscle fibers See **multicore myopathy.**

congenital myopathy with muscle spindle excess A single case of congenital hypotonia and arthrogryposis with diffuse weakness, areflexia, and respiratory and cardiac failure. Muscle biopsy shows atrophic muscle fibers and an excessive number of muscle spindles, especially in the deltoid and quadriceps.[4992]

congenital myopathy with trilaminar muscle fibers A congenital myopathy of unknown cause characterized by muscle rigidity, reduced spontaneous movements, raised serum creatine kinase levels, and the presence of muscle fibers with three concentric zones (trilaminar fibers). EMG and nerve conduction studies are normal.[5314]

congenital myophosphorylase deficiency See **glycogen storage diseases.**

congenital neuro-ectodermal dysplasia See **Sturge–Weber syndrome, phakomatoses.**

congenital neuromuscular disease with uniform type I fibers An inherited myopathy characterized by congenital facial, proximal, and distal limb myopathic weakness and changes in muscle biopsy specimens, as suggested by the title.[4762] The condition is likely to be allellic with central core disease.

congenital neuropathy with absence of myelin in PNS A rare, fatal disease of infants characterized by hypotonia, areflexia, minimal residual motor activity, and absence of developmental reflexes. Myelin is almost completely absent from the CNS and there is no myelin on the axons in the peripheral motor or sensory nerves.[4866]

congenital nonprogressive external ophthalmoplegia A rare syndrome of dominantly inherited III, IV, and VI cranial nerve pareses.[3993]

congenital nuclear agenesis/aplasia See **Möbius syndrome.**

congenital nystagmus (fixation nystagmus, hereditary nystagmus) A form of rhythmic pendular and/or jerk nystagmus which is usually detectable shortly after birth. It is usually horizontal, symmetrical in the two eyes, reduced by convergence, but increased by attempts at fixation and abolished in sleep. Horizontal nystagmus on upward gaze is a typical finding. The frequency and amplitude vary in different directions of gaze and there is a **null point**. In most cases, the slow phase has an increasing velocity. The patient's visual acuity is usually decreased and this may have pathogenetic importance. **Oscillopsia** is absent,[2703] but oscillation of the head is usual. It can occur idiopathically or in association with, for example, albinism, congenital cataracts, and optic nerve disease.

The nystagmus later evolves into a smaller-amplitude, lower-frequency pendular waveform, the latter itself sometimes changing to a jerky waveform before 18 months of age. The eye movements are commonly in the horizontal plane, but vertical forms are also described.[1561].

The differentiation from nystagmus acquired in infancy is difficult but may be made when pendular nystagmus occurs in the presence of evidence of visual impairment affecting the central part of the field. The several complex waveforms in this condition have been analyzed and reviewed.[1564, 6910,26]

congenital oculo-bulbar palsy Selective nonprogressive weakness of the ocular and bulbar muscles with onset before the age of 2 years, accompanied by subclinical myopathic weakness of trunk and limb muscles, not due to myasthenia, giant axonal neuropathy, or **Fazio–Londe disease.**[3201]

congenital oculo-facial paresis See **Möbius syndrome.**

congenital oculo-motor apraxia See **Cogan syndrome (definition 1).**

congenital oculoskeletal myopathy with abnormal muscle and liver mitochondria See **mitochondrial neurogastrointestinal encephalomyopathy** (MNGIE).

congenital ophthalmoplegia A very rare autosomal recessive or X-linked disorder characterized by progressive congenital ophthalmoplegia (without mitochondrial cytopathy seen in a biopsy specimen), myopia, pigmentary retinopathy, pituitary insufficiency, small stature, and muscular hypotonia.[5171]

congenital opioid syndrome A neonatal abstinence syndrome occurring in over half of the babies born to opioid-dependent women. It may not present until 3–5 days after the mother's last use of the drug. Neurologic signs occur in over 70% of cases and include excessive high-pitched or continuous crying, insomnia, tremors, hypertonia, myoclonus, or generalized tonic-clonic seizures. Respiratory and gastrointestinal symptoms and signs include sweating, severe, frequent yawning, mottled skin, nasal stuffiness with sneezing and excessive sucking, poor feeding, regurgitation or projectile vomiting, and diarrhea.

congenital optic atrophy (Thompson syndrome) See **Behr disease**.

congenital pain asymbolia Perception of sensations which would normally be expected to be painful but to which there is indifference on the part of the subject. The condition may be associated with other evidences of higher cortical dysfunction such as auditory imperception and personality disorder, but reports of minor changes on peripheral nerve biopsy and in autonomic tests in some reported cases suggest the possibility of a basis in peripheral neuropathy.

A variant is *pain asymbolia with auditory imperception*, a congenital syndrome characterized by speech delay and pain agnosia.[381] See also **hereditary sensory and autonomic neuropathy** and **congenital insensitivity to pain.**

congenital pain asymbolia with auditory imperception See **hereditary sensory and autonomic neuropathy (other)**.

congenital paramyotonia See **Eulenberg disease**.

congenital persistent myasthenia See **myasthenia gravis**.

congenital Pick cell encephalopathy A congenital neuronal inclusion disease manifesting amentia, joint contractures, respiratory distress, hypotonia, paroxysmal EEG discharges, and diffuse gliosis.[381]

congenital progressive oculo-acoustico-cerebral degeneration See **Norrie disease**.

congenital ptosis A syndrome of isolated ptosis, usually unilateral and accompanied in some cases by impairment of upward movement of the eye and due to abnormal differentiation of the levator palpebrae and/or superior rectus muscles.[658] Type I (1p32) is a dominant syndrome of symmetric or asymmetric ptosis with normal eye movements. Type II (Xq24) is an X-linked dominant syndrome of bilateral symmetrical congenital ptosis, again with normal eye movements, seen in both sexes.

congenital pure word deafness See **Worster-Drought–Allen syndrome**.

congenital rod disease See **nemaline myopathy**. The finding of rods is by itself nonspecific, as they may also be secondary to denervation.

congenital rubella embryopathy (Gregg syndrome) A syndrome consequent upon fetal infection with the rubella virus, and (in infants born alive) characterized by low birth weight, short stature, sensorineural deafness, glaucoma, microphthalmia, iris abnormalities, cataract, coarctation of the aorta, patent ductus arteriosus, hepatosplenomegaly, purpura, neonatal jaundice, microcephaly, pleocytosis in the CSF, wide anterior fontanelle and metopic sutures, mental and developmental delay, and high levels of specific rubella IgM antibodies in the blood at birth and of any rubella antibody after the age of 1 year.[1613]

congenital sensory neuropathies See **hereditary sensory and autonomic neuropathy, type II.**

congenital sensory neuropathy with selective loss of small myelinated fibers See **hereditary sensory and autonomic neuropathy.**

congenital spastic (di-) paraparesis See **Little disease**.

congenital stiff man syndrome A dominantly inherited syndrome of continuous motor neuron discharges arising in the CNS.[3476] See **startle epilepsy.**

congenital suprabulbar paresis A dominantly inherited congenital or childhood dysmorphic syndrome characterized by seizures, microcephaly, pyramidal signs, dysarthria, facial and bulbar weakness, and mental and developmental delay, sometimes complicated by deafness, seizures, and mental retardation.[379] See **Worster-Drought syndrome.**

congenital syphilis Infection *in utero* from the mother, leading to skin rash resembling that of secondary syphilis in the adult; rhinitis; osteochondritis and periostitis; and chronic meningitis. Manifestations appearing later in life include interstitial keratitis, gummas, Hutchinson teeth, mulberry molars, and numerous other neurological disturbances including vestibular dysfunction, nerve deafness, and further cortical atrophy.

congenital syphilitic paralysis See **Dennie–Marfan syndrome.**

congenital tilted disk syndrome See **tilted disks.**

congenital toxoplasmosis (chronic congenital toxoplasmosis with late degeneration) Infection by *Toxoplasma gondii*, an intracellular protozoan organism existing worldwide. Transplacental transmission may follow acute infection of the mother during pregnancy, leading to the classic triad of hydrocephalus, intracranial calcification, and chorio-retinitis, often accompanied by microcephaly or hydrocephalus in newborn infants.[122, 1791] The titer of anti-toxoplasma IgM antibodies is elevated.

In the *acquired form*, infection occurs after ingestion of cysts in undercooked meat or from contamination of food by the feces of cats.

congenital trigeminal anesthesia Unilateral or bilateral loss of sensation over the face, present from birth. When bilateral, this may be the only problem or focal brainstem signs may be associated; the cause in such cases is assumed to be primary neural hypoplasia. In a second group, congenital mesenchymal anomalies, such as oculoauriculovertebral dysplasia, are also present.[5402]

congenital tritan defects Inherited disorders of color vision characterized by normal distant and near vision, normal visual fields, normal appearing optic nerves, and tritanopia.[3565]

congenital unilateral lower lip palsy A syndrome of lower quadrant facial weakness occurring in infants who also have congenital heart disease. See **cardiofacial syndrome** and **asymmetric crying facies.**

congenital universal muscle hypoplasia A rare nonprogressive disorder characterized by generalized smallness of muscles from birth without histological evidence of inflammation or myopathy. Clinically, poor power and gait control, hyporeflexia, and easy tiring are the major findings.[3551]

congenital varicella A static **embryopathy** associated with infections of the mother with the varicella virus and characterized clinically by hypoplasia of the limbs, skin lesions, and cerebral atrophy.[836]

congenital webbed neck See **Klippel–Feil anomaly.**

congenital weakness with diarrhea and deafness A recessively inherited syndrome of congenital weakness and hypotonia at birth with feeding difficulties, myopathic facies, joint contractures, episodic diarrhea with infections, bullous skin eruptions, sensorineural deafness, and microcephaly, improving with age.[4992]

congenital word blindness (developmental dyslexia) A form of pure visual receptive dysphasia occurring as a developmental defect in the region of the left angular gyrus. Visual agnosia for objects is likely to be present as well. The term was coined in 1895 by James Hinshelwood, a Scottish ophthalmologist. See **alexia.**

congenital word deafness See **congenital auditory imperception** and **developmental dysphasia.**

congenital X-linked ataxia See **cerebellar ataxia.**

congestive brain swelling An increase in the volume of the brain as a result of an increase in the cerebral blood volume.

congophilic angiopathy (primary cerebrovascular amyloidosis, familial presenile dementia with spastic paralysis; precocious, juvenile, or atypical Alzheimer disease) A dominantly inherited form of amyloidosis confined to the cerebral blood vessels, characterized pathologically by multiple hemorrhages and softenings in the brain and abundant amyloid-containing plaques, mainly in the hippocampus and cerebellar cortex.

Clinically, the disease appears in adult life as a syndrome consisting of progressive dementia with ataxic dysarthria, spastic paralyses, and frequently multiple lobar intracerebral hemorrhages. The differentiation from **Alzheimer disease** can thus be made clinically, and the histological appearance of the amyloid-containing plaques is also different, although there are definite pathological similarities between the two conditions.[2579] See also **cerebral amyloid angiopathy.**

Congress of Neurological Surgeons A professional organization based at the University of Southern California. Web site: www.neurosurgeon.org/index.asp.

congruence (congruity) Uniformity of the visual field defect in the two eyes in cases of hemianopia. The more congruent the defects, the more posterior the responsible lesion.

congruity See **congruence.**

coning The downward descent of the medulla and cerebellar tonsils into the foramen magnum as a result of increasing intracranial pressure. The occurrence of coning is a sign of impending catastrophe, the brainstem and its blood supply being compressed and distorted which may lead eventually to ischemic necrosis.

conjugate eye deviation (Prévost sign) The lateral deviation of the two eyes in parallel, typically toward the side of a hemispheric stroke but away from the side of a stroke affecting the brainstem. The sign was first noted by Prévost in 1865. The lesion can occur at various sites in the circuit between the inferior parietal lobule and the frontal eye fields, and their projections to the superior colliculus or the paramedian pontine reticular formation.[6320]

conjugate gaze (Lat, yoked together) The harnessing of the two eyes so that they normally move with their axes parallel (except during convergence).

conjugate gaze palsy An inability to turn the eyes past the midline using any mechanism (saccadic, pursuit, optokinetic, or vestibular).

conjugate movements A term generally employed to describe the normal yoking together of the eyes in their movements so that the parallelism of the ocular axes is maintained. The same concept is relevant in regard to the front wheels of steered vehicles.

conjunctival reflex Blinking in response to conjunctival stimulation; a normal phenomenon.

Conn syndrome (primary aldosteronism) Excessive secretion of aldosterone by an adenoma or carcinoma or by a hyperplastic adrenal cortex. Hypertension and resultant stroke, hypokalemic myopathy, tetany, and polyuria and polydipsia are the features most likely to bring the patient to a neurologist.

connectivity The pattern of interconnection between specific cortical areas. The term can be used anatomically or functionally, or within the context of artificial intelligence.

Conradi–Hünermann syndrome (multiple epiphyseal dysplasia, chondrodystrophia calcificans punctata congenita, Conradi–Raap disease) A dominant, sex-linked or recessive condition characterized by facial dysmorphism; short neck, trunk, and limbs; mental deficiency; kyphoscoliosis due to asymmetry of the vertebral bodies; and craniosynostosis.

Alopecia, dry skin, muscle fibrosis, hypoplasia of the bones of the hands and feet, cataracts, rhizomelia of limbs with asymmetry, joint stiffness, paraplegia, and other systemic abnormalities may also be found.[1271]

In a *variant* congenital form, microcephaly, nystagmus, and mental and developmental delay are the major neurological manifestations.

Conradi–Raap disease See **Conradi–Hüunermann syndrome.**

conscious level The vigilance of an individual; the ability to perceive, attend to, memorize, and react to events in the internal and external environments.

consciousness 1. The awareness of being aware. The same neurological mechanisms which support this function also allow awareness of the self and the environment, as well as attention, perception, cognitive functions, motor decisions, and responsiveness. 2. The perception of what passes in a man's own mind (John Locke, 1690). 3. "Consciousness is not something which we can define in terms of anything else; we can only indicate its meaning denotatively, that is by pointing to instances of it . . . There is no such thing as consciousness apart from conscious states any more than there is a redness apart from red objects" (Lord Brain).

Yet if a thing exists, surely it is definable; since it appears undefinable to some, they have denied the concept or relegated it to the status of a semantic artifact or an epiphenomenon. The philosophical difficulties of the subject have been reviewed by Gloor.[2409]

consecutive (Lat, following after) Following in order.

consecutive optic atrophy 1. To ophthalmologists, optic atrophy occurring first in one and later in the other eye. 2. To neurologists, optic atrophy succeeding prior papilledema. 3. To other ophthalmologists and neurologists, optic atrophy following upon retinal or choroidal diseases.

consensual reflex The occurrence of a bilateral reflex response in response to a unilateral stimulus, as when both pupils constrict in response to the stimulation of one eye only. This response was first remarked upon by **Whytt**. When only one pupil is illuminated but the other one does not contract equally, a *consensual deficit* is said to exist.

Consortium of Multiple Sclerosis Centers A professional organization. Web site: www.mscare.org/.

Consortium to Establish a Registry for Alzheimer Disease (CERAD) A group of American workers combining in their aim to develop, standardize, and test the reliability of a brief clinical and neuropsychological assessment schedule for patients with **Alzheimer disease.**[4498, 4499]

constant pain caused by compression, irritation, or distortion of cranial nerves or upper cervical roots by structural lesions See **cervicogenic headaches.**

constructional apraxia A failure of visuoconstructive ability such that the subject is unable to assemble component parts into a coherent whole.[3540] This results in impairment of the ability to construct the copy of a visually presented model by means of assembling objects or drawing, normal visual acuity, and perception of the number and relationship of the items to be copied; and normal gross motor abilities are assumed. *Apractagnosia* was the term preferred by **Lord Brain** because of the visual perceptive disorder so often associated.

Despite the name (suggested by Kleist in 1923[4339] and more fully described by Mayer-Gross[4190]), the deficit is not truly an apraxia. Lesions of either parietal lobe may be responsible. See also **apraxia.**

contact point headache Head pains considered by some to be caused by contact between the nasal septum and the lateral nasal wall by referred pain involving the trigeminal nerve. This headache/facial pain syndrome results, it is suggested, from nasal septal spurs or other intranasal pathologies (not including chronic sinusitis) or abnormalities of the turbinates that cause "mucosal contacts." Criteria for the diagnosis of this very uncertain syndrome have been suggested.[6359] It may be remarked that the symptoms are identical with those of migraine without aura.

Criteria for the diagnosis of contact point headaches (adapted from ***Tosun,*** *2000)*[6359]

1. History of chronic headache
2. Lack of acute or chronic inflammatory findings on the ENT examination (clinical, X-ray, and CT)
3. Absence of any other cause of headache after a thorough evaluation by a neurologist, ophthalmologist, dentist, internist, and any other related specialist
4. Presence of contact points documented by nasal endoscopy, CT, or both
5. Failure of medical therapy for headaches (not further defined)
6. Relief of headache after applying topical anesthesia to the contact points
7. Contact points that still remain after mucosal decongestion

Contemporary Neurology Series A neurological review book series, published by Oxford University Press.

continence 1. The physiological capacity to maintain voluntary closure of the urinary or anal sphincter until evacuation of the contents of the bladder or bowel is appropriate. 2. Restriction of sexual activity to one partner.

contingent negative variation An event-related slow negative potential recorded best in the frontal regions of alert subjects during the 1 s interval between a warning stimulus and a response stimulus, the subject having been primed to make a decision concerning his motor response to the second signal.[6629]

continuous motor neuron discharges A dominantly inherited syndrome characterized by continuous motor neuron discharges with persistent twitching and episodic stiffness, mainly in the legs. It occurs first in early childhood and remits to some extent in adult life. The discharges disappear during spinal anesthesia, suggesting their generation from the proximal portion of the motor unit.[271]

Other conditions in which such continuous motor unit discharges occur may be classified as follows:

1. Central origin.
   congenital stiff man syndrome
2. Peripheral origin
   a. Without overt peripheral neuropathy
      Schwartz–Jampel syndrome[5680]
      hereditary myokymia[294]
      hereditary myokymia with episodic ataxia[6492]
      hereditary persistent distal cramps
      Associated with gold therapy; intrathoracic malignancy, or **idiopathic neuromyotonia.**
   b. With overt peripheral neuropathy
      hereditary neuromyotonia[4327]
      Sporadic; **Isaacs syndrome**; associated with exposure to toxins, with inflammatory neuropathy, or with intrathoracic malignancy
   c. Tetany
   d. Following plexus irradiation[271, 294]

continuous motor unit activity See **neuromyotonia.**

continuous muscle fiber activity See **neuromyotonia.**

continuous performance test A test of concentration span and vigilance, wherein the subject identifies a specific recurring letter randomly presented with others over a 10 min period.[5424]

continuous-wave Doppler sonography An early technique used in the diagnosis of carotid artery disease, in which a continuous-wave Doppler probe traverses the line of the carotid arteries; a shift in the Doppler frequency indicates the presence of severe stenosis.[4678]

contraction (from Lat, shorten or draw together) 1. (muscular) The reversible shortening of the distance between the origin and insertion of a muscle as a result of electrical excitation. A voluntary or involuntary reversible muscle shortening that may or may not be accompanied by action potentials from muscle. (From the 2001 Report of the Nomenclature Committee of the American Association of Electromyography and Electrodiagnosis.[19] Reproduced by kind permission of the AANEM.) cf. **contracture.** 2. (visual field) Absolute loss of the visual field, usually peripherally, such that no stimuli are seen in the affected area.

contraction fasciculation Clinical term for visible twitching of a muscle with weak voluntary or postural contraction which has the appearance of a fasciculation. More likely to occur in neuromuscular disorders in which the motor unit territory is enlarged and the tissue covering the muscle is thin, but may also be observed in normal individuals. (From the 2001 Report of the Nomenclature Committee of the American Association of Electromyography and Electrodiagnosis.[19] Reproduced by kind permission of the AANEM.)

The term is employed to refer to the repetitive twitching of the chin with pursing of the lips seen in **bulbospinal muscular atrophy** (neuronopathy), in which they are due to grouped motor discharges, activated by voluntary muscle contraction in some but not all cases.[4788]

contracture 1. Immobility of a joint due to fixed muscle shortening. 2. An electrically silent, involuntary state of semipermanent shortening of the distance between the origin and insertion of a muscle as a result of disease. 3. Fixed resistance to stretch of a shortened muscle due to fibrous connective tissue changes and loss of sarcomeres in the muscle. Limited movement of a joint may be due to muscle contracture or to fibrous connective tissue changes in the joint. Contrast with **contraction**, which is a rapidly reversible painless shortening of the muscle. 4. The prolonged, painful, electrically silent, involuntary state of temporary muscle shortening seen in some myopathies (e.g., muscle phosphorylase deficiency). (From the 2001 Report of the Nomenclature Committee of the American Association of Electromyography and Electrodiagnosis.[19] Reproduced by kind permission of the AANEM.) See also **cramp.**

contractures, muscle atrophy, and ocular lesions syndrome See **Cogan syndrome.**

contracturing granulomatous myositis A chronic granulomatous disease of muscles without systemic involvement, presenting in adult life with progressive flexion contractures of the limbs. The condition is thought to differ from **idiopathic granulomatous myositis** and sarcoidosis, mainly on the basis of the clinical features of lack of pain and the absence of systemic involvement.[5844]

contralateral abdominal proprioceptive reflex See **Tramer reflex.**

contralaterality The phenomenon of the clinical expression of a motor or sensory function (or functional deficit) on the side of the body opposite to that on which the responsible brain area is situated.

contrapulsion A disorder of saccadic eye movements due to lesions of the superior cerebellar peduncle and characterized by hypermetric horizontal saccades away from the side of the lesion, hypometric ipsilateral saccades, and diagonal movements of the globes with attempted vertical saccades.[5180] See also **saccadic lateropulsion.**

contrary movement A distortion of a normal willed movement seen characteristically in **athetosis**, whereby it begins with contraction of the antagonistic muscles.[2142]

contrast 1. A chemical substance given to a subject in order to enhance the visualization of certain structures during radiological imaging procedures such as myelograms or arteriograms, or during MRI. Water-soluble iodine-containing compounds are usually used in the former case and gadolinium in the latter. 2. (visual physiology) A change in brightness across space.

contraversive pushing (pusher syndrome) A phenomenon seen in some patients after stroke, who actively push away from the unaffected side, leading to lateral postural imbalance and a tendency to fall toward the paralyzed side as a result of an altered perception of the body's orientation in respect to gravity. It is seen in association with a lesion of the postero-lateral thalamus and the supra-thalamic white matter and is due to a disturbed perception of body posture in relation to gravity.

This usually follows a stroke, causing severe paresis of the contralateral arm and leg. The contraversive tilt of spontaneous posture occurs while sitting or standing, with abduction and extension of the nonparetic limbs, bringing about a pathological lateral tilt of the body axis. Subjects also resist passive correction of their tilted posture when the examiner attempts to move them to an upright position.[3307, 3306]

contrecoup injury (Fr, against + a blow) Contusion or laceration of the brain on the side opposite to that struck, as a result of the delay in deceleration of the brain after it is impelled away from the site of injury. The frontal and temporal poles are most commonly affected. The phenomenon was well known to the ancient Greeks.

Controlled Word Association Test A measure of semantic information in which the subject is asked to name as many words beginning with "F" as possible in 1 min. The same is asked for the letters "A" and "S" thereafter.[530]

controller signal A mechanism whereby signals from the nervous system cause a change of state of part of the effector mechanisms of the body and reset the system so that the new state is maintained. See **pulse-step control**.

contusion (Lat, a bruise) Physically inflicted injury to an organ without breach of its surface.

contusion index A semiquantitative account of the number and site of the lesions resulting from cerebral contusions.[6]

conus medullaris (Lat, a cone + marrow) The inferior tip of the spinal cord, comprising the last few sacral segments sited opposite the first lumbar vertebra.

conus medullaris syndrome The signs resulting from lesions of the lower three sacral and the coccygeal segment of the spinal cord, as by compression from local masses or resulting from infiltration.

These consist of **saddle anesthesia** and **dissociated anesthesia** in the appropriate dermatomal areas, loss of sphincter functions with urinary and fecal incontinence, impotence, wasting and flaccid paresis of the (few) muscles innervated by S3, -4, and -5, and pain in the back and perineum. The syndrome was first described by Roussy and Lhermitte in 1918.[5440]

See also **cauda equina syndrome**. It must be noted that lesions seldom affect the nervous system in this nicely classified manner, so that the features of both of these syndromes often occur together.

convergence 1. The termination of different axons upon the same postsynaptic membrane, allowing integration of activities to occur at synapses. 2. The turning inward of the eyes when focusing on an object brought near to the face; the only physiological situation in which the axes of the eyes are not parallel. This complex function, consisting of pupillary constriction, accommodation, and adduction of both eyes, can be disturbed by various neurological disorders, especially those affecting the dorsal midbrain in the tectal region.[3762]

convergence-evoked nystagmus Unusual forms of nystagmus in which the variable (up- or downbeating) abnormal movements are provoked by convergent gaze. Some cases are congenital; in others, the causative lesion (such as a multiple sclerosis plaque) is thought to be in the brainstem.[5765]

convergence insufficiency Impairment of fusional convergence, the near point of which is abnormally distant, in the presence of exophoria at near distances. The near point of accommodation, however, is typically normal.[2400]

convergence nystagmus See **convergence-retraction nystagmus**.

convergence paralysis An abnormality of the accommodation-vergence system such that there is impairment in adduction of the eyes at near gaze. This may be congenital or the result of **progressive supranuclear palsy** or **Parkinson disease**. See also **convergence insufficiency**.

convergence-retraction nystagmus (convergence nystagmus, nystagmus retractorius) Simultaneous contraction of all the extraocular muscles on attempted upward gaze or with a downward-moving optokinetic stimulus, leading to retraction of the eyes into the orbit and to nasal deviation of each eye, and due to the cocontraction of the agonist and antagonist extraocular muscles. The condition thus is not really nystagmus at all but rather an unusual form of saccadic movement.

The presence of the sign indicates a lesion in the pretectal regions of the midbrain; it comprises a part of the **dorsal midbrain-Sylvian aqueduct syndrome** in which condition it accompanies paresis of upward gaze.[5765, 5731]

convergence spasm Slow, persisting convergence movements of the eyes giving an appearance of VI nerve palsy or of gaze paresis, but voluntary in nature and accompanied by miosis and often facial grimacing and complaints of blurred vision and ocular pain. Pupillary constriction occurs when the patient attempts to look laterally, but full abduction is seen with the oculocephalic reflex.[1224]

The range of movement of each eye alone is normal when the other is occluded, which with the above features allows the diagnosis of functional eye disease.[3355] See **spasm of the near reflex**.

converse ocular bobbing See **slow-upward ocular bobbing**.

conversion The mental mechanism whereby the anxiety or conflict experienced is transformed into a physical manifestation. The nature, rationale, and purpose of such a mechanism is not hereby explained.

conversion disorder (somatoform or functional disorder, hysteria, dissociative or medically unexplained disorder) A relatively persistent loss or distortion of the regulation of affect and symbolization, not fully explained by structural or biochemical disease or pathophysiological mechanisms, with evidence for linkage of the symptoms to psychological factors whereby somatic experiences and complaints represent and convey emotional distress. In many cases assumption of the "sick role" occurs in the absence of diagnosed bodily disease (although this often comes to light eventually). A history of physical or sexual abuse in childhood is often present in such patients. The presentation with neurological symptoms of any kind is unaccompanied by physical signs.[6073]

The presence of other evidence of somatization disorder, of associated psychopathology, of a model for the symptom, and of evidence of past emotional stress may increase clinical confidence in the diagnosis, but there is almost always a need for neurological investigation in such patients, as judged by follow-up studies of eventual morbidity.[3728] See also **hysteria; somatization disorder, left-sided syndrome,** and **Hoover sign.**

convexity block Obstruction of CSF circulation due to failure of flow over the convexities of the hemisphere, considered to be due to adherence of the pial and arachnoid membranes, especially over the parietal lobes.

convolutions (from Lat, to roll together) Infolding of the surface of the cerebral cortex, causing a marked increase in its surface area. Their presence was known to the ancient Egyptians who considered that their greater complexity in humans than in animals reflected our greater intelligence, but this insight was lost thereafter and Galen denied that they had any function. They were drawn by **Leonardo da Vinci** and others to resemble the coils of the intestines.

convulsion (from Lat, to tear) 1. Violent agitation of the limbs, face, and trunk with intermittent, involuntary muscle contractions, usually as a result of epilepsy. 2. Episodes of excessive, abnormal, and involuntary muscle contractions which may be sustained or interrupted and which may be epileptic or nonepileptic in origin.

convulsive movements of the stump See **stump spasm.**

convulsive syncope Convulsive movements (usually tonic extensor spasms) occurring as components of **syncope** in susceptible individuals, due to the global cerebral hypoperfusion and resulting cerebral ischemia induced by the hypotension.[3848] See **Adams–Stokes–Morgagni syndrome.**

convulsive tonic-clonic status epilepticus See **status epilepticus.**

convulsive tremor See **paramyoclonus multiplex.**

Cooke, John (1756–1838) English physician who trained at Guy's Hospital in London and in Edinburgh and Leyden, later becoming physician to the London Hospital. His 920-page *Treatise on Nervous Disorders* (1820–1823, thus preceding **Romberg**) was the first book on neurology, although his insights were not really much of an advance on Galen. In it he remarked that the physiology of the nervous system "remains involved in impenetrable obscurity," a remark still likely to resonate with beginning medical students. This was, however, an important early attempt to provide a full description of diseases of the nervous system, although its three parts dealt only with the clinical aspects of **apoplexy**, palsy, and **epilepsy**.

Cooper, Sir Astley (1768–1841) English surgeon at Guy's Hospital who first ligated the carotid artery for the treatment of aneurysm, in 1805.

coonhound paralysis A demyelinating disease of dogs, resembling acute inflammatory demyelinating polyradiculoneuropathy.

coordination (Lat, with + order) The smooth patterning of voluntary movements. "It will not suffice to speak of coordination as a separate faculty, co-ordination is the function of the whole and of every part of the nervous system." "Half of the symptomatology of disorders of co-ordination is paralysis (i.e., loss of function) owing to that negative central lesion. But the other half is from forcing of other movements by overactivity of perfectly healthy nervous arrangements. The two elements, negative and positive, constitute the disorder of coordination" (**Hughlings-Jackson**, 1870, 1888).

Tests of coordination in the arms include the finger-nose test, rapid alternating movements of the fingers, pronation–supination of the forearms, repetitive hand patting tests, handwriting, and serial approximation of fingers to thumbs. Fisher describes an improvement, in which the patient taps the tip of the flexed index finger against the distal knuckle of the thumb.[2079] In the legs, the heel-knee test with Fisher's modification (tapping the knee with the heel of the other leg before running the heel down the length of its shin) is the only test in common usage.[2080]

cop-1 A random polymer simulating myelin basic protein, able to enhance the production of antigen-specific suppressor T cells and thus used in the treatment of **multiple sclerosis.**

coping The varying cognitive and behavioral attempts to manage those internal or external demands that strain an individual's resources.

coprolalia (Gr, filth or dung + speech) The compulsive uttering of obscene words, commonly but not exclusively as a complex vocal tic in **Tourette syndrome.**

Copper and Menkes Disease A Web site providing an explanation of the biochemical and genetic causes of this disease, found at www.research.deakin.edu.au/performance/pubs/reports/cd/1998/stories/story15.htm/.

copper deficiency myeloneuropathy (hypocupremic myelopathy) A syndrome of gait disturbance due to sensory ataxia from dorsal column dysfunction, with spasticity of the legs and polyneuropathy, thus resembling the presentation of **subacute combined degeneration of the cord**. Optic neuropathy is also recorded. Investigation shows low levels of ceruloplasmin and high serum zinc levels in those patients who have taken this metal as a supplement, precipitating the syndrome.[5441, 3597]

In a benign form of copper deficiency, seizures may occur but ceruloplasmin levels are normal. Low copper levels are also found in **Menkes syndrome, Wilson disease, ceruloplasmin deficiency,** and **Ehlers–Danlos syndrome.**

coprolaliopraxia See **signing tics.**

coprophemonena Motor activities which directly or indirectly are reminiscent of fecal functions or other unclassified filth. They include **coprolalia, copropraxia,** and **mental coprolalia**, all of which are motor or phonic tics or their substitutes, and occur in **Tourette syndrome.**

coproporphyria A dominantly inherited form of porphyria in which the excretion of coproporphyrins is greatly increased. The condition is characterized clinically by the onset in childhood of hirsutism, skin photosensitivity with the formation of bullae or vesicles, depression, sleep disorders, complex partial seizures, cerebellar signs, sensorimotor axonal peripheral neuropathy (which may be acute), and abnormal urinary color on standing.[5370, 1322]

copropraxia Obscene gesturing as a form of motor tic in **Tourette syndrome**.

Copy a Cross Test A test of visuospatial and constructional abilities in which the subject is asked to copy a line drawing of a Greek cross.[2474] Inability to do so appropriately suggests impairment of visuospatial functions.

CoQ deficiency A mitochondriopathy presenting with mental retardation and myopathy.

cor anglais players thumb An overuse syndrome or focal dystonia affecting the first digit.

cord bladder See **automatic bladder**.

cord sign The CT appearance of a clot in a dural venous sinus or a cortical vein, the thrombosed vein highlighting within an extra axial fluid collection.[5189] See also **dense triangle sign** and **empty delta sign**.

cordotomy (myelotomy) Incision of the anterolateral or central parts of the spinal cord in an attempt to reduce the central conduction of impulses allowing pain perception or regulating tone. The operation was introduced by **William G. Spiller** and **Edward Martin**, both American physicians, in 1912.[5985] See also **tractotomy**.

corectopia iridis (ectopia pupillae) Spontaneous, cyclic, independent, and eccentric dilation of the pupils, which are displaced from the center of the iris. This is most often seen in comatose patients with a midbrain lesion. The sign was first reported by **Kinnier Wilson** in 1906. The dilatation may be oval; up-gaze paresis and loss of the pupillary light reflexes are often present as well.[5717]

cores Areas lying centrally within type I myofibrils, which do not take up stains for oxidative enzymes. They are composed of Z-line and granular material. The appearance is seen in certain **congenital myopathies**, but also in denervation, malignant hyperthermia, etc. See also **target fibers**.

Cori, C.F. (b. 1896) German-American biochemist, professor of biochemistry at Washington University, St. Louis. He and his wife were awarded the Nobel Prize for their work on glycogen dysmetabolism.

Cori disease See **Cori–Forbes disease**.

Cori–Forbes disease (Cori disease) Type III glycogen storage disease, the major features of which are hepatomegaly, hypoglycemia, slight retardation of growth, and a degree of muscle weakness of late onset.[1284] See **glycogen storage diseases** and **debrancher enzyme deficiency**.

Coriolis effect Severe spatial disorientation with vertigo induced by the rotation of the head around two axes simultaneously, as in airplane stunt pilots.[819]

corneal reflex Sudden involuntary blinking as a result of stimulation of the sensitive fibers of the ophthalmic division of the V cranial nerve in the cornea, which leads to contraction of the orbicularis oculi muscles bilaterally.

The *eyelash* (**ciliary**) and the *conjunctival* reflexes are similar, travel by almost identical pathways, and are less hazardous to perform, though slightly less sensitive. On the other hand, if either of these are present, it may be taken as certain that the corneal reflex will be present as well.

Cornelia de Lange syndrome See **de Lange syndrome**.

Cornelia de Lange syndrome foundation A charitable support organization. Address: 60 Dyer Ave., Collinsville, CT 06022.

Cornell Scale for Depression in Dementia A validated scale yielding a quantitative measure of depression in demented patients, but not designed as a diagnostic instrument. A score is assigned on the basis of information obtained after interviewing the patient and a caregiver.

Mood-related signs such as anxiety, sadness, lack of reactivity to pleasant events, and irritability; behavioral disturbances including agitation, retardation, multiple physical complaints, and loss of interest; physical signs including loss of appetite, weight, and energy; cyclic functions such as diurnal variation of mood, difficulty falling asleep, multiple awakenings, and early morning waking; and ideational disturbances such as suicidal thoughts, poor self-esteem, pessimism, and mood-congruent delusions are the items rated on a 3-point scale.[120]

Cornell, Ethel L. (b. 1892) American psychologist who devised a nonverbal test of intelligence (Cornell–Coxe Performance Ability Scale).

Cornell sign A variant of the **Babiński reflex** whereby extension of the hallux is sought as a response to scratching the inner side of the dorsum of the foot.

corneomandibular reflex Closure of the mouth or deviation of the jaw away from the side of corneal stimulation. This is normally not present after infancy and represents one of the primitive or **developmental reflexes** which may appear in association with diffuse cortical dysfunction (especially in ill patients with a reduced level of consciousness, increased intracranial pressure, and trans-tentorial herniation) but which is also common with advancing age.

It was first described by **Von Solder** in 1902 but was further discussed by Wartenberg as the winking jaw or reverse **Marcus Gunn phenomenon**.[2605, 4939] See also **palpebromandibular synkinesia** and **Wartenberg winking-jaw phenomenon.**

corneo-oculogyric reflex Deviation of the eyes upward and away from a corneal sensory stimulus; a normal phenomenon.

Cornil, Lucien (1888–1959) French neuropathologist who trained in Paris. During and after World War I he worked with Roussy and Lhermitte, setting up the neuropathology laboratory at the Hôpital Paul-Brusse. He was elected professor of pathological anatomy at Marseille in 1930 and became dean of the faculty in 1937. His neuropathological publications mainly concerned the basal ganglia, cerebral tumors, and hypertrophic neuritis.

Corning, James Leonard (1855–1923) New York neurologist who trained in Germany and practiced in New York. He introduced the technique of lumbar puncture to America in 1885, 6 years before Wynter and Quincke, but his object was to inject cocaine and he did not draw any cerebrospinal fluid; it is thus uncertain whether his needle penetrated the arachnoid membrane at all.[2495]

corona radiata (Lat, a crown + rays) The term applied by Reil to the fanlike spread of the descending pyramidal fibers when traced upward from the pyramids through the internal capsules to the cerebral hemispheres.[5103]

coronal bipolar montage (transverse bipolar montage) A montage consisting of derivations from pairs of electrodes along coronal (transverse) arrays. (From the 1974 Report of the Committee on Terminology, IFCN. In: Chatrian GE, Bergamini L, Dondey M, et al. A glossary of terms most commonly used by clinical electroencephalographers. *EEG Clin Neurophysiol* 1974;37:538–48. Reproduced by kind permission of the IFCN and Elsevier Science.)

corpora amylaceae (From Lat, bodies + starch) Spherical basophilic, periodic acid-Schiff-positive structures found in astrocytic processes beneath the pia or ependyma in patients with various degenerative diseases and in increasing numbers with advancing age.[3900] See **polyglucosan bodies**, **Lafora bodies**, and **Bielschowsky bodies**.

corpora arenacea See **psammoma bodies**.

corpus callosum (Lat, a tough body) The term given by Galen to the largest (8-cm-long) inter-hemispheric commissure. It manifests topographical localization. It is sometimes partially sectioned in cases of intractable epilepsy since its presence is essential for the spread of a bilateral synchronous discharges. **Agenesis of the corpus callosum** may be asymptomatic, or may be associated with a clinical syndrome of mental deficiency, seizures, and hemiparesis, often accompanied by such developmental defects as deficiency of the septum pellucidum and microgyria.[143] See also **Shapiro syndrome**.

corpus callosum agenesis with recurrent hypothermia (Shapiro syndrome) A congenital dysmorphic syndrome also characterized by hypercalcemia, recurrent hypothermia and reduction in consciousness, seizures, and callosal agenesis.[5761]

corpus striatum (Lat, body + furrowed) The basal ganglia include the lentiform nucleus (comprising the putamen and globus pallidus) and the caudate, the claustrum, the subthalamic nucleus, the substantia innominata of Meynert, and the substantia nigra. The striped appearance of the caudate and lentiform nuclei on stained horizontal sections of the brain have led to the term *corpus striatum* (or striatum alone) for this region.

corrective catch-up saccades Brief, small-amplitude conjugate saccades correcting any positional error made in the last major saccade.

Corsi blocks test A test of nonverbal (visual) attention span/memory, wherein the subject points to a progressively greater number of blocks in the same order as previously indicated by the examiner, or in reverse. The normal forward span is 6 ± 1 and the reverse span is 2 less than that.[4387]

cortex (Lat, outer bark, rind) The outer neuronal layer of the cerebrum.

Cortex A neurological subspecialty journal devoted to the study of the interrelations between the nervous system and behavior. Web site: www.elsevier.com/wps/find/journaldescription.cws_home/714334/description#description/.

Corti, Alfonso Marchese (1822–1888) Sardinian histologist, who worked in Vienna, Berlin, Utrecht, Turin, and Rome. He held no academic appointment but was an amateur in the best sense; he described the spiral organ of the cochlea (the end-organ for hearing, which consists of specialized neuroepithelium in the inner ear aligned in rows within the cochlear canal upon the basilar membrane) and the perilymph.

cortical abscess See **subdural empyema**.

cortical anarthria See **aphemia**.

cortical blindness Loss of vision produced by lesions of the geniculo-calcarine visual pathways. Denial of such blindness is a rare accompaniment. See **Anton syndrome**. It is seldom complete and macular sparing may occur. The patient recovers poorly when the condition is due to vascular disease, better when it follows cardiac surgery or angiography.[114]

In a *variant* congenital, recessively inherited form, the cortical blindness is accompanied by postaxial polydactyly, mental retardation, and growth failure.[2873]

cortical cerebellar degeneration (Déjèrine–Thomas syndrome) A dominantly inherited form of late-onset cerebellar ataxia (olivopontocerebellar atrophy). See **Déjèrine–Thomas syndrome**. See also **cerebellar cortical degeneration**, which is a paraneoplastic syndrome.

cortical deafness The rare occurrence of inability to interpret verbal or nonverbal sounds in the presence of retained hearing, due to a lesion affecting the anterior and posterior transverse temporal gyri of Heschl or their connections bilaterally, while the peripheral pathways are intact. Both verbal and nonverbal sounds are uninterpreted, and the temporal order of sounds and their localization in space are impaired.

Pure word deafness (auditory agnosia) may occur as the result of bilateral infarctions of the superior temporal cortex.[2545]

cortical dementia Dementing diseases presenting with prominent dysphasia, agnosia, and apraxias, reflecting involvement of the association cortex in the pathological process. See also **subcortical dementia**, in which the major problems are slowness of cognition and impairment of executive function. However, although the distinction is clinically real, the degree of overlap in the presentations of the pathologies leading to dementia limits the diagnostic value of this differentiation.

cortical developmental abnormalities (malformations)

Disturbances of cell proliferation, neuronal migration, or cortical organization during the development of the brain *in utero.* These have been classified by Barkovich et al.[404] (Reproduced by kind permission of the American Academy of Neurology and Lippincott Williams and Wilkins) as follows:

1. Malformations due to abnormal neuronal and glial proliferation or apoptosis (e.g., **microcephaly** syndromes; **megalencephaly**; hamartomas and some tumors)
2. Malformations due to abnormal neuronal migration (e.g., lissencephaly, Cobblestone complex, and heterotopias)
3. Malformations due to abnormal cortical organization including late neuronal migration (e.g., **polymicrogyria, schizencephaly**, cortical dysplasias, and microdysgenesis)
4. Malformations of cortical development, not otherwise classified (e.g., mitochondrial, pyruvate, and peroxisomal disorders)

The conditions so classified are the following:

Autosomal recessive periventricular heterotopia and microcephaly (p23; 1q31)
Autosomal recessive **microcephaly** (9q34)
Autosomal recessive microcephaly (13q.12.2)

Autosomal recessive periventricular heterotopia and microcephaly (1q31)

Amish lethal microcephaly (17q.25.3)
Bilateral perisylvian **polymicrogyria** (Xq28)
Bilateral frontoparietal polymicrogyria (16q13)
Bilateral periventricular nodular heterotopia (Xq28; 5p15)
Bilateral periventricular nodular heterotopia with microcephaly (20q.13.3)
Fukuyama **congenital muscular dystrophy** (9q31)
Isolated lissencephaly sequence (Xq22.3–q23; 17p13.3)
Lissencephaly with cerebellar hypoplasia (7q22)
Miller–Dieker syndrome (17p13.3)
Muscle–eye–brain disease (1p33-34; 19q.13.3)
Seckel syndrome (3q22)
Subcortical band heterotopia (**diffuse cortical dysplasia**) (17p13.3)
Tuberous sclerosis (9q32; 16p.13.3)
Warburg microsyndrome (12q21.3)
Walker–Warburg syndrome (9q34.1; 19q.13.3; 9q31)

X-linked lissencephaly with abnormal genitalia (Xp22.13)

cortical dumbness See **aphemia**.

cortical dysarthria See **logopenia**.

cortical dysgenetic index
A method of scoring the presence of minor cortical irregularities, dysplasias, and microdysgenesis in the brain. **Leptomeningeal glial heterotopias, merged gyri**, and **gray matter heterotopias** score 5; abnormal cortical bundles of myelin, neuronal multinucleation, ballooned cells, and cortical nodules score 3; and neuronal heterotopias, subpial neurons, single-file neuronal radial patterns, abnormal neuronal clusters, large, overabundant, or misaligned neurons, and abnormal lamination or irregular gray/white matter score 2. A total score of 5 or more indicates the presence of cortical microdysgenesis.[471]

cortical dysplasia (focal cortical dysplasia, cortical dysplasia of Taylor) The presence of large dysplastic neurons and giant astrocytes in all but the first layer of discrete segments of the cortex, typically the rolandic cortex. **Macrogyria**, **lissencephaly**, **unilateral megalencephaly**, **pachygyria**, and **polymicrogyria** are recognized accompaniments.

The clinical syndrome comprises the onset in childhood of focal cortical myoclonus and severe focal motor seizures, with mild hemiparesis, widespread cognitive deficits, and a progressive course,[3620] worse in those with ballooned cells in the abnormal cortex.

cortical electrode An electrode applied directly upon or inserted within the cerebral cortex.

cortical function 1. "The whole cortex . . . has no other function but to select, abstract, differentiate, integrate and condense rhythms or patterns of nervous activity (to provide) . . . the basis for the comparison of sensory relationships; for recognition, or memory; for symbols which with notions of space, time direction and many other ideas have enabled man to create calculating machines, symphonies and poems." (Goody, 1954)[2471] 2. Those endowments which preferentially serve instrumental functions, such as language, perception, memory, and calculation. Dysfunction thus leads to aphasias, agnosias, acalculia, and amnesia.

cortical laminar necrosis
A permanent brain injury associated with hypoxia, prolonged status epilepticus, metabolic disturbances, drugs, and infections. The MRI shows high-intensity cortical lesions and pathologically there is focal destruction of the cerebral cortex with necrosis of the cerebral cortex involving all cell types and blood vessels.[1683]

cortical Lewy body disease See **diffuse Lewy body disease**.

cortical motor aphasia See **Broca aphasia**.

cortical myoclonus (focal cortical myoclonus, cortical reflex myoclonus) A form of **stimulus-sensitive myoclonus** (the other form being subcortical or reticular) seen in **progressive myoclonic epilepsy**, **(Unverricht–Lundborg–)Lafora body disease**, lipidoses, and postanoxic states, and also in **Alzheimer** and **Creutzfeldt–Jakob** diseases.

The movement can be considered as a fragment of partial epilepsy in which each myoclonic jerk typically involves only a few adjacent, usually distal, muscles, although many different areas may be involved. Triggers are sensory stimulation or voluntary limb movements. The somatosensory cortex is the likely site of the discharges. The cortical events recorded by EEG are time-locked to the jerks, which occur spontaneously or in response to somatosensory stimulation (**reflex myoclonus**) or to voluntary movement (**action myoclonus**).[2695]

In this condition, somatosensory-evoked potentials are typically of unusually high amplitude, suggesting pathological hyperexcitabilty of the motor cortex.

A variant is *familial cortical myoclonic tremor with epilepsy*, a channelopathy, the characteristics of which are adult onset, benign course, autosomal dominant inheritance, distal action tremor and myoclonus, epileptic seizures, effectiveness of antiepileptic drugs, and possibly cognitive decline. See also **reticular reflex myoclonus**, **primary generalized epileptic myoclonus**, and **myoclonus**.

cortical mantle The cerebral cortex, so named in appreciation of its position as a covering for the entire brain in the supratentorial compartment.

cortical nodules Projections of the pial surface of the brain into the subarachnoid space as a result of cortical dysgenesis.

cortical paralysis of visual fixation See **Balint syndrome**.

cortical receptive aphasia See **Wernicke aphasia**.

cortical reflex myoclonus Generalized myoclonus occurring in response to low-frequency photic stimulation, with an accompanying frontal spike discharge. The condition may complicate numerous diseases affecting the gray matter. See **photomyogenic response**.

cortical sensation Three classes of sensation were defined by **Head**:

1. Recognition of spatial relations, such as the recognition of passive movements, two-point discrimination or "spot finding" (topical localization)
2. A graduated response to stimuli of different intensity
3. Appreciation of similarity and difference in external objects, brought into contact with the surface of the body—thus appreciation of size, shape, weight, and texture

He also noted that diminution of sensitivity to pinprick and vibration may result from cortical lesions but to a lesser extent, and that hypotonia is another association. Representation of different areas is separate, so one finger may be affected while another is spared. The palm and sole have the greatest representational areas, "so a cortical lesion may disturb the sensibility of the hand and foot without of necessity affecting the elbow, shoulder or knee."[2812]

cortical sensory aphasia See **Wernicke aphasia** and **aphasia**.

cortical sensory loss Impairment of the senses of tactile localization; graphesthesia; appreciation of size, shape, weight, or texture; and bilateral simultaneous tactile stimulation.

cortical sensory syndrome An isolated loss of discriminative sensation involving one of two parts of the body and occurring with infarcts of the superior–posterior parts of a parietal lobe.[434] See also **parietal stroke**.

cortical spreading depression (of Leao) A transient, slowly moving suppression of electrical activity which propagates across (and remains confined to) the cortex at 2–5 mm/min, accompanied by a disruption of ion homeostasis, depolarization of nerve cells, and increased energy metabolism. The depression seldom moves further forward than the central sulcus.The role of this phenomenon is uncertain, but it has been suggested that the changes in cerebral blood flow in patients with migraine attacks resemble those in animals during the occurrence of spreading depression.[3715]

cortical thumb The adducted and flexed position of the thumb, often covered by the flexed fingers adopted by infants or children with hemiparesis in whom there is always a parietal lobe lesion. See also **fisting** and **dystonic toe**.

cortical tremor A variant of cortical reflex myoclonus resembling intractable **essential tremor** and presenting as action and postural tremulous finger movements. The condition is characterized by rhythmic but unsynchronized involuntary movements that occur distally, particularly in the outstretched hands and during activity.There is an occasional association with generalized or partial seizures.

The brief movements are accompanied by EMG bursts lasting about 50 ms, which result in a fine shivering-like finger twitching, provoked mainly by action and posture. The electrophysiological findings are of cortical reflex myoclonus with giant somatosensory-evoked potentials, enhanced long-loop reflexes, and premovement cortical spikes.[3074] See also **FAME** and **familial cortical myoclonic tremor with epilepsy**.

cortical word deafness See **pure word deafness**.

cortical-basal ganglionic degeneration See **corticobasal degeneration**.

corticectomy The removal of the cortex of a small or large area, usually performed in patients with intractable seizure disorders due to neuronal migration disorders or severe ischemic injury of the cortex.

corticobasal degeneration (cortical-basal ganglionic degeneration, cortico-dentato-nigral degeneration with neuronal achromasia, Rebeitz–Kolodny–Richardson syndrome) A rare, slowly progressive degenerative tauopathy of unknown cause affecting older adults who present with dementia, slowness and awkwardness of movements (limb **ideomotor apraxia**), myoclonus, blepharospasm, choreoathetosis, unilateral Parkinsonism (bradykinesia and rigidity unresponsive to levadopa), and pyramidal signs. The gait disturbances, cortical sensory loss, and stimulus-sensitive myoclonus result in a "jerky useless hand." Additional motor features include asymmetric limb clumsiness, dystonia and/or rigidity, and action tremor. It is probably a variety of frontotemporal dementia.

Progressive external ophthalmoplegia and dysphagia are other features. Cognitive disturbances due to degeneration of the cortical, striatal, and nigral neuronal pathways are also reported later in the course of the disease, language being more affected than memory. These comprise aphasia, the **alien limb** phenomenon, frontal release signs, and cortical sensory abnormalities. The spectrum of cognitive disorders includes depression, apathy, anxiety, irritability, disinhibition, delusions, and obsessive-compulsive behavior.

The condition leads to death within about 10 years of onset.[4066] The best predictors for the diagnosis have been identified as limb dystonia, ideomotor apraxia, myoclonus, and an asymmetric akinetic-rigid syndrome with the late onset of gait or balance disturbances.[3878] However, there is important clinical (and some genetic) overlap with **primary progressive aphasia** and frontotemporal dementia[3405] and also with **progressive supranuclear palsy**, with which this condition shares a common **tau** haplotype.[700] Criteria for the diagnosis have been proposed:[700]

Core features

Insidious onset and progressive course
No identifiable cause such as tumor or infarct

Cortical dysfunction includes at least one of the following: focal or asymmetric ideomotor apraxia; alien limb phenomena, cortical sensory loss; visual or hemisensory neglect, constructional apraxia, focal or asymmetric myoclonus, apraxia of speech, or nonfluent aphasia.

Extrapyramidal dysfunction is reflected by one of the following: focal or asymmetric appendicular rigidity, prominent and sustained response to levadopa, and focal or asymmetric appendicular dystonia.

The hallmarks of **corticobasal degeneration** are the various forms of apraxia affecting limb function, particularly **ideomotor** and **limb-kinetic apraxia**, although **buccofacial** and **oculomotor apraxia** may also be present. The asymmetric Parkinsonism and cortical signs (dysphasia, astereognosis, graphesthesia), the early and severe gait and balance problems, dystonia/action and postural tremor/myoclonus, and alien limb phenomena are the major features suggesting clinical diagnosis.

Supportive investigations include neuropsychometric testing which should show variable degrees of focal or lateralized cognitive dysfunction with relative preservation of learning and memory; CT or MR imaging showing focal or asymmetric atrophy typically in the perifrontal cortex; and SPECT or PET demonstration of focal or asymmetric hypoperfusion, particularly in the parietofrontal cortex.

Neuronal achromasia (swelling of the cell body and resistance to stains), gliosis, and asymmetric atrophy of the frontoparietal cortex and of the striatal and nigral neuronal pathways are notable pathological features.[5220] Pathological criteria for diagnosis have been suggested[3934] and include the following:

- Cortical degeneration with swollen neurones
- Neuronal loss in the substantia nigra (pars compacta) with corticobasal inclusions
- Variable involvement of subcortical structures
- Tau-immunoreactive lesions in neurons, glia, and cell processes
- The minimal pathologic features for CBD are cortical and striatal tau-positive neuronal and glial lesions, especially astrocytic plaques and thread-like lesions in both white matter and gray matter, along with neuronal loss in focal cortical regions and in the substantia nigra.[1635]

In a *variant* form, the clinical features exist in the presence of an *SCA8* mutation.

corticobasal syndrome The concurrence of Parkinsonism and prominent apraxia, seen in **progressive supranuclear palsy, Alzheimer disease, dementia with Lewy bodies,** and **frontotemporal dementias**. Diseases that cause the combination of apraxia and a primary movement disorder most often involve a variety of cerebral cortical sites as well as basal ganglia structures.[6943]

cortico-dentato-nigral degeneration with neuronal achromasia See **corticobasal degeneration**.

corticogram See **electrocorticogram**.

corticography See **electrocorticography**.

corticoid areas Parts of the basal forebrain (the septal region, the substantia innominata, and part of the amygdaloid complex) which form part of the limbic system. The structures are part of the cortical mantle but their organization is rudimentary.[4332]

cortico-meningeal diffuse angiomatosis See **Van Bogaert syndrome**.

corticopallido-(or striato-) spinal degeneration See **Creutzfeldt–Jakob disease**.

corticospinal tract See **pyramidal tract**.

corticosteroid myopathy A syndrome of proximal muscle weakness and wasting preferentially affecting the legs. Type II fiber atrophy is the characteristic finding on muscle biopsy. Serum creatine kinase levels are usually at the lower end of the normal range and the EMG normal or mildly myopathic.[3412]

corticotrophin releasing factor A peptide secreted by the hypothalamus that also inhibits the release from that site of gonadotrophic-releasing hormones.

costalgia Intercostal neuralgia.

costal arch reflex See **abdominal reflex**.

costal margin reflex See **abdominal reflex**.

costal periosteal reflex See **abdominal reflex**.

costal reflex (costo-abdominal reflex, costal arch reflex, costal periosteal reflex, costal margin reflex) The **abdominal reflex** obtained by tapping the costal margin medial to the nipple line. The reflex is mediated by cord segments T5–T9.

Costen, James Bray (1895–1962) American otolaryngologist practicing in St. Louis.

Costen syndrome The association of dull pain in the ear and the region of the temporomandibular joint, with burning in nose, throat, and tongue as well as vertical and occipital headache, persistent hearing disorders, tinnitus, vertigo, nystagmus, dryness of the mouth, stuffy ears, reduced mandibular movements, and clicking or snapping of the temporomandibular joint due to overbite (abnormal closure of the mouth with the lower teeth nestling inside those of the upper jaw). Costen considered that the mandibular joint pathology (posterior condylar displacement) was entirely responsible, but it is now thought to be due to occlusal dysfunction of the joint and/or spasm of the masticatory muscles.[1294]

Although such pain felt as a result of misalignment of the temporomandibular joint or overactivity of the temporalis or masseter muscles (or both) is an entity with high face validity, the putative cause has never been proved.

costoabdominal reflex See **abdominal reflex**.

costoclavicular syndrome See **thoracic outlet syndrome**.

Cotard syndrome (*délire de négations*) A delusional syndrome manifesting paranoia, nihilistic delusions, suicidal ideation, and sensory disturbances, described first in 1880 by Jules Cotard (1840–1889), a French neuropsychiatrist who had trained with **Charcot** and **Vulpian**. The syndrome probably represents the occurrence of somatic dysesthesias in psychotically depressed patients. The classic complaint of the subject is that s/he is dead or that part of his body has decayed.[6923] Although described classically in schizophrenia and bipolar disorder, physical disorders including migraine, tumor, and trauma have also been associated with the syndrome.[2279]

For an account of the accomplished but unhappy life of **Jules Cotard**, see Pearn (2002).[4957]

Coté–Katsantoni syndrome See **Katsantoni syndrome**.

cotton wool spots 1. (cytoid bodies) Aggregates composed of the swollen ends of disrupted retinal nerve fibers, occurring as a result of ischemia and healing with the formation of a glial scar. 2. Infarcts of the retinal nerve fiber layer, typically seen with fully developed **papilledema**.

Cotugno, Domenico Felice Antonio (1736–1822) Neapolitan

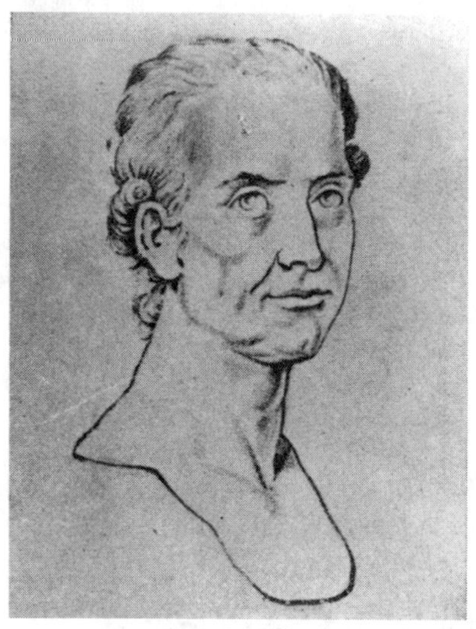

Figure C–5 Domenico Felice Antonio Cotugno.

surgeon, professor at Naples, who described the skin lesions of smallpox, the gut lesions of typhoid, the cerebrospinal and the labyrinthine fluids, and the anatomy of the inner ear (100 years before Helmholtz); he also demonstrated albuminuria, and wrote on sciatica and nephritis in his book *De Ischiade Nervosa Commentarius*, published in 1764.

Cotugno disease See **sciatica**.

cough headache An uncommon syndrome of brief severe pain in the head precipitated by coughing or by other maneuvers which raise intracranial pressure, mainly affecting middle-aged men with no organic intracranial lesion.[6175, 6176] The headaches disappear after months or years without residua. Most patients are pain-free between attacks of head pain but in some cases the paroxysms are followed by dull aching pain that may persist for hours. Since brain tumor and the **Chiari malformation** cause similar symptoms, it has been recommended that MRI of the head should be obtained in all cases.[5203] The character of the headache is the same whether there is a causal intracranial lesion or not.

cough syncope (vertige larynge of Charcot, Charcot vertigo, laryngeal epilepsy, respiratory syncope, post-tussive syndrome, laryngeal vertigo) Dizziness or actual loss of consciousness, sometimes with convulsive movements, occurring in plethoric, bronchitic middle-aged men after coughing, and in others after, for example, trumpet playing. The cough has been regarded as an aura and the whole condition thus considered to represent a form of **complex partial seizure**,[6760] although increased intrathoracic pressure and thus decreased venous return and decreased cardiac output is at first sight an obvious cause. Increased CSF pressure and induced cardiac arrhythmias may also be incriminated.[3395]

The term was applied by **Liveing** to a condition in which the patient awakens from sleep, clutches at his neck and struggles for breath, the attack subsiding in a few minutes.

counter-pressure See **geste antagonistique**.

counter-rotation A noticeable circular movement of the eyeballs in the opposite direction when the head is tilted from the upright position toward one shoulder. The movement is in the opposite direction and is maximal with the first 20° of tilt.

coup de la chaleur See heat stroke.

coup lesion The traumatic brain injury (contusion or laceration) directly beneath the point of impact.

coupled discharge See **satellite potential**.

Courtois, Adolphe (1903–1935) French psychiatrist who trained in Paris and after graduation worked for Guillain before his appointment as physician to a Parisian mental hospital.

Courtois sign Passive flexion of the head on the chest in a comatose patient with a lateralized intracranial lesion produces flexion only of the healthy leg.[1300]

Courville, Cyril (1900–1968) American neurologist and neuropathologist who trained with **Cushing** and **Bailey** before concentrating on neurology and neuropathology at the Loma Linda University School of Medicine. His most lasting works dealt with cerebral palsy, perinatal brain injuries, and cerebral tumors.[7]

Couvade syndrome (Fr, to hatch) (married man's toothache) A psychogenic disorder characterized by the occurrence of the symptoms of pregnancy in the husband during the pregnancy of the wife. Nausea, abdominal pain, bulimia or loss of appetite, toothache, and abdominal bloating are typical symptoms.[6382] The condition was first recorded by **Francis Bacon** in 1627.

cover test 1. A test of paretic ocular muscles in which the paretic (nonfixating) eye is covered first; the nonparetic eye will not move, nor does it move when the cover is taken away. When the nonparetic eye is covered, the paretic eye deviates in order to attempt fixation, and the nonparetic eye deviates excessively in the same direction (**secondary deviation**). When the cover is taken away, either the normal eye takes up fixation again or the abnormal one retains fixation and the normal eye remains in deviation—if the patient is an **alternate fixator**.[3762] 2. (*alternate cover test*) A test of paretic ocular muscles in which each of the two eyes is covered alternately every second or two, while the subject fixates on an object. The fixating eye will be positioned so that the light from the target falls on the fovea, but the occluded eye may deviate (**primary deviation**), now that it has lost its continuing stimulus to retain parallelism of the ocular axes, if it is subject to strabismus. When the normal eye is covered and the eye with defective muscle balance fixates on the object, the normal eye will deviate, this time in a direction opposite to that of the paretic eye (**secondary deviation**).

covert dyskinesia Abnormal involuntary movements (**tardive dyskinesia**), which only appear when the dose of the causal drug is reduced or when it is no longer taken.

Cowden disease See **Lhermitte–Duclos disease**.

COWS The mnemonic for the direction of the normal nystagmoid response to irrigation of the external auditory meatus with water: *C*old *O*pposite, *W*arm *S*ame. Thus, irrigation of the left ear with ice-cold water leads to nystagmus with its fast component to the right. The important ocular movement, the slow deviation, is of course in the *opposite* direction to that of the nystagmus.

crack dancing Choreoathetosis, akathisia, and Parkinsonism with tremor, associated with the repetitive use of the freebase form of cocaine as a recreational drug.[1450]

cracked-pot note (bruit de pot fêlé) The off-key sound heard when the skull of an hydrocephalic child is percussed. It is not a sign of fracture of the cranial vault, but rather of the separation of the sutures in hydrocephalus. Exactly the same sign occurs in cavitating lung disease, such as abscess or tuberculosis, when the cavity contains both air and fluid, and it is also elicited over the chests of crying children. The Scottish surgeon Sir **William MacEwen** (1848–1924) described it first in 1893.

Cram Test See **bowstring sign**.

cramp 1. Sudden involuntary painful shortening of muscle with abrupt onset, attended by visible or palpable knotting of muscle, and often leading to abnormal postures of the affected joints.[5443] 2. A painful muscle contraction with an accompanying EMG discharge comprising irregular high-frequency bursts of motor unit potentials with gradual onset and termination. See also **cramps**.

cramp discharge Involuntary repetitive firing of motor unit action potentials at a high frequency (up to 150 Hz) in a large area of a muscle usually associated with painful muscle contraction. Both discharge frequency and number of motor unit action potentials activated increase gradually during development, and both subside gradually with cessation. See **muscle cramp**. (From the 2001 Report of the Nomenclature Committee of the American Association of Electromyography and Electrodiagnosis.[19] Reproduced by kind permission of the AANEM.)

cramp-fasciculation syndrome (muscle-pain fasciculation syndrome, benign motor neuron disorder) A rare, benign, acquired and usually idiopathic syndrome characterized by the sudden onset of muscle aching, cramps, stiffness, limb muscle fasciculations or myokymia, and exercise intolerance without clinical muscle atrophy or weakness, in otherwise healthy adults, due to abnormal excitation of the distal motor axon. The serum CK level is raised and muscle biopsy specimens may show neurogenic changes. Muscle biopsy is normal or shows mild neurogenic changes. The EMG does not show continuous muscle fiber activity as in **Isaacs syndrome** (which is probably closely related) but showers of afterdischarges are recorded following motor nerve stimulation, as in that condition.[294, 6185]

The phenomenon may reflect a hyperexcitable peripheral nerve syndrome, especially if myokymia or neuromyotonia is also present, reflecting the presence of antibodies to voltage-gated potassium channels.[3643]

cramp-myalgia syndrome A nonprogressive X-linked dystrophinopathy of childhood charcterized by cramps, myalgia, exercise intolerance, and pseudohypertrophjy of the calves, without weakness. Serum creatine kinase levels are consistently raised and myoglobinuria may occur in attacks.[2515]

See also **myalgia-cramp syndrome**, **phosphofructokinase deficiency**, and **myophosphorylase deficiency**.

cramps (ordinary muscle cramps) (from Norse "cram," pinching) Sudden, severe painful, palpable involuntary contractions of muscles, most commonly experienced in the calves by elderly people during the night but potentially occurring in any healthy muscle when it is contracted voluntarily for extended periods. They may be relieved by passive stretching.

Cramps typically affect all or part of a single muscle, and are thought to follow and spread out from a zone of repetitive fasciculations at <150/s arising from nerve terminals in that muscle, followed by further fasciculations.[3725, 4379] Their biochemical basis is uncertain, but aging, dehydration, hemodialysis, hyponatremia, hypomagnesemia, hypocalcemia, dysthyroid states, adrenal insufficiency, and pregnancy are known to be associated, as are all forms of lower motor neuron disorder. Treatment with phenytoin, quinine, or calcium salts is highly effective though seldom prescribed, which is ironic when one considers that therapy for many other neurological conditions is not available.

A *variant condition* is *adolescent familial cramps*, a benign X-linked muscular dystrophy presenting with exercise-induced cramps.[2738] See also **electrically silent cramps**.

cramps, occupational See **dystonia**.

crampus syndrome The repeated occurrence of cramps without any evidence of neurological or biochemical abnormality.[5443]

Crandall syndrome The association of sensorineural deafness, pili torti, hypogonadism, and alopecia.[1312]

Crane syndrome (clefting with skeletal anomalies) A congenital dysmorphic syndrome characterized by low birth weight, hypertelorism, micrognathia, cleft upper lip and palate, segmentation defects of the spine, absent or hypoplastic clavicles, syndactyly, club foot, undermineralization of the skull, hydrocephalus, and callosal agenesis.[381]

cranial (from Gr, the skull) Pertaining to the skull.

cranial aerocele See **pneumocephalus**.

cranial arteritis See **giant cell arteritis**.

cranial dystonias (Breughel syndrome, Meige syndrome, idiopathic orofacial dystonia, spasme faciale mediane) Dystonias of adult life characterized by prolonged symmetrical contractions of the orofacial musculature with the production of any combination of **blepharospasm**, **oromandibular dystonias**, and **laryngeal** or

pharyngeal dystonias often disabling the patient.

The first account of this disorder was that of Henri **Meige** in 1910, who noted that the blepharospasm was worsened by stress and certain patterns of activity and disappeared in sleep. Extension to other muscle groups and clinical depressive illness are also common findings in such patients. Familial occurrence of the condition has been recorded.[6343] See **Meige syndrome**. In **Breughel syndrome** the classic abnormality is wide opening of the mouth rather than blepharospasm.

cranial lacunae (lückenschadel) Radiolucent defects seen on plain X-ray studies of the skulls of neonates evidencing a bony dysplasia, but of no significance in diagnosis.[2114]

cranial meningocele A developmental anomaly characterized by extracranial herniation of the meninges through a cranial defect.

cranial metaphyseal dysplasia A rare hereditary disorder of bone absorption or remodeling in which hyperostosis and sclerosis of the skull and facial bones causes narrowing of the cranial foramina which may lead to cranial nerve palsies, especially of the VII cranial nerve and which has also been associated with seizures or long tract signs.[5547]

cranial nerves The nerves issuing from the skull and emanating from the brain or brainstem.

The number of cranial nerves has never been resolved satisfactorily. **Galen** described eleven pairs, ignoring the first, which was, however, included by **Vesalius**. **Willis** in 1684 described nine pairs, the first six as they are known today, the seventh and eighth together next as the seventh, the next three included by him as the eighth, and the hypoglossal nerve as the ninth. Lensell in 1942 named sixteen pairs.

The fact that the first and second are actually clothed not with Schwann cells but with oligodendroglia would merit their classification as central rather than peripheral nervous system structures, but today we regard 12 as the correct number, as suggested by **Soemerring**.

cranial neuralgias Painful states affecting the head as a result of disease usually affecting the V, VII, or IX/X cranial nerves complex. A classification has been proposed by the International Headache Society (see Chart C–26). The individual conditions in **boldface** are entered separately.

Chart C–26. Cranial Neuralgias, Nerve Trunk Pain, and Deafferentation Pain

13.	**Cranial neuralgias and central causes of facial pain**
13.1	**Trigeminal neuralgia**
13.1.1	Classical trigeminal neuralgia
13.1.2	Symptomatic trigeminal neuralgia
13.2	**Glossopharyngeal neuralgia**
13.2.1	Classical glossopharyngeal neuralgia
13.2.2	Symptomatic glossopharyngeal neuralgia
13.3	**Nervus intermedius neuralgia**
13.4	**Superior laryngeal neuralgia**
13.5	**Nasociliary neuralgia**
13.6	**Supraorbital neuralgia**
13.7	**Other terminal branch neuralgias**
13.8	**Occipital neuralgia**
13.9	**Neck-tongue syndrome**
13.10	**External compression headache**
13.11	**Cold-stimulus headache**
13.11.1	Headache attributed to external application of a cold stimulus
13.11.2	Headache attributed to ingestion or inhalation of a cold stimulus
13.12	**Constant pain caused by compression, irritation, or distortion of cranial nerves or upper cervical roots by structural lesions**
13.13	**Optic neuritis**
13.14	**Ocular diabetic neuropathy**
13.15	**Head or facial pain attributed to herpes zoster**
13.15.1	Head or facial pain attributed to acute herpes zoster
13.15.2	Post-herpetic neuralgia
13.16	**Tolosa–Hunt syndrome**
13.17	**Ophthalmoplegic "migraine"**
13.18	**Central causes of facial pain**
13.18.1	Anesthesia dolorosa
13.18.2	Central post-stroke pain
13.18.3	Facial pain attributed to multiple sclerosis
13.18.4	Persistent idiopathic facial pain
13.18.5	Burning mouth syndrome
13.19	**Other cranial neuralgia or other centrally mediated facial pain**

cranial neuropathies Disorders which selectively or predominantly involve the cranial nerves, usually the V and VII and less commonly the bulbar (IX–XII) nerves. Autoimmune disease and mitotic lesions are the commonest causes.

cranial synostosis and fibular aplasia See Lowry Syndrome.

craniocarpotarsal dysplasia See Whistling face syndrome.

cranio-cerebral trauma Syndromes resulting directly or indirectly from head injury.[469] These include **concussion**, contusion, and laceration of the brain, **epidural (extradural) hemorrhage, subdural hemorrhage**, and **intracerebral hemorrhage**, skull fracture, **CSF rhinorrhea**, and **post-concussional syndromes**. The severity of the lesions suffered has been graded (Marshall, *J. Neurosurg.* 1992; permission sought) on the basis CT scan findings[4113] as follows:

Craniocerebral Trauma Severity Score

Diffuse injury 1.	No visible intracranial pathology.
Diffuse injury 2.	Cisterns present; shift of 0.5 mm and/or lesion densities present; no high- or mixed-density lesion >25 ml; may include bone fragments and foreign bodies.
Diffuse injury 3.	Cisterns compressed or absent; shift 0–5 mm; no high- or mixed-density lesion >25 ml.
Diffuse injury 4.	Shift >5 mm; No high- or mixed-density lesion >25 ml.
	Evacuated mass lesion
	Nonevacuated mass lesion
	High- or mixed-density lesion >25 ml; not surgically evacuated.

Other trauma severity scores[3496] and prognostic scales[6243, 3206, 6908, 5196] have also been created. See also **coma** and **coma scales**.

craniocervical dystonia That form of **dystonia** in which the muscles of the head and neck are involved, in the former case producing **oro-mandibular dystonias** and in the latter, **torticollis**, **retrocollis**, etc. The associated headaches consist of a sensation of cramp, tension, or pain in the neck, radiating to the back of the head or to the whole head.

Craniocervical Dystonia Questionnaire A validated, disease-specific questionnaire evaluating the quality of life of patients with cervical dystonia and blepharospasm. The English version is reproduced in the paper by Muller et al.,[4542] and a German version is obtainable from the authors.

cranio-cervical malformation A congenital syndrome characterized by the presence of a short neck with combinations of cerebellar and pyramidal signs. See **Chiari malformation**.

cranio-cleido-dysostosis (cranio-cleidal dysplasia) A dominantly inherited syndrome, characterized by aplasia or hypoplasia of both clavicles with variability in the size of the attached muscles; facial dysmorphisms with frontal bossing, saddle nose, and delayed ossification of the fontanelles; an abnormally wide cranium with brachycephaly; kyphoscoliosis; lax joints; and occasionally paraparesis or hemiparesis.[3424]

Syringomyelia, callosal agenesis, spinal dysraphism, and cervical ribs occasionally complicate the primary features. The condition was first described by **Pierre Marie**.[2504]

cranio-cleidal dysplasia See **cranio-cleido-dysostosis**.

cranio-diaphyseal dysplasia A group of diseases within the spectrum of craniotubular dysplasias and including at least the following:

1. A severe recessively inherited bone disorder characterized by massive generalized hyperostosis and sclerosis, especially involving the skull and facial bones, with mental and growth retardation, seizures, visual failure, and deafness.[2504]
2. A dominantly inherited syndrome manifesting hypertrophy of the membrane bones of the face and skull, leading to severe dysmorphism and to II and VIII cranial nerve palsies. Macpherson delineates a spectrum running from metaphyseal dysplasia through craniometaphyseal dysplasia and leontiasis ossea to craniodiaphyseal dysplasia and progressive diaphyseal dysplasia.[4009]

craniodigital syndrome The coexistence of mental and growth retardation, unusual facies, syndactyly, mild brachycephaly, and abnormal palmar dermatoglyphics. See also **Saethre–Chotzen syndrome**.[5686]

craniofacial dysostosis A congenital dominantly inherited dysmorphic syndrome characterized by prominent frontal bossing, absent auditory canals, hypertelorism, prominent eyes, strabismus, parrot-beaked profile of the nose, hypoplastic facial bones, high palate, oligodontia and brachycephaly, ossicle malformations and a mixed hearing loss, dwarfism, optic atrophy, micrognathia, nystagmus, hydrocephalus, craniosynostosis involving multiple sutures, callosal agenesis, and mental and developmental delay.[2499] See **Crouzon syndromes**.

craniofacial malformations Disorders of maturation characterized by abnormalities of body modelling and frequently with associated neurological defects. A classification has been achieved.[4] (See Chart C–27, adapted from **Stricker** et al. [1990][4] by kind permission.)

Chart C–27. Craniofacial Malformations

1. *Cerebrocranial dysplasias*
   (Anencephaly, microcephaly)
2. *Cerebrofacial dysplasias*
   Rhinencephalic dysplasias
   Oculo-orbital dysplasias (anophthalmia)
3. *Craniofacial dysplasias*
   a. With clefting
   b. With dysostosis
   c. With synostosis

   Craniosynostosis
   a. Craniofaciosynostosis
   b. Faciosynostosis
   c. With dysostosis and synostosis
   Crouzon syndrome
   Acrocephalosyndactyly (Apert syndrome)
   Cloverleaf skull
4. *Craniofacial dysplasias with other origin*
   a. Osseous
   b. Cutaneous
   c. Neurocutaneous (**neurofibromatosis**)
   d. Neuromuscular (Robin syndrome, **Möbius syndrome**)
   e. Muscular (glossoschizis)
   f. Vascular (haemangioma, hemolymphangioma, lymphangioma).

craniofrontonasal dysplasia A congenital dysmorphic syndrome characterized also by strabismus, syndactyly, broad hallux, sandal gap between the toes, and craniosynostosis with brachycephaly and hypertelorism.[4]

craniohypophysial xanthomatosis See **generalized xanthomatosis** and **Hand–Schüller–Christian disease**.

craniology The study of the comparative sizes and proportions of skulls.

craniometaphyseal dysplasia A dominantly or recessively inherited congenital dysmorphic syndrome characterized also by prominent eyes, thick calvarium, sclerosis of the skull with underdevelopment of sinuses, osteosclerosis or osteopetrosis, and metaphyseal splaying of the long bones, and skull abnormalities leading to headache and cranial nerve palsies (particularly deafness).[2504, 5673, 5547]

Pyle disease is similar but lacks the orofacial involvement.

craniopagus twins Infants born joined together at the head. Partial forms lack significant shared dural venous sinuses (SDVS). Total forms with SDVS exhibit more severe compressive brain distortion. A classification has been derived in order to assess the chances of success with surgical separation.[6075]

craniopathy Disease of the cranium.

craniopharyngioma Cystic or solid, benign, multiloculated tumors arising from the embryonic pouch of Rathke above the sella turcica, composed of sheets of squamous cells with calcification, keratin pearls, and granulomas, and containing glairy "machine-oil" fluid full of cholesterol crystals. They are prone to recurrence after removal.[6] The tumor arises from embryonic squamous cell rests in the site of the obliterated cranio-pharyngeal duct.

Clinically, craniopharyngiomas present most often in childhood with growth failure or complaints of headache and other evidence of raised intracranial pressure, chiasmal compression, hypopituitarism or alterations in mental status; in adults, sexual dysfunction, visual deficits, and a syndrome of progressive dementia are the usual symptoms. See also **suprasellar cysts**.

cranioschisis A severe and potentially lethal developmental defect due to failure of the cranial portion of the neural tube to close. In its most severe form (*cranioschisis aperta with encephaloschisis*, **anencephaly**) there is an absence of the cranial vault and of the cerebral cortex, the basal ganglia forming the most cephalad portion of the nervous system. In *cranioschisis occulta with encephalocele*, the brain herniates through a relatively small defect in the skull.[4078]

cranioscopy **Franz Gall**'s preferred name for **phrenology**.

craniostenosis See **craniosynostosis**.

craniosynostosis (craniostenosis) The result of premature fusion of one or more cranial sutures in infancy, leading to a reduction in the volume of the cranium and to diffuse encephalopathies as a consequence of the pressure on the brain.[1234] See Chart C–28. The sagittal suture is affected most often, while the lambdoid, metopic, or coronal sutures less commonly. Characteristic deformities of the skull (**turricephaly, brachycephaly, oxycephaly, pachycephaly**) result and may require early surgical correction, either for cosmetic reasons or because of increased intracranial pressure. The forms of craniosynostosis were first classified by **Virchow** in 1851; he also coined this term and brachycephaly, dolichocephaly, scaphocephaly, and macro- and microcephaly. A newer classification is that of **Jacobson**.[3138] The condition is not new, having been recorded in the time of the Egyptian Pharaohs.[5932]

See the syndromes of Apert, Berant, Crouzon, Christian, Carpenter, Pfeiffer, and Saethre–Chotzen, and the kleeblattschadel anomaly as well as the following *variants* listed in Chart C–28. See also **Adelaide** and **Boston craniosynostosis**, **Jackson-Weiss syndrome**, **Greig syndrome**, and **thanatophoric dysplasia**.

Chart C– 28. Variant Forms of Craniosynostosis

Armendares syndrome[245]
Baller–Gerold syndrome (craniosynostosis and radial aplasia) A recessively inherited congenital syndrome characterized by craniosynostosis and radial aplasia.[351]
Berant syndrome[539]
Christian syndrome
Complicated acrocephalopolysyndactyly (**Sakati–Nyhan–Tisdale syndrome**) A rare syndrome manifesting polydactyly, premature fusion of all cranial sutures with **acrocephaly**, giantism, and dysmorphism.[5507]
Craniosynostosis, arthrogryposis, and cleft palate syndrome (Christian–Andrews–Conneally–Muller syndrome) A recessively inherited congenital syndrome characterized by craniosynostosis, microcephaly, hypertelorism, antimongoloid slant of the eyes, ophthalmoplegia, and facial dysmorphisms.[1170]
Craniosynostosis, brachydactyly, symphalangism, strabismus, hip osteochondritis, and carpotarsal fusion A rare, probably dominantly inherited syndrome manifesting these features.[6524]
Craniosynostosis with 7p-karyotype[2504]
Craniosynostosis with foot anomalies[6705]
Fairbank syndrome
Gorlin–Chaudhry–Moss syndrome A syndrome consisting of dysmorphism with craniosynostosis, facial dysostosis, translucent teeth, congenital cardiac defects, and defective upper eyelids.[2499]
Herrmann–Pallister–Opitz syndrome (craniosynostosis, brachysyndactyly of hands, and absence of toes, Herrmann syndrome 1) A sporadic congenital malformation syndrome characterized by facial dysmorphisms including cleft lip or palate, craniosynostosis affecting the coronal suture, hypertelorism, brachysyndactyly of the hands, and absence of some toes. Mental retardation and growth failure are also present.[2878]
Lowry syndrome

1. Premature fusion of the coronal sutures with cryptorchidism.[3939]
2. Craniosynostosis and fibular aplasia (Lowry syndrome) A recessively inherited congenital syndrome characterized by these two features.[3939]

Sensenbrenner syndrome A rare syndrome manifesting premature fusion of cranial sutures with **dolichocephaly**, fine hair, impaired tooth formation, and brachydactyly.[3806]
Summitt syndrome A syndrome consisting of craniosynostosis, obesity, strabismus, and syndactyly.[6128]
Woon syndrome The congenital combination of craniosynostosis and absence of the thumbs.

---

craniosynostosis and fibular aplasia (Lowry syndrome) A recessively inherited congenital syndrome characterized by synostosis and bilateral fibular aplasia.[3939]

craniosynostosis and radial aplasia (Baller–Gerold syndrome) A recessively inherited congenital syndrome characterized by these two features:[351]

craniosynostosis, severe symmetrically deformed extremities, and cleft lip-palate syndrome See Chart C–28.

craniosynostosis with foot anomalies See Chart C–28.

craniosynostosis with 7p-karyotype See Chart C–28.

craniotabes (congenital cranial osteoporosis) Softening of the infantile skull in parasagittal, parietal, and vertical regions, considered to be caused by prolonged compression of the skull *in utero*. The condition is common, harmless, and temporary.

craniotelencephalic dysplasia A congenital dysmorphic syndrome characterized also by prominent frontal bossing, microphthalmia, hypoplasia of the optic nerves, **trigonocephaly**, **craniosynostosis**, **encephalocele**, hydrocephalus from **aqueduct stenosis**, **lissencephaly**, cerebellar atrophy, **agenesis of the corpus callosum**, and mental and developmental delay.[381]

craniotubular dysplasias Genetic hyperostotic and osteosclerotic disorders stemming from a defect in bone modeling[4045, 2501] with secondary effects upon the nervous system.

craniotubular hyperostoses Genetic hyperostotic and osteosclerotic disorders stemming from an active overgrowth of bone, and including **Camurati–Engelmann disease**.[4045]

craniovertebral anomalies (craniovertebral malformations) Congenitally determined abnormalities of the skull base and upper cervical spine. These include basilar impression, platybasia, occipitalization of the atlas, fusion of cervical vertebrae, and chronic atlantoaxial dislocation. They are common in patients with syringomyelia and cerebellar ectopias but, in other instances, may be asymptomatic or associated with postural loss in the arms, mirror movements, and vertical nystagmus with oscillopsia.[372]

craniovertebral malformations See **craniovertebral anomalies**.

cranium The membrane bones of the skull; all the skull bones above the skull base.

cranium bifidum A failure of fusion of the posterior midline portion of the skull, so that a bony cleft remains through which the brain may extrude (encephalocele).

crash migraine See **thunderclap headache** and **reversible cerebral vasoconstriction syndrome**.

creatine A muscle protein isolated in 1832 by Michel Chevreuil, a French chemist.

creatine kinase (CK) An enzyme catalyzing the reversible reaction: ATP + creatine = ADP + phosphocreatine, and thus responsible for energy production within muscle. Elevation of its levels in serum (M form) is a reliable indicator of damage to muscle membranes resulting from any cause.[4982]

creatine transporter deficiency An inborn air of metabolism caused by a defect in the X-linked creatine transporter gene mapped to Xq28. Affected males have expressive speech and language delay and mental retardation, seizures, developmental delay, and autistic behavior. Half of the female carriers also have learning disabilities.[5514]

Cree encephalitis A familial disease, possibly a viral infection, manifesting with severe mental retardation from birth, microcephaly, cerebral atrophy with white matter changes of panencephalitis with calcifications, and systemic immunological abnormalities (polyclonal hypergammaglobulinemia) leading to recurrent infections.[667]

Cree leukoencephalopathy A rapidly fatal syndrome of neonate Cree Indian children described in Quebec, and characterized by seizures, pyramidal signs, and mental and developmental delay associated with abnormal CNS myelination.[666] The brain pathology is similar to that of **central hypomyelination/vanishing white matter syndrome**.

Cree microcephaly with micromelia A congenital dysmorphic syndrome characterized by low birth weight, mesomelia of upper limbs, synostosis of the elbows, hypoplastic or absent radii and ulnae, absent fingers, and microcephaly.[3109]

creeping palsy See amyotrophic lateral sclerosis.

cremasteric reflex Contraction of the cremaster muscle with elevation of the homolateral testicle, in response to a scratch on the inside of the thigh ascending from around 3 inches (7.5 cm) below the inguinal crease and resulting from contraction of the dartos muscles in the overlying skin. This may be absent in a normal man but unilateral absence suggests a homolateral pyramidal lesion since it is a cutaneous reflex.

This superficial reflex is centered on L2 and may be lost in pyramidal tract lesions above that level, as shown by **Romberg** in 1853, as well as with scrotal pathology.

crescendo TIAs Repetitive ischemic attacks, most often due to hemodynamic phenomena in diseased small penetrating vessels. When cerebral infarction develops, it is usually lacunar and involves a single penetrating vessel, although restricted to the region of the internal capsule. The clinical manifestations usually affect the face, arm, and leg.[1687] See also **capsular warning syndrome**.

cretinism Retardation in physical and mental development due to dysgenesis or inability to synthesize thyroid hormone *in utero* or in early life.

Creutzfeldt, Hans-Gerhardt (1885–1964) German neuropsychiatrist. He studied medicine at Jena, Rostock, and Kiel and then served as a ship's surgeon. On returning to Germany, he studied psychiatry in Kiel but spent years in practice in Munich and Berlin before returning to Kiel as professor of psychiatry and neurology in 1938.

In 1920[1319] he described one case of the disease bearing his name while working with Spielmeyer in Munich. His patient, a 23-year-old woman, manifested tics, myoclonus, focal seizures, and pyramidal tract signs progressively over 1 year; this patient had two siblings who were mentally retarded and the reliability of the diagnosis is open to question, unlike the three patients of Jakob described in the following year, whose features are more in keeping with current concepts of the disease.

Creutzfeldt also published on the psychoses, multiple sclerosis, encephalitis, toxic diseases, and radioactive studies in CNS disease.[3717]

Creutzfeldt–Jakob disease (Jakob–Creutzfeldt disease, spastic pseudosclerosis, cortico-pallido-spinal degeneration, Heidenhain syndrome, subacute cerebral degeneration, human BSE, polio-encephalomyelopathy, subacute spongiform encephalopathy, subacute presenile polio-encephalopathy, subacute presenile spongy atrophy, subacute degenerative polioencephalopathy of the presenium) A rare, progressive, and fatal spongiform encephalopathy due to infection by a virus particle (**prion**).[5127]

The American Psychiatric Association (in *DSM-IV TR*)[172] suggested that the condition should be suspected in all cases of dementia that progress fairly rapidly over months to 1–2 years and that are accompanied or followed by multiple neurological symptoms, and that the triad of rapidly progressing, devastating dementia; pyramidal and extrapyramidal disease with myoclonus; and with a characteristic (triphasic wave) EEG is highly suggestive.

There usually is a progressive spastic paralysis of the limbs, accompanied by extrapyramidal signs with tremor, rigidity, and choreoathetoid movements. Numerous phenotypes are described, varying with the size of the causal virus particle. In some cases, such as the "amyotrophic" form, the neurological signs may precede the onset of the dementia. Ataxia, visual failure, muscle twitches, and upper motor neuron signs are also described, as are intrusion errors, perseveration, and periods of unresponsiveness even amounting to **akinetic mutism**.[5933]

Criteria for the diagnosis have been suggested.[4159] (See Chart C–29.) In the CSF, the presence of 14-3-3 protein (a cell surface signaling protein) is a sensitive but not a specific marker for CJD; any neurological injury such as an infarct, tumor, or infection can give a false positive result. The inclusion of this CSF protein in the criteria of Masters and colleagues (1979) improves the accuracy of clinical diagnosis. The presence of 14-3-3 protein in the CSF discriminates better between CJD and other rapidly progressive dementias than does the EEG pattern or the MRI.

In *variant* presentations, patients present with focal cortical deficits such as aphasia or visual disturbances.[5933]

Modified criteria, varying somewhat from those of Brandel and of Lanska[810] have also been suggested, as follows:

Progressive dementia over <2 years
At least two of the following:
Myoclonus
Visual or cerebellar signs
Pyramidal or extrapyramidal signs
Akinetic mutism
At least one of the two following laboratory features:
  Periodic sharp and slow wave complexes on the EEG
  14-3-3 protein present in the CSF
Pathological hallmarks are neuronal loss, spongy changes in the gray matter, and an astrocytic response.

Chart C–29. Suggested Criteria for the Diagnosis of Creutzfeldt–Jakob Disease

A. Sporadic
  1. *Definite:*
    - Neuropathologically confirmed and/or
    - Immunocytochemically confirmed PrP positive (Western blot) and/or
    - SAF (scrapie-associated fibrils)
  2. *Probable:*
    - Progressive dementia
    - Typical EEG
    - At least 2 of the following clinical features:
      myoclonus
      visual or cerebellar
      pyramidal/extrapyramidal
      akinetic mutism
  3. *Possible:*
    - Progressive dementia
    - 2 of the clinical features listed above
    - No EEC or atypical EEC
    - Duration <2 years

B. Accidental transmission
  - Progressive cerebellar syndrome in a pituitary hormone recipient
  - Sporadic CJD with a recognized exposure risk

C. Familial
  - Definite or probable CJD plus definite or probable CJD in a first-degree relative (World Health Organization)
  - Neuropsychiatric disorder plus disease-specific PRNP mutation

From Masters CL, Harris JO, Gajusdek DC, et al. Creutzfeldt–Jakob disease: Patterns of worldwide occurrence and the significance of familial and sporadic clustering. Ann Neurol *1979;5:177–88. Reproduced by kind permission of John Wiley and Sons. Inc.*

This is possibly the same condition as the **Stern–Garcin syndrome**, a rapidly progressive dementing illness described first by Dr. K. Stern in a 41-year-old patient admitted to the National Hospital under Dr. F.M.R. Walshe (and again by Raymond Garcin in 1962) with severe dementia and bilateral symmetrical degeneration of the thalamus.

Variant forms are described:

1. A form in which the cerebellar signs are preeminent initially[2465]
2. *Familial Creutzfeldt–Jakob disease*, dominantly inherited, occurring in about 10% of all cases (Baraitser[379] has summarized these reports)
3. Forms in which the duration of illness is greater than 2 years (less than 5% of all cases)
4. An *amyotrophic form* presenting with signs of upper and lower motor neuron involvement with early and conspicuous dementia[132]
5. **New variant Creutzfeldt–Jakob disease** (vCJD; **human bovine spongiform encephalopathy**) A human prion disease clinically, biochemically, and pathologically linked to bovine spongiform encephalopathy, manifesting the features of CJD and due to infection with the same strain of prion. Most patients are young adults. Neuropsychological tests show a combined cortical and subcortical dementia, with impaired performance being particularly prominent on tests of memory, executive function, speed of attention, and visuoperceptual reasoning.[3298]

   Beginning with depression and anxiety, social withdrawal, and peripheral sensory symptoms, it evolves into a syndrome of cerebellar ataxia, chorea or athetosis, and eventually dementia.. The EEG shows slow wave activity and the CSF may contain raised levels of 14-3-3 protein. MRI features include increased T2 weighted signals in the posterior thalami.[1255] See also **Alpers disease**.
6. **Heidenhain variant** A rare form with preponderant visual symptoms that may be isolated for a few weeks, before the disease develops more typical neurological features, EEG abnormalities, and evidence of 14-3-3 protein expression.[1975]

Web sites of value are http://cjddiagnosticcenter.com/, the Web site of the CJD Diagnostic and Research Center, which provides diagnostic services and information to physicians and families of CJD patients and supports research programs onthe cause of CJD; and www.ninds.nih.gov/disorders/cjd; www.who.int/mediacentre/factsheets/en//cjd.htm; and www.who.int/topics/creutzfeldtjakob_syndrome/en/, all of which provide information.

cri-du-chat syndrome (Lejeune syndrome, cat-cry syndrome) A syndrome of chromosomal dysgenesis (deletion of the short arm of chromosome 5) in which **hypertelorism**, microcephaly, severe mental and physical retardation, and facial dysmorphism are notable, and the child's cry is little more than a distant mew.[3767]

cri hydrencéphalique A brief, shrill wail intermittently uttered by children with hydrocephalus or meningitis, described first by Trousseau.[645]

cribriform (Lat, like a sieve, perforated) The ethmoid bone with its many holes merits the description—however, no more than the anterior or posterior perforated substance.

cribriform state A pathological finding, comprising dilatations of the perivascular spaces in the pallidum and putamen with smooth and clearly defined borders, containing one or more vessels which differentiates them from type I **lacunes** which are cavitating infarcts. See also **état marbré**.

Crichton-Brown, Sir James (1840–1938) Scottish physician who inherited his father's interest in psychiatry and the care of the mentally ill. He was at some time a colleague of **Hughlings-Jackson** at the West Riding Asylum, of which he was superintendent from 1866, and he established the research laboratory at Wakefield where **Ferrier** performed his early experiments in cerebral localization. He also founded the *West Riding Asylum Reports* (the first English psychiatric journal) in 1871, and with Jackson and others was a founder of ***Brain*** in 1878. He was elected a Fellow of the Royal Society in recognition of his work on mental disorders.

Crichton-Brown sign Tremor of the labial folds and the outer angles of the eyes in **general paresis of the insane**.

cricopharyngeal spasm (pharyngisimus) Spasm of the pharyngeal constrictor muscles, as in **globus hystericus** and **rabies**, and as a result of local irritation. See **pharyngisimus**.

Crighton Royal Assessment Scale A scale of use for the evaluation of patients whose mental deterioration makes clinical interviewing impossible. It is also used widely by nonmedical staff for the day-to-day assessment of change in behavior of such patients when undergoing therapy. This one combines simplicity of completion, high face validity, and interobserver reliability, but is, nevertheless, a relatively coarse measure of abilities.

Crigler–Najjar kernicterus A corencephalopathy associated with an inherited hyperbilirubinemic state. See **kernicterus**.

crises Commonly applied to acute attacks of pain in certain regions, lasting hours or days in patients with tabes dorsalis. Gastric, rectal, nephralgic, clitoral, vesical, urethral, bronchial, and laryngeal crises were described by Gowers.[2531]

Crisponi syndrome A lethal congenital syndrome characterized by contraction of the facial and neck muscles with opisthotonus, facial dysmorphism, camptodactyly, fever, and seizures, worsened by touching and with crying. See www.wustl.edu/neuromuscular.

cristae ampullaris Plumes of hair cells on the sensory neuroepithelium sited in the dilatations of the three semicircular canals.

Critchley, Macdonald (1900–1997) Incisive, insightful English neurologist with eclectic interests in neurology and its wider aspects, but specializing in the assessment of cortical functioning. His book on the parietal lobes[1329] was a classic from the day of its publication.

critical flicker fusion See **flicker fusion**.

critical illness A severe syndrome resulting from infection and with multiple organ failure. See **SIRS**.

critical illness myopathy (acute quadriplegic myopathy) Type II muscle fiber atrophy, loss of myosin-containing fibers, and muscle fiber necrosis presenting as an acute or subacute myopathy with muscle atrophy and diffuse flacid weakness, occurring in severely ill patients in status asthmaticus, following transplants, or with sepsis, all usually requiring intensive care for multiple organ dysfunction.

Three varieties of the condition are differentiated: acute necrotizing myopathy; a myopathy with selective loss of myosin filaments presenting as above; and a non-necrotizing "cachectic" myopathy.[3045] Diagnostic criteria emphasizing the electrodiagnostic features for a "probable" diagnosis and requiring histopathologic identification of myosin loss (as well as supportive nonpathologic features) for a "definite" diagnosis have been suggested for research protocols.

Suggested diagnostic criteria for critical illness myopathy are as follows (after Lacomis et al. 2000):[3634] The diagnosis of a "motor" variant of critical illness polyneuropathy should not be made without excluding myopathy with myosin loss histopathologically. Some patients may either be unable to recruit MUPs or have a preexisting or coexisting polyneuropathy and still have a myopathy. Therefore, we allow for diagnosis of "probable" or "possible" critical illness myopathy based upon a combination of major and supportive features even in the presence of low SNAP amplitudes or an equivocal needle electrode examination. Direct needle stimulation of muscle may in future be added as a major diagnostic feature and method of differentiating critical illness polyneuropathy from myopathy, perhaps even in place of histopathologic proof.

Proposed major diagnostic features for critical illness myopathy:

1. SNAP amplitudes >80 % of the lower limit of normal (LLN) in two or more nerves
2. Needle EMG with short-duration, low-amplitude MUPs with early or normal full recruitment, with or without fibrillation potentials
3. Absence of a decremental response on repetitive nerve stimulation
4. Muscle histopathologic findings of myopathy with myosin loss

Supportive features:

1. CMAP amplitudes <80 % LLN in two or more nerves without conduction block
2. Elevated serum CK (best assessed in the first week of illness)
3. Demonstration of muscle inexcitability

By definition, patients are or were critically ill and weakness should have started after the onset of critical illness. For a definite diagnosis of critical illness myopathy, patients should have all four major features. For probable critical illness myopathy, patients should have any three major features and one or more supportive feature. For possible critical illness myopathy, patients should have either major features 1 and 3, or 2 and 3, and one or more supportive feature. One may consider muscle biopsy if another myopathic process such as an inflammatory myopathy is suspected or if the histologic findings may affect management.

A second set of criteria are provided here, those of Bolton himself (2005)[729] as these are simpler in practice:

1. SNAP amplitudes more than 80% of the lower limits of normal
2. Needle EMG with short-duration, low-amplitude MUPs with early or normal. Full recruitment without fibrillation potentials
3. Abscess of a decremental response on repetitive nerve stimulation
4. Muscle histopathologic findings of myopathy with myosin loss
5. CMAP amplitudes <80% of the lower limit of normal in two or more nerves without conduction block
6. Elevated serum CK levels
7. Demonstration of muscle inexcitability

See also **acute quadriplegic myopathy**, **critical illness polyneuropathy**, **Hopkins syndrome**, and **SIRS**.

critical illness polyneuropathy A reversible, acute or subacute, generalized axonal sensorimotor peripheral neuropathy causing marked limb muscle weakness, wasting and hyporeflexia, affecting also the respiratory muscles and occurring in patients with a systemic inflammatory response (septic syndrome) and multiple organ failure, including septic encephalopathy. The necessary inducing agent is unknown.[6981]

Difficulty in weaning from a ventilator, hyporeflexia, and distal weakness are the usual presenting features. The cranial nerves are relatively spared.

EMG indicators of the condition include the presence of small polyphasic units with early full recruitment; reduced CMAP amplitudes; variable fibrillations; and occasionally reduced SNAPs or distal denervation suggesting CIDP or acquired sensorimotor axonal polyneuropathy.[4004] Such relative sural sparing (less involvement of sural SAPs than of those in the nerves of the arms) is a helpful diagnostic pointer.

The spectrum of neuromuscular disorders in such patients has been reviewed.[1075, 3045] See also **SIRS**, **Hopkins syndrome**, and **critical illness myopathy**.

Diagnostic criteria have been suggested by Bolton:[729]

1. The patient is critically ill with sepsis and multiple organ failure (SIRS)
2. There is difficulty weaning the patient from a ventilator after non-neuromuscular causes, such as heart and lung disease, have been excluded
3. Possible limb weakness
4. Electrophysiologic evidence of axonal motor and sensory polyneuropathy

critical perfusion pressure The difference between the mean systemic arterial pressure and the mean intracranial pressure; thus defining the pressure with which arterial blood is introduced into the cranial cavity.

crocodile tears

(Bogorad syndrome, gustatory lacrimation, gustolacrimal reflex)Lacrimation accompanying eating, usually as a late complication of facial palsy. The Arian theologian Asterios, seeking to explain why a crocodile sheds tears while eating, wrote in AD 340 that the animal was mourning the fact that the heads of children which he was consuming contained no meat.[5704] Hakluyt in 1600, in describing Sir John Hawkins' voyage of 1565, embarked upon a flight of fancy, claiming that the crocodile's "nature is ever, when he would have his prey, to cry and sob like a Christian body, to provoke them to come to him, and then he snatcheth at them, and thereupon came this proverb that is applied unto women when they weep, *lachrymae crocodili*, the meaning whereof is that as the crocodile . . . so doth the woman when she weeps." The syndrome was also described by Legendre.The physiological reason, adduced by the Russian physiologist F.A. Bogorad in 1928,[704] can be found in the identical innervation of the reptile's lacrimal and salivary glands. Following facial palsy in man, aberrant reinnervation may lead to the shedding of tears while eating, when salivation alone would have been appropriate. Presumably the regenerating parasympathetic fibers have been diverted through the greater superficial petrosal nerve to the otic ganglion, when they should have continued on in the chorda tympani to innervate the submandibular and submaxillary glands. The occurrence of crocodile tears thus indicates that the original lesion of the facial nerve must have been somewhat proximal.

Crohn disease

A gastrointestinal disorder associated in some cases with multiple sclerosis, cerebral vasculitis, epilepsy, myasthenia gravis, chronic inflammatory polyneuropathy, or myopathy.

Crome syndrome

(cataracts–renal tubular necrosis–encephalopathy) A fatal congenital dysmorphic syndrome characterized by cataract, seizures, microcephaly, cerebral and cerebellar atrophy, mental and developmental delay, and renal tubular necrosis.[1347]

Cross oculocerebral syndrome

(oculocerebral hypopigmentation syndrome) A recessively inherited congenital dysmorphic syndrome characterized also by generalized depigmentation of the skin and hair, cloudy corneas, microphthalmia, gum hypertrophy, high palate, nystagmus, pyramidal signs, athetosis, and mental and developmental delay.[1356]

cross talk

1. The activation of inactive nerve fibers by an action potential traveling in adjacent active fibers. The electrical transmission between fibers thus occurs at a false synapse (an **ephapse**). This has been proposed as the mechanism responsible for hemifacial spasm, and possibly for some neuralgias, gustatory lacrimation, and sweating.[2276] 2. In **kinesiologic EMG**, signals recorded from adjacent muscles.[19]

crossed adductor reflex

Contraction of the contralateral adductor muscles in response to a tap on the adductor (or quadriceps) tendon. The reflex is evidence of a pyramidal lesion above the L2 segment, but is also normally found in infants between 3 and 8 months of age.

crossed aphasia

The occurrence of aphasia and hemiplegia with a right hemisphere lesion in right-handers (or with a left hemisphere lesion in left-handers), and in subjects without a family history of left-handedness and without any clinical or imaging evidence of a left hemisphere lesion. Other right hemisphere functions may remain as usual.[2854]

This indicates either that handedness and language lateralization are not invariably linked, or that transcallosal **diaschisis** is a mechanism. The condition was known to **Hughlings-Jackson** but the term was introduced by Bramwell in 1899. The characteristics of the dysphasias are not different from those seen with lesions of the more appropriate hemisphere in other patients.

crossed cerebral-cerebellar diaschisis

Reduction of blood flow and energy metabolism in one cerebellar hemisphere following infarction of the contralateral cerebral hemisphere as a result of neuronal depression secondary to damage to the corticopontocerebellar pathways.[416, 1984] See **diaschisis**. This may be the mechanism for homolateral ataxia and crural paresis, formerly regarded as a lacunar syndrome.[2393]

crossed diplopia

That form of diplopia which is the result of **exotropia** and in which the false image is displaced away from the side of the paretic eye. See also **uncrossed diplopia** and **diplopia**.

crossed extensor reflex

(Philippson reflex) Extension of the hip and knee with plantar flexion of the ankle and toes of the opposite limb when the **flexor reflex** is being elicited. The child is placed in the supine position and the sole of the foot is stroked firmly; the opposite leg flexes and then extends, with adduction of the leg and extension and fanning of all the toes.[6898] The reflex is normally present in infancy but it disappears by 12 months of age.

crossed flexor reflex

Flexion of the hip and knee and dorsiflexion of the foot in the leg opposite to that stimulated in an attempt to elicit the ipsilateral flexor reflex.

crossed hemianopic hemispatial neglect

Failure to copy the left side of drawings and neglect of the items on the left side of the page in the **Line Bisection Test**, occurring when the subject with a severe callosal lesion holds the pencil in the right hand. These errors are not seen when the left hand is used. See also **crossed homonymous hemianopia**.

crossed hemiplegia See **pyramidal decussation syndrome**.

crossed homonymous hemianopia A varying hemianopic defect detected using static or kinetic perimetry apparatus, appearing on the side opposite that of the hand being used to push the switch of the perimeter. This (rare) condition has been described with severe callosal lesions.[3281]

crossed leg progression A peculiarity of gait whereby spasm in the hip adductors due to chronic pyramidal tract lesions (such as **spastic diplegia** and **Little disease**) leads to the subject walking with the legs tightly adducted or actually crossed one before the other.

crossed palsy See **alternating hemiplegia**.

crossed parabulbar syndrome Spastic hemiparesis, cerebellar ataxia, and trigeminal thermoanesthesia on one side and thermoanalgesia of the trunk and limbs on the other side, due to a lesion of the high cervical cord.[6340]

crossed reflexes The appearance of homologous muscle stretch reflex activity on the side opposite to that stimulated. They provide evidence of disinhibition at spinal segmental levels, and thus of bilateral pyramidal tract disease.

crossed spinoadductor reflex Adduction and inward rotation of the contralateral leg in response to the vibration set up by a tap on the anterior superior iliac spine; present in normal subjects and increased in patients with pyramidal disease.

crossed upgoing toe sign Dorsiflexion of the hallux on the abnormal side when the opposite, normal leg maintains flexion of the hip against resistance. This sign was described by Hindfelt et al. in 1976, but was only validated more recently.[6808] It represents a sign of an early or incomplete upper motor neuron lesion.

Crouzon, Octave (1874–1938) French physician with interests in pathology, genetics, and neurology who trained in Paris, where he was influenced by **Babiński**, **Marie**, and Janet. He was appointed as physician at the Hôtel Dieu and later at the **Salpêtrière**, where he investigated a range of neurological conditions including cerebellar disease, the muscle dystrophies, and topics in psychiatry. His interest in the social and legal aspects of disease led to the creation for him of a special *Chair d'Assistance medico-sociale* at the University of Paris.[2066] He first described *La Dysostose Cranio-faciale hereditaire* in 1906.[1357]

Crouzon syndromes Congenital dominantly inherited dysmorphic syndromes characterized by **craniosynostosis** affecting the coronal suture with resulting acrocephaly, prominent frontal bossing, absent auditory canals, **hypertelorism**, "parrot-beaked" profile of the nose, hypoplastic facial bones, high palate, oligodontia, malformations of the ossicles with mixed hearing loss, dwarfism, micrognathia, optic atrophy, strabismus, nystagmus, exophthalmos, hydrocephalus, callosal agenesis, and mental and developmental delay.[1358, 2499]

Five forms (maxillary, facial, cranial, and two combinations) may be differentiated according to the specific topography of the lesion.[4] The condition was first described by Oribasius (325–403) but may also have been recognized by Homer, whose hero Thersites was described as if so afflicted. See also **acrocephaly**, **oxycephaly**, **tower skull**, and **cranio-facial dysostosis**.

Crouzon–Crostophy–Gaucher syndrome See **Sturge–Weber syndrome**.

crowbar case Mr. Phineas **Gage**, an American railway foreman, was struck in the head by a tamping rod which did not kill him, but, entering the anterior cranial fossa from below, it extruded superiorly, effectively causing a frontal lobotomy. This led to the first description, by Dr. J. Harlow in 1848, of the **frontal lobe syndrome**. The changes in character and behavior of Mr. Gage as a result of the accident were severe: formerly described as pious, quiet, responsible, and hard-working, he became irreverent, profane, and unable to plan for the future or to hold down a job—he exhibited himself in a circus and was later a stagecoach driver in Chile.

crowded dens syndrome A condition of the elderly presenting with acute and severe neck pain; marked restriction of neck motion, particularly in rotation; the presence of inflammatory indicators such as an elevated C-reactive protein level; and calcium deposition around the odontoid process detected by computed tomography. There is no history of trauma and other inflammatory diseases and tumors are not present (Mula M, et al. *Neurology*, 2001;**56**:275).

crowded orbital apex syndrome The association of optic nerve lesions, retinopathy, and papilloedema secondary to intraorbital hypertension, the visual loss commonly being bilateral and progressive.

Visual-evoked responses and color perception tests are those most sensitive in diagnosis.

crowding of the optic disk Compression of the fibers of the optic nerve as the result of a small scleral canal; such horizontal crowding is considered likely to promote infarction in the case of an already compromised optic disk circulation.[4048]

Crowe, S. J. (1883–1955) American otolaryngologist who worked with **Cushing** and was later professor at Johns Hopkins.

Crowe (sign) Test 1. Swelling of the facial and retinal veins with manual compression of one jugular vein in the neck. A sign of occlusion of the contralateral jugular vein or of the transverse sinus above it. 2. Axillary freckling in **neurofibromatosis** is also known as the Crowe sign, but was described by a different physician of that name.

Crow–Fukase syndrome A **gammopathic neuropathy** manifesting polyneuropathy with lambda paraproteinemia, edema, clubbing of the digits, organomegaly, endocrinopathy, bone lesions, and hyperhidrosis.[1360] It is best regarded as part of the **POEMS** syndrome.

Cruchet, Jean-René (1875–1959) French pathologist and pediatrician, who trained and practiced in Bordeaux. His paper on 40 cases of **encephalitis lethargica** preceded by 13 days that of **von Economo**. Its clinical detail concerning initial extreme lassitude and expressionless facies, with slow recovery and motor deficits, and the types of the disease (mental, choreiform, convulsive, meningitic, hemiplegic, pontocerebellar, bulbar, and poliomyelitic) is excellent and the series was much larger than that of von Economo, who did, however, also note all the more important features of the disease. Cruchet's name has also been applied to **torticollis**, of which he gave a full account (of 357 cases!) in 1907.

cruciate hemiplegia See **pyramidal decussation syndrome**.

cruciate paralysis (alternate brachial diplegia) Disproportionate motor deficits involving both arms, with relative sparing of power in the legs, usually resulting from damage to the central part of the cervical spinal cord.[495] The syndrome is considered to result from involvement of those fibers destined for the cervical segments which decussate in the cord at a higher level than those destined for the lumbar segments.

Cruikshank, William Cumberland (1745–1800) Scottish-born surgeon, assistant to William Hunter and physician to Dr. Samuel **Johnson**. He forecast his own death from apoplexy, being aware of a thrilling sensation in the front of the left side of his head whenever he stooped forward. He had also been prone to attacks of sudden loss of memory and pallor, sneezing, and olfactory hallucinations which were precipitated by any form of strong emotional excitement.[6273]

Cruikshank disease Olfactory hallucinations, **angor animi**, and facial pallor in "complex partial" seizures. Presumably the latter features derive from the stimulation of autonomic regulating structures (amygdala) by the seizure discharge.

crural monoplegia Weakness of one leg as a result of stroke, with which a degree of mental confusion and cortical sensory loss are usually associated. The involved vessel is the paracentral branch of the anterior cerebral artery.

crural nerve The femoral nerve.

crural neuritis An acute, painful allergic motor neuropathy affecting nerves branching from the lumbar plexus. See also **acute brachial neuritis** and **lumbosacral plexopathy**.

crus (Lat, the leg or shin) A term applied to any leglike structure, often in the form of a V or an X; thus the **crus cerebri**.

crusta The lower anterior part of the crus, or cerebral peduncles, separated from the upper part (the tegmentum) by the substantia nigra.

crutch palsy Damage mainly to the lower fibers of the brachial plexus as a result of bearing excessive weight on a crutch in the axilla. The clinical impairment of function is mainly in ulnar distribution. Weir **Mitchell** described this first in emaciated U.S. Civil War veterans.

Cruveilhier, Jean (1791–1874) French surgeon and pathological anatomist who was born in Limoges and trained in Paris under **Dupuytren.** He held chairs in surgery and in descriptive and pathological anatomy, the latter at the **Salpêtrière** where he established neuropathology as a major resource upon which **Charcot** and others built further.

In so doing, he differentiated intrinsic from extrinsic cord tumors and gave the first descriptions of cerebellopontine angle tumors, the appearances of multiple sclerosis in the spinal cord, red and white infarcts, sinus thrombosis, the Chiari malformation, cerebral tumors, and brainstem hemorrhages, publishing many of these accounts in his monumental book *The Pathological Anatomy of the Human Body* (Paris, 1829–1842). He also gave a good account of **amyotrophic lateral sclerosis** (once known as Cruveilhier atrophy) in 1853, but already described in 1849 by Aran and Duchenne some 20 years before Charcot's description[2120] and published an atlas of types of cerebral atrophies, recognizing micro- and hemi-atrophy, porencephaly, hydrocephalus, and cerebral dysgenesis between 1835 and 1842.

Cruveilhier atrophy See **amyotrophic lateral sclerosis**.

Cruveilhier palsy See **amyotrophic lateral sclerosis**.

crying seizures See **dacrystic epilepsy**.

cryobulinemia Conditions characterized by the presence of a serum protein, usually IgG or IgM, which precipitates on cooling and dissolves on warming to body temperatures. In *essential cryoglobulinemia* no associated disease is present; but in the *secondary* form, the condition is associated with monoclonal or polyclonal gammopathies. Clinically, purpura, Raynaud phenomenon, arthralgia, nephropathy, and neuropathy are the commoner manifestations and encephalopathy is rare.

cryoglobulinemic neuropathy See **gammopathic neuropathy, relapsing ischemic encephalo-enteropathy**, and **cryoglobulinemia**.

cryptic vascular malformations Small arteriovenous malformations in the cortex and white matter, considered to be present in the brains of 4% of those suffering intracerebral hemorrhages, but usually destroyed by bleeding.[3561]

crypto- (Gr, hidden) Prefix denoting hidden.

cryptococcal meningitis (Busse–Buschke disease) A chronic leptomeningitis due to blood-borne infection with the yeast *Cryptococcus neoformans*, a common soil organism found in bird excrement. Granulomas may also occur. Clinically, it is marked by headache, nausea and vomiting, meningism, fever, and disturbance of balance, gait, and vision with chronically raised intracranial pressure and sometimes seizures and focal signs. The CSF shows pleocytosis and glucose levels are reduced; the yeast is shown well using india ink preparations.[1481]

The condition is unusually common and rapidly progressive among immunocompromised subjects, such as those with HIV infection, in whom the clinical features are relatively silent.[1522] See also **torulosis**.

cryptogenic drop attacks **Drop attacks** occurring as an occasional isolated symptom while walking, in perhaps 3% of adult women. They have no known cause nor associated pathology and bear a good prognosis. Matthews and Stevens noted that "extinction of the ego by intrusion of a forbidden erotic thought" had been put forward as being etiologically relevant, but they did not choose to investigate this theory.[6052]

cryptogenic epilepsies Focal (partial) or generalized unprovoked seizures or epilepsies in which no factor associated with increased risk of seizures has been identified. This group includes patients who do not conform to the criteria for the symptomatic or idiopathic categories.[1265]

cryptogenic myoclonic epilepsy

See **myoclonus**.

cryptogenic sensory polyneuropathy

A slowly progressive neuropathy of later life characterized by pain, symmetrical numbness, and paresthesias in the distal extremities (mainly the legs) without weakness and with no identified cause. The prognosis is generally favorable. Diagnosis is by exclusion of other causes; it is the residual diagnosis in perhaps one-third of patients referred for symptoms of neuropathy and there are probably many causes for this syndrome. The pathology is almost always axonal and the diagnosis is assisted using intraepidermal nerve fiber density measurement.[6848]

cryptophthalmia

A rare, recessively inherited craniofacial malformation characterized by complete fusion of the upper and lower eyelids and absence of the eyelashes, so that there is an unbroken reach of skin between the face and the forehead. The underlying eyes may be well enveloped but are frequently disorganized. Other facial dysmorphisms are commonly present. The condition was reported first by Zehender in 1872 (cited by Stricker et al.[4]).

cryptophthalmos syndrome

A recessively inherited congenital syndrome characterized by overgrowth of the skin down over the eyes, one or both of which are completely covered, with syndactyly of the fingers or toes.[6118, 6962]

CSF fistula headache

Headache resulting from leakage of CSF, with resultant traction upon the basal (and other) pain-sensitive meninges. Diagnostic criteria have been defined:

A. Headache that worsens within 15 min after sitting or standing, with at least one of the following and fulfilling criteria C and D:
   1. Neck stiffness
   2. Tinnitus
   3. Hypacusis
   4. Photophobia
   5. Nausea

B. A known procedure or trauma has caused persistent CSF leakage with at least one of the following:
   1. Evidence of low CSF pressure on MRI (e.g., pachymeningeal enhancement)
   2. Evidence of CSF leakage on conventional myelography, CT myelography, or cisternography
   3. CSF opening pressure <60 mmH_2O in sitting position

C. Headache develops in close temporal relation to CSF leakage

D. Headache resolves within 7 days of sealing the CSF leak

From the International Classification of Headache Disorders (Headache Classification Committee of the International Headache Society. *Cephalalgia* 2004;24[Suppl 1]) by kind permission of Dr. Jes Olesen, the International Headache Society and Wiley-Blackwell Publications.

See also **spontaneous intracranial hypotension**; its headache is identical.

CSF tap test

Removal of up to 100 ml of CSF as a diagnostic test and therapeutic trial in **normal pressure hydrocephalus**. Improvement in gait and intellectual functions helps in predicting improvement from shunt surgery but the reliability of the test is questioned.

CT scan

See **computerized axial tomography**.

ctenoids

See **fourteen- and six-Hz-positive burst pattern**.

C-trigonocephaly syndrome

A congenital dysmorphic syndrome characterized by strabismus, facial hemangiomas, congenital cardiac anomaly, pulmonary segmentation defects, cryptorchid testes, abnormal palmar creases, polydactyly and syndactyly of fingers and toes, joint contractures, multiple joint dislocations, hypotonia, seizures, trigonocephaly, cutis laxa, and mental and developmental delay.[381]

Cuban optic neuropathy

An epidemic neuropathy affecting both the optic and the peripheral (mainly sensory) nerves, sometimes associated with deafness, ataxia, and pyramidal signs and likely due to the combination of malnutrition and tobacco smoking in those affected.[1368] The clinical features closely resemble those of **Leber hereditary optic neuropathy**.

The United States' "Cuban Democracy Act" has been blamed for occurrence of the condition.[5362]

cubital tunnel syndrome

Compression of the ulnar nerve above, behind or just below the medial epicondyle with dysfunction of the nerve at that site due to conduction block. The signs associated are weakness and wasting of the intrinsic hand muscles supplied by the nerve (hypothenar muscles, adductor pollicis, and interossei) and numbness of the ulnar 1½ digits and palm on their anterior aspect. The flexor carpi ulnaris and the ulnar half of the flexor digitorum profundus are usually innervated by a branch of the nerve taking off above the cubital tunnel and so are likely to be spared.

Tardy ulnar palsy was the term applied by Mouchet in 1914 to the occurrence of this condition remotely following fracture of the humerus.

Cautions about anterior transposition of the nerve in cases of compression at the elbow sites have been raised and decompression advocated as a safer operation.[992] A useful Web site is www.handsurgeon.com/cubital.html.

cuff compression test

The provocation of symptoms in **carpal tunnel syndrome** by constriction of the upper arm by a blood pressure cuff inflated above systolic pressure.

Cullen, William

(1710–1790) Scottish surgeon who described the bruising behind the ear suggesting the presence of a fracture of the base of the skull.

Cumings, John Nathaniel

(1906–1974) English pathologist at the National Hospital, where he became professor of chemical pathology at the Institute of Neurology. He is best remembered for his studies of the chemical pathology of the lipidoses and leukodystrophies, and for his development of the specialty of clinical chemical pathology as a major area of research and clinical service.

cuneate fasciculus and nucleus

(Burdach's column) The lateral of the two posterior columns of the spinal cord, described in 1806 by Karl Frederich Burdach (1776–1847), a German anatomist and physiologist.[5619]

cupulolithiasis The aggregation of detached sediment from the macula of the utricle upon the cupula of the posterior semicircular canal, rendering it sensitive to changes in static head position and thus inducing positional vertigo.[819]

Current Neurology (*Curr Neurol*) A neurological review book series. Web site: www.iospress.nl/loadtop/load.php?isbn=cn.

Current Opinion in Neurology (*Curr Opin Neurol*) A neurological review/update journal. Web site: www.co-neurology.com/.

Curry syndrome See **vertebral dysplasia-spinal dysraphism**.

cursive epilepsy Seizures with a focus in the temporal lobe, in which the subject runs.[3777, 5742]

curtain sign Displacement of the whole of the posterior pharyngeal wall toward the healthy side when its mucosa is stimulated by the examiner. This is a feature of bulbar weakness, as in **Vernet syndrome**.

Curtius, Friedrich (1896–1975) German physician.

Curtius syndrome See **congenital hemihypertrophy**.

curvilinear bodies Intra-neuronal or intramuscular inclusions seen on electron microscopy in **lipofuscinosis**.

Cushing, Harvey Williams (1869–1939) American neurosurgeon, educated successively at Yale, Harvard, and Johns Hopkins, where his surgical promise led to intensive and personalized training from Halsted and where he learned his neurology from **Osler**. He also trained with Kocher in Berne. Cushing served with the British Royal Army Medical Corps and the American Army Medical Corps during World War I, when ironically he attended Osler's only son at his death in battle. His monumental work was done as Moseley Professor of Surgery at Harvard and as Sterling Professor of Neurology at Yale.

He is regarded as the father of modern neurosurgery, not only for his technical skill and practical innovations but also for his careful research into, among other topics, the pituitary gland and its diseases, cerebellopontine angle tumors, the CSF (*The Third Circulation*, 1926), classification of gliomas and meningiomas (*Intracranial Tumours*, 1932), and the history of medicine; his life of **Osler** won him a Pulitzer Prize in 1925. Nevertheless, some of his publications incorporated the observations of such associates as **Dandy** and **Bailey** without taking proper care to acknowledge them. His chapter on the "Surgery of the Head" was the first major American review of neurosurgery. He was a founder of the **Society of Neurological Surgeons** and was generally regarded as a leading citizen in medicine, not only in the Americas but throughout the world.[7] The importance of his research is indicated by the next five entries.

Cushing response (reflex) The reflex maintenance of cerebral perfusion pressure by an increase in mean arterial blood pressure in response to a decrease in medullary perfusion.[1389]

Cushing syndrome
1. Hyperadrenocorticism secondary to a chromophobe or basophil adenoma of the pituitary gland, although other causes produce similar features.[1393] *Myopathy* is a complication. See also **Nelson syndrome**.
2. Primary optic atrophy with bitemporal hemianopsia due to a sellar or suprasellar tumor. See **chiasmal syndrome**.[1392]
3. (cerebellopontine angle syndrome) Nystagmus, tinnitus, deafness, diminished corneal reflex, VI and VII cranial nerve palsies, hoarseness, dysphagia, headache, and ipsilateral cerebellar signs due to compression by a mass lesion such as an acoustic **Schwannoma**.[1390]

Cushing triad The association of systemic hypertension, bradycardia, and slow and irregular respirations seen in patients with increased intracranial pressure, at a late stage.

Cushing tumor 1. **medulloblastoma** A solid malignant cerebellar neoplasm which consists of spongioblastic and neuroblastic cells.[333] 2. See **meningioma**.[1391]

Cushing–Bailey–Cobb syndrome See **Sturge–Weber syndrome**.

cutaneocerebral angioma See **Sturge–Weber syndrome**.

cutaneomeningospinal angiomatosis A syndrome characterized by vascular malformations in the spinal cord, presenting with spasticity and other evidence of myelopathy, and brain nevi or capillary and cavernous hemangiomas, causing seizures and focal deficits. See **Cobb syndrome**.

cutaneous albinism and deaf-mutism An X-linked syndrome of sensorineural deafness and hypomelanosis of the skin.[4064]

cutaneous albinism, ataxia, and peripheral neuropathy A syndrome in which these features occur, sometimes with spastic paraparesis as well.[3867]

cutaneous allodynia Pain resulting from a nonnoxious stimulus to normal skin due to a transient increase in the responsiveness (i.e., sensitization) of central pain neurons that process information arising from intracranial structures and skin, as in migraine.[952]

cutaneous meningeal melanosis See **incontinentia pigmenti**.

cutaneous reflexes Motor activity occurring reflexly in response to stimulation of skin or mucous membranes. They include the palmar, scapular and interscapular, superficial abdominal, gluteal, plantar, and superficial anal reflexes. The first description was that of **Gowers** in 1888.[2531] See **superficial reflexes** and **cutaneous reflex**.

cutis laxa, retardation, and corneal opacity See **de Barsy syndrome**.

cutis laxa with mental and physical retardation A recessively inherited congenital dysmorphic syndrome characterized by low birth weight, dwarfism, hypertelorism, dislocation of the hips, laxity of the skin, delayed closure of the fontanelles with wide cranial sutures, and mental and developmental delay.[5258] See **Ehlers–Danlos syndrome**.

cutis verticis gyrata with acromegaloid appearance and leukoma A congenital dysmorphic syndrome characterized by tall stature, frontal bossing, cloudy corneas, prominent mandible, large hands with abnormal dermatoglyphic patterns, macrocephaly, and cutis gyrata (abnormal growth of the skin resulting in antero-posterior ridges and furrows) of the scalp.[81] The primary form is associated with a congenital statis encephalopathy and manifests chronic seizures. The secondary form occurs as a result of infiltration of the skin in the context of systemic disease without neurological disorder.

In a *variant* condition, *cutis verticis with Lennox syndrome*, seizures accompany the above findings.

cutis verticis with Lennox syndrome See **cutis verticis gyrata with acromegaloid appearance and leukoma**.

cycas circinalis The false sago palm, a tree growing in the Western Pacific, the seeds of which contain a neurotoxin considered a likely cause of **lytico-bodig**.

cycle The complete sequence of potential changes undergone by individual components of a sequence of regularly repeated EEG waves or complexes, or by physiological functions such as pupillary constriction and sleep.

cyclic eosinophilic myositis A syndrome characterized by muscular swelling, induration, and discomfort with weight gain and malaise, associated with high levels of IgE, creatine kinase, and eosinophils and with biopsy evidence of eosinophilic polymyositis. The symptoms recur on a 4- or 5-week cycle.[6171]

cyclic esotropia A rare circadian form of strabismus characterized by 1- to 3-day long periods of esotropia, followed by similar periods of normal ocular function. The condition usually occurs spontaneously in small children; its cause is not known.

cyclic insomnia Periodic and repetitive disturbances in sleeping, usually as a result of psychiatric disturbances, drug abuse, or alcoholism.

cyclic migraine The occurrence of well-regulated episodes of migraine headaches cycling over time.[4277]

cyclic oculomotor palsy (Axenfeld–Schürenberg syndrome, cyclic oculomotor paralysis) Periodic contraction and dilation of the pupil on a 1–2 min cycle. It is rare syndrome, occurring particularly in the first year of life in which a complete or partial III nerve palsy alternates with brief spasms of III cranial nerve hyperfunction.[3895]

The periodic paroxysmal unilateral III nerve paresis causes mydriasis, blurred vision, diminution or absence of eye movements, and complete ptosis, occurring for up to 3 min at a time in bouts lasting hours or days, while during the periods of overactivity there is lid retraction and miosis.[441]

The condition was first described in 1894 by Rampoldi. See also **misdirection syndrome**.

cyclic oculomotor paralysis See **cyclic oculomotor palsy**.

cyclic oculomotor spasm (springing pupil type III) A rare abnormality characterized by pupillary dilatation, ptosis, and extraocular muscle paresis after congenital or early acquired III nerve palsy, alternating after some years with periods of miosis and retraction of the upper lid during sleep and wakefulness. The cause may be aberrant regeneration.[2699]

cyclic sympathetic spasm A rare syndrome characterized by periodic dystonia of one limb with homolateral mydriasis, alternating with normal limb tone and a Horner syndrome, described in association with a spinal cord lesion.[3936]

cyclic vomiting A stereotypical childhood syndrome of recurrent episodic nausea and vomiting, often with associated pallor, lethargy, and photophobia,[406] changing into a more typical migraine syndrome with increasing age. There is complete resolution of symptoms between attacks. The condition is considered to represent a **migraine equivalent**. Diagnostic criteria have been defined:

A. At least 5 attacks fulfilling criteria B and C
B. Episodic attacks, stereotypical in the individual patient, of intense nausea and vomiting lasting from 1 h to 5 days
C. Vomiting during attacks occurs at least four times per hour for at least 1 h
D. Symptom-free between attacks
E. Not attributed to another disorder

From the International Classification of Headache Disorders (Headache Classification Committee of the International Headache Society. *Cephalalgia* 2004;24[Suppl 1]) by kind permission of Dr. Jes Olesen, the International Headache Society and Wiley-Blackwell Publications.

cyclists' palsy Distal compression of the ulnar nerve, first described in 1896 by Destot. Weakness and wasting of the muscles supplied by the deep branch of the nerve results, presumably from a prolonged period of compression of the nerve (in the region of Guyon's canal) by the handlebars.[4713] Compression more proximally, with damage to the superficial branch, leads to sensory symptoms in the ulnar 1½ fingers.

The syndrome is also known by the name of Ramsay **Hunt**, who described it (not in a cyclist) in 1908.

cyclopia A developmental malformation in which, as a result of failure of the forebrain to divide into cerebral hemispheres (**holoproscencephaly**), there is a single orbital cavity with a proboscis projecting above it.[379] The lateral ventricles are fused and midline structures may be either absent or incomplete. The malformation was described in the character Polyphemus in Homer's *Odyssey*.

cycloplegia Paralysis of both the pupilloconstrictors and the ciliary body, thus preventing miosis as a result of accommodation or light stimulation.

cyclorotation See **ocular torsion**.

cylindrocephalic Having a long (thus cylindrical) head.

cylindroma (plexiform sarcoma) An adenoid cystic carcinoma arising in the orbit and stomach, which in the former site may present with unilateral cranial neuropathy.[4145]

cylindromatosis (turban tumors) A syndrome of cystic ear pinnae, with conductive deafness and cysts and tumors of the face and scalp.[381]

cymbal-players shoulder An **overuse syndrome** presenting with shoulder pain. Deafness is not reported as associated with the syndrome.

cynic spasm (from Gr, a dog) A snarl, the muscles of one side of the face only being contracted to display the teeth.

cystathioninuria See **cystathionine deficiency**.

cystathionase deficiency (cystathioninuria) An inherited enzymatic deficiency metabolic disorder leading to a failure to break down cystathionine. The clinical features may include mental and developmental delay, signs of metabolic acidosis, and thrombocytopenia.[2780]

cystiathionine beta-synthetase deficiency See **homocystinuria**.

cystic leukoencephalopathy without megalencephaly A syndrome of nonprogressive encephalopathy with normo- or microcephaly, presenting clinically with severe psychomotor impairment. The MRI shows bilateral cysts in the anterior part of the temporal lobe and white matter abnormalities with abnormal myelination and symmetrical lesions in frontal and occipital periventricular regions.[2862]

cystic dilatation of occipital horn The occurrence of complex partial seizures associated with cystic dilatation of the posterior part of one lateral ventricle, the initial event occurring in the neonatal period as a result of occlusion of one posterior cerebral artery. The seizure disorder occurs years later.[5265]

cystic leukoencephalopathy without megalencephaly A nonprogressive, recessively inherited encephalopathy marked by normo- or microcephaly and the early onset of severe psychomotor impairment. MRI shows bilateral cysts in the anterior temporal lobes and white matter abnormalities with pericystic abnormal myelination and symmetric lesions in frontal and occipital periventricular regions.[2862]

cystic myelopathy (post-traumatic syringomyelia) Cavitations within the spinal cord following serious cord injury. The neurological features of myelopathy are not specific. Cord compression, a tense syrinx at the cervical vertebral fracture site, and kyphosis are associated with enlargement of the intraspinal cyst.[5665]

cysticercosis A systemic infection frequently causing infestation of the brain with the larvae of *T. solium*, the adult pork tapeworm, for which man is the definitive host. Infection is sometimes asymptomatic but, if the nervous system is invaded, the major clinical results are seizures, intracranial hypertension, dementia, stroke-like syndromes, myelopathy, and evidence of meningeal inflammation, usually occurring only after a long incubation period. Multiple intracranial calcifications are often demonstrable on CT scanning. The condition, although uncommon, is nevertheless the most common parasitic disease affecting the CNS and is mainly seen in Hispanic people.[4206, 4779] Diagnostic criteria for human cysticercosis have been suggested and are reproduced from Del Brutto et al. © (1996)[1331] by kind permission of Elsevier Science.

Absolute criteria
- Histologic demonstration of the parasite
- Direct visualization of the parasite by fundoscopic examination
- Evidence of cystic lesions showing the scolex on CT or MRI*

Major criteria
- Evidence of lesions suggestive of neurocysticercosis on neuroimaging studies*
- Positive immunologic tests for the detection of anticysticercal antibodies**
- Plain X-ray films showing “cigar-shaped” calcifications in thigh and calf muscles

Minor criteria
- Presence of subcutaneous nodules (without histologic confirmation)
- Evidence of punctuate soft tissue or intracranial calcifications on plain X-ray films
- Presence of clinical manifestations suggestive of neurocysticercosis***
- Disappearance of intracranial lesions after a trial with anticysticercal drugs

Epidemiological criteria
- Individuals coming from or living in an area where cysticercosis is endemic
- History of frequent travel to cysticercosis-endemic areas
- Evidence of a household contact with *T. solium* infection

*CT or MRI showing cystic lesions, ring-enhancing lesions, parenchymal brain calcifications hydrocephalus and abnormal enhancement of the leptomeninges, and myelograms showing multiple filling defects in the column of contrast medium.

**Serum immunoblot developed by the Centers for Disease Control and Prevention, and CSF immunosorbent assay.

***Epilepsy, focal neurologic signs, intracranial hypertension, and dementia.

cystinosis A recessively inherited error of metabolism (a lysosomal storage disorder) characterized by the deposition of cystine crystals in the corneas, white blood cells, and bone marrow, with impairment of water resorption by the kidney, leading to renal failure and hypophosphatemic rickets. Retinopathy, growth retardation, and distal vacuolar myopathy are also described in this condition.[1112, 5349]

cystinuria A recessively inherited inborn error of metabolism in which there is impaired intestinal and renal transport of dibasic amino acids and urinary excretion of excessive amounts of cystine with stone formation.

Neurological complications include myopathy, a syndrome resembling multiple sclerosis, mental retardation, and psychiatric disturbances; pigmentary retinopathy, pyramidal and extrapyramidal degeneration, and deaf-mutism are often associated.[670]

cystometry The graphic representation of pressure as a function of vesical volume; the patient voids and then is catheterized, after which fluid is infused into the bladder. As the fluid goes in, he reports in turn the first sensation of bladder fullness, the first urge to urinate, and the time of onset of the first severe urge to void, while the intravesical pressure is monitored throughout.

cytoarchitectonics The design of the cellular characteristics of the cortex, which varies in different brain regions and allows mapping of the cortex and some ascriptions of specialized functions to certain areas. See H. **Vogt**.

cytochrome b (complex III) deficiency A mitochondrial disease marked by deficiency of this enzyme which normally functions in the respiratory transport chain. Clinically, exercise-induced muscle pain, cramping, and weakness are present but progressive over years, with a marked increase in serum lactic acid levels following minor exertion.[4480]

cytochrome c oxidase The enzyme responsible for catalyzing the transfer of electrons from cytochrome C to oxygen, resulting in the generation of water.

Deficiency of the enzyme causes a back-up of electrons to occur, so that substances higher up the metabolic chain remain in a reduced (nonoxidized) form (e.g., NADH rather than NAD^+) and production of ATP is arrested.

cytochrome c oxidase deficiency

A mitochondrial disease marked by deficiency of this enzyme normally functioning in the respiratory transport chain. Clinically, severe hypotonia and respiratory muscle weakness affect infants with lactic acidosis, aminoaciduria, glycosuria, and proteinuria.[1645] Other phenotypes include those of **Leigh disease**, transient, chronic, or severe forms of infantile myopathy, MERRF, and **Kearns–Sayre syndrome**.

In an autosomal recessive form, stroke-like episodes have been recorded.[4489]

cytoid bodies

Retinal swellings due to axonal enlargement within the nerve fiber layer, occurring as a consequence of ischemia. See **cotton wool spots**.

cytomegalovirus infections

The organism has been described as an ubiquitous agent with protean clinical manifestations. Infection is a common condition of infants and in some cases leads to microcephaly, psychomotor retardation, seizures, chorioretinitis, or deafness. It is less commonly a cause of neurological problems in adults, but is increasing as a result of infection of the immunocompromised.[822] After childhood, acute infectious polyneuropathy, retinopathy, and meningoencephalitis are the most common neurological presentations.

The role of preceding cytomegalovirus infection in the genesis of many other neurological conditions remains unproved.[348]

cytomegalovirus polyradiculitis

See **HIV-associated lumbosacral polyradiculopathy**.

cytoplasmic bodies

Small periodic acid-Schiff-positive, eosinophilic masses of actin filaments within myofibrils in normal as well as variously diseased muscles, such as some cases of dermatomyositis and in the following conditions.

cytoplasmic body myopathies

(desmin-storage myopathy) An uncommon dominantly inherited **myofibrillar myopathy** characterized by proximal myopathic weakness and the presence of intracytoplasmic inclusion bodies originating from the Z lines in muscle biopsy specimens. The condition presents in later adult life or in childhood with facial, neck, proximal, truncal, spinal, or cardiac muscle weakness, and with a progressive course. The muscle stretch reflexes and serum creatine kinase levels may be normal. Muscle biopsy specimens show fiber variations and displaced nuclei, fibrosis, and cytoplasmic bodies.[4927] The following entries are abstracted from the Neuromuscular Web site www.neuro.wustl.edu/neuromuscular/maltbrain.html at Washington University, St. Louis, by courtesy of Dr. Alan Pestronk:

1. *Severe limb-girdle type* A recessively inherited form with onset in infancy or childhood of hypotonia and proximal weakness, skeletal abnormalities, respiratory insufficiency, and death in early adult life.
2. *Mild limb-girdle type* A dominantly inherited form with onset in adolescence of slowly or nonprogressive limb-girdle weakness.
3. *Myopathy with proximal weakness and early respiratory muscle involvement (Type I)*6 A dominantly inherited form mapped to 2q24–q31 (similar to tibial muscular dystrophy) with onset in adult life of girdle and diaphragmatic weakness with early involvement of the neck flexors. Serum CK levels are normal or slightly elevated. Muscle biopsy shows bodies containing actin in type I muscle fibers.
4. *Myopathy with proximal weakness and early respiratory muscle involvement (Type II)* A dominantly inherited form mapped to 2q21, with onset in young adult life of girdle and diaphragmatic weakness. Serum CK levels are normal. Muscle biopsy shows the presence of cytoplasmic bodies containing actin and desmin in type I muscle fibers.
5. *Distal type* A dominantly inherited form with onset of proximal and distal weakness in late adult life, progressing to respiratory failure and with cardiomyopathy producing heart block arrhythmias and congestive heart failure. Serum CK levels are normal or slightly elevated, the EMG myopathic with complex repetitive discharges, and muscle biopsy characterized by the presence of myofibrillary inclusions in the cytoplasm of type I muscle fibers.

See also **myofibrillar myopathy** and **distal myopathies**.

cytoplasmic body neuromyopathy

A sporadic chronic progressive neuromyopathy characterized by early neck weakness, weight loss, respiratory failure, fatigability, headache with increased intracranial pressure, dyspnea, somnolence, the presence of cytoplasmic bodies in type I muscle fibers, and an axonal polyneuropathy.[3213]

The difference between this condition and **cytoplasmic body myopathy** is not clear.

cytosol tyrosine aminotransferase deficiency

A rare diffuse encephalopathy resulting from this enzymatic defect, characterized clinically by midline clefting, microcephaly, and severe mental retardation.[3383]

cytosolic receptors

Receptors found on the surface of some tumor cells, able to bind sex hormones in the cytoplasm.

cytotoxic cerebral edema

Swelling of brain parenchymal cells as a result of damage to the sodium–potassium exchange pump mechanism, leading to accumulation of intracellular water. This is typically seen following hypoxia-ischemia or metabolic (toxic) damage.

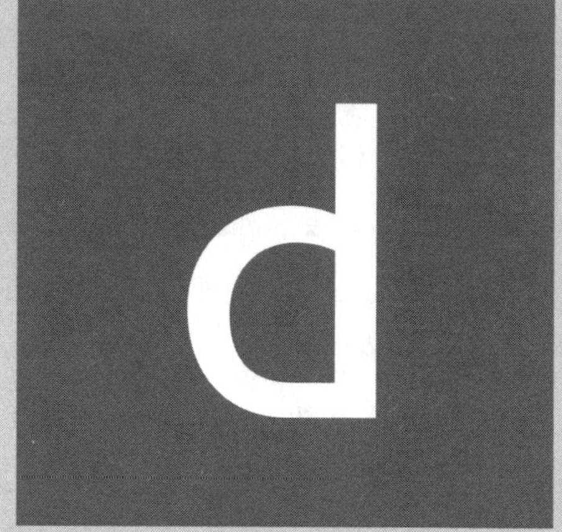

Da Vinci, Leonardo (1452–1519) Italian artist, anatomist, engineer, and writer. Analysis of his writing and drawing techniques have suggested that he is the model for disconsolate left-handers, but this may have been an effect of a right hemiparesis acquired later in life. However, most of his script was in mirror-writing, regarded by the **Vogts** as the natural form of script for sinistrals.[5641]

His anatomical drawings were lost until discovered by William Hunter, the English surgeon, in 1784.

D'Acosta disease See **altitude sickness**.

Da Costa syndrome See **chronic fatigue syndrome** and **hyperventilation syndrome**.

DACE syndrome See **dystonia**.

dacryo-(Gr, to weep) A prefix denoting the association with the lacrimal gland or tears.

dacrystic seizures (from Gr, shouting out loud) (quiritarian epilepsy) Epileptic attacks in which the patient weeps; described rarely in seizures with temporal lobe foci.[4754, 5742]

d-glyceric aciduria An aminoacidopathy causing very atypical **progressive myoclonus epilepsy**. See **glyceric aciduria**.

dactyl-(Gr, a finger) A prefix denoting an association with the finger.

DADS See **distal acquired demyelinating symmetric neuropathy**.

Daentl syndrome A congenital syndrome manifesting as short stature, blue sclerae, nephropathy, the **Chiari malformation**, and hydrocephalus.

Dagnini, G. (b. 1905) Italian physician, professor of medical pathology at Bologna.

Dagnini sign (extension-adduction reflex) Percussion of the radial aspect of the dorsum of the hand leads to extension of the wrist in patients with a pyramidal lesion of that limb.

Dale, Sir Henry (b. 1875) English physiologist and pharmacologist who differentiated the nicotinic and muscarinic effects of acetylcholine and clarified the question of the transmission of nerve impulses, demonstrated acetylcholine release at motor nerve endings, and identified oxytocin as an important secretion of the posterior pituitary gland.

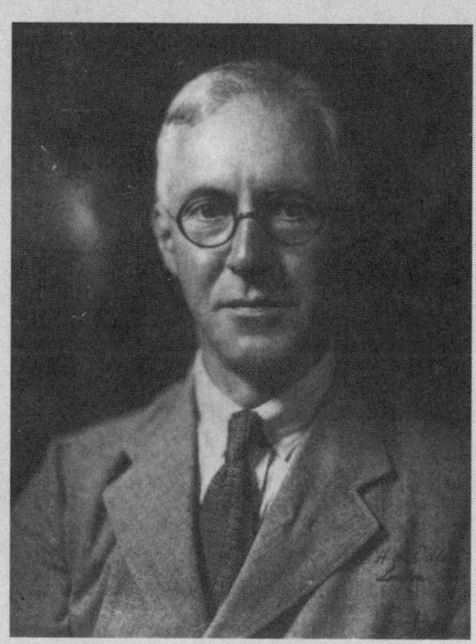

Figure D–1 Sir Henry Dale.

Dale principle Any one neuron uses but a single neurotransmitter, the same at every one of its terminals.

The principle was long considered correct but recently has been shown to have exceptions—in the corpus striatum, for example.

Dalrymple sign Widening of the palpebral fissure, mainly from retraction of the upper eyelids due to excessive sympathetic stimulation of Müller's muscle initially and later to levator fibrosis. A sign of **dysthyroid ophthalmopathy**. See **scleral show**.

John Dalrymple (1804–1852) was an English ophthalmologist.

Dalton, John (1766–1852) English chemist, who was color-blind himself but who first identified the condition (thereafter called Daltonism) in 1798.[1423] Joseph Huddart (1741–1816), however, had given an account of "persons who could not distinguish color" to Joseph Priestly, who in turn communicated it to the Royal Society in 1777.

Dana, Charles Loomis (1852–1935) New York neurologist and classicist who trained at Columbia after an early career in zoology. He became a professor of physiology and then of diseases of the mind and nervous system in New York before being appointed as professor of neurology at Cornell. He was a cofounder of the New York Neurological Institute and was president of the American Neurological Association in 1892 and again in 1928.

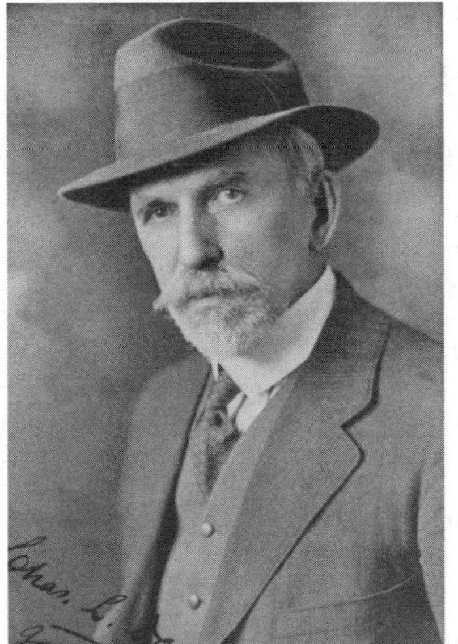

Figure D–2 Charles Loomis Dana.

Apart from identifying in 1891 the syndrome to which his name was lent (the same year as **J.J. Putnam** described it), he is remembered for having persuaded a neurosurgical colleague to resect some of the posterior spinal roots for the relief of pain and also for describing spastic pareses and amplifying Hammond's account of athetosis (1888). He was also a classical scholar with a special interest in Horace. In 1892 he published his acclaimed *Text-book of Nervous Diseases*, which went to 10 editions over the next 33 years.

Dana syndrome See **subacute combined degeneration of the cord**.

dancing eyes (dancing feet) syndrome See **opsoclonus**.

dancing larynx A variant of **palatal tremor** characterized by arrhythmic contractions of the laryngeal and pharyngeal muscles, leading to clicking sounds. The uvula is unaffected.

dancing mania (St. John dance, St. Vitus dance, danse de St. Guy, tarantism, jumpers, rollers, barkers, leaping ague, astonagaza, chorea germanorum, etc.) Probably a form of "mass hysteria" and not now reported, this consisted of epidemic propensities to dance experienced by men and women, who circled hand in hand for hours at a time. "They worked themselves up to a pitch of excitement, foamed at the mouth and fell down exhausted and half-fainting."[3113] During the dancing, some saw visions, while others appeared to convulse. As the mania spread, it became more licentious and sexually oriented. The tradition continues (in a more restrained way) on Whit Tuesday in Echternach (Luxembourg).

The condition was reported from Aix-la-Chapelle in 1374; in 1418, the Chief Magistrate of Strasbourg ordered dancers in his city to go to the chapel of St. Vitus at Zabern, a remote Alsatian village, for relief from the condition; the name of St. Vitus was thus associated with the dancing mania and by extension with the dance-like movements of chorea, until these were distinguished by Sydenham in 1675.

See also **epidemic chorea**.

Dandy, Walter Edward (1886–1946) American neurosurgeon, Professor at Johns Hopkins in Baltimore, where he had also been a student and where he trained for a time with his mentor Halsted, and then with **Cushing**, with whom he did not get on and to whom he would not speak. At Johns Hopkins, he investigated the dynamics of the CSF circulation and as a result devised operations for the relief of hydrocephalus as well as for trigeminal neuralgia (approaching the nerve roots through the posterior fossa) and for the removal of cerebellopontine angle and pineal tumors, using a transcallosal approach. He introduced the techniques of air encephalography in 1918 and of ventriculography in the following year, and was the first surgeon to clip a cerebral aneurysm.[7]

Dandy–Walker syndrome A malformation of the fourth ventricle and cerebellum, characterized by atresia of the foramina of Luschka and Magendie[1441] with failure of development of the midline structures of the cerebellum (which form instead a large cyst obstructing the CSF flow and causing hydrocephalus) and also some bulging of the occiput.[1441]

The cardinal features are malformation of the vermis, a cystic roof to the expanded fourth ventricle, and elevation of the tentorium. Clinically, the syndrome is characterized in its full expression by cleft palate, pyloric stenosis, multiple renal cysts, bilateral pyramidal and cerebellar signs, and mental and developmental delay. Dolichocephaly, scaphocephaly, or microcephaly, encephalocele or cranial meningocele, aqueduct stenosis with hydrocephalus, polymicrogyria, heterotopias, and callosal agenesis are the main pathological features. In some cases, congenital cardiac anomalies also occur[2784] and the cyst is also a feature of various other congenital malformation syndromes characterized by facial dysmorphisms, skeletal anomalies, microcephaly, etc.

A.E. Walker (b. 1907) was an American neurosurgeon, a colleague of **Dandy** at Johns Hopkins. The first description of the malformation was actually published by J.B. Sutton in *Brain* (1887).

Criteria for the diagnosis have been suggested[3475] and require all of:

1. Enlargement of the posterior fossa
2. A large median cyst is present in the posterior fossa that has a wide/broad communication with the fourth ventricle

3. The cerebellar vermis is small, rotated, and raised
4. The cerebellar hemispheres are displaced antero-laterally but otherwise are normal
5. The tentorium shows an upward displacement
6. The brainstem is normal

See **cerebellar syndromes**.

Danielssen, Daniel (1815–1894) Norwegian physician who gave the first complete clinical and pathological account of leprosy, which was at that time endemic in the coastal region where he practiced.

Danielssen–Boeck syndrome See **anesthetic leprosy**.

Danks syndrome (recessive osteodysplasty) A congenital dysmorphic syndrome manifesting also numerous skeletal malformations and recurrent infections, delayed closure of fontanelles, and hydrocephalus.[381]

Danon disease A rare X-linked dominant glycogen (lyosomal) storage cardioskeletal myopathy mapped to chromosome Xq24 and caused by lysosomal-associated membrane protein 2 (*LAMP2*) deficiency. Clinically, it is characterized by hypertrophic cardiomyopathy, cardiac conduction abnormalities, skeletal vacuolar myopathy, variable degrees of mental retardation, and peripheral pigmentary retinopathy. In men, a mild skeletal myopathy, involving facial muscles, neck flexors, and limb-girdle muscles eventually accompanies the cardiomyopathy, but distal skeletal muscles are less commonly affected. Hepatomegaly, aymptomatic hyperCKemia, and peripheral retinopathy have also been reported. The onset is in adolescence and the diagnosis caries a poor prognosis. Women are less severely affected.[1445, 4567]

Muscle biopsy shows autophagic vacuolar myopathy, with small intracytoplasmic vacuoles in muscle fibers containing basophilic granules on hematoxylin–eosin stain.

danse de St. Guy See **Sydenham chorea**.

danse du ventre A dystonic syndrome in some elderly people who make repetitive writhing movements resembling an attempt to scratch the abdomen without using the hands.

Darier disease (follicular dyskeratosis) A rare autosomal dominant disorder of childhoood or youth characterized by multiple eruptions of hyperkeratotic or crusted papules in seborrheic areas with histologic acantholysis and dyskeratosis. It is caused by mutations in the *ATP2A2* gene on chromosome 12q23–q24.1. Mood disorders, epilepsy, mental retardation, slowly progressive encephalopathy, and schizophrenia have been described as associated.[6637]

dark adaptation (dark response) Progressive improvement of vision under conditions of low illumination, largely due to widening of the pupillary aperture as a result of inhibition of the pupillary sphincter muscles and contraction of the pupillary dilators. The phenomenon was first described by Hermann Aubert (1826–1892), a German physician.[290]

dark response See **dark adaptation**.

Darkshewitsch fibers Those fibers running between the optic tract and the habenular ganglion.

Darkshewitsch, Liverij Osipovich (1858–1925) Russian anatomist at the Universities of Moscow and St. Petersburg.

Darkshewitsch nucleus (ganglion) The nucleus of the posterior commissure, situated within the third ventricle and anterior to the **Edinger–Westphal nucleus**.[1670]

Dartmouth Screening Battery for Diffuse Cerebral Dysfunction A rating scale shown to be valid and reliable in the diagnosis of diffuse cerebral dysfunction.[3198] It examines 13 functions including the **nuchocephalic** and **glabellar tap reflexes**; the **sucking** response; **pursuit eye movements**; maintenance of lateral gaze, up- and down-gaze; and **gegenhalten** both in the arms and in the legs. The battery also includes some items in the **Mini-Mental State** test (three-item recall and some knowledge questions).

dartos reflex Contraction of this muscle in response to cutaneous stimulation of the thigh, which can be used to evaluate the thoracolumbar sympathetic and genitofemoral nerve pathways. The test can also be used to assess scrotal autonomic innervation. Abnormalities of dartos innervation may affect the thermoregulation of the testis and thus spermatogenesis.[6916]

Daur–Babiński sign Dystonic permanent extreme dorsiflexion of the hallux, a sign of chronic pallidal lesions. See **dystonic toe**.

David anomaly Originally described as the congenital absence of one or both pectoral muscles with syndactyly, but now extended to include congenital absence of other muscles (e.g., the abdominals). The condition might be classified as a disorder of muscle, but it is not known whether it represents a developmental failure of the muscle only or whether whole motor units, including the anterior horn cells, are absent as well. See also **thenar hypoplasia** and **Souques syndrome**.

Davidenkow, S. (fl. 1926) Russian neurologist, practicing in Moscow.

Davidenkow syndrome See **scapuloperoneal syndrome**.

Davidsohn, Hermann (1842–1911) German physician who devised a method for illumination of the sinuses (also showing up the pupils) by shining a bright light into the mouth of the patient in a dark place.[5619]

Dawson encephalitis See **subacute sclerosing panencephalitis**.

Dawson fingers Extensions of plaques of demyelination beside blood vessels within the white matter of the brain extending perpendicularly from the walls of the lateral ventricles in **multiple sclerosis** and with small vessel disease, visible on high-T2 signal **MRI scans**.

Dax, Marc (1771–1837) French general practitioner, who in 1836 noted the relationship between left hemispheric lesions and disturbances of speech, an observation which he did not publicize and which was therefore neglected until republished in 1865 by his son Gustav.[1489]

In his graduation thesis, he described post-epileptic (now called **Todd**) paresis.

day-blindness See **nyctalopia**.

dazzling test Persistent reduction in vision after bright light stimulation; seen in subjects with optic neuritis.

De Barsy syndrome (cutis laxa, retardation, and corneal opacity) A congenital dysmorphic syndrome manifesting also short stature, sparse hair, cloudy corneas, premature aging, microcephaly with delayed closure of the fontanelles, involuntary movements, and mental and developmental delay.[1492]

De Clerambault syndrome A pathological belief that one is loved by another person, whose every action is interpreted in a way that sustains the delusion, despite the attempts of the unfortunate target of that false belief to be rid of his (more rarely her) admirer.[6382]

Dr. G.H.A.E.L.M.G. de Clerambault (1872–1934) was a French physician.

De Grouchy–Royal–Salmon–Lamy syndrome A heterogeneous entity resulting from deletion of the distal long arm of chromosome 18q and characterized variously by mental retardation, microcephaly, midface hypoplasia, abnormalities of the ears and genitalia, hypotonia, talipes equinovarus, and segmental spinal muscular atrophy.[1533, 6815] See **chromosome 18 partial deletion**.

De Lange, Cornelia (1871–1950) Dutch pediatrician, practicing in Amsterdam.

De Lange syndrome 1. (Cornelia de Lange syndrome, Brachmann-de Lange syndrome, Amsterdam dwarfism) A sporadic syndrome of growth retardation from conception with severely diminished stature (always below the third percentile) despite congenital muscular hypertrophy. The syndrome also includes microcephaly, severe mental retardation, nystagmus, initial hypertonicity, extrapyramidal disorders, facial dysmorphism, flexion contractures of the elbows, **clinodactyly**, syndactyly, transverse palmar crease and dermatoglyphic abnormalities, generalized hirsutism, and synophrys. The neck and limbs are broad and thick, the hairline low, and the skull asymmetrical due to porencephaly. Various cerebral dysgenetic malformations are also found.[1503]

Despite the attribution to de Lange, the first report was by Bruck in 1889.

2. (**Bruck–de Lange syndrome**) A syndrome of congenital symmetrical muscular hypertrophy with extrapyramidal rigidity and mental retardation, porencephaly, facial dysmorphisms, and decerebrate posturing. Death usually occurs before the end of the second year.[1504]

de Morsier syndrome 1. (posterior diencephalic autonomic epilepsy syndrome) Paroxysmal attacks of muscle rigidity of the trunk and jaws with profuse perspiration.[1511]

2. A syndrome of unilateral disorder of pain and proprioceptive impairment accompanied by photophobia, fatigability, and disturbances of memory and behavior, sometimes with disturbances of the chemical senses, hyperpathia, hallucinations, involuntary movements, and weakness. It is considered to be due to disturbances of the reticular hypothalamic system.[1509]

3. (olfacto-genital dysplasia) A rare syndrome characterized by anosmia, seizures, agenesis of the septum pellucidum, optic nerve hypoplasia, pyramidal signs, and neuroendocrine defects such as growth failure, diabetes insipidus, or panhypopituitarism.[1510] See **septo-optic dysplasia**.

De Sanctis, Sante (Carlo) (1862–1935) Italian neuropsychiatrist born in Umbria and educated in Sienna and Rome. His early career was devoted to studies of neuroanatomy, anthropology, and psychology, after which he trained in psychiatry at the **Salpêtriére** and in Rome, where he eventually became professor of neurology and psychiatry in 1929. He published over 300 papers on the normal and pathological anatomy of the nervous system and on experimental psychology; as well as describing the structure of the mamillary bodies and myelination of the cerebellum. He also studied **Down syndrome**, childhood epilepsy, and schizophrenia in the population of Italy.

De Sanctis–Cacchione syndrome (xerodermic idiocy) A recessively inherited congenital dysmorphic syndrome manifesting also skin photosensitivity with patchy pigmentation, telangiectasia, warts, and other skin tumors; seizures, microcephaly, and cerebral atrophy with ataxia, spasticity, sensory neuropathy, and mental and developmental delay.[1518] See **xeroderma pigmentosum**.

deafferentation Removal of the afferent processes normally playing upon a nerve cell or neural structure.

deafferentation pain Dysesthetic pain resulting from incomplete central or peripheral neural injury; pain felt in an area which is partially or completely anesthetic or in the region surrounding it. This implies not only a loss of input but that actual degeneration has occurred so that the spinal cord cells are free to act in a pathological way. See **causalgia**.

deafferented bladder A dilated bladder as a result of, for example, severe autonomic neuropathy, in which the reflex arc maintaining detrusor tone is interrupted on the afferent side, reflex contraction in response to stretch thus being lost.

deafness Reduction in auditory acuity, due to abnormality of either the afferent nerve pathway (*sensorineural deafness*) or the mechanically conducting tissue in the middle ear (*middle ear* or *conductive deafness*). See also **cortical deafness**, **word deafness**, entries listed in Chart D–1, other entries listed under **amyotrophic lateral sclerosis** and **cerebellar ataxia**, and the following entries.

See also the following 14 entries.

deafness-achalasia-vitiligo syndrome A congenital dysmorphic syndrome manifesting also short stature, sensorineural deafness, bulbar palsies, muscle atrophy, and patchy depigmentation of the skin.[381]

deafness–alopecia–hypogonadism syndrome See **Crandall syndrome**.

deafness and atopic dermatitis A recessively inherited syndrome of moderate congenital neural deafness with the appearance of atopic dermatitis in the second decade.[1267, 3526]

deafness and diabetes A progressive but subtotal hearing loss involving first

Chart D–1. Major Hereditary Causes of Deafness

Alport Syndrome
Dominant Albinism and Congenital Deafness
Dominant Anhidrosis and Progressive Hearing Loss
Dominant Congenital Severe Deafness
Dominant Knuckle Pads, Leukonychia, and Hearing Loss
Dominant Hand Weakness with Sensorineural Deafness
Dominant Low-Frequency Hearing Loss
Dominant Mid-Frequency Hearing Loss
Dominant Photomyoclonus, Hearing Loss, Diabetes, and Nephropathy
Dominant Preauricular Pits and Neural Hearing Loss
Dominant Progressive Nerve Deafness
Dominant Saddle Nose, Myopia, Cataract, and Hearing Loss
Dominant Unilateral Deafness
Familial Hemiplegic Migraine
Flynn-Aird Syndrome
Hereditary Motor and Sensory Neuropathy
Hereditary Motor Neuropathy
Hereditary Piebaldness and Congenital Deafness
Hereditary Photomyoclonus
Hereditary Sensory and Autonomic Neuropathy
Hereditary Spastic Paraplegia
Herrmann Disease
Hittner Syndrome
Hutchinson Triad
Hyperuricemia, Deafness, and Ataxia
Jervell–Lange–Nielsen Syndrome
Mohr–Tranebjaerg Syndrome
Mucopolysaccharidoses
Recessive Absence of Tibia and Deafness
Recessive Atopic Dermatitis and Neural Hearing Loss
Recessive Congenital Moderate Hearing Loss
Recessive Congenital Severe Deafness
Recessive Early-Onset Neural Deafness
Recessive Goiter and Deafness
Recessive Malformed Low-Set Ears and Conductive Hearing Loss
Recessive Myopia and Hearing Loss
Recessive Optic Atrophy, Hearing Loss, and Juvenile Diabetes
Recessive Pili Torti and Deafness
Recessive Retinal Changes, Deafness, Muscular Wasting, and Mental Retardation
Red-M Syndrome
Richards–Rundle Syndrome
Ruzika Syndrome
Sylvester Syndrome
Usher Syndrome
X-Linked Congenital Neural Deafness
X-Linked Early-Onset Neural Deafness
X-Linked Moderate Hearing Loss
X-Linked Pigmentary Abnormalities and Congenital Deafness

the higher frequencies in diabetic subjects. The condition is genetically determined but the association with diabetes may or may not be.[2943]

deafness and ear pits The association of congenital conductive or sensorineural hearing loss inherited as an autosomal dominant characteristic and with the presence of a small pit or sinus present in front of the anterior extremity of the helix on one or both ears.[2162] See **Wildervanck syndrome**.

deafness and goiter See Pendred syndrome.

deafness–dystonia syndrome (Mohr–Tranebjaerg syndrome) An X-linked disorder characterized by the association of progressive sensorineural deafness, cortical blindness, dystonia, dysphagia, and paranoia.[6370]

deafness, kerato-pachydermia, and digital constrictions (Vohwinkel syndrome) A rare syndrome with onset in infancy or early childhood, characterized by palmar and plantar keratoderma with keratosis of the dorsum of the hands and feet, elbows, and knees. Digital bandlike constrictions of the distal interphalangeal creases develop in childhood. High-frequency neural hearing loss is associated.[2368]

deafness, renal and digital anomalies A rare syndrome in which conductive or mixed hearing loss is associated with rudimentary distal phalanges with bifurcations at their distal ends. The condition may be inherited as an autosomal recessive trait. Some members of the single family reported had nephritis.[905]

deafness, stippled epiphyses, and goiter with elevated PBI A congenital metabolic defect characterized by resistance to thyroid hormone action, goiter, profound congenital sensory neural deafness, bird-like facies, pigeon breast, and winged scapulas. Delayed bone age with stippled epiphyses but with normal dental development are reported. The thyroid activity is not associated with high levels of free circulating thyroid hormone.[5234]

deafness-ataxia-piebaldness syndrome A congenital dysmorphic syndrome manifesting also patchy depigmentation of the skin and hair, sensorineural deafness, cerebellar ataxia, and mental and developmental delay.[6863]

deafness-diverticulosis-sensory neuropathy syndrome A congenital dysmorphic syndrome manifesting also anencephaly or craniorachischisis, sensorineural deafness, sensorimotor peripheral neuropathy, diverticulosis of the colon, and acanthosis nigricans.[381]

deafness–metaphyseal dysplasia syndrome A congenital dysmorphic syndrome manifesting also short stature, short limbs, coxa valga, genu valgum or varum, brachydactyly, conductive deafness, and mental and developmental delay.[381]

deafness–onychodystrophy-oncholysis-retardation syndrome (DOOR syndrome) A congenital recessively inherited dysmorphic syndrome manifesting the listed skeletal malformations, profound sensorineural deaf- ness, and mental and developmental delay.[2481]

In a *variant* dominantly inherited form, no seizures occur and the mental status is normal.

death, cerebral See **brain death**.

debrancher enzyme deficiency See **glycogen storage diseases**.

Debré, Robert (1882–1978) French physician.

Debré–Semelaigne syndrome (Kocher–Debré–Semelaigne syndrome) The association of generalized enlargement of muscles with slow muscle contraction and relaxation and **myoedema** in hypothyroid children.[1527] Intellectual, physical, osseous, and dental development are all retarded and the usual signs of hypothyroidism are usually marked.

The absence of pseudomyotonia and of painful spasms differentiates the condition from **Hoffmann syndrome,** which otherwise it resembles.

decerebrate rigidity An extensor posture of the neck, trunk, and limbs with hyperpronation of the arms and hyperreflexia, adopted by subjects with actual or functional transections of the brainstem below the red nucleus and colliculi but rostral to the vestibular nuclei.

It was first described by **Sherrington** in 1898. See also **decorticate rigidity**.

Dechambre, André (1812–1886) French physician and scientific journalist who graduated from Strasbourg and worked for a period at the Salpêtrière with Cruveilhier. He is remembered for being the first to use the term *lacune* for cystic cavities in the brain (in 1838) and for publication of the *Dictionnaire Encyclopedique des Sciences Medicales*, which ran to 100 volumes. He was elected a member of the French Academie de Médicine in 1875.

declarative learning The learning of facts as opposed to skills, as measured by tests that require explicit recall or recognition of prior events. It is impaired by hippocampal lesions, in **Alzheimer disease**, and as a result of scopolamine administration.

declarative memory The capacity for conscious recollection of previous events and knowledge derived from prior experience and subject to conscious recollection, verbal reflection, and explicit expression.[11] The hippocampus is critical to declarative memory in humans. See **explicit memory**.

decomposition See **automatic decomposition EMG**.

decomposition of movement 1. The performance of compound voluntary limb movements slowly, awkwardly, and without the normal flow and smoothness of execution so that the action is separated into its component parts and proceeds joint by joint, leading to the jerky performance of the same. The appearance rather resembles the movements of an unskillfully handled marionette.

It is classically a sign of a lesion of the lateral lobe of the cerebellum, in which case the mechanisms are the same as those for **dysdiadochokinesis**.

2. Delay in the initiation of one component relative to that of another, and excessive range of one element of the movement relative to another, particularly at a proximal joint.[2962]

decompression sickness (caisson disease, the bends, dysbarism) Diffuse and multifocal disease of the nervous system due to thrombogenetic nitrogen emboli forming (particularly in the epidural venous plexuses) as a result of too-rapid decompression after diving or other work done at high levels of atmospheric pressure.[3153]

The condition presents commonly with painful myelopathy but the pathology is widespread within the nervous system. Two types are defined: *type 1* is characterized by fleeting pain in the muscles or joints of the upper limbs more than the lower limbs; pruritus and vascular stasis in the skin; edema; malaise, fatigue, and anorexia; and *type 2* represents a far more serious disorder, in which the spinal cord, the brain, or the labyrinths are damaged as the result of gaseous emboli ("air embolism").

Clinical manifestations include altered consciousness, confusion, visual loss, vertigo, weakness, ataxia, sensory loss, and sphincter disturbances. The thoracic cord is the site most frequently affected.[1632]

See also **arterial gas embolism** and **Divers Alert Network**.

decorticate rigidity A state of abnormal flexion responses in the arms with or without extensor responses in the legs, resulting from a lesion of the high brainstem.

This modified extensor posture (the neck, trunk, and legs typically being thrust into extension and the arms into flexion) is adopted by subjects with actual or functional transections of the brainstem above the level of the colliculi, or possibly with lesions affecting the cortex diffusely.

decortication Removal of the cortex from a cerebral hemisophere.

decremental response See **decrementing response**.

decrementing response (decremental response) A reproducible decline in the amplitude and/or area of the M wave of successive responses to repetitive nerve stimulation. The rate of stimulation and the total number of stimuli should be specified. Decrementing responses with disorders of neuromuscular transmission are most reliably seen with slow rates (2–5 Hz) of nerve stimulation. A decrementing response with repetitive nerve stimulation commonly occurs in disorders of neuromuscular transmission, but can also be seen in some neuropathies, myopathies, and motor neuron disease. An artifact resembling a decrementing response can result from movement of the stimulating or recording electrodes during repetitive nerve stimulation (see pseudodecrement). Cf. **incrementing response**. (From the 2001 Report of the Nomenclature Committee of the American Association of Electromyography and Electrodiagnosis.[19] Reproduced by kind permission of the AANEM.)

decubitus (from Lat, to lie down) The lying or recumbent posture.

decussate (from Lat, to divide across) The crossing of fibers such as nerve fibers; the term is usually applied when it is the midline that is crossed.

de-efferented state See **locked-in syndrome**.

deep brain stimulation A neurosurgical therapeutic technique involving the insertion of wires stereotactically in order to stimulate selected basal ganglion sites, used in the management of severe **Parkinson disease**, tremor, and dystonia, and in the future possibly **Tourette syndrome**, obsessive-compulsive disorders, severe depression, and epilepsy.

deep cerebral venous thrombosis Occlusion of the deep internal cerebral vein, the vein of Galen, extending toward the straight sinus. Clinically, headache, altered consciousness, papilledema, hemisensory disturbances, and hemipareses are the usual features and the condition is often lethal. CT scans show large bilateral thalamocapsular hypodensities.[2685]

deep dyslexia (phonemic dyslexia, phonological dyslexia) An acquired reading disorder in which the patient substitutes synonyms for the written words he is reading aloud (**semantic paralexia**). Abundant word substitutions (verbal paraphasias) occur, with a difficulty in linking the visual form of words with their phonological structure as shown by the inability of affected people to read nonsense words, to identify homophones, and to appreciate rhyme. Dysphasia, dysgraphia, and a variety of parietal lobe signs such as acalculia and constructional apraxia are also commonly associated.[1259]

The syndrome reflects posterior parietal lesions of the dominant hemisphere and may appear during the recovery stage after global alexia.[1259] See also **alexia**.

deep dysphasia A disorder of language characterized by the making of semantic errors when heard speech is repeated. Errors are most pronounced when single words are repeated, less so during the repetition of phrases.[961]

deep radial nerve paralysis See **posterior interosseous syndrome**.

deep sleep 1. Sleep in nonrapid eye movement stages 3 or 4. 2. The rapid eye movement sleep state.

deep tendon reflex One of the most ubiquitous misnomers in clinical neurology, not only because it is the superficial rather than the deep tendons which are tapped in clinical practice, but because stimulation of the afferent neurons from tendons (Golgi tendon organs) causes inhibition of muscle activity rather than muscle contraction; the tendons have nothing to do with the reflex, except that they provide a site from which to stimulate the muscle stretch receptors. Either *phasic muscle stretch reflex* or *myotatic reflex* (as favored by Sherrington) would be preferable terms. See **muscle stretch reflex**.

deep toe reflex (Rossolimo reflex) Flexion and abduction of the toes in response to percussion of their ends; a minor sign, found in some patients with upper motor neuron lesions.

defecation syncope A form of situational syncope in which typically the rise in intrathoracic pressure required by those with a tendency to constipation decreases cardiac venous return, cardiac output, and thus cerebral perfusion, leading to syncope.

defense reaction Threatening, aggressive display as a result of stimulation of the amygdaloid and local limbic circuit nuclei in experimental animals.

deficient sellar diaphragm See **empty sella syndrome**.

definite multiple sclerosis See **clinically definite multiple sclerosis**.

definition A brief description of the consistent attributes of an object which allow it to be differentiated from other objects. The basis for this book.

deformation An abnormal form, shape, or position of a part of the body developing as a result of mechanical force.

degenerate Departing from the virtues of ones ancestors.

degeneration (from Lat, changing for the worse) A morbid condition of a body part which becomes less differentiated and eventually undergoes transformation to unspecialized tissue, atrophies, and dies.

degenerative dementias Disorders of the brain characterized by the decay and death of neurons leading to cognitive impairment. A listing of these has been suggested.[1998]

1. **Alzheimer disease**
2. **Dementia with Lewy bodies**
3. **Frontotemporal degenerations**
   - i. Pick disease
   - ii. Frontotemporal dementia with motor neuron disease (MND)
   - iii. Corticobasal degeneration (CBD)
   - iv. Primary progressive aphasia (PPA)
4. Vascular dementia
   - i. Lacunar disease
   - ii. Multiinfarct type (large vessel)
   - iii. **Binswanger disease**
   - iv. Watershed ischemia
   - v. Strategic infarcts
   - vi. Anoxic encephalopathy
   - vii. **Amyloid angiopathy**
   - viii. Cerebral angiitis
   - ix. **CADASIL**
   - x. Other
5. Mixed dementia (more than one of the above)
   - i. AD and VaD
   - ii. AD and DLB
6. Other degenerative dementias
   - i. **Huntington disease**
   - ii. **Progressive supranuclear palsy**
   - iii. **Parkinson disease**

degenerative spinal stenosis Narrowing of the diameter of the spinal canal, usually at multiple lumbar levels, due to local degenerative disease. Clinical features include back pain aggravated by standing and relieved by rest and forward flexion, **neurogenic claudication**, and a posture of persistent flexion of the lumbar spine.

degenerative spondylolisthesis Forward displacement of L4 on L5 without a break in the pars interarticularis; a cause of **lumbar spinal stenosis**.[2222]

deglutition (Lat, down + swallow) Swallowing.

deglutition syncope (swallow syncope) Syncope provoked by swallowing, commonly in association with esophageal lesions. Atrioventricular block and sinus bradycardia are the usual mechanisms, triggered by reflexes arising in the esophagus.[6775]

Degos syndrome See **malignant atrophic papulosis**.

Deiters nucleus The lateral vestibular nucleus of the pons, which gives rise to the lateral vestibulospinal tract, excitatory to those anterior horn cells innervating extensor muscles.

Deiters nucleus syndrome See **Bonnier syndrome**.

Deiters, Otto Frederich Karl (1834–1863) German anatomist. He studied under **Virchow** in Berlin and quickly became professor of anatomy and histology at the University of Bonn, but died young of typhoid. Deiters was the first to identify axons, in the anterior roots, which he differentiated from dendrites in 1865. He also identified astrocytes and showed that axis cylinders form the core of the nerve fiber and emanate from the nerve cells.

déjà vécu (Fr, already lived) A broader experience than **déjà vu** in which the subject falsely recalls having previously experienced a current situation. Such a symptom (usually due to epileptic discharges in a temporal lobe) is not a misinterpretation of sense impressions but an inappropriate judgment and thus is better regarded as delusional than as illusory.

déjà vu (Fr, already seen) A French phrase indicating prior awareness of an event. In neurology, it is synonymous with the aura of partial seizures with temporal lobe origin.

Phenomenologically, déjà vu can be regarded as a delusion of recognition.

Dejean syndrome (orbital floor syndrome) The occurrence of exophthalmos, diplopia, maxillary pain, and trigeminal (maxillary) sensory loss due to a mass lesion or to a **blowout fracture** of the orbital floor.[1536]

Déjèrine, Joseph-Jules (1849–1917) Parisian neurologist born in Savoy who lived his early life in Switzerland, later training in Paris under **Vulpian**, whose favorite student he became. After internship he was appointed agrégé at the faculty of medicine and eventually professor of diseases of the nervous system at the **Salpêtrière** after **Raymond**. He married Augusta (**Déjèrine-) Klumpke**, an American physician whom he met at the Salpêtrière, and she shared fully in all their clinical and research activities, continuing them after his death in 1917 as a result of exhaustion arising from his work in the wards of a military hospital.

His wide experience with neurological conditions is suggested by the following entries; he also classified **alexia** into forms with and without agraphia and that form accompanying Broca aphasia (**third alexia**).[2855] Less well known, but of even greater value, was his work on the anatomy of the nervous system, on cerebral localization, and on the clinical features of numerous neurological diseases.

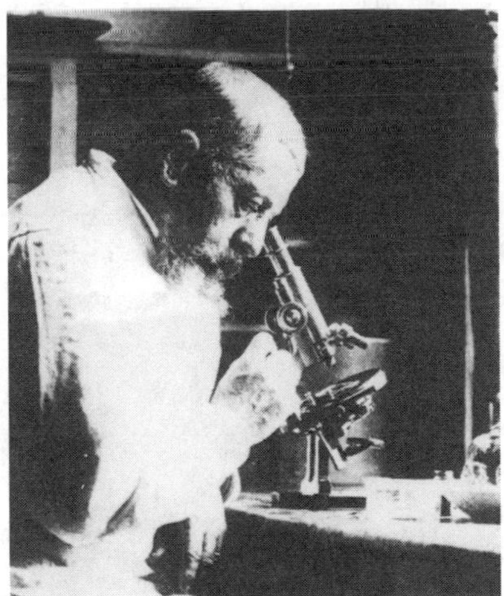

Figure D–3 Joseph-Jules Déjèrine.

Déjèrine neurotabes A form of combined anterior and posterior radiculopathy in which there is selective initial involvement of large fibers subserving deep sensibility, associated with paraparesis, in patients with syphilis.[1537] See **Déjèrine syndromes**, definition 4.

Déjèrine sign Acute pain in the neck on sneezing, as though something had torn; evidence of the precipitation of radicular pain by sudden changes in intraspinal pressure, usually, in this context, due to cervical radiculopathy.[1539]

Déjèrine syndromes 1. (anterior bulbar syndrome, pyramid-hypoglossal syndrome, alternating hypoglossal-hemiplegia, medial medullary syndrome) A brainstem syndrome due to infarction of the paramedian region of the medulla as a result of occlusion of branches of the vertebral or anterior spinal arteries. The clinical features include homolateral hypoglossal palsy, **alternating hemiplegia**, and sometimes involvement of the medial lemniscus. See also **Jackson syndrome** and **alternating hypoglossal hemiplegia syndrome**.[2923] It has also been reported in patients with meningovascular syphilis.[6239] A further complete dissection of the syndromes arising with medial medullary strokes has been published.[433]

2. (*parietal lobe syndrome*) Astereognosis and impaired tactile localization and proprioception, with retention of the senses of temperature, crude light touch, and pain.[1538]

3. Diphtheritic neuropathy.

4. (Radiculitis, **Déjèrine** *neurotabes*) A form of combined anterior and posterior radiculopathy in which there is selective initial involvement of large fibers subserving deep sensibility, associated with paraparesis in patients with syphilis.[1537]

5. **Facioscapulohumeral muscular dystrophy** (Landouzy–Déjèrine syndrome)

6. See **Verger–Déjèrine syndrome**.

Déjèrine-Klumpke, Augusta (1859–1927) American neurologist from San Francisco, the wife of J.-J. **Déjèrine**, who trained and did postgraduate work as the first woman *interne des hôpitaux* in Paris, despite initial strong resistance from the medical establishment. Her graduation thesis was on lead neuropathy.

Much of the work of her husband reflected her interest and advice; her own report of lower brachial plexus palsy was written in 1885, 3 years before her marriage. Her work on the PNS inspired **Tinel**. With **J.-J. Déjèrine**, she published an atlas of cerebral anatomy based upon their meticulous dissections, in 1894. After his death, she worked mainly on spinal cord diseases with her daughter, also a physician.[7]

Déjèrine-Klumpke palsy See **Klumpke palsy**.

Déjèrine–Mouzon syndrome See **Verger–Déjèrine syndrome**.

Déjèrine–Roussy syndrome See **thalamic syndrome**.

Déjèrine–Sottas syndrome See **hereditary motor and sensory neuropathy, type 3**.

Déjèrine–Thomas syndrome (cortical cerebellar degeneration and delayed cerebellar ataxia) A form of **olivopontocerebellar atrophy** occuring in adults, in which imbalance, gait disturbance, hyperreflexia with downgoing plantar responses, truncal ataxia, and eventual immobility develop. Cerebellar intention tremor is not seen, extraocular movements are preserved, and the posterior columns function normally. Histologically, the cerebellum and pons are atrophic.[1545]

The absence of a positive family history in the original report calls into question the familial nature of the condition. See **cerebellar ataxias**.

DeJong, Russell N. (1906–1990) American neurologist of Dutch ancestry who received his under- and postgraduate training at the University of Michigan, where he later was to become chairman of the department of neurology.

He was a founder of the **American Academy of Neurology** and was a painstaking and successful editor as well as teacher and clinician. He served as the (first) editor of ***Neurology*** for 26 years, but is even better remembered as the author of *The Neurological Examination*, a classic text which since its first publication has been the ultimate source of information on the clinical examination of the nervous system.

Delamarre, Georges French physician who described gastric crises in tabes with Pierre **Marie** in his graduating *Thèse de Paris* (1866).

delay The interval between the beginning of the horizontal sweep of the oscilloscope and the onset of an applied stimulus. See also **delay line**.[19]

delay line An information storage device used to display events which occur before a trigger signal. This is a method for displaying repetitive waveforms at the same point on a sweep on a free-running electromyogram.[19]

delayed cerebellar ataxia See **Déjèrine–Thomas syndrome**.

delayed cerebral edema Severe, possibly fatal cerebral edema following relatively minor trauma and after a lucid interval, occurring in young people. The genetic basis for this rare condition is the same as that for **familial hemiplegic migraine** and involves a mutation in the CACNA1 calcium channel subunit gene on chromosome 19.[3536]

delayed cortical cerebellar atrophy See **Déjèrine–Thomas syndrome**.

delayed cramps and fasciculation A syndrome of benign cramps, exercise-related myalgia, fasciculations, and sometimes denervation hypertrophy but without new weakness, following prior poliomyelitis or myelitis.[2014]

delayed deterioration of consciousness An unusual syndrome seen in infants and small children, characterized by progressive reduction in consciousness hours or days after a trivial head injury.[2658] See **Spät-apoplexy**.

delayed measles encephalitis The acute onset of neurological signs with intractable focal seizures and coma, with a fatal outcome occurring in children within months of an attack of measles. The anti-measles antibody titers are high and the virus is not recoverable.[3978]

delayed myotonia Myotonia that only appears after a period of muscle contraction, as in **myotonia fluctuans**.

delayed-onset cerebellar syndrome The rare occurrence of ataxia and intention tremor 3 weeks to 2 years after stroke or head injury. Dystonia and myoclonus are other complications known.[3921]

delayed posttraumatic myelitis of Gowers See **railway spine**.

delayed recall A learning test sensitive to left temporal lobe lesions.

delayed recognition span test A memory test in which the subject is required to remember a lengthening series of disks bearing various stimuli (such as words, faces, and designs) added to each other upon a board, recognizing each addition as such. The subject then tries to recall the words written thereon, both immediately and after a further 2 min. The latter part of the test differentiates between patients with **Alzheimer disease** and those with other conditions such as **Huntington disease** and **Korsakoff syndrome**.[4517]

delayed sleep phase syndrome (phase lag, phase delay, sleep-onset insomnia, morning sleepiness) A **circadian rhythm sleep disorder** characterized by a chronic disturbance of circadian sleep scheduling, manifest as a persistent and consistent delay in the times of sleep onset and of waking but with normal sleep architecture. This leads to complaints of being unable to sleep until for example, the early morning ("night people"), sleep then continuing unless interrupted for a physiological period;[6710] and of excessive daytime sleepiness when the subject's intrinsic pattern is forced into the conventional scheme. The condition affects mainly adolescents. Diagnostic criteria have been suggested.[1629]

See also http://www.sleepeducation.com/Disorders.aspx/. Another helpful Web site is at http://www.geocities.com/delayed_sleep/.

Deléage disease See **myotonic dystrophy**.

deletion 4p See **Wolf–Hirschorn syndrome**.

delirium (Lat, from + a furrow; thus, to deviate from the straight course) A transient disruption of global cognitive functioning characterized by the acute onset of alterations in attention and arousal, increased or decreased psychomotor activity, disturbed

Chart D–2. Delayed Sleep Phase Syndrome

A. A complaint of an inability to fall asleep at the desired clock time, or inability to awaken spontaneously at the desired time of awakening, or excessive sleepiness.
B. There is a phase delay of the major sleep episode in relation to the desired time for sleep.
C. Symptoms present for at least 1 month.
D. When not required to maintain a strict schedule (e.g., vacation time) patients will:
   1. Have a habitual sleep period that is sound and of normal quality and duration;
   2. Awaken spontaneously;
   3. Maintain stable entrainment to a 24-hour sleep wake pattern at a delayed phase.
E. Evidence of a delay in the timing of the habitual sleep period illustrated on daily sleep logs for a period of at least 2 weeks.
F. Laboratory evidence of a delay in the timing of the habitual sleep period by:
   1. Twenty-four-hour polysomnographic monitoring (or by means of two consecutive nights of polysomnography and an intervening multiple sleep latency test); or
   2. Continuous temperature monitoring showing that the time of the absolute temperature nadir is delayed into the second half of the habitual (delayed) sleep episode.
G. Does not meet criteria for any other sleep disorder causing inability to initiate sleep or excessive sleepiness.

From *AASM Diagnostic Classification Steering Committee.* The International Classification of Sleep Disorders Diagnostic and Coding Manual. *Rochester, MN. American Academy of Sleep Medicine 1991/2001. Reproduced by kind permission of the Academy.*

wake–sleep patterns, and disordered thinking, with a fluctuating course. The **Glasgow Coma Scale** scores will be 4-5-4. This represents an etiologically nonspecific organic cerebral syndrome characterized by concurrent disturbances of consciousness and attention, perception, thinking, memory, psychomotor behavior, emotion, and the sleep–wake schedule. The duration is variable and the degree of severity ranges from mild to very severe.

Characteristic clinical features include a disturbance of consciousness (i.e., reduced clarity of awareness about the environment); inattention with a reduced ability to focus, sustain, or shift attention; disorganization of thinking shown by rambling and irrelevant speech; perceptual disorders (hallucinations); alterations in the sleep–wake cycle and in psychomotor status; and disorientation and impairment of memory, cognition, perception, and behavior (e.g., motor restlessness). The disturbance develops over hours to days and typically fluctuates.

Nocturnal worsening, an inability to grasp and retain information for events, labile emotions, fear and restlessness, auditory and visual hallucinations, insomnia, and paranoid ideation are typical features. Celsus used the term first in this way; today a popular (if inaccurate) name for the syndrome is *confusion*.

It is caused both by primarily neurological disorders such as meningitis, brain tumor, or stroke, and by multitudinous metabolic diseases such as fever, infection, drug administration or withdrawal, vitamin deficiency, liver, lung and renal failure, hypoglycemia, and electrolyte disturbances, and is especially common in the old and those recovering from vascular surgery or in pain.[6232] More than one of these causes coexist in most instances.

The subtypes of delirium depicted in Mayne's Lexicon[5103] are numerous and include *acute* or *furiosum*, which represent mania; *cum massitania* (muttering, once regarded as specific for typhoid fever); *febrile*, in association with fevers; *ferox*, when accompanied by violent anger; *grandiosum*, in which the delusions are of personal power or riches, as in general paresis; *persecutionis*, in which the patient has delusions that others are conspiring against him; **tremens**; and *sympathetic*, the delirium occurring in the setting of acute general illness. A full description was that of Trenel.[6380] See also **confusional state**.

Two sets of diagnostic criteria have been published, in the International Classification of Diseases (at http://www.egms.de/egms/servlet/Figure?id=psm000021& figure=t2&vol=2006-3/) and by the American Psychiatric Association *DSM IV-TR* diagnostic guidelines.[172] The latter can be found at http://www.behavenet.com/capsules/disorders/dsm4TRclassification.htm/.

The *ICD-10 diagnostic criteria for delirium* are abstracted here, as follows: For a definite diagnosis, symptoms (mild or severe) should be present in each of the following areas:

a. Impairment of consciousness and attention (ranging from clouding to coma; reduced ability to direct, focus, sustain, and shift attention)
b. Global disturbance of cognition (perceptual distortions, illusions, and hallucinations—most often visual; impairment of abstract thinking and comprehension, with or without transient delusion but typically with some degree of incoherence; impairment of immediate recall and of recent memory, but with relatively intact remote memory; disorientation for time as well as in more severe cases for place and person)
c. Psychomotor disturbances (hypo- or hyperactivity and unpredictable shifts from one to the other; increased reaction time; increased or decreased flow of speech; enhanced startle reaction)
d. Disturbance of the sleep–wake cycle (insomnia or, in more severe cases, total sleep loss or reversal of the sleep–wake cycle; daytime drowsiness; nocturnal worsening of symptoms; disturbing dreams or nightmares, which may continue as hallucinations after awakening)
e. Emotional disturbances (e.g., depression, anxiety or fear, irritability, euphoria, apathy) wandering, perplexity.

delirium alcoholicum

See **delirium tremens**.

delirium cum massitania

See **delirium**.

delirium e potu

See **delirium tremens**.

delirium ferox

See **delirium**.

delirium furiosum

See **mania**.

delirium grandiosum

See **delirium**.

delirium persecutionis

See **delirium**.

delirium potatorum

See **delirium tremens**.

Delirium Rating Scale Revised-98

A scale quantitating the multiple parameters affected by delirium and containing both diagnostic and severity items. These include the temporal onset of symptoms, perceptual disturbances, long- and short-term memory, hallucination type (frequently tactile), delusions, psychomotor behavior (e.g., severe agitation or withdrawal), cognitive state during formal testing and disorders of the thought processes, the presence of a physical disorder accounting for the symptoms, sleep–wake cycle disturbances, lability of mood, and variability of symptoms.[6406]

See also **Confusional Assessment Method**.

delirium tremens

(Lat, trembling) (Saunders–Sutton syndrome, delirium alcoholicum, delirium potatorum, delirium è potu, ebriositatis) An acute organic psychosis characterized by tremors, delirium, visual hallucinations, pallor, sweating, tachycardia, restless excitement and anxiety, anorexia, and mental distress as a result of chronic alcoholism, especially following withdrawal.

Delirium tremens was possibly the basis of the Bacchanalian frenzies described by the ancient Greek writers. The first modern description was that of Samuel Burton Pearson, a physician in Newcastle (fl. 1800) in his privately circulated pamphlet *Observations on Brain Fever* (1801). Pearson advocated treatment with wine, opium, and nourishing soups together with a minimum of restraint.[6145] The English physician Thomas Sutton (1767–1835) gave a fuller description and introduced the term in 1813 for that form of delirium made worse by bleeding and improved by opium. See also **delirium**.

Delleman syndrome

(orbital cysts and cerebral malformation) A congenital dysmorphic syndrome manifesting microphthalmia, bifid ribs, hydranencephaly, callosal abnormalities, seizures, patchy aplasia of the skin, and mental and developmental delay.[381]

delta band

A frequency band under 4 Hz applied to EEG recordings

delta rhythm (Gr, the letter D, a triangle) Slow waveforms on the EEG, at or less than 3.5 Hz. Focal delta activity suggests brain pathology at that site. When diffuse, delta activity usually indicates degenerative or biochemical disease.

delta rebound An increase in the amount of **delta sleep** which occurs after deprivation of this sleep stage.

delta sleep The third and deepest stage of non–rapid eye movement sleep, characterized by the appearance of high-amplitude slow waves at 0.5–2 Hz, occupying about a fifth of the time of a nocturnal sleep recording.

delta wave An EEG wave with a duration greater than 250 ms.

deltoid reflex Abduction of the shoulder in response to a smart tap on the humerus at the level of the insertion of the deltoid. Normally this is not visible, but the amplitude of the reflex is increased in patients with a pyramidal tract lesion above C5.

delusion (Lat, a deception) An erroneous belief, tenaciously held in the face of logical counterargument. Usually, it suggests the presence of a psychiatric disorder such as schizophrenic or depressive illness, but delusions may occur in states of delirium (confusion) and other organic brain diseases causing dementia.

delusional memory 1. A false memory arising in the context of a psychosis. 2. A deluded interpretation of a true memory. In either case, the difference from spontaneous confabulation is hard to determine.

delusional parasitosis A syndrome in which a patient is convinced beyond all logic and persuasion that he or she is harboring parasites. (HJM)[3970]

delusional reduplication of body parts (pseudo-polymyelia) A condition resembling the **phantom limb** syndrome, but in which the belief that the limb is present is delusional and cannot be altered by rational argument. The phenomenon is acute, but limited in time, and is due to a large, right hemisphere lesion.

demarcation potential See **injury potential**.

dementia (Lat, out of + the mind) An acquired, persistent, more or less global impairment of intellectual, emotional, conative, and cognitive functioning due to biochemical or diffuse structural disease of the brain, occurring in the alert state, and leading to functional incapacity. Some authorities suggest that any three of language, memory, visuospatial skills, emotion, personality, and cognition should be affected in order to make the diagnosis. In mental status testing, examination of the level of arousal, orientation, recent and remote memory, language, praxis, visuospatial abilities, calculation, and judgment are necessary to make the clinical diagnosis. The American Psychiatric Association *DSM IV-TR* diagnostic guidelines for dementia[172] can be found at http://www.behavenet.com/capsules/disorders/dsm4TRclassification.htm/.

They require the presence of multiple cognitive deficits including memory impairment *and* at least one of the following:

Aphasia, apraxia, or agnosia
A disturbance in executive functioning

A loss of intellectual abilities of sufficient severity to interfere with social or occupational functioning and must represent a decline from a higher level of functioning.

Previous definitions required at least one of the following: impairment of abstract thinking as manifested by the concrete interpretation of proverbs; inability to find similarities and differences between related words and other similar tasks; impaired judgment; other disturbances of higher cortical function; personality changes; and no clouding of consciousness.

The word was first used in the modern sense by the French psychiatrist Pinel, before which time it was taken to mean all kinds of mental disease. Kraepelin (a German psychiatrist) later distinguished the schizophrenias and depressive reactions, while keeping the word *dementia* as their prefix.

The causes of dementia include numerous medical and metabolic diseases, including the effect of toxic agents as well as diseases of the CNS.[1373] **Alzheimer disease** is the commonest single cause. The first treatable form recognized was the dementia of **pellagra**.

Despite one's natural concern, it is well to recall that "Old age does not extinguish genius, provided active study be not abandoned," (Cicero, quoted by Alexander Crichton of the Westminster Hospital, London in his work *On Mental Derangement*, vol. 1, London, 1798.)

A Web site addressing dementia pathology (from the Internet Pathology Laboratory) is at http://library.med.utah.edu/WebPath/TUTORIAL/CNS/CNSDG.html/.

See also **multi-infarct dementia**.

Behavior Disturbance Scale An instrument designed to measure behavioral disturbances in patients with severe dementia.[449]

dementia guidelines New dementia guidelines released by the AAN designed to facilitate early detection, diagnosis, and treatment options for dementia patients and their families. The full text with data, tables, and summaries for physicians, patients, family, and friends is available at www.aan.com/public/practiceguidelines.

dementia infantilis See **Heller disease**.

dementia lacking distinctive histologic features (DLDH) An uncommon primary cerebral degenerative condition involving multiple sites and presenting with memory loss and personality changes, leading on to dysphagia and dysarthria after a course of between 2 and 7 years.

Pathologically, the condition is characterized by cell loss and astrocytosis in the frontoparietal cortex, striatum, medial thalamus, substantia nigra, and hypoglossal nucleus; but neuronal inclusions, neurofibrillary tangles, and senile plaques are not seen.

The degree of overlap between this condition and **frontal lobe dementia, Pick disease without Pick bodies, nonspecific degeneration, dementia with ALS**, and **dysphasic dementia** is not defined but is likely to be considerable.[3500]

dementia of frontal lobe type See **frontal lobe dementia**.

Dementia Mood Assessment Scale An objective measure of mood in cognitively impaired subjects, though not a diagnostic instrument for depression. Seven of the 24 items are concerned with providing an indication of the severity of dementia. Scores for the factors of depression, social interaction, anxiety, and vegetative symptoms can be extracted.[6131]

dementia paralytica (general paralysis of the insane, Bayle disease) Tertiary syphilis, first described by Thomas **Willis** and later by Antoine **Bayle**, a French physician in 1822. It was discovered to be a syphilitic affection by Jean Fournier, a French syphilologist in 1894. See **general paralysis of the insane**.

dementia pugilistica See **punch-drunk syndrome**.

Dementia Rating Scale (Mattis Dementia Rating Scale) A short, practical, formalized, bedside screening test instrument designed to assess cognitive dysfunction, particularly memory and behavior.[4183]

The scale is a shortened form of Mattis' much longer organic mental syndrome screening test battery, of value in the evaluation of severely demented patients. Five subscales (attention, perseveration and initiation, construction, conceptualization, and verbal and nonverbal memory) comprise the test. The perseveration item strengthens it in comparison to almost all others, although there remains a substantial false–negative rate.

Dementia Rating Scales See **Addenbrooke's Cognitive Evaluation, Alzheimer Disease Cooperative Study Activities of Daily Living Inventory, Alzheimer Disease Assessment Scale, Blessed Rating Scale, Behavioral Pathology in Alzheimer Disease, Behavioral Rating Scale for Dementia, Behavioral Rating Scale for Geriatric Patients, Brief Cognitive Rating Scale, Brief Psychiatric Rating Scale, Clinical Dementia Rating Scale, Clinician Interview-Based Impression of Change Plus (caregiver questionnaire), Cohen-Mansfield Agitation Inventory, Cornell Scale for Depression in Dementia, Dementia Rating scale, Disability Assessment for Dementia, Ferms D test, Global Deterioration Scale, Goal Attainment Scaling, Mini-Mental State Examination, Modified Ordinal Scales of Psychological Development, Neuropsychiatric Inventory, Present Behavioral Examination, Severe Impairment Battery, Test for Severe Impairment,** and **Wechsler Adult Intelligence Scale**.

Dementia Research Group A professional group based at the **National Hospital for Neurology & Neurosurgery** in London, UK. www.dementia.ion.ucl.ac.uk.

dementia screening tests Instruments designed to determine the presence of diminished cognitive function, usually in the elderly, and to chart progression of the disorder. They include the following. (See Chart D–3.) Those in boldface are those with which this author is most familiar and these are further described in this book.
A Google/PubMed search will locate most of the rest.

dementia syndrome of depression The occurrence of intermittent confusion and memory impairment in a person (usually elderly) suffering from a primary depressive illness as a complication of the early stages of **Alzheimer disease**. Although these signs are reversible with appropriate antidepressant therapy, other evidence of the underlying dementia surfaces within a year or two.[5227]

dementia, vertical gaze palsy, copper dysmetabolism syndrome See **Willvonseder syndrome**.

Dementia Web A source of information, advice, education, research findings, and support for patients and professionals supported by the Dementia Research Group, CANDID (Counselling and Diagnosis in Dementia), The **National Hospital for Neurology and Neurosurgery**, The Institute

Chart D–3. Favored Dementia Screening Tests

AB Cognitive Screen
Addenbrookes Cognitive Examination— Revised Abbreviated Mental Test
Brief Alzheimer Screen
Brief Cognitive Scale
Cognitive Abilities Screening Instrument
Cognitive Assessment Screening Test
Cognitive Capacity Screening Examination
Clock Drawing Test
Deterioration Cognitive (Observer)
Dem Tect
Dementia Questionnaire
General Practitioner Assessment of Cognition
Hopkins Verbal Learning Test
Informant Questionnaire on Cognitive Decline in the Elderly (a short form is also published)
Minnesota Cognitive Acuity Screen
Mini-Cog
Memory Impairment Screen
Mini-Mental State Examination
Modified Mini-Mental State Examination
Montpellier Screen
Neurobehavioral Cognitive Status Examination (Cognistat)
Rotterdam Version of the Cambridge Cognitive Examination
Rapid Dementia Screening Test
Short and Sweet Screening Instrument
Seven-Minute Screen
Six Item Screen
Short Memory Questionnaire
Short Orientation Memory Concentration Test (6-CIT, Short Blessed Test)
Short Portable Mental Status Questionnaire
Short Test of Mental Status
Symptoms of Dementia Screener
Three-Word Recall
Time and Change
Telephone Interview of Cognitive Status-Modified Trail Making Test
Verbal Fluency Categories
Modified WORLD Test

of Neurology and Imperial College School of Medicine at St. Mary's, London, UK.

dementia with ALS

dementia with ALS See **frontal lobe dementia**.

dementia with argyrophilic grains

dementia with argyrophilic grains A syndrome of progressive dementia resembling **Alzheimer disease** or **Pick disease** but characterized by the presence of argyrophilic grains (granular filaments staining with Alz-50 monoclonal antibody throughout the cerebral cortex) rather than senile plaques, neurofibrillary tangles, or Pick bodies characteristic in such types of dementia.[3107]

dementia with Lewy bodies

(DLB, cortical Lewy body disease, idiopathic/diffuse Lewy body disease/ dementia, Lewy body variant of Alzheimer disease, etc. A dozen other names have been given.[2733]) A clinically and genetically heterogeneous dementing disorder due to α-synuclein dysmetabolism (**synucleopathy**) in which **Lewy bodies** are found in frontal and temporal cortical and limbic regions and in the brainstem; there are also spongy changes in the medial temporal lobe and pallor in the substantia nigra. Neuronal loss also occurs in the substantia nigra, locus ceruleus, and substantia innominata. The condition is usually sporadic; dominant transmission is rare (see below). A pattern of relatively focused atrophy of the midbrain, hypothalamus, and substantia innominata with a relative sparing of the hippocampus and temporoparietal cortex is suggestive of DLB and aids in differentiation from Alzheimer disease[6761] as does the presence of frontal intermittent rhythmic delta activity on the EEG.

The features differentiating this condition from other "cortical" dementias are that the dementing features fluctuate, Parkinsonism may be present, and there are greater disturbances of attention, fluency, and information processing in this disorder.[967, 2355, 2360] The occurrence of urinary incontinence is unusually early in this condition compared with **Alzheimer disease**. *Diffuse*, *transitional*, and *brainstem* types of Lewy body disease have been differentiated on the basis of the distribution of these neuronal inclusions. Signs suggesting **amyotrophic lateral sclerosis** and **multiple-system atrophy** may also be found. Features differentiating this condition from **Alzheimer disease** are the relatively early occurrence of urinary incontinence and the

Chart D–4. Revised Criteria for the Clinical Diagnosis of Dementia with Lewy Bodies (DLB)

1. *Central feature* (essential for a diagnosis of possible or probable DLB)
   Dementia (progressive cognitive decline of sufficient magnitude to interfere with normal social or occupational functioning)
   Prominent or persistent memory impairment may not necessarily occur in the early stages but is usually evident with progression. Deficits on tests of attention, executive function, and visuospatial ability may be especially prominent.
2. *Core features* (two core features are sufficient for a diagnosis of *probable* DLB, one for *possible* DLB)
   Fluctuating cognition with pronounced variations in attention and alertness
   Recurrent visual hallucinations that are typically well formed and detailed
   Spontaneous features of Parkinsonism
3. *Suggestive features* (If one or more of these is present in the presence of one or more core features, a diagnosis of probable DLB can be made. In the absence of any core features, one or more suggestive features are sufficient for possible DLB. Probable DLB should not be diagnosed on the basis of suggestive features alone.)
   REM sleep behavior disorder
   Severe neuroleptic sensitivity
   Low dopamine transporter uptake in basal ganglia demonstrated by SPECT or PET imaging
4. *Supportive features* (commonly present but not proven to have diagnostic specificity)
   Repeated falls and syncope
   Transient, unexplained loss of consciousness
   Severe autonomic dysfunction, for example, orthostatic hypotension and urinary incontinence
   Hallucinations in other modalities
   Systematized delusions
   Depression
   Relative preservation of medial temporal lobe structures on CT/MRI scan
   Generalized low uptake on SPECT/PET perfusion scan with reduced occipital activity
   Abnormal (low uptake) MIBG myocardial scintigraphy
   Prominent slow-wave activity on EEG with temporal lobe transient sharp waves
5. A diagnosis of DLB is *less likely*
   In the presence of cerebrovascular disease evident as focal neurologic signs or on brain imaging
   In the presence of any other physical illness or brain disorder sufficient to account in part or in total for the clinical picture
   If Parkinsonism only appears for the first time at a stage of severe dementia
6. *Temporal sequence* of symptoms
   DLB should be diagnosed when dementia occurs before or concurrently with Parkinsonism (if it is present). The term "Parkinson disease dementia" (PDD) should be used to describe dementia that occurs in the context of well-established Parkinson disease. In a practice setting, the term that is most appropriate to the clinical situation should be used and generic terms such as *LB disease* are often helpful. In research studies in which distinction needs to be made between DLB and PDD, the existing 1-year rule between the onset of dementia and Parkinsonism DLB continues to be recommended. Adoption of other time periods will simply confound data pooling or comparison between studies. In other research settings that may include clinicopathologic studies and clinical trials, both clinical phenotypes may be considered collectively under categories such as LB disease or α-synucleinopathy.

From: McKeith I, Dickson DW, Lowe J, et al. Diagnosis and management of dementia with Lewy bodies. *Neurology* 2005;65:1863–1875. Reproduced by kind permission of the American Academy of Neurology and Lippincott Williams & Wilkins.

Chart D–4A. Diagnostic Criteria for Lewy Body Disease Using Neuropsychological Criteria.

A. Severe attention deficit (low total digit-span score),
B. Impaired verbal fluency affecting letter and category fluency tasks equally,
C. Severely impaired visuospatial performance on the WISC-R block design and on drawing tests, and
D. Difficulty in writing to dictation; with signs on neurological examination:

1. Mild extrapyramidal features, particularly masked facies, often combined with bradykinesia, slowing of rapid alternating movements or gait difficulty in the absence of flexed posture, resting tremor and other classical Parkinsonian signs.
2. Essential tremor.

Adapted from Hansen, L., Salmon, D., Galasko, D. et al. The Lewy-body variant of Alzheimer's disease. *Neurology* 1990;40:1–8 and reproduced by kind permission of the American Academy of Neurology and Lippincott Williams & Wilkins.

presence of fluctuating disturbances of arousal (confusion, inattention, and disorganization of speech) alternating with lucid periods. Differentiation from **Parkinson disease with dementia** (PDD) is arbitary; PDD is diagnosed if dementia occurs only after the onset of clinical Parkinson disease, while DLB is diagnosed if the motor and the cognitive signs each occur during the first year of clinical illness. Consensus guidelines for the diagnosis have been published and are given in Chart D–4.

The clinical phenotypes produced are, however, diverse; they include those of idiopathic and of (dominantly inherited) juvenile **Parkinson disease** and of **Alzheimer disease** with added features of Parkinson disease.[2435]

Other published criteria (reviewed by Mega et al.[4281]) require variously a **Clinical Dementia Rating Scale** score of 0.5–2 and extrapyramidal signs, delusions or hallucinations, unexplained falls, transient clouding of consciousness, fluctuating cognition, attention or alertness, failure to respond to L-dopa, and/or unusual sensitivity to neuroleptics. Another system[2732] requires a neuropsychological profile.

In other *variant* forms, Lewy body Parkinsonism is inherited as an autosomal dominant characteristic in adult life;[6667] in one kinship, mapping to 2q35–q36 (adjacent to the *PARK11* locus) has been accomplished.

A valuable Web site is at www.nottingham.ac.uk/pathology/lewy/lewyhome.html.

dementia with lobar atrophy and neuronal cytoplasmic inclusions

See **Pick disease**.

dementia with widespread neurofibrillary tangles

A dominantly inherited, slowly progressive neurodegenerative disease characterized by early-onset dementia resembling that of **Alzheimer disease** but with pathological features resembling **progressive supranuclear palsy**. The condition may be classified as a **tauopathy**.[5230]

demilunes of Adamkiewicz

Crescent-shaped cells lying beneath the neurilemma of medullated nerve fibers, described by **Adamkiewicz** in 1885.

DemTect

A brief cognitive screening test used in the diagnosis of dementia and able to differentiate between Alzheimer disease and minimal cognitive impairment.[3274]

demyelinating motor neuropathy

A syndrome of asymmetrical multifocal lower motor neuron lesions closely resembling **multifocal motor neuropathy with conduction block**. In fact many of the patients have anti-GM1 antibodies. Criteria for the diagnosis have been suggested:[4092]

Asymmetric lower motor neuron-type limb weakness
Chronic progressive course
Absence of pyramidal and of sensory findings
Electrical evidence of both axonal and demyelinating pathology and sometimes multifocal conduction block.

demyelinating neuropathies

One of the two major forms of peripheral neuropathy distinguished by primary and selective attack upon the Schwann cells leading to **segmental demyelination** and sometimes to the formation of **onion bulbs**. See also **axonal neuropathies**.

demyelinating polyneuropathy with IgM binding to GalNAc-GD1a and GM2 gangliosides

A rare distal symmetrical sensorimotor neuropathy of adult life presenting with gait disorder and distal pan-sensory loss, mild weakness, areflexia, and cerebellar signs. The course is slowly progressive over years. Electrodiagnostic testing shows the demyelinating neuropathy. A serum M-protein is detectable. See http://www.wustl.edu/neuromuscular and **monoclonal gammopathy of uncertain significance**.

demyelination

Loss of myelin, which in the CNS is due to disease affecting the oligodendroglia and in the peripheral nervous system to that affecting the Schwann cells. *Primary demyelination* is due to disorders which selectively damage myelin itself or the cells which form it. *Secondary demyelination* refers to the breakdown of myelin following axonal degeneration (see **Wallerian degeneration**).

The electrodiagnostic criteria[864] for demyelination in peripheral nerves are listed under **acute inflammatory demyelinating polyneuropathy**. They include complete or partial conduction block; slowed conduction; failure to transmit high-frequency impulses and the occurrence of **ephaptic transmission**.

DEND syndrome

(Developmental delay, Epilepsy, and Neonatal Diabetes) A rare neonatal disorder compromising infantile, diabetes, mild or more severe psychomotor retardation, developmental delay, therapy-resistant seizures, and muscle weakness. A mutation in a potassium ion channel has been found responsible.

dendrite

(Gr, tree or plant) The small, many-branched afferent processes leading back to the neuronal cell body.

denervation

1. The separation of a structure which is normally innervated from its nerve supply. The term is usually employed for the changes in muscle separated thus from its motor nerve supply,

which include atrophy and loss of contractile ability clinically, an increase in the number of acetylcholine receptor sites on the muscle membrane and a decrease in the resting membrane potential physiologically.
2. Electromyographically, the presence of increased insertional activity, abnormal spontaneous activity at rest (fibrillations and positive sharp waves), reduced recruitment of **motor unit potentials** with increased amplitude, abnormally long duration, polyphasia, and a high firing rate.

denervation hypertrophy An increase in the volume of partially denervated muscles, most often seen in cases of long-standing disease of the lower motor neuron, in which muscle biopsy specimens show both myofibrillar atrophy and hypertrophy. Whether this hypertrophy is due to stretch or to excessive work performed by the residual myofibrils is not known. In cases of **myokymia** or **pseudomyotonia**, continuous muscle work is considered to be the likely explanation.

denervation potential See **fibrillation potential** and **positive sharp wave**.

dengue A common mosquito-borne arboviral disease occurring in the Orient and in Africa, transmitted by mosquitoes, and due to members of the dengue group of viruses. Clinically, it is manifest by a remitting and relapsing course with severe prostrating head and eye pains, chemosis, corneal ulceration, conjunctivitis, lymphadenopathy, desquamating erysipeloid skin rashes, muscle pain, severe malaise, and flitting arthropathy. It may also cause benign acute childhood viral myositis ("myalgia cruris epidemica").

Encephalopathy with tonic–clonic seizures and periodic lateralized discharges on the EEG; severe motor weakness probably due to myositis; *dengue hemorrhagic fever* (a severe, often fatal, complication for which there is no specific treatment); ADEM; and Guillain–Barré syndrome are all rare complications.[3414, 4870] Prevention centers upon avoiding mosquito bites in areas where dengue occurs or might occur and eliminating breeding sites.

denial of illness Any condition or illness that is not acknowledged by the patient, although a healthy subject could be expected to be aware of it. This suggests an active or almost delusional process, especially since some subjects may be aware, for example, of paresis of an arm but deny any problem in their equally paretic leg. Associated sensory and/or cognitive deficits are also usually present.[1846]

The phenomenon was described first by **Anton** in 1898 with reference to his patients who were unaware of blindness. See **anosognosia**, the term suggested by **Babiński**. See also **neglect**.

Dennie, Charles Clayton (1883–1917) American dermatologist.

Dennie–Marfan syndrome (congenital syphilitic paralysis) Incomplete spastic or flaccid pareses of the legs, mental retardation, seizures, nystagmus, and cataracts occurring in children with **congenital syphilis**.[1580]

Dennis syndrome A congenital dysmorphic syndrome manifesting mental retardation, sparse hair, joint laxity, seizures, early closure of the fontanelles, and developmental delay.

Denny-Brown, Derek Ernest (1901–1981) New Zealand-born neurophysiologist and neurologist who trained in medicine at Otago and then worked under **Sherrington** at Oxford, where he developed his interest in the control of motor systems, posture, and muscle physiology. After training further in neurology at the **National Hospital** and at Guy's Hospital under **Holmes** and Symonds, he was appointed to the National and to St. Bartholomew's hospitals as neurologist in 1935, spending the following year at Yale on a Rockefeller fellowship.

He was at first unable to take up the James Jackson Putnam Chair of Neurology at Harvard, which he was offered in 1939, because of his wartime responsibility for setting up the medical side of the head injuries research unit at Oxford, but did so in 1941, returning to England in 1945 for a year to study nutritional deficits in prisoners of war. Thereafter he continued his clinical and laboratory activities at Boston City Hospital.

Among his areas of his particular research success, one may include the treatment of **Wilson disease** with British Anti-Lewisite, his description of the **hereditary sensory and autonomic neuropathies**, electromyography, **paraneoplastic syndromes**, parietal lobe functions and stroke syndromes, and continuing studies on the central and peripheral control of movement. Denny-Brown was also universally respected as a clinician and as an inspiring teacher of undergraduates and of neurologists in training.[2145, 2340]

Denny-Brown syndrome 1. **Hereditary sensory and autonomic neuropathy, type 1**. 2. **Paraneoplastic sensory neuropathy** with polymyositis.[1585]

Denny-Brown–Foley syndrome A syndrome of benign fasciculations with cramps, unassociated with other evidence of neurological disease, and of unknown cause.[1595] See **benign fasciculations and cramps**.

dens (Lat, a tooth) The tooth-like process pointing upward from the axis, covered by the transverse ligament of the atlas and helping to maintain stability of the head on the neck.

dense triangle sign An area of density seen posteriorly within the superior sagittal sinus on an unenhanced CT scan in patients with thrombosis of this sinus. See also **empty delta sign**.

dentate gyrus Three-layered archicortex on the inferomesial aspect of the temporal lobe. With the hippocampus this makes up the hippocampal formation.

dentatorubral atrophy See **dentatorubralpallidoluysian atrophy** and **Ramsay Hunt syndrome**.

dentato-rubro-olivary degeneration A form of **pallidonigral degeneration** with clinical features resembling those of **Friedreich ataxia**.

dentato-rubral-pallido-luysian atrophy (DRPLA; OMIM 125370) A group of **pallidonigral degenerations** with both dominant inheritance and sporadic occurrence at any age, reported mainly from Japan. Their onset is usually in young or mid-adult life and they are characterized by dementia, ophthalmoplegias, vertical nystagmus, cerebellar signs, choreoathetosis, ataxia, chorea, dystonia, and sometimes fasciculations and myoclonus in various combinations. Phenotypic variability is extensive and the precise diagnosis is made most often at postmortem,[3072, 6419] but a trinucleotide repeat expansion at chromosome 12q23-24-1 or 12p13.31 (*atrophin-1*) is detectable. The condition is a cause of **progressive myoclonus epilepsy**[5916, 6188] but could equally well be classified as a **cerebellar ataxia**.

The pathological changes involve mainly the dentate nucleus and the external segment of the globus pallidus and thus the subthalamic and red nuclei.

Some *variants* are described as follows:

Myoclonic form A syndrome with onset in young or mid-adult life characterized by choreoathetosis, myoclonus, and dementia.[6188]

Pseudo-Huntington form A dominantly inherited syndrome with onset in young or mid-adult life characterized by ataxia, choreoathetosis, dystonias, progressive myoclonic epilepsy, generalized seizures, and dementia.[6188] An identical *sporadic form* is also recorded.

Ataxic-choreoathetotic form A syndrome in which the initial ataxia is overwhelmed by choreoathetosis and dementia.[5916]

dentolabials Those consonants such as "F" and "V", which depend for their utterance upon pressure of the teeth upon the lips. See also **articulated labials**.

Denver Developmental Screening Test A complex assessment battery assessing personal-social, fine motor-adaptive, gross motor, and language skills in children up to the age of 6 years.[2179] A refinement has since been pubished.[2179]

deorsumduction See **ductions**.

depersonalization (cerebrocardiac neurosis, Krishaber disease) A distressing, insightful illusion of the unreality of the self in an unreal world but reversible, most easily by external stimulation; the feeling that one is not a real being, or that the mind and body are separated.[3566] A state in which the individual feels himself changed throughout in comparison with his former state. This change extends both to the self and to the outer world and leads to the individual not acknowledging himself as a personality. "His actions seem to him automatic; he observes his own actions like a spectator. The outer world seems strange to him and has lost its character of reality" (Paul Schilder, 1914).

It occurs in complex partial seizures and in some depressive and dissociated psychiatric illnesses but also occasionally as a normal phenomenon, mainly in adolescents and young adults.[5810]

depolarization The reduction of the internal negativity of the cell, normally about –90 mV, by an inward rush of sodium ions in consequence of a sufficiency of excitatory postsynaptic potentials playing upon the cell membrane. If depolarization is adequate, an action potential is generated. See **polarization**.

depolarization block Failure of an excitable cell to respond to a stimulus due to pre-existing depolarization of the cell membrane.[19]

depression 1. Sadness. 2. A morbid condition, presumably a biochemical disorder of the CNS, characterized by mental and/or physical symptoms, and signs which frequently suggest the presence of structural neurological disease. The most common forms of depressive disorders are major depressive disorder and dysthymic disorder.

Features of a depressive episode (abstracted from the NIMH site; http://www.nimh.nih.gov/health/publications/adhd/symptoms.shtml/) include the following:

Lasting sad, anxious, or empty mood
Feelings of hopelessness or pessimism
Feelings of guilt, worthlessness, or helplessness
Loss of interest or pleasure in activities once enjoyed, including sex
Decreased energy, a feeling of fatigue or of being "slowed down"
Difficulty concentrating, remembering, making decisions
Restlessness or irritability
Sleeping too much, or can't sleep
Change in appetite and/or unintended weight loss or gain
Chronic pain or other persistent bodily symptoms that are not caused by physical illness or injury
Thoughts of death or suicide, or suicide attempts

A depressive episode is diagnosed if five or more of these symptoms last most of the day, nearly every day, for a period of 2 weeks or longer.

Particular forms of depressive disorder include the following:

Major depressive disorder is characterized by a combination of symptoms that interfere with a person's ability to work, sleep, study, eat, and enjoy once-pleasurable activities. Major depression is disabling. It may occur only once in a person's lifetime, but more often it recurs.

Dysthymic disorder (dysthymia) is characterized by long-term (2 years or longer) but less severe symptoms that may not be disabling but can prevent normal functioning. One or more episodes of major depression may occur.

Psychotic depression, which occurs when a severe depressive illness is accompanied by some form of psychosis, manifesting as a break with reality with hallucinations and delusions.

Postpartum depression, the occurrence of a major depressive episode within 1 month after delivery.

Seasonal affective disorder (SAD), characterized by the onset of a depressive illness during the winter months, when there is less natural sunlight. The depression generally lifts during spring and summer.

Bipolar disorder (manic-depressive illness) is less common than major depression or dysthymia. It is characterized by cycling mood changes—from extreme highs (e.g., **mania**) to extreme lows (e.g., depression), the dramatic mood swings—overly "high" and/or irritable alternating with sad and hopeless, and then back again, often with periods of normal mood in between. Marked changes in energy and behavior go along with these changes in mood.

The American Psychiatric Association *DSM IV-TR* diagnostic guidelines[172] can be found at http://www.behavenet.com/capsules/disorders/dsm4TRclassification.htm/.

The key *DSM-IV* diagnostic criteria for major depressive disorder are that five or more of the following symptoms have been present during the same 2-week period and represent a change from previous functioning; and that at least one of the symptoms is either (1) or (2) below:

(1) Depressed mood most of the day
(2) Markedly diminished interest or pleasure in activities most of the day (anhedonia; loss of the ability to experience interest or pleasure).

The other symptoms include significant weight loss; insomnia or hypersomnia; psychomotor agitation or retardation; fatigue or loss of energy; feelings of worthlessness or excessive or inappropriate guilt; reduced ability to think or concentrate, or indecisiveness; and the presence of recurrent thoughts of death (not just fear of dying), recurrent suicidal ideation without a specific plan, or a suicide attempt or a specific plan for committing suicide. Many of these features are assessed in depression rating scales.

Depression Adjective Checklist A self-report questionnaire appropriate for the repeated assessment of depressive mood.[3942]

depression of visual acuity A loss of visual field that is relative, so that some stimuli are seen but others are not.

depression rating scales Instruments for diagnosing depression or for recording depressive symptomatology in order to assess the effect of therapy. See **Beck Depression Inventory; Cornell Scale; Depression Center for Epidemiologic Studies Depression Scale (CES-D); Depression Adjective Checklist; Geriatric Rating Scale for Depression; Hamilton Rating Scale**; Lubin Scale; and **Zung Self-Rating Depression Scale**.

depressive pseudodementia Reduction of cognitive abilities during a depressive illness. Since dementia is generally considered irreversible but these patients are likely to recover, this cognitive syndrome does not fit the standard definition. In some cases, the "dementia" is psychogenic.[586]

depth electrodes Electrodes inserted using stereotactic techniques into the substance of the brain for stimulation or recording. Fine wires inserted into the substance of the brain in order to detect and localize abnormal electrical discharges in patients with epilepsy.

depth electroencephalogram (DEEG) The electrical activity of the brain recorded by means of electrodes implanted within the brain substance itself. See also **stereotactic (stereotaxic) depth electroencephalogram**.

depth electroencephalography The technique of recording the electrical activity of the brain by means of electrodes implanted within the brain substance itself.

depth perception The ability to distinguish the relative distances of objects seen. The sense depends upon stereopsis and upon such visual clues as overlap and relative appearance of movement.

depth sense esthesiometry A simple test, invented by Dr. S. Renfrew in 1960, for assessing fingertip sensation using an acrylic plate with a sloping ridge. The subject passes a finger across the plate and sensation is measured according to his threshold of appreciation of the presence of the ridge.[5895]

deranencephalia (Gr, long + negative + the brain) (derencephalus) A malformation characterized by the total absence of the encephalon, the CNS consisting solely of the spinal cord.

Dercum, Francis Xavier (1856–1931) American neurologist and anthropologist, who succeeded C.K. Mills as head of the neurology clinic at the University of Philadelphia and was later appointed professor at Jefferson Medical College. His interests were in medical photography and hysteria and he wrote and edited successful textbooks on neurological therapeutics and on psychiatry.[5704]

Dercum disease (adiposis dolorosa, Ander disease) The association of headache and depression with voluminous and painful nodular accumulations of fat in the legs of middle-aged women. Peripheral neuropathy is said to be associated.[1601, 1602]

derealization The feeling that the world around is unreal and qualitatively different from its normal state. The causes are the same as for **depersonalization**. See also **Alice in Wonderland syndrome**.

derivation 1. The process of recording from a pair of electrodes in an EEG channel. 2. The EEG record obtained by this process.

dermal nerve sheath myxoma See **neurothecoma**.

dermatalgia Skin pain.

dermataneuria Skin anesthesia.

dermatoid (dermoid) Resembling the skin.

dermatoleukodystrophy A congenital dysmorphic syndrome manifesting also cutis laxa and excessive skin wrinkling, neurodegenerative regression, optic atrophy, grand mal seizures, cerebellar and pyramidal signs, and cerebral atrophy with diffuse gliosis and demyelination.[381]

dermatomal somatosensory-evoked potential Scalp-recorded waveforms generated from repeated stimulation of a specific dermatome. These are not the same as the **somatosensory-evoked potentials** recorded in response to stimulation of a named peripheral nerve. (From the 2001 Report of the Nomenclature Committee of the American Association of Electromyography and Electrodiagnosis.[19] Reproduced by kind permission of the AANEM.)

dermatomes The geographical areas of skin whose sensory afferents run to a single cord segment. Developmentally, the pattern can be understood as a result of outpouching of the limb buds, the trunk having a simple banded arrangement of dermatomes (although there is considerable overlap which itself varies according to the sensory modality examined). Their arrangement in the limbs is more complicated, to the extent that no two sources agree precisely. Current views are based largely on the studies of herpes zoster made by Henry **Head** and Otto **Foerster**.[2135]

dermatomyositis (Wagner syndrome, Wagner–Unverricht syndrome) An autoimmune acute, subacute, or chronic inflammatory disease of children or adults affecting muscle and skin, both of which show lymphocytic infiltration. The disease process targets the vascular endothelium, leading to ischemic tissue injury. The condition is differentiated from **polymyositis** and from **inclusion body myositis** on the bases of the frequent skin involvement and variations in the clinical and pathological findings. It is probably more common than either of these latter conditions. Various antibodies (Mi-2, Jo-1, EJ, etc., in the childhood form; Mi-2 EJ, Mi-2, or PM-Scl antibodies in adults) may be detected. The condition may be associated with malignancies and an *amyopathic form* is also described. **Childhood dermatomyositis** has different characteristics and is considered to be a separate condition, as is the form induced by penicillamine.[1038]

More females than males are affected. A mauve-colored ("heliotrope") skin eruption is seen on the eyelids and face, the extensor joint surfaces and other areas exposed to the sun. The nail beds often show erythema and scaling. Muscle fatigue, dysphagia, and respiratory muscle weakness are common, and involvement of the lungs and myocardium is usual. The distribution of weakness is proximal, the course is usually subacute, serum CK levels are usually greatly raised, and the response to treatment is good unless joint contractures occur. However, in about one-fifth of the cases, a remote carcinoma is present. Retinopathy, conjunctivitis, iritis, uveitis, and small vessel disease (Prinzmetal angina, Raynaud) are other occasional accompaniments.

In adults who are Mi-2 antibody-negative, effusions, arrhythmias, interstitial lung disease, scleroderma and rheumatoid arthritis, and an increased risk of malignancy are added problems, while those *with* this antibody have more pronounced skin involvement but associated connective tissue disorders are uncommon.

Wagner's original description was in 1863,[6591] Unverricht's in 1891.[6448] Diagnostic criteria have been suggested[3026] and are listed below.

Diagnostic criteria for dermatomyositis:

1. Clinical: Proximal muscle weakness, usually symmetrical, progressing over weeks or months, with or without muscle pain. Dermatological manifestations (rash, calcinosis) may be present.
2. Pathological: Muscle fiber necrosis and regeneration, mononuclear cell infiltration. Perifascicular atrophy may be present.
3. Biochemical: Raised serum CK (MM isoenzyme), aldolase, or myoglobin levels.
4. EMG: Multifocal EMG features of myopathy. Spontaneous activity is often present at rest.

The presence of Mi-2 or Jo-1 antibodies, myoglobinuria, and EMG evidence of an irritative myopathy with small amplitude, brief, polyphasic motor units, fibrillations, and positive sharp waves are other helpful laboratory features.

The *adult: Mi-2 antibody-negative* form is associated with other connective tissue disorders such as **scleroderma** and the **CREST** syndrome; effusions, cardiac arrhythmias, interstitial lung disease, and an increased risk of malignancy. See also http://neuromuscular.wustl.edu/antibody/infmyop.htm#pm for further descriptions.

The adult Mi-2 antibody-positive form appears acutely in adults whose skin signs tend to be severe and who all have positive ANA. The HLA type DR7 is overrepresented in this group. The form associated with malignancy is seen in adult females with advanced ovarian carcinoma; or with epithelial nasopharyngeal carcinoma in Oriental subjects.

dermatoradiculoneuromyositis See **neuromyositis**.

dermoid See **dermatoid**.

dermoid cyst (embryoma of head or neck, orbital teratoma, teratoid tumor of head or neck) Rare cysts resembling **epidermoid cysts** in their histology and site of growth in the head and neck, but containing also fragments of skin appendages. They occur almost exclusively in infants and young children.

Nasal dermoids are usually found at birth, a small midline pit on the bridge of the nose being marked by local hairiness and representing the opening of sinus tract extending back to the cribriform plate. *Orbital teratomas* are associated with unilateral exophthalmos and some degree of microphthalmos, commonly visible at birth. The mass lesion may extend into the anterior or middle cranial fossas or into the nasal cavity. *Cervical teratomas* are found in the first year of life, presenting with a mass in the neck frequently compressing the larynx or trachea and the esophagus. *Nasopharyngeal teratomas* are pedunculated or sessile tumors which are present at birth, usually in females, causing airway obstruction, rhinorrhea, and a nasal or retropharyngeal mass; they are sometimes associated with anencephaly or hemicrania.[4642]

dermotrichic syndrome (alopecia–ichthyosis–retardation and seizures) A congenital dysmorphic syndrome manifesting also alopecia, ichthyosis, megacolon or Hirschprung syndrome, aminoaciduria, seizures, and mental and developmental delay.[381] See also **alopecia-mental retardation syndrome**.

desanimania (Lat, down + the mind + madness) Mindless insanity. The term is probably obsolete.

Descartes, Renatus (Rene) (1596–1650) French philosopher and scientist. In his *magnum opus* "De Homine," he considered the pineal to be the seat of the soul whence it controlled the flow of animal spirits within the ventricles. Because he also enunciated the principle that incoming stimuli to the brain lead to specific outgoing motor effects, he may be said to be the first to delineate reflex activity; his examples were withdrawal from pain and the **menace reflex**. His comparison of the eye to a *camera obscura* and his description of accommodation as an effect of a change in the curvature of the lens in his *Dioptrica* (1637) were other prescient contributions.

Descartes reflex (retinoorbicular reflex) Involuntary blinking in response to suddenly presented visual stimuli; thus a variant of the **orbicularis oculi reflex**.

Descemet, Jean (1732–1810) French professor of anatomy and surgery in Paris. His description of the corneal membrane was actually preceded by that of Benedict Duddell, an English surgeon-oculist (1729).[1670]

Descemet membrane The posterior elastic membrane of the cornea, the site of copper deposition in **Wilson disease**.

descending paralysis Unilateral progressive descending paralysis of the trunk and limbs, first described in 1906 by Charles K. Mills (1845–1931), an American neurologist. This condition might well have been **acute inflammatory demyelinating polyneuropathy, botulism**, or **tick paralysis**.

desensitization 1. The lack of response of the receptor on the muscle membrane to persisting high levels of acetylcholine when that substance has not been hydrolyzed quickly; the muscle cell does not remain depolarized in this state, however. 2. A form of deconditioning therapy introduced by Dr. Joseph Wolpe, in which the subject creates a list of anxiety-provoking items graded in order of severity and is exposed to these in order, at lessening distances, intensities, or durations, starting with the least anxiety-provoking item. Such exposure may be either mental as a form of imagery or by actual exposure, as, for example, in the case of the agoraphobic patient who is first taken to the closed door, then the open door, then the doorstep, then the front step, etc., moving only to the next stage when the last is tolerated without excessive anxiety.[6854]

desert blindness See **photophthalmia**.

desmin The intermediate filament protein of skeletal and cardiac muscle fibers and of some smooth muscle cells.[2422] Abnormally it accumulates, as in certain myopathies—sometimes associated with cardiomyopathy—sporadically or in a familial fashion.

desmin storage myopathy See **desminopathy** and **myofibrillar (desmin-storage) myopathy**.

desminopathy (desmin "storage" myopathies) Congenital myopathies with the abnormal expression of type 3 intermediate filaments (desmin) within the subsarcolemmal regions of muscle cells, expressed clinically as a slowly progressive myopathy with cardiomyopathy. Mostly present in childhood and are familial.[6458, 2423]

Three general forms are described below, but the full range of phenotypes extends from asymptomatic hyperCKemia to **rigid spine syndrome** and the prototypes listed below as **desmin-related myopathy**. A common feature is focal dissolution of myofibrils and accumulation of multiple proteins. Links to chromosomes 2q35, 11q22, and 12 have variously been established.[4292]

Granulofilamentous type A slowly progressive, dominantly inherited form with onset in early to middle adult life, presenting with distal muscle weakness and atrophy, gait abnormalities, chest pain, and cardiac arrhythmias due to hypertrophic cardiomyopathy leading to cardiac death. The velopharyngeal muscles are also involved. Lens opacities, neuropathy, intestinal malabsorption, and pseudo-obstruction are less common features. CK levels are normal or slightly raised and the EMG shows a myopathic pattern. Muscle biopsy reveals the subsarcolemmal accumulation of granulofilamentous material containing desmin and sometimes cytoplasmic bodies. The same abnormality is present in cardiac muscles. Affected nerves show giant axons owing to the accumulation of neurofilaments.

Cytoplasmic/spheroid inclusion body type A slowly progressive, dominantly inherited or sporadic form with onset in adolescence or early adult life, presenting with variable-distributed muscle weakness and atrophy and respiratory insufficiency and infrequent cardiac involvement, exertional fatigue, and bulbar weakness.The EMG is myopathic and serum CK levels are normal or mildly elevated. Muscle biopsy reveals desmin-positive filaments in "cytoplasmic (spheroid) bodies"

A form with Mallory body-like inclusion bodies or hyaline/desmin plaques A recessively inherited form with early childhood onset and variable progression manifesting proximal or generalized weakness including respiratory failure, facial weakness, but no eye muscle involvement, high-arched palate, scoliosis, lordosis, and no cardiac involvement. The EMG is myopathic, serum CK levels are slightly raised. Muscle biopsy shows desmin-positive inclusions with granular material, intermediate filaments, and helical filaments called "Mallory body"-like inclusion bodies or hyaline plaques.

desmin-related myopathy A dominantly or recessively inherited **desminopathy** associated with mutations in desmin or B-crystallin with onset up to early adult life. Clinically, the initial leg weakness ascends to involve the trunk, face, and respiratory muscles. Cardiomyopathy with conduction block and dangerous arrhythmias and respiratory insufficiency are later developments. Lens opacities may be seen. CK levels are normal or slightly raised and the EMG is myopathic. Intracytoplasmic desmin-immunoreactive inclusions are seen on muscle biopsy.[4786, 2446] See also **distal muscular dystrophy**.

desmoid tumor (Lat, like a bundle; tumor) A large benign growth of fibrous tissue within muscle.

desmoplastic medulloblastoma See **medulloblastoma**.

desynchronization An alteration in the pattern of EEG activity as a result of external or internal stimuli. See also **blocking**, **attenuation**.

desynchronized sleep Rapid eye movement sleep, in which the regularity of the EEG waveform is disturbed by increased, irregular frequency waves. See **REM sleep**.

D'Este, Augustus (1794–1848) The unaccepted but legitimate grandson of the English King **George III**, who developed signs of **multiple sclerosis** at the age of 28 and who, in his diaries, gave a pitiful account of the progression of his symptoms until 2 months before his death.[2067]

detentio (Lat, keeping back) Catalepsy.

Determann syndrome (dyskinesia intermittens angiosclerotica) See **dystonia**.

De Toni–Fanconi–Debré syndrome Aminoaciduria resulting from dysfunction of the proximal renal tubules. See **mitochondrial cytopathy**.

detrusor (from Lat, to thrust away) The muscular coat of the bladder.

detrusor-external sphincter dyssynergia Contraction of the bladder and of its sphincter at the same time. See **dyssynergia**.

deuteranopia See **color blindness**.

deuteropathia (from Gr, second + disease) A disease induced by another.

deuteropathic lateral sclerosis An unwarranted distinction made by **Charcot** between tonic and atonic atrophy in lateral sclerosis, "the separation being based on the assumption that in such cases the primary lesion is the degeneration of the pyramidal tracts and that the affection of the grey matter is secondary or deuteropathic."[2531]

Deutsche Gesellschaft Bekampfung der Muskelkrankheiten A member society of the European Alliance of Muscular Dystrophy Societies. Web site: http://www.dgm.org/index.php?article_id=123.

Deutsche Gesellschaft für Neurologie A German professional society. Web site: http://www.dgn.org/.

developmental aphasia See **congenital auditory imperception**.

Developmental Assessment A standardized schedule for assessment of gross motor (60 items) and reflex function (18 items) in infants.[3005] Norms for posture and large movements, vision and fine movement, hearing and speech, and social behavior and play have been determined by Sheridan.[5784] See also **Denver Developmental Screening Test**.

Developmental Brain Dysfunction A pediatric neurological journal. Web site: http://content.karger.com/ProdukteDB/produkte.asp?Aktion=JournalHome&ProduktNr=224168.

developmental disabilities Chronic impairments in brain function secondary to maldevelopments or injuries to the developing brain in the perinatal or postnatal periods. The deficits are lifelong and include global cognitive deficits, motor disabilities (cerebral palsy), social and language failures, and specific cognitive deficits.

developmental dyslexia See **word blindness**.

developmental dysphasia (congenital aphasia, congenital word deafness) An isolated developmental deficit or delay in acquiring expressive and/or receptive speech and language for communicative purposes, in the absence of significant hearing loss, emotional disturbance, mental retardation, or aphasia, and resulting from focal pathological lesions usually affecting the left cerebral hemisphere.[1231] See **congenital auditory imperception**.

developmental Foix–Chavany–Marie syndrome See **bilateral central macrogyria**.

developmental indicators for assessment of learning-revised (DIAL-R) A developmental screening test designed to assess gross and fine motor activity, academic, expressive, and receptive language skills, and articulation in children aged between 3 and 7 years.

developmental learning disorders A group of conditions with their onset before puberty, characterized by difficulties in acquisition of speech or certain cognitive functions, or in anomalies of emotional development. These include stuttering, developmental dyslexia, childhood autism, hyperactivity, and possibly **Tourette syndrome**. They occur more often in males, and left-handedness is unusually common among such people.[526]

Developmental Medicine and Child Neurology A subspecialty journal. Web site: http://titles.cambridge.org/journals/journal_catalogue.asp?historylinks=ALPHA&mnemonic=DMC.

Developmental Neuroscience (*Dev Neurosci*) A basic neuroscience journal. Web site: http://www.karger.com/journals/dne/dne_jh.htm.

developmental receptive aphasia See **word deafness**.

developmental reflexes (fetal or primitive reflexes) Responses to stimulation which are normally present in the early stages of maturation of the nervous system but which disappear at various ages, reappearing when the CNS is altered by age or disease. **Sucking, snouting, palmomental, grasp, tonic foot** and **corneo-mandibular reflexes, gegenhalten**, and the ones listed in Chart D–5 are examples.[3, 4939] See also **primitive reflexes**.

Chart D–5. Developmental Reflexes

Reflex	*Age at appearance*	*Age at disappearance (months)*
Adductor spread of knee jerk	Birth	7–8
Landau reflex	10 months	24
Moro	Birth	5–6
Palmar grasp	Birth	6
Parachute	8–9 m	Persists
Plantar grasp	Birth	9–10
Rooting	Birth	3
Tonic neck response	Birth	5–6
Truncal incurvation	Birth	1–2

developmental testing The determination of certain representative motor, sensory, and psychological abilities in children in order to compare them with the average abilities of normal children of the same age.

The procedures were first rationalized by **Charles Darwin**, who described the **rooting reflex**, the cephalocaudal sequence of development, signs of emotional expression and other capabilities. **Arnold Gesell** developed the first "norms" of development in 1925 and numerous others have been published since. The **Denver Developmental Screening Test** appeared in 1967, but was based on a selected and healthy sample of children. It was followed by a briefer revised version in 1981.[2179]

deviation See **ocular motor deviation**.

deviational nystagmus See **gaze-evoked nystagmus**.

Devic, Eugene (1869–1930) French cardiologist practicing in Lyon, remembered for his complete description of **neuromyelitis optica** in 1894, in which he reviewed the reports of the same condition by 16 other authors (not including Albutt, see below).[1617]

Devic disease (Devic–Gault syndrome, neuroptic myelitis) See **neuromyelitis optica**. The condition was first described by **Albutt** in 1870,[128] followed by others, but was redescribed by **Devic** in 1894 and reviewed in detail by his student **Fernand Gault** (in his graduation thesis) in the same year.

Devic–Gault syndrome See **neuromyelitis optica**.

Devil's grippe See **pleurodynia**.

Devonshire colic Abdominal colic due to lead poisoning, described in workers in local lead mines.

dexamethasone suppression test The assessment of baseline plasma cortisol levels before and after the oral administration of 1 mg of dexamethasone. Values greater than 5 μg/dl after administration of the steroid are regarded as abnormal and suggestive of depressive illness so long as primary adrenal disease is not present.[5227]

Di Ferrante syndrome See **mucopolysaccharidosis type 8**.

diabetes insipidus (diabetes neurogenes, spurious diabetes, ureal diabetes) A condition of excessive production of urine and consequent thirst resulting from deficiency of antidiuretic hormone due to lesions of the supraoptic and paraventricular nuclei of the hypothalamus. It was distinguished from diabetes mellitus by **Willis** and shown to be due to a lesion of the posterior lobe of the hypophysis by **Alfred Frank** (b. 1884), a German physiologist. See also **Wolfram syndrome**.

The Web site http://www.diabetesinsipidus. org/ (Diabetes Insipidus Foundation, Inc.) provides information on the different forms of diabetes insipidus.

diabetes insipidus, diabetes mellitus, optic atrophy, and deafness (DIDMOAD) See **Wolfram syndrome**.

diabetes mellitus (Gr, through + to go on; and Lat, sweet) A common disorder of carbohydrate metabolism leading to high levels of blood glucose, glycosuria, and acidosis.

Apart from the neurological syndromes commonly ascribed to diabetes, it may also be noted that there are some disorders in which diabetes is a recognized associate but in which it is not thought to be causal; **myotonic dystrophy**, **Louis-Bar syndrome**, **Huntington disease**, and **progeria** are examples.

diabetes mellitus encephalopathy Organic mental deterioration, often accompanied by pyramidal signs, as a result of hypoglycemic brain damage.[1378]

diabetes mellitus-optic atrophy syndrome The occurrence of optic atrophy, sometimes with nerve deafness, vestibulopathy, hypogonadism, congenital cardiac disease, congenital cataracts, and aminoaciduria in patients with juvenile diabetes mellitus.[319] See also **Wolfram syndrome**.

diabetes neurogenes See **diabetes insipidus**.

diabetes, obesity, and hearing loss A mitochondrial disorder. See **Alström–Hallgren syndrome**.

diabetic amyotrophy See **diabetic radiculoplexus neuropathy**.

diabetic femoral neuropathy A rare form of nerve involvement mainly affecting male non-insulin-dependent diabetic patients aged over 60 years, characterized by the acute occurrence (often following a period of substantial weight loss) of severe burning, dysesthetic anterior thigh pain succeeded by quadriceps weakness and atrophy, loss of the knee jerk, and sensory loss in the painful territory. Incomplete recovery takes place over a year or more.[1277] See **diabetic radiculoplexus neuropathy**. However, a majority of diabetic patients with this syndrome actually have more extensive involvement due to **diabetic amyotrophy**.

diabetic lumbosacral radiculoplexus neuropathy See **diabetic radiculoplexus neuropathy**.

diabetic myelopathy See **diabetic amyotrophy**.

diabetic neuropathic cachexia A condition of male diabetic patients who develop anorexia, extreme weight loss, impotence, malaise, depression, and bilateral symmetrical sensorimotor neuropathy with persistent neuropathic pain, without retinopathy or nephropathy, early in the course of the diabetic disorder.[1839]

diabetic neuropathies (polyneuropathies) A heterogeneous group of peripheral somatic or autonomic neuropathies united by the common factor of their association with diabetes mellitus and characterized by degeneration of both large and small nerve fibers. They were first described by **Pitres** in 1917. Chart D–6 is based upon the classifications of Brown and Asbury,[894] Feldman et al.,[1995] and the San Antonio Conference.[1272] See also **Michigan neuropathy screening instrument**.

Diabetic neuropathies have also been classified for research purposes by the American Diabetes Association as follows:[169]

For the diagnosis of diabetic polyneuropathy, abnormalities of at least two of the following must be present:

1. Nerve Conduction (NCS);
2. Neurological Examination (NE);
3. Quantitative Motor (QME), Autonomic (QAE), or Sensory (QST) testing; or
4. Neuropathic Symptoms (NS).

Further staging is based upon the results of these assessments, as follows:[1770]

Stage 1. (Asymptomatic neuropathy) Two or more abnormalities among NC; NE; or QME, QSE, QAE but no abnormality of NS.
Stage 2. (Symptomatic neuropathy) Two or more abnormalities among NCS; NE; QME, QSE, QAE; or NS. Neuropathic symptoms are present but are of lesser severity than in stage 4.
Stage 3. (Disabling neuropathy) Two or more abnormalities among NCS; NE; QME, QSE, QAE; or NS. Disabling neuropathic symptoms are present.

Chart D–6. Classification of Diabetic Neuropathies

Class I: Subclinical neuropathy

A. Abnormal electrodiagnostic tests only
   1. Decreased nerve conduction velocity
   2. Decreased amplitude of evoked muscle or nerve action potential

B. Abnormal quantitative sensory testing (QST)
   1. Vibratory/tactile
   2. Thermal warming/cooling
   3. Other

C. Abnormal autonomic function tests (AFT)
   1. Diminished sinus arrythmia (beat-to-beat heart rate variation)
   2. Diminished sudomotor function
   3. Increased pupillary latency

In these forms, neurologic function tests are abnormal but no neurologic symptoms or clinically detectable neurologic deficits indicative of a diffuse or focal neuropathy are present. Class I "Subclinical neuropathy" is further subdivided into Class Ia if an AFT or QST abnormality is present, Class Ib if EDX or AFT and QST abnormalities are present, and Class Ic if an EDX and either AFT or QST abnormalities, or both, are present.

Class II: Clinical neuropathy

A. Diffuse neuropathy
   1. Distal symmetric sensorimotor polyneuropathy
      a. Primarily small fiber neuropathy

b. Primarily large fiber neuropathy
c. Mixed

These are the commonest major syndromes of peripheral axonal neuropathy in diabetes. They comprise:

A. *Mixed form*: An insidiously progressive axonal neuropathy producing any combination of motor, sensory, and autonomic involvement, with variable relative degrees of severity.

Clinically, this is the commonest form of diabetic neuropathy and it presents with complaints of numbness, tingling, burning paresthesia, contact hyperesthesia, aching pain, especially at night, impotence, and depression. Examination reveals loss of the ankle jerks and a symmetrical reduction in distal sensations, especially of vibration. In some cases, the manifestations are precipitated by weight loss, unstable diabetes, stress, infections, or insulin therapy.

B. *Sensory form*: An insidiously progressive symmetrical axonal neuropathy affecting large (**diabetic pseudo-tabes**), small, or mixed sensory fibers. Clinically, the pattern of sensory involvement reflects the fiber types involved. In all, paresthesias, dysesthesias, and pain are common complaints and autonomic symptoms may be present.

C. *Motor form*: An uncommon acute reversible motor polyneuropathy that may follow ketoacidosis in younger diabetic patients.

2. Autonomic neuropathy
   a. Abnormal pupillary function
   b. Sudomotor dysfunction
   c. Genitourinary autonomic neuropathy
      1. Bladder dysfunction
      2. Sexual dysfunction
   d. Gastrointestinal autonomic neuropathy
      1. Gastric atony
      2. Gallbladder atony
      3. Diabetic diarrhea
      4. Hypoglycemic unawareness (adrenal medullary neuropathy)
   e. Cardiovascular autonomic neuropathy
   f. Unawareness of hypoglycemia

These forms of selective subacutely evolving autonomic (visceral) neuropathies involve the sympathetic and parasympathetic divisions of the autonomic nervous system in the context of diabetes. Despite the name, features of motor or sensory involvement can often be detected as well. They are most commonly seen in younger insulin-dependent diabetics who present with such problems as pupillary denervation, loss of lacrimal and sweat gland secretions, postural hypotension, cardiac denervation, peripheral edema, intestinal atony, diarrhea, gustatory sweating, loss of respiratory control, bladder atony, retrograde ejaculation, impotence, and unawareness of hypoglycemia. The mortality rate is greatly increased.

B. Focal neuropathy
   1. *Mononeuropathy (peripheral entrapment neuropathy)*: Mononeuropathies occurring at the commoner sites of neural compression as in nondiabetics and carrying a fair prognosis for recovery. Whether or not this is the same as *diabetic multiple mononeuropathy* is uncertain
   2. *Multiple mononeuropathy*
   3. *Plexopathy (proximal symmetrical motor neuropathy)*: An acute, asymmetrical painful motor neuropathy affecting the lumbosacral plexus or the femoral or obturator nerves. The prognosis for eventual recovery is good. See also **diabetic femoral neuropathy** and **diabetic amyotrophy**.
   4. *Radiculopathy*: See **diabetic truncal neuropathy**.
   5. *Cranial mononeuropathy*, which reflects acute ischemic damage to a cranial nerve (usually the third) producing painful ophthalmoplegia with a tendency to spare pupillary reactivity and to abate spontaneously over weeks. The IV, VI, and VII cranial nerves may also be affected.

An alternative classification, with diagnostic criteria and easier to follow was suggested by **Dyck** in 1988 (See Chart D–8).[1770]

diabetic paralytic neuropathy
See **diabetic radiculoplexus neuropathy**.

diabetic polyradiculopathy
See **diabetic radiculoplexus neuropathy**.

diabetic proximal neuropathy
A heterogeneous condition first recognized by **Bruns** in 1890 but best described by **Garland**. See **diabetic amyotrophy**.

diabetic pseudo-tabes
The association of **Argyll Robertson pupils** with lightning pains, posterior column dysfunction, neurogenic bladder, neuropathic arthropathy, and areflexia in the legs, the whole resembling the findings in **tabes dorsalis** but in fact due to diabetic peripheral neuropathy (sensory form) and autonomic neuropathies.

diabetic radiculoplexus neuropathy
(Bruns–Garland syndrome, diabetic paralytic neuropathy, diabetic myelopathy, diabetic myopathy, diabetic amyotrophy, diabetic polyradiculopathy, proximal diabetic neuropathy, multifocal diabetic neuropathy, Garland amyotrophy, diabetic femoral neuropathy) A heterogeneous condition first recognized by Ludwig Bruns in 1890 but best described by Dr. Hugh Garland 63 years later. It is usually a subacute or insidiously progressive,

Chart D–7. Clinical Assessments of Diabetic Neuropathies for Research Purposes

	Symptom Neurologic Examination		*Abnormal physiological tests*
	Score	*Score*	
Class 1			
A	0	0	0 or AFT or QST
B	0 0		EDX or AFT and QST
C	0	0	EDX and AFT and/or QST
Class 2			
A	+	0	0 or AFT or QST
B	0/+	+	EDX or AFT and QST
C	0 or +	+	EDX and AFT and/or QST
or	+	0 or	+

[0 = Normal; + = Abnormal; AFT = Autonomic function testing; EDX = Electrodiagnosis; QST = Quantitative sensory testing.][169, 1770]

From American Diabetes Association. Report and recommendations of the San Antonio Conference on Diabetic Neuropathy. Muscle Nerve *1988; 11: 661–7: and Dyck PJ. Detection, characteristics and staging of polyneuropathy: assessed in diabetics.* Muscle Nerve *1988; 11: 21–32. Copyright 1988. All rights reserved. Reprinted by kind permission of Wiley-Blackwell Publications.)*

often sharply painful, unilateral or bilateral pure motor neuropathy producing atrophy of the quadriceps and other pelvifemoral muscles without sensory impairment, occurring in older insulin-dependent diabetic patients[2290] and in males with noninsulin-dependent diabetes, most of whom have suffered recent marked weight loss. Distal leg and proximal arm muscles may also be affected. EMG evidence of bilateral paraspinal and gluteal denervation is commonly reported. The condition tends to abate over months if diabetic control is attained but IvIg produces faster relief. The lumbosacral is the most common level, but frequently patients get combinations of involvement including thoracic and cervical sites.[5582]

Garland, an English neurologist, noted the presence of upgoing plantar responses

Chart D–8. Diabetic Neuropathy— Neurological Symptom Score[1770]

(Score 1 point for presence of a symptom)

1. Symptoms of muscle weakness
   - A. Bulbar
     1. Extraocular
     2. Facial
     3. Tongue
     4. Throat
   - B. Limbs
     5. Shoulder girdle and upper arm
     6. Hand
     7. Glutei and thigh
     8. Legs
2. Sensory disturbances
   - A. Negative symptoms
     9. Difficulty identifying objects in mouth.
     10. Difficulty identifying objects in hands.
     11. Unsteadiness in walking.
   - B. Positive symptoms
     12. Numbness, asleep feeling, "like Novocain," prickling at any site.
     13. Pain—burning, deep aching, tenderness—at any location.
3. Autonomic symptoms
     14. Postural fainting.
     15. Impotence in male.
     16. Loss of urinary control.
     17. Night diarrhea.

Abnormality of quantitative nerve tests One or more abnormal results among tests assessing muscle strength (QME), detection threshold of vibratory (VDT), cooling (CDT), or warming (WDT) sensation (QSE), or autonomic function (QAE) serve to fulfill criteria for abnormality of quantitative nerve tests.

Symptomatic neuropathy: Occurrence of any symptoms (among the 12 listed below) judged to be due to diabetic polyneuropathy but not disabling (see stage 3 below) is sufficient to fulfill the criteria for stage 2. Patients with questionable degrees of symptoms are staged as 0 or 1.

Motor

1. Symptoms of muscle weakness in acts of daily living and

Sensory

1. Absence of feeling: reported deficiency of tactile, thermal, or nociceptive sensation encountered in acts of daily living.
2. Sensory ataxia: reported unsteadiness in walking
3. Numbness or paraesthesia ("dead asleep," "prickly asleep," "like novocaine," "like hand gone asleep," "tightly bound feeling," etc.) judged by its distribution, persistence, and duration to be due to neuropathy and not due to physiologic compression as occurs in acts of daily living or entrapment, for example, carpal tunnel syndrome or to another condition.
4. Neuropathic pain: burning, aching, excessive discomfort of feet or hands with use, and lancinating pain.

Autonomic

Any of the following symptoms attributed to diabetes mellitus and not due to medications, psychologic disturbance, intercurrent illness, disease of the organ, or previous injury or surgery:

1. Gastric atony
2. Urinary retention
3. Urinary incontinence
4. Rectal incontinence
5. Diarrhoea
6. Impotence in males <65 years of age
7. Postural hypotension, light-headedness, or fainting (with postural decrease of systolic BP > 30 mmHg)

Disabling diabetic neuropathy That degree of diabetic neuropathy in which occurrence of any of the following 10 conditions occurs:

Motor

1. Symptoms of muscle weakness of such severity that the patient cannot walk independently, confirmed by examination.

Sensory

1. Symptoms of sensory loss of sufficient severity that the patient cannot walk independently because of sensory ataxia, confirmed by examination.
2. Absence of feeling in the hands such that the patient is disabled.
3. The presence of disabling neuropathic pain for which the patient has seen physicians for pain relief; work and recreational activities have been curtailed by at least 25%; and medication has been taken for pain on at least half of the preceding 42 days.

Autonomic

1. Gastric atony, as demonstrated by gastric retention tests and by exclusion of other gastric or psychiatric causes of emesis, causing emesis of retained (>18 h) food at least once weekly for at least 6 weeks.
2. Urinary retention as demonstrated by manometer evidence of detrusor hypoactivity and not due to psychiatric disturbance or urinary bladder disease, necessitating continuous use of a catheter for 6 weeks or longer.
3. Urinary incontinence due to loss of sphincter function necessitating continuous (>50% of time) use of diapers or a leg urinal for at least 6 weeks and not due to psychiatric or bladder disease.
4. Rectal incontinence due to loss of anal sphincter function of at least 6 weeks duration and not due to psychiatric or rectal disease.
5. Diarrhea to the degree that it causes weight loss (>5 kg) and steatorrhoea >10 mg/24 h, and not due to psychiatric disturbance, laxative abuse, or other bowel disease.
6. Symptomatic light-headedness or fainting due to orthostatic hypotension (>30 mmHg systolic) with concomitant blood pressure drop, present continuously (light-headedness or fainting weekly) for at least 6 weeks.

From Dyck PJ. Detection, Characteristics and staging of polyneuropathy: assessed in diabetics. Muscle Nerve *1988; 11: 21–32.*

and raised CSF protein levels in many of his patients and concluded that the disease process lay in the spinal cord,[2290] ("diabetic myelopathy"), a view no longer held.

The condition is considered to be a variety of diabetic motor neuropathy with a dysimmune vascular or axonopathic etiology[5503] and the extensor plantar responses are ignored, denied, or ascribed to a vascular lesion at a higher level. See also **diabetic neuropathies** and **nondiabetic lumbosacral radiculoplexus neuropathy** (in which latter case the clinical features are remarkably similar).

diabetic thoracic polyradiculopathy

See **diabetic radiculoplexus neuropathy**.

diabetic truncal neuropathy

(thoraco-abdominal neuropathy, diabetic thoracic radiculopathy or polyradiculopathy, truncal mononeuropathy) A common form of diabetic peripheral neuropathy affecting the truncal nerves at various sites and usually causing severe abdominal or chest pain, not always radicular in character, as well as dysesthesia, sometimes with weakness of the abdominal muscles.[6056, 3463] The condition is associated frequently with marked weight loss but carries a good prognosis for recovery.

Diagnostic Classification of Sleep and Arousal Disorders

A compilation of such disorders first prepared by the American Sleep Disorders Association[4022] but now superseded. See **sleep disorders**.

diagnostic dyspraxia Intermanual conflict occurring as an **alien hand** sign.

diagnostic interview schedule A complex interview-based, observer-rated measure of depression designed to establish the full range of the American Psychiatric Association *DSM-III* depressive disorders.[5335]

diagonal nystagmus See **circular nystagmus**.

diagonal paresis Weakness of one arm and of the opposite leg as a result of a lesion of the highest levels of the spinal cord damaging the corticospinal tract fibers supplying the arm (which at this level have crossed) and those supplying the contralateral leg (which cross one or two segments below).

dialysis cramp Painful calf cramps occurring in patients during hemodialysis, probably due to temporary hyponatremia.[3724]

dialysis dementia See **dialysis encephalopathy**.

dialysis dysequilibrium syndrome An acute delirious state lasting days to weeks, with headache, nausea, musclecramps and occasionally seizures, and due to cellular overhydration as a response to the rapid lowering of blood urea by dialysis.[5395]

dialysis encephalopathy (dialysis dementia) A subacutely progressive syndrome lasting 3–15 months in subjects on hemodialysis for over a year, and characterized by increasing dementia, a dysphasic language disorder often accompanied by hesitant, stuttering speech, and distinctive EEG patterns with **FIRDA**. Myoclonic and generalized seizures, behavioral disturbances, and confusional states are less reliable (though common) components of the syndrome.[1158]

The condition is considered to be due to toxicity from aluminum in the dialysate. Appropriate corrective steps having been taken, it is now vanishingly rare.

dialysis headache Forms of headache experienced by patients on hemodialysis, resolving within 72 h of each hemodialysis session.[2820]

diamond on quadriceps An asymmetric diamond-shaped mass in the middle of the quadriceps muscle, this muscle being wasted both above and below. It is seen when the subject stands with the knee slightly bent and is a marker for dysferlinopathies such as **limb-girdle muscular dystrophy** 2B and **Myoshi myopathy**.

diaphragm reflex of Hess The **abdominal muscle reflex**, obtained by tapping the nipple.

diaphragmatic aplasia A recessive or X-linked syndrome of uni- or bilateral diaphragmatic aplasia. The various specific syndromes are described by Dr. **Alan Pestronk** at his Web site: http://neuromuscular.wustl.edu/syncm.html#blepharophimosis.

diaphragmatic flutter (moving umbilicus syndrome, diaphragmatic tic, tremor, or chorea) Clonic contractions of the diaphragm occurring at high frequency and without any associated inspiratory sound. The syndrome is uncommon, occurs at any age, and is due either to phrenic denervation or irritation of the diaphragm itself. Patients may complain of respiratory distress, muscular fatigue, or pain in the abdominal wall or precordium, or palpitations of the chest. Presentations with recalcitrant asthma, inspiratory stridor, or difficulty in weaning from mechanical ventilation have been recorded.

The condition may represent a variant of the **palatal myoclonus syndrome**. The diaphragm contraction is at the rate 0.5–8.0 Hz but a high-frequency variant (9–15 Hz) has been reported, with symptoms of hiccups, belching, and retching. Most cases are primary or idiopathic, although postencephalitic, postviral, and tardive forms have been reported.[5085] See also **belly dancers' dyskinesia**.[3078]

diaphyseal dysplasia See **Camurati–Engelman syndrome**.

diaschisis (Gr, division or splitting) A sudden abeyance or reduction of motor function following the interruption at a remote site of an afferent pathway which normally supplied background excitation to the neurons in question, keeping them in a state of low activity. "Shock" of the nervous system.[1984]

The concept was introduced first by **von Monakow**, who described *diaschisis cortico-spinalis* (progression of functional depression of the spinal cord following an injury to the motor cortex); *diaschisis commissuralis* (functional depression of the contralateral cerebral cortex after injury to the cortex of one hemisphere); and *diaschisis associativa* (depression of function in intact cortical areas adjacent to the site of a cortical injury). The term now includes the following *varieties*:[4658]

Cortico-cerebellar diaschisis (crossed cerebral-cerebellar diaschisis, cortico-cerebellar diaschisis, transtentorial diaschisis) Reduction of metabolic activity of the cerebellar hemisphere contralateral to the side of a supratentorial ischemic infarct. Clinical signs of this are few.

Crossed hemispheric diaschisis (cerebello-cortical diaschisis, crossed cerebello-cortical diaschisis) Hypoperfusion in the contralateral cerebral hemisphere after unilateral cerebellar infarction.

Transhemispheric diaschisis Bilateral reduction of perfusion in subjects following a unilateral hemispheric infarct and dependent on continuing function of the corpus callosum.

Cortico-thalamic diaschisis Diminished metabolism and perfusion in the thalamus after an infarct or other lesion has interrupted thalamo-cortical projection pathways.

Thalamo-cortical diaschisis A reversal of the last, in which there is a reduction in metabolism of the homolateral hemisphere after subcortical/thalamic stroke.

Basal ganglion-cortical diaschisis Hypometabolism in focal or diffuse cortical regions (usually frontal) in the presence of lesions of the lenticular nucleus, globus pallidus, caudate, etc.

diastaltic (Gr, exciting) The term used by Marshall **Hall** for what is now called "reflex"; today it is seldom employed.

diastasis Separation of the cranial sutures, as may occur in children with cranial trauma, meningeal tumors, or elevated intracranial pressure.

diastematencephalacia (from Gr, to separate + the brain) A congenital maldevelopment in which the brain is divided into two by a midline cleft.

diastematomyelia (Gr, to separate + the spinal cord) (split notochord syndrome)

A congenital maldevelopment in which there is splitting of the spinal cord into two dura-enclosed tracts by a midline bony or cartilaginous spicule, usually extending over several segments in the thoracic or lumbar regions, and sometimes associated with spina bifida.

Although the condition is often asymptomatic in youth, symptoms such as gait disturbance, back pain, and motor or sensory disturbances in the legs arise when the greater growth of the vertebrae compared with that of the cord leads to traction on the cord and subsequently to myelopathy.[529]

diathesis (Gr, an arrangement) 1. A transmissible variation in the structure or function of tissues, rendering them peculiarly liable to react in a certain way to certain extrinsic stimuli. (R.J. **Ryle**, 1926) 2. A morbid tendency or susceptibility to a certain type of disease.

Yet this is still a vague term, now nearly defunct, although the underlying concept is real enough.

dicephalus A two-headed monster.

dichotic listening A procedure used to investigate selective auditory attention in which two different auditory stimuli (usually speech) are presented to the participant simultaneously, one to each ear using headphones. Participants are asked to attend to one or (in a divided-attention experiment) to both of the messages and are later asked about their content.

dichotic stimulation A psychometric localization test using auditory stimulation, whereby different sounds (e.g., numbers) are presented simultaneously to the two ears.

Dide–Botcazo syndrome A syndrome of the posterior cerebral artery in which bilateral calcarine and posterior temporal infarcts are associated with loss of immediate memory, retrograde amnesia, spatial agnosia, and temporal disorientation.[1637, 1636]

DIDMOAD See **Wolfram syndrome**.

diencephalic amnesia Deficits in anterograde visual and verbal learning and in retrograde amnesia, with retention of motor learning abilities, due to lesions involving the amygdaloid and hippocampal pathways in the anterior part of the diencephalon surrounding the floor and walls of the third ventricle and especially of the medial-dorsal thalamic nucleus.[4219, 2543]

diencephalic autonomic seizures (dysautonomia, autonomic dysfunction syndrome, autonomic storm, brainstem attack, hyperpyrexia associated with muscle contraction, hypothalamic-midbrain dysregulation syndrome, acute midbrain syndrome, Penfield syndrome, autonomic diencephalic epilepsy, tetanus-like seizures, cerebellar or tonic seizures, or minor epilepsy) An unusual variety of "seizure" in which major autonomic (sympathetic) manifestations occur due to hypothalamic lesions, such as tumors or associated with severe diffuse axonal injury and cerebral hypoxia following craniocerebral trauma. Manifestations include transient increases in blood pressure and speeding or slowing of respiration including the Cheyne–Stokes pattern, lacrimation, sweating, shivering, pupillary changes, vasodilatation, lacrimation, salivation, piloerection, tachycardia, hyper- or hypothermia, posturing, exophthalmos, and hiccuping.

Penfield's case[4975] was of a woman who died with an encapsulated tumor which was compressing the thalamus; her attacks were considered to represent epileptic discharges, but it seems more likely that they are due to a release phenomenon at the level of the upper brainstem[935] perhaps witnessing to the effects of plateau waves in patients with acute intermittent hydrocephalus. See also **de Morsier syndrome**.

diencephalic neuronal necrosis Neuronal injury limited to the thalamus, hypothalamus, and brainstem following hypoxic–ischemic injury *in utero*.[4900]

diencephalic syndrome (Batten–Russell–Collier disease) Emaciation and failure to thrive with full alertness but showing minimal neurological signs, occurring in infants or small children in association with a tumor of the diencephalon (usually an anterior hypothalamic glioma).

Alertness and increased vigor and appetite with friendliness (or even elation in the early stages) give way to vomiting, cachexia and emaciation, pallor, nystagmus, hydrocephalus, optic atrophy, and tremor although the child remains bright, cheerful, and active until a late stage. The condition was best described by Dr. A. Russell in 1951.[5471]

diencephalon (Gr, through or between + brain) The caudal end of the forebrain, continuous with the mesencephalon; the thalamus.

differential signal The difference between two unlike signals applied to the respective two input terminals of a differential EEG amplifier. (From Noachtar S, et al. A glossary of terms most commonly used by clinical electroencephalographers. *EEG Clin Neurophysiol* 1999;52[Suppl]: 21–41. Reproduced by kind permission of the IFCN and Elsevier Science.)

differentiation The process whereby tumor cells acquire unique histological characteristics differentiating them from other types of cells.

diffuse astrocytoma See **astrocytoma**.

diffuse axonal injury (diffuse degeneration of white matter, shearing injury, inner cerebral trauma, diffuse white matter shearing injury) The appearance of axonal injury with associated focal lesions in the corpus callosum and rostral brain stem and with intraventricular hemorrhage, occurring in brains subjected to severe angular acceleration but without increased intracranial pressure or hypoxia.[6] This and ischemia represent the major mechanisms responsible for neuronal damage following head injury.

This traumatic disorder of CNS axons is shown pathologically by scattered disruptions of the axons with axonal retraction, sometimes in more severe cases associated with focal petechial hemorrhages and larger areas of hemorrhagic necrosis in the dorsal lateral midbrain and corpus callosum. The condition is due to simple forces acting upon the brain and does not require that the head actually make contact with an unyielding surface. Initial coma improving through stages of mutism, hypophonia, cerebellar and pyramidal signs, and vestibular symptoms and signs are the usual clinical concomitants.

diffuse cerebellar cortical hypertrophy A rare developmental anomaly characterized by the presence of enlarged cerebellar folia with abnormal cells beneath the granule cell layer.[4806] See also **Lhermitte–Duclos disease**.

diffuse cerebral degeneration in infancy See Alpers disease.

diffuse cerebral ischemia That condition of the cerebral circulation in which the level of blood flow is not sufficient to meet the metabolic needs of the brain but is sufficient to protect against infarction.

diffuse cerebral sclerosis with pigmentary retinopathy A sporadic disorder characterized by abnormal phytanic acid storage, bilateral keratopathy, and sudanophilic leukoencephalopathy.[3348]

diffuse cortical dysplasia (double-cortex syndrome, subcortical band heterotopia, band heterotopia) A genetically determined disorder of neuronal migration characterized by diffuse band heterotopia underlying the cortical mantle and giving the appearance on MRI scans of a double cortex, as a result of the arrest of migration of a population of neurons in subcortical regions on its way to the cortex. It is due to a mutation in the doublecortin gene on chromosome X. A comprehensive review is that of Aicardi.[75]

Clinically, the disorder is usually found in females and presents with various epileptic syndromes, including drop attacks, the **Lennox–Gastaut syndrome**, and **infantile spasms**. Some degree of mental retardation is usual.[4873]

See also **lissencephaly**, in which the failure of neuronal migration is more generalized and does not show the same double-cortex appearance.

diffuse cortical sclerosis See **Alpers disease**.

diffuse degeneration of white matter See **diffuse axonal injury**.

diffuse infiltrative lymphomatosis An AIDS-related peripheral sensorimotor neuropathy in which the nerves (as well as many other tissues) are infiltrated by CD8 T lymphocytes. The condition is not a lymphoma, despite the name applied.[2347]

diffuse Lewy body disease See **dementia with Lewy bodies**.

diffuse neonatal hemangiomatosis A congenital dysmorphic syndrome manifesting also as facial capillary hemangiomas, visceromegaly, hydrocephalus, and skin papules.[381]

diffuse neurofibrillary tangles with calcification A syndrome of slowly progressive cortical dementia in adult life with temporal and/or frontal lobar atrophy, and widespread neurofibrillary tangles in the cortex.[3539]

diffuse neuronal necrosis A result of hypoxic–ischemic injury in the neonate.

diffuse poliodystrophy The condition of diffuse proliferation of microglia and astroglia with some neuronal loss within the brain, as occurs in some patients with **HIV** infection. The condition represents a subacute encephalitis, which was its former name.[4199]

diffuse progressive cerebral cortical atrophy See **Alpers disease**.

diffuse sclerosis 1. See **Schilder disease**; 2. See **leukodystrophies**; 3. Subacute encephalitis—in the classification of Poser and van Bogaert.[5096]

diffuse white matter shearing injury See **diffuse axonal injury**.

diffusion weighted imaging An MRI technique allowing visualization of stroke effects within an hour of their occurrence and also permitting aging of any stoke lesions seen. "Diffusion" refers to the random translational motion of molecules in a fluid system; in this case it is the diffusion of water itself that is imaged. An enhancement is *diffusion tensor imaging* which allows the visualization of white matter fibers on a millimeter-level multidimensional scale by measuring fractional anisotropy and mean diffusivity.

digastric line See **Fischgold line**.

DiGeorge syndrome (third and fourth pharyngeal pouch syndrome; velocardiofacial syndrome) A chromosomal anomaly (deletion of 22.q11.2) characterized by hypoplasia or absence of the thymus and parathyroid glands. Clinically, the condition presents with neonatal hypocalcemic tetany, delayed mental and neurological development, and frequent infections,[1641] as well as congenital cardiac anomalies, facial dysmorphisms, gastrointestinal malformations, and more.[3378]

digit (from Lat, a finger) 1. A finger, thumb, or toe. 2. A number from 0 to 9.

digit span test A subtest of the **Wechsler Adult Intelligence Scale** test of attention span, in which the subject repeats progressively longer lists of numbers read out at 1/s by the examiner; and then repeats similar lists but in reverse order. The normal forward span is 6 ± 1 and the reverse span is 2 less.

The test is not significantly affected by normal aging and is not very sensitive to dementia.[4332]

digit symbol test A part of the **Wechsler Adult Intelligence Scale** in which the subject is required to place the correct number under each of a line of symbols according to a key provided, over a fixed period of time.[6688] The test is sensitive mainly to right hemisphere damage.

digital reflex See **Hoffman reflex**.

digital subtraction A technique whereby X-ray information is taken from a fluoroscopic screen by photomultiplier tubes and digitalized. By obtaining information from the screen immediately before passage of the contrast material through the blood vessels, the background information can be mathematically subtracted from that obtained after injection of the dye, so that only the opacified blood vessels are visualized.

digital subtraction angiography A technique of angiography with intravenous injection of the contrast medium. Enhancement and digitalization of the initial image allows its electronic "subtraction" from the image obtained following injection, done by means of a computer.[4971, 6097]

The sensitivity of digital subtraction systems permits a great reduction in the amount of dye injected compared to that required for conventional angiography, such savings being important in patients with congestive heart failure or renal failure. The combination of smaller catheters and digital subtraction equipment may enable the examination to be performed as an outpatient procedure.[4678]

digitalgia paresthetica The term of **Wartenberg** for tingling suddenly felt in the distribution of the superficial branch of the ulnar nerve and followed by numbness without preceding trauma. Abduction of the little finger precipitates the tingling thereafter. The cause is unknown.[6660]

digiti quinti sign (fifth finger sign) Slight abduction of the little finger on one side when the arms are outstretched; a sign of mild hemiparesis rather than of cerebellar disease as differentiated by Dr. **Milton Alter**. When the finger spreads occurs bilaterally, however, the sign has no diagnostic significance.[150] See also **Souques sign, pinky finger sign** and **Léri sign**.

digitoocular maneuver See **blindisms**.

digitoocular sign The tendency of photophobic children to dig their fingers or fists into their orbits, which in time leads to atrophy of the periorbital tissues and sunken eyes.

digitorenocerebral syndrome A recessively inherited dysmorphic syndrome characterized also by absence of the distal phalanges, renal and cardiac anomalies, seizures, optic atrophy, hypotonia, and mental and motor delay.[1908]

dihydrobiopterin synthetase deficiency A congenital syndrome also manifesting as hypotonia, dystonia, spasticity, neonatal seizures, hyperphenylalaninemia, aminoaciduria, and mental and developmental delay.[3341] See **phenylketonuria**.

dihydropteridine reductase deficiency (phenylketonuria 2) A progressive congenital dysmorphic syndrome also manifesting as feeding difficulties, hypotonia, dystonia, spasticity, neonatal seizures, hyperphenylalaninemia, aminoaciduria, and mental and developmental delay,[3341] and usually leading to death within 2 years. The condition does not respond to diets with a low phenylalanine content. See also **phenylketonuria**.

dihydropyrimidine dehydrogenase deficiency A syndrome with onset in infancy or childhood, manifesting grand mal seizures as a result of this metabolic error.

dilatation (from Lat, dilato, or Fr, dilatation; to spread out or widen) Abnormal widening of a structure such as a hollow viscus or artery. The word *dilation* is perfectly adequate but the repetition of the "-at-" is for some reason now customary, though its Latin derivation is from the transitive verb, or from the noun for an implement which itself does the dilating. Dilatators are not, however, used at all today.

dilatation lag Slowness and delay in dilation of the pupil in dark conditions after a bright light stimulus is withdrawn as a result of the decreased pull of the radial dilator muscle.

There is less dilation of the affected pupil (more than 0.5 mm difference at 4 s than at 12 s) after a light flash. The lag is assessed after 5 s of darkness in comparison with the other, healthy pupil, and there should be no further lag between 5 and 10 s.[5027]

The presence of such lag is a cardinal feature of the *Horner syndrome*,[6488] although it is almost invisible to the naked eye and can only be demonstrated by in-dark or infrared pupillometry. A camera, however, can quantitate the rate of dilation accurately,[5027] science thus eclipsing art.

dilated cardiomyopathy See **limb-girdle muscular dystrophy**.

Dimitri–Parkes-Weber disease See **Sturge–Weber syndrome**.

dimorphous leprosy A form of **leprosy** with features of both the lepromatous and the tuberculoid forms, and with both skin and nerve involvement.

dimple sign The presence of a localized, concave, oval area of pressure atrophy of compressed tissues, seen over the fibular head in cases of peroneal nerve pressure palsy, below the medial epicondyle in patients with ulnar neuropathy at the elbow[1022] and in the low buttock after local trauma to fibers destined for the pudendal nerve at that site.[6026]

DIMS Acronym for **Disorders of Initiating and Maintaining Sleep**.

DIMS with atypical polysomnographic features A syndrome characterized by complaints of frequent awakenings and of non-restorative sleep. The EEG shows high voltage alpha waves superimposed on the non–rapid eye movement sleep delta activity, either persistently or as brief intrusions. See also **ASDC Diagnostic Classification**.[1629]

ding (the ding) Mild posttraumatic concussion with brief amnesia but without discernible evidence of alteration in consciousness. It is an occupational disease of professional football players[6903] but is far more frequently seen in the characters portrayed in children's animated cartoons.

dinitrophenyl hydrazine reaction (DNPH Reaction) When equal volumes of a saturated solution of DNPH in 1 N hydrochloric acid and of urine are added together, a yellow or white precipitate is formed if ketoacids or ketones are present. The test is generally requested as a screen for the presence of ketoacids in **maple syrup urine disease** but is also positive with the ketones produced in **propionic acidemia** and **methylmalonic aciduria**.

Dinno syndrome (pseudo-Marfan syndrome) A congenital dysmorphic syndrome manifesting also dislocation of the lens, arachnodactyly, macrocephaly, hydrocephalus, and osteosclerosis or osteopetrosis.[381]

Diogenes syndrome A literary allusion to the habits of the Greek philosopher who is said to have supplied all of his (minimal) needs for food and clothing by begging. His ideals included living a life according to nature, self-sufficiency, freedom from emotion, lack of shame, outspokenness, and contempt for social organization.[5704] Clark and his colleagues reported the cases of 30 people who showed gross self-neglect in old age, living in squalor and filthy domestic and personal disorder, and suggested that this state constitutes a syndrome which they labeled thus. Most had had successful careers and 15 of the group still had a mean intelligence score of 115, dementing diseases thus being ruled out as causal. Cerebrovascular disease, Parkinsonism, and malignancies were detected in some subjects, but vitamin deficiencies in almost all.

A conspicuous example of the syndrome was the nineteenth-century English aristocrat Lord Rokeby, who allowed his estate to run to seed untended, while he spent much time immersed in water, keeping a piece of meat beside him for occasional sustenance.

diphasic dyskinesia A hyperkinetic form of fluctuation in the severity of dyskinetic movements in Parkinsonian patients on long-term levadopa therapy, in parallel with the variations in the L-dopa levels in the blood.

diphasic wave (biphasic wave) A wave consisting of two components developed on alternate sides of the baseline.

diphtheria Poisoning with the toxin of *Corynebacterium diphtheriae* (Klebs–Loeffler bacillus) which induces local paralysis of the bulbar, accommodative, external ocular, respiratory, and/or limb muscles in about one in five cases due to demyelinating motor neuropathy during the third to the twelfth week after healing of the respiratory lesions. Mild sensory and potentially severe autonomic neuropathies may also occur, and optic neuritis and encephalitis have been reported, but rarely. In the majority that survives diphtheritic neuropathy, recovery is eventually complete.

Post-diphtheritic paralysis was the first neuropathy described as such, by Dr. Samuel Bard in 1771, although Hippocrates described nasal regurgitation in what was surely this disease. Lettsom gave an account of alcoholic polyneuritis 8 years after Bard's report.

diphtheritic pseudotabes The syndrome of severe proprioceptive loss with sensory ataxia occurring in some patients with **diphtheria**.[2689]

diphthongia The utterance of sounds having two different pitches during phonation, usually as the result of a local lesion of the larynx.

diplacusis 1. A sound is perceived by the two ears as having a different pitch. 2. Perception of a single sound as having two components. In each case, a disorder of the cochlear apparatus is likely to be responsible.

diplegia (Gr, two + strokes) Weakness of the corresponding part on the two sides of the body—usually of both legs or of both sides of the face. Cerebral diplegia (**Little disease**) is a form of spastic cerebral palsy with involvement of both legs.

Because we also have the term *paraplegia*, the word *diplegia* is only relevant when used to describe strokes occurring in the same site on each side of the body, for example, the arms, which is extremely rare.

In **Foerster atonic diplegia**, the legs are affected more than the arms, and a cerebellar syndrome, mental retardation, and hypotonia also occur.

diplegia with dissociation (pseudoplegia, aphemia) A term denoting dissociation of voluntary and emotional movements, such as those of the face, jaws, throat, and larynx in the **anterior operculum syndrome**.[4053] See also **oral-buccal apraxia**.

diploë The cancellous bone between the layers of compact bone forming the skull except in the cribriform plate of the ethmoid and the orbital plates of the frontal bones.

diplomyelia The longitudinal splitting of the spinal cord, as in **diastematomyelia**.

For this portion of its length, the cord is reduplicated rather than bisected; thus there are frequently two central canals.

diplopia (Gr, double + vision) The awareness of two objects with but a single stimulus, as a result of lack of parallelism of the ocular axes.

In *crossed diplopia* (double vision caused by exotropia), the false image (from the affected eye) is peripheral to that from the healthy eye. In *uncrossed* or *homonymous diplopia* (double vision caused by esotropia), the false image (from the affected eye) is on the same side as that eye; the cause is likely to be a VI nerve palsy.

In *monocular (uniocular) diplopia*, the two images are seen with one eye.[4275] *Binocular diplopia* is that condition in which one of the two images is obliterated when either eye is closed.

See also **cerebral diplopia**.

dipole localization method A technique under development whereby using computerized processing of scalp-derived recordings of induced spikes on the EEG, the dipole of origin may be localized intracerebrally.[5905]

dipping (slow-downward ocular bobbing) An abnormal ocular condition in which the eye movement is slow downward with a fast return to the mid-position. It is usually caused by anoxic encephalopathy, the area responsible being in the pons.

dipsomania (Gr, thirst + madness) (oenomania) A recurrent, overpowering desire to drink alcohol in quantity, followed by periods of abstinence.

direct current amplifier An amplifier which is capable of magnifying DC (zero frequency) voltages and slowly varying voltages. Comment: the direct-coupled amplifier and the chopper amplifier are direct current amplifiers. See also **direct-coupled amplifier** and **chopper amplifier**. (Adapted from the 1974 report of the Committee on Terminology, IFCN. In: Chatrian GE, Bergamini L, Dondey M, et al. A glossary of terms most commonly used by clinical electroencephalographers. *EEG Clin Neurophysiol* 1974;37:538–48. Reproduced by kind permission of Elsevier Science and the IFCN.)

direct-coupled amplifier An amplifier in which successive stages are connected (coupled) by devices which are not frequency-dependent.

direction-changing nystagmus That form of jerk nystagmus in which the direction of the fast component is the same as the direction of gaze. Thus the fast component will be to the left with leftward gaze and to the right with rightward gaze. See **central nystagmus**.

direction-fixed nystagmus That form of jerk nystagmus in which the direction of the fast component is to the same side, whatever the direction of gaze.

Direction-fixed positional nystagmus is a horizontal jerk nystagmus which may occur transiently in normal subjects whose heads are rotated in either direction while they lie supine in darkness, but it always beats to the same side, whereas with *direction-changing positional nystagmus* the nystagmus changes direction with head rotation, so that it either beats in the direction of the floor (*geotropic nystagmus*) or toward the sky (*apogeotropic nystagmus*). See also **peripheral nystagmus**.

direction-of-scratch test A test of posterior column (and of cortical sensory) function, wherein the examiner demonstrates the direction in which he makes a light scratch on the subject's palm (towards, away from, left, right) while the latter watches; and then asks for identification of the direction in which further scratches are made with the subject blindfolded. Rough quantitation can be attained by varying the length of the scratch stimulus.[2729]

directional akinesia (directional hypokinesia) A reluctance to move the eyes or the hands toward the (left) side, of which side there is hemispatial neglect as a result of a (right) parietal lobe lesion causing defective organization of movements toward the left half-space.[761]

directional cutaneous kinesthesia The recognition of the direction in which a cutaneous stimulus is passing; a fundamental requirement for the perception of a complex pattern drawn on the skin such as a letter or number, and a function of the posterior columns in humans.[1465] See **direction-of-scratch test**.

directional continuous-wave Doppler sonography A test employing ultrasound to assess changes in the periorbital circulation and thus to detect disease in the cervical portion of the internal carotid artery.

In normal supraorbital and frontal arteries, blood flows from within the skull to the surface of the scalp. Direction-sensing continuous-wave Doppler sonography identifies both the amplitude of the pulsations and the direction of the flow. In the presence of severe disease of the ipsilateral internal carotid artery, the direction of blood flow is reversed. The sensitivity of the test can be increased using a variety of compression maneuvers to determine whether there is a compensatory increase in blood flow from collateral vessels.

The test is relatively simple to perform but is sensitive only to severe stenosis of the internal carotid artery and cannot differentiate this from occlusion.[4678]

directional dermokinesia The awareness of the direction in which the skin is being pulled by an examiner.

directional hypokinesia See **directional akinesia**.

directional preponderance An increase in the duration or amplitude of the nystagmus beating toward one side compared with the other when induced by **caloric testing**. This lateralized difference suggests the presence of imbalance within the vestibular system but has no precise localizing value.

disability The functional consequence of impairment, reducing a patient's capacity to perform the normal activities of daily life within that person's physical and social environment. Scales for **activities of daily living** and performance scales fall within this category.

Disability Assessment for Dementia Scale A validated 40-item caregiver rating scale, measuring items concerned with activities of daily living, mostly relevant in the case of patients with dementia.[2324]

disability neurosis (posttraumatic neurosis, accident neurosis) The persistence of injury-related symptoms beyond the time expected for recovery in the absence of evidence of incapacitating illness sufficient to prevent the patient from returning to work. Such patients are convinced of the reality of their disability and their histories do not suggest previous manipulative or exploitative behavior, but they tend to retain substantial resentment against their employer and, often, their physician. In the words of Ford,[2152] "The physical symptoms are. . .worn as a badge of angry protest for the injustices which they feel they have suffered. To give up these symptoms would mean that their anger had no justification. [When seen in psychiatric consultation they] have long-established patterns of disability and like Humpty Dumpty 'all the Kings horses and all the Kings men' can't put them together again." See **compensation neurosis**.

disability scales Semiquantitative rating scales of capacity and of performance measuring disability outcomes for neurologic rehabilitation.The **Barthel Index**, **Functional Independence Measure**, the **Functional Capacity Index**, **Injury Severity Score**, **Sickness Impact Profile**, and **Functional Assessment Measure** are reliable and valid psychometrically similar measures of global disability. See also **stroke scales**.

disability status scale See Kurtzke Rating Scale.[3612]

disabling (diabetic) neuropathy See **diabetic neuropathy**.

disabling paroxysmal vertigo See **vestibular paroxysmia**.

disabling positional vertigo A syndrome of persistent positional vertigo with nausea and tinnitus, considered to be caused by ischemia of the VIII cranial nerve.[3165]

discharge An interpretive term used to designate paroxysmal EEG patterns. See **epileptiform pattern**, **seizure pattern**, and **EEG**. See also **action potential**.

discharge frequency The rate at which a potential discharges repetitively. When potentials occur in groups, the rate of recurrence of the group and rate of repetition of the individual components in the groups should be specified. (From the 2001 Report of the Nomenclature Committee of the American Association of Electromyography and Electrodiagnosis.[19] Reproduced by kind permission of the AAEE.)

discogenic pain Pain felt in radicular distribution as a result of irritation of a posterior nerve root by a protruded intervertebral disk. Its localization, lancinating quality, and association with activities that stretch the theca (such as coughing and bending over) are suggestive, but it takes a trained neuroanatomist to distinguish neurogenic pain from that due to **myofascial pain syndromes**. As a result, the diagnosis of prolapsed intervertebral disk is made in many patients when the problem is actually resulting from what is presumed to be local muscle spasm.

discography The injection of contrast medium into an intervertebral disk under fluoroscopic control, in order to visualize extrusion of the disk or other pathology such as **disk disruption** as a cause of pain in the back.

discoid In the shape of a disk or quoit.

disconnection anomia See **anomia**.

disconnection syndromes (disconnexion syndromes; transcortical syndromes, conduction syndromes) The effects of lesions of association pathways, connecting separate brain regions, either those which lie exclusively in a single cerebral hemisphere or those which join the two halves of the brain. Geschwind regarded them as higher function deficits that result from white matter lesions or lesions of the association cortices, the latter acting as relay stations between primary motor, sensory, and limbic areas.

They include **alexia (word blindness) without agraphia, pure word deafness, ideomotor apraxia, tactile aphasia, conduction,** and **transcortical dysphasias.**[2338, 2339]

Although **Wernicke** suggested that **conduction aphasia** resulted from damage to the pathways separating the posterior language comprehension center and the speech output center, the concept of disconnection as the basis for certain syndromes of cerebral damage was only fully developed by **Geschwind.**[2338] An excellent review is that of Absher and Benson.[41]

disconnexion syndromes See **disconnection syndromes**.

discrete activity See **interference pattern**.

discrete movements "A process employing a small field of musculature and producing a single phasic movement of a small movable part against the background of a phasically inert musculature, in an anaesthetized animal" (Sir Francis Walshe).

This represents a laboratory abstraction rather than a clinical reality, since all focal movements occur in association with others in more proximal areas and thus are never truly "discrete" if the word is taken to mean separate or distinct. Nevertheless, with the introduction of **transcranial magnetic stimulation** in the human, the term may have regained both relevance and currency.

disease The clinical expression of a morbid process.

disease steps An assessment schedule used in patients with multiple sclerosis, relying largely upon motor (ambulatory) functions.[2945]

disinhibition–dementia–Parkinsonism–amyotrophy complex (DDPAC) A dominantly inherited disorder with onset in mid-adult life, characterized by dementia, Parkinsonism without tremor, and amyotrophy. Personality changes, alcoholism, and hyperphagia are early symptoms, after which the usual features of frontal lobe dementia develop. The gene is mapped to 17q21–22. Pathologically, atrophy and spongy changes are found in the frontotemporal cortex and there is neuronal loss in the substantia nigra and amygdala, without Lewy bodies.[3775] See **frontotemporal dementia**.

disjunctive eye movements 1. Abnormal eye movements resulting from aberrant regeneration of one of the oculomotor nerves, its fibers being directed to the wrong nerve.[505] 2. See **vergence**.

disjunctive nystagmus Forms of nystagmus in which the eyes do not maintain their normal yoked position. See **dissociated nystagmus**.

disk disruption A syndrome of persistent low back pain following compressive spinal overload. The diagnosis is made by **discography**, which reproduces the patient's pain and demonstrates disruption of the internal architecture of the disk.[1342]

disk prolapse Backward herniation of the nucleus pulposus of an intervertebral disk as seen on a **myelogram**, to the extent that nerve roots may be compressed or the spinal canal compromised.

disk protrusion Bulging of an intervertebral disk, as seen on a **myelogram**. This is a common finding related to age and wear and tear and has no pathological significance unless it leads to operation; unlike **disk prolapse**, it is not associated with compression of a spinal nerve root. The problem lies in telling the difference.

disk reabsorption (isolated disk resorption) A variant of **degenerative spinal stenosis** in which chronic low back pain is associated with reduction of the height of the (L5/S1) disk to 3 mm or less, facet joint hypertrophy, and a trefoil appearance of the spinal canal.[1341]

disorders of excessive sleep (DOES) A group of functional and organic conditions in which the chief symptoms are the awareness of inappropriate and undesirable sleepiness during waking hours, often with decreased cognitive and motor performance, excessive tendency to sleep, unavoidable napping, and an increase in total 24-h sleep with full arousal on awakening. The classification in Chart D–9 is adapted from the 1979 Association of Sleep Disorders Centers Diagnostic Classification,[280] which although superseded by the American Sleep Disorders Association classification,[1629] still provides a useful overview of this class of disturbances.

disorders of initiating and maintaining sleep (DIMS) Heterogeneous conditions which are considered to be responsible for inducing disturbed sleep and for diminishing the amount of sleep experienced. The classification in Chart D–10 is adapted from the 1979 Association of Sleep Disorders Centers Diagnostic Classification,[280] which, although superseded by the American Sleep Disorders Association classification,[1629] provides a useful overview of this class of disturbances.

disorders of the sleep–wake cycle Conditions sharing the feature that they represent the misalignment of the subject's individual sleeping and waking patterns and the circadian pattern of that individual or society. This group represents the third class of sleep disturbances recognized in the Association of Sleep Disorders Centers Diagnostic Classification;[280](see Chart D–11; but see also the 2001 American Sleep Disorders Association Diagnostic Classification.[1629]) Reproduced by kind permission of the American Academy of Sleep Medicine.

disorganization Gross alterations in frequency, form, topography, and/or quantity of physiological EEG rhythms in (1) an individual record relative to previous records in the same subject or to the rhythms of homologous regions on the opposite side of the head or (2) relative to normal subjects of similar age and similar state of vigilance. (From Noachtar S, et al. A glossary of terms most commonly used by clinical electroencephalographers. *EEG Clin Neurophysiol* 1999;52[Suppl]:21–41. Reproduced by kind permission of the IFCN and of Elsevier Science.)

disorientation Lack of ability to define ones position vis-à-vis the environment, or

Chart D–9. Disorders of Excessive Sleep

B1. Psychophysiological

a. **Transient and situational DOES**
b. **Persistent DOES**

B2. Associated with psychiatric disorders

B3. DOES associated with use or withdrawal from drugs or alcohol

B4. DOES associated with sleep-induced respiratory impairment:

a. **Sleep apnea DOES syndrome**
b. **Alveolar hypoventilation DOES syndrome**

B5. Sleep-related myoclonus and restless legs:

a. **Sleep-related myoclonus DOES syndrome**
b. **Restless legs DOES syndrome**

B6. **Narcolepsy**

B7. **Idiopathic CNS hypersomnolence**

B8. DOES associated with other medical, toxic, and environmental conditions

B9. Other DOES conditions

a. Intermittent DOES (periodic) syndromes:
Kline–Levin syndrome
Menstrual-associated syndrome
b. Insufficient sleep
c. **Sleep drunkenness**

B10. No DOES abnormality

a. **Long sleeper**
b. Subjective DOES complaint without objective findings

Adapted from Association of Sleep Disorders Centers. Diagnostic classifications of sleep and arousal disorders. Sleep *1979; 2: 1–137 by kind permission of the American Academy of Sleep Medicine.*

Chart D–10. Classification of Disorders of Initiating and Maintaining Sleep

A1a. **Transient and situational DIMS**
A1b. **Persistent DIMS**
A2. DIMS associated with psychiatric disorders
A3. DIMS associated with use or withdrawal from drugs or alcohol
A4. DIMS associated with sleep-induced respiratory impairment;

a. **Sleep apnea DIMS syndrome**
b. **Alveolar hypoventilation DIMS syndrome**

A5. Sleep-related myoclonus and restless legs

a. **Sleep-related myoclonus DIMS syndrome**
b. **Restless legs DIMS syndrome**

A6. DIMS associated with other medical, toxic, and environmental conditions

A7. **Childhood-onset DIMS**

A8. Other DIMS syndromes

a. **Repeated REM sleep interruptions**
b. Atypical polysomnographic features

A9. No DIMS abnormality

a. **Short sleeper**
b. Subjective DIMS complaint without objective findings

Adapted from Association of Sleep Disorders Centers. Diagnostic classifications of sleep and arousal disorders. Sleep *1979; 2: 1–137 by kind permission of the American Academy of Sleep Medicine.*

Chart D–11. Classification of Disorders of the Sleep–Wake Cycle

C1. Transient

a. **Rapid time zone change syndrome** (jet lag)
b. **Work shift change** in conventional sleep–wake schedule

C2. Persistent

a. Frequently changing sleep–wake cycle
b. **Delayed sleep phase syndrome**
c. **Advanced sleep phase syndrome**
d. **Non-24-h sleep–wake syndrome**
e. Irregular sleep–wake pattern

From *AASM Diagnostic Classification Steering Committee.* The International Classification of Sleep Disorders Diagnostic and Coding Manual. *Rochester, MN. American Academy of Sleep Medicine 1991/2001. Reproduced by kind permission of the Academy.* See also http://www.sleepeducation.com/Disorders.aspx.

to localize oneself within a place such as a room, house, town, or country, usually due to a lesion in the right parietal lobe.[2091]

dissecting aneurysm See **aneurysm**.

dissection 1. Splitting of the wall of an artery due to disease of the intima, thus opening up a false channel for the passage of blood which compresses the normal channel. 2. The lesion produced by penetration of the circulating blood into the substance of the wall of a vessel with subsequent extension of the effused blood for a varying distance between its layers. They are important causes of strokes in young adults. Mechanical trauma and an inherent weakness of the arterial wall collagen are thought to be responsible. The presence of the dissection is well shown by magnetic resonance angiography.

Dissections were first recognized by Maunoir, a Swiss surgeon, in 1802. Predisposing factors include **fibromuscular dysplasia, Ehlers–Danlos type IV syndrome, Marfan syndrome, cystic medial necrosis,** polycystic kidney disease, osteogenesis imperfecta, **giant cell arteritis, polyarteritis nodosa, meningovascular syphilis**, and **moyamoya disease**. Local infections and hyperhomocysteinemia are more rare causes.

In the extracranial carotid artery, the usual clinical picture includes minor stroke-like episodes with headaches sometimes resembling **migraine** and an associated **Horner syndrome** due to dissections of the medial coat; the prognosis is commonly good. Intracranially, the dissections are usually subintimal and may lead to subarachnoid hemorrhage and to lower cranial nerve palsies, probably by direct compression at the jugular faoramen. Common carotid artery dissection causes local swelling and pain.

Dissections of the vertebral arteries extracranially are less common; they are more likely to occur in women, are often bilateral, and can lead to neck and posterior head pain and to brainstem strokes. Minor trauma is likely to play a part in causation. Intracranial vertebral dissections present with subarachnoid hemorrhage. Basilar dissections are typically lethal but fortunately are rare.

The main neurological syndrome associated with aortic dissections is that of cervical vascular myelopathy, but the cardiac complications often overshadow that.

disseminated encephalomalacia with cavity formation (familial multilocular encephalomalacia) A leukoencephalopathy of unknown cause characterized by the formation of large cavities in the white matter of infants. Seizures, progressive rigidity, and pareses lead on to stupor and early death.[1349]

disseminated intravascular coagulation A syndrome resulting from vascular damage in which there is activation of plasma coagulation factors or entry of tissue thromboplastic material into the blood. The most prominent clinical feature is bleeding, including cerebral hemorrhage, which stems from the consumption of platelets and certain coagulation factors, as a result of which severe thrombocytopenia and deficiency of fibrinogen arise. The clinical spectrum extends from insignificant laboratory abnormalities to uncontrollable and persistent hemorrhage and thrombosis.

disseminated neurogenic atrophy The occurrence of clusters of 3–6 small angulated muscle fibers of the same histochemical type in muscle biopsy specimens. The finding suggests progressive denervation without effective collateral sprouting.

disseminated sarcoid leukoencephalopathy See **neurosarcoidosis**.

disseminated vasculomyelinopathy A term encompassing the para- or post-infectious diseases of the nervous system, which takes note of the fact that there is evidence of both demyelination and damage to small blood vessels in these conditions.

Clinically, an abrupt monophasic illness follows common infections with a latent interval of days or weeks and consists of any of the syndromes of; acute brain stem (Bickerstaff) encephalitis, acute/recurrent neuromyelitis optica, acute/recurrent optic neuritis, acute/recurrent transverse myelitis, acute cerebellar ataxia, acute hemorrhagic leukoencephalopathy, acute labyrinthitis, acute toxic encephalitis/encephalopathy, acute/recurrent/multiphasic disseminated encephalomyelitis, aseptic lymphocytic meningoencephalitis, brachial plexitis, chronic progressive disseminated encephalomyelitis, Landry–Guillain–Barré syndrome, Miller Fisher syndrome, post-infectious and post-vaccinal encephalomyelitis, pseudotumor cerebri, recurrent neuromyelitis optica with endocrinopathies (Vernant syndrome), and likely clinical encephalitis, aseptic meningitis, ataxia, chorea, myelitis, cranial and peripheral neuropathies (including **acute inflammatory demyelinating polyneuropathy**), and brachial neuritis, in any combination.[5090, 840]

In the case of **acute transverse myelitis**, suggested diagnostic criteria require bilateral sensory, motor or autonomic dysfunction referable to the spinal cord, with a clearly defined sensory level progressing to a nadir at between 4 and 21 days from onset. The enhanced MRI must eliminate structural causes and show evidence of an inflammatory origin, shown by CSF findings of pleocytosis or raised IgG levels.[6264]

dissociated anesthesia Impairment of some forms of sensation with retention of others in the same area. A typical form is the loss of the thin-fiber (spinothalamic) functions of pinprick pain, light touch, and temperature sensation, with sparing of the thick-fiber functions such as discriminative light touch, position sense, and vibration, on the body below the level of a cordotomy sectioning the spinothalamic tract. The **lateral medullary syndrome**, **tabes dorsalis**, vitamin B_{12} deficiency, **diabetes mellitus**, and some forms of **hereditary sensory and autonomic neuropathy** are other examples.

dissociated aphasia See **Wernicke aphasia**.

dissociated nystagmus (disjunctive nystagmus) Those forms of nystagmus in which the movements of the eyes are not symmetrical, the oscillations being greater in amplitude, speed, or direction in one eye, or present only in one eye. Both jerky and pendular forms can occur. **Internuclear ophthalmoplegia**, **convergence-retraction nystagmus**, **spasmus nutans**, and **see-saw nystagmus** are examples. The usual cause is a brainstem lesion. See also **pseudo-abducens palsy** and **divergence nystagmus**.

dissociated vertical divergence A congenital ocular dysmotility syndrome, in which occlusion or dimming of one eye leads to the elevation of that eye. The sign has no localizing value.[1280]

dissociation (conversion) A mental mechanism whereby a subject can suppress awareness of a sensation or of mental content, or can inhibit the usual facility for movement of a body part either voluntarily or under the influence of strong emotion. Altered perceptions of the self or of the environment and depersonalization are other possible features. **Head** pointed out that neurologists employ this mechanism every time they look through an ophthalmoscope.

It is defined in ICD-10 as "a partial or complete loss of the normal integration between memories of the past, awareness of identity and immediate sensations and control of body movements." Included thus would be dissociative amnesias, fugue states, trance and possession disorders, dissociative anesthesia, sensory losses, motor disorders, convulsions (**non-epileptic seizures**), and other intercurrent and usually unnamed manifestations.[901]

dissociation cytoalbuminologique An euphonious French phrase indicating that the increases in CSF protein levels and in the CSF cell count are not always of the same magnitude; in this case, the protein level is greatly elevated but there is little or no increase in the number of white cells. Such may occur in spinal block, in **acute inflammatory demyelinating polyneuropathy**, and with **acoustic neuroma**.

dissociation of lateral gaze syndrome See **Raymond–Cestan syndrome**.

dissociation of reflexes Absence of the superficial and augmentation of the muscle stretch reflexes, as with pyramidal tract lesions.

dissociative disorder See **somatization disorder**.

dissociative speech syndromes Those varieties of dysphasia in which the relevant cortical areas are partly isolated from the remainder of the brain by virtue of the interruption of afferent, efferent, or associative pathways. **Conduction** and **transcortical dysphasias** are examples.

dissonance (from Lat, to disagree in sound) Discord.

distal (from Lat, to be distant from another thing) The term for those body parts progressively more distant from the trunk or midline—thus the hands and feet and *a fortiori* the fingers and toes—as opposed to **proximal**.

distal acquired demyelinating symmetric neuropathy (DADS) An acquired, symmetrical demyelinating neuropathy with distal sensory or sensorimotor features. The distribution of the weakness and the usual presence of an IgM kappa monoclonal gammopthy help to distinguish this condition from **chronic inflammatory demyelinating polyradiculoneuropathy**.[3330, 5526]

distal amyotrophy of predominantly the upper limbs See **monomelic amyotrophy**.

distal and segmental muscular atrophy of upper extremities See **hereditary motor neuropathy**.

distal anterior compartment myopathy A recessively inherited muscular dystrophy (a *dysferlinopathy*) mapped to the 2p13 locus. It resembles *Miyoshi* and *Nonaka myopathies* (see **distal muscular dystrophy**) but is characterized by onset in early adult life, initial weakness, and wasting in the anterior tibial muscles before rapid generalization to all muscle groups, raised serum CK levels, and sparing of the cranial muscles.[3079]

distal axonal degeneration See **distal axonopathy**.

distal axonal spheroids Swellings containing various organelles, occurring at the terminations of axons in a variety of diseases.

distal axonopathy (dying back neuropathy, distal axonal degeneration, distal lower motor neurone syndrome) Forms of neuropathy in which there is asymmetrical distal but centripetal failure of function due to impairment of the axonal transport mechanisms, in turn usually as a result of damage to the perikaryon of the nerve cell.[1060] This leads to secondary myelin breakdown.

High titers of anti-GM_1 or other antibodies are found in a majority of cases. See also **multifocal motor neuropathy** and **proximal lower motor neurone syndromes**.

distal hereditary upper limb muscular atrophy A dominantly inherited neurogenic disorder presenting with weakness and atrophy of the distal arms and hands, brisk reflexes, and minimal sensory findings. Electrophysiological studies do not suggest axonal loss. Motor nerve conduction velocities are nearly normal but distal motor latencies are prolonged.[2590]

distal latency The interval between the delivery of a stimulus to the most distal point of stimulation on a nerve and the onset of a response. A measure of the conduction properties of the most distal portion of motor or sensory nerves. (From the 2001 Report of the Nomenclature Committee of the American Association of Electromyography and Electrodiagnosis.[19] Reproduced by kind permission of the AANEM.)

distal lower motor neurone syndrome See **distal axonopathy**.

distal muscle wasting, nephritis and deafness See **hereditary motor and sensory neuropathy, type 2**.

distal muscular dystrophy (type 1 distal myopathy, Gowers syndrome, late hereditary myopathy, Welander myopathy) A heterogeneous group of genetic muscle diseases, often dominantly inherited, and characterized by progressive distal weakness and wasting. Creatine kinase levels are slightly raised and in some forms vacuolar changes are seen on muscle biopsy specimens. Cardiomyopathy is also described.[2532] Abnormalities of the genes for dysferlin and desmin are the two best decribed.

In the myopathy described by **Welander**,[6711] progressive distal weakness and wasting with onset in mature adult life affects the hands most of all. The condition is seen almost exclusively in the population of Scandinavian countries. Serum creatine kinase levels are slightly raised and vacuolar changes are seen on muscle biopsy specimens. **Gowers** described a condition such as this in 1902[2532] but his patients might equally well have had **myotonic dystrophy**. Variant forms are listed in Chart D–12.

Numerous distinct predominantly **distal myopathies** have been identified with discrete clinical and genetic patterns. The following descriptive listing owes much to the review by **Mastaglia** and **Laing** and the work of Nonaka.[4156] The entities share the common pathologic feature of rimmed vacuoles and in all but Miyoshi myopathy the serum CK levels are normal or only slightly elevated.

distal myopathy See **distal muscular dystrophy**.

distal myopathy with desmin storage A dominantly inherited distal myopathy characterized by onset in early-mid adult life, gait disturbance due to distal leg weakness, and eventual generalization to all body areas, including the heart, leading to premature death. Electrical findings include prominent spontaneous activity, short duration motor unit potentials, and polyphasia. Muscle biopsy specimens show desmin storage and autophagocytosis.[2996]

distal myopathy with onset in infancy See **distal muscular dystrophy**.

distal myopathy with proximal weakness and early respiratory failure A dominantly inherited distal myopathy presenting in mid-adult life with tibialis anterior weakness, proceeding to

Chart D–12. Forms of Distal Muscular Dystrophy[4156, 4692, 4992]

A. *Definite entities*

1. ***Welander distal myopathy*** (late adult onset, type 1), with autosomal dominant inheritance, linked to 2p13, as above.[71]
2. ***Nonaka myopathy*** (distal myopathy with rimmed vacuoles; early adult onset, type 1), with sporadic occurrence or autosomal recessive inheritance, mapped to 9p1–q1. There is striking distal weakness of the gastrocnemii and peroneal muscles and mild proximal weakness, with onset in early adult life and with slightly elevated CK levels. This is identical to *quadriceps-sparing familial inclusion body myopathy*. Progression is slow. Pathologically the condition is characterized by muscle fiber atrophy with rimmed vacuole formation in the cytoplasm. GNE mutations are responsible.[4693]
3. ***Miyoshi myopathy*** (early adult onset, type 2), with autosomal recessive inheritance, mapped to the 2p13 locus (like **limb girdle muscular dystrophy** type 2b). A *dysferlinopathy with* onset in youth or adult life with distal muscle weakness and atrophy, uniquely in this group affecting first the gastrocnemii, and with high serum CK levels. The arms are affected late but the small hand muscles are spared. Muscle biopsy changes are similar to those of **Duchenne dystrophy**.[414, 4415]
4. ***Udd/Markesbery–Griggs myopathy*** (late adult onset, autosomal dominant inheritance, onset in the anterior compartment of the legs) caused by mutations in the *titin* gene on 2q.
5. ***Tibial myopathy or Markesbery–Griggs/Type 2, late-onset hereditary distal myopathy*** (Finnish, late adult onset, type 2), with autosomal dominant inheritance and linkage to chromosome 2q31–33. This is a slowly progressive form, with onset in the anterior compartment. Serum CK levels are slightly raised.[6436, 4088, 4087]
6. ***Laing myopathy*** A dominantly inherited form with onset in infancy, of weakness and wasting of the anterior compartment of the legs, caused by mutations in a myosin gene (*MYH7*) on chromosome 14q. A *variant* is *Laing early-onset myopathy* (early adult onset, type 3), again with dominant inheritance and linkage to chromosome 14q11. Initial weakness and wasting are in the anterior compartment. Serum CK levels are slightly elevated.[3646]
7. *Autosomal dominant with tibialis anterior weakness* on 2q31 (tibial muscular dystrophy).[2745]
8. *Autosomal dominant form with infantile onset.*
9. *Hereditary distal myopathy with sarcoplasmic bodies and intermediate (skeletin) filaments.*
10. *Autosomal dominant form with late onset and with desmin storage.*[6458]
11. *Autosomal dominant inclusion body myopathy with rimmed vacuoles, ophthalmoplegia, and variable joint contractures* on 17p13.1.[4126]
12. *Juvenile onset distal myopathy.*[6977]
13. *New Finnish distal myopathy.*[4018]
14. ***Distal myopathy with proximal weakness and early respiratory failure.***[4664, 1151]
15. *Desmin-related distal myopathy.*[4357]
16. ***Desmin-related myopathy.***[6434] See **distal myopathy with desmin storage**.
17. **Desmin-related with sarcoplasmic bodies.**[1809]
18. **Oculopharyngeal distal myopathy.**[5557]
19. *Distal myopathy with onset in infancy*: An autosomal dominant form has also been described.
20. *A dominantly inherited nonprogressive form* with onset in early childhood. Clinically, distal involvement of the arms and legs with selective weakness of the deltoid muscles occurs in association with scoliosis, genu valgus, and limitation of mobility of some joints. Muscle biopsy specimens show disproportion of fibers with selective atrophy of type I fibers.[451]
21. *Distal myopathy with early adult onset*: A dominantly inherited syndrome with onset in young or middle adult life. The thenar muscles and hand flexors are affected early and pes cavus is usually present. Muscle biopsy shows sarcoplasmal bodies and an abundance of intermediate-sized skeletin filaments.[69]
22. *Double ring myopathy* A myopathy of adult life.
23. Forms with *autosomal recessive* inheritance[5685] and with more generalized weakness and earlier onset.[3559] In such cases, marked leg plantar flexor weakness is characteristic. These include *autosomal recessive form with high serum CK levels; autosomal recessive form with rimmed vacuole formation and lamellar (myeloid) bodies;* and *autosomal recessive inclusion body myopathy* on 9p1–q1.[3369]
24. *Distal myopathy (New Guinea)*: A recessively inherited syndrome of distal weakness and wasting with onset in the fourth decade leading on to oculopharyngeal symptoms within the next 10 years, reported from New Guinea.
25. *Distal myopathy affecting posterior leg and anterior upper limb muscles* A dominantly inherited slowly progressive early-onset distal myopathy, in which the tibialis anterior muscle is spared.[6797]
26. *Distal myopathy with myotilin S55F mutation* A late-onset, dominantly inherited myopathy affecting the upper and lower leg muscles.[543]
27. A recessively inherited form caused by homozygous missense mutations in the *nebulin* gene in which the weakness uniquely affects the ankle dorsiflexors, finger extensors, and neck flexors. Histologically, nemaline bodies and rimmed vacuoles are not detectable.[6612] See also the similar **Laing** distal myopathy.

B. *Forms reported only in single families*

Adult-onset distal myopathy.[2003]
Distal myopathy with pes cavus and areflexia.[5738]
Distal myopathy with vocal cord and pharyngeal signs.[1992]
Very late-onset distal myopathy.[4981]
Variable onset distal myopathy (Sumner, 1971 referenced by Udd[6434]).

ventilatory impairment and girdle weakness.[1151] Other, similar phenotypes have also been described.[6889, 4664] See **myopathy**.

distal myopathy with rimmed vacuole formation
See **distal muscular dystrophy** (*Nonaka form*).

distal small-fiber neuropathy
A form of generalized peripheral neuropathy affecting the small-diameter, thinly myelinated and unmyelinated fibers. Clinically, complaints of paresthesias, hyperesthesias and burning, aching, shooting or prickling dysesthesias, with only a minor reduction in temperature and sharp pain sensations, and reduction in distal sweating are the usual findings. Thick-fiber sensory functions, motor power, reflexes, and conventional nerve conduction studies are almost or completely normal.

Amyloidosis, monoclonal gammopathy, and **chronic inflammatory demyelinating neuropathy** are representative causes.[6057]

distal spinal muscular atrophy
A variously inherited syndrome of distal wasting without sensory change, not yet certainly classified between the hereditary motor and the hereditary motor and sensory neuropathies. The clinical manifestations appear in childhood or adolescence and resemble those of **hereditary motor and sensory neuropathy types 1 or 2** but with less arm weakness, relative preservation of the muscle stretch reflexes, and normal sensory examination.[2761] See **hereditary motor and sensory neuropathy, neuronal form**, and **hereditary motor neuropathies** (*variants*).

distal spinal muscular atrophy with a hoarse voice
See **hereditary motor neuropathy** (*variants*).

distal spinal muscular atrophy with vocal cord paralysis
See **hereditary motor neuropathy** (*variants*).

distal vacuolar myopathy
A severe generalized myopathy affecting distal muscles of the hand at first, and later the bulbar muscles. Sensory functions and muscle stretch reflexes are normal. The condition is described in patients with nephropathic cystinosis who have received renal transplants.[1112]

distance receptors
Those receptors which respond to objects at a distance and upon which the brain is constructed and has evolved. (Sherrington) Generally speaking, the channels are physical rather than chemical.

distance shortening
In patients with pyramidal lesions, the distance that the subject extends the paretic arm away from the nose in the finger-nose test progressively shortens with repeated cycles. This may be a useful early sign of an upper motor neuron lesion.[5066]

distant toe flexor reflex
(Schrijver–Bernhard reflex) Plantar flexion of the toes in response to a tap given to a distant part of the body, sometimes seen in patients with extrapyramidal but not with pyramidal lesions.[6656] The mechanism of the sign is not known and its clinical significance is dubious.

distant wounded glioma syndrome
A tumor-induced coagulopathy, leading to hemorrhage within the cavity of partially resected tumors such as multifocal glioblastoma multiforme or within distant tumor nodules following surgical resection, even though the distant sites were not directly manipulated during the surgical procedures. It is postulated that because of their rich vascularity, these distant tumor nodules are more susceptible to hemorrhage, resulting from coagulation changes after tumor resection, than are other sites.[3510]

distortion
An instrumental alteration in waveforms on EEG or EMG recordings.

disturbance
(from Lat, to put in disarray) An interference with the normal physiological functions of the body or of a part of it.

disturbance in visual orientation
See **visuomotor ataxia**.

disuse atrophy
The reduction in size of a body part when its function is impaired as a result of disease. The histological changes accompanying this are minimal, but atrophied groups of fibers may be found in some muscles.[4926]

diurna(l)
(from Lat, a day) 1. Daily. 2. In the daytime.

diurnal dystonia
(dystonia with marked diurnal variation) A dominantly inherited condition in which dystonic movements occur in the evening and night rather than in the morning and in which patients may show evidence of Parkinsonism.[4834, 5709] The condition may be a variant of **dopa-responsive dystonia** since it also responds to levadopa and to bromocriptine in low dosage. See also **dystonia**.

divaricate
(Lat, to stretch apart) Separate.

divebomber sound
The decrescendo whine of myotonic discharges heard on the EMG machine's loudspeaker. Those who have had the dubious privilege of hearing both, however, consider that the sound of a receding motor cycle provides a closer comparison.

divergence
(from Lat, apart | to incline) Separation from a common point.

divergence nystagmus
A form of nystagmus complicating congenital adduction palsy or hindbrain lesions such as the **Chiari malformation**, in which the affected eye moves into abduction on attempted adduction. The associated nystagmus is of jerk type, the fast component of the two eyes being to their respective sides.

divergence paralysis
See **dorsal midbrain syndrome**.

Divers Alert Network
(Duke University, Durham, NC) A central facility offering advice on the management of diving accidents. Tel: 919-684-8111

divination
(from Lat, to foresee) Prognostication without medical evidence.

diving headache
That headache form occurring in association with scuba and other diving activities. Diagnostic criteria have been defined as follows:

A. Headache (no typical characteristics known) fulfilling criteria C and D
B. Occurring after diving to depths below 10 m (2 atmospheres of pressure)
C. Headache develops during diving and is accompanied by at least one of the following symptoms of CO_2 intoxication in the absence of decompression illness:

1. Light-headedness
2. Mental confusion

3. Dyspnea
4. Flushed feeling in the face
5. Motor incoordination D. Headache resolves within 1 h after treatment with 100% O_2

From the International Classification of Headache Disorders (Headache Classification Committee of the International Headache Society. *Cephalalgia* 2004;24[Suppl 1]). Reproduced by kind permission of Dr. Jes Olesen, the International Headache Society and Wiley-Blackwell Publications.)

Migraine, tension-type headache, primary exertional headache, **cervicogenic headache, supraorbital neuralgia, external compression headache**, and **cold-stimulus headache** may also be precipitated by immersion in deep/cold water.

divisional paresis Weakness of the muscles supplied by the superior or by the inferior branches of the III cranial nerve.

The causal lesion will usually be found in the anterior cavernous sinus (where the two divisions separate) or in the posterior orbit, but may be in the brainstem. The superior division innervates the levator palpebrae superioris and the superior rectus (in the latter case by fibers from the contralateral side), while the inferior branch supplies the inferior and medial rectus, the inferior oblique, and the iris sphincter.[3578]

Divry–van Bogaert syndrome (familial capillary-venous leptomeningeal angiomatosis) See **van Bogaert syndrome**.

dizziness A disturbance in the sense of a person's subjective relationship to the exterior environment (subjective awareness of instability) resulting from impairment of proprioception, vision, vestibular function or global cerebral blood flow, and used in the vernacular for vertigo, light-headedness, faintness, and the awareness of being liable to fall.

DNPH reaction See **dinitrophenylhydrazine reaction**.

Doctrine of the Nerves The phrase of Thomas **Willis** denoting "neurology," adopted by Spillane for his masterly review of the history of this subject.[5978]

DOES Acronym for **d**isorders **o**f **e**xcessive **s**leep.

dogmatics An ancient Greek sect of physicians who attempted to discover the causes of disease by using reasoning and recommended the study of anatomy and the basic sciences. Their opponents, the **Empirics**, denied the value of such study.[5103]

Only when curriculum committees are composed of members of these two sects in equal numbers is a Dean able to exert some influence on the teaching methods employed within the medical school.

dolichocephaly (Gr, long + head) A developmental defect in skull shape, in which there is abnormal length of the head in its anteroposterior diameter, due to premature fusion of the sagittal suture.

In lesser degrees, this also represents one physiological skull shape as defined in 1842 by Anders Adolf Retzius (1769–1860), a Swedish anatomist, on the basis of the cranial index; the length:breadth ratios were said to be in the proportion 9:7 or more. The converse form, in which the skull is abnormally wide, is **brachycephaly**.

dolichoectasia (dilatative arteriopathy) An increase in the length and diameter of an intracranial artery (especially the vertebral and basilar arteries) with degeneration of the internal elastic laminae. Intracranial arterial dolichoectasia is a condition in which such enlargement and tortuosity exists in vessels coming off the circle of Willis, sometimes severe enough to produce fusiform aneurysms. The resulting reduced flow can lead to stagnation of blood, thrombus formation, and stroke.

Atherosclerosis is the most common cause, but it is also seen in **Fabry disease**, the **Ehlers–Danlos syndrome**, and **Marfan syndrome**. Its clinical features reflect the occurrence of stroke, local compression of neurological structures by the enlarged vessels, or increased intracranial pressure.[3082] The diameter of the descending thoracic aorta may also be increased in these patients.[1013]

Dollinger–Bielschowsky syndrome See **neuronal ceroid lipofuscinosis**.

dolls-eye movements See **oculocephalic reflex**.

doll's eye response See **oculocephalic reflex**.

dolls-eye sign See **Cantelli sign**.

doll's eyelids Reflex opening of the eyelids when the neck is briskly flexed in comatose patients; a phenomenon largely confined to cases of subarachnoid hemorrhage with stupor.[2086]

This is the only one of the commonly described "doll signs" in which the clinical phenomenon is actually the same as that seen in the toy.

doll's head response See **oculocephalic reflex**.

dolor capitis/cephalicus (Lat, pain + of the head) Headache.

Dolman–Delcato treatment An exclusive system of treatments involving passive exercises, promoted for the management of children suffering from brain damage and other conditions but condemned due to the lack of scientific substantiation provided by its proponents.[163]

dominance The particular responsibility for a function invested in one or other of the cerebral hemispheres, a concept remarked upon by Marc Dax in 1836 where even Gall was silent. (Gall had localized speech functions in the anterior part of the frontal lobes by 1819 but made no comment about lateralization.) It was introduced as a truth by Broca in 1865, who correlated aphasia, right-handedness, and lesions of the left hemisphere.[532]

Deficits which indicate dominant responsibilities of the left hemisphere are disorders of gesture; ideational and ideomotor apraxias; agnosias for reading and writing, objects, and colors; and somatognosis; bilateral asomatognosia also follows a left hemisphere lesion.

Hughlings–**Jackson** made the perceptive comment in 1864 that if "the faculty of expression resides in one hemisphere, then there is no absurdity in raising the question as to whether perception—its corresponding opposite—may not be seated in the other." Indeed, nondominant hemisphere lesions do lead to visuospatial disturbances, including unilateral **asomatognosia, dressing apraxia**, some forms of **dyslexia, dysgraphia**, and **dyscalculia**, and the inability to recognize faces (**prosopagnosia**) as suggested first by Hughlings–Jackson, who also correctly assigned to the right hemisphere a role in automatic and emotional speech. **Babiński** noted first the occurrence of anosognosia following right hemisphere lesions in 1914, while Dide[1637] considered that visuo-constructive disorders (**constructional apraxia**) reflected a posterior right hemisphere lesion.

dominant albinism and congenital deafness (Tietz syndrome) A dominantly inherited syndrome of complete albinism except for the optic fundi and irides; scanty eyebrows; and congenital severe neural hearing loss.[6319]

dominant anhidrosis and progressive hearing loss A dominantly inherited syndrome of congenital anhidrosis with progressive neural hearing loss in middle age.[2852]

dominant ataxia See **cerebellar ataxias**.

dominant basal ganglion calcification See **striatopallidal calcification**.

dominant cerebellar ataxia plus See **cerebellar ataxias** (*variants*).

dominant congenital severe deafness A dominantly inherited syndrome characterized by congenital severe deafness but normal vestibular responses.[3526]

dominant hand weakness with sensorineural deafness A rare congenital familial syndrome of unilateral or bilateral neural deafness with contractures of the digits and wasting of all the small hand muscles. Flexion creases are absent over the interphalangeal joints, and there is a single vertical palmar crease. There is no abnormality on X-ray studies of the affected hand joints.[6059]

dominant leukodystrophy with cerebellar deficits and spastic paraparesis A dominantly inherited disorder with onset in early childhood, showing progressive spastic paraparesis with cerebellar deficits and mild mental deterioration, and the subsequent appearance of limb spasticity. It results in severe disability by the fourth decade of life. Brain MRI shows diffuse white-matter involvement. No biochemical or gene deficits characteristic of other leukodystrophies are present.[2229]

dominant low-frequency hearing loss A dominantly inherited syndrome with variable penetrance, characterized by moderate low-frequency hearing loss appearing at any time in life, with slow progression to moderately severe deafness involving all frequencies but with normal vestibular function.[3526]

dominant knuckle pads, leukonychia, and hearing loss (Bart–Pumphrey syndrome) A rare, nonprogressive, dominantly inherited syndrome characterized by congenital leukonychia, childhood onset of knuckle pads, progressive neural deafness, and diminished vestibular responses.[425, 3526]

dominant mid-frequency hearing loss A dominantly inherited syndrome characterized by progressive mid-frequency hearing loss in childhood and eventually loss at all frequencies, especially high tones, but with normal vestibular function.[4115]

dominant muscular dystrophy with humero-pelvic distribution A slowly progressive myopathy presenting with humero-pelvic weakness and contractures in childhood and cardiomyopathy after the age of 20. The syndrome is dominantly inherited but otherwise resembles the **Emery–Dreifuss** form of X-linked dystrophy.[2011]

dominant myopia, hearing loss, peripheral neuropathy, and skeletal abnormalities syndrome See **Flynn–Aird syndrome**.

dominant nephritis and hearing loss See **Alport syndrome**.

dominant optic atrophy A syndrome with adult onset, characterized by ptosis, ophthalmoplegia, optic atrophy, ataxia, nerve deafness, and myopathic weakness.[6376]

dominant osteosclerosis See **hyperostosis corticalis generalisata congenita**.

dominant otofaciocervical abnormalities A dominantly inherited syndrome characterized by hypoplasia of the maxillofacial complex, preauricular pits and fistulas, hypoplasia of the cervical muscles, resulting in lowering of the shoulder girdle, and conductive hearing loss.[1963]

dominant photomyoclonus, hearing loss, diabetes, and nephropathy A dominantly inherited condition characterized by neural deafness in association with bilateral neurofibromas of the VIII cranial nerve (usually unassociated with other evidence of **neurofibromatosis**), and seizures.[2876]

dominant preauricular pits and neural hearing loss A dominantly inherited syndrome with variable penetrance, manifesting mild-to-severe progressive neural hearing loss with onset in childhood or youth, unilateral or bilateral preauricular pits, and unilateral or bilateral branchial fistulas in a few cases.[2162]

dominant progressive nerve deafness A dominantly inherited syndrome characterized by childhood onset of a progressive symmetrical neural hearing loss beginning with high frequencies and leading to moderately severe hearing loss in later life.[6033]

dominant saddle nose, myopia, cataract, and hearing loss (Marshall syndrome) A dominantly inherited syndrome consisting of myopia, cataracts, saddle nose, and early-onset progressive neural deafness.[4111]

dominant stroke-like episodes and leukoencephalopathy A dominantly inherited syndrome characterized by recurrent subcortical stroke-like episodes in adult life, and with leukoencephalopathy, muscular lipidosis, and immunological abnormalities.[6362]

dominant unilateral deafness A dominantly inherited syndrome with variable penetrance, characterized by congenital moderate to severe unilateral or bilateral hearing loss and normal vestibular function.[5900]

domoic acid encephalopathy A syndrome comprising of acute gastrointestinal upset followed by neural hyperexcitability and chronic loss of function following the ingestion of domoic acid, a naturally occurring excitatory neurotoxin which is related to glutamate and which caused an outbreak of poisoning in Canada in 1987 through the ingestion of cultivated mussels.

Initial symptoms include abdominal discomfort, vomiting, diminished consciousness, short-term memory loss, confusion, headache, seizures and myoclonus, autonomic disturbances, and variable pareses, including ophthalmopareses. In the long term, the anterograde term memory loss and chronic anterior horn cell lesions may persist.[2484, 6246]

Donaldson syndrome (nephrolithiasis-mitochondrial cytopathy) A congenital dysmorphic syndrome also manifesting as short stature, cataract, retinitis pigmentosa, strabismus, cardiomyopathy, nephropathy, diabetes, red cell abnormalities, cerebral atrophy, seizures, ataxia, and distal myopathic weakness.[381]

Donner muscular dystrophy See **congenital muscular dystrophy**.

Donohue syndrome A rare, autosomal recessive, congenital encephalopathic, and dysmorphic syndrome characterized by facial and generalized hirsutism, marasmus, hypoglycemia, hypotonia, microcephaly, prenatal growth defect, failure of bony maturation, lipodystrophy, enlarged genitalia, and mental and motor delay. It usually leads to death in infancy.[1689] See **leprechaunism**.

DOOR syndrome See **deafness–onychodystrophy-onycholysis-retardation syndrome**.[1001]

Doose syndrome See **centrencephalic myoclonic-astatic epilepsy**.

dopamine A neurotransmitter with particularly high levels in certain neurons of the neostriatum, derived from L-dopa by dopa-decarboxylase and greatly reduced in Parkinsonian syndromes.

dopamine dysregulation syndrome A condition described in some treated patients with **Parkinson disease** or in those addicted to amphetamines or cocaine, manifest by **punding**, a tendency to gamble, and hypersexual behavior.

dopamine receptors D_1 and D_2 receptors are recognized, the former stimulating and the latter inhibiting adenylate cyclase and both together thus regulating dopamine metabolism.

dopa-responsive dystonia (autosomal dominant torsion dystonia, dopa-sensitive progressive dystonia of childhood, dystonia musculorum deformans, dystonia with marked diurnal variation associated with biopterin deficiency, fluctuating dystonia, hereditary Parkinsonism–dystonia, hereditary dystonia–Parkinsonism syndrome of juvenile onset) A dominantly inherited (or recessively inherited or sporadic) variant of idiopathic (torsion) dystonia, due to a mutation of the *GCH1* locus on 14q22, manifesting lower limb dystonia and gait disorder in children before the age of 12 years, although tremor, myoclonus, axial dystonia, and cervical dystonia may be prominent clinical features too. Typically symptoms worsen as the day progresses. Unusual responsiveness of the symptoms to oral levadopa in low dosage and the frequent presence of Parkinsonian features, at least later in life, are notable.[4724] See also **dystonia** and **Segawa dystonia**.

dopa-sensitive progressive dystonia of childhood See **dopa-responsive dystonia**.

Doppler, C.J. (1803–1853) Austrian mathematician and professor of experimental physics at Vienna.

Doppler effect When a source of sound is approaching an observer, the wave length of the sound decreases and so the pitch increases. This effect is used in angiology, when ultrasound waves are reflected toward a transducer by the moving column of blood, which allows both an estimate of the speed of the blood flow and (with the aid of certain scanning devices) generation of a two-dimensional map of the anatomy of the reflecting surfaces.

Doppler's original experiments which led to the discovery of the effect were conducted with the assistance of the brass section of the Vienna Symphony Orchestra, which played while on a rolling railroad flat-car.

dorsal columns (Lat, of the back) (posterior columns, Goll columns, Burdach columns) Symmetrical pathways ascending on the posterior aspect of the spinal cord and terminating in the gracile and cuneate nuclei.

Their functional responsibilities are still disputed, but selective section in humans leads to loss of the ability to carry out tasks in which simultaneous spatial and temporal analysis of the stimulus is required, such as figure identification; however, sensations of pressure, localization, passive movement, and speed of movement remain intact.[6606]

dorsal enteric cyst See **neurenteric cyst**.

dorsal foot response (tarsophalangeal response, Mendel–Bekhterev response 1) Plantar flexion of the toes, seen in patients with pyramidal tract lesions when the lateral aspect of the dorsum of the foot is struck.

dorsal interosseous syndrome See **posterior interosseous syndrome**.

dorsal midbrain syndrome
1. (Parinaud syndrome, pretectal syndrome, Sylvian aqueduct syndrome, Koerber–Salus–Elschnig syndrome, syndrome of the posterior commissure) The association of impairment of voluntary vertical gaze, especially upward; skew deviation; paralysis of upward and sometimes of downward saccades and of pursuit; convergence-retraction nystagmus on attempted up-gaze; ptosis; eyelid retraction (**Collier sign**); **corectopia iridis**; spasm and paralysis of accommodation and convergence; and light-near dissociation of the pupillary response.[277]

The syndrome is commonly caused by tumors of the pineal region or by intrinsic lesions of the dorsal midbrain. Reflex eye movements are relatively preserved.[361] However, paralysis of up-gaze is probably a result either of bilateral lesions within the pretectum or of sectioning the posterior commissure.[4898, 4899]. The best of the original descriptions was that of Salus,[5517] a pupil of Elschnig.

2. **Benedikt syndrome** has also been known by this name.

dorsal rhizotomy Surgical section of posterior roots, used formerly for pain control and currently under investigation as a treatment in cerebral palsy.

dorsal root entry zone lesions (DREZ lesions) Surgical lesions placed in the dorsal root entry zones in order to alleviate **deafferentation pain**.[4595]

dorsal tegmental syndrome See **dorsal midbrain syndrome**.

dorso-cuboidal sign See **Mendel–Bekhterev sign** 2.

dorsolateral frontal epilepsy (Lat, of the back and of the sides) (dorsolateral region seizures) Tonic (less commonly clonic) seizure patterns with versive eye and head movements and speech arrest.[1861]

dorsolateral midbrain syndrome A vascular brainstem syndrome characterized by rubral tremor, ipsilateral **Horner syndrome**, and contralateral anesthesia for all modalities. It is due to infarction of the mesencephalon supplied by a short circumferential artery.

dorsolateral region seizures See **dorsolateral frontal epilepsy**.

dorsum The vertebral column or the back of any body part.

Dostoevsky, Fyodor Mikhailovitch (Dostoiewsky) (b. 1821) Russian novelist who suffered from epileptic seizures of various kinds, including some heralded by ecstatic auras. A number of the characters in his books (e.g., *The Idiot*) are similarly afflicted.[2306]

Dostoevsky, commenting on the pleasurable sensations as the first expression of some of his seizures, wrote that he would have given all that he had for the enjoyment of another.[94]

double athetosis Abnormal myelination of the basal ganglia due to anoxic birth injury, giving them a marbled appearance. The clinical syndrome comprises dystonia, choreoathetosis, speech disturbances, pyramidal dysfunction (cerebral palsy), seizures, and mental retardation.[4805] See also **Vogt syndrome**, **etat marbré**, **status marmoratus**, and **status dysmyelinatus**.

double cortex sign See **band heterotopia**.

double crush syndrome The coexistence of compressive lesions in tandem along the course of a nerve, theoretically producing a deficit where either of the two lesions would not have caused it alone.

An example would be compression of the C6 or the C8 nerve roots in association with a mild carpal tunnel syndrome, producing a sensory or a motor variety of the syndrome, respectively, in each case as a result of serial constraints of axoplasmic flow in nerve fibers.[6451]

Unfortunately, although it is logical and inherently likely, there is no evidence that the phenomenon exists[5284] (although absence of proof is not proof of absence).

double discharge (doublet) The appearance of two motor unit action potentials or fibrillation potentials of similar form and amplitude, occurring consistently in the same relationship to one another at intervals of 2–20 ms.[19] See also **paired discharge, multiple discharge,** and **triple discharge**.

double panda sign The presence of both the **face of the giant panda sign** and the **panda sign** on the MRI of a patient with **Wilson disease**.

double saccadic pulse A saccadic intrusion into ocular fixation characterized by the presence of two back-to-back saccades without any intervening delay, occurring in single pairs or in runs. The condition represents a diluted form of **ocular flutter**.[35]

double whammy The ability to cause protrusion of one or both of the eyes at will, the upper and lower lids being withdrawn behind the coronal equator of the eye.[577]

double-cortex syndrome See **diffuse cortical dysplasia** and **heterotopias**.

double-elevator palsy A congenital anomaly consisting of paresis of the two muscles (inferior oblique, superior rectus) controlling elevation of one eye as the result of a pretectal lesion in the brainstem on either side,[3793] causing a supranuclear paresis of monocular elevation.[496]

The same may occur in adult life as a result of a small pretectal vascular lesion.

Double Letter Cancellation Test An instrument used to evaluate the presence and severity of visual scanning deficits and to evaluate unilateral spatial neglect in near extrapersonal space.

double-stimulation evoked responses A technique for assessing cerebral cortical excitability by means of giving double stimuli at varying short interstimulus intervals; in some forms of cortical reflex myoclonus, there is marked enhancement with the second stimulus of the pair when the interval between them is 60–100 ms.

doublet See **double discharge**.

doughnut sign The ring of isotope uptake seen on radionucleide brain scans in cases of necrotic tumor, abscess, or (occasionally) cerebral infarction.

Down, James Langdon Haydon (1828–1896) English physician who trained initially as a pharmacist and so entered medical school late, but graduated with honors. He was eventually appointed to the staff of the London Hospital, where he lectured mainly on therapeutics, and to the staff of the Earlswood Asylum, where he organized a model unit for the care of the mentally retarded. He championed the cause of establishing humane and productive care for mentally retarded people for the whole of

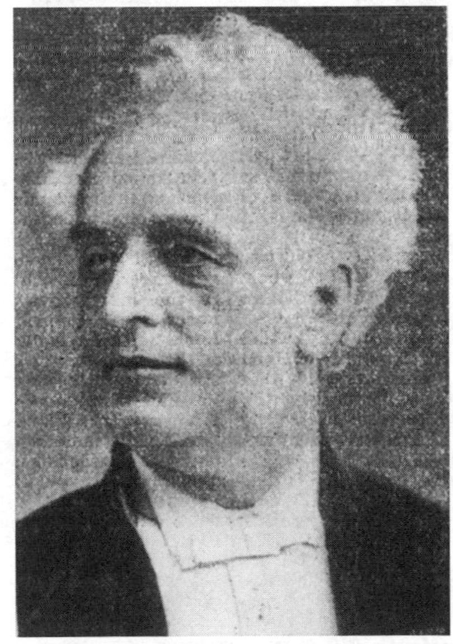

Figure D–4 James Langdon Haydon Down.

his life. The syndrome named for him was described briefly in 1866 (in the same year as a similar report on this syndrome was published by Séguin in Paris) but in full detail in his Lettsomian lectures to the Royal College of Physicians in 1887.

Down tried to classify mental defectives on the basis of their regression from one of the five ethnic groups to another and he considered that "a considerable proportion can be fairly referred to one of the great divisions of the human race other than the class from which they have sprung." Thus he tried to classify subjects as regressing to the Europoid ("Caucasian"), Ethiopian, Malay, American, or Mongolian races, substantially on the basis of their facial appearance.

Down syndrome (trisomy 21, mongolism; OMIM 190685) A genetically determined syndrome comprising amentia, growth deficiency, and abnormal morphogenesis existing as a result of either of two abnormalities—trisomy of chromosome 21 or translocation of chromosomal material (D/G or G/G) onto that chromosome.

The hallmarks of the disorder are mental retardation; a characteristic facial appearance with small skull, flat occiput, fissured tongue, epicanthic folds, short flat nose, small ears, and eyes slanting upward laterally; an increased incidence of congenital cardiac lesions; and skeletal abnormalities such as a short broad neck and limbs, broad flat hands, an incurving little finger, and a single transverse palmar crease. Hypogonadism is common. Ocular features include hypertelorism, strabismus, high myopia, **Brushfield spots** (yellow spots on the irides), and cataracts. Infantile spasms and mixed seizures are also reported.

The incidence of the trisomic form increases with maternal age. Those afflicted who live on to the fifth decade develop a syndrome that is clinically and pathologically indistinguishable from **Alzheimer disease**; the import of this for the understanding of the latter condition is appreciated.

The condition was described in 1866 by James Langdon **Down**, who named it "Mongolism."[1701]

The American National Down Syndrome Society Web page is at: http://www.ndss.org/.

downbeat nystagmus (downbeating fixation nystagmus) A form of acquired involuntary vertical jerk nystagmus overriding fixation and due to dysfunction of central vestibular systems. Clinically, the fast component beats downward. It is present in the primary position, but is typically increased by lateral gaze or convergence.

Its presence strongly suggests the existence of disease of the central vestibular connections; it may occur with the **Chiari malformation**, but other lesions at the cervicomedullary junction such as dolichoectasia of the vertebral artery; **cerebellar ataxic syndromes** such as episodic ataxia type 2, and paraneoplastic conditions and intoxications (e.g., lithium) can also be responsible.[2704, 5731] See also **ocular dipping**.

In clinical practice, patients complain of blurred vision and oscillopsia (worse on lateral gaze), unsteady gait and to-and-fro vertigo. Cerebellar signs are usually present.

In *variant* inherited forms, vertical nystagmus and ataxia are the main features[381] or the condition occurs only periodically, perhaps in association with thiamine deficiency.[1719]

downbeating fixation nystagmus See **downbeat nystagmus**.

downgaze palsy Selective impairment of downward gaze, following damage to the fasciculus retroflexus in the subthalamic region, usually due to embolic infarction in the territory of the posterior thalamosubthalamic artery.[2705] Paralysis of horizontal gaze may accompany this.

downgaze paralysis, ataxia, foam cell syndrome (DAF syndrome) See **sphingomyelin storage disorders**.

Dracula's teeth syndrome A syndrome of facial pain, ipsilateral facial dystonia, and phantom supernumerary (canine) teeth, beginning after a dental procedure.[3141]

Dracul disease See **porphyria**. The mythical Romanian character *Dracula* was depicted as suffering from this disease.

dracunculiasis A nematodal infection occurring in the poopulation of Asia and Africa in which the infestation rarely leads to mononeuropathy resulting from compression, abscesses (including extradural abscesses), and scarring.[346]

dragging monoplegic gait An abnormal gait pattern in which the whole leg is dragged as a single unit behind the patient, without circumduction of the hip but frequently with rotation at the hip and/or inversion or eversion of the ankle. The phenomenon is regarded as evidence of a **functional disorder**.[6074]

drainage headache See **post-lumbar puncture headache**.

Drake, Charles G. (1920–1998) Canadian neurosurgeon who studied at the Universities of Western Ontario and Toronto and with Fulton at Yale. Though self-described as "just a simple surgeon poking at the edges of knowledge," he was a brilliant technician, an incisive thinker, and an accomplished administrator as the first chairman of the Department of Clinical Neurological Sciences at the University of Western Ontario. He is best remembered internationally for his approaches to the management of aneurysms, particularly those in the posterior fossa, taking these procedures "from the realm of the daring to the domain of the routine" (Hachinski).

Dravet syndrome (severe myoclonic epilepsy in infancy, epilepsy with polymorphic features) An epileptic encephalopathy of infancy and childhood; a channelopathy due to a *de novo* mutation in the gene encoding the α_1 subunit of the Na^+ channel SCN1A. It is characterized by early infantile febrile clonic convulsions; afebrile generalized or unilateral clonic nocturnal seizures, myoclonic jerks, atypical absences, and complex focal seizures in the first year of life in apparently normal infants; these are later followed by myoclonus and other seizure types persisting into adulthood. Precipitants include fever, hot baths, photic and pattern stimulation, movements, and eye closure. The inter-ictal EEG shows slowing of background activity with frequent and severe generalized polyspikes-slow waves and 2 Hz spike-slow waves. Multifocal abnormalities of spikes and slow waves are common.

The seizures are usually accompanied by a slowing of psychomotor development and marked cognitive impairment and behavioral disturbances. See **severe myoclonic epilepsy in infancy**.[1711, 4882]

Myoclonic epilepsy in infancy (formerly "benign myoclonic epilepsy in infancy") is a milder but still not benign form of **Dravet syndrome**. Seizures may occasionally be reflex (i.e., touch).[1861]

Drayer syndrome A congenital dysmorphic syndrome manifesting also short stature; hirsutism; strabismus; blepharophimosis; genital, skeletal, and dermal lesions including absence of phalanges; and atrial septal defect with microcephaly and mental and developmental delay.[381]

dream A train of thoughts, images, or fancies passing through the mind during rapid eye movement (less often non–rapid eye movement) sleep. The history of mankind's attitude to and interpretation of the significance of dreams has been reviewed.[5605]

dream anxiety attacks The occurrence of an awakening from rapid eye movement sleep with full factual recall of a disturbing dream and with subjective and autonomic evidence of marked anxiety or disquiet such as tachycardia, sweating, and tachypnea. (See also **sleep disorders** and **nightmares**.)

dreamy state The epileptic manifestation described by Hughlings-**Jackson** in his paper "On a Particular Variety of Epilepsy,"[3127] in which he expanded on the "intellectual aura" (a term which he disliked) in which smell, taste, reminiscence (déja vu), and epigastric sensations may occur in company with chewing movements and a defect (though not a loss) of consciousness.

He first described this condition in 1876 in a physician, Dr. Z, who was Jackson's neighbor and patient. In 1898 Dr. Z died from an overdose of chloral, and there was found at autopsy a small patch of softening in the left uncinate region. Jackson applied the term *uncinate fits* to this form of epilepsy in 1899. See also **affective-psychic seizures**.

dressing apraxia Impairment in fitting the form of a garment to the form of the body, in the absence of significant motor or sensory impairment; and usually associated with a right-sided or bilateral parieto-occipital lesion producing neglect of left-sided space and with impairment in visuospatial judgment (**visuospatial agnosia**).[799]

Despite the name, the condition is not truly an apraxia. It was known to Hughlings-**Jackson** but was first described fully by Brain in 1941. See **apraxia for dressing**.

Drew family disease A dominantly inherited syndrome with early adult onset, characterized by progressive euphoria, optic atrophy, lost up-gaze, nystagmus, pyramidal and cerebellar signs, Parkinsonism, loss of light touch, and impaired sphincter control.[2015] The condition may be a form of **olivopontocerebellar atrophy**.

drift The tendency for a limb to sink slowly when held horizontally against gravity. The sign is examined with the patient's eyes closed and his arms held straight out in front of him. Drifting downward occurs within 15 s or so in patients with cerebellar disease, but also in those with weakness of shoulder flexion, contralateral parietal lobe disease, and disease of the shoulder joint.

Drilled Word Span Test A test of memory wherein the subject learns to criterion a list of words one shorter in length than his forward digit span; his delayed recall is tested after further unfilled or filled intervals.[4332]

dromedary gait A rolling, high-stepping gait with protrusion of the buttocks due to excessive lordosis, seen in dystonic patients.

droopy shoulder syndrome A syndrome of women characterized by the association of low-set shoulders; long neck (as shown by the appearance of T2 on lateral cervical radiographs); pain in the neck, shoulder, chest, arms, or hands made worse by downward traction of the arms and alleviated by elevation of the shoulders; and a positive **Tinel sign** over the brachial plexus.

There are no hard neurological or vascular signs and EMG and nerve conduction study findings are normal.[6167]

drop attacks Sudden weakness of the legs without loss of consciousness and causing an immediate fall to the ground; vision, hearing, and speech remain intact.The attacks may occur as a result of myoclonus, abrupt cortical inhibition, cataplexy, or impairment of the integrity of brainstem structures (vertebrobasilar insufficiency, colloid cyst, etc.), causing brief interruption of the functions of the reticular activating system. In the latter cases, brief alteration of consciousness may occur, however.

The term was introduced by Sheldon[5777] to describe a sudden, unheralded fall to the ground, usually in the elderly, without alteration in consciousness or any post-ictal residuum and with immediate righting. See also **otolithic crisis**.

drop finger Weakness of extension of a digit at the metacarpophalangeal joint due to a lesion of the posterior interosseous nerve, with resulting pareses of the extensors indicis, digitorum, and pollicis. Drop thumb and **drop wrist** have similar connotations.

drop seizure Abrupt loss of postural tone without any change in the sensorium, occurring as a manifestation of a seizure discharge ("astatic seizure" in the words of **Ramsay Hunt**).

drop wrist Inability to maintain extension of the wrist, such that it falls into a position of flexion, as with paresis of the radial extensor muscles of the wrist and fingers.

dropped head syndrome (Suarez-Kelly syndrome) Involuntary forward flexion of the neck as a result of particular weakness of the neck extensor muscles[6113] as in **myasthenia gravis**, **facioscapulohumeral dystrophy**, **polymyositis**, **amyotrophic lateral sclerosis**, **carnitine deficiency**, **nemaline myopathy**, **chronic inflammatory demyelinating polyneuropathy**, **focal steroid-responsive myositis**, and in severe hypokalemia. Some shoulder girdle weakness may also be noted. Similar weakness of the thoracic paraspinal muscles may cause "bent spine syndrome." EMG of the paravertebral muscles may suggest either neurogenic or myogenic disease.[4753] See also **camptocormia**.

Cervical **dystonias** can produce the same effect, but due to active contraction of the neck flexor muscles rather than weakness of the extensors.

dropsy (short for hydropsy: from Lat, watery) An abnormal accumulation of fluid. Thus cerebral dropsy is **hydrocephalus**.

drowsiness (Saxon; sluggishness) The earliest stage of that physiological depression of consciousness which is likely to lead on to sleep.

drug holiday A period of transient (up to 7 days) drug withdrawal during hospitalization, as used in some patients with complications of long-term levadopa therapy, in an attempt to enhance motor performance and to diminish these side effects.[6695]

Although successful to a degree in achieving these goals for a limited period after the restoration of therapy, the régime is associated with the dangers of greatly decreased mobility during the holiday and is viewed with circumspection by many physicians.

drug-induced (refractory) headache 1. See **analgesic rebound headache**, **ergotamine withdrawal headache**, and **medication-induced headache**. 2. Headaches typically and only occurring following the ingestion of certain agents such as indomethacin, nifedipine, and cimetidine, etc.

drug-induced cerebral arteritis (drug-induced vasospasm) See **reversible cerebral vasoconstriction syndrome**.

drug-induced nystagmus See **induced nystagmus**.

drug-resistant intractable seizures (OMIM 171050) A rare disorder of the p-glycoprotein mechanism characterized by multiple seizures, unresponsive to anticonvulsants.

Drummond syndrome See **blue diaper syndrome**.

drusen (from Ger, a rock cavity lined with crystal) 1. Hyaline-like pallid nodular debris derived from the pigmented retinal layers (**Brusch's membrane**), perhaps as a result of axonal degeneration.

In this dominantly inherited abnormality, the deep yellowish lesions, usually round or oval in shape, are mainly in the posterior polar region of the eye and sometimes widely spread over the retina. They possibly represent a secretion of the abnormal pigmentary epithelium. Drusen are also seen in numerous diseases of the choroid. They usually appear in early adult life and are symptomless unless there is secondary macular degeneration.[3564]

2. The same, seen on and in the region of the optic disk, where their presence causes elevation of the disk head (and thus the obliteration of the cup and the appearance of papilledema, especially if prepapillary hemorrhages are also present[2921]). Arcuate scotomas may also be found. See **pseudopapilledema**.

3. Senile plaques (in the German literature).

D-state See **REM sleep** (paradoxical sleep).

D-test A composite instrument evaluating the behavioral and functional activities of demented geriatric patients.[2018]

dualism (Lat, containing two) The system of Descartes in which he tried to explain all the phenomena of human nature based on the principles of the essential separateness of body and mind. Thus *mind* here represents more than mere expression of the function of the brain.

Duane, Alexander (1858–1926) American ophthalmologist practicing in New York.

Duane syndrome (ocular retraction syndrome, Stilling–Turk–Duane syndrome) A congenital, dominantly inherited brainstem disorder with aberrant innervation of the lateral rectus by the inferior division of the III cranial nerve in the absence of the VI n. nuclei, with maximal clinical effects upon eye movements.[1721] The major features are restriction of abduction, adduction, or both. Attempted adduction of the eyes causes globe retraction and narrowing of the palpebral fissure. Esotropia is most common. Although usually unilateral and sporadic, bilateral syndromes can occur and associated congenital malformations are common.

Three types are described: *type I*, in which there is narrowing of the palpebral fissure and retraction of the globe on adduction of the eye, with limitation of abduction; *type II*, in which there is narrowing of the fissure, retraction, and limited adduction but full abduction; and *type III*, consisting of deficiency of both ocular abduction and adduction due to fibrosis of the lateral rectus muscle, leading to retraction of the globe by 2–10 mm with narrowing of the palpebral fissure during attempted adduction.

Convergence failure and both brainstem and musculo-skeletal abnormalities may coexist. The syndrome is more common in females. It was first described by Stilling in the German literature in 1887.

Variants are as follows:

DURS1 (8q13) A sporadic multisystem disorder with weakness of abduction, retraction of the eye, and ptosis with attempted adduction and an association with C2–C3 vertebral fusion (**Klippel–Feil**), thenar hypoplasia, and deafness.
DURS2 (2q31) is a dominantly inherited congenital ophthalmoplegia with absent or reduced abduction and maybe adduction, and retraction of the eye and ptosis with attempted adduction.
Okihiro syndrome, a dominantly inherited form consists of the Duane anomaly with radial ray abnormalities and deafness, in which the typical features of Duane syndrome are also accompanied by congenital bony anomalies of the arm and cervical spine.[4781]
Sal-like 4 (20q, *SALL4*) is dominantly inherited and is characterized by added features of the **Holt–Oram syndrome**.[7720]
Sporadic Duane syndrome (chromosomes 4 or 22) The features of Wildervanck syndrome added to those of the Duane and Klippel–Feil anomalies, with congenital deafness.
Bosley–Salih–Alorainey syndrome (7p15, *HOXA1*) Recessively inherited bilateral Duane syndrome with preserved vertical gaze and convergence, but with added deafness, delayed motor development, and mental retardation. Malformations of the carotids, the skull base, and the ears are other features.

An *acquired form* is described in patients with brainstem and III cranial nerve pathology.

See also **Wildervanck syndrome** and the Web site http://www.ophthal.org/.

Dubini, Angelo (1813–1902) Italian physician, practicing in Lombardy.

Dubini disease (electric chorea) A rare and fatal form of chorea described by Dubini in 1846, but not now reported; as a result, it cannot in retrospect be classified with confidence. The disease was said to have been marked by spasmodic movements in one limb, progressing to involve others, and sometimes characterized by seizures, progressive paralysis, and muscle wasting.[1722]

The nature of the disorder remains uncertain; both a myoclonic form of epidemic encephalitis and hysteria have been suggested as its cause. Though its organicity seems dubious by description, some patients appear to have died from it (or at least with it), and it has been considered by some to be a myoclonic form of epidemic encephalitis. See also **Bergeron disease**.

DuBois-Reymond, Emil

(1818–1896) The father of modern electrophysiology who devoted his whole clinical life to this subject. He was a pupil of Johannes Müller, whom he succeeded as professor of physiology in Berlin. He demonstrated the polarized state of nerves and muscle fibers and showed that the peripheral passage of a nerve impulse was accompanied by an electrical discharge—the action potential. He was also the first to describe the electrical and mechanical properties of muscle **tetanus**.

His collection of works was translated into English and published by Charles Morgan under the title of *Electrophysiology and Therapeutics* (New York, William Wood, 1868), a book regarded by most reviewers at the time as being unreadable. His clinical contributions are less well known, but he gave good accounts of the symptoms of **migraine** from personal experience.

Dubowitz syndrome

A congenital dysmorphic syndrome manifesting also short stature, eczema, skeletal abnormalities, ptosis, blepharophimosis, microcephaly, and mental and developmental delay.[1729]

Duchenne de Boulogne, Guillaume-Benjamin Armand

(1806–1875) French neurologist born in Boulogne, who trained in Paris and returned to his home port to practice. After the death of his wife from puerperal fever when their son was 2 weeks old, he retired much from the world and devoted himself to his family practice and to exploring the benefits of electricity in medicine, although he did marry again. He relocated to Paris in 1842 but never obtained a permanent hospital appointment there, although he was accepted on to the services of many neurologists, from whose patients he gleaned and reported on cases of neurological disease in the wards of hospitals all over the city. He was highly regarded after 1849 for his use of Faradic currents to assist in diagnosis and recorded his experiences in his book *De l'electricisation localisée*, of which three editions were published (in 1855, 1861, and 1872).[1738] The title is misleading because although the book starts with a description of the method and some results, the greater part is devoted to the other areas in neurology for which Duchenne is better remembered. His presence at the Hotel Dieu and the Salpêtrière brought him into contact with all of the leading neurologists of the day and he and Charcot held each other in mutual admiration.

Duchenne described spinal muscular atrophy as a form of **amyotrophic lateral sclerosis** (but passed on publication to Aran) in 1849. He described **progressive bulbar palsy** 9 years later and **pseudo-hypertrophic muscular dystrophy** first in 1861 and more fully in 1868, the same year as he introduced the technique of needle muscle biopsy, which he had employed in the diagnosis of the boys in his paper and described also therein. The name of Aran is also linked to this condition, but that physician reported on patients with a variety of muscle disorders, some of the patients referred to him by Duchenne himself; Dr. Edward Meryon did, however, describe the condition in England in 1852.[7] In his works on muscle diseases he described the dystrophy that bears his name, at least two forms of atrophic paresis in infancy, one likely due to poliomyelitis; and a bulbar and two spinal forms of paralysis in adults. (*Guilly, J.P. Duchenne de Boulogne; Paris, Bailliere et fils. 1936.*)

In other contributions, Duchenne described upper brachial plexus palsy in 1872, some years before **Erb's** report; distinguished between upper and lower motor neuron facial palsies; described locomotor ataxia (**tabes dorsalis**), lead paralysis, and poliomyelitis; and recorded cases of what is now called **facioscapulohumeral dystrophy** in 1872, 12 years before **Landouzy** and **Déjèrine** published their description. Many of his experiments on facial expression requiring apparently painful stimulation of the facial muscles were performed on an elderly man whose face was in fact anesthetic, perhaps due to tabes dorsalis.

McHenry[4233] describes him as unworldly, naïve, absent-minded, and inarticulate, which may explain why his contributions to many areas of neurology were overshadowed so completely by those of colleagues such as **Charcot**, who nevertheless regarded Duchenne as his master in Neurology. He died, still deeply melancholy, 4 years after the death of his son, with **Charcot** at his bedside.

Duchenne disease

See **tabes dorsalis**.

Duchenne muscular dystrophy

(pseudo-hypertrophic muscular dystrophy) A progressive and still fatal X-linked recessive disorder affecting young boys in which the affected gene at Xp21.2 on the short arm of the X chromosome fails to produce dystrophin, an essential protein. The same protein is deficient in quantity or altered in composition but not absent in **Becker muscular dystrophy**, an allelic condition.

Boys with Duchenne muscular dystrophy have high levels of **creatine kinase** from birth and manifest the signs of the disease as soon as they would normally start to walk. Proximal weakness, affecting first the pelvic girdle muscles (see **Gowers sign**), and fatty replacement of the calf and tongue muscles making them firm and rubbery ("pseudohypertrophy") are the leading characteristics. Eventually kyphoscoliosis, areflexia, and cardiac failure occur.[1737] A wheelchair is needed by the time patients reach early adolescence and the patients die in their early twenties, usually of pneumonia.

The triumphant determination of the site[785] and nature of the defect gives some hope that the foregoing description may soon be out of date; if the protein can be synthesized and replaced, the fatal prognosis may be tempered.[2935] Duchenne dystrophy was described by him and Aran and by Wilhelm Griesinger (1817–1868) in 1865.[2577]

A *variant* is *autosomal recessive Duchenne-like muscular dystrophy* in which females are affected by a disease exactly mimicking Duchenne dystrophy as a result of inheritance of a different allele for a polymorphism within the dystrophin gene.[4230]

The Web site http://www.angelfire.com/band/teja/index_dmd.html reviews the causes, biology, and treatment options.

Duchenne paralysis

See **progressive bulbar palsy** and **amyotrophic lateral sclerosis**.

Duchenne sign Indrawing of the epigastrium with inspiration, a sign of diaphragmatic palsy.

Duchenne–Aran disease See **progressive bulbar palsy** and **amyotrophic lateral sclerosis**.

Duchenne–Erb palsy See **upper brachial plexus palsy**.

ductions The movements of one eye, the other being covered. The possible movements are *adduction* and *abduction* (toward or away from the nose, respectively); *sursumduction* (elevation) and *deorsumduction* (depression); *incycloduction* (intorsion with the upper pole turned toward the nose); and *encycloduction* (extorsion with the upper pole turned toward the temple).[3762] See also **forced duction** test.

dumb (Saxon; silent) Unable to make articulate sounds.

dumb rabies (paralytic rabies) A form of **rabies** producing polyneuropathy rather than encephalitis, the latter producing the "furious" form.[3724]

dumb-bell tumors (hourglass tumors) Extra- and intradural masses joined by a narrow pedicle passing through an enlarged intervertebral foramen at any level. Less commonly, tumors which are wholly intraspinal with intra- and extra-dural masses similarly joined. Many are meningiomas or neurofibromas.

dumbness The inability to make vocal sounds. The condition includes **aphthongia**, **alalia**, and a**narthria**.

Dunnigan familial partial lipodystrophy An autosomal dominantly inherited laminopathy, whose neurological features include both myopathy and tomaculous neuropathy.[6003]

Duplay syndrome (frozen shoulder, adhesive capsulitis of the shoulder) Shoulder pain due to soft tissue inflammation and fibrosis, often following cervical injury, stroke, or myocardial infarction[1755]and limiting rotation and abduction of the shoulder with consequent disuse astrophy of the periscapular muscles.

duplex ultrasonography A noninvasive scanning technique combining b-mode imaging with pulsed Doppler technology to produce an image of blood flow through a vessel.

It allows the differentiation of occluded from patent arteries and provides a method of grading the severity of arterial disease based on changes in the blood flow pattern distal to stenosis.

Continuous-wave systems give an average of the cross-sectional velocity in the area examined, while pulsed systems enable more discrete examination of the blood flow pattern in the area of disease.[4678]

duplicity theory of vision The contention that color vision is a function of the retinal cone receptors and that gray-scale tones are recognized by the rods.

Dupré, Ernest (1862–1921) French physician.

Dupré syndrome (serous meningitis, toxic encephalopathy) A syndrome of meningeal irritation, sometimes progressing to headache, convulsions, diffuse encephalopathic signs, and coma, following distant infection or as an autoimmune phenomenon after infection, more commonly seen in children.[1756, 5377] See **parameningeal infections** and **idiopathic intracranial hypertension**.

Dupuy syndrome See **gustatory sweating**.

Dupuy–Dutemps and Cestan sign Incomplete peripheral paralysis of the face; when the patient is asked to look forward and to close both eyes slowly, the upper lid on the paretic side moves upward a small amount, due to the action of the levator palpebrae superioris.[5333]

Dupuytren, Baron Guillaume (1777–1835) French surgeon. Dobson[1670] remarked that he "had a remarkable childhood, being kidnapped when three years old by a rich woman of Toulouse. Was returned by her but subsequently taken to Paris (1789) by a Cavalry officer who took a fancy to him." He was educated in Paris and became surgeon to the Hôtel-Dieu and professor at the University of Paris, publishing almost nothing and becoming a huge success.

Dupuytren's canals The diploic spaces in the cranial bones.

Dupuytren contracture Contracture of the palmar (Dupuytren's) fascia with tight bands of fibrous tissue radiating distally under the palm, causing flexion deformities of the fingers.

dura mater (Lat, hard + mother; the latter as the Arabians considered that all tissues of the body were derived from the meninges) The tough, fibrous outer layer of the meninges enveloping the brain and spinal cord.

dural arteriovenous fistula An abnormal connection between the branches of the external carotid artery and the venous sinuses, sometimes caused by sinus thrombosis. Its clinical presentations include complaints of headache, bruit, and imbalance; cranial neuropathies, ischemic, and hemorrhagic strokes may also occur. Cervical myelopathy is a rare presentation. The fistulae may disappear spontaneously or may be occluded by arterial compression or embolization.[178]

Dural Arteriovenous Fistula Scale An instrument allowing classification and prognosis of arteriovenous fistulas in dural blood vessels using two parameters; location of AV fistula drainage and the pattern of blood flow and size of the vein.[1226]

dural sinus malformation A congenital malformation in which a hugely dilated dural sinus pouch communicates with other sinuses and drains cerebral veins. Arteriovenous shunts are commonly associated.

Durand–Zunin syndrome The association of agenesis of the septum pellucidum, lacunar skull deficits, dysraphism, hydrocephalus, and pes cavus.[1762]

duration 1. The time during which something exists or acts. In electromyography, the interval from the beginning of the first deflection from the baseline to its final return to the baseline of an action potential or waveform, unless otherwise specified. If only part of the waveform is measured, the points of the measurement should be specified. For example, the duration of the M wave may be measured as the negative phase duration and refers to the interval from the deflection of the first negative phase from the baseline to its return to the baseline. 2. The interval of the applied current or voltage of a single electric stimulus. 3. The interval from the beginning to the end of a series of recurring stimuli or action potentials. (From the 2001 Report of the Nomenclature Committee of the American Association of Electromyography and Electrodiagnosis.[19] Reproduced by kind permission of the AANEM.)

Duret, Henri (1849–1921) French neurologist who trained under **Charcot**, with whom he described the lenticulostriate arteries as the "arteries of cerebral hemorrhage." He is also remembered for his precise mapping of the territories supplied by the anterior, middle, and posterior cerebral arteries[1763] and for noting the brainstem hemorrhages complicating its compression.

Duret hemorrhages Intrinsic bleeding into the upper (rostral) brainstem resulting from its compression, as by the medial part of the temporal lobe in the **uncal syndrome**.[1764]

Dutch cerebral hemorrhage (hereditary cerebral hemorrhage with amyloidosis—Dutch type) A dominantly inherited predisposition to multiple large or small cerebral or cerebellar cortical hemorrhages occurring in mid-adult life, arising from a mutation at chromosome 21q21 and leaving as residua focal and global impairments and, frequently, dementia.[2655] Subcortical hemorrhages occur later in many cases.

In a *variant* form, the similar *Icelandic form*, it is not the amyloid precursor protein but cystatin C that is mutated.

Duval's nucleus A small mass of multipolar ganglion cells situated just ventral to the hypogloossal nucleus in the medulla, described in 1883 by Mathias Marie Duval (1844–1907), a French anatomist.[5619]

dwarfism with microcephaly and hydrocephaly A congenital dysmorphic syndrome of platyspondyly, microcephaly, hydrocephalus, and callosal abnormalities.[381]

dwarfism with retinal atrophy and deafness See **Cockayne syndrome**.

Dyel phenomenon If, in a patient with papilledema, light compression of the eyeball elicits visible pulsations of the retinal arterioles at the optic nerve head, this suggests that the cause is a mass lesion rather than chronic renal disease and hypertension.[1785]

Dyggve-Melchior-Clausen syndrome A heterogeneous, congenital, recessively inherited dysmorphic syndrome manifesting skeletal abnormalities, short stature, atlanto-occipital subluxation, platyspondyly, J-shaped sella turcica, and mental and developmental delay.[1786]

dying-back The process whereby metabolic disturbances of the perikaryon of the largest and longest axons in peripheral nerves lead to a failure of the soma to maintain lines of nutrient supply first to distal and then progressively to more proximal regions of its axon.[1059] The degeneration of the axons starts with the longest fibers and the lesion progresses from distal to proximal. Empires in decay similarly lose first those of their possessions which are linked to them by the longest lines of communication.

dying-back neuropathy See **distal axonopathy**.

Dyke–Davidoff–Masson syndrome A congenital dysmorphic syndrome manifesting an asymmetrical face, thickening of the cranial vault, overdevelopment of the frontal and ethmoidal sinuses, and elevation of the petrous pyramid of the temporal bone on the side of hemispheric atrophy in children with seizures and hemiplegia.[1787]

dynamesthesia The appreciation of force or tension during the performance of a voluntary muscle contraction.

dynamic (from Gr, power) Relating to strength or force. *Sthenic* is a synonym.

dynamic aphasia (verbal adynamia) A condition in which spontaneous speech is markedly reduced in the absence of any syntactical impairment while naming. Repetition and reading skills are normal. Verbal generative and verbal planning skills are normal when the subject is asked to describe pictorial scenes and complex actions. The condition may progress to mutism when it occurs, for example, in the context of **progressive supranuclear palsy**.[5339]

dynamic axial brainstem distortion Buckling of the brainstem as a result of downward herniation of the cerebrum through the tentorial opening and a possible cause of third nerve palsy as a false localizing sign.[3700]

dynamic EMG See **kinesiologic EMG**.

dynamic overshoot (ocular quiver) 1. A form of saccadic intrusion or oscillation characterized by involuntary deviation of the eye in the direction of gaze, requiring a saccade to restore it to the appropriate position. 2. A corrective movement occurring at the end of a normal saccade and in the opposite direction, greater in degree than the normal reversal of direction that would be required to bring the eye to a halt.[3762]

dynamic saccade The fast, first part of the saccadic eye movement.

dynamic spelling alexia The occurrence of **spelling alexia** with relative sparing of writing and of the identification of letters printed in view of the patient by the clinician.

This rare condition was detected in a patient with a large left hemisphere lesion also compressing the corpus callosum.[2994]

dynamic vestibular imbalance Asymmetrical activity of the vestibular apparatus apparent only with movement. Head shaking and single, rapid head turns are used to demonstrate this. In the former case, jerk nystagmus is produced, usually with its slow phase directed toward the side of the vestibular lesion. Sudden passive turning of the head with maintained fixation will normally allow fixation to persist; with vestibular imbalance, deviation will occur and a corrective saccade will be seen.[3762]

dynamite encephalosis Headache, sweating, coughing, vomiting, fatigue, irritability, depression, and impaired concentration up to confusion as a result of chronic toxic exposure to glyceryl trinitrate.[2331]

dynamometer (Gr, power + measure) An instrument for measuring the strength of contraction of muscles. The *Mathieu dynamometer* consists of a metal ellipse, the two sides connected by a spring with a scale upon which a pointer rotates to indicate the force of manual compression applied to the ellipse. Some methods prescribe precise placement of the limbs of the examiner or the subject in the performance of the tests.[6783]

dynorphin A peptide neurotransmitter complex, containing leukoencephalins.

dys- A Greek prefix signifying bad, difficult, or painful.

dysapocatastasis (Gr, disturbance of + complete restoration) A feeling of morbid discontent with restlessness of mind.

The word is not in general usage, but, even though it has seven syllables, it is still shorter than the definition (which requires nine words). The disorder must represent one of the commoner reasons underlying visits to physicians and is otherwise unnamed.

dysarthria (Gr, difficulty + a joint) (dyslalia) 1. The indistinct pronunciation of words. 2. A group of speech disorders resulting from disturbance in the muscular control of the speech mechanisms due to damage to the central or peripheral nervous systems.

While typically evidence of either upper or lower motor neuron lesions (the latter affecting the V, VII, or the bulbar nerves, the endplates, or the muscles), it may also be caused by local mechanical problems and is heard accompanying dysphasias.[1453]

Spastic, ataxic, and hypokinetic forms are differentiated, due respectively to cortico-bulbar, cerebellar, and basal ganglion lesions. Their characteristics have been reviewed.[3490] Mechanical and flaccid forms result from local structural and lower cranial motor nerve disorders. In addition, aphasic patients also frequently manifest dysarthria.

dysarthria–clumsy hand syndrome A **lacunar syndrome** in which mild dysphagia, some dysarthria, tongue deviation on protrusion, and clumsiness of the hand are associated with slight "central" weakness of the face and arm and a positive Babiński sign. Truncal ataxia may also be present. The lesion is most often in the upper part of the internal capsule or in the basis pontis.[2085]

It may be impossible to differentiate this syndrome from **homolateral ataxia and crural paresis** or **ataxic hemiparesis** clinically except that in the latter, dysarthria is not a feature and hemiparesis and sensory changes are present.[2405] See **ataxic hemiparesis**.

dysautonomia Any disorder of the autonomic nervous system, sympathetic or parasympathetic, including hyper- as well as hypofunction. See **diencephalic autonomic seizures** and *primary dysautonomia* (comprising **pure autonomic failure, Parkinson disease** with autonomic failure, and **multiple-system atrophy**).

http://www.ninds.nih.gov/disorders/dysautonomia/dysautonomia.htm is a Web site providing links to many other sites concerned with dysautonomia.

Dysautonomia Foundation Inc. A charitable foundation. Address: 633 Third Ave., 12th Floor, New York, NY 10017-6706, USA. Tel: 212-949-6644. Web site: http://www.familialdysautonomia.org/aboutfd.htm.

dysautonomic cephalalgia A syndrome of posttraumatic headaches associated with excessive sweating and pupillary dilatation due to partial sympathetic denervation, the injury having been to the anterior triangle of the neck.[6547] See **trigeminal autonomic cephalgias**.

dysbasia lordotica progressiva See **dystonia**.

dysbarism See **decompression sickness**.

dysbulia Difficulty in the exercise of the will; mental torpor. When pathological, there is also evidence of metabolic disease or of lesions affecting the deep frontal regions. See **abulia**.

dyscalculia Disturbance in mental reckoning and in enumeration and calculation on paper, as in **Gerstmann syndrome**.

In *primary dyscalculia*, this deficit stands out in comparison to the disturbance in other skills such as language, memory, attention, or perception, which are equally or more obviously affected in *secondary dyscalculia*. A medial left frontal lesion is suggested as the necessary cause.[3946]

dyschondroplasia See **Ollier disease**.

dyschromatopsia (Gr, difficulty + color + sight) Disturbance of color vision; a distortion of the hue or color of objects seen, as though the observer were looking through a colored filter (e.g., erythropsia, xanthopsia) possibly as a result of lesions of the visual cortex or due to toxic disease.

dyscognitive aura Epileptic events in which disturbance of cognition is the prominent or most apparent feature.

dyscognitive seizures Those seizures that resemble complex partial seizures, except that there is not always impairment of consciousness and that they do not originate in limbic areas, although mesial temporal limbic areas and their immediate connections are probably involved anyway.[7735]

dysconjugate Not yoked together; or, in the case of eye movements, not moving in parallel.

dyscoria Abnormal pupillary shape, the pupil being slitlike, oval, hourglass, or irregular. The syndrome is generally benign and may be dominantly inherited.[2858]

dysdiadochokinesis (Gr, difficulty + a follower + movement) Impairment in the speed, precision, and rhythmicity of rapidly performed movements in alternating directions by virtue of irregularities in their force and an inability to change rapidly the patterns of contraction and relaxation of the muscles involved. Rapid repetitive tapping of the back of one hand alternately with the palm and the back of the other one is the test most commonly employed.

The term was originally applied by **Babiński** to such a disturbance of coordinated movement in patients with a cerebellar disorder. This is still considered to be an important sign of a cerebellar lesion on the same side, but pyramidal and basal ganglion disease and local factors may produce a similar difficulty.

dysembryoma (neuroepithelioma) A heterogeneous group of primary malignant tumors arising from peripheral nerves and characterized by the presence of spaces lined by cuboidal or columnar epithelium.[3305]

dysencephalia splanchnocystica (Gruber syndrome, Meckel–Gruber syndrome) A recessively inherited congenital **neurocutaneous syndrome** characterized by microcephaly, occipital encephalocele, meningocele, ocular abnormalities and facial clefting, and polydactyly and polycystic kidneys, liver, and pancreas.[3, 2182] Micropthalmia, congenital heart defects, cleft lip and palate, internal hydrocephalus, anencephaly, and cerebellar aplasia have also been described.[3016] See **Gruber syndrome**.

dysequilibrium syndrome 1. An unusual autosomal recessive syndrome, manifesting the combination of marked motor delay with hypotonia, nystagmus, ataxia, mental retardation, and frequent falls when at last the child attains the standing position.[2677] See **cerebellar ataxias**. 2. See **dialysis dysequilibrium syndrome**.

dysesthesia 1. Painful sensations resulting from stimuli which are not normally painful, in the presence of alterations in the quality of other sensations. They occur commonly in the territory of a partially damaged peripheral nerve. **Charcot** described under this term a distressing pain resembling vibration, which travels up and down a limb when it is touched or stimulated by cold.[5103] 2. Dullness or perversion of sensation; this, however, is an older meaning for the word and does not represent current usage. 3. Disorders of the senses (**Cullen**).

dysesthesia–dysautonomia–hypertension syndrome A syndrome with childhood onset characterized by paresthesias, spontaneous pains, and autonomic dysfunction. The cause is not known.

dysesthetic pain A form of centrally derived pain resulting from spinal pathology (such as an intrinsic or extrinsic spinal tumor, or transverse myelitis stemming from any cause) in which the dysesthesias are in the territory of one or a few dermatomes at the level of the lesion, within a region of altered skin sensation.

Dysexecutive Questionnaire A 20-item checklist, measuring cognitive, behavioral, and emotional factors, and asking for the frequency of occurrence of dysexecutive characteristics such as impaired abstract thinking, impulsivity, confabulation, and planning problems.[6812]

dysexecutive syndrome Impairment of goal formulation, planning, execution of plans, and shifting of mental set, frequently in association with dysphasic speech disturbances and impairment of new learning, changes in personality, social skills, and initiative. The syndrome is notable for the retention of general intelligence and of remote memory. It is seen in patients with orbito-frontal lobe lesions or subcortical dementias and in some patients with alcoholism in whom a loss of social control, inability to abstain, and repetitive habitual behavior are also characteristic.[3825] See also **Behavioral Assesment of Dysexecutive Syndrome** and the **Dysexecutive Questionnaire**, two tests devised to assess the magnitude of these problems.

dysferlin A membrane-based protein separate from the dystrophin-associated proteins. Its mutations are responsible for the dysferlinopathies (**LGMD2B** and **Miyoshi muscular dystrophy**).[3454]

dysferlinopathies Proximal or distal muscular dystrophies, recessively inherited and appearing in early adult life, resulting from mutations of the *dysferlin* gene at 2p12-14. Their presentations include limb-girdle dystrophy type 2B, **Miyoshi myopathy** in which, unusually for **congenital myopathies**, serum CK levels are high[3454] and distal, slowly progressive weakness. Atrophy in anterior (tibialis anterior) or posterior (gastrocnemius-soleus) regions occur. See **distal muscular dystrophy**.[5716]

dysgerminoma (atypical teratoma, ectopic pinealoma) A tumor of childhood or youth, arising from cell rests in the anterior part of the third ventricle or in the suprasellar region, and histologically resembling a seminoma or an atypical pinealoma. Typical clinical features are hypopituitarism with growth retardation, diabetes insipidus, and visual field loss.[988]

dysgeusia A distortion of the sense of taste, usually resulting from either the ingestion of toxins, or partial damage to the chorda tympani, or lesions in the brainstem. As with similar distortions of smell, the distorted taste is always interpreted as unpleasant.

dysglobulinemic neuropathy Motor neuropathies with onset in young adult life, leading to complaints of paresthesia and accompanied by paraproteinemias. See **gammopathic neuropathy**.

dysgraphia Impairment in the utilization of writing tools, usually coupled with a tendency to malform individual letters and words—a state which may include features of both dyspraxia and dysphasia, especially if there are also semantic and syntactical errors, misspellings, and neographisms.

dyshoric angiopathy See **cerebral amyloid angiopathy**.

dyskinesia (Gr, difficulty + movement) Abnormal involuntary movements, classified as **tremors**, **chorea** and **ballism**, **myoclonus**, **tics**, and **dystonias**.

Paroxysmal dyskinesias have been classified as follows:[1573]

Paroxysmal kinesigenic dyskinesia
- *Paroxysmal nonkinesigenic dyskinesia* precipitated by stress, menses, heat, and fatigue, occurring at any age and often intermixed with choreoathetosis.
- *Paroxysmal exertion-induced dyskinesia* characterized by brief episodes of dystonia induced by physical exertion.
- *Paroxysmal hypnogenic dyskinesia* characterized by intermittent attacks lasting minutes or less, with onset in early childhood and occurring both by day and at night.

dyskinetic cerebral palsy A form of cerebral palsy in which X-linked inheritance has been found occasionally.[379] See **cerebral palsy**.

dyskinetic gait (dystonic gait) No single pattern of movements can be described in patients with dystonias, the picture varying widely, although plantar flexion at the ankle and extension of the hallux are commonly found.

dyslalia See **dysarthria**.

dyslexia (from Gr, difficulty + reading) 1. An innate constitutional difficulty in learning to read; a disorder of phonemic awareness leads to impairment of reading skills in the absence of other disorders of language. 2. That variant of aphasia in which the most conspicuous feature consists of an extreme difficulty in the interpretation of verbal or literal symbols by way of visual channels.

Two definitions from the World Federation of Neurology are as follows:

dyslexia: A disorder in children who, despite conventional classroom experience, fail to attain the language skills of reading, writing, and spelling commensurate with their intellectual abilities.

specific developmental dyslexia: A disorder manifested by difficulty in learning to read, despite conventional instruction, adequate intelligence, and socio-cultural opportunity. It is dependent on fundamental cognitive disabilities which are frequently of constitutional origin.

The condition persists into adult life and is far more common in males. There is no evidence of brain damage or of perceptual defects. Left-handedness or ambidexterity is common and intelligence is normal if not high. The principal faults found include the inability to pronounce an unfamiliar word, or specific vowels or consonants; to differentiate between words that are similar in spelling; failure to read with complete understanding; the omission of phonemes or whole syllables in words; perseveration and word substitution (Critchley M. *The Dyslexic Child.* London, Heinemann, 1970). In *neglect dyslexia*, the subject with a right hemispheric lesion has difficulty reading words on the left side of the page, or even the left half of words. *Surface dyslexia* is a term applied in patients with left temporal lobe lesions who have a loss of semantic knowledge, leading to difficulties with irregular words.

This term (for what had formerly been called *word-blindness* on the supposition that it was intrinsically a visual disorder) was introduced by **Rudolf Berlin** (1833–1897) in 1887.[575] The condition is frequently familial but the transmission method not always certain. In *dyslexia-1*, however, the gene is mapped to 15q11. See **word blindness**.

A variant is *spelling dyslexia*, in which the subject with dyslexia without dysgraphia can read single letters aloud, and adopt a letter-by-letter reading strategy, spelling the word aloud.[6648]

See also **alexia without agraphia** and **deep dyslexia**.

dyslogia (from Gr, difficulty + a word) Speech which is normally formed, but the content of which indicates the presence of a disorder of thought.

dyslysis See **restless legs syndrome**.

dysmetria (from Gr, difficulty + distance) 1. The occurrence of errors in judgment of distance when a limb is made to perform a precise movement. The movements usually tested are those of extension and withdrawal of the arm with a finger outstretched, with the intention of touching successively first the examiner's finger held away from the patient at arms' length and then the patient's own nose, repetitively. Classically, the finger overshoots (*hypermetria*) or undershoots the target (*hypometria*) with disease of the cerebellum, and often shows an **action tremor**. 2. See **ocular dysmetria**.

dysmetric saccades The ocular equivalent of limb dysmetria, in which the gaze is not accurately brought to bear upon the target but over- (or under-) shooting occurs, with the need for corrective **catch-up saccades** to be made. Either cerebellar or hemispheric lesions may be responsible.[1223] When the deviation is in the line of the eye movement, the term *amplitude dysmetria* may be used; movement at right angles to that line merits the term *direction dysmetria*.[3762] See **ocular dysmetria**.

dysmnesia (from Gr, difficulty + memory) Any disturbance of memory including flashbacks, **déja vu, jamais vu, experiential hallucinations**, or panoramic experiences but not including **amnesia**.

dysmorphism (craniofacial malformations) Abnormal facial appearances, including low-set ears, flared nostrils, an antimongolian slant to the eyes, extruded lips, etc., occurring as part of a congenital, usually genetic, disorder.[1790] A classification has been suggested.[4] (See Chart D–13.)

Dysmorphology Database See **London Neurogenetic Database**.

Chart D–13. Classification of Dysmorphisms

I. *Cerebrocranial dysplasias*
- **Anencephaly**
- **Microcephaly**
- Others

II. *Cerebrofacial dysplasias*
- Rhinencephalic dysplasias
- Oculo-orbital dysplasias (anophthalmia)

III. *Craniofacial dysplasias*
- a. with clefting
- b. with dysostosis
- c. with synostosis
  - **Craniosynostosis**
  - Craniofaciosynostosis
  - Faciosynostosis
- d. with dysostosis and synostosis
  - **Crouzon**
  - **Cloverleaf skull**

IV. *Craniofacial dysplasias with other origin*
- a. Osseous
- b. Cutaneous
- c. Neurocutaneous
  - **Neurofibromatosis**
- d. Neuromuscular
  - **Pierre Robin syndrome**
  - **Möbius syndrome**
- e. Muscular
  - Glossoschizis
- f. Vascular
  - Hemangioma
  - Hemolymphangioma
  - Lymphangioma

Based upon the classification of Stricker (1990).[4]

dysmorphopsia A distortion of shape perceived.

dysmyelination An inborn error of metabolism affecting myelinogenesis that causes the process to be delayed or arrested, or the myelin to be abnormal in its constituents. The leukodystrophies, many aminoacidopathies, and the gangliosidoses are examples.[5090, 5091]

dysmyelinogenic leukodystrophy See **Alexander disease**.

dysnomia Difficulty in naming objects; a dilute form of **anomia**.

dysodia (dysodes) Hippocrates' term for smelling bad; also used as a collective term for those diseases characterized by such odors.

dysopsia algera Pain from eye movement in the absence of detectable ocular disease. As with **akinesia algera**, the condition is often considered to be functional or psychogenic, but fevers, migraine and hangovers are also possible causes.[5984]

dysorthographia Impairment in the ability to spell, as may occur in the **developmental dyslexias**.

dysosmia Distorted perception of odors, the sensation being almost invariably unpleasant. Head trauma, viral infections, and other causes of damage to the first cranial nerve, and depressive illnesses are the commoner causes.

dysosteosclerosis A congenital dysmorphic syndrome, a form of craniotubular dysplasia, also manifesting as short stature, skeletal, and dental abnormalities, blindness due to optic nerve atrophy, mental delay, and fragile bones.[2042]

dyspeptic dystonia See **Sandifer syndrome**.

dysphagia (from Gr, difficulty + to swallow) A subjective sensation that swallowing is difficult or painful. When caused by a unilateral cerebral lesion, this is usually in the lowest part of the precentral gyrus or the posterior part of the inferior frontal gyrus. In most cases with a neurological cause, however, bilateral cerebral or bulbar lesions are required to produce the symptom.[4274]

dysphasia Disturbance of communication involving language due to disturbance of specific brain regions but in the absence of primary disturbance of the subcortical motor or sensory pathways. It is manifested by difficulties, variously, in fluency, repetition, comprehension, and naming according to the type of dysphasia present. **Global aphasia; Broca aphasia; transcortical aphasias; Wernicke aphasia; conduction aphasia**; and **anomic aphasias** are those most precisely described. See **aphasia**.

dysphatic stuttering A form of dysfluency of speech related to impairment of sensory input, as with receptive dysphasia or deafness.

dysphonia (from Gr, difficulty + utterance) Abnormal production of vocal sounds, typically caused by local lesions of the larynx or of its motor nerve supply.

Dysphonia clericorum was the term given to that form of chronic laryngitis which affected those who said too much too loudly from the pulpit. In these days of shorter sermons, the condition would be more appropriately named with reference to the legislature, the racecourse, or the auction house.

dysphoria Hippocrates' term for the restlessness and anxiety which accompany disease states.

dysphrasia (from Gr, difficulty + speech) Disturbance of speech due to inadequacy of underlying ideation as in dementia.

dysphrenia (from Gr, difficulty + the mind) The term of Kahlbaum for disturbance of the intellect resulting from organic disease of the brain.

dysphrenic migraine A migrainous accompaniment characterized by confusion and amnesia for current events, but not necessarily by headache.[4948] See **confusional migraine**.

dysplasia The abnormal organization of cells into tissue as a result of abnormal histogenesis. Thus, focal cortical dysplasia is a cause of otherwise unexplained focal cortical myoclonus or other seizure types.

dysplasia of ears, sensorineural and conductive deafness, and retardation syndrome A congenital dysmorphic syndrome manifesting also psychomotor retardation.[381]

dysplastic gangliocytoma See **Lhermitte–Duclos syndrome**.

dyspnea–fasciculation syndrome: Respiratory failure occurring as an early manifestation of **amyotrophic lateral sclerosis**, presenting with exertional and nocturnal dyspnea, daytime hypersomnolence, limb fatigability, and weight loss; tachypnea, slight distal limb weakness, hyperreflexia, and prominent fasciculations are clinical signs in the absence of marked bulbar or limb weakness.[5575]

dysprosody (speech dyspraxia) Loss of the melodic intonations of cultured speech; a feature of all forms of **dysphasia** but especially of **Broca aphasia**, in which incorrect emphases, hesitations, awkward phrasing, and dysmelodic intonation are detectable.[4448]

dysproteinemic neuropathy A syndrome of acquired demyelinating motor neuropathy resembling **chronic inflammatory demyelinating polyneuropathy** but occurring in the presence of an underlying systemic illness such as plasma cell dyscrasia (including primary systemic amyloidosis), osteosclerotic myeloma, Waldenstrom macrogobulinemia, gamma heavy chain disease, cryoglobulinemia, lymphoma, systemic lupus erythematosus, Castleman disease, HIV infections, or an occult malignancy.[101] See also **paraneoplastic neuropathy** and **gammopathic neuropathy**.

dysraphism (Bremer syndrome) Axial skeletal anomalies due to improper closure of the neural tube. The severity of the resulting defect varies widely from the most minor **spina bifida occulta** to **meningomyelocele** or **cranioschisis**.

dysrhythmokinesis A disorder in the execution of regular or syncopated movements, as is seen with cerebellar lesions.

dyssomnias Disorders characterized by disturbance of the initiation or maintenance of sleep, or by excessive sleepiness. They include **intrinsic sleep disorders**, **extrinsic sleep disorders**, and **circadian rhythm sleep disorders**. See also **parasomnias** and **sleep disorders**.

dyssynergia 1. (detrusor-sphincter dyssynergia) Disturbance in the reciprocal innervation of the detrusor muscle and the internal sphincter, which should allow the former to contract while the latter relaxes, or vice versa. Sphincter-detrusor dyssynergia occurs with pyramidal lesions and leads to complaints of urgency, frequency, and dribbling of urine. 2. (asynergia) A failure of the coordination of contraction or relaxation of muscles which normally act together in a group in order to produce a smoothly programmed movement. This is classically regarded as a sign of cerebellar disease, but other disorders of motor or sensory pathways and local disease may produce similar findings. 3. A term encompassing all the disturbances of movement occurring as a result of cerebellar disease.

dyssynergia cerebellaris myoclonica (Ramsay Hunt syndrome) A rare dominantly or recessively inherited syndrome of olivodentatorubral degeneration with progressive myoclonus epilepsy and intense action and intention myoclonus, tonic–clonic seizures, cerebellar signs, and sometimes mental deterioration. It was described by Ramsay Hunt in 1921.[3050]

The main clinical features are onset in infancy or childhood, with generalized seizures, action myoclonus, truncal ataxia, and limb tremor, but no other neurological signs. A variety of EEG patterns (photosensitive responses, paroxysmal discharges, and fast polyspike discharges over central regions during rapid eye movement sleep) are found. Somatosensory-evoked responses are unusually large.[5354]

The combination of myoclonic epilepsy and cerebellar signs also occurs in storage diseases such as the **lipidoses, sialidosis,** and **lipofuscinosis, Lafora body disease, Baltic myoclonus,** and **mitochondrial encephalomyelopathy**. Another form shows dominant inheritance. Some of Ramsay Hunt's patients developed a cerebellar syndrome before, some after, the onset of myoclonic epilepsy and he did not claim that this condition was a single disease *sui generis* (although it has been convincingly distinguished from MERFF).[6221] See also **hereditary dentatorubralpallidoluysian atrophy**.[6219]

In a *variant* form, peripheral neuropathy is detected.[5925]

dyssynergia cerebellaris progressiva A clinical syndrome of chronic progressive severe, local, and later generalized intention tremors with dyssynergia, dysmetria, hypotonia, adiadochokinesis, and asthenia but without vertigo, nystagmus, optic atrophy, or dysequilibrium. The muscle stretch reflexes are normal.[3048]

It was described by **Hunt** as a pure cerebellar degeneration but it has been thought likely by others to have been **Wilson disease** (though Hunt considered this and found no corneal pigmentation), **mitochondrial encephalopathy**, or dystonic tremor.

dysthymia (Gr, bad + mind) Melancholy.

dystasia, hereditary areflexic See **Roussy–Levy syndrome**.

dysthymia (somatic) Yet another neologistic attempt, this time to name the syndrome wherein the somatic manifestations of depression are presented in the absence (or at least in the presence of denial) of affective disturbance. Thus this is possibly one of the commonest diseases presenting to neurologists.

dysthyroid orbitopathy (Graves ophthalmopathy, thyroid ophthalmopathy, endocrine exophthalmos) A varied group of symptoms which are causally related to thyroid disease but which are not always associated with systemic clinical evidence of this. They include orbital and conjunctival congestion and edema, lid retraction, lid lag, proptosis, restrictive extraocular myopathy, and optic neuropathy.[6820] Central scotomas, arcuate or inferior altitudinal defects, and generalized field constriction may be due to optic nerve compression at the orbital apex.

dystonia (idiopathic torsion dystonia, Oppenheim disease, Ziehen syndrome, tonic torsion neurosis, Gowers tetanoid chorea, paraspasm, dystonia musculorum deformans) Sustained and patterned muscle co-contractions of agonist and antagonist muscles, usually leading to twisting involuntary movements which are frequently repetitive and which may progress to fixed abnormal postures or to repetitive twisting or squeezing movements. Their speed varies from creeping to myoclonic, but their range is usually limited. Thus, the movements represent an unusually slow and persistent form of **athetosis**. Fixed dystonia also occurs, in which the muscular contraction leads the trunk, limbs, or face to assume a fixed posture. The underlying lesion is usually of the putamen, and less often of the brainstem or thalamus, and the mechanism for their production is likely to be a deficiency of the cortical inhibition of subcortical motor pathways with associated abnormalities in the somatosensory systems.[1196]

The clinical condition was first described in an M.D. thesis by Marcus Walter Schwalbe (b. 1883), a German physician, in 1908,[5669] and then by Georg Theodor Ziehen, a German psychiatrist in 1911. It was more fully delineated and named by Hermann Oppenheimer in that same year.[4804] However, subjects with what appear to be dystonic postures had been painted by Peter Breughel the younger and by William Blake, and Robert Schumann had a task-specific focal **dystonia** leading him to withdraw from the concert platform in favor of composition—though he could still improvise without the right third finger going rigid at all.

An etiological classification, recognizing *idiopathic (primary)* and *symptomatic (secondary)* forms, has been suggested,[6868] the primary dystonias being further classified as hereditary forms, those associated with other hereditary neurological diseases, and those which are sporadic. A simple clinical classification is that of Warner and Jarman,[6644] adapted here:

Another classification is based on age at onset; early-onset dystonias usually start in a leg or arm and frequently progress to involve other limbs and the trunk, while late-onset dystonias usually start in the neck, cranial muscles, or arm and tend to remain localized.

A third classification is based on the distribution of the parts affected:

- *Focal dystonias* affect a single body part. They comprise **blepharospasm**; **oromandibular dystonia**; **laryngeal** and **pharyngeal dystonias**; **spasmodic torticollis** (*cervical dystonia*); **truncal dystonia**; writers' cramp (focal hand dystonia) and other **occupational cramps**, **foot dystonia**, **adult-onset primary lower limb dystonia**, adult-onset and childhood-onset **segmental dystonias**, **generalized dystonias**, and some *symptomatic dystonias.*
- *Multifocal dystonias* affect more than one noncontiguous body part: (e.g., arm + leg, or blepharospasm with writer's cramp)

Form	Description
1. Primary dystonia	Phenotype of dystonia alone (with or without tremor; see below)
A. Dystonia-plus syndromes	Phenotype of dystonia with additional neurological features, e.g., Parkinsonism, myoclonus (**dopa-responsive dystonia** and **rapid-onset dystonia-Parkinsonism**, see below). See also **deafness–dystonia syndrome**. Plus myoclonus (myoclonic dystonia; see below)
B. Paroxysmal dystonia	**Paroxysmal kinesigenic dystonia**
	Paroxysmal dystonic choreoathetosis
2. Secondary dystonias	A. Resulting from structural CNS disease (e.g., craniocerebral trauma, drugs, encephalitis, multiple sclerosis, toxins, perinatal asphyxia, stroke)
	B. Heredo-degenerative diseases Dystonia-plus syndromes occurring in the context of an underlying neurodegenerative disease. These include **X-linked Parkinsonism–dystonia (Lubag); ataxia–telangiectasia;** biopterin-deficient states; dopamine agonist-responsive dystonia caused by decarboxylase deficiency; **dopa-responsive dystonia;** dystonic lipidosis; **gangliosidoses; glutaric academia; Hallervorden–Spatz disease (NBIA); Hartnup disease; homocystinuria; Huntington disease;** *intraneuronal inclusion disease*; **Leigh disease; Lesch–Nyhan syndrome; Machado–Joseph cerebellar ataxia; metachromatic leukodystrophy; mitochondrial encephalomyopathies** such as **Leber disease; myoclonic-dystonia; neuroacanthocytosis; neuronal ceroid-lipofuscinosis; rapid-onset dystonia-Parkinsonism;** mutations of tyrosine hydroxylase; striopallidal calcification, and **Wilson disease.**
3. Psychogenic dystonia	

- *Segmental dystonias* affect two or more adjacent body parts (e.g., neck and trunk, face and jaw, or neck and arm as with torticollis and writer's cramp). **Hemidystonia** affects the face and limbs of one side.
- *Generalized dystonias* affect two or more noncontiguous body parts.[1948]

A fourth classification is based upon age of onset: It is not reproduced here in order to preserve the composure of the reader.

However, compounding the confusion, certain forms of dystonia with unique characteristics to do with their site, precipitation or occurrence, age of onset, and speed of response to therapy are described. Thus the idiopathic dystonias include classical torsion dystonia (see Chart D–14), **paradoxical dystonia, myoclonic dystonia, diurnal dystonia**, and **dopa-responsive dystonia.**

Other dyskinesias include **dystonic dysphagia, dystonic tics, paroxysmal dystonia, hypogenic dystonia, spasmodic and axial dystonia**, and **tardive dystonia.** These are entered elsewhere.[1950, 1951, 4227] Dystonia can also be psychogenic.[3683]

A classification of the dystonias adapted from Fahn[1948] and others is provided in Chart D–14.

dystonia and basal ganglion calcification See **dystonia.**

dystonia, blepharospasm, and pigmentary retinopathy See **dystonia.**

dystonia, deafness, and mental retardation An X-linked syndrome with onset in early childhood, characterized by these features and a tendency to self-mutilation.[5695]

Dystonia Disability Scale An assessment instrument quantifying the disturbance in functioning produced by dystonic disorders.[944] The scale is reproduced as Chart D–15 by kind permission of the AAN and Lippincott Williams & Wilkins from Burke,et al. Validity and reliability of a rating scale for the primary torsion dystonias. *Neurology* 1985; 35:73–7.

Dystonia Medical Research Foundation (USA) Address: One East Wacker Dr., Suite 2430, Chicago, IL 60601-2001. Tel: 312-755-0198. (Canada) Address: 777 Hornby St. #1800, Vancouver, BC V6Z 1S4, Canada. A charitable organization, each branch seeking to determine the cause and cure of involuntary movement disorders through the provision of research funding, and undertaking patient support work and both professional and patient information services. Web site: www.dystonia-foundation.org.

Dystonia Movement Scale A rating scale used for the assessment of the scope and severity of the signs of *primary torsion dystonias*.[944] The scale is reproduced here by kind permission of the American Academy of Neurology and Lippincott Williams & Wilkins. (See Chart D–16.)

dystonia musculorum deformans See **dystonia** and **dopa-responsive dystonia.**

dystonia musculorum deformans with hyperuricemia A congenital syndrome with childhood onset, manifesting dystonia, athetosis, and hyperuricemia. See also **Lesch–Nyhan syndrome.**

dystonia rating scales The new Toronto Western Spasmodic Torticollis Rating Scale (TWSTRS) can be seen at the Web site http://www.mdvu.org/library/ratingscales/dystonia/PadwChart.11.pdf/. See also **United Dystonia Rating Scale, Burke–Fahn–Marsden Scale,** and **Global Dystonia Rating Scales.**

Dystonia Society (UK) A charitable organization. Address: 46-47 Britton St., London EC1M 5UJ, UK. Tel: 0171 490

Chart D–14. A Classification of the Dystonias

1. Primary idiopathic dystonia (No identifiable exogenous cause or other inherited or degenerative disease)

A. Inherited (*hereditary torsion dystonia*) (autosomal dominant, recessive, or pseudodominant, X-linked recessive).

The *dominant syndrome (idiopathic primary torsion dystonia)* is the most common form and is characterized by the onset in youth or young adult life of torticollis, blepharospasm, or truncal dystonia, though cranial involvement is infrequent; progressing to athetosis, dystonia, and muscle hypertrophy, starting later and of less severity than the recessive form. In this form, the younger the age of onset, the greater chance there is of generalization. It is common in Ashkenazi Jews, among whom the symptoms rather resemble those of the recessive form. The gene DYT1 maps to 9q34[938, 5159] and DYT13 to 1p36.13–36.32.

A mixed phenotype has onset in childhood or adult life, may begin anywhere, and is dominantly inherited with incomplete penetrance. Cranial involvement with dysarthria and dysphonia is common. This form is mapped to chromosome 8 in Mennonite/Amish families.

A third phenoptype has onset in adult life, with cervical, cranial, or brachial involvement and again is inherited as an autosomal dominant trait but with very reduced penetrance. The dystonia tends to remain localized. This form has been mapped to chromosome 18p but is likely to be genetically heterogeneous.

Criteria for the diagnosis of dystonia have been suggested[4102] and include the following:

The presence of dystonic movements and postures.
A normal perinatal history.
The absence of any history of precipitating illness or of exposure to drugs known to provoke torsion dystonia before the onset of the illness.
The absence of intellectual, pyramidal, cerebellar, or sensory abnormalities on examination.
A normal laboratory evaluation, including serum copper studies.

A numerical classification of the dystonias has been proposed:

DYT1 Generalized, with various presentations
DYT2 Generalized, recessively inherited, with various presentations
DYT3 Generalized, with blepharospasm and Parkinsonism
DYT4 Whispering dysphonia
DYT5 **Dopa-responsive dystonia** (DYT5). This form has been mapped to chromosome 14q22
DYT14 **Dopamine responsive dystonia** at 14q13
DYT6 A craniocervical form
DYT7 A focal form, mainly affecting cervical regions (familial torticollis) mapped to 18p
DYT8 **Paroxysmal nonkinesigenic dyskinesias** with generalized dystonia. A channelopathy.
DYT9 **Paroxysmal choreoathetosis**, ataxia, and limb dystonias. A channelopathy.
DYT0 **Paroxysmal kinesigenic dyskinesias** with generalized dystonia, chorea, athetosis and/or ballismus. A channelopathy, mapped to 16q11 or 16q13
DYT11 **Myoclonic dystonia** mapped to 7q21
DYT15 **Myoclonic dystonia** mapped to 18q11
DYT12 Rapid-onset dystonia-Parkinsonism with adult onset, mapped to 19q13. This is a dominantly inherited form occurring in youth or early adult life, in which the motor features affect bulbar and upper limbs especially, with initial onset over hours, days, or weeks, progressing only slowly thereafter.[1675, 5042]
DYT13 Generalized, with various presentations, usually with adolescent onset and mapped to 1p36
DYT16 Not yet assigned, but it will be.

For other forms of dystonia, the molecular genetics are less clear.

A *recessive form* is characterized by the onset in youth or young adult life of athetosis, dystonia, and muscle hypertrophy. Starting in one limb, symptoms extend to other limbs and the trunk at variable rates. The following *variants* (almost all conforming to the label of *dystonia-plus*, indicating the coexistence of, e.g., myoclonus, ataxia, or Parkinsonism) have been described:

Adult-onset axial dystonia, a focal dystonic syndrome mapped in some cases to 18p and which starts in adult life, does not affect the legs and progresses little. Prior trauma may be a factor in a third of cases.[610]

Deafness-dystonia syndrome

Dystonia with marked cerebellar atrophy in which dystonia is accompanied by marked cerebellar atrophy on brain MRI although the clinical signs of cerebellar disease are rather scarce. The condition may have X-linked inheritance.[3732]

Dystonia with marked diurnal variation (diurnal dystonia, Segawa disease) A dominant or recessive dystonic syndrome with onset in childhood characterized by initial involvement of one limb, deterioration during the day, abatement with sleep, and complete responsiveness to L-dopa.[5709] Like **dopa-responsive dystonia**, this condition has been mapped to chromosome 14q.

*Generalized dystonia and striatal calcifications with **lipoid proteinosis***

Hereditary myoclonic dystonia (*hereditary dystonia with lightning jerks, responsive to alcohol*) A dominantly inherited dystonic and myoclonic syndrome with onset in childhood and affecting mainly the neck and arms and sparing the legs. The lightning jerks occur spontaneously, with movement and as a response to startle, with variable symmetry and synchrony, and abate with alcohol ingestion. In some cases, abnormal EEG activity precedes the jerks.[5159]

Myoclonus-dystonia (hereditary essential myoclonus, hereditary myoclonic dystonia, DYT11) A dominantly inherited, rather benign form of idiopathic dystonia with onset in childhood or young adult life, characterized by dystonia of the face, arms, and trunk, upon which is superimposed proximal, action-induced myoclonus mainly affecting the arms and trunk and which is present at rest, worsened by exercise, and substantially relieved by alcohol.[4745] The condition has been mapped to 7q21 but also to 18p11, 11q, and (in a variant form with seizures) to the *SCGE* gene, in which condition the sexes are equally affected and the symptomsabate with alcohol.
Diagnostic criteria (adapted here) have been suggested:[3473]
Onset in the first 20 years of life, with mild dystonic features in addition to myoclonus

1. Benign course
2. Dominant inheritance with variable, severity, and incomplete penetrance
3. Absence of dementia, at a axia or other deficits
4. Normal EEG, SSEPs, and neuroimaging

Paradoxical dystonia.

Paroxysmal kinesigenic and nonkinesigenic dystonias in which dystonic attacks are precipitated by prolonged muscular exertion and last from 5 to 30 min. In some families there is an association with migraine.[4548] These conditions are sometimes dominantly inherited (mapped to chromosome 16) but may also occur sporadically.[4341] See also **dyskinesias**.

Paroxysmal nocturnal hemidystonia A syndrome characterized by the occurrence of paroxysmal dystonic-dyskinetic movements during Stages 2 and 3 of nonrapid eye movement sleep. These are actually more likely to represent seizure manifestations.

X-linked dystonia-Parkinsonism (Lubag) An X-linked recessive (Xq21) or codominant syndrome recorded originally in adult male Filipinos; elsewhere, linkage to Xq12–13.1 has been described. Clinically, this form has a gradual onset, but continues rapidly to a state of severe involvement,[379] initially with dystonia; the signs of Parkinsonism appear later in life and respond poorly to L-dopa therapy.[379, 6668] The word *lubag* is that used in the Philippines for this condition.

B. Sporadic (*idiopathic or symptomatic dystonia*)

1. Generalized.
2. Segmental or limb dystonia (usually secondary dystonias). A dominantly inherited syndrome linked in some cases to a site on chromosome 8.
3. **Hemidystonia.**
4. Multifocal dystonia.
5. Focal: *torticollis*, **occupational cramps**, **oromandibular dystonia**, **blepharospasm**, and **spasmodic dysphonia**.

Other *variants* include the following:
Benign idiopathic dystonia A dystonic state occurring in infancy and clearing by the age of 18 months.[6792]

Dystonia with multiple contractures A rare syndrome of chorea and dystonia in the setting of multiple nonprogressive contractures of muscle with childhood onset.[2010]

Determan syndrome Intermittent dystonic movements resulting from cerebrovascular disease affecting the basal ganglia.

2. Secondary dystonia

A. Associated with other hereditary neurodegenerative or metabolic disorders such as **ataxia-telangiectasia** *dystonic juvenile lipidosis*; **Huntington disease; neuronal ceroid lipofuscinosis; GM2 and GM1 gangliosidoses; glutaric aciduria type 1; Leigh disease; metachromatic leukodystrophy; Leber optic atrophy** and other **mitochondrial diseases; Hartnup disease; homocystinuria;** *Intraneuronal inclusion disease*; **juvenile dystonic lipidosis; Leigh disease; Lesch–Nyhan syndrome;** Lubag (X-linked Parkinsonism-dystonia); **Machado–Joseph disease** (SCA3); **Martha–Alma** (Hallervorden–Spatz) **disease** (NBIA); **methylmalonic academia; myoclonic dystonia; neuronal ceroid lipofuscinosis; neurovisceral storage disease; phenylketonuria** and other biopterin deficient states; **supranuclear ophthalmoplegia; tardive dystonia;**[6198] **triosephosphate isomerase deficiency; tyrosinosis;** *tyrosine hydroxylase mutations*; and **Wilson disease**.

Dystonia and basal ganglion calcification A dominantly inherited dystonic syndrome of childhood or early adult life characterized by dysarthria, dementia, resting tremors, dystonia, chorea, ataxia, and athetosis and with intracranial calcification in the basal ganglia and elsewhere.[6880] See also *DACE syndrome* (below).

Torsion dystonia with basal ganglion lucencies A slowly progressive dystonic syndrome without intellectual failure, beginning in infancy or early childhood.[4960]

Idiopathic dystonia-Parkinsonism A form of juvenile Parkinsonism with a benign and chronic course, characterized by dystonic movements and Parkinsonism with marked diurnal fluctuation of symptoms, a marked response to low doses of anti-Parkinsonian drugs, and EMG findings of continuous discharges of antagonistic muscles.[6134]

Rapid-onset dystonia-Parkinsonism A dominantly inherited disorder characterized by the rapid onset of symptoms (of dystonia more than of Parkinsonism) in youth or adult life, with little succeeding progression but with minimal response to treatment with L-dopa or dopamine agonists.[1675]

Flexion dystonia in paralysis agitans A syndrome manifesting slowly progressive persistent flexed postures of the limbs, especially the hands and wrists,[1591] accompanied by synchronous grouped discharges of antagonistic muscles.

Dystonia, blepharospasm, and pigmentary retinopathy An inherited syndrome of prominent extrapyramidal dysfunction, retinal pigmentary changes, pyramidal and cerebellar signs, and high-arched palate, with unimpaired intellect.[1278]

continued

Chart D–14. (*continued*)

DACE syndrome (Dystonia, Acanthocytosis, Basal Ganglion Calcification and Eye abnormalities) A rare syndrome with onset in childhood, characterized by the presence of these features, the dystonia being severe and progressive and the eye disorders comprising nystagmus in the primary position and limitation of vertical movements. Because the high-density signals from the globus pallidus suggest the presence of iron deposits, the condition may be a variant of **Hallervorden–Spatz disease**.[1383]

Posttraumatic cervical dystonia The occurrence of cervical dystonia following neck injury. The syndrome is said to manifest marked limitation of the range of movement of the neck, failure of relief from *gestes antagonistiques* and from sleep; tonic rather than phasic neck muscle contraction; and poor response to treatment.[5518]

B. Associated with other disorders.
C. Owing to other known acquired (?) metabolic or structural neurological disease, including Parkinsonism

Hypoparathyroidism
Encephalitis
Postinfectious states.
Toxins—manganese, carbon monoxide, carbon disulfide, L-dopa, D_2-receptor agonists.
Perinatal cerebral injury, head trauma, brain tumor, stroke.
See also **focal task-specific dystonias** (occupational cramp, musicians cramp/dystonia) In some such kinships, other dystonic disorders may occur.

D. Psychogenic

Based on Fahn S. Generalized dystonia: concept and treatment. Clin Neuropharmacol *1986;* 9 [*Suppl* 2: *S37–48) and Bressman (1998).*[831]

Chart D–15. Dystonia Disability Scale

A. Speech

0. Normal
1. Slightly involved; easily understood.
2. Some difficulty in understanding
3. Marked difficulty in understanding
4. Complete or almost complete anarthria.

B. Handwriting (Tremor or Dystonia)

0. Normal
1. Slight difficulty; legible
2. Almost illegible
3. Illegible
4. Unable to grasp to maintain hold on pen.

C. Feeding

0. Normal
1. Uses tricks; independent
2. Can feed but cannot cut
3. Finger food only
4. Completely dependent.

D. Eating/swallowing

0. Normal
1. Occasional choking
2. Chokes frequently; difficulty swallowing
3. Unable to swallow firm foods
4. Marked difficulty swallowing soft foods and liquids.

E. Hygiene

0. Normal
1. Clumsy; independent
2. Needs help with some activities
3. Needs help with most activities
4. Needs help with all activities.

F. Dressing

0. Normal
1. Clumsy; independent
2. Needs help with some activities
3. Needs help with most activities
4. Helpless

G. Walking

0. Normal
1. Slightly abnormal; hardly noticeable
2. Moderately abnormal; obvious to naive observer
3. Considerably abnormal
4. Needs assistance to walk
5. Wheelchair bound.

Adapted from Burke et al. (1985)[944].

5671. Web site: http://www.dystonia.org.uk/dystoniasocietyh.html.

dystonia with contractures and abnormal muscle An inherited congenital syndrome characterized by joint contractures, chorea, dystonia, and muscle fiber hypotrophy with ring fibers.[381]

dystonia with marked diurnal variation See **diurnal dystonia**.

dystonia with marked diurnal variation associated with biopterin deficiency See **dopa-responsive dystonia**.

dystonia with multiple contractures See **dystonia**.

dystonic choreo-athetosis induced by exercise An inherited syndrome characterized by onset in childhood or youth of athetosis and dystonia, which are precipitated by muscular activity.[2472]

This condition and **dopa-responsive dystonia** may be the same. See also **paroxysmal kinesigenic choreoathetosis**.

dystonic cramps Muscle spasms complicating manual tasks—a form of focal hand cramps.[5775]

dystonic dysphagia Focal dystonia affecting the pharyngeal muscles.

Chart D–16. Dystonia Movement Scale

Region	Severity Factor	Factor Weight	Product
Eyes	0–4 × 0–4	0.5	0–8
Mouth	0–4 × 0–4	0.5	0–8
Speech	0–4 × 0–4	1.0	0–16
Neck	0–4 × 0–4	0.5	0–8
R. Arm	0–4 × 0–4	1.0	0–16
L. Arm	0–4 × 0–4	1.0	0–16
Trunk	0–4 × 0–4	1.0	0–16
R. Leg	0–4 × 0–4	1.0	0–16
L. Leg	0–4 × 0–4	1.0	0–16

SUM (Maximum = 120)

I. *Provoking factor*

A. General

0. No dystonia at rest or with action
1. Dystonia on particular action
2. Dystonia on many actions
3. Dystonia on action of distant part of body or intermittently at rest
4. Dystonia present at rest

B. Speech and swallowing

1. Occasional, either or both
2. Frequent either
3. Frequent one and occasional other
4. Frequent both

II. *Severity factors*

Eyes

0. No dystonia
1. Slight, occasional blinking
2. Mild. Frequent blinking without prolonged spasms of eye closure
3. Moderate. Prolonged spasms of eyelid closure, but eyes open most of the time
4. Severe. Prolonged spasms of eyelid closure, with eyes closed at least 30% of the time

Mouth

0. No dystonia present
1. Slight. Occasional grimacing or other mouth movement (e.g., jaw open or clenched; tongue movement)
2. Mild. Movement present less than 50% of the time
3. Moderate dystonia movements or contractions present most of the time
4. Severe dystonic movements or contractions present most of the time

Speech and swallowing

0. Normal
1. Slightly involved; speech easily understood or occasional choking
2. Some difficulty in understanding speech or frequent choking
3. Marked difficulty in understanding speech or inability to swallow firm foods.
4. Complete or almost complete anarthria, or marked difficulty swallowing soft foods and liquids

Neck

0. No dystonia present
1. Slight. Occasional pulling
2. Obvious torticollis, but mild
3. Moderate pulling
4. Extreme pulling

Arm

0. No dystonia present
1. Slight dystonia. Clinically insignificant

continued

Chart D–16. (*continued*)

2. Mild. Obvious dystonia, but not disabling
3. Moderate. Able to grasp, with some manual function
4. Severe. No useful grasp

Trunk

0. No dystonia present
1. Slight bending, clinically insignificant
2. Definite bending, but not interfering with standing or walking
3. Moderate bending; interfering with standing or walking
4. Extreme bending of trunk preventing standing or walking

Leg

0. No dystonia present
1. Slight dystonia, but not causing impairment; clinically insignificant
2. Mild dystonia. Walks briskly and unaided
3. Moderate dystonia. Severely impairs walking or requires assistance
4. Severe. Unable to stand or walk on involved leg

Adapted from Burke et al. (1985)[944] *and reproduced by kind permission.*

dystonic foot response (striatal foot, grasp reflex of the foot, myokymia of Kny, and Schultze) Stereotyped, tonic, painful extension of the hallux with flexion of the other toes, arching of the sole, and inversion at the ankle associated with extrapyramidal disease but not with frontal lobe lesions, and worsened by L-dopa therapy.[4602] See also **dystonic toe**.

dystonic gait See **dyskinetic gait**.

dystonic juvenile lipidosis A rare syndrome comprising mental deterioration, vertical gaze palsy, seizures, dyskinesias and pyramidal signs, with hepato-splenomegaly. Sea-blue histiocytosis is found in the bone marrow. The condition may be a form of **sphingomyelin storage disorder**.[3421]

dystonic motor seizure Sustained contractions of both agonist and antagonist muscles as a seizure manifestation, producing athetoid or twisting movements which when prolonged may produce abnormal postures.

dystonic spasms Forceful and accelerated dystonic movements, with the same implications as other dystonic manifestations.

dystonic storm See **status dystonicus**.

dystonic stridor A form of **segmental dystonia** affecting the vocal cords.[1282]

dystonic syndrome of senility See **danse du ventre**.

dystonic tics See **tics**.

dystonic toe The semipermanent dorsiflexed posture of the hallux seen in some patients in whom dystonia affects the leg. See also **dystonic foot response**.

dystonic tremor Forms of **action tremor** in patients with dystonias.[1615] One form is a postural/kinetic tremor indistinguishable from **essential tremor**; a second is an irregular, jerky action tremor interposed between the involuntary dystonic movements; and a third is an irregular **task-specific tremor**.

dystroglycan A transmembrane protein, ubiquitously expressed, that connects the extracellular matrix to the cytoskeleton. Its aberrant glycosylation is a pathogenetic mechanism in several forms of congenital and late-onset muscular dystrophies.

dystrophia muscularis progressiva See **limb-girdle muscular dystrophy**.

dystrophia myotonica See **myotonic dystrophy**.

dystrophin A large intracellular protein, coded at Xp21.2, which is a component of the sarcolemmal plasma membrane (transverse tubule) system. The absence of dystrophin leads to the muscular symptoms of **Duchenne muscular dystrophy**. In **Becker dystrophy**, the protein is present but abnormal either in quantity or in composition.[2935] The dystrophin-associated proteins consist of one intracellular (*dystrobrevin–syntrophin*) and two transmembrane complexes (*dystroglycan* and *sarcoglycan-sarcospan*). Mutations or alterations in these lead to various forms of LGMD, etc.[3454]

dystrophin test A Western blot analysis of dystrophin protein from a muscle biopsy specimen, allowing characterization of the abnormal protein alleles in Duchenne and Becker muscle dystrophies.[2935]

dystrophinopathies A group of clinicopathological disorders resulting from mutations of the dystrophin gene. They include **Duchenne muscle dystrophy** (and its dilute manifestation in female carriers); **Becker muscle dystrophy**; cardiomyopathy with or without proximal weakness; a syndrome of myalgia and cramps; and hyperCKemic states.

See also **sarcoglycanopathy, desminopathy,** and **dysferlin.**

dystrophy (Gr, difficulty + nourishment; and thus bad growth) The term arbitrarily used for those (usually progressive) diseases of muscle which have a genetic basis, the remainder being called **myopathies**, which just means diseases of muscle. It would have been simpler to call them all either genetic or acquired myopathies, but it is too late now.

dysversion Congenital structural abnormalities of the eye, including tilted disks, occurring alone or in association with craniofacial syndromes.

dysynchiria The sensation of painful bilateral stimulation with a unilateral painless stimulus. This may be seen in **complex regional pain syndrome 1**.

Dzerzhinskii syndrome A familial syndrome, a form of craniomandibularfacial dysostosis, marked by acrocephaly, scaphocephaly, lordotic curvature at the base of the skull, premature closure of the cranial sutures, dysmorphism, protruding nose, and thickening of the phalanges, sternum, and clavicles.[1792]

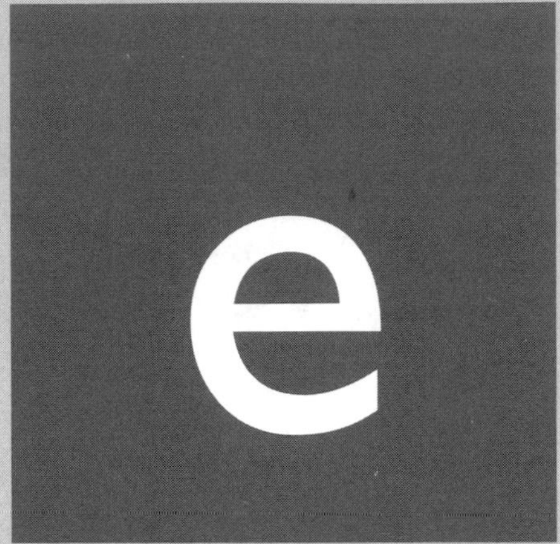

18q syndrome A leukodystrophy due to a deletion of part of the long arm of chromosome 18, which includes the region coding for myelin basic protein (18q22–3–qter). Dysmorphisms, mental retardation, hyperactivity, and aggressivity are associated. The condition has been reported to have its onset in adult life.[448]

E-1 See **recording electrode**.

E-2 See **recording electrode**.

Eagle syndrome (stylohyoid process syndrome) Pain in the face or in the floor of the mouth, supposed to be brought about by trauma to a congenitally elongated or calcified styloid process[1794] or resulting from pressure on local structures (including the carotid artery) exerted by the long styloid process.

The syndrome appears to be confined to adults, in whom the pain is brought on by jaw or neck movements, swallowing, or local pressure.[4147]

Eales, Henry (1852–1913) Ophthalmologist practicing in Birmingham, England.

Eales disease (retinitis proliferans, periphlebitis retinae, angiopathia retinae juvenalis) The occurrence of retinal periphlebitis, neovascular formation, and recurrent vitreous and retinal hemorrhages in young people.[1796] CSF pleocytosis may be found.

The acute ocular events may be followed by severe acute or subacute myelopathy, seizures, and focal neurological deficits. Eales considered that constipation was a likely cause; no better guess has been suggested since.

ear wagging See **Hassin sign**.

ear wiggling Bilateral, intermittent movements of the ears due to contractions of the auricular muscles, accompanied usually by scalp movements and considered to have a psychological basis.[3409] However, the phenomenon was also displayed by Dopey, one of the seven dwarfs in the Walt Disney movie, whose perceived stress level was likely to have been low.

earlobe reflex A normal sign in infants; rubbing the earlobe lightly causes rotation of the head toward the opposite side.[6898]

early hematoma growth Expansion of the size of an intracerebral hematoma, as after a spontaneous intracerebral hemorrhage, caused variously by continuing bleeding, vascular engorgement, and local edema produced by the irritant effects of the blood with breakdown of the blood-brain barrier. The clinical effect is further deterioration in neurologic status.

early infantile epileptic encephalopathy with suppression burst (Ohtahara syndrome) An epileptic encephalopathy of infancy (usually occurring within the first 10 days of life) characterized by frequent brief tonic spasms and a suppression burst EEG pattern in both waking and sleeping states. Hemiconvulsions and other focal seizures and generalized tonic-clonic seizures (GTCS) may occur but myoclonic seizures are rare.[4777, 690] Intrauterine seizures have been detected.

The etiology and underlying pathology are obscure but cortical dysplasia is a possible factor. The prognosis is serious, with severe psychomotor retardation and seizure intractability; often there is evolution to the **West syndrome** at age 4–6 months. (After Dreifuss FE, et al. Commission for classification and terminology, ILAE. Proposal for revised classifications of epilepsies and epileptic syndromes. *Epilepsia* 1989;30:389–99. Reproduced by kind permission of the ILAE and Wiley-Blackwell Publications.)

Electrographically, bursts of irregular spikes, sharp waves, and slow waves, lasting up to several seconds and occurring over both hemispheres, are separated by periods of marked diminution of activity on the EEG—2–6 s suppression bursts (discharges of wide amplitude spikes and polyspikes alternating with suppression of electric activity) during waking and sleep. The syndrome is caused by a variety of early and extensive brain insults, especially brain malformations, and is considered to represent a specific type of epileptic encephalopathy in the neonatal period and early infancy, resembling infantile spasms in older children.[4778] See also **Aicardi syndrome**.

Early Language Milestone Scale An instrument assessing all the components of visual and auditory language in infants from birth to 3 years of age, including auditory expressive, auditory receptive, and visual functions.[1276]

early morning akinesia A hypokinetic form of fluctuation in Parkinsonian patients on long-term levadopa therapy in which disability is increased on waking, by which time the previous night's dose has lost its effect.

early morning dystonia A dystonic form of fluctuation in Parkinsonian patients on long term levadopa therapy in which dystonic movements accompany the morning fall in levadopa levels.

early morning waking The inability to fall asleep after unusual and inappropriately early waking from nocturnal sleep. When pathological, it is usually a symptom of depressive or hypomanic illness, but it also occurs in the healthy elderly.

early multiple sclerosis A diagnostic category in the 1954 definitions of **Allison** and **Millar**, now largely replaced by the **Schumacher** or the **Poser** criteria.

early myoclonic encephalopathy A rare epileptic encephalopathy of infancy, usually with onset before the age of 3 months, characterized initially by fragmentary myoclonus and then by erratic focal seizures, massive myoclonia, and/or tonic spasms, refractory to treatment. The EEG shows suppression-burst activity, which may evolve into **hypsarrhythmia**. The course is severe as psychomotor development is arrested, and death may occur in the first year. Familial cases are frequent and this condition is likely a reflection of one or another of the congenital inborn metabolic errors, so there is no consistent genetic pattern.[4882] This seizure syndrome so closely resembles **Ohtahara syndrome** that it is possibly identical.[1861] See also **neonatal myoclonic encephalopathy**.

early-onset autosomal dominant dementia with ataxia, extrapyramidal features, and epilepsy A rare syndrome with these manifestations, not linked to currently known dementias.[2049, 2049]

early-onset spinal muscular atrophy See **hereditary motor neuropathy, type 2**.

early-onset cerebellar ataxia with retained reflexes Recessively inherited cerebellar ataxic syndromes, with onset in youth, that resemble **Friedreich ataxia** but in which areflexia, optic atrophy, heart disease, diabetes, and skeletal deformity do not occur.[2754]

A *variant* is an *X-linked recessive form*.

Other recessively inherited forms are mainly reported from Quebec;[385] their various symptoms including hypogonadism, normal muscle stretch reflexes; myoclonus (**Ramsay Hunt syndrome**); pigmentary retinal degeneration and mental retardation; optic atrophy and mental retardation; cataracts and mental retardation; deafness alone or with mental retardation; and extrapyramidal features. See also **cerebellar ataxias**.

early post-traumatic epilepsy Seizures occurring in the week following craniocerebral trauma. In adults, this is usually associated with severe or complicated cerebral injury. See also **late post-traumatic epilepsy**.

early probable (latent) multiple sclerosis See **McDonald-Halliday criteria**.[4217]

early recruitment A recruitment pattern which occurs in association with a reduction in the number of muscle fibers per motor unit or when the force generated by the fibers is reduced. At low levels of muscle contraction, more motor unit action potentials are recorded than expected, and a full interference pattern may be recorded at relatively low levels of muscle contraction. It is most often encountered in myopathy. (From the 2001 Report of the Nomenclature Committee of the American Association of Electromyography and Electrodiagnosis.[19] Reproduced by kind permission of the AANEM.)

earth See **ground electrode**.

earthbound astronaut syndrome A fanciful name applied to an acquired state of dysequilibrium.[1707]

ease-of-falling syndrome Probably the same as **thalamic astasia**[4135] in which a patient is unable to stand after a unilateral thalamic lesion or a lesion in the superior part of the internal capsule, as described by Miller Fisher.[2092, 2105] The astasia, in which the patient falls repeatedly to the side of the weakness, appears out of proportion to the mildness of the pyramidal motor deficit.

eastern equine encephalitis An uncommon mosquito-borne arbovirus infection with its reservoir among wild birds living along the American, Atlantic, and Caribbean coasts, usually occurring as sporadic infections, most commonly in children.

Clinically, the encephalitis is severe, with a mortality of up to 70%, leaving neurological sequelae in most survivors. High fevers, seizures, facial edema, signs of raised intracranial pressure, and evidence of severe progressive neurological impairment are the usual clinical features.[2447] Since the routine immunization of horses, equine infection and thus the disease in humans have become uncommon.[5135] For further information see the CDC Web site, http://www.cdc.gov/ncidod/dvbid/arbor/index.htm.

eating epilepsy (prandic epilepsy) Seizures (usually of complex partial type) provoked by the act of eating and associated with a lesion of the deep frontal lobes or rhinencephalon which appears to activate diencephalic structures involved in the cephalic phase of digestion.[5332]

The seizures represent a form of **reflex epilepsy**. There is frequently a positive family history of seizures in affected subjects. This is a disorder of young adults, especially in India, in whom some aspect of eating (hunger, site, smell, taste, chewing, or swallowing) acts as a precipitant of seizures.[3902]

Eaton, L.M. (1905–1958) American neurologist at the Mayo Clinic, where he developed an extensive interest in neuromuscular disease.

Eaton-Lambert syndrome See **Lambert–Eaton myasthenic syndrome**.

ebriositatis See **delirium tremens**.

ecchordosis physaliphora A jellylike excrescence occurring anywhere along the axial skeleton and considered to be a non-neoplastic hamartoma. The lesion is usually clinically silent and rarely leads on to the growth of a **chordoma.** Like chordomas, however, it stains positively for cytokeratin and epithelial membrane antigen.[3991]

echenne muscular dystrophy-white matter spongiosis A congenital dysmorphic syndrome characterized by feeding problems in infancy, joint contractures and arthrogryposis, grand mal and absence seizures (including reading epilepsy), dolichocephaly, scaphocephaly or macrocephaly, and myopathic weakness.[381]

Echner, Alexander (1816–1887) German anatomist in Freyburg whose precise and detailed drawings of the cortex in 1869 established the form of the sulci, gyri, and fissures (and thus the lobes) of the cerebrum.

Echner inferior parietal lobule The supramarginal and angular gyri, identified by Alexander Echner in 1869.[5619]

echo actions The precise repetition by the patient of what the examiner has just said or done. Occasionally a feature of late-stage dementias, it is more often evidence of schizophrenia.

echographia The repetition in writing of what is presented in speech or writing to a subject who is usually aphasic or (as in the first reported cases of **Pick**) is suffering from mental retardation. See **hypergraphia**.

echolalia The involuntary, automatic, precise repetition of the words or phrases said to the patient without change in pronoun, in the presence of gross difficulty in comprehension. The condition is typically due to isolation of the speech areas by a large parietal lesion.[2338]

echolaliopraxia See **signing tics**.

echopraxia The involuntary repetition of the actions or speech of another person.

EC/IC bypass surgery (extracranial–intracranial bypass) Surgical anastomosis of the superficial temporal artery with a branch of the middle cerebral artery in order to improve blood flow through the latter vessel. Theoretically and technically this is a superb operation, for which an appropriate disease is keenly being sought.

eclampsia A severe hypertensive state with widespread vasospasm, peculiar to women in the peripartum state up to 2 weeks after delivery. Evidence of hemolysis, elevated liver enzymes, and low platelets (the HELLP syndrome) may be found, associated with cerebral edema and hemorrhage in severe cases. Neurological features include grand mal seizures, headache, and other evidence of raised intracranial pressure, **posterior leukoencephalopathy**, and acutely-appearing focal deficits such as strokelike syndromes and ischemic optic neuropathy. An association with the Leiden Factor V has been shown.[6292]

Economo, Konstantin von See **Von Economo, Konstantino**.

Economo disease See **encephalitis lethargica**.

economy class syndrome The occurrence of venous thromboembolism (usually leading to pulmonary venous infarction) as a result of prolonged relative immobility in an aeroplane seat, allowing little opportunity for leg movement and requiring almost a Valsalva maneuver in order to escape from it. The migrant emboli may also pass through a patent foramen ovale to cause stroke.

ecstasies (raptures) Emotionally significant experiences at times of extreme affective arousal, the mental content often interpreted by the subject as of divine origin. Those of Teresa de Ahumada (Teresa of Jesus), Dostoevsky, and St. Paul have been interpreted as *ecstatic epilepsy* on the basis of the accompanying stereotypic movements but in one case at least attributed not to an act of God but rather to the effects of neurocysticercosis.[2272]

ecstasy 3,4-Methylenedioxymethamphetamine, an agent capable of causing the undesired effects of metabolic stimulation and muscle necrosis with hyperthermia, as well as the desired mood alterations.

ectasia, ectasis (from Gr, to stretch out) Dilation, usually applied to a hollow channel such as a blood vessel.

ectodermal calcification–basal ganglion calcification syndrome A congenital dysmorphic syndrome manifesting also short stature, alopecia, microcephaly, calcification of the basal ganglia, and mental and developmental delay. See **striatopallidal calcification**.

ectodermal dysplasia Inherited syndromes comprising abnormalities both of the skin and of the nervous system.[676, 1205, 3248, 5469, 6450] Both **neurocutaneous syndromes** and mesodermal disorders such as **Sturge–Weber syndrome** and **Lindau disease** are subsumed under this heading.

See also: **anhidrotic ectodermal dysplasia; hidrotic ectodermal dysplasia; von Recklinghausen disease; tuberous sclerosis; xeroderma pigmentosum; Rud syndrome; Berier disease; Kaposi disease; poikiloderma congenitale; progeria; Bardet-Biedel syndrome; Klippel–Trenaunay–Weber syndrome**; and **Sjögren–Larsson syndrome**.

ectodermal dysplasia-olivopontocerebellar degeneration A congenital dysmorphic syndrome with midface hypoplasia manifesting also short stature, deafness, hypogonadotrophic hypogonadism, cerebellar and pyramidal signs, and mental and developmental delay.[5469]

ectomesodermal blastomatoses See **phakomatoses**.

ectopia See **heterotopia**.

ectopia pupillae See **corectopia iridis**.

ectopic In an abnormal place.

ectopic intracranial retinoblastoma The combination of **pinealoblastoma** and **retinoblastoma**.

ectopic motor nerve behavior Ectopic discharges occur in the form of isolated **fasciculations**, **myokymia**, **neuromyotonia**, or **cramp**, with common pathophysiologic mechanisms. Cramps and fasciculations originate primarily in the most distal motor nerve terminals lacking a myelin sheath and with a porous blood–nerve barrier. With reinnervation, ionic imbalances, motor nerve disease, or pharmacologic challenge, ectopic impulses arise and create visible but sporadic fasciculations. Other circumstances, including muscle shortening and dehydration, give rise to more frequent and localized fasciculations that can erupt into a painful muscle cramp. Unusual motor ectopic phenomena involving rapidly recurrent discharges in multiple motor nerves give rise to grouped fasciculations, **myokymia**, and **neuromyotonia**.[1016]

ectopic pinealoma See **dysgerminoma**.

ectropion (Gr, a bending outward) Outward turning of the eyelids.

Eddowes syndrome See **Apert syndrome**.

Edelmann great toe phenomenon Dorsiflexion of the hallux occurring when the leg is maintained straight and the hip is flexed. This is usually a sign of meningeal irritation, but it is also present in some patients with raised intracranial pressure.

edema See **cerebral edema**.

Edinburgh syndrome A dominantly inherited, lethal congenital dysmorphic syndrome characterized by hydrocephalus, hyperbilirubinemia, and mental and motor delay.[2660]

Edinburgh-2 Coma Scale A scale measuring consciousness as manifest through the patient's best response to maximal stimuli. Subjects are asked the month and their age and to close and open their hands and eyes; their response to strong pain is also assessed.[6120]

Despite the name, the test is actually Japanese; its place in practice in relation to the **Glasgow Coma Scale** is uncertain.

Edinger, Ludwig (1855–1918) German professor of anatomy and neurology at Frankfurt, who differentiated the palaeo- and neocerebellum in 1885 on the basis of the number of cortical layers possessed by each. He also identified the **Edinger–Westphal nucleus**, 2 years before Westphal, and gave the first complete account of **thalamic pain**.

Edinger–Westphal nucleus The parasympathetic nucleus of the III cranial nerve.

EDMUS A computerized minimal descriptive record documenting clinical and laboratory data in patients with **multiple sclerosis**, developed and mainly used in Europe.[1266] (See also Confavreux C. et al. EDMUS, a European database for multiple sclerosis. *JNNP* 1992;55:671–6) A scale of impairment is incorporated. See also **COSTAR** and **Minimal Record of Disability**.

edrophonium (tensilon) A synthetic substance with a transient cholinergic effect at the motor end plate. See **Tensilon Test**.

EDS See **excessive daytime sleepiness**.

Edwards syndrome A congenital dysmorphic syndrome manifesting also generalized obesity, deafness, retinitis pigmentosa, pendular nystagmus acanthosis nigricans, hypogonadism, glucose intolerance, and mental and developmental delay.[1810] See **trisomy 18 syndrome**.

EEG Abbreviation for **electroencephalogram**.

EEG Clinical Neurophysiology See ***Clinical Neurophysiology***. A subspecialty neurological journal and the official organ of the International Federation of Clinical Neurophysiology. Web site: http://www.elsevier.com/inca/publications/store/6/0/1/5/2/8/index.htt/.

EEG coma patterns A system of grading the EEG records in comatose patients. The original form of Synek[6179] listed 165 categories; a simpler one published more recently[6927] has only nine.

Category	*Subcategory*
I. Delta/theta >50% of record (not theta coma)	
II. Triphasic waves	
III. Burst–suppression	A. With epileptiform activity
	B. Without epileptiform activity
IV. Alpha/theta/spindle coma (unreactive)	
V. Epileptiform activity (not in burst–suppression pattern)	A. Generalized
	B. Focal or multifocal
Suppression	A. $< 20\,\mu V$ but $>10\,\mu V$
	B. $\leq 10\,\mu V$

1. Burst–suppression pattern should have generalized flattening at standard sensitivity for ≥1s at least every 20s. 2. Suppression for this category; voltage criteria should be met for entire record. 3. When more than one category applies, select the most serious: Suppression is the most serious form and epileptiform activity is more serious than categories 1 or 2. See also **coma**.

EEG telemetry Techniques which enable the recording of the EEG for long periods on equipment remote from the patient, transmitted usually by cable, radio, or telephone systems.

effective osmolarity (in mOsm/L) $2[Na^+ + K^+$ (mEqL)$]$ + plasma glucose (mg/dl)/18 A value greater than 320 mOsm per liter reflects hyperosmolarity and greater than 350 mOsm per liter indicates a severe hyperosmolar state with lethal potential.

Poor outcome is related to age as well as elevated blood urea nitrogen (BUN) and sodium concentrations. The syndrome may be complicated by thromboembolic events, aspiration, and rhabdomyolysis.

efferent (from Lat, to bring out) Bearing something away from a site; as with motor nerves in which electrical impulses pass from the center to the periphery.

efferent nerve A nerve in which the direction of physiological conduction is away from the central nervous system and toward a muscle or a sweat gland.

effort headache See **benign exertional headache**.

effort syndrome See **chronic fatigue syndrome**.

Egger syndrome (Joubert syndrome with orofaciodigital anomalies) A congenital dysmorphic syndrome, manifesting also apnea or tachypnea, polydactyly, brain tumors, cerebellar ataxia, and mental and developmental delay. See also **Joubert syndrome**.

Ehlers Danlos syndrome (cutis laxa, Chernogubov syndrome) A dominantly inherited syndrome of mesodermal lesions of the collagen and elastic tissues, comprising narrow face, hyperelasticity and fragility of the skin, hypermobility of joints, easy bruising, spontaneous rupture of the heart or lung, and arterial aneurysms, such as carotid-cavernous fistulas.[1819, 2541] Among the seven subvarieties distinguished, X-linked and recessive forms are also recorded. In the genetically heterogeneous Type IV, aneurysms, dissections, and spontaneous arteriovenous fistulae are potential complications.

The first reports were by Van Meekeren in 1682 and by A.N. Chernogubov, a Russian physician, in 1892. E. Ehlers (1863–1937) was professor of clinical dermatology in Copenhagen, Denmark; H.A. Danlos (1844–1912) was a French dermatologist.

Ehret syndrome Paralysis following a painful injury, leading to the persistent assumption of the least painful posture, resulting in muscle atrophy and contractures. The condition was described by Ehret in 1898[1822] among patients with peroneal weakness after trauma. Its etiology is considered to be conditioning rather than hysteria.[3113]

Ehrlich, Paul (1854–1915) German physician who demonstrated the existence of a blood–brain barrier in 1885, when he found that every organ in the body except the brain took up vital stains injected into the blood. As a neurohistologist, he introduced methylene blue as an *intra vitam* stain for nervous tissue.

Ehrlicosis (human monocytic Ehrlicosis) A tick-borne infection due to the rickettsial bacterium *E. chaffeensis* producing clinical signs of infection, multisystem involvement, pancytopenia, elevated BUN, hepatitis and, in the nervous system, evidence of meningoencephalitis with meningism, seizures, and coma. The CSF contains increased protein and neutrophilic or lymphocytic pleocytosis. Perivascular and intramural mononuclear cell infiltrates are found in the leptomeninges and Virchow–Robin spaces.[2550]

E:I ratio In autonomic testing, the ratio of the longest electrocardiographic R–R interval during expiration to the shortest during inspiration. Primarily, it is a measure of the parasympathetic control of the heart rate. See **expiration:inspiration ratio**.

Eichorst, Herman Ludwig (1849–1921) German physician who graduated from Königsberg. After posts held in Germany, he was appointed professor of medicine at Zurich. In 1873 he described a form of peripheral motor neuropathy (Eichorst neuritis) affecting the legs only, which was probably a **hereditary motor and sensory neuropathy**.

eidetic An unusually clear mental image, perceived as though it were actually visible.

eight-and-a-half syndrome The combination of a VII nerve palsy and a **one-and-a-half syndrome** as a result of a lesion of the lower pontine tegmentum.[1817]

Eisenson examination for aphasia A clinical instrument comprising 37 subtests, designed to provide a protocol for examining the type and severity of language and related deficits.[1826]

Ekbom, Karl Axel Sr. Swedish neurologist at Uppsala.

Ekbom syndrome 1. See **restless legs syndrome**. 2. Delusional parasitosis.

Ekman–Lobstein syndrome A dominantly inherited cochleovestibular atrophy with onset in young adult life. See **Van der Hoeve phakomatosis**.

Ekiri An encephalopathy associated with shigellosis reported from Japan, but now almost eliminated as a result of public health measures. It presents in the same way as **shigella encephalopathy** and may also be fatal.

elderly gait See **cautious gait**.

electric chorea See **Dubini disease**.

electric feet syndrome See **burning feet syndrome**.

electric shock Exposure of the body to high-voltage electrical currents, which may lead in the acute phase to local burns, ventricular fibrillation, and such neurological complications as respiratory center paralysis, spinal atrophic paresis, cerebral edema, intracranial hematoma, brainstem syndromes, myelopathic spastic paraplegia,[6386] hemiplegia, radiculopathy, severe axonal neuropathy, or heat-induced myopathy,[1970] and in the longer term to syndromes resembling **amyotrophic lateral sclerosis**[3147] as well as to optic atrophy, retinopathy, cataract, involuntary movement disorders, and various patterns of upper or lower motor neuron lesions, from which latter recovery may not occur. See also **lightning encephalopathy** and **lightning polyneuropathy**.

electrical inactivity See **electrical silence**.

electrical nystagmus See **vestibular nystagmus**.

electrical silence The absence of measurable electric activity in a tissue.

electrical status epilepticus in (slow-wave) sleep (ESES, epilepsy with continuous spike-waves during sleep) An uncommon epileptic encephalopathy of infancy and childhood presenting with continuous and diffuse spike-and -slow wave complexes that persist through nonrapid eye movement sleep. The disorder is most commonly seen in children before the age of 5 years; it starts with nocturnal focal motor seizures before the appearance of one or another seizure type, including almost all forms of generalized or partial motor seizures and brief absence attacks. The EEG during wakefulness may show a combination of focal and generalized spikes, while in sleep periods of almost continuous, mainly bisynchronous 1.5–2 Hz (and 3–4 Hz) spikes and waves occur during non-REM periods.

Withdrawal, hyperkinetic behavior, impaired language development, memory and orientation, and a global reduction in intelligence are notable for a few years, after which both the electrical and the clinical features remit and the child's behavior returns toward normal.[4931] However, despite the usually benign evolution of seizures, the prognosis is guarded because of the occasional later appearance of neuropsychological disorders.[1264] Distinction from **Lennox–Gastaut syndrome** and from **Landau–Kleffner syndrome** is difficult.[6833, 4882]

This seizure syndrome results from the association of various seizure types, partial or generalized, occurring during sleep, and atypical absences when awake. Tonic seizures do not occur.

Diagnostic criteria have been suggested by the American Academy of Sleep Medicine.[1629] (See Chart E–1.)

electrically silent cramps Painful prolonged muscle contractures provoked by depletion of muscle energy stores unaccompanied by EMG activity. See **glycogenoses; rippling muscle syndrome, Brody syndrome,** and **myoedema.**

electroanalgesia The reduction of pain by stimulation of sites in the central or peripheral nervous systems.

electrocochleography A technique for assessing the electrical output of the cochlea and VIII cranial nerve in response to auditory stimulation, by means of a recording needle electrode inserted through the tympanic membrane.[5087] The test has been considered to be of value in the diagnosis of **vestibular Schwannomas** (acoustic neuromas), but **MRI scanning** and **brainstem auditory evoked responses** are much better.

electrocorticogram (corticogram) The record of EEG activity obtained by means of electrodes applied directly over or inserted into the cerebral cortex.

electrocorticography (corticography) The technique of recording the electrical activity of the brain by means of electrodes applied over or implanted into the cerebral cortex.

electrode A conducting device used to record an electric potential (recording electrode) or to deliver an electric current (stimulating electrode). In addition to the ground electrode used in clinical recordings, two electrodes are always required either to record an electric potential or to deliver a stimulus. See ground electrode, recording electrode, and stimulating electrode. See also specific needle electrode configurations: **monopolar, unipolar, concentric, bifilar recording, bipolar stimulating, multilead, single fiber, and macro-EMG needle electrodes.** (From the 2001 Report of the Nomenclature Committee of the American Association of Electromyography and Electrodiagnosis.[19] Reproduced by kind permission of the AANEM.)

electrode impedance The opposition to the flow of an AC current through the interface between an electrode and the scalp or brain, expressed in ohms (generally kilohms). This is measured between pairs of electrodes, or in some EEG machines, between each individual electrode and all the other electrodes connected in parallel. Over the EEG frequency range, because the capacitance factor is small, electrode impedance is usually numerically equal to electrode resistance. The term is not a synonym for **input impedance.**

electrode resistance The opposition to the flow of a DC current through the interface between an EEG electrode and the scalp or brain, expressed in ohms (generally kilohms). This is measured between pairs of electrodes, or in some EEG machines, between each individual electrode and all the other electrodes connected in parallel.

Measurement of electrode resistance with DC currents results in varying degrees of electrode polarization. See also **electrode impedance.**

electrodermal response See **Galvanic skin response.**

electrodiagnosis (EDX) The recording and analysis of biologic electrical potentials from the central, peripheral, and autonomic nervous systems and from muscles, for medical purposes. See also **electromyography, electroneurography,**

Chart E–1. Diagnostic Criteria for Electrical Status Epilepticus in Sleep

A. The disorder is usually asymptomatic, but there may be a complaint of difficulty in waking up in the morning.
B. Frequent, but not constant, association with epilepsy, particularly typical absences or infrequent, partial, or generalized motor seizures.
C. The age of onset is typically in childhood.
D. Polysomnographic monitoring demonstrates:
    1. Continuous, generalized spike- and slow-wave discharges persisting through nonrapid eye movement sleep stages
    2. A spike-wave (SW) index ranging from 85 to 100%
    3. Disappearance of the electrical status during REM sleep.
E. Other medical or psychiatric disorders can be present, particularly other seizure disorders.
F. Does not meet the diagnostic criteria for other sleep disorders that occur during sleep.

Adapted from the International Classification of Sleep Disorders Diagnostic and Coding Manual. Rochester, MN. American Academy of Sleep Medicine. © 1991/2001. Reproduced by kind permission of the Academy. See also **sleep disorders** and the Web site: http://www.sleepeducation.com/Disorders.aspx/.

electroneuromyography, and **evoked potential studies**.

electrodiagnostic medicine An extension of the clinical examination of the patient, wherein the physician integrates information obtained from the clinical history and physical examination of the nervous, muscular, and other systems to diagnose and treat diseases of the central, peripheral, and autonomic nervous systems, neuromuscular junctions, and muscles[19] by means of EMG and/or nerve conduction studies.

electroencephalogram The record of electrical activity of the brain made by means of electrodes placed on the scalp or from implanted electrodes. Although this represents the hallowed use of the word that will not now be changed, *electroencephalogram* is by derivation the correct term for the machine and *electroencephalograph* properly used for the printout.

electroencephalography (EEG) The procedure of recording cerebrally derived potential changes, using electrodes placed either on the surface of the scalp, upon the dura, or within the brain, with huge amplification.

Richard Caton (1842–1926), professor of physiology in Liverpool, England, first made recordings of the action currents from the brains of rabbits in 1875, but Johannes (Hans) Berger (1873–1941) recorded the alpha and beta rhythms from humans in 1929.[5619] He received, however, less credit than did Lord **Adrian**, who was awarded the Nobel Prize for his confirmation of "Berger rhythms" in 1934.

The basic science and clinical utilization of the EEG were succinctly reviewed in 1994.[647]

Electroencephalography and Clinical Neurophysiology (*EEG Clin Neurophysiol*) A neurological subspecialist journal published by Elsevier Scientific Publishers Ireland Ltd. See ***Clinical Neurophysiology.*** Web site: http://www.sciencedirect.com/science/journal/00134694/.

electromagnetic flowmeter A device able to measure the direction and volume of flow through blood vessels, but not now in use.[2748]

electromyelography The recording and study of electrical activity from the spinal cord and/or from the cauda equina.[162]

electromyogram Equipment used to activate, record, process, and display nerve and muscle action potentials for the purpose of evaluating nerve and muscle function. The machine used to perform **electromyography**.

As with **electroencephalogram**, the terms generally employed represent a reversal of the correct usage, *-gram* properly denoting recording equipment and the *-graph*, writing. The small lapse is regrettable but there is nothing that mere writers of books like this one can do about it.

electromyograph The record obtained in electromyography. See comment on **electromyogram**.

electromyography (EMG) Strictly defined, the recording and study of insertional, spontaneous, and voluntary electrical activity of muscle by means of mono- or bipolar needle electrodes, but commonly used to refer to nerve conduction studies as well.

The myofibrillar or motor unit action potentials are amplified and recorded on a cathode ray oscilloscope, a parallel lead to a loudspeaker allowing auditory as well as visual sampling by the electromyographer. The test is slightly painful, but, unless a vital organ or nerve is punctured by the needle, and provided absolute sterility is maintained, it represents a safe and valuable extension of the clinical examination.

The procedure can demonstrate which muscles have lost all or part of their nerve supply (thus permitting an accurate determination of the extent of the root or nerve lesion); can determine the amount of denervation or of the degree of recovery from that; and can inform about the presence of signs of end plate or primary muscle diseases. A handful of the latter present characteristic electrical features, most show nonspecific evidence of myopathy only, and some are not accompanied by electrical abnormalities. Pathological diagnosis is almost never possible with EMG alone. **Single-fiber EMG** is a refinement of the technique.[3435]

The first EMG was recorded in humans by Probster in 1928; **Adrian** introduced coaxial needles in the following year.

electroneurography The recording and study of the action potentials of peripheral nerves. See **nerve conduction studies**.

electroneurography index An index based on 12 electrophysiological parameters such as conduction velocities, F wave latencies, and amplitudes, providing an overall assessment of peripheral nerve function longitudinally.[5943]

electroneuromyography (ENMG) The combined studies of electromyography and electroneurography. ENMG is synonymous with clinical electromyography. "Electrodiagnostic medicine consultation" is the currently favored term.[19]

electronystagmography The detection and recording of the movement of the dipole normally arising from the slight electric field (1 mV) between the cornea and the retina, as a subject follows a target. This is the electrophysiologic equivalent of visual inspection of eye movements while obscuring fixation with high diopter or Fresnel lenses and is useful to confirm the presence of nystagmus in the "dizzy" patient.

electrooculogram (corneoretinal potential) A record of the standing potential between the cornea and the posterior pole of the eye, measuring a function of the photoreceptors and the pigment epithelium. The test is of some value in the determination of the state of the retina, but the **electroretinogram** gives more information.[232]

electro-olfactogram A record of the potential changes in the olfactory mucosa in response to a stream of air charged with odoriferous particles.

electroretinogram (ERG) A recording of the voltage change in the retinal cells in response to a flash (FERG) or changing pattern (PERG) stimulus. Because the FERG is not affected by ganglion cell disease and is thus normal in disorders affecting the afferent visual pathway, it is an indicator of the presence of lesions of the retinal cells. Although the PERG does appear to depend on the integrity of these cells, its clinical utility is marginal because of reduced reliability of the results. By varying the frequency or wavelength of the stimulus, the test can distinguish between disease of the rods and of the cones, or it can assess the retinal adaptation of the subject.[4854]

electrotonus The condition of a muscle caused to contract by a Galvanic current, described in 1843 by Émile du Bois-Réymond (1818–1896), a German physiologist.

elementary motor seizure A seizure manifesting as contractions of a single muscle or group of muscles that is usually stereotyped and not decomposable into phases. (However, see **tonic seizures**.)

elementary seizure A seizure comprising a single manifestation of activation of one primary sensory modality, for example, somatosensory, visual, auditory, olfactory, gustatory, epigastric, or cephalic.

elementary tics (simple tics) See **tics**.

elephant a sign The appearance on the T2-weighted MRI scan of hippocampal atrophy, fancifully described in, for example, **Alzheimer disease**.[5648]

elephantiasis anesthetica See **leprosy**.

Elevated Arm Stress Test (EAST) Elevation of the arms for 3 min (in the surrender position) induces the symptoms of **thoracic outlet syndrome**.[5375] What this means in terms of the underlying pathology is quite uncertain. See also **Wright maneuvre**.

elevator nystagmus See **optokinetic nystagmus**.

elfin face syndrome See **Williams syndrome**.

elicited repetitive daily blindness A dominantly inherited syndrome of repetitive, transient (about 10 s), uni- or bilateral visual loss recurring many times daily. The condition segregates with **familial hemiplegic migraine** and childhood epilepsy.[3735]

Elithorn Perceptual Maze Test A nonverbal intelligence test in which the subject is required to trace a pathway with a pencil through a lattice, covering as many of the dots randomly placed on the intersections as possible. Untimed, the test distinguishes subjects with right hemisphere damage; with time constraints, those with aphasia do especially poorly.[3825]

elk (*alces malchis*) A species of antelope, once thought to be especially susceptible to epileptic seizures which it was, however, able to cure by putting its left hoof into its ear. See also **prion diseases**.

Ellenberg syndrome See **diabetic neuropathies**.

Elliott syndrome A congenital dysmorphic syndrome manifesting also short stature, deafness, blepharophimosis, disordered sexual differentiation, delayed closure of fontanelles, and mental and developmental delay.

Elliptic nystagmus See **circular nystagmus**.

Ellis gargoylism See **mucopolysaccharidoses**.

Ellis–van Creveld syndrome (chondroectodermal dysplasia) A congenital, recessively inherited dysostosis (a disturbance in bone form or modeling due to a disturbance in developmental ectodermal or mesenchymal tissues).[1845] The clinical features include shortening of the tubular bones, especially distally, with resultant dwarfism; polydactyly; small, delayed, and defective teeth and nails; congenital heart disease; and cataract and strabismus. Mental delay has also been described.

The condition has been found mainly in an Old Order Amish kinship in Pennsylvania,[4243] but it has been suggested that the English King Richard III suffered from it too.[79]

eloquent cortex Those parts of the cerebral cortex concerned with the faculty of speech.

Elpenor syndrome An allegorical name for the behavior of people who become somnolent after ingesting alcohol or drugs and awaken in unfamiliar surroundings where they commit acts that are destructive, antisocial, or frankly illegal. After regaining awareness, the patients have only vague recollections of the events that transpired.

The syndrome was first described by Benjamin-Joseph Logre, a French psychiatrist who reported the case of Paul-Eugene-Louis Deschanel, the then President of the Republic of France, in the French newspaper *La Monde* (May 1–3, 1948). Decharnel had taken barbiturates on a train journey, lost consciousness, and fell out of the carriage window without noticing it; he regained consciousness in a ditch and was eventually restored to the Elysée Palace, where subsequently he presided with his customary lucidity. Logre detected a similarity between this incident and one related in the *Odyssey*—the story of Elpenor, the youngest companion of Ulysses, who according to legend fell off a terrace and broke his neck on awakening from a drunken sleep. Logre advised that hosts who offer their guests a bed for the night after a convivial evening should provide them with a ground floor room, but today the offer of a taxi is deemed adequate.

Elsahy-Waters branchioskeletogenital syndrome A congenital, autosomal, or X-linked recessively inherited dysmorphic syndrome manifesting also strabismus, ptosis, nystagmus, fusion of vertebrae, genital and skeletal maldevelopment, seizures, and mental and developmental delay.[1849]

Elsberg, Charles A. American surgeon, professor at New York University. His definitive book *Surgical Diseases of the Spinal Cord and its Membranes* (Philadelphia, Saunders) was published in 1916.

Elsberg syndrome Polyradiculitis (or radiculomyelitis) of the cauda equina, with urinary retention and CSF pleocytosis.[1850] The condition may complicate genital herpes (HSV-2), **borreliosis**, or **isolated angiitis of the nervous system**, but is probably most often a variant of **acute inflammatory demyelinating neuropathy** with particular autonomic involvement.

Ely sign A test in which the knee is flexed and the hip hyperextended with the patient lying prone. L.W. Ely (1868–1944), an American orthopedic surgeon, showed that the elicitation of pain by this maneuver indicates the presence of psoas irritation or hip joint disease. See also **femoral stretch test**.

embolalia The interposition of meaningless words into spoken speech; two subtypes are distinguished: **angiophrasia** and **logospasmus choreiformis**.

embolism (from Gr, to throw in) Vascular obstruction by a blood clot or other material (such as air, amniotic fluid, cholesterol, cardiac valvular material, fat, or tumor cells) carried to the site of obstruction in the circulation. The concept was first enunciated by **Virchow**.

embolization A technique in surgery or interventional radiology whereby inert spheres are introduced into the artery supplying an **arteriovenous malformation** in order to reduce the blood flow within it and to effect shrinkage of the lesion.[2169]

embouchure dystonia A focal task-specific dystonia affecting the embouchure (the pattern of lip, jaw, and tongue muscles used to control the flow of air into a mouthpiece) of professional brass and woodwind players. It usually develops in the fourth decade, initially unilaterally, but progresses without remission and responds poorly to oral medications and botulinum toxin injection. Embouchure tremor, involuntary lip movements, and involuntary jaw closure are other forms described.

embrace reflex See Moro reflex.

embryofoetal valproic acid syndrome See **fetal anticonvulsant syndrome**.

embryoma of head and neck See **dermoid cyst**.

eMedicine Neurology A free Internet-based neurology textbook from WebMD, but requiring registration. Web site: http://www.emedicine.com/neuro/.

emergency light reflex Constriction of the pupils, tight closure of the eyes, flexion of the neck, and sometimes elevation of the arms in response to a sudden threatening stimulus.

Emery–Dreifuss humeroperoneal muscular dystrophy See Emery–Dreifuss syndrome.

Emery–Dreifuss syndrome (Emery–Dreifuss humeroperoneal muscular dystrophy, Cestan–Lejonne syndrome) Heterogeneous, uncommon, slowly progressive X-linked muscular dystrophies (laminopathies) with childhood onset, exhibiting initially biceps and triceps, then pelvic and later pectoral girdle weakness; facial weakness; rigidity of paraspinal muscles; cardiac muscle involvement with conduction defects including complete heart block; features of the **scapulohumeroperoneal syndrome**; and early muscle contractures at the elbow, ankle, and neck without muscle pseudohypertrophy.[1854, 5444] The responsible (emerin) gene is localized at Xq28.

A neurogenic basis has been considered likely in some of the reported cases, a myopathic cause in others; the clinical pattern is constant, however.

Variant forms include the following:

benign muscular dystrophy with contractures.[335]

benign X-linked muscular dystrophy with cardiomyopathy.[6587]

Emery–Driefuss syndrome with dominant inheritance (see **autosomal dominant humeroperoneal myopathy**) A dominantly inherited proximal myopathy which in every other way resembles this condition but which is due to a mutation on the *laminin A/C* gene at 1q21.2–q21.3.[2377, 4372, 2005]

rigid spine syndrome A *forme-fruste* of the same condition, occurring sporadically.

X-linked muscular dystrophy with humeropelvic distribution, contractures, and cardiomyopathy A similar condition with infantile onset.[3239]

X-linked scapuloperoneal syndrome.

EMG Abbreviation for **electromyography**.

Emmetropia Normal ocular refraction, such that the image of an object at infinity is focused naturally and precisely on the retina.

emotion (from Lat, to move away) A moving of the mind; conscious or unconscious stimulation to perform some action. "Emotion moves us; hence its name" (Sir Charles **Sherrington**).

emotional facial palsy (mimetic facial palsy) Loss of movement of the lower quadrant of the face during emotional movements (such as laughter), although such movements can be made voluntarily. The condition is rare; it may be explainable if the descending fibers to the facial nerve nucleus and regulating emotional movements arise in the basal ganglia and descend in pathways other than the corticobulbar tracts.

emotional incontinence See **emotionalism.**

emotionalism (involuntary crying, pathologic emotionality, forced crying, pseudobulbar affect, organic emotionalism, emotional incontinence, spasmodic crying, inappropriate crying, pathological affect) The involuntary expression of emotion without the experience thereof. The use of this word is advocated in preference to the alternatives proposed.[139] Crying, laughter, and rage are the emotions most often expressed, usually in the context of brain disease from any cause affecting the descending motor pathways bilaterally and accompanying depression.

empiric (from Gr, deduced from experience alone) A practitioner whose skills are derived from experience. The Empirics were an ancient sect of physicians opposed to the Dogmatists; they admitted experience as the sole basis of medicine, this based upon chance observation or reporting, on trials and on imitation. They dismissed speculation and also rejected the value of anatomy and physiology.[5103]

emprosthotonos The converse of **opisthotonos,** in which tonic flexor rather than extensor spasms occur in patients with tetanus, leading to truncal hyperflexion.[2531]

empty delta sign (negative delta sign) The appearance on enhanced CT scans in a patient with occlusion of the superior sagittal sinus; normally the sinus represents a triangle with its base upward, but in this case the surrounding area is enhanced but the sinus fails to fill, leaving this pale triangular area in contrast. See also **dense triangle sign**.

empty sella headache Typically, a chronic, unilateral frontotemporal headache with facial and laterocervical dysesthesias,[4474] but variable in nature and differentiated from migraine and tension-type headaches by exclusion or in retrospect.

empty sella syndrome (intrasellar arachnoid diverticulum, deficient sellar diaphragm, intrasellar cyst, intrasellar cistern) Herniation of the arachnoid containing CSF through a defect in the diaphragma sella, leading to compression of the pituitary gland.[3337]

The optic nerve may also herniate, with the production of a visual field defect and there is a possible association with complaints of headache, and with papilledema and endocrine disorders,[4474] but otherwise the condition is asymptomatic and is usually detected by chance.

The primary empty sella was defined as that which admitted significant amounts of air at pneumoencephalography in the absence of prior surgery or radiation therapy.[4608]

The *secondary type* was that in which such procedures had been undertaken or in which there had been prior increased intracranial pressure or shrinkage of a pituitary adenoma. Today the demonstration of low attenuation in the sella on CT scans would suffice for the diagnosis,[1243] but while radiologically dramatic and sometimes associated with increased intracranial pressure, this appearance is also found in some normal subjects. The condition does not explain headaches unless there are other signs of increased intracranial pressure.

The condition may present in infancy or childhood, when there may also be found pituitary–hypothalamic dysfunction, short stature, facial dysmorphism, spina bifida occulta, hydrocephalus, mental or developmental delay, and delayed skeletal maturation.[5814]

empty speech That type of conversation which communicates nothing in faultless grammar. When spoken in private circumstances it is suggestive evidence of **dementia**, but it is commonplace in official utterances, in which context it has no diagnostic value. See also **cocktail party syndrome**.

enabling synkinesis The situation in which one arm can carry out an act only if the other one does the same thing. See **alien hand syndrome**.

enantesis (from Gr, to meet) The confluence of ascending and descending blood vessels, as with the internal mammary and the anterior spinal arteries.

encapsulation 1. The process whereby bits of words are fused to form a neologism.[1337] 2. The distinction and investment of a pathological lesion by a layer of tissue, either inflammatory or derived from the surrounding tissues.

encephalalgia An old term for head pain, wrongly used since the word derives from that for *brain*, which, unlike other cranial structures, is generally insensitive to pain.

Encéphale A French neurological journal. Web site: http://www.elsevier.com/wps/find/journaleditorialboard.cws_home/709657/editorialboard.

encephale isolé An experimental physiological preparation, the transverse cut being at the level of the low medulla. The EEG of the animal shows a wakeful pattern.

encephalic Within the head—through properly, within the brain.

encephalion Diminutive of **encephalon**, applied to the cerebellum.

encephalitis (Gr, brain + inflammation) 1. Inflammation of the substance of the brain, as opposed to its meninges only: A heterogeneous collection of diseases, classified by Greenfield[2564] in 1950. 2. Nonsuppurative inflammation, usually diffusely affecting the substance of the brain with emphasis on the gray matter, producing perivascular and parenchymal infiltration with inflammatory cells and neuronophagia and is due to any infectious or chemical agent or autoallergic attack.

Clinically, fever, headache, reduced levels of consciousness, seizures, and mononuclear pleocytosis in the CSF are the classic features.

Focal nonsuppurative encephalitis is also described, rarely; it is properly known as **cerebral abscess**. Diffuse infiltrations (e.g., encephalitis periaxialis diffusa) are not truly classified here, despite the name.[3233]

See also **herpes simplex encephalitis, Japanese encephalitis, shiga toxin encephalitis, Nipah virus encephalitis, West Nile encephalitis,** and **Lassa fever**.

encephalitis lethargica (von Economo disease, epidemic encephalitis, sleeping sickness) A polymorphic epidemic encephalitis which was recorded in Germany in 1712 and was widespread for a decade following the influenza pandemic of 1916–1927, affecting the population of the United Sates after 1918. Both before and since that time, sporadic cases of this disease have been recorded. von Economo's account,[6567] though based on fewer cases, is fuller than that of Jean Cruchet[1363] which was actually published 2 weeks before; priority of publication led to a regrettable dispute. The tendency for Parkinsonian signs to follow encephalitis lethargica was remarked first by Achille Alexandre **Souques** (1860–1944), a French neurologist, in 1921.[5962]

Clinically, the disease was marked by fever, pharyngitis, generalized pains, skin rashes, malaise, and gastrointestinal complaints, and by such signs as extreme drowsiness, oculomotor pareses, delirium, and catatonia. Other presentations included an acute Parkinsonian state and a hyperkinetic syndrome with chorea and myoclonus.[2686, 5169] The pathology was described by Lhermitte.[3829] There is an encephalitis of the midbrain and basal ganglia, with lymphocyte (predominantly plasma cell) infiltration.

Sequelae affect about 40% of those afflicted and includ tics, dystonias, akathisia, seizures, ataxia, and pareses; a Parkinsonian syndrome with oculogyric crises and narcolepsy, amyotrophy, emotional disturbances, and persistent sleep disorders are also recorded. About 40% of these patients succumb.[6819]

The nature of the disorder became clearer with recent examination of sporadic cases with a typical encephalitis lethargica phenotype. CSF examination showed elevated protein and OCB; MRI of the brain was normal or showed inflammatory changes localized to the deep gray matter; antistreptolysin-O titres are often elevated and almost all patients have auto-antibodies reactive against human basal ganglia antigens, indicating that this is likely to be a postinfectious autoimmune CNS disorder.[1417] See also **PANDAS** and **Sydenham chorea**.

encephalitis periaxialis concentrica See **Balo concentric sclerosis**.

encephalitis periaxialis diffusa See **Schilder disease**.

encephalitis subcorticalis chronica progressiva See **Binswanger disease**.

encephalitis tremens A rare condition described once in epidemic form in Nigeria,[6877] but not encountered since.

encephalocele (Gr, the brain + a tumor) A rare congenital maldevelopment characterized by extracranial herniation of part of the cerebral hemispheres such as the occipital lobe, or of the cerebellum, through a midline cranial defect. *Anterior encephaloceles* represent the same maldevelopment in the frontal region.[5924] See also **cephalocele**.

encephalocraniocutaneous lipomatosis A congenital syndrome consisting of localized scalp alopecia, craniofacial lipomas, eyelid papules, conjunctival nevi, porencephalic cysts, seizures, and mental retardation.[121]

encephalocutaneous lipomatosis A congenital neurocutaneous dysmorphic syndrome characterized by cerebral atrophy with intracranial calcification, hydranencephaly or porencephaly, hydrocephalus, seizures, soft tissue tumors of the cranium and eyes, and mental and developmental delay.[2661]

encephalofacial angiomatosis See **Sturge–Weber syndrome**.

encephalography A radiological method for estimating the size of the ventricles at **pneumoencephalography**; now obsolete.

encephaloid Resembling a brain.

encephalolith A calcareous structure within the brain. *Encephalolithiasis* is that condition in which such accretions occur.

encephalomalacia An area of softening of brain tissue occurring in the period immediately following its infarction.[JF] See **multicystic encephalopathy**.

encephalomyelitis 1. Inflammation of the substance of the brain and of the spinal cord. 2. A paraneoplastic syndrome presenting as limbic or bulbar encephalomyelitis or with more generalized involvement associated with dementia, occurring most often in the setting of a small cell lung carcinoma. Antibodies such as anti-Hu and anti-Yo are commonly detectable.

encephalomyelitis with carcinoma Forms of **paraneoplastic syndrome** including limbic (**limbic dementia**) and bulbar encephalitis, myelitis with predilection for the anterior horn cells, and ganglioradiculitis; usually with subacute progression and occurring in older adults with bronchogenic (and less often with stomach, breast, or ovarian) carcinomas.[2867]

Clinically, an initial painful neuropathy is usually followed by the development of any combination of dementia, cerebellar and pyramidal signs, extrapyramidal findings, and brainstem dysfunction with multifocal myoclonus, leading to death within 2 years.

encephalomyeloneuritis Usually a **paraneoplastic** syndrome (see **encephalomyelitis with carcinoma**); but an identical syndrome is reported in subjects without detectable malignancy.[3690]

encephalomyelopolyradiculopathy A febrile illness of unknown cause, characterized by evidence of involvement of all the structures suggested in the title and leading to confusion, pain, paraparesis, and loss of sphincter control.

encephalomyeloradiculitis See **acute inflammatory demyelinating polyneuropathy**.

encephalomyopathy with epilepsy, chorioretinitis, basal ganglion involvement, and muscle minicores A congenital muscular dystrophy complicated by psychomotor retardation, seizures, rigidity, chorioretinitis and bilateral basal ganglion, thalamic, cerebellar, and cerebral cortical MRI abnormalities.[309] See also **muscle-eye-brain disease** and **Fukuyama muscle dystrophy**.

encephalon (Gr, In + the head) (encephalos, encephalus, encephalum) Used synonymously with "the brain."

encephalo-ophthalmic syndrome See **Krause disease**.

encephalo-optic dysplasia See **Walker–Warburg syndrome**.

encephalopathie saturnine Lead encephalopathy.

encephalopathy/encephalopathia Disease of the brain. In general usage, diffuse disorders affecting the greater part of the cortex and/or subcortical regions.

See also **dialysis encephalopathy, Dupré syndrome, ESES, hypertensive encephalopathy, metabolic encephalopathy, mitochondrial encephalomyopathy, parainfectious noninflammatory encephalomyelitis, portosystemic encephalopathy, rejection encephalopathy, shiga toxin encephalopathy, tacrolimus encephalopathy, uremic encephalopathy, Wernicke–Korsakoff encephalopathy**, and the following entries.

encephalopathy of sepsis Diffuse cerebral disease producing depression in conscious level, multifocal EEG abnormalities, seizures, and focal neurological signs in the presence of chronic severe disseminated infection.

The underlying pathology includes bacterial invasion of the brain with the formation of disseminated microabscesses, cerebral infarction, multiple, small white matter hemorrhages, **central pontine myelinolysis**, and possibly disturbances in cerebral synaptic transmission as a direct result of toxicity from the infecting agent.[3119]

encephalopathy score A scale for evaluating neonates with encephalopathy, able to predict neurodevelopmental outcome at 30 months of age.[4376] Feeding, alertness, muscle tone, respiratory status, reflexes, and seizures are assessed daily for the first 3 days of life in the neonate who is neither sedated nor paralyzed. See also **hypoxic-ischemic encephalopathy**.

encephalopathy with fatty degeneration of the viscera See **Reye syndrome**.

encephalorrhagia Purpura of the brain, the blood damaging both myelin and axons.

encephalos See **encephalon**.

encephalosyncope (vasovagal attacks) Syncope, blurred vision, dizziness, abdominal sensations, or weakness with or without loss of consciousness, occurring in subjects with abnormal EEG records and considered to represent a minor seizure disorder triggered by cerebral ischemia.

The term was suggested by Kershman in 1949 but did not find favor.

encephalotrigeminal angiomatosis See **Sturge–Weber syndrome**.

encephalum See **encephalon**.

encephalus See **encephalon**.

enchondromatosis A dysmorphic syndrome characterized by short stature, scoliosis, platyspondyly, mental and developmental delay, sclerosis of the skull with enchondromata, and skeletal cysts or tumors. See **Maffucci syndrome**.

encycloduction See **duction**.

end artery An artery which, uniquely, supplies a volume of tissue.

end bulb (bouton terminale) The term employed by Krause for the expansions of the distal ends of sensory nerves.

endarterectomy An open surgical procedure whereby the stenotic or atheroma-encrusted lining of the cervical carotid artery is reamed out or dissected in order to reduce turbulence and future platelet deposition and to increase flow. The procedure has been shown to reduce a symptomatic patient's risk of stroke when the stenosis is between 70 and 99% of the lumen, but, with lesser degrees of narrowing and in asymptomatic people, whether or not it confers benefit is not yet determined.

endarteritis obliterans (Heubner endarteritis) An inflammatory condition of the media and adventitia of the walls of large- and medium-sized arteries, associated with fibroblastic proliferation of the intima, and thus liable to cause occlusion of the vessel and distal infarction. This is a typical finding in secondary or meningovascular syphilis.

endocranium The inner surface of the skull bones.

endocrine candida syndrome The association of candida with idiopathic hypoparathyroidism and Addison disease, together with defective delayed hypersensitivity.[2299] Neurological features include increased intracranial pressure with papilledema and intracranial calcification, seizures, mental retardation, muscle twitching, cramps, and rigidity.[3246]

endocrine exophthalmos See **dysthyroid ophthalmopathy**.

end-of-dose deterioration (wearing-off effect) A hypokinetic form of fluctuation in Parkinsonian patients on long term levadopa therapy, in which disability increases as the levadopa levels fall.

end-of-dose dystonia A form of fluctuation in Parkinsonian patients taking long-term levadopa therapy, in which dystonic movements appear as the levadopa levels fall.

endolymphatic hydrops See **Ménière disease**.

endomysium (Gr, within + muscle) The connective tissue investing each myofibril.

endoneurial area The total area of the nerve fascicles encompassed by the perineurium.

endoneurium (Gr, within + nerve) The connective tissue investing each nerve fiber within a funiculus.

endophasy The unspoken language of thought.

endorphins Opioid peptides. Among these, beta endorphin is a mediator of pain perception.

endosteal hyperostosis (van Buchem disease) A genetic craniotubular hyperostotic syndrome existing in two forms. *Autosomal dominant osteosclerosis* presents with hyperostosis and osteosclerosis of the skull, mandible, clavicles, and ribs and long bone diaphyseal hyperplasia; VII and VIII cranial nerve deficits may occur.[6874]

In the *autosomal recessive* form, the symptoms are similar but more severe.[6474]

end plate The specialized receptor area on the muscle membrane at the neuromuscular junction.

end-plate acetylcholine receptor deficiency A congenital myasthenic syndrome.[1866] See **myasthenia gravis**.

end-plate acetylcholinesterase deficiency A congenital myasthenic syndrome.[1866] See **myasthenia gravis**.

end-plate activity Spontaneous electric activity recorded with a needle electrode close to muscle end plates. These potentials may have several different morphologies.

1. Monophasic: Low amplitude (10–20 μV), short duration (0.5–1.0 ms) negative potentials occurring in a dense, steady pattern, the exact frequency of which cannot be defined. These nonpropagated potentials are probably miniature end-plate potentials recorded extracellularly. Referred to as end-plate noise or seashell sound (seashell roar or noise).
2. Biphasic: Moderate amplitude (100–300 μV), short duration (2–4 ms), initially negative spike potentials occurring irregularly in short bursts with a high frequency (50–100 Hz). These propagated potentials are generated by muscle fibers excited by activity in nerve terminals. These potentials have been referred to as biphasic spike potentials, end-plate spikes, and incorrectly, nerve potentials. They may also have a biphasic (initially positive) morphology.
3. Triphasic: Similar to biphasic potentials, but the waveforms have three phases with an initial positive deflection. Fire in an irregular fashion; contrast with fibrillation potential.

From the 2001 Report of the Nomenclature Committee of the American Association of Electromyography and Electrodiagnosis.[19] Reproduced by kind permission of the AANEM.

end-plate noise See **end-plate activity** (monophasic).

end-plate potential (EPP) The graded nonpropagated membrane potential induced in the postsynaptic membrane of a muscle fiber by release of acetyl choline from the presynaptic axon terminal in response to an action potential. (From the 2001 Report of the Nomenclature Committee of the American Association of Electromyography and Electrodiagnosis.[19] Reproduced by permission of the AANEM.)

end-plate spike See **end-plate activity** (biphasic).

end-plate zone The region in a muscle where neuromuscular junctions are concentrated.

end-point nystagmus (end-position nystagmus) A form of ill-sustained, irregular, low-amplitude, physiological, gaze-evoked, jerk nystagmus of small (0.5–3 μV) amplitude, at a frequency of 1–3 Hz, seen best in the abducting rather than the adducting eye during maintained far lateral gaze. It probably represents physiological fatigue in the oculomotor muscles.[34] If far lateral gaze is prolonged, **fatigue nystagmus**, a different phenomenon, may also ensue. See also **physiological nystagmus**.

end-position nystagmus See **end-point nystagmus**.

enervate (from Lat, to weaken) To be without energy; the state of weakness.

ENG Abbreviation for **electroneurography** and also for **electronystagmography**.

Engelhard syndrome A dysmorphic syndrome characterized by ptosis polydactyly, syndactyly, microcephaly, intracranial epidermoid and other tumors, and a liability to meningitis.[381]

Engelmann disease See **progressive diaphyseal dysplasia**.

English Malady Usually characterized as hypochondriasis but also including symptoms of depression, cramps and spasms, palsy, abnormal involuntary movements, and fainting spells; all ascribed by Cheyne (G. Strahan and Leake, London & Bath, 1783) to "weak nerves" and to the poor English climate of the time. See **Cheyne disease**.

engram 1. The permanent impression left behind by psychical experience in the brain's cellular network. A latent memory picture, a trace of things experienced. In the words of **Penfield**, "The writing left behind in the brain by conscious experience,"[4976] or, as put by Critchley,[1336] "a memory tracer in a conception of a word or phrase." 2. A functional template, directing the performance of skilled movements.

enhanced physiological tremor A physiological postural tremor of greater than normal amplitude but of rather high frequency (8–12 Hz), resulting from the unusual synchronization of motor unit discharges and frequently associated with hyperadrenergic states such as anxiety and some toxic and metabolic syndromes.[2052]

enhanced ptosis Relatively increased drooping of one eyelid when the subject with **myasthenia gravis** looks upward, while the other eyelid is also elevated but is maintained in that position by the examiner's finger.

In a variation of the response, the descending eyelid oscillates to a point of complete closure.[2493]

enkephalins A class of opioid pentapeptides (meta- and leuenkephalin) widely distributed in the brain and spinal cord (nucleus of the V nerve, substantia gelatinosa) in areas relevant to the transmission of pain impulses.

ENMG See **electroneuromyography**.

enolases A family of glycolytic dimeric enzymes. Neuron-specific enolase is usually found in ganglion cells but is not restricted to them.

enteric brain (enteric nervous system) Networks of ganglion cell bodies, preganglionic parasympathetic and postganglionic sympathetic fibers with their interneurons, arising from the neural crest and forming the myenteric and submucosal plexuses of the gastrointestinal tract. It can function independently of the central nervous system. Disorders arising from the enteric nervous system include **Allgrove syndrome**, achalasia, **familial visceral neuropathy** and myopathy, Hirschprung **disease**, **MNGIE**, acute intestinal ileus, and intestinal pseudo-obstruction.[2535]

enteric cysts See **enterogenous cysts**.

enteric nervous system See **enteric brain**.

enterogenous cysts (enteric cysts) Extrinsic intraspinal cysts containing elements of gut (such as a mucin-secreting mucous membrane), situated usually in the subarachnoid space and associated often with local defects in the vertebral bodies. See **neurenteric cyst**.

entomopia (from Gr, insect + eye) A rare form of polyopia in which the subject sees multiple reduplicated images in rows and columns, as one supposes to be the experience of those insects possessing compound eyes. The phenomenon has been reported as a result of lesions of the cornea or lens, and with lesions of the occipital lobe.[3910]

entomopia (from Gr, Insect + eye) A form of polyopia caused by occipital lobe pathology, in which a subject experiences multiple copies of the same visual impression in a gridlike pattern.[3910]

entonia (Gr, tension) Tonic spasm.

entopic images See **entoptic images**.

entoptic images (entopic images) Those images that arise from within the optic globe itself.

entorhinal cortex The parahippocampal area.

entrainment Synchronization to external time cues.

entrapment neuropathy Neural deficits consequent upon nerve compression.[3530]

entrapped temporal horn "Obstruction of the trigone of the lateral ventricle which seals off the temporal horn from the rest of the ventricular system" causing homonymous hemianopia, memory disturbances and hemiparesis due to compression of the internal capsule.[6665]

entropion Inward turning of the eyelids. Cf. **ectropion**.

enuresis Recurrent involuntary micturition occurring during sleep in the absence of any urologic, medical, or psychiatric pathology. Diurnal and nocturnal forms relate to the time of occurrence of enuresis, while paralytic and spastic forms relate to the lower or upper motor neuron lesions causing it respectively. In a more restricted sense, the word is applied only to involuntary micturition during any phase of sleep in subjects with normal daytime bladder control. It is considered abnormal in most cases after the age of 10 years.

In *primary enuresis*, the child never achieves continuous dry nights, while in *secondary enuresis* the child has had at least 3 months of dryness then reverting to the pattern of enuresis, usually in the first third of the night. The episodes can also occur during nocturnal wakefulness.

environmental dependency syndrome

environmental dependency syndrome Complex behavioral sequences in which the patient recognizes the environmental situation in which he finds himself (or accepts a suggestion as to its nature) and acts out behavior which would be appropriate in that situation, but which in fact is inappropriate for the subject to perform—such as watering someone else's garden, examining the physician's throat, etc. In a *variant* form, patients are "forced" to comment verbally on situations and activities occurring around them (*forced hyperphasia*).[6202] The syndrome is considered to represent a failure of personal autonomy, secondary to unilateral lesions of the frontal lobe.[3827]

environmental sleep disorder

environmental sleep disorder A sleep disturbance due to a disturbing environmental factor that causes a complaint of either insomnia or excessive sleepiness. Sleep efficiency and duration are normal, there are no psychological factors which induce the disturbance of sleep, and removal of the disturbing stimulus leads to eventual restoration of normal sleep patterns. The following are the AASM-suggested diagnostic criteria:[1629]

A. A complaint of insomnia or excessive sleepiness.
B. The complaint is temporally associated with the introduction of a physically measurable stimulus or environmental circumstance that disturbs sleep.
C. The physical properties of the environmental factor account for the sleep complaint; the psychological meaning of the environmental factor does not account for the complaint.
D. Removal of the causative environmental factor results in immediate or gradual restoration of normal sleep.
E. The disorder has been present for more than 3 weeks.
F. Polysomnographic monitoring demonstrates normal sleep efficiency and duration.
G. No evidence of significant underlying medical or psychiatric disorder accounting for the complaint.
H. Does not meet the diagnostic criteria for any other sleep disorder causing a complaint of insomnia or excessive sleepiness, for example, toxin-induced sleep disorder.

From AASM Diagnostic Classification Steering Committee. *The International Classification of Sleep Disorders Diagnostic and Coding Manual*. Rochester, MN. American Academy of Sleep Medicine 1991/2001. Reproduced by kind permission of the Academy). See also http://www.sleepeducation.com/Disorders.aspx.

Environmental Status Scale

Environmental Status Scale A rating scale designed to quantify the handicap experienced by patients with **multiple sclerosis**.[4296] See **socioeconomic scale**. See also **Kurtzke disability status scale**.

eosinophilia-myalgia syndrome

eosinophilia-myalgia syndrome The occurrence of joint pain, generalized myalgias which limit the subject in the activities of daily living, and eosinophilia ($>1 \times 10^9$ cells/l) in the peripheral blood and muscle infiltrates, in the absence of other (infectious or allergic) disease.[206]

Weakness, severe muscle pain, a scleroderma-like skin rash, mouth ulcers, pruritus, angioedema, fever, abdominal pains, and subcutaneous nodules also occur. Evidence of myopathy or peripheral axonal polyneuropathy is found in a quarter of the subjects and cognitive complaints (of fatigue, impaired memory and attention, representing a selective **dysexecutive syndrome**) may persist long into the recovery period. The erythrocyte sedimentation rate is normal.

The syndrome has most commonly been described in women who had taken (allegedly contaminated) oral L-tryptophan for premenstrual complaints, insomnia, or depression.[2884] See also **eosinophilic fasciitis, eosinophilic perimyositis,** and **eosinophilic polymyositis**.

eosinophilic adenoma

eosinophilic adenoma A benign tumor of the pituitary gland with a propensity to secrete growth hormone and thus the usual lesion in patients with **gigantism** or **acromegaly**.

eosinophilic fasciitis

eosinophilic fasciitis (Schulman syndrome) A syndrome occurring after a prodrome of fever, myalgia, arthralgia, and fatigue, in which there is tenderness and edema of the skin of the neck, trunk, and proximal limbs, which later becomes indurated or even leathery ("peau d'orange"), with patchy hyperpigmentation; interstitial myositis of subjacent muscles; eosinophilia; and painful distal joint contractures, synovitis, and nerve compression syndromes in many cases. The clinical features, mainly seen in adult males, may be precipitated by vigorous exercise.[5815] Accompanying symptoms of **carpal tunnel syndrome** and eosinophilia and hypergammaglobulinemia are not unusual, and anemia, lymphoma, and leukemia have also been associated. The presence of the **groove sign** strongly suggests the diagnosis.[5847] See also **eosinophilia-myalgia syndrome**.

eosinophilic granulomatous vasculitis

eosinophilic granulomatous vasculitis See **Churg–Strauss syndrome**.

eosinophilic myelitis

eosinophilic myelitis Infection of the spinal cord, usually with *Angiostrongylus cantonensis* or *Gnathostoma sphingerum*, leading to increased intracranial pressure, symptoms of meningitis, and sensory features typical of transverse myelitis with radicular pain. Obstructive hydrocephalus is also described. The infection is most often described in South Pacific or Southeast Asian regions and occurs after the ingestion of snails or fowls cooked rare.

Diagnosis is made through Giemsa staining of the CSF, which demonstrates the eosinophilia. ELISA antibody tests are available at Mahidol University in Bankok.

eosinophilic perimyositis

eosinophilic perimyositis A syndrome of relapsing myalgia accompanied by nonspecific inflammatory features with a perimysial infiltrate consisting of eosinophils in muscles, but with minimal peripheral eosinophilia. Biopsy evidence of fascitis is not found, there are no skin changes, and the response to anti-inflammatory agents is prompt, although relapses can occur.[5734] See also **eosinophilia-myalgia syndrome, eosinophilic polymyositis,** and **eosinophilic fasciitis**.

eosinophilic polymyositis

eosinophilic polymyositis A rare inflammatory disease of muscle in which systemic visceral manifestations, including encephalopathy and neuropathy, occur in conjunction with severe proximal or generalized muscle weakness or tenderness, localized painful swelling of muscles, and features of the hypereosinophilic syndrome.

Myocarditis, pericarditis, and multiple mononeuropathy have been reported to occur in association with the disorder.[3727] The condition may be a variant of the **Churg–Strauss syndrome**.[3727] It differs from **polymyositis** in the number of eosinophils in the inflamed muscles. See also **eosinophilia-myalgia syndrome** and the preceding entries.

eosinophilic vasculitis A component of the **Churg–Strauss syndrome** affecting the nervous system alone in rare cases as a focal inflammatory encephalopathy.[5950]

epaxial muscles (Gr, upon + Lat, an axis) Those muscles which lie above the central axis of the embryo, divided between dorsolateral and ventrolateral groups.

ependyma (Gr, a cloak or upper garment) The epithelial membrane lining the ventricles and the central canal of the spinal cord, named by **Virchow**.

ependymitis Inflammation of the ependyma, either as part of a generalized **meningitis** or due to specific infections with, for example, *toxoplasma.* See also **ventriculitis**.

ependymoblastoma A poorly differentiated, primary neuroectodermal tumor arising in the fourth ventricle in children, characterized by the prominent formation of perivascular **pseudorosettes**.[6]

ependymoma A primary neuroectodermal malignant but slowly growing glial tumor arising from the ependymal lining of the ventricles, spinal cord, or cauda equina occurring in childhood and occasionally in adult life. Their histological characteristics vary but include the presence of ciliated cuboidal epithelial cells, rosettes of ependymal cells, **pseudorosettes, Rosenthal fibers**, positive staining for S100 protein and **glial fibrillary acidic protein** but not carbonic anhydrase C, absence of a collagenous stroma, and, in well-differentiated forms, uniformity of nuclear morphology. **Ependymoblastoma, subependymoma**, and *well differentiated*, *poorly differentiated*, *anaplastic,* and *myxopapillary* types are distinguished, the latter arising from the filum terminale and characterized by the presence of columnar cells surrounding mucoid zones.[6] A *giant cell* variety is especially rare.

ephapse A point of abnormal communication where an action potential in one muscle fiber or axon can cause depolarization of an adjacent muscle fiber or axon, generating an action potential in it. Such abnormal electrical cross-communications formed between adjacent demyelinated axons are supposed to represent the result of prior local trauma. (From the 2001 Report of the Nomenclature Committee of the American Association of Electromyography and Electrodiagnosis.[19] Reproduced by kind permission of the AANEM.)

ephaptic transmission (axonal cross-talk) The situation in which nerve compression and the resulting local demyelination cause the spontaneous formation of a false synapse where ectopic activity may be triggered by mechanical irritation, changes in regional electrolyte concentration, or flow of extracellular current during passage of nerve impulses in adjacent fibers (an **ephapse**).This ectopic activity may then be conducted orthodromically or antidromically within the nerve fiber.

This may lead to pain (e.g., **trigeminal neuralgia, complex regional pain syndrome**) or motor manifestations (e.g., **hemifacial spasm**). It has been invoked to explain the repetitive firing of neurons in other chronic denervating states such as radiculopathy.[6345] See also **myokymic discharge** and **complex repetitive discharge**.

epi- Greek prefix, signifying "upon" or "beside."

epiblepharon A craniofacial malformation, sometimes dominantly inherited, in which there is absence of the palpebral groove, due to maldevelopment of the insertion of the levator palpebrae superioris muscle, with a horizontal fold of skin over the tarsal region, best seen on downward gaze.[4]

epicanthis See **epicanthus**.

epicanthus (epicanthis) 1. The inner angle of the eye. 2. A dominantly inherited craniofacial malformation in which a bilateral symmetrical skin fold (the *epicanthal fold*) runs vertically at the naso-orbital angle.[4]

epicrania fugax A stereotypical, strictly unilateral, shooting paroxysmal pain starting in the posterior parietal or temporal region and rapidly spreading forward to the ipsilateral eye or nose along a lineal or zigzag trajectory, the complete sequence lasting 1–10 s. Attacks can be either spontaneous or triggered by touch. The frequency ranges from two attacks per month to countless attacks per day, and the temporal pattern is either remitting or chronic.[4892]

epicranium The soft tissues attached to the outer surfaces of the skull bones below the **pericranium**.

epicritic (from Gr, discernment or judgment) Superficial sensations, capable of precise appreciation and localization. This implies cortical assessment and perception of the stimulus—for example, discriminative light touch, direction of scratch, and the recognition of the finer gradations of temperature into warm and cool. It is characterized by low threshold, short latency, high adaptability, and accurate localization and discrimination.[2864] It returns later than protopathic sensation during the process of recovery from a nerve injury.

The word was employed by Sir Henry **Head**; the other class of sensation which he defined, he called **protopathic**.

epidemic chorea See **hysteria**.

epidemic convulsions Hysterical seizure-like movements (the *Jerks* and the *Barks*) witnessed during a period of fundamental religious fervor in Tennessee and Kentucky during the mid-eighteenth century and regarded then either as tokens of divine favor or as a form of chorea.[6897] See **pseudoseizures**.

epidemic encephalitis See **encephalitis lethargica**.

epidemic myalgia See **pleurodynia**.

epidemic myalgic encephalomyelitis (epidemic myalgia) See **chronic fatigue syndrome**.

epidemic neurolabyrinthitis See **epidemic vertigo**.

epidemic neuromyasthenia See **postinfection fatigue syndrome**.

epidemic neuromyelitis An acute illness resembling ascending infectious polyneuritis, seen in Rio de Janeiro in 1931 but not reported since.

epidemic paralytic vertigo See **Gerlier disease**.

epidemic pleurodynia (Bornholm disease) A benign sporadic or epidemic localized inflammatory myopathy resulting from infection by coxsackie B viruses. Clinically, children are affected more often than adults, and they complain of headache, fever, and severe localized pain and tenderness in the muscles of the chest wall, shoulders, or back.

epidemic spastic paraparesis The sudden onset of spastic paraparesis associated with speech disturbances and visual complaints, occurring epidemically (and also sporadically) in central Africa. Recovery may be complete or dysarthria and paraparesis may remain. Both infectious and toxic causes have been suspected.[1046]

epidemic vertigo (epidemic neurolabyrinthitis) Small epidemics characterized by the sudden onset of vertigo, with accompanying nausea and vomiting which become paroxysmal but with decreasing frequency and intensity; many attacks follow upper respiratory or gastrointestinal symptoms, and a chronic asthenic phase is reported in a minority of cases. The etiology is not known.[4961] See **vestibular neuronitis**.

epidermal nevus syndrome (nevus unis lateralis, epidermal nevus, ichthyosis linearis neuropathica, Feuerstein–Mills syndrome, linear nevus sebaceus syndrome) A rare, sporadic, congenital **neurocutaneous syndrome**.

The skin lesions include raised, yellow-brown, verrucous skin lesions, and orange-brown waxy plaques; nevus unis lateralis; ichthyosis hystrix; acanthosis nigricans; midline linear sebaceous nevi on the scalp, neck, or face, with later hyperkeratosis and verrucous transformation. The associated neurological disorders are due to cortical dysgenesis and include mental retardation, cortical atrophy, seizures, hydrocephalus, hyperkinesis, and a variety of focal signs signifying cortical dysfunction, usually on the same side as any skin lesions present on the face or head.[345, 2038]

Colobomas of the iris, congenital cardiac anomalies, renal tumors, porencephaly, megalencephaly, sebaceous adenomas, skin pigmentation, asymmetrical limbs, and cerebral neoplasms are also described in this condition.

A *variant* form comprises facial epidermal nevus, ipsilateral hemimegalencephaly, and gyral malformations, mental retardation, seizures including early infantile spasms, and, sometimes, facial hemihypertrophy.[4943]

epidermoid cyst (epidermoid tumor) A cyst composed of squamous epidermal cells in a fibrous and keratinized wall containing cholesterol, situated usually in the cisterns at the skull base, in the cerebellopontine angle, at the cauda equina level, or within the substance of the cord.[558] See also **dermoid cyst**.

epidermoid tumor See **epidermoid cyst**.

epidural abscess Pyogenic infection of the cranial or spinal meninges in which the pus lies external to the dura and adjacent to the bone, mainly posteriorly and usually at thoracic levels.

The infection results from the spread of local (vertebral) disease or from hematogenous spread and occurs most commonly in immunocompromised or chronically sick people. The major clinical features are rapidly progressive myelopathy with progressive paraparesis and sphincter involvement, and severe local and radicular pain with local tenderness.

epidural ascending spinal paralysis See **hypertrophic spinal meningitis** and **Spiller syndrome**.

epidural block The injection of anesthetic solutions into the epidural space in order to produce regional anesthesia. The neurological complications of this technique have been reviewed.[3283]

epidural blood patch A technique of injecting autologous whole blood into the epidural space under sterile conditions in order to relieve postlumbar puncture headache, which it does safely and effectively in a high proportion of cases.[2509]

epidural electrode A recording electrode placed upon the dural covering of the cerebrum.

epidural hematoma See **epidural hemorrhage**.

epidural hemorrhage (epidural hematoma, extradural hemorrhage, or hematoma) Bleeding outside the outermost layer of the dura mater, which is thus stripped away from the inner table of the skull or spinal canal.

In almost all cases of *intracranial epidural hemorrhage*, the cause is traumatic, most often with rupture of the middle meningeal artery as a result of a fracture of the temporal bone.

Traumatic spinal epidural hematomas are associated with fracture-dislocations of the spine and cause acute or subacute myelopathy.

Nontraumatic (spontaneous) spinal epidural hematomas are usually venous in origin and occur in the setting of minor trauma, pregnancy, physical exertion, abnormal bleeding tendencies, etc.[3716]

epigastric aura An indescribable sensation in the pit of the stomach, sometimes rising to the head, occurring as the initial manifestation of some forms of complex partial seizure with origin in the temporal lobe. The lack of appropriate words which can be summoned up by the patient to describe his experience is a characteristic finding.

epigastric reflex Light stroking of the skin downward from the nipple normally leads to contraction of the epigastric muscles. The reflex informs on the reflex arcs T5–T7, but, being a superficial reflex, it is lost with upper motor neuron lesions above these levels.

epigenetics The study of the mechanisms of temporal and spatial control of gene activity during the development of complex organisms—thus, any aspect other than DNA sequence that influences the development of an organism.

Epilepsia A neurological subspecialty journal, the official organ of the International League against Epilepsy.

Address: Raven Press, 1185 Avenue of the Americas, Department 1B, New York, NY 10036. Web site: http://www.epilepsia.com/.

epilepsia arithmetices The precipitation of epileptic seizures as a result of performing mental arithmetic.[3090]

A similar condition occasionally affects computers.

epilepsia cursiva (running fit) See **cursive epilepsy**.

epilepsia larvata A postepileptic phenomenon which Esquirol called "masked" epilepsy, referring to the confused speech and automatic movements made following a tonic-clonic seizure, which was in those days thought to be itself a seizure manifestation.

epilepsia minoris continua See **status epilepticus**.

epilepsia nutans A discarded term for **myoclonic epilepsy**.

epilepsia partialis continua See **partial continuous epilepsy**.

epilepsie rotatoria See **tornado epilepsy**.

epilepsy (Gr, a seizure) 1. A tendency to recurrent epileptic seizures. This definition is not as silly as it sounds, because one seizure does not constitute epilepsy. 2. A condition characterized by recurrent (two or more) epileptic seizures, unprovoked by any immediate identified cause. Multiple seizures occurring in a 24-h period and an episode of status epilepticus are considered to represent a single event. Those who have had only febrile seizures or only neonatal seizures as herein defined are excluded from this category.[1265]

The condition was known to Hippocrates, who recorded it in children as "The Sacred Disease,"[2909] as epilepsy was then considered to be caused by a temporary departure of the soul from the body. Even in the past 100 years, attempts to call the soul back by waving a garment of the patient from the rooftops and banging gongs have been recorded in China. Hippocrates argued that it was a malady affecting the whole constitution and rejected the concept that it was a divine imposition. He also recognized that injury to one side of the brain may cause a seizure to occur on the other side of the body.[1253]

The word *epilepsy* was the invention of the Arab physician **Avicenna**. Previous names had included *hieron nosema*, *nosema paideon*, *morbus lunaticus*, *morbus major sonticus*, *morbus caducus*, *Herculean disease* (perhaps due to the strength of the convulsive movements) and the *great evil*. In England, Germany, and France it came to be known as the *falling evil* or the *falling sickness*.

Focal (partial or localization-related) epilepsies were described by **Bravais** and later by **Jackson**, but had actually been recorded by **Aretaeus** nearly 1800 years before.[235] The condition was well known in biblical times, accounts of the epileptic boy's presentation to Christ appearing in the Gospels of St. Luke and St. Mark (chapter 9). At this time, the condition was popularly regarded as evidence of demoniacal possession; and in Rome, gatherings were discontinued when an attender had a seizure, and Romans spat in the street when they passed an epileptic person, a custom which survived until the end of the eighteenth century in France. With medicine impotent to help, such reactions may have prompted the frequent appeals made to many saints, of whom 37 (ranging from SS Sebastian and Valentine to St. Edward the Confessor) have been considered to have an especial interest in the subject. Sauvage in 1750 collected all extant work on the subject, including Boerhaave's classification of the causes and description of the sign, in his book *Nosologie d'Epilepsie*. Pinel (who regarded epilepsy as a neurosis, i.e., something caused by a neurological disorder) established a hospital for epileptics at the **Salpêtrière** in 1795, generating a large research output on the subject. Effective treatment began with Sir Charles Locock's introduction of bromides; Hauptmann's publication on phenobarbitone occurred in 1910,[2794] and Merritt and Putnam synthesized phenytoin in 1934.

Among those claimed to have been subject to seizures (not always on good evidence) have been St. Paul, Julius Caesar, Caligula, Germanicus Brittanicus, Mahomet, Charles V, at least one Holy Roman Emperor, Peter the Great, the Duke of Marlborough, Balzac, the Emperor Napoleon, the Duke of Wellington, Lord Byron, Schiller, Handel, Mendelssohn, **Dostoevsky**, and Mozart.[1253] Among Shakespearean characters, Henry IV and Julius Caesar were depicted as suffering generalized, and Othello and Macbeth, complex focal (partial) seizures.

At least 11 genes have been shown to be causative, almost all coding for ion channel subunits.

Classification of Epilepsies and Epileptic Syndromes

A distinction is drawn between the various types of seizure and the syndromes of which such seizures are a manifestation. The former may be seen as colors on the palette of an artist, and the latter as a painting; the different epileptic syndromes are composed of various kinds of seizure.[1713] Those printed in bold face in Charts E–2 and E–3 are defined or described in the place appropriate to their alphabetization. See also the dictionary of Gastaut[2305] and the discussion of epileptic syndromes by Delgado-Escueta.[1556]

Generalized epileptic disorders are characterized by seizures in which there are symptoms suggesting bilateral cerebral involvement, reflected clinically and in the bilateral abnormalities of the EEG at the onset of the seizure. They reflect dysfunction of the whole brain or of major brain systems. In the *focal epilepsies* (formerly and strangely known as *partial epilepsies* but now more appropriately named), the clinical and electrographic features indicate that the seizure originates in one or more discrete brain regions.

An amended version of the 2006 revision of the International League Against Epilepsy's (ILAE) classification of *epileptic seizure types*, with added data from Panayiotopoulos, *Epileptic Syndromes and Their Treatment* (2007),[4882] is given in Chart E–2. It differs from the older classification designed for genetic studies[1557] and from the epilepsy syndromes and related conditions which are presented in Chart E–3.

Chart E–3 lists epilepsy syndromes and related conditions, organized following the scheme of Panayiotopoulos, *Epileptic Syndromes and Their* Treatment (2007),[4882] reproduced by kind permission and blending material from the revised (2006) ILAE classification.[1861]

Web sites relevant to epilepsy include the following:

- American Epilepsy Society A professional organization. http://www.aesnet.org
- British Epilepsy Association http://www.epilepsy.org.uk/
- Epilepsy Foundation of America http://www.epilepsyfoundation.org
- National Society of Epilepsy http://www.epilepsynse.org.uk/

Chart E–2. ILAE Classification of Epileptic Seizure Types

A. *Self-limited seizure types*

1. *Generalized seizures*

Tonic-clonic seizures (includes variations beginning with a clonic or myoclonic phase)
Clonic seizures (with or without tonic features)
Absence seizures Typical, Atypical, and Myoclonic
Tonic seizures
Spasms
Myoclonic seizures
Massive bilateral myoclonus
Eyelid myoclonia (with or without absences)
Myoclonic atonic seizures
Negative myoclonus
Atonic seizures
Reflex seizures in generalized epilepsy syndromes
Seizures of the posterior neocortex
Neocortical temporal lobe seizures

2. *Focal seizures*

Focal sensory seizures
With elementary sensory symptoms (e.g., occipital and parietal lobe seizures)
With experiential sensory symptoms (e.g., temporo-parieto-occipital junction seizures)
Focal motor seizures
With elementary clonic motor signs
With asymmetrical tonic motor seizures (e.g., supplementary motor seizures)
With typical (temporal lobe) automatisms (e.g., mesial temporal lobe seizures)
With hyperkinetic automatisms
With focal negative myoclonus
With inhibitory motor seizures
Gelastic seizures
Hemiclonic seizures
Secondarily generalized seizures
Reflex seizures in focal epilepsy syndromes

B. *Continuous seizure types*

1 *Generalized* **status epilepticus**

Generalized tonic-clonic status epilepticus
Absence status (typical, atypical, and myoclonic)
Clonic, tonic, and tonic-clonic status epilepticus
Myoclonic status epilepticus
Subtle status epilepticus

2. *Focal status*

Epilepsia partialis continua (of Kojevnikov) as with Rasmussen syndrome, focal lesions, or some inborn errors of metabolism)
Supplementary motor area status epilepticus
Aura continua
Dyscognitive focal (limbic) status epilepticus (psychomotor status); medial temporal or neocortical forms
Hemiconvulsive status with hemiparesis

Abstracted from the Web site: http://www.ilae-epilepsy.org/Visitors/Centre/ctf/seizure_types.cfm/.

epilepsy and febrile seizures-plus A benign, dominantly inherited syndrome of febrile convulsions and various other (usually generalized tonic-clonic) seizure types, occurring in children and in the absence of fever. Absences, myoclonic, or atonic seizures can also occur. Various chromosomal linkages have been determined; the condition is genetically heterogeneous.[3783]

epilepsy and mental retardation limited to females A dominantly inherited seizure disorder with onset in early childhood, in which half of the affected females are also mentally retarded.[3255]

Epilepsy Canada A national, nonprofit organization dedicated to improving the quality of life of people with epilepsy and their families. Address:1470 Peel St., #745 Montreal, Quebec H3A 1T1, Canada. Tel: 514-845-7855. E-mail: epilepsy@epilepsy.ca. Web site: http://www.epilepsy.ca/.

Chart E–3. Classification of Epilepsy Syndromes and Related Conditions

Neonatal epileptic seizures and syndromes

The main types of neonatal seizures are *subtle; tonic; clonic; and myoclonic seizures and nonparoxysmal repetitive behaviors*. The four syndromes recognized are

Benign familial neonatal seizures
Benign neonatal seizures (nonfamilial)
Early myoclonic encephalopathy
Ohtahara syndrome

Idiopathic epileptic seizures and syndromes in infancy

Benign familial and **nonfamilial infantile seizures (Watanabe–Vigevano syndrome)**
Benign myoclonic epilepsy in infancy
Febrile seizuresGeneralized epilepsies with febrile seizures plus (GEFS+)

Epileptic encephalopathies in infancy and childhood

Dravet syndrome (severe myoclonic epilepsy in infancy)
Early myoclonic encephalopathy (see neonatal syndromes)
Epilepsy with continuous spikes and waves during slow-wave sleep
Hypothalamic (gelastic) epilepsy
Landau–Kleffner syndrome
Lennox–Gastaut syndrome
Myoclonic status in nonprogressive encephalopathies
Ohtahara syndrome (see neonatal syndromes)
West syndrome

Severe neocortical epileptic syndromes in infancy and childhood

Hemiconvulsion-hemiplegia syndrome
Kozhevnikov–Rasmussen syndrome
Migrating partial epilepsy of early childhood
Partial continuous epilepsy (epilepsia partialis continua of Kozhevnikov) is a lengthy motor seizure-type or motor status epilepticus, but not an epileptic syndrome.

Benign childhood focal seizures

Benign childhood epilepsy with centrotemporal spikes (Rolandic seizures)
Gastaut-type idiopathic childhood occipital epilepsy
Panayiotopoulos syndrome

*Idiopathic-generalized epilepsies (**IGE**)(ILAE, 2006)*

Childhood absence epilepsy
Epilepsy with myoclonic absences
Epilepsy with myoclonic astatic seizures (Doose syndrome)
IG Epilepsy with GTCS only
Juvenile absence epilepsy (Janz)
Juvenile myoclonic epilepsy
Myoclonic epilepsy in infancy (see syndromes in infancy)
Other nonrecognized syndromes of IGEs include **IGE with phantom absences** and **perioral myoclonia with absences**

Familial (autosomal dominant) focal epilepsies

Autosomal dominant nocturnal frontal lobe epilepsy
Benign familial infantile seizures (See idiopathic epileptic seizures and syndromes in infancy)
Benign familial neonatal seizures (See epileptic syndromes in neonates)
Familial autosomal dominant lateral temporal lobe epilepsy
Familial focal epilepsy with variable foci
Familial mesial temporal lobe epilepsy

Symptomatic and probably symptomatic focal epilepsies

Common frontal lobe seizures depending on localization
Frontal lobe epilepsies
Occipital lobe epilepsies

Parietal lobe epilepsies
Temporal lobe epilepsy (TLE); **mesial temporal lobe epilepsy with hippocampal sclerosis;** (hippocampal epilepsy); **lateral temporal lobe epilepsy**

Reflex seizures and related epileptic syndromes

Idiopathic reading epilepsy
Photosensitive epilepsy—the most common form of reflex epilepsy, not an epilepsy syndrome
Idiopathic photosensitive occipital lobe epilepsy
Jeavons syndrome (eyelid myoclonia with absences)
Self-induced seizures
Television-induced epileptic seizures
Video game–induced seizures
Startle epilepsy

Reproduced by kind permission from Panayiotopoulos, C; Epileptic Syndromes and Their Treatment (2007),[4882] *with blending of material from the revised (2006) ILAE classification.*[1861]

Epilepsy Foundation of America A charitable organization in this field. Address: 4351 Garden City Dr., Suite 500, Landover, MD 20785-7223. Tel: 301-459-3700; 800-332-1000. E-mail: postmaster@efa.org. Web site: http://www.epilepsyfoundation.org/.

epilepsy, heterochromia iridis and deafness A rare variant of **Usher syndrome** in which the iris changes are added features.

epilepsy in remission with treatment A prevalent case of epilepsy with no seizures for 5 or more years and receiving antiepileptic drugs at the time of ascertainment.[1265]

epilepsy in remission without treatment A prevalent case of epilepsy with no seizures for 5 or more years and not receiving antiepileptic drugs at the time of ascertainment.[1265]

Epilepsy Research (incorporating the *Journal of Epilepsy*) A neurological subspecialty journal published by Elsevier Science. Web site: http://www.elsevier.com/locate/epilepsyres.

epilepsy seizure scales See **Chalfont Scale; Hague Scale;** and **VA Scale.**

epilepsy with continuous spike-waves during slow-wave sleep See **electrical status epilepticus during sleep.**

epilepsy with evoked parietal spikes An uncommon seizure disorder characterized by the presence of focal attacks without loss of consciousness, or with generalized seizures. Parietal spikes or spike-wave discharges are recorded on the EEG. In some cases, a similar EEG occurs but only when the contralateral foot is tapped. Thus, it appears that the condition may or may not find any clinical expression.[1568]

epilepsy with generalized tonic-clonic seizures on awakening A syndrome with its onset occurring mostly in the second decade of life. The seizures occur exclusively or predominantly (>90% of the time) shortly after awakening, regardless of the time of day, or in a second seizure peak in the evening period of relaxation. If other seizures occur, they are mostly absence or myoclonic, as in **juvenile myoclonic epilepsy**. Seizures may be precipitated by sleep deprivation and other external factors. Genetic predisposition is relatively frequent. The EEG shows one of the patterns of idiopathic generalized epilepsy. There is a significant correlation with photosensitivity. (After Dreifuss FE, et al. Commission for classification and terminology, ILAE. Proposal for revised classifications of epilepsies and epileptic syndromes. *Epilepsia* 1989;**30**:389–99 and reproduced by kind permission of Wiley-Blackwell Publications.)

epilepsy with infantile baldness and mental retardation A syndrome characterized by such features from birth. Both major motor and complex partial seizures are described in the few kinships reported.[4527]

epilepsy with myoclonic absences A rare syndrome clinically characterized by absences accompanied by severe bilateral, rhythmical clonic jerks, often associated with a tonic contraction, in children aged between 1 and 12 years with male preponderance. Impairment of consciousness may be mild or severe. On the EEG, these clinical features are always accompanied by bilateral, synchronous, and symmetrical discharge of rhythmical spike-waves at 3 Hz, as in childhood absence attacks. Seizures occur many times a day.[4757, 4882]

Awareness of the jerks may be maintained. Associated seizures such as GTCS or atonic fits are not uncommon. The prognosis is less favorable than in pyknolepsy owing to resistance to therapy of the seizures, mental deterioration, and possible evolution to other types of epilepsy such as **juvenile myoclonic epilepsy** or **Lennox–Gastaut syndrome**. The most recent ILAE publication, however, suggests that this may be a syndrome of unknown provenance. (See Dreifuss FE, et al. Commission for classification and terminology, ILAE. Proposal for revised classifications of epilepsies and epileptic syndromes. *Epilepsia* 1989;**30**:389–99.)

epilepsy with myoclonic-astatic seizures (Doose syndrome) An uncommon epileptic syndrome in which myoclonic-astatic seizures manifest as symmetrical myoclonic jerks immediately followed by loss of muscle tone (atonic component) and causing lightning-like falls, head nodding, or bending of the knees, with onset between the ages of 7 months and 6 years and with twice as many boys affected as girls. There is frequently a hereditary predisposition and usually a normal developmental background. The seizures comprise myoclonic, astatic, and myoclonic-astatic attacks, absences with clonic and tonic components, and tonic–clonic seizures. Status frequently occurs. Tonic seizures develop late in unfavorable cases.

The EEG, initially often normal except for 4–7 Hz rhythms, may have irregular fast spike-wave or polyspike-waves. In the event of nonconvulsive status lasting hours or more, there are continuous or discontinuous and repetitive 2–3 Hz spikes and waves. The course and outcome are variable.[4882, 1861]

epilepsy-telangiectasia syndrome A recessively inherited dysmorphic syndrome characterized by conjunctival telangiectasias, brachydactyly, seizures, and mental retardation. See **ataxia-telangiectasia-like syndrome.**

epileptic amnesia See **transient epileptic amnesia.**

epileptic aphasic syndrome (Landau–Kleffner syndrome) A syndrome of acquired temporary aphasia lasting days to months, in the absence of any detectable focal cerebral disease but associated with heterogeneous clinical seizures and with generalized spike-and-wave discharges on the EEG, and with the clinical and electrographic abnormalities abating together.[2462] Criteria for the diagnosis of *ictal aphasia* have been defined as follows:[5399]

The patient must be alert and speaking during the ictus
The speech produced must be dysphasic (dysnomic, nonfluent, and paraphasic)
Simultaneous EEG demonstrates seizure activity which comes and goes with the seizure events.

epileptic cephalea Headache occurring as the only manifestation of a seizure disorder.[2708]

epileptic discharge 1. A diffuse or localized but temporary paroxysmal change in EEG activity, characterized by high-amplitude rhythmic discharges due to excessive synchronization of potentials in an aggregation of neurons and less frequently by high-frequency, low-amplitude discharges.
2. Occasional, sudden, rapid, local and excessive discharges of gray matter (Hughlings **Jackson**).

epileptic drop attacks See **atonic seizures.**

epileptic encephalopathies 1. Syndromes comprising daytime absence-type seizures and nocturnal orofacial seizures during slow-wave sleep, mental impairment, aphasia, or speech arrest, with EEG activation during nonrapid eye movement sleep and the disappearance of the worst of the abnormalities during periods of rapid eye movement sleep.[4931] 2. A group of devastating seizure syndromes which begin in infancy and early childhood, usually resulting in intractable epilepsy. Most are associated with slowing of cognitive function and the evolution of severe behavioral disorders. The EEG demonstrates **hypsarrhythmia** in infancy and slow generalized spike-wave discharges and burst-suppression patterns later. Multiple seizure types and resistance to conventional therapies are characteristic.

The conditions include atypical benign partial epilepsy, **early infantile epileptic encephalopathy, early myoclonic encephalopathy** (neonatal), **electrical status epilepticus in slow-wave sleep, Dravet syndrome, Landau–Kleffner syndrome, Lennox–Gastaut syndrome, migrating partial epilepsy in infancy, myoclonic astatic epilepsy, Ohtahara syndrome (neonatal), severe infantile multifocal epilepsy, severe myoclonic epilepsy of infancy,** and **West syndrome. Hypothalamic (gelastic) epilepsy** also manifests with progressive severe seizures and cognitive and behavioral decline.

epileptic encephalopathy with continuous spike-and-wave during sleep An epileptic syndrome which may be identical with **Landau–Kleffner Syndrome.**[1861]

epileptic endocrine syndrome (Bondin–Barbizet syndrome) Mental retardation and precocious puberty with accelerated growth in epileptic children, due in most cases to a hypothalamic or diencephalic lesion.[733]

epileptic forced thinking See **forced thinking.**

epileptic mydriasis Temporary unilateral fixed dilatation of a pupil after an epileptic seizure.[4886]

epileptic myoclonus 1. Those forms of **myoclonus** which are related to some **epileptic syndrome.** These include **cortical reflex myoclonus; reticular reflex myoclonus;** and **primary generalized epileptic myoclonus.** In all forms, the EMG burst length is less than 50 ms, the muscles are synchronously activated by the same discharge, and a correlated discharge is recordable on the EEG.[2695] See also **nonepileptic myoclonus.**
2. (*petit mal triad*) The concurrence of absence seizures or GTCS, akinetic attacks, and myoclonus. See **myoclonus.**

epileptic negative myoclonus A phenomenon related to epileptiform discharges located in contralateral central regions, occurring in a variety of epileptic syndromes and presenting as brief postural lapses of muscle tone in a body segment time-locked to a train of spike discharges in the contralateral hemisphere and accompanied by periods of EMG silence lasting up to 400 ms. Giant somatosensory-evoked potentials (SSEPs) may be recorded in such patients.[4684] See also **asterixis.**

epileptic nystagmus (ictal nystagmus) Pendular, torsional, retraction, or **central (jerk) nystagmus** occurring in association with paroxysmal discharges from a contralateral parietal focus, as shown on the EEG.[2243] The phenomenology of the eye movements and the nature of the discharging lesion vary, so much so that no further definition is offered. The subject was reviewed by Leigh and Zee.[3762]

epileptic psychosis Functional alteration in mental status in patients with seizure disorders, usually of the partial variety. These can be classified as follows:

Chart E–4. Classification of Epileptic Psychoses

1. Brief psychoses in the context of altered consciousness related to an ictus.
   A. Nonconvulsive status
      Absence type
      Psychomotor type
   B. Postictal "twilight states" (brief, mild confusion)
   C. Postictal hypomania
   D. Fugue states
   E. Alternating psychoses with forced normalization of the EEG
   F. Transient ictal depression, dysphoria, or hypomania.
2. Chronic psychoses without immediate relationship to seizure activity and with normal conscious level:
   A. **Schizophrenia-like psychoses of epilepsy**[5890]
   B. Paranoid states
   C. Bipolar affective disorder

epileptic recruiting rhythm (fast rhythmic waves) Bursts of sinusoidal waves at 8–30 Hz, widespread over the scalp, resembling beta activity and presaging the occurrence of tonic seizures or absences.[690]

epileptic seizure 1. A paroxysmal clinical event as a manifestation of epileptic (excessive and/or hypersynchronous), usually self-limited activity of neurons in the brain reflecting the occurrence of an epileptic discharge. Such events are the building blocks of the **epileptic syndromes**. The International League Against Epilepsy classification is given in Chart E–5. 2. A clinical manifestation presumed to result from an abnormal and excessive discharge of a set of neurons in the cortex of the brain. The clinical manifestation consists of sudden and transitory abnormal phenomena that may include alterations of consciousness, motor sensory, autonomic, or psychic events, perceived by the patient or an observer.[1265] Their 1990 classification is still appropriate (though for 'partial', substitute 'focal') and is reproduced in Chart E–5.

epileptic spasm (infantile spasm) Sudden flexion, extension, or mixed extension–flexion movements predominantly of the proximal and truncal muscles, which are usually more sustained than in myoclonus but not as sustained as in a tonic seizure; that is, about 1 s. Limited forms may occur, involving, for example, grimacing or head nodding. They tend to occur in clusters and are associated with the EEG appearance known as **hypsarrhythmia** and occur in infants or children with **West syndrome** and in the **Lennox–Gastaut syndrome, tuberous sclerosis, Aicardi syndrome, lissencephaly-pachygyria**, and **focal cortical dysplasia**.

epileptic (epilepsy) syndrome An epileptic disorder characterized by an individual cluster of signs and symptoms customarily occurring together; these include such items as type of seizure, etiology, anatomy, precipitating factor, age of onset, severity, chronicity, diurnal and circadian cycling, and sometimes prognosis. A single syndrome may have different etiologies and prognoses.[72] A classification is given under **epilepsy**.

epileptic twilight state See **status epilepticus**.

Chart E–5. Classification of Epileptic Seizures.

1. *Partial seizures* (seizures beginning locally)
   - A. Simple partial seizures (consciousness not impaired)
     1. With motor symptoms
     2. With somatosensory or special sensory symptoms
     3. With autonomic symptoms
     4. With psychic symptoms
   - B. Complex partial seizures (with impairment of consciousness)
     1. Beginning as simple partial seizures and progressing to impairment of consciousness
        - a. With no other features
        - b. With features as in A. 1–4
        - c. With automatisms
     2. With impairment of consciousness at onset:
        - a. With no other features
        - b. With features as in A. 1–4
        - c. With automatisms
   - C. Partial seizures, secondarily generalized
2. *Generalized Seizures* (bilaterally symmetrical and without local onset)
   - A. 1. Absence seizures
     2. Atypical absence seizures
   - B. Myoclonic seizures
   - C. Clonic seizures
   - D. Tonic seizures
   - E. Tonic-clonic seizures
   - F. Atonic seizures
3. *Unclassified epileptic seizures* (inadequate or incomplete data)[1713]

From Driefuss FE. The epilepsies: clinical implications of the international classification. Epilepsia 1990;31: *S3–S10. Reproduced by kind permission of Dr. F. Driefuss and of Lippincott Williams and Wilkins.)*

epileptiform Resembling epilepsy—or, by extension, things that are often associated with epilepsy, such as certain EEG rhythms. The word means neither **epileptogenic** nor epileptic, in any context. In using the term "epileptiform discharges," electroencephalographers wish to convey the presence of spikes, sharp-waves or spike-wave complexes which, by their morphology, frequency, or distribution, suggests to them that such waveforms may be associated with a clinical seizure disorder.

epileptiform pattern An EEG pattern that applies to distinctive waves or complexes, distinguished from background activity and resembling those waves or complexes recorded in a proportion of human subjects suffering from epileptic disorders and in animals rendered epileptic experimentally. Epileptiform patterns include spikes and sharp waves, alone or accompanied by aftercoming slow waves, occurring singly or in bursts lasting at most a few seconds.

The term refers to interictal paroxysmal activity and not to seizure patterns. The probability of association with clinical epileptic disorders is variable. See also **seizure pattern**. (Adapted from the 1974 report of the Committee on Terminology, IFCN. In: Chatrian GE, Bergamini L, Dondey M, et al. A glossary of terms most commonly used by clinical electroencephalographers. *EEG Clin Neurophysiol* 1974;**37**:538–48. Reproduced by kind permission of Elsevier Science and the IFCN.)

epileptogenic (epileptogenous) Capable of provoking epileptic seizures.

epileptogenous See **epileptogenic**.

epileptogenous encephalopathy Intellectual deterioration and transient neurological signs occurring in children, with no past history or family history of epilepsy, after a sudden and dramatic illness marked by repeated convulsions and without current evidence of encephalitis.[833]

epileptoid Resembling epilepsy.

epiloia The term suggested by E.B. Sherlock in 1901 for **tuberous sclerosis**.

epimysium The connective tissue investing muscle fascicles.

epineurium Areolar connective tissue which loosely holds together bundles of funiculi to form a nerve trunk.

epipaxic postural tremor See **cerebellar tremors**.

epiphysis cerebri The pineal gland.

episodic ataxias Dominantly inherited channelopathies with early onset in which the recurrent bouts of imbalance and ataxia are the most obvious clinical feature. Most patients recover fully between attacks, but some may develop progressive ataxia with cerebellar atrophy. The clinical features vary with each syndrome, and there is clear genetic heterogeneity. Online Mendelian Inheritance of Man (OMIM) records six clinical phenotypes, each with unique genetic features.[3388]

Type 1 (EA1) is a potassium channelopathy, characterized by attacks of cerebellar ataxia triggered by startle or exercise lasting minutes, and continuous interictal myokymia, as a result of mutations of the voltage-gated potassium channel gene *KCNA1* on chromosome 12p.13.[1924]

Type 2 (EA2) is a calcium channelopathy mapped to chromosome 19p13, at the same locus as **familial hemiplegic migraine** and cerebellar ataxia (SCA6). It is characterized by attacks of cerebellar ataxia lasting hours to days, provoked by stress rather than by startle and by response to acetazolamide. Dysarthria, nystagmus, vertigo, diplopia, and headache also occur in the attacks. Interictal nystagmus is another feature.[1578] In this condition mutations in *CACN1A* are found.

A *variant* form is *episodic ataxia, hemiplegia, and seizures*, a syndrome with these features resulting from a heterozygous mutation in *EAAT1*, a glutamate transporter. See also **cerebellar ataxias**.

episodic autonomic dysreflexia

(autonomic storm) The occurrence in patients with severe thoracic cord lesions of excessive sympathetic discharge—manifested by flushing and sweating rostral to the level of the cord lesion, headache, hypertension, and reflex bradycardia—in response to visceral stimuli such as bladder distension.

episodic cluster headache

See **cluster headache**.

episodic hyperhidrosis

An uncommon manifestation of diencephalic dysfunction, usually associated with both hypothermia and reduction in conscious level. Causative pathologies have included primary and infiltrating tumors of the hypothalamus, epilepsy, and agenesis of the corpus callosum.[1455]

episodic memory

The mechanism whereby specific events, places, dates, faces, and facts that were personally experienced are remembered. Its substrates are the hippocampus and limbic system. As it contains information about the ordering of events in time, it equates with a good memory for personal history. This memory store is somewhat more fragile than semantic memory, perhaps because the data within it constantly change,[3470] and it is impaired early in, for example, **Alzheimer disease**. Cf. **semantic memory**, the context-independent remembering of word-meanings, objects, people, and places. See also **working memory** and **procedural memory**.

episodic nocturnal wanderings

Nocturnal behavioral disturbances characterized by abrupt arousal, followed by violent, stereotyped complex automatisms, including walking, screaming, yelling, and unintelligible speech; kicking, leaping, and head banging within the context of expressed fear; unresponsiveness to the environment; and with a tendency to semidirected violence. They occur mainly in adolescents and young adults, many of whom have interictal seizure discharges.

The attacks usually last for minutes and occur in clusters during nonrapid eye movement sleep stage 2. They are unaccompanied by pathological behavior by day.[4962] They resemble **night terrors** or **sleepwalking**, except that they are suppressed by anticonvulsants.[4139, 5989, 4451]

episodic paroxysmal hemicrania

A syndrome in which the bouts of otherwise typical **chronic paroxysmal hemicrania** last for weeks without progressing to a chronic phase. Responsiveness to indomethacin is near-complete.[3584]

episodic paroxysmal hemicrania

Repetitive daily attacks of **paroxysmal hemicrania**, the searing unilateral head pains lasting 10–20 min and occurring over a period of weeks without a tendency to become chronic.[3584]

episodic spontaneous hypothermia with hyperhidrosis

A rare condition seen at any age and characterized by unprovoked hypothermia, with diaphoresis lasting minutes to months and eventual remission. It is associated with the presence of congenital CNS anomalies or hypothalamic disorders. See **corpus callosum agenesis with recurrent hypothermia**.

episodic tension-type headache

(tension, muscle contraction, psychomyogenic, stress, ordinary, headache, idiopathic or psychogenic headache) Recurrent episodes of headache lasting minutes to days. The pain is typically pressing or tightening in quality, of mild or moderate intensity, bilateral in location, and does not worsen with routine physical activity. Nausea is absent, but photophobia or phonophobia may be present. See **tension (-type) headache**. See also **chronic daily headache, new daily persistent headache,** and **medication-induced headache**.[5832]

episodic unilateral mydriasis

A syndrome characterized by the spontaneous occurrence of unilateral fixed pupillary dilatation associated with homolateral headache, lasting from minutes to weeks in young people, without ptosis or diplopia, with eventual remission and without residua.

A similar syndrome occurs in **Horner syndrome,** with **springing pupils** and in **cyclic oculomotor paralysis**.[2699]

episodic vertigo

A feature of various conditions including **benign paroxysmal positional** and **benign recurrent vertigo,** vertebrobasilar insufficiency, **migraine**, and **episodic ataxia** type 2, as well as the following.

episodic vertigo and hearing loss

A dominantly inherited syndrome of fluctuating nerve deafness with episodic tinnitus and vertigo. See **Ménière disease**.

epistasis

(genetic interaction) The interaction between genes, occurring when the action of one gene is modified by one or several other "modifier genes." The gene whose phenotype is expressed is said to be *epistatic*, while the phenotype altered or suppressed is said to be *hypostatic*. The term is widely used in population genetics and refers especially to the statistical properties of the phenomenon.

Epley maneuver

A bedside method for repositioning the otolith particles in the semicircular canals as treatment for patients with posterior semicircular canal **benign paroxysmal positional vertigo**.[1893] The actual method is superbly demonstrated at http://www.emedicine.com/emerg/topic57.htm.

epoch A period of time in an EEG record or other physiological recording session, its duration determined arbitrarily.

EPP See **end-plate potential**.

EPSP See **excitatory postsynaptic potential**.

Epworth Sleepiness Scale A subjective tool for the evaluation of sleepiness, though it was the Maintenance of Wakefulness Test that was adopted by the U.S. Federal Aviation Administration as the standard for measuring treatment efficacy when testing pilots with sleep apnea.

EQ-5D A generic quality-of-life measure assessing self-care, mobility, usual activities, pain/discomfort, and anxiety/depression, and found valuable in the assessment of people with **Parkinson disease**.[5650]

equal loudness balance test A localizing test in auditory dysfunction, in which pure tones at various frequencies are delivered to the two ears alternately, the subject signifying when the sound in the two ears is of equal intensity. With cochlear dysfunction, the loudness in the affected ear approaches, equals, or exceeds that in the normal ear at high-intensity levels; with conductive deafness or retrocochlear lesions, no such recruitment occurs; and, with neural lesions, the sensation of loudness in the deaf ear grows more slowly than that in the normal ear, with increasing intensity of stimulation.[2165]

equine gait The "steppage" gait of drop foot due to weakness of the ankle dorsiflexor and evertor muscles.

equipotential A term which applies to regions of the head or to electrodes which are at the same potential at a given instant in time.

equipotential line An imaginary line joining a series of points that are at the same potential at a given instant in time.

equivocal signs Signs which suggest the presence of neuropathology but which either are so slight as to generate uncertainty or are inconsistently present. In other situations, the sign is not confirmed by the presence of other signs ordinarily present, given the lesion suggested by the original finding.

Eramo syndrome A dysmorphic syndrome characterized by short stature, dry skin, hyperkeratosis or ichthyosis, alopecia, absent eyebrows and sparse eyelashes, corneal ulceration and photophobia, mental and developmental delay, seizures, and nystagmus.[381]

Erb, Wilhelm Heinrich (1840–1921) The leading German neurologist of his time, Erb graduated from Munich and trained with **Friedreich** at Heidelberg, succeeding him there as professor after some years spent in Heidelberg and in Leipzig. He is remembered best for his initial classification of the muscular dystrophies which he also distinguished from spinal muscular atrophies; and for his work on the "tendon" reflexes. It was he who first employed a hammer to elicit these reflexes, the hammer formerly having been used to percuss the chests of humans and the heads of cows (in the latter case to detect the presence of echinococcal cysts).[5603]

Erb was one of the first neurologists to stress the value of the neurological examination; he and **Westphal** showed at the same time that the knee jerk was absent in **tabes dorsalis**. He succeeded in getting adequate training in neurology into the undergraduate medical curriculum in Germany, an advance which has sadly still proved hard to achieve, at least in North America. The syndromes etc. for which he is remembered (from over 270 of his publications) are listed in the following entries.

Erb dystrophy See **limb-girdle muscular dystrophy**.

Erb myotonic reaction The prolonged contraction of muscle resulting from faradic stimulation applied at the motor point.

Erb palsy See **upper brachial plexus palsy**.

Erb phenomenon The increased excitability of the peripheral motor nerves in tetany.

Erb's point That point behind the insertion of the sternomastoid muscle into the clavicle where percutaneous nerve stimulation activates the axons of the upper trunk of the brachial plexus.

Erb reaction of degeneration The persisting sensitivity of muscle to galvanic but not to faradic stimulation following denervation.

Erb sign Hyperexcitability of the nerves in tetany.

Erb spastic paraparesis See **Erb–Charcot syndrome**.

Erb–Charcot syndrome (spastic spinal paralysis, Erb spastic paraparesis, syphilitic myelitis) Syphilitic myelopathy with the usual pyramidal signs, sphincter disturbances, muscle atrophy at the level of the cord lesions, and long-tract sensory changes, due to syphilitic endarteritis of the thoracic cord.[1897] Syphilitic myelopathy can similarly be caused by pachymeningitis. The name given here is that by which the disease is better known, but Erb gave primacy to **Charcot** in its description.[1898]

Erb–Duchenne syndrome See **upper brachial plexus palsy**.

Erb–Goldflam syndrome See **myasthenia gravis**.[1899]

Erb–Landouzy syndrome See **limbgirdle muscular dystrophy**.

Erb–Westphal sign Absence of the knee jerk in **tabes dorsalis**.

Erdheim, Jakob (1874–1937) Viennese physician who described parathyroid adenoma and medial necrosis of the aorta as well as the tumor once named for him.

Erdheim syndrome Cervical spondylosis with hyperplasia of the intervertebral disks associated with acromegaly and leading to pain and restriction of cervical mobility.[1904]

Erdheim–Chester disease A rare form of systemic histiocytosis with widespread tissue infiltration, especially manifesting as metaphyseal sclerosis, and with retroperitoneal, cardiac, and pulmonary involvement. It is also capable of causing neurogenic diabetes insipidus, orbital lesions with exophthalmia, and pyramidal and cerebellar signs, the latter mainly due to extra-axial infiltration with dural granulomas.[6878]

Erdheim tumor Craniopharyngioma, described by Erdheim in 1904.

ergotamine tartrate A serotonin receptor agonist and vasoconstrictor isolated by Stoll in 1918 and first used for the treatment of migraine by Maier in 1926.

ergotamine withdrawal headache A form of **withdrawal headache** in subjects with a prior headache syndrome, its characteristics resembling both those of migraine and of tension-type headaches and occurring after chronic daily ergotamine intake (oral ≥2 mg, rectal ≥1 mg) within 48 h after withdrawal.

ergotism (from Fr, a cock spur, which resembles the spike on the fungus *Claviceps purpurea* which may infest spoiled rye grain) Poisoning by the toxin of the ergot fungus, the disease known in the Middle Ages as *Holy*, *St. Anthony's*, or *St. Martial's fire* and often then appearing in epidemics.

Neurovascular (gangrenous) and *spasmodic* or *convulsive* forms are recognized, the latter presenting with limb pain, paresthesias, intermittent strong muscular contractions, seizures, psychoses, and signs resembling those of peripheral neuropathy or tabes.[6819]

Erichsen, Sir John Eric (1818–1896) English surgeon (born in Copenhagen) who described **railway spine** (a condition which does not exist) in 1866. However, his clinical descriptions were extremely accurate for **cervical acceleration injury** and it would appear that the rampant litigation in this context today was equally well known in the nineteenth century.

Erisistratos (d. ca. 250 BC) Alexandrian anatomist, physician, and surgeon who was possibly the grandson of Aristotle. He named the cerebrum and the cerebellum and described the convolutions of the brain.

Erlanger, Joseph (1874–1965) American neurophysiologist who established the nature of the nerve action potential using a cathode ray oscilloscope and took the 1944 Nobel Prize (with H. Gasser, a former student of his) for work on the differentiation of nerve fiber functions.

Ernest syndrome A syndrome of facial pain considered to be due to inflammation of the tendon of the temporalis muscle, characterized clinically by pain felt in and about the ear, temporomandibular joint, anterior temple, mandible and adjacent teeth, throat, and/or eye. The pain is exacerbated by digital compression of the insertion of the stylomandibular ligament and relieved by local anesthetic injection at that site.

erratic seizures See **fragmentary seizures**.

erythema chronicum miograns Classically, an expanding red or bull's eye annular "target" lesion typically associated with *B. burgdorferi* tick bites and the most common manifestation of early **Lyme disease**. Variations such as uniform coloration, lesions with necrotic or vesicular centers, and lesions with shapes that are not circular or oval also occur. The lesion was first described by Arnold **Pick**.

erythism Redness of the skin, as part of the syndrome of poisoning with inorganic mercury. The term became generalized to describe the associated emotional irritability.

In retrospect, it is surprising that the similarity of the signs of **pink disease** to those of erethism was not recognized earlier.

erythrokeratodermia with ataxia A rare, recessively inherited syndrome of congenital ichthyosiform erythroderma, clearing by the age of 25 years, with adult-onset gait ataxia, pyramidal signs, and myalgia.[2394]

erythromelalgia (primary erythermalgia, familial erythromelalgia, Weir Mitchell disease) A dominantly inherited chronic condition characterized by episodic burning and erythema of the involved extremity. When the extremity is lowered, or heat is applied, the pain is intensified, while the application of cold or elevation of the extremity decreases the pain. Sympathetic vasoconstrictor responses are diminished, perhaps as a result of denervation supersensitivity causing increased vasoconstrictor responses to circulating catecholamines, leading to a reduction in skin blood flow.[2883] A sodium channel mutation. in the gene encoding the *Nav1.7* sodium channel, is the underlying cause.[6676]

In primary erythromelalgia there is no accompanying disease process. Secondary erythromelalgia is associated with myeloproliferative syndrome-related thrombocythemia. Silas Weir Mitchell first suggested the term in 1878. When affecting the face or head, the term used is **cluster headache**. See **Weir Mitchell syndrome** and **thrombocytosis**.[4708]

erythropia The abnormal perception of redness in objects seen; an occasional complication of lens extraction.

erythroprosopalgia A redundant term for **cluster headache**.

Escherich sign Periorbital and perioral muscle contraction induced by percussion of the lips or tongue; seen in tetany.[5333]

esodic Afferent.

esophoria (Latent convergent strabismus) A tendency for the visual axes to deviate medially; a predisposition to ocular convergence. See also **esotropia** and **exophoria**.

esotropia (convergent strabismus) A visible inward turning of the visual axis of an eye. See also **cyclic esotropia** and **thalamic esotropia**.

esphlasis (from Gr, a pressure inwards) A comminuted fracture of the skull.

Espildora–Luque syndrome Unilateral blindness with contralateral hemiplegia due to an embolism in the ophthalmic artery which, it is supposed, induces reflex spasm in the middle cerebral artery on the same side.[1915] See **amaurosis–hemiplegia syndrome**.

Esquirol, Jean-Etienne-Dominique (1772–1840) French physician, psychiatrist at the **Salpêtrière**, who first brought rational and humanistic ideas to the management of patients with mental disorders[1917] and who introduced the terms *grand mal* and *petit mal* to neurology in 1838.

essential anisocoria Benign pupillary inequality of unknown cause, in which the difference in sizes of the pupils is maintained under different conditions of illumination; responses to light and accommodation are present; and eye movements are full. See **anisocoria**.

essential benign myoclonus See **myoclonus**.[1469]

essential blepharospasm
A common **dystonia** in adults, presenting as blepharospasm with no known cause, often without any other dystonic manifestations.

essential chorea A rare disorder of unknown cause manifesting as nonprogressive chorea with onset in adult life, without associated neurological deficit, positive family history, or abnormality on cerebral imaging.[1949]

See also **hereditary nonprogressive chorea** and **senile chorea**.

essential headache See **episodic tension-type headache**.

essential myoclonus A disorder characterized solely by the occurrence of myoclonus. Both *hereditary* (paramyoclonus multiplex) and *acquired* forms have been described, but, even in the latter, no preceding causal event can be determined.[832]

The acquired, sporadic condition is heterogeneous and may represent a variant of idiopathic epilepsy in which myoclonus occurs in subjects with no other form of epilepsy and who show no neurological deficit. In some cases, malignancies are associated. See **myoclonus, hereditary essential myoclonus,** and **ballistic movement overflow myoclonus**.

essential tremor (benign essential familial tremor, Minor tremor, familial tremor) A dominantly inherited or sporadic syndrome of postural and kinetic tremor, worst in the arms with actions such as writing or lifting a cup but frequently also affecting the head, jaw, and vocal apparatus, but rarely the legs, in the absence of signs of **Parkinson disease** or of other causes of tremor. **Lewy body** pathology may, however, be present. Mapping to sites on chromosomes 2p24, 2p22–25, 6p23, and 3q13 has been achieved.[1576]

The tremor is absent at rest. It may affect other areas of the body as well as the arms. It is usually most pronounced distally and is present during both maintenance of posture and performance of an action. In elderly people, a rest component may be seen. Eye movement abnormalities are not present in association with this kind of tremor. As first recorded by Robert **Whytt**, alcohol consumption may relieve the tremor of the hands. "A dram of brandy, by stimulating the nerves of the stomach, will almost instantly lessen a tremor of the hands . . ." (Whytt R. *The Works of Robert Whytt*. Published by his Son, Edinburgh, in 1768, p. 681.)

The condition was first described in full by Lazar **Minor**. Hubble et al.[3020] have published a complete review. Criteria for the diagnosis of essential tremor have been suggested:

For *definite essential tremor*, the core criteria[339, 341, 1834] are the presence of bilateral tremor of the hands and forearms (but not rest tremor); the absence of other signs apart from the cogwheel phenomenon; and head tremor in the absence of signs of dystonia. The tremor is postural or kinetic in type. Secondary criteria supporting (but not required for) the diagnosis are long duration (>3 years); a positive family history; and a beneficial response to alcohol.

Exclusion criteria for this tremor, suggested by Dr. Joseph Jankowicz (personal communication, 1994; reproduced by kind permission), are the presence of: neurological signs; the causes of accentuated physiological tremor; current or recent exposure to tremorgenic drugs; direct or indirect trauma to the CNS or PNS; historical or clinical evidence of a psychogenic origin for the tremor; or convincing evidence of sudden onset or of stepwise deterioration.

A further form of classification could be whether the tremor is familial or presumed to be sporadic.

Subgroups of essential tremor were differentiated by Marsden et al.[4103]

Type 1, *benign exaggerated physiological essentialtremor* A nonfamilial postural tremor at 8–12 Hz seen in the arms and due to enhancement of the normal stretch reflex. See also **physiological tremor**.

Type 2, *benign pathological essential tremor* A frequently familial postural tremor at 5–7 Hz seen in the arms and perhaps in the head and legs also, considered to be due to dysregulation of a central oscillator.

Type 3, *severe pathological essential tremor* A frequently familial postural tremor at 5–9 Hz, more marked than the last, seen in the arms and perhaps in the head and legs also, and considered to be due to dysregulation of a central oscillator.

Type 4, *symptomatic essential tremor* A frequently familial postural tremor at 5–7 Hz, seen in the arms only, in association with peripheral neuropathy or with basal ganglion disorders.

Orthostatic and *primary writing tremor* and *tremor of the smile* are *variants* of the same condition,[2053] which is itself heterogeneous as judged by electrophysiological study.

The **International Tremor Foundation** is a clearing house for data on the condition. Web site: http://www.essentialtremor.org/.

esthesiometer A small handheld device like a compass with two arms that can be adjusted to separate its curved tips from 1 mm to about 8 cm, thus allowing the measurement of two point discrimination as part of the sensory examination.

esthesioneuroblastoma An invasive, malignant tumor of the nasal cavity derived from the olfactory mucosal receptor cells. Microscopically the tumor resembles a neuroblastoma. It occurs mostly in young adults and invades locally, giving rise to cranial nerve pareses, but may occasionally metastasize locally or may spread intracranially.[557, 1838]

état criblé 1. The normal open-weave appearance of the anterior and posterior perforated substance through which small arteries pass into the brain. 2. The abnormal sievelike appearance of the brain in areas of vascular ectasia, usually the centrum semiovale and the basal ganglia, due to dilatation of the perivascular spaces, thickening of the walls of the smaller arteries, and perivascular demyelination. This condition was recognized by Dechambre in the same paper in which he published his observations of lacunes.[1528] 3. The occurrence of multiple type 3 **lacunes** in the brain.

état lacunaire The occurrence of multiple type 1 **lacunes** in the brain, often associated clinically with progressive neurological deterioration, *marche à petits pas*, pseudobulbar palsy, and incontinence.

état marbré (Fr, marbled state) (status marmoratus) Scarring of the putamen and other basal ganglia with prominence of myelinated fibers in the gray matter, giving rise to a marbled appearance. It is seen in neonates following **hypoxic-ischemic encephalopathy** and clinically is usually associated with athetosis. See **double athetosis** and **Vogt syndrome**.

Ethan syndrome See **nystagmus-blockage syndrome**.

Chart E–6. TRIG Classification of Essential Tremor

A. *Definite essential tremor*

1. Inclusion criteria

i. Tremor: Bilateral postural tremor with or without kinetic tremor, involving hands and forearms, that is visible and persistent (Tremor of other body parts may be present in addition to upper limb tremor. Bilateral tremor may be asymmetric. It is reported by the patient to be persistent, although the amplitude may fluctuate, but it may or may not produce disability.)
ii. Duration: longer than 5 years

2. Exclusion criteria

i. Other abnormal neurologic signs (with the exception of the presence of tremor and **Froment sign**, the full neurologic examination should be normal for age)
ii. Presence of known causes of enhanced physiologic tremor
iii. Concurrent or recent exposure to tremorogenic drugs or the presence of a drug withdrawal state (Many drugs acting on the central nervous system can produce tremor as a side effect. In people, drug-induced tremor is most often in the form of action tremor. Subjects should be drug-free for a period exceeding the known biologic effect of the drug.)
iv. Direct or indirect trauma to the nervous system within 3 months preceding the onset of tremor (This includes head injury [direct or indirect] and peripheral injury, if the anatomic distribution is the same as that of the tremor.)
v. Historic or clinical evidence of psychogenic origins of tremor (The definition of psychogenic tremor is itself open to debate. Clinical features that may suggest [there] are unphysiological variations [>1 Hz] in tremor frequency, unusual and inconsistent behavioral characteristics, and spontaneous remission. Psychiatric or social factors [multiple somatization, secondary gain, litigation, or compensation pending] may support the diagnosis of psychogenic tremor.)
vi. Convincing evidence of sudden onset or evidence of stepwise deterioration

B. Probable essential tremor

1. Inclusion criteria

i. The same as those for definite essential tremor (Tremor may be confined to body parts other than hands. These may include head and postural tremor of the legs. However, abnormal posture of the head would suggest the presence of dystonic head tremor.)
ii. Duration—longer than 3 years

2. Exclusion criteria

i. The same as for definite essential tremor
ii. Primary orthostatic tremor (isolated, high-frequency [14–18 Hz] bilaterally synchronous tremor of the lower limbs on standing)
iii. Isolated voice tremor (because of the clinical difficulty of separating essential tremor of the voice from the speech disturbances of laryngeal dystonia and other dystonias of the vocal apparatus)
iv. Isolated position-specific or task-specific tremors, including occupational tremors and primary writing tremor
v. Isolated tongue or chin tremor

C. Possible essential tremor

1. Inclusions

i. Type I

a. Subjects who satisfy the criteria of definite or probable essential tremor but exhibit other recognizable neurologic disorders, such as Parkinsonism, dystonia, myoclonus, peripheral neuropathy, or restless leg syndrome
b. Subjects who satisfy the criteria of definite or probable essential tremor but exhibit other neurologic signs of uncertain significance not sufficient to make the diagnosis of a recognizable neurologic disorder. Such signs may include mild extrapyramidal features, such as hypomimia, decreased arm swing, or mild bradykinesia

ii. Type II

Monosymptomatic and isolated tremors of uncertain relation to essential tremor. This includes position- and task-specific tremors, such as occupational tremors, primary writing tremor, primary orthostatic tremor, isolated voice tremor, isolated postural leg tremor, and unilateral postural hand tremor

2. Exclusions
The exclusions are the same as items 2–4 under *definite essential tremor*

(After Deuschl G. et al. Mov Disord*1998;3:2–23.*

ethiologica (from Gr, forgetfulness + word) The inability to call to mind the correct word to express a thought, a feeling, or a fact.

ethmocephaly (from Gr, a sieve + brain) A developmental malformation in which the two orbits are placed unusually close together. The nose, when present, is normally sited between them.[379] The nasal cavities, nasal bones, ethmoid, and premaxilla are usually missing.[4]

ethmoid (Gr, resembling a sieve) A thin, cavitated, unpaired bone in the midline beneath the frontal and anterior to the sphenoid bones forming parts of the cranium, the orbits, and the nasal fossae. Its upper border forms the cribriform plate. The bone was known by Celsus and was named by Galen.

ethnology The science of the physical and mental differences between the races of man.

ethology The scientific study of the structure of animal behavior by observation; an activity, in Medawar's phrase, "which only simpletons think simple." This is a modern science, dating from the paper by Julian S. Huxley on "The Courtship Habits of the Great Crested Grebe" in the Proceedings of the Zoological Society of London in 1914.

That the behaviors of man resemble those of animals should come as no great surprise; that there are differences allows a measure of reassurance.

Étienne, Charles (1503–1564) French physician who gave the first account of the anatomy of the spinal canal.

Eulenberg, Albert (1840–1917) German professor of neurology in Greifswald and in Berlin. He described periodic attacks of myotonia and paralysis in six generations of one family in 1886,[1923] wrote extensively on the autonomic nervous system, and introduced ergot therapy for the treatment of migraine.

Eulenberg disease See **paramyotonia congenita**.

euphoria (Gr, easily carried) Originally, well-being, the perfect ease and comfort of healthy people.[5103] Now used (improperly) to refer to a state of unwarranted, insightless cheerfulness, optimism, and jollity of mood with the "appropriate" (actually inappropriate) verbal and behavioral accompaniments.

eupraxic centers Centers in the brain for the ideational combination of movements.

EuroMyasthenia A Web site that disseminates research results from the European project EuroMyasthenia and encourages communication on this disease, found at: http://www.euromyasthenia.org/cgi-bin/index.php.

European Brain Council (EBC) A coordinating council formed by European organizations in neurology, neurosurgery, psychiatry, basic brain research (neuroscience), patient organizations and industry, and thus with a constituency of physicians and other scientists, patients, and caretakers.

European Confederation of Neuropathological Societies A professional organization. Web site: http://www.euro-cns.org/start.php.

European Dystonia Federation Web site: www.dystonia-europe.org.

European Federation of Neurological Societies A professional organization with the aim of advancing the neurological sciences and clinical and experimental research within Europe and of fostering international exchange. E-mail: headoffice@efns.org. Web site: http://www.efns.org/.

European Huntington's Disease Network Web site: www.euro-hd.net.

European Journal of Neurology The official journal of the European Federation of Neurological Societies (EFNS). Web site: http://www.blackwell-science.com/~cgilib/jnlpage.asp?Journal=enc&File=ene& Page=aims.

European Journal of Neuroscience A subspecialist journal published by Blackwell Science, Oxford, UK. Web site: http://www.neurosciences.asso.fr/Annonces/A07032000_1.html.

European Neurological Society A professional organization. Web site: www.ensinfo.com.

European Neurology (*Eur Neurol*) A neurological journal published by S. Karger AG, P.O. Box 10, Allschwilerstrasse, CH-4009 Basel, Switzerland. Web site: http://www.karger.ch/journals/ene/ene_jh.htm.

European Neuromuscular Centre A centre for coordinating the various medical and scientific affairs of the European Alliance of Muscular Dystrophy Associations. The centre provides some research funding. Address: Lt. Gen. van Heutzslaan 6, 3743 JN Baarn, The Netherlands. Tel: +31 (0)35 54 80 481; Fax: +31 (0)35 54 80 499. E-mail: enmc@enmc.org. Web site: http://www.enmc.org/.

European Parkinson's Disease Association A charitable organization. Web site: www.epda.eu.com.

European Parkinson's Disease Foundation A charitable organization. Web site: www.parkinsons.org.uk.

European Society of Neuroradiology A professional organization. Web site: www.esnr.org.

European Stroke Scale. A system used to assess a patient who has recently had a stroke involving the middle cerebral artery.[2743] It scores level of consciousness, comprehension, speech, visual fields, gaze, facial movement, four upper limb and three lower limb motor tasks, and gait. See also **stroke scales**.

euroquol See **quality of life**.

euryblepharon (Gr, wide + the eyelid) A craniofacial malformation in which there is abnormal widening of the palpebral aperture due to deficiency of the palpebral skin.[4]

eurycephalous (Gr, wide + the head) Having a large, broad head.

euryopia See **Greig syndrome**.

Eustachius (Bartolommeo Eustachio, 1524–1574) Italian physician, professor of anatomy at Rome. He was a contemporary of Vesalius, whose discoveries overshadowed his, not least because Eustachius' illustrations were only discovered and published 140 years after his death. They showed that he had defined numerous anatomical structures not formerly recognized, including the optic and abducens nerves and much of the anatomy of the sympathetic chain.

Evans index The ratio of the transverse diameter of the anterior horns of the lateral ventricles measured at pneumoencephalography (PEG) to the greatest internal transverse diameter of the skull.

Since PEG is now obsolete, so is the index; the CT scan allows far better estimation of the size of the ventricles.

event-related potentials
Cortically derived voltage shifts seen when a subject is selectively attentive to a provided stimulus and is required to distinguish a specific stimulus from others. They are relatively independent of the physical characteristics of the stimulus and appear to monitor a substage of information processing. See **contingent negative variation** and **alpha rhythm**.

evoked potential (evoked response)
1. The potential shift in the cortical dendritic population underlying surface electrodes placed on the scalp, occurring in association with the arrival of impulses signifying peripheral or central stimulation. A wave or complex elicited by and time-locked to a physiological or other stimulus; for instance, an electrical stimulus delivered to a sensory receptor or nerve or applied directly to a discrete area of the brain and usually requiring computer summation techniques for their detection. (Adapted from the 1974 report of the Committee on Terminology, IFCN. In: Chatrian GE, Bergamini L, Dondey M, et al. A glossary of terms most commonly used by clinical electro-encephalographers. *EEG Clin Neurophysiol* 1974;37:538–48. Reproduced by kind permission of Elsevier Science and the IFCN.)

2. An electrical waveform elicited by and temporally related to a stimulus, most commonly an electrical stimulus delivered to a sensory receptor or nerve, or applied directly to a discrete area of the brain, spinal cord, or muscle. See also **auditory EP, brainstem auditory evoked potential, spinal evoked potential, somatosensory evoked potential, visual evoked potential** (SSEP), **compound muscle action potential,** and **compound sensory nerve action potential**. (Adapted from the 1987 Report of the Nomenclature Committee of the American Association of Electromyography and Electrodiagnosis and reproduced by kind permission of the AANEM.)[162]

In clinical practice, visual, auditory, somatosensory, and cognitive potentials are those usually recorded, and are regarded as providing reproducible information about the functional status of the relevant afferent sensory channel and as capable of showing abnormalities where none can be ascertained clinically. Their clinical value has been reviewed.[1145]

Castigated as lucrative, nonspecific, and uninformative by the unconvinced but defended as accurate, relevant, and underused by their champions, the tests in general inform about electrical disturbances within a sensory pathway, assist not at all in pathological diagnosis, and, if regarded as extensions of the clinical examination, provide data which the experienced clinician may find valuable when they confirm his or her clinical impressions, the errant excreta of machines being generally more acceptable to the naive than are the judgments of experienced physicians.

evoked potential studies The recording and analysis of electrical waveforms of biological origin elicited in response to electrical or physiological stimuli in the peripheral and central nervous system, whereas *nerve conduction studies* refers to studies of waveforms generated in the peripheral nervous system.

There are two systems for naming complex waveforms in which multiple components can be distinguished.

A. The different components are labeled P1 or N1 for the initial positive and negative potentials, respectively, and P2, N2, P3, N3, etc., for subsequent positive and negative potentials.
B. The components are specified by polarity and the average peak latency in normal subjects, to the nearest millisecond.

The first nomenclature principle has been used in an abbreviated form to identify the seven positive components of the normal brainstem auditory evoked potential, customarily given in Roman numerals for no obvious reason; thus, I–VII. The second nomenclature principle has been used to identify the positive and negative components of visual (N75, P100) and SSEPs (P9, P11, P13, P14, P20, P23). Regardless of the system of nomenclature employed, it is possible under standardized conditions to establish normal ranges of amplitude, duration, and latency of the individual components of these evoked potentials. The difficulty with the second system is that the latencies of components of evoked potentials depend upon the length of the pathways in the neural tissues.

Thus, the components of a SSEP recorded in a child have different average latencies from the same components of one recorded in an adult. Despite this problem, there is no better system available for naming these components at this time. (Adapted from the 1987 Report of the Nomenclature Committee of the American Association of Electromyography and Electrodiagnosis. AAEE glossary of terms in clinical electromyography. *Muscle Nerve* 1987;10S:G5–G23. © 1987. All rights reserved. © 1987 John Wiley and Sons. Inc. Reprinted by permission.)

evoked response See **evoked potential**.

evoked seizures (reflex epilepsies)
Those seizures regularly provoked by physiological or psychical stimuli. The specific external stimuli include sounds or lights; the internal ones, thoughts or memories.

The term was first introduced by Prochaska in the latter part of the eighteenth century, but these events were also recognized by Hughlings **Jackson** and were fully described by **Gowers** (1901). Abrupt changes in illumination, reading, music or other sounds, odors, particular movements, eating, startle, noise, pain, touch, emotional upsurges, and complex activities such as playing cards or chess have been described as precipitants.[6177] Reflex epilepsy is perhaps not the best or most precise term but is in current usage.[3881] See also **eating epilepsy**.

Various seizure types have also been described as triggered by playing or watching the traditional Chinese gambling game "Mah-Jong" in hard form or in a computer version. Anticonvulsant therapy is of moderate value only and abstention appears to be the best therapy.[6635] Evoked seizures are classified in Chart E–7.

evolution Change in form over generations; descent with modification. (Darwin)

evolution of the nervous system
A concept of Hughlings **Jackson** regarding the increasing specialization of the nervous system, both up the evolutionary scale and within a hierarchy of organized activity in

Chart E–7. Classification of Evoked Seizures

1. *Reflex epilepsy syndromes*
   - A. Simple stimuli
     - i. **Photogenic epilepsy**
       - a. Television epilepsy
       - b. Self-induced photogenic seizures
     - ii. **Startle epilepsy**
     - iii. **Hot water epilepsy**
     - iv. **Eating epilepsy**
     - v. Rubbing the skin
     - vi. Tooth-brushing
   - B. Complex stimuli
     - i. **Primary reading epilepsy**
     - ii. **Musicogenic epilepsy**
     - iii. Cognitive processing epilepsy
     - iv. Playing Mah-Jong
     - v. Speech/language
2. *Secondary epilepsy with stimulus-evoked seizures*
   - A. Simple stimuli such as visual or sound stimuli, or bodily movement
   - B. Complex stimuli such as reading or listening to music.

the human CNS. Evolution consists of a passage from the lowest, most-organized centers up to the highest centers, which are constrained by the least organization; from the most simple to the most complex; and from the most automatic to the most voluntary.[61] See also **levels of organization**.

evolving stroke (stroke-in-evolution) Stroke which is seen to be producing progressive impairment of function with time.

Ewald's Laws 1. A horizontal semicircular canal is maximally stimulated by movement of the endolymph that it contains away from its ampulla. 2. Maximal stimulation of a semicircular canal results in nystagmus with its fast component toward the side which is stimulated, but minimal stimulation produces nystagmus in the other direction.

Ewart phenomenon The elevation of a ptotic eyelid on swallowing—a synkinesis due to aberrant regeneration of fibers running from the VII to the III cranial nerve, joining those fibers innervating the levator palpebrae superioris.[464]

exercise-induced muscle pain and stiffness A sporadic condition presenting with muscle pain and cramps but with minimal weakness, affecting males more often than females. Serum CK levels are slightly raised, especially after exercise. See also the Web site: http://www.neuro.wustl.edu/neuromuscular/maltbrain.html.

Excerpta Medica; Neurology and Neurosurgery A neurological review book series. Web site: http://www.elsevier.com/wps/find/journaldescription.cws_home/505977/description#description.

excessive daytime drowsiness See **hypersomnolence**.

excessive daytime sleepiness (EDS, somnolence) Subjective difficulty in maintaining the awake state, coupled with a ready entry into sleep whenever possible.[280]

The most common cause is **sleep apnea** but, in some cases, the phenomenon represents only an augmentation of the normal tendency to be sleepy in the afternoons, though it can progress to a stage in which the need to sleep during this period is paramount. The result in all cases is lethargy, automatic behavior, fatigue, visual problems, and daytime sleep attacks. The symptom also appears in **Parkinson disease,** encephalopathies, the **Kleine–Levin syndrome**, and with other diencephalic lesions. See **hypersomnolence**.

excessive eye-blinks Repetitive blinking either as a result of local ocular irritation or as a prodromal sign of essential blepharospasm, when it is usually bilateral, variable, and associated with ocular irritation and photophobia.[1853]

excessive sleep inertia See **confusional arousals**.

excitability The capacity to be activated by or to react to a stimulus.

excitability of nerve The property of accepting and transmitting an electrical stimulus.

excitable cortex The motor and premotor regions.

excitation-contraction coupling The series of events whereby the propagated action potential on the muscle fiber surface membrane leads to the twitch contraction of the fiber.

excitatory postsynaptic potential (EPSP) A local, graded depolarization of a neuron in response to activation by a nerve terminal. Cf. **inhibitory postsynaptic potential**.

excitomotor system That part of the nervous system concerned in the production of reflex action. The term was applied by Marshall **Hall**.

excitotoxins Substances which cause neuronal death as a result of excessive prolonged membrane depolarization. Examples include glutamate, domoic acid, kainic acid, quisqualate, *N*-methyl-D-aspartame, and bicuculline, a γ-aminobutyric acid antagonist.

excyclotropia Rotation of the eye during attempted downward gaze (as with a IV cranial nerve palsy).

executive cognitive functions "The processes that orchestrate relatively simple ideas, movements or actions into complex goal-directed behaviors. Without them, behaviors important for independent living such as cooking, dressing, or self care . . . break down into their component parts."[5454] Conceptual reasoning, inhibition of over-learned patterns of behavior, inhibition of responses to salient stimuli, mental flexibility, set shifting, organizational ability, planning, regulation of working memory, and fluency of thought are examples.[3553] This therefore defines the complex cognitive processing that requires the coordination of several subprocesses to achieve a particular goal. Loss of executive control produces apathy, irritability, impaired spontaneity, and self-neglect is considered to reflect frontal lobe dysfunction either at cortical or at subcortical levels. See also **Stroop Test**.

Executive Interview (EXIT25) A 25-item instrument providing a standardized assessment of executive control functions, designed to elicit signs of frontal system pathology such as imitation, intrusions, disinhibition, environmental dependency, perseveration, and frontal release etc. Scores correlate strongly and specifically with left mesiofrontal cerebral blood flow by Single Photon Emission Computerized Tomography (SPECT) and left frontal system pathology on MRI and are significant independent predictors of level of care among elderly retirees. High scores indicate impairment. A cut-point of 15/50 is recommended.[5451, 5454] See also **CLOX** and **Behavioral Dyscontrol Scale**.

exercise (from Lat, to drive on or keep occupied) Voluntary muscular activity.

exercise test Serial electrodiagnostic measurements of the compound muscle action potential (CMAP) every 60 s after a 2–5 min period of exercise of the muscle examined. The test is performed between episodes of weakness in patients with thyrotoxic or **familial periodic paralysis**, in whom there is usually an initial increase in the amplitude of the CMAP immediately after exercise, followed by a progressive decrease.[3121]

exertional headache See **benign exertional headache**.

Exner, Sigmund (1846–1926) Austrian physiologist who described a fiber layer near the surface of the cerebral cortex.

exodic 1. Efferent. 2. (Gr, out of + a way—in this case the spinal cord) Marshall **Hall**'s preferred term for reflex motor activity. It has not found favor generally.

exogenous psychosis See **Bonhoeffer syndrome**.

exophasy Thoughts uttered; vocal, audible language.

exophoria A predisposition to ocular divergence as a result of impaired fusion, shown by the **alternate cover test**.

exophthalmic ophthalmoplegia The occurrence of proptosis and extraocular muscle pareses in hyperthyroidism. See **dysthyroid ophthalmopathy**.

exophthalmos (Gr, out + eye) Protrusion of the eye.

exotropia (Divergent strabismus) A condition in which the visual axes of the eyes diverge. See also **WEBINO syndrome**.

Expanded Disability Status Scale See **Kurtzke Scale**.

experiential aura Affective, mnemonic, or composite perceptual phenomena including illusory or composite hallucinatory events and depersonalization, appearing alone or in combination in the context of an epileptic event. They have subjective qualities similar to those experienced in life but are recognized by the subject as abnormal.

experiential hallucination The term of **Penfield** for hallucinations of things formerly seen or heard or experienced, occurring as manifestations of spontaneous epileptic seizures.[4977]

experiential illusions The vivid re-experience of past events in which, as **Penfield** puts it: "the subject discovers himself on the stage of the past as well as in the audience of the present."

These illusions were noted by Penfield during electrical stimulation of the upper and lateral parts of the temporal lobe at open operation in conscious epileptic patients, but it was also realized that they occur as components of the syndrome of **partial complex seizures**.

experiential responses The term of Penfield for hallucinations of things formerly seen, heard, or experienced, and reproduced by stimulation of the cortex at operation.[4977]

experimental allergic encephalomyelitis A monophasic but sometimes relapsing form of encephalitis induced by a combination of cell-mediated immunity to myelin basic protein and an antibody-mediated reaction to galactocerebroside, etc. in which the pathology closely resembles that of **multiple sclerosis**.

expiration:inspiration ratio (E:I Ratio) The ratio of the heart rate measured on the electrocardiogram during expiration to the rate during inspiration. This is a reliable measure of parasympathetic activity.[3085]

explicit memory (declarative memory) That form of memory which requires the conscious recall/recognition of specific information which has recently been presented. This is what is assessed by most of the traditional bedside or office memory tests. See also **implicit memory** and **working memory**.

explicit memory tests Memory tests which require conscious recall/recognition of specific information which has recently been presented. Memory instructions are usually given at the time of presentation and the time of retention testing to indicate clearly the nature of the task. These tests correspond to most traditional forms of memory tests. See also **implicit memory** and **working memory**.

exploding head syndrome The occurrence of the sensation as of a loud noise in the head during sleep onset (nonrapid eye movement sleep stages 1 and 2) in normal people. The sensation has been likened to a crack, a loud snap, or a bang, often waking the subject who is usually elderly and female. The phenomenon is sometimes familial, occurs over years, and is benign.[4950]

exploring electrode Any electrode over the scalp or within the brain substance intended to detect EEG activity. Such an electrode is customarily connected to either input terminal 1 or input terminal 2 of an EEG amplifier in bipolar derivations and to input terminal 1 of an EEG amplifier in referential derivations. See also **active electrode, recording electrode, bipolar derivation,** and **referential derivation**. (Adapted from the 1974 report of the Committee on Terminology, IFCN. In: Chatrian GE, Bergamini L, Dondey M, et al. A glossary of terms most commonly used by clinical electroencephalographers. *EEG Clin Neurophysiol* 1974;37:538–48. Reproduced by kind permission of Elsevier Science and the IFCN.)

express saccades Saccades with unusually short latencies (even of 100 ms), as may occur when the fixation target is extinguished before the new peripheral target appears.[3762]

expressive amusia Loss of a previously possessed ability to play a musical instrument, to sing, or to reproduce musical themes.

expressive aphasia See **Broca aphasia** and **aphasia**.

Extended Arms Test A test of vestibular system function, in which the subject stands with his arms outstretched and index fingers pointing at those of the examiner similarly held up. Deviation of the subject's fingers on eye closure (in the direction of the slow component of any nystagmus present) suggests vestibular system abnormality.

Extended Scale for Dementia An expanded version of the **Mattis Dementia Rating Scale.**[2880]

extensive (extended) large subcortical infarcts Large infarcts of the hemispheric white matter, internal capsule, and basal ganglia due to disease of the internal carotid and/or middle cerebral arteries. The clinical features resemble those of large, middle cerebral artery territory infarcts with dense hemiplegia and neuropsychological dysfunctions appropriate to the affected hemisphere. CT and MRI show extensive involvement of the hemispheric white matter and basal ganglia with cortical sparing.

extension-adduction reflex See **Dagnini sign**.

extensor (from Lat, to stretch out) That which stretches out; the word applies to those muscles which antagonize the flexors and in general act to lengthen the body (or a part of it) by straightening it.

extensor digitorum brevis reflex Contraction of this muscle with dorsflexion of the second to fifth toes following a tap on its tendons distally on the dorsum of the inverted and plantar flexed foot. The reflex does not discriminate between L5 and S1 radiculopathies.[4077]

extensor reflex See **extensor response**.

extensor response (extensor reflex) Extension of the hip and knee and plantar flexion of the foot with stimulation of the buttock, perineum, and upper thigh on that side.[4110] The **Babinski reflex** is actually an integral part of the flexion reflex, never occurring without reflex contraction of the proximal limb flexors. Accessory to this is reflex extension of the crossed limb, which includes plantar flexion of foot and toes.[6622]

extensor spasms An epileptic syndrome characterized by abrupt extension of the neck and trunk with extension and abduction of the arms. They are seen typically in West syndrome but are less common than flexor spasms in that condition.[72]

extensor thrust Reflex extension of the hip and knee with plantar flexion of the foot and toes in response to pressure upwards on the plantar surfaces of the toes; seen in patients with severe but incomplete spinal cord injuries. Flexion may follow each extensor movement, giving the appearance of marching.[4110]

external carotid steal Diversion of blood from the vertebral and internal carotid systems to supply the territory of an occluded external carotid artery.[412]

external compression headache (swim-goggle headache) Headache resulting from continued stimulation of cutaneous nerves by the application of pressure, for example, by a band around the head, a tight hat, or swimming goggles. Persistent compression may lead to a headache resembling **migraine.** Diagnostic criteria have been defined:

A. Headache with all of the following characteristics and fulfilling criteria C and D:
   1. Nonpulsating
   2. Increasing over minutes
   3. No accompanying symptoms
B. Continuing application of external pressure to the forehead or scalp
C. Headache develops during pressure and is maximal at the site of pressure
D. Headache resolves after pressure is relieved.

From the International Classification of Headache Disorders (Headache Classification Committee of the International Headache Society. *Cephalalgia* 2004; **24**[Suppl 1]). Reproduced by kind permission of Dr. Jes Olesen, the International Headache Society and Wiley-Blackwell Publications.

external hamstring reflex (biceps femoris reflex, lateral hamstring reflex, posterior peroneofemoral reflex) Contraction of this muscle in response to a tap on its tendon in the lateral part of the popliteal fossa. It is normally just palpable but is increased with pyramidal lesions above the L5 level. The reflex informs on the state of the L5 and S1 reflex arcs. The **fibular reflex** is similar.

external hydrocephalus Expansion of the subarachnoid space over the surface of the cortex. See also **internal hydrocephalus** and **communicating hydrocephalus.**

external malleolar sign See **Chaddock reflex.**

exteroceptive reflex myoclonus Reflex myoclonus triggered by exteroceptive rather than by proprioceptive afferent discharges, the latter being more commonly identified.[2466]

exteroceptive sensations Those sensations dependent upon receptors in the skin and comprising touch, temperature, and surface pain. The other group of sensations defined by **Sherrington** was **interoceptive,** now better known as **proprioceptive**.

extinction (from Lat, to quench or destroy) 1. The failure of sensory events from one side to reach awareness, while the subject is perfectly aware of similar events occurring simultaneously on the other side.

2. The inability to perceive both of two stimuli in the same sensory channel (visual, auditory, tactile) when they are presented simultaneously.

Although testing is usually performed by, for example, touching the patient on the same spot on each side of the body, touching two places on the *same* side (e.g., the face and the hand) may also demonstrate that only one of the stimuli can be perceived.[508] See also **sensory competition** and **simultagnosia**.

Any modality (or modalities) may be affected, both from personal and extrapersonal space. The lesion is usually of the right hemisphere, less commonly affecting the corpus callosum. Reduced motor activity on or toward the neglected side, dressing and constructional apraxias, and denial of illness are often notable when the lesion is of the right hemisphere. See **neglect**.

extra-abdominal paraganglionic system A group of cell masses associated with the autonomic nervous system and characterized by the storage of catecholamine granules and exhibiting chemoreceptor function. They may be situated in the adrenal medulla, glomus jugulare, or carotid body, around the aortic arch, or on the abdominal aorta. They are generally of low malignancy but may metastasize.[6]

extracampine hallucinations Sensations that another human being is close by, although not seen, because, in fact, not there This may occur in normal subjects under severe stress and also in **dementia with Lewy bodies.**[1087]

If pedantic about definitions, one might argue that this actually is not a hallucination at all but rather an **illusion** or possibly a **delusion,** because there is no perception—rather a *feeling* that there is something (someone) there.

extracerebral potential Any potential which does not originate in the brain and is regarded as an artifact in the EEG record. It may arise from electrical interference external to the subject and recording system, from the subject, from the electrodes and their connections to the subject and the electroencephalograph, and from the EEG machine itself. See **artifact**. (Adapted from the 1974 report of the Committee on Terminology, IFCN. In: Chatrian GE, Bergamini L, Dondey M, et al. A glossary of terms most commonly used by clinical electroencephalographers. *EEG Clin Neurophysiol* 1974;37:538–48. Reproduced by kind permission of Elsevier Science and the IFCN.)

extracranial–intracranial bypass surgery See **EC/IC bypass surgery**.

extradural hemorrhage See **epidural hemorrhage**.

extramedullary (Lat, outside + marrow) Outside the spinal cord.

extraocular palsy Paresis of the extraocular muscles as a result of damage to the III, IV, or VI cranial nerves, the motor end plates, or the muscles themselves and is commonly associated with the complaint of diplopia if vision is retained in both eyes.

extrapyramidal pathways Efferent cortical neuron systems other than the pyramidal pathways and all subcortical efferent neuron systems which subserve movement.

extrapyramidal seizures See **paroxysmal choreoathetosis**.

extrapyramidal signs and cataract See **Waardenburg syndrome**.

Extrapyramidal Symptom Rating Scale A 55-item instrument assessing such symptoms (mainly in the context of treated schizophrenia).[1165] Factor analysis differentiates six syndromes: hypokinetic Parkinsonism, orofacial dyskinesia, trunk/limb dyskinesia, akathisia, tremor, and tardive dystonia.

extrapyramidal syndromes Syndromes manifesting excessive involuntary movements (such as **chorea, athetosis, dystonia,** or **tremor**) or deficiency of movement, as in **Parkinsonism,** in which the pathology is considered to involve the basal ganglia or their connections.

Diseases of the cerebellum are arbitrarily excluded from this category.

extrapyramidal system The term of Kinnier **Wilson** for all those efferent mechanisms apart from the pyramidal tract which have to do with the control of motor activity. A complex of deep motor nuclei (the basal ganglia) including the striatum, globus pallidus, and substantia nigra, which project through the thalamus to the cortex. Less formally, he referred to these as "the dark basement of the brain."

Although the term is in very general use, the system has no rigid anatomical boundaries but extends from at least the olives to the cortex; it functions in ways other than those affecting motor control, and how these are achieved remains unknown. The very obvious contribution to motor control of the cerebellum and its pathways, nevertheless, does not gain it admittance.[4345]

extreme somatosensory evoked potential High-voltage somatosensory action potentials in response to tactile stimulation of the feet, recorded over the scalp in a small minority of apparently normal children who within 2 years may go on to suffer partial motor seizures for a limited period.[1568]

extrinsic sleep disorders Dyssomnias which are causally related to factors outside the body. They are classified by the ASDA as follows:[1629]

1. **Inadequate sleep hygiene**
2. **Environmental sleep disorder**
3. **Altitude insomnia**
4. **Adjustment sleep disorder**
5. **Insufficient sleep syndrome**
6. **Limit-setting sleep disorder**
7. **Sleep-onset association disorder**
8. **Food allergy insomnia**
9. **Nocturnal eating (drinking) syndrome**
10. **Hypnotic-dependent sleep disorder**
11. **Stimulant-dependent sleep disorder**
12. **Alcohol-dependent sleep disorder**
13. **Toxin-induced sleep disorder**
14. **Extrinsic sleep disorder not otherwise specified**

From AASM Diagnostic Classification Steering Committee. *The International Classification of Sleep Disorders Diagnostic and Coding Manual*. Rochester MN. American Academy of Sleep Medicine 1991/2001. Reproduced by kind permission of the Academy. See also http://www.sleepeducation.com/Disorders.aspx.

eyeblinks Spontaneous blinks are bilateral, paroxysmal, brief, repetitive eye closures occurring continuously and in the absence of obvious external stimuli, with their rate correlating with the level of central dopaminergic activity.[3318]

eyebrow lifting test A bedside maneuver differentiating ptosis due to facial muscle weakness from that due to paresis of the levator palpebrae superioris. When the eyebrow is pushed up by the examiner's thumb, the narrowing of the palpebral fissure is abolished only in cases of VII palsy.[4772]

eye–jaw synkinesis Movement of the jaw in the direction of gaze; often a normal phenomenon.

eyelid apraxia Difficulty in the voluntary opening or closing of the eyelids, while such movements are possible involuntarily. It is reported in extrapyramidal and motor neuron diseases.[33]

eyelid freezing See **apraxia of eyelid opening**.

eyelid myoclonia An unique entity comprising recurrent events at 5–6 Hz associated with impairment of consciousness, sometimes provoked by eye closure.[1861]

eyelid myoclonia with (typical) absences An unusual photosensitive myoclonic epilepsy of childhood and adolescence characterized by marked jerking of the eyelids with upward deviation of the eyes following eye closure in a lighted environment, in association with what is otherwise a typical absence attack, the whole sequence lasting less than 5 s. Photic stimulation is also a precipitant. Small jerks of the head and hands are occasionally seen as well. The EEG shows 3–5 Hz paroxysmal generalized bursts of mainly polyspikes and polyspike-slow waves at 3–6 Hz and irregular 3 Hz spike-and-wave complexes.[3177, 226] See also **photosensitive epilepsies**.

eyelid myoclonus Marked jerking of the eyelids, often with jerky, upward deviation of the eyeballs and the head, sometimes associated with or followed by mild impairment of consciousness lasting 1–2 s. In the *variant* condition *absences with eyelid myoclonus*, more prolonged eyelid myoclonus accompanies some forms of absence seizure.

Patients with eyelid myoclonus are prone to induce it themselves by complex repetitive self-stimulation by, for example, deliberate fluttering of the eyes and hyperextension of the head in front of a bright light source, thus experiencing intermittent photic stimulation. *Orbitofrontal photomyoclonus* is similar but is not regarded as a true seizure event.

Eyelid myoclonic status consists of repetitive and discontinuous episodes of eyelid myoclonia with mild absence. See **Jeavons syndrome**.

eyelid twitch sign See **Cogan signs**.

eye-of-the-tiger sign Marked decrease of the T2-weighted MRI signal in the pallidal nuclei, with a centrally located area of increased signal as a result of iron deposition, tissue necrosis, and edema, described in **neurodegeneration with brain iron accumulation** (pantothenate-kinase associated neurodegeneration, Hallervorden–Spatz disease) **with acanthocytosis**.[2896]

eye-winking tics Rapid, exaggerated, coordinated contractions of the orbicularis oculi muscles, under a degree of voluntary control, increased by boredom or anxiety and usually occurring in boys. They disappear after a few years.[3753]

Eysenck Personality Inventory A self-administered scale yielding scores on two dimensions of personality: neuroticism-stability and extraversion–introversion.[1941]

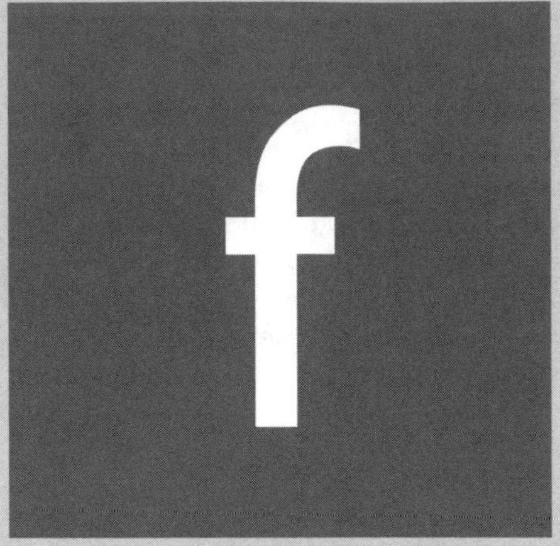

F wave A compound action potential evoked intermittently from a muscle by a supramaximal electrical stimulus to the nerve. Compared with the maximal amplitude M wave of the same muscle, the F wave has a smaller amplitude (1–5% of the M wave) and more variable configuration and latencies.

The F wave (so named by Magladery and McDougal in 1950 because they first identified it in muscles of the foot) can be found in many muscles of the upper and lower extremities, and its latency is longer with more distal sites of stimulation. It is due to antidromic activation of motor neurons. (Adapted from the 1987 Report of the Nomenclature Committee of the American Association of Electromyography and Electrodiagnosis. AAEE glossary of terms in clinical electromyography. *Muscle Nerve* 1987;10S:G5–G23. © 1987. Reproduced by kind permission of the AANEM.)

These small, variable, and delayed electrical accompaniments of the muscle potentials are evoked by stimulation of a motor nerve. They do not represent reflexes but are due to the antidromic activation of motoneuron cell bodies in the anterior horn cell pool as a result of a supramaximal electrical stimulus that passes both distally to activate the muscle and proximally back to the spinal cord, evoking the F waves irregularly. The F wave almost always evaluates more than one segmental level. It traverses only the ventral root.

Prolonged minimal latency, chronodispersion, persistence, and impersistence or absence of the wave have all been studied, but the parameter most useful in diagnosis remains undetermined[2183] and its methodology unstandardized.[4883] Although routinely performed, this appears to be a test still in search of an application.

F wave tacheodispersion The distribution of the conduction velocities of individual nerve fibers, or of small groups of nerve fibers, as estimated from repetitive recording of 30 or more consecutive F waves in a given nerve. The technique may be more sensitive than routine motor nerve conduction velocity recordings in detecting motor neuropathies.[1172]

FABERE Test (Flexion, ABduction, External Rotation, Extension) See **Patrick Test**. Pain during the performance of this test suggests sacroiliac or hip joint disease.

Fabry, Johannes (1860–1930) German dermatologist.

Fabry disease (Fabry–Anderson syndrome, angiokeratoma corporis diffusa, trihexose ceramide lipidosis, hereditary dystopic lipidosis; OMIM 301500) A progressive X-linked recessive lysosomal storage disease (a sphingolipidosis) affecting glycolipid metabolism in which there is abnormal accumulation of ceramide trihexoside in the ganglion cells, the blood vessels, kidneys, corneas, and heart due to deficiency of α-galactosidase A (GALA). The genetic defect maps to chromosome Xq21.3q22.

Its major features appear in young adult life and include a deep red papulomacular skin rash mainly involving the swim-shorts area and thighs, crises of burning pain in the limbs, edema, hyperhidrosis, fever, corneal opacities, renal impairment, strokes (mainly in the posterior circulation), and peripheral neuropathy, all due to deposition of the abnormal glycolipids.[660, 1945]

Fabry in Germany[194] and Dr. W. Anderson in England described the disease in the same year (1898).

Fabry–Anderson syndrome See **Fabry disease**.

face–hand test A test of tactile inattention in which the subject is touched on one or two points of the body simultaneously and asked to report the locations of the stimuli.[2062] Simultaneous touch stimulations of the cheek and hand on one side are normally both appreciated; children and patients with organic mental syndromes tend not to be aware of the touch on the hand (**extinction**) while they do appreciate that on the face.

In a *variant* of the test, the hand and foot are touched simultaneously. In organic mental disease, the foot "dominates" and the touch on the hand is again "extinguished."[2062]

face of the giant panda sign The appearance on the MRI scan of focal atrophy of the mid-brain tegmentum with relative hypointensity of the red nucleus and hyperintensity of the superior colliculus, as seen in axial views in **Wilson disease**.[5648] Similar appearances in the pons have led to the appellation "face of the miniature panda" sign. See also **double panda sign**.

Names such as these are somewhat fanciful but one has to bear with it.

facet (Lat, a small plane surface) A circumscribed articular surface, as in the vertebral column.

facet syndrome (facet tropism) Pain thought to arise from disease of the lumbar facet joints. A developmental or acquired degeneration of the cartilage with subluxation of the facet joints (posterior zygoapophyseal joints) of the vertebrae so that they are aligned in different planes (coronal and sagittal). This usually occurs at lumbosacral levels, leading to muscle spasm and local pain, aggravated by twisting and extension, referred to the buttocks and the posterior thigh, with stiffness and scoliosis.[2510]

Although a reputed cause of low back pain, the response to facet joint injection in such patients neither correlate with nor predict their clinical results after solid posterior lumbar fusion and this may not in fact be a reliable clinical diagnosis.[3130]

facet tropism See **facet syndrome**.

facial arthromyalgia See **temporomandibular pain and dysfunction syndrome** and **Costen syndrome**.

facial asymmetry A minor dysmorphism recognized in some healthy people and in a proportion of patients with complex partial seizures of temporal lobe origin. Unilateral facial weakness during emotional expression on the side contralateral to the cerebral lesion is the usual sign.[5264]

facial chorea (chronic chorea) See **trigeminal neuralgia**.

facial diplegia A benign variant form of the syndrome of **multiple cranial nerve palsies** in which bilateral facial weakness is associated with little if any detectable weakness of the limbs, nor with sensory loss.[1114, 5812]

Facial Grading System A simple and sensitive grading system for facial nerve injury, assessing resting symmetry, voluntary movement, and synkinesis.[5417] Nine other Facial Nerve Injury Grading systems are presented at http://www.medal.org/visitor/www/active/ch17/ch17.aspx.

facial hemangioma and cerebral corticovascular dysplasia A syndrome of dysplastic intracranial arteries and frontal polymicrogyria or dysplastic cortex associated with seizures in children with facial hemangioma.[263]

facial hemiatrophy See **Parry–Romberg syndrome**.

facial hemihypertrophy See **Friedreich disease**.

facial migraine See **carotidynia**.

facial myoclonus Generalized, sometimes bilateral facial twitches usually due to lesions of the brainstem or contralateral cortex.

facial myokymia Involuntary undulations or worm-like writhings of the facial muscles, usually in the orbicularis oculi, most commonly due to anxiety or overtiredness but sometimes associated with brainstem lesions, as in multiple sclerosis. They are usually benign, though they may be a sign of any brainstem disorder.

The definitive diagnosis is made using the EMG, which shows double discharges and brief, repetitive bursts of motor unit potentials interrupted by periods of silence for a few seconds, variably appearing in a regular pattern at 6–100 Hz.[2922]

facial nevi, anomalous cerebral venous return, and hydrocephalus A rare syndrome manifesting macrocrania, bilateral facial nevi, and anomalous intracerebral venous drainage, described in infancy and once in an adult, suggesting that the prognosis is benign.[5759]

facial onset sensory and motor neuronopathy A rare syringomyelia-like neurodegenerative syndrome reported in adult males who present with paresthesias and numbness, but in trigeminal nerve distribution; this slowly progresses to involve the scalp, neck, upper trunk, and arms in order. Cramps, fasciculations, dysphagia, dysarthria, muscle weakness, and atrophy develop later. Neurophysiological studies reveal a generalized sensorimotor axonal neuronopathy of caudally decreasing severity. The pathogenesis of the syndrome is not known.[5826]

facial palsy Weakness of the muscles of the face, including the periorbital muscles, as a result of a lesion of the VII cranial nerve, first described by Nicolaus Friedreich (1761–1836), a German physician, in 1797[655] and thereafter by Sir Charles **Bell** in 1821. In 1903 Cushing reported successful reinnervation after anastomosis with the accessory nerve. See **Bell palsy**.

Although facial palsy may recur on the same side or on the other, simultaneous biflateral facial palsy is not likely to represent Bell palsy and is more likely to be due to sarcoid, leukemia, pseudobulbar palsy, acute inflammatory polyneuropathy, or various autoimmune, malignant, metabolic, or infectious causes. See also **Melkersson–Rosenthal syndrome, Stevens–Johnson syndrome, Wernicke–Korsakoff syndrome**, and **idiopathic intracranial hypertension**.

The nerve was first noted to be a separate structure from other cranial nerves (the "portio dura") by Thomas **Willis** but was named and numbered by **Soemerring**.

Variants are a form of congenital facial palsy described with dominant inheritance but without the other features of **Mőbius syndrome**,[6538] and *emotional (mimetic) facial palsy*, a rare condition in which the facial paresis is only apparent with reflex movements of the hemi-face, as with smiling and laughing, described following a small infarction of the anterior limb of the internal capsule.

facial paraspasm See **blepharospasm**.

facial recognition test A non-memory matching task, used as a test of visual perceptual function.[533]

facial reflex Visible contraction of the orbicularis oris muscle in response to stretch applied when the examiner's finger pulling gently on the side of the mouth is tapped by a reflex hammer. The contraction is seen in patients with bilateral, diffuse lesions of the cortex and in those with damage to the corticobulbar fibers from the contralateral hemisphere.

The subject of facial reflexes was reviewed by Kugelberg.[3587]

facial tics Brief, single repetitive, coordinated, semipurposeful stereotyped movements of the facial and neck muscles, occurring physiologically or in association with diffuse encephalopathy or the use of anticonvulsants, caffeine, methylphenidate, and anti-Parkinsonian agents. Grimacing, throat clearing, and vocalizations are the usual presentations.

facial vision of the blind (fersinn, sixth sense, sense of obstacles) The unexplained ability of the blind to be at least partially aware of the presence of certain objects before them. This might be due to aural or thermal cues.

facies paralytica The facial expression encountered rather constantly in patients with **general paresis;** lack of activity in the muscles of facial expression, asymmetrical and variable facial weakness, and lack of wrinkling of the forehead were described as characteristic.

facilitation An increase in an electrically measured response following identical stimuli. It occurs in a variety of circumstances:

1. The improvement of neuromuscular transmission through the activation of previously inactive muscle fibers. This may be identified in several ways:
   - There is an increase in the amplitude and area of successive M waves during repetitive nerve stimulation.
   - Nerve stimulation studies performed within a few seconds after a brief period (2–60 s) of nerve stimulation producing tetanus or after a strong voluntary contraction may show changes in the configuration of the M wave(s) compared to the results of identical studies of the rested muscle as follows:

     a) Repair of the decrement. A diminution of the decrementing response with slow rates (2–5 Hz) of repetitive nerve stimulation;

     b) Increment after exercise. An increase in the amplitude and area of the M wave elicited by a single supramaximal stimulus. Distinguish from pseudofacilitation, which occurs in normal individuals in response to repetitive nerve stimulation at high rates (20–50 Hz) or after strong volitional contraction. It probably reflects a reduction in the temporal dispersion of the summation of a constant number of muscle fiber action potentials and is characterized by an increase in the amplitude of the successive M waves with a corresponding decrease in their duration. There is no net change in the area of the negative phase of successive M waves.

   This represents post-activation or post-tetanic facilitation.

2. An increase in the amplitude of the motor-evoked potential as a result of background muscle activation.

(From the 2001 Report of the Nomenclature Committee of the American Association of Electromyography and Electrodiagnosis.[19] Reproduced by kind permission of the AANEM.)

facilitatory paratonia A variant of **paratonia** in which the patient acts in the same direction as the passive movement, rather than in the opposite direction. Its presence predicts lower scores on tests of cognitive function.[603]

faciocardiorenal syndrome A recessively inherited dysmorphic syndrome in which numerous skeletal and visceral abnormalities are associated with mental and developmental delay.[1799]

faciolingual syndrome A clinical combination of hemiparesis affecting the lower face and the tongue with some degree of dysarthria but without any aphasia. This was first described by Déjèrine and Klumpke[1541] in 1901, who identified the presence of a small infarct in the genu of the contralateral internal capsule. See also **capsular genu syndrome**.

faciolinguopharyngomasticatory diplegia See **anterior operculum syndrome**.

facioscapulohumeral atrophy See **hereditary motor neuropathy** (*variants*).

facioscapulohumeral dystrophy (Landouzy–Déjèrine syndrome) A group of relatively common, slowly progressive, dominantly inherited muscular dystrophies with the usual onset in childhood or youth, in which the common factor is asymmetrical weakness and wasting of the muscles of the shoulder girdle (especially the periscapular and humeral muscles), the face, and the proximal leg, eventually accompanied in most cases by peroneal weakness.[3675] The smile is typically transverse and there may be marked weakness of eye closure. Scapular winging and horizontally positioned clavicles, dysarthria, and difficulties in whistling or arm raising are common initial symptoms. Variable trunkal involvement leads often to a positive **Beevor sign**. There is wide variability in age at onset, disease severity, and side-to-side symmetry. Associated manifestations include high-frequency hearing loss and retinal telangiectasias.

The responsible gene is located at chromosome 4q35 (double homeobox protein 4, *DUX4*), where there is a deletion of a fragment of DNA and an array of tandem repeat units. Despite the accepted eponyms, **Duchenne** described the condition in 1868 (as occurring congenitally).

The syndrome is clinically heterogeneous. Both neurogenic[2009] and myopathic diseases with facioscapulohumeral distribution have been identified and in some cases mitochondrial changes have been detected.[6225]

The numerous *variants* include the following:

Facioscapulohumeral muscular dystrophy 1b, also dominantly inherited but without linkage to the 4q site.
A lethal, dominantly inherited *infantile* form in which there is a severe muscular dystrophy with onset in infancy and death in adolescence. Although the disease is dominantly inherited, the parent may be only minimally affected. Facial weakness is the first sign, while bulbar dysfunction, hypotonia, progressive proximal weakness, and subsequent respiratory insufficiency follow.[336]
A form with *late exacerbation*.
Another with facial sparing.[2004]
A disputed *form with recessive inheritance*.[379]
A *childhood form* in which features of **Möbius syndrome** are also present.[2739]
Facioscapulohumeral dystrophy and deafness: A congenital myopathic syndrome characterized by proximal and facial myopathic weakness and deafness. This may be an integral part of the basic syndrome.[886]
Facioscapulohumeral dystrophy and ***Coats syndrome***: A dysmorphic syndrome with onset in infancy manifesting also sensorineural deafness, exudative retinal telangiectasia, detached retina, and tortuosity of the retinal vessels, ptosis, facial, proximal and distal myopathic weakness, and mental and developmental delay.[2370, 6233]
An early-onset form with added *epilepsy and mental retardation*.[2241]

Facioscapulohumeral Dystrophy Society A charitable organization in this field. Address: 3 Westwood Road, Lexington, MA 02420. Tel: 781-860-0501. E-mail: info@fshsociety.org/. Web site: http://www.fshsociety.org/.

facioscapulohumeral spinal muscular atrophy A variant of the usual proximal pattern of **hereditary motor neuropathy** in which dominantly inherited weakness and wasting occur in the above distribution.[2009] Nevertheless, whether this syndrome represents a neuropathic rather than a dystrophic disorder is not firmly established.

factitious disorder The conscious fabrication of symptoms and signs, whether or not the motivation to do so is perceived by the patient.Clues to the presence of this disorder have been suggested by Eisendrath.[1825]

faculty (from Lat, capability) 1. A special power or ability of the mind. 2. The academic staff of an institution of learning. The two generally correlate.

fading athlete syndrome The ascription of declining performance by skilled athletes to a neuromuscular disease, a reaction considered to be psychogenic.[5446]

Fahn–Marsden Scale An instrument rating the severity of abnormal involuntary movements, accessible at http://www.mdvu.org/library/ratingscales/dystonia/bfm_scale.pdf/.

Fahr, Theodor (1877–1945) German pathologist who graduated at Giessen and eventually became professor of pathology in Hamburg. His publications mainly concerned renal and vascular diseases. He was not the first to describe familial calcification in the basal ganglia, nor, in retrospect, have his observations been regarded as completely accurate.

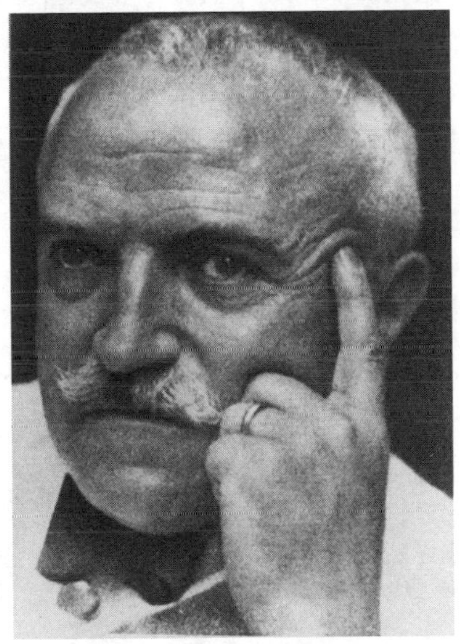

Figure F–1 Theodor Fahr.

Fahr syndrome See **striatopallidal calcification**.

failed back syndrome Continuing pain in the back following surgery, occurring almost exclusively in patients who have been operated on for the wrong reasons. Good reasons to operate on a patient with back pain presumed to be due to a herniated disc include the following:

1. Radicular pain in the appropriate distribution and under the proper conditions. (Axial pain is almost never relieved by surgery.)
2. Clinical signs of radiculopathy. If the radiculopathy is acute (e.g., sudden foot drop), the need for surgery may be urgent. Cervical myelopathy may be another indication.
3. The symptoms and signs did not remit after appropriate conservative therapy.
4. The imaging studies are consonant with the signs and symptoms.

failure of visuoconstructive ability See **constructional apraxia**.

faint 1. Weak or languid. 2. (syncope, swooning) Reduction in consciousness with loss of power of the body and the mind as a consequence of reduced cerebral blood flow.

fainting (from Gr, to cut short) A sense of impending dissolution, usually with dimming or loss of vision and eventually loss of consciousness and motor tone, leading to loss of the upright posture and due to reduction in cerebral blood flow.

Fairbank syndrome A developmental anomaly, characterized by facial dysmorphism, short hands and digits, turribrachicephaly, exophthalmos, enlarged sella turcica, and metaphyseal and epiphyseal changes.[2504] See **craniosynostosis**.

Fajersztajn crossed sciatic sign In sciatic root irritation, the hip can only be flexed when the knee is flexed, not when it is held straight, and pain is felt on the side of the root irritation during performance of the **Lasègue** manoeuvre on the healthy side.

This really amounts to the straight-leg raising test from a different aspect.

fakirism Control of the body's motor and sensory processes as a result of mental concentration. Thus, for example, pain may not be felt in circumstances which would otherwise be extremely unpleasant—classic examples being fire-walking or a lying on a bed of nails. During such times the EEG records generalized theta activity.

falciform lobe (from Lat, resembling a sickle) Schwalbe's term for the limbic lobe.

Falconer, Murray (1910–1988) Neurosurgeon, born in New Zealand. He practiced at the Guy's-Maudsley Unit in London, UK, where he specialized in the surgical treatment of epilepsy.

Falconer–Weddell syndrome See **thoracic outlet syndrome**.

fall risk index A standardized tool to assess the risk of falling in patients with dysequilibrium.[6328]

fallen fontanelle (caida de mollera) Depression of the anterior fontanelle, a sign of childhood trauma, as in the **battered baby (child) syndrome.**[2603]

falling seizures (akinetic or astatic seizures; myoclonic-astatic seizure) Epileptic seizures of which the major feature is a sudden fall to the ground forward, preceded by a jerk of the axial muscles. The EEG shows a spike–wave complex, the spike usually associated with the myoclonic jerk and the slow wave with the loss of tone. See **myoclonic epilepsies**.

Fallopius (Gabriel Fallopio, 1523–1563) Italian professor of anatomy and botany at Padua. His observations of greatest relevance to neurology were his descriptions of the facial canal in 1561 and of cranial nerves IV, V, IX, and X. His drawings demonstrate that he had noted the anatomy of the arterial circle at the base of the brain well before **Willis**.

false image The less distinct and more peripheral image, coming from the affected eye of a patient with diplopia. The mechanism responsible for the loss of clarity is the reception of light from the object by a part of the retina other than the macula.

false localizing signs Clinical neurological signs which do not arise from damage to the area of the primary lesion in question, and which suggest incorrectly that it is situated at a certain site. This may reflect dysfunction remote from the expected anatomical locus of pathology.[3700] The lesion itself is usually a tumor causing increased intracranial pressure, either the mass or more often its pressure effect leading to traction upon, or displacement or compression of, other intracranial structures, or interruption of the their blood supply.

The classic example is an unilateral VI cranial nerve palsy due to stretching of the nerve as a result of increased intracranial pressure rather than as a result of the direct compressive effect of the mass. Other examples include dementia with temporal lobe tumors; anosmia; visual field defects; anisocoria, pupillary paresis, nystagmus, ptosis, VI nerve palsy, and gaze palsies; initial contralateral mydriasis with frontal lobe hemorrhage;[1131] trigeminal paresthesia or pain; cerebellar signs; frontal ataxia, pyramidal deficits; neck stiffness; proptosis; hypothalamic disturbances and decerebrate rigidity, all being associated with increased intracranial pressure.

Signs referable to dysfunction of regions in immediate proximity to a lesion are considered to be "neighborhood" signs and not falsely localizing.[2302]

false Rombergism Wildly excessive swaying without falling, seen when the **Romberg Test** is performed by subjects with psychogenic complaints of imbalance. The remarkable gyrations without falls that are occasionally witnessed actually indicate superior balance.

false sago palm A tree growing in the Western Pacific region, the seeds of which contain the neurotoxic agent *cycas circinalis* considered responsible for **Lytico–Bodig**.

falx cerebri, falx cerebelli (Lat, sickle + brain or little brain) Condensations of the dura mater which divide and support the two lobes of each structure.

falx syndrome Acute and severe paresis and/or simple motor seizures of one or both legs as a result of an interhemispheric subdural hematoma or empyema.[3870]

fame may be considered as a variant of **progressive myoclonic epilepsy** or **juvenile myoclonic epilepsy**. It differs from these conditions in its onset in adult life and usual genetic locus but, like them, presents with variable limb myoclonus, some tonic–clonic seizures and a benign course. The disorder was reported first from Japan.[5046]

Two *variants* are *autosomal dominant cortical myoclonus and epilepsy*, a disorder characterized by complex partial seizures (and mental retardation in some cases) mapping to chromosome 2p11.1, the FAME2 locus; and *FAME3*, manifesting frequent seizures, cerebellar ataxia, dementia, and a progressive course without linkage and to the other sites for FAME.[1032]

familial acephalgic migraine The occurrence of migraine auras (usually visual and paresthetic and precipitated by bright lights) in the absence of headache. The condition has been reported as dominantly inherited.[6971]

familial acoustic neuroma See **neurofibromatosis 2**.

familial adult myoclonic epilepsy (FAME; familial cortical myoclonic tremor, familial cortical tremor with epilepsy, familial essential myoclonus and epilepsy, familial benign myoclonus epilepsy of adult onset) A dominantly inherited nonprogressive epileptic syndrome of young adults characterized by myoclonic jerks in the limbs, trembling of the fingers, cerebellar signs, and rare generalized tonic clonic seizures. It is linked to chromosome 8q24, though the condition is likely to be heterogeneous.

familial adult myoclonic epilepsy See **familial adult myoclonic epilepsy**.

familial Alzheimer disease See **Alzheimer disease**.

familial amaurotic idiocy (Tay Sachs disease) See **GM_2 gangliosidoses**.

familial amyloid neuropathy A group of inherited diseases, variously inherited, but all characterized by the extracellular deposition of fibrillar material in body tissues, predominantly in the nutrient blood vessels of the peripheral nervous system. The main precursor proteins encountered are transthyretin, apolipoprotein A1, or gelsolin, but mutations in the transthyretin protein are responsible for the sensory or autonomic neuropathies that constitute the major clinical syndromes, though ocular and cardiac manifestations are also common and leptomeningeal amyloidosis and may be manifest as a cerebral hemorrhage or

Chart F–1. Forms of Familial Amyloid Neuropathy

Amyloidosis type I, dominant (Andrade, Portuguese type) A dominantly inherited syndrome due to an abnormality of the plasma protein transthyretin (prealbumin), for which the abnormal gene maps to 18q1.2q12.1. Clinically, the condition manifests an axonal thin-fiber neuropathy that presents with spontaneous pains in youth or early adult life, and with more generalized motor, sensory, and autonomic dysfunction plus cardiac, renal, and ocular involvement later. Selective early losses of A-delta and C fibers in the peripheral nerves are characteristic.[197,196] At least 40 other transthyretin mutations producing amyloidoses are also described.

Amyloidosis type I, recessive type (Portuguese type) A recessively inherited syndrome also due to transthyretin abnormalities, characterized by the onset in mature adult life of axonal thick- and thin-fiber sensorimotor and autonomic neuropathy (often presenting as carpal tunnel syndrome) with vitreous opacities and cardiac involvement.[6948]

Amyloidosis type II (Rukavina or Indiana types) A dominantly inherited acropathic sensorimotor axonal neuropathy with adult onset, mainly affecting the arms. The early symptoms are those of **carpal tunnel syndrome**, evidence of generalized polyneuropathy appearing years later. Sclerodermatous skin thickening and both corneal and vitreous opacities are common early and cardiac involvement a late complication.[4022, 5467] Apolipoprotein-A1 is the mutated protein in this case.

Amyloidosis type III (Van Allen or Iowa type) A dominantly inherited syndrome with young adult onset of severe and widespread sensorimotor neuropathy with associated cataracts, deafness, peptic ulcer disease, and later autonomic effects, due to widespread deposition of amyloid which eventually leads to renal failure. Type III familial amyloid polyneuropathy is thus similar to type I, but has a later age of onset.[6464, 6465] The genetic defect maps to 11q23–q24.

Amyloidosis type IV (Finnish type, Gelsolin variant, cranial neuropathy) A dominantly inherited form characterized by the onset in mature adult life of facial and bulbar cranial neuropathies, followed years later by mild thick- and thin-fiber sensorimotor and autonomic neuropathy, atrophy of the skin, corneal lattice dystrophy, and renal and cardiac involvement.[4322] The genetic base substitution responsible is located at 9q33, codon 187 of plasma gelsolin complementary DNA.[3464]

Amyloidosis type V with cranial neuropathy and corneal lattice dystrophy (Jewish type) A variant due to abnormality of gelosis, for which the responsible gene maps to 9q32–q34.[2253]

Amyloidosis type VI with variant prealbumin (Appalachian type) A dominantly inherited form with late onset.[6607]

Amyloidosis type VII (oculomeningeal or Ohio type) A form characterized by the onset of cerebrovascular changes in young adult life, leading to emotional lability, abnormality in consciousness, seizures, dementia, and pyramidal and cerebellar signs.[2496]

infarction; dementia; hydrocephalus; ataxia; spastic paraparesis; or seizures.[5045]

Forms that have been identified are listed in 'Chart F–1. See also **amyloid neuropathy**. For a recent review, see Adams (2001).[49]

Other *variants* are as follows:

Trigeminal neuropathy with nasal ulceration,[5981] and *dominant familial amyloid neuropathy with severe cardiac involvement*, which is an unusually early and severe cardiomyopathy occurring in the setting of familial amyloidosis;[5568] and a *dominantly inherited form* mapping to chromosome 20.[3441] See also **Dutch cerebral hemorrhage**.

familial amyotrophic chorea with acanthocytosis See **neuroacanthocytosis**.

familial amyotrophic lateral sclerosis See **amyotrophic lateral sclerosis**.

familial antiphospholipid antibody syndrome A genetically determined disorder of blood predisposing to stroke and as yet unmapped.

familial apoceruloplasmin deficiency A rare inherited dysmetabolic state which presents with dystonias and retinal degeneration.[4413]

familial ataxic diplegia See **Fanconi–Turler syndrome**.

familial (autosomal dominant) focal epilepsies Monogenic forms of epilepsy determined by mutations in susceptibility genes, most of which code for either voltage-gated or ligand-gated ion channel subunits, and thus representing **channelopathies**. The following syndromes have been recognized: **benign familial neonatal seizures, benign familial infantile seizures, autosomal dominant nocturnal frontal lobe epilepsy, familial mesial temporal lobe epilepsy, familial lateral temporal lobe epilepsy**, and **familial focal epilepsy with variable foci**.

familial benign essential chorea See **hereditary nonprogressive chorea**. See also **Huntington disease**.

familial benign myoclonus epilepsy of adult onset See **familial adult myoclonic epilepsy**.

familial benign neonatal convulsions An inherited tendency to generalized tonic–clonic seizures in the neonatal period. The responsible gene maps to chromosome 20.

familial benign recurrent vertigo An unusual cause of attacks of uncomplication vertigo, mapped to 22q12.

familial bilateral striatal necrosis (infantile bilateral striatal necrosis, familial holotopistic striatal necrosis, juvenile Leigh disease, familial cerebral degeneration chiefly affecting the lenticular nucleus, symmetrical degeneration of the neostriatum, familial holotopistic striatal necrosis, familial striatal degeneration) A rare maternally inherited, missense mitochondrial ATPase mutation causing a pallidonigrostriatal degeneration resembling **Leigh disease** without the progression. The condition is characterized by childhood onset of an acute disturbance of consciousness followed by progressive rigidity with pyramidal signs, hyperactivity, involuntary movements such as athetosis, tremor and myoclonus, and dysphasia. Loss of spontaneous movements, seizures, mental retardation, and stereotyped responses to all stimuli are also described, as are subacutely progressive athetosis, rigidity leading on to hypotonia, dysarthria and dysphagia, and mental retardation.

Pathologically, there is with marked symmetrical neuronal loss in the caudate nucleus and putamen. The brainstem is spared.[5352, 6314, 4928] The condition might represent a form of parainfectious encephalitis[2202] but an X-linked form is considered to be a variant of **Leigh disease**.[4227]

familial brachial plexus palsy See **neuralgic amyotrophy**.

familial British dementia with amyloid angiopathy An autosomal dominant condition characterized by dementia, progressive spastic tetraparesis, and cerebellar ataxia with onset in the sixth decade and due to a point mutation in the *BRI* gene. A common ancestor has been identified between the large pedigree and a case report of "familial cerebellar ataxia with amyloid angiopathy"; neurological examination was abnormal in three, with limb and gait ataxia and mild spastic paraparesis. Three had impaired recognition and recall memory and another had mild impairment of delayed visual recall. All affected individuals had an abnormal MRI of the brain, consisting of deep white matter hyperintensity on T2-weighted scans and lacunar infarcts, but no intracerebral hemorrhage. The corpus callosum was particularly affected; in one patient it was severely atrophic.[4268]

familial calcification of the basal ganglia See **striatopallidal calcification**.

familial calcification of the brain, iron storage, and porphyria See **striatopallidal calcification**.

familial calcifying polioencephalopathy See **striatopallidal calcification**.

familial capillary-venous leptomeningeal angiomatosis See **Divry–van Bogaert syndrome**.

familial carpal tunnel syndrome See **carpal tunnel syndrome**.[1447]

familial cavernous angioma/ hemangioma of the retina (Gass syndrome) A dominantly inherited syndrome of retinal cavernous angioma and/ or skin hemangiomas.[1674]

familial cerebellar ataxia and hypogonadism The association of cerebellar ataxia with primary hypogonadism. Whether this is fortuitous or etiologically meaningful is not clear.[4182]

familial cerebellar ataxia with cerebrovascular amyloid See **cerebellar ataxias** (*variants*).

familial cerebral amyloidosis with spongiform encephalopathy A dominantly inherited infiltrative spongiform encephalopathy, also involving the peripheral nervous system and affecting mature adults who develop dementia; apraxias; ophthalmoplegia; nystagmus; pyramidal; extrapyramidal and cerebellar signs; and both sensory and autonomic neuropathies. See **Gerstmann–Straussler–Scheinker syndrome**.

familial cerebral amyloid angiopathy (Dutch type) A dominantly inherited condition mapped to 21q–21.3q22.05 and leading to cerebral hemorrhages.

familial cerebral cavernous hemangiomas See **cavernous angioma**.

familial cerebral degeneration chiefly affecting the lenticular nucleus See **infantile bilateral striatal necrosis**.

familial cerebral sarcoma The rare occurrence of cerebral fibrosarcomas in more than one family member.[2256]

familial cerebromeningeal angiomatosis See **Divry–van Bogaert syndrome**.

familial chorea with acanthocytosis See **neuroacanthocytosis**.

familial chorea with myoclonic epilepsy A dominantly inherited syndrome consisting of chorea, ataxia, myoclonus, seizures, and dementia.[6189] See **myoclonus**.

familial congenital corneal anesthesia A rare, dominantly inherited syndrome of isolated corneal anesthesia with secondary trophic lesions.[3506]

familial cortical myoclonic tremor See **familial adult myoclonic epilepsy**.

familial cortical tremor, epilepsy, and mental retardation A rare, dominantly inherited syndrome manifesting action tremor seizures and mental retardation with diffuse spike-and-wave EEG activity and photoparoxysmal responses as well as the usual features of cortical reflex myoclonus.[1837]

familial cortical tremor with epilepsy See **familial adult myoclonic epilepsy**.

familial cramps and muscle pain A syndrome with its onset in youth, characterized by muscle pain or cramps, incontinence, and the clinical and pathological features of mild myopathy. See **adolescent familial cramps**.

familial Creutzfeldt–Jakob disease See **Creutzfeldt–Jakob disease**.

familial Cushing syndrome (Swiss syndrome, Carney complex) A rare autosomal dominant disorder characterized by mesenchymal tumors including cardiac and cutaneous myxomas, and by spotty skin pigmentation, functional endocrine overactivity, and Schwannomas of the peripheral nerves.[1021]

familial cutaneous amyloidosis with systemic manifestations A congenital syndrome manifesting cloudy corneas, malabsorption, recurrent infections, hyperkeratosis, patchy skin pigmentation, seizures, and mental and developmental delay. See also **familial amyloid neuropathy**.

familial degeneration of the pallidonigral system A fatal degenerative disorder of early childhood, manifesting febrile episodes, hepatosplenomegaly, anemia, pyramidal signs, and seizures. Pathological findings include degeneration of the globus pallidus, subthalamic nucleus, and substantia nigra.[4208]

familial distal dysautonomia A familial syndrome of autonomic dysfunction affecting the hands and feet as well as vasomotor, pilomotor, and sudomotor function, without other evidence of peripheral somatic neuropathy. The condition may be dominantly inherited.[5336]

familial dysautonomia See **hereditary sensory and autonomic neuropathy type 3** and **Riley–Day syndrome**.

familial dyskinesia and facial myokymia A dominantly inherited disorder characterized by involuntary chorea-like movements and perioral and periorbital myokymia, with onset in early childhood or adolescence. The movements are paroxysmal initially but increase in frequency and severity and may become constant in the third decade, stabilizing, or even improving thereafter. The adventitious movements are worsened by anxiety but not by voluntary movement, startle, caffeine, or alcohol. The disease is socially disabling, but there is no intellectual impairment or decrease in life span. Its genetic basis is not yet determined.[2023]

familial dyslexia See **dyslexia**. The genetic abnormality in this familial form has been localized to the short arm of chromosome 15.

familial dystonic choreoathetosis (syndrome of Mount and Reback) See **familial paroxysmal dystonic choreoathetosis**.

familial encephalopathy and basal ganglion calcification See **striatopallidal calcification**.

familial epilepsy and yellow teeth A syndrome of severe seizures in infancy, with mental and motor delay, pyramidal signs, and unusually colored teeth.[3514]

familial episodic ataxia See **cerebellar ataxia**.

familial erythrophagocytic lymphohistiocytosis (Omenn syndrome) A lethal, recessively inherited, congenital dysmorphic syndrome manifesting also visceromegaly, anemia, low white blood cell and platelet counts, recurrent infections (including meningitis and encephalitis), seizures, ataxia, pyramidal signs, and neurodegenerative regression. Widespread infiltration with reticulum cells is usually found. Low-density areas due to gliosis and demyelination are seen in the white matter on CT scanning.[4793]

familial essential benign chorea See **hereditary essential chorea** and **Huntington disease**.

familial essential myoclonus A dominantly inherited syndrome of stimulus- and movement-sensitive myoclonic jerks associated with rhythmic discharges alternating with asynchronous, dysrhythmic complexes on the EEG, alleviated by alcohol consumption, and sometimes associated also with **essential tremor**.[3538]

familial essential myoclonus and epilepsy See **familial adult myoclonic epilepsy**.

familial extrapyramidal disease with polyneuropathy A dominantly inherited syndrome characterized by symptoms of **Parkinson disease** with onset in mature adult life characterized by the delayed development of an axonal or demyelinating sensorimotor peripheral neuropathy with distal weakness, ataxia, muscle wasting, and loss of reflexes.[965]

In *variant* forms, postencephalitic Parkinsonism is accompanied by amyotrophy.

familial focal epilepsy with variable foci A rare dominantly inherited genetically heterogeneous syndrome with onset at any time in life before middle age, mapped to chromosome 22q11–q12 and possibly to 2q. Clinically, family members have focal seizures emanating from different cortical locations that include temporal, frontal, centroparietal, or occipital lobe regions, often in sleep. Occasional GTCS occur in a small majority. Most often the seizures are infrequent, easily controlled, or even asymptomatic.

Focal epileptiform discharges are seen on the interictal EEG, varying in site for each affected family member but constant for each individual, and are enhanced by sleep.[4882, 1861]

familial frontotemporal dementia A dementing illness with Parkinsonism, due to mutations in the tau gene on chromosome 17.[6907] See **frontotemporal dementia**.

familial hearing loss, polyneuropathy, and optic atrophy An autosomal or X-linked recessively transmitted syndrome manifesting progressive neural deafness from childhood with polyneuropathy and optic atrophy.[2865]

familial hemiplegic migraine (cerebellar migraine) A rare, dominantly inherited or sporadic form of **migraine with aura** occurring first in youth and characterized by paroxysmal headaches, many with hemiplegia occurring before, during, or after the headache phase and lasting for hours or days. Attacks may be precipitated by head trauma. The attack is usually part of the aura of migraine and lasts less than an hour (migraine with typical aura). Typically, there is a visual aura that is followed by the onset of slowly progressive unilateral sensory or motor symptoms. Fever, dysarthria, aphasia, and reduction in consciousness are commonly associated symptoms, and in one-fifth of the cases there are permanent cerebellar signs. Rarely, symptoms can last up to a week (migraine with pronounced aura).[3004] To make the diagnosis, at least one first- or second-degree relative must have migraine auras that include motor weakness.

The condition is due to missense mutations in the *CACNA1A* gene on chromosome 19p13 (FHM1) in half the cases, and to *ATP1A2* (FHM2) and *SCN1A* (FHM3) in some others, indicating genetic heterogeneity.[3252] Various mutations at the same site are associated with **episodic ataxia** type 2, with delayed cerebral edema and with fatal coma after minor head trauma. Diagnostic criteria have been defined:

A. At least two attacks fulfilling criteria B and C
B. Aura consisting of fully reversible motor weakness and at least one of the following:
   1. Fully reversible visual symptoms including positive features (e.g., flickering lights, spots, or lines) and/or negative features (i.e., loss of vision)

2. Fully reversible sensory symptoms including positive features (i.e., pins and needles) and/or negative features (i.e., numbness)
3. Fully reversible dysphasic speech disturbance

C. At least two of the following:

1. At least one aura symptom develops gradually over ≥5 min and/or different aura symptoms occur in succession over ≥5 min
2. Each aura symptom lasts ≥5 min and <24 h
3. Headache fulfilling criteria B–D for migraine without aura.

Migraine without aura begins during the aura or follows onset of aura within 60 min.

D. At least one first- or second-degree relative has had attacks fulfilling these criteria A–E
E. Not attributed to another disorder

A *variant* is as follows:

Sporadic hemiplegic migraine
Migraine with aura including motor weakness but in which no first- or second-degree relative has an aura that includes motor weakness.

Diagnostic criteria have been defined:

A. At least two attacks fulfilling criteria B and C
B. Aura consisting of fully reversible motor weakness and at least one of the following:

1. Fully reversible visual symptoms including positive features (e.g., flickering lights, spots, or lines) and/or negative features (i.e., loss of vision)
2. Fully reversible sensory symptoms including positive features (i.e., pins and needles) and/or negative features (i.e., numbness)
3. Fully reversible dysphasic speech disturbance

C. At least two of the following:

1. At least one aura symptom develops gradually over ≥5 min and/or different aura symptoms occur in succession over ≥5 min
2. Each aura symptom lasts ≥5 min and <24 h
3. Headache fulfilling criteria B–D for **migraine without aura** begins during the aura or follows onset of aura within 60 min

D. No first- or second-degree relative has attacks fulfilling the criteria A–E
E. Not attributed to another disorder

Both of these definitions are from the International Classification of Headache Disorders (Headache Classification Committee of the International Headache Society. *Cephalalgia* 2004;**24**[Suppl 1]) by kind permission of Dr. Jes Olesen, the International Headache Society and Wiley-Blackwell Publications.

Other *variants* are follows:

Hemiplegic migraine and ataxia A dominantly inherited syndrome with onset in youth, characterized by paroxysmal headaches, ophthalmoplegia, nystagmus, ataxia, hemiplegia, and tremor.

Hemiplegic migraine, nystagmus, and deafness A rare, presumably dominantly inherited syndrome comprising these features.[6929] Associations with ataxia (cerebellar migraine), tremor, and retinal degeneration have also been reported.[6973, 379]

Hemiplegic migraine with seizures without ataxia (FHM2) due to mutations in *ATP1A2*. A form in which hemihypesthesia occurs instead of hemiplegia.

familial holotopistic striatal necrosis See **infantile bilateral striatal necrosis**.

familial horizontal gaze palsy with progressive scoliosis A rare, recessively inherited disorder characterized by congenital absence of conjugate horizontal eye movements and progressive scoliosis, developing in childhood or adolescence. The responsible gene is mapped to 11q23.[3193]

familial hyperthyroidism See **Frank syndrome**.

familial hypertrophic interstitial neuropathy See **hereditary motor and sensory neuropathy type 3**.

familial hypertrophic neuropathy with gammopathy (familial hypertrophic paraprotein polyneuritis) A dominantly inherited hypertrophic polyneuropathy with slow progression and with both motor and sensory features, accompanied by a gammopathy.

familial hyperkalemic periodic paralysis See **familial periodic paralysis**.

familial hypertrophic paraprotein polyneuritis See **familial hypertrophic neuropathy with gammopathy**.

familial hypoparathyroidism, sensorineural deafness, and renal dysplasia A rare dominantly inherited syndrome characterized by these features.[640]

familial hypoplasia of the carotid arteries (carotid hypoplasia) A developmental dysgenetic syndrome with onset in youth; a rare cause of atherothrombotic brain infarction.[381]

familial idiopathic brain calcification A dominantly inherited syndrome characterized by calcification within the basal ganglia associated with slowly progressive intellectual decline, Parkinsonism, seizures, and mild cerebellar ataxia.[3505] An X-linked dominant form is also described.

familial inclusion body myositis See **inclusion body myositis**.

familial infantile bilateral striatal necrosis A rare disorder characterized by symmetric degeneration of the caudate, putamen, and globus pallidus. Clinical features include developmental regression, choreoathetosis, dystonia, spasticity, dysphagia, failure to thrive, nystagmus, optic atrophy, and mental retardation with onset usually in the first year of life. The condition evolves through spastic quadriparesis to death.[6089]

familial infantile myasthenia A recessive variant of childhood **myasthenia gravis** in which the mother is unaffected; weakness after activity is more severe than in the classic form and leads to severe respiratory and feeding difficulties from birth but does not involve the extraocular muscles; fatigability occurs with the usual decrementing response to repetitive stimulation on EMG; and there is a tendency to later recurrence of apnea caused by crying, vomiting, or fever. There is nevertheless a trend toward spontaneous remission.

The pathogenesis is a defect in acetylcholine resynthesis. The motor end-plate potential amplitude is normal in rested muscle with stimulation, but a decrement is seen after exercise or electrical stimulation of muscle. The synaptic vesicles are abnormally small.[4465, 869, 1866]

familial infantile myopathy A **mitochondrial** disorder due to cytochrome *c* oxidase deficiency, presenting in early childhood with proximal muscle weakness and wasting.

familial intermittent ataxia An X-linked syndrome in which the intermittent ataxia is accompanied by abnormalities of pyruvate metabolism and with cerebral pathology resembling that of **Leigh disease**. There is a response to acetazolamide. It is likely that this represents more than one condition.[3883] See **cerebellar ataxias**.

familial inverted chorea A rare, dominantly inherited condition with the onset in infancy of chorea and athetosis of the legs only, with added pyramidal signs.[2109]

familial juvenile macular degeneration See **Stargardt syndrome**.

familial juvenile motor neuron disease See **amyotrophic lateral sclerosis**.

familial lateral temporal lobe epilepsy (autosomal dominant "partial" epilepsy with auditory features) A dominantly inherited non-ion channel form of idiopathic focal epilepsy with onset in adolescence, mapped to chromosome 10q24. Clinically, the focal seizures occur mainly at night and consist of simple auditory hallucinations such as ringing, humming, clicking, or unspecified noises but may progress to complex focal seizures and to GTCS. Other symptoms such as visual (lights, colors, and simple figures), olfactory, vertiginous, or cephalic perceptions are frequent with simple focal seizures while autonomic, mental, and motor symptoms are less common. Patients are neurologically and mentally normal and the seizures are generally mild, infrequent, and easily controlled.[4882] See also **familial mesial temporal lobe epilepsy** and **lateral temporal lobe epilepsy** (nonfamilial).

familial limb-girdle myasthenia A form of **myasthenia gravis** in which there is selective muscle involvement, giving the appearance of muscular dystrophy. Proximal weakness without atrophy or bulbar or ocular involvement is notable, but there is a good response to anticholinesterase drugs.[4266]

familial lipodystrophy See **lipodystrophy**.

familial lumbosacral syringomyelia See **hereditary sensory and autonomic neuropathy**.

familial lysis of type I fibers A rare form of congenital myopathy in which **cores** extend across the whole width of a muscle fiber.[6] See also **multicore myopathy** and **congenital myopathy**.

familial macrocephaly See **familial megalencephaly**.

familial Mediterranean fever An autosomal recessive disease characterized by recurrent attacks of paroxysmal abdominal pain with fever and painful episodes of sterile peritonitis, pleuritis, and/or arthritis. Febrile myalgia has also been recorded.[316]

familial megalencephaly (familial macrocephaly) A congenital syndrome of uncomplicated macrocephaly.[381]

familial meralgia paresthetica See **meralgia paresthetica**.[4143]

familial mesial temporal lobe epilepsy A dominantly inherited syndrome of youth or young adult life with heterogeneous manifestations; simple focal seizures with déjà vu, other mental illusions, and hallucinations are typical, either alone or with autonomic disturbances, fear and panic, visual and auditory illusions, and somatosensory sensations of diffuse numbness and tingling. Any of these may progress to complex focal seizures. An **epigastric aura** does not occur. Some subjects have a benign course and exhibit only simple partial seizures and infrequent complex partial seizures but in all the response to medication is good. The condition maps to chromosome 4q13.[2830, 1861]

familial methemaglobinemia A recessively inherited diffuse encephalopathy presenting with mental retardation as a result of deficiency of methemaglobin reductase.

familial migraine with vertigo and essential tremor A dominantly inherited syndrome of episodic vertigo, migraine headaches, and essential tremor, with onset in youth and with no defined genetic linkage.[356]

familial mitochondrial myopathy A dominantly inherited myopathy associated with single large or multiple deletions of mitochondrial DNA and manifesting bulbar and girdle weakness, progressive external ophthalmoplegia, and sensorineural deafness.[6970]

familial motor neuron disease A dominantly inherited syndrome of adult onset with features resembling those of acquired **amyotrophic lateral sclerosis** but with a somewhat younger onset.

Variant forms with associated sensory loss or deafness, or with onset in youth, have also been described.

familial moyamoya disease A dominantly inherited polygenic disorder mapped to 3p24.2–p26, predisposing to stroke. See **moyamoya disease**.

familial multicore disease with focal loss of cross-striations and ophthalmoplegia (familial myopathy with focal loss of cross-striations) A congenital myopathy, considered to be a subvariety of **multicore disease**, presenting with ptosis and ophthalmoplegia from birth, proximal muscle weakness with delayed motor development, hypotonia, and hyperreflexia, and with muscle biopsy findings of multicores and a focal loss of cross striations.[1872, 6158]

familial multiinfarct dementia (familial vascular encephalopathy, familial spastic paraparesis, and dementia) An inherited syndrome of young adult life characterized by vascular dementia with facial weakness, pseudobulbar and limb pyramidal signs, and cerebral atrophy. See also **familial subcortical dementia with arteriosclerotic leukoencephalopathy** and **Worster–Drought syndrome**.

familial multilocular encephalomalacia See **disseminated encephalomalacia with cavity formation**.

familial multiple symmetric lipomatosis with peripheral neuropathy (Madelung disease, Launois–Bensaude syndrome, benign symmetric lipomatosis) A rare, dominantly or recessively inherited **mitochondriopathy** mainly affecting middle-aged males and characterized by the development of large nonencapsulated lipomata on the neck, shoulders, and proximal arms, with an axonal polyneuropathy affecting mainly the larger myelinated fibers. An association with chronic alcoholism has been suggested. The condition was described first by Sir Benjamin Brodie in 1846.[1081, 4908]

familial multisystem atrophy A dominantly inherited syndrome, different phenotypes exhibiting combinations of clumsiness, spasticity, optic atrophy, and mental deterioration resembling that of **thalamic dementia**.[3324]

familial myasthenia gravis See **myasthenia gravis**.

familial myoclonic dementia (Stern–Garcin syndrome, subacute degeneration of the thalamus) A dominantly inherited form of **thalamic dementia** characterized by having a subacute course of progressive dementia (memory loss, psychotic behavior, frontal release signs, and hallucinations) occurring over a period of up to 2 years, associated with myoclonus.[3872, 6042] See **fatal familial insomnia**.

familial myoclonic epilepsy See **Unverricht–Lundborg–Lafora syndrome**.

familial myoclonus epilepsy and choreoathetosis See **hereditary dentatorubralpallidoluysian atrophy**.

familial myopathy with focal loss of cross striations See **familial multicore disease with focal loss of cross striations and ophthalmoplegia**.

familial myofibrillar inclusion body myopathy A dominantly inherited myopathy with these microscopic features. The disorder is not always symptomatic.[1189]

familial myoglobinuria See **myoglobinuria**.

familial myopathy with muscle cramps An hereditary nonprogressive muscle disorder with adult onset presenting with mild proximal muscle weakness and painless muscle cramps following exercise, associated with the finding of multiple cores in muscle biopsy specimens low in oxidative enzymes.[599]

familial myopathy with myofibrillar lysis An hereditary myopathy presenting with hypotonia in the infant and with later proximal weakness. Muscle biopsy findings are of accumulations of subsarcolemmal granules.[997]

familial myopathy with probable lysis of myofibrils in type I fibers See **hyaline body myopathy**.

familial myopathy with thrombocytopenia An hereditary nonprogressive muscle disorder with onset in childhood, comprising proximal and distal myopathic weakness and thrombocytopenia.[381]

familial myosclerosis (myodysplasia fibrosa multiplex) A condition marked by the replacement of muscle by fibrous issue, giving it a hard consistency on palpation. It is probably not a single entity, but rather represents the end stage of various primary neurogenic and primary myopathic disorders.[793]

familial myotubular myopathy A nonprogressive X-linked recessive myopathic syndrome presenting with hypotonia and respiratory difficulty in the postnatal period, with subsequent involvement of the extraocular, facial, and neck muscles and with areflexia. Muscle biopsy findings include small muscle fibers with a peripheral rim of myofibrils in the central zone containing either a single nucleus or a collection of sarcoplasmic components.[6508] See also **centronuclear myopathies**.

familial neuroacanthocytosis See **neuroacanthocytosis**.

familial neuromuscular disease with type I fiber hypoplasia, tubular aggregates, cardiomyopathy, and myasthenic features A recessively inherited syndrome comprising the aforementioned manifestations, with lordosis, joint contractures, and normal anti-acetylcholine receptor antibody levels and with onset in childhood.[1669]

familial neuropathy with dementia A slowly progressive syndrome of cerebral atrophy associated with visual loss resulting from both pigmentary retinal degeneration and optic atrophy, accompanied by the clinical features of **hereditary motor and sensory neuropathy** and by attacks of vomiting and a labile blood pressure, indicating autonomic involvement.[4845] See also **NARP syndrome**.

familial encephalopathy with neuroserpin inclusion bodies (FENIB) A severe, progressive, dominantly inherited neurodegenerative disorder with onset in youth or young adult life, in which eosinophilic neuronal inclusions of neuroserpin are found deep in the cerebral cortex and in the substantia nigra.[3903] Clinically, it is characterized by progressive myoclonic epilepsy and early-onset frontal-type dementia. It is due to mutations in the neuroserpin gene.[1487]

familial normokalemic periodic paralysis See **familial periodic paralysis**.

familial occipital calcifications, hemorrhagic strokes, leukoencephalopathy, dementia, and external carotid dysplasia (FOCHS-LADD) An inherited cerebrovascular disease with these features.[3071]

familial occipital dyspslasia See **Chiari malformation**.

familial olivopontocerebellar degenerations See **cerebellar ataxias**.[3527]

familial opticoacoustic nerve degeneration and polyneuropathy A syndrome of progressive optic atrophy and sensorineural deafness complicating **hereditary motor and sensory neuropathy type 2** and with probably X-linked inheritance.[5408]

familial orthochromic leukodystrophy A rare inherited degeneration of white matter resembling **Pelizaeus–Merzbacher disease**. Its clinical features include early-onset, psychomotor decline, pyramidal signs, progressive loss of vision, speech, and hearing, and eventual decerebration and death.

familial orthostatic hypotension See **progressive autonomic failure**.

familial paralysis of horizontal gaze A recessively inherited syndrome consisting of paretic horizontal gaze paresis and progressive scoliosis, sometimes associated with bilateral facial myokymia. Convergence, vertical gaze, and pupillary constriction are normal.[5768]

familial Parkinson disease Those forms of the disease associated with a identified genetic abnormalities. A listing of genotypes and description of phenotypes is to be found under **Parkinson disease**.

familial Parkinsonism–dementia syndrome A recessively inherited syndrome characterized by mental retardation, Parkinsonism, pyramidal signs, and external ophthalmoplegia beginning in the third decade and progressing for many years.[4162]

familial paroxysmal ataxia (familial periodic ataxia, familial vestibulocerebellar ataxia) A rare, dominantly inherited syndrome in which patients experience recurrent attacks of vertigo, nystagmus, or cerebellar incoordination in the absence of multiple sclerosis and without detectable inborn errors of metabolism.

Clinically, the attacks are accompanied by rotary, dissociated, vertical, or downbeating nystagmus, the latter suggesting the presence of a medullary lesion.[1685] See also **cerebellar ataxias** (*variants*).

In another dominantly inherited *variant* form, myokymia is associated.[6492] It responds to acetazolamide.[2582] Yet another form, in which the movements are induced by exercise, is also differentiated.

familial paroxysmal choreoathetosis See **paroxysmal kinesigenic choreoathetosis**.

familial paroxysmal dystonia See **paroxysmal kinsigenic choreoathetosis** and the following entry.

familial paroxysmal dystonic choreoathetosis (syndrome of Mount and Reback, familial paroxysmal dystonia) A rare sporadic or dominantly inherited involuntary movement disorder, usually with childhood onset, in which frequent and prolonged attacks of dystonic posturing, choreoathetosis, or ballism are induced by exercise, emotion, coffee, tea, or alcohol consumption without alteration in consciousness or on the EEG, but not induced by startle.[3654, 4521]

Attacks similarly produced but lasting less than 5 min are known as **paroxysmal kinesigenic choreoathetosis**.[3400]

Variants are similar disorders in which the attacks are induced by startle, exercise, or other stresses (*kinesigenic*[2472] and *nonkinesigenic*[4521] varieties were reviewed by Baraitser[379]); *familial paroxysmal hypogenic dystonia*, a dominantly inherited syndrome of painful dystonic flexion spasms occurring during non–rapid eye movement sleep;[3744] and a form in which myokymia also occurs and the other symptoms are relieved by brief periods of sleep.[966]

familial paroxysmal kinesigenic ataxia A familial syndrome consisting of paroxysmal ataxia, shaking, or titubation, lasting minutes and repeated many times each day, with evidence of continuous abnormal motor unit activity (**myokymia**), the impulses being generated in peripheral nerves.

familial partial epilepsy with variable foci A dominantly inherited seizure disorder with onset in youth presenting varied clinical and EEG manifestations within the same kinship, and possibly linked to a mutation on chromosome 2.[5586]

familial periodic ataxia See **familial paroxysmal ataxia**.

familial periodic paralysis Rare, dominantly inherited sodium- or calcium-channelopathies in which episodic bouts of

Chart F–2. Forms of Familial Periodic Paralysis

Type 1; hypokalemic A rare, dominantly inherited disease seldom expressed in females, manifest by episodes of flaccid paralysis of limb and trunk muscles and areflexia lasting from 12 to 24 h, in association with reduced serum potassium levels at 1.5–2.5 mEq/L, and the usual EKG changes of hypokalemia.[4959] The responsible gene is mapped to 1q32, the site of the *CACN1S* dihydropyridine receptor calcium channel α-subunit. Provocative factors include rest after exercise, carbohydrate ingestion, alcohol ingestion, physical or emotional trauma, cold, epinephrine, and steroids. Eyelid myotonia and permanent mild proximal weakness are often noted.

A similar syndrome (*thyrotoxic periodic paralysis*) is yet another type; described mainly in the Orient it may complicate hyperthyroidism, particularly in Japanese people.[4707] See also **potassium exercise test**.

Type 2; hyperkalemic (adynamia episodica hereditaria, paramyotonia congenita, Gamstorp syndrome) A dominantly inherited sodium channel disorder with onset in early childhood (abating in adult life), manifesting recurrent brief attacks of proximal muscle weakness and flaccidity and myotonia markedly increased by cold and with elevated serum potassium levels during the attacks in about half of the subjects. Cardiac rhythm disturbances may occur.[3863] The attacks are provoked by rest after exercise, hunger, exertion, or potassium administration, and are aborted by intravenous calcium, but in some cases are allayed by further activity or by eating.

As in the hypokalemic form, permanent mild proximal weakness is often noted. Myotonia of the tongue, face, and thenar muscles and lid lag may also be found. Raised serum potassium levels are characteristic during the attacks.[2267] The responsible gene maps to 17q13.1–ql3.3, where there are various SCN4A point mutations affecting the sodium channel α-subunit.

In an *acquired form*, chronic hyperkalemia produces the same clinical picture. *Myotonic periodic paralysis* may be another variant. See also **myotonia fluctuans, myotonia permanens, paramtotonia congenital**, and **Andersen–Tawil syndrome**.

Type 3; normokalemic A dominantly inherited syndrome characterized by onset during the first decade of life, episodes of often severe paralysis occurring at intervals of 1–3 months and lasting from 2 days to 3 weeks, leading to quadriplegia and weakness of the masseter muscles, but neither affecting facial expression, bladder, and bowel function nor respiratory muscles. The episodes are provoked by rest after exertion, prolonged inactivity, alcohol consumption, cold, and damp. Administration of potassium chloride brings on an attack or worsens the symptoms, but the plasma potassium level is normal during the attacks.[5097]

The position of this rare syndrome is uncertain, because its manifestations closely resemble those of the *hyperkalemic* form, and it is recognized that serum potassium levels vary according to the part of the body from which the blood is drawn.

weakness occur due to genetically determined abnormalities in potassium metabolism; these are followed by recovery of strength. (See Chart F–2.) During the paralytic episodes, muscle fibers are refractory to any form of electrical stimulation. Two (perhaps three) genetically heterogeneous major forms are described; 70% of the identified cases are due to mutations in genes encoding three ion channels, *CACN1AS, SCN4A*, and *KCNJ2*.[6523]

familial peroneal atrophy and ataxia A form of **hereditary motor and sensory neuropathy** manifesting also cataract and both cerebellar and pyramidal signs.

familial poliodystrophy, mitochondrial myopathy, and lactic acidemia A rare form of **mitochondrial encephalomyelopathy**.

familial polyradiculopathy syndrome A dominantly inherited syndrome with adult onset characterized by painful paresthesias, progressive centripetal sensory loss, fasciculations, and severe muscle wasting. The cause is unknown.[1292]

familial posterior column ataxia See **Biemond ataxia**.

familial presenile dementia with psychosis A dominantly inherited, slowly progressive dementing disease characterized by initial belligerent antisocial behavior, and later dementia, distinct from **Alzheimer disease**, with which, however, it shares some pathological features.[6125]

familial presenile dementia with spastic paralysis See **congophilic angiopathy**.

familial prion disease See **Creutzfeldt–Jakob disease** and **Gerstmann–Scheinker–Strauss** disease. The responsible gene maps to 20pter–p12.

familial progressive bulbospinal muscular atrophy See **X-linked bulbospinal neuronopathy**.

familial progressive myoclonus and ataxia A dominantly inherited syndrome of childhood, characterized by slowly progressive motor impairment (limb ataxia and tremor) with intermittent myoclonic and generalized tonic–clonic seizures but without intellectual impairment.[2374]

familial progressive subcortical gliosis See **progressive subcortical gliosis**.

familial protein intolerance (lysininuric protein intolerance, dibasic aminoaciduria II) A rare diffuse encephalopathy characterized by recurrent vomiting, diarrhea, hepatic cirrhosis, severe physical and mental retardation, mild intestinal malabsorption, and increased urinary excretion of lysine, ornithine, and arginine. Protein feeding causes hyperammonemia, asterixis, and attacks of stupor.[5843]

familial Q-T prolongation syndrome A rare syndrome with two *variants*; a *dominant form* (Romano–Ward syndrome) consisting of prolongation of the QT interval on the EKG, giving rise to syncopal attacks;[5450] and a *recessive form* (Jervell and Lange-Nielsen syndrome) which is identical to the dominant form but with the addition of congenital deaf-mutism.[3215]

familial rectal pain syndrome See **paroxysmal extreme pain disorder**.

familial recurrent brachial plexus neuropathy See **hereditary brachial plexopathy**.

familial recurrent polyneuropathy See **hereditary pressure-sensitive neuropathy**.

familial recurrent pressure palsies See **hereditary pressure-sensitive neuropathy**.

familial renal–retinal dystrophy See **Senior–Loken syndrome**.

familial restless legs syndrome See **restless legs syndrome**.

familial sleep apnea-plus syndrome A dominantly inherited syndrome consisting of sleep apnea with anosmia, color blindness, partial complex seizures, and cognitive dysfunction.

Variants of the syndrome include forms manifesting **multiple system atrophy, myotonic dystrophy, olivopontocerebellar atrophy, cervicomedullary lesions, glaucoma**, or **ophthalmoplegia**.[4046]

familial sleep paralysis An X-linked recessive syndrome seen at any age and characterized by the occurrence of **sleep paralysis** without other features of the **narcolepsy** complex.[5426] See **American Sleep Disorders Association** (ASDA) diagnostic classification and **sleep disorders**.[1629, 4904]

familial spasmodic torticollis A dystonic syndrome inherited either dominantly or recessively and characterized by the onset in youth or early adult life of torticollis without progression of the dystonia to other regions.[6315]

familial spastic ataxia A dominantly or recessively inherited syndrome characterized by the variable appearance of slowly progressive cerebellar and pyramidal signs and optic atrophy in childhood or adult life. See **cerebellar ataxias** (*variants*).

familial spastic paralysis/ paraparesis See **hereditary spastic paraplegia**.

familial spastic paraparesis and deafness See **hereditary spastic paraplegia**.

familial spastic paraparesis and dementia See **familial multi-infarct dementia** and **Worster–Drought syndrome**.

familial spastic paraparesis, peroneal neuropathy, and crural hypopigmentation See **hereditary spastic paraplegia**.

familial spastic paraplegia with amyotrophy of the hands See **hereditary spastic paraplegia**.

familial spinocerebellar ataxia See **cerebellar ataxias** (*variants*).

familial spinocerebellar degeneration with corneal dystrophy See **cerebellar ataxias** (*variants*).

familial static ophthalmoplegia A rare dominantly inherited (occasionally recessive or X-linked) syndrome of pure external ocular muscle weakness, presenting as ptosis with or without ophthalmoparesis.[3752] The cause may be either a myopathy or nuclear agenesis. See also **Möbius syndrome**.

familial stiff man syndrome See **neuromyotonia**.

familial striatal degeneration See **familial bilateral striatal necrosis**.

familial subcortical dementia with arteriosclerotic leukoencephalopathy (chronic familial vascular encephalopathy, hereditary multi-infarct dementia) A dominantly inherited syndrome of aid-adult life characterized by recurrent attacks of focal neurological deficits including **subcortical dementia** and pseudobulbar palsy, due to multiple small infarcts in the white matter, basal ganglia, thalamus, and brainstem. Their appearance resembles that of leukoencephalopathies on CT or MRI scans.[4133] See also **familial multi-infarct dementia** and **Worster–Drought syndrome**.

familial tapetoretinal degeneration and epilepsy A rare inherited childhood syndrome of pigmentary retinopathy, generalized tonic–clonic seizures, and mental and developmental delay.[1235]

familial temporal lobe epilepsy A dominantly inherited syndrome of simple (seldom complex) partial seizures with psychic and autonomic manifestations, and occasional secondary generalization, with onset in youth or early adult life. The condition appears to be genetically heterogeneous.[569] *Autosomal dominant partial epilepsy with auditory features* may represent a variant condition.

familial tremor See **essential tremor**.

familial vascular encephalopathy See **familial multi-infarct dementia**.

familial vestibulocerebellar ataxia See **familial paroxysmal ataxia**.

familial vestibulocerebellar dysfunction A syndrome characterized by motion sickness and rebound nystagmus in which the nystagmus is of the type 1 vestibular form, the slow phase of the optokinetic response is defective, and the vestibulo-optic reflex fails to be suppressed.[6268]

familial visceral myopathy (oculogastrointestinal muscular dystrophy) A group of rare genetic diseases of childhood or youth characterized by degeneration, atrophy, and fibrosis of the intestinal muscles, with or without diffuse neurological abnormalities, autonomic insufficiency, and denervation hypersensitivity of the pupil and esophageal smooth muscle. Chronic intestinal pseudo-obstruction is a common presentation. Neuronal intranuclear inclusion bodies are found in the submucosal and myenteric neurons as well as in the brain, spinal cord, autonomic nervous system, and peripheral nerves. The detrusor muscle may also be affected.[5658]

Type 1 is dominantly inherited and the upper intestine is affected; *type 2* is recessive; the stomach and small bowel are involved; *type 3*, also recessive, affects the whole length of the alimentary tract.[4406] The recessive forms have also been associated with **progressive external ophthalmoplegia** and a severe sensorimotor peripheral neuropathy.[6874]

familial visceral neuropathy A recessively inherited syndrome characterized by chronic intestinal pseudo-obstruction, with or without diffuse neurological abnormalities (especially dysphagia and peripheral neuropathy), autonomic insufficiency, and denervation hypersensitivity of the pupillary and esophageal muscles. Neuronal intranuclear inclusions are found in the submucosal and myenteric neurons and in the brain.[4189]

In a *variant* dominantly inherited form, the small bowel is affected in isolation and intranuclear inclusions are not found.

familial X-linked myalgia and cramps A nonprogressive myopathy associated with a deletion in the dystrophic gene. Clinically, the condition presents with muscle cramps and myalgia, especially following activity, and with raised serum creatine kinase levels.[2514]

Families of Spinal Muscular Atrophy A charitable organization providing support and information on these conditions. Address: P.O. Box 1465, Highland Park, IL 60035. Tel: 708-432-5551.

Family Practice Notebook A site providing medical education data. The neurology chapters are at http://www.fpnotebook.com/NEU.htm.

famous faces test A test of remote memory in which the subject is asked to name celebrities from previous years, shown in photographs.[109] See also **Wechsler Adult Intelligence Scale**.

Fanconi pancytopenia A recessively inherited, congenital dysmorphic syndrome manifesting also short stature; congenital cardiac anomalies; hematological, dermal, skeletal, and genital maldevelopments; asplenia; recurrent infections; nystagmus; strabismus; microcephaly; and mental and developmental delay.[1959]

Fanconi–Debre–DeToni syndrome A mitochondriopathy presenting with mental retardation, renal insufficiency due to tubular dysfunction with aminoacidura, glucosuria, phosphaturia, and hyperuricaemia.

Fanconi–Turler syndrome (familial ataxic diplegia) A congenital syndrome consisting of nonprogressive cerebellar ataxia, uncoordinated eye movements, and mental retardation; it is probably a form of olivopontocerebellar atrophy.[1960] See also **cerebellar ataxias**.

fantaisiste ataxia Variability of voluntary limb movement from one moment to the next, as may be seen in patients with **sensory ataxia**.

far point That most distant place from which rays of light entering the eye are focused upon the retina rather than anterior or posterior to it. In the emmetropic (normally refracting) eye, this point is at infinity; but, in myopia, it may be only inches away from the cornea. The nearer the far point, the greater the degree of myopia.

Faraday, Michael (1791–1867) English physicist who discovered inductive electricity.

Faradic nystagmus See **vestibular nystagmus**.

Faradism The term suggested by **Duchenne** de Boulogne for the application of induced currents to cause muscle excitation, in honor of Michael **Faraday**.

Farber disease (lipogranulomatosis, ceramidase deficiency, ceramide lactoside lipidosis) A rare recessively inherited lysosomal storage disease in which a deficiency of ceramidase is the key biochemical abnormality, leading to the deposition of chondroitin sulfate B. It is manifest in infants by joint swelling and stiffness, mainly at the wrists and ankles, with the development of contractures, mental retardation, short stature, skin pigmentation, hepatomegaly, respiratory distress, hoarseness, diarrhea and vomiting, inanition, and early death.[1964] Cloudy corneas or sclerocornea and a macular red spot may also be seen.

far-field A region of electrical potential where the isopotential voltage lines associated with a current source change slowly over a short distance. Some use the term far-field potential to designate a potential that does not change in latency, amplitude, or polarity over infinite distances; alternative designations include "boundary potential" and "junctional potential." The terms near-field and far-field are arbitrary designations as there are no agreed-upon criteria defining where the near-field ends and the far-field begins. Compare with **near-field**. (From the 2001 Report of the Nomenclature Committee of the American Association of Electromyography and Electrodiagnosis.[19] Reproduced by kind permission of the AANEM.)

Farnsworth–Munsell 100 hue test A test in which movable disks of different hues but with the same saturation and brightness, arranged in trays, are to be sorted along the continuum red–yellow–blue/green–blue–purple/red, as a test of color discrimination.

FAS Test A test of the ability to generate words and of controlled word association (Benton) in which the subject is asked to think of as many words as possible beginning with the letter "F," then with "A," and finally with "S." This is said to be a sensitive indicator of lesions of the frontal lobes.[3825]

fascicle See **fasciculus**.

fasciculation potential The electric activity associated with a fasciculation which has the configuration of a motor unit activation potential but which occurs spontaneously. Most commonly occur sporadically and are termed "single fasciculation potentials." Occasionally the potentials occur as a grouped discharge and are termed a "brief repetitive discharge." The repetitive firing of adjacent fasciculation potentials, when numerous, may produce an undulating movement of muscle (see myokymia). Use of the terms "benign fasciculation" and "malignant fasciculation" is discouraged. Instead, the configuration of the potentials, peak to-peak amplitude, duration, number of phases, stability of configuration, and frequency of occurrence should be specified. (From the 2001 Report of the Nomenclature Committee of the American Association of Electromyography and Electrodiagnosis.[19] Reproduced by kind permission of the AANEM.)

fasciculations 1. Clinically, spontaneous contractions of all of the myofibrils comprising a motor unit and most likely arising from the intramuscular motor nerve terminal.[3725] The twitches do not move joints but can be seen and felt by the subject or by an observer. Most arise from the distal part of the axon. Unless accompanied by wasting and weakness, they may be considered benign, and are extremely common in normal subjects. The word is presumably derived from the following entry, a bundle of muscle fibers contracting in this instance. The term was coined by **Denny-Brown**. 2. The random, spontaneous twitching of a group of muscle fibers belonging to a single motor unit. The twitch may produce movement of the overlying skin (if in limb or trunk muscles) or mucous membrane (if in the tongue). If the motor unit is sufficiently large, an associated joint movement may be observed. The electric activity associated with the twitch is termed a fasciculation potential. See also **myokymia**.[19]

So-called benign fasciculations have firing patterns suggesting two forms: one due to irritability of the distal motor nerves as in cramps and the other due to proximal irritability as in undulating **myokymia** and in **tetany**.[3477]

fasciculus (Lat, a little bundle) (fascicle) The term is synonymous with *tract, crus, column, funiculus and fillet* or *lemniscus*, all being variously employed in anatomy in order to add a little interest to an otherwise dry subject. The word *fasciculus* is usually used with reference to a bundle of nerve fibers (e.g., the spino-thalamic tract) and tends to be succeeded by geographical directions in Latin and an eponym; thus *fasciculus anterolateralis superficialis of Gowers*.

fasciculus cuneatus See **Burdach column**.

FAST See **Frenchay aphasia screening test** or **Functional Assessment Staging**.

fast alpha variant rhythm A characteristic rhythm at 14–20 Hz, detected most prominently over the posterior regions of the head which may alternate or be intermixed with **alpha rhythms**. It is blocked or attenuated by attention (especially visual) and by mental effort. (Adapted from the 1974 report of the Committee on Terminology, IFCN. In: Chatrian GE, Bergamini L, Dondey M, et al. A glossary of terms most commonly used by clinical electroencephalographers. *EEG Clin Neurophysiol* 1974;**37**:538–48. Reproduced by kind permission of Elsevier Science and the IFCN.)

fast activity (beta activity) EEG activity of a frequency higher than that of the **alpha rhythm**.

fast pain (first pain) A bright, sharp, pricking painful sensation following almost immediately upon discrete local nociceptive stimulation. This is presumably related to that sensation called **epicritic** by **Head**; the second pain felt is **protopathic pain** in Head's terminology.

fast paroxysmal rhythms See **generalized paroxysmal fast activity**.

fast spike-wave See **six-Hz slow spike-and-waves**.

fat embolism A clinical syndrome occurring 1–3 days after severe trauma in a small minority of subjects. The clinical features include skin petechiae, pulmonary insufficiency, retinal hemorrhages, and an encephalopathy with confusion, reduced conscious level, seizures, and focal signs.[1943]

fat stains Dyes such as Sudan IV and Oil Red O which preferentially stain neutral fat bright red in histological specimens.

fatal cutaneo-intestinal syndrome See **Degos syndrome**.

fatal familial infantile glycogen storage disease See **glycogen storage diseases**.

fatal familial insomnia (subacute degeneration of the thalamus, familial myoclonic dementia) A rapidly progressive, dominantly inherited prion disease of middle and late adult life beginning with difficulty in initiating sleep and leading within a few months to a total lack of non–rapid eye movement sleep, and later to spontaneous lapses from quiet wakefulness into a sleep state with enacted dreams; memory deficits with **chronotaraxis**; dysautonomia; and motor signs. Mutation of a prion protein gene at codon 178 has been detected. A sporadic form is also reported.

The above findings are accompanied by autonomic hyperactivity, with salivation, fever, hyperhidrosis, hypertension, tachycardia, and tachypnea. In late stages of the disorder, dysarthria, tremor, spontaneous and reflex myoclonus, ataxia, dystonic posturing, and pyramidal signs supervene and lead on to coma and finally to death. There is no alteration in cognitive function until the patient's alertness is impaired. Thalamic atrophy, and spongiform encephalopathy may be detected. Clinically, cerebellar ataxia and features suggesting Creutzfeldt–Jakob disease have been found in association. Diagnostic criteria are given in Chart F–3.[1629, 5421]

fatal infantile encephalomyopathy See **acute encephalopathy of infancy**.

fatal infantile leukodystrophy (childhood ataxia with diffuse CNS hypomyelination; CACH; myelinopathia centralis diffusa; vanishing white matter [VWM] disease; OMIM306896) A recessively inherited progressive leukodystrophy with a relapsing–remitting course and an unknown molecular basis, although the VWM locus has been mapped to chromosome 3q27.4.

Clinical characteristics are progressive ataxic diplegia starting between the ages of 1 and 5 years after normal early neurologic development and with rapid progression. Seizures, dysarthria, and optic atrophy are frequently found. In some patients, the disease starts acutely, progressing with recurrent episodes of neurologic deterioration and lethargy, exacerbated by febrile illness and minor head trauma.[2171]

The same condition has also been described in adults.

fatal infantile mitochondrial disease See **acute encephalopathy of infancy**.

fatal infantile mitochondrial myopathy and hepatopathy (fatal infantile myopathy) A fatal expression of inherited deficiency in cytochrome *c* oxidase (complex IV) with the complete absence of activity of this enzyme in all muscle fibers, occurring with or without cardiomyopathy and renal and hepatic dysfunction. Type I fibers have central nuclei while a focal decrease in oxidative enzymes affects mainly the larger type II fibers.[3750]

Clinically, hypotonia, myotonia, weakness, ophthalmoplegia, and both feeding and respiratory difficulties are noted shortly after birth; aminoaciduria and lactic acidosis are later detected. Death occurs before the end of the first year.[1645] See also **acute encephalopathy of infancy**.

fatal infantile muscle phosphofructokinase deficiency See **glycogen storage diseases**.

fatal infantile myopathy See **fatal infantile mitochondrial myopathy and hepatopathy**.

fatigability 1. Failure to maintain the required maximum force or output of power during sustained or repeated muscle contractions. Both central and peripheral forms are recognized. 2. Slow recovery after a period of activation of muscles.

When referring to unusually early tiring after muscular activity, this is the cardinal sign of **myasthenia gravis**; but when (and more commonly) accompanied by a feeling of lack of energy wherewith to accomplish such tasks so that they are not attempted in the first place, this is the **chronic fatigue syndrome** of which **somatic dysthymia** (masked depression) is a far more common cause. Both **central fatigue** and **psychological fatigue** are recognized.[873]

Chart F–3. Diagnostic Criteria for Fatal Familial Insomnia

A. A complaint of insomnia is initially present.
B. Autonomic hyperactivity, with pyrexia, excessive salivation, hyperhidrosis or anidrosis, and cardiac and respiratory dysfunction.
C. Familial pattern is present.
D. Progression to stupor, coma, and death within 24 months.
E. Pathological examination demonstrates degeneration of anterior and dorsomedial thalamic nuclei.
F. Polysomnographic monitoring demonstrates one or more of the following:
   1. Absence of slow-wave sleep;
   2. Dissociated rapid eye movement sleep;
   3. Myoclonus and tremor-like muscle activity.
G. Not the result of another medical or psychiatric disorder, for example, Alzheimer dementia, Creutzfeldt–Jakob disease, or schizophrenia.
H. Does not meet the diagnostic criteria for other sleep disorders, for example, REM sleep behavior disorder.[4279]

From AASM Diagnostic Classification Steering Committee. The International Classification of Sleep Disorders Diagnostic and Coding Manual. *Rochester, MN. American Academy of Sleep Medicine 1991/2001. Reproduced by kind permission of the Academy. See also* http://www.sleepeducation.com/Disorders.aspx/.

fatigue 1. A sense of weariness and inertia complicated by sleepiness, perceived weakness, and often subjective dyspnea, usually accompanying disorders of the upper motor neuron such as **Parkinson disease** and multiple sclerosis, in **chronic fatigue syndrome** and in the presence of severe systemic disease. 2. In EMG practice, a state of depressed responsiveness resulting from protracted activity and requiring an appreciable recovery time. 3. (muscle fatigue) A state of depressed responsiveness resulting from recent activity. Muscle fatigue is a reduction in contraction force following repeated voluntary contraction or electric stimulation.[19] See also **central fatigue, Piper instrument**, and the following four entries, none of which has obvious advantages over the others.

Fatigue Assessment Instrument A self-report tool used to evaluate the severity and quality of fatigue in patients with multiple sclerosis.[3575]

Fatigue Descriptive Scale A self-report tool used to evaluate the severity and quality of fatigue.

fatigue failure Fracture of a vertebral neural arch as a result of repetitive stress, as in athletes. The usual result is **spondylolysis**, presenting clinically as subacute low back pain.[2222]

Fatigue Impact Scale A self-report tool used to evaluate the severity and quality of fatigue.[3575] A 40-item inventory assessing the effects of pathological fatigue upon the physical, cognitive, and psychosocial aspects of daily living. The scale has been used mainly in studies of patients with the **chronic fatigue syndrome** and **multiple sclerosis**.[2116]

fatigue nystagmus A form of gaze-evoked **end-point nystagmus** appearing after prolonged maintenance of lateral gaze and seen with acute muscle weakness as in **myasthenia gravis** or with lesions of the brainstem.[5731] See also **physiological nystagmus**.

fatigue paresis Weakness noted at night in comparison with recovery from paresis in the morning immediately after sleep. This symptom is suggestive of **myasthenia gravis**.

fatigue recovery A phenomenon recorded in **myasthenia gravis** in which the strength of the previously fatigued levator palpebrae muscle (after prolonged upward gaze) improves after maximal contraction of the antagonistic orbicularis oculi muscles, leading to a temporary improvement in lid opening.[6365] See also **ice pack test**.

Fatigue Severity Scale A tool used to evaluate the severity and quality of fatigue in patients with multiple sclerosis.[3576]

fatigue testing Methods of testing for fatigue: 1. The output of a subject is measured while exercising at 10% of maximum capacity, the load increasing by a further 10% every minute, and 2. Direct electrical stimulation of a contracting muscle is performed, and any increase in the mechanical twitch response so produced is recorded.[873] Functional grades can be assigned to patients on the basis of their scores on these tests.

Fatty Oxidation Disorders Family Support Group A charitable patient-based organization. Web site: http://www.fodsupport.org/. See **acyl CoA dehydrogenase (MCAD) deficiency**.

faucial reflex The gag reflex.

Fazio, E. (1849–1902) Italian physician.

Fazio–Londe syndrome (progressive bulbar paralysis of childhood, bulbar spinal muscular atrophy of childhood) A dominantly inherited progressive bulbar palsy in children or young adults, presenting with facial weakness, dysphagia, drooling, dysarthria, and dysphonia, with later progression to the involvement of other cranial and spinal nerves.[5412, 4086] See **amyotrophic lateral sclerosis** and **hereditary motor neuropathy**.

The condition was described independently by the Italian and French authors in 1892–1893; it may represent a variant of amyotrophic lateral sclerosis. P.F.L. Londe (1865–1944) was a French neurologist.[1972]

Variants include a *recessive form* with onset in infancy, in which involvement of the oculomotor nerves and pyramidal system occur as well as the bulbar palsy; a form with *juvenile onset and slow progression*, which may be a genetically determined form of amyotrophic lateral sclerosis;[2874] *progressive adult-onset bulbar paresis*, a dominantly inherited syndrome of pure lower motor neuron bulbar palsy;[3926] **Vialetto–van Laere syndrome**, and *spinal muscular atrophy with optic atrophy and deafness* (See **hereditary motor and sensory neuropathy**, type 6.)[379]

febrile convulsions See **febrile seizures**.

febrile delirium See **delirium**.

febrile reflex anoxic seizures (febrile syncope) Brief tonic seizures resembling **anoxic seizures** but occurring during the course of a febrile illness at the stage of rising temperature. They can be induced by eyeball compression and are thus likely to represent the effect of an excessive vagal response. The diagnosis of **febrile convulsions** has often been made in such cases.[2313]

febrile seizures (convulsions) A "location-related" epileptic disorder characterized by the occurrence of generalized tonic–clonic seizures (seldom other phenotypes) occurring in childhood after the age of 1 month (mainly 6 months to 5 years) associated with a rising fever but not caused by an infection of the CNS; without previous neonatal seizures or a previous unprovoked seizure; and not meeting criteria for other acute symptomatic seizures.[1265]

The condition is common; some 3% of all children will have at least one febrile seizure. Simple (generalized tonic–clonic seizures lasting less than 15 min without recurrence within the next 24 h) and complex (focal, prolonged more than 15 min or occurring in a cluster of two or more convulsions within 24 h) are differentiated; the latter is less common but may be followed by transient or permanent neurological sequelae, such as the **HHE syndrome.**

Risk factors for subsequent epilepsy include seizures lasting longer than 15 min; recurrence of a seizure within 24 h; and focal neurologic features following a seizure. Although prolonged febrile seizures seem to relate to subsequent mesial temporal sclerosis and intractable temporal lobe epilepsy, that complication is exceedingly rare.

Children may also convulse as a result of brain injury caused by an infection which is also causing fever; or when fever unmasks a pre-existing tendency to suffer recurrent seizures.[72] Predisposing factors are the immature brain, the occurrence of fever, and genetic predisposition. The mode of inheritance is probably polygenic or autosomal dominant with incomplete penetrance. Dominant inheritance has been shown, with various loci on chromosomes 2, 6, 8, and 19.4565. The locus *FEB3* maps to 2q23–24.

Variant forms include one in which absence seizures occur; and generalized epilepsy with febrile seizures plus (autosomal dominant epilepsy with febrile seizures plus) in which patients have classic febrile seizures persisting beyond the age of 5 years and subsequent afebrile seizures, rarely including absences. **Dravet syndrome** probably represents the most severe end of the spectrum within the GEFS+ phenotype.[4882]

febrile seizure with neonatal seizure One or more neonatal seizures in a child who has also experienced one or more febrile seizures as herein defined.[1265]

febrile syncope See **febrile reflex anoxic seizures**.

feeling-tone See **affect**.

feer disease See **pink disease**.

Fegeler syndrome The association of a port-wine nevus in the distribution of the V cranial nerve, with weakness and hyperesthesia in the ipsilateral arm and leg. This would be diagnosed as **Sturge–Weber syndrome** were it not that the features appear for the first time following a head injury.[1972]

Fehr, Johannes Michael (1610–1688) German physician who, with Elias Schmidt, first described trigeminal neuralgia in 1671.

Feil, Andre (b. 1884) French neurologist. See **Klippel–Feil anomaly**.

Feingold syndrome 1. (*deafness–oligo/syndactyly*) A congenital dysmorphic syndrome manifesting also numerous skeletal malformations, sensorineural deafness, and plagiocephaly.[381]
2. (*microcephaly–hand abnormality–fistula*) A congenital dysmorphic syndrome manifesting also duodenal atresia, skeletal abnormalities, tracheooesophageal fistula, rocker-bottom feet, and microcephaly.[381]
3. (*retardation–short stature–cleft palate abnormal ears*) A congenital dysmorphic syndrome manifesting also short stature, hoarse voice, spina bifida occulta, brachycephaly, macrocephaly, distal and proximal myopathic weakness, and mental and developmental delay.[381]

femoral neuralgia Constant aching pain within the distribution of the femoral nerve. The character of the pain differs from that of the more classic cranial neuralgias, and unlike their presentations, motor or sensory deficits may be present. Although listed in the IASP taxonomy, the description is also accurate for any femoral neuropathy.

Depending on the severity of the damage to the nerve, weakness of the quadriceps and reduction in the knee jerk and sensory disturbances on the anterior and medial aspects of the thigh may or may not be present.

femoral neuropathy Damage to this nerve as a result of compression, stretch, direct injury, radiation, or ischemia, with resultant weakness of the quadriceps, iliacus, and sartorius muscles, and usually sensory loss in the territories of the medial and intermediate cutaneous nerves of the thigh and saphenous nerve.[3603]

femoral reflex Extension of the hip and knee in response to irritation of the skin of the upper thigh; a sign of a pyramidal tract lesion.

femoral stretch test (Ely test) Passive extension of the hip of a patient lying prone with the knee straight, or flexion of the knee of the prone patient; in each case maneuvers which put traction on the femoral nerve, causing pain in the anterior thigh in patients with L3 root irritation, but also with tight hamstring muscles. The test was described by Wassermann in 1918. See **reverse straight leg raising.** See also **bent-knee pulling**.

fenestra parietalia symmetricae See **Catlin mark**.

fenestrations Spaces between capillary cells, not present within the blood–brain barrier where these cells are joined by tight junctions.

Fenton syndrome A congenital or childhood dysmorphic syndrome manifesting ataxia, skin photosensitivity, short stature, skeletal abnormalities, ichthyosis, and mental and developmental delay.[381]

Ferguson–Critchley syndrome (autosomal dominant cerebellar ataxia, type I, hereditary spastic paraplegia with ocular and extrapyramidal symptoms) See **cerebellar ataxias**. This is the condition suffered by the Drew family of Walworth, London, UK.

Fernel, Jean-Francois (1506–1588) French physician to King Henri II, memorable because he gave the first intimation of the existence of reflex activity in the nervous system.

Fernhoff syndrome A congenital dysmorphic syndrome characterized also by microcephaly.[381]

ferric chloride reaction A urine test based upon the fact that at a pH below 7, the ferric iron reacts with a variety of drugs possessed of a cyclic structure and with ketones, to produce a color change (usually green).

ferritinopathy See **neuroferritinopathy**.

Ferrier, Sir David (1843–1928) Scottish neurophysiologist and neurologist who graduated from Edinburgh in 1868. His studies of animals and of patients at the West Riding Lunatic Asylum led to his demonstration that functions such as speech and motor activity are precisely localized in the human cerebral cortex (though not in the areas corresponding to those suggested by the phrenologists). He later moved to London, where he was a colleague of Hughlings–**Jackson** on his appointment to the **National Hospital** in 1880; he was also on the staff at Kings College Hospital where he performed new precise experiments in animals.[2031]

His localization of auditory function to the superior temporal gyrus, using faradic (alternating) currents or ablation experiments,[2833] led to his remarkable definition of the cerebral motor and sensory areas in his book *The Functions of the Brain* (London, 1876, dedicated to Hughlings–Jackson), although his conclusions were at first widely criticized. In a second book *The Localisation of Cerebral Disease* (dedicated to **Charcot**), he analyzed in some depth the case

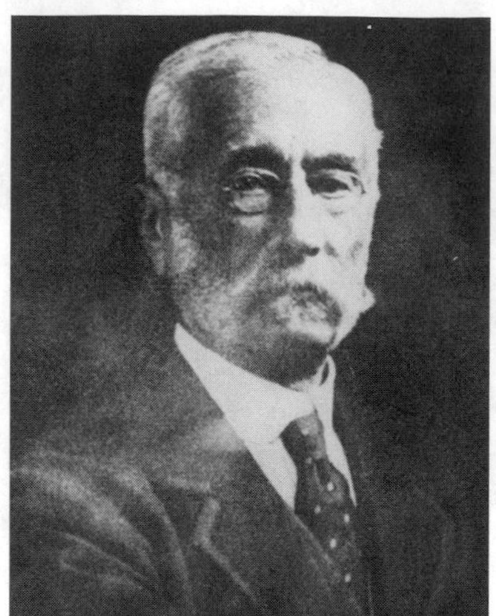

Figure F–2 Sir David Ferrier.

of Phineas **Gage** and refined his original observations on the regionalization of cerebral function in a day when, despite **Hitzig** and **Gall** or because of **Spurzheim** such considerations were not widely accepted. His cavalier attitude toward the preceding work of others was, however, a cause of controversy. Combining the results of his and Hughlings–Jackson's clinical cases, he delivered the Croonian lectures for 1890 on the topic of cerebral localization. He was elected a Fellow of the Royal Society, and continuing the tradition of the regular publication of neurological reports from the West Riding Asylum, to which he had contributed largely, was a founder of ***Brain***.

fersinn See **facial vision of the blind**.

festination (from Lat, to hurry) Acceleration of the rate of activity. In neurology, the word is usually used to describe the rapid but small paces of patients with **Parkinson disease**.

fetal akinesia deformation sequence A collection of developmental anomalies which can be associated with decreased fetal motility *in utero* as a result of any neuromuscular, connective tissue, or other diseases.[4425] See also **Pena–Shokeir phenotype**.

fetal alcohol syndrome A dysmorphic syndrome also manifesting growth retardation, hypotonia, and cardiac and skeletal abnormalities in infants born to 2–30% of mothers who have ingested excessive alcohol during pregnancy.[1195] Other neurological features include microcephaly, tremor, cavernous hemangiomas, and mental and developmental delay.[2059]

Diagnostic criteria have been suggested:[2028]

A. Growth retardation (prenatal or postnatal weight or length below the tenth centile when corrected for gestational age).
B. Central nervous system abnormalities (microcephaly with head circumference below the third centile; brain malformations; developmental delay; behavioral disorders and cognitive impairment).
C. Dysmorphisms (short palpebral fissures, elongated mid-face, long and flat philtrum, thin upper lip, flattened maxilla).

fetal aminopterin/ methotrexate syndrome The occurrence of short stature, dysplastic low-set ears, hypertelorism, prominent eyes, small mandible, cleft palate, absent fingers, syndactyly, ossification defects of the skull, and hydrocephalus in babies born to women exposed to methotrexate during pregnancy.[5770]

fetal anticonvulsant syndrome (embryofoetal valproic acid syndrome; hydantoin-barbiturate-carbamazepine embryofoetopathy) A group of syndromes seen in some children exposed to anticonvulsants *in utero*. Features variously comprise mental retardation, decreased head circumference, craniofacial dysmorphisms such as **hypertelorism**, flat nasal ridge, low-set ears, microcephaly, trigonocephaly, cleft palate and short neck, and hypoplasia of the distal phalanges or nails. Long-lasting behavioral problems and cognitive impairment are less common features. Transverse palmar creases, congenital heart disease, and neural tube defects are also described, the latter especially with valproic acid. Specific types include the following:

Fetal hydantoin syndrome (acrofacial syndrome) Characterized by hypoplasia of the distal phalanges or nails and growth deficiency, cleft lip and palate, developmental delay, mental retardation, and mid-face hypoplasia. Many other malformations are occasionally seen after gestational exposure to phenytoin, such as hypospadias, congenital heart disease, dislocation of the hip, dural epidermal cyst, pyloric stenosis, etc., short stature, generalized hirsutism, low frontal hairline, metopic ridges, small nose with a depressed nasal bridge, ptosis, mild hypertelorism, hypoplastic phalanges and nails, dislocation of the hip, delayed closure of the fontanelles, and mental and developmental delay.[3379]

Craniosynostosis affecting the sagittal and coronal sutures is also reported.

Fetal barbiturate effect Barbiturates have been linked with both pre- and postnatal growth retardation, developmental delay, and facial dysmorphisms, perhaps as a result of induced folate deficiency. Their potential for teratogenicity is uncertain.

Fetal carbamazepine syndrome Characterized by reduction in head size, spina bifida, facial dysmorphisms, microcephaly, digital anomalies, and developmental delay. An association with encephalocele has also been suggested.

Fetal trimethadione syndrome (fetal dione syndrome) Intrauterine growth retardation, microcephaly, facial and CNS malformations, congenital heart disease, and genitourinary anomalies often with delay in speech and other developmental parameters, congenital heart diseases and malformations of the kidneys, trachea, larynx, and esophagus, with an increased neonatal mortality rate. Short stature, overfolded ear helix, ptosis, epicanthic folds, small upturned nose, wide nasal bridge, micrognathia, cleft palate, and brachycephaly are also described.[1997]

Fetal valproate syndrome A prenatal syndrome seen in an infant whose mother ingested sodium valproate during pregnancy and typically comprising any of the following: neural tube defects (lumbosacral meningomyelocele) and talipes equinovarus (with intact spine); facial dysmorphisms such as infraorbital creases, deep epicanthic folds, upturned, short nose with anteverted nostrils, depressed nasal bridge, and telecanthus, long philtrum, thin vermilion border, mid-face hypoplasia, and small mouth.[1642] The digits are often thin and overlapping, and the nails hyperconvex and hypoplastic. Also described are postaxial polydactyly, triphalangeal thumbs, thumb aplasia, syndactyly, radial aplasia, various congenital cardiovascular defects, growth failure, hypospadias, cryptorchidism, bifid ribs, and psychomotor delay.

Primidone embryopathy A combination of facial hirsutism, cleft lip and palate, features of **Goldenhar syndrome**, cognitive and motor delays, and congenital heart disease in this context.

fetal barbiturate effect See **fetal anticonvulsant syndrome**.

fetal carbamazepine syndrome See **fetal anticonvulsant syndrome**.

fetal dione syndrome See **fetal anticonvulsant syndrome**.

fetal hydantoin syndrome See **fetal anticonvulsant syndrome**.

fetal nigral transplantation The instillation of nigral cells from aborted fetuses into the caudate/lenticular nuclei of patients with severe **Parkinson disease** in an attempt to relieve symptoms, especially rigidity and akinesia, tremor being unaffected by the procedure.

fetal reflexes See **developmental reflexes**.

fetal retinoid syndrome See **fetal vitamin A syndrome**.

fetal toluene syndrome The occurrence of unusual hair whorls, narrow forehead, low-set and prominent ears, deep-set eyes, short palpebral fissures, epicanthic folds, depressed nasal bridge, small mandible, simple philtrum, thin upper lip, abnormal palmar creases, hypoplastic nails, microcephaly, spasticity, and mental and developmental delay in babies born to women exposed to toluene during pregnancy.[381]

fetal trimethadione syndrome See **fetal anticonvulsant syndrome**.

fetal valproate syndrome See **fetal anticonvulsant syndrome**.

fetal vitamin A syndrome (fetal retinoid syndrome) A congenital dysmorphic syndrome that results from maternal use of retinoids, the synthetic derivatives of vitamin A, during pregnancy. It is characterized by absence of the auditory canal, microphthalmia with blindness, micrognathia, cleft palate, congenital cardiac anomalies, mental and developmental delay, microcephaly, cerebral atrophy, porencephaly, hydrocephalus and the **Dandy–Walker malformation**.

fetal warfarin syndrome A dysmorphic syndrome of mental and physical delay with optic atrophy, seizures, hypotonia, and skeletal anomalies occurring in infants born to mothers who took anticoagulants during pregnancy.[1628]

Feuerstein–Mills syndrome See **epidermal nevus syndrome**.

feverfew A herb, the leaves of which contain parthenolide, a butyrolactone which prevents the secretion of serotonin from platelets and leukocytes and suppresses prostaglandin release. This may explain why it is at present a popular herbal remedy for migraine.[310]

FG syndrome (of Opitz) A congenital X-linked recessive dysmorphic syndrome characterized by dolichocephaly or scaphocephaly resulting from synostosis affecting the sagittal suture, joint contractures, macrocephaly, hypertelorism, hydrocephalus, callosal agenesis, seizures, antimongolian slant to the eyes, strabismus, severe hypotonia, sensorineural deafness, congenital cardiac anomalies, anal atresia, and mental and developmental delay.[4800]

fiber (from Lat, a thread) An elongated cell, usually an axon or a myofibril.

fiber density 1. Anatomically, a measure of the number of muscle or nerve fibers per unit area. 2. In single fiber electromyography, the mean number of muscle fiber action potentials fulfilling amplitude and rise time criteria belonging to one motor unit within the recording area of a single fiber needle electrode, encountered during a systematic search in a weakly voluntarily contracting muscle. See also **single fiber electromyography, single fiber needle electrode**. (From the 2001 Report of the Nomenclature Committee of the American Association of Electromyography and Electrodiagnosis.[19] Reproduced by kind permission of the AANEM.)

fiber splitting A histological feature in muscle biopsy specimens in which the myofibril is split from its circumference peripherally toward an abnormally sited central nucleus. The finding is nonspecific, occurring due to age or to an excessive workload, and is seen in both primary myopathies and neurogenic atrophies.

fiber-type atrophy Selective atrophy of either type 1 or type 2 myofibrils. The former occurs in **myotonic dystrophy** and in some **congenital myopathies**, the latter with disuse and myasthenia, and with pyramidal lesions.

fiber-type grouping A finding in muscle biopsy specimens in which two or more muscle fibers of one histological type are enclosed at all points on their circumference by other fibers of the same histochemical type. In some unusually large areas, a hundred or more myofibrils are of the same fiber type, as a result of the reinnervation of myofibrils of one type by a motor axon of another. This leads to their conversion to the type determined by that motor unit. The checkerboard appearance of the normal muscle with adenosine triphosphatase or lactic dehydrogenase stains is thus lost.

The finding is evidence of denervation with reinnervation, probably by collateral axon sprouts, and is a feature of chronic motor neuropathies. See **group atrophy**.

fiber-type predominance Changes in the relative proportions of myofibrils of types I and II in a muscle biopsy specimen. The proportions vary normally in different muscles. Type II fibers predominate normally in the biceps brachii and quadriceps and to find more than 55% of type I fibers in those muscles is considered abnormal, while type II predominance is said to occur when the proportion of such fibers is greater then 80%.[1733]

fibrillary astrocytoma See **astrocytoma**.

fibrillary chorea See **Morvan chorea**.

fibrillary contractions See **myokymia**.

fibrillary gliosis Infiltration of neural tissue with hyperplastic and hypertrophied astrocytes (including **gemistocytic**

astrocytes) as seen in the plaques of **multiple sclerosis**.

fibrillation The spontaneous contractions of individual muscle fibers, not visible through the skin nor even in the tongue.

fibrillation potential The action potential of a single muscle fiber occurring spontaneously or after movement of a needle electrode and usually firing at a constant rate. The potential consists of biphasic or triphasic spikes of short duration (usually less than 5 ms) with an initial positive phase and a peak-to-peak amplitude of less than 1 mV. It may also have a biphasic, initially negative phase when recorded at the site of initiation. It has an associated high-pitched regular sound described as "rain on a tin roof."

In addition to this classic form, positive sharp waves may also be recorded from fibrillating muscle fibers when the potential arises from an area immediately adjacent to the needle electrode. (From the 2001 Report of the Nomenclature Committee of the American Association of Electromyography and Electrodiagnosis.[19] Reproduced by kind permission of the AANEM.)

While classically the result of motor neuropathy, the fracture of muscle fibers in myositis also causes one part of the myofibril to lose innervation and thus to produce fibrillations.

fibrinoid degeneration of astrocytes See **Alexander disease**.

fibroblastic meningioma See **meningioma**.

fibrocartilaginous embolism of the spinal cord A rare cause of anterior spinal artery occlusion, presenting with sudden severe pain at onset and some degree of quadriparesis or paraparesis shortly after exercise. It is supposed that an acute vertical disk herniation of nucleus pulposus material causes infarction by retrograde embolization to the central artery. An increased intradisk pressure resulting from axial loading of the vertebral column with a concomitant Valsalva maneuver may be the initiating event. The interval from pain to maximal neurologic deficit ranges from 15 min to 3 weeks. The prognosis is poor, the condition often leading to death within a year of onset (median of about 3 months).

The precipitating factors sometimes recorded include minor trauma such as falls and jumps, physical effort, and performance of the Valsalva maneuver. Pathologically, fibrocartilaginous emboli are found in the arterial and/or venous beds.[6358, 5972]

fibrodysplasia ossificans progressiva See **myositis ossificans**.

fibroma An unencapsulated benign tumor arising within peripheral nerves, fibers of which traverse the substance of the lesion. Clinically, a painful swelling in the vicinity of a nerve is the usual presenting complaint; motor and sensory deficits appropriate to the nerve ensue. Such tumors occur particularly but not uniquely in **neurofibromatosis**, in which condition they are usually multiple.

fibromatosis of the optic nerve sheath See **orbital pseudotumor syndrome**.

fibromuscular dysplasia (FMD) A segmental, nonatheromatous, and noninflammatory disorder of the muscular arteries (including the carotid and renal arteries) characterized by irregular fibrous or fibromuscular thickening of all coats of the arterial wall causing alternating rings of constriction and dilatation as seen on arteriograms. *Intimal*, *medial*, and *adventitial* forms are described.[1269, 3968]

Females are much more commonly affected; the condition may be dominantly inherited with reduced penetrance in males; it remains unmapped. Clinically, neck pain, transient ischemic attacks, and a carotid bruit are the most constant findings, sometimes due to dissection of the affected vessel. The condition is diagnosed at arteriography, which has usually been performed in the course of the investigation for transient ischemic attacks or subarachnoid hemorrhage. The arteries involved include the cervical, mesenteric, and renal vessels; irregular corrugations of the wall are noted on angiography ("*string of beads sign*"). Intracranial aneurysms are associated in a proportion of cases of cervical fibromuscular dysplasia.[4336, 5538]

fibromyalgia syndrome A common disorder of unknown etiology, affecting women more often than men, who complain that they "ache all over" and in whom areas of focal tenderness ("tender points") can be demonstrated in characteristic locations. Over half the patients with this diagnosis complain of widespread pain, areas of focal tenderness, fatigue, morning stiffness, headache, sleep disturbance, and/or paresthesias. Other common symptoms include dizziness, impaired memory and concentration, rashes, and chronic itching. There is thus a relationship with **chronic fatigue syndrome** (Dr. David Nye; personal communication).

Any patient with chronic, diffuse aching pain, and tenderness in at least 11 of 18 locations (see below) fits the diagnostic criteria. Nine "tender points" are defined on each side; such sites must be present on both sides of the body, both above and below the waist, and pain must have been present for at least 3 months. Patients typically complain of light sleep with physical discomfort, and wake up feeling tired and lethargic with discomfort and stiffness in the joints, persisting throughout the day. Diagnostic criteria have been suggested by the American College of Rheumatology:[6846]

1. History of widespread pain (indicating that pains are felt on each side of the body and both above and below the waist.) as well as axial skeletal pain (cervical spine or anterior chest or thoracic spine or low back) Shoulder and buttock pain is considered as pain for each involved side and low back' pain is considered lower segment pain.

2. Pain in 11 of 18 tender point sites on digital palpation.The sites listed are:

   Occiput: bilateral, at the suboccipital muscle insertions.

   Low cervical: bilateral, at the anterior aspects of the intertransverse spaces at C5–C7.

   Trapezius: bilateral, at the midpoint of the upper border.

   Supraspinatus: bilateral, at origins, above the scapula spine near the medial border.

   Second rib: bilateral, at the second costo-chondral junctions, just lateral to the junctions on upper surfaces.

   Lateral epicondyle: bilateral, 2 cm distal to the epicondyles.

   Gluteal: bilateral, in upper outer quadrants of buttocks in anterior fold of muscle.

   Greater trochanter: bilateral, posterior to the trochanteric prominence.

Knee: bilateral, at the medial fat pad proximal to the joint line.

This common, chronic, and often disabling disorder may be associated with neuroendocrine and immunologic changes but there is no known pathology. Central hyperexcitability of the nociceptive system and REM sleep deprivation have been suggested as relevant in pathogenesis.[1612] Whether the condition is a somatoform disorder or an organic condition that has not yet been adequately characterized remains undetermined. See also **myofascial pain syndromes**. http://www.fmpartnership.org/engmonog.htm is a site that explains the symptoms, diagnostic criteria, causes, and management of fibromyalgia.

fibromyositis See **fibromyalgia syndrome** and **myofascial pain syndromes**.

fibrosarcoma Large circumscribed tumors arising from the meninges, often characterized by necrosis, hemorrhage, and cyst formation. Histologically, long spindle cells are found in parallel rows with substantial amounts of supporting reticulin connective tissue. Various grades of malignancy occur.

In a rare *variant* form, *primary diffuse meningeal sarcomatosis*, the highly malignant tumor infiltrates the meninges widely and no single originating tumor mass can be identified.

fibrosing myositis See **myosclerosis**.

fibrositis See **fibromyalgia syndrome** and **myofascial main syndromes**.

fibrous dysplasia A nonhereditary, localized developmental disorder presenting in youth, in which dense fibrous tissue replaces bone. The craniofacial bones are involved in half of all cases.

Bone pain is a constant symptom and pathological fractures are common. When dysplasia affects the base of the skull and the temporal bones, dysmorphism, skull deformity, proptosis, optic atrophy, visual disturbance, deafness, headache, and cranial nerve compression syndromes result.[3148]

In the *polyostotic* form (McCune–Albright syndrome), skeletal anomalies leading to short stature and bone deformities, sexual precocity, and café-au-lait spots are additional features.

In another *variant* form, fibrous dysplasia of the skull is complicated by encephalopathy with seizures. See **Albright syndrome**.

fibrous dysplasia of the skull with encephalopathy See **Albright syndrome**.

fibular reflex Slight contraction of the hamstrings with resultant flexion of the knee occurring after tapping the head of the fibula. Presumably this is actually due to percussion of the lateral hamstring tendon which also inserts here. See **lateral hamstring reflex**.

fibular tunnel An arch formed by the insertion of the peroneus longus to the head of the fibula, through which the common peroneal nerve passes.

Fick, Adolf (1829–1901) German, medical physicist. He developed the principle that the blood flow of an organ can be determined if the oxygen consumption and the arteriovenous oxygen difference are known. This led to successful measurement of the rate of cerebral blood flow, initially by Kety and Schmidt.

fictitious epilepsy 1. The reporting of nonexistent seizures in a child, usually by a parent. This seems to be a form of **Munchausen syndrome** by proxy. 2. The induction of seizures by wilful abuse.[4272]

fidgety feet See **restless legs syndrome**.

field of vision (visual field) That area in space from all points of which light rays can travel to the retina of the immobile eye.

field-holding reflex A visual fixation mechanism preventing the slow drift of the eyes from a target, which would thus require corrective saccades.[3762]

fifth day seizures A benign syndrome characterized by the occurrence of repetitive seizures in full-term neonates who on examination are found to have neither detectable risk factors nor neurological abnormalities. Clonic focal or multifocal convulsions and apneic spells are the usual expressions. Bursts of alternating EEG rhythms are common and characteristic but not invariable. The syndrome may be caused by zinc deficiency.[1534]

fifth finger sign See **digiti quinti sign**.

fifth ventricle See **cava septi pellucidi et vergae**.

fight-or-flight reaction The name given by Dr. W.B. Cannon to the combined sympathetic (adrenergic) reaction that takes place in response to threatening situations.

Figueira syndrome A syndrome of subacutely developing but reversible weakness of the neck muscles with increased tone and often hyperreflexia in the legs in small children, usually following an intestinal upset. The nature of the condition is uncertain; it may be an attenuated form of acute **poliomyelitis**.[2040]

filamentopathies Disorders primarily resulting from malfunction of muscle or nerve intermediate filaments, usually genetically determined. The intermediate filaments are a family of structures interacting with actin and microtubules to impart structural resilience to cells. See **giant axonal neuropathy; hereditary motor and sensory neuropathy (type 2E); familial ALS; myofibrillar myopathy; Emery–Dreifuss muscular dystrophy, congenital muscular dystrophy with epidermolysis bullosa, amyotrophic lateral sclerosis, glue-sniffers neuropathy**, and iminodiproprionitrile neuropathy, which are other conditions affecting intermediate filaments.[2875]

Filippi syndrome (microcephaly-syndactyly syndrome) A congenital dysmorphic syndrome characterized by short stature, dysarthria, syndactyly of the fingers and toes, microcephaly, and mental and developmental delay.[381]

fillet (from Lat, a thread) A thin **lemniscus**, though usually wider than a **fasciculus** or a tract.

fine motor functions Movements performed with distal muscles, such as forming a pincer grip, finger manipulations, and the handling of small objects; a measure of both motor pathway integrity and intelligence.

Fine syndrome A congenital dysmorphic syndrome characterized by deafness, glaucoma, cataract, blindness, scoliosis, cryptorchidism, inguinal hernia, cleft palate, brachycephaly, macrocephaly, plagiocephaly, delayed closure of the fontanelles, callosal abnormalities, cavernous hemangiomas, and mental and developmental delay.[381]

finger agnosia The term employed by Gerstmann to refer to a fragment of **autotopagnosia** (the inability to indicate body parts), with the loss of ability to recognize, identify, differentiate, name, select, indicate, or orient as to the individual fingers of either hand, the patient's, or the examiner's.

Those affected are unable to appreciate the position of individual fingers among their fellows, to point to a named finger, or to move it when it is named by the examiner. The phenomenon was first described by Gerstmann in 1924 as one of the components of the syndrome of the angular gyrus, but the ability was later considered nonspecific (and indeed as evidence of dysphasia by Schilder). More recent studies suggest that "finger sense" is a real faculty and that the association of finger agnosia with the other elements of **Gerstmann syndrome** is more than coincidental,[3446] although Critchley has attacked the concept, contending that the faculty of finger gnosis does not exist.[1335]

finger flexor reflex (Wartenberg sign) Further flexion of the semiflexed fingers and of the thumb of the supinated hand in response to a tap on the examiner's fingers lying across and contacting them. The contraction is enhanced in cases of pyramidal lesions above C6 and also in states of emotional tension. See also **Rossimolo reflex, Tromner reflex,** and **Hoffmann reflex**.

finger oscillation test Part of the **Halstead–Reitan battery** of psychological tests in which the subject must press a key with his index finger as many times as possible within a specified period of time. The speed of performance of this task is slowed with aging and in the setting of dementia.[2710]

finger sign See **Gordon sign**.

finger tapping test A test of motor control (manual dexterity) in which the subject is required to tap a surface with the index finger in each hand as fast as possible.[5260, 5261] Reduction in rate compared to that of a normal age-matched control series suggests the presence of lesions of the contralateral motor areas.

fingerprint bodies An ultrastructural abnormality of muscle consisting of concentric lamellae arranged in whorls and loops, resembling fingerprints. The finding is not specific for any one disease, having been described in the setting of **congenital myopathies, oculopharyngeal muscle dystrophy, myotonic dystrophy**, and **dermatomyositis**.

fingerprint body myopathy A rare, nonprogressive recessive congenital myopathy characterized by the presence of subsarcolemmal whorled bodies on muscle biopsy specimens. Clinically, the condition presents in childhood with slowly progressive symmetrical, proximal more than distal weakness sparing the cranial nerves and with hypotonia, areflexia, and tremor but without wasting.[1869] Mental subnormality has also been associated with the disorder. Serum CK levels are variably raised. The EMG is myopathic and muscle biopsy shows arrays of parallel osmiophilic lamellae resembling fingerprints, as in **myotonic dystrophy**, some **idiopathic inflammatory myopathies**, and **malignant hyperthermia** and **central core disease**. Similar inclusions are also found in other muscle diseases.[869]

fingerprint inclusion myopathy A congenital myopathy with intracytoplasmic inclusions. See **fingerprint body myopathy**.

finger-thumb reflex Opposition and adduction of the thumb with flexion at the metacarpophalangeal joint in response to firm passive flexion of a finger. A postural rather than a muscle stretch reflex, it is normally present, disappearing in patients with pyramidal lesions.

Finkel late-onset type spinal muscular atrophy See **hereditary motor neuropathy** (*variants*).

Finnish amyloidosis See **amyloidosis**.

Finnish lipofuscinosis See **neuronal ceroid lipofuscinosis**.

FIRDA See **frontal intermittent rhythmic delta activity**.

firearm recoil palsy Symptoms resulting from entrapment of the upper fibers of the brachial plexus between the clavicle and the underlying scalene muscles as a result of backward compression exerted by the stock of a gun.[6636]

firing pattern Qualitative and quantitative descriptions of the sequence of discharge of electric waveforms recorded from muscle or nerve. (From the 2001 Report of the Nomenclature Committee of the American Association of Electromyography and Electrodiagnosis.[19] Reproduced by kind permission of the AANEM.)

firing rate The frequency of repetition of a potential. The relationship of the frequency to the occurrence of other potentials and the force of muscle contraction may be described. See also **discharge frequency**. (From the 2001 Report of the Nomenclature Committee of the American Association of Electromyography and Electrodiagnosis.[19] Reproduced by kind permission of the AANEM.)

first and second branchial arch syndrome See **oculoauriculovertebral dysplasia**.

first arch syndrome See **hemifacial microsomia**.

first pain See **fast pain**.

Fischer syndrome (hyperkeratosis-syringomyelia) A dominantly inherited congenital dysmorphic syndrome characterized by keratosis of the palms and soles, sparse hair, thickened eyelids, clubbing of the fingers, spasticity, changes resembling those of **progeria**, and physical and mental delay.[2069]

Fischgold line A line joining the lower margins of the mastoid processes on anteroposterior or transoral skull X-ray films. The line normally passes through the atlanto-occipital articulations and the tip of the odontoid is often situated on the same line; both structures are situated above it in **basilar impression**. The *digastric line* (drawn between the medial aspect of the mastoid processes at their junctions with the remainder of the skull) may be as useful,[5980] but CT scanning is much better.

fish odor syndrome A dysmetabolic, dysmorphic syndrome characterized also by a most unpleasant body smell, hydrocephalus, short stature, hypertelorism, and cortical blindness.[5780]

Fisher sign When the tip of the index finger is tapped repeatedly upon the middle joint of the thumb, the remaining fingers cannot be held still but move in synchrony; this is seen in patients with a mild corticospinal tract lesion on that side. A degree of difference is also present according to the handedness of the subject.

Fisher syndrome See **Miller Fisher syndrome**.

fissure (Lat, a cleft) A long, narrow crack or cleft such as the deeper sulci, thus delineating the cerebral or cerebellar lobes. The interhemispheric, callosal, calcarine, ectorhinal, longitudinal, and transverse fissures are some named examples.

fissure of Rolando The central fissure of the hemispheres, separating the anterior motor from the posterior sensory cortex, described by Luigi **Rolando** in 1825.

fissure of Sylvius The lateral fissure, demarcating the superior extent of the temporal lobes, and described by **Sylvius** in 1641.

fisting Persistent clenching of the fist by an infant with a hemiparesis on that side.

fist–palm–side test A test of motor control, wherein the subject is asked to tap the table repeatedly with his or her fist, then with the palm, and then with the side of his hand. Errors in the fluent repetition of this sequence suggest the presence of bilateral frontal lobe disease.

fist-ring test The subject is asked to make a fist, then to oppose the tips of the thumb and index finger, alternating between the actions; with contralateral premotor lesions, the smoothness of execution is lost and perseveration of one posture may occur. See also the **fist–palm–side test**, which is more sensitive.

fistula sign Increase or decrease in the pressure within the external auditory meatus leads to vertigo and brief horizontal nystagmus, as a result of the presence of a fistula in the bony labyrinth of the lateral semicircular canal, usually as a result of chronic otitis media. See also **superior semicircular canal dehiscence syndrome**.

fit A vernacular term for a seizure.

Fitzsimmons syndrome A congenital X-linked dysmorphic syndrome characterized by hyperkeratosis of the palms and soles, spastic paraparesis, and mental and developmental delay.[2118]

Five Word Test A serial verbal memory test with semantic cuing, allowing an estimate of cued learning, free recall, and cued recall of five words with immediate and delayed recall in people over 50 years old.[1346]

fixation Direction of the gaze upon an object so that the image of the object falls steadily upon the two foveas. See also **field-holding reflex** and **smooth pursuit system**.

fixation disparity The minimal, varying imprecision of the **fusional vergence** system in holding images precisely on the foveas of the two eyes, triggering further corrective movements initiated by that system to align the images so closely that central fusional mechanisms prevent the awareness of any blurring.

fixation index The ratio of the frequency and amplitude of the beats of nystagmus occurring when the eyes are open and when they are closed; with greater suppression, the value of the index rises. In darkness and other situations when no fixation is possible, cerebellar influences on eye movements are minimal, as the cerebellum is concerned with the control of eye movements during fixation. Fixation is the usual method by which ice skaters and ballet dancers reduce vertigo during rapid spins.[2974]

fixation instability Inability of the eyes to maintain stillness during fixation on a target, usually as a result of small horizontal saccades which result in ocular flutter when there is no delay between one saccade and the next one in the other direction, or result in square wave jerks when such a delay does exist.

fixation nystagmus The term of Gordon **Holmes** for that form of nystagmus which is enhanced by visual fixation on an object and inhibited to some degree in its absence; a characteristic of nystagmus of central origin. See **acquired nystagmus**.

fixation point The point at which the visual axes of the two eyes meet; the object of gaze.

fixation spasm A reflex fixation of gaze upon an object in space, from which the gaze cannot be transferred voluntarily. The phenomenon is described in subjects with visual impairment or with bilateral frontal or parietal lesions.[2959]

fixation suppression Suppression of the vestibulo-ocular reflex or of caloric nystagmus by visual fixation. Failure of this mechanism suggests the presence of a metabolic encephalopathy or posterior fossa disease, including tumor.[145]

fixed dystonia An unusual affliction mainly seen in young adult females in whom a peripheral injury precedes the onset and spread of **dystonia** to other body regions with few remissions. The fixed postures mainly affect the limbs, rarely the neck/shoulder region. Pain is a common complaint and a minority of subjects fulfill the criteria for **complex regional pain syndrome**, though more (but not all) appear to have psychogenic dystonia or somatization disorder with evidence of dissociative and/or affective disorders.[5651]

flaccid (Lat, flabby) Drooping or lacking in stiffness, but, in neurology, synonymous with hypotonic.

flail arm syndrome (brachial amyotrophic diplegia) Symmetrical wasting and weakness of the arms without similar involvement of other body parts, although pyramidal signs may be found in the legs. It is more commonly seen in males whose survival is prolonged. The commonest cause is a variant of **amyotrophic lateral sclerosis**, but cervical cord disease and brachial plexopathies can also present with this picture. See also **Hirayama disease** and **man-in-a-barrel syndrome**.

flail foot Loss of both dorsiflexion and plantar flexion at the ankle as a result of a sciatic nerve injury. The intrinsic foot muscle will also be paretic.

flapping tremor A bilateral but asymmetrical abnormality seen in the outstretched hands, in which involuntary repetitive brisk extension of the wrist (akin to **asterixis**) is followed by relaxation and dropping of the hand in patients with a metabolic encephalopathy, such as that due to hepatic failure.

flashbacks The recurrence of sensations formerly experienced while under the influence of lysergic acid diethylamide, now re-evoked by use of other drugs such as cannabis. A panic state often accompanies the experience.

flash-induced nystagmus See **induced nystagmus** and **flicker-induced nystagmus**.

Flatau, Eduard (1869–1932) Polish neurologist, who trained in Moscow and Berlin. After a career in neurology and comparative anatomy there, he returned to private practice in Poland. Among his many publications were important contributions on disseminated encephalitis (Flatau–Redlich disease), tumors of the neuraxis, tuberculous meningitis, and migraine, but he is best remembered for his description of torsion spasm, now known as **dystonia**.

Flatau law The greater the length of the fibers in the spinal cord, the more peripherally they are sited.[2124] This is correct for the pyramidal and spinothalamic tracts but not in the case of the posterior columns.

Flatau sign Pupillary dilation in response to stretching of the neck muscles, described in meningococcal meningitis. The genesis of the sign is unknown and its value is minimal.

flavi- (Gr, yellow) Prefix denoting yellow.

Flechsig, Paul Emile (1847–1929) Bohemian neurologist and professor of psychiatry in Leipzig, who defined the dorsal spinocerebellar tract (Flechsig's tract) in 1876, identified motor and sensory projection areas in the cortex, and named the parts of the internal capsule and the anterior and lateral "ground-bundles" (the former being the pyramidal tract).

Flechsig loop See **Meyer loop**.

Flechsig principle The primary receptive areas of the cerebral cortex have no direct neocortical connections, except with immediately adjacent parasensory (association) areas.

fleece of Stilling The interlaced fibers running to the dentate nucleus from the cerebellar cortex.

Fleischer, Bruno (1874–1965) German ophthalmologist in Erlangen, best remembered for his original account of the corneal pigmentation in **Wilson disease**, published in 1903.

flexibilitas cerea (Lat, waxy flexibility) Unvarying increased resistance to passive movement of a limb which, when overcome, is followed by the patient's maintenance of any posture in which his limb was placed by the examiner. The phenomenon is usually encountered in schizophrenics but is also a manifestation of depression or of drug-induced dyskinesia.

flexion (Lat, a bending) The state of being bent or the act of bending.

flexion dystonia in paralysis agitans See **dystonias**.

flexion reflex 1. Dorsiflexion of the hallux with flexion at the ankle, knee, and hip occurring with noxious stimulation of the skin of the foot or leg, seen in some neonates after severe perinatal asphyxia. The Babiński reflex is but a fragment of this full reflex response. 2. Tapping the long flexor tendons at the wrist leads to contraction of the long flexor muscles in patients with a corticospinal tract lesion on that side.

flexion spinal defence reflex See **flexor reflex**.

flexion-adduction sign The characteristic posture of patients with **neuralgic amyotrophy**, in which the arm is maintained in flexion at the elbow and adduction at the shoulder. Abduction and lateral rotation of the arm with the elbow extended may result in radicular pain in such patients.[6675]

flexion, adduction and internal rotation (FAIR) test When a patient lies on the unaffected side and flexes the knee of the affected leg to 90°, catching the foot behind the calf of the affected leg, the examiner swings the affected leg over the healthy one until the knee touches the examining table. The inducement of buttock pain is said to be a sign of the **piriformis syndrome**.

flexor A bender; in neurology applied to muscles which are antagonists to extensors and which tend by their action to shorten a limb or to reduce the length of the trunk.

flexor reflex (flexor withdrawal reflex, flexion spinal defence reflex, réflexe des raccourcisseurs, reflex of spinal automatism)

Flexion of the hip and knee with dorsiflexion of the ankle and toes elicited and steadily maintained by a noxious stimulus applied to the sole of the foot, particularly on its lateral side, but also from a wider area. A reflex produced by a noxious cutaneous stimulus, or a train of electrical stimuli, that activates the flexor muscles of a limb and thus acts to withdraw it from the stimulus. In humans, it is well characterized only in the lower extremity.[19]

The **Babiński response** represents part of this reflex, which is a typical finding in the lower limbs in cases of spastic paresis, especially "paraplegia-in-flexion."[4110, 6621]

When the response is bilateral, this is known as the **crossed flexor reflex**.

flexor spasms (syndrome de spasmes en flexion, jackknife convulsions, jackknife spasms, grusskrampfe) 1. A characteristic bilateral symmetrical contraction of the muscles of the neck, trunk and extremities, leading to sudden flexion of the head and trunk and abduction of the legs (**salaam attacks**). These are characteristically seen in the syndrome of **infantile spasms**. 2. Flexion of the hip and knee and dorsiflexion of the ankle in patients with spastic paraparesis when proprioceptive innervation is lacking, sometimes leading to "paraplegia-in-flexion."

In such cases the spasms are often preceded by detrusor contractions. Anal sphincter activity is generally increased in relation to detrusor contractions in patients with spinal lesions but decreased in patients with cerebral lesions.

flexor withdrawal reflex See **flexor reflex**.

flick sign Flicking or shaking of the wrists performed spontaneously by patients with **carpal tunnel syndrome** as they describe their reactions to the hand paresthesias that typically they note on waking.[5133] The specificity of the sign has been questioned.

flicker fusion (critical flicker fusion) A test of visual function and arousal in which the subject observes a flickering light, the flicker rate speeding up until he or she perceives it to shine constantly. The test and its modifications have been reported to show abnormalities in patients with multiple sclerosis in the absence of other evidence of visual disturbance.[1418]

flicker illness Symptoms of mild discomfort and headache possibly increasing to profound spatial disorientation and seizures due to photic stimulation from sunlight shining through the spinning rotor blades of a helicopter.The frequencies of flashing light thus produced range from 24 to 27 flashes/s, which is within the range reported to produce symptoms.[1395]

flicker-induced nystagmus (flash-induced nystagmus) A form of conjugate horizontal jerk nystagmus induced by intermittent photic stimulation of one eye. The slow phase beats away from the stimulated eye.[5849] See also **induced nystagmus**.

Flier syndrome A syndrome of disabling muscle pain with elevation of serum creatine kinase levels, enlargement of the hands and feet, acanthocytosis nigricans, hirsutism, and resistance of target cells to insulin.[3440]

flight of colors The perception of afterimages such as haloes or discs which repeatedly change in color following 10 s of bright-light stimulation of the eye and persisting for at least 1 min with at least two color changes in normal subjects. They are abolished or altered with disease affecting any part of the visual system concerned with central vision, and the test has been claimed to detect optic neuropathy with greater accuracy than do visual evoked responses.[2000, 5357]

flip sign Weakness in performance of quick movements of the fingers, such as flicking the finger against an object; a feature both of radial and ulnar nerve (as well as of basal ganglion and pyramidal) lesions.

flip test Straight-leg raising is performed with the patient supine, and he is then asked to sit up and to extend a leg, as if for testing of the plantar response. The ability to flex the hip in the sitting position but not when supine suggests the presence of nonorganic causes of back pain.[6580] See **Waddell signs**.

floaters Mobile vitreous opacities appearing as gray or black specks obscuring tiny arcs of vision and drifting about in the visual field, lagging behind as the individual moves the head or eyes. They represent condensations of collagen fibrils within the vitreous humor of the eye. Though quite benign, they irritate or worry some patients and indeed are sometimes evidence of retinal detachment or intraocular hemorrhage.

floating harbor syndrome A congenital dysmorphic syndrome characterized by aphasia, skeletal anomalies such as micrognathia and clinodactyly, and delay in physical maturation.[3766]

flocculus (Lat, a small tangle of wool) Part of the paleocerebellum concerned with the maintenance of posture.

floppy infant syndrome Generalized hypotonia, weakness, and lack of muscle development in neonates and small infants, usually due to central (e.g., cerebral palsy) or metabolic causes and less often to peripheral lesions such as anterior horn cell disease, myopathy, or muscular dystrophy. The causes have been reviewed.[3244] See **benign congenital hypotonia**.

floppy person syndrome See **acute quadriplegic myopathy**

Flourens, Marie-Jean-Pierre (1794–1867) Parisian, professor of comparative anatomy who suggested, on the basis of stimulation and extirpation experiments in pigeons, that functions were precisely located in many parts of the cortex, though he supposed the cerebrum to be inexcitable.[2130] He correctly identified the cerebellum as being concerned with the coordination of muscular activity (although he supposed this to be exerted contralaterally) and properly ascribed to the vestibular system responsibility for vertigo and nystagmus. He also confirmed in 1837 the presence of a center in the floor of the medulla (the *noeud vital*) controlling respiratory activity (although this had previously been suggested by Legallois); and showed that vision depends upon an intact cortex.

Flourens law Stimulation of a semicircular canal excites nystagmus in the plane of that canal.

flow void Absence of the normal flow pattern on MRI scanning in **arteriovenous malformations** or within the intracranial venous sinuses in cases of **sinus thrombosis**.

fluctuating dystonia See **dopa-responsive dystonia**.

fluctuations Variability in the severity of movement disorder in Parkinsonian patients on chronic levadopa therapy, in many instances associated with variability of the levadopa levels. Hyperkinetic forms include *peak-dose chorea* and *diphasic dyskinesia*. Dystonic forms are *early morning*, *end-of-dose*, and *peak-dose dystonias*; while hypokinetic forms include *akinetic freezing of gait*, *early morning akinesia*, *end-of-dose deterioration* (wearing-off effect), and sudden *switching-off or on–off* effects.[2749] Using a different system of classification, Quinn[5158] suggested the following categorizations:

- Short duration motor fluctuations (lasting minutes or less)
  - Sudden transient freezing (motor blocks) occurring late in the course of the disease, often provoked by external stimuli, relieved by certain rituals and related to the occurrence of "on–off" events. This is a common cause of falls in this population.
  - Paradoxic kinesis. Sudden and brief relief of the symptoms of Parkinsonism provoked by an urgent external stimulus or by rituals.
- Medium duration motor fluctuations (lasting hours or less)
  - Beginning of dose worsening
  - End of dose rebound
  - Wearing off/"on–off"/yo-yo-ing
  - Diurnal
- Long duration (days)

Slow variations in response to levadopa therapy

Fluctuations in mood, pain perception, cognitive abilities, and autonomic functions also occur.[5158]

fluent dysphasias Those forms of dysphasia characterized by empty speech which is still grammatical but in which there is a deficiency of substantive words. Many literal and paraphasic errors occur in speech, of which the patient is unaware. See **dysphasias**.

fluid attenuated inversion recovery A pulse sequence used in **Magnetic Resonance Imaging** which annulls the signal from fluids. As a result, for example, CSF effects on the image are reduced, allowing a better visualization of the periventricular hypertintense plaques of **multiple sclerosis**.

fluorescein angiography The observation of the retinal arterioles and venules following the intravenous injection of fluorescein. The morphology of the vessels, the time taken for the agent to arrive at the eye, and the subsequent appearance of the optic nerve head can be assessed safely by repetitive retinal photography, thus providing useful information in cases of retinal vessel disease, arterial occlusion, and, for example, papilledema.[4718]

fluorescent treponemal antibody test See **FTA-abs test**.

fluorosis A syndrome of bony distortion as a result of long-term excessive ingestion of fluoride. The vertebral column becomes stiff and distorted by osteophytes, which leads to compression of spinal nerves and, in time, to spinal cord compression as well.[5863]

flutter See **ocular flutter**.

flutter dysmetria A form of saccadic intrusion characterized by **ocular flutter** (back-to-back saccades) occurring at the completion of a refixational saccade in some patients with cerebellar disease.[6958]

flutterlike oscillations To-and-fro pendular oscillations of the eyes at about 10 Hz, associated with a change in fixation in patients with cerebellar disease.[1217]

flycatcher tongue Sudden irregular protrusion of the tongue, seen in subjects with dystonias or choreic states; an orobuccolingual dyskinesia.

flying saucer syndrome The tendency for those with chorea or myoclonus to lose control of, drop, or fling away the objects in their hands involuntarily. The term was first used for the matutinal domestic catastrophes of patients with **juvenile myoclonic epilepsy**, whose jerks are maximal within the first hour or so after rising.

Flynn phenomenon Constriction of the pupils in darkness. This inversion of the normal response occurs in some cases of chronic disease of the optic nerve and in congenital achromatopsia.[2177]

Flynn–Aird syndrome (cochlear deafness, myopia and oligophrenia syndrome, dominant myopia and hearing loss, peripheral neuropathy and skeletal abnormalities syndrome, neuroectodermal syndrome) A dominantly inherited syndrome consisting of progressive sensorineural deafness with myopia, painful sensorimotor peripheral neuropathy, bony cysts and osteoporosis, cataract, pigmentary retinopathy, kyphoscoliosis, mental and developmental delay, seizures, osteoporosis, and distal weakness.

Ataxia, baldness, dental caries, dermal atrophy, joint stiffness, abnormal EEG findings, and elevated CSF protein levels are also described.[2133]

FMD See **fibromuscular dysplasia**.

fMRI data center A repository of peer-reviewed fMRI studies and their underlying data sets. Web site: www.fmriclc.org/.

focal Originating from, or to do with, a particular point in space. In the context of epilepsy, a seizure whose initial semiology indicates, or is consistent with, initial activation of only part of one cerebral hemisphere. The ILAE has now properly abandoned the word "partial" to describe this concept.

focal asymmetric cortical degeneration syndromes Dementing diseases primarily affecting the cortex, still in the process of classification in the presence of different histological and clinical findings. The conditions currently subsumed are as follows:

Primary progressive aphasias (fluent, nonfluent, anomic and mixed) (See also **Pick disease**)

Perceptual-motor disorders (visual, motor, or both) (See also **cortical basalganglionic degeneration, progressive asymmetric rigidity, and apraxia syndrome**)

Frontal or frontotemporal atrophies (See also **Pick disease**)

Bitemporal atrophies[1051, 1052]

focal (asymmetric) tonic seizures Those seizures that originate from practically anywhere in the neocortex. An example is the syndrome of explosive motor seizures originating in the supplementary motor area.

focal cervical poliopathy of distal arm See **hereditary motor neuropathy** (*variants*).

focal cervical poliopathy of distal upper extremity causing juvenile muscular atrophy See **monomelic amyotrophy**.

focal clonic seizures Brief focal motor events arising from a seizure focus in the primary motor cortex and distinguished from focal myoclonic seizures only by their rhythmic repetition.

focal cortical dysplasia A malformation characterized by congregations of large, bizarre neurons and glial cells through all but the first cortical layer within the temporal lobe. The clinical presentation is usually in youth, with refractory epilepsy. A transmantle form is also described and thought to be due to abnormal stem cell development.[403]

The condition is detected in some specimens resected surgically in the management of intractable seizure disorders.[6231, 190] In the Taylor type, the histological features include cortical laminar disorganization, giant neurons, and dysmorphic and ectopic neurons. Two forms are recognized, depending on the presence or absence of abnormal glial (balloon) cells. See also **heterotopia**.

focal cortical myoclonus See **cortical myoclonus**.

focal dermal hypoplasia (Goltz syndrome) A diffuse congenital encephalopathy inherited as an X-linked dominant (lethal in males) trait characterized by linear pigmentation of the skin, focal areas of skin aplasia, mucosal papillomatosis, hypoplasia of the dental enamel and nails, alopecia, iris colobomas, microcephaly, microphthalmia, scoliosis, spina bifida, and mental retardation.[2458]

focal dystonia See **dystonia**.

focal eyelid dystonia See **apraxia of eyelid opening**.

focal inhibitory seizures See **hemiparetic seizures**.

focal levator atrophy A rare condition of ptosis as a result of disease of the levator palpebrae muscle, either uniquely or as part of a generalized myopathy.[5808]

focal motor neuron disease Weakness, wasting, and fasciculations in a discrete body region, which is progressive for some months before arresting. This is a residual diagnosis, other focal pathologies requiring exclusion before it can be considered.[5939] See also **Hirayama disease**.

focal myoclonic seizures A heterogeneous group of seizure syndromes including **progressive myoclonic epilepsy** and **Lafora body disease**.

focal myoclonus See **spinal myoclonus**.

focal myositis A rare disease characterized by focal inflammatory enlargement in a single skeletal muscle, which is usually cured without medication.[13] See also **localized nodular myositis**.

focal necrotizing myopathy Muscle necrosis, fibrosis, and calcification in the region of repeated intramuscular injections of drugs such as pentazocine or local anesthetics.[3600]

focal neuronal migration disorders A group of developmental structural lesions characterized by disorganization of the cortical architecture with an aberrant columnar and laminar neuronal arrangement, leading to macrogyria or polymicrogyria. The degree of cytoarchitectonic disorganization and the extent of the brain involved vary widely. The clinical features usually include mental retardation, intractable seizure disorders, and severe motor dysfunction in infancy; survival seldom exceeds two decades.[4873] See **heterotopias**.

focal nodular myositis A *variant* form of polymyositis.[1372] See **idiopathic inflammatory myopathy**.

focal reflex myoclonus (pyramidal myoclonus) A form of myoclonus affecting a single body part and activated by a specific stimulus such as movement. The responsible lesion is thought to involve the cortical and subcortical area of the contralateral cerebral hemisphere.[6143]

focal sensory seizures with experiential symptoms Seizures with complex, usually formed, distorted and/or multimodal, sensory symptoms implying seizure initiation in association cortices, such as the temporo-parieto-occipital junction, with connections to multiple sensory areas.[1861]

A variant is *focal sensory seizures with elementary symptoms* (visual, somatosensory, vestibular, olfactory, gustatory, or auditory) manifesting as sensory phenomena produced by activation of the primary sensory cortices.[1861]

focal steroid responsive myopathy A rare inflammatory muscle disorder that affects usually the legs, trunk, arms or neck, in which latter case it may cause the **dropped head syndrome**.[652] The presentation is typically with weakness and local muscle swelling.

focal task-specific dystonias (occupational cramps, musicians' dystonia) Dystonias affecting a single body part, usually one that has been employed in the repetitive performance of complex movements. While it affects many musicians, with a reported rate of 1:200 (Robert Schumann was an example) compared with 1:3400 in the general population, the motoric activities of many other professions and trades lead to the same condition. See also **writers' cramp**.

focal upper limb demyelinating neuropathy A form of **chronic inflammatory demyelinating polyneuropathy** restricted to the arms, usually motor or mixed motor and sensory, seldom only sensory; and with reduced motor nerve conduction velocities and conduction block and a tendency to nerve hypertrophy.[6282]

focus A limited region of the scalp, cerebral cortex, or depth of the brain displaying a given EEG activity, whether normal or abnormal.

Foerster, Otfried (1873–1941) German neurologist and neurosurgeon, born in Poland, who graduated from Breslau, studied in Paris at the Salpêtrière and returned to Breslau in **Wernicke**'s clinic, becoming professor in 1922. His clinic received funds from the Rockefeller Foundation and became an independent institute in 1934. He pioneered the methods of stimulation of the cerebral cortex at open operation in attempts to localize foci of epileptic discharge and trained **Penfield** and others in these techniques. As a result of his studies, mapping of the functions of human cortical areas was begun, previous workers such as the **Vogts** having worked on primates. He advocated section of some thoracic nerve roots to treat the lightning pains in **tabes dorsalis** and also described atonic diplegia (cerebral palsy) in 1909 and the use of tractotomy for the relief of chronic pain.

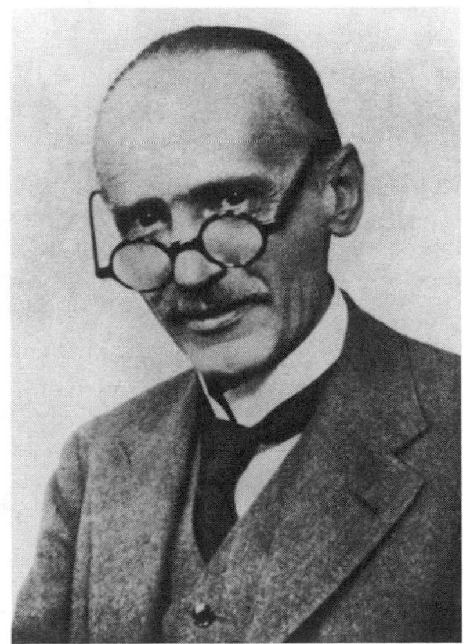

Figure F–3 Otfried Foerster.

Foerster demonstrated the effect of hyperventilation in precipitating seizures in 1925, "in showing that a row of institutional epileptics, when ordered to stand still and breathe as fast as possible, would go down one after another in a fit, like soldiers shot down by machine gun fire."[1253] He contributed over 300 papers to the literature on many neurological as well as neurosurgical topics, in which latter area his work concentrated on localization in the brain, epilepsy, and cerebral tumors.[207] His researches demonstrated the overlap in spinal nerve innervation of the dermatomes and anticipated the gate theory of pain. In his seniority he was appointed as personal physician to Lenin (d. 1924), who was then suffering from stroke-related problems.

Foerster syndrome 1. (aterioslerotic rigidity) A generalized but variable increase in tone in subjects with severe and chronic cerebral ischemia, described by Foerster (in a 169-page paper) in 1921. 2. (Foerster atonic diplegia, atonia–astasia, generalized amyotonia, cerebral atonic–astasic syndrome) A congenital hypotonic, diplegic form of **cerebral palsy** with mental and motor delay, muscle weakness, and hypotonia with laxity of ligaments, often with accompanying seizures and later mental retardation and cerebellar ataxia, described by Foerster in 1909.[2134] It is now thought that this was a form of congenital syphilis.

Foerster Test The identification by a patient of numerals traced on his skin. See **topognosis**.

Fog Test (feet–hands test) When the patient walks with the feet in different positions, abnormal associated movements (synkineses) appear in the arms.

Dr. Mogens Fog was a Danish professor of neurology and a major figure in the Danish resistance movement during World War II.

fogging effect A transitional phase in the second and third weeks after an ischemic infarct, following the early unenhanced CT scan appearance of hypodensity and prior to the late findings of **encephalomalacia**.[1080]

Foix, Charles (1882–1927) French neurologist who trained on the service of **Marie** at the **Salpêtrière**, where, after winning the gold medal in his class, he himself was later appointed. He died young, but his publications on the anatomy and pathology of **Parkinson disease**, on the syndromes of the cerebral arteries and on the following conditions witness his remarkable productivity.[1011, 2903]

Foix syndrome 1. (red nucleus syndrome) A vascular syndrome of rubral tremor and hyperkinesia in which the fibers of the III cranial nerve are spared following infarction limited to the anterior part of the red nucleus.[2137] 2. See **Foix–Jefferson syndrome**.

Foix–Alajouanine syndrome (angiodysgenetic myelomalacia, hypertrophic myelomalacia) An ischemic myelopathy leading to insidiously progressive amyotrophic paraplegia with dissociated sensory loss, areflexia, and loss of sphincter control. In the original cases, the paraparesis ascended from the lumbar regions and was at first spastic, but later flaccid.

The myelopathy is due to the primary obliterative sclerosis of abnormal, dilated intramedullary or meningeal vessels in the lower segments of the spinal cord, with thickening of the walls of the meningeal veins and often of the arteries, or it is due to thrombosis of a spinal dural arteriovenous malformation, leading in either case to an ischemic myelopathy.[2567] See also **subacute necrotizing myelopathy** and **subacute necrotizing myelitis**.

Foix–Chavany–Marie syndrome (faciolinguopharyngomasticatory diplegia or syndrome, operculum syndrome) See **anterior operculum syndrome**.

Foix–Jefferson syndrome (Foix syndrome, sphenopetrosal fissure syndrome, cavernous sinus syndrome [of Raeder], syndrome of Bonnet and Bonnet, cavernous sinus-lateral wall syndrome) The **superior orbital fissure syndrome** produced by a tumor or aneurysm in, or thrombosis of, the cavernous sinus and leading to the combination of lesions of the III, IV, V and VI nerves, exophthalmos, and eyelid edema.[2136]

Foley syndrome See **benign fasciculations and cramps**.

folie à deux Delusions shared by two people, who are usually related.

folie musculaire See **chorea**.

Fölling, Asbjorn (1888–1972) Norwegian physician who trained in Olso but, after receiving a Rockefeller Foundation award, studied metabolic disease in the United States. On his return to Norway he became professor of nutritional medicine at Olso and later professor of biochemistry at the Oslo Veterinary College, where he determined that the abnormal urinary constituent of the two retarded children of an Oslo dental colleague was phenylpyruvic acid; that this substance could be found in the urine of other mentally retarded children; and that the disorder was a recessively transmitted error of phenylalanine metabolism.

Folling disease (phenylpyruvic oligophrenia) A recessively transmitted disorder in which phenylalanine cannot be converted to tyrosine. The clinical syndrome includes fair hair, blue eyes, mental retardation, incoordination, athetosis, dystonias, and seizures. The presence of the disease can be determined by screening a urine sample at 3 weeks of life. See **phenylketonuria**.

fontanelle (Lat, a small fountain) The anterior and posterior meeting points of the cranial bones (frontal-parietal, parietal-occipital) and the same in sphenoid and mastoid regions. They are probably so named because of the welling-up which may be seen or felt there; or because, when trephined, the CSF gushes forth from such areas, which in infants are soft and pulsatile owing to the incomplete ossification of the bones at these sites at this age.

fontanelle reflex See **Grünfelder reflex**.

food allergy insomnia A disorder of initiating and maintaining sleep due to an allergic response to food allergens (usually milk products, eggs, or fish) in which the sleep disorder remits within 4 weeks of the elimination of the allergen from the diet. Psychomotor agitation, daytime lethargy, respiratory difficulties, and skin or gastrointestinal disorders are frequently present in addition.[3268]

food-elicited cataplexy A condition of dogs, best tested for by timing a dog's ability to eat all of 10 pieces of food placed in a row; cataleptic attacks will prolong the time which the affected dog takes to eat them all.

foolishness A defect of judgment in the presence of normal apprehension and memory, leading to improper inferences, often risible. (Thomas **Willis**)

foot drop Weakness of dorsiflexion of the ankle as a result of a lesion of the common peroneal nerve, or of the sciatic nerve at a higher level. In the former case, unopposed plantar flexion and function in the intrinsic muscles of the foot allow some voluntary movement at and distal to the ankle. Compare **flail foot**.

foot dystonia A rare focal dystonia, sometimes provoked by movement, in which abnormal postures of the foot are the only manifestation, unless **Parkinsonism** develops later.[3753]

footballer's migraine Vascular headaches induced by repeated mild-to-moderate head trauma, in this case from heading soccer balls for a living.[4179]

foramen (Lat) A hole.

foramen of Luschka Paired openings in the lateral recesses of the arachnoid roof of the fourth ventricle allowing egress of CSF.

foramen of Magendie A single medial opening in the arachnoid roof of the fourth ventricle allowing egress of CSF.

foramen of Monro The communication between the lateral and the third ventricles.

foramen lacerum syndrome The combination of headache, periorbital pain, palsies of cranial nerves III, IV, and VI, optic atrophy, and trigeminal anesthesia (ophthalmic division), indicating the presence of a posterior cavernous sinus lesion—in this case an aneurysm of the intradural portion of the internal carotid artery.

foramen magnum The large aperture in the base of the skull through which passes the uppermost part of the cervical spinal cord.

foramen ovale A small opening in the skull base through which passes the mandibular (third) division of the V cranial nerve.

foramen rotundum A small opening in the skull base through which passes the maxillary (second) division of the V cranial nerve.

foramina parietalia permagna See **Catlin mark**.

foramino-basilar angle See **Boorgard angle**.

Forbes disease See **glycogen storage diseases** (type 3).

Forbes Norris ALS Research Center An American academic and patient care center. Web site: http://www.cpmc.org/services/als/.

forced crying See **emotionalism**.

forced duction Mechanical traction of the globe of the eye, using forceps to grasp a fold of the anesthetized conjunctiva. The test is performed to determine the presence of any restriction to free rotation of the globe of the eye in the orbit, and is thus useful in the diagnosis of, for example, **dysthyroid ophthalmopathy** and **Brown syndrome**, in which traction in the direction of action of an apparently weak muscle may not be possible.

forced elbow extension test Passive elbow flexion with the forearm fully pronated and the wrist maximally flexed induces pain felt in the lateral part of the elbow in the presence of **lateral epicondylitis**.

forced grasping See **grasp reflex**.

forced groping See **groping**.

forced hyperphasia Compulsive, involuntary, environmentally dependent speaking; a form of **imitation behavior**.

forced normalization The tendency for patients with partial (focal) epilepsies who develop schizophrenic psychoses to achieve better seizure control; the EEG tends toward a more normal pattern at these times, reverting to its former abnormal state as the psychosis clears.[4858]

forced thinking (intellectual aura) A variety of epileptic aura comprising the experience of repetitive intrusive thoughts, ideas, or the crowding of thoughts at the beginning of a seizure and arising in most cases from a focus in the left frontal lobe.[4308]

Ford, Frank Rodolph (1892–1970) American neurologist who trained at Johns Hopkins and then at Bellvue, before returning to Baltimore, where he quickly became chief of the neurology service. His special interest in pediatric neurology was evinced by his *Diseases of the Nervous System in Infancy and Childhood*, a classic text for many years after its first publication in 1937.

forearm exercise test The measurement of venous lactate levels taken from the elbow (either with or without ischemia from compression of the arterial supply to the forearm and hand), valuable in the diagnosis of disorders of muscle glycolysis.[3352]

See also **ischemic forearm exercise test**.

forearm reflex See **brachioradialis reflex**.

forearm rolling test Asymmetry of forearm rolling (rotation of one forearm around the other in front of the body). This is a sensitive indicator or sign of unilateral cerebral dysfunction, although there may be false-positive results in **Parkinson disease**, other extrapyramidal disorders, and local musculoskeletal disorders.[5569] It was probably first described by Prof. G.H. Monrad-Krohn of the University of Oslo in the mid-twentieth century.[3335] The sensitivity of the sign is further increased if the subject is asked to roll the index fingers around each other.

forearm sign Stroking of the radial aspect of the semiflexed and semipronated arm normally leads to further flexion of the elbow and to radial deviation of the hand. With pyramidal lesions, only the elbow flexion is seen; when there is psychogenic hyperactivity of the response, elevation of the hand is the most prominent motor reaction.[1547]

foreign accent syndrome A rare speech output disorder characterized by aprosodic spoken speech with normal syntax and word choice, evolving usually after initial **aphemia**, in which the deficit in prosody (aberrations in pitch, inflection, stress, and articulation) causes speech to sound as though the patient had a foreign accent.[693] Limited motor cortex damage to the speech-dominant pre-Rolandic cortex has been considered responsible for this form of speech apraxia. Involvement also of the right cerebellum has been shown,[4075] presumably a result of **diaschisis**. The condition may also be an early sign of **primary progressive aphasia**.

Forel, August (1848–1931) Swiss psychiatrist, neurologist, and anatomist, working in Zurich. He is best remembered for his anatomical studies of sections of the basal ganglia and subthalamic region. These he performed using the technique of secondary degeneration and with the microtome newly invented by **von Gudden**.

Forel's decussation The ventral tegmental decussation between the red nuclei.[1670]

formed hallucinations Hallucinated auditory or visual images which are so structured as to have meaning.

formication A sensation as of ants crawling on the skin, experienced in the territory of regenerating nerves (when it is a microversion of **Tinel sign**), or occurring with disorders affecting the posterior columns. See also **Lhermitte sign**.

formula speech See **stereotypies**.

fornix (Lat, an arch) A long, curved fiber pathway below the corpus callosum, carrying impulses from the hippocampal formation to the mammillary bodies. Its existence was first described by Vesalius.

Forst, J-J. French neurologist who gave a modern account of sciatica in his Paris graduation thesis in 1881, including therein a description of the **Lasègue sign**.

Forster, O. See Foerster, O.

fortification spectra Common visual auras in migraine, so named (by John **Fothergill** in 1778) because the patterns seen resemble a plan of the fortifications of medieval walled cities (such as Naarden in Holland).[5044] By extension, the patterns of shimmering or flashing lights seen in the same condition have also been given this name. See **teichopsia**.

forty-five-degree test A method of standardizing muscle contraction force in order to estimate the number of motor unit action potentials firing during electromyography with reference to the values found in a normal population. The subject lies with the elbow supported and the forearm raised 45°. Recordings are made from the triceps muscle.[4996]

Foster Kennedy, Robert (1884–1952) Irish-American neurologist, whose early medical training was at Queen's University, Belfast, and then at the **National Hospital**, Queen Square. After some wartime experience, in 1915 he joined the staff of the Bellvue Hospital in New York and was appointed professor of neurology at Cornell.

In his early papers he addressed topics of current importance, such as the nature of shell shock in World War I as well as of epidemic encephalitis and other encephalopathies following an outbreak in New York. He is best remembered for his sign, described in 1911 and observed during the analysis of patients with cerebral tumors (but already described by **Gowers** 2 years before, as he acknowledged). He drew attention to the occurrence of "true" retrobulbar neuritis with a central scotoma and optic atrophy on the side of the tumor, with papilledema on the opposite side. All of his patients also had anosmia.

He died shortly after correctly diagnosing **Brown-Séquard syndrome** (secondary to polyarteritis nodosa) in himself.[4150]

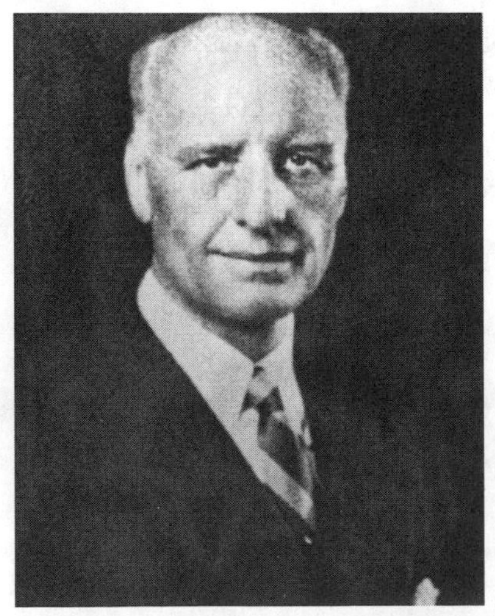

Figure F–4 Robert Foster Kennedy.

Foster Kennedy syndrome (Gowers–Paton–Kelly syndrome, basal–frontal syndrome) Unilateral optic atrophy and contralateral papilledema, commonly with anosmia, mentioned by **Gowers** in 1893 with a description published in 1909 by him and by Paton, but described more fully by Kennedy in 1911. The typical cause is a tumor on the lesser wing of the sphenoid bone that compresses the I and II nerves and induces papilledema by raising intracranial pressure,[3384] but many other tumors sited anteriorly and other nontumor pathologies can also produce the sign, however.[4150]

Fothergill, John (1712–1780) English physician and accoucheur who trained in Edinburgh (as a Quaker he was disbarred from entering any English University) and at St. Thomas' Hospital in London. He practiced with great success in London.

Fothergill was the first to give an account of **trigeminal neuralgia**, in 1776.[2157] "In a moment she would be seized with the most acute excruciating pain affecting the inner canthus of the eye; it lasted but a few seconds, forced out the tears, and gradually went off. In a few minutes the same thing happened and in like manner at unequal distances during the day, so as to occasion a great misery."

He described the **migraine** aura from personal experience in his *Remarks on that complaint commonly known under the name of sick headache* (1777 *et seq.*). He also described coronary artery sclerosis as the cause of angina; and diphtheritic sore throat.

He put into practice the teachings of his faith; he was active in prison reform and in the abolition of slavery and treated patients for nothing in the free hospital (but charged for home visits, remarking that he climbed on the backs of the poor to the pockets of the rich). He was a friend both of Lord North, the British prime minister, and of Benjamin Franklin; with them, he attempted to reconcile the political differences between England and the North American Colonies, but failed. He entertained visiting Americans after the secession of the United States and gave money and teaching materials to the Pennsylvania Hospital.[2066]

Fothergill syndrome See **trigeminal neuralgia**.

Fotopoulos syndrome The association of chorea and lower motor neuron disease (periscapular weakness and wasting) appearing in adult life.[4853] See also **neuroacanthocytosis**.

fou rire prodromique A rare form of **pathological laughter** preceding an intracranial hemorrhage[2013] or brainstem infarct. **Brissaud** suggested that spasmodic laughter and crying were due to lesions of the anterior internal capsule or the corticobulbar tract but the neuroanatomical basis for the phenomenon is still not known.[2467]

Fountain syndrome A recessively inherited congenital dysmorphic syndrome characterized by short stature, thick calvarium, seizures, sensorineural deafness, and mental and developmental delay.[2160]

FOUR score See **Full Outline of UnResponsiveness score.**

Fourier transformation A mathematical process or technique whereby any waveform is assembled by the addition or superimposition of a number of sine waves.

Fournier Test A comprehensive test of gait in which the subject is asked to stand up from a sitting position, walk, stop, and turn quickly on command.

fourteen- and six-Hz-positive burst (14- and 6 Hz-positive spikes, ctenoids) A burst of arch-shaped waves at 13–17 Hz and/or 5–7 Hz, but most commonly at 14 and/or 6 Hz, seen generally over the posterior temporal and adjacent areas of one or both sides of the head during sleep. The sharp peaks of its component waves are positive with respect to other regions and their amplitude varies but is generally below 75 μV.

Such bursts are best demonstrated by referential recording using contralateral earlobe or other remote reference electrodes. The clinical significance of this pattern is controversial. (Adapted from the report of the Committee on Terminology, IFCN,[989] © 1974, with kind permission from the IFCN and Elsevier Science.)

This EEG pattern is commonly found in normal children after the age of 3 years, in whom variable unilateral bursts of positive spikes, lasting a second or so, appear mainly over posterior temporal regions.[6126]

fourteen- and six-Hz-positive spikes See **fourteen -and six-Hz-positive burst**.

14-3-3 protein A normal neural protein, released, when there is rapid neuronal loss and found in the CSF after strokes, in encephalitis and in **Creutzfeldt–Jakob disease**.

14-3-3 test Estimation of the quantity of these acidic polypeptide proteins in the CSF in the diagnosis of sporadic **Creutzfeldt–Jakob disease**. It appears to be positive in all cases of the sporadic form, but also in some other dementing conditions including variant CJD[2557] and in **acute inflammatory polyneuropathy**. See also **tau** and **ubiquitin**.

fourth of July tetanus Tetanus contracted from the horsehair wadding of blank cartridges formerly fired off in Independence Day celebrations in the United States.[6819]

fovea (Lat, a small hollow) That part of the macula which receives light rays from the central part of the visual field and which is endowed with a high concentration of cone receptors.

foveate To bring a peripheral retinal image onto the fovea by means of a saccade, or to maintain such an image upon the fovea through pursuit movements.

foveation period A brief instant between the jerk and drift phases of nystagmus, during which time the image of the object of gaze actually lights upon the retina.

foveola (Lat, diminutive of fovea) The dark central part of the fovea at which point the retinal pigment shows through the retina.

Foville, Achille-Louis-Francois (1831–1887) French neurologist, anatomist, and physiologist, who trained at the **Salpêtrière** and practiced in the asylum in Rouen where he was appointed superintendent before becoming professor of physiology at Rouen. He later resigned from there and after a period of ill-health, went again to Paris as head of the Sharenton, succeeding Esquirol. He was dismissed during the revolution but practiced privately in Paris and finally in Toulouse. He is credited with a description of **internuclear ophthalmoplegia** (once known as *Foville–Wilson syndrome*) and with important studies of neuroanatomy including the identification of the direct spino-cerebellar tract and cranial deformities; he also contributed substantially to the psychiatric literature.[5704]

His father Achille-Louis (1799–1878) described the stria terminalis.

Foville syndrome A syndrome of infarction within the caudal tegmental pons, the major clinical features being variously described but usually including homolateral nuclear VII nerve palsy and conjugate gaze palsy toward the side of the lesion, with a contralateral hemiparesis. It is thus a form of **alternating hemiplegia**.

Foville[2164] described a VI cranial nerve palsy in his patient, whose tongue was also weak on the same side as the facial paresis, in 1858. Except for the latter two findings, the **Millard-Gubler** syndrome is thus almost identical.[5433] He also described variations, according to the involvement of the VI and the VII cranial nerves, and the presence of a conjugate gaze palsy resulting from involvement of the peripontine reticular formation.[5333]

Fowler equal-loudness balance test A test of auditory recruitment using pure tones of varying intensities delivered alternately to either ear, the patient signaling the point at which they are perceived to be equally loud; thus allowing a quantitative measure of unilateral deafness.

Fowler syndrome A recessively-inherited dysmorphic syndrome characterized by intracranial calcification and hydrocephalus.[381]

Fracastoro, Girolamo (1453–1553) Veronese physician who first applied the word syphilis in his poem *Syphilus, sive morbus Gallicus*, published in 1530. In this the poet recounted how Syphilus, a shepherd, abused the sun god when prostrated by heat and was punished by being given a foul and contagious disease.

Fracastoro was particularly interested in infectious diseases and gave the first accurate account of typhus.

fragile X syndrome (Martin-Bell syndrome, FRAXA: OMIM 309550) A relatively common X-linked neurodevelopmental disorder caused by expansion of a trinucleotide CGG repeat, the responsible gene (*FMR1*) mapping to Xq27.3 or to Xq29. Clinically, nonprogressive mental retardation, large testes, optic atrophy, cerebellar hypoplasia, mitral incompetence, flat feet, and hyperextensible fingers are the usual features. Delayed motor development, **autism**, generalized tonic–clonic seizures, myoclonus, and minor neurological signs are also sometimes present.[6835, 589] Uncommonly the clinical presentation resembles Parkinsonism, dementia, or even cerebrovascular disease.

Some 10% of female carriers manifest evidence of the disease. The name derives from the instability shown by the X chromosome when incubated in a medium deficient in folate.

A *variant* is *fragile X ataxia tremor/ syndrome* (FXTAS; OMIM 309550), a disorder seen in carriers of the fragile X premutation gene (*FMR1*) affecting males over the age of 50 who present with gait ataxia and action tremor often associated with irritability, memory loss or even dementia, Parkinsonism, global brain atrophy, peripheral neuropathy and dysautonomia. The neuropathological hallmark is the presence of intranuclear inclusions in neurons and astrocytes throughout the CNS. MRI scans show an increased T2 signal in the middle cerebellar peduncles.[3144]

It is notable that the same gene is responsible for both this syndrome, caused by excessive gene activity and production of a toxic RNA, and for the childhood-onset fragile X syndrome caused by the absence of such activity.[2681] Identification of premutations in the *FMR1* gene raises the possibility of clinical overlap with **multiple system atrophy**, although the two are unlikely to be confused clinically. Slowly progressive disease or predominant tremor are useful "red-flags" prompting the consideration of FXTAS.[3282]

See also **FRAXE** and the **National FragileX Foundation** (Web site: www.FragileX.org).

fragmentary myoclonus Brief, fine, asynchronous, and asymmetrical twitches involving the face and limbs, occurring at the onset of sleep and during all sleep stages. The phenomenon is seen in males with fragmented sleep and a variety of sleep disturbances.[881] See also **periodic limb movement disorder in sleep, hypnic jerks,** and **sleep myoclonus.**

fragmentary seizures (migratory seizures, erratic seizures) Multifocal clonic seizures occasionally seen in newborns with shifting between locations in the body. Consciousness is usually preserved.[2312]

fragmentation (of sleep architecture) The interruption of any stage of sleep due to the appearance of another sleep stage, or waking and leading to disrupted non–rapid eye movement-rapid eye movement cycles. Thus, the interruption of rapid eye movement sleep by movement arousals or by non–rapid eye movement stage 2 activity.[280]

Fragoso syndrome A congenital dysmorphic syndrome of dolichocephaly or scaphocephaly, other skeletal abnormalities resembling those of **Marfan syndrome**, strabismus, and mental and developmental delay.[381]

Framingham Disability Scale An interviewing instrument for the assessment of self-care and physical functioning in the elderly.[5415]

Franceschetti syndrome See **mandibulofacial dysostosis.**

Franceschetti–Klein–Wildervanck syndrome See **Wildervanck syndrome.**

Franceschetti–Zwahlen–Klein syndrome See **mandibulofacial dysostosis.**

Frank syndrome (familial hyperthyroidism) A congenital dysmorphic syndrome characterized by brachydactyly, clinodactyly, seizures, hyperthyroidism, and mental and developmental delay.[381]

Frankel Scale A global assessment scale for patients with spinal injury.[2178] See Chart F–4.

Frankl-Hochwart, Lothar von (1862–1915) Austrian neuropathologist who worked with Nothnagel after completing his studentship in Vienna. He became professor of neuropathology at the Vienna Polytechnic but died shortly thereafter. He wrote extensively on the neuropathology of bladder disorders, endocrinology, and **Ménière disease.**[5704]

Frankl-Hochwart syndrome 1. **Ménière disease** with unilateral polyneuritis; a rarity, seldom since detected. 2. Sexual precocity, impairment of upward gaze, evidence of raised intracranial pressure, and hypopituitarism, occurring as a result of a pineal tumor.[2180] 3. The occurrence of lesions of both divisions of the VIII, and of the V and VII cranial nerves as manifestations of early neurosyphilis.[5333]

Fraser syndrome An autosomal recessively inherited syndrome characterized by cryptophthalmos, cutaneous syndactyly, malformations of the larynx and genitourinary tract, craniofacial dysmorphism, orofacial clefting, mental retardation, and musculoskeletal anomalies.[5891]

FRAXE A variant of **fragile X syndrome** in which there is mild mental retardation.[3626]

Chart F–4. Frankel Scale

Score	Description
A	Severe cord injury has led to the absence of motor and sensor function below the level of injury.
B	Sensation only. Some sensation is preserved below the level of injury, such as sacral sparing.
C	Motor function/useless. What motor activity is retained is of no practical usefulness to the patient.
D	Motor function/useful. Some useful motor function is preserved below the level of the injury such that, for example, patients can walk, with or without mechanical assistance.
E	Recovery. Motor and sensory functions are clinically normal, although hyperreflexia may still be present.

Problems with such scales are that functions change with time and the paucity of documented prognostic value in the score at any early date of assessment. Possibly the recording of changes in grades would be more useful for this purpose.

Modified from Frankel HL, Hancock DO, Hyslop G, et al. The value of postural reduction in the initial management of closed injuries of the spine with paraplegia and tetraplegia. Paraplegia *1969;7:179–92)*

Free and Cued Selective Reminding Test A test of verbal **episodic memory**.

free fraction That portion of a drug which is not bound to plasma proteins and thus is able to cross plasma membranes.

free radicals Momentary chemical substances such as superoxide and hydrogen peroxide and hydroxyl radicals, which have an unpaired electron in their outer shell and which are highly active biologically, especially through their ability to induce the formation of lipid peroxides which damage cell membranes. They are normally produced by mitochondrial metabolism within all aerobic cells, but are quickly reduced to water by enzymes such as peroxidase, catalase, and superoxide dismutase and are scavenged by vitamins E and C. They are considered to have a role in reperfusion injury, cancer, atheroma, aging, inflammatory disease, and toxic states.

Freeman–Sheldon syndrome (whistling face syndrome) See **arthrogryposis multiplex congenita**.

freezing Brief, sudden, and complete suppression of motor functions, arising typically in patients with **Parkinson disease** and occurring at random or provoked by emotion or by the perception of obstacles to progress in walking.

Fregoli syndrome A delusional misidentification syndrome in which the subject misidentifies a person seen as somebody else, even though that person has a completely different appearance. Lesions in the fusiform gyrus, temporal cortex and hippocampus are likely to be responsible.[3029] See also **reduplicative paramnesia**.

Freiberg sign (test) Passive forceful internal rotation of the extended thigh at the hip causes pain in that area with L5, S1 radiculopathy (but also with with local structural disorders of the hip and buttock). This may also be observed in the **piriformis syndrome**.[4901] (HJM)

French Neuropathological Society A professional organization based at Laboratoire de Neuropathologie, Raymond Escourolle, Hôpital de la Salpêtrière, 47 Blvd de l'Hôpital, 75651 Paris, Cedex 13, France.

French Foundation for Alzheimer Research A charitable organization funding basic research. Address: 11620 Wilshire Blvd, Suite 270, Los Angeles, CA 90025. Web site: http://www.jdfaf.org/.

Frenchay activities index A **quality-of-life** assessment tool, assessing activities performed over the previous 3–6 months.[2948]

Frenchay Aphasia Screening Test (FAST) A simple, validated, and reliable screening test for the presence and nature of aphasia.[1857]

Frenkel sign Hypotonia of the legs in tabes dorsalis.[5704]

Frenkel-Heiden, Heinrich (1860–1931) Swiss psychiatrist who became professor of syphilology at Berlin.

frequency Number of complete cycles of a repetitive waveform in 1 s, measured in hertz (H) or cycles per second (cps or c/s).[19]

frequency analysis Determination of the range of frequencies composing a waveform, with a measurement of the absolute or relative amplitude of each component frequency. (From the 2001 Report of the Nomenclature Committee of the American Association of Electromyography and Electrodiagnosis.[19] Reproduced by kind permission of the AANEM.)

frequency response curve A graph depicting the relationships between the output pen deflection or amplifier output and the input frequency in an EEG channel, for a particular setting of low and high frequency filters. (Adapted from the 1974 report of the Committee on Terminology, IFCN. In Chatrian GE, Bergamini L, Dondey M, et al. A glossary of terms most commonly used by clinical electroencephalographers. *EEG Clin Neurophysiol* 1974;37:538–48. Reproduced by kind permission of Elsevier Science and the IFCN).

Frerichs, Friedreich (1819–1885) German physician who gave the first accounts of both **Wilson disease** (1861) and **multiple sclerosis** (1849).[5619]

Fresnel, Augustin-Jean (1788–1827) French physicist who described the use of glasses with spheres of 20 diopters in order to magnify the eye to the observer when worn as spectacles, but preventing the wearer from focusing on anything and thus from fixating, which encourages the appearance of nystagmus of peripheral (vestibular) origin.

The use of 15 diopter Fresnel prisms in patients with unilateral visual neglect or homonymous hemianopia helps visual perception but does not improve the patient's quality of life,[5422] whatever that may be.

Freud, Sigmund (1856–1939) Austrian physician, born in Moravia, who trained in medicine in Vienna and undertook studies in comparative neuroanatomy and histology until 1882, when financial circumstances drew him to clinical medicine. He combined this with human neuroanatomical studies performed in **Meynert**'s laboratory. By then his neurological diagnostic skills were of a high order, but they were further refined as the result of a period spent working with **Charcot** in 1885–1886, after which he returned to Vienna to continue his work as a lecturer in pathology and physician, by now with an interest in hysteria. His views were unacceptable to his former teachers in Vienna, however, and he entered private practice, from which he gained enough experience to write, with Joseph Breuer, *Studies in Hysteria* and 5 years later *The Interpretation of Dreams*.

By the time of his elevation to full professor of neuropathology in 1905, he had over 40 publications, mainly in the basic neurosciences, but his studies on cerebral palsy and his analysis *On Aphasia* (1891) were also notable.[6384] He was the first to distinguish ataxic cerebral palsy, and in 1897 he gave the name *cerebral diplegia* to cerebral palsies with bilateral motor involvement. Freud also translated Charcot's lectures into German, to Charcot's gratification. During the remainder of his life, he laid the foundations of psychoanalytic theory aided by such students as Adler and Carl Jung.[3185]

Frey, Lucja (1889–1944) Polish physician who was born in Lwow and trained in mathematics and philosophy before entering medical studies in Lwow. She practiced in Warsaw until her death during World War II as a victim of the Nazi régime. She described the phenomenon of gustatory sweating or sweating of the skin over the parotid gland during salivation (Frey syndrome) which she called the *auriculotemporal nerve syndrome*,[2199] although an account of the same condition had been published in 1757 in France by Dr. M. Duphenix.[954]

Frey syndrome See **gustatory sweating**.

Frey, Max von (1852–1932) German physician.

Frey's hairs Hairs of different diameters mounted on wood and pressed on the skin so that they bend slightly, thus used to determine sensory thresholds for cutaneous touch.

friable (Lat) Easily crumbled.

Fried syndrome A congenital dysmorphic syndrome characterized by syndactyly microcephaly, encephalocele or cranial meningocele, holoprosencephaly, and arhinencephaly.[381]

Friedenwald syndrome Elevation of a ptotic eyelid on turning the eyes to the right, opening the mouth wide and protruding the tongue.[3113] This must be rather uncommon. The significance of the sign is not clear.

Friedman–Roy syndrome An unusual familial syndrome consisting of retardation of both motor and psychomotor development, lalling speech, convergent strabismus, hyperreflexia, upgoing plantar responses, pes cavus, calcification of the choroid plexus, and raised CSF protein levels. The authors published their findings in a family of six feebleminded children born to normally intelligent parents (cousins) in 1944. The precise nature of the condition is unexplained.[1765]

Friedmann, Max (1858–1925) German neuropsychiatrist, working in Vienna. He described **pyknolepsy** and the following syndromes.

Friedmann syndromes 1. Fullness in the head, irritability, vertigo, insomnia, rapid fatigue, and defective memory following trauma or chronic encephalitis; a set of features which probably represent postconcussional syndrome. 2. (Friedmann–Schultze syndrome) Relapsing infantile spinal paralysis, a variant form of Erb spinal syphilis.[2204] 3. See **pyknolepsy**.[2205] 4. See **pure typical absence epilepsy of childhood**.

Friedmann–Schultze syndrome See **Friedmann syndromes**.

Friedreich, Nicolaus Anton (1761–1836) German physician who gave a complete account of facial paralysis in 1797, 24 years before that of **Sir Charles Bell**.

Friedreich, Nikolaus (1825–1882) German pathologist and physician, born in Wurzburg, where he studied medicine and came under the influence of **Virchow**. He became professor of pathological anatomy in Berlin in 1857 and of medicine at Heidelberg in the following year at the age of 32, remaining there for the rest of his life.

He made contributions in many fields of medicine, but is best remembered for his description of the hereditary ataxia which he first described in 1863[2206] and for his description of **paramyoclonus** (1881).

The independence of the ataxic condition was at first widely disputed, but **Charcot** ultimately gave the disorder the seal of his approval, referring to it as "hereditary ataxy or Friedreich disease" in 1884. Charcot–Marie–Tooth disease (**hereditary motor and sensory neuropathy**) was described by the first two and by the last of these authors 2 years later; the points on which this condition overlaps with Friedreich ataxia may have influenced Charcot to change his opinion in favor of that of Friedreich.[186]

Friedreich ataxia The archetypical, recessively inherited spinocerebellar degeneration, described in a series of papers published between 1863 and 1867.[2206] Manifestations occur by puberty and are progressive, so that patients are usually chairbound within 20 years of the onset of the disease.[3637] The defect (an unstable expansion of GAA repeats) is mapped to the frataxin site at 9q13–9q21 and leads to accumulation of iron. Mutational analysis reveals an abnormal expansion of a GAA triple repeat sequence in the frataxin gene.

The diagnostic criteria formulated by Harding[2754] are given in Chart F–5.

Pes planus, equinovarus deformities, and numerous disorders of eye movement control other than nystagmus (slow saccades, jerky pursuit) are also recorded. There is an increased incidence of diabetes and of cardiomyopathy, which is manifest by palpitations and dyspnea, in these patients.

Pathologically, nerve fiber atrophy and demyelination occur mainly in the posterior

Chart F–5. Diagnostic Criteria for Friedreich Ataxia

1. *Essential criteria for diagnosis*;
   i. Within 5 years of onset of symptoms:
      Onset before age 25 years
      Progressive ataxia of limbs and gait
      Absent knee and ankle jerks
      Extensor plantar responses
      Motor nerve conduction velocity >40 m/s, with small or absent sensory action potentials.
   ii. After 5 years since onset of symptoms.
      The above + dysarthria.
2. *Additional features present in over 60% of cases:* Scoliosis, upper motor neuron weakness of legs, leg areflexia, distal loss of proprioception and vibration, abnormal electrocardiogram (mainly inverted T-waves).
3. *Additional features present in less than 50% of cases*:
   Nystagmus, optic atrophy, deafness, distal weakness and wasting, pes cavus, diabetes.

From Harding AE. The Spinocerebellar Degenerations and Related Disorders. *Edinburgh: Churchill-Livingstone, 1983.*

columns and direct spinocerebellar and lateral corticospinal tracts. The anterior horn cells and the posterior root ganglion cells are also atrophic, the latter resulting in both the posterior column shrinkage and the loss of thick fibers in the peripheral sensory nerves—the prototypic **dying-back** process.[2752] See also **cerebellar ataxias**.

In *variant* forms, also recessively inherited, the same phenotype is associated with selective vitamin E deficiency but without fat malabsorption;[501] the condition occurs at a later age than usual; or linkage to chromosome 9 is absent.[501] A further variant form is *early onset ataxia with cardiomyopathy and retained reflexes*, which phenotypically differs from Friedreich ataxia but maps to the same locus on chromosome 9q.[4864]

The superb Web site Gene Reviews further describes this condition in depth. http://www.ncbi.nlm.nih.gov/bookshelf/br.fcgi?book=gene&part=friedreich; or http://www.geneclinics.org/profiles/friedreich/.

Friedreich Ataxia Group A charitable organization, affiliated with *Ataxia UK*. Address: 10 Winchester House, Kennington Park, Cranmer Rd., London SW9 6EJ. Tel: 020-7582-1444. E-mail: office@ataxia.org.uk/.

Friedreich's Ataxia Group in America, Inc. A charitable support organization. Address: P.O. Box 11116, Oakland, CA 94611.

Friedreich's Ataxia Research Alliance (FARA) An American charitable organization in this field providing support and information. Address: 2001 Jefferson Davis Hwy., Suite 209, Arlington, VA 22202. Tel: 703-413-4468. E-mail: fara@frda.org. Web site: http://www.frda.org/. See also **cerebellar ataxias**.

Friedreich Ataxia Research Association A charitable organization. Web site: http://www.fara.org.au/.

Friedreich disease 1. (polyclonia) A syndrome of bilateral rapid asymmetric muscle contractions which may be inhibited by voluntary muscle contraction.[2208] See **paramyoclonus multiplex**. 2. (Facial hemihypertrophy) Asymmetrical enlargement of the facial structures, either alone or with hypertrophy of the remainder of the body on that side.[3113]

Friedreich foot Pes cavus, described by Friedreich in 1863.[2206]

Fritsch, Gustav Theodor (1838–1927) German neurosurgeon, who demonstrated in 1870 that, in contradiction to currently held opinion, the cerebral cortex is indeed excitable and its stimulation may provoke movement on the other side of the body.[2214]

Fröhlich, Alfred (1871–1953) Viennese neurologist and pharmacologist who worked with **Sherrington** in Liverpool and with Langley in Cambridge, where he became interested in the autonomic nervous system which remained a major topic of his research on his return to Vienna as professor. He immigrated to the United States when Austria was invaded in 1939 and worked in Cincinnati. During his life in Europe, he was a friend of Rudyard Kipling and Anton Brückner, his talents as a writer and pianist being recognized by each, respectively.[2066]

Fröhlich syndrome (adiposogenital dystrophy) A syndrome consisting of obesity, hypogonadism, and bitemporal hemianopia resulting from hypothalamic lesions such as trauma, craniopharyngiomas, and pituitary adenomas.[2215] Despite the eponym, Berhard Mohr (a German physician) had already described the main features in 1840.[5619]

Froin, Georges (b. 1874) French physician.

Froin syndrome (Nonne syndrome) Exceptionally high protein levels in the CSF, causing **xanthochromia** and a tendency for the CSF to clot.[2216] Spinal block, the **Landry–Guillain–Barré syndrome** and vestibular Schwannomas are the commoner causes. In the complete syndrome, the CSF is under low pressure.

Froment, Jules (1878–1946) French neurologist practicing in Lyon .

Froment nerve (Froment–Rauber nerve) A branch of the radial nerve which innervates (anomalously) the first dorsal interosseous muscle.

Foment–Rauber nerve See **Froment nerve**.

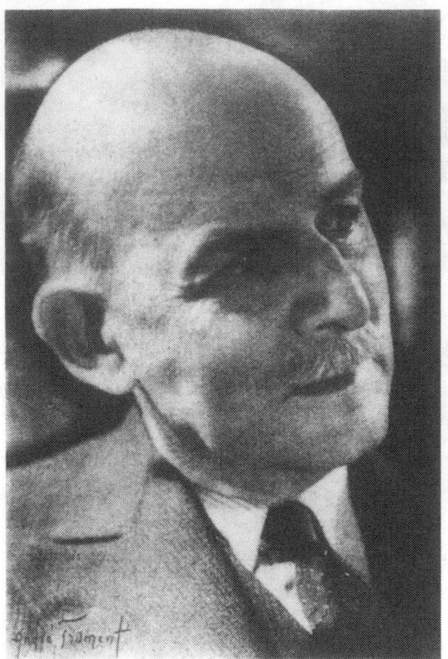

Figure F–5 Jules Froment.

Froment sign 1. (signe de journal) Involuntary flexion of the thumb when a piece of paper is held between the finger and thumb of each hand and pulled. The sign indicates ulnar nerve paresis with weakness of the adductor pollicis, for which the long flexor tries to compensate.[2217]

2. (*circle sign*) Lack of flexion at the distal interphalangeal joints of the first and second digits, as would normally be seen when a subject grips a piece of paper between his finger and thumb; a sign of weakness of the flexor digitorum profundus and the flexor pollicis longus, both of which are supplied by the anterior interosseous nerve. This sign, more or less the opposite of the first, is also attributed to Froment.

3. (*Froment maneuver*; activation or facilitation test). Resistance to passive movement of muscles about a joint specifically detected only during voluntary activity of a contralateral body part.[2218] This is not a specific sign and occurs in a number of different disorders manifesting tremor but it is mainly utilized in the diagnosis of **Parkinson disease**. Froment also showed that Parkinsonian rigidity diminishes, vanishes, or enhances depending on the static posture of the body, and proposed that in Parkinson disease "maintenance stabilization" of the body is impaired and that "reactive stabilization" becomes the operative mode of muscular tone control. Finally, he demonstrated that Parkinsonian rigidity increases during the Romberg Test, gaze deviation, and oriented attention.

Froment-Rauber nerve See **Froment nerve**.

Frommann lines Transverse striae on the axons of myelinated nerve fibers, described by Carl Frommann (1831–1892), a German obstetrician.[5619]

frons (Lat) The forehead.

front-tap contraction If the leg is extended and the sole pushed up so as to tense the gastrocnemius, tapping the tibialis anterior will lead to gastrocnemius contraction in patients with a pyramidal lesion of that limb. This is probably either due to transmitted vibration or to disinhibition at the spinal level. The phenomenon was described by **Gowers**, in his *Diagnosis of Diseases of the Spinal Cord* (3rd Edition, London, Churchill, 1884).

frontal alexia See **alexia**.

frontal apraxia See **apraxia**.

Frontal Assessment Battery A tool for the assessment of frontal lobe dysfunction, comprising questions on abstract thought, mental flexibility, motor programming, sensitivity to interference, inhibitory control, and environmental autonomy.[1723]

frontal association areas Areas 9–12 of Brodmann.

frontal ataxia A form of cerebellar ataxia resulting from lesions of the contralateral frontal cortex due to interruption of conduction in fibers of the corticopontocerebellar pathway. It represents a **false localizing sign** as a result of crossed cerebellar **diaschisis**. See **frontal disequilibrium**.

Frontal Behavioral Inventory A validated assessment instrument assisting in the diagnosis of frontotemporal dementia by examining apathy, aspontaneity, indifference, inflexibility, concreteness, personal neglect, distractibility, inattention, loss of insight, logopenia, verbal apraxia, and the **alien hand (limb) syndrome**.[3403]

frontal convexity syndrome An apathetic behavioral pattern that may occur following injury to the frontal lobe. Clinically, it is characterized by apathy and indifference, with occasional, brief, aggressive outbursts; psychomotor retardation; stimulus-boundedness; motor perseveration and impersistence; discrepant motor and verbal behavior; impaired motor programming (e.g., fist-palm-side test, rhythm tapping); poor word-list generation, abstraction, and categorization; and a segmented approach to visuospatial analysis.[6388] See also **medial frontal syndrome**.

frontal cortex The anterior major lobe of the cerebrum, comprising one-third of the hemispheres, and divisible into three zones:

1. The motor–premotor component (Brodmann areas 4 and 6, the supplementary motor area, and parts of the frontal eye fields and Broca's area 44). Lesions here result in contralateral weakness, release of grasp reflexes, altered muscle tone, incontinence, akinesia and mutism, aprosody, apraxia, some of the motor components in unilateral neglect, and **Broca aphasia**.
2. The caudal-mesial-basal part, containing the paralimbic cortex of the anterior cingulate gyrus, and the paraolfactory and caudal orbito-frontal region.
3. The rostral "heteromodal" cortex, comprising Brodmann's areas 9–12 and 45–47.

The **prefrontal cortex** comprises the latter two of these three divisions, lesions of which lead to manifestations which, taken together, constitute the **frontal lobe syndrome**. Ablation of the anterior portion leads to loss of recent memory, initiative and foresight, and indifference or euphoria; ablation of the posterior part to deficits in voluntary movements, expressive aphasia (left second and third convolutions) and motor amusia (right second and third convolutions).

frontal dementias of the non-Alzheimer type See **frontotemporal dementia**.

frontal disequilibrium (Bruns gait apraxia, frontal ataxia, astasia–abasia, frontal gait apraxia) A gait pattern dominated by disequilibrium, frequently with inappropriate or counterproductive postural and locomotor synergies. Patients cannot stand (or sometimes sit) unsupported and are unable to organize trunk and leg movements to rise; thus when trying to rise from a chair, they may lean back and do not bring their legs in, underneath their center of gravity. Nor can they walk because as they try to step, their feet frequently cross or move in an inappropriate direction.

The pattern is associated with lesions of the frontal lobes or their connections. Associated clinical signs may include dementia, frontal lobe release signs, motor perseveration, urinary incontinence, and extensor plantar responses.[4723]

frontal gait apraxia See **frontal disequilibrium** and **gait apraxias**.

frontal gait disorder (magnetic gait apraxia, arteriosclerotic Parkinsonism, Parkinsonian ataxia, lower half Parkinsonism, lower body Parkinsonism) A gait pattern characterized by a variable base (narrow or wide), short steps, shuffling, start and turn hesitation, and moderate dysequilibrium.

Patients with this gait syndrome frequently have lesions of the frontal lobes or of their connections, or have multiple hemisphere lesions due to cerebrovascular disease. Associated signs may include cognitive impairment, pseudobulbar palsy with dysarthria, frontal release signs, paratonia, pyramidal signs, and urinary disturbances.[4723] (Reproduced by kind permission of the American Academy of Neurology and Lippincott Williams and Wilkins.) See also **marche à petits pas**.

frontal intermittent rhythmic delta activity (FIRDA) A pattern of fairly regular or approximately sinusoidal waves mostly occurring in bursts at 1.5–3 Hz over the frontal areas of one or both sides of the head but not due to potential changes generated by vertical eye movements. (Adapted from the 1974 report of the Committee on Terminology, IFCN. In Chatrian GE, Bergamini L, Dondey M, et al. A glossary of terms most commonly used by clinical electroencephalographers. *EEG Clin Neurophysiol* 1974;37:538–48. Reproduced by kind permission of Elsevier Science and the IFCN.)

frontal lobe dementia See **frontotemporal dementia**.

frontal lobe epilepsies Location-related seizure disorders characterized by simple partial, complex partial, or secondarily generalized seizures or by combinations of these, emanating from a frontal lobe. This condition is the second most common type of localization-related epilepsy. Seizures often occur several times a day and frequently occur during REM (rapid eye movement) sleep.

Frontal lobe partial seizures are sometimes mistaken for psychogenic seizures. Status epilepticus is a frequent complication. In over half the patients there is focal pathology within a frontal lobe, especially malformations of cortical development. Features strongly suggesting the diagnosis include:

1. Generally short seizures (<30 s), occurring frequently and especially during sleep.
2. Complex partial seizures arising from the frontal lobe, often with minimal or no postictal confusion.
3. Rapid secondary generalization (more common in seizures of frontal than of temporal lobe epilepsy).
4. Prominent motor manifestations which can be tonic, clonic, or postural.
5. Complex gestural automatisms frequent at onset.
6. Frequent falling when the discharge is bilateral.

The attacks tend to be stereotyped and have sudden onset and termination with rapid recovery of consciousness and sometimes violent motor automatisms. Patients are at increased risk for complex partial status epilepticus. The EEG may be normal or have localizing value. Unfortunately, the response to drug therapy is not always adequate.[4882]

Many different frontal lobe seizure subtypes (**cingulate**, **orbitofrontal**, **dorsolateral**, **opercular** and **motor cortex seizures**, and **Kozhevnikoff syndrome**) are described elsewhere; however, multiple frontal areas may be involved rapidly and specific seizure types may not be discernible.[6803]

The subtypes recognized are as follows:

1. *Frontal seizures from the motor cortex*, which consist of simple focal motor clonic or tonic–clonic seizures with or without Jacksonian march to neighboring motor regions; uni- or bilateral myoclonic seizures as in **partial continuous epilepsy**; or tonic postural motor seizures with clonic movements.
2. *Frontal seizures from the supplementary sensorimotor area* presenting as frequent stereotyped hypermotor seizures with bilateral, asymmetric tonic posturing of limb girdles, often with contraversion of the eyes and head, vocalizations or speech arrest, lasting seconds, with abrupt onset and termination. They occur mainly at night and are not followed by postictal confusion but may be preceded by somatosensory and other (not epigastric) auras.
3. *Cingulate* seizure patterns are complex partial with complex motor gestural automatisms at onset. Autonomic signs are common, as are changes in mood and affect. **Gelastic seizures** of frontal lobe origin emanate from this region.
4. *Anterior frontopolar.* These seizure patterns include forced thinking or initial loss of contact and adversive movements of head and eyes, with possible evolution including contraversive movements, axial clonic jerks and falls, and autonomic signs.
5. *Orbitofrontal.* This seizure pattern is one of complex partial seizures with initial motor and gestural automatisms, olfactory hallucinations and illusions, and autonomic signs.
6. *Dorsolateral.* The patterns here may be tonic or, less commonly, clonic, with versive eye and head movements and speech arrest. Seizures characterized by unusual symptoms of "forced thinking" and "forced acts"commonly emanate from the dorsolateral intermediate frontal lobe.
7. *Opercular.* Characteristics include mastication, salivation, swallowing, laryngeal symptoms, speech arrest, epigastric aura, fear, and autonomic phenomena. Simple partial seizures, particularly partial clonic facial seizures, are common and may be ipsilateral. If secondary sensory changes occur, numbness may be a symptom, particularly in the hands. Gustatory hallucinations are particularly common.[4882]

(With my thanks to Prof. C. Panayiotopoulos for data integral to this entry).

See also **autosomal dominant nocturnal frontal lobe epilepsy**.

frontal lobe syndrome A combination of defects following upon damage to the frontal lobes. Some defects are easily classified and specific, such as aphasia and disturbance of gaze or of motor power; such functions are associated with normal activity in defined, rather more posterior frontal areas. Others, associated with normal function in the frontal association areas, are less specific and include loss of consciousness of the self and its attitude toward the future; loss of coordination and fusion of the incoming and outgoing products of the several sensory and motor areas of the cortex; loss of synthesis; loss of abstract attitude; and loss of execution of visually directed behavior, in the words of several analysts.[4339]

frontal reflex See **orbicularis oculi reflex**.

frontal release signs See **primitive reflexes**.

frontofacionasal dysostosis A recessively inherited congenital dysmorphic syndrome with hypertelorism and characterized also by ptosis, blepharophimosis, brachycephaly, and encephalocele or cranial meningocele.[2261]

frontometaphyseal dysplasia syndrome (Gorlin syndrome) A congenital, dominantly inherited dysmorphic syndrome characterized by enlarged supraorbital ridges, wide foramen magnum and other cerebral anomalies, generalized hirsutism, distal muscle wasting, and progressive mixed deafness.[2500]

frontonasal dermoid cyst A dermoid cyst in or abutting the anterior cranial fossa and presenting in childhood with seizures, anosmia, or meningitis.[381]

frontonasal dysplasia (median cleft face syndrome, median facial cleft syndrome) A congenital, sporadic or dominantly inherited dysmorphic syndrome characterized by ocular hypertelorism, anterior cranium bifidum occultum, and other inconstant defects including craniosynostosis, polydactyly, hydrocephalus, stroke syndromes, and agenesis of the corpus callosum.[2504]

frontotemporal dementia (Pick disease, frontal lobe dementia, Pick-complex disorder, frontotemporal lobar degeneration, progressive subcortical gliosis, frontal dementias of the non-Alzheimer type, dementia lacking distinctive histology, frontal lobe degeneration, disinhibition–dementia–Parkinsonism–amyotrophy syndrome, primary progressive aphasia, cortico-dentatonigral or corticobasal degeneration) This is the currently preferred term for the spectrum of non-Alzheimer type dementias characterized by focal atrophy of frontal and anterior temporal regions (but with pathological heterogeneity). Such dementing disorders are linked to chromosome 17 and are characterized by focal cerebral lobar atrophy, the actual site of this determining the clinical picture. The condition may account for about 20% of cases of dementia and is much more common in males. There is marked genetic heterogeneity but in a quarter of the cases the disorder appears to be dominantly inherited and caused by mutations in *MAPT*, which encodes **tau** protein.

Numerous clinical phenotypes are distinguished.

1. The prototype is the FTD-behavioral variant, the form once known as *Pick disease.* In this syndrome the overwhelming clinical problem is one of progressive personality change due to the nonspecific, insidiously progressive frontal lobe degeneration. It is known also as the *frontal variant* of frontotemporal degeneration, presenting with marked changes in personality and behavior, such as apathy, loss of empathy, disinhibition, change in eating patterns, ritualized or stereotypical behavior, and failure of self-care.
2. *Language variants are as follows:*

   Semantic (aphasia) dementia, in which there is major temporal lobe pathology and clinical evidence of progressive fluent aphasia with impaired understanding of the meaning of words or of the identity of objects but with little or no involvement of perception, spatial skills, praxis, or memory.

   Primary progressive aphasia or *progressive nonfluent aphasia*, a disorder of expressive language with difficulties in word-finding, but relatively preserve memory and nonverbal cognition, progressing to **logopenia**, and/or verbal apraxia.
3. *Motor variants:*

   Corticobasal degeneration and motor neuron disease, a form with added anterior horn cell loss. Clinically, cognitive, behavioral, aphasic, and extrapyramidal manifestations merge in the various subtypes of the disorder.

   Familial amyotrophic lateral sclerosis with frontotemporal dementia linked to loci on chromosome 9p13.2 and 9q21.

Other clinical subtypes have been differentiated:

An *orbitobasal* variety characterized by disinhibition, impulsiveness, confabulation, and antisocial behavior; a *dorsolateral* form with poor attention and focus, working memory deficits, poor organization, planning and word/design generation, poor insight, and abnormal expression of affect.

A *medial frontal* form is also described.

Variant familial forms, one with added Parkinsonian features and another named *hereditary dysphasic disinhibition dementia*[3775] have been mapped to 17q21–22. At least the first of these is associated with multiple tau gene mutations.[3862]

In general, the condition also overlaps with **corticobasal degeneration syndrome** and **progressive supranuclear palsy**,[3405, 3398] which are probably *variants* themselves, as is *autosomal dominant subcortical gliosis.*

Alzheimer disease is not an unusual cause of focal cortical syndromes, occurring in perhaps a third of cases of posterior cortical atrophy, corticobasal syndrome, or progressive nonfluent aphasia (but not the other forms). The focal syndrome may remain "pure" for many years. Patients with atypical AD tend to be older than those with non-AD pathology.[15]

Pick disease, cortico-basal ganglionic degeneration, progressive supranuclear palsy, and familial cases of frontotemporal dementia and Parkinsonism linked to chromosome 17 are **tauopathies**; *frontotemporal lobe dementia with ubiquitinated inclusions, dementia lacking distinctive histology, neuronal intermediate filament inclusions disease,* and *inclusion body myopathy with Paget's disease of bone and frontotemporal dementia* are **gehrigopathies**.[1482] The pathological features common to most of them are listed below. In many of the subtypes there are prominent accumulations of **tau** protein. In some cases there is evidence of ALS or EMG findings suggestive of denervation in one limb.[3907, 4605] It is likely that the philosopher Immanuel Kant died with this condition.

The Web site of an FTD support group is at www.ftdcarers.org.uk. See also **neuronal IF inclusion disease** and **progressive subcortical gliosis**.

The clinical features that best differentiate the typical condition from **Alzheimer disease** are social conduct disorders, hyperorality (see **Kluver–Bucy syndrome**), akinesia, and the relative lack of amnesia or perceptual difficulties. A more formal list has been synthesized as follows:[3349, 4362]

Onset is insidious, with slow progression
Dominant deficits in behavior and conduct appear early in the course of the disease

Loss of personal awareness (neglect of hygiene and grooming)
Loss of social graces and awareness
Disinhibition (sexually provocative or demanding, inappropriate jocularity) Impulsivity, distractibility, hyperorality (dietary changes, excessive eating, smoking, or alcohol consumption)
Withdrawal from social contact
Stereotyped or perseverative behaviors (wandering, repetitive clapping, humming or singing, ritualistic toileting, dressing)
Speech output changes
Progressive reduction of speech (late mutism)
Stereotypy of speech (few repeated phrases or themes; echolalia)
Physical signs such as early or prominent primitive or "frontal" reflexes; early incontinence; and late akinesia, rigidity, or tremor.
Deficits in social comportment, behavior, judgment, or language are out of proportion to memory deficit.

A major advance was the publication of a consensus statement on the clinical diagnostic criteria for the condition(s) reproduced in an amended form in Chart F–6 below:

frontotemporal lobar degeneration See **frontotemporal dementia**.

frontotemporoparietal encephalitic syphilis See **general paresis of the insane**.

Froriep, August von (1849–1917) German anatomist who first described a form of myositis in which connective tissue takes the place of muscle—a chronic polymyositis.[5619]

Froriep induration Chronic atrophic myositis with marked intramuscular fibrosis.[5619]

frozen shoulder See **Duplay syndrome**.

fructose 1,6-diphosphatase deficiency A rare inborn error of metabolism which may be associated with atypical **central core disease** of muscle.[3301]

fructose intolerance A diffuse encephalopathy inherited as a recessive trait and characterized by hypoglycemia (which may induce seizures) and recurrent abdominal pain, nausea, vomiting, and diarrhea resulting from the ingestion of fructose and related sugars in the presence of a deficiency of the enzyme aldolase B.[1308]

fructosemia A recessively inherited disease due to deficiency of fructose-1-phosphate aldolase and characterized clinically by the congenital onset of failure to thrive, hypoglycemic episodes, hepatic and renal impairment, and axonal motor neuropathy.[5268]

Fryns syndrome A lethal recessively inherited congenital dysmorphic syndrome manifesting also short stature, anterior chamber abnormalities, cloudy corneas, microphthalmia, ptosis, aortic stenosis, brachydactyly, and mental and developmental delay.[2224]

FTA-Abs (fluorescent treponemal antibody absorption test) A treponemal test for syphilis, which remains permanently reactive after infection.

Chart F–6. Clinical Diagnostic Features of Frontotemporal Dementia

Behavioral Disorder

Core features:

Insidious onset and slow progression
Early decline in regulation of personal conduct
Early decline in social interpersonal contact (lack of social tact, misdemeanors such as shoplifting)
Early emotional blunting despite such signs of disinhibition as unrestrained sexuality, violent behavior, inappropriate jocularity, restless pacing, etc.
Early loss of insight into the fact that the altered condition is due to a pathological change of the subject's own mental state

Supportive features:

Neglect of personal hygiene and grooming
Mental rigidity and inflexibility
Distractibility, impulsivity, and impersistence
Hyperorality (oral/dietary changes, overeating, food fads, excessive smoking and alcohol consumption, oral exploration of objects)
Stereotyped and perseverative behavior (wandering, mannerisms such as clapping, singing, dancing, ritualistic preoccupation such as hoarding, toileting, and dressing)
Utilization behavior (unrestrained exploration of objects in the environment)

Speech disorder

Progressive reduction of speech (lack of spontaneity and economy of utterance)
Press of speech
Sterotypy of speech (repetition of limited repertoire of words, phrases, or themes)
Echolalia, perseveration, or mutism

Affective symptoms

Depression, anxiety, excessive sentimentality, suicidal and fixed ideation, delusion (early and evanescent)
Hypochondriasis, bizarre somatic preoccupation (early and evanescent)
Emotional unconcern (emotional indifference and remoteness, lack of empathy and sympathy, apathy)
Amimia (inertia, aspontaneity)
NB: Spatial orientation and praxis are preserved

continued

Chart F–6. *(continued)*

Physical signs

Early appearance of primitive reflexes, incontinence
Akinesia, rigidity, tremor (late)
Low and labile blood pressure

Investigations

Normal EEG despite clinically evident dementia
Brain imaging (structural, functional, or both): predominant frontal and/or anterior temporal abnormality
Neuropsychology indicates profound failure on "frontal lobe" tests in the absence of severe amnesia, aphasia, or perceptual spatial disorder

Supportive Diagnostic Features
Onset before 65 years
Positive family history of similar disorder in a first-degree relative
Bulbar palsy, muscular weakness and wasting, fasiciculations (motor neuron disease).

Excluding Features

Abrupt onset with ictal events
Head trauma related to onset
Early severe amnesia
Early spatial disorientation, lost in surroundings, defective localization of objects
Early severe apraxia
Logoclonic speech with rapid loss of train of thought
Myoclonus
Cortical bulbar and spinal deficits
Cerebellar ataxia
Choreoathetosis
Early, severe, pathological EEG
Brain imaging (predominant postcentral structural or functional deficit. Multifocal cerebral lesions on CT or MRI)
Laboratory tests indicating brain involvement or inflammatory disorder (such as multiple sclerosis, syphilis, AIDS, and herpes simplex encephalitis)

Relative diagnostic exclusion features
Typical history of chronic alcoholism
Sustained hypertension
History of vascular disease (such as angina, claudication)
(Adapted from Brun et al.[912] *and Neary et al.* [4604] *Reproduced by kind permission of the American Academy of Neurology and Lippincott Williams and Wilkins.)*

The pathological subtypes are those with tau-immunopositive inclusions with or without Pick bodies, those with ubiquitin immunopositive inclusions (FTD with motor neuron inclusions [FTD-MND]) and those lacking distinctive histology.[2932]

Neuropathological diagnostic features of frontotemporal dementia[912]

1. *Frontal Lobe Degeneration Type*
Gross changes
These include slight symmetrical convolutional atrophy in frontal and anterior temporal lobes, neither circumscribed nor of a knife blade type; atrophy can be severe in a few cases. The ventricular system is widened frontally. Usually, there is no gross atrophy of the stratum, amygdala, or hippocampus although, in some instances, severe involvement of these regions can occur.

Distribution of microscopic changes
Changes are seen in the frontal convexity cortex, sometimes in the orbitofrontal cortex, often in the anterior third of the temporal cortex and the anterior, but rarely the posterior, cingulate gyrus. The superior temporal gyrus is conspicuously spared. The parietal cortex is mildly involved in a few patients, more so in rare, advanced cases. In some patients with pronounced stereotypic behaviors, there is less neocortical involvement, with mostly striatal, amygdala, and hippocampal changes. These may represent a possible subtype.

Microscopic characteristics, gray matter
Microvacuolation and mild-to-moderate astrocytic gliosis affecting chiefly laminae I–III are seen, sometimes one or the other change prevailing. There is atrophy/loss of neurons in laminae II and III, whereas those of lamina V are mildly affected, being atrophic rather than lost. Occasionally, there are a few dystrophic neurites. There are no Pick bodies, inflated neurons or Lewy bodies, Immunohistochemistry for tau or ubiquitin reveals no distinctive features. In the substantial nigra of some patients, there is mild-to-moderate loss of pigmented neurons.

Microscopic characteristics, white matter
White matter astrocytic gliosis, moderate to mild, is seen in subcortical U-fibers. There is very mild astrocytic gliosis in deeper white matter, sometimes with slight attenuation and loss of myelin. The distribution is related to gray matter changes. Sometimes there is also ischemic white matter attenuation.

2. *Pick type*
Gross changes
These have the same topographic localization as frontal lobe degeneration, but generally more intense and usually more circumscribed. Asymmetry and striatal atrophy are common.

Distribution of microscopic changes
These are the same as frontal lobe degeneration, in agreement with the gross distribution
Microscopic characteristics, gray and white matter
The main characteristics are the same as frontal lobe degeneration, but with intense involvement of all cortical layers. Inflated neurons and Pick bodies, which are silver positive, tau and ubiquitin immunoreactive, are present. There is more intense white matter involvement. Patients with intense astrocytosis but without inflated neurons or inclusions, or both may for the present be included.

3. *Motor Neuron Disease Type*
Gross changes
These are the same as frontal lobe degeneration, although usually less severe.

Distribution of microscopic changes and microscopic characteristics in gray and white matter
These are the same as for frontal lobe degeneration. There is spinal motor neuron degeneration, affecting cervical and thoracic levels more than lumbar or sacral. There is greater cell loss in medial than lateral cell columns. Motor neurons, layer II neurons in frontal and temporal cortex, and hippocampal dentate gyrus neurons show inclusions that are ubiquitin positive but not silver or tau reactive. Nigral cell loss is severe in many patients. There is also hypoglossal degeneration in some.

Diagnostic exclusion features
Senile plaques, diffuse amyloid deposits, and amyloid angiopathy with anti-B-protein antibodies, tangles, and neuropil threads, with anti-tau and ubiquitin antibodies more than normal for age. Prion proteins are present with anti-prion antibodies.

Synthesized from Brun A, Englund B, Mann DMA, Neary D, et al. Consensus on Clinical and Neuropathological Criteria for Fronto-Temporal Dementia. J Neurol Neurosurg Psychiatry *1994;57:416–8, and Neary D, Snowden JS, Gustafson L, et al. Frontotemporal lobar degeneration.* Neurology *1998;5157:1546–54.*

Fuchs sign 1. See **Gowers signs**. 2. Uncoordinated movements of the upper eyelid following damage to the III cranial nerve, considered to be the result of anomalous reinnervation. See **pseudo-Graefe phenomenon**.

fucosidosis A rare inherited neuronal storage disease (an oligosaccharidosis) resulting from a deficiency of α-fucosidase, which leads to the accumulation of H-isoantigen. Intralysosomal laminated structures and axonal spheroids are detectable by electron microscopy in skin biopsy specimens.[1761] Two forms of the disease are recognized:

Type 1 (infantile) is characterized by psychomotor deterioration, cloudy corneae, dry skin, telangiectasia, mucopolysaccariduria, hypotonia and later spasticity, myoclonic seizures, coarse facies, hepatosplenomegaly, cardiomegaly, and dysostoses. The sweat chloride test result is abnormal.

In *type 2 (juvenile)* the onset of similar but milder signs occurs in the first 2 years of life; the sweat chloride test result is normal.

Unnumbered is a *variant* adult form, characterized clinically by gargoylelike facies, psychomotor retardation, and angiokeratoma corporis diffusum.[3077]

fugax (Lat) Fleeing or fleeting.

Fugl-Meyer Scale A system of evaluation of motor function, balance and some qualities of sensation, and joint function in hemiplegic patients, in which a cumulative numerical score is assigned. The scale represents a stroke-specific, performance-based impairment index and was designed to assess the progressive return of physical performance following the occurrence of stroke.[2225]

fugue state See **twilight state**.

Fukada stepping test A test for vestibular dysfunction, wherein the blindfolded subject marks time for 1 min and the degree of rotation on his own axis is assessed. Normally there should be none.

Fukuyama congenital muscular dystrophy A recessively inherited α-dystroglycanopathy, frequent in Japan, where it is the second commonest muscular dystrophy after Duchenne dystrophy. It is due to mutations of the *fukutin* gene on chromosome 9q31. The classical picture is of a child with generalized muscle weakness, severe brain involvement with mental retardation, frequent seizures, and abnormal eye function. First symptoms may occur *in utero* with poor fetal movements or at birth where asphyxia is not uncommon.

Functional improvement is frequently observed and most patients achieve standing with support and occasionally are able to take a few steps with support between the age of 2 and 8 years. Enlargement of the calves, quadriceps muscles, and tongue is common. Progressive weakness then develops and respiratory failure in the middle–late teens is an invariable complication. Life expectancy averages about 15 years.

Progressive contractures of the hips, ankles, and knees are an early feature and scoliosis commonly follows the loss of independent sitting after 9 years of age. Severe weakness is usually combined with profound mental retardation, and these patients typically do not speak meaningful words, whereas the majority learns to speak short sentences and may even become able to read and write a few characters. Most patients develop seizures before 3 years of age. Cardiac involvement (dilated cardiomyopathy) is almost invariable and typically develops in the second decade of life. About 50% of cases have poor visual pursuit, strabismus, severe myopia, hyperopia, or cataracts. CNS changes are part of the type II **lissencephaly** spectrum.[4555]

The *merosin-positive* form is characterized by muscle weakness and hypotonia with delayed motor developmental milestones, severe contractures, and only mild mental retardation. CT and MRI may show some white matter lucencies and micropolygyria.[3507] The homogeneous *merosin-negative* form is characterized by marked motor disability, seizures, hydrocephalus, Dandy–Walker malformation, cerebral cortical malformations (including heterotopias and pachygyria or microgyria), and skull deformities,[2237] but mentation is relatively unaffected. Serum CK levels are raised and there are numerous areas of low signal intensity on MRI scans. It is mapped to chromosome 6q22–23 and is genetically identical to the **Walker–Warburg syndrome.** See also **congenital muscular dystrophy**.

Fukuhara syndrome See MERRF.

fukutin-related proteinopathy *FKRP* mutations manifest a range of syndromes from severe CMD (including type 1C, CMD with cerebellar cysts, and **Walker–Warburg syndrome**) to a milder adult-onset LGMD (type 2I). *Dysferlinopathies* can present as a classic LGMD phenotype (type 2B), as a distal muscular dystrophy (**Miyoshi** type) or as mixed phenotypes. Brain MRI and intelligence are normal, but dilated cardiomyopathy and respiratory failure are common complications.[3454]

Mutations in *lamin A/C* have an even wider spectrum of phenotypes associated with them. The dominant forms of LGMD have greater clinical heterogeneity, a slower course, and later onset with less elevation of serum CK levels compared with the recessive forms.

full-field stimulation Excitation of the retina by visual stimuli which occupy all or most of the visual field. Such a condition is required for the appearance of the **optokinetic reflex.**

full interference pattern See **interference pattern.**

Full Outline of UnResponsiveness (FOUR Scale) A scale assessing comatose patients, even if they are intubated. It includes brainstem reflexes and recognizes the **locked-in syndrome** and possibly the **vegetative state**. It has four parameters: eye response, motor response, brainstem reflexes, and respirations. The lower the score the deeper the coma.[6772] It is claimed to provide greater neurological detail than the **Glasgow Coma Scale** (GCS), recognizes the **locked-in syndrome**, and unlike the GCS attends to brainstem reflexes, breathing patterns, and the different stages of herniation.[6773]

FOUR score

Eye responses

Eyelids open and tracking, or blinking on command	4
Eyelids open but not tracking	3
Eyelids closed but open to loud voice	2
Eyelids closed but open to pain	1
Eyelids closed with pain	0

Motor responses

Makes sign (thumbs-up, fist, other)	4
localizing to pain	3
Flexion response to pain	2
Extension response to pain	1
No response to pain	0
Generalized myoclonus status	0

Brainstem reflexes

Pupil	*Corneal*	*Points*	
Present	Present	Present	4
One pupil wide and fixed	Present	Present	3
Absent	Present	NA	2
Present	Absent	NA	2
Absent	Absent	Present	1
Absent	Absent	Absent	0

Respiratory function

Not intubated regular		4
Not intubated	Cheyne–Stokes	3
Not intubated irregular		2
Not intubated apnea		0
Intubated	above ventilator rate	1
Intubated	breathes at ventilator rate	0

(From Wijdicks EFM, Bamler WR, et al. Validation of a new coma scale: The FOUR score. *Ann Neurol* 2005;**58**:585–93. © 2005. Reproduced by permission of John Wiley & Sons, Inc.)

full wave rectified EMG The absolute value of a raw EMG signal. It involves inverting all the waveforms below the isopotential line and displaying them with opposite polarity above the line. The technique is used to analyze kinesiologic EMG signals. (From the 2001 Report of the Nomenclature Committee of the American Association of Electromyography and Electrodiagnosis.[19] Reproduced by kind permission of the AANEM.)

fullness of the ears One of the symptoms which leads to sinking of the heart because of its nonspecificity. The complaint, however, is common in patients with **Ménière syndrome** and in those with cluster headache, so it may truly have some diagnostic value.

Fulton, John Farquar (1899–1960) American neurophysiologist born in Minnesota. After service in the World War I, he entered Harvard as a "veteran" and, in 1921, graduated with the highest honors in science, proceeding then to Oxford as a Rhodes scholar and later demonstrator in physiology. At Oxford he came under the influence of **Sherrington** which turned him in the direction of neurophysiology and medical history; while at Oxford he compiled the catalog of **Osler**'s historical library.

After further periods at Yale and Oxford, he returned to assume the Sterling Chair of Physiology at Yale, where he undertook and encouraged studies in aviation physiology, neurophysiology, endocrinology, electrocardiology, and endocrinology, and where he worked with Cushing on the study of cerebral physiology and the compilation of medical history. In 1935 he refused the appointment as successor to Sherrington at Oxford, preferring to remain at Yale. His best-known works were his *Physiology of the Nervous System* (London, 1938), *Readings in the History of Physiology*, and his biography of **Cushing**.

The personal charm and commitment which inspired so many of his students at all levels cannot be depicted adequately in a mere dictionary.

fumarase deficiency An inherited cause of mitochondrial encephalopathy in which this enzyme deficiency leads to dysfunction within the tricarboxylic acid cycle as a result of inability to convert fumaric acid to malic acid.

Clinically, this early infantile encephalopathy presents with microcephaly, failure to thrive, profound developmental delay, seizures, hypotonia, facial dysmorphisms and cerebral atrophy, and leads to death in the first year; polycythemia, lactic and pyruvic aciduria, and fumaric acidemia are other characteristic features.[6978, 3397]

fumaric aciduria A mitochondrial encephalopathy caused by a deficiency of mitochondrial cytosolic fumarase.[6978]

Functional Assessment Staging (FAST) A 16-item scale derived from the self-care axis of the **Brief Cognitive Rating Scale.** It is of use in the diagnosis and staging of patients with any type of cognitive disorder and for assessing functional capacity at the severe extreme of **Alzheimer disease.** Activities rated include memory, functioning at work and socially, self-care, and speech/language. Seven stages are defined and their dates recorded. Assessment runs from normality through complaints of forgetting the location of objects; decreased job functioning evident to coworkers; decreased ability to perform complex tasks; difficulty in choosing proper clothing; difficulty dressing; and failure in self-care and communication.[5250, 5255]

functional bent back See **camptocormia**.

Functional Capacity Index An instrument to measure functional loss 12 months after trauma.[2519]

Functional Composite An outcome measure for clinical trials of therapies in multiple sclerosis, examining arm/hand function, leg function/ambulation, and cognition.[3277]

functional disease Disturbance of body functions for which no responsible disturbance of structure can be detected. In this context, the word *structure* includes pathophysiology and abnormal chemistry within the nervous system. Other terms for the condition are "medically unexplained," "psychogenic," and "hysterical."

The similarity of this definition to that of hysteria will be remarked, but although the physician using the latter term usually considers that the patient is manifesting a disorder which is rooted in psychopathology, use of the former commonly indicates that a nonpsychiatric cause of the disease state may be incriminated, as, for example, in the case of *functional hypoglycemia.* See **hysteria**.

The term is still commonly employed, *faute de mieux*, "as a designation for those affections in which no morbid changes have been hitherto discovered . . . and from which recovery is possible." (**Gowers**) But as Gowers pointed out; "Unfortunately we have no other general term for these cases and it is to be regretted that we are compelled to make a positive term denote negative characteristics." Thus he described hysterical weakness of the legs as due to "a peculiar ungeared state of the volitional centers, which is at the root of all pure hysteric palsy." See also **Hoover sign, collapsing weakness, dragging monoplegic gait, psychogenic Romberg Test,** and **midline splitting**.

functional grading The scores assigned to patients as a result of **functional muscle testing**.[5412, 6326] The scheme of Brooke et al.[871] is given in Chart F–7. Appel et al.[218] have defined similar grades for the bulbar muscles (Chart F–8).

functional hemianopia See **hemianopia**.

functional imaging Noninvasive methods (such as SPECT, MRI, or PET scanning) that allow visualization of neural activity in brain regions during the performance of specific tasks or when treated with extraneous molecules. The most sensitive method is blood oxygen level-dependent (BOLD) functional MRI which can detect local increases in relative blood oxygenation that are most likely a direct consequence of neurotransmitter action, and thus reflect local neuronal signaling.[4177]

Functional Independence Measure An 18-item functional disability scale, of value in the determination of disability in patients with stroke, **multiple sclerosis**, or other chronic neurological conditions. The degree of dependence and independence in *personal care, sphincter control, mobility, locomotion, communication, and social cognition* are assessed, scores of between 1 (requiring full assistance) and 7 (independent) being applied.[3369]

Functional Independence measures for children A scale assessing global function in children with cerebral palsy.[4533]

Chart F–7. Functional Grades

Arms:

1. Starting with arms at the sides, patient can abduct the arms in a full circle until they touch above the head.
2. Can raise arms above head only by flexing the elbow (i.e., shortening the circumference of the movement) or by using accessory muscles.
3. Cannot raise the hands above head but can raise an 8-ounce (240 ml) glass of water to mouth (using both hands if necessary).
4. Can raise hand to mouth but cannot use hands to hold pen or pick up pennies from table.
5. Cannot raise hands to mouth and has no useful function of hands.

Hips and Legs:

1. Walks and climbs stairs without assistance.
2. Walks and climbs stairs with aid of railing.
3. Walks and climbs stairs slowly with aid of railing (over 12 s for four standard stairs).
4. Walks unassisted and rises from chair but cannot climb stairs.
5. Walks unassisted but cannot rise from chair or climb stairs.
6. Walks only with assistance or walks independently with long leg braces.
7. Walks in long leg braces but requires assistance for balance.
8. Stands in long leg braces but unable to walk even with assistance.
9. Is in wheelchair.
10. Is confined to bed.

From Brooke MH, et al. Clinical Investigation in Duchenne dystrophy: 2. Determination of the "power" of therapeutic trials based on the natural history. Muscle Nerve *1983;6:91–103.*

Chart F–8. Functional Grading for Bulbar Muscles

Swallowing	*Points*
General diet	3
Soft diet	6
Mechanical soft diet	9
Strained or pureed diet	12
Tube feeding	15
Speech	
Clear	3
Pa-Ta-Ka slightly slurred	6
Slurred	9
Unintelligible	12
None	15

From Appel V, et al. A rating scale for amyotrophic lateral sclerosis. Arch Neurol *1987;***22:***328–33.* Reproduced by kind permission of the American Medical Association.

Functional Limitations profile A British scale containing 136 questions designed to assess the limitations imposed by disease on various categories of activity, such as *ambulation, body care and movement, mobility, household management, recreation and pastimes, social interaction, affect, alertness, sleep, eating, communication, and work*. Individual scores are given on each of these items.

functional localization The localization of particular motor or sensory properties within specific cell groups within the CNS.

functional Magnetic Resonance Imaging (fMRI) A technique allowing examination of brain function during cognitive or motor tasks through the detection of an altered ratio of oxygenated and deoxygenated hemoglobin, acting as an indirect marker of metabolic activity.

functional muscle testing Techniques for evaluating the strength of muscle contractions using the subjective judgments of both the examiner and the patient as regards the capacity of the latter to perform specified motor tasks. As a result of such an evaluation, the patient is assigned a **functional grade**, which with **timed functional testing** allows accurate documentation of the course of a progressive neuromuscular disease.[4524, 201]

functional neurosurgery Nondestructive surgery, such as the implantation of neurostimulating electrodes.

Functional Rating Scale A multidimensional rating instrument derived from the **Clinical Dementia Rating Scale** with the addition of the two domains of language and behavior.[1999]

functional refractory period See **refractory period**.

functional seizures See **pseudoseizures**.

functional somatic syndromes A term applied to several related syndromes characterized more by symptoms, suffering, and disability than by consistently demonstrable tissue abnormality. These syndromes include multiple chemical sensitivity, the sick building syndrome, repetition stress injury, the side effects of silicone breast implants, Gulf War syndrome, **chronic fatigue syndrome**, irritable bowel syndrome, fibromyalgia, **railway spine**, multiple chemical sensitivity, chronic **whiplash**, chronic **Lyme disease**, candidiasis hypersensitivity, food allergies, mitral valve prolapse, neurasthenia, spinal irritation, chronic brucellosis, pinched nerves, and soldier's heart (Da Costa syndrome). Chronic carbon monoxide poisoning; chronic mononucleosis ("Royal Free disease"); and symptoms resulting from exposure to video display terminals, carbonless copy paper, mercury in dental fillings, and weak electromagnetic fields may also be subsumed here.

Common symptoms include fatigue; weakness; sleep difficulties; headache; muscle aches and joint pain; problems with memory, attention, and concentration; nausea and other gastrointestinal symptoms; anxiety; depression; irritability; palpitations and "racing heart"; shortness of breath; dizziness or light-headedness; sore throat; and dry mouth. Patients often proffer explicit, highly elaborated diagnoses, and they are often refractory to reassurance, explanation, and standard treatment of symptoms. They share similar phenomenologies, high rates of co-occurrence, similar epidemiologic characteristics, and increased prevalence of psychiatric comorbidity.

As superbly reviewed by Barsky and Borus,[424] typical patients with functional somatic syndromes have explicit and highly elaborated self-diagnoses. Their symptoms are diffuse, nonspecific and ambiguous, and include fatigue; weakness; sleep difficulties; headache; muscle aches and joint pain; problems with memory, attention, and concentration; nausea and other gastrointestinal symptoms; anxiety; depression; irritability; palpitations and "racing heart"; shortness of breath; dizziness or light-headedness; sore throat; and dry mouth. Patients are not relieved by negative findings on medical evaluation and are hardly responsive to explanation, reassurance, or palliative treatment. Associated anxiety, depressive, and somatoform disorders are common. The syndromes often begin in limited, sporadic outbreaks among small groups of people who are in close contact with each other, at first suggesting exposure to a common infectious or toxic agent, though such are never detected.

Although discrete pathophysiological causes may ultimately be found in some patients with functional somatic syndromes, the suffering of these patients is exacerbated by a self-perpetuating, self-validating cycle in which common, endemic, somatic symptoms are incorrectly attributed to serious abnormality, reinforcing the patient's belief that he or she has a serious disease. Psychosocial factors propelling this cycle of symptom amplification are the belief that one has a serious disease; the expectation that one's condition is likely to worsen; the "sick role," including the effects of litigation and compensation; and the alarming portrayal of the condition as catastrophic and disabling. Patients with functional somatic syndromes have elevated rates of psychiatric disorders, particularly anxiety, depressive, and somatoform disorders.[424] See also **factitious disease**, and **hysteria**.

Funderbunk syndrome (mesomelia and nephritis) A dysmorphic syndrome characterized by short stature and limbs, strabismus, small widely spaced teeth, nephropathy with hematuria and proteinuria, mesomelia of the upper and lower limbs, Madelung deformity, cortical hyperostosis, and mental and developmental delay.[4929]

fundus oculi (Lat, the bottom or base + eye) That portion of the retina (in the depths of the eye) visible with the ophthalmoscope.

fungal myositis The rare direct infection of muscles with fungi, particularly *Candida albicans*. Immunocompromised subjects are those most likely to be affected.

funicular pain See **central pain**.

funiculus (Lat, a small rope) A group of nerve fibers invested in a sheath of connective tissue, the perineurium, the whole varying in size from 0.04 to 3 mm. Bundles of funiculi form the nerve trunk.

funnel vision The physiological increase in the diameter of the visual field as the test object is taken farther away from the subject; a cone of vision is thus produced. See also **tunnel vision**.

Furukawa syndrome A syndrome characterized by the onset in childhood of optic atrophy, chorioretinitis, retinitis pigmentosa, kyphoscoliosis, diabetes, cerebellar ataxia, myopathic weakness, and sensorimotor neuropathy.[2249]

fusiform (from Lat) Elliptical or spindle shaped.

fusiform aneurysm See **aneurysm**.

fusimotor neurons Gamma efferent fibers which innervate **fusimotor spindles**.

fusimotor spindles Specialized muscle fibers within voluntary muscles which are sensitive to stretch and which send impulses centrally along fast-conducting Ia afferent fibers to assist in the regulation of muscle tone.

fusion (fusion reflex) A cortically mediated mechanism whereby the eyes are directed toward an object in such a manner that this image of the object falls upon the two maculas and any imbalance is corrected for through the working of the occipital cortex to suppress the awareness of blurring of the images perceived, which are now seen as one.

fusion reflex See **fusion**.

fusional adaptation A brainstem mechanism whereby the positions of the eyes are reset in order to minimize the effect of a disparity in retinal imaging, as might occur if a prism were placed before one eye.

Both *fast* and *slow* adaptive mechanisms are described.[3762]

fusional vergence (disparity-induced vergence) Movements of the eyes which rotate them in opposite directions in order to minimize any disparity in the direction of visual images on corresponding points of the foveas of the eyes.

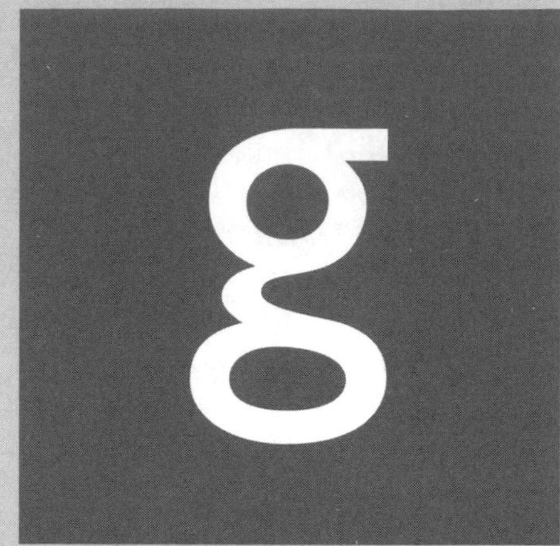

G syndrome (hypospadias–dysphagia syndrome) A rare, dominantly inherited congenital syndrome characterized by hypertelorism, slit-like palpebral fissures and other facial dysmorphisms, pigmentary retinal degeneration, hypospadias, dysphagia with aspiration and respiratory distress, anosmia, achalasia, pulmonary malformations and malformations of the alimentary tract.[3874, 4798] See also **hypertelorism–hypospadias syndrome**.

G1 See **active electrode**.

GABA Gamma-amino butyric acid, an inhibitory neurotransmitter found mainly in the central nervous system but also in the pancreas.

GABA transaminase deficiency A congenital dysmorphic syndrome manifesting also aminoaciduria, hyperpituitarism, focal CNS demyelination with diffuse gliosis, seizures, dysphagia, and mental and developmental delay.[381]

gadolinium A paramagnetic agent used in MRI scanning. It shortens the half-life of relaxation and leads to enhancement of demyelinating lesions.

gag reflex Elevation of the soft palate and contraction of the pharyngeal constrictors in response to tactile stimulation of the pharyngeal mucosa. The afferent arc of the reflex travels via the IX and the efferent via the IX and X cranial nerves.

Gage, Phineas P. An American railway foreman described as honest and industrious until in 1848 a 3-foot (0.9 m) tamping iron was accidentally blown through his frontal lobes while he was at work, effecting a frontal lobotomy from which he did not die at once; the subsequent alteration in his personality (he exhibited himself in a circus for some years and later became a stagecoach driver in Chile) provided the first clue to the highest functions of the prefrontal lobe. He died in status epilepticus 12 years after the accident.

His case was recorded in the *Boston Medical and Surgical Reporter* by Dr. J.M. Harlow, a general practitioner in the same year and further described by H.G. Bigelow, a Boston surgeon in 1850.[474]

gain The ratio of the output signal voltage to the input signal voltage of an EEG channel. For example:

$$\text{Gain} = \frac{\text{Output voltage}}{\text{Input voltage}}$$

$$= \frac{10\ \text{V}}{10\ \mu\text{V}} = 1{,}000{,}000$$

This is often expressed in decibels (Db), a logarithmic unit; thus a voltage gain of 10 = 20 Db, of 1 000 = 60 Db, or of 1 000 000 = 120 Db. See also **sensitivity**.

(Adapted from the 1974 report of the Committee on Terminology, IFCN. In Chatrian GE, Bergamini L, Dondey M, et al. A glossary of terms most commonly used by clinical electroencephalographers. *EEG Clin Neurophysiol* 1974;37:538–48. Reprinted with kind permission of Elsevier Science and the IFCN.)

gain of pursuit eye movements (pursuit gain) The relationship between the velocity of a visual target and that of the tracking eyes. It is typically reduced in

Parkinson disease, older age, and progressive supranuclear palsy and may be increased in an eye when the other eye has a paretic muscle.

gait The manner or pattern of walking. **Apraxic, ataxic, dyskinetic, hysterical, magnetic, Parkinsonian, spastic,** and **steppage** gaits are described.

Gait and Balance Scale An assessment tool comprising historical information and examination of 14 different gait and balance parameters designed to rate the severity of damage to these functional domains.[6278]

gait apraxia (frontal gait apraxia) An entity of doubtful validity in which patients fail to perform whole-body movements in response to command or on imitation, but can do so spontaneously.

Such a syndrome was dismissed by Geschwind,[2338] who emphasized that most patients so diagnosed have fixed disturbances in the performance of whole-body movements due to lesions at a lower level. However, this has been presented as an inability to stand up or move the feet along the floor while seated, in the absence of ataxia, limb apraxia, or buccofacial apraxia, and despite the retained ability to pantomime walking and pedaling movements when supine. The responsible lesion is thought to be bilateral in posterior subcortical regions or in the thalamus.[5782] See also **gait ignition failure**.

gait ignition A starting signal sent to those muscles responsible for ambulation when the appropriate preliminary shifts in the center of gravity have occurred.[4723]

gait ignition failure A term used for difficulty in initiating walking. The gait has elements of Parkinsonism with start and turn hesitation, shuffling, and freezing but is relatively normal once entrained; the posture is upright with good arm swing, a normal stride length, and no festination. Equilibrium is near normal, and when seated or lying, rhythmic leg movements are generated normally. Facial expression, upper limb mobility, and whole-body movements are well preserved. The lesions causing this syndrome include frontal lobe vascular disease and focal degeneration of the frontal lobes.[283]

galactocerebroside (from Gr, milk + brain) The abnormal substance stored in **Krabbe disease**.

galactokinase deficiency A recessively inherited syndrome resembling galactosemia but found only in the Eastern European gypsy population and characterized by hepatosplenomegaly, cataract, and sometimes seizures and mental retardation.[2397] The diagnosis is assisted by urine chromatography.

galactosemic encephalopathy A syndrome of cortical neuronal degeneration with spongy changes occurring in infants with untreated galactosemia (galactose-phosphate uridyltransferase deficiency); the gene responsible for this recessive condition maps to 9p13.

Clinically, it presents, after the introduction of milk into the diet, with jaundice and other manifestations of hepatic insufficiency, cataract, hypoglycemia, cerebral edema, and early death. Sensorineural hearing loss, mental and motor retardation, and tremors may occur in children when the delayed-onset form is treated.[133] The condition is also rarely reported in adults.

galactosialidosis (β-galactosidase-neuraminidase deficiency) An inherited condition clinically resembling **mucolipidosis type 1**. The responsible gene maps to chromosome 20.

Clinically, the condition has its onset in early adult life and manifests optic atrophy, ataxia, seizures, stimulus-sensitive myoclonus, and muscle atrophy, hypotonia, and weakness. Angiokeratomas, gargoyle facies, and vertebral changes have also been noted.[5508]

galactosidases Intracellular enzymes required for the metabolism of ceramide (α-galactosidase) or keratan (β-galactosidase) and diminished or absent in **Fabry disease** and **mucopolysaccharidosis type IVb**, respectively.

galactosylceramide lipidosis See **Krabbe leukodystrophy**.

galanin A neuropeptide, found in high concentration in the basal nucleus of Meynert, where, with choline acetyltransferase, its concentration is diminished in **Alzheimer disease**.

galant reflex (trunk incurvation) When the examiner's finger presses on one side of the back of the prone baby, the infant flexes the trunk so that the spine is concave to that side. The sign is normally present between birth and 4 months of age.

galea (Lat, a helmet) The sheet of connective tissue stretching across the scalp like a cap, into which are inserted the frontalis, temporalis, and occipitalis muscles.

Galen, Claudius (or Clarissimus) (AD 130–200) A Roman, born in Pergamum, Asia Minor, studying there and at Smyrna, Corinth, and Alexandria. He became physician to Marcus Aurelius in Venice.

Galen was the founder of the Galenical system of medicine, utilizing plants and minerals, and he reputedly published over 500 works, although many were lost when his house burned down. His studies of the nervous system were probably facilitated by his responsibility for attending to the wounds of gladiators; he described head and spinal injuries in some detail and, in the latter case, partially anticipated the description of **Brown-Séquard**. His name is given to the great vein of Galen and to the choroidal veins, but he also described and named many parts of the brain and about 300 muscles, demonstrated the origin of nerves from the brain and spinal cord, described 7 pairs of cranial nerves, and elucidated the function of the recurrent laryngeal nerve (by cutting it in a pig).

Galen considered that the choroid produced CSF, with contributions of pneuma from air passing through the cribriform plate and from the rete mirabile. He described flow from the lateral ventricles through the third and fourth ventricles to the outlet in the roof, draining thence through the cribriform plate and thence to the palate.[6353]

Galen has been regarded as the Prince of Physicians on account of his observations in almost all fields of medicine; his works constituted the leading medical authority for 1400 years. He localized mental functions in the cerebrum rather than in the ventricles[5886] and stated that seizures affecting the face were due to disease in the brain, and, when the face escaped, the lesion was in the upper part of the spinal cord. He also described the aura, the facial appearance of chronic epileptic people, the periodicity of the attacks, and focal sensory seizures.

Gall, F.J. (1758–1828) Viennese physician and neuroanatomist; the founder of the discipline of phrenology and the father of cerebral localization. As a boy he noted the different aptitudes of schoolfellows and compared these with their facial and cranial peculiarities. After completing medical studies in Strasbourg and Vienna, he continued to study the relationship between aptitudes and morphology with a series of dissections of the brain; he first described the cervical and lumbar enlargements of the cord, differentiated gray from white matter, and then described the origins of cranial nerves II, III, IV, and VI.

This work culminated in his monograph *Anatomie et Physiologie du Systeme Nerveux en Général, et du Cerveau en particulier*, published after he was prevented from further experimentation in Vienna by the offices of the Church. In this, he localized certain functions to specific brain areas—a major advance, since Cullen, in his *Practice of Physic* (1776–1784) had written "nor have we been able to perceive that any particular part of the brain has more concern in the operations of our intellect than any other. Nor have we attained any knowledge of what share the several parts of the brain have in that operation."

Gall isolated 27 cranial areas which he believed corresponded with as many mental attributes, the Propensities, the Sentiments, and the Intellectual Faculties. He was unaware of the asymmetries of brain function and many of the localizations ascribed (e.g., he considered that the cerebellum was the seat of the sexual impulse) were ill-founded, although in many ways conventional at the time. The theories which he propounded, the style with which he propounded them and the influence of his enthusiastic disciples such as J.G. **Spurzheim** led to huge popular support for the cult over some decades. It was when excessive claims were made—such as the ability of phrenology to divine character, and thus its adequacy as a method for selecting members of Parliament—that the movement fell into disrepute and attracted ridicule. Yet, as Edwin G. Boring wrote, his was "an instance of a theory which, while essentially wrong, was just right enough to further scientific thought."

Phrenology helped to move ideas concerning the mind "away from the concept of the unsubstantial Cartesian soul to the concept of the more material nerve function . . . (and thus) . . . was wrong only in detail and in the enthusiasm of its supporters." The best recent critiques of Gall's life and teaching are those of Critchley[1334] and of Temkin.[6249]

galloping tongue Episodic, involuntary, rhythmic, and wave-like tongue movements at 3 Hz and lasting 10 s with 20-s periods of rest between, starting posteriorly in the midline and extending laterally, seen rarely following pontine lesions as after head injury.[3356]

Galloway–Mowat syndrome A recessively inherited disorder, usually with infantile onset and associated with proteinuria, focal segmental glomerulosclerosis, microcephaly, and cerebellar disease.

GALOP syndrome (Gait disorder, Autoantibody, Late-age Onset Polyneuropathy)A symmetric sensorimotor demyelinating polyneuropathy of older adults producing marked gait disorder with ataxia and positive Romberg sign associated with the presence of serum IgM autoantibodies to central myelin antigen.

Galton, Francis (1822–1911) English scientist and geneticist, a cousin of Charles Darwin, who founded the statistical school of genetics. Some of his work was concerned with dermatoglyphics (fingerprints and palm prints), a subject which is again becoming of interest to geneticists.

Galton whistle A whistle with a high pitch, once used to detect high-tone hearing loss.

Galvani, Luigi or Aloysio (1737–1798) Italian physician, physiologist, and physicist, and professor of anatomy and operative surgery at Bologna. He was first impelled to study the electrical reactions of the body when his wife Lucia told him that the frog legs that she had prepared for a meal "came alive" when set upon the copper wires of the grill. By connecting the exposed spinal cord of a decapitated frog with a metallic arc to the gastrocnemius muscle, he demonstrated that animal muscles contract as a result of electrical stimulation, but erred in considering that this was derived only (as in his later experiments) from the animals' brains, conducted by the nerves to the muscles rather than from the dissimilar metals with which were constructed the apparatus from which he suspended them.[727]

Through the studies of Galvani which suggested synaptic transmission, the concept of transient electrical potentials traveling in the fibers of the nervous system replaced that of the spirits of the animal in the understanding of scientists.

It was Galvani's nephew, Aldini, who first used electricity medically on humans in attempts to revive the dead, to alleviate melancholia, or to cure paralysis. **Duchenne** was the first to use electrical stimulation for diagnostic purposes.

galvanic current That constant electrical current produced by chemical action.

galvanic nystagmus See **vestibular nystagmus**.

galvanic skin response See **psychogalvanic reflex**.

Galvanic tests (galvanic vestibular stimulation) Tests of the adequacy of labyrinthine function, involving stimulation of the standing subject using a small (5–7 mA) direct current, with the anode on the mastoid and the cathode over the sternum. Normally, mixed horizontal and rotatory nystagmus is produced, with its fast phase away from the side of the mastoid examined. The requirement for larger or smaller currents gives some indication of the state of labyrinthine excitability.[1500]

Galveston Orientation and Amnesia Test A test used in the assessment of patients after head injury. It can be administered daily. A score of 78 or more on 3 consecutive occasions is considered to indicate that the patient has recovered from **posttraumatic amnesia**.[3804]

gamma-aminoisobutyric acid A small neutral amino acid which is taken up by cerebral tumors, allowing it to be employed in the measurement of tissue permeability.

Chart G–1. Galveston Orientation and Amnesia Test

Question	Error Score	Notes
What is your name?	2	Must give both first and surname
When were you born?	4	Must give day, month, and year
Where do you live?	4	Town sufficient
Where are you now?	5	Must give actual town
What is this building?	5	Usually hospital or rehab center—actual name unnecessary
When were you admitted to this hospital?	5	Date
How did you get here?	5	Mode of transport
What is the first event you remember after injury?	5	Any plausible event is enough; record answer
Can you give some detail?	5	Must give relevant detail
Can you describe the last thing you can recall before the accident?	5	Any plausible event is enough; record the answer
Can you give some detail?	5	Any relevant detail
What time is it now?	5	–1 for each half-hour error
What day of the week is it?	3	–1 for each day error
What day of the month is it? (i.e., the date)	5	–1 for each day error
What is the month?	15	–5 for each month error
What is the year?	3	–10 for each year error
Score = (100 – total error)		

From Levin HS, O'Donnell VM, Grossman RG. The Galveston orientation and amnesia test. J Nerv Ment Dis *1979;167:675–84. Reproduced by kind permission.*

gamma-glutamylcysteine synthetase deficiency A rare aminoacidopathy of infancy mapped to 6p12 and characterized by low levels of glutamate in red blood cells, generalized aminoaciduria, and hemolytic anemia. The clinical manifestations include ataxia and peripheral neuropathy.[3529]

gammopathic neuropathy (cryoglobulinemic neuropathy) Motor, sensory, or mixed neuropathies, often complicated by Raynaud phenomenon, tremor, or ataxia, occurring in association with monoclonal proteins and plasma cell dyscrasias (dysglobulinemias, gammopathies) such as multiple myeloma, amyloidosis (light-chain type), Waldenstrom macroglobulinemia, gamma heavy chain disease, cryoglobulinemia, and benign IgM, IgA, or IgG gammopathies "of uncertain significance."[3374] The syndrome is considered to be due to the remote effects of a humoral factor secreted by neoplastic immunocytes.[5913] Presentations include selective small fiber sensory neuropathy, sensorimotor polyneuropathy, and multiple mononeuropathy, often manifesting as the first evidence of the cryoglobulinemia.

Immunoglobulin M (IgM) paraproteinemia produces a fairly characteristic syndrome of insidiously progressive chronic sensorimotor polyneuropathy in elderly people, who complain of numbness and paresthesias and who are found to have sensory ataxia, static tremor, and minor distal weakness. Both axonal degeneration and demyelination are notable in nerve biopsy specimens. The serum IgM fraction may demonstrate activity against myelin-associated glycoprotein (MAG).

Variants are the following:

Anti-MAG antibody-associated polyneuropathies, which are slowly progressive but eventually disabling with weakness, sensory loss, and gait disorder.[686]

Hereditary hypertrophic neuropathy with paraproteinemia, a dominantly inherited, slowly progressive polyneuropathy resembling **hereditary motor and sensory neuropathy type 3**, associated with some degree of nerve hypertrophy and accompanied by the presence of abnormal protein (IgD) in the serum and the CSF.[2362, 3374]

Neuropathy associated with monoclonal gammopathy of uncertain significance (MGUS), which are acquired sensorimotor polyneuropathies appearing in adult life, associated mainly with serum and urine monoclonal IgM (less often IgG or IgA) protein expression and characterized by sensory loss, ataxia, and marked nerve conduction abnormalities.[2395] See also **lower motor neuron disease**.

Gamper, E. (1887–1938) Austrian professor of psychiatry and neuropathology at Innsbruck, later working in Prague and Munich.[2066]

Gamper bowing reflex Flexion of the neck and trunk in response to extension of the hips, a response seen in infants with severe brain damage and corticospinal tract disease.[2066]

Gamstorp, Ingrid Swedish pediatric neurologist.

Gamstorp syndrome See **familial periodic paralysis** (*hyperkalemic* form).[2267]

ganglioblastoma A rare, primary malignant tumor of the CNS composed of mature ganglion cells and glial cells and occurring in childhood or youth, mainly in the region of the third ventricle.[6842]

gangliocytoma A rare primary malignant **neuronal tumor** of the CNS occurring in childhood or youth and characterized by the presence of mature neurons with Nissl substance in the cytoplasm and the nuclear characteristics of normal neurons; and supporting glial cells, mainly in the region of the third ventricle. They may stain positively for **glial fibrillary acidic protein** or neurofilament protein. Most are well differentiated.[6842]

ganglioglioma A rare, malignant, slowly growing, circumscribed tumor of the CNS containing both neoplastic astrocytes and neoplastic neuronal cells, found usually in the frontal or temporal lobes.[1057] It presents most often with seizures, and some patients have focal neurological deficits.[6969]

ganglion (Gr, a mass beneath the skin or close to tendons) 1. A swelling along the course of a nerve, normally produced by the presence of synapses in cell relay stations as in the autonomic nervous system, and abnormally by a nerve tumor or tissue laid down locally in the process of nerve regeneration. The basal ganglia are those cell masses such as the caudate and lenticular nuclei, responsible for initiating voluntary motor activity. See also **pseudocyt**. 2. A fibrous mass attached usually to tendons.

ganglion nodosum tumor See **carotid body tumor**.

ganglioneuroblastoma An uncommon primary malignant neuronal tumor occurring in the retroperitoneal or thoracic regions of children or young adults and characterized histologically by the presence of cells showing profuse fibril formation and with fibrovascular strands of tissue running through sheets of cells with small round nuclei, and frequently both astrocytes and ganglion cells.

In the *imperfect type* all stages of differentiation are seen; while in the *immature ganglioneuroblastoma*, different areas suggest **ganglioneuroma** or **neuroblastoma** histologically.[6]

ganglioneurocytoma A rare mixed neuronal and glial tumor that arises in the periventricular regions in and above the posterior fossa.

ganglioneuroma Circumscribed benign tumors consisting of a mixture of neurons, capsule cells, connective tissue, ganglion cells, Schwann cells, and reticulin. Most arise in the posterior mediastinum, on the posterior abdominal wall, or from paraspinal autonomic ganglia.[6084] See **gangliocytoma**.

ganglionitis Inflammatory disease of the dorsal root ganglia, occurring as a result of infection or autoimmune attack or as a **paraneoplastic syndrome**.

ganglionopathy A form of proximal neuropathy usually due to lesions of the small dorsal root ganglion cells and often painful. See **paraneoplastic sensory neuronopathy, Sjögren syndrome**, and **acute sensory neuropathy**. Other causes are described at http://neuromuscular.wustl.edu/antibody/sneuron.html/.

ganglioradiculitis See **subacute sensory neuropathy**.

gangliorhizolysis A technique using radiofrequency waves to induce thermocoagulative lesions in neural structures, such as the V cranial nerve in the management of chronic cluster headache. The smaller pain fibers are selectively destroyed by this method, the larger fibers subserving touch sensation being less or not at all affected.[4186]

gangliosialidosis, dysmorphic type See **sialidosis**.

gangliosides Water-soluble glycosphingolipid components of cell membranes. They have been classified as GM_1, GM_2, GM_3, etc. on the basis of their mobility on thin-layer chromatography and are normally degraded by the hexosaminidase enzymes.

gangliosidoses A group of recessively inherited **lysosomal storage disorders** in which the substances accumulating are **gangliosides** when due to deficiencies of beta-galactosidase (**GM_1-gangliosidoses**) or of *N*-acetyl galactosaminidase (**GM_2-gangliosidoses**). These lead to the accumulation of excessive amounts of ganglioside in neurons ("ballooned cells") and to the neurological manifestations.

Disorders included are **GM_1 and GM_2 gangliosidoses, sulfatide lipidosis, trihexosamide ceramide lipidosis, galactosylceramide lipidosis, glucosylceramide lipidosis, sphingomyelin lipidosis**, and **Kufs** disease.[3586] See also **neuronal ceroid lipofuscinosis**.

GANS syndrome 1. A syndrome presenting in the elderly in which the clinical features of dementia are accompanied by the pathological appearances of **Pick disease**, the atrophic process, however, being confined in this case to the frontal lobes.[5704]

2. (granulomatous angiitis of the nervous system) See **isolated angiitis of the nervous system**.

Gans-Rodiet sign Hemianesthesia of the lateral part of the sclera in cases of chronic alcoholism.[5704]

Ganser, Sigbert Josef Maria (1853–1931) German psychiatrist and neurologist, born in the Rhineland. He trained in Medicine in Wurzburg and Strasburg, and after further training in Munich and practice there and at Sorau, he succeeded **Kraepelin** as the head of the department in Dresden, where he remained for the rest of his life. Apart from the syndrome by which his name is remembered (1897), he also described the basal nucleus (named for Meynert) and twilight states and conducted studies on alcoholism.

Ganser syndrome (hysterical pseudodementia, hysterical twilight state, syndrome of approximate answers, balderdash syndrome) A manifestation of a dissociative reaction in some, of willful malingering in other patients, but not evidence of dementia.[2271] The answers given are often nonsensical but do at least have some relationship to the question, for example, how many legs has a horse?—"Four." And a cow?—"Four." And an ox?—"I don't know." Do you know any other animals?—"Elephant." How many legs has it got?—"Three." The abnormal verbal responses are always in reply to questions, not spontaneous, and indicate that the patient has actually grasped the nature and content of the question.

Ganser's patients were all criminals (or at least accused people in custody) and many also complained of headaches and manifested auditory and visual hallucinations, delusions, and patchy sensory loss. Consciousness was described as normal or clouded. Ganser noted that the syndrome was self-limited, the patients returning to normal in a few days with amnesia for the period, and he thought that this was a form of encephalitis. See also **vorbeireden**.

Ganzfeld electroretinography The recording of the electrical potential changes emanating from the retina by means of corneal surface electrodes, with the patient receiving flashes of light filtered or not according to whether rod or cone activity is sought.

GAPO syndrome See **growth retardation, alopecia, pseudoanodontia**, and **optic atrophy**.[2254]

Garcia–Lurie syndrome See **aproscencephaly**.

Garcin syndrome (syndrome paralytique unilateral global des nerfs craniens, hemi-basal syndrome, Guillain–Garcin syndrome, Bertoletti–Garcin syndrome, Guillain–Alajouanine–Garcin syndrome) Dysfunction of all or nearly all of the cranial nerves on one side, without long tract signs or evidence of increased intracranial pressure and due to infiltration by a local malignancy such as a lymphoepithelioma or sarcoma of the nasopharynx. The syndrome was described briefly by Guillain in 1926[2620] but more completely by Garcin in his graduating thesis in 1927.

gardeners' migraine Vascular-type headaches, repetitively experienced on bending down.

Gardner neuralgia See **petrous neuralgia**.

Gardner syndrome (central or type II neurofibromatosis) A syndrome of dominantly inherited bilateral vestibular neurofibromas without notable peripheral manifestations of von Recklinghausen disease.

Clinically, progressive deafness, tinnitus, and imbalance are the major features. Although the syndrome had been described before, Gardner presented a large series of cases and delineated the condition as closely resembling, but consistently different from, the more common peripheral or type 1 **neurofibromatosis**.[2277] Dr. W.J. Gardner is an American neurosurgeon.

Gareis syndrome The association of mental retardation with absence of the extensors pollices longus, the latter resulting in permanent flexion of the thumbs, with X-linked inheritance.[2283]

Garel syndrome A brainstem vascular syndrome.[421]

gargoyle A carved face on a waterspout, commonly a hideous caricature of a real or mythical being; hence the origin of the pejorative name for patients with dysmorphism due to **mucopolysaccharidoses**.

gargoylism See **Hunter syndrome** and **mucopolysaccharidosis**.

Garland, Hugh Gregory (1903–1967) English neurologist in Leeds who trained at the **National Hospital**. He set up an active neurological department in his home city, where he was recognized as an unique clinical teacher and diagnostician. He is remembered best for his description of proximal **diabetic neuropathy** (diabetic amyotrophy).

Garland amyotrophy See **diabetic neuropathies**.

Garrod, Sir Archibald English physician and chemist who introduced the concept of inborn errors of metabolism in 1908, regarding alkaptonuria, albinism, cystinuria, and pentosuria as fulfilling the criteria.

gas gangrene See **myonecrosis**.

Gaskell, W.H. English physiologist whose researches, compiled in his book *The Involuntary Nervous System* (London, 1916), helped to lay the foundations of knowledge on the functions of the autonomic nervous system.

gasoline-sniffing myopathy A subacutely progressive syndrome of proximal weakness and wasting as a result of intoxication with gasoline.[3547]

Gasparini syndrome Paralysis of cranial nerves V, VI, and VII on one side, with contralateral thermoanalgesia—a condition due to a lesion of the pontine tegmentum.[421]

Gass syndrome A neurocutaneous syndrome characterized by retinal and intracranial cavernous hemangiomas and angiomatous hamartomas of the skin.[2300]

Gasser, Johann Lorenz (1702–1777) Viennese anatomist who, in his graduation thesis, described the sensory ganglion of the trigeminal nerve.

Gasserian ganglion (semilunar ganglion) The sensory ganglion of the V cranial nerve. The appellation was bestowed in 1765 by Antonius Hirsch, an Austrian anatomist, in honor of Gasser whose student he was.

Gastaut, Henri (1915–1995) French neurologist and neurophysiologist in Marseille and University President in Aix, whose major and seminal contributions were in the realm of epilepsy and the EEG. He was the first to describe photosensitive epilepsy and **Gastaut syndrome**.

Gastaut syndrome Unilateral convulsions associated with hemiparesis and generalized seizures with epigastric, pharyngeal, or abdominal auras, occurring in children.[2304] See also **Lennox–Gastaut syndrome**.

Gastaut-type idiopathic childhood occipital epilepsy An uncommon form of benign childhood focal seizures with onset in otherwise normal children, characterized by frequent, mainly elementary, visual hallucinations, blindness, or both. The hallucinations are of small, multicolored circular patterns that appear in the periphery of a visual field, developing within seconds and lasting for up to 3 min. They may co-exist with sensory illusions of ocular movements, ocular pain, tonic deviation of the eyes, and repetitive eye closures. Complex visual hallucinations, visual illusions, and other symptoms that spread anteriorly may terminate with hemi- or generalized convulsions. Temporary ictal blindness and orbital ictal headache occur in a few cases. Consciousness is usually retained unless there is seizure progression.

The interictal EEG may show occipital paroxysms or random occipital spikes, but may be normal.

Remission within 4 years from onset is common but otherwise visual seizures and infrequent secondary generalized tonic–clonic seizures continue, especially if not treated with carbamazepine.[4882]

gastric crises (gastrodynia) Acute, severe attacks of abdominal pain occurring in **tabes dorsalis**. Neuralgia resulting from irritation of the dorsal roots by spirochetes seems the most likely cause. At thoracic levels, a similar pain occurs in some patients with postherpetic neuralgia.

gastrodynia See **gastric crises**.

gate-control theory (of pain) This theory, propounded by Melzack and Wall in 1966, accounts for the fact that, if one rubs a painful place, the pain is lessened. They postulated the existence of a functional "gate" in the region of the substantia gelatinosa of the cord, which closes during thick-fiber activity and opens with thin-fiber activity, allowing onward passage of impulses destined to induce the perception of pain. A central modulating influence was acknowledged as part of the regulatory system to accommodate the everyday observation that distraction diminishes the perception of pain. Proof of the existence of such a mechanism is still wanting, and the theory has been severely criticized but remains acceptable to a large majority of clinical neuroscientists.[4303]

Gaucher, Philippe Charles Ernest (1854–1918) French physician who trained in Paris, where as an intern he described the disease named for him. He was later professor of dermatology at the Hôpital St. Louis in Paris, his research being mainly concerned with the manifestations of tuberculosis, syphilis, and pellagra. See **glucosylceramide lipidosis**.

Gates-MacGinitie Reading Test A standardized test allowing the quantitative assessment of reading ability, used in the examination of patients with dysphasias and to form an estimate of prior intellectual functioning.[2316]

Gaucher cells Cells swollen by the intracytoplasmic accumulation of cerebrosides, giving a foamy appearance, and seen in glucosylceramide lipidosis.

Gaucher disease See **glucosylceramide lipidosis**.

Gayet, Charles-Jules-Alphonse (1833–1904) French neurologist whose description of "acute superior hemorrhagic polioencephalitis" preceded that of **Wernicke** by 6 years .

Gayet disease See **Wernicke–Korsakoff encephalopathy**.

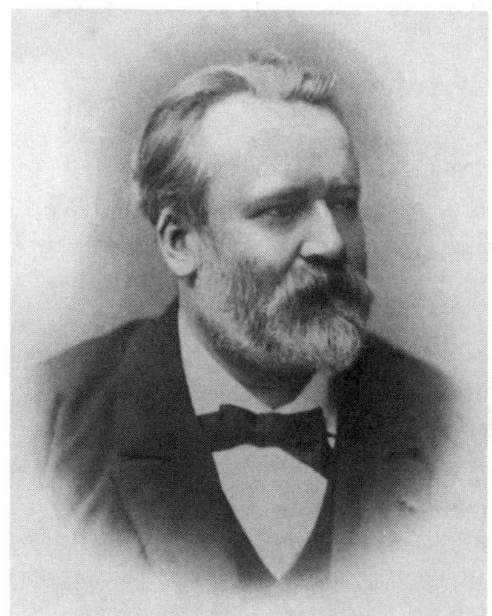

Figure G–1 Charles-Jules-Alphonse Gayet.

Gayet–Wernicke syndrome See **Wernicke–Korsakoff encephalopathy**.

gaze The persistent fixation of vision on an object.

gaze apraxia Inability to direct the eyes in response to a command or to a stimulus presented in visual space. The oculocephalic responses are preserved. The phenomenon is usually seen in the context of **Balint syndrome**, when the lesion is in posterior parietal regions bilaterally; when occurring in isolation, the lesion responsible is thought to be in the frontal eye fields.[2961]

In cases of gaze apraxia, the eyes tend to wander randomly, then either fixating poorly on the target when it is achieved or locking onto the target (*fixation spasm*); pursuit movements and convergence may also be impaired.

gaze palsy A deficit in the yoked deviation of the eyes in any direction as a result of a lesion above the cranial motor nerve nuclei.

gaze-evoked blepharoclonus Repetitive contractions of the facial muscles, with or without associated ocular nystagmus but including bilateral orbicularis spasms, occurring on lateral gaze, reported in some subjects with brainstem multiple sclerosis.[3354]

gaze-evoked nystagmus (gaze-paretic nystagmus, gaze-modulated nystagmus, deviational nystagmus, neurasthenic nystagmus, seducible nystagmus, and setting-in nystagmus) Those forms of acquired, conjugate, symmetrical, and horizontal jerk nystagmus that only appear when the eyes are deviated from the primary position (and which are thus absent in the primary position of gaze). The slow phases show a declining time course. The patients are unable to maintain eccentric fixation, the eyes drifting centrally and jerking laterally. A defect in the step function of the neural firing frequency is considered to be the pathophysiological mechanism.[5] The oscillations are jerky with a centripetal decreasing velocity exponential slow phase taking the eyes away from the fixation point so that they drift away from the desired position, this being followed by a corrective fast jerk to one or other side, depending upon gaze.[5731]

This represents the most common variety of nystagmus, in which the direction (fast phase) of the nystagmus is in the direction of gaze and which is most often due to sedative or anticonvulsant usage, or to various brainstem or cerebellar lesions. Such a nystagmus may be attributed to nerve lesions (gaze-paretic nystagmus) or to muscle disease (muscle-paretic nystagmus).

Gaze-modulated nystagmus is a form of jerk nystagmus that is present in the primary position of gaze but is increased when the subject attempts to maintain an eccentric eye position. **Vestibular nystagmus, latent/manifest latent nystagmus**, and **congenital nystagmus** are of this nature.

gaze-evoked tinnitus The occurrence of tinnitus with most or all forms of eye movement but especially far-lateral gaze and presumably stemming from abnormal new connections between the cochlear and vestibular nuclei due to aberrant sprouting of nerve fibers, since it has been reported after, for example, removal of a cerebellopontine mass with sacrifice of the VIII cranial nerve.[6604]

gaze-modulated nystagmus See **gaze-evoked nystagmus**.

gaze-paretic nystagmus (integrator nystagmus) A form of **gaze-evoked nystagmus** seen in subjects recovering from a transient central paralysis of gaze, in which the deviated eyes show fatigue, drifting toward the mid-line and then abruptly re-positioning with a laterally directed corrective saccade. See also **gaze-evoked nystagmus**.

gegenhalten (Ger, counter-holding) See **paratonia**.

gegenrucke See **square-wave jerks**.

Gehrig, Henry Louis (Lou) (1903–1941) American baseball player who succumbed to **amyotrophic lateral sclerosis** after a spectacular playing career. His name is often applied to the disease.[3319, 4599]

Gehrigopathies Conditions in which inclusion bodies containing ubiquitin are found, for example, **amyotrophic lateral sclerosis** and one form of **frontotemporal dementia**.

gelasmus (from Gr, laughter) Spasmodic or convulsive laughter.

gelastic automatisms In the context of epilepsy, bursts of laughter or giggling, usually without the appropriate affective tone.

gelastic (hypothalamic) seizures (from Gr, laughter) Seizure disorders characterized by bursts of compulsive laughter or giggling, with or without the appropriate affective tone, during the conscious state. It was recognized first by **Trousseau** in 1873.

The same phenomenon also occurs in **multiple sclerosis, amyotrophic lateral sclerosis, lacunar** states, and other causes of spastic bulbar palsy (when it appears to suggest the presence of a lesion in or near the hypothalamus[2638]); as well as in bilateral frontal lobe disease and schizophrenia. Hypothalamic **hamartomas** are characteristically associated with seizures of this type, in which situations precocious puberty and behavioral problems are often also present. They may be a manifestation of several kinds of seizure types such as partial seizures with motor symptoms, myoclonic seizures, axial tonic seizures, flexor spasms, generalized convulsive seizures, and petit mal absences.[1861]

Criteria for the diagnosis suggested by Gascon and Lombroso[2297] comprise the following: stereotyped recurrences; no external precipitants; concomitance of other manifestations generally regarded as epileptic, such as tonic or clonic movements, automatisms, or loss of consciousness; presence of interictal or ictal epileptiform discharges; and absence of neurological signs of other conditions (as above) in which pathological laughter is recorded.

A rare *variant* form is a neonatal or early childhood epileptic disorder with male predominance in which hypothalamic hamartomas manifest with brief **gelastic seizures** and in time lead on to a generalized epileptic encephalopathy with severe seizures and cognitive and behavioral decline. Clinically, mirthless, silent or loud laughter is the defining and initial manifestation. **Dacrystic** (crying) attacks may also occur in a few patients. Ictal impairment of consciousness, ictal autonomic symptoms, and tonic, atonic, generalized tonic–clonic seizures or absences are other features. Most patients develop cognitive and behavioral symptoms and most show precocious puberty. Worsening of seizures and progressive cognitive and behavioral impairment occur in many patients.

gelatio (Lat, freezing) The rigid state of the body in **catalepsy**.

Gélineau, Jean-Baptiste-Edouard (1828–1906) French surgeon and neuropsychiatrist, born near Bordeaux. He trained at the naval medical school in La Rochelle and from 1850 sailed with the French navy in the Indian Ocean as surgeon of the third class. When his thesis on diseases of Black and White people on the Comorro Islands was accepted by the University of Montpelier, he achieved naval promotion, but he relinquished his commission in 1860. Thereafter, he practiced first in southern France and later, after the Franco–Prussian War and with far more success, as a specialist in nervous diseases in Paris, whence came his numerous contributions to the literature both of medicine and of the stage. His full description of narcolepsy was published in 1880.[2325] He also wrote an autobiography and invented and marketed his own pills for epilepsy, with reported success. In 1900, wearying of the profession, he retired to his birthplace, publishing a final book on epilepsy and thereafter devoting himself to viticulture, thus completing an enviably balanced and successful career.[4923]

Gélineau syndrome See **narcolepsy**.

gemistocytic (Lat, goose-grease + cell) Cells having the appearance of goose grease, such as the plump reactive or hypertrophic astrocytes, the cytoplasm of which is filled with filaments and glial fibrillary acidic protein; the nucleus is displaced eccentrically. Such cells are seen most commonly in the white matter in early cases of demyelinating disease.

The degree to which animal husbandry has influenced neuropathology has never been recognized appropriately.

Gelle syndrome The effect of infarction of the caudal ventrolateral pons, comprising homolateral VII and VIII palsies and crossed hemiparesis.[5839]

gemistocytic astrocytoma See **astrocytoma**.

GeneClinics An online resource funded by the NIH and providing in-depth information about genetic diseases.
Web site: http://www.geneclinics.org/.

GeneReviews Peer reviewed, current disease descriptions that apply genetic testing to the diagnosis, management, and genetic counseling of patients and families with specific inherited conditions. Disorders are searchable by disease name, gene symbol, protein name, feature, author, or title and published entirely online. This free, publicly funded (University of Washington, Seattle; NIH) medical genetics information resource was developed for physicians, other healthcare providers, and researchers and is accessible at www.geneclinics.org/profiles.

general acoustic muscle reflex A startle response, manifest by widespread jerking of the body in response to a sudden and unexpected loud sound.

general adaptation syndrome The sum of all the nonspecific systemic reactions of the body which ensue upon long-continued exposure to stress; the staged responses to stress shown by an organism. The first response, the *alarm reaction*, begins with increased sympathetic and adrenal cortical activity. Selye[5719, 5720] described it as the sum of all nonspecific systemic phenomena elicited by sudden exposure to stimuli to which the organism is qualitatively or quantitatively nonadapted. The second stage is the *stage of resistance*, the third the *stage of exhaustion* in which the mechanisms called into play to resist the stress in the first place break down.

general paresis of the insane (Bayle disease, frontotemporo-parietal encephalitic syphilis) A form of subacute encephalitis occurring in patients with tertiary syphilis up to 30 years after the primary infection and characterized by dementia, irritability, a decline in self-care, and later psychotic signs. Intention tremors of the limbs, face, and tongue are common but focal signs rare. The classic grandiose delusional state occurs in no more than 20% of cases. Blood and CSF serology findings invariably confirm the diagnosis. Pathologically, cortical atrophy with gliosis and perivascular mononuclear cell infiltration are typical changes. The organism is sometimes recoverable from the brain.

The condition was first described in detail by **Bayle** in his graduation thesis of 1822,[455] although Esquirol had referred to it in his book on dementia in 1826 and Thomas **Willis** had described many of its features in *De anima brutorum* in 1672. The disease appears to have reached epidemic proportions in Northern France after the Napoleonic wars, but was probably rare before then. Guy de Maupassant and Frederich Nietzsche both suffered from this condition.

The name is a translation of the French *paralysie générale des aliénés*, the term used by Calmeil (1826)[5704]. The Germans used the term *dementia paralytica* and the English and Americans used *general paresis*. Treatment with mercury was all that was available until **Wagner von Jauregg**[6590] introduced malarial (hyperpyrexia) treatment in 1917, for which he was awarded the Nobel Prize in 1927.

General Practice Notebook—Neurology A Web site providing coverage of neurology for primary care physicians, found at: http://www.gpnotebook.co.uk/simplepage.cfm?ID=1107689483.

generalization The propagation of EEG activity from limited areas of the head to all regions of the head.

generalized (bilateral) In the context of epilepsy, a seizure whose initial semiology indicates, or is consistent with, involvement of both cerebral hemispheres.

generalized amyotonia See **Foerster syndrome**.

generalized anhidrosis A rare, congenital or acquired disorder characterized by heat intolerance and loss of sweating, often associated with autonomic peripheral neuropathies. Absent muscle stretch reflexes and pupillary abnormalities may also occur. Intrinsic sweat gland abnormalities and postganglionic sympathetic cholinergic nerve dysfunction present in similar ways, but microneurography may allow their distinction.[1680]

generalized epilepsies and syndromes Epileptic disorders with generalized seizures in which the first clinical changes indicate initial involvement of both hemispheres, and the ictal encephalographic patterns are also bilateral initially. See **absence seizures** and **generalized tonic–clonic seizures**.

A listing is to be found in the Commission for Classification and Terminology, proposal for Revised Classifications of Epilepsies and Epileptic Syndromes. *Epilepsia* 1989;**30**:389–99 (Dreifuss FE, et al.)

generalized epilepsy with febrile seizures plus (GEFS+) Dominantly inherited forms of epilepsy characterized by the first occurrence of febrile seizures around the end of the first year of life. These persist after the age of 6 and may be associated in *variant* forms with tonic–clonic seizures, myoclonus, or absences in the absence of fever. The seizures usually desist in adolescence. Various other seizure types were recorded in the original kinship.[5868]

FEB 1 (OMIM 602476) manifests myoclonus and is linked to 8q. FEB 2 (OMIM 602477) manifests atonic seizures and myoclonic astatic seizures; it maps to 19q 13.1. Yet another *variant* (OMIM 121210) manifests absences in addition to the febrile seizures.[5109] See also **febrile seizures**.

In a *variant* form the condition is associated with autosomal dominant chondrocalcinosis.

generalized gangliosidosis See **GM_1 gangliosidosis**.

generalized hyperhidrosis An abnormal tendency to sweat over the whole of the body surface, as in cases of chronic infection, hyperthyroidism, autonomic neuropathy, pheochromocytoma, carcinoid, diabetes, acromegaly, gout, or hyperpituitarism.

generalized multiple spikes (polyspikes) Multiple spikes or multiple spikes and waves occurring during wakefulness, classically seen in patients with myoclonic epilepsy.

generalized myoclonic status epilepticus Bilaterally synchronous myoclonus of the face, axial musculature, and limbs. The condition is serious; patients with myoclonic status epilepticus rarely recover consciousness.[6924]

generalized myokymia See **neuromyotonia**.

generalized paroxysmal fast activity (fast paroxysmal rhythms, generalized repetitive fast discharge, runs of rapid spikes, generalized rhythmic 15–20 Hz activity, beta band seizure pattern) A rare form of paroxysmal bilateral discharge at high frequency found during sleep in patients who have seizures of various types and who are usually mentally retarded. Clinically, tonic seizures commonly accompany this EEG pattern.[829]

generalized repetitive fast discharge See **generalized paroxysmal fast activity**.

generalized rhythmic 15–20 Hz activity See **generalized paroxysmal fast activity**.

generalized seizures A seizure is considered generalized when clinical symptomatology provides no indication of an anatomical localization and no clinical evidence of focal onset. When possible, three main seizures subtypes may be categorized:[1265]

- Generalized convulsive seizures with predominantly tonic, clonic, or tonic–clonic features.
- Generalized nonconvulsive seizures represented by absence seizure.
- Myoclonic seizures.

generalized sharp- and slow-wave discharges (slow spike-and-wave activity) The presence on the EEG of generalized sharp- and slow-wave complexes occurring at 2–2.5 Hz, frequently with some accompanying behavioral change, and seen in patients with the **Lennox–Gastaut Syndrome**.

generalized spinal muscular atrophy A variant of the usual proximal pattern of spinal muscular atrophy.[4276] See **hereditary motor neuropathy**.

generalized tics Those tics in which the movements affect more than one noncontiguous body part. The disorder may or may not involve vocal tics in a particular case. *Elementary (simple)* and *complex* tics are the other two categories.

generalized tonic–clonic seizure (grand mal seizure, major motor seizure, convulsive fit) A common form of seizure characterized typically by initial loss of consciousness with falling, followed by maximal symmetrical tonic contraction of all the somatic and autonomic muscles. This gives way to clonic contractions after 30–60 s; thereafter, a flaccid phase ensues before automatic (e.g., ventilatory) and voluntary muscle activity and consciousness are re-established over the next few minutes.

generalized xanthomatosis (Hand–Schüller–Christian disease, histiocytosis X, lipoid granulomatosis, craniohypophysial xanthomatosis) See **Hand–Schüller–Christian disease**.

generator The source of an electrical signal.

Genetic Alliance An organization devoted to promoting optimum health care for people suffering from **genetic** disorders. It represents a coalition of more than 600 advocacy organizations serving people affected by 1000 conditions. Web site: http://www.geneticalliance.org/.

Genetic and Rare Conditions Site The online resource of the department of Medical Genetics, University of Kansas Medical Center, Web site: http://www.kumc.edu/gec/support/, which lists lay advocacy and support groups, information on a large number of genetic conditions or birth defects for professionals, educators, individuals, and **National** and **International** organizations.

genetic ataxias A large complex of disorders which have in common the signs of ataxia and the pathology of degeneration of the cerebellum and/or its connections, as well as of other CNS areas in some cases. There is often pathological and phenotypic variability and overlapping, and biochemical markers are only available in a few cases. See **cerebellar ataxias** and their *variants*.

geniculate herpes See **Ramsay Hunt syndromes**. Hunt's supposition of the site of the lesion has not been verified pathologically.

geniculate neuralgia See **Ramsay Hunt syndrome**.

geniculocalcarine blindness Loss of vision due to bilateral lesions of the occipital lobes, as may result from bilateral posterior cerebral artery infarction, anoxia, trauma, migraine, demyelination, etc. See **Anton syndrome**.

geniculocalcarine pathways The fiber tracts passing from the lateral geniculate bodies to the occipital lobes, some through the temporal lobe and some through the parietal.

geniospasm (chin trembling or quivering) A rare, dominantly inherited syndrome with onset in infancy or early childhood, mapped to chromosome 9q13–q21. Clinically, it is characterized by vertical movements of the tip of the chin and quivering of the lower lip occurring spontaneously or with stress, concentration, or emotion, lasting minutes at a time. Nocturnal tongue biting may also occur. See also **oral–facial–digital syndrome**.

genital reflexes Penile erection and ejaculation produced by cerebral inducement or as a result of stimulation of the penis. Exaggeration of the reflex in response to peripheral stimulation occurs as part of the **mass reflex**.

The **superficial anal, internal anal, cremasteric, scrotal,** and **bulbocavernosus reflexes** are also so classified.

genitofemoral neuralgia See **ilioinguinal neuralgia**.

genitofemoral neuropathy A rare entrapment syndrome causing pain and paresthesia in the territory of the genitofemoral nerve, and possibly loss of the cremasteric reflex, usually as a result of tight compression from clothing, following appendicitis or with other local pathology.[4014] See also **blue jeans syndrome**.

genius (Lat, the tutelary spirit of a person—or guardian angel) 1. An inborn faculty for an aspect of mental activity; a special or peculiar characteristic. 2. A person possessed of such attributes to an exceptional degree.

Gennari, Francesco (1750–1795) A physician in Padua whose name is given to the striated occipital cortex (the Striae Genarii), which represents the outer portion of the **Baillarger** line and which he described in 1782 (while still a medical student) as the *lineola albidor*.[1670]

genomic imprinting Variability of the clinical features of a heritable disease according to which parent supplied the defective gene.

geno-neurodermatoses See **phakomatoses**.

genu (Lat, knee) A bend in part of an anatomical structure. Derivations from the word are applied to the geniculate bodies, to part of the internal capsule, and to the geniculate ganglion on account of their curvatures or their situation within another curved structure.

genu inversum See **genu valgum**.

genu recurvatum Hyperextension of the knee.

genu valgum (genu inversum, knock-knees) Lateral flexion of the knee such that the two knees approximate and the ankles are separated.

genu varum (bow-leggedness) The opposite of **genu valgum**, in which the knees are separated and the ankles approximate.

genus A class of organisms with similar characteristics within which subclasses called *species* exist.

geophagy (Gr, earth + pagein: to eat) (pica) A tendency to eat earth.

geotropic (earthward) eye and head movements Head and eye deviation remains downward with axial rotation of a subject by 180°.

geotropic nystagmus A form of nystagmus in which the direction of the fast phase is toward the center of the earth. See **vestibular nystagmus**.

Gerhardt, Karl Adolf Christian Jacob (1833–1902) German physician, professor of medicine successively at Jena, Wurzberg, and Berlin. Although he was particularly interested in croup and laryngeal lesions, he also described erythromelalgia and wrote on aspects of the physical examination.

Gerhardt law With paralysis of the vocal cords due to lesions of the recurrent laryngeal nerve, the cords assume a position midway between adduction and abduction.[3373]

Gerhardt syndrome Bilateral adductor paralysis of the larynx due to bilateral lesions of the X cranial nerve at the brainstem or skull base and leading to severe dysphonia and dyspnea.[2330] Familial forms have also been described.

In a *variant* form, cerebellar atrophy and pure motor neuropathy are associated.[387]

Geriatric Depression Scale A 30-item self-report questionnaire developed from 100 questions commonly used to diagnose depression, mainly in elderly people. The ratings are performed by the physician, the patient or an observer. A short form is also available for the subject to score himself.[6913]

A screening test for depression in the elderly is also available.[661]

Geriatric Evaluation by Relatives Rating Instrument (GERRI) A rating scale using which "significant others" can rate attributes of elderly outpatients who show symptoms of mental decline. The instrument includes 49 sentences describing potential cognitive, emotional, or behavioral abnormalities; items are rated on a 5-point frequency scale.[5674]

Geriatric Rating Scale Designed for use by nonprofessional ward staff, this reliable 31-item scale rates patients' behavior in the activities of daily living. The scale yields seven factors including confusion, memory and orientation, activity and communications, sleep, mood, eating, and psychotic symptoms and also notes disturbing behavior. It is of greatest value in the assessment of a change in behavior in severely demented inpatients.[5055]

Geriatric Self-care Scale An instrument for assessing the residual capacities of elderly infirm people.[3606]

Gerlach, Joseph von (1820–1896) German histologist in Mainz who in 1858 introduced the carmine stain for neuronal cell bodies, the first specific stain discovered.

Gerlier disease (kubisagari, paralytic vertigo) An epidemic summer disorder in Alpine areas described first by Felix Gerlier. It is manifest by transient headache; vertigo; photophobia; nerve trunk pain; and weakness of the oculomotor muscles, the neck extensors, and muscles of the face, larynx, pharynx, and back.

Its occurrence in people exposed to cattle or horses suggests that this may have been a form of brucellosis.[2332] The disease now seems to have disappeared from Europe but has been noted in Japan. See also **vertige paralysant**.

Gerlier, Felix (1840–1914) Swiss physician.

germ cell tumor Potentially malignant tumors of the pineal region, including **teratomas, germinomas, embryonal carcinomas, choriocarcinomas**, and **endodermal sinus tumors**. In each case, the tumor is characterized by an elevation of CSF α-fetoprotein and plasma β-human chorionic gonadotrophin or melanotonin levels.[669]

germinal zone (ventricular germinal zone, subependymal zone, subependymal cell plate) That part of the neural tube which generates neuronal and glial precursors destined to migrate and become the cortex and white matter, respectively.

germinoma (seminoma-like tumor, atypical teratoma) A tumor of the pineal gland or of the suprasellar space, composed of large polygonal cells with large nuclei, coarse chromatin, prominent nucleoli, and eosinophilic cytoplasm, and small T-cell lymphocytes. The tumor occurs mainly in young adult males and is capable of metastasis within the nervous system.[6]

geromarasmus (Gr, old age + decay) The muscle thinning and weakness found in many aged people.

GERRI See **Geriatric Evaluation by Relatives Rating Instrument**.

Gerstmann, Josef (1887–1969) Austrian neuropsychiatrist who studied at Vienna and then became first assistant to von Jauregg in the Viennese Psychiatric Clinic. During the World War I, he served in the medical corps in the Italian Alps, attending to a number of soldiers and others who had suffered brain damage incurred in avalanches. He later became professor and head of the neuropsychiatric unit in Vienna in 1928 but emigrated to America 10 years later to escape Nazi persecution. There he held senior posts in clinical and research psychiatry in Maryland, Washington, and New York.

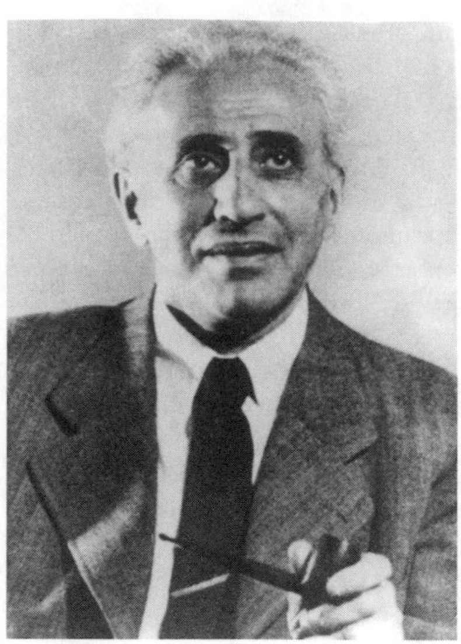

Figure G–2 Josef Gerstmann.

His earlier work was on the cerebral pathology accompanying paralyses, and he published a book on the malarial treatment of **general paresis of the insane**. He described finger agnosia in 1924, and the full syndrome, now named for him, 6 years later. The French ophthalmologist Antoine-Jules Badal (1840–1929) had reported (in 1888) on finger agnosia with inferior quadrantanopia, right-left disorientation, alexia, agraphia, and visual disorientation, but he regarded all of these as manifestations of psychic blindness.

Gerstmann also published an account of frontal gait ataxia which he considered was due to damage of the frontopontocerebellar tract. He also published descriptions of the following conditions.

Gerstmann syndromes 1. (Badal–Gerstmann syndrome, angular gyrus syndrome) The combination of right-left disorientation, acalculia, agraphia, and finger agnosia, due to a lesion of the left angular gyrus. **Asymbolia** for pain and constructional apraxia are occasionally added.

The association of these four main features has consistent localizing value to the angular gyrus, but whether the appearance of fragments of the syndrome has the same meaning is disputed.[527] Gerstmann developed the concept of a body image with visual, tactile, and somatesthetic components at the start of his 1924 paper, and considered that the cortical representation of at least part of this was in the left angular gyrus.[2334] Badal's description in 1888 was less complete but his name is sometimes added.

2. A paranoid psychosis with auditory hallucinations in patients with **general paresis of the insane**, as a result of malarial therapy, described by Gerstmann in 1924.

The Web site http://www.ninds.nih.gov/disorders/gerstmanns/gerstmanns.htm is devoted to the condition.

Gerstmann–Schilder syndrome

Gait apraxia and dysequilibrium as a result of frontal lobe lesions but resembling cerebellar ataxia. The difference between their findings and those of **Bruns** (which they acknowledge) is unclear. They ascribed the clinical disturbances to damage to the endings of the frontopontocerebellar tracts.

Gerstmann–Straussler–Scheinker syndrome

(spinocerebellar ataxia with dementia and plaque-like deposits) A rare, transmissible and usually familial spongiform encephalopathy marked by amyloid deposits associated with any one of many potential prion protein mutations and presenting in early adult life with progressive spinocerebellar ataxia, Parkinsonism, pyramidal signs, impaired smooth pursuit eye movements, and dementia. Numerous mutations are described on the prion protein gene at chromosome 20pter–p12, as in **Creutzfeldt–Jakob disease** and **fatal familial insomnia**, but in most cases there is a mutation at codon 102 of the *PNRP* amyloid gene on chromosome 20.

Pathologically, there are plaque-like deposits in the cerebral and cerebellar cortex and in the central gray nuclei. These contain the **kuru**-type amyloid protein and thus resemble the plaques of **Alzheimer disease**. This condition, described first by **Gerstmann** et al. in 1936,[2335] has also been considered to be a familial (dominantly inherited) *variant* of **Creutzfeldt–Jakob disease**.[3621] See also **cerebral amyloid angiopathy**.

In a *variant* of the condition itself, an inherited prion disease with codon 105 (Pro to Leu) mutation, progressive dementia, spasticity, and gait disturbance occur without myoclonus, cerebellar signs, or periodic synchronous discharges; amyloid plaques are found throughout the cerebral cortex but there are no spongiform changes.[3461]

Geschwind, Norman (1926–1984)

American neurologist who, before and after war service, trained in neurology at Harvard and thereafter at the **National Hospital** and in Boston, eventually being appointed James Jackson Putnam Professor of Neurology at Harvard, professor of psychology at the Massachusetts Institute of Technology, and chief of neurology at the Boston City Hospital, later at the Beth Israel Hospital in Boston.

In Boston, he established the Aphasia Research Center, thus reflecting both his administrative powers and his particular interest in behavioral neurology. The breadth of scope of his publications revealed his eclecticism and wide-ranging expertise in many areas of neurology. His particular contributions concerned the **disconnection syndromes** (which he identified and named), epilepsy, the organic basis of some psychiatric phenomena, lateralization, cerebral dominance and brain asymmetries, and the apraxias and aphasias. He revitalized the field of aphasiology in the 1960s and created the current school of behavioral neurologists in the United States. A renowned teacher with a skill for synthesis, he simplified the literature on aphasia and returned the field to its original clinicopathological methods.

In addition, he was revered in his lifetime for his personal qualities and as a teacher and clinician. He was blessed both with insatiable curiosity and the ability to nourish its fruits.[1434, 4331]

Gesner, Johann August Philipp

(1738–1801) Physician in Rothenburg who in 1769 produced the first modern account of dysphasia, which he called "speech amnesia."

gestalt An unverbalized mental impression of the totality rather than the ingredients of a situation or event, whereby the whole is seen as greater than the sum (or indeed the nature) of its parts.

gestational age Age since conception. The neurological signs allowing estimation of gestational age have been standardized by Dubowitz and Goldberg.[1728]

gestational assessment A systematized evaluation of body and neurologic characteristics, the latter including posture, **square window**, ankle dorsiflexion, arm recoil, leg recoil, popliteal angle, **heel to ear flexion, scarf sign, head lag**, and **ventral suspension** on all grades between 0 and 5.[1728]

gestational epilepsy The occurrence of seizures exclusively during (usually the first) pregnancy or in the postpartum period.

geste antagonistique

(counterpressure) Stimulation of a body part in order to reverse persistent wayward muscle contractions producing an abnormal posture, as in the expression of a focal dystonia.

An example of such a trick movement is putting a finger lightly on the chin—a maneuver which may be used to straighten the head on the neck in some patients with **spasmodic torticollis**.

gestural automatisms Often unilateral fumbling or exploratory movements with the hand directed toward the self or the environment. The movements resemble those intended to lend emotional tone to speech.

gestures Within the context of communicating information, movements used to lend further emotional tone to speech. The comprehension of the message in such movements is largely a function of the right hemisphere. In short, a movement made in order to emphasize verbal utterances, whether or not the latter are actually expressed.[1337]

geusis (Gr, tasting) The sense of taste.

Geyelin–Penfield disease

Dominantly inherited calcific endarteritis affecting the brain arterioles in the region of the junction between the gray and white matter.

Mental retardation after the age of 2 years, polymorphic seizures patterns, and pupillary constriction or dilation are the main clinical features. The condition sometimes leads to early death.[2343]

GFAP See **glial fibrillary acidic protein.**

ghost fibers Myofibrils that do not react in any histochemically stained enzyme preparations. These are occasionally seen in cases of polymyositis.

ghost image The blurred appearance of an object viewed by a person with monocular diplopia resulting from refractive errors of the ocular media.

Giacci syndrome The **mutilating acropathy** resulting from a sensory neuropathy or myelodysplasia.

Gianelli sign See **Tournay sign.**

giant axonal neuropathy A rare, recessively inherited disorder characterized by accumulations of 10-nm peripheral cytoplasmic neurofilaments within Schwann cells in peripheral nerves, giving rise to focal axonal swellings (spheroids), which may also be found in the CNS and in skin fibroblasts. The responsible gene maps to 16q 24,[1572] coding for gigaxonin.

The typical clinical presentation is in a child with gait disorder and ichthyosis, unusually kinky hair and progressive development of seizures, sensory neuropathy, ophthalmoplegia, bulbar weakness, ataxia, intellectual failure, optic atrophy, nystagmus, and pyramidal signs. A slowly progressive, mixed, axonal, and demyelinating sensorimotor peripheral neuropathy;[547] extensive white matter demyelination on MRI scans; EEG abnormalities; nephropathy; and precocious puberty are also recorded.

giant cell arteritis (cranial arteritis, temporal arteritis, Horton arteritis) A systemic vasculitis with a particular predilection for the branches of the external carotid artery and the ophthalmic and posterior ciliary arteries, which show a segmental panarteritis. Clinically, it may cause malaise, fever, weight loss, generalized or localized headaches, and permanent or temporary visual loss, diplopia, jaw muscle ischemia, neuropathies, and stroke syndromes in patients over the age of 55 years, many of whom have symptoms of **polymyalgia rheumatica.**[2478] **Ischemic optic neuritis** and central artery occlusion are potential causes of permanent blindness.[1050, 3001] In some cases, recessive inheritance is noted.

In a *variant* form, peripheral neuropathy also occurs and responds equally well to steroids.[6645]

giant cell astrocytoma See **astrocytoma.**

giant cell fibrosarcoma (monstrocellular sarcoma) See **astrocytoma.**

giant cell myositis, myasthenia, and myocarditis A rare syndrome in which these features occur in the presence of thymoma.[4588]

giant Lambl excrescences Unusually large filiform outgrowths from the free borders of cardiac valves, able to act as a source of cerebral or peripheral emboli. Normally, such outgrowths are small and innocuous.[4672]

giant motor unit action potential A motor unit action potential with a peak-to-peak amplitude and duration much greater than the range found in corresponding muscles in normal subjects of similar age. Quantitative measurements of amplitude and duration are preferable. (From the 2001 Report of the Nomenclature Committee of the American Association of Electromyography and Electrodiagnosis.[19] Reproduced by kind permission of the AANEM, which however discourages the use of the term.)

giant pyramidal cells (Betz cells) Large triangular cells in the fifth layer of the motor cortex described in 1874 by Vladimir Betz (1834–1894), a Russian anatomist.[5619]

giant somatosensory evoked potential Enlarged somatosensory evoked potentials seen as a characteristic of cortical reflex myoclonus and reflecting cortical hyperexcitability.[19] Such large cortically recorded potentials occur 40–60 ms before the EMG activity in patients with **minipolymyoclonus** or **cortical tremor** and are best revealed in frontal or parietal regions by jerk-locked averaging.[3272]

Gibbon classification A widely accepted proposal for the classification of micturition disorders on a neurological basis, adapted by Gibbon from the classification of Bors.[2363]

gibbus (Lat, a hump) The acute flexor angulation of the vertebral column in destructive diseases of the spine.

Chart G–2. Gibbon Classification of Micturition Disorders

1. *Suprasacral (upper motor neuron) lesion*
   a. *Uninhibited neurogenic bladder* The result of an incomplete lesion, leading to early detrusor contractions and desire to void with low residual urine. The sacral reflex arc is preserved.
   b. *Reflex neurogenic bladder* The result of a complete lesion, with early detrusor contractions but without a desire to void. Residual urine volumes may be high. The sensation of a full bladder may be retained through sympathetic afferent pathways. Again, the sacral reflex arc is preserved.
2. *Sacral lesion*
   a. Motor (lower motor neuron) (*motor neurogenic bladder*) There are no detrusor contractions but the desire to void and the sensation of a full bladder are retained. The residual urinary volume is large.
   b. Sensory (*sensory neurogenic bladder*) There are neither detrusor contractions nor any desire to void. Residual urine volumes may be high. The sensation of a full bladder is lost.
   c. Motor and Sensory (*autonomous neurogenic bladder*) There are neither detrusor contractions nor any desire to void. Residual urine volumes may be high. The sensation of a full bladder is retained through sympathetic afferent pathways.
3. Mixed

From Gibbon NO. Nomenclature of neurogenic bladder. J Urology *1976;8:423–31.© Elsevier. Reproduced by kind permission.* See also **Bors–Comarr** system.

Gibbs, Frederick American electrophysiologist who was the first to describe, in 1935, the 3-Hz spike-and-wave EEG pattern of petit mal epilepsy.[2367]

giddy (from Saxon, to be merry) Having the sensation of turning or unsteadiness; a popular term for many sensations including vertigo, light-headedness, imbalance, etc.

Gifford, H. (1858–1929) American ophthalmologist who trained with **Horner** in Zurich and practiced in Omaha. He described lid-lag in hyperthyroidism independently of **von Graefe**, as well as the following phenomenon.

Gifford reflex Pupillary constriction with attempted tight eye closure (a normal phenomenon). See **Westphal–Piltz phenomenon**.

Gigli, Leonardo (1863–1908) Italian surgeon and gynecologist who, in 1894, invented the flexible wire saw named for him for the performance of pubiotomy, although the saw is now used rather for craniotomy.

Gignoux syndrome A syndrome of the low brainstem.[421]

Gilford, Hastings (1861–1941) English obstetrician and pediatrician whose paper on **progeria** appeared in 1914.

Gilles de la Tourette, Georges See **Tourette**.

Gilles de la Tourette syndrome See **Tourette syndrome**.

Gillespie syndrome A congenital cerebellar ataxic syndrome due to cerebellar and brainstem hypoplasia. Associated features include dilated pupils due to partial aniridia, delayed milestones, and mental retardation.[2382] Both sporadic and dominantly inherited cases have been reported; recessive transmission is rare. See **cerebellar syndromes** (congenital ataxias).

Gilliatt, Roger William (1922–1991) English neurologist, first professor of clinical neurology in the Institute of Clinical Neurology at the **National Hospital** in London. His work centered upon the morphology and electrophysiology of the peripheral nervous system.

ginklose An Icelandic term for neonatal tetanus.[5103]

girdle (from Saxon, a waistband) 1. The parts of the body centered upon the pelvis or the shoulder, with particular reference to the muscles which move, respectively, the femur and the humerus. 2. A band around any part of the trunk, in which case the term is usually employed to describe the distribution of a radicular pain, as in diabetic truncal neuropathy, tabes dorsalis, or herpes zoster.

Giroux syndrome A dominantly inherited congenital dysmorphic syndrome manifesting also skin erythema, papules, and hyperkeratosis. Dysarthria, gait and limb ataxia, and hyporeflexia appear later, in adult life.[2394]

Gitelman syndrome A recessively inherited renal tubular disorder producing hypokalemia, metabolic alkalosis, hypomagnesemia, and hypocalciuria. Its neuromuscular symptoms include cramps, muscle weakness, and capopedal spasm.[4657]

gitterzellen See **compound granular corpuscles**.

glabella (from Lat, smooth, bald) The hairless space between the eyebrows. In **synophrys**, hair grows across this space.

glabellar tap See **orbicularis oculi reflex**.

glairy (from Lat, egg-white) Slimy. The fluid contents of some cysts (such as **craniopharyngiomas**) are so-described.

Glasgow Assessment Schedule A simple, brief, problem-oriented scale assessing impairments and disabilities in the fields of *personality change, subjective complaints, occupational functioning, cognition, neurological deficits, and activities of daily living*. The cognitive and neurological assessments are abbreviated—most items being rated only as normal, moderately severe, or severe, but are probably very reliable.[3884]

Glasgow Coma Scale A widely adopted scale for assessment of the depth and duration of impaired consciousness and coma. The features in Chart G–3 are scored.[6243]

Chart G–3. Glasgow Coma Scale

Ability to open the eyes

4 Spontaneously
3 To Speech
2 To Pain
1 None

Best motor response

6 Obeying commands
5 Localizing stimuli
4 Withdrawal
3 Flexor posturing
2 Extensor posturing
1 No movement

Best verbal response to stimulation

5 Oriented
4 Confused, Inappropriate
3 Incomprehensible words
2 Sounds only
1 None

From Teasedale G, Jennett B. Assessment of coma and impaired consciousness. A practical scale. Lancet *1974;2:81–4. Reprinted with kind permission from Elsevier Science.*

Variants of the scale include the **Glasgow–Liege Scale** and the **Reaction Level Scale**.

The scale has been modified for children as shown in Chart G–4.

Chart G–4. Modification of the Glasgow Coma Scale for Children

Best verbal response	
Appropriate words or social smiles, fixes on and follows objects	5
Cries but is consolable	4
Persistently irritable	3
Restless, agitated	2
Silent	1

The remainder of the scale is scored as for adults. See also **Children's Coma Scale**.

Glasgow Head Injury Outcome Prediction Program A prognostic tool based upon an algorithmic evaluation of the outcomes in head-injured subjects.[4682]

Glasgow–Liège Scale A variant of the **Glasgow Coma Scale** in which a 6-point scale recording the status of certain brainstem reflexes (such as the presence of vertical **doll's-eye movements**) is added to the original.[751]

Glasgow Outcome Scale A tool for categorizing the outcome in patients after severe head injuries with the following categories:

1. *Death*
2. **Persistent vegetative state**: No evidence of meaningful responsiveness
3. *Severe disability* (conscious but disabled): Patients who are dependent for daily support by reason of mental or physical disability or both
4. *Moderate disability* (disabled but independent): Patients with intellectual, personality, and neurological deficits who nevertheless are capable of traveling by public transport and who can work in a sheltered environment
5. *Good Recovery*: Resumption of normal life despite minor neurological and psychological deficits[3205]

(Reprinted from Jennett B, Bond M. Assessment of outcome after severe brain damage. Lancet 1975;1:480–2 with kind permission from Elsevier Science).

In an extended version, items 3, 4, and 5 are divided between lower and upper levels of disability or recovery, thus giving a scale with 8 levels.

glaucoma (from Gr, silvery-green) A disease characterized by increased intraocular pressures, often with vitreous opacities. Open-angle and closed-angle glaucoma are described. The word was used by Hippocrates probably to describe cataract, and it continued in that role until Brisseau defined the difference between cataract and glaucoma in 1709. Von **Graefe** devised iridectomy in 1855 for treating glaucoma.

Glees stain A silver salt method of staining axons and their terminations.

glia A term for those cells which are interspersed between the neurons within the CNS, comprising protoplasmic and fibrous astrocytes, oligodendroglia (collectively known as *neuroglia*), and microglial cells. The term was introduced by **Virchow** in 1854.

glial degenerations See **glioneuronal dystrophies.** Conditions with their onset in infancy or childhood, and characterized by seizures, myoclonus, mental deterioration, nystagmus, blindness, and deafness.[3191] The disorders subsumed under this heading include *spongy degenerations* such as **Canavan disease**; *progressive neuronal degenerations* such as **Alpers disease**; and *gliovasal diseases*, in which the process initially affects the astroglia but also engenders an inflammatory reaction leading, outside the CNS, to hepatopathy. **Zellweger disease** is an example of the last disorder.

glial fibrillary acidic protein (GFAP) Normally a protein present only within astrocytes in the CNS, but also immunohistochemically demonstrable in the cells of astrocytomas, ependymomas, papillomas, and oligodendrogliomas but not in those of brain metastases.[1860] In neuropathology, the protein is used as a marker for astroglia.

glial star Microglial ingestion of, for example, dead anterior horn cells.

glioblastoma multiforme A rapidly expanding, malignant, invasive neuroectodermal tumor of the cerebral hemispheres arising in adult life and characterized histologically by the presence of small bipolar anaplastic cells, pleomorphism, necrosis, lack of areas of differentiation of the tumor cells, **pseudopalisading**, and capillary endothelial proliferation.

Monstrocellular glioblastomas are characterized by the presence of bizarre eosinophilic giant cells in addition to the ones just described. *Gliosarcomas* are further variants in which reticulin-containing spindle cells and poorly differentiated astrocytic cells are intermixed. *Gliomatosis cerebri* is characterized by the diffuse invasion of wide areas of the brain by small spindle-shaped anaplastic glial cells.[6] In all cases, death occurs within 2 years.

In a *variant familial form*, the responsible gene maps to 10p12–q23.2.

glioma (From Gr, glue + tumor) Histologically malignant tumors of the neuroglial elements of the central nervous system, the "glue" here referring to the glial matrix of the CNS. The name was applied by Virchow in 1869.[5886]

According to Bailey,[334] the term includes astroglial gliomas (astrocytomas, anaplastic **astrocytomas, glioblastoma multiforme**, spongioblastoma multiforme, and gliosarcoma), oligodendrogliomas, gangliogliomas, ependymomas, and medulloblastomas.

See also **grading** and **brainstem glioma**.

gliomatosis cerebri A rare form of astrocytoma characterized by the diffuse cellular overgrowth of neoplastic neuroglial elements throughout the cerebral hemispheres, brainstem, and spinal cord. The architecture of the surrounding tissues is preserved. Clinical features of note are a long history of seizures, later memory loss, and eventually increased intracranial pressure but with few focal signs. This name has replaced the former term for the condition, *reticulum cell sarcoma*.[4639] See also **primary diffuse leptomeningel gliomatosis**.

gliomesodermal reaction Formation of a fibrous capsule in which there is a predominance of astrocytes, as occurs around a cerebral abscess.

gliomyosarcoma An intracranial tumor composed of mixed glial and sarcomatous elements and containing rhabdomyoblasts. The tumor constitutes some 8% of all glioblastomas.[6018, 2452]

glioneuronal dystrophies (Seitelberger disease) Conditions with onset in infancy or childhood and which are characterized clinically by seizures, myoclonus, progressive psychomotor deterioration, nystagmus, hypokinetic movements, hypotonia, limb and cranial nerve palsies, deafness, and optic atrophy with blindness. The condition may be a variant of **neuronal degeneration with brain iron accumulation**.

The prototype is a progressive neurodegenerative condition of unknown cause characterized by early delay in mental and motor milestones and the presence of myoclonic, focal, and generalized seizures. Spastic or flaccid motor weakness, abnormal movements, cerebellar ataxia, blindness, deafness, decerebration, and death before the age of 7 years are the usual features.[3191]

Pathologically, the condition is notable for spongy degeneration of the gray matter, especially of the isocortex, with neuronal loss, diffuse astrogliosis, spongy changes in the deep gray nuclei, and atrophy of the cerebellum.

Other disorders subsumed under this heading include *spongy degenerations* such as **Canavan disease**; recessively inherited *progressive neuronal degenerations* such as **Alpers disease**; and *gliovasal diseases*, in which the process initially affects the astroglia but also engenders an inflammatory reaction leading, outside the CNS, to hepatopathy. **Zellweger disease** is an example of the last disorder.

gliosis (astrocytosis, astrogliosis) The process of structural repair within the CNS whereby astrocytes produce intracytoplasmic filaments, leading to a local increase of neuroglial fibers in response to local tissue destruction. The severity of the process is in proportion to the proximity of the reacting cells to any form of brain injury. Edema and minor degrees of ischemia are also associated with swelling of the astrocytes and the formation of new neuroglial fibers.

glissade (postsaccadic drift) A slow, smooth sliding or drift of the eyes following a voluntary saccade, in which failure of the pulse part of the **pulse-step** signal leads to a hypometric **saccade**, the remainder of the required movement being engineered by the step portion of the signal.[330]

Disease of the vestibulocerebellar connections as in **internuclear ophthalmoplegia** is usually responsible, but glissades also occur in fatigued normal subjects.[330]

glissadic overshoot See **saccade**.

gloating (schadenfreude, malicious joy) An emotion reflecting one's assessment of the consequences of the (mis)fortunes of others, found to be particularly impaired in patients with ventromedial prefrontal lesions. The converse is *envy*.[5756]

global aphasia The most severe form of aphasia, characterized by severe impairment of *fluency* with sparse, short, perseverated, and stereotyped phrases and also of *naming*, *comprehension*, and *repetition*, such that the patients can neither formulate speech nor comprehend language. The features are thus those of a combination of **Broca** and **Wernicke** aphasia. Automatic speech may be preserved. The condition is due to a large lesion of the entire perisylvian region damaging both frontal and parietal language areas, as with mainstem middle cerebral artery infarction. In the classic form, there is an associated right hemiplegia.

In a *variant* subgroup, the temporal and parietal regions are unaffected, and the language disorder evolves into **Broca aphasia**.[1431]

global aprosodia See **aprosodia**.

Global Assessment of Psychiatric Symptoms A scale developed to measure changes in the symptoms and behavioral characteristics of psychiatric problems in elderly people. (Raskin A, Crook T. Psychopharmacol Bull 1988;24(4):721–5.)

Global Deterioration Scale A descriptive scale rating the severity of cognitive decline and functional impairment in normal aging and in subjects with **Alzheimer disease**, using information obtained both from the patient and from a caregiver. Strong, significant relationships between decline on this scale and numerous behavioral or investigational abnormalities have been demonstrated.

Seven levels of cognitive functioning are rated, extending from (1) no cognitive decline; (2) mild (with subjective forgetfulness); (3) moderate (early confusion—difficulty at work, in speech, or when traveling in unfamiliar areas, detectable by family, and with a subtle deficit in memory on examination); (4) moderately severe (late confusion—decreased ability to travel, to count, and to remember current events); (5) severe (early dementia—needing assistance to choose clothes, disorientation to time or place, and decreased recall of the names of grandchildren); (6) very severe decline (needing supervision in eating and toileting, incontinence, and disorientation to time, place, and perhaps person); to (7) late dementia (with incontinence, severe loss of speech and motor rigidity). For each of these stages full definitions are given. The scale is not specific for any form of dementia and is best used for staging and the followup evaluation of therapy.[5253, 5254]

Global Dystonia Rating Scale An instrument for this purpose, accessible at the Web site: http://www.mdvu.org/library/ratingscales/dystonia/gds.pdf/.

global inattention See **motor impersistence**.

globoid-cell leukodystrophy See **Krabbe leukodystrophy**.

globus hystericus (Lat, globus, a ball) A sensation of choking as if upon a ball lodged in the throat, with tightness at the level of the larynx, and sometimes accompanied by actual spasm of the pharyngeal muscles.[2531] The complaint is a classic symptom of **conversion reactions**.

glomus jugulare (Lat, a ball of thread + neck) The region below the base of the skull where chemoreceptor chromaffin cells are sited within a dilatation of the internal jugular vein.

glomus jugulare tumor A highly vascular tumor derived from the nonchromaffin chemoreceptor cells of the jugular bulb or along the IX or X cranial nerves, described by Masson in 1924.

Adult females are most often affected. Clinical features include complaints of pulsating tinnitus and pain below the ear, evidence of damage to cranial nerves VII, VIII, IX, and XII, and a mass over which a bruit may be heard. Extension of the tumor into the posterior fossa leads to evidence of cerebellar disease, a **Horner syndrome**, and/or pareses of the V and the phrenic nerves, depending upon the direction of tumor growth. A vascular polyp may be seen in the external auditory meatus.[4743, 5967] See **chemodactoma**.

glossa (Gr, the tongue) 1. The tongue. 2. The faculty of speech.

Glosso- is the usual prefix to words signifying conditions that relate to the tongue.

glossagra See **glossalgia**.

glossalgia (glossagra) Pain in the tongue.

glossodynia Pain felt in the tongue, an occasional symptom of vitamin B deficiency but sometimes a manifestation of psychopathology. See **burning mouth syndrome**.

glossolabiolaryngeal palsy See **bulbar palsy**.

glossolalia "Speaking in tongues"; the enunciation of sentences using strings of words that are not part of the subjects' normal language. This occurs in both schizophrenia and nonschizophrenic states, such as those of religious or other ecstatic experience.

glossolaryngos-capulopharyngeal hemiplegia See **Collet–Sicard syndrome**. It is this kind of compound word which provides the justification for eponyms.

glossopharyngeal nerve (Gr, the tongue + the throat) Galen's sixth pair of cranial nerves, but thought to be part of the vagus by Willis and defined as the ninth pair by **Soemerring**.

glossopharyngeal neuralgia (Reichert syndrome, tympanic plexus neuralgia) Brief paroxysms of lancinating or burning pain in the throat, posterior tongue, and ear, often intense and with trigger zones in the throat but also precipitated by talking, chewing, or swallowing. In severe cases, the subject may become emaciated on account of the pain; in even more severe cases, cardiac irregularities such as profound bradycardia may lead to loss of consciousness or even death. It is seldom seen in people aged less than 40. The pathophysiology and treatment are the same as those for **trigeminal neuralgia**.[5239]

In a partial form, the nerve of Jacobsen is involved, leading to pain felt in the external auditory meatus only. The symptomatic form was first described by Weisenberg in 1910, the idiopathic form by Wilfred Harris 11 years later.[721]

Two major forms of the complete syndrome are defined by the International Headache Society[2820] and are shown in Chart G–5.

glossoplegia Paralysis of the tongue. Apart from lesions of the XII cranial nerve, this may occur in association with a small cortical infarction in the contralateral hemisphere very close to the hand area in the inferolateral part of the precentral gyrus. Clinically, the deviation of the tongue is toward the weak side on protrusion, unlike the palate which is drawn up to the stronger side on attempted phonation.

glossoptosis The tendency for the tongue to fall back into the hypopharynx, as with hypognathism.

glossopyrosis See **burning mouth syndrome**.

glottal stop A brief audible click normally preceding a cough and following pronunciation of words ending in "a" or "e." Its loss in bulbar weakness is an early sign.

glottis (Gr) The mouth of the windpipe.

glucocerebrosidase The deficient enzyme in **Gaucher syndrome**.

glucocorticoid deficiency, achalasia, and deficient tear production A syndrome with childhood onset characterized by corneal and pupillary abnormalities, sparse tears, abnormal motility of the esophagus, achalasia, adrenal hypoplasia, hypoglycaemia, abnormality in consciousness, seizures, and diffuse depigmentation of the skin.[381]

glucosidase (β-glucosidase) An enzyme normally active in the chain of glycogen degradation to lactate, absence of which produces the features of **Pompe disease**.

glucosylceramide lipidosis (Gaucher disease, cerebroside lipidosis: OMIM 606463; 231000)

Chart G–5. Forms of Glossopharyngeal Neuralgia

Classical Glossopharyngeal Neuralgia A severe transient stabbing pain experienced in the ear, base of the tongue, tonsillar fossa, or beneath the angle of the jaw. The pain is therefore felt in the distributions of the auricular and pharyngeal branches of the vagus nerve as well as the glossopharyngeal nerve. It is commonly provoked by swallowing, talking, or coughing and may remit and relapse in the fashion of **trigeminal neuralgia**. Diagnostic criteria have been defined as follows:

A. Paroxysmal attacks of facial pain lasting from a fraction of a second to 2 min and fulfilling criteria B and C
B. Pain has all of the following characteristics:
   1. Unilateral location
   2. Distribution within the posterior part of the tongue, tonsillar fossa, pharynx, or beneath the angle of the lower jaw and/or in the ear
   3. Sharp, stabbing, and severe
   4. Precipitated by swallowing, chewing, talking, coughing, and/or yawning
C. Attacks are stereotyped in the individual patient
D. There is no clinically evident neurological deficit
E. Not attributed to another disorder

Other causes will have been ruled out by history, physical examination, and/or special investigations

Symptomatic Glossopharyngeal Neuralgia Pain as in the classical form except that aching pain may persist between paroxysms and sensory impairment may be found in the distribution of the glossopharyngeal nerve. Diagnostic criteria have been defined as follows:

A. Paroxysmal attacks of facial pain lasting from a fraction of a second to 2 min, with or without persistence of aching between paroxysms, and fulfilling criteria B and C
B. Pain has all of the following characteristics:
   1. Unilateral location
   2. Distribution within the posterior part of the tongue, tonsillar fossa, pharynx or beneath the angle of the lower jaw, and/or in the ear
   3. Sharp, stabbing, and severe
   4. Precipitated by swallowing, chewing, talking, coughing, and/or yawning
C. Attacks are stereotyped in the individual patient
D. A causative lesion has been demonstrated by special investigations and/or surgery.

From the International Classification of Headache Disorders (Headache Classification Committee of the International Headache Society. Cephalalgia 2004;24*(Suppl 1)). With the kind permission of Dr. Jes Olesen, the International Headache Society and Wiley-Blackwell Publications.*

A sphingolipidosis, in which there is generalized deposition of galactosylceramide in the nervous system, due to a deficiency in galactosylceramide β-galactosidase activity. The disease is recessively inherited, mapped to 1q23, and has three forms defined according to the onset age.[2318] All occur more commonly in Jewish people; **Gaucher cells** are detectable in all patients and all show hepatosplenomegaly.

Type 1 (*adult form*) is characterized by hypersplenism, jaundice, thrombocytopenia, anemia, arthropathy, and retinal and skin pigmentation. Dementia, generalized seizures, myoclonus, Parkinsonism, ataxia, and sensory neuropathy have been reported occasionally, but this type is not ordinarily associated with neurological dysfunction.

Type 2 (*acute infantile neuronopathic form*) is a rare form characterized by mental and motor failure, macular pigmentation, seizures or myoclonus, ataxia, extensor hypertonia, and laryngospasm, with onset at about 6 months of age; it leads to early death.

In *type 3* (*juvenile or subacute neuropathic form*), the findings include ophthalmoplegias (notably a failure of ocular adduction), pyramidal signs, generalized seizures, myoclonus, and progressive dementia, but onset is usually during the second or third decades.[4679]

An association with Parkinsonism has been defined, with relatives of those affected having an unusually high prevalence of that condition.

glucuronidase for a (β-glucuronidase) An enzyme coded for on chromosome 7. Deficiency leads to the accumulation of dermatan sulfate and heparan sulfate in the Sly syndrome (**mucopolysaccharidosis** VII).

glue-sniffer's neuropathy A progressive, mainly motor neuropathy caused by inhalation of *N*-hexane or toluene, the organic solvents in some commercial glues.[6363]

Gluszcz syndrome A congenital syndrome characterized by nystagmus, dermal abnormalities, cerebral and spinal tumors, and vascular malformations.[381]

glutamate (dicarboxylic amino acid) An excitatory neurotransmitter.

glutamate dehydrogenase deficiency A recessively inherited or sporadic progressive ataxic syndrome characterized by deficiency of this enzyme in association with the onset in young adult life of features suggesting **olivopontocerebellar atrophy**. Clinically, progressive external ophthalmoplegia, ataxia, pyramidal signs, Parkinsonism, and motor neuropathy are the main features.[1159]

glutamic acid (glutamate) An excitatory amino acid, toxic to neurones in high concentrations. Glutamic acid decarboxylase catalyses the conversion of glutamate to GABA and is the autoantigen responsible for the manifestations of **stiff person syndrome** and of insulin-dependent diabetes mellitus. (IDDM)

A related syndrome of progressive cerebellar ataxia, late-onset IDDM, and various endocrine defects is described.[5504]

glutamylribose-5-phosphate storage disease An aminoacidopathy characterized by mental deterioration, seizures, microcephaly, and proteinuria with dysmorphism. Excessive glutamylribose-5-phosphate is found in the brain and kidneys.[6799]

glutaric acidemia See **glutaric aciduria**.

glutaric aciduria (glutaric acidemia, multiple acyl-CoA/glutaryl-CoA dehydrogenase deficiency) A rare, recessively inherited disorder with onset in early childhood. It is due to a severe defect of mitochondrial oxidation of fatty acids as a result of deficiency of glutaryl coenzyme *A* dehydrogenase (type 1) or acyl-coenzyme *A* dehydrogenase (type 2) and is diagnosed by the detection of glutaric acid in plasma or urine.

Type 1 is a recessively inherited syndrome with congenital or early childhood onset due to disordered lysine and tryptophan metabolism. It is characterized by emotional lability; seizures; cerebellar, pyramidal, and extrapyramidal signs (dystonias or choreoathetosis); myoclonus; dementia; and aminoaciduria, often presenting acutely.[814, 3517] Encephalopathic crises resembling those of **Reye syndrome** may be precipitated by intercurrent febrile illnesses during a vulnerable period of brain development, resulting in acute bilateral striatal necrosis, and subsequently in a dystonic or dyskinetic movement disorder.

Biochemically, the disease is characterized by an accumulation of glutaric acid, 3-hydroxyglutaric acid, and glutarylcarnitine due to an inherited deficiency of glutaryl-CoA dehydrogenase (*GCDH* gene on chromosome 19p13.2). Radiologically, microcephaly and frontotemporal, caudate, and putaminal atrophy are described.[2523]

Type 2 presents a heterogeneous collection of phenotypes, including neonatal hypoglycemia and infantile episodic vomiting with hypoglycemia; multiple dysmorphisms; renal cysts; severe hypotonia; and lethal cardiomyopathy. Numerous developmental brain disorders are also associated. Affected children may emanate the odor of sweaty feet.[1166] This form has also been described with onset in adult life and with features of a lipid myopathy.[1521] See also **Jamaican vomiting sickness**.

Cerebral MRI shows large CSF-containing spaces (the Sylvian fissures and anterior to the temporal lobes) and basal ganglia abnormal signal. One observation showed variability of the clinical picture and course of glutaric acidemia type I in the same kindred. Systematic organic acid chromatography in all children with acute or progressive dystonia with basal ganglia abnormalities on MRI has been advised.

glutathionine synthetase deficiency See **5-oxoprolinemia**.

glutathionuria A rare, diffuse encephalopathy due to gammaglutamyl peptidase deficiency, characterized clinically by mental retardation in isolation.[2482]

gluteal compartment syndrome A rare disorder that most often occurs in conjunction with prolonged immobility in the lateral decubitus position after a sedative overdose, but also may result from direct trauma. Patients present with localized tenderness, induration, and pain with passive flexion of the gluteal muscles. Signs of sciatic nerve compression occur frequently, and rhabdomyolysis may be associated with the syndrome. If the diagnosis of gluteal compartment syndrome is suspected, intracompartmental pressures should be measured. If pressures are high or if sufficient clinical suspicion remains, the patient should undergo prompt fasciotomy. See also **blue jeans syndrome** and **ilioinguinal neuropathy**.[5130, 4840, 680]

gluteal neuropathy Damage to the superior or inferior gluteal nerves, usually occurring as a result of local distortion following a femoral fracture or a misplaced injection or due to compression by the pyriformis muscle (**piriformis syndrome**) and leading to weakness of the gluteal muscles.[5199]

gluteal reflexes 1. Stroking of the buttock of the prone subject leads to contraction of the gluteal muscles.
2. Tapping the gluteal muscles at their origin from the lateral part of the sacrum leads to their contraction. These reflexes are hard to elicit and almost impossible to interpret; their absence is not alone a sign of lesions of the L5–S1,2 reflex arcs, and their hyperactivity is never found in isolation.

gluteal syndromes Myofascial pain syndromes consisting of back pain and trigger points in the buttocks, the pain radiating in a sclerotomal distribution and unaccompanied by neurological deficits. See **piriformis syndrome** and **gluteus medius syndrome**.

Such disorders are often apparent to physicians but less so to their surgical colleagues.

gluten ataxia An immune-related, subacute, progressive cerebellar syndrome, especially manifesting gait ataxia, occurring in subjects with gluten sensitivity and clinical evidence of celiac disease in whom there may be found antibodies to Purkinje cells and to gliadin. Motor and sensorimotor axonal or demyelinating neuropathies; multiple mononeuropathy; myopathy; **leukoaraiosis; neuromyotonia**; and **stiff-person syndrome** are other neurological complications described.[2671, 2670] This may be the single most common cause of sporadic idiopathic ataxia.

gluten myopathy A neurological disorder associated with celiac disease caused by antibodies against endomysium. See also **gluten ataxia**.[2672]

gluteus medius syndrome A myofascial pain syndrome characterized by pain felt persistently in the medial aspect of the buttock (especially just below the posterior superior iliac spine), radiating to the upper thigh posterolaterally to the level of the knee, accompanied by trigger zones causing local muscle tenderness, restricted straight leg raising, and discomfort with hip and knee flexion and with medial rotation of the leg. No objective reflex or sensory changes are present.

gluts A class of stereo-specific proteins responsible for transporting glucose across tissue barriers. One form of disturbance of the system (glut-1 deficiency) is dominantly inherited and presents with seizures, developmental delay, ataxia, and low CSF glucose levels.[860]

glycerol kinase deficiency An X-linked, recessive, systemic disease manifesting as myopathy with histological changes similar to those of **Duchenne dystrophy**, accompanied clinically by psychomotor retardation, growth failure, osteoporosis, and hypoadrenalism. The serum levels of glycerol are high and those of glycerol kinase in leukocytes and cultured fibroblasts are low.[2617] The responsible gene maps to Xp21.1.

glycine encephalopathy (nonketotic hyperglycinemia) A fatal, autosomal, recessive disorder manifested in infancy in which glycine levels are high in the brain, serum, and CSF because of a defect in the glycine cleavage enzyme. The condition is characterized clinically by intractable seizures and myoclonus, lethargy, failure of mental development, and early death.[3457] The EEG shows a burst–suppression pattern. Eventually the syndrome is one of psychomotor delay with axial hypotonia in the few survivors, but peripheral spasticity, poor head control, severe seizures, and hydrocephalus are also described.[6499]

In a *variant* form, the condition is less severe because the genetic defect is partial.[2132]

glycogen storage diseases (glycogenoses) Autosomal, recessive diseases characterized by deficiency of muscle phosphorylase, an enzyme required for the breakdown of glycogen into simpler substances to be metabolized by the tricarboxylic acid cycle, with the production of that energy required for muscle contraction. As a result of the deficiency, glycogen is permanently laid down in tissues such as liver and muscle. See also **forearm exercise test**.

Ten enzyme deficiencies and thus 10 types of glycogen storage disease are recognized, among which many lead to neurological disease as described in Chart G–6. In most the onset is in adolescence with exercise intolerance, painful muscle cramps, weakness, and occasionally myoglobinuria following exercise. Rarely, the condition manifests first in later adult life with progressive generalized muscle weakness. The muscle contractures that occur are electrically silent. Myoglobinuria is common and may lead to initial presentation with acute renal failure.

The "**second wind**" phenomenon described in muscle phosphorylase deficiency has been attributed to increased utilization of free fatty acids as an energy source or increased muscle blood flow. Muscle biopsy shows the presence of excessive glycogen in subsarcolemmal vacuoles. Failure of serum lactate elevation following ischemic exercise is the usually diagnostic test but is not specific.

Other forms of glycogen storage diseases are *phosphohexoisomerase deficiency* (Satoyoshi disease), a rare variant, characterized by the late onset of myopathy with exertional muscle cramps and impaired stamina;[5558] and *glycogen synthetase deficiency*, a rare congenital variant, characterized by lethargy, coma, and seizures in recurrent hypoglycemic attacks with the later development of failure to thrive, microcephaly, and mental and motor delay.[4910] **Lactic dehydrogenase deficiency** and mixed enzyme deficiencies are other possible *variants*.

glycogen storage myopathy with cardiac involvement See *type 2 glycogen storage disease*.

glycogen synthetase deficiency See **glycogen storage diseases**.

glycogenosis The accumulation of intracellular glycogen as a result of a **glycogen storage disease**.

glycogenosome Membrane-bound sacs of glycogen (distended lysosomes) seen in patients with **glycogen storage diseases**.

glycolic aciduria See **hyperoxaluria type 1**.

Chart G–6. Types of Glycogen Storage Disease

Type 1, glycogenosis (von Gierke disease, hepatorenal glycogenosis) A syndrome due to glucose-6-phosphatase deficiency with the resultant deposition of normal glycogen in the liver and inability to process glycogen to glucose. Clinically, the condition is characterized by hepatosplenomegaly, renal enlargement, hypoglycemic attacks leading to seizures, hyperlipidemia, xanthomas, and ketoacidosis. Hypotonia is detectable but there is no evidence of myopathy.

Type 2, glycogenosis (Pompe disease, acid maltase [α-1,4-glucosidase] deficiency, idiopathic generalized glycogenosis) A recessively inherited syndrome occurring in childhood or adult life in which, due to absence of lysosomal acid α-glucosidase, failure to utilize glycogen leads to accumulation of that substance in cardiac and/or skeletal muscle, liver, kidneys, and nervous system. The condition presents with different features at different ages.[5076, 5915] The responsible gene maps to 17q23.

Infantile form (Pompe disease of infants) A fatal, recessively inherited glycogen storage myopathy of infants presenting with bulbar, proximal, and distal myopathic weakness; atrophy and pseudohypertrophy; myotonia; macroglossia; cardiomyopathy; hepatomegaly; and scoliosis.[5076, 6201] Death is usually due to cardiorespiratory failure and occurs within the first 2 years of life. The same phenotype has also been reported in children with normal levels of acid maltase.[869]

In a *variant* form the condition starts later and moves on more slowly.

Juvenile or childhood form (Pompe disease of children) A proximal glycogen storage myopathy (a lysosomal storage disease) presenting in early childhood or youth with proximal and distal myopathic weakness, atrophy and pseudohypertrophy, macroglossia, myotonia, cardiomyopathy, enlarged liver, and scoliosis.[1865] This type is more benign, but still fatal within 20–30 years.

Adult form (*acid maltse deficiency myopathy*) A slowly progressive proximal glycogen storage myopathy of adult life, presenting in the third or subsequent decades with slowly progressive proximal weakness, atrophy and pseudohypertrophy, myotonia,[1865, 5428] pain, and fatigue. The syndrome may thus resemble **polymyositis** or **myotonic dystrophy** and may also present as a **scapuloperoneal syndrome** or **rigid spine syndrome**. Typically, the patients complain of excessive daytime sleepiness with nocturnal sleep disruption resulting from intermittent apneic spells accompanied by repetitive brady-tachycardia and considered to be due to failure of the other respiratory muscles to suffice during periods of physiological sleep-related atonia in the presence of the severe myopathic weakness of the diaphragm.[1875, 2630, 2680]

The abnormal gene is located on chromosome 17. The glycogen content in muscle is only slightly increased or normal; there is no cardiomegaly; and death in respiratory failure only occurs very late. Both phenotypes may occur in the same family.[3909] A *variant form* is *acid maltase deficiency type 2* which is a lysosomal glycogenosis causing proximal muscle weakness, hypertrophic cardiomyopathy, probable intellectual impairment, and possible liver involvement occurring in the absence of any deficiency of acid maltase.[1444, 5302, 2680]

Type 3, glycogenosis (Cori–Forbes disease, amylo-1,6-glucosidase [debrancher] deficiency, limit dextrinosis) A proximal glycogen storage myopathy of infancy, childhood, or adult life, transmitted as a recessive trait (at least in infants) with a tendency to improve at puberty. This is the most common glycogen storage disease and is a relatively benign metabolic disorder due to deficiency of the enzyme amylo-1,6-glucosidase. Affected infants present with hepatomegaly, hypoglycemia, seizures, growth delay, fasting hypoglycemia and hypotonia, and cardiomyopathy may develop. In older children, cardiomyopathy and somatic muscular exercise intolerance are the main features. Adults may complain of fatigability with proximal myopathic weakness, generalized atrophy, calf pseudohypertrophy, and myotonia.[1651]

In *variant* forms, a gradually progressive polyneuropathy is caused by accumulation of glycogen within all the elements of the peripheral sensory nerves.[6438]

Type 4, brancher enzyme deficiency (Andersen disease, adult amylopectinosis, amylo transglucosidase [brancher enzyme] deficiency) A rare, recessively inherited glycogen storage disease presenting in infancy with motor delay, hypotonia, calf pseudohypertrophy, proximal myopathic weakness, and atrophy. In some cases, hepatomegaly with cirrhosis and splenomegaly are present.[2016]

A perinatal form is the *fetal akinesia deformation sequence*, characterized by multiple congenital contractures and occurs in the perinatal period. A congenital form presents with hypotonia muscle wasting new retinal involvement cardiomyopathy and death in infancy. In the childhood form cardiac or somatic myopathy are the dominant features.[914]

A fourth *variant* (adult polyglucosan body myopathy) presents in adult life with progressive asymmetrical weakness; the muscle biopsy specimen appearances are those of a vacuolar myopathy, the periodic-acid Schiff-positive vacuoles lying under the sarcolemma.

Type 5, myophosphorylase deficiency (McArdle disease) A recessively inherited glycogen storage disease with childhood or juvenile onset, due to muscle phosphorylase deficiency which results in the accumulation of unusable glycogen in muscles and leads to a failure of the muscles exercised to produce lactic acid. The clinical syndrome has its onset in childhood and comprises muscle stiffness, proximal myopathic weakness, and fatigability and pain with painful cramp-contractures on exercise, the cramp being chemically and not electrically induced. Myoglobinuria follows in severe attacks. The symptoms may be relieved during exertion by a gentle decrease in the energy expended, which leads to the "second wind" effect.[789]

This was the first of the glycogen storage diseases to be predicted (by Dr. Brian McArdle of Guy's Hospital, London) and detected.[4198] The responsible gene maps to 11q13.

The *infantile form* (fatal infantile glycogen storage disease) is an inherited multisystem storage disease presenting with mental retardation, corneal ulceration, and congenital hypotonia and severe myopathic limb weakness with respiratory distress and cardiomyopathy leading to death in childhood. Histochemistry of muscle shows a nonspecific myopathy with the subsarcolemmal accumulation of glycogen. Phosphorylase *b* kinase and phosphofructokinase-1 activities are low or absent.[181, 1444, 1650] An *intermediate* form is characterized by early childhood onset with proximal myopathic weakness and mental and developmental delay.

A *late adult* form is characterized by onset during adult life with bulbar weakness and facial and proximal myopathy.[1649, 1887]

Variants are *muscle phosphorylase b kinase deficiency* (GSD type 8) a glycogen storage disease with onset in childhood or adult life with muscle pain, exercise intolerance, cramp, and fatigability. Autosomal and X-linked recessive forms are described;[28] one form presents with late-onset cramps, stiffness, muscle swelling, and an abnormal ischemic forearm test;[3542] in others, dominant inheritance and a diffuse pattern dystrophy of the retinal pigment epithelium are described.

Type 6, Hers disease A glycogen storage disease without neurological features.

Type 7, muscle phosphofructokinase deficiency (Tarui disease) A recessively inherited proximal myopathy with young adult or late adult onset, presenting with muscle pain and decreased exercise tolerance, proximal muscle atrophy and weakness, and increased creatine kinase levels and myoglobinuria.[3726, 6214] The responsible gene maps to 1cnq32.

continued

Chart G–6. (*continued*)

Variants are *fatal infantile muscle phosphofructokinase deficiency* A congenital form characterized by corneal cloudiness and ulceration leading to blindness, high palate, club foot, joint contractures, respiratory distress in neonates, mental and developmental delay, dolichocephaly, scaphocephaly or microcephaly, pendular nystagmus, proximal and distal myopathic weakness, multifocal paroxysmal EEG discharges, and cerebral atrophy;[181, 6215] and an *inherited erythrocyte PFK deficiency* without myopathy.[1922]

Type 9, phosphoglycerate kinase deficiency An X-linked form in which both phosphoglycerate kinase and phosphorylase β-kinase are deficient; this syndrome presents in childhood with congenital limb weakness, mental retardation, and corneal ulceration, the weakness progressing to truncal weakness and respiratory insufficiency. Short stature, enlarged liver, and arthropathy are also described. The responsible gene maps to Xq13.[830]

Type 10, phosphoglycerate mutase deficiency (Thompson disease, phosphoglucomutase deficiency) A rare glycogenosis presenting in childhood or youth with tight heel cords, calf hypertrophy and muscle cramps, and pigmenturia after exercise. The forearm ischemic lactate test shows little increase in lactate production with ischemic exercise.[1655] The responsible gene maps to 7p13–p12. See also Bembi B, et al. Neurology 2008; 71 (Suppl. 2: S4–S11).

glycolytic myopathy A familial myopathy of late onset, characterized by normal work capacity for a brief period, delayed muscle pain and stiffness with exertion, absence of contractures or muscle weakness, and failure of lactate production in the blood. The condition is considered to be due to a metabolic defect occurring in glycolysis at the level of phosphohexoisomerase.[5558] See **glycogen storage diseases** (*phosphohexoisomerase deficiency*). See also DiMauro et al.[1646] on distal glycolysis.

glycopeptidosis A diffuse encephalopathy characterized by progressive myoclonic epilepsy and disorders of glycoprotein metabolism with abnormal urinary glycopeptide excretion.[1983]

glycoprotein disorders A group of inherited dysmetabolic states characterized by deficiency of glycoproteins. These include **fucosidosis types 1 and 2, mannosidosis, sialidosis** (congenital, and infantile types), and **aspartyl-glycosaminiduria**.

glycosylation disorders Genetic defects in the synthesis of the glycan moiety of glycoconjugates or in the attachment of glycans to macromolecules.[3146] Standard screening has relied upon the isoelectrofocusing of serum transferrin, but a more sensitive genetic method is now available.

Most of the phenotypes (of which there are many known and many more to be discovered) affect the nervous system: They include microcephaly; brain malformations psychomotor retardation; behavioral abnormalities; seizures; strokes; ataxia; ocular lesions; and abnormalities of eye movement, brain demyelination, peripheral neuropathy, hypotonia, and hyporeflexia.

GM_1 gangliosidosis (generalized gangliosidosis, neurovisceral lipidosis, Hurler syndrome variant, pseudo-Hurler disease, systemic late infantile lipidosis) A recessively inherited, progressive, and fatal neurovisceral storage disease due to deficiency of lysosomal acid β-galactosidases A and B, in which gangliosides accumulate in the CNS and keratan sulfate-like material in the viscera. The responsible gene maps to p3p21–p14.2. There are three main phenotypes:

The *type I infantile form* (pseudo-Hurler disease or Landing syndrome) shows mental retardation, coarse facial features, macrocephaly, multiple dysostoses, hepatosplenomegaly, seizures, severe and progressive neurological disturbance with dementia and chorea, dysostosis, and blindness. A cherry-red spot may be present. Death usually occurs within 2 years.[4585, 4726]

The *type II late-infantile/juvenile* form manifests after 6 months of age. Somatic and skeletal deformities are absent and the hepatosplenomegaly is less severe, but mental deterioration, ataxia, pyramidal signs, dysarthria, weakness, hyperekplexia, and seizures occur. Death occurs before the age of 10 years.[4726, 4727]

The *type III (adult or chronic)* form presents in infancy, childhood, or adult life with coarsening of the facial features, without visceromegaly or skeletal signs. Chorea, tics, dystonia, Parkinsonism, dementia, and spasticity are occasionally concomitant signs.[4585, 2604]

GM_2 activator deficiency See **GM_2 gangliosidosis**.

GM_2 gangliosidosis A group of **sphingolipidoses** in which there is generalized deposition of gangliosides in both neuronal and other tissues. The diseases are recessively inherited and have three forms defined according to onset; late infantile (Tay–Sachs disease), juvenile (Sandhoff disease) and adult; as well as a number of *variants*. Deficiencies of hexosaminidase A, of hexosaminidase A and B, or of the GM2 activator protein are the underlying metabolic problems. See also **hexosaminidase deficiency**.

Clinically, most forms are slowly progressive with cognitive deterioration, pyramidal and cerebellar signs, and a lower motor neuron syndrome resembling **amyotropic lateral sclerosis**. The variable phenotypes of GM_2 gangliosidosis have been reviewed[3236] and are described in Chart G–7.

GM_3 gangliosidosis A congenital dysmorphic syndrome manifesting also coarse facial features; visceromegaly; seizures; a muscular build; respiratory distress in the neonate; and spongy, cavitating, and cystic changes in the brain.[4005]

gnathalgia (from Gr, the cheek + pain) Facial neuralgia—pain in the cheek.

gnathic To do with the upper jaw or cheek.

gnathostomiasis A rare parasitic nematode infection found usually in Asia. The leading clinical features are fever, subcutaneous swellings, and abdominal pain with eosinophilia. Subarachnoid hemorrhage, myelitis, and eosinophilic encephalomyelitis with coma are the neurological syndromes most often described.[1154]

gnomes' calves Calf pseudohypertrophy as seen in **Duchenne muscular dystrophy**.

gnosanopsia The faculty of awareness without discrimination.

gnosis The faculty of knowing and comprehending the significance of what is perceived.

Chart G–7. The Phenotypes of GM_2 Gangliosidosis

1. Alpha locus mutations (deficiency of hexosaminidase A)

Type 1, infantile (classical Tay–Sachs disease, B variant, amaurotic familial idiocy) This form is due to lesions at the alpha locus on chromosome 15 (15q22–q25.1.) or at the beta locus on chromosome 5, causing total deficiency of *N*-acetyl beta-hexosaminidase A. It affects mainly Ashkenazi Jewish infants who show macrocephaly and megalencephaly, mental and motor failure, optic atrophy, spasticity, excessive startle responses, seizures, mental and developmental delay, and a cherry-red macular spot. Death occurs within years.

The macular findings were first described by Warren Tay, an English ophthalmologist in 1881,[6229] 6 years before a fuller clinical and pathological account was reported by the American Bernard Sachs[5489] who also coined the term "Amaurotic Familial Idiocy."

Partial deficiency of the enzyme leads to the later appearance of similar signs, but even more rarely; the adult form is described by O'Neill et al.[4737] The responsible gene maps to 15q22–q25.1. The condition was redescribed by Vogt in 1905.[6562]

Juvenile (partial) type A recessively inherited syndrome manifesting signs of damage to motor and cerebellar systems, dementia, convulsions, and arrest of psychomotor development from the age of 4 years, in which the enzyme deficiency is but partial.[2451] This form is characterized by more slowly progressive mental decline. The main phenotypes are syndromes of slurred speech with spasticity and ataxia,[3237] of pure ataxia; and those phenotypes resembling **hereditary motor neuropathy** type 3, **X-linked bulbospinal neuronopathy, neuronal ceroid lipofuscinosis**, and **amyotrophic lateral sclerosis**.

A late-onset form in which similar symptoms occur in youth or early-adult life.[1494]

Chronic type A heterogeneous collection of phenotypes reflecting partial deficiency of Hexosaminidase A and inherited recessively. They include a syndrome resembling **amyotrophic lateral sclerosis**;[6891] a syndrome resembling **hereditary motor neuropathy** type 3;[3236] and a variant with manifestations of each of these conditions as well as dystonia, dementia, seizures, sensory neuropathy, internuclear ophthalmoplegia, or psychiatric disorders.[409]

Atypical spinocerebellar degeneration[5194]

Normal adults[3236]

2. *Beta locus mutations (deficiency of hexosaminidase A and B)*

The *type 2 form (O Variant, Sandhoff–Jatkiewicz disease, Sandhoff variant)* resembles the late infantile form clinically (with the addition of cardiac dysfunction), but the enzyme defect is partial and of both hexosaminidases A and B; the aminoglycolipid globoside accumulates in the viscera and GM_2 ganglioside and asialo-GM_2 ganglioside accumulates in the nervous system.

This recessively inherited sphingolipidosis occurs in non-Jewish infants and is associated with total deficiency of hexosaminidases A and B with some residual hexosaminidase S activity.[5536] Otherwise it is similar to *Tay–Sachs disease* in producing hepatosplenomegaly, cardiomyopathy, bony deformities, myoclonic seizures, macrocephaly, optic atrophy with a macular red spot, pyramidal signs, and mental and motor regression, with a progressive course to death in 2–5 years. The responsible gene maps to 5q13.

Variants include the following:

Juvenile Sandhoff disease.[2451]
Chronic GM_2 gangliosidosis with Hexosaminidase A and B deficiency
A multisystem disorder with ataxia, dementia, pyramidal signs, and amyotrophy in varying combinations
Juvenile cerebellar ataxia[3237]
Adult-onset spinocerebellar ataxia[4796]
Hereditary motor neuropathy (juvenile-onset spinal muscular atrophy)[3238]
Neuromuscular disease resembling **Kennedy syndrome**.[6290]
Normal adults

3. Activator factor mutations (normal hexosaminidase A and B activity) This form of hexosaminidase deficiency may be associated with any of the following syndromes:

The *AB variant* (GM_2 activator deficiency) This form is due to deficiency of the activator protein required for the interaction of hexosaminidase A and GM_2 ganglioside. The responsible gene maps to 5q. The disorder presents in infancy with microcephaly, blindness, and a macular red spot.
Grand mal and myoclonic seizures, dementia, nystagmus, and pyramidal signs appear next[5537]
A form resembling *Tay–Sachs disease*, but milder
An adult GM2 gangliosidosis with seizures, dementia, and **normal-pressure hydrocephalus**
Normal adults[6290]

gnostic sensations Those sensations which require and implicate cortical discriminative processes. These include stereognosis; discrimination of weight, surface, form, and texture; and the senses of passive movement and of the position of joints in space and possibly of vibration.

Godfried–Prick–Carol–Prakken syndrome The combination of the signs of neurofibromatosis with mongoloid facies, areas of dermal atrophy, mental retardation, and cardiac conduction defects.[1025] See **neurofibromatosis**.

Godin syndrome Intermittent localized headache evoked by compression of the carotid arteries.

Godlee, Sir Rickman John English neurosurgeon who successfully removed a cerebral tumor in 1884, although the patient died later of sepsis.

Godtfredsen syndrome (cavernous sinus-nasopharyngeal tumor syndrome) The concurrence of oculomotor palsies and trigeminal numbness and pain due to infiltration of the cavernous sinus region by a nasopharyngeal tumor, with the addition of hypoglossal paresis due to compression of that nerve by enlarged retropharyngeal lymph nodes.[2419, 2420]

Goeminne syndrome A congenital, X-linked syndrome consisting of torticollis, facial asymmetry, keloids of the trunk and limbs, crytorchidism, renal failure, testicular failure, respiratory complaints, and renal dysplasia.[2429]

goggia Local contraction of muscle fibers when they are tapped, seen in prolonged debilitating illnesses.[5333] The origin of the term is uncertain but the condition is almost certainly **myokymia**.

gogi aphasia Selective impairment of the processing of semantic Chinese-type characters and difficulty in finding access to the lexicon in terms of both production and reception, with retention of the ability to process phonetic signs and with fluent oral repetition.[5552]

goiter headache Headache resulting from venous distension in subjects with goiters, the tumor compressing the internal jugular veins at the level of the thoracic inlet.[3657]

Golabi syndrome A congenital, X-linked dysmorphic syndrome manifesting also dwarfism, brittle hair, atrial septal defect, gastrointestinal anomalies, deafness, strabismus, microcephaly or macrocephaly, and mental and developmental delay.[2433]

Goldberg syndrome (juvenile type 2 sialidosis, mucolipidosis 1) A recessively inherited dysmetabolic state resulting from deficiency of d-*N*-acetylneuraminidase and β-galactosidase leading to the accumulation of sialyl-oligosaccharides.

Clinically, the onset is after the age of 2 years, with mental retardation, seizures, and myoclonus; a cherry-red macular spot; deafness; ataxia and short stature; angiokeratoma;and vacuolated lymphocytes in the peripheral blood.[2440] See also **sialidosis**.

Goldenhar–Gorlin syndrome See **oculoauriculovertebral dysplasia**.

Goldenhar syndrome See **oculoauriculovertebral dysplasia**.

Goldflam, Samuel Vulfovich (1852–1932) Polish neurologist who trained with **Charcot** and **Westphal** and thereafter practiced in Warsaw. He gave an early account of **myasthenia gravis** ("myasthenia pseudoparalytica," once known as Erb–Goldflam disease) in 1893, **Erb** having written on a similar topic in 1879.

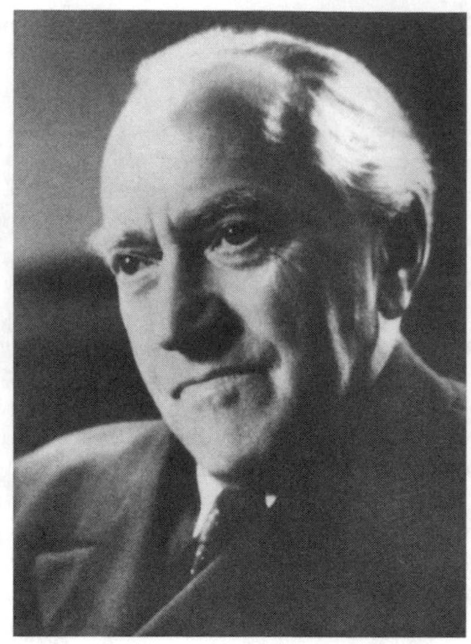

Figure G–3 Kurt Goldstein.

Goldman–Offner reference See **average potential reference**.

Goldstein, Kurt (1878–1965) German-American physician who trained with **Wernicke** and **Edinger** and later worked in Frankfurt, Berlin and after 1935, in New York. He gave the first description of the catastrophic (anxiety/outrage) reaction seen in demented patients faced with the impossibility of completing an assigned task, as well as a description of the following syndrome. He wrote widely on the topic of dysphasia; introduced a sorting test for the localization of cerebral injuries and advanced the concept of the difficulty in changing mental "sets" as a basis for understanding the cognitive problems of the brain injured.

Goldstein syndrome Acute cerebellitis—a postinfectious and probably autoallergic self-limited condition.[2454]

Goldstein–Schirer Test An instrument for the detection of right posterior parietal lesions, wherein the subject is asked to sort solid objects by their shape and color.

golf ball epilepsy Acute posttraumatic and later seizures following cranial trauma from these objects.[1077]

Golfers' elbow (medial epicondylitis) A syndrome of pain over the medial epicondyle of the elbow with marked local tenderness and pain on forearm pronation or supination.

Golgi, Camillo (1844–1926) Italian anatomist, born in Lombardy and trained in Pavia, where he eventually became, in turn, professor of histology and anatomy, dean of medicine, and Rector of the university. His staining methods allowed for the first time a full description of the morphology of the neuron. He introduced silver chromate or nitrate and osmic acid staining (to show neurons and myelin respectively) in 1873 while in practice as a hospital physician, the work being done in his kitchen; and he was the first to describe dendrites within what he wrongly considered to be a nutritive reticulum. He nevertheless shared the Nobel Prize for 1906 with **Ramon y Cajal**, who supported the rival **neuronal theory**, and with whom his relationship was poor.

Golgi also differentiated type 1 neuroglial cells with long axons from the type 2 cells with shorter axonal processes; the Golgi tendon organs; and the intracytoplasmic Golgi apparatus. His later work was largely on malaria.[2066]

Golgi apparatus A perinuclear assembly of membranes, important in the processes of excretion by the cell.

Golgi cells Golgi defined two forms of cortical cells in 1880; type 1 neurons with long axons which terminate at a distance and type 2 neurons with short axonal processes which terminate in the gray matter close to the nerve cell body; internunciate cells and the stellate cells of the cerebellar cortex are of this type.

Golgi corpuscles The cutaneous end organs for touch.

Golgi stain A silver stain for astroglia, the basis of the success of **Cajal** in neurohistology.

Golgi tendon organs Specialized stretch receptors in the tendons which discharge when stimulated by excessive tension. This causes inhibition of the α-motor neurons and thus the "give" after increasing resistance felt during assessment of tone in patients with pyramidal lesions.

Goll, Friedrich (1829–1903) Swiss anatomist, physiologist, and neurologist, who eventually became professor of anatomy at Zurich.

Goll's columns The fasciculus gracilis, the medial fasciculus of the posterior columns, described in 1860.

Gollin Incomplete Figures Test A test of right hemisphere visual perceptual processing using incomplete images to examine the subject's perceptual organizational skills.[2457]

Goltz, Friedrich Leopold (1834–1902) Professor of physiology at Halle and Strasburg, whose experimental results led him (incorrectly) to deny the theories of **Ferrier** that suggested that localization of function existed within the nervous system.

Goltz syndrome See **focal dermal hypoplasia**.

Gombault, F.A.A. (1844–1904) French neurologist.

Gombault neuritis Periaxial segmental degeneration of peripheral nerves, described in 1880; it is unlikely that this condition represents a single syndrome, but the eponym has been applied to all forms of segmental demyelination. See **hereditary motor and sensory neuropathy, type 3**.

Gomez–Lopez-Hernandez syndrome See **cerebellar syndromes** (congenital ataxias).

Gomori, Georg (1904–) Hungarian-American neuropathologist, who introduced a number of stains into pathology, the best-known of which is the "Gomori trichrome" technique for differential staining; in muscle, connective tissue stains green, muscle and cytoplasm (and myelin) red, and nuclei gray-blue.[2600]

gonadotrophin-releasing hormone A hypothalamic hypophysiotrophic hormone.

Gonda sign See **Allen sign**.

goniometer (Gr, an angle + a measure) An instrument for measuring the cranial or facial angles, now little used, although **Broca** designed one for this purpose. Such instruments are, however, still commonly employed by orthopedic surgeons and physiatrists.

go-no-go paradigm A simple clinical test of resistance to interference and thus of concentration, wherein the subject makes a simple motor response to only one of the two stimuli randomly generated by the examiner, for example, clapping in response to a single tap but not doing so in response to a double tap.

gonyalgia paresthetica (Gr, knee + abnormal sensation) **Wartenberg**'s term for tingling suddenly felt in the region of the patella when local trigger zones are lightly touched, accompanied by persistent numbness of the region supplied by the infrapatellar branch of the saphenous nerve. The cause is unknown.[6660]

Goodenough "Draw a Man" Test A test in which a child is asked to draw a man as well and as completely as he or she can, with no time limit. The items included in the child's drawing are scored—the score for the test correlating with those of intelligence tests.[5014] It can also be used to identify the presence of unilateral spatial neglect in adult patients after stroke.

goosey A chronic familial involuntary movement disorder of children seen in the southern United States in which the sudden brief movements occur in response to **startle** and are accompanied by **echolalia**.[2766]

Gopalan syndrome See **burning feet syndrome**.

Goppert sign Pupillary dilation in response to minor peripheral sensory stimulation, described in meningococcal meningitis.

Gordon, A.M. (1874–1953) French-American neurologist and psychiatrist who was born in Paris, where he graduated in medicine before emigrating eventually to Philadelphia, where he was on the staff of Jefferson Medical College. His main interest was the study of the reflexes.

Gordon extension sign See **Gordon reflex**.

Gordon reflex 1. A variant method of eliciting the **Babinski** response, in which the deep flexor muscles of the calf are squeezed; as usual, the upgoing toe indicates the presence of a pyramidal tract lesion.[2487] 2. The *tonic reflex*; the leg does not immediately fall back after the patellar tendon has been tapped.[2486] 3. (*Gordon extension sign*) Extension and perhaps fanning of the flexed fingers follows deep pressure exerted upon the radial side of the pisiform bone.[1500]

Gordon sign 1. (Souques sign, finger sign) Compression over the pisiform bone at the wrist leads to flexion of the thumb and index finger in the presence of pyramidal tract disease. 2. Spreading of the fingers and extension at the elbow when the arm is passively raised, occurring normally but to a much greater extent in patients with hemiparesis.

Gordon syndrome 1. A congenital dysmorphic syndrome manifesting also retinitis pigmentosa, sensorineural deafness, pyramidal signs, joint contractures, and mental and developmental delay.[2488] See also **Alstrom disease**. 2. Hypertension, renal tubular acidosis, and hyperkalemia with normal glomerular filtration. A syndrome of secondary **hyperkalemic periodic paralysis** may be associated.[1153]

Gordon-Hay sign The "hung-up" knee jerk, in chorea.

Gorham Proverbs Test A test of reasoning wherein the subject is required to interpret a proverb, spontaneously or by multiple choice.[2497] The instrument is used mainly to assess frontal lobe functions.

Gorlin syndrome See **frontometaphyseal dysplasia syndrome**.

Gorlin–Chaudhry–Moss syndrome A recessively inherited congenital dysmorphic syndrome manifesting craniofacial dysostosis, craniostenosis affecting the coronal sutures, brachycephaly, microphthalmia, astigmatism, corneal scarring, anti-mongolian slant to the eyes, short stature, weakness of eye closure, nystagmus on lateral gaze, dental anomalies, patent ductus arteriosus, hypertrichosis, and mental and developmental delay.[2499] See also **craniosynostosis**.

Gorlin–Goltz syndrome (Jarisch syndrome, multiple basal cell nevi syndrome) A dominantly inherited syndrome characterized by multiple basal cell nevi, hypertelorism, strabismus, vertebral anomalies with scoliosis, frontotemporal skull bossing, mandibular cysts, and a tendency to the development of medulloblastoma. The syndrome is also distinguished by a lack of responsiveness to injections of parathyroid hormone, as shown by reduced phosphate excretion.[2508] See **nevoid basal cell carcinoma syndrome**.

Gottron sign Red-purple keratotic, atrophic erythema, or macules on the extensor surfaces of joints, especially those of the hand and fingers.

Gould sign See **bowed head sign**.

gourmand syndrome A benign eating disorder associated with lesions of the right anterior cerebral hemisphere and characterized by a preoccupation with food, a passionate preference for finer quality food and a craving for food despite normal hunger and satiation signals.[5236]

Gowers, Sir William Richard (1845–1915) A leading neurologist in nineteenth-century England, he was house physician to Jenner (and later his secretary) before appointment to the staff of University College Hospital and the National Hospital, Queen Square, in 1872. He later became professor of clinical medicine at the University of London, and was elected a Fellow of the Royal College of Physicians in 1879 and of the Royal Society. He was knighted in 1897.

Despite the success of his *Diagnosis of Diseases of the Spinal Cord* (London, 1880) and of *Epilepsy and Other Chronic Convulsive Diseases* (London, 1881), his greatest work was his magnificent two-volume *Manual of Diseases of the Nervous System* (1886)[2531] in which he distilled his own and others' clinical wisdom into a work which became in successive editions the bible of neurologists worldwide and is still read with pleasure and profit for the physiological and clinical insights which it contains; it remains in print in a limited edition. He himself etched many of the illustrations, and it is likely that the original drafts were written in shorthand, of which he was a strong proponent.

His studies of epilepsy[2530] are perhaps his best known single area of clinical observation and analysis, but he also devised a hemocytometer; published an *Atlas of Ophthalmoscopy* (London, Churchill 1st edition, 1867); and described distal myopathy (1902), pseudohypertrophic muscular dystrophy, local panatrophy, **myotonic dystrophy, sleep paralysis**, and **vasovagal** attacks; differentiated choreic from dystonic forms of cerebral palsy; and defined the dorsal spinocerebellar tract.

Gowers did not publish in the journal *Brain* as he disliked the editor, who responded with a review of his textbook which offended Gowers even more.[2866]

Gowers ataxic paraplegia A myelopathy with the combination of a posterior and lateral column disorder which is nonsyphilitic[2531] and probably represents subacute combined degeneration of the cord as a result of vitamin B12 deficiency.

Gowers frontal tap An alternative method of eliciting the **ankle jerk**, in this instance by tapping the belly of the tibialis anterior muscle. It probably works by setting up vibrations transmitted to the posterior compartment of the leg.

Gowers local panatrophy Areas of wasting of the skin, subcutaneous tissues, and underlying muscles down to bone, varying in diameter from the size of a nut to that of an orange, described by Gowers in his textbook.[2531] The cause is uncertain; scleroderma may be responsible.

Gowers maneuver A method of determining that apparent paraplegia is feigned or hysterical, whereby the examiner grasps and smartly pulls the pubic hair of the seemingly paraparetic subject. When the condition is indeed not the result of a structural lesion, this leads the subject to adduct the legs at once.

Gowers paraplegia Myelopathy secondary to vertebral osteitis.[2531]

Gowers signs 1. The classic, heart-rending sign of pelvic girdle weakness in young boys who, on getting up from a recumbent position, stand with the trunk in full flexion and their hands on the floor, from which position they proceed to "walk" their hands up their legs in order to attain the erect posture. Though characteristic of every cause of pelvic muscle weakness, the sign was first described in, and still most often leads to the diagnosis of, **Duchenne dystrophy**.[2531]

2. Intermittent oscillation in pupillary size with light stimulation, occurring in early neurosyphilis.[2531]

3. Pain produced along the whole course of the sciatic nerve when the ankle is passively dorsiflexed, in cases of sciatic nerve irritation.

4. Incomplete recovery from a III cranial nerve palsy (pseudo-Graefe sign, Brixa-Koppens sign, Fuchs sign).

5. Inability of a patient with pelvic girdle weakness to rise from a sitting position with the arms outstretched.

Gowers syndromes 1. (hereditary distal muscle dystrophy) A dominantly inherited dystrophy with onset in the small muscles of the hands and feet, thereafter spreading proximally. It is more common in adults but can occur also in childhood.[2532] See **distal muscular dystrophy**.

2. (vasoconstriction syncope) Attacks of paresthesia, dyspnea, precordial discomfort, reduced pulse volume, and cramps occurring mainly in women. The resemblances to the **hyperventilation syndrome** are close.[2533]

3. **Saltatory spasm**.

Gowers tetanoid chorea See **Wilson disease** and **dystonia**.

Gowers tract (column) The superficial (anterior) spinothalamic tract, defined in Gowers' textbook *The Diagnosis of Diseases of the Spinal Cord* (London, 1880).

Gowers–Paton–Kelly syndrome See **Foster Kennedy syndrome**.

Goyer disease A dominantly inherited syndrome of children, characterized by ichthyosis, progressive deafness, and renal failure in association with hyperprolinemia.[2536]

Gradenigo, Giuseppe (1859–1926) Italian otolaryngologist who studied in Padua, Venice, Paris, London, and Berlin. He became professor at the University of Naples and wrote widely on otolaryngology. He published an account of the following syndrome in 1904.

Gradenigo syndrome (Gradenigo–Lannois syndrome, petrous apical syndrome) Painful anesthesia in the territory of the first division of the V cranial nerve with VI nerve palsy and possibly involvement of other oculomotor nerves and of the VII nerve, stemming from irritation of these structures as a result of osteitis of the petrous portion of the temporal bone or of their infiltration by a tumor at the skull base, such as a nasopharyngeal carcinoma.[2539]

The classic clinical triad consists of deep retro-orbital pain, paralysis of the ipsilateral lateral rectus muscle from involvement of the abducens nerve as it crosses the petrous bone, and otitic infection with purulent discharge from the ear. The syndrome may be associated with vertigo and hearing loss, either from a concomitant bacterial labyrinthitis or from involvement of the VIII cranial nerve in its bony canal. Radiologic evidence for infection of the petrous apex can be difficult to establish even with high resolution CT scanning, so one must be alert to this.

Gradenigo–Lannois syndrome See **Gradenigo syndrome**.

grading 1. (of reflexes) A semi quantitative score assigned to the speed and excursion of the reflex movement made in response to the percussion of tendons. The system in common usage is as follows; 0 = absent; + = reduced; ++ = normal; +++ = hyperactive; ++++ = hyperactive with sustained **clonus**. (+) is written when the reflex is obtained only with **reinforcement**. 2. (of gliomas) Methods of characterizing the attributes of tumors to achieve some idea of their prognosis.[334]

Histological methods based on the features of anaplasia, such as necrosis and mitosis, and cellular differentiation[3392] have been employed for 50 years; gliomas were divided between astrocytomas, oligodendrogliomas, and ependymomas and subdivided between four grades of malignancy. Such gradings are considered to be of utility only in the case of astrocytomas[1473] but are still employed as modern kinetic techniques are yet under development.

Graefe, Friedrich Wilhelm Ernst Albrecht von (1828–1870) German ophthalmologist who trained in Berlin and later in Prague. He studied extensively in Europe before returning to Berlin, where he became professor of ophthalmic surgery in 1857. He introduced the operation of iridectomy for glaucoma and refined the procedure of lens extraction. He is also remembered for having described sympathetic ophthalmia, retinal embolism, progressive external ophthalmoplegia, and some of the ocular signs in **dysthyroid ophthalmopathy**.[5704]

Graefe sign (lid lag) The delay in descent of the upper eyelid on looking down, as in dysthyroid ophthalmopathy and myotonic disorders.

The *pseudo-Graefe sign* consists of elevation of the upper eyelid on looking down, the result of aberrant regeneration of the III cranial nerve after injury.

Gram, Hans C.J. (1853–1938) Danish bacteriologist who invented the stain named for him in 1884.

grand mal seizures See **generalized tonic–clonic seizures**.

granular cell hyperplasia See **cerebellar ataxias** and **Lhermitte–Duclos disease**.

granular cell myoblastomas Small dermal nodules derived from Schwann cells, characterized histologically by the presence of sheets of cells with small round nuclei and copious cytoplasm containing basophilic granules.[6, 2039] They are usually benign.

granular cell Schwannomas See **granular cell myoblastoma**.

granular cell tumor of the hypophysis See **choristoma**.

granular cortical atrophy Multiple small cortical infarcts associated with narrowing of the cortical vessels and clinically accompanied by evidence of dementia.[90]

granular ependymitis A proliferative inflammatory reaction of the ependyma as a response to local viral, bacterial, or spirochetal inflammation.

granular nuclear inclusion body disease A slowly progressive multisystem disorder of the CNS and muscles, presenting clinically with dysarthria, gait disturbance, increased reflexes, akinesia, spasticity, and other pyramidal signs. Muscle and nerve biopsy specimens show hyaline nuclear inclusion bodies staining for iron. The condition may be secondary to a virus infection.[5653]

granule cell layer hypoplasia An uncommon syndrome in which this abnormality affects the cerebellum. Mental retardation, short stature, and delayed milestones accompany the limb and gait ataxia.[2754]

granulomatous angiitis See **isolated angiitis of the nervous system**.

granulomatous hypophysitis A rare, chronic (seldom acute) inflammatory disorder of the pituitary gland with no identifiable etiologic associations that presents clinically as a sellar mass lesion with pituitary insufficiency and/or hyperprolactinemia, headache, ophthalmoplegia, and possibly fever or optic neuritis. Typical MRI findings are of an intensely enhancing pituitary mass with local dural enhancement, radiologically indistinguishable from a pituitary tumor.[1140, 2122]

Variants are lymphocytic and xanthomatous hypophysitis, and the condition has been recorded as a complication of **aortic arch disease**.

granulomatous myositis Symptomatic muscle infiltration with noncaseating granulomatous tissue complicating sarcoidosis, Crohn disease, foreign-body giant-cell reaction, lymphoma, thymoma, and myasthenia gravis. Such infiltration is usually asymptomatic; but syndromes consisting of chronic myopathic weakness, painful cramps, and stiffness;[1698] and acute weakness resembling polymyositis have been described.[5840, 3736]

granulomatous neuropathy A form of multiple mononeuropathy due to sarcoidosis. The VII and VIII cranial nerves and thoracic spinal roots are most commonly involved; peripheral neuropathy is rare.[1554]

granulomatous polymyositis A slowly progressive inflammatory disorder of muscle occurring in elderly people who complain of aching and girdle weakness over the course of years. The diagnosis is made on the basis of the finding of noncaseating granulomas on muscle biopsy specimens.

The condition may be a form of sarcoidosis but also appears with Crohn disease and follows intramuscular injections.[3974, 4157] See **sarcoid myopathy**.

granulome bizarre de l'orbite See **orbital pseudotumor syndrome**.

granulovacuolar degeneration The presence of 3–5 μM argyrophilic, electron-dense intracytoplasmic granules in vacuoles within the pyramidal neurons of the hippocampus, occurring in relation to advancing age and in greater concentration in **Alzheimer disease, progressive supranuclear palsy, Down syndrome, tuberous sclerosis**, and the **ALS–Parkinsonism–dementia complex of Guam**.[6]

granulovacuolar myopathy A myopathic disease characterized by profound selective muscle wasting and weakness, electrical myotonia without clinical evidence, and muscle biopsy appearances in which a number of type I fibers show sarcoplasmic lobulation.[3256]

graphesthesia The facility of interpreting letters or figures traced upon the skin. This **gnostic** sensation is mediated by the parietal cortex.

graphogenic epilepsy A form of **reflex epilepsy** in which the seizures are triggered by writing.[261]

graphology The study of handwriting; popularly used in the divination of attributes of character.

graphomania See **hypergraphia**.

graphoreé See **hypergraphia**.

graphospasm See **writer's cramp**.

grasp reflex A stereotyped prehensile reaction of the flexors and adductors of the fingers and the flexors of the wrists induced by moving deep palmar pressure with added traction upon the flexor tendons that leads to catching and holding of the tactile stimulus—usually the hand of the examiner. This reflex is normally present on each side in babies up to 5 months old[6898] but is present asymmetrically in hemiplegia, in spastic and rigid states, and in adults with bifrontal lesions.

The reflex was first described for the adult hand by Janischewsky in 1909 and 1914 and then for the foot by Schuster in 1926. The **Hoffman** and **Tromner** signs are pathologic variations of this response.

grasp reflex of the foot (plantar grasp reflex) A reflex seen in normal infants up to the age of 1 year, consisting of tonic flexion and adduction of the toes in response to light pressure upon the ball of the big toe, whereas a scratch on the sole evokes the usual brief extensor plantar response. The foot grasp persists in patients with **Down syndrome** and in some patients with contralateral frontal lobe lesions.[801]

grasp response (forced grasping) A stereotyped prehensile reaction of the flexors and the adductors of the fingers and the flexor muscles of the wrists which can be elicited in fractional parts by appropriate localization of the stimulus. The catching phase is elicited by distally moving deep pressure over the palmar surface of the hand, the holding phase by traction on the flexor tendons. **Denny Brown** distinguished from this an *instinctive grasp reaction*, a deliberate progressive closure of the whole hand made in a series of small movements upon a stationary contact within the palm, terminating in a final complete grip and leading to pursuit (the magnet reaction) when attempts are made to remove the stimulus. Groping in response to a visual stimulus is an extension of this tactile response.[5747]

Walshe regarded the reflex as comprising the patient's closure of the hand over an object placed therein when his attention is distracted but not when it is directed to the stimulus, and considered it to represent evidence of a mild pyramidal lesion, resulting from contralateral frontal lobe pathology. The stretch of the flexor tendons leads, in his term to **tonic innervation**, over which the patient has no control; this represents the holding part of the reflex described by Denny Brown.[6626]

Grasset, Jean (1849–1918) French neurologist.

Grasset sign 1. The inability of hemiparetic patients to raise both legs together by flexion at the hip, while remaining capable of raising either one separately.[5704] 2. (Grasset–Gaussel sign, Hoover sign) When the patient with hemiparesis attempts to raise the weak leg, excessive downward pressure can be felt on the examiner's hand placed under the heel of the healthy leg. Either leg may be lifted independently but they cannot be elevated together. If the paretic leg is elevated and the normal leg is elevated next, then the paretic leg will fall back to the bed; but if the healthy leg is elevated first and the paretic leg is then passively raised, then the normal leg will remain in position.[1500]

Grasset–Gaussel sign See **Grasset sign**.

Graves, Robert James (1797–1853) Irish physician practicing in Dublin who first recognized that diseases could affect the peripheral nerves, having attended Parisian patients during an epidemic of "neuritis" in 1828.

Graves ophthalmopathy See **dysthyroid orbitopathy**.

gray matter heterotopias Nodules of neuropil, composed of astrocytes and neurons, located in the white matter of the brain.

gray rami The C fibers.

gray spinal syndrome An antique term for lesions of the central cord.

great toe phenomenon of Edelmann See **toe reflex**.

great vein of Galen A major intracerebral vein, draining into the straight sinus. It was once thought to cause hydrocephalus when occluded, but this is disproved.

greater auricular neuralgia A syndrome of intermittent painful paresthesias in the distribution of this nerve, not precipitated by touch, and likely to be caused by partial damage to the C3 nerve root.[692]

Greenfield, Joseph Godwin (1884–1958) British neuropathologist who trained in Edinburgh and at the **National Hospital**, Queen Square, where he was

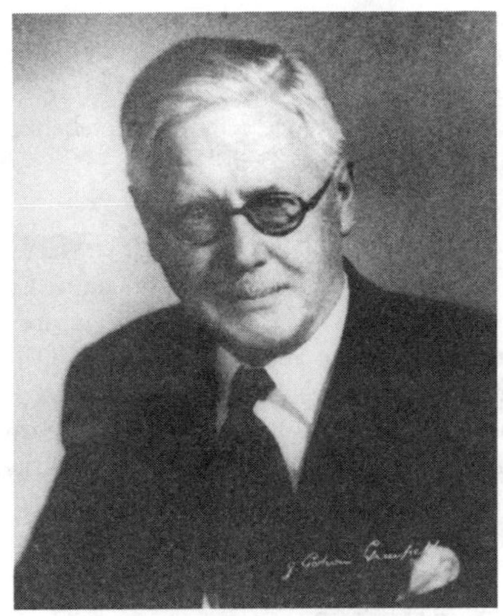

Figure G–4 Godwin Greenfield.

appointed neuropathologist in 1914. From his laboratory there emanated a steady output of important papers, their clarity enhanced by brevity, and his book on neuropathology which was the gold standard during his lifetime. As dean of the Institute of Neurology, he fostered the careers of many young physicians. His books *The Pathology of the Nervous System* (1921), *The Cerebrospinal Fluid* (1925, in collaboration), and *Neuropathology* (1958) were acclaimed for presenting the most modern information in a readable style. His contributions to the clinical practice of neurology were recognized by his presidency of the Association of British Neurologists (1954–1956).

Greenfield disease See **metachromatic leukodystrophy**.

Gregg syndrome (maternal rubella syndrome) A syndrome of multiple congenital anomalies as a result of infection of the mother with rubella during the first trimester. Characteristic findings include congenital cataract, microphthalmos, deafness, microcephaly, hydrocephalus, and congenital cardiac anomalies.[2572] See **congenital rubella embryopathy**.

Greig, David Middleton (1864–1936) Scottish surgeon working in Dundee, where he was concerned with the management of mentally retarded children as well as with a wide range of topics in clinical surgery. He was the first to describe **hypertelorism**, both isolated and as part of the **Greig syndrome**.

Greig syndrome 1. (ocular hypertelorism, euryopia) An autosomal dominant, X-linked, or sporadic syndrome of unusually wide spacing between the eyes, frequently in association with other developmental defects.[2573] 2. (cephalopolysyndactyly) A dominantly inherited congenital maldevelopment mapped to chromosome 7p and characterized by the association of hypertelorism, a vertical ridge in the forehead often with brachycephaly or scaphocephaly, flattening of the occiput and bulging of the temporal bones, optic atrophy, bilateral VI cranial nerve palsies in the event of raised intracranial pressure, polysyndactyly, and frequently mental retardation. See **hypertelorism**.

Grenet syndrome (crossed-sensory paralysis) Bilateral facial thermoanalgesia, unilateral truncal thermoanalgesia, and homolateral V cranial nerve motor involvement due to a lesion of the tegmentum of the pons such as tumor or stroke. Homolateral ataxia, a coarse tremor, and a contralateral hemiparesis may also be present.[5839]

Grey-Walter, W. English neurophysiologist at the Burden Neurological Institute in Bristol, UK, who first described **contingent negative variation**.

grid 1 (G1, input terminal 1 [E-l] active or exploring electrode) See **recording electrode**.

grid 2 (G2, input terminal 2 [E-2], or reference electrode) See **recording electrode**.

Griesinger, Wilhelm (1817–1868) German neurologist and psychiatrist who gave a good account of pseudohypertrophic muscular dystrophy well before **Duchenne**[2577] and introduced the concept of outpatient psychiatric care to clinical practice.

Griesinger sign Edema and tenderness over the mastoid process (the point of exit of an emissary vein) as evidence of thrombosis of the lateral sinus.

grip sign If the examiner's fingers are inserted between the flexed fingers of the subject, the subject's grip is normally increased by wrist extension and decreased by wrist flexion.[1500]

Grisel syndrome (nasopharyngeal torticollis) Nontraumatic, atlantoaxial dislocation with torticollis, occurring after oronasopharyngeal inflammation.[4890] The syndrome is uncommon in childhood and rare in adults.

Groll–Hirschowitz syndrome A congenital, recessively inherited maldevelopment syndrome manifesting also acanthosis nigricans, a malabsorption syndrome, sensorineural deafness, strabismus, ptosis, pes cavus, sensorimotor neuropathy (perhaps due to vitamin E deficiency), and anencephaly or craniorachischisis.[2919]

Gronblad, Ester Elizabeth (b. 1898) Swedish ophthalmologist.

Gronblad–Strandberg syndrome A rare, recessively inherited syndrome due to a widespread disorder of collagen formation and characterized by pseudoxanthoma elasticum in the skin, angioid streaks of the retina, macular and frequently gastrointestinal bleeding, accelerated atherosclerosis, and a tendency to intracranial aneurysm formation.[2585]

Groote syndrome A congenital dysmorphic syndrome manifesting also visceral maldevelopments, holoprosencephaly or arhinencephaly, polydactyly, hydrocephalus, and callosal abnormalities.[381]

groove sign Absence of dermal fibrosis overlying veins, leading to grooving over their surface when they collapse as the limb is elevated; a sign of **eosinophilic fasciitis**.

groping (instinctive grasp reaction, forced groping) The movement of pursuit of a patient's hand toward an object that has touched the hand or has crossed the patient's field of vision, as if to retain it. Further searching movements are made when the object has been removed from the palms. Like grasping, this is evidence of a mild pyramidal lesion, resulting from contralateral frontal lobe pathology.[6626] It represents an extension of the tactile response (**grasp response**) especially in response to visual stimuli.

Gross Motor and Reflex Development Test A 60-item scale for the assessment of reflex and voluntary motor functions up to the age of 5 years. See also Denver Developmental Screening Test.

Gross Motor Functional Classification System A leg functional assessment test for children with cerebral palsy.[4865]

Gross Motor Functional Measure A leg functional assessment test for children with cerebral palsy.[784]

gross motor functions Those functions that are mainly performed with the aid of proximal muscles, which allow, for example, head control, the sitting posture, and walking. See also **fine motor functions**.

Gross Motor Performance Measure A leg functional assessment test for children with cerebral palsy.[5472]

ground connection The conducting path between the subject and the EEG machine, and between the EEG machine and the earth.

ground electrode A connection from the patient to earth, used as a common return for an electric circuit and as an arbitrary zero potential reference point. (From the 2001 Report of the Nomenclature Committee of the American Association of Electromyography and Electrodiagnosis.[19] Reproduced by kind permission of the AANEM.)

group atrophy Atrophy of large groups of contiguous muscle fibers, characteristically seen in neurogenic muscle diseases. Both large groups of some hundreds of myofibrils and small groups of only a dozen or so are seen at different stages.

grouped denervation atrophy The occurrence of large groups of small angulated muscle fibers of the same histochemical type in muscle biopsy specimens. The finding suggests severe denervation. See also **disseminated neurogenic atrophy**.

grouped discharge 1. Irregular, voluntary grouping of motor unit action potentials as seen in a tremulous muscular contraction. 2. Involuntary grouping of motor unit action potentials as seen in myokymia. 3. A general term to describe repeated firing of motor unit action potentials. See **repetitive discharge**. (Adapted from the 2001 Report of the Nomenclature Committee of the American Association of Electromyography and Electrodiagnosis.[19] Reproduced by kind permission of the AANEM.)

Grove sign Abnormal resistance felt when a retracted eyelid is grasped and gently pulled downward, much as occurs with a forced duction test of the extraocular muscles. This is evidence of dysthyroid lid retraction.[2594]

growing pains Isolated nocturnal leg pains experienced by healthy children, particularly following a day of strenuous exercise. The nature of the cause is undetermined, but a family history of migraine is commonly noted.[4825]

growth cone Expansions at the head of newly sprouting axons at the site of nerve injury.

growth deficiency-clefting-retardation See **Myhre syndrome**.

growth retardation, alopecia, pseudoanodontia, and optic atrophy (GAPO syndrome) A congenital, recessively inherited dysmorphic syndrome characterized by the coexistence of Growth Retardation, Alopecia, Pseudoaniodontia, and pseudo-Optic atrophy.

Skeletal and dermal anomalies, frontal bossing, midface hypoplasia, hepatomegaly, macrocephaly, pendular nystagmus, papilledema, cerebral atrophy, and mental and developmental delay are other features described.[6333]

Grox syndrome A congenital dysmorphic syndrome manifesting also cardiac and skeletal abnormalities, seizures, microcephaly, pyramidal signs, and mental and developmental delay.[381]

Gruber syndrome (dysencephalia splanchnocystica, Meckel-Gruber syndrome) A recessively inherited congenital dysmorphic syndrome characterized by microcephaly; occipital exencephalocele; micropthalmia; hypertelorism; exophthalmos; polydactyly; polycystic kidneys, liver, and pancreas; congenital heart defects; and cleft lip and palate.[2598] Internal hydrocephalus, anencephaly, and cerebellar aplasia are also described.[3016]

Gruner–Bertolotti syndrome The association of impairment of conjugate upward gaze, loss of pain and temperature sensations, tremor and hemiparesis, and the effects of a mesencephalic lesion. Readers who enjoy eponyms will be pleased to learn that this condition has been regarded as the combination of the **Parinaud** and **von Monakow** syndromes.[1765]

Grüelder reflex (fontanelle reflex) Extension of the hallux with pressure on the fontanelle, seen in young children with increased intracranial pressure.

grusskrampfe See **flexor spasms**.

gryposis (Gr, crooked) Crookedness of a part, a term usually applied to the nails when they curve excessively or to joints (**arthrogryposis**).

Guam Parkinsonism–dementia complex (Guamanian neurodegenerative disease) A neurodegenerative disease resulting from ingestion of the seed of the neurotoxic plant *Cycas circinalis*, a traditional source of food and medicine of the Chamorro people. This causes cortical motor neural dysfunction, Parkinsonian features, and behavioral abnormalities with chromatic and degenerative changes of motor neurons in the cerebral cortex and spinal cord and an excess of cerebral neurofibrillary tangles.[5969] See **Lytico–Bodig**.

Guamanian neurodegenerative disease See **Guam Parkinsonism–dementia complex**.

guanidinoacetate methyltransferase deficiency (GAMT deficiency) A recessively inherited inborn error of creatine biosynthesis (a cerebral creatine deficiency syndrome) presenting in infancy with developmental delay, autistic features, intractable seizures and progressive extrapyramidal signs. Excretion of urinary creatinine is unusually low.[4319]

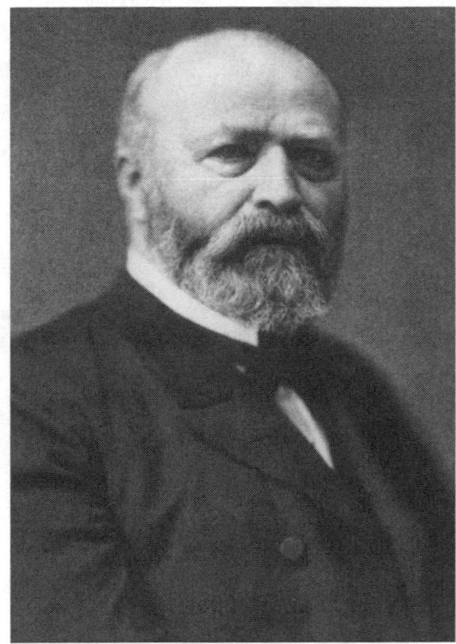

Figure G–5 Bernhard Aloys von Gudden.

Gubler, Adolphe-Marie (1821–1879) French physician and professor of therapeutics, whose first publications were on liver disease and syphilis. He recognized paralysis occurring after infections, which may have suggested the topic to **Landry**, his student. Gubler produced a series of publications on alternating hemiplegia between 1856 and 1858.[3373] See **Millard–Gubler syndrome**.

Gubler paralysis See **Millard–Gubler syndrome**.

Gudden, Bernhard Aloys von (1824–1886) Swiss psychiatrist, professor at Zurich and then at Munich. He was drowned in a lake by the actions of his patient, the insane King Ludwig II of Bavaria.[5619]

Gudden atrophy Secondary degeneration of the thalamic nuclei following destruction of certain cortical areas.[2609]

Gudden commissure A fiber tract between the inferior corpora quadrigemina and the medial geniculate bodies of the two sides, running closely with the optic tracts.

Gudden law The degeneration of the proximal end of a divided peripheral nerve proceeds centripetally.

Guerin–Stern disease See **arthrogryposis multiplex congenita**.

Guignon, Georges (1859–1932) French neuropsychiatrist, a pupil of **Charcot**, who, however, drifted away from neurology and into the specialty of tuberculosis therapy. He published a full account of convulsive tic (see **Tourette syndrome**) in 1886, a year after Tourette whose work he acknowledged, but the condition has occasionally been called Guignon disease.

Guild Memory Test A compound test including measures of immediate and delayed recall of paragraphs and paired associates and of immediate recall of designs, used to study changes in normal aging and Alzheimer disease.[2375]

Guillain, Georges (1876–1961) French physician who trained in Rouen and Paris and was intern under Raymond at the **Salpêtriére**, taking further training in America and Germany. In 1923 he became professor and chairman of neurology at the **Salpêtrière** after **Charcot, Raymond, Déjèrine**, and **Marie**, and held it until 1947 when **Alajouanine** took it over.

With Barré and Strohl, he published the classic account of **acute inflammatory demyelinating polyneuropathy**, their patients being soldiers who developed the disease during the World War I.[2621] A few years later he described the first test for CSF protein. His other areas of research were neuroanatomy, multiple sclerosis, the reflexes, brainstem vascular and other syndromes, hereditary ataxias, and the conditions described in the following entries.

Guillain sign In cases of meningitis, pinching one quadriceps muscle produces abrupt flexion of the hip and knee on the other side.[1540, 421]

Guillain–Alajouanine–Garcin syndrome See **Garcin syndrome**.

Guillain–Barré Support Group A British charitable organization providing information and support. Address: LCC Offices, Eastgate, Sleaford, NG34 7EB. Tel/Fax: +44 1529 304615. Support helpline: 0800 374 803 (UK); 0044 1529 415278 (RoI). E-mail: admin@gbs.org.uk. Web site: http://www.gbs.org.uk/.

Guillain-Barré syndrome See **acute inflammatory demyelinating polyneuropathy**.

Guillain–Barré Syndrome Foundation International A charitable organization in this field providing information and support. Address: P.O. Box 262, Wynnewood, PA 19096. Tel: 610-667-0131. E-mail: gbint@netcom.com. Web site: http://www.webmast.com/gbs/.

Guillain–Bertrand syndrome Unilateral arrhythmic myoclonus in the limbs as a result of a lesion of the dentate nucleus.[2622]

Guillain–Garcin syndrome See **Garcin syndrome**.

Guillain–Mollaret triangle A supposed brainstem pathway connecting the olive, the contralateral dentate nucleus, and the homolateral red nucleus—the circuit being completed by the posterior longitudinal bundle running between the red nucleus and the olive. Lesions of this circuit were determined by Guillain and Mollaret[2623] to result in **palatal myoclonus**. See **myoclonic triangle**.

Guillain–Thaon syndrome Spastic paraplegia as a result of meningomyelitis in tertiary syphilis.[2619]

Guinea worm (*Dracunculus medinensis*) A filarial parasite of humans which typically resides in subcutaneous tissue and protrudes through an ulcer in the skin. At this interface, the female nematode releases her larvae on contact with water and these are ingested by crustacean animalcules of the genus *Cyclops* which live in stagnant pools. When the *Cyclops* are inadvertently ingested in drinking water, the life cycle of the parasite is completed.

Aberrant migration of the parasite (dracontiasis, dracunculiasis) may rarely result in an epidural abscess with compressive myelopathy. Ocular involvement is also described.[346, 304] It is conceivable that the infestation could be eradicated globally by improvements in drinking water sanitation. (HJM)

Gulf War syndrome A selection of symptoms, sometimes bizarre and not allowing diagnosis of any known neurological disorder, occurring in some veterans of the 1991 Gulf War. Fatigue, paresthesias, numbness, headache, skin rashes, myalgia, arthralgia, chest pains or discomfort, dyspnea, impaired sleep and memory, and diarrhea are the more common symptoms. Objective signs are few, if any. The presence of a peripheral neuropathy has been suggested,[3151] but neurophysiologic analysis has discounted that.[5763]

Gull, Sir William Withey (1819–1890) Physician to Guy's Hospital, London, and a leading physician in England. He gave the first precise descriptions of anorexia nervosa, myxedema, intracranial aneurysm, and **syringomyelia** (1856–1862), and, in his Goulstonian Lectures of 1848, he dealt at length on the clinical features of cord compression and the paraplegias. Gull was also the first to recognize the lesions of **tabes dorsalis** in the posterior columns (1856).

Gull disease (adult cretinism) Acquired hypothyroidism with enlargement of the tongue, mental slowing, and the usual ectodermal and other systemic changes of **myxedema**. The condition was described by Gull in 1874;[2635] in the same issue of the Medical Society's transactions he described **anorexia nervosa**.

Gullstrand, Alivar (1862–1934) Swedish ophthalmologist who received the Nobel Prize in 1911 for his work on "the dioptrics of the eye."

Gullstrand law When a patient is made to turn the head when fixing on a distant object, if the corneal reflex (corneal light reflection) from either eye moves in the direction in which the head is turning, it moves toward the weaker muscle.[2636]

gum hypertrophy A classic sign of chronic phenytoin toxicity in those with teeth, which the overgrowth of gingival tissue may hide so that gum excision is necessary.

gumma (from Lat, gum) Inflammatory granulation tissue composed of fibrosis, mononuclear cell infiltration, and necrosis resulting from obliterative endarteritis, forming an irregular nodular tumor in the cerebral hemispheres, pons, or elsewhere in the brain or the rest of the body in patients with tertiary syphilis. The term was introduced early in the sixteenth century.

gun-barrel constriction of the visual fields (tubular constriction) Marked and usually symmetric constriction of the fields, typically found in patients with glaucoma or **pigmentary retinal degenerations**.

The term is unfortunate, because the diameter of the field perceived does in fact increase with distance from the subject in the above conditions, though not in the setting of malingering nor in hysterical visual field constriction.

Gunn, Robert Marcus (1850–1909) Scottish ophthalmologist who trained in Edinburgh and Vienna and at Moorfields Eye Hospital in London, where (as at the National Hospital and the Hospital for Sick Children) he was later appointed surgeon. He introduced substantial improvements in the methods of examination of the eyes and ocular surgery. He also wrote on the topics of the retina, optic atrophy, nystagmus, retinal vascular disease, and comparative anatomy.

Gunn pupil (Marcus Gunn pupil, relative afferent pupillary deficit) Constriction followed by re-dilation of the pupil with continued exposure to direct light stimulation in an eye affected by an optic nerve lesion (but also in the other eye consensually).[6659] When there is pathological attrition of functioning optic nerve fibers, the residual input to the pupilloconstrictor center after several seconds of constant stimulation is much the same as that resulting from the background illumination, so the pupil dilates again.

Levatin rather than Marcus Gunn described the **swinging flashlight test**; Gunn observed the reactions of both eyes to stimulation of one of them, while Levatin observed the paradoxical dilation of the pupil of the affected eye when the flashlight is swung across to it from the normal eye.

Gunn phenomenon (Marcus Gunn phenomenon, jaw winking, trigemino-ocular synkinesis) A congenital syndrome of marked unilateral ptosis with elevation of the eyelid when the mouth is opened, further increased by deviation of the jaw to the other side. Less typical clinical features include elevation of the lid on protrusion of the jaw or tongue, clenching the teeth or swallowing, and inspiration or smiling. Despite the name, the syndrome does not include a wink at all but rather ocular "mooning," to coin a phrase. It was described by Marcus Gunn in 1883.

This is thus the opposite of the **Marin-Amat syndrome** (inhibition of the levator palpebrae with jaw-opening, usually a developmental anomaly).[2640] Both conditions are usually seen as developmental anomalies, although the syndrome may be recessively inherited or occur as an irregular dominant characteristic, when a supranuclear cause is postulated. When acquired, it may indicate anomalous re-innervation of the levator palpebrae muscle after III nerve injury, but it may also occur after VII nerve lesions[2640] or as the result of abnormal innervation by the motor division of the V cranial nerve to the ipsilateral levator palpebrae superioris.[1932]

gustatory (from Lat, taste) Relating to the sense of taste.

gustatory aura A perception of taste sensations including acidic, bitter, salty, sweet, or metallic, as part of a focal seizure involving a temporal lobe. See **mesial temporal lobe epilepsy**.

gustatory lacrimation See **crocodile tears**.

gustatory piloerection Gooseflesh provoked by eating. This occasionally occurs in an upper limb following surgical injury to a cervical sympathetic ganglion. Evidently the phenomenon is the result of aberrant reinnervation. (HJM)[2886, 685]

gustatory reaction The normal infant will force the salt-coated finger away with his tongue.[6898]

gustatory sweating (Frey syndrome, Baillarger syndrome, Dupuy syndrome, auriculotemporal syndrome, Salivo-Sudipar syndrome) Localized sweating and flushing of the face in response to acid or spicy tastes, occurring after damage to the parasympathetic fibers in the auriculotemporal nerve as a result of parotid gland disease or from iatrogenic causes. The signs result from cross stimulation of sympathetic by parasympathetic fibers which have regenerated in an improper direction after injury.[2199] The syndrome was first described by Duphenix in 1757;

Dupuy in 1816 and Parkes-Weber in 1897 gave further accounts before the more modern one.

While occasionally seen in normal people (Claude **Bernard** experienced it when he ate chocolate), it is usually due to damage to the auriculotemporal nerve (auriculotemporal syndrome) when the area of sweating is localized to a small region anterior to the ear, or it is due to incomplete damage to the sympathetic pathways which still allows innervation of a region in which there is a degree of denervation hypersensitivity.[2803] Foix found the first reported description to have been that of Duphenix in 1757. A dominantly inherited *variant* is also described.[4030]

See also **gustolacrimal reflex** and **crocodile tears**.

Guttmann sign

Autonomic overactivity occurring following a high thoracic cord lesion, with piloerection, sweating, vasoconstriction, hypertension, bradycardia, mydriasis, and blockage of nasal air passages, occurring paroxysmally on the occasions of excessive stimulation of the automatic bladder by urine.

Guttmann Sweat Test

A test of sympathetic cholinergic function in which a color change is produced when quinizarin powder is placed on sweating but not on dry skin.[2648]

Guyon, Jean-Casimir-Felix

(1831–1920) French surgeon who studied in Paris, where he later became professor of surgical pathology. He described the canal named for him in 1861.

Guyon canal

A short, oblique fibro-osseous space medial to the pisiform bone in the hand and bounded by this bone, the hook of the hamate, the transverse carpal ligament, and a ligament between the hamate and the pisiform. The ulnar nerve divides into its deep palmar branch and the hypothenar motor and cutaneous sensory branches to the medial 1½ digits within the canal.

Compression of the nerve at this site is a well-recognized occupational hazard in carpenters, cobblers, cyclists, and others.

Guyon canal syndrome

(pisohamate tunnel syndrome) See **ulnar nerve palsies**.

gyrate atrophy of choroid and retina

A recessively inherited, congenital, progressive tapetoretinal degeneration manifesting also cataracts, constriction of the visual fields, night blindness, myopia, seizures, myopathic weakness with type II fiber atrophy, and hyperornithinemia resulting from an inborn error of aminoacid metabolism.[5874] Blindness is usual before the age of 60.

gyratory nystagmus

See **circular nystagmus**.

gyrus

(from Lat, a circuit or ring) The convolutions of the surface of the brain, ignored in Greek and Roman writings and only appearing in works during the Renaissance. Most are small and somewhat variable in position, but a few are constant in position, such as the hippocampal, cingulate, angular, transverse (Heschl), precentral and postcentral, subcallosal, superior, middle and inferior temporal, or cuneate and dentate gyri.

The spirals of the cochlea are so-named as well.

gyrus rectus syndrome

Compression of the optic nerve at the anterior cranial fossa by a frontal mass, with the clinical features of visual loss and papilledema.[6616]

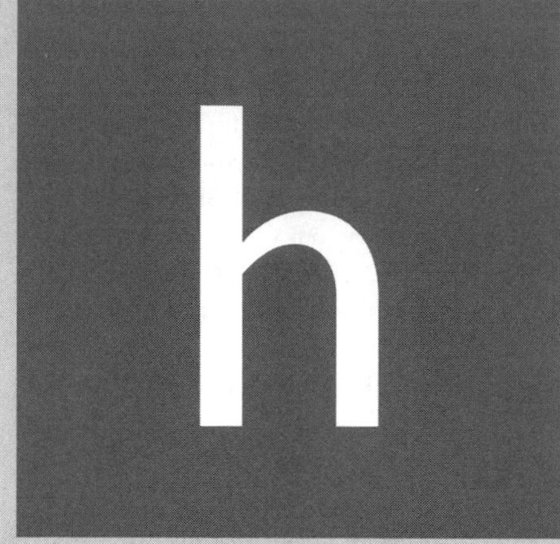

H reflex (H wave, Hoffmann reflex) A compound muscle action potential (CMAP) having a consistent latency evoked regularly, when present, from a muscle by an electrical stimulus to its nerve. It is regularly found only in a limited group of physiologic extensors, particularly the calf muscles with tibial nerve stimulation.

The H wave is most easily obtained in calf and forearm muscles with the cathode positioned proximal to the anode. Compared with the maximum amplitude M wave of the same muscle, the H wave is smaller and has a longer latency and a lower optimal stimulus intensity. The latency is longer with more distal sites of stimulation. Stimulus intensity sufficient to elicit a maximum-amplitude M wave reduces or abolishes the H wave. An abnormal H reflex results from a lesion anywhere along the reflex pathway, with either dorsal or ventral root involvement.

The H wave is thought to be a spinal reflex, with electrical stimulation of afferent fibers in the mixed nerve to the muscle and activation of motor neurons to the muscle, accomplished through a monosynaptic connection in the spinal cord. The reflex and wave are named in honor of Hoffmann, who had observed in 1918 that the CMAP associated with ankle and knee jerks were comparable in latency and configuration to those evoked by submaximal stimulation of tibial and femoral nerves and reasoned that abolition of the late response with supramaximal stimulation and brief latency (30 ms in the calf) must be a result of fast-conducting nerve fibers and a short central delay. (From the 1987 Report of the Nomenclature Committee of the American Association of Electromyography and Electrodiagnosis. AAEE glossary of terms in clinical electromyography. *Muscle Nerve* 1987;10S:G5–G23. © 1987. Reproduced by permission of the AANEM and of John Wiley and Sons. Inc.) cf. **F wave, A wave**.

The upper limit of normal is 35 ms and the normal side-to-side latency difference is less than 1.1 ms. Values corrected for height are reproduced in Chart H–1.

The reflex is hardly obtainable elsewhere, with the exception of the flexor carpi radialis.[3115]

Chart H–1. Normal Values of H-Reflex Latency According to Height

147–160 cm	163–175 cm	178–193 cm
28.46 ± 1.8	29.9 ± 2.12	31.5 ± 1.2

Haab, Otto (1851–1931) Swiss ophthalmologist, in Zurich.

Haab reflex Bilateral pupillary constriction when one eye is confronted with a bright light; the consensual pupillary reaction.

HAART Highly Active AntiRetroviral Therapy—combinations of three or more anti-HIV drugs including nucleoside and non-nucleoside reverse transcriptase inhibitors and protease inhibitors.

Haas sex-linked disease with copper metabolism defect A syndrome characterized by psychomotor retardation, seizures, low serum copper and ceruloplasmin levels, and impaired absorption of copper from the gut, but differing from **Menkes disease** in the virtual absence of pili torti, absence of hypothermia, normal birth weight at term, and later demise.[2659]

Habel syndrome A congenital dysmorphic syndrome manifesting also generalized hirsutism, skeletal maldevelopments, seizures, spasticity, hydrocephalus, and mental and developmental delay.[381]

habenula (Lat, a bridle or strap) A thalamic nucleus situated above the pineal whence it was considered by the ancients to drive and control the seat of the soul.

habituation Decrease in size of a reflex motor response to an afferent stimulus when the latter is repeated, especially at regular and recurring short intervals. (From the 2001 Report of the Nomenclature Committee of the American Association of Electromyography and Electrodiagnosis.[19] Reproduced by kind permission of the AANEM.)

habromania (Gr, graceful + madness) A form of insanity in which the patient is abnormally merry.

Hachinski Dementia Score A brief scale rating decline in the performance of everyday activities (an 8-point score) and in personal habits (up to 20 points). Although innovative in its use of a patient's easily assessed functional abilities as the basis for scoring, it has been little utilized in comparison with other similar diagnostic scales, and far less than its sibling, the **Hachinski Ischemia Score**.

Hachinski Ischemia Score A validated instrument designed to differentiate the demented patient with multiple infarcts from the patient with **Alzheimer disease**; it does this successfully, not so much as a result of any difference in mental state but on the basis of other clinical, temporal, and historical data (see Chart H–2).

Chart H–2. The Hachinski Ischemic Score

Feature	*Score*
Abrupt onset	1
Stepwise deterioration	1
Fluctuating course	2
Nocturnal confusion	1
Relative preservation of personality	1
Depression	1
Somatic complaints	1
Emotional incontinence	1
History of hypertension	1
History of strokes	2
Evidence of associated atherosclerosis	1
Focal neurological symptoms	2
Focal neurological signs	2

A score of 4 or more suggests that the patient does not have pure ***Alzheimer disease,*** *and that a vascular component is a cause of or contributing to the clinical syndrome.*[2663] *(From Hachinski VC, et al. Multi-Infarct Dementia.* Arch Neurol *1975;32:632–7. © American Medical Association 1975 by kind permission.)*

A revised and reduced *variation* of the scale has been proposed by Rosen et al.[5396] in which the assessment is limited to the following clinical features: abrupt onset, stepwise deterioration, history of stroke, focal neurological signs, emotional incontinence, and somatic complaints.

Haenel, H. (1874–1942) German neurologist who studied at Freiburg, Munich, and Berlin and graduated at Heidelberg. He practiced in Halle and Dresden.

Haenel sign Lack of pain in the eye when it is pressed by the examiner. The sign is positive in the presence of tertiary neurosyphilis. Bradycardia and hypotension, the normal responses to this maneuver, are also absent.[2673]

Haenel variant A form of muscular dystrophy affecting only the arms.

Haff disease An inflammatory myopathy resulting in **myoglobinuria** and caused by the ingestion of eels or fish contaminated by industrial toxins, probably arsenic. The first report was from the Kurische Haff (harbor) area of Königsberg, Germany.[279] **Hornet** stings may produce a similar syndrome.

hag (the old hag) An evil spirit in female form, believed in some cultures to oppress the chest in subjects with **sleep paralysis**.

Hagberg disease A *variant* of **Krabbe leukodystrophy**.

Hagberg lipofuscinosis See **neuronal ceroid lipofuscinosis**.

Hagenbach–Bing myopathy See **myopathica rachitica**.

Hague Seizure Severity Scale A 13-item self-administered scale comprising the reports of parents about their child's seizures.[1028]

Hahn sign Persistent rotation of the head from side to side in cerebellar disease.

hair-brain syndrome A congenital, recessively inherited syndrome characterized by cataract, sexual infantilism, dwarfism, nail dystrophy, brittle hair, and physical and mental delay.[3123]

Hajdu–Cheney syndrome A congenital, sporadic, or dominantly inherited dysmorphic syndrome characterized by basilar impression, craniofacial and peripheral dysostoses, spinal osteoporosis, and chondrodystrophy.[2684] See also **osteopetrosis**.

Hakim–Adams syndrome See **normal pressure hydrocephalus**.

Halal syndrome A congenital dysmorphic syndrome manifesting also pigmentary retinopathy, goiter, microcephaly, and mental and developmental delay.[381]

Hall, Marshall (1790–1857) English physician who trained in Edinburgh and after making a Grand Tour of European centers, settled to practice in Nottingham and later in London, but was never appointed to any London hospital.

As a comparative anatomist and neurophysiologist he discovered and interpreted the role of the spinal cord in reflex activity,[2692] introducing the terms **reflex arc** and **spinal shock** (1850) and demonstrating conclusively the dualistic nature of neural functioning, both volitional and reflex. He also suggested an association between epilepsy and anemia of the medulla oblongata and was the first to describe the **grasp reflex** and **spinal shock**. He published at least 15 major books, collections of lectures and tracts on neurology or

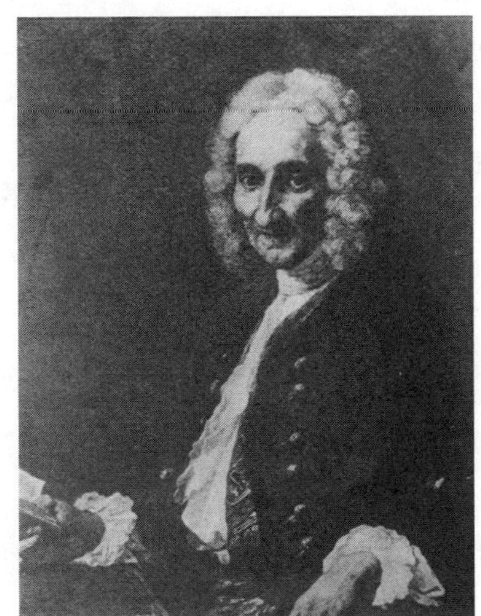

Figure H–1 Marshall Hall.

neurophysiology, and over 150 papers. His advocacy of the establishment of a hospital for people with epilepsy in 1852 (now the **National Hospital**) speeded its foundation.

Hall disease See **Wilson disease**.

Hall syndrome 1. (hydroencephaloid, spurious hydrocephalus) A syndrome thought by Marshall Hall to suggest hydrocephalus in infants or children with anemia, gastrointestinal complaints, and tachycardia. He published his comments in a volume of essays in 1825; from the descriptions given, however, dehydration following gastroenteritis seems a most likely etiology. 2. (Pallister–Hall syndrome) A sporadic, lethal, congenital dysmorphic syndrome caused by *Gli3* mutations and characterized by features of **Turner syndrome** with synostosis of the coronal suture; imperforate anus: various visceral, endocrine, and skeletal abnormalities; and a tendency for hypothalamic hamartoblastomas to develop.[2690]

Haller, Albrecht von (1708–1777) Swiss anatomist, botanist, and professor of medicine at Göttingen. He was for a time physician to the English King George II.

Haller was reputed to have had 1300 publications, among which were his demonstrations that all CSF eventually drains into the venous system, that nerves are irritable structures and that peripheral stimulation causes impulses to be sent to the brain. He was also the first to describe the foramen of Luschka.

Hallerman–Streiff–François syndrome (oculomandibular dyscephaly with hypotrichosis) A rare oculoauriculocephalic anomaly comprising short stature, brachycephaly with prominent frontal and parietal bones, long beaked nose, thin sparse hair, thin skin, microphthalmia and micrognathia, congenital cataracts, dental anomalies, nystagmus, optic atrophy, and mental delay. The dysmorphism leads to an appearance of "bird-headedness," and unilateral proptosis is also described.[2693]

Hallervorden, Julius (1882–1965) German neuropathologist who trained at Königsberg and worked as a psychiatrist in Landsberg. He described the syndrome named for him and his mentor Hugo Spatz while working in Munich in 1922. He later joined Spatz at the Kaiser Wilhelm Institute in Berlin and, after World War II, in Frankfurt.

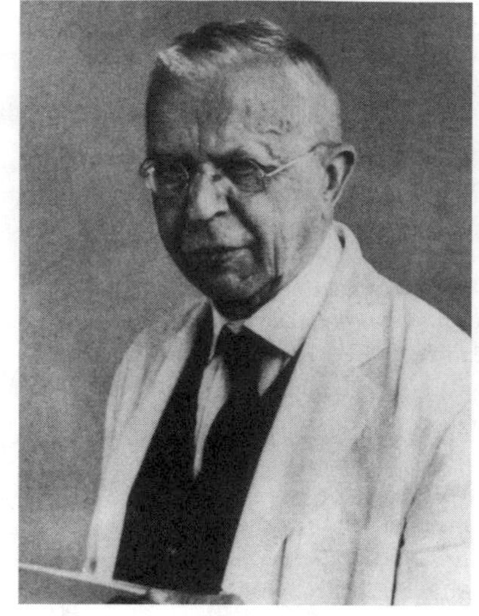

Figure H–2 Julius Hallervorden.

Hallervorden (not himself a member of the National Socialist party, but dependent upon it in wartime Germany and thus himself passively brutalized) participated actively in the Nazi-inspired euthanasia programs, thus collecting extensive data on the pathologies leading to mental illness or retardation.[5792]

Hallervorden–Spatz disease See **neurodegeneration with brain iron accumulation**.

Hallervorden–Spatz Syndrome Association A charitable organization in this field providing information and support. Address: 2082 Monaco Court, El Cajon, CA 92019-4235. Tel: 619-588-2315. E-mail: HSSA-KWPAC@msn.com. Web site: http://www.hssa.org/

Hallgren syndrome See **von Graefe–Sjögren syndrome**.

Hallipré sign Dorsiflexion of the wrist during attempted grip on the side of a radial nerve lesion.

Hallpike, Charles Skinner (1900–1979) British neuro-otologist who trained at Guy's Hospital in London. His early clinical and research interests in diseases of the ear led to his appointment to the National Hospital, Queen Square, after he defined the pathology of Ménière syndrome (endolymphatic hydrops) where he founded and directed the Neuro-otology unit, which he led until his retirement. He is best remembered for his precise definition of methods and norms for **caloric tests** and for his clinical analysis of the commoner causes of vertigo, which led to his original description of **vestibular neuronitis** and to the modern characterizations of **Ménière syndrome** and **benign paroxysmal positional vertigo**.[354]

hallucinations (from Lat, to wander mentally) Subjective perceptions without objective stimuli.

hallucinatory aura In the context of epilepsy, the creation of composite perceptions without corresponding external stimuli involving visual, auditory, somatosensory, olfactory, and/or gustatory phenomena.

hallux (from Lat, the big toe) The great toe.

Halpern syndrome See **dysequilibrium syndrome**.

Halstead Aphasia Screening Test A part of the **Halstead–Reitan Battery**.[5261] An abbreviated and amended form is also available.[2843]

Halstead–Reitan Battery An evaluative tool for a wide range of psychological activities, including parts of the **Wechsler Adult Intelligence Scale**, the category test, the Reitan **trail-making test**, an aphasia screening examination, and the **finger tapping test**. By these means, abstract thought, motor performance, rhythm and perception, gnosis, trail-making, sensory functions, grip strength, auditory perception, time perception, verbal and nonverbal memory, perceptual motor speed, spatial relations, finger gnosis, double simultaneous stimulation and personality are all assessed.[5261] An impairment score is derived from the patient's overall performance on this complex battery.

Haltia–Santavuori syndrome See **neuronal ceroid lipofuscinosis**.

HAM Acronym for HTLV 1-**associated myelopathy**. See **tropical spastic paraparesis**.

hamartoma (from Gr, to miss the goal) A collection of cells that are misplaced within the CNS as a result of faulty migration during embryonal development. They consist typically of masses of neurons, glia, and fiber bundles and may contain neurosecretory granules.

Although commonly asymptomatic, hamartomas may act as a focus for seizure discharges in certain sites, such as the temporal lobes or the hypothalamus. In the latter site they may be manifest by **gelastic seizures**. See **Hall syndrome**.

Hamilton Rating Scale (HRS) An interviewer- and observer-rated measure of psychological and somatic symptoms determining the severity of depressive illness.[2717] One of the earliest published and still probably the most widely used of the depression scales; this was not designed as a diagnostic instrument but rather as a tool for assessing change in depressed patients under treatment. This instrument scores more of the somatic symptoms of depression than do others.[2716]

hammer palsy Unilateral shoulder girdle weakness, once thought to be due to excessive use of the hammer but more probably a form of **brachial plexopathy**.

Hammersmith Motor Ability Score A scale for scoring muscle power, of particular value in the assessment of children with muscular dystrophies.[5690] (see Chart H–3)

Hammond, William Alexander (1828–1900) American neurologist, professor of anatomy and physiology at Maryland, and later Surgeon-General of the Army. He recognized the importance of the study of neurological disorders arising from the injuries sustained during the American Civil War and appointed Dr. S. **Weir Mitchell** to head a newly established neurological unit in Philadelphia. Court-martialled on trumped-up charges precipitated by his peremptory and dictatorial manner, he was dismissed after 2 years as surgeon-general but was later reinstated when Congress quashed the verdict. Meanwhile, he had returned to private practice in New York, where he was shortly afterwards appointed professor of neurology at the City University, and later at Bellvue.

His *Treatise on Diseases of the Nervous System* (New York, 1871) was the first American textbook of neurology and went to nine editions. It preceded that of **Gowers** by 10 years. His description of athetosis, contained within it,[4232] led to the eponymous labeling of that condition for over half a century. Hammond was a distinguished lecturer who also wrote novels and plays and was a founder of the **American Neurological Association** (of which both he and his son were to be presidents) and of the Army Medical Museum, now known as the Walter Reed Army Institute of Research.

Hammond syndrome See **athetosis**.

Hand, A. (1868–1949) American pediatrician. He thought that the osteolytic bone lesions that he detected in his patient were tuberculous. See **Hand–Schüller–Christian disease**.

HAND See **HIV-associated neurocognitive disorders**.

Chart H–3. The Hammersmith Motor Ability Score

1. Lifts head	11. Standing on toes
2. Supine to prone over right	12. Standing on right leg
3. Supine to prone over left	13. Standing on left leg
4. Prone to supine over right	14. Hops on right leg
5. Prone to supine over left	15. Hops on left leg
6. Gets to sitting	16. Gets off chair
7. Sitting	17. Climbing step right leg
8. Gets to standing	18. Descending step right leg
9. Standing	19. Climbing step left leg
10. Standing on heels	20. Descending step left leg

All movements are attempted and scored as follows: 2, for every completed movement; 1, for help and/or reinforcement; 0, if unable to achieve the movement. (From Scott OM, Goddard C, Dubowitz V. Quantitation of muscle function in children; a prospective study in Duchenne muscular dystrophy. Muscle Nerve *1982;5:291–301. Reproduced by kind permission of John Wiley and Sons. Inc.)*

hand cramps Focal dystonias of the hands precipitated by various skilled activities such as writing or playing musical instruments.[1230]

hand flexor reflex Flexion of the wrist in response to tapping of the flexor tendons at the wrist or the palmar surface of the fingers when the fingers are loosely supported by the examiner. The contraction is enhanced in cases of pyramidal lesions above C6, but also in states of emotional tension.

A similar extensor reflex can also be obtained.

hand washing Persistent intertwining and rotation of the hands, a characteristic motor automatism in **Rett syndrome**.

hand–arm vibration syndrome An acquired progressive disease comprising vasospasm with blanching of the fingers; neuropathy with paresthesias, numbness, impaired finger coordination, and hand dexterity; and musculoskeletal involvement. It is due to prolonged occupational exposure to high-amplitude vibrations.[4228, 1970, 6241]

See also **vibration white finger**.

handcuff neuropathy Numbness of the thumb and index finger as a result of compression damage to the superficial radial nerve resulting from the too-tight application of handcuffs, or even wristwatches. Damage to the ulnar and to the median nerve from the same cause have also been recorded.[5693]

handedness The preferential use of one hand (or foot) for motor tasks such as writing (or kicking). Such a preference is usually seen after the age of 2 years, and if present before that age suggests the presence of impairment of motor control in the opposite hand. The perception of "correctness" in using the right hand is suggested by the positive connotations of the words "right" and "dextrous" and by the pejorative "sinister," although the Book of Judges records the exploits of 700 left-handed slingers, who allegedly never missed their targets.

The dominant hemisphere for speech may be inferred from handedness—all right handers (but only *most* left handers) having speech dominance in the left hemisphere. See also **Wada Test**.

handicap 1. A disability affecting a person's social or professional activities, requiring the adoption of a change in lifestyle. 2. A disadvantage resulting from an impairment or disability, limiting or preventing the fulfilment of a role for a person. However, age and social and cultural factors must be considered when assessing a handicap. 3. The disadvantage resulting from a failure to conform with society's expectations or norms laid down for an individual. See also **disability** and **impairment**.

HaNDL See **headache with neurologic deficits and CSF lymphocytosis**.

hand–mouth reflex See **Babkin reflex**.

Hand–Schüller–Christian disease (generalised xanthomatosis, histiocytosis X, lipoid granulomatosis, craniohypophysial xanthomatosis) A disease marked by the widespread deposition of masses of cholesterol-laden histiocytes, leading to the classic triad of exophthalmos, diabetes insipidus, and osteolytic bone lesions in the orbit or in the base of the skull.

Other signs may include papilledema; extraocular palsies and nystagmus; involvement of lower cranial nerves, cerebellum, and pyramidal tracts; increased intracranial pressure; hepatosplenomegaly; pulmonary infiltration; skin eruptions; xanthelasmas and xanthomas; and lymphadenopathy.[2723] The neurological complications are variable and nonspecific, depending on the sites of accumulation of the abnormal cells.

This represents one of those conditions to which none of the usually accepted eponyms should apply, the condition having been recognized in 1865 by the English pathologist Thomas Smith (1833–1909), while Hand published a description of it in 1893, Schuller in 1915, and Christian in 1919.

A. Schuller (1874–1957) was an Austrian radiologist, who first suggested the trans-sphenoidal approach for operations on the pituitary. His description of the abnormalities to be found on skull X-ray studies was unparalleled and he was appointed professor in Vienna but fled the city, leaving his sons, when threatened by Nazism. He emigrated to Australia, where his opinions were widely sought.

H.A. Christian (1876–1951) was an American physician who was head of the medical service at Peter Bent Brigham hospital in Boston. His report covered all the important points of the disease.[2066]

Hane whistle-smile sign The failure of patients with **Parkinson disease** to smile when they are asked to whistle.[2725]

hanging leg syndrome Combined sciatic and femoral nerve palsies, leading to severe proximal leg weakness, usually in the context of nerve compression in patients with reduced consciousness due, for example, to alcohol intoxication. See also **Saturday night palsy**.

hanging sensory loss (suspended sensory loss) Altered sensation and weakness in the arms but not in the legs, occurring as a result of a central cord lesion. The pathology affects the medial portion of the descending lateral corticospinal tract, the anterior horn cells at that level, and both the crossing fibers and the more central fibers in the spinothalamic tract; these latter fibers carry impulses from the arms and upper trunk.

hangman fracture A fracture of the neural arch of the second cervical vertebra bilaterally with associated rupture of the anterior longitudinal ligament and C2–3 spondylolisthesis. The odontoid process is not displaced. This may occur as the result of a severe extension injury; the use of a submental knot in judicial hanging is intended to induce it, with immediate effective transection of the cervical cord at that level. Less severe cord injury (or occasionally none at all) may result when the fracture occurs in other traumatic conditions such as motor vehicle accidents.[796]

hangover headache See **delayed alcohol-induced headache**.

Hanhart disease Recessively inherited **hereditary spastic paraparesis** associated with mental deficiency.[5704]

Hansen, Gerhardt Henrik Armauer (1841–1912) Norwegian physician who correctly related the presence of *Mycobacterium leprae* to clinical **leprosy** in 1871.

Hansen disease See **leprosy**.

happy feet See **burning feet syndrome**.

happy puppet syndrome A congenital dysmorphic syndrome manifesting also jerky, puppet-like movements and frequent spontaneous paroxysms of laughter in retarded, often microcephalic infants or children with infantile spasms, optic atrophy, cerebellar signs, and generalized seizures.[781] See also **Angelman syndrome**.

haptic (Gr, touching) The tactile and proprioceptive image of one's own body and the recognition of external objects using touch alone. An older use of the word, now defunct, indicated mental alienation (Hippocrates).

haptodysphoria An unpleasant sensation felt in response to tactile stimuli from discrete objects; the objects creating such sensations differ between individuals.

Harada syndrome (uveomeningoencephalitic syndrome, Harada–Vogt–Koyanagi syndrome, Vogt–Koyanagi syndrome) A syndrome of bilateral uveitis, exudative choroiditis and retinal detachment, vitiligo, depigmentation and loss of the hair, and signs of meningoencephalitis, invariably with CSF pleocytosis, seen mainly in people living in the Far East and occurring most commonly in adults.[2744]

Harada–Vogt–Koyanagi syndrome See **Harada syndrome**.

Harboyan syndrome A recessively inherited syndrome characterized by nerve deafness and congenital corneal dystrophy.[4185]

hard exudates Small glistening knobs seen on the retina in patients with chronic papilledema. They are considered to be composed of axoplasmic protein, extruded with continuing damage to the retinal nerve fibers.

hard palate reflex (Hennebert sign) Protrusion of the lips with stimulation of the hard palate; a sign of diffuse cortical dysfunction.

HARD + E syndrome See **hydrocephalus, agyria, retinal dysplasia and encephalocele syndrome**, and **Walker–Warburg syndrome**.

Hardin Meta Directory—Neurology/Neurosciences A valuable, well-constructed Web site listing many neurology-related links, maintained by the Hardin Library at the Health Sciences, University of Iowa.

Harding syndrome The association of **Leber hereditary optic neuropathy** with subsequent **multiple sclerosis**.[2760]

Hardy–Wilson system A grading scale for pituitary tumors with suprasellar extension.[964]

Hare syndrome See **Pancoast syndrome**.

harelip A congenital failure of fusion producing a fissure in the upper lip, resembling that normally seen in the hare and similar animals.

harlequin syndrome The happy nomination of a condition marked by the sudden onset of loss of thermoregulatory flushing and sweating on one side of the face without associated miosis, due to local autonomic dysfunction resulting from a cervical sympathetic deficit located at the pre- or postganglionic level on the nonflushing side.

That this deficit sometimes represents a lesion of the second sympathetic neuron is suggested by the increased **gustatory sweating** on that side, but the syndrome may also follow damage to the sympathetic pathway in the brainstem. Possibly this is due to sprouting of preganglionic sympathetic fibers originally destined for the salivary glands. Impairment of sympathetic activity on one side of the face without ptosis and miosis indicates a lesion of T2–3 in the cord at the intermediolateral column or white rami, as T3 carries most vasomotor and sudomotor fibers to the head and neck. The ocular sympathetic fibers leave at the level of T1.

The lesion is usually located at the level of pre- or postganglionic sympathetic fibers, probably due to trans-synaptic postganglionic neuronal degeneration at the level of the stellate ganglion. The finding of cholinergic supersensitivity in the iris muscles of patients with this syndrome indicates a relationship with **Holmes–Adie syndrome, Ross syndrome**, and the persistent autonomic deficit occasionally associated with acute inflammatory polyneuropathy.[3663, 1717, 4457]

Harlow, J.W. American physician who cared for Phineas **Gage** and reported his findings in 1848.[2771]

harmonic A wave appearing at a frequency which is a multiple of some given fundamental frequency; an example would be alpha activity at 16 Hz.

harmonious hypersomnia See **idiopathic CNS hypersomnolence**.[4523]

harmonious oxycephaly See **oxycephaly**.

HARP syndrome See **hypoprebetalipoproteinemia, acanthocytosis, retinitis pigmentosa**, and **pallidal degeneration**.

Harris, Sir Wilfred John (1869–1960) English neurologist, educated at Cambridge and the University of London, who later trained under Hughlings-**Jackson** and Sir William **Gowers** at the **National Hospital**, Queen Square. His consultant appointments were at the Maida Vale Hospital (linked with the National) and at St. Mary's, where he organized the first department of neurology in any of the British teaching hospital. He was also the first president of the Association of British Neurologists.

He is best remembered for his studies on the trigeminal nerve, for his delineation of the features of cluster headache (the "periodic migrainous neuralgia of Wilfred Harris"), and for his successful introduction of percutaneous alcohol injection of the Gasserian ganglion in the treatment of intractable trigeminal neuralgia, on one occasion injecting the second and third division fibers before an audience of neurologists at Queen Square.

Cluster headache has been labeled with his name, on account of the full description which he provided; he later changed his own name for it to *ciliary neuralgia*.[2781]

Harris neuralgia See **cluster headache**.

Harris syndrome (functional hypoglycemia) Weakness, hunger, anxiety, and mild confusion with signs of excessive sympathetic activity due to hypoglycemia. See also **Whipple triad**.

Harrod syndrome A congenital dysmorphic syndrome manifesting visceral, genital, and skeletal malformations, dolichocephaly, and mental and developmental delay.[381]

Hart syndrome See **Hartnup disease**.

Hartmann apraxia Apraxias resulting from tumors of the frontal lobe described by Fritz Hartmann (1871–1937), an Austrian neurologist and professor at Graz.[5704, 2789]

Hartnup disease (Hart syndrome) A recessively transmitted cerebellar syndrome of childhood (5p15.33, *SLC6A19*) due to a defect in the renal tubular resorption and intestinal transport of amino acids. It is characterized by a skin rash resembling that of pellagra, optic atrophy, pyramidal signs, dystonia, tremors, episodic ataxia, and episodes of delirium. Biochemical abnormalities include severe neutral and basic aminoaciduria and the urinary excretion of indican and glycinuria, but normal ammonium levels.

The intestinal absorption of tryptophan and thus the synthesis of nicotinamide are reduced, so some of the features of the disease are not surprisingly also those of **pellagra** and treatment with nicotinamide is of some value.

The condition was named for the family in which it was first detected by Dr. Charles Dent at the Middlesex Hospital in London.[415, 6186] See also **cerebellar ataxias** (*variants*).

Hartsfield syndrome A congenital dysmorphic syndrome manifesting also skeletal maldevelopments and craniosynostosis, encephalocele, holoprosencephaly, and callosal abnormalities.[381]

Harvard Medical School: The Whole Brain Atlas A Web site offering images of a normal brain, cerebrovascular disease, neoplastic disease, degenerative disease, and inflammatory or infectious disease, found at. http://www.med.harvard.edu/AANLIB/home.html/.

Harvey, William (1578–1657) English physician and physiologist. He is remembered in neurology for his descriptions of the venous drainage from the brain, the distinctions he made between motor and sensory nerves, and for his descriptions of patients with epilepsy and with syringomyelia.

Harvey syndrome A dominantly inherited syndrome of recent description, characterized by athetosis, hypotonia, areflexia, pyramidal signs, mental retardation, and periodic attacks of fever with unconsciousness, the neurological dysfunctions having their onset in early childhood in most cases.[2790]

Hashimoto encephalopathy (SREAT; steroid responsive encephalopathy associated with immune encephalopathy, nonvasculitic autoimmune meningoencephalitis, NAIM)

A subacute condition first described by Lord Brain in 1966, affecting euthyroid subjects, mainly women. It is associated with autoimmune thyroiditis and presents with acute, stroke-like focal neurologic deficits with mild cognitive impairment, dementia or mania, focal or generalized seizures including myoclonus, psychoses, ataxia, choreoathetosis, and altered consciousness. It has been described as a relapsing form of **ADEM**.[1119] Pathologically there is lymphocytic infiltration of brainstem veins as well as perivenular lymphocytic infiltration.

Unlike the encephalopathy associated with hypothyroidism, this one responds to steroid therapy but not to thyroxine replacement. High levels of antithyroid or antithyroperoxidase auto-antibodies are characteristic though not necessarily causal. Raised liver enzyme levels, ESR and CSF protein levels, or intrathecal IgG synthesis may occur, without pleocytosis. The EEG may show rhythmic delta activity or periodic sharp-wave complexes. See also **hyperthyroidism**.[1128, 5772a]

A *variant* presentation is *Hashimoto-associated ataxia*, an acute-onset cerebellar syndrome associated with abnormal behavior and high-intensity T2 signals in the cerebellum, responding remarkably to steroids and thyroid hormone therapy.[4051]

Another form resembles **Creutzfeldt–Jakob disease** in its manifestations.[1058]

Haspeslagh syndrome A congenital dysmorphic syndrome manifesting also short stature; cardiac, thyroid, and skeletal anomalies; microcephaly; pyramidal signs; nystagmus; and mental and developmental delay.[381]

Hassin sign (Langley–Sherrington sign, ear-wagging) Protrusion of the pinna of the ear on the side of a **Horner syndrome**, of which this is an additional feature. Contraction of the anterior and posterior auricularis muscles (supplied by the posterior auricular branch of the VII cranial nerve) is responsible, but why this should be is unknown.[3689, 3688] See also **ear-wiggling**.

Hatters' shakes (paralysis agitans mercurialis) A coarse distal tremor seen in those exposed on a long-term basis to organic mercury such as the sublimate, which was used in the raising of the nap on felt hats in the nineteenth century. See also **mad as a hatter**.

Hauptmann, Alfred (1881–1948) German neurologist who introduced phenobarbitone (luminal) for the treatment of epilepsy in 1907 and described an autosomal dominant muscular dystrophy.

Hauptmann–Thannhauser muscular dystrophy See **Emery–Dreifuss muscular dystrophy**.

Hauser Ambulation Index An assessment instrument designed to determine changes in the ability of patients with **multiple sclerosis** to ambulate.[2797] The 10 levels are described in Chart H–4. See also **Rivermead Mobility Index**.

haut mal (Fr, high + illness) An old term for major epilepsy (generalized tonic–clonic seizures).

Haven syndrome Pain in the wrist progressing proximally, pallor of the hand and wrist, and loss of the radial pulse, ascribed by Haven to compression of the subclavian artery by the scaleni. Perhaps it is a form of vasogenic **thoracic outlet syndrome**.[2800]

Haver, Clopton English anatomist of the eighteenth century who described the vascular channels within bone now named for him (Haversian canals).

Haypitcher's palsy Suprascapular neuropathy. This is also an occupational hazard of baseball pitchers.

Head, Sir Henry (1861–1940) English neurologist and neurophysiologist educated at Charterhouse and Trinity College, Cambridge. He worked with Hering in Prague on respiratory physiology and continued his studies in Cambridge and London leading to graduation in medicine in 1890. His earlier posts were held at University College Hospital and at the National Hospital; he eventually was appointed physician to the London and University College Hospitals. He was fluent in French and German (which was then essential for the editorship of **Brain**, which he held from 1910 to 1925,

Chart H–4. The Hauser Ambulation Index

0. Asymptomatic; fully active
1. Walks normally, but reports fatigue that interferes with athletic or other demanding activities
2. Abnormal gait or episodic imbalance; gait disorder is noticed by family and friends; able to walk 25 ft (7.5 m) in 10 s or less
3. Walks independently; able to walk 25 ft (7.5 m) in 20 s or less
4. Requires unilateral support (cane or single crutch) to walk; walks 25 ft (7.5 m) in 20 s or less
5. Requires bilateral support (canes, crutches, or walker) and walks 25 ft (7.5 m) in 25 s; or requires unilateral support but needs more than 20 s to walk 25 ft (7.5 m)
6. Requires bilateral support and more than 20 s to walk 25 ft (7.5 m); may use wheelchair occasionally
7. Walking limited to several steps with bilateral support; unable to walk 25 ft (7.5 m); in wheelchair for most activities
8. Restricted to wheelchair; able to transfer self-independently
9. Restricted to wheelchair; unable to transfer self-independently

From Hauser SL, Dawson DM, Lehrich JR. et al. Intensive immunosuppression in progressive multiple sclerosis. N Engl Med J *1983;308:173–80.*

during which time he consolidated the prestige of that journal).

Although publishing in many fields of neurology, he wrote over 20 papers on sensation between 1905 and 1918, which comprised perhaps one of his most lasting legacies. These papers were collected together in his *Studies in Neurology* (London, 1920). He mapped the dermatomes, in one experiment having his own superficial radial nerve sectioned in order to define the resulting area of sensory loss, and described the anatomy and variations of all of the major peripheral nerves and of the brachial plexus.[5323, 2818]

The studies performed on his own nerves led to his differentiation of forms of sensation between deep sensibility (pressure and proprioception); sharp, bright, localized **epicritic** pain; and deep, persistent, unlocalized, more vivid, less acute skin pain and extreme heat and cold (**protopathic pain**)[2816] after nerve injury. Head also postulated the nature of the epicritic and protopathic systems, the functions of which are now thought to be mediated in the central rather than in the peripheral nervous system.[2864]

Many of his other studies were made possible by his post as consultant to a hospital for officers in London during and after World War I. In 1900, he localized the site of herpetic inflammation to the dorsal root ganglia.[2815] During the later years of his career, he resigned his hospital appointments on developing the earliest evidence of **Parkinson disease** and devoted the greater part of his activities to the study of aphasia. This culminated in the publication of his book *Aphasia and Kindred Disorders of Speech* (1926), in which he divided the forms of aphasia between *verbal* (inability to form words internally or externally); *syntactical* (loss of balance and rhythm of speech with retained comprehension); *semantic* (failure to recognize the intention and significance of words); and *nominal* (loss of the use of names), a scheme that others have found difficult to employ.

He has been described as erudite, obsessional, critical, original, and energetic, full of enthusiasm and vivid scientific imagination. He had a wide and devoted following as a teacher, published a volume of poetry (*Destroyers and Other Verses*, Oxford, 1919) and had the capacity to discourse with wit and profound knowledge on a range of subjects any one of which would mark out the speaker as expert.[2864, 2865]

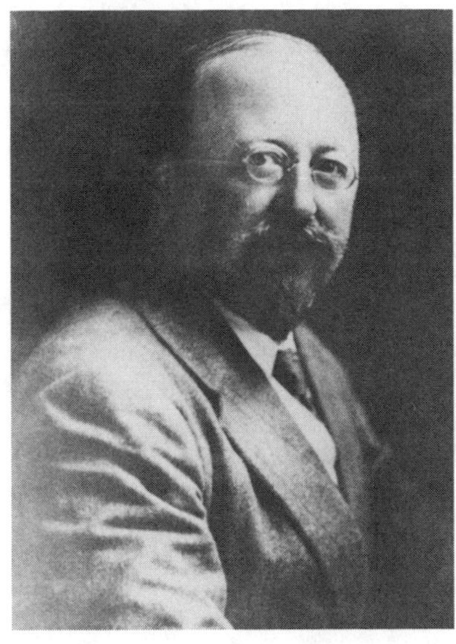

Figure H–3 Sir Henry Head.

head 1. The uppermost or anterior part of the body, including the cranium and face in vertebrates. 2. The upper end of a long bone. 3. The origin of a muscle.

head banging (jactitatio capitis nocturna) A syndrome occurring in some babies or young children during the lightest stages of non–rapid eye movement sleep, characterized by rhythmic repetitive to-and-fro rocking movements or by banging of the head on the pillow or crib side.[1929] See also the ASDC Diagnostic Classification[1629] and Chart J–1.

head circumference The greatest circumference of the head measured with the tape lying on the occiput and the frontal bones. Graphs for the normal values in males and females at different ages have been published.[4613] They are also available online at http://www.who.int/childgrowth/standards/hc_for_age/en/index.html. See also **occipitofrontal circumference**.

head drop Marked anterior curvature or angulation of the cervical spine, associated with numerous neuromuscular and extrapyramidal disorders.[6443] It is associated with increased tone of the neck flexors or weakness of the neck extensor muscles. **Myasthenia gravis, inclusion body myositis**, and **amyotrophic lateral sclerosis** are the commonest neuromuscular causes, and Parkinsonian syndromes are the most common central ones. See also **camptocormia** in which an extreme version of the same thing has a functional basis.

head extension vertigo The physiological occurrence of vertigo or postural imbalance induced when the head is maximally extended and terminating when it returns to the normal position, considered to be due to the inefficiency of otolith function in this position[819] or perhaps to vertebrobasilar insufficiency.

head flexion test (Hyndham sign) Pain in the leg experienced with passive head flexion, as a result of irritation of the lumbar roots in patients with prolapsed intervertebral disks.

head heave maneuver A test of utricular function wherein the examiner places his palms over the ears of the seated patient and makes a fast lateral translation of 1–2 inches. The appearance of corrective saccades indicates the presence of a hypometric slow-phase response, and when this is present asymmetrically, the labyrinthine lesion is likely to be on the side to which the head was pushed.[5173]

head impulse test A test examining the vestibulo ocular reflex (VOR)[2954] and a clinical method for determining the presence of canal paresis, in which the head of the gaze-fixated patient is rapidly moved in short arcs corresponding the planes of the semicircular canals, the occurrence of subsequent corrective saccades then being assessed.

It is used in the identification of acute unilateral peripheral vestibular deficits in which the VOR is abnormal, thus differentiating these from central lesions such as inferior cerebellar strokes in which it is usually retained.

head injury See **craniocerebral trauma**.

head lag Passive extension of the neck with backward drooping of the head, occurring when the supine infant is raised toward the sitting position by the examiner pulling on his or her arms; a sign of weakness of the neck flexors. The normal reaction is for the head to be maintained in the line of the body or even slightly flexed. In the case of a small infant the examiner may initially support the child's head with one hand.

Using the Dubowitz neurological criteria: one scores 0 for complete lag; 1, for partial head control; 2, for ability to maintain the head in line with the body; and 3, if the infant brings the head anterior to the body.[1728]

head nodding 1. See **spasmus nutans**. 2. An unusual seizure type described from sub-Saharan Africa, often associated with hippocampal sclerosis and in half of the reported cases manifesting also other seizure phenotypes.

head retraction reflex Brief extension of the neck in response to a tap on the maxilla when the patient's head is slightly flexed. The reflex was described by **Wartenberg**[6656] as a sign of bilateral supracervical lesions of the pyramidal tract.

head rolling See **jactitatio capitis nocturna**.

Headache The official journal of the **American Headache Society** publishing original articles dealing with headache and all aspects of pain (clinical and basic science). The journal does not use the Vancouver style of references. Web site: http://ahsnet.org/journal/.

headache (cephalalgia) Pain in the head, of numerous varieties. The International Headache Society has produced a revised International Classification of Headache Disorders II in *Cephalalgia* 2004 (Headache Classification Committee of the International Headache Society).[2820] Bolded items have their own entries elsewhere in this book. The coding numbers placed before the various headache types in this new classification are omitted elsewhere in this book. See Chart H–5 for a listing of headache types.

The Web site from the NIH devoted to this condition is http://www.ninds.nih.gov/disorders/headache/headache.htm.

Websites relevant to headache include the following:

American Council for Headache Education An expert-produced, patient-oriented organization; Web site: http://www.achenet.org/.

American Headache Society A professional organization. Web site: http://www.ahsnet.org/.

British Association for the Study of Headache A professional organization. Web site: http://www.bash.org.uk/.

International Headache Society A professional organization. Web site: http://www.i-h-s.org/.

Institute of Neurology Headache group A research-based Web site: http://www.ion.bpmf.ac.uk/~headache/headache.html/.

Migraine Trust A charitable organization. Web site: http://www.migrainetrust.org/.

Migraine Action A charitable organization. Web site: http://www.migraine.org/uk.

NINDS Web site: http://www.ninds.nih.gov/disorders/headache/headache.htm/.

Organization for the Understanding of Cluster Headache A charitable organization. Website: http://www.clusterheadaches.org.uk/.

World Headache Alliance An organization founded to reduce the burden of headache disorders by sharing information among headache organizations and by increasing the awareness and understanding of headache as a public health concern with profound social and economic impact. Web site: http://www.w-h-a.org/.

Chart H–5. International Classification of Headache Disorders (ICHD II)

ICHD-II code	*Diagnosis*
1.	**Migraine**
1.1	**Migraine without aura**
1.2	**Migraine with aura**
1.2.1	Typical **aura** with migraine headache
1.2.2	Typical aura with nonmigraine headache
1.2.3	Typical aura without headache
1.2.4	**Familial hemiplegic migraine**
1.2.5	Sporadic hemiplegic migraine
1.2.6	**Basilar-type migraine**
1.3	**Childhood periodic syndromes** that are commonly precursors of migraine
1.3.1	**Cyclical vomiting**
1.3.2	**Abdominal migraine**
1.3.3	**Benign paroxysmal vertigo of childhood**
1.4	**Retinal migraine**
1.5	Complications of migraine
1.5.1	**Chronic migraine**
1.5.2	**Status migrainosus**
1.5.3	**Persistent aura without infarction**
1.5.4	**Migrainous infarction**
1.5.5	**Migraine-triggered seizure**
1.6	Probable migraine (formerly "migrainous disorder")
1.6.1	Probable migraine without aura
1.6.2	Probable migraine with aura
1.6.3	Probable chronic migraine
2.	**Tension-type headache** (TTH)
2.1	Infrequent episodic tension-type headache
2.1.1	Infrequent episodic tension-type headache associated with pericranial tenderness
2.1.2	Infrequent episodic tension-type headache not associated with pericranial tenderness
2.2	Frequent episodic tension-type headache
2.2.1	Frequent episodic tension-type headache associated with pericranial tenderness
2.2.2	Frequent episodic tension-type headache not associated with pericranial tenderness
2.3	Chronic tension-type headache
2.3.1	Chronic tension-type headache associated with pericranial tenderness
2.3.2	Chronic tension-type headache not associated with pericranial tenderness
2.4	Probable tension-type headache
2.4.1	Probable infrequent episodic tension-type headache
2.4.2	Probable frequent episodic tension-type headache
2.4.3	Probable chronic tension-type headache
3.	**Cluster headache and other trigeminal autonomic cephalalgias**
3.1	**Cluster headache**
3.1.1	Episodic cluster headache
3.1.2	Chronic cluster headache
3.2	**Paroxysmal hemicrania**
3.2.1	Episodic paroxysmal hemicrania
3.2.2	Chronic paroxysmal hemicrania (CPH)
3.3	**Short-lasting Unilateral Neuralgiform headache attacks with Conjunctival injection and Tearing** (SUNCT)
3.4	Probable trigeminal autonomic cephalalgia
3.4.1	Probable **cluster headache**
3.4.2	Probable **paroxysmal hemicrania**
3.4.3	Probable SUNCT
4.	**Other primary headaches**
4.1	**Primary stabbing headache**
4.2	**Primary cough headache**
4.3	**Primary exertional headache**
4.4	**Primary headache associated with sexual activity**
4.4.1	Preorgasmic headache
4.4.2	Orgasmic headache
4.5	**Hypnic headache**
4.6	**Primary thunderclap headache**
4.7	**Hemicrania continua**

4.8 **New daily-persistent headache (NDPH)**
5. **Headache attributed to head and/or neck trauma**
5.1 Acute posttraumatic headache
5.1.1 Acute posttraumatic headache attributed to moderate or severe head injury
5.1.2 Acute posttraumatic headache attributed to mild head injury
5.2 Chronic posttraumatic headache
5.2.1 Chronic posttraumatic headache attributed to moderate or severe head injury
5.2.2 Chronic posttraumatic headache attributed to mild head injury
5.3 Acute headache attributed to whiplash injury
5.4 Chronic headache attributed to whiplash injury
5.5 Headache attributed to traumatic intracranial hematoma
5.5.1 Headache attributed to epidural hematoma
5.5.2 Headache attributed to subdural hematoma
5.6 Headache attributed to other head and/or neck trauma
5.6.1 Acute headache attributed to other head and/or neck trauma
5.6.2 Chronic headache attributed to other head and/or neck trauma
5.7 **Postcraniotomy headache**
5.7.1 Acute postcraniotomy headache
5.7.2 Chronic postcraniotomy headache
6. **Headache attributed to cranial or cervical vascular disorder**
6.1 Headache attributed to ischemic stroke or transient ischemic attack
6.1.1 Headache attributed to ischemic stroke (**cerebral infarction**)
6.1.2 Headache attributed to **transient ischemic attack**
6.2 Headache attributed to nontraumatic **intracranial hemorrhage**
6.2.1 Headache attributed to **intracerebral hemorrhage**
6.2.2 Headache attributed to **subarachnoid hemorrhage**
6.3 Headache attributed to unruptured vascular malformation
6.3.1 Headache attributed to saccular **aneurysm**
6.3.2 Headache attributed to **arteriovenous malformation**
6.3.3 Headache attributed to **dural arteriovenous fistula**
6.3.4 Headache attributed to **cavernous angioma**
6.3.5 Headache attributed to **encephalotrigeminal** (or leptomeningeal) **angiomatosis** (Sturge Weber syndrome)
6.4 Headache attributed to arteritis
6.4.1 Headache attributed to **giant cell arteritis**
6.4.2 Headache attributed to **primary central nervous system angiitis**
6.4.3 Headache attributed to secondary central nervous system angiitis
6.5 Carotid or vertebral artery pain
6.5.1 Headache or facial or neck pain attributed to **arterial dissection**
6.5.2 **Post-endarterectomy headache**
6.5.3 **Carotid angioplasty headache**
6.5.4 Headache attributed to intracranial endovascular procedures
6.5.5 Angiography headache
6.6 Headache attributed to **cerebral venous thrombosis**
6.7 Headache attributed to other intracranial vascular disorder
6.7.1 **Cerebral Autosomal Dominant Arteriopathy with Subcortical Infarcts and Leukoencephalopathy** (CADASIL)
6.7.2 **Mitochondrial Encephalopathy, Lactic Acidosis, and Stroke-like episodes**
6.7.3 Headache attributed to benign angiopathy of the central nervous system
6.7.4 Headache attributed to **pituitary apoplexy**
7. **Headache attributed to nonvascular intracranial disorder**
7.1 Headache attributed to high CSF pressure
7.1.1 Headache attributed to **idiopathic intracranial hypertension**
7.1.2 Headache attributed to intracranial hypertension secondary to metabolic, toxic, or hormonal causes
7.1.3 Headache attributed to intracranial hypertension secondary to hydrocephalus
7.2 **Headache attributed to low CSF pressure**
7.2.1 **Postdural puncture headache**
7.2.2 **CSF fistula headache**
7.2.3 Headache attributed to idiopathic low CSF pressure (**spontaneous intracranial hypotension**)
7.3 Headache attributed to noninfectious inflammatory disease
7.3.1 Headache attributed to **neurosarcoidosis**
7.3.2 Headache attributed to **aseptic meningitis**
7.3.3 Headache attributed to other noninfectious inflammatory disease
7.3.4 Headache attributed to lymphocytic **hypophysitis**
7.4 Headache attributed to intracranial neoplasm
7.4.1 Headache attributed to increased intracranial pressure or hydrocephalus caused by neoplasm
7.4.2 Headache attributed directly to neoplasm
7.4.3 Headache attributed to carcinomatous meningitis
7.4.4 Headache attributed to hypothalamic or pituitary hyper- or hyposecretion
7.5 Headache attributed to intrathecal injection
7.6 Headache attributed to epileptic seizure
7.6.1 **Hemicrania epileptica**
7.6.2 **Postseizure headache**
7.7 Headache attributed to **Chiari malformation** type I
7.8 Syndrome of transient **Headache and Neurological Deficits with cerebrospinal fluid Lymphocytosis** (HaNDL)
7.9 Headache attributed to other nonvascular intracranial disorder
8. **Headache attributed to a substance or its withdrawal**
8.1 Headache induced by acute substance use or exposure
8.1.1 **Nitric oxide (NO) donor–induced headache**
8.1.1.1 Immediate NO donor–induced headache
8.1.1.2 Delayed NO donor headache
8.1.2 Phosphodiesterase inhibitor–induced headache
8.1.3 Carbon monoxide–induced headache
8.1.4 **Alcohol-induced headache**
8.1.4.1 Immediate alcohol-induced headache
8.1.4.2 Delayed alcohol-induced headache

continued

Chart H–5. *(continued)*

ICHD-II code	*Diagnosis*
8.1.5	Headache induced by food components and additives
8.1.5.1	**Monosodium glutamate–induced headache**
8.1.6	Cocaine-induced headache
8.1.7	Cannabis-induced headache
8.1.8	Histamine-induced headache
8.1.8.1	Immediate histamine-induced headache
8.1.8.2	Delayed histamine-induced headache
8.1.9	**Calcitonin gene-related peptide**(CGRP)**-induced headache**
8.1.9.1	Immediate CGRP-induced headache
8.1.9.2	Delayed CGRP-induced headache
8.1.10	Headache as an acute adverse event attributed to medication used for other indications (code to specify substance)
8.1.11	Headache induced by other acute substance use or exposure
8.2	**Medication-overuse headache**
8.2.1	Ergotamine-overuse headache
8.2.2	Triptan-overuse headache
8.2.3	Analgesic-overuse headache
8.2.4	Opioid-overuse headache
8.2.5	Combination medication–overuse headache
8.2.6	Headache attributed to other medication overuse
8.2.7	Probable medication–overuse headache
8.3	Headache as an adverse event attributed to chronic medication
8.3.1	Exogenous hormone-induced headache
8.4	**Headache attributed to substance withdrawal**
8.4.1	Caffeine-withdrawal headache
8.4.2	Opioid-withdrawal headache
8.4.3	Estrogen-withdrawal headache
8.4.4	Headache attributed to withdrawal from chronic use of other substances
9.	**Headache attributed to infection**
9.1	**Headache attributed to intracranial infection**
9.1.1	Headache attributed to bacterial meningitis
9.1.2	Headache attributed to lymphocytic meningitis
9.1.3	Headache attributed to **encephalitis**
9.1.4	Headache attributed to **brain abscess**
9.1.5	Headache attributed to **subdural empyema**
9.2	**Headache attributed to systemic infection**
9.2.1	Headache attributed to systemic bacterial infection
9.2.2	Headache attributed to systemic viral infection
9.2.3	Headache attributed to other systemic infection
9.3	**Headache attributed to HIV/AIDS**
9.4	**Chronic post-infection headache**
9.4.1	Chronic post-bacterial meningitis headache
10.	**Headache attributed to disorder of homeostasis**
10.1	Headache attributed to hypoxia and/or hypercapnia
10.1.1	**High-altitude headache**
10.1.2	**Diving headache**
10.1.3	**Sleep apnea** headache
10.2	**Dialysis headache**
10.3	Headache attributed to arterial hypertension
10.3.1	Headache attributed to **pheochromocytoma** (benign or malignant)
10.3.2	Headache attributed to hypertensive crisis without hypertensive encephalopathy
10.3.3	Headache attributed to **hypertensive encephalopathy**
10.3.4	Headache attributed to pre-eclampsia
10.3.5	Headache attributed to **eclampsia**
10.3.6	Headache attributed to acute pressor response to an exogenous agent
10.4	Headache attributed to hypothyroidism
10.5	Headache attributed to fasting (**hypoglycemic** headache)
10.6	**Cardiac cephalalgia**
10.7	Headache attributed to other disorder of homeostasis
11.	**Headache or facial pain attributed to disorder of cranium, neck, eyes, ears, nose, sinuses, teeth, mouth, or other facial or cranial structures**
11.1	Headache attributed to disorder of cranial bone
11.2	Headache attributed to disorder of neck
11.2.1	**Cervicogenic headache**
11.2.2	Headache attributed to **retropharyngeal tendonitis**
11.2.3	Headache attributed to craniocervical **dystonia**
11.3	Headache attributed to disorder of eyes
11.3.1	Headache attributed to acute glaucoma
11.3.2	Headache attributed to refractive errors
11.3.3	Headache attributed to heterophoria or heterotropia (latent or manifest squint)
11.3.4	Headache attributed to ocular inflammatory disorder
11.4	Headache attributed to disorder of ears
11.5	Headache attributed to rhinosinusitis (**sinus headache**)
11.6	Headache attributed to disorder of teeth, jaws, or related structures
11.7	Headache or facial pain attributed to **temporomandibular joint disorder**
11.8	Headache attributed to other disorder of cranium, neck, eyes, ears, nose, sinuses, teeth, mouth, or other facial or cervical structures
12.	**Headache attributed to psychiatric disorder**
12.1	Headache attributed to somatization disorder
12.2	Headache attributed to psychotic disorder
13.	**Cranial neuralgias and central causes of facial pain**
13.1	**Trigeminal neuralgia**
13.1.1	Classical trigeminal neuralgia
13.1.2	Symptomatic trigeminal neuralgia
13.2	**Glossopharyngeal neuralgia**
13.2.1	Classical glossopharyngeal neuralgia
13.2.2	Symptomatic glossopharyngeal neuralgia
13.3	**Nervus intermedius neuralgia**
13.4	**Superior laryngeal neuralgia**
13.5	**Nasociliary neuralgia**
13.6	**Supraorbital neuralgia**
13.7	Other terminal branch neuralgias
13.8	**Occipital neuralgia**
13.9	**Neck–tongue syndrome**
13.10	**External compression headache**
13.11	**Cold-stimulus headache**
13.11.1	Headache attributed to external application of a cold stimulus
13.11.2	Headache attributed to ingestion or inhalation of a cold stimulus
13.12	Constant pain caused by compression, irritation, or distortion of cranial nerves or upper cervical roots by structural lesions
13.13	Optic neuritis

13.14	Ocular diabetic neuropathy
13.15	Head or facial pain attributed to herpes zoster
13.15.1	Head or facial pain attributed to acute herpes zoster
13.15.2	**Postherpetic neuralgia**
13.16	**Tolosa–Hunt syndrome**
13.17	**Ophthalmoplegic "migraine"**
13.18	Central causes of facial pain
13.18.1	**Anesthesia dolorosa**
13.18.2	**Central poststroke pain**
13.18.3	Facial pain attributed to **multiple sclerosis**
13.18.4	Persistent idiopathic facial pain
13.18.5	**Burning mouth syndrome**
13.19	Other cranial neuralgias or other centrally mediated facial pain
14.	**Other headache, cranial neuralgia, central or primary facial pain**
14.1	Headache not elsewhere classified
14.2	Headache unspecified

From the ICHD. Headache Classification Committee of the International Headache Society. Cephalalgia 2004;24*(Suppl 1). By kind permission of Dr. Jes Olesen, the International Headache Society, and Wiley-Blackwell Publications.*

headache associated with refractive errors An overestimated cause of headache, described as mild, frontal, and aggravated by prolonged focusing in subjects with refractive errors, astigmatism, or presbyopia. However, the great majority of those with such ocular problems do not have headaches.

Headache attributed to acute glaucoma and *headache attributed to heterophoria or heterotropia (latent or manifest squint)* are also defined in the International Classification of Headache Disorders (ICHD).[2820]

headache attributed to cranial or cervical vascular disorder Headache, usually mild to moderate in severity, in association with (usually posterior circulation) ischemic stroke with focal neurological deficit. Such headaches are seldom associated with **lacunar infarcts** but are extremely common with arterial **dissection**. Diagnostic criteria have been defined for many varieties. The following entries are based upon the ICHD (Headache Classification Committee of the International Headache Society. *Cephalalgia* 2004; 24[Suppl 1]):

Angiography headache An acute, severe, diffuse, and burning headache occurring during intra-arterial carotid or vertebral angiography in patients with prior migraine and having the features of migraine but resolving within 72 h.

Headache attributed to cerebral venous thrombosis is a new headache, developing in close temporal relationship with cerebral venous thrombosis with or without neurological signs.

Headache attributed to intracerebral (including intracerebellar) hemorrhage A new acute headache that develops simultaneously with or in very close temporal relation to intracerebral hemorrhage. Such headaches are more often due to associated subarachnoid blood and to local compression than to intracranial hypertension. They may also present as **thunderclap headache**.

Headache attributed to ischemic stroke (cerebral infarction) A new acute headache that develops simultaneously with or in very close temporal relation to signs or other evidence of ischemic stroke.

Headache attributed to subarachnoid hemorrhage A severe headache of sudden onset (**thunderclap headache**) due to nontraumatic subarachnoid hemorrhage with or without other clinical signs, normally resolving within a month. A similar headache may also indicate the presence of an unruptured saccular aneurysm, especially in the presence of localizing signs such as painful III nerve palsy.

Headache attributed to transient ischemic attack A new acute headache that develops simultaneously with the onset of a focal neurological deficit of ischemic origin lasting <24 h, resolving also in that time.

Postendarterectomy headache An acute headache occurring de novo after that operation. The types of pain experienced include a mild and diffuse pain; a unilateral pain like cluster headache occurring once or twice a day in attacks lasting 2–3 h; or a unilateral pulsating severe pain, developing within a week of the surgery, and resolving within a month. Similar headaches may follow *intracranial endovascular procedures* such as intracranial angioplasty or embolization, usually developing within seconds of the procedure and resolving within 24 h. After balloon inflation or embolization of an arteriovenous malformation or aneurysm, a severe pain of abrupt onset, localized to specific areas according to the artery involved, may occur within a few seconds of the procedure but disappears rapidly.

Arteriovenous malformations and **giant cell arteritis** can cause similar headaches; headaches are also a feature of arterial hypertension, **cerebral autosomal dominant arteriopathy with subcortical infarcts and leukoencephalopathy** (CADASIL), and of benign (or reversible) angiopathy of the CNS.[2820]

See also **central post-stroke pain** and **dissection**.

headache attributed to disorder of teeth, jaws, or related structures For diagnosis, the ICHD criteria[2820] require evidence of a disorder of teeth, jaws, or related structures with headache and pain occurring in close temporal relation and resolving within 3 months of successful treatment.

headache attributed to external application of a cold stimulus See **cold stimulus headache**.

headache attributed to infection An example is *chronic postbacterial meningitis headache* which is a diffuse continuous pain associated with dizziness, difficulty in concentrating, and/or loss of memory, occurring after previous intracranial bacterial infection, representing a direct continuation of *headache attributed to bacterial meningitis* and persisting for more than 3 months after resolution of the infection.

See also **aseptic meningitis** and the ICHD criteria.[2820]

headache attributed to intracranial neoplasm Headache attributed to increased intracranial pressure or hydrocephalus caused by a neoplasm. The ICHD criteria are

A. Diffuse nonpulsating headache with at least one of the following characteristics and fulfilling criteria C and D:
   1. Associated with nausea and/or vomiting
   2. Worsened by physical activity and/or maneuvers known to increase intracranial pressure (such as Valsalva maneuver, coughing, or sneezing)
   3. Occurring in attack-like episodes

B. Space-occupying intracranial tumor demonstrated by CT or MRI, causing hydrocephalus
C. Headache develops and/or deteriorates in close temporal relation to the hydrocephalus
D. Headache improves within 7 days after surgical removal or volume reduction of tumor.

From the ICHD (Headache Classification Committee of the International Headache Society. Cephalalgia 2004;24(Suppl 1)) by kind permission of Dr. Jes Olesen, the International Headache Society, and Wiley-Blackwell Publications. See also **thunderclap headache** and **colloid cyst of the third ventricle**.

Headache attributed to carcinomatous meningitis may be either localized or diffuse.

Headache attributed to hypothalamic or pituitary hyper- or hyposecretion is similar, but in this case the ICHD indicates that the pain is bilateral, frontotemporal, and/or retro-orbital and is accompanied by at least one of the following: prolactin, growth hormone, and adrenocorticotropic hormone (ACTH) hypersecretion associated with microadenomas <10 mm in diameter; or a disorder of temperature regulation, abnormal emotional state, altered thirst and appetite, and change in level of consciousness associated with a hypothalamic tumor.

headache attributed to intrathecal injection See **postdural puncture HA** *(variant)*.

headache attributed to ischemic stroke or transient ischemic attack See **headache attributed to cranial or cervical vascular disorder**.

headache attributed to ocular inflammatory disorder The diagnostic criteria for this disorder suggested by ICHD[2820] are the presence of pain in the eye and behind or around it, in the presence of documented ocular inflammation diagnosed by appropriate investigations and resolving within 7 days after relief of the inflammatory disorder.

headache attributed to other noninfectious inflammatory disease The ICHD criteria[2820] require evidence of headache in close temporal relation with one of the inflammatory diseases known to be associated with headache and resolving within 3 months of successful treatment.

See also **acute demyelinating encephalomyelitis, systemic lupus erythematosus, Behçet syndrome, anti-phospholipid antibody syndrome**, and **Vogt–Koyanagi–Harada syndrome**.

headache attributed to pre-eclampsia Diagnostic criteria have been defined as follows:[2820]

A. Headache with at least one of the following characteristics and fulfilling criteria C and D:
   1. Bilateral
   2. Pulsating quality
   3. Aggravated by physical activity
B. Pregnancy or puerperium (up to 7 days postpartum), and pre-eclampsia defined by both of the following:
   1. Hypertension (>140/90 mmHg) documented on two blood pressure readings at least 4 h apart
   2. Urinary protein excretion >0.3 g per 24 h.
C. Headache develops during periods of high blood pressure
D. Headache resolves within 7 days after effective treatment of hypertension
E. Appropriate investigations have ruled out vasopressor toxins, medications, or phaeochromocytoma as causative factors

From the ICHD (Headache Classification Committee of the International Headache Society. Cephalalgia 2004;24(Suppl 1)) by kind permission of Dr. Jes Olesen, the International Headache Society, and Wiley-Blackwell Publications.

The suggested criteria for *headache attributed to* **eclampsia** are similar, except that there are added two criteria: # 3. A seizure has occurred and F. Stroke has been excluded

headache attributed to psychiatric disorder The ICHD[2820] recognizes the following two forms within this category:

Headache attributed to somatization disorder

A. Headache, no typical characteristics known, fulfilling criterion C
B. Presence of somatization disorder fulfilling *DSM-IV* criteria:
   1. History of many physical complaints beginning before age 30 that occur over a period of several years and result in treatment being sought and/or in significant impairment in social, occupational, or other important areas of functioning
   2. At least four pain symptoms, two nonpain gastrointestinal symptoms, one sexual or reproductive symptom, and one pseudoneurological symptom
   3. After appropriate investigation, each of these symptoms cannot be fully explained by a known general medical condition or the direct effects of a substance or medication; or, if there is a related medical condition, the complaints or impairment are in excess of what would be expected from the history, examination, or laboratory findings
C. Headache is not attributed to another cause

Headache attributed to psychotic disorder (delusional headache)

A. Headache, no typical characteristics known, fulfilling criteria C–E
B. Delusional belief about the presence and/or etiology of headache occurring in the context of delusional disorder, schizophrenia, major depressive episode with psychotic features, manic episode with psychotic features or other psychotic disorder fulfilling *DSM-IV* criteria
C. Headache occurs only when (the subject is) delusional
D. Headache resolves when delusions remit
E. Headache is not attributed to another cause

From the ICHD (Headache Classification Committee of the International Headache Society. Cephalalgia 2004;24(Suppl 1)) by kind permission of Dr. Jes Olesen, the International Headache Society, and Wiley-Blackwell Publications.

headache attributed to substance withdrawal Diagnostic criteria have been defined[2820] for the following:

Caffeine-withdrawal headache

A. Bilateral and/or pulsating headache fulfilling criteria C and D
B. Caffeine consumption of ≥200 mg/day for >2 weeks, which is interrupted or delayed
C. Headache develops within 24 h after last caffeine intake and is relieved within 1 h by 100 mg of caffeine
D. Headache resolves within 7 days after total caffeine withdrawal

Opioid-withdrawal headache

A. Bilateral and/or pulsating headache fulfilling criteria C and D
B. Opioid intake daily for >3 months, which is interrupted

C. Headache develops within 24 h after last opioid intake
D. Headache resolves within 7 days after total opioid withdrawal

The ICHD criteria[2820] for *headache attributed to withdrawal from chronic use of other substances* are almost the same.

Estrogen-withdrawal headache

A. Headache or migraine fulfilling criteria C and D
B. Daily use of exogenous estrogen for ≥3 weeks, which is interrupted
C. Headache or migraine develops within 5 days after last use of estrogen
D. Headache or migraine resolves within 3 days

From the ICHD (Headache Classification Committee of the International Headache Society. Cephalalgia 2004;24(Suppl 1)) by kind permission of Dr. Jes Olesen, the International Headache Society, and Wiley-Blackwell Publications.

Withdrawal from ergot is another variety.

headache attributed to traumatic intracranial hematoma

See **headache attributed to head and/or neck trauma**.

headache attributed to unruptured vascular malformation

See **headache attributed to cranial or cervical vascular disorder**.

headache induced by acute substance use or exposure

The ICHD[2820] defines a number of headache types in association with exposure to various agents. Representative types are

Nitric oxide (NO) donor-induced headache (immediate) (nitroglycerine headache, dynamite headache, hot dog headache) Diagnostic criteria have been defined as follows:

A. Headache with at least one of the following characteristics and fulfilling criteria C and D:
   1. Bilateral
   2. Frontotemporal location
   3. Pulsating quality
   4. Aggravated by physical activity
B. Absorption of a NO donor
C. Headache develops within 10 min after absorption of NO donor
D. Headache resolves within 1 h after release of NO has ended

Carbon monoxide–induced headache (warehouse workers' headache) Bilateral and/or continuous headaches occurring within 12 h of carbon monoxide intoxication, resolving within 72 h after its elimination.

Cocaine-induced headache ICHD criteria[2820] are

A. Headache, no typical characteristics known, fulfilling criteria C and D
B. An appropriate agent or toxin has been administered or ingested and an acute rise in blood pressure has occurred
C. Headache develops in close temporal relation to the acute rise in blood pressure
D. Headache resolves within 24 h after normalization of blood pressure
E. No other mechanism for the headache

From the ICHD (Headache Classification Committee of the International Headache Society. Cephalalgia 2004;24(Suppl 1)) by kind permission of Dr. Jes Olesen, the International Headache Society, and Wiley-Blackwell Publications.

Cannabis-induced Bilateral stabbing or pulsating feelings of pressure in the head following the use of cannabis within 12 h, resolving within 72 h.

Delayed NO donor–induced headache A *variant* of the foregoing, in which people who suffer from primary headaches experience their typical headache after absorption of a NO donor but only after the NO is cleared from the blood; it resolves within 72 h of a single exposure.

Dietary headache (headache induced by food components and additives) Bilateral, frontotemporal, pulsating headaches aggravated by physical activity, developing within 12 h and resolving within 72 h after ingestion of a minimum dose of phenylethylamine, tyramine, or aspartame.

Histamine-induced headache The two forms defined by the ICHD[2820] are immediate headache in nonheadache sufferers and immediate and/or delayed headaches in migraine sufferers. The *immediate histamine-induced headache* is bilateral, frontotemporal, pulsating, and aggravated by physical activity; it develops within 10 min after absorption of histamine and resolves within 1 h The *delayed histamine-induced headache* fulfils criteria for **migraine without aura** in people who suffer from primary headaches.

Immediate calcitonin gene-related peptide (CGRP)–induced headache This *variant* has at least one of the following characteristics: bilateral, frontotemporal, pulsating, and aggravated by physical activity, developing within 10 min after absorption of CGRP and resolving within 1 h after absorption of CGRP has ceased. The *delayed CGRP-induced headaches* occur in people who suffer from primary headaches after the CGRP is cleared from the blood and resolving within 72 h. Migraineurs experience an attack of migraine without aura, tension-type headache sufferers develop tension-type headaches, both typically after 5–6 h, and those with cluster headache develop a cluster headache attack typically after 1–2 h.

Monosodium glutamate-induced headache Bilateral, frontotemporal headaches, aggravated by physical activity following ingestion of monosodium glutamate (MSG) within 1 h and resolving within 72 h. See also **Chinese restaurant syndrome**.

Headache as an acute adverse event attributed to medication used for other indications Headache may occur after ingestion of atropine, digitalis, disulfiram, hydralazine, imipramine, nicotine, nifedipine, or nimodipine. Most of these headaches are dull, continuous, diffuse, and moderate to severe.

Phosphodiesterase (PDE) inhibitor–induced headache Bilateral, frontotemporal, pulsating headaches, aggravated by physical activity, occurring within 5 h after a single dose of a phosphodiesterase inhibitor and resolving within 72 h.

headache induced by food components and additives

See *dietary headache* and *monosodium glutamate–induced headache* above.

headache associated with sexual activity

(benign sex headache, coital cephalalgia) Headache precipitated by masturbation or coitus, usually starting as a dull bilateral ache while sexual excitement increases and suddenly becoming intense at orgasm, in the absence of any intracranial disorder. Dull, explosive, and postural types are defined. See also **thunderclap headache**.

headache associated with substances but with uncertain mechanism This category would include headache in association with ingestion of estrogens and other substances.

Headache Disability Inventory
A validated 25-item scale assessing the effects of daily living in terms of disability suffered by people with recurrent headaches.[3136] See also **MIDAS** and **Headache Impact Test**.

Headache Impact Test
A validated tool assessing the burden of disability suffered by people with migraine, either in a six-question paper-based form or by accessing it on the Internet. Web site: http://www.headachetest.com/. See also **Headache Disability Inventory** and **MIDAS**.

headache scale A list of 30 adjectives (pulling, tight, tiring, dull, splitting, sharp, stabbing, throbbing, etc.) used to describe pain by headache sufferers.[3149]

Based upon such a list, clusters of headache descriptions have been defined, but different analyses have identified 2, 5, or 7 clusters, and the purpose of the scale appears to assist in the qualitative determination of the characteristics of head pains rather than in diagnosis or management.

headache with neurologic deficits and CSF lymphocytosis (HaNDL, migraine with cerebrospinal pleocytosis; pseudomigraine with lymphocytic pleocytosis) A benign and transient syndrome with these added manifestations. Characteristic features include the presence of severe headaches resembling migraine with aura, neurological deficits lasting for less than 3 days on each occasion, CSF lymphocytosis of 16–350 cells/mm^3, and limitation of the condition to less than 3 months. Additional features include a modest rise in CSF protein and pressure, transient focal nonepileptiform EEG changes, and sometimes a viral prodrome or fever.[550] Mollaret cells are absent from the CSF but the condition does otherwise resemble **Mollaret meningitis**. Conventional cerebral angiography can provoke a similar condition. (HJM) Diagnostic criteria have been defined[2820]

A. Episodes of moderate or severe headache lasting hours before resolving fully and fulfilling criteria C and D
B. Cerebrospinal fluid pleocytosis with lymphocytic predominance (>15 cells/ml) and normal neuroimaging, CSF culture, and other tests for etiology
C. Episodes of headache are accompanied by or shortly follow transient neurological deficits and commence in close temporal relation to the development of CSF pleocytosis
D. Episodes of headache and neurological deficits recur for over 3 months.

From the ICHD (Headache Classification Committee of the International Headache Society. Cephalalgia 2004;24(Suppl 1)) by kind permission of Dr. Jes Olesen, the International Headache Society, and Wiley-Blackwell Publications.

Head–Holmes syndrome The sensory deficits resulting from cortical lesions.[2816] The utility of retaining this eponymous syndrome may now be expended, but the original paper is a treasure.

headphone neuralgia A syndrome resembling glossopharyngeal neuralgia, thought to be caused by compression of the aural branches on that nerve by the hard earpieces of, for example, personal entertainment devices, stethoscopes, or hearing aids, or by idiopathic craniofacial polyneuritis.[5885]

Head–Riddoch syndrome (autonomic hyperreflexia syndrome) Sweating, flushing, pilomotor erection, nasal stuffiness, blurred vision, headache, and occasionally generalized seizures occurring as a result of excessive autonomic activity following extrinsic or intrinsic stimulation of quadriplegic patients below the level of their high spinal lesions.[2817]

Head's areas (Head's zones) The dermatomes, precisely delineated by Head as his graduation thesis at Cambridge and published in ***Brain*** in 1893.[2810]

The term has also been applied to the areas of hyperalgesia occurring in association with disease of the underlying viscera, but in effect these are also the dermatomes.

Head's principles

1. "When any level of activity is attacked, the most complex functions, and those that have appeared most recently, are the first to suffer; they are also disturbed to a greater degree and to a wider extent than those which are simpler or more inevitable in their expression."
2. "The negative manifestations of a lesion appear in terms of the affected level." (Thus, lesions of the speech area produce disturbances of speech.)
3. "A negative lesion produces positive effects by releasing activities normally held under control by the functions of the affected level." The mass reflex and thalamic pain are examples given.
4. "The functions of the nervous system have been slowly evolved by a continuous process of development. The methods by which this gradual process from lower to higher efficiency have been reached are still manifest in the phenomena of its normal activity . . . [thus] what at lower levels appeared a variable response became with the progress of evolution, voluntary control."
5. "Integration of function within the nervous system is based on a struggle for expression between many potentially different physiological activities." (Thus, a warm stimulus may be perceived as warm, cold, or painful according to its position on the skin and the state of the receptors.)[2813]

Head's zones See **Head's areas**.

head-shaking nystagmus
A provoked horizontal jerk nystagmus appearing for at least 5 s after vigorous head shaking about the vertical axis for 15 s, suggesting the presence of a brainstem lesion or of **dynamic vestibular imbalance**. See also **vestibular nystagmus**.

head-thrust response A baby is held in the sitting position with the body leaning slightly forward. When a hand placed against the back of the head thrusts the head forward, the normal infant opposes the movement.[6898]

head-tilt test See **Bielschowsky Test**.

head-turning sign The action of patients with dementing diseases, who repeatedly turn to ask their spouse the answers to questions put by the examiner (Dr. Rémi Bouchard, personal communication).

health 1. The ability of all parts of the body to perform their respective functions without giving rise to awareness of incapacity or discomfort. 2. The absence of disease. 3. A state of mental, physical, and emotional well-being.

The Healthy Brain Project A program designed to increase awareness of the brain and its importance in the overall health and longevity of the human being.

Heart and Stroke Foundation of Canada A charitable organization. Web site: http://ww2.heartandstroke.ca/splash/.

heat hematoma An artifactual extradural hematoma subjacent to a fissure fracture of the skull, found in some victims of death in extreme heat.[6]

heat stroke (coup de la chaleur) Hyperpyrexia following exposure to unusually high temperatures and associated with coma, delirium, agitation, and rigidity with pupillary constriction, complex automatisms, and raised serum creatine kinase values. The mortality rate is 40% but, in those who survive, a syndrome of akinetic mutism, anarthria, subcortical dementia cerebellar signs, sensorimotor axonopathy, and severe wasting signs are the usual sequelae.

heat-flow disk A method of assessing changes in skin blood flow by measuring the rate of heat loss from a disk placed on the skin.[1776]

heautognosis (Gr, "of oneself" + knowledge) Self-knowledge.

heautoscopy A multimodal reduplicative hallucination of one's own person; a combination of autoscopy and an out-of-body experience, resulting in the perception of a **doppelgänger**; a primary somesthetic illusion of being separated from, and outside, one's own body. It is most commonly a manifestation of complex partial seizures arising from parietal or deep temporal foci.[910] It may also be an occasional experience of normal children.

heaviness Not itself a primary sensory mode, but rather the sense of the movement required to lift a mass, or the discrimination of relative pressures (depending upon whether or not the limb is allowed to move). Gordon **Holmes** stated that "Every paretic limb exaggerates the load it carries, if sensation be normal"—that is, objects feel heavy when lifted by paretic muscles, a "sense of effort" being used to estimate the weight of a lifted object.[2270]

Hebb, Donald (1904–1985) Pre-eminent Canadian psychologist at McGill University. He is remembered in particular for his postulate, building on the work of William James, that when the axon of a neuron is close enough to excite a particular cell and does so repeatedly, the threshold for further such excitations is reduced. Thus synapses are modified by pre- and postsynaptic activity.

hebephrenia (from Gr, puberty + the mind) A variety of schizophrenia, occurring mainly in young people and unaccompanied by major paranoid ideation. The affect is changeable and "silly"; the thought disorder and hallucinations exuberant.

Heberden, William (1710–1801) English physician and classical scholar who trained at Cambridge and practiced in London. His clinical skills and his writings on rheumatism, angina, and varicella placed him in the forefront of the profession, and he was elected to fellowship both of the Royal College of Physicians and of the Royal Society. He also described night blindness (nyctalopia).

His son, William Heberden, Jr., published in 1804 a book on pediatrics said "to have been of such superlative excellence that it might well be attributed to the father"—which must be the most backhanded compliment that any medical author has received.

Hebetude (from Lat, to make blunt) Dullness of intellect as with a slight reduction in conscious level.

Hebold syndrome See **encephalotrigeminal angiomatosis**.

Hecaen, Henri (1912–1983) French neurologist, psychiatrist, neuropsychologist, and a founding father of behavioral neurology and neuropsychology. His medical training was at the University of Bordeaux, and he later studied with Jean Lhermitte and Henri Ey before joining the French Centre National de la Récherche Medicale. He was in turn director of the language pathology laboratory and of the research laboratory for neuropsychological studies at the Institut National de la Santé.

Hecaen's important clinical research on brain–behavior relationships complemented his political organization of the discipline, through the founding of the journal *Neuropsychologia* (of which he was the founding editor-in-chief) and indirectly of the International Neuropsychological Society. His best-known studies were of apractagnosia, aphasia, visual agnosia, and cerebral lateralization.[105]

heel-(knee)-shin test A test of coordination wherein the subject is required to run one heel smoothly down the other shin. Miller **Fisher**[2080] suggested a modification (shin-tapping) whereby the subject also taps the heel repetitively on the shin before continuing to slide it down toward the foot.

heel reflex Plantar flexion or spreading out of the toes in response to a tap in the heel, seen in patients with pyramidal lesions. In babies, this normally leads to extension of the leg.[6898]

heel-to-ear maneuver A test forming part of the battery used in **gestational assessment**. The heel of the supine baby is gently drawn up toward its head, and the distance between them is measured. Normally the foot will get as far as the chest but any further flexion is a sign of immaturity or hypotonia.[1727, 1728]

Heerfordt syndrome (uveoparotid fever) Bilateral facial paralysis (and occasional pareses of the V, VIII, and bulbar cranial nerves) with bilateral uveitis, fever, and parotid enlargement occurring as a manifestation of **sarcoidosis**.[2832] Both optic and peripheral neuropathies have also been reported.

C.F. Heerfordt (b. 1871), a Danish ophthalmologist, described the syndrome in 1909.

Heidenhain, Adolf (b. 1893) German neuropsychiatrist and pathologist.

Heide syndrome A congenital dysmorphic syndrome manifesting also macrocephaly, frontal bossing, osteoporosis, acral defects, optic atrophy with blindness, and mental and developmental delay.[381]

Heidenhain disease An insidiously progressive spongy degeneration of the adult cortex with neuronal loss and gliosis, leading to severe dementia, cortical blindness, rigidity, athetosis, ataxia, dysarthria, cerebellar signs, and myoclonus and causing death within months of the onset of the illness.[2837, 4340]

Heidenhain noted that the condition strongly resembles **Creutzfeldt–Jakob disease** but that the latter manifests a slower course with more pyramidal and extrapyramidal features; his patients showed mainly involvement of the occipital lobes, the frontal lobes being relatively spared. See **Creutzfeldt–Jakob disease**.

height vertigo A visually induced physiological syndrome of subjective instability in postural balance and locomotion, coupled with a fear of falling and with vegetative symptoms, which occurs when the distance between the observer and visible stationary objects becomes critically large.[819] It often appears to be enhanced with age.

Heilbronner sign Flattening of the thigh on the side of a pyramidal lesion.

Heimann–Bielschowsky phenomenon Instability of gaze in a blind eye, with uni- or bidirectional drifting or nystagmus occurring in that eye during fixation of an object by the other eye.[5921]

Heine, Jacob von (1800–1879) German physician, who trained at Wurzburg and, as a result of family connections, was asked to set up an orthopedic institute near Stuttgart. He published his report on poliomyelitis (infantile paralysis) in 1840,[2844] noticing almost all the clinical features of the disease, localizing the pathology correctly to the anterior horn cells, demonstrating its epidemic nature, showing that a single infectious agent could produce different syndromes in different people, and dealing at length with methods of management and rehabilitation.

Heine–Medin disease See **poliomyelitis**. Oskar Medin (1874–1928) studied the epidemic form of the disease.

helicopodia (Gr, circling + leg) Circumduction of the leg during walking, as is seen in hemiparetic patients.

heliotrope rash The mauve discoloration of the eyelids in some patients with **dermatomyositis**. A memorable term, but not as memorable as the alternative Victorian phrase "violaceous hue," which for some reason (certainly not accuracy) has been retained in this context where neither word is normally used by any of us from year to year in any other.

helix (Gr, a spiral) The outer border of the pinna, the external ear.

Heller, Theodor (1869–1938) Austrian psychiatrist. Born in Vienna into a family with a tradition of service to the blind, he also began training appropriate for that task, diverting to the study of the problems affecting all handicapped children. His life was largely spent in training the mentally handicapped, but he also wrote on a wider field of child psychiatry.

Heller disease (dementia infantilis, childhood schizophrenia, Heller–Zappert syndrome) A disease of unknown cause in which, after normal infancy, behavioral disturbances with overactivity, tics, immature behavior, and stereotypic movements lead on to progressive dementia with eventual speech regression and mutism, withdrawn helplessness ("separated from his surroundings by a glass wall"), and incontinence in the second or third year of life, despite a lack of focal neurological findings. No pathology was described by Heller in his major paper,[2845] nor in his brief report in 1909.

It is uncertain that this is a single condition. Julius Zappert[6952] described further cases of dementia infantilis and proposed the eponym now used. The condition is probably akin to, if not identical to, infantile **autism**,[2845] but it is also possible that the cause is a subacute encephalitis.

Heller–Zappert syndrome See **Heller disease**.

HELLP syndrome A complication of pre-eclampsia manifesting severe edema and proteinuria, upper abdominal pain, and a reduced thrombocyte count but not always with a marked rise in blood pressure.[2773]

Hellsing syndrome See **hereditary facial spasm**.

Helmholtz, Hermann Ludwig Ferdinand von (1821–1894) German physicist and physiologist, professor of anatomy and physiology variously at Konigsberg, Bonn, Heidelberg, and Berlin. Of interest to neurologists were his studies on the speed of neural transmission (1850), his pioneering books on optics and acoustics,[3373] and his invention of the ophthalmoscope in 1851.[2851] The English mathematician Charles Babbage had produced a similar instrument 4 years previously but published no report of it until 1854.

He put forward the resonance theory of hearing, stating (in 1862) that vibrations in the stapes are transmitted to the perilymph and thus to the basilar membrane, each basilar fiber responding at its own particular frequency.

Helweg-Larsen disease A dominantly inherited hereditary cochleovestibular atrophy manifesting progressive hearing loss from early adult life and anhidrosis as a result of the nondevelopment of sweat glands.[2852]

hem- Greek prefix indicating blood.

hemangiectatic hypertrophy See **Klippel–Trenauny–Weber syndrome**.

hemangioblastoma A benign, circumscribed, cystic tumor of blood vessels usually occurring in adults and arising in the cerebellum or spinal cord from unknown cell origins.

Histologically, it is characterized by cells with uniform nuclei and foamy cytoplasm containing lipid, surrounded by a fine reticulin network and many thin-walled blood vessels. Some produce erythropoietin, leading to polycythemia. In the cerebellum, the tumors eventually cause signs of posterior fossa compression and obstructive hydrocephalus.[3182]

The tumors are familial in **von Hippel–Lindau disease**, in which condition the gene maps to the short arm of chromosome 3.

hemangioma calcificans Slowly growing calcified hemangiomas usually found within one temporal lobe close to the fissure of Sylvius and frequently associated with complex partial seizures.

Tuberculomas, hemangiomas, and hematomas are other calcified lesions found in this region.[4978]

hemangiomas Vascular tumors of bone that may occur in the spinal column, leading to compression of the spinal cord. See also **cavernous angioma**.

hemangiopericytic meningioma (hemangiopericytoma) A rare, primary, potentially malignant tumor of the nervous system with histological similarities to angioblastic meningiomas. See also **meningioma**.

hemangiopericytoma See **hemangiopericytic meningioma**.

hematoencephalon Intracranial bleeding.

hematoma A mass of blood; a blood clot.

hematomyelia Hemorrhage into the spinal cord, with a tendency to spread longitudinally over several segments, particularly within the gray matter, and usually due to trauma or (when spontaneous) rupture of an occult arteriovenous malformation. The name was first applied by Ollivier d'Angers in 1827.

hematorrachis Hemorrhage into the spinal canal.

hematosidosis (anabolic GM_3 gangliosidosis) A polioencephalopathy. See also **GM_3 gangliosidosis**.

hemeralopia (Gr, day + obscure + vision) Impaired vision in bright illumination.

hemi- (Gr, half) The Latin equivalent word is **semi-**, the French word, **demi-**.

hemi-3 syndrome (**h**emihypertrophy, **h**emiparesthesias, **h**emiareflexia) A sporadic developmental syndrome consisting of hemihypertrophy, hemihypesthesia, hemiareflexia, and progressive scoliosis, perhaps due to a defect of the dorsal lip of the neural tube or neural crest. The hemihypertrophy may be quadrantic and it spares the face; the muscles are large and strong. The hypesthesia affects the modalities of pain and temperature. An increased prevalence of neural tube defects in the family is notable.[4720] Mental retardation and seizures are further complications.[5316]

hemiachromatopsia Loss of color vision in one half-field, all colors appearing as gray, while perception of white objects is unaffected.

hemiagnosia for pain A rare manifestation of a right hemisphere lesion described by Pierre **Marie**. Although the patient is hyperpathic on the left, he is unable to localize the source and to define the nature of the severe discomfort.

hemiakinesia See **inattention**.

hemianhidrosis (from Gr, half + derivative + sweating) Lack of sweating on one side of the body, usually due to a lesion of the sympathetic fibers within the CNS.

hemianopia (hemiopia, hemianopsia) Loss of vision in one half of the field of each eye. Such a loss is usually to one or the other side. The various types of hemianopia are listed in Chart H–6.

See also **congruence**.

hemianopic color blindness Residual color blindness (shown by inability to match colors) in a field which was formerly hemianopic.

hemianopic hallucinations Pure visual hallucinations within a hemianopic half-field (or in the area of a lesser visual field defect), the lesion involving the visual cortex. Migrainous visual hallucinations are an example.[2101, 3520]

hemianopsia See **hemianopia**.

hemiasomatognosia See **Anton–Babinski syndrome**.

hemiataxia See **hemiataxy**.

hemiataxia–hypesthesia An unusual, lateral thalamic stroke syndrome due to infarction in the territory of the thalamogeniculate artery, characterized clinically by isolated hemiataxia and ipsilateral sensory loss involving any modalities.[4298]

hemiataxy (hemiataxia) Unilateral motor incoordination.

hemiathetosis Athetosis occurring on one side of the body only.

hemiatrophia cerebri Severe acquired atrophy of one cerebral hemisphere in children, following an initial acute insult and associated partial seizures. See also **HHE syndrome**.[6200]

hemiatrophy Unilateral shrinkage of a body part due to various degrees of involvement of skin, subcutaneous tissue, fat, and/or bone. Though classically the sequel to infantile cortical lesions, it is also described in association with acquired neurological diseases and it also occurs idiopathically.[5407]

Chart H–6. Types of Hemianopia

Homonymous hemianopia The deficits are of the corresponding fields, right or left, in each of the two eyes.

Bitemporal hemianopia The loss is in the right half-field in the right eye and in the left half-field in the left eye. It is characteristically associated with a mid-line lesion compressing the optic chiasm.

Altitudinal hemianopia The visual field defect may also be of the upper or the lower half if the deficit is demarcated by the equator.

Sectoral hemianopia A homonymous altitudinal field defect with a linear horizontal edge, produced by lesions of the nonstriatal visual pathways.[3002]

Binasal or bitemporal hemianopias The nasal or the temporal fields are lost, respectively, in each eye. Because the field defect is a mirror image in the two eyes, such forms of hemianopia may be known as *heteronymous hemianopias*.

Complicated hemianopias The hemianopia is complicated by the presence of an oculomotor palsy.

Quadrantic hemianopia The condition in which the deficit is of one quarter of the field only; it may be bitemporal or binasal, and above or below the visual equator.

Functional hemianopia Hemianopia in the absence of organic disease of the visual pathways. This form has been reviewed by Gittinger.[2396]

hemiballism(us) (half and Gr, jumping) (hemichorea) An uncommon hyperkinetic disorder characterized by sudden, violent, persistent, unilateral, proximal flinging movements of an arm or leg due to a lesion (usually a **lacunar infarct**) involving the contralateral subthalamic nucleus of Luys.[2110] The term was first applied by **Economo**. See **ballism**.

In a *variant form*, the condition is inherited as a recessive trait.

hemibasal syndrome See **Garcin syndrome**.

hemibulbar syndrome See **Babinski–Nageotte syndrome**.

hemichorea See **hemiballism(us)**.

hemiclonic seizures Forms of seizure with little localizing value, occurring early in development, before myelination of the corpus callosum. They can affect both hemispheres alternately, as in **Dravet syndrome** and ischemic encephalopathy, or only one hemisphere in the case of focal disturbances.[1861]

hemiconvulsions, hemiplegia, epilepsy syndrome See **HHE syndrome**.

hemicrania (Gr, half + the head) (megrim) Headache affecting one side only; classic migraine. *Hemicrania alternans* affects the two sides alternately; *angioparalytic (or neuroparalytic) hemicrania* is **complicated or hemiplegic migraine**.

hemicrania alternans See **hemicrania**.

hemicrania epileptica Headache occurring in association with partial seizures. Diagnostic criteria have been defined

A. Headache lasting seconds to minutes, with features of migraine, fulfilling criteria C and D below
B. The patient has had a 'partial' epileptic seizure
C. Headache develops synchronously with the seizure and is ipsilateral to the ictal discharge
D. Headache resolves immediately after the seizure

From the ICHD (Headache Classification Committee of the International Headache Society. Cephalalgia 2004;24(Suppl 1)) by kind permission of Dr. Jes Olesen, the International Headache Society, and Wiley-Blackwell Publications.

hemicrania continua A rare, benign, unilateral headache of continuous type and moderate severity, for which no precipitants are identified and which is absolutely responsive to indomethacin. It is more common in females. The pain may or may not pulsate but tends to fluctuate in intensity, with severe exacerbations (stabbing headaches) sometimes superimposed on background pain of moderate severity felt mainly in frontal, temporal, and orbital regions. The side on which it is felt seldom changes between attacks. Cycles persist over weeks to years.[4644] There are few accompanying autonomic signs compared to those occurring in **chronic paroxysmal hemicrania**, which this headache otherwise resembles,[747, 5882, 4643] but ipsilateral lacrimation, ptosis, rhinorrhea, and nasal congestion and conjunctival injection are occasional accompaniments.

Diagnostic criteria suggested by Goadsby and Lipton[2415] and by Pareja et al.[4893] are extant, but the ICHD criteria are reproduced here:

A. Headache for >3 months fulfilling criteria B–D
B. All of the following characteristics:
   1. Unilateral pain without side-shift
   2. Daily and continuous, without pain-free periods
   3. Moderate intensity, but with exacerbations of severe pain
C. At least one of the following autonomic features occurs during exacerbations and ipsilateral to the side of pain:
   1. Conjunctival injection and/or lacrimation
   2. Nasal congestion and/or rhinorrhea
   3. Ptosis and/or miosis
D. Complete response to therapeutic doses of indomethacin
E. Not attributed to another disorder

From the ICHD (Headache Classification Committee of the International Headache Society. Cephalalgia 2004;24(Suppl 1)) by kind permission of Dr. Jes Olesen, the International Headache Society, and Wiley-Blackwell Publications.

hemicranianosis See **Brissaud–Lereboullet syndrome**.

hemidystonia Involuntary sustained posturing of the arm, leg, and face of one side. In most cases, the responsible lesion is situated in the contralateral putamen, caudate, or thalamus, disconnecting the thalamus from the striatum. The corticospinal pathways are essentially preserved. The possible etiologies are many.[5006, 4104]

hemidystonia–hemiatrophy syndrome A syndrome of adolescence in which unilateral bodily and cerebral hemiatrophy due to perinatal complications or stroke are, after some years, complicated by hemidystonia. The condition may be a static encephalopathy.[6774]

hemifacial atrophy See **Parry–Romberg syndrome**.

hemifacial microsomia (first arch syndrome, mandibular dysostosis) A congenital anomaly of unknown cause, manifesting unilateral hypoplasia of the facial soft tissues and underlying bones, with failure of formation of the mandibular ramus and condyle and ipsilateral microtia.[2503] The condition may be a *variant* of **oculoauriculovertebral dysplasia**. See also **Goldenhar syndrome**.

hemifacial spasm (Brissaud–Meige syndrome) An acquired, progressive syndrome characterized by frequent, repetitive, unilateral, involuntary tonic, or tonic–clonic spasm of the facial muscles due to compression of the VII cranial nerve at the root exit zone. Aberrant vessels have been identified on contrast-enhanced CT scans (Digre et al. 1988), MRI, and modified magnetic resonance angiography studies in 80%–100% of cases.

There are two forms. In the first, brief twitches occur simultaneously in several facial muscles, often with blinking and accompanied by isolated bursts of 20–40 repetitive motor unit discharges on the EMG at up to 400 Hz and lasting for about 0.5 s. In the second form, prolonged spasms occur erratically with electrical discharges at a slower rate.[2922]

The syndrome is likely to be caused by ephaptic transmission after nerve injury and the appearance of a new trigger in the nerve trunk which would give rise to a locally generated electrical discharge. The abnormal activity is generated at the exit zone, probably at the facial nucleus. Aberrant afferent activity generated at the site of vascular compression causes reorganization of the facial nucleus by a mechanism similar to the "kindling" phenomenon.

Some consider the basis to be a form of segmental myoclonus, while others believe that impingement of local dilated or redundant arteries upon the facial nerve exit zone is responsible, which has led to the institution of surgical procedures designed to achieve separation. Though criticized as simplistic, the theory of electrical crosstalk or chatter between artery and nerve has electrical validity,[2776] and the procedure, though potentially hazardous, has at least the merit of cure in numerous instances.[3164] The theory of vascular compression of the nerve is not new; it was propounded also by Brissaud in 1895.

In a *variant form*, autosomal dominant inheritance has been reported.[6066]

hemifield slide Diplopia with deviation of images either horizontally or vertically as an effect of bitemporal hemianopia, which prevents binocular fixation and suppression of the false image which is necessary in the presence of slight imbalance of motor input to the eyes.[3453]

hemihypertrophy–hemianesthesia–hemiareflexia–scoliosis See **hemi-3 syndrome**.

hemihypertrophy-nevi-hamartoma See **Proteus syndrome**.

hemimasticatory spasm A rare facial movement disorder (a form of segmental myoclonus) characterized by isolated, involuntary, unilateral, painful contractions of the masticatory muscles (masseter, temporalis, and pterygoid) which tend to hypertrophy.

This paroxysmal cranial neuropathy is considered to be due to irritation leading to ectopic activity in the proximal trigeminal motor nerve root, perhaps by vascular structures; the EMG findings are similar to those observed in **hemifacial spasm**.[6304]

hemimegalencephaly A congenital dysmorphic syndrome manifesting also macrocrania, hemipareses, hemianopia, refractory grand mal and myoclonic seizures in the neonatal period, infantile spasms with hypsarrhythmia, nystagmus, heterotopias, diffuse gliosis, and high-output cardiac failure in infants. The affected hemisphere is enlarged and may show agyria or pachygyria.[400, 4965] Hemimicrencephaly may be present on the other side. A *variant* is ***hemimeganencephaly*** *(posterior quadrantic dysplasia)* A sporadic developmental malformation affecting the temporal, parietal, and occipital lobes of one hemisphere and a cause of mental retardation, infantile spasms, mild hemiparesis, visual deficits, and intractable partial seizures.[1402]

Hemimegalencephaly Support Group A group of parents and friends of children with hemimegalencephaly who provide contacts and information.

hemiopia (Gr, half + the eye) Half of the (normal) visual field. The term is, however, often used erroneously in place of **hemianopia**.

hemiparalexia An unusual dyslexic syndrome due to lesions in the left posterior callosum and characterized clinically by substitutions of left-sided (initial, beginning-of-word) letter substitutions during the oral reading of words.[641]

hemiparesis (Gr, half + want of strength) Weakness of one side of the body. The term is used interchangeably with **hemiplegia**.

hemiparetic cerebral palsy Congenitally derived hemiparesis, appearing in two main forms: *arm-dominant*, which is associated with relatively large cortical or subcortical lesions and clinically with epilepsy and cognitive deficits; and *leg-dominant*, in which the lesions are of the subcortical white matter and which are less often associated with these problems.[3044]

hemiparetic seizures (focal inhibitory seizures, local or unilateral atonic seizures, status hemiparalyticus, and partial seizures with subsequent hemigeneralization) Epileptic equivalents in which unilateral paresis is accompanied by paroxysmal epileptiform discharges.

This uncommon form of focal seizures is due to discharges arising from the contralateral hemisphere without disturbance of consciousness, as shown by EEG abnormalities and radionucleotide uptake in the contralateral hemisphere. Treatment of the seizures clears both the paralysis and the abnormal brain scan. The episodes represent an ictal rather than postictal event and are neither migrainous nor due to demonstrable focal pathology.[2735] See also **Todd paralysis**.[2735]

hemi-Parkinsonism-(somatic) hemiatrophy syndrome The association of early life hemispheric injury with contralateral focal hemiatrophy and pyramidal signs, with the development on that side of slowly progressive Parkinsonism unresponsive to levadopa and the early appearance of dystonias, each appearing before the ingestion of medications.[3471] The condition is a rare form of secondary **Parkinsonism**.[6774]

hemiplegia (Gr, half + striking) Severe weakness, as due to a stroke, affecting any part of the upper motor neuron pathway, on one side of the body.

In **alternating** or *crossed hemiplegia,* the weakness affects the ocular movements or face on one side and the trunk and limbs on the other. See also **Weber syndrome**, **Millard–Gubler syndrome**, **Foville syndrome**, and **Jackson syndrome**.

hemiplegia alternans superior peduncularis See **Weber syndrome**.

hemiplegia cruciata (crossed hemiplegia, syndrome of the decussation) Corticospinal tract damage leading to a pyramidal syndrome affecting the arm on the same side and the leg on the other. The lesion must be at the cervicomedullary junction on the side of the arm weakness, at which site the fibers destined to cross to the corticospinal tract on the other side of the cord have not yet crossed (unlike those destined for the arm, which have).

hemiplegic amyotrophy (hemiplegic atrophy) Wasting of muscles in a limb affected by an upper motor neuron lesion. Such wasting is considered due to a combination of disuse, trans-synaptic degeneration, and loss of central trophic influences upon the lower motor neuron.[1160]

hemiplegic atrophy See **hemiplegic amyotrophy**.

hemiplegic epilepsy The term of Hughlings-**Jackson** for **partial seizures**.

hemiplegic gait Characteristically, that gait requiring an exaggeration of the upward pelvic tilt with rolling circumduction of the affected leg during the phase of weight-bearing on the opposite leg, in order to compensate for the lengthening effect of the paretic leg's posture. This is held extended at the hip and knee, the ankle being plantar flexed. The adducted, pronated, and flexed posture of the arm is a further diagnostic clue.

hemiplegic migraine See **familial hemiplegic migraine**.

hemipontine syndrome Hemorrhage into the lateral part of the pons; it is an unusual occurrence, most hemorrhages being central and bilateral. The major signs include alternating hemiparesis and thermoanalgesia, as well as **skew deviation** of the eyes. Consciousness is preserved and many patients make reasonable functional recoveries. See also **dorsal tegmental syndrome**.

hemi-seesaw nystagmus A rare variant of **seesaw nystagmus** in which one half-cycle of seesaw nystagmus alternates with a quick phase in the other direction.[2701]

hemisensory syndrome 1. A **lacunar syndrome** (see **pure sensory stroke**). 2. See **left sided syndrome**.

hemisomatic spasms A syndrome of unilateral spasms affecting the face and ipsilateral arm, resulting from a lesion at the ipsilateral cerebellopontine angle.[86] Only the extension of movements to the arm differentiates this condition from **hemifacial spasm**.

hemispasm A dystonic or convulsive movement affecting one side of the body only.

hemispatial agnosia See **neglect**.

hemispatial neglect (inattention) An abnormal relationship between the patient and the environment on the side opposite to a hemispheric lesion (usually the right hemisphere) in which objects and events on that side, including that half of the patient himself, are ignored to a greater or lesser extent.[4917]

hemisphere (Gr, half + a ball or sphere) Half a sphere—thus the cerebral and cerebellar hemispheres so named due to their shape.

hemispherectomy Surgical removal of most or all of one cerebral hemisphere, rarely performed but of value in children with intractable epilepsy.[48]

hemispheric epilepsy A syndrome of childhood or adolescence manifesting an intractable seizure disorder (tonic–clonic, myoclonic, tonic, atonic, or absencelike) with generalized ictal features that are focal in most cases; without demonstrable etiology or related structural abnormality of the CNS. Diffuse unilateral spike-waves are seen on EEG consistently appearing over the same hemisphere. The etiology is seldom determined.[689]

Hemispheric Stroke Scale An instrument for assessing and quantitating deficits following ischemic stroke, under the headings *level of consciousness* (derived from the **Glasgow Coma Scale**); *language*; *other cortical functions and cranial nerves*; *motor examination and gait*; and *sensory function*.[53] See also **stroke scales**.

hemivertebra A congenital anomaly characterized by the failure of normal development of one half-side of a vertebra. While the condition may be symptomless, some degree of scoliosis is the usual result.

hemodilution A technique for lowering the hematocrit, usually by about 30%, in order to increase cerebral blood flow and maximize tissue oxygenation, as following stroke. Methods may either increase blood volume (hypervolemic) or, by bloodletting at the same time as cell-free fluids are administered, allow it to remain normal (isovolemic). The method is of unproven value in the treatment of stroke.

hemoglobinopathic encephalopathy A diffuse encephalopathy occurring in children possessed of hemoglobin H and who present with mental retardation. The responsible gene maps to 16pter–p13.5.

hemophilic encephalopathy A diffuse encephalopathy.[1789]

Hemophilus influenzae meningitis A dangerous form of meningitis most commonly affecting children less than 5 years old and immunocompromised adults.

hemorrhagic leukoencephalitis See **acute disseminated encephalomyelitis**.

Hennebert, Richard (1868–1962) German neurologist who gave early accounts of **metachromatic leukodystrophy** and the **hard palate reflex**.

Hennebert sign 1. Induction of vertigo and nystagmus in subjects with a fistula of a semicircular canal by the examiner's fingertip pressure over the patient's external auditory meatus.[2861] 2. See **hard palate reflex**.

Hennebert syndrome (luetic-otitic-nystagmus syndrome) The occurrence of nystagmus and vertigo with alterations of pressure within the external auditory meatus; a feature of congenital syphilis, often accompanied by interstitial keratitis and chorioretinitis.[2860] The phenomenon was described by Camille Hennebert (1867–1962), a Belgian otologist.

Increased vertigo and/or nystagmus also occur when the pressure in the external auditory meatus is increased, as by manual pressure on the tragus, in patients with a fistula between the perilymph and the middle ear resulting from any cause.

Henoch, Eduard Heinrich (1820–1910) German physician.

Henoch–Schönlein purpura A hypersensitivity vasculitis of children in which both stroke and **subarachnoid hemorrhage** may occur apart from the gastrointestinal and renal manifestations.

Henoch syndrome The disease was called "electrical chorea" by Henoch, who noted it in children with asymmetrical and variable lightning-like twitches in the shoulder and neck muscles which disappear in sleep but which later become generalized and chronic. The term was later appropriated for the syndrome described by **Dubini**, which is probably quite different. See **paramyoclonus multiplex**.

Henzschell syndrome See Apert syndrome.

hepatic carnitine palmityl transferase deficiency A syndrome with onset in infancy, characterized by fasting hypoglycemia. As a result of lack of carnitine palmityl transferase activity, long chain fatty acid oxidation, ketogenesis, and gluconeogenesis are all impaired. No muscle disorder is associated.[763]

hepatic decerebration The occurrence of decerebrate rigidity in hepatic encephalopathy. The pathophysiology is not known.[3260]

hepatic encephalopathy A severe neuropsychiatric syndrome characterized by abnormal mental and other neurological status, occurring in patients with severe acute or chronic hepatic insufficiency or primary biliary cirrhosis. The clinical features range from mild cognitive impairment to coma and may include **asterixis**, tremor, ataxia, ophthalmoplegia, myelopathy, neuropathy, and autonomic insufficiency, usually in the presence of high levels of blood ammonia.[1491, 2181] **Triphasic waves** are commonly found on the EEG in each of the two forms described:

1. Acute hepatic insufficiency causes rapidly raised intracranial pressure with deepening drowsiness leading to coma as a result of cytotoxic brain edema; death may ensue.
2. *Porto-systemic encephalopathy*, in which the clinical development is slower, passing from personality change and altered sleep patterns through ataxia and asterixis to stupor and coma. See **acquired hepatocerebral encephalopathy**.

Hepatic Encephalopathy An online resource that reproduces sections of GI textbook, providing definition, causes, and treatments. Tables include a grading scale and common causes by type. Web site: http://www.clevelandclinicmeded.com/medicalpubs/diseasemanagement/gastro/henceph/henceph.htm.

hepatic neuropathy A mild, demyelinating, sensorimotor peripheral neuropathy due either to the metabolic disorder which induced hepatic insufficiency or to the metabolic consequences of the organ failure.[1491]

Acute inflammatory demyelinating polyneuropathy may complicate viral hepatitis,[3792] and a mild but painful sensory neuropathy is described in biliary cirrhosis.[6287]

hepatocerebral degeneration A condition resembling **Wilson disease**, which was described 2 years later. The clinical features are those of cortical and basal ganglion disturbances. See **acquired hepatocerebral encephalopathy** and **Alpers syndrome**.

hepatocerebral syndrome See **acquired hepatocerebral encephalopathy**.

hepatolenticular degeneration See **Wilson disease**.

hepatorenal glycogenosis See **glycogen storage diseases**.

hepatosplenomegaly and adrenocortical deficiency A rare, recessive congenital musculoskeletal disorder manifesting diarrhea and vomiting during the first year of life, followed by sensorineural hearing loss and pigmentary retinopathy, subnormal mentality, distal progressive muscular atrophy, hepatosplenomegaly, and adrenal insufficiency. There are reduced levels of tissue arachidonic and other polyunsaturated fatty acids; prostanate and phosphate are identified in the plasma. The condition may be a disorder of phytanic acid metabolism distinct from Refsum disease.[1784]

Heracles A Greek god (Hercules in Latin) whose name was applied to epilepsy by Hippocrates, due to the strength and violence of the motor movements of the seizures.

herald hemiparesis The occurrence of mild hemiparesis when brain-stem signs may be absent or few, prior to the massive deficit produced by a succeeding basilar artery occlusion. There is nothing about the hemiparesis, however, which allows the subsequent events to be predicted.[2098]

hereditary acrolabial telangiectasia A dominantly inherited syndrome characterized by blue discoloration of the lips, nails, and nipples, widespread telangiectasias of the skin, and migraine headaches.[4383]

hereditary adult-onset leukodystrophy A dominantly inherited, chronic progressive neurological disorder of unknown nature characterized by the appearance of cerebellar, pyramidal, and autonomic symptoms and signs in mid-adult life, clinically and radiologically similar to X-linked **adrenoleukodystrophy** but with a different pattern of transmission and to multiple sclerosis except for the symmetry of radiological findings.[1836]

hereditary amyloid neuropathy See **Andrade neuropathy**.

hereditary angiopathy, nephropathy, aneurysms, and muscle cramps (13q34; *COL4A1, collagen type IV α1*) A dominantly inherited syndrome characterized by nephropathy with renal cysts and hematuria, angiopathy with leukoencephalopathy, retinal arteriolar tortuosity and intracranial aneurysms, paroxysmal painful cramps triggered by exercise and alcohol, and proximal weakness. Serum CK levels are high.[4992]

hereditary anhidrotic sensory neuropathy See **hereditary sensory and autonomic neuropathy** (recessive).

hereditary areflexic dystasia See **Roussy–Levy syndrome**.

hereditary arthro-ophthalmopathy See **Stickler syndrome**.

hereditary ataxia See **cerebellar ataxias** and **Friedreich ataxia**.

hereditary benign chorea See **hereditary nonprogressive chorea**.[3611]

hereditary branchial myoclonus with spastic paraplegia A dominantly inherited condition with adult onset, manifesting rhythmic myoclonus-like movements of the palate, pharynx, larynx, and face; truncal ataxia; and pyramidal signs, and leading to death in 5–10 years.[1523] See also **branchial myoclonus**.

hereditary brachial plexopathy (familial recurrent brachial plexus neuropathy) A dominantly inherited syndrome of young adult life, characterized by unusual sensitivity of fibers of the brachial plexus to intercurrent stretch or pressure, probably as a result of a subclinical inflammatory polyneuropathy, and leading to temporary but still prolonged conduction block.[6240] Clinically, it presents with attacks of pain and weakness with atrophy of the muscles of the shoulder girdle and proximal arm. See also **neuralgic amyotrophy**.

Cranial mononeuropathies and **Horner syndrome** are also occasionally found in such patients.[794]

hereditary bulbar atrophy (Fazio–Londe atrophy) See **juvenile motor neuron disease**.

hereditary carnitine deficiency See **carnitine deficiency**.

hereditary cerebellar ataxia See **cerebellar ataxias**.

hereditary cerebellar ataxia with mental deficiency See **cerebellar ataxias** (*variants*).

hereditary cerebral hemorrhage with amyloidosis–Dutch type See **Dutch cerebral hemorrhage**.

hereditary cerebral vasculopathy A dominantly inherited leukoencephalopathy appearing first in the third decade, characterized by dysarthria, progressive visual loss, dementia, and gait disturbance, thus resembling multiple sclerosis except that there is also visible retinal vasculopathy.[2548]

hereditary ceruloplasmin deficiency (hereditary ferroxidase deficiency) An autosomal recessive disorder characterized by subcortical dementia, involuntary movements, retinal degeneration, and diabetes mellitus in association with onset in adult life. Low serum levels of ceruloplasmin and iron overload, especially in the brain, pancreas, and liver, are characteristic. Serum ferritin levels are high. The mutation is mapped to chromosome 3q.[4491]

hereditary chin trembling See **hereditary quivering of the chin**.

hereditary continuous motor neuron discharges with neuropathy A familial syndrome of distal weakness and atrophy with myokymia or fasciculations and delayed relaxation after voluntary contraction.[3662]

hereditary coproporphyria An uncommon, dominantly inherited form of **porphyria**. Neurological features complicate some acute attacks and include the occurrence of proximal motor neuropathy affecting the arms more than the legs (often asymmetrically) and also the face and autonomic system, in the setting of other features of the disease, including photosensitivity, abdominal pain, vomiting, tachycardia, hypertension, and often seizures and delirium.[5370]

hereditary demyelinating neuropathy of infancy A demyelinating peripheral neuropathy with onset in infancy, clinically resembling type III **hereditary motor and sensory neuropathy** (Déjèrine–Sottas disease) sometimes with bulbar and diaphragmatic involvement. Four point mutations in the peripheral myelin protein 22 (*PMP22*) gene have been found; the disease is genetically heterogeneous.[6431]

hereditary dentatorubralpallidoluysian atrophy (familial myoclonic epilepsy and choreoathetosis, progressive pallidal atrophy, dentatorubral atrophy, dyssynergia cerebellaris myoclonica) A combined systemic degeneration of the dentatofugal and pallidofugal pathways, clinically manifesting chorea, dystonia, athetosis, ballism, and/or ataxia.

Criteria for diagnosis are the presence of a dominantly inherited myoclonic epilepsy syndrome with or without cerebellar signs or choreoathetosis in the presence of dentatorubralpallidoluysian atrophy.[6188]

hereditary diffuse leukoencephalopathy with spheroids A rare, dominantly inherited progressive leukoencephalopathy characterized by giant neuroaxonal swellings within the CNS white matter, presenting with dementia in adult life.[2722]

Hereditary Disease Foundation A charitable organization providing information and support. Address: 11400 West Olympic Blvd., Suite 855, Los Angeles, CA 90064-1560. Tel: 310-575-9656. E-mail: cures@hdfoundation.org. Web site: http://www.hdfoundation.org/.

hereditary distal muscle dystrophy See **Gowers syndromes** and the following entry.

hereditary distal myopathy Genetically determined syndromes of distal muscle weakness and wasting, first described by **Gowers**.[2532] Two forms are recognized as follows: (1) The autosomal dominant *distal late hereditary myopathy* of Welander[6711] with onset after the age of 20 years, and with slow progression of symptoms starting in the hands and wrist extensors in both sexes; and (2) Another dominantly inherited form, characterized by the infantile onset of bilateral foot drop, weakness later affecting the hands and wrists but with no further progression after the age of 18 years.[4013]

hereditary distal spinal muscular atrophy A syndrome of progressive symmetrical wasting and weakness presenting in childhood or adolescence. It resembles a form of peroneal muscular atrophy (**hereditary motor and sensory neuropathy** types 1 or 2), but there is less arm weakness, relative preservation of the muscle stretch reflexes, and normal clinical sensory examination and motor and sensory conduction study findings.

Other *variants* are *scapuloperoneal, facioscapulohumeral*, and *generalized* forms.[2761]

hereditary dysphasic dementia A dominantly inherited dementing disorder of later adult life with prominent nonfluent dysphasia and Parkinsonism. Pathologically, features of **Pick, Alzheimer**, or **Parkinson diseases** are found in association with spongy degeneration of the cortex.[4497] See also **primary progressive aphasia**.

hereditary dysphasic disinhibition dementia See **frontotemporal dementia**.

hereditary dystonia with contractures and abnormal muscle A congenital syndrome characterized by joint contractures, chorea, dystonia, and muscle fiber hypotrophy with ring fibers.[381]

hereditary dystonia with lightning jerks, responsive to alcohol See **hereditary myoclonic dystonia**.

hereditary dystonia–Parkinsonism syndrome of juvenile onset See **dopa-responsive dystonia**.

hereditary dystonic lipidosis See **Fabry disease**.

hereditary endotheliopathy with retinopathy, nephropathy, and stroke (HERNS) A dominantly inherited vasculopathy mapped to 3p21, leading to subcortical leukoencephalopathy and manifesting the features suggested by the appellation. It presents clinically with visual impairment, migrainelike headaches, dysarthria, hemiparesis, and apraxias in young adult life. Funduscopy shows a characteristic retinal vasculopathy involving the maculae. The presence of contrast-enhancing subcortical lesions indicates that this is a multi-infarct syndrome, though separate from **CADASIL**.[3192]

hereditary essential myoclonus A dominantly inherited myoclonic disorder with onset before the age of 20 years, characterized by involuntary contractions of single muscles or groups of synergic muscles, resulting in jerks of various amplitudes. The movements involve arms, legs, trunk, and neck (particularly the arms and neck) and are most frequent and intense proximally. Movements are always rapid and brief and are sometimes asynchronous; accompanying EMG activity lasts less than 500 ms. The movements are increased by activities requiring fine coordination, such as writing, and by conscious attempts to inhibit them. No other neurological deficits are found; the course is benign and the condition does not decrease the lifespan.[4021]

Distinction from paramyoclonus multiplex is made mainly on the basis of the family history and exacerbation with activity.[1469] See also **paramyoclonus multiplex, myoclonus, essential myoclonus**, and **hereditary myoclonic dystonia**.

hereditary facial spasm (Hellsing syndrome) A slowly progressive complicated polyneuropathy, dominantly inherited and manifesting uni- or bilateral hemifacial spasm, with facial weakness, **Argyll Robertson pupils**, gaze disturbances, reduced caloric reactions, optic atrophy, hyporeflexia, and mild lower motor neuron paresis in the legs with pes cavus and trophic foot ulcers but normal distal sensation. To date, the condition seems to have been reported only from Sweden.[3963] The syndrome is probably a form of hereditary hypertrophic neuropathy, resembling Déjerine–Sottas neuropathy (**hereditary motor and sensory neuropathy** type 3).

hereditary ferroxidase deficiency See **hereditary ceruloplasmin deficiency**.

hereditary fructose intolerance A congenital dysmetabolic state due to the absence of fructose-1-phosphate aldolase B, the enzyme responsible for the assimilation of dietary fructose, and characterized in infancy by failure to thrive, vomiting, and hypoglycemia. In adults, the symptoms are those of hypoglycemia, including convulsions after fructose ingestion.[1308]

In a *variant* form, fructose 1:6-diphosphatase activity is deficient. The clinical features are similar.

hereditary hemorrhagic telangiectasia (Rendu–Osler–Weber hemangiomatosis) A dominantly inherited disorder characterized by the presence of multiple dermal, mucosal, and visceral telangiectasias which bleed recurrently. Neurologically, emboli resulting from pulmonary arteriovenous fistulas, intracranial aneurysms with hemorrhage, and telangiectasias within the CNS are the major complications.[5363]

Hereditary Hemorrhagic Telangiectasia Foundation International Inc. A charitable, patient-centered organization concerned with this condition. Address: P.O. Box 8087, New Haven, CT 06530. Tel: 1-800-HHT-NETW (USA) or 313-561-2537 (Canada) Web site: http://www.hht.org/.

hereditary hypertrophic neuropathy, trigeminal neuralgia, and deafness See **hereditary motor and sensory neuropathy, type 1**.

hereditary hypertrophic neuropathy with paraproteinemia See **gammopathic neuropathy**.

hereditary inclusion body myopathy (distal myopathy with rimmed vacuoles, quadriceps sparing myopathy, *GNE*-related muscle disease) A group of rare/orphan genetic disorders caused by genetic variations in *GNE* and leading to progressive muscle wasting and weakness that begins in young adulthood and can lead to very severe disability within 10–20 years. Major features are progressive muscle weakness and wasting, the latter usually starting around the age of 20–30 years, often leading to severe disability within 10–15 years, and confining many patients to a wheelchair.

The progressive weakness and severity vary from person to person. In some, weakness in the legs is noticed first. In a few others, the hands are weakened more rapidly than the legs. This disorder spares the brain, internal organs, and sensation. The quadriceps remain strong until the late stages of disease. See also **inclusion body myopathy**.

hereditary infantile hemiparesis, retinal arteriolar tortuosity, and **leukoencephalopathy** A dominantly inherited condition characterized by retinal arteriolar tortuosity and recurrent retinal hemorrhages. Infantile hemiparesis and migraine with aura are added features.[6456]

See also **hereditary endotheliopathy with retinopathy, nephropathy**, and **stroke**, and **hereditary vascular retinopathy**.

hereditary kinesthetic reflex epilepsy See **paroxysmal kinesigenic choreoathetosis**.

hereditary late-onset chorea A variant of **Huntington disease** with onset over the age of 50 years.[854]

hereditary leukoencephalopathy and palmoplantar keratoderma A recessively inherited neurocutaneous syndrome with childhood onset, manifesting spastic quadriparesis and cognitive impairment in adult life.[3918]

hereditary liability to pressure palsies See **hereditary pressure-sensitive neuropathy**.

hereditary macular dystrophies with encephalopathy

(cerebroretinal degeneration) Thars **sphingolipidoses** or **mucolipidoses**, usually recessively inherited, associated with cone or rod-cone dystrophies or with pigmentary retinopathy. See also **neuronal ceroid lipofuscinosis**.

hereditary mirror movements

A dominantly inherited syndrome with childhood onset, characterized by the performance of movements with one limb mirroring those voluntarily performed in the other, and by mental and developmental delay.[5647] See **mirror movements**.

hereditary motor and sensory neuropathies (HMSN)

A heterogeneous group of familial disorders characterized by the onset in childhood of denervation affecting the feet and legs before the hands and arms, and leading to slowly progressive weakness and muscle atrophy. The prototype was described by **Charcot** and **Marie**[1109] in France and independently by **Tooth** in England in the same year. The first-identified responsible gene lies on chromosome 1, but at two sites, with and without linkage to the Duffy locus. Other genes implicated include peripheral myelin protein-22, early growth response myelin protein zero, connexin, and the neurofilament light chain.[5688] Many *variant forms* have been identified (see Chart H–7).

Some order was brought to the classification of the hereditary mixed neuropathies when nerve conduction studies showed that, in most families, the motor conduction velocity was grossly reduced but in others it was reduced only to a figure still greater than 70% of the normal or 38 M/s. Both this syndrome and the next (HMSN 1 and HMSN 2) are also known by the names of Charcot, Marie, and Tooth, and as *peroneal muscular atrophy*.[2762] Despite the advances of recent years, the classifications below are best

Chart H–7. Classification of the Hereditary Motor and Sensory Neuropathies

Hereditary motor and sensory neuropathy type 1 (Charcot–Marie–Tooth disease, demyelinating form; peroneal muscular atrophy, CMT 1; HMSN type 1, Hoffmann disease, Roussy–Lévy syndrome) A class of relatively common, dominantly or recessively inherited, slowly progressive hypertrophic demyelinating motor, and sensory neuropathies. Mutations in the early growth response gene have been found here and in subjects with congenital hypomyeliniating neuropathy (see below).

The usual clinical onset is in childhood; widespread segmental demyelination of the peripheral nerves is found and the motor nerve conduction velocities (MNCVs) in the median nerves are below 38 M/s in the arm and <34 M/s in the leg. Secondary axonal loss reduces CMAP amplitudes and leads to abolition of sensory nerve action potentials. Distal weakness and wasting, especially in the legs, areflexia, nerve thickening, and reduction of all forms of sensation distally are commonly detected and pes cavus, scoliosis, essential tremor (*Roussy–Lévy syndrome*), or ataxia may be present. Acute or subacute deterioration of genetically proven CMT diseases may occur after a long period of stabilization due to a superimposed inflammatory polyneuropathy.[2390]

CMT1 (Classical Charcot–Marie–Tooth [CMT] disease) This dominant form is due to a duplication of DNA on the short arm of chromosome 17 (Type 1A at 17p11.2–p.12; the *PMP-22* gene) The Roussy–Lévy syndrome is a subtype of this and of the next entry. This condition is associated with an increased prevalence of obstructive **sleep apnea**.

CMT1B (mapped to 1q22; *MPZ* gene) A more severe distal sensorimotor axopathy with juvenile onset associated with distal motor weakness and sensory loss but with preserved ankle reflexes.[2631]

CMT1C (mapped to 16p13; *LITAF* gene); this resembles CMT1 clinically.

CMT1D A severe form due to mutations of the early growth response gene and mapped to 10q21 (*EGR2* gene).

CMT1E It is mapped to 1q22.

CMT1F (neurofilament light chain, mapped to 8p21) is also differentiated, based on its genetic locus.

This group also includes *Déjèrine–Sottas neuropathy* (*HMSN3*; see below) with early onset and very slow MNCVs. Although most cases are sporadic the genetic forms map to the same loci. A defect of peripheral myelin protein (*PMP-22*) is responsible. **Hereditary neuropathy with liability to pressure palsies** might well be included here as well.

Other *variant* forms classifiable here are:

Hereditary relapsing thermosensitive neuropathy A dominantly inherited relapsing form with onset from childhood to adult life in which the weakness and sensory losses are only exposed by fever.

Hypomyelination in the CNS and PNS characterized by hypopigmentation and enteric aganglionosis and mapped to 22q13. Inheritance is dominant or sporadic. It is due to a *SOX10* gene mutation.

Bilateral high-frequency hearing loss with sensory polyneuropathy A dominantly inherited variant due to a mutation of *connexin-31*, mapped to 1p35.1.

Asymptomatic congenital hypomyelinating neuropathy

A form with giant axons

Charco–Marie–Tooth disease X-linked (CMT-X) It comprises X-linked and X-linked dominant *variants* of *HMSN1*, for which, in some kinships, the responsible gene maps to Xq11–q13.[3095, 5455]

CMTX1 An X-linked dominant form of CMT (Xq13.1, mutations in the gap junction protein-β-1 gene *GJB1*, *connexin 32*). The clinical features resemble those of CMT1-affected males who show slowly progressive sensorimotor neuropathy associated with foot drop, pes cavus, and distal limb atrophy from childhood or adolescence. Affected females may be asymptomatic. Three varieties are differentiated.

Pathologically, this is an axonopathy with secondary demyelination, although a mixed picture (myelinopathy/axonopathy) may be identified by electrodiagnostic studies. NCVs of affected males are typically faster (20–30 M/s) than those of individuals affected by CMT1, but there is an overlap in NCV ranges between the two types. Mild slowing of NCVs is typical in affected females. Forms with mental retardation and spasticity have been described.

CMTX2 An X-linked recessive form (Xq22.2) characterized by the childhood onset of distal weakness and mental retardation. Both axonal and demyelinating elements are present.

CMTX3 An X-linked recessive form of axonal sensorimotor neuropathy (Xq26.3) with spasticity in some cases.

CMTX4 (Cowchock) A recessive form of axonal sensorimotor neuropathy of childhood (Xq24) with deafness and often mental delay. It may be allelic to *Charcot–Marie–Tooth X1*.

CMTX5 A recessive form of axonal sensorimotor neuropathy with deafness and optic atrophy (Xq22.3), allelic with **Arts syndrome**.

X-linked sensory neuropathy with deafness (AUNX1) A recessive form, mapped to Xq23–27.3.

X-linked motor and sensory neuropathy with pyramidal signs and cerebral white matter lesions. A variant form (possibly X-linked) with pyramidal signs and involvement of the central motor, somatosensory, and auditory pathways with diffuse white matter lesions on brain MRI.[4774]

Yet other *variant* forms include the following:

HMSN with optic atrophy The latter feature may be of the **Leber** type.[4250] See also *HMSN6*, below.

HMSN with spasticity The association of typical type 1 HMSN with pyramidal signs and abnormal auditory brainstem-evoked responses. See *HMSN5*, below.

HMSN with ataxia The association of congenital, dominantly inherited type 1 HMSN with cerebellar signs and sometimes choreoathetosis.[5977] This probably is the Roussy–Levy syndrome, misplaced.

Hereditary hypertrophic neuropathy, trigeminal neuralgia, and deafness A demyelinating sensorimotor neuropathy with onset in infancy or childhood, manifesting also sensorineural deafness and facial pain.[381]

HMSN with continuous motor unit activity A rare, dominantly inherited *variant* form of type 1 HMSN with associated fasciculations, myotonia, myokymia, and cramps.[6518]

HMSN with corneal dystrophy A congenital demyelinating sensorimotor peripheral neuropathy manifesting also cloudy corneas, hypotonia, multiple fractures, and cutaneous ulcers.[381]

Hypertrophic neuropathy with facial involvement A sensorimotor axonal and demyelinating neuropathy with onset in childhood or youth, manifesting also kyphoscoliosis, trigeminal neuralgia, facial spasm, and dysmyelination with onion-bulb formation in the peripheral nerves.[381]

HMSN with nephropathy A syndrome of progressive muscle wasting in a distribution characteristic of peroneal muscular atrophy associated with severe nephritis and neural deafness. This may be a variant of **Alport syndrome**.[2736]

Hereditary motor and sensory neuropathy with excessive myelin outfolding A recessively inherited hypomyelinating but hypertrophic sensorimotor peripheral neuropathy with onset in youth and with this unusual pathological finding.[388] Confusingly (because the standard classification of Dyck is still in the process of amendment), this is also known as CMT4B. Juvenile onset glaucoma has been associated with this form.[3466]

Hereditary motor and sensory neuropathy with features of Noonan syndrome Typical HMSN type 1a with giant proximal nerve hypertrophy, not linked to neurofibromatosis.[5834]

HMSN-Lom A recessively inherited demyelinating neuropathy with early axonal loss associated with sensorineural deafness and mapped to chromosome 8q24.[6284]

Congenital cataract–facial dysmorphism–neuropathy syndrome There are added microcorneas, mental retardation, small stature, and a predominantly motor neuropathy, sometimes pyramidal signs[1091] and mild chorea. It maps to chromosome 18qter.

Hereditary motor and sensory neuropathy type 2 (Charcot–Marie–Tooth disease, neuronal form; peroneal muscular atrophy) Slowly progressive, usually dominantly inherited motor and sensory neuropathies with onset at any age but mainly during the second decade. Their clinical features resemble those of type I but tend to be less severe and involve the hands less often. The nerves are not thickened, tremor and ataxia are uncommon accompaniments; the MNCVs in the median nerves are above 38 M/s and nerve biopsy specimens show neuronal atrophy.[4897, 634]

CMT2A A dominantly inherited axonal form, with normal or low normal MNCVs, and onset in young adult life. CMT2A1 and 2 (1p35–p36) (slightly different mutations) are distinguished.

CMT2B (3q13–q22) This type shows distal weakness but there is sensory predominance. The CMTB1 form (1q21, *LMNA* mutations) is an early-onset recessively inherited axonal form with later periscapular wasting.

CMT2B (19q13.3) presents in early adult life and is also axonal.

CMT2C (dominant, at 12q.33) is associated with paralysis of the diaphragm and vocal cords.[1781]

CMT2D (7p15, mainly affecting the hands and arms) and CMT2E (8p21) Another dominantly inherited form present in early adult life with variable conduction velocities. They have missense mutations in the neurofilament light chain gene (*NEFL*) and are differentiated only on the basis of their genetic loci.

CMT2E Mutations of the neurofilament light chain gene (*NEFL*) cause autosomal dominant neuropathies that are classified either as axonal Charcot–Marie–Tooth type 2E or demyelinating CMT type 1F (CMT1F) by causing a profound alteration of the cytoskeleton possibly related to defective targeting of NF.[1944]

CMT2F (at 7q11) characterized by young adult onset and notable trophic changes.

CMT 2G (at 12q12) presents in adult life with sensory loss, deafness, lancinating pain, pupillary abnormalities, and pharyngeal dysfunction.

CMT2H (607731), CMT4C2, ARCMT2C is a severe recessively inherited axonal form (8q21) with early childhood onset, reported from Tunisia.

CMT2I and CMT2J (each on 1q22) and CMT2L (on 12q24) Dominantly inherited axonal *variants* with similar but differentiated phenotypes

CMT2K (*GDAP1*) A recessively inherited *variant,* sometimes accompanied by vocal, cord paresis.

Hereditary neuropathy with liability to pressure palsies (perhaps a variant of HMSN1) A dominantly inherited neuropathy that presents in early adult life with episodes of localized numbness, weakness, and muscular atrophy without pain as a result of recurrent focal neuropathies. Electrodiagnostic studies show mildly slowed NCVs and conduction blocks at entrapment sites. Its clinical presentations resemble those of **multifocal motor neuropathy** and **chronic inflammatory demyelinating polyneuropathy**. Dominant or sporadic, types A and B are differentiated. One form is linked to Xp11.2; another to 17p.12. A defect of peripheral myelin protein (deletion of *PMP-22*) is responsible.

A *variant* is **hereditary neuralgic amyotrophy** in which the problem affects the brachial plexus only. Inheritance is autosomal dominant (chr. 17q25)[3590]

continued

Chart H–7. (*continued*)

Other *variants* include the following:

Benign HMSN type 2 with ptosis, Parkinsonism, and dementia. The combination of **multiple system atrophy** (ptosis, Parkinsonism, orthostatic hypotension, hyperreflexia, and mild dementia) with HMSN 2, dominantly inherited, and carrying a remarkably benign prognosis for life.[6204]

HMSN type 2 with Parkinsonism Another rare familial variant with adult onset.[965]

HMSN type 2 with neurofilamentous accumulations: A dominantly inherited sensorimotor axonal and demyelinating neuropathy with onset in childhood or youth, also characterized by pes cavus and cardiomyopathy, but without kinky hair. Nerve biopsy specimens show the presence of neurofilamentous accumulations and axonal swellings.[6559]

HMSN type 2 with deafness: (CMT4D) A sensorimotor axonal and demyelinating neuropathy with congenital or childhood onset, manifesting also sensorineural deafness.[379]

HMSN type 2 with acrodystrophy and severe limb weakness.[6283]

HMSN type 2 with optic atrophy and deafness A sensorimotor, axonal, and demyelinating neuropathy with congenital or childhood onset manifesting also sensorineural deafness, optic atrophy, and nystagmus.[5408]

HMSN type 2 with mental retardation, optic atrophy, and pyramidal signs A recessively inherited, severe but slowly progressive sensorimotor axonal neuropathy with onset in childhood, manifesting the above signs and retinal colloid bodies.[3990]

HMSN with myopathy Typical HMSN with the added histological features of myopathy, presumably as the result of repeated de- and reinnervation.

HMSN with dementia and dysautonomia A dominantly inherited syndrome consisting of slowly progressive limb weakness due to sensorimotor axonal neuropathy, attacks of vomiting, labile blood pressure, attacks of altered consciousness, mental retardation, and cerebral atrophy.[4845]

Parkinsonism with cerebellar ataxia and peripheral neuropathy A rare *variant* with adult onset.

Charcot–Marie–Tooth disease related to spinal muscular atrophy, distal type.

Charcot–Marie–Tooth peroneal muscular atrophy and ***Friedreich ataxia***. An X-linked *variant*.

Other variants listed here are dominantly inherited axonal motor and sensory neuropathies. They include *HMSN-proximal* mapped to 3q13; **HMSN 5** with pyramidal signs; *HMSN with deafness* (*P_o*, *connexin*, and eye and ear dysfunction); **HMSN 6** *HMSN with optic atrophy*; *HMSN with ulceromutilation*; **HSAN I**; *HSMN with ataxia* and **HMN** 5B.

Recessively inherited forms of axonal sensorimotor neuropathy (CMT2) are also described. These include the following:

AR-CMT2A, mapped to 1q21 *(lamin A/C)* which is allelic with **Emery–Driefuss muscular dystrophy** 2;

Autosomal dominant dilated cardiomyopathy with A–V block (CMD1A), familial partial lipodystrophy (Köbberling-Dunnigan syndrome) **LGMD 1B** and **quadriceps myopathy**.

AR-CMT2B, mapped to 19q13.3

AR-CMT with hoarseness (CMT 2K, mapped to 8q21) (*GDAP1*)

AR-CMT with pyramidal signs (CMT 2H), mapped to 8q21.3

Axonal CMT with acrodystrophy

Andermann syndrome (HMSN with agenesis of the corpus callosum) Is mapped to 15q13 *(KCC3)*

Ataxia with neuropathy mapped to 14q31 *(TDP1)*

Giant axonal neuropathy 16q24 (gigaxonin)

HMSN with optic neuropathy and/or deafness

Infantile axonal polyneuropathy with respiratory failure

Lethal neonatal sensorimotor neuropathy

Neuroaxonal dystrophy

Ouvrier variant with early childhood onset and slow progression.

Other genetically heterogeneous *variants* with late onset.[517]

Hereditary motor and sensory neuropathy type 3 (Déjèrine–Sottas syndrome, progressive hypertrophic interstitial neuropathy, onion-bulb neuropathy) A severe, congenital axonal, and demyelinating motor and sensory neuropathy with abnormal motor development and gross slowing of MNCV. There is proximal limb and trunk weakness, especially of the arms, with prominent sensory ataxia, areflexia, and hypertrophic nerves. Facial weakness is also described. Skeletal abnormalities can be a prominent feature. Nerve biopsy reveals profound demyelination and prominent onion-bulb formation.

In some cases, this may be no more than the homozygous expression of a dominant gene for HMSN1,[3973] but in most the condition is transmitted as a recessive characteristic[4835] or occurs sporadically. The multiple genotypes (1q22–q23, 17p11.2, 10q21–q22, 9q13) indicate the heterogeneity of the disorder.

Pupillary changes, optic atrophy, deafness, pigmentary retinal degeneration, hoarse voice, hypotonia, and bulbar weakness have been variously described in some kinships with HMSN 3.[2762] The condition has been subdivided according to the presence of hypomyelination and onion bulbs, the absence of myelin and a congenital neuronal form.[379, 1544]

The first postmortem examination in this condition was performed by **Déjèrine** on one of his patients who had died and had been buried for 4 days before he arranged her exhumation; the weather at the time being extremely cold, he found the body in a perfect state of preservation, allowing him to confirm the nerve enlargement.[5560]

Numerous genetic forms are identified: CMT 3A is due to mutations in the *PMP22* gene at 17p, CMT 3B has mutations in the *Po* gene on 1q, CMT 3C has mutations in *EGR2* at 10q, and CMT 3D is mapped to 8q23.

Clinical variants are as follows:

Congenital hypomyelination neuropathy A form with congenital onset, severe hypomyelination, and with the presence of atypical onion bulbs.[2653] Clinically, hypotonia, arthrogryposis, and severe weakness are seen. In yet other cases, neither myelin nor onion bulbs are present.

Hypertrophic neuropathy with facial weakness and kyphoscoliosis A form with onset in early adult life, presenting with trigeminal neuralgia, facial spasm, and palsy in addition to the usual findings.

Hereditary auditory, motor, vestibular, and sensory neuropathy in which complex condition with these features linkage to 8q24 has been achieved.[959]

Hereditary motor and sensory neuropathy type 4 (Refsum disease, heredo-ataxic hemeralopic polyneuritis, heredopathia atactica polyneuritiformis, phytanic acid storage disease) A recessively transmitted inborn error of metabolism marked by the accumulation of exogenous phytanic acid due to a defect of the alpha oxidation mechanism of beta-methyl-substituted fatty acids.

Clinically, the onset is in childhood with hypertrophic sensorimotor neuropathy, pigmentary retinal degeneration with concentric constriction of the visual fields and night blindness, cerebellar ataxia, ichthyosis, and increased CSF protein and blood phytanic acid levels. Pupillary abnormalities, cataract, anosmia, nerve deafness, epiphyseal abnormalities, and electrocardiographic abnormalities are sometimes associated.[5235]

CMT4 A recessive (seldom dominant) demyelinating, and rare syndrome. It presents in infancy or childhood with severe neuropathies resulting in delayed motor milestones as a result of progressive (mainly distal) weakness, with areflexia, mild sensory loss, and scoliosis leading to severe disability.[765]

CMT 4A Also recessively inherited, but linked to mutations in the ganglioside-induced differentiation-associated protein-1 (*GDAP1*) on 8q21.[528] A *variant* (8q13) is a severe autosomal recessive form with axonal degeneration and demyelinating features due to mutations in the ganglioside-induced-differentiation-associated protein 1 (*GDAP1*) gene which starts in the neonatal period or early infancy with weakness and wasting of the feet, subsequently involving the hands, marked distal atrophy causing severe disability. By the late teens, some patients develop a hoarse voice due to vocal cord paresis. Nerve biopsy shows depletion of myelinated fibers and axonal atrophy with onion bulbs. The unmyelinated fiber population is markedly increased.[5744]

CMT 4B (Includes CMT 4B1, European form) with congenital hypomyelination due to mutations in the myotubularin-related protein-2 (*MTMR2*) and CMT 4B2 (11q22 or 11p15, *MTMR13* gene). Both are severe types.

CMT 4C A severe recessive *variant* that clinically resembles CMT 1 but maps to 5q32 (*KIAA1985* gene).

CMT 4D (HMSN Lom) A recessive form in which the typical sensorimotor neuropathy with typical distal weakness and sensory loss is complicated by sensorineural hearing loss. A mutation of the N-myc gene-1 (*NDRG1*) on 8q24 has been shown.

CMT 4E A severe, recessively inherited, demyelinating form with onset of severe distal weakness in infancy. Conduction velocities are severely reduced, between 3 and 8 M/s, and nerve biopsy shows a virtual absence of myelin. It is linked to mutations in the *EGR2* gene on chromosome 10q21.1–q22, similar to CMT 1D.

CMT 4F presents with severe CMT 1-like signs in the legs by age 10 and in the arms by age 15. Affected individuals may have mildly delayed motor milestones. Biopsy shows onion-bulb formation with mixed demyelinating and axonal features. It is a recessive form, linked to mutations in the periaxin gene (*PRX*) on 19q13. Motor nerve conduction velocities are very slow.

CMT4G (hereditary motor and sensory neuropathy Russe) A recessively inherited syndrome characterized by severe leg and distal arm weakness, distal pan-sensory loss, foot and hand deformities, and Charcot joints, mapped to chromosome 10q23.[6284]

CMT 4H A recessive *variant* mapped to 12q11 (*FGD4*) with severe slowing of nerve conductions.

CMT 4J A recessive *variant* mapped to 6q21 (*FIG4*).

CCFDN A recessive *variant* mapped to 18q23 (*CDTP1* mutation) with hypomyelination and congenital cataracts, short stature, and dysmorphisms.

Variants are *hypertrophic interstitial neuropathy with cataracts* A congenital sensorimotor demyelinating hypertrophic neuropathy with cataract and kyphosis. *Adult Refsum disease variant with impaired pipecolic acid oxidation* A rare syndrome with the Refsum disease phenotype but with evidence of both mitochondrial and peroxisomal disorders, such as raised levels of pipecolic as well as of phytanic acid.[6369]

Other recessive variants as listed and described at http://neuromuscular.wustl.edu/naltbrain.html are given below:

CMT intermediate A (18q13, *GDAP1* mutations) A mild form reported from Turkey with axonal and demyelinating elements.

HMSN + Juvenile glaucoma

A form with cataracts mapped to 18qter

Cockayne syndrome

Congenital hypomyelinating neuropathy

Farber disease (lipogranulomatosis)

Glycosylation deficient, Ia

Krabbe disease

Metachromatic leukodystrophy

Refsum disease (PMP-22 point mutations) Infantile, childhood, adolescent, and adult forms

HMSN with CNS involvement; heterogeneous forms.

Hereditary motor and sensory neuropathy type 5 (HMSN with spasticity) A dominantly inherited sensorimotor demyelinating hypertrophic neuropathy with onset in infancy, childhood, or youth, also characterized by marked involvement of the hands, spasticity, and pes cavus.[1779, 2213, 2763]

Hereditary motor and sensory neuropathy type 6 (HMSN with optic atrophy) A recessively inherited sensorimotor axonal or demyelinating hypertrophic neuropathy with onset in early childhood, complicated by deafness, nystagmus, and optic atrophy.[4357] Features of HMSN 5 and 6 may coexist.[1644] In a variant form, the neuropathic element is minimal, and lancinating pain suggests the presence of a sensory neuropathy.[1084]

Hereditary motor and sensory neuropathy type 7 (HMSN with pigmentary retinopathy) A syndrome of HMSN with onset in childhood or adult life and with the added features of ataxia, pigmentary retinopathy, and sometimes sensorineural deafness and radiological evidence of cerebellar atrophy. The cases reported thus resemble *HMSN type* 4 (Refsum disease) but lack a detectable biochemical abnormality and peripheral nerve hypertrophy. Biopsy specimens show a reduction in the numbers of myelinated fibers without onion-bulb formation.[6414]

continued

Chart H–7. (*continued*)

To this classification may be added certain other *variant* forms:

A form mapping to Xq13 (*X-linked HMSN type 2 with deafness and mental retardation*). The onset is in infancy or childhood and sensorineural deafness and mental and developmental delay are present.[381]
HMSN with peripheral neurofibromatosis A hypertrophic demyelinating sensorimotor neuropathy with onset in infancy or childhood, manifesting also sensorineural deafness, seizures, café-au-lait spots, and neurofibromas.[381]
HMSN with epilepsy A form of HMSN with congenital onset, manifesting developmental delay, cerebellar ataxia, chorea, athetosis, and seizures.[381]
HMSN with arthrogryposis A rare *variant* form of HMSN with congenital onset.[6938]
HMSN with heart block A rare *variant* form of HMSN complicated by cardiomyopathy.[3706]
Nantahala neuropathy, due to an MPZ mutation (myelin adhesion protein) with cranial nerve involvement.
(Synthesized from Dyck and others,[1769] Ouvrier[4833] and Reilly[5245]and with data from Dr. Alan Pestronks Web site:[4992] http://neuromuscular.wustl.edu/synmot.html/) with his kind permission

regarded as work in progress. Another complication is that while the original classification of Dyck employed the term *hereditary motor and sensory neuropathy,* there has recently been a reversion to the eponymous *CMT* label.

Dyck[1769] suggested a classification for the whole group, and Chart H–7 is based thereon. The organization of the many entities is difficult today, however, because other classifications are also extant.[6510, 5597, 2756] Chart H–7 (above) is an abbreviated listing of the conditions that are further defined below, much assisted by data from the Web site of Dr. Alan Pestronk, (http://neuromuscular.wustl.edu/naltbrain.html/), which provides an expanded listing and descriptions.

See also **scapuloperoneal syndrome**, hereditary neuropathy with liability to pressure palsies, and **congenital hypomyelination neuropathy** for which both dominant and recessive forms are described with linkages to 1q22 and 10q21.

hereditary motor and sensory neuropathy with continuous motor unit activity See **hereditary motor and sensory neuropathy**, type 1.

hereditary motor and sensory neuropathy with corneal dystrophy See **hereditary motor and sensory neuropathy**, type 1.

hereditary motor and sensory neuropathy with dementia and dysautonomia See **hereditary motor and sensory neuropathy**, type 2.

hereditary motor and sensory neuropathy with myopathy See **hereditary motor and sensory neuropathy**, type 2.

hereditary motor and sensory neuropathy with optic atrophy See **hereditary motor and sensory neuropathy**, type 6.

hereditary motor and sensory neuropathy with pigmentary retinopathy See **hereditary motor and sensory neuropathy**, type 7.

hereditary motor and sensory neuropathy with spasticity See **hereditary motor and sensory neuropathy**, type 5.

hereditary motor neuropathies (distal hereditary motor neuronopathies, spinal muscular atrophies) Mainly dominant (a few recessive or X-linked recessive) disorders presenting in young adult life and characterized by insidiously progressive distal weakness and wasting with hyporeflexia, mainly in the legs, due to selective degeneration of the anterior horn cells or motor neurons, with EMG evidence of denervation. The first four major forms defined were all thought to be allelic on chromosome 5q (5q11.2–13.3.), but there are many variants and new forms continue to be detected. High arches and hammer toes are commonly seen. The term *spinal muscular atrophy* has been applied to many of these conditions, as shown in Chart H–8, but in this book that term will be used with reference to the acquired rather than to the inherited forms. See also **amyotrophic lateral sclerosis** (progressive muscular atrophy).

The terminology is again confusing in this context. Despite the neat and logical classification of hereditary neuropathies by Dyck (hereditary motor, hereditary sensory and autonomic, and hereditary motor and sensory), the obtuse term *spinal muscular atrophy* is still often preferred for *hereditary motor neuropathy*; though not here.

See also **Vialetto–van Laere syndrome**, **Fazio–Londe disease**. Other acquired forms are noted under **spinal muscular atrophy**.

Chart H–8. Classification of the Hereditary Motor Neuropathies

Hereditary motor neuropathy (HMN) type 1 (SMA1, severe/acute Werdnig–Hoffman disease, acute infantile spinal muscular atrophy type 1, infantile neuronal degeneration, amyotonia congenita, hereditary poliodystrophy) A recessively inherited, fatal, degenerative disease affecting bulbar and spinal motor nuclei with onset at birth or in the first 6 months of life, and manifesting generalized symmetrical (proximal > distal) weakness and fasciculations but with sparing of type 1 fibers in muscle biopsy specimens using ATPase stains. The first identified responsible gene maps to 5q11.2. The major forms are recessively inherited with mainly proximal involvement. Dominant distal forms are heterogeneous; their gene mutations are mapped variously to chromosomes 2q14, 12q24, 7p, and 12q23–q24. X-linked forms are also described and segregated below. At the time of writing, 28 loci including 10 causative genes had been described; Access the Web site of the HUGO Gene Nomenclature Committee at http://www.gene.ucl.ac.uk/nomenclature for updates and that of OMIM at http://www.ncbi.nlm.nih.gov/omim for further descriptions.[4812]

The disease was first described by Werdnig in 1891; Hoffmann later reported its familial nature.[6724, 2938] Instances of adult-onset **amyotrophic lateral sclerosis** have been recorded in the same families.

Criteria for the diagnosis of *spinal muscular atrophy, type 1* have been suggested[1209, 4992] and are as follows:

1. Clinical symptoms of anterior horn cell disease: areflexia or hyporeflexia; muscle atrophy; fasciculations.
2. Early onset and progressive course with an age at onset, less than 1 or 2 years and age at death less than 4 years. The children are never able to sit unsupported.
3. Creatine kinase levels are normal or up to 10 times higher than the reference value.
4. EMG study shows evidence of anterior horn cell involvement.
5. Muscle biopsy findings compatible with those of anterior horn cell disease.
6. Exclusionary findings are as follows: Symptoms referable to other neurological systems, such as sensory loss, central motor pathway signs, mental retardation, arthrogryposis, evident facial involvement, and other major organ involvement.

Variant forms include:

1. A lethal recessive form with atrial and ventricular septal defects and joint contractures.[4407] mapped to 5q. The next entry may be identical.
2. *Congenital Werdnig–Hoffman disease with glial bundles in the spinal roots* Whether this is a distinct variant is uncertain, since any form of HMN 1 may be associated with these glial bundles, but the bundles are not necessarily the cause of the disease, which is an anterior horn cell degeneration.[4407]
3. A form with pathological evidence of sensory fiber involvement.[5126]
4. *Cervical spinal muscular atrophy* A variant considered to be due to a restricted form of hereditary motor neuropathy resulting in progressive muscle wasting of the arms but generalized hyporeflexia and EMG evidence of widespread denervation.[2526]
5. A nonprogressive congenital variant considered to be due to an infarct or malformation of the lower cervical spinal cord, resulting in muscle wasting and contractures of the arms.[1464, 2916] (**Hirayama disease**) The placement of this syndrome here as an hereditary motor neuropathy is speculative.
6. *Infantile neuronal degeneration* A recessively inherited form clinically resembling HMN 1, in which there is additional widespread neuronal loss and gliosis in both the gray and white matter in the thalamus, pons, cerebellum, and spinal cord and segmental demyelination in the peripheral nerves,[6031] as in **infantile neuroaxonal dystrophy**.
7. *Dominant congenital benign spinal musular atrophy* A nonprogressive form of neurogenic weakness with leg contractures.[2210]
8. *Infantile spinal muscular atrophy with respiratory distress* A recessive form linked to a mutation on chromosome 11q13 with diaphragmatic paralysis and peripheral neuropathy.[2586]
9. A recessive or sporadic form with osteopenia, congenital bone fractures, and joint contractures.
10. *Pontocerebellar hypoplasia with spinal muscular atrophy* A lethal recessive form of hypotonia and weakness and ataxia with onset before or at birth. *(distal forms)*
11. *Autosomal dominant distal hereditary motor neuropathy I* (distal HMN I) presenting in juvenile to mid-adult life with distal symmetrical weakness and atrophy.
12. *Distal hereditary motor neuropathy with upper motor neuron signs* A dominantly inherited form characterized by pes cavus and the onset in childhood or adult life of distal weakness in all limbs with hyperreflexia; mapped to 9q34. *(senataxin)*.

Hereditary motor neuropathy type 2 (SMA2, early-onset spinal muscular atrophy, chronic or arrested Werdnig–Hoffmann disease, intermediate spinal muscular atrophy, infantile spinal muscular atrophy, arrested; chronic infantile form.) A recessively inherited, degenerative disease affecting bulbar and spinal motor nuclei with onset at or after 6 months of age and manifesting progressive, symmetrical, mainly proximal weakness and fasciculations, mild distal tremor, pes cavus, kyphoscoliosis, and contractures leading to crippling but with survival at least to 3 years and sometimes even into adult life.[2632] Mapping to 12q24 has been achieved in one dominant distal form.

Variant forms include[379]

1. A slowly progressive chronic motor neuropathy with more pelvic than shoulder girdle involvement and with dominant inheritance.[6966]
2. *Infantile spinal muscular atrophy, arrested* A nonprogressive form complicated by contractures.[2128]
3. Distal forms which can be recessively or dominantly inherited and with early or adult onset, mapped variously to 12q.24 or 9q34.

Hereditary motor neuropathy type 3 (juvenile or pseudomyopathic spinal muscular atrophy, [Wohlfart–] Kugelberg–Welander disease, chronic juvenile amyotrophic lateral sclerosis) A slowly progressive degenerative disease affecting spinal more than bulbar motor nuclei with usual onset between the ages of 5 and 15 years and manifesting progressive, symmetrical, mainly proximal weakness with fasciculations, ophthalmoplegia, and eventually kyphoscoliosis, cardiomyopathy, and contractures, but with survival into middle age or later, and without sensory signs.[6840, 3588] The responsible gene maps to 5q11.2.

When the disease is purely of the lower motor neuron type and has its onset before 24 months, the transmission is usually dominant; after that age, transmission is usually recessive. When the disease shows both upper and lower motor neuron features, inheritance is recessive.

Variant forms include

1. *Juvenile spinal muscular atrophy with hexosaminidase A deficiency (GM_2 ganglioside)* A recessively inherited form with the particular features of onset in youth, cognitive dysfunction, postural tremor, muscle pain or cramps and neuronal inclusions.[4409, 6966]
2. A form in which the signs involve both proximal and distal muscles and the course is rapid. This has only been reported from Papua New Guinea.[5696]
3. *Juvenile spinal proximal muscular atrophy* Usually recessively inherited, but both dominant[4956] and X-linked forms[6412] have been reported.
4. A form in which progressive external ophthalmoplegia is associated.

Further *variants* include;

1. The **monomelic** form which is usually sporadic;[5939] spinal muscular atrophy with **facioscapulohumeral distribution**,[2009] of which there is an X-linked variety. (Skre syndrome);[5888]
2. A distal form mapped to 11q13.3.

continued

Chart H–8. (*continued*)

3. A form with the early childhood onset of distal leg and quadriceps weakness.
4. (HMNJ, Jerash type) A recessive form mapped to 9p21 with childhood onset of distal leg more than arm weakness and some pyramidal signs.
5. *X-linked distal SMA* in which there is slow progression of distal weakness, initially of the legs, and pes cavus, reported once from Brazil.
6. *Distal hereditary motor neuropathy* A recessively inherited condition mapped to 11p reported from southern Italy.
7. *Distal hereditary motor neuropathy* A dominantly inherited condition mapped to 7q11 and allelic with *CMT 2F.*
8. *Distal hereditary motor neuropathy* A dominantly inherited condition of childhood affecting the distal legs and mapped to 7q34.

Hereditary motor neuropathy type 4 (juvenile onset) An uncommon dominantly inherited variant in which the onset occurs between the ages of 6 months and 15 years, the course is slow and the outcome benign.[4956]

Hereditary motor neuropathy type 5 (adult spinal muscular atrophy with upper limb predominance) A form with autosomal recessive (seldom dominant) inheritance and onset in early childhood or adult life, presenting with cramps, atrophy, and neurogenic weakness mainly in the arms, complicated variously by such features as truncal ataxia, myotonia, hydrocephalus *ex vacuo* or external hydrocephalus. Mapping of dominant forms to 7p.15 or 11q13 (the latter allelic with **Silver syndrome**) has been achieved.

In another dominant form described in adolescents there is weakness only in the distribution of the median or ulnar nerves.

Hereditary motor neuropathy type 6 (spinal muscular atrophy with respiratory distress) An infantile form caused by mutations in the immunoglobulin μ-binding protein-2 gene (*IGHMBP2*), mapped to 11q13.2 Diaphragmatic paralysis causes the respiratory failure.

Hereditary motor neuropathy type 7 A dominant *variant* linked to chromosome 2q14. Type 7A is described in teenagers who present with gait disorder due to the distal weakness and with evidence of vocal cord paralysis. Type 7B is similar but is mapped to 2p13.

*Other variant*s are

A *proximal spinal muscular atrophy* which may have dominant, recessive, or X-linked inheritance[5285] and another form presenting in the context of **GM2 gangliosidosis**[4603]

Hereditary motor and sensory neuropathy, proximal (HMSN-P; CMT 2*G*) A dominant form appearing in youth or adult life with added thick-fiber sensory loss and raised creatine kinase levels, described from Japan. It is mapped to 3q13.1

A congenital form, dominantly inherited, with contractures and normal nerve conductions *A distal form* with predominant involvement of the legs

Other *variants* of the above syndromes include

1. *Forms with Associated Lesions of the Nervous System:*

Anterior horn cell disease with cerebellar hypoplasia in infants A syndrome consisting of severe mental retardation, cortical blindness, and extensive peripheral paralysis of the lower motor neuron type and representing a combination of HMN 1 with extreme hypoplasia and atrophy of the cerebellum and of the ventral part of the pons.[2525]

Anterior horn cell disease with pontocerebellar hypoplasia: *bulbar palsy with olivopontocerebellar atrophy* (see **cerebellar ataxias**) A congenital form, recessively inherited, with the particular features of contractures; facial, bulbar, trunk, and limb weakness; abnormal motor conduction speeds with segmental demyelination; and pathological changes in the cerebellum, pons, medulla, and basal ganglia.

Amyotrophic dystonic paraplegia[2385]

Amyotrophic lateral sclerosis and *variants*

Amyotrophic lateral sclerosis–Parkinsonism–dementia complex of Guam

Amyotrophic lateral sclerosis *with dementia*[5036]

Amyotrophic lateral sclerosis *with autosomal dominant familial Parkinsonism.*[805]

Amyotrophic lateral sclerosis *with Pick disease*[1512]

Arthrogryposis multiplex congenita The neurogenic form with distal involvement.[2691]

Arthrogryposis multiplex congenita The neurogenic form with pulmonary hypoplasia

Arthrogryposis multiplex congenita A recessive form with renal and hepatic abnormalities and rarefaction of the anterior horns[4656]

Arthrogryposis multiplex congenita A distal, X-linked form including one type with anterior horn cell disease;[2691] other forms are attributed to nonprogressive intrauterine myopathy or connective tissue disease

Bulbar spinal muscular atrophy of childhood (See **Fazio–Londe syndrome**)

Bulbar palsy with deafness (See **Vialetto–van Laere syndrome**)

Bulbar palsy with deafness and pigmentary retinopathy

Chronic asymmetrical spinal muscular atrophy A form with onset in young adult life and with the particular features of asymmetrical muscle atrophy, muscle pain or cramps, fasciculations, and neurogenic weakness.[2757]

Chronic spinal muscular atrophy with pallidonigral degeneration A recessively (occasionally dominantly) inherited form with the addition of resting tremor, akinesia, and cogwheel rigidity without myoclonus or dementia, with severe degenerative lesions in the pallidum and substantia nigra.

Clinically there are fasciculations, proximal limb weakness, hyporeflexia or areflexia, and extrapyramidal syndromes including resting tremor, akinesia, and cogwheel rigidity. Evidence of neurogenic atrophy is obtained from EMG and from muscle biopsy spepcimens. Neurofibrillary degeneration is not present and there is no pathology resembling that of **amyotrophic lateral sclerosis**. The condition is regarded as a chronic spinopallidonigral degeneration because of the neuronal loss in the anterior horns, the globus pallidus and the substantia nigra without **Lewy bodies** or neurofibrillary degeneration.[5736]

Congenital lower motor neuron disease with arthrogryposis A form with the particular features of lordosis, scoliosis, club foot, varus joint contractures, and neurogenic trunk and limb weakness.

Adult proximal spinal muscular atrophy (Finkel late-onset type of spinal muscular atrophy included) Clinically this is not different from recessive and X-linked forms.

Hereditary muscular atrophy with ataxia, retinitis pigmentosa and diabetes mellitus A syndrome inherited as a dominant characteristic, with onset in adolescence and a slowly progressive course.[2249] See also **NARP**.
Hereditary motor and sensory neuropathy, type 2 (neurogenic form)
Kuskokwim disease
A lower motor neuron syndrome with childhood onset A recessively inherited condition of childhood with both proximal and distal weakness and wasting and with contractures, mapped to 1p36
Progressive spinal muscular atrophy with chorea and deafness
Progressive muscular atrophy with chorea and optic atrophy
Spinal muscular atrophy with amyotrophic lateral sclerosis Both recessive[2763] and dominant forms are described, the latter malignant, progressive, and resembling typical severe **amyotrophic lateral sclerosis**.[4049]
Spinocerebellar ataxia and deafness
Spinal muscular atrophy, optic atrophy, and deafness
Spinal muscular atrophy with deafness
Distal spinal muscular atrophy with vocal cord paralysis[6930]
Spinal muscular atrophy with Joseph disease (Azorean ataxia, **Joseph disease**, spinopontine atrophy, nigrospinodentatal degeneration)[5406]
Spinal muscular atrophy with ***olivopontocerebellar atrophy*** *type IV*[3672]
Spinal muscular atrophy with bulbar palsy[1668]
Spinal muscular atrophy with ophthalmoplegia
Spinal muscular atrophy with retinitis pigmentosa
Spinal muscular atrophy with retinitis pigmentosa and hereditary spastic paraplegia.
Spinal muscular atrophy with microcephaly and mental retardation A form with the particular features of microcephaly, deafness, mental and developmental delay, and onset in infancy[5991]
Spinal muscular atrophy with mental retardation
Spinal muscular atrophy, mental retardation, seizures, and orofacial dysplasia
Spinal muscular atrophy with myoclonus A slowly progressive form of spinal muscular atrophy also manifesting stimulus-sensitive myoclonus[3163]
Spinal muscular atrophy with oculopharyngeal muscular atrophy A form with onset in young adult life and with the particular features of ptosis, ophthalmoplegias, bulbar weakness, myopathic face, fasciculations, neurogenic muscle weakness, raised creatine kinase levels, and with variable fiber diameter and increased endomysial connective tissue on muscle biopsy
Spinal muscular atrophy with recessive spinocerebellar degeneration (***Friedreich ataxia***)[6471] The condition may be due to peripheral neuropathy (**hereditary motor and sensory neuropathy** type 2) rather than to anterior horn cell disease
Spinocerebellar ataxia with rigidity and peripheral neuropathy A variant form with fasciculations and Parkinsonism as well as signs of peripheral motor neuropathy.[6972] See also **hereditary motor and sensory neuropathy** type 2 *with* Parkinsonism
Troyer syndrome See **hereditary spastic paraplegia**
Neuronal intranuclear hyaline inclusion disease A single sporadic case, manifest by amyotrophy, dementia, seizures, choreoathetosis, and sphincter disorder
Spastic paraplegia with amyotrophy of hands (Silver syndrome) A rare, dominantly or recessively inherited variant with childhood or early adult onset and slow course manifesting pyramidal signs in the legs and global wasting of the small hand muscles without fasciculations. It has been mapped to chromosomes 4p and 11q12–q14 and there is likely further genetic heterogeneity.[4813] Other neurological signs have also been recorded.[5835]
Distal spinal muscular atrophy Sporadic or recessive forms which may be confined to the hands[4740]
Spinal muscular atrophy in **xeroderma pigmentosum**
Spinal muscular atrophy in **infantile neuroaxonal dystrophy** (Seitelberger disease)
Spinal muscular atrophy in amyotrophic choreoacanthocytosis (See **neuroacanthocytosis**) Both autosomal recessive and autosomal dominant inheritance patterns are described
Spinal muscular atrophy with **Huntington disease**[2159]
Spinal muscular atrophy with lysosomal enzyme deficiencies A recessively inherited syndrome.[2518]
Spinal muscular atrophy with **phenylketonuria** A recessively inherited syndrome[4287]
Spinal muscular atrophy with **hydroxyisovaleric aciduria**: A recessively inherited syndrome[1835]
Amyotrophic lateral sclerosis *with luysopallidonigral atrophy.*[2555]
Spinal muscular atrophy with pallidonigral degeneration[5736]

2. *Forms with Distinct Regional Involvement*

Hereditary motor neuropathy affecting the arms A slowly progressive demyelinating motor neuropathy affecting only the distal motor nerves of the arms.[3669]
Chronic neurogenic quadriceps amyotrophy
Distal and segmental muscular atrophy of upper extremities A form with the particular features of fasciculations, muscle atrophy, neurogenic weakness, and sensory neuropathy with paresthesias, lacking a typical inheritance pattern.[4958]
Distal spinal muscular atrophy: A form with onset at any age, from infancy to adult life, and with the particular features of high arches of the feet, bulbar as well as distal involvement, retention of muscle stretch reflexes, and resting tremor. Both dominant and recessive inheritance has been described. MNCVs suggest primary neuronal involvement.[2761] See **hereditary motor and sensory neuropathy** type 2.
Distal spinal muscular atrophy with a hoarse voice A form with the particular features of onset in childhood, youth, or young adult life and presentation with hoarseness as a result of recurrent laryngeal nerve involvement.[6930] In such a syndrome, ragged red fibers have been detected[379]

continued

Chart H–8. (*continued*)

Facioscapulohumeral atrophy A dominantly inherited neurogenic form resembling facioscapulohumeral dystrophy, with onset in childhood or youth[2009]

Familial **amyotrophic lateral sclerosis**

Fazio-Londe syndrome.[1976]

Focal cervical poliopathy of distal arm (juvenile muscular atrophy of unilateral upper extremity) A condition with a benign course, usually reported from Japan, in which the anterior horns of the spinal cord between C5 and T1 show shrinkage and necrosis of large and small nerve cells and mild gliosis. A circulatory disorder is considered the likely cause.[2915]

Infantile spinal muscular atrophy in **incontinentia pigmenti** An X-Linked dominant form, lethal in males[3705]

Juvenile bulbar spinal muscular atrophy See **Fazio–Londe syndrome**

Monomelic spinal muscular atrophy

Multiple contracture syndrome See **Pena–Shokeir phenotype**

neuropathy-motor neuron disease with visual pathway disorder

oculopharyngeal spinal muscular atrophy A rare, dominantly inherited variant manifesting external ophthalmoplegia, bulbar signs, and distal weakness and wasting, manifesting first in early adult life.[4174]

Progressive ophthalmoplegia in Kugelberg–Welander disease A form with the particular features of ptosis, ophthalmoplegias, and bulbar weakness, with onset in early childhood.[38]

Scapuloperoneal atrophy (Stark–Kaeser syndrome); A dominant, recessive, or X-linked syndrome characterized by slowly progressive neurogenic weakness and wasting in this distribution.[3267] The phenotypes have been reviewed by Baraitser.[379]

Scapuloperoneal atrophy, cardiopathy, and inflammatory myopathy The neurogenic status of this form is not certain, as there is a definite myopathic component.[3200] See also **Emery–Dreifuss syndrome** (autosomal dominant form).[4372]

Spinal muscular atrophy and pallidonigral degeneration A form with the particular added features of pyramidal signs, rigidity, and rest or postural tremor, with onset in mature adult life

Spinal muscular atrophy, ***Ryukyuan type***

Spinal muscular atrophy {HMSN} with calf hypertrophy A form with the particular features of onset in young adult life, muscle hypertrophy, pain and cramp, raised creatine kinase levels, and slow progression.[778] Duplication of 17p.11.2 has been reported in this condition.

Forms with limb girdle or peroneal distribution

X-linked varieties

Kennedy disease (spinobulbar muscular atrophy) A form mapping to Xq21.3–q12, presenting clinically in young adult life with bulbospinal weakness and atrophy and with testicular failure. See **X-linked bulbospinal muscular atrophy**.

Infantile spinal muscular atrophy with arthrogryposis (XL-SMA) A congenital or infantile form mapped to Xp11 with proximal weakness, joint contractures and facial dysmorphisms.

Autosomal dominant varieties

Adult onset with typical proximal weakness and atrophy, mapped to 20q13

Benign congenital with contractures, mapped to 12q23

A *bulbospinal* form resembling **X-linked bulbospinal muscular atrophy** but dominantly inherited

A congenital form with leg weakness A nonprogressive form, mapped to 12q23

HMSN-P (Okinawa type) Dominantly inherited and mapped to 3q13

Scapuloperoneal syndromes See **Emery–Dreifuss muscular dystrophy, acid maltase deficiency**, and **centronuclear myopathy**

A *facioscapulohumeral phenotype with ragged red fibers and cardiomyopathy* is also described

X-linked distal hereditary motor neuropathy A form with adult onset, mapped to Xq13.1–q21.

Other varieties

Spinal muscular atrophy due to mitochondrial disease A form in which the picture of spinal muscular atrophy is accompanied by cardiomyopathy and cytochrome oxidase (COX) deficiency.[5461]

Recessively inherited forms with weakness and atrophy of the legs and pyramidal features, onsetting in childhood and linked to a mutation at chromosome 9p21.1–p12;[1171] and *(SPG 30)*. A form with spastic paraparesis and peripheral neuropathy associated with mild ataxia and cerebellar atrophy on CT scan; it is mapped to chromosome 2q37.3.[3472]

(*After the work of the late Profs. Anita Harding and PK Thomas*[2762] *and with data from Pestronk*[4992] *(http://neuromuscular.wustl.edu/synmot.html/); by his kind permission; and from recent literature.*)

hereditary motor neuronopathy affecting the arms

See **hereditary motor neuropathy** (*variants*).

hereditary motor system disease

(chronic juvenile amyotrophic lateral sclerosis) A recessively inherited, slowly progressive syndrome with the onset in childhood or youth of bilateral pyramidal and lower motor neuron signs affecting bulbar and spinal muscles and without sensory loss.[2715]

hereditary multi-infarct dementia

See **familial subcortical dementia with arteriosclerotic leukoencephalopathy.**[5952]

hereditary multiple exostoses

A dyschondroplasia, usually dominantly inherited, characterized clinically by the development of multiple osteogenic exostoses from the metaphyses of long bones more often than from other bones. Neurological involvement may include paraparesis resulting from cord compression.[2026] The condition was first described by Stanley in 1894.

hereditary muscular atrophy with ataxia, retinitis pigmentosa, and diabetes mellitus See **hereditary motor neuropathy** (*variants*).

hereditary myoclonic dystonia (hereditary dystonia with lightning jerks responsive to alcohol, hereditary essential myoclonus, inherited myoclonus dystonia) A dominantly inherited benign syndrome incomplete penetrance starting in childhood and characterized by dystonia and myoclonus affecting mainly the neck and arms. There are seldom other neurological deficits and both EEG and SSEP recordings are normal. Both kinds of abnormal movement respond dramatically to alcohol ingestion.[5159]

A similar syndrome (but with onset in adult life) was reported by Davidenkow in 1926.

hereditary myoclonic encephalopathy A recessively inherited **mitochondrial encephalomyelopathy**. See **Unverricht–Lundborg–Lafora syndrome**.

hereditary myoclonus and progressive distal muscular atrophy A dominantly inherited multifocal neuronal degeneration of adult life characterized by **stimulus-sensitive myoclonus** and slowly progressive distal neurogenic muscle atrophy. Bulbar weakness, extrapyramidal signs, myoclonus, neurogenic muscle atrophy and weakness, raised serum creatine kinase levels, and paroxysmal EEG discharges are other features described.[3163]

hereditary myokymia (normocalcemic tetany) A dominantly inherited syndrome of generalized myokymia and muscle cramping without evidence of peripheral neuropathy, typically with spontaneous, regularly recurring bursts of motor unit potentials arising distally in the nerve fibers.[294, 5773]

hereditary myokymia and muscle stiffness A syndrome of continuous involuntary quivering of muscles causing movements in the eye, face, and limbs. In cases of generalized muscle stiffness and delayed relaxation, the term **neuromyotonia** has been applied. (See **idiopathic neuromyotonia** and **myokymia**.[294, 2649, 2268, 3944]) Most cases are without familial occurrence; familial cases usually have an associated peripheral neuropathy.

hereditary myokymia with periodic (episodic) ataxia (Van Dyke Hanson syndrome) A rare, dominantly inherited syndrome of childhood onset paroxysmal ataxia lasting 1–2 min and induced by vestibular stimulation, movement, or shock; the movements probably represent an epileptic manifestation. Other features include persistent widespread myokymia which supervenes in youth and affects the face, hands, arms, and legs; truncal shaking or jerking movements of the head, arms, and legs; carpopedal spasms; and lower motor neuron disease without overt peripheral neuropathy. The condition is considered to represent a form of motor neuropathy on the basis of muscle biopsy findings.[6492]

hereditary myopathy limited to females A slowly progressive dominantly inherited limb-girdle type of muscular dystrophy with onset in childhood or early adult life and expression limited to females, in which muscle biopsy specimens reveal isolated muscle fiber necrosis and phagocytosis.[2870]

hereditary myosin myopathies A group of myopathies with highly variable clinical features with onset during fetal development, childhood, or adult life and caused by dominantly inherited mutations in skeletal muscle myosin heavy chain (*MyHC*) genes. The phenotypes diseases may be mild in childhood but progressive in adult life, the proximal muscle weakness impairing ambulation. Presentation with hypertrophic or dilated cardiomyopathy without evidence of skeletal myopathy is recorded, while other mutations are associated with distinct skeletal myopathies without cardiomyopathy (e.g., **Laing** early onset distal myopathy affecting the dorsiflexor muscles of the toes and ankles and *myosin storage myopathy* (MSM) affecting proximal or scapuloperoneal muscles with subsarcolemmal accumulation of myosin in type I fibers).[4782]

hereditary nephritis and nerve deafness (distal muscle wasting, nephritis and deafness) A syndrome featuring evidence both of **hereditary motor and sensory neuropathy** and **Alport syndrome**.[2736]

hereditary neuralgic amyotrophy See **neuralgic amyotrophy**.

hereditary neurocutaneous vascular malformation The association of intracranial arteriovenous malformations with cutaneous hemangiomas, in the absence of retinal lesions. The condition has been reviewed by Baraitser.[379]

hereditary neuromyotonia See **neuromyotonia**.

hereditary neuropathy with liability to pressure palsies See **hereditary pressure-sensitive neuropathy**.

hereditary nonprogressive athetotic hemiplegia A congenital syndrome, dominantly inherited and nonprogressive after childhood, characterized by congenital left-sided hemihypoplasia, hemiparesis, and hypertonicity; left-hand athetosis after the age of 8 years and right-sided cerebral atrophy or hypoplasia.[2656]

hereditary nonprogressive chorea (hereditary benign chorea, benign familial chorea; OMIM 118700) A rare, dominantly inherited, nonprogressive, and eventually self-limiting syndrome characterized by the appearance in childhood or adult life of chorea, athetosis, and gait and limb ataxia without current or subsequent intellectual or neurological impairment. It is linked to chromosome 14q.[2022]

The condition is associated with striatal hypometabolism,[2675] but no abnormality is detected on cerebral imaging.[1949] In *variant forms*, **essential tremor** or some intellectual deficits do occur.[3769] See **chorea** and **Huntington disease**.

hereditary nystagmus See **congenital nystagmus**.

hereditary Parkinsonism and neuropathy See **hereditary motor neuropathy** (*spinocerebellar ataxia with rigidity and peripheral neuropathy*), **hereditary motor and sensory neuropathy**, *type 2 with Parkinsonism*, and **Parkinsonism-plus**.

hereditary Parkinsonism-dystonia See **dopa-responsive dystonia**.

hereditary paroxysmal ataxia A dominantly inherited syndrome characterized by the onset in childhood of paroxysmal bouts of ataxia, dysarthria, and nystagmus, lasting 1–6 h on a weekly basis and responsive to acetazolamide.[2582]

hereditary persistent distal cramps A dominantly inherited syndrome of muscle cramps involving distal muscle groups with accompanying continuous muscle discharges which wax and wane. Clinically, the condition is marked by intermittent painful stiffness of the intrinsic hand muscles and the calves. The cause is unknown.[3263]

hereditary photomyoclonus A dominantly inherited syndrome consisting of deafness, diabetes mellitus, nephropathy, and light-sensitive seizures with dementia. The pathological features resemble those of **subacute spongiform encephalopathy**.[2876]

hereditary piebaldness and congenital deafness An autosomal or sex-linked recessive disorder manifesting depigmentation of the head and arms with pigmented spots, congenital neural deafness, and normal vestibular function.[6863]

hereditary poliodystrophy See **hereditary motor neuropathy**.

hereditary polycystic osteodysplasia with progressive dementia A rare, recessively inherited syndrome characterized by the onset in young adult life of bone pain, ankle and wrist swelling, pyramidal signs, myoclonic and other seizures, and dementia.[58]

hereditary polyneuropathy, oligophrenia, premature menopause, and acromicria A syndrome of slowly progressive paresis in the hands and feet, starting in childhood and leading to moderate incapacity, areflexia, reduced motor nerve conduction velocity, oligophrenia, premature menopause without hypophyseal failure, and disproportionate smallness with short arms and legs and acromicria.[3962]

hereditary pressure-sensitive neuropathy (hereditary recurrent pressure palsies, hereditary neuropathy with liability to pressure palsies, tomaculous neuropathy, familial recurrent pressure palsy, familial recurrent polyneuropathy)[4969, 5736] A dominantly inherited syndrome of young adult life characterized by unusual sensitivity of the peripheral nerves to intercurrent pressure (probably as a result of subclinical polyneuropathy), leading to painless, temporary but still prolonged conduction block.[1798, 4011, 6240] A deletion at 17p11.2–12 has been detected, the same site as that involved in **hereditary motor and sensory neuropathy** type 1A, but the condition is genetically heterogeneous.

There may be associated electrophysiological evidence of a generalized neuropathy as well as local conduction block at the site of nerve compression. A wide range of symptoms is described, from numbness, paresthesias or absent reflexes to paralysis and objective sensory loss. The ulnar, median, radial, and common peroneal nerves are those most commonly affected, but any nerve is at risk, including the V and VIII cranial nerves. Even such trivial compressive traumas as using scissors, knitting, squatting, plaster casts, and wearing tight shoes have been incriminated.

Biopsy specimens show a **tomaculous neuropathy** with axonal loss. The syndrome of **familial (or hereditary) neuralgic amyotrophy** may be associated but is not the same condition.[1498, 2522]

In *variant* forms, the syndrome is manifest as recurrent brachial plexus palsies,[6067] or is sporadic.[5256]

hereditary proximal spinal muscular atrophy See **hereditary motor neuropathy**.

hereditary putaminal necrosis A dominantly inherited degenerative syndrome characterized by bilateral isolated necrosis of the putamen and globus pallidus with vascular proliferation and gliovascular lesions in the thalamus. Clinically, the syndrome is first expressed in infancy, the major findings being psychomotor retardation and increasing apathy with seizures, inability to lift the head from the pillow, difficulties with swallowing and eating, and apparent blindness. Various movement disorders are described in some kinships, including pyramidal syndromes, athetosis, and ataxia.

The disorder has also been described with onset in later life.[1718] See also **infantile bilateral striatal necrosis**.

hereditary quivering of the chin (geniospasm, hereditary chin trembling, trembling chin) A congenital, dominantly inherited syndrome (chromosome 9q) characterized by transient fine tremors of the mentalis muscles occurring during emotional stimulation; they disappear in calmness and sleep and go away with increasing age.[2198, 5403, 6813]

In *variant forms*, nystagmus and nocturnal myoclonus have also been described.[2504] In fact the disorder may be a form of localized myoclonus.[1614]

hereditary recurrent focal neuropathy See **hereditary pressure-sensitive neuropathy**.

hereditary recurrent pressure palsies See **hereditary pressure-sensitive neuropathy**.

hereditary sensory and autonomic neuropathy (HSAN) A group of similar sensory neuropathies which may be classified as shown in Chart H–9 (after Dyck[1769] and Donaghy[1682]).

In yet other *variant forms*, motor neuropathy, mental retardation, **Friedreich ataxia**, cerebellar degeneration, hypotonia, skeletal dysplasias, and dysmorphism are variously associated. See also **congenital asymbolia**, **Fabry disease**, and **Tangier disease**.

Chart H–9. The Hereditary Sensory and Autonomic Neuropathies

Autosomal Dominant Inheritance

HSAN1 (dominantly inherited sensory neuropathy, HSAN1 of Dyck, Denny Brown or Hicks, hereditary sensory radicular neuropathy, hereditary perforating ulcers of the feet, familial mutilating ulcerative acropathy, hereditary lumbosacral syringomyelia, familial neurogenic osteoacrolysis, hereditary sensory neuropathy with peroneal muscular atrophy, acrodystrophic neuronopathy)[1585, 2890] A dominantly inherited (9q22.1, *SPTLC1*, *serine palmitoyltransferase*), slowly progressive sensory > motor neuropathy with onset in childhood, youth, or early adult life. Clinical features include lancinating pains or painful burning paresthesias affecting the legs; autonomic signs such as distal anhidrosis and sometimes sensorineural deafness, neurogenic muscle atrophy, particular loss of pain and temperature rather than other sensations, multiple fractures, and mutilating acropathy.[1586, 1891] Muscle strength is usually normal.

This is the most common form of HSAN. Nerve conduction studies show significantly reduced or absent SNAPs with normal MNCVs. The sensory findings are often disassociated with prominent pain and temperature loss. Neurophysiology shows evidence of a sensory axonal neuropathy but in many individuals there is also electrical evidence of demyelination. Sural nerve biopsies show mainly axonal loss.[3006]

Observations of kinships in Newfoundland (and in France[1726]) indicate that there may also be notable lower motor neuron involvement, so differentiation from the axonopathy **hereditary motor and sensory neuropathy** type 2 may be difficult.

Variants are

HSAN1 with spastic paraplegia A dominantly inherited sensory neuropathy with congenital or childhood onset of loss of pain, temperature, and touch sensations leading to mutilating acropathy, neurogenic bladder, spasticity, and both myelinated and unmyelinated fiber loss.[1062]

Hereditary sensory neuropathy with deafness A form with sensorineural deafness. Dementia[2995] and ataxia have also been recorded as complications but in such cases, widespread cell loss and gliosis in other areas suggest that this may represent a form of **familial multisystem atrophy**. In a related form, loss of gastric motility is also described.

Ulcerative mutilating acropathy with abnormal CSF aminoacids An inherited sensory neuropathy with onset in youth, manifesting also loss of pain, temperature, and touch sensations; incontinence; and generalized skin atrophy.

Hereditary ataxia with thermoanalgesia and loss of fungiform papillae A *variant* with these features and added ataxia, alacrimia, impaired taste, and temperature control.

Hereditary sensorimotor neuropathy with ulcero-mutilation A dominantly inherited form with onset in adult life, similar to the prototype above but without genetic linkage to it.[4992]

See also **Madelung syndrome**.

Autosomal Recessive Inheritance

HSAN 2 (congenital sensory neuropathy, lumbosacral syringomyelia, congenital insensitivity/indifference to pain) A slowly progressive form of HSAN in which *all* modes of sensation are affected from the earliest years and in which lancinating pains are less frequent than in HSAN1.[4560, 4776] It is mapped to 12p13.

The phenomenon of *congenital insensitivity to pain* (CIP) resembles this neuropathy in its manifestations but a central origin seems more likely,[2153] especially because the sensory nerve action potentials are missing in $HSAN_2$ but not in CIP, spontaneous pains are common, and there is in HSAN2 a graded reduction of sensation centrifugally in the limbs, the trunk remaining sensitive until very late.

Variants with **tonic pupils** or with dominant inheritance have also been described.

HSAN3 (familial dysautonomia, Riley–Day syndrome, congenital insensitivity to pain with dysautonomia) A recessively inherited sensory and autonomic axonal neuropathy with congenital onset. The major clinical features include low birth weight, failure to thrive, feeding difficulty, and autonomic dysfunction, short stature, sparse and depigmented hair, absent or sparse tears, optic atrophy, nerve deafness, smooth tongue with loss of the fungiform papillae, kyphoscoliosis, hyporeflexia, loss of pain and temperature sensations, impaired temperature control, hyperhidrosis, orthostatic hypotension, and loss of the histamine flare in the skin. Nerve biopsy specimens show both myelinated and unmyelinated fiber loss.[69, 5303] It occurs almost exclusively in Ashkenazi Jews. Mapping to 9q31–q33 has been achieved. CMAP amplitudes are reduced, MNCVs are slowed and SNAPs are much reduced in amplitude if recordable at all.

A *variant dominant form* with onset in the fifth decade manifesting added ataxia is also described. (www.wustl.edu/neuromusculatr/sensory-small.html)

HSAN4 (congenital insensitivity to pain with anhidrosis, hereditary anhidrotic sensory neuropathy, syndrome of the neural crest, familial dysautonomia type II) A recessive sensory neuropathy (1q21–q22, *NTRK1*) with congenital or early childhood onset. The major clinical features are loss of pain, temperature, and touch sensation with self-mutilation, poor temperature control, multiple fractures, hypohidrosis, cutaneous ulcers, and intellectual impairment. Nerve biopsy specimens show loss of both small myelinated and of unmyelinated fibers.[6152]

Variants are described with dominant inheritance, or with a nonprogressive course.[4695]

HSAN5 (congential insensitivity to pain without anhidrosis) A rare, recessive disorder of young children, resembling HSAN IV and also due to mutations in the *NTRK1* gene on chromosome 1. Nerve biopsy shows the loss of small myelinated Aδ fibers with relative preservation of unmyelinated fibers.

HSAN with spastic paraplegia (Cavanagh variant) A recessively inherited sensory neuropathy with congenital or childhood onset of loss of pain, temperature, and touch sensations, neurogenic bladder, spasticity, and both myelinated and unmyelinated fiber loss. This condition resembles the dominantly inherited variety but is more severe.[1062] It maps to 5p15.

HSAN with loss of pain perception A rare recessive variant due to lack of nerve growth factor-b, mapped to 1p13.1 and resembling *HSAN2* except that sweating is retained.

HSAN with neurotrophic keratitis A congenital syndrome of loss of pain and temperature sensations with mutilating acropathy, corneal ulceration, and opacification and anhidrosis.[1682]

HSAN with predominant loss of small myelinated fibers.

continued

Chart H–9. (*continued*)

X-linked Inheritance Pattern

HSAN, X-linked An otherwise typical form of sensory neuropathy with onset in infancy, childhood or youth of loss of pain, touch, and temperature sensations, complicated by neuropathic deformity and ulceration of the feet, joint stiffness and arthritis, and abnormal sensory conductions. Pathologically there is a loss of myelinated fibers. The condition is marked by minimal involvement of the muscle stretch reflexes and absence of autonomic involvement.[3217] The gene lies in the dxys 1–p58–1 region of the X-chromosome.[5455]

Other Forms

Congenital insensitivity to pain A dominantly inherited congenital syndrome consisting of cloudy corneae, hyperactivity, and self-mutilation. Paroxysmal headaches, loss of pain and temperature sensations, paresthesia, and flushing are other features.[453, 3220]

Congenital pain asymbolia with auditory imperception A congenital syndrome consisting of auditory agnosia, loss of pain sensation, and speech delay.

HSAN with dysautonomia and corneal insensitivity A congenital syndrome comprising loss of pain sensation, poor temperature control, absent or sparse tears, flushing, corneal ulceration, and myelinated fiber loss. See **hereditary sensory and autonomic neuropathy** (recessive).

HSAN with tonic pupils A sensory neuropathy with childhood onset in which there is loss of pain and temperature sensations associated with features of the **Holmes–Adie syndrome**.[4373]

Sensory neuropathy with hereditary ataxia (congenital sensory neuropathy with selective loss of small myelinated fibers, congenital insensitivity to pain, HSAN5) A congenital, recessively inherited sensory neuropathy with onset in childhood, manifesting loss of pain and temperature sensations and acropathy, and also cloudy corneas, pupillary abnormalities, hyperactivity, self-mutilation, paroxysmal headache, paresthesias and flushing, and both myelinated and unmyelinated fiber loss in peripheral nerves.[3927] It is due to mutations in the *NTRK1* gene on chromosome 1.

hereditary sensory and autonomic neuropathy with deafness See **hereditary sensory and autonomic neuropathy** (dominant).

hereditary sensory and autonomic neuropathy with dysautonomia and corneal insensitivity See **hereditary sensory and autonomic neuropathy** (other).

hereditary sensory and autonomic neuropathy with neurotrophic keratitis See **hereditary sensory and autonomic neuropathy** (recessive).

hereditary sensory and autonomic neuropathy with spastic paraplegia See **hereditary sensory and autonomic neuropathy**.

hereditary sensory and autonomic neuropathy with tonic pupils See **hereditary sensory and autonomic neuropathy** (other).

hereditary sensory radicular neuropathy See **hereditary sensory and autonomic neuropathy**, type 1.

hereditary small vessel diseases of the brain (SVDB) The most common form is **cerebral autosomal dominant arteriopathy with subcortical infarcts and leukoencephalopathy** (CADASIL), caused by mutations in the *NOTCH3* gene. This systemic arteriopathy is responsible for recurrent ischemic strokes and progressive subcortical dementia in middle-aged adults. Prominent clinical manifestations also include migraine with aura and mood disorders. See also **cerebral autosomal recessive arteriopathy with subcortical infarcts and leukoencephalopathy** (CARASIL), cerebroretinal vasculopathy, **hereditary endotheliopathy with retinopathy, nephropathy, and stroke syndrome** (HERNS), and **familial amyloid angiopathies**.

hereditary spastic ataxia A dominantly inherited hereditary cerebellar ataxic syndrome of adult life with added pyramidal signs and sometimes retinal degeneration and vestibular impairment.[563] See also **familial spastic ataxia** and **cerebellar ataxias**.

hereditary spastic dystonia An inherited dystonic syndrome manifesting also optic atrophy, dystonias, and rigidity with evidence of putaminal necrosis on MRI or CT scans. The condition may be a form of **mitochondrial encephalopathy**.[926]

hereditary spastic paraparesis See **hereditary spastic paraplegia**.

hereditary spastic paraparesis with wasting and growth retardation See **Troyer syndrome**.

hereditary spastic paraplegia (HSP, hereditary spastic paraparesis, familial spastic paraplegia, Strümpell–Lorrain syndrome.) A heterogeneous group of degenerative diseases, usually dominantly inherited, with particular effects on the pyramidal tracts and occurring in pure and in complicated forms. The condition was first described by Seeligmüller in 1876 and Strümpell[6098] in 1880. Mutations in the *alastin* and *spastin* genes SPG3A or SPG4 are found in most cases, including in some of the variants listed below but nearly 40 genetic loci and 10 identified and 17 unidentified genes may also be responsible.[4213] Genetic loci are designated Spastic ParapleGia 1 (SPG1) through SPG20 in order of their discovery.

The *pure form*, in which there are no other neurological findings, has been mapped variously to chromosomes 2p22–p21(SPG4, OMIM 182601); 14q11.2q–24.3 (SPG3, OMIM 182600); 15q11.1 (SPG6, OMIM 600363); 8q232–q24 (SPG8, OMIM 603563); 10q23–q24.1 (SPG9, OMIM 601162); 12p13 (SPG10, OMIM 604187); 19q13 (SPG12, OMIM 604805); 2q24 (SPG13, OMIM 605280). Autosomal dominant is far more common (70%) than autosomal recessive (AR) transmission (8p12–q13, SPG5, OMIM 270800; 16q24.3, SPG7, OMIM 602783; 15q13–15, SPG 11, OMIM 604360; 3q27–q28, SPG14, OLMIM605229; AR symmetrical spastic cerebral palsy, 2q24–25, OMIM 603513; AR Charlevoix-Saguenay spastic ataxia, 13q12 OMIM 270550) or X-linked (Xq22). Over 16 loci had been mapped to 2005 and the number is rising.[6195, 2057, 2058]

Clinically, the onset is at any age; children show delay in the development of motor skills while adults complain of easy tiring, tripping, and stiffness. In all, insidiously progressive pyramidal signs are found (mainly in the legs), typical except that spasticity is unusually marked in comparison to the relative preservation of strength. Pes cavus is seen in about a quarter of affected subjects. Sensory complaints are generally lacking, but autopsy findings show posterior column degeneration in some cases.[777, 1766] Cognitive decline appears to be associated with the 2p and 8q mutations.

Dominant forms are Spastic ParapleGia (SPG) 3A (14q, *atlastin*) often associated with an axonal sensorimotor neuropathy; SPG 4 (2p22, *spastin*, the commonest single mutation); SPG 6 (15q11; *NIPA1* mutations; adolescent/adult-onset, a severe, slowly progressive, pure HSP); SPG 8 (8q23); SPG 9 (10q23); SPG 10 (12q13); SPG 12 (19q13); SPG 13 (2q24), SPG 17 (11q12); and SPG 19 (9q33). Most are uncomplicated, though SPG 9 is associated with cataracts, neuropathy, and gastroesophageal reflux. SPG4 has its onset at any age presenting with spastic paraparesis of any severity, and adds loss of bladder and bowel control, cognitive impairment seizures, and peripheral neuropathy. SPG19 is a pure dominant form. SPG 12 has early onset and rapid progression and is accompanied by sensory disturbances. *Kinesin heavy chain* and heat shock protein (*chaperonin*) are rare mutations. There is much overlap between cerebellar ataxias and spastic paraplegia, emphasizing the marked clinical heterogeneity of HSP associated with *spastin* mutations.[4665]

Recessive forms are SPG5 (8q); SPG 7 (16q); (*SPG7/papaplegin*) presenting as either pure or complicated forms of HSP; SPG11 (15q) often with thin corpus callosum, cognitive decline, and lower motor neuron degeneration;[6048] SPG 14 (3q27) with added neuropathy; SPG 15 (14q) with thin corpus callosum; SPG21 (13q14) with childhood onset; and SPG20 (13q, *spartin*–spastin-related autosomal recessive Troyer protein) which underlies **Troyer syndrome**. These have numerous phenotypes, including pure HSP with early onset; pure HSP with late onset; HSP with mental retardation; HSP with both mental retardation and peripheral neuropathy; and HSP with cerebellar ataxia; other CNS and PNS disturbances have also been reported.[1303, 6195] The first gene identified for the recessive forms was *paraplegin*.

X-linked forms (SPG1 on Xq28, OMIM 308840; SPG2 on Xq22, OMIM 312920; and SPG16 on Xq11, OMIM 300266) also have numerous additional clinical features.[6195] *Proteolipid protein gene duplications* and point mutations that cause **Pelizaeus–Merzbacher disease** and *L1 Cell Adhesion Molecule (L1CAM)* mutations are responsible for many X-linked neurologic disorders, including complicated spastic paraplegia, hydrocephalus, and **mental retardation aphasia, shuffling gait, and adducted** thumbs (MASA) syndrome.

Numerous kinships with clear additional features complicating hereditary spastic paraplegia have been described. In these *complicated forms*, amyotrophy resembling that of **hereditary motor and sensory neuropathy**, distal involvement, mental retardation, deafness, optic atrophy, pigmentary retinal degeneration, extrapyramidal features, ataxia and dysarthria, sensory neuropathy, and skin lesions have been detected variously.

A complete review has been published.[4214] The compilation in Chart H–10 is based upon Harding's[2754] and Baraitser's[379] reviews of the major *variants*. See also the Web site of the Spastic Paraplegia Foundation http://www.hspinfo.org/ for evolving information. See also the **Spastic Paraplegia Rating Scale** and the Web site http://www.med.umich.edu/hsp/, which provides data on genetic analysis and clinical features.

Diagnostic criteria for family members of HSP subjects have been suggested as shown in the table.

Alternative diagnoses should first be excluded, and the family history should be consistent with autosomal dominant, autosomal recessive, or X-linked recessive inheritance. These criteria are perhaps most useful for standardization in a research setting and are open to criticism. Many definitely affected individuals lack grade 4 hyperreflexia. The criteria for the definitely unaffected category are insufficiently rigorous in view of the wide range in age at onset that may occur in some families.

See also the Web site http://www.hspinfo.org/ for further information from the **Spastic Paraplegia Foundation**.

hereditary spastic paraparesis with cognitive loss An autosomal dominant form of hereditary spastic paraparesis (HSP), manifesting late-onset cognitive impairment (subcortical dementia) and with genetic linkage to the SPG4 locus on chromosome 2p as reported in pure HSP.[6681] See also the entries above.

hereditary spinal arachnoid cyst, distichiasis, lymphedema syndrome A congenital dysmorphic syndrome manifesting also vertebral abnormalities, kyphosis, spinal tumors, congenital cardiac malformations, pyramidal signs, and thick fiber sensory neuropathy.[381]

hereditary stiff baby syndrome The earliest, infantile expression of **hyperekplexia**. See also **startle epilepsy**.

hereditary striatal degeneration (holotopistic striatal degeneration) A dominantly inherited syndrome characterized by apathy and psychomotor retardation appearing in infancy or childhood. Dysarthria, rigidity,

Suggested diagnostic criteria for family members from families with pure HSP[2060]

Status	Criteria
Definitely affected	Progressive gait disturbance and frank corticospinal tract involvement of lower limbs, including grade 4 hyperreflexia and extensor plantar reflexes.
Probably affected	Individuals lacking history of progressive gait disturbance, or asymptomatic individuals with signs of spastic paraparesis, examined only once and so not proven to have a progressive gait disturbance and frank corticospinal tract involvement of lower limbs, including grade 4 hyperreflexia and extensor plantar reflexes. (Serial examinations may allow recategorisation as definitely affected.)
Possibly affected	Asymptomatic + normal gait + questionably abnormal corticospinal tract signs,for example, mild hyperreflexia, unsustained clonus but downgoing plantar reflexes.
Definitely unaffected	Asymptomatic + normal neurological examination + age greater than maximal age of symptoms in family.
Probably unaffected	Asymptomatic + normal neurological examination + age younger than maximal age of symptoms in family.

Chart H–10. Variant (Complicated, not "Pure") Forms of Hereditary Spastic Paraplegia

Complex forms of hereditary spastic paraplegia (HSP) are rare and usually recessively transmitted. Co-existing ataxia, dysarthria, unipolar depression, epilepsy, migraine, and cognitive impairment variably expressed and linked to the *SPG4* locus on chromosome 2p as for pure HSP. There is marked clinical heterogeneity of HSP associated with spastin mutations.[4666] The following compilation is from the literature and with assistance from Dr. Alan Pestronk, with many thanks.

Variants include:

Adult onset leukodystrophy A dominantly inherited form with its onset in the third or fourth decade, presenting with gait instability, pyramidal signs, and autonomic abnormalities.

Andermann syndrome

Autosomal recessive spastic ataxia associated with white matter changes A form with onset at any age, manifesting cerebellar ataxia and spasticity and mapped to 2q33–34. The more severe cases show spasticity from birth, scoliosis, dystonia, and cognitive impairment and are usually diagnosed as having cerebral palsy. Brain MRI shows cerebellar atrophy, sometimes associated with cortical atrophy, leukoencephalopathy, and thinning of the corpus callosum.[6271]

Charlevoix-Saguenay syndrome A form which is slowly progressive and recessively inherited with its onset in childhood, characterized by dysarthria, nystagmus, ataxia, pyramidal and posterior column signs, and impaired vertical pursuit movements of the eye and sphincter involvement, reported from Quebec.[762] It is mapped to 13q.11.

Familial spastic paraparesis and deafness A rare, X-linked syndrome characterized by short stature, hypogonadism, elevated CSF protein levels, and in some cases pigmentary retinopathy and lens opacities.[1278]

Familial spastic paraparesis and dementia Forms that are usually dominantly inherited. See **familial multi-infarct dementia** and **Worster–Drought syndrome**.

Familial spastic paraplegia with amyotrophy of the hands (Silver disease, hereditary spastic paraparesis with amyotrophy) A rare, dominantly or recessively transmitted variant with childhood or early adult onset, manifesting pyramidal signs in the legs and global wasting of the small hand muscles. Various other neurological features have also been described in this condition.[2289, 5835]

In further *variants,* the onset is in childhood, and leukodystrophy, cerebellar deficits, and mild mental retardation are other features;[2252] or the condition is recessively inherited with mental retardation, brainstem dysraphism, and cerebellar atrophy, mapped to 14q12.[6051]

Spastic paraplegia type 2 with dystrophic axonal peripheral neuropathy and apparent proteolipid protein gene (PLP1)[3747]

Hereditary spastic paraparesis with ataxia A dominantly inherited form appearing in adult life, in which the spastic syndrome is accompanied by pathological evidence of degeneration of the pyramidal and spinocerebellar tracts and of the posterior columns, with the expected clinical features.[5634] In still other forms, extrapyramidal features are also found.[2015] See also **hereditary spastic ataxia, familial spastic ataxia**, and **cerebellar ataxias**.

Hereditary spastic paraparesis with deafness An X-linked degenerative disorder with onset in late childhood, manifesting nerve deafness, spastic paraparesis, tremor, ophthalmic abnormalities, sensory deficits, short stature, cataract, hypogonadotrophic hypogonadism, elevated CSF protein levels, and absent or delayed somatosensory evoked potentials. Except for the normal levels of very long chain fatty acids, the condition resembles **adreno-myelo-neuropathy**.[6717]

Hereditary spastic paraparesis with brachydactyly and cone-shaped epiphyses A congenital or childhood variant with brachydactyly and epiphyseal dysplasia, reported once.

Hereditary spastic paraparesis with dementia A dominantly inherited adult *variant* characterized by the occurrence of dementia late in the course of the disease.[6873] The 2p and 8q mutations appear most liable to induce this syndrome.

Hereditary spastic paraparesis with optic atrophy, dementia, and cardiac involvement Forms in which any of these features complicate the spastic paraparesis.[6140] Further variants are reviewed by Baraitser.[379] Inheritance patterns vary.

Hereditary spastic paraparesis with seizures A dominantly inherited form with a tendency to seizures and with familial associations with multiple sclerosis due to a frame shift in the spastic (*SPG4*) gene.[4269]

Hereditary spastic paraparesis, mental retardation, and precocious puberty A childhood variant with dysarthria, early puberty, paraparesis, and mental and developmental delay.

Hereditary spastic paraparesis with oligophrenia (X-linked) A congenital *variant* with added mental retardation, facial palsy, athetosis, and ataxia.[317]

Hereditary spastic paraparesis with dysarthria and cutaneous lesions An infantile variant with dysarthria, pigmentary disturbances, and abnormal EEG. One such form maps to 1q24.

Hereditary spastic paraparesis with extrapyramidal features A childhood variant, usually dominantly inherited, characterized by athetosis or dystonia, rigidity, and hyperreflexia.[1633]

Hereditary spastic paraparesis and macular degeneration (Kjellin syndrome) A variant form presenting in youth with pigmentary retinal degeneration, distal motor neuropathy, spasticity, and mental and developmental delay. Another recessive form that is typical but with severe dysarthria has been linked to the *SPG15* locus on 14q.[3035]

Hereditary spastic paraparesis with peroneal neuropathy and crural hypopigmentation A dominantly inherited childhood **neurocutaneous syndrome** with high palate, dysarthria, lordosis, pes cavus, patchy depigmentation of the skin, and peroneal motor neuropathy.[6061]

Hereditary spastic paraparesis with peripheral retinal degeneration A recessively inherited *variant* occurring in young adult life, manifesting pigmentary retinopathy, spasticity, and mental impairment.[5888] Forms with dominant inheritance or with sensory losses have also been reported.[379]

Hereditary spastic paraparesis with sensory neuropathy A dominantly or recessively inherited *variant* with onset in childhood or early youth, characterized by the addition of a neuropathy resembling **hereditary sensory and autonomic neuropathy**, type 2.[3413, 5577]

Hereditary spastic paraparesis with mental impairment and thin corpus callosum A recessively inherited *variant* characterized by these features and mapped to 15q13–15.[5800] It is, however, both clinically and genetically heterogeneous *SPG11* and *SPG15* are the major loci.

Hereditary spastic paraparesis with epilepsy and thin corpus callosum mapped to 8p12.[89]

Hereditary spastic paraparesis with syndactyly A *variant* with onset in youth or early adult life, characterized by sensorineural deafness, osseous syndactyly of the fingers, spasticity, and incontinence.

Kjellin syndrome

Leber hereditary optic neuropathy

MASA syndrome An X-linked recessive *variant* with onset in youth, characterized by Mental retardation, Adducted thumbs, Shuffling gait (due to paraparesis), and Aphasia.[614]

Mast syndrome A static form with onset in young adult life, characterized by spastic paraparesis, athetosis, dysarthria, and dementia, described in the Pennsylvanian Amish people.[1354]

A form with features of peroneal muscular atrophy.

A form resembling **amyotrophic lateral sclerosis**.

Spinal muscular atrophy with spastic paraplegia, mental retardation, and ichthyosis See **Sjögren–Larsson syndrome**.

Spastic paraparesis, ataxia, mental retardation (SPAR) A dominantly inherited disorder manifesting these features, with marked atrophy of the spinal cord.[2692]

Spinal muscular atrophy with retinitis pigmentosa and ***hereditary spastic paraplegia***.

Troyer syndrome (hereditary spastic paraparesis with wasting and growth retardation) A static form with onset in childhood, characterized by pseudobulbar palsy, athetosis, short stature, speech defect, and mental and developmental delay, described in some Pennsylvanian Amish people.[1355]

Yet other variants with added **cerebellar signs**, **dystonia** or **choreoathetosis**, sensory neuropathy, abnormal skin pigmentation, **hyperekplexia**, or with seizures are also described.[5241]

---

and chorea are the main features in older individuals.[4416]

hereditary thermosensitive neuropathy A dominantly inherited demyelinating neuropathic syndrome characterized by reversible episodes of ascending muscle weakness, paresthesias, and areflexia triggered by elevations of body temperature above 38.5°C.[4017]

hereditary torsion dystonia See **dystonia**.

hereditary transcobalamin II deficiency A congenital dysmorphic syndrome characterized also by red blood cell abnormalities, hypotonia, microcephaly, seizures, cerebellar and pyramidal signs, cerebral atrophy, and neurodegenerative regression.[381]

hereditary tyrosinemia A recessively inherited deficiency of fumarylacetoacetate, an enzyme required in the final step of tyrosine metabolism. The disorder is manifest in infancy. The clinical features largely reflect the presence of slowly progressive hepatic failure and of a renal Fanconi syndrome; abrupt episodes of vomiting, painful peripheral neuropathy, muscle weakness, and self-mutilation are also described.[4400]

hereditary vascular retinopathy A dominantly inherited occlusive microangiopathy of the retina associated with migraine, Raynaud's phenomenon, mild cognitive decline, and depression.[6456]

hereditary vertical nystagmus A dominantly inherited syndrome with congenital onset characterized by vertical nystagmus which may be associated with mild ataxia and titubation.[2156]

hereditary vitamin E deficiency A rare, metabolic disorder of infancy manifesting tremor, ataxia, head titubation, and loss of vibration sense.

hereditary whispering dysphonia A dominantly inherited condition characterized by inability to speak above a whisper except under strong emotion, often accompanied by involuntary movements.[4903]

heredity (from Lat; inheritance) The laws whereby the characteristics of humans tend to repeat themselves in their descendants.

heredoakinesie paroxystique douloureuse A rare, familial disease characterized by paroxysmal attacks of paralysis with severe limb pains. The condition was described by Koulkov in the early 1900s but seems to have disappeared.[645]

heredoataxic hemeralopic polyneuritis See **hereditary motor and sensory neuropathy**, type 4.

heredofamilial mononeuritis multiplex with brachial predilection A dominantly inherited condition in which there are recurrent episodes of painful acute brachial plexus neuritis, although cranial and other spinal nerves have also been described as affected.[6240]

heredofamilial optic atrophy See **Leber optic atrophy**, **optic atrophy**, and **Behr disease**.

heredofamilial tremor A dominantly inherited condition in which the tremor is symmetric and affects the hands and arms first. See **essential tremor**.

heredofamilial tremor and epilepsy See **familial cortical myoclonic tremor with epilepsy**.

heredopathia atactica polyneuritiformis See Refsum disease (**hereditary motor and sensory neuropathy, type** 4).

Hering, Heinrich Ewald (1866–1948) Austrian physiologist at Cologne who is remembered for his identification of the nerve of the carotid sinus and his studies on respiratory reflexes. Henry **Head** and **Bielschowsky** were his pupils.

Hering's Law Each member of a yoked pair of ocular motor muscles must receive equal innervation, so that they move in parallel. While this is true in the normal state, small differences in innervation can occur in the presence of unilateral ocular muscle weakness.

Hering nerve A branch of the IX cranial nerve, afferent from the carotid sinus, described by Hering in 1923.

Herman Pallister Opitz syndrome A congenital syndrome characterized by synostosis of the coronal suture, hypertelerism, severe mental retardation, facial dysmorphism, and skeletal deformities.[2878] See also **craniosynostosis**

hernia A swelling produced by the protrusion of a viscus through an aperture in the walls of the cavity which contains it.

herniation 1. Abnormal protrusion of part of the brain (or of other structures such as intervertebral disks) outside their normal boundaries. Herniation of the cingulate gyrus across the mid-line below the falx, of the brainstem vertically down through the tentorial opening, of the uncus down over the tentorial free edge, of the cerebellum upward, and of the cerebellar tonsils down through the foramen magnum are examples of the reaction of the brain as a whole to major increases in intracranial pressure. The **central syndrome** and the **uncal syndrome** are the most clinically important examples. Lateral shift of the brainstem is, however, likely to be the factor causing most of the clinical signs.[2102]

2. Protrusion, displacement, or extrusion of a fragment of disk material independent of its relationship to the spinal ligaments or nerve roots; that degree of disk herniation in which there is the extrusion of a fragment from the disk space. See also **disk prolapse** and **disk protrusion**.

heroin-induced leukoencephalopathy A progressive spongiform leukoencephalopathy presenting with varying degrees of lethargy, dysarthria, bradykinesia, and cerebellar dysfunction. Imaging studies indicate extensive white matter damage shown to be due to vacuolar degeneration with axonal sparing. The cause is inhalation of heated heroin vapor, a practice known among addicts as "chasing the dragon."

Herophilus of Chaldecon (335–280 BC) A Greek physician, a teacher at the Ptolemaic school in Alexandria. Although he is credited with the first recorded descriptions of the brain, its membranes and sinuses, and noted the origin of motor and sensory nerves from the spinal cord, as well as many other anatomical and physiological facts, none of his works actually survive.[1670]

He considered that the brain was the organ of intelligence and the fourth ventricle the seat of the soul (300 BC). The *torcular Herophili* (Gr, cellar) is the name given to the confluence of the superior sagittal, straight and both transverse cerebral venous sinuses at the posterior edge of the tentorium, regarded by Herophilus as a reservoir of blood.

herpes (Gr, creeping) Hippocrates used this word for a spreading skin eruption, especially one which runs around the body. The word was subsequently used for many other forms of dermatosis.

herpes simplex encephalitis A necrotizing encephalitis with a particular predilection for the medial temporal and inferior frontal lobes. It is the commonest cause of severe sporadic encephalitis in the Western world, affecting subjects at any age. Subjects presenting with behavioral and personality changes, evidence of raised intracranial pressure, and meningism and focal neurological signs, occurring subacutely or acutely, are usually treated with acyclovir without resorting to brain biopsy, the former standard for diagnosis.[3118] Focal EEG changes and MRI demonstration of uni- or bilateral edema deep in the temporal lobes are, in this context, strongly suggestive markers for the disease.

herpes viruses Viruses of the class include herpes simplex and zoster, the Epstein–Barr virus, and cytomegalovirus.

herpes zoster (Gr, Creeping + a girdle) The clinical expression of infection with the herpes zoster virus. Infection may have no consequence or may lead, after a period of latency, to inflammation of the dorsal root ganglia or the ganglia on the afferent cranial nerves, as described by Sir Henry **Head** in 1900. This is most commonly manifest as pain, an erythematous vesicular rash next appearing within 3–4 days and leaving with either no residua or with skin atrophy and further longlasting pain. In some cases, the virus attacks the anterior horn cell pool at the same levels as it affects the posterior roots, causing wasting, weakness, and reflex loss at those segmental levels.

Herpes was first described as an infectious condition by **Landouzy** in 1884. The term *shingles* derives from the Latin word *cingulum*, a belt, presumably referring to the distribution of the rash even though it is unilateral.

herpes zoster myelopathy The rare occurrence of transverse myelitis at the level of an herpetic infection of the dorsal root ganglia, causing motor and sensory long tract signs below that level and due to direct infection of the cord.[2941]

herpetic neuralgia Continuous aching, burning, or itching pains experienced during the eruption of the herpetic rash, sometimes with superimposed lancinating pains.[5083] See also **postherpetic neuralgia**.

Herrick syndrome 1. A congenital dysmorphic syndrome manifesting also skeletal maldevelopments, microcephaly, seizures, spasticity, cerebral and cerebellar atrophy, hydrocephalus, and skin telangiectasia.[2874] 2. (Dresbach disease, sickle-cell anemia) Chorioretinal disease, retinal venous thrombosis, and secondary glaucoma, occurring in patients with sickle-cell disease.[2874]

Herrmann disease A dominantly inherited syndrome characterized by photomyoclonus, deafness, diabetes, and nephropathy, and, in some cases, progressive cerebral neuronal degeneration with periodic acid-Schiff positive glycolipid storage.[2876] Seizures, dementia, nystagmus, and pyramidal and cerebellar signs are also described in such cases.

Herrmann–Opitz syndrome See **craniosynostosis**.

Hers disease A condition in which glycogen accumulates in tissues due to lack of hepatic phosphorylase; hepatosplenomegaly, hypoglycemic attacks, mild ketosis, and retardation of growth are the main clinical features.[2879] See **glycogen storage disease** type 6.

Dr. H.G. Hers is a Belgian biochemist.

Hersh syndrome A congenital dysmorphic syndrome manifesting also sensorineural deafness, retinitis pigmentosa with visual impairment, strabismus, nystagmus, and mental and developmental delay.

Hertwig–Magendie syndrome See **skew deviation.**

Hertz (Hz) Units of frequency, equivalent to cycles per second.

Heschl, Richard L. (1824–1881) Austrian physician who became, in succession, professor of anatomy at Olmutz, of pathology at Krakau, and of clinical medicine at Graz.

Heschl gyri (transverse temporal gyri) The gyri immediately behind the insula on the mesial and superior aspect of the superior temporal gyrus, thought to be concerned with the elaboration of auditory sensation.

Hess, Walter Rudolf (1881–1973) Swiss physiologist who studied the control of autonomic system functioning. For this work he was awarded the Nobel Prize in 1949.

hetero- (Gr, different. The other one of two) Prefix denoting different.

heterochromia iridis (Gr, different + color + irises) (heteroglaucos) An alteration in the color and structure of the iris; in which the color of all or a part of one iris differs from that of the other, associated with hypo- or hyperplasia of the iris. The color change may be complete or partial and uni- or bilateral.

Simple heterochromia is thought to be due to genetic mosaicism, *complicated heterochromia* to ocular disease, and *sympathetic heterochromia* to damage to the superior cervical ganglion at birth. Although many other diseases have been reported as occurring in association (Gladstone[2399] references 77 such), the condition itself is of no pathological significance and the simple form is by far the most common; anxious parents may be reassured that it was manifested by Alexander the Great. However, deafness has been described in association.[381]

See also **Waardenburg syndrome** and **Horner syndrome**.

heterogeneous system degeneration See **Steele–Richardson–Olszewski syndrome**.

heteromodal (polymodal) association areas Cortical regions which are not devoted to any single modality and which receive convergent input from several sensory association areas and from limbic–paralimbic areas. The prefrontal cortex, posterior parietal cortex, and inferior temporal lobe are examples.[4332]

heteronymous hemianopia Binasal or bitemporal hemianopia. cf. **homonymous hemianopia**.

heteronymous reflexes Reflex contractions of muscles not supplied directly by the nerve stimulated (on the same or the opposite side) as a result of facilitation of transmission in interneuronal pathways coactivated by group I and group II afferents, and due to alterations in suprasegmental control. An example is contraction of the biceps brachii in response to stimulation of the median nerve in the cubital fossa. The phenomenon is relevant in the control of posture and balance.[4377]

heterophoria That condition in which both globes are directed normally during fixation upon near or far objects, but one or both deviate when one eye is occluded and the other eye fixates. Thus, a latent tendency for deviation of the eyes. See also **cover test** and **phoria**.

heterotopia (Gr, different + position) (ectopia) Misplacement of a part of the body during development. Within the nervous system, the occurrence of cortical cells in places other than the cortex as a consequence of arrest of normal neuronal migration during embryogenesis—thus malformations due to abnormal neuronal migration. Subependymal, subcortical, and band heterotopia (double cortex) are distinguished. In all cases, the diagnosis is made best with MRI.[5214] Most commonly, islands of gray matter are found in the subcortical white matter. Both X-linked dominant and autosomal recessive forms are described.

With subependymal (periventricular) heterotopias, the presentation is likely to be with temporal or occipital lobe-type seizures in the first two decades of life. *Bilateral nodular periventricular heterotopia* (subependymal heterotopia) is an error of neuronal migration in which subependymal clumps of gray matter protrude into the lumen of the ventricles; it is sometimes associated with cerebellar hypoplasia or with other disorders of CNS development such as the Chiari malformation, frontonasal dysplasia, and gastrointestinal and renal anomalies. Mental retardation is common but seizures are the main manifestation. The condition appears to be lethal in males and is seen almost exclusively in females. It is mapped to Xq28, but autosomal linkage is also described.

In a *variant* form, also mapped to Xq28, these features are accompanied by seizures, mental retardation, and partial syndactyly in the hands and feet. See also **Zellweger syndrome**.

Band heterotopia (double cortex syndrome) is characterized by the presence of a demarcated layer of neurons in the white matter, where they are arrested during migration to their cortical sites. Mutations at 17p13.3 or Xq22.3–q23 are sometimes found. Mental and developmental delay and partial or generalized seizures are the usual clinical accompaniments, other seizure types appearing in due course.[402] A major review has been published,[404] and a classification of heterotopia proposed

Heterotopia

1. Subependymal (periventricular) heterotopia
   a. Periventricular nodular heterotopia (PNH)
      i. Bilateral PNH with *FLN1* mutations
      ii. Other PNH
      iii. PNH with abnormal overlying cortex
   b. Periventricular laminar/ribbon heterotopia
2. Subcortical heterotopia (other than band heterotopia)
   a. Large subcortical heterotopia with abnormal cortex and hypogenetic corpus callosum
   b. Single subcortical heterotopic nodule
   c. Excessive single neurons in white matter
3. Marginal glioneuronal heterotopia.

From Barkovich AJ, Kuzniecky R, Jackson GG, et al. Classification system for malformations of cortical development. Neurology

2001;57:2168–78. Reproduced by kind permission of the American Academy of Neurology and Lippincott Williams and Wilkins.

See also **microcephaly, megalencephaly, lissencephaly, cobblestone complex,** and **poilymicrogyria**.

heterotropia (tropia) Eye deviations manifest during binocular vision. *Esotropia* indicates the adduction and *exotropia* the abduction of one eye. See also **strabismus, cover test,** and **heterophoria**.

heterotypic granular cortex Those regions of visual, auditory, or general sensory neocortex where the usual six layers are ill-defined because small stellate cells overflow into the second and fifth layers.

Heubner, Otto Johann Leonhard (1843–1926) German pediatrician, professor of medicine at Leipzig. He demonstrated the presence of a leptomeningeal anastomotic circulation in 1874.

Heubner arteritis See **Heubner disease**.

Heubner disease (Heubner arteritis) Syphilitic arteritis of the cerebral vessels, described by **Heubner** in 1874.

Heubner endarteritis See **endarteritis obliterans**.

Heubner recurrent artery An early branch of the anterior cerebral artery, supplying the superior and anterior part of the internal capsule.

Heubner–Möbius syndrome See **Möbius syndrome**.

hexosaminidase deficiency Inherited deficiencies of β-D-*N*-acetylhexosaminidase, leading to the abnormal accumulation of gangliosides and related substances within neurons. See also **GM_2 gangliosidosis**.

The hexosaminidase isoenzymes (A, B, and S) are part of a complex system metabolizing GM_2 gangliosides and related substances; when they fail, the gangliosides accumulate within the nervous system. The B form of the enzyme is coded for on chromosome 5. The numerous phenotypes have been defined by Johnson[3236] and are given in Chart H–11. (Reproduced with kind permission of the American Academy of Neurology and Lippincott Williams and Wilkins.)

Ataxia, excessive startle responses, dementia, seizures, involuntary movements, pyramidal signs, and cherry-red spots on the retina are recorded variously in these conditions, and phenotypes resembling **amyotrophic lateral sclerosis** or **hereditary motor neuropathy type 3** also represent expressions of hexosaminidase deficiency.[3236] See also **cerebellar ataxias**.

Chronic hexosaminidase A and B deficiency is a *variant* condition in which progressive dystonia and pyramidal and cerebellar signs occur during childhood.[2451]

HHE Syndrome (hemiconvulsions, hemiplegia, epilepsy syndrome; acute acquired postconvulsive hemiplegia, Gastaut syndrome) An epileptic syndrome characterized by persistent unilateral clonic motor seizures in the limbs and face, accompanied by high-voltage delta activity and spikes on the EEG and followed by flaccid hemiplegia lasting over a week, with suppression of EEG activity on the appropriate side. In three-quarters of all cases, complex partial clonic or other seizures begin, usually within 2 years. Most affected children have evidence of intellectual failure.

This uncommon syndrome is described in infants and young children following acute unilateral cerebral lesions[2304] such as tumor or herpetic encephalitis, or after febrile seizures.

HHH syndrome 1. (Hyperornithemia, Hyperammonemia, Homocitrullinemia syndrome) See **ornithinemia**. 2. (*hemiparesis, hemiatrophy and hemiathetosis*) A dominantly inherited nonprogressive athetotic hemiplegic syndrome.[2656]

HHHO syndrome (Hypotonia, Hypomentia, Hypogonadism, Obesity syndrome) See **Prader–Willi syndrome**.

hiccoughs (hiccups, singultus) Intermittent, rhythmic, chronic, spasmodic contractions of the diaphragm accompanied by similar contractions of the accessory muscles of respiration. The sudden inspiration is terminated almost immediately by abrupt closure of the glottis, producing the audible sound. The cause may lie in structural or functional disorders of the medulla affecting the region of the vagal nuclei and the nucleus tractus solitarius, or in damage to the vagi or to the afferent or efferent nerves of the respiratory muscles.

The functional utility of this involuntary respiratory reflex has not been determined.

Chart H–11. Hexosaminidase Deficiency Phentotypes

Infantile encephalopathies	
Alpha locus	Tay–Sachs disease and variant
Beta locus	Sandhoff disease and variants
Activator locus	AB variant
Late infantile/juvenile	
Alpha locus	Juvenile Tay–Sachs disease and variant
Beta locus	Juvenile Sandhoff disease
Cerebellar ataxia	
Alpha locus	Atypical spinocerebellar ataxia
Beta locus	Juvenile ataxia (Ramsay Hunt phenocopy)
Motor neuron diseases	
Alpha locus	Amyotrophic lateral sclerosis phenocopy **Hereditary motor neuropathy**, type 3 phenocopy
Adult-onset encephalopathy	
Activator locus	Adult GM2 gangliosidosis
Asymptomatic or presymptomatic adults	
Alpha locus	Total or near-total hexosaminidase deficiency
Beta locus	Hexosaminidase A and B or B deficiency

Adapted from Johnson WG. The clinical spectrum of hexosaminidase deficiency diseases. Neurology *1981;31:1453–6 with new material.*

In 1883, Short first recognized the relationship between hiccoughs and phrenic nerve irritation. The condition is usually self-limiting but in protracted cases, Hippocrates advised apnea, which is sound because an increase in the arterial carbon dioxide tension does have an inhibitory effect. Over 100 other therapies have been suggested, including digital or chemical stimulation of the pharynx; ocular compression; prayers to St. Jude; phrenic crush; and drugs such as phenothiazines, demerol, metoclopramide, carbamazepine, nifedipine, meperidine, quinidine, and orphenadrine; and digital rectal massage, recalling the comment of Dr. Charles Mayo: "The amount of knowledge on any subject such as this can be considered as being in inverse proportion to the number of different treatments suggested and tried for it."[4225]

hiccups See **hiccoughs**.

Hicks disease See **hereditary sensory and autonomic neuropathy type 1**.

Hidden Figures Test (Gollin Test) A figure-matching task testing visuo-perceptual functions, in which the stimuli to be matched are embedded in more complex figures. Like other similar tests, it is sensitive to damage localized to the parietal cortex.[2521]

hidrotic ectodermal dysplasia A familial syndrome comprising cataract, hyperpigmentation of the skin with telangiectasias, hyperkeratosis, and nail dystrophy. See also **neurocutaneous syndromes** and **Clouston disease**.

high-altitude cerebral edema (HACE) A vasogenic encephalopathy due to low ambient partial pressures of oxygen, presenting with altered sensorium, ataxia, headache, retinopathy, and cognitive impairments. MRI scans show intense T2 signals in the white matter and reversible vasogenic edema with a predilection for the splenium of the corpus callosum. Lacunar infarcts and cerebral venous sinus thrombosis are other complications.

This potentially fatal condition is considered to be due to movement of fluid and protein out of the vascular compartment.[2667]

high-altitude headache (hypoxic headache, altitudinal headache) Headache is a major symptom of **acute mountain sickness** (AMS), developing within 24 h after ascent to above 3000 m. It is associated with at least one other symptom typical of AMS including Cheyne–Stokes respirations at night, a desire to overbreathe and exertional dyspnea. Nausea, anorexia, fatigue, dizziness, and sleep disorders are typical accompanying symptoms. Diagnostic criteria have been defined[5831, 2820]

A. Headache with at least two of the following characteristics and fulfilling criteria C and D:
   1. Bilateral
   2. Frontal or frontotemporal
   3. Dull or pressing quality
   4. Mild or moderate intensity
   5. Aggravated by exertion, movement, straining, coughing, or bending
B. Ascent to altitude above 2500 m
C. Headache develops within 24 h after ascent
D. Headache resolves within 8 h after descent

From the ICHD (Headache Classification Committee of the International Headache Society. Cephalalgia 2004;24(Suppl 1)) by kind permission of Dr. Jes Olesen, the International Headache Society and Wiley-Blackwell Publications.

See also **acute mountain sickness**.

high-density lipoprotein deficiency See **Tangier disease**.

high-frequency filter A circuit which reduces the sensitivity of the EEG channel to relatively high frequencies. For each position of the high-frequency filter control, this attenuation is expressed as a percent reduction in output pen deflection at a given frequency, relative to frequencies unaffected by the filter, i.e in the mid-frequency band of the channel.

At present, high-frequency filter designations and their significance are not standardized for instruments of different manufacture. For instance, for a given instrument, a position of the high-frequency filter control designated at 35 Hz may indicate a 30% (3 Db), or other stated percentage reduction, in sensitivity at 35 Hz compared to the sensitivity, for example at 10 Hz. (Adapted from the 1974 report of the Committee on Terminology, IFCN. In: Chatrian GE, Bergamini L, Dondey M, et al. A glossary of terms most commonly used by clinical electroencephalographers. *EEG Clin Neurophysiol* 1974;37:538–48. Reproduced with kind permission from Elsevier Science.)

high-frequency response The sensitivity of an EEG channel to relatively high frequencies, determined by the high-frequency responses of the amplifier–writer combination and of the filter used and expressed as a percentage reduction in the output pen deflection at certain specific high frequencies, relative to other frequencies in the mid-frequency band of the channel. (Adapted from the 1974 report of the Committee on Terminology, IFCN. In: Chatrian GE, Bergamini L, Dondey M, et al. A glossary of terms most commonly used by clinical electroencephalographers. *EEG Clin Neurophysiol* 1974;37:538–48. Reproduced with kind permission from Elsevier Science.)

high median neuropathy See **pronator syndrome**.

Hilger syndrome See **carotidynia**.

hill of vision A three-dimensional representation of visual acuity in which the horizontal and vertical parameters representing the dimensions of visual space are joined by another representing the differential sensitivity to light of different parts of the retina. The fovea is most sensitive, and it would be shown as forming the summit of the hill, slightly removed from the bottomless crater, which is the optic nerve head or blind spot.

Hillig syndrome A congenital dysmorphic syndrome manifesting also hepatosplenomegaly, skeletal maldevelopments, macrocephaly, and mental and developmental delay.[381]

Hill-Lowenberg syndrome See **Pelizaeus–Merzbacher disease**.

Hilton, John (1804–1878) English anatomist, surgeon to Guy's Hospital, London and sometime president of the Royal College of Surgeons. He described his law in his famous book *Rest and Pain* (London: Bell, 1863).

Hilton's law "The same trunks of nerves whose branches supply the groups of muscles moving a joint, furnish also a distribution of nerves to the skin over the insertions of the same muscles . . . and the interior of the joint."

hindbrain That part of the developing brain which separates into the medulla oblongata and the cerebellum and which contains the fourth ventricle.

Hines, Edgar Alphonso, Jr.
(b. 1906) Physician at the Mayo Clinic, the originator (with Dr. G.E. Brown) of the **cold pressor test** in 1932.

Hippel, Eugen von (1867–1939)
German ophthalmologist who trained in Heidelberg and Göttingen, studied further with Leber, and later became professor at Halle and then Göttingen. Apart from describing the syndrome named for him, he published on numerous eye deformities, cataract, optic nerve lesions, and sympathetic ophthalmia.

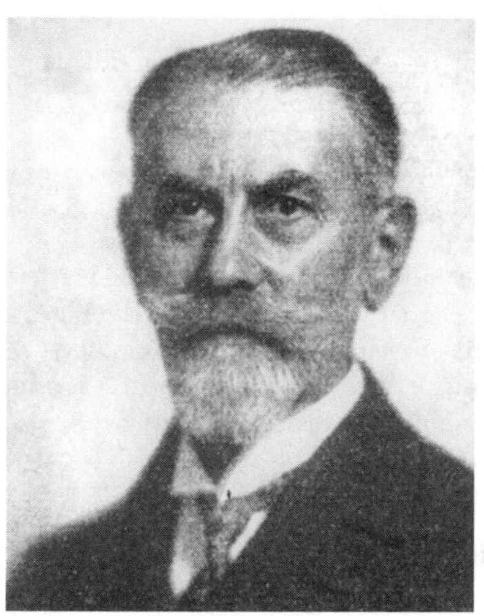

Figure H–4 Eugen von Hippel.

hippocampal (and parahippocampal) seizures
Seizures arising from the insula, amygdala, hypothalamus, or other limbic structures and depending upon local spread for their clinical manifestations. Symptoms include a sensation of epigastric rising, emotional experiences (usually intense fear), dysmnesias, focal sensory seizures with olfactory or gustatory symptoms, and paresthesias or other bilateral sensory phenomena.[1861]

hippocampal sclerosis Severe neuronal loss and gliosis of the hippocampal CA1 sector and subiculum, uni-or bilaterally; a major cause of partial seizures, arising as a developmental defect or due to febrile seizures in childhood or in association with various forms of dementia in adult life.

hippocampal theta activity
Regular, high-amplitude waves recorded by subcortical electrodes during rapid eye movement during sleep and wakefulness in animals and occasionally in man.[2255]

hippocampus (Gr, a horse and Lat, a field or racetrack) A curved cell mass with distinct zones lying in the inferomesial part of the temporal lobe, covered by the gyrus of the same name; a way-point on the pathways for smell, emotion, and memory.

hip-pocket sciatica (neuropathy) Alleged irritation of the sciatic nerve as a result of carrying a wallet in the back pocket of the trousers. A more likely diagnosis is **piriformis syndrome**.

The condition is likely to be more prevalent during times of high inflation.

Hippocrates (460–370 BC) Greek physician from the island of Cos in the Aegean; the Father of Medicine. The Hippocratic writings are almost certainly a collection of manuscripts by a number of authors, though presumably based on his books. It is said that Hippocrates taught beneath a sycamore tree (*Plantanus orientalis*) that stands to this day on Cos; scions of this tree populate many medical campuses (HJM).

Hippocrates described numerous neurological conditions as well as some neuroanatomy, based in part upon dissections performed on goats as well as man. He identified thought, intelligence, and dreams as functions of the brain but also considered that it changed pneuma into animal spirits and excreted the residua. Diseases identified by him included both focal and generalized tonic–clonic seizures, pupillary inequality, nerve palsies, ophthalmoplegia, myelopathy, apoplexy (including both subarachnoid and intracerebral hemorrhages), mental disorders, and aphasia. His comment that epilepsy was not any more sacred than other diseases was ignored for the next 2000 years.

Hippocrates phrenitis An acute, febrile, fatal syndrome consisting of severe nausea and vomiting, acute cachexia, profound mental confusion, and intense generalized motor agitation. Hippocrates also included under *Phrenitis* other causes such as malaria, typhoid, and alcoholic crises.

The term was derived from the belief that the diaphragm was the organ of mind, so in delirium (which is what Hippocrates was describing in the cases he reported with the diagnosis of phrenitis) there must be irritation of the diaphragm.[6380] The actual condition may have been encephalitis.

hippus (from Gr, hippos-continual winking) Physiological oscillation of the size of the pupils. The irregular pupillary constriction and dilatation occur continuously in dim, diffuse lighting with a cycle time of 660 ms or longer and is of variable amplitude. The phenomenon is normal but its cause is not known.

Hirano bodies Eosinophilic cylindrical structures up to 30 μm long, containing filaments derived from cytoskeletal proteins and found within the cytoplasm of hippocampal neurons in relation to advancing age, but with increased frequency in patients with numerous dementing and degenerative diseases, including **Alzheimer** and **Pick diseases**, **kuru**, and **amyotrophic lateral sclerosis**.

Dr. Asao Hirano is a contemporary American neuropathologist.

Hirayama disease (juvenile muscular atrophy of the distal upper limb[s]) A rare cervical myelopathy described mainly in young Japanese males who present with distal weakness and wasting, usually of only one arm, initially progressive and then static after years.[2916] Cold paresis and postural tremor are also described. Ischemic changes in the anterior horns of the cervical cord indicate that this is a cervical ischemic poliomyelopathy between C6 and T1, which appears to be induced by neck flexion. Nerve conduction studies are normal except for decrease in the CMAP in affected muscles. See also **Marie–Foix disease**. Requirements for the diagnosis are as follows:[6217]

1. Distally dominant muscle weakness and atrophy of the forearm and hand
2. Onset between the ages of 10 and early 20s
3. Unilateral or unilaterally dominant symptoms and signs

4. Insidious onset with gradual progression for the first several years, followed by arrest of progression
5. Lack of sensory disturbance and reflex abnormalities; no symptoms or findings in the legs
6. Other diseases of the cervical cord are excluded.

Although this entry is the definitive one, this condition might have a genetic basis and is therefore also included under **hereditary motor neuropathy** above.

See also **lower motor neuron disease**.

Hirano Parkinsonism-dementia See **Lytico–Bodig**.

Hirano–Kurland–Sayre combined neurological degeneration A dominantly inherited disease resembling **amyotrophic lateral sclerosis** but with the added features of degeneration of the posterior columns, spinocerebellar tracts, and Clarke's column and the presence of intracytoplasmic argyrophilic inclusions (**Lewy bodies**) in the anterior horn cells.[2911]

Hirano–Lewy body disease See **amyotrophic lateral sclerosis** and **Hirano–Kurland–Sayre combined neurological degeneration**.

Hirayama juvenile muscular atrophy See various entries under **hereditary motor neuropathy** type 3

Hirschberg sign See **adductor reflex of the foot**.

Hirschsprung Disease A disorder characterized by absence of ganglion cells in the intestine. The condition is most commonly seen in males and usually presents with constipation in the first 3 months of life. In three quarters of the cases the involvement is limited to the rectosigmoid region. The condition is sometimes associated with **Down syndrome, neurofibromatosis** or **neuroblastoma**.[1821] Harald Hirschprung (1830–1916) was a Danish pediatrician at Copenhagen.

A *variant* is *Hirschsprung (cleft palate, mental retardation) syndrome*, a congenital dysmorphic syndrome manifesting also speech delay, Hirschprung syndrome, microcephaly, cerebellar signs, and mental and developmental delay.[381]

His, Wilhelm (1831–1904) Swiss anatomist from Basel, a student of Remak. He originated the terms *dendrite*, *neuropil*, *neuroblast*, and *spongioblast*. His main interest was the embryogenesis of the nervous system.

histamine flare test The subcutaneous injection of 0.1 ml of a 1:1000 solution of histamine acid phosphate, with assessment of the area of erythema (the flare) produced through local axon reflexes. Once used for localization of the site of a sensory nerve lesion (normal flare size with proximal radicular lesions; reduced flare size with distal plexus or other lesions), it has been largely supplanted by nerve conduction studies.

histaminic cephalgia See **cluster headache**. Horton incriminated histamine in the pathogenesis of this condition in part because of the provocative role of histamine in precipitation of the attack. He has still not been proved right or wrong.

histidinemia A recessively inherited syndrome resulting from a deficiency of l-histidase and characterized clinically by motor and behavioral delay in some cases.[5697]

histiocytosis (systemic histiocytosis, Erdheim–Chester disease) A rare systemic disorder seen mainly in males with onset in later adult life, characterized by fever, cardiovascular and dermal features, metaphyseal cortical thickening of the long bones, and hypothalamic or orbital infiltration, the former associated with diabetes insipidus.[5923]

histiocytosis X See **generalized xanthomatosis**.

histoplamosis Infection by this dimorphic fungus, usually presenting as pulmonary infiltrations but able to disseminate in immunocompromised people, in which case meningoencephalitis is a potential complication.

History of Neuroscience A listing of milestones in the advancement of neurology, compiled by Dr. Eric H. Chudler of the University of Washington.

History of Neurosurgery A Web site that provides historical data and access to the **Cyber Museum of Neurosurgery**, found at http://www.neurosurgery.org/cybermuseum/index.html/.

histrionic palsy A synonym for **Bell palsy**, so known in the nineteenth century on account of the resultant loss of the power of facial expression.

Hittner syndrome A congenital dysmorphic syndrome manifesting also deafness, microphthalmia, retinal and iris colobomas, and mental and developmental delay.[381]

Hitselberg sign Hypoesthesia of the posterior wall of the external auditory meatus as a result of a proximal lesion affecting the VII cranial nerve (which is not purely a motor nerve).

Hitzig, Eduard (1838–1907) German neuropsychiatrist, eventually professor of psychiatry at Zurich and later at Halle. He described girdle zones and, by animal experiments performed in his home during 1870–1874 in conjunction with Fritsch, a zoologist, defined the extent of the motor areas in primates using electrical stimulation of the cortex.

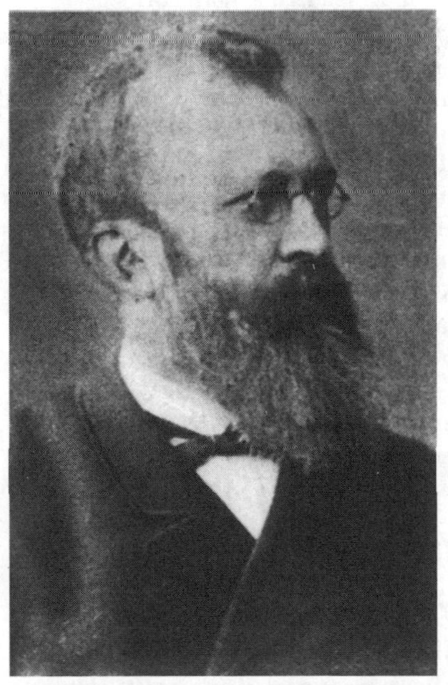

Figure H–5 Eduard Hitzig.

Hitzig girdle (zone) Analgesia in the T3–T6 regions in early **tabes dorsalis**.[5704]

HIV encephalopathy See **HIV-1-associated nervous system diseases**.

HIV meningoencephalitis (giant cell encephalitis, multinucleated cell encephalitis, subacute encephalitis) The *acute form* is an uncommon complication occurring early in the course of HIV infection and characterized by altered consciousness, seizures, mental dysfunction, evidence of inflammation in the CSF and diffuse changes on the EEG, leading on to ultimate recovery from the acute illness.

The *chronic form* (chronic HIV meningitis) is a frequent complication of HIV infection, occurring often prior to the appearance of AIDS and (if symptomatic at all) characterized by headache and mild meningeal signs, cranial neuropathies, and chronic inflammatory changes in the CSF.[2071]

HIV myelopathy See **HIV-associated myelopathy**.

HIV myopathy A proximal myopathy complicating human immunodeficiency virus type 1 (HIV) infection or (less often) its treatment with zidovudine, characterized by weakness, elevated serum creatine kinase levels and muscle biopsy appearances of myofiber degeneration, variable inflammatory infiltrates, inclusion bodies, and mitochondrial abnormalities.[6883]

HIV neuropathy See **HIV-associated multiple mononeuropathy, HIV-associated progressive polyneuropathy, HIV-associated autonomic neuropathy, HIV-associated predominantly sensory neuropathy, HIV-associated acute inflammatory demyelinating polyneuropathy,** and **HIV-associated lumbosacral polyradiculopathy. Radiculopathies** (cytomegalovirus, herpes zoster), vasculitic neuropathy, lymphomatous neuropathy, and forms associated with drug therapy are also described in patients with HIV infections.

HIV wasting disease See **HIV-associated myopathy**.

HIV-associated acute inflammatory demyelinating polyneuropathy (HIV-1-associated Guillain–Barré Syndrome) A neuropathic syndrome resembling **acute inflammatory demyelinating polyneuropathy** complicating HIV infection. The following diagnostic criteria have been suggested. (From American Academy of Neurology AIDS task force. Nomenclature and case definitions for neurological manifestations of HIV type 1 infection. *Neurology;43:*625–7. Reproduced by kind permission of the American Academy of Neurology and Lippincott Williams and Wilkins.)

Probable Patients must have 1. Guillain–Barré syndrome by previously published criteria except that the CSF cell count can be as high as 50 cells/mm^3.

Possible Patients must have one of the following:

1. Other potential etiology present (must have each of the following):
   a. As above No. 1.
   b. Other potential etiology is present and the cause of No. 1 is uncertain.
2. Incomplete clinical evaluation (patients must have each of the following):
   a. As above No. 1.
   b. Etiology cannot be determined (appropriate laboratory investigations not performed).

HIV-associated aseptic meningitis An acute aseptic meningitis with headache, meningism, cranial neuropathies, and fever occurring at the time of seroconversion (AIDS-related complex), reflecting the initial response of the nervous system to the infection. The CSF shows a monocytic pleocytosis.[4200]

HIV-associated autonomic neuropathy The occurrence of such autonomic symptoms as fainting due to orthostatic hypotension, cardiac irregularities, hypohidrosis, impotence, diarrhea, and urinary dysfunction occurring in patients suffering the later stages of HIV infection. Whether it is the disease or its treatment which is responsible is not yet determined.[5858]

HIV-associated cognitive/motor complex See **HIV-associated neurocognitive disorders**.

HIV-associated lumbosacral polyradiculopathy (cytomegalovirus polyradiculitis, myeloradiculitis) A severe but reversible cauda equina syndrome manifesting bilateral leg weakness, areflexia, and loss of sphincter function with rapid progression of the paraplegia over days. A mononuclear pleocytosis is notable in the CSF. Although cytomegalovirus infection is a common cause, lymphoma, toxoplasmosis, and syphilis can produce the same syndrome.[5937]

HIV/AIDS headache Diagnostic criteria have been defined in the ICHD.[2820] Essentially, in a person with confirmed HIV infection the headache has variable modes of onset, site, and intensity, develops in close temporal relation to the HIV/AIDS-related pathophysiology, and resolves within 3 months after the infection subsides.

HIV-associated leukoencephalopathy (progressive diffuse encephalopathy) A syndrome characterized by diffuse damage to the cerebral white matter with loss of myelin and reactive astrogliosis, and presenting in the same way as **progressive multifocal leukoencephalopathy** but with a particular tendency to cause dementia.[4199]

HIV-associated multiple mononeuropathy A multifocal sensory axonal inflammatory neuropathy presenting rarely with multiple sensory complaints, often in association with fever, cachexia, and cytomegalovirus retinopathy, within the context of HIV infection.[5858]

HIV-associated myelopathy (vacuolar myelopathy, HIV myelopathy) A vacuolar myelopathy presenting with a syndrome of motor and sensory deficits characteristic of spinal cord disease and due to direct infection of the cord with HIV. It is found to occur in a quarter of all patients dying from AIDS.[5004, 2071] Gait disturbance, leg weakness, and urinary incontinence are the major clinical features. Diagnostic criteria have been suggested by the AAN Task Force and are given in Chart H–14. (Reproduced by kind permission of the American Academy of Neurology and Lippincott Williams and Wilkins.)

HIV-associated myopathy (HIV wasting disease) A myopathic syndrome complicating HIV infection.[5857] Diagnostic criteria have been suggested and are given in Chart H–15.

Chart H–12. Diagnostic Criteria for HIV-Associated Myelopathy

Probable (must have each of the following):

1. Acquired abnormality in lower-extremity neurological function disproportionate to upper-extremity abnormality, verified by reliable history of lower-extremity weakness, incoordination and/or urinary incontinence and neurological examination (paraparesis, lower extremity spasticity, hyperreflexia or the presence of Babinski sings, with or without sensory loss).
2. Disturbance in No. 1 is severe enough to require constant unilateral support for walking.
3. Although mild cognitive impairment may be present, criteria for HIV-1-associated dementia complex are not fulfilled.
4. Evidence of another etiology, including neoplasm, compressive lesion or multiple sclerosis, must be sought from history, physical examination, and appropriate laboratory and radiological investigation (e.g., lumbar puncture, neuroimaging, myelography). If another potential etiology is present, it is not the cause of the myelopathy. This diagnosis cannot be made in a patient infected with both HIV-1 and HTLV-1; such a patient should be classified as having possible HIV-1 associated myelopathy.

Possible (must have one of the following):

1. Other potential etiology present (must have each of the following):
   a. As above Nos. 1, 2, and 3.
2. Incomplete clinical evaluation (must have each of the following):
   a. As above Nos. 1, 2, and 3.
   b. Etiology cannotbe determined (appropriate laboratory or radiological investigations not performed).

From American Academy of Neurology AIDS task force. Nomenclature and case definitions for neurological manifestations of HIV type 1 infection. Neurology 43:625–7. *Reproduced by kind permission of the American Academy of Neurology and Lippincott Williams and Wilkins.*

Chart H–13. Diagnostic Criteria for HIV-Associated Myopathy

Probable (must have each of the following):

1. Symptoms of proximal lower- and/or upper-extremity weakness, documented by physical examination.
2. No other etiology (including toxic exposure to zidovudine). EMG and muscle biopsy may be necessary to rule out certain other etiologies.

Possible (must have one of the following):

1. Other potential etiology present (must have each of the following):
   a. As above No. 1.
   b. Other potential etiology is present and the cause is uncertain.
2. Incomplete clinical evaluation (must have each of the following):
   a. As above No. 1.
   b. Etiology can not be determined (appropriate laboratory investigations not performed).

From American Academy of Neurology AIDS task force. Nomenclature and case definitions for neurological manifestations of HIV type 1 infection. Neurology 43:625–7. *Reproduced by kind permission of the American Academy of Neurology and Lippincott Williams and Wilkins.*

Chart H–14. The HIV-Associated Nervous System Diseases

HIV-associated cognitive motor complex.

1. *Severe manifestations*
   HIV-associated dementia complex.
   Acute **HIV meningoencephalitis.**
   HIV-associated myelopathy.
   HIV associated leukoencephalopathy
   Opportunistic infections (toxoplasmosis, cryptococcosis, cytomegalovirus encephalitis, primary CNS lymphoma, progressive multifocal leukoencephalopathy, and mycobacterial infections).
2. *Mild manifestations*
   HIV-1 associated minor cognitive-motor disorder.
   HIV-1 associated neurocognitive disorder.
   HIV-1 associated neurobehavioral abnormalities.
   HIV-associated acute inflammatory demyelinating polyneuropathy.
   HIV-associated autonomic neuropathy.
   HIV-associated multiple mononeuropathy.
   HIV-associated myopathy.
   HIV-associated predominantly sensory neuropathy.
   HIV-associated progressive encephalopathy of childhood.
   HIV-associated progressive polyneuropathy.

Chart H–15. HIV-Associated Asymptomatic Neurocognitive Impairment (ANI)

1. Acquired impairment in cognitive functioning, involving at least two ability domains, documented by performance of at least 1 SD below the mean for age-education-appropriate norms on standardized neuropsychological tests. The neuropsychological assessment must survey at least the following abilities: verbal/language; attention/working memory; abstraction/executive; memory (learning; recall); speed of information processing; and sensory-perceptual, motor skills
2. The cognitive impairment does not interfere with everyday functioning
3. The cognitive impairment does not meet criteria for delirium or dementia
4. There is no evidence of another pre-existing cause for the ANI.

If there is a prior diagnosis of ANI, but currently the individual does not meet criteria, the diagnosis of ANI in remission can be made.

If the individual with suspected ANI also satisfies criteria for a major depressive episode or substance dependence, the diagnosis of ANI should be deferred to a subsequent examination conducted at a time when the major depression has remitted or at least 1 month after cessation of substance use.

From J Infect Dis 1988;158:1079–83. Price RW, Brew BJ. The AIDS-Dementia complex. Reproduced by kind permission of the Univ. Chicago Press.

HIV-associated nervous system diseases The complex of disorders affecting the nervous system in patients with clinical expression of HIV infection. The conditions are listed in Chart H–16.

The syndromes of **amyotrophic lateral sclerosis** and of pure sensory neuropathy may also be related to HIV infection. Malignancies of the CNS (primary CNS lymphoma, Kaposi sarcoma) and opportunistic infections (*toxoplasma*, viruses, fungi, bacteria) are other complications.[2071]

HIV-associated neurocognitive disorders (HAND, HIV-1-associated dementia complex, chronic AIDS encephalopathy, AIDS-dementia complex, AIDS-related dementia, subacute encephalitis) A group of dementing or motor system disorders due to primary infection of the nervous system by the HIV; the most common neurological manifestation of AIDS, present in up to 75% of those affected with the disease.[2071]

Clinically, it presents with insidious mental slowing with impaired concentration, memory loss, depression, loss of libido, social withdrawal, and mild motor deficits (unsteady gait, leg weakness, tremor) with frontal release signs, advancing to a state of apathy, abulia, mutism, and profound mental failure.[4200] All of the following diagnoses require laboratory evidence for confirmation of systemic HIV-1 infection; (enzyme-linked immunosorbent assay confirmed by Western blot, by polymerase chain reaction, or by culture). Various diagnostic criteria have been suggested;[5119] those in the following entries are the revised research criteria for HIV-associated neurocognitive disorders (HAND) modified from HIV Neurobehavioral Research Center criteria.[210] and are reproduced by kind permission of the American Academy of Neurology and Lippincott Williams and Wilkins.

HIV dementia generally, but not invariably, progresses over weeks, months, or years to severe global dementia, mutism, and death.[172]

HIV-associated predominantly sensory neuropathy (distal symmetrical polyneuropathy) A painful axonal neuropathy, the most common peripheral neuropathy in patients with HIV infection. Diagnostic criteria are listed in Chart H–17. A similar neuropathy occurs in this context as a result of exposure to neurotoxins or Vitamin B12 deficiency.

HIV-associated progressive encephalopathy of childhood A dementing syndrome complicating HIV infection in children. The major clinical features include loss of developmental

Chart H–16a. HIV-1-Associated Mild Neurocognitive Disorder (MND)

1. Acquired impairment in cognitive functioning, involving at least two ability domains, documented by performance of at least 1 SD below the mean for age-education-appropriate norms on standardized neuropsychological tests. The neuropsychological assessment must survey at least the following abilities: verbal/language; attention/working memory; abstraction/executive; memory (learning; recall); speed of information processing; and sensory-perceptual, motor skills. Typically, this would correspond to an MSK scale stage of 0.5–1.0.
2. The cognitive impairment produces at least mild interference in daily functioning (at least one of the following):
   a. Self-report of reduced mental acuity, inefficiency in work, homemaking, or social functioning.
   b. Observation by knowledgeable others that the individual has undergone at least mild decline in mental acuity with resultant inefficiency in work, homemaking, or social functioning.
3. The cognitive impairment does not meet criteria for delirium or dementia.
4. There is no evidence of another pre-existing cause for the MND!

If there is a prior diagnosis of MND, but currently the individual does not meet criteria, the diagnosis of MND in remission can be made.

If the individual with suspected MND also satisfies criteria for a severe episode of major depression with significant functional limitations or psychotic features, or substance dependence, the diagnosis of MND should be deferred to a subsequent examination conducted at a time when the major depression has remitted or at least 1 month after cessation of substance use.

From J Infect Dis 1988;158:1079–83. Price RW, Brew BJ. The AIDS-Dementia complex. Reproduced by kind permission of the Univ. Chicago Press.

Chart H–16b. HIV-1-Associated Dementia (HAD)

1. Marked acquired impairment in cognitive functioning, involving at least two ability domains; typically the impairment is in multiple domains, especially in learning of new information, slowed information processing, and defective attention/concentration. The cognitive impairment must be ascertained by neuropsychological testing with at least two domains 2 SD or greater than demographically corrected means. (Note that where neuropsychological testing is not available, standard neurological evaluation and simple bedside testing may be used, but this should be done as indicated in algorithm; see below.)
   Typically, this would correspond to an MSK scale stage of 2.0 or greater.
2. The cognitive impairment produces marked interference with day-to-day functioning (work, home life, social activities).
3. The pattern of cognitive impairment does not meet criteria for delirium (e.g., clouding of consciousness is not a prominent feature); or, if delirium is present, criteria for dementia need to have been met on a prior examination when delirium was not present.
4. There is no evidence of another, pre-existing cause for the dementia (e.g., other CNS infection, CNS neoplasm, cerebrovascular disease, pre-existing neurologic disease, or severe substance abuse compatible with CNS disorder)

If there is a prior diagnosis of HAD, but currently the individual does not meet criteria, the diagnosis of HAD in remission can be made.
If the individual with suspected HAD also satisfies criteria for a severe episode of major depression with significant functional limitations or psychotic features, or substance dependence, the diagnosis of HAD should be deferred to a subsequent examination conducted at a time when the major depression has remitted or at least 1 month has elapsed following cessation of substance use. Note that the consensus was that even when major depression and HAD occurred together, there is little evidence that pseudodementia exists and the cognitive deficits do not generally improve with treatment of depression.
Children may also develop an *HIV-associated neurodevelopmental disorder,* characterized by developmental delay, hypertonia, microcephaly, and basal ganglia calcification. The neurological involvement most often occurs in the absence of opportunistic infections and neoplasms, which is not the case in adults.

From J Infect Dis 1988;158:1079–83. Price RW, Brew BJ. The AIDS-Dementia complex. Reproduced by kind permission of the Univ. Chicago Press.

Chart H–17. Diagnostic Criteria for HIV-Associated Predominantly Sensory Neuropathy

Probable (must have each of the following)
1. Distal limb sensory symptoms (feet > hands) of a peripheral nature, with numbness, burning or pain.
2. Neurological examination confirming a distal, relatively symmetrical polyneuropathy in which sensory abnormalities predominate.
3. Electrodiagnostic studies indicative of a polyneuropathy with features of both axonal loss and demyelination.
4. Normal CSF cell count and only minimal, if any, elevation of protein level, with negative VDRL.
5. No other etiology (including toxic exposure to dideoxyinosine). Nerve biopsy may be indicated to rule out certain etiologies such as amyloid, but is not a requirement.

Possible (must have each of the following):
1. Other potential etiology present (must have each of the following):
   a. As above Nos. 1, 2, and 3.
   b. Other potential etiology is present and the cause is uncertain.
2. Incomplete clinical evaluation (must have each of the following):
   a. As above Nos. 1 and 2.
   b. Etiology can not be determined (appropriate laboratory investigations not performed).

From American Academy of Neurology AIDS task force. Nomenclature and case definitions for neurological manifestations of HIV type 1 infection. Neurology *43:*625–7 *and Reproduced by kind permission of the American Academy of Neurology and Lippincott Williams and Wilkins.*

attainments or failure to achieve them and acquired symmetrical motor deficits such as pareses, hypertonia, hyperreflexia, ataxia, and gait disturbance. Diagnostic criteria have been suggested and are given in Chart H–18.

HIV-associated progressive polyneuropathy

HIV-associated progressive polyneuropathy (HIV-associated polyradiculomyelitis) A rapidly progressive, painful syndrome of leg and sacral paresthesias, moving on to areflexic paraparesis with ascending sensory loss producing saddle anesthesia and both peripheral muscle and bladder denervation, in the context of severe immunosuppression and occurring in patients suffering the later stages of HIV infection.[1823] The usual causative organism is cytomegalovirus.

An alternative system of classification based on the underlying pathology has been suggested[932] and is given in Chart H–19.

HIV-1-associated distal symmetrical polyneuropathy

See **HIV-associated predominantly sensory neuropathy**.

HIV-1-associated Guillain–Barré syndrome

HIV-1-associated Guillain–Barré syndrome See **HIV-associated acute inflammatory demyelinating neuropathy**.

Chart H–18. Diagnostic Criteria for HIV-Associated Progressive Encephalopathy of Childhood

Probable (must have each of the following):

1. Evidence for systemic HIV-1 infection:
   a. Infants and children <15 months.
      i. Virus in blood or tissues, or
      ii. Presence of HIV-1 antibody and evidence of cellular and humoral deficiency or other conditions meeting Center for Disease Control case definition for AIDS.
2. At least one of the following progressive findings present at least 2 months.:
   a. Failure to attain or loss of developmental milestones or loss of intellectual ability, verified by standard development scale or neuropsychological tests.
   b. Impaired brain growth (acquired microcephaly or brain atrophy demonstrated on serial CT or MRI scans).
3. Evidence of another etiology, including active CNS opportunistic infection or malignancy must be sought from history, physical examination, and appropriate laboratory and radiological investigation (e.g., lumbar puncture, neuroimaging). If another potential etiology is present, it is not thought to be the cause of the above cognitive/motor/ behavioral/developmental symptoms and signs.

Possible (must have one of the following):

1. Other potential etiology present (must have each of the following):
   a. As above, Nos. 1 and 2.
   b. Other potential etiology is present but the cause of No.2 is uncertain.
2. Incomplete clinical evaluation (must have each of the following):
   a. As above, Nos. 1 and 2.
   b. Etiology cannot be determined (appropriate laboratory or radiologic investigations not performed).

From American Academy of Neurology AIDS task force. Nomenclature and case definitions for neurological manifestations of HIV type 1 infection. Neurology *43:625–7 and Reproduced by kind permission of the American Academy of Neurology and Lippincott Williams and Wilkins.*

Chart H–19. Proposed Neuropathology-Based Terminology of HIV-Associated Disease of the Nervous System Recommended in a Consensus Report

Central nervous system

HIV encephalitis.
HIV leukoencephalopathy.
Vacuolar myelopathy and vacuolar leukoencephalopathy.
Lymphocytic meningitis.
Diffuse poliodystrophy.
Cerebral vasculitis, including granulomatous angiitis.

Peripheral nervous system

(HIV-1-associated) acute inflammatory demyelinating (poly-radiculo) neuropathy.
Chronic inflammatory demyelinating poly-radiculoneuropathy.
HIV-1-associated predominantly sensory axonal neuropathy.
Ganglionitis, ganglioradiculitis,
[poly]-[radiculo] -neuritis
Necrotizing vasculitis, vasculitic neuropathy

Myopathies

(Poly) myositis.
Necrotizing myopathy.
Nemaline rod myopathy.
Vesicular myopathy, mitochondrial myopathy.
Necrotizing vasculitis.

From Budka H. Cerebral Pathology in AIDS. Curr Opin Neurol Neurosurg *1992:5:917–23. Reproduced by kind permission.*

Chart H–20. Hoehn and Yahr Scale for Parkinson disease (Modified)

0.	No signs of disease
1.	Unilateral disease, usually with minimal or no functional impairment
1.5.	Unilateral disease + axial involvement
2.	Bilateral or mid-line disease without impairment of balance
2.5.	Mild bilateral disease with recovery on **Pull test.** (The first sign of impaired righting reflexes, here made evident by unsteadiness when the patient turns or when he is pushed from standing equilibrium with the feet together and eyes closed; it indicates mild to moderate disability.)
3.	Mild to moderate bilateral disease; some postural instability; physically independent.
4.	Severe disability. Still able to stand and walk unassisted, but markedly incapacitated
5.	Wheelchair-bound or bedridden unless aided

From Hoehn MH and Yahr MD. Parkinsonism: onset, progression and mortality. Neurology *1967;17:427–42. Reproduced by kind permission of the American Academy of Neurology and Lippincott Williams and Wilkins.*

HIV-1-associated minor cognitive-motor disorder See **HIV-associated acute inflammatory demyelinating neuropathy**.

HIV-1-associated peripheral nervous system disorders See **HIV-associated myopathy, HIV-associated predominantly sensory neuropathy,** and **HIV-associated acute inflammatory demyelinating polyneuropathy**. All of these diagnoses require laboratory evidence for systemic HIV-1 infection (enzyme-linked immunosorbent assay confirmed by Western blot, by polymerase chain reaction, or by culture).

See also the Web sites http://www.aegis.com/topics/oi/oi-neuropathy.html and http://www.aegis.com/topics/oi/oi-neuropathy.html.

Hobson–McCarley model A model system of the neural basis of sleep which hypothesizes an aminergic, rapid eye movement–off state controlled by the locus ceruleus and raphé nuclei, and a cholinergic rapid eye movement–on system in opposition controlled by the giganticocellular field of the pons.

Hochsinger sign Closure of the fist in response to pressure exerted on the inner side of the biceps brachii in tetany,[5704] presumably as a result of ischemia induced distally by compression of the brachial artery proximally. The sign was described by Carl Hochsinger (1869–1942), an Austrian pediatrician.[2928]

hockey stick sign Bilateral hyperintensities seen in the pulvinar and dorsomedial thalamic nuclei, leading to this appearance on MRI scans in variant **Creutzfeldt–Jakob disease**.

hocquet diabolique Intractable hiccups, recorded as a complication of numerous central (CNS) and peripheral (chest, abdomen) causes. The most prolonged case of hiccups was one lasting 8 years, during which time the patient was estimated to have "hic'ed" 100 million times. He sought assistance from any source and received, it is said, 60,000 suggestions for cure but only one of these (prayer to St. Jude) succeeded.[4225] See **hiccoughs**.

Hodgkin disease A localized or systemic lymphoma. Neurological complications include epidural compression of the spinal cord, cranial nerve palsies, progressive multifocal leukoencephalopathy, and parenchymal sarcomas.

Hoehn and Yahr Scale The original scale rating the overall level of impairment in **Parkinson disease**[2933] and still preferred by many. See Chart H–20.

Hoffmann, Johann (1857–1919) German neurologist who graduated from Heidelberg with a thesis on acute ascending paralysis. There he worked at first under **Friedreich** and then **Erb**. In 1910 he was elected full professor of medicine and, shortly before his death, professor of neuropathology.

His many clinical contributions include those next listed, his differentiation of **myotonic dystrophy** and **myotonia congenita**, the **H-reflex** and an accurate description of **hereditary motor neuropathy type 1**, acknowledging the previous report of **Werdnig**.

Hoffmann–Charcot–Marie–Tooth syndrome See **hereditary motor and sensory neuropathy**, types 1 and 2.

Hoffmann disease See **hereditary motor neuropathy**, type 1.

Hoffmann reflex 1. (Hoffmann–Tromner reflex, digital reflex) Sudden release of the flexed distal phalanx of the second, third, or fourth digits leads to flexion of the terminal phalanx of the thumb and of the last two interphalangeal joints of other fingers of that hand in the case of pyramidal tract disease affecting that limb.[1387] The phenomenon has the same significance as the **finger flexion reflex**, of which it is a variant. The first account of it was actually published by Curschmann (one of Hoffmann's students) in 1911, 10 years after he had described it orally. 2. See **H reflex**.

Hoffmann sign Increased mechanical irritability of the sensory nerves in tetany.

Hoffmann syndrome (hypothyroid myopathy) Stiffness, slowed contraction and relaxation, and persistent painful muscle contractions following effort, made worse by exertion and associated with muscle hypertrophy in adult hypothyroid patients.[2936, 2939] See **pseudomyotonia**. **Kocher–Debré–Sémélaigne syndrome** is only different by virtue of the lesser amount of pain felt and its original description in cretinoid patients. See **hypothyroid myopathy** and **pseudomyotonia**.

Hoffmann, Paul (1884–1962) German physician who described the following sign independently of Tinel.

Hoffmann sign Increased irritability of regenerating sensory nerves in response to mechanical stimuli. See also **Tinel sign**.

Hoffmann–Tromner reflex See **Hoffman reflex**.

Hollenhorst plaque A visible cholesterol embolism in the retinal arterioles accompanied sometimes by **amaurosis fugax**. It suggests the presence of atherosclerosis in the carotid system.

Hollenhorst syndrome Permanent or temporary blindness as a result of chorioretinal infarction which results from persistently increased ocular pressure. This might be caused by malpositioning of a patient lying face down during surgery with the head supported in a head rest. Ophthalmoplegias, proptosis, chemosis, corneal edema, and retinal detachment are other features reported.[2953]

hollow hand sign (of Garcin) Adduction and flexion of the thumb when the fingers are extended voluntarily. This is a sensitive sign indicating a pyramidal lesion affecting the upper limb.

Holmes, Oliver Wendell (1809–1894) American literary figure and physician, practicing in Boston. In the latter rôle, he introduced the terms *anesthesia* and *anesthetic* to medicine.

Holmes cerebellar ataxia An **autosomal dominant cerebellar ataxia**. See **Holmes disease**.

Holmes disease 1. (cerebello-olivary degeneration, Holmes cerebellar ataxia) Originally described as a recessively inherited cerebellar ataxia with hypogonadism,[2956] the appellation has been given to various forms of ataxias, including some dominantly inherited, on the basis of similar pathology. The condition is now classified as an **autosomal dominant cerebellar ataxia**.[2753] Added features may include choroidal dystrophy, ectodermal dysplasia, short stature, developmental delay, sensorineural deafness, and polyneuropathy. 2. (visual disorientation) Disorders in the perception of space, with inability to recognize the position, distance, or size of objects seen, accompanied by disorders of accommodation and of convergence, impairment of visual fixation and absence of the blink reflex.[2958]

Holmes rebound sign See **rebound**.[6062] The rebound is normally present but is exaggerated in spastic limbs and lost in cerebellar disease.

Holmes, Sir Gordon Morgan (1876–1965) Irish neurologist who trained in Dublin and in Germany (with Weigert and Edinger) before taking up junior positions at, and then becoming physician to, the **National Hospital**, Queen Square, between 1909 and 1941. He was elected a fellow of the Royal Society in 1933.[825]

Gordon Holmes, as much as Hughlings-**Jackson**, could be called the father of British neurology and has been described as "the outstanding neurological exponent of the World." Well-grounded in neuroanatomy and neurophysiology after his extensive training in Germany, his life's work reflected his preoccupation with the pathophysiology of disease; the huge advances which he made were the result of close clinical observation and accurate reporting as in the case of the seminal paper on sensation that he wrote with **Head** in 1911, and his papers on signs of spinal cord injury in 1915, on cerebellar disease in 1922, and on neuro-ophthalmology in 1919.

His most triumphant work was performed in field hospitals on the battlefields of northern France where, despite appalling conditions, he and Sir Percy Sargent, his neurosurgical colleague, made painstaking observations which led to numerous papers on neurological localization—studies only made possible by the ambient carnage. They showed, for example, that the upper retina was represented in the upper part of the visual area and the macular area at the pole; and then wrote a landmark paper on cerebellar injuries.[2957, 2965] The collected papers of Holmes have been published.[2964]

A precise and exacting man, he expected from others the standards of observation of which he himself was a master. In the opinion of this author, his book *An Introduction to Clinical Neurology* (Edinburgh, 1946) remains the finest text yet written for those beginning their studies in neurology.

Holmes syndrome A congenital dysmorphic syndrome of modern description, characterized by pes cavus, microcephaly, delayed closure of the fontanelles and mental and developmental delay.[381] See **visual disorientation**.

Holmes tremor See **rubral tremor**.

Holmes–Adie syndrome (Adie syndrome, Kehrer–Adie syndrome, Markus syndrome, Markus–Adie syndrome, Weill–Reys syndrome) The combination of **Adie pupil** and loss of the muscle stretch reflexes, either in the legs or universally, usually occurring in young women.[2960] Adie had also noted the association in his 1931 paper in the *British Medical Journal*.

A *variant* is *Holmes–Adie syndrome with segmental hypohidrosis* (**Ross syndrome**).

Holmes-Logan infantile CNS degeneration An hereditary dysmorphic syndrome of infancy, characterized also by growth failure, optic atrophy, ophthalmoplegia, areflexia, choreoathetosis, and severe mental and motor retardation, noted over the first 3 years of life.[2967]

Holmes–Stewart syndrome See **Jackson cerebellar "fits."**

Holmgren, Alarik Frithiof (1831–1897) Norwegian ophthalmologist and professor of physiology at Uppsala who introduced the wool-skein sorting test for the diagnosis of color-blindness in 1874.

holocarboxylase deficiency 1. (Biotin-responsive multiple carboxylase deficiency) A neonatal disorder due to a deficiency in three biotin-dependent mitochondrial carboxylase enzymes. Onset of symptoms occurs in the neonatal or infantile periods, with metabolic (lactic) acidosis, tachypnea, hypertonia, irritability, lethargy, and coma, responsive to biotin therapy.[4849]

2. Juvenile or late-onset form. See **biotin-responsive encephalopathy**.

holokinetic movements Extensive jerky, abrupt, rapid, and awkward movements of extensive parts of the body, as may occur in some dystonic and dyskinetic states.[4723]

holoprosencephaly (Gr, whole + front + brain) (holotelencephaly, arhinencephaly, telencephalosynapsis) A congenital, heterogeneous but sometimes dominantly inherited dysmorphic anomaly in which the forebrain is not divided by a mid-line fissure. The basal ganglia and thalami may be fused, and the pyramidal tracts are absent in some forms. Clinical manifestations also include hypotelorism, microcephaly, and mental and developmental delay. At least four separate gene mutations are known to be associated. The condition is subdivided according to the degree of completeness of the fusion of the two frontal lobes.[2441]

In the *alobar* form there is a small cerebrum with but a single ventricle, and there are no lobes nor fissures. In the *semilobar* form, there is an incomplete mid-line fissure but the cerebral cortex is in continuity across the mid-line, at least anteriorly. In the *lobar* form, the hemispheres are joined by a band of neocortex at the frontal pole or the orbital surface or over the corpus callosum (**cingulosynapsis**), or are separated but the corpus callosum is absent.

The terminological difficulties of this classification have been discussed.[3508] Various chromosomal syndromes may be associated with this anomaly.[2504]

holoprosencephaly and limb defects See **Steinfeld syndrome**.

holoprosencephaly with congenital heart disease and polydactyly A congenital dysmorphic syndrome characterized by skeletal, genital, and cardiac abnormalities; hydrocephalus; and holoprosencephaly.

holoprosencephaly with endocrine dysgenesis A congenital dysmorphic syndrome characterized by adrenal hypoplasia, hypopituitarism, small sella turcica, and holoprosencephaly.

holotelencephaly See **holoprosencephaly**.

holotopistic striatal degeneration See **hereditary striatal degeneration** and **infantile symmetrical necrosis of the neostriatum**.

Holter valve A pair of stainless steel valves connected by tubing and used in procedures to reduce intracranial pressure by drainage into another body part such as the peritoneum.

Holtermüller syndrome See **cloverleaf skull**.

Holtermüller–Weidermann syndrome See **cloverleaf skull**.

Holt–Oram Syndrome A dominantly inherited syndrome (12q24.1; *TBX5*) characterized by atrial or ventricular septal defects, AV block, skeletal anomalies such as the absence of a thumb or of the radius; or phocomelia; contractures at the elbows or wrists; and absent or hypoplastic muscles such as the thenar, trapezius, and shoulder girdle musculature.

Holzer stain A glial stain using phosphomolybdic acid and crystal violet, useful for showing fibrous astrocytic processes.

Homen, Erst Alexander (1851–1926) Finnish pathologist, professor at Helsingör. His major interest was the pathological anatomy of neurological infections and inherited diseases.

Homen syndrome Generalized rigidity, vertigo, amnesia, apraxia, speech disorders, and progressive dementia occurring with lesions of the lenticular nucleus.[2972]

Homeric laughter A literary allusion to Homer: "Where unextinguished laughter shakes the skies . . ." referring here to episodic outbursts of irrepressible hearty laughter not provoked by any merry ideas, occurring with pseudobulbar palsy resulting from any cause (such as multiple sclerosis or Kuru), and occasionally after prefrontal lobotomy or as an epileptic manifestation. Such **emotionalism** is, however, more usually seen as weeping.[668] See **spasmodic laughter**.

homocarnosinosis A recessively inherited syndrome with onset in childhood or adult life and characterized by hepatosplenomegaly, spastic paraplegia, mental deterioration, and markedly elevated levels of homocarnosine in the CSF.[5878]

homocysteine An essential amino acid, high blood levels of which have been implicated as risk factors for silent brain infarcts and white matter lesions. (Vermeer S, et al. *Ann Neurol* 2002;51:285–9.)

homocystinuria (cystiathionine β-synthetase deficiency, Field syndrome, Carson syndrome) A recessively inherited dysmorphic syndrome with infantile onset, the responsible gene (for cystathionine l: I-synthase) mapping to 21q22.3.

Clinical characteristics include fine fair hair, pale skin with facial flushing, myopia, cataract, dislocation of the lens, optic atrophy and a tendency for multiple cerebrovascular, coronary, and renal arterial occlusions to develop. Mental retardation, various psychiatric disorders including schizophreniform psychosis, seizures, pyramidal signs, dystonias, hepatomegaly, and osteoporosis are also described, as is dislocation of the lenses. Excessive amounts of homocystine are present in the blood and urine.[6749]

Variants are

N-Methylene-tetrahydrofolate methyltransferase deficiency type, in which decreased blood methionine levels occur and megaloblastic anemia is reported, each due to deficiency of this enzyme which is required for the metabolism of homocysteine and for activation of vitamin B12. Clinically, the phenotypes are diverse, but mental retardation, impaired memory, hallucinations, features of **Marfan syndrome**, nystagmus, and ataxia may occur.[1409]

N-Methylene-tetrahydrofolate reductase type, in which there is a failure of homocysteine metabolism in childhood, associated clinically with any combination of pyramidal signs, seizures, myopathy, chorea, and psychosis.[2189]

Homocystinuria with methylmalonic aciduria A combination of the two defects, leading to a syndrome of dystonia with associated megaloblastic anemia.

homolateral ataxia and crural paresis Originally considered to be a **lacunar syndrome** manifesting cerebellar ataxia, weakness, and pyramidal signs involving the limbs of the same side, the leg more than the arm, due to a supratentorial lesion in the capsular–corona region or in the paracentral area supplied by the anterior cerebral artery.[709, 2105] See **ataxic hemiparesis**. The condition may actually be a crossed cerebral–cerebellar **diaschisis**.[2393]

homolateral imitative synkinesis A condition in which voluntary movement of the hand leads to involuntary movement of the homolateral leg, or *vice versa*. The mechanism whereby a contralateral motor pathway lesion causes this is uncertain. See also **mirror movements**.

homologous (Gr, agreeing) The same in value, structure, or position.

homonomous (Gr, subject to the same law) The same on the two sides of the body; similarly constituted.

homonymous (Gr, the same + name) Having the same name, but possibly a different meaning.

homonymous diplopia See **diplopia**.

homonymous hemianopia Loss of vision in the same half-field in each eye due to a lesion at a point in the visual pathway in or behind the lateral geniculate bodies. See also **bitemporal hemianopia, binasal hemianopia**, and **paracentral scotoma**. cf. **bitemporal hemianopia** and **binasal hemianopia**.

homonymous hemianoptic paracentral scotoma A syndrome characterized clinically by difficulty in reading and fixation of objects located close to the central field on the side of the defect, normal visual acuity, and a homonymous scotoma that does not include the macula. There is maintenance of the peripheral field so that vision is retained in that portion of the field that lies between the periphery and the scotoma. The condition usually has a sudden onset and may be due to vascular lesions in or near the lateral geniculate bodies.[135]

homunculus (diminutive of Lat, man) A caricature representing the cortical regions for the various body parts overlying the motor and sensory cortices. The name was adopted despite the ancient assertion of the disciples of **Paracelsus** that a figure so named was produced by digesting semen in a glass, incubated within a dunghill.

Hooft syndrome A recessively inherited disorder of tryptophan metabolism characterized by tapetoretinal degeneration, physical and mental retardation, microcephaly, skin rashes, hypoglycemia and hypolipidemia, and abnormalities of the nails and teeth.[2975]

Hooke, Robert (1635–1703) English scientist who in his *Micrographia* wrote of seeing "little boxes or cells, distinct from one another" under the microscope, thus introducing the concept of the cellular structure of the body.

Hooper, Robert (1773–1835) English physician, practicing in London. Spillane[5978] relates that he performed over 4000 autopsies, gathering his observations into a book *The Morbid Anatomy of the Human Brain* in 1828, which was the first atlas of neuropathology.

Hooper Visual Organization Test A complex, modern, nonverbal test of perceptual processing, wherein the subject is required to assemble mentally the separated parts of a line drawing and to name the object depicted; right hemisphere functions are thus examined.[2977]

Hootnick–Holmes syndrome See **acrocephalopolysyndactyly**.

Hoover, Charles Franklin (1865–1927) American neurologist who diverted to medicine after training for the Methodist ministry. On graduation from Ohio Wesleyan University, he trained in Europe and on his return to America was quickly appointed as physician and teacher of physical diagnosis at Cleveland City Hospital, and later professor of medicine at Western Reserve University. Most of his publications were on cardiorespiratory medicine. He described the Hoover sign in 1908.

Hoover Sign A test of feigned weakness in the legs. It can be elicited in two ways.[242]

1. When a normal subject is asked to *raise*, for example, the right leg off the bed, the left foot will be felt to press down with a similar force as is required to raise the right one. In simulated hemiparesis, when the "normal" leg is raised the "paralysed" leg will show this downward pressure but, in the setting of organic hemiparesis, it will not. In "hysterical" weakness of one leg, the lack of downward pressure by the other (normal) leg suggests that no effort is being made to elevate the affected one. See also **Grasset sign**.

2. A patient's firm voluntary pressure of the sound leg *downward* upon the bed leads to a slight lifting of the other one in normal and also in hemiparetic patients, but such elevation does not occur in patients with hysterical or simulated weakness.[242]

The sign has some validity, but is not always reliable, although Hoover claimed to prefer it to the **Babiński trunk-thigh test**, which he found "unsatisfactory."[2980]

Hopkins Symptom Checklist An assessment tool assessing symptoms in a 57-item questionnaire and providing data on both mental and physical health.

Hopkins syndrome The occurrence of acute flaccid paralysis, resembling poliomyelitis, following an attack of asthma. This is a rare condition, more commonly described in children. Flaccid paralysis, atrophy and fasciculations of one limb, without pain or sensory change, are the typical findings.[1496] An enterovirus other than poliovirus is presumably responsible for both the lower motor neuron lesions and the lower respiratory tract infection which triggered the asthma attack, but the combination of muscle relaxants and steroids is also under scrutiny as a cause.[2988]

The occurrence of **acute myopathy** following treatment of acute asthma with steroids and/or pancuronium has also been reported.[3633] See also **critical care neuropathy** and **postventilatory paretic syndrome**. See **acrodermatitis chronica atrophicans**.

Hopkins Verbal Learning Test A simple, recently developed test of learning and recent memory with six alternate forms, allowing assessment of free recall, recognition, discrimination, and semantic versus serial clustering.[812]

hopping nystagmus See **square-wave jerks**.

horizontal gaze palsy Inability to turn the eyes conjugately to one side, due to a lesion of the pons and the peripontine reticular formation on the same side or to a lesion of the frontal eye field on the other. See also **Vulpian sign**.

horizontal gaze palsy and progressive scoliosis A rare, recessively inherited disorder characterized by absence conjugate lateral eye movements with preserved vertical gaze and progressive scoliosis,[756] but the homozygotic mutations in the *ROBO3* gene have been detected.

horizontal insomnia Back pain made worse by recumbency, requiring that the patient sit up to sleep. The usual cause is the presence of a mobile cauda equina neoplasm which causes complete myelographic block in the supine position.

horizontal nystagmus Nystagmus in which the abnormal eye deviations occur in the horizontal plane.

horn players palsy An **overuse syndrome** presenting with mononeuropathy in the arm.

Horner, Johann Friedrich (1831–1886) Swiss ophthalmologist who trained with von Graefe and was professor in Zurich. In 1869, he gave the first complete description of the ocular changes that occur with sympathetic denervation[2993] (though Claude Bernard had described the same changes in animals 7 years before) and demonstrated that color blindness was a sex-linked characteristic.[2066]

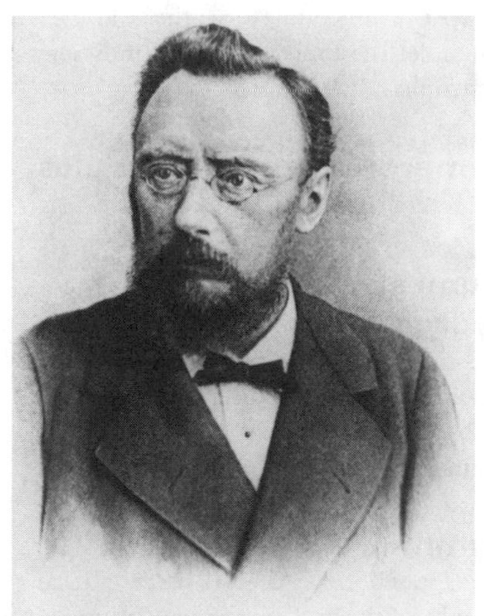

Figure H–6 Johann Friedrich Horner.

Horner syndrome (Bernard–Horner syndrome, oculosympathetic palsy) Reduction in the size of the pupil, both in light and in dark, with narrowing of the palpebral fissure due to ptosis of the upper lid and elevation of the lower due to a lesion at any point along the homolateral sympathetic pathway. Acute lesions affecting the third neuron in the wall of the common carotid artery may also produce temporary flushing and anhidrosis of the same side of the face. Enophthalmos is an associated clinical sign encumbered by subjectivity.

Pharmacological testing assists in localizing the site of the lesion; thus, a brisk constriction with 4% cocaine drops is seen due to denervation hypersensitivity when the lesion affects the third (postganglionic) neuron.

The syndrome was described in animals by Francois **Pourfoir du Petit** in 1727. E.S. Hare[2993] in England (in 1838) and later Claude **Bernard** [582] in France gave precise accounts of the changes before Horner's report in 1869.[2767] An American origination by **Weir Mitchell** is also claimed.[3456]

A *variant* is *dominant congenital Horner syndrome*, in which the lesion is partial and is thought to lie in the middle fossa.[2678]

hornet-sting myopathy An acute myopathy with myoglobinuria due to the venom from the bite of this insect.[5803] See also **Haff disease**.

horopter A set of points in space which pass through the fixation point in a semicircle, concave toward the observer.

Horsley, Sir Victor (1857–1916) Pioneering British neurosurgeon who trained at, and later was on the staff of, University College Hospital and the **National Hospital**, Queen Square from 1886. He performed experiments using brain stimulation in humans[2997] and, in his first year on the staff of the National Hospital, became the first ever to attack an epileptogenic lesion surgically (in a Scottish man of 22 years with scarring after a local infection that had complicated a depressed skull fracture. It was on this occasion that Dr. Hughlings-**Jackson** remarked that Horsley had missed the opportunity of putting a joke into a Scotsman's head).

Horsley also introduced bone wax to seal off the edges of a craniotomy and pioneered other methods of ensuring antisepsis; he attempted to relieve trigeminal neuralgia by posterior fossa exploration, was the first to remove a pinealoma and also to operate in the region of the pituitary, and was a coinventor of a prototype stereotactic frame for intracranial surgery.[2999]

The procedure in 1886 was a spectacular success, as was another he performed in the following year when he successfully removed a spinal fibromyxoma clinically localized by Jackson, but, after another few dozen operations (including one performed on his son who had also developed seizures), Horsley appeared to lose interest in such surgery and turned to medical politics. It was much due to his pressure that regulations were adopted which led to the elimination of **rabies** in England, and he made devoted efforts to improve the regulation of the medical profession, to encourage female suffrage, and to stop vivisection. He was a founder member of the Neurological Society of London and was elected a Fellow of the Royal Society. He volunteered (and was accepted) for military service at the age of 57 and died in Mesopotamia, probably of typhoid or heat stroke, in 1916.[3980, 3981, 6234]

Hortega, Pio del Rio (1882–1945) Spanish neuroanatomist who trained with **Cajal**, in whose laboratory he identified microglial cells and oligodendroglia as a result of improvements which he had made to Cajal's staining techniques. Rio Hortega delayed publication of his findings because they contradicted Cajal's opinions, and, when he did publish, he was dismissed. For

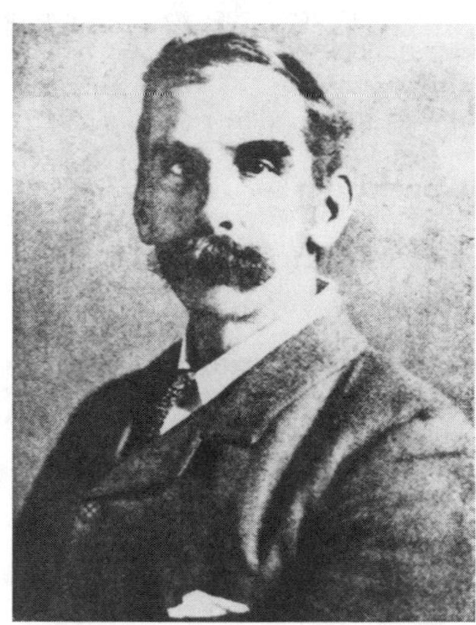

Figure H–7 Sir Victor Horsley.

the remainder of his career he worked elsewhere in Madrid, and (having taken the Republican side in the Spanish Civil War) he went on to work in Paris, Oxford, and Buenos Aires.[2066]

Horton arteritis See **giant cell arteritis**.

Horton, Bayard Taylor (b. 1895) American neurologist at the Mayo Clinic. Apart from his description of **cluster headache**, he is remembered for his identification of the syndrome of **giant cell arteritis**.

Horton headache (syndrome) See **cluster headache**.

hospital addiction See **Munchausen syndrome**.

hot cross bun skull (Parrot sign) Bossing of the frontal bones in congenital syphilis.

hot feet See **burning feet syndrome**.

hot (and dry) foot sign Erythema of the lateral part of the sole of the foot in association with an S1 radiculopathy, which is commonly due to neoplastic lumbosacral plexopathy.

hot water epilepsy (immersion epilepsy) The occurrence of reflex seizures (usually of complex partial type) after the heads of children aged 6 months to 10 years have been bathed in very hot water. Water at colder temperatures or hot water applied to other parts of the body has also been recorded as initiating seizures.[5376] The condition has usually been reported from India.

hot-bath sign See **Uhthoff symptom**.

hour glass tumors See **dumb-bell tumors**.

House classification An arm functional assessment for children with cerebral palsy.[3007]

Houssay syndrome Relief from the signs of diabetes mellitus by naturally occurring extirpation of the anterior pituitary, as by a pituitary adenoma.

The name follows the demonstration that hypophysectomy relieves the hyperglycemia, ketonuria, and fluctuating blood sugar levels and allows survival without insulin for months in pancreatectomized animals.[985]

Howship, J. (1781–1841) An English surgeon.

Howship syndrome See **obturator neuralgia**.

Howship–Romberg syndrome Pain referred to the inside of the knee resulting from irritation of the obturator nerve at the hip, as by a hernia. See **obturator neuralgia**.

Hoyeraal–Hreidarsson syndrome See **cerebellar syndromes** (congenital ataxias).

Hozay–van Bogaert syndrome See **van Bogaert syndrome**.

HRS See **Hamilton Rating Scale**.

HSAN See **hereditary sensory and autonomic neuropathy**.

HTLV See **human T-cell lymphotropic virus**.

HTLV 1-associated myelopathy See **tropical spastic paraparesis**.

Huber, Johann Jacob (1707–1778) Swiss professor of anatomy and botany in Göttingen and later at Cassel.

Huber's ganglion A ganglion in the posterior root of C1, not always present.

Huc–Alajouanine–Gopcevitch syndrome See **Alajouanine syndrome**.

Huchard ataxia Forms of gait disturbance seen in hysterical patients.[3023]

Hughes, C.H. (1839–1916) American neurologist and psychiatrist, professor in St. Louis.

Hughes reflex Downward movement of the penis when the prepuce is pulled upward. The significance of this phenomenon is unclear.

Hughes Scale A rating scale allowing the determination of improvement in patients with acute polyneuropathy, devised by Prof. R.A.C Hughes, a contemporary English neurologist.[3041]

Hughlings-Jackson, J. See **Jackson, J.H-**. Jackson adopted the hyphen and preferred its use in his name.

Huguenin edema Acute congestive cerebral edema.

human African trypanosomiasis (HAT) See **sleeping sickness**.

human pincushion A Bohemian from Prague who had some form of congenital insensitivity to pain and who, in the nineteenth century, staged performances in which objects were thrust through parts of his anatomy to his complete indifference. His performances were temporarily halted by decree when many members of his American audience were cast into a swoon, unable to tolerate his faithful re-enaction of the Crucifixion. See **congenital indifference to pain**.

human T-cell lymphotropic virus (HTLV) A RNA retrovirus with at least three types, capable of inducing human "slow virus" neurological disease. Visna, AIDS, and HTLV-1-associated myelopathy (**tropical spastic paraparesis**) are representative disorders.

humeroperoneal myopathy A dominantly inherited form of proximal myopathy which in every other way resembles the **Emery–Dreifuss muscular dystrophy**.[2377]

humeroradial synostosis plus See **Keutel syndrome**.

Humes melanosis and hydrocephalus syndrome A congenital dysmorphic syndrome manifesting also microcephaly, hydrocephalus, and patchy skin pigmentation.[381]

hummingbird sign (penguin sign) The appearance on the MRI scan of focal atrophy of the mid-brain tegmentum as seen in a lateral view in **progressive supranuclear palsy**.[5648]

humors The four fluids, yellow and black bile, phlegma and blood, which were thought in Galenical medicine to produce disease when present in abnormal proportions or when themselves abnormal.

Humpty-Dumpty syndrome A form of disability neurosis, the subject appearing unable to believe in his recovery.[2152]

hung-up reflexes Persistent contraction of a muscle stimulated by a tap on its tendon; this is seen both in chorea when involuntary contraction of the muscle interrupts the relaxation phase and also in hypothyroidism.

hunkering A test of virility in parts of the southern United States, the competitors trying to remain longest in the squatting position. See **sciatic neuropathy**.

Hunt, James Ramsay See **Ramsay Hunt, J.** Hunt did not assume a hyphen and it would be reasonable to place entries concerning him here, except that the compound name is so universally employed.

Hunt juvenile paralysis agitans See **Parkinsonism plus** and **juvenile Parkinsonism syndromes**.

Hunt epilepsy Pyridoxine-dependent seizures, described by Dr. A.D. Hunt and others in 1954.[3046]

Hunt paralysis See **juvenile Parkinsonism syndromes**.

Hunter, C.H. (1872–1955) Scottish-Canadian physician, professor of medicine at Manitoba. His single description of two Canadian brothers with the disease named for him was published in 1917 while he was in England, 2 years before the report of Gertrud Hurler from Munich.

Hunter oculoencephalohepatorenal syndrome A congenital dysmorphic syndrome of recent description, characterized by retinal colobomas, strabismus, cerebellar, and extrapyramidal signs, and mental and developmental delay.[381]

Hunter syndrome Deficiency of iduronate sulfatase, inherited as a sex-linked recessive trait. Severe and mild forms are distinguished, with optic atrophy, pigmentary retinal degeneration, deafness, and nodular skin lesions; mental retardation, spinal flexion deformities, and cataracts are not seen until later, if at all.[3055] See **mucopolysaccharidoses**.

Hunter–McAlpine syndrome A congenital dysmorphic syndrome manifesting also short stature, ptosis, skeletal malformations, microcephaly, craniosynostosis affecting the coronal sutures, and mental and developmental delay.[3054]

Hunt–Hess Scale A scale in common use for recording the status of patients with **subarachnoid hemorrhage**, introduced in 1968.[3052] See chart H–21.

Huntington, George Sumner (1851–1916) A general practitioner who was born into a family tradition of care for the people of East Hampton, Long Island. After receiving a classical education and medical training at the New York College of Physicians and Surgeons, he described the familial dementia now named for him, briefly but completely[3056] within a year of graduation, while practicing in Ohio. Here, apart from 2 years spent in North Carolina (for the good of his health) he remained for the rest of his professional life without making any further notable contributions to the medical literature.

Huntington Association (International) A federation of national voluntary health agencies that share common concern for individuals with Huntington Disease and their families. Each agency promotes lay and professional education; individual and family support; psycho-social, clinical and biomedical research; and ethical and legal considerations related to the disease in its respective country. Web site: http://www.huntington-assoc.com/.

Huntington disease A progressive, autosomal dominantly inherited neurodegenerative disorder due to expansion of a CAG trinucleotide repeat in exon 1 of the gene coding for the huntingtin gene on chromosome 4p16.3, while another Huntington-like syndrome is mapped to 20p.[4065] Mutations are rare and penetrance is complete. ("Unstable and whimsical as the disease may be in other respects, in this it is firm, it never skips a generation to again manifest itself in another; once having yielded its claims, it never regains them."[3056])

The clinical features are usually manifest in the third to fifth decades; they include abnormal movements (chorea), deterioration in personality and in cognitive abilities, and psychiatric disturbances. Neuropsychological deficits include slowness of thought, learning failures, and inability to shift mental set or attention, traditionally regarded as cortical functions but now shown to correlate better with atrophy of the caudate nucleus. Explosive dysarthria, impaired eye movement control, hypotonia with hyperreflexia, and later bradykinesia with rigidity, cachexiadysphagia, and urinary incontinence are other unwelcome manifestations.

Pathologically, there is loss of neurons from the neostriatum and cortex, especially the frontal cortex.

Chart H–21. Status of Patients with Intracranial Aneurysm with and without Subarachnoid Hemorrhage. (Hunt–Hess Scale)

Grade	Symptoms and Signs
0.	Unruptured aneurysm–no history nor other manifestation of subarachnoid hemorrhage.
1.	Asymptomatic or minimal headache and slight nuchal rigidity.
1a.	No acute meningeal or brain reaction, but fixed neurological deficit.
2.	Moderate to severe headache, nuchal rigidity, no neurological deficit other than cranial nerve palsy.
3.	Drowsiness, confusion, or mild focal neurological deficit.
4.	Stupor, moderate to severe hemiparesis; may also include early decerebrate rigidity and vegetative disturbances.
5.	Deep coma, decerebrate rigidity, moribund appearance.

From Hunt HE, Hess RM. Surgical risks as related to time of intervention in the repair of intracranial aneurysms. J Neurosurg *1968;28:14–20. Reproduced by permission.*

The disease had been known to many generations of the family that Huntington described and was known as "magrums" or "megrims" to the people of colonial New England; many affected subjects were burnt as witches, as it was popularly believed in those days that the families in which the disease appeared were cursed because they had dared to pantomime Christ's sufferings on the cross in this derisory manner. Thilenius reported a case in 1816, Rufs another in 1834, and Waters yet another, published in Robley Dunglison's *Practice of Medicine* in 1842 (Vol 2, p. 312). It formed the subject of an inaugural thesis (now lost) by Charles Rollin Gorman of Lucerne, Pennsylvania in 1848 and was again reported by Irving Lyon in the *American Medical Times* of 1863. References to Huntington disease appeared in the German literature in 1885 and 1887, since when the eponym has been firmly established.[6741] The disease was imported to America from Bures in Suffolk, UK, by the wife of a young Englishman in 1630; the match was disapproved of by his family (her father was choreic), but he married her anyway and emigrated.

Diagnostic criteria have been defined as follows:[2149]

Definite Huntington disease: 1. Chorea or the characteristic impairment of voluntary movement, which was not present at birth, was insidious in onset, and had gradually become worse; and 2. A family history of at least one other member with these typical symptoms of the disease. Dementia and emotional symptoms are usually present but are not required and are not alone sufficient for the diagnosis.

Probable Huntington disease: The clinical features as above, but with a family history that is unobtainable because of adoption or unknown parentage.

In early cases, impairment of movements requiring rhythm and speed, slow voluntary (saccadic) eye movements, mild speech abnormalities, impaired balance on tandem walking, and bradykinesia occur. In advanced cases, severe slowing or absence of both saccades and pursuit eye movements, severe dysarthria or mutism, inability to walk, long tract motor signs, and extreme slowing of all movements are evident. *Variants* are listed in Chart H–22.

The Web site http://neuroregeneration.org/ provides information on Huntington disease and other neural degenerations with full text research papers and other publications.

Chart H–22. Variants of Huntington disease

hereditary nonprogressive chorea (*hereditary nonprogressive chorea without dementia*) A dominantly inherited syndrome characterized by the onset in childhood of chorea in the face and arms, with the later appearance of dysarthria and axial dystonia and without dementia, rigidity, seizures, or cerebellar ataxia.[2675, 3611] In a further subgroup, progression does occur.[5576]

Familial essential benign chorea A dominantly inherited syndrome of nonprogressive chorea, sometimes with added **essential tremor**.[656, 5033] This and the last condition listed are not clearly distinguished.

Huntington chorea, myoclonic variant A cause of very atypical **progressive myoclonic epilepsy**.

Juvenile Huntington disease (rigid or Westphal variant) A form characterized by the onset in youth of a rigid-akinetic syndrome with minimal chorea, but with bradykinesia and severe cognitive impairment. Seizures and myoclonus are also described. The clinical course thereafter resembles that of the later-onset form. This *variant* is more likely to occur in cases with paternal transmission.[2426]

Spinal muscular atrophy with ***Huntington disease*** See **motor neuronal diseases**.

A Huntington-like syndrome mapped to 20p.

Huntington disease-like 2 (HDL2) A condition that may present as dominant **chorea-acanthocytosis**, with which it appears to overlap since both have a CTG trinucleotide repeat expansion mutation of the *junctophilin-3* gene.[6601]

Huntington sign

When a patient is asked to cough forcibly when lying supine with the legs over the side of the bed, the hip will flex and the knee extend on the side of a pyramidal lesion.

Huntington Society of Canada

A charitable organization. Address: 151 Frederick, St. Suite 400 Kitchener, Ontario N2H 2M2. Tel: 519-749-7063. Web site: http://www.hsc-ca.org/.

Huntington Study Group

An international professional organization. Web site: www.huntington-study-group.org/.

Huntington's Disease Association

A UK-based charitable organization.Address: 108, Battersea High Street, London SW11 3HP, UK. Tel: 0171-223-7000. Web site: http://www.hda.org.uk/.

Huntington's Disease Society of America

A charitable organization. Address: 158 West 29th St., 7th Floor New York, NY 10001-5300. Tel. 212-242-1968; 1-800-345-HDSA. Web site: http://www.hdsa.org/.

Hunt–van Bogaert syndrome

See **pure pallidal atrophy**.

Hurler, Gertrud

(1889–1965) German pediatrician who trained at Munich and worked in Neuhauser.

Hurler syndrome

See **mucopolysaccharidoses**.

Hurler syndrome variant

See **neurovisceral lipidosis**.

Hurler–Scheie syndrome

See **mucopolysaccharidoses**.

Hurst disease

(hemorrhagic leukoencephalitis) See **acute hemorrhagic encephalomyelitis**.

Hutchinson, Sir Jonathan

(1828–1913) English surgeon, dermatologist, and ophthalmologist at the London Hospital and professor at the Royal College of Surgeons. He was elected a fellow of the Royal Society in 1882 and was knighted 5 years before his death. His interests were legion, as may be deduced from the following entries, but he was especially interested in syphilis and was said to have gained experience from a million patients with that disorder;[2066] but even assuming 40 years in practice, 50 weeks a year, and 5 days a week, this translates into 100 patients per day, which is ridiculous.

Hutchinson facies

Extension of the neck and contraction of the frontalis muscles in an attempt to compensate for the ptosis of **tabes dorsalis**.

Hutchinson–Gilford syndrome

See **progeria**.

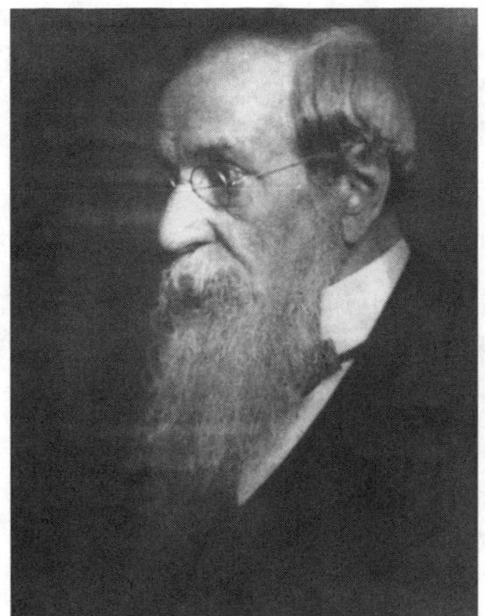

Figure H–8 Sir Jonathan Hutchinson.

Hutchinson pupil Unilateral dilatation of a pupil with impaired light and accommodation reactions due to compression of the parasympathetic fibers in the III cranial nerve, as caused by a swollen herniating temporal lobe. Initially the affected pupil may constrict due to irritation of the nerve, dilating later and finally becoming fixed.

The same pattern of events may occur with a time lag in the other eye as a result of the stretching of its III nerve as the brainstem also herniates downward.

Hutchinson teeth Notching of the permanent incisors in congenital syphilis.[3062] With interstitial keratitis and bilateral nerve deafness, this constitutes the **Hutchinson triad**.

Hutchinson triad Interstitial keratitis, notching of the central incisors and nerve deafness, occurring in congenital syphilis.[3061]

Hutchinson, Sir Robert (1871–1943) Scottish radiologist, who investigated the use of radium implants in the management of bladder cancers.

Hutchinson tumor Neuroblastoma of the left adrenal gland with a secondary deposit in the orbit, less often in other cranial areas, occurring in infants and young children who present with proptosis, papilledema or optic atrophy, and frequently extraocular palsies.

The right-sided tumor metastasizes to the liver.[3064]

hyaline body myopathy (myopathy with lysis of type I myofibrils, myosin storage myopathy) (14q11, *myosin-cardiac β heavy chain MYH7* mis-sense mutations) A sporadic or dominantly inherited set of slowly progressive myopathies, characterized by the early onset of hypotonia and delayed motor milestones, proximal more than distal symmetrical scapuloperoneal weakness, sometimes with cardiac arrhythmias. The serum creatine kinase is normal or slightly elevated and the EMG myopathic. Muscle biopsy shows subsarcolemmal eosinophilic hyaline bodies, mostly in type I fibers.[4161] See also **scapuloperoneal muscular dystrophy** and **myosin storage myopathy**.

hyalinosis cutis et mucosae See **Urbach–Wiethe disease**.

hyaloid remnants Residua of the embryonic vascular channels in the eye which may overlie the optic disk, causing apparent blurring on ophthalmoscopy.

Hyams cerebral palsy and glaucoma syndrome A congenital syndrome manifesting short stature, buphthalmos, spasticity, and mental and developmental delay.[381]

hydantoin-barbiturate-carbamazepine embryofoetopathy See **fetal anticonvulsant syndrome**.

hydranencephaly (hydroanencephaly) An uncommon congenital abnormality consisting of more or less complete replacement of the cerebral hemispheres by fluid, contained within a thin-walled capsule composed of glial tissue and meninges. The normally sized skull thus transilluminates brilliantly. It occurs as the result of a severe ischemic cerebral lesion, usually in carotid territory, during the fifth month of intrauterine development. **Cruvheilier** gave the first description in 1829.[1366]

hydrargyria Mercury poisoning.

hydrencephaloid See **Hall syndrome**.

hydro-anencephaly See **hydranencephaly**.

hydrocephalus (Gr, water + brain) (hydrocrania) Dilatation of the cerebral ventricles, first described by Vesalius in 1550 but known to the Hippocratic authors. In *internal hydrocephalus*, there is an obstruction to the flow of CSF somewhere between its site of production in the ventricles and the subarachnoid space in the posterior fossa. In *external hydrocephalus*, the obstruction is between the roof foramina of the fourth ventricle and the arachnoid granulations in the dural venous sinuses.

Although grossly, though accurately, described by Vesalius, it was Morgagni (1682–1771) who in 1769 noted the occurrence in young children, comprising cranial enlargement, separation of the sutures, thinning of the skull, dilatation of the lateral ventricles, and a normal cerebellum and brainstem. One of his patients undoubtedly had a **Chiari malformation**.[6354]

In a *variant X-linked form*, the responsible gene maps to Xq28.

See also the Web site: http://www.ninds.nih.gov/disorders/hydrocephalus/hydrocephalus/.

Hydrocephalus Association A charitable organization in this field. Address: 870 Market St. Suite, 705, San Francisco, CA 94102. Tel: 415-732-7040; 888-598-3789. E-mail: hydroassoc@aol.com. Web site: http://www.hydroassoc.org/.

hydrocephalus, agyria, retinal dysplasia, and encephalocele syndrome (HARD+E syndrome, Warburg syndrome) See **Walker–Warburg syndrome**.

hydrocephalus ex vacuo (external hydrocephalus) An increase in the volume of CSF resulting solely from independent atrophy of brain tissue. See **normal pressure hydrocephalus**.

Hydrocephalus Support Group, Inc. A charitable organization in this field providing information and support. E-mail: dhydrobuff@aol.com. Web site: http://www.ninds.nih.gov/find_people/voluntary_orgs/volorg870.htm/.

hydrocephalus with polydactyly (Biemond syndrome, definition 2) A syndrome of hydrocephalus, iris colobomata, hypogenitalism, polydactyly, mental retardation, and obesity.[630]

hydrocephalus-costovertebral dysplasia with Sprengel deformity See **Waaler anomaly**.

hydrocrania See **hydrocephalus**.

hydrolethalus syndrome A recessively inherited dysmorphic syndrome characterized also by hydrocephalus; cardiac, renal, genital, and skeletal malformations; and a tendency to die in utero or shortly after birth.[5515]

hydromyelia (Gr, water + marrow) The term applied by Olliver d'Angers in 1827 to cystic dilatation of the central canal of the spinal cord. The condition is usually congenital and results from increased pressure of CSF in the fourth ventricle and hypertrophic arachnoiditis of its roof, as with a **Chiari malformation**.

hydrophobia (Gr, water + fear) The repulsion for water or any fluid to drink, manifest by those about to die from **rabies**, owing to the violent paroxysms of muscle contraction which the sufferer now knows will follow any attempt to swallow.

hydrops (Lat, dropsy) See **idiopathic intracranial hypertension**.

hydrostatic cerebral edema Excessive water content of the brain extracellular space, usually as a result of increased intravascular pressure, as in hypertensive encephalopathy.

hydroxyamphetamine test (paredrine test) One drop of 1% hydroxyamphetamine solution is instilled into the eye. A normal pupil will not respond by dilating, but the pupil on the side of a lesion of the first- or second-order sympathetic neuron will.

The drug releases vesicles of stored norepinephrine from the healthy nerve terminals of the long ciliary nerves, but at 1% it is insufficient to result in dilatation of the pupil in normal subjects and those with a first-order sympathetic neuron lesion but will do so in those with a lesion of the third-order neuron in the sympathetic pathway to the eye. See also **cocaine test**.

hydroxyisovaleric aciduria A disorder of branched-chain amino acid metabolism considered due to deficiency of dimethylacrylyl coenzyme A-carboxylase, characterized clinically by the features of hereditary motor neuropathy, and notable for the infant's strong odor of cat urine.[6069]

hydroxykynureninemia A rare syndrome in infancy characterized by mental retardation, hemolytic anemia, and hepatosplenomegaly in the presence of excessive urinary excretion of xanthenuric acid and hydroxykynurenine.[1409]

3-hydroxy-3-methyl coenzyme A lysase deficiency A rare disorder resulting from a failure of leucine catabolism, and characterized clinically by acidosis, hypoglycemia, hypotonia, seizures, and progressive reduction of consciousness in infancy or childhood.[1974]

hygroma A fluid-filled cavity. Those in the subdural space have usually followed trauma or meningitis.

Hyndham sign See **head flexion test**.

hyp- (Gr, A diminution) Prefix denoting diminution.

hypacusis Diminution in hearing.

hypalgesia (Gr, under + sense of pain) (hypalgia) A diminution in the perception of pain.

hypalgia See **hypalgesia**.

hyper- (Gr, over, in excess of) Prefix denoting excess.

hyperabduction syndrome See **thoracic outlet syndrome**.

hyperacusis Abnormal perception of sounds as being loud. Increased keenness of hearing for quiet sound stimuli is not associated. This is a common symptom in patients with migraine attacks and with any disease causing cerebral irritability such as meningitis.

hyperaldosteronism Increased production of aldosterone, usually due to an adenoma of the adrenal cortex in adults. A neurological complication is a myasthenia-like syndrome appearing as intermittent severe weakness or paralysis, associated with tetany, paresthesias and hypertension. Raised sodium and reduced potassium and magnesium serum levels are also present and a vacuolar myopathy may also be associated.[1927]

hyperalgesia (hyperalgia) An abnormally increased response to a stimulus which normally is indeed painful. In the primary form, it is due to sensitization of the C-fibers and occurs within the area of injury while the secondary form is caused by sensitization of dorsal column neurons and occurs remote from the injured site.

hyperalgia See **hyperalgesia**.

hyperammonemia-orthinemia-homocitrullinuria (HHH) syndrome (OMIM 238970) A recessively inherited inborn error of metabolism in which there is impairment of transport of ornithine across the inner mitochondrial membrane. Clinically it is expressed in childhood and characterized by vomiting, irritability, seizures, and ataxia in the first year of life and by hyperammomnemia, homocitrullinuria, gyrate atrophy of the choroid and retina with visual field constriction, myopia, pyramidal signs, ataxia, myoclonic seizures, episodic disturbances of consciousness due to intermittent hyperammonemia, and mental retardation.[379, 5802] The responsible affected *ORNT1* gene maps to chromosome 13q14.[6410] See also **ornithinemia**.

hyperammonemias A group of inherited disorders involving any of the five enzymes of the urea cycle and presenting as intermittent ataxic syndromes associated with elevated serum ammonia levels and leading to diffuse encephalopathies. **Arginase deficiency**, **argininosuccinuria**, **citrullinemia**, **carbamyl-phosphate synthetase deficiency**, **hyperornithinemia**, and **ornithine transcarbamoylamase deficiency** are described.[5935, 442] Levels of ammonia are also raised in **pyruvate carboxylase deficiency**.

The usual presentation is of a catastrophic illness in the first week of life with poor suck, hypotonia, vomiting, lethargy, and hyperventilation, progressing to seizures and eventually to coma. The EEG shows low voltage with theta and delta activity. Imaging suggests the presence of cerebral edema.

Individuals with partial syndromes present later in childhood with anorexia, ataxia, behavioral disturbances, and hyperactivity. In adult life the features include migrainous headaches, nausea, dysarthria, confusion, hallucinations, papilledema, visual impairment, episodic ataxia, pyramidal signs, decerebrate/decorticate posturing, and coma. Hyperammonemic episodes tend to be precipitated by high protein meals, infections, surgery, and pregnancy or delivery.[442]

hyperammonemic syndromes See also **cerebellar ataxias** (*variants*).

hyperaphia Increased sensibility to touch.

hyper-β-alaninemia An aminoaciduria due to deficiency of β-alanine α-ketoglutarate transaminase, characterized by infantile seizures and by elevations in the plasma and urine levels of β-alanine and β-immunoisobutyric acid.[5698]

hypercapnic headache (mixed hypoxia and hypercapnia) A metabolic cause of headache resembling **migraine** included in that category of the International Headache Society's Classification (see Chart H–5) as are **hypoglycemic** and **dialysis headaches**.

hypercolumn The alternating arrangements of the columns of cells in the cortex, each column having a specific receptivity to inputs at different orientations.

hyperconvergence Spasm of the muscles producing convergence.[2086]

hyperCKemia Elevation of serum creatine kinase levels above 500 UI/l.This may reflect the presence of a neuromuscular disorder, endocrinopathy, alcoholism, prolonged exercise, muscle trauma, infections, or malignancy. It also occurs in healthy people,among whom 40% remain undiagnosed.[2020]

hyperdense MCA sign Unusual density of the middle cerebral artery on neuroimaging, highly suggestive of embolic or atherothrombotic MCA occlusion in the appropriate clinical context but not specific when present in isolation. It is likely due to calcium or to the hemorrhagic components of the acute plaque. False-positive hyperdensity may be seen in asymptomatic patients with a high hematocrit or calcific atherosclerotic disease.

hyperdense Sylvian fissure branch sign Hyperdensity on CT scans of the more distal branches of the middle cerebral artery in the Sylvian fissure within hours of their embolic occlusion.

hyperdynamia Abnormally increased strength.

hyperechogenic rim The appearance on carotid ultrasound of a hyperintense rim surrounding an adherent internal carotid artery thrombus after treatment with intravenous heparin.[3304]

hyperekplexia (stiff baby syndrome) A rare, dominantly (seldom recessively) inherited syndrome with incomplete penetrance which in its major form comprises an excessive **startle response** to unheralded sensory stimuli and generalized stiffness and transient hypertonia from early infancy; falling attacks ("falling like a log") without unconsciousness, often leading to injuries such as concussion; nocturnal leg jerking; episodic generalized shaking resembling generalized spontaneous clonus or repetitive myoclonus; generalized hyperreflexia; an insecure and hesitating or puppetlike gait due to fear of falling, all in the absence of gross brain pathology. The episodes are maximal at night. Seizures and mental retardation are inconstant features.[2766] There is an increased incidence of associated neurologic and electroencephalographic abnormalities

The pattern of muscle recruitment suggests that the condition represents a widespread elevated gain of the vestigial withdrawal reflexes in the brainstem and spinal cord due to increased excitability of the reticular neurons.[4171] The condition has been mapped to 5q33–q35, involving the glycine receptor α-1 subunit, binding strychnine.

Excessive startle was identified as leading to seizures by Alajouanine and Gastaut, but it was later recognized that a nonepileptic surprise reaction also exists.

In *variant* minor forms, an inconstant excessive startle response brought out by a febrile illness and in adults by emotional stress and improving with time is the only feature,[189] or the clinical manifestations first appear in youth.

hyperemesis gravidarum A syndrome of recurrent vomiting occurring in the first trimester of pregnancy, but occasionally persisting thereafter and liable to be complicated by vitamin deficiency and **Wernicke–Korsakoff syndrome**.

hyperendorphin syndrome of necrotizing encephalopathy A *variant* of **subacute necrotizing encephalomyelopathy** characterized by attacks resembling acute morphine poisoning with prolonged apnea and unconsciousness, temporarily reversible with nalorphine. The postmortem brain changes are the same as those of the parent syndrome.[815]

hyperesthesia 1. The term of Henry **Head** for a most unpleasant prolonged stinging sensation felt in areas sensitive to pinprick but not to light touch; it follows peripheral nerve injury and is due to a loss of the normal inhibitory effects of local touch receptors. 2. An increased sensitivity to sensory stimuli, often with an added unpleasant quality. **Hyperpathia** has the same meaning. 3. Increased sensitivity (decreased threshold) to a stimulus.

hyperflexion-hyperextension syndrome See **acceleration injury syndrome**.

hypergeusia A morbid sensitivity to taste sensations—more a disorder of reaction than one of sensation, as taste thresholds are not necessarily affected.

hyperglycinemia An inborn error of metabolism causing both a primary organic acidemia and a secondary defect in the metabolism of glycine. The *nonketotic* form is due to a primary error in the metabolism of glycine; the *ketotic* form (see **proprionic academia**) is due to an error in proprionic acid metabolism, but their features are similar.

Micrencephaly, severe hypomyelination of those systems which myelinate only after birth, and spongy degeneration of the brain are the pathological characteristics; lethargy, myoclonus and epileptic seizures, and progression to decerebration and death after only one or two days of normal development after birth are the usual findings.[5816] The condition may also occur as a response to therapy with sodium valproate.

In a *variant* form, the hyperglycinuria is paroxysmal and associated with **paroxysmal kinesigenic dystonia**.

hypergraphia (echographia, graphomania, anosognosic graphopmimia, graphoreé, phonographie) 1. A disturbance of writing seen in patients with right hemisphere lesions, characterized by writing on the right side of the paper only, inability to maintain a straight line, and the repetition of letters.[6896, 6507] This syndrome is known as *multiple loop agraphia*. 2. Unusually detailed and copious but graphically normal writing observed as a compulsive phenomenon in patients with complex partial seizures[6677] or with frontal lobe dementia.[3347]

A distinction between hypergraphia as defined here and "automatic writing behavior" has been suggested,[6507] although the value of this remains unproven.

hyperhidrosis Morbidly increased sweating. See also **episodic hyperhidrosis**.

hyperhomoctstinemia A monogenic disorder with genetic heterogeneity, mapped to 1p36.3; predisposing the subject to stroke[2669] and to dementia.

hyperinsulin neuronopathy A motor axonal neuropathy associated with excessive insulin production.[4536]

hyperkalemic periodic paralysis See **familial periodic paralysis**.

hyperkalemic periodic paralysis with dysrhythmias (Andersen syndrome) See **familial periodic paralysis**.

hyperkeratosis–syringomyelia See **Fischer syndrome**.

hyperkinesia (Gr, above + movement) A condition in which a subject makes excessive and even continuous movements, these themselves not necessarily being abnormal. Examples are **paroxysmal kinesiogenic choreoathetosis, paroxysmal nonkinesiogenic choreoathetosis,** and **stiff person syndrome**.

hyperkinetic automatism In the context of epilepsy, irregular sequential ballistic movements such as pedaling, pelvic thrashing, or rocking movements, predominantly of proximal limbs or of the axial muscles.

hyperkinetic seizures (hypermotor seizures) Seizures of frontal lobe origin, manifesting bilateral forceful limb movements, sometimes with vocalizations.[1861]

hyperkinetic state A condition of childhood in which the patient manifests stimulus-oriented behavior, distractibility, shortened attention span, lack of tolerance of frustration, and lack of fear. See **attention deficit disorder**.

hyperkinetic tremor See **cerebellar tremors**.

hyperlexia 1. The presence of outstanding reading ability in brain-damaged children before having had formal instruction, who otherwise manifest retardation in the normal development of language, with failure of spontaneous speech, dysarthria, echolalia, and evidence of a hyperkinetic syndrome. Its occurrence is part of the continuum of **autism**. An associated to-and-fro rocking movement during reading is nearly invariable and the childs drive to examine and read written material is at times compulsive.[4282] 2. The acquisition of reading skills at an unusually early age.[11] 3. The protracted, quasi-obsessional reading of written material, as evidenced by writers of books like this.

hyperlysinemia A hyperammonemic syndrome characterized by failure to thrive, hypotonia due to lax ligaments, and seizures occurring in infancy.[2346] Mental retardation is common but not invariable, and a few normal children with this condition have been reported.

hypermetamorphosis The tendency to change behaviors unusually quickly; a feature of the **Kluver–Bucy syndrome**.

hypermethioninemia A rare, fatal, diffuse encephalopathy occurring in infancy, probably a variant of hereditary tyrosinemia. It is characterized clinically by irritability, lethargy, and intracranial hemorrhage.[1409]

hypermetria An excessive range of movement of a limb due to a delay in starting and then in completing the arrest of a limb in its trajectory toward a target.[2962] It appears to be based upon misjudgment of the required point of arrest of a limb during extension (overshoot) which is a sign of cerebellar disease affecting the lateral lobes.

hypermetric saccades A normal single saccade which only stops past the point of fixation of the desired target (overshooting), requiring thus a further small corrective saccade in order to place the image of the target back on the fovea (a refixation eye movement). See also **hypometric saccades** and **pulse dysmetria**.

hypermnesia A rare condition of abnormally enhanced memory, met with occasionally in *idiots savants*.

hypermotor seizures See **hyperkinetic seizures**.

hypernormal CT scans CT scan images in which the sulci are narrow and the ventricles small, not because the brain is normal but because of the presence of chronic bilateral isodense subdural hematomas.[3137]

hyperopia (Gr, above + the eye) Far-sightedness (in the ophthalmological sense), in which the entering rays are focused behind the retina due to inadequate refraction by the media.

hyperopsia Abnormally acute vision.

hyperornithinemia A rare, hyperammonemic syndrome of childhood presenting with irritability, ataxia, constriction of the visual fields, and myoclonus. The precise biochemical abnormality is unknown.[2754] See **HHH syndrome**.

In a *variant* form, there is associated gyrate atrophy of the retina with optic atrophy.

hyperornithinemia, hyperammonemia, homocitrullinemia syndrome See **HHH syndrome**.

hyperosmia 1. Abnormal sensitivity in the realm of odor detection. 2. Increased sensitivity to the qualities of odors without any decrease in the threshold for their detection. This latter definition represents the current usage of the word.

hyperosmolar diabetic nonketotic coma A life-threatening endocrine emergency characterized by drowsiness passing into coma with severe fluid depletion, electrolyte disturbance, and profound hyperglycemia, usually in older type 2 diabetics. Diagnostic criteria include extreme hyperglycemia with serum glucose >33 mmol/l, increased serum osmolality >320 mmol/kg, mild ketoacidosis with <3+ urinary ketones, and serum ketones <5 mmol/l. The arterial pH is >7.2 and bicarbonate >15 mmol/l, unlike in diabetic ketoacidosis in which there is significant metabolic acidosis.

The lack of ketogenesis is due to the presence of low levels of endogenous insulin, sufficient to inhibit lipolysis but not gluconeogenesis. Precipitants include infection, stroke, intercurrent illness, noncompliance with diabetic treatment, alcohol abuse, myocardial ischemia, acute gastrointestinal illness, and surgically induced stress.[6329]

hyperostosis 1. Bony overgrowths or excrescences. 2. Thickening of normal bone as in **hyperostosis frontalis interna**.

hyperostosis corticalis generalisata congenita (dominant osteosclerosis, Caffey Silverman syndrome) The milder, dominantly inherited form of **endosteal hyperostosis** characterized by hyperostosis and osteosclerosis of the skull, mandible, and other parts of the skeleton, and commonly complicated by VII and VIII cranial nerve deficits.[6874] See also **hyperostosis corticalis generalisata familiaris**.

hyperostosis corticalis generalisata familiaris (van Buchem syndrome, chronic hyperphosphatemia tarda) The severe autosomal recessive form of **endosteal hyperostosis** characterized by hyperostosis and osteosclerosis of the skull, mandible, and other parts of the skeleton, commonly complicated by VII and VIII cranial nerve deficits, and occasionally by increased intracranial pressure and optic nerve involvement.[928, 6474]

hyperostosis cranialis interna A dominantly inherited hyperostotic and osteosclerotic disease with onset in youth, manifesting intracranial hyperostosis, osteosclerosis of the calvaria, and skull base only, recurrent facial palsy and variable involvement of cranial nerves I, II, and VIII.[4045]

hyperostosis frontalis interna (Morgagni–Stewart–Morel syndrome, calvarial hyperostosis) Thickening and condensation of the frontal bones, seen almost exclusively in females. Obesity and hypertrichosis but no neurological deficits accompany this phenomenon, although all manner of troubles were ascribed to it by Morgagni (1761).

A *variant* is *hyperostosis frontalis interna with cataracts*, a congenital dysmorphic syndrome characterized also by skeletal deformities, cataract, strabismus, short neck, thick calvarium, fasciculations, and mental and developmental delay.[381]

hyperoxaluria type 1 (glycolic aciduria) A recessively inherited **peroxisomal disorder** resulting from a deficiency of alanine glyoxalate aminotransferase and characterized by hyperoxaluria, hyperglycolic aciduria, the formation of calcium oxalate stones in the urine, and nephrocalcinosis.[1446]

Combined axonal and demyelinating polyneuropathy, causing painful paresthesias or weakness, is a noted complication.[2688] Renal failure usually leads to death before the end of the second decade.

hyperparathyroid myopathy A syndrome consisting of fatigue, wasting, quadriceps weakness with intact reflexes, and skeletal pain, occurring in the presence of a parathyroid adenoma.[1163]

hyperparathyroidism Overactivity of the parathyroid glands, leading to proximal and bulbar muscle weakness, wasting, aching, and fatigue with hyperactive muscle stretch reflexes. The findings in osteomalacia are similar.[5927] More severe neurological disturbances, including ataxia, **internuclear ophthalmoplegia**, and pyramidal signs have also been reported.[4932]

hyperpathia (Gr, excessive + pain) 1. Great torment of mind. 2. Delay in the perception of a stimulus with an after-sensation and overreaction to the painful stimulus, as frequently occurs in association with **causalgia**. **Hyperesthesia** has the same meaning and represents the current usage of the term. 3. A painful syndrome of increased reaction to a stimulus in association with a raised threshold for perception of that stimulus.

hyperphagia Pathological overeating, as may result from some hypothalamic lesions. See **bulimia**.

hyperphenylalaninemia Diffuse encephalopathies occurring in a number of conditions, such as **phenylketonuria, dihydropteridine** and **dihydrobiopterin synthetase deficiency, persistent hyperphenylalaninemia,** and **phenylalanine transferase deficiency**, in all of which there is an abnormality of the phenylalanine hydroxylase enzymic system.[1409]

hyperphoria A latent tendency for one eye to deviate to a position above that assumed by the other.

hyperpipecolic academia A recessively inherited peroxisomal disorder with onset in infancy, characterized clinically by hypotonia, hepatomegaly, and nystagmus; thereafter, progressive quadriparesis and mental retardation occur as a result of demyelination in the CNS. Elevated serum pipecolate levels are found.[2317] See **Zellweger disease** and **neonatal adrenoleukodystrophy**.

hyperpolarization A change in the existing membrane potential to a more negative value. See also **polarization**.

hyperpraxia Excessive activity, as in manic conditions.

hyperprolinemia A metabolic error characterized by a deficiency of proline oxidase or of a related dehydrogenase. The syndrome is regarded as a diffuse encephalopathy which in some cases causes renal and ocular disease, seizures, mental retardation, and various CNS disorders, or which may be asymptomatic.[4440]

hyperpyrexia associated with muscle contraction See **diencephalic autonomic seizures**.

hyperschematia A disproportionate enlargement and embellishment of the left side of objects drawn by patients with a right hemispheric lesion; a disorder of representation of extrapersonal space.[5346]

hypersensitivity raking Unusual responsiveness to the visual environment, considered to be a manifestation of **Parkinson disease** and a factor leading to **freezing** of gait.[4329]

hypersensitivity vasculitis A group of vasculitic syndromes resulting from abnormal responses to foreign antigens. In **serum sickness** and **Henoch–Schönlein purpura**, neurological complications are reported.

hypersexuality The increased sexual display and attentiveness manifested by animals (and occasionally by humans) suffering from the **Klüver–Bucy syndrome**.

hypersomnia (excessive daytime somnolence) A climate of sleepiness; enhanced proclivity toward sleep punctuated by spells in which awareness of environmental stimuli is actually lost. It is a feature of the **Kleine–Levin, Pickwickian**, and various psychiatric syndromes.[735] See also **hypersomnolence** and **idiopathic hypersomnia**.

hypersomnia with increased CSF 5-HIAA A syndrome characterized by a high normal sleep time of 12–14 h/day over several consecutive days, the raised serotonin levels presumably reflecting hyperactivity of serotonergic mechanisms.

hypersomnia-bulimia See **Klein–Levin syndrome**.

hypersomnolence (excessive daytime somnolence, excessive daytime sleepiness, hypersomnia) The condition of experiencing prolonged nocturnal sleep and long periods of gradual and resistible non–rapid eye movement stage 1–2 sleep (subwakefulness) during waking hours, especially in the morning and when sleep is neither desired nor anticipated. *Essential hypersomnolence* is defined[4904] as "chronic persistent daytime drowsiness without obvious organic cause."

Physiologic functions reflecting hypersomnolence include pupil diameter and fluctuation, other autonomic functions, and EEG activity. The most commonly used objective measures of hypersomnolence are the **Multiple Sleep Latency Test** and the **Stanford Sleepiness Scale**.

Variants include

Secondary hypersomnolence which results from some metabolic or structural disorder of the nervous system.

Neurotic hypersomnolence, a condition consisting of lifelong fatigue, hypersomnia, and sometimes sleep reversal as a complication of neurotic or depressive disease.

Nocturnal hyperkinesis with daytime hypersomnolence, which is the occurrence of severe myoclonus, restlessness, bruxism, and frequent arousals during the night, with daytime drowsiness.

Sleep apnea.

Long-cycle hypersomnia, a condition of recurrent hypersomnolence occurring at intervals longer than a day. It is also seen in the **Kleine–Levin syndrome;** secondary to drug or alcohol abuse; and in shift workers.

hypertelorism (orbital hypertelorism, ocular hypertelorism, teleorbitism) A craniofacial anomaly in which there is unusual widening of the space between the eyes, and thus increased interorbital and interpupillary distances, due to maldevelopment of the lesser wings of the sphenoid bones. Mental retardation is sometimes associated even when the condition is present in isolation,[2573] but it is also a feature of numerous other developmental syndromes. The condition is usually sporadic but may be inherited as a dominant or recessive trait.[4, 1168, 2504] In adults, the normal distance between the inner canthi is 30–33 mm, and between the pupils it is more than 64 mm.

Orbital hypertelorism exists when there is true lateralization (i.e., out-turning) of the orbits; *interorbital hypertelorism* is the term used when there is no such lateralization, as is commonly the case in **craniosynostosis**.[4] The term was originally coined by Dr. David Greig, conservator of the Edinburgh museum, in 1924. See also **Greig syndrome**.

hypertelorism–hypospadias syndrome (BBB syndrome, Elsahy–Waters syndrome) A dominantly inherited developmental syndrome with incomplete penetrance and variable expressivity, so that males are mainly affected. Clinically, it is characterized by wide-spaced inner canthi (telecanthus), hypospadias, cryptorchidism, mental retardation, cranial asymmetry, and strabismus.[1168] Coarctation of the aorta, cleft lip and palate, and micrognathia may also be associated.

hypertensive encephalopathy An acute syndrome due to a rapid rise in blood pressure, occurring primarily in patients with chronic, poorly controlled hypertension. Clinically there are altered states of consciousness and severe headaches, in the setting of ophthalmoscopic alterations of malignant hypertension. Uremia, obtundation, seizures, and sometimes transient neurological deficits are common, but nausea, vomiting, seizures, focal signs, and visual disturbances are less so. The level of consciousness is relatively more depressed than the severity of the neurological signs might lead one to expect. Papilledema, flame-shaped hemorrhages, and retinal exudates are almost invariable. The diastolic blood pressure is usually >130 mmHg, but there is no gross bleeding into or around the brain on imaging or as detected by lumbar puncture. The CSF pressure is usually increased.[1662, 4678]

Neuropathologic changes consist of fibrinoid necrosis of arterioles, thrombosis of arterioles and capillaries, and parenchymal lesions such as microinfarcts and petechial hemorrhages secondary to the vascular lesions, which are not confined to the brain but affect also the eyes, kidneys, and other organs. In the CNS the brainstem is most severely affected. Cerebral edema is not observed, even in patients with increased CSF pressure and papilledema.[1139] See also **eclampsia** and **posterior leukoencephalopathy**.

Diagnostic criteria for *hypertensive encephalopathy headache* are defined below:

A. Headache with at least one of the following characteristics and fulfilling criteria C and D:

1. Diffuse pain
2. Pulsating quality
3. Aggravated by physical activity

B. Persistent blood pressure elevation to >160/100 mmHg with at least two of the following:

1. Confusion
2. Reduced level of consciousness
3. Visual disturbances (other than those of typical migraine aura) including blindness
4. Seizures

C. Headache develops in close temporal relation to blood pressure elevation

D. Headache resolves within 3 months after effective treatment and control of hypertension
E. Other causes of the neurological symptoms have been excluded

From the International Classification of Headache Disorders (Headache Classification Committee of the International Headache Society. Cephalalgia 2004;24(Suppl 1)) by kind permission of Dr. Jes Olesen, the International Headache Society, and Wiley-Blackwell Publications.

A *variant* is *headache attributed to hypertensive crisis without hypertensive encephalopathy.* The ICHD criteria[2820] suggest that this is a headache that is bilateral, pulsating, or precipitated by physical activity during a hypertensive crisis (a paroxysmal rise in systolic [to >160 mmHg] and/or diastolic [to >120 mmHg]) blood pressure without the features of hypertensive encephalopathy, developing during such a hypertensive crisis and resolving within 1 h after normalization of blood pressure. Vasopressor toxins or medications should have been excluded as causative factors.

hypertensive headache The popular perception of high blood pressure as a cause of headache, for which there is no good evidence except in association with **hypertensive encephalopathy**.

hyperthyroid myopathy A syndrome of proximal muscle weakness with atrophy and myopathic EMG abnormalities complicating nearly all cases of hyperthyroidism. See also **acute thyrotoxic myopathy** and **familial periodic paralysis**.

hyperthyroid neuropathy (Basedow paraplegia) An acute flaccid proximal neuropathy or plexopathy complicating hyperthyroidism.[1986]

hyperthyroidism See **amyotrophic lateral sclerosis, endocrine exophthalmos, myasthenia gravis**, and **familial periodic paralysis**.

hypertonia (Gr, excessive + tone) Increased muscle resistance to passive stretching, as occurs with upper motor neuron lesions.

hypertonia of opposition Rigidity in neurodegenerative diseases associated with a general attitude of flexion, particularly of the neck muscles, and with a positive limb placement sign.[6428, 6429] The association of hypertonia in the upper limbs with dyspraxia. See also **arteriosclerotic rigidity**.

hypertonic bladder See **Bors Comarr classification**.

hypertrichosis and gingival fibromatosis A congenital dysmorphic syndrome manifesting also generalized hirsutism, seizures, and mental and developmental delay.[381]

hypertrichosis–mental retardation–seizures A congenital dysmorphic syndrome characterized by generalized hirsutism, coarse facial features, gum hypertrophy, seizures, and mental and developmental delay.

hypertrophia (hypertrophy) (Gr, above + nourishment) See **hypertrophy**.

hypertrophia musculorum vera A dominantly inherited syndrome with the onset in youth or adult life of muscle hypertrophy with muscle pain, cramps, and often paresthesias, but without weakness.[5056]

A *variant* is *hypertrophia musculorum vera and ataxia*, which is a congenital syndrome characterized by painful muscle hypertrophy, fasciculations, and neurogenic weakness, cerebellar ataxia, raised serum creatine kinase levels and sensory neuropathy.[4732]

hypertrophic brachial plexus neuritis A dominantly inherited disorder linked to 17q24, possibly a form of **neuralgic amyotrophy** or a painless manifestation of hereditary pressure-sensitive neuropathy. In yet other cases it appears to be due to localized chronic autoallergic or viral inflammation, producing marked hypertrophy of the nerves of the plexus.[1396, 6479] See **multifocal inflammatory demyelinating neuropathy**.

hypertrophic branchial myopathy A syndrome of isolated enlargement of the masseter and/or temporalis muscles, either sporadically or in association with hypothyroidism.[3840] See **branchial myopathy**.

hypertrophic cervical pachymeningitis Chronic inflammation of the spinal meninges, including the leptomeninges, producing compression of the spinal cord and nerve roots.[1100] Whether this is due to infections or autoimmune disease is not certain.

hypertrophic granulomatous cranial pachymeningitis Inflammatory swelling of the intracranial dura mater as a result of **Wegener granulomatosis** or infection.[2017]

hypertrophic inflammatory neuropathy involving bilateral brachial plexus See **multifocal inflammatory demyelinating neuropathy**.

hypertrophic interstitial neuritis (Déjèrine–Sottas syndrome) See **hereditary motor and sensory neuropathy**, type 3.

hypertrophic interstitial neuropathy with cataracts See **hereditary motor and sensory neuropathy**, type 1.

hypertrophic mononeuritis, focal upper limb demyelinating neuropathy See **multifocal inflammatory demyelinating neuropathy**.

hypertrophic myelomalacia See **Foix–Alajouanine syndrome**.

hypertrophic myopathy Generalized enlargement of muscles which are strong.[2207] When not physiologically induced, this is probably **Thomsen disease**. See **hypertrophia musculorum vera**.

hypertrophic neuropathy Neuropathies in which there is visible or palpable thickening of the cutaneous (anterior tibial, supraclavicular, greater superficial petrosal, radial sensory) or other superficial nerves such as the ulnar or peroneal. This occurs for example, in **hereditary motor and sensory neuropathies** types 1, 3, and 4, **amyloid** and **diabetic neuropathies, neurofibromatosis, Roussy–Cornil syndrome**, and **Marie syndrome**.

hypertrophic neuropathy with facial involvement See **hereditary motor and sensory neuropathy, type 1**.

hypertrophic neuropathy with facial weakness and kyphoscoliosis See **hereditary motor and sensory neuropathy, type 3**.

hypertrophic pachymeningitis A meningitic syndrome arising secondary to an inflammatory retropharyngeal pseudotumor, manifesting as severe headache and multiple cranial nerve palsies. MRI and CT scans reveal pachymeningeal enhancement and obstructive hydrocephalus attributable to the marked dural thickening around the foramen magnum.[4172]

Many inflammatory conditions, chronic subdural hematoma, and intracranial hypotension also present in a similar manner.[3604]

hypertrophic spinal meningitis (Charcot–Joffroy syndrome, epidural ascending spinal paralysis) A syndrome clinically resembling **syringomyelia** or **amyotrophic lateral sclerosis** but with pain in the neck and back and often sphincter disturbances and vasomotor changes in the limbs, and associated with chronic granulomatous inflammation of the cervical spinal meninges.[1108] See **Spiller syndrome**.

hypertrophy (hypertrophia) Abnormal enlargement of a tissue or organ.

hypertropia Vertical strabismus, one eye being elevated with respect to the other.

hypertryptophanemia An aminoacidopathy characterized by elevated serum tryptophan levels with the massive urinary excretion of indoleacetic, lactic, and pyruvic acids and characterized clinically by ataxia, spasticity, mental retardation, and pellagrinoid skin rash. The responsible enzymatic defect might be of tryptophan transaminase.[5930]

hyperuricemia, deafness, and ataxia A rare syndrome of elevated blood uric acid levels appearing in late childhood with progressive spinocerebellar ataxia, sensorineural deafness, weakness, and renal insufficiency occurring after puberty. The condition is probably dominantly inherited but the biochemical lesion is unknown.[5400]

hypervalinemia A diffuse encephalopathy characterized by vomiting, nystagmus, hyperkinesias, ataxia, and failure to thrive in infancy. The EEG shows a pattern of sharp waves and spikes.[6182]

hyperventilation syndrome (Da Costa syndrome, overbreathing) The state in which the ventilatory activity is greater than that which is physiologically required, leading to a lowering of P_aCO_2 and consequent cerebral vasoconstriction. This then causes a variety of symptoms (paresthesias, loss of consciousness, giddiness, weakness, tetany, and transient visual loss) which are often accompanied by other symptoms of anxiety. For confident diagnosis, the symptoms must be reproduced in the office when the patient hyperventilates for 30–60 s. The condition is most commonly seen in the context of a chronic anxiety state.[4193]

hyperventilation-epilepsy syndrome The occurrence of seizures as a result of hyperventilation was described by Rosett in 1924, and in the following year Foerster showed that seizures could be induced thus in many epileptic patients. If overbreathing leads to seizures, surely underbreathing should stop them; and Durham recounts the use of artificial pneumothorax as a treatment modality, noting that between the two World Wars it was recorded that patients with tuberculosis treated thus had far fewer "seizures."[1765]

hyperviscosity syndrome See **Waldenstrom macroglobulinemia**.

hypesthesia Decreased sensitivity to sensory stimuli, usually applied to common sensory modes. **Hypoesthesia** has the same meaning.

hyphema The presence of red blood in the anterior chamber of the eye due to infection or hemorrhage.

hypnagogic jerks (from Gr, sleep + leading) See **sleep starts**.

hypnagogic hallucinations The occurrence of vivid, waking auditory or visual perceptions incorporated into dreamlike periods during the lightest stages of nonrapid eye movement sleep (or immediately upon awakening–**hypnopompic hallucinations**) in normal people and in the rapid eye movement sleep periods of narcoleptics. They represent the sleep–dream imagery of rapid eye movement sleep occurring inappropriately and include a recall of scenes from recent waking experience. They may be accompanied by visual, auditory, or somesthetic sensory illusions. When combined with sleep paralysis, the subject experiences a true nightmare.

See also **hypnopompic hallucinations, narcolepsy**, and Chart S–6.

hypnagogic imagery Vivid sensory images occurring at the onset of sleep, both in rapid eye movement sleep-onset periods[280] and in nonrapid eye movement sleep awakenings, when they are briefer and less affectively charged.

hypnagogic startle A sudden bodily jerk observed commonly at the onset of sleep and resulting in at least momentary awakening.[280]

hypnic headache (alarm clock headache, clockwise headache) A rare, benign, regularly occurring, diffuse, and self-limited nocturnal headache affecting patients usually over the age of 60 years during rapid eye movement sleep and lasting up to an hour. The mild-to-moderate head pain lasts from 15–60 min and is typically generalized, although it may be unilateral. Nausea, photophobia, phonophobia, lacrimation, nasal congestion, and ptosis are rare accompaniments.[5202] It is distinct from **cluster headache** by virtue of its diffuse site and relative lack of severity and by the absence of ocular and nasal symptoms. A lesion of the suprachiasmatic nucleus is postulated as causative.[1520] Diagnostic criteria have been defined as follows:

A. Dull headache fulfilling criteria B–D
B. Develops only during sleep and awakens patient
C. With at least two of the following characteristics:
   1. Occurs >15 times per month
   2. Lasts ≥15 min after waking
   3. First occurs after age of 50 years
D. No autonomic symptoms and no more than one of nausea, photophobia, or phonophobia

From the International Classification of Headache Disorders (Headache Classification Committee of the International Headache Society. Cephalalgia 2004;24(Suppl 1)) by kind permission of Dr. Jes Olesen, the International Headache Society, and Wiley-Blackwell Publications.

hypnic jerks (sudden bodily jerks on falling asleep) Shocklike starts, affecting the whole body, occurring in nonrapid eye movement sleep stages 1 and 2 and thus at sleep onset in normal people. See **sleep starts**.

hypnogenic paroxysmal dystonia Episodes characterized by coarse, violent movements of the limbs with tonic spasms, vocalization, or laughter, occurring mainly or only at night. A familial form is recognized.[3954] See **nocturnal paroxysmal dystonia**.

hypnopompic hallucinations The occurrence of vivid waking auditory or visual perceptions incorporated into dreamlike periods immediately upon awakening.

hypnosis A state of altered awareness induced by suggestion and associated with further abnormal suggestibility, focused awareness, loss of critical judgment, amnesia and possibly anesthesia, time regression, and ability to maintain fixed postures. The condition can be induced at least to some extent in all humans, and in some animals.[4904]

hypnotic-dependent sleep disorder Insomnia or excessive sleepiness associated with tolerance to or withdrawal from hypnotic medications.[1629]

hypo- (Gr, below, under, less than).

hypobaropathy See **altitude insomnia**.

hypobetalipoproteinemia A dominantly inherited syndrome manifest in youth or young adult life by low levels of cholesterol, β-lipoproteins and triglycerides, sometimes with **acanthocytosis**. The responsible gene maps to 2p24–p23.

The neurological features are extremely variable, if any occur at all; seizures, multifocal lesions of white matter, myelopathy, sensorimotor neuropathy, and ataxia have all been reported in different kinships. The most common symptom complexes are spinocerebellar degeneration or peripheral neuropathy.[2754, 4098] See also **cerebellar ataxias** (*variants*).

hypobetalipoproteinemia, acanthocytosis, retinitis pigmentosa, and pallidal degeneration (HARP syndrome; OMIM 200150) An encephalopathy characterized by the onset in childhood of orofacial dyskinesias, dystonia, pigmentary retinopathy, progressive dementia, prominent facial dyskinesias, and dystonias with associated hypo-pre-betalipoproteinemia, abundant acanthocytosis, and evidence of iron deposition in the basal ganglia.[2896] The **eye of the tiger sign** may be present on MRI scans. The condition is allelic with pantothenate kinase–associated neurodegeneration (PKAN; **neurodegeneration with brain iron accumulation**).

hypoceruloplasminemia A dominantly inherited syndrome characterized by low serum ceruloplasmin levels in the absence of other evidence of **Wilson disease**.[1305]

hypochondriasis A morbid concern with one's health, generally manifested as a belief that one is or is about to be affected by a disease. The problem may be a manifestation of chronic anxiety or of depression.

hypocretins Hypothalamic excitatory neuropeptides concerned with the regulation of feeding, sleep, and arousal. See **orexins**.

hypocupremic myelopathy See **copper deficiency myeloneuropathy**.

hypoesthesia Decreased sensitivity to sensory stimuli, usually applied to common sensory modes. **Hypesthesia** has the same meaning.

hypogastric reflex of Bekhterev See **abdominal reflexes**.

hypogenic dystonia See **familial paroxysmal dystonic choreoathetosis** (*familial paroxysmal hypogenic dystonia*).[3954]

hypoglossal nerve (Gr, beneath + the tongue) The XII cranial nerve, containing purely motor fibers, all of which pass to the tongue muscles.

hypoglossal-alternating hemiplegia syndrome A vascular syndrome of the medulla due to a paramedian lesion which damages the pyramid and the fasciculus of the XII cranial nerve on one side to produce the **alternating hemiplegia**. See also **Jackson syndrome**.

hypoglossal-facial anastomosis An operation performed to normalize facial movement in people with hemifacial spasm or in those who have lost facial nerve function as a result of surgery for the treatment of cerebellopontine angle tumors.

Autogenous nerve grafts may produce better results because functional reinnervation from the stump of the divided VII cranial nerve leads too often to synkinetic mass action of the facial muscles during attempts to move the tongue.

hypoglycemic amyotrophy A syndrome of distal muscle wasting associated with hypoglycemia, probably due to damage to the anterior horn cells or motor roots. Recovery occurs clinically with evidence of reinnervation accomplished by axonal sprouting.[2782]

hypoglycemic headache (headache attributed to fasting) Diagnostic criteria have been defined as follows:

A. Headache with at least one of the following characteristics and fulfilling criteria C and D:
   1. Frontal location
   2. Diffuse pain
   3. Nonpulsating quality
   4. Mild or moderate intensity

B. The patient has fasted for >16 h

C. Headache develops during fasting

D. Headache resolves within 72 h after resumption of food intake

*From the International Classification of Headache Disorders (Headache Classification Committee of the International Headache Society. Cephalalgia 2004;***24***(Suppl 1)) by kind permission of Dr. Jes Olesen, the International Headache Society, and Wiley-Blackwell Publications.*

hypoglycorrachia An unnecessary term meaning low glucose levels in the CSF.

hypokinesia Poverty of willed movement. See **akinesia**.

hypokinetic automatism In the context of epilepsy, a decrease in the amplitude and/or the rate of, or the arrest of, ongoing motor activity.

hypokalemic myopathy Muscle membrane damage with resulting weakness and myoglobinuria, complicating chronic potassium depletion.

hypokalemic periodic paralysis A familial syndrome of attacks of flaccid weakness of the trunk and limbs, precipitated by food and sometimes relieved by exercise. See **familial periodic paralysis**.

hypomagnesemia Tremors, twitches, and seizures, often with mental confusion, agitation, and hallucinations and a positive **Chvostek sign**, as a result of magnesium deficiency.[2129]

hypomania A state judged to be more intense than simple euphoria (or unwonted cheerfulness) but less intense than mania, the etiologies of which it shares. It represents a mild to moderate level of mania that may actually be pleasurable and can be associated with good functioning and enhanced productivity. However, hypomania can progress to mania (or to depression).

A manic episode is diagnosed if elevated mood occurs with three or more of the other symptoms listed below for most of the day, nearly every day, for 1 week or longer. If the mood is irritable, four additional symptoms must be present. The clinical features of mania (From the NIMH Web site: http://www.nimh.nih.gov/health/publications/) include a lasting period of behavior that differs from normal by virtue of the following:

- Increased energy, activity, and restlessness with reduced need for sleep
- Excessively "high," euphoric mood with lack of insight (denial that anything is wrong)
- Extreme irritability
- Racing thoughts and rapid speech output, jumping from one idea to another
- Distractibility, poor concentration
- Impaired judgment; unrealistic beliefs in the subjects' abilities and powers
- Provocative, intrusive, aggressive, or unregulated behavior (e.g., spending sprees, asocial manifestations of an increased sexual drive)
- Abuse of drugs, particularly cocaine, alcohol, and sleeping medications

hypomelanosis of Ito (incontinentia pigmenti achromicans, systemic achromic nevus) An uncommon, sporadic, or dominantly inherited congenital multisystem neuroectodermal disorder described by Ito in Japan in 1952. The responsible gene maps to 9q33-qter. It is characterized by the presence of a whorled or swirling pattern of skin hypopigmentation, shown up by viewing the skin under Woods light. Heterotopias of the white matter lead to mental retardation, convulsions, disturbances of language, and hypotonia or pyramidal signs in most affected children.[233, 5465]

Short stature, skeletal abnormalities, cloudy corneas, microphthalmia, myopia, retinitis pigmentosa, strabismus, nystagmus, macrocephaly, alopecia, and low densities in the white matter on CT scans as well as many other complications may also be associated.[3639]

hypometria A reduction in the amplitude of limb movements which are otherwise normally formed. A lesion of the contralateral **supplementary motor area** has been incriminated.[4271]

hypometric saccade A normal single saccade which stops before fixation of the desired target is achieved (undershooting), requiring thus a further small corrective saccade in order to place the image of the target on the fovea (a refixation eye movement). See also **hypermetric saccades, pulse dysmetria,** and **postsaccadic drift**.

hypomimia Reduced facial expressivity, as seen in Parkinsonism or depressive states.

hypomyelinating leukoencephalopathies A heterogeneous group of childhood genetic disorders, characterized by a reduced formation of brain myelin and presenting with nystagmus, hypotonia, motor delay, cerebellar ataxia, and spasticity. The clinical progression is usually slow, with motor handicap being greater than intellectual impairment. Numerous patients of both genders who fail to show *PLP* mutations may have a slowly progressive disease with clinical and MRI features indistinguishable from PMD. Given the phenotypic homogeneity, these patients are referred to as affected by a PMD-like disorder (PMLD). Loci on Xq, mutations in the autosomal *GJA12* gene connexin have been discovered in some cases.[933]

See **Cockayne syndrome type II, Salla disease, Tay syndrome, PCWH (peripheral demyelinating neuropathy, central dysmyelinating leukodystrophy, Waardenburg syndrome, and Hirschsprung disease), 18q-syndrome** (MIM 601808), **brain hypomyelination with atrophy of the basal ganglia and cerebellum,** and **Pelizaeus–Merzbacher disease**.

hyponatremia Low serum sodium levels, frequently developing in patients on neurologic intensive care units and complicating the course of acute neurologic disorders. Two pathophysiological mechanisms have been suggested to cause noniatrogenic hyponatremia: **cerebral salt-wasting syndrome** (CSWS) and inappropriate secretion of antidiuretic hormone (**SIADH**).

hyponatremic encephalopathy A combination of brain swelling and increased intracranial pressure, leading to increased pressure on the brain, decreased cerebral blood flow, and sometimes cerebral herniation, due to the retention of free water and an osmotic imbalance between the extracellular fluid and neural tissues. **Central pontine myelinolysis** is not necessarily a feature.[6318]

hypo-osmotic brain edema Excessive water content of the brain's extracellular space as a result of hypo-osmolality of the blood, as seen in patients with the **syndrome of inappropriate ADH secretion** or after the massive replacement of blood with hypotonic fluids.

hypoparathyroidism Impaired activity of the parathyroid glands, leading to the neurological complications of increased intracranial pressure, seizures, and tetany in a few cases. Other complications occasionally reported include the features of Addison disease, ptosis, blepharospasm, increased intracranial pressure, superficial moniliasis, proximal myopathy, seizures, and tetany.[3972, 2299, 5757]

hypoperfusion syndrome A rare and potentially devastating complication of carotid endarterectomy, angioplasty or stenting, and due to acute focal edema of the brain or acute hemorrhages, causing seizures and focal deficits in 24 h after the procedure.

hypophosphatasia (phosphoethanolaminuria) A fatal, recessively inherited neonatal syndrome characterized by craniostenosis, skeletal deformities, and hypercalcemia.

Variants include forms occurring in later years with a syndrome resembling rickets and the occurrence of low levels of serum alkaline phosphatase without symptoms.[1957]

hypophosphatemia A condition of reduced serum phosphate levels below 2 mmol/l, as may occur in diabetes mellitus, alcoholism, renal tubular acidosis, hepatic disease, excessive alkali ingestion, etc.

Profound hypophosphatemia can produce severe proximal and respiratory flaccid weakness resembling that in **acute inflammatory demyelinating polyneuropathy**. The condition may be due to the decreased absorption of phosphate or its increased renal excretion cellular uptake. It also occurs in association with abnormalities of vitamin D metabolism.

Clinically, the condition is marked by anorexia, proximal muscle weakness and waddling gait, irritable paresthesias, dysarthria, and seizures,[5646] while, with extreme reduction of phosphate levels (<0.5 mg/dl), an encephalopathy ensues with irritability, dysarthria, confusion, seizures, and coma. Acute rhabdomyolysis is a further complication.

hypophysial nanism See **Burnier syndrome**.

hypophysitis (*lymphocytic hypophysitis*) A rare, destructive autoimmune inflammatory disease of the pituitary often causing severe hypopituitarism.[2121] It occurs mainly in females, usually during or after a pregnancy and is thus difficult to differentiate from **Sheehan syndrome**.

Granulomatous hypophysitis presents similarly with pituitary enlargement, hypopituitarism, and diabetes insipidus. Various granulomatous diseases may be responsible and the condition may also be idiopathic.

Diagnostic criteria have been defined for *headache attributed to lymphocytic hypophysitis*

A. Headache, no typical characteristics known, fulfilling criterion C
B. Hypopituitarism fulfilling the following criteria:
   1. MRI demonstrates symmetrical pituitary enlargement with homogeneous contrast enhancement
   2. Biopsy confirmation of lymphocytic hypophysitis
C. Headache develops in close temporal relation to hypopituitarism

From the International Classification of Headache Disorders (Headache Classification Committee of the International Headache Society. Cephalalgia 2004;24(Suppl 1)) by kind permission of Dr. Jes Olesen, the International Headache Society, and Wiley-Blackwell Publications.

hypopituitarism Failure of the pituitary gland to produce normal amounts of some or all of its hormones such as adrenocorticotropic hormone (ACTH); antidiuretic hormone (ADH); follicle stimulating hormone (FSH); growth hormone (GH); luteinizing hormone (LH); oxytocin, prolactin, and thyroid stimulating hormone (TSH). In hypopituitarism, the lack of one or more of these hormones leads to loss of function in the gland or organ that it controls.

Causes include brain surgery, tumor, head trauma, local infections, radiation, and stroke (including subarachnoid hemorrhage). See the Web site: http://www.nlm.nih.gov/medlineplus/ency/article/000343.htm/.

hypoplasia of the cerebellum and pons See **Paine syndrome**.

hypoplasia of the thenar eminence A congenital condition characterized only by thenar muscle Hypoplasia, with malformation of the underlying bones.[1063] See also **Souques syndrome.**

hypopyon The presence of pus in the anterior chamber of the eye as a result of anterior uveitis.

hypospadias-dysphagia syndrome See **G syndrome**.

hypothalamic crossroads syndrome See **hypothalamique carrefour syndrome**.

hypothalamic ganglionic hamartoma A developmental defect consisting of a mass of redundant gray matter, usually attached to the mammillary bodies. Compression of the hypothalamus may lead to excessive gonadotropin production, resulting in precocious puberty. The condition is commoner in males.

hypothalamic hamartoma See **hamartoma**.

hypothalamic hypophysiotrophic hormones Synaptically active peptide molecules released from the hypothalamus with effects upon the release of other hormones.

hypothalamic syndrome The clinical syndromes resulting from various hypothalamic disorders. They include disturbances of appetite, sleep, water metabolism, sexual function, thermoregulation, and behavior. See also **syndrome of inappropriate ADH secretion, Fröhlich syndrome, Kleine–Levin syndrome**,[5054] and **diabetes insipidus**.

hypothalamic–midbrain dysregulation syndrome See **diencephalic autonomic seizures**.[4161]

hypothalamique carrefour syndrome (hypothalamic crossroads syndrome) A stroke syndrome characterized by the association of sudden visual loss, hemiplegia, hemianesthesia, apraxia, astereognosis, and asynergias.[5175]

hypothermia A state in which the core body temperature is below 34 °C. As temperatures fall to 32.2 °C., there is a linear depression of cerebral metabolism, with shivering, ataxia, apathy, dysarthria, impaired judgment, and maladaptive behavior. Between that level and 28 °C there is a progressive depression of the level of consciousness with EEG slowing, reduction in shivering, and muscle rigidity. Hallucinations may occur and there is mydriasis. Below 28 °C. no movements are made and there are a loss of cerebral autoregulation, reduction in cerebral blood flow, loss of ocular and muscle stretch reflexes, and progressive attenuation of the EEG.[1449]

hypothyroid encephalopathy See **myxedema coma**.

hypothyroid headache The diagnostic criteria defined in the ICHD[2820] include the presence of bilateral, nonpulsatile, continuous headaches developing within 2 months after other symptoms of hypothyroidism become evident and resolving within 2 months after its effective treatment.

hypothyroid myopathy

1. (Hoffmann syndrome) A syndrome of stiffness, slowed contraction and relaxation (**pseudomyotonia**), and persistent painful muscle contractions following effort, made worse by exertion and occurring in hypothyroid patients.[2939] See also **Kocher–Debré-Semelaigne syndrome**. 2. Girdle muscle hypertrophy with weakness.[4706]

hypothyroid neuropathy

A symmetrical, distal, sensorimotor, demyelinating polyneuropathy complicating primary hypothyroidism and presenting with cramps, hyporeflexia, distal pain, and paresthesias. The symptoms remit slowly with thyroid replacement.[1780] The same condition may occur due to thyrotropin deficiency.[2538] Axonal polyneuropathy is also described.[4625]

Mononeuropathies such as the **carpal tunnel syndrome** due to mucinous compression of the nerve in hypothyroidism were also described; but are uncommon now because of earlier diagnosis of the thyroid disorder.

hypotonia 1. Decreased resistance to the passive stretching of a limb muscle, as interpreted by an observer from the feel of the limb manipulated by the examiner or from an increase in the to-and-fro movements of the leg when the knee jerk is tested with the patient in the sitting position and the legs hanging freely (the pendular knee jerk). It occurs in association with lesions of the extrapyramidal pathways, the cerebellar system, or the reflex arc. If "the outstretched arms rest lightly on a bar, the normal limb keeps its position or sags a little when the bar is suddenly removed, but the hypotonic arm falls through a greater angle and may fail to maintain its new posture. This is more striking if the hand carries even a moderate weight . . . When the arms are extended horizontally, the affected limb is more easily displaced by a tap on the wrist . . . When shaken, the distal segments of the limbs swing more passively and through a greater range" (Sir Gordon **Holmes**).

Determination of the existence of hypotonia is difficult and comprises part of the artistic quality of this discipline. Holmes described increased drooping (flexion) of the wrist when the flexed elbows are placed on a level surface as a characteristic sign of hypotonia; in the case of the upper limb, this is perhaps one of the signs most easy to interpret.

The traditional view that hypotonia is due to a reduction in stretch reflexes now appears incorrect, reduction in tone being the result of weakness preventing voluntary activity.[1599]

2. The resistance to stretch of a muscle forming part of a damaged reflex arc or of muscles on the side of a lesion of the cerebellum or its connections.

hypotonia-hypomentia-hypogonadism-obesity syndrome See **Prader–Willi syndrome**.

hypotonic cerebral palsy A form of cerebral palsy mimicking generalized lower motor neuron disease, recognized by Otfried **Foerster** in 1909. See **cerebral palsy**.

hypotrophy Failure of growth to a normal size.

hypotropia Manifest vertical deviation of an eye.

hypovolemia Reduction in the volume of the intravascular compartment.

hypoxanthine The oxidation of hypoxanthine forms superoxide radicals which may cause postischemic damage.

hypoxic degenerative polioencephalopathy A diffuse encephalopathy. See **hypoxic-ischemic encephalopathy**.

hypoxic headache (high-altitude headache, altitudinal headache) Hypoxia is associated with three headache varieties. They are

Hypoxic headache (low pressure environment, pulmonary disease causing hypoxia) Occurs within 24 h after the acute onset of hypoxia with arterial oxygen tensions of $\leq$70 mg Hg or in chronic hypoxic patients with arterial oxygen tension persistently at or below this level.

Sleep apnea headache Headaches resulting from hypercapnia, mixed hypoxia and hypercapnia, hypoglycemia, **dialysis**, and other metabolic disorders are also included in this category of the International Headache Society's Classification. Headache is also a major symptom of **acute mountain sickness** developing within 24 h after ascent to above 3000 m. It is associated with at least one other symptom typical of AMS including Cheyne–Stokes respirations at night, a desire to overbreathe and exertional dyspnea. Nausea, anorexia, fatigue, dizziness, and sleep disorders are typical accompanying symptoms.

hypoxic neuropathy Focal or multifocal central fascicular or sector axonal fiber degeneration, leading to endoneurial hypoxia—the basis of most diabetic and some other neuropathies.[1772]

hypoxic-ischemic encephalopathy (hypoxic degenerative polioencephalopathy) A syndrome of diffuse neuronal destruction involving primarily the cerebral cortex, basal ganglia, and thalamus. It is most commonly seen in neonates after complicated deliveries and is characterized clinically by reduced Apgar scores, hypotonia, seizures, or coma initially, with mental and motor delay, seizures (including **infantile spasms**), and spastic or athetotic cerebral palsy developing in those infants who survive.[6]

Hypoxic-Ischemic Encephalopathy (FATES) Score

A system rating Feeding, Apgar scores at birth, muscle Tone, Extubation (need for respiratory support), and Seizure activity after the first week to grade the severity of the encephalopathy and provide a prognosis.[6183]

hypoxic-ischemic injury Changes in the CNS following trauma or a severe reduction in cerebral blood flow, usually after cardiac arrest. The condition is characterized by widespread cortical neuronal loss, small areas of patchy infarction in the watershed interarterial zones, cerebral infarction in the territory of a major vessel, or any combination of these. Clinically, patients suffering such injury frequently show evidence of increased intracranial pressure and episodes of systemic hypotension, often secondary to severe systemic injury as a result of the initial trauma. The territory of the posterior cerebral artery is that most frequently involved.

hypsarrhythmia (from Gr, high + lack of + rhythm) An age-related EEG pattern consisting of random, multifocal, high-voltage (>200 μV), arrhythmic, chaotic slow waves at 1–3 Hz interspersed with multifocal spike discharges, without consistent synchrony between the two sides of the head or between different areas on the same side during wakefulness and between seizures. The pattern may disappear during rapid-eye-movement sleep. Many variations are also described.[690] These findings are usually associated with infantile spasms (**West syndrome**) but may also be noted in neurofibromatosis and in certain metabolic diseases of the nervous system.

Hyrtl's loop Small recurrent branches between the two hypoglossal nerves in the geniohyoid muscle recorded by Joseph Hyrtl (1810–1894) the Hungarian anatomist, in 1842.[5619]

hyster- (Gr, uterus) Hysteria was considered from ancient times to be a condition of the womb because it was only recognized in females; it was supposed that the womb (considered to be an animal endowed with the faculties of sensation and motion) wandered indignantly through the body when dissatisfied in its ardent desire to bear children. Pregnancy was determined to be the most effective remedy. The author exhorts his readers to suggest a better explanation.

hysteria (psychogenic disease, conversion syndrome, abnormal illness behavior, somatoform disorder) 1. A condition in which the mental mechanism of **dissociation** is used as if to protect the subject from the awareness of painful mental content, also considered to be an instinctual response to threat. 2. A form of mental depression (of highest cerebral functions) characterized by the retraction of the field of personal consciousness and a tendency for dissociation and emancipation of the systems of ideas and functions that constitute personality. (Janet P. The Major Symptoms of Hysteria New York, Macmillan 1920). The first two of the alternative terms for the condition given above are those usually employed;[3992] others are modified newspeak. There is no hysterical symptom that cannot be produced by well-defined nonhysterical causes. The word was introduced by William Cullen in 1766.

Within neurology, it is manifest as symptoms and signs which can be ascribed to abnormal function (or loss of function) in any parts of the nervous system, for which no chemical, electrical, or structural cause can be determined; but because perhaps half of the patients so diagnosed do in fact turn out to have such "organic" disease after prolonged follow-up, it might be best to make the diagnosis only in retrospect after 5 years or more.

The reader will by now have noticed that neither this author nor any other[5889, 6620] can frame a satisfactory definition of hysteria (although classic *descriptions* were given by Thomas **Willis** in 1671 and by Henry **Head** in 1922). Perhaps this is because, in the words of Charcot: "Bear well in mind, and this should not exact too great an effort, that the word hysteria means nothing." However, "The figure of Hysteria shrinks in proportion as the various forms of organic disease acquire greater solidity and sharper definition."[963]

Eames[1797] classified the presentations as follows: *hysterical personality disorder,*[1200] *Briquet syndrome* (the stable syndrome of hysteria), *conversion hysteria* (focal presentations), and *Charcot syndrome* ("gross hysteria", seen also in patients with prior diffuse brain insults such as hypoglycemia or hypoxia). In this context it is fair to note that in functional paralysis the primary motor cortex is not activated, but right orbitofrontal and right anterior cingulate cortex activity appears to be responsible for inhibiting the prefrontal willed movement.[4108] See also **functional disease**.

hysterical flutter See **psychogenic flutter**.

hysterical gait No single abnormality is subsumed here, but characteristic findings are the variability of the deficits with time and circumstance, their unphysiological nature, and the absence of physical findings of neurological examination in the bed, although none of these is unique to this gait disorder.

hysterical neurosis See **somatization disorder**.

hysterical nystagmus See **psychogenic flutter**.

hysterical personality (psychopathy) A set of traits described as including the clinical pointers listed in Chart H–23.[1200]

hysterical pseudodementia See **Ganser syndrome**.

hysterical seizures (pseudoseizures, nonepileptic seizures) Attacks resembling epileptic seizures in which there is a wide range of events, including bizarre behavior. The EEG is normal during and after the attack and there is no relationship to medication. The attacks may start gradually. Tongue biting, incontinence, abnormal neurological signs, and nocturnal occurrence are rare, and postseizure drowsiness and confusion are absent. The patient frequently retains vivid recollections of the attack[1609, 4148] (and of one or more episodes of sexual abuse during childhood).

Chart H–23. Traits Described as Associated with the Hysterical Personality

1. Superficial charm and "intelligence."
2. Absence of delusions and other signs of irrational thinking.
3. Absence of nervousness or psychoneurotic manifestations.
4. Unreliability.
5. Untruthfulness and insincerity.
6. Lack of remorse and shame.
7. Inadequately motivated antisocial behavior.
8. Poor judgment and failure to learn by experience.
9. Pathologic incapacity to love.
10. General poverty in major adjective reactions.
11. Specific loss of insight.
12. General unresponsiveness in interpersonal relations.
13. Fantastic and uninviting behavior with drinking, sometimes without.
14. Suicide threats are seldom carried out.
15. Sex life is impersonal, trivial, and poorly integrated.
16. Failure to follow any life plan.

From Cleckley H. The Mask of Sanity. *St. Louis, Mosby, 1964.*

hysterical sensory loss Subjective abnormalities of sensation, seldom conforming to the anatomical distribution of a nerve or a root, commonly involving all modes of sensation, and considered to reflect the use of the mental mechanism of dissociation. See also **Waddell signs** and **hysteria**.

hysterical signs Clinical signs suggestive of nonorganic pathology. There follows a clinically derived compendium; no single one of these signs is itself sufficient to make the diagnosis with any confidence.

Sensory

1. Vibration is felt when the tuning fork is placed on one side of the sternum, forehead, or incisor teeth but not when it is placed across the mid-line on the other side, which is unphysiological.
2. During sensory testing, the patient may be asked to say "yes" if she or he feels the touch, pin, etc. and "no" if not.
3. Distal arm anesthesia ends precisely at the shoulder line, as if it were the top of the sleeve.
4. Psychogenic hemiparesis is often complicated by hemianesthesia that extends to the mid-line, affects all modalities of sensation, and may be accompanied by an ipsilateral decrease or loss of vision, hearing, taste, and smell. Anesthesia of the affected half of the body is rare in organic hemiparesis. If present, the cause is usually a cerebral lesion. In both psychogenic and organic paralyses, secondary contractures and vasomotor changes occur.

Formal Motor Testing

5. Collapse during toe walking, always toward the "good" side.
6. Give-way weakness on testing the abductor digiti quinti and palpating the tendon of the flexor carpi ulnaris.
7. See the **forearm rolling test**.
8. In organic hemiparesis there is sparing only of the upper portion of the face; in psychogenic paralysis there is also sparing of the face, tongue, platysma, and sternocleidomastoid muscles. In organic hemiparesis the muscle stretch reflexes are exaggerated, the abdominal reflexes are diminished or absent, the Babinski and other corticospinal tract responses are present and there may be clonus. However, in psychogenic paresis the muscle stretch reflexes are normal or increased in range but have normal speed, the abdominal reflexes are normal or increased, there are no corticospinal tract responses, and there is no persistent clonus. In organic hemiparesis the gait is of the unilateral spastic variety with circumduction of the leg; in psychogenic paralysis the gait is bizarre and there may be dragging of the foot.
9. See **Hoover sign, Babinski trunk-thigh sign, Neri sign** of combined flexion of the thigh and leg, **Bechterew sign,** and **Raimiste** arm and leg **signs**.
10. Asynchronous leg and arm movements occur in tonic–clonic seizures (although bilateral asynchronous movements without loss of consciousness may be accompanied by EEG findings of 6 Hz spike and wave).
11. Any hyperactivity of the muscle stretch reflexes is characterized by an increase in the range of movement rather than in the speed of response.
12. Pseudoclonus at the knee or ankle is irregular and poorly sustained and is not stopped by plantar flexion of the foot.
13. Subjects with nonorganic weakness of one lower extremity may use a cane on the wrong side.
14. Cutaneous reflexes are not affected in psychogenic paralyses, but the abdominal reflexes may be increased.
15. The Babinski sign and the related dorsiflexor and fanning responses are seen only in organic conditions.
16. Tests for power, tone, and coordination may be normal if carried out while the patient is lying down.

Gait

17. On testing stance, any body swaying occurs from the hips rather than from the ankles; trembling and shaking occur without signs of fear or pain. The truly ataxic patient makes every effort to maintain the erect posture and to avoid falling, whereas the simulator or hysteric usually reels from side to side or falls en masse without trying to maintain equilibrium. The patient may appear to be about to fall to the floor, but either catches himself or herself, if he or she does fall, does so in a theatrical manner, without injury.
18. If a subject with either hysteria or malingering is asked to carry out various commands, such as touching a finger to the nose or alternately pronating and supinating the hands while standing with feet together, she or he may cease to sway and fall.
19. The patient with organic ataxia can usually maintain an upright position with very slight support from a wall or table, or by lightly touching the examiner's hand, watching the floor, or placing the feet a short distance apart; the patient with psychogenic ataxia is not aided by these measures.
20. In hysterical astasia-abasia, although the subject seems unable to stand or walk, she or he may be able to move the limbs for other purposes and may skip, jump, run, or walk backward without difficulty.
21. Locomotion is accompanied by superfluous movements of other parts of the body.

Cranial Nerves

22. A large mirror moved in front of the face of a patient who claims to be blind leads to eye movements because patients cannot avoid moving their eyes when the mirror is moved. Note, however, that because patients with cortical blindness can perceive objects (although making no sense of them) they will also move their eyes when confronted with a moving mirror.
23. The complaint of restriction of the visual fields turns out to be tunnel vision rather than restricted funnel vision on bedside testing and on perimetry.
24. Subjects may be unable to find their own hand in the peripheral field, but this is a function of proprioception rather than of vision.
25. Subjects simulating deafness may react to the sound of coins thrown to the floor after saying goodbye.

General

26. Pelvic/coital rocking in pseudoseizures, especially if the subject grabs a bed rail to obtain more effective rocking.
27. Puffed-up cheeks with breath holding.
28. Events occurring just after the change of nursing shifts.
29. The presence of wrist scars from previous suicidal gestures.
30. Detection of a Medic-Alert or similar bracelet stating "see wallet card."

hysterical twilight state See **Ganser syndrome**.

hysteroepilepsy The simulation of epileptic seizures by those who do not suffer from them. The differentiation has been aided by video monitoring, but in the nineteenth century, **Charcot** considered that in hysteroepilepsy the onset of the seizure was preceded by a peculiar mental state and gradual flexion of one limb; violent limb movements preceded the tonic spasm; attacks were brought on or arrested by compression of the ovaries or other "hysterogenic areas"; and standard treatment failed to stop the attacks.[4148] See also **hysterical seizures**.

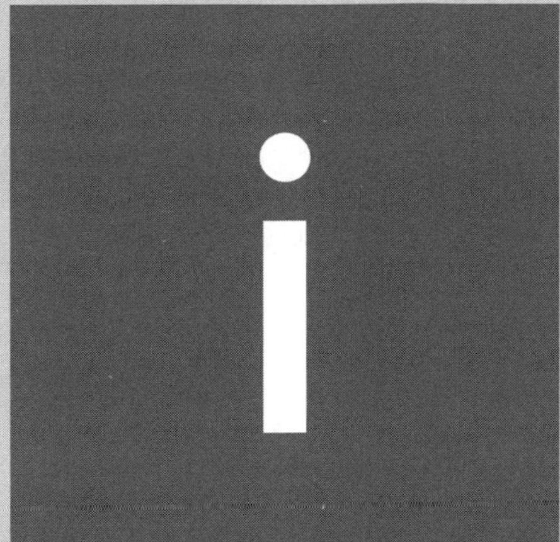

iatros (Gr, physician) Used as iatro-, a prefix signifying a relationship with physicians or with the art of medicine.

ice-cream headache See **cold stimulus headache**.

ice-cream cone sign A sign seen in subjects with a sterile abscess in the gluteal muscles as a result of receiving multiple injections at that site. The swelling is visible and palpable as a conical, fluctuant mass with a line of needle marks leading to it (the late Dr. Asa Wilbourn, personal communication, 1993).

Iceland amyloid angiopathy A form of **familial amyloidosis** with involvement of the cerebral vessels, as in **cerebral amyloid angiopathy**.

Icelandic disease See **chronic fatigue syndrome** and **postinfection fatigue syndrome**.

I-cell disease (inclusion cell disease and **mucolipidosis, type 2**) An inherited condition of deficiency of intracellular lysosomal hydrolases in which large cytoplasmic inclusions are detectable in cultured skin fibroblasts.

The clinical manifestations are seen in infancy and include gingival hyperplasia and both psychomotor and growth retardation, as well as facial telangiectasias, kyphosis, skeletal and vertebral abnormalities, arthritis, and seizures, with the slow development of corneal opacities; abnormal excretion of mucopolysaccharides is not a feature. The condition resembles both **Hurler** and **pseudo-Hurler syndromes**. A major review is that of Kolodny and Cable.[3522]

ice-on-eyes test See **ice-pack test**.

ice-pack test (ice-on-eyes test) A bedside diagnostic maneuver in **myasthenia gravis** in which a small bag of crushed ice is held over one closed eye while the myasthenic patient who is currently experiencing diplopia looks upward. The ice pack is removed after 2 min and the degree of diplopia and speed of opening of the eyelids are assessed. In a positive test, the ptosis will have improved by 2 mm or more from the baseline level and when compared to the other one. A lack of fatigability in the cooled eye relative to the other eye and faster opening of that eyelid also suggests the diagnosis.[5741]

ice-pick pains Recurrent twinges of sharp needlelike pains in the head, lasting for a second or so and occurring mainly in patients with migraine.[5204] See **idiopathic stabbing headache**.

It is a puzzle that something so characteristic and common should not have been recognized until the last decade.

ice water test Introduction of 100 ml of ice cold water into the bladder leads to its immediate contraction if the bladder is uninhibited, with detrusor instability. With the patient in the supine position, 100 ml of sterile saline water at 4–8°C is injected manually. If cystometric capacity was $<$200 ml, a volume of about half the individual cystometric bladder capacity is used. The fluid is left within the bladder for 3 min. The test is considered positive if an involuntary bladder contraction $\geq$15 cm H_2O is registered. Autonomic hyperreflexia, manifested as systolic blood pressure increase $\geq$50 mmHg within 3 min of ice-water instillation occurs commonly.[1090]

ICH Score A prognostic instrument for patients with intracerebral hemorrhage. The

Glasgow Coma Scale is the most significant factor, while age of at least 80 years, infratentorial origin of ICH, the volume of the ICH, and the presence of intraventricular hemorrhage are independent factors associated with the 30-day mortality.

GCS Score—2 points if 3–4 and 1 point if 5–12. ICH volume—1 point if at least 30 ml. IVH—1 point if intraventricular hemorrhage. Infratentorial—1 point if origin is infratentorial. Age—1 point if 80+ years old. Thirty Day Mortalities for total ICH Scores: 0 = 0%; 1 = 13%; 2 = 26%; 3 = 72%; 4 = 97%; 5 and above = 100%[2853]

ichthyosis (Gr, fishiness) Scaliness of the skin (reptilian skin); a feature in **Rud** and **Refsum syndromes** and with **Sjögren–Larsson syndrome**.

Variants of the last are an ichthyotic condition appearing in adult life that is associated with progressive spastic paraparesis but without mental impairment; and a neurocutaneous syndrome resembling **myotonic dystrophy** but inherited as an X-linked characteristic.[4263]

Ichthyosis and neutral lipid storage disease is a congenital dysmorphic syndrome manifesting also sensorineural deafness, cataract, retinal dysplasia, myopathic weakness, and mental and developmental delay.[381]

ichthyosis linearis neuropathica See **nevus unis lateralis**.

ichthyosis-alopecia-photophobia See **Eramo syndrome**.

ichthyosis-Little disease See **Sjögren–Larsson syndrome**.

ictal amaurosis A rare **inhibitory seizure** disorder of childhood, in which temporary blindness is associated with occipital EEG paroxysms and succeeded by headaches and nausea.[2384]

ictal bradycardia Any degree of bradycardia up to asystole, occurring during a seizure, with temporal lobe origin. It is suggested by marked pallor during the attack and diagnosed by monitoring of the EEG and EKG, the former having little localizing value.[853] See also **sudden unexplained death in epilepsy patients**.

ictal catatonia A syndrome of nonconvulsive status epilepticus characterized by catalepsy, waxy flexibility, mutism, muscle rigidity, psychotic negativism, stereotypies and **verbigeration**, associated with concurrent abnormal discharges on the EEG.[3847]

ictal deafness A rare, **inhibitory seizure** disorder associated with a left posterior temporal focus.[2351]

ictal eye closure A sign suggesting that the event is a psychogenic, nonepileptic seizure.[1175] Normal responses to cold caloric testing and retention of the oculocephalic reflex are other signs of the same condition.

ictal nystagmus See **epileptic nystagmus**.

ictal paralysis (inhibitory seizure paralysis, somatic inhibitory seizure) A form of nonconvulsive seizure presenting as transient paralytic attacks involving the face, hand, and/or leg, usually lasting anything from 2 min to a day. Serious structural pathology is commonly absent.

ictal stuttering A finding strongly suggestive of psychogenic, nonepileptic seizurelike events rather than true epileptic seizures.

ichthyotocicosis See **scombroid**.

ictus (Lat, a blow or stroke) A sudden neurological happening, such as a cerebrovascular event or a seizure.

ictus emeticus Paroxysmal vomiting as an epileptic event. The causative lesion was right sided in most but not all of the cases described. Two features suggesting that the symptom is in fact ictal are the patient's unawareness of the act of vomiting and the association of this with other ictal events.[3554]

Idaho syndrome A craniofacial malformation characterized by scaphocephaly, strabismus, and skeletal abnormalities such as ulnar deviation of the fingers, congenital heart malformations, and physical and mental delay.[4]

ideation Thoughts and feelings generated spontaneously, in the absence of obvious extrinsic stimuli.

ideational agraphia A selective inability to write letters or words in the absence of any difficulty in copying them.[452]

ideational apraxia A defect in the actual handling of common objects or a loss of conceptual knowledge relating to the use of tools, on account of spatiotemporal errors; however, the subject retains the correct intent and the gross motor power and coordination required for these purposes. The error patterns include perseveration, omission, or incorrect ordering of those acts that are components of multistage complex actions requiring the manipulation of objects, in company with a loss of pantomime ability in response to command or imitation.

The diagnostic clue is that the patient can do things spontaneously which he cannot manage when he is asked to do them, although he understands the command itself. Usually the phenomenon is seen in the left limbs in association with left-sided deep parietofrontal and occipitofrontal and anterior callosal lesions—so dysphasia and a right hemiparesis coexist in most cases. The condition may be considered as a **disconnection syndrome**.

The causative lesion, in dextrals, is in the dominant parietal lobe; but in **callosal apraxia**, there is disconnection of the engrams for skilled movement in the right hemisphere from the speech centers on the left.[6671] See **apraxia**.

ideomotor apraxia See **apraxia**.

ideomotor prosodic apraxia A condition in which spontaneous everyday speech has normal prosody, but the subject cannot produce the same acoustical features underlying prosody to command, described in the context of **Alzheimer disease**.[3273]

idioglossia 1. Severe retardation of articulatory development, often accompanied by congenital auditory imperception or retardation of language development and leading to a form of abnormal speech in which the subject uses individual words for objects, persons, and affective states.[131] 2. A private language developed by two or more people, particularly twins, which is unintelligible to others.

idiomuscular Peculiar to muscle.

idiomuscular contraction See **myotatic irritability**.

idiopathic (Gr, of itself, individual + disease) Now used to refer to disease arising spontaneously, with no known cause.

idiopathic acute lethal catatonia See **acute lethal catatonia**.

idiopathic adult hydrocephalus See **normal pressure hydrocephalus**.

idiopathic autonomic neuropathy See **autonomic neuropathy**.

idiopathic axonal polyneuropathy A gradually progressive sensory or sensorimotor neuropathy causing mild to moderate disability. Toxic exposure and hypertriglyceridemia are risk factors but glucose intolerance and alcohol overuse are not. A history of peripheral neuropathy in first- or second-degree relatives and the presence of pes cavus in many of these subjects may suggest a familial origin.[3043]

idiopathic brachial plexopathy See **neuralgic amyotrophy**.

idiopathic calcification of the basal ganglia A syndrome inherited in either dominant or recessive modes, with the onset in childhood or adult life of spasticity, rigidity, bradykinesia, tremor, dystonia, chorea, and dementia,[3938] accompanied by evidence of basal ganglion calcification on MRI or CT scans. In a few cases, there are no clinical features of the calcification at all.

In a *variant* form, familial ataxia and pigmentary macular degeneration are found.[6092] The differences from so-called Fahr disease are subtle at best. See **striatopallidal calcification**.

idiopathic cranial polyneuropathy The association of self-limited facial pain and involvement of (mainly motor) cranial nerves such as the III, V, and VII and the bulbar nerves (or either of these features in isolation) with diverse etiologies. The condition was first recognized by **Gowers** and is hardly separable from the **superior orbital fissure syndrome** or the **Tolosa–Hunt syndrome** (which themselves may be identical).[3259]

idiopathic dementia/autism See **infantile autism**.

idiopathic epilepsy syndrome A syndrome that only comprises seizures and in which there is no underlying structural brain lesion nor other neurological signs or symptoms. These are presumed to be genetic and are usually age dependent.[1861]

idiopathic enuresis See **sleep-related enuresis**.

idiopathic familial intracerebral arterial calcification See **striatopallidal calcification**.

idiopathic generalized epilepsies (IGEs; OMIN 600669) Forms of generalized epilepsy in which all seizures are initially generalized, with an EEG pattern of bilateral, synchronous, and symmetrical discharges (as is described in the seizure classification of the corresponding type). The patient usually has a normal interictal state, without neurological or neuroradiological signs. In general, interictal EEGs show normal background activity and generalized discharges, such as spikes, polyspikes, spike wave, and polyspike waves of >3 Hz. The discharges are increased in slow-wave sleep. Seizure-precipitating factors such as hyperventilation, sleep deprivation, and intermittent photic stimulation are common.

The term *idiopathic* as defined by the ILAE is reserved for certain focal or generalized epileptic syndromes with particular clinical characteristics and with specific EEG findings, and should not be used to refer to epilepsy or seizures without obvious cause.[1265]

The various syndromes of idiopathic generalized epilepsies comprise about a third of all epilepsies and include absence, generalized tonic-clonic, and myoclonic seizure disorders alone or in combination, differing mainly in the age of onset.[4083] Most if not all are genetically determined; in some cases mapping to 8q24 has been achieved.

The IGEs recognised by the International League Against Epilepsy (ILAE) are

Childhood absence epilepsy
Epilepsy with myoclonic absences
Epilepsy with myoclonic astatic seizures
IG Epilepsy with GTCS only
Juvenile absence epilepsy (Janz)
Juvenile myoclonic epilepsy
Myoclonic epilepsy in infancy

Other nonrecognized IGE syndromes include **perioral myoclonia with absences** and **IGE with phantom absences**.

A *variant* is *adult-onset idiopathic generalized epilepsy* which is relatively frequent and benign. The seizures are usually provoked, but easy to control. Absences and myoclonus may accompany the GTCS.[4083] See also **benign neonatal familial convulsions, benign neonatal convulsions, benign myoclonic epilepsy in infants, childhood absence epilepsy, epilepsy with tonic-clonic seizures on awakening,** and **eyelid myoclonia with typical absences**.

idiopathic generalized epilepsy with generalized tonic-clonic seizures (GTCS) only A genetically determined seizure syndrome with onset between childhood and mid-adult life. Linkage to the *EJM1* locus for GTCS on awakening but not with GTCS at other times has been established. Clinically, GTCS most often occurs within an hour or so of awakening. Sleep deprivation, fatigue, and excessive alcohol consumption are precipitants. The interictal EEG is usually normal but generalized spike/ multiple spike wave discharges are often recorded and the condition is photosensitive. The manifestations are usually lifelong but are responsive to current treatments.

idiopathic generalized epilepsy with phantom absences An uncommon form in which occasional GTCS occurs after adolescence in otherwise healthy people, accompanied by myoclonic jerks and subclinical absences which are detectable only with video-EEG recordings but which can be provoked by hyperventilation. Absence status could be a significant social problem since the condition is clinically undetectable.

The interictal EEG may show focal paroxysmal bursts of localized slow or sharp waves or spikes while brief generalized 3–4 Hz spike/multiple spike waves are seen during spells.

idiopathic generalized glycogenosis See **glycogen storage diseases.**

idiopathic headache See **episodic tension-type headache.**

idiopathic hypercalcemia See **Williams syndrome.**

idiopathic hyperCKemia A benign condition without neurological abnormalities and with normal or nonspecific findings on other (necessary) laboratory studies, including EMG and muscle biopsy. The frequency of diagnosis of the condition has diminished since the development of knowledge regarding the variable presentations of dystrophinopathies and recognition that β-blockers, antipsychotics, and cholesterol-lowering drugs may also be responsible.[66] Unexplained persistently increased creatine kinase (CK) levels in an otherwise healthy patient should alert the anesthesiologist to the possibility of **malignant hyperpyrexia** and/or myopathy.

In the more serious cases, raised serum CK levels are a presentation of **dystrophinopathies**, seen mainly in males, in a minority of whom clinical and/or histopathologic evidence of a neuromuscular disorder develop between 1 and 7 years after detection of hyperCKemia. Such conditions include distal myopathy, **myoadenylate deaminase deficiency**, subclinical hypothyroidism, **polymyositis**, mitochondrial myopathy, sarcoid myopathy, McArdle disease, **central core disease, multicore disease, inclusion body myopathy**, and **Duchenne muscular dystrophy** carrier status.

idiopathic hypersomnia A disorder of presumed CNS cause that is associated with normal or prolonged major sleep episodes and excessive sleepiness, consisting of prolonged sleep episodes lasting 1–2 h which are composed of nonrapid eye movement sleep. Diagnostic criteria have been suggested (see Chart I–1).[1629]

Chart I–1. Diagnostic Criteria for Idiopathic Hypersomnia

A. A complaint of prolonged sleep episodes, excessive sleepiness, or excessively deep sleep.
B. Presence of a prolonged nocturnal sleep period or frequent daily sleep episodes.
C. The onset is insidious and typically before the age of 25 years.
D. The complaint is present for at least 6 months.
E. The onset does not occur within 18 months of trauma.
F. Polysomnography demonstrates one or more of the following:
   1. A sleep period that is normal or prolonged in duration
   2. Sleep latency less than 10 min
   3. Normal REM sleep latency
   4. An MSLT that demonstrates a sleep latency less than 10 min
   5. Less than two sleep-onset REM periods.
G. Absence of any medical or psychiatric disorder that could account for the symptom.
H. Does not meet the diagnostic criteria of any other sleep disorder causing excessive sleepiness, e.g., narcolepsy, obstructive sleep apnea syndrome, or post-traumatic hypersomnia.

MSLT = Multiple sleep latency test; REM = rapid eye movement.

From AASM Diagnostic Classification Steering Committee. The International Classification of Sleep Disorders Diagnostic and Coding Manual. *Rochester, MN. American Academy of Sleep Medicine 1991/2001. Reproduced by kind permission of the Academy.* See also http://www.sleepeducation.com/Disorders.aspx/.

idiopathic hypertrophic cranial pachymeningitis A rare, chronic fibrotic, granulomatous, inflammatory condition of the dura mater, presenting usually with severe headache, papilledema, visual losses, diplopia, cranial nerve palsies, ataxia, seizures, confusion, and hydrocephalus,[3605] more commonly occurring in the Far East. The CSF may or may not show evidence of chronic inflammation with raised protein and white cell counts. MRI and CT images show the thickening of the basal dura. No specific organism has been implicated as responsible in the cases reported to date. The signs usually dissipate after the institution of steroid therapy. See also **Tolosa–Hunt syndrome**.

A similar syndrome has been described in patients with rheumatoid arthritis, syphilis, Wegener granulomatosis, tuberculosis, or cancer.

idiopathic inflammatory myopathies A heterogeneous group of inflammatory muscle diseases from which no infectious agent can be isolated but sharing the features of the presence of inflammatory infiltrates within skeletal muscles and muscle fiber destruction. Disturbances of the immune system are considered responsible in many cases. **Polymyositis** and **dermatomyositis** are the classic phenotypes, in which typical clinical findings include proximal girdle weakness, muscle pain and tenderness with or without skin rash; elevated serum CK levels; multifocal myopathic changes with spontaneous, small, short duration, polyphasic motor unit potentials with or without increased insertional activity as shown by EMG; and a necrotizing inflammatory process with muscle fiber necrosis, regeneration, and perivascular and intrafascicular mononuclear cellular infiltrate with or without perifascicular atrophy on muscle biopsy. Many atypical presentations are, however, recorded.

Chart I–2 is constructed using data from Mastaglia (1985)[4153] and from the Web site: http://neuromuscular.wustl.edu/antibody/infmyop.htm/. Reproduced by kind permission of Dr. Alan Pestronk.

idiopathic insomnia A lifelong inability to obtain adequate sleep, presumably due to an abnormality of the neurological control of the sleep-wake mechanism. The suggested AASM diagnostic criteria[1629] are given in Chart I–3.

idiopathic intracerebral vascular calcification A rare, probably dominantly-inherited disorder characterized by pigmentary retinal degeneration, calcification of the basal ganglia, thumb deformities, pectoralis muscle hypoplasia and peroneal muscular atrophy with mental retardation.[5031]

idiopathic intracranial hypertension (spontaneous intracranial hypertension, pseudotumor cerebri, serous meningitis; toxic, minor, or pseudo-meningitis; meningismus; Julien-Marie-See syndrome; increased

Chart I–2. Classification of the Idiopathic Inflammatory Myopathies

Generalized

Polymyositis (idiopathic immune myopathy)

Dermatomyositis

Inclusion body myositis

Angiopathic myopathy An inflammatory myopathy associated with **Churg–Strauss syndrome, Wegener granulomatosis**, or **polyarteritis nodosa**.[4158]

Anti-Jo-1 antibody syndrome An immune myopathy with perimysial pathology presenting with weakness, myalgias, or cramps and with Raynaud phenomenon, hyperkeratosis of the hands, and often interstitial lung disease. Perimysial inflammation is seen on muscle biopsy.

Anti-MAS antibody syndrome An acute disease of young adults with rhabdomyolysis related to alcohol ingestion and characterized by myalgias and palpitations. Serum CK levels are high and anti-Mas antibodies are detectable.

Anti U1-small nuclear ribonucleoprotein syndrome An adult onset disorder characterized by proximal muscle weakness, dysphagia, and myalgia, with interstitial pneumonitis, distal, arthritis, Raynaud phenomenon, lymphadenopathy, and sometimes lymphocytic meningitis. Serum CK levels are high and an antibody binding to snRNP is detectable.

Brachiocervical inflammatory myopathy A syndrome with the phenotype of **polymyositis** or **dermatomyositis** occurring in later adult life, in which shoulder–girdle and posterior neck weakness are accompanied by dysphagia and sometimes ptosis or ophthalmoplegia. The EMG is myopathic and a decrement may be recorded with repetitive nerve stimulation.[4994]

Chondroitin sulfate c deficiency A rare syndrome of adults who present with diffuse, symmetrical, proximal weakness, and respiratory failure with dysphagia, but with normal serum CK levels. Muscle biopsy shows absence of staining for chondroitin sulfate.[6890]

Collagen vascular diseases; **polymyalgia rheumatica, lupus, scleroderma**.

Drug-induced myositis as with penicillamine or statins

Eosinophilia myalgia syndrome

Eosinophilic perimyositis[5734]

Eosinophilic fasciitis

Eosinophilic polymyositis The presence of an inflammatory myopathy as a complication of a systemic hypereosinophilic syndrome characterized by eosinophilia, anemia, hypergammaglobulinemia, cardiac and pulmonary involvement, skin changes, peripheral neuropathy, and encephalopathy.[3727]

Graft-versus-host disease A cell-mediated immune reaction mediated by donor cytotoxic T-cells (e.g., following bone marrow transplant) and leading to multiorgan involvement, including the phenotypes of myasthenia, myositis, neuropathy, or fasciitis.

Granulomatous myositis A syndrome with the phenotype of polymyositis with dysphagia, sometimes associated with flexion contractures in the arms. The serum CK is normal or raised and the underlying pathology is the presence of noncaseating granulomas in muscles anywhere in the body. **Sarcoidosis** is one cause.

Hemophagocytic lymphohistiocytosis An uncommon inherited systemic disease in which activated macrophages engulf erythrocytes, leukocytes, and platelets. Neurological complications include cerebral edema, seizures, and myalgias. Type I is recessively inherited (9q21) and lethal in early childhood; type 2 (10q22) is less clearly defined.

Inflammatory myopathy with abundant macrophages

Interstitial myositis

Infections: protozoa (**toxoplasmosis**, malaria etc.) cestodes (e.g., **cysticercosis**) and nematodes (**trichinosis**); **benign viral myositis, Coxsackie B infection, HIV** infection, **Lyme disease, leptospirosis, pyomyositis, Sarcocystis** etc.

Macrophagic myofasciitis

Mitochondrial myopathies

Multinodular polymyositis

Myositis complicating **myasthenia gravis**

Myositis with OJ antibodies An adult-onset syndrome characterized by interstitial lung disease and the phenotype of polymyositis without skin involvement.

Necrotizing myopathy with pipestem capillaries A syndrome with the phenotype of **dermatomyositis** distinguished by its onset in late adult life with subacute or episodic weakness after exercise, myalgias, and an association with cerebral infarctions. Its unique pathology is an enlargement of capillary walls that are thickened due to the deposition of amorphous PAS material and complement.[304]

Neonatal perifascicular myopathy A nonprogressive syndrome of infancy presenting with diffuse weakness and later with hypotonia, accompanied by cognitive delay. The child's motor skills may improve with time.

Paraneoplastic necrotic myopathy A severe and progressive syndrome of later life, in which the phenotype of polymyositis occurs in association with an underlying malignancy.

Perimyositis

Signal recognition particle antibody syndrome A disorder of adult life characterized by the acute or subacute onset of severe girdle weakness more than distal weakness with myalgia, Raynaud phenomenon, and very high CK levels. It is differentiated from dermatomyositis only by the presence of antisignal recognition particles.

TNF receptor–associated periodic syndrome (TRAPS) A dominantly inherited syndrome of children who develop recurrent high fevers with focal areas of myalgia and an erythematous skin rash overlying sites of localized myositis or fasciitis on the trunk or limbs. It is mapped to 12p13.2.

continued

Chart I–2. *(continued)*

Localized

Benign acute childhood myositis A self-limiting syndrome of childhood, more common in males, associated with influenza in which following a prodrome of fever with cough and headache the child complains of calf pain and tenderness with slight weakness and difficulty in walking. Serum CK levels are increased in the acute phase of the disorder.[3999]

Focal myositis A syndrome occurring at any time of life, characterized by the appearance of a solitary, painful mass in the large leg muscles or occasionally in the arms, trunk, or tongue without generalized weakness, slowly regressing over months to years. Muscle biopsy shows thickening of the perimysial connective tissue and changes of degeneration and regeneration.[5901, 1372]

Idiopathic **orbital myositis** An acute, relapsing or chronic idiopathic syndrome occurring mainly in young adults and due to inflammation of one or more extraocular muscles. Clinical features include proptosis and periorbital edema, conjunctiva injection and frequently the complaint of diplopia since eye movements are paretic or at least restricted by the involvement of individual muscles.

Masticator myopathy A syndrome of pain and swelling in the masseter and temporalis muscles that is sometimes seen in large dogs but is rare in humans.

Monomelic myositis (Gr, single + limb)

Myositis associated with **linear scleroderma**

Myositis associated with panniculitis

Proliferative myositis

Diagnostic criteria for the idiopathic inflammatory myopathies have been suggested[2976] as follows:

Polymyositis (PM)

Definite polymyositis

1. All clinical criteria with the exception of rash
2. Elevated serum CK
3. Muscle biopsy criteria include *b* and exclude *c*, *d*, *h*, *i*.*

Probable polymyositis

1. All clinical criteria except rash
2. Elevated serum CK
3. Other laboratory criteria (1 of 3)
4. Muscle biopsy criteria include *b* and exclude *c*, *d*, *g*, *h*, *i*.*

Dermatomyositis (DM) Definite dermatomyositis

1. All clinical criteria
2. Muscle biopsy criteria include *c**

Probable dermatomyositis

1. All clinical criteria
2. Muscle biopsy criteria include *d* or **e* or elevated serum CK or other laboratory criteria (1 of 3)

Amyopathic dermatomyositis

1. Rash typical of DM: Heliotrope, periorbital edema, V-sign*, shawl sign*, holster sign*
2. Skin biopsy demonstrates a reduced capillary density, deposition of MAC on small blood vessels, along the dermal epidermal junction and variable keratinocyte decoration for MAC
3. No objective weakness
4. Normal serum CK
5. Normal EMG
6. Muscle biopsy does not reveal features compatible with definite or probable DM

Possible dermatomyositis without dermatitis

1. All clinical criteria with the exception of rash
2. Elevated serum CK
3. Other laboratory criteria (1 of 3)
4. Muscle biopsy criteria include *c* or *d**

Nonspecific myositis

1. All clinical criteria with the exception of rash
2. Elevated serum CK

3. Other laboratory criteria (1 of 3)
4. Muscle biopsy criteria include *e* or *f** and exclude all others.

Immune-mediated necrotizing myopathy

1. All clinical criteria with the exception of rash
2. Elevated serum CK
3. Other laboratory criteria (1 of 3)

Muscle biopsy criteria include *g** and exclude all others.
When all four criteria are satisfied, a diagnosis of *definite* PM or DM can be made. The presence of three criteria would allow a diagnosis of *probable* PM or DM and it would be reasonable to treat such patients provided that the clinical features of the illness are compatible (i.e., criterion 1 is present), and that other genetic, metabolic, toxic, and infective causes of myopathy have been adequately excluded.

* See original text

*From Hoogendijk JE, Amato AA, Lecky B. Trial design in adult idiopathic inflammatory myopathies with the exception of inclusion body myositis. Neuromuscul Disord. 2004;***14***:337–45. Reproduced with permission from Elsevier Science.*

Chart I–3. Diagnostic Criteria for Idiopathic Insomnia

A. A complaint of insomnia, combined with a complaint of decreased functioning during wakefulness.
B. The insomnia is long-standing, typically beginning in early childhood, if not at birth.
C. The insomnia is relentless, unvaried through periods of both poor and good emotional adaptation.
D. Polysomnography demonstrates one or more of the following:

1. An increased sleep latency;
2. Reduced sleep efficiency;
3. An increased number and duration of awakenings;
4. Often a reversed first night effect.

E. No medical or psychiatric disease can explain the early onset of insomnia
F. Other sleep disorders producing insomnia can occur simultaneously, for example, adjustment sleep disorder.

From AASM Diagnostic Classification Steering Committee. The International Classification of Sleep Disorders Diagnostic and Coding Manual. *Rochester, MN. American Academy of Sleep Medicine 1991/2001. Reproduced by kind permission of the Academy.* See also http://www.sleepeducation.com/Disorders.aspx/.

intracranial pressure without localizing signs; and Dupré syndrome) First described by Quincke (an originator of lumbar puncture) in 1891,[5155] this condition is characterized by a rise in intracranial pressure (greater than 200 mm CSF) in the absence of an intracranial mass lesion or of hydrocephalus and with normal CSF contents. It usually represents a disorder of CSF dynamics resulting from increased intra-abdominal and intra-pleural pressure, leading to increased cardiac filling and jugular venous pressures.[6119, 6603] Although bilateral sinovenous stenoses were found in almost all of one series, the condition is also a complication of vitamin A poisoning, drug side effects, and renal disease. Increased venous pressure may be secondary to increased CSF pressure in this condition.

Clinically, it presents with papilledema, visual obscurations and occasionally a VI cranial nerve palsy without other clinical signs, most often in female subjects. The condition causes blindness in 10% of cases. Over 120 disorders have been described as associated with it, the most common being obesity, but in 30 percent of the cases in which such clinical features are noted, a different pathology is finally detected.[6700] See also **otitic hydrocephalus**.

Diagnostic criteria[5917] (modified from those originally suggested by **Dandy**) include

1. Clinical features of increased intracranial pressure (e.g., headache and papilledema)
2. Increased intracranial pressure at lumbar puncture (>250 mm CSF)
3. Absence of localizing findings on CNS examination. False localizing signs may be present.
4. Normal neurodiagnostic studies (apart from CSF pressure >220 mm in the nonobese and >250 mm CSF in the obese). No evidence of venous obstructive disease.
5. No disturbance of consciousness
6. Normal CSF constituents
7. Benign course apart from visual deterioration
8. No other cause of increased intracranial pressure is found.

(Reproduced from Smith JL.[5898] *Whence pseudotumor cerebri? J Clin Neuro-Ophthalmol 1985;5:55–6 by kind permission.)*

Another set of criteria requires that the symptoms and signs are only those of generalized intracranial hypertension or papilledema; there is documentation of raised intracranial pressure; the CSF composition is normal; no hydrocephalus, mass, structural, nor vascular lesion is found on MRI or MRV (except perhaps for an empty sella); and the condition cannot be ascribed to another cause.[2203]

Variant forms are *fulminant/malignant idiopathic intracranial hypertension*, in which the presentation is acute with rapidly progressive visual loss. This is most commonly associated with venous sinus thrombosis or a meningeal process; and *paroxysmal intracranial hypertension* which is characterized by headache and severe papilledema caused by paroxysms of raised intracranial pressure.[3420]

For *headache attributed to idiopathic intracranial hypertension*, diagnostic criteria have been defined as follows:

A. Progressive headache with at least one of the following characteristics and fulfilling criteria C and D:
   1. Daily occurrence
   2. Diffuse and/or constant (nonpulsating) pain
   3. Aggravated by coughing or straining
B. Intracranial hypertension fulfilling the following criteria:
   1. Alert patient with neurological examination that either is normal or demonstrates any of the following abnormalities:
      A) Papilledema
      B) Enlarged blind spot
      C) Visual field defect (progressive if untreated)
      D) VI nerve palsy
   2. Increased CSF pressure (>200 mmH_2O in the non-obese, >250 mmH_2O in the obese) measured by lumbar puncture in the recumbent position or by epidural or intraventricular pressure monitoring
   3. Normal CSF chemistry (low protein is acceptable) and cellularity
   4. Intracranial diseases (including venous sinus thrombosis) ruled out by appropriate investigations
   5. No metabolic, toxic or hormonal cause of intracranial hypertension
C. Headache develops in close temporal relation to increased intracranial pressure
D. Headache improves after withdrawal of CSF to reduce pressure to 120–170 mm H_2O and resolves within 72 h of persistent normalization of intracranial pressure

(From the International Classification of Headache Disorders (Headache Classification Committee of the International Headache Society. Cephalalgia 2004;24(Suppl 1)) by kind permission of Dr. Jes Olesen, the International Headache Society and Wiley-Blackwell Publications.)

Headache attributed to intracranial hypertension secondary to metabolic, toxic or hormonal causes represent a *variant* for which the diagnostic criteria are virtually identical except that criterion C requires that the headache develops after weeks or months of endocrine disorder, hypervitaminosis A or intake of substances (other than medications) that can elevate CSF pressure; and criterion D that the headache resolves within 3 months after removal of the cause.

idiopathic late-onset cerebellar ataxias A heterogeneous group of ataxic syndromes which were generally reported as *olivopontocerebellar atrophies* (OPCAs) by Déjèrine and Thomas in 1900 but first described by Menzel in 1891. Clinically, the onset is usually around 40 years of age with gait ataxia, cerebellar and spastic speech, some arm incoordination, impassive facies, and hypertonia. The muscle stretch reflexes are brisk and the plantar responses upgoing. Dementia and nystagmus are more marked in the OPCAs than in the cortical cerebellar atrophies (see below) but pursuit movements and optokinetic nystagmus are much affected in both forms.

Numerous *variant* forms of OPCA are recognized, usually with dominant inheritance and associated with various other problems. Linkage to chromosome 6 has been found in some kinships but not in others. These conditions closely resemble *parenchymatous or cortical cerebellar atrophy* (CCA), but, in the latter, the olivary and pontine changes are less marked and optic atrophy, pigmentary retinal degeneration, and ophthalmoplegia do not occur. See **cerebellar ataxias**.

idiopathic leg pain Chronic deep mild muscular pain felt especially during rest after exercise. Both the cause and the cure are unknown.

idiopathic Lewy body disease See **Lewy body disease**.

idiopathic localization-related epilepsies Childhood epilepsies with focal ("partial") seizures and focal EEG abnormalities. They are age related, without demonstrable anatomical lesions, and are subject to spontaneous remission. Clinically, the patients have neither a neurological nor an intellectual deficit, and there is no history of antecedent illness, but they frequently do have a family history of benign epilepsy. The seizures are usually brief and rare, but may be frequent early in the course of the disorder. The seizure patterns may vary from case to case but usually remain constant in the same child. The EEG is characterized by normal background activity with localized high-voltage repetitive spikes, which are sometimes independently multifocal. Brief bursts of generalized spike-waves can occur. Focal abnormalities are increased by sleep and are without change in morphology. *(After Dreifuss FE, et al. Commission for classification and terminology, ILAE. Proposal for Revised Classifications of Epilepsies and Epileptic syndromes.* Epilepsia *1989;30:389–99 by kind permission of the ILAE and Wiley-Blackwell.)*

idiopathic lumbosacral plexitis See **lumbosacral plexitis**.

idiopathic neonatal convulsions Focal clonic or multifocal clonic seizures and minimal seizures including tonic deviation, eyelid blinking, lip smacking, sucking or swallowing, or alterations in muscle tone with assumption of bizarre postures occurring in the neonatal period, and most commonly due to **hypoxic-ischemic encephalopathy**. Myoclonic seizures also occur less commonly.

idiopathic neurogenic anorectal incontinence A syndrome of adult life, characterized by weakness or the anal sphincter with loss of the anal reflex, usually occurring in women among whom it is often due to denervation of the puborectalis muscle resulting from prolonged constipation or from the process of childbirth.[4907]

idiopathic neuromyotonia (continuous muscle fiber activity, neurogenic benign fasciculations, pseudomyotonia and pseudotetany, chronic or sporadic tetany, acquired myotonia, pseudomyotonia, generalized myokymia, quantal squander, Isaacs syndrome, Isaacs–Mertens syndrome) A sporadic, probably autoimmune syndrome of abnormal spontaneous distal motor unit activity of neural origin (**neuromyotonia**) manifesting benign fasciculations, generalized myokymia, delayed muscular relaxation (pseudomyotonia), pseudotetany, hyperhidrosis, painful spasms, cramps, and stiffness at rest and in sleep (but exacerbated by exercise); muscle hypertrophy; and abnormal motor nerve conduction velocities. The face and branchial muscles may be affected. The condition is heterogeneous in nature and causation; most cases are sporadic and a few are paraneoplastic or autoallergic.[3662, 6619]

The condition may be of any degree of severity and in some cases is permanent; in others, the symptoms are worsened by voluntary muscle contraction but abate after repetitive effort. The lesion is localized to the distal part of the motor unit and may represent motor axonal hyperexcitability, but its nature is obscure.[1212]

Variant forms are **neurogenic Isaacs syndrome**, characterized by onset in youth, pes cavus, myotonia, pseudohypertrophy, myokymia, fasciculation, neurogenic weakness, and loss of pain sensation with neural myelinated fiber loss; an inherited form; and forms associated with **hereditary motor and sensory neuropathy**,[3662] *chronic inflammatory polyneuropathy*, *squamous cell carcinoma of the lung*,[6619] and *exposure to* 2,4-D *or to penicillamine*.

idiopathic ophthalmoplegia (Collier syndrome) A syndrome reported from the Far East resembling the superior orbital fissure syndrome with involvement of the III, IV, VI, and the first two divisions of the V cranial nerves. The optic nerve may also be involved. The erythrocyte sedimentation rate is typically raised.

Clinically, diplopia, ptosis, giddiness, headache, facial numbness, chemosis, retro-orbital pain, proptosis, conjunctivitis, and/or progressive blindness are the usual features. The signs clear within 2 months, in some cases requiring steroids to do so.[6228] See also **superior orbital fissure syndrome**.

idiopathic orofacial dystonia See **cranial dystonia**.

idiopathic orthostatic hypotension See **progressive autonomic failure**.

idiopathic painless brachial plexopathy A syndrome resembling neuralgic amyotrophy with neurogenic muscle weakness and atrophy but without pain. See also **neuralgic amyotrophy**.

idiopathic Parkinsonism A syndrome characterized by resting tremor, rigidity, bradykinesia, and impairment of postural reflexes. See **Parkinson disease**.

idiopathic photosensitive occipital lobe epilepsy A rare form of reflex epilepsy with onset between infancy and 19 years characterized by the experience of elementary visual hallucinations, blurring of vision, or blindness, alone or in combination, as in spontaneous occipital lobe epilepsy. Deviation of the eyes and head, eyelid fluttering, and orbital pain are less common. Myoclonic jerks, absences, GTCS, and bizarre ictal symptomatology mimicking hysterical attacks, and autonomic symptoms as in **Panayiotopoulos syndrome** are sometimes described. Postictal symptoms include headache, nausea, and vomiting. Flickering lights (including TV monitors) are precipitants, especially if combined with such facilitating factors as excitement, fatigue, or sleep deprivation.

The ictal EEG shows occipital discharges of fast spikes ending spontaneously, spreading to temporal regions or progressing to GTCS. Visually evoked responses are abnormally large. See also **Jeavons syndrome, television epilepsy**, and **Pokemon syndrome**.[4882]

idiopathic postural orthostatic tachycardia syndrome A form of autonomic neuropathy seen mainly following a viral illness in women who complain of the acute onset of fatigue and light-headedness, postprandial bloating, or vomiting and tachycardia, exaggerated with tilting. The condition is considered possibly due to decreased plasma volume or red blood cell mass or to adrenergic hypersensitivity resulting from postganglionic sympathetic denervation.[5637] See also **pandysautonomia** and **postural orthostatic tachycardia syndrome**.

idiopathic pure motor neuropathy A syndrome of later life characterized by insidiously progressive asymmetrical, distal weakness, and atrophy, mainly in the legs, with hyporeflexia but with normal sensation. The deficits advance to paraplegia and upper limb involvement eventually, but respiratory and bulbar muscles tend to be spared. Electrodiagnostic studies suggest an axonal neuropathy without conduction block. CSF protein is modestly elevated ($<$100 mg/dl) but blood studies including ganglioside antibodies are normal.

idiopathic reading epilepsy A rare, rather benign reflex epilepsy syndrome with an unknown genetic basis, affecting adolescents and characterized by myoclonic jerks of the masticatory and orofacial muscles (perceived as clicking) following or during prolonged reading. If that stimulus continues, the jerks may spread to the trunk and limb muscles before a generalized seizure develops. Talking fast or argumentatively and reading music are also precipitants. In a similar condition (graphogenic epilepsy) myoclonic jerks of the hands occur with writing.

idiopathic recurrent myoglobinuria See **myoglobinuria** (*variant*).

idiopathic recurring stupor A rare syndrome characterized by the occurrence of transient episodes of stupor or coma in the absence of toxic or structural brain disease and with accompanying 14-Hz activity on the EEG, as a result of a disturbance of the gamma amino butyric acidergic systems.[6331, 6332]

idiopathic sensory neuronopathy (chronic sensory ataxic neuropathy) An acute, subacute, or chronic asymmetrical sensory neuropathy affecting large rather than small fibers in the extremities, face, and trunk, occurring mainly in females aged between 40 and 60 years. Patchy areflexia is notable but there is no motor weakness. All sensory modes may be affected and the Romberg test is usually positive. Progression is variable but usually slow. Antineuronal antibodies are not detected. The condition is not associated with distant carcinoma nor with abnormalities of the CNS or the CSF, and the cause is unknown.[3339, 6192] See also **cryptogenic sensory polyneuropathy** and **idiopathic axonal polyneuropathy**.

idiopathic small fiber neuropathy The most common subset of small fiber neuropathies, usually presenting in mid-adult life with burning pain in the feet, and with lancinating pains, numbness, paresthesias, and autonomic failure. Involvement of the arms is late if present at all. The QSART, cardiovagal tests, and abdominal fat and skin biopsies assist in diagnosis.[3931]

idiopathic stabbing headache See **primary stabbing headache**.

idiopathic steroid responsive chronic lymphocytic meningitis A steroid responsive chronic meningitis for which an etiological cause is seldom found. Leptomeningeal biopsy and long-term follow-up seldom identify the underlying cause.[1110]

idiopathic stimulus-sensitive myoclonus See **stimulus-sensitive myoclonus**.

idiopathic subcortical degeneration See **pallidonigral degenerations**.

idiopathic torsion dystonia See **dystonia**.

idiopathic vertebral sclerosis Narrowing of a disk space with diffuse sclerosis of the anterior inferior part of the vertebral body, usually of L4. The condition can only be diagnosed radiographically. The condition mainly affects women and is a cause of severe low back pain.[6745]

idiospasm Cramp or spasm occurring only in one area.

idiosyncrasy (Gr, one's own + mixing together) 1. The special or peculiar temperament or body habit of a person whereby he or she differs from the ordinary. This peculiarity extends to susceptibility to certain disease and to the actions of different drugs.[5103] 2. Exceptional responses on the part of exceptional individuals to stimuli that are insufficient to produce any conspicuous effects in the great majority of the human race. (Sir Archibald Garrod) More pithily, "individuality run mad" (Jonathan Hutchinson).

idiotic aphasia See **Worster-Drought-Allen syndrome**.

iduronate sulfatase The enzyme deficient in mucopolysaccaridosis Type 2 (Hunter disease), leading to the accumulation of dermatan and heparan sulfate.

iduronidase The enzyme deficient in **mucopolysaccharidoses** Types 1 and 1A (Hurler disease), leading to the accumulation of dermatan and heparan sulfate.

Ilheus encephalitis A rare form of encephalitis due to a flavivirus member of the togavirus group of arboviruses, occurring occasionally in South America.

iliac reflex Contraction of the lower abdominal muscles in response to a tap on the iliac crest, seen occasionally in patients with pyramidal lesions above T10.

iliohypogastric neuralgia Continuous burning or lancinating pain felt in the distribution of this nerve, usually following partial injury to it.

The pain is felt in the midline above the pubis but may also radiate to the hip; hypoesthesia may be noted in the same region.

ilioinguinal neuralgia Continuous burning or lancinating pain felt in the distribution of this nerve, usually following its partial injury. The pain is felt in the groin and pudenda and hypesthesia may be noted in the same region. The pain of **genitofemoral neuropathy** is practically indistinguishable from this condition.[3531]

Illinois Test of Psycholinguistic Abilities A test profile designed to delineate communication deficits in children and to suggest remedial programs. Tests of **cognitive closure**, visual memory, and visual and auditory reception are also of value in adults. The test is reviewed by Lezak.[3825]

Illness Severity Score A modified form of the **disability status scale** for **multiple sclerosis** with weighting added to stress pyramidal and cerebellar dysfunction and incorporating additional areas of disease activity and a further factor reflecting the phase of illness. The score is proposed as a useful method for evaluating progression in clinical trials of multiple sclerosis therapy.[4351]

illusions Misperceptions of objective environmental stimuli, affecting any sensory modality.

illusory aura In the context of epilepsy, an alteration of percepts involving the visual, auditory, somatosensory, olfactory, or gustatory systems.

illusory splitting Fragmentation of visual perception, such that the parts of an object or person seen appear to be fractured and displaced from one another. It has been described as a feature of migraine auras.[5057]

illusory visual spread A form of visual perseveration in the spatial sense, wherein the object appears to extend beyond its normal boundaries; or its colors may similarly extend such that the colors of a dress may appear to expand onto the face or arms of the wearer. It is an unusual manifestation of disease of the visual cortex.[1328, 1333]

iminoglycinuria A benign inborn metabolic disorder presenting with nerve deafness and sometimes mental retardation, in which there is increased urinary excretion of proline, hydroxyproline, and glycine.[5401]

imitation behavior A disturbance in motor response wherein patients imitate the gestures and behavior of the examiner despite the fact that they have not been asked to do so, and continue with such imitations although asked to stop. It represents an early stage of **utilization behavior** and is interpreted as demonstrating impairment of the frontal lobe's normal function of inhibiting parietal lobe function.[3826]

imitation synkinesis Involuntary, symmetrical movements tending to reproduce on one side of the body those movements executed by the other. The condition is usually associated with thalamic or parietal lesions and sometimes with lesions of the posterior columns or the PNS and thus is seen in body regions where lemniscal sensation is lost or diminished but motor function is at least relatively intact.[986] A *cerebellar* form is also distinguished.[6400]

immediate memory See **short-term memory**.

immersion epilepsy See **hot water epilepsy**.

immersion foot Cold-induced **Wallerian degeneration** of peripheral nerves.

immune-mediated inflammatory myopathies A group of immune-mediated or infective disorders ranging from focal varieties confined to a single muscle or group to forms with widespread involvement of the skeletal muscles The three major forms are **dermatomyositis, polymyositis**, and **inclusion-body myositis,** each with distinctive clinical features, although muscle biopsy is always needed to confirm the diagnosis histopathologically.[4154]

Proposed classification of idiopathic inflammatory myopathies

1. **Dermatomyositis** (juvenile or adult)
2. **Polymyositis** T-cell mediated (α/β, γ/δ), eosinophilic, or granulomatous
3. Overlap syndromes with polymyositis, dermatomyositis, or inclusion-body myositis
4. Cancer-associated myositis
5. **Inclusion-body myositis**
6. Focal: orbital myositis, **localized nodular myositis**, and inflammatory pseudotumor
7. Diffuse: macrophagic myofasciitis, necrotizing myopathy with pipestem capillaries, and infantile myositis

immune-mediated neuropathies Those neuropathies associated with high titers of auto-antibodies directed against a specific neural antigen. These are listed in Chart I–4. See also **acute inflammatory and demyelinating polyneuropathy** and **gammopathic neuropathies**.

immunoblastic sarcoma See **primary CNS lymphoma**.

immunodeficiency syndromes with encephalopathy Microcephaly, encephalopathy, developmental delay, incoordination, and basal ganglion calcification in infants with AIDS.[500]

immunophilins A family of proteins that act as receptors for the immunosuppressant drugs CsA and FK506 in immune tissue and are highly enriched in the nervous system. They regulate the mitochondrial permeability transition pore, modulate the stability and function of ion channels, and act as molecular chaperones for a variety of proteins.

CsA and FK506 and their derivatives inhibit the function of the immunophilins and provide neuroprotective and neuroregenerative actions in experimental models of stroke, Parkinson disease, neuropathies, etc.

Impact of Event Scale A series of questions assessing the degree of mental trauma experienced following an accident. Both intrusion items and avoidance items are scored.

Presentation: "Below is a list of comments made by people after stressful life events such as your recent accident. Please check each item, indicating how frequently these items were true for you during the past 7 days; Not at all/Often/Sometimes/ Rarely. If they did not occur at all, please mark the 'not at all' column."

1. I thought about it when I didn't mean to
2. I avoided letting myself get upset when I thought about it or was reminded of it
3. I tried to remove it from memory
4. I had trouble falling asleep or staying asleep because of pictures or thoughts about it that came into my mind
5. I had a wave of strong feelings about it
6. I had dreams about it
7. I stayed away from reminders of it
8. I felt as if it hadn't happened or wasn't real
9. I tried not to talk about it
10. Pictures about it popped into my mind
11. Other things kept making me think about it
12. I was aware that I still had a lot of feelings about it but I didn't deal with them
13. I tried not to think about it
14. Any reminder brought back feelings about it
15. My feelings about it were kind of numb

(Reproduced by kind permission of the Rivermead Rehabilitation Centre, Abingdon Rd, Oxford, OXI 4XD UK)

impaired sleep-related penile tumescence The inability to attain or sustain a penile erection during sleep as a result of organic disease affecting the CNS. Such impairment in penile expansibility is a marker for the presence of organic impotence.[6641] It represents a non-event rather than a symptom.

impairment 1. Any loss or abnormality of psychological, physiological, or anatomical structure or function. (WHO) 2. The disturbance of a specific function at the level of an organ; for instance, the elements of the neurological examination that make up stroke scales. Stroke scales are typical examples of impairment scales.

impersistence The inability to maintain a particular activity. This can be considered abnormal only with reference to the concept of the "reasonable person," but does resemble that lack of attention and concentration commonly found in the confused and demented as well as the interruption of static postures by such abnormal movements as chorea. Impersistence of eyelid closure is also a feature of acute (usually right) hemispheric disease.[1604]

Chart I–4. The Immune-Mediated Neuropathies

Multifocal motor neuropathy with persistent conduction block.

Anti-MAG-associated neuropathy A syndrome of paresthesias in the legs, progressing slowly to a distal symmetrical demyelinating sensorimotor peripheral neuropathy, accompanied by high levels of anti-MAG (myelin-associated glycoprotein) IgM antibodies.[3713]

Paraneoplastic sensory neuronopathy associated with small cell lung cancer and anti-Hu antibodies A subacute, progressive paraneoplastic syndrome characterized by paresthesias and painful distal dysesthesias, sensory deficits affecting all modalities, and asymmetrical proximal sensory signs accompanied by high levels of IgG anti-Hu antibodies which bind to neuronal nuclei. In some cases, **limbic encephalitis**, seizures, diplopia, bulbar signs, and autonomic dysfunction are also found.[1585, 2554]

Acute axonal motor neuropathy with anti-Gm1 antibodies and campylobacter infection (Chinese paralytic disease) An acute, life-threatening axonal motor neuropathy resembling **acute inflammatory demyelinating polyneuropathy** but with early and severe axonal damage, associated with infection by *Campylobacter jejuni* and accompanied by high titres of anti-GM_1 antibodies.

Painful sensory neuropathy with antisulfatide antibodies A syndrome characterized by slowly progressive distal sensory loss involving both large and small fibers, accompanied by pain and paresthesias and with detectable IgM and IgG antibodies to sulfatide.[4993]

Tests for impersistence include examining the ability of the patient to maintain the tongue protruded, the eyes closed, or the arms outstretched; and those in the **Dartmouth battery**, particularly with regard to gaze. See also **perseveration**.

implicit memory Knowledge without awareness of the possession of that knowledge; the unconscious retention of learned material; memory where retention is implicit in the performance of tests, although it is not explicitly requested. Frontal and temporal cortices (rather than the hippocampi and perirhinal areas) appear essential for this capacity.[1743]

Tests are usually administered as an evaluation of some function other than memory (such as reading or the learning of motor skills), and memory is assessed indirectly from changes in the performance of the task in question. See also **explicit memory tests** and **working memory**.

impotence (Gr, want of power) Inability to generate or sustain a satisfactory penile erection; sexual incapacity such that the spirit is willing but the flesh is weak.

impulse (from Lat, to push against) A force communicated suddenly, such as the passage of a wave of depolarization through tissues.

impulse blocking See **blocking**.

impulse control disorders Pathological gambling, kleptomania, and compulsive buying, yielding somewhat to treatment with serotonin reuptake inhibitors, opioid antagonists, mood stabilizers, or atypical antipsychotics. [6820] Pathological gambling is a complication of treatment with dopamine agonists or with levadopa itself.

impulsive petit mal See **benign juvenile myoclonic epilepsy**.

imubacco See **Tourette syndrome**, for which this is the Japanese term.

inactivity (record of electrocerebral) The absence over all regions of the head of identifiable electrical activity of cerebral origin, whether spontaneous or induced by physiological stimuli or pharmacological agents.

The determination of electrocerebral inactivity requires advanced instrumentation and stringent technical precautions. Tracings of electrocerebral inactivity should be held in clear contradistinction to low-voltage EEGs and records displaying low amplitude delta activity. *(Adapted from the 1974 report of the Committee on Terminology, IFCN. In Chatrian GE, Bergamini L, Dondey M et al. A glossary of terms most commonly used by clinical electroencephalographers. EEG Clin Neurophysiol 1974;37:538–48. Reproduced by kind permission of Elsevier Science and the IFCN.)*

inadequate sleep hygiene A sleep disorder due to the performance of daily living activities that are inconsistent with the maintenance of good quality sleep and full daytime alertness. These include practices that produce arousal, and those which are inconsistent with the principles of sleep organization.[1629] Diagnostic criteria have been suggested and are given in Chart I–5.

inapperceptive agnosia That form of **agnosia** in which the subject is unable to copy objects visualized.

Chart I–5. Diagnostic Criteria for Inadequate Sleep Hygiene

A. Complaints of either insomnia or excessive sleepiness
B. Presence of at least one of the following:

1. Daytime napping at least two times each week
2. Variable wake-up times or bedtimes
3. Frequent periods (2–3 times per week) of extended amounts of time spent in bed
4. Routine use of products containing alcohol, tobacco, or caffeine in the period preceding bedtime
5. Scheduling exercise too close to bedtime
6. Engaging in exciting or emotionally upsetting activities too close to bedtime
7. Frequent use of the bed for nonrelated activities (e.g., television watching, reading, studying, snacking, etc.)
8. Sleeping on an uncomfortable bed (poor mattress, inadequate blankets, etc.)
9. Allowing the bedroom to be too bright, too stuffy, too cluttered, too hot, too cold, or in some way not conducive to sleep
10. Performing activities demanding high levels of concentration shortly before bed
11. Allowing such mental activities as thinking, planning, reminiscing, etc. to occur while in bed

C. Polysomnography demonstrates one or more of the following:

1. Increased sleep latency
2. Reduced sleep efficiency
3. Frequent arousals
4. Early morning awakening
5. A multiple sleep latency test that shows excessive sleepiness

D. No evidence of psychiatric or medical disorder that accounts for the sleep disturbance
E. Absence of other sleep disorder either producing difficulty in initiating or maintaining sleep or excessive sleepiness

From AASM Diagnostic Classification Steering Committee. *The International Classification of Sleep Disorders Diagnostic and Coding Manual.* Rochester, MN. American Academy of Sleep Medicine 1991/2001. Reproduced by kind permission of the Academy. *See also http://www.sleepeducation.com/Disorders.aspx/.*

inappropriate ADH syndrome

See **syndrome of inappropriate ADH secretion**.

inappropriate crying

See **emotionalism**.

inattention

Lack of response to stimuli for which the primary perceptive mechanism and pathways are intact.

This is usually a phenomenon detected unilaterally (**neglect**) when the subject fails to perceive a stimulus in the presence of competing stimuli from the opposite side (normally within the same sensory modality, *sensory inattention*). Many or all sense channels may be so involved, or the condition may affect one (e.g., vision or touch) selectively. With unimodal inattention, the responsible lesion is of the right inferior parietal lobe; while with multimodal inattention, lesions of the centrum semiovale may also be responsible.[2035]

Motor inattention (hemiakinesia) is the term used to describe a disinclination for direct motor activity, or for using the limbs on one side, in the absence of any detectable motor deficit; in such cases, normal power can be demonstrated, at least briefly, with encouragement. Premotor cortical and thalamic lesions are considered to be responsible. See also **hemispatial neglect**.

Global inattention is synonymous with **motor impersistence**.

Incapacity Status Scale

See **Kurtzke scales**.

inching

A technique used in sensory nerve conduction studies, whereby the median nerve is stimulated at points separated by 1–2 cm along its course in the palm. A record of the sensory nerve action potential is made from the finger distally, or from the wrist proximally, in an attempt to define precisely the site of compression of the nerve in **carpal tunnel syndrome**.[902]

incidentaloma

An asymptomatic pituitary adenoma shown on CT or MRI scans to the surprise of the physician and the likely consternation of the patient when informed.

incisura

(from Lat, to cut into) A cleft. The term formerly applied to the cerebral or cerebellar fissures.

incisura scapulae syndrome

Atrophy and weakness of the infraspinatus muscle as a result of compression of the distal extension of the suprascapular nerve at the level of the scapular notch.

incisural sclerosis

The term of **Penfield** for the mesial temporal lobe gliosis occurring as a remote effect of temporal lobe ischemia resulting from difficulties during parturition. [RMS]

inclusion body encephalitis

See **subacute sclerosing panencephalitis**.

inclusion body myopathy

(vacuolar myopathy sparing the quadriceps, myopathy with congenital joint contractures, ophthalmoplegia, and rimmed vacuoles) A (usually) dominantly inherited proximal syndrome with these features, the contractures normalizing in later childhood.[1452]

Suggested diagnostic criteria are (1) A primary skeletal muscle disease presenting usually with distal muscle weakness in the legs. (2) Sustained quadriceps sparing, despite marked weakness of all other hip muscles. (3) Onset in late teenage years or early adult life. (4). The presence of at least two affected family members. (5) Modest elevation of serum CK levels. (6) Numerous rimmed vacuoles with few other pathologic changes in muscle fibers. (7) Detection of numerous filamentous inclusions without inflammation on muscle biopsy.[2581, 237] Variants are IBM1 (dominant); IBM2 (recessive; 9p12, *GNE*); IBM3 (17p13, *MyHC-IIa*, dominant) and IBM with Paget disease (9p13, dominant).

inclusion body myositis (sporadic)

(sIBM) A benign, usually slowly progressive inflammatory myopathy resembling chronic polymyositis, most common in males over the age of 50 years. The condition presents with painless asymmetrical proximal and distal weakness especially of the flexor digitorum profundus (more than sublimis) and finger extensors, quadriceps and glutei, with foot-drop from affection of the tibialis anterior, and loss of the knee jerks. Occasionally dysphagia, skin or ocular, facial or respiratory muscle involvement, fatigue or arthralgias are noted. The weakness does not respond to steroid therapy.[3258, 5312] The condition is slowly progressive to a state of marked disability. Serum CK levels are normal or slightly raised.[2292] This is the most common inflammatory myopathy in older adults.

Three distinct subsets of IBM have been recognized

(a) *sporadic IBM* An inflammatory vacuolar myositis with the distinct clinical phenotype described above
(b) *familial inflammatory IBM* An inflammatory vacuolar myositis occurring in several family members of the same generation with clinical and histological phenotype identical with the sporadic form
(c) *hereditary inclusion body myopathy* A group of noninflammatory vacuolar myopathies of recessive or dominant inheritance. The recessive disease is usually characterized by quadriceps sparing and is linked to chromosome 9p. The dominant form comprises a heterogeneous group of vacuolar myopathies not all of which have been genetically identified yet[1410] and includes Finnish and Swedish forms, **oculopharyngeal muscular dystrophy**, and **Welander distal myopathy**.[1882]

Confirmation of the diagnosis is pathological; biopsy specimens show the presence of ragged red fibers, rimmed vacuoles, and intranuclear filaments, as well as many of the usual changes of myositis.[3310] Both myopathic and neurogenic EMG patterns may be found. The condition is unresponsive to current treatments. Adenovirus has been isolated from a few cases.

The entity has been reviewed[1882] and diagnostic criteria have been proposed.[2581] For a full examination of the disorder, visit the following Web site:

http://www.ninds.nih.gov/disorders/inclusion_body_myositis/inclusion_body_myositis.htm.

Variant forms include *familial inclusion body myositis*, a dominantly inherited form of the disease;[4637] a form presenting with dysphagia;[5308] late juvenile sIBM; and sIBM features in association with **HTLV1** infection, **post-polio syndrome** or neuropathy. One set of diagnostic criteria for inclusion body myositis proposed is given in Chart I–6.

Chart I–6. Proposed Diagnostic Criteria for Inclusion Body Myositis

1. Characteristic features and inclusion criteria
   A. Clinical features
      1. Duration of illness >6 months
      2. Age of onset >30 years old
      3. Muscle weakness
         Must affect proximal and distal muscles of arms and legs *and* Patient must exhibit at least one of the following features:
         a. Finger flexor weakness
         b. Wrist flexor more than wrist extensor weakness
         c. Quadriceps muscle weakness (≤ grade 4 MRC)
   B. Laboratory features
      1. Serum creatine kinase < 12 times normal level
      2. Muscle biopsy
         a. Inflammatory myopathy characterized by mononuclear cell invasion of nonnecrotic muscle fibers
         b. Vacuolated muscle fibers
         c. Either *(i)* Intracellular amyloid deposits (must use fluorescent method of identification before excluding the presence of amyloid) *or* *(ii)* 15–18-nm tubulofilaments by electron microscopy.
      3. Electromyography must be consistent with features of an inflammatory myopathy (however, long-duration potentials are commonly observed and do not exclude diagnosis of sporadic inclusion body myositis). Also, confusingly, as well as brief, small, abundant potentials with an excess of polyphasics, both fibrillations, and positive sharp waves may be found on the EMG.
   C. Family history
      Rarely, inclusion body *myositis* may be observed in families. This condition is different from hereditary inclusion body *myopathy* without inflammation. The diagnosis of familial inclusion body *myositis* requires specific documentation of the inflammatory component by muscle biopsy in addition to vacuolated muscle fibers, intracellular (within muscle fibers) amyloid, and 15–18-nm tubulofilaments.
2. Associated disorders
   Inclusion body myositis occurs with a variety of other, especially immune-mediated conditions. An associated condition does not preclude a diagnosis of inclusion body myositis if diagnostic criteria (below) are fulfilled.
3. Diagnostic criteria
   A. *Definite* inclusion body myositis
      Patients must exhibit all muscle biopsy features including invasion of nonnecrotic fibers by mononuclear cells, vacuolated muscle fibers, and intracellular (within muscle fibers) amyloid deposits or 15–18-nm tubulofilaments. None of the other clinical or laboratory features are mandatory if muscle biopsy features are diagnostic.
   B. *Possible* inclusion body myositis.
      If the muscle shows only inflammation (invasion of nonnecrotic muscle fibers by mononuclear cells) *without* other pathological features of inclusion body myositis, *then* a diagnosis of possible inclusion body myositis can be given if the patient exhibits the characteristic clinical (Al, 2, 3) and laboratory (B1, 3) features.

(From Griggs RC, Askanas V, DiMauro S, et al. Inclusion body myositis and myopathies. Ann Neurol 1995;38:705–13. Reproduced by permission of Lippincott, Williams and Wilkins.. Alternative diagnostic criteria are presented at http://www.enmc.org/pdf/emery81.pdf.)

Inclusion Body Myositis Association A nonprofit educational organization with a mandate to support research into this disease. Tel: 703-433-7686. Web site: http://www.myositis.org/about_myositis/inclusion-body_myositis.cfm.

Inclusion Body Myositis Functional Rating Scale An assessment tool designed for this condition that rates swallowing, handwriting (with dominant hand prior to IBM onset), cutting food and handling utensils, fine motor tasks (such as opening doors, using keys and picking up small objects), dressing, hygiene (bathing and toileting), turning in bed and adjusting covers, sit-to-stand capability, and walking and climbing stairs, each on a five-point scale.[3122]

inclusion cell disease See I-cell disease.

incomplete activation Motor unit action potentials firing, on requested maximal effort, in decreased numbers at their normal physiological rates, within the basal firing range of 5–10 Hz. Causes include upper motor neuron syndrome, pain on muscle contraction, hysteria or conversion reaction and malingering. Contrast with reduced recruitment. (From the 2001 Report of the Nomenclature Committee of the American Association of Electromyography and Electrodiagnosis.[19] Reproduced by kind permission of the AANEM.)

incontinence Inability to contain the natural evacuations, leading to the inadvertent or uncontrolled passage of urine or feces or both.

incontinentia pigmenti (Bloch–Sulzberger syndrome, cutaneous meningeal melanosis) An X-linked (or autosomal) dominant mesodermal and ectodermal dysplastic condition causing a variety of pigmented skin lesions, including vesical and bullous eruptions, hyperkeratosis, warts, dermal atrophy, and alopecia, with additional problems such as microphthalmia, cataract, dental and retinal dysplasia, blue sclerae, hemivertebrae with scoliosis, and other skeletal malformations; and, in a third of the cases, neurological disorders, including optic atrophy, chorioretinitis, nystagmus, mental retardation, microcephaly, cerebellar atrophy, hydrocephalus, spastic pareses, and seizures, rarely with anterior horn cell degeneration.[1023, 3703, 3704] The condition is lethal in utero for hemizygous males, and so is seen to excess in female infants. Franceschetti and Jadassohn distinguished Naegeli syndrome from incontinentia pigmenti (Bloch-Sulzberger syndrome) by the equal frequency of the disorder in males and females.

The differentiation between the syndromes of Naegeli and of Bloch is based on the fact that while the former disease occurs in both sexes, the latter affects only females.[683]

Variants are *incontinentia pigmenti achromicans* (See **hypomelanosis of Ito**) and *infantile spinal muscular atrophy* with incontinentia pigmenti.[3705]

incontinentia pigmenti achromicans See **hypomelanosis of Ito**.

increased intracranial pressure (ICP) A syndrome due to the presence of a solid or fluid mass in the intracranial cavity, characterized by bradycardia, headache, drowsiness, photophobia, adducted eyes, and dilated pupil(s) (usually due to III nerve palsy, but the dilatation may also be attributed to loss of vision), ptosis, vomiting, and bradypnea.

increased intracranial pressure without localizing signs See **idiopathic intracranial hypertension**.

increment Increase in the size of a compound motor action potential during repetitive motor nerve stimulation, due to an increase in the number of muscle fibers responding to the stimuli. See also **decrement**, **potentiation**, and **pseudofacilitation**.

incremental exercise test A procedure whereby the force of muscular contraction required to perform motor tasks is correlated with the force expended by the patient at different levels of required exertion. There should be a precise correlation between the force demanded and that expended; when this is not the case, the presence of "strength withheld" or other forms of noncompliance is likely. *Incremental ergonometry* is a further development of the same principle.

incrementing response A reproducible increase in amplitude and/or area of successive M waves to repetitive nerve stimulation. The rate of stimulation and the number of stimuli should be specified. It is commonly seen in two situations. In normal subjects the configuration of the M wave may change in response to repetitive nerve stimulation so that the amplitude progressively increases as the duration decreases, leaving the area of the M wave unchanged. This phenomenon is termed **pseudofacilitation**. Also, in neuromuscular transmission disorders, the configuration of the M wave may change with repetitive nerve stimulation so that the amplitude and the area of the M wave progressively increase. This phenomenon is termed facilitation. Cf. **decrementing response**. (From the 2001 Report of the Nomenclature Committee of the American Association of Electromyography and Electrodiagnosis.[19] Reproduced by kind permission of the AANEM.)

incubus (from Lat, to lie down upon) A male devil, thought in the Middle Ages to be seeking sexual intercourse with women during their sleep. The word is now used occasionally for the sense of extreme pressure on the chest. See also **night terror**, **sleep terrors**, and **succubus**.

incurvation reflex With the infant held in ventral suspension, the examiner runs his finger along the paravertebral area, close to the spine. This normally induces a firm swinging of the baby's pelvis toward the stimulation.[6898]

incycloduction See **duction**.

indeterminate leprosy An early stage in the development of leprosy, manifest by no more than the presence of an anesthetic, depigmented macule which has the potential for resolution or for progression to either the tuberculoid or the lepromatous forms of the disease.

indeterminate tremor syndrome Bilateral postural or kinetic tremor of the hands and forearms, or isolated head tremor associated with equivocal neurological signs or concomitant neurological signs of doubtful significance (such as a slightly unsteady gait, mild dementia in an elderly person, hypomimia, reduced arm swing, or mild bradykinesia).[1834, 1615] See **essential tremor**, of which this is likely to be a *variant*.

index (From Lat, to point out) 1. A pointer; the second digit, next to the thumb. 2. Numerous measurements and ratios of measurements between the points of the body, and especially of the head, used mainly by anthropologists but not of great value in medicine. See **cephalic index**.

index of suspicion The clinician's awareness of the relative likelihood of one pathological condition as opposed to another within the context of his or her work.

Indian Agarwal megalencephalic leukodystrophy with cysts A recessive syndrome of megalencephaly, cognitive decline, slowly progressive spasticity, ataxia, occasional seizures, and extensive white matter changes with temporal cysts on imaging studies, seen in the Northern Indian ethnic group called Agarwal.[2511] See also **megalencephalic leukodystrophy with cysts**.

indifferent electrode (reference electrode) See **reference electrode** and **recording electrode**.

Individualized Quality of Life questionnaire (INQoL) An instrument designed to assess **quality of life** in patients with neuromuscular disease. It consists of 45 questions in 10 sections focusing on weakness, myotonia, pain, and fatigue, and the impact that muscle disease has on particular areas of life, as well as the effects of treatment.[6552]

induced nystagmus (flash-induced, drug-induced nystagmus, provoked nystagmus) Forms of **vestibular nystagmus** appearing in normal subjects only in response to some exciting external event. See also **arthrokinetic nystagmus, audiokinetic nystagmus, vestibular nystagmus** (caloric nystagmus), **optokinetic nystagmus, pseudocaloric nystagmus**, and **anticipatory nystagmus**.

infant Hercules syndrome See **Kocher-Debré-Semelaigne syndrome**.

infant sleep apnea is characterized by central or obstructive apneas that occur during sleep. The proposed diagnostic criteria are as follows:[1629]

A. The clinical presentation of infant sleep apnea includes one or more of the following:
    1. An episode of cessation of breathing during sleep
    2. An episode characterized by
        a. Color change (pallor or cyanosis)
        b. Tone change (limpness, rarely stiffness)
    3. Noisy breathing during sleep

B. Central or obstructive apneas occur during sleep.

C. The age of infant at presentation can be either
    1. Less than 37 weeks postconceptional age (for AOP)
    2. Greater than 37 weeks postconceptional age (for AOI)

D. Polysomnographic monitoring demonstrates one or more of the following:
    1. Prolonged central apnea, longer than 20 seconds
    2. Obstructive apnea, longer than 10 seconds
    3. An apnea accompanied by cyanosis
    4. An apnea accompanied by transient bradycardia (defined as a drop in heart rate to levels below 50 bpm, a heart rate below 60 bpm lasting more than 10 s or a drop below 60 bpm with a duration exceeding 30 s below baseline heart rate)
    5. Arterial oxygen saturation less than 85% during sleep
    6. Sustained hypoventilation (e.g., PETCO2 >45 mm Hg) during sleep

E. An identifiable cause for the apnea was either
    1. Found following a thorough diagnostic evaluation and is believed to be the cause of the apnea (ALTE with apnea, OSAS)
    2. Not found following a thorough diagnostic evaluation (AOP, AOI)

From AASM Diagnostic Classification Steering Committee. *The International Classification of Sleep Disorders Diagnostic and Coding Manual*. Rochester, MN. American Academy of Sleep Medicine 1991/2001. Reproduced by kind permission of the Academy. See also http://www.sleepeducation.com/Disorders.aspx/.

infantile adrenoleukodystrophy A recessively inherited, rapidly progressive syndrome characterized by severe neuropathy from birth, seizures, and hepatomegaly.[2402] See also **adrenoleukodystrophy**.

infantile ascending hereditary spastic paraparesis A genetically heterogeneous syndrome characterized by spastic paraplegia stopping in the first 2 years of life and progressing to tetraplegia with anarthria, dysphagia, and slow eye movements but with long survival and preservation of intellectual capacity.[3790] See **hereditary spastic paraparesis**.

infantile amaurotic familial idiocy See **gangliosidosis** (Tay–Sachs disease).

infantile autism (idiopathic autism) A syndrome characterized by failure to establish communication with others, an obsession to continue "sameness," failure of language communication, aloofness, preoccupation with handling small objects, and an inability to anticipate with appropriate body positioning the likelihood of being picked up.[3287]

Clinically, the condition usually presents toward the end of the first year of life with diminution in crying, motor activity, feeding, language, and response, although motor milestones are normal. Stereotypic movements and gestures are common. The condition is likely to be multifactorial; no single biochemical or structural abnormality is typically associated and there is no characteristic abnormality on laboratory examination. See also **autism** and **Heller disease**.

infantile bilateral striatal necrosis See **familial bilateral striatal necrosis**.

infantile botulism A syndrome consisting of constipation, cranial nerve deficits, pupillary involvement (dilatation), and hypotonic weakness with an EMG pattern of brief small abundant (for power exerted) motor unit potentials, considered to be due to damage to the motor end plate resulting from botulinus toxin.[1199] See **botulism**.

infantile cerebellar ataxia See **acute cerebellar ataxia**.

infantile CNS degeneration A syndrome characterized by optic atrophy, ophthalmoplegia, areflexia, hypotonia, dysmorphic facies, and severe mental and motor retardation. Microcephaly and seizures may also occur. The course is slowly progressive, but the full-blown syndrome appears within the first 3 years of life. The cause is unknown.[2967]

infantile CNS spongy degeneration See **Canavan leukodystrophy**.

infantile convulsions and choreoathetosis The occurrence of **benign familial infantile seizures** with the subsequent development of choreoathetosis.

infantile cortical hyperostosis (Caffey–Silverman syndrome) A dominantly inherited infantile syndrome characterized by facial swelling due to the formation of new bone (especially of the mandible), excessive bone formation in long bones with pain and pseudoparalysis, fever, and irritability. The condition resolves slowly within a year or two.[973]

infantile epileptic dyskinetic encephalopathy A syndrome caused by a trinucleotide repeat expansion in ARX, consisting of profound mental retardation, early onset infantile spasms, and severe generalized dystonia beginning in late infancy and progressively worsening. MRI eventually shows multifocal cystic changes in the basal ganglia with mild ventricular dilatation.[2616]

infantile facioscapulohumeral dystrophy A more malignant variant of **facioscapulohumeral dystrophy**, also dominantly inherited, with onset in infancy and death in adolescence.[336]

infantile hexosaminidase deficiency A cause of very atypical progressive myoclonus epilepsy. See also **GM2 gangliosidoses**.

infantile lactic acidosis with failure to thrive A form of **mitochondrial encephalomyopathy**.

infantile metachromatic leukodystrophy See **metachromatic leukodystrophy**.

infantile muscular atrophy See **hereditary motor neuropathy**.

infantile myasthenia See **myasthenia gravis**.

infantile myoclonic petit mal See **centrencephalic myoclonic-astatic epilepsy**.

infantile myoclonic encephalopathy with hypsarrhythmia See **West syndrome**.

infantile myopathy and lactic acidosis A mitochondrial disease, presenting in the first year of life with feeding and respiratory problems. A fatal form is associated with cardiomyopathy.

infantile neuroaxonal dystrophy (**Seitelberger disease**)A recessively inherited, fatal primary axonopathy of infancy affecting multiple tracts in the CNS. It is characterized by extrapyramidal dysfunction and often by the involvement of optic, cerebellar, and spinal systems. Failure of mental and motor growth, dystonia, dementia, spasticity, areflexia, generalized analgesia, optic atrophy, pendular nystagmus, deafness, and other cranial nerve palsies and peripheral neuropathy result; the affected children never walk nor talk, and eventually die decerebrate before the age of 10 years.[3065] Diagnostic criteria are as follows:[4593]

1. Unequivocal histologic evidence in the form of axonal swellings and spheroid bodies in skin biopsies
2. Onset of symptoms before the age of 3 years
3. Clinically, psychomotor deterioration, with increasing pyramidal tract signs and with marked truncal hypotonia
4. Relentlessly progressive course leading to spastic tetraplegia, blindness, and dementia by the age of 4 years.

(From Nardocci N, Zorzi G, Farina L, et al. Infantile neuroaxonal dystrophy. Neurology *1999;52:1472–8. Reproduced by kind permission of the American Academy of Neurology and Lippincott, Williams and Wilkins.)*

Pathologically, the presence of dystrophic axons containing spheroid bodies is notable throughout the CNS and in peripheral tissues. The condition was first reported by Seitelberger.[5712] It runs a shorter course and starts at an earlier age than does **neuronal degeneration with brain iron accumulation** which it otherwise resembles and from which distinction may be impossible. The question is reviewed by Baraitser.[379]

Variants include

Neuroaxonal dystrophy with tubular acidosis, a rare congenital dysmetabolic syndrome characterized by renal tubular acidosis, axonal neuropathy, cerebral and cerebellar atrophy with ataxia and pyramidal signs, resting tremor, and mental and developmental delay.[3985]

Juvenile neuroaxonal dystrophy, a rare dementing illness in children, with axonal spheroids.[1695]

Forms with *neonatal onset* or *X-linked inheritance*.

Spinal muscular atrophy in infantile neuroaxonal dystrophy.

infantile neuronal ceroid lipofuscinosis A recessively inherited form of neuronal ceroid lipofuscinosis, characterized by psychomotor retardation, hypotonia, trunk and limb ataxia, severe visual deficits due to retinal dystrophy and optic atrophy, myoclonic jerks, and microcephaly, with onset in infancy.[5543] See also **neuronal ceroid lipofuscinosis**.

infantile neuronal degeneration A variant form of **hereditary motor neuropathy type 1** (which it resembles clinically). It is recessively inherited and there is additional widespread neuronal loss and gliosis in both the gray and white matter in the thalamus, pons, cerebellum, and spinal cord as well as segmental demyelination in the peripheral nerves.[6031]

infantile Niemann–Pick disease See **sphingomyelin storage diseases**.

infantile onset spinocerebellar ataxia with sensory neuropathy A recessively inherited ataxic syndrome, presenting with ataxia, hypotonia, athetosis, and areflexia between the ages of 9 and 18 months, with later-developing ophthalmoplegia and sensorineural hearing loss.[3541]

infantile osteopetrosis and neuronal storage disease A recessively inherited congenital neuroaxonal storage disease characterized by osteopetrosis; osteosclerosis with multiple fractures; enlarged liver and spleen; anemia; cerebral atrophy and macrocephaly; optic atrophy; pyramidal signs; mental and developmental delay; and neuronal inclusions.[160]

infantile paralysis (infantile palsy) See **poliomyelitis**.

infantile phytanic acid storage disease A recessively inherited peroxisomal disease characterized by elevated plasma phytanic acid levels with minor facial dysmorphism, sensorineural deafness, cataract, pigmentary retinopathy with visual failure, ichthyosis, electrocardiographic abnormality, enlarged liver, myoclonus, nystagmus, cerebellar ataxia, painful sensorimotor peripheral neuropathy, and developmental delay.[6714] See also **hereditary motor and sensory neuropathy** type 4.

infantile polymyoclonia See **myoclonic encephalopathy of infancy**.

infantile Refsum disease See **infantile phytanic acid storage disease**.

infantile sleep apnea See **sleep apnea**.

infantile spasms See **West syndrome**.

infantile spasms, hemimegalencephaly, and hemihypsarrhythmia See **West syndrome**.

infantile spasms, X-linked See **West syndrome**.

infantile spinal muscular atrophy, arrested See **hereditary motor neuropathy, type 2**.

infantile striatonigral degeneration A progressive familial neurodegenerative disorder characterized by degeneration of the cerebellum, dentate nucleus, substantia nigra, globus pallidus, inferior olives, and intermediolateral columns of the spinal cord, and clinically associated with mental and motor regression starting from the latter part of the first year of life, seizures and myoclonus, ataxia, pyramidal signs and neuropathy, all progressing to death within the first 5 years of life.[2831]

infantile subacute necrotizing encephalopathy See **Leigh disease**.

infantile sudanophilic leukodystrophy See **adrenoleukodystrophy**.

infantile symmetrical necrosis of the neostriatum See **infantile bilateral striatal necrosis**.

infantile tremor syndrome A syndrome described in India comprising the abrupt onset in summer of a rapid high-intensity tremor, apathy, and hypokinesia in children between the ages of 6 months and 2 years. The tremors mainly affect the face and arms, the latter being abducted at the shoulders and flexed more distally, like a bird drying its wings. The illness is self-limiting over a few weeks, but the children may then show developmental retardation. Anemia is the only constant pathological finding.

The cause is unknown,[5062] but it is thought to be a meningoencephalitis, as about half the affected children have fever. Apart from the tremor and an expressionless pallid facies, there are no accompanying physical signs.[6205]

infantile X-linked ataxia and deafness A familial syndrome comprising progressive cerebellar dysfunction, dementia, deafness, hypotonia, optic atrophy, esotropia, and later vomiting, dysphagia with choking, increasing weakness, lethargy, and death. Pathologically, the maximum neuronal loss is in the dentate and olivary nuclei.[5615]

infarct Ischemic coagulative necrosis of tissue resulting from obstruction of the lumen of the artery supplying the infarcted area. The concept was formulated initially by **Virchow**.

infectious chorea See **Sydenham chorea**.

infectious hepatitis A systemic viral infection with a particular tendency to damage the liver. Neurological complications such as meningitis, encephalitis, and polyneuropathy occasionally occur.[3792]

infectious mononucleosis A disease due to the Epstein–Barr virus, preferentially affecting children and young adults and causing fever, lymphadenopathy, pharyngitis, and splenomegaly. Neurological complications include lymphocytic meningitis, encephalomyelitis, facial palsy, polyneuropathy, and mononeuropathy, but they occur in less than 10% of the cases.[2320] In the context of CNS involvement, however, the classic features of mononucleosis mentioned above need not be present.[1606]

infectious polyneuritis See **acute inflammatory demyelinating polyneuropathy**.

infective endocarditis Bacterial infection of the cardiac valves with an incidence of neurologic complications of 30%, almost all occurring in patients with left-sided valvular disease and when the endocarditis is caused by virulent organisms such as *S. aureus* and the *enterobacteriaceae*. The clinical presentation is dependent on the area of the CNS involved by infected (micro) emboli. A complication is intracranial mycotic aneurysm.[6422]

inferior calcaneal neuropathy Compression of this nerve, presenting usually with heel pain. The associated weakness and wasting of the abductor digiti quinti are seldom clinically apparent.[4902]

inflammatory bowel disease neuropathy Forms of neuropathy often resembling **chronic inflammatory demyelinating neuropathy** or **multifocal motor neuropathy** complicating Crohn disease or ulcerative colitis, mainly seen in adult males. Both small- and large-fiber sensory axonal neuropathies and large-fiber axonal sensorimotor neuropathies are described, all with a likely response to immunotherapy.[2468]

inflammatory myopathy See **dermatomyositis**, **polymyositis**, and **inclusion body myositis**.

inflammatory myopathy, scapuloileoperoneal atrophy, and cardiomyopathy A dominantly inherited syndrome with onset in adult life, characterized by slowly progressive muscle weakness in a scapuloileoperoneal distribution and by cardiopathy. Muscle biopsy specimens show both neurogenic and myopathic changes with inflammatory cell reactions and perivascular cuffing, the latter considered to be a manifestation of a secondary polymyositis.[3200]

inflammatory sensory polyganglionopathies Disorders affecting primarily the spinal sensory ganglion cells, posterior roots, and peripheral nerves and leading to prominent sensory deficits. Both **paraneoplastic** and nonmalignant inflammatory disorders are responsible. In the *malignant form*, ataxic and/or hyperalgesic syndromes occur with or without accompanying dysautonomia. Progression is usually subacute. The most striking clinical features are paresthesias, dysesthesias and eventually anesthesia, loss of reflexes with retained strength, and constipation. Antineuronal nuclear antibodies are present in the serum. Small-cell carcinoma of the lung is the commonest association.

In the *nonmalignant form*, ataxic and/or hyperalgesic syndromes occur, usually with subacute or chronic progression. The clinical features resemble those of the other form, but autonomic signs are not detectable. Extractable nuclear antigen is present in the serum. Other dysimmune conditions such as **Sjögren syndrome**, connective tissue disease, HIV or other viral infections[5903] are commonly associated. This form may thus be regarded as a variant of **acute inflammatory demyelinating polyneuropathy**.

influenza A viral infection due to many evolving strains, some capable of causing a wide range of neurologic manifestations ranging from minor symptoms such as increased fatigue to coma and death. The more serious forms include febrile and nonfebrile seizures, confusion, lethargy or coma, acute inflammatory demyelinating polyneuropathy, acute disseminated encephalomyelitis, transverse myelitis, abnormal involuntary movements, acute psychosis, frontal lobe syndromes, mutism, visual hallucinations, and recently **acute necrotizing encephalopathy**.[4067, 3184]

Information Centre for Rare Diseases and Orphan Drugs

A Bulgarian Web site in English, offering an internet portal and including data on rare diseases and orphan drug information. Web site: http://www.raredis.org/modules/mylinks/.

Information-Memory-Concentration Test The forerunner of most of today's scales for diagnosing or rating dementia; it was originally combined with pathological measurements. The test items concern orientation (name, age, temporal items), awareness of site, recognition of people, recall of personal factors, recall of significant dates and persons, tests of 5 min recall, counting, and reversed sets (20 to 1, months of the year). Though validated in the original papers, this test appears to have been superseded by those of more recent origin.[681] See also **Blessed Roth dementia scale** and **Addenbrookes Cognitive evaluation** .

infra- (Gr, beneath) Prefix denoting beneath.

infraorbital neuralgia Pain felt in the distribution of that nerve with a persistent quality, unlike the stabbing pain of **trigeminal neuralgia**, although the same treatments may give relief. The cause is seldom determined.

infraspinatus reflex Exaggerated contraction of the infraspinatus when it is tapped; a sign of minimal clinical value even with lesions of the corticospinal pathway above C5 level.

ingravescent apoplexy The slow rather than abrupt onset of a stroke syndrome. This is usually due to thrombosis of a major artery or a dural venous sinus as opposed to embolism or hemorrhage.

inherited erythermalgia See **erythromelalgia**.

inherited ion channel disorders

Channelopathies (disorders caused by mutations in genes encoding ion channels). **Hyperkalemic periodic paralysis, paramyotonia congenita**, and **potassium-aggravated myotonia** are skeletal muscle sodium channelopathies; **hypokalemic periodic paralysis, malignant hyperthermia**, and **central core disease** are skeletal muscle calcium channelopathies, while **Thomsen** and **Becker myotonia** are skeletal muscle chloride channelopathies. The **generalized epilepsy febrile seizures plus syndrome** is a neuronal sodium channelopathy; **familial benign neonatal convulsions** and **episodic ataxia type 1** are neuronal potassium channelopathies. **Episodic ataxia type 2, familial hemiplegic migraine**, and **spinocerebellar ataxia type 6** are neuronal calcium channelopathies. A neuronal glycine receptor channelopathy is **hyperekplexia**. Muscle ACh receptor channelopathies underlie the congenital **myasthenic syndromes**.

Some forms of epilepsy (e.g., autosomal dominant frontal lobe nocturnal epilepsy), the Lambert–Eaton **myasthenic syndrome, Alzheimer disease, Parkinson disease**, and schizophrenia may result from dysfunction of voltage-gated sodium, potassium, and calcium channels, or acetylcholine- and glycine-gated channels. Vision disorders, for example, **congenital stationary night blindness** and total **color-blindness** may also be linked to mutations in ion channels.[6136, 1067]

inherited myoclonus dystonia

See **myoclonus dystonia**.

inherited prion disease See **Jakob–Creutzfeldt disease**.

inherited tendency to pressure palsies See **hereditary pressure-sensitive neuropathy**.

inhibition (from Lat, to hold in) The arrest of functional activity of an organ or structure as an effect of a restraining influence exerted by a neuronal system.

inhibitional palsy of Chavasse

Apparent paresis of the contralateral yoke muscle (a) in response to hypoactivity of that muscle (b) which is normally antagonistic to the action of a paretic muscle (c). Thus with a right lateral rectus palsy (c), there will be overaction of the left medial rectus (the yoke muscle) and contracture of the ipsilateral antagonist (the right medial rectus). This latter muscle (b) is now hypoactive, which leads to the paresis of its contralateral yoke muscle, the left lateral rectus (a), especially if the paretic eye is used for fixation.[2400]

inhibitory epilepsy Rare seizure types in which it is surmised that inhibitory impulses originating from higher centers act on the upper motor neuron itself leaving the anterior horn cell and possibly the upper motor neuron input to the gamma efferents is switched off. Differentiation from postepileptic paralysis is difficult because both may have associated seizures.[5871] Inhibitory simple partial (nonconvulsive) seizures also occur, presenting as focal neurological deficits with EEG evidence of appropriate focal seizure activity, for example, after neurosurgical procedures.[247]

Epileptic aphasic seizures, ictal deafness, ictal amaurosis, epileptic **negative myoclonus, Todd paresis**, and *brief focal atonia* are other forms described. See also **chalastic fits**.

inhibitory nerve A nerve capable of slowing, restraining, or preventing secretion or contraction of the gland or muscle which it innervates.

inhibitory phenomenon A rare form of seizure disorder in which attacks of paralysis are not preceded by convulsive movements in the same territory.[2735] See also **Todd paralysis**.

inhibitory postsynaptic potential (IPSP) A local graded hyperpolarization of a neuron in response to activation at a synapse by a nerve terminal. Cf. **excitatory postsynaptic potential**. (From the 2001 Report of the Nomenclature Committee of the American Association of Electromyography and Electrodiagnosis.[19] Reproduced by kind permission of the AANEM.)

inion The apex of the external occipital protuberance. The name derives from the Greek word for the tendon at the back of the neck.

injection myopathy Local inflammation following needling of a muscle, especially when antibiotics, digoxin, penicillin, or narcotic analgesics are injected through it. If such inflammation is widespread, it may induce a transient rise in the serum creatine kinase levels.[3724]

injection paralysis Poliomyelitis in a single limb into which an injection had been given for any reason in the last 2–3 weeks.[6885]

injury potential 1. The potential difference between a normal region of the surface of a nerve or muscle and a membrane region that has been injured; also called a "demarcation" or "killed end" potential. It approximates the potential across the membrane because the injured surface has nearly the same potential as the interior of the cell. 2. In electrodiagnostic medicine, the term is also used to refer to the electrical activity associated with needle electrode insertion into muscle. (From the 2001 Report of the Nomenclature Committee of the American Association of Electromyography and Electrodiagnosis.[19] Reproduced by permission of the AANEM.) See also **fibrillation, insertion activity**, and **positive sharp wave**.

inner cerebral trauma See **diffuse axonal injury**.

inner speech (endophasy) "The totality of processes and experiences which occur when we are going to express our thoughts, etc. in external speech and when we perceive heard sounds such as language. Inner speech is, on the one hand, in relation to the nonlanguage mental processes: on the other hand, to the external instrumentalities (external speech)."[2455]

Thus, a central language process coming between nonverbal thought and expressed speech or, in short, the silent processes of thought.[1337]

innervation The nerve supply of a structure.

Innsbruck Coma Scale An assessment instrument with excellent predictive value as regards poor outcome in patients with severe head injuries. (see Chart I–7)[537]

Chart I–7. The Innsbruck Coma Scale

Neurological Assessment	*Score*
Reaction to acoustic stimuli	
Turning towards stimuli	*3*
Better-than-extension movements	*2*
Extension movements	*1*
None	*0*
Reaction to pain	
Defensive movements	*3*
Better than extension movements	*2*
Extension movements	*1*
None	*0*
Body posture	
Normal	*3*
Better-than-extension movements	*2*
Extension movements	*1*
Flaccid	*0*
Eye Opening	
Spontaneous	*3*
To acoustic stimuli	*2*
To pain stimuli	*1*
None	*0*
Pupil size	
Normal	*3*
Narrow	*2*
Dilated	*1*
Completely dilated	*0*
Pupil response to light	
Sufficient	*3*
Reduced	*2*
Minimum	*1*
No response	*0*
Position and movements of eyeballs	
Fixing with eyes	*3*
Sway of eyeballs	*2*
Divergent	*1*
Divergent fixed	*0*
Oral automatisms	
Spontaneous	*2*
To external stimuli	*1*
None	*0*

From Benzer A, Mitterschliffthaler G, Marosi M, et al. Prediction of nonsurvival after trauma: Innsbruck coma scale. Lancet *1991;*338*:977–8. Reproduced by kind permission of Elsevier Science.*

input circuit A system consisting of the EEG electrodes and intervening tissues, the electrode leads, jack box, input cable, and electrode selectors. (Adapted from the 1974 report of the Committee on Terminology, IFCN. In: Chatrian GE, Bergamini L, Dondey M et al. A glossary of terms most commonly used by clinical electroencephalographers. *EEG Clin Neurophysiol* 1974;37:538–48. Reprinted with kind permission from Elsevier Science.)

input impedance The impedance that exists between the two inputs of an EEG amplifier, measured in ohms (generally megohms), with or without the additional specification of input shunt capacitance (measured in pico-farads [pF]). This is not a synonym for **electrode impedance**.

input terminal 1 (recording, active, or exploring electrode) The input terminal of a differential amplifier at which negativity, relative to the other input terminal, produces an upward deflection. (From the 2001 Report of the Nomenclature Committee of the American Association of Electromyography and Electrodiagnosis.[19] Reproduced by kind permission of the AANEM.)

input terminal 2 (reference electrode) The input of a differential amplifier at which negativity, relative to the other input terminal, produces a downward deflection. (From the 2001 Report of the Nomenclature Committee of the American Association of Electromyography and Electrodiagnosis.[19] Reproduced by kind permission of the AANEM.)

input voltage The potential difference between the two input terminals of a differential EEG amplifier.

insensitivity to pain See **pain asymbolia** and **hereditary sensory and autonomic neuropathy**.

insertion activity Electrical activity from myofibrils caused by insertion or movement of a needle electrode within a muscle. See also **fibrillation** potential and **positive sharp wave**.

integrated EMG The mathematical integration of the full wave rectified EMG signal that reflects the cumulative EMG activity of a muscle over time.[19]

insertions The appearance in speech of material related to thoughts at a remote time—a form of perseveration, but with excessive delay. A sign in demented patients who sometimes make inapposite use of words which would have been in context half an hour before.[2097]

Inside MS A neurological journal devoted to **multiple sclerosis**, and the official publication of the National Multiple Sclerosis Society. Address: National Multiple Sclerosis Society, 205 East 42nd St., New York, NY 10017. Web site: http://www.nationalmssociety.org/InsideMS.asp/.

insistence A useful term suggested by Miller Fisher for stubborn ideational perseveration along a track of thought from which the demented patient's mind is not to be derailed. The patient ignores all inducements to change the subject or to desist from the repeated utterance and may become overtly hostile if pressed to do so or if ignored.[2097]

insomnia The subjective impression of inadequacy in the quantity or quality of sleep. The condition may be transient or chronic and is due to nonpsychiatric factors in perhaps one in four cases. The types of insomnia as suggested by Parkes[4904] are as follows:

Sleep onset insomnia
Sleep maintenance insomnia
Early morning waking
Phase-shift disorders
Cyclical insomnia

In *persistent psychophysiological insomnia*, the lack of sleep represents a learned pattern.[2796] Total absence of sleep (*agrypnia*) in a man with Morvan fibrillary chorea and **vesperal hallucinations** has been reported.[2073]

inspiratory gasp A clinical test of autonomic vasomotor control in which brief dermal vasoconstriction is sought when a subject takes a sudden inspiratory gasp.

inspiratory speech See **spasmodic dysphonia**.

instinctive grasp reaction/response A deliberate, involuntary progressive closure of the whole hand, made in a series of small movements but terminating in complete grip when the palm is stimulated by variable pressure. See **grasp response** and **groping**.

instructional deficit Inability to perform a test satisfactorily or at all because of the lack of ability to comprehend the instructions.

Instrumental Activities of Daily Living Scale An assessment instrument by which eight functions (telephoning, shopping, preparing food, housekeeping, doing laundry, traveling, taking medication, and handling finances) are evaluated on 3 to 5 point rating scales completed by family members on the basis of the capacity of a family member living with them to cope unaided with such activities.[3722] See **activities of daily living**.

instrumental phase reversal Simultaneous pen deflections in opposite directions caused by a single wave recorded in two bipolar derivations. This inversion is purely instrumental in nature, that is, due to the same signal being simultaneously applied to the input terminal 1 of the other amplifier.

When observed in two linked bipolar derivations, phase reversal indicates that the potential field is maximal or less frequently minimal at or near the electrode common to such derivations, so the phenomenon can be used to localize EEG activities, whether normal or abnormal. See also **true phase reversal, bipolar montage**, and **differential amplifier**. (From the 1974 report of the Committee on Terminology, IFCN. In: Chatrian GE, Bergamini L, Dondey M et al. A glossary of terms most commonly used by clinical electroencephalographers. *EEG Clin Neurophysiol* 1974;37:538–48. Reproduced by kind permission of Elsevier Science.)

insufficient sleep syndrome A disorder occurring in an individual who persistently fails to obtain sufficient nocturnal sleep required to support normal alert wakefulness. Diagnostic criteria are given in Chart I –8.[1629]

insula (Lat, island) (Island of Reil) That area of cortex lying deep in the Sylvian fissure, covered by the opercula of the frontal and parietal lobes.

insular sclerosis The first name applied to **multiple sclerosis** by Moxon, who first described the condition in England.

insular strokes Relatively small strokes that are restricted to the insular cortex and presenting with the following clinical features:

A transient contralateral pseudothalamic sensory syndrome
Transient painful syndromes
Deficits in taste recognition
An acute pseudovestibular syndrome with dizziness, gait instability, difficulty remaining upright, and a nonlateralized tendency to fall, but without nystagmus or cerebellar dysfunction, *or*
Distortion of body image
Language deficits are also described with left-sided insular strokes[1070]

integrative action of the nervous system The term of **Sherrington** for the coordination of movements as a response to sensory stimuli, the coordination being regarded as the simultaneous and successive compounding of simple reflexes; the cooperation of reflexes with allied or harmonious tendencies; and the prevention of simultaneous activity in

Chart I–8. Diagnostic Criteria for Insufficient Sleep Syndrome

A. A complaint of excessive sleepiness or (in prepubertal children) of difficulty in initiating sleep.
B. Habitual sleep episodes shorter in duration than expected for the age of the individual.
C. When the habitual sleep schedule is not maintained (e.g., on weekends or in vacation time), patients will have a sleep episode that is greater in duration than the habitual sleep episode and will awaken spontaneously.
D. The abnormal sleep pattern is present for at least 3 months.
E. A therapeutic trial of a longer sleep episode eliminates the symptoms.
F. Polysomnographic monitoring performed over the patient's habitual sleep period demonstrates
   1. Sleep latency less than 15 min longer, a sleep efficiency greater than 85%, and a final awakening of less than 10 min
   2. A multiple sleep latency test that demonstrates excessive sleepiness
G. No evidence of significant underlying medical or psychiatric disorder to account for the symptoms
H. Does not meet the criteria for any other sleep disorder producing either insomnia or excessive sleepiness

From AASM Diagnostic Classification Steering Committee. The International Classification of Sleep Disorders Diagnostic and Coding Manual. *Rochester, MN. American Academy of Sleep Medicine 1991/2001. Reproduced by kind permission of the Academy.* See also http://www.sleepeducation.com/Disorders.aspx/.

reflex arcs which have antagonistic functions.[5787]

integrator nystagmus See **gaze-paretic nystagmus**.

integument (Lat, upon + to cover) A covering, such as the skin.

intellect (from Lat, perceiving or choosing between) The power of reasoning and of understanding.

intellectual aura See **dreamy state**.

intelligence 1. The faculty of using means to attain ends, with understanding. 2. A set of (cognitive) abilities comprising the senses, gnosis, and reflection.[2823] 3. That set of abilities measured by intelligence tests. At least two forms of intelligence are recognized: *fluid intelligence* is that required for the solution of new problems, while *crystallized intelligence* refers to the manipulation of previously learned information.[2992]

intention An end which a subject decides to attain.

intention myoclonus See **action myoclonus**.

intention rigidity The occurrence of "freezing," often leading to falling, when a patient with **myotonia congenita** has to do something suddenly.

intention spasm The simultaneous contraction of agonists and antagonists during performance of a precise voluntary movement, rendering correct execution of the movement impossible. A form of dystonia.

intention tremor A form of kinetic tremor due to an oscillation of a limb during the performance of a voluntary goal-directed movement that requires precision in the final placement of part of that limb on a distant target. Such to-and-fro movements, increasing in amplitude as the limb approaches the distant target, are taken as a sign of cerebellar disease on the same side. See also **cerebellar tremors** and **tremor**.

inter- (Lat, between) Prefix denoting between.

intercalated nodes Nodes of Ranvier with an unusually short internodal distance, occurring in the course of remyelination after previous segmental demyelination of peripheral nerves.

intercostal neuralgia (segmental neuralgia) Paroxysmal, sharp pain in the distribution of an intercostal nerve, precipitated by spinal movements, usually with cutaneous tenderness. The primary form is rare, and local spinal or generalized (infectious or metabolic) causes are more often incriminated as causal agents, although the mechanism is usually unclear.

interdigital neuralgia See **Morton metatarsalgia**.

interdigital neuropathy See **Morton metatarsalgia**.

interdischarge interval The time between corresponding points upon consecutive discharges of the same potential. (Adapted from the 2001 Report of the Nomenclature Committee of the American Association of Electromyography and Electrodiagnosis.[19] Reproduced by kind permission of the AANEM.)

interdose withdrawal headache See **analgesic rebound headache**.

interelectrode distance The spacing between pairs of electrodes. The distances between adjacent EEG electrodes placed according to the standard 10–20 system or more closely spaced electrodes are frequently referred to as *short* or *small interelectrode distances*. Larger distances such as the double or triple distance between standard electrode placements are often termed *long* or *large interelectrode distances*. (From the 1974 report of the Committee on Terminology, IFCN. In: Chatrian GE, Bergamini L, Dondey M, et al. A glossary of terms most commonly used by clinical electroencephalographers. *EEG Clin Neurophysiol* 1974;37:538–48. Reprinted with kind permission from Elsevier Science.)

interference Unwanted electric activity recorded from the surrounding environment.

interference pattern Electric activity recorded from a muscle with a needle electrode during maximal voluntary effort. A full interference pattern implies that no individual motor unit action potentials can be clearly identified. A reduced interference pattern (intermediate pattern) is one in which some of the individual motor unit action potentials may be identified while others cannot due to superimposition of waveforms. The term *discrete activity* is used to describe the electric activity recorded when each of several different motor unit action potentials can be identified in an ongoing recording due to limited superimposition of waveforms. The term *single unit pattern* is used to describe a single motor unit action potential, firing at a rapid rate (should be specified) during maximum voluntary effort. The force of contraction associated with the interference pattern should be specified. See also **early recruitment, recruitment pattern**, and **reduced recruitment pattern**. (From the 2001 Report of the Nomenclature Committee of the American Association of Electromyography and Electrodiagnosis.[19] Reproduced by kind permission of the AANEM.)

interference pattern analysis The quantitative analysis of the interference pattern. This can be done either in the frequency domain using fast Fourier transformation (FFT) or in the time domain and can be done using a fixed load (e.g., 2 kg), at a given proportional strength or at random strengths. Both the number of turns per second and the amplitude, defined as the mean amplitude between peaks, can be measured.[19]

interictal That period intervening between acute events affecting the nervous system—for example, the time after one seizure and before the next.

Interlocking Finger Test A task in which the patient is required to imitate the examiner's finger configurations in which the fingers are interlocked in different postures, without symbolic meaning. Results correlate highly with other standard measures of parietal lobe dysfunction and this can be used as a screening test.[4458]

intermanual conflict A state in which one hand performs an action that is undone by the other hand. See also **alien hand syndrome**.

intermediary coup contusions Single or multiple contusion hemorrhages in the deeper structures of the brain.[6]

intermediary nerve of Wrisberg The small sensory component of the seventh cranial nerve, conveying common sensation from the anterior wall of the external auditory meatus.

intermediary sleep stage Nonrapid eye movement sleep stage 2.[280]

intermediate filaments Fibrous proteins that mediate cell-type-specific features of cytoarchitecture, including α-internexin, cytokeratins, desmin, lilensin, glial fibrillary acidic protein (GFAP), lamins, nestin, neurofilaments, paranemin, peripherins, phakinin, synemin, and vimentin. Intermediate filament-associated proteins responsible for other disorders include αB-crystallin, desmoplakin, emerin, gigaxonin, and plectin.

(This entry is abstracted from the neuromuscular Web site at Washington University, St. Louis, [http://www.neuro.wustl.edu/neuromuscular/maltbrain.html] by courtesy of Dr. Alan Pestronk.)

intermediate interference pattern See **interference pattern**.

intermediate petit mal seizures An epileptic syndrome characterized by features of both classic typical absence attacks and the **Lennox–Gastaut syndrome**. The clinical seizure patterns include typical absences and tonic-atonic seizures, but motor phenomena including automatisms and change in muscle tone may occur, as may generalized tonic-clonic seizures, or tonic seizures during sleep. The attacks can be precipitated by hyperventilation. The patients frequently show a degree of mental impairment. EEG discharges consist of slow spike-wave complexes, but the frequency of the complexes varies during short periods of time.[3959]

intermediate spinal muscular atrophy See **hereditary motor neuropathy, type 2**.

intermetamorphosis The delusion that known or unknown people have altered their physical or mental identity.

intermittent ataxias Cerebellar syndromes, usually recessively inherited and with an early age of onset. Most are associated with a metabolic deficit.[2754]

intermittent branched-chain ketoaciduria A recessively inherited, intermittent ataxic syndrome, a variant of **maple syrup urine disease**. Various stresses such as infections and surgery may lead to attacks of lethargy, hyporeflexia, ataxia, vomiting, coma, and possibly death. In such attacks, the urinary levels of ketoacids are high.[2754] See also **cerebellar ataxias**.

intermittent claudication of the cord The occurrence of pain, leg weakness, and ascending sensory deficits during exercise, relieved by rest and lumbar spinal flexion, and resulting either from steal of the blood supply from the lower cord segments and cauda equina or from compression of lumbosacral roots at many levels as a result of extension during activity in the setting of spinal stenosis.

The term was introduced by **Déjèrine**, as his patients had pyramidal signs on walking and thus their gait was disturbed. Verbiest detected radicular symptoms on exercise and the condition was subsequently called *intermittent claudication of the cauda equina* or *neurogenic claudication*. Since the term is derived from the Latin word for limping, and it is the patient rather than the cord that limps, it is an obvious misnomer. See **lumbar spinal stenosis**.

intermittent oculosympathetic paresis See **periodic miosis**.

intermittent painful ophthalmoplegia See **superior orbital fissure syndrome**.

internal anal sphincter reflex Contraction of the sphincter in response to dilatation, as from a gloved finger. The reflex is mediated by the presacral (sympathetic) nerves. See also **external anal sphincter reflex**.

internal arousal insomnia See **persistent DIMS**.

internal auditory artery occlusion An arterial occlusion leading to labyrinthine infarction and to the syndrome of acute vertigo and unilateral hearing loss.[3431]

internal border-zone (subcortical junctional infarcts) Small infarcts in paraventricular regions or high in the internal capsule resulting from distal middle cerebral artery occlusion beyond the takeoff of the perforating vessels but before the bifurcation of the artery, or from severe extracranial carotid occlusive disease. Clinically, hemiparesis and hemisphere-specific neuropsychological dysfunction are the usual findings.

internal carotid artery web A linear filling defect in the proximal part of the internal carotid artery, seen in the arteriogram of some patients with **fibromuscular dysplasia**.[4486]

internal hamstring reflex (semitendinosus reflex, semimembranosus reflex, posterior tibiofemoral reflex) Contraction of the hamstrings in response to a tap on the tendons of these muscles, on the medial aspect of the popliteal fossa. The reflex informs on the state of the L4–5 and S1–2 reflex arcs.

internal hydrocephalus Expansion of the ventricles, assumed to be due to increased intracranial pressure. This term and **noncommunicating hydrocephalus** are interchangeable.

internal purulent pachymeningitis See **subdural empyema**.

International Academy for Child Brain Development A professional society. Web site: http://www.iahp.org/.

International Alliance of ALS/MND Associations The central body for national organizations that support people living with **amyotrophic lateral sclerosis** (motor neuron disease). Web site: http://www.alsmndalliance.org/whatsnew.html.

International Association for the Study of Pain (IASP) A charitable association in this field. Web site: http://www.iasp-pain.org//AM/Template.cfm?Section=Home.

International Brain Research Organization A public charity that serves as a platform for funding leading neuroscientists and research institutions around the world. The objective is to maximize the potential benefits derived from basic research and translate it into clinically useful treatments for those afflicted with disorders of the brain. It was founded by H.H. Jasper in 1960 to promote international cooperation in research on the nervous system. Web site: http://www.ibro.org/.

International Center for Types A and B Niemann–Pick Disease A nonprofit organization whose Web site offers information on the prevention and treatment of this disorder for patients and physicians. Web site: http://www.mssm.edu/niemann-pick/.

International Child Neurology Association A professional organization. Web site: www.child-neuro.net.

International Classification of Diseases of the Nervous System A neuropathologic group particularly concerned with dementing disorders. Web site: http://www.ICDNS.org.

International Cooperative Ataxia Rating Scale A 100-point semi-quantitative scale quantifying postural and stance disorders, limb ataxia, dysarthria, and oculomotor disorders, in order that subscores concerning these symptoms may be separately studied.[6401]

International Continence Society Classification A system of classifying neurogenic bladder disorders.[3093]

Detrusor: Normal, overactive, and underactive
Urethra: Normal, overactive, and incompetent
Sensation: Normal, hypersensitive, and hyposensitive

See also **Bors-Komarr classification** and **Krane–Siroky classification**.

International Essential Tremor Foundation A charitable organization in this field. Address: 7046 West 105th St., Overland Park, KS 66212-1803. Tel: 913-341-3880; 888-387-3667. E-mail: staff@essentialtremor.org/. Web site: http://www.essentialtremor.org/.

International Federation of Clinical Neurophysiology (Formerly the International Federation of Societies for Electroencephalography and Clinical Neurophysiology, IFCN). A professional organization concerned with the practice of clinical neurophysiology, teaching, and research worldwide, equal representation being accorded to EEG and EMG. National societies from 36 countries are affiliated. The journal *Clinical Neurophysiology* is the official publication of the federation. Web site: www.ifcn.info.

International Federation of Multiple Sclerosis Societies A professional organization to which all national societies are affiliated, concerned with cooperation in multiple sclerosis research, the publicizing of research information, and the standardization of materials and methodologies in multiple sclerosis research. Web site: http://findarticles.com/p/articles/mi_m0850/is_1_21/ai_97115891.

International Foundation for Alternating Hemiplegia of Childhood (IFAHC) A charitable organization in this field. Address: 239 Nevada St. Redwood City, CA 94062. Tel: 650-365-5798. E-mail: LAEgan@aol.com. Web site: http://www.ahckids.org/.

International Headache Society A professional organization, particularly notable for its classification of headaches and facial pain. Its official journal is **Cephalalgia**. Web site: http://www.i-h-s.org/.

International Joseph Disease Foundation A charitable organization concerned with this condition. Address: P.O. Box 994268, Redding, CA 96099. Tel: 530-246-4722. Web site: http://www.shasta.com/bastiana/.

International Multiple Sclerosis Support Foundation A charitable organization in this field. Address: 9420 East Golf Links Rd., PMB# 291, Tucson, AZ 85730-1340. E-mail: jean@imssf.org/. Web site: http://www.msnews.org/.

International Neurotoxicology Association A professional organization in this field. Web site: http://www.neurotoxicology.org/.

International Polio Network/ Gazette International Networking Institute A charitable organization providing support and information on this condition. Address: 4207 Lindell Blvd. #110, St. Louis, MO 63108-2915. Tel: 314-534-0475. E-mail: gini_intl@msn.com. Web site: http://www.post-polio.org/.

International Research Council of Neuromuscular Disorders A professional society, the members of which are active in research into diseases of nerve and muscle. Address: P.O. Box 41, New Bremen, OH 45869.

International Rett Syndrome Foundation A nonprofit organization for parents of children with **Rett syndrome**, interested professionals, and others. It offers information and referral service and support groups and supports research. Address: 9121 Piscataway Rd., Suite 2-B, Clinton, MD 20735. Tel: 301-856-3334; 1-800-818-7388. E-mail: irsa@rettsyndrome.org. Web site: http://www.rettsyndrome.org/.

International Society of Neuropathology A professional organization for members of national societies of neuropathology publishing the quarterly journal *Brain Pathology*. Web site: http://www.intsocneuropathol.com/.

international 10–20 system A system of electrode placement on the scalp in which electrodes are placed at sites either 10 or 20% of the total distance on a line on the skull between the nasion and inion in the sagittal plane and between the right and left preauricular points in the coronal plane.[1117]

International Tremor Foundation A charitable organization publishing information for patients with essential tremor or Parkinson disease, as well as for physicians involved in their care. Address: 833. West Washington Blvd., P.O. Box DR, Chicago, IL 60607. Tel: 312-733-1893. Web site: http://www.essentialtremor.org/.

Internet Handbook of Neurology A comprehensive information source compiled by the University of Debrecen, Hungary, with superb illustrations of the neuroanatomy and neuropathology of many neurological diseases as well as links to other resources. The Web sites include www.neuropat.dote.hu/movement.htm and www.neuropat.dote.hu/dementia.htm/.

Internet Journal of Neurology A free, online journal publishing reviews and original material. Web site: http://www.ispub.com/ostia/index.php?xmlFilePath=journals/ijn/front.xml.

Internet stroke center A useful informational site at http://www.strokecenter.org/.

internodes The portions of nerve fibers between nodes of Ranvier.

internuclear ophthalmoplegia (ataxic nystagmus, Bielschowsky–Lutz–Cogan syndrome) A term introduced by **Lhermitte** to describe the clinical phenomenon of horizontal jerk nystagmus in the abducting eye and impaired adduction of the other eye on lateral gaze, the lesion being in the medial longitudinal fasciculus on the side of the adduction failure. Lutz (a Cuban ophthalmologist in Havana) defined the following two varieties: in his *anterior form*, the lateral rectus functions normally but the medial rectus is paralyzed on movement toward the side of the lesion, though it supports convergence. In his *posterior form*, the lateral rectus is paralyzed, but the medial rectus functions normally. The validity of this definition is questioned, and the absence of convergence in the affected medial rectus would suggest that the lesion is higher—that is, more anterior. Dissociated optokinetic nystagmus and ocular dysmetria are also commonly present.[5918]

The syndrome may be bilateral,[6093] in which case **multiple sclerosis** is the commonest cause, but any brainstem pathology and even **myasthenia gravis** can be responsible.[628, 5433]

internuncial cells/fibers Those which relay impulses between major tracts, such as the corticospinal, and target neuronal cell bodies, such as the anterior horn cells.

intraoperative monitoring The use of electrophysiological stimulating and recording techniques in the operating room, in order to detect injury to nervous tissue during surgery or to guide the surgical procedure.[19]

interossei phenomenon When the arm is stretched out, the fingers abduct in the presence of a pyramidal lesion. See **fifth finger sign**.

interparietal sulcus A horizontal sulcus separating the superior and inferior parietal lobules.

interpeak interval Difference between the peak latencies of two components of a waveform.

interpotential interval The time elapsing between the corresponding points on two different potentials.[19]

interpretative cortex The term of **Penfield** for those parts of the temporal cortex which, when stimulated spontaneously or exogenously, lead to the occurrence of experiential hallucinations or illusions or interpretative responses.[4977]

interpretative illusions The term of **Penfield** for illusions of things formerly seen or heard or experienced, occurring as manifestations of spontaneous epileptic seizures. Such phenomena include auditory and visual illusions, illusions of recognition (déjà vu), and illusional emotions.[4977]

interscapular reflex (scapular reflex) Contraction of the periscapular muscles in response to a tap on the spine between the scapulae, described as present in the case of a lesion of the corticospinal tracts above C5.

Intersocietal Commission for the Accreditation of Vascular Laboratories A nonprofit organization established with the support of 11 medical organizations to provide a mechanism for the accreditation of facilities that perform comprehensive testing for vascular disease using noninvasive modalities. Tel: 301-881-8744. Web site: http://www.icavl.org/icavl/index.htm.

interstitial brain edema Increase in the amount of water in the extracellular space adjacent to the ventricles, as a result of increased intraventricular pressure, as occurs with acute obstructive hydrocephalus.

interstitial cells As classified by Cajal, astrocytes and oligodendroglia of epiblastic origin and microglia of mesoblastic origin.

interstitial radiotherapy (brachytherapy) A technique for the focusing and collimation of intense beams of gamma radiation in the treatment of deep-seated, inoperable brain lesions.

interventional neurology The subspecialty comprising the performance of therapeutic maneuvers for neurological conditions which rely upon technical procedures (such as CT or MRI, arteriography or electromyography) for the proper direction of the intervention. Nerve blocks, biopsy, angioplasty, thrombolysis, local delivery of chemotherapy, botulinus toxin injection, and trigger-point injection are examples. Most such procedures are not commonly performed by neurologists.[3535]

intestinal neuronal dysplasia A condition characterized pathologically by hyperganglionosis in the myenteric and submucosal plexuses of the colon or small bowel with giant ganglia, isolated heterotopic ganglion cells in the lamina propria, and increased acetylcholinesterase activity in the parasympathetic fibers of the lamina propria and circular muscle. The clinical condition presents in infancy with obstinate constipation resembling that of **Hirschsprung disease**, megacolon, or rectal bleeding.[2859]

Multiple endocrine neoplasia syndrome type 2b, **Hirschsprung disease**, or **neurofibromatosis** are sometimes associated.

intestinal pseudo-obstruction The occurrence of repeated episodes of small-bowel dilatation, the clinical picture suggesting obstruction but without any lesion detectable at operation. The causes include both neuropathic and myopathic disorders. See **intestinal neuronal dysplasia, familial visceral neuropathy, megacystis-microcolon-intestinal hypoperistalsis syndrome**, and **Hirschsprung disease**.

A *variant* is the occurrence of the condition as a **paraneoplastic syndrome** usually associated with small-cell carcinoma of the lung and presenting with intestinal obstruction due to degeneration of the myenteric plexus.

intra- (Lat, inside) Prefix denoting inside.

intracerebral hemorrhage (intraparenchymal hemorrhage) Bleeding into the substance of the brain or its ventricles. Depending on the cause, this may be in the putamen, thalamus, pons, cerebellum, or elsewhere in the subcortical white matter, as is most usual in patients with hypertension; or in the cortex or subcortical regions, as in those with arterial diseases such as **cerebral amyloid angiopathy**, etc. Arteriovenous malformations, aneurysms, cavernous and venous angiomas, tumors, dural sinus thromboses, coagulopathy and vasculitis are other causes.[5162]

The clinical diagnosis is suggested by the rapid onset of focal neurological deficits with clinical evidence of raised intracranial pressure, such as reduction in consciousness, headache, or vomiting. Diagnosis is further suggested by (1) the demonstration of an intracerebral hematoma by CT or MRI scan, *and* (2) at least one of the following: depression of conscious level, unilateral or bilateral paresis, unilateral or bilateral sensory deficit, visual field deficit, impairment of speech or dysphagia or ataxia, and/or the occurrence of sudden severe headache, in the context of acute stroke.

intracerebral steal When there is diminution of response to metabolic factors, for example CO_2, a rise in P_aCO_2 may lead to a fall in regional cerebral blood flow (RCBF). Here, blood is directed away from the diseased brain with abnormal reactivity to the normally reactive brain which can dilate with CO_2, or RCBF may be increased in areas of hypocarbia, which is termed *intracerebral counter-steal.*

intracranial arteritis with spontaneous benign outcome See **isolated benign cerebral vasculitis**.

Intracranial Hypertension Research Foundation A charitable organization in this field. Address: 6517 Buena Vista Dr., Vancouver, WA 98661. Tel: 360-693-4473. E-mail: IHRF@aol.com. Web site: http://www.IHRFoundation.org/.

intracranial hypotension See **spontaneous intracranial hypotension**.

intracranial pressure The pressure inside the cranial cavity, normally 0–10 mmHg and always less than 15 mmHg.

intracranial pressure monitoring Constant assessment of the intraventricular pressure by means of a catheter introduced into the frontal horn of a lateral ventricle and connected to an external transducer, requiring thus puncture of the brain; or by inserting a hollow metal screw subdurally through a burr hole.

The normal intraventricular pressure ranges between 0 and 15 mmHg (lower in children). Continuous monitoring, although an invasive procedure with some hazards, is the only reliable way of ascertaining intracranial pressure and thus assists in the management of patients with increased pressures, as that due to Reye syndrome, coma following subarachnoid hemorrhage or intracerebral hematoma, hypoxia, encephalitis, and head injury, with the aim of preventing brain death, which is the typical result of a great increase in such pressure.[4366, 4654, 5381]

intracranial pressure waves Three principal varieties are described as follows:

A waves (plateau waves) are sustained increases in intracranial pressure lasting from 5–20 min, followed by a fall to normal levels and are due to episodes of cerebral vasodilation without an increase in blood flow, as during rapid eye movement sleep periods. They indicate poor compliance (or "venting") in response to slight increases in pressure.

B waves are much briefer and occur every 1–3 min, in association with phasic changes in respiration.

C waves correspond with spontaneous alterations in arterial perfusion pressure and indicate decreased cerebral vascular resistance.[3961]

intractable headache Persistence of headache despite an adequate trial of regulatory approved, conventional treatments according to local national guidelines. An appropriate dose should have been taken for an appropriate length of time and medication overuse excluded, but despite this there will have been no satisfactory therapeutic effects nor intolerable side-effects. In the case of migraine, failure of at least four classes of drug (β-blockers, anticonvulsants, calcium channel blockers, tricylic drugs, other treatments with at least one positive randomized controlled trial, nonsteroidal anti-inflammatory drugs, and metabolic enhancers such as vitamin B2 or coenzyme Q10) should be documented. In the case of cluster headache, failure of at least four of verapamil lithium, methysergide, melatonin, topiramate, and gabapentin should have been recorded.[2417]

intradural enterogenous cyst A spinal malformation leading to a myelopathic syndrome of spasticity and loss of pain and touch sensations in infancy or childhood. See also **neurenteric cyst**.

intradural meningeal cyst See **arachnoid diverticula**.

intramedullary (Lat, within + marrow) Situated within the brainstem or spinal cord. Even though the lesion may thus be far from the medulla oblongata, the word is still often used in this confusing manner. However, **intrinsic** is preferable.

intranuclear rod myopathy A pure intranuclear **rod body myopathy** caused by mutations in the skeletal actin gene (*ACTA1*).[1679]

intraparenchymal hemorrhage See **intracerebral hemorrhage**.

intrasellar arachnoid diverticulum See **empty sella syndrome**.

intrasellar cistern See **empty sella syndrome**.

intrasellar cyst The presence of an arachnoid cyst within the sella turcica, causing focal erosion of bone, unlike the situation in **empty sella syndrome**, which does not lead to this finding.

intrauterine seizures Abnormal movements assumed to be a form of epilepsy occurring toward the end of pregnancy, in that the fetus is suffering from pyridoxine dependency or any form of brain dysplasia.[489]

intravascular lymphoma(tosis) (primary intravascular lymphoma, malignant angioendotheliomatosis, proliferating angioendotheliomatosis, angiotropic large-cell lymphoma, malignant angioendotheliomatosis fulminans, and neoplastic angioendotheliomatosis) A rare multifocal angiotrophic large-cell B cell and less commonly T cell lymphoma leading to vascular occlusion of arterioles, capillaries, and venules due to the proliferation of neoplastic lymphoid cells. It may be either systemic or confined to the CNS (including the lower spinal cord). Pathologically, the intravascular collections of large lymphoid B cells are instrumental in causing the multiple microinfarcts[2404]

Typical presenting syndromes are of multiple subcortical infarcts; paraparesis, pain, and incontinence; subacute encephalopathy; or cranial and/or peripheral neuropathy, all accompanied by nonspecific constitutional symptoms. Patients usually present with progressive encephalopathy, focal neurologic deficits, and seizures associated with skin petechiae or purpura. Other involved organs include the adrenal glands, lungs, heart, spleen, liver, pancreas, genital tract, and kidneys. Anemia, elevated ESR, CSF protein, and serum LDH are commonly found. The mean survival is 6 months from the onset of symptoms. The administration of steroids can cause brief remissions.

intravenous digital subtraction angiography An invasive radiological test in which a large volume of contrast material is injected rapidly, so that the dye travels as a bolus through the pulmonary system, the left heart, and the aorta to the brachiocephalic vessels.

Such studies are successful only if the cardiac output is normal, so that the dye travels as a dense bolus. The injection of large volumes of dye may precipitate congestive heart failure or renal failure, and the technique is being supplanted by intra-arterial digital arteriography[4678] or magnetic resonance angiography.

intrinsic (from Lat, on the inside) Within, inherent, special to.

intrinsic sleep disorders Sleep disorders that either originate or develop within the body or arise from causes within the body. They are classified as follows:[1629]

1. **Psychophysiological insomnia**
2. **Sleep state misperception**
3. **Idiopathic insomnia**
4. **Narcolepsy**
5. **Recurrent hypersomnia**
6. **Idiopathic hypersomnia**
7. **Post-traumatic hypersomnia**
8. Obstructive **sleep apnea**
9. Central **sleep apnea** syndrome
10. **Central alveolar hypoventilation syndrome**
11. **Periodic limb movement disorder**
12. **Restless legs syndrome**
13. **Intrinsic sleep disorder not otherwise specified.**

From AASM Diagnostic Classification Steering Committee. *The International Classification of Sleep Disorders Diagnostic and Coding Manual.* Rochester, MN. American Academy of Sleep Medicine 1991/2001. Reproduced by kind permission of the Academy. See also http://www.sleepeducation.com/Disorders.aspx/.

intron A segment of a gene.

intrusions The inappropriate recurrence of a response or of a type of response following a preceding test item or procedure due to proactive inhibition; or the recall of information learned previous to that which was most recently learned and which is now requested.

The resemblance to **perseveration** is close; the difference lies in the fact that the intrusion error occurs not immediately following the first response but even minutes later. In each case, diffuse organic brain disease is likely.[2238] In speech, these are known as **insertions**.

inv dup (15) syndrome A chromosomal disorder resulting in tetrasomy or partial tetrasomy of 15q. The phenotypes are variable but multiple types of seizure, motor delay, hypotonia, facial dysmorphism, and lack of social interaction are common; and mental retardation is always present. See also **Prader–Willi syndrome.**[443]

inverse bobbing See **ocular dipping**.

inverse cerebellum (ventral cerebellum) Grossly abnormal development of the cerebellum such that the folia project ventrally, covering the basilar artery, as a result of inability of the cerebellum to grow in the appropriate direction because of the presence of an occipital encephalocele. The malformation is usually accompanied by other anomalies.[5924]

inverse jaw-winking See **Amin-Amat syndrome**.

inverse latent macro square wave jerks An unusual variety of **square-wave jerks** that are present with binocular vision at a distance but which cease with monocular fixation (i.e., when one eye is closed).

inverse Marcus Gunn pupil See **Amin-Amat syndrome** and **Wartenberg winking-jaw phenomenon**.

inverse myasthenia See **Lambert–Eaton myasthenic syndrome**.

inverse Uhthoff symptom See **Uhthoff symptom**.

inversion of the radial reflex (inverted supinator reflex) A phenomenon described first by **Babinski** in 1910, comprising the replacement of the brachioradialis reflex by finger flexion. This is taken to indicate the presence of a cord lesion at the C6 level. An increase in the triceps jerk is usually detectable as well.[1918]

inversion recovery (IR) An MRI pulse sequence which begins by inverting the magnetization of the nucleus with a 180° pulse and then, after a time (T1), measures the recovery of the magnetization to equilibrium.[4510] This sequence provides an image with twice the T1-weighting discrimination of the spin-echo sequence, at the expense of a longer imaging time.

inverted ocular bobbing See **reverse ocular bobbing**.

inverted optokinetic nystagmus (inverted pursuit) A variant of the normal pattern, in which the fast component of the optokinetic nystagmus is in the direction of the movement of the visual stimulus. This may be seen in some patients with **congenital nystagmus**.

inverted pursuit See **inverted optokinetic nystagmus**.

inverted reflexes Occasional variant forms of the usual muscle stretch reflexes, modified in certain conditions by the underlying pathology and the method of elicitation.[6656] Contraction of the muscles supplied by an adjacent segment below that stimulated by the tendon hammer when a reflex is sought in the normal way.

Thus, tapping the biceps tendon (C5) leads to contraction of the brachioradialis muscle (C6) when there is a cord lesion at C5 which produces signs of a lower motor neuron lesion at that level but of an upper motor neuron lesion as seen from C6 (Babinski's inversion of the radial reflex), or tapping the quadriceps tendon (L3, 4) leads to contraction of the hamstrings (L5–S1) with a lesion at L3–4.

Despite the inherent logical confusion, the former is known as the *inverted supinator reflex*, the latter as the *inverted knee jerk*.[787]

inverted supinator reflex See **inversion of the radial reflex**.

involuntary crying See **emotionalism**.

involuntary (EMG) activity Spontaneous or reflex motor unit action potentials, not under volitional control. cf. **spontaneous activity**.[19]

inward fits The term of Dr. J. Hughlings-**Jackson** for laryngismus stridulus (stridor due to **tetany** in rickets).

ion channels Transmembrane proteins that allow ions to flow in or out of the cell. Sodium and potassium channel activation and inactivation are the basis of action potential's production and conduction. Over 30 mutations of the muscle channel gene SCN4A, which encodes the muscle voltage-gated sodium channel, have been described and associated with neuromuscular disorders like hypo- and hyperkalemic periodic paralyses, paramyotonia congenita, sodium channel myotonias, and congenital myasthenic syndrome.

ion channel diseases (channelopathies) A group of disorders caused by mutations in genes encoding ion (sodium, potassium, calcium, chloride) or ligand (glutamate, GABA, glycine, acetylcholine) channels and with clinical expression in any tissue, but predominantly skeletal muscle or the central nervous system. "Channels" are macromolecular protein complexes within the lipid membrane, forming functional pores in the cell membrane through which ions flow to depolarize or hyperpolarize the cell.

Iowa Neuroradiology Library A neuroradiology teaching Web site of the Department of Neurology, University of Iowa Hospitals and Clinics, found at: http://www.uiowa.edu/~c064s01/.

ipsilesional neglect The unusual situation in which there is impairment of processing of stimulus data originating from the side ipsilateral rather than contralateral to a hemispheric lesion. An example is that of patients with a right hemispheric lesion who deviate their responses *to the left* in a **line bisection** task.[3623]

ipsipulsion See **saccadic lateropulsion**.

IPSP See **inhibitory postpsynaptic potential**.

IR See **inversion recovery**.

iridoplegia Paralysis or immobility of the iris; thus, loss of all pupillary reflexes.

iridoplegia interna See **Adie syndrome**.

iris (Gr, a bright-colored circle) The pigmented contractile organ demarcating the pupil of the eye.

irregular generalized spike-wave activity (atypical or rapid spike-wave activity) The occurrence of generalized bursts of spike and spike-wave complexes, occurring irregularly at about 3.5–6 Hz, commonly found in patients with idiopathic generalized epilepsy.

irregular potential See **serrated action potential**.

irregular sleep–wake pattern A condition characterized by variable temporal disorganization of sleep and waking behavior which occur at irregular intervals for irregular durations. Nocturnal sleep is interrupted and total sleep time is maintained at a normal level only by the individual taking irregular naps by day. Diagnostic criteria are given in Chart I–9:[1629]

irritability (from Lat, to provoke) 1. Abnormal excitability. 2. The property of movement in response to a stimulus, possessed by muscles only (Robert **Whytt**).

irritable legs See **Ekbom syndrome**.

Isaacs syndrome See **idiopathic neuromyotonia**.

Isaacs-Mertens syndrome See **idiopathic neuromyotonia**.

Chart I–9. Diagnostic Criteria for Irregular Sleep–Wake Pattern

A. A complaint of either insomnia or excessive sleepiness
B. Irregular pattern of at least three sleep episodes during a 24-h period
C. Presence of the sleep pattern for at least 3 months
D. Total average sleep time per 24-h period is normal for age
E. Evidence of disturbed chronobiological rhythmicity can be noted by either
   1. demonstration of loss of the normal sleep–wake pattern by continuous polysomnographic monitoring for at least 24 h, or
   2. demonstration of loss of the normal temperature pattern by continuous temperature monitoring for at least 24 h
F. Absence of any medical or psychiatric disorder that would account for the symptom
G. Does not meet criteria for any other sleep disorder causing insomnia or excessive sleepiness

From AASM Diagnostic Classification Steering Committee. The International Classification of Sleep Disorders Diagnostic and Coding Manual. *Rochester, MN. American Academy of Sleep Medicine 1991/2001. Reproduced by kind permission of the Academy.* See also http://www.sleepeducation.com/Disorders.aspx/.

ischemia (Gr, staunching of blood) Reduction of the blood supply to a region. The term was introduced by **Virchow**.

ischemia test A method of increasing the sensitivity of repetitive nerve stimulation in the diagnosis of **myasthenia gravis**, in which the ulnar nerve is stimulated supramaximally at 3 Hz for 4 min, after which the nerve is again stimulated at 3 Hz for brief periods every 30 s. The decrement in the ulnar-supplied muscles is assessed; if none occurs, the arm is made ischemic by a blood pressure cuff inflated above the systolic pressure at a point above the site of stimulation, and the procedure is repeated.

In even mild generalized myasthenia, the first part of the procedure usually induces a marked decrement in the amplitude of the muscle action potential; and even if it does not, such a decrement is highly likely under ischemic conditions.[3435] See also **regional curare test** and **single fiber electromyography**.

ischemic cerebrovascular disease Cerebral ischemia or infarction resulting from reduction of blood flow to part or all of the brain, as opposed to hemorrhage into the brain or its coverings.

ischemic chiasmal syndrome Binasal field defects due to ischemia of the optic chiasm, as a result of atheroma of the cervical or intracranial carotid artery or of the anterior cerebral arteries.[6301]

ischemic conduction resistance Hypoxia may lead to the down-regulation of enzymes, decreased Na-K-adenine triphosphatase activity and consequently reduced oxygen requirements. This may explain the phenomenon in which damaged nerves (in diabetes) continue to conduct despite induced ischemia.

ischemic forearm exercise test A standardized test of muscle glycogenolysis in which the forearm is made ischemic by occlusion of the brachial artery and blood is sampled from the draining veins before, during, and after work is done with the forearm muscles, sometimes measured by ergometry. In normal subjects, peak lactate levels (3–5 times the resting levels) are found at 3 min after cessation of work; both decreases in lactate production (in the **glycogen storage diseases**) and increases in production (in certain metabolic myopathies) may be found in abnormal cases.[4553] See also **myoadenylate deaminase deficiency**.

A nonischemic form of the test in which the isometric exercise is performed at 70% of the maximal voluntary contraction for 30 s has also been proposed.[2944]

ischemic monomelic neuropathy The occurrence of multiple axonal neuropathies in a single limb, occurring abruptly, simultaneously, and without evidence of muscle necrosis, as a result of acute occlusion of, or shunt placement within, a major limb artery.[6779]

ischemic muscular necrosis syndrome See **Bywaters syndrome**.

ischemic myopathy A syndrome characterized by changes in muscle which histologically resemble those of **Duchenne muscular dystrophy**, but which are due to peripheral vascular disease.[1889]

ischemic neuropathy Any injury of peripheral nerves caused by compromise of their bloody supply.

ischemic oculopathy A syndrome of periorbital pain and transient or persistent visual loss resulting from chronic ocular ischemia, as may occur with acute or chronic carotid artery occlusion. Clinically, the major features include tenderness of the globe, episcleral vascular congestion, conjunctival injection, hyperemia, and cellular deposits in the anterior chamber, neovascularization of the iris (rubeosis iridis), a mid-dilated sluggish pupil, increased intraocular pressure, attenuated or dilated retinal vessels, and **venous stasis retinopathy**.[3502]

ischemic optic neuropathy A condition of older people who develop sudden segmental monocular visual field defects (**scotomas**) as a result of infarction of the anterior, retrolaminar part of the optic nerve, in the absence of inflammation, nerve compression, demyelination, or generalized hypoperfusion. **Crowding** of the disk is said to predispose to the condition. In most cases the cause is not apparent, but, in a few, **cranial arteritis**, hypertension, diabetes, or atherosclerosis is diagnosed. The other eye may be affected subsequently.[703]

In *variant* forms, the condition follows cataract extraction[1037] or complicates collagen vascular disease, migraine, uremia, or severe ocular ischemia.

ischemic papillopathy Swelling of the optic disk in association with **ischemic optic neuropathy**.

ischemic penumbra A marginal zone of tissue surrounding a brain infarct within which the cells are functionally impaired since they are perfused at a level between the thresholds of functional impairment and morphological integrity. Such metabolically challenged cells are, however, still viable and able to survive and to recover function if perfusion improves.[282]

ischemic vascular dementia Dementia resulting from cerebrovascular disease. See **vascular dementia**.

ischuria paradoxa Dribbling incontinence in **tabes dorsalis**.

Ishihara, Shinobu (1879–1959) Japanese professor of ophthalmology at Tokyo, who in 1917 developed isochromatic plates for the detection of various forms of color blindness.[3101]

Ishihara plates See **pseudoisochromatic plates**.

island of vision The term of **Traquair** for the variable sensitivities of different parts of the retina to light and contrast, the use of different illuminations of the stimuli yielding a set of values which chart these sensitivities over a large area of the retinal surface. The resultant chart is thus drawn in three dimensions—two for area and one for sensitivity.[1840]

-ismus A suffix indicating spasm—thus pharyngismus, laryngismus, esophagismus, etc.

isocortex The greater part of the six-layered cortex, consisting of two kinds of cortical structure: (1) The *idiotypic* cortex (**koniocortex**) of the primary motor and primary sensory areas which represents the most highly developed part of the cortical mantle, and (2) The *homotypical* cortex which is the **association cortex** some of which is *unimodal* and some *heteromodal* (polymodal, multimodal, supramodal, polysensory, or high-order association cortex) in its response to differing kinds of stimulation.

isoeletric focusing A technique used to separate IgG on the basis of different charges or isoelectric points. It is the most sensitive test for detecting humoral immune responses, and when followed by IgG specific antibody staining, it is employed in the detection of oligoclonal bands in the CSF.[195]

isoelectric line In electrophysiologic recordings, the display of zero potential difference between the two input terminals of the recording apparatus. See **baseline**. (From the 2001 Report of the Nomenclature Committee of the American Association of Electromyography and Electrodiagnosis.[19] Reproduced by kind permission of the AANEM.)

isokinetic dynamometry A method of quantitating muscle power which requires subjects to exert their maximum force against that of a hydraulic or motor-driven instrument, which then measures the torque produced at the anatomical joint tested.[1560]

isolated benign cerebral vasculitis (benign distal cranial arteritis, intracranial arteritis with spontaneous benign outcome) A disease of intracranial vessels unassociated with other primary pathological processes and demonstrating segmental narrowing on angiography.

Clinically, the condition typically affects young adults who present with headache, nausea, and focal deficits. Whether this is truly an inflammatory disease or a manifestation of arteriospasm is uncertain.[5728] See also **Aβ angiitis** and **reversible cerebral vasoconstriction syndrome**.

isolated disk reabsorption See **disk reabsorption**.

isolated finger flexion A rare syndrome due to **neuromyotonia** of the flexor digitorum sublimis muscles, causing progressive, painless, involuntary flexion of the fourth and fifth fingers and eventually leading to contractures. The cause is unknown but may be related to chronic pulmonary obstructive disease or its treatment.[4422]

isolated gait ignition failure (gait apraxia, magnetic gait, slipping clutch gait, lower-half Parkinsonism, arteriosclerotic Parkinsonism, trepidant abasia, Petren gait) A gait pattern characterized by marked difficulty with initiating gait (*start hesitation*) and maintaining locomotion (*turn hesitation*, **freezing**) in the absence of impairment of equilibrium, cognition or limb praxis. Once locomotion is initiated, steps are short and barely clear the ground, giving the gait a shuffling appearance. However, with continued stepping, the stride lengthens, foot clearance becomes normal, and the arms swing as they should.

Diversion of the patient's attention while negotiating narrow passages or turning may precipitate freezing and a resumption of shuffling. Certain tricks (such as kicking the bottom of a cane) may be employed by the patient in order to maintain progress. Postural responses and stance base are normal, and falls are rare.

The pattern is associated with lesions of the basal ganglia, or of the frontal lobes or their connections. (Adapted from Nutt JG, Marsden CD, Thompson PD. Human walking and high-level gait disorders, particularly in the elderly. *Neurology* 1993;43:268–79. Reproduced by kind permission of the American Academy of Neurology and Lippincott, Williams and Wilkins.)

isolated generalized polymyoclonus Acquired generalized repetitive myoclonus with subacute onset in adult life, resembling whole-body tremor and usually impairing gait. Malignant or other neurologic dysimmunity and ingestion of opioids or selective serotonin reuptake inhibitors may be causally related.[4239]

isolated hemihypertrophy A congenital dysmorphic syndrome characterized by multiple renal cysts and tumors, asymmetrical limb hypertrophy, and mental and developmental delay.[381]

isolated lissencephaly sequence A developmental anomaly characterized by type 1 **lissencephaly** of variable severity, bitemporal hollowing with a prominent occiput, severe or profound mental retardation with minimal developmental progress, early hypotonia and subsequent hypertonia, decreased spontaneous movements, feeding difficulties, and seizures including **infantile spasms**.

Numerous other anomalies may accompany the above, which represent minimal diagnostic criteria.[1672]

isolated neck extensor myopathy An important cause of the dropped head syndrome in elderly people.[3326]

isolated polymyositis See **primary idiopathic polymyositis**.

isolated speech deafness See **pure word deafness**.

isolated trigeminal neuropathy Chronic persistent sensory disturbance of the face, usually numbness in one or more divisions of the trigeminal nerve, affecting responses to pain, temperature, and light touch rather than other sensory modes, but sparing motor functions and without demonstrable pathology or evidence of any lesion compressing the trigeminal nerve fibers.[5982]

isolated voice tremor Tremulousness of the voice in the absence of tremor in any other body part. Both dystonia of the vocal cords and **essential tremor** appear to be capable of causing this.[1615]

isolation aphasia A form of aphasia in which the subject can repeat but cannot speak spontaneously, nor comprehend. See **transcortical aphasias** (*mixed form*).

isometric contraction Muscle contraction which occurs without any change in the length of the muscle fibers (and thus without movement at a joint), as when pushing against an immovable object.

isometric tremor That form of tremor occurring normally when muscle activity is exerted at maximal force against an unyielding object, or against the antagonists of the muscle in question. See also **tremor**.

isopter 1. The extent of the visual field that is plotted with a given stimulus. 2. Retinal zones of equal visual sensitivity.

isothermagnosia The perception of thermal stimuli at all temperatures as being warm—an occasional finding in patients with high spinal cord lesions.

isotonic contraction Muscle contraction which occurs with shortening of the muscle fibers but without any further increase in the tension within them after the initial contraction has occurred, as is the case when an object is lifted from off the ground.

isotope cisternography A diagnostic technique for studying the flow of the CSF, useful in the diagnosis of **normal-pressure hydrocephalus** and in identifying the site of a CSF leak. Radioactive-labeled albumin is injected into the lumbar subarachnoid space and the patient is scanned repeatedly over the next 72 h. Normally, the isotope will be seen to ascend to the basal cisterns in 4–6 h, collecting around the superior sagittal sinus in 24 h, after which it is reabsorbed.

isovaleric acidemia A rare organic aciduria due to deficiency of isovaleryl-coenzyme *A* dehydrogenase, leading to a block in the pathway of leucine catabolism. The condition is characterized clinically by an intermittent ataxic syndrome in infants, who present with vomiting, ketosis, ataxia, hyperreflexia, and coma, and in whom cardiomyopathy, congenital heart disease, simple partial seizures, intracerebral hemorrhage, and mild mental and motor delay may also be found.

Most affected infants die before they are a year old. Aminoaciduria, hyperammonemia, and gliosis and spongy changes in the CNS are characteristic pathological findings. The condition is notable for the odor of stale sweat given off by the child, especially during the acute attacks.[931, 2754]

Israeli Vertebrobasilar Stroke Scale A valid and reliable score-sheet rating level of consciousness, gaze, visual fields, diplopia, dysarthria or dysphonia, dysphagia, motor functions in the arms and legs, ataxia, sensory functions, and gait.[2641]

itch An unpleasant sensation that provokes the desire to scratch. Although relief of itch by contralateral ventrolateral cordotomy suggests that the spinothalamic tract is involved in the transmission of itch-related information, there is persuasive evidence that itch and pain are independent sensory modalities.[5432] The subject has been reviewed.[6418] (HJM) See also **mitempfidungen**.

iter cerebelli (Lat, a passage + cerebellum) The cerebral aqueduct (of Sylvius).

iterative discharge See **repetitive discharge**.

ivory osteomas Slowly growing solid tumors which arise within the nasal sinuses and may extrude into the orbit or the anterior cranial fossa.

Iwashita syndrome A syndrome comprising polyneuropathy, skin hyperpigmentation, edema, hepatosplenomegaly, and hypertrichosis complicating myelomatosis.[3111] See also POEMS.

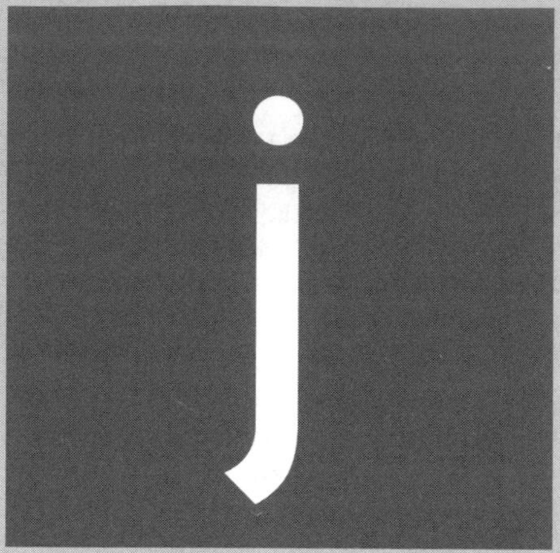

J receptors Receptors lying in the walls of pulmonary capillaries, which when excited cause apnea, hypotension, and bradycardia through vagal stimulation.

jabs and jolts syndrome A syndrome of head pain in which brief stabbing pains lasting a second or a few seconds appear in various locations, or sometimes in a single localized area. The jabs may occur in isolation or in association with other headaches such as migraine or cluster headaches. The phenomenon is probably the same as a prolonged **ice-pick pain**.[5877]

jack-in-the-box phenomenon The appearance as though objects were jumping about; a distortion of vision due to aberrations produced by wearing strong plus lenses.

jack-knife convulsions See **jack knife spasms**.

jack knife spasms (jack-knife convulsions, infantile spasms, salaam attacks) Massive myoclonic jerks with trunk flexion as seen in **West syndrome**. See **flexor spasms**.

Jackson, James (1777–1867) American physician, professor at Harvard, who described alcoholic polyneuropathy in 1822.

Jackson, John Hughlings (1835–1911) One of the greatest figures in the history of neurology. He was born in Yorkshire and apprenticed to a physician in York before further training at St. Bartholomew's Hospital in London. Thereafter he worked in a Poor-Hospital in York and then at the London Hospital and Moorfields Eye Hospital. **Brown-Séquard** helped to secure his appointment as assistant physician to the **National Hospital** in 1862 and he joined the staff of the London Hospital in the following year. He was elected a fellow of the Royal Society in 1878, the same year in which he, with others, founded the journal ***Brain***. He retired from practice at the London Hospital in 1894 and from the National Hospital in 1906.

It was by his work at these hospitals that Hughlings-Jackson, out of the chaos of speculative and descriptive medicine, organized and laid the foundations of modern neurology and became himself, without doubt, the greatest neurologist and scientific clinician of the nineteenth century in England.

Jackson described the intellectual *aura* (he disliked the term) or dreamy state-smell, taste, reminiscence (déjà vu) and epigastric sensations with chewing movements, and a defect (not a loss) of consciousness, which he had first described in 1876. He applied the term *uncinate fits* in 1899. His best-studied patient was a physician, Dr. Z., who lived close by Jackson's house[6235] and who later died from an overdose of chloral; at autopsy a small patch of softening was found in the left uncinate region. His description of the basis of epilepsy—occasional, sudden, rapid, local, and excessive discharge of gray matter—has never been bettered.

He introduced the routine use of the ophthalmoscope; described a patient with **Tourette syndrome** in 1865; expounded his system of **levels of organization** in *Brain* (1887); and divided speech into the propositional and emotional, regarding aphasia as a loss of propositional speech. His studies of epilepsy, aphasia, apraxia, stroke, functional localization, and levels of organization within the nervous system were made without his ever performing a laboratory experiment.[6155] Jackson's contributions in the area of speech were summarized by Head[2811] as follows: The differentiation between speechlessness and plentiful words wrongly used, between *internal* and *external speech* and between *intellectual* and *propositional* speech; the statement of the principle that the loss of power of performance varies with the complexity of the act; the recognition of the power of intellectual expression by movements of any kind; and the characterization of agnosia as nonlanguage aphasia.

Jackson also described the evolution and dissolution of the nervous system, noting that the symptoms observed after a lesion could not be produced by the part which has been destroyed but must be the result of the activity of surviving parts of the brain which in many cases are to be regarded as having been released from some form of higher control.

In his *Selected Writings* (Oxford, Oxford University Press, 1931) there are 32 papers relating to seizure disorders in the first volume, and 37 on dissolution in the brain, brain tumors, speech, optic neuritis, disorders of other cranial nerves, and other subjects in the second.

His contributions in ophthalmology were summarized by Taylor in 1915,[6238] who noted Jackson's recognition of the importance of the use of the ophthalmoscope; the nature of optic neuritis and atrophy; the occurrence of headache as a result of refractive errors; ocular vertigo; and the anatomical innervation of levator palpebrae superioris by the fifth as well as the III cranial nerve in the Marcus **Gunn syndrome**.

Walshe[6625] considered that the areas most influenced by Jackson were: (1) The nature of the relationship between mind and brain, noting that Jackson adopted the doctrine of psychophysical parallelism—mental states arose during but not from the activities of the brain; (2) on movements and their organization; (3) speech and loss of speech; (4) the duality of symptoms—positive and negative; (5) the hierarchy of levels in the nervous system; (6) the meaning of the term *representation*; and (7) evolution and dissolution in the nervous system. Broadbent[856] published a full review of Jackson's work during his lifetime. The work *An Introduction to the Life and Work of John Hughlings Jackson with a Catalogue Raisonne of His Writings.* York GK, Steinberg DA. 2006. (London: Wellcome Trust Centre for the History of Medicine) represents yet more recent scholarship.

Jackson cerebellar "fits" (Stewart–Holmes syndrome, Holmes–Stewart syndrome) A form of movement disorder in which the head is drawn back, the spine extended, the forearms and hands flexed with the arms kept to the sides, and the legs extended. A persistent hyperextended posture remains present between the attacks.

Originally described by Jackson in 1871 as resembling seizures, the invariable presence of posterior fossa pathology causing raised intracranial pressure suggests that this rather resembles tonic decerebrate posturing.[3128] Wurffbain had described the same entity in 1671.

Holmes' name is also applied to this syndrome, but in his paper he made it plain that he had never seen what Jackson had described.[6062]

Jackson's laws 1. Those neural functions that are most lately developed are also the first to be lost. This is restated in a variation as Jackson's rule: After epileptic attacks, simple nervous processes are more quickly regained than are complex ones.

2. "The study of the causes of things must be preceded by the study of things caused."

Jackson syndrome (Jackson–MacKenzie syndrome, alternating hypoglossal hemiplegia) A brainstem disorder, the main clinical features being homolateral IX, X, and XII cranial nerve palsies, producing anesthesia of the pharynx and larynx, paresis of the soft palate, sternomastoid and trapezius muscles and of the tongue, and contralateral hemiparesis, usually occurring as a result of a medullary tegmental stroke or tumor.[3125, 6147]

Some indicate that the XI nerve is also affected, but the condition of the trapezius and sternomastoid muscles was only mentioned by Jackson in an earlier report of his case, a patient who also had syphilis or tuberculosis and who had suffered a number of prior vascular events as a result of severe and generalized atheroma. This is thus another type of **alternating hemiplegia**. The syndromes of **Tapia** and of **Schmid** are *variants*.

Sir Stephen Mackenzie (1844–1909) trained at the London Hospital and in Berlin, returning to join the staff of the London Hospital, where he worked as a pathologist and dermatologist. He reported two cases of unilateral bulbar paresis in 1886.[4003] The two syndromes are considered sufficiently alike as to allow their fusion.

Jackson–MacKenzie syndrome See **Jackson syndrome**.

Jackson-Weiss syndrome A dominantly inherited form of craniosynostosis also characterized by large, broad toes and fusions of the tarsal bones. It is mapped to chromosome 10q.

Jacksonian epilepsy See **Jacksonian march**.

Jacksonian march (Jacksonian epilepsy, Bravais–Jackson epilepsy) The spread of tonic-clonic epileptic movements through contiguous body parts on one side of the body as the causative epileptic discharge successively excites adjacent cortical regions.[3124, 16]

Dr. L. Bravais had described the same events in his graduation thesis of 1827 for the University of Paris, but contributed no analysis of their cause.

Jacob disease (spastic pseudosclerosis) See **Wilson disease**.

Jacobsen, Ludwig Levin (1783–1843) Danish physician and anatomist. His name is appended to the tympanic plexus and canal as well as to the nerve.

Jacobsen nerve The tympanic branch of the IX cranial nerve.

Jacobsohn reflex Flexion of the fingers in response to a tap on the lower end of the radius. When enhanced, this may be evidence of a pyramidal tract lesion or of heightened emotional tone, or it may be normal.[6656]

Dr. L. Jacobsohn was a German neurologist in Berlin.

Jacod syndrome (triad) (Negro–Jacod syndrome, petrosphenoidal space syndrome) Dysfunction of cranial nerves II, III, IV, V, and VI in the retrosphenoidal space, due to compression or infiltration by tumors of the middle cranial fossa such as nasopharyngeal carcinomas. Unilateral visual loss, progressive ophthalmoplegia, and trigeminal pain and numbness are the presenting features.[3139]

Negro described the syndrome from Italy in 1921, and Jacod from France in the same year.

Jacod-Rollet syndrome

Dysfunction of the optic nerve with exophthalmos, due to optic gliomas or other tumors at the orbital apex or aneurysm of the internal carotid artery.

jactitatio capitis nocturna

(headrolling, body rocking, body rolling, rhythmie du sommeil) A form of **ritualistic movement** performed by some infants and young children and consisting of rhythmic movements of the head, frequently persisting through the night. A group of stereotyped, repetitive movements involving large muscles, usually of the head and neck, typically occurring immediately prior to sleep onset and sustained into light sleep. See also **headbanging.** Diagnostic criteria have been suggested and are given in Chart J–1.[1629]

Chart J–1. Diagnostic Criteria for Jactitatio Capitis Nocturna

A. Rhythmic body movements occurring during drowsiness or sleep.
B. At least one of the following types of disorder is present:
   1. The head is forcibly moved in an anterior–posterior direction—*head-banging type*
   2. The head is moved laterally while in a supine position—*head-rolling type*
   3. The whole body is rocked while on the hands and knees—*body-rocking type*
   4. The whole body is moved laterally while in a supine position—*body-rolling type*
C. Onset typically occurs within the first 2 years of life.
D. Polysomnographic monitoring during an episode demonstrates:
   1. Rhythmic movements during any stage of sleep or in wakefulness *and*
   2. Absence of seizure activity in association with the disorder
E. Absence of any other medical or psychiatric disorder that causes the symptom, e.g., epilepsy.
F. Does not meet the diagnostic criteria for other sleep disorders producing abnormal movements during sleep, e.g., sleep bruxism. See also **head banging**.

From AASM Diagnostic Classification Steering Committee. The International Classification of Sleep Disorders Diagnostic and Coding Manual. *Rochester, MN. American Academy of Sleep Medicine 1991/2001. Reproduced by kind permission of the Academy.* See also http://www.sleepeducation.com/Disorders.aspx/.

jactitation

(Lat, to pour forth frequently) Originally a restless tossing of parts of the body; but now the word is used for repetitive movements resembling myoclonus.

Jadassohn nevus phakomatosis

See **epidermal nevus syndrome.**[3145]

Jaeger, Eduard Ritter von Jaztthal

(1818–1884) Austrian ophthalmologist who, in 1860, introduced the test types still in occasional use today.

Jaeger test types

A visual test card using the printers' designation of type sizes. Jaeger 1+ is equivalent to 20/20 vision.

Jaffe–Lichtenstein syndrome

See **fibrous dysplasia.**[3148]

Jahnke syndrome

A *variant* of **Sturge–Weber syndrome** in which glaucoma does not occur. See **encephalofacial angiomatosis.**

jake paralysis

(Jamaica ginger paralysis) A clinical syndrome due to poisoning by triorthocresyl phosphate, a chemical introduced as a contaminant by the American makers into an (illicit) alcoholic extract of ginger sold in the Southern United States around 1929, and later by others into cooking oil sold in Algeria and Vietnam. At least three notorious outbreaks resulted.

Symptoms include cramping leg pains and weakness proceeding to quadriparesis due to a severe motor neuropathy and later due to an upper motor neuron syndrome, which improves only minimally.[4477]

Jakob, Alfons Maria

(1884–1931) German neuropathologist. He studied medicine at Munich, Hamburg, and Berlin, graduating at Strasbourg in 1908 and later worked with Kraepelin, Nissl, and Alzheimer. After World War I he returned to Hamburg where he practiced academic and private neuropsychiatry and headed the anatomical laboratory of the university psychiatric clinic until his early death.

His most important contributions concerned cerebral trauma, demyelination, neurosyphilis, extrapyramidal diseases, and brain anatomy and histology. **Alpers** described the disease bearing Jakob's name, having worked on the case with him in his laboratory. The paper on three patients with this form of dementia was received 9 months after that of **Creutzfeldt** and was published in the following year.[3150]

Jakob–Creutzfeldt disease

See **Creutzfeldt–Jakob disease.**

Jamaican ginger paralysis

See **Jake paralysis.**

Jamaican neuritis

See **Strachan syndrome.**

Jamaican neuropathy

A form of tropical myeloneuropathy of unknown cause(s), manifesting spastic and ataxic variants. Clinically the disease has its onset in adult life and leads to weakness, sensory ataxic gait, numbness or dysesthesias in the legs, distal loss of proprioception and vibration, and decreased muscle stretch reflexes (*ataxic form*) or to a radicular back pain, spastic gait, bladder disturbances, increased muscle stretch reflexes, and upgoing plantar responses with few sensory complaints (*spastic form*). (See also **tropical spastic paraparesis.**) Optic atrophy, deafness, and an axonal peripheral neuropathy may occur in either form.[396]

Jamaican optic neuropathy

A rapidly progressive bilateral optic neuropathy of unknown cause, resulting in dense central scotomas, reported so far only among West Indian and West African people.[1971]

Jamaican vomiting sickness

A severe metabolic encephalopathy due to poisoning with hypoglycine A (present in unripe akee fruit) and characterized by anorexia, vomiting, progressive encephalopathy, and elevation of serum ammonia levels, thus resembling **Reye syndrome**[6180, 4453] or **glutaric acidemia type 2.**

jamais vécu

(Fr, never + lived) The sensation that although the current situational experience is in fact well known, it appears strange, as if it were completely unfamiliar. This is occasionally a normal percept but is typically considered to be a feature of complex partial seizures arising from a lesion in the mesial temporal neocortex.[4977]

See also **jamais vu**.

jamais vu An awareness that although the visual percepts are well known, they appear strange as if they were completely unfamiliar. This is occasionally normal, but it is typically considered also to be a feature of complex partial seizures arising from a lesion in the mesial temporal neocortex.[4977] See also **déjà vu** and **jamais vécu**.

James–Lange theory The hypothesis that emotion merely represents the perception of the autonomic changes induced by exciting causes.[3154] "Anger, fear, love, hate, joy, grief, shame, pride, and their varieties, may be called the coarser emotions, being coupled, as they are, with relatively strong bodily reverberations.

Our natural way of thinking about these coarser emotions is that the mental perception of some fact excites the mental affection called the emotion, and that this latter state of mind gives rise to the bodily expression. My theory, on the contrary, is that the bodily changes follow directly the perception of the exciting fact, and that our feeling of the same changes as they occur is the emotion."

But, one might ask, what evokes the bodily changes in the first place?

Janin tetanus See **Rose disease**.

Jannetta procedure Microvascular decompression of branches of the basilar artery impinging on emerging cranial nerves, as in **trigeminal neuralgia** or **hemifacial spasm**. The risks of posterior fossa surgery are significant, although uncommon in the hands of an experienced surgeon, but the results of this procedure can be life-enhancing.

Dr. P.J. Jannetta is a contemporary American neurosurgeon.

Jansky-Bielschowsky lipofuscinosis See **neuronal ceroid lipofuscinosis**.

Janz syndrome See **juvenile myoclonic epilepsy of Janz**.

Japanese encephalitis Direct infection of the brain with a *flavivirus* member of the togavirus group of arboviruses, occurring in India, China, and adjacent countries of the Far East and borne by mosquitos.

Clinically, the condition is most likely to cause disease in children and the elderly, in whom a syndrome of aseptic meningitis with headache, malaise, fever, headache and added confusion, muscle weakness, extrapyramidal and other focal signs, and sometimes convulsions occur, progressing in severity. Acute flaccid paralysis is a variant presentation. The disease carries a mortality of up to 40%.[6858]

Other neurotropic flavivirus encephalitides include St. Louis, West Nile, Murray Valley, Russian Spring-Summer, Western and Far-Eastern tick-Borne, and louping ill.[5948]

See also the home page of CDC Japanese Encephalitis. http://www.cdc.gov/ncidod/dvbid/jencephalitis/facts.htm.

Jarcho–Levin syndrome A recessively inherited congenital developmental disorder characterized by facial dysmorphisms, short stature, hemivertebrae, block vertebrae, missing vertebrae, and spina bifida.[2326]

In a *variant* form, the condition is dominantly inherited.

jargon 1. (undifferentiated jargon) Recurrent, stereotypical utterances which are not in context with the current subject of conversation. 2. A form of speech containing many neologisms but with a preserved syntactical framework, the use of some grammatical words, phonemic variability, and the preservation of appropriate intonation and stress. 3. Specialized terms relating to a profession or occupation that are appropriately used by only professionals in conversation with each other. Although jargon is sometimes used as a pejorative, this definition nevertheless reflects the philosophical basis of this book.

jargon aphasia Fluent, paraphasic speech which is grammatical and profuse but so distorted by phonetic and phonemic errors as to be incomprehensible. The phenomenon is usually evidence of a posterior hemispheric lesion.

Jarisch syndrome See **Gorlin–Goltz syndrome**.

Jasper, Herbert Henri (1906–1999) American-born neurologist, electroencephalographer, and experimental neurophysiologist who worked with **Penfield** at the Montreal Neurological Institute in Canada, investigating brain function using electrical clues. His pioneering work on brain stimulation in the conscious patient contributed hugely to our understanding of cerebral localization and to the successes of **Penfield** in epilepsy surgery. He was Penfield's coauthor in their landmark book *Epilepsy and the Functional Anatomy of the Human Brain*. From 1960 he was executive secretary of the International Brain Research Organization.[1990]

jaw jerk See **jaw reflex**.

jaw reflex (masseter reflex, mandibular reflex, jaw jerk) Contraction of the masseter and temporalis muscles in response to a brisk downward tap on the lower teeth or on a finger placed on the mental region.

Usually invisible, the movement of the jaw can be seen and felt in cases of bilateral suprapontine disease (spastic bulbar palsy). The reflex was first described by de Watteville in 1886.[6656, 2982]

jaw winking See **Gunn phenomenon**.

jaw-closing spasm Involuntary paroxysmal contractions of the masseter muscles causing sudden opening, deviation, or closing of the jaw, and probably representing an unusual focal dystonia.

Jeanne sign Hyperextension of the metacarpophalangeal joint of the thumb in patients with partial paralysis of the flexor pollicis longus muscle due to an ulnar nerve lesion, this nerve often assisting the median nerve in supplying that muscle.

Jeavons syndrome (eyelid myoclonia with absences) An uncommon, genetically determined reflex idiopathic generalized epilepsy syndrome with onset in childhood or youth, seen especially in girls who exhibit brief but very frequent attacks of **eyelid myoclonia** with or without absences, eye closure–induced seizures, EEG paroxysms, and photosensitivity. Spontaneous or photic-induced GTCS are sparse and avoidable but more common in the presence of sleep deprivation, alcohol, and inappropriate AED modifications. Myoclonic jerks of the limbs are infrequent features. Video-EEG shows frequent and brief high-amplitude 3–6 Hz generalized spike and wave discharge of mainly polyspikes, which generally occur after eye closure, frequently associated with eyelid myoclonia.

Photoparoxysmal responses occur in all untreated young patients.

Dr. Peter Jeavons was a psychiatrist and clinical neurophysiologist in Birmingham, England, practicing in the second half of the twentieth century.

Jefferson, Sir Geoffrey (1886–1961) English neurosurgeon at Manchester. He described the syndromes resulting from aneurysms of the internal carotid artery in the cavernous sinus, pointing out that the trigeminal nerve is variably involved, that anterior aneurysms involve the first division only, that those in the middle of the sinus affect the first and second divisions, and that posterior aneurysms affect all three divisions.[3179, 3180] See **cavernous sinus syndrome**.

Jefferson syndrome See **cavernous sinus syndrome**.

Jendrassik, E. (1858–1921) Hungarian neurologist in Budapest.

Jendrassik maneuver The induction of sustained voluntary contraction of distant muscle groups in order to enhance the muscle stretch reflex responses, described by Jendrassik in 1883.[3195]

Jennings syndrome (endocardial fibroelastosis with neurological dysfunction) A congenital dysmorphic syndrome manifesting genital maldevelopments, cardiomyopathy, hypoglycemia, seizures, plagiocephaly, and mental and developmental delay.

Jensen syndrome A mitochondrial disorder (Xq22, *DDP protein*) presenting with optic atrophy causing blindness, sensorineural hearing loss, dementia, and muscle wasting.

jerk nystagmus That form of nystagmus in which the speed of the deviations of the eyes differs in the two directions, and in which the speed of eye deviation in one direction (drift) is slower than that of the restitution phase (correction).

jerking stiff-man (person) syndrome A syndrome with onset in young adult life, characterized by progressive scoliosis, cerebral atrophy, cerebellar and pyramidal signs, downbeat nystagmus, axial rigidity, leg rigidity, stimulus-sensitive myoclonus, and muscle cramps.[99] See also **stiff person syndrome**.

jerk-locked averaging A technique for back-averaging the EEG with respect to a myoclonic discharge recorded on the simultaneously recorded EMG. It is used to study the scalp distribution of myoclonus-related spikes or the time interval separating an EEG spike and a myoclonic discharge, and for the detection of myoclonus-related EEG spikes which may be undetectable on the usual polygraphic record.[5795] Time-locking is seen with cortical but not with reticular reflex **myoclonus**.

jerk-locked evoked potentials A technique for studying cortical excitability following a myoclonic jerk. The stimulus is presented at varying times in relation to a myoclonic discharge and the EEG and EMG are back-averaged using the EMG pulse as a trigger. In cortical reflex myoclonus, cortical excitability can be demonstrated thus.

Jervell–Lange-Nielson syndrome A recessive disorder characterized by sensorineural deafness, mutism, heart block (prolonged Q-T interval), recurrent syncope, and a tendency to sudden death.[2066]

Jervis syndrome A congenital familial syndrome of inconspicuous and nonprogressive cerebellar signs and mental deficiency, occurring in both sexes but leading to death in the first year of life in the more severe cases. Degeneration of the granular layer and Purkinje cells of the cerebellum and of the inferior olives is noted.[3216]

jet lag See **rapid time zone change**.

Jeune asphyxiating thoracic dystrophy See **Jeune syndrome**.

Jeune syndrome 1. (Jeune–Tommasi syndrome) A recessively inherited disorder of childhood, characterized by the presence of pigmented spots on the skin, polydactyly, short limbs and ribs, severe nerve deafness, optic atrophy, hypotonia and ataxia, and mental retardation. The condition is progressive to death due to myocardial sclerosis or renal failure.[3219]

2. (Jeune asphyxiating thoracic dystrophy, thoracic-pelvic-phalangeal dystrophy) A recessively inherited syndrome characterized by cone-shaped phalangeal epiphyses; pigmentary retinopathy; pelvic bony changes; and small, shortened ribs, which may cause death from respiratory insufficiency during infancy as a result of thoracic constriction.[4742] Hepatic or renal failure leads to death in childhood in those who escaped that fate earlier.

Jeune–Tommasi syndrome See **Jeune syndrome**.

Jewish Genetic Diseases An informational site on genetic diseases more commonly seen in Jewish populations. Web site: http://www.mazornet.com/genetics/index.htm.

jiggle Shape variability of motor unit action potentials recorded with a conventional EMG needle electrode. A small amount occurs normally. In conditions of disturbed neuromuscular transmission, including early reinnervation and myasthenic disorders, the variability can be sufficiently large to be easily detectable by eye. Quantitative methods for estimating this variability are not yet widely available. (From the 2001 Report of the Nomenclature Committee of the American Association of Electromyography and Electrodiagnosis.[19] Reproduced by kind permission of the AANEM.)

jimpy mice A strain of mouse affected by a mutation of the X chromosome affecting the proteolipid gene and leading to a form of demyelination, which provides an animal model for **Pelizaeus–Merzbacher disease**.

jimson weed *Datura stramonium*, a plant whose pods, stems, and leaves contain atropine and scopolamine. Ingestion leads to an acute anticholinergic syndrome with pupillary dilatation, psychosis, hyperpyrexia, and hallucinosis.

jitter The variability of consecutive discharges of the interpotential interval between two muscle fiber action potentials belonging to the same motor unit. Usually expressed quantitatively as the mean value of the difference between the interpotential intervals of successive discharges (the mean consecutive difference, A/CD). Under certain conditions, it is expressed as the mean value of the difference between interpotential intervals arranged in the order of decreasing interdischarge intervals (the mean sorted difference, MSD). See **single fiber electromyography**. (From the 2001 Report of the Nomenclature Committee of the American Association of Electromyography and Electrodiagnosis.[19] Reproduced by kind permission of the AANEM.)

jittery legs See **burning feet syndrome**.

Joffroy, Alexis (1844–1908) French physician, practicing in Paris.

Joffroy reflex Contraction of the glutei with pressure on the buttocks, seen in patients with paraparesis.

Joffroy signs 1. Failure of the forehead to wrinkle on upward gaze in dysthyroid ophthalmopathy.[3224] 2. Impairment in tests of simple arithmetic as an early sign of **general paresis of the insane**.[5333]

Jogger's foot See **medial plantar neuropathy**.

Johnson, Dr. Samuel (1709–1784) English lexicographer and author. James Boswell's invaluable biography and other descriptions, as perceptively analyzed by Prof. T.J. Murray of Dalhousie University, Canada, have made it clear that he suffered from **Tourette syndrome**. His mannerisms, vocal utterances, and habits were recognized by Johnson himself as abnormal and by others as bizarre or frightening, but the brilliance of his intellect and the wit of his conversation diminished, within the minds of his companions, the relevance of such eccentricities. He described poignantly the effects upon his speech of the left hemispheric stroke which he suffered in the last year of his life.

Johnson syndrome (adherence syndrome, oculomotor pseudoparalysis) Fibrosis of any of the oculomotor muscles in early childhood (but usually the lateral or superior recti), leading to the appearance of palsy but distinguished by the results of **forced duction tests**, which are abnormal. **Duane syndrome** is similar but affects both lateral recti.[3230]

joint position sense (conscious and unconscious proprioception) The faculty of being able to localize the position of stationary body parts without the aid of vision. The pathways ascend to the thalamus in the posterior columns of the spinal cord. cf. **kinesthesis**, the discernment of movement at joints. The afferent pathways are the same at peripheral and spinal levels but diverge at the thalamus.

Jolliffe syndrome The encephalopathy of **pellagra**.

Jolly, Friedrich (1844–1904) German neurologist.

Jolly sign The position of abduction of the shoulder and flexion of the elbow adopted by people with C7 root lesions. When bilateral, the sign is also known by the names of Bradburne or Thorburn.

Jolly test A technique described by Dr. Friedrich Jolly,[3243] who applied an electric current to excite a motor nerve while recording the force of muscle contraction. The method was layer refined by recording the M waves evoked by repetitive supramaximal nerve stimulation (at 2–50 Hz) to detect a defect of neuromuscular transmission. (Adapted from the 1987 Report of the Nomenclature Committee of the American Association of Electromyography and Electrodiagnosis. AAEE glossary of terms in clinical electromyography. *Muscle Nerve* 1987;10S:G5–G23. Copyright 1987 by John Wiley and Sons. Inc. Reprinted by permission.) The term was formerly used for repetitive nerve stimulation.

jolt accentuation Worsening of a headache when the patient's head is rotated to-and-fro by the examiner 2–3 times each second. The phenomenon is commonly present in patients with intracranial pathology of many kinds, including migraine, and in those conditions causing cerebrospinal fluid pleocytosis.[6432]

Jones syndrome A congenital dysmorphic syndrome characterized by short trunk and neck, lordosis, scoliosis, skeletal deformities, platyspondyly, dolichocephaly, J-shaped sella turcica, and mental and developmental delay.[381]

Joplin "neuroma" Interdigital neuropathy of the foot comprising isolated compression of the medial plantar nerve, causing pain and numbness of the medial aspect of the hallux. Though called a neuroma, the tissue expanding and compressing the nerve is actually fibrous.[3245]

Jorgenson syndrome A congenital X-linked or autosomal dominant dysmorphic syndrome also manifesting short stature, strabismus, ptosis, blepharophimosis, xerophthalmia, and often resulting blindness, various skeletal maldevelopments, microcephaly, cortical hyperostosis, and mental and developmental delay.[3248]

Joseph disease 1. (SCA 3, Machado–Joseph disease, Azorean neuropathy, nigrospinodentatal degeneration, ataxia plus, autosomal dominant cerebellar atrophy with optic atrophy, dementia, extrapyramidal signs and lower motor neuron lesions, Azorean ataxia, nigro-spino-dentatal degeneration, dominant striatonigral degeneration; OMIN 109150) A dominantly inherited multisystem disorder with differing phenotypes, manifesting variously progressive cerebellar ataxia, dystonia, progressive external ophthalmoplegia, and peripheral neuropathy and mapped to 14q24–q32, where there is expansion of an unstable trinucleotide CAG repeat. The disease is seen in descendants of William Machado, once a resident of Sao Miguel in the Portuguese Azores Islands. The name "Joseph" is the surname of the Portuguese–Californian family in which this disease was described in 1976.[5410, 5987]

The condition is best classified with the progressive late-onset cerebellar ataxias of unknown cause until the underlying biochemical defect is ascertained. Three overlapping phenotypes have been described[1302] and all three have been recorded in each of the separate families affected; the major clinical features are as follows:[4584]

1. *Nigrospinodentatal degeneration with nuclear ophthalmoplegia* (Joseph phenotype) A form with onset in the second or third decade, with ophthalmoplegia, pyramidal and extrapyramidal signs (chorea, dystonia, rigidity), facial myoclonus, face and tongue fasciculations, prominent eyes due to lid retraction, and death by the age of 45 years.
2. *Dominant striatonigral degeneration* A form with onset in adult life (20–45 years) and characterized by the same ophthalmoplegia, face and tongue fasciculations, pyramidal and extrapyramidal signs, and marked ataxia.
3. *Machado disease* A late-onset variant, beginning after the third decade and characterized by progressive cerebellar gait ataxia, hyporeflexia, hypotonia, distal atrophy, and distal sensory loss.

Eventually, peripheral neuropathy is common to all types, but initially the presentations tend to be with ataxia, progressing to ataxia with peripheral neuropathy, and eventually to ataxia with peripheral neuropathy and striatal signs.[2166] Rapid eye movement sleep disturbance is a common problem, especially in patients with the Joseph phenotype.

Variants include forms with pigmentary retinal degeneration, myoclonus and deafness, essential tremor, late onset (usually over 50 years), periodic expression, and features of spinal muscular atrophy. See **motor neuronal diseases.**

2. A recessively inherited congenital syndrome consisting of mental retardation; renal disease; urogenital malformations; sensorineural deafness; convulsions with hyperprolinemia; and the increased urinary excretion of proline, hydroxyproline, and glycine.[3249]

A relevant Web site (http://www.ijdf.net/) is that of the International Joseph Disease Foundation, which provides medical referrals, updates, and support to those interested in Machado–Joseph disease.

Joubert syndrome A rare, recessively inherited congenital malformation characterized clinically by episodic tachypnea and apnea, hypotonia, colobomas of the iris and retina, pigmentary retinopathy with blindness, ptosis due to congenital ocular fibrosis, torsional nystagmus, ocular apraxia, skew deviation of the eyes, renal lesions, syndactyly, microcephaly, cerebellar vermis hypoplasia with ataxia, **Dandy-Walker malformation**, cranial meningocele, and global developmental delay. Many other associated abnormalities have been described, including hypersensitivity to noise, autism, low-set ears, polydactyly, retinal dysplasia, renal cysts, soft tissue tumor of the tongue, liver disease, and duodenal atresia.[3594] The condition is genetically heterogeneous.[6945]

Although the disease is nonprogressive, most affected children die at an early age as the result of their neurological and other problems.[3251] MRI studies show displacement and agenesis of cerebellar structures and very deep interpeduncular fossae at the level of the midbrain (**molar tooth sign**).

The following seven *variants* are recognized:[4992]

Type 1 (9q34.3) A form characterized by the infantile onset of ataxia, nystagmus, vertical gaze paresis, oculomotor apraxia, ptosis, pigmentary retinopathy with colobomas, rhythmic tongue protrusion, episodic hyperpnea or apnea, and mental retardation.

Type 2 (cerebello-oculo-renal syndrome) (11p12) A variant characterized by the infantile onset of ataxia, hydrocephalus, and episodic hyperpnea or apnea, to which are added visual impairment (colobomas), renal cysts, and facial dysmorphism with depressed nasal bridge, hypertelorism, and a high-arched palate.

Type 3 (6q23.2) A form with neonatal onset, manifesting breathing problems, hypotonia with motor delay, impaired vision, and kyphoscoliosis, as well as the features common to all forms as above.

Type 4 (2q13) A mild form of the syndrome.

Type 5 (12q21) A form presenting with mild motor delay and hypotonia, head tilt, breathing abnormalities, and retinal dystrophy.

Type 6 (8q21) A *variant* characterized by early onset of mild to severe disability.

Type 7 (16q12) A form showing ataxia, developmental delay, ptosis; nystagmus, scoliosis, polydactyly, and renal failure later in childhood.

See also **cerebellar syndromes** (congenital ataxias).

Joubert syndrome with orofaciodigital anomalies See **Egger syndrome**.

Journal of Child Neurology (*J Child Neurol*) An interdisciplinary subspecialty journal examining aspects of nervous system disorders in children and adolescents. Web site: http://bcdecker.combcdecker/soc3.asp?bjid=69.

Journal of Clinical Neuromuscular Disease A subspecialty journal published by Lippincott Williams and Wilkins. Web site: http://www.jcnmd.com/.

Journal of Clinical Neurophysiology A specialist journal. Web site: www.clinicalneurophys.com.

Journal of Clinical Neuroscience The official journal of the Neurosurgical Society of Australasia, the Australian Association of Neurologists, the Australian and New Zealand Society for Neuropathology, the **Taiwan Neurosurgical Society, and the Asian/Australian Society of Neurological Surgeons**, published by Harcourt Brace. Web site: http://www.harcourt-international.com/journals/jocn/.

Journal of Cognitive Neuroscience A neurological subspecialist journal. Web site: http://jocn.mitpress.org/.

Journal of Communication Disorders A neurological subspecialist journal. Web site: http://www.elsevier.com/wps/find/journaldescription.cws_home/505768/description#description.

Journal of Comparative Neurology (*J Comp Neurol*) A neurological/neuroscience journal. Web site: http://eu.wiley.com/WileyCDA/WileyTitle/productCd-CNE.htm.

Journal of Epilepsy (*J Epilepsy*) A neurological subspecialist journal. Address: Butterworth Heinemann, 80 Montvale Ave., Stoneham, MA 02180. Web site: http://www.ingentaconnect.com/content/els/08966974.

Journal of Geriatric Psychiatry and Neurology (*J Geriatr Psychiatry Neurol*) The official journal of the **Alzheimer Foundation**. Web site: http://jgp.sagepub.com/.

Journal of Nervous and Mental Disease (*J Nerv Ment Dis*) A private publication founded by James S. Jewell of

Chicago in 1874 and owned at one time by Dr. Bernard **Sachs** of New York. The journal emphasized psychiatric rather than neurological articles, although in part this was due to the relative numbers of articles submitted, and in 1919 turned further toward psychiatry with the founding of the rival **Archives of Neurology and Psychiatry**. Web site: http://www.jonmd.com/pt/re/jnmd/home.htm;jsessionid=Lh1X6noz XRLDJYbBZKhnbZR47pfbwTVW24y2D LmRHyT362hCYzhS!834597482!181195 629!8091!-1.

Journal of Neuroimmunology A professional research-based journal. Web site: http://www.elsevier.nl/locate/jneuroim.

Journal of Neurology (*J Neurol*) The official journal of the European Neurological Society and organ of the Deutsche Gesellschaft für Neurologie. Address: Springer-Verlag GmbH & Co. KG, Heidelberger Platz 3, D-100 Berlin 33 Germany. Web site: http://link.springer.de/link/service/journals/00415/http://link.springer-ny.com/link/service/journals/00415/index.htm.

Journal of Neurology, Neurosurgery, and Psychiatry (*J Neurol Neurosurg Psychiatr*) A British journal of the neurosciences, published monthly, which was founded in 1920 by Alexander Bruce as the *Review of Neurology and Psychopathology* (1903–1918), and which became the *Journal of Neurology and Psychopathology* (edited first by Ninian Bruce and then by Kinnier **Wilson** until his death). It has been published by the British Medical Journal group since 1926. A new series began in 1938, as the *Journal of Neurology and Psychiatry* with Dr. E.A. Carmichael as the editor until 1947. Dr. W Ritchie Russell, Prof. J. Simpson, Prof. David Marsden, Prof. R.A.C. Hughes, Prof. Charles Warlow and Prof. Martin Rossor have been editors subsequently. The present name was taken in 1944. Web site: http://jnnp.bmjjournals.com/.

Journal of Neuropathology and Experimental Neurology A professional journal. Web site: http://neur.allenpress.com/neuronline.

The Journal of Neuroscience Online The official journal of the Society for Neuroscience.

Journal of Neurosurgery (*J Neurosurg*) A neurosurgical journal. Address: Waverly Press Inc., 428 East Preston St., Baltimore MD 21202. Web site: http://www.thejns.org/?cookieSet=1.

Journal of Neurotrauma (*J Neurotrauma*) A neurological subspecialist journal. Web site: http://www.liebertpub.com/Products/Product.aspx?pid=39.

Journal of Sleep Research A professional subspecialty journal. Web site: http://www.blacksci.co.uk/~cgilib/jnlpage.asp?Journal=JSR&File=JSR&Page=aims.

Journal of Speech and Hearing Disorders (*J Speech Hear Disord*) A neurological subspecialist journal. Address: American Speech Language and Hearing Association, 10801 Rockville Pike, Rockville MD 20852. Web site: http://jshd.asha.org/.

Journal of Stroke and Cerebrovascular Diseases (*J Stroke Cerebrovasc Dis*) A neurological subspecialist journal. Web site: http://www.strokejournal.org/scripts/om.dll/serve?action=searchDB&searchDBfor=home&id=jscd.

Journal of the History of the Neurosciences (*J Hist Neurosci*) A quarterly publication sponsored by the World Federation of Neurology History of Neurosciences Research Group, containing contributions relating to the development of basic neuroscience and clinical neurology from the remote and more recent past. Web site: http://home.earthlink.net/~dgjoseph/jhn/jhn.html.

Journal of the Neurological Sciences (*J Neurol Sci*) A neurological journal. Editors: Drs. G.W. Bruyn and J.M.B.V. de Jong. Elsevier Science Publishers B V, P.O. Box 211, 1000 AE Amsterdam, The Netherlands. Web site: http://www.elsevier.nl/locate/jns.

Journal of Tropical and Geographical Neurology (*J Trop Geogr Neurol*) The official journal of the World Federation of Neurology Research Group on Tropical Neurology, founded in 1991.

Journal Watch Neurology A site publishing reviews of papers relevant to neurology appearing in over 150 medical journals. Web site: http://neurology.jwatch.org/.

J-shaped sella The appearance seen when the tuberculum sella and the anterior clinoids are eroded. This is a typical feature in patients with gliomas of the optic nerve but is also found in subjects with **Down syndrome** and gangliosidoses, and occasionally in normal subjects.[2955]

Juberg–Hayward syndrome A recessively inherited congenital dysmorphic syndrome manifesting also short stature, hypoplastic or absent radii, clinodactyly, microcephaly, cleft palate, and mental and developmental delay.[3254]

Judgement of Line Orientation Test A test for perceptual disturbances involving the posterior part of the right hemisphere, wherein the subject is required to match the orientation of a line drawn on a paper with a standard set of other lines arranged like spokes on a protractor.[533]

jugular (from Lat, the throat) So translated by the Benedictine monk who made the first medieval translations of Galen's works, Galen having called it the "sacrificial vein."

jugular foramen syndrome Involvement of various combinations of cranial nerves IX, X, and XI by a lesion at the jugular foramen. If the XII nerve is also involved, the condition is known as the **Collet–Sicard** or posterior lacerocondylar syndrome. See **Vernet syndrome**.

Variant syndromes described and separately named (with the cranial nerves involved)[6147] include the following:

- **Avellis** (X; some have contralateral spinothalamic loss)
- **Collet–Sicard** (IX, X, XI, XII)
- **Jackson** (Complete X, XI, XII; no comment on taste)
- **Lannois-Jouty** (IX, X, XI, XII)
- **Mackenzie** (IX, X, XI, XII)
- **Schmidt** (X, XI)

Tapia (XI, XII)
Vernet (VII, IX, X, XI, XII)
Villaret (Collet–Sicard syndrome with cervical sympathetic palsy)

Cervical sympathetic palsy, hemiparesis, and other signs may, however, accompany any of these.

Julien-Marie–See syndrome See **idiopathic intracranial hypertension**.

jumpers See **dancing mania**.

jumping Frenchmen of Maine (goosey) A familial syndrome seen mainly in males, characterized by brief involuntary movements occurring from infancy, precipitated by startle without alteration in consciousness, and sometimes accompanied by echolalia, echopraxia, and automatic obedience. It was described in 1878 by George Beard among French–Canadian workers in Maine and is still present in their descendants living in Quebec.[460]

Tourette translated the article and compared this condition to **tics** in 1881. **Latah** and **myriachit** are similar conditions to jumping and were described first in English by **Hammond** in 1884.[6053]

jumpy stump Involuntary twitching of an amputation stump, usually associated with lancinating pain, often seen in the postoperative period but occasionally becoming chronic. Voluntary movement and local cutaneous stimuli may act as precipitants.[3754]

junctional infarct Infarction in the border zone between the territories of the superficial (pial) perforating medullary branches of the middle cerebral artery and the deep perforators from the MCA trunk, carotid siphon, anterior choroidal artery, anterior cerebral artery trunk, Heubner's artery, and posterior communicating artery. More plainly, they are for the most part infarcts in between superficial and deep territories supplied by the middle cerebral artery.

junctional scotoma (junctional visual field loss) That visual field defect due to a lesion present at the point where the optic nerve runs back into the chiasm, compressing both and leading to total visual loss or field constriction in the homolateral eye and an upper quadrantic temporal field defect in the other; the latter is due to compression of those optic nerve fibers from the contralateral inferior nasal retina looping forward in von Willebrand's knee. See **Traquair scotoma**.

junctional visual field loss See **junctional scotoma**.

juster reflex Finger flexion with stimulation or irritation of the palm. The normal response is extension.

juvenile absence epilepsy (OMIM 600131) An uncommon idiopathic epilepsy syndrome of childhood and youth in which myoclonic jerks and GTCS usually begin 1 to 10 years after the onset of absences.

It is genetically determined but its mode of transmission and relation to other forms of IGE have not yet been established. The syndrome may be possibly mapped to chromosomes 8, 21, 18, and 5.

Clinically, frequent, severe absence seizures lasting up to 30 s are accompanied in most cases by occasional GTCS and sometimes by sporadic myoclonic jerks as in childhood absence epilepsy. Hyperventilation and arousal are the main precipitants for the absences, while sleep deprivation, fatigue, alcohol, excitement, and lights (alone or usually in combination) precipitate the GTCS. Clinical photosensitivity is exceptional. While the absences are the same as occur in **pyknolepsy**, those accompanied by retropulsive movements are less common. The ictal EEG shows generalized 3 Hz spike or polyspike slow-wave complexes.[4882] The response to therapy is excellent.

A family history of epilepsy is not unusual. Juvenile absence epilepsy, childhood absence epilepsy, **juvenile myoclonic epilepsy**, and epilepsy with grand mal seizures on awakening seem to have a close relationship, since more than one of these often appear in a single family. Onset in adult life is also described.[1749]

juvenile acute nonherpetic encephalitis A condition resembling **limbic encephalitis** mediated by an antibody-associated immune response against the NMDA receptor and associated with ovarian teratoma.[3073].

juvenile Alzheimer disease See **congophilic angiopathy**.

juvenile amaurotic familial idiocy See **GM2 gangliosidoses**.

juvenile amyotrophic lateral sclerosis See **amyotrophic lateral sclerosis**.

juvenile amyotrophy of distal upper extremity See **monomelic amyotrophy**.

juvenile bulbar palsy 1. See **Fazio–Londe Syndrome**. 2. See **Vialetto-van Laere syndrome**. 3. See **amyotrophic lateral sclerosis**.

juvenile bulbar spinal muscular atrophy See **Fazio–Londe syndrome**.

juvenile cerebromacular degeneration A clinical syndrome of dementia and visual loss, with diverse causes.

juvenile Creutzfeldt–Jakob disease See **Creutzfeldt–Jakob disease**.

juvenile dermatomyositis See **childhood dermatomyositis or polymyositis associated with vasculitis**.

juvenile distal and segmental atrophy of upper extremities See **monomelic amyotrophy**.

juvenile distal (nonprogressive) muscular atrophy A syndrome of insidiously progressive asymmetrical muscle atrophy in the hands and forearms with a self-limiting clinical course, usually reported in males from the Orient. A neurogenic etiology is probable.[5867]

Of clinical interest is the usual sparing of the brachioradialis muscle. Bladder, pyramidal, and sensory signs are absent, and the EMG shows evidence of both myopathic and neurogenic disease.

juvenile distal spinal muscular atrophy of upper extremities See **monomelic amyotrophy**.

juvenile dystonic lipidosis A juvenile variant of Niemann–Pick disease type C, itself a heterogeneous group of disorders generally manifesting dementia, epilepsy, and vertical gaze pareses in infancy or adult life, and in which sea-blue histiocytes and foam cells are found in the bone marrow. The nature of the primary biochemical defect remains unknown. See **sphingomyelin storage disorders**.[3314]

juvenile epilepsy See **juvenile myoclonic epilepsy of Janz**.

juvenile galactosialidosis (type 2 juvenile sialidosis) A lysosomal storage disease in which sialyloligosaccharides are stored. The onset is in youth or young adult life and the condition is characterized by mental retardation, coarse facies, corneal clouding, a macular cherry-red spot, deafness, seizures, and myoclonus. See **salidosis**.

juvenile global tremor A slow tremor at 1–1.5 Hz seen throughout the body, reportedly associated with bilateral olivary disease and with a likely metabolic basis.

juvenile GM_2 gangliosidosis with hexosaminidase A deficiency A recessively inherited syndrome characterized by ataxia, loss of speech, spasticity, athetosis, and minor motor seizures in early childhood with death by age 15. Late pigmentary retinopathy is also described.[4727] See **GM_2 gangliosidosis**.

juvenile head trauma syndrome See **traumatic spreading depression syndrome**.

juvenile Leigh disease See **infantile bilateral striatal necrosis**.

juvenile lipofuscinosis See **neuronal ceroid lipofuscinosis**.

juvenile motor neuron disease (hereditary bulbar atrophy) A sporadic variant of **amyotrophic lateral sclerosis** most commonly seen in the people of southern India. It is characterized by slower progress than the classical form; the lower motor neuron lesions of the limbs and bulbar muscles are accompanied by fasciculations and hearing loss; and the stretch reflexes are increased asymmetrically. The highest cerebral functions are spared.[6583]

juvenile muscular atrophy of the upper extremity See **monomelic amyotrophy**.

juvenile muscular atrophy of unilateral upper extremity (distal chronic spinal muscular atrophy affecting the hands) A benign syndrome of distal, segmental muscular atrophy of the upper limb with juvenile onset, affecting mainly the intrinsic hand muscles and those of the forearms.[2916] It usually occurs sporadically, but familial cases have also been recorded. See **Hirayama syndrome**, **hereditary motor neuropathy** (*variants*), and **monomelic amyotrophy**.

juvenile muscular atrophy simulating muscular dystrophy Forms of **hereditary motor neuropathy** in which the neurogenic nature of the disorder is not initially apparent.[869]

juvenile myasthenia Clinically, electrophysiologically and immunologically, typical **myasthenia gravis** occurring in childhood. It always has its onset after the age of 1 year and usually after 10 years.. All degrees of severity occur, as with adults, including an acute fulminating form.[2007]

juvenile myoclonic epilepsy of Janz (impulsive petit mal, Janz syndrome, JME, myoclonic epilepsy of adolescents, benign myoclonic juvenile epilepsy; OMIM 254770) A distinct group of diseases in which there are generalized, idiopathic, and age-related seizures with onset around puberty, characterized by clusters of seizures with bilateral single or repetitive, arrhythmic, irregular myoclonic jerks, predominantly affecting the arms and occurring characteristically within half an hour of awakening. The jerks may cause some patients to fall suddenly without noticeable disturbance of consciousness (but their intensity is usually so mild that only the patient can perceive them). Sleep deprivation, fatigue, and excessive alcohol intake are major precipitants; photosensitivity and mental and psychological arousal are less effective stimuli.

Generalized seizures also occur often, absences less frequently. These also usually occur shortly after awakening and are often precipitated by sleep deprivation, fatigue, and photic stimulation. Interictal and ictal EEG have rapid, generalized, often irregular spike waves and polyspike-waves; there is no close phase correlation between the EEG spikes and the jerks. The response to appropriate drugs is good. (After Dreifuss FE, et al. Commission for classification and terminology, ILAE. Proposal for Revised Classifications of Epilepsies and Epileptic syndromes. *Epilepsia* 1989;**30**:389–99. By kind permission of Wiley-Blackwell Publications.)

Classic JME (as above) is by far the most common variety, but **childhood absence epilepsy** evolving to JME and JME with adolescent absence or with **astatic seizures** are other phenotypes described.[4124]

The disorder was first described as being recessively inherited through an abnormal gene at chromosome 6p.21[3167] and was initially mapped to 6p21.2–p11 and to 15q.14; both dominant and recessive transmission are described. Generalized tonic-clonic seizures, myoclonus, and absences may all occur.[1749] but now seven chromosome loci, three epilepsy-causing mutations, and two genes with single nucleotide polymorphisms associating with JME have been identified.

In summary, this is a rather benign form of seizure disorder, in which nocturnal or early morning tonic-clonic epileptic seizures and repetitive attacks of myoclonus on awakening begin in adolescence but remain as a life-long trait, and in which the neurological and mental state of those affected is normal.

juvenile neuroaxonal dystrophy A rare variant of **neuroaxonal dystrophy**, characterized by the onset in childhood or young adult life of progressive myoclonic epilepsy, cerebellar ataxia, and intellectual deterioration. Dysarthria, pyramidal and extrapyramidal signs, resting tremor, incontinence, and axonal neuropathy are other features.[1695] See also **infantile neuroaxonal dystrophy**.

juvenile neurogenic muscle atrophy with lysosomal enzyme deficiencies A syndrome of childhood onset characterized by mental retardation, features of Marfan syndrome, neurogenic muscle atrophy and hyporeflexia, multiple epithelial dysplasia, increased urinary secretion of dermatan sulphate, and decreased lysosomal enzyme activities (β-galactosidase, β-glucuronidase and *n*-acetyl β-D-glucose amylidase).[2518]

juvenile nonprogressive muscular atrophy localized in hand and forearm See **monomelic amyotrophy**.

juvenile-onset Parkinsonism with dystonia See **juvenile Parkinsonism syndromes** and **young-onset Parkinson disease**.

juvenile Parkinsonism syndromes (corpus striatum syndrome, Hunt paralysis, pallidopyramidal disease) A pure **system disease** of unknown cause, causing Parkinsonian syndromes of bilateral rigidity and tremor with diurnal variation and paralysis of certain automatic and associated movements before the age of 21 years. The disease is associated with lesions of the efferent motor neurons of the globus pallidus. The response to levadopa is gratifying.[6918] Missense mutations of ATP13A2 have been found in some cases.

There tends to be a high familial incidence in these varieties and Lewy bodies are absent in patients examined before the age of 20 years. The condition was first noted by Ramsay **Hunt** in 1917.

A *variant* is *juvenile-onset Parkinsonism with dystonia*, an uncommon dominantly inherited disease characterized by the onset in the first two decades of life of levadopa responsive Parkinsonism with prominent dyskinesias, such as equinovarus posturing of the feet, on-off oscillations, and slow progression of symptoms. The presence of motor fluctuations distinguishes this from **Segawa dystonia**, which it otherwise closely resembles.[2355, 3049]

juvenile progressive spinal muscular atrophy See **hereditary motor neuropathy**.

juvenile Sandhoff disease A syndrome of progressive cerebellar disorder and mental and motor delay with onset in childhood, associated with total deficiency of hexosaminidase.[4008] See **GM_2 gangliosidosis**.

Other *variant* forms include partial deficiency of the enzyme producing the same clinical picture, and a syndrome of tremor, cherry-red spots, and mild truncal ataxia without dementia, associated with total deficiency of hexosaminidase B.[3236]

juvenile segmental muscular atrophy See **monomelic amyotrophy**.

juvenile spinal muscular atrophy See **hereditary motor neuropathy, type 3**.

juvenile spinal muscular atrophy with hexosaminidase A deficiency (GM_2) See **hereditary motor neuropathy** (*variants*).

juvenile type of distal and segmental atrophy of upper extremities See **monomelic amyotrophy**.

Juvenile Unknown Mitochondrial Problems (JUMP Foundation) A charitable organization. Address: 2232 South Main St., Suite 130, Ann Arbor, MI 48103. Tel: 313-327-5070. Web site: http://www.umdf.org/ (**United Mitochondrial Disease Foundation**).

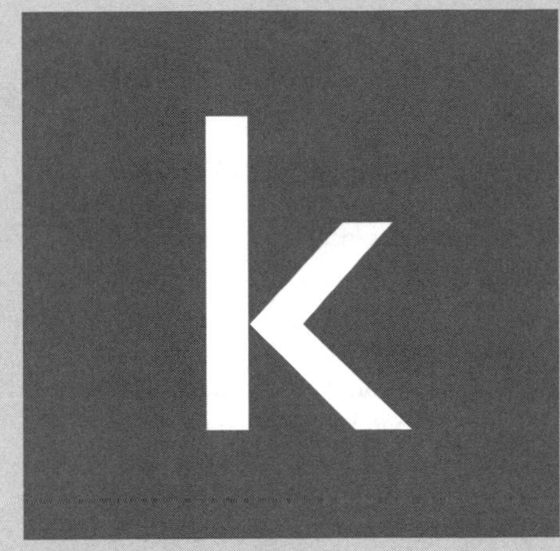

K complex A burst of waves on the EEG of variable appearance, consisting most commonly of a high-voltage diphasic slow wave frequently associated with a **sleep spindle**. Its amplitude is generally maximal in proximity of the vertex. K complexes occur during sleep, apparently spontaneously or in response to sudden sensory stimuli and are not specific for any individual sensory modality. See also **vertex sharp transients**. (Adapted from the 1974 report of the Committee on Terminology, IFCN. In: Chatrian GE, Bergamini L, Dondey M, et al. A glossary of terms most commonly used by clinical electroencephalographers. *EEG Clin Neurophysiol* 1974;37:538–48. Reproduced by kind permission of Elsevier Science and the IFCN.)

Such EEG waveforms are recorded from all head regions during non–rapid eye movement sleep stages 2–4 at 2–3/min, and are characterized by an initial slow negative wave followed 700 ms later by a positive wave. They may represent nonspecific evoked potentials because they are sometimes induced by external stimuli.[3228]

Kabuki make-up syndrome A dominantly inherited congenital dysmorphic syndrome characterized by depression of the tip of the nose, short stature, ectropion, congenital cardiac anomalies, brachydactyly, recurrent infections, and mental and developmental delay, seen mainly in Japan.[4675]

The name derives from the supposed resemblance of the affected subjects' faces to those of a class of Japanese traditional actors.

Kaeser syndrome See **scapuloperoneal syndrome** (*scapuloperoneal muscular atrophy without sensory disturbance*). Although Kaeser's name is given to this condition, his description came 25 years after that of Davidenkow.

kainic acid An excitotoxic amino acid.

Kakke The Japanese name for **beriberi**.

Kahlbaum, Karl Ludwig German psychiatrist who described **catatonia** in 1868.

Kahlbaum syndrome (catatonia) The association of at least one motor sign of catatonia (catalepsy, posturing, or waxy flexibility) and at least one sign of psychosocial withdrawal or excitement and/or bizarre repetitions (mutism, negativism, impulsiveness, grimacing, stereotypies, mannerisms, command automatism, echopraxia or echolalia, verbigeration).

The syndrome was first described by Kahlbaum in 1868, but catatonia itself is nonspecific with a range of psychiatric and organic neurological causes.[411]

Kahler disease A solitary plasmacytoma, rarely located in the cranial vault and usually observed in elderly patients. Progression to multiple myeloma is recorded.

kainate receptors Glutamate receptors, modulators of GABAergic synaptic transmission in the hippocampus. Their activation reduces GABAergic synaptic transmission at principal interneuron cell synapses in the CA1 layer of the hippocampus.

Kallmann syndrome (olfactogenital dysplasia) A syndrome of (usually) X-linked dominant hypogonadotrophic hypogonadism with olfactory agenesis and consequent hyposmia, sometimes associated with color blindness.[3278] The responsible gene maps to Xp22.3.

Other features found have included mental retardation, hypotelorism, scoliosis, renal agenesis, pes cavus, spasticity, and sensory neuropathy. The disease has also been reported in females.

Kanzaki disease A lysosomal storage disorder with angiokeratoma corporis diffusum due to deficiency of lysosomal α-*N*-acetylgalactosaminidase activity. Clinical features include an axonal sensorimotor polyneuropathy and mild impairment of intellectual functions, attacks of vertigo, and sensorineural hearing impairment.[6444]

kappa rhythm A rhythm consisting of bursts of alpha or theta frequency occurring over the temporal areas of the scalp of subjects engaged in mental activity.

The cerebral origin of this rhythm is unproven. It is best recorded between electrodes located lateral to the outer canthus of each eye. (Adapted from the 1974 report of the Committee on Terminology, IFCN. In: Chatrian GE, Bergamini L, Dondey M, et al. A glossary of terms most commonly used by clinical electroencephalographers. *EEG Clin Neurophysiol* 1974;37:538–48. Reproduced by kind permission of Elsevier Science and the IFCN.)

Karnofsky Scale See **quality of life**.

Karsch syndrome A rare, recessively inherited congenital syndrome consisting of nystagmus, strabismus, pigmentary retinal degeneration, and splitting of the hands and/or feet.[3317]

Kashida sign The appearance of muscle spasms and tingling in response to warming of cooling the skin, reported to occur in tetany.[421]

Katsantoni syndrome (Coté–Katsantoni syndrome) A congenital dysmorphic syndrome manifesting also sparse, brittle hair and nails, ptosis, torticollis, nystagmus, osteosclerosis, atrial septal defect, abnormal immunoglobulins, and mental and developmental delay.[676]

Katz activities of daily living scale A well-known and reliable instrument for evaluating a patient's ability to perform six activities in the realm of basic self-care (*bathing, dressing, toileting, transferring, continence, and feeding*) independently, requiring some assistance or requiring total assistance, and thus of value in the assessment and management of elderly demented people.[3332–3334]

Kaufman Assessment battery for Children A diagnostic test for cognitive impairment in children.[3]

Kaufman syndrome (oculocerebrofacial syndrome) A congenital dysmorphic syndrome manifesting also fusion of vertebrae with scoliosis, myopia, pendular nystagmus, strabismus, ptosis, brachycephaly, microcephaly, intracranial calcifications, and mental and developmental delay.[3340]

Kawasaki disease (mucocutaneous lymph node syndrome) An acute febrile illness of unknown cause, usually affecting young children and manifest by cervical and hilar adenopathy, thrombocytosis, and coronary artery aneurysms. Encephalopathy and aseptic meningitis with increased intracranial pressure, muscle tenderness and weakness, and elevated CK levels[3546] have also been described.

Kayser, Bernard (1869–1954) German ophthalmologist practicing in Stuttgart.

Kayser–Fleischer ring An orange, gold, or greenish deposit, about 2 mm wide, around the limbus of the cornea and due to copper deposition within the Descemet membrane. It is found in cases of **Wilson disease,** for which it is pathognomonic, but it may not be visible to the naked eye (it was not described by Wilson), requiring the use of a slit lamp to exclude its presence.[3351]

Kearns–Sayre syndrome (Kearns–Shy syndrome, Kearns–Sayre–Daroff syndrome, oculocraniosomatic neuromuscular disease with ragged red fibers) A laudable coalescence of two conditions (progressive external ophthalmoplegia and the Kearns–Sayre syndrome) through the demonstration that a deficiency of cytochrome *c* oxidase and the usual demonstration of deletions of mtDNA in muscle and sweat glands are factors common to patients with various combinations of progressive ophthalmoplegia, pendular nystagmus, heart block, pigmentary retinal degeneration, cerebellar ataxia, pyramidal signs, mild facial and somatic muscle weakness, retarded somatic growth, and raised CSF protein levels.

The syndrome as initially described has its onset in youth and is characterized by choroidal atrophy and retinal changes resembling **retinitis pigmentosa**, external ophthalmoplegia, small stature, deafness, an elevated CSF protein level, and cardiac conduction block,[3364] with which proximal and distal lipid storage myopathy, cerebellar ataxia, deafness, dementia, hypoparathyroidism, and basal ganglion calcification may be associated. Familial factors play an undefined role in its genesis.[3313]

See also http://www.ninds.nih.gov/disorders/kearns_sayre/kearns_sayre.htm, an informational site from the NIH.

Kearns–Sayre–Daroff syndrome See **Kearns–Sayre syndrome**.

Kearns–Shy syndrome See **Kearns–Sayre syndrome**.

Keating syndrome See **glycogen storage disease** *type 9, phosphoglycerate kinase deficiency*.

Kehrer, Ferdinand Adalbert (1883–1966) German neurologist. He described the auriculopalpebral reflex (closure of the eyes in response to various stimuli such as sudden noise, in the presence of increased intracranial pressure).

Kehrer–Adie syndrome See **Adie pupil, Holmes–Adie syndrome**.

Keipert syndrome An X-linked or autosomal recessively inherited dysmorphic syndrome characterized also by digital anomalies (broad terminal phalanges), hydrocephalus, mental retardation, and deafness.[3368]

Keith–Wagener Scale A classification of hypertensive retinopathy developed by Keith, Wagener, and Barker. It combines the clinical findings of atherosclerosis and hypertension and is that most generally employed. The four levels comprise:

1. Mild-to-moderate narrowing or sclerosis of the arterioles

2. Moderate-to-marked arteriolar narrowing, local and/or generalized, with exaggeration of the light reflex and compression of the venules at arteriovenous crossings
3. The same retinal arteriolar narrowing with focal constriction, retinal edema showing as "cotton-wool patches," and/or hemorrhages into the retina
4. The changes listed in point 3 with added papilledema

Other schemes for classification (Schie, Leishman) are also presented at the following Web site: http://www.medal.org/ch19.html/.

Kemp sign Reduction in back pain with flexion of the lumbar spine, seen in patients with prolapsed intervertebral disks.

Kennedy, Robert Foster See **Foster Kennedy, Robert**.

Kennedy syndrome 1. (Foster Kennedy sign) See **Foster Kennedy syndrome**. 2. See **bulbospinal muscular neuronopathy**.

Kennedy's Disease Association A nonprofit organization working to increase public awareness about this disease. The multilingual Web site includes discussion forums, support, research, and resources. http://www.kennedysdisease.org/.

Kenney–Alter–Sung syndrome See **progressive proximal spinal and bulbar muscular atrophy of late onset**.

Kenny self-care scale An instrument for the assessment of a patient's abilities in self-care and ambulation, of particular value in the elderly.[808]

Kent Waldrep National Paralysis Foundation A charitable organization in this field. Address: 16415 Addison Rd., Suite 550, Addison, TX 75001. Tel: 972-248-7100; 800-925-2873. E-mail: kwaldrep@spinalvictory.org. Web site: http://www.spinalvictory.org.

keratan sulfate One of the glycosaminoglycans, forming part of the mucopolysaccharide which accumulates and is excreted in the **mucopolysaccharidoses**.

keratic precipitates Deposits of inflammatory and epithelioid cells on the posterior surface of the cornea.

keratoconjunctivitis sicca See **Sjögren syndrome**.

keratoconus A conical forward projection of the cornea due to corneal dystrophy as occurs in **Marfan syndrome**, trisomy 21 syndrome, **Leber amaurosis**, and other keratopathies. The condition may also occur in isolation as a dominantly or recessively inherited malformation. See also **Munson sign**.

keratosis follicularis A dominantly inherited diffuse encephalopathy characterized by dwarfism, alopecia, and hyperkeratosis.[6750] Microcephaly, cerebral atrophy, seizures, and mental and developmental delay have also been described in association.

keraunoparalysis (from Gr, A thunderbolt + paralysis) A transient state of paralysis particularly affecting the legs that may occur after being struck by lightning. Cardiac arrest is probably a more common result of this event, however. See **lightning encephalopathy**.

The phenomenon was described first by James **Parkinson** and later by J.-M. **Charcot**, but the name was applied by Macdonald **Critchley**.

kernicterus (bilirubin encephalopathy, nuclear jaundice) A syndrome of hypotonia, lethargy, and poor sucking response, leading on to spasticity, opisthotonos, seizures, and eventually mental retardation, sensorineural deafness, choreoathetosis, dystonia, ataxia, and a pyramidal syndrome. Vertical gaze palsy is also described. Brainstem auditory evoked potentials are abnormal or absent (auditory neuropathy) although inner ear function is normal.

The condition is a toxic effect of unconjugated bilirubin which crosses the immature blood–brain barrier unimpeded in children with hemolytic disease of the newborn or other hyperbilirubinemic syndromes, damaging the globus pallidus most severely.[6505, 141] The condition was first described by Johannes Orth (1847–1923), a German physician, in 1875.

Kernig, Vladimir Mikhailovich (1840–1917) Russian neurologist, born in Latvia, who became director of the Obohovsk Hospital in St. Petersburg until his retirement in 1911.

Kernig sign The classic test for meningeal irritation, as in meningitis, described by Kernig in 1882, but a full description of it was only published 23 years later.[3391] To elicit the sign, the hip is flexed on the pelvis and the knee flexed also; the knee is then gradually extended by the examiner. Resistance due to involuntary hamstring contraction suggests irritation of the L5 and S1, 2 roots.

The test is now almost invariably done with the patient supine, but in his original paper, Kernig described its elicitation in the sitting position as well.

Kernohan, J.W. (b. 1897) Irish neuropathologist who emigrated to America and worked at the Mayo Clinic. He introduced a grading system for gliomas as well as describing the following syndrome.

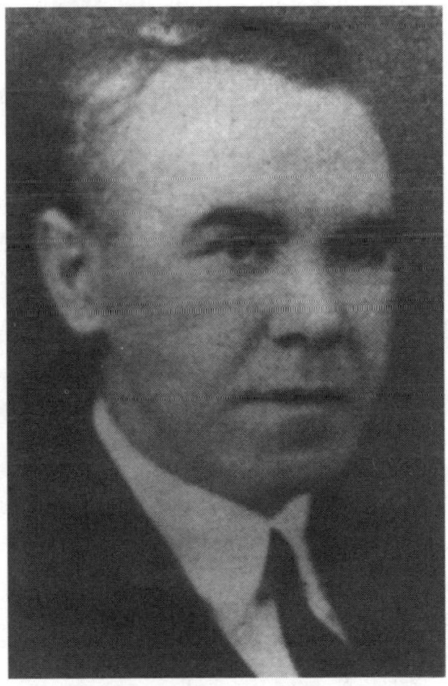

Figure K–1 James Watson Kernohan.

Kernohan notch syndrome (clivus edge syndrome) Unilateral or bilateral pyramidal signs resulting from direct compression of a cerebral peduncle in the **uncal syndrome**, and further indirect compression of the contralateral peduncle as a result of its displacement across the midline to abut the contralateral tentorial free edge, indenting ("notching") the peduncle.[3393]

The name of H.W. Woltman, a colleague of Kernohan at the Mayo Clinic, has also been applied to this syndrome.

Kerr syndrome Stiffness and dryness of the skin for a few segments below a spinal cord lesion.

Kestenbaum number A rough measure of the relative afferent pupillary defect, obtained by comparing the size of each pupil while the other one is in darkness.

Kestenbaum also counted the vessels crossing the edge of the optic disk and believed that a substantial reduction was an indication of optic neuropathy, though this has not been confirmed as a valid marker for that condition.

Kestenbaum syndrome See **Sylvian aqueduct syndrome**.

ketoacidosis Accumulation of ketones in the blood, resulting from, for example, glucose dysmetabolism or **mitochondriopathies**, in which short stature, ataxia, deafness, and episodic coma are notable accompaniments.

ketogenic diet A high-fat, high-protein diet used in the management of intractable generalized or partial seizure disorders in children and adults. As over three-quarters of the calories are derived from fats, chronic ketoacidosis results and this appears to have anticonvulsant activity.

3-ketothiolase deficiency (β-ketothiolase deficiency) A congenital metabolic aminoaciduric syndrome manifesting an abnormality in consciousness, neonatal respiratory distress, and mental and developmental delay.[381]

ketotic hyperglycinemia A recessively inherited primary organic acidemia presenting in infancy with failure to thrive, seizures, hypertonia, cerebellar ataxia, and mental and motor delay, induced by the ingestion of milk protein (casein).[1148] See **proprionic acidemia, cerebellar ataxias** (*variants*).

ketotifen A drug that blocks the secretion of mast cells, which are thought to contribute to the origin and growth of neurofibromas.

Keutel syndrome (humeroradial synostosis plus) A recessively inherited congenital dysmorphic syndrome manifesting also skeletal and genital abnormalities, microcephaly, meningocele, deafness, and mental and developmental delay.[3410]

keyhole aqueduct syndrome (pure **syringobulbia**) The occurrence of a syrinx in the midbrain and upper pons communicating with the aqueduct and fourth ventricle without associated syringomyelia. The condition is associated with gliosis of the cerebellum, and presents clinically with signs and symptoms of cerebellar and brainstem dysfunction with dysarthria, nystagmus, deafness, and **internuclear ophthalmoplegia**.

The syrinx may be a centimeter or more in its widest diameter, and is in the shape of an old-fashioned keyhole.[1502]

Kienbock, Robert (1871–1953) Austrian radiologist, professor at Vienna, who described both the following condition and that of osteochondritis of the semilunate bone.

Kienbock disease Posttraumatic **syringomyelia**.[3422] See also **hematomyelia**.

Killian–Pallister mosaic syndrome (chromosome 12p tetrasomy) A congenital dysmorphic syndrome characterized by facial dysmorphism and skeletal abnormalities, brachycephaly, strabismus, ptosis, hypotonia, cerebral atrophy, seizures, and mental and developmental delay.[4869]

Kiloh–Nevin syndromes
1. **anterior interosseous syndrome**.[3426]
2. **ocular myopathy**. A syndrome of dominantly inherited progressive weakness of the external ocular muscles with adult onset. The difficulty of distinguishing myopathic from neuropathic changes in these muscles has led to uncertainty as to the actual pathology, but, in many cases, further spread of the weakness to the facial and bulbar and ultimately to the girdle muscles, coupled with the frequent finding of **ragged red fibers** on muscle biopsy specimens, has swung the balance in favor of a myopathy (probably mitochondrial), as originally described.[3425]

This condition and **Kearns–Shy syndrome** are presumably the same.

kindling The progressive and permanent reduction in seizure threshold that occurs when certain brain regions are stimulated repeatedly. Initially stimulus-bound, the seizures later occur spontaneously and eventually become intractable.[4262]

kinesia paradoxica The remarkable ability of some patients with akinetic Parkinsonism to regain normal motor freedom for a short time, usually when under acute emotional stress (as when their hospital ward catches fire, and they are capable of short-lived but useful movement, such as running out of the building).

kinesics 1. The complex of all of an individual's gestural activity, conscious or unconscious, replacing or embellishing speech.[1337] 2. The study of limb, body, and facial movements associated with nonverbal communication.

kinesigenic choreoathetosis An uncommon paroxysmal movement disorder characterized by the onset in childhood or youth of dystonic spasms, chorea, and athetosis precipitated by walking or other muscle activity, and seizures but without succeeding dementia.[3400] Whether this is a form of reflex epilepsy or a movement disorder with basal ganglion origin is undetermined. See **paroxysmal kinesigenic choreoathetosis, familial kinesigenic choreoathetosis**.

kinesin One of a family of proteins found within axons, which are able to translocate axoplasmic vesicles along the microtubules, and thus are responsible for axoplasmic transport.

kinesiologic EMG (dynamic EMG) The muscle electrical activity recorded during movement, giving information about the timing of muscle activity and its relative intensity. Either surface electrodes or Intramuscular fine wire electrodes are used. (From the 2001 Report of the Nomenclature Committee of the American Association of Electromyography and Electrodiagnosis.[19] Reproduced by kind permission of the AANEM.)

kinesiology The study of movement.

kinesiometer An instrument for measuring the range of motion of a joint.

kinesthesis (Gr, to move + perception) The sense of movement determined by conscious and unconscious awareness of the current state of extension (and thus the length) of the muscles, so in turn of the varying positions of a limb. The afferent impulses actually come from tendon organs and the older term *muscular sense* for the senses both of movement and of static position is not therefore appropriate.

This, the sixth or "muscular" sense or sense of movement, was known to Aristotle but was described precisely by Sir Charles **Bell** in 1826 and assigned by him to the posterior columns. Bastian introduced the term in its current usage.

kinetics The internal and external forces affecting the moving body.

kinetic cerebellar tremor See **cerebellar tremors**.

kinetic deviation See **past pointing**.

kinetic nystagmus See **optokinetic nystagmus**.

kinetic perimetry That (conventional) form of perimetry in which a test spot of given size and contrast is moved from the periphery into the center of the subject's visual field.[1840]

kinetic tremor Tremor occurring during a voluntary movement.[1615] When the amplitude of the tremulous movements is increased at the end of the movement of a limb toward a target, the terms *intention* or *terminal tremor* may be used. When a kinetic tremor occurs only during certain activities, such as writing, it is also known as **task-specific kinetic tremor**. See **tremor**.

kinetopsia The illusion of movement all objects in the visual environment, likely due to a lesion in the region of the temporo-parieto-occipital junction.[3640]

King–Denborough syndrome A congenital myopathy complicated by malignant hyperthermia occurring in children with short stature, generalized muscle weakness, dysmorphism with anti-Mongolian slant to the eyes, and multiple congenital skeletal abnormalities.[3438] See **malignant hyperthermia**.

kinking Acute-angle tortuosity of an artery, such as the carotid. The pathological significance of such a directional change is disputed, unless it is associated with stenosis.

kinky hair syndrome See **Menkes disease**.

kinky hair–photosensitivity–mental retardation See **Calderon syndrome**.

Kinsbourne–Warrington syndrome See **opsoclonic meningoencephalitis**.

kippdeviationen/kippnystagmus Horizontal conjugate large-amplitude oscillations of the eyes which are suppressed by visual fixation at a rate of 2.5 Hz.[1459] See also **square-wave pulses**.

Kisch, B. (b. 1890) German physiologist who, like **Kehrer**, described the **auriculopalpebral reflex**.

Kit test Upward movement of the umbilicus of the supine patient with a cord lesion at T 10, on saying the word "KIT" loudly. This is due to the retained activity of the upper but not of the lower fibers of the rectus abdominis muscle which contract during the expiration required to say the word.

See also **Beevor sign**, in which the same movement is produced (rather more reliably) by neck flexion.

Kitamura syndrome See **thyrotoxic periodic paralysis**.

Kjellin syndrome A recessive form of **hereditary spastic paraplegia** complicated by muscular atrophy, mental retardation, and pigmentary retinal degeneration.[3467]

klazomania Paroxysmal shouting. Although described as a chronic vocal tic disorder, it is also a distressing feature of severe dementia.

kleeblattschadel anomaly (cloverleaf skull) A combination of anomalies based on the presence of craniosynostosis, leading to a trilobar skull with associated hydrocephalus. Retraction of the upper lids and proptosis lead on to the **sunset sign**, and both strabismus and visual failure due to optic nerve compression are common.

Associated features include bony ankylosis of the limbs, hydrocephalus, EEG abnormalities, motor and mental retardation, cerebellar deformities, and polymicrogyria, while numerous other developmental defects have been reported less commonly.[2970]

Klein syndrome A dominantly inherited dysmorphic syndrome, characterized also by hypertelorism, blepharophimosis, partial albinism, deafness, syndactyly, and bone dysplasias.[3474] See **mandibulofacial dysostosis**.

Klein–Lisak syndrome See **Andersen syndrome**.

Kleine, Willi German neuropsychiatrist who published a series of five cases of periodic somnolence, two of which also showed morbid hunger, in 1925. He considered hypothalamic pathology as a possible basis for it. Four years later, Max Levin, an American neurologist, reported a further case and in 1936 he summarized the features of seven cases reported as a new syndrome of periodic somnolence and morbid hunger. See **Kleine-Levin syndrome**.

Kleine-Levin syndrome (hypersomnia-bulimia) A syndrome characterized by recurrent periods of excessively prolonged sleep in adolescent males, intermixed with periods of normal sleep architecture lasting for a few days or weeks, occurring every few months, and eventually ending with recovery. During the abnormal sleep phases, apathy, irritability, confusion, hyperphagia (compulsive eating), and sexual disinhibition may occur (see also Chart S–6).

A confusional state, hallucinosis, irritability, or a schizophreniform state may occur around the time of the attacks. Thalamic rather than hypothalamic disease was detected in the only case so far to come to postmortem examination. The syndrome was reported by Antimoff in 1898, more fully (in German) by Kleine in 1925,[3478] and in English by Levin 4 years later. The subject was reviewed by Critchley in 1962.[1332]

Variants of the syndrome include forms due to hypothalamic pathology, **menstruation-related hypersomnia**, and cyclical depression, and a form characterized by insomnia rather than by hypersomnia.[4904] See also **recurrent hypersomnia**.

http://med.stanford.edu/school/Psychiatry/narcolepsy/KLS.html is a relevant university-based informational resource.

Klemm tetanus See **Rose disease**.

Klippel, Maurice (1858–1942) French neurologist at the **Salpêtrière**. He described the following two conditions as well as a familial form of frontal cranial hypertrophy resembling that seen in craniocleidodysostosis.[3486]

Klippel–Feil anomaly (congenital cervical synostosis, congenital webbed neck, congenital brevicollis) Fusion of two or more cervical vertebrae, with or without occipitalization of the atlas, and basilar impression. Three types are described: 1. Complete fusion of the cervical vertebrae; 2. A decreased number of cervical vertebrae; and 3. Subtotal fusion of some cervical vertebrae. In all cases, the neck is short, the hairline low, and neck movements limited.

The major neurological complications are myelopathy and radiculopathy, resulting from the bony or associated neural malformations[5980] but synkineses, pyramidal signs, and a syringomyelic syndrome have also been described.[4507] Some patients have other skeletal abnormalities, including **dysraphism** with hydrocephalus, scapular winging, cleft palate, micrognathia, deafness, and spinal tumors.[2504, 3485]

A *variant* is **Wildervanck syndrome**.

Klippel–Trenaunay–Weber syndrome (Parkes–Weber syndrome, hemangiectatic hypertrophy) A congenital **neurocutaneous syndrome**, characterized by spinal vascular malformations with dermal hemangiomas of the trunk and limbs, telangiectasias, arteriovenous communications, varices and nevi at the same segmental levels, and asymmetrically hypertrophic limbs.[3487, 3923] Irregular dominant inheritance is suggested.

Macrocephaly, hypertrophy of other areas, subcutaneous calcification, syndactyly, malabsorption, seizures, glaucoma, and other ocular abnormalities are other features described. Weber's paper in 1907 referred to the account of the condition by Kallischer in 1899 but not to that of Klippel and Trenaunay, which had been published in 1900.

Manifestations of other neurocutaneous disorders such as **tuberous sclerosis** and **neurofibromatosis** have been described in association.[379]

Klippel–Weil sign When the contracted fingers of the patient are quickly extended by the examiner, flexion and adduction of the patient's thumb indicate the presence of pyramidal disease.[3484]

Kloepfer syndrome A recessively inherited syndrome with onset in infancy, characterized by amentia, cortical blindness, deafness, infantilism, and a photosensitive erythematous skin rash. Pathologically, there is subcortical demyelination and marked loss of cortical neurons. The biochemical basis for the condition is not known.[3489]

Klumpke, Augusta Déjèrine (1859–1927) Parisian neurologist, the wife of Dr. Jules Déjèrine. She was born in San Francisco and studied medicine in Paris, becoming the first woman Interne des Hopitaux in Paris (in the face of substantial opposition on the grounds of her gender, as might then have been expected).

Klumpke palsy (Déjèrine–Klumpke palsy) Lower brachial plexus injury, with consequent weakness and wasting of the C8–T1 musculature. When due to violent physical abduction/stretch injury, the sympathetic fibers may also be damaged with consequent **Horner syndrome**. The syndrome usually follows birth injury (traction of the after-coming arm with breech delivery), arrest of a fall by grabbing on to a projection, or motor vehicle accidents.

Klüver–Bucy syndrome A disconnection syndrome of the temporal lobes from midline structures. Clinically, this is characterized by hyperphagia, loss of the ability to make correct choices under visual control (visual agnosia, "psychic blindness"), restlessness, excessive oral exploratory behavior and appetite, overattentiveness to visual stimuli (hypermetamorphosis), sexual libertarianism, and loss of the ability to learn new skills. The syndrome was first described in monkeys following lesions of both hippocampi.[3491]

In humans, bilateral temporal lobe damage (usually in the context of head trauma, encephalitis, or dementia, or with dysfunction of one remaining temporal lobe) may lead to a blunted, affectless, apathetic state with inability to learn new data, occasional arousing to hypersexuality, bulimia, and a tendency to hypermetamorphosis.[3846]

Knapp streaks Angioid streaks on the retina, as seen in pseudoxanthoma elasticum. See **angioid streaks, Grondblad–Strandberg syndrome**. Dr. Herman Knapp (1832–1911) was an American ophthalmologist.

knapsack palsy Brachial plexopathy as a result of compression by the straps of a knapsack or a hod.[5295] See also **Rieder paralysis, cadet palsy, upper brachial plexus palsy**.

knee flexor reflex Contraction of the flexor muscles of the knee and of others in the leg in response to a tap behind the calcaneum, either as part of a generalized (increased) flexor response or as the result of vibrations set up by the tap.

knee jerk (patellar reflex, quadriceps reflex) Contraction of the quadriceps muscle when its tendon is percussed; like other muscle stretch reflexes, it is augmented in pyramidal tract disease above that level and reduced with damage to the reflex arc, in this case at L3–4.

The *contralateral quadriceps reflex* (tapping one patellar tendon leads to extension of the other knee as well) is part of a generalized mass movement (a crossed-extensor response) in patients with severe pyramidal disease.

knee-bending sign Slight flexion of one knee occurring while the subject is standing. The sign indicates root irritation at L5 or S1.[1306] See **Neri sign** No. 1.

Knobloch-Layer syndrome A recessively inherited congenital syndrome consisting of cataract, macular degeneration, detached retina, myopia, cardiac situs inversus, lung hypoplasia, pendular nystagmus, and occipital encephalocele.[1233]

knock-knees See **genu valgum**.

Kny disease See **paramyoclonus multiplex.**[3504]

Kocher, E.T. (1841–1917) Swiss surgeon who became professor of surgery at Berne and advanced the techniques of thyroidectomy (an operation commonly required in those days in the iodine-deficient, goitrous regions of Switzerland). He was awarded the Nobel Prize in 1909 for his contributions to the understanding of thyroid disease.[2066]

Kocher reflex Contraction of the abdominal wall when the patient's testicles are squeezed by the examiner. The utility of the reflex is hard to discern.

Kocher sign (globe lag) The delay in ascent of the eyeball relative to the upper eyelid on looking upwards in dysthyroid ophthalmopathy.

Kocher–Debré–Sémelaigne syndrome (muscular hypertrophy in cretins, infant Hercules syndrome, hypothyroid myopathy) The association of general enlargement of muscles with slow muscle contraction and relaxation and **myoedema** in patients with cretinism or adult hypothyroidism.[1527] Painful muscle spasms are not a feature but aching pain, stiffness, and slow muscle contractions, with "hung-up" reflexes and a stiff gait, dysarthria, and paramyotonia are other features.[3509] The only differences between this and **hypothyroid myopathy** (Hoffmann syndrome) appear to be the absence of pseudomyotonia and the amount of pain felt, as both states may occur in the same patient at different times.

The condition was described first by Kocher in 1882.[3509] The contribution of Debré and Sémelaigne was to demonstrate the response of the symptoms to treatment with thyroid extract, in 1935. The underlying mechanism is uncertain, but possibly an increased intracellular potassium concentration makes the end-plate less sensitive to acetylcholine and the cell less excitable; or it may reflect the failure of myosin heavy-chain switching from the neonatal to the adult IIb form of myosin as a result of the absence of thyroxine.

Koenen tumor Periungual or subungual fibromas occurring after puberty and diagnostic of tuberous sclerosis.[2460]

Koerber–Salus–Elschnig syndrome Retraction nystagmus and failure of up-gaze, described in patients with a pineal tumor or a cysticercus cyst in the region of the Sylvian aqueduct. The best of the original descriptions was that of Salus,[5517] a pupil of Fleshnig. See **dorsal midbrain syndrome.**

Kofferath syndrome A combination of **Duchenne–Erb palsy** (upper brachial plexus palsy) and phrenic nerve paresis following birth injury.[6983]

Koh blocks A set of cubes bearing designs in four colors which the subject is asked to arrange to match a printed pattern. The test was used to assess posterior right parietal function but because of its complexity has now been superseded by the block design test on the **Wechsler Adult Intelligence Scale.**

Kohler syndrome A congenital dysmorphic syndrome manifesting also cataract; congenital heart disease; pulmonary, renal, genital, and endocrine abnormalities; and cerebellar atrophy.[381]

Kohlmeier–Degos disease See **malignant atrophic papulosis.**

Kohlschutter syndrome A congenital X-linked or autosomal recessive inherited dysmorphic syndrome, manifesting also hypohidrosis, myopia, abnormality of the dental enamel, intractable seizures, pyramidal signs, and mental and developmental delay.[3514]

Kojewnikow, A. See **Kozhevnikoff.**

koniocortex (Gr, dust + Lat, bark) The primary receptive areas of the cortex; the granular primary sensory cortex. It includes the primary visual cortex, the primary auditory cortex on Heschl's gyrus, the primary somatosensory cortex on the post central gyrus, and the primary motor cortex on the precentral gyrus.

Konzo An abrupt-onset, nonprogressive, epidemic upper motor neuron disease (tropical myelopathy) presenting as spastic paraparesis. It occurs in children and young adults in central African countries such as Zaïre. The cause is considered to be cyanide intoxication due to excessive consumption of improperly processed cassava.[3014]

Kopf tetanus Cephalic tetanus, the wound often being cranial and the onset occurring with trismus.

Kornzweig, Abraham Leon (b. 1900) American ophthalmologist who practiced at the Mt. Sinai hospital in New York. See **abetalipoproteinemia.**

Koro (Indonesian; shrinking tortoise) An acute anxiety reaction occurring in oriental males who fear that their penis is receding into the abdomen and insist that it be grasped firmly, by themselves or others.[2066] One cause of such a fear, in some cultures, is the belief that ghosts (who of course lack penises) disguise themselves in order to steal those of the living.

Korsakoff, Sergei Sergeyovich (1854–1900) Russian neuropsychiatrist who studied at the University of Moscow, receiving his MD degree with a thesis on alcoholic paralysis in 1887. He later took charge of the university psychiatric clinic. His contributions, apart from the syndrome of which he summarized the findings and which he described as an entity between 1887 and 1889, included a classification of mental diseases and works on paranoia and memory disturbances. He also wrote a major textbook of psychiatric disease.

It is of interest that while Korsakoff noted that the syndrome often follows an episode of **delirium tremens**, he also reported 16 cases of nonalcoholic origin.

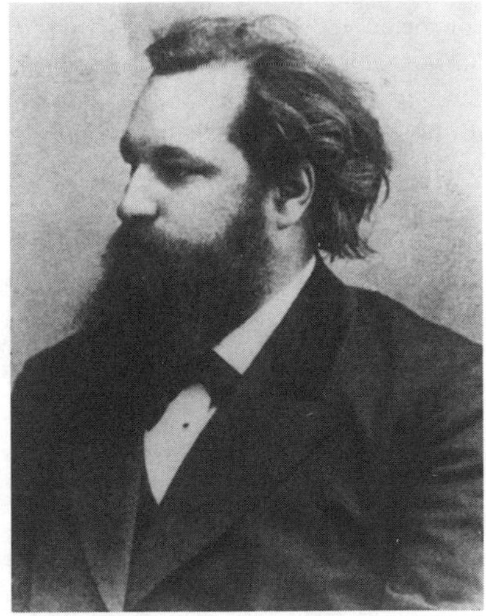

Figure K–2 Sergei Sergeyovich Korsakoff.

Korsakoff psychosis See **Wernicke–Korsakoff encephalopathy**.

Korsakoff syndrome (Korsakoff psychosis) See **Wernicke–Korsakoff encephalopathy**.

Kousseff syndrome A recessively inherited congenital dysmorphic syndrome characterized also by short stature, facial hemangiomas, webbed neck, sacral meningomyelocele, arthropathy, congenital cardiac disease, and distal weakness.[3545]

Kozhevnikoff, Aleksei Yakovlyevich (Kojewnikow, A.Y.) (1836–1902) Russian neuropsychiatrist who graduated from Moscow and studied further in Paris, London, and Germany before returning to Moscow. He was eventually elected professor of nervous and mental disease there. He described the form of epilepsy described in the next entry,[3548] as well as **lathyrism**, the microanatomy of the cerebral and cerebellar cortices, the neuropathology of myasthenia and bulbar paralyses, **amyotrophic lateral sclerosis**, and familial spastic diplegia (reported when studying with **Charcot** in Paris). He was the author of a successful textbook of neurology. In Moscow, **Korsakoff** was at one time his pupil and later his assistant.

Kozhevnikoff syndrome 1. (partial continuous epilepsy, Kozhevnikoff–Rasmussen syndrome) A rare form of Rolandic partial epilepsy of unknown etiology occurring in both adults and children but related to some lesion of the motor cortex. Its principal features are the initial appearance of simple focal motor or somatosensory seizures or **epilepsia partialis continua**, complex focal seizures without automatisms, or GTCS. Postictal and later permanent hemiparesis is a residuum. As the condition progresses, the seizures become longer, more frequent and more generalized, and hemihypesthesia, hemianopia, and intellectual/language impairment develop over years until the process starts to burn out. The MRI shows progressive Hemiatrophy that usually starts in the temporoinsular region and focal or multifocal spikes and slow waves are recorded on the EEG. See also **Rasmussen encephalitis** and Dreifuss FE, et al. Commission for classification and terminology, ILAE. Proposal for revised classifications of epilepsies and epileptic syndromes. *Epilepsia* 1989;30:389–99.

The condition may also result from **mitochondrial encephalopathy** (MELAS).
2. Atrophy of the neck and shoulder muscles and later of the muscles of mastication, attributed by Osler to a lesion in the region of the mesencephalon (Osler, 1928 quoted by Durham[1765]).

Kozlowski syndrome A recessively inherited dysmorphic syndrome, characterized by generalized skin atrophy with excessive wrinkling, short stature, dislocation of the hips, microcephaly, seizures, and mental and developmental delay.[3549]

Krabbe, Knud Haraldsen (1885–1961) Danish neurologist who trained at Copenhagen and studied in London and with **Marie** in Paris, where he developed an interest in the pineal gland. He became head of the neurology department in Copenhagen. His full account of the following condition was published in 1916; other major contributions were his complete description of **Sturge–Weber syndrome** in 1934 and his description of **congenital universal muscular hypoplasia** in 1947. The journal **Acta Neurologica et Psychiatrica Scandinavica** was founded in 1926, largely at his instigation.

His colleague Viggo Christensen was professor of neurology at Copenhagen.

Krabbe leukodystrophy (globoid cell leukodystrophy, Christensen–Krabbe syndrome, galactosylceramide lipidosis; OMIM 245200) A recessively inherited lysosomal degenerative disorder of myelin (leukodystrophy) occurring in infancy or later childhood with a fatal course, characterized by a deficiency of galactosylceramide β-galactosidase, the deposition of galactocerebroside, and the presence of **globoid cells**. The responsible gene for galactosylceramidase maps to chromosome 14q31.

Clinically, *early and late infantile* and *juvenile* forms are distinguished. The former accounts for 90% of cases and is characterized by fevers, psychomotor regression, irritability, optic atrophy, tonic seizures, opisthotonos, deafness, cortical blindness, basal ganglion and pyramidal signs, demyelinating sensorimotor peripheral neuropathy, and a raised CSF protein level with onset after 4 months of age. The disease progresses to decerebration and death within 2 years.

The *late infantile* type is characterized by optic atrophy, dysarthria, dementia, hypotonia, cerebellar signs, spasticity, myoclonus, and motor neuropathy with onset after 6 months of age.[3550]

Juvenile and *adult* forms are described with dementia, cortical blindness, optic atrophy, and pyramidal signs that resemble hereditary spastic paraplegia,[342] and often peripheral neuropathy is also recognized .[1348]

The diagnosis is made by finding the characteristic multi-nucleated globoid cells with severe astrocytic gliosis in an almost totally demyelinated brain and in nerve biopsy specimens.[3550]

Other *variants* are *Hagberg disease* (prolonged floppy infant syndrome), which is characterized by the late onset of the usual clinical features,[379] and a form with added *congenital fiber type disproportion*.[1535]

See also **National Tay–Sachs and Allied Diseases Association**.

Krabbe syndrome See **Sturge–Weber syndrome**.

Krabbe universal muscular hypoplasia A wasting disease of infancy, probably a form of **hereditary motor neuropathy**.

Kraepelin dementia A dementing syndrome with onset in early adult life, manifesting behavioral disturbances, extrapyramidal rigidity, and cerebral atrophy with gliosis and spongy changes.

Kraepelin, Ernst (1856–1926) German psychiatrist, professor at Dorpat, Heidelberg, and later Munich. His major contributions were in the classification of mental symptoms and diseases, the descriptions of schizophrenia, and the provision of an academic milieu wherein assistants such as **Nissl**, Jakob, **Barany**, and Spatz flourished.

Krane–Siroky classification A system for classifying disorders of micturition based on urodynamic data.[3556]

Detrusor Hyperreflexia

Coordinated sphincters
Striated sphincter dyssynergia
Smooth sphincter dyssynergia
Nonrelaxing smooth sphincter

Detrusor Areflexia

Coordinated sphincters
Nonrelaxing striated sphincter
Denervated striated sphincter
Nonrelaxing smooth sphincter

See also **Bors–Komarr classification, International Continence Society classification**.

Kratschmer reflex Inhibition of breathing when a baby encounters a bad smell. The reflex appears not to persist, however.

Krause, Wilhelm Johann Friedrich (1833–1910) German, professor of anatomy at Göttingen and later at Berlin.

Krause corpuscles Rounded end-bulbs on sensory nerves in such sensitive areas as the lips and glans penis.

Krause syndrome (retinal dysplasia, congenital encephalo-ophthalmic dysplasia, encephalo-ophthalmic syndrome) The combination of retinal and cerebral dysplasia with microphthalmos, malformations of the retina, choroid and optic nerve, persistent remains of the hyaloid artery, and microcephaly. Affected children, who are usually born prematurely, show failure of mental development and hydrocephalus and are blind. Oxycephaly and encephalocele may also be found.[3560]

The condition was described by Dr. A.C. Krause, an American ophthalmologist, in 1946. Trisomy 13–15 may be responsible for the syndrome.

Kraus–Ruppert syndrome A congenital dysmorphic syndrome, characterized by hypogonadotrophic hypogonadism, small testes, microcephaly, syndactyly, and mental and developmental delay.[381]

Kretschmer, Ernst (1888–1964) German neuropsychiatrist.

Kretschmer syndrome See **apallic syndrome**.

Krishaber, Maurice (1836–1883) Hungarian-French physician who studied medicine at Vienna, Prague, and Paris, graduating from the last in 1864. He settled and practiced in Paris. His original publication on depersonalization recorded 38 cases, representing a huge range of mental and neurological symptoms, but linked by the common thread of, at some time, loss of the sense of personal identity. Krishaber considered this to be a neurological condition due to focal pathology, but this view is not now held.[5810]

Krishaber disease See **depersonalization**.

Kristiansen syndrome Progressive dissociated anesthesia, hyperpathia, spontaneous pain, hemiballismus, diplopia, seizures, and behavioral changes leading on to bulbar palsies, as a result of an intrinsic thalamic/brainstem lesion.[5333]

Kubisagari See **vertige paralysant, Gerlier disease**.

Kufor–Rakeb syndrome (autosomal recessive, levodopa-responsive Parkinsonism with pyramidal degeneration, supranuclear gaze palsy, and dementia) A pallido-pyramidal disorder first described in Brazil. It is characterized by subacute juvenile-onset, partially levodopa-responsive Parkinsonism, pyramidal signs, dementia supranuclear palsy of vertical gaze, visual hallucinations; levadopa-provoked motor fluctuations, and widespread cerebral atrophy on neuroimaging. Late features are facial-faucial-finger mini-myoclonus, visual hallucinations, and oculogyric dystonic spasms.[6796] The condition is mapped to 1p36 (*ATP13A2*)[4579] but was formerly assigned the label *PARK9*.

Kufs, Hugo Frederich (1871–1955) German neuropathologist, who practiced in Leipzig.

Kufs disease (late or adult amaurotic familial idiocy, adult ganglioside lipidosis) The dominantly inherited adult form of **neuronal ceroid lipofuscinosis**, in which there is deposition in neurons and other cells of an abnormal lipoprotein with characteristic ultrastructural patterns.

Clinically, it presents with photosensitive progressive myoclonic epilepsy or with progressive mental deterioration, seizures, and facial dyskinesias, but without pigmentary retinal degeneration.[567, 3586]

Kugelberg–Welander disease See **hereditary motor neuropathy type 3**.

Kulenkampff–Tarnow syndrome (cervicolinguomasticatory syndrome) A drug-induced dyskinetic syndrome. See **tardive dyskinesia, cervicolinguomasticatory syndrome**.[3592]

Kurtzke, John F. Contemporary American neurologist.

Kurtzke scales (Expanded Disability Status Scale, EDSS; Disability Status Scale, incapacity status scale) Clinical rating scales for evaluating the disabilities of patients with multiple sclerosis. The Expanded Disability Status Scale[3612] extends the older (1955) scale, which had been widely adopted in clinical and research settings. The EDSS is now half of a bifid rating system, assessing overall disability, while the remainder (the functional scale) represents "a series of grades in each of eight functional groupings . . . In each portion there is a numerical rating which is mutually exclusive in its category, and the higher the number, the greater is the dysfunction. Only objectively verifiable defects due to multiple sclerosis as elicited upon neurological examination are included. Symptoms are discarded." The scale is given in Chart K–1 and the EDSS in Chart K–2.

Kuru (laughing death syndrome) See **Lytico–Bodig.** The term is derived from the local word meaning "to shiver." See also **Creutzfeldt–Jakob Foundation Inc.**, a charitable organization in this field providing information and support. Address: P.O. Box 611625, Miami, FL 33261-1625. Tel: 954-704-0519. E-mail: crjakob@aol.com. Web site: http://cjdfoundation.org/.

Kushtha See **leprosy**.

Kuskokwim syndrome A recessively inherited congenital syndrome characterized by multiple joint contractures, mainly affecting the knees and ankles, hypoplasia of the lumbar vertebrae with spondylolisthesis, and atrophy (less often hypertrophy) of local muscles.[4998]

Kussmaul, Adolf (1822–1902) Peripatetic German physician, sometime professor or professor emeritus of medicine at Heidelberg. He made advances in a number of areas of medicine, including the invention of the stomach pump, and he was the first to describe the following; polyarteritis nodosa

Chart K–1. The Kurtzke Scale

A. Functional Systems

Pyramidal functions

0. Normal
1. Abnormal signs without disability
2. Minimal disability
3. Mild or moderate paraparesis or hemiparesis; severe monoparesis
4. Marked paraparesis or hemiparesis, moderate quadriparesis, or monoplegia
5. Paraplegia, hemiplegia, or marked quadriparesis
6. Quadriplegia

V. Unknown

Cerebellar functions

0. Normal
1. Abnormal signs without disability
2. Mild ataxia
3. Moderate truncal or limb ataxia
4. Severe ataxia, all limbs
5. Unable to perform coordinated movements due to ataxia

V. Unknown

X. Is used throughout after each number when weakness (grade 3 or more on pyramidal) interferes with testing

Brainstem functions

0. Normal
1. Signs only
2. Moderate nystagmus or other mild disability
3. Severe nystagmus, marked extraocular weakness, or moderate disability of other cranial nerves
4. Marked dysarthria or other marked disability
5. Inability to swallow or speak
6. Unknown

Sensory functions (revised 1982)

0. Normal
1. Vibration or figure-writing decrease only, in one or two limbs
2. Mild decrease in touch or pain or position sense, and/or moderate decrease in vibration in one or two limbs; or vibratory (with or without figure writing) decrease alone in three or four limbs
3. Moderate decrease in touch or pain or position sense, and/or essentially lost vibration in one or two limbs; or mild decrease in touch or pain and/or moderate decrease in all proprioceptive tests in three or four limbs
4. Marked decrease in touch or pain or loss of proprioception, alone or combined, in one or two limbs; or moderate decrease in touch or pain and/or severe proprioceptive decrease in more than two limbs
5. Loss (essentially) of sensation in one or two limbs; or moderate decrease in touch or pain and/or loss of proprioception for most of the body below the head
6. Sensation essentially lost below the head

V. Unknown

Bowel and bladder functions (revised 1982)

0. Normal
1. Mild urinary hesitancy, urgency, or retention
2. Moderate hesitancy, urgency, retention of bowel or bladder, or rare urinary incontinence
3. Frequent urinary incontinence
4. In need of almost constant catheterization
5. Loss of bladder function
6. Loss of bowel and bladder function

V. Unknown

Visual (or optic) functions

0. Normal
1. Scotoma with visual acuity (corrected) better than 20/30
2. Worse eye with scotoma with maximal visual acuity (corrected) of 20/30 to 20/59
3. Worse eye with large scotoma, or moderate decrease in fields, but with maximal visual acuity (corrected) of 20/60 to 20/99
4. Worse eye with marked decrease of fields and maximal visual acuity (corrected) of 20/100 to 20/200; grade 3 plus maximal acuity of better eye of 20/60 or less

5. Worse eye with maximal visual acuity (corrected) less than 20/200; grade 4 plus maximal acuity of better eye of 20/60 or less
6. Grade 5 plus maximal visual acuity of better eye of 20/60 or less
V. Unknown
X. Is added to grades 0 to 6 for presence of temporal pallor

Cerebral (or mental) functions

0. Normal
1. Mood alteration only (does not affect disability status scale score)
2. Mild decrease in mentation
3. Moderate decrease in mentation
4. Marked decrease in mentation (chronic brain syndrome—moderate)
5. Dementia or chronic brain syndrome—severe or incompetent
V. Unknown

Other functions

0. None
1. Any other neurological findings attributed to multiple sclerosis (specify)
V. Unknown

From Kurtzke JF. Rating neurological impairment in multiple sclerosis: an expanded disability scale (EDSS). Neurology 1983;33:1444–52. *Reproduced by kind permission of the American Academy of Neurology and Lippincott Williams and Wilkins.*

Chart K–2. Expanded Disability Status Scale (EDSS)

0. Normal neurological examination (all grade 0 in FS; cerebral grade 1 acceptable)
1.0. No disability, minimal signs in one FS (i.e., grade 1 excluding cerebral grade 1)
1.5. No disability, minimal signs in more than one FS; disability, minimal signs in more than one FS (more than one grade 1 excluding cerebral grade 1)
2.0. Minimal disability in one FS (one FS grade 2, others 0 or 1)
2.5. Minimal disability in two FS (two FS grade 2, other 0 or 1)
3.0. Moderate disability in one FS (one FS grade 3, others 0 or 1), or mild disability in three or four FS (three/four FS grade 2, others 0 or 1), though fully ambulatory
3.5. Fully ambulatory but with moderate disability in one FS (one grade 3) and one or two FS grade 2; or two FS grade 3; or five FS grade 2 (others 0 or 1)
4.0. Fully ambulatory without aid, self-sufficient, up and about some 12 h a day despite relatively severe disability consisting of one FS grade 4 (others 0 or 1), or combinations of lesser grades exceeding limits of previous steps. Able to walk without aid or rest some 500 m.
4.5. Fully ambulatory without aid, up and about much of the day, able to work a full day, may otherwise have some limitation of full activity, or require minimal assistance; characterized by relatively severe disability, usually consisting of one FS grade 4 (others 0 or 1) or combinations of lesser grades exceeding limits of previous steps. Able to walk without aid or rest for some 300 m.
5.0. Ambulatory without aid or rest for about 200 m; disability severe enough to impair full daily activities (e.g., to work full day without special provisions). (Usual FS equivalents are one grade 5 alone, others 0 or 1; or combinations of lesser grades usually exceeding specifications for step 4.0.)
5.5. Ambulatory without aid or rest for about 100 m; disability severe enough to preclude full daily activities. (Usual FS equivalents are one grade 5 alone, others 0 or 1; or combinations of lesser grades usually exceeding those for step 4.0.)
6.0. Intermittent or unilateral constant assistance (cane, crutch, or brace required to walk about 100 m with or without resting.) (Usual FS equivalents are combinations with more than two FS grade 3+.)
6.5. Constant bilateral assistance (canes, crutches, or braces) required to walk about 20 m without resting. (Usual FS equivalents are combinations with more than two FS grade 3+.)
7.0. Unable to walk beyond about 5 m even with aid, essentially restricted to wheelchair; wheels self in standard wheelchair and transfers alone; up and about in wheelchair some 12 h a day. (Usual FS equivalents are combinations with more than one FS grade 4+; very rarely, pyramidal grade 5 alone.)
7.5. Unable to take more than a few steps; restricted to wheelchair; may need aid in transfer; wheels self but cannot carry on in standard wheelchair a full day; may require motorized wheelchair. (Usual FS equivalents are combinations with more than one FS grade 4+.)
8.0. Essentially restricted to bed or chair or perambulated in wheelchair, but may be out of bed itself much of the day; retains many self-care functions; generally has effective use of arms. (Usual FS equivalents are combinations, generally grade 4+ in several systems.)
8.5. Essentially restricted to bed much of the day; has some effective use of arm(s); retains some self-care functions. (Usual FS equivalents are combinations, generally 4+ in several systems.)
9.0. Helpless bed patient; can communicate and eat. (Usual FS equivalents are combinations, mostly grade 4+.)
9.5. Totally helpless bed patient; unable to communicate effectively or eat/swallow. (Usual FS equivalents are combinations, almost all grade 4+.)
10.0. Death due to MS.

FS, functional systems. From Kurtzke JF. Rating neurological impairment in multiple sclerosis: An expanded disability scale (EDSS). Neurology 1983;33:1444–52. *Reproduced by kind permission of the American Academy of Neurology and Lippincott Williams and Wilkins.*

(1866); progressive bulbar paralysis (1873); diabetic coma with the respiratory pattern now bearing his name (1874); and pulsus paradoxus, thoracentesis, gastroscopy, and mesenteric thrombosis. He was the first to use the term *poliomyelitis* and, for aphasia, "word-blindness."

Kussmaul aphasia (aphrasia paranoica) Voluntary mutism, simulating aphasia, in cases of paranoia; a clinical syndrome of stupor followed by overtalkativeness, described by Kussmaul in 1877. ("The insane often remain for months and years in absolute silence; they would be taken for aphasics if they did not begin to speak unexpectedly at a given moment.")[3616]

Kussmaul respirations Deep and rapid breathing in acidotic states, such as diabetic ketosis or uremia.

kwashiorkor (M'Bwaki, red boy, plurideficiency or malignant malnutrition syndrome) Depigmentation of hair and skin, edema, growth failure, lassitude, apathy, photophobia, and fatty infiltration of the liver with hypoalbuminuria as a result of starvation in children, who develop the signs after weaning in countries afflicted by family, regional, or national famine.[6403]

Kwok quease Poisoning by monosodium glutamate. See **Chinese restaurant syndrome**.

kyphosis (from Gr, bent) Flexion curvature of the spine, either *regular* over a large number of segments, or *angular*, affecting one or two levels only.

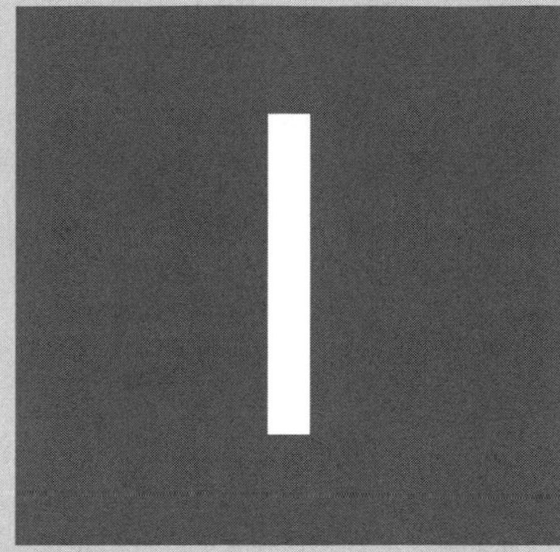

L-nystagmus A form of nystagmus that occurs during prolonged linear (or translational, not rotational) movements of the head. The receptors for such movements are the otolithic organs.[5887] See also **vestibular nystagmus**.

L-2-hydroxyglutaric acidemia A rare recessively inherited chronic leukodystrophic syndrome characterized by microcephaly, mental retardation, pyramidal and extrapyramidal signs, ataxia, organic acidemia and hyperlysinemia, subcortical leukoencephalopathy, and cerebellar atrophy.[428] Nerve biopsy shows a reduction in the size of myelinated axons.

la belle indifférence The lack of emotional expression in the presence of an overt bodily disorder, shown by patients with hysterical conversion syndromes (when it is regarded as culpable) and by Stoics (when it is regarded as laudable). Physicians who can tell the difference are called *psychiatrists*; those who cannot, *cynics*.

Brave, ignorant, agnosic, Parkinsonian, and depressed patients may also decline to wear their emotions on the sleeves of their hospital gowns, but the tempting phrase will nevertheless often lead to their inclusion with the hysterics until an experienced physician examines them.

la crampe des écrivains See **writer's cramp**.

la main étrangère See **alien hand (limb) syndromes**.

la rage See **rabies**.

Labbé, Charles (1852–1889) French anatomist at the medical faculty in Paris.

Labbé's vein The posterior anastomotic vein, crossing the temporal lobe about 5 cm behind its tip.

labials (Lat, pertaining to the lips) Those consonants such as "B," "M," and "P" requiring use of the lips for articulation. See also **articulated labials, modified labials**, and **dentolabials**.

laboratory-supported multiple sclerosis Diagnostic categories of **multiple sclerosis** in which two previous attacks occurred, separated both in time and in the location of the lesions; one clinical or one paraclinical feature is present; and the results of CSF oligoclonal banding are positive (*laboratory-supported definite*). Other categories are also defined.

In the *laboratory-supported probable* category, there have been two prior attacks and the results of CSF oligoclonal banding are positive.[5094] See also **Poser criteria**.

labyrinth (from Gr, a place with many turnings) The internal ear, composed of the cochlea, vestibule, and the semicircular canals, both osseous and membranous.

labyrinthine apoplexy Acute vertigo and vomiting with succeeding permanent vestibuloparesis, probably resulting from occlusion of a branch of the artery of the internal auditory meatus.

labyrinthine fistula Leakage of perilymph from the inner ear into the middle ear, disruption of the bone of the labyrinth caused by cholesteatoma or other manifestations of chronic otitis media, and **superior semicircular canal dehiscence syndrome**. It is caused by abnormal communications between the inner ear and its surrounding structures, sometimes as a result of barotraumas; and causes sudden sensorineural hearing loss.

labyrinthine nystagmus See **vestibular nystagmus**.

labyrinthine reflex The sign is most easily elicited in infancy; the child is held up by, and facing, the examiner, who then rotates about his own axis several turns to the right and then to the left. The baby will look ahead in the direction of the rotation and, after stopping, will look back in the opposite direction.[6898] See also **vestibulo-oculogyric reflex**.

labyrinthine righting reflex See **righting reflexes**.

labyrinthine Romberg sign When the subject with unilateral labyrinthine disease stands with his feet together and eyes closed, he feels a sensation of being drawn to one side and there is slow lateral flexion of his neck to that side.

labyrinthitis See **acute peripheral vestibulopathy**.

La Crosse encephalitis A mosquito-borne arboviral cause of potentially severe encephalitis or aseptic meningitis, characterized often by hyponatremia, seizures, focal neurological signs, and increased intracranial pressure.[4235] See also the CDC Fact sheet on La Crosse encephalitis at http://www.cdc.gov/ncidod/dvbid/arbor/lacfact.htm

Fact Sheet: La Crosse Encephalitis

Lacheretz–Allain syndrome A congenital dysmorphic syndrome characterized by female pseudohermaphroditism, nephropathy, multiple synostoses, acrocephaly, and craniosynostosis.[3632]

lacrimal (Lat, a tear) Pertaining to lacrimation; weeping.

lactate dehydrogenase deficiency A rare recessively inherited metabolic myopathy in which this muscle isoenzyme is missing, thus causing incomplete block of glycolysis. The responsible gene maps to chromosome 11p15. Clinically, the condition is marked by fatigue, exercise intolerance, muscle cramps, and myoglobinuria following heavy exercise, without detrimental storage of excess glycogen.[1649, 3288]

lactate stress testing Estimation of serum lactate levels following exercise rather than at rest, and used in the diagnosis of mitochondrial diseases. Abnormally increased levels reflect impairment of function of respiratory chain enzymes in muscle so that anaerobic replaces aerobic metabolism and shifts the pyruvate/lactate equation toward lactate. The addition of exercise enhances the diagnostic yield of the test.[2056]

lactic acidemia A metabolic acidosis due to a failure in pyruvate catabolism, in which lactate levels exceed 2.2 mmol/l. The causes include many inborn errors of metabolism, mitochondrial disorders, systemic diseases, and intoxications. An idiopathic congenital form also exists.[3106] See also **pyruvate dehydrogenase deficiency, pyruvate carboxylase deficiency, Leigh disease, mitochondrial diseases**, and **carnitine deficiency**.

lactosylceramidosis A rare neurovisceral glycolipid storage polioencephalopathy characterized by intracellular accumulation of lactosylceramide and clinically by the appearance in infancy of cerebellar and pyramidal signs and optic atrophy with a progressive course to death in the vegetative state.[1488]

lacunar dementia A form of dementia associated with multiple small infarcts in the subcortical brain regions as a result of occlusive hyalinosis of the small penetrating vessels.[90] See also **Binswanger disease**.

lacunar infarcts Infarcts in the deep white matter of the brain, presumed to be due to occlusion of single perforating arteries supplying the internal capsule, striatum, thalamus, pons, or cerebellum. The classic syndromes are pure motor hemiparesis, sensorimotor stroke, pure sensory stroke, dysarthria–clumsy hand syndrome, and ataxic hemiparesis. See also **striatocapsular infarcts, thalamic infarcts, white matter medullary infarcts**, and **extended large subcortical infarcts**.

lacunar skull (lükenschädel) The "soap-bubble" radiological appearance of the inner table of the skull seen in some newborn infants with spina bifida and other developmental anomalies. Although this resembles copper-beating, it is not associated with increased intracranial pressure and it tends to go away within the first 6 months of life.

lacunar state The presence of multiple small cavitating infarcts in the white matter, due to multiple **lacunes**. The term was introduced by Déchambre in 1838 and amplified by Durand-Fardel 4 years later, but the clinical correlations were made with greatest effect by Pierre **Marie** in 1901 and by Dr. C. Miller **Fisher** between 1953 and 1982.

lacunar syndromes Constellations of more or less constant clinical signs considered to arise from the presence of **lacunes** in certain areas of the cerebral white matter.[3892] The syndromes defined at present are listed in Chart L–1.[2092]

Hachinski[2662] has suggested diagnostic criteria (see Chart L–2).

Lacunar transient ischemic attacks are also described, in which isolated motor or sensory symptoms involve at least two of the three areas, namely, face, arm, and leg.[3670]

lacune (from Lat, a pond; or Fr, a small lake) The term used by Pierre **Marie** in 1901 and reintroduced by Miller Fisher in 1965 to describe small (less than 1 cm) deep cystic cavities in the white matter of the cerebrum, brain stem, and cerebellum, representing healed infarcts resulting from occlusion of deep penetrating cerebral arterioles.[2076] For larger lesions he suggested the term *giant lacune*; others prefer *lagoon*.

Three forms have been described: type 1—small areas of cerebral infarction; type 2—cystic scars, which are the residue of small hemorrhages; and type 3—areas of perivascular dilatation not associated with infarction.[4174]

Lacunes are associated with a prior history of hypertension, with atherosclerosis of the cerebral vessels, and with cerebral hemorrhages. When numerous, they produce the **état criblé** (from Lat, a sieve). Over 20 clinical syndromes have been identified as resulting from lacunes in various sites (see **lacunar syndromes** above), but most are probably asymptomatic.[2092] In some cases, the clinical diagnosis is plain, but in most cases, the differentiation from other stroke pathologies is impossible.

The underlying lesion is said to be ischemic infarction resulting from lipohyalinosis, or occlusion of the mouth of the branching vessel, but the sites of the

Chart L–1. Lacunar Syndromes

1. **Pure sensory stroke.**
2. **Pure motor hemiparesis.**
3. **Ataxic hemiparesis** (homolateral ataxia and crural paresis, however, is an example of crossed cerebral–cerebellar **diaschisis**).
4. **Dysarthria–clumsy hand syndrome.**
5. *Modified pure motor hemiparesis with aphasia*, characterized by pyramidal signs mainly in the face and hand, with initial dysarthria and due to a lesion of the genu and anterior limb of the internal capsule.
6. *Pure motor hemiparesis sparing the face*, in which unilateral pyramidal signs in the limbs with initial nystagmus and vertigo are due to an infarct of the medullary pyramid.
7. *Mesoencephalothalamic syndrome* characterized by III cranial nerve palsy, impairment of upward gaze and abulia, and due to bilateral paramedian infarcts of the subthalamic and thalamic region or of the midbrain. See also **top o' the basilar syndrome.**
8. **Thalamic dementia.**
9. *Pure motor hemiparesis with horizontal gaze palsy* in which a transient **one-and-a-half syndrome** is associated with hemiparesis; this is due to a paramedian pontine infarct.[2092]
10. *Pure motor hemiparesis with crossed III nerve palsy* (**Weber syndrome**).
11. *Pure motor hemiparesis with crossed VI nerve palsy* in which these findings are due to a low paramedian pontine infarct.[2092]
12. *Pure motor hemiparesis with confusion*, a rare syndrome due to a small deep infarct interrupting the thalamofrontal connections, in which the hemiparesis is associated with acute confusion and a memory deficit.
13. Cerebellar ataxia with crossed III nerve palsy (**Claude syndrome**).
14. **Sensorimotor stroke** (thalamocapsular).
15. **Hemiballism** or hemichorea.
16. **Lower basilar branch syndrome.**
17. **Lateral medullary syndrome.**
18. **Lateral pontomedullary syndrome.**
19. *Acute loss of memory* due to an infarct of the corpus callosum.
20. **Locked-in syndrome.**
21. Miscellaneous:

    Weakness of one leg with ease of falling.
    Pure dysarthria; a presumed **lacunar syndrome** characterized by the sudden onset of dysarthria without any angiographic or CT abnormality.
    Acute dystonia of thalamic origin, a presumed **lacunar syndrome.**
    Other lacunar syndromes identified[4811] include III nerve palsy, nuclear and prenuclear syndromes of the III nerve, vertical gaze palsy, **internuclear ophthalmoplegia, one-and-a-half syndrome**, focal **dystonia** of the arm, and unilateral **asterixis.**

Adapted from Fisher CM. Lacunar strokes and infarcts; a review. Neurology 1982;**32**:871–6.

Chart L–2. Diagnostic Criteria for Lacunar Syndromes

Component	*Diagnostic Criteria*	*Exclusions*
Etiology	Hypertension (present on past history or prescribed for)	Seizures, severe unusual headache, vomiting, loss of consciousness
Deficit	Pure motor hemiplegia in face, arms, or leg	Abnormal higher functions (aphasia, neglect apraxia, agnosia)
	Pure sensory stroke in face, arms, or leg	Hemianopia
	Motor sensory stroke in face, arms, or leg	
	Ataxic hemiparesis	
	Dysarthria–clumsy hand syndrome	
CT	Compatible with a small deep infarct or normal (or normal isotope brain scan)	Superficial CT lesion Deep lesion greater than >1cm Focal abnormality
EEG	Normal or symmetrically abnormal	
Angiography	No tight stenosis of the internal carotid, middle, cerebral, vertebral, or basilar arteries	

(Based upon Hachinski VC. Classification of stroke for clinical trials. *Stroke* 1990;21:**Suppl II.** 27–9.)

lacunes (exactly the same as the sites of primary intracerebral hemorrhage), the presence of hematin-laden macrophages around them, the absence of pathological reports of recent acute lacunes, and the occasional CT image of small deep hemorrhages in the appropriate areas suggest that to incriminate ischemic infarction in every case is not warranted.

The wholesale ascription of clinical presentations to the collection of lacunar states has been criticized.[3665]

As criteria for *possible lacunar stroke* it has been suggested[4381] that all of the following must be met:

1. Clinical presentation of lacunar syndrome, which includes pure motor hemiparesis, pure sensory stroke, ataxic

hemiparesis, or the dysarthria–clumsy hand syndrome.

2. Age ≥60 years or a history of hypertension or diabetes.
3. CT or MRI performed ≥72 h after stroke shows appropriate subcortical lesion <2 cm in diameter or demonstrates no lesion appropriate to the stroke.
4. No obvious other cause of small vessel disease (e.g., vasculitis).
5. Arterial imaging shows no evidence of significant occlusive disease.

Laehr reflex (Laehr–Henneberg reflex, hard palate reflex) Contraction of the orbicularis oculi and lowering of the upper lip when the hard palate is tickled. This sign may be found in cases of pseudobulbar palsy.

Laehr–Henneberg reflex See **Laehr reflex**.

Lafora, Gonzalo Rodriguez (1886–1971) Spanish neurologist, neuropathologist, and psychiatrist who graduated from Madrid, taking further training there with **Cajal** and then in a number of German centers. While working in Washington DC, he described the amyloid bodies known by his name. After a further period as an exile in Mexico during the Spanish Civil War, he returned to Cajal's laboratory in Madrid for the remainder of his career.

Lafora bodies (amyloid bodies, myoclonus bodies, polyglucosan bodies) Rounded periodic-acid-Schiff-positive, argyophilic intracytoplasmic inclusion bodies with a dense central basophilic core and a rim that takes up less stain, found in the larger neurons of the thalamus, dentate nuclei, and substantia nigra, in progressive myoclonic epilepsy (**Lafora body disease**) and less abundantly in normal aged brains.

Lafora body disease (progressive myoclonic epilepsy with Lafora bodies; OMIM 254780) A recessively inherited polioencephalomyelopathy of late childhood or early adult life, characterized clinically by progressive dementia, dysarthria, visual loss, pyramidal and cerebellar signs, and photoconvulsive progressive myoclonic and other seizure types, leading to death in 2–10 years from the onset of symptoms. Many patients present with an apparently benign seizure disorder but the emergence of myoclonus and rapidly progressive dementia identify it as one of the PMEs. It is mapped to 6q24 but there is more than one locus.

The EEG shows generalized and focal or multifocal posterior discharges, photoconvulsive responses, and slowing of the background rhythms. The diagnostic pathological finding of basophilic intracytoplasmic PAS-positive inclusions in cells of the dentate nucleus, thalamus, and brain stem was described by Lafora in 1911,[3641] 20 years after Unverricht's original identification of progressive myoclonic epilepsy.[6449] The diagnosis is made by detecting **Lafora bodies** within neuronal processes in the central nervous system. Similar accumulations occur in the liver, heart, skin, and skeletal muscles. In practice, the method of choice for confirming the diagnosis is axillary skin biopsy.[1246]

Lafora body disease differs from **Unverricht–Lundborg–Lafora syndrome** in its slightly later mean age of onset, less severe myoclonus, and earlier and relentless cognitive decline, but this does not mean that the underlying abnormality is not the same. See also **adult polysaccharidosis**. The following *variants* are described

Progressive myoclonic epilepsy without Lafora bodies—a precisely similar clinical condition in which the Lafora bodies are not detected.[4181]

Juvenile neuronopathic Gaucher disease, type III—a cause of progressive myoclonus epilepsy, with the added clinical features of horizontal and vertical supranuclear gaze palsies, hepatosplenomegaly, and cerebellar signs.[4679]

laforin A protein with unknown function, seemingly relevant in the pathogenesis of **Lafora body disease**.

lag-in-pulse sign Delay in the re-establishment of the radial pulse after manual compression of the radial artery proximally—seen in the vasogenic form of the **thoracic outlet syndrome**.

lagophthalmos (from Gr, a hare + the eye) Inability to close one or both eyes fully while at rest, as may occur with bilateral VII cranial nerve palsies or myopathy affecting the facial muscles. The name derives from the ancient belief that hares sleep with their eyes open. Iritis and corneal nodules are predictable complications.

Laing distal myopathy See **limb-girdle muscular dystrophy**.

lalling (from Lat, to sing a lullaby) 1. The earliest speech sounds made by infants, varying between cooing and the repetitive utterance of consonants. The name was formerly used for that mode of speech in which the R sound is replaced by that of L. 2. The imperfect pronunciation of letters or words as by small children or by the inebriated. It includes slurring, **mogilalia**, and **paralalia**.

lambda The Greek letter "L," written as an inverted "V" and thus appropriately applied to the cranial posterior suture separating the parietal and occipital bones. Hence also *lambdoid* (of this shape).

lambda wave A sharp transient on the EEG, mainly electropositive relative to other areas and occurring over the occipital regions of the head of waking subjects during visual exploration. It is time-locked to saccadic eye movement and its amplitude varies but is generally below 50 μV. (Adapted from the 1974 report of the Committee on Terminology, IFCN by kind permission of Elsevier Science.)

These bi- or triphasic waves are recorded in parieto-occipital regions with intermittent stimulation and are absent in darkness or with a neutral visual field.

lambdoid wave See **positive occipital sharp transient of sleep**.

Lambert–Brody syndrome An X-linked disorder of childhood characterized by electrically silent muscle contractions with impairment of relaxation, similar to myotonia clinically but without percussion myotonia and electrically silent. It is due to impairment of calcium re-uptake by the sarcoplasmic reticulum as a result of calcium-adenosine triphosphatase deficiency in type 2 myofibrils.[293, 3316]

Lambert–Eaton myasthenic syndrome (Eaton–Lambert syndrome, inverse myasthenia, LEMS) An autoimmune disorder of presynaptic neuromuscular transmission affecting the voltage-gated P/Q Ca^{2+} channels, resulting from the impaired release of acetylcholine from the motor end plate due to blockade of functional calcium channels in the presynaptic membrane by autoantibodies; a **paraneoplastic syndrome** associated with carcinoma (usually small cell carcinoma of the lung) is the cause in at least

60% of all cases.[5232] Thus, the syndrome can occur either with or without malignant disease. See also **neuromuscular transmission disorders**.

Clinically, the condition is manifested by mild girdle weakness, especially of the hips and thighs, transiently improving with brief sustained exercise; muscle aching and cramps; paresthesias; and hyporeflexia. Oculobulbar signs such as ptosis, diplopia, hypometric saccades, dysarthria and dysphagia, and dryness of the mouth and eyes are present in many cases. Other features of autonomic involvement include impotence. Despite the name, fatiguability is not a prominent feature; in fact, there is augmentation of strength during initial voluntary activation. Both the weakness and the depression of reflexes abate with repeated effort due to the augmented mobilization of acetylcholine quanta, as seen by the post-tetanic potentiation recorded with 20 Hz and by the paradoxical lid elevation that occurs with sustained upward gaze. Electrophysiologic testing also demonstrates small compound muscle action potentials, amplified with continuing activity.[3651, 4061] The weakness results from a reduction in the quantal release of acetylcholine from motor nerve terminals, caused by autoantibodies to P/Q-type voltage-gated calcium channels of the paraneoplastic variety; the stimulus in other forms is not known.[4649]

A serum test for voltage-gated calcium channel antibodies is commercially available, but 15% of the cases are seronegative.

The same condition had been described by Anderson and others in England 3 years before the report of Lambert and Eaton, but they did not perform repetitive stimulation and did not describe the nature of the defect in full.

lamellated cytoplasmic inclusion disease A neuronal storage disease characterized by the childhood onset of cerebral atrophy with spasticity, rigidity, chorea, and mental and developmental delay with sensorimotor neuropathy. Nerve or rectal biopsy specimens show inclusions and cytoplasmic bodies.[381]

lamin A/C A multifunctional intermediate filament of the inner nuclear membrane involved in **Emery–Dreifuss muscular dystrophy**, cardiopathy with conduction system disease, **autosomal recessive axonal polyneuropathy** (CMT2), mandibuloacral dysplasia, **Hutchinson–Gilford progeria syndrome**, and atypical **Werner syndrome**, as well as rare cases of autosomal dominant **limb-girdle muscular dystrophy**.[3454]

lamina papyracea (Lat, a thin plate + made from papyrus).

laminin-2 (*merosin*) The most important extracellular ligand of α-dystroglycan in muscle. Mutations in the gene encoding the laminin-α2 chain cause **congenital muscular dystrophy** *1A*, or the form with *primary merosin deficiency*. Mutations in collagen VI underlie **Bethlem myopathy** and **Ullrich dystrophy**.

laminopathies Conditions due to mutations in the A/C lamin gene. They include **Emery–Dreifuss** muscular dystrophy, autosomal dominant limb-girdle muscular dystrophy with cardiac conduction disturbances, autosomal dominant dilated cardiomyopathy with conduction system disease, and familial partial lipodystrophy of the Dunnigan type. See **limb-girdle muscular dystrophy**.

Lamy–Maroteaux syndrome (diastrophic dwarfism, cherub dwarfism) A recessively inherited dysmorphic syndrome characterized by extreme short stature due to shortness of the limbs, kyphoscoliosis, joint contractures, hand deformities, and bilateral club foot.[4096]

The neurological Maroteaux–Lamy syndrome is different, and a **mucopolysaccharidosis**.

Lancaster red–green test A quantitative test measuring the degree of diplopia, in which red and green filters are placed successively over the subject's eyes, and the subject and the examiner each project a light (one red, one green) onto a screen in the nine cardinal positions of gaze. The separation of the images as seen by the subject is measured in each case.[5274] The test has been found valuable in demonstrating even small improvements of ocular motility in myasthenic patients given edrophonium.

Lance–Adams syndrome (chronic posthypoxic myoclonus) Multifocal cortical **action myoclonus** with cerebellar ataxia and a degree of mental slowing, due to subcortical ischemic anoxia,[3660] as following cardiorespiratory arrest. Clinically it presents with multifocal cortical action myoclonus, which may be stimulus-sensitive, and with mild cognitive deficits. An exaggerated startle response and brain stem reticular reflex myoclonus are also described.[6725]

Lancet One of the longest established medical journals, publishing also neurological papers. Web site: http://www.lancetneuronet.com/.

Lancet Neurology A specialty review publication in print and electronic format. Web site: http://www.lancetneuronet.com/.

lancinating pain Pain of a sharpness resembling that of a stab with a needle or scalpel. The pain of **trigeminal neuralgia** is typically described thus.

Landau reflex Extension of the neck, spine, and legs when the normal infant is held in ventral suspension, but flexion of the legs and trunk when the head is flexed by the examiner.

The reflex normally appears between the third and sixth month, and is lost at the end of the first year. Children with spastic states may show exaggeration of the reflex, while those with neuromuscular disease may not exhibit it at all and instead droop listlessly from the examiner's hands.[4401] See also **developmental reflexes**.

Landau syndrome A syndrome of retarded mental development with psychomotor seizures, dysplastic facial changes resembling acromegaly, and later generalized amyotrophy, slowly progressing and leading to early death. The pathogenesis is unknown.[3668]

Landau–Kleffner syndrome (acquired verbal auditory agnosia with convulsive disorder, acquired epileptic aphasia, Andermann syndrome) An epileptic encephalopathy of infancy and childhood[6833] more common in males and characterized by the acute or subacute appearance of regression of previously acquired language skills, leading eventually to mutism in young children whose former language development was proceeding normally. Verbal auditory agnosia and a rapid reduction in spontaneous speech are typical. Often associated are auditory agnosia and behavioral disorders, without intellectual deterioration. Nonverbal skills are unaffected. Generalized tonic-clonic or partial motor seizures and behavioral and psychomotor disturbances occur in two-thirds of the patients; the EEG findings include spike-wave discharges, especially during slow-wave sleep. Both the seizures and the EEG abnormalities are likely to remit somewhat before the age of 15 years and the language and neuropsychological disturbances gradually improve eventually. (Adapted from the revised ILAE Classification [Dreifuss FE, et al. Commission for classification and terminology, ILAE. Proposal for Revised Classifications of Epilepsies and Epileptic Syndromes. *Epilepsia* 1989;**30**:389–99 by kind permission of Wiley-Blackwell Publications] and from Panayiotopoulos [2007][4882]).

The condition responds poorly to anticonvulsant drugs, but steroids lastingly correct both the regression in higher functions and the EEG abnormalities.[3667]

In a *variant* form, there is associated selective gait disorder and paroxysmal dystonia.[4636]

Landing syndrome See **GM$_1$ gangliosidosis**.

Landing–Oppenheimer disease See **neuronal ceroid lipofuscinosis**.

Landouzy, Louis-Theophile-Joseph (1845–1917) French physician, professor of therapeutics and later dean of the faculty of medicine in Paris. His description of **facioscapulohumeral muscular dystrophy**[3675] was his only important contribution to neurology, most of his work being on tuberculosis. However, he also described muscle atrophy in association with sciatica, which some have called *Landouzy syndrome* or *Landouzy sciatica*.[3673]

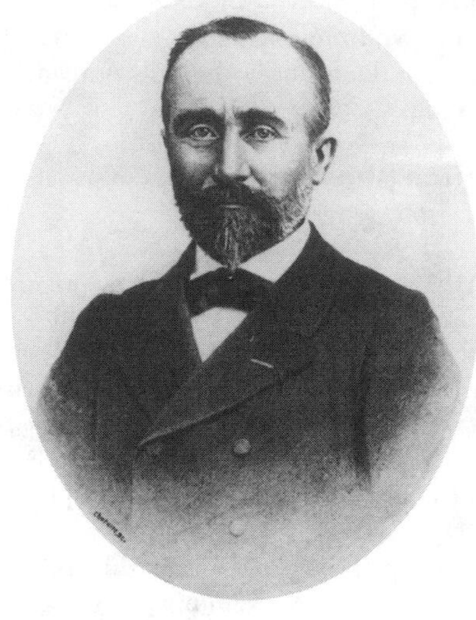

Figure L–1 Louis-Théophile-Joseph Landouzy.

Landouzy camptodactyly Irreducible contractures at the interphalangeal joints of the fingers (especially the fifth) due to fibrosis of the tendon sheaths.[3676]

Landouzy–Déjerine syndrome See **facioscapulohumeral dystrophy**.

Landouzy–Grasset law When a unilateral cerebral lesion produces hemiplegia, the head is turned to the side of the lesion if the paralysis is flaccid and to the side of the affected limbs if it is spastic.[3674] See also **Vulpian sign** and **Prevost sign**.

Landry de Thezillat, Jean-Baptiste-Octave (1826–1865) French neurologist, born in Limoges, whose description of acute infectious polyneuropathy in 1859[3678] (making most of the important clinical points and henceforward leading to the names *acute ascending* or *Landry paralysis*) preceded that of Guillain, Barré, and Strohl by nearly 60 years, although **Kussmaul** also described two cases in the same year.

His original account emphasized the sensory as well as the motor findings, but obviously omitted reference to the CSF as lumbar puncture had not then been introduced . Following this report, he left Paris for financial reasons and devoted the remainder of his professional life to the management of patients at the Auteuil spa.

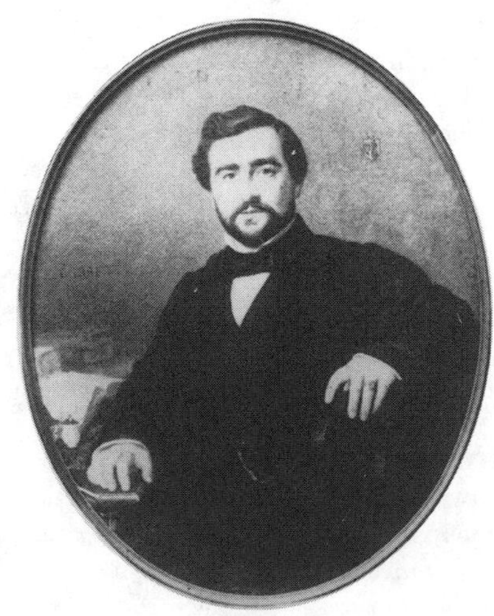

Figure L–2 Jean-Baptiste-Octave Landry de Thezillat.

He returned to Paris in 1865 to help in the care of patients during a cholera epidemic, and died from the disease despite the attention of **Charcot**.[2066]

Landry-Guillain-Barré (–Strohl) syndrome See **acute inflammatory demyelinating polyneuropathy**.

Langdon-Down, J.L.H. See Down, J.L.H.L.

Lange, Cornelia Catherina de (1871–1950) Dutch pediatrician who graduated from Amsterdam and worked in Zurich before returning, eventually becoming professor of pediatrics.

de Lange syndrome 1. (*de Lange–Brachmann syndrome*, Cornelia de Lange syndrome, Amsterdam dwarfism) A sporadic dysmorphic syndrome, characterized by growth retardation from conception and postnatally, with severely diminished stature, always below the third percentile, severe mental retardation, facial dysmorphism, antimongoloid slant to the eyes, syndactyly, flexion contractures of the elbows, **clinodactyly**, microbrachycephaly, transverse palmar crease, synophrys, and generalized hirsutism.[1503]

2. (*Bruck–de Lange syndrome*) Congenital muscular hypertrophy, mental retardation and extrapyramidal disorders (hypertonia) with broad and thick neck and limbs, low hairline, and asymmetrical skull due to porencephaly. Various cerebral dysgenetic malformations are also found.[1504]

Despite the attribution to de Lange, the first report (acknowledged by her) was that of Dr. Franz Bruck in 1889.

Lange, Karl (b. 1883) German physician, inventor of the colloidal gold test in the diagnosis of neurosyphilis.

Langer–Gierdon syndrome (thoracic–pelvic–phalangeal dystrophy) A dysmorphic syndrome characterized by microcephaly, polydactyly, hypotonia, deafness, an unusually bulbous nose, redundant folds of skin in cervical regions, and both physical and mental retardation, and due to a chromosomal deletion at 8q24.[4556]

Langerhans cell histiocytosis A rare granulomatous disease with predilection for the pituitary gland and hypothalamus, typically presenting with skull lesions, proptosis, and diabetes insipidus. See also **hypophysitis**.

Langley, John Newport (1852–1925) English physiologist, professor of physiology at Cambridge. He devoted most of his research to the study of the autonomic nervous system, differentiating the sympathetic and parasympathetic systems by 1894. Both these names and *orthosympathetic* were suggested by him, and he also differentiated and named the pre- and postganglionic fibers.[3688]

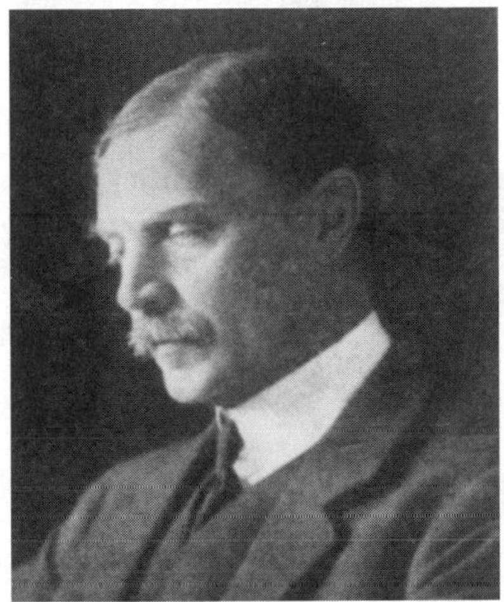

Figure L–3 John Newport Langley.

Langley nerves Pilomotor nerves.

Langley–Sherrington sign Protrusion of the pinna of the ear on the same side as a **Horner syndrome**. See also **Hassin sign**.

language 1. An essentially human method of expressing ideas and feelings by way of a system of visual or auditory symbols; the expression and reception of ideas and feelings.

2. Expression of mental content through muscular activity with the intention of communicating it to another person. The symbolic representation of many forms of sensory experience, the symbols taking the form of written or spoken words and of gestures (including *body language*) used for the expression and communication of thoughts or feelings.[2455, 5247]

language disorder Disturbances of reading, writing, spelling, calculation, and verbal memory or learning as well as dysphasia.

language-induced epilepsy A reflex seizure disorder in which the seizures are triggered by multiple language-related functions, including reading, speaking, and writing.[2342]

Lannois–Jouty syndrome A syndrome of paresis of cranial nerves IX, X, XI, and XII, indicating a lesion of the skull base. See also **Avellis syndrome**.

Lantermann, A.J. German anatomist whose paper reporting what are now known as **Schmidt–Lantermann clefts** in myelin followed that of Schmidt by 3 years.

lardaceous hegemony The term used by Dr. H.L. Parker for the fatty imperatives of the antiepileptic **ketogenic diet**.

Larrey, D.-J. (1766–1842) French surgeon who headed the medical services in Napoleon's armies. His experiences gained from the military carnage he witnessed led to numerous original descriptions of diseases or of methods for their management and (apart from surgical topics) included accounts of **Jacksonian seizures**, contralateral paresis with cerebral injury, homolateral paresis with cerebellar injury, and aphasia with cerebral lesions.[2066]

Larsen disease A congenital dysmorphic syndrome manifesting also sensorineural deafness, optic atrophy, retinal cone dystrophy with night blindness, hepatic disorder, hypertension, diabetes, hypothyroidism, and a large sella turcica.[381]

larval discharges Runs of abnormal activity on the EEG, such as are frequently associated with clinical seizure activity, but which in these cases are unaccompanied by seizures.

larval epilepsy (Lat, a mask + seizures) An antique name for **complex partial seizures**, in which the evidence for epilepsy is masked by the atypical nature of its manifestations.

laryngeal abductor paralysis An X-linked congenital syndrome of dysphonia with stridor and mental retardation, due to agenesis of the nucleus of the nerve in the medulla. A VI cranial nerve palsy may be associated.[6674]

Laryngeal adductor paralysis is also described as a dominantly inherited abnormality.[3993]

laryngeal dystonia Dystonic spasms of the vocal cords which adduct on phonation, resulting in **spastic dysphonia**. The cause is not known.[179] See also **Meige syndrome**.

laryngeal epilepsy See **cough syncope**.

laryngeal nystagmus See **ocular myoclonus**.

laryngeal vertigo See **cough syncope**.

laryngisimus stridulus Laryngeal spasm in children with hypocalcemia (usually as a result of rickets), which causes arrest in inspiration followed by relaxation of the vocal cord adduction and resulting in a crowing inspiratory sound.

Lasègue, Ernest-Charles (1816–1883) Parisian neuropsychiatrist who had already held a chair of rhetoric when he entered the University of Paris. He graduated in 1846, became a student of **Trousseau** and eventually became physician at the **Salpêtrière** and later at the Pitié Hospital. It was his student J.-J. Forst who published Lasègue's 1864 observations on straight-leg raising (in his doctoral thesis in 1881), although the same sign had already been described by Lazarevic in 1880.

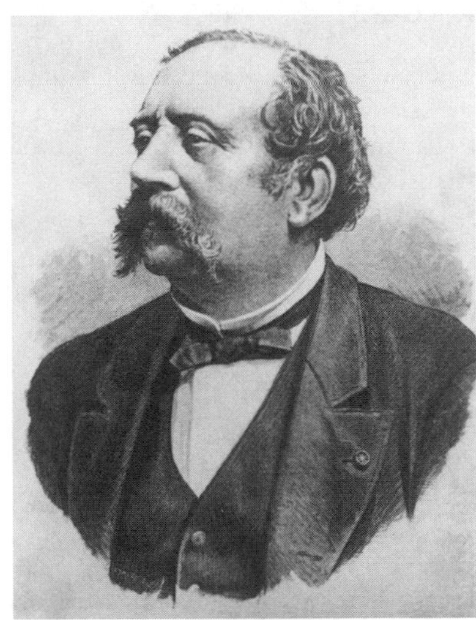

Figure L–4 Ernest-Charles Lasègue.

Lasègue also gave a superb description of paranoid dementia praecox (schizophrenia) in 1852 and of anorexia nervosa (hysterical anorexia) in 1873,[3709] just after the first note by **Gull** in the *Lancet* of 1868.

"It is interesting to note the extraordinary differences in the descriptions of the same condition by the two men. While Gull's comments are as direct and precise as a pathological report, Lasègue conveys a sense of the spirit and feeling of these people, the nuances of their disturbed relationships and the subtleties of their psychiatric upheaval."[5704]

Lasègue's acquaintance with such cases sprang from his appointment as physician to the Paris prefecture in 1849, whither all persons arrested on a charge of lunacy were brought. He was chef de clinique under Trousseau, whose favorite pupil he was, from 1852 to 1854. In the remainder of his career, he published over 115 papers on subjects as diverse as cretinism, hysteria, alcoholism, migraine, vertigo, typhoid, rheumatism, and syphilis.[5704]

Lasègue signs 1. (straight-leg raising) A sign of lumbosacral root irritation. Pain and limitation of further movement occur when the patient's hip is slowly, passively flexed with the knee extended, but not when the hip is flexed with the knee flexed also. The test can be augmented by passive dorsiflexion of the ankle, which causes more pain in the back in positive cases.

Lasègue originally likened the stretching of the sciatic nerve over the ischium when the leg is elevated to the tuning of a violin string by his son-in-law, but thought that the pain came from compression of the nerve by muscles.[3707] **Wartenberg**[6661] noted that the sign (and a more correct interpretation of its genesis) was described by Lazarevic, a physician in Belgrade, in 1880, a year before the thesis of Forst.

2. **Lasègue syndrome** In hysterical anesthesia, the patient will be unable to move the limb when the eyes are closed, but can do so when they are opened.[3708, 3709]

Lashley, Karl (1890–1958) American neurophysiologist and psychologist. He defined the law of mass action, noting that the degree of impairment in maze learning by rats was proportional to the volume of brain removed but was not dependent on the site of the ablation, thus giving support to those who believed in the functional equivalence of the cortex. He later modified his view, considering such equipotentiality to exist only within regions.[3710]

Lassa fever An acute severe nosocomially spread hemorrhagic disease caused by an arenavirus and characterized by the insidious onset of influenza-like symptoms followed, in severe cases, by a generalized bleeding diathesis, encephalopathy, and death. It is endemic in central Africa. Early diagnosis may be possible using polymerase chain reaction technology. The Junin and Machupo arenaviruses are responsible for the similar conditions of Argentine and Bolivian hemorrhagic fever, respectively.[1379]

lata See **latah**.

latah (lata) A chronic condition manifest by excessive startle responses to noise or touch with involuntary mimicry, tics, striking out, coprolalia, and automatic obedience to commands, occurring mainly in adult females in Africa and the Far East.[5854]

It was recorded first in the 16th century, but in modern times was described in 1883 by Beard among Malaysians.[6901] See also **Jumping Frenchmen of Maine**.

late amaurotic familial idiocy See **GM_2 gangliosidoses** and **neuronal ceroid lipofuscinosis**.

late component (of a motor unit action potential) See **satellite potential**.

late cortical cerebellar atrophy See **olivopontocerebellar atrophy**, **autosomal dominant cerebellar ataxias**, and **Marie–Foix–Alajouanine syndrome**.

late distal myopathy A form of muscular dystrophy appearing in mature adult life, affecting first the hands but later also the feet.[6711] See also **distal myopathy**.

late hereditary myopathy See **distal muscular dystrophy**.

late infantile amaurotic familial idiocy See **GM_2 gangliosidoses** and **neuronal ceroid lipofuscinosis**.

late infantile metachromatic leukodystrophy See **metachromatic leukodystrophy**.

late post-traumatic epilepsy Seizures occurring more than a week after craniocerebral trauma. They are more likely to recur than those occurring within the first week.

late response A general term used to describe an evoked potential in motor nerve conduction studies having a longer latency than the M wave. Examples include **A wave**, **F wave**, and **H wave**. (From the 2001 Report of the Nomenclature Committee of the American Association of Electromyography and Electrodiagnosis.[19] Reproduced by kind permission of the AANEM.)

late-life muscular dystrophy See **chronic polymyositis**.

late-onset ataxia, rigidity, and peripheral neuropathy A dominantly inherited degenerative disease of late onset, characterized by cerebellar ataxia, muscular rigidity, bradykinesia, dysarthria, muscle atrophy, and spasticity in various combinations in affected individuals.[6972] See also **cerebellar ataxias** (*variants*).

late-onset cerebellar ataxias See **cerebellar ataxias** (*variants*).

late-onset childhood occipital epilepsy (Gastaut type) A rare condition without adequate confirmatory reports to allow confident identification, according to the ILAE (2006).

late-onset proximal myopathy with diabetes mellitus A syndrome with onset in later adult life, comprising muscle pain and cramp, cataract, diabetes, and proximal myopathic weakness.[381]

late-onset proximal riboflavine-responsive myopathy with combined multiple acyl CoA dehydrogenase and respiratory chain deficiency A rare syndrome resulting from the impaired oxidation of fatty acids with onset in later adult life and comprising lipid storage myopathy with severe proximal weakness.[214]

An *infantile variant* in which the presentation is with nonketotic hypoglycemia, hypotonia, failure to thrive, and acute attacks resembling **Reye syndrome**; and a *juvenile* form with progressive limb-girdle and axial myopathy and secondary carnitine deficiency, are also described.

latency The interval between a stimulus and the response to it. The onset latency is the interval between the onset of a stimulus and the onset of the evoked potential. The peak latency is the interval between the onset of a stimulus and a specified peak of the evoked potential. (From the 2001 Report of the Nomenclature Committee of the American Association of Electromyography and Electrodiagnosis.[19] Reproduced by kind permission of the AANEM.)

latency of activation The time required for an electric stimulus to depolarize a nerve fiber (or bundle of fibers as in a nerve trunk) beyond threshold and to initiate an action potential in the fiber(s). This time is usually in the order of 0.1 ms or less. (From the 2001 Report of the Nomenclature Committee of the American Association of Electromyography and Electrodiagnosis.[19] Reproduced by kind permission of the AANEM.)

latent Concealed, not yet manifest.

latent convergent strabismus See **esophoria**.

latent nystagmus (monocular "fixation" nystagmus, unimacular nystagmus) A congenital form of jerk nystagmus that appears (in both eyes) only when one eye is occluded and in which the slow phase has a decreasing-velocity exponential curve. The fast phase is in the direction of gaze of the viewing eye. Strabismus is always present as well. The condition is a disorder of tonic innervation that is precipitated by an inability to adjust properly to the differences between monocular and binocular perceptual domains.[1562] It is seen in association with a lack of normal binocular development and childhood strabismus.[5731]

Manifest latent nystagmus is similar, occurring in both eyes of subjects with image suppression due to squint or amblyopia, who for this reason are actually viewing with one eye only, even though both are open.[1562]

latent period See latency.

latent tetany See **spasmophilia**.

lateral (Lat, belonging to the side)

lateral antebrachial cutaneous neuropathy Compression of the terminal cutaneous branch of the musculocutaneous nerve at its point of exit beside the biceps tendon, resulting in pain and sensory deficit in the territory of that nerve.[3112]

lateral bulbar syndrome See **lateral medullary syndrome**.

lateral cervical puncture Percutaneous insertion of a needle into the spinal cord through the C1–2 interspace under fluoroscopic control, performed in order to interrupt the spinothalamic tracts as a method of pain control.

In an adaptation, the needle is advanced only into the subarachnoid space for the collection of CSF.[6979]

lateral epicondylitis (tennis elbow) A common syndrome of adults characterized by pain in the region of the lateral epicondyle, which is exacerbated by gripping with the hand (and perhaps caused by overuse of that function in the arm), and associated with tenderness over the origin of the extensor carpi radialis brevis at the lateral humeral epicondyle.

The **forced elbow extension test** result is usually positive.[6588]

lateral femoral cutaneous nerve An independent branch of the lumbar plexus; this long nerve runs into the thigh, passing beneath the lateral part of the inguinal ligament. There it may be entrapped by the ligament itself or by a pad of fat beneath it, leading to complaints of pricking pain and numbness in its distribution, which is equivalent to an area about the size of a hand located on the lateral part of the thigh. The precise diagnosis is seldom aided by nerve conduction studies. Decompression of the nerve may relieve symptoms in intractable cases but the condition is usually self-limiting.

lateral femoral cutaneous neuropathy See **meralgia paresthetica**.

lateral foot reflex (von Monakow reflex) Eversion of the foot in response to light stroking of the lateral edge of the sole, seen in patients with pyramidal lesions.

lateral hamstring reflex See **external hamstring reflex**.

lateral hypothalamic syndrome A rare syndrome characterized by loss of appetite amounting to aphagia, resulting from lesions of the lateral hypothalamus.

lateral inferior pontine syndrome Deafness, facial palsy, homolateral facial numbness, and cerebellar ataxia, usually due to a small pontine vascular lesion.

lateral medullary nystagmus See **Bruns nystagmus**.

lateral medullary syndrome (Wallenberg syndrome, lateral bulbar syndrome, syndrome of the posterior inferior cerebellar artery) The syndrome resulting from occlusion of the vertebral artery or its branch, the posterior inferior cerebellar artery, and manifested by acute vertigo, vomiting, hiccups, dysarthria, dysphagia and dysphonia, homolateral cerebellar ataxia, Horner syndrome, and alternating thermoanalgesia (loss of temperature and pinprick sensation on the same side of the face and on the trunk and limbs on the opposite side).

The syndrome was described in detail by **Wallenberg** in 1895.[6608] He encountered it in a young man who perhaps had herpetic angiitis when he was first seen but whose arteries were severely and generally diseased when Wallenberg performed the autopsy 4 years later, at which time the stenoses of the posterior inferior cerebellar arteries confirmed his predictions.

The classic syndrome is of inestimable value to teachers of neurology because of the precise clinicopathological correlations that it allows,[1386] but it may also occur as a **lacunar syndrome.**[2092, 2106] Further downward extension results in the **Opalski syndrome.**

In *variant* forms, *face–arm–trunk–leg sensory loss* occurs on the contralateral side,[6576] or there is a *pontomedullary sulcus infarct* which presents with mainly sensory features.

lateral plantar neuropathy Damage to this nerve within or just distal to the tarsal tunnel, producing pain and numbness of the lateral plantar surface of the foot. See also **tarsal tunnel syndrome.**[4767]

lateral pontomedullary syndrome A **lacunar syndrome** with features resembling the **lateral medullary** or **Foville syndromes**. Clinically, it is characterized by vertigo, vomiting, facial weakness, dysarthria, dysphagia, tinnitus, ataxia, nystagmus, **Horner syndrome**, and **alternating thermoanalgesia**.[2092, 4954, 5015]

The usual pathology is a small occlusion of one of the short circumferential branches of the vertebral artery, but the same features may also occur as a result of local compression or infiltration. See also **lower basilar branch occlusion**.

lateral temporal lobe epilepsy See **temporal lobe epilepsy**.

lateral transtentorial herniation See **uncal herniation**.

lateralization 1. Specialization of cerebral function within one or other hemisphere. 2. Localization of disease to one or other part of the neuraxis.

The concept that there was specialization in the function of one hemisphere was introduced by Dax in 1836, countering the older idea of organic duality with functional unity, but it was **Broca** who developed the idea to the point of effective proof, leading to his dictum that we speak with the left hemisphere. Hughlings-**Jackson** took the hypothesis on to the next stage; if the left hemisphere is specialized for speech, what is the special function of the right hemisphere?

Geschwind showed that cerebral dominance is founded upon asymmetries of structure, for speech, particularly of the posterior part of the superior temporal gyrus—the planum temporale.[2341]

A test for determining the side of a brain lesion was suggested by Heimburger and Reitan:[2843] the subject is asked to copy a square, a Greek cross, and a triangle, to name each of the figures, to spell each name, and to repeat the phrase "He shouted the warning." Pierre **Marie** had previously suggested a similar brief test.

lateralized Involving mainly the right or the left side of the body.

lateralizing (Todd or Bravais) phenomenon Any unilateral postictal dysfunction relating to motor, speech, somatosensory, and/or integrative functions including visual, auditory, or somatosensory neglect phenomena.[16]

laterocollis A focal dystonia characterized by sustained involuntary contractions of the neck muscles, which result in abnormal lateral flexion of the head on the neck. See also **cervical dystonia**.

lateropulsion (Lat, to the side + to push) Involuntary drawing of the body or veering of the gait toward one side; a characteristic sign after cerebellar, paramedian pontine, or lateral medullary infarction.[1638]

Latham–Munro disease A recessively inherited syndrome consisting of congenital deafness and both myoclonic and grand mal epilepsy.[3712]

lathyrism (from Gr, the vetch) An ancient neurodegenerative syndrome mostly seen in males on the Indian subcontinent, who develop subacutely progressing muscle cramps, paresthesias, urgency and frequency of micturition, and nocturnal erections and ejaculations proceeding to pyramidal weakness and spasticity following chronic consumption of the seeds of the chickling or grass pea (*Lathyrus sativus*) in times of war, famine, or pestilence. This substance contains an excitotoxic amino acid (B (n) oxalyl aminoalanine) that may be responsible for causing this **central-distal axonopathy**.[3950, 4392] Little or no recovery occurs. See also **epidemic spastic paraplegia**.

latissimus dorsi reflex A tap on the examiner's finger placed upon the tendon of the muscle (which forms the posterior wall of the axilla) leads to its contraction, causing adduction and internal rotation of the shoulder. The maneuver informs (a little) about the status of the C6–C8 reflex arcs.

laughing death (kuru) See **Lytico-Bodig**.

Launois syndrome See **pituitary gigantism**.

Launois–Bensaude syndrome See **familial multiple symmetrical lipomatosis with peripheral neuropathy**.

Laurence, John Zachary (1828–1870) English ophthalmologist who was a founder of the Royal Eye Hospital and editor of the first journal of ophthalmology published in English.

Laurence–Moon–Biedl syndrome A recessively inherited diffuse encephalopathy, characterized by the combination of obesity, spastic paraparesis, mental deficiency, pigmentary retinal degeneration with severe rod degeneration leading to blindness, and renal anomalies suggesting abnormal maturation.[3714] Polydactyly is unusual in this form of the disorder, but is common in the variant **Bardet–Biedl syndrome**.[2774]

The first description (by Laurence and Moon) was in 1866, Bardet's report appearing in 1920. R.C. Moon (1844–1914) was an American ophthalmologist and A. Biedl (1869–1933), a Czech physician.

law of denervation See **Cannon's law**.

law of dynamic polarity The observation (of Ramon y **Cajal**) that the nerve impulse passes from the dendrite through the cell body to the axon.

law of motor correspondence See **Hering law**.

law of reciprocal innervation Agonist and antagonist muscles do not normally contract against each other (Sir Charles **Sherrington**).

law of regression see **Ribot law**.

law of specific nerve energies The concept of Johannes Müller (1838) that there is an intrinsic difference between the nervous mechanisms subserving the five senses, such that the same stimulus applied to different nerves would evoke different sensations. Thus, different nerve fibers subserving, for example, touch, cold, and tickle would exist. This "specific fiber" theory has now given way to the "pattern" theory.

Lawford syndrome A variant of **Sturge–Weber syndrome** in which glaucoma occurs without any increase in the volume of the globe.[3720]

Laxova syndrome A lethal congenital recessively inherited dysmorphic syndrome manifesting also strabismus, seizures, microcephaly, lissencephaly, muscle atrophy, tremor, syndactyly, and mental and developmental delay. Agenesis of the corpus callosum may also be present.[3723] See also **Neu–Laxova syndrome**.

lazaroids Cytoprotective steroid derivatives, of possible value in patients with cerebral ischemia or with physical or chemical injury of the brain.

Lazarus complex A term applied by Thomas Hackett in 1972 to those symptoms affecting the survivors of cardiac arrest who have, as it were, been "raised from the dead." These include anxiety, depression, nightmares, insomnia, a sense of alienation, and occasionally a delusional state.

Such symptoms usually occur as a result of anoxic brain damage, but are nevertheless based on the normal mental mechanisms of denial and isolation (inhibition) of the affective response, projection, and displacement.

Lazarus movements (Lazarus sign) A Moro-like automatism comprising spontaneous flexion of the arms, occurring (rarely) in brain-dead people, perhaps as a result of spontaneous discharge of cervical motor neurons.[5380]

le main en griffe See **claw hand**.

le pied en griffe See **claw foot**.

lead colic Cramping abdominal pains as a result of lead poisoning, best described by George Baker (1722–1809), who realized that the lead was coming from the glaze inside the cider presses used in his Devonshire village.

lead encephalopathy A syndrome of headache, irritability, tremulousness and giddiness, progressing to seizures, raised intracranial pressure, stupor, and coma, due to lead poisoning.

The direct neurotoxic actions of lead include apoptosis, excitotoxicity, and influences on neurotransmitter storage and release, mitochondria, and on neurons and glial cells. Lead can substitute for calcium (and perhaps zinc), which may account for some of its toxic actions, many of which may depend on its ability to cross the blood–brain barrier by substituting for calcium ions. Inside and outside the CNS, lead may induce neuronal death through apoptosis; D2 receptors and astroglial function are especially vulnerable to even low levels. The damaging effects of lead on the development of the nervous system are responsible for cognitive impairments in exposed children, while specific effects on glutamatergic transmission, which is critically involved in both development and neuronal plasticity, presage impairments in learning and memory. Disruption of dopaminergic functioning may be responsible for such behavioral problems as **attention-deficit hyperactivity disorder** as well as cognitive impairments.

The 5-week half-life of lead in the blood determines that high blood levels are only an indicator of recent exposure; lead poisoning from chronic exposure to low levels is more common and may lack definitive physical signs, although some children have stomach pains, anorexia (loss of appetite), and anemia. Impairment of cognitive skills and behavioral problems are described even with low (15 μg/dl) lead levels.[3841]

lead hyperesthesia Excessive hyperexcitability of the sensory nerves giving rise to paroxysmal pain, as a result of lead poisoning. *Lead neuralgia* has the same meaning.

lead neuralgia See **lead hyperesthesia**.

lead palsy (cyder palsy) A focal motor neuropathy most prone to affect the radial nerve, first described by Thomas Cadwalader (1708–1779), an American physician. Benjamin Franklin later showed that the lead had come from the pipes leading off the distillate (Jamaica rum), a favored beverage of New Englanders at that time, while the same etiology in southwest England led to what was called *cyder palsy*. Clinically, colic, constipation, indigestion, muscle weakness, and atrophy mainly in the extensor muscles of the arms are the major features. Mild sensory and autonomic symptoms may also occur. The pathophysiology may involve the precipitation of lead-induced porphyria.[5456] See also **Remak paralysis**.

lead pipe rigidity A type of increase in muscle tone in which the resistance of the patient's limb is constant in magnitude throughout the range of passive excursion. In keeping with modern advances in plumbing technology, the term *plastic rigidity* is nowadays often substituted.

lean spastic dwarfism See **Coffin syndrome**.

Leao, Aristide A contemporary Brazilian neurophysiologist.

leaping ague See **dancing mania**.

learning 1. The modification of thought, feeling, or action as a result of experience. 2. The body of (usually considered exceptional) knowledge possessed by an individual.

Learning Disabilities Association A charitable association in this field. Address: 4156 Library Rd., Pittsburgh, PA 15234. Tel: 412-341-1515.

Learning Disabilities Association of Canada A charitable organization based at 3 Chapel St., Ottawa, Ontario KIN 7Z2, Canada .

Leber, Theodor Karl Gustav von (1840–1917) German ophthalmologist who graduated from Heidelberg and trained further in France and Germany. He was elected professor of ophthalmology at Göttingen and then Heidelberg, where he remained for the rest of his life, describing the hereditary optic neuropathy named for him in 1871. He first proposed the term *tapetoretinal degenerations*.

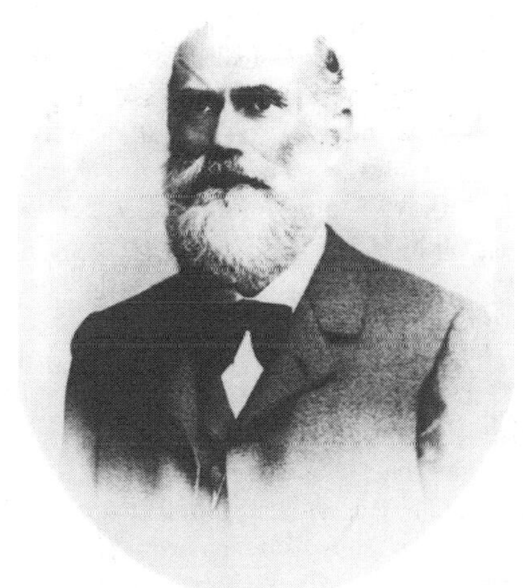

Figure L–5 Theodor Leber.

Leber congenital amaurosis (hereditary retinal aplasia, retinal abiotrophy) A recessively inherited congenital syndrome of near-blindness due to abnormalities of the retinal photoreceptors, with absent electroretinographic potentials. The clinical features include pendular nystagmus, photophobia, pigmentary retinal degeneration, optic atrophy, chorioretinitis, keratoconus, and cataract. Multiple renal cysts, intellectual failure, seizures, hypotonia, morphological abnormalities of muscle, and deafness have been recorded in some cases.[3739, 4531] These features resemble those of **neuronal ceroid lipofuscinosis**.[5032]

In a *variant* form, diffuse CNS demyelination is associated and the affected individuals show psychomotor retardation.[1382]

Leber disease, dystonia, and basal ganglia low densities

See **hereditary spastic dystonia**.

Leber miliary aneurysms

Telangiectasia and varicosity of the retinal capillaries, which become unusually permeable as a result. This may represent the pathological basis of **Coats disease**.

Leber optic atrophy

(Leber hereditary optic neuropathy, LHON) An acute, sequentially bilateral optic neuropathy causing painless permanent visual loss and occurring mainly in young males (>80%) over the age of 10; women are affected much less frequently. The condition affects the second eye within 3 months. Pseudoedema of the retinal nerve fiber layer, peripapillary microangiopathy, and tortuosity of the retinal vessels are characteristic signs. There is an absence of peripapillary staining on fluorescein retinal angiography. Clinically, loss of acuity, contrast sensitivity, and of color vision and centrocecal visual field defects are accompanied by temporal pallor of the disk and loss of the papillomacular bundle in the retinal nerve fiber layer.

Though familial and following a transmission pattern resembling that of X-linked recessive disorders, being maternally transmitted, this transmission does not follow the usual Mendelian principles[3738, 3739] and is a **mitochondrial encephalopathy**, usually resulting from point mutations at 11778, 3460, or 14484 in the mitochondrial genome,[5317] all of which affect genes that encode subunits of the respiratory chain in Complex I. It is considered to reflect both this abnormality of respiratory chain enzymes and also the operation of an exogenous factor such as cyanide or folate deficiency. The diagnosis is proven by mtDNA analysis. In the typical form, the triad listed above is present. Similar but acquired mitochondrial damage is likely to be responsible for **Cuban optic neuropathy**, **tobacco–alcohol amblyopia**, and certain toxic optic neuropathies. In *variant* forms,

> The clinical presentation is compatible with Leber disease but the microangiopathy is not seen in the subject (although it may be present in family members).[3911]
>
> Other evidence of neurological disease (such as headaches, emotional instability, myoclonic and other seizures, mental retardation, tremor, dystonia, hypotonia, peripheral neuropathy, or pyramidal signs), cardiac arrhythmias, or **broad band** disease may also be present (*Leber-plus syndrome*).[4530, 4677]

Leeuwenhoek, Antonius van

(1632–1723) Dutch draper and biologist, who was the first to describe the striations in muscle and the sarcolemma as well as spermatozoa and many other structures, based on his observations made with the microscope,[3755] for which he was elected a corresponding Fellow of the Royal Society.

He also described respiratory myoclonus (**diaphragmatic flutter**) as the cause of paroxysms of epigastric pulsation and dyspnea in himself, differentiating the problem from one of cardiac origin, as his diaphragmatic contractions were not in time with his pulse.

left-handedness

(sinistrality) A preference for using the left side of the body for performing fine motor tasks such as writing, using scissors, a knife, or a sporting implement. It occurs in some 10% of the population, and more often in males. Left-eyedness also occurs.

Except for the nuisance value of being left-handed in a world run mainly by and for the right-handed majority, there is little that is negative about the preference, although there is a statistical excess of subjects with autism, stuttering, dyslexia, migraine, allergies, and immune diseases in a population of strong sinistrals.

A major review of cerebral lateralization and hypotheses as to its nature was presented in the last paper of Norman **Geschwind**.[2341]

left–right confusion

Impairment of the ability to differentiate the two sides, usually as a result of right parietal lobe disease. See also Gerstmann syndrome.

left-sided syndromes

1. Weakness of the left arm and leg (but of the right side of the face), left optic atrophy, loss of auscultatory blood pressure in the left arm, and staggering gait with a tendency to fall to the left, all occurring in the presence of renal failure and generalized atherosclerosis.[6679]

2. The complaint of both positive and negative painless sensory symptoms, felt on the left side of the body (face, neck, and arm >leg) mainly by females, in whom no objective physical signs can be found and no underlying structural pathology demonstrated.[6025] In some cases, anxiety with hyperventilation appears relevant in causation, but why unilateral *right*-sided symptoms are only a tenth as likely to be evidenced than those on the left is unexplained.[5435]

leg jerks

See **periodic limb movement disorder**.

leg phenomenon

See **Pool–Schlesinger sign**.

leg sign

(Barré sign) With the patient prone, the knees are flexed so that the lower leg is vertical. Return of a leg to the extended position (on the bed) suggests the presence of a pyramidal lesion (but also argues in favor of gravity).

Legallois, Julien-Jean-César

(1770–1814) French physiologist, notable for his isolation of the medullary respiratory center and for demonstrating neurogenic influences on the heart.

Legionnaire disease

A widespread infection by organisms of the class Legionnairaceae, most commonly occurring in epidemics and producing mainly respiratory tract disease. The latter is associated with weakness, headache and myalgia, cough, and high fever. Gastrointestinal symptoms are also common. Neurological signs, including emotional lability, confusion, delirium, or CNS depression, occur in about one-third of the cases.

leg-straightening reflex

The legs and body normally straighten when the sole of an infant's foot is pressed onto the surface of the examining table. See also **developmental reflexes**.

Leichtenstern, Otto Michael Ludwig

(1845–1900) German physician in Cologne. He had a particular interest in infectious diseases, but also gave a good account of subacute combined degeneration of the cord in 1884.

Leichtenstern phenomenon Hyperalgesia when any bone is pressed; found in patients with meningitis.[3757]

Leigh disease (subacute necrotizing encephalomyelopathy) A fatal, recessively inherited mitochondrial disease of infancy or childhood (rarely occurring in adults, in whom the disease may be relatively mild), of unknown cause but with a major biochemical defect in the deficiency of cytochrome *c* oxidase and thus in the oxidation of pyruvate.[3758] Serum lactate and pyruvate levels may be raised. Abnormalities of the pyruvate dehydrogenase complex and (rarely) of the NADH–CoQ reductase system have also been described.[1152]

Clinically, it is characterized by psychomotor retardation, weakness, hypotonia, feeding difficulties with failure to thrive, and dystonias, seizures, myoclonus, visual deterioration due to optic atrophy, metabolic acidosis with vomiting, tachypnea, apneic spells, reduced consciousness, nystagmus and other ocular signs, pyramidal and cerebellar signs, and hepatomegaly. The eye signs and the histological appearances are similar but not identical to those of **Wernicke disease** and, as in that condition, abnormalities of liver function and of cardiac and skeletal muscle may also be found.[2425, 6493] However, the response to vitamin B therapy is usually disappointing.

Dr. A. Denis Leigh (1915–1998) was a consultant psychiatrist at the Bethlem-Maudsley Hospital in London, UK.

The following *variants* have been identified:

See **Alpers disease**. The differentiation of this condition from Leigh disease is uncertain.

Acute neonatal Leigh disease—A fatal recessively inherited syndrome with rapid progression, characterized by hypotonia, oacidosis, and cardiomyopathy with sudanophilic leukoencephalopathy.[5714]

Juvenile Leigh disease—A sporadic syndrome of adolescence characterized by weakness, exercise intolerance with dyspnea, Parkinsonism, pyramidal and cerebellar signs, and dementia.[6493]

Adult Leigh disease—A sporadic pleomorphic condition, usually diagnosed initially as multiple sclerosis but with no MRI abnormalities in the initial stages, despite clinical evidence of brain stem involvement (respiratory failure, nystagmus, oculomotor palsies, palatal myoclonus, reticular myoclonus, etc.), visual failure, ataxia, and spasticity. Coma and paroxysmal brain stem failure with apnea may occur.[2556]

See also **Association for Neuro-Metabolic Disorders**, a charitable organization in this field providing information and support. Web site: http://www.kumc.edu/gec/support/neuro-me.html. Leigh Disease is an information sheet compiled by the NINDS. Web site: http://www.ninds.nih.gov/disorders/leighsdisease/leighsdisease.htm.

leiodystonia A chronic but intermittent disturbance of regulation of the autonomic nervous system manifesting as hypotension, pallor, dilated pupils, perspiration, and impotence, described in the 1930s in Europeans living in the tropics and probably representing a combination of dehydration and depression.[4876, 6884]

leiomyoma (Gr, smooth + muscle + tumor) A benign tumor of unstriated muscle, as in the uterus or prostate gland.

Leishmaniasis (kala-azar) Infection with *Leishmania donovani*, resulting from the bite of a sandfly and causing a parasitic reticuloendotheliosis. Peripheral neuropathy is a complication, perhaps reflecting the nutritional deficiency that results from anorexia in this condition.[5724]

Leiter International Scale (Arthur adaptation) A nonverbal test of cognitive ability, used in children and young people. See http://portal.wpspublish.com/ portal/page?_pageid=53,114601&_dad=portal&_schema=PORTAL.

leitungaphasie See **conduction aphasia**.

Lejeune disease See **cri-du-chat syndrome**.

Lejonne–Lhermitte disease (olivorubrocerebellar atrophy) A syndrome of adult onset, characterized by atrophy and gliosis of the olives, cerebellar cortex, dentate nucleus, and both superior and inferior cerebellar peduncles.[3768]

Lemierre, André-Alfred (1875–1956) French physician in Paris who specialized in infectious diseases.

Lemierre syndrome (postanginal septicemia) Septic thrombophlebitis of the internal jugular vein and metastatic infections involving especially the lungs, following an acute oropharyngeal infection. The syndrome was described by Lemierre in 1936.

Lemierre–Boltanski–Justin–Besançon syndrome (tuberculous alcoholic polyneuritis) Regarded by the original authors as a specific variety of polyneuropathy with twin etiologies, it seems likely that this condition represents the occurrence of both polyneuropathy and tuberculosis as complications of alcoholic malnutrition, although it is singular that the cases reported initially were all in relatively young women with marked cachexia, cirrhosis, and miliary tuberculosis. The condition has not hitherto been reported from the Western world.[3771]

Lemieux–Neemeh syndrome A congenital syndrome, perhaps recessively transmitted, manifesting sensorineural deafness, nephropathy, and sensorimotor neuropathy, resembling **hereditary motor and sensory neuropathy**.[3772]

lemniscal system (from Gr, bandage or woolen strand) One of two somatosensory systems (the other is the **spinothalamic**) comprising the ascending fiber pathway, which transmits tactile and kinesthetic impulses from the large myelinated fibers in the peripheral nerves and posterior columns to the medullary gracile and cuneate nuclei, from which arise second-order afferents, which decussate and pass to the ventrobasal thalamic nuclei. Nerve cells from here project to the primary somatosensory area of the postcentral cortex.

The system is highly adaptive, rapidly conducting, and mode- and place-specific, and appears to provide the anatomical base for the discriminative and localizing functions of the nervous system.

LEMS See **Lambert–Eaton myasthenic syndrome**.

lengthening reaction 1. When a tonic muscle is stretched, it assumes, by virtue of its proprioceptive arc, a new tonic length that is approximately the length to which it has been stretched.[5788]

2. **Sherrington** later wrote that in trying to bend the knee of a decerebrate animal, "the attempt causes further accentuation of the stretch reflex in muscles which are already highly responsive to stretching. If the attempt to flex the joint is maintained, there comes a point and time at which the muscle suddenly gives way and allows any degree of flexion to be imposed on it (the clasp-knife reaction). This is the lengthening reaction and it marks the partial or total abolition of the stretch reflex."[5164]

Lennox, William Gordon (1884–1960) American humanitarian, clinical neurophysiologist, and epileptologist who trained at Harvard and, after a period spent in China at the Rockefeller Medical School, satisfying in part his missionary zeal, returned to Harvard and began his lifelong studies of the cerebral circulation and later the nature and treatment of epilepsies.

He collaborated with Stanley Cobb, H.G. Wolff, F.A. Gibbs, E.L. Gibbs, and others during the long period of his research output. Prominent among the studies completed and published as a large series of papers was his investigation of the electrical activity of the brain, using the newly introduced EEG. His major book *Epilepsy and Related Disorders* (written in association with his daughter, Dr. Margaret Lennox-Buchthal) was immediately hailed as a classic.

In addition to his important laboratory studies, he built up a major epilepsy service and taught widely on all aspects of epilepsy, not the least being the importance of the education of the patient, the family, and the community.

Lennox disease See **Lennox–Gastaut syndrome**.

Lennox–Gastaut syndrome (severe myokinetic epilepsy of childhood with slow spike and wave, childhood encephalopathy with diffuse slow spike-waves, Lennox syndrome, minor motor seizures, myoclonic–astatic seizures)[1] An epileptic encephalopathy of infancy and childhood—a polioencephalopathy, characterized by the association of slow spike-wave activity in the EEG, mental retardation, and various types of intractable seizure (including tonic-axial, atypical absence, atonic, myoclonic and generalized tonic-clonic seizures, head drops, and falls) in children aged 1–8 years. The seizure frequency is high, and status epilepticus is frequent (stuporous states with myoclonic, tonic, and atonic seizures).[3777, 6833]

The EEG usually shows abnormally slow background activity, slow spike-waves (1–2.5 Hz), and often multifocal abnormalities. During sleep, bursts of fast rhythms appear. Seizures are difficult to control, and their development is mostly unfavorable. In 60% of the cases, the syndrome occurs in children suffering from a previous encephalopathy, but is primary in other cases. Known causes are metabolic and dysgenetic and many peri- or postnatal acquired disorders can also precipitate the syndrome.[1398] The prognosis is poor, severe neurological and mental deficits persisting for the remainder of the patient's life.

The term has been used to refer to a number of conditions, indicating that the precise delineation of the syndrome has not yet been achieved.

1. A syndrome of epilepsy in childhood accompanied by diffuse slow spike-wave patterns on the EEG (see above). In this childhood epileptic encephalopathy, there are diffuse interictal slow spike-wave complexes and multiple seizures including tonic seizures as well as atonic and myoclonic attacks, atypical absences, and even absence, tonic, or myoclonic status. The classic EEG feature is a diffuse slow spike-wave pattern originally described as a "petit mal variant." Secondary or symptomatic forms of the syndrome are common. Aicardi defines the syndrome as one limited to those cases characterized clinically by brief tonic and atonic seizures and atypical absences as the predominant types of attacks and from the EEG viewpoint by at least some 2-Hz (slow) diffuse spike-wave activity. Myoclonic seizures may also occur, as may 3-Hz (fast) spike-wave activity.[72] 2. **Myoclonic epilepsies**. In such *variants*, the frequency and intensity of the myoclonic jerks are both unusually high. The EEG is typical except that it is activated by overbreathing.[72] 3. An epileptic syndrome secondary to diffuse or mild focal brain damage and characterized by astatic and myoclonic seizures, mental retardation, the presence of neurological signs, and in most cases neuroradiological abnormalities.

See also **Epilepsy Foundation**, a charitable organization in this field providing information and support. Web site: http://www.epilepsyfoundation.org/ and Dreifuss FE, et al. Commission for classification and terminology, ILAE. Proposal for Revised Classifications of Epilepsies and Epileptic syndromes. *Epilepsia* 1989;30:389–99.

Lenoble–Aubineau syndrome (nystagmus–myoclonus syndrome) An X-linked congenital nonprogressive syndrome of nystagmus with myoclonic contractions of the extraocular and limb muscles occurring in response to cold and muscle percussion. Pigmentary retinopathy, tremor of the head and arms, muscle fasciculations, hyperactive reflexes, and vasomotor disturbances made worse by cold are also described.

The syndrome was described first in 1898 in the residents of Brittany[3778] and appears to be confined to Breton and British Celts.

lenticular, lenticulate (from Lat, a lens or a lentil)

lentiginosis–deafness–cardiopathy syndrome See **LEOPARD syndrome**.

Lenz micropthalmia syndrome An X-linked recessive or autosomal dominant syndrome characterized by micropthalmia; skeletal abnormalities of the hands; renal, genital, and dental abnormalities; and mental retardation with microcephaly.[3779]

Lenz–Majewski syndrome (hyperostotic dwarfism) A congenital dysmorphic syndrome manifesting also short stature, polysyndactyly, dental and dermal abnormalities, delayed closure of the fontanelles, a thick calvarium, sclerosis of the skull, osteoporosis, and spasticity.[4034]

Leonardo da Vinci (1452–1519) Italian artist, anatomist, and scientist. A brilliant contributor in many areas of science, art, and medicine, he himself dissected corpses and was probably the illustrator for Vesalius. He published in these pictures many structures that others proclaimed in prose only centuries later. There exists dispute as to his handedness, some suggesting that he was left-handed, others that he used the left hand only after he suffered a right hemiparesis.

Leonhard syndrome An acquired syndrome characterized by a disturbance in the sense of time, constructional apraxia, dysgraphia, and dyscalculia.[1335, 3781]

leontiasis ossea Bilateral hypertrophy of the bones of the cranial vault, leading to a lion-like appearance; first described by Marcello Malpighi (1628–1694), an Italian anatomist.

LEOPARD syndrome (dominant lentigines and congenital deafness, lentiginosis–deafness–cardiomyopathy syndrome) A dominantly inherited neurocutaneous syndrome consisting of multiple **l**entigines over the entire body, **e**lectrocardiographic conduction defects (due to hypertrophic cardiomyopathy), **o**cular hypertelorism giving a triangular shape to the face, **p**ulmonary stenosis, **a**bnormal genitalia, growth **r**etardation, and congenital severe neural **d**eafness with normal vestibular function.[2302] Scoliosis, spina bifida, dwarfism, and scapular winging are also described inconsistently. See also **multiple lentigenes syndrome**.

leopard skin appearance Hypointense punctate areas within the regions of demyelination on the MRI in **leukodystrophies**. See also **tigroid appearance**.

leprechaunism See **Donohue syndrome**.

lepromatous leprosy (nodular leprosy, cutaneous leprosy) That form of the disease in which the bacterial proliferation in the skin and peripheral nervous system proceeds unabated, leading to multiple mononeuropathies, the nerve territories involved being those in the distal, cooler parts of the body, where also the skin nodules and macules are most abundant.

The clinical features include those of a predominantly thin-fiber hypertrophic neuropathy with patchy sensory loss that eventually becomes confluent; mutilating acropathy; Charcot joints and autonomic involvement.[5485]

leprosy (from Gr, scaly) (Hansen disease, elephantiasis anesthetica, Kushtha) A mildly contagious disease with a long incubation period, caused by infection with the *Mycobacterium leprae* (Hansen bacillus), which has an affinity for cells originating from the neural crest. **Tuberculoid, lepromatous, dimorphous**, and **indeterminate** forms are described.

Leprosy was Hippocrates' name for psoriasis; later what we know today as leprosy was called *leontiasis* by Arateus of Cappadocia, while Lucretius and Celsus called it *elephantiasis*.[5886] *Kushtha* (in the Indian Vedas MS of 1300 BC) was probably the same disease, but English biblical translators, using bridging Arabian medical texts as well as Hebrew sources, rendered the Hebrew word tsara'ath ("zaraath"), meaning any variety of skin disease requiring separation from the tribe, as *leprosy*, which led to use of the term for **Hansen disease**,[2731] the leprosy that we recognize. There is good evidence that syphilis, not leprosy, was a more likely cause of the contagions referred to in Mosaic texts. (EWM)

This age-old condition was known in India at least 2500 years ago but was also found throughout Europe at least since the return to the Mediterranean shores of Alexander the Great. While it was taught that this was the commonest cause of neuropathy worldwide, limited control of the disease has meant that diabetes is now likely to be more prevalent as a cause. The various forms of leprosy are listed in Chart L–3.

leptocephaly (from Gr, thin + head) A malformation due to premature fusion of the anterior fontanelle and the metopic suture, leading to elongation of the skull and narrowing of the forehead.[4]

leptomeningeal carcinomatosis A rare metastatic complication of solid tumors, usually of the breast or lung or of melanoma. It usually presents with headache, altered level of consciousness, and focal neurological deficits. Imaging shows meningeal enhancement and the CSF contains malignant cells.[31]

leptomeningeal cyst See **arachnoid diverticula**.

leptomeningeal glioneuronal heterotopias Irregular nodules of glial tissue, sometimes containing neurons, budding from the pial surface or forming nests within the leptomeninges.[471]

leptomeninges (Gr, thin + membrane) The pia and arachnoid—the delicate as opposed to the coarse (dural) meninges.

leptomeningitis Inflammation of the arachnoid and pia mater. Although the term was originally used to refer to inflammation

Chart L–3. The Forms of Leprosy

The *tuberculoid* form indicates the presence of increased resistance, as is seen mainly in African patients, in whom classically there are a few asymmetrical lesions, the skin is dry, scaly, and anesthetic in places, and there is evidence of a thin-fiber neuropathy in such areas. The lepromin test result is strongly positive and the nerves are enlarged and granulomatous. Acid-fast bacilli are not found.

In an *intermediate form (BT type)*, the clinical features are the same, but the number of lesions is markedly increased and there is more scaling induration of the skin and less evidence of neuropathy and sensory loss.

In the second major form (*borderline, intermediate dimorphic or BB type*), the skin lesions consist of rounded red papules that are not anesthetic. Intermediate between this and the third major form is a type characterized by the presence of macular, popular, or nodular lesions that are asymmetrical (BL type) and which contain substantial numbers of acid-fast bacilli.

In the third major *lepromatous* form (LL type), there is decreased resistance or even no resistance to the acid-fast bacilli. The Lepromin test result is negative and mycobacteria are abundant.

In a diffuse *variant*, the whole skin is thickened; this has given rise to the name *pretty leprosy* as facial wrinkles are abolished; and in a nodular lepromatous form, nodules form plaques in the skin in all regions, although less upon the scalp and in the axillae and groins. A late finding in this form is the presence of generalized symmetrical polyneuropathy.

In a *variant* form (*neural leprosy*), only the nerves are involved and the skin is unaffected; however, anesthetic patches are detected, mainly distally and in the colder acral parts. Dementia is a rare complication. See also **mutilating acropathy** and **ocular leprosy**.

of these thinner meninges, it has now been replaced by the simpler **meningitis** to embrace all forms of infection of the meninges .

Léri, André (1875–1930) French physician who trained in Paris and took further training with **Charcot** and **Marie** at the **Salpêtrière**. He practiced in Paris, writing mainly on rheumatic and neurological topics.

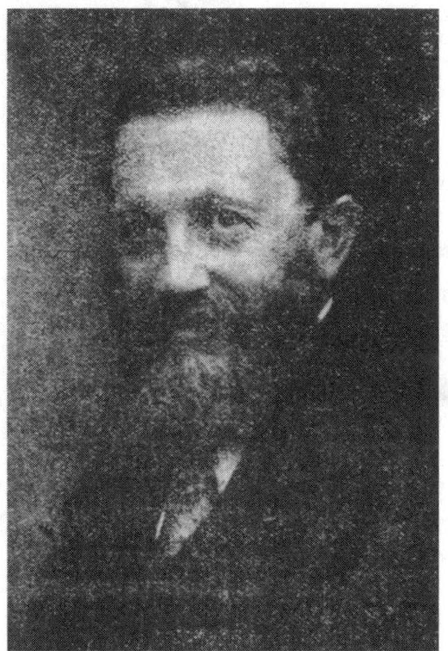

Figure L–6 André Léri.

Léri reflex See **Léri sign**.

Léri sign (Léri reflex) Flexion of the elbow of the patient's relaxed arm in response to forceful and painful passive flexion of the fingers and hand on that side; said to be increased in subjects with lesions of the pyramidal tracts or of the frontal lobes.[3784] The difference between this and the **bending reflex** is not easy to discern.

Léri syndrome (pleonosteosis) A dominantly inherited congenital osteodystrophy with premature ossification of the epiphyses, leading to dwarfism, corneal opacities, and cataract, and often to compression of the median nerve in the carpal tunnel.[5809]

Lériche syndrome Occlusion of the aorta or iliac arteries causing ischemic pain in the buttocks and legs, as well as, variably, either **impotence** or **priapism**.[3785]

Lermoyez, M. (1858–1929) French otolaryngologist.

Lermoyez syndrome Tinnitus, nausea, vomiting, and deafness with temporary improvement in hearing after the onset of vertigo. The attacks complicate a condition of gradually increasing deafness, as in **Ménière syndrome**, but generally occur in younger adults.[3788]

Leroy, Raoul (b. 1868) French psychiatrist.

Leroy syndrome (Lilliputian hallucinosis) The perception of hallucinations of small people, animals, etc., against a background of normal size. The phenomenon thus differs from **micropsia**, in which everything is seen in miniature.

The occurrence of such hallucinations was recorded by Macarius in *The Lives of the Saints* (4th century AD) who dismissed them with the words "Arise, Oh Lord, that your enemies might be dispersed, that they may flee before Thy face; for our soul is full of illusions."[5704] Henceforward, they were usually documented in religious mystics, in those suffering from systemic infections or in those exposed to toxic substances such as ether, hashish, cocaine, hyoscine, or caffeine. Organic brain diseases held responsible have been many and various—**general paralysis of the insane**, seizures, temporoparietal tumors, and lobar hematomas, for example—and these hallucinations have also been reported in dementing states and in schizophrenia.

Finally, they have also been recorded in healthy people, including Ben Jonson (the playwright), who regarded them as products of his "overheated imagination."

Les Turner ALS Foundation, Ltd. A charitable organization based at 3325 West Main Street, Skokie, IL 60076. Web site: http://www.lesturnerals.org/

Lesch–Nyhan syndrome A congenital X-linked recessive syndrome with the abnormal locus situated at chromosome Xq26, characterized clinically by choreic, dystonic, and athetoid movements, pyramidal signs, hyperuricemia with urinary stone formation, mental retardation, and compulsive, recurrent self-injurious behavior such as biting the lips, cheeks, and fingers. Deficiency of hypoxanthine-guanine phosphoribosyltransferase,[3791] overproduction of uric acid, and low levels of immunoglobulin E are commonly found.[3222, 3886]

As a *variant*, some forms present late with choreiform movements, dysarthria, and renal stones.

lethal catatonia A rare syndrome resembling the **neuroleptic malignant syndrome**, characterized by prolonged mental and physical excitement and agitation leading on to stupor and hypotension with muscle rigidity, hyperpyrexia, increased serum CK levels, and death. The condition was first described by Calmeil in 1832. Typically, the patient becomes rigid and mute, with periods of intense agitation and bizarre repetitive movements. This condition occurs in the setting of a major psychiatric disturbance with labile mood, insomnia, anorexia, increasingly disorganized thought processes, auditory and visual hallucinations, as well as bizarre delusions. Violence is occasionally a feature, and there may be unprovoked assaults and attempts at suicide. High fever, tachycardia, and fluctuations in blood pressure develop and can be followed after several days by exhaustion, coma, cardiac arrest, and death.

The autonomic features and abnormal movements characteristic of the **neuroleptic malignant syndrome** are not seen in this condition.[4044]

lethal multiple pterygium syndrome A congenital recessively inherited dysmorphic syndrome characterized by low birthweight, dwarfism, hypertelorism, cleft upper lip and palate, webbed neck often with a cystic hygroma, fusion of vertebrae, hydranencephaly, congenital hernia of the diaphragm, congenital cardiac anomalies, lung hypoplasia, webbing of the elbows and knees, radioulnar synostosis, symphalangism of the fingers, and neurogenic muscle weakness.[4195]

lethargic encephalitis See **encephalitis lethargica**.

lethargy (Gr, forgetful) The ancient meaning has given way to that of a state of drowsy inertia.

letter fluency test A test of language in which subjects are asked to name verbally as many words beginning with the letters "F," "A," and "S" as they can within 1 min, proper names and different forms of the same word being disallowed.[2732] See also **Category Fluency Test** and **FAS Test**.

Letterer-Siwe histiocytosis A diffuse encephalopathy of infants, who also manifest osteolytic bone lesions, hepatosplenomegaly, a reduction in all blood cell types with hemorrhage, and skin infiltration. The condition is a disseminated form of histiocytosis.

Lettsom, John Coakley (1744–1815) A popular and successful English Quaker physician working in the Virgin islands, where he was the first to describe alcoholic peripheral neuropathy.[3373] He later returned to practice in London, where he probably became aware of **delirium tremens** and of the **Wernicke–Korsakoff** syndrome too.

leucine encephalin An opioid peptide in the brain with a role in the mediation of pain perception.

leukemia A systemic hematological malignancy with neurological complications including intracerebral hemorrhages, the accumulation of leukemic cells within the brain, **progressive multifocal leukoencephalopathy**, and infiltration of the meninges.

leukoaraiosis (from Gr, white + rarefied) A modern descriptive term for the presence of lucencies (patchy diffuse areas of low attenuation) in the deep white matter surrounding the frontal and occipital horns and in the centrum semiovale.[2665] It is clinically associated with advancing age, a history of hypertension, motor weakness, upgoing plantar responses, and signs of the multi-infarct rather than of the Alzheimer type of dementia. The condition is a descriptive label and is associated with numerous pathologies including lacunar strokes, cerebral amyloid angiopathy, CADASIL, and possibly migraine.

Diffuse confluent white matter abnormalities showing low density on CT and high intensity on T2 weighted or FLAIR MRI scans, often with irregular margins, are notable imaging findings.

leukocytoclastic angiitis See **Churg–Strauss syndrome**.

leukodysplasia, microcephaly, and cerebral malformation An autosomal recessive congenital microcephaly mapped to chromosome 2p16 with severe failure of postnatal brain growth, the neonatal onset of intractable seizures, lack of developmental progression, and death within 3 years. Cerebral imaging shows simplified gyration, a nonthickened cortex, severe hypoplasia of the corpus callosum, a small flattened brain stem, and specific cystic lesions in the white matter around the temporal and occipital horns.[1092]

leukodystrophies A group of progressive genetically determined demyelinating disorders selectively affecting the myelin of the cerebral or peripheral nervous system. The main disorders and their subgroups were classified by Baraitser.[379] Some additions are made in Chart L–4.

leukodystrophy, cerebellar deficits, and spastic paraparesis A dominantly inherited disorder with onset in early childhood characterized by progressive spastic paraparesis, cerebellar deficits, and mild mental deterioration, resulting in severe disability in the third to fourth decades of life. Brain MRI shows diffuse white matter involvement but no biochemical or genetic deficits have been determined.[2229]

leukodystrophy with brain stem and spinal cord involvement and high lactate A syndrome of slowly progressive pyramidal, cerebellar dysfunction, often with dorsal column dysfunction and with an MRI pattern showing heterogeneous cerebral white matter abnormalities and selective tract involvement over their lengths. Onset is in childhood or youth, with spasticity and ataxia mainly affecting the legs.[6486]

leukoencephalopathy Any disease primarily affecting the white matter of the brain. See also **posterior leukoencephalopathy, toxic leukoencephalopathy, hereditary adult-onset leukoencephalopathy**, and **polycystic lipomembranous osteodysplasia with sclerosing leukoencephalopathy** as well as the preceding and succeeding entries.

Chart L–4. The Leukodystrophies

Aicardi–Goutières syndrome
Alexander disease

X-linked forms:

Adrenoleukodystrophies
Adrenoleukomyeloneuropathies
Infantile sudanophilic leukodystrophy
Cerebrotendinous xanthomatosis
Cockayne syndrome
18q syndrome

Glial or glioneuronal degenerations

Alpers disease
Canavan disease
Glioneuronal degeneration
Globoid-cell leukodystrophy (Krabbe disease)
Infantile neuroaxonal dystrophy
NBIA (Neurodegeneration with Brain Iron Accumulation)
Menkes disease
Metachromatic leukodystrophy
Multiple sulfatidase deficiency (Austin disease)
Pelizaeus–Merzbacher disease
Polycystic lipomembranous osteodysplasia with sclerosing leukoencephalopathy
Reye syndrome
Sjogren–Larsson syndrome

Orphan genetic leukodystrophies

Adult-onset autosomal dominant leukodystrophy
Cystic leukoencephalopathy without megalencephaly
Dominantly inherited leukodystrophy with cerebellar deficits and spastic paraparesis
fatal infantile leukoencephalopathy (CACH, vanishing white matter disease)
Hereditary diffuse leukoencephalopathy with spheroids
Leukoencephalopathy, cerebral calcifications, and cysts
Leukoencephalopathy with metaphyseal chondrodysplasia
Ovarioleukodystrophy
Vacuolating megalencephalic leukodystrophy with subcortical cysts

Modified from Baraitser M. *The Genetics of Neurological Disorders*. Oxford, Oxford University Press, 2nd edition, 1990; and Berger, et al. (2001)[554]

leukoencephalopathy, cerebral calcifications, and cysts A rare, probably recessively inherited microangiopathic syndrome of childhood manifesting these features, some of which overlap with those of **Coats disease**.[4574]

leukoencephalopathy with ataxia, hypodontia, and hypomyelination A hypomyelination syndrome of childhood characterized by the early onset of slowly progressive ataxia, short stature, hypodontia, hypomyelination, and cerebellar atrophy.[6843]

leukoencephalopathy with metaphyseal chondrodysplasia A slowly progressive X-linked syndrome of childhood characterized by the onset after the age of 2 of spastic paraparesis, tremor, ataxia, optic atrophy, and eventually spastic tetraparesis and metaphyseal chondrodysplasia.[4630]

leukoencephalopathy with neuroaxonal spheroids A rare, dominantly inherited progressive, diffuse white matter disorder with onset in adult life, characterized by seizures, evidence of frontal lobe dysfunction, pyramidal signs, ataxia, and mild extrapyramidal signs. MRI shows cortical atrophy and multifocal white matter changes especially in frontal regions. Biopsy reveals the presence of axonal spheroids in the white matter.[6483]

leukoencephalopathy with ragged red fibers See MERRF.

leukoencephalopathy with vanishing white matter (CACH) A chronic progressive and episodic disease of childhood and youth, probably recessively inherited, manifesting episodes of deterioration following infections and minor head traumas that result in unexplained coma. The MRI findings are of changes such that the signals from the white matter resemble those of CSF as a result of extensive cystic degeneration of the cerebral white matter, the cortex being preserved.[6484] See also **fatal infantile leukodystrophy**.

leukoma A corneal scar.

levator (from Lat, to lift up) The first name of those muscles elevating, for example, the eyelids, the pelvic floor, and the scapula.

levator dehiscence–disinsertion syndrome Separation of the levator palpebrae superioris muscle from its origin as a result of inflammation, also described after local surgical procedures and in the elderly; a cause of ptosis.

levels of organization A concept of Hughlings-**Jackson** in which he postulated the existence of separate hierarchically ordered brain regions that function together to produce a motor effect. The *highest level* is made up of centers of the prefrontal lobes and governs the most complex movements of all parts of the body from the eyes to the perineum. ("The central nervous system knows nothing of muscles, it only knows movements . . . There are, shall we say, thirty muscles in the hand, these are represented in the nervous system in thousands of combinations—that is, as very many movements. It is just as many chords, musical expressions and tunes, can be made out of a few notes.") The *second level* is composed of centers of the rolandic region (so-called motor regions of the cerebral cortex) and possibly of the ganglia of the corpus striatum as well. It is responsible for mediating complex movements of all parts of the body from the eyes to the perineum. The *lowest level*, corresponding to the pons, medulla, spinal cord, and motor units, represents the simplest movements of all parts of the body mediated by a series of lower motor centers.[61, 800] In fact, at this last level, the CNS structures mainly function as lines of communication.

The analogy of an army is appropriate; at the highest level, the general determines the strategy, namely what is to be accomplished by military means; the staff determine the mechanisms whereby that goal is to be accomplished; and, at the lowest level of organization (corresponding to the motor unit), the soldiers try to do it.

Levic syndrome See **progressive nuclear ophthalmoplegia syndrome**.

Levin, Max (b. 1901) American neuropsychiatrist, born in Latvia, who graduated from Johns Hopkins and worked in neurology and psychiatry in Philadelphia and Pittsburg before returning to Johns Hopkins and eventually becoming clinical professor of neurology at the New York Medical College. He is best remembered for his description of the **Kline–Levin syndrome** in 1936; his other publications chiefly focused on toxic psychoses and delirium.

Levine syndrome See **neuroacanthocytosis**.

Lévy, Gabrielle (1886–1935) French neurologist who collaborated with Roussy in describing the **Roussy–Lévy syndrome**.

Lewis–Besant dystrophy A rare congenital muscular dystrophy localized to the diaphragm and pectoralis muscles and leading to early death.[3817]

Lewis–Sumner syndrome (multifocal acquired demyelinating sensory and motor neuropathy/MADSAMN; multifocal motor sensory demyelinating neuropathy/MMSDN) An immune-mediated form of neuropathy with slow progression presenting with asymmetrical weakness (predominantly distal, asymmetric weakness mainly affecting the upper limbs but involving the cranial nerves in a few patients) with sensory impairment and atrophy and impaired sensation in the distribution of specific peripheral nerves. There is evidence of persistent multifocal conduction block over short segments of the affected nerves. Muscle cramps and fasciculations are common complaints. The CSF protein is raised in a third of cases. The condition can be distinguished from multifocal motor neuropathy by the presence of sensory involvement, the absence of serum anti-GM_1 antibodies, and, in some cases, a positive response to steroids.[6540]

Whether this condition is the same as or distinct from **multifocal motor neuropathy with conduction block** or **chronic inflammatory demyelinating polyneuropathy** (into which state the condition occasionally evolves) is unresolved.[4915, 5548] See also **multifocal inflammatory demyelinating neuropathy**.

Lewy (Lewey) Fritz Heinrich (1885–1950) German neuropathologist, neurologist, and psychiatrist who left Germany urgently in 1934 to live in the United States, where he held academic appointments at the University of Pennsylvania.

Lewy bodies Intracytoplasmic, eosinophilic, hyaline inclusions staining for α-synuclein and ubiquitin, signifying the presence of neuronal injury and found in the cortex, substantia nigra, autonomic nervous system, basal nucleus of Meynert, and brain stem nuclei in patients with **Parkinson disease, NBIA, dopa-responsive dystonia**, idiopathic **dementia with Lewy bodies**, and some other disorders affecting the basal ganglia.[3822]

They are also found in the anterior horn cells in **amyotrophic lateral sclerosis** and have been found in asymptomatic elderly people. The most consistent association is with dementia in patients with Parkinson disease.[2359] Lewy bodies are detected more frequently with increasing age.[2355]

Lewy body disorders Conditions comprising **Parkinson disease, Parkinson disease with dementia**, and **dementia with Lewy bodies**, or pure autonomic failure, linked by their shared basis as disorders of α-synuclein metabolism. As the Lewy bodies and the neurites and oligodendroglial inclusions in **multiple system atrophy** are composed of α-synuclein, these disorders are named **synucleopathies**.

Lewy neurites Nerve cell processes containing α-synuclein seen in **Parkinson disease with dementia, Parkinson disease**, and **dementia with Lewy bodies**.

lexical agraphia A form of agraphia marked by the impairment of writing of words but not of speech, of spelling without impairment of phoneme–grapheme conversion, nor of reading. There is thus a specific difficulty in spelling words with irregular phoneme–grapheme transformations. The condition has been reported in the context of a left parieto-occipital lesion.[465]

lexical system One of two reading method systems (the other being the phonological system) in which reading is considered to be performed by lexical or semantic processing. This system is affected when *surface dyslexia* occurs, in which subjects can read pronounceable nonsense words but not orthographically irregular words.

lexicon The words contained in a language and their semantic definitions.[3949]

Leyden, Ernst Victor von (1832–1910) German physician who became professor of medicine in Berlin after Frerichs. He was most successful in his practice, in which he concentrated on tuberculosis and neurological diseases, especially poliomyelitis, tabes, and muscular dystrophy. He also described a form of ataxia (pseudotabes), periodic vomiting, and the following disorders.

Leyden ataxia See **acute cerebellar ataxia**.

Leyden neuritis (lipomatous neuritis) Neuropathy with fatty replacement of the degenerating nerve fibers. Leyden's paper was entitled [*On Poliomyelitis and Neuritis*] and this condition may be a variant of that viral motor neuropathy.

Leyden paralysis 1. See **Weber syndrome**. 2. Quadriplegia associated with pontine hemorrhage, described by Leyden in 1875.

Leyden syndrome (cerebral peduncle syndrome) See **Weber syndrome**.

Leyden–Möbius muscular dystrophy A recessively inherited muscular dystrophy affecting the pelvic girdle initially and beginning in adult life.[3823] The classification of this among similar syndromes is in flux. See also **limb-girdle muscular dystrophy** and **scapulo humeral dystrophy**.

Lhermitte, Jean-Jacques (1877–1959) French neurologist who trained in Paris and after graduation became chef de clinique under Raymond at the Salpêtrière. Later, he emphazised psychiatry in his practice and held the chair of mental diseases at the Hôpital Ste. Anne. He coined the term **internuclear ophthalmoplegia** (sometimes known as *Lhermitte syndrome*), described the sign described in the next entry and **peduncular hallucinosis**, and made significant contributions to the study of **narcolepsy**,[3828] **encephalitis lethargica**, herpes, neuropathies, **Huntington disease**, sleep, phantom limb, and disturbances of the body image.[1198, 5704]

Lhermitte sign (barber's chair sign) Described in 1924 by Lhermitte (but before him by **Babinski**), this is more properly a symptom, comprising a sensation as of an electric shock or paresthesia that shoots down the back and/or into the limbs when the neck is flexed or with coughing or neck flexion or rotation.[3834]

Although Lhermitte regarded the sign as diagnostic of **multiple sclerosis**, any cervical cord lesion, intrinsic or extrinsic, is capable of inducing it.

Lhermitte syndrome 1. See **peduncular hallucinosis**.[3832] 2. See **internuclear ophthalomoplegia**.

Lhermitte–Cornil–Quesnel syndrome (progressive pyramidopallidal degeneration) A rare syndrome of slowly progressive degeneration of the pyramidal and pallidal systems, manifest as pathological emotionality, generalized muscle rigidity, pseudobulbar palsy, Parkinsonian signs, and chorea. Pathologically, there is cell loss in the basal ganglia and dentate nucleus with calcium deposition.[3830, 3833]

Dr. Lucien Cornil (1888–1952) was a French physician who trained in Paris and worked with Roussy and Lhermitte during the First World War on spinal cord injuries. He later became professor of experimental medicine at Marseille.

Lhermitte–Duclos disease (granular cell hypertrophy, cerebrellar hamartoma, dysplastic gangliocytoma of the cerebellum, Purkinjeoma, Cowden disease, diffuse cerebellar cortical hypertrophy, striated cerebellum) A sporadic or dominantly inherited hamartomatous condition of cerebellar hypertrophy with onset in childhood or adult life, characterized by hypertrophy of the ganglion cells in the granular and molecular layers and excessive myelination of axons in the molecular layer. The gyri are "coarse." Whether the condition represents a neoplasm, a malformation, or a hamartoma remains undetermined.

Clinical manifestations include macrocephaly, increased intracranial pressure, and mental and developmental delay.[4850, 6553] See also **Cowden disease**, which may indeed be a *variant* of this condition.

Lhermitte–McAlpine syndrome A syndrome of gradual onset and slow progression affecting adults and characterized by Parkinsonism and choreic movements of the face and bulbar muscles with pseudobulbar and pyramidal signs and marked hypertonia, with only slight weakness. Pathological examination shows lesions in the putamen, globus pallidus, and pyramidal tracts.[3833]

Lichtenstein–Knorr syndrome A rare, congenital, recessively inherited ataxic syndrome characterized also by progressive deafness and skeletal anomalies.[3837]

Lichtheim, Ludwig (1845–1928) German pathologist and neurologist who graduated from Zurich and eventually succeeded **Quincke** as professor of medicine at Berne. He later removed to Königsberg.

Lichtheim made important contributions to the study of aphasia, describing subcortical aphasia in 1885, and also wrote on the topics of pseudobulbar palsy, brain tumors, meningitis, the spinal cord in pernicious anemia (once known as *Lichtheim syndrome*), and oculomotor palsies, as well as on general pathology.[5704]

Lichtheim aphasia (subcortical sensory aphasia) A form of expressive dysphasia in which the patient is mute but able to indicate with his fingers the number of syllables in the word he would like to utter.[3838]

Lichtheim syndrome See **subacute combined degeneration of the cord**.[4060]

lid apraxia See **apraxia of eyelid opening**.

lid lag Abnormal delay in descent of the eyelid when the globe of the eye rotates downward. This classic sign was described by **von Graefe** in hyperthyroidism. See **Graefe sign**.

lid nystagmus Type 1—Jerky vertical movements of the eyelids, mimicking (but exceeding the amplitude of) an underlying vertical nystagmus.[277] Type 2—Rapid, phasic twitches of the eyelids occurring with lateral deviation of the eyes in patients with horizontal jerk nystagmus, as in the **lateral medullary syndrome**. Type 3—Similar movements to the last, occurring on convergence in the presence of cerebellar or medullary lesions.[1460, 5535] Type 4—The association of type 3 lid nystagmus with neck extension movements during attempts at upward gaze.[2400] This is described in the **Miller Fisher syndrome**.

lid retraction Elevation of the upper lid, giving rise to a staring gaze and occurring in association with the **dorsal midbrain syndrome**. See also **Collier sign**.

lid twitch sign See **Cogan twitch sign**.

Liepmann, Hugo Karl (1863–1925) German psychiatrist and humanitarian who graduated in philosophy and then in medicine from Berlin and who then studied further under Weigert and **Wernicke**. He directed a mental hospital for some years but then entered private practice since he was excluded from a chair in psychiatry because of his Jewish birth. He showed in 1904 that the left hemisphere is dominant for praxis in right-handed people; other topics to which he contributed were alcoholic delirium, agnosias, and the effects of callosal lesions.

During the final blockade of Germany in 1918, he refused to eat any better than did his patients and as a result lost 60 lb, but it was his **Parkinson disease** that led him to suicide in 1925.

Liepmann disease Motor apraxia—the inability to perform skilled acts in the presence of normal motor power and coordination, differentiated by Liepmann into three varieties: ideational, ideomotor, and limb-kinetic.[3845] See also **apraxia**.

ligature neuropathy Severe ischemic damage to peripheral nerves, described in association with the detention of prisoners by their adversaries using tight cables to bind the limbs for prolonged periods. See also **handcuff neuropathy**.

light blindness Episodic binocular visual impairment related exclusively to exposure to light. The cause is usually bilateral stenosis or occlusion of the internal carotid arteries causing delay in the regeneration of visual pigment in the relevant epithelial layer of the retina.[6769]

light reflex Constriction of the pupil stimulated by light, the first modern description of which was that of **Robert Whytt** in 1751.

light sleep stage Non-rapid eye movement sleep stages 1 and 2.[280]

light stress test (photostress test) A method of assessing the degree of macular disease as opposed to optic nerve disease, based upon the impairment of photochemical processes in the retina as a result of local disease. The function tested is the delay in the regeneration of visual pigment after retinal "bleaching" with the light; optic nerve disease is not associated with any delay in the return of visual acuity in this test.[2401]

The best-corrected vision is assessed in each eye, and then bright light is shown into one eye for 10 s. The amount of time elapsing before the patient can read one line larger than he could prior to the light stimulation is recorded, and the process is then repeated in the opposite eye. Normally, the recovery takes less than 1 min (usually less than 30 s) but in the presence of macular disease, recovery takes longer than a minute, while in the presence of optic nerve disease, the recovery time should be normal.[2401]

light-near dissociation Pupillary constriction occurring when a person focuses on a close object, but not in response to light stimulation. The mechanism is more likely to be found in the much more extensive innervation of the ciliary muscle than of the sphincter; after infection or other injury to the ciliary ganglion, some of the nerves passing to the ciliary muscle sprout into channels destined for the sphincter muscle instead.

lightning encephalopathy Syndromes exhibited by victims of lightning strikes. In the acute stage, these include immediate but transient unconsciousness, amnesia, headache, and temporary pareses (**keraunoparalysis**), most likely due to circulatory arrest with hypoxic encephalopathy, less commonly due to intracranial hemorrhage or cerebral infarction. Delayed syndromes can also occur; these are progressive and include Parkinsonism, myelopathy, and a syndrome resembling **amyotrophic lateral sclerosis**.[1136, 1137]

Electrical currents delivered by Tasers© ("stun guns") also appear able to cause some of these short-term effects and even death.

lightning eye movements Uncommon fast horizontal ocular dyskinesias of small amplitude, which represent disordered saccadic deviations and which may be seen with lesions of the Parapontine reticular formation.[284] See also **square-wave jerks**, **opsoclonus**, and **ocular myoclonus**.

lightning eyes See **opsoclonus**.

lightning pains Sudden lancinating pains. occurring chiefly in the legs but also in the trunk, arms, or even head. They are paroxysmal, lasting some hours or a day or two, and represent irritation of the dorsal roots, typically seen in **tabes dorsalis**.[1107] Similar pains occur in **trigeminal neuralgia**.

lightning polyneuropathy An acute polyneuropathy resulting from extensive peripheral nerve damage as a result of being struck by lightning. Apart from death, cataract, autonomic dysfunction, renal failure, **rhabdomyolysis**, and respiratory distress syndrome are also documented complications of this mishap.[2801]

lightning streaks (Moore lightning streaks) Brief, alarming but benign luminous visual impressions arising as a result of separation of the vitreous from the surface of the retina.[4462]

lightning stroke A syndrome of subtle cognitive impairment described in survivors of a lightning strike, manifest as loss of consciousness with subsequent amnesia, fatigue, loss of energy, irritability, and emotional lability with associated impairments in attention, memory, and visual reaction times.[6509] The similarity to **chronic fatigue syndrome** is obvious.

Lihastautiliitto R.Y. A member society of the European Alliance of Muscular Dystrophy Societies based at De Muskelhandikappades Forbund RF, Lantinen Pitkakatu 35, SF-0100 Turku, Finland.

Lille Apathy Rating Scale A 33-item scale assessing manifestations of apathy such as reduction in everyday productivity, lack of interest, lack of initiative, extinction of novelty-seeking and motivation, blunting of emotional responses, lack of concern, and poor social life. It has been validated for use in **Parkinson disease**.[5940]

Lilliputian hallucinations The hallucinated perception of small people, alone or with small animals. The beings are mobile, colored, and generally multiple and are seen by the subject within real external space (which itself is of normal size). The Lilliputian people occasionally speak, not surprisingly in small voices.

The phenomenon occurs in toxic encephalopathies such as those due to alcohol, cocaine, or marijuana abuse and (rarely) as an aura in migraine.[3789] See also **Leroy syndrome**.

limb apraxia See **apraxia**.

limb placement reaction When a healthy baby is supported and the anterior aspect of the tibia or of the ulna is brought into contact with the edge of a table, the leg or the arm is lifted and placed on the surface of the table. See also **placing reaction**.

limb shaking The occurrence of brief, irregular, coarse, and wavering movements of an arm or leg, or both; it is evidence of a transient ischemic attack in the carotid territory[2081] and occurs as a result of **cerebrovascular insufficiency**.[376]

limb-girdle muscular dystrophy (LGMD, Erb–Landouzy syndrome, Erb dystrophy, dystrophia muscularis progressiva) A heterogeneous group of diseases, sporadic or variously inherited, which share the common characteristic of slowly progressive girdle and proximal limb weakness (often sparing the deltoid muscles at first) with later spread to the pelvic girdle and limbs[1901] and which are not caused by a primary dystrophin deficiency. Only heel-cord contractures are commonly found. Myopathic features are notable on muscle biopsy specimens and serum CK levels are very high.[4709]

The condition starts at variable ages between birth and later adult life, and it is unlikely that it represents a single entity, a number of conditions formerly so diagnosed now being classified as, for example, **congenital myopathies**. Fifteen forms are known, 10 autosomal recessive and accounting for over 90% of cases, and 5 autosomal dominant.

A complete classification of limb girdle muscle dystrophies (and of all other neuromuscular diseases) is provided by Dr. Alan Pestronk at his Web site http://www.neuro.wustl.edu/neuromuscular/musdist/lg.html.

Genotype–phenotype correlations in this group are poor. Forms of autosomal recessive LGMD include calpainopathy, *caveolinopathy*, *telethoninopathy*, *and dysferlinopathy.* Some LGMDs share pathogenetic mechanisms with other forms of muscular dystrophy, such as the *sarcoglycanopathies* (LGMD2C–F) and the *dystrophinopathies* (Duchenne and Becker muscular dystrophy) and some are allelic with other forms of muscular dystrophy. Thus LGMD1B is allelic with autosomal dominant muscular dystrophy and LGMD2H is likely due to mutations affecting the *ubiquitin–proteasome* pathway.

Chart L–5. Forms of Limbe-Girdle Muscular Dystrophy

Dominant limb-girdle dystrophies: Much of the following information is derived from the Web site of Dr. Alan Pestronk (http://neuromuscular.-wustl.edu/musdist/lg.html) with kind permission.

LGMD1 subtypes present with weakness and atrophy, which are roughly symmetrical, and in some cases there are complaints of stiffness and myalgias. Bulbar signs may be present. There is occasionally evidence of cardiomyopathy. Progression is usually slow. The forms described include the following:

LGMD1A (**5q22, myotilin**) Onset is in adult life. Dysarthria is added to the usual features. **Spheroid body myopathy** is a variant.

LGMD1B (1q11–21, **lamin A/C gene**) Onset is in childhood or youth with symmetrical proximal leg weakness, contractures and frequently rigid spine, and cardiomyopathy.[3454] **Quadriceps myopathy** is a variant. This condition is allelic with dominant Emery–Dreifuss dystrophy.

LGMD1C (3p25, **caveolin**) Onset is from childhood to late adult life with pelvic girdle weakness and possibly calf pseudohypertrophy. **Idiopathic hyperCKemia, rippling muscle disease**, and distal myopathy are associated.

LGMD1D (7q; 6q23?) A form with adult onset.

LGMD(?1E) **familial dilated cardiomyopathy** (7q) Onset is in youth or adult life without cranial involvement but with significant arrhythmias, later cardiac failure and sometimes sudden death.

continued

Chart L–5. (*continued*)

LGMD1F (7q32) The onset of distal weakness is in youth or adult life.
LGMD1G (4q21) A form with adult onset and with notable leg cramps. Biopsy shows rimmed vacuoles.

Other dominantly inherited *variants* are:

Autosomal dominant cardiomyopathy with conduction system disease
Bethlem myopathy (21q22 and 2q37, *collagen VI*) A form allelic with **Ulrich muscular dystrophy**, usually presenting in infancy or early childhood with hypotonia, proximal and distal weakness, and contractures, especially in the hands. Its course is relatively benign.
Multiple epiphyseal dysplasia with mild myopathy (20q13.3, *collagen 9*) A form with childhood onset of joint pains and symmetrical proximal girdle, including neck, weakness.
Dominant myopathy with bone fragility (9p21–p22) A rare variant presenting in young adult life with proximal weakness, a tendency to bone fractures with poor healing, premature gray hair, and hernias.
Dominant myopathy with cardiomyopathy Possibly the same condition as *LGMD1*; it presents in childhood or adult life with proximal symmetrical girdle weakness, which leads to the development of cardiomyopathy and the potential for sudden death.
Dominant myopathy with ankle contractures and high CK levels A form with onset in adolescence or early adult life with proximal symmetric weakness, ankle contractures, and eventual severe disability. CK levels are very high.
Barnes myopathy This is possibly the same condition as *LGMD1*.
Other *variants* with *earlier onset or later onset with dominant inheritance*,[869, 1179] the dominant form mapping to 5q22.
Laing early-onset distal myopathy A form presenting with initial weakness of the hallux and of ankle dorsiflexion but with the later development of weakness of finger extension and neck flexion. Age of onset is before the age of 30 and progression is slow. The condition is due to mutations within the slow skeletal muscle heavy chain gene *MYH7* and is allelic with **hyaline body myopathy**.[3653]

Other dominantly inherited myopathies include

Central core disease
Cytoplasmic body myopathy
Centronuclear myopathy
Distal myopathies
Emery–Dreifuss muscular dystrophy
Facioscapulohumeral dystrophies
Hyperkalemic periodic paralysis
Myofibrillar (desmin storage) myopathy
Myotonic dystrophy
Oculopharyngeal dystrophy
Proximal myotonic myopathy
Rippling muscle syndromes (some *variants*)
Scapuloperoneal syndrome (most *variants*)

Recessive limb-girdle dystrophies

Much of the following is taken from the Web site of Dr. Alan Pestronk (http://neuromuscular.wustl.edu/musdist/lg.html) with kind permission.
Most of the forms of LGMD2 are recessively inherited. The numerous chromosomal mutation sites variously encode for calpain-3, dysferlin, sarcoglycans, and telethonin.[1660, 1732, 4166, 6954]

LGMD2A (15–*q*15.1, *calpain-3*) Onset is in childhood or youth (Leyden–Möbius dystrophy) or later (Erb dystrophy) with scapular, pelvic girdle, and trunk weakness with sparing of the face and hip abductors. CK levels may be normal or grossly raised.
LGMD2B (2*p*13.3, *dysferlin*) Onset is in youth or young adult life with weakness affecting the legs (especially the gastrocnemii) earlier than the arms. Progression is slow and CK levels are very high. The condition is allelic with Miyoshi distal myopathy.
LGMD2C (13*q*12, *γ-sarcoglycan*) A severe childhood form with macroglossia, resembling Duchenne or Becker dystrophy but with sparing of the quadriceps. Cardiomyopathy is an occasional complication.
LGMD2D (17*q*12, *α-sarcoglycan*) A mild or occasionally severe childhood form with very high CK levels. Cardiomyopathy and ventilatory insufficiency are occasional complications.
LGMD2E (4*q*12) A severe form with onset in early childhood or youth and with very high CK levels. Cardiomyopathy may ensue.
LGMD2F (5*q*33–*q*34, *δ-sarcoglycan*) A severe form with onset in childhood, with very high CK levels. Cardiomyopathy and ventilatory insufficiency may ensue.
LGMD2G (17*q*11–*q*12, *telethonion*) A variety reported from Brazil that presents in youth with proximal and distal weakness and atrophy, often progressing to cardiomyopathy.
LGMD2H (9*q*31–*q*33, *TRIM32 mutation, as in sarcotubular myopathy*) A form with mainly pelvic girdle and quadriceps weakness and wasting, and with slow progression, reported from Canada.
Sarcotubular myopathy (9*q*31–*q*33, *TRIM32*) A variant of the above with onset at any time with mild facial and girdle weakness and calf hypertrophy and with exercise-induced myalgias.
LGMD2I (19*q*13.3, *fukutin-related protein gene FKRP*) A relatively mild form presenting in infancy or youth with girdle weakness progressing to calf hypertrophy and with eventual cardiac and respiratory muscle involvement. Serum CK levels may be grossly raised.[4555, 5077]
An allelic *variant* is *myopathy with abnormal merosin (laminin-2)* (19*q*13.3) characterized by onset in youth or adult life of cranial, neck, shoulder, and pelvic girdle weakness and wasting, with calf hypertrophy.
LGMD2J (2*q*13, *titin*) This type, reported from Finland, is allelic with a distal myopathy *variant* and with dilated cardiomyopathy and presents in childhood with proximal and anterior tibial weakness and wasting. CK levels are high.

LGMD2K (*9q34.1, POMT1*) Allelic with **Walker–Warburg syndrome**; this type presents in childhood with proximal weakness, often with contractures and with mental retardation. CK levels are very high.

LGMD2L (*11p13*) An adult-onset form with marked quadriceps wasting and with complaints of muscle pain.

LGMD2M (*9q31, fukutin*) Allelic with **Fukuyama congenital muscular dystrophy**, this form presents in infancy with proximal and distal weakness and hypotonia and very high CK levels.

LGMD4 A geographically restricted condition, possibly a variant of LGMD2E.

A recessive or sporadic form with pelvi-femoral involvement.[6107]

Adult-onset autophagic vacuolar myopathy with multiorgan involvement A sporadic disorder described once in Japan, characterized by the adult onset of proximal weakness with achromatopsia, retinal pigmentary degeneration, optic atrophy and subsequent blindness, exertional pain, cardiomyopathy, and pulmonary fibrosis.

Autosomal recessive dystrophy of childhood, resembling **Duchenne dystrophy**, but more benign and affecting both sexes. The condition is more common in Tunisia and in parts of the Middle East.[502]

Childhood autophagic vacuolar myopathy A rare variant described in the UK with the onset in youth of neck and girdle weakness and knee contractures.

Familial partial lipodystrophy with associated somatic and/or cardiomyopathy.

Infantile autophagic vacuolar myopathy Described in Japan; a form presenting with congenital hypotonia, developmental delay, and cardiomyopathy, leading to early death.

Late-onset limb-girdle muscular dystrophy with diabetes A myopathic syndrome with onset in adult life, characterized by proximal myopathic weakness with cataracts and diabetes.[6157]

LGMD with quadriceps femoris asymmetrical atrophy A recessive variant (11p12) characterized by atrophy and weakness of the hamstrings and adductor magnus in which there is fatty infiltration. Serum CK values vary from normal to very high.[3171]

Limb-girdle muscular dystrophy and Wolff–Parkinson–White syndrome A myopathic syndrome with onset in adult life, characterized by proximal myopathic weakness and cardiomyopathy.[6709]

Limb-girdle myasthenia

Quadriceps myopathy

X-linked limb-girdle dystrophies (myopathies)

Much of the following is taken from the Web site of Dr. Alan Pestronk (http://neuromuscular.wustl.edu/musdist/lg.html) with kind permission.

Barth syndrome (X-linked dilated cardiomyopathy) (Xp28, tafazzin) characterized by the onset in infancy of hypotonia due to a mild and nonprogressive proximal myopathy and later cardiomyopathy, which is eventually lethal. The serum CK levels are normal.

Becker muscular dystrophy A dystrophinopathy (Xp21) A *variant* is *partial dystrophin deficiency* (Xp21) a recessively inherited form.

Danon disease (X-linked vacuolar cardiomyopathy and myopathy) (Xq24, *LAMP-2*)

Duchenne muscular dystrophy A dystrophinopathy (Xp21)

Emery–Dreifuss syndrome (Xq28, *emerin*)

McLeod Syndrome (Xp21.1, XK)

Other *variants* are

Barth-like syndrome with mitochondrial mtRNA Leu mutation, which has a similar presentation; and a form with scapulohumeral, pelvic-femoral muscle, and cardiac muscle involvement (atrioventricular conduction blocks and dilated cardiomyopathy).[503]

X-linked myopathy with excessive autophagy (Xq28) A form with onset in the first 20 years of life, presenting with slowly progressive, mild girdle weakness and with the development of cardiomyopathy. Mental retardation, hepatomegaly, and retinopathy are also described. Female carriers present the same phenotype in a milder form. In one *variant* form, there is no mental retardation and onset may not occur until mid-adult life. Another *variant* is *scapuloperoneal muscular dystrophy with mental retardation and lethal cardiomyopathy.*

---

limb-girdle myasthenia A rare syndrome of abrupt onset, manifesting proximal weakness and fatigability without involvement of the bulbar or extraocular muscles, occurring in childhood or adult life. It is likely that this is a heterogeneous group of conditions.[1862, 2007]

limb-kinetic apraxia See apraxia.

limbic (Lat, edged, a border, or fringe—hence "limbo," the suburbs of hell)[5886]

limbic dementia A rare amnestic syndrome with cognitive and behavioral changes including marked confabulation, denial of illness, distractibility, and change of affect, resulting from complete, selective **limbic lobe** destruction in a previously normal nervous system.

The functions primarily lost, however, are not those cognitive abilities usually associated with intelligence, but those that add an affective quality to all perceptions. Clinically, the presentations resemble both the **Wernicke–Korsakoff** and the **Klüver–Bucy** syndromes. Herpes simplex encephalitis is a typical cause.[2296]

limbic encephalitis A **paraneoplastic syndrome** of the CNS occurring in adult life and due to sterile inflammatory or degenerative changes in the temporal parts of the limbic system gray matter, resembling those of a viral encephalitis and complicating small cell lung carcinoma in most cases.

The clinical manifestations include personality changes, irritability, depression, and seizures followed within weeks by an abrupt permanent impairment of recent memory leading to clinical dementia, variable focal neurological signs stemming from medullary, spinal, or peripheral nerve disease, and subsequently altered consciousness and death.[1290, 2296]

The diagnosis of PLE requires neuropathological examination or the presence of the following four criteria: (i) a compatible clinical picture; (ii) an interval of <4 years between the development of neurological symptoms and tumor diagnosis; (iii) exclusion of other neuro-oncological complications; and (iv) at least one of the following:

CSF with inflammatory changes but negative cytology;
MRI demonstrating temporal lobe abnormalities;
EEG showing epileptic activity in the temporal lobes.[2637]

Commonly associated neoplasms are small cell carcinoma of the lung (50%), and carcinomas of the testis and breast. Neurological symptoms precede the cancer diagnosis in most patients by a median of 3 months or so. Antineuronal antibodies (anti-Hu, anti-Ta, CRMP5, ANNA-3) are present in most cases. Pathologically, perivascular inflammatory infiltrates, microglial nodules, neuronal loss, and gliosis are the major features seen especially in Ammon's horn and the amygdala but also in the hypothalamus, orbitofrontal cortex, and cingulate gyri.

See also **juvenile acute nonherpetic encephalitis**.

limbic epilepsy Epileptic syndromes in which complex focal ("partial") seizures involving the medial aspect of the temporal lobe are associated with behavioral disturbances and evidence of psychopathology, such as the **schizophrenia-like psychoses**.[6375, 6702]

limbic lobe Also known as the *gyrus fornicatus* (Lat, arched gyrus), the lobe on the medial aspect of the cerebral hemispheres was so called by **Thomas Willis**, who noted that the structures comprising it encircle the gray matter of the thalamus and basal ganglia. These structures include the cingulate and parahippocampal gyri, the hippocampal formation, fornix, amygdala, mammillary bodies, mammillothalamic tract, and the dorsomedial and other thalamic nuclei.

limbic P3 potentials Event-related potentials normally recorded with depth electrodes placed in limbic structures. The absence of such potentials predicts with high sensitivity the presence of a local epileptogenic focus.[5139]

limbic system A C-shaped circuit defined first by James **Papez** in 1939, comprising the hippocampus, fornix, mammillary bodies, bundle of Vicq d'Azir, anterior thalamic nucleus, cingulate gyrus, and cingulum. Its cortex is of the four-layered variety and it is younger in phylogeny than the archicortex of the temporal lobe. The complete role of the system is not confidently defined, but the functions of smell, emotion, and memory are almost certainly dependent upon this region.

limit dextrinosis See **glycogen storage diseases**.

limit-setting sleep disorder A childhood disorder characterized by the inadequate enforcement of bedtimes by a caretaker, with the child's resultant stalling or refusal to go to bed at an appropriate time.[1629]

limited chronic focal encephalitis A likely variant of **Rasmussen syndrome**, more limited and less malignant than the original.[2266]

limp man syndrome A rare syndrome characterized by intermittent attacks of hypotonia with failure to maintain posture as a result of continuous, partial, fluctuating **cataplexy**.[6009]

Lindau, Arvid (1892–1958) Swedish pathologist who trained at Lund and in Europe and America before returning to Lund, where he was eventually appointed professor of pathology.

Lindau disease Cavitating myelopathy due to spinal hemangioblastoma.

Lindenov–Hallgren syndrome A syndrome of infancy characterized by the combination of pigmentary retinal degeneration, congenital deafness, and vestibulocerebellar ataxia, often with mental retardation.[3853]

Lindstrom syndrome A congenital dysmorphic syndrome, characterized also by low birthweight, short stature, short neck, skeletal malformations, nevi, cryptorchidism, cerebral atrophy, seizures, hydrocephalus, and pyramidal signs.[381]

line bisection test A diagnostic maneuver to detect evidence of visual **neglect**, in which the subject is asked to draw vertical lines bisecting each of several horizontal lines randomly printed on the right- or the left-hand side of a sheet of paper. In the presence of neglect, the point marked will veer toward the damaged, nondominant hemisphere, and thus away from the neglected side. The lines on the right-hand side of the paper may also be ignored. By using multiple lines, the test discriminates between right and left hemisphere lesions, whereas to ask a patient to bisect a single line is unlikely to yield such information.[5596]

linear envelope EMG Moving average of the full wave rectified EMG, obtained by low-pass filtering. See also **integrated EMG**.

linear scleroderma ("scleroderma en coup de sabre") A rare sporadic form of localized scleroderma characterized by an atrophic band-like region of induration as a result of collagen deposition in the forehead and scalp, extending deeply to involve also the underlying muscles and bone, and leading to local atrophy as in the **Parry–Romberg syndrome** of idiopathic progressive facial hemiatrophy. The condition may be a neurocutaneous syndrome of vascular dysplasia similar to the **Sturge–Weber syndrome**.

Neurological complications include complex partial seizures, headache, and focal neurological signs. Brain MRI may show predominantly ipsilateral relapsing and remitting gray and white matter lesions, cerebral atrophy, ventricular enlargement, and parenchymal calcifications which with CSF and brain biopsy results provides evidence of an underlying inflammatory process.[6072]

Although the condition overlaps with some collagen vascular diseases, it is more likely to be a developmental or focal inflammatory disorder.[1174, 5466]

linear sebaceous nevus syndrome of Jadassohn See **epidermal nevus syndrome**.

lingual dystonia Dystonia affecting the tongue. See also **dystonia**.

lingual seizures A rare form of stimulus-sensitive epilepsy, characterized by the occurrence of painful involuntary tongue movements, with head turning and clonic movements of the corner of the mouth; the EEG shows a centrofrontal spike discharge.[4631]

lingual syndrome See **benign childhood epilepsy with centrotemporal spikes**.

linguals Speech sounds formed with the aid of the tongue. "D," "L," "N," "R," "T," and "Th" are also known as *tongue-point* or *alveolar sounds*; "S," "Sh," "Z," "Zh," "Ch," and "J" are also known as *dentals*, *tongue-blade*, or *palatoalveolar sounds*. "K," "G," and "Ng" are articulated between the back of the tongue and the palate; they are also known as *velars*, *gutturals*, or *tongue-back sounds*.

linkage The connection of a pair of electrodes to the two respective input terminals of a differential EEG amplifier. (From the 1974 report of the Committee on Terminology, IFCN. In: Chatrian GE, Bergamini L, Dondey M, et al. A glossary of terms most commonly used by clinical electroencephalographers. *EEG Clin Neurophysiol* 1974;37:538–48. Reproduced by kind permission of Elsevier Science and the IFCN.)

linked potential See **satellite potential**.

Linnaeus, Carolus (Charles Linné) (1707–1778) Swedish physician and botanist practicing in Stockholm, where he was professor of medicine and physician to the Swedish court and later professor of botany. He was the first to give a full description of aphasia.

lipid myopathies (lipid storage myopathies) Inherited disorders of muscle leading to a syndrome of proximal and distal myopathic fatigue, weakness, pain, and cramping after prolonged exercise, usually in muscular adult men who cannot run (but, paradoxically, who *can* lift weights).

In some cases, true myotonic discharges are recorded on the EMG. The muscle free carnitine levels are normal or depressed. Muscle biopsy specimens show evidence of lipid storage, mainly in the type I muscle fibers, brought about by failure of the enzyme systems responsible for the metabolism of free fatty acids within the muscle. Borderline delayed ketosis is found with fasting.[1371]

The prototype is **carnitine palmityl transferase deficiency**;[1657] other conditions await delineation[869] and are likely to be genetically diverse with multiple etiologies.[5934] These include **glycogen storage disease, mitochondrial myopathy, arthrogryposis, multisystem triglyceride storage disorder,** and **pyruvate decarboxylase deficiency**. See also **carnitine deficiency**. *Variants* are listed in Chart L–6.

lipid neuromyopathy A dominantly inherited mitochondrial myopathic syndrome, characterized by proximal weakness, loss of vibration sensation, myelinated fiber loss, and excess lipid in muscle fibers, due to a systemic defect in fat metabolism.[275]

Chart L–6. Variant Forms of Lipid Myopathy

Alpha-glycerophosphate dehydrogenase deficiency, a mitochondrial disorder presenting as a glycogen storage disease with progressive ophthalmoplegia.[1656]

Congenital ichthyosis with lipid storage myopathy (Chanarin–Miranda syndrome), a lipid storage myopathy characterized by proximal limb weakness, congenital ichthyosis, ectropion, and steatorrhea. Abnormal lipid accumulations are found in muscle, skin, leukocytes, and liver.[1089] The subject has been reviewed by Di Mauro, et al.[1657]

Lipid (storage) myopathy with congenital onset, a syndrome of generalized hypotonia with the development of nonprogressive proximal muscle weakness with easy fatigability. Muscle biopsy specimens show a lipid storage myopathy. Serum carnitine levels are normal.[3214]

Lipid (storage) myopathy with joint contractures, a congenital recessively inherited syndrome, characterized by proximal myopathic weakness, hypotonia and fatigability, muscle pain and cramps, myotonia, cleft palate, scoliosis, clubfoot, joint contractures, abnormal levels of plasma lactate, and normal or mildly depressed muscle free carnitine levels, with borderline delayed ketosis accompanied by neutral lipid storage in muscle biopsy specimens.[5934]

Riboflavin-responsive lipid myopathy with carnitine deficiency.[446]

See also http://www.neuro.wustl.edu/neuromuscular/html for further discussion.

lipid storage diseases See **lipidoses**.

lipid storage myopathies See **lipid myopathies**.

lipidoses (lipid storage diseases) Lysosomal storage diseases characterized by the accumulation of abnormal amounts of lipid within neurons and macrophages within the nervous system. Those involving myelin in the white matter are termed **leukodystrophies**. Those in which the nature of the material stored is known are known as **sphingolipidoses**. Representative disorders are **Gaucher** and **Nieman–Pick** diseases, **Krabbe** globoid leukodystrophy, **metachromatic leukodystrophy, Fabry** disease, **Tay–Sachs** disease and its variants, and GM_1 **gangliosidosis**.

lipodystrophic muscular hypertrophy with encephalopathy (Beradinelli syndrome) A rare condition of childhood, characterized by a deficiency of fatty tissue; hirsutism; muscular hypertrophy and excessive linear growth; enlarged hands, feet, and liver; and hyperpigmentation without endocrine dysfunction. Diabetes and hyperlipidemia are also occasionally found.[538]

lipodystrophies Diseases characterized by altered body fat repartition and major metabolic alterations, with insulin resistance. Dominantly inherited partial lipodystrophies present as subcutaneous lipoatrophy with preserved or increased fat at the level of face and neck (Dunnigan syndrome or FPLD due to LMNA mutations) and/or the abdomen (PPAR gamma-linked forms). FPLD is further characterized by muscular hypertrophy, hyperandrogenism, acanthosis nigricans, hepatomegaly with steatosis and, at the biological level, marked hypertriglyceridemia, low HDL cholesterol, insulin resistance, and altered glucose tolerance or diabetes.

Clinical signs occur after puberty and are more marked in females. Most LMNA mutations are heterozygous substitutions. Features of **limb-girdle muscular dystrophy**, Hutchinson–Gilford **progeria**, or acromandibular dysplasia occur in patients with FPLD with unusual frequency.[6546]

Familial lipodystrophy associated with neurodegeneration and congenital cataracts is a dominantly inherited *variant* also exhibiting spinal cord and cerebellar dysfunction.[555]

lipodystrophy Atrophy of the subcutaneous fat; when occurring on one side of the face only, this is part of the **Parry–Romberg syndrome**.

lipofibromatous hamartoma Extensive fatty infiltration of a nerve (usually the median nerve at the wrist and seen most often in children) causing a compression mononeuropathy.[3232]

lipofuscin (ceroid, wear-and-tear pigment) A pale yellow-brown periodic-acid-Schiff-positive sudanophilic pigment, accumulating in the cytoplasm of nerve and muscle cells with increasing age and acting as a marker of the wear and tear of life. The substance is particularly notable in the thalamus and the hippocampus, and more diffusely in aged brains in Parkinsonism, in **Alzheimer disease**, and in certain **lysosomal diseases**.

lipofuscinosis (juvenile cerebroretinal degeneration) A chronic lipid storage disease resembling Tay–Sachs disease in its clinical manifestations, but not biochemically. See also **neuronal ceroid lipofuscinosis**.

lipogranulomatosis See **Farber disease**.

lipohyalinosis The characteristic pathological change in the intracerebral arterioles of patients with hypertensive vascular disease, consisting of segmental arterial disorganization associated with the presence of macrophages laden with hemosiderin, indicating that some extravasation of erythrocytes has occurred.

lipohyalinotic aneurysm See **microaneurysm**.

lipoid granulomatosis See **Hand–Schüller–Christian disease** and **generalized xanthomatosis**.

lipoid proteinopsis (hyalosis cutis et mucosae; OMIM 247100) A recessively inherited congenital dysmorphic syndrome of childhood mapped to 1q21. It manifests also alopecia; hyperkeratosis; nasal, facial, and other skin tumors; leukoplakia; hoarse voice; intracranial calcification; memory impairment or even mental retardation, behavioral disturbances, and seizures. See also **Urbach–Wiethe disease**.

lipomas Intracranial or intraspinal midline developmental abnormalities consisting of masses of adipose tissue, usually sited above the corpus callosum, in relation to the cerebellum, within the spinal canal (see also **spinal epidural lipomatosis**) or extrinsically at the level of the cauda equina. The masses, although benign and often asymptomatic, may be responsible for seizures, headaches, behavioral disturbances, and cranial nerve palsies.[6915]

lipomatosis with proximal myopathy A rare lipid storage myopathy, sometimes with a mitochondrial 8344 mutation. See also **multiple symmetric lipomatosis**.

lipomatous neuritis See **Leyden neuritis**.

lipomembranous osteocystic osteodysplasia (brain, bone, and fat disease) An unusual recessively inherited cystic disease of bone characterized by pathological fractures, progressive dementia, seizures, calcifications of the basal ganglia, and death in the fourth to sixth decades.[657]

lipomeningomyelocele A subcutaneous lipoma that extends intradurally through a defect in the posterior vertebral arch, extending thus down as far as the conus medullaris. The lesion is large and may compress the lowest spinal nerve roots. Cutaneous manifestations such as an angioma, a patch of hair, or an open sinus tract may be notable. See also **dysraphism**.

lipopigments Autofluorescent materials that stain with Sudan black, but which are insoluble in conventional lipid solvents. They are found in various types of juvenile cerebromacular degeneration, but also represent normal aging pigment (lipofuscin) and include the material known as *ceroid*.

Lisch nodules Clear, yellow or brown melanocytic hamartomas that appear as well-defined, dome-shaped elevations projecting from the surface of the iris in **neurofibromatosis** type 1.[3945]

Lissauer, Heinrich (1861–1891) German neuropsychiatrist who trained in Heidelberg, Berlin, and Leipzig and practiced as a psychiatrist in Breslau,[1670] publishing on the topics of **general paralysis of the insane**, pharmacology, and pathological anatomy (Lissauer tract, 1885) before his early death.

Lissauer atrophy See **Lissauer paralysis**.

Lissauer dementia See **Lissauer paralysis**.

Lissauer paralysis (Lissauer atrophy, Lissauer dementia) A variety of **general paralysis of the insane** marked by diffuse atrophy of the cerebral cortex, leading to seizures, strokes, and prominent focal neurological syndromes.

The condition was described in a note edited posthumously by one of Lissauers pupils. Although diffuse cortical loss and subcortical demyelination were detected, the major lesion appears to be that caused by a widespread vasculopathy.[6078]

Lissauer tract (dorsolateral tract, marginal tract) A fiber pathway in the root entry zone of the spinal cord containing mainly unmyelinated fibers running in both directions. The fibers terminate within one or two segments of their entry level within the root entry zone or cross the midline to ascend in the contralateral spinothalamic tract. Lissauer published his description of this tract in 1885.

lissencephaly (from Gr, smooth + brain) (agyria) A rare developmental disorder of neuronal migration, characterized by the complete or partial failure of gyral formation in the cerebral hemispheres (agyria, pachygyria) and by increased thickness of the cortical gray matter. In some cases, the responsible gene maps to 17p13.3, indicating a mutation in the doublecortin gene. The diagnosis is best made using MRI. A scheme of types, subtypes, and diagnostic criteria for lissencephaly is offered in Chart L–7. See also **cerebellar syndromes** (congenital ataxias).

Other conditions that lissencephaly may accompany are listed by Dobyns[1672] and an exhaustive classification system for malformations of cortical development is provided by Barkowicz, et al.[404]

Chart L–7. Types of Lissencephaly and Their Diagnostic Criteria

Classic or *type 1 lissencephaly* (agyria–pachygyria spectrum; OMIM 601545; subcortical band heterotopia) is the commonest form, is recessively inherited (17p.13.3), and is characterized by agyric and macrogyric regions composed of four layers and resulting from failure of neuronal migration at 10–14 weeks gestation. Infantile spasms and mixed seizure types, mental retardation, and facial dysmorphisms are typical features. Abnormalities of *LIS1* at Xq22–q23 (*DCX*, doublecortin) have been detected.

Subtypes include the following:

Miller–Dieker syndrome (OMIM 247200) in which the agyric and pachygyric regions of the cortex have only four layers. Clinical features include congenital cardiac anomalies, craniofacial anomalies, enlarged liver, seizures, hypotonia, microcephaly, and camptodactyly.

Minimal diagnostic criteria that have been suggested are as follows:

A. Type 1 lissencephaly.
B. Bitemporal hollowing, midface hypoplasia, short nose with upturned lip, and micrognathia.
C. Profound mental retardation, feeding problems, decreased spontaneous movements, early hypotonia with later hypertonia, and seizures including **infantile spasms**. In some cases, there are *LIS1* or *DCX* mutations.

Isolated lissencephaly sequence, characterized by lissencephaly, microcephaly, enlarged ventricles, and heterotopias, presenting clinically as mental retardation, spasticity, and seizures but with minimal facial dysmorphism.[1676]

X-linked lissencephaly with subcortical band heterotopia in carrier females.

X-linked lissencephaly with absent corpus callosum and ambiguous genitalia (XLAG) with trilayered cortex, enlarged ventricles, dysplastic basal ganglia and hypothalamus, spongy white matter, intractable seizures, hypotonia, and early death. Mental retardation and seizures are common among related females.[736]

Type 2 lissencephaly comprises variants of this syndrome usually accompanied by microcephaly, absence of the corpus callosum, cerebellar hypoplasia, etc. See also **muscle eye brain disease**.

Type 3 lissencephaly is characterized by a thick and disordered cortex with fibroglial proliferation and without obvious cell layers. Clinically, this form is associated with hydrocephalus and other major malformations. See **cobblestone complex**.

Walker lissencephaly (Walker–Warburg syndrome, **HARD+E syndrome**) is one such type, in which there is also hydrocephalus due to an arachnoid cyst of the posterior fossa, obliteration of the subarachnoid space, cerebellar hypoplasia, and unilateral microphthalmia. This condition is thought to result from an intrauterine infection.[401, 1086] Minimal diagnostic criteria that have been suggested are as follows:[1672]

A. Type 3 lissencephaly.
B. Cerebellar dysplasia with vermis hypoplasia.
C. Retinal malformations, with hypoplastic ganglion cells, nerve fiber layer, and optic nerves.
D. Congenital muscular dystrophy.
E. Profound mental retardation, feeding problems, decreased spontaneous movements, early hypotonia with later hypertonia, and seizures including **infantile spasms**.

Type 4 lissencephaly is characterized by its association with extreme microcephaly.

An alternative classification is that of Aicardi (1994)[75]

Lissencephalies/subcortical band heterotopia (SBH) spectrum

1. Classical lissencephaly (agyria–pachygyria) and subcortical band heterotopia (SBH)
    a. Miller–Diecker syndrome with deletions of LISl and telomeric genes
    b. Lissencephaly or SBH with LIS1 mutations
    c. Lissencephaly or SBH with DCX (XLIS) mutations (an X-linked dominant form, OMIM 300067, linked to Xq22–q23 with multiple seizure types and mental retardation)
    d. Baraitser–Winter syndrome
    e. Other lissencephaly and SBH loci
2. Lissencephaly with agenesis of the corpus callosum (LACC)
    a. LACC with neonatal death
    b. LACC
    c. X-linked LACC with abnormal genitalia (XLAG)
3. Lissencephaly with cerebellar hypoplasia (LCH)
    a. LCH identical to classical LIS except moderate vermis hypoplasia
    b. LCH with AP gradient, malformed hippocampus, and globular cerebellum
        i. LCH with RELN mutations
        ii. Other loci
    c. LCH with severe brain stem and cerebellar hypoplasia, and neonatal death
    d. LCH with brain stem and cerebellar hypoplasia
    e. LCH with abrupt AP gradient
    f. LCH with agenesis of the corpus callosum, brain stem, and cerebellar hypoplasia
4. Lissencephaly, NOC
    a. Lissencephaly with T-cell deficiency
    b. Winter–Tsukahara syndrome (WTS)

Lissencephaly Network A charitable organization in this field providing information and support. Address: 10408 Bitterroot Court, Ft. Wayne, IN 46804. Tel: 219-432-4310. E-mail: lissnet@lissencephaly.org. Web site: http://www.lissencephaly.org/.

List syndrome See **Chiari malformation**.

listeriosis Infection with *listeria monocytogenes*, capable of producing neurologic syndromes of leptomeningitis, rhomboencephalitis, syningomyelia, and multiple cerebral microabscesses, most often seen in patients with underlying disease or immunocompromise. Cerebritis and abscess can also occur.[431]

Listings law Under normal conditions, there are no torsional eye movements during voluntary saccades (up/down, right/left) when the head is stationary. (This is not always true, however.[2849])

literal alexia An inability to recognize written letters,[759] as seen in patients with lesions of the dominant angular gyrus.

literal paraphasia The selection of wrong words by patients with dysphasias.

Little, William John (1810–1894) English general practitioner and later orthopedic surgeon who trained in London and later practiced at the London Hospital and at the orthopedic institution that he helped to found. He himself was afflicted with an equinus deformity of the left foot as a result of infantile paralysis, for which he obtained some surgical relief while in training in Germany with Stromeyer. It is perhaps ironic that spastic diplegia, the disease that he described in *Treatment of Deformities in the Human Frame* (1853), is associated with a similar foot deformity.

His major interest was the diagnosis and management of cerebral palsies, and he classified the different types of cerebral palsies as generalized rigidity, paraplegia (cerebral diplegia, Little disease), hemiplegic rigidity, and a form with abnormal movements (1861), later called *athetosis* by **Hammond**. Nicholas André in France had reported on cerebral diplegia in 1741.

Little was the first to demonstrate the importance of perinatal injury in the causation of the conditions. Other contributions included his advocacy of saline injections or transfusions in cases of cholera and the performance of tenotomy of the Achilles tendon for contractures, he himself having obtained relief from that operation.

Little club A group of pediatric neurologists and others constituting a medical advisory board for the British Spastics Society, holding annual conferences and publishing occasional studies on cerebral palsy over the last 40 years. The name of the club honors Dr. W.J. **Little**.

Little disease Congenital spastic paraparesis, a form of **cerebral palsy**, which Little recognized to be the result of birth injury and most likely to occur in children who had had convulsions in the postpartum stage.[3875] He acknowledged the recognition of asphyxia neonatorum, infantile hemiplegia, and infantile apoplexy by others such as Duges and **Cruveilher**, but emphasized the types of abnormal labor (unnatural presentations, delayed labor, cord around the neck, breech presentations, instrumentation, etc.) and postpartum injuries that could produce cerebral injury. His second paper contained descriptions of spasticity, hemiparesis, torticollis, mental retardation, and cranial deformities, all resulting from perinatal injury.[3876]

little Broca aphasia See **Broca aphasia**.

little toe reflex of Puusepp See **toe reflex**.

Liveing, Edward (1832–1919) English physician, migraineur, and migrainologist. His book *On Megrim, Sick-Headache and some Allied Disorders* (London, 1873) established the unique nature of migraine headaches and gave a very complete account of their manifestations.

liver flap See **asterixis**.

liver-lover's headache The headache of increased intracranial pressure resulting from **idiopathic intracranial hypertension** and due to excess consumption of liver. The liver is supposed to contain large amounts of vitamin A, a known precipitant of idiopathic intracranial hypertension, but this is mainly true of the livers of polar bears, which are becoming decreasingly available.

Liverpool Seizure Severity Scale A tool to assess seizure severity (not frequency) through the comments of the patient rather than family or attendants.[344] See also **VA scale**, **Chalfont Scale**, and **Hague Scale**.

Livingston, Samuel (1908–1984) American neurologist and epileptologist who graduated in medicine from Vanderbilt University. He practiced privately but also directed the epilepsy clinic at Johns Hopkins, from which he published a stream of important papers on the social and pharmacological management of seizures. His popular book *Living with Epileptic Seizures* (1963) made him a household name in nearly 2% of the Western world.

livresse du sommeil See **confusional arousals**.

loa-loa A filarial nematode whose larvae are transmitted to the human host by the bite of a fly of the genus *Chrysops*. These larvae mature to the adult parasites, which migrate through subcutaneous tissue including the conjunctivas, whence the popular name "eyeworm" is derived. Fertile adult females release microfilaria into the bloodstream diurnally, and biting flies then become infected to complete the life cycle. Loiasis is endemic in central and western Africa, but most residents are asymptomatic in spite of high microfilarial burdens. Eosinophilia is prominent. Visitors are prone to develop symptoms including itching, urticaria, and a fugitive form of angioedema known as the Calabar swelling, which occasionally causes compressive neuropathy. The most serious complication of loa-loa infection is encephalitis, which may occur following attempted treatment with antihelminthic agents such as diethylcarbamazine. As this is likely to be a reaction to the destruction of the parasites, pretreatment with steroids is advisable. (HJM)

lobar atrophy Acquired focal cortical atrophy, leading to syndromes such as **primary progressive aphasia** and **posterior cortical atrophy**.

lobar cerebral hemorrhage Bleeding into the cerebrum outside the basal ganglia and thalamus, neither due to arteriovenous malformation nor to trauma.

This is less common than hypertensive hemorrhage in the ganglionic–thalamic region, the brain stem, and cerebellum and has a better prognosis. The clinical features of the hemorrhages in different lobes have been summarized.[5384] Hypertension, **cerebral amyloid angiopathy**, and fibrinolytic therapy are important antecedents.[4436]

lobar holoprosencephaly A developmental forebrain disorder in which the cerebral hemispheres are only partially separated by a fissure, which is deepest posteriorly. Mental and developmental delay without hydrocephalus is the usual result.[1571] See also **holoprosencephaly**.

lobar sclerosis See **Pick disease**. The term was employed because of the massive astroglial proliferation within the cortex sometimes seen in that condition.

lobotomy "Partial separation of the frontal lobes from the rest of the brain [which] results in the reduction of disagreeable self-consciousness, abolition of obsessive thinking, and satisfaction with performance, though that performance is inferior in quality. The emotional 'nucleus' of the psychosis is removed . . . "[2193] The procedure was introduced by Egaz **Moniz** but was enthusiastically adopted by Freeman and Watts in the United States, who also advised it for chronic pain and for schizophrenia.

Lobstein, Jean Georges Chretien Martin (1777–1835) French neurologist who gave an early description of **Apert syndrome** in 1833.[3888]

Lobstein syndrome See **Apert syndrome**.

lobular sclerosis See **multiple sclerosis**.

local atonic seizures See **hemiparetic seizures**.

local epilepsy See **localization-related epilepsies** and **syndromes**.

local tetanus That form of **tetanus** in which the symptoms appear first in a single limb, from which they may or may not spread to other areas.

localization A cortical function relating the site of a stimulus to the entire remainder of the body schema; there is no pathway in the cord for this purpose.

The localization of functions within the nervous system was remarked indirectly by Hippocrates, but this insight gave way to error, in the idea that the whole brain was considered equipotential with regard to sensation and activity, forming altogether the seat for overall sensation—the **sensus communis**. The concept of functional localization was, however, further supported when in 1809 **Rolando** stimulated animal brains and produced lateralized responses, but the flowering of the concept only came when **Gall** and **Spurzheim** published their studies in **phrenology** and claimed that certain faculties of the mind resided in particular areas of gray matter.

These studies led them to generate maps of ridiculous complexity, but for a time their concepts held sway, untempered by persisting criticism and (in time) apparent experimental disproof; thus, **Flourens** and others failed to elicit motor activity by stimulation of the hemispheres of animals, although **Todd** had done so successfully before, and Bouillaud also had shown earlier in the 19th century that speech disorders followed lesions of the frontal lobe.

It was the work of Hughlings-**Jackson** in the field of focal seizures, however, that established a degree of cerebral localization, especially his demonstration that cortical discharging lesions lead to focal motor seizures. By this, he contradicted the opinion then held that motor activity originated only from the brain stem and basal ganglia. Further studies by **Hitzig, Ferrier, Horsley**, and others, using electrical stimulation of the cortex, confirmed the existence of localization of function.

localization-related epilepsies and syndromes (focal, local, or partial epilepsy) Epileptic disorders in which seizure semiologic studies or investigation findings disclose a localized origin of the seizures. This includes not only patients with small circumscribed, constant epileptogenic lesions (anatomical or functional), that is true focal epilepsies, but also patients with less well defined lesions, whose seizures may originate from variable loci. In most symptomatic localization-related epilepsies, the epileptogenic lesions can be traced to one part of one cerebral hemisphere, but in idiopathic age-related epilepsies with focal seizures, corresponding regions of both hemispheres may be functionally involved. (After Dreifuss FE, et al. Commission for classification and terminology, ILAE. Proposal for Revised Classifications of Epilepsies and Epileptic Syndromes. *Epilepsia* 1989;30:389–99 by kind permission of Wiley-Blackwell Publications.)

localized adhesive spinal arachnoiditis See **arachnoid diverticula**.

localized hypertrophic neuropathy A focal sensorimotor neuropathy with many characteristics of **hereditary motor and sensory neuropathy**, type 3 except that it is localized to one or more peripheral nerves such as the radial.[224] The nerves are enlarged with the formation of perineuronal whorls, despite a loss of myelinated axons. The condition is sustained usually as the result of trauma. See also **perineurinoma**.

localized nodular myositis (focal nodular myositis) A condition of slowly increasing, painful, localized inflammatory swelling, initially of the thigh or calf muscles but sometimes extending to other sites or becoming generalized, in the presence of elevations in the serum creatine kinase levels and the erythrocyte sedimentation rate.[4157] The disease affects young and middle-aged adults, sometimes evolving into a diffuse proximal myopathy accompanied by dysphagia and resembling the "facioscapulohumeral syndrome," but sometimes with eosinophilic infiltration. Recurrence is rare after excision, but in a few cases polymyositis develops.

Muscle biopsy specimens show intense interstitial polymorphic infiltration of muscle with scattered foci of fiber destruction and regeneration. The condition is considered to be an unusual presentation of polymyositis.[1377] See also **proliferative myositis**[2835] and **eosinophilic perimyositis**.

localized scleroderma See **linear scleroderma, morphea**, and **Parry-Romberg syndrome**.

locked-in syndrome (pseudocoma, the de-efferented state, ventral pontine syndrome [or state], ventral brain stem syndrome, Monte Cristo syndrome, cerebromedullary disconnection, pontopseudocoma, akinetic mutism, pontine locked-in syndrome, pontine disconnection syndrome) A term proposed by Plum and Posner[5053] for the near-total motor paralysis resulting from lesions of both cerebral peduncles or of the ventral pons at or above the abducens nuclei, with retained though inexpressible consciousness. Only eye opening, vertical (not lateral) eye movements, and convergence remain in the full form of the syndrome; the patients are truly mute and akinetic. The EEG shows the pattern of wakefulness. The **Glasgow Coma Scale** scores will be 4-2-1 or less.

Major pontine lesions sparing the ascending reticular activating system are the commonest causes, but any condition that deprives the patient of motility—**myasthenia gravis, poliomyelitis, acute inflammatory demyelinating neuropathy**, and muscle relaxant administration, for example—can do the same thing. The syndrome may also occur as a **lacunar syndrome** (bilateral **pure motor hemiparesis**).[2092, 2106]

Essential for the diagnosis are

full consciousness and self-awareness;
severe paralysis of voluntary muscles with quadriplegia, pseudobulbar palsy, and aphonia, though vertical eye movements and blinking are usually preserved sufficiently to allow for limited communication;
retention of sleep–wake cycles and preservation of respiratory, auditory, and visual function and of emotional experience.[4546]

Darolles first described the syndrome in 1875, in a patient who had sustained a basilar artery occlusion. In 1941, **Cairns** described **akinetic mutism** in a patient with an epidermoid cyst in the third ventricle, who neither spoke nor moved but who followed the observer with her eyes, could be made to carry out simple commands, and would withdraw from painful stimuli. This suggests a different condition, perhaps **abulia** as the patient *could* move, but did not do so. A complete review of the syndrome and the etiologies encountered has been published.[4934] In Alexandre Dumas' novel *The Count of Monte Cristo*, the elderly M. Noirtier communicated only by eye blinks signifying yes or no, but retained perfect understanding. More recently, others afflicted have actually produced books using this means of communication, as poignantly depicted in the film *The Diving Bell and the Butterfly*.

lockjaw Tonic spasm of the masseter muscles, classically seen in **tetanus**, for which this was an alternative name.

Locock, Sir Charles (1799–1875) English obstetrician who, noting in 1857 that impotence had been reported as a side effect of bromide treatment and believing that seizures were a manifestation of abnormal sexual tendencies including masturbation, suggested the use of bromides as treatment for epilepsy.[3890] Serendipitously, it worked.

locomotor ataxia (ataxy) An antique term for **tabes dorsalis**.

locus ceruleus (Lat, place + dark or sky blue) Medullary adrenergic nuclei situated bilaterally in the floor of the fourth ventricle, involved in sensory, autonomic and perhaps motor functions, arousal, and attention.

Loewi, Otto (1873–1961) German-American physiologist who detected the presence of cholinesterase in motor end-plate regions, demonstrating that it was inhibited by eserine (1924–1926). He showed that the vagus nerves liberate acetylcholine, establishing the theory of chemical transmission in the nervous system, and he isolated both cholinesterase and physostigmine, an anticholinesterase. He shared the 1936 Nobel Prize with Sir Henry Dale.

logical memory A form of verbal memory tested by getting the patient to recall details of a trite story, each successful recollection (either immediately or after a filled interval) adding to the subject's score. The model is used in the **Wechsler Memory Scale**. Typical examples are the story of the donkey and the salt, and of the Boston woman who lost her purse.

logopathy (Gr, word + disease) A morbid affection of speech.

logopenia (cortical dysarthria, anarthria, aphemia, pure motor aphasia) A difficulty in word finding, but the patient's phrase length is still longer than four words and syntax is preserved.[3398]

logopenic progressive aphasia A subgroup of **primary progressive aphasia** in which there is a progressive decrease in speech output with anomia and impairment of short-term verbal memory.[5393]

logorrhea (Gr, word + flow) Uninhibited speech output, occurring in schizophrenia and in confusional states.

logospasmus choreiformis The pathological insertion of the same word into sentences, when it is out of context with regard to the patient's otherwise normal speech.

lollipop sign The appearance on CT scans of swelling of the inferior rectus muscle in **dysthyroid ophthalmopathy**.

Lombard sign Elevation of the pitch of the voice when a normal subject reads with his normal ear subjected to white noise, compared to its pitch when he reads without such stimulation. The test is of value in the detection of feigned unilateral deafness.

Lomtadse sign Dorsiflexion of the hallux when the examiner's knuckles are pressed upon and run distally down the tibial spine. Lomtadse believed that the sign indicated the presence of both a cortical and a capsular lesion causing hemiparesis, but it can equally well be interpreted as yet another form of stimulation leading to the Babinski response. The **Soederbergh phenomenon** is very similar.

London Dysmorphology Database See **Winter-Baraitser Dysmorphology Database**.

London Handicap Scale A validated six-question health outcome measure designed to assess disadvantage as a result of ill health. The questions concern the items contributing to handicap as defined by the WHO, namely mobility, physical independence, occupation, social integration, orientation, and economic self-sufficiency.[2792]

London Neurogenetics Database A comprehensive, computerized, menu-driven database assisting in the recognition of over 2400 defined neurogenetic syndromes by means of a listing of selected features; allowing a search for a differential diagnosis of specific clinical features; reviewing the clinical manifestations of named disorders; and providing references to recent or seminal papers.

The database was conceived and written by Dr. Michael Baraitser and Dr. Robin Winter, and is published by Oxford University Press, Walton St., Oxford OX2 6DP, UK. See also **Winter-Baraitser Dysmorphology Database**.

lone status epilepticus The abrupt presentation of status epilepticus in a previously healthy adult with no past history of neurological disease. There is good recovery from the attack, but it is nevertheless most likely to have been caused by a cerebral tumor.[4843]

long Q-T syndrome Syncope or cardiac arrest following unexpected stimuli and resulting from prolongation of cardiac cell repolarization due to dysfunction of ion channels. Sudden, alerting adrenergic stimuli such as an unexpected loud noise cause tachycardia and new depolarization that occurs prior to the complete repolarization of the cardiac myocyte. The resultant reduction in cerebral blood flow may trigger syncope, seizures, or even sudden death. The arrhythmia classically associated is the *torsade des pointes*. A gene mutation affecting a potassium channel expressed in cardiac muscle is the likely cause. EKG shows a QTc >460 ms (normal <420 ms).

long sleeper A variant of the normal sleep patterns, characterized by a perceived need to sleep for longer than is usual in a subject's age group and accommodation of this perception. The sleep architecture is normal.[2788] See also the American Academy of Sleep Disorders *International Classification of Sleep Disorders Diagnostic and Coding Manual*;[1629] **sleep disorders** (Chart S–6) and **short sleeper**.

long thoracic nerve of Bell The nerve supply to the serratus anterior muscle, arising from C5–7. It was identified by Sir Charles **Bell** in 1821 as the "external respiratory" nerve.[493] Palsy resulting from damage to the nerve is usually the result of neuralgic amyotrophy or direct trauma but may be familial.[5017]

long-chain acyl-coenzyme A dehydrogenase deficiency A rare, genetically determined enzyme defect resulting in episodic juvenile-onset recurrent myoglobinuria, hypoketotic hypoglycemic coma, and hypertrophic cardiomyopathy, triggered by fasting.[6244]

long-cycle hypersomnia See **hypersomnolence**.

long-latency reflex A reflex with many synapses (polysynaptic) or a long pathway (long-loop) so that the time for its occurrence is greater than the time of occurrence of short-latency reflexes. See also **long-loop reflex**. (From the 2001 Report of the Nomenclature Committee of the American Association of Electromyography and Electrodiagnosis.[19] Reproduced by kind permission of the AANEM.)

long-latency somatosensory evoked potential That portion of a somatosensory evoked potential normally occurring more than 100 ms after stimulation of a nerve in the upper extremity at the wrist, or the lower extremity at the knee or ankle.[162]

long-loop reflex A reflex thought to have a circuit that extends above the spinal segment of the sensory input and motor output and may involve the cerebral cortex. It should be differentiated from reflexes arising from stimulation and recording within a single or adjacent spinal segments (i.e., a segmental reflex). See also **long-latency reflex**. (From the 2001 Report of the Nomenclature Committee of the American Association of Electromyography and Electrodiagnosis.[19] Reproduced by kind permission of the AANEM.)

longitudinal bipolar montage An EEG montage consisting of derivations from pairs of electrodes along longitudinal, usually anteroposterior arrays. (Adapted from the Committee on Terminology, IFCN. © 1974, with kind permission from Elsevier Science.)

look nystagmus A wide-amplitude, slow variety of **optokinetic nystagmus** induced by having a patient follow a succession of moving vertical stripes presented before him. The nystagmus is faster and of smaller amplitude when the subject stares through the striped stimulus (*stare nystagmus*).[3762]

Looser syndrome See **Apert syndrome**.

Lopez–Hernandez syndrome A congenital dysmorphic syndrome characterized by fusion of the vermis and pons with resulting cerebellar ataxia and trigeminal anesthesia, and manifesting also short stature, parietal alopecia, cloudy corneas, craniosynostosis, and mental and developmental delay.[3912]

lordosis (Gr, bent backward) An extended posture of the spine, usually as an exaggeration of the normal lumbar curve, so that the small of the back is hollowed and the chest prominent.

Lorente de No, Rafael American neurobiologist who described the role of the internuncial pool in reflex sympathetic dystrophy and the CA 1, 2, 3, 4 regions of the hippocampus.

Lorenzo's oil A 4:1 combination of glycerol trioleate and glycerol trierucate, formerly used with uncertain success in the treatment of **adrenoleukodystrophy**.[5676]

loss of memory Isolated amnesia occurring as a **lacunar syndrome**.[2092, 2106]

lotus footdrop Sciatic neuropathy in the thigh, sustained as a result of prolonged meditation in the customary yoga position.[6558] See also **yoga footdrop**.

Lou Gehrig disease See **amyotrophic lateral sclerosis**. Gehrig (1903–1941) was an acclaimed American baseball player (New York Yankees) whose eventual, originally inexplicable, decline in performance on the field was the result of this disease.

loudness recruitment A sign of cochlear or of brain stem disease, characterized by the perception of a great increase in the loudness of sounds, which are actually only slightly more intense than sounds previously presented below that threshold. See also **Equal Loudness Balance Test**.

Louis-Bar, Denise A Belgian neuropathologist who described the syndrome named for her (see the next entry) in 1941,[3922] although there had been a report of the same condition in 1926.

Boder and Sedgwick published a more detailed account in 1958 and noted the frequent infections; selective deficiency of IgA was found in one patient 3 years later.

Louis-Bar syndrome (ataxia-telangiectasia, Boder–Sedgwick syndrome) A rare, recessively inherited syndrome of neurological deterioration and failure of DNA repair in which there are breaks on chromosome 11 at 11q22–q23. See also **ataxia-telangiectasia**.

louping Ill An encephalitic illness due to direct infection by a flavivirus member of the togavirus group of arboviruses, occurring in Scotland and Northern Ireland and responsible for a form of ataxia in sheep, but only occasionally affecting humans.[6858]

low-affinity fast channel syndrome A variant metabolic disorder underlying the clinical phenotype of congenital myasthenia gravis.

low-frequency filter (high-pass filter) A circuit that reduces the sensitivity of the EEG channel to relatively low frequencies. For each position of the low-frequency filter control, this attenuation is expressed as a percentage reduction of the output pen deflection at a given stated frequency relative to frequencies unaffected by the filter, that is, in the midfrequency band of the channel.

Low-frequency filter designations and their significance are not standardized for instruments of different manufacture. For instance, in a given instrument, a position of the low-frequency filter control, designated 0.5 Hz, may indicate a 30% (or 3 decibel) or other stated percentage reduction in sensitivity at 0.5 Hz, compared to the sensitivity, for example, at 10 Hz. The same position of the low-frequency filter control may also be designated by the time constant. See also **time constant**. (Adapted from the 1974 report of the Committee on Terminology, IFCN. In: Chatrian GE, Bergamini L, Dondey M , et al. A glossary of terms most commonly used by clinical electroencephalographers. *EEG Clin Neurophysiol* 1974;37:538–48. Reproduced by kind permission of Elsevier Science and the IFCN.)

low-frequency response The sensitivity of an EEG channel to relatively low frequencies, determined by the low-frequency response of the amplifier and by the low-frequency filter (time constant) used, and expressed as the percentage reduction in the output pen deflection at certain stated low frequencies relative to other frequencies in the midfrequency band of the channel. See also **low-frequency filter** and **time constant**. (Adapted from the 1974 report of the Committee on Terminology, IFCN. In: Chatrian GE, Bergamini L, Dondey M, et al. A glossary of terms most commonly used by clinical electroencephalographers. *EEG Clin Neurophysiol* 1974;37:538–48. Reproduced by kind permission of Elsevier Science and the IFCN.)

low-pressure headache See **postlumbar puncture headache**.

low-pressure hydrocephalus See **normal pressure hydrocephalus**.

low-voltage EEG A waking EEG record characterized by activity with an amplitude not greater than 20 μV over all head regions. With appropriate instrumental sensitivities, this activity can be shown to be composed primarily of beta and theta (and to a lesser degree delta) waves, with or without alpha activity over the posterior area.

Low-voltage EEGs are susceptible to change under the influence of certain physiological stimuli, sleep, pharmacological agents, and pathological processes. They should be held in clear contradistinction to the tracings of **electrocerebral inactivity** (which are records consisting primarily of delta waves of relatively low voltage) and to tracings that display low voltages over limited regions of the head. (Adapted from the 1974 report of the Committee on Terminology, IFCN. In: Chatrian GE, Bergamini L, Dondey M, et al. A glossary of terms most commonly used by clinical electroencephalographers. *EEG Clin Neurophysiol* 1974;37:538–48. Reproduced by kind permission of Elsevier Science and the IFCN.)

Lowe oculocerebrorenal syndrome See **oculocerebrorenal syndrome**.

Lowenberg–Hill syndrome A dominantly inherited syndrome of tremor associated with patchy demyelination of the cerebral white matter; a variant of the **Pelizaeus–Merzbacher** form of leukodystrophy.[3935]

Lowenthal sclerosis A hereditary syndrome of congenital generalized muscle hypotonia, joint hyperextensibility, kyphoscoliosis, blepharoptosis, hyperhidrosis, and skeletal deformities in which biopsy specimens show firm adhesion of the muscles to the overlying subcutaneous adipose tissues.[3937]

lower basilar branch syndrome A **lacunar syndrome** characterized clinically by dizziness, diplopia, gaze palsy, dysarthria, cerebellar ataxia, and numbness of the face.[2092, 2106] See also **lateral pontomedullary syndrome**.

lower body Parkinsonism See **frontal gait disorder**.

lower brain stem (bulbar) encephalitis A chronic, progressive **paraneoplastic syndrome** most likely associated with carcinoma of the prostate and characterized by loss of voluntary horizontal gaze and later by spasms of the bulbar muscles. Notable pathological features are the presence of perivascular round-cell infiltrates and of microglial nodules in the brain stem.[360]

Lower Extremity Rating Scale A leg functional assessment test for children with cerebral palsy.[1289]

lower level seizures (pontobulbar seizures) Positive electrical events arising from lesions of the brain stem or spinal cord. The modern concept that this could occur was that of Hughlings-**Jackson**, based upon his delineation of a hierarchy of functional levels within the brain, although others such as Galen, Rolando, and Fourens had considered the same possibility before him.[3573]

lower motor neuron disease Sporadic syndromes in which adult subjects display only lower motor neuron signs in two or more regions. Many develop upper motor neuron and bulbar signs characteristic of **amyotrophic lateral sclerosis** after 6 years, but the determination of the disorders suffered by those who, in retrospect (e.g., after 4 years), do *not* have signs allowing that diagnosis is difficult. It has, however, been assisted by the designation of the syndrome(s) as *lower motor neuron disease*.

The clinical presentations in such conditions indicate male predominance, onset of weakness most frequently in one upper limb, distally; weakness associated with muscle wasting; absent or decreased reflexes; and sometimes the presence of elevated titers of IgM anti-GM1 ganglioside antibodies. The prognosis appears to be favorable, since clinical abnormalities are still confined to one limb in most cases after a median disease duration of 12 years. The differential diagnosis is wide; see also **hereditary motor neuropathy, amyotrophic lateral sclerosis, Hirayama syndrome, multifocal motor neuropathy, gammopathic neuropathy, spinobulbar muscular atrophy (Kennedy disease), and monomelic amyotrophy**.

Three major categories are distinguished, all showing evidence of restricted lower motor neuron involvement with slow progression:[6476]

1. *Slowly progressive spinal muscular atrophy*, presenting with initially asymmetric generalized weakness (more in the legs than in the arms) and with an older age at onset, but progressing to severe weakness and muscle atrophy, slow reflexes, marked functional impairment, widespread abnormalities on concentric needle EMG, eventual respiratory insufficiency, and serum M-protein.
2. *Distal spinal muscular atrophy* with symmetrical, distal muscle weakness. Sporadic cases with symmetrical and distal muscle weakness in both arms and legs.

3a. *Segmental distal spinal muscular atrophy* This amounts to **Hirayama syndrome** with weakness of the hand and forearm, starting unilaterally and often with eventual involvement of the legs. Again there is a marked male preponderance.

3b. *Segmental proximal spinal muscular atrophy* in which there is ipsilateral muscle weakness and wasting of the shoulder and proximal arm muscles. It carries a favorable prognosis for life but there is considerable functional impairment.

lower motor neuron lesion Any pathology that affects the cell body of the motor neuron, its axon and branches, or the motor end plate. Diseases of the muscle are sometimes included, mainly because they also may lead to hypotonia, wasting, weakness, and depressed muscle stretch reflexes, although the muscles can hardly be regarded as neurons.

lower motor neuron syndrome The presence of muscle weakness, atrophy, and/or fasciculations with evidence of denervation on EMG examination, in the absence of upper motor neuron signs. This may represent the initial stage of **amyotrophic lateral sclerosis** or can be sporadic (progressive spinal muscular atrophy or an adult-onset **hereditary motor neuropathy**). **Multifocal motor neuropathy** and **postpoliomyelitis syndrome** may also mimic LMNS.

A biological marker for early detection of ALS is Nogo-A, a protein mainly involved in preventing neurite outgrowth and nerve regeneration in the CNS. Detection of Nogo-A in muscle biopsy samples from LMNS patients reliably identifies patients who will further progress to ALS.[5105]

lower-half headache Another term for **cluster headache**. It certainly draws attention to the site of the pain, but by no means are all headaches affecting the lower part of the face due to that condition, and the term is now seldom employed.

lower-half Parkinsonism A gait disturbance resembling that of **Parkinson disease** but with few or no other signs of the full syndrome. Whether this is due to that disease or is merely associated with periventricular ischemia in older people is uncertain. See also **isolated gait ignition failure** and **frontal gait disorder**.

Lowry syndrome (Lowry–MacLean syndrome, cranial synostosis, and fibular aplasia) A recessively inherited congenital craniofacial malformation syndrome characterized by short stature, beaked nose, bilateral fibular aplasia, proptosis, glaucoma, **Brushfield spots**, atrial septal defect, intestinal malrotation, seizures, microcephaly, callosal abnormalities, hydrocephalus, craniosynostosis affecting all sutures, and mental and developmental delay.[3939] See also **craniosynostosis**.

Lowry–MacLean syndrome See **Lowry syndrome**.

lubag (DYT3) An X-linked recessive syndrome characterized by dystonia (initially blepharospasm or limb dystonia) and Parkinsonism, described only in Filipinos.[6784]

Lubarsch–Pick disease See **amyloidosis**.

Luciani, Luigi (1842–1919) Italian neurophysiologist and Rector of the University of Rome who performed ablation experiments on the cerebellum and was the first to conclude that it serves as the regulatory center for tonic, static, and voluntary movement functions.

Luciani triad Asthenia, atonia, and ataxia, three major manifestations of cerebellar disease. See also **Charcot triad** of nystagmus, ataxia, and slurred speech.

lucid dreaming The awareness of dreaming while it is occurring, coupled with a limited ability to control the script.[4027]

lucid interval That period commencing with the awakening of a patient following concussion and the onset of coma due to brain compression by a resulting intracranial (usually extradural) hemorrhage.

The patient who awakens following concussion from severe head trauma, and whose conscious level shortly thereafter declines again, probably has a fracture of the squamous temporal bone with laceration of the middle meningeal artery, causing an epidural hematoma. The latter is the cause of the delayed coma, through rapid brain compression. In this interval, the patient is likely to be fully conscious, and his thinking may be lucid.

The phenomenon was first described by H.-F. le Dran in 1731.

lückenschädel See **lacunar skull**.

Lucky syndrome A congenital dysmorphic syndrome manifesting also tall thin stature, skeletal deformities including arachnodactyly, erythema, strabismus, ptosis, facial telangiectasia, hypotonia, muscle atrophy, and mental and developmental delay.[4929]

lucubration (from Lat, to work by the light of a lamp) Insomnia.

lues (Lat, a pestilence or a criminal) See syphilis The word was used in previous centuries meaning an expiation, such as epilepsy; an epidemic, such as dysentery; and as a contagion, such as syphilis.[5103] Only the last meaning survives.

luetic otitic-nystagmus syndrome See **Hennebert syndrome**.

Luft disease (nonthyroidal hypermetabolism) A rare hypermetabolic **mitochondrial myopathy** due to the uncoupling of oxidative phosphorylation in the mitochondria of skeletal muscles. Patients complain of fever, heat intolerance, sweating, dyspnea at rest, polyphagia, polydipsia and polyuria without weight gain, and sometimes with slight muscle weakness. Muscle biopsy specimens demonstrate a profusion of ragged red fibers.[3953]

Dr. Rolf Luft introduced the concept of mitochondrial myopathies in 1962.

Lujan syndrome A congenital X-linked dysmorphic syndrome manifesting also tall stature, atrial septum defect, arachnodactyly, macrocephaly, joint laxity, callosal malformations, and mental and developmental delay.[381]

lumbago (Lat, pain in the loins) Etymologically, a very proper word for back pain, but it has lost its respectability because of popular usage, and is no longer commonly employed in medicine.

lumbar (from Lat, the loins) Of or belonging to the loins or low back.

lumbar puncture An invasive procedure (insertion of a needle between the lumbar vertebra into the subarachnoid space for the purpose of obtaining cerebrospinal fluid), introduced in the living with great bravery by **Quincke** in Germany and Walter Essex Wynter in England,[6888] both in 1891.

Cotugno had obtained CSF from the dead a century before, and **Corning**, a physician in New York, put a needle into the spinal column in 1889, but there is evidence that he did not attempt to withdraw spinal fluid.[2495] Despite the introduction of the procedure in England, it was not performed at the **National Hospital** until after the retirement of Sir William **Gowers**, who disapproved of it, perhaps because all four of Wynter's meningitic patients died.

Practice parameters regarding the indications, contraindications, and methodology of lumbar puncture (diagnostic, therapeutic and incidental and in adults and children) have been reviewed by the American Academy of Neurology.[167]

lumbar spinal stenosis (Verbierst syndrome, pseudoclaudication syndrome) Narrowing of the lumbar spinal canal over several segments as a result of multiple disk protrusions or other pathology; pain, weakness, and ascending numbness in the legs as a result of exercise, relieved by rest and by flexion of the spine, are typical symptoms.[6525]

Such a syndrome is sometimes improperly called *intermittent claudication of the cord*, but it is probably the spinal nerve roots that are ischemic and, anyway, the spinal cord cannot limp.[3344]

The Shuttle Walking Test, the Swiss Spinal Stenosis Questionnaire, the Oxford Claudication Score, and the Oswestry Disability Index are described as useful assessment tools and have been reviewed.[5110]

lumbarization The fusion of the S1 vertebra with that at L5, effectively producing a state of having six lumbar vertebrae separated from the remainder of the sacrum by a disk and joint capsule.

Low-back pain may result, but in many cases there are no adverse effects at all.[2222]

lumbosacral plexopathy (lumbosacral plexus neuritis) An acutely or subacutely evolving monophasic syndrome of painful neurogenic muscle weakness in the legs with areflexia, atrophy, and sensory disturbances such as paresthesias in the distribution of the spinal nerves and the plexus at and below L1, usually unilaterally. The numerous causes include microvasculitis and less often compression, malignant infiltration, and diabetes; often no cause is ascertainable, in which case there is a tendency for slow recovery.[5529, 6530] The criteria for diagnosis resemble those for **neuralgic amyotrophy**, except that it is the lumbosacral rather than the brachial plexus that is involved.

A *variant* syndrome of *painful lumbosacral plexopathy* has been described, which presents with acute pain, weakness, hyporeflexia, and muscle atrophy in the legs with slow recovery, occurring as a manifestation of ischemic axonal neuropathy in the absence of evidence of cancer, vasculitis, or other autoimmune disease (although an autoimmune etiology is assumed and the erythrocyte sedimentation rate is high).[791] In other variant forms, *lower lumbosacral plexopathy* occurs postpartum, producing perineal sensory disturbances and sphincter failure without leg weakness; or an upper plexopathy occurs as a rare obstetric complication in the third trimester or in the intra- or postpartum periods, and is associated with upper (L2–S1) lesions causing obturator, femoral, or sciatic nerve palsies.[3104]

lumbosacral plexus neuritis See **lumbosacral plexopathy**.

lumbosacral radiculoplexus neuropathy (LSRPN; nondiabetic) A subacute asymmetrical, painful, and debilitating neuropathy of the lower limbs associated with weight loss, beginning focally in the thigh or leg but usually extending to local regions and to the other side. Morbidity is prolonged due to pain, paralysis, autonomic involvement, and sensory loss, and recovery is usually delayed and incomplete. In biopsied distal nerves, changes are found similar to those found in the diabetic form and are typical of ischemic injury and of microvasculitis.

Although LSRPN mirrors the diabetic variety in its clinical features, course, pathological findings, and long-term outcome, few patients actually go on to develop diabetes mellitus.[1782]

lumbosacral syringomyelia See **hereditary sensory and autonomic neuropathy** (recessive).

lumbrical (Lat, like a worm) Small intrinsic hand muscles, named in the seventeenth century for their resemblance to (rather fat) worms.

lunacy (from Lat, lunaticus, from luna, moon) denotes a link between madness and the phases of the moon, between which there is little evidence for any causal association. It has however been suggested that the phase of the moon may in the past have had an effect on bipolar patients by providing light during nights that would otherwise have been dark, and affecting susceptible patients through the well-known route of sleep deprivation.

In England and Wales, the Lunacy Acts (1890–1922) referred to "lunatics," a term later changed to "Persons of Unsound Mind" and subsequently to "mental illness."

Lundberg syndrome 1. (hereditary neurological disease with facial spasm, myopathy–oligophrenia–cataract) The occurrence of slowly progressive peripheral paresis in the hands and feet, starting in childhood with areflexia and reduced conduction velocities; moderate oligophrenia; multiple cranial nerve lesions (optic atrophy, pupillary abnormalities, facial spasms or palsy, cataract, speech delay); ataxia; premature menopause; and disproportionate smallness of the limbs. The condition is considered to be related to **hereditary motor and sensory neuropathy**.[3962]

2. *Acromicria, mental retardation, polyneuropathy*, a congenital recessively inherited syndrome characterized by short stature, hypogonadotrophic hypogonadism with premature menopause at 20–25 years of age, small hands and feet, ophthalmoplegias, nystagmus, oculomotor apraxias, bulbar palsies, a slowly progressive motor peripheral neuropathy resembling hereditary motor and sensory neuropathy type 1, and mental and developmental delay.[3962]

3. **Benign acute childhood myositis** (myalgia cruris epidemica) A syndrome of transient pain and tenderness in the calves and elevated serum creatine kinase levels occurring in children within a week of an upper respiratory infection.[3960]

lupoid sclerosis The clinical condition in which **systemic lupus erythematosus** presents in a manner suggestive of **multiple sclerosis**.

lupus anticoagulant A circulating immunoglobulin autoantibody (IgG, IgM, or both) directed against phospholipids, which interferes with the *in vitro* phospholipid-dependent tests of coagulation such as the activated partial thromboplastin time, producing an anticoagulant effect; paradoxically, its presence is associated clinically with thrombocytopenia, prothrombin deficiency, pulmonary emboli, deep vein thromboses (type 1), arterial thromboses (type 2), cerebrovascular thrombotic disease leading to ocular or focal cerebral deficits, mainly in younger women (type 3), or any combination of these (type 4).

Although initially detected in subjects with **systemic lupus erythematosus**, it is also sometimes found in normal subjects and those with complicated migraine, seizures, or chorea; those with viral infections including HIV infection; those with malignancy or lymphoproliferative disorders; or those taking chlorpromazine, procainamide, etc. Suspicion as to its presence is aroused by finding an increased partial thromboplastin time or elevated levels of anticardiolipin antibodies.[3810]

lupus cerebritis Complications of **systemic lupus erythematosus** presenting with, for example, neuropsychiatric features, headaches, seizures, stroke, and/or chorea. Nineteen such syndromes have been defined and diagnostic criteria provided by the American College of Rheumatology.[46]

Lupus Foundation of America A charitable organization in this field. Address: 1300 Piccard Dr. Suite 200, Rockville, MD 20850-4303. Tel: 301-670-9292; 800-558-0121. E-mail: info@lupus.org. Web site: http://www.lupus.org/.

Luria, Aleksander Romanovich (1902–1977) Russian aphasiologist who distinguished six aphasic syndromes: efferent (Broca aphasia), afferent apraxic, amnesic, sensory, semantic, and dynamic.

Luria-Nebraska battery A complex timed instrument for the assessment (by neuropsychologists) of perseveration and other functions that may be affected in states of cognitive decline. The battery is derived from the techniques used by **Luria**, but is itself a North American creation[2442] and its validity and reliability are not unquestioned.[3825]

Luschka, Hubert von (1820–1875) German physician, Professor of Anatomy at Tübingen.

Luschka foramen The paired lateral foramina in the meningeal roof of the fourth ventricle.

Luschka joints Originally described as narrow joint cavities between a small bony eminence on the posterior rim of the superior surface of the bodies of the C3–7 and T1 vertebrae (the uncus), forming part of the medial wall of the adjacent intervertebral foramen, and the inferior facet of the superjacent vertebra—the lateral intervertebral joints. These "joints," however, probably represent nothing more than fissures in the lateral part of the cervical disks.[4946]

Luschka syndrome See **Sturge–Weber disease**.

Lust phenomenon (peroneal sign) Eversion and dorsiflexion of the ankle in response to tapping the common peroneal nerve; a sign of **tetany**.

luxury perfusion Abundant cerebral blood flow in a region with impaired ability to extract oxygen, as a result of ischemic or other damage.[3711] This localized reactive hyperemia is due to a local chemical effect of lactic acidosis in and around ischemic tissue, and also occurs following trauma and seizures.

A reduction in oxygen and glucose uptake larger than the drop in perfusion is known as *relative luxury perfusion*.

Luys, Jules-Bernard (1828–1897) French neurologist who became chief of the Neurology Service of the **Salpêtrière** and the Charité hospitals. He first described the subthalamic nucleus in 1865, but is also remembered for his demonstration of the degeneration of the anterior horn cells in progressive muscular atrophy.[4896]

luysopallidonigral atrophy and amyotrophic lateral sclerosis A rare variant, characterized by anterior horn cell loss and corticospinal tract degeneration in association with dystonias, rigidity, and hyperkinesias.[2555]

In a further *variant* form, signs of spinal muscular atrophy are also found. See also **motor neuronal diseases**.

Lyle syndrome 1. See **cortical blindness**. 2. See **syndrome of the mesencephalic gray matter**.

Lyme disease (Garin–Bujadoux–Bannwarth syndrome, Bannwarth syndrome; neuroborreliosis) A tick-borne, seasonal, spirochetal disease endemic in North America, Europe, and Australia with cutaneous manifestations such as spreading red papules and erythema chronicum migrans, occurring initially at the site of a tick bite. Later, neurological and finally arthropathic symptoms and signs may appear.[6029] In addition, atrioventricular conduction defects are described.

The neurological features of importance are nonspecific chronic malaise, headache, and pains, progressing over perhaps 6 months in about 15% of the cases to become a chronic cranial and spinal meningoencephalitis, myelitis, or encephalitis accompanied by painful polyradiculopathies and neuropathies, both cranial and peripheral. The VII cranial nerve is most often affected, often bilaterally. A lymphocytic pleocytosis and raised protein levels are found in the CSF.[994, 4050, 5244] The spirochaete *Borrelia burgdorferi* was first isolated from patients living in Lyme, Connecticut, but the first reports of the disease were from southern France in 1922 and from Germany by Bannwarth in 1941.[375] The various clinical syndromes have been reviewed.[4820]

Criteria for the diagnosis of definite nervous system Lyme disease have been suggested[2707] (reproduced by kind permission of the American Academy of Neurology and Lippincott, Williams and Wilkins) and the place of the polymerase chain reaction defined.[4847]

1. Possible exposure to appropriate ticks in an area where Lyme disease occurs.
2. One or more of the following:
   i. Erythema migrans, the pathognomic rash, or histologically proven borrelia lymphocytoma or acrodermatitis.
   ii. Immunologic evidence of exposure to *B. burgdorferi* (e.g., positive serologic test).
   iii. Culture, histologic, or PCR proof of the presence of *B. burgdorferi*.
3. Occurrence of one or more of the (typical) neurological disorders (such as lymphocytic meningitis with or without cranial neuritis or painful radiculoneuritis; encephalomyelitis; peripheral neuropathy; or encephalopathy) after exclusion of other potential etiologies. Additional testing is indicated based on the likelihood that a given neurological disorder is causally related to Lyme borreliosis. If CNS disease is suspected, CSF should be examined for intrathecal antibody production, culture, or PCR.

Lyme Disease Foundation A charitable organization in this field. Address: One Financial Plaza, 18th Floor, Hartford, CT 06103-2601. Tel: 860-525-2000; 800-886-5963. E-mail: lymefnd@aol.com. Web site: http://www.lyme.org/.

lympho- (Gr, water).

lymphocytic choriomeningitis See **aseptic meningitis**. The condition was first described by Arvid Johan Wallgren in 1924.

lymphocytic hypophysitis A rare inflammatory disease of the pituitary gland presenting with mass effect, hypopituitarism, and raised prolactin levels, usually in pregnancy or postpartum.[3742]

lymphocytic meningoradiculitis See **Bannwarth syndrome**.

lymphogranuloma inguinale See **lymphogranuloma venereum**.

lymphogranuloma venereum (lymphogranuloma inguinale) A chlamydial infection that occasionally progresses to cause aseptic meningitis or encephalitis.[1760]

lymphoma A generic term for Hodgkin disease, lymphosarcoma, reticulum cell sarcoma, and follicular lymphoma. Neurologic complications include the effects of local deposits on the brain, spinal cord, and the cranial (oculomotor, V and VII cranial nerves) and peripheral nerves: **progressive multifocal leukoencephalopathy**, peripheral neuropathy, cauda equina compression, **polymyositis**, and infections such as **herpes zoster** and **cryptococcosis**. See also **primary CNS lymphoma**.[4254]

lymphomatoid granulomatosis A lymphoreticular proliferative and granulomatous disorder with polymorphic cellular infiltrates, mainly affecting the lungs and skin, but also capable of causing central or peripheral nervous system abnormalities, the former usually presenting as a neoplasm or multifocal disease, the latter as a sensorimotor neuropathy.[2942, 3842]

lymphomatous leptomeningitis See **neurolymphomatosis**.

lymphomatous neuropathy See **neurolymphomatosis**.

lypemania (Gr, grief + madness) Esquirol's term for depressive illness.

lypothymia (Gr, grief + the spirit) Great sadness.

lysine cystinurnia with benign myopathy A rare congenital familial disorder presenting with severe muscular hypotonia, respiratory failure, and feeding difficulties, but with eventual improvement in most cases. The condition is accompanied by dwarfism but there is no mental defect. Aminoaciduria and mild renal acidosis are also present.[1188]

lysine intolerance A rare diffuse encephalopathy due to a failure in the intestinal transport of dibasic amino acids and a resulting deficiency of available arginine, ornithine, and lysine. Clinically, the condition is characterized by cataract, short stature, hepatosplenomegaly, and weakness, with aminoaciduria.[4985]

lysinuric protein intolerance See **familial protein intolerance**.

lysis The destruction of an object; in medicine, usually a cell or a chemical substance such as an enzyme.

lysis of myofibrils in type 1 fibers A rare congenital myopathy presenting with severe weakness and hypotonia, with lumbar lordosis, and characterized pathologically by small type 1 myofibrils, within which oxidative activity is absent but adenosine triphosphatase activity is increased in some peripheral zones.[5500]

lysosomal enzyme defects See **lysosomal storage diseases**.

lysosomal glycogen storage disease A dominantly inherited disease that presents with vacuolar myopathy, cardiomyopathy, and weakness in infants, and proximal limb weakness and diaphragmatic paralysis but no cardiac involvement in adults. A deficiency of lysosomal alpha 1,4 amyloglucosidase is usually detected at all ages. See also **Pompe disease**.

lysosomal storage diseases (lysosomal enzyme defects) Genetically determined disorders in which the intracytoplasmic enzymes that normally metabolize peptide and glycosidic linkages are deficient, so that the substances normally degraded accumulate within and cause swelling of the lysosomes, which contain undigested metabolic products in various types of cells.[1409] Their overall frequency may be 1 in 5000 live births. Confident diagnosis requires skin biopsy.[5108]

Disorders affecting the nervous system include **sphingolipidoses** (Niemann–Pick and variants), **mucopolysaccharidoses, mucolipidoses, glycoproteinoses, cystinosis,** and some **glycogenoses**. In all, over 40 such diseases are known. See also **GM$_1$ gangliosidosis, GM$_2$ gangliosidosis** (Tay–Sachs and Sandhoff disease, AB variant), **sulfatidoses, metachromatic leukodystrophy** and *variants*, and **mucosulfatidosis, Gaucher disease** Types 1, 2, and 3, **Krabbe disease, sphingomyelin storage disorders, Fabry disease, Jansky–Bielschowsky disease** (Types A, B, C, and D), **Spielmeyer–Vogt disease, mucopolysaccharidoses** (Hurler; Hunter; Sanfilippo Types A, B, C, and D; Morquio; Maroteaux–Lamy; and beta-glucuronidase deficiency), **glycogen storage disease type** 2, oligosaccharidoses (**fucosidoses, mannosidosis**, and **aspartylglucosaminuria**), **Wolman disease, sialidoses, saposin defects, adrenoleukodystrophy, neuronal ceroid lipofuscinosis**, and **acid phosphatase deficiency**.[2407, 3522, 6720] In most of these, the clinical features include progressive psychomotor retardation and abnormal facial appearances.

lysosomes Membrane-bound intracytoplasmic bodies containing the hydrolytic enzymes required for the degradation of lipids, proteins, and nuclides, which form an integral part of the structure of normal cells.[2407]

lyssa See **rabies**.

lyssophobia (Gr, rage or canine madness + fear) Pseudohydrophobia. A condition resembling **rabies** without true respiratory muscle spasm.

Lytico-Bodig (Hirano Parkinsonism–dementia, laughing death) The vernacular term for the amyotrophic lateral sclerosis–Parkinsonism–dementia complex occurring in the Chamorro people of Guam and Rota in the Western Pacific.[2257, 5969] Cerebellar ataxia is another feature. See also **amyotrophic lateral sclerosis**.

M wave A compound muscle action potential evoked from a muscle by an electric stimulus to its motor nerve. By convention, the M wave elicited by a supramaximal stimulus is used for motor nerve conduction studies. Ideally, the recording electrodes should be placed so that the initial deflection of the evoked potential from the baseline is negative. Common measurements include latency, amplitude, and duration. Also referred to as the motor response. Normally, the configuration is biphasic and stable with repeated stimuli at slow rates (1–5 Hz). See repetitive nerve stimulation. (From the 2001 Report of the Nomenclature Committee of the American Association of Electromyography and Electrodiagnosis.[19] Reproduced by kind permission of the AANEM.)

MAAP Services (for Autism, Asperger Syndrome, and PDD) A charitable organization in this field. Web site: http://www.maapservices.org/index.html.

Mabry muscular dystrophy An X-linked muscular dystrophy with incomplete penetrance, in which muscle weakness and wasting appear between the ages of 5 and 35 years, the pelvic muscles being affected first.

Later clinical features include calf pseudohypertrophy, EKG abnormalities, and very slow progression, such that ambulation is still possible until mature adult life, and survival to late middle age is usual.[3983] See **X-linked muscular dystrophy**.

MacCormack, W. (1836–1901) Irish surgeon, practicing in Belfast.

MacCormack reflex Adduction of the contralateral thigh after tapping the patellar tendon, due to reflex disinhibition in patients with bilateral pyramidal tract disease.

MacEwen, Sir William (1848–1924) Scottish surgeon who trained with Lord Lister in Glasgow. He became Regius professor of surgery in Glasgow, was elected a Fellow of the Royal Society in 1895, and was knighted in 1902. Even before this honor was bestowed, however, he used to speak of himself in the first person plural.

His 1879 paper in the *Glasgow Medical Journal* "Tumour of the dura mater—convulsions—removal of tumour by trephining—recovery" was not only an account of a spectacular surgical *tour de force*, but combined within the title the introduction, patient and methods, results, and conclusions sections, while the discussion seems superfluous. His later publications concerned above all his treatment of cerebral abscesses and sinus thrombosis, summarized in his book *Pyogenic Diseases of the Brain and Spinal Cord* (1893).

MacEwen pupil See **MacEwen signs**.

MacEwen signs 1. Increased resonance on combined percussion and auscultation of the head. When the parietal region is tapped with the finger, a short high-pitched note can be heard with the stethoscope placed over the frontal region in children with increased intracranial pressure, so long as the fontanelles are closed. The sound becomes quieter when the tapping finger approaches the stethoscope.[3996, 5333] This is a form of auscultatory percussion and is not the same as the **cracked-pot note** heard without a stethoscope in similar conditions.
2. (MacEwen pupil) The pupil of a patient comatose due to alcohol intoxication dilates briefly when the patient is stimulated but not awakened, while that of a patient comatose due to structural disease does not dilate with such mild stimulation.[3995]

MacEwen triangle (suprameatal triangle) A space bounded by the lower part of the posterior end of the zygoma, the superior posterior edge of the external auditory meatus, and the mastoid process, a landmark for identifying the position of the underlying middle meningeal artery.

Machado–Joseph Azorean disease See **Joseph disease**.

Machado–Joseph disease A Web site describing the origins of the disease and the Jewish connection, etc. It is found at http://www.mazornet.com/genetics/machado.htm/.

Another information site (Machado–Joseph Disease Fact Sheet) provides data developed by the National Institute of Neurological Disorders and Stroke (NINDS). This is found at http://www.ninds.nih.gov/disorders/machado_joseph/detail_machado_joseph.htm.

Mackenzie, Sir Stephen (1844–1909) British physician.

Mackenzie syndrome Dysfunction of cranial nerves IX, X, XI, and XII with a Horner syndrome, resulting from infiltration by a tumor of the retroparotid space below the base of the skull.[4003]

macro- (Gr, long or large).

macro–creatine kinase Variant forms of creatine kinase, including CK-BB with immunoglobulin, and aggregates of mitochondrial creatine kinase.[3686]

macro motor unit action potential (macro-MUAP) The average electric activity of that part of an anatomic motor unit that is within the recording range of a macro-EMG electrode. Characterized by consistent appearance when the small recording surface of the macro-EMG electrode is positioned to record action potentials from one muscle fiber. The following characteristics can be specified quantitatively: (1) maximal peak-to-peak amplitude, (2) area contained under the waveform, (3) number of phases. (From the 2001 Report of the Nomenclature Committee of the American Association of Electromyography and Electrodiagnosis.[19] Reproduced by kind permission of the AANEM.)

macro-MUAP See **macro motor unit action potential**.

macrophagic myofasciitis A rare disease of adults, mainly reported in France, in patients injected with aluminum-containing vaccines (hepatitis, tetanus) in the previous year and who complain of muscle pain and discomfort, arthralgias, and mild proximal weakness. Also described in some cases are pyramidal signs, hemisensory and cerebellar signs, visual loss, and fatigue somewhat suggestive of multiple sclerosis except for the additional presence of fever, dyspnea, and cough, although the MRI does sometimes show single or multifocal regions of demyelination, sensory evoked potentials may be abnormal and the CSF contains raised protein levels and oligoclonal bands. The definitive status of the disorder remains to be established.[303]

macrosaccadic oscillations Sequences of large- or small-amplitude square wave saccadic jerks (1–30°) which oscillate with increasing and decreasing amplitude, bypassing the fixation point with each reversal. They are absent in darkness. Such oscillations reflect excessive gain within the saccadic system and typically occur in patients with lesions of the deep midline cerebellar structures.[5718, 5731]

Adaptive changes made to muscle activation during periods of weakness may become maladaptive, with return of strength as when edrophonium chloride is given to patients with myasthenia gravis, in which condition these oscillations may also be found.

macro square-wave jerks (kippdeviationen/kippnystagmus) Unwanted saccadic movements (saccadic intrusions) appearing as large-amplitude square-wave jerks (10–40°), followed by corrective saccades after an interval.

These bursts of square-wave jerks of large amplitude occur at about 2 Hz during fixation. Both eyes suddenly and conjugately move off the target with a saccade, but after a latent period of about 80 ms a nonvisually evoked reflex saccade returns them to the target. They may, however, be present in darkness. They have been described in patients with acute cerebellar lesions and with chronic ataxic syndromes, including **multiple sclerosis**.[1563] See also **square-wave pulses**.

macrocephaly (macrocrania) Enlarged head circumference, greater than 2 standard deviations above the mean for the person's age and sex. Although this is a frequent feature of numerous named clinical syndromes, macrocrania may also exist in isolation, when it is a factor increasing the risk of perinatal brain damage but is otherwise harmless.

macrocephaly and callosal agenesis See **Young syndrome**.

macrocephaly with angiomatosis A congenital syndrome comprising asymmetrical limbs, macrocephaly, and capillary and cavernous hemangiomas with papilledema,[381] presumably due to raised intracranial pressure with obstructive hydrocephalus.

macrocrania See **macrocephaly**.

macrodactyly (Gr, macros, long + dactylos, finger) Enlargement of a digit, as may occur rarely in **neurofibromatosis**, with arteriovenous malformations, with **localized hypertrophic neuropathy**,[224] or in the syndrome described in the next entry.

macrodactyly with connective tissue nevi and hemihypertrophy A congenital neurocutaneous syndrome, characterized by scoliosis, asymmetrical limbs, macrodactyly, calcification of muscle and subcutaneous tissues, and patchy depigmentation of the skin.[381]

macrodystrophia lipomatosa A condition occurring in young people, characterized by hypertrophy of the finger or part of the hand as a result of infiltration of the soft tissues (including the nerves traversing the region) by fat.

The disorder may be a form of **neurofibromatosis**, but there is very little disturbance in the function of the nerves affected.

macroelectromyography (macro-EMG) A general term referring to the technique and conditions that approximate recording of all muscle fiber action potentials arising from the same motor unit. See **macro motor unit action potential**. (From the 2001 Report of the Nomenclature Committee of the American Association of Electromyography and Electrodiagnosis.[19] Reproduced by kind permission of the AANEM.)[6010]

macro-EMG See **macroelectromyography**.

macro-EMG needle electrode A modified single fiber electromyography electrode insulated to within 15 mm of the tip and with a small recording surface (25 μm in diameter) 7.5 mm from the tip.

macroglobulinemia A group of conditions characterized by a marked increase in the amount of IgM in the blood. This may occur as an isolated condition, or may complicate lymphomas, collagen vascular diseases, or some hemolytic anemias. Clinically, malaise, fatigue, weakness, and the usual features of a demyelinating sensorimotor peripheral neuropathy are the most prominent features; when this presents acutely, the overall picture is that of **acute inflammatory demyelinating polyneuropathy**.[2516] See **Bing-Neel syndrome**.

macroglossia (Gr, long + tongue) Enlargement of the tongue to the extent that it protrudes beyond the teeth or alveolar ridge at rest. It occurs with hypothyroidism, lymphangioma, hemangioma, and muscle dystrophies (primary form) and as a result of infiltrations such as amyloid and benign and malignant masses (secondary form).

macrogyria A rare neuronal migration disorder consisting of an increase in the width (and therefore a decrease in the number) of the cerebral cortical gyri. This is sometimes combined with **microgyria**. In its most extreme form, it is associated with complete absence of the gyri.[6024]

macroprolactinoma A prolactin-secreting pituitary adenoma greater than 10 mm in diameter and liable to compress local structures such as the optic chiasm.

macropsia The apparent magnification of objects seen—a perceptual distortion in which objects appear too large to the subject. Both retinal lesions and complex partial seizures may be responsible.

macrotia (Gr, macros, long + otos, ear) Enlargement of the ears, occasionally dominantly inherited.

macula lutea (Lat, a small spot + yellow) The portion of the retina to the temporal side of the optic disk, about 1 mm in diameter, which contains the greatest concentration of cone receptors and where the blood vessels are all of capillary size. At its center is the fovea, where even capillaries are absent.

macular degeneration Hereditary or acquired absence or degeneration of the cone cells of the retina (**pigmentary retinopathy**) or of both cones and rods. The former presents with bilaterally diminished visual acuity, impaired color vision, and photophobia by day (**hemeralopia**). Various degenerative or metabolic neurological disorders are frequently associated.

macular dystrophy–deaf-muteness syndrome See **Amalric syndrome**.

macular ischemia Focal ischemia of the macula, resulting usually from presumed embolism or hematological disorders such as sickle cell disease, and manifest clinically by the presence of a central scotoma.[6348]

macular sparing That condition in which the macular representation on the involved side is wholly or partly unaffected despite the presence of homonymous visual field defects, leaving an island of central vision within a sea of blindness. It occurs probably as a result of the large area of the visual cortex devoted to the representation of the macula. See also **sparing of fixation**.

macular star The glistening sheen upon the retina radiating around the fovea or between the fovea and the optic disk, indicating the presence of retinal edema.

maculoanesthetic leprosy See **tuberculoid leprosy**.

maculopapillary fibers The bundle of nerve fibers running from the macula to the optic nerve head. These are especially, but not selectively, susceptible to damage from demyelination; in such cases, a striped appearance (*retinal slits*) is sometimes seen when they are viewed with red-free (i.e., green) light through the ophthalmoscope.

mad as a hatter An opprobrious term popularized by the fiction of Lewis Carroll, but with a root in truth, in that sublimate of mercury was once used to rub up the nap on the felt used in making hats. The resultant encephalopathy (with visual field constriction, neuropathy, depression, and tremor) suffered by the hatters led to the name.

mad cow disease See **bovine spongiform encephalopathy**. http://www.mad-cow.org/ is a Web site providing data on mad cow disease, **Creutzfeldt-Jacob disease**, prions, spongiform encephalopathies, scrapie, BSE, CWD, TME, and TSE.

madarosis Loss of the outer part of the eyebrow as occurs in **leprosy** and hypothyroidism.

MADD See **myoadenylate deaminase deficiency syndrome**.

Maddox rod A test instrument comprising a disk composed of parallel red glass cylinders which can be employed in estimating the degree of diplopia in the nine cardinal positions of gaze. The presence of the rod placed before one eye prevents fusional vergence. When the disk is placed over one eye (by convention, the right), a bright white light source is seen as a red line with that eye, and its position and orientation can be compared with the white image seen by the unoccluded eye.[3762] See also **red glass test** and **Lancaster red-green test**.

Madelung disease See **familial multiple symmetrical lipomatosis with peripheral neuropathy**.

Madras neuropathy A variant of **amyotrophic lateral sclerosis** in which VIII cranial nerve involvement and bulbar palsy, with slowing of motor nerve conduction velocities, are commonly found. The condition, reported from Madras, India, may be either dominantly or recessively inherited.[244]

Maffucci syndrome A rare sporadic neurocutaneous syndrome of unknown cause characterized by multiple enchondromas, visceral and cutaneous hemangiomas, bony malformations, and phlebolithiasis.

It was described by Dr. Angelo Maffucci, an Italian physician, in 1881. Primary brain tumors and syndromes consequent upon compression of the CNS by the bony abnormalities are the usual neurological complications.[3] This condition and **Ollier disease** may be the same.[4297]

Magendie, François (1783–1855) French physician, born in Bordeaux, who trained in Paris and eventually became professor of physiology and pathology at the Collège de France and physician at the Hôtel-Dieu. Among his earliest work was the demonstration of the effects of what turned out to be strychnine. He confirmed the report of **Bell** (published in 1811) that the anterior spinal roots were motor, but was the first to show that the posterior roots were sensory (the Bell-Magendie law) in 1822, although his report was somewhat hesitant. He described the CSF in 1827,[4015] and the **foramen** in the fourth ventricular roof which bears his name in 1842. He was also the first to describe **decerebrate rigidity**. Claude **Bernard** was his most famous pupil, and later his successor.

His claim to have discovered CSF (which he thought was secreted by the pia-arachnoid membrane at the surface of the brain and flowed into the ventricles through the midline foramen which he had described in 1828) was false. Key and Retzius restored a correct understanding of the formation, direction of flow, and absorption of CSF in 1876, Luschka redescribed the lateral foramina, and Magendie's errors were forgotten; but the name lives on.[6353]

MAGIC syndrome (mouth and genital ulcers with inflamed cartilage) A rare variant of **Adamtiades-Behcet syndrome** with these features.

magnet reaction See **grasp response**.

magnet reflex When the examiner's finger pushes the sole of a baby's foot so that the knee and the hip flex, and then slowly withdraws his finger, the baby's leg normally extends so that the foot remains in contact with it.

magnetic apraxia Bimanual grasping of objects seen or felt, occurring in patients with orbital frontal-lobe lesions, perhaps through release of parietal-lobe activity.[3826]

magnetic foot See **tonic foot response**.

magnetic gait See **isolated gait ignition failure**.

magnetic gait apraxia See **frontal gait disorder**.

magnetic gaze attraction Persistence of a subject's gaze upon one object among a number presented, especially within the remaining normal homonymous half-field, seen in subjects with right hemispheric lesions. The phenomenon is commonly associated with unilateral spatial neglect.[1241]

magnetic resonance angiography (MRA) A development of MRI scanning, allowing accurate visualization of arterial anatomy.

magnetic resonance imaging (MRI, nuclear magnetic resonance) A technique adapted for neuroimaging that studies the absorption or emission of electromagnetic energy by nuclei in a static magnetic field after excitation by a suitable radiofrequency stimulus.[875]

The method uses the principles of nuclear magnetic resonance and the same computer techniques as are used for CT scanning to produce a map of the body's soft (water-containing) tissues. This requires high-strength magnetic fields, in which the magnetic properties of hydrogen atoms (protons) and the sensitivity of the spin of those nuclei to radiofrequency signals are studied. There are no known side effects, and the technique complements and often replaces CT scanning as a means of imaging inaccessible structures. Thus, it has been estimated that MRI has 10 times the power of CT in the resolution of the lesions of multiple sclerosis.[6856] A review of its nature and diagnostic value has been published.[1805]

Diffusion weighted imaging is a refinement of MR technique that measures the Brownian motion of water; it is of value in the diagnosis of ischemic disease, producing increased signals in ischemic tissue. *Perfusion weighted imaging* measures the relative blood flow in tissues using the patients own blood or injected contrast agents such as gadolinium.

magnetic resonance spectroscopy A technique based upon the principles of **magnetic resonance imaging**, but which also examines the concentration and distribution of elements other than the hydrogen proton, such as ^{31}P, thus informing on the metabolism of tissues without such intervention as biopsy. To date, such examinations have yielded information of the greatest value in primary muscle diseases and in cerebral ischemic states.

magnetization transfer ratio The magnitude of the exchange of magnetization between free water (which is normally visible on conventional T1- and T2-weighted MRI images) and bound water (which being fixed within lipid membranes and proteins is normally invisible on conventional MRI scans) following selective saturation of the bound water pool. The ratio gives an indication of the amount of macromolecular material present in a unit of brain.

Myelin is the most prevalent complex macromolecule present in the brain and MTR may thus indicate the extent of demyelination.[2298]

magnetoencephalography (MEG) The measurement, recording, and display of magnetic fields mainly perpendicular to the skull (and thus emanating from the sulci) produced by ionic flow across active neuronal membranes, which are the same ionic currents as are produced by EEG signals. This is a technique still in its infancy with regard to clinical diagnosis, but currently under scrutiny as to its ability, usually in combination with EEG, to localize abnormal electrical discharges within the brain.[168, 1228]

magnetometer A device capable of measuring the smallest magnetic fields of the brain, and which is thus able to detect the location, depth, orientation, and polarity of intracerebral spike discharges.

Magnus, Rudolf (1873–1927) Dutch professor of pharmacology and neurophysiologist at Utrecht. He demonstrated the existence of the antidiuretic factor in pituitary extracts, but is best known for his studies of postural, tonic labyrinthine, righting, and neck reflexes in the decerebrate animal, which led to huge advances in understanding of the activity of the vestibular apparatus.

The *Magnus-de Kleijn reflex* consists of extension of the limbs and rigidity on the side to which the head is turned passively, with flexion of the limbs with decreased tone on the other side; it is seen in subjects with decerebration.

Magoun, H.W. Neurophysiologist who with **Moruzzi** delineated the reticular activating system.

Maida Vale Hospital for Nervous Diseases Formerly the London Hospital for the Paralysed and Epileptic. A division of the **National Hospital**, Queen Square, London.

main d'accoucheur (Fr, obstetrician's hand) See **carpopedal spasm**.

main de fakir (Fr, fakir's hand) A minor **dystonia**, not uncommon in the elderly, in whom this may be the first or only sign of a basal ganglion disorder. Flexion at the metacarpophalangeal joints, extension of the interphalangeal joints, and adduction of the thumb are the postures producing this appearance.

main en griffe (Fr, hand in the shape of a claw) The manual posture seen in the setting of most lower motor neuron lesions chronically affecting the C8-T1 roots and thus those fibers destined for the median and ulnar nerves. In this condition the metacarpophalangeal joints are extended and the interphalangeal joints flexed; contractures of the long flexors also play a part in causing this. **Duchenne** first used the term in describing the appearance of the hands in **amyotrophic lateral sclerosis**, but it is more commonly seen with severe ulnar nerve pareses.

main en pince (Fr, hand + claw) Partial flexion of the first two digits and full flexion of the remaining fingers, the posture of the hand thus slightly resembling a crab's claws; seen in some patients with severe motor neuropathies or **syringomyelia**. The name was applied by Pierre **Marie** and **Guillain**.

main en poing fermée (Fr, hand with the fist clenched) Clenching of the fist, as the first or only sign of a minor **dystonia**, as is not uncommon in the elderly. See also **fisting**.

main succulente (Marinesco hand sign) The term applied by **Marinesco** to the cold, edematous, shiny, and livid appearance of the hand in some cases of **syringomyelia**. It may also be a feature of **complex regional pain syndrome**.

maintenance of wakefulness test A variation of **polysomnography**, wherein subjects with complaints of excessive sleepiness are assessed.[4405]

Mainzer-Saldino syndrome A congenital dysmorphic syndrome characterized by short stature, retinitis pigmentosa, hepatic and renal insufficiency, broad hands with arachnodactyly and cone-shaped phalangeal epiphyses, cerebellar signs, and mental and developmental delay.[381]

Majewski syndrome See **short rib–polydactyly type 2**.

major causalgia See **reflex sympathetic dystrophy**.

major motor seizure See **generalized tonic-clonic seizure**.

make/break test An extension of the technique of hand-held dynamometry, in which the patient's power is tested isometrically (power being generated against immovable resistance; "make") and compared with that generated isotonically (power generated up to a maximum against increasing resistance; "break"). An increase of more than 20% in the force exerted can be generated by patients with functional weakness tested with the "break" rather than the "make" technique.[6487]

mal (Fr, evil, pain or sickness) Hence *mal d'amour* for toothache (married man's toothache, part of the **Couvade syndrome**); *mal de mer* for seasickness; *mal de montagne* for mountain sickness; *mal de tête* for headache; *grand and petit mal* epilepsies; *mal Saint, mal sacre, mal de terre, mal de St. Jean, and mal haut* for forms of epilepsy; and many other secular (*mal Francais, mal des Allemands, mal Neapolitain, mal Espagnol, mal de Brunn, mal de chien*) or saintly (e.g., *mal divin, mal de SSt. Mervuis, Sement, Homme, Job, or Euphemie*) attributions for syphilis.[5103]

mal de débarquement A persisting sensation of imbalance, swaying, or rocking (as if trying to walk on a trampoline) that occurs after disembarking from a ship after a sea voyage. In rare cases it persists for months or years. The illusory floor movement may be accompanied by nausea, gaze instability, or visual disturbances whereby objects jump and shimmer ahead but there is no rotational vertigo. The cause and therapy are unknown. See also **space motion sickness**.

mal perforant Painless perforating ulcers of the digits, most commonly seen in patients with **hereditary sensory and autonomic neuropathy type 2** but also in **tabes dorsalis** or **syringomyelia**.

malabsorption encephalopathy Fatigue, weakness, and physical and mental retardation, usually with evidence of subacute combined degeneration of the spinal cord and polyneuropathy, resulting from chronic malnutrition with steatorrhea.[5725]

maladie des tics compulsifs/impulsifs See **Tourette syndrome**.

malaise The subjective awareness that one is not perfectly well. In its mildest form, Miller Fisher[2099] noted as typical symptoms tiredness, a wish to sleep longer, disinclination for activity, loss of enthusiasm and cheerfulness, diminished appetite, and a disinclination to clear thinking. In more severe degrees of affliction, lack of strength, energy, initiative, appetite, alertness, and intellectual effort may be disabling. These symptoms are a part of the effort syndrome, and also of depression, but they are not usually accompanied by notable affective change and are closely linked temporally with organic diseases, both serious and trivial. Their neural substrate remains elusive and in fact no pathology may exist.

malar (Lat, of the cheek bone).

malaria Infection with *Plasmodium vivax, malariae, falciparum, or ovale*, as a result of transfer of the sporozoites of the organism resulting from a mosquito bite. Congestion of cerebral capillaries with *P. falciparum*-laden red blood cells is the cause of the multifocal encephalopathy, perhaps the commonest nontraumatic encephalopathy in the world, presenting with fever, seizures, and focal cerebral signs and known as *cerebral malaria*.[1458]

Diagnostic criteria for cerebral malaria have been suggested as follows:[4651]

> A deep level of unconsciousness (such that a painful stimulus is not localized) in the presence of a *P. falciparum* asexual parasitemia, after the correction of hypoglycemia and exclusion of other encephalopathies, especially bacterial meningitis and locally prevalent viral encephalitides.

Other neurological complications include mononeuropathy and perhaps radiculopathy.

malformation A defective part of an organ or of a region of the body resulting from an abnormality of development.

malignant (from Lat, to act spitefully) Disposed to harm.

malignant angioendotheliomatosis (malignant intravascular lymphoma, malignant systematized angioendotheliomatosis, neoplastic angioendotheliomatosis) A rare, rapidly fatal disorder of adult life, characterized by the intravascular proliferation of atypical mononuclear cells, leading to ischemic damage to many organs, but especially the CNS. Clinically, a subacute progressive dementing syndrome is the most typical presentation; cortical blindness; disturbances of gait, the special senses, and speech; and motor and sensory deficits progress to cause death within a year.[456, 3498]

The same term is applied to a condition of intravascular malignant metastasis or lymphomatous spread occurring in adults.

malignant atrophic papulosis (Kohlmeier-Degos disease, Degos syndrome, fatal cutaneointestinal syndrome) A rare fatal cutaneous and systemic vaso-occlusive disease of unknown cause. The numerous painless skin lesions (the effects of the vasculopathy) are papular or atrophic and are scattered all over the trunk, while small infarcts also occur in the gastrointestinal tract and conjunctivae and occasionally in the CNS.[1531]

The condition occurs mainly in adult males; occasional involvement of the CNS has been reported, with nonspecific signs of disseminated disease (ptosis, ophthalmoplegias, dysarthria, bleeding diatheses, seizures, multifocal cerebral infarctions, venous thrombosis, subdural hematoma, and rarely myelopathy and neuropathy) resulting from vascular thrombosis.[4222] CSF examination shows pleocytosis and elevated protein. Brain biopsy reveals extensive small vessel occlusions and thrombosis with intimal proliferation.

malignant brain edema Increased cerebral blood flow with fluid extravasation as a result of a failure of autoregulation. This is typically seen in children after severe head injury.[4919]

malignant fasciculation Large, polyphasic fasciculation potentials firing at a slow rate. This pattern has been seen in progressive motor neuron disease, but the relationship is not exclusive. (From the 2001 Report of the Nomenclature Committee of the American Association of Electromyography and Electrodiagnosis.[19] Reproduced by kind permission of the AANEM.)

malignant hyperpyrexia See **malignant hyperthermia**.

malignant hypertensive headache (accelerated hypertensive headache) See **hypertensive encephalopathy**.

malignant hyperthermia (malignant hyperpyrexia and, in animals, capture myopathy) A dominantly inherited defect in the transmembrane transport of calcium, which may lead to muscle rigidity, hyperthermia, tachycardia, tachypnea, and hypertonicity but hyporeflexia, with acidosis, raised serum creatine kinase levels hypercapnia, hypoxemia, and **rhabdomyolysis** with myoglobinuria and potentially renal failure. The condition occurs within ½–24 h of exposure to depolarizing muscle relaxants, inhalational anesthetics, or tricyclic drugs.[3682] In cases with ryanodine receptor disturbance, the responsible gene maps to chromosome 19q12-q13.2. At least six varieties are defined, as follows: MHS1 (19q13, *ryanodine* receptor); MHS2 (17q11, Na^+ channel *SCNA4*); MHS3 (7q21, Ca^{2+} channel *CACNL2A*); MHS4 (3q13); MHS5 (1q32, Ca^{2+} channel *CACNA1S*); MHS6 (5p) to which may be added carnitine palmitoyl transferase 2 deficiency (1p32).

King-Denborough syndrome was the original form described but is now considered a *variant.* It presents mainly in young males in whom the syndrome is triggered by heat or anesthesia and who show proximal symmetrical weakness, slowing of motor development, slight facial dysmorphism, scapular winging, and mild chest and spinal deformities.

Screening is possible in those with a suspected family history (usually of death related to anesthesia), as baseline serum CK levels are usually elevated, but a firmer diagnosis can be achieved by an *in vitro* test on a muscle biopsy specimen activated with caffeine.[1925]

The original syndrome was characterized by short stature, mandibular hypoplasia, ptosis, spinal deformity, and pectus carinatum,[3438] but the condition also complicates various other subclinical, dominantly inherited or myotonic myopathies[2779] and **Noonan syndrome**. See also **neuroleptic malignant syndrome** (which is clinically similar but pharmacologically distinct) and **ecstasy**. See also http://neuromuscular.wustl.edu/msys/myoglob.html#mother for a full listing of differential diagnostic possibilities.

Malignant Hyperthermia Association A Canadian charitable organization at. Address: 200 Elizabeth St., Room ES3-403A, Toronto, ON M5G 2C4. Tel: 416-340-3128. Web site: www.mhaus.org/. Sister sites exist in the UK (http://www.bmha.co.uk/) and the United States (http://medical.mhaus.org/).

malignant inflammatory sensory polyganglionopathies (See also **nonmalignant inflammatory sensory polyganglionopathies**) A group of dysimmune disorders of dorsal root ganglia and autonomic and CNS structures affecting adults usually with small cell carcinoma of the lung and presenting with ataxic and/or hyperalgesic syndromes, with or without autonomic dysfunction and cerebral, cerebellar, or other CNS involvement. Women may be more prone to these conditions than men. The presence of antineuronal nuclear antibodies (ANNA or anti-Hu) strongly suggests the presence of the small cell carcinoma. The condition was originally described by **Denny-Brown** in the 1940s. See also **inflammatory sensory polyganglionopathies**.

malignant intravascular lymphoma See **malignant angioendotheliomatosis**.

malignant malnutritional syndrome See **kwashiorkor**.

malignant melanoma See **melanoma**.

malignant meningioma See **meningeal sarcoma** and **meningioma**.

malignant meningitis (neoplastic meningitis) Diffuse infiltration of the meninges and CSF by malignant cells, producing encephalopathy, evidence of raised intracranial pressure, seizures, focal signs including cranial neuropathies, and neck rigidity. The condition can complicate almost any kind of tumor, but especially cancers of the breast and lung, lymphoma, and leukemia. Among primary brain tumors that can spread through the intracranial and intraspinal cavities are ependymoma and medulloblastoma.

malignant monophasic multiple sclerosis (Marburg disease) A fulminant monophasic demyelinating disease of unknown cause usually affecting young adults and leading to severe disability (blindness, paraplegia, etc.) and early death; and with pathological features characteristic of multiple sclerosis but with unusually extensive axonal loss.[4056]

malignant neurofibroma See **neurofibromas**.

malignant Schwannoma See **Schwannoma**.

malignant sensory neuropathy See **subacute sensory neuronopathy**.

malignant systematized angioendotheliomatosis See **malignant angioendotheliomatosis**.

malignant tumors Tumors that are rapidly growing and often invasive, and that histologically show frequent mitoses, necrosis, vascular proliferation, and endothelial hyperplasia.

malignant vasovagal syncope See **neurocardiogenic syncope**.

malingering The conscious, motivated simulation of disease.

Mallory body myopathy See **myofibrillar (desmin-storage) myopathy**.

Mallory stain (PTAH stain) A method of demonstrating glial fibers histologically, using mercuric chloride, phosphotungstic acid, and alcohol. Muscle fibers, myelin, and astroglia stain blue; collagen stains brown.

malnutrition syndrome A syndrome described in black African infants in the month or two following treatment of severe malnutrition. Clinically, the findings include Parkinsonian tremor and rigidity with hyperreflexia, and sometimes myoclonus, opisthotonos, and insomnia. The condition may result from relative deficiency of some essential dietary factor such as a trace element or vitamin in the context of sudden replenishment of protein stores.[3269]

Malta syndrome The association of hydrocephalus, encephalopathy, or retinal dystrophy and renal cysts.

maltase deficiency myopathy See **glycogen storage diseases**.

malum vertebrale suboccipitale Tuberculous caries of the atlanto-occipital region.

mandibular dysostosis See **hemifacial microsomia**.

mandibular reflex Tapping the chin causes elevation of the mandible in the normal newborn.[6898] See also **jaw jerk**.

mandibulofacial dysostosis (Franchescetti syndrome, Franchescetti–Zwahlen–Klein syndrome, Treacher Collins syndrome) A dominantly (or X-linked recessively) inherited congenital dysmorphic syndrome, characterized by anti-Mongolian slant of the eyes, malar and mandibular hypoplasia, colobomas of the lower lids, ocular malformations, prominent low-set ears with deformed pinnas, absent auditory canals, a flat malar region, cleft palate, webbed neck, pulmonary stenosis, cryptorchidism, microcephaly, dwarfism, and mental and developmental delay. Cervical vertebral anomalies and various other systemic abnormalities may also occur.[1256]

The condition was well described by Dr. E. Treacher-Collins,[1256] an English ophthalmologist at Moorfields Eye hospital, but the very first account was that of Allen Thompson, professor of physiology at Edinburgh in 1847. Franchescetti and Klein analyzed 65 cases in 1949 and integrated many unrelated observations into one logical clinical complex.

mandibulofacial syndromes A group of genetically determined malformations in which abnormal formations of the facial bones represent a common factor.

mandrake (*Atropa mandragora*) A plant whose root has anesthetic properties, used in ancient days to alleviate pain before amputations; and also as an enchantment, because it was considered capable of rendering a person invisible.

mands Self-limiting statements concerning the needs of the speaker.[1337] See also **tacts**.

manganism (manganese madness) Chronic manganese intoxication, usually from inhalation in a metal workshop, presenting as a syndrome resembling **Parkinson disease** but with hallucinations, cognitive impairment, flight of ideas, compulsive behavior and progression of gait disturbance, rigidity, flexed body posture, and distal tremor even for some time after cessation of exposure.[3018, 4259]

mania (Gr, violent madness) (delirium furiosum) A psychosis characterized by both mental and physical excitement. The term is still employed to refer to one aspect of bipolar depressive illness, and occasionally dipsomania (morbid alcoholic ingestion), but is seldom used in other contexts in modern medical parlance. The dancing mania (tarantism) came and went in 1374. Many other descriptive Latinisms to do with mania are also no longer current.

mania à potu (mania inebriosa) Alcoholic delirium. See **delirium tremens**.

mania inebriosa See **mania à potu**.

manifest latent nystagmus Conjugate horizontal, jerky eye movements seen in subjects with impaired vision (or visual deprivation) from birth, in which the movements are of decreasing exponential velocity and in which the fast phase always beats toward the viewing eye. It is associated with the presence of strabismus, is strongly visually driven and depends on the attentional state of the subject.[26] See also **latent nystagmus**.

man-in-the-barrel syndrome The association of weakness of the arms with intact leg power, as though the patient were constrained within a barrel. Brainstem functions are retained. The usual cause of this unusual syndrome is cerebral hypoperfusion, such as may occur after myocardial infarction. Bilateral infarction of the motor cortices, in the "watershed" areas, is also a cause.[4428] See also **amyotrophic lateral sclerosis, flail arm syndrome, lower motor neuron disease,** and **Hirayama disease**.

Mann syndrome The association of a positive Romberg sign, diminution of the corneal reflex, past pointing, and loss of arm swing on the same side as a contusion of the brain, with restricted movement of the eyes to that side.

The syndrome, which has uncertain validity and which does not permit localization of the responsible lesion to a single site, was described by Dr. Ludwig Mann (1866–1936), a German neuropathologist and professor of neurology in Breslau.[4042]

Mannkopf sign Pressure over a painful area usually causes an increase in the pulse rate of 10–30 per minute, but this increase does not occur in subjects with feigned pain, though it may do so in those in hysterical states.[1500]

mannosidosis 1. A rare congenital lysosomal storage disease due to deficiency of α-mannosidase, leading to the deposition of excessive amounts of glycoprotein (mannosyl-oligosaccharides). The responsible gene maps to chromosome 19p13.2-q12.

The clinical features, particularly the dysmorphism, resemble those of **Hurler syndrome** and include mental retardation, corneal opacities, nerve deafness, hepatosplenomegaly, osteoporosis, vertebral anomalies, short stature, sensorineural deafness, cataract, umbilical hernia, jaundice, mucopolysaccariduria, immunoglobulin deficiency, thickening of the calvarium, pyramidal signs, and mental and developmental delay. As *variants*, both rapidly progressive infantile and more lenient juvenile forms occur.[3459]

A rare *variant* is *adult α-mannosidosis*, presenting with late-onset ataxia and retinal degeneration, hearing loss, intellectual impairment, and dysostosis. The MRI shows cerebellar atrophy and parieto-occipital white matter changes.[2651]

2. **β-Mannosidosis (OMIM 25841)** is a rare congenital lysosomal storage disease of glycoprotein catabolism due to deficiency of β-mannosidase. Deafness and other neurological signs and facial dysmorphisms are the usual features; peripheral neuropathy has also been described. The diagnosis is made by finding severe reduction in β-mannosidase activity and elevation of urinary disaccharides.[3718]

Manta syndrome A rapidly progressive asymmetrical tetraparesis, ending fatally due to denervation as a result of rapidly progressive anterior horn cell disease without any involvement of the upper motor neuron.[4049] The cause is not determined.

mantakassa A form of acquired spastic paraplegia due to cyanide toxicity from cassava consumption in the residents of Mozambique.

Manto syndrome The unusual association of **spasmodic torticollis** and **thoracic outlet syndrome**.[1665]

manual automatism (pedal automatism) Bilateral or unilateral fumbling, tapping, or manipulating movements that indicate principally distal muscle activation.[16]

manual muscle testing Clinical techniques for evaluating the strength of muscle contractions semi-quantitatively, using the subjective judgments of the examiner, who provides the resistance to the patient's limb movement. The modified **Medical Research Council Scale** represents one such system.[4306]

Kendall's grading system[3381] expands on the MRC Scale:

10. Holds test position against strong pressure
9. Holds test position against moderate to strong pressure
8. Holds test position against moderate pressure
7. Holds test position against a slight to moderate pressure
6. Holds test position against slight pressure
5. Holds test position without pressure
4. Gradual release from test position
3. Moves through <100% range of motion against gravity or through full range of motion, gravity eliminated against resistance, or through full range of motion, gravity eliminated, and holds against resistance
2. Moves through full range of motion, gravity eliminated
1. Moves through <100% range of motion, gravity eliminated; trace of visible or palpable muscle contraction
0. No contraction palpable

maple syrup urine disease A recessively inherited leukoencephalopathy due to a block in the oxidative decarboxylation of leucine, isoleucine, and valine.[4315] The responsible gene maps to chromosome 19p13.1-q13.2. See also **branched-chain ketoaciduria**.

Clinically, drowsiness, vomiting, seizures, ataxia, and spasticity with intermittent opisthotonos are the usual signs, occurring first when protein is introduced into the infant's diet. Most infants die within a month of birth after rapid cerebral deterioration. The serum leucine levels are raised and hypoglycemia is common. Boiled urine assumes a yellow cast in the DPNH test.[4313]

A *variant* is *thiamine-dependent maple syrup urine disease*, which is characterized by similar but milder symptoms in the presence of some residual branched-chain ketoacid dehydrogenase activity and which is responsive to thiamine treatment.[1759]

marasmus (Gr, wasting) Emaciation of the body with stunting of growth, as in **protein-calorie malnutrition** and the **diencephalic syndrome**.[2287]

marble-bone disease See **Albers–Schönberg disease** and **osteopetrosis**.

marble brain disease See **carbonic anhydrase II deficiency**.

Marburg disease See **malignant monophasic multiple sclerosis**.

March of Dimes Birth Defects Foundation A charitable organization based at 1275 Mamaroneck Ave., White Plains, NY 10605. Web site: http://www.marchofdimes.com/.

march syndrome See **anterior tibial syndrome**.

marche à petits pas (Fr, gait with little steps) A feature of Parkinsonism and also of diffuse cerebral dysfunction, as in **Alzheimer disease**. See **frontal gait disorder**.

Marchi, Vittorio (1851–1908) Italian physician and anatomist. After graduation at Modena, he was assistant to **Golgi** for a time, and later worked in Florence and Modena. His name is occasionally given to the spinothalamic tract, but he is best remembered for the staining technique that he described in 1886.

Marchi stain A method of staining a block of neural tissue, achieved by immersing it in a mixture of osmium tetroxide and an oxidizing agent; degenerating myelin products stain black.

Marchiafava, Ettore (1847–1935) Italian physician who graduated from the University of Rome, where he eventually became professor of pathology and of clinical medicine. He published important work on malaria, vasculitis, and pathological anatomy as well as on the following condition.

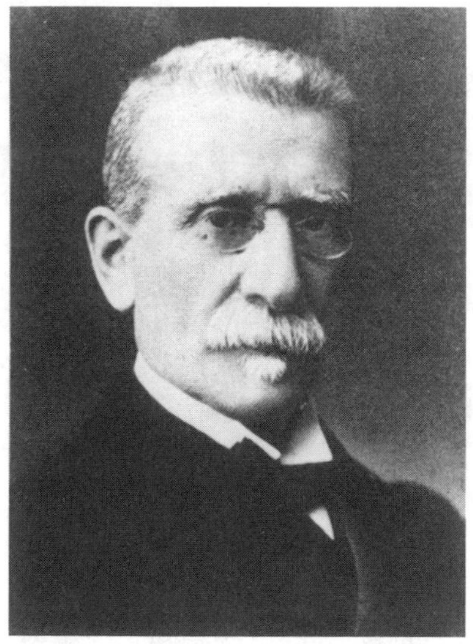

Figure M–1 Ettore Marchiafava.

Marchiafava–Bignami disease (corpus callosum degeneration, progressive alcoholic dementia) Degeneration of the middle layer of the corpus callosum throughout its extent, occurring classically in male Italian drinkers of red wine, but also described among alcoholics in other lands, drinking different wines. The anterior and hippocampal commissures, cerebellar peduncles, optic chiasm, and deep white matter pathways may also be affected. Clinically, confusion, seizures, dementia, aphasia, apraxias, pyramidal signs, rigidity, disconnection syndromes, mutism, and coma result; death follows shortly.[4058]

The mellifluous names of the original describers have fixed this syndrome in the minds of neurologists, almost none of whom will ever encounter it.

Marchiafava–Micheli syndrome Paroxysmal nocturnal hemoglobinuria, a potential cause of cerebral venous thrombosis and more often of back pain.[3234]

Marcus Gunn, Robert (1850–1909) Scottish ophthalmologist who trained in Vienna and at Moorfields Eye Hospital in London. See **Gunn, R.M.**

Marcus Gunn Phenomenon See **Gunn phenomenon**.

Marcus Gunn Pupil See **Gunn pupil**.

Marden–Walker syndrome A recessively inherited dysmorphic syndrome characterized by blepharophimosis, kyphoscoliosis, arachnodactyly, micrognathia, cleft palate, and multiple joint contractures present during the first year of life, and cataract.[4059] Pectus carinatum, congenital cardiac anomalies, camptodactyly, clubfoot, joint contractures, neurogenic muscle atrophy with hypotonia and hyporeflexia, agenesis of the corpus callosum, and mental and developmental delay are also occasionally described.

Marden–Walker-like syndrome See **Suliman syndrome**.

Marek disease A demyelinating neuropathy of poultry caused by a herpes virus with pathological similarities to **acute inflammatory polyneuropathy**.

Marfan, Antonin-Bernard-Jean (1858–1942) French pediatrician who trained in Toulouse and Paris, working for most of his life in the latter city as professor of therapeutics in one or another of the children's hospitals. The topics on which he published most often were tuberculosis, diphtheria, and nutrition, but he is best remembered for describing the following syndrome.

Marfan syndrome A polygenic, dominantly inherited disorder of connective tissue, the responsible gene mapping to 15q21.1, where the gene *FBN1* codes for fibrillin, a component of extracellular microfibrils. Its variable manifestations affect the eyes and the cardiovascular and skeletal systems.

The major clinical features include displacement of the lens, myopia, blue sclerae, dolichocephaly, high-arched palate, scoliosis with chest deformity, pectus carinatum or excavatum, inguinal hernia, flat arches of the feet, abnormally long limbs (the span of the body being greater than its height), arachnodactyly, laxity of joints, aortic and mitral valve lesions, and aortic dissecting aneurysm.[4062, 5148] The lower-segment (pubis to sole) measurement is greater than that of the upper segment (vertex to pubis), the ratio averaging 0.85 (normal, 0.93).[2504] A brief but comprehensive handbook has been published for the National Marfan Foundation of New York.[5147] Revised diagnostic criteria have been suggested.[1514]

In a *variant* form (*Marfan myopathic syndrome*), a slowly progressive myopathy is associated with early weakness in girdle distribution.[2428]

marginal gliosis See **Chaslin gliosis**.

marginal tract See **Lissauer tract**.

Marie, Pierre (1853–1940) French neurologist who trained in law before entering medicine. After his internship, he became a pupil of **Charcot** and eventually chef de clinique at the age of 65, after many years at the Bicêtre. He gave original descriptions of hypertrophic pulmonary osteo-arthropathy, achondroplasia, **primary lateral sclerosis**, and **craniocleidodysostosis** and, in 1886, with Charcot, described what is now known as **hereditary motor and sensory neuropathy** (peroneal muscular atrophy or Charcot–Marie–Tooth disease). In 1885 he had described acromegaly and later noted its association with a pituitary tumor. In 1893, he identified the hereditary ataxia now named for him (see next entry) and later described ankylosing spondylitis. His classification of the aphasias in 1906[4072] was notable for his vehement contradiction of **Broca** in its denial of any special role for the left third frontal convolution in speech.[804] He also questioned the existence of Aran–Duchenne progressive muscular atrophy in a paper in 1897.

Marie was a founder of the *Revue Neurologique* with Brissaud in 1893. He did not succeed **Charcot** as professor of diseases of the nervous system on the latter's death, but only in 1917 after the deaths of **Raymond** and then **Déjèrine**. Within 6 years, his closest family having died, he resigned and retired to the south of France.[7]

Marie ataxia (Nonne–Marie syndrome) A dominantly inherited spastic–ataxic syndrome with gaze palsies, which is probably not different from the olivopontocerebellar atrophy type 1 of Menzel, but may not comprise a single entity. Marie distinguished the condition from **Friedreich ataxia** on the grounds of later age of onset and the presence of hyperreflexia and pyramidal signs; oculomotor pareses; a reduction in visual acuity, and of the visual fields and of color vision; and the absence of Rombergism, of pes cavus, and of scoliosis.[4070] Optic atrophy, and in some cases mental deterioration, may occur late in the course of the disease.

One may remark a tendency to put most non-Friedreich ataxic patients into this category, which is what Marie seems to have done. However, a modern classification places this condition with the late-onset autosomal dominant **cerebellar ataxias**.[2753]

Marie syndrome See **pituitary gigantism**.

Marie–Foix retraction sign In patients with pyramidal lesions, pressure on the toes or vigorous plantar flexion at the ankle leads to flexion at the hip and knee and to attempts to dorsiflex the ankle.

Marie-Foix sclerosis Nonprogressive lesions of the white matter with sclerosis following perinatal encephalopathy or associated with acquired multifocal cerebrovascular disease.[4073] The condition has been mistaken for a form of **Schilder disease** and as a result the eponym *Schilder–Foix disease* was coined.

Marie–Foix syndrome Unilateral cerebellar ataxia with contralateral hemiparesis and thermoanalgesia, resulting from a rostral lateral pontine lesion. See **lateral pontomedullary syndrome**, which is almost if not exactly the same thing.

Marie–Foix–Alajouanine syndrome (late cortical cerebellar atrophy) A sporadic, adult-onset cerebellar syndrome with atrophic changes limited to the cerebellum and inferior olives, resembling Holmes cerebellar atrophy, except that the latter is dominantly inherited. It is occasionally accompanied by dementia, pyramidal signs, or absent ankle jerks. See **autosomal dominant cerebellar ataxias** and **olivopontocerebellar atrophy**.

Marie–Léri syndrome Acromegaly, described by Marie in 1886, by von Recklinghausen in 1890 and by Leri in 1913.

Marie–Sée syndrome The occurrence of **idiopathic intracranial hypertension** in children, here due to vitamin A intoxication. The condition was originally described in 1951[4069] by Dr. J. Marie.

Marin-Amat syndrome (inverted Marcus Gunn phenomenon) Abnormal synkinetic movements following facial nerve paresis and manifesting as eye closure when the jaw is opened wide. The condition has been described as the opposite of the **Gunn phenomenon** (jaw-winking)[4076, 5179] but probably represents a normal associated movement rather than the manifestation of any abnormal trigeminofacial anastomosis. It may be noted in passing that, when the mouth is opened unusually wide, as in yawning, the eyes close anyway.

Dr. Marin-Amat was a Spanish ophthalmologist.

Marinesco, Georges (Marinescu, Georghe) (1863–1938) Romanian neurologist who trained under **Charcot** and Weigert and later became professor of neurology at Bucharest. He identified and named **chromatolysis**, the lesions of the substantia nigra in **Parkinson disease**, and **neuronophagia** (which he so named). He also wrote on salvarsan therapy for syphilis, painful amputation neuromas, pathological anatomy, diseases of muscle, and conditioned reflexes, and published a number of books on neurology and pathology. See also **Marinesco–Sjörgen (–Garland) syndrome**.

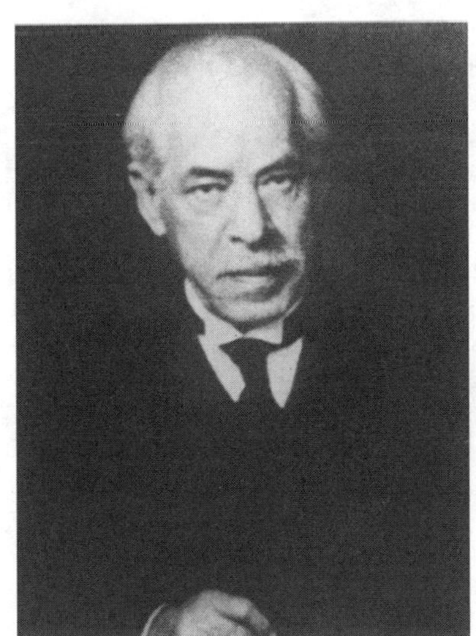

Figure M–2 Georges Marinesco.

Marinesco bodies Eosinophilic intranuclear inclusions found in the pigmented brainstem nuclei and substantia nigra, in numbers proportional to the subject's age; also found mainly in the substantia nigra in elderly people and in those with hepatic encephalopathy.

Marinesco hand sign (main succulente) The cold, livid, and edematous hand in **syringomyelia**, resulting from sympathetic irritation. This was the subject of Marinesco's graduation thesis.[4081]

Marinesco–Sjögren(–Garland) syndrome A rare recessively inherited congenital degenerative disorder, characterized clinically by progressive cerebellar ataxia, nystagmus, and cataract occurring at any age but usually in early childhood, and a variable degree of mental retardation.

Skeletal anomalies such as dwarfism, kyphoscoliosis, and pes cavus; pigmentary retinopathy, hypertension, hypergonadotropic hypogonadism, delayed motor development, dysarthria, myopathy,[436] pyramidal signs, and peripheral neuropathy with inclusions seen on nerve biopsy specimens have also been described in this condition.[5737]

The first report of the syndrome was in 1904. Marinesco published in 1931 and Sjögren emphasized the genetic nature of the disease in 1950.[4082] See also **Gillespie syndrome**, in which aniridia is present rather than cataract but which is otherwise identical. The Web site http://www.marinesco-sjogren.org/ provides information and support for families affected with this syndrome.

Marinescu–Radovici reflex See **palmomental reflex**.

Mariotte spot The blind spot.

Markesbery–Griggs disease A late-onset dominantly inherited titinopathy with distal myopathic symptoms and signs, mapped to 2q31 and allelic with **tibial muscular dystrophy**.[4088]

Markus syndrome See **Adie pupil**, **Holmes–Adie syndrome**.

Markus–Adie syndrome See **Holmes–Adie syndrome**.

Maroteaux–Lamy syndrome 1. mucopolysaccharidosis type VI See

mucopolysaccharidoses. 2. pyknodysostosis; from Gr, dense + bone + condition
A recessive syndrome of mental retardation, dwarfism, delayed closure of the fontanelles, skull and spinal dysplasia with deformity, a double row of teeth, and blue sclerae.[4095]

Marsden, C. David (1938–1998)
Pre-eminent British neurologist and neurophysiologist, professor and chairman of neurology at the *National Hospital*, Queen Square, and prolific contributor to knowledge, especially in the fields of movement disorders and genetics. He described such syndromes as *painful legs and moving toes*, *reticular reflex*, *cortical* and *propriospinal myoclonus*, and *abdominal dyskinesias*, and in the words of Stanley Fahn, "brought order into the spectrum of dystonia." He was elected a Fellow of the Royal Society in 1983.

Marshall criteria
A scoring system for the severity of head injuries based on the results of cranial CT scans.[4114]

Marshall syndrome
See **dominant saddle nose, myopia, cataract**, and **hearing loss**.

Martha–Alma disease
See **neurodegeneration with brain iron accumulation**.

Martin–Albright syndrome
See **pseudohypoparathyroidism**.

Martin–Bell syndrome
See **fragile X syndrome**.

Martin–Gruber anastomosis
A common anomalous connection between the median and ulnar nerves, usually in the upper forearm. In the most common form, fibers of the median nerve leave the trunk of that nerve and run with the ulnar nerve to the hand where they branch off to innervate the thenar muscles as usual. The anomaly occurs in between 10 and 30% of humans and may be dominantly inherited.

Variants on the common pattern have been identified[6005] and electrical criteria for anomalous innervation suggested, as follows:[183]

A. Median to ulnar

1. The compound muscle action potential (CMAP) is higher over the abductor pollicis brevis (APB) with stimulation of the median nerve at the elbow than with stimulation at the wrist.
2. The CMAP of the first dorsal interosseous is higher with elbow than with wrist stimulation of the median nerve.
3. Recording of a negative potential over the abductor digiti minimi (ADM) on stimulation of the median nerve at the elbow.

B. Ulnar to median

1. The CMAP over the APB is higher on stimulation of the median nerve at the wrist than at the elbow.
2. The CMAP over the ADM is lower on stimulation of the ulnar nerve at the wrist than at the elbow, and there may be an additional recording of a CMAP from the ADM with stimulation of the median nerve at the wrist (the Riche–Cannieu anastomosis, leading fibers from the median to the hypothenar muscles). A proximal Martin–Gruber anastomosis may mimic ulnar neuropathy at the elbow.

Martsolf syndrome
See **cataract-spasticity–mental retardation syndrome**.

MASA syndrome
(Mental retardation, Aphasia, Shuffling gait, Adducted thumbs) A congenital syndrome inherited as an X-linked trait and characterized by short stature, aphasia, adducted thumbs, spasticity, and psychomotor retardation.[614] See **hereditary spastic paraplegia**.

masked epilepsy
A nineteenth-century term for what are now known as **complex partial seizures**.

masking
The stimulation of one ear with white noise or with a band of sound at frequencies close to the test frequency, while the acuity in the other ear is tested; a technique designed to prevent the perception of the test sound by the ear not being studied.

mass lesions
(space-occupying lesions) Pathological collections of abnormal material which are (but should not be) inside the cranium where they act to increase intracranial pressure. The alternative term is rejected, as this author cannot think of any lesions apart from psychiatric disorders and amputations which do not occupy space.

mass reflex
(Riddoch mass reflex) Diffuse activity of the disinhibited spinal cord below the level of a complete or near-complete lesion of the descending motor pathways, appearing after the period of **spinal shock**. The clinical manifestations include flexor spasms and autonomic discharge, the latter leading to detrusor contraction, hypertension, bradycardia, sweating, and piloerection. The reflex occurs in response to external (painful or tactile) or internal (infections, full bladder) stimuli below the level of the lesion.[2817, 5291]

Massachusetts General Hospital Neurology chatrooms
A neurology discussion forum. Web site: www.BrainChat.org.

masseter inhibitory reflex
Inhibition of contraction of the muscle bilaterally resulting from unilateral trigeminal sensory stimulation, especially of the mental nerve. Electrophysiologically, the reflex has both early and late phases.[2982]

masseter reflex
See **jaw reflex**.

masseteric hypertrophy
(masticatory muscle hypertrophy) Uni- or bilateral hypertrophy of the masseters, usually in subjects prone to grinding their teeth (**bruxism**).[2646] Such enlargement of the temporalis and masseter muscles is due to reactive muscle fiber hypertrophy with type 1 fiber predominance. The condition may also occur as a familial condition,[4121] as a manifestation of **branchial myopathy**, or from unknown causes.[2777]

massive infantile spasms
See **West syndrome**.

Masson stain
A trichrome connective tissue stain which colors astrocytes, myofibrils, and myelin red-brown and collagen blue-green.

mast syndrome
1. A recessive form of hereditary spastic paraparesis with extrapyramidal features, dementia, and pyramidal signs found in an Old Order Amish kinship in Pennsylvania.[1354] See **hereditary spastic paraplegia**. 2. A compression mononeuropathy resulting from the wearing of Medical AntiShock Trousers.

mastication reflex
See **Wolfing reflex**.

masticator myopathy
A rare, reversible syndrome of pain and swelling of the masticatory muscles following coxsackie

or echo virus infection, accompanied by low serum IgG levels and eosinophilia.[6895]

masticatory dysfunction Persistent or repeated clenching of the masseter muscles, usually seen in patients under stress and causing pain felt diffusely over the side of the face, usually unilaterally, extending from the temple down to the jaw.

masticatory muscle hypertrophy See **masseteric hypertrophy**.

masticatory palsy Weakness of the muscles supplied by the V cranial nerve.

mastocytosis (systemic mastocytosis) A syndrome characterized by urticaria pigmentosa, spinal anomalies; platyspondyly; malabsorption; dizziness; seizures; recurrent migraine-like headaches with hypotension; osteoporosis; osteosclerosis or osteopetrosis; and distal myopathic weakness. Intracerebral hemorrhage has also been reported. Hives, flushing, lacrimation, and anaphylaxis are the more visible features; hepatosplenomegaly and anemia, abdominal cramps, and respiratory distress the main systemic manifestations. The benign localized form affects the skin only (urticaria pigmentosa).[3533, 3617]

Mastroiacovo syndrome A congenital dysmorphic syndrome characterized by thinness, micrognathia with an open-mouth appearance, scoliosis, cryptorchidism, arachnodactyly, joint contractures, hypotonia, seizures, muscle atrophy, strabismus, and mental and developmental delay.[381]

masturbation (from Lat, the hand + licentious conduct) Stimulation of erogenous zones by means other than contact with the erogenous zones of another person. This solitary activity was widely regarded as a cause of neurological disease during the nineteenth century, but is not now considered to have any such long-term effects. Ladame (1890) wrote that is was likely to "favour the evolution of . . . disease by exhausting an already enfeebled spinal cord."[3637] *Autres temps, autres moeurs*.

Matas Test See **carotid compression test**.

maternal rubella syndrome See **Gregg syndrome**.

Mathew Scale A popular neurological scoring system designed for the evaluation of stroke patients[4164] (Chart M–1).

Chart M–1. The Mathew Scale: Neurological Evaluation in Patients with Acute Stroke

Factor	*Score*
Mentation	
Level of consciousness	
Fully conscious	8
Lethargic but mentally intact	6
Obtunded	4
Stuporous	2
Comatose	0
Orientation	
Orientated × 3 modalities	6
Orientated × 2	4
Orientated × 1	2
Disorientated	0
Speech	
Reitan test	0–23
Cranial nerves	
Homonymous hemianopsia	
Intact fields	3
Mild	2
Moderate	1
Severe impairment	0
Conjugate deviation of eyes	
Intact	3
Mild	2
Moderate	1
Severe impairment	0
Facial weakness	
Intact	3
Mild	2
Moderate	1
Severe impairment	0
Motor power (each limb separately)	
Normal strength	5
Contracts vs. resistance	4
Elevates against gravity	3
Gravity eliminated	2
Flicker	1
No movements	0
Performance on disability status scale	
Normal	28
Mild impairment	21
Moderate impairment	14
Severe impairment	7
Death	0
Reflexes	
Normal	3
Asymmetrical/pathological	2
Clonus	1
No reflexes elicited	0
Sensation	
Normal	3
Mild sensory abnormality	2
Severe sensory abnormality	1
No response to pain	0

After Mathew NT, Meyer JS, Rivera VM, et al. Double blind evaluation of glycerol treatment in acute cerebral infarction. Lancet *1992;2:1327–9. Reproduced by kind permission.*

Mattis Dementia Rating Scale A screening instrument designed to detect the presence of brain pathology in impaired geriatric patients. Consciousness, insight, affective tone, attention, memory, verbal and motor perseveration, constructional ability, conceptual ability, and naming are examined.[4183] See also **Extended Scale for Dementia**.

matutinal vertigo That common form of vertigo in which symptoms are commonly precipitated, *inter alia*, by arising from bed in the morning. It occurs with both central and peripheral causes of the vertigo and it has no localizing value, but is seldom present in **Ménière disease**.[572] See **benign positional vertigo**.

Maurois syndrome See **pituitary gigantism**.

Mauthner, Ludwig Wilhelm Hungarian pediatrician who trained and worked in Vienna, where he founded and ran a hospital for sick children; in 1844 he published the first textbook of pediatric neurology.[7]

maximum volumetric isometric contraction A valid technique for evaluating the strength of muscle contractions against unyielding resistances, and thus a method of estimating motor unit loss.[201] See also **Tufts Quantitative Neuromuscular Examination**.

May–White syndrome (autosomal dominant cerebellar ataxia, ataxia with myoclonus and deafness) A dominantly inherited multisystem degeneration causing progressive myoclonic epilepsy, sensorineural deafness, ataxia, sensorimotor peripheral neuropathy, and muscle atrophy beginning in adolescence.[4187] In some cases, changes typical of mitochondrial disease have been reported.

Mayer, K. (1862–1931) Austrian neurologist.

Mayer finger-thumb reflex (Mayer sign) Adduction of the thumb, with extension at the interphalangeal joint and flexion of the metacarpophalangeal joint, in response to forcible flexion of digits 2, 3, and 4 when the patient's hand is in full supination. Normally present, it disappears in the presence of a pyramidal lesion.[4188]

Mayer disease See **neuronal ceroid lipofuscinosis**.

Mayer sign 1. See **Mayer finger-thumb reflex**. 2. See **Wartenberg sign**.

Mayer-Gross, Willi (b. 1889) German psychiatrist.

Mayer-Gross apraxia See **constructional apraxia**.[4190]

Mayer-Gross sign See **closing-in phenomenon**.

Mayo Clinic Scale for Reflex Assessment A scheme enumerating the activity of muscle stretch reflexes, with 9 points ranging from absent (−4) through normal (0) to continuous clonus (+4) but not improving inter-rater agreement.[4047] See also **MRC Scale** and **NINDS Scale**.

Mayou, Marmaduke Stephen (b. 1876) English ophthalmologist who described familial cerebromacular degeneration (Batten–Mayou disease) in 1904. See **gangliosidoses**.

M'Bwaki See Kwashiorkor.

McArdle disease See **glycogen storage diseases**.

McArdle sign Increase in pyramidal leg weakness produced by neck flexion and relieved by extension, probably due to conduction block in demyelinated segments of the cervical cord. The mechanism for this is likely to be ischemia induced by the flexion when the spinal canal is narrowed by degenerative joint disease.

Dr. M.J. McArdle was a neurologist at Guy's Hospital, London, in the latter half of the twentieth century. His brother Dr. Brian McArdle (**McArdle disease**) was a biochemist.

McCarthy, D.J. (1874–1965) American neurologist who published two papers on the supraorbital reflex in 1901 (in German).

McCarthy reflex (McCarthy sign) Percussion of the superior orbital region causes blinking of the homolateral eyelid; a normal finding in infants.[6898] See **orbicularis oculi reflex**.

McCarthy sign See **orbicularis oculi reflex**.

McCrae syndrome A syndrome consisting of X-linked mental retardation and deafness with mental and developmental delay.[381]

McCune–Albright syndrome (polyostotic fibrous dysplasia) A sporadic congenital syndrome of progressive fibrous dysplasia of the long bones and skull, leading to complaints of bone pain, fractures, and cranial nerve palsies; irregular brown-pigmented patches are found on the skin, their outline said to resemble that of the coast of Maine; and various endocrine disturbances occur, especially precocious puberty in girls.

The syndrome was first reported by McCune in 1936 but a fuller paper[4211] and an extensive review by Albright both appeared in the following year. *Jaffé–Lichtenstein syndrome* is similar, but the endocrine and dermal abnormalities are not present.

McDonald–Halliday criteria A system of criteria for the diagnosis of multiple sclerosis, published in 1977 and introducing the concept of isolated spinal involvement.[4217] See Chart M–2. A recent revision of these criteria is reproduced under **multiple sclerosis**. See Chart M–21. See also **Schumacher panel criteria, Poser criteria**, and **multiple sclerosis**.

See also **multiple sclerosis** (revised McDonald criteria).

McGill Pain Inventory A questionnaire consisting primarily of three classes of word descriptors—sensory, affective, and evaluative—that are used by patients who describe the pains from which they suffer; and containing also a scale of the intensity of the pain. A background history also forms part of the questionnaire, as do enquiries about accompanying symptoms, the timing and geography of the pain, the pain modifying activities used, and the effect of the pain upon sleep and sexual activity.[4301]

McGregor's line The line drawn from the upper surface of the posterior edge of the hard palate to the most caudal point of the occipital curve in the true lateral X-ray of the skull.

Although originally thought to be of value in the diagnosis of **basilar impression**, CT scanning or anteroposterior (AP) tomography of the foramen magnum are now preferred.[5980]

McHenry, Lawrence Chester (1929–1985) American neurologist, born

Chart M–2. McDonald–Halliday Criteria for the Diagnosis of Multiple Sclerosis

Proved

Diagnosis established at necropsy

Clinically Definite

Some physical disability
Remitting or relapsing course
History of two or more episodes and
Evidence of lesions at two or more necessarily separate sites in the CNS and
Lesions predominantly in the white matter and
Age at onset of symptoms 15–50 years and
History of signs or symptoms for 1 year or longer, and
No better explanation.

Early Probable or Latent

Slight or no disability
Single episode suggestive of multiple sclerosis and
Evidence of lesions at two or more sites in the CNS OR
Remitting and relapsing course, and
Evidence of one or more lesions associated with multiple sclerosis.

Progressive probable

Progressive history of paraplegia and
Evidence of lesions at two or necessarily separate sites in the CNS, and
Other causes excluded.

Progressive possible

Progressive history of paraplegia and
Evidence of only one lesion, and
Other causes excluded.

Suspected

Single episode suggestive of multiple sclerosis without evidence of any lesion or with evidence of a single lesion only, OR
Recurrent optic neuritis (unilateral or bilateral) with one additional episode not involving the optic nerve but without evidence of lesions outside the eye.

in Oklahoma, where he later trained in medicine, afterwards receiving his neurological training in Boston. During his army service, he became interested in cerebral blood flow and published extensively in that field over many years, from the Army Institute of Research and from Jefferson Medical College Hospital, Philadelphia; but his abiding interest was medical—specifically neurological—history. He entitled his *magnum opus Garrison's History of Neurology*, even though he was revising what was originally a book chapter into a whole book, some five times as long as the original.

In 1972 he became professor of neurology at the Bowman Gray School of Medicine and for the remainder of his life continued in the teaching and practice of his specialty and the encouragement of further historical research into its past, an area in which he had become internationally pre-eminent.

McLellan classification A system for the classification of voiding dysfunction. Spastic and atonic forms were defined, the latter reclassified by Lapides into motor paralytic and sensory paralytic forms.

McLeod syndrome (benign X-linked myopathy with acanthocytes, Xp21 myopathy; OMIM 314850) A rare X-linked recessive multisystem disorder presenting in adult life and characterized by acanthocytosis, anisocytosis, and weakened blood cell antigenicity in the Kell blood group system, due to a mutation of the *XK* gene.[6160] Clinically, psychiatric disturbances are common presenting signs;[3261] subclinical myopathy with areflexia and raised serum CK levels, seizures, dystonia, chorea, peripheral sensorimotor axonal neuropathy, cardiomyopathy, and caudate atrophy seen on MRI scans are variable other manifestations.[1442]

The name comes from that of the blood donor (a dental student) in whom the disorder was first detected. The responsible gene maps to Xp21.2–p21.1 on the short arm of the chromosome, close to that of **Duchenne dystrophy**. Although originally regarded as a benign condition, longer follow-up shows that it is rather a progressive multisystem disorder sharing many features with **Huntington disease**.[2888]

In a *variant* form, a limb-girdle muscular dystrophy (LGMD2A, a calpainopathy) co-exists.

McQuarrie syndrome (idiopathic infantile or neonatal hypoglycemia) Hypoglycemia causing convulsions and nonlocalizing signs in small children in whom no pathological abnormality is consistently detected.[4265]

MCTD Abbreviation for medium-chain triglyceride disease.

mean consecutive difference See **jitter**.

mean sorted difference See **jitter**.

measles inclusion body encephalitis A fatal encephalitic illness seen in some immunocompromized patients exposed to measles virus. It is characterized clinically by obtunded delirium and myoclonus, and pathologically by the finding of measles antigen within neurons and by the presence of eosinophilic intranuclear inclusions.

meat ingestion headache Headache occurring in patients with a tendency to hyperammonemia as a result of a disorder of the urea cycle. See **Aguecheek syndrome**.

MEB disease See **muscle, eye,** and **brain disease**.

mechanical hyperalgesia A decrease in the threshold but an increase in the suprathreshold magnitude of pain induced by mechanical stimulation of the skin. A *static form* (tested by gentle skin pressure and mediated by unmyelinated fibers) and a *dynamic form* (tested by light skin stroking and mediated by myelinated fibers) have been defined.[4748]

Meckel, Johann Freidrich (the elder; 1724–1774) German anatomist who described the sphenopalatine ganglion (Meckel ganglion) and the dural space lodging the Gasserian ganglion (Meckel cave) in 1748.[4502] He also defined the syndrome named for him in 1822.

Meckel cave The dural sac overlying the medial tip of the petrous portion of the temporal bone, in which lies the Gasserian ganglion of the V cranial nerve.

Meckel syndrome See **dysencephalia splanchocystica**.

Meckel–Gruber syndrome See **dysencephalia splanchnocystica**.

medial brachial fascial compartment syndrome A potential complication of axillary artery angiography, the result of hematoma formation with damage to the lower brachial plexus and presenting as a median and/or ulnar neuropathy.[5906]

medial epicondylitis (golfers' elbow) A syndrome of pain on the medial aspect of the elbow, radiating distally. It results from tendinitis of the long wrist and finger flexors occasioned by excessive use of those muscles.

medial forebrain bundle A complex collection of ascending and descending fibers running through the lateral hypothalamus, including noradrenergic fibers from the medulla and dopaminergic fibers of the nigrostriatal pathway.

medial frontal syndrome
An akinetic behavioral pattern that may occur following injury to the frontal lobes. It is characterized by paucity of spontaneous movement, gesture, and verbal output; weakness and loss of sensation in the legs and urinary incontinence.[6388]

See also **frontal convexity syndrome**.

medial medullary syndrome See **Déjèrine syndromes**.

medial pectoral neuropathy
An entrapment syndrome in which the nerve is compressed as it passes through the pectoralis minor, leading to wasting of the inferior sternal part of the pectoralis major muscle.[5420]

medial plantar neuropathy
(jogger's foot) A focal neuropathy resulting from compression of this nerve in the tarsal tunnel, giving rise to local tenderness and distal sensory loss.[4769]

medial pterygoid reflex A stretch reflex elicited in the EMG laboratory with needle electrodes in this muscle that is stimulated by performing the jaw jerk. The reflex may be useful in the localization of brainstem or peripheral trigeminal nerve lesions.[2982]

medial tegmental paralysis See **Babinski–Nageotte syndrome**.

median cleft face syndrome See **frontonasal dysplasia**.

median facial cleft syndrome See **frontonasal dysplasia**.

median longitudinal bundle
(fasciculus) A fiber bundle running between the oculomotor nuclei in the medulla and mesencephalon, first described by Benedict Stilling in 1846, but named by His in 1895.

median pubic reflex Tapping the symphysis pubis leads to contraction of the muscles of the abdominal wall and adduction of the leg in patients with hyperexcitability of the spinal cord resulting from lesions of the corticospinal tracts above T11.

Medical Matrix-Neurology
A collection of neurology Home Pages and Resource Directories hosted by Medical Matrix Guide to Internet Clinical Medicine Resources. Web site: http://www.medmatrix.org/_SPages/Neurology.asp.

Medical Outcomes Study 20-item Scale An instrument for measuring aspects of **quality of life**.

Medical Research Council Scale
A popular nonlinear scale for the clinical grading of the strength of individual muscles. The defined grades (in a modified form) are given in Chart M–3.

Despite the increase of the number of steps from 5 to 10 through the expansion of the 5th, 4th, and 3rd grades, the scale is still bottom-heavy, grades 4 and 5 representing over 90% of the potential strength of a muscle. See also **Mayo Clinic Scale** and **NINDS Scale**.

Medical Research Council scale for grading sensory recovery
A scale assessing progress after injury to a peripheral nerve.[2898]

S0 No sensibility (no sensation)
S1 Recovery of deep cutaneous pain sensibility
S2 Some degree of superficial cutaneous pain and tactile sensibility
S3 Return of superficial cutaneous pain and tactile sensibility throughout the autonomous area with disappearance of overreaction
S4 Return of superficial cutaneous pain and tactile sensibility with some recovery in 2-point discrimination
S5 Complete recovery

medication induced headache
(analgesic rebound headache) A form of **chronic daily headache** occurring in those with pre-existing migraine or tension-type headaches for which they have taken analgesics, aspirin, acetaminophen, opioids, benzodiazepines, ergot preparations, or triptans on a regular basis for their headaches (usually 3 days/week or more). The new headache usually has the same qualities as the previous ones, but occurs characteristically on waking and is partially relieved (but not removed) by further ingestion of the usual remedy. A re-setting of the tolerances of pain receptors in the brain is supposed to underlie the problem. Treatment demands abstention from the causative drug, but the "rebound" headaches resulting may last up to 2 weeks.

medication overuse headache
The ICHD[2820] defines forms of headache occurring in association with excessive use of migraine therapies and of other medications.

Ergotamine-overuse headache

A. Headache present on >15 days/month with at least one of the following characteristics and fulfilling criteria C and D:

Chart M–3. Modified Medical Research Council Scale

5	Normal strength
5−	Barely detectable weakness
4+	Same as 4, but stronger
4	Muscle is weak but moves the joint against a combination of gravity and some resistance
4−	Same as 4, but weaker
3+	The muscle is capable of transient resistance but collapses abruptly
3	Muscle cannot move against resistance but moves the joint fully against gravity. With the exception of knee extensors, the joint must be moved through the full mechanical range against gravity. If a patient has contractures that limit movement of the joint, the mechanical range will be to the point at which the contractures cause a significant resistance to the movement.
3−	Muscle moves the joint against gravity but not through the full extent of the mechanical range of the joint
2	Muscle moves the joint when gravity is eliminated
1	A flicker of movement is seen or felt in the muscle
0	No movement[4306]

From Mendell JR, Florence J. Manual muscle testing. Muscle Nerve 1990;13:S16–20. © *1990, John Wiley and Sons. Inc. Reproduced by permission.)*

1. Bilateral
2. Pressing/tightening quality
3. Mild or moderate intensity

B. Ergotamine intake on ≥10 days/month on a regular basis for ≥3 months
C. Headache has developed or markedly worsened during ergotamine overuse
D. Headache resolves or reverts to its previous pattern within 2 months after discontinuation of ergotamine

Triptan-overuse headache

A. Headache present on >15 days/month with at least one of the following characteristics and fulfilling criteria C and D:

1. Predominantly unilateral
2. Pulsating quality
3. Moderate or severe intensity
4. Aggravated by or causing avoidance of routine physical activity (e.g., walking or climbing stairs)
5. Associated with at least one of the following:

a, nausea and/or vomiting
b. Photophobia and phonophobia

B. Triptan intake (any formulation) on ≥10 days/month on a regular basis for ≥3 months
C. Headache frequency has markedly increased during triptan overuse
D. Headache reverts to its previous pattern within 2 months after discontinuation of triptan.

From the International Classification of Headache Disorders (Headache Classification Committee of the International Headache Society. *Cephalalgia* 2004;**24**[Suppl 1]) by kind permission of Dr. Jes Olesen, the International Headache Society and Wiley-Blackwell Publications.

See also **analgesic overuse headache**.

For *opioid-overuse headache combination medication-overuse headache* and *exogenous hormone-induced headache,* broadly similar diagnostic criteria have been defined. Thus, for ***opioid-overuse headache***

A. Headache is present on >15 days/month and fulfills criteria C and D
B. Opioid intake on ≥10 days/month for >3 months
C. Headache has developed or markedly worsened during opioid overuse
D. Headache resolves or reverts to its previous pattern within 2 months after discontinuation of the opioid.

For *combination medication-overuse headache*, it is suggested that a mild or moderate, bilateral, pressing/tightening (nonpulsating) headache is present for >15 days/month in subjects taking combination medications on ≥10 days/month for >3 months, leading to development or marked worsening. The headache resolves or reverts to its previous pattern within 2 months after discontinuation of combination medication.

For *exogenous hormone-induced headache*, the suggested criteria are that the headache or migraine develops or markedly worsens within 3 months of commencing exogenous hormones but resolves or reverts to its previous pattern within 3 months after total discontinuation of exogenous hormones.

Based on the International Classification of Headache Disorders (Headache Classification Committee of the International Headache Society. *Cephalalgia* 2004;**24**[Suppl 1]).

Medin, Oskar (1874–1928) Swedish physician in Stockholm. He described the Stockholm poliomyelitis epidemic of 1887 in great detail, and the disease was accordingly known for some time by the name of Medin and of **Heine**.

medioplantar reflex (of Guillain and Barré) Tapping the heel or the middle of the sole elicits plantar flexion of the ankle in patients with pyramidal lesions. This represents merely an alternative method of eliciting the ankle jerk.

medium chain acylCoA dehydrogenase deficiency See **acylCoA dehydrogenase deficiency**.

MEDLINEplus A US Government site that provides extensive information about diseases for patients. Web site: www.nlm.nih.gov/medlineplus/neurologicdiseses general.html.

MedLink Neurology A neurology on-line textbook, available by paid subscription. Web site: www.medlink.com/.

Medscape A commercial Web site covering many areas of medicine, including neurology. http://www.medscape.com/neurologyhome/.

medulla oblongata (Lat, marrow + oblong shape) That part of the brainstem between the pons and the spinal cord. Formerly, according to **Willis** and others, the word signified the entire brainstem, but it has been restricted to its present extent since Haller's text published in 1750.[5886]

medullary respiratory centers Dorsal and ventral nuclear masses (the solitary nucleus and tract, and the nucleus ambiguus) which act as pattern generators for respiratory activity.

medullary satiety Diminution in appetite and early satiety, thought to be due to a lesion of the area postrema in the medulla.[4137]

medullary sheath The Schwann cell layer of peripheral nerves; the investment of myelin-containing Schwann cells surrounding the axons.

medullary tegmental paralysis See **Babinski–Nageotte syndrome**.

medullary tube The tube formed by the closure and union of the laminae dorsales in the embryo, and from which the brain and spinal cord develop. Its walls constrict to become the forebrain or proscencephalon, the interbrain or thalamencephalon, the midbrain or mesencephalon, the hindbrain or epencephalon, and the afterbrain or metencephalon. The tube itself becomes the cerebral ventricles of the brain and the central canal of the spinal cord.

medullated (myelinated) nerve fibers (myelinated nerve fibers) Those nerve fibers which are individually surrounded by myelin-containing Schwann cells and which are thus greater in diameter, visibility, and conductive ability than the nonmedullated fibers which are invaginated into nonmyelin-containing Schwann cells.

medulloblastoma (Cushing tumor, medullomyoblastoma) A malignant **primitive neuroectodermal tumor** arising from the cerebellum (in children, from the vermis or medullary velum) and composed of sheets of small, round cells with oval hyperchromatic nuclei and small amounts of fibrillary cytoplasm, frequently arranged in rosettes with the nuclei at the periphery of the cells. Local invasion of the cerebellum and brainstem is usual, and the tumor seeds throughout the spinal subarachnoid space in many cases. This is the commonest primary brain tumor in childhood. Unbalanced translocations, with loss of chromosome 17q and changes in chromosome 1, are the commonest karyotypic abnormality described.

Clinically, it presents with signs of midline cerebellar and medullary dysfunction and ultimately leads to signs of raised intracranial pressure.[1364]

Variants include *desmoplastic medulloblastoma*, in which local invasion of the meninges leads to the occurrence of an intense fibrous reaction; *medullomyoblastoma* in which striated muscle and epithelial cells appear; and *medulloepithelioma*, characterized by the tubular arrangements of cells resembling the "epithelial" cell pattern in the primitive neural tube.[6]

medulloepithelioma A primitive, highly malignant tumor of the cerebral hemispheres containing a columnar epithelial layer resembling that of the primitive neural tube,[3305] lacking cellular differentiation and frequently hemorrhage and necrotic. It occurs in the first 5 years of life. See **medulloblastoma**.

medullomyoblastoma See **medulloblastoma**.

Mees lines Single solid white bands across the finger- and toenails, a sign of arsenic intoxication at least 2 months before (on appearance) and 5 months before if the bands have reached the free edge of the nails. Multiple episodes of arsenic ingestion lead to multiple bands.

meeting badge neuropathy Superficial radial (sensory) nerve injury as a result of compression against this personal label when the arms were crossed for a prolonged period. See also **cheiralgia paresthetica**.

MEG See **magnetoencephalography**.

megaconial myopathy A familial muscular disorder presenting with slowly progressive weakness from infancy and associated with an excess of giant mitochondria and morphological inclusions within such organelles.[5822] This is a member of the group of benign, nonprogressive congenital myopathies presenting in infancy with weakness and hypotonia which result in significant motor delay.

megacystis–microcolon–intestinal hypoperistalsis syndrome (Berdon syndrome) A congenital visceral myopathy with two variant types: *type 1* is dominantly inherited and is characterized by esophageal dilatation, megaduodenum, redundant colon, and megacystis; *type 2* is recessively inherited and is characterized by dilatation of the stomach and the small intestine with external ophthalmoplegia and ptosis.[642]

megadolichobasilar anomaly (S aneurysm) A rare condition consisting of the abnormal elongation and widening of the basilar arteries, usually in adult males, first described by **Dandy** in 1947. The distortion may be so great that aqueductal and cranial nerve compression syndromes result.[699]

megalencephalic leukodystrophy with cysts A rare recessively transmitted disorder mapped to 22qtel and characterized by macrocephaly, slow progressive delay in development and mild mental deterioration followed by slowly progressive ataxia, pyramidal tract involvement, and seizures. MRI shows diffuse cerebral white matter lesions and subcortical temporopolar and frontal cysts.[6352, 3544]

megalencephaly (Gr, big + brain) (macrocephaly) Enlargement of the brain with or without histological abnormalities, as shown by a rapid increase in the occipitofrontal circumference of the head above the 98th percentile during the first year of life. This occurs with such infiltrative or storage diseases as **GM_2 gangliosidosis, Niemann–Pick disease,** sulfatidosis, **tuberous sclerosis,** and **glioblastomatosis**, and also as a familial characteristic without associated disease. The primary form is developmental or it can be associated with other inherited disease. In the secondary form, the brain enlargement results from the accumulation of excessive lipid. See also **macrocephaly, megalobarencephaly, megalocephaly,** and **microcephaly**. A Web site providing data on these subjects, compiled by NINDS, is found at: http://www.ninds.nih.gov/disorders/megalencephaly/megalencephaly.htm.

Anatomic and *metabolic* forms are recognized. In the former, the brain is enlarged because of an increase in the number or size of its cells. In the latter, the enlargement reflects the accumulation of a metabolic product without any increase in the number of cells. Diagnostic criteria are given in Chart M–4.

In a *variant* form, megalencephaly is associated with polymicrogyria and hydrocephalus.[404]

megalobarencephaly An abnormal increase in the weight of the brain. This is a more accurate term than the foregoing, in that a brain may be enlarged as a result of hydrocephalus, but it remains susceptible to misinterpretation in the presence of brain edema.

megaloblastic madness Cognitive and emotional symptoms resulting from deficiency of vitamin B12.

megalocephaly The word usually employed to indicate enlargement of the head, although the derivation suggests rather enlargement of the brain. See also **megalencephaly**.

Chart M–4. Diagnostic Criteria for Asymptomatic (Benign) Familial Anatomic Megalencephaly[1575]

1. Occipitofrontal circumference (OFC) more than 2 standard deviations above the mean or above the 98th percentile.
2. No clinical evidence of increased intracranial pressure in the form of bulging fontanelles, palpably split sutures, or persistent vomiting.
3. Normal developmental and neurological examination findings.
4. Absence of any neurocutaneous signs, or craniofacial, or somatic anomalies that may identify a specific syndrome.
5. At least one parent or sibling has a large occipitofrontal circumference but is neurologically normal, or the increased OFC can be traced through several generations.
6. Follow-up visits establish the normality of the patient's developmental course, and the OFC curve levels off and, although it remains high, begins to parallel the normal curve.
7. Radiographic demonstration of normal or only slightly enlarged ventricles in one of the family members with an enlarged OFC, establishing that the condition is megalencephaly, not arrested hydrocephalus or some other lesion.
8. Negative chemical screening test results for metabolic disorders or lysosomal enzyme deficits in those patients lacking some of the other criteria.

Adapted from DeMyer W. Megalencephaly; types, clinical syndromes and management. Pediatr Neurol *1986;2:321. Reproduced by kind permission of Elsevier Science.*

megalocornea with skeletal abnormalities A congenital dysmorphic syndrome characterized by frontal bossing, low-set posteriorly rotated ears, hypertelorism, macrocornea, micrognathia, open-mouth appearance, gibbus, kyphoscoliosis, camptodactyly, clubfoot, macrocephaly, and mental and developmental delay.[381]

megalocornea-mental retardation See **Neuhauser syndrome**.

megalopapilla Congenital enlargement of the optic disk, sometimes associated with midline cranial defects, dysmorphism, and midline clefting.[2450]

megalopsia Exaggerated **macropsia**, a condition in which everything looks abnormally big. A word generated by neologismophiles for neologismophiles.

megaphagia Excessive ingestion of food without inducing hunger; often a compulsion. The condition should be distinguished from morbid hunger. The word was suggested by Critchley as more precisely derived than *hyperphagia* in the context of the **Kleine–Levin syndrome**.

megaseme The term of **Charcot** for a skull with an orbital index greater than 90, but this measurement is not now considered to be of practical usefulness.

megasthenic Possessed of great muscular power. The necessity for the word must be limited, but it is reassuring to come across an exaltation of the normal in a work otherwise devoted to the abnormal.

megrim (from Middle English and Fr, a headache; derived from Gr, a pain on one side of the face) An obsolete term for **migraine**, but applied still to a staggering disease in horses.

Meige, Henri (1866–1940) French neurologist who trained in Paris and studied with **Charcot**. He gave the first good description of the symmetrical dystonic spasms of the facial muscles occurring in oromandibular dystonia, and of **Munchausen syndrome**. He was cofounder of the Revue Neurologique and of the Société de Neurologie in Paris.

Because some paintings by Pieter Breughel the Elder (1525–1569) depict faces in similar dystonic postures, the name of Breughel has been added to that of Meige (see next entry) but unaccountably those of Stanley Spencer and William Blake (British artists of the distortive school) have not.[4290]

Meige syndrome (idiopathic orofacial dystonia, Breughel syndrome) A segmental cranial dystonia of adult onset characterized by blepharospasm, oromandibular dystonia, apathy, depression, tics, bulbar weakness, rigidity, chorea, and tremor at rest. See **cranial dystonias**.

Meinecke syndrome A congenital dysmorphic syndrome characterized by brachydactyly (short, broad thumbs), wide-spaced teeth, speech delay, patchy pigmentation of the skin, seizures, and mental and developmental delay.[381]

Meissner, Georg (1829–1905) German anatomist, professor of physiology and anatomy at Basle, later at Freiburg and Göttingen.

Meissner's corpuscles Expansions of sensory nerve endings, sensitive to touch-pressure.

Meissner's plexus The submucous plexus of the intestine, described in 1853.

melancholy See **chronic fatigue syndrome**.

melanocytoma (cellular blue nevus) A rare, relatively benign pigmented nevoid tumor of the meninges or elsewhere, presenting as an intradural, extrinsic mass lesion. The histological patterns resemble those of Schwannoma, dermal nevi, and neuroblastomas, and the tumor shows positive immunochemical reactions for the S-100 protein.[3630]

melanodermic leukodystrophy See **adrenoleukodystrophy**.

melanoma A tumor usually arising from neural crest tissues and skin, commonly malignant and with likely autosomal dominant inheritance, mapped in some cases to 9p. In familial cases, other family members may have at least multiple dysplastic nevi of the skin. Cerebral or optic gliomas appear to be associated. Multiple secondary metastases to the brain are common.[3338]

melanomatosis (primary diffuse meningeal melanomatosis) A rare variant of primary malignant melanoma of the CNS with extensive leptomeningeal invasion, presenting with intracranial hypotension and nonspecific neurological deficits. CT scans show hydrocephalus with effacement of the cerebral convexity sulci and abnormal contrast enhancement in the fissures, while MR shows diffuse dural and leptomeningeal contrast enhancement.[5037]

MELAS (Mitochondrial Encephalopathy, Lactic Acidosis, and Stroke; OMIM 540000) A maternally transmitted mitochondrial disease with onset in infancy or childhood, characterized by recurrent migraine-like headaches, vomiting, hemiplegia ("stroke-like episodes" not conforming to known vascular territories), and hemianopia.

Other features include dementia, partial seizures, cortical blindness, ataxia, deafness, short stature, intracranial calcification, and cardiomyopathy. Increased lactate levels in the blood and CSF, ragged red fibers/abnormal mitochondria in muscle biopsy specimens, and spongy degeneration of the cortex with basal gangion calcification are the laboratory abnormalities usually detected.[1645, 4941] Noninsulin-dependent diabetes mellitus may also develop. Myoclonus, cerebellar lesions, retinal pigmentary changes, and heart block are not present. Diagnostic criteria have been suggested as follows:[2914]

1. Stroke before the age of 40
2. An encephalopathy characterized by seizures, dementia, or both
3. Blood lactic acidosis or ragged red fibers in skeletal muscle, or both.

Diagnostic criteria for the associated headache[2820] suggest that this resembles migraine with or without aura in association with stroke-like episodes and seizures in the presence of the 3243 point mitochondrial DNA mutation in the tRNA Leu gene or other DNA MELAS point mutation. See also **MERRF** and **mitochondrial diseases**.

Melkersson–Rosenthal syndrome The unusual combination of recurrent facial palsies with facial edema, migraine headaches, and fissuring of the tongue (lingua plicata).[4295] Ocular complications are also described. *Miescher cheilitis* is considered to be the same thing.[3113]

The syndrome is usually sporadic, but dominant inheritance has been recorded. Hubschmann described it in 1894, Melkersson in 1928, and Rosenthal in 1931.

melodic intonation therapy The utilization of the retained capacity of some aphasic patients to sing when they cannot speak, whereby short phrases are incorporated first into a musical recitative and thereafter into progressively less and less intonational speech. One recalls the epigram of Dr. Samuel Johnson: "That which is too silly to be said may yet be sung," but that was in the context of opera.

The success of the method is thought to indicate the recruitment of the undamaged right hemisphere into the process of language production.[108, 24]

membrane instability The tendency of a cell membrane to depolarize spontaneously, with mechanical irritation or after voluntary activation. It may be used to describe the occurrence of spontaneous single muscle fiber action potentials such as fibrillation potentials during needle electrode examination. (From the 2001 Report of the Nomenclature Committee of the American Association of Electromyography and Electrodiagnosis.[19] Reproduced by kind permission of the AANEM.)

memory (from Lat, memoria, memory) The ability to retain and recall experiences; a physical system by which a record or representation of organized spatiotemporal events is made which thus can be carried forward in time. One mechanism (explicit memory) deals with those memories for which there is conscious awareness and is dependent upon frontotemporal cortex, hippocampal, and perirhinal function. In the other form (**implicit memory**) the memory is acquired without intention, is maintained without awareness, and does not depend on hippocampal function.[1743] See also **episodic memory, working memory, semantic memory,** and **procedural memory**.

Memory Assessment Clinics Test Battery A complex memory test instrument assessing also attention and psychomotor speed, and designed to assess memory function in normal elderly subjects and patients with **age-associated memory impairment** or **Alzheimer disease**.[3702]

Memory for Designs Test An instrument for assessing visual recall and reproduction,[2544] and thus right hemisphere function.

Memory Impairment Screen A validated, sensitive, and specific 4-min, four-item delayed free- and cued-recall test of memory impairment, usable as a screening test for dementias.[958]

Memory Loss Scale An abbreviated test of mental status emphasizing orientation, but also assessing attention, abstraction, mental tracking, language, memory, and praxis.[4091]

memory tests See **Computerized Everyday Memory Battery, Wechsler Memory Scale,**[6686] **Memory Assessment Clinics Test Battery, Memory for Designs Test, Memory Impairment Screen, Mini-Mental State Examination, Recognition Memory Test, Buschke** selective reminding tests, **Babcock sentence,** and **Rey** tests. Lezak[3825] has provided a critique and compendium of the tests available.

menace reflex See **palpebral reflex**.

Mendel, Kurt (b. 1874) German neurologist.

Mendel–Bekhterev sign
1. (dorsocuboidal reflex, tarsophalangeal reflex, dorsal foot response) Percussion over the dorsal aspect of the cuboid bone leads to plantar flexion of the toes in patients with pyramidal lesions. The normal response is dorsiflexion.[4305] See **dorsal foot response**.
2. (carpometacarpal reflex, carpophalangeal reflex) In the hand, percussion over the carpal bones causes flexion of the wrist and fingers in patients with pyramidal lesions.

Mengel syndrome A recessively inherited syndrome characterized by early-onset severe neural hearing loss, leading to complete deafness after the age of 6 years, but normal vestibular responses.[4311]

Ménière, Prosper (1799–1862) French otologist who trained in Angers and Paris and initially was assistant to Baron Dupuytren at the Hötel Dieu. He failed in his attempt to become professor of medicine in Paris, but instead directed the Institute for Deaf-Mutes, which provided him greater experience in the diagnosis and management of otological problems, and also more time to devote to the study of literature, of which he was passionately fond.

The syndrome that he described was certainly that known today by his name, but the only evidence which he adduced for his belief that the lesion affected the inner ear was a brief mention of vertigo in patients who died suddenly and had had a blood-tinged or grayish exudate in the semicircular canals; the cause of this was not given, but Ménière considered tuberculosis was the likely cause in one patient.[6083]

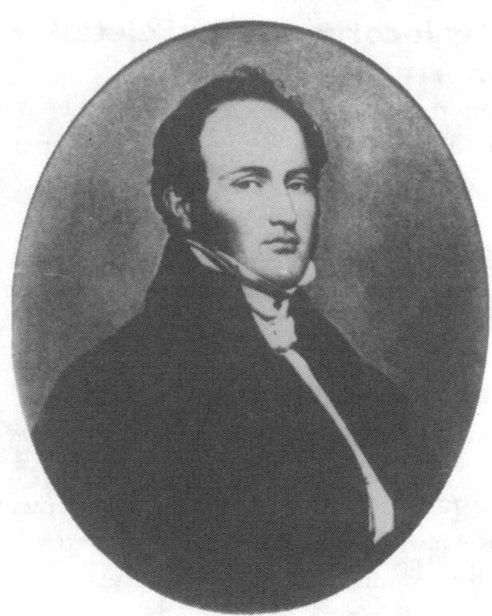

Figure M–3 Prosper Ménière.

Ménière disease Idiopathic, symptomatic, endolymphatic hydrops leading to a syndrome of intermittent aural vertigo with nausea, vomiting, progressive tinnitus, and low-tone deafness with increased endolymphatic pressure. The name was once applied to suppurative or hemorrhagic labyrinthitis as well.

This relatively common syndrome was first described in 1861,[4312] but Ménière followed this with a further series of papers on the same subject. Hallpike and Cairns showed in 1938 that dilatation of the membranous labyrinth was commonly associated.[4887] Jonathan Swift had given a good personal description of the condition 100 years before the medical description.

meningeal angiomatosis See **Sturge–Weber syndrome** (*van Bogaert–Divry* form).

meningeal apoplexy An ancient term for **subarachnoid hemorrhage**.

meningeal carcinomatosis See **carcinomatous meningitis**.

meningeal gliomatosis Diffuse or multifocal invasion of the cranial and/or spinal leptomeninges by malignant glioma.

The condition was considered rare before more recent studies showed otherwise.[6940]

meningeal hemorrhage An old term for **extradural hemorrhage**.

meningeal hydrops See **idiopathic intracranial hypertension** and **arachnoid diverticula**.

meningeal sarcoma An uncommon malignant tumor arising from the arachnoid and resembling a fibrosarcoma or malignant fibrous histiocytoma histologically, but liable to recur, invade, and metastasize.

meninges (from Gr, a membrane) The membranous coverings of the CNS, comprising the dura mater, arachnoid, and pia mater.

meningioangiomatosis without neurofibromatosis An uncommon cerebral dysplasia characterized by the localized proliferation of fibrous tissue in the arachnoid membrane and by perivascular fibrous tissue infiltration of the subjacent cortex. Clinically, the condition presents with seizures.[3601]

meningioblastoma See *anaplastic meningiomas* in Chart M–5.

meningioma (dural endothelioma, fungus durae matris) The most common benign and slow-growing brain tumor of adult life arising from the meningoepithelial arachnoid cells of the arachnoid membrane or from the choroid plexus. Multiple deletions of chromosome 22 (22q12.3-qter) are frequently found in its rare familial forms, almost all these patients having neurofibromatosis (NF2). An extracranial origin is rare and metastasis quite exceptional, but recurrence not uncommon. They represent about 20% of all intracranial tumors. Their slow growth leads to late detection in most cases; although headache, visual disturbances, loss of intellectual functions, and memory disturbances are common presentations, certain features are typical at different sites. Olfactory groove meningiomas sometimes cause uni- or bilateral anosmia.

The histological appearances vary and numerous variant subtypes are differentiated (see Chart M–5).

The tumor was first described by Felix Platter in his book *Observationem in Hominis Affectibus* (1614) but first fully documented by Cushing,[1391] who noted their origin from cell rests in the arachnoid; their appearance as solid masses or *en plaque*; the associated cranial hyperostosis; and the particular sites whence they arise, which he listed as intraspinal, foraminal, suprasellar, olfactory groove, sphenoidal ridge, sylvian cleft, convexity (including parasagittal, falx, and true convexity tumors), transverse sinus, and cerebellopontine angle. They may also occur (rarely) in the lateral ventricles.

Chart M–5. Varieties of Meningioma Pathology

Meningoepithelial (syncytial) meningiomas are characterized histologically, by the uniformity of nuclei with prominent nucleoli, the formation of whorls of cells, the presence of desmosomes between adjacent cells and of fibrous collagenous bands within the tumors, and by the absence of reticulin in most forms.

Fibroblastic meningiomas are characterized by the presence of sheets of elongated spindle cells with arachnoid cell nuclei; they contain **psammoma bodies**.

Transitional meningiomas combine features of both fibroblastic and meningoepithelial meningiomas.

Psammomatous meningiomas contain numerous **psammoma bodies**.

Angiomatous meningiomas resemble syncytial or transitional forms but contain many blood vessels, around which reticulin is prominent.

Angioblastic meningiomas comprise *hemangioblastic* forms that resemble **hemangioblastomas** located elsewhere in the body; and the *hemangiopericytic* variety, which contains numerous thin-walled blood vessels and which has a strong tendency to invade locally and to recur after removal.

Papillary meningiomas contain collagenous cores of papillae comprised of sheets of uniform cells; pseudorosettes are common. These tumors are aggressive in their growth.

Anaplastic meningiomas are malignant tumors with the usual histological features thereof, and may invade locally, recur, and metastasize.[6] See also **meningeal sarcoma**.

Forms in which bone, fatty tissue, cartilage cells, or melanin are present.

meningioma en plaque The appearance of a **meningioma** that forms a flattened mass, usually adjacent to the dura mater at the skull base or over the convexity.

meningiomatosis The presence of multiple meningiomas arising due to contiguous spread through the CSF to other locations. This happens in less than 10% of the population with meningiomas.

meningism (meningismus) A clinical syndrome resembling mild meningitis, and due to irritation without direct infection of the meninges. See **serous meningitis**.

meningismus See **meningism**.

méningite de voisinage See **parameningeal infections**.

meningitis Inflammation of the meninges by bacterial, viral, fungal, or other infectious agents or as a result of chemical irritation or malignant invasion. **Leptomeningitis** is the usual alternative term, indicating that the finer meninges are affected. **Pachymeningitis** indicates inflammation of the dura. **Basal meningitis** is that form in which the meninges of the skull base are maximally affected; **chronic lymphocytic** and **carcinomatous** (malignant) meningitis and **spinal arachnoiditis** are entered elsewhere.

meningitis circumscripta spinalis See **chronic spinal meningitis**.

meningitis serosa circumscripta Nonpurulent meningitis with focal signs, resulting either from subjacent cortical infarcts or from the presence of loculated arachnoid, forming cysts and giving rise to signs appropriate to an expanding mass lesion. For the spinal form *meningitis serosa circumscripta spinalis*, see **spinal arachnoiditis**.

meningitis tuberculosa chronica circumscripta A subacute or chronic variety of tuberculous meningitis in which the tubercles elicit a jelly-like exudate upon the meninges, in which there is but a limited mesodermal reaction.[6819]

meningocele A defect of neural tube closure at any level of the neuraxis, leading to the exposure of meninges, which do not contain nervous tissue. There is no associated neural deficit.[4358]

meningocerebral angiodysplasia A developmental anomaly of the cerebral vasculature, characterized by the presence of multiple tortuous and dilated vessels on the surface of the cerebral cortex, with subjacent infarcts and calcification.

meningococcal meningitis (cerebrospinal fever) An acute meningitis seen mainly in youth, resulting from infection with *Neisseria meningitidis*, a gram-positive diplococcus.

The condition was described first by Thomas **Willis** in his book *The London Practice of Physick* (1684) and next by Gaspard Vieusseux (1746–1814), a Geneva physician in 1805.[5619] The organism was first discovered by Anton Weichselbaum (1845–1920), a German pathologist, in 1887.

meningoencephalitis Inflammation of the meninges and of the underlying substance of the brain.

meningoencephalocele (hernia cerebri) A developmental anomaly (a **craniofacial malformation**), characterized by the presence of a sessile or pedunculated swelling in the glabellar region, composed of glial tissue and fibrous tissue, protruding through a skull defect. Telecanthus and elongation of the nose are invariably present, and hydrocephalus due to atresia of the foramen of Monro, agenesis of the corpus callosum, cortical atrophy, seizures strabismus, and mental retardation are common accompaniments.[4]

meningoencephalomyelitis Inflammation of the meninges, brain tissue, and spinal cord.

meningoepithelial meningioma See **meningioma**.

meningomyelitis Inflammation of the meninges and of the underlying substance of the spinal cord.

meningomyelocele A severe defect of neural tube closure occurring at any level of the neuraxis, leading to the exposure of both the meninges and the neural contents of the spinal canal to the outside. These represent the commonest physically disabling birth defects in humans. The relative roles of genetic and of environmental causes have not yet been determined.

The condition is associated with severe motor and sensory deficits in the legs, and frequently with the **Chiari malformation** and resulting **hydrocephalus**. The presence of the disorder is suggested antenatally by the finding of high levels of α-fetoprotein in the amniotic fluid and in maternal blood.

meningovascular syphilis A form of tertiary **syphilis**, characterized by cerebral arteritis and by lymphocytic infiltration of the meninges with or without **gummas**. The clinical effects result from a basal meningitis with optic and lower cranial nerve involvement, and from multiple small cerebral infarcts resulting from obliterative endarteritis.

Pachymeningitis cervicalis hypertrophicans is a variant in which the cervical meninges are matted together, leading to compressive and vascular myelopathy.

Menkes disease 1. (trichopoliodystrophy, kinky-hair disease, steely-hair disease) An X-linked recessive degenerative disorder due to a deficiency of copper as a result of its impaired absorption, leading to failure of function of copper-dependent enzymes such as cytochrome *c* oxidase. The responsible gene maps to chromosome Xq12-q13.

The main clinical features are failure to thrive with seizures in infancy, severe mental retardation, dysmorphism, ivory-white and brittle hair that feels like steel wool (pili torti), short stature, bony changes, poikilothermia, poor feeding, abnormal temperature control, and arterial tortuosity from the age of 2 months. Generalized seizures, cerebral atrophy, callosal dysgenesis, and demyelination accompany these features. The disorder leads eventually to decerebration and death within 2 years. It was first defined by Dr. Milton Alter[4314] while he was a junior resident.

In a *variant* form, chorea, athetosis, hypotonia, seizures, and psychomotor retardation are associated with low copper and ceruloplasmin levels, and intestinal copper absorption is reduced.[2659] 2. See **branched-chain ketoaciduria**.[4315]

Menkes disease A Web site providing information and images at: http://themenkesfoundation.org.

Menkes Support Group At eGroups A support group open to anyone interested in making friends, sharing information, and providing support for persons affected by Menkes syndrome. Web site: http://www.healthinforum.org/Menkes-Support-Group-info-23006.html.

menopausal muscular dystrophy See **chronic polymyositis**.

menstrual-associated sleep disorder A disorder of unknown cause, characterized by a complaint of either insomnia or excessive sleepiness temporally related to the menses or menopause. Three forms are delineated: premenstrual insomnia, premenstrual hypersomnia, and menopausal insomnia.[1629]

menstrual-associated syndrome A syndrome characterized by marked hypersomnolence in association with menstruation.[639]

menstrual migraine (pure) Attacks of migraine that occur on days −2 to +3 of the menstrual cycle and at no other time. The headache is associated with increased circulating prostaglandin levels.[473]

A *variant* is *menstrually associated {or related} migraine*, in which the attacks occur at any time of the cycle but with increased frequency at period times.

mental 1. (from Lat, the mind) Relating to the mind. 2. Relating to the chin.

mental coprolalia The unwanted intrusion of obscene words into the thoughts of patients with **Tourette syndrome**.

Mental Health Inventory A 31-question multiple-choice self-assessment instrument designed to survey experience of anxiety, depression, behavior/emotional control, general positive affect, and emotional ties in response to life events experienced by the subject.[6520]

mental neuropathy Numbness of the chin, most commonly due to malignant infiltration of the mental nerve.[4149]

mental retardation A state of abnormal development manifested by impaired intelligence and inadequate ability to learn. Nonspecific X-linked forms without other distinguishing neurological features have been mapped to chromosome Xq11-q12 or Xp22.

mental retardation, aphasia, shuffling gait, adducted thumbs See **MASA syndrome**.

mental retardation, diabetes mellitus, hypogonadism, and nerve deafness A rare recessive syndrome characterized by these features, in which pigmentary retinal degeneration has also been described.[1810]

mental retardation–epilepsy See **cerebellar syndromes** (congenital ataxias).

Mental Status Questionnaire (MSQ) A widely used, formalized bedside screening test of cognitive function. Like the many others developed in the last quarter-century, it is brief (requiring only 5 min or so to put the 10 questions on orientation, memory, and general knowledge) to the patient; focuses on cognitive factors rather than on affect, thought-disorder or behavioral features; and is valid, reliable, and simple both to give and to score. However, it is rather insensitive.[3270] See also **Mini-Mental Status Examination**.

mentation Use of the mind, or intellect.

Menzel disease A dominantly inherited form of **cerebellar ataxia** causing pyramidal, cerebellar, and posterior column dysfunction.[1793, 4317] See **olivopontocerebellar atrophy** and **autosomal dominant cerebellar ataxia**.

MEPP See **miniature end-plate potentials**.

meralgia paresthetica (Gr, the thigh + pain) (lateral femoral cutaneous neuralgia, Roth–Bernhardt disease, Bernhardt–Roth {Rot} paresthesia) Paresthesias, hypoesthesias, numbness, and often pricking or burning pain in the distribution of the lateral cutaneous nerve of the thigh, supposedly often caused by compression of the nerve by a fat pad under the lateral part of the inguinal ligament and most commonly seen in middle-aged men.[583, 5425] Lumbar plexus or L2, 3 lesions can cause the same picture. A *familial form* has been described.[4143]

Despite the usual eponyms, the condition was first described by **Remak**.

meranesthesia (Gr, part + deprivative + feeling) Partial anesthesia.

mercuric encephalopathy See **pink disease** and **Minamata disease**.

mercuric neuropathy A syndrome resembling **amyotrophic lateral sclerosis** or **lead** neuropathy resulting from the ingestion of organic mercury. Headache, loss of the teeth, tremor, weakness initially of the arms, wasting, fasciculations, hyperreflexia, and up-going plantar responses are found, and a blue line on the gum margins is noted in some patients.[3290] See also **Hatters shakes**.

Meretoja syndrome Dominantly inherited generalized **amyloidosis** with lattice dystrophy of the cornea, progressive cranial neuropathies, and late peripheral neuropathy.[4321]

merged gyri A cortical dysplasia, characterized by fusion of the gyral surfaces of the brain; a *forme fruste* of **polymicrogyria**.[471]

meridrosis Localized sweating.

Merkel, Karl Ludwig (1812–1876) German anatomist.

Merkel disks A form of sensory nerve ending, sensitive to touch.

merlin A molecule protective against the excessive replication of cells; alterations in the neurofibromatosis-2 gene coding for merlin cause all of the benign tumors that occur in patients suffering from that condition, all spontaneous Schwannomas and most meningiomas.[2726]

mermaid syndrome See **caudal regression syndrome**.

meropia Partial dullness or obscuration of vision.

Merrill Palmer scales of mental development A composite nonverbal test of perceptual and motor skills designed for children under the age of 5 years.

MERRF (Myoclonic Epilepsy with Ragged Red Fibers, Fukuhara syndrome, leukoencephalopathy with ragged red fibers; OMIM 545000) A maternally transmitted mitochondrial disorder with onset in infancy, childhood, or early adult life, characterized by short stature, myoclonus, nerve deafness, generalized tonic–clonic seizures, ataxia, myopathy with ptosis and mental and developmental delay, with lactic acidosis, spongiform encephalopathy, and the presence of ragged red fibers in muscle biopsy specimens.[2232, 3780] In short, it presents as a typical progressive myoclonic encephalopathy with myoclonus, tonic-clonic seizures, progressive ataxia, and dementia.

Optic atrophy, Parkinsonism, deafness, pyramidal signs, peripheral neuropathy resembling HMSN, myopathy migraine, and hypoventilation are other inconstant features described. See also **MELAS** and **mitochondrial myopathies**.

Merritt, H. Houston (1902–1979) A leading American neurologist who was educated at Chapel Hill and at Vanderbilt and Johns Hopkins, then at the Boston City Hospital and in Munich. His professional life was spent first at Harvard (where with Tracy Putnam he was first to complete clinical studies of diphenylhydantoin in 1937),[4325] and then in New York at Columbia University where he became professor and chairman of the Department of Neurology and established model Departments of Neurology at Montefiore and the New York Neurological Institute. He was also sometime dean of the medical school and vice president for medical affairs.

Merritt was an outstanding clinician, a superb teacher (his *Textbook of Neurology* went through six editions before his death), and a productive researcher, but he also was active on the boards of charitable organizations in the neurological field and of the National Institute of Neurological Diseases.

As one of the most influential neurologists in the United States, he promoted neurology as an independent clinical discipline and fostered the organization of dedicated neurological training programs with a strong basic science component. His residency program trained a remarkable proportion of those physicians who today are most influential in American neurology. Merritt was also instrumental in the foundation of the National Institute of Neurological and Communicative Disorders and Stroke and as a research worker himself, published over 200 papers, particularly on the topics of epilepsy, syphilis, cerebrovascular disease, and nutritional disease.

Merwarth syndrome See **Rolandic vein occlusion**.

Merzbacher, Ludwig (1875–1942) German physician who trained in Strasbourg and practiced mainly in Argentina. In 1910 he added to the 1885 description by Friedrich **Pelizaeus** of the syndrome now known by both of their names, having re-studied members of the same family.

mesaticephalic Broca's term for a skull with a **cephalic index** between 75 and 80. The significance of the shape is not known.

mesencephalic artery syndrome See **top o' the basilar syndrome**.

mesencephalitis and rhombencephalitis A syndrome of subacute progression, manifesting drowsiness; oculomotor, facial, and bulbar palsies; anarthria; and cerebellar ataxia without limb weakness. There may be mild pyrexia. The CSF contains increased numbers of mononuclear cells.

Despite severe bulbar failure occurring at some time during the course of the disease, eventual recovery may be complete.[621] See **Bickerstaff brainstem encephalitis**.

mesencephalon (Gr, the middle brain) (mesocephalon) That part of the brain derived from the middle cerebral vesicle and comprising the brainstem structures below the hypothalamus and above the pons.

mesial temporal lobe epilepsy syndrome See **temporal lobe epilepsy**.

mesial temporal sclerosis (Ammon's horn sclerosis, hippocampal sclerosis, incisural sclerosis, and pararhinal sclerosis) Loss of nerve cells with gliosis in Sommer's sector of the hippocampus, usually with additional abnormality elsewhere in the temporal lobe.

After many years of uncertainty as to whether such changes were the cause or the effect of complex focal (partial) seizures, Falconer concluded that they signified prior anoxia due to repetitive seizures in infancy, were themselves epileptogenic, and were the commonest lesions found in tissue specimens removed after anterior temporal lobectomy for the management of drug-resistant epilepsy.[1954, 1955] However, the issue remains unsettled and the seizures may in some cases at least be the result rather than the cause of the sclerosis.[6513]

mesiobasal limbic seizures See **amygdalohippocampal seizures**.

Mesmer, Franz Anton (1734–1815) Austrian physician and metaphysician who trained originally for the priesthood and then for law before changing to medicine, the subject in which he graduated from Vienna in 1765. He was earlier interested in the effect of the planets on the human body, which he considered similar to their effects on each other; this formed the subject of his dissertation and led to his proposition of the existence of animal magnetism (*gravitas animalis*), a mysterious fluid permeating all organic and inorganic substances. Mesmer considered that obstruction to the flow of this fluid was the basis of disease, and that such obstructions could be relieved by putting the patients into a trance and then inducing a convulsion.

His ideas were rejected by orthodox physicians in Vienna and he left for Paris, in which city his success was phenomenal, thanks to adept stage management, the innocuous nature of the treatments, and the high prevalence of naïveté and ignorance at that time. By 1784, these had diminished enough to allow the creation of a commission of inquiry into the basis of Mesmer's system, of which Benjamin Franklin, Antoine Lavoisier, and Dr. Armand Guillotin were members. Their conclusions that mesmeric fluid did not exist and that the effects of Mesmer's treatments were but the result of imagination led to his departure from Paris and to his further demonstrations being given in a traveling format.

Mesmer considered that he was dealing with physical rather than with mental forces. It was James **Braid** who introduced the term *hypnotism* for the trance-like state induced in his subjects by Mesmer, and who regarded this as a mental state of heightened suggestibility.

mesocephalon See **mesencephalon**.

mesoencephalothalamic syndrome Isolated bilateral internal and external ophthalmoplegias with vertical gaze paresis and **abulia** resulting from a vascular lesion in thalamic and high brainstem regions. This may occur as a **lacunar syndrome**.[2092, 2106] See **syndrome of the mesencephalic gray matter**.

mesolimbocortical dementia A rare, insidiously progressive dementing syndrome of unknown cause, characterized pathologically by nonspecific neuronal loss and gliosis in the limbic system and also in the mesencephalic dopaminergic fields, their terminal fields in the cortex and the caudate nuclei, substantia nigra, and inferior olive. Clinically, late-onset, slowly progressive personality changes; loss of memory, insight, judgment, and self-care skills; behavioral disturbances such as those in the **Klüver–Bucy syndrome**; and sometimes Parkinsonism, all giving rise to features of **subcortical dementia**, are the most prominent features.[6356, 6529]

mesomelia and nephritis syndrome See **Funderbunk syndrome**.

meta- Greek prefix, signifying "beyond."

metabasis The changing over from one thing to another—as suggested by its derivative *metabolism*. However, a change in the appearance of symptoms of disease is also an acceptable, if somewhat archaic, meaning.

metabolic craniopathy See **Morel–Stewart–Morgagni syndrome**.

metabolic headache See **headache** (*headache associated with disorders of homeostasis*).

metabolic myopathy See **lipid myopathies; carnitine deficiency, riboflavin responsive; acid maltase deficiency; glycogen storage disease;** and **myopathy**.

metabolic poliodystrophy Anterior horn cell disease due to chemical disorders, such as hypoglycemia or lead poisoning.

metabolic syndrome A group of interrelated risk factors linked to insulin resistance (atherogenic dyslipidemia, abdominal obesity, raised blood pressure, raised serum glucose, and a prothrombotic state) that affect about a quarter of the adult population and together increase a person's risk of cardiovascular disease. Leukoaraiosis and intellectual decline are clinically associated.

metachromasia A change in color.

metachromatic leukodystrophy (Greenfield disease, Scholtz syndrome, van Bogaert–Nijssen–Pfeiffer disease, sulfatide lipidosis; OMIM 250100) A group of recessively inherited lysosomal storage diseases caused by deficiency of leukocyte arylsulfatase A and leading to intralysosomal storage of cerebroside sulfate in the white matter of the CNS and peripheral nerves. The resulting demyelination causes a variety of neurological features including loss of cognitive function or behavioral abnormalities and neuromuscular weakness with impaired nerve conduction. The responsible gene maps to chromosome 22q13.13-qter or, when there is a lack of sphingolipid activator protein, to 10q21-q22.

The usual presentation is of a slow progressive symmetrical and severe demyelination of the cerebral and cerebellar hemispheres occurring as a result of damage to oligodendroglia, and leading to axonal damage; pyramidal degeneration with isomorphic gliosis; and loss of myelin in the peripheral nerves with sparing of the subcortical U-fibers. Sulfatide (a cerebroside sulfuric acid ester, which is a metachromatic material causing a brown stain in the presence of acidic cresyl violet) is deposited in white matter, nerves, neurons such as the anterior horn cells; in the dentate and other nuclei;[2563] and in the liver, kidney, testes, and pituitary gland. CT scanning shows bilateral white matter lucencies in the cerebrum and cerebellum, with cortical atrophy.

There are three types of arylsulfatase: A and B are lysosomal; C is microsomal. The A form is deficient in the late infantile, juvenile, and adult forms of metachromatic leukodystrophy. Some allelic types of the disease are recognized. Clinically the disease is heterogeneous, and different forms are classified according to the age at onset of symptoms (late infantile, juvenile, and adult) (Chart M–6).

Chart M–6. Allelic Forms of Metachromatic Leukodystrophy

The *late infantile* form is commonest. Clinically, it presents at the age of 1–2 years with irritability, poor eating, gait disorder, floppy posture, loss of motor skills, optic atrophy, squint, and nystagmus. With further decline, spasticity takes over, despite evidence of a peripheral neuropathy, and seizures, myoclonus, cortical blindness, mental deterioration, decerebration, and opisthotonos lead on to death.

In the *juvenile* form, the onset is between 3 and 16 years of age with gait disturbance and behavioral change. The neuropathy is less prominent, but mental changes, dystonia, and incontinence may be severe.[2713]

The *adult* form is rare; clinical features include insidious dementia, psychoses, optic atrophy, ataxia, pyramidal and extrapyramidal signs, and neuropathy with onset after the age of 16 years.[6634] The neuropathy has been reported as occurring in isolation.

Other *variants* include the following:

Metachromatic leukodystrophy due to cerebroside sulfatase activator defect: A phenotype resembling the juvenile form, in which the enzyme activity is reduced but not absent.[5760]

The *Austin variant* (O Variant, multiple sulfatase deficiency): A recessively inherited mucosulfatidosis—a nonallelic variant. The features are similar to the *late infantile* variety, with progressive motor and intellectual deterioration, ichthyosis, and hepatosplenomegaly, progressing to blindness, deafness, decerebrate rigidity, and dementia; but the biochemistry resembles that of some of the gangliosidoses and mucopolysaccharidoses, with storage of gangliosides in the cortical neurons.[302]

Adult onset form of metachromatic leukodystrophy with nor-aryl sulfatase: A form characterized by the onset in adult life of dementia, ataxia, spasticity, orthostatic hypotension, diffuse demyelination, and low-density lesions in the white matter on CT scans.

Metachromatic leukodystrophy with heterozygous compound allele (pseudodeficiency): A form characterized by the onset in infancy of gaze palsy, dysarthria, ataxia, spasticity, psychomotor arrest, cerebral atrophy, and diffuse gliosis and demyelination. The same apparent deficiency may also occur in healthy people.

Metachromatic leukodystrophy with early juvenile onset: A form characterized by the onset in childhood of optic atrophy, seizures, ataxia, pyramidal and extrapyramidal signs, sensorimotor peripheral neuropathy, and dementia.

Metachromatic leukodystrophy without arylsulfatase deficiency: A form characterized by dementia, pyramidal signs, hypertrophic demyelinating sensorimotor peripheral neuropathy, neurogenic bladder, and developmental delay.

Metachromatic leukodystrophy with retinitis pigmentosa: A form characterized by the onset in infancy of pigmentary retinal degeneration, dysarthria, dysphagia, dystonia, ataxia, pyramidal signs, demyelinating sensorimotor peripheral neuropathy, diffuse demyelination with low-density lesions in the white matter on CT scanning, and mental and developmental delay.

metacognition The diverse processes of self-knowledge, self-monitoring, and self-regulation that contribute to adaptive behavior in complex and changing environments.[1913] It is especially disturbed in the **frontotemporal dementias**. Such patients are unable to follow the dictum of the philosopher Michel de Montaigne; "Know thyself" so that they can neither monitor nor regulate their behavior. See also **dysexecutive syndrome**.

metamorphopsia Distortion (alteration of size, shape, or angulation) of objects seen. When persistent, it is usually due to ocular disease or to bilateral occipital or occipitotemporal lesions. In some cases, the distortion affects only one or two quadrants of the visual field, making the environment appear grotesque.

metamorphosis The change in an object from one form or structure to another.

metaphyseal dysplasia A **craniotubular dysplasia** with cranial bone sclerosis, associated sometimes with muscle weakness, scoliosis, or optic atrophy.[6250] See **Pyle disease**.

metastatic Shifting of disease from one place in the body to another.

metencephalon That part of the brain derived from the posterior part of the third cerebral vesicle during embryonic development and comprising the medulla oblongata, the VIII cranial nerve and the fourth ventricle.

methacholine test Instillation of one drop of 2.5% methacholine into the conjunctival sac normally has no effect, but produces miosis within 15 min, lasting for up to 2 h, in states of parasympathetic denervation with denervation hypersensitivity, as with the **Adie pupil**. See also **pilocarpine test**.

methemoglobinemia (recessive hereditary methemaglobinemia) An inborn error of metabolism. The type II recessive form is due to deficiency of generalized NADH-cytochrome b5 reductase and results in mild cyanosis but severe neurological impairment—severe encephalopathy, microcephaly, generalized dystonia, and other movement disorders, with early death. Never do the children either speak or walk.[1934]

methionine malabsorption syndrome See **oasthouse disease**.

methioninemic myopathy A rare inborn metabolic error manifest in infants by high circulating levels of methionine; it presents as a proximal myopathic syndrome with hyporeflexia and mental retardation.[2319]

methyl crotonyl-coenzyme A-carboxylase deficiency A congenital metabolic disorder characterized by neonatal seizures, hypotonia, spinal muscular atrophy, alopecia, patchy skin abnormalities, neurodegenerative regression, and organic aciduria with metabolic acidosis.[381]

5-10 methylenetetrahydrofolate reductase deficiency A rare inherited error in the pathway for synthesis of methionine, presenting as an infantile dysmorphic syndrome of pyramidal signs with spasticity, cognitive deterioration, myoclonic seizures, microcephaly, sensory ataxia, rigidity, tremor, motor neuropathy, neurogenic bladder, cerebral atrophy, and diffuse cerebral demyelination with aminoaciduria.[6598]

3-methylglutaconic aciduria A rare, congenital, dominantly inherited syndrome characterized by chorea, truncal and limb ataxia, optic atrophy, retinal aplasia, sensorineural deafness, severe hypotonia giving way to spasticity by the age of 6 years, and mild mental retardation, with excessive excretion of 3-methylglutaconic acid (MGA) in the urine. The clinical features closely resemble those of **Behr syndrome**.

Three syndromes are differentiated according to the amounts of MGA excreted, in which the same features, and also macrocephaly, seizures, pigmentary retinal degeneration, and cataracts, are seen in varying combinations.[1293]

methylmalonic acidemia A group of rare congenital inborn metabolic errors, usually manifesting neonatal seizures, dystonias, feeding problems, apneic attacks, and mental and developmental delay, but occasionally with minor signs only. Organic aciduria, hyperammonemia, and raised plasma lactate levels are characteristically found.[3534]

methylmercuric encephalopathy See **Minamata disease**.

metopic (Gr, between the eyes) Relating to the forehead. An antique term for the frontal bone. A *metopic suture* is a persistent sagittal suture between the right and left sides of the frontal bone.

metopion (Gr, the forehead) An alternative term for the glabella or interorbital region.

metrizamide encephalopathy A syndrome of asterixis, sometimes with generalized seizures and with severe stuttering speech, occurring as a toxic manifestation of metrizamide myelography. It is considered that impaired brain glucose metabolism may be responsible for some of these effects.

Metrizamide is a nonionic contrast agent derived from glucose and metrazoic acid, widely used for imaging of the CSF spaces.[592]

mevalonate kinase deficiency A disorder due to mutations in the mevalonate kinase gene, associated with the following two phenotypes: 1. *HyperIgD and periodic fever syndrome,* an autoinflammatory disease characterized by lifelong recurrent episodes of fever, abdominal distress, lymphadenopathy, and skin rash starting in infancy. 2. *Mevalonic aciduria,* also starting in infancy but manifesting psychomotor retardation, failure to thrive, dysmorphisms, cataracts, and ataxia.[5846]

Meyer, Adolf (1866–1950) Swiss-American neurologist and psychiatrist born in Zurich, who became professor of psychiatry at Cornell after emigration and later went to Johns Hopkins. Although outstanding as a psychiatrist, his early neurological and pathological studies led to his identification of the following anatomical fact.

Meyer loop (Fleschig loop) The lowermost fibers of the geniculocalcarine (optic) radiation, which pass through the temporal lobe and loop around the tip of the temporal horn on their way to the calcarine cortex. These carry impulses from the inferior nasal quadrant of the retina, and thus lesions of the temporal lobe may produce a superior quadrantanopia.[1219]

Meyer phenomenon Mydriasis in response to abdominal pressure, described in psychiatric patients.

For a sign so trite the word *phenomenon* seems overstated; perhaps *happening* would be more appropriate?

Meyer–Betz disease Paroxysmal myoglobinuria, unassociated with other evidence of muscle disease, but occurring after heavy exertion or during infections, with associated muscle pain and swelling. The myoglobinuria can lead to renal impairment.[3532, 4344]

Meynert, Theodor Hermann (1833–1892) German professor of psychiatry and later of neurology in Vienna, where he combined neurological science with psychiatric research, convinced that diseases of the mind must reflect disease of its substrate, the brain. His anatomical studies revealed the central projections of the sensory fields onto the cortex, the functional topography of which he mapped out, differentiating between the association fields and the primary receptive areas. He also studied the morphology of the brainstem in detail.

Meynert amentia An acute confusional psychosis. See **Wernicke–Korsakoff encephalopathy**.

Meynert decussation The decussation of the dorsal tegmental tract.

Meynert fasciculus (habenulopeduncular tract) A small bundle passing from the habenula of the thalamus to the interpeduncular region, described by Meynert in 1867.

MGUS See **monoclonal gammopathy of uncertain significance**.

Michael J. Fox Foundation for Parkinson's Research A charitable organization in this field. Address: Grand Central Station, P.O. Box 4777, New York, NY 10163. Tel: 212-213-3525. Web site: http://www.michaeljfox.org/.

Michel defect A developmental defect comprising the absence of the otic capsule and the VIII cranial nerve.

Michel syndrome (clefting with ocular anomalies) A congenital dysmorphic syndrome characterized by sensorineural deafness, telecanthus, hypertelorism, iris adhesions, corneal opacities, strabismus, impairment of upward gaze, ptosis, blepharophimosis, epicanthic folds, cleft upper lip and palate, and mental and developmental delay.[4]

Michigan Diabetic Neuropathy Score A protocol used to evaluate peripheral neuropathy in diabetic patients. It is based both upon clinical examination (sensory: vibration in great toe touch with 10 g filament, pin prick to great toe); (muscle strength; finger spread, great toe extension, ankle dorsiflexion); (reflex testing; biceps and triceps brachii, quadriceps, ankle jerk) and median, ulnar, and sural sensory and median and peroneal motor nerve conduction studies.[1994]

Mickey Illness Severity Score A weighting system providing an overall score of functional disability in patients with **multiple sclerosis**, based upon **Kurtzke's** functional systems score and his disability status scale.[4351]

Mickey Mouse sign The appearance on the MRI scan of atrophy of the mid-brain tegmentum as seen on axial views in **progressive supranuclear palsy**.[5648]

micrencephaly Reduction in brain weight to a value less than a figure 2 standard deviations below the mean for a given age, with any size of cranium. **Broca** considered that brain weights below 1049 g in males and below 907 g in females were abnormal. **Microcephaly** is also commonly present.

micro- Greek prefix signifying smallness.

microbleeds Small, homogeneous, round foci of low signal intensity seen on MRI gradient echo (GRE) sequences, due to hemosiderin deposition. If deep they are closely correlated with the presence of hypertension and are possible markers for microangiopathy;[1283] when lobar, they are associated with **cerebral amyloid angiopathy**.

micro border-zone infarct The distribution of lesions occurring after arterial occlusion.

micro syndrome Microphthalmia and cerebellar and callosal hypoplasia, usually with X-linked inheritance.[4944]

microadenoma A functioning adenoma within the pituitary gland which has caused no detectable expansion of the gland by virtue of its size, arbitrarily defined as less than 10 mm in diameter.

microaneurysm 1. (lipohyalinotic aneurysm) Focal bulging of the wall of an arteriole damaged by **lipohyalinosis** and arteriolosclerosis with an increase in the diameter of the vessel's lumen. This is seen mainly in the putamen, caudate, and thalamus, and to a lesser extent in the cerebral cortex. 2. (saccular miliary aneurysm) Focal bulging of the wall of an arteriole, its new wall being composed of fibrin thrombus and organized red blood cells resulting from prior bleeding from the arteriole. **Charcot–Bouchard aneurysms** are considered to include both of these forms.

microangiopathic encephalopathy and hearing loss A syndrome with onset in young adult life, characterized by sensorineural deafness, vascular abnormalities of the retina, dysarthria, dementia, aggressive behavior, cerebellar ataxia, and spasticity. See **RED-M syndrome**.

microcephalic primordial dwarfism A congenital dysmorphic syndrome characterized by low birthweight, dwarfism with short (or absent) limbs and metacarpal bones, alopecia, beaked nose, micrognathia, short neck, rhizomelia of the upper limbs, dislocation of the elbows and hips, Perthes disease, delayed skeletal maturation, hyperkeratosis, **microcephaly** due to early closure of the fontanelles, and mental and developmental delay.[381]

microcephaly A reduction in the circumference of the head, the occipitofrontal circumference measuring less than 2 standard deviations below the mean for the person's **gestational age**, sex, and race. This may be due to failure of development of the underlying brain or of the skull bones themselves during the first 4 months of gestation, or may result from premature fusion of the cranial sutures. The result is usually severe psychomotor delay.

In familial cases, recessive, dominant, and X-linked inheritance have all been described. In such cases, the cerebrum is small and contains evidence of multiple neuronal migration defects, but the cerebellum is usually of normal size. Sporadic cases are also common.[4244]

In *primary microcephaly*, anomalies of induction and migration have occurred during the first 7 months of intrauterine life; in the secondary form, the reduction in brain size is due to infectious, traumatic, metabolic, or anoxic lesions incurred in the last 2 months of gestation or in the perinatal period.[4313]

A classification of the congenital microcephalies has been suggested.[404]

1. Microcephaly with normal to thin cortex
   a. Primary microcephaly (microcephaly vera)
   b. Extreme microcephaly with simplified gyral pattern
2. Microlissencephaly (MLIS: extreme microcephaly with thick cortex)
   a. MLIS with thick cortex (**Norman–Roberts syndrome**)
   b. MLIS with thick cortex, severe brainstem, and cerebellar hypoplasia (Barth MLIS syndrome)
   c. MLIS with intermediate cortex, abrupt AP gradient
   d. MLIS with mild-to-moderate cortex whose thickness is 6–8 mm.
3. Microcephaly with polymicrogyria or other cortical dysplasias
   a. Extreme microcephaly with diffuse or asymmetric polymicrogyria
   b. Extreme microcephaly with agenesis of the corpus callosum and cortical dysplasia.

From Barkovich AJ, Kuzniecky R, Jackson GG, et al. Classification system for malformations of cortical development. Neurology 2001;57:2168–78. Reproduced by kind permission of the American Academy of Neurology and Lippincott Williams and Wilkins.

Variant forms are listed in Chart M–7.

See also **COFS** and the syndromes of **Aicardi, Cockayne, Coffin and Siris, de Lange, dysencephalia splanchnocystica, Dubowitz, Hallermann–Streiff–Francois, Meckel, Pen–Shokeir phenotypes, Rett, Rubinstein and Taybi, Seckel,** and **Smith, Lemli,** and **Opitz**.

microcephaly with basal ganglion calcification See **Aicardi–Goutières syndrome**.

Chart M–7. Variant Forms of Microcephaly

Microcephaly and chorioretinal dysplasia: A dominantly inherited anomaly characterized by microphthalmia, dysplasia of the optic nerve and retina, detached retina, pigmentary retinopathy with blindness, strabismus, early closure of the fontanelles, microcephaly, and psychomotor retardation.[6252]
Microcephaly-chorioretinopathy: A recessively inherited syndrome of dwarfism, microphthalmia, optic atrophy, aplasia or dysplasia of the retina, pigmentary retinopathy, microcephaly, and cutis marmorata.[999]
Microcephaly, motor neuron disease, and nigral degeneration: A congenital dysmorphic syndrome characterized by the onset in early childhood of dysarthria, dementia, microcephaly, tremor at rest, dystonias, fasciculations, neurogenic muscle atrophy, and cerebral atrophy.[381]
Multiple epiphyseal dysplasia–microcephaly–nystagmus: A congenital syndrome characterized by short stature, small pelvis, epiphyseal dysplasia, microcephaly, nystagmus, and mental and developmental delay.[3940]
Microcephaly with spasticity and seizures: A congenital dysmorphic syndrome characterized by tonic–clonic and myoclonic seizures, microcephaly, spasticity, and cerebral atrophy.[937] See **Paine syndrome**.
In other *variant* forms, lymphedema, retinopathy, cervical spine anomalies, intracranial calcification and/or pyramidal signs are associated. These and a summary of syndromes in which microcephaly also occurs are reviewed by Baraitser.[379]

microcephaly–absent phalanges–short stature–retardation syndrome See Drayer syndrome.

microcephaly-albinism-limb defects See **Castro–Gago syndrome**.

microcephaly–syndactyly syndrome See **Filippi syndrome**.

microcompression An operative technique in which a small balloon is inflated in a position where it will compress a nerve, such as the trigeminal nerve in Meckel's cave in cases of trigeminal neuralgia resistant to medical treatment.

microcoria A synonym for **miosis**.

microdeletion syndromes Inherited conditions caused by the deletion of small segments of chromosomes at a variable number of contiguous loci.

microdiskectomy Microsurgical excision of prolapsed intervertebral disks, of value in patients with segmental signs who have not responded to conservative treatment, including **chemonucleolysis**, and in those with osseous **spinal stenosis**.

microdrift Dysconjugate slow eye movements of less than 1 degree in amplitude, occurring during fixation of an object. They are of no known pathological significance.

microdysgenesis Disturbances of focal cortical architecture from the presence of nests of ectopic neurons and glia in the first layer of the cerebral cortex. This is often associated with focal dysplasia of adjacent cortical layers, including focal microgyria, and with superficial excrescences known as *brain warts* representing abnormalities of cortical development. Clinically, the abnormality may either be asymptomatic or associated with dyslexia or seizures[3343] (**cortical dysplasias**). Variable usage of the term, however, has led to its abandonment.

microflutter See **ocular flutter** and **microsaccadic flutter**.

microglia (Gr, small + glue) The smaller supporting neuroglial cells in the CNS; interstitial cells of mesoblastic origin representing the reticuloendothelial system in the CNS, having both the morphology and staining characteristics of macrophages. They were first described by Rio **Hortega** in 1921. See **primary CNS lymphoma**.

microglial stars Clusters of activated microglia around damaged or dead neurons.

microglioma (microgliomatosis, reticulum cell sarcoma) A form of reticulosis affecting the brain and producing clinical signs of a fast-advancing intracranial tumor.[5473] See **primary CNS lymphoma**.

microgliomatosis See **microglioma**.

microglossia Smallness of the tongue, congenital or acquired.

micrognathia Congenital smallness of the jaw.

micrographia Smallness of the handwriting; a classic sign in Parkinsonism.

microgyria (hemiatrophy of the brain) A developmental abnormality of prenatal origin, characterized by a decrease in the cell population of the middle cerebral cortical layer leading to decreased width and therefore an increased number of cerebral cortical gyri focally. It is sometimes combined with **macrogyria**. Such laminar destruction of the middle layer only is considered evidence of an acquired injury rather than of a neuronal migration defect.[3] Clinically, seizures and a degree of mental impairment are commonly present.[5904, 5909]

micromelia Small limbs.

microneurography The technique of recording peripheral nerve action potentials in humans by means of intraneural electrodes.

micropapilla See **optic nerve hypoplasia**.

microphthalmia A congenital ocular malformation in which the presence of some ocular development can be determined by clinical means. Microcephaly and other brain malformations are occasionally associated. See **Walker–Warburg, Meckel,** and **Neu-Laxova syndrome**.

micropsia The illusion of reduction in the size of objects seen, as in some forms of complex partial seizure.

microsaccades Small-amplitude, rapid saccadic oscillations of the eyes contributing to ocular "noise" in normal subjects and suppressed during the performance of close work.[3762]

microsaccadic flicks See **microsaccadic flutter**.

microsaccadic flutter (microflutter, microsaccadic flicks) The rare phenomenon of conjugate saccadic horizontal ocular oscillations at 15–30 Hz, invisible to the naked eye and inconsistently associated with neurological disease, although considered to reflect abnormal function of the brainstem omnipause neurons.[266]

The perplexed lexicographer notes the high validity but the slight importance of this phenomenon but recalls with relief:

A symbol said "I represent
The meaning someone else has meant.
I personally have no leanings
Toward any of the many meanings."

micro-saccadic oscillations and limb tremor A familial disorder manifest by tiny saccadic oscillations of the eyes and tremor of the hands.

microscopic polyangiitis (overlap syndrome) A vasculitis affecting arterioles, capillaries, and venules with skin manifestations and frequently with neuropathy.[5582]

microsleeps Brief periods in which the EEG activity is that of stage 1 or 2 nonrapid eye movement sleep activity but lasting less than 10 s, interrupting wakefulness and impairing sustained attention. They occur in normal people after sleep deprivation and may be associated with **excessive daytime sleepiness** and with automatic behavior.[280]

microsomia Smallness of the whole body—head, trunk, and limbs.

MICROSTROKE A computer-based system designed to use the clinical features of a patient's case to diagnose the type of stroke suffered.[5995] See also TOPOSCOUT.

microsurgery Surgical procedures utilizing the operating microscope and small instruments for meticulous operations within a confined space. Microvascular decompression of the V cranial nerve in the cerebellopontine angle for relief of **trigeminal neuralgia** is an example.

microtia Small ears. A sporadic congenital syndrome of middle ear anomalies, ear atresia, and conductive hearing loss.[3]

microtremor Dysconjugate, low amplitude, high-frequency ocular vibrations, of no known pathological significance except in the case of a rare familial disease of saccadic oscillations and limb tremor.[5751]

microtropia Divergence of the ocular axes, leading to a manifest deviation so small that the **alternate cover test** fails to reveal it. A degree of diplopia may result.[2400]

microtubules Cytoskeletal structures within axons synthesized within the cell body, consisting of polymerized dimers of tubulin protein forming a hollow tube, about 20 nm in diameter and 1 mm long. They are longitudinally oriented and are linked by cross-bridges to neurofilaments, and move centrifugally within the axoplasm at up to 3 mm/day.

microvasculitic neuropathy Neuropathy due to a small vessel disease, as with hematological malignancies and rarely as a **paraneoplastic** manifestation, usually with B-cell lymphomas.

miction (from Lat, to pass water) The act of passing water. The word is hardly used now, but it appears to be the better derivation to describe normal urinary functioning.

micturition (Lat, a desire to pass water) 1. A constant inclination to urinate. 2. The act of passing water—the modern, but slightly incorrect meaning. See also **miction**.

micturition syncope Syncope which occurs during or after voiding, usually in the case of elderly men who rise from their beds at night for this purpose, and thus are at risk by virtue of attaining the upright posture when peripherally vasodilated, and also because of the Valsalva maneuver required to overcome the effects of prostatism.[1225]

MIDAS (Migraine Disability Assessment Scale) A tool for the evaluation of the effects of headaches upon those that suffer from them. A pediatric version is also available. Web site: http://www.migraine-disability.net/home.asp/.

See also **Headache Impact Test**.

midbrain The **mesencephalon**.

midbrain corectopia A shift in the geometric center of a pupil, which becomes oval, in association with disease of the brainstem.

midbrain deafness Total deafness as a result of degeneration of the lateral lemnisci and inferior colliculi, described following a head injury.[3011]

midbrain infarction Localized posterior circulation infarctions, usually in the territories of paramedian branches of the basilar artery supplying the midbrain and presenting with overt eye movement disorders such as those due to oculomotor nerve palsies, vertical gaze palsies, pure motor hemiparesis, and/or four-limb ataxia but with few other localizing findings. Infarcts in the territories of the mesencephalic branches of the posterior cerebral artery and of the superior cerebellar artery are distinctly less common.[708]

midbrain "myasthenia" The occurrence of some ocular signs of myasthenia (fatigable ptosis, lid twitch, ophthalmoparesis) as a result of a midbrain tumor.[5168]

midbrain pseudo-sixth Impairment of ocular abduction as a result of **convergence spasm** without any lesion of the VI cranial nerve.[1007]

midbrain tremor (cerebellar outflow tremor, red and black tremor) A predominantly unilateral tremor at 1.5–3 Hz, involving both proximal and distal muscles, present at rest but successively increased by maintenance of a posture and by volitional movement. Occasional large-amplitude tremor bursts may induce a quasi-myoclonic component.[2052] See **rubral tremor**.

midcervical central cord syndrome Numbness of the fingertips and clumsiness of the hands with tightness felt at midthoracic levels resulting from midline cervical disk protrusions at C3–4.[4583]

middle cranial fossa syndrome See **Raeder paratrigeminal syndrome**.

middle finger test The patient extends his elbow, wrist, and middle finger and holds them against resistance. Increase of pain in the region of the lateral part of the elbow indicates pressure on the posterior interosseous nerve, as with compression underneath the arcade of Frohse.[3871]

midfacial hypoplasia Dominantly inherited or sporadic malformations (dysmorphisms) occurring in **holoproscencephaly**, or in **Apert** or **Crouzon syndromes**, characterized by maldevelopment of the parts derived from the frontonasal process. Deafness and facial dysmorphisms (hypotelorism, flattening of the nose, **cebocephaly**, **ethmocephaly**, **cyclopia**, an indistinct philtrum, palatal deformity, mandibular hypoplasia, malformations of the temporomandibular joints and tongue, fusion of the jaws, and other anomalies of the cranial bones) may be associated.

midlatency SEP That portion of the waveforms of a somatosensory evoked potential normally occurring within 25–100 ms after stimulation of a nerve at the wrist, within 40–100 ms after stimulation of a nerve at the knee, and within 50–100 ms after stimulation of a nerve at the ankle. (Adapted from the 1987 Report of the Nomenclature Committee of the American Association of Electromyography and Electrodiagnosis. AAEE glossary of terms in clinical electromyography. *Muscle Nerve* 1987;10S:G5–G23. © 1987. Reproduced by kind permission of the AANEM and John Wiley and Sons Inc.)

midline fusion defect syndrome See **Wolf–Hirschorn syndrome**.

midline hyperplasia with malformation of the fornical system A congenital dysmorphic syndrome characterized by meningocele, hydrocephalus, and cerebellar atrophy.

midline nevus flammeus with intracranial vascular disease See **Sturge–Weber syndrome**.

midline spikes An encephalographic finding during interictal periods, consisting of the appearance of spikes with maximal amplitude at the Fz, Pz, and Cz positions, with phase reversals in the waking or sleeping states. They correlate well with the presence of various forms of epilepsy, including generalized tonic–clonic and focal motor seizures and less commonly myoclonic or atonic attacks.[1818]

midline splitting The precise change from abnormal to normal sensation across the midline of the trunk. While this is usually considered to be evidence of a **functional disorder**, it has also been reported in patients following a thalamic stroke.[6074]

midwinter insomnia A seasonal form of the **delayed sleep phase syndrome** encountered in the "Land of the Midnight Sun."[3859]

Mietens syndrome A recessively inherited congenital dysmorphic syndrome manifesting also strabismus, corneal clouding, horizontal and rotary nystagmus, short limbs with flexion contractures, and mental retardation.[4354]

migraine (from Gr, half + skull, through Lat, hemicrania to Fr, migraine) A familial systemic syndrome encompassing various forms of head pain or evidence of focal disturbance of the nervous system. The condition was known to Hippocrates, Celsus, Arateus, and Galen, but the first modern account was that of Thomas **Willis** and a more formal description was provided by John **Fothergill** in a pamphlet "*Remarks on that complaint commonly known under the name of sick headach*" published in 1777.[4502] The history of the development of thought in the area has been recounted by Pearce,[4948] who quotes Liveing's definition of 1873: "A form of centrencephalic seizure, the activity of which is projected rostrally upon the cerebral hemispheres and peripherally via the autonomic nervous system," and notes that we are little wiser now.

The classification of the International Headache Society,[2820] is reproduced in Chart M–8. Definitions or descriptions of the various subtypes reproduced elsewhere in this book are as shown in bold below.

Our knowledge of the pathophysiology of migraine has advanced since the second edition of this book, though not far enough to allow confident mapping of the whole underlying chain of events. Cortical hyperexcitability, evidenced by laboratory techniques and by the persistence of the after-image following fundoscopy[1519] and the activity of a brain-stem generator of impulses activating the trigemino-vascular complex and thus leading to the liberation of vasoactive peptides in the extra- and intracranial arterial walls, in turn causing progressive pain perception through other brainstem mechanisms appear to be the major elements of the process.

Chart M–8. Classification of Migraine

1. Migraine
   - 1.1 *Migraine without aura*
   - 1.2 *Migraine with aura*
     - 1.2.1 Typical **aura** with migraine headache
     - 1.2.2 Typical aura with nonmigraine headache
     - 1.2.3 Typical aura without headache
     - 1.2.4 **Familial hemiplegic migraine**
     - 1.2.5 Sporadic hemiplegic migraine
     - 1.2.6 **Basilar-type migraine**
   - 1.3 *Childhood periodic syndromes that are commonly precursors of migraine*
     - 1.3.1 **Cyclical vomiting**
     - 1.3.2 **Abdominal migraine**
     - 1.3.3 **Benign paroxysmal vertigo of childhood**
   - 1.4 *Retinal migraine*
   - 1.5 *Complications of migraine*
     - 1.5.1 **Chronic migraine**
     - 1.5.2 **Status migrainosus**
     - 1.5.3 **Persistent aura without infarction**
     - 1.5.4 **Migrainous infarction**
     - 1.5.5 **Migraine-triggered seizure**
   - 1.6 *Probable migraine*
     - 1.6.1 Probable migraine without aura
     - 1.6.2 Probable migraine with aura
     - 1.6.5 Probable chronic migraine

migraine accompagnée See **migrainous accompaniments**.

migraine accompaniments (migraine accompagnée) Transient and reversible neurological deficits occurring in the absence of a current headache and of any other detectable cause, supposed to be occurring on the same basis as the rest of the migrainous syndrome, whatever that may be. Not all patients who have such problems have migraine headaches as well.

Clinically, scintillating scotomas, blindness, blurred vision, numbness, paresthesias, aphasia, dysarthria, and motor weakness are the commoner symptoms. Clues to the migrainous nature of the syndrome are

A. The presence of visual symptoms
B. A gradual build-up and migration of any scintillating display
C. **A march of paresthesias**
D. The serial progression of symptoms

E. The occurrence of two or more identical spells
F. Accompanying headache
G. A duration of 15–25 min
F. The occurrence of a flurry of accompaniments
I. Recurrence of similar spells over a period of years
J. The exclusion of cerebral thrombosis, subclavian steal, epilepsy, thrombocythemia, polycythemia, hyperviscosity, and lupus anticoagulant; and
K. Normal cerebral arteriographic findings.[2095]

migraine angiitis See **reversible cerebral vasoconstriction syndrome**.

migraine-anxiety related dizziness (MARD) The concurrence of migraine, balance disorder, and anxiety, suggested as occurring with more than chance frequency.[2242]

migraine-associated vertigo See **migrainous vertigo**.

migraine aura A recurrent disorder manifesting in attacks of reversible focal neurologic symptoms that usually develop gradually over 5–20 min and last for less than 60 min.

migraine aura status Frequent but separate auras over a prolonged period of time (at least two auras per day for 5 consecutive days).

migraine aura without headache (migraine equivalents, acephalgic migraine) A condition diagnosed when focal neurological symptoms come on gradually and spread or intensify over a period of minutes; positive visual symptoms occur classically as in migraine; headache is absent or mild if present; and the patient has not had similar symptoms previously in the context of classical migraine or in association with a more severe headache.[1582] For the ICHD criteria, see **aura**.

migraine–cluster headache syndrome The occurrence of headaches which are predominantly of one of these types, but with at least one major timing factor (random vs. clustering, frequency, duration, hour of onset) or three other major features of the other (prodrome; aura; nausea and vomiting; incapacitation leading to bed, etc., with migraine; and with eye redness and tearing; Horner syndrome; rhinorrhea; and physical mobility with cluster headache).[5947]

migraine coma (meningitic migraine) A repetitively occurring, self-limited, generalized encephalopathy with delirium, rarely reported in patients with prior classic or familial migraine, but sometimes following head trauma.[1281] The attacks are preceded by severe headache and vomiting and lead through clouding of consciousness to pyramidal signs, often accompanied by fever and further reduction in consciousness, with recovery in about 2 days. Despite the alternative title the CSF is usually normal, although pleocytosis may occur some days after admission.

migraine complications See **chronic migraine, status migrainosus, persistent aura without infarction, migrainous infarction**, and **migraine-triggered seizure**.

migraine equivalents See **migraine aura without headache**.

Migraine Foundation A Canadian charitable association. Web site: http://www.migraine.ca/.

migraine madness Psychosis occurring in temporal association with migraine in subjects known to have that condition in the past without such mental abnormality. The state may last days or weeks and recur over many years. Delusions, both paranoid and other, visual hallucinations, **reduplicative paramnesia** and speech disturbances are described. Migraine-induced ischemia of the nondominant hemisphere is considered to be responsible.[2239] See also **dysphrenic migraine**.

migraine stroke See **migrainous infarction**.

migraine-triggered seizure A seizure triggered by a migraine aura.

migraine with acute-onset aura The full development of an attack of **migraine with aura** in less than 5 min in Which a thromboembolic transient ischemic attack and other intracranial lesions are ruled out by appropriate investigations.

migraine with aura (classic migraine, classical migraine, ophthalmic migraine, hemiparesthetic migraine, hemiplegic migraine, aphasic migraine, migraine accompangneé, complicated migraine) An idiopathic, recurring disorder manifesting with attacks of neurological symptoms unequivocally localizable to the cerebral cortex or brainstem, usually gradually developed over 5–20 min and usually lasting less than 60 min.

Headache, nausea, and/or photophobia usually follow neurological aura symptoms directly or after a free interval of less than an hour. The headache usually lasts 4–72 h but may be completely absent. This definition and the following diagnostic criteria are suggested by the Headache Classification Committee of the International Headache Society (Chart M–9). See also **migraine without aura**.

A *variant* is *migraine with aura, flushing spells, myalgias, asthma, and advanced sleep phase syndrome.*

migraine with interparoxysmal headache A condition in which occasional but increasingly frequent episodes of migraine headache are separated by periods during which further headaches occur, similar to but not identical with the patient's usual migraine and which occur daily and chronically. The condition has been considered a "transformational syndrome" between migraine and chronic daily headache.[5546] See **rebound headache**.

Chart M–9. Diagnostic Criteria for Migraine with Aura

migraine with aura (classic or classical migraine, ophthalmic, hemiparesthetic, hemiplegic or aphasic migraine) A recurrent disorder manifesting in attacks of reversible focal neurological symptoms that usually develop gradually over 5–20 min and lasts for less than 60 min; and headache with the features of migraine without aura. The head pain usually follows the aura.

A. At least two attacks fulfilling criterion B
B. Migraine aura fulfilling criteria B and C for one of the subforms 1.2.1–1.2.6
C. Not attributed to another disorder

From the International Classification of Headache Disorders (Headache Classification Committee of the International Headache Society; Cephalalgia *2004;24(Suppl 1)) by kind permission of Dr. Jes Olesen, the International Headache Society and Wiley-Blackwell Publications.*

migraine with prolonged aura

Migraine with one or more aura symptoms lasting more than 60 min and less than a week. Neuroimaging findings are normal. According to the International Classification of Headache Disorders, the diagnostic criteria are that the syndrome fulfils criteria for (**migraine with aura**, as above) but at least one symptom lasts between 60 min and 7 days. If neuroimaging reveals a relevant ischemic lesion, migrainous infarction should be diagnosed, regardless of symptom duration.

migraine with typical aura

(ophthalmic, hemiparesthetic-, hemiparetic-, hemiplegic-, or aphasic migraine, migraine accompagnée) Migraine with an aura consisting of homonymous visual disturbances, hemisensory symptoms, hemiparesis or dysphasia or combinations thereof. Gradual development, duration under 1 h and complete reversibility characterize the aura which is associated with headache.

Chart M–10. Diagnostic Criteria for Migraine without Aura

migraine without aura (common migraine, hemicrania simplex) A recurrent headache disorder manifested by attacks lasting 4–72 h. Typical characteristics of the headache are unilateral location, pulsating quality, moderate or severe intensity, aggravation by routine physical activity and association with nausea and/or photophobia and phonophobia. Diagnostic criteria have been defined as follows:

A. At least five attacks fulfilling criteria B–D
B. Headache attacks lasting 4–72 h (untreated or unsuccessfully treated)
C. Headache has at least two of the following characteristics:

1. unilateral location
2. pulsating quality
3. moderate or severe pain intensity
4. aggravation by or causing avoidance of routine physical activity (e.g., walking or climbing stairs)

D. During headache at least one of the following:

1. nausea and/or vomiting
2. photophobia and phonophobia

E. Not attributed to another disorder

From the International Classification of Headache Disorders (Headache Classification Committee of the International Headache Society. Cephalalgia 2004;24(Suppl 1)) by kind permission of Dr. Jes Olesen, the International Headache Society and Wiley-Blackwell Publications.

migraine with unilateral motor symptoms

A sporadic form of migraine in which patients complain of weakness on one side (usually the same side as the headache) with a "give-way" character. Such weakness may be accompanied by sensory symptoms and tends to "march" up the limbs. It is also often present between attacks. The face is seldom involved. Other symptoms include language disturbances and dizziness.[6934] See also **familial hemiplegic migraine**.

migraine without aura

(common migraine, hemicrania simplex) An idiopathic, recurring headache disorder manifesting in attacks lasting 4–72 h. Typical characteristics of headache are unilateral location, pulsating quality, moderate or severe intensity, aggravation by routine physical activity, and association with nausea, photophobia, and phonophobia. This definition and the diagnostic criteria in Chart M–10 are suggested by the Headache Classification Committee of the International Headache Society.

A *variant* is **familial migraine with vertigo and essential tremor**.[356]

migrainous disorder not fulfilling criteria

are those headache attacks that are believed to be a form of **migraine**, but which do not quite meet the operational diagnostic criteria for any of the forms of migraine (nor of **tension-type headaches**).

migrainous dysautonomia

Autonomic disturbances resulting in labile hypertension and sometimes alternating with postural hypotension with tachycardia, reported in peri-menopausal women during acute headache episodes.

migrainous infarction

(complicated migraine; migraine stroke) The condition in which one or more migrainous aura symptoms are associated with relevant ischemic lesions as demonstrated on neuroimaging studies. Compare persistent aura without infarction (aura symptoms persisting for more than 1 week without radiographic evidence of infarction).

A combination of (possibly migraine attack-related) hypoperfusion and embolism is the likeliest mechanism rather than atherosclerosis or small-vessel disease.[3571, 714] The occipital lobe is most commonly affected, producing a homymous field loss. Diagnostic criteria have been defined as follows:

A. The present attack in a patient with **migraine with aura** is typical of previous attacks except that one or more aura symptoms persists for >60 min
B. Neuroimaging demonstrates ischemic infarction in a relevant area
C. Not attributed to another disorder.

From the International Classification of Headache Disorders (Headache Classification Committee of the International Headache Society. *Cephalalgia* 2004;**24**(Suppl 1]) by kind permission of Dr. Jes Olesen, the International Headache Society and Wiley-Blackwell Publications.

migrainous neuralgia

See **cluster headaches**.

migrainous vasospasm

(crash migraine) See **reversible cerebral vasoconstriction syndrome**.

migrainous vertigo

A common cause of episodic vertigo in migrainous subjects who present with attacks of spontaneous or positional vertigo lasting seconds to days with nystagmus and imbalance but without hearing loss. It can present both as a central and as a peripheral vestibular disorder.[6565] The occurrences of the headache and the vertigo are not necessarily at the same time. Diagnostic criteria have been suggested;[4633, 972] and also by the IHS.

1. Recurrent vestibular symptoms (rotatory/positional vertigo, other or illusory self or object motion, head motion intolerance) of at least moderate severity.
2. Migraine according to IHS criteria.
3. At least one of the following symptoms during two vertiginous attacks; migrainous headache; photophobia; phonophobia; visual or other auras.
4. Other causes are excluded by appropriate investigations.[6565]

See also **basilar-type migraine**.

Benign paroxysmal positional vertigo and **Ménière disease** are statistically related to migraine, but the possible pathogenetic links have not been established. Moreover, migraineurs suffer from motion sickness more often than controls.[4632]

migralepsy The association of features of migraine and of epilepsy in the same attack. The term was suggested by Sir William **Gowers**.

migrant sensory neuritis (of Wartenberg) A self-limiting condition characterized by the repetitive brief occurrences of a sudden searing pain in the territory of a sensory nerve, precipitated by movement of a limb and leading sometimes to sensory deficits. It has been considered that this may occur because of stretching resulting from movements of a limb[4180] or from compression (as in the case or **meralgia paresthetica**) but **multiple sclerosis** is sometimes a more acceptable explanation.

migrating focal seizures in infancy A rare epileptic encephalopathy of infancy characterized by frequent and then almost continuous intractable, multifocal seizures with motor and autonomic components. The EEG records multifocal spikes, particularly in the Rolandic and temporal areas, and diffuse background theta activity.[6833, 4882] The disorder is devastating and often fatal.

migration abnormalities See **heterotopias, lissencephaly** and Chart L–6.

The main pathological types of migration abnormality have been defined as follows:[75, 1673]

Major Abnormalities

1. Type I lissencephaly-agyria: A smooth brain possessed of a 4-layer cortex with a thick layer of arrested heterotopic neurons, resembling a fetal brain at 13 weeks of gestation.
2. Type II lissencephaly (Walker–Warburg syndrome): A totally disorganized cortex divided by gliomesenchymal trabeculae into glomeruli with disoriented cells.
3. Pachygyria: few, thick gyri, similar to lissencephaly with less numerous heterotopic neurons.
4. Polymicrogyria: Multiple small gyri with "cauliflower" appearance; 4-layer cortex without heterotopic neurons but paucicellular layer in continuity with normal layers 4–5. Other types include unlayered microgyria.
5. Localized cortical dysplasia. (The term dysplasia is used both in a general sense to designate all developmental cortical abnormalities or in the restricted sense of focalized defect of cortical organization). Absent lamination, anarchic distribution of neurons and glial cells are typical. In one type, "balloon cells" similar to those in tuberous sclerosis are found.

Minor Abnormalities That May Exist Alone or in Association with Major Anomalies

6. Glioneuronal heterotopias: A verrucous cortex with excess cell migration into the molecular layer and the meninges.
7. Microdysgenesis: An excessive number of neurons in the molecular layer, irregular thickness of neuronal layers, and the presence of heterotopic neurons in the outer white matter.

migratory recurrent cranial neuritis A syndrome of repetitive cranial nerve palsies lasting a few weeks and affecting the same or different nerves (usually the cranial nerves II to VI), with headache.[6228] See also **acute painful ophthalmoplegia**.

migratory seizures See **fragmentary seizures**.

Mikulicz–Gougerot–Sjörgren syndrome See **Sjögren syndrome**.[4478]

Milan Overall Dementia assessment A composite tool for the assessment of cognitive impairment, composed of an autonomy scale measuring everyday coping skills; four items concerning orientation; and nine neuropsychological tests assessing attention, intelligence, memory, language, space cognition, and visual perception.[1145]

mild Broca aphasia See **Broca aphasia**.

mild cognitive impairment (benign senescent forgetfulness, age-associated cognitive decline, age-associated/consistent memory impairment; minimal cognitive impairment, MCI) An operational definition for a heterogeneous collection of disorders causing a measureable degree of cognitive decline in elderly people, which however is not definable as dementia by current criteria. The essential complaint is of subjective memory impairment (relative to the performance of others matched by age and education). General cognitive functions are relatively unimpaired and activities of daily living are carried out normally. Criteria for the diagnosis of clinical dementia are not fulfilled.

Pathologically, patients with *amnestic MCI* show the early changes of **Alzheimer disease**. Conversion rates from amnestic MCI to Alzheimer disease are about 15% per year. However, scores below the expected level for any subject could reflect the normal attainment level for that individual; the effect of the earliest stages of Alzheimer or another disease, or the effects of some intercurrent influence, such as drug or alcohol ingestion, recent/current morbidity from other disease, other psychological stresses, etc.[3183] Thus reversible causes of MCI include depression, upper airway obstruction, and a variety of metabolic, nutritional, or sensory impairments. Control of vascular risk factors such as systolic hypertension, hypercholesterolemia, diabetes mellitus, atrial fibrillation, transient ischemic attacks, and strokes may delay progression to dementia.[4089] Examining the cognitive domains of speed/attention, memory and learning, visuo-spatial function, language and executive function, rather few subjects actually have pure, isolated, memory impairment;[4696] however, the relative sparing of cognitive domains other than memory does distinguish the condition from diagnosable Alzheimer disease. Diagnostic criteria have been suggested as follows:[5000]

Complaint of memory loss (by patient or an informant)
Normal activities of daily living (no impairments)
Normal general cognitive functioning
Abnormal memory for age (score more than 1.5 SD below mean for age)
Failure to meet current criteria for dementia.
These criteria were only minimally changed by an European Working Group in 1995. It has been suggested that four subcategories (amnestic or not, and with single or multiple domains) can be differentiated, but the value of this is uncertain.

mild head injury (mild traumatic brain injury) A traumatic incident resulting in loss of consciousness for less than 30 min, or in dazing without loss of consciousness at all; an initial **Glasgow Coma Scale** score of

13–15 without subsequent deterioration; and an absence of focal neurological deficits, depressed skull fracture, intracranial bleeding, or other pathology.[1931]

Symptoms such as headache, dizziness, fatigue, irritability, impaired concentration, memory, and the ability to perform mental tasks, insomnia, depression, and reduction in tolerance to stress, alcohol, and excitement are however common, and are remarkable for their transience in the presence of verbal motivation.[3370]

mild postural cerebellar tremor See **cerebellar tremors**.

mild traumatic brain injury See **mild head injury**.

milestones The motor skills acquired, in order, by the developing infant. These are listed in Chart M–11.

See also **Denver Developmental Screening Test**.

Milgram Test When the supine patient raises both legs a few inches off the bed for 30 s, back pain suggests the presence of radiculopathy, caused by the increased intrathecal pressure induced by the maneuver.

miliary aneurysms (from Lat, millet seeds) The term of **Charcot** (1866) and of **Bouchard** (1872) for the tiny dilatations of arterioles now known by the names of both. See **Charcot-Bouchard aneurysm**.

milk-alkali syndrome See **Burnett syndrome**.

milkmaid sign Variability in the isometric force exerted by the wrist and by individual fingers during attempts to grasp an object. The sign is positive in choreic states.[6789]

Millard, Auguste (1830–1915) French physician who graduated from Paris, where he practiced and published extensively in the areas of pediatrics and internal medicine.

Millard–Gubler syndrome (Gubler paralysis) A pontine lesion affecting the VII nerve nucleus and the descending pyramidal fibers on one side of the ventral pons, causing homolateral facial paresis and contralateral hemiplegia.[2608] The syndrome may also include a VI nerve palsy. Credit for localization of the syndrome belongs to Gubler, Millard having his anecdotal contribution (a letter) published immediately after it in the same issue of the *Gazette hebdomadaire médicine et chiurgerie* although he had previously described the same condition, but without any useful analysis.[4359]

Chart M–11. Developmental Milestones

Months (The latest date by which the milestones are normally first attained)	
1	Watches mother
1–2	Smiles
1	Extends neck in prone position, raising head briefly
2	Vocalizes, apart from crying
3	Lifts head prone when held in ventral suspension
4	Laughs; turns head toward meaningful sound
5	Grasps with whole; hands come together in play; rolls over alone
6	Head held erect while sitting; raises upper body on arms in prone position; transfers objects between hands; drinks from a cup (held); looks at own hands; stretches arms out to mother
7	Simple sounds (Ba, Da, Goo, etc.)
8	Double-syllable words (DaDa, MaMa etc.)
9	Sits supported
10	Responds to own name
11	Crawls; pulls up to standing; walks while holding-on
12	Pincer (finger-thumb) grasp
14	Says at least one meaningful word
15	Builds a tower of two cubes; Walks unsupported
16	Picks up, and drinks from, a cup
24	Builds a tower of 6 cubes; uses pronouns (I, me, you)
36	Builds a tower of 9 cubes; copies a circle
48	Copies a cross
60	Copies a triangle
60–96	Dry at night

Miller, Henry (1913–1976) English neurologist. After completing medical studies at the University of Newcastle-upon-Tyne, he trained in psychiatry and neurology in Newcastle and London, returning to northern England for the rest of his clinical career, except for wartime service.

His teaching and almost prescient clinical skills were legendary. The clinical research topics he explored included multiple sclerosis, accident neurosis, and numerous other topics in neurology and psychiatry, not all of the latter being welcomed by psychiatric colleagues, perhaps in part because in his writing he displayed readability, irreverence, individuality, courage, and common sense. Some of his *obiter dicta* are not to be forgotten; "The best instrument for obtaining the plantar response is the ignition key of a Bentley" and "Hemiplegic multiple sclerosis is a rarity and only to be diagnosed by me" are classic examples.

He was professor of neurology, dean of the medical school, and later vice-chancellor of his University, secretary-general of the World Federation of Neurology, and visiting professor in numerous universities. He also held many other positions in national or international neurology by election or acclamation. The book *Remembering Henry* (BMJ Publications) was compiled within a decade of his death by those who knew him and displays a true renaissance figure who enhanced the form as well as the substance of neurology.

Miller–Dieker syndrome (OMIM 247200) The association of lissencephaly with facial dysmorphism, hypertelorism, cloudy corneae, congenital cardiac and renal anomalies, enlarged liver, polydactyly, syndactyly, seizures (infantile spasms), decerebrate posturing, and microcephaly, described by Dr. J.Q. Miller.[4367] The responsible chromosomal deletion is of a band on 17p13.3. See **lissencephaly**.

Miller Fisher syndrome (Fisher syndrome, ophthalmoplegia–ataxia–areflexia syndrome, acute oropharyngeal palsy, brainstem "encephalitis") A self-limited syndrome in which truncal and limb ataxia, ptosis, and conjugate gaze palsies leading on to ophthalmoplegia, the involvement of other cranial nerves, and hyporeflexia without significant motor or sensory deficits in the limbs are the leading signs. There is often a history of recent antecedent infection. Other features include acellular CSF with high protein levels and occasionally internal ophthalmoplegia.[2077] IgG antibodies to GQ1b and GT1a have been detected.[6807] Sensory loss is unusual. Electrodiagnostically, sensory and motor conduction velocities are normal but sensory nerve action potentials may be small.

Long considered to be a variant of the **acute inflammatory demyelinating polyneuropathy** syndrome, it has now been suggested that it is actually a manifestation of brainstem encephalitis;[83] but whether this represents a central or a peripheral lesion (or both) is still debated. Anti-GQ1b IgG antibodies have been found in both of these conditions and in acute ophthalmoparesis. IgG anticerebellum (anti-Purkinje cell) antibodies may also be found, the latter perhaps explaining the central nervous system involvement.[970]

A similar condition was reported by Collier in 1932. See also **multiple cranial nerve palsies syndrome, mesencephalitis, rhombencephalitis,** and **Bickerstaff brainstem encephalitis**.

Variants include absence of the ophthalmoplegia; a syndrome of bilateral ptosis, ataxia, and areflexia;[6917] and an ataxic form of **acute inflammatory polyneuropathy** resulting from damage to the brainstem or cerebellum.

Diagnostic criteria in Chart M–12 have been suggested by Ropper et al.[5387]

http://www.ninds.nih.gov/disorders/miller_fisher/miller_fisher.htm is a relevant Web site from the NIH.

Chart M–12. Diagnostic criteria for Miller Fisher syndrome

Clinical Features:

A. Bilateral, relatively symmetrical weakness of several extraocular muscles, and ptosis
B. Limb and gait ataxia with cerebellar tremor
C. Areflexia in all limbs by 1 week
D. Progression of the aforementioned three features over several days to 3 weeks
E. Minimal or no limb, facial or oropharyngeal weakness, or paresthesias
F. Normal alertness, no cerebellar dysarthria except as a result of the previous feature; no Babinski signs

Laboratory abnormalities that confirm the diagnosis:

A. Variable, usually slight, elevation of CSF protein concentration
B. Abnormal motor nerve conduction and late responses in the legs

From Ropper AH, Wijdicks EFM, Truax BT. Guillain–Barré Syndrome. *Philadelphia, F.A. Davis, 1991 by kind permission of Oxford University Press.*

Milles syndrome A variant of the **Sturge–Weber syndrome** in which an angioma of the choroid occurs without glaucoma.

Millikan–Siekert syndrome See **vertebrobasilar insufficiency**.

Mills, Charles Karsner (1845–1931) American neurologist, the first professor of neurology in the United States, who operated the first neurological ward, at Philadelphia General Hospital. (Later neurological wards were created at Bellvue in 1898 for Dana, at Mount Sinai in 1900, and at Boston City Hospital in 1909. By 1923, eight independent neurological departments existed in the United States.)

Mills described ascending and descending forms of progressive paralysis, alcoholic polyneuropathy, and geniculate ganglion neuralgia. His classic and highly popular textbook *The Nervous System and its Diseases—A Practical Treatise on Neurology* (Philadelphia) was published in 1898 and was notable for its inclusion of sections on the neurological examination and on functional localization.

Mills syndrome A rare chronic, unilateral progressive ascending or descending paralysis with wasting but also hyperreflexia, usually starting in the leg and later affecting the arm and eventually the other side as well without significant sensory involvement. The bulbar muscles are spared.[4384]

It is an entity of uncertain nature, but probably represents a form of **amyotrophic lateral sclerosis** (primary lateral sclerosis). Some have considered it to represent **acute inflammatory demyelinating polyneuropathy** or a form of **gammopathic neuropathy**, although the latter presents with a lower motor neuron syndrome.[3631]

mimetic (Gr, imitative) Apt to imitate. 1. Applied to diseases which resemble others in their manifestations, such as syphilis, AIDS, and systemic lupus erythematosus. 2. Human actions which copy those of others.

mimetic automatism In the context of epilepsy, a facial expression suggesting an emotional state such as fear.

mimetic palsy See **emotional facial palsy**.

mimetic smile Retention of the ability to contract the lower facial muscles on the hemiparetic side during the spontaneous act of smiling or laughing, while voluntary contraction of these muscles is impossible on command; and due to an upper motor neuron lesion above the pons.

The disparity results from the anatomical situation; while the corticobulbar tract mediates the volitional "smile," the mimetic smile depends on the functional integrity of fibers from the central tegmental tract derived from the hypothalamus, thalamus, and globus pallidus. Thus, the subject with a high supranuclear lesion may laugh symmetrically even though the lower facial quadrant is paretic when attempting voluntary, nonemotional movements.

mimic palsy Facial palsy. See **Bell palsy**.

mimic spasm Facial muscle spasm, probably due to **dystonia**.

mimo-causalgia See **reflex sympathetic dystrophy**.

Minamata disease A toxic encephalomyeloneuropathy due to chronic mercury poisoning, which occurred between 1953 and 1956 in people living by a bay in southern Japan, methyl mercury in the seawater having been concentrated in the fish that they caught and ate. Salivation, cerebellar signs, numbness due to sensory neuropathy, deafness, concentric constriction of the visual fields, and delirium or dementia were the major signs recorded.[4197] Low-level exposure is under investigation as a factor reducing motor skills and auditory and visual functions in the young.

mind (Middle English, from Saxon; to remember) 1. The power of human intelligence. 2. The sum total of the phenomena of the functional activity of the brain, subdivided into feeling, will or volition, and thought, through which all subjective and objective experience is derived.

miner's nystagmus A form of pendular nystagmus accompanied by light intolerance and oscillations of the head in people who have worked for years in darkness. Whether this entity really exists is questionable.

Mingazzini maneuver With the patient lying supine, the hips are actively flexed to about 80° and the knee is held at a 100° angle so that the lower leg is horizontal, parallel to the bed. The ankles are then dorsiflexed to 90° and this position is held as long as possible, up to a maximum of 30 s. The test is positive (for a pyramidal lesion) if the hip or the leg begin to fall or if there is a loss of foot dorsiflexion.[6245]

miniature end-plate potential (MEPP) The postsynaptic muscle fiber potentials produced through the spontaneous release of individual acetylcholine quanta from the presynaptic axon terminal. As recorded with monopolar or concentric needle electrodes inserted in the end-plate region, MEPPs are monophasic, negative, short duration (<5 ms), and generally <20 μV in amplitude.

minicore–multicore myopathy (MMM) A benign, congenital, recessively inherited nonprogressive myopathy in which the muscle fibers have histochemical defects of both oxidative and myofibrillar adenosine-triphosphatase enzymes and show disorganization of myofilaments.[1873]

Clinical phenotypes include marked axial weakness, scoliosis, and severe respiratory impairment; the same with ophthalmoplegia; a form with predominant hip girdle involvement with or without arthrogryposis; and another with marked distal weakness and wasting, mainly in the arms. The second of these forms may be caused by mutations in the ryanodine receptor type I gene.[3262]

minimal brain damage See **minimal brain dysfunction**

minimal brain dysfunction (minimal brain damage, Struwwelpeter syndrome, hyperkinetic syndrome) A syndrome of incoordination, overactivity, impulsivity and emotional lability, reduced attention span, and often specific learning deficits, apparent when the child first attends school.[1203] See **attention deficit disorder**.

minimal change myopathy Weakness of presumably congenital origin associated with normal or near-normal muscle biopsy.[1966] See **benign congenital myopathy**.

minimal ice water caloric test A test of labyrinthine function using 0.2 ml of ice-cold water with the head elevated 30° and tilted toward the opposite side for the first 10 s. The patient should wear +20D (Frenzel) lenses.

The standard test popularized by **Bárány** used 10–20 ml, which induces nystagmus, past-pointing, and drift, but also nausea and vomiting in many cases. This modification results in nystagmus for a shorter period, but without the unpleasant accompaniments.[4619]

minimal record of disability (MRD) A rating scale published by the U.S. National Multiple Sclerosis Society, designed to quantitate the effects of **multiple sclerosis**. It was last modified in 1983.[3094] The record was designed to follow the three-tier classification of dysfunction developed by the World Health. Organization. As applied to neurological disorders these are

1. *Impairment*: clinical signs and symptoms produced by damage to the nervous system.
2. *Disability*: the personal limitations imposed upon the activities of daily living by the neurologic impairment.
3. *Handicap*: the social and environmental effects of the disability.

minimal seizures (subtle seizures) An epileptic seizure pattern in newborns, characterized by tonic deviation; jerking of the eyes or eyelids; lip smacking, sucking, or swallowing; abnormal limb movements; and brief alterations of muscle tone with assumption of bizarre postures. Seizures presenting as autonomic dysfunction only also fall into this category. Clonic jerks of the eyelids or limbs are occasionally seen in the later stages.[72]

minimally conscious state A condition of reduced consciousness characterized by inconsistent but discernible, sustained, and reproducible evidence of consciousness/awareness, retention of sleep–wake cycles, ability to localize sounds and noxious stimuli and to fixate visually, and with some ability to vocalize and to show emotional facial movement.[2353] Thus patients may purposefully track objects visually and even communicate; sleep–wake cycles are retained; the subject can localize noxious stimuli and sounds, are capable of sustained visual fixation, and may vocalize, smile, or cry in response to environmental stimuli. It is related to dysfunction of the forebrain and medial thalamus.

Surveying the diagnostic criteria suggested[2352, 2064] it seems agreed that at least one of the following must be present:

1. The subject can follow simple commands, though perhaps inconsistently, and
2. Can respond with gestures or yes/no answers (regardless of accuracy).
3. Intelligible verbalization is retained (to some degree)
4. Purposeful behaviors (contingent smiling or crying, vocalization or gestures, reaching for, holding, or touching objects) are present and contingent upon environmental stimuli rather than being reflexive.
5. Sustained visual pursuit or sustained visual fixation occurs in direct response to moving or salient stimuli.

Patients are said to emerge from this state when able to show functional recovery of verbal or nonverbal communication.

The major purpose of defining this condition appears to be its differentiation from the wakeful unresponsiveness of the **(persistent) vegetative state** with which it can easily be confused, but in that condition there is no awareness of self, of others, or of the environment. To make the diagnosis of the minimally conscious state, one must demonstrate limited but clearly discernible evidence of self- or environmental awareness on a reproducible or sustained basis by one or more of the behaviors listed above. See also **akinetic mutism**, in which patients may also show visual tracking and other responses (and which may in fact be the same condition). A useful review is found at the Web site: http://www.kurzweilai.net/articles/art0161.html? printable=1/.

Mini-Mental State Examination (MMSE) A standardized and formal 11-item examination of certain mental functions, including orientation, concentration, data retention, registration, calculation ability, recall, language, visuospatial functions, and praxis. It is used as a screening test for dementia and for the serial assessment of geriatric patients. The original test[2147] has been expanded (see **Modified Mini-Mental State Test**[6254]) by the addition of items including date and place of birth, some abstract thought items, and more memory and naming tasks so that the maximum score is now 100, and a cutoff point of 76 is suggested as distinguishing between normal and abnormal. See also the newer (free online) **Addenbrooke's Cognitive Evaluation**, which has usefully expanded the MMSE yet further.

minimum conduction velocity The nerve conduction velocity measured from slowly conducting fibers in motor or sensory nerves, requiring special techniques not commonly employed in clinical practice.

minipolymyoclonus Subtle, small-amplitude multifocal movements, once considered to represent myoclonic jerks but more likely due to fasciculations of enlarged motor units causing twitching predominantly in the fingers and hands, and preceded by a synchronous, frontocentrally predominant negative slow wave in the condition of **primary generalized epileptic myoclonus**.[6785] The movements resemble small-amplitude coarse tremors, and may also be seen in patients with anterior horn cell disease.[3074, 5990] See also **cortical tremor**.

Minnesota Child Development Inventory A questionnaire for parents, assessing general development, gross and fine motor activity, language, comprehension, and personal and social skills, etc. in their infants.

Minnesota Multiphasic Personality Inventory A comprehensive self-administered inventory allowing an assessment of personality factors.[2793]

Minnesota Test for the Differential Diagnosis of Aphasia An aphasia battery.[5657] See also **Western Aphasia Battery**, **Boston Diagnostic Aphasia Examination**, and **Porch Index**.

Minnesota thermal disks A set of mounted disks made of copper, stainless steel, glass, and polyvinyl chloride, respectively, which are placed upon prepared areas of skin and which, due to the different rates of heat transfer between such materials and the skin, will feel relatively warmer or cooler than one another to the normal subject.

The disks have been used for the semi-quantitative assessment of temperature sensation.[1776]

Minor, Lazar Salomavitch (1855–1942) Russian neurologist and neuropathologist, professor in Moscow, who described hematomyelia (**Minor disease**) in 1892 and thereafter **serous meningitis** (Minor pseudomeningitis), the **Minor method**, the **Minor sign**, and **Minor tremor**.

Minor causalgia See **reflex sympathetic dystrophy** and **causalgia**.

Minor disease A syndrome resembling **syringomyelia**, occurring after blunt stretching or compressive trauma to the spinal cord, usually at cervical levels.[4393] See **central hematomyelia**.

minor epileptic status See **status epilepticus**.

minor head injury A cranial trauma producing an initial loss of consciousness limited to 20 min or less, a **Glasgow Coma Scale** score of over 13–15 on admission and requiring hospitalization for less than 48 h.[5307]

minor hemisphere syndrome See **apractagnosia**.

minor intervertebral disorder Mechanical lesions of the **mobile segment** of the spine (particularly of the facet joints) without demonstrable pathology, but leading to pain referred to the appropriate dermatomal territory.[4029]

minor ischemic stroke An acute ischemic disturbance of focal neurological function with symptoms lasting more than 24 h and less than 1 week.

minor meningitis See **idiopathic intracranial hypertension**.

Minor method The use of an iodine-alcohol-castor oil application to demonstrate areas of sweat production, invented by Dr. L. **Minor**.

minor motor epilepsy See **Lennox–Gastaut syndrome**.

minor motor seizures Myoclonic, astatic, or brief atonic seizures, or any type of seizure of limited expression regardless of clinical and EEG features.[72] The term is honored more in the breach than in the observance. See **absence seizures**.

Minor pseudomeningitis See **serous meningitis**.

Minor sign The patient with sciatica arises by putting weight on the healthy leg, bending the other one, placing one hand on the back, and flexing the spine.[5333]

minor status See **absence status**.

Minor tremor A familial tremor with childhood onset, described by Dr. L. **Minor** in 1925; it is increased by stress, is unassociated with other neurological problems, and is properly known as **essential tremor**.

miosis (Gr, lessening) Constriction of the pupil to a diameter of 3 mm or less as a result of accommodation (physiological), of decreased sympathetic or increased parasympathetic activity, or of the effects of drug administration.

miotics Agents that produce pupillary constriction, many also causing contraction of the ciliary muscle and thus disturbing accommodation. Eserine (physostigmine), pilocarpine, and opioids are examples.

mirror agnosia See **Ramachandran sign**.

mirror focus Excessive electrical activity arising in a contralateral homologous site to a primary epileptic focus as a result of repetitive transmissions across the corpus callosum.

mirror movements Symmetrical involuntary movements of the opposite side of the body involving the use of the homologous contralateral muscles, very commonly seen in childhood but thereafter generally suppressed except in some left-handers, hemiparetics (see **Leonardo Da Vinci**), especially if congenital, and dyslexic children. Reports of increased left-handedness and mirror writing among children in mental defective institutions are of uncertain merit. The basis is likely to be abnormal branching of crossed fast-conducting fibers from the undamaged primary motor cortex to homologous motor neuron pools.[1183] See also **alien hand syndrome**.

In a *variant* form, *hereditary mirror movements*, an anatomical variation of the corticospinal tracts has been considered to be the basis of the phenomenon.[2674, 3555, 3289]

mirror test

If a large mirror is moved to and fro in front of the face of a subject who claims blindness, movements of the eyes indicate that vision is in fact retained.

mirror writing

(spiegelschrift) Reversed writing, sometimes performed by mentally retarded people and more easily performed in normal subjects by those who are left handed.[5645] **Da Vinci**, paretic in his right hand in later life, wrote with his left in this manner.

miscellaneous headaches unassociated with structural lesion

A category of headache recognized by the International Headache Society (Classification of headache disorders, cranial neuralgias, and facial pains; and diagnostic criteria for primary headache disorders. *Cephalalgia* 1988;8[Suppl]):1–96); and comprising

- 4.1 **Idiopathic stabbing headache**
- 4.2 **External compression headache**
- 4.3 **Cold stimulus headache**
  - 4.3.1 External application of a cold stimulus.
  - 4.3.2 Ingestion of a cold stimulus.
- 4.4 **Benign cough headache**.
- 4.5 Benign exertional headache.
- 4.6 **Headache associated with sexual activity**.
  - 4.6.1 Dull type.
  - 4.6.2 Explosive type (benign sex headache).
  - 4.6.3 Postural type.

misdirection syndrome

Adduction and depression of the eye on attempted vertical gaze, elevation of the eyelid and miosis, all due to abnormal mass discharges in aberrant regenerating fibers of the III cranial nerve after injury. These features, occurring periodically, thus resemble those of **cyclic oculomotor paralysis**.[6615]

misery perfusion

Locally increased oxygen extraction occurring in an area of chronic reduction of cerebral blood flow. It may follow a small focal infarct or may itself lead to symptoms of **transient ischemic attacks**.

miso-

Greek prefix denoting hatred of something.

misoplegia

(Gr, hate + stroke) Behavior suggesting hatred of a paralyzed limb, as seen occasionally in patients with a left hemiplegia due to a right hemispheric infarct, who reject, push away, or curse their offending members.

misplaced objects task

A visuospatial recall task in which the subject places cardboard cutouts of household items into the rooms of a two-dimensional representation of a seven-room house, and after a delay is asked to recall in which rooms of the house the objects now are.[1351]

Mitchell, Silas Weir

See **Weir Mitchell, S.W.**

Mitchell treatment

A method for the treatment of neurasthenia introduced by **Weir Mitchell**. As it consisted of removal from the responsibilities of home, rest in bed, massage, electrical stimulation of the limbs twice daily, and somewhat excessive feeding, it proved most popular and it was deemed successful in many cases.

mitempfidungen

(Ger, with sympathy) See **referred itch**.

mitochondrial cytopathy

A heterogeneous group of multisystem disorders mainly affecting cardiac and skeletal muscle and the CNS, many with added features. Some examples are

1. (*Fanconi–Toni–Debré form, cystinosis*) A rare, recessively inherited congenital syndrome comprising short stature, sensorineural deafness, cloudy corneas, cataract, retinitis pigmentosa, cardiomyopathy, renal tubular acidosis, glycosuria, aminoaciduria, cystinuria, and mental and developmental delay or dementia with widespread excessive storage of cystine.

   Seizures, ophthalmoplegia, intermittent ataxia, pyramidal and extrapyramidal signs, sensorimotor peripheral neuropathy, and proximal myopathic weakness are other clinical features recorded. Raised levels of lactate and the presence of ragged red fibers and abnormal mitochondria in muscle biopsy specimens are markers indicating that this is a **mitochondrial disease**.
2. *Late-onset optic atrophy, ataxia, and myopathy*, which is associated with a mutation of a Complex II gene.[653]
3. In other *variant* forms, onset occurs in childhood or youth; or the features are predominantly or exclusively those of a muscle disease;[5007] or of a disorder of the CNS.

mitochondrial diseases

(mitochondriopathies) A heterogeneous group of progressive multisystem disorders usually presenting in young adult life, in which an impairment in mitochondrial functions due to single- or multiple-point deletions of mtDNA or nDNA are considered to be the basic defects.[3450, 2056] Disturbed activity of the respiratory chain protein complexes is the major mechanism, leading to impaired oxygen utilization and reduced energy production. The peripheral nervous system (myopathy, polyneuropathy, and lactacidosis) and the brain (leukoencephalopathy, calcifications, stroke-like episodes, atrophy with dementia, epilepsy, upper motor neuron signs, ataxia, extrapyramidal manifestations, and fatigue) are often involved. The endocrine system does not escape (short stature, hyperhidrosis, diabetes, hyperlipidemia, hypogonadism, amenorrhoea, delayed puberty), and nor does the heart (impulse generation or conduction defects, cardiomyopathy, left ventricular failure), the eyes (cataract, glaucoma, pigmentary retinopathy, optic atrophy), the ears (deafness, tinnitus, peripheral vertigo), the GI system (dysphagia, vomiting, diarrhoea, hepatopathy, pseudo-obstruction, pancreatitis, pancreas insufficiency), the kidney (renal failure, cysts), or the bone marrow (sideroblastic anemia).[2065]

Aside from the clinical presentations, diagnosis may be assisted by the results of a **lactate stress test**, rather more than resting serum lactate levels. For further elaboration, see also the Web site: http://www.neuro.wustl.edu/neuromuscular/mitosyn.html/.

mitochondrial encephalomyopathies

A genetic classification includes disorders due to defects of mitochondrial DNA (mtDNA) and disorders due to defects of nuclear DNA (nDNA) recently reviewed.[1652]

Two main groupings of the phenotypes can be made (Chart M–13).

Accompanying these disorders, or in isolation, there may be cardiomyopathy, growth retardation, endocrinopathy, a malabsorption syndrome, and abnormal liver function test results. Pathological abnormalities suspicious for these conditions include an increase in the CSF pyruvate–lactate ratios, systemic lactic acidosis, and the presence of abnormal mitochondria, with or without inclusions, in biopsy specimens. Provisional diagnostic criteria have been suggested[584] and are reproduced in Chart M–14 by kind permission of the American Academy of Neurology and Lippincott Williams and Wilkins.

Chart M–13. Mitochondrial Diseases Affecting the Nervous System

Presentation as myopathy

Carnitine palmitoyl transferase deficiency
Chronic progressive myopathy
CoQ deficiency (mental retardation, myopathy)
Fatal infantile myopathy
Kearns–Sayre syndrome (Kearns–Shy syndrome)
Lethal infantile cardiomyopathy/infantile myopathy and lactic acidosis
Luft disease
Malignant hyperthermia
MERFF
MELAS
MIMYCA (mitochondrial myopathy with cardiomyopathy)
mitochondrial encephalomyopathy with elevated methylmalonic acid
MNGIE
Progressive external ophthalmoplegia (CPEO)
Transient neonatal myopathy

Presentation as encephalopathy

Acute encephalopathy of infancy
Alpers disease (subacute poliodystrophy)
Aminoglycoside-associated deafness
ARCO (sensory neuropathy, dysarthria, and ophthalmoparesis)
Autosomal recessive ataxia with polymerase mutations
Canavan disease
CPEO
Diabetes with deafness
Familial multiple symmetrical lipomatosis
Fanconi–Debre–DeToni syndrome
Fumarase deficiency
Glutaric aciduria II
Ketoacidotic coma (short stature, ataxia, deafness)
2**Late-onset encephalopathy** (with seizures status epilepticus, hemiparesis, and lactic acidosis)
Leber optic atrophy
Leigh disease (subacute necrotizing encephalopathy)
May–White syndrome
Menkes disease
Mitochondrial cytopathy
NARP
NIDDM (maternally inherited noninsulin-dependent diabetes)
PDC deficiency
Pyruvate decarboxylase deficiency
Pyruvate dehydrogenase deficiency
Wolfram syndrome

Based upon Jackson MJ, Schaefer JA, Johnson MA, et al. Presentation and clinical investigation of mitochondrial respiratory chain disease. Brain *1995;118:339–57. By kind permission of Oxford University Press.*

mitochondrial disease, X-linked

A congenital syndrome comprising cardiomyopathy, respiratory difficulties, abnormality in consciousness, proximal myopathic weakness and hypotonia, and the usual biochemical and muscle biopsy hallmarks of mitochondrial disease.[381]

Mitochondrial Disorders Foundation of America

A charitable organization at 5100-1b Clayton Rd., Suite 187, Concord, CA 94521. Tel: 510-798-8798. Web site: http://www.familyvillage.wisc.edu/lib_mito.htm. See also **United Mitochondrial Disease Foundation**.

mitochondrial electron transport chain

A composite set of energy-producing metabolic pathways in the body comprising the following enzymes:

Complex I	NADH:CoQ oxide reductase
Complex II	Succinate CoQ reductase DHO-QO dihrotate CoQ oxidoreductase
Complex III	CoQ cytochrome idoreductase ETF-QO electron transfer flavoprotein
Complex IV	Cytochrome *c* oxidase ANT (adenine nucleotide translocater)
Complex V	ATPsynthase

mitochondrial encephalomyopathies

Members of a clinically and biochemically heterogeneous group of complex sporadic inborn errors of metabolism, affecting the energy pathways of mitochondrial metabolism in many systems, in particular defects of the respiratory chain and other enzyme systems involving the citric acid cycle or electron transport systems, and due to abnormal structure or function of the mitochondria.[1645] These are inherited through the maternal line. In such cases, both muscle and the CNS, at least, are affected.

Failure to thrive, seizures, ataxias, psychomotor regression, hypotonia, and organ failure, including visual failure, are typical effects when the condition

Clinical features useful in identifying patients with respiratory chain disease.[3129]

Rank 1	*Rank 2*	*Rank 3*
PEO	Myoclonic epilepsy	Failure to thrive
Elevated lactate in blood/CSF	Ataxia	Small stature
Maternal inheritance	Myopathy	Dementia
Low density in putamen on CT scan	Stroke-like episodes after seizures	Metabolic acidosis
SSAM in muscle biopsy	Deafness	Developmental regression
Retinal pigmentation		
Cardiomyopathy		
Optic atrophy		

Rank I: features which alone are highly suggestive of respiratory chain disease;
Rank 2: features which in combination are suggestive of respiratory chain disease;
Rank 3: features which are commonly associated with respiratory chain disease but not suggestive of it unless associated with category 1 (or possibly 2) features.

After Jackson MJ, Schaefer JA, Johnson MA, et al. Presentation and clinical investigation of mitochondrial respiratory chain disease. Brain *1995;118:339–5, reproduced by kind permission of Oxford University Press.*

The numerous pathogenic mutations of mitochondria reported can be found at the Web site: www.mitomap.org.

Chart M–14. Major Diagnostic Criteria for Respiratory Chain Disorders

Clinically complete respiratory chain (RC) encephalomyopathy (such as **Leigh disease, Alpers disease, lethal infantile mitochondrial disease, Pearson syndrome, Kearns-Sayre syndrome, mitochondrial encephalomyopathy, lactic acidosis, and stroke-like episodes** [**MELAS**], **myoclonic epilepsy with ragged-red fibers** [**MERRF**], **neuropathy, ataxia, and retinitis pigmentosa** [**NARP**], **mitochondrial neuro-gastro-intestinal encephalomyopathy** [**MNGIE**], **and Leber's hereditary optic neuropathy** [**LHON**)]) or a mitochondrial cytopathy defined as fulfilling all three of the following conditions:

1. Unexplained combination of multisystemic symptoms that is essentially pathognomonic for an RC disorder.
2. Symptoms must include at least three of the organ system presentations described elsewhere, namely neurologic, muscular, cardiac, renal, nutritional, hepatic, endocrine, hematologic, otologic, ophthalmologic, dermatologic, or dysmorphic.
3. A progressive clinical course with episodes of exacerbation (e.g., following intercurrent illnesses) or a family history that is strongly indicative of a mtDNA mutation (at least one maternal relative other than the proband whose presentation predicts a probable or definite RC disorder).

Other possible metabolic or nonmetabolic disorders will have been excluded by appropriate testing, which may include metabolite, enzyme, or mutation analyses, imaging, electrophysiological studies and histology.
Histology: >2% ragged red fibers in skeletal muscle
Enzymology: >2% COX-negative fibers if <50 years of age; >5% COX-negative fibers if >50 years of age; <20% activity of any RC complex in a tissue; <30% activity of any RC complex in a cell line; <30% activity of the same RC complex activity ≥2: two tissues
Functional: *Fibroblast ATP synthesis rates >3 SD below mean*
Molecular: *Identification of a nuclear or mtDNA mutation of undisputed pathogenicity.*
Minor diagnostic criteria have also been suggested by these authors.

A genetic classification of human mitochondrial disorders has been constructed[1152] and is adapted here

Chart M–14a. A Genetic classification of Human Mitochondrial Disorders.

1. *Mitochondrial genetic disorders*

Rearrangements (large-scale deletions and duplications)

chronic progressive external ophthalmoplegia; **Kearns–Sayre syndrome**; diabetes and deafness

Point mutations

Protein encoding genes (The tRNA genes and rRNA genes associated with neurological and other disorders are also listed.)
LHON, NARP/Leigh syndrome

2. *Nuclear genetic disorders*

Disorders of mtDNA maintenance (all with various mutations)
Autosomal dominant **progressive external ophthalmoplegia; mitochondrial neuro-gastrointestinal encephalomyopathy;** myopathy with mtDNA depletion; encephalopathy with liver failure.

Primary disorders of the respiratory chain (variously Complex I and II deficiencies)
Leigh syndrome; leukodystrophy and myoclonic epilepsy; cardioencephalomyopathy; optic atrophy and ataxia

3. *Disorders of mitochondrial protein import*

Dystonia–deafness

4. *Disorders of assembly of the respiratory chain*

Leigh syndrome; cardioencephalomyopathy; hepatic failure and encephalopathy; tubulopathy, encephalopathy, and liver failure.

Criteria for the diagnosis of mitochondrial disease in children have been suggested by Morava et al. (2006).[4469] Their scoring system (a simplified version for bedside use) is reproduced in an amended form here

I. *Clinical signs and symptoms* (1 point/symptom to max. 4 points)

- A. Muscular presentation (max. 2 points) Ophthalmoplegia, myopathic facies, exercise intolerance, muscle weakness, rhabdomyolysis, abnormal EMG.
- B. CNS presentation (max. 2 points) Developmental delay, loss of skills, stroke-like episode, migraine, seizures, myoclonus, cortical blindness, pyramidal signs, extrapyramidal signs, brainstem involvement.
- C. Multisystem disease (max. 3 points) Hematology, GI tract, endocrine/growth, heart, kidney, vision, hearing, neuropathy, recurrent/familial.

II. *Metabolic/imaging studies* (max. 4 points) Elevated lactate, lactate/pyruvate ratio, alanine, CSF lactate, protein or alanine, urinary tricarbon acid (TA) excretion, ethylmalonic aciduria, stroke-like picture or Leigh syndrome on MRI, elevated lactate on MRS.

III. *Morphology* (max. 4 points) Ragged red/blue fibers, COX- (cytochrome *c* oxidase) negative fibers, reduced COX staining, reduced succinate dehydrogenase (SDH) staining, SDH-positive blood vessels, abnormal mitochondria visualized under the electron microscope.

Scoring: 1 = mitochondrial disorder unlikely; 2–4 = possible mitochondrial disorder; 5–7 = probable mitochondrial disorder; 8–12 = definite mitochondrial disorder.

presents in infancy; they are usually due to cytochrome *c* oxidase deficiency and are often fatal. Three main symptom complexes are reported (Chart M–15).

Certain syndromes such as **MERRF, MELAS, maternally inherited myopathy and cardiopathy,** and **Leber hereditary optic neuropathy** are maternally transmitted and due to point mutations in mitochondrial DNA. In all of these conditions, the hallmark is the presence of **ragged red fibers** in muscle biopsy specimens stained with Gomori trichrome, a marker suggesting that the primary abnormality is of the mitochondria, although the finding is not always present and is not specific for any primary mitochondrial disease.[5580] Described syndromes include the following:

1. Ataxia, intellectual impairment, myoclonic jerks, seizures, and small stature accompanied by muscle biopsy findings of abnormal accumulations of mitochondria and lipid droplets, with decreased cytochrome *c* reductase activity in the mitochondrial respiratory chain.[5301]
2. Hepatic failure, hypotonia, and failure to thrive in infancy with early death.[6390]

Chart M–15. The Mitochondrial Encephalomyopathies

1. Muscle weakness with severe exercise intolerance, including the hypermetabolic state **Luft disease** and *mitochondrial myopathy with nonsense mutation of the COX 1 gene*[3303]
2. The same as No. 1, complicated by chronic progressive external ophthalmoplegia, etc. The best-studied of these are

   A. Congenital/neonatal onset:

   Alpers disease
   Canavan disease
   Familial myoclonic epilepsy with ragged red fibers
   Fatal infantile myopathy with cytochrome *c* oxidase deficiency
   Leigh disease
   Menkes disease (trichopoliodystrophy)
   Methylmalonic acidemia
   NARP (neuropathy, ataxia, and retinitis pigmentosa).
   Myopathy with multiple deletions of mitochondrial DNA
   Ramsay Hunt syndrome (dyssynergia cerebellaris myoclonica)
   Zellweger syndrome

   B. Onset in childhood, youth, or adult life:

   Kearns–Sayre syndrome
   Adult-onset mitochondrial myopathy with progressive external ophthalmoplegia, *presenting usually with fatigue and mild muscle weakness with elevated serum lactate levels.*[1577]
   MELAS
   MERRF
   mitochondrial neurogastrointestinal encephalomyopathy (MNGIE)
   mitochondrial encephalomyopathy with sensorimotor polyneuropathy, ophthalmoplegia and pseudo-obstruction. See **mitochondrial neurogastrointestinal encephalomyopathy** (*MNGIE*)

3. Various combinations of CNS syndromes, such as seizures, dementia, deafness, headache, somnolence, vomiting, pigmentary retinopathy, optic atrophy, ataxia, myoclonus and/or involuntary movements, short stature and psychomotor retardation, often with myopathy or neuropathy,[4482] and sometimes with involvement of other organ systems.[1938, 5007]

3. Progressive dementia, chorea, cerebellar ataxia, deafness, and peripheral neuropathy without myopathy.[4618]
4. Parkinsonism, deafness, and peripheral neuropathy.[6313]

mitochondrial encephalomyopathy with elevated methylmalonic acid

A recessively inherited mitochondrionopathy mapped to chromosome 13q14 (*SUCLA2 gene*) and presenting with hypotonia, muscle atrophy, hyperkinesias, severe hearing impairment, and postnatal growth retardation. Neuroimaging shows demyelination and central and cortical atrophy, including atrophy of the basal ganglia. Some patients fulfill the criteria for **Leigh syndrome**. Urine and plasma methylmalonic acid levels are high.[4826]

mitochondrial encephalopathy, lactic acidosis, and stroke

See MELAS.

mitochondrial–lipid–glycogen disease of muscle

A spontaneously reversible syndrome of muscle weakness, hypotonia, and hyporeflexia, with hepatomegaly and macroglossia, in infants with evidence of excessive storage of mitochondria, lipids, and glycogen in muscle biopsy specimens.[3211] See **benign infantile mitochondrial myopathy**.

mitochondrial myelomyopathy

(3-M syndrome) A progressive myelopathy described in adult males, with associated myopathy and the usual evidence of excessive storage of mitochondria, lipids, and glycogen in muscle biopsy specimens.[4759]

mitochondrial myopathies

Neurological diseases with maternal inheritance (Chart M–16) in which 4% or more of the fibers in a muscle biopsy specimen show peripheral mitochondrial accumulations (using the Gomori trichrome and succinate dehydrogenase stains)[4479] and with deficiencies in oxidative phosphorylation enzymes, mutations in mitochondrial DNA, elevated resting serum lactate levels, abnormal ^{31}P magnetic resonance spectra of resting muscle, and a lowered anaerobic threshold. (At least three of these features should be present for the diagnosis to be made.)

Three overlapping syndromes have been identified, encompassing the conditions listed in the entries for **mitochondrial-lipid-glycogen disease of muscle, mitochondrial myelomyopathy**, and **mitochondrial peripheral neuropathy**.

1. Ophthalmoplegia and limb weakness (**Kearns–Sayre syndrome**).
2. Proximal weakness and fatigability.
3. **Mitochondrial cytopathy**.

Mitochondrial Myopathies

An information sheet compiled by NINDS (the National Institute of Neurological Disorders and Stroke) accessible at the Web site: http://www.ninds.nih.gov/disorders/mitochondrial_myopathy/mitochondrial_myopathy.htm/.

mitochondrial neurogastrointestinal encephalomyopathy

(MNGIE; congenital oculoskeletal myopathy with

Chart M–16. The Mitochondrial Myopathies

Benign reversible infantile myopathy—cytochrome oxidase deficiency (complex IV deficiency): A syndrome with onset in infancy comprising proximal hypotonia and weakness also affecting the face, macroglossia, and severe lactic acidosis, remitting within the first 2 years of life.

Mitochondrial myopathy—complex I deficiency: A syndrome comprising optic atrophy, neurodegenerative regression, ophthalmoplegia, rigidity, dystonia, proximal and distal myopathic weakness, muscle pain and cramps, fatigability, and cardiomyopathy, and the usual biochemical and biopsy hallmarks of mitochondrial disease. In this category is included **fatal infantile encephalomyopathy**, which is a similar encephalopathy of later onset. **MELAS** and **Alpers disease** are other manifestations of complex 1 deficiency.[4483]

Mitochondrial myopathy—complex III deficiency: A syndrome with onset in childhood or adolescence, comprising myoclonus, pigmentary retinopathy, ptosis, progressive external ophthalmoplegia, nerve deafness, ataxia, pyramidal signs, proximal and distal myopathic weakness, muscle pain and cramps, fatigability, and cardiomyopathy, with the usual biochemical and biopsy hallmarks of mitochondrial disease.[4483]

Mitochondrial myopathy—complex IV deficiency: See **fatal infantile mitochondrial myopathy**.

Mitochondrial myopathy with multiple deletions of mitochondrial DNA: A dominantly inherited form, characterized by progressive external ophthalmoplegia, dysphagia, cataract, lactic acidosis, exercise intolerance, and early death. Ragged red fibers are found on muscle biopsy specimens; muscles also contain diminished amounts of mitochondrial enzymes, and mitochondrial deletions are detected in muscle cells only.[5739]

Mitochondrial myopathy with myotonia: A syndrome with onset in childhood, comprising dwarfism, kyphoscoliosis, high arches of feet, ophthalmoplegia, myopathic muscle atrophy or hypertrophy, myotonia, hypertrophic motor neuropathy, glycogen storage, basal ganglia calcification, and the usual biochemical and biopsy hallmarks of mitochondrial disease.[381]

Mitochondrial myopathy, encephalopathy, lactic acidosis, and stroke: The commonest mitochondrial encephalomyopathy. See **MELAS**.

Mitochondrial myopathy, myoclonic epilepsy, and ragged-red fibers: See **MERRF**.

Respiratory chain complex I deficiency: an underdiagnosed energy generation disorder.[3450]

Further *variant* forms are described as follows:

A form associated with a mild axonal or demyelinating *sensorimotor peripheral neuropathy*.[6914] The onset may be in youth or adult life; the sensory peripheral neuropathy is associated variously with cerebral atrophy, optic atrophy, ophthalmoplegia, proximal neurogenic and myopathic weakness and atrophy, and the usual biochemical and biopsy hallmarks of mitochondrial disease.

A form associated with *cardioskeletal myopathy* and chronic magnesium-losing nephropathy.[5300]

A rare metabolic myopathy presenting in young adult life with *exercise-induced muscle pain*, myoglobinuria, and elevated serum creatine kinase levels, due to a failure of oxidative metabolism involving mitochondrial transport systems.

A form with onset in late adult life, presenting with insidious progressive muscle weakness, often axial and accompanied by fatigability.[3241]

abnormal muscle and liver mitochondria; polyneuropathy, ophthalmoplegia, leukoencephalopathy, intestinal pseudo-obstruction syndrome [POLIP]; oculogastrointestinal muscular dystrophy, mitochondrial encephalomyopathy with sensorimotor polyneuropathy, ophthalmoplegia, and pseudo-obstruction) A rare, recessively inherited mitochondrial syndrome with early childhood onset, due to multiple deletions of mitochondrial DNA (thymidine phosphorylase mutations).

Clinically, it is characterized by progressive external ophthalmoparesis; deafness; ptosis; leukoencephalopathy; recurrent nausea; vomiting or diarrhea with resultant cachexia due to visceral neuropathy; intestinal dysmotility; and peripheral neuropathy. Histologically, abnormal mitochondria are seen in muscle. Serum lactate levels are raised.[6446, 2348]

A variant is *mitochondrial encephalomyopathy with sensorimotor polyneuropathy, ophthalmoplegia, and pseudo-obstruction.*

mitochondrial peripheral neuropathy A syndrome with onset in youth or adult life, comprising optic atrophy, ophthalmoplegia, proximal neurogenic and myopathic weakness and atrophy, sensory peripheral neuropathy, cerebral atrophy, and the usual biochemical and biopsy hallmarks of mitochondrial disease.[381]

mitochondrion An intracellular organelle concerned with the synthesis of ATP from ADP and phosphate by oxidative phosphorylation, the pathway using reducing potential generated by several oxidative systems, in particular the citric acid cycle; and possessing its own DNA.[2806]

mitral valve prolapse with ophthalmoplegia A progressive mitochondrial disease characterized by ataxia, ophthalmoplegia, ptosis, and myopathy, including cardiomyopathy manifested as heart block or mitral valve prolapse with regurgitation. Muscle biopsy specimens show the usual ragged red fibers, or congenital fiber-type disproportion.[1462] The condition is likely to represent a *variant* of **Kearns-Sayre disease**.

mitten hand A hand affected by **syndactyly** of the second through fifth digits.

mixed connective tissue disease An overlap syndrome, with features of **systemic lupus erythematosus, progressive systemic sclerosis,** and **polymyositis**, and characterized by the presence of high titers of speckled-pattern fluorescent antinuclear antibody. Neurological complications occur in half of all cases, and include **aseptic meningitis**, paranoid psychosis, trigeminal neuropathy, peripheral neuropathy, and seizures.[516]

mixed dementia Dementing illnesses for which more than one etiology can be adduced. A diagnosis of mixed dementia should be made when one or more other systemic or brain disorders are present and are thought to be causally related to the dementia. The degree of confidence in the diagnosis of **ischemic vascular dementia** (IVD) should be specified as possible, probable, or definite, and the other disorder(s) contributing to the dementia should be listed—for example, mixed dementia due to probable IVD and possible Alzheimer disease, or mixed dementia due to definite IVD and hypothyroidism.

mixed headache (chronic daily headache) Headache with the characteristics both of **migraine** and of **muscle contraction headaches** and which tend to occur on a near-daily basis in patients with added symptoms of sleep disturbance, depression or anxiety, and a tendency to ingest excessive quantities of analgesic medications.[5545] See also **rebound headache** and **medication overuse headache**.

mixed hypoxia and hypercapnia See **hypercapnic headaches**.

mixed nerve A nerve containing both motor and sensory axons.

Miyoshi myopathy A "congenital" myopathy caused by mutations in the membrane protein *dysferlin*. See also **distal muscular dystrophy**.

A *variant* is sporadic isolated calf atrophy and weakness with onset after age 30 years, associated with only moderately elevated serum CK, presenting with calf and shin muscle wasting before the age of 30 years with a myopathic pattern on EMG, moderately high serum CK levels, and absence of dysferlin with immunohistochemical staining.[3328]

MMM See **minicore-multicore myopathy**.

MNCV Abbreviation for motor nerve conduction velocity.

mnemonic aura Components that reflect ictal dysmnesia such as feelings as familiarity (déjà-vu) and unfamiliarity (jamais-vu).[16]

mnemonist One possessed of an extraordinary capacity for the memorization of data.[3966]

mobile segment The segment between two vertebrae including the intervertebral disk, the articular facets, and all the muscles and ligaments related to them, believed by Maigne to act as a unit so that any pathology affecting one also affects the others.[4029]

mobile spasm "Tonic spasm, slowly varying in relative degree in different muscles, causing slow, irregular movements, chiefly conspicuous in the hand, and slow irregular incoordination . . . A disorder of movement seen after hemiplegia." (Gowers)

Möbius, Paul Julius (Moebius) (1853–1907) German neurologist who graduated in philosophy and then in

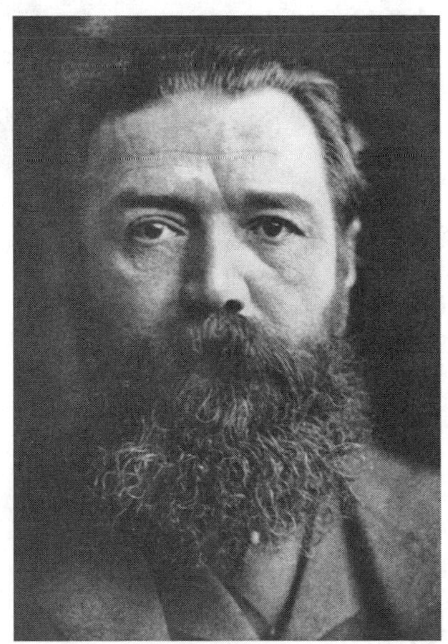

Figure M–4 Paul Julius Möbius.

medicine from Leipzig, and became assistant to Strumpell in Heidelberg. He described ophthalmoplegic migraine in 1884[4420] and the syndrome named for him 4 years later.[4421]

Möbius is also remembered for his differentiation of exogenous and endogenous disease states, but not for his publications on the weak-mindedness of women.[2066]

Möbius sign

The inability to maintain ocular convergence in hyperthyroidism.

Möbius syndrome

1. **ophthalmoplegic migraine**. 2. (congenital facial diplegia, oculofacial paralysis, congenital oculofacial paresis, nuclear agenesis, congenital facial-abducens paralysis, congenital nuclear agenesis/aplasia, congenital facial palsy, congenital bulbar palsy, agenesis of cranial nerve nuclei; OMIM 157900)

A complex regional developmental disorder of the brainstem with absent or impaired facial nerves and possibly an added supranuclear defect.[6537] The major features are congenital aplasia of the VI and VII nerve nuclei, leading to inability to abduct the eyes from the midline, loss of facial movements with dysarthria and drooling, poor eye closure, and resultant exposure keratopathy. Strabismus may result if there are associated III or IV nerve palsies. Malformations of the skeleton or limbs, atrophy of the tongue, micrognathia, weakness of the muscles of mastication and of the soft palate, clubfoot, syndactyly or absence of fingers or toes, aplasia of the sternomastoid and pectoral muscles, and congenital dislocation of the hips may also be found in association,[4421, 2150] as may developmental delay.

Denervation of the spinal musculature due to anterior horn cell lesions and cerebellar and hypothalamic anomalies are also described. The MRI may show medullary hypoplasia and flattening of the floor of the fourth ventricle.[4963]

Möbius first described this syndrome in a 50-year-old man, though the condition is congenital and static in nature. Despite the eponym, the first description was by von **Graefe** in 1880. While the VI nerve palsy is the main cause of the oculomotor disorder, supranuclear influences are also responsible.[6463]

In a progressive *myopathy resembling* **facioscapulohumeral dystrophy**, congenital facial diplegia may be a presenting sign, giving rise to diagnostic confusion.[2739]

Variant forms[4371] include *Möbius syndrome with hypogonadotrophic hypogonadism*;[4791] a form with *hypogonadism* of hypothalamic/pituitary origin and an acute peripheral neuropathy;[39] a form with *absence of the pectoral muscles* (see **Souques syndrome**); and *Levic syndrome* (**progressive nuclear ophthalmoplegia**).[3799] 3. See **akinesia algera**.

modality

A variety of sensation. It was considered by Sinclair (1955) that for every sensation there exists a specific nervous apparatus terminating in a specific type of nerve ending, rather in keeping with Müller's doctrine of the specific irritability of nerves, but today the synthesis of pattern theory and specific irritability has left acceptable only the concept that there is a degree of functional specificity of the receptors.

It is supposed that impulse patterns arising peripherally enable central cells to define the stimulus; the significant characteristics of these patterns depend on such factors as the specificity, adaptation, threshold, and location of the various receptors called into action.[983]

modality-specific anomia

See **anomia**.

modified labials

Those vowels (primarily "O" and "U") which depend for their utterance upon intact lip function. See also **articulated labials** and **dentolabials**.

Modified Mini-Mental State Examination

(3MS) See **Mini-Mental State Examination**.

Modified Motor Assessment Scale

A system for measuring the recovery occurring in patients with stroke, in the areas of movement from the supine position to side lying or to sitting on the side of the bed; balanced sitting; movement from a sitting to a standing position; walking; upper arm function; hand movements; and advanced hand activities.[3894] See also **Barthel index of activities of daily living**.

modified pure motor hemiparesis with "aphasia"

A **lacunar syndrome** with these features, resulting from a thalamic-parathalamic lacune.[2092, 2106]

modified radius reflex

Flexion of the fingers in response to a tap on the radius, occurring in patients with a pyramidal lesion. If the normal elbow flexion response to brachioradialis stretch is also not seen, the presence of a lesion at C5 in the cord is likely (inversion of the radial reflex).

Moebius

See Möbius.

Moebius Syndrome Foundation

A charitable organization in this field. Address: P.O. Box 147, Pilot Grove, MO 65276. E-mail: vmccarrell@mid-mo.net. Web site: http://www.moebiussyndrome/.

Moerman syndrome

A lethal congenital dysmorphic syndrome, characterized by dwarfism; kyphoscoliosis; vertebral and limb anomalies; skeletal, cardiac, pulmonary, and renal anomalies; **Dandy-Walker malformation;** and callosal agenesis.[381]

Moersch-Woltman syndrome

A condition of progressive fluctuating muscular rigidity and spasm described in 1956.[4424] See **stiff person syndrome**.

mogigraphia

(Gr, with painful effort + to write) An old name for **writers cramp**.

mogilalia

The imperfect pronunciation of a single letter such as "G," "K," "L," "R," or "S."

Mohr syndrome

1. See **orofaciodigital syndrome II**. 2. Circumscribed left posterior cerebral artery infarction with right hemianopia and deficits in color perception and memory.[4430]

Mohr-Tranebjaerg syndrome

(deafness-dystonia syndrome) A rare X-linked neurodegenerative deafness syndrome associated with dystonia, myoclonus, and other neurological abnormalities. The clinical course typically involves early-onset sensorineural hearing loss and progressive dystonia in adolescence. Symptoms may include myopia, constricted visual fields, cortical blindness, retinal change, dystonia and mental deficiency, spasticity, cognitive impairment, and psychiatric symptoms. The gene defect is located within the deafness-dystonia peptide (*DDP1*) gene on Xq22.[6370]

molar tooth sign An appearance on MRI scans described in patients with **Joubert syndrome** and some other congenital anomalies in which the brainstem has the shape of a molar tooth. This results from hypoplasia of the cerebellum vermis, distorted superior cerebellar peduncles, and an abnormally deep interpeduncular fossa.[6945]

Mollaret meningitis A recurrent form of aseptic lymphocytic meningitis characterized by marked pleocytosis of the CSF and lasting for a few days. The condition occurs abruptly usually in adults with fever and meningism, who return to normal over a few days but suffer recurrences over years. It was described by Dr. Pierre Mollaret, a French physician, in 1944.[4439] Herpes simplex type II has been incriminated as the causal organism. Diagnostic criteria have been suggested as follows:

1. Recurrent attacks of fever with clinical evidence of meningeal irritation.
2. The attacks last several days, are accompanied by myalgias, and are separated by symptom-free intervals lasting weeks or months.
3. During the attacks, there is CSF pleocytosis, including the presence of numerous polymorphonuclear cells and large mononuclear endothelial cells (Mollaret cells) with irregular nuclear and cytoplasmic membranes; these disappear after 24 h, leaving a CSF picture of lymphocytic meningitis.
4. The disease remits spontaneously.
5. No causative microorganisms have been found. (This may now be incorrect, as herpes simplex virus has been isolated in some cases.)[925]

molluscum fibrosum The subcutaneous papular, nonplexiform neurofibromas in **neurofibromatosis**.

molybd- Latin prefix signifying the metal lead. Thus the terms molybd-amaurosis, -amblyopia, -epilepsia, -ocolic, -oparesis, -spasmus, etc. refer to various symptoms complicating lead poisoning. The name was perhaps bestowed before the discovery of molybdenum, an essential trace element in humans.

molybdenum cofactor deficiency (OMIM 252150) A rare, recessively inherited progressive neurodegenerative disorder caused by a deficiency in sulfite oxidase, which induces severe neuronal loss, astrogliosis, and spongiform encephalopathy.[5513]

Mona Lisa syndrome Contracture of the facial muscles after **Bell palsy**, leaving an enigmatic (half-)smile on the patient's face.[60]

Monakow, Konstantin von (1853–1930) Russian-German neurologist whose noble family emigrated from Russia for political reasons. He trained in Zurich, where he was later appointed professor. He is remembered best for his definition of **diaschisis**, but also showed the connections between the lateral geniculate nuclei and the occipital cortex and isolated two anatomical parts: **Monakow's bundle**, the rubrospinal tract (1909), and **Monakow's nucleus**, the external cuneate fasciculus.

Something of an eccentric, he left instructions in his will that his spinal cord be examined to determine the cause of his chronic **thenar hypoplasia**, but this was not done.[2066]

Monakow syndromes
1. Hemiplegia, hemianesthesia, and hemianopia due to occlusion of the contralateral anterior choroidal artery; Monakow showed that the artery supplies part of the lateral geniculate body and gave some clinical details.[4442] Further descriptions of the anatomy and clinical significance of the artery have been published.[29] 2. Dysmorphic microcephaly, the very large nose and ears being the main facial characteristics. The brain weighed 25 g in the original case, the cerebral and cerebellar hemispheres being almost absent and the pons, thalamus, and hypothalamus also small.[4443]

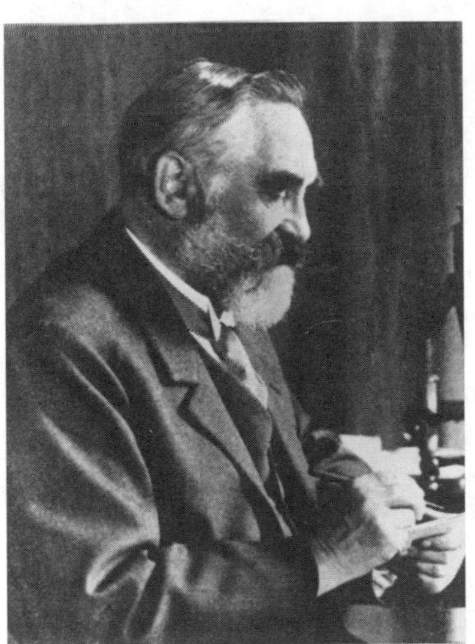

Figure M–5 Konstantin von Monakow.

Monbrun-Benisty syndrome Severe unilateral orbital and cranial pain radiating to the occiput and accompanied by facial vasodilatation, sweating, and hyperesthesia and by lacrimation, without the pathology of sympathetic ophthalmia. The condition follows ocular injury or removal, and the eye pain is considered to be a form of **causalgia**[4444] or, perhaps more likely, a **trigeminal autonomic cephalgia**.

Mondini defect A developmental disorder characterized by deafness, due to aplasia of the bony and membranous labyrinths of the inner ear. It was first described by Dr. C. Mondini, an Italian anatomist, in 1791 but more fully in 1972.[4888] The congenital deformity of the bony labyrinth can be linked to a fistulous tract communicating it with the intracranial subarachnoid with the risk of recurrent bacterial meningitis.[6515]

Mondonesi reflex See **bulbomimic reflex**.

Monge disease See **mountain sickness** and **high-altitude headache**.

mongolism See **Down syndrome**.

Moniz, Antonio Caetano de Egas (1874–1955) Portuguese neurosurgeon, sexologist, gambler, biographer, parliamentarian and diplomat, professor of neurosurgery, and sometime dean of medicine at Lisbon, who introduced arteriography in 1927, using 25% sodium iodide.[1815] and prefrontal leucotomy in 1936.[1816] He won the Nobel Prize in 1949, oddly enough for the latter, which is the less useful of the two procedures.

Moniz reflex A variant method of eliciting the Babinski response, the stimulus being passive ankle plantar flexion.

monoamine oxidase inhibitors Drugs that inhibit the enzymes responsible for breaking down serotonin, monoamines and norepinephrine in the body. See also **serotonin syndrome**.

monochromatopsia The tinting of all perceptions with a specific color—yellow in digitalis poisoning, for example; perhaps rose in euphoria?

monoclonal gammopathy of uncertain significance (MGUS)

A generally benign monoclonal gammopathy (IgG, IgA, IgD, IgM) frequently associated with sensory or motor neuropathy.[2395, 3374] The IgG-MGUS and IgM-MGUS conditions differ, in that an insidious course, raised CSF protein level, more sensory loss, slower nerve conduction velocities, and antimyelin-associated glycoprotein (anti-MAG) antibodies are found in the latter, which is also the more common of the two. In the IgG form, weakness is the predominant feature.

In the motor form, the weakness is predominantly distal, asymmetric, and slowly progressive. Conduction block is not present.[4995]

Criteria for the diagnosis of MGUS (as opposed to multiple myeloma) have been suggested:[3624]

A. Monoclonal serum protein, <2 g/l.
B. Normal serum albumin levels
C. Marrow plasma cells, <5%
D. Absence of bone lesions, anemia, and monoclonal urine protein
E. Observation shows no change over 3 years.

See **dysglobulinemic neuropathy** .

Criteria for demyelinating polyneuropathy associated with MGUS have also been suggested. (See Chart M–17) See also **multiple myeloma** and **POEMS Syndrome**.

monocular (from Lat, relating to one eye)

monocular diplopia (uniocular diplopia) See **diplopia**.

monocular elevation failure A deficit in up-gaze in one eye, despite the supranuclear level of the causative lesion.[3793]

monocular "fixation" nystagmus See **latent nystagmus.**

Chart M–17. Criteria for demyelinating polyneuropathy associated with MGUS.[4712]

A causal relation between demyelinating polyneuropathy and MGUS should be considered in a patient with:

1. Demyelinating polyneuropathy according to the electrodiagnostic MN criteria for idiopathic CIDP
2. Presence of an M protein (IgM, IgG, or IgA), without evidence of malignant plasma cell dyscrasias-like multiple myeloma, lymphoma, Waldenstrom macroglobulinemia, or amyloidosis
3. Family history negative for neuropathy
4. Age >30 years.

The relation is *definite* when the following is present:

1. IgM M protein with anti-MAG antibodies

The relation is *probable* when at least three of the following are present in a patient without anti-MAG antibodies:

1. Time to peak of the neuropathy >2 years
2. Chronic slowly progressive course without relapsing or remitting periods
3. Symmetrical distal polyneuropathy
4. Sensory symptoms and signs predominate over motor features.

A causal relation is *unlikely* when at least three of the following are present in a patient without anti-MAG antibodies:

1. Median time to peak of the neuropathy is within 1 year
2. Clinical course is relapsing and remitting or monophasic
3. Cranial nerves are involved
4. Neuropathy is asymmetrical
5. Motor symptoms and signs predominate
6. History of preceding infection
7. Presence of abnormal median SNAP in combination with normal sural SNAP.

After Notermans NC, Fransses H, Eurelings M, et al. Diagnostic criteria for demyelinating plyneuropathy associated with monoclonal gammopathy. Muscle Nerve 2000;23:73–9. *Reproduced by kind permission of John Wiley and Sons. Inc.*

monocular nystagmus An unusual dissociated motor ocular sign in which involuntary oscillations of only one eye in any direction(s) are present in the primary position of the gaze. In the presence of visual loss, the nystagmus is pendular in the affected eye. It has been reported in numerous neurological conditions and is not a localizing sign.[3142]

monogenic neuromuscular disorders A user-friendly gene table of the monogenic neuromuscular disorders (nuclear genome only); an interactive site linked to major databases and regularly updated between the appearances of printed versions.[17] The data are freely available online at http://www.musclegenetable.org and http://194.167.35.195/, a site devised, developed, and maintained by Dalil Hamroun and Christophe Béroud at the Institut Universitaire de Recherche Clinique (IURC) 34093 Montpellier Cedex 5, France. E-mail: hamroun@igh. cnrs.fr.

monogenic Parkinsonism Forms of Parkinson disease induced by any of several PARK genes, including parkin, PINK-1, LRRK2, ATP13A2 (PARK9), and Omi/HtrA2 (PARK13), all of which are enzymes involved in normal protein and mitochondrial function.

monomania A form of mental illness in which the subject is irrational on one subject only, appearing quite normal in other areas of mental activity.

monomelic amyotrophy (benign focal amyotrophy; benign focal atrophy; benign juvenile focal muscular atrophy of upper extremities; benign monomelic amyotrophy; distal amyotrophy of predominantly the upper limbs; focal cervical poliopathy of distal upper extremity causing juvenile muscular atrophy; juvenile amyotrophy of distal upper extremity; juvenile distal spinal muscular atrophy of upper extremities; juvenile muscular atrophy of the upper extremity; juvenile nonprogressive muscular atrophy localized in hand and forearm; juvenile segmental muscular atrophy; juvenile type of distal and segmental atrophy of upper extremities; monomelic atrophy; monomelic spinal muscular atrophy; nonfamilial juvenile central neurogenic muscular atrophy; nonfamilial juvenile distal spinal muscular atrophy of the upper extremity; nonfamilial spinal segmental muscular atrophy in juvenile and young subjects; spinal monomelic amyotrophy; unilateral juvenile muscular atrophy of the upper limbs) A rare sporadic lower motor neuron syndrome affecting the arms only, presenting as asymmetric, painless atrophy, and weakness of the distal upper limbs of young oriental adults, seldom accompanied by pyramidal signs.[1688] The occurrence of this condition and the next listed mainly in oriental males suggests that they may be identical with each other and with **Hirayama disease.** See also **lower motor neuron disease**.

monomelic atrophy (benign focal amyotrophy, monomelic spinal muscular atrophy) A sporadic syndrome of progressive wasting of a limb, usually the arm, with evidence of spinal cord atrophy at the appropriate levels and with clinical and electrical evidence of chronic anterior horn cell disease. Most often reported from the Orient, the condition usually affects young men and is benign and after a year or two, becoming nonprogressive.[2524] See **Hirayama disease** and **monomelic amyotrophy**.

monomelic myopathy A rare congenital syndrome characterized by hypertrophy of muscle and bone, confined to a single extremity.[1068] Percussion myotonia may also be detectable.

monomelic myositis A form of **polymyositis** in which the weakness and atrophy are confined to a single limb.

monomelic spinal muscular atrophy See **monomelic amyotrophy**.

monomyositis Eosinophilic infiltration and painful inflammation of one muscle or a part of one muscle.

mononeuritis multiplex See **multiple mononeuropathy**.

monophasia An extreme degree of loss of expressive language due to localized brain disease, whereby the patient is unable to emit anything more than extremely few stereotyped utterances, either verbal or nonverbal, despite insight into the occurrence of the problem.[1336] See **stereotypy**.

monophasic wave An EEG waveform developed on one side of the baseline only.

monoplegia (Gr, one + a stroke) 1. Paralysis of one muscle or of a group of muscles only. 2. Paralysis of a single limb. The latter is the preferred usage today. Brachial (arm), crural (leg), and faciolingual forms are seen and are "more common in disease of the cortex." (Sir William **Gowers**) Crural monoplegia also occurs with thoracic or lumbar cord disease, but any peripheral lesion can cause monoplegia.

monoplegia anesthetica See **Morvan disease**.

monoplegia masticatoria Unilateral weakness of the muscles supplied by the trigeminal nerve, usually without accompanying sensory changes.[5980]

monopolar needle recording electrode A solid wire, usually made of stainless steel and coated with an insulating material except at its tip. Variations in the voltage between the tip of the needle (the active electrode) positioned in a muscle and a reference electrode on the skin surface or in subcutaneous tissue are measured (*monopolar needle electrode recording*).[19]

monotherapy The philosophy that one medication is better than two for treating a single complaint. Though not always achievable, this is accepted as desirable in the management of epilepsy, but not necessarily in that of other conditions.

Monrad-Krohn, Georg Herman (1884–1964) Norwegian neurologist from Bergen who trained in Oslo and thereafter at the National Hospital and the Salpêtrière before returning to Oslo as physician to the neurological clinic and then professor of neurology. His book *Clinical Examination of the Nervous System* (London, 1921) quickly became the classic in many translations, by which he is better remembered even than for his clinical research publications on leprosy, facial palsies, and aphasia.

Monrad-Krohn sign Paradoxical emotional hypermimia occurring in bilateral upper motor neuron facial weakness, regarded as a release from some normal suppression—the phenomenon of liberation—by Monrad-Krohn in 1924.

Monro, Alexander (*primum*; 1697–1767) Professor of anatomy at Edinburgh. He first noted that the nerves of the body were ". . . composed of small parallel threads."

Monro, Alexander (*secundum*; 1733–1817) Scottish anatomist, holding the chair at Edinburgh in succession to his father of the same name. He first described the interventricular foramen in 1753; his son (also Alexander, and thus known as *tertius*, and also subsequently professor of anatomy at Edinburgh) wrote in his *Elements of the Anatomy of the Human Body* (Vol. 2, p. 363) "Hence at this place the lateral ventricles of the brain communicate with each other, and with the third ventricle. This aperture has been very particularly described by my Father in his work in the Nervous System."

Of this Monro, the third of the line (1773–1859), it is said[5886] that he contributed little that was new himself, but relied extensively upon the notes of his grandfather, even including such statements as "When I was a student at Leyden in 1719."

Monro-Kellie hypothesis Since the brain is incompressible and the cranial cavity inelastic, compensation for an increase in the volume of any one of the intracranial contents must be attained through diminution in the volume of the others. This insight was first expressed in 1783 but was repeated by Kellie in 1824.

monstrocellular sarcoma (giant cell fibrosarcoma) See **glioma**.

montage The particular arrangement or pattern of placement of electrodes on the scalp, allowing the simultaneous display of potential changes at numerous sites on the EEG record.

Monte Cristo syndrome See **locked-in syndrome**.

Montgomery-Asberg Depression Rating Scale A 10-item rating scale assessing the features of depression, shown to have high validity and an ability to demonstrate changes in depressive symptomatology.[4454]

Montreal Cognitive Assessment A brief screening tool for **mild cognitive impairment**.[4596]

Mood Assessment Scale See Geriatric Depression Scale.

Mood Scales—Elderly A set of 50 adjectives referring to five factors (tense-irritable, considerate, cognitive disturbance, inept helpless, depressed) to be rated by the caregivers of elderly subjects.[5201]

Moon molars Mulberry-shaped molar teeth, seen in patients with congenital syphilis, described by H. Moon (1845–1892), a dental surgeon at Guy's Hospital in London.

Moore, M.T. (b. 1901) American neuropsychiatrist, professor at the University of Pennsylvania.

Moore, Robert Foster (b. 1878) London ophthalmologist who described the **pseudo-Argyll Robertson pupil** in 1924.[4461]

Moore lightning streaks Flashes of light (phosphenes) perceived by normal patients with eye closure when brief pressure is exerted on the globe and occasionally perceived by those with intraocular pathology. They are named for R.F. **Moore**. See **lightning streaks**.

Moore syndrome Abdominal pain as a manifestation of a seizure. The recurrent attacks of abdominal pain occur in children and young adults and are associated with abnormal EEG changes and occasionally are followed by generalized tonic-clonic convulsions.[4459] They are named for M.T. **Moore**. See **abdominal epilepsy**.

morbid (Lat, sickly) Of or belonging to disease; unhealthy.

morbid hunger (bulimia) Excessive appetite with decreased satiety after eating.

morbidity Predisposition to disease.

morbific Causing disease.

morbus (Lat, disease) A sickness. Hence a large number of alternative names for certain diseases such as *morbus celsi* (catalepsy); *M. aphrodisius, gallicus, hispanicus, and indicus* for syphilis; *M. astralis, attonitus, caducus, comitialis, convivialis, daemonicus, deificus, divinus, foedus, herculeus, infantilis, insputatus, interlunis, lunaticus, magnus, major, mensalis, popularis, puerilis, sacer, sancti johannes or valentini, sclestus, seleniacus, viridellus, and vitriolatus* for epilepsy; *M. cerebralis whytii* (meningitis); and *M. gesticulatorius, lascicus, and saltatorius* for chorea.

Such names allow a measure of understanding of ancient views of the disease in question. In the case of epilepsy one may understand from the above that it is a frightful disease, has major and minor forms, occurs in children and in company, leads to stunning of the mind, and to falling to the ground with strong movements, is influenced by God, the gods or devils and by that lesser light, the moon (at least when it recurs regularly on a monthly cycle); breaks up a meeting by its occurrence and leads others to spit upon the sufferer.

morbus gallicorum (Lat, the French disease) Syphilis. So-called by those other than the French, who regarded it as an English disease.

morbus medicorum The disease of patients who "seek advice from many physicians, trusting those who pander to their apprehensions . . . For the best chance of recovery, [they] should keep away from doctors." (Gowers) The dangers of the condition include susceptibility to **Ulysses syndrome**.

morbus sacer (Lat, disease + holy) The term of Linnaeus for a disorder involving continuous distortion of the limbs without affection of the mind. It is probably the same as the mobile spasms described by **Hammond**, and thus **athetosis**.

Morel, Benedict Augustin (1809–1873) Austrian-French psychiatrist who trained at the **Salpêtrière** and practiced in northeastern France. He introduced the terms *dementia praecox* (which was later popularized by Kraepelin) and *obsession*, and published widely on psychiatric disorders and their history and on forensic psychiatry.[6407]

Morel, Ferdinand (1868–1957) Swiss psychiatrist, born in Geneva, who trained in medicine in Paris after early studies in philosophy. He trained under **Charcot** and returned to graduate in Geneva, where he remained for most of the rest of his life, becoming professor of psychiatry and director of Bel Air psychiatric hospital in 1938.

Morel disease (alcoholic laminar cortical sclerosis) Symmetrical neuroglial proliferation in the third cortical layer occurring in alcoholics, mainly in the frontal regions, and combined with generalized astrocytic hyperplasia. Clinically, the syndrome comprises dementia, dysarthria, weakness, gait disturbance, and tremor.[4471]

Morel-Stewart-Morgagni syndrome (metabolic craniopathy) Frontal hyperostosis, obesity, hirsutism, hypertension, amenorrhea, diabetes mellitus and insipidus, headache, vertigo, lethargy, somnolence, seizures, and psychiatric manifestations, occurring in adult women.[4470] The condition was originally considered to be due to a diencephalic lesion, but its identity is now in question, the association of any endocrinopathy with the skull changes being at best suspect. See **hyperostosis frontalis interna**.

Morel-Wildi syndrome Asymptomatic disseminated nodular dysgenesis of the frontal cortex, manifest as small, pearl-like prominences.[4472]

Moreno syndrome A congenital dysmorphic syndrome characterized also by gigantism, high birth weight, tall stature, advanced skeletal maturation, epiphyseal dysplasia, micrognathia, scoliosis, brachydactyly, joint contractures, macrocephaly, early closure of the fontanelles, ridged cranial sutures, ossification defects of the skull, umbilical hernia, spasticity, wide metaphysis, and cutis laxa.[381]

Morgagni, Giovanni Battista (1682–1771) Italian physician born in Forli (Bologna) who was a pathological anatomist and professor at Padua. He was the first to give an account of **subarachnoid hemorrhage** and to note that hydrocephalus in children (but not in adults) caused enlargement of the head. He described cerebral gummas, aneurysm of the aorta, and heart block, and was the first to show that the cerebral lesion in apoplexy resulted in contralateral paralysis. His book *De sedibus et causis morborum per anatomen indagatis* published in 1761[4475] was started when he was 79. In it he applied the anatomical method to achieve disease localization, based on over 600 autopsies.

Morgagni-Stewart-Morel syndrome See **hyperostosis frontalis interna**.

Morgagni syndrome See **hyperostosis frontalis interna**.

moria (Gr, silliness) Naïve childish excitement, a behavioral pattern sometimes seen with prefrontal-lobe lesions.

Morin's pathway An ascending pathway in the dorsomedial portion of the lateral funiculus of the cat, relaying in the dorsal horn and lateral cervical nucleus before crossing to join the medial lemniscus. Ascending fibers probably take a similar route in humans and may have a role in the perception of vibratory stimuli.[983]

morning/evening comparison test A simple test for the diagnosis of **myasthenia gravis** which involves measuring the difference in the width of the palpebral fissures between morning and night.[5616]

morning glory syndrome A dysmorphism of the optic disk, characterized by a deep funnel-shaped pit surrounded by heaped-up glial tissue, the retinal vessels radiating out in all directions. The anomaly is associated with enlargement of the blind spot, but other visual disturbances may not be present.[3436] The name springs from a fanciful resemblance to the shape of the flower.

morning paralysis See **poliomyelitis**.

morning sleepiness See **delayed sleep phase syndrome**.

Moro, E. (1874–1951) Austrian pediatrician who described the reflex named for him in 1918.

Moro reflex (embrace reflex, body startle reflex) Abduction and extension of the arms and opening of the hands followed by adduction of the arms, in response to sudden withdrawal of support from the head of the normal baby (aged <3–4 months) held up at 45°, the head being allowed to fall back for an inch or two. This is also elicited by any sudden stimulus, such as a loud noise, sudden displacement of the body of the infant or a blow to the bed on which the infant lies.[6898] The reflex can be elicited after 30 weeks of gestation and is normally lost by 5 months of age.

The reflex is inhibited in hypertonic states and asymmetrical in hemiplegia and with local disease of the arms.[4909] See also **developmental reflexes**.

moron (from Gr, sluggish) A term selected by **Binet** for that class of the intellectually deprived with a mental age of 0–2 years.

morphea (localized scleroderma) A slowly progressive atrophic inflammatory process, pathologically resembling **eosinophilic fasciitis** but without the eosinophils and involving a localized area of skin and subjacent tissues. Such focal scleroderma may rarely affect the brain, resulting in focal deficits and perhaps partial seizures.

In some cases, it leads to facial, limb, or generalized hemiatrophy.[5681]

morpheme The smallest meaningful unit of language, which occurs either as a word or part of a word.

Thus, *troubleshooting* contains three morphemes: trouble-, shoot-, and -ing. The acceptable use of words depends upon the morphemes they contain. Morphemes may be appended to words; for example, verb endings, *-ed*, *-ing*; noun modifiers, *-es*, *-s*; adverb endings, *-ly*; and adjective modifiers, *-er*, *-est*.[3949]

morphology The morphemes contained in a language and the system of rules followed by speakers when combining morphemes into phrases.[3949]

morphosynthesis The physiological process underlying the perception of both visual and tactile form, making possible accurate localization in space.

Morquio, Luis (1867–1935) Uruguayan professor of pediatrics at Montevideo, who also trained in Paris in neurology with **Charcot**.

Morquio disease See **mucopolysaccharidosis type 4**.

Morquio-Brailsford syndrome See **mucopolysaccharidosis type 4**.

de Morsier syndromes 1. A syndrome comprising mental fatigability, memory disturbances, hallucinations, disorders of perception, hyperosmia and hyperacusis, and gait disturbances, considered by de Morsier to result from damage to the hypothalamus, but not now known to have any specific pathology.[1509] See **posttraumatic syndrome**. 2. See **sensorimotor psychological syndrome**.[1511] 3. (olfacto-genital dysplasia) A congenital dysmorphic syndrome manifesting also agenesis of the olfactory lobe and corpus callosum, and eunuchoidism.[1510]

Morton, Thomas (1835–1903) American surgeon who trained at Pennsylvania and, after further training there, became a member of its staff as well as of other hospitals in the region, some of which he had helped to found. He was the first to ligate the common carotid artery (for the treatment of orbital aneurysm) in 1864.

Morton metatarsalgia (interdigital neuralgia) A syndrome of constant aching pain with lancinations felt in the sole of the foot and due to compression of a digital neuroma by the heads of the 2nd/3rd or the 3rd/4th metatarsals.

The syndrome usually occurs in older women, mainly while standing or walking, and can be relieved surgically.[4503]

Morvan, Augustin-Marie (1819–1897) French physician in Brittany, whose writings were praised by **Charcot**. He is remembered for the two conditions named for him, but produced nothing else remembered in medicine, perhaps because as a fervid republican his life was greatly occupied in the management of current political and social problems.

Morvan chorea (fibrillary chorea, chorea fibrillaris) A disorder of very uncertain provenance, first described by Morvan in 1890 as the combination of fibrillary chorea of the calf and other leg muscles (**myokymia** or **neuromyotonia**) with shooting pains, hyperhidrosis, albuminuria, and encephalopathy with delirium, terminating fatally in one patient with severe insomnia that later led to delirium and coma.[4506] Cramps, weakness, and pruritis have also been recorded as part of the syndrome. Most patients have an underlying thymoma, but the condition has also been associated with carcinoma, autoimmune diseases, and the presence of voltage-gated, potassium channel antibodies.

S. A. K. **Wilson** was confident that it was "neither chorea nor myoclonus" and regarded it as "a meaningless term except as synonymous for flickering contractures of muscles." The condition went unremarked for 40 years after Morvan's publication until **Mollaret** described another case in 1930 (*Rev Neurol* 2:552). See also **myokymia** and **Isaacs syndrome**.

In *variant* forms, the condition exists in association with a rare brain disease (**agrypnia**) which is characterized by total abolition of the ability to sleep;[2072, 2073] or is associated with a myasthenia-like syndrome as a paraneoplastic manifestation of a thymoma.[3745]

Morvan disease (monoplegia anesthetica) Dissociated analgesia with severe trophic changes and paralysis of the limbs (usually the arms). The sense of touch may be retained but pain and temperature sensations are much affected and may be entirely lost.

Regarded as synonymous with **syringomyelia** during the first half of the last century, this disease could equally well have been a form of **hereditary sensory and autonomic neuropathy**, perhaps type 2, as the losses of pain and of common sensation distally (mutilating acropathy) occur in both conditions.[4505]

Moschowitz disease (thrombotic thrombocytopenic purpura, thrombotic microangiopathy) A rare, acute, and often lethal systemic autoimmune vasculopathy with widespread effects, such as fever, purpura, thrombocytopenia, and hemolytic anemia. In the nervous system, the main features are delirium, various focal neurological signs, and seizures.[4508]

MOSES See **Multidimensional Observation Scale For Elderly Subjects**.

Moskowskij sign Right-sided mydriasis in patients with acute appendicitis or other abdominal sepsis. Why this should occur (if it is indeed confirmed) is not known.

Mosso, Angelo (1846–1910) Italian physiologist.

Mosso's ergometer An early device for measuring muscle force in fatigable and other states. Mosso also remarked in 1884 on a patient whose symptoms suggest **paroxysmal choreoathetosis**.

moth-eaten fibers The biopsy appearance of myofibrils (especially those of type 1) in which the normally regular myofibrillary network seen in the oxidative enzyme preparation is disturbed, giving rise to a whorled appearance and lack of reactivity to NADH as a result of a loss of mitochondria. The change is not specific but is commonest in inflammatory myopathies. The significance of this finding is that of **cores**, of which it may represent a stage in development.[6158]

motility (from Lat, movement) The power of movement or of contractility.

motion sickness Nausea and vomiting induced by unfamiliar bodily accelerations or intersensory mismatch during passive locomotion in vehicles, and reduced or inhibited by visual perception of a static environment.[819]

motivation A force based upon personality, reflexes, and the totality of individual experience, inclining one toward a course of action.

motor (Lat, a mover) Giving, imparting, or producing movement.

Motor Activity log-28 An instrument assessing the spontaneous use of a hemiparetic arm outside the treatment setting.[6455]

motor agrammatism The term of Goldstein for the speech in motor aphasia, with suppression of the "little tools of language" such as articles, pronouns, and connectors, such that speech is ultimately reduced to nouns, infinitives, and names.

motor and sensory demyelinating mononeuropathy multiplex, See **multifocal inflammatory demyelinating neuropathy**.

motor and sensory neuropathy, dementia, and dysautonomia A rare autosomal recessive syndrome with adult onset, also marked by pigmentary retinal degeneration, described in a single family.[4845]

motor aphasia See **aphasia**.

motor apraxia See **apraxia**.

motor aprosodia A condition characterized by the loss of melody in vocal output with an associated decrease in the use of gesture. The monotonous verbal output lacks emotional quality. The underlying lesion is of the right inferior motor cortex. See **aprosodia**.

motor area See **motor cortex**.

motor asynergy (Lat, motor + Gr, not affording assistance) Ataxia.

motor block See **freezing**.

motor centers Those areas of the cortex which, when stimulated, produce coordinated movement of a limb.

motor cortex (motor area, precentral area, Brodman's area 4, area giganto-pyramidalis) An arbitrary term for that part of the precentral convolution lying adjacent to the fissure of Rolando, in which are found the giant cells of Betz. The anterior border is ill-defined, and its functions and those of the **premotor cortex** overlap or may even be the same except that damage to this area leads to contralateral hemiparesis and later to hyperreflexia and hypertonia.

motor cortex seizures Epilepsies which are mainly characterized by simple partial seizures, their localization depending on the side and topography of the area involved. In the case of seizures involving the lower pre-Rolandic area, there may be speech arrest, vocalization or dysphasia, tonic-clonic movements of the face on the contralateral side, or swallowing. Generalization of the seizure frequently occurs.

In the Rolandic area, partial motor seizures without march or Jacksonian seizures occur, particularly beginning in the contralateral upper extremities. In the case of seizures involving the paracentral lobule, tonic movements of the ipsilateral foot may occur as well as the expected contralateral leg movements. Postictal or **Todd paralysis** is frequent. (From Dreifuss FE, et al. Commission for classification and terminology, ILAE. Proposal for revised classifications of epilepsies and epileptic syndromes. *Epilepsia* 1989;**30**:389–99 by kind permission of the ILAE and Wiley-Blackwell Publications.)

motor end plate A specialized area on the surface of the myofibril where it is unusually responsive to depolarization by packets of acetylcholine arriving from the motor nerve terminal.

motor end point (motor point) The site where a motor nerve enters a muscle, which is also the point over a muscle where its contraction may be elicited by a minimal-intensity, short-duration electric stimulus. These sites were first noted and defined by **Remak** and have recently regained prominence because they are the regions where injections of botulinum toxin are most effectively placed in order to alleviate unwanted muscle contractions.

motor-evoked potentials The electrical events accompanying muscle contraction recorded by electrodes placed over or within the muscle in question and best assessed following magnetic stimulation of the motor cortex.

The magnetic stimulation technique may one day be found useful in monitoring spinal cord function in the awake patient, but the potentials are lost during anesthesia.

motor extinction Inhibition of activity in one limb during voluntary movement in the other.[6672]

Motor Function Measurement Scale A reliable scale in neuromuscular diseases comprising 32 items to do with standing position and transfers, axial and proximal motor function, and distal motor function. It does not require any special equipment and is well-accepted by patients.[4945]

motor hyperactivity Excessive involuntary muscle contraction as a result of lesions of the central or peripheral nervous systems. Its causes include **spasticity; stiff man syndrome**, which is probably an autoimmune syndrome due to the presence of antibodies to alpha-glutamic acid dehydrogenase, leading to a decrease in the amount of gamma aminobutyric acid present; **tetanus**, in which condition the toxin reduces levels of glycine/gamma aminobutyric acid; **segmental myoclonus;** and increased motor neuron excitability, as with **fasciculations**, **myokymia**, and **neuromyotonia**.

motor impersistence (global inattention) A term introduced by Miller Fisher[2078] to describe an inability to sustain simple acts such as conjugate gaze, tongue protrusion, mouth opening, or the exertion of steady manual grip pressure, all in the absence of a detectable motor deficit. The sign suggests right hemispheric damage.[3406] Compare with **perseveration**.

motor inattention See **inattention**.

motor latency The interval between the application of a stimulus and the onset of the resultant compound muscle action potential (M-wave). The term may be qualified as either *proximal* or *distal,* depending upon the relative position of the stimulus.[162]

motor negativism A consistent increase in resistance to the passive stretch of a muscle, occurring bilaterally as a sign of diffuse cerebral dysfunction and unilaterally as a result of a focal lesion of the contralateral hemisphere. See **paratonia**.

motor nerve conduction velocity The speed of conduction of the nerve impulse down a motor nerve (varying normally in different nerves between 45 and 55 m/s), first measured by von **Helmholtz** in 1850.

motor nerve involvement syndrome A congenital storage disorder manifesting osteoporosis, lytic lesions of bone, demyelinating motor neuropathy, and inclusions on nerve or rectal biopsy specimens.[381]

motor neuron A neuron with its cell body in the anterior horn of the spinal cord, its single axon passing out in the anterior root to innervate the myofibrils within that **motor unit**.

motor neuron disease See **amyotrophic lateral sclerosis**.

motor neuron disease with dementia A disorder resembling **frontotemporal dementia** with added features of **amyotrophic lateral sclerosis**.

motor neuronal diseases Disorders primarily affecting the anterior horn cells, the motor roots or the motor nerves of the body, cranial or spinal. The classification in Chart M–18 is based upon that of the World Federation of Neurology.[6869] See also **radiculopathy** (*disorders of motor nerve roots);* **neuropathy** (*disorders of peripheral nerve*); **neuromuscular transmission disorders;** and **myopathy** (*disorders of muscle*). The term has also been used to include disorders with upper motor neuron involvement.[1681]

motor neuronopathy A disorder of the anterior horn cells and/or of the cranial nerve motor nuclei, as in **amyotrophic lateral sclerosis**, some dysimmune polyneuropathies, **paraneoplastic syndromes, diabetic amyotrophy, porphyria**, postradiation neuropathies, and **lead poisoning**. Cf. **multifocal motor neuropathy with conduction block**.

motor neuronopathy predominantly affecting the hands A dominantly inherited condition mapped to gene 7p (but heterogeneous) with the onset in youth of asymmetric distal weakness and wasting of the hands more than of the feet in the absence of sensory disturbances or of pyramidal signs.

motor neuropathy predominantly affecting the arms A neuropathy with onset in childhood, characterized by neurogenic brachial muscle atrophy and weakness. See also **hereditary motor neuropathy, amyotrophic lateral sclerosis**.

motor paralytic bladder A dilated and flaccid bladder resulting from detrusor weakness and lack of tone due to damage to its motor nerve supply, as in lesions of the conus medullaris or severe autonomic neuropathy. As a result, the bladder stretch reflex fails and it becomes a large urine-containing sac with dribbling incontinence resulting.

motor persistence The ability to sustain motor activity, diminished in patients with an attention deficit-hyperactivity disorder.

motor persistence of the OO muscles Prolonged activity of the orbicularis oculi muscles, causing **apraxia of lid opening**.[6367]

motor point See **motor end point**.

Chart M–18. Spinal Muscular Atrophies and Other Disorders of Motor Neurons

A1. Autosomal recessive, biochemical abnormality unknown

1. Spinal muscular atrophy type 1. **Hereditary motor neuropathy, type 1** (Werdnig-Hoffman).
2. Spinal muscular atrophy type 2. **Hereditary motor neuropathy, type 2** (Kugelberg-Welander).
3. Spinal muscular atrophy type 3. **Hereditary motor neuropathy, type 3** (Kugelberg-Welander).
4. Proximal spinal muscular atrophy of adults, indistinguishable from recessive and X-linked forms. (**Hereditary motor neuropathy, type 4**)
5. Scapuloperoneal muscular atrophy. See **hereditary motor neuropathy**
6. (Distal) spinal muscular atrophy of childhood. See **hereditary motor and sensory neuropathy, type 2**
7. **(Distal) spinal muscular atrophy** (of adults). See **hereditary motor neuropathy** (*variants*)
8. Spinal muscular atrophy with microcephaly and mental retardation
9. Spinal muscular atrophy, **Ryukyuan** type
10. Progressive muscular atrophy with chorea and optic atrophy
11. **Arthrogryposis multiplex congenita** neurogenic type
12. **Arthrogryposis multiplex congenita** with pulmonary hypoplasia
13. Multiple contracture syndrome, Finnish type; see **Pena–Shokier phenotypes**
14. **Kuskokwim disease** (arthrogryposis-like disorder)
15. Charcot–Marie–Tooth disease, progressive ataxia and tremor. See **hereditary motor and sensory neuropathy, type 2**
16. Charcot–Marie–Tooth disease (same as 15?)
17. Progressive bulbar palsy of childhood. See **Fazio–Londe disease**
18. Progressive bulbar palsy with deafness. See **progressive bulbar palsy** (*Vialetto–van Laere syndrome*)
19. Bulbar palsy, with deafness and retinitis pigmentosa
20. Bulbar palsy with olivopontocerebellar atrophy. See **cerebellar ataxias** (unknown etiology and late onset)
21. Spinal muscular atrophy with amyotrophic lateral sclerosis, spinocerebellar ataxia and deafness. See **amyotrophic lateral sclerosis**
22. Spinal muscular atrophy with optic atrophy and deafness
23. Spinal muscular atrophy with deafness
24. Spinal muscular atrophy with ophthalmoplegia
25. Spinal muscular atrophy with retinitis pigmentosa
26. Spinal muscular atrophy with retinitis pigmentosa and **hereditary spastic paraplegia**
27. Troyer syndrome. See **hereditary spastic paraplegia**
28. Spinal muscular atrophy and mental retardation. See **hereditary motor neuropathy** (*variants*)
29. Spinal muscular atrophy, mental retardation, seizures, and orofacial dysplasia
30. Spinal muscular atrophy, restricted forms (e.g., one or both hands or quadriceps)
31. Spinal muscular atrophy with recessive spinocerebellar degeneration or **Friedreich ataxia**
32. Spinal muscular atrophy with spastic paraplegia, mental retardation, and ichthyosis. See **Sjögren–Larsson syndrome**
33. **Neuronal intranuclear hyaline inclusion disease** (single sporadic case, manifest by amyotrophy, dementia, choreoathetosis, seizures, and sphincter disorder)
34. Spinal muscular atrophy or axonal neuropathy in **xeroderma pigmentosum** (spinal cord may be found abnormal at autopsy)
35. Spinal muscular atrophy in **infantile neuroaxonal dystrophy**
36. Spinal muscular atrophy in **NBIA**
37. Spinal muscular atrophy in amyotrophic **choreoacanthocytosis**

A2. Autosomal recessive, biochemical abnormality known

1. Spinal muscular atrophy with hexosaminidase deficiency. See **GM_2 gangliosidosis**
2. Spinal muscular atrophy with lysosomal enzyme deficiencies
3. Spinal muscular atrophy with **phenylketonuria**
4. Spinal muscular atrophy with **hydroxyisovaleric aciduria**

A3. Autosomal dominant, biochemical abnormality unknown

1. Spinal muscular atrophy, ataxia, retinitis pigmentosa, and diabetes mellitus
2. Spinal muscular atrophy, juvenile, proximal type (usually autosomal recessive, but dominant forms are reported) (Tsukagoshi)
   Variants include the **monomelic** form, which is usually sporadic and spinal muscular atrophy of **facioscapulohumeral distribution**
3. **Progressive muscular atrophy with malignant course**, a form which is fatal within 1 year, but which is not clearly different from autosomal dominant **amyotrophic lateral sclerosis**
4. Progressive muscular atrophy with amyotrophic lateral sclerosis. See **amyotrophic lateral sclerosis**. This entity is not clearly different from "peroneal muscular atrophy with pyramidal features."
5. **Amyotrophic dystonic paraplegia**
6. **Madras** type
7. **Amyotrophic lateral sclerosis–Parkinsonism–dementia complex of Guam**
8. Spinal muscular atrophy with olivopontocerebellar atrophy. See **cerebellar ataxias** (unknown etiology and late onset)

9. Amyotrophic lateral sclerosis with dementia. See **amyotrophic lateral sclerosis**
10. Distal spinal muscular atrophy with vocal cord paralysis
11. Spinal muscular atrophy with bulbar palsy. See **amyotrophic lateral sclerosis**
12. **Arthrogryposis multiplex congenita**, distal, type 1 (neurogenic or myopathic)
13. Charcot–Marie–Tooth disease, neuronal type. See **hereditary motor and sensory neuropathy, type 2**
14. Scapuloperoneal atrophy with cardiopathy. See **Emery–Dreifuss syndrome**
15. Scapuloperoneal amyotrophy. See **Kaeser syndrome**
16. Spastic paraplegia with amyotrophy of hands. See **amyotrophic lateral sclerosis**
17. **Distal spinal muscular atrophy** confined to the hands (See **hereditary motor neuropathy**, *hereditary motor neuropathy affecting the arms*)
18. Spinal muscular atrophy, facioscapulohumeral type (see **hereditary motor neuropathy**)
19. Proximal spinal muscular atrophy, adult type (Finkel late-onset type). See **hereditary motor neuropathy, type 5**
20. Spino**cerebellar ataxia** with Parkinsonian rigidity and peripheral neuropathy and fasciculations
21. Spinal muscular atrophy with myoclonus. See **hereditary motor neuropathy**
22. Spinal muscular atrophy with **Joseph disease**
23. Scapuloperoneal atrophy with cardiopathy and inflammatory myopathy. See **hereditary motor neuropathy**
24. Amyotrophic lateral sclerosis with **Pick disease**
25. Amyotrophic lateral sclerosis with autosomal dominant familial **Parkinsonism**. See **amyotrophic lateral sclerosis**
26. Spinal muscular atrophy with **Huntington disease**
27. Amyotrophic lateral sclerosis with **pallidonigroluysian atrophy**
28. Spinal muscular atrophy with **pallidonigral degeneration**
29. **Motor neuronopathy predominantly affecting the hands**

A4. X-linked recessive, biochemical disorder unknown

1. Spinal and bulbar muscular atrophy (**Kennedy disease**)
2. X-linked proximal juvenile spinal muscular atrophy. See **Kennedy syndrome**
3. X-linked scapuloperoneal muscular atrophy with cardiomyopathy. See **Emery–Dreifuss syndrome**
4. Charcot–Marie–Tooth peroneal muscular atrophy and **Friedreich ataxia**. See **hereditary motor and sensory neuropathy, type 2**
5. X-linked spinal muscular atrophy with facioscapulohumeral distribution. See **hereditary motor neuropathy**
6. **Arthrogryposis multiplex congenita** with renal and hepatic abnormality
7. **Arthrogryposis multiplex congenita**, distal, X-linked.

A5. X-linked dominant, lethal in males

Infantile spinal muscular atrophy in **incontinentia pigmenti**.

B. Congenital and developmental abnormalities

1. **Möbius syndrome**
2. Congenital absence of muscles. See **David anomaly**
3. Amyotrophy with developmental anomalies of the spinal cord or nerve roots: **hydromyelia, syringomyelia,** or **syringobulbia** (often with **Chiari malformation**); **spinal dysraphism; meningomyelocele**; aplasia of the spinal cord (amyelia)
4. Spinal muscular atrophy with **pontocerebellar hypoplasia**[2525]
5. **Arthrogryposis multiplex congenita** of non-neural, nonmyopathic origin

C. Disorders of motor neurons attributed to physical causes

1. Trauma: direct injury of the spinal cord (birth injury, spinal fracture); traumatic **hematomyelia**
2. Amyotrophy due to destruction, compression, or compressive ischemia of anterior horn cells
3. **Progressive vascular myelopathy** (amyotrophy due to ischemia of anterior horns)[3189]
4. Amyotrophy after electrical injury[1970]
5. Amyotrophy after radiotherapy[3645]

D. Disorders of motor neurons attributed to toxins, chemicals, or heavy metals

The following agents have been incriminated: tetanus toxin, strychnine; **botulinum toxin** (adult and infantile forms),[1199] lead,[990] **mercury**, organic phosphates (triorthocresyl phosphate, **jake paralysis**), saxitoxin and related marine toxins, dapsone[2971] and phenytoin.[1664]

E. Disorders of motor neurons attributed to viral infection

E1. Acute disorders

1. Paralytic acute anterior **poliomyelitis**: due to poliomyelitis or to other enteroviruses
2. Amyotrophy in **Russian spring–summer encephalitis**
3. **Herpes zoster**[6274]
4. Amyotrophy with acute hemorrhagic conjunctivitis[3528]

continued

Chart M–18. *(continued)*

5. Amyotrophy with asthma.[476] See **Hopkins syndrome**
6. Amyotrophy in acute transverse myelitis, cause not determined

E2. Subacute or chronic disorders

1. Amyotrophy in **Creutzfeldt-Jakob** disease[132]
2. Amyotrophy due to human immunodeficiency virus.[2937] See **HIV infection**
3. Persistent infection by poliovirus in agammaglobulinemia
4. Late **postpoliomyelitis muscular atrophy (postpolio syndrome)**[1413]
5. Syndrome of benign fasciculation and cramps in survivors of paralytic poliomyelitis or other forms of acute myelitis[2037]
6. Amyotrophy after **encephalitis lethargica**[2566]
7. **Delayed cramps and fasciculation after poliomyelitis or myelitis**

F. Disorders of motor neurons with immunological abnormality

1. Motor neuron diseases with monoclonal paraproteinemia (including Waldenstrom macroglobulinemia, multiple myeloma, chronic lymphatic leukemia)[5825]
2. Amyotrophy with Hodgkin disease[5632] or non-Hodgkin lymphoma
3. Carcinomatous motor neuron disease.[4399] See **amyotrophic lateral sclerosis** (paraneoplastic ALS)

G. Disorders of motor neurons of undetermined etiology

1. **Amyotrophic lateral sclerosis**, including **monomelic** and the sporadic and both adult- and childhood-onset inherited forms[2791, 3615]
2. Juvenile **amyotrophic lateral sclerosis**[4620]
3. Amyotrophy in **Shy-Drager syndrome**
4. Amyotrophy in sporadic **Pick disease**[4391]
5. **Quadriceps amyotrophy** (sporadic, neurogenic)[2248]
6. Muscle pain-fasciculation syndrome

H. Disorders of motor neurons in endocrine disorders

1. **Tetany** (hypocalcemia, hypomagnesemia, alkalosis)
2. Amyotrophy in hypoglycemic hyperinsulinism
3. Amyotrophy, fasciculation, and upper motor neuron signs (amyotrophic lateral sclerosis) in **hyperthyroidism**[2108]
4. Amyotrophy in **hyperparathyroidism**[4932]

I. Disorders of motor neurons manifest by hyperactivity

1. **Ordinary muscle cramps**
2. **Benign fasciculation-cramp syndrome** (syndrome of Foley and Denny-Brown)
3. **Occupational cramps** and writer's cramp
4. **Isaacs syndrome**[6619]
5. **Tetanus**
6. Strychnine intoxication
7. **Stiff man syndrome**
8. **Satoyoshi syndrome**[5559]
9. Myelopathy with rigidity, spasm, or continuous motor unit activity
10. Myokymia with hyperhidrosis and impaired muscle relaxation[2268]
11. Black widow spider bite
12. **Tetany**
13. **Spinal myoclonus**
14. **Facial myokymia**
15. **Hemifacial spasm**
16. **Painful legs and moving toes**[5979]
17. **Ekbom syndrome**. See **restless legs syndrome**[2778]

This classification is amended and updated from that of the World Federation of Neurology (World Federation of Neurology Classification Subcommittee. Classification of neuromuscular diseases. J Neurol Sci *1988;86:333–60) and is reproduced by kind permission of the late Prof. P.K. Thomas, Lord Walton, and the World Federation of Neurology.*

motor response 1. The compound muscle action potential (M wave) recorded over a muscle with stimulation of the nerve to that muscle. 2. The muscle twitch or contraction elicited by stimulation of the nerve to a muscle. 3. The muscle twitch elicited in the muscle stretch reflex. (Adapted from the 1987 Report of the Nomenclature Committee of the American Association of Electromyography and Electrodiagnosis. AAEE glossary of terms in clinical electromyography. *Muscle Nerve* 1987;10S:G5–G23. Reproduced by kind permission of the AANEM)

motor system degeneration A dominantly inherited syndrome resembling

Azorean neuropathy, but occurring in people without Portuguese ancestry.[2821]

motor system diseases See **amyotrophic lateral sclerosis**.

motor tics Irregularly repetitive, involuntary, abrupt, rapid, purposeless, coordinated movements of multiple muscle groups, occurring in stereotyped sequences, preceded often by a conscious urge to perform the movement but persisting in sleep; in the awake state they can be suppressed for a period by an effort of will.

Those involving an isolated body part, such as shrugging or eye-blinking, are known as *simple tics*; those comprising a more coordinated movement pattern such as jumping or touching are known as *complex tics*. *Phonic tics* (vocalizations) may also be simple or complex, the latter comprising perceptible words or phrases. Brief, jerky movements merit the label *clonic tics*, but slower, prolonged forms occur as well (**tonic** or **dystonic tics**). See also **sensory tics**.

motor unit The anatomical unit of an anterior horn cell, its axon, the neuromuscular junctions, and all of the muscle fibers innervated by the axon.

motor unit action potential (MUAP) An action potential reflecting the electrical activity of a single anatomical motor unit; the compound action potential of those muscle fibers within the recording range of an electrode.

With voluntary muscle contraction, the MUAP is characterized by its consistent appearance with, and relationship to, the force of contraction. The parameters listed in Chart M–19 should be specified, quantitatively if possible, after the recording electrode is placed so as to minimize the rise time (which by convention should be less than 0.5 ms).

Chart M–19. Parameters of the Motor Unit Action Potential

1. *Configuration*
   - A. Amplitude, peak-to-peak (μV and mV)
   - B. Duration, total (ms)
   - C. Number of phases (monophasic, biphasic, triphasic, tetraphasic, polyphasic)
   - D. Sign of each phase (negative, positive)
   - E. Number of turns
   - F. Variation of shape, if any, with consecutive discharges
   - G. Presence of satellite (linked) potentials, if any
2. *Recruitment characteristics*
   - A. Threshold of activation (first recruited, low threshold, high threshold)
   - B. Onset frequency (Hz)
   - C. Recruitment frequency (Hz) or recruitment interval (ms) of individual potentials

From the 1987 Report of the Nomenclature Committee of the American Association of Electromyography and Electrodiagnosis. AAEE glossary of terms in clinical electromyography. Muscle Nerve *1987;10S:G5–23.* © *1987. Reproduced by kind permission of the AANEM and of John Wiley and Sons Inc.*

motor unit estimation An electrophysiological technique in which threshold and then increasing electrical stimuli are given to a motor nerve, the sizes of the muscle-evoked potentials being measured and the average divided into the size of the evoked potential recorded with maximal stimulation to provide an estimate of the number of functioning motor units in that muscle.[4204]

motor unit territory The area in a muscle over which the muscle fibers belonging to an individual motor unit are distributed.[162]

motricity index A scoring system for the power of selected movements which can be derived for the upper and lower limbs or for one side of the body after the motor evaluation of patients with vascular hemiplegia.[1570] The first group of tests is performed with the patient sitting. It includes measurements of *arm function* (pinch grip, elbow flexion, and shoulder abduction) and of *leg function* (hip flexion, knee extension, and ankle dorsiflexion).

A *trunk control test* may be added, in which the subject is assessed on his ability to roll over to the weak or to the strong side, to sit up from the supine position and to maintain balance while sitting on the side of a bed. Scores for the arms, for the legs, and for one side may be derived.

Mott, Sir Frederick Walker (1853–1916) English physician and pathologist, who proved conclusively the relationship between **syphilis** and **general paresis** by finding spirochetes in the brain of paretic patients. He also described the pathology of neuronal degeneration in his Croonian lectures of 1900.

Mouchet syndrome Ulnar nerve paresis resulting from a distal fracture of the humerus. This is worthy of note only because the original description was of a fracture of the *condyle externe*, suggesting the lateral epicondyle rather than the medial, as was actually the case. Dr. Albert Mouchet was a French physician, born in 1869.

mounding phenomenon A focal contracture of a skeletal muscle in response to a direct tap on the muscle. It was first observed (in recently-dead animals) by Schiff in 1858; its genesis has been determined to be calcium liberation from the sarcoplasmic reticulum.[4419]

Mount Fuji sign The CT scan appearance in the supine patient in the presence of a large amount of subdural air that compresses both frontal lobes (tension pneumocephalus).[5491]

Mount–Reback syndrome See **paroxysmal kinesiogenic choreo-athetosis**.

mountain sickness 1. (acute mountain sickness) Cerebral edema and pulmonary symptoms developing within hours of arriving at altitudes above 2500 m. Headache, anorexia, nausea, vomiting; and dyspnea at rest, cough, pink frothy sputum, and audible râles are typical clinical features. Retinal hemorrhages may accompany these findings. See also **high-altitude headache**. The pulmonary problems at least are responsive to steroids. 2. (Monge disease, chronic mountain sickness) The occurrence of polycythemia and pulmonary hypertension in subjects living at high altitudes for long periods (years), the clinical effects of note comprising fatigue and mental slowing.[6144]

mouthing Repetitive chewing and licking throughout wakefulness with tongue protrusions, seen in edentulous elderly patients and inhibited briefly by eye closure or by a touch on the face. Midline cerebellar lesions are considered responsible.[222] See also **oromandibular dystonia**.

movement arousal A body movement associated with arousal or awakening.[280]

Movement Disorder Society A professional organization dedicated to disseminating information on recent advances in both clinical and basic sciences related to movement disorders, and to the education of physicians and the public. Tel: 414-276-2145. Web site: http://www.movementdisorders.org/.

movement disorders Those neurological conditions in which the major clinical expressions involve reduced normal movements or excessive or abnormal involuntary movements of the limbs, face, or trunk, and which in most instances are considered to reflect disease of the extrapyramidal system.

***Movement Disorders* (*Mov Disord*)** The offical journal of the **Movement Disorder Society**, published by John Wiley & Sons, and available online via Wiley InterScience. Web site: http://www.movementdisorders.org/.

movement-induced seizures A questionable variety of seizure in which the actual voluntary movement of a limb induces a motor response resembling that in **startle-induced seizures**.

movement phosphenes Those **phosphenes** induced by movement of the eyes; an occasional accompaniment of **optic neuritis**.[1483]

moving ear Slow semi-rhythmic movements of the auricle; likely a focal dyskinesia.

Moving Forward A charitable organization in the field of **myoclonus**. Address: 2934 Glenmore Ave., Kettering, OH 45409. Tel: 937-293-0409.

Moxon, William Eighteenth-century physician to Guy's Hospital, London who gave the first account of **multiple sclerosis** ("insular sclerosis") in the English literature.

moyamoya disease (Jpn, hazy, like a puff of smoke) (Nishimoto-Takeuchi-Kudo disease) A form of large-vessel occlusion affecting the intracranial supraclinoid carotid artery, in which a secondary network of proliferating collateral arterioles is seen to arise from the carotid artery proximal to the occlusion.[6146] The posterior circulation is rarely involved.

Children or young adults with such an abnormality usually present with hemiplegia; adults present with subarachnoid hemorrhage, although dementia, dysphasia, pyramidal or extrapyramidal signs, and cerebral atrophy have all been recorded.[3582] The angiographic appearances (described first by Takeuchi in 1961) resemble a mist or puff of smoke arising from the floor of the skull; a similar appearance can occur in disease of the posterior circulation. Moyamoya disease is the most common vascular etiology of childhood stroke.

The clinical picture is that of bilateral basal vascular occlusive disease with telangiectasias involving the basal ganglia as a result of occlusion of the internal carotid artery.[6138] A few patients also manifest signs and symptoms of **neurofibromatosis**, sickle-cell anemia, or **Down syndrome**.

In *variant* conditions, the disorder is dominantly inherited (17q25.3) while in *moyamoya disease and Ollier disease* there are associated enchondromatosis and lytic lesions of bone, skeletal cysts, or tumors leading to multiple fractures. Linkages to chromosomes 3p, 6q, 17q, 8q, and 12p have been found.

Moynahan syndrome A recessively inherited syndrome characterized by alopecia, hypohidrosis, seizures, and mental retardation.[4527] Dr. E.J. Moynahan was a British dermatologist at Guy's Hospital.

Mozart effect Slight and transient improvement in spational reasoning skills detected in normal subjects as a result of exposure to the music of Mozart, specifically his sonata for two pianos (K448). Such music (as also that of JS Bach and of his son JC Bach) has been shown to contain long-lasting periodicities and repetition of melodic lines, considered somehow responsible for the effect.[3197]

A decrease in the manifestations of neurological disease such as seizure activity has also been described as an extension of the effect; the fact that some patients showing it are in coma indicates that an emotional reaction to the beauty of the music is not itself the relevant mechanism.

MPTP (methyl-phenyl-tetrahydropyridine) A substance synthesized in the illicit, nonprofessional but highly commercial production of heroin, and which is intensely toxic to the nigrostriatal pathways in man and some monkeys to the extent that ingestion leads inexorably and quickly to a **Parkinsonian** syndrome.

MRA See **magnetic resonance angiography**.

MRD See **minimal record of disability**.

MRI See **magnetic resonance imaging**.

MS Neuropsychological Screening Questionnaire A brief self-report procedure that garners data from both the patient and an informant that predicts cognitive impairment with reasonable accuracy.[512]

MSLT See **minimal sleep latency test**.

MSQ See **Mental Status Questionnaire**.

mu rhythm (arceau rhythm, wicket rhythm, comb rhythm) An EEG rhythm at 7–11 Hz composed of arch-shaped waves occurring over the centroparietal regions of the scalp during wakefulness. Its amplitude varies but is mostly below 50 μV. It is blocked or attenuated most clearly by contralateral movement, the thought of movement, readiness to move or tactile stimulation. (From the 1974 report of the Committee on Terminology, IFCN. In: Chatrian GE, Bergamini L, Dondey M, et al. A glossary of terms most commonly used by clinical electroencephalographers. *EEG Clin Neurophysiol* 1974;37:538–48. Reproduced by kind permission of Elsevier Science and the IFCN.)

The rhythm is seen in Rolandic regions and is of no known pathological significance.

MUAP See **motor unit action potential**.

Muckle-Wells syndrome

(dominant urticaria, amyloidosis, nephritis, and hearing loss) A dominantly inherited cochleovestibular syndrome of childhood, characterized by progressive renal impairment due to amyloidosis, recurrent urticarial rashes, fever, and neural deafness.[4535]

mucocele Benign cysts composed of mucus-secreting epithelium situated within the nasal sinuses, but capable of eroding into the orbit or cranial cavity.

mucocutaneous lymph node syndrome See **Kawasaki disease**.

mucolipidoses Sphingolipid and mucopolysaccharide lysosomal storage diseases in which lipid-like and polysaccharide-like material is deposited in the tissues. See **sialidosis**.

Mucolipidosis IV Foundation

ML4 Foundation, originally known as CHARM (Children's Association for Research on Mucolipidosis). A charitable organization. Web site: http://www.ml4.org/.

mucopolysaccharidoses (Ellis gargoylism, Pfaundler-Hurler syndrome) A group of lysosomal disorders of mucopolysaccharide metabolism resulting from deficient activity of the enzymes which degrade mucopolysaccharides; they are usually autosomal recessively inherited, and involve the storage of glycosaminoglycans (mucopolysaccharides) in the lysosomes of various tissues. The catabolism of dermatan sulfate, heparan sulfate, and/or ketaran sulfate is thus blocked, and in some cases, that of chondroitin sulfate as well. The types are listed in Chart M–20.

Other *variant* conditions are *O'Brien mucopolysaccharidosis*, characterized by short stature, gibbus, mucopolysaccariduria, rhizomelia of the upper limbs, bowed radius and ulna, skeletal and joint anomalies, and mental and developmental delay;[381] and a form form presenting with multiple nerve entrapments.[3311]

Chart M–20. The Types of Mucopolysaccharidosis

Hurler syndrome (type 1-H): A lethal, recessively inherited systemic disease appearing within the first year of life, due to α-L-iduronidase deficiency, which leads to the deposition of dermatan and heparan sulfate in the joints, liver, spleen, and skin. Clinically, the syndrome is characterized by short stature, gargoyle-like facies, prominent lips and tongue, cataract, hypertelorism, psychomotor retardation, macrocephaly, thickened skin, hepatosplenomegaly and cardiomegaly, arthropathy, kyphoscoliosis, and sometimes spastic quadriparesis due to C1–2 subluxation.[3058] Entrapment neuropathies are also often found. The children usually die of respiratory or cardiac failure.

Hurler–Scheie syndrome (type 1-H/S): A recessively inherited syndrome in which deficiency of α-L-iduronidase leads to the accumulation of dermatan and heparan sulfate and in which the clinical features resemble both the syndromes suggested by its name. The responsible gene lies on chromosome 22.

Scheie syndrome (type 1-S or 5): A recessively inherited systemic mucopolysaccharidosis due to deficiency of the enzyme α-L-iduronidase, in which dermatan sulfate and heparan sulfate are deposited. Diffuse congenital corneal haziness and the later development of pigmentary retinopathy, cataract, dwarfism, joint ankylosis, mild dysmorphism, skeletal defects, carpal tunnel syndrome, coarctation of the aorta, and hepatosplenomegaly are the main clinical features. Urinary levels of chondroitin sulfate B are high.[5588] The condition differs from most other mucopolysaccharidoses in that the physical and mental statures of the patients are not diminished. It is allelic with Hurler syndrome.

Although the term *Hunter-Hurler syndrome* is also applied, these and **Hunter** diseases are separate, though similar, mucopolysaccharidoses.

Hunter syndrome (type 2): An X-linked form due to deficiency of iduronate 2-sulfate sulfatase appearing in childhood and characterized by short stature, enlarged nose with a depressed nasal bridge, coarse facial features, delayed tooth eruption, kyphosis, beaked vertebrae, platyspondyly, pectus carinatum, thick ribs, inguinal and umbilical hernias, enlarged liver, joint stiffness, mucopolysaccharhiduria, oligosaccariduria, macrocephaly, J-shaped sella turcica, epiphyseal dysplasia, and psychomotor retardation. Mild and severe forms are distinguished on the basis of the degree of mental impairment and on the course of the disease. The responsible gene maps to chromosome Xq27.3.

Sanfilippo syndrome (types 3 A, B, C, D):(OMIM 252940): Recessively inherited systemic mucopolysaccharidoses of young children due to the absence of any one of the three sulfamidase enzymes that are responsible for the degradation of heparan sulfate, which is therefore accumulated.The four subtypes are caused by deficiency of different enzymes: heparan *N*-sulfatase (type A), α-*N*-acetylglucosaminidase (type B), acetyl coenzyme A:α-glucosaminide acetyltransferase (type C), and *N*-acetylglucosamine-6-sulfatase (type D; autosomal recessive, caused by mutations in the GNS on chromosome 12q14).

Clinically, the conditions are similar and are marked by severe mental deterioration with aggressive behavior, coarse facial features, cataract, dwarfism, joint ankylosis, skeletal defects, hepatosplenomegaly, vertebral abnormalities, joint stiffness, seizures, ataxia, mucopolysacchariduria, and abnormal lysosomal enzymes. In the B form, there is striking visceral involvement. Urinary levels of heparan sulfate are high.[5541] Clinically, it is characterized by severe CNS degeneration but relatively mild somatic disease, manifesting in childhood and leading to death before the age of 30 years.[3166]

In a *variant* form, the disorder presents as a dementing disease in early adult life.

Morquio disease (type 4 A and B, Morquio–Brailsford syndrome): An autosomal recessive metabolic disease presenting in early childhood, due to deficiency of *N*-acetyl-galactosamine 6 sulfate sulfatase (Type A) or β-galactosidase (Type B), in which keratan sulfate and chondroitin-6-sulfate are deposited in tissues and excreted in the urine. The clinical manifestations include coarse facial features, corneal opacities, deafness without mental deterioration, dwarfism, hyperextensible joints, aortic valve anomalies, epiphyseal dysplasia, platyspondyly, and osteoporosis, the latter leading to widespread skeletal deformities. In the case of the spine, these may cause vertebral subluxation such as atlanto-axial dislocation and cord compression.[3494, 4494, 4493] The responsible gene for Morquio syndrome B maps to chromosome 3p21–p14.2 J.F. Brailsford (1888–1961) was an English radiologist practicing in Birmingham.

In related *variant* forms, neuronal storage or corneal opacities occur as well.

Maroteaux-Lamy syndrome (type 6): A recessively inherited lysosomal storage disease (mucopolysaccharidosis type VI) with deficiency of arylsulfatase B and accumulation of dermatan sulfate. It exists in severe, intermediate, and mild forms, the latter appearing in adult life.

continued

Chart M–20. (*continued*)

The main clinical features are dwarfism, facial dysmorphism with prominent lips and tongue, severe skeletal deformity, deafness, corneal opacities, hepatosplenomegaly and cardiomegaly, kyphoscoliosis and sometimes spastic quadriparesis due to C1–2 subluxation. Hydrocephalus and carpal tunnel syndrome are the other main neurological complications. The urine contains large amounts of chondroitin sulfate B.[4096] Mental retardation is not a feature. A milder *variant* is also described.

β-Glucuronidase deficiency (type 7, Sly disease): A rare, recessively inherited disorder of mucopolysaccharide metabolism due to a defect on chromosome 7 with deficiency of β-glucuronidase and the accumulation of dermatan and heparan sulfate. Clinically, it presents with short stature, mental retardation, macrocephaly, corneal clouding, hepatosplenomegaly, and polymorphic skeletal malformations.[5894]

Di Ferrante syndrome (type 8): A rare, recessively inherited disorder of mucopolysaccharide metabolism due to a defect on chromosome 7 with deficiency of glucosamine-6-sulfate sulfatase. Clinically it presents in childhood with psychomotor delay, hepatomegaly, coarse hair, and odontoid anomalies.[2389]

mucormycosis A rare, severe infection with the fungus *Phycomycetes* which may be manifested in pulmonary, disseminated, intestinal, and rhinocerebral forms. Debilitated or immunocompromised subjects with systemic illnesses such as diabetes, leukemia, organ failure, renal acidosis, etc. are the most susceptible.

The rhinocerebral manifestations include the orbital apex syndrome, cavernous sinus syndrome, and carotid occlusion. A nasopharyngeal form that includes multiple cranial nerve palsies is also described. Depression of consciousness may occur in association with any of these.[5185]

mucosulfatidosis A diffuse encephalopathy with onset in infancy and due to deficiency of arylsulfatases and other enzymes, leading to the accumulation of sulfatide, heparan, and dermatan sulfate. The condition is regarded as a variant form of **metachromatic leukodystrophy**.

Muenchmeyer syndrome See **myositis ossificans**.

MuLiBrEy syndrome A rare recessively inherited dysmorphic syndrome characterized by **Mu**scle, **Li**ver, **Br**ain and **Ey**e anomalies. **Nanism**, hypotonia, hypertelorism, hepatomegaly, pigmentary retinopathy, cerebral ventricular enlargement, pericarditis, and skeletal malformations are the most constant clinical features.[4984]

Müller, Eduard (1876–1928) German, neuropsychiatrist in Breslau.

Müller sign Early loss of the abdominal reflexes in **multiple sclerosis**,[4541] named after **Eduard Müller**.

Müller, Heinrich (1820–1864) German, professor of anatomy at Wurzburg.

Müller's muscle Smooth muscle fibers in the upper eyelid, weakly assisting the levator palpebrae superioris. It is named after **Heinrich Müller**.

Müller, Johannes (1801–1858) German, professor of physiology at Berlin who in 1826 propounded the law of specific nerve energies, which states that each sense organ responds to any stimulus with impulses giving rise to its particular sensation and is supplied by nerves sensitive only to that one form of stimulation. Thus, specific sense organs are responsible for specific modalities of sensation.

In 1831, Müller published accounts of his stimulation experiments on frogs and finally demonstrated without doubt the sensory functions of the posterior roots and the motor functions of the anterior roots, thus sealing the observations of **Bell** and of **Magendie** in this area.

Müller's Law (law of specific nerve energies) Every nerve fiber subserves one modality of sensation, whatever stimulation its end-organ receives, propounded by Johannes Müller in 1826.

multicore myopathy (myopathy with multicore and central nuclei, congenital myopathy with multifocal degeneration of muscle fibers) A group of congenital myopathies resulting from various genetic abnormalities affecting variously the *ryanodine* receptor (19q13.1, recessive); *selenoprotein N*, 1 (1p35-p36, recessive or sporadic); short-chain acyl–CoA dehydrogenase deficiency; *titin*; etc. Overall, this is a benign and nonprogressive myopathy with multiple, small, randomly distributed areas of myofibrillar disorganization with a local decrease in mitochondrial oxidative enzyme activity found on muscle biopsy. Multicores, a focal loss of cross striations and a failure of fiber-type differentiation are also noted, as in **central core disease**, but they occur only patchily within the muscle biopsy specimens.[1871, 1873, 6158] Multicore and minicore diseases are nosologically identical but many prefer the term minicore disease for both disorders, as multiple cores are also present in both **central core disease** and minicore disease.

Clinically, lifelong (proximal more than distal) limb and facial weakness, delayed motor development, ptosis, dolichocephaly, ophthalmoplegias, and slightly raised creatine kinase levels are the only constant associations.[1874] The respiratory muscles and myocardium are rarely affected. A case has been reported with onset in adult life.[741] Motor milestones are delayed and typically there is hypotonia, axial, girdle and limb weakness, severe scoliosis, and respiratory insufficiency, though milder phenotypes occur, some with pelvic girdle weakness; motor delay is usual in all forms. Ptosis and ophthalmoplegia are occasionally present. The EMG is myopathic but serum CK levels are not raised. *Variants* include the following:

Minicore disease with ophthalmoplegia with dominant or recessive inheritance, due to mutations of the *RYR1* or *SEPN1* genes. The onset is in the first year of life.

Antenatal onset with arthrogryposis, associated with generalized arthrogryposis, dolichocephaly and facial dysmorphisms, severe kyphosis or kyphoscoliosis, and mild proximal weakness.

A mild *"central core-like" phenotype* is recessively inherited and usually due to mutations of the ryanodine receptor.

Congenital myopathy with fatal dilated cardiomyopathy is recessively inherited and due to *titin* mutations. It causes early general motor weakness, hypotonia, and delayed milestones. Pseudohypertrophy may be seen in the thighs and calves. A progressive dilated cardiomyopathy with rhythm disturbances appears in later childhood, with the potential for sudden death. The condition is allelic with *Finnish distal myopathy, dilated cardiomyopathy 1G* and **limb girdle muscular dystrophy** 2J.

Multicore Myopathy is a relevant Web site: http://home.cogeco.ca/~famadio/.

multicystic encephalopathy (polyporencephaly) Multiple areas of cavitation in the cerebral cortex and in the subcortical white matter, found in infants following **hypoxic-ischemic encephalopathy**, usually in the territory of the anterior or middle cerebral arteries. See also **porencephaly** and **encephalomalacia**.

Multidimensional Observation Scale for Elderly Subjects (MOSES) A scale designed for observers to evaluate aspects of functioning in elderly residential patients in five areas of functioning, including self-care, disoriented behavior, depressed or anxious mood, irritable behavior, and withdrawn behavior. These factors are determined after rating the subject on 40 areas of function.[2850]

Multidimensional Pain Inventory An instrument for assessing cognitive, behavioral and affective aspects of pain, yielding scores for pain severity; interference; life control; affective distress; support; punishing, solicitous, and distracting responses; household chores; outdoor work; activities away from home; and social activities.[3394]

multifidus syndrome A myofascial pain syndrome with the trigger point below the posterior superior iliac spine.[3882]

multifocal acquired demyelinating sensory and motor neuropathy (Lewis-Sumner syndrome, MADSAM) 1. A slowly progressive, or relapsing distal, asymmetrical neuropathy of adult life, the weakness affecting mainly the arms. A proximal syndrome is also described affecting mainly the phrenic and suprascapular nerves. Any sensory loss is mild and distal. Electrophysiology shows multifocal conduction blocks, variably slow NCVs and long distal latencies. CSF protein is raised, usually up to <100 mg/dl and MRI shows swollen nerves in the brachial plexus. The pathology is patchy nerve demyelination with some axonal loss.[5526]

2. An asymmetric, acquired chronic sensory and motor polyneuropathy with an immune-based etiology. Electrophysiological changes are consistent with axonopathy and do not fulfill the criteria for demyelinating neuropathies.[5526] See also DADS and **sensory CIDP**.

multifocal demyelinating neuropathy with persistent conduction block See **multifocal motor neuropathy (with persistent conduction block)**.

multifocal diabetic neuropathy See **diabetic radiculoplexus neuropathy**.

multifocal giant-cell encephalitis A chronic encephalitis associated with HIV infection, characterized by the perivascular accumulation of microglia, monocytes, and macrophages, with virus-containing multinucleated giant cells.[6]

multifocal inflammatory demyelinating neuropathy (MIDN) An asymmetric sensory or sensorimotor demyelinating neuropathy not fulfilling criteria for **multifocal motor neuropathy with persistent conduction block** nor for **chronic inflammatory demyelinating polyneuropathy**. Clinically, the disorder starts in one limb, slowly progressing asymmetrically. Electrically there is evidence of multifocal demyelination and conduction block in motor and sensory nerves. MRI may show swelling of nerves in the brachial plexus and biopsy shows inflammatory changes.[6478]

The condition known as **multifocal motor sensory demyelinating neuropathy** is possibly the same condition, as may be **idiopathic sensory neuropathy**.

multifocal interstitial myositis with localized lipoatrophy An inherited myopathy characterized by the young adult onset of proximal and distal myopathic weakness with inflammatory cells in muscle.[381]

multifocal motor and sensory demyelinating neuropathy See **multifocal inflammatory demyelinating neuropathy**.

multifocal motor neuropathy (with persistent conduction block) (MMN) An uncommon, acquired, chronic, progressive, asymmetrical, sensorimotor, or pure motor demyelinating immune-mediated neuropathy occurring in adult life, clinically resembling **amyotrophic lateral sclerosis** or **multiple mononeuropathy**, but most pronounced distally in the arms, in which at least two nerves show persistent, asymmetrical, multifocal, persistent but partial motor **conduction blocks** away from the usual sites. The condition is more common in males and wrist- and foot-drop, and weakness of grip are the most common presenting features. Atrophy is relatively mild, fasciculations and cramps are common, stretch reflexes are often depressed in the affected areas, and myokymia is occasionally noted. Sensory symptoms are not to be expected. Optic neuritis and phrenic nerve involvement are associated in some cases, but other cranial nerves and the pyramidal system are seldom involved. Electrodiagnostic studies show focal segmental distal nerve conduction blocks as evidenced by >50% reduction of CMAP amplitudes with proximal vs. distal stimulation sites; axonal loss is a late finding.

In sural nerve biopsy specimens the pathological findings include both demyelination and remyelination, and there is a variable degree of fiber loss. High titers to anti-GM1 or NP-9 lipid antigen IgM antibodies are detected in over 90% of cases.[3821]

Numerous sets of diagnostic criteria have been suggested. Unfortunately, the correlation between fulfillment of diagnostic criteria and response to, e.g., IVIg therapy is imperfect. See also **lower motor neuron disease**.

Proposed diagnostic criteria for Multifocal Motor Neuropathy

Clinical criteria

1. Slow or stepwise progressive limb weakness
2. Asymmetrical limb weakness
3. Fewer than seven affected limb regions (upper arm, lower arm; upper leg, or lower leg on both sides of the body; maximum 8)
4. Muscle stretch reflexes in the affected limbs are decreased or absent

5. Signs and symptoms are more pronounced in the arms than in the legs
6. Age 20–65 years at onset
7. No objective sensory abnormalities except for vibration sense
8. No bulbar signs or symptoms
9. No upper-motor-neuron features
10. No other neuropathies (e.g.; diabetic, lead, porphyric, or vasculitic neuropathy, CIDP, Lyme neuroborreliosis, postradiation neuropathy, hereditary neuropathy with liability to pressure palsies, Charcot-Marie-Tooth neuropathies, meningeal carcinomatosis)
11. No myopathy (e.g., facio-scapulo-humeral muscular dystrophy, inclusion-body myositis)

Suggested laboratory criteria

1. CSF protein <1 g/l
2. High anti-GM1 titers
3. High signal intensity on T2-weighted MRI of the brachial plexus.

Electrodiagnostic criteria

1. *Definite motor conduction block*: CMAP area reduction on proximal vs. distal stimulation of at least 50% over a long segment between Erb's point and axilla, upper arm, lower arm; lower leg); or a CMAP amplitude reduction on proximal vs. distal stimulation of at least 30% over a short distance (2.5 cm) detected by inching. CMAP amplitude on stimulation of the distal part of the segment with motor conduction block of at least 1 mV.
2. *Probable motor conduction block:* MAP amplitude reduction on proximal vs. distal stimulation of at least 30% over a long segment of an arm nerve. CMAP amplitude on stimulation of the distal part of the segment with motor conduction block of at least 1 mV.
3. Slowing of conduction compatible with demyelination: MCV <75% of the lower limit of normal; distal motor latency or shortest F wave, latency >130% of the upper limit of normal; or absence of F waves after 16–20 stimuli. CMAP amplitudes on distal stimulation of at least 0.5 mV.
4. Normal sensory nerve conduction in arm segments with motor conduction block. Normal SNAP amplitudes on distal stimulation.

Scoring:
Definite MMN
1–11 on clinical criteria, 1 on laboratory criteria, and 1 and 4 on electrodiagnostic criteria.
Probable MMN
1–3 and 6-11 on clinical criteria, 1 on laboratory criteria and 2 and 4 on electrodiagnostic criteria.
Possible MMN
1 and 7–11 on clinical criteria, 2 or 3 on laboratory criteria and 3 and 4 on electrodiagnostic criteria.

A slightly shorter set of criteria have been produced by the AANEM more recently;[4789] that publication also contains more detailed criteria for diagnosing conduction block which will not be reproduced here.

From Van den Berg et al. (2000)[6477]. Reproduced with kind permission of the American Academy of Neurology and Lippincott Williams and Wilkins.

Alternative criteria for the diagnosis of multifocal motor neuropathy (AANEM; slightly amended; reproduced by kind permission.)

Definite

1. Weakness without objective sensory loss in the distribution of two or more named nerves. During the early stages of symptomatic weakness, the historical or physical finding of diffuse, symmetric weakness *excludes* multifocal motor neuropathy.
2. Definite conduction block is present in two or more nerves away from common entrapment sites. (Median nerve at wrist; ulnar nerve at elbow or wrist; peroneal nerve at fibular head.)
3. Normal sensory nerve conduction velocity across the same segments with demonstrated motor conduction block.
4. Normal results for sensory nerve conduction studies on all tested nerves, with a minimum of three nerves tested.

Probable

1. Weakness without objective sensory loss in the distribution of two or more named nerves. During the initial weeks of symptomatic weakness, the presence of diffuse, symmetric weakness excludes multifocal motor neuropathy.
2. The presence of either
   a. Probable conduction block in two or more motor nerve segments that are not common entrapment sites, or
   b. Definite conduction block in one motor nerve segment and probable conduction block in a different motor nerve segment, neither of which segments are common entrapment sites.
3. Normal sensory nerve conduction velocity across the same segments with demonstrated motor conduction block, when this segment is technically feasible for study (i.e., this is not required for segments proximal to the axilla or popliteal fossa).
4. Normal results for sensory nerve conduction studies on all tested nerves (a minimum of three nerves tested).

For the diagnosis of both probable and definite forms, upper motor neuron signs such as spastic tone, clonus, extensor plantar response, and pseudobulbar palsy must be absent.

The condition may be considered a variant of **chronic inflammatory demyelinating polyneuropathy**, differing in its distal and asymmetric presentation, the rarity of sensory symptoms, localized electrophysiological findings, and lack of the inflammatory signs and onion bulbs seen in the widespread peripheral nerve demyelination of that condition.

In *variant* forms, the condition presents with ophthalmoplegia;[5123] no conduction block is found;[4860] or there are neither conduction block nor evidence of demyelination in an immune-related and presumably associated form. A third possible form is *multifocal acquired motor axonopathy*, which appears to be an axonal MMN variant.[3329]

Further definitions or descriptions of this and other neuromuscular syndromes are superbly presented at Dr/ Alan Pestronk's Web site: http://www.neuro.wustl.edu/neuromuscular.

multifocal motor and sensory demyelinating neuropathy (MADSAMN) A multifocal inflammatory demyelinating polyneuropathy. See **Lewis-Sumner syndrome**.

multifocal pseudohypertrophic neuropathy See **multifocal inflammatory demyelinating neuropathy**.

multifocal sensorimotor demyelinating neuropathy A likely variant of **multifocal motor**

neuropathy with persistent conduction block in which there are also sensory complaints, raised CSF protein levels, a shorter course, a better steroid response and sensory nerve conduction abnormalities.[4760]

multifocal sensory demyelinating neuropathy

Yet another likely variant of **multifocal motor neuropathy with persistent conduction block**, here presenting with sensory complaints, raised CSF protein levels, a response to IvIg and evidence of demyelinating sensory neuropathy on near-nerve conduction studies only.[4761]

multi-infarct dementia

A relatively common and partially reversible form of dementia due to multiple focal cortical infarctions.[2664] However, subcortical strokes, many of which occur without noticeable clinical symptoms, may also be responsible. See **leukoaraiosis**.

Symptoms include confusion, problems with short-term memory; wandering, or getting lost in familiar places; walking with rapid, shuffling steps; losing bladder or bowel control; frontal-lobe syndromes (laughing or crying inappropriately); difficulty in following instructions; and problems in handling money, gadgets, organizations etc. Mild pyramidal signs are often also present. Diagnostic criteria have been suggested (http://www.mentalhealth.com/dis1/p21-or02.html/).

A. The development of multiple cognitive deficits manifested by both:
   1. Memory impairment (impaired ability to learn new information or to recall previously learned information) and
   2. One or more of **aphasia, apraxia, agnosia**, and disturbance in executive functioning (i.e., planning, organizing, sequencing, abstracting).

B. These cognitive deficits cause significant impairment in social or occupational functioning and represent a significant decline from a previous level of functioning.

C. Focal neurological signs and symptoms (e.g., exaggeration of muscle stretch reflexes, extensor plantar response, pseudobulbar palsy, gait abnormalities, weakness of an extremity) or laboratory evidence indicative of cerebrovascular disease (e.g., multiple infarctions involving cortex and underlying white matter) that are judged to be etiologically related to the disturbance.

D. The cognitive deficits do not occur exclusively during the course of a delirium.

In the ICD-10 it is also pointed out that the impairment of cognitive function is commonly uneven, so that there may be memory loss, intellectual impairment, and focal neurological signs while insight and judgement may be relatively well preserved. An abrupt onset or a stepwise deterioration, as well as the presence of focal neurological signs and symptoms increases the probability of the diagnosis; in some cases, confirmation can be provided only by CT scans or neuropathological examination. Associated features include hypertension, carotid bruit, emotional lability with transient depressive mood, weeping or explosive laughter and transient episodes of clouded consciousness or delirium, often provoked by a further infarction. The personality is relatively well preserved, but personality changes may be evident in a proportion of cases with apathy, disinhibition, or accentuation of previous traits such as egocentricity, paranoid attitudes, or irritability.

The **Hachinski Ischemic Scale** was devised to reflect the clinical features of this and other **vascular dementias**. The presence of brainstem and pyramidal signs, of gait disorder and of depression are features not specifically rated on the Hachinski Scale that suggest multi-infarct dementia rather than **Alzheimer disease**. Dementia occurring as a result of multiple cerebral emboli, or following cardiac arrest or cardiac surgery might also be included under this heading. See also **vascular dementia**.

A *variant* is *multi-infarct dementia, familial type* (familial vascular encephalopathy, Worster-Drought Syndrome), which is a syndrome of adult onset characterized by cerebral atrophy with dementia, facial palsy, pyramidal signs, and arteriopathy, described in Sweden and in England.

multilead electrode

A metal cannula through which any small number of insulated wires are inserted to extrude through apertures in it, their bared tips flush with the cannula's outer surface and thus recording from fibers that are members of a number of motor units within a muscle.[19] See **electrode**.

multi-minicore disease

A recessively inherited benign congenital myopathy associated with multifocal zones of degeneration of sarcomeres, with lack of oxidative activity.[1886] Weakness is axially predominant and severe respiratory difficulty, scoliosis are common features, but the phenotype is variable.[2028]

multi-MUP analysis

A template matching, decomposition EMG method used for MUAP analysis. (From the 2001 Report of the Nomenclature Committee of the American Association of Electromyography and Electrodiagnosis.[19] Reproduced by kind permission of the AANEM.)

multiple acyl–coenzyme A dehydrogenation disorders

Mitochondrial disorders including **glutaric aciduria type 2**, characterized by a deficiency in the electron transfer flavoprotein or its dehydrogenase. In the *severe* (MAD: S) form, infants present with seizures and are found to have nonketotic hypoglycemia and metabolic acidosis. In the *mild* form (MAD: M) the **sudden infant death syndrome**, an illness resembling **Reye syndrome** or a lipid storage myopathy (see next entry) may occur; such conditions may respond to riboflavine.[6387]

multiple acyl–coA dehydrogenase-deficient myopathy

A carnitine-deficient lipid storage myopathy with organic aciduria due to an inborn error of the enzymes catalyzing the oxidation of straight- and branched-chain acyl coenzyme A and glutaryl coenzyme A. Muscle weakness with recurrent episodes of hypoglycemia and an odor of sweaty feet are the leading features. Both mild and severe (lethal) forms occur. In some cases, the condition, a mitochondrial disorder, is remarkably responsive to large doses of thiamine.[1625] See also **glutaric aciduria type 2**.

Multiple Affect Adjective Checklist

A self-report questionnaire appropriate for the repeated assessment of disturbed mood states.[6985]

multiple basal cell nevi syndrome

See **Gorlin-Golz syndrome**.

multiple carboxylase deficiency A neonatal metabolic syndrome due to a deficiency in biotin holocarboxylase synthetase,[4849] and characterized clinically by alopecia, sensorineural deafness, conjunctivitis, hypotonia, seizures, cerebellar ataxia, tremor, eczema, erythema, psychomotor delay, and eventually death in coma. High plasma ammonia and lactate levels and organic aciduria are found.[6312]

In the *neonatal* form the deficiency is of numerous carboxylase enzymes including pyruvate carboxylase and holocarboxylase synthetase, while in the *late-onset* form, biotinidase is deficient.

multiple cerebral/retinal arteriovenous malformations See **Wyburn-Mason syndrome**.

multiple congenital articular rigidities See **arthrogryposis multiplex congenita**.

multiple congenital contractures (multiple-contracture syndrome) A lethal autosomal recessive syndrome characterized by intrauterine growth retardation with multiple contractures and facial abnormalities.

The condition is a variant of the **Pena-Shokeir phenotype**, differentiated by the presence of severe fetal hydrops and the increased severity in this condition. See also **multiple pterygium syndrome**.[2885]

multiple cranial nerve palsies syndrome 1. A variant of **acute inflammatory demyelinating polyneuropathy**, described first by Guillain in 1937, in which a number of cranial nerves (usually at least four, including the oculomotor nerve) are affected bilaterally. The CSF protein level is elevated and ataxia or areflexia may also be found, but limb strength and sensation are typically unaffected. The prognosis for recovery is excellent.[5812] See also **Miller Fisher syndrome; facial diplegia; ataxia, areflexia,** and **facial diplegia**.

2. Painful ophthalmoplegia related to a granulomatous inflammatory process in the cavernous sinus, preceded by facial palsy; an extended form of **Tolosa-Hunt syndrome**.[6259]

multiple discharge Four or more motor unit action potentials of the same form and nearly the same amplitude occurring consistently in the same relationship to one another and generated by the same axon. See **double and triple discharge**. (From the 2001 Report of the Nomenclature Committee of the American Association of Electromyography and Electrodiagnosis.[19] Reproduced by kind permission of the AANEM.)

multiple endocrine neoplasia Type 1 is a dominantly inherited syndrome characterized by pituitary, pancreatic, adrenal, and/or parathyroid hyperplasia or adenomatosis. Chromophobe, basophil, or eosinophil pituitary adenomas may also complicate the syndrome.[6726]

Type 2 (Sipple syndrome) is a dominantly inherited disorder characterized by carcinoma and/or hyperplasia of the adrenal or thyroid glands; parathyroid hyperplasia uncommonly; a physique resembling that of **Marfan syndrome**; neuromas of the tongue, lips, and eyelids; autonomic symptoms due to ganglioneuromatosis in the alimentary tract; pheochromocytoma; and signs of **hereditary motor and sensory neuropathy**.[1774]

Type 2b is a rare autosomal dominant condition linked to chromosome 10q.11.2, in which medullary carcinoma of the thyroid, pheochromocytoma, ganglioneuromatosis, or various skeletal disorders are associated with pes cavus, atrophy of the peroneal muscles, lingual tumor-like excresences, and thickened lips.[1020]

multiple epiphyseal dysplasia-microcephaly-nystagmus See **Conradi-Hünermann syndrome**.

multiple epiphyseal dysplasia with mild myopathy A dominantly inherited myopathy mapped to 20q13.3 and presenting with knee pain in childhood, mild symmetric weakness of neck flexion, shoulder abduction and elbow extension and with pelvic girdle weakness. Evidence of osteoarthritis with joint space narrowing, osteophytes, and femoral condylar bony flattening appears in mid-adult life. The serum CK is mildly elevated and muscle biopsy shows mild myopathic changes.

Multiple Errands Test A test of frontal-lobe planning function, wherein the subject has to complete a number of errands, such as shopping in an unfamiliar mall, according to a set of pre-learned guidelines.[5754]

multiple evanescent white spot syndrome The presence of small white dots deep to the retina and causing transient visual impairment. This may be a variant of the **big blind spot syndrome**; it is considered likely to be due to a virus infection.[1678]

multiple exercise-related mononeuropathies with colic A dominantly inherited syndrome characterized by painful motor neuropathies with abdominal pain, occurring after strenuous exercise.[6392]

multiple exostosis A rare, sporadic or dominantly inherited syndrome characterized by cartilaginous and bony protuberances, most often involving the metaphyseal regions of tubular long bones and capable of causing pressure on local nerves or myelopathy.[2026]

multiple lentigenes syndrome See **LEOPARD syndrome**.

multiple lipomatosis with chronic encephalopathy 1. The presence of benign intracranial lipomas in the corpus callosum or elsewhere. The symptoms in such patients are frequently the result of other brain malformations rather than of the lipomas.[343] 2. See **encephalocraniocutaneous lipomatosis**.

multiple mononeuropathy (mononeuritis multiplex) Acute haphazard infarction of various nerves, usually occurring asymmetrically, with resultant rapid motor and reflex loss, pain, and some sensory deficits adopting the sensory and/or motor topography of the nerves involved.

The sequential involvement of several nerves may, over the course of development, yield a clinical picture that gives a false appearance of symmetrical polyneuritis. The causes comprise any of the numerous systemic diseases, particularly the systemic vasculitides,[1773] Lyme disease, AIDS, and leprosy; diabetes; and multiple Schwannomas, and they also develop following dialysis.[1984] Each of these pathologies causes **persistent conduction block** at the usual sites of nerve compression.

multiple myeloma A gammopathy frequently complicated by slowly progressive neuropathies of various types. These include a mainly distal amyloid deposition with sensory and autonomic neuropathy; a distal axonal polyneuropathy; a sensory neuronopathy; or a neuropathy resembling **chronic inflammatory demyelinating polyneuropathy**. See also POEMS and **monoclonal gammopathy of uncertain significance**.

multiple nevoid basal cell carcinoma syndrome A dominantly inherited syndrome characterized by frontal and temporal skull bossing, the presence of multiple nevoid basal cell carcinomas in childhood or early adult life, and skeletal malformations including kyphoscoliosis.[2507]

Hydrocephalus, blindness due to corneal cataract, glaucoma, coloboma of the choroid and optic nerve, strabismus, a Marfanoid build, and numerous other endocrine, oral, and muscular abnormalities may be associated.[2504]

multiple peripheral nerve entrapments A syndrome which represents an unusual phenotypical variant of the Hunter Syndrome (**mucopolysaccharidosis**, type 2), in which multiple peripheral entrapments occur, particularly of the median and ulnar nerves.[3311]

multiple pterygium syndrome A rare, recessively inherited dysmorphic syndrome, characterized also by microcephaly, ptosis, vertebral fusion defects, scoliosis, and mental retardation.[1911, 1911]

multiple sclerosis (insular sclerosis, lobular sclerosis, polysclerosis, sclérose en plaques, MS) A disease of unknown cause most frequently affecting young adults and characterized by the presence of islands of perivascular demyelination anywhere in the central nervous system which give rise to intermittent or progressive neurological signs with highly variable presentations and courses. Most cases start with a relapsing-remitting course leading on eventually to a "progressive" phase but acute, benign, and subclinical forms also occur.

Following Charcot's written description, his student L. Ordenstein gave a fuller account of eight patients with this condition in his doctoral thesis (Martinet, Paris, 1867) in which he compared and contrasted the features of MS and of Parkinson disease, based upon the observations of Charcot and Vulpian. A superb engraving of the macroscopic appearance of MS affecting the spinal cord and brainstem was published by Robert Carswell in 1838 (printed privately in London) under the title "A peculiar diseased state of the chord and pons."

The clinical signs are characteristically more pronounced than the patient's symptoms would have suggested. In nearly half of all cases the disease begins monosymptomatically, the most frequent complaints being unilateral ocular pain and impaired vision, imbalance, sensory disturbances, weakness, and disturbances of micturition. Worsening of symptoms tends to follow infections, pregnancy, trauma, spinal anaesthetics, and increased body temperature from any cause.

The range of possible examination findings is almost unlimited, but some of the more common ones are as follows:

Optic nerve

- Retrobulbar neuritis, papillitis. This is the commonest of all manifestations of MS and produces a central more often than an arcuate scotoma or sectoral loss. More than half of the patients have other lesions shown on MRI scans.
- Perivenous sheathing (periphlebitis retinae) is a marker of increased disease activity.
- Retinal fiber layer slits, seen with red-free (i.e., green) light
- Impaired color vision
- Relative afferent pupillary defect (Marcus Gunn pupil)
- Field defects with chiasmal lesions.

Involvement of extraocular nerve function is shown as the following:

- III, IV, VI nerve palsies
- Gaze palsies
- Vertical, horizontal, pendular nystagmus, and impaired pursuit
- Cogwheel saccades
- Internuclear ophthalmoplegia.

Other cranial nerve involvement causes are

- Trigeminal pain (symptomatic **trigeminal neuralgia**)
- Facial palsy, facial myokymia
- Bulbar signs

Involvement in the remainder of the nervous system leads to the following:

- Cerebellar ataxia (see **Charcot triad** of nystagmus, ataxia, and slurred speech)
- Pyramidal (weakness, abnormal postures, spasticity, muscle spasms, hyperreflexia, abnormal reflexes)
- Posterior column sensory losses (much more than spinothalamic involvement)
- The **Lhermitte** symptom
- The **Uhtoff** (hot bath) sign due to the fact that conduction increases block at higher temperatures
- Hesitancy, urgency, incontinence, impotence with involvement of the autonomic nervous system.

Cortex

- Usually rather late in the course of the disease, cognitive impairment is commonly found, though it is not always remarked.
- *Facial pain attributed to multiple sclerosis* may be uni- *or* bilateral, with or without dysesthesias, and tends to remit and relapse. Pain may be tic-like, as in **trigeminal neuralgia**, or continuous. Trigeminal neuralgia occurring in young people or affecting one and then the other side should arouse the suspicion of multiple sclerosis.

The diary of Augustus **D'Este** and WNP Barbellion's *Diary of a Disappointed Man* (London, Chatto and Windus, 1919) poignantly recount their experiences of the disease.

Various defining diagnostic criteria have been drawn up. (See **Schumacher panel criteria, McDonald-Halliday criteria, Poser criteria** and [revised] **McDonald criteria**; Chart M–21.)[5094] **Charcot**'s criteria were published in 1868.[1097] The first descriptions of the disease were by Jean Cruveilhier 1835, Carswell in 1838 and **Frerichs** in 1849. A checklist of symptoms in multiple sclerosis[2633] and an **Illness Severity Score**[4351] have been created. See also **primary progressive multiple sclerosis;** *relapse;* and **pediatric multiple sclerosis**.

An "attack" of multiple sclerosis is an episode of neurologic disturbance that lasts for at least 24 h with either objective observation or a historical report with objective findings. The prognosis in an early case may be suggested by the age at onset, the initial presentation (optic neuritis, sensory symptoms, progressive weakness, and the presence of cerebellar signs), the annual attack frequency and the level of disability at 5 years being considered to be the best predictors.[6697]

A new set of clinical diagnostic criteria was suggested by McDonald and colleagues;[4216] revisions of these were suggested by an International Panel 4 years later. The revised criteria emphasize objective clinical findings, the demonstration of dissemination of lesions in space and time, use of supportive or confirmatory paraclinical examinations such as MRI, CSF analysis, and visual-evoked potentials, and the elimination of alternative clinical explanations. Chart M–21 provides an adapted summary.

Multiple Sclerosis Association of America A nationwide, nonprofit health agency providing patient and educational services and research support. Address: 706 Haddonfield Rd., Cherry Hill, NJ 08002. Tel: 856-488-4500; 800-532-7667. E-mail: msaa@msaa.com. Web site: http://www.msaa.com/. See also **National Multiple Sclerosis Association**.

Primary progressive multiple sclerosis is the term used for a distinct clinical phenotype of the disease that is progressive from its onset.[6296] Patients with this variety comprise some 10–15% of all of those with multiple sclerosis. The major presentations are motor deficits, sensory impairment, or cerebellar or brain stem symptoms. The peak age of onset at 40 years is a decade later than that of the classical variety of MS and progression is slightly slower.[6378]

Characteristics of primary progressive multiple sclerosis (disease with progression from its onset) are as follows:

Insidious neurologic progression suggestive of multiple sclerosis

– *One* year of disease progression (retrospectively or prospectively determined) and two of the following:

Positive brain MRI (nine or more MRI T2 lesions, or four or more T2 lesions) + positive VEP findings

Positive spinal cord MRI (i.e., two focal T2 lesions)

Positive CSF (see note 1 below)

In all cases, no better explanation for the clinical presentation can be shown. If the criteria are not completely met, but the clinical picture is suspicious, the diagnosis is "possible multiple sclerosis."

Note 1. The *CSF abnormalities supporting a diagnosis of multiple sclerosis* are the presence of oligoclonal bands detected by isoelectric focusing that are different from any bands in the serum, and an increased IgG index. (They are also present in tears, which are easier to harvest.)

Note 2. *MRI criteria for the demonstration of dissemination of MS lesions in time* are

Detection of gadolinium enhancement at least 3 months after the onset of the initial clinical event at a location different from that corresponding to the initial clinical event.

Detection of a new T2 lesion that was not present on a previous scan done at least 30 days after the onset of the initial clinical event.

The "new" lesion must be sufficiently large and located appropriately so that it is clear that it was not simply missed previously for technical reasons, such as slice orientation, thickness or spacing, patient motion, or other artifacts. T2 lesions developing in the first few weeks after onset of a first clinical episode are not considered to be a separate new event meeting criteria for dissemination in time.

The revised MRI criteria to demonstrate dissemination of the lesions in space are any three of the following:

An enhancing lesion or sufficient T2 hyperintense lesions

1. At least one gadolinium-enhancing brain or spinal cord lesion, or nine T2 hyperintense brain or spinal cord lesions (if there is no gadolinium-enhancing lesion).
2. At least one infratentorial or spinal cord lesion.
3. At least one juxtacortical lesion.
4. At least three periventricular lesions.

Various other sets of MRI criteria have also been suggested: one set is reproduced here (*Offenbacher et al*, 1993).[4755] At least three areas of increased signal,

Chart M–21. The 2005 Revisions of the McDonald Criteria for Multiple Sclerosis (after Polman et al. 2005)[5073]

For the diagnosis of multiple sclerosis one of the following is required:

A. In the case of two or more attacks with objective clinical evidence of two or more lesions, additional diagnostic tests are not required.
B. With two or more attacks but when there is objective clinical evidence of only one lesion, evidence of dissemination in space is required. This may be demonstrated either by MRI (see note 2 below) *or* by the presence of two or more. MRI-detected lesions consistent with MS *and* positive CSF findings (see note 1 below). Alternatively, a further clinical attack implicating a different site would allow the diagnosis.
C. When there has been only one attack but clinical examination reveals evidence of two or more lesions, evidence of dissemination in time is required—*either* by MRI (see note 2 below) *or* by the occurrence of a second clinical attack.
D. Where there has been only one attack and there is objective clinical evidence of only one lesion (the so-called "clinically isolated syndrome"), additional data required for the diagnosis of MS are:
   Evidence of dissemination in *space* as demonstrated by MRI *or* by the presence of two or more MRI-detected lesions consistent with MS, *and* positive CSF findings (note 1 below)
   and also
   Evidence of dissemination in time as shown by the MRI or by the occurrence of a second clinical attack
E. In the case of insidious neurological progression suggestive of MS, the additional data required are;
   Evidence that the disease has progressed over at least a year (determined retrospectively or prospectively) *and* two of the following;
   a. The presence of at least nine T2 MRI lesions or four or more T2 lesions *and* positive VEP results
   b. Two focal T2 MRI lesions in the spinal cord
   c. Positive CSF results (see note 1 below)

If additional diagnostic tests (e.g., MRI and lumbar puncture) are performed and are negative, extreme caution should be used in making a diagnosis of multiple sclerosis and alternative explanations should be carefully considered. (After Polman et al., 2005,[5073] reproduced by permission.)

with two of the following characteristics in addition:

1. Abutting the body of the lateral ventricles,
2. Infratentorial lesion location, and
3. Size >5 mm

and three of the following:

1. One gadolinium-enhancing lesion or nine T2-weighted hyperintense lesions if there is no gadolinium-enhancing lesion
2. At least one infratentorial lesion
3. At least one juxtatentorial lesion
4. At least three periventricular lesions

Secondary progressive multiple sclerosis indicates that the condition has become progressive after an initial relapsing–remitting course. The pathogenesis and eventual prognosis of these two forms is not known to differ, but they do exhibit differences in their MRI appearances, the former group developing fewer new lesions with less gadolinium enhancement over an observed period.

A possible variant is *transitional progressive multiple sclerosis (MS)* with an unusual presentation and course of disease.[2048] See also **benign multiple sclerosis** and ***chronic progressive multiple sclerosis***.

Guidelines for the diagnosis of multiple sclerosis in children have also been drawn up and are shown below under **pediatric multiple selerosis.**

It is difficult to assess minor cognitive impairment, but this is a problem in the early stages of multiple sclerosis. The first functions to be impaired are verbal memory, abstract reasoning, and linguistic processes. Appropriate assessment tools include the **MS Neuropsychological Screening Questionnaire** and the **Neuropsychological Screening Battery for Multiple Sclerosis**.

Multiple Sclerosis Clinical and Laboratory Research A subspecialty journal published by Arnold. Web site: http://www.arnoldpublishers.com /journals/pages/mul_scl/13524585.htm.

Multiple Sclerosis Foundation A charitable organization in this field. Address: 6350 North Andrews Ave., Ft. Lauderdale, FL 33309. Tel: 954-776-6805; 888-673-6287. E-mail: support@msfocus.org. Web site: http://www.msfocus.org/.

Multiple Sclerosis Functional Composite A test battery comprising three timed tests of neurologic function; a 25-foot walk, the nine-hole peg test, and a 3-s version of the **PASAT**. The battery correlates with the **EDSS**, MRI lesion load, and self-reported quality of life.[5464]

Multiple Sclerosis Impact Scale (MSIS-29) A reliable and sensitive, psychometrically designed, patient-reported measure of the effects of multiple sclerosis on their activities of daily living, of potential use as an outcome measure.[2925] It is accessible through www.jnnp.com.

Multiple Sclerosis Quality of Life Inventory An instrument addressing all of the functions covered by the SF-36 but also fatigue, pain, sexual satisfaction, bladder and bowel control, visual impairment, cognitive function, and social support. It calculates a number for the burden of illness suffered by individual MS patients.[5322]

Multiple Sclerosis Rating Scale A system for quantitating the findings noted on physical evaluation of patients with **multiple sclerosis**.[5873]

Multiple Sclerosis Severity Score An instrument that relates the Expanded Disability Status Scale and the distribution of disability in MS patients with comparable disease durations. It is offered as a powerful method for comparing disease progression using single assessment data.[5448]

Multiple Sclerosis Society of Canada A Canadian charitable organization dedicated to enhancing the quality of life of people coping with multiple sclerosis through specific assistance and funded research. Tel: 416-922-6065. Fax: 416-922-7538. E-mail: info@mssociety.ca. Web site: http://www.mssociety.ca/.

Multiple Sclerosis Spasticity Scale A reliable and valid 88-item patient-based measure of the impact of spasticity in multiple sclerosis.[2925]

Multiple Sclerosis Symptom and Impact Diary An instrument measuring the outcomes of MS in clinical trials, assessing, mobility, fatigue, and the overall impact of MS.[2568] It can be viewed at www.jnnp.com/supplemental/.

multiple sclerosis stages Arbitrary gradings of multiple sclerosis according to the temporal pattern of the disease.

1. Stable multiple sclerosis.
2A. Infrequent relapses (less than 1/year).
2B. Slowly progressive (deterioration in the expanded disability status scale of <0.5/year).
3A. Frequent clinical relapses (more than one attack/year).
3B. Rapidly progressive (deterioration in expanded disability status scale of >0.5/year).

multiple sensory neuritis See **Wartenberg sensory neuritis**.

multiple sleep latency test (MSLT) A standardized test of sleepiness carried out in a sleep laboratory by day, wherein the subject is allowed to fall asleep but is awakened shortly after each successful attempt; the latency to the onset of sleep is measured on each occasion while the usual parameters assessed during **polysomnography** are recorded. The test is of value in determining the premature onset of rapid eye movement sleep in patients with narcolepsy.[1043] See also **maintenance of wakefulness test**.

multiple sulfatase deficiency (Austin disease) A rare, recessively inherited metabolic disorder (a *variant* of **metachromatic leukodystrophy**), due to the deficiency of expression of at least seven distinct lysosomal sulfatases. Deficiency of arylsulfatases A, B, and C, as well as of other enzymes, leads to the accumulation of sulfatides, sphingolipids, glycolipids, and other substances in the tissues and body fluids. Clinical phenotypes resemble either **mucopolysaccharidoses** with the addition of ichthyosis, hypotonia and later hypertonia, minor ataxia, myoclonus, sensorineural deafness, pigmentary abnormality of the macula, optic atrophy, cerebellar and pyramidal signs, and mental and developmental delay; or they resemble **metachromatic leukodystrophy** (late infantile form).[301]

multiple symmetric lipomatosis

(Madelung disease) A rare sporadic or inherited mitochondriopathy presenting in adult life, characterized by the development of multiple lipomas of the neck and shoulder regions, frequently associated with peripheral neuropathy, proximal myopathy, and/or deafness.[4552] See **familial multiple symmetrical lipomatosis with peripheral neuropathy**.

multiple system atrophy

A term introduced by Graham and Oppenheimer in 1969 to include all of the adult-onset degenerative conditions of unknown cause showing selective involvement of various combinations of defined nuclei and long tracts within the CNS, as first described by Déjèrine and Thomas in 1900. Such structures have included the retinas; the optic, thalamic, and pyramidal pathways; the cerebellar cortex and deep nuclei; the inferior olives; the vestibular nuclei; the posterior columns; the spinocerebellar and spinothalamic tracts; and the anterior horn cells.

Clinically, any combination of extrapyramidal, pyramidal, cerebellar, and autonomic features may occur, and both gaze palsies and other disturbances of eye movements are described, as has the phenotype of **amyotrophic lateral sclerosis**.[5842] Onset is usually after the age of 45 years. The response to levadopa is transient and incomplete.

Pathologically, the hallmarks of the conditions are the distribution of the lesions in the olivopontocerebellar, pyramidal, and striatonigral systems and in the nuclei of Onuf, innervating the external sphincter muscles; the presence of argyrophilic intracellular cytoplasmic and nuclear inclusions in oligodendrocytes, neuronal cell bodies and axons; and the absence of neurofibrillary tangles and (usually) of Lewy bodies. The cellular pathology has been reviewed.[3697] The **olivopontocerebellar atrophies**,[1545] **striatonigral degeneration**,[51] and the **Shy-Drager syndrome**[5819] are all subsumed under this general heading. The characteristics of the two major forms have been summarized.[5157]

Striatonigral degeneration type (predominant Parkinsonism): Sporadic, adult-onset Parkinsonism, nonresponsive or poorly responsive to levadopa, without dementia, but manifesting down-gaze progressive supranuclear palsy with severe symptomatic autonomic failure, with or without cerebellar or pyramidal signs and areflexia.

The features distinguishing this from other causes of the Parkinsonian syndrome include the presence of autonomic symptoms, the occurrence of falls, a poor response to levadopa, the presence of speech or bulbar dysfunction and the absence of dementia and of levadopa-induced confusion.[6722]

Olivopontocerebellar atrophy type (predominantly cerebellar): A sporadic, adult-onset cerebellar, and/or pyramidal syndrome with severe symptomatic autonomic failure and/or Parkinsonism, manifest by mild bradykinesia or rigidity.

In a further *variant* form, the progression of the disease to death is rapid.[5842] http://www.nlm.nih.gov/medlineplus/ency/article/000757.htm provides further data from the NIH.

More recently, consensus criteria for the diagnosis of multiple system atrophy have been defined as in Chart M–22[2388] and future data are supplied in Charts M–23 and M–24.

multiple-contracture syndrome

See **multiple congenital contractures**.

multiple-spike complex

(polyspike complex) A sequence of two or more spikes recorded on the EEG.

multiple-step hypometric saccades

Refixations of the eye upon a target requiring more than two saccadic steps. This is occasionally present in normal subjects when fatigued but is always abnormal if dominantly present in one or other direction. In such cases, pyramidal or cerebellar disease may be the cause.

multiple-step saccadic refixations

Eye movements composed of multiple dynamic steps and pulses (**saccades**).

multiple-tic syndrome

See **Tourette syndrome**.

multiplex

(Lat, plaited or folded many times) A derivation ill-employed within the term *mononeuritis multiplex*, in which nothing of the sort happens. See **multiple mononeuropathy**.

multisensory syndrome

The effect of a mismatch between the visual, vestibular, and proprioceptive inputs informing a subject about his orientation in space, occurring as a result of disease affecting any two or all of them; thus a form of physiological vertigo.

Clinically, it is a condition characterized by the sensation of severe imbalance occurring as a result of deficits in conscious or unconscious proprioception, visual acuity, peripheral vision, dark adaptation, contrast sensitivity, and accommodative capacity, usually seen in elderly people.[1707]

multisystem atrophies

A heterogeneous group of diseases characterized by cell loss and variable amounts of gliosis occurring in one or more neuronal groups.[3324, 4801] See **system degenerations**.

multisystem disorder with cerebellar atrophy

A recessively inherited syndrome with adult onset, characterized by ophthalmoplegias,

Chart M–22. Diagnostic Criteria for Multiple System Atrophies[2387]

SND type	*Degree*	*OPCA type*
Sporadic onset, non/poorly responsive parkinsonism	Possible	—
The above ± severe symptomatic autonomic failure ± cerebellar ± autonomic signs	Probable	Sporadic adult-onset cerebellar ± pyramidal syndrome with severe symptomatic autonomic failure and/or Parkinsonism
Post-mortem confirmation	Definite	Post-mortem confirmation

In each case, autonomic failure is defined as postural syncope or presyncope and/or marked urinary incontinence or retention not due to other causes.
From Gilman S, et al. Consensus statement on the diagnosis of multiple system atrophy. 1989;163(1) reproduced by permission of Elsevier Ltd. © 1999.

Chart M–23. Diagnostic Categories of MSA

I. Possible MSA: one criterion plus two separate features from other domains. When the criterion is Parkinsonism, a poor levodopa response qualifies as one feature (hence only one additional feature is required).
II. Probable MSA: criterion for autonomic failure/urinary dysfunction plus poorly levodopa responsive Parkinsonism or cerebellar dysfunction.
III. Definite MSA: pathologically confirmed by the presence of a high density of glial cytoplasmic inclusions in association with a combination of degenerative changes in the nigrostriatal and olivopontocerebellar pathways.

Exclusion criteria for the diagnosis of MSA

I. History
   Symptomatic onset under 30 years of age
   Family history of a similar disorder
   Systemic diseases or other identifiable causes for features listed in Chart M–24
   Hallucinations unrelated to medication

II. Physical examination
   DSM criteria for dementia
   Prominent slowing of vertical saccades or vertical supranuclear gaze palsy.
   Evidence of focal cortical dysfunction such as aphasia, alien limb syndrome, and parietal dysfunction.

III. Laboratory investigation
   Metabolic, molecular genetic, and imaging evidence of an alternative cause of the features of the condition.

Chart M–24. Clinical Domains, Features, and Criteria Used in the Diagnosis of MSA

A feature (A) is a characteristic of the disease and a criterion (B) is a defining feature or composite of features required for diagnosis

I. Autonomic and urinary dysfunction
   A. Autonomic and urinary features
      1. Orthostatic hypotension (by 20 mmHg systolic or 10 mmHg diastolic)
      2. Urinary incontinence or incomplete bladder emptying
   B. Criterion for autonomic failure or urinary dysfunction in MSA. Orthostatic fall in blood pressure (by 30 mmHg systolic or 15 mmHg diastolic) or urinary incontinence (persistent, involuntary partial, or total bladder emptying, accompanied by erectile dysfunction in men) or both

II. Parkinsonism
   A. Parkinsonian features
      1. Bradykinesia (slowness of voluntary movement with progressive reduction in speed and amplitude during repetitive actions)
      2. Rigidity
      3. Postural instability (not caused by primary visual, vestibular, cerebellar, or proprioceptive dysfunction)
      4. Tremor (postural, resting, or both)
   B. Criterion for Parkinsonism in MSA; bradykinesia plus at least one of the items 2–4

III. Cerebellar dysfunction
   A. Cerebellar features
      1. Gait ataxia (wide-based stance with steps of irregular length and direction)
      2. Ataxic dysarthria
      3. Limb ataxia
      4. Sustained gaze-evoked nystagmus
   B. Criterion for cerebellar dysfunction in MSA. Gait ataxia plus at least one of the items 2–4

IV. Corticospinal tract dysfunction
   A. Corticospinal tract features
      1. Extensor plantar responses with hyperreflexia
   B. Corticospinal tract dysfunction in MSA: no corticospinal tract features are used in defining the diagnosis of MSA

Adapted from Gilman S, Low PA, Quinn N, et al. Consensus statement on the diagnosis of multiple system atrophy. J Aut Nerv Syst *1998;74:189–92, with permission from Elsevier Science.*

cerebellar and pyramidal signs, athetosis, anterior horn cell involvement, and sensory and autonomic neuropathy. See **multiple-system atrophies**.

multisystem mitochondrial cytopathy A rare syndrome consisting of ophthalmoplegia, pigmentary retinal degeneration, cardiac lesions, and dystonias.[306]

multisystem neuronal degeneration A syndrome of infancy characterized by pigmentary retinal degeneration, optic atrophy, failure to thrive, nerve deafness, progressive distal muscular atrophy with adrenal cortical hormone deficiency, hepatosplenomegaly, and mental and developmental retardation. Tissues show a consistent reduction in the contents of arachnidonic acid and other polyunsaturated fatty acids, but not of phytanic acid.

The syndrome resembles **adrenoleukodystrophy**, but that condition is not apparent at birth, tends to have a defined subacute onset, and is unassociated with retinitis pigmentosa, deafness, or hepatosplenomegaly. Generalized **gangliosidosis** is ruled out by finding an absence of deposited gangliosides, and phytanic acid levels are normal, thus excluding **hereditary motor and sensory neuropathy** type 4 (Refsum disease).[1784]

multisystem triglyceride storage disorder A recessively inherited congenital dysmorphic syndrome due to a defect in the degradation of endocellularly synthesized triglycerides; a neutral lipid storage disorder.

Clinically, it is characterized by microcephaly, short stature, lordosis, enlarged liver and spleen, vacuolated granulocytes, ichthyosis, diffuse depigmentation of the skin, proximal lipid storage myopathy, neurogenic atrophy, and mental and motor delay.[1624] Nystagmus, retinopathy, opacities of the lens and corneas, and nerve deafness are other features described. The underlying biochemical deficit is not yet determined.

Mulvihill progeria-like syndrome A congenital dysmorphic syndrome characterized by thinness, short stature, sparse fine hair, metopic ridges, sensorineural deafness, myopia, premature aging, micrognathia, dental anomalies, wide-spaced nipples, hypospadias and small penis, diabetes, deficient adipose tissue, hypohidrosis, skin atrophy and telangiectasia, microcephaly, bulbar weakness, and mental and developmental delay.[381]

Munchausen syndrome (hospital addiction, peregrinating problem patient syndrome, chronic factitious disorder with physical symptoms) The repetitive, factitious simulation of severe organic disease leading to numerous hospital consultations, admissions, and unnecessary operations. The patients also give false names, addresses, occupations, and histories. When recognized, or when apparently bored with their hospital experience, they discharge themselves, usually against forceful medical advice if their operation was recent. Their underlying motives have been listed as a desire to be the center of interest, a grudge against physicians and hospitals, which is satisfied by such deceptions, a desire for drugs, a desire to escape from the police, and a need for board and lodging.

The title has literary allusions. Henri **Meige** was actually the first to describe the syndrome, in his graduation thesis (University of Paris, 1893) but it was Dr. Richard Asher,[268] who defined the condition recently and dedicated the syndrome to Karl Friedreich Hieronymous, Baron Munchhausen (1720–1797), whose dramatic accounts of his exploits as an army captain serving with the Russian army against the Turks in the 1763–1772 war were similarly fabulous; it was thought that, at times, he seemed to lie merely for the sake of lying, according to the German writer and geologist Rudolph Erich Raspe in his fictional work *Baron Munchausen's Narrative of his Marvellous Travels and Campaigns in Russia* (London, 1785), published without the consent of the (real) Baron Munchhausen (sic).

Asher defined three varieties of the syndrome: the acute abdominal type (*laparotomophilia migrans*), which is the most common; the hemorrhagic type; and the neurological type, this last presenting with complaints of paroxysmal headache, loss of consciousness, or peculiar fits. He noted the consistent pattern of behavior, with no obvious motive or gain from it, but found no consistent psychiatric abnormality. The syndrome can also occur by proxy, as when a parent claims that a child has symptoms and may go on to contaminate samples collected and repeatedly presents the child for medical attention, while there is recovery when the child is separated from that parent or guardian.[4273]

Munchmeyer, Ernst (1846–1880) German physician who first described **myositis ossificans**,[4549] although "a woman who has become as hard as wood" was mentioned by Dr. Patin in a letter to Dr. Falret, a physician in Troyes, in 1648.[5704]

Munchmeyer syndrome See **myositis ossificans**.

Munch–Petersen encephalomyelitis See **Redlich encephalitis**. Dr. Carl Julius Munch-Petersen was a Danish physician who described this form of encephalomyelitis in 1932.

Munich Coma Scale A tool for the assessment of behavioral arousal (or depth of coma) using two additive scales which measure *susceptibility to stimulation* by electrical, tactile, acoustic, and optical stimuli, and *reactivity*, for which motor, mimic, orienting, and communicative movements are assessed. Verbal responses are not examined.[843]

Despite the sensitivity of this instrument, the **Glasgow Coma Scale** has been utilized more widely.

Munk, Hermann German anatomist who suggested the presence of a post-Rolandic sensory cortex in 1868.

Munson sign Protrusion of the lower lid on downward gaze as a result of pressure from **keratoconus**.

Munzer-Rosenthal syndrome See **Rosenthal syndrome**.

Muratov syndrome Hemichorea following a cerebrovascular episode, the lesions being in the mesencephalon and thalamus.[4557]

Murdoch syndrome A congenital dysmorphic syndrome characterized by sensorineural deafness, telecanthus, hypertelorism, colobomas and atrophy of the iris, detached retina, myopia, antimongolian slant, dental enamel abnormalities, inguinal hernia, recurrent infections, seizures, and mental and developmental delay.[381]

Murray valley encephalitis (Australian X disease) Direct infection of the brain (polioencephalitis) by a flavivirus member of the togavirus class of arboviruses occurring endemically in Victoria (Australia) and New Guinea. The clinical features resemble those of Japanese encephalitis.[519, 1201]

Murri, Augusto (1841–1932) Italian physician.

Murri syndrome A generalized parenchymatous cerebellar atrophy of late adult onset, presenting with slowly progressive signs of vermis involvement and probably caused by chronic alcohol abuse in the original cases reported.[4561]

muscae volitantes Vitreous floaters, composed of collagen fibrils and leading to the perception of specks drifting around in the visual field, lagging behind but restituting in position after a voluntary eye movement. Unlike some other phenomena pertinent to aging, these are benign (unless harbingers of retinal detachment). See **floaters**.

muscle (dim. of Lat, a little mouse) The contractile organ of the body.

***Muscle & Nerve* (*Muscle Nerve*)** A specialist scientific journal published monthly since 1977 by John Wiley and Sons, New York. The journal has been adopted as the official organ of the **American Academy of Neuromuscular and Electrodiagnostic Medicine** and publishes original contributions in the field of neuromuscular disease with an emphasis on electrodiagnosis. Web site: http://www.interscience.wiley.com/muscleandnerve/.

muscle action potential See **compound muscle action potential**.

muscle aplasia Inherited developmental anomalies characterized by the failure of formation of certain muscles or muscle groups; the congenital absence of certain muscles or groups of muscles. Syndromes include the absence of the glutei, of the thenar muscles, of the trapezii, and of the pectoralis major either alone (**Poland anomaly**) or with the absence of the serratus and latissimus dorsi (a dominantly inherited syndrome).[379] See also **blepharophimosis, cardiofacial syndrome, CHILD syndrome, David anomaly, diaphragmatic aplasia, Duane syndrome, Möbius syndrome, congenital ptosis, Holt-Oram syndrome, palmaris longus aplasia, peroneus tertius aplasia, Poland syndrome, prune belly syndrome, Souques syndrome, thenar aplasia**, and **trapezius aplasia**.

muscle atrophy Reduction in the size or number of the myofibrils, and thus of the fascicles within muscles, as a result of disuse or disease.

muscle carnitine palmitoyl transferase deficiency (CPTase deficiency) A myopathy characterized by cramps and myoglobinuria, usually related to exercise but also induced by fasting or a high-fat diet, and due to a defect in the utilization of the long-chain fatty acids by skeletal muscle resulting from a deficiency of muscle CPTase.[1648]

muscle-contraction headache See **episodic tension-type headache**.

muscle cramp syndrome A dominantly inherited syndrome charaterized by neurogenic muscle cramps at rest, in sleep and with exertion.[1147]

muscle cramps Painful involuntary contractions of muscles, usually associated with electrical activity (cramp discharge). Muscle cramps may be accompanied by other types of repetitive discharges, and, in some metabolic myopathies such as McArdle disease (a **glycogen storage disease**), the painful contracted muscle may show **electrical silence**.[162]

muscle disease See **myopathies** for general classification.

muscle–eye–brain disease (MEB disease, Santavuori syndrome) A congenital, recessively inherited dysmorphic syndrome characterized by congenital myopia, glaucoma and retinal hypoplasia, mental retardation, and structural brain involvement (pachygyria, flat brainstem, and cerebellar hypoplasia). The mutant gene is mapped to 1p32-p34. Patients present in the neonatal period with profound muscle hypotonia and poor visual alertness.

Patients at the severe end of the spectrum remain bedridden, never achieve sitting, head control, or visual contact. These patients may die during the first years of life. Moderately affected patients usually show high myopia, but have some preserved vision enabling them to establish contact. Their maximum motor ability is to sit unsupported, and occasionally speak a few words. Muscle enlargement can be present. Patients at the milder end of the spectrum may acquire ambulation for a number of years. Often their functional abilities are more impaired by the coexistence of spasticity and ataxia than muscle weakness. Vision is preserved in these patients and limited verbal communication skills possible. Seizures are common. The ocular problems include high myopia, retinal dysplasia, persistent hyperplastic primary vitreous, glaucoma, and cataracts. Giant visual-evoked potentials are typical.

Associated CNS malformations range from pachygyria/polymicrogyria/agyria, partial callosal agenesis, hypoplasia the pyramidal tracts and obstructive hydrocephalus to mere flattening of the brainstem, vermis hypoplasia, and cerebellar cysts.[4555] See also **Fukuyama congenital muscular dystrophy**[5544] and **Walker Warburg syndrome**, both of which are also characterized by congenital muscle dystrophy and cerebral malformations based on migration disorders, with differing genetic locations.[1286]

muscle fiber action potential An action potential recorded from a single muscle fiber.

muscle fiber conduction velocity The speed of propagation of a muscle fiber action potential, expressed in meters per second (M/s).[19]

muscle hypertrophy Enlargement of a muscle due either to an increase in the size of its myofibrils or (pseudohypertrophy) replacement or displacement of the myofibrils by material such as fat or amyloid. Myofibrils increase in size physiologically in response to repetitive, strong voluntary contraction or pathologically as the result of abnormal electrical activity, such as **myotonic** or **complex repetitive discharges**.

muscle-paretic nystagmus (myasthenic nystagmus) A form of gaze-evoked nystagmus resulting from abnormal fatigability of the extraocular muscles (as in **myasthenia gravis**) in which a slow drift of the tiring, deviated eyes toward the primary position is corrected by brief saccadic movements resembling genuine nystagmus.[5618]

muscle pain-fasciculation syndrome See **cramp-fasciculation syndrome**.

muscle phosphofructokinase deficiency See **glycogen storage diseases**.

muscle phosphorylase b kinase deficiency See **glycogen storage diseases**.

muscle quantitation Methods for determining the power of muscle on a prospective basis. These have included the **Medical Research Council Scale**, muscle strength myometry using an instrument to measure the voluntary strength of muscle groups, and assessments of motor ability (**Hammersmith Motor Ability Score**).[5690] See also **quantitative neuromuscular examination**.

muscle sense The term of Sir Charles **Bell** for *position sense* (proprioception) or *sense of movement* (kinesthesis). These are, however, derived from information transmitted from tendon and joint receptors and not from any receptors within muscles themselves.

muscle stretch reflexes (phasic muscle stretch reflexes) Reflex muscle contraction in response to a sudden lengthening or vibratory stimulus. Oblique early descriptions of the phenomenon were provided by Robert **Whytt** and by S. **Weir Mitchell**. These reflexes were called *tendon reflexes* by Erb in 1875, who published his paper in a journal edited by Westphal, whose own observations on the knee phenomenon were printed in a paper adjacent to that of Erb. **Gowers** revised this term to *knee jerk*, which is prosaic and restricted but memorable.

The term *deep tendon reflex* is rejected, both because the tendons struck must obviously be superficial and because the response to afferent discharges emanating from the Golgi tendon organs actually inhibits contraction. Scales for reflex activity have been designed. See NINDS **myotatic reflex scale**.

muscle tone (tonus) The constant slight tension characteristic of healthy muscle, which offers a steadily maintained resistance to passive stretching; thus the amount of resistance to passive stretch is supplied by muscles. It is recognized by the resistance experienced when the limbs are moved or displaced by the examiner. (Sir Gordon **Holmes**).

In the case of postural muscles, it is also defined as "the steady contraction of muscles dependent on the activity of spinal reflexes but modifiable by supra-segmental mechanisms, the function of which is the maintenance of posture or postural adaptation" (Sir Charles **Sherrington**).[5788]

In healthy states, tone is related to the inherent elasticity of the muscles, but in disease states it reflects a reduction in supraspinal influences upon the reflex arc or is due to damage to the reflex arc itself.

MuscleNet from The World Muscle Society—WMS A site providing information on neuromuscular disorders, cardiomyopathies, and the recent advances of the scientific research on these subjects. It also contains a study companion in muscle biology and various links in this field. Web site: http://www.worldmusclesociety.org/.

muscles of fixation Muscles which stabilize neighboring joints and thus assist in the efficient performance of the contraction of other muscles. See also **agonists, antagonists**, and **synergists**.

muscular atrophy, diabetes mellitus, and ataxia A rare dominantly inherited syndrome characterized by the onset in childhood or adolescence of the features listed in the title, together with pigmentary retinal degeneration. The intellect is unaffected and the phytanic acid levels are normal.[4845]

muscular atrophy in cretins See **Debré-Sémélaigne syndrome**.

muscular dystrophies Inherited progressive disorders of muscle. Those that are assigned to this heading[6869] are listed in Chart M–28 (Disorders of Muscle; A. Heritable Myopathies).

The terminology used in this area is imprecise. Traditionally, the term "muscular dystrophy" has been used to denote those inherited disorders of muscle that are progressive, while "myopathy" was applied either to all disorders of muscle or just to those that are acquired. The traditional definition of muscular dystrophy is used in this book, while myopathies are regarded simply as disorders of muscle of any nature. Thus, all muscular dystrophies are myopathies, but not all myopathies are muscular dystrophies. See also the NINDS Muscular Dystrophy Information Page Web site at http://www.ninds.nih.gov/disorders/md/md.htm/.

Muscular Dystrophy Association (MDA) A charitable association providing support and information on this condition, amyotrophic lateral saclerosis, etc. National Office: 3300 E. Sunrise Drive, Tucson, AZ 85718. Tel: 520-529-2000; 800-572-1717. E-mail: mda@mdausa.org. Web site: http://www.mdausa.org. Also at 10 East 40th Street, Room 4110, New York, NY 10016. Tel: 212-689-9040 and at 3561 East Sunrise Drive, Tucson, AZ 85718. Tel: 1-800-572-1717. Web site: http://www.als-mda.org/disease/als.html/.

Muscular Dystrophy Association of Canada A Canadian charitable organization in this field. Web site: http://www.muscle.ca/.

Muscular Dystrophy Family Foundation An American charitable organization in this field. Address: 2330 North Meridien St., Indianapolis, IN 46208. Tel: 317-923-6333; 800-544-1213. E-mail: mdff@mdff.org. Web site: http://www.mdff.org/.

Muscular Dystrophy Group of Great Britain and Northern Ireland A British charitable organization and member society of the European Alliance of Muscular Dystrophy Societies. Web site: http://www.touchlondon.co.uk/business/list/bid/99053.

muscular infarction A rare complication of diabetes in which thrombotic occlusive disease of the small muscular arteries of the quadriceps leads to infarction of that muscle.[371]

muscular pain-fasciculation syndrome A chronic neuromuscular syndrome characterized by muscle aching and burning pain, fasciculations, cramps, fatigue and occasional paresthesias affecting the legs more than the trunk, girdle muscles and arms, worsened by physical activity, and due to a mild axonal motor neuropathy.[3028]

Musella Foundation for Brain Tumor Research and Information A charitable organization in this field. Address: 1100 Peninsula Blvd., Hewlett, New York, NY 1155.7. Tel: 516-295-4740. E-mail: musella@virtualtrials.com. Web site: http://www.virtualtrials.com/.

mushroom myopathy A subacute myopathic syndrome caused by *Amanita phalloides* mushroom ingestion.[2469] The onset of symptoms generally occurs >6 h after ingestion. Massive rhabdomyolysis associated with respiratory failures and myocarditis, acute tubulopathy, **erythromelalgia**, and encephalopathy have also been described as complications of the ingestion of certain types of wild mushroom.[475]

music The art or science of arranging sounds in notes and rhythms to give a desired pattern or effect (Jacobs, 1967, quoted by Brust[922]) (See also Critchley and Henson[1340]).

musical alexia and agraphia Inability to comprehend or reproduce musical notation (as opposed to verbal language); a function still unlateralized as well as inexactly localized, despite the popular belief that receptive amusia follows damage to the language-dominant side and expressive amusia follows nondominant frontal-lobe damage.[922]

musical hallucinations Hallucinated music occurring in association with deafness, or with lesions of the brainstem, or of the frontal or temporal regions.[4289]

musician overuse syndrome (musicians' cramp) Painless focal task-specific dystonia of the hand occurring as an occupational dystonia.[2220] There is a positive family history of dystonia in up to 10% of cases.

Strict union regulations prevent overuse of the musicians themselves.

musicogenic epilepsy (musicolepsy, musicolepsia, sonogenic reflex epilepsy, audiogenic epilepsy) A form of reflex epilepsy occurring in young adults who suffer simple or complex partial seizures, more rarely secondary generalized atonic-clonic seizures precipitated by certain musical airs or sometimes by music played by certain combinations of instruments. However, thinking about, remembering, or playing music may also act as a precipitant.[1325] The first description has been attributed to Merzjejeuvski who presented a case in St. Petersburg in 1884.

The seizure may originate from either side in this condition (even though music function is considered to be lateralized to the right hemisphere, at least in nonmusicians) and the stimulus may be exquisitely specific; for example, in Sutherling's patient,[6142] the seizures were triggered only by playing a specific hymn ("*Nun danket*; Now Thank We All Our God") on the organ. Critchley and Henson[1340] reviewed the reports to 1977.

musicolepsia See **musicogenic epilepsy**.

musicolepsy See **musicogenic epilepsy**.

Muskelsvindfonden A member society of the European Alliance of Muscular Dystrophy Societies based at Vestervang 41, DK-000 AARHUS C, Denmark. Web site: http://www.muskelsvindfonden.dk/.

Musset sign A rhythmic nodding of the head as a consequence of ballistic (vascular) forces resulting from severe aortic incompetence. The name remembers the French novelist and poet Alfred de Musset (1810–1857), who was thus affected as a result of a syphilitic aortic aneurysm.

Mutchinick syndrome A congenital dysmorphic syndrome characterized by dwarfism, fine hair, hypertelorism, blepharophimosis, antimongolian slant, high-arched palate, brachycephaly, microcephaly, spasticity, and mental and developmental delay.[381]

mutilating acropathy See **ulceromutilating acropathy** and **hereditary, sensory** and **autonomic neuropathy**.

mutism 1. Loss of power of making sounds with the larynx. 2. Loss of power of making articulate sounds or speech; absence of verbal output.

mutism and subsequent dysarthria See **cerebellar mutism**.

myalgia Pain arising from muscles, especially following exertion. Pathologies such as tumor, infection, ischemia, or infarction are important causes, but for neurologists, **polymyositis**, and other inflammatory diseases of muscle such as **polymyalgia rheumatica**, and almost all metabolic muscle diseases such as **cramps, chronic fatigue syndrome, lipid myopathy, myalgia cruris epidemica, myoadenylate deaminase deficiency, glycogen storage disease, mitochondrial encephalomyopathy**, and **hypothyroid myopathy** are of particular interest.

A *variant* is *exercise-induced pain, stiffness, and tubular aggregations in skeletal muscle* with a persistent elevation of the serum creatine kinase levels but normal EMG and forearm ischemic exercise test results. A muscle biopsy specimen shows aggregations of tubular structures in most fibers.[911]

myalgia cruris epidemica See **benign acute childhood myositis**.

myalgic encephalomyelitis See **postinfection fatigue syndrome** and **chronic fatigue syndrome**.

myasthenia (Lat, muscle + debility) Muscle fatigability.

myasthenia gravis (Erb-Goldflam syndrome) An autoimmune disorder, commoner in women, in which antibodies to the acetylcholine motor end-plate receptors (AChRs) lead to loss of their structure and function. The pathogenic effects on neuromuscular transmission are mediated by antibody-induced antigenic modulation of end-plate AChR, end-plate membrane destruction through complement fixation and recruitment of inflammatory cells, and antibody-induced blockade of the function of the remaining AChR molecules. See also **neuromuscular junction disorders**.

Clinically, it is characterized by impairment of neuromuscular transmission, leading to fluctuating weakness and fatigability of, in order of severity, the ocular, bulbar, and limb muscles. The deficit is lessened by cooling and increased with warmth,[748] which may be of value during electrical testing. See **ice-pack test, Tensilon Test**, and **single fiber EMG**. Assay of AChR antibodies however, is considered to be the gold standard, if slightly impure by virtue of the fact that there are some cases in which the titer is low.

The generalized *adult* form is that generally recognized; it was described in an Amer-Indian in 1644 and by Thomas **Willis** in 1672,[6805] but the first modern descriptions were those of **Erb**[1899, 1900] and of Sir Samuel Wilks (1824–1911), who described the manifestations as part of a treatise on bulbar paralysis in 1877.[6788] The clinical features are described variously among the entries in Chart M–25.

Two subgroups are differentiated; a *severe* (or even *acute fulminating*) type, most common among young women, is associated with the HLA8 antigen; and another form, occurring mainly among older patients, is associated with thymoma and with the presence of the HLA2 or A3 antigens.

Physostigmine, the first effective treatment, was introduced by Dr. Mary Walker, an intern at St. Alfege's Hospital, Greenwich, UK, who tried it in a 56-year-old woman with myasthenia, having discussed the similarity of myasthenia and curare poisoning with the visiting neurologist, Dr. **Denny Brown**. She published the result as a letter in the *Lancet* on June 2, 1934 (cited by Keynes G[3411]).[5286]

Presynaptic pathologies lead to defects in the evoked release of acetylcholine (ACh) quanta or ACh resynthesis (ChAT mutations). Lesions at the synaptic basal lamina are usually caused by mutations in the collagen tail of AChE; and postsynaptic pathologies are caused by mutations in subunits of AChRs. Presynaptic defects include congenital myasthenia with episodic apnea (familial infantile); a form due to paucity of synaptic vesicles and reduced quantal release; and *congenital Lambert-Eaton-like syndrome* and **episodic ataxia** 2. Postsynaptic defects include disorders of the acetylcholine receptor (AChR) with or without kinetic abnormalities in AChR function with a reduced number of AChRs at neuromuscular junctions (NMJs) and with either increased or reduced responses to ACh: with a normal number of AChRs at NMJs or with an increased number of AChRs at NMJs, or with rapsyn mutations or plectin deficiency. See also Dr. Alan Pestronk's Web site: http://neuromuscular.wustl.edu/synmg. html#scs/.

A listing of the types of myasthenia gravis is presented in Chart M–25.

A scale rating the severity of myasthenia gravis, based on that of Osserman,

Chart M–25. Forms of Myasthenia Gravis

Adult form, as above

Myasthenia gravis and dystonia with diurnal fluctuation, characterized by congenital ptosis, ophthalmoplegias, dystonia, tremor, and muscle fatigability varying by time of day

A. *Heritable varieties*:

Familial myasthenia gravis (recessive form) is characterized by strabismus; ptosis; enlarged thymus; ophthalmoplegias; facial, distal, and proximal myopathic weakness and fatigability with onset before the age of 2 years. In a similar form with later onset (2–20 years) there is no recognizable pattern of inheritance.[936]

Familial infantile myasthenia (congenital MG with episodic apnea) A presynaptic syndrome of myasthenia (10q11.2) inherited as a recessive trait and characterized by fluctuating ptosis and ophthalmoplegia; feeding difficulties in infancy; facial, distal, and proximal myopathic weakness and fatigability after exercise; and attacks of apnea precipitated by crying, vomiting, or fever. Enlargement of the thymus and unusually small synaptic vesicles in the nerve terminals are found.[4465, 4587] The condition responds to anticholinesterases and may remit in time.

Familial limb-girdle myasthenia A heterogeneous group of recessive myasthenic syndromes manifesting progressive weakness in a proximal limb-girdle distribution that begins in the first or second decade of life with a decremental EMG response on 3 Hz stimulation and a favorable response to anticholinesterases. The oculobulbar muscles are spared except for slight facial weakness and ptosis in some patients. Short-term fatigability induced by exercise is not a feature and anti-AChR antibodies are absent. Pathologically, the neuromuscular junctions are small.[1862] Diagnosis is achieved with repetitive nerve stimulation and single fiber EMG. Tubular aggregates are sometimes seen in skeletal muscle in the familial form.[4766, 5348] Mild elevations of serum CK levels may be found and the EMG findings usually suggest a myopathy. An arrhythmogenic cardiomyopathy sometimes occurs in association.[4266] Linkage to chromosome 4 has been established. A *variant* is

Congenital myasthenia with DOK7 mutations. A recessively inherited condition that presents between birth and the third decade with limb-girdle weakness, a waddling gait, respiratory insufficiency, and ptosis but without ophthalmoparesis. Patients do not benefit from therapy with cholinesterase inhibitors. The neuromuscular junctions are small and simplified (*synaptopathy*) but acetylcholine receptor (AChR) and acetylcholinesterase functions are normal.[4544, 4861] Some cases have mutations in the gene coding *rapsyn*, a postsynaptic molecule which stabilizes AChR aggregates at the neuromuscular junction. The phenotypes are as follows: a severe neonatal form; more benign cases starting during infancy; and cases with arthrogryposis and/or facial malformations.[1939] In some cases, linkage to chromosome 11p.11 has been established.

Congenital myasthenia gravis: A recessively inherited group of myasthenic syndromes occurring in infants, in which anti-AChR-Abs are absent. Thymectomy, immunosuppression, and plasmapheresis are ineffective and spontaneous remissions do not occur. Presynaptic (impaired resynthesis or packaging of ACh); synaptic (absence of acetylcholinesterase from the end-plate); and post-synaptic (abnormal receptor) varieties are defined; various mutations are responsible.

The clinical patterns described include the following (adapted from Beeson, Palace et al. 1997).[478] In the *typical form*, in which infants are born to nonmyasthenic mothers, the disease resembles the typical postsynaptic form, except that anti-AChR-Abs are absent, the external ocular muscles are prominently involved, and the usual forms of treatment are ineffective. At least three subgroups are described in this category.[936] One form (endplate acetylcholinesterase [AChE] deficiency, see below) is mapped to 3p25.

Congenital myasthenia with ptosis, ophthalmoplegia, proximal weakness, and fatigability unresponsive to anticholinesterases.[6385]

Congenital MG with MuSK mutations A recessive form (9q31.3–q32, *MuSK*) in which there is reduced expression of AChRs. Onset is in the neonatal period with respiratory involvement and later bulbar involvement, ptosis, upgaze limitation, mainly proximal limb weakness also affecting the neck extensors, and fatigue. The signs may improve during childhood.

Other presynaptic syndromes include *familial infantile myasthenia with tetanic facilitation*, and *congenital Lambert–Eaton syndrome;*[4138] *abnormality of synaptic vesicles* with reduction in quantal release;[4465] and *familial immune myasthenia,* recessively inherited with the onset between 2 and 20 years of features similar to those of nonfamilial adult myasthenia, but usually without anti-AChR antibodies.

A form in which the ophthalmoplegia is mild and nonprogressive, and there is proximal, distal, and facial myopathic atrophy and weakness with fatigability. Muscle biopsy shows group atrophy and fiber-type predominance. Anti-AChR antibodies are absent and treatment with immunosuppressants is ineffective.[2007]

A recessively transmitted form in which facial malformations such as prognathism and high-arched palate are associated with a postsynaptic neuromuscular transmission defect.[5492]

Juvenile myasthenia gravis An acquired autoimmune disorder in which circulating antibodies to ACh receptors and complement together reduce the number of functioning ACh receptors available on the motor end plate, and thus interfere with normal neuromuscular transmission.[202] The clinical features are the same as those in #1 above, but with slightly earlier onset.

Recurrent congenital ***arthrogryposis***, which occurs in children born to women with myasthenia, usually untreated. See also **Pena–Shokeir** syndrome.

Myasthenia gravis with myotonic dystrophy, in which myotonia complicates otherwise typical adult myasthenia.

Pseudocholinesterase deficiency (suxamethonium paralysis).

Congenital end-plate ACh receptor deficiency: A rare postsynaptic, recessively inherited form occurring in the neonatal period or in infancy, in which there is a deficiency of ACh receptors due to their abnormal synthesis or reactivity. Clinical features include congenital ptosis, kyphoscoliosis, lordosis, and myopathic distal and proximal weakness, atrophy, and fatigability.[1876, 1877, 1870] Decrementing responses can be found in all voluntary muscles and, due to the prolonged interactions of ACh and its receptors, a single supramaximal stimulus to a motor nerve elicits more than one compound muscle action potential.[477] Various mutations at 2q24, 17p.113, 2q33, and 17p13 have been identified.[4992]

End-plate acetylcholinesterase deficiency, a relatively common, recessive, postsynaptic form (3p25) in which acetylcholinesterase is absent or markedly deficient at the neuromuscular junction. It presents in infancy (rarely) or later with severe fatigue, weakness, episodes of respiratory distress, lack of response to anticholinesterases, and repetitive CMAPs in response to a single stimulus.[4775, 478]

Slow-channel congenital myasthenic syndromes: Dominantly inherited or sporadic postsynaptic disorders presenting in childhood or young adult life with selective weakness, fatigability, and atrophy of the muscles of the neck, shoulder girdle, and forearms, with variable involvement of the extraocular and other muscles, due to abnormally slow closure of the ACh receptor ion channel.[1878] An acquired form, presenting in later adult life, is also described.[6832] Linkages to chromosomes 2 and 17 (involving variously α, β, δ, or ϵ ACh receptor subunits) have been defined.[4992]

Decreased amplitude of the miniature end-plate potential without ACh receptor deficiency is a putative defect in ACh synthesis or packaging.[1870]

Congenital persistent (neonatal persistent) myasthenia, a syndrome characterized by congenital ptosis, ophthalmoplegia, and distal and proximal myopathic weakness and fatigability.

Infantile myasthenia, characterized by ptosis and respiratory distress in the neonate, with muscle fatigability.

ACh receptor channel fast closure: A congenital myasthenic syndrome characterized by ocular and limb weakness and fatigability from birth, with later improvement. High conductance and fast closure of the ACh receptor channel are demonstrable.[1879]

Forms with *abnormal interaction between ACh and the ACh receptor*[6433] or with presynaptic disorders involving the resynthesis or packaging of ACh.[4464]

Fast channel syndrome[1879] A recessively inherited form with neonatal onset in which there is a reduced affinity of the ACh receptor for ACh molecules. At least three other fast-channel variants are also described.[4992]

B. *Toxic varieties:*

1. **Botulism**
2. **Tick paralysis**
3. **Puffer-fish paralysis** (tetrodotoxin)
4. Magnesium intoxication
5. Unwanted effects of kanamycin and other antibiotics[4267]
6. *Myasthenia due to penicillamine*: A disorder mimicking idiopathic myasthenia gravis, even including the detection of anti-ACh receptor antibodies, occurring in subjects taking penicillamine.[2291] Anticonvulsants and quinidine have also been implicated as causing the same problem.

C. *Autoimmune varieties*:

1. **Myasthenia gravis** (see above)
   a. *Transient neonatal myasthenia*. A form in which the affected infant is born of a woman with myasthenia; within 72 h of birth, feeding difficulties, generalized weakness, respiratory difficulties, and facial weakness with ptosis are seen, lasting a few days. Pharmacological tests are frequently positive and the condition responds to anticholinesterase medication and respiratory support.[4586]
   b. Ocular myasthenia with peripheral neuropathy and spastic paraparesis[924]
   c. Generalized myasthenia:
      i. severe, especially in young women, correlated with HL-A8
      ii. in older patients, often with thymoma and with HL-A2 or A3
   d. Myasthenia with thyrotoxicosis
   e. Myasthenia with hypothyroidism[6190]
   f. Myasthenia with other autoimmune diseases
   g. Myasthenia combined with **Lambert–Eaton myasthenic syndrome**[4763]
   h. Myasthenia with the **Satoyoshi syndrome**[5554]

D. **Lambert-Eaton (myasthenic) syndrome**

anti-AChR-Abs = antibodies to acetylcholine motor end-plate receptors; ACh = acetylcholine; HLA = human lymphocyte antigen

Based upon Verma P, Oger J. Treatment of acquired autoimmune myasthenia gravis. Can J Neurol Sci 1992;*19:*360–75;[6531] *search of recent literature; and data from Dr. Alan Pestronk's Web site*: http://neuromuscular.wustl.edu/synmg.html#lgm/.

recognized five degrees of severity but a more modern scale has been devised.[3169] These authors also provide a table for the quantitation of disease severity based on assessment of 13 single functions.

Myasthenia Gravis Foundation of America Clinical Severity Classification[3168]

Class I Any ocular muscle weakness; may have weakness of eye closure but strength in other muscles' is normal.

Class II Mild weakness affecting other than ocular muscles. May also have ocular muscle weakness of different degrees of severity.

IIa Predominantly affecting limb, axial muscles, or both; may also have lesser involvement of oropharyngeal muscles.

IIb Predominantly affecting oropharyngeal, respiratory muscles, or both. May also have lesser or equal involvement of limb, axial muscles, or both.

Class III Moderate weakness affecting other than ocular muscles; may also have ocular muscle weakness of different degrees of severity.

IIIa Predominantly affecting limb, axial muscles, or both; may also have lesser involvement of oropharyngeal muscles.

IIIb Predominantly affecting oropharyngeal, respiratory muscles, or both; may also have lesser or equal involvement of limb, axial muscles, or both.

Class IV Severe weakness affecting other than ocular muscles; may also have ocular muscle weakness of different degrees of severity.

IVa Predominantly affecting limb and/or axial muscles; may also have lesser involvement of oropharyngeal muscles.

IVb Predominantly affecting oropharyngeal, respiratory muscles, or both; may also have lesser or equal involvement of limb, axial muscles, or both.

Class V Defined by the need for intubation, with or without mechanical ventilation, except when employed during routine postoperative management. The use of a feeding tube without intubation places the patient in class IVb.

(Reproduced by kind permission of the American Academy of Neurology and Lippincott Williams and Wilkins.)

See also **midbrain myasthenia**.

Myasthenia Gravis Association A charitable organization in this field. Address: 77 Nottingham Rd., Derby DE1 3QS, UK. Tel: +44-332-290219. Web site: http://www.mgauk.org/.

Myasthenia Gravis Foundation of America Inc. A voluntary organization dedicated to the conquest of myasthenia through programs of research, education, and information and patient services, including support, diagnostic, and therapeutic services. Web site: http://www.myasthenia.org/.

Myasthenia Gravis Society A charitable organization providing support and information on this condition. Address: 25 Caravan Drive, Don Mills, Ontario, Canada M3B 1M9. Tel: 416-444-8357.

Myasthenia Severity Scale A scale for assessing impairment in myasthenic crisis.[5161]

Dyspnea:	1 = intubated; 2 = dyspnea at rest; 3 = dyspnea on exertion; 4 = no dyspnea.
Cough:	1 = intubated; 2 = weak; 3 = normal.
Ocular:	1 = weakness at rest; 2 = weakness on fatigue; 3 = none.
Bulbar:	1 = weakness at rest; 2 = weakness on fatigue; 3 = none.
Extremities:	1 = worst affected muscle 3/5 or less; 2 = worst affected muscle 4/5 motor strength or weakness on fatigue; 3 = no detectable weakness.

myasthenic crisis Abrupt deterioration in strength in a myasthenic patient, due to exacerbation of the defect in neuromuscular transmission, either as a result of the natural progression of the disease or because of the effects of drugs which further reduce the availability of acetylcholine to the end plate.

myasthenic myopathy 1. The occurrence of fatigability in patients with primary myopathic diseases; the symptoms may be partially responsive to anticholinesterase medication. 2. Persistent proximal weakness and wasting complicating longstanding **myasthenia gravis**.

myasthenic nystagmus An asymmetric gaze-evoked nystagmus which may be in any direction and which is relieved by intravenous edrophonium chlopride. See **muscle-paretic nystagmus**.

myasthenic syndrome See **Lambert-Eaton myasthenic syndrome**.

myasthenic syndrome in hypothyroidism A *variant* which may resemble the **Lambert-Eaton myasthenic syndrome** but which is considered to be due to conduction block in the fine terminals of the motor axons.[6190]

Mycoplasma pneumoniae An organism capable of widespread infection usually causing non-neurologic disease in young people, but rarely able to cause a heterogeneous spectrum of clinical manifestations such as meningoencephalitis, acute disseminated encephalomyelopathy (ADEM), transverse myelitis, seizures, PNS involvement, and stroke. Concomitant postinfectious hemorrhagic encephalitis and peripheral or central demyelinating disorders have also been described.[5957]

mycotic aneurysm (septic aneurysm) An aneurysm developing due to weakening of an arterial wall as a result of infection. Bleeding into the substance of the brain or into the subarachnoid space may result. See **aneurysm**.

mydriasis Pupillary dilatation, usually accepted as being greater than 6 mm in diameter. It is due to paresis of the iris by drugs (mydriatics) or disease or is due to emotion. This use of the word is attributed to Galen, but Areteus used it to refer to pupillary constriction and Hippocrates is said to have used the word *mydros* for the cautery tool that he employed—an instrument likely to produce fear and its attendant sympathetic manifestations. See also **Pourfour du Petit syndrome**.

mydriatic A drug which paralyzes the iris and thus causes pupillary dilation. Atropinic derivatives, ephedrine, cocaine, and some synthetic agents are examples.

myelencephalon The term of Huxley for **metencephalon**.

myelin (from Gr, marrow) The insulating fatty substance ensheathing axons, so named by Virchow in 1854.

myelin basic protein An immunogenic structural component of myelin, of which it forms about 40% of the total protein. When injected with Freund's adjuvant into animals, it induces experimental allergic encephalomyelitis, a paralytic disease. There is evidence that it appears in a higher concentration in the blood of **multiple sclerosis** patients during exacerbations.

myelin-associated glycoprotein (MAG) A component of myelin, metabolites of which can be detected in the CSF but which cannot be linked to active demyelination. Patients with high serum IgM antibody levels to MAG may present with gait ataxia and polyneuropathy.

myelin stains Histological enhancement methods which preferentially stain myelin. They include the Weigert-Pal, Spielmeyer, Weil, and Marchi methods, variously employing hematoxylin, osmium tetroxide, Luxol fast blue (a copper-containing dye staining myelin bright blue) and metallic salts with borax ferricyanide, iron alum, lithium, and/or alcohol. See also **axon stains**.

myelinated nerve fibers Fibers bearing myelin and also myelinated and also nonmyelinated and demyelinated fibers, the diameter of which is in the range of the normal population of myelinated fibers.[2653] See **medullated (myelinated) nerve fibers**. In the retina this is a developmental anomaly occurring in 1% of the population in which myelination extends beyond the lamina cribrosa or the optic nerve head, appearing as striated white patches with feathery borders and caused by differential myelination of individual axons. It is bilateral in 20% of cases and is continuous with the disk in almost all. Usually, visual acuity is normal and the condition is benign.

myelination The process of myelin accumulation around axons during pre- and postnatal development, and following de-myelination.

myelinoclastic disease Conditions in which normally formed myelin is damaged, as opposed to **dysmyelinating** diseases, in which the myelin itself is abnormally constituted.[5090]

myelinopathia centralis diffusa See **vanishing white matter disease**.

myelinopathy A pathological process affecting peripheral nerves in which there is paranodal or segmental demyelination. Cf. **neuronopathy, axonopathy**.

myelinosclerosis centralis diffusa See **fatal infantile leukodystrophy**.

myelitis Originally this was defined as "Inflammation of the Central Nervous System with Particular Effects upon the Myelin" (Marshall Hall), but this definition has been discarded in favor of one which regards myelitis as inflammation of the spinal cord only, inflammation of the brain being called **encephalitis** and both together, **encephalomyelitis**.

Classifications have been based upon the following categories: *topical* (transverse, ascending or descending, central, marginal, or funicular), *structural* (poliomyelitis, leukomyelitis), or *etiological*. **Neuromyelitis** indicates the combined involvement of the spinal cord and cranial or peripheral nerves. See **acute intrinsic myelopathy, acute transverse myelitis, encephalomyelitis,** and **paraneoplastic syndromes**.

myelitis with predilection or anterior horn cells resembling motor neuron disease A **paraneoplastic syndrome** associated with carcinoma, usually of the lung, breast, or stomach, and manifesting muscle weakness and atrophy with fasciculations and pyramidal signs affecting the bulbar and/or spinal muscles and resembling typical **amyotrophic lateral sclerosis** in everything but a slower course to death.[803]

myelocele (Gr, marrow + a cavity) A form of failure of closure of the neural tube in which the protruding sac contains meninges and CSF, but no nervous tissue.

myelodysplasia Developmental abnormalities of the spine and spinal cord. These include **diplomyelia, myeloschisis, hydromyelia, syringomyelia,** and **diastematomyelia**.

myelography The introduction of a solution of iodinated substances into the subarachnoid space at lumbar levels in order to outline the extent of the space by radiography as a diagnostic test for intrinsic or extrinsic spinal cord or root disease. A useful but unpleasant test, now giving way to MRI scanning where it is available.

myeloma See **multiple myeloma**.

myelomalacia Noninflammatory softening of the spinal cord.

myelomeningitis Inflammation of the spinal cord and the meninges surrounding it.

myelomeningocele See **meningomyelocele**.

myeloneuropathy A disorder affecting both the spinal cord and the peripheral nerves or nerve roots. **Tabes dorsalis** was a classic example but other conditions are probably (in aggregate) more prevalent today. See **Cuban** and **Tanzanian epidemic neuropathy, recurrent optic neuromyelitis with endocrinopathy,** and **HTLV-1 myelopathy. Vernant disease,** tuberculous neuropathy, and hemorrhagic fevers are other listed causes.

myelopathic muscular atrophy See **amyotrophic lateral sclerosis**.

myelopathy Disease of the spinal cord. See also **progressive necrotic myelopathy; myelitis; myeloneuropathy; pseudocervical cord syndrome**; and **copper deficiency myelopathy**.

myelopathy complicating diabetes mellitus See **diabetic myelopathy**.[2371]

myelopathy with optic neuritis See **neuromyelitis optica**.

myeloplegia Paralysis resulting from a lesion of the spinal cord.

myeloradiculitis See **HIV-associated lumbosacral polyradiculopathy**.

myelosclerosis (Gr, marrow + induration).

myelotomy See **cordotomy**.

myenteric (Gr, muscle + the intestines) The smooth muscle in the wall of the intestines.

myenteric plexus (Gr, myenteric + weaving) Auerbach's plexus of autonomic nerve fibers within the muscular wall of the intestines.

Myerson, Abraham (1881–1948) Lithuanian-American psychiatrist and neurologist who trained at Tufts and became professor of neurology and psychiatry at Harvard. Most of his major publications were on psychiatric topics, but he is remembered for the following signs.

Myerson reflex Contraction of the biceps and pectoralis on both sides or only on the opposite side, when the clavicle is tapped. The reflex is present in patients with pyramidal lesions.[4563]

Myerson sign See **orbicularis oculi reflex**.

myesthesia Muscle sense; the sense of the position of the parts of the body as a result of afferent impulses from muscle receptors and thus a form of proprioception.

Myhre syndrome (growth deficiency-clefting-retardation) A congenital dysmorphic syndrome characterized by muscular build, high birth weight, short stature, cleft upper lip, cleft palate, platyspondyly, constrictive pericarditis, thick ribs, duodenal ulcers, hypoplastic iliae, hypospadias, cryptorchidism, arthropathy, deafness, hypermetropia, spina bifida occulta, thick calvarium, muscle hypertrophy, facial weakness, and mental and developmental delay.[381]

myo- Greek prefix signifying relationship with a muscle.

myoadenylate deaminase (MADA) A muscle enzyme responsible for catalyzing the deamination of adenosine monophosphate, producing energy and ammonia.

myoadenylate deaminase deficiency syndrome (MADD) A common familial or acquired metabolic myopathy which is often asymptomatic, but in some cases is expressed clinically as a syndrome of muscle pain, cramp, and fatigue induced by exercise, sometimes with fixed proximal weakness and wasting, hyporeflexia, paresthesia, and repeated infections in childhood or young adult life.[869] Using the **ischemic forearm exercise test**, serum ammonia levels increase absolutely by 100 uG/dl in normals but by less than this amount in those with MADD. The lactate/ammonia ratio is high in this condition but low in the glycogenoses.

The *acquired form* is associated with a range of other muscle disorders. Adenosine monophosphate deaminase activity is undetectable in the muscle biopsy specimens of such patients.[1654]

myoatrophy Muscle atrophy; a more proper but less euphonious term than amyotrophy.

myoclonia (Gr, muscle + confused motion) Intermittent convulsive jerks of muscles. See **myoclonus**.

myoclonic absence attacks (clonic absence attacks) An epileptic syndrome characterized by rhythmic jerks occurring at 3 Hz throughout the body, but most obviously seen in the shoulder girdle, frequently leading to elevation of the arms and backward tilting of the head. The attacks occur in infancy, childhood, or youth, and are accompanied by 3-Hz spike-and-wave discharges on the EEG. Mental deterioration is a feature in some patients. See **myoclonus**.

myoclonic absence status epilepticus Proximal, predominantly upper extremity myoclonic jerks corresponding with 3 Hz spike-wave discharges on the EEG, lasting hours or even days and usually resistant to therapy.[1861]

myoclonic astatic seizures (akinetic seizures, Doose syndrome, static seizures, minor motor epilepsy, propulsive petit mal, akinetic petit mal, severe myokinetic epilepsy of childhood with slow spike-and-wave) A generalized epilepsy syndrome of infancy and childhood presenting in the first 5 years of life and characterized by daily myoclonic, astatic, or myoclonic-astatic seizures that are increased in the drowsy state, and by mental and developmental delay. The last may be due to a static encephalopathy. Treatment resistance is common, the family history often positive for epilepsy. Despite this definition, it has been suggested that this syndrome may not be unique but rather representative of atonic seizures.[1861] The course is variable with regard to seizure outcome, both complete remission and persistent epilepsy being recorded. Cognitive development may be normal or delayed.[6441]

The EEG typically records background theta activity and slow (2-4 Hz) spike–wave activity between seizures, and generalized multiple spike–wave bursts during them.[4757, 3423] See **Lennox-Gastaut syndrome, myoclonus, myoclonic epilepsies,** and **absence seizures**.

myoclonic encephalopathies A collection of cerebral diseases in which **myoclonus** occurs. Mitochondrial encephalopathies, malabsorption syndromes, multiple-systems atrophy and the various causes of the **Ramsay-Hunt syndrome** are examples.

myoclonic encephalopathy of infancy (infantile polymyoclonia, dancing eyes syndrome, dancing eyes-dancing feet, opsoclonus, ataxic conjugate movements of the eyes, Kinsbourne-Warrington syndrome) A generalized, recurrent but nonprogressive, self-limiting, and benign myoclonic disorder of late infancy. Clinical features of diagnostic value include the acute onset of opsoclonus and somatic myoclonus (especially of the trunk and head) in a previously normal infant, often following a minor infection or complicating aseptic meningitis. The condition runs a fluctuating but protracted course, but may remit with steroid therapy.[1788, 3443] No laboratory abnormalities are found. See **opsoclonus**.

In *variant* forms, the condition is associated with **neuroblastoma**[6642] or with progressive cranial nerve palsies.

myoclonic encephalopathy with progressive cranial nerve palsies See **Unverricht-Lundborg-Lafora syndrome**.

myoclonic epilepsy in infancy (formerly *benign myoclonic epilepsy in infancy*) See **benign** and **severe myoclonic epilepsy (Dravet syndrome)** in infancy.

myoclonic epilepsy of adolescents See **juvenile myoclonic epilepsy**.

myoclonic epilepsies (myoclonic astatic epilepsy) Seizure syndromes of infancy and childhood characterized by various types of tonic, atonic, absence, and myoclonic seizures, leading to repeated falls. The conditions are resistant to therapy. See **early myoclonic epilepsy, benign myoclonic**

epilepsy in infants, severe myoclonic epilepsy in infants, myoclonic absences,[6220] **juvenile myoclonic epilepsy of Janz,** and **Unverricht-Lundberg-Lafora syndrome.**[6833] The term is considered by some to be interchangeable with **Lennox-Gastaut Syndrome.**

myoclonic epilepsy with ragged-red fibers (Fukuhara syndrome)[2233] See **MERRF** and also **mitochondrial diseases.**

myoclonic epilepsy with supranuclear ophthalmoplegia See **myoclonus.**

myoclonic ocular jerks See **ocular myoclonus.**

myoclonic seizure A seizure type in which EMG records during the attacks show biphasic or polyphasic potentials, lasting between 20 and 100 ms, followed by a tonic contraction of the affected muscles or by a transient suppression of normal tonic activity lasting up to 350 ms; EEG findings include generalized burst or polyspike-and-waves or spike–wave activity.[72]

These single, or irregularly recurrent motor events resemble clonic seizures, which are rapid, rhythmically recurrent events. See **juvenile myoclonic epilepsy.** Localized reflex myoclonus can also occur.[1861]

myoclonic status epilepticus The occurrence of irregular bilateral or generalized myoclonic jerking without impairment of consciousness, lasting hours or days and most often seen in infants with nonprogressive encephalopathies such as poorly controlled **juvenile myoclonic epilepsy, Dravet syndrome, lissencephaly,** or **nonprogressive myoclonic epilepsy in infancy,** particularly **Angelman syndrome.** In **myoclonic-astatic epilepsy,** it predominates in the extremities of the upper limbs and around the mouth, the areas most represented in the precentral gyrus.[1861, 4882]

myoclonic triangle That part of the brainstem bounded by the inferior olivary nuclei, the cerebellar dentate nucleus and the red nucleus, with their interconnections in the central tegmental tract and the superior and inferior cerebellar peduncles. The term recognizes that lesions of any of these structures may give rise to ocular (and sometimes to reticular) **myoclonus.**[2623] See **Guillain-Mollaret triangle.**

myoclonic variant of Lennox-Gastaut syndrome A form of the syndrome in which the frequency and intensity of the myoclonic jerks are both unusually high. The EEG is typical, except that it is activated by overbreathing.[72] See **Lennox-Gastaut Syndrome.**

myoclonic writer's cramp The occurrence of repetitive myoclonic jerks precipitated by writing.[5212]

myoclonique de la calotte See **palatal myoclonus.**

myoclonus Sudden regular or irregular brief, jerky, or shocklike involuntary contractions of muscle fibers, muscles or muscle groups, as a manifestation of hyperexcitability in the nervous system at any level between the cerebral cortex and the spinal cord, and unassociated with alteration in consciousness.

The term derives from **Friedreich** in 1881, who called such movements "paramyoklonus multiplex." Two major subdivisions of myoclonus are defined, according to whether or not the movements are fragments of an epileptic syndrome.

Epileptic myoclonus is said to be focal, elicited by stimuli, accompanied by large somatosensory-evoked potentials and enhancement of long-loop reflexes, and responsive to anticonvulsants. *Cortical reflex myoclonus* is considered to represent a fragment of **partial epilepsy;** *reticular reflex myoclonus* and *primary generalized epileptic myoclonus* are fragments of types of **generalized epilepsy.**

Nonepileptic myoclonus consists of massive spontaneous bodily jerks, with normal somatosensory-evoked potentials and long-loop reflexes and with a poor response to anticonvulsants.[4247]

Using an anatomical basis for classification, **spinal/propriospinal, segmental, brainstem-reticular,** and **cortical** forms can be defined. *Essential myoclonus* is the term used when none of the above appear appropriate. The existence of *psychogenic myoclonus* attests to the astounding variety of responses of which the stressed human is capable.

Hallett[5798] has shown that with *cortical* myoclonus the movements are shock-like, occurring with maintenance of a posture or during movement. They are irregular, but may appear rhythmic, and are highly sensitive to stimuli. *Subcortical* myoclonus is less shock-like, occurs at rest, may be periodic, and is not sensitive to stimuli. *Spinal myoclonus* can be shock-like, occurs at rest, can be either periodic or rhythmic, and can be stimulus-sensitive.

Positive myoclonus refers to abnormal involuntary movements produced by single motor units or groups of motor units discharging synchronously but not rhythmically for about 100 ms in many or all of the muscles of a limb. *Negative myoclonus* (see **asterixis**) is also described. The electrical characteristics of myoclonus have been reviewed.[5796]

Myoclonus may also be classified according to whether it is triggered by stimuli (**stimulus-sensitive [reflex] myoclonus**) or is spontaneous (**non-stimulus-sensitive myoclonus**)[2696] or again by whether it is *rhythmic* (see **palatal** and **ocular myoclonus**), *oscillatory* (see **ballistic movement overflow myoclonus**), or *arrhythmic* (most forms). The palatal form, characterized by fast-recurring small-amplitude movements of the palate, probably represents **myokymia.** See also **photomyogenic response.**

Jerks of massive bilateral myoclonus mainly involve the upper limbs, with elevation of the shoulders producing slight contraction of the trunk. See also **myoclonic-astatic epilepsy, progressive myoclonic epilepsy, startle, hyperekplexia, benign myoclonic epilepsy,** and **Dravet syndrome.**

In a typical **myoclonic motor seizure** there are sudden, brief (<100 ms) involuntary single or multiple contraction(s) of muscles(s) or muscle groups of variable topography (axial, proximal limb, distal).[1861] A listing of forms of myoclonus is presented in Chart M–26.

See also **paramyoclonus multiplex; photomyogenic response; palatal myoclonus; myoclonus-dystonia;** and **opsoclonus.** The Myoclonus Fact Sheet is a useful data resource compiled by the National Institute of Neurological Disorders and Stroke. Web site: http://www.ninds.nih.gov/disorders/myoclonus/myoclonus.htm/.

myoclonus bodies See **Lafora bodies.**

myoclonus, deafness, and cerebellar ataxia See **myoclonus.**

Chart M–26. A Listing of Causes of Myoclonus

1. *Epileptic myoclonus*. Myoclonic syndromes in which rapid bursts of action potentials occur as neurons discharge synchronously, detectable as spikes on the EEG. The EMG burst length associated with the muscle jerk is usually <50 ms; muscles active in the same jerk are activated synchronously and an EEG correlate can be identified.[2695] Such epileptic myoclonic syndromes include the following:

   a. *Fragments of epilepsy:*

   Isolated epileptic myoclonic jerks
   Epilepsia partialis continua
   Idiopathic stimulus-sensitive myoclonus
   Photosensitive myoclonus and myoclonic absences in petit mal
   Cortical reflex myoclonus
   Reticular reflex myoclonus
   Photic reflex myoclonus
   Primary generalized epileptic myoclonus
   Unverricht–Lundborg–Lafora syndrome

   b. *Childhood myoclonic epilepsies:*

   Benign myoclonus of infancy (cryptogenic myoclonic epilepsy[72]). An idiopathic syndrome characterized by the onset in the first year or two of life of myoclonic and generalized tonic–clonic seizures that disappear in adolescence. The affected children are otherwise neurologically unimpaired; but the EEG shows spike/polyspike-and-wave activity.[5353]
   Early myoclonic encephalopathy: An idiopathic, probably recessively inherited syndrome characterized by the onset in the first month of life of massive myoclonic seizures, progressing to infantile spasms during the first 6 months of life.[72]
   Juvenile myoclonic epilepsy (of Janz): A syndrome with onset in youth, characterized by myoclonic and generalized tonic or tonic–clonic seizures, especially upon waking from sleep. The EEG typically shows polyspike and wave discharges.
   Myoclonic absences: A syndrome with onset in childhood or youth, characterized by the absence of attacks with myoclonus, associated in some cases with progressive intellectual decline. The EEG shows 3 Hz spike-and-wave discharges.[6220]
   Myoclonic astatic epilepsy (**Lennox–Gastaut syndrome**).
   Myoclonic astatic epilepsy of early childhood: An idiopathic syndrome characterized by the onset in the first 5 years of life of myoclonic, astatic, absence, and generalized tonic–clonic seizures. The affected children are neurologically unimpaired at onset, but the prognosis is variable. The EEG shows spike/polyspike-and-wave activity.[1692]
   Severe myoclonus of infancy: An idiopathic syndrome characterized by the onset in the first year of life of myoclonic and clonic seizures with progressive neurological deterioration. The EEG shows spike/polyspike-and-wave activity.[5353] See also **neonatal myoclonic encephalopathy**.
   West syndrome (infantile spasms).

   c. **Benign familial myoclonic epilepsy** (Rabot).

   Other *variant* forms include the following:
   Myoclonus and chorea: A syndrome of infancy or childhood characterized by myoclonic seizures, cerebellar ataxia, and chorea.[3611]
   Myoclonus, deafness, and cerebellar ataxia: A syndrome of childhood characterized by sensorineural deafness, cerebellar ataxia, and myoclonus. See **May–White syndrome**.[4187]
   Myoclonus–dystonia
   Familial chorea with myoclonic epilepsy: An apparent association of these two syndromes.[6189]
   Myoclonus epilepsy with Lafora bodies: A degenerative disease with onset in childhood or youth, manifesting dysarthria, dementia, seizures and myoclonus, cerebellar ataxia and spasticity, and neuronal inclusions (Lafora bodies).
   Myoclonic epilepsy with signs of spinal muscular atrophy.
   Myoclonus epilepsy with supranuclear ophthalmoplegia: A rare, recessively inherited syndrome of ataxia followed years later by epilepsy, myoclonus, mild dementia, and supranuclear ophthalmoplegia. Pigmentary retinopathy has also been recorded in this condition.[3897]

2. *Nonepileptic myoclonus*: Myoclonic syndromes in which the underlying disorder is not characterized as epileptic on the basis of the EEG and in view of the lack of accompanying clinical events. The EMG burst length associated with the muscle jerk is usually 50–300 ms; muscles active in the same jerk are usually activated asynchronously and may be alternating; and no EEG correlate can be identified.[2695] This class includes the following:

   1. *Physiological myoclonus*: Sleep jerks (**hypnic jerks**), sneezing, hiccough, and myoclonus induced in otherwise normal subjects by anxiety or exercise.
   2. *Essential myoclonus*: A sporadic or familial syndrome characterized by the occasional occurrence of isolated myoclonic jerks in the absence of other neurological deficits. This syndrome also includes **periodic movements of sleep** or nocturnal myoclonus.
   3. **Ballistic movement overflow myoclonus**.
   4. *Exaggerated* ***startle***.
   5. *Segmental myoclonus* See **spinal myoclonus; propriospinal myoclonus;** and **palatal myoclonus**.
   6. *Symptomatic myoclonus*: Syndromes in which a progressive or static encephalopathy dominates the clinical picture, and in which myoclonus is a characteristic clinical feature. Classes of disease associated include storage diseases; spinocerebellar degenerations; basal ganglion degenerations; dementing diseases; viral, metabolic, toxic, and physical encephalopathies; and other conditions involving focal CNS damage. See **Lafora body disease; dyssynergia cerebellaris myoclonica; lipidoses; MELAS;** and **MERFF**.

myoclonus-dystonia A rare, dominantly inherited syndrome with clinical and genetic heterogeneity, characterized by the onset in childhood or adolescence of myoclonic and dystonic muscle contractions, mainly of the neck and arms, in the absence of other signs of neurological disease and with a relatively benign course. The movements are often responsive to alcohol and both alcohol dependence and obsessive-compulsive disorders may be associated.[5563] Other features are mild dystonias such as torticollis and writer's cramp. Dementia, ataxia, and seizures are not associated.

The course of the disease is variable, both progression and spontaneous remission of the motor symptoms having been described.[4592] The unusual irregular, tremor-like dystonic movements of subcortical origin last 50–200 ms and are often superimposed upon sustained dystonic contractions. Time-locked EEG discharges do not precede the movements.[4745]

The condition has been mapped to 7q21-q31 (mutations in the *epsilon-sarcoglycan* [*SGCE*] gene)[4725] but also to other loci, indicating that the disorder is genetically heterogeneous. It has been suggested that myoclonic dystonia, **hereditary dystonia with lightning jerks, essential myoclonus,** and **benign hereditary chorea** can be grouped into one entity, *inherited myoclonic dystonia*.[1055]

In *variant* forms, the onset is very early; or distal myoclonus and involvement of the legs are found.

myoclonus epilepsy with Lafora bodies See **myoclonus**.

Myoclonus Research Foundation, Inc. A public charity supporting research in myoclonus, investigating its basic mechanisms, and developing new therapies. Address: 200 Old Palisade Rd., Suite 17D, Fort Lee, NJ 07024. Tel: 201-585-0770. See also the Web site: http://www.myoclonus.com/.

myodynamometer An instrument for measuring muscle power.

myodynia Muscle pain. The term has now been replaced by **myalgia**.

myodysplasia fibrosa multiplex See **familial myosclerosis**.

myodystrophia fetalis deformans See **arthrogryposis multiplex congenita**.

myoedema Slow dimpling and then elevation of a muscle due to localized contraction following percussion, the contraction spreading across the muscle surface. It resembles myotonia except that it is electrically silent, but is classically seen in some hypothyroid patients and also in **cachexia**.[4663]

myofascial pain dysfunction See **Costen syndrome**.

myofascial pain syndromes (fibromyalgia, fibromyositis, myo-fibrositis, fibrositis, myofascial pain, myospasm; "fibrositis" was Gowers' term in 1904) Syndromes of enduring localized muscle aching or pain, stiffness, fatigue and local tenderness without definite pathology, muscle biopsy, or EMG abnormalities, known cause or cure. Weakness of muscle is however a real feature.[4703] The condition is a common cause of prolonged pain and disability.

Certain muscles are particularly vulnerable—such as the upper fibers of the trapezius, gluteus medius, piriformis, spinati, deltoid, and sartorius. Prolonged stress, spinal degenerative disease, irritable bowel disturbances, a sensation of joint swelling, anxiety, paresthesias, skin-fold tenderness, and certain features of somatic dysthymia such as nonrestorative sleep are all associated.

The condition is commonly and appropriately diagnosed by those who believe in it, but is ignored or derided by others.[6942] The criteria of the American College of Rheumatology require symptoms of generalized pain for at least 3 months and pain by palpation at 4 kg at more than 11 out of 18 specified tender point locations, ignoring the usual systemic symptoms.[6847] Diagnostic criteria for fibromyalgia are to be found at the Web site: http://www.rheumatology.org/publications/classification/fibromyalgia/fibro.asp?aud=mem/.

myofibrillar (desmin-storage) myopathy (desmin storage myopathy, familial desminopathy, spheroid body myopathy, cytoplasmic body myopathy, Mallory body myopathy, familial cardiomyopathy with subsarcolemmal vermiform deposits, myopathy with intrasarcoplasmic accumulation of dense granulofilamentous material) Hereditary myopathies presenting in mid-adult life with proximal, distal, and respiratory muscle weakness; a scapuloperoneal syndrome and/or cardiomyopathy; and a myopathic EMG with abnormal electrical irritability and either normal or elevated serum CK levels. Pathologically, focal degradation primarily affects the myofibrils, which may contain vacuoles and hyaline spheroid cytoplasmic inclusions reacting intensely for actin, and in which numerous proteins such as desmin, lamin-B, gelsolin, ubiquitin, dystrophin, g-sarcoglycan, and a1-antichymotrypsin as well as amyloid may accumulate.[159, 5715] Mutations in the filamin C gene (*FLNC*) are considered responsible. See also **inclusion body myositis, intermediate filament disorders**, and **myopathy**.

The following entries concerning subtypes are based upon the Neuromuscular Web site at Washington University, St. Louis (http://www.neuro.wustl.edu/neuromuscular/maltbrain.html) by courtesy of Dr. Alan Pestronk.

Myofibrillar myopathy with desmin mutations (OMIM 601419) Dominant or recessively inherited myopathies mapped to chromosome 2q35 and resulting from a mutation in the desmin gene.

The *dominant form* produces early distal progressing to proximal weakness and wasting leading to wheelchair use eventually in most cases. Cardiac involvement is common with right bundle branch block, ST segment depression, and syncopal episodes, sometimes requiring a pacemaker. The serum CK levels are normal or mildly elevated, and the EMG and biopsy findings myopathic.

A *variant is familial hypertrophic cardiomyopathy*, also dominantly inherited and characterized by a desmin point mutation causing cardiomyopathy. This form has also been mapped to chromosome 10q.[4292]

In the *recessive form*, the syndrome is dominated by cardiomyopathy with onset in early childhood, progressing to facial, girdle, and respiratory muscle weakness within a decade or two. High-arched palate and scoliosis are associated features. Biopsy shows hyaline/desmin plaques resembling Mallory bodies and amorphous subsarcolemmal material, immunoreactive for desmin and dystrophin.

Myofibrillar myopathy: aB-crystallin mutations (Type 1) A dominantly inherited condition due to a missense mutation at

11q22.3-q23.1. Clinically, the onset is in early adult life with slowly progressing proximal and distal, facial, and bulbar weakness, but cardiac death can occur as a result of cardiac arrhythmias, conduction block, or congestive failure. Associated signs include lens opacities and intestinal malabsorption. Serum CK levels are somewhat elevated, and the EMG and muscle biopsy findings myopathic with loss of the intermyofibrillar network in type I fibers, accumulations of granulofilamentous material containing phosphorylated desmin, and autophagocytosis (http://www.neuro.wustl.edu/neuromuscular/maltbrain.html).

Myofibrillar myopathy with arrhythmogenic right ventricular cardiomyopathy (ARVC) A dominantly inherited condition due to a mutation at 10q22.3. Clinically, the onset is in adult life of mild axial, distal, or generalized muscle weakness with cardiomyopathy and rhythm disturbances. The EMG is myopathic and biopsy findings include myofibrillar disorganization, rimmed vacuoles, and accumulation of desmin.

In another *variant* form, also dominantly inherited, the onset of proximal and distal weakness with dysphagia occurs at any time, and cardiac findings are less common. Muscle biopsy shows the presence of cytoplasmic or spheroid bodies associated with desmin.

myofibrositis See **myofascial pain syndromes**.

myogelosis See **myofascial pain syndromes, fibromyalgia**.

myoglobin A respiratory pigment with a low renal threshold, found in muscles; it is capable of binding oxygen, which it releases only under conditions of low partial pressure of oxygen, as with sustained exertion and in certain diseases, as mentioned under **myoglobinuria**.

myoglobinuria The excretion of myoglobin into the urine as a result of necrosis of muscle membranes, with the subsequent liberation of all of their contents into the circulation. Clinically, the affected muscles are weak, swollen, and tender during attacks and the urine may be pink, red, or black, depending on the degree of myoglobinemia. The condition results from impairment of fuel usage by skeletal muscle in numerous conditions and causes proximal more than distal weakness, muscle pain and swelling, and often fever.

Hereditary and acquired causes of the syndrome are numerous;[5442, 5446] metabolic disorders such as the **glycogen storage diseases, malignant hyperthermia, lipid myopathies,** and others with an unknown metabolic basis are in the former group; overexertion, muscle ischemia, electric shock, crush injury, **polymyositis**, and metabolic and toxic causes (e.g., alcohol, drugs, *hornet venom*,[502] and **quail myopathy**) account for most of the latter. Renal failure is a well-recognized complication of myoglobinuria from any cause. For a full listing of potential causes see the Web site: http://neuromuscular.wustl.edu/msys/myoglob.html#general.

Variant forms include the following:

Idiopathic recurrent myoglobinuria, in which limb weakness and elevated creatine kinase levels persist between the attacks, the EMG shows a myopathic pattern, and neither an enzyme deficiency nor a biochemical abnormality is demonstrable.[580]

Familial myoglobinuria, which is a severe intermittent myoglobinuria in which attacks are precipitated by exercise or by infection.[5565]

myograph An instrument for recording the attributes of muscular contraction. See **electromyogram**.

myohypertrophia kymoparalytica A syndrome of muscular hypertrophy, cramps, wave-like muscular contractions and pareses of unknown nature. It was described by Oppenheim, but is not now reported; possibly the condition represented a form of **dystonia**.

myoid cell A thymic cell somewhat resembling a myofibril which may express acetylcholine receptors on its surface.

myo-inositol Disturbed metabolism of myo-inositol is associated with a reduction in nerve conduction velocities, presumably through an effect on the Na–K–ATPase system. Impaired axonal conduction results and axonopathy follows, from which it has been considered that the disturbance of myo-inositol in diabetes mellitus is a cause of the peripheral neuropathy. This is as yet unproven.

myokinetic epilepsy See **absence seizures**.

myokymia (from Gr, muscle + wave) (fibrillary contractions) Involuntary, localized, writhing, undulating, persistent quivering contractions of a muscle due to a process arising in the peripheral portion of its motor nerve and leading to spontaneous, synchronous, repetitive discharges of motor unit potentials. Electromyographically, continuous, repetitive, brief discharges of groups of 2-6 motor unit potentials, recurring rhythmically or semi-rhythmically at 5–60 Hz and usually several times per second, are recorded. The differential diagnosis has been discussed.[294, 2649] See **neuromyotonia, myokymic discharge, fasciculations,** and **fasciculation potential**. Neuromyotonia and myokymia appear to represent loci on a spectrum of abnormal activity in muscle due to aberrant neural input.[2650]

Myokymia often accompanies motor nerve lesions of any type, but can also occur without demonstrable pathology; in such cases, the commonest site is the orbicularis oculi muscles of people who are tired or anxious. Irritation of the fasciculus of the VII cranial nerve within the brainstem by a plaque of **multiple sclerosis** or a brainstem neoplasm are rarer causes. The lesion is of the dorsolateral pontine postgenu portion of the facial nerve. Elsewhere in the body, Guillain-Barré syndrome, **radiation plexopathy**, brainstem tumor and timber rattlesnake envenomation are possible, if uncommon, causes. The condition may also be hereditary[5773] or toxic.[4410] The review of Albers et al. remains current and complete.[100]

Superior oblique myokymia is a misnomer as that condition is really a microtremor. See also **Isaacs syndrome (neuromyotona); cramp-fasciculation syndrome; episodic ataxia**; and **Morvan disease**. *Variant* forms are listed in Chart M–27.

myokymic discharge A form of involuntary activity in which motor unit action potentials fire repetitively and may be associated with clinical **myokymia**. Two firing patterns have been described: (1) Commonly, the discharge is a brief, repetitive firing of single motor unit action potentials for a short period (up to a few seconds) at a uniform rate (2-60 Hz) followed by a short period (up to a few seconds) of

Chart M–27. Variant Forms of Myokymia

Generalized myokymia and muscle cramping without peripheral neuropathy: EMG findings are of spontaneously recurring regular bursts of motor unit potentials, termed **myokymic discharges**, with normal motor and sensory nerve conduction velocities. Repetitive discharges follow each motor nerve stimulus.[294]

Hereditary myokymia and paroxysmal ataxia: A dominantly inherited syndrome mapped to chromosome 12p with a missense mutation in the *KCNA1* gene. The attacks of ataxia with slowed movements and tremor last up to 15 min, are precipitated by kinesigenic stimuli, exertion, and startle, and are responsive to acetazolamide. The myokymia may lead to generalized stiffness or be simply minimal contractions of distal muscles.[3941] See also **cerebellar ataxia**. (*variants*)

Idiopathic generalized myokymia. See **neuromyotonia**.

Morvan fibrillary chorea: A form of generalized myokymia, probably occurring as a toxic effect of gold therapy.

Myokymia and ataxia with continuous muscle discharge: A congenital degenerative disease characterized by clubfoot, joint contractures, cerebellar ataxia, tremor at rest, myokymia, and raised creatine kinase levels.[381]

Myokymia and impaired muscle relaxation with continuous muscle discharge: A disorder of peripheral nerves characterized by generalized muscle twitching, weakness, stiffness, cramping and hyperhidrosis, persistent during sleep, and initial fatigue, followed by increasing strength with continued effort. Nerve conduction velocities are reduced.[3944, 3944]

silence, with repetition of the same sequence for a particular potential at regular intervals. (2) Rarely, the potential recurs continuously at a fairly uniform firing rate (1-5 Hz). Myokymic discharges are a subclass of grouped discharges and repetitive discharges. See also ephapse and ephaptic transmission. (From the 2001 Report of the Nomenclature Committee of the American Association of Electromyography and Electrodiagnosis.[19] Reproduced by kind permission of the AANEM.)

myolemma (sarcolemma) The connective tissue layer investing myofibrils.

myoleukoencephalopathy A mitochondrial disease presenting with overlapping features of MERRF and MELAS, and in addition severe myopathy and seizures.[1532]

myology The study of the nature, structure, function, and pathology of muscles.

myoma A tumor consisting of muscle fibers. If these are striated, the name **rhabdomyoma** is applied; if they are unstriated, it is known as a **leiomyoma**.

myomesin The major structural protein of the M-line in vertebrate muscle.

myonecrosis (gas gangrene) Infection and subsequent decomposition of muscle, usually by *Clostridium perfringens* or *welchii*, the exotoxin of which causes large areas of muscle necrosis with marked systemic reaction. *S. pyogenes* and *Group B Streptococcus* may do the same thing. Clinically, pain out of proportion to the appearance of the wound, extensive edema of the overlying skin, watery or purulent exudates, fever, and skin necrosis are in succession the main findings, leading on to hypovolemic shock, intravascular hemolysis, and organ failure.

myoneural junction The structures comprising the mechanism for the transmission of nerve impulses from nerve to muscle. These include the axon terminal, the synaptic cleft, and the **motor end plate**.

myoneurogastrointestinal encephalopathy (MNGIE) A rare mitochondrial disorder of young adult life comprising external ophthalmoplegia, muscle atrophy, polyneuropathy, gastrointestinal dysmotility and hyperdensities of the cerebral white matter, associated with acidosis. The condition is a mitochondrial multi-system disorder that is considered due to a partial defect of the cytochrome *c* complex of the respiratory chain.[391]

myopalmus (Gr, muscle + swinging) Twitching of muscle.

myopathic carnitine deficiency See **carnitine deficiency**.

myopathic motor unit potential Low amplitude, short duration, polyphasic motor unit action potentials. The use of the term is discouraged because it incorrectly implies specific diagnostic significance of a motor unit action potential configuration. See **motor unit action potential**. (From the 2001 Report of the Nomenclature Committee of the American Association of Electromyography and Electrodiagnosis.[19] Reproduced by kind permission of the AANEM.)

myopathic recruitment An increase in the number and firing rate of motor unit action potentials compared with normal for the strength of muscle contraction. (From the 2001 Report of the Nomenclature Committee of the American Association of Electromyography and Electrodiagnosis.[19] Reproduced by kind permission of the AANEM.)

myopathica rachitica (Hagenbach-Bing myopathy) A severe hypotonic myopathy occurring in infants with rickets.

myopathies Diseases in which the structure or function of muscles is compromised. Many (but not all) of those that are inherited are subsumed under the heading of **muscular dystrophies**, but the term myopathy is all-encompassing and all dystrophies are myopathies, though not all myopathies are dystrophies. Some of them are considered under the heading **congenital myopathy**, others under, e.g., **mitochondrial myopathies**, or by name when listed in bold print; the remainder are dealt with as shown in Chart M–28. See also **distal myopathy** and the Web site: http://www.hibm.org/arm/index.html from Advancement for Research into Myopathies.

myopathy and chronic renal failure Proximal weakness and wasting of myopathic type in association with severe osteomalacia secondary to renal disease, mainly affecting the flexors and other proximal leg muscles, commonly asymmetrical and partially responsive to vitamin D therapy.[2131]

Chart M–28. A Listing of the Muscular Dystrophies and Other Myopathies

A. Heritable myopathies

a. **X-linked forms**:

1. X-linked recessive (severe) **Duchenne muscular dystrophy**
2. Myopathy in manifesting Duchenne carriers
3. X-linked Duchenne dystrophy due to chromosomal translocation in females or to **Turner syndrome**[785]
4. X-linked recessive form. See **Becker muscle dystrophy**
5. X-linked recessive myopathy (Xp21) with **glycerol kinase deficiency**
6. X-linked myopathy (Xp21) with **McLeod syndrome**
7. X-linked recessive dystrophy with contractures and cardiomyopathy
8. X-linked recessive congenital muscle fiber hypotrophy with central nuclei
9. X-linked dominant lethal myopathy in hemizygous boys
10. X-linked **myotubular myopathy**, lethal in neonates
11. X-linked **scapuloperoneal muscular dystrophy** with lethal cardiomyopathy
12. X-linked vacuolated myopathy[6549]
13. **X-linked myopathy with excessive autophagy**

b. **Facioscapulohumeral muscular dystrophy**:

1. Autosomal dominant involving face, scapulohumeral, and anterior tibial muscles
2. Severe infantile form
3. Childhood form with **Möbius syndrome**
4. With sensorineural deafness alone, or with **Coats disease** of the retina or tortuosity of retinal vessels

c. **Scapuloperoneal muscular dystrophy**:

1. Autosomal dominant
2. X-linked (may be Emery–Dreifuss type) (see A.11 above)
3. With inflammatory changes and cardiopathy

d. **Limb-girdle muscular dystrophy** (LGMD)

1. Quadriceps myopathy
2. LGMD with Wolff–Parkinson–White syndrome
3. Late-onset proximal myopathy with diabetes mellitus

e. **Autosomal recessive dystrophy of childhood**:
Resembling **Duchenne dystrophy** but more benign and affecting both sexes. The condition is reported from Tunisia and parts of the Middle East·

f. **Distal muscular dystrophy**:

g. **Autosomal dominant dystrophy with humeropelvic distribution and cardiomyopathy**.[2011]

h. **Emery–Dreifuss dystrophy** with dominant inheritance

i. **Benign muscular dystrophy with contractures** but without cardiomyopathy[335]

j. **Myositis ossificans** (autosomal dominant fibrodysplasia ossificans progressiva)

k. **Ocular myopathies** (progressive external ophthalmoplegias):

1. Isolated (autosomal dominant) with or without ragged red fibers
2. With pigmentary retinal degeneration (dominant or sporadic)
3. **Kearns–Sayre syndrome** (with retinal degeneration, short stature, heart block, ataxia, and high CSF protein)
4. With curare sensitivity
5. **Oculopharyngeal muscular dystrophy**, usually autosomal dominant, sometimes recessive
6. Oculopharyngeal myopathy with distal myopathy and cardiomyopathy, and other varieties of **oculopharyngodistal myopathy**
7. **Familial multicore disease** with ophthalmoplegia
8. Progressive ophthalmoplegia with mental retardation
9. Congenital ophthalmoplegia in the **Goldenhar–Gorlin syndrome**
10. X-linked recessive ophthalmoplegia and myopia
11. **Neonatal ophthalmoplegia with microfibers**
12. **Nemaline myopathy** with ophthalmoplegia and mitochondrial abnormalities
13. **Nemaline myopathy** with cardiomyopathy
14. **Familial paralysis of horizontal gaze**
15. Late-onset **oculogastrointestinal muscular dystrophy**
16. **Familial static ophthalmoplegia**

Unlisted *variants* include the following:
Manitoba variant muscular dystrophy A recessively inherited muscular dystrophy with onset in early childhood of proximal muscle atrophy and weakness, and **benign X-linked muscular dystrophy** (Waida). See **Becker muscular dystrophy**. See also **myofibrillar (desmin-storage) myopathy**.

2. *Myopathies of unknown etiology, usually congenital*

A. **Congenital muscular dystrophy**, including some cases of **arthrogryposis multiplex congenita** with infantile cataract
B. Congenital muscular dystrophy with severe mental retardation
C. **Benign congenital myopathy** without specific features
D. **Benign congenital or infantile hypotonia**
E. **Central core disease**
F. **Nemaline** (rod-body) myopathy
G. Myotubular (**centronuclear**) myopathy and variants
H. **Familial myosclerosis** (Myodysplasia fibrosa multiplex)
I. Myopathy in **Marfan syndrome**, and variants; centronuclear myopathy with type 1 fiber hypotrophy, and "fingerprint" inclusions with Marfan syndrome.
J. **Marinesco–Sjögren syndrome** (familial congenital myopathy with cataract, gonadal dysgenesis, and oligophrenia)
K. Myopathies with characteristic histochemical abnormalities:

1. **Type 1 fiber hypotrophy**
2. **Congenital fiber-type disproportion**
3. **Congenital myopathy with uniform fiber type** (type 1)
4. Congenital fiber-type disproportion in **Krabbe disease**
5. **Reducing body myopathy**
6. **Congenital myopathy with trilaminar muscle fibers**
7. **Congenital myopathy with multifocal degeneration of muscle fibers**

L. **Rigid spine syndrome**[5061]
M. Myopathy with features of both centronuclear myopathy and multicores. See **myofibrillar myopathy**
N. Myopathies with cytoplasmic[3750] or with "fingerprint" inclusions.[1869] See **myofibrillar myopathy**
O. **Multicore disease**
P. **Sarcotubular myopathy**
Q. **Tubular aggregate myopathy**
R. Familial neuromuscular disease with type 1 fiber hypoplasia, tubular aggregates, cardiomyopathy, and myasthenic features[1669]
S. Congenital myopathy with type 2 fiber hypoplasia[872]
T. Myopathy with crystalline intranuclear inclusions.[3196] See **myofibrillar myopathy**
U. Autosomal dominant "spheroid body" myopathy. See **myofibrillar myopathy**
V. **Hypertrophic branchial myopathy**
W. **Monomelic hypertrophic myopathy**
X. **Cytoplasmic body neuromyopathy** with respiratory failure and weight loss. See **myofibrillar myopathy**
Y. **Zebra body myopathy**
Z. Myopathy with absence of muscle glycogen and neutral lipid in the **neuroleptic malignant syndrome**
AA. **Benign myopathy**
BB. **Myopathy with merosin-deficient fibers**. See **myofibrillar myopathy**
CC. *Vocal cord and pharyngeal muscular dystrophy* on 5q31[1992]
DD. **Late-onset riboflavin-responsive myopathy with multiple acyl CoA dehydrogenase deficiency** A lipid-storage myopathy presenting with weakness and wasting of the trunk and limbs in late adult life.[214] See also **lipid myopathy**
EE. *Fatal infantile hypertonic muscular dystrophy* A progressive myopathy appearing soon after birth with continuous muscle activity and progressive weakness to death before the age of 18 months, described in Canadian aboriginal infants. The pathology shows fibrosis, necrosis, and regeneration.[3636]
FF. *Myopathy with intrasarcoplasmic accumulation of dense granulofilamentous material* See **myofibrillar (desmin-storage) myopathy**
GG. **Myopathy with cardiomyopathy** A dominantly inherited condition similar to LGMD 1B with the onset in childhood or young adult life of proximal symmetrical weakness affecting mainly the pelvic girdle and the occurrence of dysrhythmias and conduction disturbances potentially leading to sudden death. Serum CK levels are somewhat elevated and the EMG and muscle biopsy are myopathic. See http://www.neuro.wustl.edu/neuromuscular/maltbrain.html/.
HH. *Dominant myopathy with ankle contractures & high serum CK* A dominantly inherited condition characterized by proximal symmetric weakness with onset in youth or young adult life and joint contractures. Serum CK levels are very high and muscle biopsy findings typically myopathic. See http://www.neuro.wustl.edu/neuromuscular/maltbrain.html/.
II. *Myopathy with abnormal merosin* (laminin-2) 4 A progressive form with likely autosomal recessive inheritance characterized by onset in youth or adult life, female preponderance, facial, neck, and shoulder girdle weakness without scapular winging, weakness of the hamstrings and hip adductors and flexors and ventilatory impairment. Hypertrophy of the calves and brachioradialis is reported. Serum CK levels are greatly increased and the EMG and biopsy findings are myopathic.
JJ. *Recessive myopathy with external ophthalmoplegia* A myopathy mapped to chromosome 17p13.1–p12, with early onset and slow progression. It is characterized by prominent external ophthalmoplegia (conjugate, nonrestrictive ocular motility impairment greatest on upgaze, and without ptosis), mild facial and proximal arm weakness and atrophy, facial dysmorphisms, and scoliosis. Orbital MRI shows atrophy of the oculorotatory muscles and muscle biopsy shows type I fiber predominance with core-like formations.[3916]
KK. *Surplus protein myopathy* A mild myopathy with elevated serum CK levels, distinguished by the presence of myofibrillar inclusions constituted by an excess of proteins normally present in the terminal cisternae of sarcoplasmic reticulum.[6347]

continued

Chart M–28. *(continued)*

LL. An autosomal recessive congenital muscular dystrophy with hyperlaxity, described in Quebec, presenting with muscle weakness, proximal contractures, and distal joint hyperlaxity, mapped to chromosome 3p23–21.[6260]
For current updates, see http://www.neuro.wustl.edu/neuromuscular/maltbrain.html.

3. Myotonic disorders

A. **Myotonic dystrophy** type 1
B. Myotonic dystrophy type 2 (proximal myotonic myopathy)
C. **Myotonia congenita** (autosomal dominant form, Thomsen disease)
D. **Myotonia congenita** (autosomal recessive form)
E. **Schwartz-Jampel syndrome**: Myotonia, dwarfism, facial dysmorphism, and diffuse bone disease
F. **Paramyotonia congenita** (Eulenburg): Clinical paramyotonia and electrical myotonia.
G. **Paramyotonia** without paralysis on exposure to cold
H. *Familial granulovacuolar lobular myopathy with electrical myotonia*. See **myotonia congenita**.
I. *Myotonia with painful cramps*. See Chart M–29.
J. **Familial (hyperkalemic) periodic paralysis**: Clinical paramyotonia and electrical myotonia.
K. **Acid maltase deficiency** (electrical myotonia without clinical myotonia)
L. Uncommon causes: denervation, myopathy, drug-induced hypothyroidism[4378]
See also http://www.ninds.nih.gov/disorders/myotonia/myotonia.htm.

B. Trauma to muscle by external agents

B1. Physical

1. **Crush syndrome**
2. Ischemic infarction or atrophy
3. **Volkmann contracture**
4. **Compartment syndromes**:
   a. **Anterior tibial syndrome**
   b. Posterior compartment (tibial) syndrome
   c. Lateral (peroneal) compartment syndrome
   d. Triceps surae compartment syndrome
   e. Extensor compartment syndrome of the forearm
   f. Rectus abdominis compartment syndrome
5. Congenital or idiopathic **torticollis**

B2. Toxic

1. **Haff disease**
2. Snake-bite by *Enhydrina schistosa*
3. Saxitoxin poisoning
4. **Myoglobinuria** caused by hornet venom
5. **Quail myopathy**

B3. Drugs

C. Inflammatory myopathies
C1. Infections of muscle

1. **Viral myositis**
   a. **Benign acute myositis**
   b. Acute myopathy with **rhabdomyolysis**
   c. **Epidemic pleurodynia** due to Coxsackie B5 (also B1, B3, and B4)
   d. **Postviral fatigue syndrome** (benign postinfection «myositis»).
2. Bacterial infections
3. Fungal myositis (e.g., disseminated candidiasis)
4. Protozoal myositis
5. Cestode myositis
6. Nematode myositis

C2. Other inflammatory disorders of muscle

1. **Dermatomyositis**
2. **Polymyositis** (possibly an organ-specific autoimmune disease):
   a. Acute polymyositis with myoglobinuria
   b. Subacute polymyositis
   c. Chronic polymyositis (including chronic myositis fibrosa)

3. **Polymyositis** in the context of autoimmune disease, including systemic lupus erythematosus; rheumatic fever; rheumatoid arthritis, systemic sclerosis, scleroderma (morphoea), polyarteritis nodosa or giant cell arteritis, Sjögren disease, Werner disease, localized nodular myositis, chronic graft-versus- host disease, benign acute childhood myositis, acne fulminans with inflammatory myopathy.
4. **Polymyositis** or dermatomyositis with malignant disease
5. **Polymyositis** with associated virus particles
6. Acute fulminant myoglobinuric **polymyositis** with picornavirus-like particles
7. **Eosinophilic polymyositis**
8. Cyclic eosinophilic **polymyositis** and hyperimmunoglobulin E
9. **Inclusion body myositis** and variants
10. Orbital myositis (**pseudotumor orbiti**)
11. Polymyositis with **HIV** infection

C3. Inflammatory disorders of muscle of unknown etiology

1. **Sarcoidosis** with myopathy
2. **Granulomatous polymyositis** and giant cell myositis
3. **Polymyalgia rheumatica**
4. Localized **myositis ossificans**
5. **Fibrositis** and nodular fasciitis; myositis proliferans or pseudotumor
6. Myopathy in relapsing panniculitis (**Weber–Christian Syndrome**)
7. Myositis with **necrotizing fasciitis**
8. **Psoriatic myopathy**
9. Myopathy in **Reye syndrome**

D. Metabolic myopathies

D1. Muscle disorder associated with endocrine disease

1. Hyperthyroidism (See **acute thyrotoxic myopathy**)
2. Hypothyroidism (Girdle myopathy; **Debré-Sémélaigne syndrome; Hoffmann syndrome; pseudomyotonia**, neuromyopathy following iodine^{131} therapy
3. **Hypopituitarism** with myopathy
4. **Acromegaly** with muscle hypertrophy or myopathy
5. **Exophthalmic ophthalmoplegia** (infiltrative ophthalmopathy or ophthalmic Graves' disease)
6. **Cushing disease** myopathy (and iatrogenic corticosteroid myopathy)
7. ACTH myopathy in **Nelson syndrome**
8. **Addison disease** with myopathy
9. **Primary aldosteronism** (with hypokalemic periodic paralysis)
10. **Hyperparathyroidism** with myopathy
11. **Hypoparathyroidism** with myopathy
12. Myopathy in other forms of metabolic bone disease such as **osteomalacia**
13. Myopathy with calcitonin-secreting medullary carcinoma of the thyroid

D2. Heritable metabolic myopathies with known biochemical abnormality

1. **Glycogen storage disease** involving muscle

   a. **Glycogenosis** type I (von Gierke disease)
   b. Glycogenosis type II (Pompe disease)

      1. Infantile form
      2. Adult or late-onset variety

   c. Glycogenosis type III (Cori-Forbes disease)
   d. Glycogenosis type IV (Andersen disease, adult polyglucosan body myopathy)
   e. Glycogenosis type V (McArdle disease)

      1. Usual form, with onset in childhood or adolescence
      2. Infantile form
      3. Late-onset **myophosphorylase deficiency**

   f. Glycogenosis type VII (Tarui disease) due to phosphofructokinase deficiency:

      1. Typical form, lack of M-subunit
      2. Hemolysis with myopathy, lack of L-subunit

   g. **Phosphoglycerate kinase deficiency**
   h. **Phosphoglycerate mutase deficiency**

continued

Chart M–28. (*continued*)

i. **Lactate dehydrogenase deficiency**
j. Lysosomal glycogen storage disease without acid maltase deficiency
k. Mixed enzyme deficiencies (e.g., phosphofructokinase and phosphorylase kinase)

2. Other inherited disorders of carbohydrate metabolism

a. Muscle fructose 1,6-diphosphatase deficiency with atypical **central core disease**
b. Myopathy due to glycolytic abnormality involving phosphohexoisomerase

3. **Myoadenylate deaminase deficiency** (with cramps and exertional myalgia)
4. **Familial periodic paralysis** and related syndromes:

a. Hypokalemic periodic paralysis
b. Hyperkalemic periodic paralysis (adynamia episodica hereditaria), sometimes with cardiac arrhythmia
c. Normokalemic periodic paralysis
d. Myotonic periodic paralysis (paramyotonia congenita; possibly a variant of b.)
e. Thyrotoxic periodic paralysis

5. **Mitochondrial myopathies** and **lipid storage myopathies**

a. Lipid storage myopathies of uncertain origin:

1. Lipid storage myopathy and congenital ichthyosis (Chanarin–Miranda syndrome)
2. Congenital myopathies with lipid storage
3. Associated with recognized disease (glycogenosis type l, hyper β-lipoproteinemia, pyruvate decarboxylase deficiency, arthrogryposis)
4. Autosomal recessive lipid storage myopathy with electrical myotonia, lipid in leukocytes, and defect in long-chain fatty acid utilization
5. Autosomal dominant lipid storage neuromyopathy with systemic abnormality of fat metabolism
6. Idiopathic lipid storage myopathies with glycogen storage, and structurally abnormal mitochondria

b. α-glycerophosphate dehydrogenase deficiency. See **lipid myopathy**
c. Deficiencies involving the carnitine acyl-carnitine carrier system:

1. Muscle **carnitine deficiency**
2. **Systemic carnitine deficiency** with cardiomyopathy
3. Partial muscle carnitine deficiencies
4. **Carnitine palmitoyl transferase deficiency**; CPT II deficiency with normal CPT I, CPT deficiency with myoglobinuria and respiratory failure
5. Combined carnitine and CPT deficiencies

d. Defects of mitochondrial substrate utilization:

1. Pyruvate decarboxylase deficiency
2. Dihydrolipoyl transacetylase deficiency
3. Dihydrolipoyl dehydrogenase deficiency
4. Pyruvate dehydrogenase phosphatase deficiency
5. Pyruvate carboxylase deficiency
6. Carnitine acetyltransferase deficiency

N.B. Many disorders in this group cause myopathy but the clinical picture is often dominated by progressive encephalopathy, hypotonia, lactic acidosis, and respiratory insufficiency.

e. Defects of the respiratory chain:

1. Defects of NADH oxidation
2. Cytochrome *b* deficiency
3. Cytochrome *c* oxidase (aaa3) deficiency
4. Combined cytochrome deficiencies (aaa3 + b)
5. Encephalomyopathy with decreased succinate-cytochrome *c* reductase deficiency

f. Defects of energy conservation and transduction:

1. Hypermetabolic mitochondrial myopathy (**Luft disease**)
2. Other **mitochondrial myopathies** with "loose coupling"
3. Mitochondrial ATPase deficiency
4. Myopathy due to a malate-aspartate shuttle defect[2807]

N.B. The mitochondrial myopathies in e. and f. are associated with diverse clinical syndromes that include ophthalmoplegia, severe hypotonia, cramps, myoglobinuria, exercise-induced myalgia, and limb weakness, occurring at different stages of life. **Fukuhara syndrome** comprises myoclonic epilepsy and ragged red fibers (MERRF). The controversies about the delineation of specific disorders have been reviewed by Petty et al.[5007]

6. **Malignant hyperpyrexia** (halothane, suxamethonium, ketamine, psychotropic agents, etc.)
7. Progressive muscle spasm, alopecia, diarrhoea, and malabsorption (**Satoyoshi syndrome**)
8. Myopathy in **lysine-cystinuria**
9. **Xanthenuric myopathy**.
10. Myopathy in **Lafora disease**
11. **Tubular aggregate myopathy** often associated with myalgia
12. **Cytoplasmic body myopathy**
13. Benign **reducing body myopathy**

D3. Other metabolic myopathies

1. **Alcoholic myopathy**
   a. Acute, with myoglobinuria
   b. Subacute or chronic proximal
   c. Hypokalemic
2. **Nutritional myopathy**
   a. Protein deficiency; malnutrition due to anorexia nervosa or malabsorption
   b. Human myopathy due to vitamin E deficiency
   c. Chronic myopathy with hypocalcemia and hypophosphatemia
3. Myopathy in chronic renal failure: See **uremic myopathy**
4. **Acute polymyopathy** during total parenteral nutrition
5. Potassium depletion myopathy
6. **Carnitine deficiency** induced during hemodialysis
7. Riboflavin-responsive **lipid myopathy** with carnitine deficiency
8. **Myoglobinuria** (other than that due to glycogen storage disease, mitochondrial or lipid storage myopathies, and CPT deficiency)
   a. Exertion (including military training, running, skiing, anterior tibial syndrome, status epilepticus, electric shock, myoclonus, and severe dystonia)
   b. Crush or ischemic injury to muscle (see above)
   c. Metabolic depression or distortion (including carbon monoxide or drug intoxication, diabetic ketoacidosis, hyperosmolar states, renal tubular acidosis, hyper- and hyponatremia, hypokalemia and hypophosphatemia)
   d. Due to drugs and toxins (see above) including the ingestion of **quail**
   e. Abnormalities of body temperature (including hypothermia due to cold or hypothyroidism, or fever due to toxins, vaccines, heat stroke, malignant hyperpyrexia, or the malignant neuroleptic syndrome)
   f. Infections (including viral, bacterial, and *Mycoplasma* infections, and the toxic shock syndrome).
   g. Autoimmune muscle disease (polymyositis and dermatomyositis)
   h. Idiopathic recurrent myoglobinuria, sometimes leading to myopathy with persistent weakness
   i. Chronic myopathy due to drugs (chloroquine, emetine, steroids, penicillin, vincristine, colchicine; repeated intramuscular injections of meperidine or pentazocine)
   j. Proximal myopathy in diabetes mellitus[6161]

E. Myopathy associated with malignant disease

1. **Carcinomatous myopathy** (other than polymyositis)
2. **Lambert-Eaton syndrome**
3. **Carcinomatous embolic myopathy**
4. Proximal myopathy due to discrete carcinomatous metastases in muscle
5. Myopathy in the **carcinoid** syndrome

F. Myopathy associated with myasthenia gravis
G. Myopathy in ***thalassemia***
H. Other disorders of muscle of unknown or uncertain etiology

1. Acute muscle necrosis of unknown cause, or complicating chronic alcoholism, carcinoma, or intensive care treatment. See **acute quadriplegic myopathy**
2. **Amyloid myopathy**
   a. Primary familial
   b. Primary sporadic (sometimes causing pseudohypertrophy of muscle)
   c. In myelomatosis
   d. With angiopathy
3. **Disuse atrophy**
4. Muscle **cachexia** (in wasting diseases and in the elderly)
5. Muscle wasting in contralateral cerebral lesions (particularly of parietal lobe)
6. **Granular nuclear inclusion body disease** affecting skeletal muscle and the nervous system

continued

Chart M–28. *(continued)*

I. Tumors of muscle

1. **Rhabdomyoma**
2. **Rhabdomyosarcoma**
   a. Adult pleomorphic type
   b. Embryonal botryoid type
   c. Embryonal alveolar type
3. **Desmoid fibroma**
4. **Alveolar sarcoma**
5. Angioma
6. Other connective tissue tumors occasionally occurring in muscle

J. Unclassified myopathies

Familial myopathy with thrombocytopenia
Myopathy complicating methioninemia
Myopathy complicating **mucolipidosis** type 4
CPT = carnitine palmityl transferase.

The classification above is based upon that of the World Federation of Neurology[6869] *and the continuously updated Web site of Dr. Alan Pestronk at Washington University; http://www.neuro.wustl.edu/neuromuscular/maltbrain.html; but much adapted.*

myopathy (Bender type) A congenital myopathic syndrome, comprising proximal and facial muscle atrophy, weakness and hypotonia, ptosis, ophthalmoplegia, kyphoscoliosis, feeding problems in infants and the presence of fiber hypotrophy, central nuclei, fiber-type predominance, and central core-like lesions in muscle biopsy specimens.[381]

myopathy following adrenalectomy A condition of proximal weakness and wasting with unusual pigmentation in patients prescribed adrenocorticotrophic hormone following adrenalectomy for Cushing disease.[5122]

myopathy with characteristic sarcoplasmic bodies and skeletin (desmin) filaments See myofibrillar myopathy.

myopathy with cylindrical spiral inclusions A myopathic syndrome with onset in childhood, comprising proximal weakness and atrophy, lordosis, myotonia, and muscle pain and cramps.[381]

myopathy with exercise intolerance and weakness A limb-girdle myopathic syndrome presenting at any time of life, sometimes with ophthalmoplegia.[4483]

myopathy with focal loss of cross striations and multicores A congenital myopathic syndrome, comprising proximal and facial muscle atrophy, weakness and hypotonia, ptosis, ophthalmoplegia and lordosis, and central nuclei, and with the finding of central core-like lesions on muscle biopsy specimens.

myopathy with inclusion bodies See **myofibrillar myopathy**.

myopathy with lysis of myofibrils in type I fibers See **type 1 fiber hypotrophy with central nuclei**.

myopathy with Mallory body-like inclusions See **myofibrillar myopathy**.

myopathy with merosin-deficient fibers A syndrome of rapidly evolving and severe weakness leading to incapacity and respiratory insufficiency, reported in subjects following severe illness and steroid administration. Serum CK levels are normal or mildly elevated and the EMG myopathic. Pathology shows lack of myosin-ATPase staining in many small angular fibers with marked loss of myosin. Slow recovery is usual.[85]

myopathy with mucolipidosis type 4 A congenital myopathic syndrome, a *variant* of **mucolipidosis** type 4, characterized by cloudy corneas, optic atrophy, retinitis pigmentosa, joint contractures, spasticity, athetosis, proximal and distal weakness, hypotonia, and mental and developmental delay.[381]

myopathy with multicore and central nuclei See **multicore disease**.

myopathy with myosin-deficient fibers A syndrome of rapidly evolving and severe weakness leading to incapacity and respiratory insufficiency, reported in subjects following severe illness and steroid administration. Serum CK levels are normal or mildly elevated and the EMG myopathic. Pathology shows lack of myosin-ATPase staining in many small angular fibers with marked loss of myosin. Slow recovery is usual.[85]

myopathy with tubular aggregates Proximal myopathic syndromes characterized by the presence of cytoplasmic aggregates of membranous tubules derived from the sarcoplasmic reticulum, mainly in type II fibers. Three *variants* are described as follows:

1. *Autosomal dominant (or recessive)*, presenting with slowly progressive proximal weakness in childhood or early adult life, sometimes with extraocular muscle weakness or ankle contractures and with normal serum CK levels.
2. *Autosomal dominant*, a slowly progressive form with onset in adult life of proximal and sometimes distal weakness, muscle pain, cramps, and exertional stiffness.

Serum CK levels are normal or slightly raised. Muscle biopsy shows the presence of tubular aggregates in type II muscle fibers and type II muscle fiber atrophy.

3. *Sporadic*, a slowly progressive form with onset in adolescence of proximal weakness. The serum CK levels are normal or mildly elevated. Muscle biopsy reveals the presence of tubular aggregates in type I & II muscle fibers.

Many of the above entries were abstracted from the Neuromuscular Web site at Washington University St. Louis, http://www.neuro.wustl.edu/neuromuscular/maltbrain.html by courtesy of Dr. Alan Pestronk.

myopathy with tubulomembranous inclusions

An inherited myopathic syndrome with onset in youth, characterized by high-arched palate and by facial, proximal, and distal myopathic weakness. See **tubular aggregate myopathy**.

myopathy–oligophrenia–cataract

See **Lundberg syndrome**.

myophosphorylase deficiency

The biochemical cause of McArdle disease (type V glycogenosis), leading to a metabolic myopathy characterized by the deposition of subsarcolemmal glycogen in skeletal muscles and occasionally in endothelial cells. See **glycogen storage diseases**.

myopia

(from Gr, to close + eye; thus to close the eye) Shortsightedness; the condition in which rays of light entering the eye are brought to focus anterior to the retina, within the vitreous humor. The eye is thus adapted for near-vision.

myopic crescent

A pale crescent surrounding part of the optic disk in myopes, due to choroidal atrophy in this region.

myorhythmia

(skeletal myoclonus) A coarse, rhythmic or irregular alternating tremor of small amplitude, which may be intermittent or continuous and present at rest, but is intensified by posture and voluntary activity, occurring at 1–4 Hz (usually about 2 Hz) in the limbs ipsilateral to a dentate or superior cerebellar peduncle lesion or contralateral to a lesion of the inferior olive;[4160] it disappears in sleep.

Muscles such as the superior oblique or those of the palate may also be involved; this phenomenon is variously regarded as myoclonic (implying a central origin) or myokymic (when the origin is presumed to be peripheral). Brainstem and cerebellar diseases, **Hashimoto encephalopathy**, and Hodgkin lymphoma have been associated with this movement disorder. Progressive supranuclear ophthalmoplegia with oculomasticatory myorhythmia or oculofacioskeletal myorhythmia are movement disorders seen in **Whipple disease** complicated by neurological involvement. The phenomenon is sometimes associated with **branchial myoclonus**.[4160] See also **midbrain tremor**.

myosclerosis

(fibrosing myositis) A heterogeneous condition, in which the consistency of muscles is increased to a woody hardness. Dystrophic, neurogenic, and inflammatory causes are recognized.[793]

myosin

A major muscle protein, selectively absent in certain myopathies as above and in critical illness myopathy.

myosin (storage) myopathy

(hyaline body myopathy, familial myopathy with probable lysis of myofibrils in type I fibers) A rare, chronic nonprogressive congenital myopathy with variable patterns of inheritance, presenting with proximal limb weakness, calf hypertrophy, aching pain, myopathic features on EMG, and modest elevations of serum CK. Muscle biopsy shows fatty infiltration of skeletal muscle fibers and an increased number of fibers with internal nuclei. Subsarcolemmal well-delineated hyaline areas are seen in type I fibers. The condition may persist into adult life.[5167] It is allelic with **Laing distal myopathy**.[3653]

myosis

See **miosis**.

myositis

(polymyositis) Inflammatory myopathies due to infection by viruses, bacteria, fungi, or parasites or occurring as manifestations of autoallergic disease (**idiopathic inflammatory myopathies**).

Viral infections may produce the syndromes of **benign acute myositis, acute rhabdomyolysis** or **epidemic pleurodynia,** and possibly **chronic myopathy**. Bacterial infections lead to **acute suppurative myositis. Fungal myositis** is considered separately. Protozoa, cestodes, and nematodes are the agents leading to **parasitic myositis.**[4157] Numerous other forms of inflammatory myopathy are considered under **polymyositis.** See **also focal steroid responsive myositis.**

Myositis Association of America

A charitable organization providing information and support. Web site: http://www.myositis.org/template/index.cfm/.

myositis of chronic graft-versus-host disease

A rare complication of bone marrow transplantation presenting with severe proximal weakness. Muscle biopsy specimens show necrotic fibers with anti-IgG deposits and interstitial inflammation.[5280]

myositis ossificans

(Munchmeyer syndrome, fibrodysplasia ossificans progressiva, myositis ossificans progressiva, Patin syndrome) A rare dominantly inherited severe disabling disorder of childhood characterized by painful swelling due to fibrosis and ossification of affected muscles and of local fascia and other fibrous tissues. The proximal limb muscles are most affected, but the heart and intercostal muscles may also be involved, a situation eventually incompatible with life in some cases.[4549] Spinal anomalies and malformations of the hallux may be associated.[5040] Radiologically, the mass is encircled by a rim of calcification and is separated from underlying bone.

The same condition was probably that described by Guy Patin in 1648 and again by John Freke (1688–1756), an English physician in 1740 as a case of "Extraordinary Exostoses on the Back of a Boy."[2197, 5619] *Variants* include the following:[2772]

Myositis ossificans traumatica, a condition of localized calcification in muscle damaged in the remote past and the commonest form, in which the lesions arise following trauma.

Pseudomalignant "non-traumatic" myositis ossificans, a form of **proliferative myositis**[3642] occurring in response to repeated minor muscle traumata even if no major injury is recalled.

A familial form in which the mass is sited within the paravertebral muscles.[2772]

Heterotopic bone formation occurring within muscles in patients with prior poliomyelitis, polymyositis, burns, paraplegia, infections, etc. without obvious cause.[2772]

myositis ossificans progressiva

See **myositis ossificans.**

myositis proliferans See **nodular fasciitis**.

myospasm See **myofascial pain syndromes**.

myospasm gravis See **Satoyoshi syndrome**.

myospasmus (Gr, muscle + contraction) Muscle cramp or spasm.

myostatin A member of the *transforming growth factor-β* family of signaling molecules. Deletion results in excessive growth of skeletal muscle, while inhibition of its activity results in increased force production and better tissue architecture.

myotalgia senilis An uncommon syndrome occurring in elderly people who suffer darting or aching pains, undiagnosable neuralgias, dysesthesias, and painful cramps in the legs associated with movement. The underlying pathology is not elucidated.

myotatic (Gr, muscle + a stretching) Resulting from muscle stretching.

myotatic irritability 1. (goggia) Mounding or dimpling of a muscle tapped by the finger or tendon hammer, common in chronic debilitated states but classically evidence of **myotonia**. 2. Excessive reactivity of the muscle stretch reflexes (Sir William **Gowers**).

myotatic reflexes The term of **Gowers** for the phasic muscle stretch reflexes. The myotatic unit comprises muscle stretch receptors and their afferents, the intraspinal connections which these make with the α-motor neuron, the motor neurons themselves, and the muscle fibers of that motor unit.[3839]

myotatic reflex scale Adopted by the American NINDS, this 5-point scale rates the activity of muscle stretch reflex responses as follows:[2697]

- 0 Reflex absent
- 1 Reduced reflex response, including a trace response or one only evident with reinforcement
- 2 Response in lower half of the normal range
- 3 Response in upper half of the normal range
- 4 Response enhanced, maybe including clonus.

The scale is thus bottom-heavy; the need for two gradings for normal responses and of only one to include all levels of hyperreflexia is not easily comprehensible, but reliability has been claimed.[3879]

myotatic unit The reflex arc—all of the neural and muscular structures required for the occurrence of a muscle stretch reflex; thus, the muscle receptors and their afferent fibers, the segmental spinal pathways, the alpha motor neuron, and the muscle.

myotilinopathy A disease characterized adult onset of weakness in distal or proximal leg muscles, eventually spreading to other muscle groups of the lower and upper extremities. Cardiomyopathy, respiratory failure, and peripheral neuropathy are sometimes described in association. Pathologically, focal myofibrillar destruction resulting in intracytoplasmic deposits strongly immunoreactive to myotilin, multiple rimmed and centrally or subsarcolemmally located nonrimmed vacuoles, and streaming Z-lines are characteristic.

Mutations in the myotilin gene (*MYOT*) are also associated with **limb girdle muscular dystrophy** type 1A (LGMD1A) and a subgroup of **myofibrillar myopathy**.[4785]

myotome 1. (metamere) A segment of the muscular system of the vertebrate embryo. The word dates from Goodsir's use of it in 1857. The muscles comprising a particular myotome are all those which are innervated by one spinal nerve root. 2. An instrument for cutting muscle sections.

myotomy The division of a muscle to release contractures.

myotonia 1. The clinical observation of delayed relaxation of a muscle after voluntary contraction or percussion. Such delayed relaxation may be electrically silent, or may be accompanied by propagated electrical activity such as **myotonic discharge, complex repetitive discharge**, or **neuromyotonic discharge**. 2. Repetitive discharges of muscle fiber action potentials, at 20–80 Hz, resembling fibrillations or positive sharp waves and occurring with decreasing frequency and amplitude, each run having a duration between 0.1 and 30 s. Myotonic discharges wax and wane;[4380] runs are initiated by needle insertion, needle movement, muscle contraction, or muscle percussion. The phenomenon of prolonged after-contraction of a muscle after voluntary effort has ceased, usually diminishing with continuing muscle activity. The basis for this is abnormal muscle fiber contraction associated with abnormal and continued sarcolemmal membrane excitation and with a reduction in the potential difference across the membrane, the precise mechanism of which is still uncertain. The increased muscle activity produces muscle stiffness that improves with repeated activity. 3. Muscle tension (obsolete).

Paradoxical myotonia (in paramyotonia) worsens with repeated activity. *Delayed myotonia* appears after a period of muscle contraction; see **myotonia fluctuans**.

An historical review is that of Thomasen.[6293]

The following genetic classification of the myotonias has been suggested[5138] and is adapted here

1. *Sodium channel diseases: SCN4A mutations*

   Hyperkalemic periodic paralysis (with clinical paramyotonia and electrical myotonia)
   Paramyotonia congenita (with clinical paramyotonia and electrical myotonia)
   Myotonia fluctuans
   Myotonia permanens
   Potassium-aggravated myotonias
   Acetazoleamide-responsive myotonias

2. *Protein kinase-related disease*

   Myotonic dystrophy type 1
   Proximal myotonic myopathy type 2

3. *Chloride-channel diseases*

   Myotonia congenita (Thomsen; autosomal dominant)
   Myotonia congenita (Becker; autosomal recessive)

4. *Unknown cause*

   Schwarz-Jampel syndrome (chondrodystrophic myotonia)
   Hyperkalemic periodic paralysis with dysrhythmias
   Dominantly inherited painful myotonia[3915]
   Myotonia complicating toxic, metabolic, or inflammatory myopathies.

(Based upon Ptacek LJ, et al. New Engl J Med *1993;328:482–89.*

In **acid maltase deficiency** there is electrical but no clinical myotonia. **Paramyotonia** produces a similar symptom, but the stiffness paradoxically increases with activity. Myopathy, denervation, and drug-induced hypothyroidism are other uncommon causes of myotonia.

myotonia acquisita Transient **myotonia**, which is not of genetic origin and which is precipitated by exercise, or as a result of trauma, infectious, or metabolic disease (such as poisoning with diazocholesterol or 2.4-D), or polyneuropathy.[6196] See **pseudomyotonia** and **Talma disease**.

myotonia atrophica See **myotonic dystrophy**.

myotonia congenita (Thomsen disease) A nonprogressive, nondystrophic myopathy with infantile or childhood onset, marked by abnormal electrical afterdischarges in muscles subjected to voluntary contraction and leading to a failure of relaxation which is made worse by rest and cold. The resultant cell membrane hyperexcitability results in reduction in sarcolemmal chloride conductance. Both dominant (mapped to 7q35) and (less commonly in North America) recessive inheritance (*Becker myotonia*) are recorded, the former having an earlier onset but lesser severity, the latter sometimes associated with muscle dystrophic changes and periodic paralysis. This is the commonest genetic skeletal muscle ion channelopathy and is caused by mutations in *CLCN1* on chromosome 7q35, which alter the function of the major skeletal muscle voltage-gated chloride channel.

Clinically, painful, electrically silent muscle contractions, action and percussion myotonia, paradoxical myotonia in the cold, and severe cold-insensitivity affecting especially the face are other notable symptoms. The EMG findings that repetitive muscular contractions do not alter the recruitment pattern and that, after cooling of the hand, the myotonic activity increases, differentiate this condition from **paramyotonia congenita**.[4669]

Dr. Thomsen himself was thus affected and there was a strong family history of it (affecting at least four generations), but he was stirred to publish on the subject only because his affected son was being accused of malingering in an attempt to escape military service.[6305] Ernst von Leyden (1832–1910) gave an account of the disease in the same year.

Variant myotonic syndromes in this class are described,[6090] as listed in Chart M–29.

See also **paramyotonia congenita** and **myotonic dystrophy** and the WUSTL Web site: http://www.neuro.wustl.edu/neuromuscular/maltbrain.html/.

myotonia congenita and painful muscle contraction See **myotonia congenita**.

myotonia congenita with severe cold sensitivity See **myotonia congenita**.

myotonia fluctuans (sodium-sensitive myotonia) A rare skeletal muscle sodium channel disease (SCN4A sodium channel α-subunit) presenting as a variant form of **myotonia** and characterized by dominant inheritance, exercise-induced delayed-onset myotonia variable from day to day and the absence of weakness. Symptoms are made worse with potassium loading but are minimally affected by cold.[5288] The responsible gene is mapped to 17q23.

A *variant* is *acetazolamide-responsive myotonia* (see above).

myotonia, myokymia, hyperhidrosis, and muscle wasting See **myotonia congenita**.

myotonia permanens A syndrome of continuous myokymia with marked muscle hypertrophy and superimposed attacks of marked muscle stiffness as a result of sodium channel impairment.[3756]

myotonia with centronuclear myopathy See **myotonia congenita**.

myotonia with dwarfism and bone disease A rare dysmorphic syndrome with these characteristics.[37]

myotonic chondrodystrophy See **Schwartz-Jampel syndrome**.

myotonic discharge Repetitive discharge which occurs at rates of 20–80 Hz. There are two types: (1) Biphasic (positive-negative) spike potentials less than 5 ms in duration resembling fibrillation potentials. (2) Positive waves of 5–20 ms duration resembling positive sharp waves. Both potential forms are recorded after needle electrode insertion, after voluntary muscle contraction or after muscle percussion, and are due to independent, repetitive discharges of single muscle fibers. The amplitude and frequency of the potentials must both wax and wane. This change produces a characteristic musical sound in the audio output of the electromyogram due to the corresponding change in pitch, which has been likened to the sound of a dive bomber (but that is incorrect as the sound of an approaching dive bomber is characterized by increasing pitch, while myotonic discharges sound more like the whine of a rapidly departing motor cyclist), Cf. waning discharge. (Adapted from the 2001 Report of the Nomenclature Committee of the American Association of Electromyography and Electrodiagnosis.[19] Reproduced by kind permission of the AANEM.)

myotonic dystrophy (DM1; Batten-Gibb disease; Batten-Steinert-Curschmann disease; Steinert disease; Deleage disease; dystrophia myotonica; myotonica atrophica; OMIM 160900) A dominantly inherited multisystem disease, the gene mapping to l9ql3.3, considered to be due to an expansion of an unstable cytosine-thiamine-guanine trinucleotide repeat. There is marked anticipation. The mutation is identified by the p5B1.4 probe. This is the most prevalent genetic dystrophy in the Western world, although **Duchenne dystrophy** has a higher incidence. Onset is at any age between birth and late adult life. Fragments of the syndrome may occur in isolation.[5134]

The main features of the full syndrome include distal, centripetal, and cranial muscular atrophy with weakness, including respiratory muscle weakness; myotonia, shown best in the distal hand and faciobulbar muscles after percussion or voluntary contraction; cardiomyopathy; endocrinopathy with frontal balding, diabetes, and hypogonadism; and multiple tiny posterior subcapsular polar specks (*Christmas-tree cataracts*), reduced intraocular pressure and slow pupillary reactions as well as diminished insight into the gravity of the condition. A "circumflex" or tented upper lip in children and sternomastoid and temporalis wasting in adults are characteristic. Excessive daytime sleepiness, mental torpor, and reduced cognitive function are other notable features.

Chart M–29. Variant Myotonic Syndromes

Acetazolamide-responsive myotonia A dominantly inherited disorder of the sodium channel mapped to 7q35 and characterized by muscle hypertrophy without weakness, "paradoxical" myotonia made worse by repeated activity, muscle pain and stiffness, aggravation by potassium, and response to acetazolamide.

Becker variant A recessively inherited disorder of the muscle chloride channel (CLCN1) at chromosome 7q35. Clinically, the symptoms are more severe than in the dominant form. The onset is in childhood, presenting with myotonia of the leg muscles, improving with continuing activity (the "warm-up" phenomenon). Muscle hypertrophy may be seen in the leg and gluteal muscles. Initially, strength is normal but with brief exercise there is rapid occurrence of weakness, returning to normal with further activity. Some permanent distal weakness may be apparent. EMG findings include distal more than proximal myotonia, reduced with maximal contraction, and other features of mild myopathy. A decremental response occurs, especially at 30 Hz stimulation frequency.

Familial granulovacuolar lobular myopathy with electrical myotonia.[3256]

Familial hyperkalemic periodic paralysis with myotonia.

Myotonia congenita and painful muscle contraction (type 2) (myotonia with painful cramps): A congenital syndrome of hypothyroidism, myotonia, and muscle pain.[5531]

Myotonia congenita with severe cold sensitivity (type 3): A dominantly inherited syndrome in which the abnormal muscle contractions are markedly increased at low temperatures.

Myotonia with centronuclear myopathy: An inherited syndrome characterized by cataract, ptosis, ophthalmoplegia, torticollis, pes cavus, joint contractures, and proximal and distal myopathy with myotonia.

Myotonia, myokymia, hyperhidrosis, and muscle wasting: A benign syndrome of young men, manifesting these features. The EMG and muscle biopsy findings are generally normal.[2569]

Paramyotonia congenita: A rare dominantly inherited nonprogressive syndrome with onset in childhood and characterized by muscle stiffness worsened in cold temperatures, with increased and prolonged weakness after exercise (especially of the hand, facial, and bulbar muscles).[1923] Delayed eye opening after tight closure is characteristic. Independent attacks of paralysis also occur in some cases, precipitated for example by potassium loading.

Recessive generalized myotonia: A progressive myotonic syndrome characterized by childhood onset with marked muscle stiffness, especially in the legs, and only mild proximal muscle weakness.

Recessive myotonia congenita with dystrophic features.[4575]

The above is based upon, but modified from the classification of Streib (1987).[6090]

An *infantile* form with hypotonia, weakness, and respiratory insufficiency occurring in the children of affected mothers (not of affected fathers) is unusually severe in the neonatal period, seems to modify the degree of affliction during childhood, but reappears in serious form in youth. Hydramnios is often recorded during pregnancy.

The first descriptions were those of C.L. **Dana** in 1888 and of Francisque Deléage (b. 1862) in his graduation thesis for the Université de Paris, 1890 (although he thought that it was a variety of **Thomsen disease**). Hoffmann gave a partial description in 1900 and Steinert a fuller one in 1904. It is also of interest because the Ypsilante brothers, leaders of the Greek revolution of 1821 in which Greece was successfully wrested from the control of the Ottoman Empire, suffered from it.[2775] The condition was the first disease in which the phenomenon of anticipation was proven.

Defined *variants* of the syndrome are expanding in number, but all multisystem myotonic disorders are subsumed under the heading of myotonic dystrophies. They include the following:

Myotonic dystrophy and hypertrophic neuropathy, characterized by neurogenic muscular atrophy and demyelinating sensorimotor neuropathy in addition to the usual signs of the disease.[381]

Myotonic dystrophy and axonal-demyelinating polyneuropathy, characterized by the presence of a severe sensorimotor polyneuropathy in addition to the usual signs of the disease.[6570]

Myotonic dystrophy with hypersomnia and alveolar hypoventilation, in which the typical signs of myotonic dystrophy are accompanied by excessive somnolence and alveolar hypoventilation.

Proximal myotonic myopathy (DM2; PROMM) and its subvariants

Unclassified familial myopathy resembling Steinert disease, a proximal myopathy with the usual non-neurological findings of myotonic dystrophy but without clinical or electrical evidence of myotonia.[6247]

See also **action myotonia, percussion myotonia**, and **paradoxical myotonia**.

Myotonic Dystrophy Foundation A charitable organization providing support and information on this condition. http://www.myotonic.com/go/mdf/.

myotonic periodic paralysis See **paramyotonia congenita**.

myotonic (Adie) pupil See **Holmes–Adie syndrome**.

myotonic pupillary reaction See **Adie pupil**.

myotonica atrophica See **myotonic dystrophy**.

myotubes Multinucleated cell structures seen early in fetal development (7 weeks) and composed of fused myoblasts. In postnatal life, myotube-like structures are found in one form of congenital myopathy.

myotubular myopathy See **centronuclear myopathies**.

myriachit A familial tic-like disorder affecting both sexes, occurring epidemically in Siberia, the movements precipitated by startle and lasting hours, sometimes accompanied by echolalia. It was described by **Tourette** in 1884.

mythomania The psychological "need" to tell lies, described by **Charcot** among patients diagnosed with **hysteria** at the **Salpêtrière**.

myxedema (Gull disease, hypothyroidism)[2635] The painless, nonpitting edema of the shin described in hypothyroidism. Such edema was considered so specific that its name was also used for the whole syndrome of hypothyroidism.

myxedema cerebellar syndrome Ataxia and incoordination complicating hypothyroidism, remitting with successful treatment of that condition.[3187]

myxedema coma (hypothyroid encephalopathy) A recurrent acute encephalopathy with confusion leading on to coma with pyramidal signs and seizures or myoclonus, and a low-voltage EEG marked by generalized slow–wave activity. It is seen in myxedema in the context of **Hashimoto** encephalopathy and results from a marked depression of the hypoxic respiratory drive, leading to further hypoxia, hypercapnia, and coma resulting from CO_2 narcosis. Hyponatremia due to inappropriate antidiuretic hormone secretion, hypothermia, and hypoglycemia may also contribute, and pituitary and adrenal insufficiencies are also incriminated. The mortality rate ranges up to 30%.[3770]

The illness is usually precipitated by cold, chest infections, stroke, congestive heart failure, or sedative drugs, typically in patients with a history of thyroid disease, and often with evidence of dementia or **myxedematous madness**. The condition was first recognized in 1879 by William Ord.

myxedematous madness The colorful term used by Richard Asher in 1949 for a syndrome (also well described by A.J. Cronin in *The Citadel*, 1937) comprising disturbances in mentation often accompanying severe hypothyroidism. These include delirium, melancholia, paranoid psychoses, and sometimes restless violence, hallucinations, depression, dementia, extreme somnolence, and sometimes hypothermia. No one of these manifestations is predominant. There are no focal signs except for localized EEG changes. See **myxedema coma**.[267]

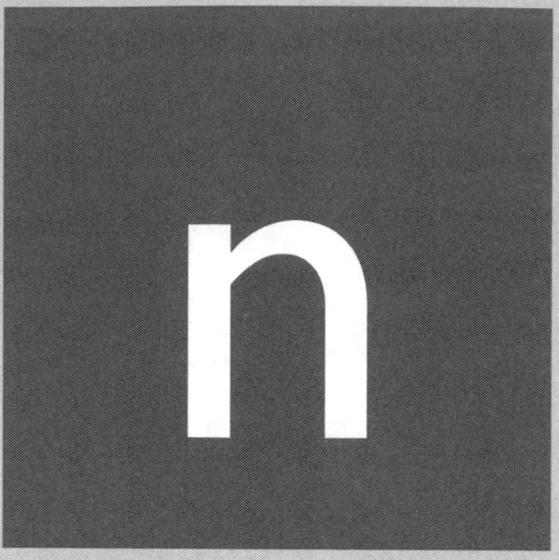

_N_-acetylaspartic aciduria A congenital syndrome resulting from aspartoacylase deficiency and manifesting spasticity, macrocephaly, tremor, diffuse cerebral demyelination, and mental and developmental delay with organic aciduria.[381]

NADH-coenzyme Q reductase deficiency An inherited mitochondrial myopathy characterized by Complex 1 defects that lead to exercise-induced fatigue, acute attacks of weakness provoked by exercise, alcohol or fasting, and lactic acidosis.[4481]

Naegeli syndrome See **incontinentia pigmenti**.

Naffziger, Howard Christian (1884–1961) American neurosurgeon who trained and saw war service with **Cushing**. Later, he became professor at the University of California at San Francisco.

Naffziger signs 1. Compression of both jugular veins increases CSF pressure, which, being transmitted to the lumbar theca, stretches both the meninges and the attached nerve roots and causes (or increases) pain in patients with root irritation at those levels.[4750] 2. Pressure on the scalenus anterior muscle above the clavicle leads to paresthesias of the hand in patients with **thoracic outlet syndrome**. 3. Shift of the pineal gland (visible on skull X-ray when calcified) as a sign of an expanding intracranial mass, such as a subdural hematoma.

Naffziger syndrome (scalenus syndrome) See **thoracic outlet syndrome**.

Nagel anomaloscope A device for detecting defects in color vision, in which the subject has to match the appearance of a monochromatic yellow field to one of a number of mixtures of red and green lights.[4954]

Nageotte, Jean (1866–1948) French neurologist, born in Dijon. He graduated from the University of Paris, where he was appointed as physician at the Bicêtre hospital and later at the **Salpêtrière**. He succeeded Ranvier as professor of comparative histology at the Collège de France.

Nageotte was a friend of **Babiński**, with whom he collaborated in studies of the CSF and in describing medullary tegmental paralysis, and he was also the first correctly to ascribe the lesion in **tabes dorsalis** to the dorsal roots.

Naidech scale A nomogram for predicting the risk of rebleeding from an intracranial aneurysm, based on the Hunt–Hess grade for the initial subarachnoid hemorrhage and the diameter of the aneurysm.[4577]

Naidu variant See **adrenoleukodystrophy**.

naked axons Nonmyelinated nerve fibers or demyelinated fibers of usually myelinated axons; the axons of the Remak fibers.

NAME syndrome (nevi, atrial myxoma, myxoid neurofibromata, epiphelides) A congenital dysmorphic syndrome characterized also by gynecomastia; tumors of the breast, testes, and heart; abnormal genital pigmentation; adrenal hyperplasia; large sella turcica; osteoporosis; acanthosis nigricans; nevi; cavernous hemangioma; skin cysts; and neurofibromas.[5233]

Name–Face test A test of visual–verbal associations in which names appear with photographs.[2033]

Nance–Sweeney dwarfism A recessively inherited congenital chondrodystrophy characterized by dysmorphism; short stature; calcification of the ear cartilage, subcutaneous tissue, and muscle; macrocephaly; conductive and sensorineural deafness; brachydactyly, scoliosis, and other skeletal anomalies.[4589]

nanism Dwarfism.

nanocephaly (from Gr, a dwarf + the head) Abnormal smallness of the head; the same as microcephaly.

Nantahana neuropathy A dominantly inherited sensorimotor neuropathy resembling CMT1A but with the added features of trigeminal neuralgia and hemifacial spasm, found in a North Carolina kinship (Dr. James B. Caress, personal communication).

narcolepsy (from Gr, numbness + a seizure) A disorder of excessive sleepiness often associated with the occurrence of manifestations of rapid eye movement (REM) sleep, such as **hypnagogic hallucinations**, **cataplexy**, and **sleep paralysis**, during waking periods.

Clinically, in its fullest expression, the syndrome is characterized by excessive daytime sleepiness, **hypnagogic hallucinations**, **cataplexy**, **sleep paralysis**, microsleep lapses, amnesic automatisms, memory blackouts, diplopia, and disturbed nocturnal sleep. In early cases, the disorder may be monosymptomatic. The onset is generally in youth or young adult life. The above symptoms along with the sleep attacks make up a tetrad of narcoleptic symptoms occurring more often in association with **REM-onset sleep patterns** as seen on the EEG, whereas patients who have **idiopathic CNS hypersomnolence** have sleep attacks with non-rapid eye movement sleep (NREM) onset. **Sleep apnea** may also complicate the syndrome, which characteristically begins in youth.

A quarter of the patients have only sleep attacks, 70% have both narcolepsy and cataplexy, and the remainder experience all four symptoms of the tetrad.

A positive family history is common, and tight linkage to HLA DQB1 0602 has been demonstrated, but the responsible gene maps to chromosome 6p21.3. The pathophysiology appears to involve acquired damage to hypothalamic cells secreting the peptide hypocretin.

While Gélineau[2325] gave the first modern account of the syndrome in 1880 (his patient had sleep attacks and cataplexy), he acknowledged Caffé's earlier identification of the disorder in 1862, but not that by H.B. Schindler, an ophthalmologist in Breslau, in 1829. In fact, Thomas **Willis** had recounted his treatment of patients with excessive sleepiness 200 years before in *De Anima Brutorum* and **Westphal** described it 3 years before Gélineau, but the latter named it. The American general "Stonewall" Jackson probably suffered from this condition, but it did not seem to diminish his military effectiveness.

See also Chart S–6, **sleep disorders**.[1629, 2625]

Diagnostic criteria were first suggested by Yoss and Daly,[6922] but newer ones have been suggested and are listed in Chart N–1.[1629]

Variants include the following:

Secondary narcolepsy (symptomatic), in which some symptoms of the condition appear in patients with various diseases affecting the brain stem
Narcolepsy with congenital oculomotor pareses
Narcolepsy with congenital cataract
Narcolepsy with diplopia and strabismus[4904]

See also **idiopathic hypersomnia**.

Narcolepsy Network A charitable organization providing support and information on this condition. Address: 10921 Reed Hartman Highway, Cincinnati, OH 45242. Tel: 513-891-3522. Web site: http://www.websciences.org/narnet/.

narcosis (from Gr, benumbing) The condition of those under the influence of sedative agents.

narcotic abstinence headache See **rebound headache** in which headaches on withdrawal from other substances are included.

NARP syndrome (Neurogenic weakness with Ataxia and Retinitis Pigmentosa) A sporadic, X-linked or autosomal recessive mitochondrial disorder characterized by sensory peripheral neuropathy resembling Refsum syndrome (**hereditary motor and sensory neuropathy**, type 4) but with normal serum phytanic acid and lipoprotein levels, and including ataxia and retinitis pigmentosa. The biochemical abnormality is not known. Sensorineural deafness and evidence of cerebellar atrophy have also been detected in such patients.[4151, 5748, 6414]

Chart N–1. Diagnostic Criteria for Narcolepsy

A. A complaint of excessive sleepiness or sudden muscle weakness
B. Recurrent daytime naps or lapses into sleep that occur almost daily for at least 3 months
C. Sudden bilateral loss of postural muscle tone in association with intense emotion (cataplexy)
D. Associated features include the following:
   1. Sleep paralysis
   2. Hypnagogic hallucinations
   3. Automatic behaviors
   4. Disrupted major sleep episode
E. Polysomnography demonstrates one or more of the following:
   1. Sleep latency less than 5 min
   2. REM sleep latency less than 20 min
   3. A multiple sleep latency test that demonstrates a mean sleep latency of <5 min
   4. Two or more sleep-onset REM periods
F. HLA typing demonstrates DQB1*0602 or DR2 positivity
G. Absence of any medical or psychiatric disorder that could account for the symptoms
H. Other sleep disorders may be present, but are not the primary cause of the symptoms, for example, periodic limb movement disorder or central sleep apnea syndrome

From AASM Diagnostic Classification Steering Committee. *The International Classification of Sleep Disorders Diagnostic and Coding Manual*. Rochester, MN. American Academy of Sleep Medicine 1991/2001. Reproduced by kind permission of the Academy.) See also http://www.sleepeducation.com/Disorders.aspx/.

See also **Cockayne syndrome, Hallgren syndrome, von Graefe–Sjörgren syndrome, lipidoses,** and **cerebellar ataxias.**

nasal reflex 1. (sternutatory reflex, sneeze reflex) Sneezing in response to nasal tickle. 2. (nasal reflex of Bechterew) Contraction of the ipsilateral facial muscles in response to nasal tickle. An abrogation of No. 1.

nasal reflex of Bechterew See **nasal reflex.**

nascent (from Lat, to be born) In the process of being born.

nascent motor unit potentials Very low-amplitude, short-duration, highly polyphasic motor unit action potentials observed during the early stages of reinnervation. The use of the term is discouraged, as it incorrectly implies diagnostic significance of a motor unit action potential configuration. See also **motor unit action potential.** (After the 2001 Report of the Nomenclature Committee of the American Association of Electromyography and Electrodiagnosis.[19] Reproduced by kind permission of the AANEM.)

nasion The median point of the junction between the two frontal and the two nasal bones; thus, the center point above the bridge of the nose.

nasociliary neuralgia (Charlin neuralgia) A rare condition in which touching the outer aspect of one nostril causes a lancinating pain radiating to the medial frontal region. Diagnostic criteria have been defined as follows:

A. Stabbing pain lasting seconds to hours in one side of the nose, radiating upward to the medial frontal region and fulfilling criteria B and C.
B. Pain is precipitated by touching the lateral aspect of the ipsilateral nostril.
C. Pain is abolished by block or section of the nasociliary nerve, or by the application of cocaine to the nostril on the affected side.

From the International Classification of Headache Disorders (Headache Classification Committee of the International Headache Society. *Cephalalgia* 2004;24[Suppl 1]) by kind permission of Dr. Jes Olesen, the International Headache Society and Wiley-Blackwell Publications.

nasolacrimal reflex The secretion of tears in response to chemical stimulation of the nasal mucosa.

nasomental reflex See **buccal reflex** and **orbicularis oris reflex.**

nasopalpebral reflex (glabellar tap, orbicularis oculi reflex) Blinking in response to tapping on the bridge of the nose.[6898] See also **McCarthy reflex.**

nasopharyngeal electrode An EEG electrode introduced through the nasal passages to lie against the nasopharyngeal wall, its tip thus close to the body of the sphenoid bone.

nasopharyngeal torticollis See **Grisel syndrome.**

Nasu-Hakola lipodystrophy (polycystic lipomembranous osteodysplasia with sclerosing leukoencephalopathy; OMIM 221770) A recessively inherited dysmorphic syndrome with juvenile or young adult onset, characterized by bony cysts and multiple fractures, progressive frontal-type dementia with dyspraxia, agnosia and dysphasia, seizures, myoclonus, pyramidal signs, frontal lobe atrophy, and calcifications of the basal ganglia.[4875] Three genetic forms are differentiated. It is mapped to19q13.1 (*DAP 12*, functioning in microglial activation and in the differentiation of macrophages and osteoclasts).

nasute (from Lat, nose) Having a keen sense of smell.

nates (Lat, the rump) The buttocks. The *nates cerebri* are the corpora quadragemini, from their supposed resemblance to the foregoing.

Nathalie syndrome A congenital syndrome characterized by short stature, sensorineural deafness, cataract, absent or hypoplastic breasts, EKG abnormality, and axonal motor neuropathy.[381]

National Adult Reading Test A measure of premorbid cognitive function, achieved by assessing the subject's pronunciation of 50 irregular English words. Its value is in the fact that the scores achieved are not affected by progressing cognitive impairment.[4617]

National AIDS Information Clearinghouse A government-sponsored service in the United States. Address: 1600 Research Blvd., Rockville, MD 20850. Tel: 1-800-458-5231.

National AIDS Network A charitable association. Address: 1012 14th Street, NW, Suite 601, Washington, DC 20005. Tel: 202-347-0390.

National ALS Association A charitable association in this field. Address: 15300 Ventura Blvd., Suite 315, Sherman Oaks, CA 91403.

National Aphasia Association A charitable organization. Web site: http://www.aphasia.org/.

National Association for Down Syndrome A charitable organization. Web site: http://www.nads.org/.

National Association for Hearing and Speech See **American Speech and Hearing Association.** http://www.asha.org/default.htm/.

National Ataxia Foundation A nonprofit organization established in 1957 with the primary mission of encouraging and supporting research into hereditary ataxias. Address: 750 Twelve Oaks Center, 15500 Wayzata Blvd., Wayzata, MN 55391. Tel: 612-473-7666. Web site: http://www.ataxia.org/.

National Brachial Plexus/Erb's Palsy Association, Inc. A charitable organization in this field. Address: P.O. Box 23, Larsen, WI 54947. E-mail: erbspalsy@usa.net. Web site: http://www.nbpepa/.

National Brain Injury Information Center A resource providing brain injury information only. Tel: 1-800-444-6443.

National Brain Research Association See **International Brain Research Foundation.**

National Brain Tumor Foundation A charitable organization. Address: 785 Market Street, Ste. 1600, San Francisco, CA 94103. Tel: 1-800-934-CURE and at 323 Gear St., Suite 510, San Francisco, CA 94102. Web site: http://www.braintumor.org/.

National Chronic Pain Outreach Association A charitable organization in this field. Address: P.O. Box 274, Millboro, VA 24460. Tel: 540-862-9437. Web site: http://www.ijdf.net/.

National Committee for Research in Neurological and Communicative Disorders An organization composed of representatives of voluntary health agencies and professional societies concerned with neurological diseases, and aiming to stimulate public information and to enlist continuing support for increased training in research into these diseases.

National Disability Sports Alliance A charitable organization in this field. Address: 25 West Independence Way, Kingston, RI 02881. Tel: 401-792-7130. E-mail: info@ndsaonline.org. Web site: http://www.ndsaonline.org/.

National Down Syndrome Society A charitable association in this field. Web site: http://www.ndss.org/main.html.

National Dysautonomia Research Foundation An organization concerned with these conditions. E-mail: ndrf@ndrf.org/. Web site: http://www.ndrf.org/. A patient-support network is at http://www.medhelp.org/network.htm.

National Easter Seal Society A charitable organization based at 2023 West Ogden Ave., Chicago, IL 60612.

National Epilepsy Library See **Epilepsy Foundation of America**.

National Eye Institute A government health research organization. Address: National Institutes of Health, Bldg. 31, Rm. 6A32, Bethesda, MD 20892-2510. Tel: 301-496-5248: Professionals 800-869-2020. E-mail: 2020@b31.nei.nih.gov. Web site: http://www.nei.nih.gov/.

National Foundation for Brain Research A charitable organization that collects, organizes, and disseminates information relating to the *Decade of the Brain*. Web site: http://www.brainnet.org.

National Foundation for Jewish Genetic Diseases A charitable association in this field providing information and support. Address: 250 Park Ave., Suite 1000, New York, NY 10177. Tel: 212-371-1030. Web site: http://www.nfjgd.org/.

National Fragile X Foundation A patient support group and charity. Web site: www.FragileX.org.

National Gaucher Foundation A charitable organization in this field providing information and support. Address: 5410 Edson Lane, Suite 260, Rockville, MD 20852-3130. Tel: 301-816-1515; 800-428-2437. E-mail: ngf@gaucherdisease.org. Web site: http://www.gaucherdisease.org/.

National Head Injuries Association A charitable association in this field. Address: 17 Climber Ave., Sherwood Rise, Nottingham NG5 1AG, UK.

National Head Injury Foundation A charitable association in this field. Address: 1776 Massachusetts Ave., NW, Suite 100, Washington, DC. Tel: 202-296-6443. See also **Brain Injury Association of America**.

National Headache Foundation A charitable organization in this field providing information and support. Web site: http://www.headaches.org/.

National Hospital, Queen Square The first hospital dedicated to the care and cure of patients suffering from neurological diseases; it was opened in Queen Square, London, England, in 1860 largely due to the efforts of Miss Joanna Chandler, who saw the great need for such an institution and determined to devote her life to supply such a place for the treatment of the paralyzed and epileptic. The stated object of the hospital was to "give relief to such persons as are disqualified for the duties of life by either paralysis or epilepsy and are proper objects of charity. Those who need only partial relief . . . will be treated as outdoor patients . . ." The appointment to its staff of some of the best-known London practitioners saved the hospital from the hostility of the medical profession and it flourished, although existing almost totally upon the proceeds of charitable appeals. New buildings were added, the Rockefeller Foundation contributing funds for the erection of research laboratories in 1934, and for over 100 years, the hospital, with the Institute of Neurology built later, was preeminently the center for the study of neurological disorders in Great Britain, receiving referrals from all parts of the United Kingdom.

Dr. J. Hughlings-**Jackson**, Sir William **Gowers**, Dr. **Brown-Sequard**, Sir David **Ferrier**, Sir Gordon **Holmes**, Sir Victor **Horsley**, Dr. Marcus **Gunn**, Dr. S. A. K. **Wilson**, Sir Francis **Walshe**, Sir Charles **Symonds**, and Dr. W. J. **Adie**, among others, were members of the staff of the hospital during its first hundred years of its operation.[2963]

National Huntington's Disease Association A charitable organization supporting medical research and providing educational guidance services. Address: 128A East 74th St., New York, NY 10021. See also the NINDS Web site: http://www.ninds.nih.gov/disorders/huntington/huntington.htm/.

National Hydrocephalus Foundation A charitable organization in this field. Address: 12413 Centralia Rd., Lakewood, CA 90715-1623. Tel: 562-402-3523; 888-857-3434. E-mail: hydrobrat@earthlink.net. Web site: http://nhfonline.org/.

National Institute of Aging An American government organization based at 9000 Rockville Pike, Bethesda, MD 20205. Tel: 301-496-4000. Web site: http://www.nia.nih.gov/.

National Institute of Child Health and Human Development A government health research organization. Address: National Institutes of Health Bldg. 31, Rm. 2A32,

Bethesda, MD 20892-2425. Tel: 301-496-5133; 800-370-2943. E-mail: NICHDClearinghouse@mail.nih.gov. Web site: http://www.nichd.nih.gov/.

National Institute of Deafness and Other Communication Disorders A government health research organization. Address: National Institutes of Health Bldg. 31, Rm. 3C35, Bethesda, MD 20892-2320. E-mail: nidcdinfo@nidcd.nih.gov. Tel: 301-496-7243. Web site: http://www.nidcd.nih.gov/.

National Institute of Mental Health A government health research organization. Address: 6001 Executive Blvd., Rm. 8184, MSC 9663, Bethesda, MD 20892-9663. Tel: 301-443-4513. Depression Info: 800-421-4211. Anxiety Info: 88-88-ANXIETY (269-4389). Panic Info: 888-64-PANIC (64-72642). E-mail: nimhinfo@nih.gov. Web site: http://www.nimh.nih.gov/.

National Institute of Neurological and Communicative Disorders and Stroke See National Institute of Neurological Disorder and Stroke.

NINDS—National Institute of Neurological Disorders and Stroke (National Institute of Neurological Disease and Blindness, National Institute of Neurological and Communicative Disorders and Stroke) An American government organization established in 1951 as an institute for research in neurological diseases. Its name was changed to the National Institute of Neurological and Communicative Disorders and Stroke in 1968 and subsequently to the current one. The institute functions to increase study in the basic sciences; to initiate research in targeted areas, such as neonatal brain damage, stroke, and neurogenetics; and to provide research and training fellowships in the neurological disciplines. It is an excellent source of factsheets on many neurological disorders, genetic and acquired. Address: 31 Center Drive 8A07 Bethesda, MD 20892-2540. Tel: 301-496-5751; 800-352-9424. Fax: 301-402-2186. E-mail: braininfo@ninds.nih.gov. Web site: http://www.ninds.nih.gov/.

National Institute of Neurological Disorder and Stroke myotatic reflex scale
A standardized scale adopted in that center for the assessment of muscle stretch reflexes

0. Absence of the reflex.
1. Reduced responsiveness, or presence only with reinforcement.
2. Responsiveness assessed as in the lower half of the normal range.
3. Responsiveness assessed as in the upper half of the normal range.
4. Hypereflexia, including clonus.

Adapted from Hallett M. *Neurology* 1993;43:2723.

The scale is bottom-heavy, and any level of reflex activity, from 1 to 4, may actually be present in a normal subject.

National Institutes of Health
A vital US Government agency. Web site: www.nih.gov.

National Institutes of Health Office of Rare Diseases
A governmental agency. Web site: http://rarediseases.info.nih.gov/.

National Leigh's Disease Foundation An organization providing information about and support for people with this condition, with brief discussion about the organization and contact details. See the Web site: http://www.health.gov/nhic/NHICScripts/Entry.cfm?HRCode=HR2524/.

National Mental Health Association A charitable organization at 1021 Prince Street, Alexandria, VA 22314. Tel: 1-800-969-NMHA.

National Migraine Foundation
A charitable organization based at 5252 North Western Ave., Chicago, IL 60625. Tel: 301-496-4000. Web site: http://www.migraines.org/.

National Mucopolysaccharidosis Society
A charitable organization concerned with mucopolysaccharidoses. Address: 102 Aspen Dr., Downingtown, PA 19335. Tel: 610-942-0100. E-mail: info@mpssociety.org. Web site: http://www.mpssociety.org/.

National Multiple Sclerosis Society An American charitable organization devoted to supporting research into the causes and treatment of multiple sclerosis, and to providing support for those affected by the disease through the formation of chapters for education, counseling, referral, and advocacy. Address: 733 Third Ave., New York, NY 10017-3288. Tel: 212-986-3240 or 1-800-FIGHT MS (344-4867). E-mail: nat@nmss.org. Web site: http://www.nationalmssociety.org/.

National Neurofibromatosis Foundation Inc. A charitable organization devoted to supporting research into the causes and treatment of neurofibromatosis, promoting the development of diagnostic protocols and clinical centers, publishing educational materials, and supporting those affected by the disease through the formation of chapters for education, counselling, referral, and advocacy. Address: 95 Pine St., 16th Floor, New York, NY 10005. Tel: 800-323-7938; 212-344-6633. E-mail: nnff@nf.org. Web site: http://www.nf.org/.

National Neurological Research Specimen Bank
A research organization. Address: VA Medical Center, Wilshire and Sawtelle Blvds., Los Angeles, CA 90073. Tel: 310-824-430.

National Niemann-Pick Disease Foundation, Inc. A charitable organization in this field. Address: P.O. Box 49, Ft. Atkinson, WI 53538. Tel: 920-563-0930; 877-287-3672. E-mail: nnpdf@idcnet.com. Web site: http://www.nnpdf.org/.

National Organization for Rare Disorders, Inc. Address: P.O. Box 1968, 55 Kenosia Ave., Danbury, CT 06813-1968. Tel: 203-744-0100; 800-999-6673. E-mail: orphan@rarediseases.org. The Web site: http://www.rarediseases.org/ provides information about NORD, its programs, special events, and the variety of services offered. Includes a rare disease, organization, and orphan drug database. Diseases are listed alphabetically.

National Parkinson's Foundation A charitable organization in this field. Address: 710 West 168th St.,

New York, NY 10032-9982. Tel: 212-923-4700; 800-457-6676. E-mail: info@pdf.org. Web site: http://www.parkinsons-foundation.org/.

National Parkinson Foundation, Inc. A charitable association in this field. Address: 1501 NW 9th Avenue/Bob Hope Road, Miami, FL 33136. Tel: 1-800-327-4545. Web site: http://www.parkinson.org/.

National Pediatric Myoclonus Center SIU School of Medicine, Dept. of Neurology, Div. of Ped. Neurology, P.O. Box 19643, Springfield, IL 62794-9643. Tel: 2175457635. E-mail: oms@siumed.edu. Web site: http://www.omsusa.org./

National Rehabilitation Information Center A health research and support organization. Address: 4200 Forbes Blvd., Suite 202, Lanham, MD 20706. Tel: 800-346-2742; 301-459-5900. E-mail: naricinfo@heitechservices.com. Web site: http://www.naric.com/.

National Reye's Syndrome Foundation A charitable organization in this field. Address: P.O. Box 829, 426 North Lewis, Bryan, OH 3506-0829. Tel: 419-636-2679; 800-233-7393. E-mail: nrsf@reyessyndrome. org. Web site: http://www.reyessyndrome. org/.

National Sleep Foundation A charitable organization in this field. Address: 1522 K Street, NW, Suite 500, Washington, DC 20005. Tel: 202-347-3471. E-mail: nsf@sleepfoundation.org. Web site: http://www.sleepfoundation.org/.

National Society for Epilepsy A British organization providing information about and support for people with this condition. The society also runs (in conjunction with the National Hospital for Neurology and Neurosurgery) an inpatient epilepsy treatment center and epilepsy outpatients clinic and organizes respite care and sheltered workshops. Web site: http://www.epilepsynse.org.uk/.

National Society to Prevent Blindness A charitable organization. Address: 500 East Remington Rd., Schaumburg, IL 60173.

National Spasmodic Dysphonia Association A charitable association providing support and information on this condition. Address: P.O. Box 1574, Birmingham, MI 48009-1574. Tel: 810-646-6885. Web site: http://www.dysphonia.org/.

National Spasmodic Torticollis Association A charitable organization in this field. Address: 9920 Talbert Ave., Suite 233, Fountain Valley, CA 92708. Tel: 714-378-7837; 800-487-8385. E-mail: NSTAmail@aol.com. Web site: http://www.torticollis.org/.

National Spinal Cord Injury Association A charitable organization providing support and information on this condition. Address: 600 West Cummings Park, Suite 2000, Woburn, MA 01801. Tel: 617-935-2722; 1-800-962-9629. E-mail: NSCIA2@aol.com. Web site: http://www.spinalcord.org/.

National Spinal Cord Injury Hotline An informational and support service. Tel: 1-800-962-9629. Web site: http://www.proneuron.com/Links/index.html.

National Stroke Association A charitable organization committed solely to stroke prevention, treatment, rehabilitation, and community reintegration. It provides packaged training programs; on-site assistance; and physician, patient, and family education materials to acute care and rehabilitation hospitals; organizes workshops; operates the Stroke Information and Referral Center; and produces professional publications (*Stroke: Clinical Updates and Journal of Stroke and Cerebrovascular Disease*). Address: 8480 East Orchard Road, Suite 1000, Englewood, CO 80111-5015. Tel: 303-839-1992; 1-800-STROKES. Also at 300 East Hampden Ave., Suite 240, Englewood, CO 80123-2654. Tel: 303-762-9922. E-mail: info@stroke.org/. Web site: http://www.stroke.org/; www.strokejournal.org/.

National Tay–Sachs and Allied Diseases Association A charitable organization providing support and information to families affected by Tay–Sachs disease and many other degenerative genetic disorders. Address: 2001 Beacon St., Suite 204, Boston, MA 02135. Tel: 617-277-4463; 800-906-8723. E-mail: NTSAD-boston@worldnet.att.net. Web site: http://www.ntsad.org/.

National Tremor Foundation A British Foundation offering information, support, and advice to people of all ages with tremor. It is situated at Harold Wood Hospital (DSC), Gubbins Lane, Romford, Essex RM3 OBE, UK. Tel: 01708-378-050. Web site: http://www.tremor.org.uk/.

National Tuberous Sclerosis Association A charitable association in this field. Address: 8000 Corporate Dr., Suite 120, Landover, MD 20785. Tel: 1-800-225-NTSA. Web site: http://www.pslgroup.com/dg/1fefe.htm.

natural killer neuropathy A widespread multifocal, axonal, inflammatory neuropathy attacking roots and peripheral nerves, in association with CSF pleocytosis, in the context of natural killer cell leukemia.[694]

Nature Neuroscience A leading basic science journal. Web site: http://www.nature.com/neuro/.

nausea The desire or urge to vomit, unaccomplished.

NBIA See **neural degeneration with brain iron accumulation**.

NCS See **nerve conduction studies**.

near-constant-frequency trains See **complex repetitive discharge**.

near-death experience (NDE) A feeling of detachment from the world or the body, usually in a situation of severe ischemia or hypoxia and interpreted as a response to danger with or without neurological impairment during the time of danger. It is composed of several elements, classified by Nelson et al.[4622] as follows:

- Cognitive (altered sense of time, accelerated thought processes, life review, sense of sudden understanding)
- Affective (feeling of peace, joy, cosmic unity)
- Purportedly paranormal (vivid senses, parasensory perception, precognitive vision, a sense of being out of one's physical body, seeing/feeling as if surrounded by light)

In some cases, the subject is immobilized while alert to the surroundings and "aware of being dead." Such observations resemble the REM sleep state; REM intrusion may well underlie some of the subjective experiences of both NDE and syncope.

near-field A region of electrical activity where the isopotential voltage lines associated with a current source change rapidly over a short distance. The terms near-field and far-field are arbitrary designations, as there are no agreed-upon criteria defining where the near-field ends and the far-field begins. Cf. **far-field**. (From the 2001 Report of the Nomenclature Committee of the American Association of Electromyography and Electrodiagnosis.[19] Reproduced by kind permission of the AANEM.)

near-field potential Electrical activity of biological origin generated near the recording electrodes. The AANEM discourages the use of the terms *near-field potential* and *far-field potential* because, as they point out, all potentials in clinical neurophysiology are recorded at some distance from the generator and there is no consistent distinction between the two terms.[19]

near infrared (NIR) A form of functional imaging like fMRI, allowing examination of brain function during cognitive or motor activation tasks.

near point The closest place in front of the eyes at which an object is still in focus.

near reflex See **near triad**.

near response Pupillary constriction (accommodation) with vergence of the eyes during gaze upon an object near to the face. See also **near triad**.

near synkinesis See **near triad**.

near triad (near response, near reflex, near synkinesis) The three mechanisms whereby the eye disposes itself to allow focused close vision. They comprise **convergence**, **miosis**, and pupillary constriction (**accommodation**).

neck All that part of the body that lies between and connects the head and the thorax.

neck phenomenon See **Brudzinski signs**.

neck rigidity Active reflex resistance to passive flexion of the neck; a sign of meningeal irritation from any cause and of increased intracranial pressure. Increased tone of the neck extensors is also a feature of **progressive supranuclear palsy**, and increased resistance to flexion occurs in subjects with cervical spinal disease, but in such cases other signs of meningeal irritation (**Kernig sign** and **Brudzinski sign**) should be absent.

neck torsion nystagmus See **cervical nystagmus**.

neck–eye loop See **cervico-ocular reflex**.

neck-righting reflex See **righting reflex**.

neck-righting response A variation of the **tonic neck reflex**, seen in the first 10 months of life, wherein rotation of the infant's head to one side induces rotation of the shoulder and pelvis and eventually of the whole body to that side. The reflex may be induced clinically in order to compare motor activity on the two sides of the body.

neck–tongue syndrome The occurrence of pain in the occiput or upper neck and numbness on one side of the tongue induced by turning the head and likely to be due to irritation of the C2–3 cervical roots as they course between the axis and atlas. Diagnostic criteria have been defined as follows:

A. Pain lasting seconds or minutes, with or without simultaneous dysaesthesia, in the area of distribution of the lingual nerve and second cervical root and fulfilling criteria B and C.
B. Pain has acute onset.
C. Pain is commonly precipitated by sudden turning of the head.

From the International Classification of Headache Disorders (Headache Classification Committee of the International Headache Society. *Cephalalgia* 2004;**24** [Suppl 1]) by kind permission of Dr. Jes Olesen, the International Headache Society and Wiley-Blackwell Publications.

Repeated minor subluxations of the C1–2 articulatory process with compression and stretch injury of adjacent nerves such as the C2 ramus may be responsible. Afferent fibers from the lingual nerve join the hypoglossal nerve and then enter the upper cervical rami, which accounts for the tongue symptoms. The pain is thought to be due to stretching of the joint capsule of the lateral articulating process.[3661, 4815]

necrosis (from Gr, a state of death) Irreversible destruction of some or all of the cellular elements of a tissue.

necrotizing fasciitis An uncommon, severe and potentially lethal condition manifesting gross swelling of an affected part with severe fever and necrosis of the overlying skin, with fever, shock, and multisystem involvement resulting from bacterial infection.[4293] Type 1 is caused by mixed anaerobes, enterococci, and gram-negative aerobes and tends to destroy fat and fascia, while Type 2 is caused by group A streptococcus and is characterized by severe local pain, systemic toxicity and shock, organ failure, and extending necrosis of skin and subcutaneous tissues.[662]

In a *variant* form, *necrotizing fasciitis with polymyositis*, the infection is considered secondary to the immunosuppression associated with the polymyositis.[1042] See also **myonecrosis**.

necrotizing granulomatous angiitis with a predilection for the CNS See **allergic angiitis** and **granulomatosis**.

necrotizing leukoencephalopathy Rapidly progressive necrosis of the white matter of the brain as a complication of the combined treatment of leukemia with methotrexate and cranial irradiation. Clinically, confusion, ataxia, and quadriparesis lead to seizures, stupor, and eventual death. See also **somnolence syndrome**.

necrotizing leukoencephalopathy with CNS vasculitis A fatal dysimmune condition and a rare complication of celiac disease, presenting with progressive cerebellar ataxia, epilepsy, myoclonus, peripheral neuropathy, pyramidal tract signs, tremor, and evidence of brain stem involvement. Pathologically, there is extensive gliosis and neuronal loss in the cortex, cerebellum, brain stem, and deep gray matter.[5468]

necrotizing myelopathy A rare **paraneoplastic syndrome** occurring in patients with a variety of malignancies and characterized by the subacute onset of painless motor, sensory, and sphincter dysfunction with evidence of a transverse cord lesion at a defined level, with accelerating progression. Pathologically, there is massive transverse cord necrosis at that level.[2724]

necrotizing myopathy Moderate and scattered necrosis of muscle fibers occurring as a toxic effect of drugs such as clofibrate, statins, and epsilon-aminocaproic acid. Clinically, myalgia, muscle tenderness, and muscle weakness are the main complaints. The serum CK levels are raised and the electrical and pathological findings are those of nonspecific degeneration of myofibrils.[3600, 3724]

needle electrode A metallic device used for recording from or stimulating tissues into which it has been inserted. Specific electrode types include bifilar (bipolar) needle recording electrodes, concentric needle electrodes, macro-EMG needle electrodes, monopolar needle electrodes, multilead electrodes, single fiber needle electrodes, and stimulating electrodes.[19]

needle-in-the-eye syndrome The occurrence of repetitive, sudden, brief, lancinating pains felt in one eye. No pathology is known to be associated and the condition is benign.[4947]

See also **ice-pick pains**, **benign paroxysmal cranial neuralgia**, and **exploding head syndrome**.

needle-like occipital spikes Innocuous, unusually brief spikes recorded over the occipital regions in congenitally blind children. They disappear during adolescence and are considered to reflect only functional deafferentation.[3647] See also **benign occipital spikes**.

Neftel, W.B. (1830–1906) Russian-American physician who trained in Moscow and, after service in the Crimean War, emigrated to New York.

Neftel disease (hysterical astasia–abasia) Inability to walk, although all appropriate leg movements can be made in the supine position.

negative afterimages The ephemeral complementary image of a bright object, which remains for a while when darkness supervenes, as with eye closure, so that what was bright is now seen as dark and vice versa.

negative delta sign See **empty delta sign**.

negative myoclonus Silent periods of 35–200 ms duration that interrupt voluntary background EMG activity and result in jerky myoclonus-like movements such as asterixis.[6931] See also **myoclonus** and **asterixis**.

A *variant* is *epileptic negative myoclonus* in which brief postural lapses of a body segment are time-locked with EEG spike activity in contralateral central areas, where almost continuous paroxysmal activity is recordable. The syndrome occurs in subjects with partial epilepsies of various etiologies, who complain of action-activated jerks of an arm, each jerk being related to a silent period on the EMG lasting 100–400 ms. Motor neglect and impaired awareness of the disorder are commonly associated.[2615]

negative symptoms Those clinical features (such as paresis or sensory loss) that appear due to the removal of a normal state of tonic activation of part of the nervous system. They may be compared with **positive symptoms** (such as most epileptic events) that occur due to abnormal activation within the nervous system. (Negative phenomena however can also occur in epilepsy–speech arrest, amaurosis, **aphasia**, **amnesia**, numbness, deafness, neglect, and atonic seizures–just as they do in **asterixis**.) The distinction was made first by Hughlings-**Jackson**.

neglect 1. (hemispatial agnosia) The phenomenon whereby objects or occurrences in one half-field are perceived but to which responses are inhibited. This has been interpreted as a defect in the orienting response, either due to hemispatial hypokinesia restricted to acts that have to be performed on the side of the inattention or due to a hemispatial memory defect.[2841] See also **paralexia** and **paragraphia**.

2. Inability to direct the focus of awareness toward behaviorally relevant sensory events in one direction of extrapersonal space.[4332] The phenomenon is most often found with right hemisphere lesions, sensory events occurring within the left extrapersonal hemispace having a diminished or no impact upon awareness. See also **extinction**. The processes preventing neglect in healthy subjects are mediated by the posterior parietal cortex, prefrontal cortex, and the cingulate gyrus; damage to any of these may give rise to the syndrome of unilateral neglect. See also **visual neglect**.

3. (*representational neglect*) Neglect of space that is not actually seen but only imagined. Neglect of the space that is seen is known as *perceptual neglect*. The phenomenon is seldom considered in daily neurological practice.

neglect syndrome Hemi-inattention, extinction of double simultaneous stimuli, hemiakinesia, allesthesia, hemispatial neglect, anosognosia, and anisodiaphoria[6076] probably due to impairment of attention–arousal systems induced by dysfunction of those neuronal networks that form the basis of cortico-limbic-reticular interaction,[2842] that is, there is dysfunction in the heteromodal cortex (usually in the parietotemporal or prefrontal regions) or in the thalamus.

Inability to use the limbs in the absence of paralysis or of severe sensory loss is also subsumed under this heading.

Negri, Adelchi (1876–1912) Italian physician and pathologist who trained at Pavia and was assistant to Golgi. He became professor of microbiology at Pavia, writing mainly on hematology, dysentery, malaria, and rabies.[2066]

Negri bodies Eosinophilic intracytoplasmic inclusions composed of virus particles, seen in the Purkinje cells of the cerebellum and in the hippocampal pyramidal cells in **rabies**, described by Negri in 1905 (although he thought that they were parasitic protozoa).[5333]

Structures that are similar but without the core are known as **Lyssa bodies** and are not specific for rabies.[4360]

Negro, Camillo (1861–1927) Italian neurologist in Turin.

Negro sign (phenomenon) 1. (toothed trochlea phenomenon) Cogwheel rigidity, described by Camillo Negro in 1901 in his Parkinsonian patients. In **Gowers'** words, "The least degree of tremor is felt

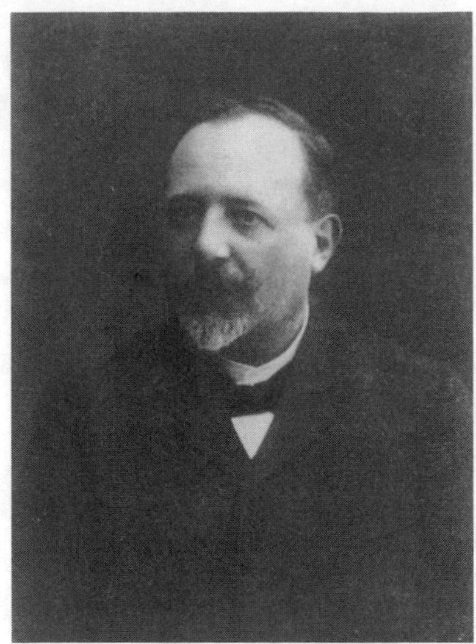

Figure N–1 Camillo Negro

during passive movement of a rigid part." 2. Apparent decrease in the upward excursion of the globe on the affected side when the patient with a lower motor neuron lesion of the facial nerve attempts to look up.[4609]

Negro–Jacod syndrome See **Jacod syndrome**.

Neill–Dingwall syndrome
A recessively inherited syndrome manifesting signs similar to those of **Cockayne syndrome** (dwarfism, microcephaly, pigmented chorioretinitis, cerebellar signs, and short trunk), but with the absence of cataract and the presence of hepatomegaly and intracranial calcifications.[4610]

Nelson syndrome 1. The excessive secretion of ACTH and MSH by a chromophobe pituitary adenoma, developing after adrenalectomy and leading to hyperpigmentation and features of Cushing syndrome. Myopathy is a potential complication.[4615] 2. See also **acrocallosal syndrome**.

nema (Gr, a thread).

nemaline myopathy (rod body myopathy, congenital rod disease)
A dominantly or recessively inherited or sporadic congenital myopathy characterized by the presence of **rod bodies** composed of actin and α-actinin in muscle biopsy specimens. The responsible dominant gene maps to chromosome 1q21–q23. Mutations in five separate genes (*a-tropomyosin-3, nebulin, a-actin, troponin T1*, and *b-tropomyosin*) have been described; all encode for protein components of muscle thin filaments. Mutations in the ryanodine receptor gene (*RYR1*) have also been associated with core-rod myopathy.

The clinical pictures vary. In the classical *recessive* form, infants with the severe form have progressive hypotonia, weakness, and atrophy in proximal muscles with feeding and respiratory difficulties and the condition is sometimes fatal; in milder forms, this is a mild progressive myopathy with hypotonia, small muscles, feeding problems, generalized weakness, and some face, trunk, and limb dysmorphisms. A *dominant* form is nonprogressive when presenting in early childhood. In adults, the course can resemble either of the foregoing.[5820] The greatest involvement is found in the facial, trunk flexor, ankle dorsiflexor, and toe extensor muscles.

The diagnosis is suggested when this clinical picture is encountered in a subject with features resembling **Marfan syndrome** (high-arched palate, arachnodactyly, and span greater than height) and it is confirmed by light and electron microscopy of a muscle biopsy specimen that shows characteristic rod bodies within the myofibrils (mainly of type 1).[4123] Diagnostic criteria have been suggested[5482]and a clinical classification proposed,[6611] (See Table.)

Variants are

1. An *adult-onset* form, characterized by cardiomyopathy and proximal and distal myopathic weakness with the typical microscopic findings just described.[4288] Many such cases are associated with the presence of a monoclonal gammopathy.
2. *Autosomal dominant nemaline myopathy with onset in infancy with hypotonia and motor delay* in which weakness involves the neck flexors and the abdominal and proximal limb muscles without bulbar, respiratory, or foot dorsiflexion weakness and with no slowness in movement. High-arched palate, feeding problems, joint contractures, and severe facial and proximal myopathic weakness are also described. Nemaline rods are present in <5% of muscle fibers.[3176]
3. *A severe congenital* form marked by lack of movements and by respiratory insufficiency, occasionally associated with contractures or even **arthrogryposis**.
4. An *intermediate congenital* form with clinical problems apparent only in early childhood.
5. A *mild childhood or adolescent type*, the classic form, without facial weakness.
6. Forms with *ophthalmoplegia and mitochondrial abnormalities* are described, in some cases, as well as the myopathy that affects the face, neck, limbs, and trunk.[2234]
7. *A group with diverse features* such as cardiomyopathy, ophthalmoplegia, or rigid spine.
8. A variant with associated core-like lesions presenting with muscle weakness and slowness of movements, mapped to chromosome 15q21–q23 (tropomyosin-1?).[2464] See also **central core disease**, with which this condition may overlap.

See also http://www.neuro.wustl.edu/neuromuscular/maltbrain.html and (a support group) http://www.davidmcd.btinternet.co.uk/.

nemaline rods Intramyofibrillar material found in the foregoing myopathy but scattered reports have recorded them in many other conditions, mainly involving neurogenic muscle disease.

nematodes Worms of the class **Nemathelminths**, including the hairworms and threadworms, with a body cavity. Examples of neurological relevance are *Ascaris, Trichina*, and *Filaria*.

neo- Greek prefix denoting new.

neocortical death See **persistent vegetative state**.

neocortical temporal lobe epilepsies Seizures characterized by elementary or complex hallucinations, complex psychic phenomenon such as hallucinations and delusions, dreamy states, emotional manifestations, and visceral sensory disturbances. They include primary rhinencephalic, frontal, opercular, frontobasal cingulate, temporal pole and posterior neocortical seizures.[72] See also **temporal lobe epilepsy**.

neologism (from Lat, new + word)
1. A word newly created, either in response

Clinical classification of Nemaline Myopathies.[6611]

Clinical categories of nemaline myopathy

A.1. Severe congenital nemaline myopathy

Inclusion criteria:

- No spontaneous movements at birth
- No spontaneous respiration at birth
- Contractures at birth
- Fractures at birth

Exclusion criteria:

- Associated features:
- Cardiomyopathy
- Ophthalmoplegia
- Unusual distribution of weakness
- Intranuclear nemaline bodies

A.2. Intermediate congenital nemaline myopathy

Inclusion criteria:

- Infantile onset
- Breathing and moving at birth, but later in early childhood unable to achieve respiratory independence or unable to achieve sitting or unable to achieve walking
- Contractures developing in early childhood
- Use of wheelchair before the age of 11 years

A.3. The typical form of congenital nemaline myopathy

Inclusion criteria:

- Onset in early childhood
- Weakness especially pronounced in the facial, bulbar and respiratory muscles, and in the neck flexors
- Proximal > distal weakness initially
- Milestones delayed, but reached
- Later distal involvement
- Slowly progressive or nonprogressive course

Exclusion criteria:

- No spontaneous movements at birth
- No spontaneous respiration at birth
- Contractures at birth
- Fractures at birth
- Unable to establish independent respiration
- Unable to learn to sit or walk
- Use of wheelchair before the age of 11 years
- Adult or late childhood onset
- Associated features include cardiomyopathy, ophthalmoplegia—an unusual distribution of weakness, and the presence of intranuclear nemaline bodies

A.4. Mild childhood- or juvenile-onset nemaline myopathy

Childhood or juvenile onset
No facial weakness
No foot drop

A.5. Adult-onset forms of nemaline myopathy

Inclusion criterion:

- Adult onset

A.6. Other forms of nemaline myopathy

Inclusion criteria:

- Cardiomyopathy
- Ophthalmoplegia
- Unusual distribution of weakness
- Intranuclear nemaline bodies

From Wallgren-Pettersson C, Laing NG. *Report of the 70th ENMC International Workshop: Nemaline Myopathy.* 1999, Naarden, The Netherlands. *Neuromusc Disorders* 2000;**10**(4–5):299–306, with permission from Elsevier Science.

to a communicative need within a category of intellectual activity or as a result of disease of the brain. In the latter case, the word cannot be defined by the inventor and represents a failure of production of normal speech. Shakespeare invented many such words that have entered common parlance, but in neurology their production is usually an evidence of psychosis, dysphasia, or delirium. 2. The replacement of a desired word with an articulate sound devoid of conventional meaning.

neologistic jargon A form of **jargon aphasia** in which more than 80% of the words enunciated are unintelligible. The causative disease is usually in the left superior temporal and inferior parietal regions.[3402]

neonatal adrenoleukodystrophy See **adrenoleukodystrophy**.

neonatal cerebellar atrophy with retinal dystrophy A rare and fatal congenital syndrome of retinal dystrophy, arthrogryposis, vomiting, and generalized edema with postmortem evidence of cerebellar atrophy.[2765]

neonatal endotoxin encephalopathy A form of **periventricular leukomalacia** occurring in the perinatal period, considered to be due to the effect of endotoxins.[2381]

neonatal familial hyperparathyroidism A congenital dysmetabolic syndrome manifesting also constipation, hepatosplenomegaly, hypercalcemia, hypotonia, seizures, osteoporosis, and multiple fractures.[381]

neonatal herpes simplex infection Infection by herpes simplex virus (type 2), usually acquired by the infant during passage through the maternal genital tract.

Clinically, a disseminated form of the disease damages the liver and adrenal glands, while neurological symptoms and signs include seizures, cranial nerve palsies, lethargy, and coma due to diffuse encephalitis as a result of direct infection of the brain by the virus. The disease is often fatal; in those who survive, the long-term consequences include seizures, microcephaly, blindness, and pyramidal signs.[6758]

neonatal myasthenia The occurrence of the features of **myasthenia gravis** in the infants of mothers with that condition.[6065] Immunosuppressants and plasma exchange are effective therapies, if required at all, although they are not effective in **congenital myasthenia**.

neonatal myoclonic encephalopathy (early myoclonic encephalopathy) A syndrome characterized clinically by the occurrence of erratic fragmentary myoclonus of early onset usually in association with other seizure types and with the EEG finding of a suppression-burst pattern. Associated seizures include partial motor seizures, massive myoclonus, and atonic spasms.

All affected infants have severe neurological impairment and the disease is frequently fatal before the age of 6 months. In some cases, recessive inheritance is considered likely.[72]

neonatal ophthalmoplegia with microfibers A congenital myopathy characterized by nonprogressive hypotonia, weakness, and hoarseness; permanent external ophthalmoplegia; and, on muscle biopsy, marked variation in fiber size, some being less than 3 μm in diameter.[2737]

neonatal perifascicular myopathy A nonprogressive neonatal syndrome of hypotonia and weakness with cognitive delay, although there is subsequent improvement in motor skills. Muscle biopsy shows perifascicular atrophy and immature type 2C fibers and perivascular inflammation.[4992]

neonatal persistent myasthenia See **myasthenia gravis** (*congenital or developmental*).

neonatal seizures Epileptic seizures occurring in the first 4 weeks of life.[1265] Such forms of seizure differ from those of older children and adults. The most frequent neonatal seizures are described as subtle, because the clinical manifestations are frequently overlooked. These include tonic, horizontal deviation of the eyes with or without jerking, eyelid blinking or fluttering; sucking, smacking, or other buccal-lingual oral movements; swimming or pedalling movements; and occasionally apneic spells.

Other neonatal seizures occur in the form of tonic extension of the limbs, mimicking decerebrate or decorticate posturing. These occur particularly in premature infants. Multifocal clonic seizures characterized by clonic movements of a limb, which may migrate to other body parts or other limbs, or focal clonic seizures, which are much more localized, are also described. In the latter, the infant is usually not unconscious. Rarely, myoclonic seizures occur, when the EEG pattern is frequently that of suppression-burst activity.[4192] The tonic seizures have a poor prognosis because they frequently accompany intraventricular hemorrhage. The myoclonic seizures also have a poor prognosis because they are frequently a part of the early myoclonic encephalopathy syndrome. (From Dreifuss FE, et al. Commission for classification and terminology, ILAE. Proposal for revised classifications of epilepsies and epileptic syndromes. *Epilepsia* 1989;30:389–99 by kind permission the ILAE and Wiley-Blackwell Publications.)

neoplasm (Gr, new + to form) An abnormal, independent proliferation of cells characterized by histological diversity from the matrix from which it takes its origin (Bland-Sutton); a tumor.

neoplastic angioendotheliosis See **malignant angioendotheliomatosis**.

neoplastic meningitis Invasion of the meninges and CSF by malignant cells, especially from cancers of the breast and lung.

neovascularization The formation of a new system of blood vessels within a tissue, such as the retina in diabetes.

nephrogenic diabetes insipidus (vasopressin- or ADH-resistant diabetes insipidus) An inherited condition characterized by inability to concentrate the urine, which results in polyuria and polydipsia. Affected untreated infants usually have poor feeding and failure to thrive with the rapid onset of severe dehydration. Short stature and secondary dilatation of the ureters and bladder from the high urine volume are common. The responsible genes are *AVPR2* (X-linked) and *AQP2* (autosomal recessive and autosomal dominant). See also the Web site http://www.geneclinics.org/profiles/ndi/.

nephrolithiasis-mitochondrial cytopathy See **Donaldson syndrome**.

nephropathy with retinitis pigmentosa, cerebellar ataxia, and skeletal abnormalities A recessively inherited syndrome reported once; juvenile nephronophthisis is a feature.[4031]

nephrosialidosis (Gr, kidney + saliva) (severe infantile sialidosis) A congenital lysosomal storage disease due to deficiency of beta-galactosidase, leading to storage of sialo-oligosaccharides and presenting with a nephrotic syndrome, coarse facies, corneal clouding, multiple dysostoses, a cherry-red spot at the macula, seizures, and mental and developmental delay. See also **sialidosis**.

Neri, Vincenzo (b. 1882) Italian neurologist who trained at the **Salpêtrière**.

Neri signs 1. Flexion of the knee with forward bending of the trunk indicates lumbar root irritation on that side. The same knee flexion occurs in patients with a pyramidal tract lesion on the affected side. 2. (Pronation sign) In hemiparesis or monoparesis, flexion of the sound arm lying pronated and extended leads to supination of the contralateral paretic arm. 3. In organic hemiparesis, with the patient lying supine, spontaneous bending of the knee occurs when the leg is passively lifted.[4628]

nerve (Middle English, from Lat, a tendon) Anatomical collections of bundles of nerve fibers and their supporting connective tissue and vascular and lymphatic elements, with their origin in nuclei situated within or beside the brain stem or spinal cord. Over 250 have been named.

The early Greeks did not distinguish between nerves and tendons (hence the word aponeurosis) until this was achieved at Alexandria by **Eristratus** and **Herophilus**.

nerve action potential (NAP)

Strictly defined, refers to an action potential recorded from a single nerve fiber. The term is commonly used to refer to the compound nerve action potential. See also **compound nerve action potential**. (From the 2001 Report of the Nomenclature Committee of the American Association of Electromyography and Electrodiagnosis.[19] Reproduced by kind permission of the AANEM.)

nerve agents Organic esters of phosphoric acid derivatives capable of inactivating acetylcholinesterase by permanent binding and thus leading to syndromes of cholinergic excess, both nicotinic and muscarinic. Clinically, weakness, circulatory and respiratory depression, seizures, and coma occur at the time of exposure; delayed effects include anxiety symptoms, giddiness, memory disturbances, headaches, insomnia, confusion, and ataxia.[2639]

nerve compression syndromes

Combinations of motor and sensory deficits, often with positive **Tinel signs** during the recovery phase, caused by compression and thus ischemia of peripheral nerves.

The median, ulnar, radial, suprascapular, axillary, femoral, sciatic, common peroneal and posterior tibial nerves and (where appropriate) their cutaneous branches are those most often affected.

nerve conduction study (NCS, electroneurography) Recording and analysis of electric waveforms of biological origin elicited in response to electric or physiologic stimuli. The waveforms are compound sensory nerve action potentials, compound muscle action potentials, or mixed nerve action potentials. The compound muscle action potentials are generally referred to by letters that have historical origin: M wave, F wave, H wave, T wave, A wave, and Rl, R2 waves. It is possible under standardized conditions to establish normal ranges for amplitude, duration, and latency of the waveforms and to calculate the maximum conduction velocity of sensory and motor nerves. The term generally refers to studies of waveforms generated in the peripheral nervous system, whereas evoked potential studies refer to studies of waveforms generated in both the peripheral and central nervous systems. (From the 2001 Report of the Nomenclature Committee of the American Association of Electromyography and Electrodiagnosis.[19] Reproduced by kind permission of the AANEM.)

nerve conduction velocity (NCV) The speed of propagation of an action potential along an axon, assumed to refer to the maximum speed of propagation. The speed of conduction of nerve impulses (normally as a result of saltatory conduction) in both motor and sensory nerves at normal temperatures in adults ranges between 45 and 65 m/s. These values apply to the fastest conducting, most heavily myelinated A or alpha fibers, which also have the largest axons; B and C fibers conduct at substantially slower rates but cannot normally be measured in the clinical laboratory because the action potentials they induce are overshadowed by those produced by the faster-conducting fibers. In the newborn, the rates are about one-third of the speeds given above, rising to adult values by about the age of 8 years.

The velocity of nerve conduction was first measured by Helmholtz in 1850.

nerve deafness–optic atrophy–dementia syndrome

An X-linked syndrome manifesting sensorineural deafness, optic atrophy, and neurodegenerative regression with onset in early adult life.[3208]

nerve fiber The axon and its sheath, its outer limit being the endoneurial membrane; the Schwann cells investing the fiber may be myelinated or not.

nerve fiber action potential

Action potential recorded from a single axon.

nerve fiber-bundle defect A visual field defect occurring with either a retinal or optic nerve lesion, which follows the pattern of loss of retinal nerve fibers. Examples are altitudinal defects, temporal sector defects, steps, and nasal scotomas.

nerve growth factor A substance synthesized in the Schwann cells of the peripheral nervous system and transported retrogradely to the perikaryon.

nerve injury The three-heading classification of Seddon (**neurapraxia**, **axonotmesis**, and **neurotmesis**) was criticized by Sunderland, who defined five forms, given in Chart N–2; the Seddon schema, however, has found so much favor by clinicians that it is generally preferred.

Chart N–2. Sunderland's Five Groups of Nerve Injury

First degree: (interruption of conduction with preservation of anatomical continuity) Conduction is blocked at the site of injury, but the continuity of all components comprising the nerve trunk, including the axon, is preserved. There is no Wallerian degeneration and the disturbance that is responsible for blocking the conduction is fully reversible, so that the function is rapidly and completely restored.

Second degree: (disintegration with regeneration of axons) Disintegration of the axon occurs with distal Wallerian degeneration, but the general arrangement of the axon sheath and the other neural structures is retained, so that regeneration of the axons is down the appropriate endoneurial tube in all cases.

Third degree: (disorganization of the contents of the funiculi, with loss of continuity of the endoneurial tubes). The bundles of funiculi remain in continuity, but there is disorganization of their internal structure, so that the continuity of the endoneurial tubes is lost and there is distal axonal disintegration and Wallerian degeneration. As a result of interfunicular fibrosis, the regenerating axons do not sprout down their original endoneurial tubes.

Fourth degree: (complete disorganization of the internal structure of the nerve) Breaching and disorganization of the funiculi with preservation of continuity of the anatomical nerve trunk. The involved segment becomes a tangle of connective tissue, Schwann cells, fibrosis, and axon sprouts, and the chance that an axon will grow back down its own endoneurial tube is remote.

Fifth degree: Severance of the nerve trunk.[6130]

From Sunderland S. A classification of peripheral nerve injuries producing loss of function. *Brain* 1951;74:491–516.

nerve potential Equivalent to **nerve action potential.** Also commonly, but inaccurately, used to refer to the biphasic form of end-plate activity observed during needle electrode examination of muscle. The latter use is incorrect, because muscle fibers, not nerve fibers, are the source of these (From the 2001 Report of the Nomenclature Committee of the American Association of Electromyography and Electrodiagnosis.[19] Reproduced by kind permission of the AANEM.)

nerve roots The nerve fiber bundles entering and leaving the spinal cord and brain stem. The motor function of the anterior roots and the sensory function of the posterior roots were detected by Georg Prochaska in 1779, but the first (and partial) account in English was that of Sir Charles **Bell** in 1811, published 10 years later, while **Magendie** completed the differentiation in the following year.

nerve sheath myxoma See **pseudocyt**.

Nervenzart A leading German neurological journal. Its Web site is found at http://link.springer.de/link/service/journals/00115/index.htm/.

nervi erigentes The pelvic parasympathetic nerves leaving the cord at S2,3,4. They were described by Carl Ludwig in 1866.

nervous system The compilation of the whole of the central and peripheral nervous systems, thus comprising in humans the cerebral hemispheres and their ascending, descending, and commissural connections, the thalamus, basal ganglia and limbic system, the brain stem and cerebellum, the cranial nerves, the spinal cord with its spinal nerves, and the autonomic nervous system.

The differentiation between the central and peripheral nervous systems is made on the basis of the type of cells investing the axons; these are oligodendroglia in the former and Schwann cells in the latter.

nervus intermedius The name given by Wrisberg to that part of the VII cranial nerve that runs as a separate bundle, lying between the remainder of the VII and the VIII nerves.

nervus intermedius neuralgia
A rare disorder characterized by brief paroxysms of pain felt deeply in the auditory canal. The following diagnostic criteria have been defined:

A. Pain paroxysms of intermittent occurrence, lasting for seconds or minutes, in the depth of the ear.
B. Presence of a trigger area in the posterior wall of the auditory canal.
C. Not attributed to another disorder. Other causes, in particular a structural lesion, have been ruled out by history, physical examination, and special investigations.
D. Disorders of lacrimation, salivation, and/or taste sometimes accompany the pain. There is a common association with herpes zoster. In view of the sparse innervation of the affected area by the nervus intermedius, some patients may have an otalgic variant of **glossopharyngeal neuralgia**.

From the International Classification of Headache Disorders (Headache Classification Committee of the International Headache Society. *Cephalalgia* 2004;**24**[Suppl 1]) by kind permission of Dr. Jes Olesen, the International Headache Society and Wiley-Blackwell Publications.

Neuhauser syndrome
(megalocornea-mental retardation) A congenital dysmorphic syndrome characterized also by abnormalities of the cornea and iris, seizures, hypotonia, and mental and developmental delay.[381]

Neu–Laxova syndrome A lethal congenital dysmorphic syndrome characterized also by microphthalmia, cataract, ascites, edema of hands, syndactyly, joint contractures, microcephaly, intracranial calcification, lissencephaly, and cerebellar and callosal anomalies.[4629]

Neumann type dementia See **subcortical gliosis**.

neural Of or belonging to a nerve or the nervous system.

neural amyotrophy with familial retinitis pigmentosa See **NARP syndrome**.

neural crest A line of epiblastic cells situated on the dorsal lips of the neural tube, from which cells migrate to form some cranial nerves (III, V, VII, VIII, IX, and X), peripheral sensory ganglia and satellite cells, autonomic ganglia and plexuses, the Schwann cells, some endocrine glands or parts of them (e.g., thyroid, parathyroid, and thymus), much of the meninges, the skin and bones of the face, the tooth-enamel organs, and almost all pigmented cells in the body, though not those of the retina.[3733]

A *syndrome of the neural crest* arising from a failure in its differentiation has been proposed to consist of loss of superficial or deep pain sensibility, autonomic dysfunction, dysplasia of dental enamel, meningeal thickening and cystic change, mild mental retardation, hyporeflexia, blond hair, blue-green eyes, and a pale complexion.[893]

neural induction The process of the formation of primitive neural elements as the first part of the process of organogenesis, leading to differentiation of the neural plate and then to formation of the neural tube.

NeuraLinksPlus A Web page of links to neuroscience, psychology, and other general science pages, created by Prof. Mark Dubin of the University of Colorado.
Web site: http://spot.colorado.edu/~dubin/bookmarks/index.html/.

neural myxedema bodies Round, granular, glycogen-containing bodies in the dorsal root entry zone of the spinal cord and in the cerebellar vermis of patients with myxedema.[5120]

neural tube The infolding of the dorsal ectoderm forming a tube from which develop the brain and spinal cord. It was first noted by Remak and confirmed by Huxley.[5886]

neural tube defects A group of developmental disorders occurring due to failure of normal closure of the neural tube between 22 and 29 days after conception. The most severe forms are **anencephaly** and **meningomyelocele** (spina bifida).

neuralgia (Gr, nerve + pain) Pain felt in the distribution of a nerve or nerve root, due usually to a proximal lesion of that nerve. The characteristics of such pains tend to constancy in their intermittency, brevity, severity and explosive onset and in the usual finding of normal function in the territory supplied by the nerve in between attacks, but these criteria do not hold for **postherpetic neuralgia**. The pain may be sharp, even lancinating when affected by **ephaptic transmission** but is burning and constant in inflammatory conditions.

Further comments are entered for the particular varieties of neuralgia; **trigeminal**, **geniculate**, **glossopharyngeal**, **occipital**, **vagal**, and **superior laryngeal** forms are described. While **tabetic crises** could also be considered to be neuralgias using the preceding criteria, they are not usually so classified. The history of the term has been reviewed.[95]

neuralgic amyotrophy (Spillane syndrome, Parsonage–Turner syndrome, shoulder-girdle syndrome, shoulder-girdle neuritis, brachial neuritis [idiopathic], brachial plexopathy, brachial plexus neuropathy, acute brachial plexitis/plexopathy/neuritis/neuropathy, hereditary peripheral neuropathy predominantly affecting the arms) A syndrome characterized by the acute onset of pain in the shoulder and arm followed by variable weakness and atrophy of muscles, usually unilaterally and most often in the C5–6 (upper trunk of the brachial plexus) distribution, but any upper limb muscles can be affected as can the diaphragm. The cause is unknown.[4916]

Sensory functions are much less affected. Sometimes a single nerve (usually the long thoracic) or multiple unrelated nerves (e.g., the phrenic, axillary, anterior interosseous, and/or suprascapular) are involved. The syndrome is more common in males in early adult life, and is often preceded by a variety of infectious, traumatic, or immunological events. Laboratory studies other than EMG are unhelpful in diagnosis. The prognosis for eventual recovery is good.

Spillane actually described the entity 5 years before Parsonage and Turner. Diagnostic criteria have been reviewed as follows:[5529]

A. Acute onset over the course of hours or days.
B. Pain in the shoulder girdle and arm, often severe.
C. Subsequent weakness and atrophy in the territory of individual nerves arising from the brachial plexus.
D. Little or no sensory loss.
E. Eventual recovery.
F. EMG findings consistent with axonal neuropathy.
G. Normal CSF.
H. Frequent antecedent viral infection, vaccination, or serum sickness.

Variants are

A *dominantly inherited* form with predilection for the brachial plexus (OMIM 162100) described in 1887, presenting with recurrent attacks of pain and weakness lasting for a few days and leading to muscle atrophy. It is mapped to 17q24–qter. This condition is nearly identical with the classic picture in affecting the brachial plexus most often but the lesions are more extensive and may involve the recurrent laryngeal nerves, isolated limb nerves, or the lumbosacral plexus.[253, 481, 2323] Dysmorphic features such as hypotelorism, syndactyly, short stature, and epicanthic folds may accompany the neural problems.

A chronic painless form[5642] and another occurring postpartum.

In rare cases, a multifocal relapsing sensory neuropathy occurs, resembling **sensory perineuritis**.[6285]

See also **hereditary pressure-sensitive neuropathy**, **multiple exercise-related neuropathy with colic**, **carpal tunnel syndrome** (familial variant), **meralgia paresthetica**, **giant axonal neuropathy**, and **lumbosacral plexopathy**.

neuralgic osteopathy See **Camera syndrome**.

neurapraxia (Gr, nerve + lack of + action) (transient block) A minimal lesion of a peripheral nerve usually due to compression or stretch injuries, producing paralysis that is usually incomplete, unaccompanied by peripheral axonal degeneration and with rapid, spontaneous and complete recovery. This is one of three types of nerve injury described by Seddon.[5705] See also **conduction block**, **axonotmesis**, and **neurotmesis**.

neurasthenia (Gr, nerve + weakness) Nervous exhaustion, a fashionable diagnosis by any of its many names. A condition that it is polite to regard as possibly organic but without demonstrable pathology; a refuge for physicians and patients.

First described by Jean-Antoine-Eugène Bouchat (1818–1891) in a monograph entitled "De l'état nerveux aigu et chronique ou nervosisme" (Paris, 1860), it was more fully detailed by George **Beard** in 1869[459, 461] and described by him as a "want of nervous force . . . most frequently met with in civilized, intellectual communities. They are part of the compensation for our progress and refinement." Symptoms identified included "general malaise, debility of all the functions, poor appetite, abiding weakness in the back and spine, fugitive neuralgic pains, hysteria, insomnia, hypochondriasis, disinclination for consecutive manual labour, severe and weakening attacks of sick headache . . . and other analogous symptoms and at the same time gives no evidence of anemia or of other organic disease. We have reason to suspect that the central nervous system is mainly at fault and that we are dealing with a typical case of neurasthenia."

Beard treated the condition with general electrization, the patients' feet being placed on a sheet of copper to which the "negation pole" was attached; the positive pole was a large sponge applied to the (moistened) head. Violent muscular contractions were produced. He also used hypnotism and "air, sunlight, water, food, rest, diversion, muscular exercise and . . . strychnine, phosphorus, arsenic etc. which directly affect the nervous system." Beard's practice flourished and the diagnosis and treatment were each so convenient that alternatives seldom required consideration. The treatment employed by Weir **Mitchell** was similar and produced equally good results. See also **chronic fatigue syndrome**.

neurasthenic nystagmus See **gaze-evoked nystagmus**.

neurectasy (Gr, nerve + stretch) Manual traction on a nerve exposed at operation in an attempt to relieve pain and numerous other neurological symptoms. Early scepticism in the late 18th century gave way to later incredulity and the procedure has now been abandoned.[3360]

neurenteric Relating to the nerves and to the intestines.

neurenteric cyst (dorsal enteric cyst, archenteric cyst, or enterogenous cyst) A congenital defect due to herniation of the ventral yolk sac and its adherence to the dorsal ectoderm, resulting in the presence of an intraspinal cystic mass with an endodermal epithelial lining. Secondary spinal cord or nerve root compression may occur at any age.

A classification of such developmental disorders has been achieved by Smith.[5914] See also **intradural enterogenous cyst**.

neurilemma (Gr, nerve + covering) Described originally by **Schwann** and named for him, thus indicating the Schwann cell sheath, although the intent was to label the connective tissue covering of nerve fibers, the epi- and the perineurium.

neurites (nerve sprouts) Small axon sprouts, regenerating from the tip of a severed axon at a node of Ranvier.

neuritic plaques (senile plaques) Spherical argyrophilic structures, 5–200 μm in diameter, comprising a dense central core of amyloid fibrils surrounded by a clear halo, outside which is a ring of neurofilamentous and mitochondrial material derived from degenerating dendritic and axonal nerve terminals. They are found in the cerebral cortex, hippocampal regions, and gray matter, and relate in number to the age of the subject, although they are not always present even in the brains of very elderly people.[6] Such plaques are also characteristic findings in **Alzheimer disease**.

neuritis Inflammation of nerves from any cause. However, the word has been used in a far less specific way in the past century to include almost any nerve disorder other than tumor. It should be retained for inflammatory disease, unsullied by association with noninflammatory diseases that affect nerve conduction.

neuroacanthocytosis (choreoacanthosis, Levine–Critchley syndrome, familial neuroacanthocytosis, familial amyotrophic chorea with acanthocytosis, familial chorea with acanthocytosis) A heterogeneous (recessively or dominantly inherited or sporadic) progressive multisystem degenerative disorder caused by mutations in the VPS13A gene (9q21–22). It is seen in children or young adults and characterized by movement disorders (chorea, motor and phonic tics, dystonias, and orofacial dyskinesias causing dysphagia and dysarthria with lip and tongue biting) followed by orolingual ("eating") dystonia, generalized chorea, proximal or distal muscle weakness and atrophy, and personality changes or cognitive impairment. The chorea is slowly progressive and involves the bulbar muscles first and most. Psychoses, behavioral disorders with self-mutilation, Parkinsonism, vertical ophthalmoparesis, seizures, and occasionally lower motor neuron signs, myopathy, and cardiac involvement have also been recorded. Dystonia, Parkinsonism, seizures, depression, and psychosis have rarely been the initial features.[3919]

Other features that have been reported include evidence of a sensorimotor axonal neuropathy affecting the larger myelinated fibers, the occurrence of cerebellar or pyramidal signs, and CT evidence of cortical atrophy.[2750] Bulbar involvement and sphincter disturbances are additional but inconstant features.[3157, 3160] Caudate atrophy and hypometabolism have been detected. Neuronal loss and gliosis are particularly prominent in the striatum and pallidum but may also affect the thalamus, substantia nigra, and anterior horns of the spinal cord.

The clinical picture and pathological findings of striatal degeneration with caudate atrophy may resemble those of Huntington disease,[177] but to this are added neuropathy and myopathy and the serum CK levels are high.[3809] Wet blood or Wright-stained fast dry smears usually reveal that over 15% of red blood cells are acanthocytes. The multisystem neurological involvement in this disorder has been reviewed.[2750, 6602]

Three forms of neuroacanthocytosis have been differentiated as follows:[6602]

1. Core syndromes with basal ganglion degeneration, including recessively inherited choreoacanthocytosis and **McLeod syndrome**.[6838] The core autosomal recessive form (OMIM 200150) is due to mutations of *VPS13A*, which encodes the protein chorein and is characterized by the appearance in young adulthood of involuntary movements, usually chorea and dystonia.
2. Conditions with decreased lipoprotein levels, including **abetalipoproteinemia** and **hypobetalipoproteinemia**.
3. Conditions in which acanthocytosis is occasionally seen, including **Huntington disease-like** 2, PKAN, and some mitochondrial disorders.

Other *variants* are

Spinal muscular atrophy in choreoacanthocytosis and *hypoprebetalipoproteinemia*, each of which may present similarly.[6054]

Neuroanatomy & Neuropathology on the Internet An excellent anatomical and pathological resource from the Neuropathology Laboratory, Department of Neuroscience, University Medical School, Debrecen, Hungary. Web site: http://www.neuropat.dote.hu/.

neuroaxonal dystrophies A group of sporadic or recessively inherited conditions characterized by neuronal degeneration and fragmentation of the axon with the formation of homogeneous round eosinophilic bodies, at first in the distal part of the nerve, in which numerous spheroids are present in distal axons and throughout nerve cell processes. These conditions include **neurodegeneration with brain iron accumulation**, nutritional disorders, old age, and **infantile neuroaxonal dystrophy**. Clinically, affected children show rigidity, chorea, dystonia, tremor, seizures, dementia, and pigmentary retinopathy; in adults, the inheritance pattern is dominant and there is evidence of Parkinsonism with dementia and dystonias.[6771]

Neurobehavioral Rating Scale (revised) A structured 20 min interview, of use in the assessment of patients after head injury. It provides scores for agitation, anxiety, articulation, blunting of affect, calculation, conceptual thought, comprehension, depression, disinhibition, emotional withdrawal, excitement, guilt, hallucinatory behavior, hostility, attention, difficulties in mental flexibility, irritability, reduced alertness, insight, judgment, memory, mood lability, orientation, planning, repetition of speech, retardation, somatic concern, suspicion, thought content, and word-finding/naming.[3803, 4203]

neuro-Behçet disease The occurrence of predominantly neurological features in Behçet disease, an idiopathic multisystem inflammatory disease of young adults. Diagnostic criteria are the presence of recurrent aphthous stomatitis with at least two of genital aphthous ulcers, uveitis, cutaneous or large-vessel vasculitis, synovitis, and meningoencephalitis.[2882]

neuroblastoma An uncommon solid, soft, malignant tumor of the central or peripheral nervous systems, arising from undifferentiated sympathetic neuroblasts of the adrenal medulla or from sympathetic ganglia (neural crest cells); a type of **primitive neuroectodermal tumor**. Such tumors are dominantly inherited in a fifth of the cases and usually occur in infants or children in either location,[3000] in which population they are the most common solid tumors found.

Apart from the usual focal neurological signs of a mass lesion and of raised intracranial pressure, such tumors are remarkable for the **opsoclonus**, which is often present.[816]

Cerebral neuroblastomas occur mainly in children within the cerebral hemispheres. Histologically, they are characterized by sheets of cells with small and hyperchromatic nuclei with little cytoplasm, and occasionally they show focal glial or neuronal differentiation and rosette formation. *Olfactory neuroblastomas* (**esthesioneuroblastomas**) are rare *variants* arising in the anterior cranial fossa and consisting of small cells with fibrillary cytoplasm containing cytokeratin and staining positively for protein S100. *Abdominal neuroblastomas* arise from the chromaffin cells of the adrenal gland or from the sympathetic chain. *Differentiated neuroblastomas* (central neurocytomas) are rare *variants* of the above, usually occurring in young adults and with a good prognosis. They are characterized by the presence of vesicles or of synaptic structures. See also **ganglioneuroblastoma**.

Relevant Web sites include that of the Neuroblastoma Society (http://www.nsoc.co.uk/), an organization dedicated to raising funds for British research in this disease but also providing resources, support, and information for families and patients, and the NCI site http://www.cancer.gov/cancerinfo/types/neuroblastoma/, which offers information about treatment options, screening, clinical trials, and research.

neuroborreliosis See **Lyme disease**.

neurobrucellosis The occurrence of predominantly neurological features in patients suffering from brucellosis, a zoonosis. Clinically, headache, fatigue, and myalgia are the usual early features and transient ischemic attacks, strokes, acute confusional or psychotic states, myelopathy, anterior horn cell disease, multisystem degenerations, polyradiculopathy, sciatica, **neuralgic amyotrophy**, mononeuritis, and **cauda equina syndromes** at later stages are the commoner presentations.[82, 5752, 1125]

neurocardiogenic syncope (neurally mediated syncope, vasovagal syncope, ventricular syncope) A condition characterized by bradycardia, hypotension due to profound generalized vasodilatation and peripheral venous pooling of blood and thus decreased venous return to the heart with consequent decrease in cerebral blood flow, often leading to reduction in consciousness—all resulting from a failure of the normal autonomic compensatory responses to the assumption of the upright posture, but in the absence of serious cardiac disease. The paradoxical withdrawal of sympathetic activity (and increased parasympathetic activity) occurs, probably due to excessive activation of cardiac mechanoreceptors. Norepinephrine levels are high, accounting for the presence of pallor and sweating.[30] The hypotension and bradycardia are sufficiently profound that transient loss of consciousness may ensue. Misdiagnosis as epilepsy is common.

Presyncopal symptoms include weakness, lightheadedness, sweating, visual blurring, headache, nausea, and feelings of warmth or cold. Signs include pallor, yawning, and dilatation of the pupils—all occurring from half a minute up to a few minutes before the syncopal episode (if they occur at all). Seizure-like movements can occur during an episode (*convulsive syncope*).[2595] Normally, recovery is rapid, without confusion on awakening, except in those with pre-existing cerebral pathology.

Less dramatic falls in blood pressure may not cause full syncope, but can cause near-syncope, with vertigo, dizziness, and TIA-like episodes. During baseline tilt table testing, such patients demonstrate an increase in heart rate of $\geq$30 beats/min (or a maximum heart rate of 120 beats/min) within the first 10 min upright (unassociated with profound hypotension), reproducing their symptoms.[2596]

The **postural orthostatic tachycardia syndrome** is a neurocardiogenic variant identified during head-up **tilt testing**, which procedure suggests the following categories of hypotension, only the first representing true neurocardiogenic syncope:

1. Malignant vasovagal syncope, in which there is an abrupt drop in systolic blood pressure (mean drop over 100 mmHg) with severe bradycardia and maybe loss of consciousness after a mean of 18 min.
2. Orthostatic hypotension with a drop of systolic pressure of more than 20 mmHg within a minute of tilting.
3. Delayed orthostatic hypotension, with a mean drop of 40 mmHg after 20 min.

Neurocase A journal of the Oxford University Press dealing with single case studies and reviews of brain–behavior relationships. Web site: http://neurocase.oupjournals.org/.

neurocentral (Gr, nerve + the center of a circle) Relating to the centrum and the neural arch of a vertebra.

neurocirculatory asthenia See **chronic fatigue syndrome**.

neurocristopathy A neurological disorder due to abnormal development of structures arising from the neural crest. **Neurofibromatosis** is an example.[722]

neurocutaneous angiomatosis See **Sturge–Weber syndrome**.

neurocutaneous melanosis A rare, sporadic, congenital neurocutaneous syndrome characterized by numerous benign pigmented nevi (giant hairy nevus) mainly in the cycle-shorts area of the skin, with widespread deposits of pigmented cells in the leptomeninges and in the cerebral and cerebellar white matter. For the diagnosis to be made, no malignant melanoma may be present in other organs. The affected children have seizures, hydrocephalus, and brain hamartomas; they are also mentally retarded and show a variety of neurological deficits.[6468]

neurocutaneous syndromes (choristoma) A group of heterogeneous disorders involving both the skin and the nervous system and marked by a tendency to neoplasia. See also **phakomatoses**. In all, over 35 different forms are known,[2176] and these are listed in Chart N–3.

neurocysticercosis Infestation of the CNS by the encysted larvae of *Taenia solium*, the pork tapeworm, representing the commonest cause of cystic lesions in the brain worldwide and probably the commonest cause of acquired seizures. Cysts in the brain parenchyma and subarachnoid space lead to psychiatric symptoms, variably raised intracranial pressure, focal signs, and cognitive impairment, but the first clinical

Chart N–3. A Compilation of Neurocutaneous Syndromes

Dominantly inherited: Hypomelanosis of Ito; lentiginosis–deafness–cardiopathy; neurofibromatosis; nevoid basal-cell carcinoma syndrome; Sturge–Weber syndrome; tuberous sclerosis; von Hippel–Lindau syndrome; and Waardenburg syndrome.
Recessively inherited: Argininosuccinic aciduria; ataxia-telangiectasia (Louis–Bar syndrome); biotin-responsive multiple carboxylase deficiency; Chediak–Higashi disease; citrullinuria; Cockayne syndrome; fucosidosis; homocystinuria; giant axonal neuropathy; hereditary motor and sensory neuropathy type 4 **(Refsum disease); hereditary sensory and autonomic neuropathy,** type 3 **(familial dysautonomia); neuroichthyosis; phenylketonuria; Sjörgen–Larsson syndrome;** Werner syndrome **(progeria);** and **xeroderma pigmentosum.**
X-linked inheritance: **Adrenoleukodystrophy; Fabry disease; incontinentia pigmenti;** and **Menkes kinky-hair disease.**
Uncertain transmission: **Albright syndrome; Cobb syndrome; van Bogaert syndrome; dysencephalia splanchnocystica; focal dermal hypoplasia; hereditary hemorrhagic telangiectasia;** linear nevus sebaceous; **neurocutaneous melanosis,** peroneal neuropathy with crural hypopigmentation; **poikilodermia congenitale; progeria; Rud syndrome;** and **Sturge–Weber syndrome.**

Table. Diagnostic Criteria for Neurocysticercosis

Absolute

1. Histological demonstration of the parasite from biopsy of a brain or spinal cord lesion
2. Cystic lesions showing the scolex on CT or MRI
3. Direct visualization of subretinal parasites by funduscopic examination

Major

1. Lesions highly suggestive of neurocysticercosis on neuroimaging studies[a]
2. Positive serum EITB[b] for the detection of anticysticercal antibodies
3. Resolution of intracranial cystic lesions after therapy with albendazole or praziquantel
4. Spontaneous resolution of small single enhancing lesions[c]

Minor

1. Lesions compatible with neurocysticercosis on neuroimaging studies[d]
2. Clinical manifestations suggestive of neurocysticercosis[e]
3. Positive CSF ELISA for detection of anticysticercal antibodies or cysticercal antigens
4. Cysticercosis outside the CNS[f]

Epidemiologic

1. Evidence of a household contact with Taenia solium infection
2. Individuals coming from or living in an area where cysticercosis is endemic
3. History of frequent travel to disease-endemic areas

[a] CT or MRI showing cystic lesions without scolex, enhancing lesions, or typical parenchymal brain calcifications.
[b] Enzyme-linked immunoelectrotransfer blot assay using purified extracts of *Taenia solium* antigens, as developed by the Centers for Disease Control and Prevention (Atlanta, GA).
[c] Solitary ring-enhancing lesions measuring less than 20 mm in diameter in patients presenting with seizures, a normal neurologic examination, and no evidence of an active systemic disease.
[d] CT or MRI showing hydrocephalus or abnormal enhancement of the leptomeninges and myelograms showing multiple filling defects in the column of contrast medium.
[e] Seizures, focal neurologic signs, intracranial hypertension, and dementia.
[f] Histologically confirmed subcutaneous or muscular cysticercosis, plain X-ray films showing "cigar-shaped" soft-tissue calcifications, or direct visualization of cysticerci in the anterior chamber of the eye.
ELISA = enzyme-linked immunosorbent assay.

manifestation is usually intractable seizures.[6519]

In a spinal form, the cysts may be extra-or intramedullary and lead to an increase in the CSF protein content, pressure, and cell count, with eosinophilia. Laboratory (CT and pathology) results in acute, transitional, and inactive stages have been described.[1031] Diagnostic criteria have been suggested[1550] and are reproduced in the Table above by kind permission of the American Academy of Neurology and Lippincott Williams and Wilkins.

neurocytoma A benign tumor derived from neuronal cells, usually presenting in young adults, and usually found in the lateral ventricles. The very vascular mass contains neurotubules, neurosecretory granules, clear vesicles, and well-developed intercellular junctions; it resembles neuroblastoma, but is better differentiated. It may cause sudden death, acute hydrocephalus, or a frontal lobe syndrome.[6904] The prognosis is generally good after removal but recurrence can occur.[1126]

Neurodegeneration A journal devoted to neurodegenerative disorders, neuroprotection, and neuroregeneration. Web site: http://www.academicpress.com/en/

neurodegeneration with brain iron accumulation (Hallervorden–Spatz disease, Martha–Alma disease, progressive pallidal degeneration, adult amaurotic idiocy, pantothenate kinase deficiency, NBIA type 1) A rare, clinically heterogeneous group of recessively inherited progressive degenerative neurological movement disorders, in most cases due to mutations in the gene on 20p12–3t,[643] leading to deficiency of the enzyme pantothenate kinase and causing iron accumulation in the globus pallidus and substantia nigra. MRI shows this accumulation in the globus pallidus, red nucleus, and substantia nigra (**eye-of-the-tiger sign**). Within this group, the recognized forms include an early-onset, rapidly progressive, extrapyramidal syndrome often associated with pigmentary retinopathy; a late-onset syndrome with prominent behavioral difficulties and slower progression (atypical PKAN); and **HARP** (hypoprebetalipoproteinemia, acanthocytosis, retinitis pigmentosa, and pallidal degeneration).

In HARP syndrome, there is a specific lipoprotein abnormality, but it has a mutation in the PKNA2 gene, thus including it within this diagnostic category. **Neuroferritinopathy** and **aceruloplasminemia** are other disorders without the *PANK2* mutation that are part of the NBIA spectrum.

Clinical signs are usually first evident in infancy, childhood, or young adult life, with dystonia (which is often bulbar), cognitive impairment, cerebellar ataxia, dystonia, chorea or rigidity and sudden involuntary movements accompanied by progressive night blindness and loss of peripheral vision due to pigmentary retinal degeneration or optic atrophy.[1024, 2694] In some cases, there is also evidence of a motor neuropathy. The condition ends in death after 5–20 years. When this condition occurs in early childhood at least, it and **infantile neuroaxonal dystrophy** are identical.[6771] See also **neuroaxonal dystrophies**.

Neuropathologically, there is neuronal loss, gliosis, and iron deposition as above. The hallmark pathological lesions are axonal spheroids, but Lewy body-like intraneuronal inclusions containing synuclein, glial inclusions, and neurofibrillary tangles also occur.

Diagnostic criteria have been suggested by Swaiman[6148] as follows:

Obligatory features:

- Onset before the age of 20
- Progressive course
- Presence of extrapyramidal signs

Corroborative features:

- The presence of pyramidal signs, progressive dementia, pigmentary retinopathy, optic atrophy, and/or seizures
- Autosomal recessive transmission
- Hypodensities on MRI scanning
- Presence of sea-blue histiocytes

Excluding features:

- Abnormal copper, ceruloplasmin, hexosaminidase, or GM_1 levels.
- Neuronal ceroid lipofuscinosis
- Severe retinal abnormality
- Dominant inheritance
- Caudate atrophy
- Absence of extrapyramidal features

From Swaiman, K. *Arch Neurol* 1991;48:1285–93. © American Medical Association. Reproduced by kind permission of the American Medical Association.

Variants are a *late-onset* form with dysarthria, dementia, extrapyramidal rigidity, tremor, and incontinence accompanying the cerebral atrophy and striatal gliotic changes,[3161] and an *infantile* form with features similar to those of the late-onset form. One *variant* that occurs after the age of 10 is less severe and progresses more slowly. Presenting symptoms include palilalia, rapid speech (tachylalia), dysarthria, and psychiatric symptoms such as impulsive behavior, depression, and lability of mood. In another, individuals who do not fit the diagnostic criteria have radiographic or pathologic evidence of increased basal ganglion iron deposition. The **"eye-of-the–tiger" sign** is unusual in this form; hypointense signals in the globus pallidus are more common.[3492]

neurodegenerative disease A collective term for the numerous atrophic symmetrical diseases of unknown etiology and pathogenesis that progressively damage specific systems within the nervous system following at least some period of apparently normal functioning. See also **tauopathies**, **synucleinopathies**, and **amyloidopathies**.

neurodynia An obsolete term signifying pain from nerve disease. See also **causalgia**.

neuroectodermal dysplasia A disorder of the development of structures of ectodermal origin; **incontinentia pigmenti**, **hypomelanosis of Ito**, and **basal cell nevus syndrome** are examples.

neuroectodermal melanolysosomal disease (Elejalde syndrome) A congenital dysmorphic syndrome manifesting also short stature, depigmentation of skin and hair, myopia, seizures, and mental and developmental delay.[381]

neuroectodermal tumors Primary intracranial tumors that arise from neuroectoderm. They include **astrocytomas**, **glioblastoma multiforme**, **oligodendrogliomas**, **ependymomas**, **choroid plexus papillomas**, **primitive neuroectodermal tumors**, and **neuronal tumors**.

neuroectomesodermoses See **phakomatoses**.

Neuroendocrinology A subspecialty medical journal. http://www.karger.com/journals/nen/nen_jh.htm/.

neuroepidemiology The study of the natural history of neurological disease, including its frequency of occurrence, severity, and course; the context in which it occurs; and the characteristics of those who suffer from it.[3613]

Neuroepidemiology A subspecialty medical journal. Web site: http://www.karger.com/journals/ned/ned_jh.htm.

neuroepithelial cyst (colloid cyst) A congenital cyst originating from neuroepithelial folds, including those in ectopic, endothelium-lined structures, or originating from the cleft of Rathke's pouch, and found in or beside the third ventricle or intraspinally. Their clinical expression occurs through the obstruction of CSF flow or compression of local structures.

neuroepithelial tumors of the central nervous system The new WHO classification provides the standard for communication between different centers and around the world. The basics of this classification are as follows:

Various systems are used for tumors of

Chart N–4. WHO Classification of Neuroepithelial Tumors of the CNS

1. *Astrocytic tumors* (glial tumors—categories I–V, in original). They may be invasive or noninvasive. The non-invasive tumor types are indicated below. Categories in italics are not recognized by the new WHO classification system, but are in common use.
   1. Astrocytoma (WHO grade II) (protoplasmic, gemistocytic, fibrillary, and mixed types)
   2. Anaplastic (malignant) astrocytoma (WHO grade III) in *hemispheric, diencephalic, optic, brain stem, or cerebellar sites*
   3. Glioblastoma multiforme (WHO grade IV) (giant cell glioblastoma and gliosarcoma)
   4. Pilocytic astrocytoma (noninvasive, WHO grade I) in *hemispheric, diencephalic, optic, brain stem, or cerebellar sites*
   5. Subependymal giant cell astrocytoma (noninvasive, WHO grade I)
   6. Pleomorphic xanthoastrocytoma (noninvasive, WHO grade I)
2. *Oligodendroglial tumors*
   1. Oligodendroglioma (WHO grade II)
   2. Anaplastic oligodendroglioma (WHO grade III)
3. *Ependymal cell tumors*
   1. Ependymoma (WHO grade II) (cellular, papillary, epithelial, clear cell, and mixed types)
   2. Anaplastic ependymoma (WHO grade III)
   3. Myxopapillary ependymoma
   4. Subependymoma (WHO grade I)
4. *Mixed gliomas*
   1. Mixed oligoastrocytoma (WHO grade II)
   2. Anaplastic (malignant) oligoastrocytoma (WHO grade III)
   3. Other (e.g., ependymoastrocytoma)
5. *Neuroepithelial tumors of uncertain origin*
   1. Polar spongioblastoma (WHO grade IV)
   2. Astroblastoma (WHO grade IV)
   3. Gliomatosis cerebri (WHO grade IV)
6. *Tumors of the choroid plexus*
   1. Choroid plexus papilloma
   2. Choroid plexus carcinoma (anaplastic choroid plexus papilloma)
7. *Neuronal and mixed neuronal-glial tumors*
   1. Gangliocytoma
   2. Dysplastic gangliocytoma of the cerebellum (Lhermitte–Duclos)
   3. Ganglioglioma
   4. Anaplastic (malignant) ganglioglioma
   5. Desmoplastic infantile ganglioglioma (*desmoplastic infantile astrocytoma*)
   6. Central neurocytoma
   7. Dysembryoplastic neuroepithelial tumor
   8. Olfactory neuroblastoma (esthesioneuroblastoma); olfactory neuroepithelioma is a *variant*.
8. *Pineal parenchyma tumors*
   1. Pineocytoma
   2. Pineoblastoma
   3. Mixed pineocytoma/pineoblastoma
9. *Tumors with neuroblastic or glioblastic elements (embryonal tumors)*
   1. Medulloepithelioma
   2. Primitive neuroectodermal tumors with multipotent differentiation
      i. Medulloblastoma (*variants* are medullomyoblastoma, melanocytic medulloblastoma, and desmoplastic medulloblastoma)
      ii. Cerebral primitive neuroectodermal tumor
   3. Neuroblastoma (ganglioneuroblastoma is a *variant*)
   4. Retinoblastoma
   5. Ependymoblastoma

astrocytic lineage (i.e., astrocytomas, anaplastic astrocytomas, and glioblastomas). Grades assigned are based on the microscopic appearance of the tumor. The numerical grade assigned for a given tumor, however, can vary depending on which grading system is used. The St. Anne/Mayo grading correlates better with survival than does the Kernohan system. It can only be applied to invasive tumors of astrocytic lineage; it is otherwise similar to the WHO grading system.

These comments are taken with kind permission from a web page created by Dr. S.B. Tatter at http://neurosurgery.mgh.harvard.edu/newwhobt.htm/.

neuroepithelioma See **dysembryoma**.

neuroepithelium The epithelial layer of the sense organs which contain the endings of the nerves of special sense such as the second and the eighth cranial nerves.

NeuroExam.com An interactive online guide to the neurological examination with streaming video demonstrations.

neurofaciodigitorenal syndrome A recessively inherited congenital dysmorphic syndrome, characterized also by short stature, renal agenesis, digital anomalies, megalencephaly, hypotonia, and mental and developmental delay. (Freire-Maia, Am J Med Genet. 1982;11:329–336)

neuroferritinopathy A progressive, dominantly inherited adult-onset movement disorder clinically resembling torsion dystonia, **Parkinson disease**, or **Huntington disease**, caused by mutations in the ferritin light chain gene (*FTL1*). A family history of movement disorder is common. The condition becomes overt in adult life and generalizes over a few years, leading to chorea, an akinetic-rigid syndrome, aphonia, dysphagia, action-specific facial dystonia, and/or other severe motor disabilities (often asymmetrical) with eventual frontal cortical or subcortical cognitive impairment.

Gradient echo brain MRI is always abnormal. Depressed serum ferritin levels are common except in premenopausal females and can be used as a screening test.[1150] See also **neurodegeneration with brain iron accumulation**.

Chart N–4A. Other (Non-Neuroepithelial) Tumors of the CNS

1. *Tumors of the sellar region* (pituitary adenoma, pituitary carcinoma, and craniopharyngioma)
2. *Hematopoietic tumors* (primary malignant lymphomas, plasmacytoma, granulocytic sarcoma, etc.)
3. *Germ cell tumors* (germinoma, embryonal carcinoma, yolk sac tumor [endodermal sinus tumor], choriocarcinoma, teratoma, and mixed germ cell tumors)
4. *Tumors of the meninges*:
   1. Meningioma (*variants* are meningothelial, fibrous [fibroblastic], transitional [mixed], psammomatous, angiomatous, microcystic, secretory, clear cell, chordoid, lymphoplasmacyte-rich, and metaplastic subtypes)
   2. Atypical meningioma
   3. Anaplastic (malignant) meningioma
5. *Nonmeningothelial tumors of the meninges*
   1. Benign mesenchymal (osteocartilaginous tumors, lipoma, fibrous histiocytoma, and others)
   2. Malignant mesenchymal (chondrosarcoma, hemangiopericytoma, rhabdomyosarcoma, meningeal sarcomatosis, etc.)
   3. Primary melanocytic lesions (diffuse melanosis, melanocytoma, maliganant melanoma, and the variant meningeal melanomatosi)
   4. Hematopoietic neoplasms (malignant lymphoma, plasmacytoma, and granulocytic sarcoma)
   5. Tumors of uncertain histogenesis (hemangioblastoma [capillary hemangioblastoma])
6. *Tumors of cranial and spinal nerves*
   1. Schwannoma (neurinoma and neurilemoma) with cellular, plexiform, and melanotic subtypes
   2. Neurofibroma (circumscribed [solitary] neurofibroma, plexiform neurofibroma)
   3. Malignant peripheral nerve sheath tumor (malignant Schwannoma); epithelioid, divergent mesenchymal or epithelial differentiation, and melanotic
7. Local extensions from regional tumors; paraganglioma (chemodectoma); chordoma; chondroma; chondrosarcoma; and carcinoma
8. Metastatic tumors
9. Unclassified tumors
10. Cysts and tumor-like lesions; Rathke cleft cyst, epidermoid, dermoid, colloid cyst of the third ventricle, enterogenous cyst, neuroglial cyst, granular cell tumor (choristoma, pituicytoma), hypothalamic neuronal hamartoma, nasal glial heterotopia, and plasma cell granuloma

neurofibrillary degeneration (tangles) Intraneuronal basophilic masses composed of paired helical filaments in tangles that displace the nucleus. They are found in the hippocampal regions, the frontotemporal cortex, and the pigmented nuclei of the brain stem in relation to advancing age. They were described first by **Alzheimer**. Their presence is described after cerebral trauma; in **Alzheimer disease, postencephalitic Parkinsonism**, the **ALS–Parkinsonism–dementia complex of Guam**, in **subacute sclerosing panencephalitis**, in adults with **Down syndrome**, and in normal aged brains.

Variant (straight) filaments are seen in **progressive supranuclear palsy** and in sporadic **motor neuron disease.**[6]

neurofibromas Benign, unencapsulated tumors of the nerve sheath of mixed composition, containing fibroblasts, Schwann cells, and other cells, which infiltrate the nerve from which they arise, as well as local tissues, and thus are frequently multiple, as in **neurofibromatosis**.

Histologically, they are characterized by the presence of loosely packed spindle cells seen separating the axons of a nerve, with collagen bands and mucoprotein located interstitially. Malignant change is rarely described.[6]

neurofibromatosis (von Recklinghausen syndrome, central neurofibromatosis, NF) A dominantly inherited or sporadic neurocutaneous syndrome manifesting genetic heterogeneity. Both NF1 and NF2 may also occur in mosaic forms.

Neurofibromatosis-1 is a dominantly inherited neurocutaneous syndrome due to a genetic abnormality at 17q11.2, the site of a gene coding for *neurofibromin*. It is characterized by scoliosis; bifid ribs; early puberty in males; renal artery stenosis; renal tumors; absent or hypoplastic patella; adrenal tumors; mental and developmental delay; seizures; macrocephaly; arterial disorders in the CNS; brain tumors; pseudoarthrosis; patchy depigmentation of skin; café-au-lait spots and axillary, groin or submammary freckles; dermal fibromas; and nodules in the iris (**Lisch nodules**). Lipomas and other pedunculated skin lesions are also found.

Complications include plexiform neurofibromas, cerebral tumors such as cerebral and optic gliomas and meningiomas, vestibular Schwannomas, spinal neurofibromas, neurofibrosarcomas, aqueduct stenosis, learning disabilities, and scoliosis. Visceral and endocrine tumors are also associated.[5224] Evidence of axonal or demyelinating neuropathies of any degree of severity, somewhat correlated with the presence of subcutaneous neurofibromas, may also be detectable.

Neurofibromatosis-2 (central [bilateral acoustic] neurofibromatosis) is due to a genetic abnormality at 22q11.21–q13.1. It is characterized clinically by sensorineural deafness; facial weakness; cerebellar signs; cerebral, brain stem, and optic nerve gliomas; meningiomas, sarcomas, or neurofibromas; and café-au-lait spots. The bilateral acoustic Schwannomas may be the only features, however. The excessive frequency of benign and malignant neuroectodermal tumors in neurofibromatosis is likely due to the defective production of neurofibromatin, an antioncogene.

The condition was first described by Robert Smith, an Irish physician, in 1849, 33 years before von Recklinghausen's account.

Criteria for the diagnosis have been suggested[4129] and one set (from the National

Chart N–5. Diagnostic Criteria for Neurofibromatosis

Neurofibromatosis-1 may be diagnosed when two or more of the following are present:

A. Six or more café-au-lait macules whose greatest diameter is more than 5 mm in prepubertal patients and more than 15 mm in postpubertal patients
B. Two or more neurofibromas of any type, or one plexiform neurofibroma
C. Freckling in the axilla or inguinal region
D. Optic glioma
E. Two or more Lisch nodules (iris hamartomas)
F. A distinctive osseous lesion such as sphenoid dysplasia or thinning of long bone cortex, with or without pseudoarthrosis
G. A parent, sibling, or child with neurofibromatosis-1, according to the above criteria

Neurofibromatosis-2 (definite) may be diagnosed when one of the following is present (https://www.ctf.org/about-nf/diagnosis-of-nf2/menu-id):

A. Bilateral vestibular schwannomas or
B. A parent, sibling, or child with NF2 *and* either a unilateral vestibular schwannoma or any two of the following: neurofibroma, meningioma, glioma, schwannoma, or juvenile posterior subcapsular lenticular opacity, plus
   1. Unilateral vestibular schwannoma <30 years or
   2. Any two of the following: meningioma, glioma, Schwannoma, juvenile posterior subcapsular lenticular opacity, or juvenile cortical cataract

(From Martuza RL, Eldridger R. Neurofibromatosis 2. N Engl J Med. 1988;318:684–688. © 1988. With kind permission from the Massachussetts Medical Society.

Neurofibromatosis Foundation) is given in Chart N–5. For NF2, various sets of criteria are available including those from the NIH, and from Manchester.

Relevant Web sites include those of the following:

British Columbia Neurofibromatosis Foundation http://bcnf.bc.ca/, an organization that empowers individuals with NF and their families to reach their full potential by providing support, education, and research funding.

The Children's Tumor Foundation is an organization dedicated to improving the health and well-being of individuals and families affected by neurofibromatosis. Web site: http://www.ctf.org/.

The National Neurofibromatosis Foundation (*NNFF*) http://www.nf.org/, which is a patient-based site.

http://www.ninds.nih.gov/disorders/neurofibromatosis/neurofibromatosis.htm, is an information page compiled by the National Institute of Neurological Disorders and Stroke.

Neurofibromatosis Association of Australia Inc. http://www.nfaa.org.au/, a support group for Australian people with neurofibromatosis.

The Neurofibromatosis Association UK http://www.users.zetnet.co.uk/neurofibromatosis/, is a support group for people with neurofibromatosis in Britain.

M.D. Anderson Cancer Center http://www.mdanderson.org/departments/ provides information about neurofibromatosis and details of diagnosis, treatment, patient education, and relevant research.

Variant conditions are

Noonan features with neurofibromatosis, a dominantly inherited congenital dysmorphic syndrome, characterized also by short stature; ptosis; short webbed neck; vertebral and other skeletal, dermal, and congenital cardiac anomalies; seizures; macrocephaly; mental and developmental delay; and the usual features of neurofibromatosis[5413]

Segmental neurofibromatosis, in which there is restriction of the cutaneous and neoplastic features to a few adjacent segments of the body[4374]

Spinal and cutaneous neurofibromatosis, in which the occurrence of multiple schwannomas has been described as sporadic but which probably represents a variant of NF2[1928]

Godfried–Prick–Carol–Prakken syndrome, in which dermal atrophy, Mongoloid facies, mental retardation, and cardiac conduction disturbances are added features[1025]

Schwannomatosis (multiple schwannomas, multiple Schwannomatosis, neurilemmomatosis) A third major form of the condition causing multiple schwannomas without those vestibular tumors that allow the diagnosis of NF2. Suggested diagnostic criteria[3987] are

Definite

Age over 30 years *and* two or more known intradermal schwannomas, at least one having histological confirmation, *and* no evidence of vestibular tumor on high-quality MRI scan *and* no known constitutional NF2 mutation

or

One pathologically confirmed nonvestibular Schwannoma plus a first-degree relative who meets the above criteria

Possible

Age over 30 years *and* two or more nonintradermal Schwannomas, at least one with histological confirmation, *and* no evidence of vestibular tumor on high-quality MRI scan *and* no known constitutional NF2 mutation

or

Age over 45 years *and* two or more nonintradermal schwannomas, at least one with histological confirmation *and* no symptoms of VIII nerve dysfunction *and* no known constitutional NF2 mutation

or

Radiographic evidence of a nonvestibular schwannoma *and* a first-degree relative who meets criteria for definite Schwannomatosis

Segmental Schwannomatosis

Meets criteria for either definite or possible Schwannomatosis but limited to one limb or five or fewer contiguous segments of the spine

Neurofibromatosis, Inc. (NF Inc.) A charitable organization in this field. Address: 8855 Annapolis Rd., Suite 110, Lanham, MD 20706-2924. Tel: 301-577-8984. E-mail: nfinc1@aol.com. Web site: http://www.nfinc.org/.

neurofilament inclusion body disease A clinicopathological entity presenting in mid-adult life with a rapidly progressive course manifesting either as frontotemporal dementia or as a corticobasal degeneration syndrome leading to loss of ambulation and mutism with premature death. Pathologically it is characterized by spongiosis affecting the frontal lobes and severe caudate atrophy with extensive eosinophilic or basophilic intracytoplasmic neurofilament protein inclusions.[3250]

neurofilaments Small (10-nm) organelles that exist within the axoplasm, determining its diameter. The filaments are especially notable in larger axons and move centripetally at up to 3 mm per day.

Neurogastroenterology and Motility A subspecialty medical journal. Web site: http://www.blacksci.co.uk/~cgilib/jnlpage.asp?Journal=NGEM&File=NGEM &Page=aims/.

neurogenesis 1. The continued generation of new neurons, as in the hippocampus and the olfactory bulb in adult mammals, suggesting that neuronal stem cells persist throughout the entire lifespan. Surprisingly, the cells that give rise to the new neurons in the adult brain express markers for radial glial cells, which can give rise not only to astrocytes but also to oligodendrocytes, ependymal cells, and neurons and which are the precursors of neuronal stem cells in the adult brain.[241] 2. See the Web site http://neurogenesis.iord.org/ for an introduction to neurodegenerative disorders and to neurogenesis treatments.

Neurogenetics A subspecialty medical journal. Web site: http://link.springer-ny.com/link/service/journals/10048/index.htm.

neurogenic acroosteolysis See **ulceromutilating acropathy**.

neurogenic arthropathy (Charcot joints) A clinical syndrome of painless joint enlargement with crepitus, effusions, laxity of ligaments, and excessive mobility leading to dissolution of the joint, and associated with a loss of nocioceptive sensation, as in **hereditary sensory and autonomic neuropathy**, **tabes dorsalis**, **diabetic or amyloid neuropathies** and **leprosy**.

neurogenic benign fasciculations See **idiopathic neuromyotonia**.

neurogenic bladder The condition of the bladder after interruption of its motor or sensory nerve supply. See also **reflex neurogenic bladder**, **autonomous neurogenic bladder**, **motor paralytic bladder**, and **deafferented bladder**.

neurogenic claudication The complaint of ascending numbness and weakness of the legs that occurs in association with postural extension of the lumbar spine, as during shaving, and both with standing and exercise in patients with lumbar **spinal stenosis**. The similarities with vasogenic claudication are many but, in the neurogenic form, the absence of cramps and paresthesias and the procurement of relief by the adoption of flexed posture are differentiating points.

The term *claudication* is derived from the Latin word *claudicare*, to limp; perhaps deriving also from that deficit of the Roman Emperor Claudius. The word is poorly applied here, because, when patients with lumbar spinal stenosis become symptomatic, they do not limp but rather stop walking and bend forward, a maneuver that enlarges the internal dimensions of the spinal canal. Such people should rely on bicycles for local transport.

neurogenic diabetes insipidus Transient reduction in the secretion of antidiuretic hormone following head injury or cranial surgery.

neurogenic fever See **neurogenic hyperthermia**.

neurogenic hyperthermia ("neurogenic fever") Fever reflects the action of pyrogens upon the intact hypothalamus. Lesions of the anterior hypothalamus may impair the body's ability to dissipate heat, leading to hyperthermia, but they do not change the hypothalamic set point. The hypothalamus contains two areas involved in maintaining temperature homeostasis, one located anteriorly, concerned with heat dissipation and containing the "hypothalamic thermostat," and the other located posteriorly and involved in heat generation. Electrical stimulation of the posterior area produces shivering, piloerection, peripheral vasoconstriction, and behaviors raising body temperature. Lesions of this area prevent the normal response to cold.

In true fever, pyrogens such as interleukin 1 act on anterior hypothalamic neurons to raise the set point of the hypothalamic "thermostat" through a prostaglandin E2-mediated system. Sensing a difference between the current and desired temperatures, these neurons stimulate activity in the posterior thalamic center to increase thermogenic activities. Once the body temperature has reached the new set point, these activities normally subside.

In most cases, there is a history of trauma, infarct, or tumor in the hypothalamus, spinal cord injury, familial dysautonomia, or autonomic neuropathies, but the syndrome may also be seen in late stages of neurodegenerative disorders. Helpful in diagnosis are relative bradycardia, maintenance of the fever with little diurnal fluctuation, absence of sweating, and lack of efficacy of antipyretics. Reduction of the fever may be accomplished by external cooling, unless rigidity produces a large internal heat load.

Subarachnoid blood, air, or iodinated contrast may cause a low-grade fever due to an inflammatory response in the subarachnoid space, but there is accompanying evidence of inflammation in the CSF. Diencephalic epilepsy and complex partial status epilepticus may be associated with temperature elevations thought to be secondary to episodic hypothalamic dysfunction.[1659, 1905, 4975]

neurogenic inflammation An early response to tissue injury. In the context of migraine, the term applies to the vasodilatation and extravasation of plasma that occur following stimulation of the unmyelinated afferent C-fibers supplying dural and scalp blood vessels.

neurogenic pulmonary edema The occurrence of pulmonary edema as a complication of generalized tonic-clonic seizures, first reported by Shanahan in 1908. The precise mechanism of this effect remains uncertain.[6256]

neurogenic sarcoma An uncommon malignant tumor of the peripheral nerve sheath.

neurogenic thoracic outlet compression syndrome An uncommon lower trunk brachial plexopathy predominantly damaging the T1 fibers in the median motor nerve fibers to the thenar muscles and in the medial antebrachial cutaneous nerve fibers.[3805] See also **thoracic outlet syndrome**.

neuroglia (Gr, nerve + glue) The name applied by Virchow (1846) to the supporting cells (as opposed to the neurons) of the CNS; the differentiation was achieved without benefit of special stains, which had not then been invented.

neuroglioma See **glioma**.

neuroichthyoses Genetically determined diffuse encephalopathies, including **Sjögren–Larsson syndrome**, **Rud syndrome**, keratitis–ichthyosis–deafness syndrome, ichthyosis with neutral lipid storage, and **Refsum syndrome**.

NeuroImage A journal of diagnostic neuroradiology. Web site: www.elsevier.com/inca/publications/store/6/2/2/9/2/5/.

Neuroimmunomodulation A subspecialty medical journal. Web site: http://www.karger.com/journals/nim/nim_jh.htm.

neuroimmunophilins A family of proteins expressed in the nervous system that act as receptors for some immunosuppressant agents and with a likely rôle in neuroprotection and regeneration.[2139]

neurokinin A peptide substance discovered by Wolff, with a possible rôle in the genesis of **migraine**.

neurolabyrinthitis See **acute peripheral vestibulopathy**.

Neuroland A valuable Web site maintained by Dr. Charles Tuen, containing current data on numerous neurological diseases including multiple sclerosis, headache, pain, stroke, polyneuropathy, seizures, anticonvulsants, low-back pain, Parkinson disease, infectious diseases, and Internal Medicine. Web site: www.neuroland.com/.

neuroleptic malignant syndrome (lethal catatonia) An uncommon, fulminant, life-threatening and unpredictable idiosyncratic reaction in response to (mainly) neuroleptic medications (dopamine receptor-blocking agents) in adults, described by Delay and Deniker in 1960 and due to imbalance of 5HT and dopamine, or to withdrawal of dopaminergic drugs, causing a relatively hypodopaminergic state. Agents incriminated include haloperidol, metoclopramide, phenothiazines, tetrabenazine, tricyclics, SSRIs, and lithium.

The clinical features that develop over 1–3 days and last for up to 10 days include hyperthermia, autonomic instability (labile blood pressure, pallor, sweating, tachycardia, or bradykinesia), intense plastic muscular rigidity, altered consciousness with delirium, and elevated muscle enzyme levels in almost all cases. Mutism, tremor, choreic or dystonic movements, and incontinence occur in a majority and oculogyric crises, opisthotonos, seizures, and trismus are seen in a few. Shock, respiratory failure, and rhabdomyolysis with myoglobinuria can occur with serious renal consequences.[3798, 6521] ICU management with aggressive fluid and electrolyte management, and supportive care usually lead to recovery; the value of dantrolene sodium, amantadine, and bromocriptine as treatments[54] is disputed. Cardiac failure and cerebellar degeneration are potential late complications.

The condition occurs at some time in 0.5% of subjects (especially young males) exposed to neuroleptic agents and is considered to have a central (presynaptic) origin.[2652] It is also described following withdrawal of levadopa therapy in the treatment of idiopathic **Parkinson disease**, while an identical syndrome may be seen rarely in untreated catatonic schizophrenia. The following diagnostic criteria have been defined:

major criteria: fever, rigidity, and elevated serum CK levels;
minor criteria: tachycardia, labile blood pressure, tachypnea, altered consciousness, sweating, and leukocytosis.

The presence of three major signs or two major and four minor signs makes the diagnosis probable.[54]

In a *variant* form, an absence of muscle glycogen and neutral lipid is found on muscle biopsy specimens.[4117] Partial syndromes are also seen. See also the Web site: http://www.neuro.wustl.edu/neuromuscular/index.html/ and **serotonin syndrome** and **malignant hyperthermia**.

neurolipidoses Hereditary metabolic disorders in which abnormal lipid accumulations occur, such as in the **gangliosidoses**. Myoclonic epilepsy is often a prominent clinical feature.

Neurolist An international E-mail discussion forum for neurologists run from the Medical College of Georgia. Web site: www.neurolist.com/site.

Neurologic Clinics of North America (*Neurol Clin North Amer*) A quarterly periodical reviewing neurology topics, published by W.B. Saunders. Address: Independence Square West, Philadelphia, PA 19106-3399. Web site: http://www.us.elsevierhealth.com/fcgi-bin/displaypage.pl?isbn=07338619/.

Neurologic Disorder Information and Glossary An NIH site providing brief description, treatment, prognosis, and links for a long list of neurological disorders. Web site: http://www.ninds.nih.gov/disorders/disorder_index.htm.

Neurological Alliance A British alliance of charities devoted to neurological disorders. Web site: www.neurologicalalliance.org.uk/.

Neurological Disability Score A semiquantitative method of assessing the disability produced by diseases of the *peripheral* nervous system, in which the degree of abnormality in clinical tests of the cranial nerves (6 items), muscle weakness (16 movements or muscles), muscle stretch reflexes (5), and sensation in the index finger and hallux (4 modalities in each site) on each side is scored between 0 (no deficit) and 4 (complete absence of function or severest deficit). The summed score is used to obtain a raw score to evaluate progression of diabetic neuropathic symptoms.[1770, 1783]

Deficits produced by lesions of the *central* nervous system are not considered in this scale.

neurological examination A complex learned skill possessed by some physicians.

Neurological Institute of New York An institution founded in 1909 by Joseph Collins and Pearce Bailey, later attracting Ramsay **Hunt**, Charles **Dana**, Elsberg, and Sachs as members. It moved to Columbia Presbyterian Medical Center in 1929 and has expanded greatly since. Address: Columbia-Presbyterian Medial Center, New York, NY 10032-3784. Tel: 212-305-8551.

Neurological Rating Scale A simple assessment tool in **multiple sclerosis** in which dysfunction is scored in the categories of mentation and mood; cranial nerves (visual acuity, fields, discs and pupils, eye movements, and nystagmus); lower cranial nerves; motor and reflex functions in each limb; Babinski signs; sensory functions in each limb; cerebellar function in the upper and the lower limbs; gait; and bladder/bowel/sexual dysfunction—the whole yielding a total impairment score. The maximum (normal) score is 100.[4351]

Neurological Society of London An institution founded in 1885 with Hughlings-**Jackson** as the Founding president, and Samuel Wilks, **Bastian**, Crighton-Browne, Broadbent, **Ferrier**, **Galton**, Bucknill, and others as councillors. Two years after its founding, it created the journal **Brain** as its organ.

Neurological Symptoms Score A checklist of symptoms assisting in the diagnosis of the presence of a neuropathy.[1771] The items assessed are

Muscle weakness, bulbar: extraocular/facial/tongue/throat
Muscle weakness, limbs: shoulder girdle and upper arm/hand/glutei and thigh/legs
Sensory disturbances, "negative" symptoms: difficulty in identifying objects in the mouth or hands/unsteadiness in walking
Sensory disturbances, "positive" symptoms: complaints of numbness, "asleep feeling," "like Novocain," "prickling"—at any site/burning, deep aching pain or tenderness at any location
Autonomic symptoms: postural fainting/impotence in males/loss of urinary control/nocturnal diarrhea

Neurological Teaching Videos A digital video of the neurological examination, requiring free online registration by Wright State University. Web site: http://www.ntv.wright.edu/.

Neurologiskt Handikappades Riksforbund A member society of the European Alliance of Muscular Dystrophy Societies, based at Kungsgatan 32, S-11 35 Stockholm, Sweden.

neurologist (Gr, a nerve + a discourse) 1. One who is occupied with the study of the nerves and the nervous system. 2. A physician who is trained in the diagnosis and management of patients suffering from diseases of the nervous system, or their symptoms.

The Neurologist —A review journal focusing on clinically relevant issues, published by Lippincott Williams and Wilkins. Web site: http://www.theneurologist.org/.

neurology The study of the nervous system in health and disease. The term was originally that of Thomas **Willis**, who also described this labor as "The doctrine of the nerves." This phrase was taken by Spillane for his superb review of the history of the subject.[5978]

Neurology A professional journal founded as the official publication of the **American Academy of Neurology** in 1951 with Dr. R. de Jong as the first editor. The journal was published monthly since 1953 but now weekly. Web site: http://www.neurology.org/.

Neurology and Neurosurgery An Excerpta Medica abstract journal providing a current awareness service, published by Elsevier. Web site: http://www.elsevier.com/inca/publications/store/5/0/5/9/7/7/.

Neurology and Neurosurgery Forum An interactive medical question-and-answer site from the Cleveland Clinic providing an explanation of various neurological conditions for laypeople at http://www.medhelp.org/perl6/neuro/archive/6454.html/.

Neurology Channel.com A site offering patient information, clinic web design, and member services.

Neurology Links A professional resource. Web site: www.neurologylinx.com/.

Neurology Resources A site listing various data sources and organizations relevant to neurological disorders compiled by the Neurodegeneration Research Group. Web site: http://www.asahi-net.or.jp/~QB8M-AMGS/neurology.html/.

neurolymphomatosis (reticulosis of the nervous system, polyradiculitis with cellular infiltrates, lymphomatous neuropathy, lymphomatous leptomeningitis) Lymphomatous infiltration of the peripheral nerves producing various clinical pictures of sensorimotor peripheral and cranial neuropathies. These include those of acute inflammatory polyneuropathy, mononeuropathy, subacute or relapsing neuropathy, and cauda equina syndrome.

The condition is analogous to Marek disease, which afflicts Orpington roosters.[1631]

neuroma (Gr, nerve + tumor) A benign tumor of nerves, first described by William Wood, a Scottish physician, in 1828.

neuroma sign In patients with severe proximal brachial plexus lesions, if the side of the neck is tapped and paresthesias are felt in the distribution of a dermatome, the nerve root is likely to have been ruptured.

Neurometer A commercial device for quantifying sensory thresholds, thus potentially of value in the diagnosis and/or follow-up of patients with neuropathies. Web site: http://www.neurotron.com/site/index.html/.

neuromics The analysis of genomic DNA for risk association with a neurological disease. An increased risk for conditions such as **amyotrophic lateral sclerosis**, **Alzheimer disease**, **restless leg syndrome**, or **multiple sclerosis** has been associated with polymorphisms in specific genes.

neuromodulator A substance altering the receptivity of a neuron to stimulation, as by altering the resting potential or changing synthesis in the cell for receptors, etc. Examples include secretin, bombesin, neuropeptide Y, substance P, vasoactive intestinal peptide, and glucagon.

neuromuscular blockade Impairment of the passage of acetylcholine from the nerve ending, across the synapse to the motor end plate, or reduction of the effect of acetylcholine at the latter site.

Neuromuscular Disease Center (Washington University, St. Louis) A superb resource maintained by Dr. Alan Pestronk. It provides complete data for physicians on the clinical and laboratory aspects of all neuromuscular disorders and ataxias. Web site: http://www.neuro.wustl.edu/neuromuscular/index.html.

neuromuscular diseases The range of disorders affecting the peripheral nervous system. An overview of the classification provided by the World Federation of Neurology is used as the framework presented in Chart N–6.

Neuromuscular Disorders An international multidisciplinary journal covering all aspects of the neuromuscular disorders of childhood and adult life. The journal publishes original research, reviews, short communications, and book reviews. Web site: http://www.elsevier.nl/locate/nmd.

Chart N–6. Classification of Neuromuscular Disorders

1. *Spinal muscular atrophies and other disorders of motor neurons* (for further descriptions, see **motor neuronal disorders** and specific diseases)

   A. Inherited muscle atrophies (**hereditary motor neuropathies**)

      A.1. Autosomal recessive, biochemical abnormality unknown
      A.2. Autosomal recessive, biochemical abnormality known
      A.3. Autosomal dominant, biochemical abnormality unknown
      A.4. X-linked recessive, biochemical disorder unknown
      A.5. X-linked dominant, lethal in males

   B. Congenital and developmental abnormalities (see Chart M–17, **motor neuronal diseases** for further consideration of groups B, C, D, E, F, G, H, and I)
   C. Disorders of motor neurons attributed to physical causes
   D. Disorders of motor neurons attributed to toxins, chemicals, or heavy metals
   E. Disorders of motor neurons attributed to viral infection

      E.1. Acute disorders
      E.2. Subacute or chronic disorders

   F. Disorders of motor neurons with immunological abnormality
   G. Disorders of motor neurons of undetermined etiology
   H. Disorders of motor neurons in endocrine disorders
   I. Disorders of motor neurons manifest by hyperactivity

2. *Disorders of motor nerve roots* (for further descriptions, see **radiculopathy**)

   A. Congenital
   B. Acquired

3. *Disorders of peripheral nerve* (for further descriptions, see **neuropathy** and entries for specific diseases)

   A. Heritable, biochemical abnormality unknown
   B. Congenital
   C. Traumatic
   D. Infections
   E. Guillain–Barré syndrome (**acute inflammatory demyelinating polyneuropathy**) and related disorders
   F. Neuropathy associated with connective tissue disorder
   G. Metabolic neuropathy
   H. Neuropathy in malignant disease
   I. Neuropathy associated with other systemic or nonhereditary degenerative diseases
   J. Chronic neuropathy with no known cause or association
   K. Tumors of nerves

4. *Disorders of neuromuscular transmission* (for further descriptions, see Charts N–5A and B, **neuromuscular transmission disorders**)

   A. Heritable
   B. Congenital or developmental **myasthenia**
   C. Toxic
   D. Autoimmune
   E. **Lambert–Eaton syndrome**
   F. Cholinergic paralysis

5. *Disorders of muscle* (for further description and subclassification, see **myopathies**)

   A. Heritable myopathies

      A.1. The muscular dystrophies
      A.2. Congenital myopathies of unknown etiology
      A.3. Myotonic disorders

   B. Trauma to muscle by external agents

      B.1. Physical
      B.2. Toxic
      B.3. Drugs

C. Inflammatory

C.1. Infections of muscle
C.2. Other inflammatory disorders of muscle
C.3. Inflammatory disorders of muscle of unknown etiology

D. Metabolic myopathies

D.1. Muscle disorder associated with endocrine disease
D.2. Heritable myopathies, biochemical abnormality known
D.3. Other metabolic myopathies

E. Myopathy associated with malignant disease
F. Myopathy associated with **myasthenia gravis**
G. Myopathy in thalassemia
H. Other disorders of muscle of unknown or uncertain etiology
I. Tumors of muscle

6. *Disorders of supraspinal tonal regulation which may mimic neuromuscular disorders*

This listing is compiled from that of the World Federation of Neurology Classification Subcommittee (*J Neurol Sci* 1988;**86**:333–60); on reports from the more recent literature and from Dr. Alan Pestronk's comprehensive Web site http://www.neuro.wustl.edu/neuromuscular/maltbrain.html with his kind permission

Chart N–6A. Disorders of Neuromuscular Transmission

A. Heritable

1. Hereditary **myasthenia gravis**

a. Congenital and juvenile[936]
b. Myasthenia with myopathy[4266]

2. **Pseudocholinesterase deficiency** (suxamethonium paralysis)

B. Congenital or developmental myasthenia

1. Putative defect in acetylcholine synthesis or packaging
2. **Congenital end-plate acetylcholinesterase deficiency**
3. **Slow-channel syndrome**
4. **Congenital end-plate acetylcholine receptor deficiency**
5. Decrease of miniature end-plate potential amplitude without acetylcholine receptor deficiency
6. Abnormality of synaptic vesicles[4465]

C. Toxic

1. **Botulism**
2. **Tick paralysis**
3. **Puffer-fish paralysis** (tetrodotoxin)
4. Magnesium intoxication
5. Kanamycin and other antibiotics[4267]
6. Penicillamine-induced myasthenia, also anticonvulsants, quinidine[2291]

D. Autoimmune

1. **Myasthenia gravis**

a. Transient neonatal myasthenia[2362]
b. Ocular myasthenia, with peripheral neuropathy and spastic paraparesis[924]
c. Generalized myasthenia

(i) Severe, especially in young women, correlated with HLA-8 antigen
(ii) In older patients, often with thymoma and with HLA-2 or A3 antigen

d. Myasthenia with thyrotoxicosis
e. Myasthenia with hypothyroidism[6190]
f. Myasthenia with other autoimmune diseases
g. Myasthenia combined with **Lambert–Eaton syndrome**[4763]
h. Myasthenia with **Satoyoshi syndrome** (muscle cramps, alopecia, and diarrhea)

E. Lambert–Eaton syndrome (a facilitating disorder of neuromuscular transmission)

1. With malignant disease
2. Without malignant disease

F. Cholinergic paralysis (e.g., due to poisoning with anticholinesterase compounds such as nerve gases, depolarizing drugs, or black widow spider venom)

(Compiled from various sources but based upon the the World Federation of Neurology Classification Subcommittee. *Classification of Neuromuscular Diseases. J Neurol Sci* 1988;**86**:333–60.)

neuromuscular transmission disorders Clinical disorders primarily affecting synaptic transmission at the neuromuscular junction, associated with pathology affecting its structure and function. Charts N–6A and N–6B show two alternative classifications. The first of these is closely based upon that of the World Federation of Neurology and is an overview of all forms, hereditary and acquired.

A more recent system for classifying the congenital and familial disorders of neuromuscular transmission, based upon the underlying pathophysiology, has been constructed by Dr. Alan Pestronk (Web site: http://neuromuscular.wustl.edu/synmg.html) and is reproduced in Chart N–6B with his kind permission.

neuromyasthenia See **chronic fatigue syndrome**.

neuromyelitis Originally signifying "inflammation of the nervous or medullary substance,"[5103] the word is now used to indicate the coexistence of inflammation of the spinal cord and a nerve, usually the optic nerve.

Chart N–6B. Alternative Classificatuion of Disorders of Neuromuscular Transmission

Presynaptic defects
Congenital MG with episodic apnea (familial infantile): ChAT; 10q11
Paucity of synaptic vesicles and reduced quantal release
Congenital **Lambert–Eaton**-like syndrome
Episodic ataxia 2: CACNA1A; 19p13
Reduced quantal release

Synaptic basal lamina defects
Acetylcholinesterase (AChE) deficiency at NMJs: ColQ; 3p25

Postsynaptic defects: AChR disorders; α, β, δ, e subunits
Kinetic abnormalities in AChR function
Reduced numbers of AChRs at NMJs

Slow AChR channel syndromes: increased response to ACh
Delayed channel closure: AChR mutations
Repeated channel reopenings: AChR mutations

Fast-channel syndromes: reduced response to ACh
Mode-switching kinetics disorder: AChR e subunit
Gating abnormality: AChR α or e subunit
Arthrogryposis: AChR δ subunit
Also see e subunit disorders
Normal numbers of AChRs at NMJs: reduced response to ACh
Fast-channel syndrome: low ACh affinity of AChR; AChR e subunit
Fast-channel syndrome: reduced channel openings; AChR α subunit

---

continued

Chart N–6B. *(continued)*

High conductance and fast closure of AChRs
Increased numbers of AChRs at NMJs
Slow AChR channel syndrome: AChR subunit βL262M
No kinetic abnormalities in AChR function
Reduced numbers of AChRs at NMJs
AChR mutations
Usually e subunit: 17p13
Rarely other subunits: α; 2q24, β; 17p12, δ; 2q33
Arthrogryposis syndromes
Recurrent congenital MG: maternal antibodies vs fetal AChRs
Multiple pterygium syndrome (Escobar): AChR γ subunit mutations

Postsynaptic defects: other
MuSK: 9q31
Plectin deficiency: plectin; 8q24
Rapsyn: 11p11
Weakness + episodic apnea and bulbar dysfunction: SCN4A; 17q35

Other hereditary MG syndromes
Congenital myasthenia gravis
Benign congenital MG with facial malformations: rapsyn
Congenital and acquired myasthenia gravis
Other
Familial immune
Limb-girdle myasthenia gravis. Familial: Dok-7; 4
Limb-girdle myasthenia gravis with tubular aggregates

neuromyelitis optica

neuromyelitis optica (Devic disease, Devic–Gault syndrome, myelopathy with optic neuritis, optic myelitis, Schilder myelinoclastic diffuse sclerosis) A necrotizing and demyelinating immune-modulated disease with its attack targeted upon the spinal cord and both optic nerves, described from France by M.E. Devic in 1894[1617] and before him by Chisholm in England.

The disease, which may be a variant of (though distinct from) **multiple sclerosis**,[2683] is uncommon in the Western world but not in Japan. Clinically, subacute visual failure is followed within days by signs of longitudinally extensive myelopathy, but brain stem, cerebellar, and cognitive disturbances do not occur. NMO-IgG is a marker antibody useful in confirming the diagnosis. Secondary progressive disease is uncommon.

Suggested diagnostic criteria,[6825] modified here, are

Absolute criteria:

1. Optic neuritis
2. Acute myelitis
3. No evidence of clinical disease outside of the optic nerve or spinal cord

Major supportive criteria:

1. Negative brain MRI at onset (does not meet criteria for MS)
2. Spinal cord MRI showing signal abnormality that extends over at least three segments
3. CSF pleocytosis of at least 50 WBC/mm^3 or at least 5 neutrophils/mm^3

Minor supportive criteria:

1. Bilateral optic neuritis
2. Severe optic neuritis with fixed visual acuity worse than 20/200 in at least one eye
3. Severe, fixed, attack-related weakness (MRC grade 2 or less) in one or more limbs

The diagnosis requires *all* absolute criteria and *one* major supportive criterion *or* two minor supportive criteria.

A briefer set[3574] modifies the above so that subjects must have optic neuritis and acute myelitis as major criteria, and must either have a spinal MRI lesion extending over three or more segments or be *NMO* positive on antibody testing. Information on the condition may be found at the Web site http://devicsnotes.blogspot.com/.

A *variant* form is recurrent neuromyelitis optica with endocrinopathies (**Vernant syndrome**).

Neuromyelitis optica can also be caused by **systemic lupus erythematosus**, **Sjögren disease**, and **antiphospholipid syndrome**. See also **disseminated vasculomyelinopathy**.

neuromyopathy

neuromyopathy Clinical disorders resulting from pathology affecting both nerve and muscle fibers.See **carcinomatous neuromyopathy** and **cachectic myopathy**.

neuromyositis

neuromyositis (dermatoradiculoneuromyositis) The rare concomitant association of polyneuropathy and polymyositis, first described by Senator in 1888, and probably representing the chance concurrence of **acute inflammatory demyelinating polyneuropathy** and **polymyositis**.[4221]

neuromyotonia

neuromyotonia 1. (Isaacs syndrome, continuous muscle fiber activity, hereditary myotonia, continuous muscle fiber activity, continuous motor unit activity, idiopathic generalized myotonia, Isaacs–Mertens syndrome, quantal squander, generalized myokymia, normocalcemic tetany, neurotonia) A nonprogressive syndrome of continuous, generalized involuntary twitching or quivering in several muscles with impaired relaxation after contraction (**myokymia**) but without a true myotonic response. It is due to hyperexcitability of the peripheral motor axons, possibly as a result of autoimmune disease[3099, 6643] mediated by IgG antibodies to voltage-gated potassium channels, although familial occurrence has been recorded.[4327] Electrically, there are irregular and abrupt spontaneous bursts of single motor unit potentials at a rate of between 2 and 300 Hz, prolonged over up to 30 s, and associated with and provoked by persistent muscle contraction. The situation is complicated by the coexistence of **myotonia**in some cases.[3155] See also **pseudomyotonia**, **myokymia**, **Morvan disease**, **limbic encephalitis**, and **cramp–fasciculation syndrome**, in all of which autoimmunity is implicated in the pathogenesis.

Clinically, the condition presents at any age with continuing contraction of muscles at rest or following voluntary effort, leading to a delay in relaxation, and with fasciculations, muscle stiffness, cramps, weakness and often twitching, and increased warmth and sweating. The accompanying electrical activity may be intermittent or continuous.

The phenomenon resembles **myotonia** clinically, but, in this case, may be the result of many disorders of motor nerves that lead to ectopic or ephaptic neural discharges, as with myokymia following plexus irradiation. It responds to phenytoin and to carbamazepine. Lung and thymic neoplasms and myasthenia with anti-AChR antibodies have been reported in association. See also **Schwartz–Jampel syndrome**.

2. A combination of subjective muscle stiffness and myokymia, sometimes with added muscle hypertrophy, supervening in some patients with **chronic inflammatory demyelinating polyneuropathy**.

3. (*ocular neuromyotonia*) Recurrent episodes of sustained contraction of the muscles supplied by a paretic III cranial

nerve, both spontaneously and following eccentric gaze. The condition appears usually in the context of recent pituitary radiation therapy.[3794] Ephaptic neural transmission is the likely underlying mechanism.[6324]

Variants include the following:

acquired neuromyotonia, an autoimmune cause of motor hyperexcitability presenting with cramps, muscle stiffness and twitching, sweating, and impaired relaxation after muscle contraction.[5232] Many patients have antibodies to voltage-gated potassium channels and some a thymoma.

A syndrome of muscle stiffness associated with a bronchial carcinoma, the stiffness precipitated by movement and accompanied by bizarre high-frequency motor unit discharges appearing during and after voluntary contraction. The features are abolished by nerve block and reduced by phenytoin. HIV infection, thymus cancer, and Hodgkin disease are also associated. See also **stiff person syndrome**.[6619]

Morvan "chorea" (neuromyotonia, hyperhidrosis, and encephalopathy)

Familial stiff person syndrome, manifesting hypertonia at birth, which regresses, only to return in adolescence.[5528] See also **limp man syndrome** and **idiopathic neuromyotonia**.

See also **continuous muscle fiber activity syndrome, Isaacs syndrome, Isaacs–Merten syndrome, quantal squander, generalized myokymia, pseudomyotonia, normocalcemic tetany**, and **neurotonia**, and the Web site: http://www.neuro.wustl.edu/neuromuscular/maltbrain.html.

neuromyotonic discharge

Bursts of motor unit action potentials that fire at high rates (150–300 Hz) for a few seconds, often starting or stopping abruptly. The amplitude of the waveforms typically wanes. Discharges may occur spontaneously or be initiated by needle electrode movement, voluntary effort, ischemia, or percussion of a nerve. The activity originates in motor axons. Distinguish from myotonic discharges and complex repetitive discharges. One type of electrical activity recorded in patients who have clinical neuromyotonia. (From the 2001 Report of the Nomenclature Committee of the American Association of Electromyography and Electrodiagnosis.[19] Reproduced by kind permission of the AANEM.)

neuronal ceroid lipofuscinosis

(Gr, nerve + wax + fat) (cerebroretinal lipofuscinosis, Batten–Vogt disease, Batten–Mayou disease, Batten disease, Landing–Oppenheimer disease, NCL) Conditions that, with the **gangliosidoses**, were formerly classified together under the pejorative rubric "familial amaurotic idiocy." They are a group of recessively inherited lysosomal storage diseases (the commonest group of neurodegenerative storage diseases in childhood) and are characterized by the accumulation of abnormal amounts of ceroid lipofuscin (an autofluorescent lipopigment) in the lysosomes and by the presence of characteristic curvilinear or fingerprint inclusions in brain, skin, muscle, or rectal mucosa; an excessive accumulation of granular lipopigment in neuronal perikarya; neuronal loss; and elevated levels of urinary sediment dolichols.

Clinically, all forms manifest progressive encephalopathy with psychomotor deterioration, visual failure with pigmentary retinal degeneration, seizures with visual sensitivity, psychiatric disturbances, spasticity, ataxia, and movement disorders. Death usually occurs within 10 years of the onset. Increased autofluorescent lipopigment is detectable in neuronal cells.

For the many known mutations in NCL, see http://www.ucl.ac.uk/ncl/. Although the gene for the disorder has been cloned, the function of the encoded protein CLN3P (a palmitoyl-protein-9 desaturase) remains uncertain.[4591] A mutation in the cathepsin D gene may underlie all cases of congenital NCL.[5830]

Five clinical varieties were described variously by Batten (1903), Mayer (1904), Vogt (1904), Spielmeyer (1904), Jansky (1908), Bielschowsky (1913), and Sjögren (1931). Others have been added more recently (Chart N–7). See also **Unified Batten Disease Rating Scale**.

Berkovic suggests the following diagnostic criteria:[567]

Onset of phenotypes resembling **progressive myoclonic epilepsy** or of behavioral change, dementia, and motor disturbances, there being no visual failure in either case, at around the age of 30 years. The clinical course leads to death with dementia in about 12 years. Elevated urinary sediment dolichol levels are found; a marked photoparoxysmal response on the EEG is seen in the first of the two phenotypes; and ultrastructural studies reveal fingerprint profiles or granular osmophilic deposits.

Variant forms have been reported as follows:

Early juvenile form: A neuronal inclusion/storage disease with juvenile onset, characterized by dementia; seizures; cerebellar, pyramidal, and extrapyramidal signs; myoclonus; multifocal paroxysmal discharges; and abnormal electroretinogram.

Pigment form: A neuronal inclusion/storage disease with dementia, ataxia, spasticity, resting tremor, and myoclonus.

An *atypical* form: One in which the features of retinal abnormalities or visual symptoms are absent.[2570]

Ceroid lipofuscinosis storage, sea-blue histiocytes, and posterior column dysfunction.[6149]

neuronal heterotopias

A form of dysplasia characterized by accumulations of clumps of neuronal cell bodies within the white matter of the brain.

neuronal intermediate filament inclusion disease (NIFID)

A variant of **frontotemporal dementia** in which there are accumulations of intermediate neurofilaments containing α-internexin in cortical neurons. Its manifestations are heterogeneous, but distinguishing clinical features are its early onset, the absence of a family history, supranuclear ophthalmoplegia, and pyramidal as well as extrapyramidal signs, all occurring at a young age.[978] Other features include memory loss, cognitive impairment, language deficits, atypical dementia with perseveration, executive dysfunction, and the presence of frontal release signs, while buccofacial apraxia and limb dystonia are infrequent.

Pathologically, there is focal atrophy of the frontal lobes and to a lesser degree of the temporal and parietal lobes. The caudate is frequently affected. Neuronal intermediate filament inclusions staining for α-internexin are the neuropathological signatures of NIFID and are detected in the cortex, deep gray matter, cerebellum, and spinal cord. These contain neither tau nor alpha-synuclein but are variably ubiquitinated.

neuronal intestinal dysplasia

A visceral neuropathy characterized by hyperganglionosis of the bowel with hyperplasia of the submucosal and myenteric plexus and the formation of giant ganglia; isolated heterotopic ganglion cells in the lamina propria and between the muscle fibers of the muscularis mucosae; and an increase in acetylcholine activity in the parasympathetic fibers of the laminar and circular muscle. The condition may be confined to the colon or may involve more diffuse regions of the small bowel.

Chart N–7. Forms of Neuronal Ceroid Lipofuscinosis (after Wisniewski, 2001)[6836]

1. *Infantile (Haltia-Santavuori, Hagberg or Finnish type; OMIM 256730)* A form beginning at the end of the first year of life up to mid-adult life, mapped to 1p32. Clinically it is characterized by microcephaly, psychomotor deterioration, hypotonia and ataxia (giving way later to spasticity and rigidity), myoclonus and seizures, optic atrophy and retinal dystrophy, accompanied by severe diffuse brain atrophy due to neuronal destruction and demyelination.[5543] Visual evoked responses are lost and there is marked slowing on the EEG. In a *variant* form, onset is delayed for a few years.
2. *Late-infantile (Jansky–Bielschowsky, late amaurotic familial idiocy)* A recessive form mapped to 11q15 in which myoclonic and tonic-clonic seizures, atonic attacks, and atypical absences present between the age of 2 and 8 years, after which stimulus-sensitive myoclonus, ataxia, psychomotor failure, pigmentary retinopathy, and optic atrophy with visual failure occur. Intractable seizures and myoclonus, relentless dementia, and progressive ataxia and spasticity lead to death within 5 years.[568, 629] This is the second most common form of this disorder. See also **Weil-Cornell LINCL Scale**.

   A *Finnish variant* of this form maps to 13q31 and presents in childhood with cognitive and motor decline, seizures, and visual loss. It is distinguished from the typical form on the basis of pathological findings.

   A third ([*Gypsy/Indian/Costa Rican*] *late infantile variant*) maps to 15q21 and presents in infancy or childhood with cognitive and motor decline, seizures, and visual loss.
3. *Juvenile (Batten, Mayer, Speilmeyer–Vogt, Spielmeyer–Sjögren)* A recessively inherited syndrome mapped to 16p11.2–12.1 and presenting with visual failure occurring between the age of 4 and 10 years, sometimes with tonic-clonic and myoclonic seizures and followed by psychomotor regression, seizures, stuttering dysarthria, pyramidal signs, ataxia, and extrapyramidal dystonic rigidity. Optic atrophy, pigmentary macular degeneration, attenuation of the retinal vessels, and cardiac conduction defects[2491] are other typical findings.[444] The disease has no ethnic predilection.

   Earlier and more severe cases contrast with the slower course of those with later onset, known as the *chronic juvenile (Batten)* form, in which visual failure occurs in later childhood, sometimes with tonic-clonic and myoclonic seizures, followed by the slow development of psychomotor regression, seizures, stuttering dysarthria, pyramidal signs, ataxia, and extrapyramidal rigidity. Optic atrophy, pigmentary macular degeneration, and attenuation of the retinal vessels are characteristic findings.
4. *Adult (Kufs* or *Parry)* A recessively inherited (rarely dominant) variety in which hexosaminidase A is not absent but is severely decreased in content. The disease is characterized clinically by variable cerebellar, extrapyramidal (dystonic), cognitive and psychiatric disturbances, lower motor neuron lesions, and often myoclonic or other seizures, usually with their onset in early adult life, with only minor, if any, dementia and without visual symptoms. The optic fundi are normal.[238, 379, 3586]
5. A *Turkish variant* presenting in early childhood with motor decline, seizures, and visual loss, distinguished from other forms on the basis of pathological findings and mapping to 8p23, the same site as the next *variant*.
6. *Northern epilepsy* (OMIM 600143) presenting in childhood with cognitive decline and seizures and mapped to 8p23.[3685]
7. A *congenital form* mapped to 15p15.5 is also described.

Clinically, the disease presents with megacolon and pseudo-obstruction, resembling that seen in **Hirschsprung disease**. Associations with multiple endocrine neoplasia syndrome type 2b, **neurofibromatosis**, and **Hirschsprung disease** are well described.[5581]

neuronal intranuclear hyaline inclusion disease A rare, slowly progressive, inherited neuronal storage disorder with onset in childhood, characterized pathologically by the presence of round, eosinophilic antifluorescent inclusion bodies in neuronal nuclei in both the central and peripheral nervous systems.[2712, 4551]

The variable phenotypes include cerebellar, extrapyramidal, and pyramidal signs; seizures; oculogyric spasms; lower motor neuron lesions; kyphoscoliosis; pes cavus; behavioral disturbance; tics; seizures; microcephaly; ophthalmoplegia; sensory and autonomic neuropathy; cerebral atrophy; and mental and developmental delay or (later) dementia.[4551]

In a *variant* form, the disorder presents in adult life with dementia, amyotrophy, choreoathetosis, seizures, and sphincter disorder[6133] or with peripheral neuropathy resembling HMSN.[5951]

neuronal migration disorders Disorders that result from specific derangements in fetal neuronal development. Such developmental structural lesions are characterized by disorganization of the cortical architecture with an aberrant columnar and laminar neuronal arrangement. When severe, they present with severe seizure disorders, mental retardation, and incapacitating motor dysfunction, but minor *formes frustes* produce only syndromes of diluted severity.

The conditions encompassed by this term include **lissencephaly** (agyria), **Miller–Diecker syndrome**, **pachygyria** (macrogyria), **polymicrogyria**, **schizencephaly**, and other **heterotopias** of the gray matter.[190, 3619] See also **focal neuronal migration disorders**.

neuronal storage diseases Inherited conditions such as **GM_2 gangliosidosis**, **metachromatic leukodystrophy**, and **gangliosidoses**, in which abnormal material accumulates within neuronal cell bodies.

neuronal tumors Uncommon tumors showing histological features of neuronal differentiation to a variable extent and occurring mainly in the cerebral hemispheres of children and young adults or in the sympathetic system. **Gangliocytoma**, **ganglioglioma**, **ganglioneuroblastoma**, **neuroblastoma**, **paraganglioma–ganglioneuroma**, **anaplastic gangliocytoma**, and **esthesioneuroblastoma** are examples.

neuron(e) A nerve cell and all of its processes; the unit structure of the nervous system. The name was first applied by Heinrich Wilhelm Waldeyer (1837–1921), a German anatomist who showed that all nerve fibers, axons and dendrites, are outgrowths of the neuronal cell bodies.

The word was formerly used by Hippocrates to mean a tendon.

neurone doctrine The cells in the cerebrum are linked by contact, not by continuity and thus there is physiological autonomy of the nerve cell and its branches. This point of view was supported by **Remak** against the **reticular theory**, which held that the cerebral gray matter formed a huge reticulum or nerve net, as was believed by **Gerlach**, **Golgi**, and **Weigert**. Using the Golgi silver stain, Ramon y **Cajal** showed that the neuron doctrine was correct, although Golgi was not converted to this view, even as they shared the Nobel Prize in 1906.

NeuroNet An online resource center that addresses information needs in the fields of dementia, acute stroke, epilepsy, and multiple sclerosis. Access to NeuroNet is limited to physicians only and preregistration is required. Web site: http://www.neuro-net.net/.

neuronopathy 1. A disease of the peripheral nervous system in which the primary neuropathological changes appear in the nerve cell body rather than the axon or the myelin sheath. 2. A motor neuropathy in which the anterior horn (or cranial nerve motor nucleus) cells or a sensory neuropathy in which the dorsal root ganglion cells (or cranial nerve sensory nuclei) are the site of the pathology.[6038] See also **subacute motor neuronopathy**.

neuronophagia (from Lat, nerve cell + to swallow) The ingestion and removal of dead neuronal tissue by phagocytic macrophages.

Neuro-ophthalmology atlas A free public online database, endorsed by the International Council of Ophthalmology. Web site: http://www.atlasophthalmology.com/atlas/folder.jsf;jsessionid=E72B0B6DC3C0366B05F156B295EB6560?node=3404&locale=en/.

neuroparalytic hemicrania See **migraine with aura** and **familial hemiplegic migraine**.

neuroparalytic keratitis Corneal ulceration developing as a result of corneal anesthesia and consequent failure of the protective **blink reflex**.

neuropathic motor unit potential Abnormally high-amplitude, long-duration, polyphasic motor unit action potential. Use of the term is discouraged as it incorrectly implies a specific diagnostic significance of a motor unit action potential configuration. See also **motor unit action potential**. (From the 2001 Report of the Nomenclature Committee of the American Association of Electromyography and Electrodiagnosis.[19] Reproduced by kind permission of the AANEM.)

neuropathic pain Chronic burning, smarting, shooting, aching, or pricking pain resulting from damage either to the peripheral or the central nervous system and characteristically unrelenting, not self-limiting, persistent for years after the initial injury, refractory to multiple treatment modalities, and often accompanied by chronic anxiety, fear, depression, sleeplessness, and impaired social functioning. It is felt in areas with sensory abnormality, often with added dysaesthesias and tingling. In spinal cord injury, it can be spontaneous or stimulus-evoked, the latter presenting as **allodynia** and **hyperalgesia**.

Other common features are **wind-up** (abnormal temporal summation of pain), after-sensations (pain continuing after stimulation has ceased), and unusual referral patterns (referred pain).

In the case of spinal cord injury, it is often divided into above-level, at-level, and below-level types, where "level" refers to the level of the spinal cord that was injured. Above-level neuropathic pain also includes pain due to compressive mononeuropathies and **complex regional pain syndromes**. Below-level pain is considered to be a central pain caused by the spinal cord trauma and it develops months or years after spinal injury. At-level pain may have both nerve root and central (cord) components.

Neuropathic Pain Questionnaire-Short Form A validated tool discriminating between pain that is and that which is not neuropathic, using the subject's responses to three questions related to the presence of numbness, tingling pain, and increased pain with light touch.[328]

Neuropathic Pain Scale A five-question scale designed to assess distinct pain qualities associated with neuropathic pain.[2259]

neuropathic recruitment A recruitment pattern characterized by a decreased number of motor unit action potentials firing at a rapid rate. Use of the term is however discouraged. See also **reduced interference pattern**, **discrete activity**, and **single unit pattern**. (From the 2001 Report of the Nomenclature Committee of the American Association of Electromyography and Electrodiagnosis.[19] Reproduced by kind permission of the AANEM.)

neuropathic tremor A form of coarse tremor at 3–6 Hz with both postural and action components, usually affecting the arms and associated with the presence of thick-fiber peripheral sensory neuropathy.

See also **Roussy–Levy syndrome** (**hereditary motor and sensory neuropathy**).

Neuropathies An American charitable organization providing support and education and funding research into the causes and cure of peripheral neuropathies. E-mail: info@neuropathy.org. Web site: http://www.neuropathy.org/.

neuropathy (Gr, nerve + disease) A disorder of one or more peripheral nerves, more correct than *neuritis* (the word more commonly used) because relatively few disorders of nerves are actually accompanied by inflammation. The word *neurosis* for this condition is obsolete. Disorders of the cell body are also known as neuronopathies; of the axon, axonopathies; and of the myelin sheath, demyelinating neuropathies. Motor, sensory, or autonomic nerves may be uniquely affected or the neuropathy may involve these elements in any combination. The classification in Chart N–8 is based upon that of the World Federation of Neurology[6869] with more recent data from a review of the literature and from the Web site of Dr. Alan Pestronk (http://www.neuro.wustl.edu/neuromuscular/index.html) from which more complete information about all neuropathies can be accessed.

neuropathy associated with ataxia and retinitis pigmentosa See **NARP syndrome**

Chart N–8. Classification of the Neuropathies

A. Heritable, biochemical abnormality unknown

1. See **hereditary motor and sensory neuropathy**
2. See **hereditary sensory and autonomic neuropathy**
3. Hereditary neuropathies associated with specific biochemical abnormalities

   a. **Familial amyloid neuropathy**

      Type 1—Portuguese type (transthyretin abnormality)
      Type 2—Indiana type
      Type 3—Iowa type
      Type 4—Finnish type
      Type 5—Jewish type
      Type 6—Appalachian type

   b. **Porphyria**
   c. Analphalipoproteinemia. See **Tangier disease**
   d. **Abetalipoproteinemia**
   e. **Metachromatic leukodystrophy**
   f. Globoid cell leukodystrophy; see **Krabbe leukodystrophy**
   g. **Niemann–Pick disease**
   h. **Adrenoleukodystrophy** and **adrenomyeloneuropathy**
   i. **Fabry disease**
   j. **Refsum syndrome**. See **hereditary motor and sensory neuropathy**
   k. Glycogen storage diseases. See **glycogen storage diseases** types 2 (Pompe) and 3 (Forbes–Cori disease)
   l. **Primary hyperoxaluria**

4. Miscellaneous hereditary neuropathies

   a. **Hereditary liability to pressure palsies**
   b. **Familial recurrent brachial plexus neuropathy**
   c. **Giant axonal neuropathy**
   d. **Ataxia-telangiectasia**
   e. **Cockayne syndrome**
   f. **Mitochondrial myopathies**
   g. **Neurofibromatosis** (von Recklinghausen disease)
   h. Hereditary hypertrophic neuropathy with paraproteinemia. See **gammopathic neuropathy**
   i. **Hereditary polyneuropathy with oligophrenia**, **premature menopause**, and **acromicria**
   j. Neuropathy in **neuroectodermal dysplasias**
   k. **Subacute necrotizing encephalomyelopathy**
   l. Peripheral neuropathy associated with **xeroderma pigmentosum**
   m. **Marinesco–Sjögren syndrome**
   n. Hereditary Parkinsonism and neuropathy
   o. Neuropathy in spinocerebellar and cerebellar degenerations. See **cerebellar ataxias**
   p. Neuropathy with **familial lipomatosis**
   q. **Distal hereditary upper limb muscular atrophy**
   r. **Hereditary thermosensitive neuropathy**
   s. Neuropathy in thalassemia

B. Congenital

1. Congenital neuropathy with **arthrogryposis multiplex congenita**
2. **Congenital neuropathy with absence of myelin** in the peripheral and central nervous systems
3. **Congenital hypomyelination neuropathy**

C. Traumatic
C.1. Physical

1. Laceration, contusion, compression, or distraction of nerves or plexuses
2. Birth trauma to brachial plexus. See **upper brachial plexus palsy** and **Klumpke palsy**
3. Compression neuropathies

   a. Of cranial nerves

      (i) **Bell palsy**
      (ii) **Clonic facial spasm**
      (iii) Recurrent familial facial palsy (**Melkersson syndrome**)

b. Of the upper extremity

(i) Cervical rib or **cervical band syndrome**
(ii) Median nerve in the forearm (**pronator syndrome**)
(iii) Median nerve under supracondylar process or **Struther's ligament**
(iv) Median nerve in the forearm (**anterior interosseous syndrome**)
(v) Median nerve at the wrist (**carpal tunnel syndrome**)
(vi) Ulnar nerve at the elbow (**cubital tunnel syndrome**)
(vii) Ulnar nerve at the elbow (the medial epicondyle)
(viii) Ulnar nerve at the wrist or its deep branch in the palm
(ix) Radial nerve in the spiral groove
(x) Radial nerve in the forearm
(xi) Posterior interosseous nerve in the forearm
(xii) Suprascapular nerve at the shoulder
(xiii) Long thoracic nerve at the shoulder
(xiv) Axillary nerve at the shoulder
(xv) Musculocutaneous nerve in the upper arm

c. Of the lower extremity

(i) Sciatic nerve at the pelvic exit
(ii) Obturator nerve in the obturator canal
(iii) Ilioinguinal nerve at the groin
(iv) Genitofemoral nerve
(v). Femoral nerve in the groin or upper thigh
(vi) Lateral cutaneous nerve of the thigh (**meralgia paraesthetica**)
(vii) Common peroneal nerve
(viii) Deep peroneal nerve (including compression terminally under the cruciate ligament on the dorsum of the foot)
(ix) Tibial nerve
(x) Posterior tibial nerve in the tarsal tunnel
(xi) Medial plantar nerve
(xii) Digital nerve (**Morton neuroma**)

d. Of the trunk

(i) Intercostal neuropathy
(ii) Lesions of dorsal branches or thoracic and lumbar spinal nerve (**notalgia paraesthetica**)

e. Multiple entrapments in **mucopolysaccharidosis**

4. Electric shock
5. Cold injury (**trench foot, immersion foot**)
6. Burns
7. Vibration injury (vibrating tools)
8. Radiation injury
9. Ischemic neuropathy

a. Vasculitis[3417]

(i) Polyarteritis nodosa
(ii) Neuropathy in **systemic lupus erythematosus**
(iii) **Churg–Strauss syndrome**
(iv) **Diabetes mellitus**
(v) Giant cell arteritis
(vi) Cryoglobulinemia
(vii) Hypersensitivity angiitis
(viii) Neuropathy in **rheumatoid arthritis**
(ix) Neuropathy in **sarcoidosis**
(x) **Wegener granulomatosis**
(xi) Neuropathy in **Lyme disease**

b. Arteriosclerotic occlusive disease
c. Thromboangiitis obliterans (Buerger disease)
d. Embolic infarction of nerve trunks
e. Hemorrhage into nerve trunks
f. Occlusion of large arteries by compression, for example, tourniquet and trauma
g. **Volkmann ischemic contracture**
h. Anterior tibial **compartment syndrome**
i. **Ischemic monomelic neuropathy**
j. **Vasculitic neuropathy**

continued

Chart N–8. *(continued)*

C.2. Toxic (e.g., drugs, inorganic substances, organic substances, or toxins derived from bacteria)
C.3. Of uncertain etiology (? toxic, ? nutritional)

1. Neuropathy and amyotrophy in

   a. **Jamaican** and other tropical neuropathies
   b. **South Indian paraplegia**
   c. Neuropathy in Nigerian **tropical ataxia** and **tropical spastic paraparesis**

2. **Cryptogenic sensory polyneuropathy**
3. Neuropathy in the **Spanish toxic oil syndrome**

D. Infections

1. Direct infection of nerves

   a. **Leprosy**
   b. **Herpes simplex**
   c. **Herpes zoster**
   d. Lymphoadenopathy-associated virus/HTLV III in AIDS
   e. Trypanosomiasis
   f. Nosematosis

2. Neuropathies occurring in other infections

E. Guillain–Barré syndrome and related disorders (probably immunologically mediated)

1. **Acute inflammatory demyelinating polyneuropathy**
2. **Miller Fisher syndrome**
3. **Chronic inflammatory demyelinating polyradiculoneuropathy**

   With CNS demyelination

F. Neuropathy associated with connective tissue disorder
G. Metabolic neuropathy

1. Nutritional

   a. Specific deficiencies
   b. Of uncertain etiology (probably B_1, B_2, and B_6 vitamin deficiency)

2. Neuropathies associated with endocrine disorder

   a. **Diabetes mellitus**
   b. Thyroid disorders
   c. Neuropathy in organic hyperinsulinism
   d. In **acromegaly**

3. Neuropathy in blood dyscrasia

   a. Polycythemia vera
   b. Myelofibrosis
   c. Leukemia—acute and chronic
   d. Bleeding disorders—hemorrhage into nerves
   e. In sickle cell disease

4. Neuropathy in renal failure

   a. Uremic polyneuropathy
   b. Mononeuritis multiplex following dialysis
   c. **Carpal tunnel syndrome** due to amyloid deposition

5. Neuropathy in acute and chronic liver disease, including primary biliary cirrhosis
6. Neuropathy associated with paraproteinemia and dysproteinemia (see **gammopathic neuropathy**)

   a. Multiple myeloma
   b. **Macroglobulinemia** (Waldenstrom)

c. Cryoglobulinemia
d. Benign monoclonal gammopathy—IgA, IgG, IgM
e. Amyloidosis
f. Paraproteinemia
g. **Neuropathy with IgM binding to myelin-associated glycoprotein** (MAG)
h. **Neuropathy with IgM binding to sulfatide**

H. Neuropathy in malignant disease

1. **Carcinomatous neuropathy**
2. Neuropathy in reticulosis—lymphoma, leukemia, myeloproliferative disorders. See **subacute motor neuronopathy** and **subacute sensory neuronopathy**

I. Neuropathy associated with other systemic or nonhereditary degenerative diseases

1. Sarcoidosis
2. Chronic obstructive pulmonary disease
3. **Total lipodystrophy**
4. **Acrodermatitis chronica atrophicans**
5. **Critical illness polyneuropathy**
6. Neuropathy with **retinitis pigmentosa and ataxia**

J. Chronic neuropathy with no known cause or association

1. **Chronic sensorimotor neuropathy of undetermined cause**
2. **Chronic idiopathic ataxic neuropathy**

K. Tumors of nerves

1. Arising from supporting structures and/or axons
   a. **Plexiform neuroma**
   b. **Traumatic neuroma**
2. Arising from supporting structures
   a. **Schwannoma** (neurinoma, neurofibroma), including acoustic neuroma
   b. Fibroma
   c. **Neurogenic sarcoma**
   d. Hemangioma
   e. Lipoma
   f. Neuroepithelioma (**dysembryoma**)

Neuropathy Impairment Score
A scale used in the assessment of neuropathic symptoms assigning grades of normal, moderate, moderately severe, or severe deficits, especially in the legs. See http://content.karger.com/ProdukteDB/produkte.asp?Doi=52074.

neuropathy in acute and chronic liver disease
A demyelinating neuropathy associated with acquired chronic hepatic insufficiency.[1491]

neuropathy in chronic obstructive pulmonary disease
A chronic demyelinating sensorimotor peripheral neuropathy due either to malnutrition or some unknown metabolic disorder affecting Schwann cells.[225]

neuropathy in hereditary Parkinson disease[965]
See Parkinson disease.

neuropathy in Nigerian tropical ataxia
See Nigerian neuropathy.[6793]

neuropathy in spinocerebellar and cerebellar degenerations
See **cerebellar ataxias**.

neuropathy of critical illness
See **critical illness polyneuropathy**.

Neuropathy Screening Instrument
A 15-item questionnaire and a brief structured examination protocol for use together in the diagnosis and follow-up of patients with diabetic neuropathy.[1996]

Neuropathy Symptom profile
A formal method of assessing the range and severity of symptoms of neuropathy, employing a true-or-false type of questionnaire that asks questions dealing with subjective weakness, functional weakness, cramps, abnormal sensation, prickling, deadness, burning, thermal insensitivity, pain on use of a limb, coldness, and aching. The profile gives rise to scores dealing in general with weakness and with sensory and autonomic functions.

The instrument is thought to be suitable for screening a population at risk for neuropathy, for detecting and characterizing symptoms of neuropathy, and for controlled trials of therapy.[1770, 1777]

Neuropathy Symptom Score

A formal method of assessing the range and severity of symptoms of neuropathy obtained by history, designed initially for use with patients suffering from diabetic neuropathies but also appropriate for use in patients suffering from neuropathies of other etiologies.[1778](See Chart N–9).

Other questions are added to assess completeness, reliability, and the presence of "neurasthenia." See also **peripheral neuropathy symptom questionnaire**.

neuropathy with IgM binding to GalNAc-GD1a and GM_2 gangliosides A rare distal symmetrical sensorimotor demyelinating neuropathy of adult life presenting with gait disorder and distal pan-sensory loss, mild weakness, areflexia, and cerebellar signs. The course is slowly progressive over years. Electrodiagnostic testing shows the demyelinating neuropathy. A serum M-protein is detectable. See the Web site: http://www.neuro.wustl.edu/neuromuscular/index.html.

neuropathy with IgM binding to myelin-associated glycoprotein (MAG) A rare distal symmetrical sensorimotor neuropathy of adult life presenting with weakness, gait disturbance, and tremor. and slowly progressive over years. Electrophysiology shows evidence of a demyelinating neuropathy with prolonged distal latencies, slow NCV, and temporal dispersion of CMAPs, without conduction block. Evidence of axonal loss is eventually found. Serum IgM autoantibodies vs MAG protein are detected, sometimes with anti-MAG titers >30,000. **Waldenström macroglobulinemia** may coexist. Nerve pathology shows demyelination and subsequent axonal loss.

In a variant syndrome, the anti-MAG antibody titers are <10,000 and the clinical picture is dominated by sensory loss affecting small rather than large fiber modalities, without motor involvement. See http://www.neuro.wustl.edu/neuromuscular/index.html.

Chart N–9. Neuropathy Symptom Score

I. Symptoms of muscular weakness

A. Bulbar
B. Limbs

1. Extraocular
2. Facial
3. Tongue
4. Throat
5. Shoulder girdle and upper arm
6. Hand
7. Glutei and thigh
8. Legs

II. Sensory disturbances

A. Negative symptoms

9. Difficulty in identifying objects in the mouth
10. Difficulty in identifying objects in the hands
11. Unsteadiness in walking

B. Positive symptoms

12. "Numbness," "asleep feeling," "like novocain," "pricking" at any site
13. Pain—burning, deep aching, tenderness—at any location

III. Autonomic symptoms

14. Postural fainting
15. Impotence in male
16. Loss of urinary control
17. Night diarrhea[1783]

(From Dyck PJ, Kratz KM, Lehman KA, et al. *The Rochester Diabetic Neuropathy Study. Neurology* 1991;41:799–807. Reproduced by kind permission of the American Academy of Neurology and Lippincott Williams and Wilkins.)

neuropathy with IgM binding to sulfatide A rare distal symmetrical sensorimotor neuropathy of adult life presenting with distal paresthesias and weakness, gait disorder, and tremor. Electrodiagnostic studies show prolonged distal latencies and slowed NCV, with eventual evidence of axonal loss. A serum IgM autoantibody to sulfatide is detectable. See also the Web site http://www.neuro.wustl.edu/neuromuscular/index.html.

neuropathy with IgM paraproteinemia See **gammopathic neuropathy**.

neuropathy–dementia–retinitis pigmentosa–dysautonomia syndrome See **hereditary motor and sensory neuropathy**, type 7.

neuropathy–motor neuron disease with visual pathway disorder A neuropathic syndrome characterized by the onset in childhood or youth of neurogenic muscle atrophy and weakness, demyelinating peripheral sensory neuropathy, hypohidrotic skin, and pyramidal signs. See also **hereditary motor and sensory neuropathy** (*HMSN type 2 with mental retardation, optic atrophy, and pyramidal signs*).

Neuropediatrics (formerly *Neuropediatrie*) A German journal of child neurology. Web site: www.thieme.de/neuropediatrics.

neuropeptide Y A neurotransmitter found in the basal ganglia that stimulates appetite.[1]

neurophobia A fear of the neural sciences and clinical neurology among medical students. Its causes are various and disputed but are likely to include inadequate time given to the subject in medical schools; its effects include the difficulty in recruiting young physicians to the specialty and the reluctance of physicians who are not neurologists to manage patients with neurological presentations (Jozefowicz RF. *Arch Neurol*. 1994;51:328–9).

neurophysins Precursors of vasopressin and oxytocin.

neuropil The complex mesh of myelinated and unmyelinated axons and dendrites and the processes of oligodendroglia, astrocytes, and microglia within the nervous system.

neuropore (Gr, nerve + a passage) An opening from the neural tube in the developing nervous system. The *anterior* aspect connects the cavity of the brain with the epiblast; the *posterior* portion is the aperture of the neurenteric canal into the body cavity.

Neuropsychiatric Inventory A validated tool evaluating the frequency and severity of 12 domains often found in patients with cognitive disturbance, including aberrant motor behavior, agitation, anxiety, apathy, delusions, depression, disinhibition, euphoria, hallucinations, and irritability.[1375]

neuropsychiatry 1. An approach to the study of psychiatric disorders, whereby a neurological basis for them is presumed and sought; that aspect of psychiatry that seeks to advance the understanding of clinical problems through increased knowledge of brain structure and function.[3865] 2. A branch of psychiatry involving the study of organic psychosyndromes (such as the dementias, disorders resulting from toxic, traumatic, or developmental brain diseases, the psychological complications of the epilepsies, and memory disorders).

Neuropsychological Screening Battery for Multiple Sclerosis A measure assessing spatial and verbal memory, short-term and long-term recall, attention, and verbal fluency.[5191]

Neuropsychology Central A directory devoted exclusively to the subject of Human Neuropsychology, although several links are out of date.

neuroptic myelitis See **Devic disease**.

Neuroradiology A neuro-radiological Journal. Springer-Verlag GmbH & Company KG, Heidelberger Platz 3, D-1000 Berlin 33, Germany. Web site: http://link.springer.de/link/service/journals/00234.

neuroregeneration The Web site http://neuroregeneration.org/ provides information on **Parkinson**, **Huntington**, and **Alzheimer diseases** with full text research papers and other publications.

Neurorehabilitation A neglected and underfunded neurological subspecialty dedicated to making the best of a bad job. The **World Federation for NeuroRehabilitation** at http://www.wfnr.co.uk/ is a multidisciplinary organization based in the United Kingdom that publishes the journals *Neurorehabilitation* and *Neural Repair and Developmental Neurorehabilitation.*

neuroretinal rim The edge of the optic cup.

neuroretinitis 1. The appearance of the retina when there has been leakage of edema fluid at the macula. The optic disk is swollen and a macular star figure is produced in the outer plexiform layer of the retina by the lipid-containing exudates derived from the capillaries at the disk head. The condition is not associated with multiple sclerosis. Clinically, central visual loss occurs over hours and is associated with a central scotoma and a macular star on ophthalmoscopy. Faster-progressing syndromes carry a worse prognosis. In some cases, evidence of vasculitis or infection (such as Lyme disease) may be found. 2. Inflammation of both the retina and the optic nerve.

neuroretinoangiomatosis See **Bonnet syndrome** (#3).

neurosarcoidosis (disseminated sarcoid leukoencephalopathy) A rare disorder in which any part of the nervous system is affected with the lesions of sarcoidosis—comprising some 5% of all such cases. Meningeal, parameningeal, facial, and other cranial nerve lesions (especially the VII nerve); hypothalamic and pituitary infiltration; myelopathy; involvement of the conus medullaris and many forms of peripheral neuropathy and plexopathy are described, and periventricular parenchymatous infiltration can also occur, leading to hydrocephalus and lymphocytic meningitis.[6040, 6944] However, muscle biopsy findings suggest that granulomatous myositis is even more common, though often subclinical.[5692] Spinal MR may show leptomeningeal enhancement throughout the spinal cord and asymptomatic enhancing cauda equina lesions.[695]

In a *variant* form, evidence of angiitis is detected.[4626]

neuroschisis A developmental abnormality characterized by splitting of the closed neural tube.

Neuroscience Links to Neurology and Neuroscience Journals An internet site (based in the United Kingdom) providing information about/access to neurological journals. Web site: http://www.uku.fi/neuro/links2.htm/.

Neuroscience page from BUBL (UK) A site providing a selection of subject-indexed links, with evaluative descriptions. Web site: http://bubl.ac.uk/Link/n/neuroscience.htm.

Neurosciences on the Internet A comprehensive professional resource referencing a large number of Web sites relevant to clinical neurologists and others. It was created and is still maintained by Dr. Neil Busis, an American neurologist, whose expertise has ensured that the content is valid and appropriate. Web site: www.neuroguide.com.

Neurosciences Virtual Library A site listing links to scores of neuroscience-based organizations. Web site: http://neuro.med.cornell.edu/.

Neurosensory Center Comprehensive Examination for Aphasia An aphasia battery.[5998, 5999] See also **Boston Diagnostic Aphasia examination**, **Western Aphasia battery**, **Frenchay Aphasia Screening test**, **Token test**, **Reporters test**, and **Porch index of Communicative Ability**.

neuroserpins A family of serine proteinase inhibitors, including α-antitrypsin and antithrombin, with an uncertain role in the nervous system. Mutations are responsible for various conditions including **familial encephalopathy with neuroserpin inclusion bodies**.

neurosis In the 19th century, a physical disease without apparent or discernible cause; now a pejorative term for disease without physical signs, for which the patient is usually blamed.

neurosonology The study of the physical characteristics of the nervous system using high-frequency ultrasound.

Neurosurgery Clinics A periodical reviewing neurosurgical topics, published by W.B. Saunders. Web site: http://www2.us.elsevierhealth.com/scripts/om.dll/serve?action=searchDB&searchDBfor=home&id=cnsu.

Neurosurgical Society of America A professional association of young specialists in neurological surgery. Address: 7703 Floyd Curl Drive, San Antonio, TX 78229. Web site: http://www.neurosurgicalsociety.com/.

neuro-Sweet disease (complicated acute febrile neutrophilic dermatosis) The association of benign recurrent encephalitis with the features of Sweet syndrome, the latter characterized by malaise, fever, leukocytosis, mucosal ulceration, and symmetrical, tender, and dull-red skin plaques due to dermal cellular infiltrates that heal without scarring. The condition thus resembles **Behçet syndrome** but is associated with HLA B54, which is rare in the latter condition. Suggested diagnostic criteria[2920] are adapted here as follows:

1. *Neurologic features*
   Confusion, depression, seizures, myoclonus; recurrent encephalitis or meningitis; usually with fever, responsive to systemic steroids.
2. *Dermatologic features*
   Painful or tender, dull-red, erythematous plaques or nodules, mainly on the face, neck, upper limbs, and upper trunk. Predominantly neutrophilic infiltration of the dermis with sparing of the epidermis and without vasculitis.
3. *Other features*
   Absence of cutaneous vasculitis and thrombosis and of uveitis.
4. *HLA association* with HLA Cw1 or B54, while HLAB51 is negative.

All of 1, 2, and 3 make the diagnosis *probable*. With a neurological manifestation, either 2 and 4 and one item or more of 3 make the diagnosis *possible*.

neurosyphilis Those forms of secondary or tertiary syphilis in which there is involvement of the CNS, usually 2–18 months after the primary infection.[5852] Specific entities included are

Meningovascular (**asymptomatic neurosyphilis, acute syphilitic meningitis**, and **cerebrovascular neurosyphilis**) and
Parenchymatous (**tabes dorsalis, general paresis** ["of the insane"], **optic neuritis**, and *variants* with myelopathic or VIII nerve involvement)

neurotensin An oligopeptide found in the hypothalamus and in the dorsal horn of the spinal cord, where it may act as a modulator in pain pathways.

neurothecoma (dermal nerve sheath myxoma) A benign skin tumor consisting of nests of large stellate or spindle cells with a mucous matrix.

neurotic fatigue A state of disinclination or incapacity to indulge in muscular exertion as a result of a generalized feeling of heaviness, tiredness, or stiffness of the muscles, for which no organic or biochemical reason can be detected. See also **chronic fatigue syndrome**.

neurotic hypersomnolence See **hypersomnolence**.

neurotmesis (Gr, nerve + a cutting) Complete anatomical division of a peripheral nerve with disruption of the axons, their myelin sheaths, and the supporting connective tissue, resulting in Wallerian degeneration of the axons distal to the injury site. This represents the most severe of the three types of nerve injury described by Seddon.[5705] Cf. **axonotmesis** and **neurapraxia**.

neurotomy Section or dissection of nerves.

neurotonia (pseudomyotonia) Delay in the relaxation of a muscle following voluntary contraction, due to electrical hyperexcitability of its motor nerve.[6643] See also **neuromyotonia**.

neurotonic discharges Repetitive motor unit action potentials recorded from intramuscular electrodes during intraoperative monitoring. Thought to arise from irritation or injury of nerves supplying the muscle from which the recording is made. (From the 2001 Report of the Nomenclature Committee of the American Association of Electromyography and Electrodiagnosis.[19] Reproduced by kind permission of the AANEM.)

neurotoxic shellfish poisoning A syndrome resembling **paralytic shellfish poisoning** occurring mainly in the Caribbean and caused by the dinoflagellate *Gymnodinium brevis*. Bronchoconstriction is another effect if the toxin is inhaled.[2484]

neurotoxic signs In the context of envenomation, these include ptosis, ophthalmoplegia, dysphoria, inability to protrude the tongue, and facial and generalized weakness. Both presynaptic and postsynaptic forms are described.[2484]

neurotropic calcergy Selective calcification of the nerves of the autonomic nervous system, produced in rats by the injection of lead acetate and histamine.[5721]

neurotropism The theory of **Cajal** that neural growth is oriented by both generic and specific stimuli, the former from Schwann cells and the latter from motor end plates and sensory receptors, all producing some factor attracting the axon.[6819]

neurotuberculosis Tuberculous infection of the nervous system, classified by Kinnier **Wilson**[6819] (Chart N–10).

neurovisceral lipidosis See **GM$_1$ gangliosidosis**.

neurovisceral storage disease with vertical supranuclear ophthalmoplegia A genetic disorder of metabolism presenting between the age of 1 and 15 years and characterized by vertical supranuclear ophthalmoplegia, limited convergence with normal pupillary functions, dementia, hearing loss, ataxia, rigidity, seizures, and hepatosplenomegaly. The bone marrow shows foamy histiocytes. See also **sphingomyelin storage disorders**, type 3 and **GM$_1$ gangliosidosis**.

neutral state syndrome A subwakefulness syndrome in which patients complain of excessive daytime sleepiness (hypersomnolence) without an

Chart N–10. Classification of Neurotuberculosis

I. Tuberculosis of bone
  A. Skull (cranial osteitis)
  B. Spine
    Spinal caries
    Radicular compression
    Paraplegia
II. Tuberculosis of the meninges
    Pachymeningitis
    Leptomeningitis
    Tuberculous meningitis
      Acute, subacute, serous
    Meningeal tuberculosis
      Miliary
      Solitary pial tubercle
      Chronic meningeal tuberculosis
III. Tuberculosis of brain and cord
    Tuberculomas
    Encephalitis, myelitis
    Ocular
IV. Tuberculous neuritis
V. Psychoses of tuberculosis

From Wilson SAK. *Neurology*. London: Edward Arnold and Co. (1940).

increase in the total sleep time. The complaint is associated with a lack of nocturnal stage 3–4 non-rapid eye movement sleep, frequent daily microsleeps, and episodes of automatic behavior.[2629]

nevi–atrial myxomas, myxoid neurofibromata-epiphelides See **NAME syndrome**.

Nevin, Samuel (1905–1979) British neuropathologist, born in Belfast, where he took his medical training at Queen's University. After some years in junior positions at the **National Hospital**, he became director of the research laboratory in the Institute of Psychiatry at the Maudsley Hospital and at Maida Vale, and professor of mental pathology in the University of London. A distinguished neuropathologist, most of his published work concerned the presenile dementias. His description with D.P. Jones of "progressive spongy encephalopathy" (**Creutzfeldt–Jakob disease**) defined that condition more clearly than any other report had done so to that date, although his conclusion favoring a vascular etiology was incorrect.[4640]

Nevin syndrome A progressive dementing illness with visual failure, pyramidal signs, speech disturbance, cerebellar signs, myoclonus, and accelerated death. In the original papers, the authors considered that a vascular etiology underlay the rapidly progressive cerebral degeneration (a subacute spongiform encephalopathy) and that it was distinct from **Creutzfeldt–Jakob disease**, but that view is not held today.[4641]

nevoid basal cell carcinoma syndrome (Gorlin–Goltz syndrome) A dominantly inherited **neurocutaneous syndrome** characterized by hypertelorism, frontal bossing, poly- and brachydactyly, kyphoscoliosis, and mental retardation. Pigmented papules appear between 12 and 35 years of age and undergo malignant transformation. There is also an increased incidence of **medulloblastoma**, squamous cell carcinoma, and odontogenic keratocysts.[2508]

nevus flammeus (Lat, a mole + fiery) (salmon patch, capillary nevus, capillary hemangioma) The port-wine stain that is characteristically present in the distribution of the trigeminal nerve in patients with **Sturge–Weber syndrome**, but also sometimes in the skin of the trunk or limbs. It can also occur as a dominantly inherited disorder without neurological features.[5781]

See also **midline nevus flammeus with intracranial vascular disease**.

nevus linearis sebaceous (of Jadassohn) See **epidermal nevus syndrome**.

nevus of Ito Pigmentation (melanoderma) of the lateral cervical area, shoulder, and thorax.[3108]

nevus of Ota (Ota syndrome) Localized periorbital pigmentation (melanoderma), which is especially marked on the eyelids, zygoma, and frontal regions, and sometimes extending to the lips, buccal cavity, and eyes. Heterochromia iridis is common. Ballooning of the posterior cranial fossa has also been described. The syndrome is more common in the Black and the Asiatic races. Neurological complications include malignant tumors of the nervous system, sensorineural deafness, the **Sturge–Weber syndrome**, spinocerebellar degenerations, and vascular malformations, including those sited intracranially.[1018, 4146]

nevus unius lateris (linear nevus, ichthyosis linearis neuropathica) A linear group of brown papules in the skin, usually present at birth and found in any part of the body. Cortical dysgenesis with epilepsy and mental retardation are commonly associated.[2950] See also **epidermal nevus syndrome**.

new daily-persistent headache (de novo chronic headache) Headache that is daily and unremitting from very soon after onset (within 3 days at most). The pain is typically bilateral, pressing or tightening in quality and of mild to moderate intensity. There may be photophobia, phonophobia, or mild nausea. Diagnostic criteria have been defined as follows:

A. Headache for >3 months fulfilling criteria B–D
B. Headache is daily and unremitting from onset or from <3 days from onset
C. At least two of the following pain characteristics:
  1. Bilateral location
  2. Pressing/tightening (nonpulsating) quality
  3. Mild or moderate intensity
  4. Not aggravated by routine physical activity such as walking or climbing stairs
D. Both of the following:
  1. No more than one of photophobia, phonophobia, or mild nausea
  2. Neither moderate or severe nausea nor vomiting
E. Not attributed to another disorder

From the International Classification of Headache Disorders (Headache Classification Committee of the International Headache Society. *Cephalalgia* 2004;**24**[Suppl 1]) by kind permission of Dr. Jes Olesen, the International Headache Society, and Wiley-Blackwell Publications.

Headaches resembling migraine also occur in such patients and a similar headache syndrome also occurs with raised or decreased CSF pressures. The **Melkersson–Rosenthal syndrome** has been reported in association.

new variant Creutzfeldt–Jakob disease A degenerative inflammatory disease of the nervous system resembling both Creutzfeldt–Jakob disease and **bovine spongiform encephalopathy**, of which it may itself be a variant. The diagnostic criteria suggested by Will[6791] are reproduced by kind permission.

1.

A. Progressive neuropsychiatric disorder (depression, anxiety, apathy, withdrawal)
B. Duration of illness >6 months
C. Routine investigations do not suggest an alternative diagnosis
D. No history of potential iatrogenic exposure

2.

A. Early psychiatric symptoms
B. Persistent painful sensory symptoms
C. Ataxia
D. Myoclonus or chorea or dystonia
E. Dementia

3.

A. EEG does not show the typical appearance of sporadic CJDc (or no EEG performed)
B. Bilateral pulvinar high signal on MRI scan

Definite: lA (progressive neuropsychiatric disorder) *and* neuropathological confirmation of new variant Creutzfeldt–Jakob disease
Probable: I *and* 4/5 of II *and* IIIA *and* IIIB (see original text)
Possible: I *and* 4/5 of II *and* IIIA (see original text)
In young children, the condition may well be diagnosed as **Alpers syndrome**.

New York Rating Scale

An assessment instrument designed to provide a semiquantitative score of the impairments and disabilities suffered by patients with **Parkinson disease**.

As with many other similar scales, the battery provides a template for the neurological examination, including thus an appraisal of eye movements, blink rate, emotional and voluntary facial movements, swallowing, tongue movements, motor speech, neck rotation, shoulder and arm elevation, lying supine, writing, rising from a chair, normal and heel-toe walking, climbing stairs, sit-ups, trunk turning, straight-leg raising, foot movements, rigidity, general mobility, tremor, and contractures.[97]

New York University computerized test battery

A computerized evaluation designed to assess cognitive changes in normal elderly subjects and those with dementia or **age-associated memory impairment**. The battery contains 12 subtests evaluating immediate and recent memory, language, concept formation, and psychomotor speed and attention. Use of the computer allows a simulated situation to be presented to the subject, whose reactions can then be directly assessed on the basis of their computer-interactive responses. The test is sensitive to drug effects and to changes in dementia.[2034]

Newcastle Dementia Scale

See **Blessed Roth dementia instrument**.

NGIE

A mitochondrial disease characterized by **n**euromyopathy with **g**astro**i**ntestinal symptoms and **e**ncephalopathy. See also **MNGIE**.

n-hexane neuropathy

A subacute axonal sensorimotor peripheral neuropathy, with secondary demyelination, resulting from persistent exposure to *N*-hexane in the workplace. Optic neuropathy and involvement of the CNS are uncommon.[1094]

nicotinic acid deficiency encephalopathy

An acutely evolving and often fatal syndrome of stupor or delirium with cogwheel rigidity of the limbs, sometimes with grasping and sucking reflexes, often with clinical evidence of pellagra and in some cases with oculomotor and polyneuropathic features like those in Wernicke–Korsakoff syndrome.[3242] Though commonly diagnosed (and apparently relieved by nicotinic acid) in the years after World War II, it is now seldom seen.

nictitating spasm

See **blepharospasm**.

nictitatio

See **spasmus nictitans**.

Nielsen syndrome

1. A condition of generalized weakness with fasciculations seen in states of terminal exhaustion.[4670]

2. (cingulate gyrus syndrome)
Apathy, akinesia, mutism, and incontinence in the awake patient with bilateral damage to the cingulate gyri.[4667] Presumably the syndrome was described in patients in whom this damage was as a result of a tumor, which was also affecting other areas, because bilateral surgically created lesions of the cingulate gyri lead to only minimal similar findings.

Niemann, Alfred

(1880–1921) He gave a short account of **Niemann–Pick disease** in 1914, but the account by Ludwig Pick (also a German pediatrician) 12 years later was more substantial.

Niemann–Pick cells

Foamy storage cells derived from macrophages, found in **sphingomyelin storage disorders**.

Niemann–Pick disease

See **sphingomyelin storage disorders**.

Nigerian neuropathy

(tropical ataxic neuropathy, tropical nutritional ataxia)
A slowly progressive posterior column myelopathy and painful symmetrical demyelinating sensorimotor neuropathy (leading to severe proprioceptive loss) with bilateral optic atrophy and nerve deafness. The condition is considered to be due to the ingestion of cyanide-containing foods such as cassava, and is conditioned by vitamin deficiency.[4827, 6793] It is seen mainly in central and west African countries.[2668]

A *variant* condition is *Nigerian acute seasonal ataxia* (encephalitis tremens), an acute cerebellar ataxic syndrome described in low-income Nigerians. The ataxia progresses in some cases to ophthalmoplegia and a reduction in consciousness, and is possibly due to acute thiamine deficiency resulting from the ingestion of thiamine-binding glycosides in certain foods consumed locally.[47]

night starts

See **periodic limb movement disorder**.

night terrors

(pavor nocturnus, incubus, and sleep terror) A **parasomnia** characterized by the sudden waking of the subject from sleep, screaming with terror and violently mobile, with marked autonomic arousal, confusion, and great and inconsolable distress. Complete amnesia follows restoration of normal functioning.[4025] Such an attack of acute panic with screaming occurs during a spontaneous arousal from the first NREM sleep (stage 3 or 4) period of the night, with succeeding amnesia for the episode. The condition is more common in children between the age of 4 and 12 years but may also occur in young adult life.[2311] See also **dream anxiety attacks**.

nightmare (Middle English, night + a crushing thing) (dream anxiety attack, REM nightmare) A vivid and frightening dream, often provoking a feeling of dread, oppression on the chest, or the conviction of paralysis, occurring during the middle third of the night during rapid eye movement sleep periods and leading to awakening with a normal sensorium. Diagnostic criteria have been suggested,[1629] and are reproduced in Chart N–11.

nightwalkers A name self-applied by those who suffer from **restless leg (limb) syndrome**.

nigrospinodentatal degenerations (nigrostriatal degenerations) Hereditary disorders classifiable as progressive **cerebellar ataxias** (autosomal dominant forms of late onset) but not homogeneous in nature, in some cases the major extrapyramidal and/or cerebellar features being accompanied by, for example, nuclear ophthalmoplegia, pyramidal signs, sensory disturbances, muscle atrophy, or pes cavus.

Their final apportionment will have to await the detection of the underlying biochemical deficits.[6861] See also **Joseph disease**.

nigrostriatal degenerations See **nigrospinodentatal degenerations**.

NIH Stroke Scale A relatively short but valid, reliable, and reproducible instrument for the semiquantitative assessment of deficits following stroke, used in numerous clinical trials[2456] (Chart N–12). It is available online at http://www.ninds.nih.gov/doctors/NIH_Stroke_Scale.pdf. Some training is required in order to administer it correctly; this is available at http://www.ninds.nih.gov/doctors/stroke_scale_training.htm.
A descriptive booklet with the required pictures, word lists, etc. is available at http://www.ninds.nih.gov/doctors/NIH_Stroke_Scale_Booklet.pdf.

See also **Canadian Stroke Scale**, **Orgogozo Scale**, **Stroke Scales**, **Mathew Scale**, and **Nottingham 10-point ADL Index**.

NINCDS Stroke Data Bank A prospective observational study designed to provide a resource for research questions on the characteristics, clinical course, and outcome of patients hospitalized with acute stroke.

Within the study, a research classification scheme was developed to establish uniform diagnostic subgroups based on supporting data from angiography, from brain imaging using CT scanning, and from Doppler ultrasonography, and based on the nature of clinical syndromes and related medical conditions.

NINDS See **National Institute of Neurological Disorders and Stroke**.

NINDS Scale A 5-point system for grading muscle stretch reflexes, ranging from absent (0) to normal (+2 and +3) to clonus (+4). The scale does not seem to enhance inter-rater reliability.[4047] See also **Medical Research Council scale** and **Mayo Clinic scale**.

Nine-Hole Peg Test A simple and portable method for the evaluation of fine motor performance, sensitive in patients with slight but not severe disability.

The equipment required consists of nine wooden dowels (9 mm in diameter and 12 mm long) and a wooden base in which there are nine holes (10 mm in diameter and 15 mm deep) spaced 15 mm apart in three rows of three holes. The patient sits at a table and is asked to place the pegs in the holes, while the observer times his performance from start to finish (but can stop at 50 s), recording the number of pegs correctly placed. The normal subject can place the pegs correctly within 18 s.[6129]

Nipah encephalitis A form of encephalitis caused by a paramyxovirus, reported from south Asia. Clinically, severe encephalitis is accompanied by fever, headache, segmental myoclonus, areflexia, hypertension, and tachycardia and is often fatal. Relapse of the disorder after initial recovery is described. See also **encephalitis**.

Nishimoto disease See **moyamoya disease**.

Nishimoto–Takeuchi–Kudo disease See **moyamoya disease**.

N-methyl-D-aspartate (NMDA) An excitatory amino acid, the receptors of which mediate relatively slow and long-lasting responses as compared to the non-NMDA receptors L-glutamate and L-aspartate. The amino acid is epileptogenic in animals by virtue of its power to depolarize neurons and to allow the generation of repetitive epileptiform discharges.[3563]

Chart N–11. Diagnostic Criteria for Nightmares

A. At least one episode of sudden awakening from sleep with intense fear, anxiety, and feeling of impending harm
B. Immediate recall of a frightening dream context
C. Alertness is full immediately upon awakening, with little confusion or disorientation
D. Associated features include at least one of the following:
   1. Return to sleep after the episode is delayed and not rapid
   2. The episode occurs during the later half of the habitual sleep period
E. Polysomnographic monitoring demonstrates the following:
   1. An abrupt awakening from at least 10 min of rapid eye movement sleep
   2. Mild tachycardia and tachypnea during the episode
   3. Absence of epileptic activity in association with the disorder
F. Other sleep disorders such as sleep terrors and sleepwalking can occur
   See also **hag** and **dream anxiety attack** and cf. **night terror**

From AASM Diagnostic Classification Steering Committee. *The International Classification of Sleep Disorders Diagnostic and Coding Manual*. Rochester, MN. American Academy of Sleep Medicine 1991/2001. Reproduced by kind permission of the Academy. See also http://www.sleepeducation.com/Disorders.aspx/.

Chart N–12. The NIH Stroke Scale

Each examination is assessed independently from previous examinations. A response must be checked for each item, using the following headings:

1.a. Level of Consciousness
1.b. Level of Consciousness—Questions
1.c. Level of Consciousness—Commands
2. Gaze
3. Visual Field
4. Facial Movement (Facial Paresis)
5. Motor Function—Arms (Left and Right Arm)
6. Motor Function—Legs (Left and Right Leg)
7. Limb Ataxia
8. Sensory
9. Best Language
10. Dysarthria
11. Neglect (Extinction and Inattention)

1.a. **Level of Consciousness:** The investigator must choose a response if a full evaluation is prevented by obstacles such as an endotracheal tube, language barrier, and orotracheal trauma/bandages. A 3 is scored only if the patient makes no movement (other than reflexive posturing) in response to noxious stimulation.

0 = **Alert**; keenly responsive.
1 = **Not alert**; but rousable by minor stimulation to obey, answer, or respond,
2 = **Not alert**; requires repeated stimulation to attend, or is obtunded and requires strong or painful stimulation to make movements (not stereotyped).
3 = Responds only with reflex motor or autonomic effects or totally unresponsive, flaccid, and areflexic.

1.b. **LOC Questions:** The patient is asked the month and his/her age. The answer must be correct—there is no partial credit for being close. Aphasic and stuporous patients who do not comprehend the questions will score 2. Patients unable to speak because of endotracheal intubation, orotracheal trauma, severe dysarthria, from any cause, language barrier, or any other problem not secondary to aphasia are given a 1. It is important that only the initial answer be graded and that the examiner not "help" thepatient with verbal or nonverbal cues.

0 = **Answers** both questions correctly.
1 = **Answers** one question correctly.
2 = **Answers** neither question correctly.

1.c. **LOC Commands:** The patient is asked to open and close the eyes and then to grip and release the nonparetic hand. Substitute another one step command if the hands cannot be used. Credit is given if an unequivocal attempt is made but not completed due to weakness. If the patient does not respond to command, the task should be demonstrated to him or her (pantomime) and the result should be scored (i.e., follows none, one, or two commands). Patients with trauma, amputation, or other physical impediments should be given suitable one-step commands. Only the first attempt is scored.

0 = **Performs** both tasks correctly.
1 = **Performs** one task correctly.
2 = **Performs** neither task correctly.

2. **Best Gaze:** Only horizontal eye movements will be tested. Voluntary or reflexive (oculocephalic) eye movements will be scored, but caloric testing is not done. If the patient has a conjugate deviation of the eyes that can be overcome by voluntary or reflexive activity, the score will be 1. If a patient has an isolated peripheral nerve paresis (CN III, IV, or VI), score a 1. Gaze is testable in all aphasic patients. Patients with ocular trauma, bandages, pre-existing blindness, or other disorder of visual acuity or fields should be tested with reflexive movements and a choice should be made by the investigator. Establishing eye contact and then moving about the patient from side to side will occasionally clarify the presence of a partial gaze palsy.

0 = **Normal.**
1 = **Partial gaze palsy**; gaze is abnormal in one or both eyes, but forced deviation or total gaze paresis is not present.
2 = **Forced deviation**, or total gaze paresis not overcome by the oculocephalic maneuver.

3. **Visual:** Visual fields (upper and lower quadrants) are tested by confrontation, using finger counting or visual threat, as appropriate. Patients may be encouraged, but if they look at the side of the moving fingers appropriately, this can be scored as normal. If there is unilateral blindness or enucleation, visual fields in the remaining eye are scored. Score 1 only if a clear-cut asymmetry, including quadrant-anopia, is found. If patient is blind from any cause, score 3. Double simultaneous stimulation is performed at this point. If there is extinction, patient receives a 1 and the results are used to respond to item 11.

0 = **No visual loss.**
1 = **Partial hemianopia.**
2 = **Complete hemianopia.**
3 = **Bilateral hemianopia** (blind including cortical blindness).

4. **Facial Palsy:** Ask or use pantomime to encourage the patient to show teeth or raise eyebrows and close eyes. Score symmetry of grimace in response to noxious stimuli in the poorly responsive or noncomprehending patient. If facial trauma/bandages, orotracheal tube, tape, or other physical barriers obscure the face, these should be removed to the extent possible.

0 = **Normal** symmetrical movements.
1 = **Minor paralysis** (flattened nasolabial fold, asymmetry on smiling).
2 = **Partial paralysis** (total or near-total paralysis of lower face).
3 = **Complete paralysis** of one or both sides (absence of facial movement in the upper and lower face).

5. **Motor Arm:** The limb is placed in the appropriate position: extend the arms (palms down) 90° (if sitting) or 45° (if supine). Drift is scored if the arm falls before 10 s. The aphasic patient is encouraged using urgency in the voice and pantomime but not noxious stimuli. Each limb is tested in turn, beginning with the nonparetic arm. Only in the case of amputation or joint fusion at the shoulder, the examiner should record the score as untestable (UN) and clearly write the explanation for this choice.

0 = **No drift**; limb holds 90° (or 45°) for full 10 s.
1 = **Drift**; limb holds 90° (or 45°), but drifts down before full 10 s; does not hit bed or other support.
2 = **Some effort against gravity**; limb cannot get to or maintain (if cued) 90° (or 45°), rifts down to bed, but has some effort against gravity.
3 = **No effort against gravity**; limb falls.
4 = **No movement.**
UN = **Amputation** or joint fusion, explain

5a. **Left arm**
5b. **Right arm**

6. **Motor Leg:** The limb is placed in the appropriate position: hold the leg at 30° (always tested supine). Drift is scored if the leg falls before 5 s.The aphasic patient is encouraged using urgency in the voice and pantomime but not noxious stimulation. Each limb is tested in turn, beginning with the nonparetic leg. Only in the case of amputation or joint fusion at the hip, the examiner should record the score as untestable (UN) and clearly write the explanation for this choice.

0 = **No drift**; leg holds 30° position for full 5 s.
1 = **Drift**; leg falls by the end of the 5 s period but does not hit bed.
2 = **Some effort against gravity**; leg falls to bed by 5 s, but has some effort against gravity.
3 = **No effort against gravity**; leg falls to bed immediately.
4 = **No movement.**
UN = **Amputation** or joint fusion, explain

6a. **Left leg**
6b. **Right leg**

7. **Limb Ataxia:** This item is aimed at finding evidence of a unilateral cerebellar lesion. Test with eyes open. In case of visual defect, ensure testing is done in intact visual field. The finger–nose–finger and heel–shin tests are performed on both sides, and ataxia is scored only if present out of proportion to weakness. Ataxia is absent in the patient who cannot understand or is paralyzed. Only in the case of amputation or joint fusion, the examiner should record the score as untestable (UN) and clearly write the explanation for this choice. In case of blindness, test by having the patient touch nose from extended arm position.

0 = **Absent.**
1 = **Present in one limb.**
2 = **Present in two limbs.**
UN = **Amputation** or joint fusion, explain

8. **Sensory:** Sensation or grimace to pinprick when tested, or withdrawal from noxious stimulus in the obtunded or aphasic patient. Only sensory loss attributed to stroke is scored as abnormal and the examiner should test as many body areas (arms [not hands], legs, trunk, face) as needed to accurately check for hemisensory loss. A score of 2, "severe or total sensory loss," should be given only when a severe or total loss of sensation can be clearly demonstrated. Stuporous and aphasic patients will, therefore, probably score 1 or 0. The patient with brain stem stroke who has bilateral loss of sensation is scored 2. If the patient does not respond and is quadriplegic, score 2. Patients in a coma (item 1.a.= 3) are automatically given a 2 on this item.

0 = **Normal**; no sensory loss.
1 = **Mild-to-moderate sensory loss**; patient feels pinprick is less sharp or is dull on the affected side; or there is a loss of superficial pain with pinprick, but patient is aware of beingtouched.
2 = **Severe to total sensory loss**; patient is notaware of being touched in the face, arm, and leg.

9. **Best Language:** A great deal of information about comprehension will be obtained during the preceding sections of the examination. For this scale item, the patient is asked to describe what is happening in the attached picture, to name the items on the attached naming sheet, and to read from the attached list of sentences. Comprehension is judged from responses here, as well as to all of the commands in the preceding general neurological exam. If visual loss interferes with the tests, ask the patient to identify objects placed in the hand, repeat, and produce speech. The intubated patient should be asked to write. The patient in a coma (item 1.a.=3) will automatically score 3 on this item. The examiner must choose a score for the patient with stupor or limited cooperation, but a score of 3 should be used only if the patient is mute and follows no one-step commands.

continued

Chart N–12. *(continued)*

0 = **No aphasia**; normal.
1 = **Mild-to-moderate aphasia**; some obvious loss of fluency or facility of comprehension, without significant limitation on ideas expressed or form of expression. Reduction of speech and/or comprehension, however, makes conversation about provided materials difficult or impossible. For example, in conversation about provided materials, examiner can identify picture or naming card content from patient's response.
2 = **Severe aphasia**; all communication is through fragmentary expression; great need for inference, questioning, and guessing by the listener. Range of information that can be exchanged is limited; listener carries the burden of communication. Examiner cannot identify materials provided from patient response.
3 = **Mute, global aphasia**; no usable speech or auditory comprehension.

10. **Dysarthria:** If patient is thought to be normal, an adequate sample of speech must be obtained by asking patient to read or repeat words from the attached list. If the patient has severe aphasia, the clarity of articulation of spontaneous speech can be rated. Only if the patient is intubated or has other physical barriers to produce speech, the examiner should record the score as untestable (UN) and clearly write an explanation for this choice. Do not tell the patient why he or she is being tested.

0 = **Normal.**
1 = **Mild-to-moderate dysarthria**; patient slurs at least some words and, at worst, can be understood with some difficulty.
2 = **Severe dysarthria**; patient's speech is so slurred as to be unintelligible in the absence of or out of proportion to any dysphasia, or is mute/anarthric.
UN = **Intubated** or other physical barrier, explain
0 = **No abnormality.**
1 = **Visual, tactile, auditory, spatial, or personal inattention** or extinction to bilateral simultaneous stimulation in one of the sensory modalities.
2 = **Profound hemi-inattention or extinction to more than one modality**; does not recognize own hand or orients to only one side of space.

11. **Extinction and inattention (formerly " 'neglect' "):** Sufficient information to identify neglect may be obtained during the prior testing.If the patient has a severe visual loss preventing visual double simultaneous stimulation, and the cutaneous stimuli are normal, the score is normal. If the patient has aphasia but does appear to attend to both sides, the score is normal. The presence of visual spatial neglect or anosagnosia may also be taken as evidence of abnormality. Since the abnormality is scored only if present, the item is never untestable.

From *Arch Neurol* 1989;46:660–2. Goldstein LB, et al. *Interrater reliability Reliability of the NIH stroke Stroke scaleScale.*

Nissl, Franz (1860–1919) German neurologist and neuropathologist working in Frankfurt, Heidelberg, and finally in Munich. He noted that, within the swollen VI cranial nerve neurons after section of the nerve, there was a loss of chromophilic granules that no longer stained with basic dyes such as methylene blue (an agent that he had introduced for this purpose in 1858).

A clinician as well as laboratory-based physician, he enthusiastically adopted the technique of lumbar puncture and was known to his students as "punctator maximus."

Nissl bodies Blocks of intranuclear granular endoplasmic reticulin composed of protein, DNA, and RNA.

Nissl degeneration Swelling of neuronal cell bodies with loss of chromophilic granules, occurring after nerve injury.

Nissl granules Described in 1894, these consist of granular basophilic material within the cytoplasm of perikarya. In chromatolysis, they break down to yield free ribosomes.

Nissl stains Methods of enhancement of histological specimens, using thionine, toluidine blue, cresyl violet, or chrome-alum reagents with alcohol. The cresyl violet stains rough endoplasmic reticulum.

nitric oxide (NO) An inorganic gas synthesized endogenously by endothelial cells and capable of relaxing arterial walls and thus with a function in cardiovascular control but also contributing to the role of macrophages as killers of pathogens, reducing platelet activation, and acting as a diffusible messenger within the nervous system where it modulates neuronal firing and regulates blood flow, among other functions. Excessive NO concentrations can destroy CNS neurons.[604]

nitroblue tetrazolium dye test A laboratory test based on the ability of this dye to enter white blood cells in the presence of bacterial inflammatory products, where it is reduced and turns black.

It was origiinally used on CSF samples, where it was thought to be capable of differentiating aseptic from septic meningitis, but is now not much employed.

NMDA See **N-methyl-D-aspartate**.

NMO-IgG An immunofluorescence antibody binding to aquaporin-4, a water channel, and staining some CNS tissues in patients with **neuromyelitis optica**.

NMR Acronym for **nuclear magnetic resonance**, generally euphemized to **magnetic resonance imaging** in order to quiet an excitable populace.

nodose Knotty or possessed of swellings.

no-reflow Impairment of postischemic reperfusion of the brain, most often seen following transient arterial occlusion. It is mainly due to the accumulation of neutrophils within the lumen of the vessel.

No to Hattatsu (Brain and Development) A Japanese journal of child neurology, founded in 1969. Address: Japan Publishing Co. Ltd., P.O. Box 5030, Tokyo International, Tokyo, Japan.

Noack syndrome A form of mild acrocephaly (type 1) without neurological features. See also **acrocephalopolysyndactyly**.

Nobel e-Museum A Web site offering more than 7000 documents about Nobel Prize winners, including portraits and biographies of laureates.

Nobile-Orazio Ataxia Scale An observer-rated scale for gait ataxia.[4686]

0 Normal—stands on one foot with eyes closed.
1 Stand/walk normally with eyes closed.
2 Stand/walk normally with minor swaying with eyes closed, normally with eyes open.
3 Stand/walk with some swaying with eyes open.
4 Stand/walk on a wide base with eyes open.
5 Stand/walk impossible without support.

nocardiosis Infection with the fungus *Nocardia asteroides*, usually of the lungs in immunosuppressed people, with a tendency to spread to the brain as granulomatous meningitis or abscess.

The organism was first described by E.-I.-E. Nocard (1850–1903), a French veterinary pathologist.

nocioception (from Lat, to hurt or damage + perception) The awareness of pain.

nocioceptive pain A pain that fulfills its most appropriate function, namely warning that a tissue or organ is damaged or diseased. Examples include sprains, muscle stretch, fractures, burns, bruises, and inflammation (from an infection or arthritic disorder). Nociceptors sense and respond to tissue irritation and to impending or actual injury; when activated, they transmit signals leading to the perception of pain, that is, pain is typically well localized, constant, and often with an aching or throbbing quality. Visceral pain, however, is more likely to be episodic and poorly localized. Cf. **neuropathic pain**.

nociceptive reflex (Lat, to hurt or damage + to take) (Riddoch reflex, Buzzard reflex) With pyramidal tract lesions, painful stimulation of the inner aspect of the arm or of the upper chest leads to abduction and external rotation of the shoulder with flexion at all joints of the arm. With quadriplegia, especially when due to high cervical cord lesions, the same stimuli induce adduction, internal rotation, and elevation of the shoulder; pronation of the elbow; extension of the elbow and wrists; and adduction and extension of the fingers and thumb.[1500]

This is considered to be an associated postural reaction in patients with loss of supraspinal inhibitory control of spinal reflex activity.

nociceptor A receptor that is activated by injury and which warns the subject by transmitting impulses leading to the sensation of pain. The term was introduced by **Sherrington** in 1906.

nocturnal arm dysesthesias See **Wartenberg cheiralgia paresthetica**. However, the symptom is usually due to **carpal tunnel syndrome**.

nocturnal cardiac ischemia (angina decubitus) Evidence of cardiac ischemia occurring during sleep, usually associated with similar evidence during the day.

nocturnal eating (drinking) syndrome The condition characterized by recurrent wakening with the inability to return to sleep without eating or drinking. This is primarily a problem in infancy and early childhood but can also occur as a conditioned response in adult life.[6109]

nocturnal frontal lobe epilepsy See **autosomal dominant nocturnal frontal lobe epilepsy**.

nocturnal hemidystonia See **dystonia**.

nocturnal hemiplegia See **sleep paralysis**.

nocturnal hyperkinesis with daytime hypersomnolence See **hypersomnolence**.

nocturnal leg cramps Painful sensations of muscular tightness or tension usually felt in the calf but occasionally in the foot during sleep. The cramp frequently results in arousal and is accompanied by electrical evidence of muscle fiber contraction in the affected muscles.[1629]

Such cramps occur without other signs of peripheral neuropathy, usually in elderly people and in subjects of any age suffering from chronic renal failure or after vigorous treatment with diuretics. They represent a nightly curse to many aged people, but can often be prevented by oral calcium salts, quinine, or phenytoin.

nocturnal leg myoclonus See **periodic limb movement disorder**.

nocturnal myoclonus See **periodic limb movement disorder**.

nocturnal paroxysmal dystonia (hypnogenic paroxysmal dystonia, non-REM sleep-related dystonic or dyskinetic episodes) A **parasomnia** characterized by repeated stereotyped dystonic or dyskinetic (choreoathetoid and ballistic) episodes during non-rapid eye movement sleep, lasting 15–60 s and preceded by EEG evidence of arousal. Severe sleep disruption may result. The following diagnostic criteria have been suggested:[1629]

A. Abnormal motor activity during sleep.
B. Dystonic or dyskinetic episodes occur mainly during sleep.
C. Short-duration episodes typically last 15–60 s. Prolonged-duration episodes typically last 60 min.
D. Polysomnography demonstrates dystonic or dyskinetic movements occurring out of NREM sleep.
E. Not associated with any medical or psychiatric disorder that can account for the symptom, for example, frontal lobe epilepsy.
F. Does not meet the diagnostic criteria for other sleep disorders, such as **REM sleep behavior disorder** or **sleep terror**.

From AASM Diagnostic Classification Steering Committee. *The International Classification of Sleep Disorders Diagnostic and Coding Manual*. Rochester, MN. American Academy of Sleep Medicine 1991/2001. Reproduced by kind permission of the Academy.) See also http://www.sleepeducation.com/Disorders.aspx/.

The following *variant* forms have been described:

Typical attacks, but with dominant inheritance.[3957]

Nocturnal paroxysmal dystonia with long-lasting attacks: The attacks are similar but are more protracted, lasting between 2 min and an hour.[3955]

Nocturnal paroxysmal dystonia with intermediate-duration attacks: The attacks last between 2 and 5 min and consist of brief jerky movements affecting the limbs or trunk alternately, but are precipitated by arousal from sleep or by physical exercise-induced wakefulness.[3955]

Nocturnal paroxysmal dystonia with nocturnal wandering: See **episodic nocturnal wandering**.

Behavioral arousals with abnormal motor pattern: Presenting with complaints of sudden nocturnal awakenings, which occur due to dystonic–dyskinetic movements following sudden awakening.[3955]

Atypical periodic movements in sleep: A syndrome characterized by sudden repetitive nocturnal awakenings from non-rapid eye movement sleep, occurring every 1–2 min, accompanied by fragmentary dystonic posturing or dyskinetic movements lasting 2–5 s.[3955]

Nocturnal paroxysmal hemidystonia: See **dystonia**.

nocturnal psychogenic dissociative intrusion The occurrence of protracted dissociative episodes including multiple-personality disorder occurring upon awakening from rapid eye movement sleep or non-rapid eye movement sleep. The condition is usually described in patients who have experienced childhood physical or sexual abuse and who in many cases have manifested sleepwalking or sleep terror.[5595]

nocturnal sleep epilepsy Generalized seizures, restricted to, or predominantly occurring during periods of sleep.

nocturnal start See **periodic limb movement disorder**.

nocturnal tooth-grinding See **bruxism**.

nocturnal vertigo "The sensation of falling from a height when falling asleep or just after going to sleep" (Sir William **Gowers**).

nodes of Ranvier Interruptions in the axon's myelin sheath; places where the Schwann cell cytoplasm is in contact with the axon.

nodose ganglion (Lat, a knot + Gr, a tumor) A relay station attached to the vagus nerve just below the base of the skull, which contains the cell bodies of the afferent fibers from the pharynx, larynx, trachea, esophagus, and the thoracic and abdominal viscera.

nodular fasciitis (myositis proliferans) A localized inflammatory pseudotumorous swelling in muscles mainly of the shoulder and arms resulting from local injury.[3390] It is most often seen in the forearm.

nodular leprosy See **lepromatous leprosy**.

Noguchi, Hideyo (1876–1928) Pathologist who, with J. W. Moore, isolated *Treponema pallidum* from the brain of a patient with general paresis in 1913.

noise 1. Properly, artifactual potentials produced by electrodes, cables, the amplifier, or storage media, unrelated to the potentials of biological origin. 2. Colloquially in electromyography, physiological **end-plate activity**.

Noise thus refers to electric activity not related to the signal of interest. In electrodiagnostic medicine, it refers to waveforms generated by electrodes, cables, amplifier, or storage media and unrelated to potentials of biological origin. The term has also been used loosely to refer to one form of end-plate activity. (From the 2001 Report of the Nomenclature Committee of the American Association of Electromyography and Electrodiagnosis.[19] Reproduced by kind permission of the AANEM.)

nominal aphasia (nominal dysphasia) The term used by Sir Henry **Head** for that form of speech disorder in which there is defective use of names and want of comprehension of words as names or indicators. Reading is difficult, writing affected, and copying often impossible.[2814]

A graded naming diagnostic test has been described.[4237] See also **anomia**.

nominal dysphasia See **nominal aphasia**.

nona A form of sleeping sickness described by Gayet in 1875, in which mesencephalic and hypothalamic lesions were identified. Whether or not it was the same as **encephalitis lethargica** is impossible to tell.[4904]

noncommunicating hydrocephalus That form of hydrocephalus in which there is obstruction to the circulation of CSF between the sites of its formation in the ventricles and brain, and the roof of the fourth ventricle. See also **obstructive hydrocephalus**.

nonconcomitant deviation Misalignment of the visual axes, which varies with the position of gaze, changing according to which eye is fixating. In most cases, muscle paresis is responsible.

nonconvulsive seizure paralysis Transient paralysis of one or more limbs possibly due to migraine, transient ischemic attacks, or inhibitory seizures. The syndrome has been analyzed superbly[2089] but a final conclusion is not always possible in a particular patient. See also **nonconvulsive status**.

nonconvulsive status (NCSE) An epileptic condition lasting more than 30 min in which continuous or recurrent seizure activity on the electroencephalogram (EEG) is responsible for diverse clinical symptoms including alteration of mental state, abnormal behavior, disturbances of perception, and/or impairment of consciousness. Such variable seizure syndromes may resemble dementia, delirium, sleepiness, or clouding of consciousness, but motor and postural abilities are preserved and there is little or no visible evidence of motor seizure activity. The condition is seen in patients of any age with a past history of generalized or partial seizures and may persist for hours, days, or even months, in association with EEG evidence of persistent seizure discharges. It is thus a form of absence status or "complex partial status," and is usually precipitated by infection, low anticonvulsant levels, or withdrawal from benzodiazepines.

NCSE can be most usefully viewed as a form of cerebral response that is dependent largely on the level of cerebral development of the individual (age and cerebral integrity/development/maturity), epilepsy syndrome, and the anatomical location of the epileptic activity.[5811]

The commoner clinical appearances include clouded consciousness with confusion, disorientation, and diminished responsiveness; myoclonic or clonic movements of the eyes, face, or jaw, and automatisms in absence status; and more severe but variable clouded consciousness, less-frequent facial movements, and episodic adversive movements of head and eye. Slow recovery occurs after treatment but prolonged memory dysfunction may be a sequel.[1754] The condition may complicate hypoxic–anoxic encephalopathy, malignancies, drug toxicity, autoimmune disorders, **Creutzfeldt–Jakob disease**, chromosomal alterations, peritoneal dialysis, infections, cerebral **hamartomas**, or head trauma.

Absence status (epilepsia minor continua, petit mal status, spike-wave stupor) is characterized by confusion or diminished responsiveness with occasional blinking or twitching, lasting hours to days, with generalized spike and slow-wave discharges on the EEG.

Complex partial status consists of prolonged or repetitive complex partial seizures (with a presumed focal onset) and produces an "epileptic twilight state" with fluctuating lack of responsiveness or confusion. In this group, the presence of some physical signs is more likely than in the last.

Other confused, stuporous, or comatose patients with rapid, rhythmic, epileptiform discharges on the EEG may have "electrographic" status and should be considered in the same diagnostic category. While generalized convulsive status epilepticus produces lasting neuropathologic hippocampal damage, absence status epilepticus (SE) appears to cause no lasting effects. Complex partial SE is less uniform.[1714] See also **absence status**.

nonepileptic myoclonus

Those forms of **myoclonus** that have no relationship to any **epileptic syndrome**. These include **dystonic myoclonus**; **ballistic movement overflow myoclonus**; exaggerated startle; physiological phenomena such as hiccups, sneezing, and **sleep jerks**; **periodic movements of sleep**; and **segmental myoclonus** such as spinal and palatal myoclonus.

In such cases, the EMG burst length is between 50 and 300 ms, muscle jerking during the discharge may be asynchronous, and there is no correlated discharge recordable on the EEG.[2695] See also **epileptic myoclonus** and **myoclonus**.

nonepileptic seizures

1. (pseudoseizures, psychogenic nonepileptic seizures, functional/pseudoepileptic seizures, dissociative or psychogenic seizures, nonepileptic "attacks") Episodes of altered movement, sensation, or experience resembling epileptic seizures but without a causal epileptic mechanism and considered to have a psychogenic basis. The clinical manifestations are presumed to be unrelated to an abnormal and excessive discharge of a set of neurons of the brain but they may coexist with true epileptic seizures.[1265] Recent important commentaries have been published.[901, 3572, 5275] The prognosis is worse in patients with maladaptive personality disorders, in whom the problem may be persistent. Although more common in women aged less than 50 years, later occurrence has also been recorded.

Clinical clues to these events include their relatively slow onset, motor activity that is undulating rather than abrupt in onset/offset, the variability of motor activity the patterns of which are atypical for recognized seizure types, the partial preservation of consciousness and its quick recovery after the end of the episodes, increased motor activity lasting more than 90 s, tight closure of the eyes, retained downgoing plantar responses, and the lack of efficacy of intravenous benzodiazepines. There are no abnormalities on the EEG, and posterior background activity is present during states of unresponsiveness to stimulation. Moreover, the EEG together with closed circuit TV monitoring shows no correlation between physical seizure activity and any epileptiform discharges recorded.

Unresponsiveness without motor manifestations may be the most common presentation, but partial seizure simulations are often seen, in which any motor activity exhibited is usually coordinated. Side-to-side head movements, out-of-phase limb jerking, and pelvic thrusting are typical patterns, while bizarre and incongruous movement patterns are probably less common.[3765] Such attacks are rare in subjects who do not suffer from true epileptic seizures as well. They do not respond to anticonvulsant medication.

2. Seizures of any type provoked by intercurrent disease (such as anoxia or head trauma) in a subject not formerly subject to recurrent seizures.

nonfamilial juvenile central neurogenic muscular atrophy

See **monomelic amyotrophy**.

nonfamilial juvenile distal spinal muscular atrophy of upper extremity

See **monomelic amyotrophy**.

nonfamilial spinal segmental muscular atrophy in juvenile and young subjects

See **monomelic amyotrophy**.

nonfluency

Effortful, dysmelodic speech with impairment of both articulation and grammar. Some call this *telegraphese*. Dysprosody (speech that lacks normal rhythm) is notable.

nonfluent aphasia

See **Broca aphasia** and **agrammatism**.

nonhypertrophic muscular dystrophy

See **Emery–Dreifuss syndrome**.

noninfantile Gaucher disease

A cause of Ramsay Hunt syndrome (cerebellar). See also **glucosylceramide lipidosis**.

noninfectious granulomatous angiitis with a predilection for the nervous system

See **isolated angiitis of the nervous system**.

nonketotic hyperglycinemia

(OMIM 238300) A recessively inherited (9p22) inborn error of the glycine cleavage system, causing ataxia and myoclonus and usually fatal within the first few weeks of life. See also **cerebellar ataxias** (*variants*) and **glycine encephalopathy**.

nonketotic hyperosmolar syndrome

Severe hyperosmolarity (>320 mOsm/l), hyperglycemia (>600 mg/100 ml), and dehydration occurring as a result of an inability to drink enough fluid to keep pace with the osmotic diuresis caused by hyperglycemia, usually in elderly patients with mild or undiagnosed type II diabetes. The resultant impaired renal function reduces glucose loss leading to elevations in blood glucose.

The onset is typically insidious with deterioration over weeks; severe acidosis and ketosis are not features. The level of consciousness generally correlates with the severity and duration of hyperosmolarity. Ten percent of patients present in coma, and an equal number have clear consciousness. Generalized or focal seizures, focal neurological signs, delirium, exacerbation of any pre-existing organic mental syndrome, and profound dehydration are the main features. The laboratory picture is of uncontrolled diabetes and dehydration, renal functional impairment, raised hemoglobin, abnormal liver function tests, and hypertriglyceridemia yielding falsely low serum sodium levels ("pseudohyponatremia").

non-length-dependent small fiber neuropathy A frequent cause of neuropathic pain in patients with **burning feet syndrome**. It is probably in fact a ganglionopathy in which the small fibers are selectively damaged and is often the result of an underlying metabolic or immune process. Major clinical features are early involvement of the face, trunk, and proximal limbs, neuropathic pain in the affected areas, and loss of thin fiber function (scratch, temperature, and pinprick) in the affected regions with preservation of large fiber sensibility.[2512]

nonmalignant inflammatory sensory polyganglionopathies (see also **malignant inflammatory sensory polyganglionopathies**) A group of uncommon dorsal root ganglion cell and autonomic neuronal disorders presenting as a sensory ataxic or hyperalgesic syndrome or both. Sensory nerve action potentials are small or absent. The CSF protein level is not raised. Sometimes, positive tests for antinuclear antibodies, antibodies to extractable nuclear antigens, or rheumatoid factor suggest that connective tissue diseases are etiologically relevant.

non-Menkes-type copper deficiency with regression, lactic acidosis, and granulocytopenia A rare syndrome of early childhood comprising low serum copper and ceruloplasmin levels, low granulocyte count, lactic acidosis, truncal ataxia, and neurodevelopmental regression considered due to impaired copper transport across the intestinal wall and across the blood–brain barrier.[2226] See also Haas et al.[2659]

nonmetastatic syndromes See **paraneoplastic syndromes**.

nonmigrainous vascular headaches Headache with some characteristics of **migraine** but induced by specific circumstances, such as fever, hangover, or stroke (see also **Willis headache**).

non-neuroepithelial tumors of the CNS See **neuroepithelial tumors of the CNS** (Chart N–4A).

nonoptic aphasia A form of aphasia due to malfunction of the semantic system in which there is impairment of spontaneous speech and of the generation of word lists, and reduction in semantic knowledge, but preservation of visual confrontation naming.[5818] The phenomenon is most often reported in **Alzheimer disease**.

nonprogressive congenital neuromuscular disease with uniform type 1 fibers A congenital myopathy in which more than 99% of the muscle fibers are of type 1. Clinically, the disease is characterized by delayed motor development, the early onset of mild proximal weakness, hyporeflexia, normal serum muscle enzyme levels, EMG changes of myopathy, and a nonprogressive course.[4762]

nonprogressive encephalopathy The current term for cerebral palsy, also called *infantile cerebral paralysis* by **Freud**. See also **static encephalopathy**.

non-rapid eye movement sleep (quiet sleep, synchronized sleep, deep sleep, delta sleep, NREM sleep) A slow, steady metabolic state characterized by low cardiac output, blood pressure, cerebral blood flow, and respiratory rate. Four stages are defined in Chart N–13.

See also **sleep stages** and **rapid eye movement sleep**.

non-rapid eye movement sleep-related dystonic dyskinetic episodes See **nocturnal paroxysmal dystonia**.

nonspecific degeneration See **frontal lobe dementia**.

nonspecific EEG abnormalities Abnormal EEG activity, such as patterns of theta or delta activity occurring in bursts or rhythmic trains during wakefulness. Such activity may be produced by a wide variety of pathologies and alone has no diagnostic value.[5583]

nonspecific granuloma of the orbit See **orbital pseudotumor syndrome**.

nonspecific lipid myopathy A rare familial myopathy characterized by the deposition of lipid droplets in the muscle. Clinically, muscle weakness, abdominal cramps, and nausea following consumption of a fatty meal were described as the leading symptoms. Muscle carnitine levels are normal.[275]

nonspecific poliodystrophy and lactic acidosis A mitochondrial

Chart N–13. Stages of Non-Rapid Eye Movement Sleep

NREM stage 1. A stage of sleep following directly upon wakefulness and characterized by the EEG appearance of low-voltage activity with alpha activity less than 50%, beta activity and vertex spikes, and with slow rolling eye movements. This usually comprises some 5% of the total sleep time

NREM stage 2. A stage of sleep characterized by the appearance of sleep spindles and K complexes on a low-voltage, mixed-frequency background and with delta activity comprising up to 20% of the stage. This stage usually comprises some 50% of the total sleep time

NREM stage 3. A stage of sleep characterized by the appearance of high-amplitude delta waves (>75 μV, <2 Hz) for a period of 20–50% of the time, which occurs in the first third of the sleep period

NREM stage 4. A stage of sleep characterized by the appearance of high-amplitude delta waves (>75 μV ,<2 Hz) for more than 50% of the time and comprising, with NREM stage 3, slow-wave (SWS) or delta sleep

encephalomyelopathy causing atypical **progressive myoclonic epilepsy**.

non-stimulus-sensitive myoclonus

Myoclonus occurring spontaneously at rest and periodic, rhythmic, or irregular in occurrence. See also **myoclonus**.

nonsyndromic mental retardation

A recessively inherited developmental disability, mapped to 3p25–pter. Clinically, it is manifest as delay in the acquisition or maturation of language and social rather than of motor skills in children with no past history of hereditary or acquired disease known to be associated with mental retardation, no dysmorphism, normal vision and hearing, and no evidence of autism.[2897]

nonsystemic vasculitic neuropathy

A chronic multiple mononeuropathy (seldom a distal polyneuropathy) affecting only the peripheral nerves without involvement of joints, skin, or viscera, lacking constitutional signs, and due to an indolent necrotizing vasculitis. Diagnosis requires at least three of the first five of the following criteria; criterion 6 is also mandatory for systemic vasculitis.[1773]

1. Clinical presentation typical for a vasculitic neuropathy
   - Asymmetric or multifocal, painful, sensorimotor neuropathy
   - Acute/subacute relapsing, progressive, or relapsing progressive course
   - No spontaneous remission
2. Elevated sedimentation rate or other laboratory evidence of a systemic inflammatory state
3. Electrodiagnostic evidence of an active, asymmetric, axonal, sensorimotor neuropathy
4. Suggestive neuromuscular pathology
   - Vascular thickening or sclerosis, narrowing or obliteration of the vascular lumen, thrombosis, periadventitial capillary proliferation, hemosiderin deposits, nonrandom nerve fiber loss, or Wallerian-like degeneration
5. Clinical response to immunosuppressive therapy
6. Clinicopathologic evidence of a systemic/secondary etiology
   - Concurrent condition known or suspected to predispose to vasculitis (connective tissue diseases, certain infections, certain drugs, malignancies/paraproteinemias, cryoglobulinemia)
   - Simultaneous multiorgan, nonperipheral nerve involvement
   - Biopsy-proven vasculitis in other tissues

non-24-hour sleep–wake syndrome

A condition characterized by a chronic steady pattern comprising 1- to 2-h daily delays in sleep onset and wake times in an individual living in society. As a result of these persistently incrementing delays in the times of sleep and waking over successive days, the subject is at most times out of phase with the sleep–wake cycle of others in his environment. The commonest pattern is of prolongation of the individual's sleep–wake cycle to 25 h. The condition is seen particularly in males, often those with schizoid tendencies, and in the blind.[6682] Diagnostic criteria have been suggested.[1629] (See Chart N–14).

nonthyroidal hypermetabolism

See **Luft disease**.

nonvasculitic autoimmune inflammatory meningoencephalitis (NAIM)

A syndrome of progressive cognitive decline, psychosis, and unsteady gait occurring in adults due to a steroid-responsive nonvasculitic autoimmune inflammatory meningoencephalitic syndrome. CSF shows elevated immunoglobulin (Ig)G index and IgG synthesis rates, and brain biopsy reveals perivascular lymphocytic infiltrates without vessel wall invasion.[1049]

nonversive movements

See **versive seizures**.

non-Wilsonian extrapyramidal disease with copper dysmetabolism

A rare syndrome of hepatic copper metabolism characterized by hepatic copper accumulation, low levels of ceruloplasmin, and normal or low serum copper levels, but normal or raised urinary copper levels.

Clinically, extrapyramidal signs including dystonia and chorea occur in the absence of **Kayser–Fleischer rings** and without hepatic cirrhosis.[2828]

non-Wilsonian hepatocerebral degeneration

See **acquired hepatocerebral encephalopathy**.

Nonne, Max

(1861–1959) German neurologist, who trained with **Erb** in Hamburg, where he was later a colleague of **Jakob**.

Nonne syndrome

See **Froin syndrome**.

Nonne–Marie syndrome

Congenital cerebellar disease due to agenesis. See also **cerebellar ataxias** and **Marie ataxia**.

Nonne reaction

A qualitative test for excess globulin in the CSF.

Chart N–14. Diagnostic Criteria for Non-24-hour Sleep–Wake Syndrome

A. Primary complaint of difficulty in initiating sleep or difficulty in awakening
B. Progressive delays of sleep onset and offset with the inability to maintain stable entrainment to a 24-h sleep–wake pattern
C. Presence of the sleep pattern for at least 6 weeks
D. Evidence of a progressive sequential delay of the sleep period revealed by
   1. Polysomnography performed over several consecutive days on a fixed 24-h bedtime and waketime schedule or
   2. Continuous 24-h temperature monitoring over at least 5 days shows a progressive delay of the temperature nadir
E. Does not meet criteria for any other sleep disorder causing inability to initiate sleep or excessive sleepiness

From AASM Diagnostic Classification Steering Committee. *The International Classification of Sleep Disorders Diagnostic and Coding Manual*. Rochester, MN. American Academy of Sleep Medicine 1991/2001. Reproduced by kind permission of the Academy. See also http://www.sleepeducation.com/Disorders.aspx/.

nonverbal auditory agnosia Difficulty in interpreting musical or nonlanguage environmental sounds, due to lesions of the auditory association cortex.

Noonan syndrome (Ullrich–Noonan syndrome, chromatin-positive Turner syndrome) A dominantly inherited or sporadic congenital dysmorphic syndrome mainly seen in girls, and characterized by ptosis, anti-Mongolian slant of the eyes, broad nose, small jaw, hypertelorism, webbed neck, high-arched palate, low hairline, short stature, cubitus valgus, hypogonadism, seizures, sensorineural deafness, mild mental retardation, and congenital heart defects.[4694] The chromosome pattern XO is present. See also **neurofibromatosis**.

nootropic drugs A class of psychotropic drugs that raise levels of ATP in the brain, enhance the acquisition of new data, and reverse learning impairments in experimental animals with virtually no physiological effects in other bodily areas. The prototypical example was piracetam, a gamma-amino butyric acid analogue, with diverse effects on brain chemistry, facilitating performance on various learning and memory paradigms in humans and animals.[2398]

Nordic myoclonus See **Unverricht–Lundborg–Lafora syndrome** and **Baltic myoclonus**.

normal-pressure hydrocephalus (adult occult hydrocephalus or low-pressure hydrocephalus, hydrocephalus ex vacuo, cerebral enlargement, brain distension, Hakim–Adams syndrome, idiopathic adult hydrocephalus syndrome) An uncommon syndrome of adult life, characterized by the presence of grossly enlarged cerebral ventricles under normal pressure, urinary incontinence, gait apraxia, pyramidal signs, and mild "subcortical" dementia. The quality of the gait disorder suggests bifrontal damage. A fourth criterion should be perceptible behavioral decline over a period of weeks to months varying from mild apathy to severe psychomotor retardation.[52] The condition was probably firstidentified by Riddoch in 1936.

It results from impairment of CSF flow and episodes of slightly raised CSF pressure with a pressure gradient between the ventricles and subarachnoid space, coupled with widespread reduction in cerebral blood flow. The impairment of CSF flow is usually at the level of the basal cisterns.

Radioimmunosorbent assay scans may demonstrate reflux of the isotope into the ventricles after lumbar intrathecal injection and ventricular decompression sometimes leads to significant improvement in gait, but little in cognitive function. Neither the CSF tap test nor CSF conductance measurements provide information distinguishing patients whose conditions will or will not respond to shunting.[4036] However, a short history, any known cause of hydrocephalus, a predominance of the gait disorder, and CT or MRI evidence of hydrodynamic hydrocephalus are somewhat predictive of a good response to shunting, as is a positive response to external lumbar CSF drainage over a few days.[6514] The latter involves prolonged external lumbar drainage in excess of 300 ml, which has a high sensitivity (50–100%) and a positive predictive value (80–100%). The "therapeutic" lumbar puncture has too low a yield to be worth doing.

Diagnostic criteria have been suggested.[466] If these criteria are satisfied, a shunt operation may be indicated.

1. The presence of two or more of progressing gait disturbance, dementia, and urinary urge incontinence
2. Ventricular enlargement on brain CT scan
3. Increased R out (≥10 mmHg/ml/min) with or without B-wave activity ≥50% of the monitoring period

The disorder may also occur in children who present with decreasing scholastic performance, delay in walking or frequent falls, and impaired bladder control (Bret et al. *JNNP* 2002;73:9–12).

normal-volume hydrocephalus The occurrence of **slit ventricles** in children who formerly had suffered increased intracranial pressure and whose shunts had blocked.[1881]

Norman leukodystrophy (Norman–Tingey syndrome) A familial form of sudanophilic leukodystrophy with microcephaly, striate calcification, and pachygyria. Dwarfism, paraplegia, mental retardation, and the appearance of **progeria** are inconstant but notable features.[4699]

Norman Wood congenital amaurotic familial idiocy A congenital syndrome of extreme micrencephaly with gliosis and free neutral fat and the massive deposition of intracellular lipoid and cholesterol throughout the white matter of the brain.[4701]

Norman–Roberts lissencephaly A rare, recessively inherited congenital dysmorphic syndrome, characterized also by microcephaly, heterotopias, **lissencephaly**, microcephaly, and ventricular dilatation.[4698]

Norman–Tingey syndrome See **Norman leukodystrophy**.

normocalcemic tetany See **hereditary myokymia** and **neuromyotonia**.

normokalemic familial periodic paralysis See **familial periodic paralysis**.

Norrbotten disease See **glucosylceramide lipidosis**.

Norrie disease (oculoacousticocerebral degeneration) A developmental disorder inherited as an X-linked recessive trait, in which the eyes shrink and develop retrolental opacities, optic atrophy, and retinal phakomas in early childhood. Other features include short digits, psychomotor regression, deafness, behavioral disturbances, and hallucinations.[4704] The responsible gene maps to chromosome Xp11.4.

North American Chronic Pain Association (Canada) A charitable organization providing support and information on this condition. Tel: 905-793-5230. Web site: http://www.chronicpaincanada.com/.

Northwestern University Disability Scale One of the original instruments designed for the assessment of patients with **Parkinson disease** and providing scores in the categories of *walking, dressing, hygiene, eating and feeding, and speech*.[998] See also **Hoehn and Yahr Scale**, **Columbia rating scale**, **Unified rating scale for Parkinson disease**, and **New York rating scale**.

northern epilepsy See **neuronal ceroid lipofuscinosis**.

nosocomial (Gr, hospital) Of or belonging to a hospital—for example, unusual infections acquired during hospitalization.

nosology (Gr, disease + a discourse) The practice of naming and classification of diseases.

notalgia paresthetica A benign and self-limiting syndrome of burning paresthesia, pruritus, and hypoesthesia felt in the interscapular region, considered to be a consequence of dorsal spinal root compression at T2–6.[5048]

notch filter A filter that selectively attenuates a very narrow frequency band, thus producing a sharp notch in the frequency response curve of an EEG channel. A 60 (50) Hz notch filter is used in some EEG machines to provide attenuation of 60 (50) Hz interference under extremely unfavorable recording conditions. (Adapted from the 1974 report of the Committee on Terminology, IFCN. In: Chatrian GE, Bergamini L, Dondey M, et al. A glossary of terms most commonly used by clinical electro-encephalographers. *EEG Clin Neurophysiol* 1974;**37**:538–48. Reproduced by kind permission of Elsevier Science and the IFCN.)

Nothnagel, Carl Wilhelm Hermann (1841–1905) German internist, neurologist, and pathologist who trained with Virchow and Leyden. He became professor of medicine at Freyberg, Jena, and later Vienna. He described the syndrome named for him in patients with tumors.

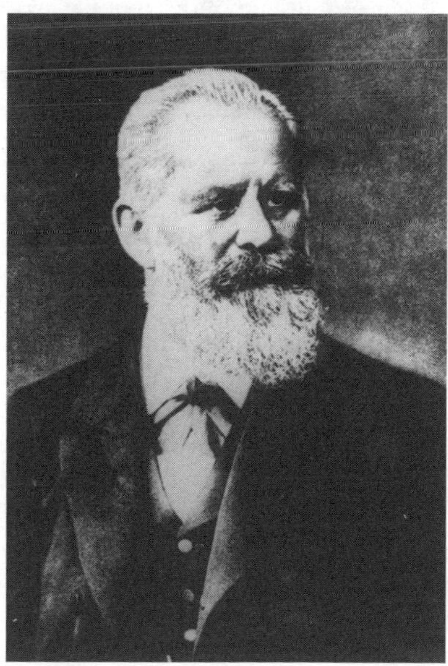

Figure N–2 Carl Wilhelm Hermann Nothnagel

Nothnagel disease 1. "Vasomotor acroparesthesiae"; tingling, cyanosis, blanching, edema, and even gangrene of the digits. A severe form of Raynaud phenomenon, described by Nothnagel in 1867.[4714] 2. Angina pectoris.

Nothnagel sign Loss of emotional but not voluntary facial movements with thalamic tumors.

Nothnagel syndrome (ophthalmoplegia-ataxia syndrome) Damage to the oculomotor nerves on one or both sides, and to the superior cerebellar peduncle, caused by a tumor in the mesencephalic tectum or by a mesencephalic vascular accident. Oculomotor nerve and vertical gaze palsies, depressed consciousness, and cerebellar ataxia are the clinical results.[4715]

The syndrome may be regarded as a variant of the **dorsal midbrain syndrome** or as **Benedikt syndrome** with an added paresis of vertical gaze.

notochord (Gr, back + string) The primitive skeletal axis of vertebrates, which forms a template for the differentiation of the vertebral column. It was discovered by Karl von Baer, a German embryologist (1792–1876)

Nottingham 10-point ADL Index A scale assessing the functional capacity of subjects after stroke or cerebral trauma.[1802] The items assessed are the patient's ability to

1. Drink from a cup
2. Eat
3. Wash face and hands
4. Transfer from bed to chair
5. Walk or use wheelchair indoors
6. Use the toilet
7. Undress
8. Dress
9. Make a hot drink
10. Get in and out of a bath

Nougaret night blindness A dominantly inherited syndrome of absence of the rod receptors of the retina.

Dr. J. Nougaret (1637–1719) was a French physician.

Nova Scotia variant See **sphingomyelin storage disorders**.

NREM intrusion The interposition of non-rapid eye movement sleep or of a component of NREM sleep such as increased EMG activity, or K-complexes, sleep spindles, or delta waves on the EEG, during rapid eye movement sleep periods.[280]

NREM narcolepsy See **idiopathic CNS hypersomnolence**.

NREM period The non-rapid eye movement sleep portion of the REM–NREM sleep cycle, consisting usually of stages 3 and 4 early in the night and stage 2 later.[280]

NREM sleep See **non-rapid eye movement sleep**.

nuchal Of or belonging to the nape of the neck.

nuchocephalic reflex (Gr, neck + head) A sign of diffuse cortical dysfunction elicited by rapidly turning the shoulders of a subject (standing with his eyes closed) to the right and left. The reflex is inhibited (normal) if the subject turns his head in the direction of the rotation—usually with a fraction of delay—and uninhibited if the original position of the head is maintained.[3199]

nuclear agenesis See **Möbius syndrome**.

nuclear jaundice See **kernicterus**.

nuclear magnetic resonance scanning (NMR) A variant of **magnetic resonance imaging**, allowing the study of nuclei other than that of hydrogen (e.g., fluorine, carbon, sodium).

When magnetic nuclei such as ^{1}H, ^{31}P, ^{13}C, ^{23}Na, ^{19}F, or ^{15}N are placed in a strong magnetic field, they line up like tiny compass needles, even if they are incorporated in the molecules of a living organism. They precess about the flux lines of the field at characteristic resonant frequencies that vary with their chemical structure; such frequencies can be used to identify particular compounds.

NMR measurements are made by perturbing nuclear precession with radiofrequency energy and then recording the similar radio waves the perturbed nuclei emit as they "relax" back to their equilibrium state. Magnetic nuclei in small molecules that tumble rapidly—water, lactate, and ATP, for instance—produce strong enough radio signals from within the brain to be detected.

Magnetic resonance spectroscopy (MRS) is the general term for the measurement of specific substances by detection of their characteristic resonant frequencies. MRI uses some strong signal—usually from water protons—to make pictures based on differences in the intensity and relaxation rates of the signal between different anatomical regions. The much weaker signals from sources such as ^{1}H in lactate, ^{31}P in ATP, and ^{13}C in glycogen can also be made into anatomical images that map the distribution of specific compounds. Of necessity, these are less detailed than water proton images, but they do provide chemically specific information.[5121]

nucleus A concentration of neuronal cell bodies within the brain or spinal cord. The term was first applied by J. C. **Riel** to the basal ganglia in 1808 but was first used by Benedict **Stilling** in 1846 in connection with the cells of origin of the cranial and spinal nerves.

nucleus basalis of Meynert A clump of neurons in the substantia innominata below the globus pallidus, the cells of which provide most of the cholinergic innervation of the cerebral cortex. The nucleus suffers marked cell loss and a reduction in choline acetyltransferase activity in patients with **Alzheimer disease**.

nucleus of Perlia A median group of nerve cells situated between the oculomotor nuclei, the postulated center for ocular convergence. This hypothesized function, however, has been strongly criticized and, if the nucleus exists as a separate anatomical entity, it is more probably the origin of neurons innervating the inferior oblique and superior rectus muscles.[6662]

null point That position of the eyes in which a congenital nystagmus, present with gaze in some direction, disappears or shows the least amplitude.

numb and clumsy hands The presence of such symptoms occurring in association with midline cervical disk protrusions at C3–4 and thus definable as a **false localizing sign**.[3700]

numb cheek syndrome The occurrence of infraorbital neuropathy with numbness of the cheek and of the gums at the level of the upper incisor and canine teeth, usually as a result of malignant infiltration of the nerve.[991]

numb cheek-limp lower lid syndrome The association of the **numb cheek syndrome** with drooping of the homolateral lower eyelid and also of the upper lip, due to damage to the infraorbital nerve and some distal branches of the facial nerve, and caused by the same processes as those that cause the following syndrome.[824]

numb chin syndrome The occurrence of mental neuropathy with numbness in the distribution of the nerve, usually as a result of malignant infiltration of the nerve or atrophy of the mandible.[2247] The condition was first reported by Sir Charles **Bell** in 1830.

numbness The subjective awareness that stimuli applied to the skin or mucosae are not perceived. A positive feeling from the numb area, which cannot be verbalized, is also often present.

nummular headache A chronic, often continuous, self-limited, mild-to-moderate unilateral head pain usually felt in the parietal regions with occasional lancinating bursts, without accompanying clinical or investigational abnormalities. The cause is unknown, but is probably a localized neuralgia of a terminal branch of the trigeminal nerve. The pressure-like pain is felt in a circumscribed area of 2–6 cm in diameter in which there may also be paresthesias. Some patients also have more common primary headache syndromes.[4894]

Although uncommon and when recognized a reassuring diagnosis, one case has been reported in which the same headache was associated with underlying tumor.

nurse's contracture tetany This name was proposed by **Trousseau** because of the frequency of the condition in nursing mothers, suffering undoubtedly from hypocalcemia.

Nursing Tips for People Living with ALS A site providing information on how to deal with some of the medical complications faced by ALS patients. See also the Web site: http://www.alsa.org/files/cms/Resources/FYI_07_Bill%20of%20Rights.pdf.

nutritional amblyopia Slowly progressive visual failure with retro-ocular discomfort; optic atrophy and bilateral central or centrocecal scotomas are the usual findings.[4741] The condition may appear as a paraneoplastic nutritional deficiency state. See also **tobacco–alcohol amblyopia** and **Obal syndrome**.

nutritional deficiency with encephalopathy Intellectual retardation resulting from specific or generalized nutritional deficits during gestation or infancy and associated with a reduction in brain weight.

nutritional myopathy 1. Cachexia in association with starvation and protein malnutrition. 2. Myopathy in association with chronic deficiency of vitamin E,[4638] **hypocalcemia**, or **hypophosphatemia**.

nutritional neuropathy A severe but reversible thick fiber sensory neuropathy occurring in a state of general nutritional deprivation with minimal motor involvement, but with no evidence of a specific deficiency of vitamins or other food factors. Most cases have been recorded after gastric stapling for obesity; deficiency of which nutrient or other substance is responsible for the syndrome is uncertain.[1991] Riboflavin is one likely culprit.

See also **beri-beri**, **Strachan syndrome**, **Wernicke–Korsakoff encephalopathy**, **pellagra**, **alcoholic neuropathy**, and **burning feet syndrome**.

nutritional optic neuropathy See **tobacco–alcohol amblyopia**.

nyctalopia (from Gr, night + sight) Impairment of twilight or night vision as occurs with deficiency of vitamin A, pigmentary retinal degeneration, or color blindness. The original Greek meaning was actually the opposite—the ability to see by night only, but it seems to have been reversed by Galen and the present meaning was that intended by Heberden (1768).[2824] Compare with **hemeralopia** (day blindness).

nyctophonia Elective mutism during the day, vocal communication occurring only at night. Seldom exhibited by humans, it is however a common attribute of cats.

Nylen-Bárány test The patient who is seated on a table is quickly laid back into supine position with the neck extended 45° over the end of the table and the head rotated 45° to one side and is observed for vertigo, nausea, and nystagmus (onset, direction, and duration). After a period of restitution while sitting up, the maneuver is repeated with the head rotated to the other side.

Lesions of the central and peripheral portions of the vestibular system induce the above physical signs, which are not seen in normal subjects.[1707] See also **central nystagmus** and **peripheral nystagmus.**

Nyquist theorem Accurate digital representation of an EEG signal requires that the sampling rate is at least twice the highest frequency of the signal; thus a frequency of 50 Hz requires at least a sampling rate of 100 Hz. (After Noachtar S, et al. A glossary of terms most commonly used by clinical electroencephalographers. EEG Clin Neurophysiol 1999;52[Suppl]:21–41. Reproduced by kind permission of the IFCN and Elsevier Science.)

Nyssen–van Bogaert syndrome See **metachromatic leukodystrophy** and **opticocochleodentate degeneration**.

nystagmus (from Gr, to nod in sleep) Involuntary rhythmic oscillations of the eyes about one or more axes; biphasic ocular oscillations with an initial slow component responsible for their genesis and continuation. **Vestibular nystagmus** was first described by Erasmus Darwin, the grandfather of Charles Darwin, in 1794. **Optokinetic nystagmus** was first noted by **Purkinje** in people looking out of train windows.

Normally, there are three control mechanisms that maintain steady gaze, fixation, the vestibulo-ocular reflex, and a gaze-holding system (the neural integrator)—all of which operate when the eyes are required to hold an eccentric gaze position. Failure of any of these control systems disrupts steady fixation and either nystagmus or saccadic intrusions/oscillations result. The difference between these lies in the initial movement that takes the line of sight off the object of regard. In the case of nystagmus, it is a slow drift (slow phase), while with saccadic intrusions or oscillations, it is an inappropriate fast movement that moves the eyes off target.

Congenital, acquired, and physiological forms are recognized; these are further classified by the degree of conjugacy, the various planes of the oscillation, the direction(s) of gaze at which it is present, and the waveform, its amplitude, and its frequency.

Dell'Osso[1561] lists 47 types, with subgroups, and suggests a clinical classification, reproduced in modified form in Chart N–15.

Chart N–15. Listing of Forms of Nystagmus

Congenital, **latent**, **manifest latent**, and **spasmus nutans** (infancy and childhood)
Acquired pendular
Acquired horizontal jerk (**vestibular**, **gaze-evoked**, and **gaze-paretic**)
Special types: **cervical**, **circular/elliptical/oblique**, **convergence-evoked**, **dissociated**, **downbeat**, **lid**, **muscle-paretic** (myasthenic), **periodic/aperiodic alternating**, **physiological**, **rebound**, **rotary**, **see-saw**, **upbeat**, and **voluntary**
Induced: **arthrokinetic**, **audiokinetic**, **caloric**, **drug-induced**, **optokinetic**, **positional**, and **rotational**

See also other terms referable to nystagmus: **anticipatory**, **arthrokinetic-induced**, **associated**, **ataxic**, **Bartel**, **bow-tie**, **Bruns**, **central**, **centripetal**, **convergence-retraction**, **direction-changing**, **direction-fixed**, **dissociated**, **divergence**, **downbeat**, **epileptic**, **flicker-induced**, **horizontal**, **induced**, **jerk**, **lateral medullary**, **manifest latent**, **miner's**, **optokinetic after-induced**, **pendular**, periodic downbeat, **peripheral**, **pursuit defect**, **rebound**, **reflex**, **retraction**, **somatosensory**, **spontaneous**, **torsional**, **uniocular**, upbeat, and **vertical**. See also **oscillations**.

nystagmus retractorius See **convergence-retraction nystagmus**.

nystagmus-blockage syndrome (Ethan syndrome, compensation syndrome) The suppression of congenital nystagmus through the development of esotropia and with head turning[3762, 2400] or with forced convergence while fixating a distant object.

nystagmus–myoclonus syndrome See **Lenoble–Aubineau syndrome**.

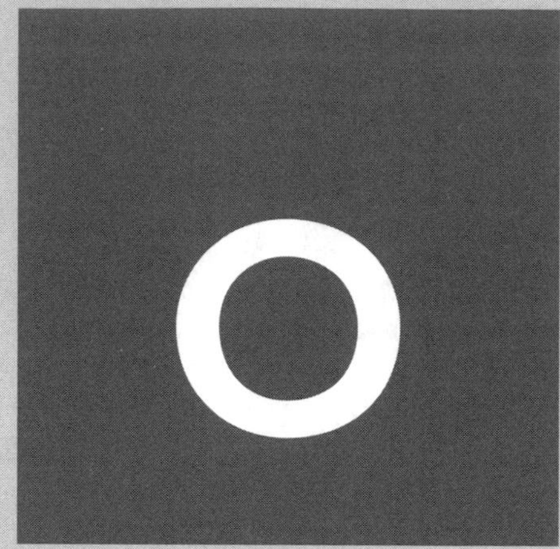

oasthouse disease (methionine malabsorption syndrome) A rare, recessively inherited diffuse encephalopathy of infancy, characterized by malabsorption of amino acids, particularly methionine, and the excretion of alpha-hydroxybutyric acid, giving a delightful smell of hops to the urine. The major clinical features are seizures, diarrhea, and mental retardation.[5902]

ob- (Lat, against) A prefix indicating before, about, against, toward, or over.

Obal syndrome Relative central or ring scotomas, nyctalopia, impaired color vision (especially for green), and frequently evidence of peripheral sensorimotor polyneuropathy occurring in those starved for long periods, such as prisoners of war. See **nutritional amblyopia**.[4741]

obelion (Gr, sagittal) A cranial index marker point between the two parietal foramina, employed by **Charcot** but not now in common use.

Ober test A method of assessing the degree of tightness in the tensor fascia lata (TFL). With the patient lying in the lateral decubitus position at the edge of the examination table, the superior thigh is flexed slightly and dropped off the edge of the table toward the floor with the knee extended. A tight TFL will not allow the thigh and leg to drop below the table edge. Comparison is made between the two sides.

Obersteiner, Heinrich (1847–1922) Austrian professor of neurology at Vienna whose textbooks of neuroanatomy (1888) and neuropathology (1897) were regarded as classics in their day. His own neurological Institute was opened in 1878, the first of its kind.

Obersteiner sign Perception of a stimulus given to one side of the body as if coming from the other side. See **allocheiria**. The phenomenon has been described in **tabes dorsalis, multiple sclerosis,** and **hysteria**.[4744]

obesity–polydactyly–iris coloboma See **Biemond syndrome**.

obfuscation (from Lat, to darken) 1. A darkening or obscuration of vision, as in the case of **amaurosis**. 2. Speech, the content of which clouds its purported meaning (if any).

object agnosia The inability of a subject to name or recognize an object by sight, due to lesions in the visual association areas.

objective tinnitus See **tinnitus**.

obligate grasp reflex See **palmar grasp reflex**. This should diminish between 3 and 6 months of age and disappear after 6 months; its persistence suggests corticospinal tract dysfunction.

oblique nystagmus See **circular nystagmus**.

oblongata crises Episodes of apnea and coma occurring in tertiary syphilis and resembling gastric crises, although their pathophysiology is unknown.[3836] They were first described by Dusser de Barenne in 1913.

obmutescence Loss of speech.

obnubilation (Lat, clouding) Clouding of consciousness.

O'Brien mucopolysaccharidosis See **mucopolysaccharidoses**.

obscuration 1. Transient dimming or blacking-out of vision, typically experienced by patients with papilledema due to increased intracranial pressure, or with heat in the case of preceding optic neuropathy. 2. Diminution (rather than extinction) of the perception of a stimulus applied to the side of the body or visual half-field opposite the side of a hemispheric lesion, such that the subject reports that the stimulus looks darker or feels weaker when presented at the same time as a similar stimulus given to the other side than when it is presented alone.[535]

obsessional slowness Significant slowness in preparation for the execution of a movement. This is commonly accompanied by stooped posture and such signs as a positive **glabellar tap** in the absence of the other typical signs of **Parkinson disease**. Cognitive difficulties, such as in shifting set and in spatial orientation, may also be detected by neuropsychological testing.[3068]

obstetrical paralysis 1. Any nerve or spinal cord injury suffered by the fetus during delivery. Brachial plexopathy (**Erb palsy** or **Klumpke palsy**) (for a recent review, see van Dijk et al., 2001)[6490] and spinal cord crush injury due to C3–4 fracture-dislocation sustained during breech delivery are examples. 2. Lumbosacral plexopathy suffered by the mother as a result of compression by the fetal head of the lumbosacral trunk (L4–5) and S1 root where they join and pass over the pelvic rim, or as a result of traction on the sciatic nerve or compression of the common peroneal nerve during a prolonged period in which the legs are held flexed in "stirrups" at the hip and knee. Small maternal size, a large fetus, midforceps rotation, and fetal malposition may place the mother at special risk of this nerve injury.[1978]

obstructive hydrocephalus Increased intracranial pressure with dilatation of the ventricles of the brain, as a result of obstruction to the flow of CSF anywhere between its site of origin in the ventricles and brain substance and the roof foramina of the fourth ventricle. See **noncommunicating hydrocephalus, communicating hydrocephalus**.

obstructive sleep apnea syndrome Cessation of airflow during sleep while thoraco-abdominal effort continues, as a consequence of narrowing and closure of the upper airway leading to (in order) oxygen desaturation, snorting or snoring, arousal, resaturation of blood oxygen, and a return to sleep. Sleep fragmentation, hypoxemia, and cardiac and hemodynamic alterations such as bradycardia, increased pulmonary arterial pressures, and cardiac arrhythmias result.

The clinical features include the complaint of excessive daytime sleepiness and the occurrence of loud nocturnal snoring followed by periods of silence, usually reported by the bed partner; enuresis; morning headaches; excessive movements in sleep; automatic behavior; poor memory; morning headaches; and intellectual deterioration. The condition is particularly common in overweight men. Polysomnographic monitoring demonstrates that more than five obstructive apneas lasting more than 10 s occur during each hour of sleep, accompanied by at least one of the following conditions: frequent arousals from sleep associated with the apneas, bradytachycardia, and arterial oxygen desaturation during the apneic episodes. See also **polysomnogram**.[3434]

obtundation (from Lat, blunting or dulling) A condition of mild to moderately reduced consciousness, the subject being rousable with verbal or slightly painful stimuli but tending to slip back into sleep after the stimuli cease.

obtundation status A long-lasting decrease in the level of consciousness in the context of **severe myoclonic epilepsy of infancy** (a variety of complex partial status epilepticus)[6490, 6592, 767]

obturator (from Lat, to stop up) The obturator foramen is more or less occluded by a fascial sheet; the obturator nerve derives its name by benefit of proximity.

obturator neuralgia (Howship–Romberg syndrome, obturator neuropathy) Constant pain in the distribution of the obturator nerve, felt in the groin and the medial aspect of the thigh, often with hypoesthesia in that region and weakness of the adductors and rotators of the hip, due to a lesion of the nerve as after hip replacement or damage to the nerve during labor,[3015] or as a result of infiltration of the nerve by a pelvic tumor.

obturator neuropathy See **obturator neuralgia**.

occasional seizure A seizure occurring only in response to provocation by a definable external or internal event. **Febrile convulsions** represent a form of occasional seizure in which the attack is precipitated by a rapid rise in body temperature.

occipital apoplexy Hemorrhage and hematoma formation in the occipital lobe as a result of bleeding from an **arteriovenous malformation**. Clinically, sudden intense headache and homonymous hemianopia are the major features.[6395]

occipital intermittent rhythmic delta activity Fairly regular or approximately sinusoidal waves, mostly occurring in bursts at 2–3 Hz over the occipital areas of one or both sides of the head and frequently blocked or attenuated by opening the eyes. (Adapted from the 1974 report of the Committee on Terminology, IFCN. In: Chatrian GE, Bergamini L, Dondey M, et al. A glossary of terms most commonly used by clinical electroencephalographers. *EEG Clin Neurophysiol* 1974;**37**:538–48 by kind permission.)

occipital lobe The paired posterior lobes of the brain, continuous with the parietal and temporal lobes anteriorly.

occipital lobe epilepsies Seizure syndromes usually presenting with visual hallucinations which indicate an occipital focus. They are usually characterized by simple focal and secondarily generalized seizures. Complex partial seizures may also occur when the discharge spreads beyond the occipital lobe. The clinical seizure manifestations usually, but not always, include visual manifestations. Elementary visual seizures are characterized by fleeting visual manifestations, which may be either negative (scotoma, hemianopia, amaurosis) or, more commonly, positive elementary visual hallucination (sparks or flashes, phosphenes). Such sensations appear in the visual field contralateral to the discharge in the specific visual cortex, but can spread to the entire visual field. Perceptive illusions, in which the objects appear to be distorted, may occur. Blindness and field defects, dizziness, and the epigastric aura are diminishingly less common.[3748]

The following varieties can be distinguished: a change in size (macropsia or micropsia) or a change in distance, an inclination of objects in a given plane of space and distortion of objects, or a sudden change of shape (metamorphopsia). Visual hallucinatory seizures are occasionally characterized by complex visual perceptions (e.g., colorful scenes of varying complexity). In some cases, the scene is distorted or made smaller, and, in rare instances, the subject sees his own image (**heautoscopy**). Such illusional and hallucinatory visual seizures result from an epileptic discharge in the temporoparieto–occipital junction.

The initial signs may also include tonic and/or clonic contraversion of the eyes and head or the eyes only (oculoclonic or oculogyric deviation), palpebral jerks, and forced closure of the eyelids. Sensations of ocular oscillation or of oscillations of the whole body may occur. The discharge may spread to the temporal lobe, producing seizure manifestations of either lateral temporal or mesial temporal seizures. When the primary focus is located in the supracalcarine area, the discharge can spread forward to the suprasylvian convexity or the mesial surface, mimicking those of parietal or frontal lobe seizures. Spread to the contralateral occipital lobe may be rapid. Occasionally the seizure becomes secondarily generalized. (After Dreifuss FE, et al. Commission for classification and terminology, ILAE. Proposal for Revised Classifications of Epilepsies and Epileptic syndromes. *Epilepsia* 1989;**30**:389–99 by kind permission of Wiley-Blackwell Publications).

Major causes are malformations of cortical development and vascular disorders, including epilepsy with bilateral occipital calcifications associated with celiac disease, and mitochondrial, metabolic, and idiopathic syndromes. The idiopathic occipital epilepsies comprise identifiable electroclinical syndromes of childhood and adolescence.[6237] The frequent association of occipital lobe seizures and migraine is complicated, controversial, and ill-defined.

Variant symptoms within the syndrome have been described.[3057, 3956]

occipital lobe epilepsy and intercalated migraine (benign focal epilepsy with occipital lobe spike waves, benign epilepsy with occipital paroxysms) A syndrome of childhood characterized by the sudden onset and resolution of visual disturbance accompanied by severe headache, nausea, and vomiting; the attacks are often followed by loss of consciousness, automatisms, or generalized seizure activity. The neurological examination and CT scan findings are normal, but the EEG shows continuous occipital or posterior temporal high-voltage slow-and-sharp wave EEG activity that is suppressed by eye opening.[72]

Gustave Flaubert, the French novelist, suffered from this condition, which has also been regarded as a type of **basilar artery migraine**.

occipital lobe partial epilepsy, occipital cortical and subcortical calcification, and celiac disease A recently described variant in which bilateral occipital calcification without physical signs, and in particular without evidence of **Sturge–Weber syndrome**, is associated with seizures and celiac disease.

occipital needle-sharp spikes An EEG pattern consisting of brief occipital spikes in visually impaired children, having but a weak association with clinical epileptic seizures.[3469]

occipital neuralgia A paroxysmal jabbing pain in the distribution of the greater or lesser occipital nerves or of the third occipital nerve, sometimes accompanied by diminished sensation or dysesthesias in the affected area. It is commonly associated with tenderness over the nerve concerned. The pain may mimic that of **thunderclap headache**. Diagnostic criteria have been defined:

A. Paroxysmal stabbing pain, with or without persistent aching between paroxysms, in the distribution(s) of the greater, lesser, and/or III occipital nerves
B. Tenderness over the affected nerve
C. Pain is eased temporarily by local anes thetic block of the nerve.

From the International Classification of Headache Disorders (Headache Classification Committee of the International Headache Society. *Cephalalgia* 2004;**24**[Suppl 1]) by kind permission of Dr. Jes Olesen, the International Headache Society, and Wiley-Blackwell Publications.

occipital spikes Repetitive spikes or sharp-and-slow wave EEG complexes recorded by occipital electrodes, mainly during eye closure.[4879]

occipitalization Synostosis of the atlas to the occiput, affecting the anterior or posterior arches, or lateral masses, or any or all of them.[5980] The term *assimilation* is best used when all the bony elements of the atlas are fused.

occipitofrontal circumference The circumference of the head when the tape measure lies upon the forehead and the occiput. A table of normal head circumferences for boys and girls has been prepared.[4613]

occiput The posterior part of the head, lying behind the posterior fontanelle.

occlusion (from Lat, to close up) Blockage of a hollow viscus; usually applied to pathological closure of an artery, but also referring to the covering of the eyes.

occult Secret, hidden, unknown, and undiscoverable.

occupational cervicobrachial disorder Functional and/or organic disturbances that result from neuromuscular fatigue due to work in a fixed position and/or to a repetitive movement of the upper extremities.[4012]

occupational cramp (occupational dystonias, craft palsies) A nonprogressive focal activity-specific dystonic syndrome presenting as muscle spasm or inability to execute a specific complex motor action by those who need to do so repetitively. Writers, pianists, bowlers (in cricket), telegraphists, violinists, and many others have been reported as afflicted.

Originally described by Kinnier Wilson[6819] and considered to be a central phenomenon, peripheral mechanisms may also be relevant.[4648]

occupational dystonias See **occupational cramps**.

occupational nystagmus See **miners' nystagmus**.

Ochsner, A.J. (b. 1896) American surgeon, professor at Tulane University, who with Dr. M. DeBakey suggested a link between cigarette smoking and lung cancer in 1941. The proof of this link was obtained by Sir Richard Doll in England nearly 20 years later.

Ochsner sign When the hands are clasped together, the index finger on the side of a high median nerve injury does not flex.

O'Connell test Straight leg raising is performed, first of the sound leg, next of the affected leg, and finally of both together. An increase in the permissible flexion of the affected hip when both hips are flexed together, compared with the angle of flexion obtainable when the affected leg is flexed alone, suggests the presence of root irritation.

If both hips are flexed to a point short of that which induces pain, and the sound leg is lowered, pain felt on the side of the affected leg further indicates the presence of root irritation.[1500]

ocular (from Lat, oculus) To do with the eyes.

ocular agitation See **restless eyes**.

ocular albinism An inherited deficiency of retinal and ocular pigment, accompanied usually by abnormalities in smooth pursuit and by nystagmus of various types.[1958] See also **oculocutaneous albinism**.

ocular and visual reflex The eyes of the newborn close under strong light.[6898] This observation appears somewhat trite. The author wonders whether the *failure* to close the eyes in strong light might be a more useful observation, as an indication either of impaired vision or of facial power.

ocular angina Periorbital pain due to ocular ischemia.

ocular apraxia A congenital syndrome of dyspraxic eye movements with callosal abnormalities.[1216] See **Cogan syndrome**.

A *variant* is ataxia-ocular apraxia 2, a recessively inherited ataxic syndrome mapped to 9q34 (encoding for *senataxine*). The ataxia has its onset in adolescence and is associated with an axonal sensorimotor neuropathy.

ocular bobbing A form of saccadic oscillation characterized by fast, repetitive, irregular, nonrhythmic, downward movements of both eyes, which return more slowly to the primary position. It is seen in patients with severe pontine dysfunction from any cause, who typically are unresponsive and have paralysis of horizontal lateral gaze. The initial phase of the eye movement is usually downward and fast, with a slower return to the primary position after a brief latent period. The condition was recognized and named by Fisher.[2082]

In *reverse ocular bobbing*, seen in pontine lesions and metabolic encephalopathy, the initial phase of the eyes' movement is fast upwards with a slow return to the mid position. With *inverse bobbing (ocular dipping)*, the primary eye movement is slow and downward, with a fast return to the mid position; anoxic encephalopathy is the usual cause.[2082, 4285] *Converse ocular bobbing* leads to a slow upward eye movement with a fast return to the mid position, and again is usually a result of pontine disease. Reports of *perverse* and *obverse bobbing* are eagerly awaited.

ocular counter-rolling A slight compensatory movement made reflexly by the eyes when the head is persistently tilted to the side. The receptors are in the otolithic organs.

ocular dipping (inverse ocular bobbing) Abnormal cyclic spontaneous eye movements along the vertical axis, usually seen in the course of coma due to anoxia or following seizures. The downward eye movement is slow and the upward return fast (the inverse appearance of ocular bobbing), and spontaneous roving horizontal eye movements are often noted. The responsible lesions are considered to be in the cortex and basal ganglia.[5378]

In *reversed ocular dipping* the primary movement is upward and slow. In this condition, metabolic encephalopathy is a more likely cause. See also **ocular bobbing**.

ocular dysmetria An inaccurate saccadic eye movement characterized by over- or undershooting at the end of a saccade which requires a correction to be made. The term is also employed to denote the presence of pathological ocular hypermetria.[1217] See also **dysmetric saccades, flutter dysmetria**.

ocular fibrillation See **psychogenic flutter**.

ocular flutter A brief run of spontaneous, intermittent, binocular horizontal ocular oscillations (repetitive saccadic oscillations) occurring during fixation on a point straight ahead or with re-fixation[266, 1217] without a saccadic interval. Damage to the pause cells in the brainstem is considered to be responsible. Ocular flutter may present as the first sign of **multiple sclerosis**.[2173] A unidirectional form has also been described.

Microflutter represents the same, but the movements are of high frequency and low amplitude and are only seen during ophthalmoscopy. It may not indicate disease.

Ocular dysmetria and other signs of cerebellar disease are usually associated. See also **oscillations**.

ocular hypertelorism See **Greig syndrome, hypertelorism**.

ocular ischemic syndrome (carotid artery syndrome) Acute ocular inflammation associated with decreased ocular perfusion as a result of carotid occlusive disease (usually atherosclerotic). Clinically, corneal edema, neovascularization of the iris or disk, clouding of the lens, venous stasis retinopathy, and central retinal artery occlusion are the usual presenting signs.[2952]

ocular leprosy Corneal ulceration (exposure keratitis) resulting from anesthesia caused by facial and trigeminal neuropathies in **leprosy**.

ocular microtremor A high-frequency, low-amplitude physiological tremor of the eyes at rest, due to excessive discharge of brainstem oculomotor mechanisms. The frequency of the microtremor is slowed with brainstem disease such as multiple sclerosis.[723]

ocular motor deviation Drift of an eye from the primary position to take up another position so that the two visual axes are no longer aligned. These may occur when only one eye is viewing (**phorias**) or during binocular vision (**tropias**). They are shown well by the **cover test** or, in the case of vertical deviations, by the **Bielschowsky head tilt test**.

ocular myoclonus (laryngeal nystagmus, lightning eye movements, pharyngeal nystagmus) A form of oscillation from the primary position of gaze, characterized by continuous, rhythmic, pendular, vertical oscillations of the eyes at 40–200 Hz, with dissociation between them, and unaffected by attempts to fixate, converge, or gaze.[6194] They are accompanied by slower (1–3 Hz) rhythmic movements of other branchial arch structures (**palatal myoclonus**) and of the trunk.

The condition is due to lesions of the dentatorubrothalamic pathway (Guillain–Mollaret triangle), especially the inferior olive, as after brainstem hemorrhage. See also **oscillations, square-wave jerks**.[3762]

Ocular myoclonus and **palatal myoclonus** can occur simultaneously, occasionally with similar myoclonus involving the pharyngeal and extraocular muscles, the diaphragm, neck, and (rarely) the shoulder muscles. The vascular, neoplastic, or inflammatory lesion is usually ipsilateral to the myoclonia, somewhere within the Guillain–Mollaret triangle. Unlike most other involuntary movements, this persists during sleep.

ocular myopathy A muscular dystrophy inherited variously, with onset in youth or adult life and characterized by slowly progressive weakness of the external ocular muscles producing ptosis and external ophthalmoplegia, and slowly progressive weakness of the face. In some cases, weakness of the bulbar and eventually of the limb girdle muscles also ensues. Patients with this condition manifest extreme sensitivity to curare. The commonest form is dominantly inherited. Ragged red fibers are frequently found on muscle biopsy specimens.

The condition was first reported by von **Graefe** in 1868.[6573] Further reports by **Gowers, Hutchinson, Möbius,** and others led to dispute as to whether the disease was primarily neurogenic or myopathic, but it has been concluded on balance that the latter is more often correct[3425] although both may be, because mitochondrial diseases have multiple effects. Variant forms are listed in Chart O–1.

Chart O–1. Variant Forms of Ocular Myopathy

A sporadic form with added *pigmentary retinal degeneration*.
Familial multicore disease with ophthalmoplegia.[6158]
Familial paralysis of horizontal gaze.
Familial static ophthalmoplegia.
Goldenhar–Gorlin syndrome (oculoauriculovertebral dysplasia) with congenital ophthalmoplegia.[117]
Kearns–Sayre syndrome.[3364]
Nemaline myopathy with cardiomyopathy.[4288]
Nemaline myopathy with ophthalmoplegia and mitochondrial abnormalities.
Neonatal ophthalmoplegia with microfibers.
Oculogastrointestinal muscular dystrophy See **familial visceral myopathy.** (Ionasescu, *V. Am J Med Genet*. 1983; 15:103–112)
Oculopharyngeal muscular dystrophy (usually autosomal dominant, sometimes recessive.)[3873]
Oculopharyngeal myopathy with distal myopathy, cardiomyopathy, and other varieties of **oculopharyngopdistal myopathy.**
Ophthalmoplegia and myopia with X-linked recessive inheritance.
Progressive ophthalmoplegia with mental retardation.

ocular neuromyotonia Intermittent spasm of some of the ocular muscles supplied by the III cranial nerve (rarely the IV of VI nerves), resulting in episodic diplopia due to noncomitant strabismus and **oscillopsia**, lasting up to half a minute, occurring either spontaneously or with sustained adduction of the affected eye, and sometimes painful. Almost all cases are unilateral.

The problem may occur following damage to the III nerve in the cavernous sinus,[5289] as after pituitary irradiation. See **neuromyotonia**.

ocular oscillation and truncal myoclonus See **opsoclonus**.

ocular quiver See **dynamic overshoot**.

ocular retraction syndrome (Stilling syndrome) Congenital paresis or deficiency of convergence with impaired abduction and sometimes adduction, and with retraction of the affected eye(s) into the orbit on attempts to adduct.[3021] See also **Duane syndrome**.

ocular shuddering See **psychogenic flutter**.

ocular tilt reaction A transient postural abnormality following unilateral labyrinthine damage, consisting of the triad of ipsilateral head tilt, conjugate ocular torsion, and skew deviation (ipsilateral eye lower) due to a unilateral otolithic lesion in the utricle or to a lesion of the mesencephalic tegmentum.[2702, 6737]

ocular torsion (cyclorotation) Abnormal position of the eyes in the roll plane (about the line of sight), occurring as a feature of a peripheral or central **ocular tilt reaction**.[1639]

ocular torticollis An abnormal head posture, adopted in order to minimize the effect of congenital nystagmus (by attaining the **null-point**), or that of paresis of oculomotor muscles (by turning the head in the direction of action of the paretic muscle).[5459]

ocular vertigo That form of vertigo which occurs only as a result of diplopia.

oculoacousticocerebral degeneration See **Norrie disease**.

oculoauriculocutaneous syndrome (Burns syndrome) A rare congenital syndrome characterized by ichthyosis (erythroderma), deafness, and keratitis.[950]

oculoauriculovertebral dysplasia (Goldenhar syndrome, Goldenhar–Gorlin syndrome, first and second branchial arch syndrome) Usually sporadic, but variably a dominant or a recessive syndrome; the main features include facial dysmorphism with auricular appendages and pretragal blind fistulas; hemivertebrae; visceral maldevelopments; epibulbar dermoid cysts, upper lid colobomas, microphthalmia, and strabismus; encephalocele; hydrocephalus; and macrostomia, microtia, and micrognathia due to asymmetrical cranial bone dysgenesis.

Cranial muscle hypoplasia (as may result from failure of development of the trigeminal nerve), conductive deafness, and cardiac defects may also occur, and many affected children are mentally retarded.[2445, 3113] Incomplete manifestations are common.[2503] See also **hemifacial microsomia**.

In a *variant* form, paralysis of various extraocular eye movements are described, as a result of hypoplasia or agenesis of the extraocular muscles or nerves.[117]

oculobuccogenital syndrome See **Behçet syndrome**.

oculocardiac reflex (Aschner cardiac phenomenon) A brainstem reflex mediated via the first division of the trigeminal nerve and the vagus such that ocular compression normal characteristically leads to vagally mediated increase in the R-R interval on the **EKG** such that the rate slows by 5–10 bpm. Subjects with **reflex anoxic seizures** characteristically show a much reduced latency in the first measurable R-R interval increase with 6 s or more of asystole. Painful stimulation of the skin of the neck may also induce this response as well as the **ciliospinal reflex**.

Bernard Aschner (b. 1883) was an Austrian gynecologist;[5619] his recognition of the sign is remarkable, unless he had become aware of the previous report by Dagnini.

oculocephalic reflex (doll's eye response, doll's head response, doll's eye movements, Puppenkopfphänomenon) Lateral deviation of the eyes (in parallel) in the direction opposite to that of sudden passive rotation of the neck. The reflex is normally present but inhibited after a few hundred milliseconds so that there is almost immediate restitution of the eyes to the primary position of gaze (straight ahead). In comatose patients, the restitution is seen late if the pathogenesis is diffuse cortical depression, not at all in cases of primary brainstem pathology, and asymmetrically if coma is due to, for example, a lesion producing an **uncal syndrome** and thus a III cranial nerve palsy.

Reflex upward deviation of the eyes with sudden neck flexion represents the same reflex, turned 90°. These may be the only vertical movements possible in patients with supranuclear or collicular lesions preventing voluntary upward gaze, and indicate that the infranuclear mechanisms for vertical gaze are intact. Absence of the movements in a comatose patient suggests a severe degree of brainstem damage or depression of function stemming from toxic causes.

In most dolls marketed today, only vertical movements are present, and then only in the more expensive ones. Even these typically show movements of the eyelids rather than of the eyes. Bielschowsky introduced the term in 1939, dolls with lateral eye movements perhaps then being more populous than they are today.[5328] See also **vestibulocerebral response**.

oculocerebellar tegmental syndrome A mesencephalic lacunar syndrome characterized by internuclear ophthalmoplegia, bilateral cerebellar ataxia, and contralateral hemiparesis.[5350]

oculocerebellomyoclonic syndrome The occurrence of rapid irregular movements of the eyes and limbs (**dancing eyes [dancing feet] syndrome**) in children with neuroblastoma.[4877]

oculocerebral hypopigmentation syndrome See **Cross oculocerebral syndrome**.

oculocerebral malformative syndrome See **Walker–Warburg syndrome**.

oculocerebrocutaneous syndrome A rare, dominantly inherited congenital dysmorphic syndrome, characterized by microphthalmia with orbital cysts, facial skin tags, cerebral atrophy, seizures, and mental delay.[1565]

oculocerebrofacial syndrome See **Kaufman syndrome**.

oculocerebrofacial-skeletal syndrome See **Pena–Shokeir phenotype**.

oculocerebrorenal syndrome (Lowe oculocerebroretinal syndrome) An X-linked recessive metabolic disorder manifesting cataract, glaucoma, rickets and osteomalacia, retardation of physical and mental development, and eventually renal failure.[3933] The main neurological features are craniosynostosis, pyramidal and lower motor neuron signs, nystagmus, **buphthalmos**, and seizures. Periodic metabolic acidosis with urinary excretion of organic acids and variable aminoaciduria are the usual chemical findings. The responsible gene maps to chromosome Xq24–q26 or Xq25.

Defective renal and intestinal aminoacid transport and disturbances in excretion of glycosaminoglycan may be the basis for the aminoaciduria and organic aciduria.

oculocraniosomatic dystrophy with ragged red fibers See **Kearns–Sayre syndrome, mitochondrial myopathies**.

oculocutaneous albinism 1. Type 1a (tyrosinase-negative), the classic X-linked recessive syndrome characterized by nystagmus, sensorineural deafness, hypopigmentation of the fundus, and cutaneous albinism (piebaldness).[5231]

2. Tyrosinase-positive oculocutaneous albinism is a recessively inherited condition mapped to 15q11–q13, in which the biosynthesis of melanin is reduced in the skin, hair, and eyes. It may complicate the **Prader–Willi** and **Angelman** syndromes, each involving deletions of chromosome 15q.

A *variant* is *oculocutaneous albinism with deafness* (Woolf syndrome).

oculocutaneous (Delleman) syndrome A disorder of the midbrain associated with congenital fibrosis of the extraocular muscles and other congenital anomalies of cranial nerve nuclear function caused by abnormal migration of the brainstem nuclear neurons or abnormalities of axonal pathway navigation.[405] See also **Harada disease**.

oculodentodigital syndrome A rare, dominantly inherited congenital disorder manifesting ocular and facial abnormalities, defects in tooth enamel, and type III syndactyly, occasionally with added spastic paraparesis. Its genetic basis is unknown.[4659]

oculodento-osseous dysplasia See **osteopetrosis**.

oculofacial paralysis See **Möbius syndrome**.

oculogastrointestinal muscular dystrophy See **familial visceral myopathy (mitochondrial neurogastrointestinal encephalomyopathy)**.

oculogyric crises Paroxysmal tonic or clonic contractions of the external ocular muscles deviating the eyes in any direction, but usually upward, and lasting seconds on each repeated occasion, preceded by an emotional upsurge and accompanied by an attentional disorder in which obsessive forced thinking occurs.

The episodes may be precipitated by psychical or sensory stimuli. They were first described in 1921 as complications of **encephalitis lethargica**, but now are more usually the result of poisoning by major tranquillizers.[3759]

oculogyric-auricular reflex

Retraction of the auricle and curling-back of the helix of the ear on far lateral gaze to the other side. Sometimes both auricles retract. The reflex is a curiosity of no known pathological significance.

oculomandibular dyscephaly with hypotrichosis

See **Hallerman–Streiff–François syndrome**.

oculomandibulofacial syndrome

See **Hallermann–Streiff–François syndrome**.

oculomasticatory myorhythmia

The association of continuous, rhythmic, pendular vergence oscillations of the eyes with synchronous jaw movements, at about 1 Hz, reported only in **Whipple disease**.[5677] Ocular pareses may also occur.

oculomotor and facial palsy

A syndrome of early adult life manifesting III, IV, V, and VI and/or VII cranial nerve palsies; diabetes; and red blood cell abnormalities.[381] The condition is probably a microangiopathy.

oculomotor apraxia

See **Cogan syndrome**.

oculomotor nerve

The III cranial nerve, which divides into two branches at the cavernous sinus. The superior branch supplies the superior rectus and levator palpebrae superioris, while the inferior branch supplies the medial and inferior recti and the inferior oblique muscles and carries the parasympathetic fibers to the pupil.

Causes of neurologically isolated, relative pupil-sparing III nerve palsy include compression by tumors or aneurysms and miscellaneous disorders such as diabetes, but sparing of pupillary function, once thought to indicate a noncompressive cause, can occur with compression as well, so neuroimaging for mass lesions is indicated in all patients.[18]

oculomotor psychoparalysis

See **Johnson syndrome**.

oculomotor synkinesis

Inappropriate elevation of the eyelid, movement of the eye, or changes in pupil size following remote damage to the III cranial nerve and presumed to be due to aberrant regeneration of its nerve fibers. The form occurring with slowly growing parasellar lesions is said to be *primary*; that occurring with acute acquired disorders of the nerve, such as trauma or aneurysmal compression, is termed *secondary*.

In *variant* forms, such synkineses occur without evidence of prior trauma, or in muscles innervated by both the superior and the inferior divisions of the nerve when only the former had been damaged, or bilaterally, or as a result of abnormal connections between the III and the VI cranial nerves.[5]

oculopalatal myoclonus

The combination of **palatal myoclonus** with jerky oblique and rotatory nystagmoid movements and sometimes with pendular oscillations. This is known as the *lateral form*. A *mid-line* form is characterized by vertical to-and-fro pendular eye movements with symmetrical bilateral palatal myoclonus.[4581]

oculopalatocerebral syndrome

A recessively inherited, congenital dysmorphic syndrome, characterized by short stature, microcephaly with cerebral atrophy, spasticity, mental retardation, conductive deafness, cleft palate, cloudy corneas, glaucoma, retinal phakomas, microphthalmia, and abnormalities of the vitreous.[2221] Cryptorchidism may also be present.

oculopharyngeal muscular dystrophy

(OMIM 164300) An unusual, dominantly inherited systemic myopathy affecting people of European descent in later life. Clinical features include ptosis, external ophthalmoplegia, upper facial weakness, dysphagia, and proximal lower leg weakness, but all voluntary muscles are affected eventually (although smooth and cardiac muscles are not). Muscle involvement is specific and symmetrical and involves, in order, the extraocular, tongue, diaphragm, pharynx, somatic, and limb muscles. The only characteristic diagnostic feature of the disease is the presence of rimmed vacuoles.[3873]

The condition is mapped to chromosome 14q11–2.q13, where there is a stable trinucleotide repeat expansion in exon 1 of the poly(A)-binding protein 2 gene (*PABP2*). It is a distinct disease entity although overlapping with **oculopharyngodistal myopathy.**

Morphological abnormalities of mitochondria are commonly detected on systemic muscle biopsy specimens, and the relationship of this condition to the **Kearns–Sayre syndrome** is close.[4559] Whether one regards this and **ocular myopathy** as the same or different conditions reflects more a frame of mind than a judgment based on scientific evidence.

Variants include a neurogenic form;[4174] a recessively inherited form; and *oculopharyngeal myopathy with distal myopathy and cardiomyopathy*, in which the usual features of slowly progressive ptosis, facial weakness, dysphagia, and atrophy are accompanied by distal weakness and cardiomyopathy with conduction system disorders. EMG suggests a myopathic disorder. Both familial and sporadic cases are described;[2517] see also **oculopharyngodistal muscular dystrophy.**

oculopharyngeal spinal muscular atrophy

A rare *variant* of **hereditary motor neuropathy**, type 3 in which the peripheral signs are accompanied by ophthalmoplegia and bulbar signs.[4174]

oculopharyngodistal muscular dystrophy (myopathy)

(OMIM 164310) An unusual dominantly or recessively inherited systemic myopathy of adult life, characterized by progressive ptosis and extraocular palsy with eventual weakness of the facial and bulbar muscles and distal limb weakness.[5557] See **Satoyoshi syndrome, oculopharyngeal dystrophy**.

In *variant* forms, the muscle involvement progresses distally and cardiomyopathy and platybasia are associated;[2517] or intestinal pseudo-obstruction complicates the disorder.[158]

oculoplethysmography

An investigational technique that indirectly assesses carotid blood flow (and thus the patency of the arterial lumen) by determining the amount of externally applied ocular pressure required to collapse the retinal arterioles and by recording the timing and amplitude of the pressure pulses in the eye occurring with each cardiac cycle. With the availability of **magnetic resonance arteriography**, the test is threatened with redundancy.

oculorenalcerebellar syndrome A recessively inherited syndrome characterized by pigmentary retinal degeneration with optic atrophy, pyramidal and cerebellar signs, nephropathy, mental and developmental delay, and progressive glomerulopathy.[4929, 3053]

oculosensory reflex Dilation of the pupil in response to painful stimulation of the eye or of adjacent structures; a **pain reflex** mediated by the sympathetic pathways. See **ciliospinal reflex**.

oculosympathetic palsy See **Horner syndrome**.

oculovestibular reflex Deviation of the eyes toward the side of cold stimulation of a lateral semicircular canal, with a fast correcting saccade in the opposite direction in the conscious healthy subject. If such nystagmus is not elicited but only a tonic deviation of the eyes to the irrigated side occurs, the brainstem may be considered to be intact, but freed from suprabulbar control. A dysconjugate response (or none at all) indicates the presence of serious brainstem damage. See **caloric tests, vestibuloocular reflex**.

oculus (Lat, an eye.) *Ocular* is thus derived).

odontoid (Gr, like a tooth. The Latin form is *dens*) The peg-like odontoid process of the axis which projects superiorly and is retained by the transverse ligament; it does not resemble a tooth very closely in form.

odontotrichomelic-tetramelic ectodermal dysplasia A congenital dysmorphic syndrome characterized also by abnormalities of the hair, skin, teeth, and skeleton, as well as by aminoaciduria and seizures.[4929]

oenomania (Gr, wine + madness) (oniomania) 1. Severe alcohol addiction; "A peculiar form of insanity excited by a drinking tendency." (Sir William **Gowers**) 2. A term for **delirium tremens**. 3. A compulsion to make purchases. See also **punding**.

Office of Rare Diseases A site providing information on more than 6,000 rare diseases, including current research, publications from scientific and medical journals, completed research, ongoing studies, and patient support groups. Web site: http://rarediseases.info.nih.gov/.

Oguchi syndrome A recessively inherited syndrome characterized by night blindness (hemeralopia), described in 1912 by Dr. C. Oguchi, a Japanese ophthalmologist, among others.

OHAHA syndrome A rare, recessive form of ophthalmoplegic migraine occurring in infancy and characterized by Ophthalmoplegia, Hypotonia, Ataxia, Hypacusis, and Athetosis, as well as any of a selection of focal neurological deficits such as hemiparesis, athetosis, chorea, nystagmus, and strabismus.[6862]

ohmmeter An instrument used to measure electrical resistance.

Ohtahara syndrome A rare, sporadic primary generalized seizure disorder occurring in infancy and characterized by burst suppression on the EEG.[4777] See **early infantile epileptic encephalopathy with suppression burst**.

OKT3 encephalopathy A syndrome of aseptic meningoencephalitis with obtundation, quadriparesis, and CT evidence of cerebral edema ascribed to the use of OKT3 (Muromonab-CD3), a murine immunoglobulin monoclonal antibody (IgG2a), and immunosuppressant drug.[1245]

Oldendorf, William H. (1925–1992) American neurologist, physicist, and physiologist who took the first conceptual and practical steps toward the realization of computerized tomographic scanning. For these insights, as well as for those regarding the nature of the blood–brain barrier, he was honored in the United States and abroad, though perhaps not to the extent that many thought appropriate. His book *A Quest for an Image of the Brain* is a classic in its time.

older-onset benign occipital epilepsy An epileptic syndrome with onset in childhood or youth, characterized by frequent seizures accompanies by visual hallucinations or occipital blindness in which the occipital lobe discharges on the EEG are blocked by visual fixation. The condition usually remits in the late teens.[4039]

olecranon reflex See **paradoxical triceps reflex**.

olfactogenital dysplasia See **Kallmann syndrome, de Morsier syndromes**.

olfactory groove meningioma See **meningioma**.

olfactory nerve The I cranial nerve in today's classification, proposed by Soemerring, although it was not included as such by Galen (who was actually right because the I and II "nerves" are invested with oligodendroglia and not Schwann cells, and so are properly regarded as extensions of the central rather than as parts of the peripheral nervous system).

The function of the nerves was recognized by Alessando Achillini (1463–1512), the Italian anatomist. The derivation is from Latin or Greek roots with the expected meaning.

olfactory reference syndrome The perception of (hallucinated) foul personal body odors by sensitive and obsessional depressed people, who thus exhibit secondary delusions that others are offended, indeed outraged, by their "smell" and whose contrite behavior includes excessive attention to self-cleanliness, self-isolation, and (in some cases) suicide.[5132]

Diagnostic criteria have been published but they do not emphasize depression

oligoastrocytoma See **oligodendroglioma**.

oligoclonal banding A technique of protein immunoelectrophoresis, commonly used on CSF samples, whereby bands of immunogammaglobulin G with different migratory characteristics can be demonstrated using appropriate staining.

Normally, a single broad area is present, but the finding of such bands suggests the diagnosis of any chronic inflammatory disease of the nervous system; **multiple sclerosis** is the classic example. The technique is also applicable to serum, and when bands are found in serum as well as in CSF samples, the usefulness of the test as a diagnostic aid in neurological disease is compromised.[6967]

oligodendroglia (Gr, few + branches + glue) Neuroglial cells of the supporting substance of the brain containing small oval nuclei and few fine processes. These are the myelin-forming cells of the CNS, and were first described by Rio del **Hortega** in 1921.

oligodendroglioma A form of primary infiltrative intracranial glioma, first described by Bailey and **Cushing** in 1926, with defined histological criteria.[3951] This usually well-differentiated malignant neuroectodermal tumor is composed of uniform small round cells with few fibrillary processes. It usually arises in the cerebral hemispheres of adults and is normally slow growing, though, in less common anaplastic forms (showing necrosis, vascular proliferation, high cellularity, and obvious mitotic activity), it is capable of diffuse invasion through the cortex and white matter. Positive staining for **glial fibrillary acidic protein** is usual.[6] *Oligoastrocytomas* are mixed gliomas in which a prominent astrocytic component accompanies the features of oligodendrogliomas just mentioned.

Clinically, the mean age at presentation is about 40 years. The sexes are equally affected, and clinical features such as headache, seizures, nausea, dementia, focal neurological signs, and increased intracranial pressure have often been present for some 5 years before the diagnosis is made. The tumor is most commonly sited in the frontal lobe, and causes frontal ataxia in a high proportion of patients; intracranial bleeding, stroke syndromes, and meningismus due to leptomeningeal spread are other notable characteristics. In children, seizures are the most common presenting features.[3951, 6786]

oligohydramnios syndrome See **Potter syndrome**.

oligophrenia, epilepsy, and ichthyosis syndrome See **Rud syndrome**. Rud's description was, however, translated inexactly, and it is not certain that he described the condition known by his name.[962]

oligosaccharidoses Inherited storage diseases of childhood, including **fucosidosis, mannosidosis,** and **aspartylglucosaminuria**.

olivary hypertrophy Enlargement of the inferior olivary nuclei as a result of transsynaptic degeneration following ischemic or other damage to the central tegmental tract, its principal afferent pathway.[36]

The classic clinical accompaniment is **palatal myoclonus**.

olivopontocerebellar atrophies (Déjèrine–Thomas syndrome, parenchymatous cortical cerebellar atrophy, late cortical cerebellar atrophy, Marie–Foix–Alajouanine syndrome, Thomas atrophy) A collective term embracing a heterogeneous group of neurodegenerative syndromes characterized by severe cerebellar ataxia and other complicating manifestations (dementia, Parkinsonism, cramps, pigmentary retinal degeneration, optic atrophy, myoclonus, spasticity, posterior column dysfunction, musculoskeletal deformities, etc.), tenuously united by the common finding of neuronal loss in the basis pontis, inferior olives, and cerebellar cortex.[541]

The conditions are usually either dominantly inherited, as described by Menzel (1891), or sporadic (Déjèrine and Thomas, 1900).[1545, 6272] A definitive synthesis and categorization was achieved by Konigsmark (1970), who defined five categories, but Harding[2753, 2754] fitted them equally neatly into the group of autosomal dominant **cerebellar ataxias** of late onset. Complicating this, however, is the fact that prion disorders, mitochondrial encephalomyopathies, and hereditary metabolic diseases may also present with these phenotypes.[542]

The classic *Menzel type* is dominantly inherited with onset in youth or adult life and with a course of between 4 and 10 years to death. Gait ataxia, limb ataxia, dysarthria, dysphagia, and various abnormal movements such as tics, chorea, and Parkinsonian features are sometimes recorded, as are the presence of bulbar palsies, internal and external ophthalmoplegias, pyramidal signs, and impairment of intellectual function.[1793] Posterior column dysfunction and demyelinating sensorimotor neuropathies have also been described. See also autosomal dominant **cerebellar ataxias, hereditary spastic paraparesis**. Transition from typical sporadic olivopontocerebellar atrophy into **multiple system atrophy** with autonomic failure and Parkinsonism has been recorded.[2386]

Variants are *olivopontocerebellar atrophy with velolaryngeal paralysis*, a cerebellar syndrome appearing in late life and complicated by bulbar palsy due to atrophy of the bulbar nuclei,[3698] and *olivopontocerebellar atrophy with liver cirrhosis and retinal dystrophy*.

The Web site http://www.ninds.nih.gov/disorders/opca/opca.htm provides further information from the National Institute of Neurological Disorders and Stroke.

olivorubrocerebellar atrophy See **Lejonne–Lhermitte disease**.

Ollier disease (enchondromatosis, dyschondroplasia) A chondrodysplasia with maximal effects within the long bones, but also a potential cause of optic nerve compression and of ophthalmoplegia.[1254, 4297]

Dr. L.X.E.L. Ollier (1830–1900) was a French surgeon. See also **Maffucci syndrome**.

Ollivier d'Angers, Charles-Philippe (1796–1845) French neurologist. His book on the spinal cord and its maladies was the first in this area upon its publication in 1824, when he was 28 years old. In it he described spina bifida, **diastematomyelia**, and both compression and atrophy of the cord. In the third edition (1837), he coined the term **syringomyelia** but did not note the **dissociated anesthesia**. He also gave an account of the clinical features of cases of **multiple sclerosis** (recording the deterioration of function with heat) and of **acute inflammatory demyelinating polyneuropathy** (reviewed by Spillane.[5978])

Ollivier disease Diffuse primary meningeal sarcomatosis.[596]

-oma The modern clinicopathological equivalent of the Galenic conception of "tumors against nature," a term introduced by Hooper in 1828.

Omenn syndrome See **familial erythrophagocytic lymphohistiocytosis**.

omnipause neurons Neurons receiving impulses from the frontal cortex and superior colliculus, which exert inhibitory influences on saccadic mechanisms on those occasions that saccades are not required.[5294]

Onanoff, Jacques (b. 1859) Franco-Russian physician who studied at the University of Paris, graduating in 1892. He published papers with Paul Blocq on the diagnosis of neurological disease, but is thenceforward lost to history; presumably he returned to Russia.

Onanoff reflex See **bulbocavernosus reflex**.[4795]

Onanism Strictly speaking, this refers to *coitus interruptus*, but the present meaning of the word is masturbation. "Judah commanded Onan, the son of Juda and the Canaanite Shua, to take Tamar, the widow of Er, in a leverite marriage. Onan withdrew during intercourse with Tamar and God slew him for this evil" (Genesis 38:8–10). The word was first employed by a profiteering surgeon, John Marten, who was the author of a work entitled *Onania, or the heinous sin of self-pollution, and its frightful consequences, in both sexes* (ca. 1710). A formerly, incorrectly cited author was a Dr. Bekkers, a clergyman turned quack but not an MD; he advertised secret pills (half-a-guinea a box) that were alleged to provide a remedy for masturbation, impotence and sterility. The Swiss physician **Tissot** took up the name in his antimasturbatory diatribe *L'Onanisme* (translated by Alexander Hume, 1781), their combined reputations coloring medical thought to the degree that the belief that masturbation leads to "debility of the brain and nervous system" is only just now disappearing.[5704] (I am grateful to Dr. Robert Daroff, MD for his assistance with this entry).

onchocerciasis (river blindness) A metazoal infestation endemic in many parts of West Africa, leading to optic atrophy and blindness. See **Guinea worm infestation**.

onco- (Gr, bulk) Prefix denoting bulk or mass.

oncocytoma A nonfunctioning pituitary neoplasm.

oncogene A group of genes with the power, when activated by unknown factors, to release cell systems from the ordinary constraints to multiplication and differentiation, thus stimulating normal cells to undergo malignant transformation.

oncosphere Developed embryos of parasites such as cysticercosis, as may lodge in muscle and brain.

Ondine's curse A rare congenital syndrome resulting from the primary failure of medullary automatic respiratory centers, leading to cessation of ventilation in sleep, almost permanent cyanosis, and eventually to hypoxic cerebral ischemia. Bulimia, central diabetes insipidus, or other evidence of hypothalamic disturbance may be associated in some cases. Insensitivity of the central chemoreceptors is held responsible for the failure in respiratory drive.[2112, 4294]

Severinghaus coined the name with reference to the unlikely story of Ondine (a water nymph in a novel of that name by Giraudoux), who punished her unfaithful mortal husband (Hans, a knight) by depriving him of the ability to perform all automatic functions—such as breathing while asleep.[5743] (I am grateful to Dr. Robert Daroff, MD for his assistance with this entry.)

In *variants* of the condition, Hirschsprung disease is associated; dysautonomic features are added; or it is acquired as a result of a medullary lesion in adults.

one-and-a-half syndrome A clinical disorder of extraocular movements characterized by ipsilateral horizontal conjugate gaze palsy (the "one") associated with **internuclear ophthalmoplegia** on contralateral gaze (the "half"). The lesion is in the dorsal tegmentum of the pons, affecting the VI nerve nucleus or the parapontine reticular formation (the "center" for lateral gaze) *and* the medial longitudinal fasciculus (leading to failure of adduction of the ipsilateral eye).[6605]

Brainstem infarction and **multiple sclerosis** are the commoner causes. The condition was so named by Miller Fisher in 1967.[2086]

oneirism (from Gr, dreaminess) The positive aspects of disordered consciousness, including hallucinations, terrifying fantasies, and intense emotional experiences.

oneirodynia (Gr, dream + pain) Unpleasant dreams.

oniomania See **oenomania**.

onion bulbs Superimposed reduplications of an axon's Schwann cell processes, with intermixed fibroblasts and collagen, leading to microscopical appearances that resemble the lamellations of an onion. This process occurs after repeated cycles of axonal swelling and regression with division of Schwann cells and the production of excessive amounts of myelin, which becomes redundant.

onion bulb neuropathy See **hereditary motor and sensory neuropathy**, type 3.

onion-peel sensory loss Facial anesthesia or hypoesthesia that is complete centrally, around the nose and mouth, but shades off peripherally, originally described by **Déjèrine** in 1914.[1540] It is seen in **tabes dorsalis** and with medullary lesions.

on–off effect The rapid alteration in motility (improving or worsening) shown by patients with Parkinson disease who are taking levadopa, as a result of rapidly changing levels of the drug in the brain. The off periods are frequently accompanied by depressive mood swings.[2749]

Online Mendelian Inheritance in Man An invaluable U.S. government professional genetics resource, updated daily. Web site: www.ncbi.nlm.nih.gov/omim/.

Online Neurology A list of resources in neurology and other medical specialties. Web site: http://www.emedicine.com/neuro/index.shtml.

onset frequency The lowest stable firing rate for a single motor unit action potential that can be voluntarily maintained by a subject.

ontogenesis (Gr, things which exist + origin) The process of development, from the ovum to the adult condition.

Opalski, Adam (1897–1963) Polish neurologist.

Opalski cells Large astrocytes with small, eccentric, pyknotic, densely staining nuclei displaced to the periphery, found in the cortical and subcortical regions of the brains of people with **Wilson disease** and **acquired hepatolenticular degeneration**.

Opalski syndrome (submedullary syndrome) An extended form of the **lateral medullary syndrome**, in which there are also homolateral pyramidal signs due to downward extension of the ischemic lesion into the upper part of the cervical cord, there damaging the corticospinal tract, which at that level has crossed to the side of the medullary lesion.[4797]

open opercular sign Bilateral wide enlargement of the Sylvian fissures, exposing the insulas, seen on CT scans of some children. A measurement of more than 3 mm between the caudal part of the frontal edge and the most rostral part of the temporal edge of the fissure is taken as abnormal.

The sign suggests that a patient's neurological impairment is due to arrested development,[6224] but it may also occur in other conditions and in normal infants.

open ring imaging sign Contrast enhancement of a brain lesion shaped as an open ring or as a crescent circumscribed to the white matter on MRI or CT imaging. The sign is reported to be highly specific for demyelination.[4136]

opercular seizures Seizures characterized by mastication, salivation, swallowing, laryngeal symptoms, speech arrest, epigastric aura, fear, and autonomic phenomena. Simple partial seizures, particularly partial clonic facial seizures, are common and may be ipsilateral. If secondary sensory changes occur, numbness may be a symptom, particularly in the hands. Gustatory hallucinations are particularly common in this area. (After Dreifuss FE, et al. Commission for classification and terminology, ILAE. Proposal for Revised Classifications of Epilepsies and Epileptic syndromes. *Epilepsia* 1989;**30**:389–99 by kind permission of Wiley-Blackwell Publications.)

operculum (Lat, a lid or cover) Those parts of the cortex of the frontal, parietal, and temporal lobes which cover the insula.

operculum syndrome See **anterior operculum syndrome**.

ophthalmia (Gr, disease of the eyes).

ophthalmic migraine See **migraine with aura**.

ophthalmodynamometry 1. The forerunner of **oculoplethysmography**, this test was designed to assess stenosis of the carotid artery by measuring blood pressure in the ophthalmic arteries by applying pressure to the globes using either a compression or suction apparatus; both diastolic and systolic blood pressures can be obtained. The technique is good at demonstrating but bad at excluding carotid disease.[4678] 2. Originally, the use of an instrument to measure the strength of ocular convergence. (Landolt)

ophthalmodynia Pain in the eyes.

ophthalmopathic hallucinations (syndrome of Charles **Bonnet**) Pure visual hallucinations associated with visual impairment resulting from disease of the ocular globes, optic nerves, or optic tracts.[2101]

ophthalmoplegia (Gr, eye + stroke) Paresis of eye movements. The many causes have been summarized.[544]

ophthalmoplegia, demyelinating neuropathy, leukoencephalopathy, myopathy, and gastrointestinal dysfunction See **mitochondrial encephalomyopathy**. See also MNGIE.

ophthalmoplegia, facial contraction, and progressive scoliosis A rare syndrome characterized by the onset in infancy of ophthalmoplegias, scoliosis, and myokymia.[381]

ophthalmoplegia interna Pupillary paralysis. The term was introduced by Jonathan **Hutchinson** in 1878. *Iridoplegia* is an alternative term.

ophthalmoplegia–ataxia See Nothnagel syndrome.

ophthalmoplegia–ataxia–areflexia syndrome See Miller Fisher syndrome.

ophthalmoplegia–hypotonia–ataxia–hypacusis–athetosis syndrome See OHAHA syndrome.

ophthalmoplegia-retinal degeneration See Barnard–Scholz syndrome.

ophthalmoplegic "migraine" A rare inflammatory cranial neuropathy mainly seen in children,, presenting with recurrent attacks of migrainous headache associated with paresis of one or more ocular cranial nerves (commonly the III nerve) in the absence of any demonstrable intracranial lesion other than MRI changes within the affected nerve. Clinical features include transient migraine-like headaches lasting hours to months, accompanied by painful and often long-lasting III, IV, or VI neuropathy and (if the oculomotor nerve is involved) pupillary abnormalities and ptosis. Symptoms almost always resolve, but after several episodes some deficits may persist. There is no demonstrable intracranial lesion.[3800]

Migraine-like headaches associated with total unilateral external ophthalmoplegia (with pupillary involvement) which outlasts the headache were first described by Paul **Möbius**[4420] in 1884. The criteria for the **superior orbital fissure syndrome**[2734] may also be satisfied by the features of ophthalmoplegic migraine. Diagnostic criteria have been defined:

A. At least two attacks fulfilling criterion B
B. Migraine-like headache accompanied or followed within 4 days of its onset by paresis of one or more of the III, IV, and/or VI cranial nerves
C. Parasellar, orbital fissure, and posterior fossa lesions ruled out by appropriate investigations.

MRI may show gadolinium uptake in the cisternal part of the affected cranial nerve, which suggests that the condition may be a recurrent demyelinating neuropathy. (From the International Classification of Headache Disorders [Headache Classification Committee of the International Headache Society. *Cephalalgia* 2004;**24**(Suppl 1)] by kind permission of Dr. Jes Olesen, the International Headache Society, and Wiley-Blackwell Publications.)

ophthalmoplegic neurolipidosis A congenital syndrome characterized by strabismus, an enlarged liver and spleen, seizures, ataxia, and trigeminal nerve abnormalities.[4929]

ophthalmoplegia plus The term of Drachman for cases of idiopathic progressive external ophthalmoplegia (PEO) occurring in association with any combination of retinal, brainstem, auditory system, vestibular system, hypothalamic, pyramidal, endocrine, cardiac, and/or muscular involvement.[1705]

In the same paper, Drachman noted reports of 14 different syndromes in which ophthalmoplegia had been described, and the overlapping features in many of them; he therefore questioned the utility of designating disease entities merely on the basis of their clinical presentation, and discussed principles of nosology of relevance when this is done.

The syndrome of PEO thus is heterogeneous, although the **Kearns–Sayre syndrome** has been separated out as showing a more-or-less constant association of signs, and a common etiology in the presence of mitochondrial disease appears at least possible.

ophthalmoscope A device for examining the interior of the eye, the observer's gaze running down the center of a beam of light angled by a mirror. The earliest instrument consisted merely of a tube that passed through a candle flame. It was invented by the English polymath Charles Babbage 4 years before Helmholtz in 1851 described the machine that, adapted and refined, is still in use today. The concept was enthusiastically adopted by Hughlings **Jackson** while working as an assistant to **Hutchinson** at Moorfields Eye Hospital in London.

opioid peptides (Gr, poppy juice + digest) Endogenous morphine-like oligopeptides having a role as modulators in the transmission and processing of pain information.

opisthotonos (Gr, stretched backward) Strong extensor muscular contractions occurring in the patient lying supine and leading to a bridge-like posture (Fr, *arc-en-cercle*), seen characteristically in the context of **rabies**, brainstem hemorrhage, posterior fossa tumor, meningitis, or encephalitis, but rather more commonly in dystonias or hysterical states. The phenomenon was called *dolor inflexibilis* by Pliny.

Opitz trigonocephaly syndrome See **C syndrome**.

Opitz–Frias syndrome (hypospadias–dysphagia syndrome) A congenital dysmorphic syndrome manifesting also hoarse voice and stridor due to bulbar weakness; congenital gastrointestinal, cardiac, and lung anomalies; hypospadias; and mental and developmental delay.[4798]

Oppenheim, Hermann (1859–1919) German neurologist and psychiatrist, initially assistant to **Westphal** in Berlin but not succeeding him as professor of neurology for political reasons.[2066] Both his private practice and his 1894 two-volume textbook of neurology were extremely successful.

Oppenheim is credited with introducing the term **dystonia musculorum deformans** (1911), and with realizing that this is an organic rather than a neurotic disease. He also related hyperreflexia and spasticity.

Oppenheim disease 1. (amyotonia congenita) Congenital muscle weakness and hypotonia with the potential for recovery. His report contained no pathological data and the nature of the condition is uncertain;[4802] it was probably **hereditary motor neuropathy** or **benign congenital hypotonia**, or both. 2. Dystonia musculorum deformans (Oppenheim–Ziehen disease). See **dystonia**. 3. (pseudo-tabes, Sternberg–Cushing–Oppenheim syndrome) Optic atrophy, pupillary disturbances, impotence, and loss of the knee and ankle reflexes in association with a pituitary neoplasm but considered by Oppenheim and others to resemble tabes dorsalis with respect to these clinical features.[4607]

Oppenheim–Ziehen disease See **dystonia**.

Oppenheimer reflex A variant of the **Babinski reflex** in which the hallux extends in response to a scratch on the inner side of the tibia or in response to firm finger pressure, sliding down the tibial spine.[4803]

opsoclonic meningoencephalitis (Kinsbourne–Warrington syndrome) See **opsoclonus–myoclonus syndrome**.

opsoclonus (lightning eye movements, ataxic conjugate movements, acute ocular oscillations, saccadomania, polymyoclonia, infantile polymyoclonia, ocular oscillations and truncal myoclonus, myoclonic encephalopathy of infancy). Ocular oscillations characterized by unpredictable, large-amplitude, irregular, rapid, involuntary, repetitive, multidirectional, and more or less conjugate saccades, which are increased by visual fixation and with eyelid closure but which occur both in the sleeping and waking states. Dysfunction of pontine pause cells is considered to be responsible, often increased.[5731]

Opsoclonus is one feature of a syndrome complicating viral infections characterized by myoclonus, cerebellar signs, **hyperekplexia**, and vomiting.[3443, 4877]. The underlying lesion of the dentate nucleus may thus be postinfectious, but it may also be associated with local or distant malignancies such as **neuroblastoma** or other malignancies with neural crest origin, and breast, lung, or uterine carcinoma. The anti-Ri antibody may be detectable in subjects with cancer, particularly cancer of the breast. See also **opsoclonus–myoclonus syndrome; oscillations**.

The word was introduced by Orzechowsky in 1913.[4819]

opsoclonus–myoclonus syndrome (sporadic myoclonic encephalopathy, opsoclonic meningoencephalitis, dancing eyes, dancing feet syndrome) A self-limiting syndrome characterized by **opsoclonus** with oscillopsia and myoclonus, mainly of the legs with ataxia, dysarthria, learning and behavioral disorders, and mental retardation.[5107] When occurring in the setting of **neuroblastoma** or of small cell or breast carcinoma in adults, it constitutes a **paraneoplastic syndrome**, but in as many cases the condition appears following a presumed viral infection and may be a postinfectious encephalopathy. See also **myoclonus**.

Opsoclonus Myoclonus Support Network, Inc. A charitable

organization in this field. Address: c/o 420 Montezuma Way, West Covina, CA 1791. E-mail: sandragreenberg@hotmail.com. Web site: http://www.geocities.com/opso-myoclonus/.

See also *Dancing Eye Syndrome Support Trust* (http://www.dancingeyes.org.uk/).

optacon An electronic device measuring the sensation of vibration on the fingertips.[236]

optic (Gr, relating to sight).

optic ataxia (misreaching) Severe impairment of visually guided movements, most evident when a patient tries to reach for an object, when his manual groping resembles that of a normal person whose sight is distorted by a prism.[726]

The condition was originally described in 1909 by Balint as occurring in the context of severe oculomotor impairment. The same problem resulting from parietal lobe disease was named *visual disorientation* by **Holmes**. The condition has been regarded as a disconnection syndrome between the visual and motor systems. See also **Balint syndrome**.

optic atrophy Demyelination of the optic nerve as a result of hereditary or acquired disease. The prototypical dominantly inherited syndrome has its onset in childhood or youth. The mild reduction in visual acuity and blue-yellow dyschromatopsia are unaccompanied by other evidence of neurological impairment. *Variant* syndromes are listed in Chart O–2.

optic chiasmal neuritis Inflammation of the optic chiasm with swelling, well shown on MRI scans and usually due to demyelinating disease.[4645]

optic disk drusen Hyaloid bodies situated in front of the lamina propria of the optic nerve head and sometimes visible within the optic disk, which appears swollen. Any associated field defects follow a nerve fiber-bundle pattern. Small hemorrhages on or beside the disk may be associated. Drusen become more prominent with age and may be inherited as an autosomal dominant characteristic.[3914] See **drusen**.

optic disk vasculitis See **papillophlebitis**.

optic fixation reflex Persistence of gaze directed upon an object despite passive rotation of the head. A sign suggesting the presence of a destructive frontal lobe lesion. Paresis of voluntary gaze may be associated.

optic myelitis See **neuromyelitis optica**.

optic nerve aplasia See **optic nerve hypoplasias**.

Chart O–2. Variant Syndromes of Optic Atrophy

Adrenoleukodystrophy

A *dominantly inherited juvenile form* (DOA) in which the visual defects are similar to those seen in patients with congenital tritan defects. It is characterized by retinal ganglion cell degeneration leading to optic neuropathy. A subset of DOA is caused by mutations in the *OPA1* gene, encoding for a dynamin-related GTPase required for mitochondrial fusion.[6950]

The following diagnostic criteria have been suggested by Smith;[5907]

A. Autosomal dominant inheritance.
B. Insidious onset between 4 and 8 years.
C. Moderately reduced visual acuity to 6/20–6/60.
D. Temporal pallor of the optic disks.
E. Centrocecal enlargement of the blind spot.
F. Full peripheral fields in response to white.
G. Inverted peripheral fields in response to colors.
H. Acquired blue-yellow dyschromatopsia.

Mitochondrionopathy A dominantly inherited form presenting with visual failure and optic atrophy in childhood, followed by progressive external ophthalmoplegia, ataxia, deafness, and a sensorimotor polyneuropathy in adult life.[3031]

Conditions in which optic atrophy is part of a more widespread neurological disorder, including **Friedreich ataxia, late-onset cerebellar ataxias, hereditary motor and sensory neuropathy** (HMSN Type 6), and conditions characterized by **osteopetrosis**.[5408]

Early infantile recessive optic atrophy A rare recessive form characterized by severe but nonprogressive visual impairment with nystagmus and severe dyschromatopsia seldom discovered before the fourth year of life. The electroretinogram is normal. A similar *dominant form* is also described.[3468]

Familial bilateral optic nerve hypoplasia A rare association, reported both sporadically and with dominant or recessive inheritance.[379]

Leber optic atrophy, which is either an X-linked condition or a **mitochondrial cytopathy**.

Optic atrophy and tritanopia A rare association.[3565]

Optic atrophy-ataxia syndrome See **Behr syndrome**.

Optic atrophy, congenital cataract, and ataxia A congenital syndrome characterized by cataract, optic atrophy, cerebellar ataxia, and extrapyramidal signs.[2274]

Optic atrophy, deafness, and sensory ataxia A syndrome with the onset in childhood of nerve deafness, optic atrophy, and cerebellar ataxia.[3209] Optic atrophy may also occur as a dominant trait in association with deafness alone.[3526]

Optic atrophy, diabetes mellitus, and diabetes insipidus (Wolfram syndrome)

The rare combination of these disorders as a recessively inherited disorder, sometimes accompanied by nerve deafness, and with onset in childhood. The condition is progressive, and leads to severe reduction in visual acuity and dyschromatopsia. The association has been reviewed by Baraitser.[379]

Optic atrophy with spastic paraparesis An X-linked syndrome with the onset in childhood of optic atrophy, speech defects, scoliosis, pectus excavatum, ophthalmoplegias, VII cranial nerve and bulbar palsies, pyramidal and cerebellar signs, athetosis, neurogenic muscle atrophy, and loss of pain and touch sensation.[3964]

optic nerve dysplasia See **coloboma, morning glory syndrome, optic pits, optic nerve hypoplasia**.

optic nerve gliomas A heterogeneous collection of primary malignant tumors of the optic nerve. Their clinical expressions include visual failure, visual field defects, optic atrophy, papilledema, and evidence of hypothalamic or other local infiltration, including increased intracranial pressure.[154] The optic canal is characteristically enlarged. The features of **neurofibromatosis** are present in half of the children affected. The tumors are substantially less common and more malignant (glioblastoma) in adults.

optic nerve hypoplasia (micropapilla, partial optic aplasia, optic nerve aplasia, optic nerve dysplasia) A rare, sometimes dominantly inherited reduction in the number of axons in an optic nerve with a consequent reduction in the area of the optic nerve head, giving a horizontal optic disk diameter of less than 3.4 mm.

The causes of this abnormality are many and involve the eyes, the nervous system, or other systems; various malformations may be associated, especially when the hypoplasia is bilateral. The usual clinical presentation is of an **altitudinal field defect**, but visual acuity may be normal.[4623] Astigmatism and nystagmus may be associated.

optic neuritis (optic neuropathy) Inflammation of the optic nerve as a result of any of numerous etiologies. Clinically, the syndrome presents most commonly in young women who present with rapidly progressive (over a day or so), unilateral loss of central vision revealed by perimetry, ocular pain on movement of the eyes, tender globes, and homolateral head pain. A central or centrocecal scotoma is demonstrable and acuity (especially to color and contrast) is almost always much decreased. A relative afferent pupillary defect will be present in unilateral or asymmetric optic neuropathies. Papillitis and flame hemorrhages are commonly seen when the inflammation is anterior, but the fundi appear normal with retrobulbar neuritis. In a third of the cases, swelling of the optic head is visible. The **Uhthoff phenomenon** is usually present.

Visual function generally spontaneously improves over weeks, and 95% of patients attain a visual acuity of at least 20/40 within a year. Initial magnetic resonance imaging helps to stratify the risk of multiple sclerosis in patients with acute isolated optic neuritis.[287] Optic disc pallor will be apparent at least 4 weeks after the onset.

Bilateral involvement is etiologically and prognostically diverse, but children do not seem to develop **multiple sclerosis**, although some adults do at a rate which is not agreed upon by any two authors and which ranges between 13 and 85%, varying with the duration of follow-up. Whether optic neuritis not obviously due to another cause is a *forme fruste* of multiple sclerosis or is a separate entity is not agreed upon either.[1800, 3614]

A *variant* is *chronic relapsing inflammatory optic neuropathy*, a steroid-responsive inflammatory form which is frequently bilateral and often painful, characterized by relapses and remissions. MRI scans of the brain are normal, but those of the optic nerves often show enhancing high signal abnormalities. The syndrome behaves like granulomatous optic neuropathy but without evidence of sarcoidosis.[3418] See also **ischemic optic neuropathy**,[564] **papilledema, relative afferent pupillary defect**, and the private patient-based Web site http://www.mult-sclerosis.org/opticneuritis.html.

optic neuropathy Disease of the optic nerve(s). See **optic neuritis; Cuban optic neuropathy; Leber hereditary optic neuropathy; multiple sclerosis**.

optic nystagmus See **optokinetic nystagmus**.

optic pits A congenital optic disk dysplasia characterized by depression of the disk margin on the temporal side with nerve fiber loss, causing arcuate field defects and enlargement of the blind spot.[888]

optical apraxia Impairment in performing saccadic eye movements on command[3540]. Impairment of hand–eye coordination results, although patients affected may perform such tasks as the finger-nose test better with the eyes closed than with them open. The condition is a feature of **Balint syndrome**. See **apraxia**.

optical coherence tomography A noninvasive diagnostic tool measuring the thickness of the retinal nerve fiber layer (NFL) using low-coherence light. The images produce high-resolution cross-sectional images of the retina. In **multiple sclerosis** a reduction in NFL thickness has been used to assess overall neuronal loss because the thickness of the retinal NFL correlates with the volume of CSF and with the amount of parenchyma making up the total brain volume.

opticocentral syndrome See **opticocerebral syndrome**.

opticocerebral syndrome (opticopyramidal syndrome) A syndrome of simultaneous optic nerve and watershed cerebral infarctions, usually with occlusion of the ipsilateral internal carotid artery and reversal of flow in the ophthalmic artery.[715, 716]

opticocochleodentate degeneration (Nyssen–van Bogaert syndrome) A congenital dysmorphic syndrome, characterized also by sensorineural deafness, optic atrophy, skeletal deformities, cerebral atrophy with seizures and pyramidal signs, and mental and developmental delay.[4543]

opticofacial reflex See **orbicularis oculi reflex**.

opticoopyramidal syndrome See **opticocerebral syndrome**.

opticospinal multiple sclerosis An uncertain entity because it does not share the biomarker for **neuromyelitis optica** but otherwise behaves in the same way.

optokinetic after-induced nystagmus (reverse postoptokinetic nystagmus). A physiological, brief reversal of the direction of nystagmus occurring after normal optokinetic nystagmus has been elicited.

optokinetic inversion A sign seen in **congenital nystagmus**; when the subject watches a rotating drum, the quick phase is the same direction as the motion of the drum.[5731]

optokinetic nystagmus (railway nystagmus, elevator nystagmus, kinetic nystagmus, optomotor nystagmus, optic nystagmus, panoramic nystagmus, sigma nystagmus or train nystagmus, optokinetic after-induced nystagmus) A physiological form of reflex horizontal or vertical nystagmus induced by fixation on a series of moving visual targets in the environment.

The *subcortical* or *field* type requires stimulation of most of the visual field and is followed by an after-nystagmus; it is impaired by brainstem or labyrinthine lesions. The *cortical* or *object* type resembles visual smooth-pursuit tracking, is not succeeded by an after-nystagmus, and is impaired with posterior cortical lesions.

With routine clinical testing, employing a striped tape, the optokinetic response is normally symmetrical in both directions. In the presence of a frontal lobe lesion, the patient's eyes tend to drift slightly and slowly in the direction of tape movement. In the setting of parietal lesions, the response is lost when the object moves in the direction of the diseased lobe. There is a dissociated response in **internuclear ophthalmoplegia**.

The test was introduced as a clinical tool by Bárány in 1921, although the phenomenon was noted by **Purkinje**, among onlookers during a cavalry parade in 1825. A very complete review is that of David.[1477]

optomotor nystagmus See **optokinetic nystagmus**.

oral dysesthesias See **burning mouth syndrome**.

oral reflex See **buccal reflex, orbicularis oris reflex**.

oralbuccal apraxia (pseudoplegia, aphemia, diplegia with dissociation) A term denoting the dissociation of voluntary and emotional movements, such as those of the face, jaws, throat, and larynx in the **anterior operculum syndrome**.[4053]

oralfacialdigital syndrome (Mohr Syndrome) See **orofaciodigital syndrome**.

orbi- Gr, A sphere.

orbicularis oculi reflex (naso-palpebral reflex, blink reflex, McCarthy reflex, supraorbital reflex, frontal reflex, trigeminofacial reflex, glabellar reflex, Meyerson sign)

Bilateral contraction of the orbicularis oculi and relaxation of the levator palpebrae superioris in response to visual, auditory, or tactile stimuli, the latter causing vibration in the muscle. It is tested clinically by tapping over the forehead as far back as the hairline (blink reflex), or by stretching the muscle itself by tapping the examiner's thumb which, with the index finger, is drawing back a fold of skin at the lateral angle of the patient's eye. Normally a single blink is elicited in response to each of the first five or so repetitive taps, the reflex fatiguing thereafter. In patients with diffuse cerebral cortical dysfunction, either acute (delirium) or chronic (dementia), the blinking persists.

The reflex was first described by Overend in England in 1896 and further by McCarthy 5 years later. It is unique by virtue of the number of types of stimuli that induce it, and its low threshold, enhancing thus its efficiency in protecting the cornea. It is enhanced in the presence of upper motor neuron facial weakness and Parkinsonism.[6656] See also **glabellar tap**.

orbicularis oris reflex (oral reflex, buccal reflex, nasomental reflex) Contraction of the levator muscles of the angle of the mouth when the upper lip or the side of the nose are percussed. The mentalis may also contract, adding wrinkling of the chin to the above signs.

The reflex is lost after the first year of life, but reappears in subjects with bilateral corticobulbar tract lesions and in those with parkinsonism.[6656] See **perioral reflex**.

orbicularis sign The patient is unable to close the eye on the paretic side without closing the other eye as well.[5333]

orbit (Lat, a track or circuit) Applied to the bony eye socket sometime in the Middle Ages.[5886]

orbital apex syndrome See **superior orbital fissure syndrome**.

orbital blowout fracture See **blowout fracture**.

orbital cysts and cerebral malformation See Determan **syndrome**.

orbital fibrositis See **orbital pseudotumor syndrome**.

orbital fissure syndromes See **orbital apex syndrome, superior orbital fissure syndrome, Foix syndrome, Jacod syndrome**, and **pseudotumor orbiti**.

orbital floor syndrome See **Dejean syndrome**.

orbital hypertelorism See **hypertelorism**.

orbital lipogranuloma See **orbital pseudotumor syndrome**.

orbital lymphomatosis See **orbital pseudotumor syndrome**.

orbital myositis Acute, persistent, painful focal inflammation of one or more extraocular muscles in adolescents or young adults, leading to ophthalmoplegias, redness of the eye, and chemosis without proptosis, but with a normal orbital CT image (thus differentiating the condition from the myositis of hyperthyroidism).[5997] See **orbital pseudotumor syndrome.**

orbital periostitis See **orbital pseudotumor syndrome**.

orbital pseudotumor syndrome (pseudotumor orbiti, orbital myositis, orbital periostitis, pseudoblastoma, orbital lymphomatosis, periostitis or fibrositis, granulome bizarre de l'orbite, chronic dacryo-adenitis, fibromatosis of the optic nerve sheath, superior orbital fissure syndrome, syndrome of Rochon-Duvigneau, orbital lipogranuloma, nonspecific granuloma of the orbit, Tolosa–Hunt syndrome, painful ophthalmoplegia) Mass lesions of the orbit not due to common inflammations, specific granulomas, simple vascular lesions, hematomas, neoplasms nor lymphomas, nor to endocrine exophthalmos, but in which there is edema and cellular infiltration of the orbital contents.

The condition usually presents with malaise, unilateral ocular pain, visual loss, and proptosis, usually of one eye, and frequently there is evidence of a trigeminal sensory disturbance. The course is remitting, progressive, or chronic and the pathogenesis autoimmune.[3186] See also **superior orbital fissure syndrome.**[3815]

orbital teratoma See **dermoid cyst**.

orbitofrontal seizures Complex "partial" seizures with initial motor and gestural automatisms, olfactory hallucinations and illusions, and autonomic signs. (After Dreifuss FE, et al. Commission for classification and terminology, ILAE. Proposal for Revised Classifications of

Epilepsies and Epileptic syndromes. *Epilepsia* 1989;30:389–99 by kind permission of Wiley-Blackwell Publications).

orbitofrontal syndrome
A behavioral pattern that may occur following injury to the frontal lobe. It is characterized by emotional lability, distractibility, disinhibition with impulsive behaviors, inappropriate jocular affect or euphoria, and poor insight and judgment.[6388]

order of activation The sequence of appearance of different motor unit action potentials with increasing strength of voluntary contraction. See **recruitment**. (From the 2001 Report of the Nomenclature Committee of the American Association of Electromyography and Electrodiagnosis.[19] Reproduced by kind permission of the AANEM.)

ordinary headache See **episodic tension-type headache**.

orexins (hypocretins) Excitatory neuropeptide transmitters found only in the lateral hypothalamus. They are relevant in control of sleep, arousal, and energy metabolism. Mutations of their genes are associated with narcolepsy in animal models and the ligand is likely to be defective in human **narcolepsy**.[4680, 447]

organic acidemia (organic aciduria)
Inborn errors of metabolism characterized by the presence of organic acids in the blood. Clinically, the presentations are similar: Failure to thrive in infancy, hypotonia, vomiting, hypoglycemia, seizures, and eventual coma are the common features. In some cases, psychomotor arrest occurs.[813]

Conditions of neurological importance are **proprionic acidemia, methylmalonic aciduria, isovaleric acidemia, betamethylcrotonylglycinuria, glutaric aciduria** type 1, **glutathione synthetase deficiency, maple syrup urine disease, multiple carboxylase deficiency**. See also **hyperammonemias**.

Biotin-unresponsive 3-methylcrotonyl-CoA carboxylase deficiency, 3-hydroxy-3-methylglutaryl-CoA (HMG-CoA) lyase deficiency, and ketothiolase deficiency are other organic acidemias. See also the comprehensive review of Seashore, MR at the Web site: http://www.ncbi.nlm.nih.gov/bookshelf/br.fcgi?book=gene&part=oa-overview.

Organic Acidemia Association
A charitable organization. Tel: 612-559-1797. E-mail: oaanews@aol.com. Web site: http://www.kumc.edu/gec/support/organic.html.

organic aciduria See **organic acidemia**.

organic brain syndrome
A euphemism for "a chemical or structural brain disease producing delirium or dementia." The only justification for its use is induced compliance with the dictates of expert professional committees.

organic dementias Those dementing illnesses associated with the presence of morphological alterations in the brain.

organic emotionalism See **emotionalism**.

organic mental syndromes
Disorders affecting cognition or other aspects of mentation. They have been grouped into six categories by the American Psychiatric Association[171] (Chart O–3).

Such a listing is of some value, but one wonders what the underlying cause could be for any single psychological manifestation (other than a maladaptive effect of learning) if it is not based on some "organic" malfunction.

organic mercury cerebellar degeneration See **Minamata disease**.

organization 1. The degree to which physiological EEG rhythms conform to certain hypothesized ideal characteristics displayed by a proportion of subjects in the same age group, free from a personal and family history of neurological and psychiatric diseases, and free also from other illnesses that might be associated with dysfunction of the brain.

2. The organization of physiological EEG rhythms progresses from birth to adulthood. Poor organization of such EEG rhythms as the alpha rhythm does not necessarily imply abnormality. (Adapted from the 1974 report of the Committee on Terminology, IFCN. In: Chatrian GE, Bergamini L, Dondey M, et al. A glossary of terms most commonly used by clinical electroencephalographers. *EEG Clin Neurophysiol* 1974;37:538–48.)

organoid nevus syndrome
A disorder of neuroectodermal proliferation characterized by unilateral facial linear sebaceous nevi and neurological manifestations such as asymmetrical macrocephaly, hemiparesis, seizures, cognitive impairment, developmental delay, and focal or lateralized EEG abnormalities of the hypsarrhythmia or Lennox–Gastaut types, all appearing and progressing after birth.[1187]

orgasmic epilepsy Nocturnal somatosensory seizures arising from a central parietal focus and leading to complaints (?) of orgasm.[982]

Chart O–3. Categories of Organic Mental Syndrome

1. **Delirium** and **dementia**, in which cognitive impairment is relatively global (and in which the underlying organic [structural or biochemical] lesion can be ascertained)
2. **Amnestic syndrome** and organic hallucinosis, in which selective areas of cognition are impaired
3. *Organic delusional, mood, and anxiety syndromes*, which have features resembling schizophrenia, as well as mood and anxiety disorders. (However, the morphological or chemical bases of such conditions are seldom known and their organicity sometimes is only inferred.)
4. *Organic personality syndrome*, in which the personality is affected
5. *Intoxication and withdrawal*, in which the disorder is associated with the ingestion of or reduction in use of a psychoactive substance and does not fulfill the criteria for any of the previous syndromes. (Strictly speaking, these two organic mental syndromes are etiologically rather than descriptively defined.)
6. *Organic mental syndrome not otherwise specified*, a residual category for any other organic mental syndrome not classifiable above.

orgasmic headache See **headache associated with sexual activity**.

Orgogozo Scale A simple, brief, and rather reliable method of estimating the impairments suffered by patients with stroke (see Chart O–4).[4809] See also **stroke scales**.

orientation (Fr, to determine the East) Thus to position oneself in space and, by extension, with relation to other people, places, structures, or events.

Chart O–4. The Orgogozo Scale

Consciousness

15 Normal; awake and responsive to stimuli
10 Drowsiness; can be woken to remain awake through examination
5 Stupor; localizes and responds to painful stimuli
0 Coma; nonpurposeful response to painful stimuli

Verbal Communication

10 Normal/not restricted; can sustain informative conversation
5 Difficult; limited to essential ideas, dysarthria included
0 Extremely difficult/impossible; for any reason

Eyes and Headshift

10 Normal symmetrical horizontal eye movements
5 Gaze failure/unilateral neglect; gaze restricted on one side
0 Forced/tonic deviation; unable to gaze beyond midline

Facial Movements

5 Normal/slight weakness; only minimal asymmetry at most
0 Paralysis, or marked paresis

Arm Raising

10 Possible; can raise above horizontal against some resistance
5 Incomplete; only against gravity, not horizontally
0 Impossible; arm abduction impossible

Hand Movements

15 Normal; no disability
10 Skilled; restriction of fine movements, slow/clumsy use
5 Useful; gross movements possible, can hold a walking stick
0 Useless; cannot hold or carry objects even if the hand moves

Arm Tone

5 Normal/near normal
0 Severe spasticity or flaccidity

Leg Raising

15 Normal; can be elevated from bed almost as other side
10 Possible against resistance; can be elevated, but weak
5 Possible against gravity; not against resistance
0 Impossible; cannot be lifted off bed

Foot Dorsiflexion

10 Possible against resistance; even if weaker than normal
5 Possible against gravity; can raise tip of foot off floor
0 Foot drop; active dorsiflexion impossible

Leg Tone

5 Normal/near normal
0 Overt spasticity or flaccidity

Total (out of 100)

(From Orgogozo JM. Evaluation of treatments in ischemic stroke patients. In Amery WK, Bousser MG, Rose FC, eds. Clinical Trial methodology in Stroke. *London: Baillière Tindall; 1989, 35–53, reproduced by kind permission of Prof. Orgogozo.)*

Orientation Memory Concentration Test A brief screening test of cognitive functioning pre-dating the **Addenbrookes Cognitive evaluation, MMSE, 3MS,** and **IMC** tests.

The items used are:

What year is it now? What month is it now?
Repeat this address: Arthur/Jones/42/ West Street/Witney **OR**
Philip/Smith/ 92/Columbia Road/ Banbury
About what time is it? (within 1 h)
Count backwards 20 to 1
Say the months in reverse order
Repeat the address given.

ornithinemia See HHH **syndrome**.

ornithine transcarbylamase deficiency (OTC deficiency) A congenital intermittent ataxic syndrome (Xp21.2) inherited as an X-linked dominant trait and characterized by the accumulation of circulating neurotoxins, hyperammonemia, low levels of citrulline and orotic aciduria, due to deficiency of OTC, a mitochondrial urea cycle enzyme. Urinary orotic acid levels are high; blood levels of glutamine and alanine are high, but citrulline, arginine, and arginino-succinic acid levels are low or normal.[989, 442, 3843] The responsible gene maps to chromosome Xp21.1.

Clinically, lethargy, ataxia, vomiting, migraine-like headaches, ptosis, dysarthria, involuntary movements, seizures, and confusion occur from early infancy, with liver failure precipitated by dietary protein and fever. The children are mentally retarded. Cerebral atrophy and edema are noted terminally.

In a *variant* incomplete form, similar features do not present until later childhood and with a partial enzyme defect they may not occur until adult life.

ornithosis See **psittacosis**.

oroalimentary automatism In the context of epilepsy, the occurrence of lip smacking, lip pursing, chewing, licking, tooth grinding, or swallowing, suggesting a mesial temporal lobe focus.

orobuccolingual dyskinesia (orofacial dyskinesia) The occurrence of complex and often asymmetrical facial, oral, and lingual contortions including grimaces, tongue protrusion, licking movements, mouth opening, and vocalization.[2281] The movements may represent a form of **tardive dyskinesia**, may occur spontaneously in the edentulous aged, and may occur in the context of various structural disorders of the basal ganglia.[152]

orofacial apraxia Impairment in performing mouth or face actions on verbal command or imitation.[3540] See **apraxia, buccofacial apraxia**.

orofacial dyskinesia See **orobuccolingual dyskinesia**.

orofaciodigital dysostosis See **orofaciodigital syndrome** (I).

orofaciodigital syndrome Inherited dysmorphic syndromes of three (rather similar) kinds (Chart O–5).

orolingual tardive dyskinesia A form of **tardive dyskinesia** in which there is involvement of the mouth and tongue.[2281]

orolingual tremor A rhythmic, involuntary oscillatory movement of the jaw, tongue, pharynx, and/or lower face occurring predominantly at rest or during jaw activation.[5837]

orolingual-buccal dystonia An unusual movement disorder in which there are persistent involuntary movements of the lower face, mouth, and tongue, particularly, including forceful extrusion of the tongue. Secondary or "heredo-degenerative" dystonias are the most likely cause.[5627]

oromandibular dysfunction A collective term for abnormalities of dental occlusion and of the temporomandibular joints, which involves **bruxism**. See also **temporomandibular pain and dysfunction syndrome**.

oromandibular dystonia (Meige syndrome) A form of focal uni- or bilateral dystonia of unknown cause in which repetitive, strong spasmodic contractions affect the masticatory muscles and thus the mouth, jaw, and tongue. Jaw-opening and jaw-closing forms are described.[6303, 6198] **Meige syndrome** is the same but with added blepharospasm. See also **Breughel syndrome**.

oropharyngeal palsy See **Miller Fisher syndrome**.

Oroya fever (Carrion disease, bartonellosis, verruga peruana, sitki) An infectious disease caused by *Bartonella bacilliformis* and transmitted by the bite of sandflies. Hemolytic anemia with vasculitis, disseminated hemorrhages, and meningoencephalitis are the major features. Clinically, these lead to acute fever, headache, and myalgias which are typically intense, and to vertigo, seizures, delirium, visual and auditory deficits, cranial and spinal nerve palsies, and frequently death.

The transmission and nature of the disease were determined by Carrión, a Peruvian medical student, who died as a direct result of his research.[6377]

orphan diseases Rare conditions that are potentially susceptible to treatment, if only economic factors allow the commercial search for it.

Orphanet Database A portal for rare diseases and orphan drugs. Web site: http://www.orpha.net/consor/cgi-bin/index.php?lng=EN.

Orshansky sign The knee-angle phenomenon in **tabes dorsalis.**[4816]

ortho (Gr, straight) Prefix denoting straight.

orthochromatic leukodystrophy (pigmented orthochromatic or nonmetachromatic leukodystrophy) A rare, sporadic or dominantly or recessively inherited dementing syndrome of adults presenting with initial depression, behavioral disorder, and inability to function prior to the appearance of severe dementia.

Pathologically, the findings include severe homologous demyelination, axonal loss, and gliosis in cerebral white matter, sparing the brainstem and cerebellum, the U-fibers, and peripheral nerves. Abundant lipofuscin granules are found in the microglia, macrophages, and astrocytes.[3501] The enzyme deficiency is not known. See also **leukodystrophy**.

orthodromic (Gr, straight + run) Propagation of an impulse in the direction which is the same as that of physiologic conduction: for example, conduction along sensory nerve fibers toward the spinal cord or of motor fibers away from it and toward the muscle innervated. cf. **antidromic**.

orthoses Devices for straightening limbs, preventing contractures, stabilizing joints (*static orthoses*) or for assisting weak muscles in order to improve functional capacity (*dynamic orthoses*).

orthostatic headache Headache occurring on attaining the upright position, usually because of resultant intracranial hypotension (less than 6 mm water) in the presence of CSF hypovolemia.[1176] Spinal surgery including shunting, lumbar puncture, cranial trauma, dehydration,

Chart O–5. The Orofaciodigital Syndromes

Orofaciodigital syndrome (orofaciodigital dysostosis) An X-linked dominant syndrome, lethal in males, characterized by high-arched palate and sometimes a hypoplastic mandible, polydactyly, syndactyly, brachydactyly, lobulation of the tongue, conductive deafness, facial and palatal clefts, lingual hamartomas, polycystic kidneys, alopecia, hydrocephalus, porencephaly, agenesis of the corpus callosum, and mental retardation.[378, 2505]

Orofaciodigital syndrome II (Mohr Syndrome, Mohr–Majewski syndrome, acrofacial dysostosis) A recessively inherited dysmorphic syndrome characterized by high-arched palate, cleft lip, hypoplastic mandible, polydactyly, syndactyly, brachydactyly, lobulation and hamartomas of the tongue, conductive deafness, tibial hypoplasia, the **Dandy–Walker malformation, hydrocephalus,** and mental and developmental delay. The condition was first recognized by O.L. Mohr in 1822.[380, 4432]

Orofaciodigital syndrome III is characterized by facial dysmorphisms, a lobulated tongue, mental retardation, myoclonus, skeletal abnormalities, and often abnormal eye movements.[6119]

diabetic coma, uremia, infection, pseudo-Chiari malformations, skull-base tumors, and sexual intercourse have variously been considered as causative. See **idiopathic intracranial hypotension**.

orthostatic hypotension Reduction in arterial blood pressure on attaining the upright posture. Numerous criteria have been suggested.[5157] A typical example is a consistent and persistent fall of 30 mmHg or more in the systolic pressure and 15 mmHg or more in the diastolic pressure, accompanied by clinical symptoms (on attaining the upright position). While this was classically required to occur within 3 min, there is good evidence that such falls may take 10 min to occur on tilt table testing.[2365]

Falls of 20 mmHg systolic, 10 mmHg diastolic, or 20 mmHg mean blood pressures have been considered sufficient for this diagnosis. See **progressive autonomic failure**.

orthostatic myoclonus Nonrhythmic muscle jerks in multiple leg muscles that appear or increase immediately upon standing. The underlying muscle discharges have burst durations of $\leq$75 ms, which is diagnostic of myoclonus. **Gait ignition failure** may be associated.[2403]

orthostatic tremor (primary orthostatic tremor, shaky legs syndrome) A clinical syndrome seen in elderly people, characterized by a feeling of unsteadiness when standing (but not when walking, sitting, or lying) and rapid, regular, and asynchronous quivering of the legs and trunk, especially when the subject is standing quietly. Patients often show evidence of essential tremor, of which this is considered by some to be a *forme fruste*. Other complaints include leg cramps and dystonia.[2838] It may coexist with essential tremor in the arms.

Electrophysiological findings are of a rapid (frequency around 16 Hz) fast-firing burst discharges causing regular leg tremor in weight-bearing muscles, presumed to be generated by a central oscillator. It is not influenced by peripheral feedback and is synchronous between homologous leg muscles. The fast frequency of this muscle activity causes unsteadiness when standing (presumably due to partially fused muscle contractions), but only a fine ripple of muscle activity is visible. EMG studies show burst activity at 13–18 Hz in weight-bearing muscles. The major differences from essential tremor are the frequency of electromyographic burst firing, the invariable involvement of lower limb and paraspinal muscles, and the task-specific nature of the tremor in orthostatic tremor.[4256]

A related Web site is: http://orthostatictremor.org/, which provides information on treatment, coping, and experiences related to orthostatic tremor.

Ortner, N. (1865–1935) Austrian professor of medicine at Vienna.

Ortner syndrome (cardiovocal syndrome) Compression of the left recurrent laryngeal nerve by an enlarged left atrium, leading to dysphonia.[4818]

Orzechowski syndrome Opsoclonus, incapacitating postural tremor and fever, sometimes with signs suggesting encephalitis complicating a recent viral upper respiratory infection. This is probably a form of postinfectious encephalomyelitis.[1221]

OSAS Collapse of the pharynx and cessation of airflow while the diaphragm continues the breathing effort. See **obstructive sleep apnea syndrome**.

oscillations (saccadic oscillations) Repetitive involuntary ocular **saccades** without intervening slow phases, thus differing from **nystagmus**.

Dell'Osso[1561] reviewed the following varieties: **convergence-retraction "nystagmus"; double saccadic pulses; dynamic overshoot; flutter dysmetria; macro-saccadic oscillations; macro-square-wave jerks; ocular bobbing; ocular dipping; ocular dysmetria; ocular flutter; ocular myoclonus; opsoclonus; psychogenic flutter; saccadic lateropulsion; saccadic double pulses; saccadic pulses; square-wave jerks; superior oblique myokymia; and voluntary "nystagmus"**.

oscillopsia A subjective illusion of the rhythmic movement of the surrounding stationary world. This may be horizontal, vertical, or oblique and may vary. It is the result of movement disorders affecting one or both eyes, stemming from lesions affecting the visual, oculomotor, or vestibular systems; but it can also occur with mechanical displacement of an eye (*chewing oscillopsia*). When unilateral, **superior oblique myokymia** and **palatal myoclonus** are likely associations.[507]

Osler, Sir William (1849–1919) Canadian physician who trained at the University of Toronto and in Montreal at McGill University and after graduation, spent some years in Europe. On his return to Canada at the age of 25, he was made professor of the "Institutes of Medicine" (physiology) at McGill and lectured on pathology and physiology with such success that he removed to the University of Pennsylvania and then 5 years later became the first professor of medicine at Johns Hopkins, Baltimore. Here he established an institution that revolutionized the teaching of medicine in North America by combining the British tradition of bedside teaching with the European tradition of the coordination of the wards and the laboratories. He accepted the Regius Chair of Medicine at Oxford in 1904, where he was also curator of the Bodleian Library.

From Johns Hopkins he published *On Chorea and Choreiform Affections* (Philadelphia, 1884) and *The Cerebral Palsies of Children* (1889) and the first editions of his classic textbook *The Principles and Practice of Medicine* (1892), in which 300 pages were devoted to neurological topics. He contributed many chapters on neurology to the textbooks of internal medicine edited by others. He also published the first or the best current accounts of intracerebral hemorrhage, cerebral embolism, meningitis, and acute infectious polyneuropathy, noted the relationship of chorea and (rheumatic) heart disease, and recognized that jaundice may predispose to athetosis (1894). He also contributed many clinical reports on other neurological subjects. In later life, he published his reflective books *Aequanimitas* and *A Way of Life*, each of which had wide appeal as a result of their depiction of his own philosophy of medicine. He was described as "the greatest personality in Medicine at the time of his death" at Oxford in 1919.

An excellent biography is that of Bliss, M. *William Osler: A Life in Medicine*. Toronto, Univ. Toronto Press, 1999.

osmotic demyelination syndromes Encephalopathies resulting from the treatment of acute severe hyponatremia (serum sodium <120 mEq/l) or chronic hyponatremia (serum sodium

Chart O–6. Variant Forms of Osteopetrosis

Acroosteolysis with osteoporosis (Hajdu–Cheney syndrome) A congenital dysmorphic syndrome characterized by basilar impression, optic atrophy, and abnormal skull shape.[6713]

A type in which renal tubular acidosis and cerebral calcifications are associated.[5893]

Oculodento-osseous dysplasia A congenital dysmorphic syndrome characterized by microphthalmia, syndactyly, and cranial hyperostosis with a tendency to cranial and spinal nerve palsy as a result of compression.[488]

Osteoporosis, pseudoglioma, and mental retardation A congenital syndrome characterized by joint laxity, osteoporosis with multiple fractures, cloudy corneas, microphthalmia, pseudoglioma of the retina, blindness, and mental and developmental delay.

<134 mEq/l for over 48 h). Cellular edema results, due to an osmotic gradient caused by extracellular fluid dilution (for example, that due to hyponatremia), and leads on to extrusion of intracellular cations as a corrective response. If the hyponatremia is quickly corrected, then the extracellular hyperosmolarity may lead to cell damage; swelling and reciprocal compression of interdigitating nerve fiber bundles crossing the midline is a likely result.

The prototype is **central pontine myelinolysis**, which is characterized by a single confluent focal area of myelin destruction in the central pons with relative preservation of axons, in the absence of inflammatory changes It has been associated with various metabolic abnormalities such as alcoholism and too rapid correction of profound hyponatremia (faster than 12 mmol/l per day), and may reflect swelling of the interdigitated crossing fibers in the pons; however, lesions are also found in the pontine tegmentum, the mesencephalon, the deep cerebral nuclei, and the subcortical white matter. Clinically, coma, seizures, and acutely evolving signs of corticospinal, cerebellar, and lower cranial nerve dysfunction are the major features,[4697, 5117] sometimes even progressing to a **locked in syndrome**.

In some cases the condition is due to hypoxia rather than to abnormalities of sodium regulation. An acute demyelinating polyneuropathy has been described in association.

osteitis deformans See **Paget disease**.

osteochondromuscular dystrophy See **Schwartz–Jampel syndrome**.

osteogenesis imperfecta (van der Hoeve syndrome, Ekman syndrome, Spurway syndrome, Lobstein syndrome, Eddowes syndrome) A dominantly inherited disorder of collagen which leads to thin, brittle, osteoporotic, and easily fractured long bones, abnormal teeth, loose ligaments, and a tendency for the sclerae to show a blue tinge.

Neurological complications include hydromyelia and communicating hydrocephalus; myelopathy due to spinal deformity; macrocephaly; basilar invagination with brainstem compression; seizures; conductive deafness; spina bifida, platyspondyly, thin calvarium; and the consequences of accelerated atherosclerosis.[1113] Arachnodactyly, syndactyly, keratoconus, cataracts, growth retardation, and osteopenia are other features described. The condition was first described in Sweden in 1788.[2504]

osteoglophonic dwarfism syndrome A congenital dysmorphic syndrome characterized by short stature, dental and metaphyseal deformities, craniosynostosis, and enlargement of the sella turcica.[487]

osteomalacic myopathy An acquired proximal myopathy characterized by muscle and bone pain, proximal muscle weakness without wasting, and normal serum creatine kinase levels but with typically myopathic muscle biopsy and EMG findings, occurring in patients with osteomalacia from any cause, except the X-linked form of type 1 hypophosphatemic rickets. Muscle biopsy and EMG findings are typically myopathic. The unusual finding in myopathy of retained brisk muscle stretch reflexes is characteristic here.[3724, 4106]

osteopetrosis (Albers–Schönberg disease, marble bones) A rare recessively (rarely dominantly) transmitted condition manifesting generalized sclerosis of bone with thickening of cortical and spongy bone as well as increased fragility; hepato-splenomegaly, anemia, thrombocytopenia, and susceptibility to infections; and thickening of the skull base, macrocephaly, and frontal bossing.

Neurological consequences may include optic atrophy with blindness, nystagmus, deafness, hydrocephalus, strabismus, facial palsy, intracranial hemorrhage, headache, mental retardation, seizures, basal ganglia calcification, and involvement of cranial nerves I and V.[3483, 3526] *Variant* forms are listed in Chart O–6.

osteophyte Ossified portions of the intervertebral disks which splay out posterolaterally, thus tending to impinge on the spinal nerves and the spinal cord.

osteoporosis Low bone mass and microarchitectural deterioration of bone tissue, leading to enhanced bone fragility and consequent increase in fracture risk.[6762] Dual-energy X-ray absorptiometry scanning is the best investigative tool allowing a confident diagnosis.

Steroid, phenobarbitone, and dilantin therapy and immobility resulting from any paretic disorder are the more important potential causes of interest to neurologists, and both bone pain and fractures as a result of falling are the commoner consequences.[3887]

osteosclerosis fragilis See **Albers–Schönberg disease**.

osteosclerosis–microcephaly–cataracts A congenital syndrome characterized by cataract, congenital cardiac anomaly, microcephaly, and multiple fractures.[381]

osteosclerotic myeloma See POEMS.

Osterreichische Gesellschaft zur Bekampfung der Muskelkrankheiten A member society of the European Alliance of Muscular

Dystrophy Societies, based at Lazarettgasse 14, Postfach 23 A-097, Wien, Austria.

Ostrum–Furst syndrome The association of platybasia, congenital synostosis of the neck, and a Sprengel deformity of the shoulder with mild facial weakness and some disturbances of the arm reflexes, reported in 1942.[1765, 2246]

Osuntokun syndrome Congenital asymbolia for pain (although the differentiation between sharp and dull sensations is retained) and auditory imperception of the significance of spoken words, without deafness.[4828]

Ota syndrome See **nevus of Ota**.

otitic hydrocephalus (sinus thrombosis causing intracranial hypertension) A syndrome of raised intracranial pressure with headache and often vomiting and diplopia, bilateral papilledema, normal ventricular size, and a normal neurological examination except for VI nerve palsy, occurring as a result of thrombosis of the lateral dural venous sinuses following otitis media. The findings would be similar for thrombosis of the superior sagittal sinus, which is less common.

The condition is classed as a variety of **idiopathic intracranial hypertension**.[2144] It was first described by Quincke,[5155] but this term was introduced (and later withdrawn) by Sir Charles **Symonds**. See also **Battle sign**.

otoconia Crystals of calcium carbonate within the utricles, floating in the endolymph and thus sensitive to gravitational forces. When they settle in the cupula of the posterior semicircular canal, they may be responsible for causing position-related sensations of imbalance by stimulating the hair cells also within the fluid.

otofaciocervical syndrome A congenital dysmorphic syndrome, characterized also by skeletal deformities, conductive deafness, winged scapulae, and mental and developmental delay.[4929]

otolithic catastrophe Acute episodes of vertigo with abrupt atonia and falling, without loss of consciousness, considered to reflect an undetermined inner ear disorder.[6420]

otoliths Small calciferous granules in the semicircular canals of the inner ear. Their gravitational effect upon the hair cells leads to afferent responses signaling acceleration in the various dimensions of space.

otopalatodigital syndrome A recessively inherited dysmorphic syndrome characterized by dwarfism, broad nasal root, hypertelorism, frontal and occipital bossing, small mandible, cleft palate, digital anomalies, abnormal bony ossification, conductive deafness, and mental and motor delay.[1741] See **Taybi syndrome**.

otosclerosis A dominantly inherited syndrome with variable penetrance, characterized by the onset of slowly progressive conductive symmetrical hearing loss of variable severity in the second or third decade, with tinnitus but normal vestibular responses.[3526]

outliers Motor unit action potentials that have values for amplitude, duration, or number of phases far outside the mean; their analysis providing information of diagnostic value in both neuropathic and myopathic muscle diseases.[6011]

out-of-phase signals Two waves of opposite phases.

oval pupils A transient sign of damage to the oculomotor nerve or nucleus in the setting of acute severe intracranial vascular disease, as a result of which there is nonuniform paresis of the sphincter pupillae.[2090]

Overall Neuropathy Limitations Scale A measure of handicaps in peripheral neuropathy.[2547] Instructions for administering it are available at http://www.jnnp.bmjjournals.com/supplemental/

overbreathing See **hyperventilation**.

overflow myoclonus See **ballistic movement overflow myoclonus**.

overlap myasthenic syndrome The coexistence of **myasthenia gravis** and **Lambert–Eaton myasthenic syndrome**.[4763]

overlap neuropathy The coalescence of the areas of motor or sensory deficit resulting from multiple mononeuropathies, which may give the appearance of a peripheral polyneuropathy at first sight. See **vasculitic neuropathy**.

overlap syndrome 1. (polymyositis or dermatomyositis associated with connective tissue disorder, microscopic polyangiitis) The concurrence of signs of polymyositis or dermatomyositis with evidence of one of the connective tissue disorders, such as **systemic lupus erythematosus**, mixed connective tissue disease, rheumatoid arthritis, **Sjögren syndrome**, rheumatic fever, or progressive systemic sclerosis. The only clinical difference from typical polymyositis is the frequent concurrence of sclerodactyly and Raynaud phenomenon.[4157] 2. A vasculitis in which the features combine those of **polyarteritis nodosa, allergic angiitis and granulomatosis,** and **hypersensitivity vasculitis**.[1972, 5582]

overuse syndromes (repetitive overuse syndrome, repetition strain syndrome).

Injuries presumed to be caused by the cumulative effects on tissues of repetitive physical stress that exceeds physiological limits. These usually affect the muscle-tendon unit in the arms, and are common in, for example, musicians, but spinal and other joint disease, pulmonary disease, nerve entrapment syndromes, and dystonias are other examples.[3743, 3889]

Oxford stroke classification A neat differentiation of the four clinically identifiable subgroups of cerebral infarction; large anterior circulation infarcts with both cortical and subcortical involvement with a large or medium-sized cortical infarct or a large subcortical infarct in the middle cerebral artery territory (*total anterior circulation infarcts*); restricted and predominantly cortical infarcts or a large subcortical infarct in the anterior or middle cerebral artery territories (*partial anterior circulation infarcts*); infarcts clearly associated with the vertebrobasilar arterial territory (*posterior circulation infarcts*); and small infarcts confined to the territory of the deep perforating arteries (*lacunar infarcts*).[368, 6640]

5-oxoprolinemia (glutathionine synthetase deficiency) A diffuse encephalopathy due to a deficiency of glutathione synthetase and characterized by metabolic acidosis with mental retardation and increased urinary excretion of 5-oxoproline.[6716]

oxycephaly (Gr, sharp + head)
1. A congenital deformity of the skull which is high and conical due to too early closure of the posterior part of the sagittal, of the metopic, or of the sagittal and both coronal sutures, such that it resembles a wedge with the long axis lying above the sagittal suture. The term was first used by Aristophanes. The *tête en poire* of King Louis XVI was presumably so caused. Increased intracranial pressure, optic atrophy, and exophthalmos are commonly found. 2. A late appearing synostosis affecting the coronal sutures and leading to recession of the supraorbital rim backward, including the forehead, and to elevation of the top of the head.

In *harmonious oxycephaly*, the suture is fused but the shape of the head remains normal.

oxytocin A hormone secreted by the magnocellular cells in the supraoptic and paraventricular nuclei of the posterior pituitary.

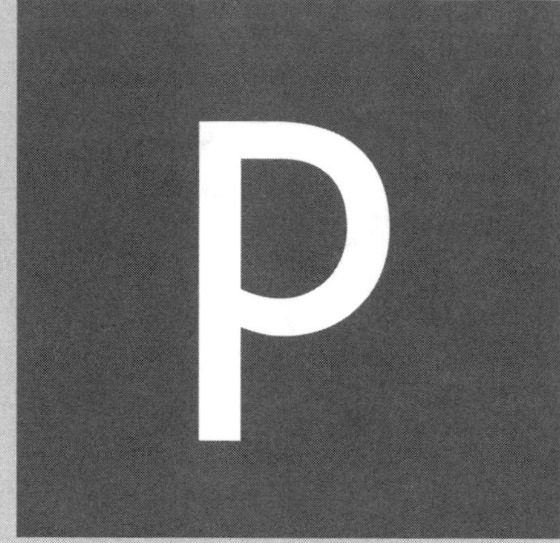

P 300 evoked potential A high-amplitude, positive waveform (an event-related potential) of limbic origin, recorded over the parietal regions following detection of a sensory event in any channel for which the individual has been primed. The waveform increases in latency and diminishes in amplitude with age and in dementing states.[2476]

Pacchioni, Antonio (1665–1726) Italian professor of anatomy at Rome, who in 1705 described the granulations named for him, and who described the anatomy of the meninges in 1724. He erred in considering the granulations to have lymphatic functions[5886] and was corrected by Fantoni in 1738.

Pacchionian granulation seizures A syndrome of uncertain validity, reported as occurring in early life and characterized by focal convulsions beginning in the leg or shoulder which occur chronically over many years without associated neurological signs. Anomalous Pacchionian granulations extending into the precentral gyrus or primary motor areas are considered to be the cause.

The original description recounted the performance of an operation to divide the anomalous granulations; an attendant reduction in seizure frequency was claimed.[5574]

Pacchionian granulations The larger arachnoid villi projecting into the superior sagittal sinus, constituting a lock on the "canal" of CSF circulation and filtering the CSF from the subarachnoid space to the venous circulation. Hypertrophy of the granulations is described secondary to raised CSF pressure, sometimes producing local lytic lesions of the overlying skull.

The radiological differences from sagittal sinus thrombosis have been listed; the occurrence of hypertrophic granulations in the lateral transverse sinuses, normal dural sinus blood flow, and local bony lysis are the most useful distinguishing features.[2391]

Pace sign Weakness, faltering, and reproduction of pain when the patient abducts the thigh and externally rotates the hip against resistance while seated or lying with the painful side up, the painful leg being semiflexed. This is observed in the **piriformis syndrome**.[4846, 462] (HJM)

Paced Auditory Serial Addition task A test of the efficiency of information processing in which the subject hears 60 single numbers presented at various speeds and is required to sum the last 2 numbers heard, over 4 trials. There is thus both a need to recall the previous number, adding it to the new one without distraction from the mental operation of successive addition.[2588] The test has been used particularly in patients with **postconcussional syndrome** and **multiple sclerosis**.

pachycephaly (Gr, thick + head) A rare craniofacial dysplasia in which there is hypoplasia and flattening of the occiput due to premature fusion of the lambdoid sutures, with or without the involvement of other sutures. When occurring alone, it is seldom of consequence.[4]

pachyencephalia Abnormal thickness of the vault of the skull. A misnomer, but it is hardly ever used anyway.

pachygyria A developmental disorder due to abnormalities of neuronal migration, characterized by abnormally few, thickened and wide cerebral gyri, and the presence of histological abnormalities in the claustrum, medulla, and cerebellum. The condition is also associated with both **agyria** and **microgyria**.[2721]

pachymeninges (Gr, thick + membrane) The dura mater, the thicker meningeal covering of the brain which separates it from the skull and the spinal cord from the spine.

pachymeningitis A term (now seldom used) to refer to inflammation of the thicker outer coverings of the brain. *Pachymeningitis externa* is such inflammation resulting from local infection in the cranial bones; *pachymeningitis interna* is due to infections spreading outwards from the arachnoid; *pachymeningitis serosa* is the term for a subdural serous effusion. *Pachymeningitis hemorrhagica interna* (Virchow) represents a **subdural hematoma**, and *pachymeningitis externa spinalis* or *peripachymeningitis* constitutes an inflammatory process (usually syphilitic) occurring outside and around the spinal dura mater, sometimes causing hyperplasia and secondary compression of the nerve roots or the spinal cord.

Syphilis, sarcoidosis, and tuberculosis are the most common identified causes, and headaches, cranial nerve palsies, and ataxia are the leading clinical features, along with inflammatory changes in the CSF. In *idiopathic intracranial pachymeningitis*, no cause is found.[4152]

A local form also occurs in the **superior orbital fissure syndrome** (Tolosa–Hunt syndrome). Inflammation of the other meninges may be referred to as **arachnoiditis** or as **leptomeningitis**, but meningeal inflammation usually affects all three layers, at least to some extent.

pachymeningitis cervicalis hypertrophica Thickening of all the meninges in the cervical region as a result of **meningovascular syphilis**.

pachymeningitis externa See **spinal epidural abscess**.

pachymeningitis hemorrhagica interna See **chronic subdural hematoma**.

Pacini, Filippo (1812–1883) Italian anatomist who re-described the sensory organs described by Vater, but now bearing his name.

Pacinian corpuscles The sensory endings of some cutaneous and other nerves, which had been mentioned by Vater a century before their description by Pacini, although the data had been lost.[5886] They are widely distributed in the skin, especially of the hands and feet, but also are found in the periosteum, the joints, and many other areas. Steady mechanical pressure leads to a rapidly adapting response, although they were at first thought (by **Adrian**) to be organs for signalling static pressure.

pack palsy See **rucksack palsy**.

PADL See **Performance of Activities of Daily Living test**.

Page syndrome Blotchy red areas on the face, neck, and upper trunk, seen usually in young women who are embarrassed. Other sympathetic evidence of anxiety, including transient elevations of blood pressure, may accompany the rash.[4851] The condition has been elevated beyond its dignity by the term *hypertensive diencephalic syndrome*; the latter term is also used for **Penfield syndrome**, which is an accepted entity with few similar features.

Paget, Sir James (1814–1899) English surgeon.

Paget disease (osteitis deformans) A dominantly inherited disease with variable penetrance, characterized by variable degeneration and regeneration of the membrane bones of the skull and of the bones of the limbs. The condition is manifested in later life and leads to bony softening, overgrowth, and deformity due to absorption and rarefaction, and sometimes to sarcomatous change.

Compression of nervous tissue at cranial or spinal levels results in a proportion of cases, leading on to deafness, hemifacial spasm, trigeminal neuralgia, pyramidal signs resulting from basilar invagination, or myelopathy.[1190] Basilar impression may also cause other cranial nerve palsies, compression of the cerebellum and medulla, and hydrocephalus with dementia, while shallow orbits may be responsible for proptosis. Paget described the disease in 1876.[3526]

pagophagia The eating of ice; a form of pica which may indicate an iron deficiency state. (HJM)

pain 1. An unpleasant subjective sensory and emotional experience associated with or described in terms of actual or potential tissue damage. Varieties can be classified as *neuropathic*, *nocioceptive*, or *psychogenic*.[5082]

This definition, however, ignores the point made by Galen that pain may also have a protective function—as witnessed by the acropathies suffered by patients with **hereditary sensory and autonomic neuropathy** type II, **leprosy** or **syringomyelia**. Leriche disagreed with that point of view, however, and stated that most diseases attack us without warning, and that when pain develops it is too late, so the pain has only made more distressing and more sad a situation already lost: "pain is always a baleful gift, which reduces the subject of it and makes him more ill than he would be without." 2. A localized form of sorrow. (Spinoza)

Pain The Journal of the International Association for the Study of Pain, published by Elsevier. Web site: http://www.halcyon.com/iasp/journal.html/.

pain asymbolia (insensitivity to pain) The term of Schilder for loss of the psychic reaction to pain despite retention of the sensation of painful stimuli.[3220, 5602] Such loss of the affective-motivational component of pain occurs nevertheless with preserved sensory discrimination. It is likely due to central lesions of the parietal lobe, anterior cingulate, or insular cortex. See **also congenital pain insensitivity**.

pain asymbolia with auditory imperception See **congenital pain asymbolia**.

pain density A measure of the severity of chronic pain, in which numerical values are assigned to severity and frequency and are then multiplied to yield a score.[198]

pain disorder A persistent syndrome in which significant pain is appreciated despite the absence of continuing demonstrable pathology considered adequate to cause it, and is accompanied by behavioural changes relevant to the perception, including mental distress or impairment in social, occupational, or other important areas of functioning.

The diagnosis can be supported when pain has existed for at least 6 months and there is strong evidence that psychological factors have caused or are maintaining the pain. Many of these patients have depressive illnesses. Additional diagnostic criteria are that psychological factors seem important in the onset, maintenance, severity, or worsening of the pain; other psychiatric disorders do not explain the symptoms better, the patient does not meet criteria for dyspareunia, and the patient is considered not to be consciously feigning the symptoms for material gain (which is malingering), nor to occupy the sick role ("factitious disorder").

How this judgment is made, however, is not explained.

The American Psychiatric Association *DSM IV-TR* diagnostic guidelines[172] are accessible at http://www.behavenet.com/capsules/disorders/dsm4TRclassification.htm/. See also http://www.action-on-pain.co.uk/ and http://www.psychnet-uk.com/dsm_iv/pain_disorder.htm/ for further descriptions.

pain reflex Dilation of the pupil in response to painful stimuli. See **ciliospinal reflex**.

pain spots Areas in the skin where pain can be appreciated, surrounded by areas in which it cannot. The existence of such places was proposed by **von Frey**, but the idea was discredited by those who did not try hard enough to find them.

Paine syndrome (hypoplasia of the cerebellum and pons) An X-linked syndrome of recessive microcephaly, seizures, psychomotor retardation, various skeletal deformities, and spasticity occurring in the presence of brain stem and cerebellar hypoplasia and accompanied by generalized aminoaciduria.[2754, 4856]

Paine–Efron syndrome A spinocerebellar degeneration characterized by the onset of mild but slowly progressive cerebellar signs in childhood or adult life. Diffuse telangiectasia or pigmented nevi also appear but the other features of **Louis-Bar syndrome** are not found.[4857]

painful arms and moving fingers A syndrome of pain in the arm with discontinuous, involuntary, irregular, repetitive contractions of the small hand muscles, producing a writhing, pseudoathetotic appearance, described in the setting of brachial plexus neuritis following radiotherapy[6528] or following relatively slight arm trauma.

painful feet See **burning feet syndrome**.

painful hand and moving finger A syndrome seen in patients with radiation-induced brachial plexopathy, presenting with complex sequences of flexion/extension and abduction/adduction of the fingers with deep, aching pain in the hand.[6527] See also **painful legs and moving toes**.

painful jumping amputation stumps See **stump spasm**.

painful legs and moving toes A chronic syndrome characterized by deep, pulling, gnawing, or aching pains of variable severity in the feet or legs, accompanied by spontaneous, purposeless, wriggling movements of the toes. The pain is worsened by movement but is sometimes relieved temporarily by sympathetic block.[5979] The underlying pathology is not understood, but the phenomenon has been recorded after root or nerve lesions, following minor trauma to the legs and with lateral plantar nerve lesions. The nature of the central or peripheral cause is at present unknown.

Along with **painful arms and moving fingers**, this condition should probably be subsumed under the heading of *painful limbs and moving digits*. See also **cramp-fasciculation syndrome**.

painful lumbar plexopathy A syndrome of painful deficits in lumbar or sacral regions associated with an elevated ESR and cuffing of epineurial blood vessels by mixed inflammatory cells on sural nerve biopsy specimens, in the absence of other evidence of an autoimmune disorder and of vasculitis or cancer.[791] See also **idiopathic lumbosacral plexopathy**.

painful ophthalmoplegia syndrome See **superior orbital fissure syndrome**.

painful penile erections Awakenings from rapid eye movement sleep periods occasioned by painful sensations resulting from normal rapid eye movement sleep-related penile erections.[4176, 3302] (See also Chart S–6 and ASDA Diagnostic Classification,[1629] **sleep disorders**.)

painful sensory neuropathy with antisulfatide antibodies See **immune-mediated neuropathies**.

painless legs and moving toes The occurrence of painless semicontinuous involuntary movements of the toes of the foot similar to those seen in **painful legs and moving toes**. EMG and nerve conduction studies show only a predominant co-contraction of the foot flexors and extensors at 0.6–1.2 Hz in a pattern sometimes seen in painful legs and moving toes. The etiology is undetermined.

painless whitlows (panaris analgésique de Morvan) Infection of the terminal parts of the digits in limbs that have lost their thin-fiber sensory innervation, as in **hereditary sensory and autonomic neuropathy** or **syringomyelia**.

paintbrush sign The myelographic appearance in the case of extradural compression at the level of the cauda equina. The column of contrast becomes less and less homogeneous as it is followed from above downward to the level of the compression; the dye is drawn out into vertical lines similar to those left by a paintbrush, its paint progressively yielded up to the surface along which it is drawn.

painters' palsy Radial nerve palsy. See **lead palsy**.

paint-sniffer's encephalopathy (glue-sniffer's neuropathy) An irreversible syndrome resulting from long-term toluene inhalation and characterized by cerebellar ataxia, tremor, and cognitive defects and by disturbances in very long–chain fatty acid metabolism.[2991]

Paired Associated Learning Test A traditional test of new learning in which subjects are required to associate the two words of a pair presented, so that, when one is given after an interval, the other will be recalled and reproduced. The test is sensitive to early changes in short-term memory function.[6687, 6688]

paired discharge Two action potentials occurring consistently in the same relationship with each other. Cf. **double discharge.**[162]

paired stimuli Two consecutive stimuli delivered in a time-locked fashion. The time interval between the two stimuli and the intensity of each stimulus can be varied but should be specified. The first stimulus is called the *conditioning stimulus* and the second stimulus is the *test stimulus*. The conditioning stimulus may modify tissue excitability, which is then evaluated by the response to the test stimulus. (From the 2001 Report of the Nomenclature Committee of the American Association of Electromyography and Electrodiagnosis.[19] Reproduced by kind permission of the AANEM.)

Pal, Jakob Budapest physician and neuropathologist who with Weigert introduced a staining reaction for myelinated fibers.

palatal fricative A consonant made by partially blocking the air flow between the palate and tongue, causing air turbulence and resulting in a sound; for example, /sh/ as in shoe.[3949]

palatal myoclonus (bulbar myoclonus, myoclonique de la calotte, palatal myokymia, ocular palatal tremor, oculopalatal myoclonus) An uncommon, irreversible, involuntary movement disorder characterized by continuous, rapid, regular, and rhythmic quivering of the soft palate, larynx, and other structures derived from the embryonic branchial arches (face, neck, and diaphragm) occurring at about 10 Hz and probably due to denervation hypersensitivity of the inferior olive. The movements persist in sleep. Audible clicks may be the presenting symptom.[2623, 4175] **Ocular bobbing** may accompany the palatal movements,[6900] in which case the condition is known as **oculopalatal myoclonus/tremor**. *Essential* and *symptomatic* forms have been differentiated.

Despite the usual name, this is not true myoclonus at all, but is a form of **myokymia**. The pathology is usually infarction involving the **Guillain–Mollaret triangle**, particularly the contralateral inferior olivary nuclei, which may be hypertrophic. *Variants* are as follows:

Palatal myoclonus and ataxia A dominantly inherited syndrome with adult onset characterized by dysarthria, branchial (palatal) myoclonus, nystagmus, cerebellar ataxia, and spastic paraparesis.[1523] Further association with brainstem or pontine atrophy, Parkinsonism, autonomic dysfunction, or corticospinal tract abnormalities leads to a picture that resembles **multiple system atrophy**.[5520]

Complicated palatal myoclonus A progressive, dominantly inherited disorder with onset in the third decade, characterized clinically by palatal myoclonus, ataxia, bulbar weakness, and spastic quadriparesis and pathologically by the presence of **Rosenthal fibers** and myelin loss. Differentiation from the last entry is speculative.[3010]

palatal myokymia See **palatal myoclonus.**

palatal tremor See **palatal myoclonus.**

palatopalpebral reflex Blinking in response to palatal stimulation, described by Imperartori in 1930. See **palpebral reflex.**

paleo- (Gr, ancient).

palencephalography (Gr, to shake + the brain) A technique for recording cephalic vibrations at 1–20 Hz. in an attempt to localize intracranial lesions.[389] It is now superseded by more precise methods.

paleocerebellar syndrome Ataxic gait, limb ataxia, and disturbance of postural reflexes with muscle hypotonia, due to a lesion of the anterior lobe of the cerebellum.[332]

paleocerebellum The anterior lobe of the cerebellum, consisting of the vermis and the paravermian cortex.

paleocerebrum The second oldest part of the cerebellum (the archicerebellum is phylogenetically more ancient), differentiated from the **neocerebrum** by Edinger in 1885.

paleostriatal syndrome See **dyssynergia cerebellaris myoclonica.**

paleostriatum The globus pallidus, caudate, and putamen situated lateral to the internal capsule.

paligraphia (Gr, again + to write) Perseveratory writing of a word or phrase that has already been written once.[1336]

palilalia (from Gr, again + language) 1. The phenomenon whereby the patient repeats the last word or two of a verbal statement, the words tailing off in a diminuendo fashion and with increasing rapidity.[1330] 2. Repetition by the patient of a phrase spoken by the examiner, with or without a change in pronoun; a morbid, obsessive, involuntary reiteration of spoken words, both spontaneously and in reply to questions. It is not heard when the patient recites or reads aloud, nor in singing.

The condition which **Brissaud** called *autoecholalia* is probably the same as palilalia, the name supplied in 1908 by **Souques** in a lecture to the Société de Neurologie in Paris.[5961] It is observed especially in demented patients, and in the settings of postencephalitic Parkinsonism, paramedian thalamic infarcts, and diffuse cerebrovascular disease.

palilaliopraxia See **signing tics.**

palilogia An oratorical device whereby emphasis is attained by repetition.

palinacousis An auditory hallucination in which sounds heard persist or recur after the initial stimulus has ceased. It is usually seen in patients with temporal lobe lesions. See also **palinopsia.**

palindromic (from Gr, a running back) Relapsing.

palinesthesia The persistence or recurrence of tactile sensations after the exciting stimulus has been withdrawn.

palinopsia (paliopsia) (Gr, again + vision) The persistence or brief recurrence of a visual image for minutes or hours after the exciting stimulus has been extinguished. This may occur in either seeing or blind fields.

The phenomenon has been considered to be a form of release hallucination and suggests the presence of a structural lesion in the parieto-occipital cortex, but many other causes have been implicated.[5075] See also **visual perseveration, polyopia, allesthesia.**

paliopsia See **palinopsia.**

palipraxia Complex hyperkinesias including psychomotor forms, in which small, patterned fragments of movement are performed stereotypically (patting the hands, touching or stroking objects, and so on), and others in which the movement appears to be a deliberate volitional action that is perseverated long after the initial stimulus has passed.

palipsychism (from Gr, again + soul) The superimposition of mental activities that are normally processed sequentially, such that a subject may offer biographical information while working on a calculation test.[2350]

pallanesthesia Loss of the appreciation of vibration.

Pallbearer's palsy A brachial plexus lesion resulting from compression of its upper fibers from the weight of the coffin borne on the shoulder. See **rucksack palsy**.

pallesthesia The appreciation of vibration. See **vibratory sensation**.

pallid breath-holding spells See **breath-holding spells**.

pallidal atrophies A group of hereditary or sporadic diseases characterized clinically by various movement disorders, including Parkinsonism, chorea, and dystonia. They include **pure pallidal atrophy, pallidonigral degenerations**, and combinations of pallidal atrophy with other system degenerations.

pallidal degeneration It is doubtful whether this condition exists as an entity separate from **pallidal atrophies** or the next entries.[2355]

pallidal polyglucosan bodies in cerebral palsy One of the group of **pallidonigral degenerations** in which cerebral palsy due to perinatal hypoxia presents in childhood with chorea and dystonia, accompanied by the finding of polyglucosan bodies in the neuronal cytoplasm of cells in the pallidum.[6892]

pallidoluysian atrophy (pure pallidoluysian atrophy) A system degeneration presenting in adult life and characterized by generalized dystonia, dysarthria, loss of postural reflexes, gait disorder, supranuclear vertical gaze palsy, and bradykinesia without either tremor or rigidity. Pathologically, atrophy of the lateral segment of the globus pallidus and of the subthalamic nucleus are the only notable features.[6865]

pallidonigral degeneration with spinal muscular atrophy One of the group of pallidonigral degenerations in which these two findings coincide.[5736]

pallidonigral degenerations (idiopathic subcortical degenerations) A group of rare conditions united by this singular abnormality and their production of complicated akinetic-rigid syndromes. They include **dentatorubropallidoluysian degeneration, neurodegeneration with brain iron accumulation, hereditary (holotopistic) striatal degeneration, idiopathic calcification of the basal ganglia, infantile neuroaxonal dystrophy, pallidal polyglucosan bodies in cerebral palsy**, and **pallidonigroluysian atrophy**.[2355]

Other *variants* are **pallidonigral degeneration with spinal muscular atrophy** and *amyotrophic lateral sclerosis with pallidonigroluysian atrophy*.[2355] See **motor neuronal diseases**.

pallidonigroluysian atrophy One of the group of **pallidonigral degenerations** in which akinesia, rigidity, dystonia, tremor, and dementia appear sporadically in adults. In some cases the picture resembles **progressive supranuclear palsy**; in others, **amyotrophic lateral sclerosis** has been associated.[2355] See **pallidonigral degenerations** (*variants*).

pallidopyramidal disease See **juvenile Parkinsonism syndrome**.

pallidostriatonigral degeneration See **system degenerations, pallidonigroluysian atrophy**.

Pallister syndrome An X-linked recessive, congenital dysmorphic syndrome manifesting also skeletal anomalies, seizures, pyramidal signs, and mental and developmental delay.[4868]

Pallister–Hall syndrome See **Hall syndrome**.

Pallister–Hawes–Landon syndrome A disorder due to vitamin B deficiency, probably identical to **Strachan syndrome**.

Pallister–Killian syndrome A rare, sporadic, genetic disorder characterized by dysmorphic features, learning disability, and drug resistant epilepsy, and associated with a mosaic supernumerary isochromosome 12p, present in skin fibroblasts. The onset is late but the condition persists beyond infancy.[5525]

pallium (Lat, cloak) The cerebral cortex, covering the rest of the brain like a cloak.[5886]

palmar grasp See **palmar reflex, developmental reflexes**.

palmar-plantar erythrodysesthesia A syndrome of dysesthesias and tenderness of the hands and feet with swelling and redness of the skin, described as a complication of 5-fluouracil therapy and usually responsive to pyridoxine.[370]

palmar reflex (palmar grasp) Flexion of the fingers in response to gentle stroking of the palm of the hand. The sign is present at birth and normally disappears by 2 months of age. When enhanced, it forms the basis of the **grasp reflex**.

palmaris brevis sign Wrinkling of the ulnar side of the palm due to spontaneous repetitive contractions of the palmaris brevis, which is spared in the case of lesions of the ulnar nerve at the pisohamate ligament (Guyon's canal), but not with those at more proximal sites.[5049] The **palmaris brevis spasm syndrome** may accompany this.

palmaris brevis spasm syndrome Isolated, spontaneous, brisk, tonic, painless involuntary contractions of this muscle leading to dimpling of the ulnar side of the hand and usually seen in older males with proximal ulnar nerve or root lesions. The syndrome is benign and slowly progressive over years.[5733] It may occur as a complication of radiculopathy or as an occupational condition with distal ulnar nerve damage.

palmaris longus aplasia A dominantly inherited syndrome with incomplete penetrance, in which this muscle is absent.

palmomental reflex (Marinesco–Radovici reflex) Contraction of the mentalis muscle causing wrinkling of the chin with elevation and protrusion of the lower lip when the skin over the thenar eminence is scratched.[4841, 5248] This is a nonspecific sign of diffuse cerebral dysfunction (although often detectable in infancy and in the normal elderly), first described by Marinesco and Radovici in 1920.

palmus See **Bamberger disease**.

palpebra (Lat, an eyelid)

palpebral reflex (menace reflex) Blinking in response to a variety of stimuli, such as loud noises, menace, bright lights, or sensory stimulation of the face or buccal mucosa. See **orbicularis oculi reflex**.

palpebromandibular synkinesis (spontaneous corneomandibular reflex) A centrally initiated synkinesis characterized by the association of bilateral eyelid closure with anterolateral deviation of the mandible to the opposite side, in response to spontaneous eye-blinks, in patients with bilateral cerebral or brainstem disease.[5140, 5141]

palpebro-oculogyric reflex See **Bell phenomenon**.

palsy (derived from Middle English, *parlesie*, and from French, *paralysie*[5886]) Lack of power, paralysis.

Palthe reflex Arrest of respiratory and of swallowing movements in response to cold stimulation of structures supplied by the second division of the trigeminal nerve, such as a sudden cold stimulus to the face. It is presumed to have a protective function that serves to discourage the ingestion of harmful substances into the pharynx.[4876]

palytoxic fish poisoning A form of seafood poisoning occurring in Indo-Pacific and Caribbean regions, clinically indistinguishable from **ciguatera** fish poisoning.[2484]

pamplegia (from Gr, all + a stroke) (panplegia) Generalized weakness following a stroke.

Pan-African Association of Neurological Sciences An organization seeking to further neurological sciences and the exchange of ideas for neurologists in Africa and worldwide. Address: P.O. Box 20413, Nairobi, Kenya. Web site: http://www.paans.org/.

PanArab Union of Neurological Sciences A professional society with aims similar to the above and publishing the journal *Neurosciences*. Web site: http://www.neurosciencesjournal.org/.

panaris (Fr, a whitlow)

panaris analgésique de Morvan See **painless whitlows**.

panautonomic failure See **pandysautonomia**.

Panayiotopoulos syndrome (benign age-related focal seizure disorder occurring in early and mid-childhood) A common idiopathic childhood-specific autonomic seizure disorder defined as "a benign age-related focal seizure disorder occurring in early and mid-childhood characterized by seizures that are often prolonged, with predominantly autonomic symptoms, and by an EEG that shows shifting and/or multiple foci, often with occipital predominance."

The cardinal clinical manifestations consist of clusters of autonomic epileptic seizures that are may last over half an hour (thus constituting autonomic status epilepticus). The major autonomic symptom is emesis but also any other episodic disturbance of autonomic function can occur, such as pallor (less often, flushing or cyanosis), mydriasis (less often, miosis), cardiorespiratory and thermoregulatory disturbances, loss of sphincter control, hypersalivation, and modifications of intestinal motility. These may be the only features of the seizure, but in a fifth or so of cases the child becomes unresponsive and flaccid (ictal syncope) before or often without convulsions. Cardiorespiratory arrest is exceptional. More conventional cortical seizure symptoms often appear after the onset of autonomic manifestations such that the child becomes confused and later unresponsive. The eyes turn to one side or stare. Half the seizures end with brief hemiconvulsions or generalized convulsions, but convulsive status epilepticus is rare. Half of the seizures last for >30 min (autonomic status epilepticus) which is the more common afebrile nonconvulsive status epilepticus in normal children. Two thirds of seizures occur during sleep.

The EEG shows multiple, shifting, mainly occipital, spikes.[4881] Remission usually occurs within 2 years. There are no residual neurologic deficits and the risk of epilepsy in adult life is not increased. However, autonomic seizures are potentially life-threatening in the rare event of cardiorespiratory arrest.[4882]

This syndrome probably affects 13% of children aged 3–6 years who have had one or more afebrile seizures and 6% of such children in the 1–15-year age group. It is probably an early-onset form of Rolandic epilepsy in which ictal discharges, irrespective of their location at onset, activate autonomic disturbances, and thus is an early-onset phenotype of a maturation-related benign childhood seizure-susceptibility syndrome, complementing Rolandic epilepsy at a later age. (CP)

The symptoms/sequence of autonomic seizures and autonomic status epilepticus in Panayiotopoulos syndrome are only seen in children. (CP) (The author is indebted to Prof. Panayiotopoulos for his assistance with this entry). See also **childhood epilepsy with occipital paroxysms**.[546]

Pancoast, Henry Khunrath (1875–1939) American radiologist and radiotherapist, occupant of the first American chair in radiology, at the University of Pennsylvania, and the leader of that branch of the profession in his lifetime.

Pancoast syndrome (Pancoast–Tobias–Ciuffini syndrome, Hare syndrome) A painful lower brachial plexopathy with an added **Horner syndrome** occurring as a result of infiltration of these nerve trunks by an apical carcinoma of the bronchus or other malignancy.[4884]

Pancoast–Tobias–Ciuffini syndrome See **Pancoast syndrome**.

pancreatic encephalopathy A complication of acute pancreatitis characterized by focal signs, cognitive impairment, seizures, hallucinations, and sometimes acute axonal neuropathy. Sudden blindness can occur, resulting from a retinopathy (Purtscher syndrome) or from optic neuritis. With concurrent renal failure and thrombotic microangiopathy, confusion and seizures may occur.[1618]

PANDAS See **postinfectious (pediatric) autoimmune neuropsychiatric disorders associated with streptococcal infection**.

pandiculation (from Lat, to stretch oneself) A compound automatic movement consisting of extension of the legs, elevation and stretching of the arms, and extension of the head and trunk with yawning. It is generally physiological and related to drowsiness and waking, but may occur preceding a paroxysm of malaria.[5103]

Pandy test A test for the concentration of globulin in the CSF; it is not of current value.

pandysautonomia (panautonomic failure) A syndrome of acquired failure of both sympathetic and parasympathetic functions; it is most often due to **multiple system atrophy, primary autonomic failure**, or **hereditary motor and sensory neuropathy** type III. when slow in onset; it occurs rather more acutely in **acute inflammatory demyelinating polyneuropathy** and as a **paraneoplastic syndrome**. The pathogenesis is unknown. It is seen most commonly in adults and is characterized clinically by widespread autonomic failure involving the pupils, skin, and blood pressure, with added trigeminal and bulbar weakness, dysarthria, sensorimotor peripheral neuropathy, and spontaneous pain. See also **postural tachycardia syndrome, neurocardiogenic syncope, multiple system atrophy, familial amyloid neuropathy, diabetic neuropathy, Shy–Drager syndrome**, POLIP (pseudo-obstruction) syndrome, heat intolerance. A relationship to chronic fatigue syndrome has also been suggested.

panoramic looking Overall gaze that precedes seeing.[1592] Its pathway involves posterior parietal area 7, an area dominantly important in visual attention.

panoramic nystagmus See **optokinetic nystagmus**.

panplegia See **pamplegia**.

Pansini, Sergio (1860–1918) Italian neurologist who trained at Naples and practiced there, eventually as professor of clinical semeiology. His publications covered numerous areas including myotonia, acromegaly, the innervation of the diaphragm, and infectious diseases.

Pansini syndrome A cerebellar syndrome with marked dysarthria, reported as a complication of malaria.[4885]

pantanencephalia (Gr, complete + absence + the brain) A synonym of **anencephaly**.

pantomime 1. Movements made for semeiotic or referential purposes within the context of communicating information.[1327] 2. Movements carried out in silence with strict deliberation in order to express an idea or feeling.[1330]

Disturbances in the comprehension of such activity is another result of damage to the dominant hemisphere.

pantomime agnosia The ability to imitate pantomimes that are however not comprehended, reported as accompanying amnesia and alexia and associated with a lesion of the inferior visual association cortex.[5431]

pantothenate kinase deficiency See **neurodegeneration with brain iron accumulation**.

Panum's fusional area That part of space encompassing the **horopter**, where binocular vision is preserved (although always containing points that have some retinal disparity).

paper test A test of verbal comprehension introduced by Pierre **Marie**. "Here are three papers, a big one, a medium sized one and a small one. Take the biggest and rumple it up and throw it on the ground. Take the medium one and give it to me. Put the smallest one in your pocket."

Papez, James Wenceslaus (1883–1958) American neurophysiopsychologist at Cornell, whose insights led to the realization of the functions of the limbic system in 1937.[4889] The "Papez circuit" (hippocampus–fornix–mammillary body–anterior nucleus of the thalamus–bundle of Vicq d'Azir–cingulate gyrus) is essentially synonymous with the limbic system. This, Papez considered, through its connections with the hypothalamus, was a central regulator of the autonomic nervous system and of sexual and emotional experience and expression.

papill- (Gr, projection) Prefix denoting projection.

papillary meningioma See **meningioma**.

papilledema (Lat, teat + Gr, swelling) Swelling of the optic nerve head due both to axonal swelling and the presence of extra-axonal fluid, and occurring as a result of increased intracranial pressure.[486] **Jackson** defined four stages (Chart P–1).

papillitis Inflammation of the head of the optic nerve, thus visible with the ophthalmoscope. The swelling may be mistaken for **papilledema**, but in papillitis the visual acuity is significantly reduced and a central scotoma is present rather than enlargement of the blind spot with or without constriction of the outer fields.

papillomacular bundle The tract of myelinated fibers running from the macula

Chart P–1. The Four Stages of Papilledema

Early, characterized by blurring of the nerve fiber layer with indistinctness of the superior and inferior disk margins, retinal venous distention, loss of spontaneous venous pulsations, splinter hemorrhages in the nerve fiber layer at or close to the disk margin and retention of the optic cup.

Fully developed, in which there occur opacification of the nerve fiber layer, which prevents visualization of vessels crossing the rim of the disk; elevation and expansion of the disk, with an increase in the size of the blindspot; flame hemorrhages; infarcts of the nerve fiber layer; retinal edema (**macular star**); marked venous distention; and hyperemia of the disk.

In the *chronic* stage, the optic cup is obliterated and the disk takes on the shape of a button mushroom, surrounded often by hard exudates. Eventually the disk becomes gliotic, *atrophic* (secondary optic atrophy), pallid and flattened, with associated field defects due to damage to the retinal nerve fiber layer.[5]

to the optic nerve head, visibly pallid when demyelinated, as in some patients with **multiple sclerosis**. Because the tract enters the optic disk on the temporal side, that side appears paler than the nasal side in such cases, leading to the appearance of temporal pallor, but this is also the case in normal subjects and the determination of abnormal pallor is sometimes an artistic judgment.

papillophlebitis (optic disk vasculitis) A benign and self-limited condition characterized by mild, protracted, monocular visual impairment, swelling of the optic disk, retinal venous engorgement, and perivenous retinal hemorrhages in young people, without evidence of optic neuropathy. The other eye is normal and the cause is unknown.[1841] See also **retinal vasculitis, big blind-spot syndrome**.

pa-ping An endemic form of periodic paralysis with hypokalemia and vacuolar myopathy described in China, where it was due to barium poisoning.[3724]

papulosis atrophicans maligna A severe progressive atrophic and necrotic skin disease, rarely associated with features of necrotizing cerebral and spinal vasculitis.[1182]

para- (Gr, beside)

paraabducens center The brainstem center for lateral gaze, situated ventral to the median longitudinal fasciculus and lateral to the abducens nucleus.

paraballism 1. Bilateral hemiballism, caused in some cases not by lesions of the subthalamic but of the caudate nucleus and putamen; a rare and possibly lethal condition, most often occurring as a lacunar syndrome.[3253, 3891] See **ballism**. 2. A form of chorea in childhood induced by oral contraceptive ingestion.

Paracelsus (Gr, beside Celsus) Aureolus Threophrastus Bombastus von Hohenheim (1493–1541), an eccentric Swiss physician from Zurich who trained first in Vienna and then in medicine at Ferrara. He adopted the name of Aulus Celsus, a Roman historian, in a (successful) attempt at self-glorification. The name Bombastus was a similar addition, but he did not actually use the name "Paracelsus" himself.

He attacked the teachings of Galen, advocating the replacement of these mythologies with a new, scientific and empirical system, and encouraged scientific experiment. On the basis both of experiment and cogitation, he introduced the use of mercurials for the treatment of syphilis and he was the inventor of Laudanum, an extract of morphia. Paracelsus also described congenital syphilis and the manifestations of hysteria; linked endemic goitre and cretinism; produced anesthetic ether; and described **chorea**. His collected writings, published in 1658, spurred the investigative approach of such English physicians as Boyle, **Willis**, and **Sydenham**.[3028]

paracentral scotoma A scotoma, the edge of which passes through the fixation point, bisecting the line of central vision.

parachiasmal mass lesions Tumors of the sphenoid or petrous temporal bones or of the overlying meninges, an aneurysm of the internal carotid artery, granulomas, or other masses in the region of the cavernous sinus that may compress the chiasm on its medial aspect.[1392]

parachute reflex (parachute response) Extension of the arms of an infant suspended prone and dropped, still in the examiner's hands, toward a table below, the movement made as if to grab onto something to break the fall. This appears at 5–9 months and normally persists, but is absent in the setting of neuromuscular disease, spastic diseases, and mental retardation. Asymmetry of the response suggests the presence of a local upper or lower motor neuron lesion. See also **developmental reflexes**.

parachute response See **parachute reflex**.

paraclinical evidence (of a multiple sclerosis lesion) Demonstration by means of various tests and procedures of the existence of a lesion of the CNS which has not produced *signs* of neurological dysfunction but which may or may not have caused *symptoms* in the past. Such tests and procedures include the **hot bath test**, evoked response studies, oligoclonal banding in the CSF, tissue imaging procedures (MRI), and expert urological assessment.[5094, 5095]

paracrusis (Gr, playing a discord) Mild delirium.

paracusis (Gr, next to + hearing) 1. Distortion of the loudness of sounds heard. 2. Paradoxical improvement in hearing in the presence of background noise, as recorded by Thomas **Willis**.

paracusis of Willis (paracusis Willisiana) The state of only being able to hear in the presence of loud background noise, as in the case of the deaf woman who could only hear while a drum was beating, described by Thomas **Willis** in his *De Anima Brutorum*. The phenomenon is a feature of otosclerosis.

paracusis Willisiana See **paracusis of Willis**.

paradigm of Sternberg A memory test, wherein the subject is required to determine whether a word presented by the examiner was or was not included in word lists presented immediately before.[6047]

paradoxical ankle reflex (of Bing) Tapping the extensor (dorsal) aspect of the ankle between the malleoli produces plantar flexion of the foot in patients with pyramidal lesions, presumably due to vibrations transmited to the gastrocnemius.

paradoxical dystonia Dystonia at rest with improvement on exercise. See **dystonia**.

paradoxical flexor reflex See **Gordon reflex**.

paradoxical foot phenomenon of Westphal Involuntary and persistent contraction of the tibialis anterior, extensor digitorum longus, and peronei when the ankle is passively dorsiflexed; a dystonic feature seen in some patients with Parkinsonism.[645]

paradoxical myotonia Myotonia that increases with repeated muscle contractions, unlike the more common finding of a reduction or improvement in the myotonia in that situation. This phenomenon represents a major feature of **paramyotonia congenita**.

paradoxical pain Pain generated as a result of neural dysfunction, not following classical pain pathways and without any stimulation of peripheral nociceptors. Chronic nociceptive pain of this nature does not respond to morphine.[4492]

paradoxical patellar reflex Contraction of the thigh adductors in response to a tap on the quadriceps tendon, as a result of disinhibition of the spinal cord at levels adjacent to L2,3 in the presence of pyramidal tract lesions above those sites, or in response to transmitted vibration to the adductor muscle.

paradoxical pupil phenomenon See **Westphal–Piltz phenomenon**.

paradoxical pupillary dilatation (of Byrne) The pupil with sympathetic denervation, especially of the third neuron, exhibits **denervation hypersensitivity** to circulating catecholamines and thus may dilate under stress (when the levels of such substances are increased). Thus the pupil is usually smaller than its fellow in **Horner syndrome**, but may be larger in stressful conditions. The phenomenon represents a **pain reflex** mediated by sympathetic pathways. See also **Westphal–Piltz phenomenon**.

paradoxical reflexes Occasional *variant* forms of the usual muscle stretch reflexes, modified in certain conditions by the underlying disorder and the method of elicitation[6656] as with the **paradoxical triceps reflex**.

paradoxical sleep Rapid eye movement sleep, so called because the EEG resembles that of wakefulness but the subject is asleep. See **rapid eye movement sleep**.

paradoxical triceps reflex (olecranon reflex) Contraction of the elbow flexors when the triceps tendon is tapped, as a result of a lesion at C7 (8), which is causing depression of the triceps response; the tap leads to a slight stretch of the biceps, which is followed by contraction of that muscle.[6656]

parafoveal region The region of the macula immendiately about the fovea contralis.

paraganglioma 1. A neuronal tumor, usually arising in the cauda equina and characterized by the presence of neurons within the uniform mass of polygonal cells.[6] 2. (chemodactoma) See **glomus jugulare tumor**.

paraganglioma-ganglioneuroma A neuronal tumor.

parageusia See **dysgeusia**.

paragonimiasis A trematodal infestation characterized clinically by meningoencephalitis, seizures, focal neurological deficits, visual disturbances with optic atrophy, and dementia. Intracerebral calcifications are common.[2893]

paragraphia A syndrome characterized by writing errors that occur when one half of a word is neglected; thus *bus-stop* may be written as *stop*. It may occur in patients with right hemispheric neglect syndromes. See also **paralexia, neglect syndromes**.

parainfectious inflammatory encephalomyelitis A form of encephalitis clinically indistinguishable from direct viral encephalitis, but in which the organism (such as Epstein–Barr virus, *mycoplasma* or influenza virus) cannot be cultured from the brain but is detected as a result of a rise in antibody titers. The CSF contains an increased number of white cells.[5377] See also **acute disseminated encephalomyelitis, opsoclonus-myoclonus syndrome**.

parainfectious noninflammatory encephalomyelitis (acute toxic encephalopathy, acute nonsuppurative encephalitis, acute brain swelling) A form of encephalopathy characterized by acute brain swelling without inflammation or glial reaction, occurring usually in children who present with acute confusion, coma, and seizures, and who manifest a marked increase in intracranial pressure due to cerebral edema, without cells in the CSF.[5377] The condition was first described by Dr. James **Putnam**. See also **Reye syndrome, acute disseminated encephalomyelitis**.

paralalia The substitution of other distinct sounds for those which cannot be pronounced as a result of **mogilalia**. The pronunciation of "Th" for "S" (lisping) and of "W" for "R" are examples.

paralanguage Nonverbal methods of communication, including gesture and music.[1330]

paraleresis Mild delirium.

paralexia 1. The occurrence of substitutions in reading aloud. 2. Inability to attend to the words on one side of a page, as may be seen in **neglect syndromes**. The reading errors occur because one half of a word is neglected; thus *tenant* may be read as *ant*. This may occur in patients with right hemispheric neglect syndromes.[4112] See also **paragraphia**.

paralgesia Diminished sensibility of painful stimuli.

paralimbic areas Mesocortical areas better differentiated than **allocortex** but still lacking the six-layered structure of the **neocortex**. These areas include the insula, orbitofrontal cortex, temporal pole, the parahippocampal and cingulate gyri, and the paraolfactory areas.

paralinguistic communication The use of gestures and facial expressions to enhance verbal understanding.

paralysie des amants Radial nerve paralysis following prolonged compression of the nerve by the head or body of an actual or intended sexual partner. The lesion usually involves that portion of the radial nerve below the upper arm, so that triceps function is spared and the other individual can be pushed away.

paralysis (from Gr, weakness, disabling) Loss of motor function—formerly (until the late eighteenth century) also used for loss of sensation—thus paralysis of sight, smell, and so on.

paralysis agitans Dr. James **Parkinson**'s name for the disease now bearing his.[4906] See **Parkinson disease**.

paralysis agitans mercurialis Basal ganglion disease due to chronic mercury poisoning. See **hatters' shakes**.

paralysis vacillans (from Lat, paralysis + to stagger) Chorea.

paralytic pontine exotropia An **internuclear ophthalmoplegia** with paralytic monocular exotropia of the eye on the other side; the combination of an unilateral horizontal gaze palsy and internuclear ophthalmoplegia, caused by a single paramedian lesion of the pons. In the acute phase, one eye deviates laterally while the other is immobile in the primary position of gaze.[5767] See also **one-and-a-half syndrome**.

paralytic postural syncope Syncope due to impairment of autonomic reflexes, including the vasovagal reflex, which leads to impairment in the redistribution of blood flow with alterations in posture, such that venous return to the heart (and so cardiac output) is reduced.

paralytic pupil A dilated and unreactive pupil, occurring as a result of damage to the preganglionic parasympathetic nerves running with the III cranial nerve and supplying the pupillary sphincter.

Ptosis and either complete or partial III nerve extraocular palsy are usually present as well. See also **pupillary sparing**.

paralytic rabies See **dumb rabies**.

paralytic shellfish poisoning A severe illness resulting from inhibition of the voltage-dependent sodium channel due to saxitoxin poisoning. The condition occurs mainly (in North America) on the northern and Alaskan coasts. After an incubation period of ½–3 h, patients experience paresthesias of the mouth, face, and limbs, usually with headache, nausea, vomiting, and diarrhea and a "floating" sensation. Severe intoxication leads to dysphonia, ataxia, and systemic weakness progressing to ventilatory failure within 2–12 h. Symptoms persist for about 3 days. The case fatality rate varies from 1 to 12%.[3396, 2484] Most deaths occur within the first 12 h; those surviving 24 h will recover.

paralytic strabismus Those forms of strabismus which result from a lesion of cranial nerves III, IV, or VI.

Paralyzed Veterans of America A charitable organization also concerned with advocacy for its members. Tel: 202-872-1300. Web site: http://www.pva.org/site/PageServer/.

Paralyzed Veterans of America Spinal Cord Research Foundation A charitable organization providing support and information on this condition.

paramagnetic Possessed of an uneven number of particles (nucleons). When placed in a magnetic field that is sufficiently intense, some of the paramagnetic nuclei in a substance align themselves with that field and are susceptible to further alterations of their axes when a radiofrequency signal is applied to them, returning to their former position at various rates when it ceases. This represents the basis of MRI scanning.

paramagnetic agents Chemical substances which, when injected into the patient, enhance the quality of the images produced by **magnetic resonance imaging**.

paramedian diencephalic syndrome (syndrome of the thalamoperforating pedicle of Foix and Hillemand, thalamosubthalamic infarction syndrome, syndrome of the basilar communicating artery of Percheron, syndrome of the mesencephalic artery, thalamosubthalamic infarction syndrome) The combination of fluctuating hypersomnolent apathy, an amnesic syndrome, impaired vertical (mainly downward) gaze, and often aphasia and palilalia, resulting from bilateral diencephalic infarctions.[4291] See also **top of the basilar syndrome**.

paramedian infarction Bilateral thalamic infarctions resulting from occlusion of the thalamosubthalamic arteries, producing a syndrome of acute transient coma, followed by drowsiness, asterixis, hypersomnia, vertical gaze paresis, and, in some cases, persistent amnesia.[2607] See also **paramedian diencephalic syndrome** above.

paramedian pontine infarction One of three types of pontine infarction described by Foix in 1926 (the others being *short circumferential* and *tegmental*) producing hemiplegia worse in the arm, with mild dysarthria and due to either one large or numerous small lacunes, sometimes bilateral.[2106]

paramedian thalamic syndrome A state resulting from bilateral vascular, paramedian thalamic lesions, causing subwakefulness with slowing of background EEG activity and a lack of both deep sleep and alert wakefulness.[4450]

parameningeal infections (meningite de voisinage, Dupré syndrome) Infectious processes situated within the dura mater (sinus thrombophlebitis) or outside the meninges completely (epidural abscess, otitis, sinusitis) but which cause a meningeal reaction by virtue of their proximity.[1756]

Some authorities would also include intracerebral abscesses within this category.

paramnesia (Gr, beside + memory) A psychiatric condition characterized by the misinterpretation of events or locations. See also **reduplicative paramnesia**.

paramyoclonus multiplex (Kny disease, convulsive tremor) (from Gr, beside + a muscle + a tumult) A dominantly inherited myoclonic disorder characterized by involuntary contractions of single muscles or groups of synergic muscles, resulting in sudden, paroxysmal, symmetrical, clonic spasms at 10–50 Hz, occurring mainly in males and at any age. Voluntary movements and alcohol intake may suppress them, but they persist in sleep and are increased by activities requiring fine coordination such as writing and by conscious attempts to inhibit them.[2208] See also **Friedreich disease, hereditary essential myoclonus**.

The movements involve the arms, legs, trunk, and neck, but particularly the arms and neck, and are most frequent and intense proximally; the diaphragm may be involved. They are always rapid and brief and are sometimes asynchronous. The accompanying EMG electrical activity lasts less than 500 ms.

This was the original term applied by **Friedreich** in 1881 and by Kny 7 years later[3504] to a condition characterized by bursts of irregular myoclonus in the trunk and limbs lasting several minutes. It has been been suggested[4020] that the onset of paramyoclonus (bilaterally symmetrical jerks often inhibited by movement) before the age of 20 years in the presence of dominant inheritance and with a benign course, in the absence of generalized seizures, dementia, and ataxia and a normal EEG, constitute appropriate diagnostic criteria.

paramyotonia Intermittent myotonia induced by repetitive use of muscles and increased by exposure to cold or (rarely) to heat. It is most obvious in the face, neck, and distal extremities. Attacks usually last for hours.

Compare this with **myotonia**, in which the abnormal muscle contraction tends to lessen with exercise or with warmth, and with **paradoxical myotonia. Paramyotonia congenita** and hyperkalemic periodic paralysis are each associated with both clinical paramyotonia and electrical myotonia.

paramyotonia congenita

(Eulenberg disease, myotonic periodic paralysis, congenital myotonia) A rare, dominantly inherited sodium channelopathy with the onset in infancy of intermittent, nonprogressive tonic contraction (myotonia) of the facial, bulbar, and distal muscles precipitated by exposure to cold for short periods, with episodic flaccid weakness of the limbs and areflexia occurring after longer exposure. The responsible gene maps to chromosome 17q13.1–q13.5. The physiological basis is disruption or inactivation of the fast sodium channel (the SCN4A subunit), though some mutations also disrupt the slow Na^+ channel. Numerous point mutations of the *SCN4A* gene have been held responsible.

There are no dystrophic features, but a tendency to muscle hypertrophy is notable clinically, as is a variation in muscle fiber size histologically. No other laboratory abnormalities coexist, but EMG reveals that repetitive muscular contractions lead to a decreasing recruitment pattern, and after cooling the hand in ice water, the myotonia disappears and the hand enters a state of electrically silent contracture.[4669, 1546] **Paradoxical myotonia** may also occur.[6309]

The disease was described in 1886 by Eulenberg, who was aware of its occurrence in six generations of the family that he studied.[1923] Becker suggested the term *paralysis periodica paramyotonica*[472] to refer to those patients in whom the weakness is associated with hyperkalemia, and in whom prolonged, repeated movements stimulate the myotonia and fatigability is noted. *Variant* conditions are as follows:

Acetazolamide-responsive myotonia
Myotonia fluctuans
Myotonia permanens

Paramyotonia congenita without cold paralysis, a dominantly inherited myotonic syndrome in which the symptoms begin in childhood. The myotonia is easily provoked by exercise and elicited by percussion, but not by cold.[1499]

Paramyotonic periodic paralysis, a dominantly inherited syndrome of percussion and paroxysmal myotonia induced by exercise, warmth, and cold, and associated with weakness and easy fatigability.[221] This may or may not the the same condition as paramyotonia congenita. See **familial periodic paralysis**.

Potassium-aggravated myotonia, in which the attacks are precipitated by a potassium load, and in which there is no weakness. Weakness precipitated by hypokalemia resembles paramyotonia congenita but without the cold paralysis.

Temperature-sensitive sodium channelopathy with heat-induced myotonia and cold-induced paralysis, a rare dominantly inherited syndrome with these findings and due to a mutation in the skeletal muscle sodium channel.[6121]

paraneoplastic acute ascending polyneuropathy

An illness indistinguishable from **acute inflammatory demyelinating polyneuropathy** occurring in some patients with **Hodgkin disease**.

paraneoplastic acute necrotizing myopathy

A rare complication of remote carcinoma, characterized by rapidly or subacutely progressive symmetrical proximal muscle weakness and atrophy due to both neuropathy and muscle inflammation.[6154]

paraneoplastic amyotrophic lateral sclerosis

A disorder almost indistinguishable from amyotrophic lateral sclerosis except for its potential for improvement following the elimination of the malignancy. See **amyotrophic lateral sclerosis** (*variants*).

paraneoplastic antibodies

See **anti-Yo, anti Hu, anti-Ri**.

paraneoplastic autonomic neuropathy

Sympathetic and parasymptathetic failure as a result of remote malignancy. Varieties include the following:[6106]

a. Acute pandysautonomia (see **autonomic neuropathy**)
b. Paraneoplastic intestinal pseudo-obstruction
c. Dysautonomia complicating **paraneoplastic encephalomyelitis**
d. Impaired sweating and postural hypotensiion with **paraneoplastic sensorimotor peripheral neuropathy**
e. Local autonomic dysfunction with root infiltration
f. Autonomic effects as a result of therapy (e.g., vincristine) or in the **Lambert–Eaton syndrome**.

paraneoplastic cerebellar degeneration

A rapidly progressive syndrome characterized by unsteady gait and later a full range of cerebellar symptoms and signs with downbeat nystagmus and often oscillopsia. MRI scans show cerebellar atrophy. Gynecological, breast, and small cell lung carcinomas and Hodgkin disease are defined causes. Anti-Yo, anti-Hu, anti-Tr, and anti-nGluR antibodies are variously detectable.[5232]

paraneoplastic dementia

An acute or slowly developing dementing syndrome usually accompanying other paraneoplastic disorders. See also **paraneoplastic limbic encephalitis**.

paraneoplastic dermatomyositis

(paraneoplastic polymyositis) The appearance of clinical signs of polymyositis or dermatomyositis in the presence of overt or latent malignancy, especially small cell carcinoma of the lung or alimentary carcinomas in men and carcinomas of the ovary or breast in women.[4157]

paraneoplastic encephalomyelitis

(with/without rigidity) Diverse subacute syndromes affecting almost any part of the nervous system, central or peripheral, complicating remote malignancy (usually bronchogenic carcinoma), and listed under **paraneoplastic syndromes** (carcinomatous encephalo-myeloneuropathy). Lymphocytic infiltrates in the meninges and parenchyma, glial nodules, and perivascular lymphocytic cuffing are characteristic pathological findings[1694] and both motor and sensory neuronopathies may be associated. Anti-Hu antibodies may be detected.

In the form with rigidity, this affects the trunk and limbs and is associated with stimulus-sensitive myoclonus. Anti-amphiphysin antibodies are undetectable in the serum.

paraneoplastic encephalomyelitis with bulbar involvement

A syndrome of meningoencephalitis with subacute cerebellar degeneration, myelitis, ganglioradiculitis, ophthalmoplegia, nystagmus, and peripheral neuropathy, occurring mainly in males with an underlying malignancy (usually oat-cell carcinoma of the bronchus),[1694] but also in women with breast or uterine carcinomas. Clinically, marked memory loss, seizures, and agitation are the most notable features.

Various paraneoplastic neuronal autoantibodies may be detected.

paraneoplastic limbic encephalitis A subacute amnestic dementing syndrome complicating small cell carcinoma of the lung or other malignancies in which there are varying degrees of anxiety, confusion, and memory impairment. Pathologically, amygdaloid and hippocampal degenerative changes and widespread inflammation in other parts of the CNS are usually detected;[1290] antineuronal antibodies are also detectable.

paraneoplastic motor neuronopathy A syndrome of slowly developing lower motor neuron-type weakness without sensory changes in patients treated with irradiation for **Hodgkin disease** or other lymphomas. A potential for recovery after successful treatment of the malignancy has been described. See **subacute motor neuronopathy, amyotrophic lateral sclerosis** (*variants*).

paraneoplastic myopathy Muscle disease occurring as a remote effect of malignancy. Varieties include the following:[6106]

1. **Dermatomyositis**
2. **Acute (necrotic) myopathy**
3. **Carcinoid myopathy**
4. **Steroid nyopathy**
5. **Cachectic myopathy**

paraneoplastic myeloradiculoneuropathy A mixed syndrome with elements of both **paraneoplastic subacute necrotic myelopathy** and **paraneoplastic sensorimotor peripheral neuropathy**. Clinically, radicular pain, sensory loss, lower motor neurone disease, and areflexia are typical findings and the CSF is almost always abnormal.

paraneoplastic myopathies Muscle disorders occurring in association with a remote carcinoma. These include **paraneoplastic dermatomyositis/polymyositis, Lambert–Eaton myasthenic syndrome, paraneoplastic acute necrotizing myopathy**, and **cachectic myopathy**.

paraneoplastic neuropathies Disorders of the peripheral nervous system occurring as remote effects of a distant malignancy. These include the following:[6106]

1. Motor neuron disorders
   a. **Amyotrophic lateral sclerosis**-like syndrome
   b. **Paraneoplastic motor neuronopathy**
   c. Anterior horn cell disease with **paraneoplastic encephalomyelitis**
2. Radiculopathies
   a. **Paraneoplastic myeloradiculoneuropathy**
   b. Neuritis, e.g., herpes zoster
3. Plexopathies
   a. Neoplastic **plexopathies**
   b. **Radiation-induced plexopathies**
4. Other neuropathies
   a. **Paraneoplastic sensory neuronopathy**
   b. **Paraneoplastic sensorimotor peripheral neuropathy**
   c. Autonomic neuropathies
   d. Mononeuropathies, especially of the median and common peroneal nerves
   e. Radiation-induced schwannomas
   f. Neuropathies coomplicating chemotherapy (vincristine, platinum, cytosine arabinoside, procarbazine, etc.)

See also **dysproteinemic neuropathy, amtoineuronal antibodies**.

paraneoplastic opsoclonus/myoclonus See **opsoclonus**.

paraneoplastic optic neuritis A rare complication of remote carcinoma, presenting with progressive visual loss and swelling of the optic nerve head.

paraneoplastic polymyositis See **paraneoplastic dermatomyositis**.

paraneoplastic retinopathy (cancer-associated retinopathy) A syndrome of retinal photoreceptor degeneration leading to rapid visual deterioration, accompanied by narrowing of the retinal arterioles, visual field defects, nyctalopia, and absence of the electroretinographic response, and occurring in association with small cell lung, breast, uterine, or renal carcinomas.[3481] See **visual paraneoplastic syndrome**.

paraneoplastic sensorimotor peripheral neuropathy A mixed acute, subacute, or chronic axonal peripheral neuropathy, often with secondary demyelination, complicating carcinomas of the lung, breast, and gastrointestinal tract and associated with raised CSF protein levels and with the presence of antimyelin antibodies in the serum.[2868] This is perhaps the commonest of the neuropathies due to distant malignancy.[1344, 1345, 6106] Raised CSF protein levels are usual.[2869] The appearance of symptoms may precede evidence of the malignancy by years or may follow it. See also **gammopathic neuropathy**.

Variants are *acute inflammatory demyelinating polyneuropathy* seen with Hodgkin disease or lung cancer; a form of **chronic acute inflammatory demyelinating polyneuropathy;** and a vasculitic form of polyneuritis. Cachectic neuropathy may also occur. See also **paraproteinemia**.

paraneoplastic (carcinomatous) sensory neuronopathy (or ganglionopathy, or ganglionitis) A severe, immunologically mediated, acute or subacute, painful, pure sensory neuronopathy, most commonly seen in female patients with small cell lung cancer and presenting with distal paresthesias, dysesthesias and numbness, severe proprioceptive loss, pain, and hyporeflexia. Later features include generalized sensory loss, pseudoathetosis, and sensory ataxia. Even though anti-Hu antibodies staining neuronal nuclei may be detected, the usual small cell lung or other cancer may not appear until up to 3 years after the time of presentation of the neuropathy. Other paraneoplastic syndromes such as limbic encephalitis may coexist.[6106]

The spinal ganglion cells are destroyed as a result of a presumed autoimmune attack.[1585, 3003] The CSF protein levels are raised and other cerebellar, autonomic, or cerebral paraneoplastic syndromes are also present in about half the cases.[1082] The sensory nerve action potentials are small or absent and SEPs delayed or absent.

In a *variant* form, the same condition occurs with added **polymyositis**.

paraneoplastic stroke Stroke (affecting any vessel) occurring in association with mucin-induced coagulopathy in patients with carcinomas which are not necessarily mucin secreting.[175]

paraneoplastic subacute cerebellar degeneration with bulbar involvement A rare complication associated with ovarian, small cell lung, or breast carcinomas, or with **Hodgkin disease**, and presenting with ptosis, ophthalmoplegia, **opsoclonus**, and facial weakness.[803] Deafness due to degeneration of the cochlear nerve may also occur as a component of the syndrome. Anti-Purkinje cell antibodies are detectable in the serum. See also **subacute cortical cerebellar degeneration**.

paraneoplastic subacute necrotic myelopathy A rapidly progressive syndrome of myelopathic motor and sensory loss ascending to thoracic levels in some patients with carcinoma of the bronchus.[2724]

paraneoplastic syndromes (nonmetastatic syndromes) Autoimmune diseases resulting from the expression of autoantibodies to onconeural antigens by tumor cells which are identical or antigenically related to molecules whose expression is normally restricted to neurons; from cellular immune reaction against onconeural antigens; from monoclonal paraproteins; or from other other poorly understood immune mechanisms.

These rare, distant, nonmetastatic complications of underlying malignant disease (such as small cell carcinomas of the lung or ovarian carcinomas) are not caused by direct tumor invasion, metastasis toxicity of cancer therapy, cerebrovascular disease, coagulopathy, infection, or toxic or metabolic causes. The neurologic symptoms are commonly the presenting feature of an undiagnosed tumor. In part they may be due to the immunological response of the host to the tumor protein, the immunoglobulins cross-reacting with antigens on certain subsets of neurons. See the preceding 19 entries, **paraneoplastic vasculitis**, and **hyperviscosity syndromes**. The clinical syndromes described are listed in Chart P–2.

Chart P–2. The Paraneoplastic Syndromes

1. *Carcinomatous encephalomyeloneuropathy*

Subacute cortical cerebellar degeneration (small cell Ca. lung, etc.)
Paraneoplastic subacute cerebellar degeneration with bulbar involvement (Hodgkin disease etc.)
Lower brainstem (bulbar) encephalitis (small cell Ca. lung, Ca. breast or testicle, etc.)
Paraneoplastic limbic encephalitis or encephalomyelitis (small cell Ca. lung, testicular, breast carcinomas, thymoma, ovarian teratoma)
Acute intrinsic (necrotizing) in myelopathy (small cell Ca. lung, thymoma)
Paraneoplastic subacute necrotic myelopathy (necrotizing myelitis with predilection for anterior horn cells)
Psychological disorders
Opsoclonus-myoclonus syndrome (neuroblasstoma, testicular carcinoma, small cell Ca. lung)
Paraneoplastic dementia.
Neuromyotonia, stiff person syndrome (thymoma, small cell Ca. lung)
Extrapyramidal syndromes (small cell Ca. lung, thymoma)

2. *Myopathic-myasthenic syndromes*

Lambert-Eaton myasthenic syndrome (small cell Ca. lung)
A syndrome resembling **myasthenia gravis**
Paraneoplastic polymyositis/dermatomyositis
Acute necrotizing myopathy
Myotonia

3. ***Progressive multifocal leukoencephalopathy***

4. *Ophthalmological disorders*

Cancer-associated retinopathy (**paraneoplastic retinopathy**, CAR syndrome) (melanoma, small cell Ca. lung CLC, others)
Nutritional amblyopia
Uveomeningitic syndrome
Paraneoplastic optic neuritis. (small cell Ca. lung)

5. *Neuropathies* (reviewed by Grisold and Drlicek, 1999)[2584]

Paraneoplastic sensory neuronopathy and subacute sensory neuropathy (small cell Ca. lung, etc.)
Paraneoplastic sensorimotor neuropathy (small cell Ca. lung, plasma cell dyscrasias etc.)
Subacute pure **motor neuronopathy**
Paraneoplastic vasculitis with multiple mononeuropathy
Monoclonal **gammopathic neuropathy**
Neuropathy with insulinoma
Paraneoplastic acute ascending polyneuropathy
Paraneoplastic **amyotrophic lateral sclerosis** (small cell Ca. lung etc.)
Pandysautonomia (small cell Ca. lung)
Stiff person syndrome (Ca. breast, small cell Ca. lung, etc.)

Diagnostic criteria for paraneoplastic neurological syndromes (PNS) have been suggested[2553] and are reproduced by kind permission of the BMJ Publishing Group.

Definite PNS

1. A classical syndrome of cancer that develops within 5 years of the diagnosis of the neurological disorder.
2. A nonclassical syndrome that resolves or significantly improves after cancer treatment without concomitant immunotherapy, provided that the syndrome is not susceptible to spontaneous remission.
3. A nonclassical syndrome with onconeural antibodies (well characterized or not) and cancer that develops within 5 years of the diagnosis of the neurological disorder.
4. A neurological syndrome (classical or not) with well-characterized onconeural antibodies (anti-Hu, Yo, CV2, Ri, Ma2, or amphiphysin) and no cancer.

Probable PNS

1. A classical syndrome without onconeural antibodies or detected cancer, but at high risk for an underlying tumor.
2. A neurological syndrome, classical or not, with partially characterized onconeural antibodies but no detected cancer.

3. A nonclassical syndrome without onconeural antibodies in which cancer presents within 2 years of diagnosis.

paraneoplastic vasculitis A multiple mononeuropathy in which Wallerian degeneration is associated with microvasculitis, usually complicating a small cell carcinoma of the lung.[3231] Clinically, the disorder presents as a mixed sensorimotor neuropathy with autonomic signs.

paraneurons Endocrine brothers of neurons which produce substances that are either the same as or related to neurotransmitters or neurohormones; they possess neurosecretory-like and/or synaptic vesicles or granules and have receptosensory functions.[2227]

paranoia (from Gr, beside + mind; hence out of one's mind) From ancient Greek times to the Middle Ages, it was the term for all forms of madness, being restricted to the endogenous psychoses in the nineteenth century and then incorporated as a type of *dementia praecox* by Kraepelin early in the last century. The term is now used for the delusional belief that one is the target of unwarranted hostility.

paraphysial cyst Colloid cysts arising from the ependyma of the paraphysis, a vestigial third ventricular structure.

paraparesis 1. Weakness of the legs, usually as a result of bilateral pyramidal tract lesions. 2. Incomplete paraplegia.

paraphasia (Gr, beside + speechlessness) 1. The tendency to utter words that are distorted although similar to the correct words sought; the incorrect use of words, within the context of a dysphasic condition. The phenomenon is a manifestation of patients with aphasias whose utterances are distortions of normal words. *Literal* and *phonemic* forms are distinguished. In *verbal paraphasias*, whole words or phrases are substitutes for those intended. 2. The evocation of an inappropriate sound in place of a desired word or phrase; the replacement of a desired word with an articulate sound which is devoid of conventional meaning.

paraphilia (Gr, beside + love) 1. Intense fantasies, aberrant urges, or behaviors involving sexual arousal by nonhuman objects. 2. Unusual sexual practices, not necessarily implying deviance; or the awareness of sexual feelings toward otherwise nonsexual objects.

paraphonemia An inability to distinguish between phonemes that are somewhat similar in their acoustic properties.[1330]

paraphrasia Incoherent or disordered speech.

paraphrenesis Dementia or delirium (eighteenth century).

paraphrenia A paranoid state occurring in the elderly.

paraplegia (from Gr, beside + a stroke) (paraplexia) "A palsy which seizeth all parts of the Body below the Head" (Blancard's *Dictionary*, 1693; quoted by Skinner[5886]). Now taken to mean complete paralysis of the legs, as from a spinal cord lesion or severe neuropathy.

paraplegia dolorosa Paraplegia with pain, usually due to spinal cord compression from spinal tumors, described by **Cruveilhier**.

paraplegia-in-extension A posture of the legs consequent upon a pyramidal lesion, in which resting tone is greater in the extensor muscles than in the flexors; usually an entity in which the severity of the lesion is less than that which occurs in cases of **paraplegia-in-flexion**.[4110]

paraplegia-in-flexion The result of unantagonized flexor reflex action giving rise to a rigid posture of the legs, which is intermittent and thus gives rise to involuntary movements; it is consequent upon a pyramidal lesion. In this state, resting tone is greater in the flexor muscles than in the extensors. Absent or reduced knee and ankle jerks and an extensor response accompany these findings.

Its presence usually indicates that the severity of the lesion is greater than that occurring in cases of **paraplegia-in-extension**.[4110, 6622] The term was introduced by **Babinski**.

paraplegin A mitochondrial metalloproteinase, a mutation of which is responsible for a recessive form of **hereditary spastic paraparesis**.

paraplexia See **paraplegia**.

paraplexy A state of paralysis due to apoplexy or perhaps to other causes. The word was used by early Greek physicians and is probably synonymous with the term **paraplegia** as we use it.[1191]

paraproteinemia The presence of elevated amounts of abnormal immunoglobulins in the plasma, due either to plasma cell malignancies or to nonmalignant conditions. Polyneuropathies complicate the syndrome in up to a third of cases.[3724] See **gammopathic neuropathy**.

pararhinal sclerosis See **mesial temporal sclerosis**.

parasagittal In a plane parallel to the anteroposterior midline axis.

parasagittal cerebral injury A syndrome of usually bilateral and symmetrical cortical and subcortical ischemic injury in the **watershed zones** of the brain as a result of a reduction in cerebral perfusion pressure. In the newborn, the clinical characteristics include hypotonia and weakness in the arms and legs, later developing into spastic quadriparesis.[1301]

parasellar lesions Those lesions that are sited alongside the pituitary fossa, such as those within the cavernous sinus, and including meningiomas, aneurysms, etc.[1392] See **parachiasmal mass lesions**.

parasite potential See **satellite potential**.

parasomnias Recurrent physiological or abnormal motor, behavioral, or experiential phenomena representing disorders of arousal, partial arousal, and sleep transition, which intrude into the sleep process and reflect activation of the CNS. In Chart P–3 are listed the four groups as originally classified by the American Sleep Disorders Association.[1629]

Restless limb syndrome, periodic limb movements in sleep, and **hypnagogic and hypnapompic hallucinations** could equally well be included in this list. *Secondary parasomnias* include nocturnal epilepsy syndromes, various headache disorders, nocturnal muscle cramps, nocturnal panic

Chart P–3. The [Primary] Parasomnias

A. *Arousal disorders*
Manifestations of partial arousal that occur during sleep. These are the "classic" arousal disorders that appear to be primarily disorders of normal arousal mechanisms and comprise;
1. **Confusional arousals**
2. **Sleepwalking**
3. **Sleep terrors** (pavor nocturnus)

B. *Sleep-wake transition disorders*
Disorders that occur mainly during the transition from wakefulness to sleep or from one sleep stage to another.
1. **Rhythmic movement disorder**
2. **Sleep starts**
3. **Sleep talking**
4. **Nocturnal leg cramps**

C. *Parasomnias usually associated with rapid eye movement sleep*
1. **Nightmares** (dream anxiety attacks)
2. **Sleep paralysis**
3. **Impaired sleep-related penile erections**
4. **Sleep-related painful erections**
5. **Rapid eye movement sleep-related sinus arrest**
6. **Rapid eye movement sleep behaviour disorder**

D. *Other parasomnias*
1. Sleep **bruxism**
2. Sleep **enuresis**
3. **Sleep-related abnormal swallowing syndrome**
4. **Nocturnal paroxysmal dystonia**
5. **Sudden unexplained nocturnal death syndrome**
6. Primary **snoring**
7. Infant **sleep apnea**
8. **Congenital central hypoventilation syndrome**
9. **Sudden infant death syndrome.**
10. **Benign neonatal sleep myoclonus**
11. Sudden onset of sleep in Parkinson disease.
12. **Catathrenia**
13. Other parasomnias not otherwise specified.

attacks, and certain respiratory and gastrointestinal conditions.[6079]

paraspinal mapping An electromyographic technique wherein the EMG needle probes in many directions from each of five specified paraspinal sites, in order to sample activity from multifidus muscles at different levels in the precise diagnosis of radiculopathy.[2682]

parasympathetic system The procreative, vegetative division of the autonomic nervous system, comprising the unmyelinated fibers of the vagus nerve and the sacral outflow at S2, 3, 4. See **autonomic function tests**.

parathymia Brain exhaustion (nineteenth century).

paratonia (paratonic or arteriosclerotic rigidity, pure motor negativism, gegenhalten) An increase in muscle tone proportional to the amount of force used to achieve passive movement of a limb (usually the leg), and often worsened by exhortations made to the patient to relax; such resistance to movement may be a consequence of a dyspraxia.[6428] See **Foerster syndrome**.

It occurs as a result of diffuse bifrontal disease (when the legs are involved) and in association with dyspraxias (when it occurs in the arms).[3479]

paratonic rigidity An inability to relax a group of muscles, occurring together with brisk reflexes and extensor plantar responses. (Dupré) See also **paratonia**.

paratrigeminal oculosympathetic syndrome The presence of oculosympathetic loss shown by miosis, ptosis, or both, with normal forehead sweating and evidence of trigeminal involvement (sensory change or neuralgic pain), are likely to have a lesion in the middle cranial fossa sited medial to the trigeminal ganglion.[2413] See **Raeder paratrigeminal syndrome**.

paredrine test See **hydroxyamphetamine test**.

parencephalis An antique term for the cerebellum.

parencephalocele A congenital malformation in which there is herniation of a cyst of the posterior fossa through a defect in the occipital bone.

parenchymatous cortical cerebellar atrophy (late cortical cerebellar atrophy, Thomas atrophy)[199] See **olivopontocerebellar atrophy, autosomal dominant cerebellar ataxias, Marie–Foix–Alajouanine syndrome**.

parenchymatous syphilis That form of tertiary syphilis affecting the substance of the nervous system directly, as opposed to **meningovascular syphilis. General paresis, tabes dorsalis,** and syphilitic optic atrophy are the three varieties of this form.

paresis (Gr, a slackening) Partial paralysis or weakening of muscle power.[5886] The word is used almost interchangeably with **paralysis**, but is generally used to indicate a less severe degree of weakness than the latter.

paresthesias (Gr, beside + sense perceptions) 1. Abnormal sensations as of tingling or burning in regions to which the nerve supply is impaired but not lost, and due to the generation of ectopic nerve impulses in dysfunctional axons.

The contraction of *paraesthesia* to *paresthesia* is usual in North America, but the dipthong is retained in the United Kingdom. To retain a certain quasi-authenticity, the plural may be written *paresthesiae*, but the -*s* ending is used here for simplicity, the author having little Latin and less Greek.

2. An illusion of sensation, affecting any sense channel (nineteenth century).

paretic Of or belonging to a **paresis**.

paretic nystagmus Nystagmus that occurs when a subject attempts to deviate the eyes voluntarily in the direction of action of a weak extraocular muscle. The same phenomenon may occur in subjects with conjugate gaze paresis.

parietal (from Lat, concerning a wall) The wall of a cavity, or, in neurology, the covering of the ventricles; thus the parietal lobe or (relating to the wall or side of a cavity) the parietal bone. The syndromes of the parietal lobe have been reviewed by Critchley.[1329]

parietal apraxia See **apraxia**.

parietal ataxia (parietal kinetic ataxia, pseudocerebellar ataxia) Ataxia resembling that due to cerebellar disease, occurring in the absence of clinical weakness or any sensory deficit and due to a lesion of the contralateral parietal lobe.[223, 1329] The original report of **Claude** and **Lhermitte** in 1918 documented gait ataxia resulting from bilateral parietal lobe lesions, but pathological studies were not performed.

parietal foramina-cleidocranial dysplasia A congenital dysmorphic syndrome manifesting also absent auditory canals, hypertelorism, absent clavicles, dolichocephaly, and macrocephaly with parietal foramina, but the foramina can also be present in isolation.

parietal kinetic ataxia See **parietal ataxia**.

parietal lobe epilepsies Uncommon focal epileptic syndromes usually characterized by simple partial and secondarily generalized seizures. Most events are simple partial seizures lasting up to 2 min, but complex "partial" seizures may occur with spread beyond the parietal lobe. Typical clinical features include somatosensory disturbances of body image (somatic illusions), vertiginous or visual illusions, or complex formed visual hallucinations or **palinopsia**. Tingling and electric shock sensations may be confined or spread in a Jacksonian manner. There may be a desire to move a body part or a sensation as if a part were being moved. Muscle tone may be lost. The parts most frequently involved are those with the largest cortical representation (e.g., the hand, arm, and face). There may be tongue sensations of crawling, stiffness, or coldness, and facial sensory phenomena may occur bilaterally. Occasionally an intraabdominal sensation of sinking, choking, or nausea may occur, particularly in cases of inferior and lateral parietal lobe involvement. Superficial burning pain or vague but severe pains and dysesthesias are felt uncommonly.

Parietal lobe visual phenomena include formed hallucinations and **metamorphopsia** (somatic illusions, such as sensations of a distorted posture, limb position, or movement, or of an extremity or body part being alien) and mainly arise from the non–language dominant hemisphere. Inability to move one extremity or a feeling of weakness in the hand contralateral to the epileptogenic zone with sensations of distortion, foreshortening, or elongation may occur, more frequently in cases of nondominant hemisphere discharges.

Negative phenomena include numbness, a feeling that a body part is absent, and a loss of awareness of a part or a half of the body, known as *asomatognosia*, particularly with nondominant hemisphere involvement. Severe vertigo or disorientation in space suggests an inferior parietal lobe focus. Seizures in the dominant parietal lobe result in a variety of receptive or conductive languages disturbances. Some well-lateralized genital sensations may occur with paracentral involvement, and some rotatory or postural motor phenomena are described. Seizures of the paracentral lobule frequently show secondary generalization. Postictal symptoms include **Todd paralysis** (22%) and dysphasia (7%). (Adapted from Panayiotoupolos [2007][4882] by kind permission; and Dreifuss FE, et al. Commission for Classification and Terminology, ILAE. Proposal for Revised Classifications of Epilepsies and Epileptic syndromes. *Epilepsia* 1989;**30**:389–99 by kind permission of Wiley-Blackwell Publications.)

The more common of these experiences are somatosensory (occasionally painful) sensations, disturbances of body image, visual illusions, vertiginous sensations, aphasic auras, feeling of inability to move one extremity, complex visual or auditory hallucinations, elementary visual hallucinations, conscious confusion, and cephalic or epigastric sensations.[5509]

In addition, complex partial seizures with loss of contact and automatisms, or asymmetric tonic seizures may occur.[6802] Ictal SPECT studies are a preferred way of localizing the originating discharges.[2924]

parietal lobe syndrome See **Déjèrine syndromes**.

parietal stroke Infarcts of a parietal lobe, often producing one of three sensory syndromes; the **pseudothalamic sensory syndrome**, the **cortical sensory syndrome**, or an **atypical sensory syndrome** in addition to or in place of the **Déjèrine syndromes**.[434]

Parinaud, Henri (1844–1905) French neuro-ophthalmologist whose doctoral thesis (Université de Paris) was on the subject of papilledema in meningitis. He described the syndrome named for him (in a paper describing many forms of gaze paresis) in 1883, localizing the lesion to the pons and midbrain without autopsy verification. This article concerned convergence and divergence impairment as well as horizontal and vertical gaze abnormalities, but he was not certain about the localization of the lesion (whether in the ocular motor nuclei or the corpora quadrigemina). He later suggested that the center for vertical gaze is in the frontal lobes, but also that the lesion causing failure of upward gaze was of the quadrigeminal plates.

His professional appointment at the **Salpêtrière** gave him access to the patients of **Charcot** and so provided him with huge experience in disorders of eye movement, strabismus, and binocular vision, on all of which subjects he wrote extensively. He is properly regarded as the father of neuro-ophthalmology.

Parinaud syndrome 1. A supranuclear paresis of vertical gaze. See **dorsal midbrain syndrome**. 2. The oculoglandular syndrome in cat-scratch disease.

Parkes–Weber syndrome See **Klippel–Trenaunay–Weber syndrome**.

Parkes–Weber–Dimitri disease See **Sturge–Weber syndrome**.

parkin One of half a dozen gene products identified in monogenic forms of **Parkinson disease**, considered to be responsible for autosomal recessive juvenile Parkinsonism in Japanese families. In forms associated with this mutation, Lewy bodies are seldom found.[4418]

Parkinson, James (1755–1824) English physician, social activist, ethicist, and amateur paleontologist, practicing in Hoxton in the East End of London. He was apprenticed to his father, and at the age of 29, his name appeared on a list of surgeons approved by the Corporation of that city. Parkinson's career was overshadowed by his involvement in a variety of social and philanthropical, even revolutionary, causes, and he wrote many pamphlets, most appearing under the pseudonym "Old Hubert," in his radical capacity. Perhaps because he was a member of the London Corresponding Society, a genteel club devoted both to gastronomy and to revolution, he was haled before the Privy Council as an agitator on more than one occasion, but it appears was not punished. In keeping with his strong religious beliefs, he spent a considerable time attempting to ease the burden of the poor, to regulate the conduct of mental asylums, to provide more Sunday schools, and to reform the method of parliamentary representation.[4949, 6893]

His medical works included books on family medicine for lay audiences (one of which at least went to six editions), a handbook of chemistry, a textbook of geology, and memoirs of his days as a hospital pupil, as well as works on trusses, fevers, appendicitis (written with his son), and the gout. His *Essay on the Shaking Palsy* (**Parkinson disease**) was published in 1817; he referred to the preceding descriptions of the condition by Galen, Boetius, and others in the first chapter. In this work, he paid little attention to rigidity and claimed that the senses and intellects were uninjured (both errors being corrected later by Trousseau), wrote that the tremor was severe in sleep, and considered that the likely lesion was in the cervical cord, but otherwise his observations have stood the test of time.

It is of some interest that the first of the cases he described, and that one in the greatest detail, would now be classified as a case of **multiple system atrophy**. Half of the patients he reported on had been seen only on the street and never examined, but his description of the progression of the disease over years is so convincingly accurate that he must have had further experience of it either within his practice or in that of his father.

Parkinson also noted that paralysis from stroke inhibited the tremor, anticipating later attempts at surgical relief.[5704, 6893]

Parkinson disease The name applied by **Charcot** to the prototypical form of Parkinsonism; a chronic progressive degenerative disease initially described by James **Parkinson** under the rubric "shaking palsy," and manifesting the triad of tremor, bradykinesia, and rigidity, with a shuffling, festinating, or propulsive gait; stooped posture; and (in its advanced stages) loss of postural reflexes and torsion spasms, **hypophonia**, dysphagia, cachexia, and dementia. Additional (nonmotor) manifestations include cognitive impairment, seborrhea, bladder and bowel disturbances, and other autonomic problems and sleep disturbances. Impulse control disorders such as **punding**, problem gambling, binge eating, compulsive shopping, and hypersexuality affect a minority of patients with Parkinson disease (especially those on dopaminergic therapy) and can be a cause of marked morbidity.[1120]

Neuronal degeneration in the perikaryon of surviving neurons in the substantia nigra is the main histological feature. Lewy bodies may be found both there and in neurons in the peripheral autonomic ganglia, the Auerbach and Meissner plexuses, the intermediolateral cell column of the thoracic spinal cord, the hypothalamus, the amygdala, the hippocampus, and, in some cases, the cerebral cortex diffusely.

In patients with diffuse cortical Lewy bodies (and in those without, at a late stage), dementia may be the predominant clinical manifestation (see below).

A screening questionnaire for community use has been developed.[1088] An excellent review is found at www.aafp.org/afp/990415ap/2155.html.

The etiology is unknown; most cases are apparently sporadic but familial occurrence has been reported, and both exogenous environmental and genetic factors are suspected [RCD]. At May 2008, 11 genetic variants are recognized, some autosomal dominant (AD) (1, 3, 4, 5, 8) and others recessive (AR) (2, 6, 9).

PARK 1 4q21–q23/ *α-synuclein.* Autosomal dominant, with younger age at onset, low prevalence of tremor, and a more rapid clinical deterioration. Concomitant dementia, myoclonus, and central hypoventilation are described.

PARK2 6q25 2q–27/*Parkin.* Autosomal recessive, often with early onset and slow progression. Presentations range from classical Parkinsonism to foot or other dystonias and dyskinesias with dopaminergic treatment. Cognition is normal and Lewy bodies are seldom present. There is an excellent response to levadopa. Atypical forms manifest psychosis, panic attacks, depression, hypersexuality, and obsessive-compulsive behavior.

PARK3 2p–13. Autosomal dominant (the gene not yet identified) levadopa-responsive Parkinsonism with early or late onset. Additional features described include exercise-induced dystonia; an atremulous bilateral akinetic rigid syndrome; focal dystonias such as writer's cramp or torticollis; autonomic or peripheral neuropathy; and cerebellar/pyramidal tract dysfunction.

PARK4. See PARK1—they are probably the same.

PARK5 4p14/*UCHL1.* An autosomal dominant form of levadopa-responsive idiopathic Parkinson disease.

PARK6 1p35–p36/*PINK1.* Autosomal dominant or recessive. This is an early-onset form with slow progression, predominant tremor, and usually no dystonia. There is a good response to levodopa but also the frequent appearance of levodopa-induced dyskinesias and of dystonias. Some patients exhibit foot dystonia at onset and sleep benefit, thereby resembling *parkin*-associated PD. The gene is not identified.

PARK7 1p.36q/DJ1. Autosomal dominant or recessive. Characteristic is the variable severity of disease and slow progression of symptoms, with sustained response to levodopa treatment. This entity accounts for much early-onset Parkinsonism. Behavioral and psychic disturbances and focal dystonias such as blepharospasm have been reported early in the disease course.

PARK8 12p12 2p–13 1. Autosomal dominant, typical Parkinson disease with a good response to levodopa. The mean age at onset is 51 years. Neuropathological examination in four cases revealed "pure nigral degeneration" lacking the Lewy bodies. The gene is not identified.

PARK 9 1p36. Autosomal recessive; see **Kufor–Rakeb syndrome**. This is a juvenile-onset neurodegenerative disorder presenting as atypical Parkinson disease with a good response to levodopa but with spasticity, dementia, and supranuclear gaze paralysis. The gene is not identified.

PARK10 1p32. Gene not identified. A syndrome of typical late-onset sporadic Parkinson disease.
PARK 11 2q36. Another typical late-onset sporadic Parkinson disease phenotype.
PARK13 2p12.
PARK 15 *Autosomal recessive early-onset Parkinsonian-pyramidal syndrome* (pallido-pyramidal disease) due to an *FBXO7* mutation.
NR4A2. Mutations (*NURR1* gene) cause typical late-onset Parkinson disease.
SCA2 12q34 (*ATX2*). Autosomal dominant, presenting with combinations of ataxia and typical Parkinson disease.
SCA3 (Machado–Joseph) 14q24.3–q31. Autosomal dominant. Presents with combinations of ataxia and typical Parkinson disease. See **Joseph disease**.
FTDP-17, chr. 17. *(tau)*. Autosomal dominant, presenting with personality changes, cognitive decline and Parkinsonism.

In addition, GBA at 1q21 is a susceptibility factor and NA/synphilin at 5q23, POLG at 15q25, and NA at 2q22 are also identified but not enumerated. PARK 2, 6, and 7 are most relevant to *early-onset Parkinson disease*. Many of these are enzymes involved in normal protein and mitochondrial function. The clinical phenotype of the monogenic forms is similar to that of sporadic Parkinson disease. *SNCA* on chromosome 4 codes for α-synuclein, a protein found in synaptic vesicles with neurotransmitters but here a constituent of Lewy bodies.

Many other disorders also give rise to one or more of these manifestations as well as other features, including **oculogyric crises**, depression, ophthalmoplegia, motor neuropathy, and ataxic syndromes; such conditions are subsumed under the general heading of **Parkinsonism-plus**.

Numerous assessment scales are used to evaluate patients with Parkinson disease; these have been reviewed by Chaudhuri et al.[1120] See **SCOPA-Aut, Braak staging, Parkinsonism**. A neat classification scheme for Parkinsonism has been proposed:[2262]

Classical Parkinsonism

Sporadic

Idiopathic Parkinson disease

Genetic

LRRK2 mutations
SNCA mutations, duplications
Parkin. mutations
PINKl mutations
DJ-l mutations
Others (e.g., SCA2)

Atypical Parkinsonism

Sporadic

Dementia with Lewy bodies
Multiple system atrophy
Progressive supranuclear palsy
Corticobasal degeneration
Others

Genetic

Frontotemporal dementia and Parkinsonism linked to chromosome 17 (FTDP-17)
SNCA mutations, triplications
Others

Many diagnostic algorithms for Parkinson disease have been published over the years. Chart P–4 provides an accepted modern set of clinical criteria.[1855]

A simpler set of diagnostic criteria was proposed by Calne et al.[984] and another by Hughes and colleagues (2001)[3034] as follows:

Akinesia and one of tremor or rigidity, *plus*
Asymmetric onset, *plus*
No atypical features, such as early marked autonomic disturbance or dementia; Corticospinal tract dysfunction or supranuclear gaze palsy, *plus*
No history of an alternate cause such as ingestion of neuroleptic drugs, strokes, and encephalitis at onset.

(Reproduced by kind permission of the American Academy of Neurology and Lippincott Williams and Wilkins.)

Chart P–4. UK Parkinson's Disease Society Brain Bank Clinical Diagnostic Criteria for Parkinson disease

Inclusion criteria

Bradykinesia (slowness of initiation of voluntary movement with progressive reduction in speed and amplitude of repetitive actions) and at least one of the following:

Muscular rigidity
4–6 Hz rest tremor
Postural instability not caused by primary visual, vestibular, cerebellar, or proprioceptive dysfunction

Supportive criteria (Three or more required for diagnosis of definite PD)

Unilateral onset
Rest tremor present
Progressive disorder
Persistent asymmetry affecting side of onset most
Excellent response (70–100%) to levodopa
Severe levodopa-induced chorea
Levodopa response for 5 years or more
Clinical course of 10 years or more

Exclusion criteria

History of repeated strokes with stepwise progression of Parkinsonian features
History of repeated head injury
History of definite encephalitis
Oculogyric crises
Neuroleptic treatment at onset of symptoms
More than one affected relative
Sustained remission
Strictly unilateral features after 3 years
Supranuclear gaze palsy
Cerebellar signs
Early severe autonomic involvement
Early severe dementia with disturbances of memory, language and praxis
Babinski sign
Presence of cerebral tumor or communicating hydrocephalus on CT scan
Negative response to large doses of levodopa (if malabsorption excluded)
MPTP exposure

From Emre M, Aarsland D, Brown R, et al. Clinical diagnostic criteria for dementia associated with parkinson's disease. Mov Disord 2007;22. (Reproduced by kind permission of John Wiley Publications)

Other sets of criteria have also been published, such as those of Gibb and Lees (1988)[2357] and of Koller.[3519]

Variant forms of Parkinson disease include the following:

A *dominantly inherited* form with numerous Lewy bodies[6667] and due to a mutation in the *α-synuclein* gene.

A *familial autosomal dominant* form in which signs of **amyotrophic lateral sclerosis** are also found. See **motor neuronal diseases**.

Autosomal recessive juvenile Parkinsonism with diurnal fluctuation linked to 6q25.2–27.

Autosomal recessive juvenile Parkinsonism, due to degeneration of the substantia nigra, is not accompanied by Lewy body formation. The condition has its onset between the ages of 6 and 35 years. The phenotype resembles that of typical Parkinson disease and results from a mutation of the *parkin* gene at 11p.[4418]

Benign early-onset Parkinson disease

Dominantly-inherited early-onset Parkinsonism: A form with onset in the third decade, characterized by the typical clinical features of Parkinson disease with the frequent addition of dystonias and without Lewy bodies or neurofibrillary tangles in the brain and mapped to 4q21–23.[1768, 2435]

Segawa dystonia

Despite this clear classification, it should be appreciated there are at least six autosomal dominant and three autosomal recessive genes responsible for dopa-responsive Parknsonism.[4522]

For other *variants*, see **Parkinsonism-plus**. See also **American Parkinson Disease Association, Michael J. Fox Foundation for Parkinson's Research, National Parkinson Foundation, Parkinson Alliance, Parkinson's Action Network, Parkinson's Institute, and Parkinson's Resource Organization**.

Features of dementia may be associated with Parkinson disease as well as with Lewy body dementia; one description of these is as follows,[1855] reproduced by kind permission of John Wiley and Sons. Inc.

I. Core features

1. Diagnosis of Parkinson's disease according to Queen Square Brain Bank criteria (see above, Chart P–4)
2. A dementia syndrome with insidious onset and slow progression, developing within the context of established Parkinson disease and diagnosed by history, clinical, and mental examination, defined as
   - Impairment in more than one cognitive domain
   - Representing a decline from premorbid level
   - Deficits severe enough to impair daily life (social, occupational, or personal care), independent of the impairment ascribable to motor or autonomic symptoms

II. Associated clinical features

1. Cognitive features:
   - Attention: Impairment of spontaneous and focused attention, poor performance in attentional tasks; performance may fluctuate during the day and from day to day
   - Executive functions: Impairment of tasks requiring initiation, planning, concept formation, rule finding, set shifting, or set maintenance; impaired mental speed (bradyphrenia)
   - Visuo-spatial functions: Impairment of tasks requiring visual-spatial orientation, perception, or construction
   - Memory: Impairment of free recall of recent events or in tasks requiring learning new material, memory usually improves with cueing, and recognition is usually better than free recall
   - Language: Core functions largely preserved. Word finding difficulties and impaired comprehension of complex sentences may be present
2. Behavioral features:
   - Apathy: Decreased spontaneity; loss of motivation, interest, and effortful behavior
   - Changes in personality and mood including depressive features and anxiety
   - Hallucinations: Mostly visual, usually complex, formed visions of people, animals or objects
   - Delusions: Usually paranoid, such as infidelity, or phantom boarder (unwelcome guests living in the home) delusions
   - Excessive daytime sleepiness

III. Features that do not exclude Parkinson disease–dementia (PD-D), but make the diagnosis uncertain

- Co-existence of any other abnormality which may by itself cause cognitive impairment, but judged not to be the cause of dementia, eg., presence of relevant vascular disease in imaging
- Time interval between the development of motor and cognitive symptoms not known

IV. Features suggesting other conditions or diseases as cause of mental impairment, which, when present, make it impossible to diagnose PD-D reliably

- Cognitive and behavioral symptoms appearing solely in the context of other conditions such as

  Acute confusion due to

  a. Systemic diseases or abnormalities
  b. Drug intoxication

  Major Depression according to *DSM IV*.
- Features compatible with "Probable Vascular dementia" according to the NINCDS-AIREN criteria in the context of cerebrovascular disease as indicated by focal signs on neurological examination such as hemiparesis, sensory deficits, and evidence of relevant cerebrovascular disease by brain imaging *and* a relationship between the two as indicated by the presence of one or more of the following: onset of dementia within 3 months after

Criteria for the diagnosis of probable and possible PD-D

Probable PD-D

A. Core features: Both dementia and Parkinson disease must be present
B. Associated clinical features:
   - Typical profile of cognitive deficits including impairment in at least two of the four core cognitive domains (impaired attention that may fluctuate, impaired executive functions, impairment in visuo-spatial functions, and impaired free recall memory which usually improves with cueing)
   - The presence of at least one behavioral symptom (apathy, depressed or anxious mood, hallucinations, delusions, excessive daytime sleepiness) supports the diagnosis of Probable PD-D; lack of behavioral symptoms, however, does not exclude the diagnosis
C. None of the group III features present
D. None of the group IV features present

Possible PD-D

A. Core features: Both dementia and Parkinson disease must be present
B. Associated clinical features:
   - Atypical profile of cognitive impairment in one or more domains, such as prominent or receptive-type (fluent) aphasia, or pure storage-failure type amnesia (memory does not improve with cueing or in recognition tasks) with preserved attention
   - Behavioral symptoms may or may not be present *or*

C. One or more of the group III features are present
D. None of the group IV features are present.

Parkinson Alliance A charitable organization in this field. Address: 211 College Rd. East 3rd Floor, Princeton, NJ 08540. Tel: 609-688-0870; 800-579-8440. E-mail: admin@parkinsonalliance.net. Web site: http://www.parkinsonalliance.net/.

Parkinson Disease Disability Scales Rating scales designed to record changes in patients with Parkinson disease. The **Hoehn and Yahr scale**,[2933] UCLA disability scale, New York University Parkinson disease disability scale, Columbia scale,[1942] the **Parkinson Disease Impairment Index**, and the Northwestern University disability scale are commonly used; unfortunately, the correlations between them are imperfect.[1630]

Parkinson Disease Impairment index An instrument designed to quantitate the impairment suffered by patients with Parkinson disease, including arbitrary scores as to the presence of depression and of dementia.[4218]

Parkinson Disease Sleep Scale An instrument assessing many aspects of sleep and nocturnal disability in Parkinson disease.[1121]

Parkinson Disease society A British charitable organization based at 36, Portland Place, London W1N 3DG. Web site: http://www.parkinsons.org.uk/.

Parkinson Education program A charitable educational trust. Address: 1800 Park #302, Newport Beach, CA 92660.

Parkinson Foundation of Canada See Parkinson Society Canada.

Parkinson Society Canada A national charitable organization dedicated to raising funds for research into the cause and treatment of Parkinson disease, to providing a wide range of services which support Parkinsonians and their families, and to disseminating information to individuals and organizations across Canada. Web site: http://www.parkinson.ca/.

Parkinson–ALS–dementia complex of Guam See Lytico–Bodig.

Parkinsonian ataxia See **frontal gait disorder**.

Parkinsonian gait Walking that is delayed and slowed, with a tendency to accelerate and to fall forward, the subject often taking many little steps (*marche à petits pas*) on tiptoe and showing a posture of flexion affecting the upper and lower limbs as well as the trunk. The arms swing less than normally or not at all. **Freezing** is common, especially at a doorway or when an obstacle has to be negotiated. **Propulsion** and **retropulsion** are occasionally seen.

Parkinsonian hand The resting posture of the hand in some patients with Parkinsonism, characterized by wrist dorsiflexion, flexion at the metacarpophalangeal joints, extension of the fingers with adduction, and ulnar deviation of the wrist.

Parkinsonian syndromes Parkinsonism may also occur as complications of **Sjögren syndrome, HIV** infection, **syphilis, Japanese B encephalitis**, and **West Nile** diseas, and in some toxic states (manganese, mercury, etc.). See the following entry.

Parkinsonism A clinical syndrome of tremor, bradykinesia, rigidity, stooped posture, and impaired postural reflexes due to degeneration or dysfunction of the nigrostriatal neuronal system, or to pharmacological blockade or loss of striatal dopamine receptors; thus, a syndrome of striatal dopamine deficiency. Most commonly it is due to **Parkinson disease**, but the syndrome may also occur as part of the clinical expression of many other disorders such as **progressive supranuclear palsy, multiple-system atrophy**, various types of cerebral vascular disease, **Lytico–Bodig, Wilson** and **Huntington diseases**, and as a sequel to encephalitis (**postencephalitic Parkinsonism**). It may also be produced by various pharmacological agents, notably the neuroleptic drugs, and by the dopaminergic neurotoxin **MPTP**. [RCD] Yet other causes have been listed.[3519, 2927, 6341]

Parkinsonism–dementia The combination of some features of these two syndromes, as occurs in **Alzheimer disease, communicating hydrocephalus, corticobasal degeneration, dementia with Lewy bodies, Lytico–Bodig, NBIA**, variants of **Pick disease, progressive subcortical glial dystrophy, progressive supranuclear palsy, sporadic amyotrophic lateral sclerosis**, and **vascular dementia**.[2356] See above under **Parkinson disease**.

A *variant form* is *dominantly inherited dementia and Parkinsonism with non-Alzheimer amyloid plaques*; a dominantly inherited syndrome of adult onset characterized by severe dementia and Parkinsonism with extracellular hyaline eosinophilic and congophilic amyloid plaques in the cerebral cortex, basal ganglia, thalamus, and substantia nigra.[5409]

Parkinsonism–hyperpyrexia syndrome A syndrome indistinguishable from **neuroleptic malignant syndrome** seen after a reduction in the dose or withdrawing dopaminergic drugs in patients with Parkinson disease. It can also develop after withdrawal of nondopaminergic drugs used to treat Parkinson disease.

Parkinsonism-plus A group of disorders in which the signs of Parkinsonism are accompanied by others, including myoclonus, pyramidal signs, dementia, autonomic failure, and cerebellar signs.

The conditions are listed in Chart P–5.

Such associations are also found in **corticobasal ganglionic degeneration; diffuse Lewy body disease; Lytico–Bodig; Huntington disease; neuroacanthocytosis; neuronal ceroid lipofuscinosis; neurodegeneration with brain iron accumulation; normal pressure hydrocephalus; olivopontocerebellar degeneration; Parkinsons-motor neurone disease; progressive pallidal atrophy; progressive supranuclear palsy; Shy–Drager syndrome; striatal necrosis; strianonigral degeneration**; and **Wilson disease**.

Chart P–5. Disorders Comprising Parkinsonism-Plus

A syndrome of **amyotrophic lateral sclerosis** accompanying Parkinsonism without dementia, dominantly-inherited. See also **Creutzfeldt-Jakob disease.**[805]

Familial extrapyramidal disease with peripheral neuropathy A dominantly-inherited sensorimotor peripheral neuropathy with distal weakness, muscle atrophy and areflexia, and stocking hypoesthesia occurring in association with Parkinson disease. Axonal degeneration is more common than demyelination as the underlying pathology.[965]

Familial parkinsonism-dementia (Lewy body) syndrome: See **dementia with Lewy bodies.**

Fatal parkinsonism, alveolar hypoventilation and depression: A rare syndrome of adults manifesting respiratory difficulties, depression, bulbar pareses, tremor, seizures and early death.[5142]

Juvenile parkinsonism: A rare syndrome in which pyramidal signs, rigidity, dystonia and tremor occur before the age of 20 years.[2361] See also **young-onset Parkinson disease**. The autosomal recessive for of juvenile is mapped to 11p.

Parkinsonism with anosmia: A rare dominantly-inherited syndrome of young adult onset characterized by anosmia in association with rigidity and tremor. See **Kallmann syndrome**.

Parkinsonism with cerebellar ataxia and peripheral neuropathy: See **hereditary motor and sensory neuropathy**, type 2.

Parkinsonism with cerebellar ataxia: A rare association of unknown significance.

Parkinsonism, depression and taurine deficiency: A rare dominantly-inherited syndrome of adult onset characterized by these features.[4990]

Parkinsonism-dystonia: See ***juvenile parkinsonism syndromes***.

Rapid onset dystonia-Parkinsonism A dominantly-inherited disorder characterized by the rapid onset of Parkinsonian signs and dystonia, involvement more of the bulbar and arm muscles than of the legs, lack of response to levadopa and normal cranial imaging.[5042]

Rapidly-progressing autosomal dominant parkinsonism and dementia with pallidopontonigral degeneration: A progressive syndrome of parkinsonism with dystonia, frontal release signs, pyramidal features, urinary incontinence and perseverating vocalizations.[6881] Linkage to 4q21–23 has been established in at least one kinship.

Tic, Parkinson disease, motor neuron disease and acanthocytosis: A syndrome with childhood onset, characterized by acanthocytosis with self-mutilation, rigidity, motor neuropathy and a burst-suppression pattern on the EEG. See **neuroacanthocytosis**.

X linked dystonia parkinsonism (Lubag) A complicated form mapped to XqI2–13.1

Parkinson's Action Network

A charitable organization in this field. Address: 300 North Lee St., Suite 500, Alexandria, VA 22314. Tel: 800-850-4726; 703-518-8877; 707-544-1994. E-mail: info@parkinsonsaction.org. Web site: http://www.parkinsonsaction.org/.

Parkinson's Disease Foundation, Inc.

A charitable organization based at William Black Med Research Bldg. 640 W. 168th St. New York, NY 10032. Tel:212-923-4700. Web sites: http://www.pdf.org/; and http://www.parkinson.org/medications.htm/.

Parkinson's Disease Society

A British charitable organization. Web site: http://www.parkinsons.org.uk/

Parkinson's Institute

A charitable organization in this field. Address: 1170 Morse Ave. Sunnyvale, CA 94089-1605. Tel: 408-734-2800; 800-786-2958. E-mail: outreach@parkinsonsinstitute.org. Web site: http://www.parkinsonsinstitute.org/.

Parkinson's Resource Organization

A charitable organization in this field. Address: 74-090 El Paseo, Suite 102, Palm Desert, CA 2260-4135. Tel: 760-773-5628: 310-476-7030: 877-775-4111. E-mail: info@parkinsonsresource.org. Web site: http://www.parkinsonsresource.org/.

Parkinson Study Group

A nonprofit, cooperative group of Parkinson' disease experts in the United States and Canada who are dedicated to improving treatment for persons affected by Parkinson disease. Web site: www.parkinson-study-group.org/.

Parkinsonism & Related Disorders

The official journal of the World Federation of Neurology Research Committee on Parkinsonism and Related Disorders, published by Elsevier. Web site: http://www.elsevier.com/homepage/sah/wfn-rced/doc/main_frm.html/.

paroniria

The disturbance of sleep by disagreeable dreams.

parosmia

Distortion of the sense of smell, almost invariably interpreted as unpleasant.

paroxysm

(from Gr, to excite, hence a severe attack of disease) A periodic fit or attack of a disease, or of certain symptoms that occur periodically; the increase of symptoms to a maximum, with succeeding decline, their severity being less emphasized than their tendency to abrupt recurrence.

paroxysmal aphasia

Intermittent language disorders classified as *dysphasic seizures* (paroxysmal posterior aphasia) and *phonatory seizures* (paroxysmal anterior aphasia), almost always due to a discharging lesion in the left hemisphere.[63]

paroxysmal ataxia and vertigo

A dominantly inherited cerebellar ataxia; a *variant* of **May–White syndrome.**[4187]

paroxysmal autonomic instability with dystonia

(after brain injury) Episodic hyperthermia, tachycardia, tachypnea, diaphoresis, and hypertension in conjunction with catatonic posturing such as that described by **Charcot** as *"arc on cercle."* This can evolve into **malignant catatonia** and is most often hyperactive, although a hypoactive form is known. A mortality rate of 60% has been reported, hence the prior term **lethal catatonia**.

paroxysmal choreoathetosis

(extrapyramidal seizures) A syndrome of abnormal involuntary movements resembling chorea, athetosis, or dystonia, variously considered to be due to dystonia or, in the past, to subcortical seizures. They were first described by Mount and Reback[4521] but were also known to **Gowers** as "reflex epilepsy." The *variants* were classified by Lance,[3654] amended here:

A. *Familial paroxysmal dystonic choreoathetosis*, a dominantly inherited syndrome with onset in childhood in which the movements occur in prolonged attacks lasting between 2 min and 4 h and may be complicated by spasticity. They are only seldom triggered by voluntary activity.[4521] The condition has been mapped to chromosome 1p.
B. *Intermediate form*, a dominantly inherited syndrome in which the attacks of abnormal movements last between 5 and 30 min after precipitation by heavy exertion.
C. **Paroxysmal kinesigenic choreoathetosis**.
D. *Paroxysmal choreoathetosis after craniocerebral trauma*.[1710]

paroxysmal choreoathetosis and spasticity

A dominantly inherited variant of **paroxysmal dystonic choreoathetosis** in which the attacks are precipitated by exercise and in which spastic paraplegia, perioral paresthesias, diplopia, headache, and myoclonus are associated features.[289]

paroxysmal depolarization shift

An alteration in the charge of a neuronal cell body causing a sudden, high amplitude burst of high-frequency action potentials and producing locally synchronous sustained depolarization and prolonged after-hyperpolarization. If this occurs synchronously in a number of adjacent neurons, an isolated spike may be recorded on the EEG and this may be the basic neurophysiological abnormality underlying the production of focal spikes in epilepsy. The term was introduced by Ajmone-Marsan in 1964.

paroxysmal dyskinesias

A heterogeneous group of acute, transient movement disorders, seven of which have been differentiated. They include **paroxysmal dystonic choreoathetosis, paroxysmal exertion-induced dyskinesia, nocturnal hypogenic paroxysmal dyskinesia, paroxysmal choreoathetosis and spasticity,** infantile convulsions, paroxysmal choreoathetosis and Rolandic epilepsy, paroxysmal exercise-induced dystonia and writer's cramp.[6543]

paroxysmal dystonia

See **familial paroxysmal dystonic choreoathetosis, nocturnal paroxysmal dystonia**.

paroxysmal dystonic choreoathetosis

(paroxysmal nonkinesigenic dyskinesias, PDC/PNKD) A channelopathy presenting as attacks of abnormal involuntary movements such as ballism, chorea, and dystonic postures, sometimes triggered by voluntary activity and occurring first in childhood.[611, 1710] The attacks are of long duration (up to 6 h) and are induced by variety of factors including coffee, tea, alcohol, and fatigue but not by sudden movement. The gene for familial PDC has been linked to chromosome 2q34, but sporadic cases also occur. See **familial paroxysmal dystonic choreoathetosis, paroxysmal kinesigenic choreoathetosis**.

In a *variant* dominantly inherited form, there is added spasticity.[607]

paroxysmal exertion-induced dystonia

A rare, dominantly inherited condition in which the movements, mostly affecting the feet, are induced by prolonged or sustained exercise such as walking or running. The attacks last from a few minutes to up to 2 h. Patient ages at onset range from 2 to 30 years. Hemidystonic attacks, bilateral leg involvement, and single leg involvement have all been described.[611]

paroxysmal extreme pain disorder

(familial rectal pain syndrome; submandibular, oral, and rectal pain with flushing) A dominantly inherited lifelong syndrome starting in infancy and characterized by brief episodes of burning rectal pain followed by flushing of the legs, face, and eyelids. In infants, tonic attacks with apnea and bradycardia may also occur, as may cardiac asystole in adults. The attacks are especially provoked by defecation. Associated features include ocular pain (caused by cold wind or other irritants), jaw pain, triggered by the sight of food, and limb pain; less often, harlequin color changes and nonepileptic seizures (sometimes associated with cardiac asystole). The neurological examination and all laboratory studies including EEG are normal.

The cause is not known; the attacks could represent forms of **dysautonomia, migraine**, or epilepsy,[5656] but mutations in the sodium channel *SCN9A* have been identified, confirming the disorder as a sodium channelopathy.[2036]

paroxysmal hemicrania (chronic paroxysmal hemicrania)

A rare **trigeminal autonomic cephalgia** manifesting frequent short-lasting (2–40 min) attacks of severe unilateral pain, usually in the orbital, supraorbital, or temporal regions, but sometimes spreading further afield.[1185] The attack frequency usually ranges from 5 to 40 attacks per day. The pain is associated with autonomic symptoms such as conjunctival injection, lacrimation, nasal congestion, facial flushing, rhinorrhoea, ptosis, or eyelid oedema. Almost all reported cases respond to treatment with indomethacin. There is a distinct female preponderance. Diagnostic criteria have been defined:[2820]

A. At least 20 attacks fulfilling criteria B–D
B. Attacks of severe unilateral orbital, supraorbital, or temporal pain lasting 2–30 min
C. Headache is accompanied by at least one of the following:
   1. Ipsilateral conjunctival injection and/or lacrimation
   2. Ipsilateral nasal congestion and/or rhinorrhea
   3. Ipsilateral eyelid edema
   4. Ipsilateral forehead and facial sweating
   5. Ipsilateral miosis and/or ptosis
D. Attacks have a frequency above 5 per day for more than half of the time, although periods with lower frequency may occur
E. Attacks are prevented completely by therapeutic doses of indomethacin
F. Not attributed to another disorder

From the International Classification of Headache Disorders (Headache Classification Committee of the International Headache Society. *Cephalalgia* 2004. 24[Suppl 1]) by kind permission of Dr. Jes Olesen, the International Headache Society and Wiley-Blackwell Publications.

Variants are as follows:

Episodic paroxysmal hemicrania Attacks of paroxysmal hemicrania occurring in periods lasting 7 days to 1 year separated by painfree periods lasting 1 month or longer.

Chronic paroxysmal hemicrania Attacks of paroxysmal hemicrania occurring for more than 1 year without remission or with remissions lasting less than 1 month, for which diagnostic criteria have been defined:

A. Attacks fulfilling criteria A–F for 3.2 **paroxysmal hemicrania**
B. Attacks recur over >1 year without remission periods or with remission periods lasting <1 month.

Other forms of headache with marked autonomic activation include **chronic** and **episodic paroxysmal hemicrania, short-lasting unilateral neuralgiform headache with conjunctival injection and tearing** (SUNCT syndrome), and **cluster headache**. Those without autonomic activation include **hypnic headache** and persistent headache with milder autonomic features such as **hemicrania continua**.

paroxysmal hypnogenic dyskinesia See **paroxysmal hypogenic dystonia**.

paroxysmal hypogenic dystonia (paroxysmal hypnogenic dyskinesia) The occurrence of multiple brief tonic flexor or extensor spasms in several extremities, waking the patient from nonrapid eye movement sleep and not diminishing consciousness. The ictal and interictal EEG record is normal but some patients also have seizures. The condition may be either familial or sporadic.[3744] See **dyskinesias**.

paroxysmal kinesigenic choreoathetosis/dyskinesia (PKC/PKD; Mount-Reback syndrome, familial paroxysmal choreoathetosis, paroxysmal dystonic choreoathetosis, periodic dystonia, reflex epilepsy, seizures induced by sudden movement, conditionally responsive extrapyramidal syndrome, hereditary kinesthetic reflex epilepsy) A sporadic or dominantly inherited syndrome of frequent uni- or bilateral dystonic posturing of the trunk, eyes, and limbs without alteration of consciousness, occurring in the waking state and usually lasting 5 min but possibly up to 2 h (the "reflex epilepsy" of **Gowers**). These choreoathetotic or ballistic movements are provoked by startle or by sudden movement and may be suppressed by anticonvulsant drugs.[3400, 3654, 607] The condition has been mapped to 2q33–35. Proposed diagnostic criteria[916] are as follows, reproduced by kind permission of the American Academy of Neurology and Lippincott Williams and Wilkins.

A kinesigenic trigger for the attacks can be identified.
Attacks last less than a minute.
There is no loss of consciousness, nor pain during the attacks.
Other organic diseases are excluded and the neurologic examination is normal.
Attacks can be controlled with phenytoin or carbamazepine.
Age at onset between 1 and 20 years if there is no family history.

In a *variant* of this condition, a focal brain lesion is present and in addition, secondary forms are described conjugating, for example, multiple sclerosis, metabolic derangements, and cerebrovascular disease.

Despite some of the names attached, this is not an epileptic syndrome at all; it could be an ion-channel disorder. It was first described by **Gowers** in the second edition of his book *Epilepsy and other Chronic Convulsive Diseases* (London, 1801), but was then forgotten for 40 years until re-described in 1940.[4521] See also **paroxysmal choreoathetosis, paroxysmal dystonic choreoathetosis**.

paroxysmal kinesigenic and nonkinesigenic dystonias See **dystonia**.

paroxysmal kinesigenic dyskinesia See **dyskinesias**.

paroxysmal lacrimation syndrome See **crocodile tears**.

paroxysmal motor disorders of sleep These have been reviewed and classified.[1608] They include **parasomnias** such as **confusional arousals, sleepwalking,** and **sleep terrors**, all of which are NREM arousal disorders; and those associated with REM sleep, including **REM sleep behavior disorder**, parasomnia overlap disorder, and **sleep paralysis. Catathrenia** (nocturnal groaning) may also be classified here.

The sleep-related movement disorders with paroxysmal expression are **periodic limb movements of sleep, sleep bruxism, nocturnal leg cramps,** and **rhythmic movement disorder** (jactacio capitis nocturna).

Other paroxysmal nocturnal events which are neither **parasomnias** nor movement disorders are **sleep starts, somniloquy,** benign sleep myoclonus of infancy, and nocturnal psychogenic nonepileptic seizures (**pseudoseizures**).

paroxysmal movement disorders See **paroxysmal kinesigenic dystonic choreoathetosis, paroxysmal exertion-induced dystonia, paroxysmal hypogenic dystonia, multiple sclerosis,** and **Sandifer syndrome** as well as adjacent entries.

paroxysmal myoclonic dystonia with vocalizations A movement disorder characterized by paroxysmal bursts of involuntary, regular, repetitive, rhythmic, bilateral, stereotypical, and severe myoclonus with vocalizations, often associated with tonic movements and interfering with voluntary activity. Mild **attention deficit disorder**, hyperactivity, learning disabilities, and resistance to treatment with haloperidol are other features of the condition.[1989]

paroxysmal nocturnal dyskinesia A form of **frontal lobe epilepsy** which may be familial with autosomal dominant inheritance (ADNFLE).

paroxysmal nocturnal dystonia (dyskinesia) A syndrome characterized by sleeptalking, stereotypical movements in sleep with autonomic excitation, and transient arousals leading to the complaint of excessive daytime sleepiness.[3986] In some cases dominant inheritance is suggested with a mutation of the neuronal acetylcholine receptor gene (*CHRNA4*) on chromosome 20q. This may be the same condition as **autosomal dominant nocturnal frontal lobe epilepsy**. See also **dystonia**.

paroxysmal nocturnal hemidystonia See **dystonia**.

paroxysmal nocturnal hemoglobinuria (Marchiafava–Micheli syndrome) A rare sporadic hematological disorder characterized by a deficiency in blood cell membrane glycoproteins, causing intravascular hemolysis, pancytopenia, and frequently intravascular (cerebral arterial or venous sinus) thrombosis.[84]

paroxysmal nonkinesigenic dyskinesia (PNKD, paroxysmal dystonic choreoathetosis, familial paroxysmal choreoathetosis) Mount and Reback reported the first family who had autosomal dominant paroxysmal attacks of chorea and athetotic movements. (See **paroxysmal kinesigenic choreoathetosis/dyskinesia**) Mutations in the myofibrillogenesis regulator 1 (*MR-1*) gene on chromosome 2 have been reported. Suggested clinical criteria for PNKD with MR-1 mutation are as follows.[915] See also **dyskinesias**.

1. Hyperkinetic involuntary movement attacks, with dystonia, chorea, or combination of these, typically lasting 10 min to 1 h, but possibly up to 4 h
2. Normal neurologic examination results between attacks, secondary causes excluded
3. Onset of attack in infancy or early childhood
4. Precipitation of attacks by caffeine and alcohol
5. Family history of movement disorder meeting the above criteria.

paroxysmal polyspike activity aith arousal See **pure tonic seizures with arousal**.

paroxysmal positional nystagmus See **benign positional vertigo**.

paroxysmal positional vertigo A common and benign symptom of peripheral vestibular dysfunction occurring spontaneously or following head trauma, and probably due to **cupulolithiasis**. See **benign positional vertigo**.

paroxysmal tonic upgaze A benign neuro-ophthalmological syndrome of infancy characterized by prolonged episodes of sustained tonic upward deviation of the eyes, often with incomplete downward saccades (resembling nystagmus) on downgaze and sometimes accompanied by ataxia, speech and learning disability, and developmental delay. The ocular condition is worsened by fatigue and remits during sleep. It usually follows infection or vaccination but is likely heterogeneous.[2809]

paroxysmal torticollis in infancy See **benign paroxysmal vertigo of childhood**.

paroxysmal vertical ocular dyskinesia Paroxysmal, spontaneous, rapid, involuntary, vertical, and pendular eye movements lasting some 5 min, suppressed by horizontal movement, depressed by eye opening, made more regular with eye closure and maximal in the midposition of gaze.

They are thought to be due to a supranuclear defect in vertical gaze control, the lesion resembling that of the **sylvian aqueduct syndrome**.[4006]

Parrot, Joseph-Marie-Jules (1829–1883) French physician and anthropologist, who trained in Paris, where he later became professor of medical history and then of pediatrics. He described syphilitic pseudoparalysis (characterized by a disinclination to move because of osteitic pain, occurring in infants[4911]) as well as achondroplasia and the following two signs.

Parrot nodes Frontal and parietal bossing of the skull in congenital syphilis, leading to a "natiform" skull shape rather resembling that of a hot-cross bun.[4912]

Parrot sign 1. See **hot-cross bun skull**. 2. Dilation of the pupil when the skin of the neck is pinched, a normal response though once thought diagnostic of meningitis.[4913] See **ciliospinal reflex**.

Parry, Caleb Hillier (1755–1822) English physician who practiced in Bath. He was the first to describe facial hemiatrophy (**Parry–Romberg syndrome**), his notes being published posthumously in 1825, while **Romberg**'s account appeared in 1846. His notes also contained excellent descriptions of Hirschsprung disease, exophthalmic goiter, and angina.[2066]

Parry syndrome A congenital dysmorphic syndrome of sparse, prematurely gray hair, sensorineural deafness, pigmentary abnormalities of the iris, cataract, abnormal teeth and nails, hypogonadotropic hypogonadism, arthritis, hyperkeratosis, depigmented skin, and psychomotor retardation.[381]

Parry–Romberg syndrome (Romberg disease, [progressive] hemifacial atrophy, localized linear scleroderma, Wartenberg syndrome) A rare syndrome of unknown cause, in which atrophy of the skin and subcutaneous tissues of one side of the face occurs during the second (seldom the first) decade of life. The tongue, gums, and soft palate, and the cartilage of the nose, ear, larynx, and eyelid are all affected. Brain MRI may show hyperintense cortical and subcortical lesions with calcification and focal cortical atrophy. The condition may represent localized scleroderma,[269] but in cases with intractable seizures, the cerebral pathology is that of **Rasmussen encephalitis**.

Associated abnormalities have included heterochromia iridis, alopecia, vitiligo, pigmented facial nevi, facial pain, optic atrophy, enophthalmos, strabismus, ptosis, miosis, uveitis, ataxia, and focal motor epilepsy.[5368] Cerebral lesions (cystic encephalomalacia) demonstrable by CT scan, ophthalmoparesis, involvement of other cranial nerves, and numerous other neurological signs appear less commonly.[4914] Some patients have café-au-lait spots, although this condition has nothing to do with **neurofibromatosis**. Migraine-like headaches, trigeminal neuralgia, or seizures affecting the contralateral side of the body have also been associated.

Parry described it in 1825, Romberg in 1846, and Wartenberg in 1945.[6655] See also **linear scleroderma**, a likely *variant*.

Parsonage–Turner syndrome See **neuralgic amyotrophy**.

Parsons, Sir John (1868–1957) English physician, who introduced the word **papilledema** to refer to the appearance of the swollen optic disk in patients with raised intracranial pressure—properly displacing the term *optic neuritis*, previously applied by **von Graefe**.

partial complex seizures See **complex partial seizures**.

partial continuous epilepsy (epilepsia partialis continua of Kozhevnikov) A rare form of focal status epilepticus characterized by the association of variable, repetitive, clonic, focal, asymmetrical muscular twitching or jerks localized to a limited area on one side of the body without alteration of consciousness, lasting hours, days, or months and often associated with Jacksonian seizures.[3548] They are almost always the result of lesions involving the Rolandic cortex.

Nearly all patients also have other seizures such as focal motor seizures in the same side and secondarily generalized tonic–clonic seizures (GTCS). The *mesial temporal* type predominantly involves the mesial limbic structures and presents with repeated dyscognitive focal ictal events without a return of clear consciousness in between.

The *neocortical* type originates in various neocortical regions, presenting with various unpredictable clinical patterns such as absence status, generalized tonic–clonic status or repetitive discrete behavioral seizures.[4882, 1861]

The EEG may show spike activity with high-amplitude focal or diffuse slow waves or other nonspecific abnormalities. The seizure episodes sometimes occur as a result of encephalitis of acute or chronic types, of inborn errors of metabolism or mitochondrial encephalopathies.[369] See also **Kozhevnikoff–Rasmussen syndrome syndrome**.

Since the (appropriate) discarding of the word "partial" in the context of focal epilepsies, it is likely that a better name will be found for this condition. It is retained here because the original Latinism is so familiar.

partial convulsive status epilepticus See **status epilepticus**.

partial epilepsy See **epilepsy, localization-related epilepsies and syndromes**.

partial epilepsy with auditory features An unusual localization-related epilepsy syndrome, probably a variant of lateral temporal lobe epilepsy, characterized by auditory hallucinations and other sensory symptoms and linked to a mutation at 10q22–24.[6822]

partial epilepsy with pericentral spikes A benign familial epilepsy syndrome linked to chromosome 4p15, and characterized by many variable seizure types (hemiclonic, hemitonic, generalized tonic–clonic and complex partial) with onset in or after the first decade and manifesting spikes or sharp waves in the pericentral regions on the EEG.[3448]

partial epilepsy with variable foci (OMIM 600512) A dominantly inherited localization-related epileptic disorder of childhood manifesting various seizure types and deafness, with normal cognition, mapped to 10q22–q24.[5109]

partial nonconvulsive status epilepticus See **status epilepticus**.

partial optic aplasia See **optic nerve hypoplasia**.

partial seizures A term now discarded, but in use for many years in the recent past to denote seizures with a focal origin within the brain as opposed to generalized or centrencephalic seizures which are considered to have their origin in deep central brain regions, with bilateral, synchronous clinical and electrical manifestations. The older use of the word "partial" suggests that the committee selecting it operated under a communal linguistic challenge. The word would have been equally incorrect appearing in the definitions of other such absolute entities as, for example, pregnancy or death. "Focally" or "locally originating seizures" would have been more appropriate.

In the remainder of this entry the word "partial" used by the ILAE Commission of Epidemiology and Prognosis[1265] has been replaced by "focal" or "local." The following was originally published in Epilepsia 1993;**34**:592–6 and is reproduced by kind permission of Wiley-Blackwell Publications and the ILAE.

A seizure should be classified as focal when there is evidence of a clinical local onset, regardless of whether the seizure is secondarily generalized. The aura (the first clinical signs of a seizure) has high localizing value and results from the anatomical or functional neuronal activation of part of one hemisphere.

- When alertness and ability to interact appropriately with the environment are maintained, the seizure is classified as a *simple focal seizure*.
- When impairment of consciousness, amnesia, or confusion during or after a seizure is reported, the seizure is classified as a *complex focal seizure*.
- When a seizure becomes secondarily generalized, the seizure is classified as *focal seizure, secondarily generalized (simple or complex)*.
- When the distinction between simple and complex focal seizures cannot be made from information provided by the history and medical records, the seizure is classified as a focal epileptic seizure of unknown type.

partial syndrome Incomplete, minor manifestations of typical dominantly inherited **myotonic dystrophy** carrying the same prognosis for transmission of the disorder. Isolated cataracts, few colored lens specks (**Christmas-tree specks**), or minor EMG abnormalities are typical of these isolated manifestations.[5134]

Partington syndrome (Russell–Silver-like syndrome) A congenital dysmorphic syndrome, an X-linked dominant trait due to mutations in the *ARX* gene, manifesting low birth weight, short stature, patchy skin pigmentation, facial weakness, and delayed closure of the fontanelles and dystonic movements of the hands.[381]

parturition palsy Compressive neuropathy of the femoral nerve due to prolonged hyperflexion of the hips during childbirth. See also **obstetric palsy**.

parvo- (Gr, small) Prefix denoting small.

PAS stain (periodic acid–Schiff stain) A stain used to demonstrate the glycogen in, for example, muscle biopsy specimens. When the sample is stained using PAS stain with and without diastase, the glycogen content is both displayed and quantified. However, mucoproteins, mucolipids, glycoproteins, and glycolipids are also stained purple in histological preparations using this method.

Pascual–Castroviejo syndrome (cerebrofaciothoracic dysplasia) A congenital dysmorphic syndrome manifesting also short neck, hypertelorism, brachycephaly, flat occiput, kyphoscoliosis, vertebral anomalies, a high or Sprengel shoulder, strabismus, intracranial calcifications, callosal abnormalities, and mental and developmental delay.[381]

passibility (from Lat, to suffer + able) Unpleasant sensations; a term used in the nineteenth century for **hyperesthesia**.

Passow syndrome The association of **Horner syndrome** with **heterochromia iridis**, kyphoscoliosis, cervical rib, and spina bifida. Optic atrophy, facial hemiatrophy, trigeminal sensory loss, and generalized muscle weakness may also be found.

Dr. Arnold von Passow (1888–1966) was a German ophthalmologist.

Passwell syndrome The association of congenital ichthyosis, erythroderma, mental retardation, dwarfism, and generalized aminoaciduria. Spastic paraparesis may also occur.[4924]

past pointing 1. (kinetic deviation) The subject (with his eyes closed) extends his arm to touch the examiner's finger with his own, and repeatedly lowers and raises his arm again; progressive deviation to one side may be seen in patients with labyrinthine disease. 2. In the **finger–nose–finger test**, the subject's finger repeatedly veers off to one side of the target, and thus fails to come to a stop when the target is reached. This sign usually indicates disease of a cerebellar hemisphere.

Pasteur, Louis (1822–1895) French bacteriologist and physiologist who determined that **rabies** was an infectious disease, although he never saw it. He also introduced preventive vaccination at a time when such prevention only existed for smallpox, his vaccine experiments having shown that the virulence of the virus was reduced with successive passage through a tribe of monkeys, or through rabbits. He later used a drying technique to reduce the virulence of the organism.

His therapy was at first controversial, partly on account of the immune reactions caused by the injection of foreign neural tissue; but the huge reduction in mortality resulting from use of the vaccine eventually quieted doubts, if not anxieties.

Patau syndrome See **trisomy 13 syndrome**.

patellar clonus Repetitive contraction of the quadriceps muscle after elicitation of its muscle stretch reflex in states of reflex hyperexcitability. The absurd name is derived from the fact that it is the movements of the patella that are the most obvious, at least to the untrained eye.

patellar reflex Another misnomer; if the patella is struck moderately, the result is slight pain. It is struck hard enough to shorten the quadriceps muscle the reflex may or may not appear but the pain level will be significant. See **knee jerk**.

patent foramen ovale A cardiac anomaly linked epidemiologically to migraine with aura, which condition, however, is not ameliorated by closure of the defect.[775]

Paterson–BrownKelly syndrome See **sideropenic dysphagia**.

pathoclisis (Gr, disease + a tendency) An unusual vulnerability of certain neuronal systems to specific pathogenic agents.

pathological affect See **emotionalism**.

pathological emotionality The expression of strong emotion without the appropriate experience of joy or sadness; usually evidence of diffuse lesions affecting the brainstem and occasionally the cortex. See **emotionalism**.[139]

pathological fall An unintended change in position occurring when unhealthy homeostatic mechanisms fail to preserve normal postural integrity. This typically occurs in **Parkinson disease**.

pathological hypersexuality A state in which sexual thoughts or behaviors are excessive or represent an atypical change from baseline (assuming normality at baseline, though this is not defined).

Diagnostic criteria have been suggested in the context of **Parkinson disease**.[6574] They include a maladaptive preoccupation with sexual thoughts; inappropriate quest for sex; habitual promiscuity; compulsive masturbation; use of the media for sexual purposes; and the presence of **paraphilias**. Such behavior must have persisted for at least a month and shall have caused marked distress, especially, when the subject attempts to control it unsuccessfully. In addition, such activities should be time consuming and should interfere with social occupational functioning, and the behavior should not occur exclusively during periods of hypomania or mania.

pathological laughter Involuntary recurrent, episodic, and inappropriate laughter occurring as a result of cerebral disease. Three varieties are defined; *forced laughter* (or crying) may occur in patients with pseudobulbar or bulbar palsies, with or without awareness of the affect portrayed. **Gelastic** *laughter* is an epileptic manifestation, and *inappropriate laughter* may occur in psychotic patients,[668] one hopes in accord with their inner feelings.

The exact mechanism by which this condition develops is currently unknown although obviously injury to pathways controlling emotional expression has occurred.

Patin syndrome See **myositis ossificans**.

Paton–Gowers–Kennedy syndrome See **Foster Kennedy syndrome**.

Patrick, H.T. (1860–1938) American neurologist and psychiatrist, and professor at Northwestern University, Chicago. He was a founder and editor of the *Archives of Neurology and Psychiatry*.[2066]

Patrick sign (FABERE test) Pain felt in the hip when the painful leg is flexed at the hip and knee, the heel placed on the opposite knee and pressed downward and laterally, causing thus abduction and external rotation. This maneuver does not cause pain in patients with root irritation, but is intensely painful in those with hip joint disease. The acronym FABERE is derived from flexion, abduction, external rotation, and extension.

Patrick trigger areas Trigger points in the distribution of the trigeminal nerve which, when touched, induce paroxysms of pain in patients with **trigeminal neuralgia**.

pattern 1. A waveform recognizable by contrast with its background. A model or standard from which other models may be made or recognized by exact reproduction. 2. Within neurology, it may be regarded as the space–time relationships of theoretically deducible and operationally detectible changes in the nervous system.[2470]

pattern theory The theory that there are neither specific fibers nor receptors for sensation; what leaves the skin as a result of cutaneous stimulation is a complex spatially and temporally dispersed pattern of impulses, and this, or something like it, is what arrives in the brain.[5860]

pattern-sensitive seizure An epileptic syndrome characterized by the occurrence of absence, myoclonic, or other seizures upon viewing a contrasting pattern. Most subjects also show clinical and electrical sensitivity to flicker.[72]

Patterson pseudoleprechaun syndrome A congenital dysmorphic syndrome also manifesting low birthweight, dwarfism, hirsutism, cutis laxa, bronzed skin, a Cushingoid appearance, kyphoscoliosis, genu valgum, osteoporosis, delayed skeletal maturation, wide metaphyses, and seizures.[4933] See also **leprechaunism**.

pause (omnipause) neurons Neurons which, with burst neurons, are found in the paramedian pontine reticular formation and whose tonic high-frequency activity, which normally inhibits the burst neurons, is interrupted before saccades occurs either in a specific direction or in any direction.

Pavlov, Ivan Petrovich (1849–1936) Russian physiologist who trained in medicine at St. Petersburg, where he later became professor at the army medical academy and director of the institute of experimental medicine.

He is best remembered by neurologists for his studies of reflex action, particularly conditioned reflexes. He also enunciated the law of dynamic localization, which introduced the concept of graded or variable localization of function in the cortex, allowing different areas the potential for more than one function (pluripotentiality). He was awarded the Nobel Prize in 1904, largely for his studies of the autonomic nervous system.

Pavlov reflexes Conditioned reflexes (learned behavior patterns displayed in response to a stimulus repeatedly presented in association), first fully described by Pavlov in his *Lectures on Conditioned Reflexes* (New York, 1928).

pavor nocturnus One or 2-min episodes of **night terror** occurring in children more often than in adults, which occur within the first half hour of nocturnal sleep (in non–rapid eye movement stages 3 or 4). The child awakens screaming or moaning with the usual autonomic accompaniments of extreme fear.

PCB neuropathy A toxic sensory polyneuropathy accompanied by headache and dysequilibrium and resulting from exposure to polychlorinated biphenyls.[1143]

PDQ-39 A questionairre used in **Parkinson disease**, examining mobility, activities of daily living, emotional well-being, stigma, social support, cognition, communication, and bodily dysfunction.[5005]

Peabody picture vocabulary test A test of comprehension, wherein the subject is supplied with a word and is required to identify the corresponding picture from among four choices at different levels of complexity.[1753] As a test of receptive vocabulary, it is used in children over the age of 2 years and in adults.

peacock trunk A form of focal or axial dystonia affecting the truncal muscles and leading to a gait pattern resembling that of the peacock.

peak-dose chorea A hyperkinetic form of fluctuation in Parkinsonian patients on long-term levadopa therapy, in whom choreic movements occur as the drug levels rise.

peak-dose dyskinesia See **peak-dose dystonia**.

peak-dose dystonia (peak-dose dyskinesia) A dystonic form of fluctuation in Parkinsonian patients on long term levadopa therapy in which dystonic movements appear as the drug levels rise to their maximum values.

peak latency The interval between the onset of a stimulus and a specified peak of the evoked waveform.

pectoral reflex Contraction of the pectoral muscle when its tendon is tapped in the anterior axillary line, or when the tap is on the seventh rib. The reflex is normally present but is palpable rather than visible. It is enhanced in the setting of pyramidal lesions sited above the C5 cord level.

pectoralis minor syndrome Weakness and discomfort precipitated by manual labor, due to compression of the axillary veins below the pectoralis minor which causes a syndrome in the arm (*venous claudication*) resembling intermittent claudication in the legs.[4580]

pedal Relating to the foot.

pedialgia Pain in the foot. See **Morton metatarsalgia**.

pediatric autoimmune neuropsychiatric disorders associated with streptococcal infections (PANDAs) See **postinfectious (pediatric) autoimmune neuropsychiatric disorders associated with streptococcal infections**.

Pediatric Evaluation of Disability Inventory A scale assessing global function in children with cerebral palsy.[1993]

Pediatric MIDAS Scale A questionnaire designed to assess the disability suffered by children with migraine.[2881] See also **Headache Impact test**.

Pediatric Neurology A subspecialty journal published by Elsevier. Web site: http://www.elsevier.nl/inca/publications/store/5/2/4/9/0/4/.

pediatric multiple sclerosis Consensus definitions have been published[3574] and are amended here:

The diagnosis of MS in children requires multiple episodes of CNS demyelination separated in time and space as specified for adults, but eliminating any lower age limit.

The MRI can be used to meet the dissemination in space requirement if the (2004 revision of the) McDonald criteria for a positive MRI are applied: The MRI must show three of the following four features:

1. nine or more white matter lesions or one gadolinium enhancing lesion
2. three or more periventricular lesions
3. one juxtacortical lesion
4. An infratentorial lesion.

The combination of an abnormal CSF (either oligoclonal bands or an elevated IgG index) and two lesions on the MRI, of which one must be in the brain, also meeting criteria for dissemination in space, supports the diagnosis.

As in adults, the MRI can satisfy criteria for dissemination in time. Following the initial clinical event, even in the absence of new clinical signs of demyelination, new T2 or gadolinium enhancing lesions must develop within 3 months.

However, the authors state that an episode consistent with the clinical features of ADEM cannot always be considered as the first event of MS—see Krupp et al. (2007)[3574]

Pediatric Musculoskeletal Functional Health questionnaire An instrument measuring quality-of-life in children with cerebral palsy.[1425]

PedsQL4.0 An instrument measuring quality-of-life in children with cerebral palsy.[6517]

peduncle (from Lat, a foot stalk) A stalk like process by which an anatomical part is joined to the main organ. Such an appearance led to the terms *cerebral* and *cerebellar peduncles*.

peduncular hallucinosis (red nucleus hallucinatory syndrome) The occurrence of vivid, colored, variable, nonthreatening visual **pseudohallucinations** of patterns, places, or moving images, in association with lesions of the mesencephalon, pons, thalamus, or cerebral peduncles. They are accompanied in most cases by paresis of upward gaze, skew deviation, horizontal gaze paresis, nystagmus, choreoathetosis, cerebellar signs, sleep disturbance, or other signs of posterior fossa dysfunction[3832] and may be regarded as an expression of dissociated sleep associated with release of dream images.

The phenomenon was first described by J.-J. **Lhermitte** in 1922 in a 75-year-old woman with a mesencephalic infarct who saw animals and people in the room with her, especially at nightfall (*vesperal hallucinations*); they appeared absurd to her, but aroused neither psychic nor motor reactions. Lhermitte regarded these as manifestations of diurnal dreaming (rapid eye movement dream material during wakefulness),[3831] an interpretation which is not much different from their current explanation as a release phenomenon related to damage to the ascending reticular activating system. The name was supplied by van Bogaert in 1924.[2101] See also **cerebellar tremors**.

peek sign Myasthenic fatigue leads to weakening of the orbicularis oculi muscle during sustained tight eye closure, so that the subject's eyes open a little and he or she "peeks" through half-open lids.[4821]

PEHO syndrome (progressive encephalopathy with edema, hypsarrhythymia, and optic atrophy) An X-linked syndrome of mental retardation, with Marfanoid habitus, microcephaly, epilepsy, hypsarrhythmia, blindness due to optic atrophy, and coarse facial features. The basis of the disorder appears to be an increase in the endogenous production of nitric oxide leading to atrophy of most cerebral structures.[6512] Peripheral edema is another notable finding.

Peiper optic reflex The occurrence of **opisthotonos** in response to stimulation with bright light; a normal response in the newborn.

Pel, Pieter Klazes (1852–1919) Dutch physician, professor of pathology and medicine at Amsterdam, who in 1898 described the crises now named for him.[5619]

Pel crises (tabetic ciliary neuralgia) Paroxysmal crises of orbital pain with lacrimation and photophobia, eventually leading to glaucoma and occurring in **tabes dorsalis**.

pelagic paralysis See **paralytic shellfish poisoning, scombroid, ciguatera**.

Pelizaeus, Friedrich (1847–1929) German neurologist who in 1885 first described the features of the syndrome named for him.

Pelizaeus–Merzbacher disease (OMIM 312080) A rare, X-linked recessive degenerative myelinopathy (a sudanophilic **leukodystrophy**) in which there is preservation of some myelin islands among widespread demyelination, with sparing of the cortical U-fibers, due to mutations of the proteolipid protein (*PLP*) gene.

Clinically, the condition appears in infants or young children who manifest slowly progressive mental deterioration, arrhythmic nystagmus, bradylalia, choreoathetosis, seizures, spastic paraparesis, and both Parkinsonian and cerebellar signs.[4967] A syndrome of spinal muscular atrophy (see **hereditary motor neuropathy**) is also described. The original gene location was to chromosome Xq21.2–q22. See also **Merzbacher E.**

Six varieties have been differentiated[5711] (Chart P–6).

Pelizaeus–Merzbacher-like disease A recessively inherited hypomyelinating leukoencephalopathy with onset in early infancy characterized by nystagmus, cerebellar ataxia, and spasticity due to permanent lack of myelin deposition in the brain. It differs from the classic form in slower progression, the retention of cognitive functions, and partial myelination of the corticospinal tracts.[933]

pellagra (It, skin + rough) (mal de rose, maidism, mal de sole, malattia della miseria) A syndrome of vitamin B (nicotinic acid) deficiency, characterized by a red, scaly,

Chart P–6. Varieties of Pelizaeus-Merzbacher Disease

Pelizeus-Merzbacher disease type 1 (classic form): A congenital syndrome, usually-inherited as an X-linked recessive trait and manifesting short stature, optic atrophy, nystagmus, dysarthria, microcephaly, pyramidal and cerebellar signs, choreoathetosis and psychomotor delay. White matter hypodensities are seen on CT scans. Death occurs by the age of 25 years.[6664]

Pelizaeus-Merzbacher type 2: (Seitelberger disease, connatal disease) A congenital recessive or X-linked syndrome in which there is severe CNS dysmyelination to the extent that there may be no stainable myelin, although the axons are spared. Clinically, the condition is characterized by cataract, absent phalanges, hypotonia, microcephaly, nystagmus, spasticity, extrapyramidal signs and severe psychomotor delay or arrest. White matter hypodensities are seen on CT scans.[5711]

Pelizaeus-Merzbacher type 3: (transitional form) A sporadic syndrome in which the findings are transitional, resembling both of the above two types.

Pelizaeus-Merzbacher type 4: (adult form, Lowenberg-Hill disease) A dominantly-inherited syndrome characterized by tremor, ataxia, pyramidal signs and dementia with onset in mature adult life.[3935]

Pelizaeus-Merzbacher type 5: A *variant* in which there is only patchy demyelination.

Pelizaeus-Merzbacher type 6: A form characterized by microcephaly, dwarfism, mental retardation, ataxia, retinal pigmentation, cataract, facial thickening, joint contractures and peripheral neuropathy. See **Cockayne syndrome**. "Jimpy" mice probably suffer from this condition.

photosensitive dermatitis; dementia; depression; diarrhoea; glossitis; insomnia; irritability; fatigue; depression; optic atrophy; tremors and rigidity; myelopathy; and anorexia. The rash is first seen in a necklace distribution—the "*Casal collar.*"

The condition was first described by Gaspar Casal (1691–1759) and is still seen in alcoholics, patients with **Hartnup disease**, and in people who subsist upon a diet of maize, from which the nicotinic acid may not be easily extractable. The myelopathy and skin rash respond to treatment with nicotinic acid; when present, an accompanying sensory neuropathy responds to thiamine.

pellagra encephalopathy A syndrome of confusion, paratonia, and myoclonus, seen in patients with chronic alcoholism and multiple vitamin B deficiencies, in this case particularly of niacin.[6542] See also **Wernicke–Korsakoff encephalopathy, Marchiafava–Bignami disease, acquired hepatocerebral encephalopathy**.

pellagrinoid Suffering from **pellagra**.

Pellizzi disseminated cortical dysplasia See **tuberous sclerosis**.

Pellizzi–Bourneville disease See **tuberous sclerosis**.

pelvic floor syndromes Myofascial pain syndromes affecting the muscles of the pelvic floor and causing pain in the buttocks, coccyx, hip, and posterior thigh regions. Per-rectal massage has been recommended as treatment.

pelvic thrusting Repetitive forward pelvic jerks resembling those characteristic of sexual activity but clinically manifested as evidence of underlying frontal or temporal lobe or pseudo- (nonepileptic) seizures.[2344]

Pena–Shokeir phenotype (Pena–Shokeir 1 syndrome; OMIM 208150) A lethal, recessively inherited congenital syndrome, characterized by camptodactyly, severe fetal hydrops, multiple ankyloses, facial anomalies, pulmonary hypoplasia, hypokinesia *in utero*, and resulting arthrogryposis.[4973] See also **fetal akinesia malformation sequence**[4423] and **cerebro-oculofacioskeletal syndrome**.

The *multiple contracture syndrome, Finnish type* is probably the same condition, except that it is fatal in the neonatal period.

Pena–Shokeir 1 syndrome See **Pena–Shokeir phenotype**.

Pendred syndrome (deafness and goiter) The association of congenital bilateral sensorineural deafness, mutism, and goiter, inherited recessively.[4974]

pendular knee jerk See **hypotonia**.

pendular macro-oscillations See **square-wave pulses**.

pendular nystagmus (undulatory nystagmus, talantropia; [from Gr, to oscillate]) That form of nystagmus in which there are two back-and-forth, equal-velocity slow phases of the abnormal deviations of the eyes, with no jerk component.

In the commoner *congenital* form, the movements are usually horizontal and complaints of **oscillopsia** are rare; the lesion is considered to involve the dentate-rubro-olivary pathway. In the less common *acquired* form, the movements are omnidirectional and rapid at 2–6 Hz and oscillopsia is usual. Numerous disorders of the brain and brainstem or cerebellum (especially demyelinating diseases) represent the most common causes.[3762]

pendular pseudonystagmus Spontaneous pendular oscillations of the eyes, made worse by reading, concentration, or trivial head movement and leading to complaints of blurred and shimmering vision or of oscillopsia. The **vestibulo-ocular reflex** is absent. The condition is considered to reflect an imbalance in ocular compensation for an **essential tremor** affecting the head.[866]

Penfield, Wilder (1891–1973) American-Canadian neurosurgeon who was an undergraduate at Princeton and was awarded a Rhodes scholarship, after which he graduated in medicine from Johns Hopkins in 1918 and later trained in surgery at Harvard, New York, Edinburgh, and London. He practiced in New York for some years before moving to Montreal in 1928, when he was appointed professor of neurology and neurosurgery at McGill University. An internationally respected figure, he was honored by governments and universities in many countries.

The advances in neurosurgical technique that he made over the few years after his arrival in Montreal led the Rockefeller Foundation to provide funds to establish the Montreal Neurological Institute with Penfield as its first director. Over his professional life, his researches particularly concerned cerebral cortical localization, epilepsy, and the surgical approaches to its treatment. As well as numerous papers, he published books on the cytology of the CNS, military surgery, *Epilepsy and Cerebral Localization* (1941), *The Cerebral Cortex of Man* (1950), and *Epilepsy and the Functional Anatomy of the Human Brain* (1954) authored alone or in conjunction with colleagues at the institute. He also wrote popular works of fiction.

Penfield syndrome (autonomic diencephalic epilepsy) An unusual variety of seizure in which major autonomic (sympathetic) manifestations occur due to hypothalamic lesions.

Penfield's original case was of a woman who died with an encapsulated tumor that compressed the thalamus. Intermittent episodes of vasodilation, lacrimation, sweating, salivation, hypertension, piloerection, tachycardia, hypothermia, exophthalmos, hiccuping, shivering, and Cheyne–Stokes respirations were clinical features of the attacks recorded. Most other cases have occurred in young males, among whom headache, abdominal pain, and evidence of autonomic arousal are the manifestations most frequently recorded.[4975] See also **diencephalic autonomic seizures**.

Penfield–Ward syndrome Calcifying cerebral hemangiomas.[4978]

penguin sign See **hummingbird sign**.

PEP syndrome See POEMS.

Pepper syndrome See **Hutchinson tumor**.

peptides (Gr, digest) Single-chain, low-molecular-weight aminoacid compounds distributed widely throughout the CNS in selective neuronal pathways. Over 30 such compounds are known to act as neurotransmitters; *vasoactive intestinal peptide* exerts influence on the cerebral circulation, *substance P* and *opioid peptides* on pain pathways, *cholecystokinin* on appetite control, and *vasopressin* and *adrenocorticotrophic hormone* on memory functions.

Perceived Deficits questionnaire A subjective measure of cognitive function designed for assessment of mental activity in patients with **multiple sclerosis**.[6124]

perception The qualitative experience of a conscious person, evoked by a series of events including the unconscious reception, selection, differentiation, and integration of afferent stimuli. It depends upon alterations in the strength and rate of impulses derived from a peripheral organ and transmitted centrally.[2470]

Perception thus denotes the identification of the source, significance, and emotional connotation of sensory stimuli. A percept stripped of meaning is merely a sensation.

perceptual cortex The name given by **Penfield** to the upper lateral portion of the temporal lobe, stimulation of which led to **perceptual illusions** in the subjects he studied.

perceptual speed test A digit cancellation task dependent upon psychomotor speed and sensitive to brain damage.[4466]

percussion myotonia Contraction of muscle fibers with delayed relaxation, not under voluntary control, induced by tapping the muscle. This is a constant feature in myotonic syndromes.

percutaneous rhizotomy Blind surgical section of posterior nerve roots, usually performed in an attempt to relieve spasticity or pain.

percutaneous transluminal angioplasty A surgical technique for clearing an artery of a stenotic obstruction, employing a double lumen balloon catheter that is inflated within the vessel at the site of the obstruction.

peregrinating problem patients See **Munchausen syndrome**.

Perez reflex Pressure upward along the spine of the normal neonate lying prone leads to flexion of the limbs, extension of the neck, and crying.

Performance of Activities of Daily Living test (PADL) An objective instrument used especially in the elderly at home for determining physical functional abilities such as self-care, mobility, and transfers, with regard to their future management and need for care, and assessing some aspects of cognitive capacity.[3570]

Performance scales A self-report tool used in multiple sclerosis research, inquiring into the patient's perception of their capacities in mobility, hand function, fatigue, cognitive functions, bladder–bowel control, and sensory and spasticity symptoms.[5672]

perfusion pressure (cerebral) The difference between the mean systemic arterial pressure and the cerebral venous pressure.

peri- (Gr, around) Equivalent to the Latin *circum*.

periarteritis See **polyarteritis nodosa**.

periaxin A constituent protein of neural plasma membranes, its mutations causing a wide range of genetically determined neuropathies.

pericranium The membranous covering of the skull (the periosteum), first described by Galen.

perifascicular atrophy The presence of myofibrils with an abnormally reduced diameter in the peripheral rather than the central parts of a muscle fascicle. Such an appearance is a characteristic of **dermatomyositis**.

periictal hyperorality A rare ictal–postictal mental disturbance representing an incomplete **Klüver–Bucy syndrome** usually associated with bilateral or left-sided epileptic activity.

perikaryon The cell body.

perilymphatic fistula An abnormal connection between the inner and middle ear that allows escape of perilymph into the middle ear compartment. Rupture of the round window membrane after changing pressure levels is a cause of abrupt deafness, vertigo, and tinnitus, but it can also occur spontaneously. Vertigo and hearing loss[4033] are the major symptoms[4394] See also **superior semicircular canal dehiscence syndrome**.

perimetry The mapping of visual fields, introduced in 1856 by **von Graefe** and subsequently refined by **Holmes** and **Traquair**. The subject fixates upon a central point and responds when first becoming aware of a stimulus emanating from some peripheral point well outside the area of fixation. See also **static perimetry, kinetic perimetry**.

perimyositis A chronic syndrome of exercise-related myalgias, with normal EMG and serum CK levels: but usually with eosinophilia. Muscle biopsy discloses an inflammatory response in the perimysium and epimysium.[6980]

perinatal telencephalic leukoencephalopathy A condition due to damage to the white matter in neonates, possibly inflicted by endotoxins, and marked by the presence of hypertrophic astrocytes or acutely damaged glial cells in the neonatal telencephalon.[3813]

perineurial cysts Tarlov cysts found on MRI of the spine, commonly in the sacral region. They may be entirely asymptomatic or may present with back pain. The few cysts large enough to cause localized deficits can be surgically removed.

perineurioma 1. A solitary intramuscular tumor composed of perineurial cells, but containing neither nerve fibers nor onion-bulb lesions and unattached to a nerve trunk. 2. Perineurial cell accumulations within the nerves in **localized hypertrophic neuropathy**.[4408]

perineuritis Inflammation of the perineurium with thickening of that membrane and degeneration of its cells with an associated lymphocytic inflammatory reaction; a well-recognized finding in older patients with dysimmune sensory or sensorimotor multiple neuropathy of various etiologies[5954] including **diabetes mellitus,**

CIDP, and **cryoglobulinemia**. See also **sensory perineuritis**.

periodic acid–Schiff stain See **PAS stain**.

periodic alternating gaze (ping-pong gaze) A disorder of ocular movement usually noted in patients in coma due to structural cerebral damage or drug toxicity. It consists of slow, rhythmic, and pendular conjugate horizontal deviations of the eyes that alternate from one extreme of gaze to the other every 3–7 s.[5726] Compensatory head turning to the opposite side for 1–2 min also occurs, followed by a midline changeover period lasting 15 s or so.

The phenomenon is seen in some comatose patents with severe bilateral hemispheric[5726] or with hindbrain disease.

periodic alternating nystagmus (and aperiodic alternating nystagmus) Most commonly an acquired horizontal or oblique jerk nystagmus, present in the primary position and occurring in cycles lasting between 1 and 2 min, in which the direction of the fast component changes after a few seconds pause, persisting in this alternation.[6956] Posterior fossa lesions of all kinds (usually sited in the dorsal medulla or cerebellum) and drug toxicity have been incriminated as causes. The phenomenon reflects disordered activity within a γ-amino butyric acid inhibitory pathway, as confirmed by its inhibition by baclofen. An elegant elucidation of the mechanisms has been presented by Leigh et al.[3760]

In a *variant* form, the phases are irregular and occur in association with bilateral severe visual loss, which is usually congenital.

periodic alternating skew deviation A variant form of **skew deviation** in which the direction of the ocular deviations reverses spontaneously. It is sometimes associated with **periodic alternating nystagmus**.[3819]

periodic ataxia A dominantly inherited syndrome characterized by episodes of ataxia, vertigo, nystagmus, and dysarthria responsive to acetazolamide. The same problem can occur as a complication of **multiple sclerosis**, in which case they are frequent and brief but do not cease with acetazolamide treatment.[1685, 2269]

periodic downbeat nystagmus An unusual complication of hypomagnesemia, reported as 1.5 min of downbeating nystagmus separated by a period of 2 min.[1719]

periodic dystonia See **paroxysmal kinesigenic choreoathetosis**.

periodic hypersomnia (recurrent hypersomnia) A disorder characterized by recurrent episodes of hypersomnia that typically occur weeks or months apart. Diagnostic criteria have been suggested[1629] and are given in Chart P–7.

periodic hypersomnia associated with menstruation Intervals of severe excessive daytime sleepiness and elevated total sleep time lasting for about a week after the onset of menstruation, sometimes also associated with depression.[2626]

periodic lateralized epileptiform discharges (PLEDs) Recurrent uniform spike- or sharp-wave discharges localized to part of one hemisphere on the EEG, occurring regularly at 0.5–2 Hz or irregularly. In adults they involve a large area of one hemisphere and are associated most commonly with acute destructive lesions of the brain caused by tumors or cerebral infarct; in children, chronic diffuse lesions of the CNS are most often responsible. They are often accompanied by disturbed consciousness and focal motor seizures.[1118]

When there are additional high-frequency, low-voltage polyspike rhythms (PLEDS-Plus), clinical seizures and status epilepticus are even more likely.

periodic leg movements See **periodic limb movement disorder**.

periodic limb movement disorder (periodic leg movements, nocturnal myoclonus, periodic limb movements in sleep, leg jerks, sleep myoclonus, periodic sustained anterior tibial contractions with arousal, night starts, sudden bodily jerks on falling asleep) A disorder characterized by periodic episodes of repetitive, stereotyped, semi-purposeful limb movements that occur during stages 1 and 2 of non–rapid eye movement sleep or in the period of relaxed wakefulness immediately prior to sleep,[1248, 1249, 6173] consisting of single body-wide jerks of unknown cause, unassociated with known neurological disease and immediately

Chart P–7. Diagnostic Criteria for Periodic Hypersomnia

A. A complaint of excessive sleepiness.
B. The episodes of somnolence last for at least 19 h a day.
C. The excessive sleepiness recurs at least once or twice a year, lasting a minimum of 3 days and up to 3 weeks.
D. The disorder occurs predominantly in males, with an age of onset typically in adolescence.
E. Associated features during the episodes include at least one of the following:
   1. Voracious eating.
   2. Hypersexuality.
   3. Disinhibited behaviors such as irritability, aggression, disorientation, confusion and hallucinations;
F. Polysomnographic monitoring during an episode demonstrates:
   1. A high sleep efficiency;
   2. Reduced NREM stages 3 and 4 sleep;
   3. Reduced sleep latency and rapid eye movement latency; and
   4. A multiple sleep latency test that demonstrates a mean sleep latency of less than 10 min.
G. Not associated with other medical or psychiatric disorders, such as epilepsy or depression.
H. The symptom is not associated with other sleep disorders, such as narcolepsy, sleep apnea syndromes or periodic limb moment disorder.

Adapted from AASM Diagnostic Classification Steering Committee. The International Classification of Sleep. *Disorders Diagnostic and Coding Manual. Rochester, MN. American Academy of Sleep Medicine 1991/2001. Reproduced by kind permission of the Academy.* See also http://www.sleepeducation.com/Disorders.aspx/

restoring the subject to wakefulness. Extension of the hallux, dorsiflexion of the ankle, and flexion of the knee and hip are the usual movements recorded (a pattern reminiscent of the **Babinski reflex**).

The bursts of electrical activity underlying them last 2–15 s (unlike other forms of positive **myoclonus**) and recur with marked periodicity during NREM sleep or daytime drowsiness.[1249] A disorder of the CNS dopaminergic systems producing increased excitability of segmental spinal flexor reflexes is considered to be the underlying pathophysiology.

Despite the alternative names, these movements are seldom as fast as true myoclonus. They are associated both with **narcolepsy** and with the **restless limbs syndrome**. Daytime somnolence and nocturnal insomnia may also result. See also **sleep myoclonus**. Diagnostic criteria have been suggested;[5012, 1629] the more recent are abstracted in Chart P–8.

periodic migrainous neuralgia of Wilfred Harris Yet another term for **cluster headache**, but this one more comfortably euphonious if rather lengthy. At least it recognizes the uncertainty which yet remains as to whether the pathogenesis of this condition is neural, vascular, or both.

periodic miosis (intermittent oculosympathetic paresis) Periodic pupillary constriction with conjunctival injection, lasting from minutes to months.[6141]

periodic movements in sleep See **periodic limb movements of sleep**.

periodic paralysis Rare, dominantly inherited inherited channelopathies that manifest as episodic bouts of abnormal, often potassium-sensitive muscle membrane excitability leading to episodic flaccid paralysis mainly in the limbs and lasting hours to days, with areflexia.[6522] The attacks can follow a carbohydrate load or exertion, or insulin or adrenalin administration. Depolarization of the muscle fibers and impaired Na^+–K^+ activity in muscle may predispose. In the setting of hyperthyroidism, the condition is mainly recorded in Japanese males. See **familial periodic paralysis**.

periodic somnolence with morbid hunger see **Kleine–Levin syndrome**.

periodic sustained anterior tibial contractions with arousal See **periodic limb movement disorder**.

periodic syndromes 1. A childhood syndrome of typical adult migraine or a combination of one or more of the following: cyclic vomiting or repeated bilious attacks; recurrent vague abdominal pain; recurrent headaches; dizzy spells; periodic attacks of fever; and periodic attacks of limb and joint pains or stiffness ("growing pains"). The prevalence of this condition alone may be 4.5%. The syndrome most likely includes many cases of juvenile **migraine**, particularly when headache is present.[406]

2. Recurrent episodes of neurological deficit in children, which may be precursors of or associated with migraine (migraine equivalents). There are three varieties; see **alternating hemiplegia of childhood, benign paroxysmal vertigo of childhood**, and **cyclical vomiting**.

periodic vestibulocerebellar ataxias Dominantly inherited conditions of adult onset manifested by diplopia and intermittent attacks of vestibular dysfunction and ataxia. See **cerebellar ataxias**.

periodic/aperiodic nystagmus See **periodic alternating nystagmus**.

perioptic neuritis (optic perineuritis) An inflammatory disorder of the optic nerve sheaths; when explained, it is usually due to syphilis, sarcoidosis, or other inflammatory conditions.[4063]

perioral myoclonia with absences A rare epilepsy syndrome, a variant of typical absences, occurring especially in girls, many of whom have a positive family history of idiopathic generalized epilepsies.

Clinically, the typical absence seizures lasting a few seconds are accompanied by perioral myoclonia (protrusion of the lips, twitching of the corners of the mouth, or jaw jerking); there is some degree of impairment of consciousness. Their frequency is very variable but hyperventilation is a strong precipitant. All patients suffer from generalized tonic–clonic seizures that are typically infrequent and which are often preceded by clusters of absences or absence status.

The inter-ictal EEG shows generalized 3–7 Hz spike/multiple spike wave discharges that are usually asymmetrical, and focal abnormalities, including single spikes, spike–wave complexes, or slow waves, are common; this pattern is enhanced with hyperventilation.[4882]

perioral reflexes Contraction of various facial and cervical muscles in response to a tap on the lips or the perioral

Chart P–8. Diagnostic Criteria for Periodic Limb Movement Disorder

A. The patient has a complaint of insomnia or excessive sleepiness but may occasionally be asymptomatic, the movements only being noticed by an observer.
B. Repetitive, highly stereotyped limb muscle movements are present. In the leg, characterized by extension of the big toe with partial flexion of the ankle, knee, and sometimes the hip.
C. Polysomnographic monitoring demonstrates repetitive episodes of muscle contraction (0.5–5 s) separated by an interval of typically 20–40 s. Arousals or awakenings may be associated with the movements.
D. Thre is no evidence of another medical or mental disorder that can account for the primary complaint.
E. Other sleep disorders present do not account for the movements. (Minimal criteria: A + B)

After Phillips B. Diagnostic criteria for periodic limb movement disorder. Neurology 2004;62:S9–S16. Reproduced by kind permission of the AAN and Lippincott, Williams and Wilkins.

regions, or as a result of other stimuli to the face. Both proprioceptive and nociceptive stimulation produce such responses, which are present in most normal subjects but which may be exaggerated in the presence of diffuse cortical dysfunction.[1832, 6656] See also **corneomandibular reflex, orbicularis oris reflex**.

periosteal reflexes A misnomer, the periosteum having no receptors stimulation of which leads to reflex muscle contraction. The numerous "reflexes" described with this suffix are phasic muscle stretch reflexes and are only entered as such in this book. See **muscle stretch reflex**.

peripheral neurofibromatosis and peroneal muscular atrophy See **hereditary motor and sensory neuropathy** (*variants*).

peripheral neuropathy A disorder of the motor and/or sensory nerves, as opposed to the fiber tracts within the CNS. Involvements of cranial nerves below the optic nerve and of the autonomic nervous system are subsumed.

Primary disease of the cells of the motor nuclei of cranial and spinal nerves might be supposed to indicate the presence of a CNS disorder, but the effects are the same as those of other, more distal, neural pathologies and are generally classified under the heading of peripheral neuropathy.

peripheral neuropathy affecting the arms A dominantly inherited syndrome of distal neurogenic arm weakness and wasting with early adult onset.[3669]

(Peripheral) Neuropathy Association A charitable organization providing support and information on peripheral nerve disorders. Web site: http://www.neuropathy.org/site/PageServer. See also http://www.ninds.nih.gov/disorders/peripheralneuropathy/peripheralneuropathy.htm.

Peripheral Neuropathy Symptom questionnaire A validated tool for the detection of neuropathy in neuroepidemiological studies.[2191] The following questions are asked:

How often have you had any of the following conditions in the past 4 weeks?
Cramps in the muscles of the arms or legs.
Twitching in the muscles of the arms or legs.
Need for help getting out of a chair.
Difficulty in opening screw top lids on jars.
Tingling or pins and needles sensations in the hands, arms, feet, or legs.
Numbness.
A burning sensation in the arms or legs.
Pain in the arms after work, when resting.
A need to strain in order to start urine flowing.
A need to push on the abdomen to start or to keep the urine flowing.

peripheral neuropathy with hepatic disease A demyelinating peripheral neuropathy complicating cirrhosis, portosystemic shunt, or hepatic necrosis, considered most likely to be due to a toxic metabolite or to disordered insulin metabolism as a result of the hepatic damage.[1491]

peripheral nystagmus A form of conjugate, direction-fixed nystagmus often with both horizontal and rotatory components, caused by a lesion of the vestibular system outside the CNS. When it is induced by head movements (**Bárány test**), there is a delay of some seconds before it occurs, and it fatigues with time and with repetition. Unlike **central nystagmus**, its amplitude is lessened by visual fixation. See also **direction-fixed nystagmus**.

peripheral osmotic demyelination syndrome The rare occurrence of demyelination in the peripheral nervous system in the setting of an **osmotic demyelination syndrome**.

peripheral vertigo That form of vertigo due to a lesion of the end-organ of the vestibular system or of the vestibular nerve, giving rise to **peripheral nystagmus**.

peripheral vestibular paroxysmia (disabling peripheral vertigo) A tentative syndrome considered likely due to neurovascular crossovers between the VIII nerve and a brainstem artery such as the AICa. Clinically, it presents as as a series of short attacks or a series of rotational or to-and-fro vertigo, sometimes related to changes in head position and often with hypacusis and tinnitus.[6104]

peripheral vestibulopathy A syndrome of single or recurrent episodes of vertigo lasting for hours to days, unassociated with hearing loss or other neurological dysfunction.The clinical syndrome encompasses various nonspecific disorders, the most notable being **vestibular neuronitis**.[1707]

periphlebitis retinae Sheathing or cuffing of the retinal veins by lymphocytes and plasma cells. See **Eales disease, multiple sclerosis**.

perisylvian syndrome A congenital syndrome characterized by bilateral perisylvian micropolygyria with multiple seizure types, cognitive deficits, and pseudobulbar (facio-pharyngo-masticatory) palsy.[3618]

perithelial small cell sarcoma See **primary CNS lymphoma**.

perivascular plaques (Scholz plaques) Amyloid deposits in the walls of cerebral arterioles.

perivascular sarcoma See **primary CNS lymphoma**.

periventricular heterotropia A condition characterized by neuronal nodules in the wall of the lateral ventricles. It is a heterogeneous disorder often inherited as an X-linked dominant due to mutations of *FLNA*. Female patients present with seizures, but have normal intelligence, but the condition may be lethal for hemizygous males. An autosomal recessive form is also described mapped to chromosome 5p.[5776]

periventricular leukomalacia (periventricular lucencies) Damage to the white matter, particularly in the occipital radiation and close to the foramen of Monro, involving the centrum semiovale at the junction of the corpus callosum and the internal and external capsules. They are typically caused in infants by **watershed infarcts** of the (as yet unmyelinated) white matter. When occurring as a result of hypoxic-ischemic injury some form of **cerebral palsy** with motor deficits, cognitive and visual impairment and seizures usually result. The condition is common in the brains of neonates of low birth weight who survive severe clinical insults in the perinatal period for only a few days.[5817] **Leukoaraiosis** has a similar distribution in adults.

periventricular lucencies See **periventricular leukomalacia**.

Perlia, Richard XIX Century German ophthalmologist.

Perlia nucleus A small group of cells medial to the III cranial nerve nuclear complex, described in 1889. They probably represent a center for the control of ocular convergence, but the existence, let alone the function, of this "nucleus" has been called into question.

permanent global amnesia A rare, severe, selective, and stable memory disorder of adult life affecting both new learning and recall, and associated with selective hippocampal atrophy, probably on an ischemic basis.[3568] See also **transient global amnesia**.

permanent persistent postconcussive syndrome The prolonged experience of symptoms that are common in the immediate phase after mild traumatic brain injury (concussion) including dizziness, headache, unusual sensitivity to most or all sensations, impairment of memory, attention, and executive functions, and emotional symptoms such as irritability, depression, and resentment.[118]

permanent unconsciousness See **persistent vegetative state**.

peroneal compartment syndrome Ischemic necrosis of the muscles with resultant compression of the nerves in the peroneal compartment, either as a result of primary vascular occlusion or following overexertion, which may lead to muscle swelling beneath the strong fascial membrane delimiting the compartment, thus inducing secondary occlusion of the blood vessels within it. Clinically, pain, swelling, weakness, and sensory loss in the territory of the common peroneal nerve are the major findings.[5272]

peroneal muscle reflex Contraction of the anterior compartment muscles when the examiner's finger, placed on the dorsum of the foot, is tapped with a reflex hammer. The contraction is increased in the presence of pyramidal lesions and decreased with lesions of the L5 or S1 reflex arcs[574] but is often hard to detect in healthy people.

peroneal muscular atrophy See **hereditary motor and sensory neuropathy, types 1 and 2**.

peroneal sign See **Lust phenomenon**.

peroneus (from Gr, a leg bone; the same as the Latin word *fibula*, which bone the peroneal nerve and muscles overlie. The relationship of the tibia to the fibula was considered similar to that of a brooch and its pin) A word applied to neural and muscular structures in the anterior compartment of the lower leg.

peroneus tertius aplasia A recessively inherited anomaly with this feature.

peroxidase deficiency A dominantly inherited form of **neuronal ceroid lipofuscinosis**; a corencephalopathy.[698]

peroxisomal disorders Inborn errors of metabolism affecting multiple organ systems and caused by disorders of these intracellular organelles in which the enzymatic utilization of oxygen and the production of hydrogen peroxide occur.[5212, 3730, 4447] Disorders involving these entities are due to absence of a specific peroxisomal enzyme or to a failure to form peroxisomes, resulting in a generalized deficiency of these enzymes (peroxisomal biosynthesis disorders). Peroxisomes are responsible for the catabolism of very-long-chain fatty acids, dicarboxylic acids, and pipecolic and phytanic acids, and for the biosynthesis of bile acids.[3]

Clinically, severe mental retardation and both visual and auditory defects are constant symptoms in those peroxisomal diseases with congenital presentations, as in Group 1 in Chart P–9, which lists those of neurological interest identified to date.

A benign *variant* is *ataxia and peripheral neuropathy*, a childhood syndrome of ataxia, hyporeflexia, and hypotonia with panperoxisomal dysfunction in the plasma, fibroblasts, and liver.[3988, 4512]

peroxisomal polydystrophy syndromes The syndromes of **infantile Refsum disease**, neonatal **adrenoleukodystrophy**, and **hyperpipecolic acidemia**.[3377]

peroxisomes Subcellular organelles that generate H_2O_2 in the course of oxidizing a large number of substrates including immunoacids, hydroxyacids, and fatty acids. They also contain catalase, an enzyme that breaks down H_2O_2.

These ubiquitous organelles house the proteinaceous *impedimenta* of numerous metabolic pathways, most involving brain more than peripheral nervous system functioning. Chemical abnormalities associated with peroxisomal defects include elevated concentrations of very-long-chain fatty acids, excessive pipecolate in blood and

Table: Clinical features suggesting the possible presence of a peroxisomal disorder include:

Invariable;	Psychomotor retardation	
Over 75% of cases	Low, broad nasal ridge	Neonatal hypotonia
	Encephalopathy	Seizures
	Impaired hearing	Abnormal electroretinogram
	Hepatomegaly	
50%–70% of cases	Large fontanelles	Shallow orbital ridges
	Epicanthus	Pigmentary retinopathy
	Congenital cataracts	
	Peripheral neuropathy in early childhood	
	Failure to thrive after 6 months of age.	

Precise listings of symptoms related to age are presented by Baumgartner [450] and by Theil et al. cited by Moser. [4512]
The genetic correlations of the various disorders were fully reviewed by Barth et al. [427] and by Raymond.[5216]

Chart P–9. The Peroxisomal Disorders

1. *Single-enzyme defects with normal peroxisomal structure and abnormalities of a single peroxisomal function.*
   Examples are:

   Acatalasemia
   Acyl CoA oxidase deficiency (pseudo-neonatal adrenoleukodystrophy)
   Adult Refsum disease (**hereditary motor and sensory neuropathy** type 4)
   Glutaric aciduria type 3
   Hyperoxaluria type 1.
   Mevalonic aciduria; Hyper IgD syndrome [427]
   Other adult-onset polyneuropathy
   Pseudo-**Zellweger disease**
   Rhizomelic chondrodysplasia and variant phenotypes
   X-Linked adrenoleukodystrophy and the *Naidu variant*.
   X-linked adrenomyeloneuropathy
   A form involving accumulation of pristanic acid (a derivative of phytanic acid) presenting with pigmentary retinopathy, peripheral neuropathy and hypogonadism. [4248]

2. *Disorders of peroxisomal dysgenesis*: Disorders in which peroxisomes are present but two peroxisomal functions are disturbed, and there are multiple enzyme disorders. These devastating diseases are characterized by failure to thrive, mental retardation, seizures, blindness, deafness and liver failure due to deficiency in multiple peroxisomal enzymes. [3988]
   Examples are

   Infantile Refsum disease.
   Leber optic atrophy
   Neonatal **adrenoleukodystrophy**.
   Pseudo-Zellweger disease.
   Rhizomelic chondrodysplasia punctata
   Zellweger syndrome.

urine, and reduced tissue concentrations of plasmalogenes.[2448]

per-rotational response

Nystagmus induced by the onset of a velocity-step stimulus.[3762]

perseverance (persistence) The laudable ability of an individual to stick to a task in hand.

perseveration The involuntary continuance or recurrence of a purposeful response that is more appropriate to a preceding stimulus than to the succeeding one just given, which is essential to provoke it.[137] More simply, the continuation or recurrence of an experience or activity without the appropriate stimulus.

It is not spontaneous; two or more stimuli are required to demonstrate it. It is seen in normal subjects at the extremes of age, but is also a sign of any kind of diffuse or focal organic brain disease.

Three varieties have been defined:[5539]

1. Recurrence of a previous response with a subsequent stimulus within the context of an established set (*recurrent perseveration*). This is most closely associated with left hemisphere lesions.
2. Inappropriate maintenance of a category or framework of activity (*stuck-in-set perseveration*), associated with frontal-subcortical and mesolimbic lesions.
3. Abnormal prolongation or the continuation without cessation of current behavior (*continuous perseveration*), for which right hemisphere lesions are most commonly responsible.

The term was introduced by Neisser in 1895. As described by Wilson, "The persistence of certain impressions may become a fertile source of error in the execution of complex movements; a patient may recognise an object and use it correctly, but be unable to prevent himself from repeating this act when a different object is shown to him."[6819]

Perseveration is a reliable sign of organic mental dysfunction at any time after infancy.[2192]

persistence See perseverance.

persistent aura without infarction Aura symptoms persisting for more than 1 week without radiographic evidence of infarction. The ICHD committee suggests as diagnostic criteria that the present attack in a patient with **migraine with aura** is typical of previous attacks except that one or more aura symptoms persists for >1 week and that the condition cannot be attributed to another disorder. See **aura**.

persistent conditioned insomnia See **persistent** DIMS.

persistent DIMS (disorders of initiation or maintenance of sleep) (persistent conditioned insomnia, internal arousal insomnia, psychophysiological arousal) A disorder of sleep initiation and maintenance (i.e., falling asleep and staying asleep) as a result of chronic somatized tension combined with conditioned reinforcers of sleeplessness. (See also ASDA/AASM Diagnostic Classification.[280])

persistent DOES (disorders of excessive sleep) Chronic sleepiness following a prolonged period of emotional stress. See also **General adaptation syndrome** and the ASDA/AASM Diagnostic Classification.[280]

persistent idiopathic facial pain (atypical facial pain) Persistent facial pain that does not have the characteristics of the cranial neuralgias and is not attributed to another disorder. Diagnostic criteria have been defined:

A. Pain in the face, present daily and persisting for all or most of the day, fulfilling criteria B and C
B. Pain is confined at onset to a limited area on one side of the face, and is deep and poorly localized
C. Pain is not associated with sensory loss or other physical signs
D. Investigations including X-ray of face and jaws do not demonstrate any relevant abnormality

Adapted from the International Classification of Headache Disorders (Headache Classification Committee of the International Headache Society. *Cephalalgia* 2004;**24**[Suppl 1]) by kind permission of Dr. Jes Olesen, the International Headache Society and Wiley-Blackwell Publications.

persistent idiopathic hyperCKemia Unexplained persistently increased CK levels in an otherwise healthy patient without symptoms, without physical or electrical evidence of muscle disease and in the absence of such potential causes as recent strenuous exercise; hypokalemia, hypothyroidism, or parathyroid disease; a family history of neuromuscular disease; excess alcohol or certain drug ingestion; or recent intramuscular injections. The continued presence of such raised levels should alert anaesthesiologists to the possibility of **malignant hyperthermia** or myopathy.[6692]

persistent infantile sleep apnea Congenital failure of the automatic control of respiration, leading to alveolar hypoventilation in the presence of normal function of the lungs and heart and normal metabolism; one likely cause of the sudden infant death syndrome.

persistent pain of cranial nerve origin Diagnostic criteria were suggested by the Headache Classification Committee of the International Headache Society[2820] and are reproduced in Chart P–10 by kind permission. See also the review of Portenoy.[5083]

persistent primitive trigeminal artery An embryonic carotid-basilar anastomosis continuing into adult life in up to 1% of the population, sometimes associated with **trigeminal neuralgia**.

persistent vegetative state (wakefulness without awareness, akinetic mutism, apallic state, alpha coma, chronic coma, coma vigil[e], irreversible coma, neocortical death, permanent unconsciousness) A form of eyes-open permanent unconsciousness in which the patient has periods of wakefulness and physiological sleep/wake cycles within 1–2 weeks following the initial coma, but is at no time aware of the self or the environment, although blinking may occur in response to threat or loud noises. Cognition, recognition, and meaningful interaction with the environment are absent, and thought, reason, memory, speech, and affect (as well as any other qualities which are conventionally characteristic of human nature or personhood) are lost. As far as can be determined, neither pain nor suffering is experienced. Wandering, conjugate eye movements return but sustained visual pursuit does not occur. Brainstem functions such as breathing, chewing, swallowing, and cranial/spinal reflexes are preserved and occasional nonpurposive movements may be performed. Sphincter control is lost.

The condition results from diseases that lead to the total loss of cerebral cortical functions, while those of the brainstem are retained. Most commonly, it follows severe anoxic or traumatic brain disease, but it can also occur as an end-stage in chronic dementing or other neurological disorders. Its characteristics have been defined by committees of the American Academy of Neurology.[165] and of the American Neurological Association,[170] the latter being reproduced in Chart P–11 in a slightly adapted form. A further major review has ben published.[6262]

Despite such confident assertions, a problem is that one can only say that the condition is actually persistent in retrospect, because we do not yet have the power of accurate prognosis for this condition. How long it takes for this syndrome to be labeled "persistent" with justification is a question removed from the practice of medicine and best left to the family, the lawyers, the ethicists, and the administrators of the hospital where the metabolising patient lies dead to the world. Some suggest 1 year; this author's living will specifies 1 week. The simpler term "vegetative state" avoids the issue, but at least makes fewer assumptions.

Chart P–10. Diagnostic Criteria for Persistent Pain of Cranial Nerve Origin

A. Pain in the distribution of one or more cranial nerves and/or cervical roots 2 and 3, with or without projection to neighboring areas.
B. Demonstration of a relevant lesion.
C. Onset of pain temporally related to the onset of a cranial nerve lesion.
D. If the lesion can be effectively treated or remits spontaneously, pain abates or disappears.

Compression or distortion of cranial nerves and second or third cervical roots: Headache or facial pain caused by a lesion directly compromising one or more of the afferent nerves supplying pain sensation to the head and neck (namely the trigeminal, nervus intermedius, glossopharyngeal, vagus and cervical roots 2 and 3).

Optic neuritis (retrobulbar neuritis).

A. Pain is felt.
B. Central vision becomes impaired due to a central or paracentral scotoma.
C. No extrinsic lesion can be demonstrated.

Infarction of cranial nerves.

Diabetic neuritis: Pain around the eye and forehead associated with an oculomotor (III cranial nerve) palsy of diabetic origin.

A. Pain is felt around the eye on the affected side.
B. Pain is of acute onset, developing over a few hours.
C. There is a partial or complete oculomotor nerve palsy.
D. The patient suffers from diabetes mellitus.
E. No extrinsic lesion can be demonstrated.

Inflammation of cranial nerves.

Chronic **post-herpetic neuralgia:** Facial pain developing during the acute phase of herpes zoster infection and persisting more than 6 months thereafter.

A. Pain is restricted to the distribution of the affected cranial nerves or divisions thereof.
B. Pain persists more than 6 months after the onset of herpetic eruption.

See also **trigeminal neuralgia, glossopharyngeal neuralgia, occipital neuralgia, superior laryngeal neuralgis, nasociliary neuralgia**.

From: Headache Classification Committee of the International Headache Society. Classification of headache disorders, cranial neuralgias and facial pains; and diagnostic criteria for primary headache disorders. Cephalalgia 1988;8(Suppl):1–96. Reproduced by kind permission of Elsevier Science and the IHS.

persistent wakefulness A disorder of sleep (dyssomnia) characterized by an inability to sleep, and due to a pre-trigeminal midpontine lesion or to psychophysiological mechanisms.[2796]

perte de la parole (Fr, loss of words) The earliest term for what we now know as **aphasia**, used by Bouillaud in 1825.[766]

Chart P–11. Diagnostic Criteria for Persistent Vegetative State

To allow the diagnosis, the following slightly adapted criteria must be met:

A. The patient displays no evidence of awareness of self or surroundings, although reflex or spontaneous eye opening may occur.
B. No meaningful and consistent auditory or written communication between the examiner and the patient can be established. (Target stimuli are not usually followed visually, but visual tracking can occasionally occur.) The patient shows no emotional response to verbal input.
C. There is no comprehensible speech nor mouthing of words.
D. Smiling, frowning and crying can occur, but are inconsistently related to any apparent stimulus.
E. Sleep-wake cycles are present.
F. Brainstem and spinal reflex activity is variable. Sucking, rooting, chewing and swallowing reflexes may be preserved. Pupillary reactivity to light, oculocephalic reflexes, grasp reflexes and muscle stretch reflexes may be present.
G. The presence of voluntary movements or behavior, no matter how rudimentary, is a sign of cognition and is incompatible with the diagnosis of persistent vegetative state. There is no motor activity suggesting learned behavior and no mimicry. Rudimentary movements (such as withdrawal or posturing) may be seen with noxious or disagreeable stimuli.
H. Blood pressure control and cardiorespiratory functions are usually intact. Incontinence of bladder and bowel is present.

Adapted from American Neurological Association Committee on Ethical Affairs. Persistent vegetative state. Ann Neurol 1993;33:386–90. © 1993. Reproduced with permission of John Wiley and Sons. Inc.)

pertussis neurotoxic syndrome A supposed neurological complication following the adminstration of whole-cell pertussis vaccine. It is characterized clinically by screaming, ataxia, irritability, convulsions, or coma, occurring several hours after injection of the vaccine into an infant.[5115]

pervasive developmental disorders (PDDs) A group of conditions characterized by delays in the development of socialization and communication skills, usually manifesting before the age of 3 years. Symptoms may include problems with using and understanding language; difficulty relating to people, objects, and events; unusual play with toys and other objects; difficulty with changes in routine or familiar surroundings, and repetitive body movements or behavior patterns.

Autism (a developmental brain disorder characterized by impaired social interaction and communication skills, and a limited range of activities and interests) is the most characteristic and best studied PDD. Other types include **Asperger syndrome**, childhood disintegrative disorder, and **Rett Syndrome**. Children with PDD vary widely in abilities, intelligence, and behaviors. Some do not speak at all, others speak in limited phrases or conversations, and some have relatively normal language development. Repetitive play skills and limited social skills are generally evident. Unusual responses to sensory information, such as loud noises and lights, are also common.

perverse pupillary reaction Pupillary dilation on attempted near-gaze. It is thought to be a psychosensory response to the examiner's enthusiastic encouragement.[6617]

perverted nystagmus Vertical nystagmus resulting from unilateral caloric stimulation.[3762] See **vestibular nystagmus**.

pes cavus A common congenital or acquired deformity of the foot, in which the anteroposterior measurement is decreased, the arch high, and the toes flexed at the distal, and extended at the proximal interphalangeal joints.

In a third of the cases the abnormality is not associated with any neurological deficits, but it is a frequent finding in patients with **spinocerebellar degenerations** and with the **hereditary motor and sensory neuropathies** and other genetically determined neuropathies.[834]

pes planus Flat foot, either mobile or fixed in that position.

Pescia epileptogenic encephalopathy A congenital syndrome manifesting seizures, microcephaly, cerebral atrophy, callosal agenesis, and mental and developmental delay.[381]

PET scan A test of regional cerebral metabolic function. See **positron emission tomography**.

petalias Indentations on the inner table of the skull due to asymmetrical compression by the asymmetrical brain during development.

Petges syndrome See **dermatomyositis**.

petit mal See **three-Hz spike-and-slow waves, atypical repetitive spike-and-slow waves**.

petit mal epilepsy See **absence epilepsy** (minor seizures).

petit mal seizures with focal components Attacks differing from other forms of typical absence attack by virtue of a later age of onset, the frequent presence of cerebral lesions (usually frontal), and a poor response to treatment.[1416]

petit mal status See **status epilepticus, absence status**.

petit mal triad The combination of akinetic and absence seizures with myoclonus.

petit mal variant See **atypical repetitive spike-and-slow waves**.

Petren gait A disorder of motility in which the patient becomes unable to continue walking after the first few steps have been taken. The condition is usually considered to indicate the presence of frontal lobe pathology.

The phenomenon is a version of **astasia trépidante**. See also **isolated gait ignition failure**.

petrosal ganglion A ganglion associated with the IX cranial nerve, which contains the cell bodies of fibers which pass to the nucleus solitarius.

petrosphenoidal space syndrome See **Jacod syndrome (triad)**.

petrous apical syndrome See **Gradenigo syndrome**.

petrous neuralgia (Gardner neuralgia) Intermittent bouts of severe pain in the cheek and lateral parts of the eyebrow, with lacrimation and rhinorrhea. The condition resembles, and is probably a variant of, **cluster headache**, but also contains elements of **trigeminal neuralgia**.

Pfaundler–Hurler syndrome See **mucopolysaccharidoses**.

Pfeiffer scale A short portable mental status questionnaire for the assessment of organic brain deficit in elderly patients.[5009]

Pfeiffer syndrome (acrocephalosyndactyly type IV, congenital ataxia with choroidal coloboma) A congenital dysmorphic syndrome characterized by craniosynostosis affecting the coronal suture, with turri-brachycephaly and kleeblattschädel (cloverleaf malformation of the skull), ocular hypertelorism, broad thumbs, syndactyly, proptosis, strabismus, deafness, elbow joint synostosis, and developmental delay.[4127] See **acrocephalopolysyndactyly**.

PGO waves See **pontogeniculo-occipital waves**.

PHACES syndrome The association of posterior fossa brain malformations such as the Dandy–Walker syndrome, or cerebellar hypoplasia; hemangiomas, arterial, cardiac, or eye abnormalities and sternal clefting or a supraumbilical raphe.

phakomatoses (from Gr, mark on the skin) (neurocutaneous syndromes, neuroectomesodermoses, genoneurodermatoses, ectomesodermal blastomatoses, congenital neuroectodermal dysplasias) A heterogeneous collection of inherited ectodermal disorders which have in common the involvement of the skin and of the nervous system.

The name was bestowed by van der Hoeve (1923). See **neurocutaneous syndromes**.

Phalen sign Compression of the median nerve by the exertion of finger pressure over the carpal tunnel leads to the complaint of paresthesias in the median nerve distribution in many patients with **carpal tunnel syndrome**. The incidence of positive results with this sign varies rather widely between different series.[5010] See also **Tinel sign, flick sign**.

Dr. George Phalen was an orthopedic surgeon who practiced at the Cleveland Clinic.

phantom (from Gr; to make invisible) A mental illusion.

phantom eye syndrome The illusory sensation that an eye that has been removed is still present, most commonly occurring when the diseased eye was painful prior to its removal.[5955]

phantom limb The subjective perception of the presence of a body part when it is in fact absent, either due to amputation or to congenital absence. The size of the limb perceived may slowly diminish over the years following amputation, or may remain unaltered, sometimes enlarging during intercurrent illnesses.

In *variant* forms, a patient with sensory or motor loss may feel the paretic limb moving when it is not doing so, or may experience a phantom as part of a sensory seizure.

Such a perception might well have been regarded as evidence of possession in medieval times, but it was recognized as a medical problem by Ambrose Paré (1551), Réne Descartes, and Sir Charles **Bell**. Admiral Lord Nelson believed that his awareness of the phantom fingers of his amputated arm provided direct proof of the existence of the soul. More modern descriptions are those of **Weir Mitchell**,[4402, 5293] drawing from his experiences in the American Civil War, and of Herman Melville ("a dismasted man never loses the feeling of his old spar but it will still be pricking him at times").

A variant is *supernumary phamtom limb*, in which the subject has the sensation of an extra limp, described after brain injury—such as pontine hemorrhage.

phantom (limb) pain Persistent but variable cramping, burning, or aching pain, made worse by any emotional or physical stimuli and by attempted "movement" and felt in a phantom part, especially the arm, and also especially by patients who had experienced severe protracted pain in their limb prior to its removal.

Such pain is experienced, fortunately, by less than 5% of all amputees. It is sometimes relieved by sympathetic block, suggesting a peripheral origin.[2857]

phantom optic nerve An artifact on CT scanning, whereby an optic nerve that has been removed nevertheless appears to be present in horizontal sections of orbital scans.[5791]

phantom petit mal See **phantom spike and wave**.

phantom spike and wave (phantom petit mal, wave-and-spike phantom) Generalized, bilateral, brief bursts of low-voltage spike-and-wave discharges on the EEG which run at about 6 Hz, mainly in frontocentral regions (but occasionally seen posteriorly) and which are activated by diphenhydramine.[6628]

The appearance is rare, although it is more common in adult women and has been linked, with incomplete confidence, to various other EEG abnormalities and to the occurrence of clinical seizures, headaches, and some psychiatric disorders. The discharge is, however, probably physiological and no more than an electrophysiological curiosity.[4057] See **six-Hz spike-and-slow waves**.

phantom tics The extracorporeal projection of the premonitory sensations preceding motor tics in Tourette syndrome as a result of mental projection of sensory impression to other people, inanimate objects, or even nonexistent objects, partially relieved by touching those that do exist.[3309]

phantom vision The transient belief that visual sensations are present, received by an eye that is in fact absent.[1240]

pharmacological pupillary testing The use of drugs in low concentrations to assess the innervation of the pupils. Thus, 4% *cocaine* dilates the pupil so long as postganglionic sympathetic activity is intact; 0.1% *adrenaline* has no effect on a normal pupil but causes dilatation when there is postganglionic failure, due to denervation supersensitivity; 1% *hydroxyamphetamine* dilates a normal pupil by releasing norepinephrine, while its failure to do so signifies a lesion of the second or third neuron; and both 2.5% *methacholine* and 0.125% *pilocarpine* have no effect on a normal pupil but constrict one with pre- or postganglionic parasympathetic denervation, again due to supersensitivity. See **autonomic function tests**.

pharyngeal dystonia A rare, idiopathic dystonic syndrome presenting in adult life with dysphagia.[4099]

pharyngeal nystagmus See **ocular myoclonus**.

pharyngeal-cervical-brachial variant of acute inflammatory polyradiculoneuropathy See **acute inflammatory demyelinating polyneuropathy**.

pharyngisimus Spasm of the pharyngeal constrictor muscles. While this is usually a psychogenic problem (**globus hystericus**), it is also seen in **rabies** and as a result of local irritation. See also **cricopharyngeal spasm**.

phase 1. (In electromyography) That portion of a waveform that occurs between the departure from and the return to, the baseline. 2. The time or angular relationships between a point on a wave and the onset of the cycle of the same wave. This is usually expressed in degrees or radians. (Adapted from 1974 report of the Committee on Terminology, IFCN. In: Chatrian GE, Bergamini L, Dondey M, et al. A glossary of terms most commonly used by clinical electroencephalographers. *EEG Clin Neurophysiol* 1974;**37**:538–48. Reproduced by kind permission of the IFCN and of Elsevier Science.)

phase advance The movement of a subject's period of sleeping or waking to a position earlier in the 24-h cycle.

phase delay The movement of a subject's period of sleeping or waking to a position later in the 24-h cycle. See **delayed sleep phase syndrome**.

phase lag See **delayed sleep phase syndrome**.

phase reversal The opposite polarity of the spike discharge on each side of an electrically discharging lesion in the CNS. This site, where no spike at all is seen, is regarded as **equipotential**. See **true phase reversal, instrumental phase reversal**.

phase transition The two junctures of the major sleep and wake phases in the 24-h cycle.

phasic muscle strectch reflexes A brief burst of muscular activity evoked by a tap on its tendon, which both transmits a vibratory stimulus to the intrafusal fiber nerve endings and imparts a sudden stretch to them, eliciting a volley of impulses in the afferent fibers. These make monosynaptic connection with the anterior horn cells in the cord at that level in which there is an evoked efferent volley, causing reflex contraction of the muscle.

phasic reflexes Those reflexes which chiefly employ the limb flexor muscles and which give rise to phasic (or clonic) reflex movements. Their origin is at the spinal level (Sir Charles **Sherrington**). The hind-limb flexion response reflex is an example.

phase-shift disorders Conditions arising as a result of mismatch between the real time and the personal body-clock time, as after a journey across numerous time zones and in certain experimental situations.

phenobarbitone The first drug for the treatment of epilepsy possessing an acceptable therapeutic ratio, introduced by Alfred Hauptmann (1881–1948) in 1912.

phenylketonuria (Fölling syndrome, phenylpyruvic oligophrenia: OMIM 261600) A recessively inherited dysmetabolic syndrome due to lack of phenylalanine hydroxylase. As a result of this, the subject cannot oxidize phenylalanine to tyrosine. The gene responsible is mapped to chromosome 12q–24.1. Clinically, the condition typically manifests neonatal feeding problems, mild microcephaly, fair hair, hyperkinesia, and irritability; seizures, spasticity, aminoaciduria, and mental and developmental delay are evident by the end of the first year of life. The condition was described by **Fölling** in 1934. A recent complete review was by Pietz in 1998.[5024] *Variants* of the syndrome are as follows:

Dihydropteridine deficiency (PKU II), a rare condition characterized by high phenylalanine levels in which feeding disturbances from infancy lead rapidly to death.[5912] Seizures and both physical and mental retardation are notable. The gene responsible for the lack of dihydropteridine reductase maps to chromosome 4q16.1–p15.1.

Biopterin deficiency, a progressive degenerative disorder of infants characterized by rigid hypertonia and later hypotonia, Parkinsonism, myoclonus, seizures, and upper and lower motor neuron signs.[2231,3342]

Spinal muscular atrophy with phenylketonuria.

Progressive spastic paraparesis with dementia, a rare adult phenotype.[3322]

phenylpyruvic oligophrenia See **phenylketonuria**.

pheochromocytoma A benign tumor of the adrenal medulla secreting norepinephrine. It usually occurs in isolation but may also be a feature of **neurofibromatosis** and of the pluriglandular syndrome (**multiple endocrine neoplasia**). Intermittent discrete attacks of headache accompanied by sweating, palpitations, anxiety, and pallor are characteristic, occurring in association with an abrupt rise in blood pressure.

Philippson reflex See **crossed extensor reflex**.

Phillips thoracic dysplasia with retinal aplasia A congenital dysmorphic syndrome manifesting also optic atrophy; retinal aplasia with pigmentation and macular colobomas, leading to blindness; nystagmus; pectus carinatum; cleft palate; digital abnormalities; and mental and developmental delay.[5013]

phobic postural vertigo A form of psychogenic vertigo with dizziness and subjective disturbance of balance while standing or walking despite normal clinical balance tests such as Romberg, tandem walking, balancing on one foot, and routine posturography. Its clinical characteristics have been defined by Brandt[817] as follows:

1. Fluctuating unsteadiness in episodes lasting seconds to minutes or momentary

perceptions of illusory body perturbations.

2. Although the attacks can occur spontaneously, there is usually a perceptual stimulus (bridge, staircase, empty room, street) or social situation (department store, restaurant, concert, crowd) from which the patients have difficulty withdrawing and which they recognize as a provoking factor. There is a tendency for rapid conditioning, generalization, and avoidance behavior to develop.
3. Anxiety and distressing vegetative symptoms often occur during or after the vertigo. Most patients have attacks both with and without anxiety.
4. Obsessive-compulsive type personality, labile affect, and mild depression are common.
5. The onset of the condition frequently follows a period of particular emotional stress, a serious illness, or an organic vestibular disorder.

(Reproduced by kind permission of the American Academy of Neurology and Lippincott Williams and Wilkins.)

phonation (from Gr, the sound of the voice) The expression of sounds by the larynx.

phone The actual sound produced in speech.

phoneme The minimum distinctive sound feature into which any given flow of speech can be separated;[1330] a distinct sound unit recognized by speakers of a language, and the most elementary unit of speech, existing only as constituents of words.
A phoneme is a category of sounds which embraces all **phones** (since different people pronounce each different phoneme differently). There are 46 phonemes in the English language: 9 vowels and 37 consonants.[3949]

phonemic dyslexia See **deep dyslexia**.

phonemic errors Disturbances of speech consisting of substitutions of *words* (*literal paraphasias*) and/or *syllables* (*verbal* **paraphasias**).

phonetic errors Disturbances of speech affecting the formation and articulation of the words themselves; errors are thus **dysarthrias**.

phonetic palsy Aphonia due to disease affecting the X cranial nerve.

phonetics The science of spoken speech.

phonographie See **hypergraphia**.

phonological agraphia The condition resulting from damage to the **phonological system** in which patients cannot spell nonwords such as CHOSP but can spell those with which they are already familiar. The lesion is thought to be in the left precentral gyrus.[5753]

phonological dyslexia See **deep dyslexia**.

phonological memory One of two postulated passive auditory–verbal short-term memory storage systems concerned with the memorization and repetition of lists, as opposed to the other (lexical) system which is concerned with the comprehension of language.[4202]

phonological system One of two functional systems used by human beings for spelling. It employs sound-letter (phoneme) conversion rules, and is used when spelling unfamiliar words or pronounceable nonwords.

The other is the **lexical** system, which compares what is read or heard to a bank of previously acquired visual word-images of learned word spellings in order to achieve comprehension. Either can be damaged in isolation. Damage to the phonological system leads to an inability to spell nonwords, although the ability to spell known real words remains (**deep dyslexia**).

phonological–syntactical syndrome A mixed expressive-receptive disorder resembling Broca **aphasia** in which the speech is nonfluent, the articulation faulty, and the syntax simplistic.

phonology The speech sounds of a language and the rules followed by speakers when combining and pronouncing speech sounds.[3949]

phoria The normal tendency for a slight misalignment of the visual axes of the two eyes during monocular viewing. This is normally overcome by fusion mechanisms when the eyes are both viewing; thus, a phoria is a latent, not usually overt, deviation of the visual axes of the eyes. See **heterophorias**.

phosphatide A combination of phosphoglyceric acid with fatty acids and a base such as choline or ethanolamine.

phosphenes Positive visual sensations (light spots or patterns) perceived in the absence of visual (luminous) stimuli. They may occur in the presence of disease of the striate cortex or optic nerve and may be triggered by alerting stimuli.[4824, 4852] See also **movement phosphenes**.

phosphoethanolaminuria See **hypophosphatasia**.

phosphofructokinase deficiency (Tarui disease) A recessively inherited form of glycogen storage disease due to complete or partial deficiency of this enzyme, leading to complaints of fatigability, exertional muscle weakness, cramps, and pain and in some cases to hyperuricemia and hemolytic anemia.[3726] See **glycogen storage diseases**.

phosphoglucomutase deficiency See **glycogen storage disease**.

phosphoglycerate kinase deficiency An X-linked recessive disorder due to the presence of a phosphoglycerate kinase variants (*pgk New Jersey, PGK North Carolina*[6411]) that impair the second stage of the glycolytic process within muscle. This leads to the clinical complaints of weakness and exercise-induced muscle pain with myoglobinuria, as occur in **McArdle disease**, but with the added features of mental retardation and hemolytic anemia.[1647] See **glycogen storage disease** (type 9).

phosphoglycerate mutase deficiency A recessive syndrome with onset in youth, in which lack of the enzyme impairs the glycolytic process within muscle and leads to the clinical complaints of weakness and exercise-induced muscle pain with myoglobinuria as occur in **McArdle disease**.[1655] However, lactate production is maintained during aerobic exercise. See **glycogen storage diseases** type 10.

phosphohexoisomerase deficiency See **glycogen storage diseases**.

phosphorylase An enzyme with numerous isoenzymes, existing in both active and inactive forms. For its normal function in active form, adenyl cyclase, cyclic AMP, protein kinase, and phosphorylase kinase are necessary enzymes.

Myophosphorylase cleaves glucose from glycogen within muscles, thus allowing the use of glycogen as a source of energy. Its absence may be due to a condition inherited either as a dominant or as a recessive characteristic. See **glycogen storage diseases**.

phosphorylase b kinase deficiency A rare deficiency of an enzyme initiating glycogenolysis, leading to the clinical syndrome of weakness, exercise-induced muscle pain, and myoglobinuria in adults, and to weakness and hepatomegaly in children.[1202] See **glycogen storage disease**.

photic driving (photoentrainment) A physiological response recorded on the EEG, consisting of rhythmic activity elicited over the posterior regions of the head by repetitive photic stimulation at frequencies of about 5–30 Hz. It is suggested that the term should be limited to refer to activity time-locked to the stimulus and at a frequency identical to, or harmonically related to, the stimulus frequency. Photic driving should be held in contradistinction to the visual evoked potentials elicited by isolated flashes repeated at very low frequencies. (From the 1974 Report of the Committee on Terminology, IFCN. In: Chatrian GE, Bergamini L, Dondey M, et al. A glossary of terms most commonly used by clinical electroencephalographers. *EEG Clin Neurophysiol* 1974;**37**:538–48. Reproduced with permission from Elsevier Science.)

photic-induced seizures Seizures provoked by intermittent visual stimulation. See idiopathic photosensitive occipital lobe epilepsy, childhood absence epilepsy (CAE), juvenile-onset absence epilepsy, juvenile myoclonic epilepsy, Lafora body disease, myoclonus epilepsy with ragged red fibers (MERRF), epilepsy with myoclonic–astatic seizures, and epilepsy with GTCS on awakening.

photic reflex myoclonus A form of stimulus-sensitive myoclonus of cortical origin, manifest as myoclonic jerks elicited at a fixed latency by photic stimulation.[3289] See **myoclonus**.

photic sneeze reflex (Autosomal Dominant Compelling Helio-Ophthalmic Outburst syndrome [ACHOO], photosternutatory reflex)

Sneezing when a bright light is shone into the eyes; a normal reflex in infants, but seen in adults, too. It is likely to be dominantly inherited. Parasympathetic overactivity has been suggested as a mechanism,[1933] but the cause is not known.[6759]

The acronym is slightly forced but remains, in the author's opinion, the best of the last few decades.

photic stimulation Delivery of intermittent flashes of light to the eyes of a subject as an EEG activation procedure.

photisms Transient "positive" anomalies of vision consisting of simple but brightly colored spectral phenomena, often of a geometrical character, and occurring in the context of epilepsy and migraine.

photoconvulsive response A generalized paroxysmal EEG discharge, usually at 3 Hz, evoked by intermittent photic stimulation. See **photoparoxysmal response**.

photoelectric oculography Techniques for measuring the displacement of the ocular globe, using a light source directed upon the cornea and equipment responsive to the light reflected therefrom.

Horizontal rather than vertical ocular deviations are measured because of eyelid interference in recordings of the latter. See also **electrooculogram**. An infrared method is also available.[5]

photoentrainment See **photic driving**.

photogenic epilepsy A tendency to recurring seizures triggered only by exposure to a flickering light source.[379] See also **photosensitive epilepsies, photoparoxysmal response**.

photomotograph A photoelectric device for recording the speed of muscle contraction and relaxation, usually applied to the ankle jerk.[5785] It was most often employed in the assessment of hypothyroidism, in which condition slowness of relaxation (the "hung-up" reflex) is common, but it is not now in general clinical use.

photomyoclonic response (photomyoclonus) An anteriorly located EEG discharge accompanied by facial, periocular, and occasionally arm myoclonic jerks and time-locked to flashes of light during intermittent photic stimulation.[625] See **photomyogenic response**.

photomyoclonus See **photomyoclonic response**.

photomyoclonus, diabetes mellitus, nephropathy, and deafness A dominantly inherited syndrome characterized by these features and by dementia. This condition may be a lipidosis.[379]

photomyogenic response (photomyoclonic response, photomyologic response) A response to intermittent photic stimulation, characterized by brief, repetitive spikes derived from muscle over the anterior regions of the head. These often increase gradually in amplitude as stimuli are continued and cease promptly when the stimulus is withdrawn.[3740]

This response is associated frequently with flutter of the eyelids and vertical oscillations of the eyeballs and sometimes with discrete jerking mostly involving the musculature of the face and head. (Adapted from the 1974 Report of the Committee on Terminology, IFCN. In: Chatrian GE, Bergamini L, Dondey M, et al. A glossary of terms most commonly used by clinical electroencephalographers. *EEG Clin Neurophysiol* 1974;**37**:538–48. Reproduced with permission from Elsevier Science.)

photomyologic response See **photomyogenic response**.

photo-oculodynia Pain in the eye out of proportion to the stimulus of the light; an alternative term for **photophobia**.

photoparoxysmal response (photoconvulsive response) An abnormal response to intermittent photic stimulation characterized by spike-and-slow wave and polyspike-and-slow-wave complexes. (From Noachtar S, et al. A glossary of terms most commonly used by clinical electroencephalographers.[4686a] Reproduced by kind permission of the IFCN and Elsevier Science.) These are bilaterally synchronous, symmetrical, and generalized and may outlast the stimulus by a few seconds. They may be associated with impairment of consciousness and brisk jerks involving the musculature of the whole body, most prominently that of the upper extremities and head.

photophobia (Gr, light + dread) (photo-oculodynia) Pathological discomfort experienced as eye pain and excessive glare in light conditions which, by definition, are comfortable for others. Photophobia is evidence of inflammation or irritation of ocular structures including the optic nerve, but is also extremely common with migraine and related headaches.

photophthalmia (snow blindness, desert blindness, ultraviolet keratitis) The occurrence of photophobia, burning ocular pain, itching, lacrimation, blepharospasm, and blurred vision following ocular exposure to intense ultraviolet radiation.

photoplethysmography A method of detecting the volume of pulsation in the frontal and supraorbital arteries using an infrared photosensor placed over the area of skin they supply. Compression maneuvers of the facial, temporal, and carotid arteries can be used to increase the sensitivity of the test, which is otherwise not as accurate as more sophisticated methods; it is now rarely used.[4678]

photopsias Visual disturbances which accompany migraine attacks.

photoreceptor degeneration See **visual paraneoplastic syndrome**.

photosensitive epilepsies (visual sensitive epilepsies) Heterogeneous seizure disorders in which the convulsion is associated in time with photic (visual) stimulation. Abnormal EEG responses to light or pattern stimulation occur in up to 3% of the population, especially in youth, but this does not correlate with clinical photosensitivity. Females are more susceptible. Autosomal dominant (less often recessive) inheritance with probable linkage to 7q32 and 16p13 has been shown. The usual manifestations are myoclonic jerks, generalized seizures, and absences, alone or in combination. The resting EEG is usually normal but 20–30% of cases show eye closure-related paroxysms. Intermittent photic stimulation elicits abnormal photoparoxysmal responses that may be posterior (the mildest form) or generalized, which are highly associated with clinical photosensitivity.[4882]

Four types of photosensitive epilepsy are distinguished.[72, 72] (Chart P–12)

See also **juvenile myoclonic epilepsy, Dravet syndrome, Unverricht-Lundborg disease**, and other **progressive myoclonic epilepsies, photic-induced seizures**.

photosensitive epilepsy with spontaneous seizures See **photosensitive epilepsies**.

photosensitive myoclonic epilepsy A syndrome in which myoclonic absences, myoclonic jerks, and generalized clonic convulsions all occur.[1712]

photosensitivity Genetically determined precipitation of neurological phenomena (such as generalized seizures) by flashing light stimuli.[6845] See also **visual-sensitive seizures**.

Chart P–12. The Photosensitive Epilepsies

Eyelid myoclonia with absences: A syndrome characterized by upward jerking of the eyes and eyelids on eye closure in well-lit surroundings. Spike (or polyspike)-and-wave patterns are seen on the EEG with eye closure in the dark.[3177]

Photosensitive epilepsy with spontaneous seizures (**Jeavons syndrome**): A variant of the above, in which seizures also occur without such provocation.[3178]

Pure (idiopasthic) photosensitive epilepsy: The occurrence of seizures (usually of the generalized tonic–clonic variety) exclusively as a result of environmental flicker stimulation. *Television epilepsy* and *space-invaders epilepsy* are forms of this, in which the attacks are precipitated when the subject (usually an adolescent) sits too close to a television screen.[3178]

Self-induced photosensitive epilepsy: A syndrome of absence seizures or myoclonic epileptic attacks as a consequence of self-induced flicker stimulation, as accomplished by oscillating the hands with the fingers outstretched in the line of sight to a bright light-source.

photosternutatory reflex See **photic sneeze reflex**.

photostress test See **light stress test**.

phrenesis An ancient term for any affection capable of inducing delirium.

phrenic (from Gr, the seat of the mind; the diaphragm) The techniques for electrophysiological study of the phrenic nerves supplying the two sides of the diaphragm have been described.[1130]

phrenitis (Gr, the seat of the mind + Lat; inflammation) The term of Celsus and of Galen for what we know colloquially as madness. The term *phrenopathia* is synonymous. Both are defunct.

phrenology (cranioscopy) A system introduced by Franz **Gall**, an anatomist in the latter part of the eighteenth century, who postulated that the brain was the organ of mind, with its mental and moral faculties localized to various parts of the cortex. A deficiency or a surfeit of each faculty could be determined by palpating the bumps on the cranium, and maps were published showing the positions of the relevant area for each. As Clarke and Dewhurst[1193] remark, it is curious that the faculties are all represented by bumps, because deficiency in one of them should presumably have led to a depression. Neither the system of faculties nor the localizations of those which are acceptable to us today have stood the test of time.

The organs (faculties) that Gall identified as common to man and animals are listed in Chart P–13.

phthinodes (from Gr, to waste away + form) Tissue wasting.

physaliphorous cells (Gr, bubble + cary) (bubbly cells) Tumor cells found in **chordomas** which contain "bubbles" of nonstaining material.

physical ADL See **activities of daily living**.

Physical and Mental Impairment of Function Evaluation A 77-item scale providing a comprehensive behavioral assessment of institutionalized geriatric patients and allowing scores on 10 factors, including

Chart P–13. Gall's Organs ('Faculties')

1. Instinct for reproduction
2. Love of offspring
3. Friendship
4. Self-defence and courage
5. Carnivorous instinct, tendency to murder
6. Cunning, cleverness
7. Ownership, covetousness, tendency to steal
8. Pride, love of authority
9. Vanity, ambition, love of glory
10. Caution, forethought
11. Memory of things and facts
12. Sense of places and space
13. Memory and sense of people
14. Memory of words
15. Sense of language and speech
16. Sense of color
17. Sense of sound, music
18. Sense of numbers, mathematics
19. Sense of mechanics, architecture

Those occurring only in man he listed as:

20. Wisdom.
21. Sense of metaphysics.
22. Satire, witticism.
23. Poetical talent.
24. Kindness, compassion, morality.
25. Mimicry.
26. Religion.
27. Firmness of purpose, obstinacy or constancy.

self-care, dependency, confusion, anxiety, behavioral deterioration, withdrawal, paranoia, etc.[2643]

Physical Self-Maintenance Scale

An instrument on which an observer rates toileting, feeding, dressing, grooming, physical ambulation, and bathing on a 5-point scale. A 3-point scale is used when these functions are self-rated by the patient.[3721]

physiological hypnic myoclonus

Small-amplitude, irregular, and asynchronous twitches, mainly affecting the orofacial and the distal muscles during stage 1 non–rapid eye movement and during rapid eye movement sleep and relaxed wakefulness. Electrically, they may be composed of isolated simple potentials or of brief tonic discharges.[1507]

physiological myoclonus

See **myoclonus**.

physiological nystagmus

(end-point nystagmus, fatigue nystagmus) That form of nystagmus induced in normal subjects by rotation, caloric irrigation, or optokinetic stimuli, representing an automatic resetting of the position of the eyes to compensate for their normal reflex tendency to move in a direction contrary to, and during, bodily movement with the purpose of maintaining clear vision. This form of horizontal jerk nystagmus is commonly elicited by sustained lateral deviation of the eyes and lasts for 15–25 s. Some subtypes are as follows:

1. *Fatigue nystagmus*: A form of jerk nystagmus seen in both eyes symmetrically in normal subjects who maintain far-lateral deviations of the eyes. This tends to be of greater amplitude in the adducting eye.
2. Micro-oscillations of the eyes occurring during precise high-resolution eye movement recordings. See **ocular flutter**.
3. *End-point nystagmus*: A few lateral jerks of the eyes normally occurring on far-lateral gaze.
4. *Sustained end-point nystagmus*: Persistent lateral jerks of the eyes normally occurring on far-lateral gaze.[5]

Other varieties of physiological nystagmus listed under **vestibular nystagmus** are *positional alcohol*, *positioning*, *post-rotational*, and *pseudo-caloric* forms.

physiological tremor

A normal and usually asymptomatic small-amplitude oscillation of all body parts. When a limb is supported, cardioballistic thrust is the most important mechanism, combined with the mechanical resonance of that body part. During maintenance of a posture, the tremor depends on the initial firing rate of motor units, which is usually around 8 Hz. Such oscillations are made worse by fatigue, recent physical exercise, or increased adrenergic tone, as occurs with emotion or in hyperthyroidism. **Essential tremor** is an exaggerated form.

physiological vertigo

Those forms of vertigo induced by external stimulation of the normal vestibular, visual, or somatosensory systems. **Motion sickness, space sickness,** and **height, visual, somatosensory, auditory, head-extension,** and **bending-over vertigo** are examples.

physostigmine

An inhibitor of cholinesterase which can cross the blood–brain barrier, having no quaternary amine group.

phytanic acid

(3,7,11,15 tetramethylhexadecanoic acid) A fatty acid found in dairy products, meat, and fish oils that accumulates in Refsum disease (**hereditary motor and sensory neuropathy** type 4), **infantile Refsum disease, Zellweger disease,** neonatal **adrenoleukodystrophy,** and **rhizomelic chondrodysplasia punctata**.

phytanic acid storage disease

See **hereditary motor and sensory neuropathy, type 4**.

pia mater

(Lat, soft + mother; *mater* because of the ancient Arabian belief that the meninges gave rise to all the body's membranes.[5886]) The innermost and thinnest of the three membranes (meninges) covering the brain.

Pianist's cramp

An **overuse syndrome** or focal occupational/ task-specific **dystonia,** in which the performer's digits cease to obey his or her will and take up an extended position for a few seconds.

piblokto

(arctic hysteria) Screaming, removal of clothing, and wild running with succeeding amnesia, considered to be a dissociative state. The similarity to **amok** in the Malays is notable.[839]

pica

(Lat, a magpie) Depraved appetite; abnormal eating behavior in which the subject ingests objects which are not acceptable food substances.

Pick, Arnold

(1851–1924) Austrian-Czechoslovakian neuropathologist and psychiatrist. He was born in Moravia and studied in Iglau, Vienna, Berlin, and Prague, where he was eventually elected professor of psychiatry in 1886, retaining that position until his retirement in 1921. He published over 350 contributions to the medical literature, but is best known for his studies on early-life dementia (Pick disease; **fronto-temporal dementia**). His first patient seems to have been suffering from primary progressive aphasia but he reported no microscopic findings.

Pick was both the first to put **Wernicke**'s ideas of aphasia on a sound anatomicopathological basis and to demonstrate the origin of the fibers of the spinocerebellar tract in the axis-cylinder processes of the cells of Clarke's column. He also described various spinal cord abnormalities, established with Kohler the clinical picture of combined systemic disease, associated hemichorea and hemiathetosis with thalamic and lenticular lesions, and conducted important studies on apraxia and agrammatism.[5704]

Pick bodies Spherical neurofilamentous argyrophilic and eosinophilic intracytoplasmic inclusions, found in hippocampal neurons (**Pick cells**) in some cases of **Pick disease**.

Pick cells Swollen eosinophilic neuronal cell bodies with a peripherally displaced nucleus and argyrophilic inclusions, found in the neocortex, hippocampus, basal ganglia, and brainstem in **Pick disease**.

Pick complex disorder See **frontotemporal dementia**.

Pick disease (Pick lobar atrophy, Pick-complex disorder, lobar sclerosis, circumscribed cortical atrophy, dementia with lobar atrophy and neuronal cytoplasmic inclusions) See **frontotemporal dementia**.

Pick disease Internet websites of value are: www.picksdisease.org/Pick, www.bhoffcomp.com/coping/picks.html and www.pdsg.org.uk, the last a Pick disease support group.

Pick disease type 2 See **progressive subcortical gliosis**.

Pick disease without Pick bodies See **frontal lobe dementia**.

Pick lobar atrophy See **Pick disease**.

Pick sign Lid nystagmus induced by convergence movements of the eyes; an uncommon feature in some posterior fossa lesions.[1460]

Pick syndrome See **aphasia–agnosia–apraxia syndrome**.

Pick, Ludwig (1868–1944) German physician who graduated from Königsberg and later trained further in pathology in Berlin, where he was eventually elected professor of pathological anatomy. His paper, distinguishing what we know as **Niemann–Pick disease** from **Gaucher disease**, was published in 1927. He died in a concentration camp for Jews in 1944.

Pick cells Foam cells in the brain, named for Ludwig Pick.

Pickwickian syndrome Somnolence, periodic respiration, polycythemia, pulmonary hypertension, cor pulmonale, diminished respiratory drive in response to increases in pCO_2, and excessive appetite with obesity as complications of the obstructive sleep apnea syndrome. The somnolence can be traced to alveolar hypoventilation. The syndrome takes its name (applied by **Osler**) from Charles Dickens' character Joe, the fat boy in *The Pickwick Papers*.[955]

pico- (Gr; small) Prefix denoting small.

Pictorial test of Intelligence A cognitive test appropriate for children with severe motor and speech impairment.

picture arrangement A subtest on the **Wechsler Adult Intelligence scale** sensitive to disturbances of function of the right parietal lobe.

picture completion A subtest on the **Wechsler adult Intelligence scale** (revision) sensitive to parietal lobe disorders.

pied en griffe (Fr, claw foot) Weakness with atrophy of the intrinsic muscles of the foot leads to unopposed action of the long toe extensors, which causes dorsiflexion of the proximal phalanges while the long flexors shorten the foot and produce plantar flexion at the distal interphalangeal joints.

P-I-E-N-O Tremor Information Index A site carrying advertisements and offering articles on tremors for patients, caregivers, students, and professionals.

Piepkorn short rib-polydactyly syndrome A congenital dysmorphic syndrome manifesting also skeletal and visceral anomalies, brachydactyly and polydactyly, brachycephaly, craniosynostosis, delayed closure of fontanelles, and ossification defects of the skull.[381]

Pierre Robin syndrome A congenital syndrome of mental retardation, cleft palate, facial dysmorphism (notably a small receding chin causing glossoptosis), flattening of the nasal bridge, low-set ears, microphthalmos, congenital glaucoma, cataract, myopia, and a tendency to congenital heart disease.[5334]

Pierre Robin (1867–1950) was professor of dental surgery in Paris.

pierres de la peau See **Proficher syndrome**.

Pietrantoni syndrome The occurrence of **infraorbital neuralgia** and facial hypoesthesia as a complication of infiltrating nasopharyngeal tumors.[5023]

Pietrowski, A. (b. 1878) German neurologist.

Pietrowski sign See **anterior tibial sign**.

pigment variety of amaurotic idiocy A variety of **neuronal ceroid lipofuscinosis**, characterized by the onset in childhood of progressive mental and neurological deterioration with ubiquitous lipid infiltration of neurons and extracellular pigmentation of the globus pallidus and substantia nigra.[5713]

pigmentary retinal degeneration See **pigmentary retinopathy**.

pigmentary retinopathy (pigmentary retinal degeneration) A hereditary noninflammatory degenerative retinal dystrophy marked by gliosis and the deposition of melanin derived from the retinal pigmented epithelium within the walls of blood vessels in the neurosensory retina. Clinically, the condition is characterized by marked constriction of the visual fields with retention of some central vision, arteriolar narrowing, disk pallor, and frequently (but not invariably) pigmentary deposition in the retina.

Central and *sectorial* types are described, as is another *variant* in which the same changes occur without any pigment deposition (*retinitis pigmentosa sine pigmento*). In a further *variant* form, only certain sectors of the retina are affected.

See also **cone dystrophy, retinitis pigmentosa**.

pili torti Kinky hair. When combined with deafness this is known as *Björnstadt syndrome*.[664] Otherwise, see **Menkes syndrome**.

pill-rolling tremor See **resting tremor**. This is a classic error in terminology, because early pharmacists did not make pills by rolling the ingredients between their fingers and thumbs but between two flat wooden boards, much as in the same way as butter balls are fashioned still in expensive restaurants. The term was used neither by **Parkinson** nor by **Gowers** but appeared in the early part of this century.[2185]

pilocarpine test Instillation of a drop of 0.1% pilocarpine into the conjunctival sac of the normal eye has no effect; constriction of the pupil within 15 min, lasting for up to 2 h, suggests the presence of denervation hypersensitivity resulting from a lesion of the parasympathetic supply to the iris, as with the **Adie pupil**.

See also **methacholine test, pharmacological pupillary testing**.

pilocytic astrocytoma See **astrocytoma**.

pilomotor seizure A rare manifestation of partial seizures in which paroxysmal piloerection ("gooseflesh") occurs following an **epigastric aura**, without alteration in consciousness.[863] A right hemisphere lesion has been responsible in the few cases reported.[2558]

pilomyxoid astrocytoma (PA) A type of brain tumor formerly grouped with pilocytic astrocytoma; a slow-growing and benign tumor now shown to demonstrate unique histological features that allow its differentiation. It tends to behave aggressively and carries a poor prognosis, with significantly shorter survival than typical PA, as well as a high rate of metastasis throughout the nervous system.

Pilotto syndrome A congenital dysmorphic syndrome manifesting also short stature, scoliosis, fusion of vertebrae, hemivertebrae, patent ductus arteriosus, brachycephaly, microcephaly, and pyramidal signs.[381]

Piltz, Jan (1870–1931) Polish neurologist who studied in Switzerland and Russia and, after graduation, studied psychiatry and neurology at the **Salpêtrière** and in Zurich. He concluded his career as professor of neurology and psychiatry at Krakow.

Piltz reflex 1. The consensual light reflex. 2. Constriction of the pupil when a person's attention is drawn to an object, not necessarily requiring ocular convergence.[5029]

pincer grasp Use of the thumb and forefinger to grasp a small object. This skill is normally present by 7–10 months of age, and persists.

pinch sign When the patient is asked to make a hollow square by putting the tip of the index finger onto the tip of the thumb, he or she cannot do so because of weakness of the long flexors of the finger and of the thumb, and makes a triangle instead. The sign is typically positive in the **anterior interosseous nerve syndrome**. See also **Froment sign**.

pinch-press test A test of the sense of passive movement of the skin in which the examiner variously pinches or presses upon the skin and the patient reports which sensation is felt.[1500]

pincushion effect A distortion of vision caused by the wearing of **Freznel glasses**.

pineal (from Lat, a pine-cone) Resembling a pine-cone.

pineal apoplexy An acute hemorrhagic upper brainstem lesion in the pretectal region.[227]

pineal cyst A cyst containing fluid with the density of CSF, located within the pineal gland, regarded as a normal variant when detected on MRI scanning.[1623]

pineal gland A dorsal midline outgrowth of the diencephalon. In lower vertebrates it was light sensitive; its function in man is still not understood, although it may have a role in modifying skin pigmentation through the production of melanotropin. Descartes proposed it as the seat of the soul, in which resided the imagination.

The tendency of the gland to calcify relatively early in life was useful as a sign of midline shift before the advent of echoencephalography, a test which itself is redundant since the development of CT and MRI scanning.

pineal shift A radiological sign, indicating shift of the hemispheres across the midline, thus pushing the (calcified) pineal gland with them. It was first described by Arthur Schüller.

pinealoblastoma A malignant, invasive **primitive neuroectodermal tumor** resembling the **medulloblastoma** histologically as well as in its aggressive local and metastatic spread.

pinealocytoma A rare tumor arising in the pineal gland in young adult life and composed of small cells arranged in ribbons or lobules, often with argyrophilic and eosinophilic polar cytoplasmic processes.[6]

pinealoma Any tumor of the pineal gland.

Pinel, Philippe (1755–1826) French psychiatrist at the Bicêtre and later at the **Salpêtrière**, who established new standards for the humane care of the mentally ill and who made the first systematic attempt to classify mental illness. He wrote repeatedly that he owed most of his experiences and insights into the dynamics of insanity to the French Revolution, which showed him the tremendous wealth of reactions that the human may show under the stress of exceptional situations. Initially, however, he had taken to psychiatry after a friend lost his reason and ran into the woods, where he was eaten by wolves.[2066, 5035]

ping-pong ball depression A small depressed skull fracture resulting from compression by forceps or with molding during delivery.

ping-pong gaze (short-cycle periodic alternating gaze deviation) A disorder of ocular movement consisting of rhythmic and pendular conjugate horizontal deviations of the eyes which alternate from one extreme of gaze to the other every 3–8 s. This is usually noted in patients in coma due to structural cerebral damage, drug toxicity, or other causes of metabolic encephalopathy.[5726] See **periodic alternating gaze**.

pinhole test A simple method of correcting for, and in doing so, diagnosing the presence of refractive errors. The subject reads from a test card, first without and then with a cover pierced by a small hole placed in front of the pupil; an improvement in acuity suggests the presence of a refractive error, because the focal length of a lens system is increased as its aperture is diminished, and the elimination of light coming in from an angle with retention of that coming straight (and thus subject to little or no refraction anyway) allows more precise focusing on the macula. Subjects with macular disease will see nothing at all through the pinhole.

The test was devised by Christoph Scheiner (1575–1650), a German physicist, in 1619.[5619]

pink disease (acrodynia, Feer disease, mercuric encephalopathy) A syndrome of scaly erythema of the skin with coldness and redness of the cheeks and extremities, perspiration, alopecia, insomnia, irritability, convulsions, peripheral sensorimotor neuropathy, tachycardia, stomatitis, pruritus, tremor, hypotonia, a flexed posture, and photophobia, resulting from mercury encephaloneuropathy in infants. The cause was chronic mercury poisoning, coming from the calomel in teething powder which loving parents placed on the gums of their physiologically unwell babies.[4929] The condition was described by Dr. E. Feer (1864–1911), a Swiss pediatrician, but he did not recognize its etiology.[2066]

pinky finger sign Reflex movements of the fifth finger that are elicited when the subject extends and abducts the fingers of one hand, after which the 2nd, 3rd, and 4th fingers are flexed at the metacarpophalangeal (MCP) joints against the examiner's resistance. Normal subjects and patients with a pyramidal lesion affecting the limb hyperextend the fifth finger at the MCP joint while patients with pseudodementia (depression), psychogenic hemiparesis, and whiplash-induced upper limb monoparesis flex the fifth finger at the MCP joint during resisted finger flexion.[4758]

Pinocchio syndrome A rare form of reflex epilepsy in which partial seizures are triggered by the enunciation of terminological inexactitudes.

pinpoint pupils The term for pupils which are each about 1 mm in diameter but still react to light. Such extreme pupillary constriction occurs with morphine poisoning and with complete loss of sympathetic innervation of the pupil, as with pontine lesions.

pinwheel photopsias Visual hallucinations resembling fireworks, occurring in patients with irritative temporal lobe lesions.[1219]

Piotrowski sign (antagonistic anterior tibial reflex) Percussion of the tibialis anterior muscle leads to plantar flexion of the toes in the presence of pyramidal lesions, presumably as a result of vibrations transmitted to the gastrocnemius muscle. This response was described by Piotrowski in 1912. See also **anterior tibial sign**.

A variant stimulus is percussion of the external malleolus, described by Balduzzi in 1925. The (slight) utility of both signs has been reviewed.[5499]

pipecolic acidemia See **hyperpipecolic acidemia**.

pipestem capillaries Thickening of the capillaries in muscles affected by necrotizing myopathy complicating underlying carcinoma or arteritis.[1856]

piriformis syndrome (Lat, a pear + shape) (wallet neuritis, hip pocket neuropathy) 1. A sciatica-like syndrome considered to be due to periarthritis involving the anterior sacroiliac ligament, the piriformis muscle, and the adjacent sciatic nerve.[6912, 2196, 5337] The buttock pain radiates down the thigh and lower leg and is thought to be caused by compression of the sciatic nerve at the pelvic outlet by the piriformis muscle. The pain is exacerbated by prolonged sitting (as while driving or cycling) or during activity that requires hip adduction and internal rotation but is relieved with standing or walking. The pain is usually accompanied by point tenderness in the buttock near the sciatic notch. Paresthesias in the buttock and/or in a patchy sciatic nerve distribution may occur. Dyspareunia in women and pain with bowel movements are other common symptoms. There are no localizing physical signs, but patients may walk with the affected leg externally rotated and there may be piriformis tenderness on rectal or pelvic examination. Slight wasting of the gluteus maximus due to entrapment of the superior gluteal nerve is occasionally noted. Back pain and objective weakness are not features.[2113, 6511]

The similarity of symptoms to those of lumbar radiculopathy, including a positive **Lasègue** sign, can lead to misdiagnosis and ineffective lumbar surgery. Correct anatomic localization is indicated by the consistent occurrence of sciatic notch tenderness. The **Freiberg** and **Pace** signs may also be present.[4918] (HJM)

Nerve conduction studies and needle EMG are usually normal; but H-reflex prolongation by flexion, adduction, and internal rotation (**FAIR test**) beyond 1.86 ms (3 SD) of the mean is reported as of diagnostic value. In the occasional case with true denervation the findings are those of a mild axonal sciatic mononeuropathy at the level of the sciatic notch, with or without an inferior gluteal mononeuropathy.[2111] In such cases there may be a fibrous band or aberrant artery compressing the sciatic nerve in the region of the piriformis muscle. The validity of the syndrome is considered to be controversial by those who have not experienced it themselves. (Moore HJ. Personal communication, 2002; Yuen.[6937]) See also **Trendelenburg sign**.

2. A myofascial pain syndrome manifested by external rotation of the leg and some response to local anesthetic injection into the piriformis muscle. The buttock pain may be referred to the thigh and there is exquisite point tenderness over the sciatic notch elicited externally and on rectal or pelvic examination, with or without back pain.[3579] The pain is maximal during prolonged sitting (such as while driving or cycling), bending at the waist, or activity that require hip adduction and internal rotation such as cross-country skiing. The Trendelenberg test is positive. Weakness, reflex changes, and definitive sensory loss are absent. Rotation or abduction of the hip joint causes pain (but this is not specific for this condition). Lumbar MRI does not show disc disease.

Although the first of these two definitions is thought to reflect neuropathy and the second "myofascial pain," the distinction between the two is at best blurred. The inordinate space here accorded to the entity reflects its frequency of occurrence rather than of diagnosis.

Pisa syndrome (pleurothotonos) An axial dystonia first described by Ekbom in 1972 and usually seen as a side effect of neuroleptic drugs or due to anticholinergic medications in patients with **Alzheimer disease, Parkinson disease,** or **multiple system atrophy**. It is characterized by truncal rotation and lateral flexion, unaccompanied by other dystonic signs. The name reflects the leaning position of the subject.[6906, 3754]

pisohamate tunnel syndrome See **ulnar nerve palsies**.

pitcher's arm An electrodiagnostic anomaly probabably representing the result of repetitive strain to the brachial plexus of professional baseball pitchers, characterized by a reduction in the amplitude of sensory nerve action potentials in the throwing arm. There appears to be no deficit in performance as a result, however.[3908]

pithiatism (from Gr, suggestion + curable) The term coined by **Babinski** for diseases which are curable by persuasion; it was used by **Charcot** to replace the word **hysteria**, but it failed to do so.

Pitres, Albert (1848–1928) French neurologist and histologist, professor of medicine at Bordeaux, who trained with **Charcot** and Ranvier and whose major works concerned cortical localization and aphasia. His book on neuroanatomy and physiology with Testut, "*Les nerfs en schemas*" (Paris, 1925), was quickly regarded as a classic.

Pitres sign Loss of deep pain sensation, assessed by the response to squeezing of the testicles. The sign was described in patients with **tabes dorsalis**, some of whom benefited financially as a result of winning bets on their capacity to tolerate such insults.

Pitres' law (1895) The language that the patient used most before onset of aphasia will be recovered best. The rule has not been validated.

Pitt syndrome A recessively inherited congenital dysmorphic syndrome manifesting also short stature, respiratory difficulties, clubbing of the fingers, abnormal skin creases, pes cavus, seizures, microcephaly, and mental and developmental delay.[5038]

Pitt–Hopkins syndrome See **cerebellar syndromes** (congenital ataxias).

Pittsburgh Brain Stem Score A scale that can be used in a comatose patient to assess brainstem reflexes such as the eyelash, corneal, and doll's eye responses, ice water calorics, R and L pupil reactions to light, and the gag and/or cough reflexes.[5667]

pituitary (from Lat, phlegm [mucous secretion], one of the humors) The pituitary gland was first described in 1524 by Berengarius, and was thought by Vesalius to secrete mucus into the nose, an opinion held until the seventeenth century.[5886]

pituitary adenomas Circumscribed benign tumors arising from cells within the pituitary gland and in many cases extending upward or eroding laterally, and thus causing clinical effects by compression. Secreting and nonsecreting forms are defined. The former usually secrete prolactin; less commonly they secrete growth hormone, FSH and LH.

http://www.ninds.nih.gov/disorders/pituitary_tumors/pituitary_tumors.htm is an informational Web site from the NIH.

pituitary apoplexy A rare, life-threatening syndrome resulting from acute infarction of the pituitary gland, usually in the presence of an adenoma or as a component of **Sheehan syndrome**.

The clinical manifestations include a history suggesting dyspituitarism; severe retro-orbital headache (see below) with meningism; ocular palsies; rapidly advancing visual impairment, especially bitemporal field loss; altered consciousness; and involvement of the first division of the trigeminal nerve. Vasospasm or compression of the internal carotid may lead on to seizures or focal deficits. However, the condition may also occur silently after asymptomatic hemorrhage into a pituitary adenoma. Surviving patients show evidence of pituitary failure with loss of lactation, amenorrhea, lethargy, and sometimes diabetes insipidus. The syndrome and its many predisposing causes have been reviewed.[5242]

The IHS-ICHD[2820] describes the associated headache as severe, acute, retro-orbital, frontal, or diffuse, accompanied by at least one of the following: nausea and vomiting, fever, diminished level of consciousness, hypopituitarism, hypotension, and ophthalmoplegia or impaired visual acuity, with neuroimaging evidence of acute hemorrhagic pituitary infarction and resolving within a month.

pituitary gigantism (Launois syndrome, Maurois syndrome, Marie syndrome)

Increased growth due to excessive production of growth hormone by a pituitary adenoma prior to closure of the epiphyses, first described by Launois in 1904, but described in greater detail by the other authors whose names are variously attached to the syndrome.

Pituitary Network Association An international nonprofit organization for patients with pituitary tumors and disorders and those who treat them.

The Pituitary Society An organization of basic scientists and clinicians dedicated to furthering the understanding of diseases of the pituitary gland.

pituitary tumor without acromegly but with genital arrest See **Frölich syndrome**.

placing reaction When the normal infant is lifted up and the dorsum of the foot brought into contact with the underside of, for example, a table top, the infant's leg flexes at the hip and knee so that the foot is lifted and placed on the upper surface of the table.[4001] The sign is present after the 34th week of gestation and disappears at 2 months of age.

plagiocephaly (from Gr, sideways + the head) (wry head) 1. A craniofacial malformation resulting from asymmetrical premature fusion of a coronal or lambdoid suture on one side, causing the skull to have its longest axis on the diagonal.[4] There is, thus, abnormal flattening of one side of the head (and compensatory bulging of the other side) with flattening of the forehead on the affected side and elevation of the orbit and distortion of the root of the nose. Radiologically, the orbits are obviously asymmetrical, the affected orbit being triangular in its upper and outer part, producing a "devil's eye" or "harlequin" appearance. 2. Also given this name is the persistent deviation of the head to one side in infancy, due to the posture assumed by a child lying supine for most of the day.

planotopokinesia The term suggested in 1922 by Pierre **Marie** for **visuospatial agnosia**.

plantar grasp reflex (Lat, sole of the foot) Stroking of the palmar surface of the foot causes flexion of the toes.[6898] The sign is present from birth until 2 months of age. See also **grasp reflex of the foot, developmental reflexes**.

plantar muscle reflex (Rossolimo reflex) Extension of the hallux when the sole is tapped with a reflex hammer, a toe is flicked upward, or the plantar surfaces of a number of toes are percussed with the ankle dorsiflexed.

This is a muscle stretch reflex, the counterpart of the **finger flexion reflex** in the arm and not a true variant of the **Babinski response**. Tapping on the heel may also elicit toe flexion as the result of vibration transmitted to the plantar muscles.

plantar neuroma See **Morton metatarsalgia**.

plantar reflex (plantar response) See **Babinski signs**.

plantar response See **Babinski signs**.

planum temporale The isthmus of the temporal lobe—the region on the superior surface of the temporal lobe between Wernicke's language area and Heschl's gyrus.

plaques 1. (in **multiple sclerosis**) Zones of demyelination within the white matter of the CNS, most common in the periventricular and periaqueductal regions, the optic nerve and the spinal cord.

Histologically, acutely formed plaques are characterized by the presence of intact axons, myelin breakdown products within foamy macrophages, a proliferation of hypertrophic reactive astrocytes, local and circumferential round cell infiltration, and perivascular cuffing; as well as by a paucity of oligodendrocytes. Chronic "burnt-out" plaques are circumscribed regions within the white matter which lack myelin but show intense gliosis without inflammatory cells.

2. (in **Alzheimer disease**) Various forms are defined:

Classic plaques (senile, amyloid, or discrete plaques) are areas close to the capillaries in the neuropil, consisting of a densely stained core of amyloid surrounded by argentophilic rods and granules derived from dystrophic neuronal processes.

Primitive plaques (amorphous or neuritic plaques) are small clusters of distended neurites without a discrete central core. See **neuritic plaques**.

Burnt-out plaques (compact plaques) are amyloid deposits in the neuropil without other distinguishing features.

Diffuse plaques comprise a network of fibrillar or granular material without amyloid content.[90]

3. See **perivascular plaques**.

plasma exchange See **plasmapheresis**.

plasmapheresis (Gr, form + removal) (plasma exchange) The mechanical separation of certain protein fractions of plasma from whole blood by centrifugation, followed by the replacement of the blood without such elements but with the addition of volume expanders. The procedure is established as beneficial in **myasthenia gravis**, presumably due to the removal of anti-acetylcholine receptor antibodies; in **acute inflammatory demyelinating polyneuropathy** and in some **gammopathic neuropathies**. Its value in the treatment of **Lambert–Eaton myasthenic syndrome, amyotrophic lateral sclerosis, multiple sclerosis, polymyositis, Fabry disease,** and other conditions has remained under study since at least 1984.[1467]

plasticity Alterations in structure and function at synapses as a result of sustained inputs, leading to long-term potentiation that fulfills many of the criteria for a neural correlate of memory. This process is virtually the same as sensitization. Thus, as peripheral nociceptors are sensitized during inflammation, peripheral nerve fibers begin to discharge ectopically, evoking a complex neuronal response in the spinal cord where neurons in the substantia nigra also become hyperexcitable and a new balance is set between their excitation and inhibition. The spinal processes are normally influenced by brainstem circuits that inhibit or facilitate nociceptive processing but such modulation may be insufficient to prevent pain perception in the face of the long-term potentiation/sensitization referred to above.[1274, 5579]

plateau waves See **intracranial pressure waves**.

platelet-activating factor An endogenous phospholipid with a role in the mediation of many physiological reactions, including vasoconstriction and hemostasis. In the brain, where it is released after injury, it may act directly or through other mediators to cause vasospasm, disruption of the blood–brain barrier, and cerebral edema.[3857]

platy- (Gr, flat). Prefix denoting flatness.

platybasia An increase in the breadth (obtuseness) of the basal angle of the skull (the angle made by the intersection of the plane of the sphenoid with the plane of the clivus) to more than 150°. The term is attributed to **Virchow** and has been used by anthropologists interested in craniometry for over 100 years. It is not the same thing as **basilar impression**.[5980]

platycephaly (Gr, flat + the head) An abnormal skull shape in which the vertical height of the skull is reduced.

platysma phenomenon (signe de Peaucier) Failure of the platysma muscle on the side of a hemiparesis to contract when a subject opens his mouth widely against resistance.

PLEDs See **periodic lateralized epileptiform discharges**.

pleoconial myopathy A familial muscular disorder presenting with slowly progressive weakness, attacks of flaccid paralysis, and a craving for salt from infancy. The characteristic pathological feature is an excess of mitochondria and morphological inclusions within such organelles.[5822]

pleocytosis A pathological overabundance of cells.

pleomorphic xanthoastrocytoma See **astrocytoma**.

pleonosteosis A dominantly inherited diffuse encephalopathy characterized by abnormal unusually early ossification of the epiphyses, with dwarfism, broad digits, flexion contractures, a mongoloid facial appearance, and mental retardation. See **Leri syndrome**.

pleurodynia (Gr, side + pain) (Devil's grippe, epidemic myalgia, Bornholm disease) A syndrome of chest wall and often other myalgic pain (the former made much worse by deep breathing) and fever, without the clinical or radiological features of pleurisy. Infection with the Coxsackie B virus is the usual cause.

pleurothotonos An unusual form of axial dystonia, the muscular spasm leading to lateral flexion of the trunk. See **Pisa syndrome**.

plexiform neuroma Peripheral neural tumors which resemble Schwannomas and which appear in childhood and adolescence, increasing in size and number during pregnancy and with aging.

plexiform sarcoma See **cylindroma**.

plexitis Inflammation of the brachial or lumbosacral plexuses.

plexopathy Any disease of the brachial or, less commonly, of the lumbosacral plexus. *Neoplastic plexopathies* affect mainly the lower brachial plexus, causing pain in the shoulder girdle and medial aspect of the forearm and hand and often a **Horner syndrome**. Arm lymphedema is uncommon. See also **Pancoast syndrome**. **Lumbosacral plexopathy** is most often due to diabetes, vasculitis, or direct extension of a tumor of the colon or cervix, and presents mainly with pain and sensory and motor findings according to the level of the plexus infiltrated. Sphincter disturbance is uncommon. See also **radiation plexopathy**.

plexus (from Lat, a braid or weaving; to intertwine) The complex rearrangements of the nerve roots into peripheral nerves. The term is also applied to networks of blood vessels.

Plicz sign Tight eye closure leads to constriction followed by dilation of the pupils. Presumably this is determined by infrared photography.

PLO-SL See **polycystic lipomembranous osteodysplasia with sclerosing leukoencephalopathy**.

Plott laryngeal abductor paralysis–retardation syndrome A congenital syndrome of optic atrophy, facial weakness, stridor, tracheolaryngeal anomalies, and mental and developmental delay.[381]

plumbism (Lat, lead) Lead poisoning. See **Remak paralysis**.

Plummer–Vinson syndrome See **sideropenic dysphagia**.

pluridefi ciency malnutrition syndrome See **kwashiorkor**.

plus-minus lid syndrome Unilateral ptosis with contralateral retraction of the eyelid, due to a small lesion in the paramedian mesencephalon causing damage to the III cranial nerve nucleus involving the ipsilateral levator palpebrae fascicles as they emerge from the central caudal nucleus. Overactivation of the contralateral levator palpebrae muscle accompanies this due to a failure of inhibition.[2321]

PNET See **primitive neuroectodermal tumors**.

pneumatic nystagmus See **vestibular nystagmus**.

pneumatic tourniquet paralysis See **tourniquet paralysis**.

pneumocele The presence of air within the cranium, usually as the result of trauma.

pneumocephalus (cranial aerocele) Gas (usually air) within the head, resulting from skull fractures, infection, tumor, or surgical trauma.[1401]

pneumococcal meningitis Neurological infection by *S. pneumoniae*, causing not only meningitis but potentially also cerebral vasculitis with intracranial hemorrhage, cerebral edema, cerebral necrosis, hydrocephalus, and myelitis. Disseminated intravascular coagulation is a further acute complication, while hearing loss is a common residuum in adults and in children.[1485]

The condition mainly occurs in adults with chronic debilitating conditions such as chronic alcoholism, malignancies, chronic immunosuppressive therapy, or poorly controlled diabetes mellitus; patients with asplenia; and previously healthy adults with acute infections such as otitis, sinusitis, pneumonia, or endocarditis.

pneumoencephalocele A gas-containing cyst within the brain.

pneumoencephalography The introduction of air into the lumbar subarachnoid space in order to visualize radiographically the basal cisterns and ventricular system which are outlined by the air after it has ascended through the CSF. The test, introduced in 1919, was pitifully unpleasant for most patients though diagnostically valuable in its day.[1440] Fortunately, that day has passed.

pneumogastric nerve The **vagus nerve**.

pneumorrachis The presence of intraspinal air, which may occur after prolonged and violent coughing.

pneumotaxic and apneustic centers Cell collections within the pons responsible for the synchronization and modulation of respiratory effort.

pNN50 A parameter that indicates the proportion of differences in consecutive normal-to-normal R-R intervals on the EKG longer than 50 ms. It calculates the percentage of such intervals in comparison to the total number of analyzed intervals and reflects parasympathetic activity.[2906]

pocket sign The ability of patients with pseudokyphosis (due to severe weakness of the thoracic muscles) to attain spinal extension by bracing their extended arms against their upper thighs.[6849]

Why this term was chosen remains a mystery to this author.

POEMS (Polyneuropathy, Organomegaly, Endocrinopathy, Monoclonal gammopathy, and Skin changes; PEP syndrome, Crow–Fukase syndrome, Tatasuki syndrome, osteosclerotic myeloma) A rare, dominantly inherited plasma cell dyscrasia of adult life manifesting recurrent episodes of flaccid weakness and areflexia due to partial depolarization of the muscle fiber membrane in the context of symmetric demyelinating sensorimotor polyneuropathy, sparing the cranial nerves but progressing centrally from its initial distal location. Hepatosplenomegaly and lymphadenopathy are found; hypogonadism, hypoadrenalism, hypothyroidism, and diabetes are the main endocrine features, and hypercalcemia is present in those cases in which the condition complicates osteosclerotic myeloma. The skin is thickened and hyperpigmented, with hirsutism and angiomas. The associated neoplasm is more often an osteosclerotic than an osteolytic myeloma, and it can sometimes cause myelopathy. The associated dysproteinemia is sometimes polyclonal (IgG, IgA).

Suggested minimal criteria to establish the diagnosis are the presence of a demyelinating and axonal polyneuropathy associated with an IgA or IgG monoclonal gammopathy, the light chain being almost always lambda, and at least two of the eight other features: sclerosing plasmocytoma, endocrinopathy, skin changes, organomegaly, Castleman disease, anasarca, papillary edema, or thrombocytosis.[3644]

Intracranial hypertension with papilledema, infiltrative orbitopathy, peripheral edema, pleuritis, and bone lesions may also accompany the findings indicated by the acronym.[392] The condition has been reported mainly from the Orient. The Mayo Clinic Web site http://www.mayoclinic.org/poems/ provides further infomration.

poikiloderma congenitale (Rothmund–Thompson syndrome) A recessively inherited diffuse encephalopathy manifesting mental retardation, juvenile cataract, small genitalia, short stature, macrocephaly, abnormal hands and feet, atrophy and pigmentation of the skin with photosensitivity, and later hyperkeratosis.[6306]

point apophysiaire A tender spot overlying the spinous process of a vertebra corresponding (roughly) to the level of irritation of a nerve root, described by **Trousseau**. See also **cellulalgia**.

pointe-onde (Fr, spike and wave).

pointing test See **Barany test**.

Poisoned Food Problem task (of Arenberg) A test measuring problem-solving skills.

Poland anomaly See **Poland syndrome**.

Poland syndrome (Poland anomaly) Congenital unilateral absence of part of the sternomastoid or of one or both pectoral muscles, usually with scoliosis, syndactyly, and hypoplasia of the ipsilateral arm and hand, occurring sporadically but perhaps dominantly inherited in some cases. Other shoulder muscles may also be aplastic and ipsilateral syndactyly and short fingers are often noted. Other associated signs include absence of some digits, herniation of the lung, and absence or hypoplasia of the breast.[1478]

The condition was described in 1841 by Alfred Poland of Guy's Hospital.[5063] See also **muscle aplasia, Souques syndrome**.

In *variant* forms, the features of **Möbius syndrome** are also found[2990] or other craniofacial anomalies including ptosis; skeletal anomalies such as scoliosis, hemivertebrae, and the **Klippel–Feil** syndrome; and systemic anomalies of the urogenital and gastrointestinal tracts and the heart are also described, as are neoplasms including leukemia and lymphoma.

polar spongioblastoma A **primitive neuroectodermal tumor** which resembles an astrocytoma, but differentiates along the lines of neuroglia. It tends to occur in early life, arising close to the ventricles and spreading through CSF pathways.

polarization In clinical neurophysiology, the presence of an electrical potential difference across an excitable cell membrane. The potential across the membrane of a cell when it is not excited by an input or spontaneously active is termed the *resting potential*; it is at a stationary nonequilibrium state with regard to the electrical potential difference across the membrane. *Depolarization* describes a reduction in the magnitude of the polarization toward the zero potential. *Hyperpolarization* refers to an increase in the magnitude of the polarization relative to the resting potential. *Repolarization* describes an increase in polarization from the depolarized state toward, but not above, the normal resting potential. (From the 1987 Report of the Nomenclature Committee of the American Association of Electrodiagnostic Medicine. AAEE glossary of terms in clinical electromyography. *Muscle Nerve* 1987;10S:G5–G23. Reproduced by kind permission of the AANEM.)

POLG mutations The clinical spectrum of recessive POLG mutations is expanded by sensory ataxic neuropathy, combined with variable features of involvement of CNS and other organs. Progressive external ophthalmoplegia, myopathy, ragged red fibers, and Southern blot abnormalities of muscle mitochondrial DNA also are not mandatory features associated with POLG mutations.[6498] See also **ataxia with OLG mutations**.

policeman's tip See **porter's tip position**.

polio- (Gr, gray—hence gray matter).

Polio Connection of America A charitable organization in this field. Address: P.O. Box 182, Howard Beach, NY 11414. Tel: 718-835-5536. E-mail: w1066polio@hotmail.com. Web site: http://www.geocities.com/w1066w/.

Polio Survivors Association A charitable organization providing support and information on this condition. Address: 12720 La Reina Ave., Downey, CA 90242. Tel: 310-862-4508.Web site: http://www.polioassociation.org/.

polioencephalitis (from Gr, gray + brain + inflammation) Inflammation of the gray matter of the brain.

polioencephalitis hemorrhagica superior See **Wernicke–Korsakoff encephalopathy**.

polioencephalomyelopathy See **Creutzfeldt–Jakob disease**.

poliomyelitis (from Gr, gray + marrow + inflammation) (Heine–Medin disease, acute anterior poliomyelitis, infantile paralysis, morning paralysis) An acute systemic viral illness caused by the polio picornavirus types 1, 2, or 3, usually spread by the fecal–oral route. The gene responsible for susceptibility to poliomyelitis maps to chromosome 19q12–13.2.

Clinically, it only sometimes affects (but then often devastates) the nervous system. The greatest effects of the disease are on the anterior horn cells or cranial nerve motor nuclei in the gray matter of the spinal cord or brainstem, respectively. Most commonly a febrile *minor illness* occurs without progression to neurological involvement; but, in some 2% of the cases, this is followed by a *major illness*, characterized by features of **aseptic meningitis**, which in some cases progresses further to a paralytic stage, typically affecting the limbs proximally and asymmetrically with myalgia, tenderness, weakness, fasciculations, loss of muscle stretch reflexes, and eventual muscle atrophy. Bulbar involvement occurs in some 10% of the cases of paralytic disease.[445] Signs of autonomic involvement and of encephalitis, meningitis, or cerebellar ataxia are also described, but rarely.

The first modern description was that of Jacob Heine in 1840,[2844] but Dr. Michael Underwood (1737–1820) gave a very adequate account in his *Treatise on the Diseases of Children* in 1789 and the effects of the disease were carved in Egyptian relicts in 1500–1400 BC. The name of Karl Medin, a Swedish physician (1847–1927), also used to be associated with this disease, following his observation that the disease ran in epidemics. That the virus has a particular predilection for the anterior horn cells of the cord and for the cranial nerve motor nuclei was first demonstrated by **Charcot**. Major epidemics occurred in the United States in 1890, in 1907, and in the following few decades, but ceased after an effective vaccine was introduced by Salk in 1955.[4938]

In *variant* forms, a polio-like syndrome occurs in association with infection by enteroviruses 70 and 71. *Enterovirus 71 infection* may also cause an aseptic meningitis, *hand, foot, and mouth disease*, or a poliomyelitis-like illness with encephalitic signs.[6858]

In *acute hemorrhagic conjunctivitis*, a severe painful peripheral neuropathy with acute paralysis of the legs, areflexia, and sensory loss are the usual neurological findings. The enterovirus-70 responsible appears to attack the lumbar anterior horn cells or these and the anterior and posterior roots preferentially.[6585]

poliosis Premature graying of the hair.

POLIP syndrome A progressive and potentially fatal neurological disorder characterized by sensorimotor Peripheral neuropathy, external Ophthalmoplegia, Leukoencephalopathy, deafness, and chronic Intestinal Pseudo-obstruction due to visceral neuropathy.[5850]

Pollitt syndrome A recessively inherited congenital dysmorphic syndrome manifesting also low birthweight, dwarfism, sparse fine brittle hair, cataract, premature aging, hypogonadotropic hypogonadism, microcephaly, seizures, cerebellar signs, spasticity, osteosclerosis or osteopetrosis, ichthyosis, and mental and developmental delay.[1299]

poly- (Gr, many) Prefix denoting many.

polyarteritis nodosa (periarteritis, systemic necrotizing vasculitis) An inflammatory disease of the large and medium-sized arteries described by Adolf Kussmaul (1822–1902) and Rodilg Maier (both German physicians) in 1866.[5619] Three conditions are regarded as variants; the classic form, the **Churg-Strauss syndrome**, and an **overlap syndrome**.[2728]

The classic form is complicated by painful asymmetric multiple mononeuropathies, cutaneous neuropathies, or sensorimotor polyneuropathies, and (less often) by radiculopathies or brachial plexopathies. Focal or multifocal cerebral or spinal cord lesions and diffuse encephalopathies are also common.[2728] It is often associated with hepatitis B infection.

polyclonia See **Friedreich disease**.

polycystic lipomembranous osteodysplasia with sclerosing leukoencephalopathy (PLO-SL; Nasu-Hakola disease; OMIM 221770) A recessively transmitted disorder characterized by the onset of bone pain and fractures in the twenties or thirties, frontal type dementia and successively agnosic-aphasia-apraxic syndromes and seizures, and death occurring during the following two decades. CT scans reveal atrophy with calcification of the basal ganglia. Plain X-Ray studies show cysts in the small hand bones.[657] See **Nasu Hakola disease**.

polydactyly The presence of six or more digits on a limb. In *preaxial polydactyly*, the extra digit is on the radial side of the hand, the thumb or index finger being duplicated, and in *postaxial polydactyly* it is on the ulnar side of the hand or the fibular side of the foot. The malformation is usually dominantly inherited.

polyglucosan bodies Small, non–membrane-bound cytoplasmic structures, composed of unusual polymers of glucose. Lafora bodies, Bielschowsky bodies, and corpora amylacea are all composed of such polymers[6892] and are found within neuronal and astrocytic processes in various pathological conditions such as **Lafora body disease**, adult **polyglucosan body disease**, and many others, as well as in normal aged brains.[3900]

polyglucosan body disease An inherited storage disease with onset in adult life, manifesting cerebral atrophy with dementia, pyramidal signs, sensorimotor peripheral neuropathy with loss of pain, vibration and proprioception, axonal neuropathy (nerve conduction studies also show myelinated fiber loss), neurogenic bladder, myopathy, and hypodensities in the white matter on CT scanning.[3917] See **adult polyglucosan body disease**.

polyglutamine expansion degenerative disorders DNA triplet repeat expansions leading to the expression of expanded glutamine amino acid repeat tracts in the affected proteins. See **Kennedy syndrome** (spinobulbar muscular atrophy), **Huntington disease, Joseph disease, dentatorubrropallidal atrophy**, and some autosomal dominant **cerebellar ataxias**.

polygraphic recording The simultaneous monitoring of multiple physiological functions such as the EEG, the EKG and EMG, respirations, eye movements, galvanic skin resistance, and blood pressure.

polygyria A developmental abnormality of the cerebrum, characterized by the presence of many small but true gyri.

polymicrogyria A congenital developmental of neuronal migration within the cerebrum or cerebellum, in which the number of gyri is increased but their size is reduced. It may be focal or widespread. **Schizencephaly** is likely to be associated. Cytomegalovirus infection has been incriminated as a cause.

Clinically, the anomaly is associated with disordered intellectual maturation. Bilateral opercular or perisylvian polymicrogyria constitutes a part of the **Foix–Chavany–Marie syndrome;** bilateral parasaggital (parieto-occipital) polymicrogyria is a localized and sporadic condition. Bilateral frontal polymicrogyria is symmetrical and asociated clinically with developmental delay, mild spastic quadriparesis, language impairment, and occasionally seizures.[2612] A classification has been suggested[404] and is reproduced (amended) by kind permission of the American Academy of Neurology and Lippincott Williams and Wilkins.

Classification of the polymicrogyrias and schizencephalies

1. Bilateral polymicrogyria syndromes
   a. Bilateral diffuse polymicrogyria
   b. Bilateral frontal polymicrogyria (recessive if fronto-parietal, mapped to 16q12)[1093]
   c. Bilateral perisylvian polymicrogyria (autosomal dominant [22qll.2 and others], recessive or X-linked)
   d. Bilateral parieto-occipital polymicrogyria
   e. Bilateral mesial occipital polymicrogyria
2. Schizencephaly (polymicrogyria with clefts)
   a. Isolated schizencephaly
   b. Septo-optic dysplasia—schizencephaly syndrome
   c. Other rare schizencephaly syndromes
3. Polymicrogyria with other brain malformations or abnormalities
   a. Polymicrogyria with abnormal white matter
4. Polymicrogyria or schizencephaly as part of Multiple Congenital Anomaly/Mental Retardation syndromes
   a. Adams-Oliver syndrome
   b. **Aicardi syndrome**
   c. Arima syndrome
   d. Delleman syndrome (oculocerebrocutaneous syndrome)
   e. Galloway–Mowat syndrome
   f. Micro syndrome

polymodal nociceptor

A sensory nerve ending that signals the presence of any of the various potentially damaging stimuli to tissue such as extreme temperature, physical insults, or chemical damage, along C fibers.

polymyalgia rheumatica

A systemic disease marked by inflammation of the intramuscular septa and restricted to people over the age of 50 years, who complain of stiffness of the girdle muscles (which is much worse in the mornings), fatigue, malaise, anorexia, weight loss, and low-grade fever. The ESR is almost always greatly raised. The syndrome is at one end of a spectrum, at the other end of which is **giant cell arteritis**, but it responds to a lower dose of steroids and is eventually self-limiting.[386] Diagnostic criteria have been suggested:[4687]

1. Bilateral muscle pain lasting for more than 2 weeks in more than two of the following areas: neck, shoulders or shoulder girdle, upper arms, hips or pelvic girdle, and thighs.
2. Normal serum muscle enzyme (CK) levels.
3. ESR >40 mm/h.
4. No swelling of the joints of the hands.

The presence of all four of these is practically diagnostic of the condition.

polymyoclonia

See **opsoclonus**.

polymyositis

(idiopathic immune myopathy) Acquired, subacutely progressive, idiopathic, inflammatory, noninfectious, nongranulomatous proximal myopathies of adults. When a skin rash is associated, the term **dermatomyositis** is used. The condition was first described by Wagner in 1863. The definition of the term is currently in evolution, while once all generalized inflammatory myopathies of presumed autoimmune, paraneoplastic, or collagen-vascular etiology were subsumed under the heading, two major categories of **infective myopathies** and **idiopathic inflammatory myopathies** are now recognized, the latter including both *generalized* and *localized* varieties. Polymyositis is included in the "generalized" category.

Classification of the varieties of polymyositis or dermatomyositis has been achieved[718, 719] and amended.[4157, 4158] The classification in Chart P–14A, however, is taken from the Web site of Dr. Alan Pestronk,[4992] http://neuromuscular.wustl.edu/antibody/infmyop.htm#pm, with his kind permission.

The typical clinical features of polymyositis and of most of the nonfocal members of this class are the onset in adult life of symmetrical, proximal more than distal, painful muscle weakness, sometimes selectively affecting the bulbar muscles, the neck extensors, and the quadriceps. Cardiac arrhythmias or inflammatory cardiomyopathy, respiratory muscle weakness, and esophageal paresis are less common findings. Serum CK levels may be raised to 100 × normal. The EMG shows myopathic changes with evidence of active denervation, such as fibrillations, resulting from the fracture of myofibrils by the inflammatory process.

In both polymyositis and sporadic inclusion body myositis, mononuclear cells in the endomysium surround and invade non-necrotic muscle fibers, but this is not the case in dermatomyositis, which is a different condition on histopathologic grounds. On this basis, polymyositis is actually rather uncommon.[1078]

For a classification of such conditions, see **idiopathic inflammatory myopathies** (Chart I–2, Classification of the Idiopathic Inflammatory Myopathies).

Criteria for the diagnosis of polymyositis and dermatomyositis have been formulated and are given in the first part of Chart P–14B. They are based on Hudgson P, Peter JB. Classification (of polymyositis) *Clin Rheum Dis* 1984;10:3–8 by kind permission of the WB Saunders Company.

Chart P–14A. Forms of Polymyositis and Dermatomyositis

Immune myopathies (**Polymyositis** + . . .)
Brachio-Cervical Inflammatory Myopathy
Collagen vascular disease
Complement: C2 deficiency
Drug-induced
Graft-vs-host disease
Idiopathic
t-RNA synthetase antibodies (Jo-1, OJ)
Malignancy-associated
MAS antibody
PM + Mitochondrial disorder (PM/COX-)
Sarcoidosis
Signal recognition particle antibodies
Systemic disorders & Myositis
U1-snRNP antibodies

Dermatomyositis

Childhood
Adult: Mi-2 antibody –
Adult: Malignancy-associated
Adult: EJ antibody +
Adult: PM-Scl antibody +
Adult: Amyopathic
Mi-2 antibody +

Inclusion body myositis

Chart P–14B. Criteria for the Diagnosis of Polymyositis and Dermatomyositis

1. Clinical.

   A. Proximal muscle weakness, myalgia and muscle tenderness, usually symmetrical, progressing during weeks or months, with or without muscle pain. The bulbar and neck muscles are typically involved.
   B. Arthralgia, fever and the Raynaud phenomenon are commonly present and in cases of dermatomyositis, dermatological manifestations will be present.

2. Pathological.

   Muscle fiber necrosis and regeneration, mononuclear cell infiltration. Perifascicular atrophy is sometimes present.

3. Biochemical

   Raised ESR and serum CK (MM isoenzyme), aldolase or myoglobin levels; frequently polyclonal hypergammaglobulinemia is found.

4. EMG.

   Multifocal EMG features of myopathy; spontaneous activity is often present at rest.

   A more recent but somewhat more complicated set of classification criteria for the idiopathic inflammaory myopathies (except IBM), proposed by Dr. Anthony A. Amato, was approved at an international workshop in 2004.[2976]

Inclusion criteria for idiopathic inflammatory myopathies

1. Clinical criteria

   a. Onset usually over 18 years (post-puberty) Onset may be in childhood in dermatomyositis and in non-specific myositis.
   b. Subacute or insidious onset
   c. Pattern of weakness symmetric, proximal > distal, neck flexors > extensors
   d. Rash typical of dermatomyositis: heliotrope (purple) periorbital edema; violaceous papules or macules, scaly if chronic, at metacarpophalangeal and interphalangeal joints and other bony prominences. Erythema of chest and neck (V-sign) and upper back (shawl sign)

Exclusion criteria

   a. Clinical features of inclusion body myositis; asymmetric weakness, wrist/finger flexors same or worse than deltoids; knee extensors and ankle dorsiflexors same or worse than hip flexors.
   b. Ocular weakness, isolated dysarthria, neck extensor > neck flexor weakness
   c. Toxic myopathy (e.g., recent exposure to myotoxic drugs) active endocrinopathy (hyper- or hypothyroid, hyperparathyroid), amyloidosis, family history of muscular dystrophy or proximal motor neuropathies.

2. Elevated serum CK levels
3. Other laboratory criteria

   a. Electromyography

   Inclusion criteria:

      Increased insertional and spontaneous activity (fibrillation potentials, positive sharp waves or complex repetitive discharges)
      Morphometric analysis reveals predominantly long-duration large amplitude MUAPs
      Decreased recruitment pattern of MUAPs

   Exclusion criteria
      Myotonic discharges
      Morphometric analysis reveals predominantly long-duration large amplitude or decreased recruitment of MUAPs

   b. MRI: diffuse or patchy increased signal within muscle disuse on STIR images
   c. Myositis-specific antibodies detected in serum

4. Muscle biopsy inclusion and exclusion criteria

   a. Endomysial inflammatory cell infiltrate (T-cells) surrounding and invading non-necrotic musclefibers
   b. Endomysial CD8 + T cells surrounding, but not definitely invading non-necrotic muscle fibers or ubiquitous MHC-1 one expression
   c. Perifascicular atrophy
   d. MAC depositions on small blood vessels, or reduced capillary density or tubuloreticular inclusions in endothelial cells on EM or MHC-1 expression of perifascicular fibers
   e. Perivascular perimysial inflammatory cell infiltrate
   f. Scattered endomysial CD8 + T cells infiltrate that does not appear to surround or invade muscle fibers
   g. Many necrotic muscle fibers as the predominant abnormal histological feature. Inflammatory cells are sparse or only slight perivascular; perimysial infiltrate is not evident. MAC deposition on the small blood vessels, or pipestem capillaries on EM may be seen, but tubuloreticular inclusions in endothelial cells are uncommon or not evident.
   h. Rimmed vacuoles, ragged red fibers, COX negative fibers that would suggest IBM
   i. MAC deposition on the sarcolemma of non-necrotic fibers and other indications of muscular dystrophies with immunopathology.

Reprinted from Hoogendijk JE, Amato AA, Lecky B. Trial design in adult idiopathic inflammatory myopathies with the exception of inclusion body myositis. Neuromuscul Disord 2004;14: 337–45 with permission from Elsevier Science.

Variant forms are as follows:

Acute myoglobinuric polymyositis with virus-like crystals: An acute, degenerative, necrotic muscle disease presenting with fever and muscle hypotonia and accompanied by myoglobinuria, probably due to influenza B6 virus infection.[1164, 2236]

Chronic focal polymyositis: A chronic, sporadic inflammatory myopathy of adult life with insidious onset, affecting the quadriceps, the forearm flexors, and the brachioradialis muscles, associated with raised serum CK levels and with typical muscle biopsy specimen appearances.[606]

Inflammatory myopathy with COX negative muscle fibers: A slowly progressive proximal myopathy affecting mainly the quadriceps.[3812]

An overlap syndrome with the features of both polymyositis and **inclusion body myositis** is also described.

See also **inclusion body myositis, scapuloileoperoneal atrophy with cardiomyopathy and inflammatory myopathy, congenital inflammatory myopathy, acne fulminans with inflammatory myopathy**.

polyneuritis cranialis
1. A demyelinating disorder affecting the lower cranial nerves (V, VII, IX, X, and XII), and considered to represent a localized form of **acute inflammatory demyelinating polyneuropathy**. In some cases, ophthalmoplegias, ataxia, or weakness of the limbs and trunk are also present. The CSF protein level is raised.[5074] 2. See **superior orbital fissure syndrome**.

polyneuropathy, ophthalmoplegia, leukoencephalopathy, intestinal pseudo-obstruction syndrome (POLIP) See **mitochondrial neurogastrointestinal encephalomyopathy** (MNGIE).

polyneuropathy, organomegaly, endocrinopathy, monoclonal gammopathy, and skin changes See POEMS.

polyneuropathy with acromicria A recessively inherited demyelinating peripheral neuropathy accompanied by retardation of intellectual function, premature menopause, unusual smallness of the extremities, and shortness of stature.[3962]

polyneuropathy–skin pigmentation–hepatosplenomegaly syndrome A syndrome with onset in early adult life, characterized by papilledema, gynecomastia, hepatosplenomegaly with ascites, lymphadenopathy, demyelinating sensorimotor neuropathy, edema, skin hyperpigmentation, and cavernous hemangiomas.[381]

polyopia The perception of multiple images with a single visual stimulus. This occurs occasionally in patients with right-sided occipital lobe disease who see multiple images of moving targets in the defective field of vision. In such cases, the polyopia closely resembles, and may actually represent, **visual perseveration**. See also **cerebral diplopia**.

polyosotic fibrous dysplasia See **McCune–Albright syndrome**.

polyphagia Excessive ingestion of food without hunger; often a compulsion, to be distinguished from morbid hunger.

polypharmacy The practice of prescribing more than one drug for the same condition, notably the use of multiple anticonvulsant agents in the treatment of intractable forms of epilepsy.

polyphasic action potential An action potential with four or more baseline crossings, producing five or more phases. See **phase**. Cf. **serrated action potential**. (From the 2001 Report of the Nomenclature Committee of the American Association of Electromyography and Electrodiagnosis. Reproduced by kind permission of the AANEM.) See also **diphasic wave, triphasic wave**.

polyporencephaly See **multicystic encephalopathy**.

polyradiculitis (polyradiculopathy, polyradiculoneuropathy) Disorders affecting the spinal nerve roots at many levels. Most are inflammatory, often as a result of autoimmune attack, as in the case of **acute inflammatory demyelinating polyneuropathy**.

polyradiculitis with cellular infiltrates See **neurolymphomatosis**.

polyradiculoneuritis See **acute inflammatory demyelinating polyneuropathy**.

polyradiculoneuropathy See **polyradiculopathy**.

polyradiculopathy 1. Any disease involving numerous spinal roots. 2. An EMG diagnosis made in patients with clinical evidence of disease affecting multiple roots and with normal or near-normal motor and sensory nerve conduction study findings but EMG evidence of **denervation** in a multiple-root distribution, either bilaterally or in three or more levels on one side.

polysclerosis See **multiple sclerosis**.

polysomnogram (polysomnography) The concurrent recording during sleep of such physiological variables as EEG, EOG, EKG, ear oximetry, respiratory rate and excursion, nasal air flow, and surface EMG of the anterior tibial and submental muscles.

polysomnography See **polysomnogram**.

polyspike complex See **multiple spike complex**.

polyspikes See **generalized multiple spikes**.

polysynaptic reflex arc A spinal reflex arc in which interneurons are involved between the afferent and efferent neurons. Most nociceptive reflexes and some postural reflexes are of this type.

polytoxic fish poisoning A form of seafood poisoning in Indian, Pacific, and Caribbean waters with clinical features indistinguishable from **ciguatera** fish poisoning.[2484]

Pompe, J.C. (1901–1945) Dutch pathologist who described the disease named for him in his Amsterdam graduation thesis. He was shot by the German occupying forces for his resistance activities.

Pompe disease (glycogenosis type 2) See **glycogen storage diseases**.

Pompe disease of children See **glycogen storage diseases**.

Pompe disease of infants See **glycogen storage diseases**.

pons (or pons varioli) (Lat, a bridge) The section of the brain stem between the medulla and the midbrain. The first published description was that of **Variolus** in 1573.

pontine disconnection syndrome See **locked-in syndrome**.

pontine locked-in syndrome See **locked-in syndrome**.

pontine tegmental cap dysplasia A brainstem and cerebellar embryonic defect in which on MRI shows vermal hypoplasia, subtotal absence of the middle cerebellar peduncles, flattening of the ventral pons, a vaulted pontine tegmentum, a **molar tooth sign**, and absence of the inferior olivary prominence. Clinical features include peripheral hearing impairment in all patients and horizontal gaze palsy, dysphagia, bilateral V and VII nerve involvement, ataxia, and bony vertebral anomalies in some cases.[429]

pontobulbar palsy with deafness (Brown–Vialetto–Van Laere syndrome) A rare recessive syndrome of bilateral nerve deafness and nonfunctioning labyrinths with progressive weakness of all the muscles supplied by the cranial nerves below the fifth, occurring in early childhood. Spinal motor neurons and the pyramidal tract are also affected[2260] such that the condition may be considered as a motor neuron disease.

pontocerebellar hypoplasia (pontoneocerebellar hypoplasia) A group of hereditary neurodegenerative disorders of uncertain etiopathogenesis, though possibly mitochondrionopathies. These rare congenital disorders are characterized by hypoplasia mainly of the lateral lobes of the cerebellum and the brainstem, manifested clinically in neonatal life with feeding problems and respiratory distress, microcephaly and brachycephaly, seizures, optic atrophy, ataxia, hypotonia with hyperreflexia, and mental and developmental delay. Callosal agenesis is commonly found as well. This condition is similar to **olivopontocerebellar degenerations** in that spastic paraparesis may also be found; it is incompatible with life after a few years.[4700] One form maps to 7q11–21. See **cerebellar ataxias** (*variants*), **Paine syndrome**.

Variants are *pontocerebellar hypoplasia type 1*, a recessively inherited form characterized by hypoplasia of the pons and the cerebellum in association with an axonal motor neuropathy and gross developmental delay without extrapyramidal features; *spinal muscular atrophy with* pontocerebellar hypoplasia; and *pontocerebellar hypoplasia type 2*, also recessively inherited and associated with microcephaly and extrapyramidal dyskinesia.[426]

pontogeniculo-occipital waves (PGO waves) Cortical signals recorded in animals during rapid eye movement sleep, accompanied by muscular twitching, autonomic changes, and irregular respirations.These electrical discharges arise from the giganticocellular field in the pons and pass to many brain areas, as a result of disinhibition during rapid eye movement sleep. They have been considered to underlie the desynchronization of the EEG, the eye movements, and the instability of the autonomic nervous system during rapid eye movement sleep.[280] They are also occasionally recorded in the human EEG immediately before the onset of rapid eye movement sleep.[2255]

pontomedullary sulcus infarct See **lateral medullary syndrome**.

pontoneocerebellar hypoplasia See **pontocerebellar hypoplasia**.

pontopseudocoma See **locked-in syndrome**.

pontosubicular necrosis Neuronal injury limited to the pontine nuclei and hippocampus occurring in premature infants born between 26 and 36 weeks gestation who suffer hypoxia and acidosis and who are subsequently exposed to high oxygen concentrations.[407]

ponytail headache A pure extracranial headache arising from pericranial muscle fascia and traction on tendons by the weight of hair within a ponytail.[678]

Pool, James Lawrence (b. 1906) New York neurologist who described myeloscopy (in 1942) and the following sign.

Pool-Schlesinger sign (leg phenomenon) A sign of latent **tetany**; the induction of painful spasms in the knee extensors and ankle plantar flexors when the hip is maintained in flexion with the knee extended. The same phenomenon occurs in the forearm and hand when the shoulder is held in a position of elevation and forced abduction.

Popeye effect The appearance of the wasted proximal part of the arm compared with the less-affected forearm in certain forms of muscular dystrophy, notably **facioscapulohumeral** dystrophy. The phenomenon is named for the cartoon character depicted thus.

Popeye syndrome A form of brachial plexus palsy in which there is proximal (upper arm) muscle atrophy with retention of muscular bulk more distally, as may occur with C5–6 lesions. A similar finding is occasionally seen in patients with **limb-girdle muscular dystrophy**.

popliteal angle Part of Dubowitz' battery of tests for assessing **gestational age**.[1728] With the infant supine and the pelvis flat on the examining couch, the thigh is held in the knee-chest position by the examiner's left index finger and thumb supporting the knee. The knee is then extended by gentle pressure from the examiner's right index finger behind the ankle, and the popliteal angle (between the femur and the lower leg) is measured—the smaller the angle, the greater the degree of hypertonia.

Popplelreuter task A test of right hemispheric visual perceptual processing, wherein the subject is required to identify each of two superimposed line drawings of common objects.[5078]

Porch index of communication ability A standardized and reliable (but complex) instrument for the assessment of a sample of language functions, praxis, and other communication skills, requiring substantial training on the part of the interviewer, in which a patient is made to see, hear, or feel common objects, and his spoken and written naming responses are recorded.[5080]

porencephaly The replacement of cerebral tissue by fluid, usually as the result of a localized ischemic lesion in the pre- or perinatal periods (type 1) or as a familial developmental disorder (type 2). The condition was recognized by **Cruveilhier**, but was so named by **Heschl** in 1859. Clinically, hemiparesis, seizures, and intellectual impairment are the usual features. Radiological criteria have been defined.[1842]

See also the NIH Web site: http://www.ninds.nih.gov/disorders/porencephaly/porencephaly.htm.

poriomania Wandering, as a manifestation of a clouded or confused state in complex partial seizures. The term was introduced by Emil Kraepelin.[4191]

porphyrias Dominantly inherited disorders in the biosynthesis of heme, leading to the excessive production and excretion of porphyrins. Hepatic and erythropoietic forms are differentiated, neurological complications occurring only in the former. See **acute intermittent porphyria, variegate porphyria,** and **hereditary coproporphyria**.[410, 1322]

Doss porphyria is a very rare *variant*, presenting with abdominal pain. Excessive excretion of porphobilinogen and of λ-aminolevulinic acid is characteristic.

In a classic exercise in medical detection, Macalpine and Hunter[3984] concluded that porphyria has affected members of the royal houses of the United Kingdom (and their European relatives), back at least to Mary, Queen of Scots, but most prominently to King George III.

porter's tip position That position of the arm assumed by patients with Erb palsy (C5–6 or upper trunk brachial plexopathy). The arm hangs adducted and pronated, with the fingers in slight flexion due to weakness of the shoulder abductors, the elbow flexors and supinators, and the long extensors of the wrist.

In previous eras, porters were available to carry luggage. Today, regrettably, the alternative name of *policeman's tip* has gained favor.

Porteus maze test A test of planning behavior assessing largely the function of the frontal lobes, wherein the subject is required to trace with a pencil the paths through progressively more complicated printed mazes.[5086]

portmanteau word The fusion of part or whole of two or more words to form a hybrid neologism.[1330]

portosystemic shunt encephalopathy See **acquired hepatocerebral encephalopathy**.

Porto-Systemic Encephalopathy Index A scale used to evaluate the severity of the encephalopathy by scoring asterixis, the mental state, trailmaking test time, EEG changes, and arterial ammonia levels.[1268]

Portuguese neuropathy See **Andrade neuropathy**.

Portuguese Society of Clinical Neurophysiology A professional organization based at Laboratoria de EEG, Centro de Estudos Egas, Moniz Hospital, Santa Maria 1699, Lisboa Codex, Portugal.

Poser criteria Criteria for the diagnosis of **multiple sclerosis**, the first to introduce the concept of laboratory evidence as support for the clinical diagnosis.[5094] Dr. Charles M. Poser is a contemporary American neurologist.

positional alcohol nystagmus The occurrence of nystagmus and vertigo in the presence of levels of blood alcohol above 0.4 gm/l. This occurs due to the diffusion of alcohol into the cupula within the ampulla of the semicircular canals, where it alters the relative densities of the cupula and the endolymph, transforming the semicircular canals into gravity-sensitive receptors.[819] See also **vestibular nystagmus**.

positional nystagmus Nystagmus induced by changes in the position of the head, usually tested by getting the patient to move quickly from an upright to a head-down position. It may have either *central* (brainstem) or *peripheral* (VIII cranial nerve and vestibular apparatus) causes. The phenomenon was regarded by Nylen as the surest and simplest sign of disturbance of the vestibular system.

Most cases have a peripheral cause (**benign paroxysmal positional vertigo**). In such cases there is a latency of 5–30 s before the nystagmus appears with assumption of the provocative position, the nystagmus fatigues after some seconds, habituation occurs on re-testing, the direction of the nystagmus is always to one side only (although a torsional component may be present), and the accompanying vertigo may be severe. None of these features is present when the lesion is central.

In a variant form, *persistent direction-changing positional nystagmus*,[358] fatigue does not occur but the nystagmus persists as long as the position is held but changes direction with different head positions.

positional vertigo See **benign positional vertigo**.

positioning nystagmus A common form of nystagmus occurring as a result of rapid head movement, seen in many patients with lesions of the vestibular system of any type and at any site. See **vestibular nystagmus**.[5]

positive myoclonus See **myoclonus**.

positive occipital sharp transients of sleep (lambdoids) Sharp, transient, single, or repetitive EEG waves with maximal amplitude over the occipital regions, positive relative to other areas, and occurring apparently spontaneously during sleep. Their amplitude varies but is generally below 50 μV. (Adapted from the 1974 Report of the Committee on Terminology, IFCN[1117] and reproduced by kind permission of Elsevier Science and the IFCN.)

positive sharp wave A biphasic, initially positive action potential from a single muscle fiber. It may be initiated by needle electrode movement (insertional or unsustained positive sharp wave) or may occur spontaneously. Typically the discharge is in a uniform, regular pattern at a rate of 1–50 Hz; the discharge frequency may decrease slightly just before it ceases. The initial positive deflection is rapid <1 ms), its duration is usually less than 5 ms, and its amplitude is up to 1 mV. The negative phase is of low amplitude with a duration of

10–100 ms. It is assumed that the discharge emanates from a damaged area of a muscle fiber. This configuration may result from the position of the needle electrode, which is believed to be adjacent to the depolarized segment of a muscle fiber injured by the electrode.

This waveform is not specific for muscle fiber damage as it may also occur in association with fibrillation potentials which are equivalent discharges. Some motor unit action potentials and potentials in myotonic discharges may have the configuration of positive sharp waves.

(This is an edited version of the entry in the 2001 Report of the Nomenclature Committee of the American Association of Electromyography and Electrodiagnosis.[19] Reproduced by kind permission of the AANEM.)

positive supporting reaction
A postural reflex consisting of extension of the leg in response to pressure applied upward on the sole of the foot, said to be increased in primates after resection of the anterior lobe of the cerebellum but normally present at birth and persisting for about 6 months thereafter.

positive symptoms Those symptoms caused by abnormal electrical activity within the nervous system as opposed to those due to the cessation of normal electrical activity. Hughlings-**Jackson** pointed out that destructive lesions never cause positive effects, but may induce a negative condition permitting positive symptoms to appear.[4339] Those positive symptoms arising from peripheral motor axons include fasciculations, cramps, and spasms; those from sensory axons, pricking or tingling (paresthesias) and sensations of tightness, crawling, heat and cold, and pain.[1770] Seizure activity in the CNS usually produces positive symptoms, though negative ones (such as atonic seizures) also occur.

positive wave See **positive sharp wave**.

positron emission tomography (PET) An investigational technique for the creation of images using radioactive isotopes that decay with the emission of positively charged electrons (positrons) as tracers to map the physiological, biochemical, hemodynamic, and pharmacological processes of the body.

Radioisotopes emitting positrons, produced in a cyclotron, such as the isotopes of oxygen, carbon, nitrogen, and fluorine are incorporated into molecules with known biological behavior, and tomographically produced cross-sectional images of the distribution of these agents within the body are produced, making use of the same principles as in CT scanning. Such images indicate underlying biochemical or pharmacological processes in defined anatomical loci. Over 500 compounds have been labeled with these isotopes for use as PET tracers. Ideally, all will have short half-lives.

Brain metabolic variables that can be mapped regionally by PET include blood flow and volume, pH, the oxygen extraction fraction, and the rates of consumption of glucose and oxygen. Tracers are also available for measuring the transport and metabolism of amino acids, free fatty acids, and glucose metabolites, and for the assessment of protein synthesis and molecular diffusion. Specific receptor ligands labeled with positron emitters have been used to map dopamine, serotonin, benzodiazepine, cholinergic, opioid, and adrenergic binding sites. Positron emitting–labeled medications including antiepileptics, neuroleptics, and agents suitable for mapping enzyme distribution can also be produced.[5121]

Cerebral glucose metabolism has been the most studied using, for example, fluorine-^{18} labeled fluoro-2-deoxyglucose, but oxygen^{15}-labeled water or gases such as C^{15}-labeled carbon dioxide also allow assessments of cerebral blood flow, oxygen utilization, etc. Neurotransmitters may also be labeled to allow mapping of their distribution and activity. The technique has been employed in the preoperative evaluation of patients with refractory seizures, and in subjects with dementia, movement disorders, and brain tumors.[168, 877]

possible multiple sclerosis
A diagnostic category in the 1954 definitions of Allison and Millar,[138] now largely replaced by the **Schumacher** or the **Poser criteria**.

post- (Lat, after)

Post, Wright (1766–1822) American surgeon who was the first to ligate the carotid artery, in a patient with aneurysm (1814).

postactivation The period following voluntary activation of a nerve or muscle. Contrast with posttetanic. (From the 2001 Report of the Nomenclature Committee of the American Association of Electromyography and Electrodiagnosis.[19] Reproduced by kind permission of the AANEM.)

postactivation depression
A reduction in the amplitude and area of the M wave(s) in response to a single stimulus or train of stimuli which occurs within a few minutes following a 10–60 s strong voluntary contraction. (From the 2001 Report of the Nomenclature Committee of the American Association of Electromyography and Electrodiagnosis.[19] Reproduced by kind permission of the AANEM.)

postactivation exhaustion
A reduction in the safety factor (margin) of neuromuscular transmission after sustained activation at the neuromuscular junction. The changes in the configuration of the M wave due to postactivation exhaustion are referred to as postactivation depression. The term is also used to describe the reduction of the M wave following a tetanus, which should logically be termed posttetanic depression. (From the 2001 Report of the Nomenclature Committee of the American Association of Electromyography and Electrodiagnosis.[19] Reproduced by kind permission of the AANEM.)

postactivation facilitation See **facilitation**.

postactivation potentiation An increase in the force of contraction (mechanical response) after a strong voluntary contraction. See also **facilitation**.

postanesthetic apnea Prolonged depolarization of muscles following succinylcholine usage during anesthesia, leading to flaccidity and weakness, most prominently manifest as apnea. The responsible gene maps to chromosome 3q21–q26. See **succinylcholine sensitivity**.

postanoxic myoclonus see **Lance–Adams syndrome**.

postchalastic fits See **sleep paralysis**.

Postconcussion questionnaire

A checklist of postconcussional symptoms[3439] generously made available by the Rivermead Rehabilitation Centre, Abingdon Rd, Oxford, OXI 4XD UK.

The introduction is as follows: *After a head injury or accident some people experience symptoms which can cause worry or nuisance. We would like to know if you now suffer any of the symptoms given below. As many of these symptoms occur normally, we would like you to compare yourself now with before the accident. For each one please circle the number closest to your answer.*

Compared with before the accident, do you now (i.e. over the last 24 h) suffer from headaches, feelings of dizziness, nausea or vomiting, hypersensitivity to noise or to light, easy tiring, irritability, depression, frustration or impatience, forgetfulness/poor memory, impaired concentration, slow thinking, impaired vision, restlessness, more energy, or other difficulties?

Please specify, and rate as above: Scoring—0 = Not experienced at all/1 = No more a problem/2 = A mild problem/3 = A moderate problem/4 = A severe problem.

The problem of suggestibility arises in this as in all other such questionairres. The scale is available at http://www.wsib.on.ca/wsib/wsibobj.nsf/lookupfiles/pocmtbirivermead/$file/mtbi_rivermead.pdf/. See also **CogSport**, **Impact of Event Scale, Orientation–Memory–Concentration Test**.

Postconcussion syndrome checklist

Postconcussion syndrome checklist An instrument recording the experience of cognitive, emotional, and physical symptoms of subjects following concussion.[2345]

postconcussional syndrome (PCS)

postconcussional syndrome (PCS) A persistent constellation of physical, cognitive, and emotional/behavioral symptoms commonly following head trauma (not always severe enough to result in loss of consciousness) and including such disparate somatic symptoms as headache; fatigue; diplopia; convergence insufficiency; dizziness (seldom true vertigo); tinnitus; hearing loss or hyperacusis, insomnia, reduced tolerance to stress, emotional excitement, and alcohol; blurred vision and photo- and phonophobia; cognitive disturbance such as difficulty in concentrating and performing mental tasks (especially those involving information processing); impairment of memory and of judgment; slowed thinking and reaction times; and emotional disturbances including irritability, lack of spontaneity, reduced initiative and both anxiety and depression, all occurring in the absence of physical signs.[2084, 4905, 5481] In addition, imbalance may be present due to "vestibular concussion"[5385] and there is usually intolerance of stress, emotion, and alcohol.

Symptoms usually last for less than 3 months, but in about 15% of cases they are prolonged. The presence of headache, dizziness, or nausea in the emergency room after mild traumatic brain injury is strongly associated with the severity of posttraumatic symptoms 6 months later.

The emergence and persistence of the postconcussional syndrome are associated with social adversity before the accident. However, in a Lithuanian matched control study, scores of visual analogue scales of symptoms attributed to PCS showed no significant differences between injured and uninjured people except that depression, alcohol intolerance, and worry about brain injury were more frequent in the concussed group. Such findings might question the validity of the condition as a useful clinical entity.[4350]

It is asserted that the complaints are not typically motivated by thoughts of compensation. Marginal premorbid achievement and pre-existing social adverity may be risk factors for the later development of postconcussion syndrome and likelihood of litigation; it is also suggested that depression, not head-injury status, largely accounts for the reports of cognitive and other symptoms.[6122, 1501]

Diagnostic criteria suggested in the International Classification of Disease (10th Revision) (found at http://www.nimh.nih.gov/health/publications/adhd/symptoms.shtml/) include the following:

Interval between head trauma with loss of consciousness and development of symptoms is less than 4 weeks
Symptoms in at least 3 of the following categories
Headache, dizziness, fatigue, noise intolerance
Irritability, depression, anxiety, emotional lability
Subjective concentration, memory, or intellectual difficulties without neuropsychological evidence of marked impediments
Insomnia
Reduced alcohol tolerance
Preoccupation with the above symptoms, fear of brain damage, hypochondriacal concern, and adoption of the "sick rôle."

Refinement of the PCS diagnostic criteria of the *DSM-IV* and the ICD-10 is needed before either can be recommended for routine use because of the discrepancies between them.

Evaluation with EEG, brainstem evoked potentials, brain imaging, or oculonystagmography may yield objective evidence to substantiate the symptoms but results are often negative. PET scanning during cognitive challenge may, however, show distant hypometabolic regions. See also **Paced Auditory Serial Addition Task, postconcussion questionnaire, Glasgow Coma Scale,** and **chronic fatigue syndrome,** the symptoms of the latter being similar in nature.

postcontusion seizure syndrome

postcontusion seizure syndrome See **traumatic spreading depression syndrome**.

postconvulsive palsy

postconvulsive palsy See **Todd paralysis**.

postcraniotomy headache

postcraniotomy headache See **posttraumatic headaches**.

postdural puncture headache

postdural puncture headache See **postlumbar puncture headache**.

postencephalitic Parkinsonism

A Parkinsonian syndrome occurring years after the illness **encephalitis lethargica**, and characterized by especially severe rigidity and facial impassivity, by the occurrence of **oculogyric crises**, by psychiatric features such as dementia, personality change, psychosis, and akinetic states, and by the remarkable feature of the return to active mobility for short periods under extreme emotional stimulation.[5169] It is recounted that when there was a fire in a London hospital, the patients in the postencephalitic ward were independently the first that ran out of the building.

postencephalitic Parkinsonism with amyotrophy

postencephalitic Parkinsonism with amyotrophy The occurrence of progressive atrophy of the spinal muscles many years after the onset of Parkinsonism of the postencephalitic type. There is degeneration in the pons, oculomotor nuclei, and anterior horn cells of the cervical and dorsal levels of the spinal cord, without tract degeneration.[2566]

postencephalitic syndrome

A syndrome of residual behavioral change following recovery from either viral or bacterial encephalitis. Symptoms are nonspecific and vary from individual to individual, from one infectious agent to another, and, most consistently, with the age of the individual at the time of infection. The principal difference between this disorder and the organic personality disorders is that it is often reversible.[172]

A previous (*DSM-III R*) American Psychiatric Association diagnostic guideline noted that the manifestations may include general malaise, apathy, or irritability, some lowering of cognitive functioning (learning difficulties), altered sleep and eating patterns, and changes in sexuality and in social judgment. There may be a variety of residual neurological dysfunctions, such as paralysis, deafness, aphasia, constructional apraxia, and acalculia.

Chart P–15. Clinical Features of the Posterior Cerebral Artery Syndromes

Proximal occlusions may lead to:

Visual signs, including III cranial nerve palsy, **Parinaud syndrome**, vertical gaze paresis, paralysis of downward gaze, bilateral ptosis, oval pupils, blepharospasm, **retraction nystagmus**, tucking of eyelids, anterior **internuclear ophthalmoplegia**, pseudo-paralysis of the VI cranial nerve, decreased or absent spontaneous blinking with retained reflex blink to light and sound, absence of slow roving eye movements, absence of horizontal saccades, delayed eye closure on falling asleep and ocular tremor; and to other signs including: **abulia**, drowsiness, brief wake-sleep cycles, coma, dementia, **tachyphemia**, hemiparesis, **decerebrate posture**, **Horner syndrome**, cerebellar ataxia, **rubral tremor**, **Weber**, **Claude** or **Benedikt syndromes**, **hemiballismus**, **asterixis** and **Cheyne-Stokes respirations**.

Distal occlusions may lead to:

Visual signs, including hemianopia, unilateral and bilateral; **Anton syndrome**, **alexia without agraphia**, color anomia, **dyschromatopsia**, simple, complex, formed and unformed hallucinations; **central photophobia**; **visual perseveration**; **polyopia**; tilted vision; visual spread; migrainous features (scintillations, blindness and blurring); **prosopagnosia**; **topographic agnosia**; **visual agnosia**; **peduncular hallucinosis**; checkerboard fields and **metamorphopsia**; and to other signs, including sensory deficits, the **Déjèrine-Roussy syndrome** of thalamic pain; choreoathetosis; confusion; agitation; impairment of memory; anomia for proper names; isolated **dysgraphia**; unsteadiness or lightheadedness; and hemorrhagic infarction secondary to brain herniation.

Adapted from Fisher CM. The Posterior Cerebral Artery Syndrome. Can J Neurol Sci *1986;13:232–9, reproduced by kind permission.)*

postepileptic headache

A migraine-like headache following generalized tonic–clonic seizures experienced by many epileptic patients.[5635]

postepileptic paralysis See **Todd paralysis**.

posterior agraphia See **agraphia**.

posterior aprosodia A receptive form of **aprosodia**, in which the subject is unable to discern the emotive content of the spoken speech heard. The lesion is situated in the posterior right temporoparietal area or in the thalamic and adjacent regions.[5418]

posterior canal benign positional vertigo The commonest form of **benign positional vertigo**.

posterior cerebral artery syndrome(s) Clinical syndromes resulting from occlusion of the posterior cerebral artery by embolism or thrombus. The clinical features, visual and nonvisual, resulting from occlusions at proximal and distal sites have been summarized by Fisher[2096] and are given in Chart P–15.

posterior cervical sympathetic syndrome A constellation of subjective complaints including occipital head pain, vertigo resulting from head turning, tinnitus, hazy vision without objective abnormality, and fatigability. The condition was considered by Barré[420] to result from cervical joint disease. See **cervical migraine, Barré syndrome**.

posterior column ataxia see **Biemond syndrome**.

posterior column sensations

Déjèrine wrote that with posterior column lesions, "Even if tactile sensibility is almost normal, the sense of localization, the notion of weight, the sense of tactile discrimination (two-point) are greatly altered; and finally astereognosis is frequent." Wartenberg noted that the posterior columns mediate spatial functions such as the recognition by feeling of forms (e.g., numerals) traced on the skin.

There is now evidence that the posterior columns and the anterolateral tracts together subserve at least touch and pressure sensibility, and that the disturbance of position sense leads to many of the other impairments of discrimination.[4598] Other authorities consider that **directional cutaneous kinesthesia** is the only sensation properly named.[509]

posterior columns (Wall)[6606] See **dorsal columns**.

posterior compartment syndrome of the thigh A sciatic neuropathy recorded as complicating prolonged sitting (e.g., during craniotomy). A CT scan may assist in diagnosis. Prompt decompression of the nerve has been advised.[5079]

posterior cortical atrophy

(posterior cortical dementia, De Renzi–Benson syndrome) A rare syndrome of slowly progressive dementia with initial alexia, anomia, asomatognosia, and visual object agnosia, followed by a **Balint** or a **Gerstmann syndrome, constructional apraxia**, visuospatial disorientation, and transcortical sensory aphasia, due to bilateral, asymmetrical parieto-occipital atrophy.[524, 1515] Memory, insight, and judgment are relatively preserved.The onset is usually before the age of 65 years.

The syndrome may be seen in patients with **Alzheimer disease** (the commonest pathology) but also in those with **frontotemporal dementias** (Pick disease), **progressive subcortical gliosis**, or **Creutzfeldt-Jakob disease**. It was described first by Rosenfeld in 1909, but more completely by Benson and by De Renzi in the last decade. See also **progressive biparietal atrophy**.

posterior cortical dementia See **posterior cortical atrophy**.

posterior diencephalic autonomic epilepsy syndrome See **de Morsier syndrome**.

posterior femoral cutaneous neuralgia A syndrome of pain in the scrotal and perineal area, radiating to the adjacent thigh, associated with damage to the posterior femoral cutaneous nerve.[1178]

posterior fossa compression syndrome The occurrence of apnea and coma with continuous cardiac function due to a primary failure of the respiratory center, as a result of compression as a result of posterior fossa disease.[5355]

posterior fossa stare See **Collier sign**.

posterior inferior cerebellar artery syndrome See **lateral medullary syndrome**.

posterior internuclear ophthalmoplegia Conjugate gaze palsy recovering to leave paresis of the lateral rectus on that side, while the contralateral medial rectus regains its function. One cause is an infarct of the brainstem just above the abducens nucleus.[5433]

posterior interosseous syndrome (supinator channel syndrome, radial tunnel syndrome, deep radial nerve paralysis, dorsal interosseous syndrome) Deficits in this major terminal branch of the radial nerve, which supplies the extensor muscles of the forearm.

Compression of the nerve in the arcade of Frohse by lesions at the level of the radioulnar joint or due to repeated pronation-supination hand movements leads to complaints of proximal forearm pain, worsened by forced supination and resembling that of tennis elbow or tenosynovitis; weakness of wrist, finger, and thumb extension and of thumb abduction with a radial drift; and occasionally wasting of the forearm extensor muscles.[6727] Most cases are idiopathic, but trauma or local mass lesions may be responsible. Surprisingly about 50% of the nontraumatic cases also show some sensory disturbance in the forearm, wrist, or hand. The diagnosis is suggested if there is exacerbation of pain when the middle finger is extended against the examiner's resistance, or when the affected arm is passively flexed at the elbow, the forearm maximally supinated, and the wrist abruptly flexed by the examiner.

Lateral epicondylitis (tennis elbow) shows somewhat similar symptoms, but in that condition the site of maximal tenderness is directly over the lateral epicondyle; in the posterior interosseous syndrome the maximal tenderness is at about 4 cm below that point.

The **supinator syndrome** is considered to be a special form of this syndrome.[1017, 1967, 1313]

posterior lacerocondylar syndrome Involvement of the XII cranial nerve, usually with involvement of nerves IX, X, and XI as well, due to a lesion such as a primary or secondary tumor at the base of the skull. See **Collet–Sicard syndrome**.

posterior reversible leukoencephalopathy syndrome See **reversible posterior leukoencephalopathy syndrome**.

posterior peroneofemoral reflex See **external hamstring reflex**.

posterior quadrantic dysplasia See **hemi-hemimegancncephaly**.

posterior retroparotid syndrome See **Villaret syndrome**.

posterior retropharyngeal syndrome See **Villaret syndrome**.

posterior scarf sign See **scarf sign**.

posterior temporal lobe epilepsy A seizure syndrome arising from a focus usually in the basal region of the temporal lobe, seen most often in children and characterized clinically by initial behavioural arrest followed by tonic contraversive movements and then motor signs. Automatisms are late appearing and a minor feature only.[1739]

posterior thalamic syndrome See **thalamic syndrome**.

posterior tibial neuropathy A syndrome of weakness and wasting of the gastrocnemius–soleus and of the intrinsic muscles of the foot as a result of damage to the posterior tibial nerve fibers, either while still a part of the sciatic nerve in the pelvis or more distally in isolation. Lesions of the main trunk of the nerve in the thigh are usually a result of compression, trauma, or ischemic disease and cause sural sensory and lower motor neurone lesions in the gastrocnemius, soleus, and plantar muscles. Distally the problem could be sited at any point along its course, but, due to the protection afforded by overlying structures at higher levels, it is usually at a point below the medial malleolus, in which case only the foot muscles and sensation in the sole of the foot are affected. See **tarsal tunnel syndrome**.

posterior tibiofemoral reflex See **internal hamstring reflex**.

posterior vermal split syndrome Impairment of tandem gait with relative retention of other cerebellar functions, following surgical transection of the posterior inferior cerebellar vermis.[438]

posterolateral sclerosis See **subacute combined degeneration of the cord**.

postfixation An anatomical variant of the optic chiasm such that it lies posteriorly in relation to the sella turcica, and above the dorsum sella.

postfixational blindness Loss of vision distal to a point of close fixation in patients with bitemporal hemianopia, due to the approximation of the blind half-fields that occurs as the eyes converge. The subject thus retains a cone of vision immediately anterior to the face, but can see nothing behind this.

postganglionic cholinergic dysautonomia The rare occurrence of pure postganglionic cholinergic dysfunction which presents as internal ophthalmoplegia, impaired secretion of tears and saliva, anhidrosis, and hypertension without the sympathetic involvement present in **autonomic neuropathy** (def. 1). The condition may have an autoimmune or postinfectious etiology.[2768]

postganglionic fibers Those neurons of the parasympathetic and sympathetic systems arising from the peripheral ganglia and passing to their respective end-organs. The name was bestowed by J.N. **Langley**.

posthemiplegic chorea (postparalytic chorea) Chorea following stroke, first described by Silas Weir **Mitchell** in 1874.

posthemiplegic dystonia The occurrence of dystonic movements (or athetosis) years after a stroke. The responsible lesions are of the contralateral caudate nucleus, the thalamus, or both.

postherpetic neuralgia A chronic painful condition in which burning and jabbing pain persists for longer than 3 months in the distribution of the skin eruptions of prior herpes zoster—such as a thoracic dermatome or a division of the trigeminal nerve (usually the first).

The pain, which can be either burning hyperesthesias or lancinating stabs, occurs both spontaneously and following any stimulus to the affected skin and may be intractable. It is commoner in females and increases both in severity and in frequency with advancing age. In the initial acute stage the pain precedes the herpetic skin eruption by up to a week and may persist for months or years, especially in older patients. Hypesthesia, hyperalgesia, and/or allodynia are usually present in the territory involved. Scarring of the skin and sensory loss are also common in the affected regions.

Based upon the International Classification of Headache Disorders [Headache Classification Committee of the International Headache Society. *Cephalalgia* 2004; **24**(Suppl 1)] by kind permission of Dr. Jes Olesen, the International Headache Society, and Wiley-Blackwell Publications.

posthyperventilation apnea A period of apnea not normally exceeding 12 s, occurring after a period of voluntary hyperventilation, such as five deep breaths. When it lasts longer, bilateral hemispheric disease is suggested.[5052]

Such cessation of breathing following hyperventilation is due to removal of the hypercapneic drive to breathe. A mechanism linked to vigilance and to the respiratory control centers acts to prevent this apneic pause in normal, awake people, but is disturbed itself in states of diminished consciousness, leading to a prolonged period of apnea.

postictal headache Headache with features of tension-type headache or of migraine, following closely upon a seizure but resolving within 3 days.

postictal hemiplegia Weakness of one side of the body lasting for periods of up to days, usually following prolonged somatomotor seizures but also occurring after partial seizures without motor manifestations. See also **Todd paralysis**.

postictal hemisyndrome See **Todd paralysis**.

postictal nose rubbing A behavioral pattern strongly suggesting an ipsilateral temporal lobe location of seizure origin.[6721]

postictal phenomenon A transient clinical abnormality of central nervous system function that appears or becomes accentuated after clinical signs of the ictus have ended.[1861, 16]

postictal psychosis Paranoid or schizophrenia-like psychoses developing after a flurry of complex partial or generalized seizures, and also seen sometimes following right temporal lobectomy performed for the control of intractable partial seizures.[4038] The EEG does not show seizure activity during such psychotic episodes.[3899]

postinfection fatigue syndrome (myalgic encephalomyelitis, benign encephalomyelitis, chronic Epstein–Barr virus infection, Icelandic disease, epidemic neuromyasthenia, Royal Free disease) A syndrome of persistent profound fatigue precipitated by minimal physical exertion, occurring after a viral or other infection, almost invariably associated with some emotional disturbance. There is little or no objective abnormality revealed by EMG, isometric strength testing, or muscle biopsy.[3885]

The syndrome may be episodic or sporadic. What combination of organic and functional factors interact to cause it remains the subject for intermittent dispute, except among its sufferers, who reject angrily any hint of a psychological etiology. Despite this, their symptoms much resemble the somatic complaints of patients with depressive illnesses.

Criteria for diagnosis have been suggested[3885] and are given in Chart P–16.

postinfectious autoimmune neuropsychiatric disorders associated with streptococcal infection (PANDAS) A spectrum of childhood behaviors such as the occurrence of tics and/or obsessive-compulsive disorder following group A β-hemolytic streptococcal infections in children or adolescents, mostly those with normal pre-morbid personalities.[2294] The likely pathophysiology is the development of antistreptococcal antibodies that cross-react with antigens in the basal ganglia of genetically susceptible hosts (molecular mimicry). See also **Sydenham chorea**.

The clinical manifestations include fragments of **Tourette syndrome**, including obsessive-compulsive features, **myoclonus**, and **attention-deficit hyperactivity disorder**.[3609] Proposed diagnostic criteria[6163] are adapted here:

1. Pediatric onset: Symptoms of the disorder first become evident abruptly, usually between the ages of 3 years and the beginning of puberty.
2. The presence of tics and/or OCD: Symptoms must meet lifetime diagnostic criteria for OCD and/or a tic disorder. (The tics may be severe, involving head, limb, or whole body jerks with no history of the more typical eye-blinking or facial movements.)
3. An episodic clinical course: The onset of a specific symptom's exacerbation can often be assigned to a particular day or week, at which time symptoms seemed to "explode" in severity. Symptoms may resolve completely between episodes, or continue at lesser severity.
4. Symptom exacerbations must be associated with a group A β hemolytic streptococcus (GAS) infection. Because both such infections and tics are common in childhood, confirmation of an association between them can only be made by following the children over time, observing at least two exacerbations occurring shortly after GAS infections.
5. During symptom exacerbations, patients may have adventitious movements (motor hyperactivity and/or choreiform movements).

Chart P–16. Criteria for the Diagnosis of Postinfection Fatigue Syndrome

To fulfill the criteria, the patient must have chronic persisting or relapsing fatigue of a generalized nature, causing disruption of usual daily activities, present for greater than 6 months, AND two major criteria OR one major and three minor criteria, as follows:

1. Symptoms: Persistent for at least 6 months continuously, or relapsing on three or more occasions with a similar pattern, over 6 months or more;

Major	*Minor*
Concentration or memory impairment	Myalgia
Arthralgia	
Headaches	
Depression	
Tinnitus	
Paresthesias	

2. Signs: Present on at least one occasion subsequent to the initial illness;

Major	*Minor*
Lymphadenopathy	Pharyngitis
Localized muscle tenderness	

3. Immunological assessment:

Major	*Minor*
T4 or T8 lymphopenia (absolute count)	
Cutaneous anergy or	Hypoergy

Adapted from Lloyd et al., 1988; reproduced by kind permission of BMJ Publishing Group.

postinfectious cerebellar ataxia (acute benign cerebellar ataxia) An uncommon self-limiting syndrome of limb and gait ataxia, nystagmus or opsoclonus following viral infections such as measles and varicella in children.[3482]

postinfectious encephalomyelitis A multifocal immunological, inflammatory, and demyelinating polioencephalopathy considered to result from allergy to an infectious agent. The syndrome evidences widespread acutely or subacutely evolving cerebral and spinal cord disease following a viral or other infection, such as measles, mumps, varicella, or rubella; and presents with fever, headache, seizures, and focal neurological signs, alteration in consciousness, slow activity on the EEG, and modestly increased CSF protein levels and mononuclear cell counts, while signs of meningeal irritation are less common.[3382, 5377] The patients usually recover. See also **postvaccinial encephalomyelitis, disseminated vasculomyelinopathy**.

postinfectious encephalopathy See **toxic hydrocephalus**.

postinfectious polyneuropathy See **acute inflammatory demyelinating polyneuropathy**.

postinfective See **postinfectious**.

postinfluenzal myositis (benign acute childhood myositis) A mild necrotizing inflammatory myopathy occurring in epidemic or sporadic forms, and manifesting pain, tenderness, and swelling of calf and thigh muscles in the week following an attack of influenza or parainfluenza A or B, with spontaneous resolution.[4067]

See also **influenza**.

postirradiation myelopathy See **radiation myelopathy**.

post–lumbar puncture headache (low-pressure headache, post–dural puncture headache, postmyelogram headache, drainage headache) Headache peristing after a dural puncture and causing a reduction in CSF pressure. Diagnostic criteria have been defined:

A. Headache that worsens within 15 min after sitting or standing and improves within 15 min after lying, with at least one of the following and fulfilling criteria C and D:
   1. Neck stiffness
   2. Tinnitus
   3. Hypacusis
   4. Photophobia
   5. Nausea
B. Dural puncture has been performed
C. Headache develops within 5 days after dural puncture
D. Headache resolves either
   1. Spontaneously within 1 week or
   2. Within 48 h after effective treatment of the spinal fluid leak (usually by epidural blood patch). In 95% of cases this is so. When headache persists, causation is in doubt.

Adapted from the International Classification of Headache Disorders (Headache Classification Committee of the International Headache Society. *Cephalalgia* 2004;24[Suppl 1]) by kind permission of Dr. Jes Olesen, the International Headache Society, and Wiley-Blackwell Publications.

A *variant* is *headache attributed to intrathecal injection*, a diffuse headache in the recumbent position developing within 4 h after an intrathecal injection has been given and resolving within 14 days.[2820]

postmyelogram headache See **post–lumbar puncture headache**.

postoptokinetic nystagmus See **optokinetic afterinduced nystagmus**.

postparalytic chorea See **post hemiplegic chorea**.

postpartum cerebral angiopathy A true inflammatory vasculitis or transient vasoconstriction related to the hormonal events of pregnancy and the postpartum period and a cause of hemorrhagic stroke in young women. Cerebral angiography demonstrates diffuse irregularity of branches of the middle cerebral arteries consistent with a diffuse vasospastic process or classic vasculitis. Neurological deficits resolve after high-dose corticosteroids.[6453] See **reversible cerebral vasoconstriction syndrome** (Call–Fleming syndrome).

postpertussis encephalopathy A potentially fatal polioencephalopathy characterized by fever, alterations in consciousness, seizures, and focal neurological signs,occurring rarely during the paroxysmal stage of pertussis, usually in young children. Whether the cause is hypoxic or immunological is uncertain.[6858]

postpolio syndrome See **postpoliomyelitis muscular atrophy**.

postpoliomyelitis muscular atrophy (postpolio syndrome) A condition characterized by slowly progressive, asymmetrical impairment of muscle function after a documented attack of poliomyelitis with succeeding functional stability or recovery which has lasted at least 15 years. Residual atrophy, fasciculations, weakness and areflexia in at least one limb, normal sensation, a combination of acute and chronic denervation changes on EMG testing, and the presence of new muscle weakness and neuromuscular symptoms unrelated to other intercurrent disorders are other suggested criteria. The muscle pain and cramping are noted where not present previously.

Clinically, the new weakness occurs 30–40 years after the original illness and in most cases is asymmetrical and predominantly focal. Fatigue, myalgias, and atrophy are common. Fasciculations are occasional accompaniments, but are increased by exercise. The course is slow, stepwise, and unpredictable, but the weakness and decreasing levels of function are progressive, although there are long periods of subjective stability. Upper motor neuron signs are not present.[1412] See also **postpoliomyelitis syndromes**.

post-pump chorea The development of choreic and athetoid movements in up to 18% of small children within 2 weeks of cardiopulmonary bypass operations when deep hypothermia is used. The clinical accompaniments range from mild learning disability to profound hypotonia and lethal obtundation.[4278]

postrotational nystagmus See **vestibular nystagmus**.

postrotational response Nystagmus induced by sudden cessation of a velocity-step rotation.[3762]

postsaccadic drift See **glissade**.

post sino-cibal syndrome See **Chinese restaurant syndrome**.

poststroke depression The occurrence of long-lasting depression as diagnosed using the *DSM IV(TR)* criteria and present in about a third of subjects following a stroke. The criteria may be found at: http://www.behavenet.com/capsules/disorders/dsm4TRclassification.htm/. The site of the lesion seems to have little effect in determining the occurrence of the depression.[1027]

postsympathectomy neuralgia A pain syndrome appearing within 2 weeks of sympathectomy, characterized by deep boring pain in the proximal part of the affected limb with local tenderness and lasting a few weeks.[418]

posttetanic The period following a tetanus.

posttetanic depression See **postactivation depression**.

posttetanic facilitation See **facilitation, potentiation**.

posttetanic potentiation 1. The incrementing mechanical response of muscle during and after repetitive nerve stimulation. 2. In central nervous system physiology, enhancement of excitability or reflex outflow ofneuronal systems following a long period of high-frequency stimulation. See also **facilitation, potentiation**. (From the 2001 Report of the Nomenclature Committee of the American Association of Electromyography and Electrodiagnosis.[19] Reproduced by kind permission of the AANEM.)

posttraumatic amnesia A period of time following a concussion during which the subject is unable to make a permanent record of his experiences. The period ends when his capacity to retain information continuously is regained. Its duration is regarded as a crude but reliable indicator of the severity of the cerebral trauma sustained.

posttraumatic angiospasm See **reflex sympathetic dystrophy**.

posttraumatic apoplexy The occurrence of an intracerebral hematoma days after cerebral trauma.

posttraumatic dysesthesia A neurogenic dysesthetic pain syndrome occurring some months after paraplegia caused by trauma at any level of the cord, including cordotomy.[6752]

posttraumatic edema See **reflex sympathetic dystrophy**.

posttraumatic encephalopathy A prolonged period of impaired intellectual functioning with variable somatic complaints occurring after craniocerebral trauma.[3190]

posttraumatic epilepsy The occurrence of seizures related to a previous episode of head injury sustained more than a week before. Factors identified as increasing the risk of subsequent seizures include dural penetration or loss of consciousness at the time of the original trauma; the occurrence of neurological deficit; wounds in the centro-parietal area; intracerebral, extradural, or subdural hemorrhage; and seizures occurring during the first week after the injury.[1985]

Two forms are defined: *early*, the commoner form, in which partial motor or generalized tonic–clonic seizures occur within a week of head trauma and usually in the first 24 h and *late*, in which generalized tonic–clonic, complex partial or partial motor seizures occur after that time. Either penetrating or nonpenetrating injuries may be responsible in either case.[3203, 3204]

postpoliomyelitis syndrome (PPS)

A slowly progressive neuromuscular disease occurring in individuals who have recovered from paralytic poliomyelitis and manifesting as new weakness, muscle fatigability, general fatigue, and muscle or joint pain. Less commonly new muscular atrophy, respiratory insufficiency, sleep abnormalities including sleep apnea, dysarthria, dysphagia, muscle cramps, cold intolerance, fasciculations, and new or progressive joint deformities occur. The usual latency following prior poliomyelitis is more than a quarter of a century.

The primary criteria necessary for the diagnosis are a history of paralytic poliomyelitis with partial or complete recovery of neurological function followed by a period of stability (usually several decades); persistent new muscle weakness or abnormal muscle fatigability; and the exclusion of other causes of new symptoms. The etiology is likely due to a distal degeneration of enlarged postpoliomyelitis motor units, while contributing factors may be aging (with motor neuron loss), overuse, and disuse.[6393] A persisting intrathecal immune response to the poliovirus is frequently present.[5762] The condition probably represents the exhaustion of overstressed motor neurons as they try to maintain innervation of the unusually large number of myofibrils in each of the few remaining motor units.[1414]

A synthesis of suggested diagnostic criteria[2709, 4539, 1965] follows:

1. A confirmed prior episode of paralytic poliomyelitis with residual motor neuron loss
2. A period of neurologic recovery, followed by an interval of stability (partial to fairly complete neurologic and functional recovery, usually for ≥15 years)
3. The gradual or abrupt onset of two or more of the following health problems since achieving a period of stability:
    - Unaccustomed fatigue, muscle, and/or joint pain
    - New weakness in muscles previously affected and/or unaffected
    - Functional loss
    - New muscle atrophy
    - Cold intolerance
4. Exclusion of other conditions that could explain the findings in point 3 above.

See also the NINDS informational Web site: http//www.ninds.nih.gov/disorders/post_polio/post_polio.htm/.

posttraumatic headache

Those headaches that follow upon some form of craniocerebral trauma. Various forms are differentiated in the 2004 International Classification of Headache Disorders (ICHD).[2820] The criteria for the acute types are given in Chart P–17, and those for the chronic type in Chart P–18.

Related is *acute posttraumatic headache attributed to mild head injury* for which the criteria are the same as the foregoing except that the loss of consciousness lasted for less than 30 min; the GCS score was 13 or higher; and the headache resolves within 3 months after head trauma.

For *acute headache attributed to other head and/or neck*, the ICHD criteria are very similar.

A related form is *acute headache attributed to whiplash injury*. The IHS committee pointed out that the term *whiplash* commonly refers to sudden acceleration/deceleration of the neck (usually due to a motor vehicle accident). The clinical manifestations include symptoms and signs that relate to the neck, as well as somatic extracervical, neurosensory, behavioral, cognitive, and affective disorders whose appearance and modes of expression and evolution can vary widely over time. Their diagnostic criteria specify that any kind of headache syndrome can occur following sudden and significant acceleration/deceleration movements of the neck, associated at the time with neck pain and developing within a week of whiplash injury. It usually resolves within 3 months. (Adapted from the International Classification of Headache Disorders [Headache Classification Committee of the International Headache Society. *Cephalalgia* 2004; **24**(Suppl 1)] by kind permission of Dr. Jes Olesen, the International Headache Society, and Wiley-Blackwell Publications.)

Closely-related to this is *chronic headache attributed to whiplash injury* for which the ICHD criteria are the same as the foregoing except that criterion D now reads, "Headache persists for >3 months after whiplash injury."

An unusual variant is *acute postcraniotomy headache*, a headache of variable intensity, maximal in the area of the craniotomy, developing within a week of the craniotomy and commonly resolving in less than 3 months, although persistence is recognized.

The ICHD Classification[2820] recognizes the following varieties: acute and chronic posttraumatic headache (attributed to moderate or severe head injury); acute or chronic headache attributed to whiplash

Chart P–17. Diagnostic Criteria for Acute Post-Traumatic Headache

Acute post-traumatic headache attributed to moderate or severe head injury. Diagnostic criteria have been defined:

A. Headache, no typical characteristics known, fulfilling criteria C and D
B. Head trauma with at least one of the following:
    1. Loss of consciousness for >30 min.
    2. Glasgow coma scale [score] <13
    3. Post-traumatic amnesia for >48 h
    4. Imaging demonstration of a traumatic brain lesion (cerebral hematoma, intracerebral and/or subarachnoid hemorrhage, brain contusion and/or skull fracture)
C. Headache develops within 7 days after head trauma or after regaining consciousness following head trauma
D. One or other of the following:
    1. Headache resolves within 3 months after head trauma
    2. Headache persists but 3 months have not yet passed since head trauma

Adapted from the International Classification of Headache Disorders (Headache Classification Committee of the International Headache Society. *Cephalalgia* 2004;**24**[Suppl 1]) by kind permission of Dr. Jes Olesen, the International Headache Society and Wiley-Blackwell Publications.)

Chart P–18. Diagnostic Criteria for Chronic Posttraumatic Headache

Chronic headache attributed to other head and/or neck trauma, for which the ICHD criteria are the same as those for the acute form except that criterion D now reads: "Headache persists for >3 months after the head and/or neck trauma".

Headache attributed to epidural hematoma Diagnostic criteria have been defined:

A. Acute-onset headache, no other typical characteristics known, fulfilling criteria C and D
B. Neuroimaging evidence of epidural hematoma
C. Headache develops within minutes to 24 h after development of the hematoma
D. One or other of the following:
   1. Headache resolves within 3 months after evacuation of the hematoma
   2. Headache persists but 3 months have not yet passed since evacuation of the hematoma.

Related to this is *headache attributed to subdural hematoma* for which the ICHD criteria are the same as the foregoing except that criterion B now reads; "Neuroimaging evidence of subdural hematoma".

Adapted from the International Classification of Headache Disorders (Headache Classification Committee of the International Headache Society. Cephalalgia 2004;**24** *{Suppl 1} by kind permission of Dr. Jes Olesen, the International Headache Society and Wiley-Blackwell Publications.)*

injury; headache attributed to traumatic intracranial hematoma (epidural hematoma, subdural hematoma); acute or chronmic headache attributed to other head and/or neck trauma; and acute and chronic **postcraniotomy headache**.

posttraumatic syndrome A condition of asthenia, irritability, diminished concentration, depression, and frequently headache following head trauma that was severe enough to have caused at least a brief period of unconsciousness.

posttraumatic hypersomnia A dyssomnia that occurs as a result of a traumatic event involving the CNS, characterized clinically by complaints of excessive sleepiness and frequent daily sleep episodes, their onset temporally associated with head trauma, and with normal timing, quality, and duration of sleep. The **minimal sleep latency test** shows a mean latency of less than 10 min and less than two sleep-onset REM sleep periods as recorded by polysomnography.[1629]

posttraumatic movement disorders Tremors, Parkinsonism, and generalized or segmental axial dystonias of central or peripheral origin, occurring either as a direct result of the trauma on the nervous system or by acceleration of a pre-existing condition.[3158]

posttraumatic neuralgia (cold pain) Intense, deep throbbing pain in the hand or foot, referred proximally and resembling the normal person's sensation of intense cold, brought on by cold or by deep pressure in the area bordering the zone of complete anesthesia following a peripheral nerve injury. It is a variant of Head's **hyperesthesia**, but differs from **causalgia** in its restriction to the innervation territory of the affected nerve and in the response to cooling.[1590]

posttraumatic neurosis See **disability neurosis**.

posttraumatic osteoporosis See **reflex sympathetic dystrophy**.

posttraumatic pain syndrome See **reflex sympathetic dystrophy**.

posttraumatic Parkinson disease Criteria for the diagnosis have been suggested by Crouzon,[1359] who considers that the trauma shall have been sufficiently violent to cause concussion; the time between the trauma and the onset of Parkinsonism must be short, and that an uninterrupted course of Parkinson disease should follow.

posttraumatic paroxysmal choreoathetosis A syndrome characterized by the occurrence of attacks of typical paroxysmal choreoathetosis within a month or two after recovery of consciousness from a head injury without abnormal EEG activity or imaging evidence of lesions of the basal ganglia. The reported response to anticonvulsants suggests that the condition may have an epileptic basis.[1710]

posttraumatic stress disorder (shellshock, nostalgia) A multisymptom complex occurring in some subjects following severe and distressing physical or emotional trauma outside the range of normal human experience. The disturbance causes clinically significant distress or impairment in social, occupational, or other important areas of functioning. It has also been defined in the ICD-10, accessible at http://www.nimh.nih.gov/health/publications/adhd/symptoms.shtml/ as an anxiety disorder that can develop after exposure to a terrifying event or ordeal in which grave physical harm occurred or was threatened. The traumatic events that may trigger PTSD include violent personal assaults, natural or human-caused disasters, accidents, or military combat.

People with PTSD have persistent frightening thoughts and memories of their ordeal and may experience sleep problems, feel detached, or be easily startled. The person who develops PTSD may have been the one who was harmed but alternatively the harm may have happened to a loved one or the person may have witnessed a harmful event. Though first brought to public attention in relation to war veterans, it can also result from a variety of traumatic incidents such as mugging, rape, torture, being kidnapped or held captive, child abuse, car accidents, train wrecks, plane crashes, bombings, or natural disasters such as floods or earthquakes.

People with PTSD may startle easily, become emotionally numb (especially in relation to people with whom they used to be close), lose interest in things they used to enjoy, have trouble feeling affectionate, be irritable, become more aggressive, or even become violent. They avoid situations that remind them of the original incident, and anniversaries of the incident are often very difficult. PTSD symptoms seem to be worse if the event that triggered them was deliberately initiated by another person, as in a mugging or a kidnapping. Most people with PTSD repeatedly relive the trauma in their thoughts during the day and in nightmares when they sleep. These are called flashbacks. Flashbacks may consist of images, sounds, smells, or feelings, and are often triggered by ordinary occurrences, such as a door slamming or a car backfiring on the street. A person having a flashback may lose touch with reality and believe that the traumatic incident is happening all over again.

Not every traumatized person develops full-blown or even minor PTSD. Symptoms usually begin within 3 months of the incident but occasionally emerge years afterward. They must last more than a month to be considered PTSD. The course of the illness varies. Some people recover within 6 months, while others have symptoms that last much longer. In some people, the condition becomes chronic.

The major indices are that there shall have been exposure to a traumatic event that is persistently re-experienced in any of several ways; the subject avoids reminders of the event and displays a numbness of feeling to it; and has symptoms of increased arousal such as insomnia, mood swings, impaired concentration, and increased startle reactions.

The American Psychiatric Association *DSM IV-TR diagnostic guidelines*[172] can be found at http://www.behavenet.com/capsules/disorders/dsm4TRclassification.htm/.

posttraumatic syndrome

A condition of asthenia, irritability, diminished concentration, depression, and frequently headache following head trauma that was severe enough to have caused at least a brief period of unconsciousness. See also **de Morsier syndrome**.

posttraumatic syringomyelia

The occurrence of a syrinx, usually at thoracic or cervical levels, months or years after spinal cord injury.[1833, 5665]

posttraumatic tremor Postural and kinetic tremor of the hands and head occurring 1–4 weeks after mild head injury, often accompanied by myoclonic-like jerking. The shaking resembles that of **essential tremor**.[615]

posttussive syndrome See **cough syncope**.

postural deviation Tilting or movement of the whole body in the direction of the flow of endolymph provoked by caloric testing or by intrinsic disease of the vestibular system. This is noted when the subject walks heel-to-toe or along a straight line on the floor.

postural motor seizure The adoption of a posture which may be bilaterally symmetrical or asymmetrical (as in a "fencing posture") during a seizure.[16]

postural orthostatic tachycardia syndrome (POTS)

(neuro-mediated cardiogenic syncope) A mild and treatable form of autonomic dysfunction presenting with modest falls in blood pressure that are insufficient to cause actual syncope, but produce near-syncope with vertigo, dizziness, atrial tachycardia, disabling fatigue, exercise intolerance, and lightheadedness accompanying postural tachycardia. It usually is seen in young people who experience recurrent episodes leading to neurocardiogenic syncope that occur without warning. Diagnosis is facilitated by head-upright tilt table testing, which demonstrates a heart rate increase of $\geq$30 beats/min (or a maximum heart rate of 120 beats/min) within the first 10 min upright (unassociated with profound hypotension), reproducing the symptoms.

Central serotonergic mechanisms appear to participate in the pathogenesis of such recurrent neurally mediated syncope. Aside from the secondary risks of sudden syncope, the condition is usually not life-threatening.[2597]

postural reflexes Involuntary patterns of muscle contraction designed to compensate for shifts in gravity with alterations in body position. Such neural equilibratory mechanisms are of two kinds:

Anticipatory postural responses are truncal adjustments made immediately preceding a limb movement in order to preserve balance.

Reactive postural responses are sequential postural reactions to a shift of the center of gravity of the body when standing.[4723] (Reproduced by kind permission of the American Academy of Neurology and Lippincott Williams and Wilkins.)

Postural control declines with age, as assessed by counting the number of steps a (forewarned) patient takes backward in response to a modest thrust on the sternum; two to four steps are considered evidence of moderate impairment.[2596, 6696, 6266] See also **rescue reactions, protective reactions**.

postural syncope (areflexic syndrome) Reduction in consciousness as a result of reduced cerebral perfusion after attaining the upright posture. The mechanisms of this may be either vasovagal, or an impairment of autonomic reflex function.

postural tremor Tremor present when the subject voluntarily maintains a position against gravity. When it appears, usually during the performance of visually guided tasks, it may be called *position-specific postural tremor*. See **cerebellar tremors, tremor**.

posturography A standardized quantitative laboratory method of studying vestibulo-ocular function, in which patients with dysequilibrium stand on a platform and the amount of body sway is analyzed when standing level or with anteroposterior or lateral tilt of the platform and with the eyes open and closed.[2046, 23]

postvaccinal encephalomyelitis

See **disseminated vasculomyelinopathy**.

postvaccinial encephalomyelitis

A potentially lethal multifocal immunological, inflammatory, and demyelinating polioencephalopathy occurring as a complication in subjects who have received primary vaccination. In children younger than 2 years, encephalitis may develop abruptly in the first 10 days after vaccination, presenting with any combination of fever, malaise, irritability, headache and vomiting, hyperactivity or somnolence or coma, apnea, **Jacksonian seizures**, aphasia, VI nerve palsy, hemiplegia, Guillain–Barré syndrome, stiff neck, and **opisthotonos**. Survivors are usually left with mental impairment and paralysis.

In older children, the encephalitis occurs 10 days after vaccination, with fever, vomiting, malaise, lethargy, personality changes, paraparesis, headache, anorexia, confusion and drowsiness, generalized and focal motor seizures, and coma. The brain is hyperemic, with lymphocytic infiltration of the meninges and degeneration of the ganglia. Mortality is 10–35% within 7 days of onset. Survivors are often left with upper motor neuron paralyses and mental impairment. Except for its causation, the condition is identical with **post infectious encephalomyelitis**.

postventilatory paretic syndrome An acquired syndrome of unknown cause occurring in adults or in children, characterized by neurogenic or myopathic weakness due to axonal neuropathy developing after a period of assisted ventilation for asthma or other severe pulmonary or meningitic illness. See **Hopkins syndrome, acute myopathy**, and **critical illness polyneuropathy**, the conditions variously considered to be responsible.[2913, 3633]

postviral asthenia See **chronic fatigue syndrome**.

potassium-aggravated myotonia A sodium channelopathy presenting with muscle stiffness after exercise.

potassium exercise test A standardized exercise test designed to show that increases in serum potassium levels as a result of exercise (80–100 W on a bicycle ergometer) are less than normal in subjects with the hypokalemic variety of **familial periodic paralysis**.[3291]

potassium depletion myopathy An acute myopathy associated with endogenous or drug-induced potassium loss, and presenting with flaccid muscle weakness without sensory loss, myalgia, polyuria, and polydipsia. Serum CK levels are markedly raised. Atrophy of type 2 fibers is observed on muscle biopsy specimens. The condition reverses with potassium repletion.[1262]

potassium-sensitive myotonia See **myotonia fluctuans**.

potential 1. A difference in charge (measured in volts) that exists between two points. Most biologically produced potentials arise from the difference in charge between two sides of a cell membrane. 2. A physiologically recorded waveform. (After the 2001 Report of the Nomenclature Committee of the American Association of Electromyography and Electrodiagnosis.[19] Reproduced by kind permission of the AANEM.)

potential field The amplitude distribution of an EEG wave at the surface of the head or of the cerebral cortex or in the depth of the brain, measured at a given instant in time, and usually represented in diagrams by equipotential lines. (Adapted from the 1974 report of the Committee on Terminology, IFCN. In: Chatrian GE, Bergamini L, Dondey M, et al. A glossary of terms most commonly used by clinical electroencephalographers. *EEG Clin Neurophysiol* 1974;**37**:538–48. Reproduced with kind permission from the IFCN and Elsevier Science.)

potentiation Physiologically, the enhancement of a response. The convention is to use the term to describe the incrementing mechanical response of muscle elicited by repetitive nerve stimulation, e.g., **posttetanic potentiation**, whereas the term **facilitation** is used to describe the incrementing electrical response elicited by repetitive nerve stimulation, e.g., postactivation facilitation. (From the 2001 Report of the Nomenclature Committee of the American Association of Electromyography and Electrodiagnosis.[19] Reproduced by kind permission of the AANEM.)[6325] See also **incrementing response**.

potomania An abnormal desire to drink. (HJM)

Pott, Sir Percival (1714–1788) English surgeon at St. Bartholomew's Hospital. Pott's fracture was that of the fibula, originally described in himself following a fall from a horse. He also described cancer of the scrotum in chimney-sweep children and wrote on hernias and head injury as well as the following condition, in 1779.

Pott paraplegia Paraplegia due to compressive myelopathy, the latter resulting from tuberculous spondylitis (caries of the vertebral column), local accumulations of tuberculous pus or granulation tissue, or as a result of vertebral collapse or dislocation.[5099] See also **chronic spinal meningitis**.

Potter syndrome (oligohydramnios syndrome) A recessively inherited congenital dysmorphic syndrome, characterized by oligohydramnios prior to birth, and thereafter by growth retardation, lung hypoplasia, bilateral renal agenesis, dry skin, micrognathia, limb deformities, defects of neuronal migration with cerebellar heterotopias, and, in some cases, hydrocephalus.[2601]

Potzl, Otto (1877–1962) Austrian psychiatrist who graduated from Vienna, where he spent most of his professional life, latterly as professor of neurology and psychiatry.

Potzl syndrome Word blindness with hemianopia and disturbance of the recognition of colors.[5100]

Pourfour du Petit, Francois (1664–1741) French ophthalmologist, anatomist, and army surgeon who described contralateral innervation as a result of the decussation of the pyramids in his *Lettres d'un médecin des hospitaux* (Naumur, 1710) as well as the anatomy of the sympathetic chain and the ocular signs resulting from damage to it, as in the following syndrome which he observed in soldiers wounded by sabres.

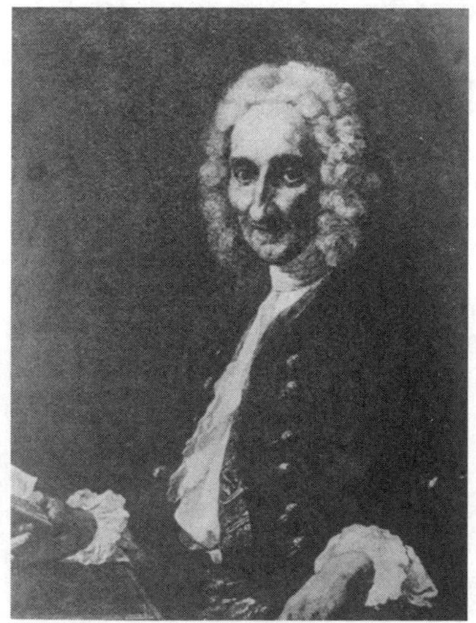

Figure P–1 Francois Pourfour du Petit

Pourfour du Petit syndrome (cervical sympathetic irritation syndrome) Mydriasis, exophthalmos, widening of the palpebral fissure, and increased intraocular pressure as a result of irritation of the sympathetic chain in the neck. This represents the inverse of **Horner syndrome**.[1720]

Powassan encephalitis A tick-borne direct infection of the brain by a flavivirus member of the togavirus group of arboviruses, and representing another member of the **Russian spring-summer encephalitis** complex but characteristically causing only sporadic (but severe) encephalitis with convulsions, respiratory failure, coma, and frequently death. The condition is described rarely, mainly affecting children, in all parts of the Northern United States and Southern Canada.[6816]

Practical Neurology A neurology digest journal covering current research, practice, and thinking in neurology, published by BMJ Journals and complementing the *Journal of Neurology, Neurosurgery and Psychiatry*.

Prader syndrome (pseudodeficiency rickets) A congenital dysmorphic syndrome manifesting also short stature, dental and skeletal anomalies, aminoaciduria and renal tubular acidosis, hypocalcemia, multiple fractures, hypotonia, seizures, and delayed closure of the fontanelles.[381]

Prader–Willi syndrome (hypotonia, hypomentia, hypogonadism, obesity syndrome, HHHO syndrome) A complex multisystem chromosomal disorder. The diagnostic features (present in over 90% of cases) include congenital mental retardation; cerebellar ataxia; infantile hypotonia; short stature; obesity after infancy; cryptorchidism; hypogonadism; diabetes, strabismus, and various musculoskeletal and dysmorphic deformities, including ocular hypertelorism; low-set ears with overlapping helix; high-arched palate; micrognathia; microdontia; defective dental enamel; and partial syndactyly of the toes. Most affected subjects have a deletion at 15q11.[1054, 1236]

prae- (pre-) (Lat, in front of, before) Prefix denoting before.

pragmatic decoding The utilization of non language cues to assist in decoding verbal meaning.

prandic epilepsy See **eating epilepsy**.

praxis The function of performance, as of a manual task; the execution of a learned movement in response to an appropriate stimulus, in the presence of normal afferent and efferent functions and without lack of attentiveness or of cooperation. This may be assessed formally by, for example, the **Block Design test**, using patterned cubes; by constructional tasks; and by having the patient perform complex movements on command or in imitation.

preacher's hand (main de prédicateur) Extension of the metacarpophalangeal joints, flexion of the interphalangeal joints, and extension of the thumb as a result of combined median and ulnar nerve pareses, which put the hand into the position traditionally assumed by priests during the act of blessing.

preangular alexia (anterior alexia) See **alexia**.

precentral area See **motor cortex**.

prechiasmal syndrome (Lat, before + Gr, decussation) Compression of an optic nerve and of the olfactory, as by a presellar meningioma, which later grows back to involve the optic chiasm. Initially there is involvement of one optic nerve, including the fibers within **von Willebrand's knee**; at a later stage, a **Foster Kennedy syndrome** may be also present.

preclinical multiple sclerosis A speculative diagnosis made in asymptomatic patients with a normal neurological examination whose MRI scans fulfill the Barkhof–Tintoré criteria for multiple sclerosis. About a third of them do in fact develop MS after a mean delay of 6 months.[3740]

precocious Alzheimer disease See **congophilic angiopathy**.

precognition See **prescience**.

precommunal posterior cerebral artery That segment of the artery proximal to the posterior communicating artery.

precordial catch syndrome See **Texidor twinge**.

predormital myoclonus See **sleep starts**.

prefixation An anatomical variant in which the optic chiasm is situated unusually far forward with reference to the sella turcica, such that it lies above the tuber cinereum.

prefixation blindness The inability to see objects introduced into the space between the subject and the point of fixation, as the result of overlap of the two blind hemifields when the eyes of a patient with binasal hemianopia converge.[5027]

prefrontal leukotomy See **prefrontal lobotomy**.

prefrontal lobotomy (prefrontal leukotomy) An operation introduced by Egas **Moniz**, designed to free schizophrenic patients from the torment of their disordered thinking. Latterly it was found of some use in the management of obsessive-compulsive states and of depressive illnesses, but its wide use, frequently in cases where the blunting of affect and the dilution of personality characteristics were more troublesome than the original disorder of mentation, led to its vilification and eventual disuse.[1816, 2194]

preganglionic neurons Those neurons of the parasympathetic and sympathetic systems arising from the CNS and passing to the peripheral ganglia. The name was attached by J.N. **Langley**.

preherpetic neuralgia Severe, burning radicular pain felt in those dermatomal regions destined to bear the acute lesions of herpes zoster between a week and 3 months later.[2379]

preictal pseudosleep A state behaviorally resembling normal sleep in that the subject is motioness with the eyes closed, although the EEG shows a persisting alpha rhythm. It is recorded as preceding the appearance of **pseudoseizures** (nonepileptic seizures).[504]

premature aging with telangiectasias See **Breathnach syndrome**.

premature senility syndrome (Hutchinson–Gilford syndrome) See **progeria**.

premaxillary agenesis A congenital, sporadic, dominantly or recessively inherited dysmorphic syndrome reflecting disordered embryonal differentiation and characterized by midline cleft lip, microcephaly, flattened nose, hypotelorism, mental and developmental delay, seizures, spastic quadriparesis, and impaired vision with colobomas. Hypopituitarism is commonly associated. The chromosomal abnormalities include trisomy 13 or 18, deletions at 18p- and 13q-, etc.[1235]

premotor area An arbitrary term for that area of brain lying immediately anterior to the **motor cortex;** its posterior border is ill-defined and its functions and those of the motor cortex overlap or may even be the same, except that damage to this region leads to motor **apraxia** rather than to hemiplegia. Damage to the areas immediately anterior to it gives rise to slowness of movements and perseveration.

premotor syndrome According to **Fulton**, a syndrome bearing witness to the effects of lesions of the premotor cortex. This syndrome has four main components: inability to perform skilled movements, particularly with the digits, without gross impairment of motor power; spasticity and an increase in the muscle stretch reflexes; forced grasping; and vasomotor disturbances, often with Jacksonian seizures in addition. **Walshe,**[6623] however, criticized this formulation and considered that apraxia of movement was the only important consequence of such lesions.

presbyacusis Deafness occuring with advancing age.

presbyophrenia Dementia occurring with advancing age.

presbyopia (from Gr, old man + eye) Impairment of the power of accommodation with aging.

prescience A profound sense of "knowing" what is going to happen in their environment in the immediate future, experienced as an aura by some patients with temporal lobe epilepsy.[5493]

"presenile" dementia A term with no useful meaning, there being no notable difference either in the characteristics of a disease attacking mankind after as opposed to before the age of 65 years or indeed in the people themselves. The term is best reserved as a pejorative for political opponents rather than as one bundling together such entities as early-onset **Alzheimer disease,** the **frontotemporal dementias, dementia with Lewy bodies**, and prion disorders such as **Creutzfeldt–Jakob disease**.

"presenile" dementia–motor neuron disease (ALS–Parkinson–dementia syndromes) A dementing syndrome of adult onset manifesting behavioral and speech disturbances, bulbar palsies, pyramidal signs, and cerebral atrophy with gliosis and spongy changes in the cerebral cortex. See **amyotrophic lateral sclerosis**.

Present Behavioral examination A semistructured examination with 121 main questions assessing mental health and abnormal behavior in patienst with dementia, administered to a caregiver.[2981]

Present State examination A semistructured psychiatric interview used mainly in the diagnosis of dementia.[6824]

presque vu (Fr, almost seen) An internal feeling of patients with visual field defects that they are going to see something within the blind field; a feeling not borne out by subsequent experience.

pressor nerves Those sympathetic nerves which, when stimulated, lead to arteriolar vasoconstriction and thus to an increase in blood pressure.

pressure palsy Weakness as a result of conduction block occurring in a peripheral nerve compressed as a result of internal derangements caused by external forces; the loss of function of a peripheral nerve due to incidental compression. The compression has presumably led to ischemia with local conduction block; it is usually reversible within months unless the severity of compression has led to **axonotmesis**.

A *variant* familial form occurs, with onset at any age, in which weakness and sensory loss with autonomic dysfunction occur randomly in peripheral nerves in the presence of relatively minor compressive lesions.

pressure sensation The awareness of deep, nonpainful compressive distortion of a body part. This function is mediated by the same pathways as subserve discriminative touch sensation, and uses the larger myelinated fibers in the peripheral and in the posterior columns of the CNS. The term *touch-pressure sensation* underscores the similarity of the two modalities, which indeed may form a continuum.

pressure–volume index That volume of CSF required to produce a 10-fold increase in CSF pressure; a calculation of value physiologically in assessing CSF formation and absorption rates and clinically in prognosticating the outcome after severe head injuries.[4140]

pretectal pseudobobbing Involuntary, repetitive, rapid, arrhythmic, downward, and inward eye movements with a faster downstroke than upstroke, occurring at slow rates and associated with pretectal rather than with pontine lesions, such as acute obstructive hydrocephalus. A blink precedes most of the movements, which may represent a form of spontaneous convergence nystagmus.[3357]

pretectal syndrome A collection of ocular changes associated with lesions of the dorsal brainstem at the level of the superior colliculus, characterized by limitation of downward gaze; retraction of the upper lid; convergence–retraction eye movements; paralysis of convergence; dysjunctive eye positions including esotropia and skew deviation; and nystagmus. The pupillary abnormalities include diminished light response, **light-near dissociation**, and **anisocoria**.[3361] See **dorsal midbrain syndrome**.

pretraumatic amnesia See **retrograde amnesia**.

pretrigeminal neuralgia A mild "toothache" or "sinus-like" pain felt in the distribution of the trigeminal nerve, triggered by jaw movement or drinking hot or cold liquids and preceding by days or years acute episodes of **trigeminal neuralgia** in the same facial region.[2219]

Preus syndrome A congenital dysmorphic syndrome characterized also by low birth-weight, small mouth, cleft palate, dwarfism, coarse hair, hernias, skeletal anomalies, sensorineural deafness, cryptorchidism, hypotonia, myoclonic seizures and mental and developmental delay.[381]

Prevention and Treatment of Wernicke–Korsakoff Syndrome An informational site of the Medical Council on Alcohol. Web site: http://www.medicouncilalcol.demon.co.uk/.

Prévost sign (Vulpian sign) Conjugate deviation of the head and eyes toward the side of an acute cerebral lesion and away from the paralysed side.[5116] See also **conjugate eye deviation, Vulpian sign**.

priapism (from Lat, Priapus—the god of procreation) Sustained penile erections, as may occur in men with incomplete spinal cord lesions or on walking, when it may be a sign of **spinal** (canal) **stenosis**.

primary adhalinopathy See **myopathy** (*severe childhood muscular dystrophy*)

primary alcoholic dementia A non-entity.[6542] See instead **Wernicke–Korsakoff encephalopathy, pellagra encephalopathy, Marchiafava–Bignami disease,** and **acquired hepatocerebral encephalopathy**.

primary aldosteronism See **Conn syndrome**.

primary alveolar hypoventilation syndrome See **congenital central hypoventilation syndrome**.

primary amnesia A monosymptomatic cognitive disorder in which there is slowly developing amnesia in the absence of other signs of cortical functional impairment such as that of language, praxis, perception, or calculation.[3947]

primary angiitis of the central nervous system See **Aβ-related angiitis**.[1314]

primary antiphospholipid syndrome The occurrence of clinical thrombotic disease and/or fetal loss in association with thrombocytopenia and the presence of antiphospholipid antibodies in the blood. Young adults are predominantly affected; noninflammatory thrombotic occlusion of large or small arteries or veins causes, variously, spontaneous abortion, migraine, seizures, multi-infarct dementia, chorea, **amaurosis fugax** or retinal artery occlusion, cardiac murmurs, mitral valve lesions, and livedo reticularis.[2887]

primary autonomic failure See **progressive autonomic failure**.

primary basilar impression A bony deformity characterized by indentation of the floor of the posterior fossa by the atlas, diminishing its volume, and not due to bone disease such as osteomalacia or Paget disease. The condition may be asymptomatic or associated with features suggesting the **Chiari** malformation.

primary cerebrovascular amyloidosis See **congophilic angiopathy**.

primary chronic cluster headache See **chronic cluster headache**.

primary chronic insomnia An idiopathic syndrome of lifelong fragmentation of sleep with daytime fatigue, tension, and depression, sometimes associated with signs of minimal brain damage.

primary CNS lymphoma (reticulum cell sarcoma, perivascular sarcoma, microglioma, perithelial small cell sarcoma, primary [malignant] cerebral lymphoma, immunoblastic sarcoma) A potentially fatal primary neurological malignancy characterized by the presence of multiple deep intracerebral (periventricular) or sub-meningeal lymphomatous masses, their histological appearance similar to that of systemic non-Hodgkin lymphoma, and consisting of large lymphoid cells, perivascular histiocytes, microglia, plasma cells and various (mainly B) forms of lymphocytes with multiplication of the basement membranes of those blood vessels involved by the lymphomatous process. The B-cell and T-cell types can be differentiated by immunocytochemistry.[4739] It can also appear in the eye, the spinal cord, and the peripheral nerves.

Clinically, the tumor presents as a supratentorial solitary lesion in 80% of cases, producing the clinical syndromes of confusion, dementia, increased intracranial pressure or focal CNS signs, and seizures; uveocyclitis is unusually common. Both progressive and relapsing-remitting courses are described. Such features are increasingly seen in this decade as a complication of immunosuppression, as in **AIDS**,[4200] as well as of congenital immunodeficiency syndromes, drug therapy, and collagen vascular diseases, but in the past the tumor was found to affect mainly males during later adult life. Enhancement of a mass in the gray matter or the corpus callosum without surrounding edema, and contrast-enhancing lesions in contact with the subarachnoid space and without necrosis are characteristic findings on CT or MRI scans. They sometimes appear well before the clinical manifestations of the disease (*sentinel lesions*).[6860] The tumor is exquisitely sensitive to steroid treatment, which induces lysis of its cells.

Lesions are located in deep structures only in one-third of the cases, and rarely involve the posterior fossa. Most are hyperdense or isodense on CT scans, hypointense or isointense on T1 weighted MRI images. Nearly all enhance. Meningeal or ventricular enhancement is rare but suggestive.[1297] See also **intravascular lymphomatosis** (primary intravascular lymphoma).

primary cough headache (benign cough headache, Valsalva-maneuver headache) Headache of sudden onset and lasting from 1 s to 30 min resulting from temporary impaction of the cerebellar tonsils below the foramen magnum due to the pressure difference between the ventricles and the lumbar subarachnoid space during coughing, etc. but in the absence of any intracranial disorder. **Idiopathic intracranial hypotension** is another cause.

The headache occurs only in association with coughing and/or sneezing, straining, e.g., during bowel movements, laughing, or stooping or any other activity that induces a Valsalva maneuver. Because possible etiologies include **Chiari** malformation type

1, posterior fossa mass lesions, basilar impression, intracranial hemorrhage, and brain tumours, MRI of the brain must be performed to exclude possible structural lesions.[1132]

primary degeneration of the granular layer of the cerebellum A congenital developmental abnormality leading to cerebellar ataxia. See **Lhermitte–Duclos disease**.

primary degenerative dementia Those forms of dementia caused by disease processes that primarily affect the CNS but which are neither infectious nor due to vasculopathy.[6871] Other organs may also be affected. The disease causes progressive dysfunction and degeneration of neurons and other cells. Four subgroups are defined (Chart P–19):[2647]

primary dementias Those dementing conditions due to degenerative disease of the brain affecting primarily the nerve cells.

primary deviation A phenomenon observed during the performance of the **alternate cover test** in a patient with a lesion of one of the oculomotor nerves causing muscle paresis. When patients direct their gaze in the direction of action of the affected muscle, deviation of the covered paretic eye away from the target is known as *primary deviation.* When they direct their gaze so that the paretic eye fixes on the target, the deviation of the covered normal eye is known as *secondary deviation*. The latter is of greater amplitude. See **Cover test**.

primary diffuse leptomeningeal gliomatosis A rare, fatal syndrome characterized by extensive basal and chronic infiltration of the meninges by tumor cells arising from heterotopic cell nests, without parenchymal involvement. The clinical presentation is typically with headache, raised intracranial pressure, and encephalopathy. Elevated CSF levels of protein and low glucose with moderate mononuclear pleocytosis are usual and in the absence of direct evidence of neoplasia commonly lead to a diagnosis of chronic meningitis. Meningeal biopsy may assist in making the diagnosis.[463]

primary diffuse meningeal melanomatosis See **melanomatosis**.

primary generalized epilepsies Seizure disorders without macroscopic pathological features, inherited either as polygenic or as autosomal dominant characteristics with age-dependent penetrance and characterized by **generalized tonic–clonic, myoclonic,** or **generalized absence** seizure types, either alone or in combination.

primary exertional headache (benign exertional headache, "weight-lifters' headache") Headache precipitated by any form of exercise. Diagnostic criteria have been defined:

A. Pulsating headache fulfilling criteria B and C.
B. Lasting from 5 min to 48 h.
C. Brought on by and occurring only during or after physical exertion.
D. Not attributed to another disorder.

From the International Classification of Headache Disorders (Headache Classification Committee of the International Headache Society. *Cephalalgia* 2004;24[Suppl 1]) by kind permission of Dr. Jes Olesen, the International Headache Society and Wiley-Blackwell Publications.

Exercise-induced **migraine** may also occur in such subjects.

primary generalized epilepsy of adolescence See **typical absence epilepsy of adolescence**.

primary generalized epileptic myoclonus A fragment of primary generalized epilepsy usually manifesting as small focal muscle jerks (**minipolymyoclonus**) or as generalized and precisely synchronized bodily jerks. The origin of the electrical discharge is considered to be an area of hyperexcitable cortex driven to synchrony by ascending impulses from subcortical regions.[2695]

primary headaches The ICHD[2820] lists these as **migraine, tension-type headache, cluster headache,** and **trigeminal autonomic cephalalgias;** also **hemicrania continua; hypnic headache; new daily-persistent headache; primary cough headache; primary exertional headache; primary headache associated with sexual activity; primary stabbing headache; primary thunderclap headache**.

primary headache associated with sexual activity (benign sex headache, coital cephalalgia, benign vascular sexual headache, sexual headache) Headaches precipitated by sexual activity, usually starting as a dull bilateral ache as sexual excitement increases and suddenly becoming intense at orgasm, in the absence of any intracranial disorder. Two forms are recognized:

Preorgasmic headache, for which diagnostic criteria have been defined:[2820]

A . Dull ache in the head and neck associated with awareness of neck and/or jaw muscle contraction and fulfilling criterion B
B . Occurs during sexual activity and increases with sexual excitement
C . Not attributed to another disorder

Chart P–19. Subgroups of Degenerative Dementia

Frontotemporal cortical predominance

- **Pick disease**.
- **Frontal lobe dementia**.
- ALS with dementia.
- Atypical **Alzheimer disease.**
- Rare familial forms.

Temporoparietal cortical predominance

- **Alzheimer disease** with early onset.
- **Alzheimer disease** with late onset.
- **Down syndrome** with dementia of Alzheimer type.

Subcortical Dementias.

Other forms

- **Parkinson disease with dementia.**
- **Diffuse Lewy body disease.**

After Gustafson L. Clinical classification of dementia conditions. Acta Neurol Scand ***Suppl*** *1992;*139:*16–20.*

Adapted from the International Classification of Headache Disorders (Headache Classification Committee of the International Headache Society. *Cephalalgia* 2004;**24**[Suppl 1]) by kind permission of Dr. Jes Olesen, the International Headache Society and Wiley-Blackwell Publications.

Orgasmic headache, a postural headache resembling that of low CSF pressure, developing after coitus.

primary hyperaldosteronism

(Conn syndrome) Excessive secretion of aldosterone by the adrenal cortex, leading to hypertension, sodium retention, hypokalemic alkalosis, muscle weakness, tetany, and, in some cases, to features of **familial periodic paralysis** (hypokalemic form).

primary hyperoxaluria

Two rare recessive disorders of glyoxalate metabolism characterized clinically by recurrent calcium oxalate nephrolithiasis leading to chronic renal failure with death from uremia. The pathological mechanism responsible is the deposition of calcium oxalate crystals within the kidney and within the walls of arterioles and venules in other organs. An associated neuropathy with both axonal degeneration and segmental demyelination has been reported rarely.[2688]

primary idiopathic dermatomyositis

A form of **idiopathic dysimmune inflammatory myopathy** in adults, resembling **primary idiopathic polymyositis** but showing in addition various skin changes including erythema affecting the butterfly area of the face and extensor limb surfaces and trunk, violet discoloration of the eyelids with periorbital edema, periungual hyperemia, telangiectasia, sclerodactyly, keratosis, and skin edema. See **dermatomyositis**.

primary idiopathic polymyositis

(isolated polymyositis) An acute inflammatory myopathy due to a disorder of the immune mechanisms. Clinically, the condition is characterized by acute, subacute, or chronically progressive proximal weakness and Raynaud phenomenon, with maximal incidence in childhood and again in mid-adult life. Arthralgia, bulbar and respiratory muscle involvement, and muscle pain are unusual and the skin is not involved.

Muscle biopsy specimens show little vascular change, but there is marked invasion of myofibrils by cytotoxic lymphocytes and macrophages and scattered muscle fiber necrosis is notable.[3310] The presence of skin changes should dictate the diagnosis of **dermatomyositis**.

The diagnostic criteria in Chart P–20 have been suggested by Hudgson (1984).[3026]

Chart P–20. Diagnostic criteria for Primary Idiopathic Polymyositis

A. Predominantly or exclusively proximal, usually symmetrical muscle weakness, progressive over weeks or months, with or without myalgia and with or without compatible dermatological features.
B. Biopsy evidence of muscle fiber necrosis, regeneration and mononuclear cellular infiltrate (perifascicular and intrafascicular) with or without perifascicular atrophy.
C. Elevated serum CK (MM isoenzyme), aldolase or myoglobin levels.
D. Multifocal EMG changes typical of myopathy (small, short-duration polyphasic motor potentials), with or without increased insertional activity and spontaneous potentials.

Definite polymyositis is diagnosed when all four criteria are satisfied; three criteria allow a diagnosis of *probable polymyositis*.

Adapted from Hudgson P, Peter JB. Classification (of Polymyositis). Clin Rheum Dis *1984;10:3–8, reproduced by permission.)*

primary intravascular lymphoma

See **intravascular lymphomatosis**.

primary intraventricular hemorrhage

The uncommon occurrence of hemorrhage into the ventricles without periventricular extension, usually as a result of bleeding from an arteriovenous malformation in a lateral ventricle, or as a result of **moyamoya disease**.[1451]

primary lateral sclerosis (PLS)

A syndrome of adult life with slowly progressive generalized, asymmetric spasticity starting most commonly in the legs, but sometimes in the arms or with speech, and resulting from circumscribed atrophy of the precentral gyrus where there is eventually a complete loss of Betz cells, decreased numbers of pyramidal neurons, and laminar gliosis in the external and internal pyramidal cell cortical layers. There are no lower motor neurone lesions and there is no cognitive impairment, though emotional lability does occur. Severe spastic dysarthria progressing to anarthria is usual.

Signs start most commonly in the legs, but can start in the arms, or with speech in the form of a progressive spastic dysarthria which all patients eventually develop. Other features include saccadic breakdown of smooth pursuit eye movements (in most), and urinary incontinence (in about half).

Patients become wheelchair bound after several years, but the rate of progression is variable. Cognitive impairment is absent but emotional lability common. MRI scans may show atrophy of the precentral gyrus.

Pathologically there is highly circumscribed atrophy of the precentral gyrus with complete loss of Betz cells, decreased numbers of pyramidal neurons, and laminar gliosis in the external and internal pyramidal cell cortical layers. No lower motor neuron abnormalities are found in hypoglossal or spinal nuclei and the substantia nigra is unaffected. Pathology in these cases sometimes shows the nonspecific degenerative changes of **frontotemporal dementia**. Degeneration of motor neurons in the motor cortices is a hallmark feature of motor neuron disease, and primary lateral sclerosis (PLS) has been thought by many to represent a pure upper motor neuron form of MND. Pathological confirmation of the diagnosis has seldom been achieved in life and confusion with cervical spondylotic myelopathy, stroke, **multiple sclerosis**, or **hereditary spastic paraparesis** is likely in many of the reported cases.[457] A genetic locus has been identified at 4ptel–4p16.1.[6460]

Erb in 1875 considered this is a rare variant of **amyotrophic lateral sclerosis** characterized by the isolated appearance of slowly progressive upper motor neuron lesion signs affecting all four limbs in the absence of any lower motor neurone signs and of disorder of cognition; that view is still disputed.

A categorization of PLS has been proposed (Gordon et al.),[2492] equating PLS with amyotrophic lateral sclerosis. This work is reproduced in Chart P–21 by kind permission of the American Academy of Neurology and Lippincott Williams and Wilkins.

Chart P–21. Diagnostic Categories of Upper Motor Neurone-Predominant Motor Neurone Disease

Autopsy proven primary lateral sclerosis (PLS)

Clinically diagnosed PLS with degeneration in motor cortex and corticospinal tracts, no loss of motor neurons, no gliosis in anterior horn cells and no **Bunina bodies** nor ubiquitinated inclusions.

Clinically pure PLS

Evident upper motor neuron signs, no focal muscle atrophy or visible fasciculation and no denervation on EMG within 4 years from onset of symptoms. Age at onset >40 years. Secondary and mimicking conditions are excluded by laboratory tests and neuroimaging.

UMN-dominant ALS

Symptoms present for less than 4 years. or disability due predominantly to UMN signs but with minor EMG denervation or LMN signs on examination, not sufficient to meet diagnostic criteria for ALS.

PLS plus

Predominant UMN signs accompanied by clinical, laboratory, or pathologic evidence of dementia, Parkinsonism or sensory tract abnormalities. (If cerebellar signs, urinary incontinence, or orthostatic hypotension are evident, **multiple system atrophy** should be considered.)

Symptomatic lateral sclerosis

Clinically diagnosed PLS with evident possible cause (e.g., a paraneoplastic syndrome).

Suggested diagnostic criteria are adult onset; negative family history; a duration of at least 3 years and normal. blood, CSF, EMG, and MRI results.[3030]

A more extensive set of diagnostic criteria has also been proposed by Singer (2007)[5862] and is adapted here.

Clinical features

Presence of: 1. Findings of UMN disorder (spasticity, pathologic reflexes, weakness, when present, in UMN distribution) 2. Regions of involvement: Limb (legs, arms, or both); Bulbar; Mixed limb and bulbar. 3. Time course >4 years; 4. Progressive; 5. Age of onset: adult >20 years; 6. Bladder symptoms due to UMN dysfunction may be present.

Absence of LMN disorder such as fasciculations or atrophy; sensory signs on examination; family history of a similar disorder

Laboratory features supporting the diagnosis;

1. Transcranial magnetic stimulation: Increased CMCT, decreased cortical excitability (e.g., MEP cannot be obtained)
2. Magnetic resonance spectroscopy findings in motor cortex of decreased NAA/Cr ratio or NAA/Cho ratio
3. Diffusion tensor imaging findings in posterior limb of internal capsule such as decreased FA or increased ADC.

Exclusionary findings: Serologic evidence for etiology of myelopathy; abnormal CSF; evidence of structural abnormality or demyelinating disorder on MRI of brain or spine; EMG findings of abnormal motor or sensory nerve conductions; the finding of any known HSP or *alsin* gene mutations.

Classification of PLS

Clinical PLS fulfils the above clinical and laboratory inclusionary and exclusionary features.

Suspected PLS fulfils above clinical and laboratory inclusionary and exclusionary features except: 1. < 4-year duration; and 2. The finding of EMG evidence of minimal denervation that does not satisfy EI Escorial criteria for ALS.

Complicated PLS (PLS plus) is that condition in which patients fulfil the criteria for clinical or suspected PLS but also have evidence of dementia, parkinsonism, or sensory abnormalities.

Frontal lobe patterns of dementia have been associated on rare occasion with amyotrophic lateral sclerosis. Excellent reviews are those of Pringle and of Milller Fisher.[5124, 1051, 2088] See also **amyotrophic lateral sclerosis**.

primary leukodystrophies Rare, usually genetic metabolic disorders resulting from deficits of myelin sphingolipids or specific proteins, with clinical onset mainly in infancy or childhood. See **leukodystrophies**.

primary malignant (cerebral) lymphoma See **primary CNS lymphoma**.

primary memory See **short-term memory**.

primary orthostatic tremor (supermarket tremor, cocktail party tremor, **orthostatic tremor**) A high-frequency, synchronized tremor in the legs and axial muscles occurring within seconds after standing up and increasing in amplitude over time until relieved by walking, sitting, or lying down again. The patients usually complain of unsteadiness or imbalance. The frequency of the tremor is between 14 and 18 Hz.[2838] It is sometimes possible to see and to hear with a stethoscope (or detect with EMG) a 16-Hz tremor in the quadriceps muscle after the patient has been standing for a few seconds. The condition may occur alone or in association with cerebellar disease.

primary pallidal atrophy A basal ganglion syndrome characterized by involvement of the subthalamic nucleus, globus pallidus, and cerebellum.[3049] See **pure pallidal atrophy**.

primary parasomnias Sleep disorders occurring without associated pathology. Sleep and wakefulness are not mutually exclusive; for example, **sleep drunkenness**, **microsleeps**, and automatic behaviour. Rapid eye movement sleep has both tonic and phasic components, and these may persist into wakefulness; such disorders are subsumed under this heading.

primary partial epilepsies Focally originating, age-dependent seizure disorders of congenital or childhood origin without macroscopic pathology. The group includes **benign rolandic epilepsy, benign partial epilepsy with occipital sharp waves, benign sensorimotor epilepsy with parietal spikes,** and **atypical benign parietal epilepsy of childhood**. See also **primary generalized epilepsies**.

primary position The position of the eyes at rest, looking directly forward in parallel. See also **secondary position**.

primary position upbeat nystagmus A downward drift of the eyes when the patient attempts to maintain the primary position of gaze, interrupted by saccadic movements that correct the position of the eye back toward the primary position. It is due to intra-axial lesions, usually of the pons or of the superior cerebellar vermis.[2075]

primary progressive aphasia A focal cerebral cortical degenerative syndrome characterized by a slow but relentless deterioration of language abilities with sparing of cognitive and behavioral functions for 2 years or so, and due to focal spongiform degeneration in the left perisylvian region, confirmed by imaging techniques.[4330] Although usually sporadic, an autosomal dominant form has been described.[1095]

Three subvarieties are distinguished: **semanatic dementia, progressive nonfluent aphasia,** and **logopenic progressive aphasia.**[5393]

The language deficit most often resembles **Broca aphasia** in its agrammaticism and nonfluency, but other dysphasic types are also described. The difference between this condition and **slowly progressive aphasia**, in which dementia eventually supervenes, appears to be largely a function of time. The relationship with **Alzheimer disease** is unclear, but, on the basis of current neuropathological data, seems unlikely to be close,[3455] and the pathology may resemble that of Pick disease;[3404] thus it is best regarded as an **asymmetric cortical dengeneration syndrome**.

Diagnostic criteria have been proposed[4334] and are reproduced in Chart P–22 by permission.

See also **Pick disease, corticobasal ganglionic degeneration**.

Chart P–22. Diagnostic Criteria for Primary Progressive Aphasia

1. Insidious onset and gradual progression of word finding, object-naming, or word-comprehension impairments as manifested during spontaneous conversation or as assessed through formal neuropsychological tests of language
2. A limitation of daily living activities attributable to the language impairment, for at least 2 years after onset
3. Intact premorbid language function (except for developmental dyslexia)
4. Absence of significant apathy, disinhibition, forgetfulness for recent events, visuospatial impairment, visual recognition deficits or sensory-motor dysfunction within the initial 2 years of the illness. (This criterion can be fulfilled by history, survey of daily living activities or formal neuropsychological testing.)
5. Acalculia and ideomotor apraxia may be present even in the first 2 years. (Mild constructional deficits and perseveration [as assessed in the **go no-go** paradigm] are also acceptable as long as neither visuospatial deficits nor disinhibition influences daily living activities.)
6. Other domains possibly affected after the first 2 years faster than other affected domains
7. Absence of "specific" causes such as stroke or tumor as ascertained by neuroimaging.

primary progressive freezing gait A neurodegenerative syndrome that causes gait freezing during the first 3 years and later results in postural instability and a wheelchair-bound state. Bradykinesia, rigidity, postural tremor, hyperreflexia, and dementia are sometimes associated. The condition does not respond to dopaminergic medications.

It has been described in association with **pallidonigroluysian degeneration, dementia with Lewy bodies, progressive supranuclear palsy,** and **cortico-basal degeneration.**

primary progressive multiple sclerosis (PPMS) That form of **multiple sclerosis** in which the disease manifests a slowly progressive course from its onset. It usually presents in later life (about 10 years later than the mean for relapsing–remitting MS) with asymmetrical spastic paraparesis (or quadriparesis) although visual distubances, ataxia, hemiparesis, or brainstem syndromes are also described in this form. Sensory changes are minimal if present at all but early bladder involvement (spastic bladder) is ususal and some cognitive impairments are described.[4364]

PPMS may manifest a reduced number of MRI lesions and be associated with a specific heterozygous Taq 1 HLA DQ ß restriction fragment, unlike **secondary progressive multiple sclerosis.**[6296] This form represents 10–15% of all cases of multiple sclerosis. Linkage to the DR2 haplotype *DRB1**1501 (Class II MHC, chromosome 6), has been established. MRI scans usually show atrophy of the cervical cord in addition to cerebral lesions as in relapsing-remitting multiple sclerosis. A late-onset form may in fact be due to **Pelizaeus–Merzbacher disease.**[6650]

Diagnostic criteria have been suggested:[6301] and are reproduced with permission of Lippincott Williams and Wilkins.

Definite PPMS

1. Clinical progression for at least 1 year *and*
2. Positive CSF evidence *and*
3. Positive MRI evidence *or* equivocal MRI evidence *and* a delayed visual evoked potential (VEP)

Probable PPMS

Either:

1. Clinical progression for at least 1 year *and*
2. Positive CSF evidence *and*
3. Equivocal MRI evidence *or* delayed VEP

or:

1. Clinical progression for at least 1 year *and*
2. Positive MRI evidence *or* equivocal MRI evidence *and* a delayed VEP (but CSF evidence either unavailable or negative)

Possible PPMS

1. Clinical progression for at least 1 year *and*
2. Equivocal MRI evidence *or* delayed VEP

The revised McDonald criteria[5073] are similar, requiring progression for at least a year and two of the following:

Nine MRI brain lesions or at least four brain lesions and abnormal visual evoked potentials
At least two MRI spinal cord lesions
Positive CSF oligoclonal banding or increased IgG index

primary reading epilepsy

A dominantly inherited form of **reflex epilepsy** with symptoms beginning in the second decade, in which seizures are triggered by reading or by the eye or jaw movements commonly associated with that activity. If reading continues, a generalized convulsion may occur. A family history of epilepsy is common. The developmental history, neurologic examination, interictal EEG, and CT scan are normal, but EEG paroxysmal activity may be seen in the attacks with paroxysmal rhythmic theta activity or spikes evoked by reading over one or both frontocentral, centroparietal, or temporoparietal regions in association with jaw jerks.

More prolonged reading-induced partial seizures with ictal dyslexia or alexia, possibly speech arrest, and reading-induced bilateral myoclonic seizures and absences have also been reported. Increased task difficulty, increased complexity of different types, and long duration of reading increase the chance of an attack. Most patients respond well to anticonvulsant therapy.

An EEG pattern of left frontotemporal wave discharges is a common concomitant. See **reading epilepsy**.

primary rhinencephalic epilepsy

Seizure disorders with initial involvement of the hippocampal and amygdaloid structures. Their clinical features include olfactory hallucinations, visceral motor symptoms, elementary automatisms, apnea, cardiovascular changes, tonic somato-motor manifestations, and disturbances of memory.[72]

primary sensory area

The principal somatosensory area of the cerebral cortex comprising Brodmann's areas 3, 2, and 1.

primary sensory neuropathy

See **subacute sensory neuronopathy**.

primary stabbing headache

(ice-pick pains, jabs and jolts, ophthalmodynia periodica) An indomethacin-responsive headache syndrome of mature adults (mainly women), now included as a separate entity in the IHS classification under "other primary headaches." It is a paroxysmal disorder of short duration manifested as head pain involving the area supplied by the first division of the trigeminal nerve and occurring as a single stab or a series, lasting seconds, recurring irregularly from once to many times per day, with no underlying attributable disorder. The ICHD criteria[2820] describe head pain occurring as a single stab or a series of stabs lasting up to a few seconds and recurring irregularly, exclusively or predominantly felt in the distribution of the first division of the trigeminal nerve (orbit, temple, and parietal area).

primary subcortical gliosis

A dementing syndrome of adult life with progressive and insidious course, differing from **Pick disease** only in the general atrophy of the cortex and in the absence of Pick cells.

The usual histological features of **Alzheimer disease** are also absent, but there is widespread gliosis of the brainstem, basal ganglia, and subcortical white matter.[4634] See also **frontal lobe dementias**.

primary suppurative myositis

See **pyomyositis**.

primary systemic amyloidosis

See amyloid.

primary thrombocythemia

See **thrombocythemia**.

primary thunderclap headache

A high-intensity headache with an abrupt onset mimicking that of ruptured cerebral aneurysm. Diagnostic criteria have been defined:

A. Both of the following characteristics:
   1. Sudden onset, reaching maximum intensity in <1 min
   2. Lasting from 1 h to 10 days
B. Does not recur regularly over subsequent weeks or months
C. Not attributed to another disorder

Adapted from the International Classification of Headache Disorders (Headache Classification Committee of the International Headache Society. *Cephalalgia* 2004;24[Suppl 1]) by kind permission of Dr. Jes Olesen, the International Headache Society, and Wiley-Blackwell Publications.

See also **primary cough headache, primary exertional headache,** and **primary headache associated with sexual activity,** which can all present as thunderclap headache too.

primary trochlear headache

Orbital pain emanating from the trochlear area in the absence of trochleitis or other orbital or systemic disease and possibly acting as a trigger point for migraine attacks. The condition appears to be more common in women, who complain of chronic unilateral moderate pain in the trochlear area with acute exacerbations and frequently with extension to other cranial sites.

The diagnosis requires:[6899]

1. Unilateral headache with intense pain in the periorbital area appearing at the same time as soreness of the trochlea itself
2. Clear tenderness and exacerbation of the pain on examination of the trochlear region
3. Pain is exacerbated when the patient abducts the eyes fully
4. Lack of abnormal radiological and blood findings

primary writing tremor

A task-specific tremor; a variant of essential tremor in which the unwanted movement appears only with attempts to write or on assuming the writing position.[3265, 4745, 5434] Dystonia may be associated.

prime movers

(agonists, protagonists) Those muscles whose action is to perform precisely a movement in question. See also **antagonists, synergists, muscles of fixation**.

primidone embryopathy

See **fetal anticonvulsant syndrome**

primitive neuroectodermal tumors (PNETs)

Rare, highly malignant embryonal neuroectodermal tumors found in children and young adults and characterized histologically by small cells with a high nuclear–cytoplasmic ratio; fine fibrillary processes; small, oval hyperchromatic nuclei; frequent mitotic figures; and evidence of glial, neuronal, or ependymal differentiation. They usually occur above the tentorium and seed widely through the neuraxis.[2783] **Medulloblastoma, medulloepithelioma, cerebral** and **abdominal neuroblastoma, esthioneuroblastoma, retinoblastoma, medulloblastoma, pinealoblastoma, ependymoblastoma,** and **polar**

spongioblastoma have been regarded as examples of PNETs.[6]

primitive reflexes (frontal release signs, release symptoms) "A mechanism by which a particular type of response is brought about by either the activity of a single nervous arc or several nervous arcs, such reflexes as have been observed in embryonic and later life in lower forms of animals and in human beings . . . The reflexes appearing earliest in the order of functional development are apt to be the last to disappear in the process of functional disintegration. In a similar manner, the last to be acquired are likely to disappear early in the course of the dementia" (Buckley, 1927, quoted by Landau.[3666])

Swallowing, sucking, grasp, palmomental, corneomandibular, glabellar, nuchocephalic, and flexor reflexes are considered to be examples,[3134] but these are not usually present in patients who had had frontal lobotomies, and to attribute such reflexes to lack of inhibition resulting from a single lesion is inappropriate. See also **developmental reflexes**.

Primrose syndrome A congenital dysmorphic syndrome manifesting also calcification of the ear cartilages, cataract, joint contractures, hydrocephalus, proximal and distal myopathy with atrophy, and mental and developmental delay.[381]

principle of compensation A theory of Hughlings-**Jackson**: When any loss of function ensues from a lesion of the nervous system, recovery takes place, not because other units have taken on functions they never had before, but because those units, having functions closely similar to those of the units destroyed, can perform nearly as well for the functions of both. On this basis, compensation can never be absolute, as is clinically obvious.

Pringle, J.J. (1855–1932) English dermatologist on the staff of the Middlesex Hospital, London.

Pringle–Bourneville disease See **tuberous sclerosis**.

prion diseases (transmissible spongiform encephalopathies, slow virus diseases) Dementing illnesses involving the transmission of an aberrant isoform of prion protein, which also makes up the content of amyloid plaques. Although transmissible; they are not contagious.

Such human transmissible, noninflammatory, neurodegenerative conditions include **kuru; iatrogenic**, familial, variant, and sporadic **Creutzfeldt–Jakob disease** (CJD); **Gerstmann–Straussler–Scheinker syndrome; fatal familial insomnia**; and some other atypical dementing diseases (*prion dementia without characteristic pathology; dementia with spastic paraparesis*), while in animals, **scrapie**, chronic wasting disease of elk, feline spongiform encephalopathy, transmissible mink encephalopathy, and **bovine spongiform encephalopathy** are examples. Two recent major reviews were those of Prusiner[5128, 5129] and of Colinge.[1255]

Rare inherited forms may cause early onset dementia and ataxias.

prions Small proteinaceous infectious particles that contain little or no nucleic acid and in which a host protein is a major and necessary component. The molecular properties of these unconventional agents distinguish them from viruses.

pro- (Gr, and Lat, before, for or on behalf of) Prefix denoting before or for.

probable multiple sclerosis That form of **multiple sclerosis** characterized by relapsing–remitting symptoms with only neurological signs commonly associated with multiple sclerosis, or a documented single episode with signs of multifocal white matter disease and with signs of partial recovery; with no better explanation.[5663]

This diagnostic category is now largely replaced in the **McDonald criteria**.

Probst bundle An anomalous bundle of fibers which would normally have crossed in the corpus callosum but which pass rostrocaudally, parallel to the cingulate bundle, in cases of agenesis of the corpus callosum.

procedural learning (procedural memory) The learning of manual skills rather than of words and facts. These skills are lost early in patients with lesions of the caudate nuclei. The differentiation is made because patients with dementing conditions such as **Alzheimer disease**, and those given scopolamine, may retain these abilities even though **declarative learning** and other memory forms are severely impaired.

Procerus sign An "astonished," "reptile-like," or "worried" facial expression shown by subjects with progressive supranuclear palsy, likely resulting from focal dystonia of the procerus muscle, reduced blinking, spasticity, lid retraction, and gaze palsy. The muscle originates on the nasal bone and inserts into the skin of the central forehead.

Prochaska, Georg (1749–1820) Professor of anatomy and of ophthalmology variously at Prague and Vienna. He was the first to ascribe different (motor and sensory) functions to the anterior and posterior nerve roots, in 1812. He also made one of the earliest suggestions that reflexes occur in considering that the cerebrum acts as the *sensorium commune* in receiving afferent impulses, which it reflects into the periphery again to the motor nerves (1780–1784).

proctalgia fugax (Gr, anus + pain and Lat, fleeting) Severe brief episodic pain arising irregularly in the anal region as a result of cramp of the levator ani, often during sleep, and lasting 5–30 min with spontaneous resolution and without known cause or treatment. The condition was first described by MacLennon in 1917.

prodrome 1. Clinical events that herald worse clinical events, with which they share a common cause. 2. A preictal phenomenon consisting of a subjective or objective experience, e.g., ill-localized sensation or agitation that heralds the onset of an epileptic seizure but does not form part of it.[16]

Profichet syndrome (calcinosis universalis, pierres de la peau) The slow development of widespread subcutaneous calcifications in adults. Muscle atrophy and sensory changes are the usual neurological features.[1765]

Profile of Mood states A self-report questionnaire evaluating mood states in psychiatric patients and assessing changes in affective status.[4261]

Profile of Nonverbal Sensitivity Test A test of the ability to comprehend nonverbal, emotional aspects of human communication, wherein the subject describes the message portrayed in a set of standard videotapes.[5414] Patients with right hemisphere lesions are likely to do poorly on this test.

profile perimetry See **static perimetry**.

progeria (Lat, before + Gr, old age) (Hutchinson–Gilford syndrome, Variot–Pironneau senile dwarfism; in adults, **Werner syndrome**) Recessively inherited dwarfism with accelerated aging, supervening after a normal early childhood. Apart from the changes in physical appearance which suggest advanced age (such as gray hair, baldness, thinness, arthritis, loss of eyebrows and teeth, cataract, a seemingly small face, atrophic skin, loss of subcutaneous fat, and narrow chest), premature atherosclerotic changes lead to angina and strokes.[3063] Myopathy,[1894] spastic paraparesis, and polyneuropathy are yet other complications.

A *neonatal* form exists as a congenital dysmorphic syndrome, manifesting also low birth weight, muscular build, sparse hair, premature aging, delayed closure of fontanelles, and deficient/absent adipose tissue.[381] **Cockayne syndrome** (trisomy 10, Neil-Dingwall syndrome) is similar.[1210]

progressive adult-onset bulbar paresis See **Fazio–Londe syndrome**.

progressive alcoholic dementia See **Marchiafava–Bignami disease**.

progressive amusia and aprosody A focal cortical degeneration syndrome.[1266]

progressive anarthria A focal cortical degeneration syndrome.[885]

progressive aphasia without dementia See **primary progressive aphasia**.

progressive apraxia A focal cortical syndrome characterized by isolated apraxia or visual agnosia, which may progress to dementia but which has been distinguished from **Alzheimer disease**.[1515, 314]

progressive ascending spinal paralysis (Mills disease) See **amyotrophic lateral sclerosis**.

progressive ataxia and palatal myoclonus A rare primary neurodegenerative disease (a tauopathy) with these features and olivary hypertrophy.

progressive ataxia, retinal degeneration, peripheral neuropathy, myopathy, and mental subnormality See **cerebellar ataxias** (5. Of unknown etiology).

progressive autonomic failure (PAF) (idiopathic orthostatic hypotension, primary or pure autonomic failure, Bradbury–Eggleston sundrome) A part of the sporadic syndrome of **multiple system atrophy** (MSA) characterized by idiopathic degeneration of the central, peripheral, and autonomic nervous systems in elderly people. However, a more distal site of pathology has also been suggested in some cases, Lewy bodies being present also in the autonomic nervous system.

Clinically, orthostatic hypotension with drop attacks, dizziness, weakness, anhidrosis, sphincter disturbances, and impotence are the most prominent features, but forms with associated Parkinsonism (PAF-P) or typical multiple system atrophy (PAF-MSA, Shy–Drager syndrome[5819]) also occur. There is evidence that this represents a postganglionic failure, both of sudomotor and of other adrenergic fibers.[6276, 4251, 6277] There is also an opinion that such patients go on to develop signs of multiple system atrophy; the pathology is much the same even though the time course of progression differs—the prognosis is better for PAF.

A *variant* is *familial orthostatic hypotension* characterized by autonomic failure, upper and lower motor neuron signs, ataxia, and Parkinsonism.[3820, 6277]

progressive axial muscle rigidity of infancy A syndrome characterized by rigidity of the axial and proximal limb muscles, occurring in infancy and leading on to ventilatory failure. EMG studies reveal continuous muscle firing in apparently normal motor units, unaffected by neuromuscular blockade and without evidence of CNS abnormality.[4052] See also **stiff person syndrome**.

progressive biparietal atrophy A focal cortical dementing syndrome considered to precede the more typical manifestations of **Alzheimer disease** and likely to represent the dorsal form of **posterior cortical atrophy**. Clinical manifestations are early visuospatial problems, peripheral or apraxic agraphia, and difficulties with bimanual tasks, but with only minor impairments of memory or language in the early stages, although these do supervene later and a full Alzheimer-type dementia picture may develop eventually. MRI and SPECT studies reveal local biparietal involvement.

progressive bulbar palsy (Duchenne paralysis) A form of **amyotrophic lateral sclerosis** described by **Duchenne** in 1858 as "labioglossolaryngeal paralysis," of which the earliest features are lower motor lesions of the bulbar muscles, and in which the prognosis tends to be worse than that in the forms with predominant upper motor neuron lesions.[1736] In rare instances, ophthalmoplegia or deafness has been associated. See also **motor neuronal diseases**. *Variants* are as follows:

- **Fazio–Londe disease** (progressive bulbar palsy of children).
- *Vialetto–van Laere syndrome* (progressive bulbar paralysis and nerve deafness), which is a recessively inherited syndrome characterized by the onset of progressive deafness in childhood followed by visual loss and amyotrophy of cranial and upper limb muscles; signs of corticospinal tract involvement appear later.[98]
- *Progressive pure bulbar paralysis*, a dominantly inherited syndrome characterized by the occurrence of progressive bulbar paralysis in advanced adult life without other evidence of neurological dysfunction.[3926]

progressive bulbar paralysis of childhood See **Fazio–Londe syndrome**.

progressive cerebral poliodystrophy See **Alpers disease**.

progressive CNS deterioration A slowly progressive deterioration of CNS function seen in some premature infants treated with ventilatory assistance and continuous positive airway pressure for over 28 days, and characterized by loss of developmental milestones, increasing hypotonia, EEG changes, and death; or by progressive apnea, bradycardia, and sudden death.[1847] Pulmonary hypertension, hypoxemia, hypercapnia, and acidosis are probably the most relevant etiological factors.

progressive cramp Increasing difficulty in performing new tasks due to the presence of hand cramps.[1230]

progressive dementia with photosensitivity See **neuronal ceroid lipofuscinosis**.

progressive diaphyseal dysplasia (Engelmann Disease) A recessively inherited syndrome characterized by increased density of the bones of the skull and thickening of the diaphyseal cortex of the limb bones, the former leading to optic atrophy and deafness in youth or young adult life.[4243] A waddling gait due to proximal myopathy is another common feature. See **Camurati–Engelmann syndrome**.

progressive diffuse encephalopathy A neurological complication of HIV infection, characterized pathologically by diffuse demyelination, astrocytic proliferation, and multinucleated giant cells.

progressive dystonia with diurnal fluctuation A dystonic syndrome of childhood or early adult life, characterized by emotional lability, pyramidal signs, rigidity, dystonias, chorea, and resting tremor, all of which are worse during the daytime.[5709] See **Segawa dystonia**.

progressive encephalomyelitis with rigidity (PEWR, subacute myoclonic spinal neuronitis) A rare progressive, incapacitating, and ultimately fatal syndrome of tonic muscular rigidity producing abnormal postures, accompanied by myoclonus and painful stimulus-sensitive muscle spasms (thus resembling the **stiff-person syndrome**), but associated also with changes in the brainstem and cervical cord suggesting encephalomyelitis with destruction of spinal internuncial neurons.[6755]

progressive external ophthalmoplegia (chronic progressive external ophthalmoplegia, von Graefe syndrome, PEO) A heterogeneous syndrome appearing in adult life, comprising progressive symmetrical ptosis, and limitation of ocular motility, as shown by a reduction in the velocity of the saccadic movements (if any are possible at all).

The syndrome may occur in isolation or in association with other neurodegenerative disorders including ataxia, pigmentary retinopathy, mitochondrial myopathy, optic atrophy, cardiac conduction defects, spasticity, deafness, organic mental changes, small stature, and elevated CSF protein levels.[6572] Ragged red fibers are found in muscle biopsy specimens. Mutations of *POLG1* are responsible. See also **Kearns–Sayre syndrome, myotonic dystrophy, oculopharyngeal muscular dystrophy, centronuclear myopathy, mitochondrial diseases**.

Variants are as follows:

Autosomal dominant PEO (OMIM 157640),[3649] with typical features, mapped variously to 4q34, 10q24, and 15q25.

Autosomal dominant progressive external ophthalmoplegia with multiple deletions of mtDNA, which has been mapped variously to 10q23.3–24.3 and to 3p 14.1–21.2. Clinically, muscle weakness, depression, and personality disorders accompany the usual features of the condition.[6135]

Autosomal recessive PEO3649

Progressive external ophthalmoplegia with floppy mitral valve, a progressive cardioneurological syndrome characterized by the concurrence of mitral valve prolapse and ophthalmoplegia.[1461]

Progressive external ophthalmoplegia with horizontal gaze palsy and scoliosis (11q23, *ROBO3*), a congenital recessive trait manifesting horizontal gaze paresis (only), esotropia, pendular nystagmus, scoliosis, and often mental retardation.

Progressive external ophthalmoplegia with immunological abnormality, a syndrome of adult life comprising ophthalmoplegias and myopathic muscle atrophy, with ragged red fibers present in muscle biopsy specimens.

progressive facial hemiatrophy See **Parry–Romberg syndrome**.

progressive familial encephalopathy A syndrome with congenital or infantile onset, comprising bilateral spasticity and dystonia, microcephaly, a rapid course to death, basal ganglion calcification, and persistent CSF lymphocytosis.[77]

progressive familial myoclonic epilepsy See **Unverricht–Lundborg–Lafora syndrome**.

progressive hemifacial atrophy See **Parry–Romberg syndrome**.

progressive hereditary diaphyseal dysplasia See **Camurati–Engelman syndrome**.

progressive hypertrophic interstitial neuropathy (Déjèrine–Sottas syndrome) See **hereditary motor and sensory neuropathy**, type 3.

progressive infantile poliodystrophy See **Alpers disease**.

progressive juvenile bulbar palsy A rare syndrome manifesting ocular, facial, and bulbar weakness in childhood, leading on to weakness and atrophy of the trunk and limb muscles with selective degeneration of the bulbar and spinal motor nuclei.[2461] See **Fazio–Londe disease**.

progressive lenticular degeneration See **Wilson disease**.

progressive multifocal leukoencephalopathy An acquired fatal demyelinating disease of adult life, caused by a papovavirus and characterized by widely disseminated small perivascular foci of myelin sheath destruction, these foci becoming confluent. Astrocytic hypertrophy and basophilic staining of the nuclei of oligodendrocytes are other pathological features. The condition appears to be a complication of disturbed cellular immune systems.

Clinically, the presentations include progressive cognitive and personality changes and focal neurological signs such as hemiparesis, facial paresis, incoordination, language, visual deficits, and occasionally seizures. The condition has been reported as a **paraneoplastic syndrome** in association with systemic Hodgkin disease and leukemia, and as a complication of sarcoidosis, tuberculosis,[281] and now **HIV/AIDS**,[6416] in which situation progression to death is usually rapid.

In those patients with HIV infection, diagnostic criteria include rapid onset (<2 weeks) of multifocal neurological signs and symptoms, advanced immunosuppression, and asymmetric uni- or multifocal white matter lesions without mass effect, contrast enhancement, or cortical atrophy on MRI. Mean survival is a few months. Human polyoma virus JCV polymerase chain reaction in the cerebrospinal fluid demonstrates a considerable rate of possible cerebral co-infection with HIV-1 as well as subclinical infection with JCV. Routine stereotactic brain biopsy is not necessary to confirm the diagnosis.[6569] Thus the label *JCV encephalopathy* might be more appropriate.

progressive muscle spasms, alopecia, and diarrhea

See **Satoyoshi syndrome**.

progressive muscular atrophy

See **amyotrophic lateral sclerosis**.

progressive (spinal) muscular atrophy

1. (Aran–Duchenne disease) A form of **amyotrophic lateral sclerosis** in which the earliest features are lower motor neuron lesions of the spinal musculature.[229] *Variants* are as follows:

Progressive muscular atrophy with malignant course, a form which is fatal within 1 year, but which is not clearly different from autosomal dominant **amyotrophic lateral sclerosis**.

Progressive muscular atrophy with amyotrophic lateral sclerosis; this entity is not clearly different from "peroneal muscular atrophy with pyramidal features." See **amyotrophic lateral sclerosis**.

2. See **hereditary motor neuropathy**, type 1.

progressive muscular rigidity

See **stiff-person syndrome**.[4424]

progressive myelopathy

See **chronic myelopathy; progressive necrotic myelopathy**.

progressive myoclonic ataxia

A mitochondrial encephalopathy syndrome presenting with myoclonus and progressive "cerebellar" ataxia. Epileptic seizures are infrequent and cognitive decline is not notable.[4107] The condition overlaps **progressive myoclonic epilepsy**.

progressive myoclonic ataxia with celiac disease

A progressive myoclonic ataxic syndrome dominated by action and stimulus-sensitive myoclonus of cortical origin with mild ataxia and infrequent seizures, following the gastrointestinal and other manifestations of celiac disease while on a gluten-free diet, in the absence of overt features of malabsorption or nutritional deficiency. The brain shows selective symmetrical atrophy of the cerebellar hemispheres with Purkinje cell loss and Bergmann astrocytosis, and preservation of the cerebral hemispheres and brainstem.[609]

progressive myoclonic epilepsy

(OMIM 254800) A rare group of recessively inherited neurodegenerative conditions presenting with myoclonus and generalized seizures, in which there is progressive neurological decline taking the form of ataxia, visual loss, and/or dementia.[4107, 5353] Abnormalities of somatosensory evoked potentials are commonly demonstrable.[5799] The responsible gene maps to chromosome 21q22.3. The commonest form is EPM1, a recessively inherited disorder.

Such stimulus-sensitive cortical reflex myoclonic diseases include some that are recessively inherited and some that are acquired, and are either degenerative or metabolic in pathogenesis. **Unverricht–Lundborg disease** (Baltic myoclonus), **Lafora body disease, sialidosis,** dominant **cerebellar ataxia** (SCA2), **neuronal ceroid lipofuscinosis,** the **encephalomyelopathies** (Fukuhara syndrome), **sialidosis, dentatorubral-pallidoluysian atrophy,** and **May–White syndrome** are examples.

A *variant* is *progressive myoclonic epilepsy, seizures, scoliosis, pes cavus, retinopathy, cardiac involvement, ophthalmoplegia, and dementia,*[3897] which in almost every way resembles **mitochondrial cytopathy** except for the absence of ragged red fibers.

progressive myoclonic epilepsy with Lafora bodies

See **Lafora body disease**.

progressive necrotic myelopathy

A disease of unknown cause affecting adults who present with paresthesias, and burning in the limbs or ill-defined pains in the trunk, worsening subacutely over months and culminating in para- or tetraplegia. CSF protein levels are increased, with or without pleocytosis, but oligoclonal bands are not detected. The condition does not respond to immunomodulation.

Clinical diagnostic criteria have been suggested[3327] and comprise the regional loss of reflexes with flaccidity and muscle atrophy; a shrunken or cavitated cord on MRI scans, without evidence of arteriovenous malformation; denervation over several cord segments as shown by EMG, while sensory nerve action potentials may be retained; and the absence of evidence of systemic disease, including malignancy. See also **Devic disease**.

progressive neuronal degeneration of childhood

See **Alpers disease**.

progressive neuronal degeneration of childhood with liver disease

See **Alpers disease**.

progressive, nonfamilial hypertrophic neuritis

See **Roussy–Cornil syndrome**.

progressive nonfluent aphasia

A form of frontotemporal dementia with insidious onset and gradual progression, in which spontaneous speech is not fluent and shows agrammatism, phonemic paraphasias, and/or anomia. Other supportive diagnostic features suggested by Neary et al.[4606] include stuttering or oral apraxia; impaired repetition; alexia, agrammatism with preservation of word meaning, and late mutism. Behavioral criteria are the early preservation of social skills, but late behavioral changes as in frontotemporal dementia. Physical signs, occurring late in the process, include the presence of primitive reflexes contralaterally, akinesia, rigidity, and tremor.

progressive nuclear ophthalmoplegia syndrome

(Levic syndrome, nigrospinodentatal degeneration with nuclear ophthalmoplegia) A genetically determined, extensive degenerative process, characterized by bilateral facial weakness, congenital external near-complete ophthalmoplegia with ptosis (but sparing the pupil), scrotal tongue, progressive chorioretinal sclerosis, and intellectual deficit.[3799, 6861] Motor neuron involvement, ataxia, spastic paraplegia, dystonia, retinitis pigmentosa, and peripheral neuropathy have also been described in a few cases; the condition is unlikely to consist of a single entity.

progressive ophthalmoplegia, glycogen storage, and abnormal mitochondria

A mitochondrial disease presenting with facial and proximal limb weakness in childhood and with progressive ophthalmoplegia. See also **glycogen storage diseases**.

progressive ophthalmoplegia in Kugelberg-Welander disease See **hereditary motor neuropathy** (*variants*).

progressive pallidal atrophy A basal ganglion syndrome presenting with Parkinsonian features, of which at least four variants are recorded; **pure pallidal atrophy;** *pallidal atrophy with atrophy of the sub-thalamic nucleus*, consisting of extended pallidal atrophy with striatal and nigral involvement; *pallidal atrophy in association with degeneration of other neuronal systems*;[3188] and *progressive pallidal degeneration with pigmentary retinopathy*.[6826]

See also **hereditary dentatorubralpallidoluysian atrophy**.

progressive pallidal degeneration See **neurodegeneration with brain iron accumulation**.

progressive pontobulbar palsy with deafness See **Vialetto–van Laere syndrome, progressive bulbar palsy**.

progressive possible multiple sclerosis See **McDonald–Halliday Criteria**.[4217]

progressive proximal spinal and bulbar muscular atrophy See **bulbospinal neuronopathy**.

progressive proximal spinal and bulbar muscular atrophy of late onset (Kennedy–Alter–Sung syndrome) An X-linked recessive anterior horn cell disease manifesting after the age of 30 years and characterized by cramps, low backache, proximal muscle weakness and wasting, fasciculations, and bulbar muscle weakness, with hyporeflexia but without pyramidal tract or sensory involvement. The course is only slowly progressive and life span is not diminished.[3385] See **bulbospinal muscular neuronopathy**.

progressive pseudorheumatoid arthropathy of childhood A syndrome of childhood manifesting irregular end-plates to vertebrae, platyspondyly, arthropathy, proximal and distal myopathic weakness, and stippled or fragmented epiphyses.[381]

progressive pure anomia A form of progressive fluent aphasia in the presence of selective atrophy of the left temporal cortex, presenting as a profound progressive anomia while semantic knowledge is unaffected.[2546]

progressive pyramidopallidal degeneration A slowly progressive degenerative condition manifesting a pseudobulbar palsy, mild pyramidal signs in the limbs, and postural rigidity with akinesia and chorea, and with cell loss and gliosis in the putamen, globus pallidus, and pyramidal tracts.[3833] The condition appears to resemble **neuronal degeneration with brain iron accumulation**. See also **Lhermitte–Cornil–Quesnel syndrome**.

progressive rigidity with apraxia See **corticobasal degeneration with neuronal achromasia**.

progressive rubella panencephalitis A severe progressive encephalitis, clinically resembling **subacute sclerosing panencephalitis** apart from the presence of clinical cerebellar involvement and of histological evidence of vasculitis and an absence of detectable viral antigen.[1309]

progressive senile scoliosis Increasing scoliosis documented in elderly women. In the absence of osteoporotic vertebral body crush fractures, the common underlying mechanism appears to be asymmetric loading of the spine which can be caused by a previously established scoliosis, spondylolysis/spondylolisthesis, lumbosacral anomalies, or leg length discrepancy. Subsequent factors causing increasing curvature include degenerative disc disease with lateral disc space narrowing, soft tissue failure, and osteoporosis.[2380]

progressive sensory neuropathy See **subacute sensory neuropathy**.

progressive sensory radiculopathy A benign and reversible syndrome due primarily to lesions of the preganglionic sensory roots, characterized by slowly progressive pansensory loss spreading proximally to involve the whole body, with mild weakness, incoordination, and areflexia. CSF protein levels are raised; electrodiagnostic studies suggest the presence of an axonal motor neuropathy and sural nerve biopsy findings are normal.[1184] The condition appears to be responsive to steroid therapy and may be presumed to have a similar etiology to that of **chronic inflammatory demyelinating polyneuropathy** and of **chronic idiopathic ataxic neuropathy**.

progressive spatial disorientation A focal cortical syndrome resulting from right hemisphere degeneration and leading to loss of memory for people.[5192]

progressive spinal muscular atrophy with chorea and deafness See **hereditary motor neuropathy** (*variants*).

progressive subcortical arteriosclerotic encephalopathy See **Binswanger disease**.

progressive subcortical glial dystrophy (progressive subcortical gliosis, Pick disease type 2) A rare, slowly progressive, sporadic, or dominantly inherited dementing illness with onset between 35 and 50 years resembling **Pick disease** and mapped to chromosome 17.[5002] Personality change and impaired social abilities with disinhibition and depression and delusions appear first, with memory impairment and depression, leading on to progressive dementia, disturbances of visual perception, reduced speech output, echolalia, auditory hallucinations, and features of the **Kluver–Bucy syndrome** following.[4631, 3694] The condition may be indistinguishable in life from **progressive supranuclear palsy** and may represent a variety of **frontotemporal dementia**.

Distinctive neuropathologic features include fibrillary astrocytosis in the subcortical white matter and in the subpial and deeper layers of the cortex especially in the fronto-temporal lobes, without amyloid deposits or neuronal inclusions.

progressive supranuclear palsy (Steele–Richardson–Olszewski syndrome) A slowly progressive dementing syndrome of later adult life exhibiting ocular and neurological signs, the cause of which is unknown, although the condition is a **tauopathy**. The cardinal clinical features include those of **subcortical dementia**,[106] with early axial rigidity, supranuclear vertical gaze parese, frequent falls due to impaired otolithic function, and a poor response to levadopa therapy. Moderate to severe postural instability and falls during the first year after onset of symptoms and bradykesia and dysphagia are typical features. Defects in fixation, saccades, pursuit, convergence, and vestibulo-ocular reflexes are also notable.[6028, 1767] Apathy is a common manifestation but irritability, agitation, and anxiety are not. Segmental dystonia and myoclonus are described but aphasia and alien limb syndrome are not. The eponymous title recalls the syndrome's more recent descriptors, although a similar condition was described by W. C. Posey in 1904. Linkage to chromosome 1q31.1 has been reported.[5388]

The clinical picture of progressive supranuclear palsy (PSP) in its full-blown form is readily recognized; the patient has a fixed "Mona Lisa stare" with a very low blink frequency, the head is retracted, and speech is reduced to a distinctive slurred growl. The patient walks clumsily and unsteadily, with a marked tendency to fall backwards. Clothes are soiled with spilled food because the patient is unable to look at the plate when eating and has dysphagia. Motor recklessness, personality change, and behavioural disturbances are also early features. Within the class, however, two clinical phenotypes can be distinguished:[6794]

Richardson syndrome is characterized by early onset of postural instability and falls, supranuclear vertical gaze paresis, and cognitive dysfunction, thus resembling classic PSP as described above.

PSP-P, in which the disease duration is more benign and presents with asymmetrical onset, tremor, and a moderate initial response to levodopa. The condition is frequently confused with Parkinson disease.

The unstable gait, absence of tremor-dominant disease, and absence of a response to levodopa differentiate PSP from **Parkinson disease;** however, notable pathological evidence differentiates the two conditions. Clinically, the supranuclear vertical gaze palsy, gait instability, and the absence of delusions distinguish it from **diffuse Lewy body disease;** the supranuclear vertical gaze palsy and increased age at symptom-onset distinguish it from **multiple system atrophy;** the gait abnormality, severe upward gaze palsy, bilateral bradykinesia, and absence of **alien limb** syndrome separate it from **corticobasal degeneration;** and the postural instability separates it from **Pick disease.**[3878] Nevertheless, PSP, corticobasal degeneration (CBD), an extrapyramidal variety of Pick disease, frontotemporal dementia, and primary progressive aphasia all show pathological or clinical overlaps, such that the syndromes of frontotemporal dementia/Pick disease can be produced by underlying CBD, PSP, or Pick pathology and share a spectrum of different tau mutations.[3399]

A *Progressive Supranuclear Palsy Rating Scale* comprising 28 items in 6 categories (daily activities by history; behaviour; bulbar; ocular motor; limb motor; and gait/midline) has been constructed.[2436] See the Web site: http://www.mdvu.org/library/ratingscales/psp/psp_rs.pdf/. Other valuable Web sites are www.psp.org/ and (from the Baylor College of Medicine); http://www.bcm.edu/neurology/patient_education/pdcmdc/psp.html.

Criteria for the neuropathologic[2798] and clinical diagnosis of PSP have been defined (Chart P–23).

Chart P–23. NINDS-SPSP Criteria for the Diagnosis of Progressive Supranuclear Palsy[3877]

Definite PSP

Clinically probable or possible PSP and histologically typical PSP

Probable PSP

Mandatory inclusion criteria:
Gradually progressive disorder
Onset at age 40 or later
Vertical supranuclear (either upward or downward gaze abnormalities) ophthalmoparesis and prominent postural instability with tendency to falls in the first year of symptom onset

Possible PSP

Mandatory inclusion criteria:
Gradually progressive disorder
Onset at age 40 or later and either:

(a) Vertical supranuclear (either upward or downward gaze abnormalities) ophthalmoparesis or
(b) Slowing of vertical saccades and prominent postural instability with falls within 1 year of symptom onset.

Mandatory exclusion criteria (for both probable and possible PSP)

A history compatible with **encephalitis lethargica**
Alien hand syndrome, cortical sensory deficits, focal frontal or temporoparietal atrophy
Hallucinations or delusions unrelated to dopaminergic therapy
Cortical dementia of Alzheimer type (severe amnesia and aphasia or agnosia)
Prominent cerebellar symptomatology or unexplained **dysautonomia** (early, prominent incontinence, impotence, or symptomatic postural hypotension)
Severe asymmetry of **Parkinsonian** signs (bradykinesia)
Neuroradiologic evidence of relevant structural abnormality (basal ganglia or brainstem infarcts, lobar atrophy)
Whipple disease, confirmed by polymerase chain reaction, if indicated

Supportive features (not required for diagnosis)

Symmetric akinesia or rigidity, proximal more than distal
Retrocollis
Poor, absent or transient response of Parkinsonism to levodopa therapy
Early dysarthria and dysphagia
Early cognitive impairment, including at least two of the following: apathy, impaired abstract thought, decreased verbal fluency, "imitation" behavior or frontal release signs

A diagnostic algorithm has been suggested[1258] in which prerequisites for the diagnosis are: onset age over 40 years; no family history; insidious onset and progressive course; no relevant structural lesions on neuroimaging and the presence of supranuclear downgaze paralysis and three of the following signs, prominent early postural instability with frequent falls and five of the foillowing signs, or both of these and two of the following signs, all in the absence of exclusionary criteria (below). The added required signs are:

Bradykinesia	Rigidity in the neck > arms
Staring, non-blinking facies	Wide-based, shuffling gait

Retrocollis or dystonic arm
Babinski signs
Sitting *en bloc*
Dementia or personality change

Pseudobulbar signs (two of dysarthria, dysphagia, pathological emotionality)
Verification is obtained with a history of 2 years of minimal or unsustained response to levadopa.
Exclusionary criteria are:

Prominent and early dysautonomia, especially orthostatic hypotension
Prominent polyneuropathy
Pronounced rest tremor
Cortical sensory loss
Alien limb sign
Unilateral presentation or pronounced asymmetry.

A simpler set of eight criteria has also been compiled: The disease has a progressive course over <10 years, manifesting Parkinsonism (hypertonia and akinesia) that is not responsive to levadopa; vertical voluntary gaze palsy; falls; and pseudobulbar palsy or dysarthria without evidence of a focal lesion. The diagnosis is probable in a patient with all eight clinical criteria and possible if six or seven criteria are met.

Variants of the syndrome are listed in Chart P–24.

Progressive Supranuclear Palsy Association A charitable organization in this field. Address: The Old Rectory, Wappenham, Nr. Towcester, Northamptonshire, UK. NN12 85Q. Tel: + 44 1327 861007. E-mail: psp.eur@virgin.net. Web site: http://www.pspeur.org/. See also **Society for Progressive Supranuclear Palsy**.

progressive systemic sclerosis See **scleroderma**.

progressive unilateral hypertrophic myopathy A condition characterized by the occurrence of complex repetitive discharges within a group of muscles, the histological appearances of which suggest the presence of myopathy.

Clinically, stiffness and cramps occur within the hypertrophied muscles.[5026]

progressive vascular myelopathy A syndrome of progressive amyotrophy due to ischemia of the anterior horns of the spinal cord.[3189]

projected patterns Abnormal EEG activities believed to result from a disturbance at a site remote from the recording electrodes. (Adapted from the 1974 report of the Committee on Terminology, IFCN. In: Chatrian GE, Bergamini L, Dondey M, et al. A glossary of terms most commonly used by clinical electroencephalographers. *EEG Clin Neurophysiol* 1974;37:538–48. Reproduced with kind permission from Elsevier Science.)

projected rhythms An EEG pattern showing intermittent bursts of bilaterally synchronous rhythmic slow waves, seen in the frontal or occipital regions in patients with metabolic disease, diffuse cerebral diseases, or deep midline cerebral lesions.[3469] See **frontal intermittent rhythmic delta activity, occipital intermittent rhythmic delta activity**.

projection (tactile projection) The sensation of a touch in a place distant from that place which was actually touched by the examiner. See also **alloesthesia**.

prolactinoma (Lat, before + milk + tumor) A prolactin-secreting benign pituitary basophil adenoma.

proliferating systematized angioendotheliomatosis See **malignant angioendotheliosis**.

proliferative myositis A syndrome with a benign course characterized by the appearance of a rapidly growing, localized painless muscle swelling at any site, lasting up to 2 months without ossification. Histologically, bundles of degenerating and muscle fibers with excessive fibrous reaction are found. The cause is unknown.[3390]

The myositis seldom recurs after excision.[1892] See also **focal nodular myositis** and **pseudomalignant myositis ossificans**.

prolonged exercise test 1. A standardized exercise test involving 2 h of exercise on a bicycle ergometer set at half the subject's maximal tolerated work load. Measurements of serum lactate, serum CK and fatty acid levels allow the differentiation of metabolic and mitochondrial myopathies from psychogenic states.[870]

2. A mode of demonstrating paresis in **paramyotonia congenita** or **familial hyperkalemic periodic paralysis**. The patient spreads his fingers maximally for 20 s at a time, then relaxing them for 2–3 s after each contraction repetitively over about 4 min. In normal control subjects, there may be a small decline or a small increase (pseudofacilitation) in the compound muscle action potential following the exercise, but the potentials return to their normal shape within several minutes. In those with periodic paralysis, a progressive decline of the compound muscle

Chart P–24. Variants of Progressive Supranuclear Palsy

Progressive supranuclear palsy with action myoclonus and seizures: A progressive neurological disease characterized by dysarthria, facial action myoclonus with correlated EEG spikes, generalized convulsions, pseudobulbar signs and late eye movement disorder. The condition differs from typical progressive supranuclear palsy by the conspicuous presence of action myoclonus and seizures, the late appearance of the eye movement disorder and the absence of rigidity and conspicuous dementia. The pathological characteristics include neuronal loss, gliosis, loss of neurofibrils and secondary demyelination with occasional perivascular cuffing with lymphocytes mainly affecting the cerebral cortex but not the globus pallidus, subthalamic nuclei, substantia nigra nor red nuclei.[3607]

Recessive progressive supranuclear palsy-like syndrome: A condition resembling the classic disease, except for the presence of neurofibrillary tangles, predominantly in the limbic system.[4771]

Autosomal dominant progressive supranuclear palsy-like syndrome: A form in which the clinical and pathological lesions are those of the sporadic variety, but in which dominant inheritance is postulated.[890]

action potential occurs for 20–40 min after the exercise.[4255]

prolonged Q–T syndrome A cardiac condition associated with ventricular tachyarhythmias and sudden death. It may also present as epilepsy.[4848] See **syncope**.

pronation sign See Neri **signs**.

pronation–supination test The patient is asked to make rapid repetitive rotatory movements of the forearm. Such movements cannot be performed fluently in a subject with a cerebellar lesion affecting the arm because of slowness of movement, lack of rhythm, irregularity of range, loss of postural tone, and imperfect timing of the arrest of movement.

pronator (from Lat, turned or inclined forward) Each of the two forearm muscles (pronator teres and quadratus) which function to rotate the arm internally on the elbow.

pronator catch A temporary resistance to passive pronation, evidencing hypertonia of the muscles in an arm affected by a pyramidal lesion.

pronator drift Slow movement of the outstretched arm downwards and laterally, with pronation of the forearm and slight flexion of the elbow, wrist, and fingers; a sign of mild pyramidal weakness of the arm, but also recorded in the setting of chorea and with cerebellar lesions.[1500, 6245]

pronator reflex Pronation of the forearm in response to a tap on the volar aspect of the radius, the arm lying in the neutral position. The contraction is enhanced in the presence of pyramidal lesions and states of increased emotional tension, and is reduced by lesions at C6.

pronator sign The tendency of the arms to rotate into a pronated position when extended above the head or while in recumbency. In the former case, this is a nonspecific sign of basal ganglion disease; in the latter, it suggests pyramidal disease. See also **pronator drift**.

pronator teres syndrome (high median neuropathy) Compression of the median nerve at the level of the pronator teres muscle at the elbow (between the two heads of which it passes), leading to weakness of the forearm muscles supplied by the anterior interosseous nerve and of the median-supplied hand muscles, and also to paresthesias in the hand.

The clinical diagnosis is confirmed by EMG studies and decompression may relieve the symptoms.[4496] See also **anterior interosseous nerve syndrome**.

propagation velocity of a muscle fiber The speed of transmission of a muscle fiber action potential.

propaxic postural tremor See **cerebellar tremors**.

propositional language Aspects of verbal communication, including lexicon, grammar, and articulation; a left hemisphere function.

propositional speech Speech containing a judgment; a term and concept important within Aristotelian logic. Though a sentence is a significant portion of speech, not every sentence is a proposition; propositions are those which have in them either truth or falsity. Such speech may be internal and unenunciated or external and enunciated, but the two forms are different only in degree. Propositions and thought have been considered identical, leading to the classification of aphasia as a thought disorder by Hughlings-**Jackson**.[5299]

propping reaction Extension of the arm toward the side to which the sitting normal infant of 5–6 months is pushed.

proprioception (from Lat, one's own + to receive) The term of **Sherrington** (1900) for the ability to recognize the position of ones joints and therefore limbs in space. It depends upon a reduplicated system (one pathway reaching consciousness, the other not) informing the brain as to the angulation of joints and therefore the position of body parts, also contributing to the individual's image of his or her own body—the body schema. Alternative terms are *enteroception* and *eomesthesis*, the latter especially pointing out peoples awareness of their own bodies. Both static and kinetic types of proprioception exist—the former giving information on the momentary position of limbs, and the latter informing about the movement at joints (kinesthesia). Their afferent pathways are identical.

proprioceptive ataxia See **sensory ataxia**.

proprioceptive, exteroceptive (Lat, self + receive: Lat, outside + receive) The terms of **Sherrington** denoting the sense organs whose adequate stimuli come from inside and from outside the body, respectively. See also **proprioception**.

Interoceptive sensations are those mediated by sense organs, in this case within the alimentary canal with relationships to local musculature. *Exteroceptive* sensations are subdivided between those stimulated by objects in contact with the body and those stimulated by distance receptors such as the eyes and ears.

proprioceptive tricks Maneuvers which, as patients suffering from dystonia have learned, may inhibit the abnormal posture. Thus, a touch on the face or head may restore the cranial posture to normal in a patient with spasmodic torticollis. See also **geste antagonistique**.

proprionic acidemia A lethal, recessively inherited syndrome characterized by episodic vomiting, lethargy, coma, seizures, chorea, hypertonia, and respiratory insufficiency with ketotic hyperglycinemia, occurring in neonates and infants as a result of deficiency of proprionyl coenzyme A carboxylase. The responsible gene for the B form maps to chromosome 3q13J.3q22, that for the A form to chromosome 13.

Hypoglycemia, platelet abnormalities, hyperammonemia, organic aciduria, and low densities in the white matter on CT scans are also found.[811] See **ketotic hyperglycinemia**.

propriospinal myoclonus That form of focal and segmental spinal myoclonus in which the abnormal movements in axial muscles originate from discharges in slowly conducting spinal tracts, such as the long propriospinal pathways.

Clinically, the movements are limited to the thoracoabdominal muscles, predominantly on one side and especially at times transitional between wakefulness and sleep. See also **segmental myoclonus** (that form of spinal myoclonus in which the discharges originate in a few adjacent spinal segments).[1161]

proptosis (Lat, forward + Gr, falling) Protrusion of the eye, most commonly due to dysthyroid ophthalmopathy in adults.

propulsion Forward inclination of the body in **Parkinson disease**, leading to a tottering, almost running gait, as though the patient were trying to chase his or her own center of gravity.

propulsive petit mal See **myoclonic astatic seizures**.

proscencephalon Those parts of the brain formed from the foreparts of the anterior cerebral vesicle, thus including the cerebral hemispheres, corpora striata, and olfactory lobes.

prosody (Gr, modulation) 1. (chanson de parler) The timing, stress, intonation, accent, and overall individual melodic quality of spoken speech, conveying both linguistic and affective information. Impairment of this function is known as *dysprosodia*, while absence of such melody in speech (as in Parkinsonism) is *aprosodia*. Excessive use of speech inflections, etc., is *hyperprosody*, as is heard in some patients with Broca aphasia and in many Shakespearean actors.

The right hemisphere plays a dominant role in the modulation of the affective components of language. Affective language is tested by examining spontaneous speech and the patient's enunciation of speech in different affective styles, and by his or her comprehension and identification of affectively charged speech and pantomime. 2. The fluctuations in rhythm and timbre of articulated speech.

prosopagnosia An unusual impairment of perception, characterized by the inability to recognize known faces or individual members of a group, always in association with some visual field deficit. Thus, a farmer may lose the ability to identify his cows, or any person his own belongings or even his own face. Lord Salisbury, an English prime minister, is reported once to have failed to recognize the face of his own son. The cause is the presence of bilateral lesions of the central visual system, often in mesial occipitotemporal rsgions and more marked on the right side, but right or left hemisphere lesions have also been held responsible. Dressing apraxia, topographic agnosia, unilateral spatial agnosia, achromatopsia, **Balint syndrome**, visual neglect, and impairment of nonverbal learning are often present as well.[1432, 1433]

The word was coined by Bodamer in 1947, although the phenomenon had been recognized by **Jackson** and by **Charcot** at the end of the nineteenth century.[1242] Prosopagnosia is not specific for faces, but relates to all visual items and to topography; but the patient may be able to read unless there is a lesion of the deep left occipitotemporal and occipital white matter. The commonest cause is a vascular (embolic) lesion; tumors and **herpes simplex encephalitis** are others. See also **agnosia**.

prosopalgia (Gr, the face + pain) (prosopodynia) Facial pain.

prosopodiplegia (Gr, face + double + blow) Bilateral facial paralysis.

prosopodynia See **prosopalgia**.

prosopoplegia Unilateral facial paralysis.

protagonists See **prime movers**.

protective reactions Automatic limb responses brought into play to prevent injury when falling is occurring as a result of the failure of other mechanisms to maintain equilibrium.[4723] (Reproduced by kind permission of the American Academy of Neurology and Lippincott Williams and Wilkins.)

protein C deficiency A dominantly inherited anomaly mapped to 2q13–q14 and associated with an increased tendency to stroke.

protein S deficiency A dominantly inherited anomaly mapped to 3p11.1–q11.2 and associated with an increased tendency to stroke.

protein-calorie malnutrition Marked growth retardation as a result of prolonged starvation. See **kwashiorkor**.

proteus syndrome (hemihypertrophy-nevi-hamartoma) A dominantly inherited combination of plantar hyperplasia ("moccasin feet"), macrocephaly, exostoses, asymmetrical limbs and lipomas, hemangiomas, epidermal nevi, and varicosities, leading in some cases to a fearful appearance. Tall stature, thick calvarium, macrocephaly, strabismus, ptosis, asymmetrical hypertrophy of arms and legs, hypocalcemia, osteoporosis, seizures, and muscle atrophy are other features described.

Tibbles and Cohen[6316] have suggested that this was the condition from which Joseph Merrick (the "Elephant Man" befriended by Sir Frederick Treves) suffered. The syndrome is named for the Greek God who appeared in polymorphous guises.

proto- (Gr, the first) Prefix denoting first.

proton magnetic resonance spectroscopy A magnetic resonance spectroscopy technique providing signals for phospholipids, creatine, n-acetyl aspartate, etc. and allowing estimation of the relative amounts of demyelination and axonal injury in brain regions.

protopathic pain The term of **Head** for more vivid but less acute sensation of superficial skin pain coupled with more extreme heat and cold sensation, as may be experienced after incomplete nerve injury.[2818]

protopathic sensory loss A disorder of superficial sensation in the area between that in which there is total thermoanesthesia and the surrounding area in which sensation is normal, following peripheral nerve injury. In this area, cotton wool touch is not perceived, discrimination of small changes in temperature and in two-point sensation is diminished, and pinprick leads to a most unpleasant ill-localized and persistent sensation.

Head originally proposed that this group of sensory modalities was subserved by a distinct system of sensory nerve fibers, but in fact the problem is a qualitative reduction in sensitivity, not a separate system.

protopathic system The sensory system envisaged by Henry **Head** as capable of responding to painful cutaneous stimuli and to extremes of heat and cold; it is characterized by high threshold, long latencies, poor localization, an inability to adapt, and an intense response to stimulation.

protoplasmic astrocytoma See **astrocytoma**.

protracted febrile myalgia syndrome Severe, paralyzing myalgia with high fever, abdominal pain, diarrhea, arthritis/arthralgia, and transient vasculitic rashes mimicking Henoch–Schonlein purpura, and possibly associated with recent streptococcal infection.[5964] See also **familial Mediterranean fever**.

Proust–Lichtheim maneuver A method whereby the patient, who is unable to evoke an appropriate word, can nevertheless indicate how many syllables are entailed—for example, by squeezing the examiners hand or by tapping the table the appropriate number of times.

proven multiple sclerosis That form of the disease in which the diagnosis is established at autopsy.

provoked nystagmus See **induced nystagmus**.

provoked seizures (acute symptomatic seizures) Seizures occurring in close temporal association with an acute systemic, metabolic, or toxic insult or in association with an acute CNS insult (infection, stroke, cranial trauma, intracerebral hemorrhage, or acute alcohol intoxication or withdrawal). They are often isolated epileptic events associated with acute conditions, but may also be recurrent seizures or even status epilepticus when the acute conditions recur—for example, in alcohol withdrawal seizures. See also **situation-related seizures**.

proximal chronic inflammatory polyneuropathy with multifocal conduction block See **multifocal inflammatory demyelinating neuropathy**.

proximal diabetic neuropathy See **diabetic radiculoplexus neuropathy**.

proximal intentional neglect A failure to move toward or in proximal space, associated with a right parietal lesion.[2438]

proximal lower motor neuron syndrome An acquired proximal motor axonal neuropathy with adult onset, initially affecting the arms, and frequently associated with the presence of antibodies to asialo-GM1 and to galactose β-1-3GaINAc-disaccharide.

proximal myotonic myopathy (PROMM) (myotonic dystrophy type 2, proximal myotonic myopathy, OMIM 600109) A dominantly inherited multisystem disorder resulting from an abnormality at a locus similar to **myotonic dystrophy** (3q21, zinc finger protein 9, ZNF9) but without the CTG repeat found in that condition; rather there are CUG or CCUG expansions at the RNA level. Clinically, the onset is in childhood or adult life with asymmetric muscle enlargement and weakness affecting the hip flexors and extensors and distal arms early on (facial and distal leg strength are normal), which can vary over hours and is worse with warming; stiffness (**myotonia**) with muscle contraction and percussion; and muscle pain. Muscle atrophy and cognitive failure are not features. Cataracts, testicular atrophy, diabetes, hypogammaglobulinemia, and cardiac arrhythmias are only described late in the course of the disease, if at all. MRI may show white matter hyperintensities on T2 weighted images. Serum CK levels are modestly raised and muscle biopsy findings are nonspecific. There is no congenital form.

Electrically, the myotonia shows no decrement. Repetitive stimulation may provoke "myopathic" motor unit potentials.[5287] The exercise test reveals that there is no decrement in CMAP amplitude or area immediately following exercise, unlike the situation in classical myotonic dystrophy.[5527]

Further *variants* are *proximal myotonic myopathy with both myotonic and myopathic features*,[4318] *proximal myotonic dystrophy* characterized by the same and added dystrophic features,[6435] and *myotonic dystrophy type 2* (OMIM 602688), another multisystem myotonic disorder clinically closely resembling classic myotonic dystrophy, but again without the CAG repeat.

proximal symmetrical motor neuropathy See **diabetic neuropathies**.

prune belly syndrome (triad syndrome) A rare autosomally inherited condition characterized by the absence of abnormal abdominal musculature, megaureter, and undescended testicles. Associated anomalies include polydactyly and syndactyly; malformations of the jaw, intestines, heart, eyes, ears, and nose; spina bifida or meningomyelocele; patent ductus arteriosus, congenital dislocation of the hip; and congenital myopathy.[65]

pruritis See **itch**.

psammoma bodies (Gr, sand + tumor) (corpora arenacea, acervuli) Small spheres composed of concentric layers of calcification within collagen, seen within some **meningiomas** and in the normal pineal gland. The resemblance of these calcific deposits to sand was noted by **Virchow**. *Pseudopsammoma bodies* are intra- or extracellular periodic acid–Schiff positive protein droplets secreted by meningothelial cells.

psammomatous meningioma See **meningioma**.

pseudo (Gr, false)

pseudoabducens palsy 1. Impairment of lateral deviation of a sound eye in the presence of a lesion of the III cranial nerve nucleus.[4134] 2. Impairment of lateral deviation of the eye due to **convergence spasm**, in which case the accompanying miosis suggests the diagnosis.[6396] 3. Paresis of voluntary ocular abduction while abduction is possible with, for example, ice-water caloric stimulation and thus not due to a lesion of the VI nerve. A rostral mesencephalic lesion is the usual cause.

pseudoaneurysm (fibrous globes, fibrin globes) Arteriolar outpouchings in the deep white matter and basal ganglia, consisting of a platelet plug at the end of an occluded arteriole and limited by a condensation of fibrin and white cells.

pseudo-anterior interosseous syndrome The production of the usual features of compression of the anterior interosseous nerve by a partial lesion of the main trunk of the median nerve at a point above its branching.[6734]

pseudo–Argyll Robertson pupil see **Holmes–Adie syndrome**.

pseudoathetosis Random slow, writhing involuntary movements of a limb deficient in proprioceptive sensory function but without any primary involvement of motor control systems. The afferent lesion may be at any site in the sensory pathway from peripheral nerve to cortex.[5764] The movements are clinically indistinguishable from **athetosis** but are due to loss of proprioception, whereas in true athetosis sensation is normal.

pseudo–Babinski sign Permanent dorsiflexion of the hallux, seen in some basal ganglion disorders such as the later stages of Parkinsonism and of pallidal degenerations. See also **dystonic foot response**.

pseudoblastoma See **orbital pseudotumor syndrome**.

pseudobobbing See **pretectal pseudobobbing**.

pseudobulbar affect See **emotionalism**.

pseudobulbar palsy 1. Bilateral upper motor neuron lesions affecting the bulbar musculature, and thus sited at or above the level of the pons. 2. A form of **amyotrophic lateral sclerosis** in which the earliest features are those of upper motor neuron lesions affecting the bulbar musculature.[1108]

The term is regrettable, for, as **Wartenberg** pointed out, there is nothing "pseudo" about the paralysis. *Spastic bulbar palsy* would be a far better term.

pseudobulbar palsy and mental retardation See **bilateral central macrogyria**.

pseudocaloric nystagmus Horizontal jerk nystagmus of mild intensity, beating in the appropriate direction (away from the irrigated ear) in response to caloric irrigation of an ear in which vestibular function has, however, been lost. The fast phase beats away from the diseased ear, regardless whether warm of cold stimuli are used. The cause is unknown, but it may represent unmasking of **latent nystagmus** by the alerting effect of the stimulation.[470]

pseudo–carpal tunnel syndrome (sublimis syndrome) A neuropathy of the median nerve proximal to the carpal tunnel, caused by compression of the nerve by the lateral border of the belly of the sublimis muscle, clinically mimicking the true syndrome.[2275] This might explain why 5% of patients who clinically have a carpal tunnel syndrome have normal electrodiagnostic findings.

pseudocataplexy Transient loss of muscle tone immediately following laughter, but not other emotional perturbations, occurring as a seizure manifestation (*gelastic-atonic seizures*) in subjects without any other features of the **narcolepsy** tetrad.[3143]

pseudocele See **cava septi pellucidi et vergae**.

pseudocerebellar ataxia See **parietal ataxia**.

pseudocervical cord syndrome A central cord pattern of weakness resembling paraparesis, reported in the context of **hepatic encephalopathy**.[4215]

pseudocholinesterase deficiency See **myasthenia gravis**.

pseudoclaudication syndrome See **lumbar spinal stenosis**.

pseudocoma See **locked-in syndrome**.

pseudocyst (nerve sheath myxoma) A benign intracranial tumor characterized by its mucinous content. It usually occurs on the common peroneal or ulnar nerves, suggesting a traumatic etiology. See also **ganglion**.

pseudodecrement An artifact produced by movement of the stimulating or recording electrodes during repetitive nerve stimulation. The amplitude and area of the M wave can vary in a way that resembles a decrementing response; however, the responses are generally irregular and not reproducible. (From the 2001 Report of the Nomenclature Committee of the American Association of Electromyography and Electrodiagnosis.[19] Reproduced by kind permission of the AANEM.)

pseudodeficiency rickets See **Prader syndrome**.

pseudodementia Cognitive disorders resulting from functional disorders; a group of conditions in which features suggesting dementia are not associated with any organic illness.[5487]

The following characteristics are usually described:

1. The impairment of memory, learning, and related cognitive functions is caused by a psychiatric illness.
2. The impairment is nonprogressive and is likely to be reversible if the primary illness is treated.
3. Any neuropathological process present is considered to be minor and insufficient to explain the severity of the cognitive defects.

Depression, mania, and malingering are the usual antecedents. See also **Ganser syndrome**.

pseudodrusen Multiple refractile bodies, representing degenerated axons, situated close to the optic nerve head and sometimes seen in patients with chronic papilledema.[2921] See also **drusen**.

pseudoepileptic seizures See **pseudoseizures**.

pseudoepileptiform patterns EEG patterns containing spikes which occur in bursts or trains, and which are not associated with clinical seizures. Such abnormalities are more likely to occur in non–rapid eye movement sleep stages 1 or 2.

pseudofacilitation See **incrementing response**.

pseudo–Foster Kennedy syndrome Unilateral optic atrophy with contralateral optic nerve swelling as a result of conditions other than tumors compressing that eye with the atrophic optic nerve.[2327] See also **pseudo-pseudo–Foster Kennedy syndrome**.

pseudoglaucoma A dominantly inherited syndrome with onset in young adult life, characterized by a deep optic cup and slowly progressive visual loss with constriction of the visual fields in a pattern resembling that seen in glaucoma, but with normal intraocular pressure.[5540]

pseudo–Graefe phenomenon (Fuchs sign) Elevation of the upper eyelid on downward movement of the eyes; a synkinesis wherein the action of the levator palpebrae is linked with that of the inferior rectus as a result of aberrant regeneration of the III cranial nerve after injury. Miosis on down-gaze may be associated.[6618, 6578] See also **Gowers signs**.

pseudohallucinations Vivid, usually visual, hallucinations, into the unreality of which the patient retains insight.Those hallucinations which result from organic brain disease and which are without any alteration in consciousness are commonly of this type.

pseudo–Horner syndrome Unilateral miosis with lid drooping, not due to sympathetic damage as pharmacological testing yields normal results. The condition may have no underlying pathology or may be due to any of numerous causes of miosis and of ptosis, as reviewed by Thompson et al.[6298]

pseudo–Huntington disease A rare variant of **dentatorubropallidoluysian atrophy** characterized by dementia and chorea.[379]

pseudo–Hurler disease See **GM1 gangliosidosis**.

pseudo–Hurler polydystrophy See **sialidosis**.

pseudohydrophobia An infectious bulbar paralysis described in Hungary and in Brazil, where it is known as the "scratching pest."[295]

pseudohypertrophic muscular dystrophy See **Duchenne muscular dystrophy**.

pseudohypertrophy Increase in the size of an organ despite a loss in the size or number of its constituent cells, which is usually due to the replacement of normal components by exogenous infiltrates, fat, or other connective tissue.

pseudohypoparathyroidism (Martin–Albright syndrome) A rare metabolic disorder due to end-organ unresponsiveness to parathyroid hormone. Neurological features include seizures, headache, photophobia, blurred vision, weakness, lethargy, muscle cramps, paresthesias, and numbness; the **Trousseau** and **Chvostek** signs are positive. Classically, the patients have round faces and short, wide digits with an absence of knuckles.[111]

A normocalcemic form (pseudo-pseudohypoparathyroidism) was also described by Albright, but the two conditions are now considered to be but *variants* of each other.

pseudohypoparathyroidism with Parkinsonism A rare autosomal or X-linked dominant syndrome resulting from end-organ resistance to parathyroid hormone and characterized by the above features, without calcifications of the basal ganglia.[1926]

pseudoinsomnia See **subjective DIMS complaint without objective findings**.

pseudoisochromatic plates (Isihara plates) Colored surfaces printed with dots reflecting a mixture of wavelengths that appear different in color to a normal ("trichromatic") observer, who can thus read numbers, etc., on the surfaces, but which appear identical to a dichromatic person suffering a defect in the retinal cones' pigment, so that no numbers, etc., can be discerned. This is the standard portable test for **color blindness**.[4954]

pseudokyphosis Trunkal flexion resulting from severe weakness of the thoracic musculature.

pseudolarval electrographic seizure of the elderly See **subclinical rhythmic discharges of adults**.

pseudolymphoma Generalized lymphadenopathy, joint swelling, hepatosplenomegaly, and skin rash due to an idiosyncratic reaction to long-term treatment with diphenylhydantoin. Lymph node biopsy specimens show replacement of the normal architecture by large reticulo-endothelial cells and the presence of germinal centers. The condition usually abates when the offending drug is withdrawn.[5652]

pseudomalignant myositis ossificans Rapidly growing, localized painless swelling in a muscle, due to inflammation and thus resembling **proliferative myositis** except that, in this condition, the process leads on to ossification.[5186] See **proliferative myositis**.

pseudo–Marfan syndrome See **Dinno syndrome**.

pseudomeningitis See **idiopathic intracranial hypertension**.

pseudomigraine with temporary neurological symptoms and lymphocytic pleocytosis A migraine variant most commonly seen in young males, some with a history of migraine and some after a viral-like illness up to 3 weeks prior to the onset of the syndrome. The clinical picture consists of episodes of changing variable neurological deficits accompanied by moderate to severe headache and sometimes fever. The headaches are typically throbbing and bilateral, lasting less than a day, while the transient neurological deficits last a mean of 5 h. Sensory symptoms are most common, followed by aphasia and motor symptoms. Visual symptoms appear rarely. Patients are asymptomatic between episodes. The pleocytosis ranges from 10 to 760 lymphocytes/mm^3 CSF (mean, 199), and CSF protein is increased in almost all cases. Brain CT and MRI are normal but the EEG frequently shows focal slowing.[2463]

pseudomyasthenic syndrome See **Lambert–Eaton myasthenic syndrome**.

pseudomyelia paresthetica Sensations perceived as though coming from phantom extremities.[6698]

pseudomyoclonic seizures Tonic or atonic seizures in which the patient suddenly falls to the ground as a result of lack of tone or generalized abnormal contraction of those muscles normally responsible for the maintenance of posture.

pseudomyopathic spinal muscular atrophy See **hereditary motor neuropathy**, type 3.

pseudomyotonia (myotonia acquisita, Hoffman syndrome) 1. The association of muscle hypertrophy with painful stiffness, worse in the cold; electrically silent **myoedema**; presence of the Woltman sign (hung-up reflexes); and affection of speech and gait more than of the face.

The slow, weak, painful sustained contractions and slow relaxation of muscles reflect a reduction in myosin ATPase activity and impaired calcium uptake by the sarcoplasmic reticulum. On muscle biopsy specimens, type 1 fiber atrophy, decreased oxidative enzyme activity, and increased glycogen content are the usual findings.

This condition is not the same as **paramyotonia**. The complex rhythmic discharges are pseudomyotonic and thus are not worse with rest, nor better with exercise, and there is no percussion myotonia but rather silent myoedema. Hyperparathyroidism may also contribute to the proximal weakness and fatigability, which abate with restoration of normal parathyroid hormone levels and vitamin D replacement. See also **acid maltase deficiency, neuromyotonia**. 2. See **pseudomyotonic discharge**.

pseudomyotonia and pseudotetany See **idiopathic neuromyotonia**.

pseudomyotonic discharge See **complex repetitive discharge**.

pseudoneurogenic thoracic outlet syndrome The occurrence of the typical clinical features of the **thoracic outlet syndrome** including focal atrophy and weakness, resulting however from disease of the contralateral cerebral hemisphere.[5856]

pseudonystagmus 1. A rare form of psychogenic eye movement disorder characterized by rapid, fine, pendular horizontal movements, accompanied by blepharospasm, convergence spasm, and miosis in almost all cases. 2. Abnormal pendular eye movements described in patients with vestibular failure and head tremor.

pseudoophthalmoplegia See **Roth–Bielschowsky syndrome**.

pseudopalisading The radial arrangement of the adjacent nuclei of tumor cells around areas of necrosis; a characteristic appearance in **glioblastoma multiforme**.[6]

pseudopapilledema (pseudoswelling of the disk) A benign congenital anomaly characterized by elevation and enlargement of the optic nerve head on each side, not due to increased intracranial pressure but rather to excessive myelination at the margins of the optic disk, so that the nerve fibers appear to be elevated and the disk edge blurred. The finding may be dominantly inherited and may occur without accompanying features or in the presence of hyperopia or skull deformities. Clinical manifestations (if they occur at all) may include transient visual obscurations, retinal hemorrhages, or arcuate field defects. The area of the blind spot is commonly increased. Venous pulsations are present. Hyaline bodies in the disk are a common cause. See **drusen**.

Criteria for differentiating true and pseudopapilledema have been defined by Glaser,[5] from which the following in Chart P–25 is adapted.

pseudoparalysis Apparent weakness of ocular muscles, the appearance being produced not by nerve lesions but by mechanical problems with certain muscles, such as fibrosis of the inferior rectus in **dysthyroid orbitopathy**, of the lateral rectus in **Duane syndrome** and of any of the ocular muscles after years of strabismus. Convergence spasm is another possible cause.

pseudoparalytic syndrome See **myasthenia gravis**.

pseudophakia The presence within the eye of an artificial lens in place of the natural one.

pseudoplegia A term denoting dissociation of voluntary and emotional movements, such as those of the face, jaws, throat, and larynx in the **anterior operculum syndrome**.[4053] See **diplegia with dissociation, oral-buccal apraxia**.

pseudopolymyelia The delusion of reduplication of parts of the body, usually occurring in those with left hemiparesis. The condition is regarded as a syndrome of parietal lobe origin involving disruption of the body schema.[6698]

pseudopolyneuropathy Sensory disturbances in a pattern resembling that of peripheral neuropathy but found in patients with cervical spondylotic myelopathy at C5–7 and in **multiple sclerosis**. Nerve conduction studies and F-wave latencies are normal. The anatomical substrates for this type of sensory impairment could be caused by combination of the dorsal horn/anterior commissure lesions for the upper limbs, and the anterolateral funiculi lesions for the lower limbs.[6920]

pseudopolyphasic action potential See **serrated action potential**.

pseudoprogeria A congenital dysmorphic syndrome manifesting also short stature, atrophy of the skin, glaucoma, ptosis, skeletal anomalies, osteoporosis, seizures, microcephaly, pyramidal signs, and mental and developmental delay.[381]

pseudopsammoma bodies See **psammoma bodies**.

pseudo-pseudo–Foster Kennedy syndrome The clinical picture of progressive visual loss suggesting pseudo–Foster Kennedy Syndrome due to nonarteritic anterior ischemic optic neuropathy, but here due to a compressive lesion situated posteriorly.[2327]

pseudo-pseudohypoparathyroidism See **Albright syndrome**.

pseudo-pseudoulnar claw hand The appearance of **pseudoulnar claw hand** but in this case due to cervical radiculopathy at C8 or to other proximal lesions.[993]

Chart P–25. Diagnostic Features of Pseudopapilledema

A. The central cup is absent and the disk diameter tends to be small;
B. Hyperemia is not present;
C. Vessels arise from the central apex of the disk;
D. Anomalous branching of vessels, an increased number of major disk vessels and venous pulsations are present;
E. The disk may be transilluminated, with a glow appearing from hyaline bodies (if they are present);
F. The disk margins are irregular, with derangement of the peripapillary retinal epithelium;
G. The nerve fiber layer is not opaque;
H. Superficial capillary telangiectasias, hemorrhages, exudates and **cotton-wool spots** are absent;
I. Retinal folds are uncommon and choroidal folds absent.

Adapted from Glaser JS. Neuroophthalmology, *2nd edition. Philadelphia, J.B. Lippincott, 1990.*

pseudoptosis 1. The appearance of unilateral ptosis in an eye that is in fact healthy, because of the presence of proptosis (with consequential eyelid retraction) of the other. 2. See **apraxia of eyelid opening**.

pseudoradicular syndrome Numbness and paresthesias felt in an apparent radicular distribution such as C8, in association with a lesion of the contralateral sensory cortex or thalamus.

pseudorelapse A temporary deterioration in the clinical status of a patient with **multiple sclerosis** as the consequence of a concurrent (usually febrile) illness.

pseudorosettes Clear rings around blood vessels due to the centripetal extension of fine fibrillary processes from the ependymal tumor cells surrounding them.

pseudo–Schnabel cavernous degeneration of the optic nerve Degeneration of the optic nerve occurring in glaucoma; the "pseudo" form is that in which a similar appearance is found in association with local silicone injections.[5801]

pseudosclerosis The term of Westphal for a disease (actually **Wilson disease**) in which the signs resemble those of **multiple sclerosis** but the pathology does not.

pseudoseizures See **nonepileptic seizures; factitious epilepsy**.

pseudosixth Failure of ocular abduction, not due to a lesion of the abducens nerve but rather to a mesencephalic lesion. The sign is frequently bilateral and is accompanied by **hyperconvergence**. See **pseudoabducens palsy, Duane syndrome, ocular myasthenia. Graves orbitopathy**, old squint, medial rectus entrapment, and convergence spasm also enter the differential diagnosis.

pseudospasticity An increase in muscular resistance to passive stretch and in muscle activity, leading to the adoption of abnormal postures, as a consequence of peripherally generated continuous motor unit discharges. The pathogenesis may involve a reduction of ionized calcium levels in the presence of an axonal motor neuropathy.[5114]

pseudo–status epilepticus Simulated status epilepticus, differentiated from the true condition by the frequent occurrence of retained consciousness; pelvic thrusting; flailing, asynchronous, or rolling limb movements; tight eye closure or gaze aversion; resistance to passive movements; frequency of induction by suggestion; gradual onset; and prevention of hand falling onto the face. Cyanosis, tongue, and other injuries and abnormal ictal or postictal EEG records are uncommon.[3013]

pseudoswelling of the disk See **pseudopapilledema**.

pseudotabes (peripherica) A syndrome in which the clinical features (sensory ataxia, pupillary changes, **Charcot joints**, etc.) resemble those of tabes dorsalis, but their cause is not syphilis. Diabetes mellitus is the classic example, but alcoholic and diphtheritic neuropathies may do the same. See **Oppenheim disease**.

pseudotabetic pupillotonia The preferred term of **Wartenberg** for **Adie syndrome**, which did not find favor, perhaps in part because of the decline in the incidence of **tabes dorsalis**.

pseudotabetic syndrome The occurrence of **Argyll Robertson pupils** with areflexia and proprioceptive disturbance, occurring either as a complication of diabetes or in the **Holmes–Adie syndrome**.

pseudo-tetanus of d'Espine Tonic spasm of all limbs or opisthotonos in children with markedly increased intracranial pressure, who cry or who are stimulated externally. It may be due to spasmodic decorticate posturing.

pseudothalamic syndrome Unpleasant radiating sensations resembling thalamic pain, but in this case due to lesions of the opercular part of the postcentral gyrus.[1594] Touch, pain, temperature, and vibration sensations in the contralateral face, arm, and leg are lost when the lesion (which is usually a stroke) involves the anterior–inferior part of the parietal lobe. See also **parietal stroke**.

pseudothalidomide syndrome A recessively inherited syndrome of symmetrical reductive limb defects, flexion contractures, scanty blond hair, hypoplastic ears and nose, and sometimes seizures and mental retardation.[2877] See **Roberts syndrome**.

pseudotonic pupillotonia See **Adie pupil**.

pseudotumor cerebri See **idiopathic intracranial hypertension**.

Pseudotumor Cerebri Society A charitable organization in this field. Address: 750 East Adams St. c/o Dr. D. Friedman, Syracuse, NY 13210. Tel: 315-464-3937. Web site: http://www.pseudotumorcerebri.com/.

Pseudotumor Cerebri Support Network A charitable organization in this field. Address: 8247 Riverside Dr. Powell, OH 43065. Tel: 614-794-0442. E-mail: sondra@sprynet.com/.

pseudotumor orbiti An autoimmune disorder in which inflammation of the orbital contents with striking edema and round cell infiltration is associated with proptosis, painful ocular palsies, and visual deterioration. See **orbital pseudotumor syndrome**.

pseudoulnar claw hand Hyperextension at the fourth and fifth metacarpophalyngeal joints with distal flexion, due to a partial lesion of the radial or posterior interosseous nerves.[4074]

pseudoxanthoma elasticum (Gr, false + yellow + tumor + driven) A rare, recessively inherited disorder characterized by loosening of the skin, abnormalities of blood vessels such as early calcification, and the formation of aneurysms and **angioid streaks** of the retina with hemorrhages.

Neurologically, intracranial hemorrhages, infarcts, dementia, calcification of the falx, and seizures have all been reported.[3096]

pseudo–Zellweger syndrome A **peroxisomal disorder** that clinically and biochemically is identical to **Zellweger syndrome** but in which there are abundant liver peroxisomes and it is β-ketothiolase that is defective. Clinically, it is characterized by dysmorphisms, expressionless face due to facial weakness, a cat-like cry, ventricular septal defect, enlarged liver and kidneys, multiple renal cysts, adrenal hypoplasia, recurrent infections, and seizures.[2448]

psittacosis (Gr, parrot) (ornithosis) Infection with *Chlamydia psittaci*, an unique form of intracellular parasite, following the inhalation of dust from dried bird excreta. The disease mainly affects the lungs, but, in some cases, fever, chills, diffuse headaches, myalgia, and eventually encephalomyelitis with coma have been described.[1034]

psoas insufficiency syndrome A syndrome of tightness and weakness of the psoas muscles, found almost exclusively in gymnasts and dancers and resulting from the use of the muscles mainly to pull the lumbar spine into a position of flexion and lordosis.[5480]

psoriatic myopathy A chronic proximal myopathy; an unusual complication of the skin disease.[4441]

psychiatric dizziness (space and motion discomfort) Both the occurrence of anxiety symptoms as a result of imperfect procressing of environmental clues and the precipitation of the sensation of imbalance as a result of anxiety, each witnessing the close functional association of the vestibular and limbic systems. Furman and Jacob (1997) have reviewed the subject.[2245]

psychic akinesia Hypoactive–hypoalert behavior with loss of psychic autoactivation, **apathy**, and stereotyped activity, that are reversible with external stimulation. The condition may be a manifestation of lesions of the brainstem, basal ganglia, or frontal lobes and has been described with **spontaneous intracranial hypotension**.

psychic paralysis of visual fixation See **Balint syndrome**.

psychic pillow The appearance of some patients with schizophrenia or **Parkinson disease** who lie supine in bed with the neck flexed off the mattress, as though there were a pillow supporting the head.

psychic variant See **affective-psychic seizures**.

psychical hallucinations Those formed hallucinations produced by stimulation of the temporal or parietal cortex anterior to area 19, and considered by Penfield and Jasper to be re-evocations of prior perceptions elicited from the experiential cortex.

Psychnet-uk A site designed as a major UK psychology link resource for mental health professionals, students, or others wanting to know more, offering academic software, etc.

psychogalvanic reflex (electrodermal response, sympathetic skin response, Tarchanov phenomenon) A test of sudomotor function, measuring the change in skin resistance to the passage of a constant current with psychic (or with sensory) stimuli. It can normally be evoked by electrical stimulation of a peripheral nerve in subjects less than 60 years old. The presence of the reflex indicates that pre- and postganglionic sympathetic functional innervation of sweat glands is intact.[3638] See **galvanic skin response**.

Charles Féré[2012] noted in 1888 that the electrical resistance in the body, measured with a galvanometer, was variable with emotional fluctuations, as did Ivan Romanovich Tarchanov (1848–1909), a Russian physiologist, in 1890, but the first mention was by **Waller**, who thought that it was an artifact.

psychogenic "coma" a state of voluntary unresponsiveness, considered to be due to severe emotional stress, in which the eyes are kept closed and resist passive opening. Caloric testing leads not only to the expected nystagmus, but sometimes to restoration of an interactive state. The EEG shows patterns consistent with normal wakefulness.

psychogenic disease See **hysteria**.

psychogenic dystonia Atypical dystonia without response to the usual medications and with a protracted course. The legs are most affected. Additional features include give-way weakness, nonanatomic sensory changes, excessive slowness, marked resistance to passive movements, and multiple somatizations.[4414] See also **causalgia-dystonia syndrome**.

Differences between this entity and structurally based torsion dystonia have been summarized.[3683] Chart P–26 interprets these criteria.

Chart P–26. Comparison of Psychogenic and Idiopathic Torsion Dystonia

Psychogenic Dystonia	*Idiopathic Torsion*
Dystonia	
Onset with resting dystonia	Onset with action dystonia
Adult-onset leg involvement common	Leg involvement rare with adult-onset
Often fixed spasm	Mobile spasms
Rapid progression and spread to maximum disability early in the course	Slow progression
Dystonic movements inconsistent over time	Consistent over time (*rarely patients with cervical dystonia may change the direction of dystonia after a remission*)
No *geste antagonistique*	*Geste* is frequent
Selective disabilities or abilities inconsistent with fixed spasms	Surprising abilities despite severe movements and postures (*Action dystonia may however result in selective disabilities; patients with* ***paradoxical dystonia*** *improve with action*)
Painful (often with pronounced tenderness to touch and exaggeration with passive movement)	Usually painless. (*But patients with cervical dystonia do have pain*)
No improvement after sleep	Symptoms often improve briefly after sleep

continued

Chart P–26. *(continued)*

Attempted voluntary movement to command may activate antagonists with little apparent action in agonist muscles (limb or digit may do the opposite of what is requested by the examiner)	Voluntary movement and attempts to overcome the dystonia often result in further co-contraction of agonists and antagonists with variable changes in the dystonic posturing.
Paroxysmal dystonia (isolated or mixed with persistent dystonia) and/or other paroxysmal movements.	Paroxysms not a feature *(caution: exclude other causes of paroxysmal dystonia/dyskinesias)*
Other psychogenic movement disorders Other nonorganic neurological features	Other movements possible e.g., tremor, myoclonus *(caution: important to consider a psychogenic movement disorder or other psychogenic features superimposed on an organic movement disorder)*
Precipitant common	Precipitant uncommon
Remissions: spontaneous or with nonphysiological treatments	*(caution: spontaneous remissions occasionally espec occur ially in cervical dystonia)*
No family history	Family history not uncommon.

After Lang AE. Psychogenic dystonia: a review of 18 cases. Can J Neurol Sci *1995;***22:***136–43, reproduced by kind permission.)*

psychogenic flutter (psychological nystagmus, hysterical flutter, hysterical nystagmus, voluntary flutter, ocular fibrillation, ocular shudderings) A form of saccadic intrusion or oscillation characterized by back-to-back saccades occurring at high frequency, usually induced voluntarily during attempted convergence.[3762] See also **voluntary nystagmus**.

psychogenic gait Gait disorders, without underlying structural abnormality characterized by hesitation, excessive slowness of movements, fluctuations in symptomatology, a pattern as though "walking on ice," and a psychogenic Romberg test. Inconsistent, but helpful diagnostic features include knee buckling without falls, astasia, tremor, a strained facial expression, and grasping of the leg, with hyperventilation.[4414]

psychogenic headache See **episodic tension-type headache**.

psychogenic movement disorders Abnormal motor activity resulting from functional (nonstructural, not biochemical) disorders. These take many forms (see above and below). Pointers to their diagnosis are incorporated in the following list, which synthesizes the data provided by a number of sources:[1952, 5804, 1946, 5238]

Psychotherapy or suggestion accords persistent relief, and the subject does not usually manifest the movement disorder when feeling free of observation.

The presence of astasia-abasia or of selective disability; abrupt onset; entrainment of tremor to the frequency of repetitive movements; the co-contraction sign (agonists and antagonists work together) in tremor; an atypical response to a pharmacological agent; atypical stimulus sensitivity; paroxysmal nature of the movements or periods of spontaneous remission*; false sensory signs or weakness; movements that are inconsistent over time or incongruent with a classical movement disorder; the presence of false neurological signs; the presence of an obvious psychiatric disturbance; unusual distractibility; deliberate slowness in executing movements; the patient's actions are inconsistent or incongruent; other false neurological signs or multiple somatizations (complaints involving at least three different organ systems other than pain and fatigue) are observed; there is a pre-movement Bereitschaftspotential on EEG (myoclonus only); complaints of pain or fatigue are judged excessive; the subject has had previous exposure to a disease model; there is a potential for secondary gain (including the continuing attention of a devoted "significant other").

*However, see entries under **paroxysmal**. Moreover, somatization and psychiatric disturbance should be somewhat discounted because many patients with, for example, **Parkinson disease** or **Tourette syndrome** also have concomitant neuropsychiatric disease. A response to placebo is a feature of both structural and functional disorders and is of no value in diagnosis.

See also **Waddell signs**.

psychogenic myoclonus Segmental, generalized, or focal myoclonus for which neither structural nor biochemical causes can be elucidated. Clinically, incongruous clinical presentations of the myoclonus or of associated motor or sensory features, evidence of underlying psychopathology, and improvement with distraction or placebo have been suggested as useful points in diagnosis.[4445] The problem occurs at rest but it worsened by exercise. Tremor, focal dystonia, and gait disturbances may also be present.[4414]

Electrodiagnosis is helpful, as these patients do not show a **bereitschaftpotential** and have variable and inconsistent muscle activation patterns, while stimulus-induced responses habituate, as seen in the normal startle response but not with stimulus-induced myoclonus.[4414]

psychogenic nonepileptic attacks See **nonepileptic seizures**.

psychogenic palatal tremor A movement disorder presenting with intermittent audible ear clicking, disappearing with mouth opening, and under a degree of voluntary control.[6795]

psychogenic Parkinsonism The appearances of **Parkinson disease** in young or middle-aged adults, whose symptoms occur suddenly and bilaterally with features suggesting **psychogenic tremor**. The tremor persists with posture and during activity, and it lacks the dampening effect associated with movement as is normally seen in Parkinson disease. Excessive slowness and rigidity resembling voluntary resistance are also notable and the gait may be bizarre.[4414]

psychogenic pseudoneuropathy A syndrome comprising positive and negative motor and sensory complaints and vascular symptoms and considered to result from psychological dysfunction. The incorrect diagnosis of **reflex sympathetic dystrophy** is commonly made.[4747]

psychogenic seizures Attacks in which geotropic (earthward) eye and head movements occur even when the body is turned 180°. Other features suggesting the presence of this entity include asynchronous movements of the legs and arms, pelvic thrusting or rocking, holding on to a bed-rail, puffed-out cheeks with breath-holding, and the preferred occurrence, in hospital, at times of nursing shift change.

In such cases the shaking, jerking, or thrashing occur with retained awareness; there is usually a history of psychiatric comorbidity (somatoform, dissociative, affective, personality disorders) or abuse (physical and/or sexual) and/or of recent stress. The typical attacks display nonphysiologic features and can sometimes be induced or stopped by suggestion. See also **nonepileptic seizures** which, though differently named, must surely be the same thing.

psychogenic tremor Abnormal repetitive movements (tremors) starting abruptly with maximal deficit at onset, present at rest, maintained both with posture and in action, with a static or fluctuating course and unassociated with demonstrable CNS lesions. One limb is initially affected in most cases but diffusion occurs. Spontaneous resolution and recurrence, distractibility, response to suggestion, and lack of response to conventional therapies are other common features.[3430, 4414] However, after prolonged follow-up, many such patients turn out to have organic neurological disease Diagnostic criteria have been suggested, adapted as follows:[2583, 3387]

Sudden onset or remission or both.
Unusual clinical combinations of rest and postural/intention tremor.
Decrease of tremor amplitude and/or frequency during distraction (e.g., by alternate finger tapping or mental concentration tasks) and exacerbation with hyperventilation.
Varying frequency of the tremor during distraction or during voluntary movements of the other side.
Coactivation sign (resistance to passive movement when a trembling limb is tested for rigidity. The tremor depends on there being an increase in tone and it disappears when the voluntary increase in resistance ceases.)
A positive history of somatization.
The appearance of additional and unrelated neurologic signs.

psychogenic unresponsiveness A nonorganic coma-like state. Physical signs helpful in making the diagnosis include; opposition to eye opening; the presence of Bell's phenomenon; retention of corneal reflexes; inhibition of eye movement with oculocephalic maneuvers as a result of visual fixation (in true coma, the eyes "roll" with oculocephalic maneuvers, unless there is a brainstem lesion); when the subject's passively elevated hand is dropped so as to hit the patients face, it is steered away; the patient placed in uncomfortable postures spontaneously assumes a more natural and comfortable resting posture; breath holding when spirits of ammonia are kept under the nostril; nystagmus, not just tonic deviation of the eyes, in the cold caloric test; retention of optokinetic nystagmus; an avoidance reaction when a vibrating tuning fork is touched to the nostrils or air is blown up the nostril with a syringe; and a normal alpha pattern with the eyes closed that attenuates when the eyelids are elevated.

psychogenic vertigo A common diagnosis but an uncommon syndrome, most patients with a psychogenic basis to their symptoms having basic organic (structural) lesions as well, either demonstrable at the time or subsequently. The subject has been reviewed.[2245]

psychological fatigue Failure of motivation to perform a muscular task with the full power available.[873]

psychological nystagmus See **psychogenic flutter**.

psychomotor retardation Slowing of the thought processes and of the initiation and execution of voluntary movements, either in the context of a depressive reaction or of generalized depression of cortical function stemming from any cause.

psychomotor seizures A term introduced by **Gibbs** in 1937 for those seizures originating within a temporal lobe, with alteration in consciousness and affective upsurges as components. See **pseudoseizures, affective-psychic seizures, complex partial seizures**.

psychomotor variant Rhythmic mid-temporal bursts of theta activity which are benign and not associated with an epileptic process. See **rhythmic temporal theta burst of drowsiness**.

psychomyogenic headache See **episodic tension-type headache**.

psychopathy See **hysterical personality**.

psychophysiological arousal See **persistent DIMS**.

psychophysiological insomnia A disturbance of initiating or maintaining sleep which is not due to an underlying structural or to a major psychiatric cause, in which tension and anxiety insufficient to allow a diagnosis of anxiety state lead on to a learned pattern of sleep disorder through the association of poor sleep with the habitual sleeping environment. Although most commonly transient (*adjustment sleep disorder*), a persistent variety also occurs.[2796] Diagnostic criteria have been defined[1629] and are listed in Chart P–27.

psychosis A class of mental illness in which there is gross impairment of reality testing, usually evidenced by such features as delusions, hallucinations, or seriously disorganized behavior. The individual with gross impairment revealed by reality testing incorrectly evaluates the accuracy of his or her perceptions and thoughts, and makes incorrect inferences about external reality, even in the face of contrary evidence. Two forms are usually differentiated: the *organic psychoses*, in which physical disease (primarily or secondarily of the brain) is present; and the *functional psychoses*, which include schizophrenia and manic-depressive psychosis.[6633]

The term is, however, loosely used and, in the absence of complete understanding of causes, it could well be dropped from the vocabulary.

PTAH stain See **Mallory stain**.

ptarmus See **sneezing**.

pterygocorneal reflex See **Wartenberg winking jaw phenomenon**.

pterygoid reflex (Gr, wing-like) Contraction of the medial pterygoid muscle in response to a downward tap on the chin. The reflex can only be assessed electrically with an EMG needle in the muscle. It is said to inform about the status of neuronal pools

Chart P–27. Diagnostic Criteria for Psychophysiological Insomnia

A. A complaint of insomnia combined with a complaint of decreased functioning during wakefulness.
B. Indications of learned sleep-preventing associations are found:
   1. Trying too hard to sleep, suggested by an inability to fall asleep when desired, but ease of falling asleep during other relatively monotonous pursuits, such as watching television or reading.
   2. Conditioned arousal to bedroom or sleep-related activities, indicated by sleeping poorly at home, but sleeping better away from home or when not carrying out bedtime routines.
C. Evidence for increased somatized tension, e.g., agitation, muscle tension, increased vasoconstriction.
D. Polysomnographic monitoring demonstrates:
   1. An increased sleep latency.
   2. Reduced sleep efficiency.
   3. An increased number and duration of awakenings.
E. No evidence of other medical or psychiatric disorder that would account for the sleep disturbance.
F. Other sleep disorders can coexist with the insomnia, e.g., inadequate sleep hygiene, obstructive **sleep apnea** syndrome, etc.

Adapted from AASM Diagnostic Classification Steering Committee. The International Classification of Sleep Disorders Diagnostic and Coding Manual. *Rochester, MN. American Academy of Sleep Medicine 1991/2001. Reproduced by kind permission of the Academy.* See also http://www.sleepeducation.com/Disorders.aspx/.

in the pontomesencephalic region,[2984] but the clinical utility of the technic requires further study.

pterygopalatine ganglion The ganglion in association with the glossopharyngeal nerve within the fossa of the same name, through which pass fibers conducting taste impulses from the palate.

pterygopalatine fossa syndrome 1. Pain in the second and later the third divisions of the trigeminal nerve, numbness in the territory of the infraorbital nerve, paresis of the soft palate and of the pterygoid muscles, deafness resulting from compression of the Eustachian tube, blindness resulting from optic nerve compression, and lateral rectus, pterygoid, and palatal palsies, all occurring as a result of malignant infiltration of the fossa, usually by a nasopharyngeal tumor.[270] See also **Trotter syndrome**. 2. See **cluster headache**.

ptosis (from Gr, a falling) (blepharoptosis) Drooping of the upper eyelid, as with myasthenia gravis, myopathy, or III nerve palsy. In **Horner syndrome**, the lower lid rises a little as well and the ptosis is not severe; while in the other conditions, the upper lid may descend completely, occluding the eye.

Cerebral (supranuclear) ptosis is uni- or bilateral and is thought to be due to damage to cortico-bulbar fibers rather than to the oculomotor nerve or due to damage to the sympathetic fibers supplying the eye.[1006]

pubic reflex The **abdominal reflex**, obtained in this case by tapping the symphysis pubis. The induced vibration also leads to contraction of the hip adductors in some cases.

pudendal (from Lat, shameful) The parts of the body that should normally be covered; the genitalia.[5886]

pudendoanal reflex Contraction of the external anal sphincter in response to stimulation of the dorsal nerve of the penis or the clitoris, with a normal latency of around 40 ms. This latency is increased in subjects with neurogenic lesions affecting the external anal sphincter.[6516] The bulbocavernosus muscle is similarly stimulated to contract by this maneuver.

Pudenz valve A plastic valve placed subcutaneously under the scalp and attached to a slit valve, allowing the bubble to be pumped in order to check intracranial pressure and to clear partial obstructions.

puerperal hemiplegia The sudden onset of headache, convulsions, coma, and hemiplegia in a woman days to weeks after delivery, as a result of **cerebral venous sinus thrombosis**.

puffer fish toxin See **tetrodotoxin**.

pugilistic encephalopathy See **punch-drunk syndrome**.

Pulfrich phenomenon When an observer views a pendulum swinging in a plane perpendicular to the line of vision (i.e., side to side) with one of his eyes covered by a filter or smoked glass, the pendulum appears to trace an elliptical path, coming toward him as it goes one way and away from him as it goes the other, the direction varying according to which eye is covered. The illusion is due to delayed perception in the covered eye, as with **optic neuritis**.[1814]

pull test A method of assessing postural instability, mainly used in the context of **Parkinson disease**. The examiner abruptly pulls the informed patient backwards by the shoulders, who is expected to prevent falling by retreating a step or two in response. A standardized method of performing the test has been published.[4550] For accurate evaluation, one or two practice trials should be performed.

The *sternal push test* also measures the righting reflex but adds the risk of injury and litigation unless there is a competent catcher behind the patient being tested.

pulsatile tinnitus An intracranial murmur synchronous with the heartbeat and due to disorders of the arterial or venous systems in the cranium or to idiopathic intracranial hypertension.[6597]

pulse A burst of neuronal activity with precise onset and offset.

pulse dysmetria An abnormality of saccadic control in which the rapid initial (pulse) part of the saccade is too great or too small. See also **glissade**.

pulse-delay oculoplethysmography A technique for measuring the arrival of pulses in the vessels of the eye and the earlobe. Severe internal carotid artery stenosis is suggested by a delay in arrival of the pulse wave between the eye and ipsilateral ear, or in the different times of arrival of the pulse wave in the two eyes. External carotid artery stenosis is documented by a delay in arrival of the ear pulse compared with the ocular pulse.[4678] **pulse sequence** A set of radiofrequency (and/or gradient) magnetic field pulses and time spacings between these pulses used in conjunction with gradient magnetic fields and MRI signal reception to produce magnetic resonance images.

pulse-step control A motor neuronal control signal comprising initially a phasic, high-frequency burst of activity in the motor nerve leading to the activation of agonist and the inhibition of antagonist muscles (the pulse), followed by a steady-state or tonic neuronal firing rate (the step), as seen in the extraocular muscles, in which the duration of the pulse is normally half that of the whole saccade.[330] These represent two components of the **controller signal** managing eye movements.[331]

pulseless disease See **aortic arch disease**.

pulseless saccade See **hypometric saccade**.

PULSES profile A global assessment of disability in which *physical condition, upper and lower limb functions, sensation and bladder and bowel functions* are rated on 4-point scales. The instrument's limitation in scope is offset by its reliability in usage.[1041]

pulvinar (from Lat, a cushion) The elevated posterior projection of the thalamus; the largest and most posterior of the thalamic nuclei, having a role in motor functions and also in the processing of certain sensory signals.

pulvinar sign The presence of T2 weighted MRI hyperintensities in the posterior thalamus relative to that of other deep gray matter nuclei and cortical gray matter. It is recorded in patients with new variant **Creutzfeldt–Jakob disease**.[2212]

punch-drunk syndrome (dementia puglistica, pugilistic encephalopathy) A chronic encephalopathy presenting as a dementing illness, usually with added Parkinsonian features and evidence of cerebellar and pyramidal disease, resulting eventually from the cumulative effect of repeated head injuries as incurred in professional **boxing**.[3247] It is characterized pathologically by perforation of the septum cavum, lesions of the substantia nigra, and the presence of scattered neurofibrillary tangles in the cortex and brainstem, and by diffuse cerebral atrophy on CT scans.

punding Stereotyped motor behavior in which there is a protracted occupation with repetitive purposeless activity such as disassembling mechanical objects, jotting down figures, sorting or arranging of common objects (e.g., lining up pebbles, rocks, or other small objects), or hoarding objects. It is often accompanied by a tendency to gamble and by hypersexual behaviour. Punding is observed among stimulant abusers and may be a result of excess dopamine stimulation. (HJM)[2021, 5483] See also **dopamine dysregulation syndrome**.

pupil (from Lat, pupilla, an orphan girl) The aperture of the eye, surrounded by the iris. It has been said to be so-called because a tiny image of the beholder is therein reflected (Trevisa, 1398).

pupil campimetry An objective test of the visual field in which a pupillary light response is elicited by focal light stimuli from different locations within the visual fields and measured by infrared pupillography. The method correlates reasonably well with automated perimetery. In the case of functional loss of visual field sensitivity, the pupil reacts normally even when light is shone from the "blind" field.[5614]

pupil cycle time The time taken between constriction and dilation of the pupil stimulated with a light beam shone through a slit-lamp. The light causes the pupil to constrict, reducing the retinal stimulus so the pupil re-dilates; this leads to the repeated light stimulation of the retina and so to pupillary constriction, and so on. The duration in seconds of a hundred such cycles is recorded and the mean determined; the average cycle time is 840 ms.

Abnormal slowing indicates a lesion of the parasympathetic efferent pathway in the absence of an afferent pathway defect.[4130] The test is of value in cases of bilateral compressive optic neuropathy in which the optic nerves are symmetrically affected, so that a relative afferent pupillary defect is not easily demonstrated.[4375] See also **hippus**.

pupillary dilatation lag See **dilatation lag**.

pupillary escape The re-dilation of the pupil on the side of an afferent defect (a lesion of the optic nerve or retina) elicited by the swinging flashlight test. The mechanism, as explained by Levatin, is diminished stimulation of the pupilloconstrictor center when the light swings across from the normal to the abnormal eye, and thus diminished constriction. The phenomenon also occurs with continued light stimulation of an eye in the presence of an afferent defect. The clinical utility of the test is not established.[1307]

pupillary reflex Constriction of the pupils in response to light stimulation.

pupillary sparing The retention of normal pupillary reactions to light in the presence of a III cranial nerve palsy causing paresis of the extraocular muscles. Small-vessel disease is determined as the cause in three-quarters of such patients, but aneurysms and tumors can also, though rarely, be responsible.[4568]

pupillography A technique whereby infra-red light is used to record the size of the pupils in such conditions as sleep.

pupillotonia The tonic pupillary reaction as seen in the **Adie pupil**.

pupillotonic pseudotabes See **Adie pupil**.

puppenkopfphänomenon See **oculocephalic reflex**.

puppet-like gait A stiff, uncoordinated, and jerky gait adopted by some patients with leg spasticity in association with the myelopathy of hepatic disease.

puppy sign The MRI appearance in axial oriented sections seen in some patients with bilateral internal carotid artery dissection, the appearances somewhat resembling a cartoon picture of the face of a small dog.[1980]

pure affective deafness (pure prosodic deafness) A rare syndrome comprising motor aprosodia, loss of emotional gesturing, impaired repetition, and comprehension of affective prosody but normal comprehension of emotional gesturing, due to an anterior right hemisphere lesion.[5418]

pure agraphia See **agraphia**.

pure akinesia syndrome A rare syndrome characterized by freezing of gait, speech, and handwriting without accompanying limb rigidity, tremor, dementia, or ophthalmoplegia, unresponsive to levadopa therapy but strikingly responsive to treatment with L-threo-3,4 dihydroxyphenylserine (L-DOPS).[4590] The condition may represent an atypical presentation of **progressive supranuclear palsy**.

pure alexia A modality-specific disconnection syndrome. See **alexia without agraphia, pure word blindness**.

pure autonomic failure See **progressive autonomic failure**.

pure autonomic variant of acute inflammatory polyradiculoneuropathy See **autonomic neuropathy**, definition 1.

pure axonal neuropathy A syndrome with the onset in youth of axonal motor and both thick-fiber and thin-fiber sensory neuropathy, accompanied later by dementia and pyramidal and cerebellar signs, and with spongy/cavity/cystic changes in the CNS. This condition may be a *variant* of **hereditary motor and sensory neuropathy**, type 2.

pure cholinergic dysautonomia See **autonomic neuropathy**.

pure dysarthria Dysarthria (usually with obvious lower-quadrant facial weakness) occurring as a **lacunar syndrome**.[2092, 2106]

pure midbrain infarction Infarction usually of the middle of the midbrain, mainly in the paramedian territory and presenting typically with nuclear or fascicular III nerve palsies often in isolation. Vertical gaze pareses, pure motor hemiparesis, four-limb ataxia from unilateral lesions, and hypesthetic ataxic hemiparesis are also described. Patients with isolated upper or lower midbrain infarcts may have no localizing clinical findings.[705]

pure motor aphasia See **logopenia**.

pure motor demyelinating neuropathy See **chronic inflammatory demyelinating polyneuropathy**.

pure motor hemiparesis (pure motor stroke) A **lacunar syndrome** manifesting complete or incomplete paralysis of the face, arm, and leg on one side, unaccompanied by sensory disturbances, visual deficits, aphasia, or apractagnosia. In the case of brainstem lesions, the patient will be free of vertigo, tinnitus, deafness, diplopia, cerebellar ataxia, and gross nystagmus.[2106] In 15% of cases, however, another stroke cause is detected. The disorder is due to a small infarct of the basis pontis, in the middle part of the cerebral peduncle or in the posterior limb of the internal capsule.

Various degrees of involvement are described ranging from those due to extensive lesions (pure motor hemiplegia) to incomplete basilar-pontine syndromes and restricted deficits such as ataxic hemiparesis, dysarthria–clumsy hand syndrome, dysarthria–dysmetria and dysarthria–facial paresis. The syndromes are not discrete and are only distinguished by their relative severity.

Variant forms include the following:

Pure motor hemiparesis sparing the face: See **lacunar syndromes**.[2092, 2106]
Pure motor hemiparesis with confusion: See **lacunar syndromes**.[2092, 2106]
Pure motor hemiparesis with crossed III nerve palsy: (Weber syndrome) See **lacunar syndromes**.[2092, 2106]
Pure motor hemiparesis with crossed VI nerve palsy: (Foville syndrome) See **lacunar syndromes**.[2092, 2106]
Pure motor hemiparesis with horizontal gaze palsy: See **lacunar syndromes**.[2092, 2106]

pure motor monoparesis Isolated corticospinal deficits in one limb only, of sudden onset and usually due to a mass lesion in the contralateral cerebral hemisphere.[272]

pure motor negativism See **paratonia**.

pure motor stroke A **lacunar syndrome** usually due to a lesion in the basis pontis or in the internal capsule. See **pure motor hemiparesis**.[2092]

pure motor variant of acute inflammatory polyradiculoneuropathy See **acute inflammatory demyelinating polyneuropathy**.

pure pallidal atrophy (Hunt–van Bogaert syndrome) A progressive familial degenerative system disease of young adult life, manifesting Parkinsonian features, the tremor later disappearing and the rigidity and hypokinesia remaining. Pathologically, there is degeneration of the motor neurones of the pallidal system.[3049] See also **progressive pallidal atrophy**.

pure pandysautonomia Virtually complete but reversible paralysis of both sympathetic and parasympathetic functions in the absence of other features of neurological disease.[6932] See **acute autonomic neuropathy**.

pure photosensitive epilepsies Epileptic syndromes in which the seizures are induced exclusively by exposure to light, no attacks occurring spontaneously.[72] See **photosensitive epilepsies**.

pure posterior column ataxia See **Biemond ataxia, posterior column ataxia, and retinitis pigmentosa (PCARP)**.

pure progressive aphemia Severe anarthria or apraxia of speech, reported as a manifestation of **primary progressive aphasia** or vascular lesions affecting the inferior left premotor cortex.[1229]

pure prosodic deafness See **pure affective deafness**.

pure sensory stroke (hemisensory syndrome) A common **lacunar syndrome** characterized by complaints of intermittent or persistent numbness occurring unilaterally in the face, arm, and leg without other complaints. The lesion was originally described as being in the ventroposterolateral thalamic nucleus,[2083] but posterior cerebral artery infarctions and lacunes in the thalamocortical pathways may also produce the syndrome.

pure sensory variant of acute inflammatory demyelinating polyneuropathy See **acute inflammatory demyelinating polyneuropathy**.

pure tone audiometry
A quantitative test of auditory function employing electrically generated pure tones delivered by air or bone conduction. The threshold of acuity is determined at different frequencies and compared to an arbitrary standard.

pure tonic seizures with arousal
(paroxysmal polyspike activity with arousal)

Nocturnal seizures presenting solely with arousal from sleep but with **excessive daytime sleepiness** as a related complaint. Daytime seizures seldom occur in such patients.[4966]

pure typical absence epilepsy of childhood (pyknolepsy) A syndrome characterized by the daily occurrence of frequent simple and complex absence attacks, with onset between the ages of 3 and 9 years. Typical spike and wave complexes are recorded on the EEG during the attacks.[906]

pure visual associative agnosia
Failure to recognize or demonstrate the functions of objects seen but without any impairment of verbal facility.

pure word blindness (agnosic alexia, pure alexia, subcortical visual aphasia)
A condition in which there is an inabilty to read but writing and oral language are preserved. Essentially, language activities are normal except for the recognition of written symbols, so that reading is somewhat impaired, although letters can be comprehended.[93] See also **alexia, pure alexias**.

pure word deafness (subcortical auditory aphasia, isolated speech deafness, auditory verbal agnosia) A rare aphasic disconnection syndrome in which the pathway from the auditory area to the Wernicke area is interrupted, leading to lack of auditory comprehension and of being able to write from dictation or to repeat spoken language, but with normal fluent spontaneous speech, reading, and comprehension ability, both of written language and of all nonverbal sounds.[521] In some cases, auditory agnosia is also present. Cortical deafness may precede the development of the problem.

The condition is due to disconnection (isolation) of Wernicke area (the posterior part of area 22 in the posterior part of the dominant superior temporal gyrus) from the left auditory radiation and from the callosal fibers from the opposite auditory region, within the temporal lobe, thus preventing it from receiving auditory stimulation. This may occur with bilateral lesions in the auditory association areas or a with unilateral left-sided lesion interrupting transcallosal input. The syndrome was first described by Liepman in 1898.[2338, 2339]

pure word dumbness See **aphemia**.

Purine Research Society
A charitable organization in this field providing information and support. Address: 5424 Beech Ave. Bethesda, MD 20814-1730. Tel: 301-530-0354. E-mail: purine@erols.com. Web site: http://www2.dgsys.com/~purine/. See also **Lesch Nyhan syndrome**.

Purkinje, Johannes Evangelista von (Purkyne, Jan) (1787–1869) Bohemian priest and professor of physiology at Breslau and Prague. He was known as the "gypsy physiologist" perhaps both because of his race and because his areas of research were eclectic—the effects of poisoning by various agents; digestive and visual physiology; fingerprints; the use of the microtome, Canada balsam, and glass slides; staining methods with potassium bichromate and carmine; vertigo; deafness; ciliary movement and both cardiac and CNS histology being areas in which he made important contributions, for example, the identification in 1837 of the cerebellar cortical neurons named for him.

His enthusiasm for the experimental method led him to induce seizures in himself by the administration of camphor in 1835.[1253] After years of ostracism on account of his fervid nationalism and his individualistic approach to medicine, he was appointed professor of physiology at Prague and thereafter to the Czech parliament, while still holding an appointment as newspaper editor, thus contemporaneously combining service to the third and the fourth estates.

Purkinje cells Constituents of the middle layers of the cerebellar cortex, described by Purkinje in 1837.[5886] Pure atrophy of the cells was described by André-Thomas.[199]

Purkinje images The shadows of one's own retinal vasculature, visible to the subject in a dark environment when a bright light is shone onto the conjunctiva.

Purkinje phenomenon Fields of equal brightness but with different colors, appearing unequally bright when the intensity of the illumination is decreased.[3373]

purple glove syndrome A rare, generally benign, and self-limited syndrome of distal limb edema with discoloration and local pain, recorded following the administration of dilantin intravenously, less often orally. Skin necrosis and limb ischemia resulting from the compression of vascular structures have also been documented in this condition.[4729]

pursuit Ocular deviations performed in order to maintain fixation upon a moving target.

pursuit defect nystagmus A form of horizontal jerk nystagmus seen in patients with a hemispheric lesion, in which there is a constant drift of the eyes toward the intact hemisphere and a failure of pursuit movements toward the damaged one. The nystagmus occurs with the fixation of moving and static objects. It is thought to be due to an imbalance in drives from the smooth pursuit system.[5766]

pursuit eye movements Smooth, reflexly controlled eye movements with speeds of up to 60° to 70° per second which maintain the image of a moving target upon the fovea after it has been placed there by a refixation saccade. Disturbances in this function in all directions (*omnidirectional pursuit paresis*) suggest the presence of diffuse cerebral disease; disturbances in one direction only suggest the existence of a lesion of the cortical, subcortical, or cerebellar structures on the same side. See also **smooth pursuit system**.

pursuit gain See **gain of pursuit eye movements**.

pursuit imbalance nystagmus Conjugate drifting of the eyes toward the side of the intact hemisphere, seen in patients with parietal lobe disease during the performance of **pursuit movements**.

pursuit rotor test An instrument for the quantification of motor skills, wherein the subject is required to follow a moving target with a hand-held stylus.[1285]

Purtscher syndrome See **pancreatic encephalopathy**.

Purves–Stewart sign Spontaneous flexion of the toes of one foot while walking—an early sign of **Parkinson disease**.[5143]

pusher syndrome See **contraversive pushing**.

pushing palsy Self-induced bilateral peroneal palsies incurred during natural childbirth (without instrumentation or analgesia) as a result of compression of the nerves caused by the patient's pulling the hips and knees into maximal flexion.[59] See also **obstetric palsy**.

putamen (Lat, a paring—hence rind or tree bark) The outermost portion of the lenticular nucleus.

Putnam, James Jackson (1846–1918) An American neurologist who trained at Harvard and studied thereafter in Germany and in England with Hughlings-**Jackson**. He was the first neurologist appointed to the Massachusetts General Hospital (1872), and one of the first professors of neurology at Harvard. He was a founder of the American Neurological Association and one of its early presidents. Putnam described subacute combined degeneration of the cord,[5145] athetosis, and hypothyroidism following hyperthyroidism, and published with G.A. Waterman *Studies in Neurological Diagnosis* (Boston, 1902) and a book on ethics in 1915.

Putnam acroparesthesia See **carpal tunnel syndrome**.

Putnam sign Apparent lengthening of the involved limb occurring with hysterical weakness.

Putnam syndrome Delirium following spinal injury; usually a fatal sign.[5146]

Putnam–Dara syndrome See **subacute combined degeneration of the cord**.

Puusepp, Ludwig Martinovich (1879–1942) Russian-Estonian neurologist who trained in St. Petersburg and, after military service, with Bekhterev. He became professor of clinical neurology but moved to Estonia after the Russian Revolution and to Germany at the start of the World War II. His publications covered topics in both neurology and neurosurgery.

Puusepp little toe reflex Slow abduction of the little toe when the outer border of the foot is lightly stroked; a phenomenon said to occur in disorders of the extrapyramidal system, especially of the striatum. Puusepp's original patients had tumors or epidemic encephalitis.[5704]

pyknodysostosis (Maroteaux-Lamy syndrome) A recessively inherited congenital dysmorphic syndrome of macrocephaly with frontal and occipital bossing of the skull, delayed closure of the fontanelles, osteoporosis, multiple fractures, micrognathia, and underdevelopment of the facial bones, deformed teeth, dwarfism due to defective and shortened long bones, and sometimes kyphoscoliosis. About a quarter of the affected subjects show a degree of mental retardation as well.[4095]

pyknolepsy (Gr, frequent + seize) A term not currently employed but originally used to refer to the frequent brief spells of unawareness observed in childhood petit mal epilepsy (simple absence seizures). It was introduced by Max Friedmann, a German neurologist in 1906.[2205] See **pure typical absence epilepsy of childhood, absence seizures, childhood absence epilepsy**.

Pyle disease A dominantly inherited cochleovestibular atrophy in which progressive neural or conductive deafness occurs in infancy, accompanied by metaphyseal dysplasias and sometimes optic atrophy and facial palsy.[5149] See **craniometaphyseal dysplasia**.

pyocephalus See **ventriculitis**.

pyomyositis (Gr, dischagre +muscle + inflammation) (primary suppurative myositis, tropical pyomyositis) Acute or subacute infection of muscles by pyogenic bacteria giving rise to the usual systemic and focal signs of inflammation; a rare condition in temperate climates.[3724] See **acute suppurative myositis**.

pyramidal (Gr, conical; a pyramid: "a solid resting on a plane base with three or more sides, each of which is triangular and rises to an apex"[5886]) The pyramidal tract was described by Paul Emil Fleschig in 1876, and its functions most critically discussed by **Walshe**.[6624]

pyramidal decussation syndrome (crossed hemiplegia syndrome, cruciate hemiplegia) Paresis of one arm and the other leg with sparing of the face, due to a lesion within the pyramid at a point below the decussation of the fibers destined for the arm and above that of the fibers destined for the leg.[1123]

pyramidal lesion See **upper motor neurone lesion**.

pyramidal myoclonus See **focal reflex myoclonus**.

pyramidal pathways All those corticospinal fibers which arise from the pyramidal cells in the fifth layer of the precentral cortex and, traversing the medullary pyramid, decussate or remain uncrossed and make up the crossed or uncrossed pyramidal tracts, respectively, of the spinal cord. Functionally, this is the pathway whereby the sensory system initiates and continuously directs willed movements.[6624]

pyramidal tract (corticospinal tract) A fiber pathway comprising a bundle of about a million descending fibers which arise from the Betz cells of the motor cortex and traverse the medullary pyramids *en route* to the anterior horn cell pools in the spinal cord. Despite this, the term *pyramidal* is conventionally applied to all descending motor pathways, even those which play on the cranial motor nerve nuclei, which obviously do not pass though the pyramids. Moreover, the term is used synonymously with *corticospinal*, although some of the fibers traversing the pyramids do not arise from the motor cortex.

In monkeys at least, lesions of the pyramids in the medulla cause flaccid paralysis of the appropriate limbs and an upgoing plantar response; the remainder of what is generally called the *pyramidal syndrome* must, in humans, be due to associated lesions of other other descending pathways.

The tract was discovered by Ludwig Turck in 1851, its decussation by Duverney.

pyramid-hypoglossal syndrome See **Déjèrine syndromes**.

Pyramids and Palm trees A test of semantic access from pictures and words requiring subjects to imagine semantically associated items.[3009]

pyridoxine deficiency A potential cause of seizures (Hunt epilepsy) and peripheral neuropathy.[3046]

pyridoxine dependency seizures (pyridoxine responsive seizures, OMIM 266100) A recessively inherited syndrome linked to 2q31, characterized by increased fetal movements and intractable neonatal seizures due to glutamate acid decarboxylase deficiency and responsive to high-dose pyridoxine therapy, required for life.[1194]

pyridoxine overdose neuropathy A severe sensory neuropathy resulting from a massive overdose of vitamin B6; a milder form is characterized by paresthesias, hyperesthesias, bone pains, muscle weakness, numbness, and fasciculations, all of which are most marked in the extremities and usually bilateral. It is also seen in women who take lower doses of up to 200 mg per day. The symptoms remit when the ingestion ceases.[1424]

pyruvate decarboxylase deficiency A rare recessive disorder usually manifesting in the first year of life and characterized by episodic anorexia, nausea, and vomiting with failure to thrive, ataxia, respiratory difficulties, hypoglycemia, hypotonia, microcephaly, seizures, CNS demyelination, aminoacidemia, disturbances of lactate and pyruvate metabolism with severe lactic acidosis, lipid myopathy, and mental and developmental delay.[285, 4207] The responsible gene maps to chromosome 11q. Neuropathy (including optic neuropathy), choreoathetosis, and abnormal eye movements are other features reported.[2754] See also **cerebellar ataxias**.

pyruvate dehydrogenase (PDH) deficiency An inherited mitochondriopathy presenting with an intermittent ataxic syndrome due to a failure of the PDH complex of enzymes responsible for the conversion of pyruvate to acetyl coenzyme-A and involved in the synthesis of acetylcholine and lipids. Depending on the severity of the enzyme deficiency, different phenotypes include fulminant neonatal acidosis, **Leigh disease**, chronic ataxic encephalopathy, hypotonia and weakness, and mental and motor delay. Clinically, the deficiency presents congenitally or during infancy with combinations of optic atrophy, feeding problems, lethargy, hypotonia, apneic spells, seizures, microcephaly, ophthalmoplegia, ataxia, spasticity, chorea and athetosis during fevers, accompanied by organic acidosis with high pyruvate and lactate levels. Dysmorphic features are usually evident. Many of the children also develop a peripheral neuropathy[2754] and cerebral atrophy: Callosal agenesis, absence of the pyramids, ectopic inferior olives, and heterotopias may also be present.[675]

A *variant* is *familial intermittent ataxia*, an X-linked ataxic syndrome with onset in infancy of dysarthria and neurodegenerative regression triggered by carbohydrate feeding and with abnormal lactate and pyruvate metabolism.[381]

pyruvic acidemia Abnormal levels of serum pyruvate, found in some cerebellar ataxic syndromes and in **Leigh disease**.

Pythagoras Greek mathematician who was the first to record his opinion that the brain was charged with the power of reasoning.

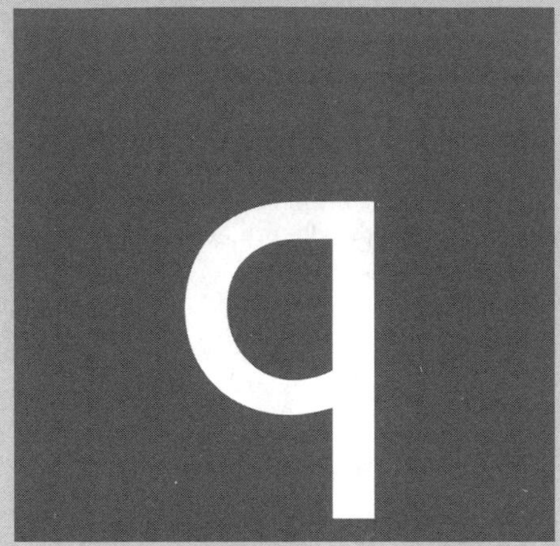

QDIRT (quantitative direct and indirect reflex testing of sudomotor function) An alternative methodology to **QSART**, here employing high-resolution digital photography in the assessment of sudomotor system function.[2366]

Q-fever An acute self-limited febrile illness due to infection with *Coxiella burnetii*. The primary infection is occasionally complicated by the **Miller Fisher syndrome**, encephalitis, meningitis, or myelopathy. Chronic endocarditis, hepatitis, and osteomyelitis are other reported associations.[3066] The "Q" derives from Queensland, the Australian state where the disease was first defined.

qNP See **quantified neurophysiology**.

Q-SART See **quantitative sudomotor axon reflex test**.

quadrantanopia (Lat, quarter + Gr, loss of vision) Loss of vision in one-quarter of the visual field. This occurs with parietal (inferior quarter-field loss) or with temporal (superior quarter-field loss) lobe lesions, because of the differing courses of the various fibers from the retina that pass through these two lobes, respectively. See **Meyer loop**.

Restricted occipital lobe lesions may also produce quadrantanopia.

quadrantic hemianopia See **hemianopia**.

quadraplegia See **quadriparesis**.

quadriceps myopathy A dominantly or recessively inherited, slowly progressive syndrome of myopathic weakness and wasting solely of the quadriceps muscles, with adult onset.

Late spread to other regions in some cases suggests that this condition is a variant of **limb-girdle muscular dystrophy**[6157] or, when there is abnormal staining for **dystrophin**, a *forme fruste* of **Becker muscular dystrophy**.

Variants are a neurogenic form with juvenile onset, and sporadic *chronic neurogenic atrophy of the quadriceps*.

quadriceps reflex See **knee jerk**.

quadrilateral space An anatomical artifact described as bounded by the teres major muscle below, the long head of the triceps medially, the neck of the humerus laterally, and the subscapularis muscle above, while the teres minor lies behind. The axillary nerve passes through this space.

quadrilateral space syndrome Compression of the axillary nerve in this space, sometimes associated with compression of the posterior circumflex artery and presenting clinically with deltoid weakness and wasting and hypoesthesia in C5 distribution.[4863]

quadriparesis (quadriplegia) Weakness of all four limbs. By common usage, this term is used when the degree of that weakness is incomplete and "quadriplegia" (quadriplegia) when the weakness is total.

quadriparesis, deafness, and mental retardation A rare syndrome, probably with autosomal recessive inheritance but possibly X-linked, characterized by facial weakness, mental retardation, spastic quadriparesis, impaired hearing, and diffuse coarse pigmentary retinopathy.[2489]

quadripedal reflex See **brain reflex**.

quadriplegia (quadraplegia) More or less complete paralysis of all four limbs, due either to an upper or to a lower motor neuron lesion.

quadriplegic myopathy (acute necrotizing myopathy of intensive care, floppy person syndrome, thick filament myopathy, acute quadriplegic myopathy) An acute, generalized myopathy occurring in patients admitted to intensive care units with nonneuromuscular problems and treated with steroids and nondepolarizing muscle blockers.[6982, 2946] The pathological characteristics are muscle fiber atrophy (often type 2), vacuolar muscle necrosis, and loss of myosin thick filaments. See **acute quadriplegic myopathy**. See also **postventilatory paretic syndromes**.

quadruple sectoranopia A visual deficit in which a thin strip of visual activity is spared around the horizontal meridian of a blind field. This is noted in some patients with infarction in the territory of the anterior choroidal artery and is considered to be diagnostic of infarction of the lateral geniculate body.[2211]

quail myopathy An acute myoglobinuric syndrome associated with the eating of quail, perhaps as a result of the prior ingestion of hemlock (the plant that was used to kill Socrates) by the birds, for which it appears to be nutritious.

It has also been suggested that the plague affecting the Jews during their exodus from Egypt was of this nature.[4836]

quality extinction test A method of determining hemisphere malfunction which evaluates the verbal answers of a blindfolded subject to the simultaneous brushing of the palm of each hand with two different common materials which he has examined previously.[5671]

quality of life (quality of life index, quality of well-being scale) An attempt to express in a single statement a composite of all of those factors which determine the extent to which a person is able to participate in activities capable of providing pleasure or fulfillment. These might include relationships with family and friends, the health of the person and of those important to him/her, finances, housing, independence, leisure activities, religion, and social life.

Disease- and treatment-related symptoms; self-care, mobility, and physical activity levels; cognitive and emotional factors (including a sense of physical and psychological well-being); and social activity are the four areas considered central to this assessment.

Ten of the instruments currently most favoured for this purpose are reviewed by de Haan, et al.[1496] There follows a selection of scales with a similar purpose.

Frenchay Activities Index A measure of disability and functional handicap in stroke patients, assessing the following:

1. (In the last 3 months) Abilities related to preparing main meals; washing-up; washing clothes; light and heavy housework; local shopping; social outings; walking outside for longer than 15 min; actively pursuing a hobby or interest; and driving.
2. (In the last 6 months) Ability to go on outings; gardening; household or car maintenance; reading books; and gainful work.[2948]

Nottingham Ten-point Activities of Daily Living Index A simple rating scale of items of daily living, used originally in stroke patients, to assess such activities as eating and drinking from a cup; transferring; washing; dressing; and preparing simple foods.[1802]

Nottingham Extended Activities of Daily Living Index A rating scale of items of daily living, used originally in stroke patients, to assess activities under the headings of mobility, kitchen work, domestic tasks, and leisure.[4716]

Karnofsky Performance Scale A simple if arbitrary score, given in percentages, reflecting the overall ability of a subject to cope with working and domestic or self-care activities.[3308] However, at all levels below 50% the subject is so greatly in need of assistance that the sensitivity of the scale, and thus its value, is lessened.

Sickness Impact Profile A reliable and valid inventory assessing best the effects of illness upon day-to-day functions. Its physical dimension contains three subscales measuring ambulation, mobility, and body care and movement, which have been used especially in the determination of disability in subjects with multiple sclerosis.[5976]

Whatever the scales may indicate, patients themselves rate the quality of their life mainly on such criteria as employability, ability to perform domestic tasks and to care for themselves, balance and gait, and their ability to communicate with others.

quality of life index See **quality of life**.

Quality of the Upper Extremities skills An arm functional assessment test in children with cerebral palsy.[1569]

quality of well-being scale See **quality of life**.

quantal squander See **neuromyotonia**.

quantified neurophysiology (qNP) Topographic EEG mapping; a computerized technique using the waveforms recorded over different areas of the scalp to produce a composite picture of the electrical activity of different brain regions.

How much this represents a technical advance and how much an expensive (but professional) toy, is disputed.

quantitative cisternography A technique for the indirect measurement of CSF flow using intrathecally injected radio-iodinated albumin and repetitive scintigraphic scanning.

quantitative electromyography (QEMG) A systematic method for measuring the recordings made by an intramuscular needle electrode. Measurements include motor unit action potential characteristics such as amplitude, duration, and phases, or interference pattern characteristics. See **turns-amplitude analysis**. (Adapted from the 2001 Report of the Nomenclature Committee of the American Association of Electromyography and Electrodiagnosis.[19] Reproduced by kind permission of the AANEM.)

quantitative muscle testing Techniques for evaluating the strength of muscle contractions, in which a mechanical myometric system is employed to allow objective measurement of the muscular force generated.[5690] See **quantitative neurological examination**.

Quantitative Myasthenia Gravis score A validated measure of disease severity in this condition. The items assessed are diplopia on lateral gaze, timed in seconds (s); the presence of ptosis on upward gaze (s); facial muscle power, assessed by strength of eyelid closure; bulbar function, assessed by the subject's ability to swallow half a cup of water and by speech after counting aloud up to 50; duration maintaining a horizontal arm position on each side (s); vital capacity (% predicted); left- and right-hand grip strength; ability to keep one and then the other leg elevated at 45° (s); and the ability to maintain the head flexed when in the supine position (s).[3169]

Quantitative Neurological Examination A structured clinical examination emphasizing the findings in the motor system[1475] (Chart Q–1).

Quantitative Neuromuscular Examination A protocol that examines total muscle strength in terms of the MRC (Medical Research Council Scale) score, based on a clinical assessment of 32 groups of muscles using the 6-point MRC grading; the force of 8 selected muscle groups measured on a myometer; a motor ability score based on 20

Chart Q–1. The Quantitative Neurological Examination

Lateral Gaze

Pursuit. Hold index finger or pointer about 18 inches from the patient's eye and ask him to follow it as it is slowly moved laterally.

A. Range

0 = Normal
1 = Incomplete
2 = No pursuit

B. Smoothness of movement

0 = One continuous movement
1 = "Catch" or jerky; may stop mid-movement and look the other way
2 = No pursuit

Vertical Gaze

Pursuit. As the patient moves his eyes up and down, it is useful for the examiner to hold the eyelids up for a better view of smoothness.

A. Extent

0 = Normal
1 = Incomplete
2 = No pursuit

B. Smoothness of movement

0 = One continuous movement
1 = "Catch" or jerky
2 = No pursuit

Saccades

Examiner holds up both index fingers about 18 inches (45 cm) from the patient at the extremes of lateral gaze and asks the patient to look from one finger to the other as quickly as possible.

A. Speed

0 = Normal
1 = Slow
2 = Patient cannot execute command

B. Blink suppression: If the patient blinks while performing saccades, ask him to stop.

0 = Does not blink or can stop
1 = Cannot stop
2 = Patient cannot execute command

C. Smoothness of movement

0 = One smooth lateral movement
1 = Attains goal by series of short movements
2 = Patient cannot execute command

D. Head moves laterally (ask not to move head)

0 = None
1 = Head moves with eyes
2 = Patient cannot perform saccades

Gaze Holding

Ask the patient to keep his eyes on a target at the lateral extreme of gaze, several meters away.

0 = Keeps eyes firmly on the target
1 = Eyes keep wandering off the target
2 = Patient cannot execute command

Forceful Eye Closure

Ask patient to close his eyes tight, burying the eyelids. Score normal if patient does so even momentarily.

0 = Buries lids
1 = Cannot bury lids
2 = Patient cannot execute command

Facial Mimicking

Ask the patient to mimic the examiner's performance of the following movements.

0 = Can perform
1 = Cannot perform

a. Blow out both cheeks at once, keeping mouth closed.
b. Put tongue in cheek with enough force to make the cheek "pouch out."
c. Frown (knit brows).
d. Wink (non-winking eye may move but not close).
e. Rapid tongue movements.

(Ask the patient to touch the tip of his tongue to each corner of his lips alternately. There should be at least 4 touches/sec. performed smoothly to score 0.)

Motor Impersistence

(This item rates the patient's ability to sustain voluntary movement.)

a. Eye closure. Ask the patient to close his eyes and to keep them closed.

0 = Maintains eyes closed 20 s.
1 = Opens before 20 s.
2 = Patient cannot execute command.

b. Tongue. Ask the patient to protrude the tongue. He may not hold it out by using his teeth.

0 = Maintains tongue out for 20 s.
1 = Retracts before 20 s.
2 = Cannot execute command.

Speech: Repeated Syllables

Ask the patient to repeat the following syllables after the examiner.

Rhythm (rh): 0 = Regular
1 = Irregular
Rate (ra): 0 = > 4 syllables/sec.
1 = 4 syllables/sec.
Clarity (cl): 0 = Each syllable clear
1 = Syllables run together.
Add 1 to each category if the patient is mute (total = 12).

a. La-la-la ...
b. Go-go-go ...
c. Kitty-kitty-kitty ...
d. Attenuation (ask the patient to count to 20—or may be scored if noted in conversation)

0 = No
1 = Yes
2 = If mute

Conversational Speech

This should be rated as the interview and examination progress.

continued

Chart Q–1. *(continued)*

Rhythm

0 = Smooth with expected pauses and transitions
1 = Unexpected pauses; speech comes in bursts
2 = Mute

Rate

0 = Normal
1 = Speech is either too fast or too slow
2 = Mute

Note: This seems subjective but is easily noted when present.

Clarity

0 = Speech is normally understandable
1 = The examiner must listen carefully but does not need to ask the patient to repeat himself if speech is "jerky."
2 = The patient must often try more than once, but can be understood.
3 = Speech is almost or entirely incomprehensible.
4 = Mute.

Tone

(Examine tone in wrists and elbow and neck. Code arms and neck separately.)

0 = Normal
1 = Decreased
2 = Increased

Strength

Test biceps and strength of grasp, unless more extensive examination is indicated by clinical symptoms.

0 = Normal
1 = Decreased
2 = Cannot test due to advanced disease

Muscle Stretch Reflexes

Assess the composite score of the biceps, knee, and ankle jerks.

0 = Normal
1 = Absent
2 = Very brisk but no clonus
3 = Brisk with clonus at the ankle (or throughout)

(If asymmetrical, draw a diagram on the coding sheet showing the findings).

Plantar Response

(Score the left and right responses separately).

0 = Flexor
1 = Extensor

Asymmetry: Tone, Strength, and Reflexes

0 = Symmetrical
1 = Asymmetry present

Finger–Nose

(Ask the patient to make a pointer with his finger and to touch the examiner's finger and then his own nose. The examiner's finger should be held far enough away so that the patient must completely extend his arm).

0 = Quick, smooth, accurate (finger–nose-finger in 1 s)
1 = Slow but accurate
2 = Dysmetria.
3 = Cannot execute command.

Finger–Thumb Tap

(Ask the patient to tap his index or third finger with his thumb quickly. Score each hand separately.)

0 = >4 taps/sec. smooth
1 = 3 taps/sec. or faster but arrhythmic
2 = < 2 taps/sec.
3 = Cannot perform

Diadochokinesis

(Ask the patient to pronate and supinate his hand alternately, patting the other palm on the ipsilateral knee. Score each hand separately.)

0 = <3 pats/sec. smoothly executed
1 = 2 pats/sec. or faster but arrhythmic
2 = <2 pats/sec.
3 = Cannot perform

Also ask the patient to stand with his feet together, eyes closed, arms out 90°, palms down, and fingers apart. Note balance as well as any tremor or chorea of the finger tips. Score tremor or chorea.

Tremor

(If the patient cannot stand, ask him to hold his arms at 90° while sitting. Tremor will not be scorable in patients with severe chorea.)

0 = None
1 = Mild
2 = Marked
3 = Cannot test because of chorea or poor concentration

Chorea

(Notice all body parts and make a summary rating. Chorea is a fairly quick jerky movement which is not as stereotyped as a tic. It may be of any amplitude. It is not as quick as ballismus which is also not usually symmetrical.)

0 = Absent
1 = Mild, occasional
2 = Frequent but low amplitude
3 = Frequent or continuous with moderate amplitude
4 = Continuous, severe, but patient can carry out some voluntary movements
5 = So severe as to be totally incapacitating

Note: All patients should have chorea scored at rest and with stress. Score as above in the following situations:

a. With arms out at 90°
b. Ask patient to hold as still as he can while sitting, hands in lap, or lying in bed
c. During conversation
d. During voluntary movement (e.g., walking)
e. During stress (e.g., calculating)

Posture

(Rate standing or seated if unable to stand)

0 = Normal
1 = Somewhat stooped
2 = Very stooped with downward gaze or rigid and extended

Standing

(Observe for 10–15 s)

0 = Normally still or slight weaving
1 = Widened base to stay in one place
2 = Cannot stand still for 10 s or cannot stand

Walking

0 = Normal gait, narrow base (heels should approximate a straight line)
1 = Wide base

continued

Chart Q–1. *(continued)*

2 = Wide base with deviation from a straight line
3 = Walks with assistance (person, walker, leans on wall)
4 = Unable to walk

Stopping

0 = Stops on command
1 = Stops but body lurches forward or takes a step
2 = Takes 2 or more steps before stopping
3 = Unable to walk

Turning

0 = Pivots on a narrow base
1 = Hesitates, widens base, or moves feet
2 = Turns slowly and awkwardly
3 = Cannot walk

Tandem Walk

Four practice steps, then 10 paces, heel touching toes at each stop.

0 = No deviations or weaving after practice
1 = 1–3 deviations or excessive truncal weaving
2 = More than 3 deviations, but completes 10 paces
3 = Cannot complete the task although tries.
4 = Cannot attempt task

Snout

Tap middle of closed lips with reflex hammer. Do not score random choreic movement.

0 = Absent
1 = Present

Grasp

Stroke patient's palm, with patient's palm down. Ask the patient not to grasp the examiner's hand.

0 = Absent
1 = Patient grasps the examiner's hand

Bradykinesia

0 = Voluntary movements normal speed
1 = Mild slowness or gait, speech, task completion
2 = Marked slowness
3 = In bed without movement

Motor Impairment Scale

Eye closure (0–2)
Clarity or repeated syllables (0–4)
Finger–nose (0–3)
Diadochokinesis
right (0–3)
left (0–3)
Plantar response (0–2)
Gait (0–4)
Tandem walk (0–4)
Bradykinesia (0–3)
Maximum score = 28

From David AS, et al. Voluntary movement dysfunction in Huntington's disease and tardive dyskinesia. Acta Neurol Scand *1987;*75:*130–39. Reproduced by kind permission of Wiley-Blackwell Publications.*

consecutive motor activities; walking times over 28 and 150 ft; and a recording of muscle contractures. See also **Hammersmith Scale**.

quantitative oculopneumoplethysmography

A method of measuring absolute ophthalmic systolic blood pressure and the amplitude of the pulsations, capable of identifying stenoses reducing the diameter of the arterial lumen by more than 60%.

The technique employs scleral cups to raise the intraocular pressure and to interrupt the circulation; when the vacuum is removed; returning pulsations are detected by a sensor in the cup. Severe stenosis is suggested when the ophthalmic and brachial systolic blood pressures, the intraocular systolic blood pressures of the eyes, or the relative amplitudes of the ocular pulsations are abnormal.

This is the most widely used of the oculoplethysmographic tests and is the most accurate, but it does suffer from deficiencies in distinguishing occlusion from severe stenosis, and bilateral severe disease may also be difficult to identify with this method.[4678]

quantitative phonoangiography

A technique whereby the frequency content of bruits is analyzed and related to the residual lumen diameter of the internal carotid artery. It does this accurately in patients who have bruits, but suffers from the fact that about half of all patients with severe disease do not have one, and it provides no information about the features of the vessel wall itself.

quantitative sensory testing

The instrumented techniques used to measure the intensity of stimuli needed to produce specific sensory perceptions; methods of testing absolute sensory thresholds, designed for the assessment of the deficits in patients with peripheral neuropathy.

Vibratory detection thresholds, thermal perception, light touch, pain thresholds, and autonomic functions can all be quantitated using current methods,[1770, 1778, 8] but standardization has not yet been achieved.[4986] The techniques may be useful in identifying small fiber neuropathies.

Quantitative Somatosensory Thermotest

A mechanical method of assessing the function of the A delta and C fibers responsible for transmitting impulses concerned with the appreciation of temperature sensation, using a technique for determining warming and cooling thresholds.[6526]

quantitative sudomotor axon reflex test (QSART)

A method of measuring sweat production in a specific skin area in response to acetylcholine iontophoresis, in order to assess postganglionic sympathetic cholinergic function.[3929] The drug should induce sweating in preganglionic but not in postganglionic sympathetic disorders and is thus useful in the estimation of C-fiber function.

Antidromic transmission of the impulse from the nerve terminals reaches a branch point, then travels orthodromically to release acetylcholine from the nerve terminals, inducing a sweating response. In small fiber polyneuropathy, the response may be reduced or absent. In painful neuropathies, and in reflex sympathetic dystrophy, the response may be excessive and persistent or reduced. (Adapted from the 2001 Report of the Nomenclature Committee of the American Association of Electromyography and Electrodiagnosis.[19] Reproduced by kind permission of the AANEM and of Wiley-Blackwell Publications.)

Queckenstedt, Hans Heinrich Georg

(1876–1918) German physician who graduated from Leipzig and practiced in Heidelberg and at Rostock. He became head of the German army medical services in Hamburg during World War I. His life was ended suddenly when he was thrown off his horse and under a munitions truck, 2 days before the end of the War and 1 year after his two publications, one on changes in CSF pressure with coughing, straining, and jugular vein compression and the other on high protein levels in acellular CSF in cases of **acute inflammatory demyelinating polyneuropathy** and sciatica.[5153, 5154]

Queckenstedt Test

Compression of the jugular veins causes elevation of the intraspinal fluid pressure as measured by a manometer, the pressure falling again when compression ceases. These pressure changes are dampened or absent in the presence of spinal block.[5153] The sign was doubtless valuable in its day; the rationale for performing it now that safer and far more precise diagnostic tests are available is doubtful at best.

In the *reversed Queckenstedt Test*, saline is injected into the lumbar theca and the consequent pressure changes are monitored through a needle placed in the cisternal space. Failure of the pressure to increase indicates an obstruction to the flow of CSF between the lumbar and cervical regions.

quiet sleep

See **non–rapid eye movement sleep**.

Quincke, Heinrich Irenaeus

(1842–1922) German physician who trained at Berlin, Wurzurg, and Heidelberg and who quickly became professor of medicine, first at Bern and later at Kiel and Frankfurt. He made contributions in all fields of internal medicine and was the first to describe angioneurotic edema, but he is remembered in neurology for having successfully performed lumbar puncture in 1891, describing both the pressure changes and the constituents of CSF.[5155] He was not the first to do so, however, as Walter **Wynter** had published an account of lumbar puncture in the ***Lancet*** in the same year, while Corning in New York had described the operation in 1889.[6661]

Unlike **Wynter**'s patients who all had meningitis and all of whom died, many of Corning's patients lived (one at least probably having meningism rather than meningitis and others having hydrocephalus; however, it is not certain that Corning actually entered the subarachnoid space). Quincke also published on the topics of cerebral palsy, the physiology of the choroid plexus, and puncture of the anterior fontanelle in infants.

Quincke meningitis

See **idiopathic intracranial hypertension**.

quinolinic acid

A neurotoxic endogenous tryptophan metabolite that acts through the *N*-methyl-D-aspartate set of glutamate receptors to produce axon-sparing lesions similar to those in **Huntington disease**.

Quinquaud, Charles-Eugène French hematologist and dermatologist who studied in Limoges and Paris where he became chief of service at the Hôpital St-Louis. A "modest, honest, indulgent, sympathetic and great savant" (Maridort), he was elected a member of the French Academy of Medicine in 1891, by which time he had become well known as a brilliant dermatologist and for his publications on many topics in dermatology, pathology, and hematology, in the latter applying the principles of physics and chemistry to medicine. He died prematurely, "a victim of overwork."[5704]

Quinquaud sign Tremor felt by the examiner when the patient's abducted fingers are firmly placed vertically on the examiner's palm. The sign was first described in alcoholics; a description of it was published by Quinquaud's pupil Dr. P. Maridort, 6 years after Quinquaud's death. He recounted that "the Master forcibly applied the palm of his right hand to the tip of the extended fingers of his pupils. He looked at two of them (a point there is no need to labour) with a slight irony and made a negative sign to the others. Early in the ensuing month the beloved professor died and no one after him could determine what pressure on the tip of the extended fingers could reveal . . . He carried his secret to the grave."

Maridort, however, determined that "little shocks, as if the bones of each finger were being pushed back suddenly and were striking your palm" indicated that the patient suffered from alcoholism.[4068]

quisqualic acid An excitotoxin.

quitarian epilepsy Seizures in which the subject weeps. Quiritian was a Roman citizen, but the word quitarian probably derives from the Latin, to shout out loud. See **dacrystic epilepsy**.

quiver eye movement (postsaccadic glissade) A backward drift of the eyes, interrupting the completion of a saccade as a result of fatigue of the myofibrils in the extraocular muscle.[3762]

quix test The patient stands with both arms extended horizontally, and the fingers pointing at the examiner's shoulders. Drift of both hands consistently in any direction when the patient's eyes are closed is abnormal and suggests disease of the vestibular apparatus.[1707]

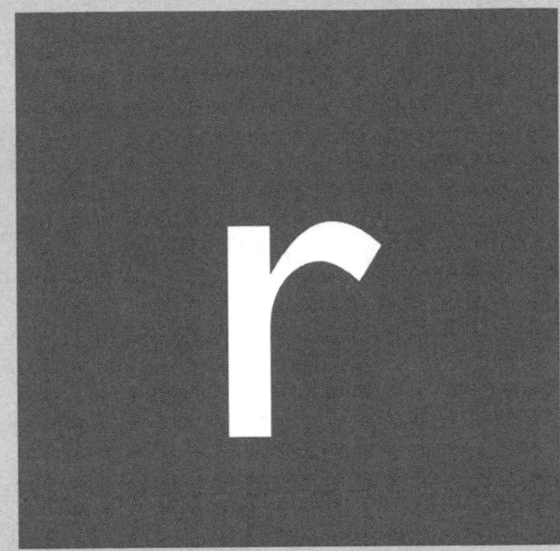

R1, R2 waves See **blink responses**.

rabbit syndrome See **rabbit tremor**.

rabbit tremor (rabbit syndrome) Fast, chittering movements of the lips and jaw with the mouth held slightly open; a feature in some cases of **tardive dyskinesia**, but also occurring at rest in some patients with Parkinsonism. However, it is most often seen as a complication of neuroleptic treatment.[3754]

rabies (from Lat, rage) (hydrophobia, lyssa, la rage, St. Hubert disease) An acute viral encephalomyelitis resulting from infection by a member of the rhabdovirus family transmitted by foxes, wolves, raccoons, and dogs in Europe; by wolves, jackals, and small carnivores in Asia and Africa; and by vampire bats in the Caribbean and South America. Transmission is almost always the result of the bite of an infected animal, the virus being found in its saliva, but airborne transmission is also described.

The incubation varies from a week to several years, but is usually less than 3 months after an animal bite, and the occurrence of the disease in *spelunkers* (facultative cave dwellers) suggests that the virus may infect after inhalation through the olfactory mucosa; this is followed by prodromal symptoms of a flu-like illness, pain, and paresthesias at the site of the bite; later by anxiety, agitation, and insomnia, and then by either the *furious* or the *dumb* form of rabies. Three cases of rabies have been reported in which the patient lived. The remainder of the 15,000 or more cases occurring annually in the word dic as a result of the disease.[6858] **Negri bodies** are found in the brain in most cases. The condition was recognized in the third century BC, but the usual term used to refer to it up to the seventeenth century was *hydrophobia*.

The *furious* form is an encephalopathy with at least some mental disturbance, but this is overshadowed by the intermittent inspiratory and pharyngeal spasms and attacks of terror which are precipitated by attempts to drink (or even the thought of doing so), and which may lead to seizures and respiratory arrest. Cranial nerve palsies, pyramidal signs, involuntary movements and meningism, and autonomic disturbances are also typical. Laryngeal spasm may lead to respiratory arrest and death. Hyperexcitability with hallucinations and delirium occurs, interspersed with periods of normal cognitive functioning. Meningism and bulbar palsies precede coma and eventual death.

The unusual *dumb (paralytic)* form closely resembles **acute inflammatory demyelinating polyneuropathy** and is characterized by progressive pareses beginning in the limb that was bitten, but ascending to produce respiratory and bulbar weakness.[4360] Muscle spasms and hydrophobia develop terminally in these patients prior to death.

Vaccination is possible using a human diploid fibroblast culture vaccine, which is safe and effective, having been successful even when used after exposure.

Rabot epilepsy A form of benign familial myoclonic epilepsy due to a hereditary error of metabolism.

raccoon eyes Periorbital bruising, occurring bilaterally in most cases after fractures of the anterior cranial vault.

racemose aneurysm See **arteriovenous malformation**.

racemose angioma See **arteriovenous malformation**.

rachialgia (Gr, the spine + pain) "Spinal irritation . . . local pain and tenderness referred to the spinal column itself" (Sir William **Gowers**).

rachischisis (Gr, the spine + splitting) (dysraphism) Disorders of fusion of the dorsal midline structures of the primitive neural tube. **Spina bifida, meningocele, meningomyelocele, tethered cord**, and **diastematomyelia** are examples.

rad The basic unit of absorbed radiation in tissue.

radial aplasia See **Baller–Gerold syndrome**.

radial bending reflex An enhancement of the normal reflex contraction of the flexors of the elbow with forced passive flexion of the wrist, such that it is produced by even mild passive radial deviation of the wrist, as with parasagittal precentral lesions. See **bending reflex**.

radial deviation Inclination of the hand toward the radial side when the subject with a posterior interosseous nerve lesion attempts to make a fist. Sparing of the extensor carpi radialis longus (innervated by the radial rather than by the posterior interosseous nerve) is responsible for this.[2917]

radial neglect A visual vertical neglect syndrome in which the subjects fail to bisect accurately radial lines extending from a midpoint.[3451] See also **line bisection test**.

radial reflex See **brachioradialis reflex**.

radial tunnel syndrome Entrapment of the posterior interosseous nerve by an abnormal fibrous band or by the edge of the extensor carpi radialis brevis tendon or its origin, causing pain in the lateral part of the elbow and forearm.[5359] See **posterior interosseous syndrome**.

radialis sign Inability to make a fist without marked extension of the wrist. The sign was described by **Strumpell** and is present with pyramidal lesions and in tetany.

radian An arc or segment of a circle with a length equal to the radius of the circle. The term is included because it has been suggested that cerebral concussion, in the absence of impact, approximates 330 radians/s over at least 20 ms and about half of that with concussive injuries.[2918]

radiary nystagmus See **circular nystagmus**.

radiation damage to the nervous system Transient or permanent neurotoxicity resulting from direct or incidental irradiation of the nervous system. The neurological complications of such radiotherapy have been reviewed and classified by Keime-Guibert et al. (1998).[3367]

Acute (minutes to 1 week)	*Early-delayed (4–16 weeks)*	*Late-delayed (4 months to years)*
Acute encephalopathy	Somnolence syndrome Increased focal signs, worsening MRI findings **Rhombencephalopathy**	Radiation necrosis Late cognitive dysfunction, dementia Endocrinopathy Radiation arteriopathy Radiation-induced tumor
Paraesthesias	Transient cognitive dysfunction **Ageusia** **Lhermitte** sign **Anosmia** Hearing loss Brachial or lumbosacral reversible **plexopathy**	Transverse myelopathy (see **radiation encephalomyelopathy** Hemorrhagic myelopathy Motor neuron syndrome Visual loss Hearing loss, hair cell damage Lower cranial nerve paralysis Brachial or lumbosacral late plexopathy Radiation-induced tumors

From Keime-Guibert F, Napolitano M, Delattre J-Y. Neurological complications of radiotherapy and chemotherapy. J Neurol *1998;245:695–708. ©Springer Science + Business Media. Reproduced by kind permission.*

radiation encephalomyelopathy (postirradiation myelopathy) Insidiously progressive evidence of damage to the spinal cord occurring 3 months to 5 years after its irradiation. Slowly progressive paraparesis with spinothalamic sensory loss or a **Brown-Séquard syndrome** are the usual syndromes developing after cervical irradiation. A painless motor neuropathy may occur when the cauda equina was included in the field but almost any syndrome of myelopathy can be produced. In the commonest form, with cervical disease, pain in the neck and shoulders, and sensory disturbances such as numbness, paresthesias, **Lhermitte** symptom, and thermoanalgesia in the legs are the usual presenting complaints.[5219]

These features may be *early and transient* (in the first 6 months after irradiation) or may go on to the *chronic (late-delayed) progressive* form in which after 6 months there appear typical motor and sensory signs of partial cord transection with sphincter involvement; these are irreversible.

Variant syndromes such as *arrested radiation myelopathy*, *disseminated demyelination in the CNS causing encephalopathy*, *acute paraplegic*, and *lower motor neuron* types have also been recorded.[4872, 3599]

radiation-induced peripheral neuropathy See **radiation plexopathy**.

radiation of pain The experience of pain at a distance from the site from which it is perceived to emanate, but within the distribution of the sensory nerve or root supplying the painful part. See also **referred pain**.

radiation plexopathy (radiation-induced peripheral neuropathy) A syndrome of paresthesia in the fingers, hypoesthesia, and weakness, the last affecting mainly muscles innervated by C5 through C7, occurring months or years after irradiation with 6000 cGy or more to a field including the brachial plexus, usually for the treatment of breast cancer. A **Horner syndrome** is seldom seen.[6070] Lymphedematous swelling of the arm is a common associated sign and, electrically, myokymia is often found in the affected muscles.

Lumbosacral plexopathy is a less common result of radiation therapy. Other causes of plexopathy have been reviewed.[6108]

radiation radiculopathy A subacute or slowly progressive syndrome of muscle atrophy and weakness with paresthesias occurring between 3 months and 3 years after irradiation of the spinal column, particularly at lumbosacral levels.[792]

radicular compression The result of degenerative changes of the spinal column, whereby spinal nerve roots are distorted or compressed. The clinical criteria establishing the diagnosis comprise a local muscle spasm causing stiffness of the neck or a decrease in straight-leg raising, postural and gait disturbances, and motor or sensory neurological deficits appropriate to the roots compressed.

radicular deficit See **radiculopathy**.

radicular myelopathy associated with spinal neuronitis See **chronic spinal meningitis**.

radicular reflex myoclonus A myoclonic disease in which the jerks appear to originate from the brainstem reticular substance. See **myoclonus**.

radiculitis (spinal neuritis) Inflammation of the roots of the spinal nerves. This occurs with viral infections such as herpes zoster, and may also be due to toxic agents. The word is also sometimes used to describe the state of the nerve roots irritated by local mechanical disease, such as occurs with a prolapsed intervertebral disk.

radiculomeningitis Inflammation of the spinal arachnoid meninges with consequent compression and inflammation of the nerve roots traversing these, usually due to collagen vascular diseases such as **ankylosing spondylitis** or rheumatoid arthritis. Clinically, lumbar pain, atrophy, and weakness or a full **cauda equina syndrome** are the more common presentations.

radiculomyelopathy The association of long-tract signs due to cervical cord disease with evidence of root lesions at higher cervical levels, in conjunction with anomalies of the spinal column such as **atlantoaxial dislocation**; a disorder reported from India.[6584]

radiculoneuritis See **acute inflammatory demyelinating polyneuropathy**.

radiculopathy (radicular deficit, root lesion) A clinical syndrome resulting from lesions of the anterior or posterior spinal nerve roots. Motor features include complaints of weakness, with wasting and hyporeflexia in the territory of the roots affected; sensory symptoms include pain and sensory dysfunction such as hypoesthesias, dysesthesias, and paresthesias, again restricted typically to the appropriate territory. The pathophysiology, clinical manifestations, and diagnostic methodologies have been reviewed.[6778]

From the viewpoint of electrodiagnosis, axonal and/or demyelinating disorder affecting the nerve fibers exclusive to one spinal nerve root or spinal nerve may affect the anterior (motor) or posterior (sensory) spinal nerve roots, or both, at one spinal cord segment level. The resulting clinical syndrome may include pain, sensory loss, parethesias, weakness, fasciculations, and muscle atrophy. If more than one spinal root is involved, the term *polyradiculopathy* may be used as a descriptor. (Adapted from the 2001 Report of the Nomenclature Committee of the American Association of Electromyography and Electrodiagnosis.[19] Reproduced by kind permission of the AANEM and of John Wiley-Blackwell Publications.)

The classification in Chart R–1 is based on that of the World Federation of Neurology. See also **neuromuscular diseases**.

Radiology Education A professional resource. Web site: http://www.radiologyeducation.com.

radioperiosteal reflex A misnomer. See **brachioradialis reflex**.

radiosurgery A therapeutic method in which intense beams of gamma radiation are collimated and focused on deep-seated inoperable brain lesions such as arteriovenous malformations in a single session.

Chart R–1. Classification of Radiculopathies

Disorders of Motor Nerve Roots

A. *Congenital*

1. Associated with **meningomyelocele** and other anomalies
2. **Arthrogryposis multiplex congenita** (radicular type)

B. *Acquired disorders*

B1. *Physical causes*

1. Laceration, contusion, distraction, or avulsion of roots
2. Compression of roots by vertebral osteoarthritis, prolapsed intervertebral disk, **Paget disease**, tumor in the spinal canal or intervertebral foramina, or vertebral collapse

B2. *Ischemia*

B3. *Radiation*

B4. *Toxic agents* (injected local anesthetics, phenol, etc.)

B5. *Infective* (e.g., radiculopathy in meningitis, syphilis, AIDS,[1288] granulomatous arachnoiditis from other causes (including spinal tuberculosis and sarcoidosis), bilharziasis

B6. *Postinfective, allergic, or immunologically mediated*

1. **Acute inflammatory demyelinating polyneuropathy** (polyradiculoneuropathy)
2. Polyradiculoneuropathy after inoculation
3. **Serum neuropathy**
4. **Neuralgic amyotrophy**
5. Radiculopathy of **Lyme disease**
6. Radiculopathy in **HIV Infection**[1288]

B7. *Neoplastic* (e.g., neurofibroma, meningioma, metastases, reticulosis)

B8. *Vascular malformation*

Adapted from the World Federation of Neurology Classification Subcommittee Classification of neuromuscular diseases. J Neurol Sci *1988;86:333–60. The classification used here is based on that of the World Federation of Neurology, from which it was adapted by kind permission of Lord Walton, the late Professor P.K. Thomas, and the World Federation of Neurology.*

radius (Lat, a ray, hence the spokes of a wheel[5886]) The name for the smaller of the two bones of the forearm, applied by Celsus.

Radovici sign The **palmomental reflex**, first described by J. Radovici (b. 1868), a Romanian neurologist and a pupil of **Marinesco**.[2066]

Raeder paratrigeminal syndrome (middle cranial fossa syndrome, paratrigeminal [oculosympathetic] syndrome, POSS) The occurrence of oculosympathetic paresis with evidence of trigeminal sensory loss or motor weakness, the trigeminal involvement usually presenting with facial or temporal pain in the distribution of the first (but occasionally the second) division of the V cranial nerve.[5166] The retention of sweating over the forehead despite evidence of trigeminal involvement suggests the presence of a lesion in the middle cranial fossa medial to the trigeminal ganglion.[2413] Thus this is not just a painful **Horner syndrome**.

The presence of head or face pain was not regarded originally as part of the syndrome, although sometimes it is considered so today. If pain were to be included as a criterion, it should be neuralgic rather than, for example, vascular in type. The sign localizes a lesion to the middle cranial fossa.

Dr. G. Raeder was a Norwegian ophthalmologist. In his patients, diplopia and systemic features such as vomiting and anorexia also occurred; tumor and trauma were the only defined etiologies.[4434]

In *variants* of the syndrome, optic nerve involvement, oculomotor pareses, or dysgeusia occur with the signs just described.

ragged-red fiber mitochondrial disease See **mitochondrial encephalopathy**.

ragged red fibers An appearance on muscle biopsy specimens stained with Gomorri trichrome, in which subsarcolemmal clumps of red-staining mitochondria impart an uneven, granular appearance to the edge of the type 1 myofibrils. The biochemical defect in the muscle is also expressed in the brain. The condition is a marker for the presence of mitochondrial oxidation defects, especially in those diseases associated with a clinical myopathy such as **cytochrome c oxidase deficiency**,[1645] but is not invariably present and is not a criterion for the diagnosis of **mitochondrial diseases**.

railway nystagmus See **optokinetic nystagmus**.

railway spine (delayed posttraumatic myelitis of Gowers) Symptoms supposed to result from concussion of the brain and spinal cord as a result of traveling in railway carriages in the nineteenth century. Such a problem was accepted as genuinely organic in the early days of railway travel and received much support in England and the United States from the writings of **Erichsen**, who, however, did note that "railway spine" was described years before the invention of railways. In his book descriptions of direct cord injuries are given first. He also noted that recent railway collisions were fertile sources of litigation.

The symptoms of cervical acceleration injury following even relatively trivial and even remote concussion to the spine were recounted, some of these persisting for years even after trivial injury. There was often a delay before the appearance of symptoms. He described a woman who gave "a lengthened and minute history of her ailments" and noted the disproportion between the trifling degree of injury and the severity of the succeeding symptoms, many patients thinking initially that they had not sustained any significant injury at all; and he also observed that these diffuse symptoms are not seen when there has been direct spinal or cord injury. The absence of reports of such symptoms stemming from travel in stagecoaches appears not to have been remarked, but his observations paralleled exactly those that are seen today in patients with cervical acceleration ("**whiplash**") injury.

Raimistes signs 1. Flexion at the wrist in an arm affected by pyramidal tract lesion, when extended. 2. When the hemiparetic patient lies prone with his legs separated and tries to adduct or abduct the sound leg against resistance, the paretic leg adducts or abducts also.[5333]

Rainbow Foundation for Brain Tumor Research, Inc. A charitable association in this field. Address: Box 327 Highland Mills, New York 10930. Tel: 914-928-8683.

Ramachandran sign (mirror agnosia) When a subject with a right parietal lesion is asked to look into a mirror held to his right side and to reach out to grasp a pen held up on his left side, he reaches repeatedly into the mirror, thus mistaking the mirror for the object even though aware of the nature and properties of the mirror itself.[5172]

Ramon y Cajal, Santiago (1852–1934) Spanish anatomist and neurohistologist who trained at Saragossa. He was appointed professor of anatomy at Valencia at the age of 29, but transferred to Bologna and then returned to Spain as professor of histology and morbid anatomy in Madrid. His major work, *Histologie du système nerveuse de l'homme et des vertebres* (Paris, 1909–1911), established him as the father of neurohistology, although some of the credit belongs to Camillo **Golgi**, a modification of whose silver stain Cajal used, and with whom he shared the Nobel Prize in 1906.

He also introduced a silver nitrate stain to show the content of neuronal cytoplasm; this stain was used by **Alzheimer** to demonstrate neurofibrillary tangles. Among his students or collaborators were **Lorento de No, Lafora**, and Wilder **Penfield**.

Cajal used the brains of small immature animals such as embryonic mice, bats, and rats for study, because in them the relative lack of myelin allowed better staining of the cellular elements. With these techniques, he revolutionized the understanding of the form and nature of the cell populations of the nervous system. He was the first to show that the processes of cells are not linked indiscriminately within a reticulum, but have specific sites of termination on the dendrites or bodies of other cells. He enunciated his neuronal theory in three parts: First, nerve cells are independent elements that do not anastomose (as in a synctium) but make contact with others only at specific points. Second, nervous impulses are always transmitted from the cell body out to the axon. And third, the axon conducts away from the cell body.

His collected opinions appeared in his *Manual de anatomia patologica general* (Madrid, 1909) and in the translated *Studies on Degeneration and Regeneration in the Nervous System* (London, 1928). His autobiography has recently been published.

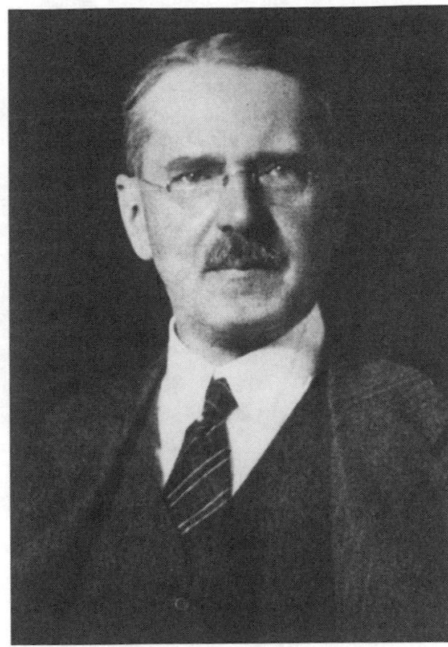

Figure R–1 James Ramsay Hunt

Ramsay Hunt, James (1872–1937) American neurologist who trained in Philadelphia and then in Paris and Berlin, returning to Cornell and later becoming professor of nervous diseases at Columbia. He was the first to describe in detail the effects of internal carotid artery occlusion and of damage to the deep palmar branch of the ulnar nerve, as well as to report the following conditions.

Ramsay Hunt paralysis See **juvenile Parkinson disease**.

Ramsay Hunt syndromes

1. **dyssynergia cerebellaris myoclonica**, a recessively inherited cause of **progressive myoclonic epilepsy** producing the clinical triad of severe action and stimulus-sensitive myoclonus, progressive ataxia, and grand mal seizures, with onset in childhood or youth.[3050] Other clinical features include dysarthria and pes cavus. The EEG and polygraphic findings include normal background activity in most patients, spontaneous fast generalized spike-and-wave discharges, photosensitivity, no activation during slow sleep, and vertex and rolandic spikes during rapid eye movement (REM) sleep.[6218]

Variants include the following:

A *dominantly inherited* form with seizures, chorea, dementia, and mental and physical delay.

Ramsay Hunt syndrome with peripheral neuropathy A rare variant of the preceding entry, with the onset in youth of speech defects, dementia, seizures and myoclonus, cerebellar signs, and peripheral neuropathy. Spongy changes, demyelination, and gliosis in the brain are the pathological hallmarks.[381]

Other forms complicated by central neurogenic hypoventilation, mental retardation, and morphological mitochondrial changes in skeletal muscle. See **MERRF**.

This syndrome is not a single entity; **Unverricht–Lundborg progressive myoclonic epilepsy, neuronal ceroid lipofuscinosis, sialidosis, biotin-responsive encephalopathy,** malabsorption secondary to celiac disease, **action myoclonus–renal failure syndrome, mitochondrial encephalopathies,** and many of the **multiple-system degenerations** are all causes.

2. *Geniculate herpes*. Herpes zoster of the external ear and the oral mucosa with homolateral facial paralysis, due to infection of the facial nerve (actually distal to the geniculate ganglion) causing severe lancinating pains felt deep in the external auditory canal.[3047] The peripheral ganglia of cranial nerves VIII, IX, and X may also be infected, with resulting dysfunction. Tinnitus, hearing loss, nausea, and vomiting may be associated. The prognosis for recovery in this form of facial palsy is worse than in the case of the more common **Bell palsy**.

In a small number of cases, the rash does not appear.[6164] See also **geniculate neuralgia**.

3. **Dentatorubral atrophy**.[3049]

4. Juvenile paralysis agitans. Progressive atrophy of the globus pallidus producing a Parkinsonian syndrome in young people. Both dominant and recessive inheritance patterns have been described.

ramus communicans (Lat, a branch + communicating) The sympathetic fibers running between the spinal roots and the sympathetic chain in the thoracolumbar outflow. White rami are lightly myelinated efferent fibers; gray rami are scantily myelinated and afferent.

Rancho Los Amigos levels of cognitive functioning A scale of cognitive functioning applicable to head-injured patients. Eight levels are defined:

1. No response to stimuli
2. Generalized response to stimuli
3. Localized response to stimuli
4. Confused, agitated
5. Confused, inappropriate—not agitated
6. Confused, appropriate
7. Automatic, appropriate
8. Purposeful, appropriate

random epilepsy Generalized seizures occurring independently of the sleep–wake cycle.

Rankin Scale A popular scale for the assessment of the burden of stroke[5186] in which the first and last points are objective, the remainder rather subjective. It runs from 0 (no symptoms) to 6 (death). Minor symptoms that do not interfere with activities of daily living rate 1; minor handicap in the form of symptoms that restrict lifestyle but do not interfere with the patient's capacity for self-care rates 2, while handicaps that significantly restrict lifestyle and prevent independent existence, although the patient can walk without assistance ("moderate handicap") rate 3; symptoms that prevent independent existence such that the patient cannot walk unaided and needs assistance with personal bodily needs (though not requiring constant attention) are regarded as "moderately severe handicap" and rate 4; while "severe handicap" is defined as the condition of being totally dependent and likely bedridden and incontinent, requiring constant attention, and it rates 5.

See also **stroke scales**.

Ranvier, Louis-Antoine (1835–1922) French histologist, who trained in medicine in Paris and was selected by Claude **Bernard** to lead the histological service at the Collège de France. Ranvier was soon appointed professor of general anatomy there and published on many areas of histology. In 1878, he described the **nodes** named for him.[5886]

RAPD See **relative afferent pupillary defect**.

raphe (Gr, a seam) A place where it appears as though adjacent structures had been sewn together.

Rapid Disability Rating scale An instrument for assessing the activities of daily living, disabilities, and special problems in elderly subjects.[3860]

rapid eye movement sleep
See **REM sleep**.

rapid-onset dystonia–Parkinsonism
(DYT12) A dominantly inherited movement disorder characterized by the onset over hours to days of Parkinsonism and dystonia, together with a subsequently stable course. There is only minimal response to dopamine agonists or other therapies. Dysarthria and bradykinesia are prominent features, and the condition affects the bulbar and arm muscles more than those of the legs. Focal or segmental dystonia precedes the onset of the disorder in some cases.[1675, 5441] It is caused by mutations in the *ATP1A3* gene.

The phenotype includes a rostrocaudal gradient and sometimes the absence of tremor at onset, occasional mild limb dystonia before the primary onset, lack of response to dopaminergic medications, rare abrupt worsening of symptoms later in life, stabilization of symptoms within a month, and minimal improvement overall. Tremor at onset of symptoms, a reversed rostrocaudal gradient, and significant limb pain exclude a diagnosis of rapid-onset dystonia–Parkinsonism (RDP).[821] Diagnostic criteria have been suggested,[820] and are reproduced by kind permission of the American Academy of Neurology and Lippincott Williams & Wilkins:

Typical RPD

- Autosomal dominant inheritance
- Sudden onset of combined dystonia and Parkinsonism with stabilization in less than 4 weeks
- Bulbar symptoms including dysarthria and dysphagia
- Bulbar and arm involvement greater than that of the legs
- Moderate to no response to levodopa/carbidopa or dopamine agonists
- Normal brain CT or MRI
- Low CSF HVA levels (not required for diagnosis)

Other RDP Phenotypes

- Family history of classical RDP
- Gradual or sudden onset of dystonia (± subtle Parkinsonism)
- Moderate or no response to levodopa/carbidopa or dopamine agonists
- Normal brain CT or MRI
- Low CSF HVA levels (not required for diagnosis)

rapid time zone change syndrome
(jet lag, acute phase shift of sleep) A transient desynchronization of an individual's sleep–wake cycle as a result of rapid travel across multiple time zones. Clinically, excessive sleepiness and irritability with impaired memory occur during waking periods, and insomnia during the normal sleep period of the new environment. The normal circadian patterns for cortisol levels and temperature are also affected.[4223]

Readjustment occurs at the rate of 88 min/day going west and 55 min/day going east. (See also ASDC Diagnostic Classification.[1629])

rapidly progressive aphasic dementia and motor neuron disease
A rare syndrome characterized by the occurrence of speech and language impairment, including severe nonfluent dysphasia, as the initial features of rapidly progressing **amyotrophic lateral sclerosis**.[1053]

rapidly progressive Parkinsonism and dementia with pallidopontonigral degeneration
An autosomal dominant neurodegenerative disease characterized by progressive Parkinsonism with dystonia unrelated to medications, as well as dementia, abnormal ocular motility, pyramidal tract dysfunction, frontal lobe release signs, perseverative vocalizations, and urinary incontinence. The course is exceptionally aggressive, with symptom onset and death consistently occurring in the fifth decade.

Rappaport disability rating scale
A rating scale designed for the continuing assessment of patients with severe head injury throughout the course of recovery. Three items in the scale reproduce the **Glasgow Coma Scale**, while others deal with *toileting*, *grooming*, *feeding*, *overall level of functioning*, and *employability*.[5196]

rapsyn
A postsynaptic protein essential for anchoring and clustering acetylcholine receptors (AChRs) at the endplate. Mutations in the rapsyn gene cause a postsynaptic **congenital myasthenic syndrome**.[1863]

RAS
See **reticular activating system**.

Rasdolsky syndrome
Contracture and paresis of the masseter and facial muscles as a result of a neoplasm of the homolateral pontine tegmentum.[5198]

Rasmussen, Theodor
(1910–2002) American-Canadian neurosurgeon and neuroscientist who, following war service, was appointed to McGill University, working with Wilder **Penfield**. He was for a time professor of neurosurgery at the University of Chicago before returning to McGill and, like Penfield, hugely advancing the specialty of epilepsy surgery. He defined the following condition. He also played jazz clarinet.

Rasmussen encephalitis
(chronic unilateral encephalitis of Rasmussen; OMIM 30-59915) A chronic, progressive, smoldering rare but severe immune-mediated brain disorder presenting (usually in children but also rarely in adult life) with intractable epileptic seizures (**epilepsia partialis continua**), dementia, and varied neurological and psychiatric disturbances.[5207] These lead to unilateral hemispheric atrophy, associated progressive neurological dysfunction, and intractable simple or complex partial seizures or secondarily generalized tonic–clonic seizures; status epilepticus can be the presenting manifestation.

Rasmussen described the condition in 1958. Its etiology is autoimmune, but even that remains as uncertain today as when Wilder **Penfield**, doubting a primary inflammatory cause in 1956, offered a new hat to anyone who could prove him wrong. Whether this is a chronic viral infection, an acute viral infection leading to a local immune response, or an independent autoimmune process not linked to infection is uncertain, but the response to IVIg suggests at least an immune basis. However, the early occurrence of uveitis may indicate a role for a viral pathogen, and about half the patients have a history of some infectious or inflammatory illness prior to the onset of their seizures; cytomegalovirus has been particularly incriminated.[4246]

Stages of development of the condition have been defined. Stage 1 involves the evolution of a hemiparesis on the afflicted side. Seizures usually are simple partial or complex partial with occasional episodes of epilepsia partialis continua. The usual duration of this stage is about 3 years. During stage 2, there continues a steady deterioration of neurologic function. Seizures may tend to generalize more frequently. This stage has an average duration of 4 years. Stage 3 indicates an end stage of function. Typically, there is a hemiparesis or hemiplegia with hemianopia, and while the seizures tend to be less severe but still intractable, there is overt loss of intellectual function.

The CSF either is normal or contains a few lymphocytes/monocytes with or without elevation of protein. The EEG reveals focal slowing over the affected hemisphere with multifocal epileptiform discharges and/or periodic lateralized epileptiform discharges (PLEDs) interictally. CT and MRI eventually show perisylvian atrophy. There are abnormal T2-weighted signal abnormalities in the white matter early in the course of the illness. Single-photon emission tomography and positron emission tomography demonstrate decreased blood flow and metabolism in the affected area. Pathologically, frontotemporal cortical areas show chronic inflammatory changes with microglial nodules, neuronal loss, gliosis, and cortical dysplasias in the affected areas and with perivascular collections of round cells without inclusions.[5207] *Diagnostic criteria* have been proposed[633] and are reproduced in Chart R–2 by kind permission of Oxford University Press.

Chart R–2. Criteria for the Diagnosis of Rasmussen Encephalitis

The condition can be diagnosed if either all three criteria of Part A or two out of three criteria of Part B are present. Check first for the features of Part A and then, if these are not fulfilled, of Part B.

If no biopsy is performed, MRI with administration of gadolinium and cranial CT need to be performed to document the absence of gadolinium enhancement and calcifications, in order to exclude the differential diagnosis of a unihemispheric vasculitic disease.

Part A:

1. Clinical—focal seizures (with or without epilepsia partialis continua) and unilateral cortical deficit(s)
2. EEG—unihemispheric slowing with or without epileptiform activity and unilateral seizure onset
3. MRI—unihemispheric focal cortical atrophy and at least one of the following: gray or white matter T2/FLAIR hyperintense signal, hyperintense signal, and atrophy of the ipsilateral caudate head

Part B:

1. Clinical—epilepsia partialis continua or progressive* unilateral cortical deficit(s)
2. MRI—progressive* unihemispheric focal cortical atrophy
3. Histopathology—T–cell dominated encephalitis with activated microglial cells (typically, but not necessarily forming nodules) and reactive astrogliosis. Numerous parenchymal macrophages, B cells or plasma cells, or viral inclusion bodies exclude the diagnosis of RE.

** "Progressive" means that at least two sequential clinical examinations or MRI studies are required to meet the respective criteria. To indicate clinical progression, each of these examinations must document a neurological deficit, and this must increase over time. To indicate progressive hemiatrophy, each of these MRIs must show hemiatrophy, and this must increase over time.*

raster A method of displaying a free-running sweep on the cathode ray oscilloscope by off-setting each successive sweep below the last.

Rathke, Martin H. (1793–1860) German anatomist and physiologist, professor at Dornat and then at Konigsberg, who described the anatomy of the pituitary region and the "pouch" in 1838.

Rathke cleft cyst Cysts within the sella turcica derived from Rathke's pouch, pathological in humans but common in certain other species. They are usually asymptomatic but may rarely cause chiasmal compression or hypophysial dysfunction.[5309]

Rathke's pouch A diverticulum from the embryonic buccopharyngeal area which gives rise to the anterior part of the pituitary gland.[5886]

Raven Progressive Matrices A standard nonverbal test of visual perception and analogue reasoning, wherein the subject is required to determine which of a set of alternative patterns completes the sequence of patterns printed on a card.[5209]

A variant is the simpler **colored progressive matrices.**[5210] A more difficult set has been designed for those of high native intelligence.

raw EMG Unprocessed EMG signals recorded with surface or intramuscular electrodes.

Raymond, Fulgence (1844–1910) French neurologist with a strong interest in neuropathology, practicing in Paris at the **Salpêtrière,** where he succeeded **Charcot** as professor for a few years before handing over to **Marie.**

He continued the Tuesday demonstrations, filling those of the first 6 months following the death of **Charcot** with a biography of the Master. Apart from describing the syndromes in the following, entries, he wrote extensively on the topic of spinal diseases and collaborated with Pierre Janet in studies of the neuroses.

Raymond syndrome See **Raymond-Cestan syndrome.**

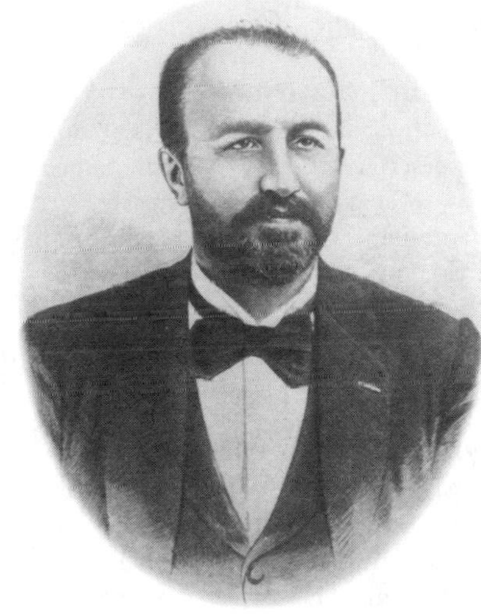

Figure R–2 Fulgence Raymond

Raymond-Cestan syndrome 1. (dissociation of lateral gaze, superior Foville syndrome, alternating abducent hemiplegia) A syndrome seen with lesions of the rostral-tegmental pons, characterized by homolateral VI nerve palsy with contralateral hemiparesis. It has also been also described as the combination of paralysis of conjugate gaze horizontally or vertically with internuclear ophthalmoplegia, contralateral hemiparesis, hemianesthesia, and athetosis.

These signs were considered by the original authors to indicate the presence of lesions of the paramedian regions of the pons and upper medulla[5215] as they originally reported the case of a young woman with syphilis whose illness began with dysphasia and right hemiparesis affecting the lower face and limbs, but who later showed prosopagnosia and both partial left III and VI cranial nerve palsies. Raymond localized the disease to the lower pons and considered that a VI nerve palsy and alternating hemiplegia were the hallmarks of the condition, in this case due to a gumma. The syndrome now known by this eponym is thus somewhat suspect, although MRI scanning has confirmed that a lesion at the mesial pontomedullary junction can indeed produce homolateral VI nerve palsy with contralateral hemiparesis.

2. Lateral rectus palsy with crossed hemiparesis, resulting from a lesion of the caudal-ventral pons.[5839]

Raymond–Foville syndrome See **Foville syndrome**.

Raynaud, Maurice (1834–1881) French physician who in his Paris graduation thesis described the phenomenon named for him as "local syncope," and correctly ascribed it to autonomic dysfunction. He did not have a particularly notable professional career thereafter, although he was regarded as a fine clinician and was elected to the French Academy of Medicine.

Raynaud phenomenon The successive appearance of pallor, cyanosis, and redness of the extremities (in that order), lasting minutes or hours, the final phase being extremely painful. It is a result of excessive sympathetic vasoconstrictor activity. The syndrome is especially common in women who are otherwise generally healthy. Its occurrence is stimulated by exposure to cold and tobacco use, and by the use of vibrating instruments, but it may also be symptomatic of small vessel disease such as the collagen vascular diseases or cryoglobulinemia.[2562, 5217]

RBANS (Repeatable Battery for the Assessment of Neuropsychological Status) A brief, commercially available test in two forms that measures cognitive decline in adults who have neurologic injury or disease such as dementia, head injury, or stroke. Twelve subtests allow sampling of immediate memory, visuospatial/constructional ability, attention, language, and delayed memory.[4236]

Reaction Level Scale (RLS 85) An eight-point scale rating patients on factors included in the **Glasgow Coma Scale** and adding an overall assessment of drowsiness and orientation.[6022]

1. Alert; no delay in response
2. Drowsy or confused; responsive to light (gentle) stimulation
3. Very drowsy or confused; responsive to strong stimulation
4. Unconscious; localizes but does not ward off pain
5. Unconscious; withdrawal movements on pain stimulation
6. Unconscious; stereotyped flexion movements on pain stimulation
7. Unconscious; stereotyped extension movements on pain stimulation
8. Unconscious; no response to pain stimulation

See also **coma scales**.

reaction time The interval between a stimulus (such as a click) and a learned manual response to it. Such an interval is increased in both hands with cerebral lesions, especially those of the nondominant hemisphere.

reactive myotonia Local myotonia produced by muscle percussion.

reactivity The susceptibility of individual rhythms or the EEG as a whole to change following sensory stimulation or other physiologic actions. (Adapted from the 1974 report of the Committee on Terminology, IFCN. In: Chatrian, G.E., Bergamini, L., Dondey, M., et al. A glossary of terms most commonly used by clinical electroencephalographers. *EEG Clin Neurophysiol* 1974;37:538–48. Reproduced by kind permission of Elsevier Science and the IFCN.)

reading epilepsy (primary reading epilepsy) An induced seizure disorder in which the subject complains that his jaw snaps or opens when he reads, especially aloud. Abnormal focal or generalized EEG discharges accompany the myoclonus-like movements of the mouth and throat, which progress to a generalized seizure if the subject persists in reading thereafter.[624, 626] The mechanism may lie in afferent stimulation derived from the neural mechanisms controlling eye movements. Sporadic and likely dominantly inherited cases have been described.[1427]

Rebeitz–Kolodny–Richardson syndrome See **corticobasal degeneration**.

rebound A phenomenon remarked by Sir Gordon **Holmes;** when the extended arm is depressed by the examiner against the patient's resistance and the pressure is suddenly removed, the normal subject's arm travels upward for a short distance and then recoils downward. This last correction is the rebound or **check reflex**.

Although the upward excursion is greater in patients with cerebellar disease, the real rebound is actually the final downward corrective movement and is normally present, being reduced or lost in the presence of cerebellar disease and increased in spastic limbs.[6062]

rebound headache (medication induced headache, analgesic rebound headache, narcotic abstinence headache, refractory headache, ergotamine headache, drug-induced headache) A common, persistent, daily-occurring headache afflicting chronic migraine or tension-type headache sufferers who have, over the long term, taken to consuming acetylsalicylic acid, acetaminophen, nonsteroidal anti-inflammatory agents, benzodiazepines, ergot compounds, caffeine, narcotics, barbiturates, triptans or combinations of these agents in increasing doses and on a regular basis, usually daily or near-daily.[5195]

The headaches have the clinical characteristics both of **migraine** and of **tension-type headaches**, and are frequently increased in the mornings on waking. They are partially relieved by ingestion of the subject's usual medication. Their mechanism is unknown, but the morning accentuation of the symptom would support the existence of chemical dependence, such that headaches are triggered by falling levels of the offending drug. This perpetuates and worsens instead of alleviating the headaches and is assumed to be the result of some alteration in the setting of serotonin 1_D receptors occasioned by frequent use of the serotonergic drugs listed.

rebound nystagmus 1. A form of horizontal jerk gaze–paretic nystagmus usually associated with cerebellar disorders. The nystagmus is seen on sustained lateral gaze; it fatigues and reverses the direction of its fast component after some seconds; on return to the center, jerk nystagmus appears with its fast component in the direction opposite to the previous direction of gaze and lasting several seconds.[2973]

2. A form of gaze-evoked horizontal jerk nystagmus which is not present in the primary position but which beats transiently in the opposite direction after relaxation of sustained lateral gaze to one side. The first of these types may be followed by the second. A lesion in the cerebellum and phenytoin intoxication are the most common causes.[2973]

rebound phenomenon See **rebound headache**.

receptive amusia Defects in the perception and recognition of tones and melodies, due to disease of one or other temporal lobe.[922]

receptive field That region of the skin, position of a joint or location of an initial stimulus, which, when stimulated appropriately, give rises to activity within a particular neuron.

recessive absence of tibia and deafness A recessively inherited syndrome characterized by congenital absence of one or both tibias and severe deafness.[1035] See also **Berant syndrome**.

recessive atopic dermatitis and neural deafness A nonprogressive, recessively inherited syndrome manifesting moderate neural deafness associated with atopic dermatitis involving only the trunk and arms. Vestibular function is normal.[3526]

recessive congenital moderate deafness A recessively inherited syndrome characterized by congenital symmetrical, nonprogressive, moderate neural hearing loss, but normal vestibular function.[3526]

recessive congenital severe deafness A recessively inherited syndrome characterized by congenital severe neural hearing loss and normal vestibular function.[3526]

recessive deafness, mental deficiency, ataxia, and hypogonadism See **Richards–Rundle syndrome**.

recessive distal muscular dystrophy A recessively inherited myopathic disorder with onset in young adult life, characterized by conspicuous distal muscle weakness and atrophy affecting especially the calf muscles but spreading proximally. The arms are affected late but the small hand muscles are spared. Serum CK levels are raised and the muscle biopsy specimen changes are similar to those of **Duchenne dystrophy**.[4415]

recessive early-onset neural deafness A recessively inherited syndrome characterized by early-onset severe neural hearing loss, in which essentially no hearing remains after 6 years of age, but the vestibular responses are normal.[1311]

recessive generalized myotonia See **myotonia congenita**.

recessive goiter and deafness A recessively transmitted disease manifesting severe sensorineural deafness and goiter due to a failure of iodination of tyrosine.[3526] See **Pendred syndrome**.

recessive malformed low-set ears and conductive deafness A recessively inherited disease characterized by uni- or bilateral malformed pinnae, mild to severe conductive hearing loss and low-set ears in about half of those affected.[3526]

recessive distal muscular dystrophy An inherited myopathy with onset in young adult life, characterized by conspicuous muscle atrophy and weakness in the calves and mild proximal muscle weakness. The arms are affected late but the small hand muscles are spared. Serum CK levels are raised and the muscle biopsy appearance is that of massive fiber necrosis with active fiber regeneration, as in **Duchenne dystrophy**.[4415]

recessive mitochondrial ataxic syndrome A progressive disorder that starts with episodic symptoms such as migraine-like headache or epilepsy. Ataxia and ophthalmoplegia develop later and there is a high risk of status epilepticus. The commonest seizure pattern is focal, involving the occipital lobes, but myoclonus is also common. MRI typically shows signal changes in the central cerebellum, olivary nuclei, occipital cortex, and thalami. Multiple mtDNA deletions have been identified in all patients so studied.

Mutations in *POLG* cause a recessively inherited syndrome with episodic features and progressive ataxia. Characteristic changes on MRI are seen and although skeletal muscle may appear morphologically normal, multiple mtDNA deletions can be detected using real-time PCR.[6830]

recessive myopia and deafness A recessively inherited syndrome of congenital severe myopia, nonprogressive neural deafness, and mild intellectual impairment.[4773]

recessive optic atrophy, hearing loss, and juvenile diabetes A recessively transmitted syndrome manifesting progressive optic atrophy, neural deafness, and diabetes mellitus from the time of childhood.[394]

recessive osteodysplasty See **Danks syndrome**.

recessive pili torti and deafness A recessively inherited syndrome characterized by congenital pili torti and neural deafness.[5231]

recessive retinal changes, deafness, muscular wasting, and mental retardation A recessively transmitted syndrome manifesting congenital deafness, retinal detachment, marked mental retardation, severe muscle wasting and weakness, and the retinal changes characteristic of **Coates disease**.[5896]

recessive retinal degeneration See **Alström–Hallgren syndrome**.

recessive retinitis pigmentosa with congenital deafness See **Usher syndrome**.

recessive split-hand and foot syndrome A recessively inherited syndrome characterized by the congenital absence of phalanges or syndactyly, severe deafness, and impaired vestibular function.[6782]

reciprocal contralateral leg sign See **Brudzinski signs**.

reciprocal inhibition Inhibition of a motor neuron pool secondary to the activation of the motor neuron pool of its antagonist. It is one of several important spinal mechanisms of motor control that help to make movements smoother and utilize less energy. There are multiple mechanisms for reciprocal inhibition, including one mediated by the la inhibitory intemeuron that activates la afferents and disynaptically inhibits the muscle that is antagonist to the source of the la afferents. (Adapted from the 2001 Report of the Nomenclature Committee of the American Association of Electromyography and Electrodiagnosis.[19] Reproduced by kind permission of the AANEM.)

Recklinghausen German pathologist who trained in Berlin and was then assistant to **Virchow**, later becoming professor of pathological anatomy, in order, at Konigsberg, Wurzburg, and Strasbourg. He described the disease now bearing his name in 1882, although a Scottish physician, Robert Smith, had published an excellent illustrated account of the same condition in 1849.[5619]

Recklinghausen also described osteitis fibrosa cystica, hemochromatosis, the periostitis of congenital syphilis and fibroids.

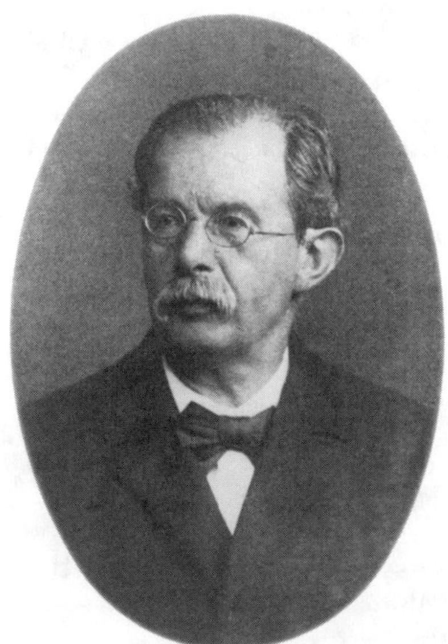

Figure R–3 Friedrich Daniel von Recklinghausen

Recklinghausen disease See **neurofibromatosis**.

recognition memory test An instrument for assessing visuoverbal and nonverbal memory, in which the subject is asked to recall which of a set of printed letters or photographs of people had been shown to him on a previous run.[6647]

recording electrode A device used to record electric potential difference. All electric recordings require two electrodes. The electrode close to the source of the activity to be recorded is called the active or exploring electrode, and the other recording electrode is called the reference electrode. Active electrode is synonymous with input terminal 1, or E-l (or older terms whose use is discouraged, grid 1 and Gl). Reference electrode is synonymous with input terminal 2, or E-2 (or older terms whose use is discouraged, grid 2 and G2). In some recordings, it is not certain which electrode is closer to the source of the biologic activity, e.g., recording with a bifilar needle recording electrode, or when attempting to define far-field potentials. In this situation, it is convenient to refer to one electrode as input electrode 1, or E-l, and the other as input electrode 2, or E-2. By present convention, a potential difference that is negative at the active electrode (input terminal 1, E-l) relative to the reference electrode (input terminal 2, E-2) causes an upward deflection on the display screen. The term "monopolar recording" is not recommended, because all recordings require two electrodes; however, it is commonly used to describe the use of one type of intramuscular needle electrode. A similar combination of needle electrodes has been used to record nerve activity and also has been referred to as monopolar recording. (Adapted from the 2001 Report of the Nomenclature Committee of the American Association of Electromyography and Electrodiagnosis.[19] Reproduced by kind permission of the AANEM.)

recovery nystagmus A form of spontaneous nystagmus seen to change direction as the initial stimulus producing the nystagmus (e.g., otolithic stimulation) diminishes with time.

recruitment The successive activation of the same and additional motor units with increasing strength of voluntary muscle contraction. (From the 2001 Report of the Nomenclature Committee of the American Association of Electromyography and Electrodiagnosis.[19] Reproduced by kind permission of the AANEM.)

recruitment frequency The firing rate of a motor unit action potential (MUAP) at the time that a different MUAP first appears with gradually increasing voluntary muscle contraction. This parameter is essential to the assessment of recruitment pattern. (From the 2001 Report of the Nomenclature Committee of the American Association of Electromyography and Electrodiagnosis.[19] Reproduced by kind permission of the AANEM.)

recruitment interval The interdischarge interval between two consecutive discharges of a motor unit action potential (MUAP) when a different MUAP first appears during gradually increasing voluntary muscle contraction. The reciprocal of the recruitment interval is the recruitment frequency. See also **interdischarge interval**. (From the 2001 Report of the Nomenclature Committee of the American Association of Electromyography and Electrodiagnosis.[19] Reproduced by kind permission of the AANEM.)

recruitment pattern A qualitative and/or quantitative description of the sequence of appearance of motor unit action potentials during increasing voluntary muscle contraction. The recruitment frequency and recruitment interval are two quantitative measures commonly used. (Adapted from the 2001 Report of the Nomenclature Committee of the American Association of Electromyography and Electrodiagnosis.[19] Reproduced by kind permission of the AANEM.) A reduction in the number of motor units available to generate a muscle contraction for the interference pattern reduces its amplitude and possibly its duration. See **interference pattern, recruitment pattern**.[19]

recruitment spasm The spread of tonic spasm from one muscle to adjacent muscle groups, as in **tetanus**.

rectal crises Paroxysmal rectal pain in tabetic patients.

rectocolic reflex Distension of the rectum prior to evacuation precipitates the colonic contractions designed to refill it.

rectosphincteric reflex Contraction of the external sphincter in response to rectal distension.

rectus abdominis syndrome
1. Abdominal wall pain made worse by head elevation in the supine position, and thought to be due to compression of the intercostal nerves by the rectus abdominis muscle.[3524]
2. Acute rhabdomyolysis of the rectus muscles following excessive use, as with the performance of repetitive sit-ups. Local pain, rigidity, and tenderness with an increase in serum CK values are the main findings.[5621]

recurrent (Lat, turning or running back) Turned back so as to lie or run in a direction opposite to the former one.

recurrent brachial neuritis and cleft palate A dominantly inherited syndrome characterized by sudden attacks of pain in the shoulder, arms, and hands, with persisting paresthesias and weakness, winging of the scapulas, and some sensory loss in association with facial asymmetry and hypotelorism.[1906]

recurrent hypersomnia See **periodic hypersomnia**.

recurrent inhibition Decreased probability of firing of a motor neuron pool mediated by Renshaw cells. Renshaw cells are activated by recurrent collaterals from the axons of α-motoneurons. Such inhibition influences the same cells that originate the excitatory impulses and their neighbors. (From the 2001 Report of the Nomenclature Committee of the American Association of Electromyography and Electrodiagnosis.[19] Reproduced by kind permission of the AANEM.)

recurrent laryngeal nerve That branch of the vagus nerve which innervates almost all of the intrinsic laryngeal muscles. The name acknowledges the long course of the nerve, which on the left side runs below the aorta before ascending again to the larynx.

recurrent optic neuromyelitis and endocrinopathies A demyelinating syndrome of uni- or bilateral optic neuropathy and acute or subacute myelopathy in the cervical and thoracic segments causing dissociated sensory loss, the whole culminating in blindness and paraplegia. Amenorrhea, galactorrhea, diabetes insipidus, hypothyroidism, or hyperphagia are associated problems. See also **Devic disease**.[6532]

recurring utterances See **stereotypy**.

red boy See **kwashiorkor**.

red ear syndrome (auriculo-autonomic cephalgia) A disorder first described by Prof. James Lance[3658] that is characterized by attacks of migraine-like headache with or without aura accompanied by redness and burning of the ear. Upper cervical disorders, temporomandibular joint dysfunction, atypical trigeminal and glossopharyngeal neuralgia, and local axon reflexes have been implicated in this syndrome, whose pathophysiological explanation is still not completely elucidated but it may be caused by antidromic discharges of nerve impulses in the third cervical root and greater auricular nerve in response to a local pain-producing lesion, vasodilatator peptides being released during activation of the trigeminovascular system.

It can be primary (commonly in association with migraine) or secondary, in association with an upper cervical abnormality. The pain is the most prominent feature and the localized vasodilator relatively minor. This appears to be a **trigeminal-autonomic cephalalgia** mediated by the auriculotemporal nerve.

red-eyed shunt syndrome Vascular dilatation of the scleral and conjunctival vessels in the presence of a **caroticocavernous fistula**.[5011]

red glass test Assessment of vision with a red screen placed before one of the patient's eyes. In the presence of diplopia, both a red and a white image of the light are seen by the subject, allowing in turn determination of the muscles, which are paretic according to the **rules for diplopia**.

red-green test See **Lancaster red-green test**.

red migraine See **cluster headache**.

red muscles The dark-colored striated muscles, best seen in animals or birds, composed mainly of type 1 myofibrils. They contain substantial amounts of myoglobin and oxidative enzymes, and have a slow-twitch capacity and tonic contraction functions. Compare with **white muscles**. The back muscles in humans are representative of this type.

red nucleus hallucinatory syndrome See **peduncular hallucinosis**.

red nucleus syndrome See **Foix syndrome**.

red nucleus tremor See **rubral tremor**.

red orbit syndrome The association of redness of the eye and of the periorbital tissues with proptosis, accompanied by diplopia and/or visual loss.[5730]

red reflex The red color normally visible through the pupil when the eye is examined with the ophthalmoscope from a distance. The presence of a cataract or of another lesion obstructing light obliterates the reflex, which is thus used for quick determination of the transparency of the ocular media.

red-and-black tremor See **midbrain tremor**. The term derives from the supposition that the tremor is caused by damage to both the red nucleus and the substantia nigra.

Redlich, E. (1866–1930) Austrian neurologist practicing in Vienna. He described **narcolepsy** independently of **Gelineau**, and his name has also been attached to that disorder.

Redlich encephalitis (Redlich–Flatau syndrome, Munch-Petersen encephalomyelitis) A poorly defined entity, either a mild but protracted form of epidemic disseminated encephalomyelitis[5704] or a presentation of **encephalitis lethargica**. Redlich and Flatau described it in the populations of Poland and Austria during 1927–1928. The nature of the infectious agent is speculative.[2125]

Redlich-Fischer plaques "Senile" plaques found in the brain in patients with **Alzheimer disease** and **Down syndrome**.

Redlich–Flatau syndrome See **Redlich encephalitis**.

RED-M syndrome The combination of Retinopathy, Encephalopathy, and Deafness with Microangiopathy; a condition of unknown cause.[4142]

redressement du tronc Extension of the hips and elevation of the trunk when pressure is placed on the soles of a baby seated with his back to the examiner.

reducing body myopathies A group of congenital myopathies characterized by the presence of sarcoplasmic inclusion bodies possessed of sulfhydryl groups, RNA, and glycogen, which stain positively with menadione-nitroblue-tetrazolium and with the following phenotypes: *severe infantile onset* manifesting more proximal than distal weakness, rapidly progressing to death in cardiorespiratory failure before the age of 5 years. Other types described are a *congenital myopathic* form with delayed developmental milestones but a benign course;[4770] a form with childhood onset; another in which the myopathy is nonprogressive and benign or occurs at a later age, in association with mitral valve prolapse and scoliosis;[4691] and a fifth, with dominant inheritance and onset in adult life (Xq26, *FHL1*).[874] The condition is allelic with **scapuloperoneal (hyaline body) myopathy**, type I. See also Pestronk (2008).[4992]

Clinically, early development is normal but with asymmetric scapuloperoneal weakness; sometimes **rigid spine syndrome** and dilated cardiomyopathy appear later. Muscle biopsy shows cytoplasmic reducing bodies (as in *acid maltase deficiency* and distal myopathies with rimmed vacuoles). See also **congenital myopathies** and the neuromuscular Web site: http://neuromuscular.wustl.edu/musdist/masym.html.

redundant carotid artery syndrome The condition in which transient ischemic attacks occur, leading to the performance of arteriography which in turn demonstrates tortuosity of the carotid artery, without ulceration or stenosis. This deviation from the assumed normal has thus been regarded as pathological.[5320] Whether it is or not is quite unproved.

redundant nerve roots Tortuous, elongated, and enlarged roots of the cauda equine, seen mainly in elderly people presenting with evidence of lumbar spinal stenosis.[4389]

reduplicative paramnesia A specific memory disturbance (a "delusional misidentification syndrome") characterized by the subject's certainty that a familiar place, person, object, or body part has been duplicated; hence, the confabulation of the existence of two or more places with almost similar attributes, although only one exists in reality. The syndrome was first described by Arnold **Pick** in 1903.[5019]

Reduplication of time is also described and may accompany any other form, all reduplicative phenomena having as their basis diffuse dysfunction of the cerebrum.[6698] The causative lesions were considered to involve the right hemisphere (altering spatial coding of the environment) bifrontally (preventing awareness of this deficit), but specific lesions of the anterior part of the right fusiform gyrus have now been shown capable of causing the syndrome.[3029]

The same mechanism is likely to exist when an individual believes that he has a double (a *Doppelganger*); see **Frégoli syndrome, Capgras syndrome**.

reference electrode (grid 2, G2) The recording electrode farthest from the source of the biological activity to be recorded; in general, any electrode against which the potential variations of another electrode are measured. Specifically, a suitable reference electrode is any electrode customarily connected to the input terminal 2 of an EEG amplifier and so placed as to minimize the likelihood of its picking up the same EEG activity as that recorded by an exploring electrode usually connected to the input terminal 1 of the same amplifier, or its picking up other activities.

Whatever the location of the reference electrode, the possibility that it might be affected by appreciable EEG potentials should always be considered. A reference electrode connected to the input terminal 2 of all or several EEG amplifiers is called a **common reference electrode**. See also **recording electrode, input terminal 2**. (Adapted from the 1974 report of the Committee on Terminology, IFCN. In: Chatrian GE, Bergamini L, Dondey M, et al. A glossary of terms most commonly used by clinical electroencephalographers. *EEG Clin Neurophysiol* 1974;37:538–48 by kind permission of the IFCN and Elsevier Science.)

referential derivation A recording made from a pair of electrodes consisting of an exploring electrode generally connected to the input terminal 1 and a reference electrode usually connected to the input terminal 2 of an EEG amplifier. See also **exploring electrode, reference electrode, referential montage, common reference montage**. (Adapted from the 1974 report of the Committee on Terminology, IFCN. In: Chatrian GE, Bergamini L, Dondey M, et al. A glossary of terms most commonly used by clinical electroencephalographers. *EEG Clin Neurophysiol* 1974;37:538–48 by kind permission of the IFCN and Elsevier Science).

referential montage An EEG montage consisting of referential derivations. A referential montage in which the reference electrode is common to multiple derivations is called a **common reference montage**. (Adapted from the 1974 report of the Committee on Terminology, IFCN by kind permission. In: Chatrian GE, Bergamini L, Dondey M, et al. A glossary of terms most commonly used by clinical electroencephalographers. *EEG Clin Neurophysiol* 1974;37:538–48 by kind permission of the IFCN and Elsevier Science)

referred headache (headache or facial pain associated with disorders of the cranium, neck, eyes, ears, nose, sinuses, teeth, mouth, or other facial or cranial structures) The descriptions in Chart R–3 are based upon those suggested by the Headache Classification Committee of the International Headache Society (1988).

Chart R–3. Features of Referred Headache

There is clinical and/or laboratory evidence of disorder in the cranium, neck, etc. responsible for a headache located in the affected facial or cranial structure and radiating to surrounding close or more distant areas of the head. The headache disappears within a month of successful treatment or spontaneous remission of the underlying disorder. Osteomyelitis, Paget disease, and multiple myeloma are possible causes of such headaches.

Pain from the *cervical spine* is localized to the neck and occipital region but may project to the forehead, orbital region, temples, vertex, or ears. It is precipitated or aggravated by special neck movements or sustained neck posture and is associated with at least one of the following: resistance to or limitation of passive neck movements; changes in neck muscle contour, texture, and tone, or response to active and passive stretching and contraction; and abnormal tenderness of neck muscles. Radiological examination reveals at least one of the following: movement abnormalities in flexion/extension; abnormal posture; local pathology such as fractures, congenital abnormalities, bone tumors, rheumatoid arthritis.

In the case of pain from the eyes, *acute glaucoma* causes pain in, behind, or above the eye; uncorrected refractive errors such as *hypermetropia*, *astigmatism*, *presbyopia*, or the wearing of incorrect glasses may lead to mild frontal and ocular headache which is absent on awakening but is aggravated by prolonged visual tasks at the distance or angle where vision is impaired.

Heterophoria or *heterotropia* (latent or manifest squint) may be responsible for mild to moderate constant headache in the frontal region that occurs or worsens especially during a prolonged visual task, with intermittent blurred vision or diplopia and difficulty adjusting focus from near to distant objects or vice versa. Closing one eye relieves or reduces these symptoms.

Headache can also be referred from middle ear disease and from the nose and sinuses. See **sinus headache** and **contact point headache**.

Temporomandibular joint disease is associated with mild to moderate pain in the temporomandibular joint precipitated by movement and/or clenching, a decreased range of jaw movement, often with crepitus, and tenderness of the joint capsule. X-ray and/or isotope scintigraphic findings should be positive.

referred itch (Fr, synalgies; Ger, *mitempfidungen*: [associated feelings]) 1. The induction of another itch somewhere else in the body (but almost always on the same side) when an inflamed itching spot is scratched. The first modern description was that of Kovalesky, professor of physiology in Kazan, in 1885,[1930] but the original phenomenon was first described in 1733 by the English cleric and experimental physiologist, Rev. Stephen Hales.

The sensations of the stimulus and the response differ, but are ipsilateral. The response is pinpoint, immediate, transient, and reproducible, and is usually experienced at a higher segmental level than the stimulus. The mechanism is unknown. (HJM)

2. The peculiar sensation of referred itching wherein a sensory stimulus in one part of the body is followed by awareness of an ipsilateral sensation akin to a sudden itch elsewhere, possibly as a result of impulses traveling through the variable spinocervical tract.[5640, 1930]

referred pain Pain felt at a distance from the site of nociceptive stimulation, in an area innervated at the same segmental levels, first described by Benjamin Brodie.[861] Such pain is felt deeply rather than superficially, and is often accompanied by hyperalgesia of the skin at the referred site and sometimes by muscle spasm and tenderness.[2929]

referred trigeminal syndrome A syndrome of constantly lateralized pain lying entirely within the sensory cutaneous territory of the trigeminal nerve, in association with evidence of pathology at the level of the craniovertebral junction (Dr. C.J.F. Davis, personal communication).

reflex (Lat, to turn back) Stereotyped, unlearned, involuntary motor responses to stimuli. Erb described "Tendon reflexes" in 1875. **Westphal** published his account of the phenomenon in the same issue of the same journal (of which he was the editor), but he rejected **Erb**'s contention that the responses were reflexes.

reflex acoustic nystagmus Jerk nystagmus induced by sudden loud noise.

reflex action The mechanism whereby a sensory stimulus elicits a motor response without conscious participation or influence. Reflexes were known to Descartes, Stephen Hales, and Robert **Whytt**, but the concept of reflex action was further realized by Prochaska in 1784, who stated (in his essay on the functions of the nervous system) that "the impressions of the sensitive nerves are reflected into the motor nerves." **Marshall Hall** further developed the concept for clinical use. The word was used first by Johann August Unzer (1727–1799) of Halle.

reflex anoxic seizure (pallid breath-holding attacks, reflex asystolic syncope, white breath-holding attacks) Nonepileptic attacks occurring mainly in healthy infants or young children and due to an abrupt interruption in the supply of energy to the cerebral cortex, as with a reduction in cerebral perfusion by oxygenated blood. Causes include a brief noxious stimulus such as a minor bang on the head, sudden fright, vasovagal and cardiac syncope, breath-holding attacks, cardiac arrhythmias or structural cardiac disease, hyperventilation, hyperekplexia, and familial rectal pain syndrome. Recovery is often rapid, but the event can trigger an anoxic-epileptic seizure.

Two types have been defined: type 1 corresponds to (blue) breath-holding spells while type 2 represents hypoxic crises due to a period of vagally induced cardiac asystole.[6036]

See also **syncope,** postural tachycardia syndrome, **oculocardiac reflex, breath-holding spells, febrile reflex anoxic seizures.**

reflex asystolic syncope See **reflex anoxic seizure**.

reflex atrophy The rapid and severe wasting of muscles around an inflamed or tender joint, associated with hyporeflexia.

reflex dystrophy See **causalgia**.

reflex epilepsies See **evoked seizures, paroxysmal choreoathetosis, paroxysmal kinesiogenic choreoathetosis, stimulus-sensitive epilepsies**. See also **idiopathic photosensitive occipital lobe epilepsy,** and other visual sensitive epilepsies, and **startle epilepsy**.

reflex hammer The trademark of the neurologist, much as the mirror is to the ENT surgeon and the couch to the psychiatrist. The hammer was introduced by J. Madison Taylor and S. **Weir Mitchell** in the 1880s and a similar version (the rubber "tomahawk") is still made. **Babinski** coated a metal disk on a short handle with rubber in 1912. The hammer used by Sir Gordon **Holmes** was a disk of ivory circled by a rubber pessary, mounted upon a hollow ebony stem, allowing its alternative use as a stethoscope. The Queen Square hammer was devised in 1925 by a nursing sister at the **National Hospital** and is the standard one used in English neurology, while the German Troemner hammer is that favored on the European continent and the Taylor tomahawk finds favor in the United States. A history of the reflex hammer has been published.[3693]

reflex incontinence The passage of urine due to contraction of the bladder wall in response to stretch, occurring in patients with severe or complete upper or lower motor neuron lesions. This forms the basis of automatic micturition. See **automatic bladder**.

reflex muscle atrophy Unusually rapid atrophy of muscles adjacent to an inflamed or painful joint, often with loss of their stretch reflexes and due to an unidentified mechanism operating in the spinal cord.

reflex myoclonus See **stimulus-sensitive myoclonus, cortical myoclonus**.

reflex neurogenic bladder See **autonomous bladder**.

reflex neurovascular dystrophy See **reflex sympathetic dystrophy**.

reflex of spinal automatism See **flexor reflex**.

reflex seizures (seizures with specific modes of precipitation, stimulus-sensitive seizures, triggered or evoked seizures) Epileptic seizures that are consistently elicited by a specific stimulus. "Reflex" is the preferred name in the new ILAE diagnostic scheme. The afferent stimuli can be *elementary*, i.e. unstructured (light flashes, startle, a monotone) or *structured*. Activities may be elementary (e.g., a movement); elaborate, such as reading or playing chess; or both (e.g., reading aloud). In this syndrome, seizures are precipitated by sensory stimuli. Those that occur in focal and generalized epilepsy syndromes that are also associated with spontaneous seizures are listed as seizure types.[4882]

Reflex seizures may be generalized (absences, myoclonic jerks, or GTCS) or focal (visual, motor, or sensory). Examples are as follows:

Photosensitive epilepsy, the most common form of reflex epilepsy, is not an epilepsy syndrome.
Hot water epilepsy
Idiopathic photosensitive occipital lobe epilepsy
Jeavons syndrome (eyelid myoclonia with absences)
Primary reading epilepsy
Self-induced seizures
Startle epilepsy
Television-induced epileptic seizures
Video game-induced seizures

reflex sensory nystagmus Jerk nystagmus induced by painful cranial stimulation.

reflex sympathetic dystrophy See **complex regional pain syndrome**.

Reflex Sympathetic Dystrophy Syndrome Association An organization founded to promote awareness of the condition, distribute information, finance research, collect data, and organize support groups in the United States. The organization also provides referral services and publishes a quarterly newsletter. E-mail: jwbroatch@aol.com. Web site: http://www.rsds.org/.

reflex syncope Brief fainting due to a vagal reflex inducing dilation of intramuscular capacitance vessels and thus reducing venous return to the heart, cardiac output, and cerebral blood flow. This is the commonest form of syncope, and is usually precipitated by pain, standing for a long period, hot surroundings, or coughing. Graying of vision, collapse, pallor, sweating, cold skin, and muscular flaccidity with occasional brief myoclonic jerks are the usual features and recovery is quick without confusion. See also **vasovagal syncope**.

Breath-holding attacks in children are considered to be a form of reflex syncope.

reflexe des raccourcisseurs See **flexor reflex**.

reflexes (conditioned reflexes) "The elemental units in the mechanism of perpetual equilibration" (Pavlov). He described conditioned reflexes and their dependence on the cortex; thus "If food or some rejectable substance finds its way into the mouth, a secretion of saliva is produced. The purpose of the secretion is, in the case of food, to alter it chemically, in the case of a rejectable substance to dilute and wash it out of the mouth. This is an example of a [simple] reflex . . . But . . . a similar reflex secretion is evoked when these substances are placed at a distance from a dog and the receptor organs affected are only those of smell and sight. Even the vessel from which the food has been given is sufficient to evoke the alimentary reflex . . . [which] may also be provoked even by the sight of the person that brought the vessel or by the sound of his footsteps. All these innumerable stimuli falling upon the several finely discriminating distance receptors lose their power for ever as soon as the hemispheres are taken from the animal, and [only those] that have a direct effect on mouth and tongue still retain their power."[4942]

reflexive memory Probably the same as **procedural memory**—a noncognitive learned motor response, similar to learned habits.

reflexology A system of alternative medicine, the practitioners of which believe that, by digital compression of certain regions of the soles of the feet, beneficial changes can be induced in distant organs.

refractory period The general term for the time following an action potential when an excitable membrane cannot be stimulated to produce another action potential—i.e., a nerve cannot conduct a second potential. The *absolute refractory period* is the time following an action potential during which no stimulus, however strong, evokes a further response. The *relative refractory period* is the time following an action potential during which a stimulus must be abnormally large to evoke a second response. The *functional refractory period* is the time following an action potential during which a second action potential cannot yet excite the given region. (Adapted from the

2001 Report of the Nomenclature Committee of the American Association of Electromyography and Electrodiagnosis.[19] Reproduced by kind permission of the AANEM.)

refrigeration palsy So called because of a supposed association between exposure to cold or drafts and the onset of the VII cranial nerve paresis. See **Bell palsy**.

Refsum, Sigvald (1907–1991) Norwegian neurologist who studied medicine at Oslo, where he went on to train in neurology and psychiatry. He was professor of neurology successively at Bergen and Oslo, and president of the World Federation of Neurology for 8 years. His major academic contribution was the description and elucidation of much of the abnormal biochemistry of the hereditary neuropathy named for him, but he also published widely on other aspects of neurology, especially hereditary diseases and migraine, and on electroencephalography.

Refsum disease A recessively inherited syndrome of polyneuropathy, pigmentary retinopathy, and cerebellar ataxia. See **hereditary motor and sensory neuropathy**, *type 4*.

Infantile Refsum disease is a neonatal variant of this condition and is a **peroxisomal disorder** with features resembling a mild form of **Zellweger syndrome**, such as facial dysmorphism, failure to thrive, hypotonia, pigmentary retinopathy, nerve deafness, seizures, hepatomegaly, and developmental delay. The possibility that adult Refsum disease may also be a peroxisomal disease thus arises. **Hyperpipecolic acidemia** is probably the same condition.[2317]

regeneration The restoration of anatomical and physiological integrity through the regrowth of nerve elements following injury. It occurs to a minimal degree in the CNS; that it occurs at all in the peripheral nervous system was first recognized in 1776 by William Cruickshank (1745–1800), who worked as a dissector for John Hunter and who sectioned the vagus nerves serially in dogs; when the dogs did not die following the second (delayed) section, he deduced that nerve regeneration had occurred, and went on to demonstrate the nerve swelling and repair at the site of the first section.[4749]

regional curare test A diagnostic maneuver for **myasthenia gravis**, in which a small dose of curare is injected into the veins of the wrist and allowed to diffuse regionally, the local circulation being occluded. Standard electrical end-plate testing is then performed; in the presence of myasthenia, unusual sensitivity to the curare results in abnormal test results (**decrementing response**) where they were normal before.[2141]

Reichert syndrome See **glossopharyngeal neuralgia**.

Reid's baseline A line drawn from the lateral canthus of the eye to the top of the external auditory meatus, being exactly horizontal. Originally used for pneumoencephalography measurements, it is now defunct.

Reil, Johann Christian (1759–1813) Danish physiologist, anatomist, and psychiatrist who was professor of medicine at Halle and later at Berlin. He first described the insula or island of Reil, the triangular area forming the floor of the space within the insula in 1796. He is also remembered for his descriptions of the lobes of the cerebellum and for applying the term *vegetative nervous system* to the **autonomic nervous system**.

reinforcement The augmentation of muscle stretch reflex responses as a result of slight contraction within the muscle before the stimulus is applied. This can be achieved by getting the subject to tighten other muscles (**Jendrassik maneuver**), or to cough, do mental arithmetic, grasp the examiner's arm, or concentrate on anything; or it can be elicited by applying any sensory stimuli to the patient immediately before the necessary stimulus.

reinforcement sign (of **Babinski**) Extension of the paretic leg when the subject sits with the legs hanging free and pulls the hands against each other; a sign of a pyramidal tract lesion affecting that side.

rejection behavior Strong withdrawal or refusal to be touched on the face or head even though this would not produce pain; a behavioral pattern resulting occasionally from lesions involving temporoparietal regions bilaterally.[4487]

rejection encephalopathy A syndrome of headache, confusion, seizures, and evidence of increased intracranial pressure occurring in renal transplant recipients during rejection episodes. The severity of the encephalopathy parallels the severity of the rejection, as estimated by serum CK levels.[2592]

relapse In the context of *multiple sclerosis*, the new occurrence of symptoms or signs or the recurrence or worsening of those previously existing, lasting more than 24 h and then stabilizing or resolving, and not resulting from intercurrent fever.

relapsing corticosteroid-dependent polyneuritis See **chronic inflammatory demyelinating polyneuropathy**.

relapsing eosinophilic perimyositis A syndrome of relapsing muscle pain with biopsy and EMG findings of myositis, the latter demonstrating a perimysial infiltrate, sometimes with peripheral blood eosinophilia. The condition differs from **eosinophilic fasciitis** in the absence of pseudosclerodermic skin changes, its prompt response to anti-inflammatory agents, and the occurrence of relapses.[5734]

relapsing fever See **neuroborreliosis**.

relapsing hypertrophic neuritis See **chronic inflammatory demyelinating polyneuropathy**.

relapsing inflammatory polyradiculoneuropathy A form of **acute inflammatory demyelinating polyneuropathy** in which recurrences occur.[249]

relapsing ischemic encephaloenteropathy and cryoglobulinemia A rare complication of cryoglobulinemia characterized by recurrent encephalopathy and symptoms of gastrointestinal ischemia. The cryoglobulinemia is seldom ascertained in life. Autopsy examination shows diffuse cerebral, enteral, and systemic small vessel lesions immunoreactive for immunoglobulins and typical of mixed essential cryoglobulinemia.[3083]

relative afferent pupillary defect (RAPD) An impaired light response in one pupil relative to the other, although the consensual response is normal. This latter finding rules out an efferent lesion as the cause, and so allows a diagnosis of optic nerve disease on the side of the defective pupil response. See **Gunn pupil, swinging flashlight test**.

Relative Assessment of Global Symptomatology A rating instrument for use by a close relative or a friend of a patient, assessing the latter's behavior in the community. In this assessment, the caregiver determines to what extent the subject needs help in certain activities of daily living, participates in activities, or shows evidence of abnormal psychopathology or of cognitive disturbance. In all, 21 items are rated.[5200]

relative refractory period See **refractory period**.

relaxation times (MRI) After excitation, the spins tend to return to their equilibrium distribution, in which there is no transverse magnetization and the longitudinal magnetization is at its maximum value oriented in the direction of the static magnetic field. In the absence of an applied radiofrequency, the transverse magnetization decays toward zero with a characteristic time constant (T2), and the longitudinal magnetization returns to the equilibrium value with a characteristic time constant (TI).

release hallucinations Visual hallucinations occurring in areas of visual loss stemming from any cause.[923]

release symptoms See **primitive reflexes**.

REM atonia The lack of muscle activity (other than respiratory and eye muscle activity), characteristic of rapid eye movement (REM) sleep.

REM density A measurement of the frequency of eye movements during REM sleep.[280]

REM intrusion The isolated and inappropriate intrusions of components of REM sleep (such as eye movements or inhibition of EMG activity) into non-REM (NREM) sleep or wakefulness, accounting for many of the symptoms of **narcolepsy**, such as **cataplexy** and **sleep paralysis**. NREM sleep intrusions (e.g., automatic behavior in patients with narcolepsy) may also occur.[280]

REM nightmare See **nightmare**.

REM percent The proportion of the total sleep time that is constituted by REM sleep.

REM rebound (REM sleep recovery) A lengthening and increase in the frequency and density of REM sleep periods following a period of REM sleep deprivation.

REM recovery See **REMS rebound**.

REM sleep (active sleep, desynchronized sleep, paradoxical sleep, D-state) A sleep period occurring three to six times nightly, during which the brain's metabolism is increased as physiological activity is enhanced (as shown by cortical activation and EEG desynchronization); rapid saccadic eye movements (REMs) and pontogeniculo-occipital (PGO) waves are recordable discontinuously, but EMG activity in most other muscle groups is inhibited, and there is total relaxation of postural muscles with dropping of the head.[265]

EEG activity in this sleep stage is characterized by low voltage, fast (not alpha) activity, and saw-toothed waves. REM sleep occupies some 20–25% of the total sleep time. *Tonic* stages (paralysis with muscle atonia, increased cerebral blood flow, high arousal threshold, penile erections, cortical EEG desynchronization, and hippocampal theta activity) and *phasic* stages (muscle twitching, bursts of eye movements, hypopnea, variable pulse and blood pressure, and pontogeniculo-occipital spike activity) are differentiated. **Dreaming** and **nightmares** also occur during REM sleep.

REM sleep behavior disorder A **parasomnia** characterized by abnormal complex activity during REM sleep in which muscle tone is restored even though the patient is in the REM phase of sleep; this facilitates the release of stereotypic behavior during dreaming.

Such behavior occurs during the middle third of nocturnal sleep at any age, but mainly in elderly men with brainstem disease. The bizarre behavior, which may lead to physical injury of others, may represent the acting-out of dreams. The responsible lesion is considered to be in the pontomesencephalic tegmentum, perhaps leading to dopamine deficiency. In a few patients, **narcolepsy** is associated.[4026, 5593] In some cases the disorder is an early marker for **synucleopathies**.[1962] In others it may be a manifestation of an evolving neurodegenerative disorder. Minimal diagnostic criteria have been suggested and are given in Chart R–4.

REM sleep intrusions The isolated and inappropriate occurrence of components of REM sleep during wakefulness.[4027] They include components of the narcolepsy tetrad and REM dreaming during the transition between wakefulness and sleep.

Chart R–4. Diagnostic Criteria for REM Sleep Behavior Disorder[4026]

A. *Polysomnographic abnormality*. At least one of the following must be noted during REM sleep:
   1. Excessive augmentation of chin EMG tone
   2. Excessive chin and/or limb phasic EMG twitching, irrespective of chin EMG tone

B. *Documentation of abnormal REM sleep behaviors*. At least one of the following must be observed:
   1. Excessive limb and/or body jerking
   2. Complex behaviors
   3. Vigorous or violent behaviors, *or*

History of problematic sleep behaviors. At least one of the following must apply:
   1. Harmful or potentially harmful behaviors
   2. Behaviors disruptive of sleep continuity

C. *Lack of evidence for seizure activity on EEG*

From Mahowald MW, Schenck CH. REM sleep behavior disorder. In Kryger MH, Roth T, Dement WC (eds). Principles and Practice of Sleep Medicine. *Philadelphia: W.B. Saunders, 1989. Reproduced by permission.*

REM sleep phasic events Rapid eye movements, middle ear muscle activity, and somatic muscle twitching.[4027]

REM sleep recovery See REM **rebound**.

REM sleep tonic events Desynchronization of the EEG, muscle atonia, and penile tumescence.[4027]

REM sleep-related sinus arrest A cardiac rhythm disorder that is characterized by sinus arrest during REM sleep in people without cardiac, medical, or other sleep disorders. No sleep complaints occur, but the person may have vague chest discomfort during the day and infrequently syncope at night, should they get up.[4520]

Remak, Ernest Julius (1848–1911) German neurologist, son of Robert **Remak**. He graduated from Berlin and practiced there for most of his life, finally as professor of neurology. He remarked (but did not appreciate) the plantar response before **Babinski**. He is best remembered for his studies on peripheral nerves.

Remak, Robert (1815–1865) German physiologist and professor of neurology in Posen. In his graduating thesis (University of Berlin, 1838), he described nonmedullated fibers, the axis cylinder, and the origin of axons from the nerve cell, thus introducing the modern concept of the autonomic nervous system. He was also the first to define the endoderm, mesoderm, and ectoderm (in 1851), and was a pioneer of electrotherapy. He also described the **Horner syndrome** in animals, although the first description in humans was that of Claude **Bernard** in 1852.

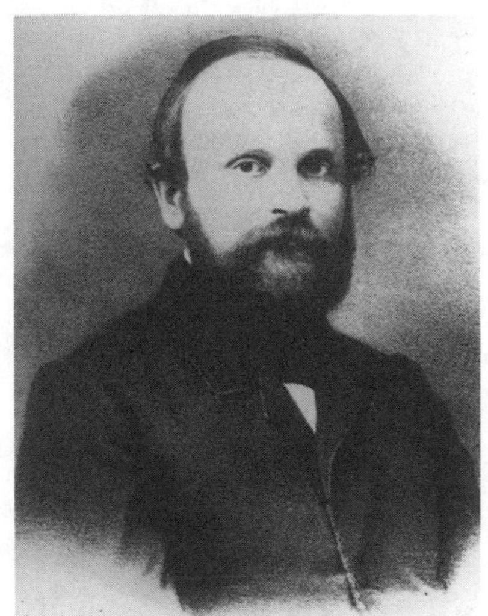

Figure R–4 Robert Remak

Remak cells Cells with functions similar to those of **Schwann cells**, the cytoplasm of which, however, surrounds numbers of unmyelinated axons. They are named for Robert **Remak**.

Remak fibers Nonmedullated fibers described by Robert **Remak** in 1838.

Remak paralysis (plumbism, saturnine palsy) A peripheral motor neuropathy named after E.J. **Remak**, affecting the nerves/muscles most used, thus usually the radial forearm extensors producing wrist-drop; potentially any muscle group could be involved, however. Tremor, delirium, and somnolence witness the presence of an associated encephalopathy due to the chronic lead poisoning.[5263] See **lead palsy**.

Remak reflex Extension of the knee and plantar flexion of the toes on the side on which the thigh is stroked. This is a sign of pyramidal disease and is named after E.J. **Remak**.

Remak sign A double sensation experienced with a single peripheral painful stimulus in the setting of **tabes dorsalis**. It is named after E.J. **Remak**.

reminiscence The process of remembering events and activities, usually discursively.

remission (of multiple sclerosis) A definite abatement of signs, symptoms, or both that has been present for at least 24 h; but a remission must last for at least 1 month to be considered significant.[5094]

remote atrophy Lower motor neuron signs in the arms and hands in association with a lesion of the level of the foramen magnum without evidence of cervical cord involvement; thus a false localizing sign.[3700]

Remote Memory Questionnaire A multiple-choice recognition test containing questions about news items dating between 1930 and 1970, grouped by decade. The test is sensitive to dementia and assesses its severity.[6004]

remote memory tests See **retrograde memory tests**.

renal tubular acidosis with periodic paralysis, optic atrophy, or calcification of the basal ganglia A syndrome characterized by these features and due to carbonic anhydrase deficiency II, the responsible gene mapping to chromosome 8q32.

Renaut bodies Loosely textured whorled structures containing few cells, found in the subperineurial space of normal peripheral nerves, especially at sites of compression.[257]

Rendu tremor A coarse tremor of the limbs, increased by attempted movement and thus resembling that of cerebellar disease, but in this case hysterical in origin. It was described in 1888 by Henri-Jules-Louis Rendu (1844–1902), a French physician at the Hôpital Necker in Paris.

Rendu–Osler–Weber hemangiomatosis A dominantly inherited syndrome of facial hemangiomas and telangiectasias in the skin, lung, and brain with cerebral arteriovenous malformations. See **hereditary hemorrhagic telangiectasia**.

Renier syndrome (adrenal hypoplasia with mental retardation and muscular dystrophy) The occurrence of short stature, adrenal hypoplasia, mental and developmental delay, and proximal and distal myopathic weakness in the presence of muscle hypertrophy.[381]

Renshaw cells Small neurons in proximity to the anterior horn cells, recurrent collaterals of which activate them to inhibit the parent motor neuron pool and the 1a inhibitory interneurons that are responsible for the reciprocal inhibition of the antagonist muscles. The cells thus dampen agonistic contraction, both directly and indirectly. They were described by

Birdsey Renshaw (1911–1948), an American neurophysiologist.

reo- (Gr; behind, backward) Prefix denoting behind.

repeated dream arousals See **repeated REM sleep interruptions**.

repeated REM sleep interruptions (repeated dream arousals) A pattern of insomnia in which the subject awakens for 2–3 min or more during at least 75% of all nocturnal REM sleep periods and with less than 20% of occurrences during non-REM sleep periods.[2560] (See also AASM Diagnostic Classification.[1629])

reperfusion nerve injury An acute inflammatory response occurring when ischemic tissues are re-perfused, as a result of the enhanced production of inflammatory mediators, increased adherence, and emigration of leukocytes in postcapillary venules and leakage of proteins from the vessels. Local nerve demyelination results.[4721]

repetition A faculty allowing the rehearsal of speech that has been heard, dependent upon normal functioning in an "arch," suggested by **Wernicke** and comprising the primary auditory reception area, Wernicke's area, Broca's area, and the primary motor area. Repetition is faulty in all forms of aphasia apart from the anomic and transcortical forms.

repetitive discharge A general term for the recurrence of an action potential with the same or nearly identical form. It may refer to recurring potentials recorded in muscle at rest, during voluntary contraction, or in response to a single nerve stimulus. See **double discharge, triple discharge, multiple discharge, myokymic discharge, complex repetitive discharge, neuromyotonic discharge,** and **cramp discharge**.

repetitive nerve stimulation The technique of repeated supramaximal stimulation of a nerve while recording successive M waves from a muscle innervated by the nerve, commonly used to assess the integrity of neuromuscular transmission. The number of stimuli and the frequency of stimulation should be specified. Activation procedures performed as a part of the test should be specified, e.g., sustained voluntary contraction or contraction induced by nerve stimulation. If the test includes an activation procedure, the time elapsed after its completion should also be specified. For a description of specific patterns of responses, see **incrementing response, decrementing response, facilitation,** and **postactivation depression**. (Adapted from the 2001 Report of the Nomenclature Committee of the American Association of Electromyography and Electrodiagnosis.[19] Reproduced by kind permission of the AANEM)

repetitive overuse syndrome See **overuse syndrome**.

repetitive stimulation test See **repetitive nerve stimulation**.

repetitive strain injury A clinical disorder unsupported by demonstrable pathology, thought to be characterized by musculotendinous injuries caused by overload of a particular muscle group as a result of repeated use or by the maintenance of contraction. It mainly affects the distal upper limbs. The chief clinical features are pain (which is usually aching, burning or boring, and which leads to easy fatigue and a decline in work performance), subjective swelling, cramping, tightness, stiffness, numbness and tingling, and impairment of dexterity and finger control, accompanied by marked tenderness to palpation and increased discomfort with limb manipulation or voluntary use.[904] See also **chronic fatigue syndrome**.

replay phenomenon The spontaneous intrusion into consciousness of the recollection of part of a melody recently heard, silently but with exact precision; similarly, some seconds of recent scenes witnessed may be re-enacted within the inner imagination just before the onset of sleep at night.[2099]

repolarization A return in membrane potential from a depolarized state toward the normal resting level. See also **polarization**.

Reporters test A sensitive test to detect expressive language disturbances in aphasic patients.[1516, 1603]

representation 1. The assignment of responsibility for directing motor or sensory functions of an anatomical part to a region of the brain. Thus, the function of speech is represented in the left speech area, and of discriminatory sensations in the left arm in the right parietal sensory cortex. 2. An aspect of knowledge, corresponding to the way in which this information is recorded, stored, or expressed; a coded form of information. Thus, the printing of this sentence *represents* the meaning that is to be conveyed. The next stage is to *process* the information in order to use it in cognitive tasks. 3. The mental and physiological trace of a psychological or physiological event. See **engram**.

reptilian stare An imaginative name applied to the unblinking gaze of the patient with **Parkinson disease**.

rescue reactions Automatic limb responses brought into play when **anticipatory** or **reactive postural reflexes** fail to maintain equilibrium.[4723] (Reproduced by kind permission of the American Academy of Neurology and Lippincott Williams & Wilkins).

Research Group on Motor Neuron Diseases The World Federation of Neurology Research Group on motor neuron diseases. Membership is open to physicians with an interest in clinical or scientific aspects of motor neuron diseases, including amyotrophic lateral sclerosis. Membership provides the Research Group's official journal *Amyotrophic Lateral Sclerosis and Other Motor Neuron Disorders*.

residual latency The calculated time difference between the measured distal latency of a motor nerve and the expected latency, calculated by dividing the distance between the stimulating cathode and the active recording electrode by the maximum conduction velocity measured in a more proximal segment of the nerve. It is due in part to neuromuscular transmission time and to slowing of conduction velocity in terminal axons due to decreasing diameter and the presence of unmyelinated segments. (From the 2001 Report of the Nomenclature Committee of the American Association of Electromyography and Electrodiagnosis.[19] Reproduced by kind permission of the AANEM.)

resistance–capacitance coupled amplifier An amplifier in which successive stages are connected (coupled) by networks consisting of capacitors and resistors.

resistant tennis elbow Pain in the region of the lateral epicondyle that does not respond to rest, anti-inflammatory drug therapy, or local injections of anesthetics because it is due (in most cases) to entrapment of the posterior interosseous nerve at a point just below the epicondyle.

respirator brain (brain death with autolysis) The changes characteristic of cerebral autolysis in subjects whose vital support systems are artificially maintained following the death of brain cells, due to anoxia/ischemia. Swelling or congestion of the cerebral cortex, softening of the brain, and cerebellar and pituitary destruction are typical features.

Arrest of the cerebral circulation due to extremely high intracranial pressure is the supposed basis for the initial cell death.[4511]

respiratory alternans A ventilatory pattern occurring when there is a reduction in central respiratory drive and characterized by alternation of rib cage and abdominal movements.

respiratory apraxia Selective abnormalities of voluntary breathing due to increased respiratory center responsiveness to CO_2, suggesting that medullary centers are disinhibited, as may occur in patients with bilateral cerebrovascular disease.[4650]

respiratory chain An intracellular metabolic pathway comprising four functional units (complexes), disorders of which are common forms of inborn errors of metabolism, leading to heterogeneous syndromes ranging from isolated myopathy to severe multisystem disease with death in the neonatal period. Four complexes are presently defined:

Complex I (NADH-coenzyme Q reductase), defects of which lead to myopathy with exercise intolerance and weakness with onset in youth, or to encephalomyopathy or liver disease. Syndromes include **MELAS, Leber optic neuropathy, Leigh disease, Alpers disease, Huntington disease, Parkinson disease, dystonia, Kearns-Sayre syndrome,** cardiomyopathy, cataracts, hepatopathy, and tubulopathy.[3450]

Complex II (succinate-coenzyme Q reductase).

Complex III (reduced coenzyme Q–cytochrome *c* reductase), deficiency of which leads to myopathy or encephalomyopathy. Multiple phenotypes exist, including confusional states, **progressive external ophthalmoplegia**, pyramidal signs, and exercise intolerance.

Complex IV (cytochrome *c* oxidase) Defects of this pathway are those most commonly detected. They are found in **benign** and in **fatal infantile mitochondrial myopathies; Menkes disease; Leigh** and **Alpers diseases;** and in the **Kearns–Sayre syndrome**.[1645]

The clinical features most useful in identifying patients with respiratory chain disease have been defined by Jackson et al.[3129]

First-rank features that alone are highly suggestive are **progressive external ophthalmoplegia** (PEO); elevated lactate in blood/CSF; ataxia; maternal inheritance; low densities in the putamen on CT scans; metabolic acidosis; and ragged red fibers on muscle biopsy.

Second-rank features that in combination are suggestive of the diagnosis include myoclonic epilepsy; small stature; myopathy; stroke-like episodes after seizures; deafness; and cardiomyopathy.

Third-rank features are commonly associated but only suggest it if associated with category 1 (or possibly 2) features. These include developmental regression; failure to thrive; dementia; retinal pigmentation; and optic atrophy.

respiratory patterns Characteristic patterns of ventilatory activity, such as **Cheyne-Stokes, Biot** and **Kussmaul** breathing, and **central neurogenic hyperventilation**.

respiratory syncope See **cough syncope**.

response An activity elicited by a stimulus.

response-to-next-patient stimulation Perseveratory verbal or gestural activity in response to the stimulation of other patients in the immediate environment, the patient replying to questions or obeying commands when the physician has actually addressed these to, for example, the patient in an adjacent bed. The syndrome suggests severe right hemisphere damage in dextrals.[710]

resting membrane potential Voltage across the membrane of an excitable cell in the absence of a stimulus. See **polarization**.

rest(ing) tremor Tremor occurring in a distal part of the body despite complete relaxation and physical support; a characteristic feature in Parkinsonism. See **tremor**.

restiform body (Lat, a rope + a shape) The inferior cerebellar peduncle, named by Humphrey Ridley, an English anatomist, in 1665.

restless eyes (ocular agitation) Rapid, violent, and abrupt oscillations of the eyes at up to 100 Hz as a result of released brainstem activity following bilateral hemispheric lesions.[2086]

restless (limbs) legs syndrome (Ekbom syndrome, fidgety feet, irritable legs, dyslysis, anxietas tibiarum, restless legs DIMS syndrome, Wittmaack–Ekbom syndrome, Allison leg jitters) An exasperating intermittent compulsion to move the legs, usually occurring sporadically but sometimes in association with iron deficiency or peripheral neuropathy. The unpleasant nocturnal paresthesias or creeping sensations of the legs absolutely require the subject to move them. Weakness or clumsiness while walking and a sensation of cold in the legs are other occasional symptoms, all occurring in the absence of physical signs.[1828, 1829, 2778] In the elderly, coronary artery disease appears to be associated.

Urges such as these crop up variously; when suppressed they are known (at least by psychiatrists) as *obsessions*, but when acted out as *compulsions*. Neurologists naturally subclassify them; compulsions to move the legs are called the *restless legs syndrome of Ekbom*; compulsions to utter and to make facial or limb movements signify that the patient has **Tourette syndrome**.

The fully developed syndrome comprises irresistible restlessness; paresthesias, prickling, tension, or aching of the legs, from which relief is gained only by moving the limbs; accentuation of the symptoms at night with resulting sleep disturbance; **periodic limb movements of sleep;** and dyskinetic or myoclonic movements while awake. The family history is often positive.[4456] A disorder of central dopaminergic systems appears to be responsible, because relief is often obtained by treatment with dopamine agonists.

Two forms are recognized; *asthenia crurum paresthetica*, which is painless, and *asthenia crurum dolorosa*, which is not. Although many diseases have been associated, no causal connection has been proved. Clinically, patients complain of an unpleasant sensation in the legs at night with difficulty in initiating sleep. The disagreeable sensations of "creeping" inside the calves are often associated with general aches and pains in the legs but are relieved by movement of the limbs. **Periodic limb movements in sleep** are commonly associated. To a much lesser extent, the same symptoms can occur in the arms as well.

Diagnostic criteria have been suggested and are reproduced below, somewhat adapted from those of Walters:[6630]

A desire to move the limbs, usually associated with uncomfortable or unpleasant sensations in the legs (para- or dysesthesias) and partially or totally relieved by movement such as walking or stretching, at least as long as the activity continues.
They begin or worsen during periods of rest or inactivity such as lying or sitting.
There is accompanying motor restlessness.
Symptoms are worse or exclusively present at rest; partial or temporary relief occurs with activity.
Symptoms are worse in the evenings or at night.
Additional features include sleep disturbance, periodic limb movements in sleep, normal CNS examination findings, a positive family history, response to dopaminergic drugs, and chronicity of symptoms with exacerbations and remissions. Daytime drowsiness is an understandable complication.[6381, 134]

In addition, a low (<45–50 μg/l) serum ferritin level may be found.

Although Ekbom[1829] is to be credited with the fullest modern description in 1945, the condition was also well reported by Thomas **Willis** in 1685, thus "Wherefore to some, when being abed, they betake themselves to sleep, presently in the Arms and Leggs, Leapings and Contractions of the Tendons and so great a Restlessness and Tossings of their members ensue that the diseased are no more able to sleep than if they were in a Place of the greatest Torture."[6805] Which actually they are.

Excellent Web sites are http://www.rls.org/NETCOMMUNITY/Page.aspx?&pid=471&srcid=-2 and http://www.rls.org/ and http://www.restlesslegs.org.uk/, the last being a British academic group promoting research into and awareness of RLS and offering teaching slides, diagnostic details, and information about clinical trials.

Variants include *familial restless legs syndrome*, a dominantly inherited form in which the typical symptoms begin in childhood, and a form in association with lipomas, ataxia, and MERRF.[981] In (different?) forms, linkages to 20p13, 9p, and 12q have been shown. One dominantly inherited form has been mapped to 14q13–21.

restless legs DIMS syndrome

See **restless legs syndrome**. (See also ASDC Diagnostic Classification.[1629])

restless legs DOES syndrome

The equivalent (near-identical) syndrome as **restless legs DIMS syndrome**, except for the patient's leading complaint, which here is of excessive daytime sleepiness rather than of insomnia. See ASDC Diagnostic Classification.[1629]

restless red legs syndrome

The association of the **restless legs syndrome** with arborizing telangiectasia of the limbs, of unknown cause.[4335]

Restless Legs Syndrome Foundation

A charitable organization providing support and information on this condition. Tel: 919-834-0821. Web site: http://www.rls.org.

restrictive ophthalmopathy

The prevention of full and free ocular excursions within the orbit as a result of disease of the extraocular muscles, which either prevent their relaxation or reduce their elasticity. See also **Brown syndrome, forced duction**.

ret

A measure of the biologic effect of ionizing radiation, derived from the total dose of radiation in rads, the number of fractions in which it was given, and the time over which this irradiation took place.

retardation–hyperkeratosis–spastic paraplegia syndrome

See **Fitzsimmons syndrome**.

rete mirabile

(Lat, a net + wonderful) 1. Galen's term for the network of blood vessels at the base of the brain in ungulates, which was also known as the *marvellous net* by Herophilus. It was considered by Galen to receive pneuma from the lungs and heart by way of the internal carotid artery, which it refined to animal spirits, the life force, for storage in the ventricles, while the unrefined material (*pituita*) was excreted into the nose and pharynx. From the ventricles the animal spirits were thought to be transported inside hollow nerves throughout the body.

The rete is not normally present in rodents, nor in primates such as humans, but, because Galen's dissections were mainly performed on sheep, he was not to know that. **Vesalius'** pictures showed it in 1538, but he accepted the earlier opinion of Berengarius in denying its existence in humans 5 years later.

2. A fine network of new blood vessels emanating from the inner retinal surface.

reticular activating system

(RAS) Those parts of the lower brainstem which in the myelin-stained preparation are characterized by an interlacing network of fiber bundles, thus including all the gray masses of the tegmentum of the medulla, pons, and midbrain which do not belong either to the normal nerve nuclei or to the relay nuclei of the lemniscal systems.[4504] The system is neither an anatomical unit nor a physiological entity, although it has complex and varied relationships with consciousness. Functionally, its direct stimulation desynchronizes the EEG in a manner simulating wakening from sleep or alerting to attention. Collaterals from all afferent paths to the cortex turn into this subcortical system and EEG arousal induced by afferent stimulation can be shown to be mediated through it.

reticular reflex myoclonus

(subcortical reflex myoclonus)
A fragmentary type of generalized epilepsy, in which myoclonic jerks typically affect the whole body or a segment of it, spontaneously or with movement or somatic stimulation. Muscles that are proximal or flexor are affected more than those that are distal or extensor. The origin of the abnormal movement may lie in hyperexcitability of the caudal brain stem reticular formation.

When provoked by stimulation, the condition is regarded as one form of

stimulus-sensitive myoclonus (the other being **cortical reflex myoclonus**). It is seen most commonly in **postanoxic states** and in **progressive myoclonic epilepsy**.[2695, 5795]

reticular theory The contention of Golgi, Gerlach, and Weigert that the cells of the cerebral gray matter were in continuity, forming a reticulum or nerve net. **Cajal's** use of Golgi's own silver stain allowed the disproof of the theory.

reticulosis of the nervous system See **neurolymphomatosis**.

reticulum cell sarcoma See **primary CNS lymphoma**.

retinal abiotrophy See **Leber congenital amaurosis**.

retinal angiomatosis See **Von Hippel–Lindau disease**.

retinal blur Imprecise images occurring as a result of the inexact focusing of light on the retina.

retinal dysplasia See **Krause syndrome**.

retinal dysplasia with hydrocephalus See **Walker–Warburg syndrome**.

retinal infarction Acute, painless, and persistent (more than 24 h) monocular loss of visual acuity or of the visual field, with the ophthalmoscopic findings consisting of pallor of all or a section of the posterior pole of the retina. Additional findings may include the presence of an afferent pupillary defect, embolic material in the retinal arteries or arterioles, and a cherry-red spot over the fovea in cases of central retinal artery occlusion.[2730]

retinal migraine Repeated attacks of (reversible?) monocular visual disturbance, including scintillations, scotomas or blindness, ipsilateral to the associated attacks of **migraine with** or **migraine without aura** that begin during the visual symptoms or follows them within an hour. The ophthalmological examination is normal between attacks.

Although the ICHD-2 criteria specify reversibility of the condition, some permanent monocular visual loss is not uncommon.[2589]

retinal slip The difference between the speed of eye movement and the speed of movement of an object viewed; this represents the input signal that controls the velocity of pursuit eye movements.

retinal slits Defects in the retinal nerve fiber layer, best visualized close to the optic nerve head through the ophthalmoscope using red-free light. They arise as a result of atrophy of several small adjacent nerve fiber bundles, as occurs in optic atrophy stemming from various causes. *Sectoral defects* are wedge-shaped areas in which the atrophy of the nerve fiber layer is yet more extensive, as in glaucoma, nutritional amblyopia, and retinal infarcts.[4646]

retinal vasculitis 1. A benign syndrome characterized by monocular visual blurring, swelling of the optic disk with enlargement of the blind spot, dilated retinal veins, and multiple small hemorrhages into the retinal nerve fiber layer, lasting a year or two and then regressing. The condition may be a *variant* form of **central retinal vein occlusion** but is not obviously an inflammatory disorder.[5524] See **big blind spot syndrome**. 2. The presence of focal or extensive retinal vascular sheathing or occlusion, retinal infiltrates or hemorrhages, cellular debris in the vitreous humor, and vascular leakage demonstrated on fluorescein angiography, in association with multiple sclerosis or autoimmune, granulomatous, or systemic inflammatory disease.[5534] See **papillophlebitis**.

retinal vein pulsations Pulsations of the retinal veins at the disk head, seen through the ophthalmoscope and present in about 90% of normal subjects. Their presence is a reliable indicator that the intracranial pressure is <180 mm CSF, while the absence of such pulsations may be found in the presence of normal intracranial pressure but usually indicates increased pressure, as with obstructed venous drainage.[3802]

retinitis pigmentosa (pigmentary retinopathy, retinal dystrophy, rod-cone dystrophy, pigmentary retinal degeneration) A heterogeneous group of noninflammatory ocular disorders, usually genetically determined and characterized by a progressive loss of photoreceptor and pigment epithelium function. All forms of genetic transmission have been described.[5797]

Clinically, the early symptoms are night blindness and clumsiness due to constriction of the visual fields. Central visual acuity is preserved in relation to peripheral acuity, but there is early impairment in color discrimination. Myopia, lens and vitreous opacities, disk pallor, and retinal arteriolar narrowing are usual, but the characteristic abnormality is the deposition throughout the equatorial region of the ocular fundus of patches of black pigment with the shape of bone spicules, although this may not appear in the early stages. Electroretinography shows defective rod responses from the earliest stages.

The following diagnostic criteria have been formulated:[1851]

1. Bilateral involvement.
2. Loss of peripheral vision.
3. Rod dysfunction, evidenced by rod final threshold on dark adaptation and/or rod responses on electroretinography that are reduced in amplitude and prolonged in implicit time, or are not detectable.
4. Progressive loss of photoreceptor function.

Retinitis pigmentosa is a feature of a large number of syndromes, including those characterized by sensorineural deafness (see **Usher syndrome**), ataxia or mental retardation; storage diseases; mitochondrial diseases; peroxisomal disorders; mucopolysaccharidoses; and skeletal dysplasias. The topic has been reviewed by Pagon.[4854]

Different forms of the pure syndrome occur according to the inheritance pattern:

Dominant: A mild and slowly progressive form with onset in youth, mapped to 3q. A peripherin-related form is mapped to 6p21.1

Recessive: The most common form; it is more severe and rapidly progressive with onset in youth, and often associated with cataract and macular degeneration. Much less common is a milder, slowly progressive recessive form that has its onset in early adult life.

X-linked: A rare type, intermediate in severity between the previous two.

In all forms the visual fields are constricted and night blindness is an early complaint. Visual fields are affected in proportion to the extent of macular involvement.

retinitis pigmentosa, ataxia, and neuropathy A sporadic autosomal or X-linked recessively transmitted condition characterized by clinical features resembling Refsum syndrome (**hereditary motor and sensory neuropathy**, type 4) but with normal serum phytanic acid levels. Sensorineural deafness and evidence of cerebellar atrophy have also been detected in such patients.[6414] See also **cerebellar ataxias** (*variants*), **NARP syndrome**.

retinitis proliferans Neovascularization extending from the retina into the vitreous. See **Eales disease**.

retinoblastoma See **primitive neuroectodermal tumor**.

retinocephalic angiomatosis See **Wyburn–Mason syndrome**.

retinocerebellar degenerations A phenotypically diverse, dominantly inherited syndrome manifesting any combination of signs consistent with retinal rod, cone, and ganglion cell atrophy; neuronal loss in the brainstem and spinal cord; pyramidal lesions; and olivocerebellar and dentatorubral pathway disease of early or late onset.[4116]

retinocochleocerebral arteriolopathy A syndrome of deafness, encephalopathy, and blindness due to retinal arteriolar occlusions. The cause is unknown.[706]

retinoic acid embryopathy A malformation syndrome characterized by hydrocephaly, dysplastic calvaria, ocular hypertelorism, micrognathia, and congenital cardiac defects.[4]

retinoorbicular reflex See **Descartes reflex**.

Retinopathy, Raynaud syndrome, and migraine A dominantly inherited syndrome characterized by these features but without apparent linkage to the *CACNA1* gene.[6258]

retinotopy The functional topographical anatomy of the retina as represented in the visual cortex.

retraction bulbs Eosinophilic or argyrophilic axonal swellings seen in the subcortical white matter and the corpus callosum in brains affected by **diffuse axonal injury**.

retraction nystagmus (retraction–convergence nystagmus, nystagmus retractorius) A form of nystagmus in which all the extraocular muscles contract synchronously and intermittently, so that the eyes retract into the orbits with each beat.[5517] The cause is usually a lesion such as a pinealoma in the region of the Sylvian aqueduct, compressing the mesencephalon. Vertical and convergence nystagmus, pupillary abnormalities, and convergence spasm may be associated (Koerber–Salus–Elschnig syndrome).[3113]

retraction–convergence nystagmus See **retraction nystagmus**.

retro- (Lat, behind or backwards) Prefix denoting behind or backwards.

retrobulbar neuritis Inflammation of the optic nerve behind the globe of the eye and thus invisible on ophthalmoscopy.

retrocollis A focal dystonia characterized by sustained involuntary contractions of the neck muscles, which result in abnormal extension of the head on the neck. See **cervical dystonia**.

retrograde amnesia 1. Loss of memory for remote events. 2. (pretraumatic amnesia) Loss of memory for events during a period which preceded a neurological event such as head injury. Its duration usually shrinks with time.

retrograde memory tests (remote memory tests) Psychological tests which assess a subject's memory for events acquired normally at times prior to the onset of the subject's illness—traumatic or other. See also **retrograde amnesia**.

retrolisthesis Backward displacement of a vertebra upon the one below as a result of degeneration of the facet joints.

retroparotid space syndrome See **Villaret syndrome**.

retropharyngeal tendinitis An aseptic inflammatory process in the longus collis tendon, triggered by deposition of calcium hydroxyapatite crystals. It presents with intense neck pain and occipital headache, the pain being aggravated by neck extension. Amorphous calcification anterior to C1–2 and prevertebral soft tissue swelling on cervical X-rays and full recovery after treatment with nonsteroidal anti-inflammatory drugs are consistent features. Diagnostic criteria for the associated headache have been defined:

A. Unilateral or bilateral nonpulsating pain in the back of the neck, radiating to the back of the head or to the whole head and fulfilling criteria C and D.
B. Swollen prevertebral soft tissues, in adults measuring >7 mm at the level between C1 and C4 (special X-ray technique may be required).
C. Pain is aggravated severely by bending the head backwards.
D. Pain is alleviated within 2 weeks of treatment with nonsteroidal anti-inflammatory drugs in their recommended doses.

From the International Classification of Headache Disorders (Headache Classification Committee of the International Headache Society. *Cephalalgia* 2004; **24**[Suppl 1]) by kind permission of Dr. Jes Olesen, the International Headache Society and Wiley-Blackwell Publications.

retropulsion The tendency for patients with **Parkinson disease** to move backward, as if unable to straighten up and thus to halt. The sign is iatrogenic, seldom occurring except when the physician pushes back on a patient who then takes small, fast steps (as is the case with the opposite but forward movement, **propulsion**) as if chasing his center of gravity.

retropulsive absences See **tonic absences**.

Rett syndrome A condition characterized by a progressive loss of cognitive and motor skills, autism, and the development of stereotypic hand movements, occurring after an apparently normal initial 6–18 months of development. It was described by Dr. Andreas Rett of Vienna in 1966 and is inherited as an X-linked dominant trait, lethal in males. An MECP2 mutation is present in all or almost all subjects with the disorder.[6462, 180]

Chart R–5. Diagnostic Criteria for Rett syndrome[6383]

A. Necessary criteria[a]

1. Apparently normal prenatal and perinatal period
2. Apparently normal psychomotor development through the first 6 months[b]
3. Normal head circumference at birth
4. Deceleration of head growth between the ages of 5 months and 4 years
5. Loss of acquired purposeful hand skills between the ages of 6 and 30 months, temporally associated with communication dysfunction and social withdrawal
6. Development of severely impaired expressive and receptive language and presence of apparent severe psychomotor retardation
7. Stereotypical hand movements such as hand wringing/squeezing, clapping/tapping, mouthing and "washing"/rubbing automatisms appearing after purposeful hand skills are lost
8. Appearance of gait apraxia and truncal apraxia/ataxia between the ages of 1 and 4 years
9. Diagnosis tentative until 2–5 years of age

B. Supportive criteria

1. Breathing dysfunction
2. Periodic apnea during wakefulness
3. Intermittent hyperventilation
4. Breath-holding spells
5. Forced expulsion of air or saliva

C. EEG abnormalities

1. Slow waking background and intermittent rhythmical slowing (3–5 Hz)
2. Epileptiform discharges, with or without clinical seizures
3. Seizures
4. Spasticity, often with associated development of muscle wasting and dystonia
5. Peripheral vasomotor disturbances
6. Scoliosis
7. Growth retardation
8. Hypotrophic small feet

D. Exclusion Criteria[a]

1. Evidence of intrauterine growth retardation
2. Organomegaly or other signs of storage disease
3. Retinopathy or optic atrophy
4. Microcephaly at birth
5. Evidence of perinatally acquired brain damage
6. Existence of identifiable metabolic or other progressive neurological disorder
7. Acquired neurological disorders resulting from severe infections or head trauma

[a]*Modified from Hagberg et al.*[2676] *and Trevathan E et al. Diagnostic criteria for Rett Syndrome. Ann Neurol 1988; 23: 425–8. © 1988.* [6383] *Reprinted by permission of John Wiley and Sons. Inc.*
[b]*Development may appear to be normal for up to 18 months.*

Repetitive movements resembling hand washing are a prominent feature of the disease, though not specific to it. The condition is not all that uncommon, but was only identified comparatively recently. Four stages of the disease have been described: an early-onset stagnation stage between 6 and 18 months, a rapid destructive stage lasting weeks to months at 1–3 years, a pseudostationary stage lasting until the school years, and finally late motor deterioration which may continue for decades.

Diagnostic criteria have been established[6383, 5273] and are given in Chart R–5. See also **International Rett Syndrome Association**.

Described *variants* include the following:[5861]

A *forme fruste* with delay in the appearance of symptoms until late childhood
A late childhood regression variant, in which there is early psychomotor delay but the major features appear only at school age
A congenital variant, without the initial period of normality
A familial variant
A variant with preserved speech
A male (Hanefeld) variant presenting in boys with failure to thrive, microcephaly, progressive encephalopathy, and one or more of respiratory insufficiency, abnormal movements or tone, and intractable seizures[3286]

Rett Syndrome Research Foundation A charitable organization in this field. Address: 4600 Devitt Dr. Cincinnati, OH 45246. Tel: 513-874-3020. E-mail: mail@rsrf.org. Web site: http://www.rsrf.org/.

Retzius, Gustav Magnus (1842–1919) Swedish anatomist whose anatomical studies of the cerebrospinal fluid pathways and physiology laid the foundations of current knowledge.

reversal sign A decrease in the CT scan density of gray matter and relatively increased density of white matter in the brain following hypoxic brain damage.[807]

reverse Chaddock sign A variant of the **Babinski response** in which the stimulus consists of stroking the dorsum of the foot from the medial to the lateral side, especially with stimulation of the sural nerve territory, while the normal and abnormal responses are the same as those elicited in the classic maneuver.[6216]

reverse Marcus Gunn phenomenon See **Wartenberg winking jaw phenomenon**.

reverse ocular bobbing (atypical ocular bobbing, inverted ocular bobbing) Abnormal spontaneous eye movements complicating metabolic encephalopathy or pontine hemorrhage, in which the fast phase is in an upward direction and the slow return in a downward direction. See also **ocular bobbing, ocular dipping**.

reverse ocular dipping See **ocular dipping**.

reverse post-optokinetic nystagmus See **optokinetic after-induced nystagmus**.

reverse straight leg raising See **femoral stretch test**.

reverse optokinetic nystagmus

That form of **optokinetic nystagmus** in which the fast phases of the eye movements beat in the same direction as the movement of the stimulus, explained as the patient's own gaze-modulated spontaneous (congenital) nystagmus which is shifted to the primary position of gaze by optokinetic stimulation.[2703]

reverse pursuit A phenomenon seen in some patients with congenital nystagmus, in whom the ocular movements stimulated by the moving visual stimulus are in the direction opposite to that normally expected.

reversible angiopathy of the CNS See **reversible cerebral vasoconstriction syndrome**.

reversible cerebral vasoconstriction syndrome

(Call–Fleming syndrome, benign [reversible] angiopathy of the CNS, benign angiopathy of the CNS, drug-induced vasospasm, postpartum angiopathy, crash migraine, migrainous angiitis) A syndrome of sudden severe headache (**thunderclap headache**) idiopathic cerebral edema and concomitant reversible vasoconstriction involving the arteries of the circle of Willis or its immediate branches. It is most commonly seen in young adult women, sometimes in association with eclampsia, the postpartum period, bathing, pheochromocytoma, and the use of some vasoactive drugs[979] including cannabis, SSRIs, and nasal decongestants. The neurologic deficits are variable and, like the angiographic findings, usually recover completely within 1–2 months.

Clinically, the onset of the diffuse and severe headache is sudden, without an accompanying seizure. The blood count and ESR are normal as is the CSF and there is angiographic evidence of segmental cerebral vasospasm (the "string of beads" appearance) involving arteries of or immediately arising from the circle of Willis, lasting weeks or months. (Vasoconstriction here indicates at least two narrowings per artery in two different cerebral arteries.) Cortical subarachnoid hemorrhage, intracerebral hemorrhage, seizures, and **reversible posterior leukoencephalopathy** are complications occurring mainly within the first week; ischemic events occur slightly later.[1740] See also **Aβ angiitis**.

In the context of headache, diagnostic criteria (ICHD-2) have been defined by the International Headache Society.:

A. Diffuse, severe headache of abrupt or progressive onset, with or without focal neurologic deficits and/or seizures and fulfilling Criteria C and D
B. "Strings and beads" appearance on angiography; subarachnoid hemorrhage is ruled out by appropriate investigations
C. One or both of the following:
   1. Headache develops simultaneously with neurologic deficits and/or seizures
   2. Headache leads to angiography and so to the discovery of the "strings and beads" appearance
D. Headache (and any neurologic deficits present) resolves spontaneously within 2 months.

reversible ischemic neurological deficit (RIND)

A minor stroke of which there remains no clinical signs after an (arbitrary) period of 3 weeks. Such stroke syndromes have a degree of severity uncomfortably situated between **transient ischemic attacks** and **ischemic infarction**, the "reversible" part of the term indicating that clinical examination demonstrates improvement in the clinical condition; an improvement which (though clinically real) may be belied by the appearances on CT or MRI scans, which sometimes show evidence of infarction that is not appreciable to even the most talented observer.

reversible posterior leukoencephalopathy syndrome

(posterior reversible leukoencephalopathy syndrome) A syndrome of vasogenic edema associated with immunosuppressive therapy, eclampsia, renal disease, or hepatorenal failure with abrupt increases in blood pressure and/or impairment of renal function. It is likely due to a failure of cerebrovascular autoregulation leading to capillary leakage. Clinically it is characterized by headache, vomiting, delirium, seizures, cortical blindness and other visual abnormalities, and motor signs. Patients may be receiving immunosuppressive therapy or have eclampsia or acute hypertensive encephalopathy. CT and MRI studies show extensive bilateral white-matter abnormalities suggestive of vasogenic subcortical edema, without infarction, in the posterior cerebral hemispheres. Such changes may also involve other cerebral areas, the brainstem, or the cerebellum.[2907] The neurologic deficits resolve with therapy. Causative agents incriminated include chemotherapeutic drugs, immunosuppressives, and cytotoxic agents. The condition is also seen in normotensive patients not receiving chemotherapeutic medications, and in acute kidney disease, with blood pressure recordings less than 140/90 mmHg.[3749]

In children, again it presents as an acute transient syndrome characterized by seizures, headache, visual disorders, decreased awareness, and anomalous neuroimages. The most frequent causes are arterial hypertension and immunosuppressive therapy. The initial symptoms are vomiting, headaches, partial or generalized seizures, and visual disorders, with decreased awareness. The condition clears within days of effective antihypertensive therapy.[12]

See also **reversible cerebral vasoconstriction syndrome** which has close similarities.

Revilliod, Jean-Leoprard-Adolf

(1835–1918) Swiss physician who trained in Geneva and Paris and became professor of clinical medicine in Geneva in 1876.

Revilliod sign (Herey–Simoneau sign) Inability to close only that eye on the affected side in the presence of upper motor neuron facial weakness.[5276]

revised behavior problem checklist An inventory scale for the assessment of child behavioral disturbances.[5152]

Revue Neurologique (*Rev Neurol*) A neurological journal. Address: Masson SA, Avenue Beauregard 12, CH-1701, Fribourg, Switzerland. Web site: http://www.info-presse.fr/fiches/revue-neurologique_1791_pro.htm/.

Rey Auditory Verbal Learning Test A complex test of learning, of the effects of interference, and of the adequacy of recognition, in which the subject is required to recall as many as possible of a list of 15 words read out, after which a second list is presented; the next task is to recall words from the first list. Finally, the subject is asked to identify whether words that the examiner reads out were or were not on the first list.[5278] The amount of proactive and retroactive interference can be assessed as the subject supplies words variously from the wrong list.

Rey–Osterreith Test (Complex Figures Test) A method of examining visual memory, perceptual organization, and constructional abilities, wherein the subject is required to reproduce on paper a complex and meaningless pattern, after having studied it for a short time.[5277, 5278]

Reye, Ralph Douglas Kenneth (1912–1977) Australian physician who graduated from the University of Sydney and became director of pathology at the Royal Alexandra Hospital for Children. He recognized the syndrome named for him in 1951 and published an account of 20 cases of it in 1963.[2066]

Reye syndrome (encephalopathy and fatty degeneration of the viscera, white-liver disease) A noninflammatory encephalopathy with cerebral edema and fatty degeneration of the liver and kidneys following a viral infection in small children, also facilitated by their exposure to aspirin. Clinically, the condition is characterized by irritability, lethargy, and persistent vomiting following upper respiratory infections with influenza B, varicella, or other viral illnesses. Coma ensues, with hypoglycemia, acidosis, hyperammonemia, and ketonuria. Increased intracranial pressure due to brain edema, hyperpyrexia, hypotension, gastrointestinal hemorrhage, pancreatitis, and seizures are other potential complications, and in some cases there is clinical evidence of myopathy.[5279] The condition is frequently fatal.

Intermyofibrillar edema, mitochondrial disruption, and swelling of the vascular endothelium are demonstrated in muscle biopsy specimens.[2741, 2740] Pan-lobar fatty metamorphosis of the liver with severe ultrastructural changes in the mitochondria also occurs.

Suggested diagnostic criteria (in the appropriate context) are as follows:

1. A clinical history of a preceding viral-like prodrome and a biphasic illness.
2. Less than 10 cells/mm^3 in the CSF.
3. Serum transaminase levels exceeding 200% of normal, and blood ammonia levels exceeding 150% of normal.
4. Exclusion of other causes of encephalitis with hepatocellular dysfunction.

Logically, fulfillment of the last criterion should be sufficient by itself. See also **ornithine transcarbamylase deficiency, systemic carnitine deficiency,** and **medium and long chain AcylCoA dehydrogenase deficiency**.

Reye's Syndrome An information sheet available from the National Institute of Neurological Disorders and Stroke. Web site: http://www.ninds.nih.gov/disorders/reyes_syndrome/reyes_syndrome.htm.

Reynolds, Russell J. (1828–1896) English physician who became professor of medicine at University College, London and later president of the Royal College of Physicians and a fellow of the Royal Society. He first came to prominence when only 30 years old, upon his publishing a clear account of the then-current knowledge of the nervous system.

rhabdo- (Gr, rod)

rhabdoid tumor A rare, highly malignant neoplasm occurring in early childhood, usually arising from the kidney but occasionally in the CNS.[4545]

rhabdomyolysis The process of breakdown of the muscle fiber membrane, resulting in a clinical syndrome characterized by pain, weakness, and swelling of skeletal muscles with myoglobinuria. The syndrome has numerous inciting causes, such as excessive exertion, toxins, ischemia, certain primary muscle disorders, and metabolic defects.

In some cases (**idiopathic rhabdomyolysis, paroxysmal myoglobinuria**) no cause can be detected, although there are forms in which the rhabdomyolysis recurs in adolescent males who have recently engaged in very strenuous exercise, and another in which it follows a benign febrile illness in childhood but is not recurrent. It involves damage to the membranes of the myofibrils, leading to spillage of the fluid contents of the myofibrils, myoglobin, and creatine kinase being the ones most easily measured.

rhabdomyoma A rare tumor of muscle composed of or containing striated muscle fibers.

rhabdomyosarcoma A rare, primary, highly malignant tumor of voluntary muscle, often metastasizing to the orbit. *Adult pleomorphic*, *embryonal botroid*, and *embryonal alveolar* types are differentiated; however, the tumor is usually seen in children.

Rhazes (869–962) Arabian Physician who recognized and described nocturnal and febrile seizures as well as **night terrors**.

rhencospasm See **snoring**.

rheobase See **strength–duration curve**.

rheoencephalography (Gr, flow + brain + write) The use of electrical impedance plethysmography to determine changes in cerebral circulation, and indirectly to monitor changes in intracranial pressure.[4231] The procedure is now obsolete.

rheumatic chorea See **Sydenham chorea**.

rheumatic palsy See **Bell palsy**.

rheumatoid neuropathy A group of peripheral neuropathies associated with this vasculitic disease, including mononeuropathies of the upper or lower limbs, digital neuropathy, distal sensory neuropathy, and distal sensorimotor polyneuropathy.[4867] Both pressure and intrinsic arthritis of the vasa nervorum are considered to be causal.[5980]

rhinencephalic seizures See **amygdalohippocampal seizures**.

rhinencephalon (Gr, nose + brain) That most anciently derived part of the cortex, functionally related to olfaction, memory, and emotion—thus the **limbic system**.

rhino- (Gr, nose) Prefix indicating nasal.

rhinolalia Nasal speech, as is heard in patients with weakness of the soft palate.

rhinorrhea Discharge of fluid from the nose. When serous, this is trivial and is usually due to sinusitis; but, when clear and with a measurable glucose content, it suggests CSF leakage and is thus an ominous finding.

rhizalgia Pain occurring due to irritation of spinal nerve roots.

rhizo- (Gr, a root) A root.

rhizomelia A congenital deformity consisting of disproportionate shortness of the proximal limb bones.

rhizomelic chondrodysplasia punctata (Spranger syndrome) A rare **peroxisomal disorder**, resulting from deficiency of DHAP-acyltransferase. The condition is recessively inherited, and is characterized by dysmorphisms, dwarfism, microcephaly, cataract, ichthyosis, vertebral coronal clefts occupied by cartilage, tracheal or laryngeal calcification, rhizomelia of the arms and legs, joint contractures, microcephaly, spasticity, and mental and developmental delay. Affected infants usually die within a year of birth.[2889]

rhombencephalitis Brainstem encephalitis, caused in some cases by *Listeria*.[1745] See also **Bickerstaff brainstem encephalitis**.

rhythm EEG activity consisting of waves of an approximately constant period.

rhythmias Coordinated, repetitive, seemingly purposeful and partly voluntary abnormal movements usually seen in young children or subjects with mental retardation. They include head rolling, shaking, or nodding, as well as swaying and rocking movements of the body which are regularly repeated. The anatomical basis for the movements is not known.

rhythmic movement disorder Sleep–wake transition **parasomnias** in which occur stereotyped movements such as head banging, head rolling, body rocking, and similar sleep-related stereotypical repetitive movements of the head, neck, or large muscle groups, often associated with rhythmic vocalization.[1629] Such features occur mainly in children during any stage of sleep. The cause and the remedy are each unknown.[4025]

rhythmic nystagmus See **jerk nystagmus**.

rhythmic temporal theta burst of drowsiness (psychomotor variant pattern) Extended runs of 4- to 7-Hz EEG activity frequently notched by faster waves, occurring over the temporal regions of the head during drowsiness. The clinical significance of this pattern would be controversial, were it important enough to be so.

rhythmie du sommeil See **jactitatio capitis nocturna**.

TheRibbon An organization offering information for the caregivers of those with Alzheimer disease. Web site: http://www.theribbon.com/index.asp.

riboflavin-responsive lipid myopathy with carnitine deficiency See **lipid myopathies**.

Ribot law (law of regression) The events that occurred closest to the onset of amnesia (as in **Wernicke–Korsakoff syndrome**) are recalled least well.[109]

Ribot's Rule (1883) The language best recovered by the polyglot after, for example, a stroke involving the dominant hemisphere, should be the mother tongue.

Richards–Rundle syndrome (ataxia-hypogonadism-deafness; recessive deafness, mental deficiency, ataxia and hypogonadism) A recessively inherited syndrome of childhood characterized by progressive hearing loss, mental deterioration, weakness, ataxia, distal muscle wasting, hyporeflexia, hypogonadism with failed development of the secondary sex characteristics, ketoaciduria, and decreased excretion of steroids.[5283]

Richardson, J. Clifford (1909–1986) Canadian neurologist, professor of neurology in Toronto, remembered internationally for his description of **progressive supranuclear ophthalmoplegia** (Steele–Richardson–Olszewsky syndrome) and nationally for his leadership of Canadian neurology during his professional lifetime.

Riche–Cannieu anastomosis An anastomosis between the median nerve in the palm and the deep branch of the ulnar nerve. As a result, the thenar muscle retain their innervation in the presence of a palmar lesion of the median nerve.[5478]

Richieri–Costa syndrome A congenital dysmorphic syndrome comprising short stature, hypotelorism, prominent teeth, brachydactyly, camptodactyly, clinodactyly or skin syndactyly, microcephaly, and mental and developmental delay.[381]

A *variant* is *Richieri-Costa Schwartz-Jampel like syndrome* that has the added features of platyspondyly and myotonia.[381]

Richner–Hanhart syndrome (tyrosinemia II) An autosomal recessive syndrome mapping to chromosome 16 q22.1–q22.3, in which a deficiency of hepatic tyrosine aminotransferase causes the subject to suffer palmoplantar keratoderma, keratitis, mental retardation, and any of a wide variety of neurological deficits.[4855]

Riddoch, George (1888–1947) Scottish physician who trained at Aberdeen and, during World War I, worked with Henry **Head** at a wartime neurological unit, where he studied traumatic brain disease and its effects on visual perception and the reflex functions of the damaged spinal cord.[5291] His administrative abilities being recognized, his research declined and the

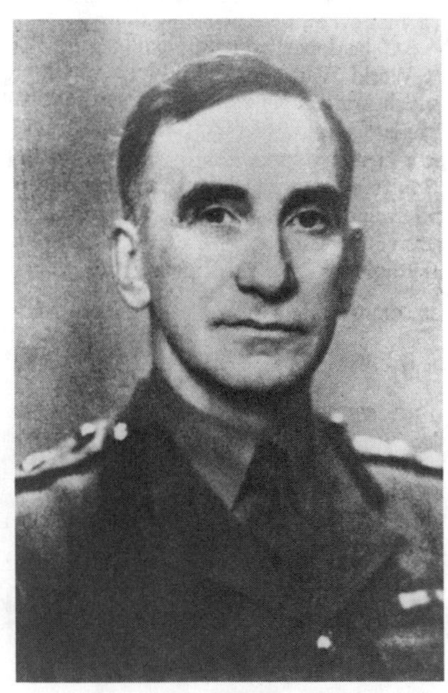

Figure R–5 George Riddoch

latter years of his career were spent in wartime clinical and governmental activities.

Riddoch mass reflex See **mass reflex**.

Riddoch reflex See **nociceptive reflex**.

Riddoch syndrome The ability to discriminate visual stimuli presented in the blind field following a lesion affecting the primary visual cortex.[5292] See **visual disorientation**.

Rieder paralysis (knapsack paralysis) Paralysis of the muscles supplied by the upper fibers of the brachial plexus due to prolonged compression, as from the straps of a knapsack or a hod.[5295] See **upper brachial plexus palsy, cadet palsy**.

Riegel, Wilhelm (fl. 1900) German neurologist and ophthalmologist, practicing in Nuremberg.

Riegel symptom (sprung pupil) Alternating constriction and dilation of one pupil with retained light and accommodative reactions between the episodes of dilatation.[5296]

Rieger syndrome A dominantly inherited congenital dysmorphic syndrome manifesting also myotonic dystrophy, iris dysplasia, glaucoma, corneal opacities, optic atrophy, and dental anomalies.[5297]

rifle-sling palsy A form of compression neuropathy of the radial nerve at the level of the axilla.

right eye closure Excessive closure of the right eye ipsilateral to the side of a middle cerebral artery infarct, with slight closure of the left also. The pathogenesis is not known.

righting reflexes Coordinated synergistic patterns of muscle contraction triggered by visual, vestibular, tactile, and proprioceptive stimuli, and designed to bring the head and the body into an upright position in order to facilitate stance and locomotion.[2750]

Such postural reflexes, normally appearing in defined order during the first year of life, are lost or suppressed in spastic states. They include the following:

1. *Neck righting reflex*: Turning of the head to one side is followed by body movements. This is present at birth and maximal by 3 months of age.
2. *Labyrinthine righting reflex*: Extension of the neck of the infant suspended prone, or flexion of the neck in the supine infant. This is present at 2 months and is maximal at 10 months of age.
3. *Body righting reflex*: A modification of the neck righting reflex, appearing at 7–12 months of age.[3080]

rigid spine syndrome A relatively benign, nonprogressive myopathy due to a deficiency of selenoprotein N, an endoplasmic reticulum protein of unknown function, affecting children who show marked limitation of flexion (and later extension) of the cervical and dorsolumbar spine due to myopathic shortening of the spinal extensor muscles. Less important signs include mild and nonprogressive proximal muscle weakness, flexion contractures, waddling gait, scoliosis, and a reduction in subcutaneous fat.[6503] Nocturnal hypoventilation is a dangerous complication recorded in some cases. EMG shows myopathic changes and serum CK levels are moderately raised.

A type 1 fiber myopathy is usually the basis of the syndrome, but that it represents a single pathological entity is unlikely. It was described first by Dubowitz in 1965.[1730] The same phenotype occurs in **nemaline myopathy, Emery–Dreifuss syndrome, acid maltase deficiency**, and **Bethlem myopathy**, and in a late-onset myopathy with spinal extensor contractures, seen in adults. It may also be included under the heading of **arthrogryposis**. See also **congenital muscular dystrophy**.

Variants include the following:

Congenital muscular dystrophy with early spine rigidity type 1 (1p35–p36; selenoprotein N, 1 [SEPN1]): The prototypical recessive syndrome presenting in infancy with symmetrical neck, face, and proximal and distal weakness, axial hypotonia, poor head control, and possible ventilatory impairment. Spinal rigidity starts in early childhood with limited neck and spinal flexion and scoliosis. Contractures occur at the elbow, hip, ankles, and knees. The serum CK is normal. Muscle biopsy shows minicores, loss of mitochondria, and type 1 fiber predominance. The condition has features in common with **minicore congenital myopathy, congenital myopathy with desmin inclusions,** and **congenital fiber type size disproportion**. Ambulation is usually maintained into adulthood unless there develops a severe progressive scoliosis that cannot be treated surgically.[4555, 4992]

An *autosomal recessive neurogenic* form with facioscapuloperoneal atrophy.[4874]

A *recessively inherited* form, characterized by the onset of symptoms in childhood as in the usual form, and by the presence of autophagic vacuoles, muscle spindle swelling, and type 1 fiber predominance in muscle biopsy specimens.[3920]

Congenital muscular dystrophy with muscle hypertrophy (19q13.3; *fukutin-related protein)*: A recessive form allelic with **limb girdle muscular dystrophy** 2I, presenting in early infancy with hypotonia, reduced movement and activity, and diffuse weakness. Most muscles are wasted but calf hypertrophy is usual. Contractures develop occasionally at the knees, ankles, elbows, and spine. Serum CK levels are very high and the EMG is myopathic. Muscle biopsy shows varied fiber size and there is a reduction in laminins and α-dystroglycan.[4992]

A form which is not benign, characterized by pronounced weakness of the vertebral column and limb girdles, severe respiratory muscle weakness, including weakness of the diaphragm, para-spinal wasting, and diffuse proximal weakness, which are accompanied by a myopathic appearance on EMG. Muscle biopsy specimens show inclusions similar to those seen in mitochondrial myopathy, with marked variability in appearance and fiber size.[6828]

Congenital muscular dystrophy with respiratory failure and muscle hypertrophy (1q42): A recessive form with generalized weakness with delayed motor milestones, but severe diaphragmatic involvement leading to respiratory failure. Generalized muscle hypertrophy is an unusual but occasional feature. Contractures are seen at the ankles and there is spinal rigidity in many cases. The serum CK levels are very high. Muscle biopsy shows dystrophic changes.[4992]

A *lethal, dominantly inherited* variety, otherwise clinically similar to the preceding form.[5061]

Familial mixed congenital myopathy with rigid spine phenotype: An autosomal dominant form characterized by the early onset of a slowly progressive myopathy and rigid spine syndrome and pathologically by cytoplasmic bodies, tubulofilamentous inclusions, increased desmin storage, and microscopic features of reducing body myopathy.[5240]

A listing and further descriptions of rigid syndromes are to be found at Dr. Alan

Pestronk's Web site: http://neuromuscular.wustl.edu/msys/contract.html#rigid/.

rigidity (from Lat, stiff) Increased involuntary resistance to passive stretching of muscles throughout the range of movement. Three major types are described: *plasticity*, in which the degree of resistance is constant and does not change throughout the range of movement tested; *cogwheel rigidity*, in which a ratchet-like sensation is transmitted to the examiner's hand; and *paratonia* (**gegenhalten**), in which the resistance increases in proportion to the stretching force applied.

From the viewpoint of electrodiagnosis, rigidity is defined as a velocity independent increase in muscle tone and stiffness with full range of joint motion as interpreted by the examiner. It is often associated with simultaneous low-grade contraction of agonist and antagonist muscles. Like muscle spasticity, the involuntary motor unit action potential activity increases with activity or passive stretch, but it does not seem to change with the velocity of stretch and, on passive stretch, the increased tone has a "lead pipe" or constant quality. It is a cardinal feature of central nervous system disorders affecting the basal ganglia. (Adapted from the 2001 Report of the Nomenclature Committee of the American Association of Electromyography and Electrodiagnosis.[19] Reproduced by kind permission of the AANEM)

rigor (Lat, stiffness. Gr, shuddering) Both meanings of the term are in use today, the Latin for continuous stiffness (**rigor mortis**) and the Greek for intermittent contractions, as with a rigors as part of a febrile illness.

Riley–Day syndrome (familial dysautonomia) A recessively inherited syndrome of sensory neuropathy with autonomic dysfunction, seen mainly in Jewish children. It is mapped to 9q31–33. The main clinical features are lack of tearing, blotchy red skin marks, postural hypotension, febrile episodes, hyperhidrosis, indifference to pain as a result of the somatic sensory neuropathy, ageusia, lack of tongue papillae, and speech disorder. Few patients survive beyond adolescence.[5303]

Nerve biopsy specimens show marked reduction in the number of unmyelinated fibers, and of large myelinated fibers above 12 μM.[69] See **hereditary sensory and autonomic neuropathy**, type 3.

Riley–Schwachman syndrome A syndrome of abnormal gait, pyramidal signs in the legs, easy fatigue, anorexia with emaciation, and symmetrical areas of increased density and dilatation of the bony shafts of the long bones with lucencies seen on X-ray films.[5304]

Riley–Smith syndrome A dominantly inherited syndrome of congenital macrocephaly, pseudopapilledema with normal vision, and multiple subcutaneous angiomata.[5306]

rimmed vacuoles Nonstorage autophagic cytoplasmic vacuoles exhibiting lipid and granular staining in their periphery and surrounded by filaments. Though characteristic of the **familial periodic paralyses**, they are also found in the settings of inclusion-body myositis, oculopharyngeal dystrophy, distal myopathy, and neurogenic muscle atrophies.[1452]

RIND See **reversible ischemic neurologic deficit**.

ring chromosome 20 syndrome A syndrome presenting with a confusional state (nonconvulsive status epilepticus) or refractory seizures lasting minutes to hours with abnormal EEG findings (bilateral slow waves with occasional spikes), mapped variously to 20p.13q3, p13q.13p, and p13q13.33.[5109]

ring scotoma A scotoma that encircles the central part of the visual field. This is most commonly seen in glaucoma and in pigmentary retinal degenerations, but may also be produced by the wearing of strong positive lenses.

ring scotoma with nasal step A ring scotoma formed by the fusion of arcuate defects that do not join perfectly at the equator, giving rise to the "step" on the nasal side of the disk.

ringebinden See **ringed fibers**.

ringed fibers (ringebinden, rinngbande) Striated myofibrils surrounded by an aberrant spiral of cross-striated myofibrils ("spiral annulets"), which in cross-section appear as a circle. They are found most commonly in muscles containing sarcoplasmic masses (e.g., **myotonic dystrophy**), but also in normal muscles.[600]

Rinne Test A bedside hearing test comparing air and bone conduction. A vibrating tuning fork (512 Hz) is held first with its foot on the mastoid process and, when the subject can no longer hear the humming, beside the ear. Normally, the subject hears the ringing more loudly when the fork is in the second of these positions (air better than bone conduction). In patients with middle ear (conductive) deafness, the sound is heard more loudly when the fork is applied to the mastoid process (so that bone is better than air conduction).

The test was described by H.A. Rinne (1819–1868), a German otolaryngologist. See also **Weber** and **Schwabach tests**.

rinngbande See **ringed fibers**.

Rio-Hortega, Pio del Spanish histologist, remembered for his stains for microglia, oligodendroglia, and nerves.

Rio-Hortega stain A glial metallic implant method using ammoniacal silver nitrate and formalin, of particular value in demonstrating astrocytes, oligodendroglia, and microglia.

Rip van Winkle syndrome The process of adaptation to major environmental change that has occurred during the subject's prolonged absence from his familiar surroundings. Refuge from that environment obtained by sleeping is a prominent feature. In the story of Washington Irving, van Winkle slept for 20 years; many patients discharged from long-term care institutions into a "caring" environment have been away longer than that, but difficulty in adaptation to home and to work with subsequent depression is also described in young patients discharged after only a few months in hospital.[5112]

A similar syndrome of hypersomnia may be familial, and is also a feature in some patients after stroke.

rippling muscle disease (OMIM 606072) A rare dominantly inherited or sporadic disorder of muscle due in some cases to a mutation at chromosome 1q41, presenting with painful muscle stiffness and cramps, mainly in the legs and worse with exercise, slowly-moving self-propagating ("rippling") contractions of these muscles in response to stretch, and painful mounding of muscles after percussion, resembling **myotonia** except for the absence of accompanying electrical discharges.[5290, 951] Serum CK levels are raised. The phenomenon may evidence stretch-activated channels in human skeletal muscle. Various mutations in the *CAV3* gene have been described.

A variant is *sporadic rippling muscle syndrome*, which is basically the same syndrome associated with thymoma and myasthenia gravis. A *caveolin-3* mutation has been detected in one case, but an immune-mediated disruption of caveolar function has been suggested as exacerbated by exposure to statins.

RISA cisternography The injection of radio-iodinated serum albumin (RISA) into the lumbar subarachnoid space, with serial scintillation scanning of the spine and cranium in order to determine the rate and pattern of CSF flow.[1622]

RISA ventriculography The injection of radio-iodinated serum albumin into the lateral ventricles, with serial scintillation scanning of the cranium in order to determine the rate and pattern of CSF flow.[1622] Many false-positive and false-negative results have led to uncertainty about the value of the test in the diagnosis of **normal-pressure hydrocephalus**.

rise time The interval from the onset of a change in polarity of a potential to its peak.

risus sardonicus Spasm of the facial muscles as in tetanus, drawing the mouth open, narrowing the palpebral fissures, and elevating the eyebrows, and thus giving the appearance of a forced smile. "A sneering grin was thought of old to resemble the effect of Sardinian ranunculus, which on being chewed, contorted the face of the eater."[6819]

Ritchie Russell, W. (1903–1980) English neurologist, professor of clinical neurology at the University of Oxford. His most respected research work was that on craniocerebral trauma, performed at the military head injury center situated in Oxford during and after World War II, and on the management of **poliomyelitis**. He was also a teacher who built up the Oxford neurological school to a position of eminence, and he served as editor of the *Journal of Neurology, Neurosurgery and Psychiatry*.

ritualistic movements Patterned movement sequences, commonly slow, squirming hand movements frequently accompanied by a blank stare and withdrawal of the child from any interaction with the environment. The ritual can, however, be interrupted by stimulation and the condition is not epileptic in origin. It is seldom seen outside the age range of 2–4 years.

river blindness See **onchocerciasis**.

Rivermead Activities of Daily Living Scale An instrument for the assessment of residual functions in patients after stroke. Sixteen items to do with self-care (e.g., shaving, washing, and combing hair) and 15 household activities (e.g., making a hot drink or a snack, making a bed, vacuuming) are scored.[3851]

Rivermead Behavioral Memory Test An instrument for assessing nonverbal memory.[6810]

Rivermead Mobility index A scale assessing overall mobility within the context of any neurological disorder such as stroke or **multiple sclerosis**. The patient is asked the questions, listed in Chart R–6 and the responses are scored.[1250]

Chart R–6. The Rivermead Mobility Index

1. Turning over in bed: Do you turn over from your back to your side without help?
2. Lying to sitting: From lying in bed, do you get up to sit on the edge of the bed on your own?
3. Sitting balance: Do you sit on the edge of the bed without holding on for 10 s?
4. Sitting to standing: Do you stand up (from any chair) in less than 15 s and stand there for 15 s (using hands and with an aid if necessary)?
5. Standing supported: Observe the patient standing for 10 s without any aid.
6. Transfer: Do you manage to move from the bed to the chair and back without any help?
7. Walking inside, with an aid if needed: Do you walk 10 m with an aid if necessary, but with no standby help?
8. Stairs: Do you manage a flight of stairs without help?
9. Walking outside (even ground): Do you walk around outside on the sidewalk without help?
10. Walking inside, with no aid: Do you walk 10 m inside, with no walker, splint, or aid and without standby help?
11. Picking off floor: If you drop something on the floor, do you manage to walk 5 m, pick it up and then walk back?
12. Walking outside (uneven ground): Do you walk over uneven ground (grass, gravel, snow, ice, etc.) without help?
13. Bathing: Do you get in and out of the bath or shower unsupervised, and can you wash yourself?
14. Up and down four steps: Do you manage to go up and down four steps with no rail, using an aid if necessary?
15. Running: Can you run 10 m without limping in 4 s? (A fast walk is acceptable.)

A score of 1 is given for each "yes" answer.

From Collen FM. Rivermead Mobility Index. Int Disabil Stud 1991;13:50–54. The ethical status of the center is gratefully recognized in its permission to all to access its productions freely.

Rivermead Motor Assessment An instrument for assessing motor function in patients who have suffered stroke. Gross motor function, leg and trunk movements, and arm functions are rated after clinical enquiry and physical examination.[3849]

Rivers, William Halse (1864–1922) English physician who experimentally sectioned a peripheral nerve of Henry **Head** (at Sir Henry's request).[5323]

Roaf sign Tilting of the neck, a posture adopted by patients with a spinal cord injury complicated by root avulsion.[5326]

Robb, James Preston (1914–2004) Professor of neurology and neurologist-in-chief at the Montreal Neurological Hospital, Quebec, Canada. One of his ancestors was Thayendanegea (Joseph Brant), the Mohawk chief who commanded the Iroquois forces allied with the British in the American Revolutionary War. He was and remains an iconic figure in Canadian neurology on account of his humanitarian, administrative, clinical, and research activities, the latter mainly in the fields of epilepsy and cerebral palsy.

Roberts syndrome

(pseudothalidomide syndrome) A congenital dysmorphic syndrome characterized by short stature, sparse depigmented hair, dysplastic ears, hypertelorism, proptosis, cloudy corneas, cataract, blue sclerae, facial hemangiomas, cleft lip and palate, congenital heart disease, multiple renal cysts, digital deformities, syndactyly, hypoplastic thumbs, microcephaly, encephalocele, cranial meningocele, hydrocephalus and mental and developmental delay.[381] See **cleft lip–palate and tetraphocomelia**.

Robertson, D.M.C.L.A. See Argyll Robertson.

Robin, Charles (1821–1885) French histologist who described the perivascular lymphatic spaces in 1868. **Virchow** demonstrated that, in the brain, these contained CSF. They are now known as **Virchow–Robin spaces**.

Robin, Pierre See Pierre Robin.

Robinson ectodermal dysplasia

A dominantly inherited congenital dysmorphic syndrome manifesting also dental anomalies, hypoplastic nails, and sensorineural deafness.[5340]

robotic speech A disorder of enunciation in which the syllables are separated, slowing the flow. It resembles the "scanning" speech described in patients with cerebellar disease.[2373]

ROCA syndrome A developmental anomaly manifesting Retardation of growth and development, Ocular ptosis, Congenital heart disease, and Anal atresia.[4992]

Rochon–Duvigneau syndrome

Dysfunction of cranial nerves III, IV, VI and the first division of cranial nerve V, with blindness, exophthalmos, and some vegetative disturbances, as a result of a tumor in the superior orbital fissure.

Nevertheless, Rochon–Duvigneau described this syndrome in patients with syphilis.[5344] See **superior orbital fissure syndrome**.

Rocky mountain spotted fever

A rickettsial infection with a tick vector, most commonly found in northern California and the eastern parts of the United States. The clinical disease is seasonal, with maximum incidence in the spring and summer, and is the result of widespread vasculitis. Clinically, fever, chills, headaches, myalgia, conjunctival injection, photophobia, skin rash and features of encephalitis with delirium, convulsions, focal neurological deficits, and coma may occur, and in many cases some of these features persist after recovery. The Weil–Felix reaction shows agglutination of strains OX 19 and OX 2, but the specific diagnosis can be made using complement fixation tests.[4368]

rod bodies Tetragonal filaments in structural continuity with thin filaments, detected within muscle fiber sarcoplasm, which originate from the Z-disk and in which the periodic lines are perpendicular and parallel to the long axis.[1864] They are seen in **nemaline myopathy, polymyositis**, and certain forms of **limb-girdle muscular dystrophy**.

rod body myopathy See **nemaline myopathy**.

rod monochromatism See **cone dystrophy**.

rod-cone dystrophy See **retinitis pigmentosa**.

Rodiet–Cans sign Corneal anesthesia occurring in chronic alcoholic patients.[5347]

Roger sign Numbness of the chin. See **numb chin syndrome**.[4149]

Rolandic seizures See **benign childhood epilepsy with centrotemporal spikes** and *variants*.

Rolandic spikes See **central-midtemporal spikes**.

Rolandic vein occlusion (Merwarth syndrome) A progressive pyramidal syndrome primarily affecting the leg, due to occlusion of this cortical vein.[4328]

Rolando, Luigi (1773–1831) Italian professor of anatomy in Sardinia and later at Turin, who first described the substantia gelatinosa, the central sulcus, or fissure in 1825 (named for him by Leurat in 1839), and the motor area lying anterior to it. However, the ascription of his name to the latter structures was in error, Leurat being unaware of their earlier description by **Vicq d'Azir**. Following animal experiments, Rolando also demonstrated the homolateral motor functions of the cerebellum in humans, in 1809.

benign focal epilepsy with centrotemporal spikes, popularly known as *Rolandic epilepsy*, is named for the anatomy, not the anatomist.[6500]

Rolex sign The effect of hypokinesia upon self-winding watches, leading to the complaint that the watch does not keep proper time. This is of occasional value in the diagnosis of early **Parkinson disease**. Presumably any supervening tremor should lead to correction of this problem.

roller coaster headache Head pain due to the generation of a chronic subdural hematoma by the gravitational stresses imposed when riding giant roller coasters.[2019] Dissection of the internal carotid or vertebral arteries represents another complication of this pursuit of temporary freedom from gravity.

rollers See **dancing mania**.

Rollet syndrome (orbital apex syndrome, Tolosa–Hunt syndrome) See **superior orbital fissure syndrome**.[5361]

rolling arm test See **forearm rolling test**.

Romano–Ward syndrome See **familial Q-T prolongation syndrome**.

Romberg, Moritz Heinrich

(1795–1873) German physician who trained in Berlin and Vienna and was later professor at the University of Berlin. He translated the works of **Bell** into German and was himself the author of the first textbook emphasizing neurological symptoms and signs (*Lehrbuch der Nervenkrankheiten des menschen,* 1840–1846), but in it classified all conditions as neuroses of sensibility or motility, a system that has not stood the test of time. Although he named **tabes dorsalis** and gave a good description of achondroplasia (in his graduation thesis), the

Argyll Robertson pupil, **facial hemiatrophy**, **cluster headache**, and numerous other disease states well recognized today, he is best remembered for his test of conscious proprioception (see **Romberg Test**). Romberg was indeed one of the first to emphasize the value of the physical examination in neurology.

The correct spelling of his surname (without an "h") is a neurological shibboleth.

Romberg disease See **Parry–Romberg syndrome**.

Romberg spasm A form of masticatory spasm of unknown cause, probably dystonic.

Romberg syndrome A syndrome that is usually sporadic, comprising facial hemiatrophy with onset in childhood, contralateral focal sensory or motor seizures, trigeminal neuralgia, and changes in the eyes and hair.[5367] See **Parry–Romberg syndrome**.

Romberg sign (test) A test of conscious proprioception, wherein the patient stands and the amount of body sway is compared when his/her eyes are open to that which occurs when they are closed. Increased sway or unsteadiness actually amounting to a tendency to fall when the eyes are closed rather than open indicates proprioceptive failure. Gross swaying *without* falling frequently has a psychogenic basis.

Romberg published his accounts of the sign in his *Lehrbuch der Nerven-Krankheiten des Menschen* between 1840 and 1846, considering it diagnostic of tabes dorsalis.[5369] The origination of the sign has been reviewed.[3695]

Rommen syndrome A congenital dysmorphic syndrome also characterized by short stature, Fallot tetralogy, thyroglossal cyst, skeletal deformities, seizures, brachycephaly, microcephaly, plagiocephaly, and mental and developmental delay.[381]

room tilt illusion The transient perception of a 90° shift in the environment following vestibular stimulation in subjects with skew deviations due to brainstem lesions.[6322]

Roos Test The patient is asked to raise the arms into the "stick-up" position, causing abduction and external rotation at the shoulder, and to open and close the hands repeatedly. Pallor and lack of pulsations in the limb suggests the presence of a vascular **thoracic outlet syndrome**. Pain and numbness in C8 distribution may accompany the vascular signs.[3855]

root lesions Lesions that impinge upon the spinal nerve roots, leading to either sensory or motor features. Prolapsed intervertebral disks and tumors are the more common examples. See **radiculopathy**.

rooting reflex (search reflex) Exploration of the mother's skin by the normal full-term baby's mouth in an effort to locate the nipple, stimulated by the touch of her skin on the baby's cheek or lips; a developmental reflex.[4939] Similarly, touching the cheek of the infant with the tip of the index finger induces opening of the mouth and turning of it toward the stimulus.[6898]

The reflex appears at 30 weeks' gestation and normally disappears at 1 year of age. See also **developmental reflexes**.

Roque sign Left pupillary dilatation and mild proptosis in association with aneurysmal dilation of the aorta. This, the opposite of **Horner syndrome**, may have been what **Pourfour Du Petit** described; it is presumably due to irritation of the sympathetic chain.

Rosai–Dorfman disease (sinus histiocytosis with massive lymphadenopathy) A histiocytic proliferative disorder usually presenting in adults with massive cervical lymphadenopathy but capable of invading, skin, sinuses, and many other sites including the intracranial and intraspinal compartments.[5008] Laboratory abnormalities include hypergammaglobulinemia and a raised ESR. Rare cases present with seizures, cord compression, or focal motor deficits and show leptomeningeal enhancement on MRI.[2174]

Rose disease (Rose–Villar syndrome, Janin tetanus, Klemm tetanus) Tetanus confined to the muscles of the head following a head wound, manifesting spasmodic dysphagia and facial paresis. It carries a prognosis even more deadly than other forms of tetanus.[5391] See **cephalic tetanus**.

Rose tetanus See **cephalic tetanus**.

Rose–Villar syndrome See **cephalic tetanus**.

Rosen neuralgia Tic-like neuralgic pain in the territory of the chorda tympani; a variant of **glossopharyngeal neuralgia**.[5394]

Rosen Scale A modification of the **Hachinski Scale**, shortened without apparent loss of reliability, which scores only the following: abrupt onset, stepwise deterioration, history of stroke, focal neurological signs, emotional incontinence, and somatic complaints.[5397]

Rosenbach, Ottomar (1851–1907) Silesian physician who trained at Berlin. After graduation he worked with Nothnagel and then practiced in Breslau, eventually as professor, until induced to go to Berlin. He analyzed the abdominal reflexes in 1876.

Rosenbach sign 1. Fine tremor of the gently closed eyelids in the presence of dysthyroid ophthalmopathy. 2. Absence of the abdominal reflexes on the side of a hemiparesis[5398] and also in the presence of acute abdominal disease.

Rosenberg–Bertstrom disease A dominantly inherited condition manifesting ataxia, deafness, renal insufficiency, and hyperuricemia.[5400]

Rosenberg–Chutorian syndrome A recessively inherited condition with onset in infancy or childhood, manifesting optic atrophy, **hereditary motor and sensory neuropathy**, and progressive nerve deafness.[5408]

Rosenthal, Curt (fl. 1930) German neuropsychiatrist at the University of Breslau. He described **sleep paralysis** in 1927, but noted that earlier reports of the same condition were known since 1903; his paper called attention to the overwhelming fear that may attend this experience.

Rosenthal–Melkersson syndrome See **Melkersson–Rosenthal syndrome**.

Rosenthal syndrome (Munzer–Rosenthal syndrome, cataleptic hallucinatory fear syndrome) See **sleep paralysis**.

Rosenthal fibers Cylindrical, hyaline astrocytic processes staining with acid dyes, found in areas of fibrillary gliosis, diffusely in the brain in **Alexander disease** and in the more indolent gliomas and ependymomas such as pilocytic astrocytomas or ependymomas.[6] See also **palatal myoclonus**.

Ross syndrome A progressive and complex disorder of thermoregulation that may be hard to differentiate from the probably pathogenetically related **Holmes–Adie syndrome** and manifesting a combination of the tonic (**Adie**) pupil, areflexia, and segmental hypohidrosis, leading to fever, tachycardia, tachypnea, and even exhaustion (heat stroke) when the patient gets very hot.[5416] The autonomic dysfunction may, however, be more widespread than this description suggests. Areflexia and tonic pupil are also rescribed as features.[4690]

This benign syndrome of cranial postganglionic parasympathetic and sympathetic dysfunction in association with more widespread autonomic failure does not usually carry severe clinical consequences.[4689] See also **Harlequin syndrome**.

A *variant* is *Ross syndrome plus*, in which there is also a **Horner syndrome**.[5805]

Rossolimo, Grigoryi Ivanovitch (1860–1928) Russian physician, who described "myotonia atrophica" in 1902,[5423] 7 years before Steinert, whose name has been given to the disease.

Rossolimo reflex 1. (Rossolimo–Goldflam reflex) See **plantar muscle reflex**. 2. The **anal reflex**. 3. (Rossolimo reflex of the hand) Percussion of the volar aspect of the flexed fingers leads to further flexion of the fingers and supination of the forearm in patients with pyramidal lesions affecting the arm.[1500]

Rossolimo–Goldflam reflex See **plantar muscle reflex**.

rostral basilar artery syndrome Rostral brainstem, diencephalic, and posterior hemisphere dysfunction as a result of vascular occlusive disease of the rostral basilar artery. Numerous named and unnamed syndromes may result; **Déjèrine–Roussy, Benedikt**, and **Weber syndromes** for example. Clinically, thalamic amnesia, visual field defects, limb anesthesia or dysesthesias, and a variety of motor signs affecting the face and arm more than the leg are all examples. An acute confusional state initially seems to be an invariable accompaniment. In many such cases the clinical features are reversible.

Subcortical aphasia, hemiballism, acute amnestic syndromes; Balint syndrome; hemispatial neglect; hemispatial agnosia; internuclear ophthalmoplegia; visual associative agnosia; color agnosia, anosognosia; dysorthographia, topographic agnosia, peduncular hallucinosis; vertical gaze paresis; delirium; and **preangular alexia** are other syndromes described.[4283]

rostral dominance Of two touches simultaneously applied to the face and the hand, it is the former that is normally more likely to be perceived in normal people but particularly in those with contralateral hemispheric disease.

rota- (Lat, Wheel)

rotary nystagmus See **torsional nystagmus**.

rotary pursuit A motor learning task in which the subject's ability to apply a stylus continually to a rotating target is measured in the two hands successively.[1285] See **pursuit rotor test**.

rotation test A method for assessing the side of a diseased labyrinth; the patient, who is seated on a revolving chair, is rotated 10 times in 20 s with the head bent forward at 30°; the nystagmus that results is assessed after such rotations in each direction. It is greater in severity and duration when the rotation occurs in the direction of the affected side.

rotational nystagmus (perrotational response, postrotational response) A physiological form of horizontal jerk nystagmus of the peripheral vestibular type induced by endolymphatic movement as a result of rotatory acceleration of the subject, which causes asymmetrical stimulation of the labyrinths. During the rotation, the fast phase of the nystagmus is in the direction of rotation; after rotation ceases, the fast phase is in the opposite direction.[5] See also **vestibular nystagmus**.

rotational vertebral artery syndrome (bow hunters syndrome) The occurrence of vertigo and downbeat/rotational nystagmus several seconds after head rotation to one side, usually in association with hypoplasia or stenosis of one vertebral artery and compression or occlusion of the dominant artery at the atlantoaxial junction while the head is turned to the other side.

This is usually associated caused by mechanical compression from degenerative changes, especially at the atlanto-axial level. The leading symptom is rotational vertigo with downbeat torsional and horizontal-beating nystagmus.[1157]

rotatory nystagmus That form of nystagmus with a torsional component about the anteroposterior axis of the eye. It is usually due to brainstem lesions but may be congenital. See **torsional nystagmus**.

rotatory seizures (circular, volvular, or gyratory seizures) Generalized or partial seizures during which the subject turns around one or more times. The direction of turning has no localizing value.[5505]

Roth spots Pale areas representing organized leukocytes and fibrin following hemorrhage in the retina, as in bacterial endocarditis, described by M. Roth (1839–1914), a Swiss pathologist in Basel. See **white-centered retinal hemorrhages**.

Roth, Vladimir K. (Rot, V.K.) (1848–1916) Russian neurologist, a pupil of **Korsakoff**.

Roth–Bernhardt disease See **meralgia paresthetica**.

Roth–Bielschowsky syndrome (pseudo-ophthalmoplegia) Paralysis of conjugate gaze in one direction, but with retention of the slow phase of conjugate deviation on caloric testing. This is evidence of a supratentorial lesion affecting the pathways for conjugate gaze in the tectum.[1222]

Rothmund–Thompson syndrome See **poikiloderma congenitale**.

Roussy, Gustave (1874–1948) Swiss-French neuropathologist who trained

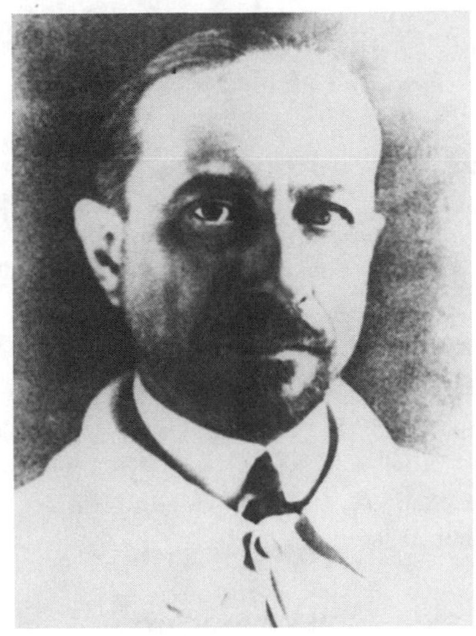

Figure R–6 Gustave Roussy

in Geneva and Paris, and became professor of pathological anatomy at the University of Paris and later dean of the faculty and Rector there. He published on the thalamic syndrome bearing his name and that of **Déjèrine** (to whom he was assistant) while he was still an intern, and wrote also on the topics of hypothalamic lesions, syringomyelia, and other spinal lesions, as well as neurophysiology. The other syndromes to which his name is attached are shown in the next two entries.

Roussy–Cornil syndrome (progressive, nonfamilial hypertrophic neuritis) A demyelinating sensorimotor peripheral neuropathy with onset usually after the third decade, affecting the upper limbs more than the lower. Sensory ataxia, lancinating pains, generalized areflexia, and intention tremor may also be evident.[5438]

This condition resembles **hereditary motor and sensory neuropathy**, for example of type 3, but has its onset in adult life and is sporadic.

Roussy–Levy syndrome (hereditary areflexic dystasia; OMIM 180800) A dominantly inherited condition associated with partial duplication at chromosome 17p11.2 and related to the spinocerebellar degenerations. It is manifested as a delay in walking with pes cavus, sensory, and gait ataxia, areflexia, awkward movements, and a mild cerebellar intention tremor without nystagmus, present from infancy. Kyphoscoliosis, sensory changes, extensor plantar response, and typical cerebellar signs are absent.

The presence of pyramidal signs was hinted at, but Roussy and Levy did not describe the pathology in their original paper in 1926.[5439] The syndrome may represent a combination of **hereditary motor and sensory neuropathy** (HMSN) and **benign essential tremor**; however, tremor was only a minor feature of two of the seven cases initially reported, though manual dexterity was generally poor. Confusion with **Friedreich ataxia** is less likely when it is recalled that the latter is inherited in an autosomal recessive manner, so that most patients have no affected relative (but a few HMSN type 1 kinships also show recessive inheritance). See **hereditary motor and sensory neuropathy**, type 1.[291]

Rowland Universal Dementia Assessment Scale A screening test for dementia developed in a multicultural setting that contains six items assessing body orientation, praxis, drawing, judgment, memory, and language.[6081]

Rowland–Payne syndrome The association of recurrent laryngeal and sympathetic nerve palsies due to their compression by lymph nodes in the neck at the level of C6.

Royal Free disease See **chronic fatigue syndrome**, **postinfection fatigue syndrome**.

R-R interval variation A measure of vagal influences upon the heart, derived from continuous electrocardiographic recordings obtained during deep breathing or with the Valsalva maneuver. With deep breathing, the variation between the maximal and minimal heart rate is normally 15 beats per minute or more; 10 beats per minute or less is definitely abnormal. With the Valsalva maneuver, the normal ratio is 1.21 or more and less than 1.20 is abnormal.[1936] See **autonomic function tests**.

RSD See **reflex sympathetic dystrophy**.

rub epilepsy A form of reflex epilepsy induced by prolonged or repetitive stimulation of the skin or (as with tooth-brushing) of mucosal surfaces. The site of excitation is usually on the left side and leads to a sensory Jacksonian march of symptoms starting at the site stimulated, but a motor march may occur with tooth-brushing. The phenomenon is considered to reflect the effect of propagation of epileptic discharges from the post-central to the supplementary motor area.[3284]

rubbing nose sign The tendency of subjects with frontal lobe tumors to rub the nose repeatedly. The same phenomenon may occur in those with temporal lobe neoplasms, and in those with caudate lesions.

rubeosis iridis Proliferation of new blood vessels on the anterior surface of the iris, leading frequently to glaucoma.

rubi- (Gr, red)

Rubinstein–Taybi syndrome A dysmorphic syndrome of broad, short thumbs and halluces, dwarfism, microcephaly, psychomotor retardation, high-arched palate, refractive error, ptosis, strabismus, antimongolian slant to the eyes, nevus flammeus in half the cases, and unusual susceptibility to chest infections.[5457, 6230] Seizures, callosal agenesis, and pyramidal signs have also been described. See also **microcephaly**.

rubral tremor (red nucleus tremor, Holmes tremor, midbrain or thalamic tremor, myorhythmia) A large-amplitude, rotatory tremor of the limbs or head, present at rest and increased when maintaining a posture and with voluntary movements, with which it interferes. Random movements of the hands and abnormal head postures may be associated. It is thought to occur as a result of damage to the red nucleus. See also **cerebellar tremors**, **midbrain tremor**, **Benedikt syndrome**.

rubrospinal tract (von Monakow bundle) A diffuse network of fibers that descend from the red nucleus, crossing in the anterior tegmental decussation to reach the lower brainstem and upper cervical spinal cord; identified in the dog by von Monakow in 1883, but small to the point of near-disappearance in humans below the cervical level.[4597]

rucksack palsy (trekkers shoulder, Erb palsy, pallbearers palsy, cadet palsy, pack palsy) The syndrome of upper brachial plexus (Erb) palsy brought about by compression from the shoulder straps of a heavy rucksack (or other compressive objects). Clinically, painless weakness, atrophy, depressed reflexes, and sensory loss are found variously in the territories of the suprascapular, axillary, radial, and musculocutaneous nerves. The median nerve is minimally affected and the ulnar nerve is spared.[1468] See **upper brachial plexus palsy**.

Rud syndrome A sporadic **neurocutaneous syndrome** characterized by congenital ichthyosis, hypogonadotropic hypogonadism, dwarfism, mental retardation, deafness, seizures, and polyneuropathy.[5463] Macrocytic anemia, pigmentary retinopathy, arachnodactyly, and muscular atrophy are associated features.[3113, 4132]

rudimentary athetosis Athetosis that can only be detected by its appearance during voluntary movements.

Ruffini, Angelo (1874–1929) Italian anatomist who trained and practiced in the Bologna-Siena-Florence region, settling down as professor of histology in Bologna.

Ruffini corpuscles Deep sensory cutaneous nerve endings, described by Ruffini in 1898.

Ruggeris' sign Tachycardia on attempted adduction of the eyes, in the setting of hyperthyroidism.

Rulandus, Martinus (1582–1602) Bavarian physician and court physician at the Ducal palace; the original descriptor of **benign focal epilepsy with centrotemporal spikes** (confusingly known as **Rolandic seizures**) in 1597.[6500]

rule of the Bs A mnemonic defining the factors requiring the closest attention in patients following a head injury—namely breathing, bleeding, brain, bladder, bowel, and bone.

rules for diplopia 1. The peripheral image is the false image. 2. The separation of images is greatest in the direction of action of the affected muscle(s). 3. The false image is less distinct that the true image.

rum thumb A mnemonic indicating that three nerves, the radial, ulnar, and median, innervate, in order, the abductor pollicis longus, the adductor pollicis, and the abductor pollicis brevis muscles of the thumb.

run See **montage**.

runners' dystonia An adult-onset focal dystonia in the lower limbs occurring during long-distance running. The clinical features overlap with those of more recognizable forms of focal dystonias, including relief with sensory or motor "tricks." The family history is usually negative and the dystonia remains focal. Injury to the affected leg within a year prior to the onset of the dystonia is sometimes recorded.[6882]

runners' headache A form of **benign exertional headache** related to this form of exercise.[3084]

running fits See **epilepsia cursiva**.

runs of rapid spikes See **generalized paroxysmal fast activity**.

rushes A **migraine** *variant* described in children, characterized by subjective distortions of time such that sounds or other perceptions of the environment appear to rush by abnormally fast. This suggests cortical dysfunction occurring as a feature of the aura.[1690] See also **Alice in Wonderland syndrome**.

Russell, Dorothy (1895–1983) Australian pathologist who was trained at Cambridge and the London Hospital where she was appointed as neuropathologist until her retirement, apart from the war years, which she spent in Oxford. Her most lasting work was in neuro-oncology. She characterized the pinealoma as a teratoma, recognized primary CNS lymphoma (to which she gave the name **microgliomatosis**) and published, with Lucien Rubinstein, the landmark *Pathology of Tumours of the Nervous System* (1959), as well as authoring important papers on hydrocephalus, methodologies in neuropathology, etc.

Russell, James Samuel Risien (1863–1939) English physician who with **Batten** and **Collier** described and named **subacute combined degeneration of the cord**[5476] although Dana had already described that condition.

Russell syndrome 1. See **diencephalic syndrome**. 2. (Russell–Batten–Collier syndrome, neuroanemic syndrome). See **subacute combined degeneration of the cord**.

Russell-Batten-Collier syndrome See **subacute combined degeneration of the cord**.

Russell, A. Contemporary English pediatrician.

Russell–Silver syndrome A dominantly inherited syndrome of dwarfism, hemihypertrophy, smallness of the facial bones (pseudohydrocephalus), short stature, and craniofacial dysostosis.[2949] Blue sclerae, facial dysmorphism, asymmetrical arms and legs, clinodactyly, finger clubbing, hypoglycemia, delayed closure of the fontanelles, and delayed skeletal maturation are other features of the condition.

Russell–Silver like syndrome See **Partington syndrome**.

Russian spring-summer encephalitis A direct infection of the brain by a flavivirus member of the togavirus group of arboviruses. The condition occurs epidemically and presents with severe headaches, fever, meningism, and extreme damage to the anterior horns and cranial nerve motor nucleus cells in the cervical cord and bulbar regions.[6858]

Rutledge cerebellar-renal-ocular-limb syndrome A congenital dysmorphic syndrome also characterized by short stature; ocular, cardiac, pulmonary, tracheal, and other visceral abnormalities; rhizomelia of the arms; polydactyly; pes cavus; craniosynostosis; hydrocephalus; and cerebellar atrophy.[381]

Rust phenomenon The use of the hands to support the head, seen in patients with high cervical spinal cord injuries (and with tuberculosis and rheumatoid arthritis). It was described by J.N. Rust (1775–1840), a German surgeon with wide experience in war injuries.[2066]

Ruvalcaba–Myhre–Smith syndrome (macrocephaly-intestinal polyps-genital pigmentation) A congenital dysmorphic syndrome characterized by high birth weight, macrocephaly, myopathic weakness, myotonia, acanthosis nigricans, ocular abnormalities including the presence of visible nerve fibers in the cornea, lobulated tongue, pectus excavatum, gastrointestinal tumors, and genital pigmentation.[5479]

Ruzika syndrome (ichthyosis-deafness-brachydactyly) A congenital dysmorphic syndrome characterized by ichthyosis, sensorineural deafness, myopia, oligodontia, extra ribs, brachydactyly, clinodactyly, thyroid tumors, and mental and developmental delay.[381]

ryanodine receptor A myofibrillar transmission site. *RYR1* mutations are associated with central core disease, multiminicore disease, and malignant hyperthermia.

Rydel–Seuffer tuning fork An instrument vibrating at 64 Hz that provides quantitative outcome measures of vibration sensation.

Ryukyuan muscular atrophy A rare, recessively inherited form of **hereditary motor neuropathy** with onset in early infancy, and characterized by proximal symmetrical muscle atrophy, more severe in the pelvic girdle. Fasciculations, kypho-scoliosis, contractures, and pes cavus are associated. The prognosis for prolonged survival is good.

The condition has been detected only in the residents of the Ryukyuan islands of northern Japan. It has been ascribed to a single mutation occurring before the fourteenth century.[3525]

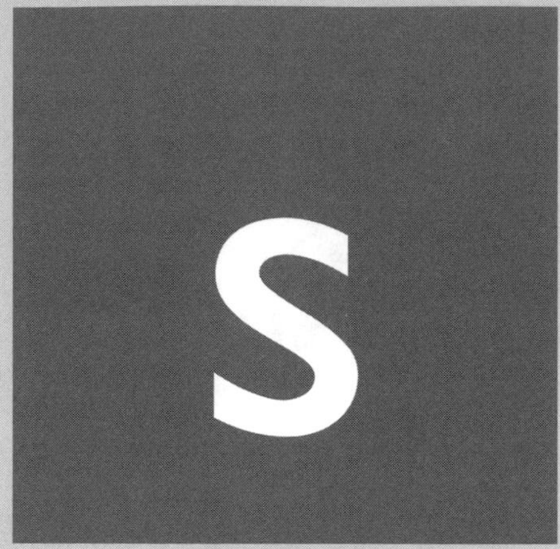

S-100 protein A soluble cytoplasmic protein present almost exclusively in neuroectodermal cells. Stains for this protein are useful in the diagnosis of **Schwannomas** and of metastatic melanocarcinomas.

Sabinas syndrome (tricho-onycho-oligophrenia–Gr, hair + nail + few + mind) A congenital dysmorphic syndrome manifesting brittle hair, dysplastic nails and skin, pigmentary retinal degeneration, and mild mental delay.[230] The condition is named after the Mexican community in which the first cases of the condition were recognized.

Sabin–Feldman syndrome An acquired infection of early childhood, leading to extensive cerebral damage with disseminated calcification, microphthalmia, optic atrophy, and chorioretinitis. The condition resembles toxoplasmosis in every way, except that the serological findings are negative.[4245]

Saccade Velocity Test A method for the rapid, quantitative measurement of saccade amplitude, duration, and velocity using DC electro-oculography. The technique is of particular value in the determination and assessment of subclinical disturbances of eye movement.[365]

saccades (from Fr, a twitch or jerk) Rapid, voluntary eye movements lasting less than 100 ms, including voluntary refixations, the fast components of optokinetic nystagmus, and vestibular nystagmus. They represent the mechanism for turning the eyes rapidly and voluntarily upon a target in any direction. This demands an initial *pulse*, which overcomes the inertia of the eyes and moves them in the required direction, followed by a *step*, which maintains the eyes in the appropriate position now achieved. *Volitional*, *reflexive*, and *spontaneous* types are described.[3762]

With a *normometric* saccade, a single-step refixation occurs because the pulse and the step signals are appropriate for the desired change in fixation. *Hypometric* single-step saccades occur when the pulse portion of the controller signal is too small for the eye to reach the target and it slides to its required new position (**glissade**) as a result of the step signal; thus the eye does not deviate as far as it should in search of the target. *Slow* saccades are hypometric saccades with a very low velocity due to absence of the pulse signal.

Hypermetric saccades are those which overshoot the target as a result of incorrect, dynamic, or glissadic steps as the eye deviates in the direction of the target. The occurrence of two or more dynamic saccadic components underlies *multiple-step dysmetric* saccades.[331]

The word was formerly applied to involuntary jerking movements occurring as part of the act of swallowing. See also **microsaccades, catch-up saccades, corrective catch-up saccades, express saccades**, and the following entries.

saccadic contrapulsion A disorder of ocular movement occurring in patients with cerebellar disease and characterized by saccades which overshoot the target on the opposite side and undershoot it on the same side as the cerebellar lesion.[3762] See also **saccadic lateropulsion**.

saccadic delay Prolongation of the latency of saccadic eye movements; a feature of congenital ocular apraxia and lesions of the visual afferent and central oculomotor systems, the cerebrum, or the basal ganglia at various sites.

saccadic double pulses Intrusions of fixation composed of two back-to-back saccades without any intervening latent period, occurring in normal subjects.

saccadic dysmetria (saccadic overshoot/undershoot) Inaccurate saccades as a result of excessive or inadequate pulses initiating them, respectively. They may be caused by lesions of the cerebellar pathways, the median longitudinal fasciculus, the end plate, or the VI cranial nerve.[6959]

saccadic intrusions Abnormal, brief, inappropriate, and involuntary saccadic eye movements which occur during, and disrupt, normal saccades and thus impair the fixation of an object by the macula. See also **square-wave jerks, square-wave pulses, ocular flutter, opsoclonus, macro square wave jerks, macro saccadic oscillations, saccadic double pulses, saccadic lateropulsion**, and **superior oblique myokymia**.

saccadic ipsipulsion See **saccadic lateropulsion**.

saccadic lateropulsion (ipsipulsion, saccadic ipsipulsion) A dramatic form of saccadic intrusion or oscillation characterized by overshoot of voluntary saccadic movements (hypermetria) toward the side of a medullary lesion, with undershoot (hypometria) in the other direction.[1321]

saccadic nystagmus A sustained conjugate horizontal ocular dyskinesia of moderate amplitude at a frequency of 2–3 Hz, dependent on visual fixation. This is one of many ocular dyskinesias which occur in the presence of brainstem or cerebellar disease.[146] See also **square-wave pulses**.

saccadic oscillations Bursts of high-frequency to-and-fro movements of the eyes, as with **voluntary nystagmus.** See also **square-wave pulses, oscillations**, and **square wave jerks**.

saccadic overshoot/undershoot See **saccadic dysmetria**.

saccadic paralysis (selective saccadic palsy) Inability to trigger saccadic eye movements in a direction away from the side of an acute cerebral lesion or toward the side of a lesion of the pontine tegmentum, due in the latter case to damage to the paramedian pontine reticular formation.

saccadic pulses (abduction nystagmus, ataxic nystagmus, saccadic intrusions, saccadic oscillations, stepless saccades) Intrusions of fixation resulting from burst cell discharges without the usual step. Saccades are off-target and are corrected by a glissade back to the desired point of fixation.[1561] Such brief intrusions that take the eye away from the fixation position with a rapid drift back are reported in patients with **internuclear ophthalmoplegia**.[5731]

saccadomania See **opsoclonus**.

saccharopinuria A defect in the catabolic pathway of lysine, resulting in a clinical syndrome consisting of short stature, mild intellectual impairment, and progressive pyramidal signs. Plasma lysine levels and urinary lysine and saccharopine levels are greatly raised.[1044]

saccular miliary aneurysm See **microaneurysm**.

saccule A statokinetic receptor in the inner ear, responsible for detecting linear displacement of the body.

Sachs, Bernard Parney (1858–1944) German–American pediatric neurologist. After obtaining a BA degree from Harvard, he studied medicine in Strasbourg. Thereafter, he did the usual rounds of European centers (Berlin, Vienna, Paris, London), and then returned to America, eventually becoming professor of medicine and neurological diseases at the New York Polyclinic and a consultant at other New York hospitals. He was at one time the owner of the ***Journal of Mental and Nervous Diseases.***

He is best remembered for his descriptions (first in 1887, and independently of Warren Tay) of the gangliosidosis which has for a century or so been named for them,[5489] which Sachs had recognized during his general practice and for which he suggested the name *amaurotic familial idiocy*. The term *cherry-red spot* was first used by Herman Knapp, a New York ophthalmologist who saw Sachs' patient. Among Sachs' most important publications were *A Treatise of Nervous Diseases of Children* (1895), the first textbook of child neurology in English, and a monograph on normal childhood development.

Sack syndrome The occurrence of cerebrovascular accidents in patients with **Ehlers–Danlos syndrome**, such as those resulting from caroticocavernous fistulas or from vertebral or carotid branch aneurysms.[3458]

sacral agenesis A syndrome characterized by aplasia of the bony structures of the lower spine and sacrum, usually associated with severe motor deficits in the pelvic and leg muscles, mild sensory losses, and visceral anomalies. Besides agenesis of the sacrum, the typical features are absence of the coccyx and aplasia of the lumbar facets and of vertebrae at higher levels.[5551] See **caudal regression syndrome**.

sacral lipomatosis (Schmidt-Voigt syndrome) An entity of doubtful provenance, said to be characterized by the presence of dense palpable lumps in the lumbar and sacral regions of women of early middle age who complain of local pains that are worse with movement. See also **myofascial pain syndromes**.[1765]

sacral sparing The absence of sensory loss in the S2–4 dermatomes in the presence of uni- or bilateral hypesthesia in, for example, L4–5, S1 territory (but no lower). The causal lesion is usually a disk or tumor which compresses the outermost fibers of the cauda equina but spares those from lower cord levels, which are situated more centrally. See also **saddle anesthesia**.

sacralization Fusion of the L5 with the S1 vertebra, thus enlarging the sacrum. This condition may cause subacute low back pain but is often asymptomatic.[2222]

sacralization-scoliosis-sciatica syndrome See **Bertolotti syndrome**.

saddle anesthesia Reduced sensation in the territory of the conus medullaris, which includes the natal cleft and buttocks and the posterior upper thighs. This is classically a sign of damage to the S2–4 segments of the cord or, less often, to those roots after they have left the cord. In clinical terms, the phenomenon represents the reverse of **sacral sparing**.

SADS See **schedule for affective disorders in schizophrenia**.

Saenger sign Return of the lost pupillary light reflex when the patient is placed in a darkened room. It is described as a sign in cerebral syphilis but is not present in **tabes dorsalis**.

Dr. Alfred Saenger (1860–1921) was a German neurologist in Hamburg.[5495, 5704]

Saenger syndrome See **Adie pupil**.

Saethre–Chotzen syndrome A dominantly inherited congenital dysmorphic syndrome manifesting also ptosis, asymmetrical craniosynostosis with plagiocephaly or brachycephaly, syndactyly, and sometimes mental delay.[5497] It is mapped to chromosome 7p. See also **acrocephalosyndactyly** type III; **craniosynostosis**.

safety factor The physiological excess in the amplitude of an electrical stimulus, in the concentration of transmitter in a chemical transmission system or in the extent of the available receptor pool. Thus, in the case of myelinated nerve fibers, the safety factor is the ratio of the current available to stimulate a given node to the minimum current required for that purpose. At the neuromuscular junction, it is the (normally) excessive number of quanta of acetylcholine released by the nerve terminal, such that a reduction in their number is nevertheless able to trigger myofibrillar contraction. It is determined by the difference in postsynaptic depolarization caused by the end-plate potential (EPP) and the depolarization required to activate the voltage-sensitive sodium channels deployed in segments of the postsynaptic membrane that line the depths of the secondary synaptic clefts. The amplitude of the EPP is determined by the amplitude of the miniature EPP and the number of quanta released by nerve impulse.[1862]

sagittal (from Lat, an arrow) The anteroposterior suture of the skull, crossing the coronal suture as an arrow sits upon a bow.

Sahs, Adolph L. (1906–1986) American neurologist, born in Iowa, where he received his medical training and where he practiced for most of his life, becoming chairman of the department of neurology in the University of Iowa in 1948. He was president of both the American Neurological Association and the American Academy of Neurology (of which latter he was a founding member) and as editor further developed *Grinker's Textbook of Neurology*. The most influential research area in which he published was intracranial hemorrhage.

Sakati–Nyhan–Tisdale syndrome (acrocephalopolysyndacytly type 2) A sporadic dysmorphic syndrome characterized by craniosynostosis affecting all of the sutures and leading to turri-brachycephaly. Acrocephalopolysyndactyly, short limbs, congenital heart disease, anomalous ears, alopecia, and atrophic skin are other features described.[4] See **craniosynostosis**.

salaam attacks The term applied by Sir Charles Clarke to the peculiar movements of children with **West syndrome**. In the words of Dr. West, the forward bobbings of his affected infant son's head "become so frequent and powerful as to cause a complete heaving of the head forwards toward his knees, and then immediately relaxing into the upright position . . . these bowings and relaxings would be repeated alternately at intervals of a few seconds and repeated from ten to twenty or more times, for two or three minutes; he sometimes has two, three or more attacks in the day . . . just before they come on he is all alive and in motion, making a strange noise, and then all of a sudden down goes his head and upwards his knees; he then appears frightened and screams out." See also **flexor spasms**.

Saldino–Mainzer syndrome A recessively inherited syndrome characterized by pigmentary retinopathy, ataxia, cone-shaped epiphyses of the digits, and short limbs.[5511]

Salih syndrome A congenital dysmorphic syndrome manifesting also pellagnoid skin lesions, cataract, cerebellar signs, microcephaly, and mental and developmental delay.[381]

Salinas syndrome A congenital dysmorphic syndrome manifesting also clefting of the mandible, face, and palate; acrocephaly; and microcephaly.[381]

Salivo-Sudipar syndrome See **gustatory sweating**.

Salla disease See **sialidosis** (*type 3*).

salmon patch See **nevus flammeus**.

salmonella encephalopathy A syndrome of altered consciousness, cognition, and personality with seizures in which nontyphoidal salmonella species are found in the stool in the absence of other viral or bacterial infections. The condition may be lethal. Clinically it is characterized by diffuse and rapidly progressive brain dysfunction and circulatory failure developing after enteritis in the absence of severe dehydration or sepsis. The CSF pressure is raised and CT scan suggests brain edema.[243] See also **ekiri**.

Salpêtrière (from Fr, Salpêtre; gunpowder) A large hospital in south east Paris, formerly an ammunition storehouse and now a general hospital attached to the Hôpital Pitié. During the nineteenth century its function as a house of asylum for the insane was changed so that it became a neurological as well as a psychiatric hospital, in large measure due to the influence of J.-M. **Charcot** who was appointed to its staff in 1862, later referring to it as "that grand asylum of human misery."

salt and pepper on the face Painful dysesthesias, or stinging or burning sensations due to damage to the quintothalamic tract at its decussation, usually as a result of ischemia.[1015]

salt wasting syndrome Hyponatremia and polyuria with substantial loss of cations, especially sodium, leading to hypovolemia and occurring as a complication of subarachnoid hemorrhage. The condition may result from excessive production of atrial natriuretic peptide, but is not the result of inappropriate ADH secretion.[4540]

saltatory spasm (Lat, a dancer + Gr, spasm) (static reflex spasm) "Applied to a rare form of clonic spasm in the legs which comes on when the patient attempts to stand, and causes springing or jumping movements, whence the name" (Sir William **Gowers**).

As a manifestation of flagrant hysteria, it was first described by Bamberger in 1859[366] but now seems to have died out. See **Bamberger disease**.

San Francisco Syncope rule A template designed to identify those patients who, after experiencing an episode of syncope, are at risk for short-term serious outcomes. It is suggested that the presence of abnormal ECG, a complaint of shortness of breath, hematocrit <30%, systolic blood pressure <90 mmHg, or a history of congestive heart failure has 96% (95% CI 92%–100%) sensitivity and 62% (95% CI 58%–66%) specificity.[5156]

Despite the name, two of the authors and many of the subjects studied were from Ottawa, Canada.

San Francisco syndrome A craniofacial malformation characterized by synostosis affecting the coronal suture, ptosis, midface hypoplasia, bulbous nose, and small ears.[4]

Sanchez–Corona syndrome A congenital dysmorphic syndrome manifesting also abnormalities of the hair, speech defects, scoliosis, cerebellar signs, and mental and developmental delay.[381]

Sanderson syndrome A congenital, dysmorphic syndrome manifesting also abnormalities of the genitalia and hair, microcephaly, and cerebral atrophy.[381]

Sandhoff–Jatkiewicz disease See **GM_2 gangliosidosis**.

Sandifer syndrome (dyspeptic dystonia) A pseudodystonic syndrome presenting with torticollis and neck extension in different directions, occurring in infants and small children as a response to the sensations arising from a hiatal hernia and the accompanying esophagitis during and after feeding. The condition was first recognized by Sandifer but was further described by Kinsbourne and others.[607, 3444, 3754]

Sandifer, Paul (1908–1964) English neurologist who trained at the Middlesex Hospital and then at the **National Hospital**, Queen Square. He practiced at the National and Royal National Orthopedic Hospitals and at the Hospital for Sick Children as a pediatric neurologist. His publications dealt mainly with the *floppy infant* syndrome, **cerebral palsy**, and cerebral degenerative diseases, and he first characterized the **opsoclonus syndrome** (dancing eyes–dancing feet) as well as **Sandifer syndrome**.

SANDO (sensory ataxic neuropathy, dysarthria, and ophthalmparesis) A mitochondrial disorder, presenting with sensory ataxic neuropathy, ophthalmoparesis, and dysarthria. It is recessively inherited and maps to 15q25, and 10q24 (*POLG*).

Sandoz Clinical Assessment Geriatrics Scale (SCAG) A reliable clinician-rated instrument designed to differentiate between early senile deterioration and depression in elderly people and to evaluate the effects of drug treatment on dementia. The scale examines a broad spectrum of cognitive, affective, and behavioral manifestations; the items deal with confusion, impaired mental alertness, impaired recent memory, disorientation, anxiety, depression of mood, emotional lability, irritability, impaired self-care, anxiety, lost motivation, bothersomeness, hostility, fatigue, appetite, responsiveness to the surroundings, sociability, cooperativeness, fatigue, and dizziness and allow an overall impression of the seriousness of the condition to be gained by the rater.[5750]

S-aneurysm See **megadolichobasilar anomaly**.

Sanfilippo disease A, B, C See **mucopolysaccharidoses**.

Sanger Brown (1852–1928) American psychiatrist and neurologist who after his initial training studied the functions of the occipital lobe with Schafer. Returning to Chicago, he eventually became professor of clinical neurology at the College of Physicians and Surgeons there but later went into private practice.[2066]

Sanger Brown ataxia (Brown ataxia) A dominantly inherited hyperreflexic spinocerebellar degeneration with juvenile or adult onset, and with added chorea, dementia, optic atrophy, and ophthalmoplegia. The condition thus resembles some of the olivopontocerebellar ataxias, but it is pathologically heterogeneous. The condition was reported by Sanger Brown in 1892 but is now classified as an **autosomal dominant cerebellar ataxia** of late onset.[2754, 2753]

Santavuori disease See **neuronal ceroid lipofuscinosis** (infantile type),[5543] See **muscle, eye**, and **brain disease**.

Sao Paulo south coast epidemic encephalitis Encephalitis caused by *Rocio flavivirus*, a B arbovirus capable of attacking the gray matter throughout the neuraxis and of producing acute encephalopathy with behavioral disturbances, cerebellar signs, intracranial hypertension, and sometimes coma.[5392]

saphenous neuropathy An uncommon entrapment neuropathy, usually presenting with pain in the distribution of the nerve on the medial aspect of the lower leg, and causing tenderness at the site where the nerve exits from the femoral canal.[6371]

saposin defects Forms of lysosomal storage disease with phenotypes resembling **metachromatic leukodystrophy** or **Gaucher disease** or extant in a more generalized form.[6720]

Sarbo sign Anesthesia in the distribution of the peroneal nerve, once thought specific for **tabes dorsalis** but not so.

sarco- (Gr, flesh) Denotes flesh, hence *sarcoma*, a fleshy tumor. The term is now restricted to describe tumors of connective tissue.

sarcocystis (sarcosporidiosis) Infection by a class of parasites (of the genus *sarcocystis*) acquired from the ingestion of beef or pork, mainly in Malaysia, where infection is common (but usually asymptomatic). Symptomatic cases have skeletal muscle involvement with myalgias and possibly cardiomyopathy, fever, weight loss, bronchospasm, and subcutaneous nodules. The illness may be either monophasic or recurrent over years. Peripheral blood eosinophilia and a raised erythrocyte sedimentation rate (ESR) are usual. Muscle biopsy discloses the encysted parasites.[250]

sarcoglycanopathies A class of slowly progressive muscular dystrophies consequent upon defects of α-, β-, δ-, and γ-sarcoglycan (limb girdle muscular dystrophy [LGMD] 2D, E, F, and C, respectively) and responsible for severe forms of LGMD without cognitive involvement. Clinical or subclinical dilated cardiomyopathy is sometimes present.[3454] The condition especially affects the gluteus maximus and thigh adductors and the pelvic and shoulder girdle muscles. Calf contractures cause toe walking. A **rigid spine syndrome**, elevated serum CK levels, and myopathic muscle biopsy findings are other features. See also **severe childhood autosomal recessive muscular dystrophy** and Dr. Alan Pestronk's Web site: http://www.neuro.wustl.edu/neuromuscular/maltbrain.html.

sarcoid myelopathy A rare subacute myelopathy with intense focal enhancement of the C6–7 cord, resembling the appearances of an intramedullary tumor.[6939]

sarcoid myopathy A chronic proximal myopathy resulting from the presence of noncaseating granulomas within the muscle in the context of systemic sarcoidosis. However, in many cases, the presence of such granulomas does not produce any symptoms.[2280]

sarcoid neuropathy Multiple fluctuating and remitting cranial nerve pareses, involving especially cranial nerve VII and less often cranial nerves I, II, V, and XI; or peripheral multiple mononeuropathy.[4178] A subacute or chronic axonal sensorimotor neuropathy without cranial neuropathy, beginning months to years after established systemic sarcoidosis, is also described, as are diaphragmatic weakness, atypical neuropathies, **acute inflammatory polyneuropathy**, unilateral lumbosacral plexopathy, and a subacute symmetric sensory polyneuropathy, all able to appear before systemic sarcoidosis becomes evident.[6987]

sarcoidosis (Besnier-Boeck-Schaumann disease) A multisystem granulomatous disorder of unknown etiology, most commonly affecting young adults and presenting most frequently with bilateral hilar lymphadenopathy, pulmonary infiltration, and skin or eye lesions. Less than 10% of cases have neurological involvement. The diagnosis is supported by histological evidence of widespread noncaseating epithelioid cell granulomas in more than one organ, and by a positive Kveim-Siltzbach skin test result.[3152, 4719] See also **neurosarcoidosis**.

sarcolemma (Gr, flesh + rind, peelings) (myolemma) The most intimate limiting membrane of the myofibril.

sarcoma A malignant tumor arising from muscle or nerve. In the latter case, the context is most often the syndrome of **neurofibromatosis**. Neural sarcomas cause pain, swelling, and motor and sensory deficits in the appropriate territory; in muscle, local pain, swelling, and weakness are the usual complaints.

sarcosinemia An aminoaciduria characterized by mental retardation in some cases, with increased levels of sarcosine and ethanolamine in the blood and urine as a result of a deficiency of sarcosine dehydrogenase.[3210]

sarcotubular myopathy A rare, benign, recessively inherited, nonprogressive myopathic syndrome characterized by onset in early childhood, myopathic facial and proximal weakness and atrophy, and the presence of multiple empty membrane-bound vacuoles in type 2 myofibrils in muscle biopsy specimens, representing dilatation of the sarcotubular system.[6, 3212]

SARS A severe respiratory infection responsible also for neuromuscular problems such as **critical-illness polyneuropathy** or **myopathy**.

sartorius (from Lat, a tailor) The tailor's muscle; it flexes the knee and laterally rotates the thigh, thus allowing the traditional cross-legged position to be adopted.

satellite potential A small action potential, separated from the main motor unit action potential by an isoelectric interval, which fires in a time-locked relationship to the main action potential. It usually follows, but may precede, the main action potential. Less preferred terms include *late component*, *parasite potential*, *linked potential*, and *coupled discharge*. (From the 2001 Report of the Nomenclature Committee of the American Association of Electromyography and Electrodiagnosis.[19] Reproduced by kind permission of the AANEM.)

satellitosis An increase in the numbers of oligodendrocytes clustering around the larger neurons of the basal ganglia and the fourth, fifth, and sixth layers of the cerebral cortex. The pathological significance of this is not known.

Satoyoshi disease A sporadic syndrome with the onset in childhood of progressive but intermittent and painful muscle spasms, diarrhea, malabsorption, short stature, slipped epiphyses, bone cysts, fatigue fractures and osteolysis, amenorrhea, and alopecia. See **glycogen storage diseases** and **oculopharygo-distal muscular dystrophy**.

Satoyoshi syndrome (progressive muscle spasms, alopecia and diarrhea, myospasm gravis) A sporadic syndrome with onset in childhood or youth characterized by frequent painful, progressive, intermittent episodes of rigid muscle cramps beginning in the legs (*myospasm gravis*), and then several years after onset, the neck, trunk, and masticatory muscles become affected.

Associated features include alopecia, diarrhea, short stature, multiple bony abnormalities, intestinal malabsorption, a flat oral glucose tolerance curve, amenorrhea, and sometimes retardation of growth. The cramps result from synchronized motor unit discharges at 40–50 Hz and 4–10 mV amplitude.[5556, 5559] Intestinal polyposis was present in the two patients originally studied. The condition is considered to be a specific variety of malabsorption.

In a *variant form*, **myasthenia gravis** is associated.

Saturday night palsy 1. Radial nerve compression palsy sited in the spiral groove of the humerus, usually therefore sparing the branches to the triceps muscle. The term is applied because the disorder is occasionally seen in young men whose chivalry has extended to supporting the head of their girlfriend for a period of an hour (or even a night), with resultant ischemic compression of the nerve. Since this is usually a neurapraxia, recovery is typically both early and complete. 2. Sciatic nerve compression palsy as a result of prolonged compression of the buttocks and thighs wedged into a toilet seat while the street-drugged subject is unconscious.[6430]

Saturday night retinopathy Unilateral visual loss related to ocular pressure caused by the person remaining in the prone position while deeply intoxicated (or from wearing an anesthetic mask).[3174]

saturnine encephalopathy (Lat, pertaining to lead) Any kind of cerebral syndrome caused by lead poisoning. Coma, delirium, toxic psychoses, aphasias, seizures, and pareses were mentioned by Kinnier **Wilson**.[6819]

saturnine palsy See **lead palsy** and **Remak paralysis**.

saturnism Weakness due to lead poisoning.

satyriasis (Gr, satyr or lewd person) 1. Exceedingly great sexual desire in a male. 2. An old term for **leprosy**—on account of the malformations thereby produced, leading the patient to resemble the mythical satyrs who were represented as being extremely ugly.

Saul syndrome 1. A congenital dysmorphic syndrome manifesting also tall stature, dislocation of the lens, ectopic pupils, arachnodactyly, seizures, and mental and developmental delay.[379] Pigmentary skin disorders, microcephaly, and extrapyramidal lesions are also described.

Saunders, William (1743–1817) British physician who was born in Scotland and trained at the University of Edinburgh, but practiced in London as physician to Guy's Hospital. He was very involved in the activities of the Royal College of Physicians. His unpublished descriptions of **delirium tremens** were recognized by Thomas **Sutton**, who named the condition thus in his tract of 1813, in which he also gave a definitive description. Saunders did publish, however, on the topics of hepatitis, other diseases of the liver, the treatment of ague, and on the dissolution of renal stones.

Saunders–Sutton syndrome See **delirium tremens**.

Sauvineau syndrome See **internuclear ophthalmoplegia**.

Sauvineau, Charles (b. 1862) French ophthalmologist in Paris who first described **internuclear ophthalmoplegia.** (Un nouveau type de paralysie associé des mouvements horizontal des yeux. Ann. Ocul., Paris 1895; 113: 363–4)

savant syndrome A precocious ability to function superbly in certain tasks, set against a background of intellectual mediocrity at best. The syndrome is classified by the nature of the skill exhibited; exceptional memory, language, mathematical skills, abilities in the visual arts, and musical talents are described.

Savez Distroficara Jugoslavije A professional organization, and a member society of the European Alliance of Muscular Dystrophy Societies. Address: UI. Radomira Vujovica 3, 11000 Beograd, Serbia.

saw-tooth bursts Sharp transients recorded over the temporal lobes of preterm infants. They occur in bursts of 3–8 sharp rhythmic waves at 4–8 Hz, often with high (1–200 µ) voltage. (After Noachtar S, et al. A glossary of terms most commonly used by clinical electroencephalographers. EEG Clin Neurophysiol 1999;52[Suppl]:21–41. Reproduced by kind permission of the IFCN and Elsevier Science.)

saxitoxin neuropathy A manifestation of **paralytic shellfish poisoning**, first recognized by Captain Vancouver in 1801. The toxin is a sodium channel blocker and is contained in certain protozoa ingested by the mollusks (mussels, oysters, clams, and scollops). The local discoloration of the water that is produced has led to the term *red tide*. Clinical symptoms include burning in the mouth, paresthesia and numbness with ataxia, and sometimes brainstem involvement. See also **ciguatera poisoning**.[140]

saxophone headache Severe episodic headache associated with an increase in intrathoracic or intra-abdominal pressure, reported in patients with **Chiari malformation** (type 1) but with the same character as the head discomfort commonly occurring as a result of performing a sustained Valsalva maneuver.[1981, 2727]

Say syndrome A congenital dysmorphic syndrome in which skeletal abnormalities and microcephaly are the other main features.[5571]

SCAG See **Sandoz Clinical Assessment Geriatrics Scale**.

scalenus anticus syndrome See **thoracic outlet syndrome**.

scallop pupils Irregularities in the edge of the pupil, usually associated with amyloidosis or other disease of the short ciliary nerves leading to sector atrophy of the iris.[3795]

scalp (Dutch, a shell) The shell or covering of the head.

scalp electrode A recording electrode held against, attached to, or inserted into the scalp.

scalp electroencephalogram The usual record of electrical activity of the brain made by means of a scalp electrode.

Scandinavian Neurological Association An association of Scandinavian neurological societies promoting research and cooperation between Scandinavian neurologists.

Scandinavian Neurological Stroke Scale A reliable instrument for the stratification of stroke patients and for the evaluation of long-term outcome. The scale rates nine factors (consciousness, eye movements, arm motor power, hand motor power, leg motor power, orientation, speech, facial palsy, and gait) and derives from these both prognostic and long-term scores. Neglect and visual field deficits are not scored, increasing the reliability of the scale.[3854]

scanning EMG A technique by which a needle electrode is advanced in defined steps through muscle while a separate single fiber EMG electrode is used to trigger both the display sweep and the advancement device. It provides temporal and spatial information about the motor unit. Distinct maxima in the recorded activity are considered to be generated by muscle fibers innervated by a common branch of an axon. These groups of fibers form a motor unit fraction. (From the 2001 Report of the Nomenclature Committee of the American Association of Electromyography and Electrodiagnosis.[19] Reproduced by kind permission of the AANEM.)

scanning speech Separation of the syllables of words so that speech sounds disjointed, somewhat resembling that of partially literate schoolchildren made to recite the work of poets, thus damaging the reputations of both. It is due to an inability to change the positions of the vocal muscles rapidly, as occurs with disorders of the cerebellum. With nystagmus and ataxia, it formed the **Charcot triad** of signs of **multiple sclerosis** (all of which are, however, merely signs of cerebellar disease).

scanpaths The pathways along which vision is directed during stereotypical visual scanning of the critical stimulus features of a studied image.[5324]

scaphocephaly (Gr, hull + head) A developmental defect in skull shape with a long and narrow configuration as a consequence of premature fusion of the sagittal suture, such that it resembles an upturned boat, the keel lying along the suture. This, the most common form of craniosynostosis, also produces lowering and narrowing of the parietal level with a compensatory projection of the frontal and occipital areas; the face is little affected and hypertelorism is absent.[4] A similar deformity occurs in premature neonates as a result of skull molding during birth.

scapular reflex Stroking of the skin overlying the scapula leads to contraction of the underlying muscles. This is usually present but invisible, although it may be felt. Augmentation of the response occurs in the presence of a pyramidal lesion above C5. See **interscapular reflex**.

scapular winging Backward protrusion, often with rotation, of the scapula as a result of lesions of the long thoracic nerve, the C7 root or the XI nerve branch to trapezius, but also occasionally due to a proximal myopathy.[4035]

scapulocostal syndrome A painful condition ascribed to myofasciitis of the shoulder muscles and thought to be caused by altered posture, prolonged immobilization of the shoulder region, or fixed scapular or spinal deformities.[6953, 4814]

scapulohumeral reflex Contraction of various muscles of the shoulder girdle, particularly those supplied by C5–6, in response to a tap on the medial border of the scapula. Unilateral absence of the reflex indicates a lesion at the level of C5.

scapuloilioperoneal atrophy with cardiopathy and inflammatory myopathy A dominantly inherited syndrome of slowly progressive muscle weakness with a scapuloilioperoneal distribution and cardiopathy, with onset in young adult life. Muscle biopsy specimens show neurogenic and myopathic changes with inflammatory cell reactions and perivascular cuffing.[3200]

scapuloperoneal atrophy (Kaeser syndrome, Stark–Kaeser syndrome) See **scapuloperoneal syndrome**.

scapuloperoneal atrophy, cardiopathy, and inflammatory myopathy See **hereditary motor neuropathy** (*variants*).

scapuloperoneal syndrome (Davidenkow syndrome) A heterogeneous syndrome of muscle weakness and wasting affecting the scapular and peroneal muscles first and most, although arm, neck, ocular, and other cranial and trunk muscles may be affected later. The onset is at any time after childhood. It is usually dominantly inherited, but all forms of inheritance patterns and also sporadic cases have been described.[5679, 6281]

The syndrome represents a combination of the features of the **hereditary motor neuropathies** (spinal muscular atrophies) and of the girdle dystrophies.[3267] The pathological findings and results of electrical studies constitute the usual features of either neurogenic or myopathic disease, or of both. The course is generally benign unless cardiac complications ensue, as in the **Emery–Dreifuss syndrome**.[6281] It was described first by Brossard in 1886, but more fully by Davidenkow in 1939,[1479] who commented that the signs in the legs resembled those of Charcot–Marie–Tooth neuropathy, while the atrophy of the shoulder girdle muscles was like that of Erb muscular dystrophy.

The typical form (scapuloperoneal muscular atrophy type 1 with sensory disturbance, adult onset scapuloperoneal myopathy) is a dominantly or recessively inherited scapuloperoneal syndrome with juvenile or young adult onset, characterized by facial, bulbar, proximal, and distal myopathic weakness, often with pseudohypertrophy, ophthalmoplegias, sensory disturbances, and pes cavus.[1479, 6911] *Variant subtypes* are listed in Chart S–1.

Other neuromuscular syndromes which may present with this distribution include **myotonic dystrophy**, various **congenital myopathies** and myopathy with **Paget disease**. See also **centronuclear myopathy, Emery–Dreifuss muscular dystrophy, McArdle disease, limb girdle muscular dystrophy** (LGMD2A), **myosin storage myopathy, benign muscular dystrophy with contractures**,[335] and **acid maltase** or **phosphofructokinase deficiency** with scapuloperoneal weakness.

scarf sign Abnormal mobility of the arms of the supine infant, as shown when the examiner is able to pull the infant's hand across the chest, around the neck, and possibly back around the opposite shoulder. Using the scoring system of Dubowitz et al.[1728] for assessing **gestational age**, score 0 if the elbow reaches the opposite axillary line; 1 if the elbow can be moved to a point between the midline and the opposite axillary line; 2 if the elbow reaches to the midline; and 3 if the elbow does not reach the midline.

In the *posterior scarf sign*, the hand is drawn toward the opposite acromion but behind the neck. In hypotonic states, the hand can be led unusually far, constituting a positive response.[3080]

Scarff syndrome A syndrome characterized by early-onset focal seizures affecting the legs first, with minimal neurological deficit. The condition was thought by the original author to be due to the large Pacchionian granulations which were detected at operation and which had extended into the primary motor areas.[5574]

Scarpa, Antonius (1747–1832) Italian professor of surgery in Modena and later of anatomy in Pavia. He traveled widely and was a fellow of the Royal Colleges of London, Edinburgh, and Ireland, as well as a fellow of the Royal Society. A superb artist, he illustrated his own work on the inner ear, ocular disease, and other subjects. He described (Scarpa's) canal in the inner ear, and the nerve, canal, fascia, and triangle to which his name is also given. He was also the first to identify disease of the medial wall of arteries as the basis of aneurysms.

Chart S–1. Subtypes of Scapuloperoneal Syndrome

Scapuloperoneal muscular atrophy without sensory disturbance (Stark–Kaeser syndrome, scapuloperoneal atrophy; OMIM #181400). An adult-onset, dominantly inherited desminopathy with a peculiar distribution of weakness and atrophy, due to heterozygous missense mutation of the desmin gene (*R350P*) mapped to 2q35. There is marked phenotypic variability, including scapuloperoneal, limb girdle, and distal forms with variable cardiac or respiratory involvement. Facial weakness, dysphagia, and gynecomastia are frequently found. There is an increased risk of cardiac death.[6627, 6020] An X-linked recessive inheritance of this condition has also been reported.[379]

Scapuloperoneal muscular atrophy without sensory disturbance, recessive form A congenital or childhood scapuloperoneal syndrome manifesting only neurogenic muscle atrophy and weakness.

Scapuloperoneal muscular dystrophy type 1, *X-linked* (hyaline body myopathy) A severe scapuloperoneal syndrome mapped to Xq26 with onset in young-to-mid-adult life and manifesting proximal shoulder girdle and distal leg muscle atrophy and weakness. Contractures and cardiomyopathy are sometimes found. It is allelic with **reducing body myopathy**. See also **Emery–Dreifuss syndrome**.

Scapuloperoneal muscular dystrophy type 2 A dominantly inherited *variant* (**hyaline body myopathy**) with onset at any time from childhood to mid-adult life and characterized by scapuloperoneal weakness and weakness of neck flexion, shoulder abduction, knee flexion, and ankle dorsiflexion, with slow progression.

Scapuloperoneal muscular dystrophy type 3 (**hyaline body myopathy**) A recessively inherited *variant,* that maps to 3p22.2. The onset is in childhood or early adult life with typical scapuloperoneal weakness and impaired neck flexion and ankle dorsiflexion, with slow progression.

Scapuloperoneal muscular dystrophy, X-linked, without contractures A severe congenital scapuloperoneal syndrome manifesting both myopathic and neurogenic muscle atrophy, weakness, and severe cardiomyopathy.[559] See **Emery–Dreifuss syndrome**.

Scapuloperoneal neuronopathy (also known as Davidenkow syndrome) A dominantly inherited form with childhood or adult onset, presenting with early distal leg weakness and later shoulder girdle involvement with hyporeflexia. Some patients also have hereditary neuropathy with liability to pressure palsies mutations (*PMP*-22 deletions).

Scapuloperoneal muscular dystrophy, cardiomyopathy, and mental retardation An X-linked myopathic syndrome manifesting in childhood with cardiomyopathy, syncope, and neurodegenerative regression[3200] due to a mutation of the *LAMP*2 gene. See also **Danon disease**.

FSH phenotype with ragged red fibers and cardiomyopathy.

Scapuloperoneal neuropathy (motor neuron disease) A dominant variant mapping to 12q24.1 (a similar locus to distal HMN 2), characterized by the congenital absence of muscles and by progressively increasing scapuloperoneal, distal, and laryngeal weakness. A recessive *variant* is also described.

Scarpa's ganglion A ganglion on the vestibular nerve in the internal auditory meatus.

scelotyrbe festinans (from Gr, leg + perturbation, and Lat, hurrying; hence *festinating gait*) The classic gait disturbance of Parkinsonism, in which (in the words of Trousseau) "his center of gravity is thus displaced, he is obliged to run after himself, as it were, so that he keeps trotting and hopping on."

SCHAD deficiency See **short-chain acyl–coenzyme A dehydrogenase deficiency**.

Schaefer reflex An alternative method of seeking the **Babinski response**, in this case by pinching the Achilles tendon or the skin overlying it.[5578] **Babinski** himself had mentioned this method in a paper the year before Schaefer's report.

Schedule for Affective Disorders in Schizophrenia (SADS) A complex interviewer- and observer-rated scale designed to establish research and other diagnostic criteria for specific depressive disorders.[1858]

Scheibe defect (membranous cochleosaccular dysplasia) An inherited dysplasia of the inner ear with atrophy of both the cochlear and the vestibular divisions of the VIII cranial nerve.

Scheie disease See **mucopolysaccharidoses**.

schema (Gr, form) 1. A preconscious phenomenon, not amounting to a mental image (which is consciously appreciated). 2. The term of Sir Henry **Head** for a pattern of response in both the realms of speech and sensation, based upon previous responses of the organism but occurring outside awareness.[1331]

Scheuermann disease A benign epiphyseal disease of the spine, causing complaints of mild pain on exercise in adolescents over the course of a few (usually 2–4) years.

Schilder disease (encephalitis periaxialis diffusa) A term for disorders with different etiologies, characterized by diffuse sclerosis of the cerebral white matter. The patients reported by Schilder[5601] suffered from different conditions; he himself pointed out that "diffuse sclerosis" was not a single entity.

Some such cases are due to **multiple sclerosis** (*demyelinating form*) and the remainder to a disturbance of abnormally constituted myelin (*dysmyelinating form*).[5089] The condition now regarded as that most likely affecting the patients described by him is **adrenoleukodystrophy**;[5091] the term *Schilder disease* is best taken to refer to diffuse sclerosis occurring as a subacute condition in children, while transitional sclerosis is most likely to be a form of multiple sclerosis. See also **diffuse sclerosis**.

Schilder myelinoclastic diffuse sclerosis See **neuromyelitis optica**.

Schilder variant of multiple sclerosis A form of multiple sclerosis characterized clinically by the presence of dementia and pathologically by the presence of cerebral atrophy, ventricular dilatation, and shrinkage of the white matter associated with the presence of multiple chronic **plaques**. See also **neuromyelitis optica**.

Schilder, Paul Ferdinand (1886–1940) Austrian neurologist and psychiatrist who trained in Vienna, where he

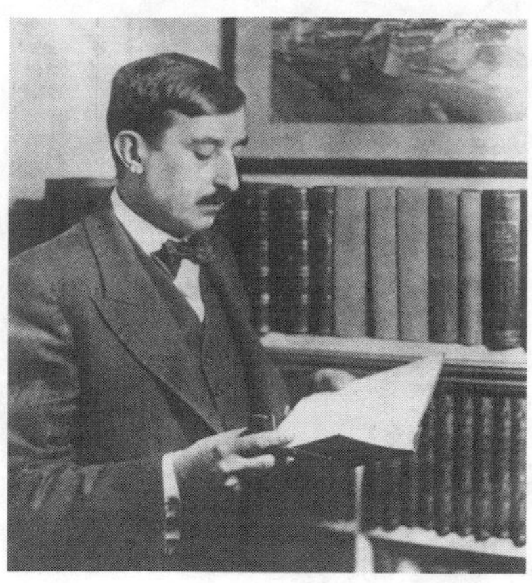

Figure S–1 Paul Ferdinand Schilder

soon obtained a staff position in the university hospital. He continued there (except for a period of war service) until he emigrated to the United States in 1929. He worked at Bellvue hospital in New York and later became associate professor of psychiatry at the New York Medical College.

His description of the syndrome named for him was published in 1912; his remaining 300 or so publications concerned psychiatric and philosophical topics, but, in neurology, his papers on involuntary movements, aphasia, other disorders of language, consciousness, and the syndromes described in the following entries were especially notable.

Schilder–Flatau disease See **Schilder–Foix disease**.

Schilder–Foix disease (Marie–Foix syndrome, Schilder–Flatau disease, intracerebral symmetrical lobar sclerosis) A nonprogressive condition due to perinatal anoxic encephalopathy, in which gliotic lesions are distributed throughout the cerebral white matter. **Marie**,[4073] Foix, and Flatau further analyzed some of the cases of Schilder and separated the condition from diffuse sclerosis.

Schimke syndrome An X-linked recessive congenital syndrome characterized by short stature, deafness, extraocular palsies, microcephaly, chorea, pyramidal signs, myopathy, and mental and developmental delay.[5607]

Schindler disease A form of lysosomal storage disease due to a defect in α-*N*-acetylgalactosaminidase and presenting with developmental delay, seizures, blindness, and psychomotor regression.[6720]

Schinzel syndrome (trisomy chromosome 13) A congenital dysmorphic syndrome also manifesting postaxial polydactyly with duplication of the halluces, macrocephaly, callosal agenesis, and severe mental and developmental delay.[5610] See **acrocallosal syndrome**.

Schiotz tonometry A method of assessing intraocular pressure by measuring the compressibility of the cornea. The normal pressure is up to 15 mmHg.

Schirmer syndrome A variant of **Sturge–Weber syndrome** in which glaucoma occurs unusually early.

Schirmer Test A test of tear formation, wherein a 5 mm wide strip of absorbent filter paper is hooked around the lower lid so that one end lies in the inferior conjunctival sac. The length of the paper wetted by normal tear formation during 5 min is measured and the two sides compared with each other and with the normal (which is 15 mm or more). In **Sjögren syndrome**, the length of the paper wetted is less than this.

Schirmer, O.W.A. (1864–1917) German ophthalmologist.

Schirmer–Sturge–Weber syndrome See **Sturge–Weber syndrome**.

schistosomiasis (bilharziasis) A common protozoal infection with *schistosoma japonicum, haematobium,* or *mansoni*, occurring in Africa, South America, and the Orient. Neurological complications are seldom the presenting problem, but seizures and myelopathy may result from the granulomas that form in reaction to the presence of the ova in the brain or spinal cord.

schizencephaly (Gr, split + brain) A congenital primary neuronal migration defect of the brain in which the cerebral mantle is not formed in the regions of the major (especially the Sylvian) fissures. The condition appears in infancy or up to early adult life and is characterized by microcephaly, hemiplegia, infantile spasms, and mental and developmental delay in association with deep symmetrical cerebral clefts with infolding of cortical gray matter along them and abnormalities of the ventricular system including hydrocephalus.[4365]

schizophrenia-like psychosis of epilepsy A chronic paranoid psychosis occurring in some patients with a long-standing history (mean: 14 years) of complex partial seizures originating in the temporal lobe. No important differences exist between the psychological symptoms of this condition and those of schizophrenia without an accompanying seizure disorder.[5890] The prevalence of schizophrenia in epileptic people is substantially higher than that in a control population.

schlaftrunkenheit See **confusional arousals**.

Schlemm, Friedrich (1795–1858) German anatomist. The canal of Schlemm is a small opening at the junction of the cornea and the sclera.

Schlesinger sign Strong passive inversion of the hip leads to extreme extension of the leg and inversion of the foot in **tetany**.[421]

Schmidt syndrome (vagoaccessory syndrome) Unilateral paresis of the muscles (vocal cords, soft palate, trapezius, and sternomastoid) supplied by the X and XI cranial nerves with contralateral hemiplegia, due to a medullary lesion which is usually vascular.[6147] It is thus a variant of the **Jackson–Mackenzie syndrome**, but without the tongue paralysis.[5617] The syndrome is named after Dr. A. **Schmidt**.

Schmidt, Adolf (1865–1918) German neurologist.

Schmidt, Henry D. (1832–1888) American pathologist practicing in New Orleans. His description of the clefts in the nerve sheaths (1874) preceded that of Lantermann by 3 years.

Schmidt, Johann Baptist (1823?–1884) German obstetrician who trained at Würzburg and whose paper on aphasia (1871) was drawn upon by **Wernicke** in his classic description of the syndrome 3 years later.[724]

Schmidt-Lantermann clefts Conical interruptions in the myelin sheath (intersegmental clefts) seen by light microscopy, named after H.D. Schmidt.

Schmidt-Rimpler Test The subject complaining of loss of vision is asked to look at his own hand.[1500] Those with true blindness will turn their eyes in the appropriate direction; those with simulated blindness will look randomly in any direction, unless they have the wit to realize that this is a test of conscious proprioception rather than one of vision. The test is named after Dr. A. **Schmidt**. See also **palpebral reflex**.

Schmidt-Voigt syndrome See **sacral lipomatosis**.

Schnabel optic atrophy Mucoid degeneration of the optic nerves occurring in patients with glaucoma, and described by Dr. Isidor Schnabel (1842–1908). See also **pseudo–Schnabel cavernous degeneration of the optic nerve**.

Schneider disease A virus infection usually occurring in the spring and fall, causing high fever, chills, nasopharyngitis, arthralgia, malaise, headache, and vomiting for about 4 days, followed by a latent period, and then either by serous meningitis and complete recovery or by a more severe meningoencephalitis with hyperkinesia, sensory disorders, tics, and seizures, but with full recovery eventually. Rarely, the meningoencephalitis produces signs resembling those of **poliomyelitis**.

The nature of the disorder is uncertain and these syndromes may in fact be nonspecific complications of different viral infections.[5624]

Scholz plaques See **perivascular plaques**.

Scholz syndrome See **metachromatic leukodystrophy**.

Scholz, Willibald (b. 1889) German psychiatrist, neurologist, and neuropathologist at Tübingen, Leipzig, and Munich, who developed the concept of glial insufficiency in **metachromatic leukodystrophy** (sulfatide lipidosis) in 1925; as a result his name has been attached to the disease.

Schrijver-Bernhard reflex Plantar flexion of the toes in response to a tap on the tibia or the overlying muscles—a sign of pyramidal tract disease and perhaps of basal ganglion disease. See **distant toe flexor reflex**.

Schroeder tetrad A child from a rural area; in good general health; with marked intracranial hypertension; and with ill-defined focal neurological signs. The presence of these four features strongly suggests the diagnosis of cerebral hydatid disease.[5654]

Schüller, Artur (1874–1957) Viennese radiologist who published the first X-ray atlas of the skull and described the signs of increased intracranial pressure on the sella turcica. He also contributed data leading to the definition of **Hand–Schüller–Christian disease**.

Schulman syndrome See **eosinophilic fasciitis**.

Schultze acroparesthesia (Schultze–Nothnagel syndrome, Putnam–Schultze syndrome) The concurrence of acroparesthesia, anesthesia, and pain in the distal arms without vasomotor symptoms. The condition probably represents a severe form of **carpal tunnel syndrome**. Dr. Frederich Schultze (1848–1934) was a German physician.

Schultze syndrome Meningeal neurofibroblastomatosis.

Schultze Test Percussion of the skin of the face overlying the facial nerve between the angle of the jaw and the zygoma. Twitching of the middle part of the face in response is a positive result, indicating the presence of latent **tetany**.[421]

A *variant* test is to tap the protruded tongue. In tetany, and in **myotonic dystrophy**, dimpling or rising-up of the part tapped may occur. See also **Chvostek Test**, of which this is but a modification, although perhaps increasing the sensitivity.

Schumacher Panel criteria Criteria for the diagnosis of definite **multiple sclerosis**, published in 1965 and, in the opinion of some physicians, still the least disputatious.[5663] The criteria are as given in Chart S–2.

Schumacher, G.A. American neurologist at the University of Vermont.

schusterkrampf (Ger, shoemaker cramps) Tetany.

Schwab, Robert S. (1903–1972) American neurologist, educated at Harvard and Cambridge Universities, who trained in neurology at the Boston City and Massachussetts General Hospitals, where he established a reputation as a clinician-researcher, becoming well-known as an expert in **Parkinson disease**, the EEG, **epilepsy**, and **myasthenia gravis**.

Chart S–2. The Schumacher Panel Criteria for the Diagnosis of Multiple Sclerosis

1. The neurological examination must reveal objective abnormalities that can be attributed to dysfunction of the CNS.
2. The case history must supply evidence that two or more parts of the CNS are involved.
3. Evidence of CNS disease must reflect predominant involvement of white matter—that is, long-tract damage.
4. Involvement of the neuraxis must have followed one of two time patterns given below
   a. Two or more episodes of worsening, each lasting at least 24 h and each at least a month apart.
   b. Slow or stepwise progression of signs and symptoms over at least 6 months.
5. At onset, the patient must be aged between 10 and 50 years.
6. A physician competent in clinical neurology should decide that the patient's condition could not be better attributed to another disease.

However, it is now clear that criterion number 5 should be discarded, as pediatric multiple sclerosis is being increasingly recognized. Moreover, criterion number 6 is highly subjective and unquantifiable. See **McDonald criteria** for the currently accepted means of making the diagnosis.

Schwabach Test The direct comparison of a patient's ability to hear a vibrating tuning fork placed on the mastoid process with the ability of the examiner to do so. The test has elements of both the **Rinne** and the **Weber** tests; if the examiner hears the sound for longer than the patient, the latter is suspected to have sensorineural deafness.

Schwalbe, Gustav (1844–1916) Professor of anatomy at Strasbourg. He gave his name to a number of anatomical features, the most memorable being the medial vestibular nucleus.

Schwalbe's nucleus The principal (medial) vestibular nucleus.

Schwann cell A macrophage, the supporting cell providing myelin insulation for the axons of peripheral nerves.

Schwann, Theodor (1810–1882) Prussian physician, professor of anatomy, physiology, and comparative anatomy at various northern European universities, notably Liège and Louvain. He was an early proponent of the neuronal theory of the nervous system and of the cellular doctrine of tissues in general; he was also the discoverer of pepsin as well as of the cell named for him (1838).

Schwannoma (neurilemmoma, neurinoma, acoustic neuroma, neurofibroma, lemmoma, perineurial fibroblastoma, endothelioma, gliofibrosarcoma) A benign, solitary, sporadic, lobulated, encapsulated tumor of the nerve sheath, arising usually from the vestibular portion of the VIII cranial nerve or from the sensory roots of other cranial or spinal nerves, usually in adult life. Histologically, these tumors are characterized by the presence of a rich reticulin network, **Antonini type A** and **B** areas, **Verocay bodies**, and positive staining for S-100 protein.

Most clinical symptoms arise as a result of compression of local structures; neural hearing loss, vertigo, facial numbness, and weakness, dysphagia, ataxia and hydrocephalus are the more common problems encountered when the tumor arises from the VIII nerve; and pain and segmental sensorimotor deficits when it arises from a spinal nerve root. Malignant transformation can occur. In rare instances, the tumor is part of the **neurofibromatosis 2 syndrome**—a dominantly inherited disorder mapping to chromosome 22.

The tumor was actually first described by Sandifort in 1777.

Schwannomatosis The occurrence of multiple Schwannomas in people whose disorder does not meet the criteria for **neurofibromatosis** type 2. The condition is manifest later and is seldom familial; the prognosis is better and the tendency for other tumors to develop is much less than in that condition.[3989]

Schwartz disease See **syndrome of inappropriate ADH secretion**.

Schwartz, Henry Gerard (b. 1909) American surgeon practicing in St. Louis. He was the first to describe the operation of medullary tractotomy for the relief of intractable pain.[5675]

Schwartz, W.B. Contemporary American physician.

Schwartz–Jampel syndrome (myotonic chondrodystrophy, chrondrodystrophic myotonia, oculochondromuscular dystrophy) A rare, recessively inherited dysmorphic condition of early childhood, mapped to chromosome 1p34–p36 and manifesting dwarfism; metaphyseal and epiphyseal dysplasias; ocular, genital, and skeletal abnormalities; blepharophimosis; and muscle weakness, stiffness, and contractures with small muscle mass despite the unique feature of the presence of myotonia and continual high-frequency muscle fiber activity, as recorded on the EMG at rest.[2168]

Type 1A is characterized by the onset in childhood of myotonia, bone dysplasia, micrognathia, platyspondyly, cleft vertebrae, small stature, contractures, myopia, hirsutism, and small testes. There is an increased risk of malignant hyperthermia. Type 1B is congenital and resembles Type 1A except that there is more severe bone dysplasia.

Type 2 is recessively inherited. This is probably the same entity as Stuve–Wiedemann syndrome (SWS) characterized by the congenital onset of hypotonia, respiratory and feeding difficulties, and recurrent episodes of hyperthermia. The EMG shows complex repetitive discharges.

In a *variant* form, the condition is dominantly inherited.[4920]

Drs. Oscar Schwartz and R. Jampel are contemporary American ophthalmologists.

Schwarz-Lelek syndrome A syndrome of massive internal bowing of the femurs (genu valgum) with radiolucent splaying of the metaphyseal area and hyperostosis and sclerosis of the skull,[5673] described by Dr. L. Schwarz in 1960. See **craniometaphyseal dysplasia**.

Schweiz Gesellschaft für Muskelkrankheiten (SGMK) A member society of the European Alliance of Muscular Dystrophy Societies. Address: Lenggstrasse 67, Ch-8008 Zurich, Switzerland. Web site: http://www.muskelkrank.ch/.

Schweizerische Gesellschaft für Neurologie A professional organization. Address: c/o Dr. A. Steck, CHUV, 8011, Lausanne, Switzerland. Web site: http://www.swissneuro.ch/Intro/WebHome.

sciatic (from Gr, the hip joint, later Lat, pains in that region) The condition of **sciatica** indicates irritation of the sciatic nerve with pain felt in the distribution of the nerve. The first description was that of **Cotugno** in 1764.

sciatic list The distance between a plumb line dropped from the cervicodorsal spine to the gluteal cleft. With radiculopathy, this deformity remains during forward bending, while psychogenic lists usually disappear with spinal flexion.[1306]

sciatic neuralgia See **sciatica**.

sciatic neuropathy Pain, weakness, wasting, and sensory disturbances in the territory of the nerve as a result of damage to it in the pelvis; but, for reasons unknown, clinically more likely to damage the peroneal rather than the posterior tibial portion.

Lesions above the piriformis muscle affect also the glutei, tensor fascia lata, and possibly the paraspinal muscles; below it but within the pelvis, the hamstrings; and below the sciatic notch, the structures innervated by the two major branches of the nerve according to the relative damage done to each branch. Presenting features include numbness and paresthesias, distal dysesthesias, subjective and objective weakness, reduced or absent ankle jerks, and elctrodiagnostic evidence of denervation in the EDB, tibialis anterior, or abductor hallucis, and reduced or absent sural or superficial peroneal sensory nerve action potentials.[6937] See also **piriformis syndrome**, **posterior tibial neuropathy**, **common peroneal neuropathy**, and **hunkering**.

sciatica (Cotugno disease, sciatic neuralgia) The popular name for pain radiating in sciatic nerve distribution as a result of root irritation.[1296] Drs. William J. Mixter and Joseph S. Barr showed in 1934 that this was frequently due to nerve root irritation by a prolapsed intervertebral disk.

The pain is sharp, continuous, or lancinating, felt in the region innervated by the damaged nerve fibers and worsened by spinal movements. It is usually accompanied by paresthesias and by motor and sensory deficits when the cause is radicular compression. However, deep, aching pain may be referred in the same distribution without paresthesias as a result of distortion or inflammation of structures close to the spinal column. See also **Cotugno, D.**[6937]

sciatique spasmodique Sciatic nerve irritation with spasm of the contralateral erector spinae muscles, leading to scoliosis. The sign was described by **Brissaud**; it is found in patients with severe sciatica and is also described with **facet syndromes**.

scintillating scotomas (Lat, spark + Gr, darkening) Areas of visual loss with superimposed positive visual phenomena such as showers of sparks and twinkling lights, occurring as a result of retinal or occipital lobe ischemia, as in migraine. These were first described by Dianon in his 1875 graduation thesis (Université de Paris), but had been recorded earlier by Fothergill, Wilks, Parry, Living, and many other migraineurs.

scintillations Hallucinated persistent or transitory shimmering or flickering lights, seen by patients with lesions of the calcarine cortex and suggesting the presence of ischemia in the territory of the posterior cerebral artery.[2086]

scleral show Sclera visible below the iris of the eye, suggesting weakness of the orbicularis oculi muscle—a sign occurring in facial nerve palsies and in those muscular dystrophies which affect the facial muscles. See **Dalrymple sign**.

sclero- (Gr, hard).

scleroderma (progressive systemic sclerosis) A multisystem collagen-vascular disease characterized by inflammation and fibrosis of small blood vessels and of the dermal layers, and by fibrosis and atrophy of smooth muscle and connective tissue. The major neurological complication is neuropathy, most evidently of the trigeminal nerve but occasionally of the peripheral nerves;[3417] while CNS complications are usually due to hypertension or to any associated vasculitis. Proximal, symmetrical myopathy, inflammatory polymyositis, and neuropathic weakness are also described.[2892]

Scleroderma *en coup de sabre* is a localized linear form displaying skin atrophy in discrete lines, usually in the frontoparietal regions of the head. It is associated with ipsilateral underlying brain atrophy with seizures.[2593] See **Parry–Romberg syndrome**, **linear scleroderma**.

scleromalacia perforans Thinning and sometimes perforation of the sclera, as may occur in rheumatoid arthritis.

sclérose en plaques See **multiple sclerosis**.

sclerosis disseminata dolorosa Neuralgic or other pains occurring in the course of **multiple sclerosis**.

sclerosis Accumulation of glial scar tissue in the brain and spinal cord, there being no fibroblasts present to produce fibrosis.

sclerostosis A recessively inherited craniotubular hyperostotic syndrome, characterized by osteopetrosis, syndactyly, severe facial dysmorphism, increased intracranial pressure, optic atrophy, and cranial nerve palsies affecting the VII and VIII cranial nerves in particular.[6405]

sclerotome The deep somatic structures which share innervation by a single spinal segment and to which pain may be referred when any part of the sclerotome is damaged. The area of referred pain is somewhat variable between subjects, and the concept of fixed sclerotomes, akin to **dermatomes**, has been criticized.

scoliosis (Gr, curvature or twisting) The word used by Hippocrates for a spinal curvature; today it signifies more specifically a lateral curvature of the spine, with rotation in cases of fixed or structural spinal disease.

scombroid A relatively common icthyotoxicosis resulting from the ingestion of fish such as tuna, marlin herring, mackerel, and skipjack (or cheese)—the fish at least having a peppery taste or a honeycombed appearance resulting from the bacterial decarboxylation of histidine to histamine. Within minutes up to an hour after ingestion, the patient complains of abdominal cramps, nausea, burning in the mouth and throat, headache, and dizziness. Flushing is usual; bronchospasm and respiratory distress are occasional. Untreated, the condition lasts but a few hours and is seldom fatal.

SCOPA (SCales for Outcomes in Parkinson disease) A collection of rating scales for the disease which addresses both motor and nonmotor domains such as sleep, depression, and anxiety, autonomic functions, pain, and psychosocial factors, not all of which are covered in the **Unified Parkinson Disease Rating Scale**. It was reviewed by Chaudhuri et al. (2006)[1120] SCOPA-Aut is an assessment tool rating autonomic outcomes in **Parkinson disease**. It is available at the Web site: http://www.scopa-propark.eu/index.php?page=1&navRight=3&doc=3 &group=Yes& taal=eng&language=eng.

scotoepilepsy A form of seizure disorder in which visual fixation can suppress the paroxysms. The clinical features resemble those of **benign occipital epilepsy**.[3956]

scotoma (Gr, darkening, an eclipse) An island of blindness in a sea of vision. An *absolute scotoma* is an area in which not even light can be perceived. A *relative scotoma* is that form in which the subject can see form or movement but not color. *Negative scotomas* are imperceptible to the patient, while *positive scotomas* are appreciated as areas of darkness, as in the case of lesions situated anterior to the retina. See also **central**, **paracentral**, **ring**, and **centrocecal scotoma**.

Scott palsy (Scott-Strachan disease) See **Strachan syndrome**.

Scott syndrome A congenital X-linked dysmorphic syndrome characterized also by obesity, short stature, acanthosis nigricans, deafness, genital and skeletal abnormalities, microcephaly, and mental and developmental delay.[5686]

Scott-Strachan disease See **Strachan syndrome**.

scrapie A chronic, naturally occurring transmissible demyelinating disease of sheep due to a subvirus particle (virion) which induces a spongiform encephalopathy. The name derives from the tendency of the sheep to scrape alongside fences and other field furniture as a result of their progressive ataxia.

Scratch 'n Sniff Test A commercial smell-identification test in which a series of familiar odors is presented in the form of impregnated cards which release different odors when abraded.

scratching pest See **pseudohydrophobia**.

Scripps Neurological Rating Scale A scale designed for the assessment of subjects with **multiple sclerosis**.[5873]

scrivener's palsy (*crampe des écrivains*) A focal (occupational) dystonia. See **dystonia** and **writer's cramp**.

scrotal reflex Vermicular contraction of the dartos muscle, not causing elevation of the testicle, normally seen in response to gentle stimulation of the perineum.

scrotal tongue A ridged appearance to the tongue, reminding some of the dermal anatomy in baser regions.

scrub typhus (tsutsumagushi fever) An infection caused by *rickettsiae tsutsumagushi*, prevalent in eastern and southern Asia and transmitted by mites. Clinically, after a one-to-three week incubation period, an eschar develops at the site of the bite and this is followed in order by the appearance of regional lymphadenopathy, fever, conjunctival injection, severe headache, myalgia, and frequently a rash. Neurological complications comprise features of encephalitis, including restlessness, delirium, tremors, seizures, and papilledema. Deafness and bulbar signs have also been described. The Weil–Felix reaction shows agglutination of O-K but the immunofluorescent test is more precise in diagnosis.[6858]

scurvy The condition resulting from deficiency of vitamin C, so demonstrated by James Lind, a ship's surgeon in the Royal Navy in 1753. His book[3852] contains one of the earliest accounts of a prospective controlled trial, in which Lind compared six of the many different treatments for scurvy then in use, selecting 12 sailors at a similar stage of the disease, who received the same basic diet and were accommodated in the same part of the ship. The results suggested that oranges and lemons were more effective than other treatments for preventing scurvy, but it was only almost half a century later that citrus fruit was made mandatory by the British Admiralty so that British sailors could benefit from the results of this research.

SDEEG See **stereotactic (stereotaxic) depth electroencephalogram**.

sea shell sound (sea shell roar or noise) The fanciful (though acceptably appropriate) name given to the continuous background activity sometimes recorded during electromyography and representing **end-plate activity**.

sea-blue histiocytosis The presence of large macrophages in which the cytoplasm is packed with granules staining blue-green or blue on Wright-Giemsa staining, particularly in the spleen, liver, and bone marrow. The granules may contain, for example, ceroid, lipofuscin, sphingomyelin, or other phospholipids. See **sphingomyelin storage disorders**. The condition has been associated with a number of neurological, hematological, and other diseases; in the former category, **albinism**, **neurodegeneration with brain iron accumulation**, **neuroaxonal dystrophies**, **Niemann–Pick disease**, peripheral neuropathy, posterior column dysfunction and a multisystem CNS and anterior horn cell disease are examples.[273]

seamstresses' cramp A focal (occupational) dystonia. See **dystonia**.

search reflex See **rooting reflex**.

Seashore Measure of Musical Talents A test of pitch, loudness, rhythm, time, timbre, discrimination, and tonal memory. The evocative name, however, is merely that of the inventor.[5700]

seatbelt injury 1. Injury to the musculoligamentous structures of the neck and shoulder due to rapid deceleration while wearing a lap–shoulder seatbelt. Chest bruising may also be notable. 2. Traction injury to the brachial plexus from the same cause; eventual recovery after a neurapraxic injury may be expected.[2947] See also **stinger syndrome.**

seatbelt syncope Syncope, mainly in the elderly, due to pressure of a seat-belt worn too high and thus pressing upon the carotid sinus.

Sebire syndrome A pediatric encephalopathy characterized by the subacute appearance of movement disorders such as orofacial dyskinesias and chorea or limb dystonias; loss of motor skills; global aphasia; CSF pleocytosis; and sometimes seizures, with spontaneous recovery.[5701]

Seckel bird-headed dwarfism (Virchow–Seckel syndrome, nanocephalic dwarfism, and birdlike face syndrome) A recessively transmitted disease of children in which the head is small, the eyes apparently large, the nose beaked, and the mandible underdeveloped, all in association with severe mental retardation.

High-arched or cleft palate, prominent low-set or lobeless ears, antimongolian slant, epicanthic folds, kyphoscoliosis, sternal defects, absent patellae, congenital dislocation of the hip, and disorders of bone maturation are other features described.[5703] Apart from the dysmorphism, and sometimes feeding problems due to temporomandibular ankylosis, the condition may be complicated by hypersomnia, periodic obstructive apneic periods during sleep, and alveolar hypoventilation.

The first description of the condition was actually that of **Virchow** in 1882.

Seckel, H.P.G. (b. 1900) Swiss pediatrician.

second impact syndrome An unusual syndrome of uncertain provenance in which diffuse brain swelling occurs with delayed deterioration in cerebral function after repeated concussions, the second event occurring before the effects of the first one have subsided. It has usually been described in the context of sports played by young people. Both a failure in cerebral vascular autoregulation and true cerebral edema have been considered responsible.

Although it is most commonly reported in football, the syndrome can occur while playing any sport that can produce head blows. Any athlete still complaining of postconcussion symptoms after a head injury must not be allowed to return to play.[1000] Diagnostic criteria have been formulated[4210] and require medical review after a witnessed first impact, the documentation of ongoing symptoms following the first impact up to the time of the second impact, and a witnessed second head impact with subsequent rapid cerebral deterioration, after which there should be neuropathologic or neuroimaging evidence of cerebral swelling without significant intracranial hematoma or other cause for edema. See also **pugilistic encephalopathy** and **ding**.

second messenger A substance mediating the transduction of a usually external cellular stimulus or signal and a given cellular response, such as muscle contraction, and neurotransmitter release, etc.

second sensory area An area of cortex lying along the upper bank of the Sylvian fissure with crude somatotopic representation, not including the face.[3948]

second sensory seizures Epileptic seizures arising from a focus within the second sensory region, characterized by pain in the trunk and limbs.[6925]

second visual system A system involving the pathway between the colliculus, the pulvinar, and the parietal lobe, which is concerned with directed visual attention (the detection of events, their location in space, and the control of orienting responses to them for subsequent identification by the first system). The control of orienting responses involves the geniculostriate pathway and is concerned with identification rather than detection.[6974]

second wind Adaptation to exercise following an initial transient period of progressive fatigue and weakness of the affected muscles, first described in myophosphorylase deficiency but to some degree a normal phenomenon.

The mechanisms of this reinvigoration include an increase in cardiac output and thus in muscle blood flow, increased EMG activity, and an alteration in the metabolic pathways such that hexose phosphates, free fatty acids, and blood-borne glucose can be mobilized to supply energy.[789]

secondary (ocular) deviation See **primary deviation** and **cover test**.

secondary bilateral synchrony The occurrence of sequential focal spikes of sharp waves on the EEG that lead on to bilaterally synchronous epileptiform paroxysms within 500 ms.[690]

secondary carnitine deficiency Low levels of carnitine in the muscles of patients suffering from generalized systemic disease, other myopathies, or renal disease. The role of the reduced carnitine levels in the genesis of weakness in such situations is unproved.

secondary chronic cluster headache See **chronic cluster headache**.

secondary dementias Those dementing conditions due to pathological conditions affecting the brain or other organs other than primary degenerations.

secondary headaches Those forms of headache with a known causative pathology, unlike **migraine, cluster headache, tension-type headache**, etc. (See **primary headaches**). They include the following:

- Headache attributed to head and neck trauma
- Headache attributed to cranial or cervical vascular disorder
- Headache attributed to nonvascular intracranial disorder
- Headache attributed to a substance or its withdrawal
- Headache attributed to infection
- Headache attributed to disturbance of homeostasis
- Headache or facial pain attributed to disorder of cranium, neck, eyes, ears, nose, sinuses, teeth, mouth, or other facial or cranial structures
- Headache attributed to psychiatric disorder

From the International Classification of Headache Disorders (Headache Classification Committee of the International Headache Society. *Cephalalgia* 2004;**24**[Suppl 1]). Reproduced by kind permission of Dr. Jes Olesen, the International Headache Society, and Wiley-Blackwell Publications. See also **headache**.

secondary hypersomnolence See **hypersomnolence**.

secondary optic atrophy Optic atrophy following previous papilledema. Unlike the stark white disk of primary optic atrophy, the appearance in this condition is of a ragged, yellowish disk, sometimes with pigmentary deposits evidencing previous hemorrhage. See **consecutive optic atrophy**.

secondary phase nystagmus See **vestibular nystagmus**.

secondary position The position of the eyes when in adduction or abduction, elevation, or depression—that is, directed anywhere away from the straight-ahead primary position.

secondary syringomyelia The formation of cavities within the spinal cord as a result of hemorrhage, tumor, or trauma.

secondary wave A visible wave of contraction slowly progressing through a healthy muscle after it has been tapped or firmly stroked. The phenomenon was first described in 1857 by Schiff in Berne.[4564]

sector defects See **retinal slits**.

sector scotoma Holmes' term for homonymous loss of vision in the ipsilateral field due to lesions of the calcarine cortex, in which the loss lies along the vertical axes through the fixation points, either above or below the meridian and generally becoming wider toward the upper or lower limits of the fields.

sectoral hemianopia See **hemianopia**.

sectoranopia (sector defects) Loss of a section of the visual field, as a result of retinal lesions or of infarcts of the lateral geniculate body. See **retinal slits**.

Sedgwick–Boder syndrome See **Louis-Bar syndrome**.

seducible nystagmus See **gaze-evoked nystagmus**.

Seeligmüller neuralgia Bilateral auriculotemporal neuralgia, in which the pain is felt from ear to ear over the vertex of the skull, especially pain elicited by pressure on the head; described in syphilis.[5707]

Seeligmüller sign Mydriasis on the side affected in **trigeminal neuralgia**. The mechanism is uncertain.

Seeligmüller, Otto Ludwig Gustav Adolf (1837–1912) German neuropathologist who graduated from the University of Halle, studied neurology in Vienna and Paris, and was an associate professor in Halle. He is best remembered for his studies on childhood spastic states[5706] and for the observations in the preceding two entries.

Seemenova syndrome A recessively inherited congenital dysmorphic syndrome, characterized also by short stature, T-cell and immunoglobulin deficiency, and microcephaly.[5708]

seesaw anisocoria See **springing pupil**.

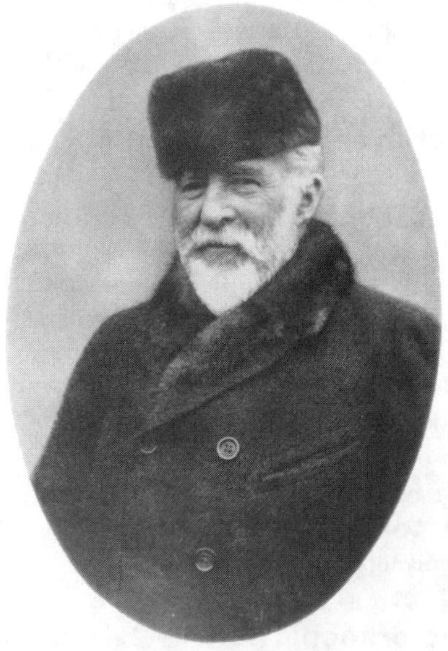

Figure S–2 Otto Ludwig Gustav Adolf Seeligmüller

seesaw nystagmus A rare ocular oscillation induced by an unstable visuovestibular interaction control system (likely due to disruption of chiasmal crossing fibers) in which there is rapid, rhythmic, opposed alternation of the vertical positions of the eyes. The movements are pendular or jerky and torsional with a vertical component, but are asymmetrical; the intorting eye rises while the other, extorting eye falls.

The condition is not actually a true nystagmus.[1561] The most common cause is a caudal diencephalic lesion, such as a parasellar tumor expanding into the third ventricle, in which case a bitemporal field defect is also commonly found. Trauma, **multiple sclerosis**, and brainstem vascular diseases are other causes.[4582] When pendular, lesions of crossing axons at the optic chiasm may be found, but when of jerk type, seesaw nystagmus is due to lesions in the region of the interstitial nucleus of Cajal.[5731]

A *congenital form* is similar, but it lacks the torsional component. See also **ocular tilt reaction** and **hemi-seesaw nystagmus**.

seesaw winking with orofaciodigital signs A congenital dysmorphic syndrome, characterized also by dental and skeletal abnormalities, strabismus, and mental and developmental delay.[381]

Segawa syndrome (dopa-responsive dystonia, hereditary progressive diurnal dystonia; dystonia 5; dyt5 dystonia; progressive dystonia with diurnal variation, dystonia-Parkinsonism with diurnal fluctuation, autosomal dominant dystonia, dopa-responsive; autosomal dominant dopa-responsive dystonia) An extrapyramidal syndrome of childhood presenting with dystonic postural disturbances showing diurnal fluctuation (symptoms are aggravated in the evening but alleviated after sleep). The onset is insidious but the condition progresses to all limbs within 5 years. Torsion of the trunk, rigidity, resting tremor, cerebellar, pyramidal or sensory changes, and cognitive impairments are not found, but Parkinsonian features may be present.

A response to low dose levadopa is a diagnostic and therapeutic test. A locus on Chr. 14q22.1–q22.2 has been identified.[1597, 5709] See also **dopa-responsive dystonia**.

Segelman syndrome A congenital dysmorphic syndrome characterized by skeletal abnormalities, multiple cavernous hemangiomas, recurrent infections, and mental and developmental delay.[381]

segmental demyelination Selective, discontinuous damage to Schwann cells, rendering them unable to maintain that segment of myelin for which they are responsible and leading to the disruption and removal of myelin in the segments between two nodes of Ranvier; loss of portions of the myelin sheath surrounding peripheral axons.

Depending on both the number of adjacent Schwann cells so affected and their position in relation to the node of Ranvier, **conduction block** may or may not occur.

segmental dystonia Dystonia that affects more than one body area, such areas being contiguous.

segmental hyperhidrosis Increased sweating in the skin supplied by one or more spinal segments uni- or bilaterally and usually indicating irritation or infiltration of preganglionic sympathetic fibers or of the sympathetic chain. See also **Ross syndrome**.[5662]

The same problem can also occur in trigeminal nerve territory.

segmental instability A spinal disorder, possibly a cause of recurrent low back pain and scoliosis, characterized by narrowing of the disk space, the presence of numerous **traction spurs**, and shifts in spinal alignment seen on radiographs taken in flexion and extension.[2223, 4566] However, the very existence of the syndrome is controversial.[2222]

segmental myoclonus Myoclonus of cranial or spinal origin, which thus affects a group of muscles innervated by one cranial nerve (as with **hemifacial spasm**) or affects one or more than one adjacent spinal segment. The movements may be irregular or periodic, and may be stimulus-sensitive. See **spinal myoclonus**.

segmental neuralgia See **intercostal neuralgia**.

segmental neurofibromatosis See **neurofibromatosis**.

segmental spinal muscular atrophy A sporadic or dominantly inherited syndrome of weakness and atrophy which affects especially the distal upper extremities.[4964] This condition may be the same as **de Grouchy syndrome**.

Séguin sign Contraction of a local group of muscles immediately before a generalized tonic-clonic convulsion,[5333] and thus evidence of a focal origin of the seizure.

Séguin, Edouard Onesimus (1812–1880) French psychiatrist who trained under Esquirol and was later an instructor at the Bicêtre. Encouraged by the example of **Itard** with the "Wild Boy of Aveyron," he espoused the cause of the mentally retarded, employing the principle that the senses could be made to compensate for each other when any one was impaired. From his unit at the Bicêtre he published his *Traitement moral, hygiene et éducation des idiots et des autres enfants arrières* in 1846, an account of his pioneering experiences in the training of mentally retarded people.

His political activities made it advisable for him to emigrate from France on the ascent of Louis Napoleon, and he chose the United States, where successively in Cleveland, Pennsylvania, and New York he introduced new methods in the management of the mentally ill and the mentally defective, using his refinements of the methods of Esquirol. The spirit of these endeavors was adopted by Mme. Montessori in her schools.

Seguin, Edward Constant (1843–1898) British physician who described the autopsy findings in **multiple sclerosis** and **papilledema**.

Seitelberger disease 1. See **infantile neuroaxonal dystrophy** and **glioneuronal dystrophies**. 2. See **Pelizaeus–Merzbacher disease**.

Seizure—European Journal of Epilepsy A subspecialty neurological journal published by Elsevier Science. Web site: http://www.harcourt-international.com/journals/seiz/.

seizure arrest The process whereby the further development of a "partial" seizure is aborted by a specific activity of the patient. **Gowers** pointed out that ligatures placed about the upper arm of one of his patients who suffered Jacksonian seizures in that arm successfully stopped his seizures at that point, with greater effect as the exercise was repeated. In other cases, strong odors have been found effective in arresting "complex partial" seizures.

seizure pattern EEG The occurrence of repetitive EEG discharges with a relatively abrupt onset and termination and with a characteristic pattern of evolution, lasting at least several seconds. The component waves or complexes vary in form, frequency, and topography. They are generally rhythmic and frequently display increasing amplitude and decreasing frequency during the same episode. When focal in onset, they tend to spread subsequently to other areas. EEG seizure patterns unaccompanied by a clinical epileptic manifestation detected by the recordist and/or reported by the patient should be referred to as *subclinical*. See also **epileptiform pattern**. (Adapted from the 1974 report of the Committee on Terminology, IFCN. In: Chatrian GE, Bergamini L, Dondey M, et al. A glossary of terms most commonly used by clinical electroencephalographers. *EEG Clin Neurophysiol* 1974;37:538–48. Reproduced with kind permission from Elsevier Science.)

seizure rating scales Attempts to quantify the impact and severity of seizures, most assessing seizure frequency, type, and duration, postictal events and their duration, automatisms, seizure clusters, known patterns, warnings, tongue biting, incontinence, resulting injuries, and functional impairment. Those in current use, reviewed by Cramer and French (2001),[1311] include the **VA, Chalfont-National Hospital, Liverpool, Hague**, and Occupational Hazard Scales.

seizures induced by movement See **paroxysmal kinesigenic choreoathetosis**.

seizures with multiple independent spike foci An epileptic syndrome seen in younger children, characterized by the frequent occurrence of polymorphic bilateral seizures, including generalized atonic-clonic seizures, myoclonic jerks, atypical absences and tonic or clonic bilateral motor seizures, or partial motor seizures, associated with neurological signs, including mental retardation. Three or more spike foci are recorded in both hemispheres on the EEG.[688]

seizures Combinations of motor, sensory, and psychical events occurring as the result of occasional, sudden, rapid, local, and excessive discharges of gray matter (after J. Hughlings-**Jackson**).

selective amnesia A restricted failure of memory resulting from unilateral damage to the limbic system. The defect resulting is material-specific (verbal or nonverbal), according to the side of the lesion.

selective attention evoked potential A negative potential shift recorded from scalp electrodes positioned at the vertex, lasting less than a second and occurring during directed attention to auditory, visual, or somatosensory stimuli presented from one side as opposed to the other.[4332]

selective neuronal necrosis Cellular damage following ischemia of selectively susceptible cells, usually due to cardiac arrest. The affected cells (for instance, of the hippocampus, striatum, or neocortex) show pyknosis, nuclear swelling, and cytoplasmic eosinophilic change.

selective neuronal vulnerability The variable response of certain neurons and of discrete areas of the brain to a generalized metabolic insult, such as hypoxia; to which, for example, the third, fifth, and sixth cortical cell layers, Sommers' sector of the hippocampus, the Purkinje, and basket cells of the cerebellum, and parts of the amygdala are especially sensitive, while the spinal cord is relatively immune.

selective saccadic palsy See **saccadic paralysis**.

selective signature dysgraphia A selective inability to sign one's name, in the absence of other cognitive disorders, first described by one of the original authors following his left parietal lesion.[5237]

selective sleep stage deprivation The process whereby the functions of rapid eye movement or nonrapid eye movement sleep are studied by repetitively waking the patient when such a stage is entered.

selenoproteins N (*SEPN1*) The structural bases of **rigid spine muscular dystrophy** and **multiminicore** disease. To establish the diagnosis, a muscle biopsy is required.[3454] See **limb girdle muscular dystrophy.**

self-grasping The grasping of one forearm with the other hand, a sign indicating the presence of a contralateral frontal or parietal lobe lesion.[5379]

self-induced photosensitive epilepsy See **photosensitive epilepsies**.

self-induced seizures Seizure precipitation employed as a displacement activity by normal or mentally impaired patients (usually children) to induce seizures in themselves, using flickering light, patterns, proprioceptive stimuli, or higher brain functions. Absences and myoclonic jerks are the seizure types most commonly self-induced; any GTCS occurring are usually accidental. The goal appears to be relief of tension and anxiety, and escape from a disturbing situation. The classic maneuver for self-induced photosensitive epilepsy is looking at a bright light source such as the sun and voluntarily passing the abducted fingers to and fro before the eyes ("*sunflower* syndrome").[4882]

sella turcica (Lat, a Turkish saddle) The fossa in the skull base within which lies the pituitary gland.

Selye syndrome See **general adaptation syndrome**.

Selye, Hans (1907–1952) Austrian physician, philosopher, and physiologist who trained in Vienna, Paris, Rome, and Prague. He emigrated to Canada and became director of the Institute of Experimental Medicine at the Université de Montréal. His philosophy was overt rather than institutional and it led (among other things) to his concept of the **general adaptation syndrome**.[5720]

semantic anomia See **anomia**.

semantic aphasia The term of Sir Henry **Head** for that form of speech disorder characterized by a disturbance in the capacity to comprehend and to retain the general significance of a word or phrase as part of a complete act of language. The single word may be understood, but its ultimate meaning within the context of the sentence is lost. It stems from a lesion of the supramarginal gyrus. The term is now seldom employed.[2814]

semantic dementia A fluent variety of **primary progressive aphasia** (**frontotemporal dementia**) in which patients lose semantic memory and the comprehension of the meaning of words but retain normal articulation and syntax, although their speech is rather "empty" due to anomia and thus reduced vocabulary. It is not modality-specific, so object naming, single-word comprehension, object categorization, identification of famous faces, environmental sound recognition, and use of objects may also be defective.[4681] Nonverbal memory is retained unless or until dementia supervenes. The most common pathological findings are those of frontotemporal degeneration with ubiquitin inclusions, often with motor neuron disease-type inclusions in the dentate gyrus and cerebral cortex.[5282]

semantic jargon Speech in which the correct words are replaced by those that are acceptable but semantically faulty in that context. This occurs in **transcortical** and **Wernicke aphasias**.

semantic memory A type of long-term memory comprising the store of all the information required in order to use language, including the words, their meanings, and what they represent; as well as grammatical, mathematical, and factual rules; and the names of objects, people, and places and related data.

semantic paralexia The substitution of synonyms for the written words read aloud.

semantic pragmatic syndrome A disorder of higher language processing leading to impairments in answering questions of the "why?" "when?" or "how?" type and in prosody and fluency, despite retention of phonological and syntactical skills, and the ability to answer questions of the yes/no variety. It was described first in hydrocephalic children.[6168]

semantic retrieval-organization syndrome A disorder of higher language processing leading to impairments in fluency due to difficulties in word finding and syntax, especially in elicited as opposed to spontaneous speech.

semantics 1. The meanings contained within words and phrases. For example, in English it would be unacceptable to say "bachelor's wife," since the phrase contains a contradiction in meaning. Further, the sentence "The baseball bat bit the girl" is unacceptable, because a baseball bat is an inanimate object.[3949, 6649] 2. The rules governing meaningful verbal dialogue; that branch of linguistics which deals with meaning.[1336]

semi- (Lat, half. The Greek form is *demi*).

semicircular canals The three curved, endolymph-containing channels situated at right angles to one another, which open into the utricle and saccule within and constitute the inner ear. They were described by Fallopius in 1561.

semilumar ganglion (Gr, half + moon) The main sensory ganglion (**Gasserian ganglion**) of the trigeminal nerve, lying on the medial end of the petrous portion of the temporal bone.

semimembranosus reflex See **internal hamstring reflex**.

Seminars in Neurology (*Semin Neurol*) A neurological review journal. Web site: http://www.thieme.com/SID1993373986839/journals/pubid2017629976.html.

seminoma-like tumor See **germinoma**.

semiotics (semantics) A system of symbols manipulated according to certain conventions, such as numbers, letters, Morse code, and chessmen.

semipurposeful automatisms See **sleepwalking**.

semitendinosus reflex Contraction of this muscle in response to a tap on its tendon on the medial side of the popliteal fossa. The reflex has little clinical importance, although the biceps femoris reflex is of value since it informs uniquely about the state of the L5 reflex arc. The tendon of this latter muscle is on the lateral side of the popliteal fossa.

Semliki forest encephalitis Direct infection of the brain by an alphavirus member of the togavirus class of arboviruses, occurring in southern and eastern Africa.

Semon, Sir Felix (1849–1921) German–English laryngologist who trained in Heidelberg and Berlin but went to England in 1875 and practiced in London, where he worked at the **National Hospital** and other hospitals and collaborated with **Horsley**. He showed that adductor paralysis of the larynx could be due to psychosomatic states, myasthenia, or other muscle diseases, and that nerve lesions affecting the larynx affected the abductors first.

Semon's law The abductor fibers of the recurrent laryngeal nerve are affected by disease sooner than the adductor fibers. Thus, with partial lesions of the vagus (recurrent laryngeal) nerve, the paretic cord tends to lie in a position of adduction.[5722]

Semont liberatory maneuver (maneuvre libératoire) A technique for relieving the symptoms of **benign positional vertigo**[5723] (see Chart S–3). See also modified **Epley maneuver**.

Senator disease See **polymyositis**.

Senator, Hermann (1834–1911) American neurologist.

Sener syndrome The co-occurrence of frontonasal dysplasia and dilated **Virchow–Robin spaces**.[3975]

Senger syndrome A congenital dysmorphic syndrome inherited as an X-linked recessive trait and characterized by obesity, short stature, hypogenitalism, hydrocephalus, and mental and developmental delay.[381]

senile chorea A rare condition of later life characterized by the appearance of generalized and progressive chorea which is unaccompanied by mental changes or any family history of **Huntington disease**,[112] although the pathological changes in the caudate nucleus are similar.

senile dementia of the Alzheimer type See **Alzheimer disease**.

senile dementia of the Binswanger type See **Binswanger disease**.

senile dementia See **Alzheimer disease**.

senile gait See **cautious gait**.

senile macular degeneration Bilateral retinal degenerative changes, including the formation of subretinal fibrovascular plaques, hemorrhages, pigmentation, and proliferative retinopathy, occurring as an age-related change in the macular region as a result of microvascular disease.

senile plaques See **neuritic plaques**. They were regarded by Rio Hortega as resembling rooks' nests in winter elms.

Chart S–3. The Semont Liberatory Maneuver

1.A. Starting with the patient sitting straight up on the examining table, swing the patient down quickly, with the offending ear down and the head "slightly declined." If the nystagmus appears (it should be torsional with the fast phase beating toward the down ear), keep the patient there until the nystagmus disappears and then wait another 2–3 min.

1.B. If the nystagmus doesn't appear in A, turn the patient's head so that the face is up 45° from the horizontal. The nystagmus should then appear. Again, keep the patient in this position for 2–3 min after the nystagmus ceases.

2. Hold the patient's head and neck with both hands and swing the patient quickly to the opposite side. The speed of the head must be zero at the moment it touches the examining table.

3.A. If you are dealing with a classic case of benign positional paroxysmal vertigo (BPPV), a rotatory nystagmus will develop with the fast phase still beating toward the offending ear (the top ear). If it is beating toward the down ear, all bets are off and you are not dealing with BPPV. The typical BPPV nystagmus generally has a greater amplitude but lower frequency than the nystagmus with the bad ear down.

3.B. If no nystagmus develops after the turn to the opposite ear, move the head slowly to 90° facing up, and then turn the head in the opposite direction 135° so that it is 45° facing down below the horizontal (with the sick ear up). The nystagmus should then occur.

3.C. Hold the patient in the nystagmus-inducing position for at least 5 min and then bring the patient back to a sitting position "very, very slowly."

4. Have the patient keep the head absolutely vertical during the next 48 h, day and night. See the instructions to patients, below.

5. After the 48-h interval, patients are prohibited from sleeping on their vertigo-generating side for a week. If the maneuver is not successful, it is performed again a week later.

There is an 84% positive success rate with one maneuver and 90% positive success rate after a second maneuver 1 week later. The recurrence rate is 4.2%.

Instructions to patients after the liberatory maneuver: Whatever the position of your body, you must keep your head vertical for the next 48 h. Imagine your head being hung by an invisible string to the ceiling. You must not bend your head forward or backward. You must not go to the barber, hairdresser, or dentist. No exercise. When men shave under their chins, they should bend the body forward in order to tense the skin and keep the head vertical. Do not instill eyedrops. Only shampoo when under the shower. At night, lie on your back with plenty of pillows to keep your head vertical while your trunk is 30°–45° elevated off the bed. Put something at the bottom of the bed in order not to slip down during the night.

From Semont A, Freyss G, Vitte E. Curing the BPPV with a liberatory maneuver. Adv Otorhinolaryngol *1988;42:290–3. Permission sought from Karger, Basel.*

senile psychosis A term which is irritating due to the use of the word *senile* and imprecise because of use of the word *psychosis*, but which is used variously to refer to the dementias of later life and for presbyophrenia (a paranoid state probably arising from a depressive illness in elderly people).

senile thenar atrophy A focal muscle atrophy described by Marie and Foix well before the delineation of the **carpal tunnel syndrome**, which is the usual cause.

senile A pejorative term of no clinical worth, there being no known physical alteration affecting people at the time of their 65th birthday. Even the euphemistic term "of later life" is preferable to this author.

Senior–Loken syndrome (familial retinal–renal dystrophy) A rare, recessively inherited syndrome characterized by pigmentary retinal degeneration with visual failure, psychomotor retardation, anemia, and renal impairment leading eventually to renal failure.[5664] Both congenital and adult forms are described—the latter of lesser severity and longer course.

sensation,cortical Modes of awareness depending upon the presence of the analytic powers of the cortex. These include **graphesthesia, stereognosis, tactile discrimination**, and **tactile localization**.

sense of obstacles See **facial vision of the blind**.

Sensenbrenner syndrome See **craniosynostosis**.

sensitivity The ratio of the input voltage to the output pen deflection in an EEG channel, measured in microvolts/millimeter (μV/mm). Thus:

$$\text{Sensitivity} = \frac{\text{input voltage}}{\text{output trace deflection}} = \frac{50\ \mu V}{10\ mm} = 5\ \mu V/mm$$

(After Noachtar S, et al. A glossary of terms most commonly used by clinical electroencephalographers. *EEG Clin Neurophysiol* 1999;52[Suppl]:21–41. Reproduced by kind permission of the IFCN and Elsevier science.)

sensitization A state of heightened activity within neural receptor pathways involving spontaneous neuronal activity, a lowered threshold for activation, and an increased response to stimuli. This is one of the pathophysiological bases for central pain, including that of migraine.

sensorimotor perineuritis A rare sensorimotor peripheral neuropathy with prominent motor deficits, accompanied by marked slowing of nerve conduction velocities, histological evidence of inflammatory perineurial thickening, and deposits of immunoglobulin G and M on perineurial cells.[772] See also **sensory perineuritis** and **gammopathic neuropathy**.

sensorimotor psychological syndrome Hemianesthesia with psychological and motor disturbances accompanied by visual, auditory, and vestibular symptoms including hallucinations, and involuntary movements, all affecting the same side of the body and considered by de Morsier to be due to some disturbance of the hypothalamic system.[1511]

sensorimotor stroke (thalamocapsular stroke) A **lacunar syndrome** characterized by the association of hemiparesis with hypesthesia or dysesthesia involving one side of the mouth and the arm on that side, or the whole of that side of the body. The site of the lesion is variable—it may be either deep in the basal ganglia or in the corona radiata.[6701]

sensorineural deafness Deafness resulting from genetic, neoplastic, inflammatory, vascular, traumatic, or other lesions of the cochlear branches of the auditory nerves. Such deafness may also complicate systemic autoimmune diseases, and autoimmunity has been proposed as the basis of some cases of **Ménière disease** and acute vertigo.

sensorium commune The entire central nervous system—the common seat of the mechanism of sensation. See also **sensus communis**.

sensory and autonomic neuropathy A rare syndrome characterized by features otherwise typical of progressing **hereditary sensory and autonomic neuropathy,** but with onset during adult life and without the appearance of the disease in other family members.[4780]

sensory aprosodia An inability to perceive the emotive content of language heard, despite retention of normal spontaneous affective prosodic variation and gesture. It is a sign of a right parietotemporal lesion[5418] (inferior divisional infarction of the right middle cerebral artery). See **aprosodia**.

sensory ataxia (proprioceptive ataxia) Awkwardness of voluntary movements as a result of impaired conscious proprioception. The syndrome is characterized by poor directional control of movement, made worse by eye closure, **fantaisiste ataxia**, and disorganization of movement rather than true incoordination. An inherited form of this condition is mapped to 8p12, *SNAX1*. See also **Biemond ataxia**.

sensory ataxia–optic atrophy syndrome A nutritional disorder resulting from vitamin B complex (B_1, B_2, B_3, B_5, and B_6) deficiency.[6583] The leading clinical features are sensory ataxia due to peripheral neuropathy and visual failure with optic atrophy.

sensory ataxic ganglionopathies See **paraneoplastic syndromes**, **Sjögren syndrome**, and **sensory ganglionitis**.

sensory ataxic neuropathy with anti-GD1b antibodies (CANOMAD—Chronic Ataxic Neuropathy Ophthalmoplegia M-protein Agglutination Disialosyl antibodies—syndrome) An acquired sensory neuropathy with adult onset characterized by slowly progressive distal, symmetrical sensory loss affecting all modalities in all four limbs, with paresthesias and areflexia but usually without weakness. A sensory ataxic gait and positive Rombergism, ophthalmoplegia (50–90%) perioral paresthesias IgM protein (κ or λ) levels are elevated, as is the ESR and CSF protein. Sensory potentials are absent and motor conduction velocities normal or mildly reduced.

A *variant* is *acute ataxic sensory neuropathy* following *C. jejuni* infection and presenting with sensory loss mainly affecting large fibers, paresthesias, sensory ataxia, and areflexia within 3 weeks of the infection. Complete recovery may occur over months. Polyclonal IgG antibodies to GD1b are detectable in the serum and the CSF protein levels may be raised. SNAP amplitudes are reduced but their conduction velocity is normal.

sensory ataxic neuropathy, dysarthria, and ophthalmparesis See SANDO. See also **chronic inflammatory demyelinating neuropathies** (*sensory ataxic neuropathy with anti-GD1b antibodies*).

sensory aura In the context of epilepsy, a perceptual experience not caused by appropriate external stimuli.

sensory chronic inflammatory demyelinating neuropathy A variant of **chronic inflammatory demyelinating neuropathy** presenting with distal painful pansensory loss, minimal if any distal weakness, and typical electrical evidence of demyelination.[5526] See Dr. Alan Pestronk's Web site at: http://www.wustl.edu/neuromuscular/.

sensory competition A sign of parietal lobe dysfunction. The inability to appreciate one of two stimuli presented simultaneously. The test is most often performed with bilateral stimulation, but double stimuli on the one side may also show an abnormality wherein only one is perceived though each is appreciated when presented in isolation. See **extinction**.

sensory dermatomes The area of skin supplied by a single sensory root. Overlap on the trunk makes the determination of the dermatomes difficult, but the areas supplied in the limbs are relatively constant, and the overlap between segments is much less.

sensory end-organ An apparatus by which a sensory nerve fiber is rendered distinctly amenable to some particular physical agent, and at the same time rendered less amenable to (i.e., is shielded from) other excitants (Sir Charles **Sherrington**). The definition thus accepts both the concepts of receptor specificity and of the adequate stimulus.

sensory fusion The ability to fuse two retinal images together using cerebral cortical mechanisms.

sensory ganglionitis (autoimmune ataxic neuropathies; sensory ataxic ganglionopathies) Immune-mediated disorders in which inflammatory changes affect the dorsal root ganglia and lead to the clinical picture of sensory axonal neuropathy. It may occur as a **paraneoplastic syndrome**, in the **sicca syndrome**, and in **idiopathic sensory neuronopathy**. Toxic, deficiency, and hereditary causes are also described. Clinically, losses of thick fiber function lead to prominent sensory ataxia with loss of motor control.[4736]

See also **Miller-Fisher syndrome, acute demyelinating neuropathy, chronic idiopathic ataxic neuropathy, chronic inflammatory dysimmune polyneuropathy, hereditary sensory and autonomic neuropathy**, and **olivopontocerebellar atrophy**.

sensory inattention See **inattention**.

sensory Jacksonian seizures Attacks of paresthesia occurring spasmodically in a certain part of the body and spreading in a certain order, not always in keeping with the accepted geography of the sensory homunculus on the postcentral gyrus. According to Arnold **Pick**, the term was first employed by Krafft-Ebing, who described sensory paralytic attacks in his book on **general paresis**.

sensory latency The interval between the onset of a stimulus and the onset of the negative deflection of the compound sensory nerve action potential. This term has been used loosely to refer to the sensory peak latency. It may be qualified as proximal sensory latency or distal sensory latency, depending on the relative position of the stimulus. (From the 2001 Report of the Nomenclature Committee of the American Association of Electromyography and Electrodiagnosis.[19] Reproduced by kind permission of the AANEM.)

sensory loss See **alternating, cortical, hysterical, suspended**, and **thalamic sensory loss**.

sensory modalities Different sensory perceptions, mediated by patterns of neuronal input which vary in time and space but which are not exclusively associated with a particular afferent pathway. The ascription of pain and temperature function to the spinothalamic tract thus is but a convenient approximation.

sensory nerve action potential (SNAP) See **compound sensory nerve action potential**.

sensory nerve conduction velocity The speed of propagation of action potentials along a sensory nerve.

sensory nerve A nerve containing only sensory fibers, composed mainly of axons innervating cutaneous and joint receptors.

sensory neuron diseases Conditions characterized by the primary degeneration of the dorsal root ganglion cells, resulting in degeneration of their short and long peripheral axons and of their afferent projections in the posterior columns. The hereditary and acquired (paraneoplastic, immune-mediated, infective, iatrogenic, vitamin-related, and idiopathic) forms have been reviewed.[5748] See **hereditary sensory and autonomic neuropathy, Fabry disease, Tangier disease, Biemond ataxia, cerebellar ataxias, NARP syndrome, SANDO**, and **PCARP**.

sensory neuronopathy See **subacute sensory neuropathy**.

sensory neuropathy with hereditary ataxia See **hereditary sensory and autonomic neuropathy** (*variants*).

sensory neuropathy A group of diseases characterized by the primary degeneration (axonal or demyelinating) of peripheral sensory nerve fibers. See also **sensory neuron diseases**.

sensory paralytic bladder Afferent denervation of the bladder, with anesthesia, dilatation, retention, and overflow incontinence but without loss of the ability to initiate micturition consciously. Lesions of the pelvic nerves or of the posterior columns may be responsible.

sensory peak latency Interval between the onset of a stimulus and the peak of the negative phase of the compound sensory nerve action potential.

sensory perineuritis A sensory peripheral neuropathy or multiple mononeuropathy with the pathological finding of chronic inflammatory and fibrotic changes limited to the perineurium of the affected nerves. Clinically, patients complain of pain and sensory loss in a glove-and-stocking distribution. No systemic disease is detected and the cause is not known,[260] but the condition may respond to steroid therapy. See also **migrant sensory neuritis** and **sensorimotor perineuritis**.

sensory starts Sudden paroxysmal awareness of stimulation of one sensory channel on falling asleep; the sensory equivalent to **hypnic jerks**.

sensory system All of the afferent pathways informing the organism about the disposition of the internal and external environments.

sensory tics Uncomfortable, involuntary, transient, and recurrent somatic sensations felt in the skin and relieved only by vocalization or other movements in **Tourette syndrome**. They are variously described as feelings of pressure, tickle, warmth, cold, or other sensations and are usually localized to the upper half of the body.[5758, 1124] See also **restless limb syndrome**.

sensory trick See **geste antagonistique**.

sensus communis (sensorium commune) A primary faculty of perception. The gathering of all specific sense impressions to allow the appreciation of magnitude, motion, and time, according to Aristotle. This overall appreciative sense was termed **coenesthesis** by Reil in 1794, who noted its obscure, immediate, compound nature and considered it to be the basis for self-awareness and personal identity, localized somewhere (he knew not where and nor do we) in the cerebrum.

sentinel headache (warning headache) An acute head pain, usually felt posteriorly and resembling the pain of **subarachnoid hemorrhage**, though less severe and commonly lasting for less time. The pathogenesis is, however, the leaking of blood into the CSF, usually from an aneurysm, and the headache demands the same attention and management as does the full-blown condition, as catastrophic rupture of an aneurysm may follow at any time.

SEPs See **somatosensory evoked potentials**.

septic aneurysm See **mycotic aneurysm**.

septic embolism An infected embolus occluding an artery. The consequences of this include infarction or septic infarction of the territory supplied by that vessel; a focal arteritis which may spread into surrounding tissues to cause (in the brain) a local cerebral abscess or focal meningitis; and weakening of the vessel wall, which may lead on to the formation of a **mycotic aneurysm**.

septic encephalopathy (sepsis-associated encephalopathy) A heterogeneous syndrome of altered consciousness with paratonia and impairments in attention, orientation, concentration, and writing, occurring early in the course of systemic (not CNS) sepsis, trauma, or burns, with multiple organ dysfunction ("critical illness") developing later. Frank delirium occurs later still. Focal or multifocal seizures, multifocal myoclonus, cranial nerve palsies, and asterixis are *not* typical clinical features of the condition. The syndrome is normally detected through CSF analysis and imaging studies but not by the EEG findings. See also **systemic inflammatory response syndrome**.

The underlying mechanisms include **central pontine myelinolysis**, microabscesses, microhemorrhages, multiple cerebral infarctions, and direct toxic or metabolic causes.[3119, 6814]

septic myopathies Disorders of muscle complicating severe septic illnesses and possibly burns and severe trauma. These include cachexia, which commonly occurs; myositis and myoglobinuria due to panfascicular muscle fiber necrosis, and **acute suppurative myositis** (a condition of multiple purulent abscesses within muscles) occur rarely.[731]

septo-optic dysplasia (OMIM 182230) A rare congenital syndrome, sometimes recessively inherited, characterized by hypoplasia of the optic nerve, hypoglycemia, hypopituitarism, seizures, small sella turcica, cavum septi pellucidi, and both physical growth retardation and psychomotor delay.[682]

Callosal abnormalities, schizencephaly, hydrocephalus, encephalocele, and cerebral atrophy have also been reported in this syndrome.[379] See **de Morsier syndrome**.

septum pellucidum (septum lucidum) A thin membrane between the fornix and the corpus callosum, first described by Galen.

sequential ultrasonic arteriography A technique whereby either pulsed or continuous-wave Doppler sonography is used to construct an image of blood vessels, disease being detected by the finding of defects in the image itself and by spectral analysis (as in duplex ultrasonography). The method accurately identifies severe disease, but is insensitive to minor lesions.[4678]

SERCA1 and calsequestrin storage myopathy A mild surplus protein myopathy, sometimes actually asymptomatic, with elevated serum CK levels. Muscle biopsy shows inclusions of different sizes and shapes.[6346]

Serial Digit Ordering Test A test of **working memory**.

serial recitation tests Tests of attention, wherein the subject is required to count in 3s, to subtract numbers serially (serial sevens), or to recite the days or months in forward or reverse order.

serial seizures A series of epileptic attacks in which consciousness is regained between each.[72]

serotonin receptors Receptors present in both cerebral blood vessels and in central pain pathways. 5-HT1a, 1b, 1c, and 5-HT2 sites are identified with certainty, and more are likely to be detected.

serotonin syndrome A syndrome resulting from central serotonergic hyperstimulation, typically as a result of combining serotonergic drugs with monoamineoxidase inhibitors (MAOIs). It may also occur when combinations of L-tryptophan, clomipramine, bromocriptine, levadopa, demerol, or dextromorphan are given at the same time as MAOIs, carbamazepine, pentacozine, or SSRIs due to enhancement of serotonin activity through blockade of its reuptake, thus increasing presynaptic release.

Clinically, it is characterized by mental status and behavioral changes (agitation, excitement, confusion, hypomania, and obtundation), motor system involvement (myoclonus, hemiballismus, tremor, hyperreflexia, motor weakness, dysarthria, akathisia, and incoordination) and autonomic symptoms (fever, chills, diarrhea, hypotension, tachycardia, sweating, and shivering). The syndrome has been reported exclusively in patients on medications for psychiatric illness and Parkinsonism, and in those taking one or more serotonomimetic agents for migraine prophylaxis (sertraline, paroxetine, lithium, imipramine, amitriptyline) or acute therapy (a triptan or dihydroergotamine). Typical combinations of drugs reported to produce the syndrome include L-tryptophan and SSRIs or MAOIs; SSRIs and carbamazepine, pentacozine, or MAOIs (or alone); venlafaxine and MAOIs; clomipramine and MAOIs (or alone); Bromocriptine and levadopa; and demerol or dextromorphan and MAOIs. Lithium worsens all features of the syndrome.

Symptoms are usually transient with full recovery on withdrawal of the responsible agents; but high fever, nystagmus, oculogyric crises, dysarthria, pyramidal syndrome, myoglobinuria, renal failure, disseminated intravascular coagulation, cardiac arrhythmias, and death have been reported, rarely.[4165, 697] The following diagnostic criteria have been determined:[6045, 6046]

1. The symptoms must coincide with the introduction or dosage increment of a known serotonomimetic agent.
2. At least three of the following signs and symptoms must be present:

Mental status changes (confusion or hypomania)	Agitation
Myoclonus	Hyperreflexia
Diaphoresis	Shivering
Tremor	Diarrhea
Poor coordination	Fever

3. Other etiologies must be ruled out, such as infection, metabolic disturbance, and substance abuse or withdrawal.
4. **Neuroleptic malignant syndrome** should be excluded from the differential diagnosis (a neuroleptic agent should not have been initiated or increased in dose prior to the onset of signs and symptoms).

serotonin 5-Hydroxytryptamine (5-HT), a vasoactive (variously constrictor or dilator) substance which is also involved in mood, appetite, sleep, and pain pathways.

serous meningitis (minor pseudomeningitis) See **idiopathic intracranial hypertension**. The term is now largely discarded, though once it was used to denote meningeal irritation without evidence of such in the CSF and so usually indicated the presence of a parameningeal focus of inflammation or a nonpurulent (lymphocytic) meningitis.

serpinopathies Malfunction of serine proteinase inhibitors (serpins) that normally inhibit proteinolysis. They are released in the CNS as part of the inflammatory response. Levels are raised in **Alzheimer disease** and in Lewy body disease.

serrated action potential A waveform with several changes in direction (turns) which do not cross the baseline. Most often used to describe a motor unit action potential. The term is preferred to complex motor unit action potential and pseudopolyphasic action potential. See also **turn** and **polyphasic action potential**.[19]

serum sickness A form of hypersensitivity vasculitis. Neurological complications may include encephalopathy with coma and seizures, brachial plexopathy, and (rarely) symmetrical peripheral neuropathy.[1702]

Set test A test of verbal fluency in which subjects are asked to name as many examples as they can recall in each of four categories—animals, colors, fruits, and towns—to a maximum of ten each; scores of under 15 are considered to indicate a loss of verbal fluency.[3098]

setting sun sign Tonic downward deviation of the eyes in association with retraction of the upper lid (**Collier sign**); a sign of compression of the dorsal midbrain, as in infants with hydrocephalus.

setting-in nystagmus See **gaze-evoked nystagmus**.

Seven Minute screen A sensitive screening tool to help identify patients who merit evaluation for Alzheimer disease, using a series of questions to assess different types of intellectual functionality and claimed to be able to distinguish between cognitive changes due to the normal aging process and those due to dementia.[4337]

Four tests are included, as follows: *temporal orientation* (awareness of the current year, month, date, day of the week, and time); *memory* (cued recall of 16 pictures presented four at a time on individual "flash cards." A cue is offered when the patient is asked to recall each set of pictures: While healthy individuals benefit from this hint, persons with Alzheimer disease do not); *clock drawing*, in which the subjects are asked to draw the face of a clock, with the hands set to 3.40 p.m.; and *verbal (category) fluency*, in which the subject is asked to name as many items as possible in a specific category (such as "vegetables") within 1 min. The test is available at http://www.7minutescreen.com/html/works.html.

Despite the name, the test takes about 12 min to complete.

severe childhood autosomal recessive muscular dystrophy (SCARMD; OMIM 253700) A polygenic, recessively inherited form of congenital muscular dystrophy (an **adhalinopathy or dystrophinopathy**) resembling **Duchenne dystrophy** except for its autosomal recessive inheritance pattern. All components of the sarcoglycan complex are absent in the muscles.[4844] The condition is mapped variously to 13q and 17q.

For a confident diagnosis, the parents of the subject should be healthy and consanguineous and their male and female children should exhibit calf pseudohypertrophy and other DMD-like symptoms. See also **autosomal recessive muscular dystrophy** and **limb–girdle muscular dystrophy**.

severe congenital encephalopathy A fatal familial disease due to a primary disorder of axonal development, leading to a reduction in interneuronal synaptic contacts. Clinically, a profound disorder of mental and motor development, hypotonia, secondary microcephaly, and agenesis of the corpus callosum are characteristic features; necrotizing myopathy, cardiomyopathy, cataracts, and failure to thrive are others.[3977]

Severe Impairment battery A scheme for assessing the retained capabilities of patients with advanced dementia using simple verbal commands with gestural reinforcement.[5570]

severe infantile multifocal epilepsy An epileptic encephalopathy associated with *SCN1A* mutations, characterized clinically by early-onset multifocal seizures and later cognitive decline.[2769]

severe infantile neuraminic acid storage disease, French type See **sialuria**.

severe infantile neuropathy with diaphragmatic weakness
1. The early onset of diaphragmatic palsy in association with a progressive neuropathy and due to mutations in a gene encoding the immunoglobulin μ-binding protein.
2. Suggestive diagnostic features are the early onset of respiratory compromise, a markedly low birth weight, very slow motor nerve conduction velocities and a decrease in the size of myelinated fibres on sural nerve biopsy.[5039]

severe infantile sialidosis See **nephrosialidosis**.

severe muscular dystrophy in girls A rare, recessively inherited condition in which there is severe muscular dystrophy presenting in infancy or early childhood with delayed motor milestones, predominant early toe-walking, more weakness of the deltoid muscles, and a slower and milder course than in the case of **Duchenne dystrophy**. There is no cardiac involvement. The distribution and nature of the other symptoms are similar to those of Duchenne dystrophy, but the serum CK levels are raised only to between 7 and 70 times the normal levels.[2278]

severe myoclonic epilepsy of infancy (Dravet syndrome) A rare, early childhood encephalopathy, the characteristics of which include normal development before onset, prolonged and repeated febrile and afebrile generalized or unilateral convulsive seizures, early photosensitivity beginning during the first year of life, and myoclonic jerks. Psychomotor development is retarded from the second year of life onward and ataxia, pyramidal signs, and interictal myoclonus appear, accompanied by psychotic or autistic traits and by hyperactivity.

This type of epilepsy is very resistant to all forms of treatment.[6851, 4882] The EEG shows generalized spike–waves and polyspike-waves, a photoparoxysmal response, and focal abnormalities. The condition is a sodium channelopathy, often with mutations of *SCN1A*. See also **myoclonus**.

severe postural cerebellar tremor See **cerebellar tremors**.

sex-linked diseases See X-Linked diseases.

Seyffrath syndrome See **pronator teres syndrome**.

SFEMG See **single fiber electromyography**.

shadow plaque Incomplete staining of newly formed myelin in a plaque of **multiple sclerosis** in the brain.

shagreen patch A roughened and pitted area of skin with an orange peel or pigskin texture, overlying a region of subepidermal fibrosis, usually in lumbosacral regions; a diagnostic finding in **tuberous sclerosis** manifesting after the age of 2 years.

shaken infant syndrome An encephalopathy resulting from shaking injuries that caused cortical and subcortical contusions, hemorrhages, hypoxic or ischemic and axonal damage, and/or severe edema. These findings, however, usually resolve within 6 months but may result in multicystic encephalomalacia, porencephaly, generalized white matter attenuation, diffuse cortical atrophy, microgyria, ulegyria, and hydrocephalus ex vacuo, progressive cortical dysplasia with cytoarchitectural disorganization, laminar obliteration, morphologic, and functional (synaptic reorganization) neurofilament immunoreactivity.[4079]

shaking palsy The term applied by Dr. James **Parkinson** to what is now known as **Parkinson disease**.

shaky legs syndrome See **orthostatic tremor**.

sham mirth Release of the controlling mechanisms for activity of the laughter centre (wherever that is) in the absence of the appropriate stimulus, usually either as a manifestation of epilepsy or in cases of bilateral pyramidal tract disease, sometimes actually before the establishment of a stroke or subarachnoid hemorrhage (*Le fou rire prodromique* of Féré, 1903). While the precise anatomy of the lesions is unclear, the hypothalamus appears to be involved in most cases.[4118] See **spasmodic laughter**.

sham rage A state in which an animal deprived of its cerebral hemispheres (or of the amygdaloid nuclei, bilaterally) reacts to all stimuli with the behavioral and autonomic manifestations of extreme anger.

Shapiro syndrome See **corpus callosum agenesis with recurrent hypothermia**.

shark mouth The appearance of the upper lip of some children with **myotonic dystrophy**, the lip being tented upward like a circumflex accent.

sharp wave A transient wave on the EEG clearly distinguished from background activity, with a pointed peak at conventional paper speeds and with a duration of 70–200 ms. Its main component is generally negative relative to other areas and its amplitude is variable. The term applies neither to distinctive physiologic events such as **vertex sharp transients, lambda waves**, and **positive occipital sharp transients of sleep** nor to sharp transients poorly distinguished from background activity, nor to sharp-appearing individual waves of EEG rhythms.

Sharp waves should be differentiated from spikes—that is, transients having similar characteristics but shorter duration—but this distinction is largely arbitrary and serves primarily descriptive purposes. Practically, in ink-written EEG records obtained at 3 cm/s, sharp waves occupy more than 2 mm of paper width and spikes 2 mm or less. See also **spike**. (Adapted from the 1974 report of the Committee on Terminology, IFCN. In: Chatrian GE, Bergamini L, Dondey M, et al. A glossary of terms most commonly used by clinical electroencephalographers.

EEG Clin Neurophysiol 1974;37:538–48. Reproduced with kind permission from Elsevier Science.)

sharp-and-slow-wave complex The sequence of a sharp wave and a slow wave recorded on the EEG, especially as a characteristic of **absence seizures**. The hyphenation facilitates the use of the term in the plural form: sharp-and-slow-wave complexes or sharp-and-slow-waves.

shawl sign Erythema of the chest, neck ("V-sign") and upper back in **dermatomyositis**.

shearing injury See **diffuse axonal injury**.

sheathing The appearance of the retinal veins in some cases of sarcoid or multiple sclerosis, in which the veins are outlined by a white streak on either side as a result of preceding periphlebitis.

Sheehan syndrome Postpartum pituitary necrosis leading to the cessation of lactation, amenorrhea, and hypopituitarism, described by H.L.D. Sheehan (b. 1900), professor of pathology at Liverpool.[5774]

shell shock (acute stress disorder) A clinical spectrum of neuropsychiatric conditions ranging from concussion to sheer funk and including confusion, "hysteria," neurasthenia (acute war neurosis), exhaustion, and malingering.[4007] See **Brissaud syndrome**.

shellfish poisoning See **paralytic shellfish poisoning, neurotoxic shellfish poisoning, amnesic shellfish poisoning**, and **dianthetic shellfish poisoning**.

Sherlock epiloia See **tuberous sclerosis**.

Sherrington, Sir Charles (1857–1952) English physiologist, linguist, philosopher, and poet, "the most profound student of the nervous system that the world has yet known" (Fulton), educated at Cambridge and St. Thomas' Hospital, and later in Spain, Italy, and Germany. His physiological studies began while he was an undergraduate working with Langley and were continued while he was on the staff at St. Thomas' Hospital in London, then at the University of Liverpool (where **Cushing** learned from him) and, from the age of 56, as Waynflete Professor of Physiology at Oxford. He was elected a fellow of the Royal Society in 1893 on the basis of his work on nerve roots and reflexes and was its president from 1920 to 1925. He was knighted in 1922 and with E.D. (Lord) Adrian, was awarded the Nobel Prize for medicine in 1932 for his studies of the physiology of the nervous system.

The central problem which motivated him was, in the words of **Denny-Brown**, "how the relationship between a network of myriads of nerve cells and fibers, each functioning in terms of transmitting nerve impulses, could develop the properties of self-awareness, mind and memory . . . . The conclusion was that a dualism between nerve function and mind is a natural mystery, insoluble by prevailing scientific knowledge." Starting with anatomical studies of dermatomes and myotomes, he quickly branched into neurophysiology, discovering or illuminating (and often naming) reciprocal innervation, decerebrate rigidity, inhibitory reflex effects, the final common pathway, cortical reactivity, synaptic activity (he coined the term *synapse* in 1897), excitation, and inhibition.

He was the first to investigate the proprioceptive system in depth. In his studies of sensory functions, he introduced the terms *exteroception, enteroception,* and *nocioception*. His analysis of **decerebrate rigidity** paralleled that of **Magnus**, while his stimulation and ablation experiments on the cortex were at least as precise as those of clinical scientists such as **Ferrier** and **Horsley**.

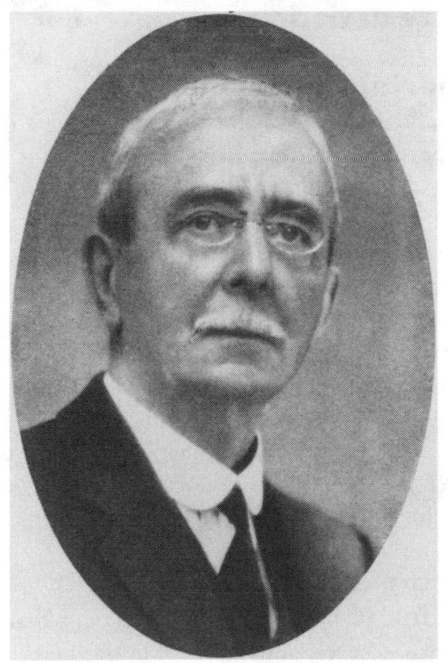

Figure S–3 Sir Charles Scott Sherrington

He regarded the brain as a manager of muscle, a thoroughfare for nerve action passing on its way to the motor animal, and an input–output signalling system.[5789] His view that the function of the brain was to coordinate the activities of the rest of the organism and his studies on decerebrate rigidity,[5786] reciprocal innervation, and cortical reactivity were all summarized in his book *The Integrative Action of the Nervous System* (published in 1906 but still a classic neurophysiology text,[5787]) as is his *Selected Writings*, edited by **Denny-Brown** (London, 1939).[5790]

At the end of his academic life and in retirement, he published books of verse and of literary criticism as well as biographies of Goethe and of Jean Fernel.[1803]

Sherrington's law The posterior spinal nerves supply their own skin territories but overlap with adjacent territories.

shift-work sleep disorder A syndrome either of insomnia or of excessive sleepiness that occurs as a transient phenomenon in relation to altering work schedules (usually night work) with loss of the normal sleep–wake pattern (i.e., disturbed chronobiologic rhythmicity).[1629]

Shiga toxin A substance produced by some *Escherichia coli* strains capable of causing hemorrhagic colitis, hemolytic-uremic syndrome, and acute encephalopathy with severe autonomic dysfunction.

shingles (from Lat, cingulum, a belt) An English corruption, denoting the dermatomal spread of the painful rash of herpes zoster.

Shipley Institute of Living Scale A compound measure of global psychological functioning. The abstraction subtest examines verbal analogic reasoning, the subject being required to complete unfinished verbal series.[5807]

Shirres, David Alexander A Scottish physician, the first neurologist appointed as such in Canada (at the Montreal General Hospital in 1902) and the first physician anywhere to attempt spinal cord transplantation (performed in a person suffering from traumatic division of the cord, without success).[5327]

shock optic neuropathy Bilateral blindness resulting from optic atrophy; an unusual complication of shock and cardiorespiratory arrest as may result from increased intraocular pressure and low systemic perfusion pressure synergistically causing ischemia of the optic nerves.[1125]

Shokeir syndrome See **Pena-Shokeir phenotype**.

Shoni No Noshinkei (*Nervous System in Children*) A Japanese journal of pediatric neurology, founded in 1976.

Short Care Scale An instrument for the brief assessment of cognitive impairment and depression performed by interview.[3570]

short ciliary nerves Small myelinated postganglionic parasympathetic nerves running from the ciliary ganglion to the iris sphincter muscle.

Short Exercise Test A method of demonstrating transient weakness following physical rest in patients with myotonic syndromes. The hand is immobilized and the ulnar nerve stimulated every minute, the compound muscle action potential (CMAP) being recorded from the hypothenar muscles.

Maximum voluntary isometric exercise is performed for 10 s, the patient spreading the fingers maximally. The ulnar nerve is stimulated again after the exercise and again every 10 s for 1 min. Both the size of the evoked CMAP and twitch tension decrease as a result of this exercise, the detriment being caused by transient inexcitability of the muscle fiber membrane in the absence of any abnormality at the motor end plate itself.[6090, 6091]

Short Portable Mental Status questionnaire A formalized, short, bedside screening test for overall cognitive impairment, containing 10 items, with emphasis being placed on orientation and personal and remote memories. It is most suitable for the detection of the more disabled subjects but like similar tests has a substantial false-negative rate.[5009]

short rib-polydactyly (Majewski syndrome) A lethal, congenital dysmorphic syndrome manifesting these anomalies, in which numerous other skeletal, genital, and ocular abnormalities occur, accompanied by macrocephaly.[4034] Other short rib-polydactyly syndromes also occur, without notable neurological features.

short sleeper The condition in which a normal subject feels adequately refreshed by shorter periods of (normal pattern) sleep than are regarded as normal for age.[2788, 1629] See also **long sleeper**.

Short Wisconsin Card Sort A modified card sorting test sensitive to frontal lobe dysfunction.[4616] See **Wisconsin Card Sorting Test**.

short-chain acyl-coenzyme A dehydrogenase deficiency (SCHAD deficiency) A rare, genetically determined enzyme disorder of infancy; the genetic defect resulting in failure to thrive, developmental delay, episodic juvenile-onset recurrent myoglobinuria, hypoketotic hypoglycemic encephalopathy, myopathy, and hypertrophic cardiomyopathy triggered by fasting.[6244]

short-chain specific 3-ketothiolase defect See **beta-ketothiolase deficiency**.

short-cycle periodic alternating gaze deviation See **ping-pong gaze**.

shortening reaction 1. The paradoxical contraction of a muscle when it is passively shortened, described first by Westphal in 1877. The phenomenon is only commonly detected in patients with Parkinsonism, athetosis, dystonia, or cerebellar disease, but it is in fact present in normal subjects as well.[203] 2. A tonic contraction supervening on the initial contraction of, for example, the quadriceps when its tendon is tapped; this checks the momentum of the falling leg. The absence of such a reaction leads to unchecked swinging of the leg—the **pendular reflex**.

Short-Increment Sensitivity Index (SISI) An auditory test in which the subject responds to small (1 decibel) increments of an intermittent tone superimposed upon a background continuous tone at the same frequency. In normal subjects and those with retrocochlear lesions, such increments cannot be identified, but they can in those with cochlear lesions.

short-lasting unilateral neuralgiform headache attacks with conjunctival injection and tearing See SUNCT **syndrome**.

short-lasting unilateral neuralgiform headache attacks with cranial autonomic features See SUNA **syndrome.** A syndrome of brief orbital, supraorbital, or temporal head pains, migrating elsewhere in the cranium. Attack types include brief stabs or groups of stabs and saw-tooth attacks lasting between 1 min and 3 h with a mean attack frequency of 59/day (2–600). Conjunctival injection or tearing (not both) and nasal blockage, rhinorrhea, eyelid edema, facial sweating or flushing, and ear flushing occur. Agitation is common in the attacks.[7621] See also **red ear syndrome** and **short-lasting unilateral neuralgiform headache attacks with conjunctival injection and tearing.**

short-latency reflex A reflex with one (monosynaptic) or few (oligosynaptic) synapses used, in contrast to long-latency reflexes.

short-latency somatosensory evoked potential (SSEP) That portion of the waveforms of a somatosensory-evoked potential normally occurring within 25 ms after stimulation of the median nerve in the upper extremity at the wrist, and 40 ms after stimulation of the posterior tibial nerve in the popliteal fossa. (From the 2001 Report of the Nomenclature Committee of the American Association of Electromyography and Electrodiagnosis.[19] Reproduced by kind permission of the AANEM.) The characteristics of SSEPs in various nerves are summarized in Chart S–4.

short-period alternating nystagmus A benign and self-limited form of **periodic alternating nystagmus** with an unusually short (4–9 s) cycle, occurring in association with ataxia and dysarthria in patients with brainstem encephalitis.[5249]

Chart S–4. Short-Latency Somatosensory Evoked Potentials

1. *Median nerve SSEPs* Normal short-latency response components to median nerve stimulation are designated P9, P11, P13, P14, N20, and P23 in records taken between scalp and noncephalic reference electrodes, and N9, N11, N13, and N14 in a cervical spine–scalp derivation. Potentials having opposite polarity but similar latency in spine–scalp and scalp–noncephalic reference derivations do not necessarily have identical generator sources.
2. *Common peroneal nerve SSEPs* Normal short-latency response components to common peroneal stimulation are designated P27 and N35 in records taken between scalp and noncephalic reference electrodes, and L3 and T12 from a cervical spine–scalp derivation.
3. *Posterior tibial nerve SSEPs* Normal short-latency response components to posterior tibial nerve stimulation are designated as the PF potential in the popliteal fossa, P37 and N45 waves in records taken between scalp and noncephalic reference electrode, and L3 and T12 potentials from a cervical spine–scalp derivation.

Adapted from the 2001 Report of the Nomenclature Committee of the American Academy of Neuromuscular and Electrodiagnostic Medicine.[19] *Reproduced by kind permission of the AANEM.*

short-term memory (primary memory, immediate memory working memory) The present content of thought; the mental tasks which a person is currently working on or thinking about. In this form of memory, seven to nine words or objects are stored for immediate access, in order to allow other mental operations to proceed. If rehearsal is not allowed, significant decay occurs. Variable amounts of the material contained may be transferred to long-term memory stores, depending on their significance and on the amount of reinforcement given.

This term is not a synonym for *recent memory*, a nonspecific phrase used clinically.

shoulder girdle disk Weakness and wasting of shoulder girdle muscles, associated with cervical spondylosis producing cord compression at C3–4 or with root compression below this level.[5015]

shoulder girdle neuritis See **neuralgic amyotrophy**.

shoulder girdle syndrome See **neuralgic amyotrophy**.

shoulder-hand syndrome See **complex regional pain syndrome**.

Shprintzen–Goldberg syndrome A congenital craniofacial malformation syndrome, characterized also by skeletal and cardiac abnormalities, optic atrophy, strabismus, craniosynostosis with dolichocephaly, mitral valve prolapse, and mental and developmental delay.[4]

shuddering attacks in infants An uncommon movement disorder characterized by frequent, paroxysmal tremors of the head, elbows, trunk, and knees, with adduction of the arms and legs, but without alteration of consciousness or EEG abnormality, occurring in infants and young children who thereafter develop normally. They occur perhaps 100 times daily.[2966, 930] The cause is unknown, but ingestion of monosodium glutamate has been incriminated.

Shulman syndrome See **eosinophilic fasciitis**.

Shy, George Milton (1919–1967) American neurologist who trained in Oregon and, after the war, at the **National Hospital**, Queen Square, and at McGill University, Montreal. After a short period on the faculty at Oregon, he became the first clinical director of the NINCDS, of which institute he was later associate director. He was professor and chairman at the University of Pennsylvania and moved, just before his untimely death, to the College of Physicians and Surgeons of Columbia University.

He is best remembered for his discoveries or descriptions of a number of congenital myopathies, **idiopathic orthostatic hypotension**, and the **Kearns–Shy syndrome**; he edited and prepared for publication the first of the important books published in the last two decades relating to clinical and basic science neurology, but died suddenly, before its publication.

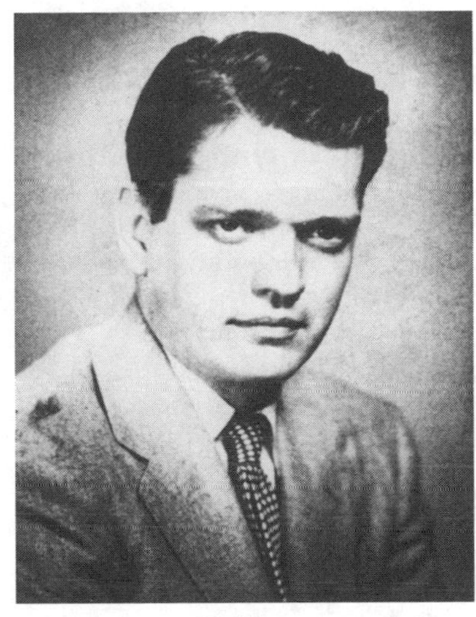

Figure S–4 George Milton Shy

Shy–Drager syndrome A constituent disorder within the group of diseases comprising **multiple system atrophy**, representing a progressive multisystem degeneration. Clinically, it presents as a combination of Parkinsonism and autonomic failure (orthostatic hypotension, anhidrosis, pupillary failure, loss of bladder and bowel sphincter function, and iris atrophy) in the presence of certain signs, such as unresponsiveness to levadopa and the existence of pyramidal or cerebellar signs, which are atypical for idiopathic **Parkinson** disease. Other signs noted include extraocular pareses, rigidity, and tremor, as well as evidence of damage to lower motor neurons.[5819] Pathologically, the condition is marked by neuronal loss in the intermediolateral cell columns, the substantia nigra, the striatum, and the cerebellum.

The syndrome is not identical to **spontaneous** (idiopathic) **orthostatic hypotension**, either alone or in combination with idiopathic **Parkinson disease** and autonomic signs.[5157, 5819] See also **progressive autonomic failure** and **Lewy body disease**.

The condition is named for the late Dr. G.M. Shy and for Dr. Glenn Drager, also an American neurologist. A review of their original paper suggests inconsistencies, leading to the suggestion that rectal incontinence, iris atrophy, gaze palsies, fasciculations, distal wasting, and evidence of lower motor neuron lesions should not be regarded as typical of the syndrome, which should encompass only autonomic failure, pyramidal and cerebellar signs, and Parkinsonism.[5160] The Web site http://healthlink.mcw.edu/article/921961623.html further describes the types, treatment, and prognosis of the condition.

Shy–Drager/Multiple System Atrophy Support Group, Inc. A charitable organization providing information and support in this field. Tel: 866-737-4999; 800-288-5582. E-mail: Don.Summers@shy-drager.com. Web site: http://www.shy-drager.com/.

Shy–Gonatas syndrome A form of complicated progressive external ophthalmoplegia with added ataxia, myopathy, and neuropathy, resembling **Kearns–Sayre syndrome**.[5821] See **mitochondrial myopathies**.

Shy–Magee syndrome See **central core disease**.

SIADH See **syndrome of inappropriate ADH scretion**.

sialidoses (Gr, saliva) (mucolipidoses, cherry-red spot myoclonus, OMIM 256550) A group of recessively inherited sphingolipid and mucopolysaccharide lysosomal storage disorders associated with α-*N*-acetyl-neuraminidase deficiency, in which excessive amounts of sialo-oligosaccharides are excreted in the urine and lipid-like and polysaccharide-like material is deposited in the tissues.[3932] They are mapped to 6p21.2

Clinical presentations, usually between the ages of 8 and 15 years include visual failure with a cherry-red macular spot, tonic-clonic seizures, and myoclonus; intelligence is normal and there are neither somatic nor bony abnormalities. A classification of the sialidoses is given in Chart S–5.

sialuria (mucolipidosis or sialidosis type 4; severe infantile neuraminic acid storage disease, French type; Tondeur syndrome) A recessively inherited congenital generalized lysosomal storage disease, characterized by corneal clouding, optic atrophy, and retinal dystrophy impairing vision; mucopoly or oligosaccariduria; pyramidal and extrapyramidal signs; and psychomotor retardation. Achlorhydria is also a feature. Levels of free sialic acid in urine and cultured fibroblasts are increased,[6349] but conjunctival or skin biopsy showing cytoplasmic inclusions is the easier diagnostic method.[2195] Mutations in the *MCOLN1* gene are responsible.

Siber syndrome A congenital dysmorphic syndrome characterized by ocular and genital abnormalities and microcephaly, seizures, cerebellar and pyramidal signs, aqueduct stenosis with obstructive hydrocephalus, callosal agenesis, and mental and developmental delay.[381]

Sicard sign Aggravation of the back pain induced during straight-leg raising as a result of passive dorsiflexion of the hallux.[421] See also **Bragard sign**.

Sicard spasm See **hemifacial spasm**.

Sicard, Jean-Athenase (1872–1929) French neurologist, born in Marseille, who trained in medicine in Paris, where he was influenced by **Brissaud** to enter neurology. He became chef-de-clinique under Brissaud and spent most of the rest of his professional career at the Hôpital Necker in Paris, where he was elected professor of pathology in 1923 and from which he made numerous basic contributions to neurology in the short time remaining before his early death.

With Jacques Forestier in 1922, he introduced radio-opaque iodized oil (lipiodol) for the investigation of intraspinal disease, and he contributed significantly to the techniques of angiography and pneumo-encephalography. He also wrote on syphilis, encephalitis, and toxic neuropathies and collaborated with others in the description of brainstem stroke syndromes, one of which is named for Collet and himself.

Sicard–Brissaud syndrome See **Brissaud syndrome**.

Sicard–Collet syndrome See **Collet–Sicard syndrome**.

Sicard–Hagueman syndrome See **Meige syndrome**.

Sicca syndrome See **Sjögren syndrome**.

sick sinus syndrome A clinical state characterized by a primary disorder of the atrial pacemaker, presenting first as sinus bradycardia and later progressing to sinus arrest or sinoatrial block. Some patients alternate between attacks of bradycardia and tachycardia. Clinically, syncope, dizziness, convulsions, and possibly sudden death in childhood are recognized neurological complications.[5689]

sickle-cell disease A sickling hemoglobinopathy of black people, which may manifest in a homo-or heterozygous form. Painful crises, jaundice, anemia, leg ulcers, and hepatomegaly are common symptoms; stroke syndromes, myelopathy, cognitive impairment, headaches, retinopathy, stupor or coma, and seizures are the main neurological complications and are due to the occlusion of small blood vessels by sickle cells.[6857] The condition has been reviewed by Prengler M. et al. in *Ann Neurol* 2002;51:543–52.

Sickness Impact profile A self-reported general health status measure of the dysfunction experienced as a result of disease. *Psychosocial factors* such as social interaction, alertness, emotional behavior, and communication; *physical factors* such as mobility, ambulation, and body care; and *other* areas of concern (communication, bodily functions, activities of daily living) are assessed through the subjects' responses to about 140 questions.[562, 5067] See also **quality of life**.

sideropenic dysphagia (Gr, iron + shortage + difficulty in eating) (Plummer–Vinson syndrome, Paterson–Brown–Kelly syndrome) An acquired syndrome of dysphagia with the usual clinical accompaniments of chronic hypochromic anemia, occurring in adult life, usually in women.[3012]

siderophilia A tendency to accumulate iron or calcium and other metals, seen in both neurons and astrocytes in the settings of **neurodegeneration with brain iron accumulation** and **Fahr** disease, and occurring in areas adjacent to leaked blood.

siderosis See **superficial siderosis of the central nervous system**.

SIDS See **sudden infant death syndrome**.

Chart S–5. Classification of Sialidoses

1. *Sialidoses with isolated sialidase deficiency*

   Congenital sialidosis
   Severe infantile sialidosis
   Nephrosialidosis
   Cherry red spot-myoclonus syndrome (sialidosis type 1) See below.

2. *Sialidosis with additional β-galactosidase deficiency*

   Goldberg syndrome (mucolipidosis 1, infantile sialidosis)

3. *Other forms*

   Fucosidosis
   Mannosidosis
   Aspartyl-glycosaminuria
   Mucolipidosis type 1 (see below)
   Mucolipidosis, other types

Sialidosis type 1 (cherry red spot-myoclonus syndrome, normosomatic type) A lysosomal storage disease in which sialo-oligosaccharides accumulate. The clinical syndrome is characterized by the onset (after the age of 10 years) of **progressive myoclonic epilepsy** with severe, progressive stimulus-sensitive action and intention myoclonus and tonic-clonic seizures.[5193] Cerebellar signs and mental deterioration are also described. Lens and corneal opacities, pyramidal signs, and a mild peripheral neuropathy are less constant signs.[1982] The retinal spot appears later. β-galactosidase levels are normal but fibroblast α-neuraminidase levels are low. The EEG shows photosensitive responses, paroxysmal discharges, and fast polyspike discharges over central regions during rapid eye movement sleep.[1880]

The association of such abnormalities also occurs in **Tay–Sachs disease, Nieman–Pick disease, GM_1 gangliosidosis, metachromatic leukodystrophy,** and the **glycogenoses.**

A *variant* is *mild infantile sialidosis* (lipomucopolysaccharidosis), an inherited lysosomal storage disease characterized by a deficiency of neuraminidase and the accumulation of sialo-oligosaccharides. The clinical features include short stature and the onset in infancy of mental retardation, ataxia, deafness, seizures, and myoclonus, with coarse facies, corneal clouding, cherry-red spot, visceromegaly, and dysostosis.

Sialidosis type 2 (mucolipidosis type 1; Goldberg syndrome; gangliosialidosis, dysmorphic type) Forms in which action myoclonus, tonic-clonic seizures, cherry-red spots, gargoyle-like coarsening of the facial features, dementia, hearing loss, mental impairment, pyramidal and cerebellar signs, multiple dysostoses, hepatosplenomegaly, and deafness occur between the ages of 10 and 30 years, mainly in subjects of Japanese ancestry. In this group, deficiency of β-galactosidase may be present in cases with juvenile onset, leading to the designation *galactosidosis*.[568] When onset is in infancy, the galactosidase levels are normal. Fibroblast α-neuraminidase levels are low.

I-Cell disease

Sialidosis type 3 (Salla disease, Finnish-type lysosomal storage disorder) A recessively inherited lysosomal storage disease due to a deficiency of oligosaccharide-specific neuraminidase, leading to lysosomal storage of sialic acid and oligosaccharides.

Clinically, the onset is in early childhood; severe and progressive mental retardation with early onset, coarse facies, speech failure, short stature, strabismus, myoclonus and other seizures and pyramidal, cerebellar, and basal ganglion signs are the most notable features. An increased urinary excretion of free sialic acid is a diagnostic pointer. The condition has been reported mainly from Finland.[296]

Sialidosis type 3a. Pseudo-Hurler polydystrophy An inherited lysosomal storage disease characterized by deficiency of β-galactosidase, α-L-fucosidase and neuraminidase, and by the accumulation of mucopolysaccharides, gangliosides, and oligosaccharides. This congenital dysmorphic syndrome is marked by the accumulation of mucolipids and sphingolipids as a result of an inherited enzyme failure. Clinically, the syndrome presents at the age of 2–5 years, with stiffness of joints and muscle contractures, carpal tunnel syndrome, bony changes, corneal clouding, mild mental retardation, coarsening of facial features, short stature, platyspondyly, arthropathy, epiphyseal dysplasia, acne, ataxia, mental and developmental delay, deafness, visceromegaly, and aortic or mitral valve disease.[6236]

Sialidosis type 4 See **sialuria.**

Berman type A recessively inherited lysosomal storage disease of Ashkenazi Jews, characterized by deficiency of ganglioside neuraminidase and the accumulation of mucopolysaccharides, phospholipids, and gangliosides. The clinical features include the onset in infancy of mild mental retardation and corneal clouding, optic atrophy, pigmentary retinopathy, hypotonia, pyramidal signs, athetosis, and dystonia in Ashkenazi Jewish children.[578]

In a *variant* form, there is an added congenital myopathy with proximal and distal weakness and hypotonia, with joint contractures, spasticity, athetosis, and mental and developmental delay.

From Celani MG, Righetti E, Migliacci R, et al. Comparability and validity of two clinical scores in the early differential diagnosis of acute stroke. *Brit Med J* 1994;308:1674–6.

Siegrist streaks Pigmented lines on the fundus, seen in some patients with chronic uremia.

Siemens syndrome A recessively inherited syndrome seen mainly in males, characterized by anhidrosis, skin pallor, hypotrichosis, cataract, corneal dystrophy, and mental retardation.[5829]

Siemens–Bloch pigmented dermatosis See **incontinentia pigmenti**.

Siemerling–Creutzfeldt disease See **adrenoleukodystrophy**.

Sierpinski-Bart syndrome A congenital dysmorphic syndrome characterized by skeletal and genital abnormalities, retinitis pigmentosa, myopia, strabismus, kyphoscoliosis, optic atrophy, microcephaly, and mental and developmental delay.[381]

Sieveking, Sir Edward H. (1816–1904) English physician at the **National Hospital**, who reported the impression of **Locock** that bromides were effective in the treatment of hysterical seizures, and so advocated their use in organic ones in his book *On Epilepsy and Epileptiform Seizures* (London, 1858).

SIF cells See **small intensely fluorescent cells**.

sigma nystagmus See **optokinetic nystagmus**.

sigma rhythm See **sleep spindles**.

signe de journal See **Froment sign**.

signe de l'éventail See **Babinski signs**.

signe de la pensée douloureuse The precipitation of headaches by intensive mental concentration, considered by Josue to be a sign of cerebral vascular insufficiency,[645] although today such disorders would probably be classified as **tension-type headaches**.

signe de Peaucier See **platysma phenomenon**.

signing tics The use of gestures to replace the usual speech accompaniments (phonic tics) of tic disorders such as **Tourette syndrome**. Such complex learned movements parallel the performance of verbal symptoms such as coprolalia, echolalia, and palilalia; the terms *coprolaliopraxia*, *echolaliopraxia*, and *palilaliopraxia* have naturally been coined for them.[3684]

signpost phenomenon If a subject with **Parkinson disease** rests his elbows on the table with the forearms vertical and lets his arms and wrists relax, the wrists nevertheless remain in partial extension and do not fall as they do normally, so that the hand assumes a position near the horizontal.

silent period A pause in the electrical activity of a muscle, such as that seen after its rapid unloading.[162] Such reflex inhibition of muscle electrical activity typically follows a twitch contraction for about 100 ms and is due to direct inhibition of the reflex arc by Renshaw cells, with withdrawal of afferent muscle spindle facilitation. It is normal in the **stiff-person syndrome** but is shortened or absent in **tetanus**.[3724]

silent pituitary apoplexy Nonsymptomatic hemorrhage within pituitary adenomas.

silent stroke The CT or MRI appearances of strokes that are unaccompanied by historical or clinical evidence of transient ischemic attacks or of persisting stroke deficit. **Leukoaraiosis** or bilateral periventricular lucencies alone are insufficient for the diagnosis.

Silk Road disease A colloquial name for **Adamantiades–Behcet syndrome** based on the geography of the disease which encompasses the route between the Mediterranean basin and Japan.

Silver syndrome (disease) See **hereditary spastic paraplegia**.

simian crease A single palmar crease.

simian hand (Lat, monkey-like) See **ape hand**.

simian stance A posture characterized by slight flexion of the knees, hips, and lumbar spine and by loss of the normal lumbar lordosis. This is seen in **lumbar spinal stenosis** and in **Parkinson disease**, but in the latter case there is also flexion of the neck and upper limbs.

similarities test A subtest of the **Wechsler Adult Intelligence Scale** in which the subject is asked in what way two items (eating–sleeping, wall-fence, pen–pencil) are alike (i.e., share common properties).

Simmerlin dystrophy See **limb–girdle muscular dystrophy**.

Simmonds syndrome Panhypopituitarism, occasionally complicating pituitary tumors or following **pituitary apoplexy**. See **Sheehan syndrome**.

Simon sign Incoordination of the intercostal and diaphragmatic movements, said to be a sign of early meningitis.[5333]

Simon–Binet tests See **Binet**, **intelligence tests**.

simple aphasia See **aphemia**.

simple central anisocoria Asymmetry in the size of the pupils, measuring a constant 0.5-mm difference or less in both bright and dim illumination. See also **Horner syndrome**.

simple cramp Difficulty in performing a single specific task due to the presence of focal hand cramps.[5775]

simple partial seizures A term now mercifully replaced by the ILAE Commission on Terminology[1861] for focal seizures, often without accompanying EEG changes, in which there are elementary symptoms, consciousness is not impaired, and later recollection is undistorted. They are further subdivided according to the nature of the symptoms; thus, motor, sensory, autonomic, cognitive, affective, and mixed components occur variously. Rapid generalization to generalized tonic-clonic seizures may sometimes occur.

simple tremor See **cerebellar tremors**.

Simpson's Test A sign in myasthenia gravis, positive when the patient staring up at the ceiling develops worsening ptosis within 1 min. An expanded form requires 3 min of upward gaze.

simultagnosia The inability to perceive more than one object in a particular sensory channel at one time, most commonly seen in patients with bilateral or right parietal lobe disease. The term was suggested by Wolpert in 1924,[4339] but the defect is better considered a form of **visual disorientation**.

sin-cib-syn (sino-cibal syndrome) See **chinese restaurant syndrome**.

sincipital At the junction of the frontal and ethmoidal bones of the skull.

sinciput The anterior protuberance of the cranium, as opposed to the occiput.

singing paraplegia Intermittent leg weakness occurring as the result of increased venous pressure transmitted to a spinal dural arteriovenous fistula during the act of singing, with resultant cord compression and ischemia.[3416] Presumably more prosaic causes of the Valsalva maneuver could do the same thing.

single (isolated) seizure One or more epileptic seizures occurring in a 24-h period.[1265]

single fiber electromyographic jitter See **jitter**.

single fiber electromyography (SFEMG) A general term referring to the technique and conditions that permit the recording of action potentials from single muscle fibers.[162] A review of the technique and its value has been published.[5532]

single fiber needle electrode A needle electrode with two small recording surfaces (usually 25 μm in diameter) which permits the recording of single muscle fiber action potentials between the active recording surface in the bevel at the tip of the cannula and that facing laterally through a side port situated more proximally.[162]

single-photon emission computed tomography (SPECT) A technique for imaging cross sections of the body and for measuring focal intracerebral blood flow, in which isotopes emitting single photons are detected using the same principles of image reconstruction as those used in CT, but employing a rotating gamma camera. Single photon-emitting isotopes of carbon, hydrogen, oxygen, or nitrogen do not exist; hence, SPECT is not directly useful for metabolic imaging based on these biologically important atoms.

At present, SPECT is used principally for brain perfusion imaging. Commonly employed tracers are ^{123}I-iodoamphetamine, ^{99m}Tc-hexamethyl-propyleneamine oxime (HMPAO), and ^{99m}Tc-bicisate. These diffuse into the brain tissue at a rate proportional to regional perfusion rates and thus to the rate of local cerebral metabolism.

SPECT tracers are highly lipophilic and therefore cross the blood-brain barrier easily. Once in the brain, some tracers such as HMPAO are metabolized to less lipophilic compounds and leave the brain slowly. Their distribution preserves a record of the regional cerebral blood flow (rCBF) at the time of injection, which can be imaged at any time within the next several hours. However, tracers that are not metabolized (e.g., xenon 133) demonstrate rCBF by the kinetics of their entry into or departure from the brain, and must be imaged at the time that these events occur.[5058, 5121]

singultus See **hiccoughs**.

sinistrality (from Lat, left-handedness) Although the word, meaning **left-handedness**, is occasionally regarded as a pejorative (sinister), the Book of Judges in the Old Testament refers to an army of 700 left-handed slingers, who never missed.

sinistrosis See **Brissaud syndrome**.

sinking pitch sign A reduction in the pitch of the voice occasioned by fatigue of the laryngeal adductor muscles in **myasthenia gravia**.[6599]

sinus arrhythmia A physiological alteration of heart rate which depends on cardiac parasympathetic activity such that the decreased vagal activity occurring with inspiration leads to an increase in the heart rate. When a subject breathes at 6 respirations per minute, the electrocardiogram should show differences of 15 bpm; less than 10 bpm change is abnormal.[3801]

Quantitation of the normal response has been achieved. The **expiratory:inspiratory ratio** (the mean of the longest R-R interval during expiration divided by the mean of the shortest R-R interval during inspiration) should exceed 1.2 in patients aged less than 40 years.[1936]

sinus headache (headache attributed to rhinosinusitis) Facial or frontal headaches often extending into the ears or teeth, due to current acute rhinosinusitis and remitting within a week of its successful treatment.

No entry is made for "chronic sinus headache" in this book because, in the opinion of this author, that condition only exists in the minds of advertising copywriters, patients so diagnosed actually having diluted attacks of **migraine,** and/or **medication-induced headaches** induced by what the advertisers are trying to sell.

sinus of Morgagni syndrome See **Trotter syndrome**.

sinus pericranii A persistent venous connection between the superior sagittal sinus and the scalp veins in the parieto-occipital region, seen in some infants. The fluctuant mass swells with crying, but this is only dangerous in the event that it should bleed.

sinus thrombosis causing intracranial hypertension See **otitic hydrocephalus**.

sinus thrombosis Partial or complete occlusion of an intracranial venous sinus, often leading to venous infarction of the subjacent brain. Septic and aseptic causes are recognized. The condition was noted by **Gowers**[2531] in association with pregnancy and wasting diseases, but it also occurs in conjunction with hematological conditions, cardiac failure, oral contraceptive therapy, and dehydration; with local infections such as mastoiditis; and sometimes without any known cause.

The clinical features of superior sagittal sinus thrombosis include headache with signs of raised intracranial pressure, seizures, nausea and vomiting, aphasia, focal deficits affecting mainly the legs, and reduced level of consciousness.

Sipple syndrome See **multiple endocrine neoplasia**.

Siriraj score A bedside instrument for assessing the likelihood of intracerebral hemorrhage in stroke patients awaiting computed tomography. It assesses consciousness, vomiting, headache within 2 h, diastolic blood pressure, and such atheroma markers as diabetes, angina, and intermittent claudication.[1066] See also **Allen Score**.

Calculation of Siriraj Score

Variable	*Clinical Feature*	*Score*
Consciousness (× 2.5)	Alert	0
Drowsy, stupor		1
Semicoma, coma		2
Vomiting (× 2)	No	0
	Yes	1
Headache within 2 h (× 2)	No	0
	Yes	1
Diastolic blood pressure (× 0.11)		
Atheroma markers (× 3)	None	0
(diabetes, angina, intermittent claudication)	One or more	1
Constant		−12

From Celani MG, Righetti E, Migliacci R, et al. Comparability and validity of two clinical scores in the early differential diagnosis of acute stroke. *Brit Med J* 1994;**308**:1674–6. © 1989. Reproduced by kind permission of the BMJ Group.

Siris–Coffin–Wegienka syndrome See **Coffin–Lowry syndrome**.

SISI See **short increment sensitivity index**.

Sisto sign Constant crying in children with congenital syphilis. Dr. G. Sisto was an Argentinian pediatrician.

site-of-injury headache A form of post-traumatic headache in which the pain is localized to the site of the original injury, probably due to local soft-tissue trauma and entrapment of sensory nerves in scar tissue.[6548]

sitki See **oroya fever**.

situational syncope The provocation of syncope by certain activities or by normal activities performed in particular situations. **Cough, swallow, micturition**, and **defecation syncope** are examples.

situation-related seizures (provoked seizures) Seizures which occur within a week of acute metabolic disorders, heavy alcohol consumption or withdrawal, or stroke or head trauma, or with cerebral tumor or infection.[3901]

six hertz spike-and-slow-waves (phantom spike-and-wave, fast spike-wave) Spike-and-slow-wave complexes at 4–7 Hz (but mostly at 6 Hz), occurring generally in brief bursts bilaterally, synchronously, symmetrically or asymmetrically and either confined to or of larger amplitude over the posterior or anterior regions of the head. Their amplitude is variable but is generally smaller than that of spike-and-slow-wave complexes repeating at slower rates. The clinical significance of this pattern is controversial. (From the 1974 report of the Committee on Terminology, IFCN. In: Chatrian GE, Bergamini L, Dondey M, et al. A glossary of terms most commonly used by clinical electroencephalographers. *EEG Clin Neurophysiol* 1974;37:538–48. Reproduced with kind permission from Elsevier Science.)

This EEG pattern is seen mainly in young adults and is not usually associated with seizures; it is more likely to be benign when it occurs in Females, predominantly Occipitally, with Low amplitude, and during Drowsiness (FOLD); but this may not be so when the pattern occurs during Waking, with High Amplitude, predominantly Anteriorly, and in Males (WHAM). Such discharges have an uncertain relationship with any clinical epileptic syndrome.[6275]

six-element test A test of planning ability in which the subject is asked to carry out six open-ended tasks in a fixed time. The tasks include dictating details of a journey, performing arithmetic, and writing down the names of pictures presented.[5754]

sixth nerve pseudopalsy See **pseudo—sixth nerve palsy**.

sixth sense See **facial vision of the blind**.

Sjäastad syndrome See **chronic paroxysmal hemicrania**.

Sjögren syndrome (keratoconjunctivitis sicca, sicca syndrome, Mikulicz–Gougerot–Sjörgren syndrome) A collagen-vascular disease characterized by dryness of the mouth and eyes, ichthyosis, keratitis, corneal ulceration, recurrent salivary gland enlargement, rheumatoid arthritis, and sometimes relapsing and remitting neurological signs.[5883] Anemia, leukopenia, and a raised erythrocyte sedimentation rate are also commonly found. The condition occurs mainly in postmenopausal women, either alone or in association with other autoimmune disorders.

Possible neurological complications include seizures; focal or multifocal CNS signs including cognitive dysfunction, meningoencephalitis or encephalopathy; psychoses; migraine; myalgias and fatigue; optic neuropathy; ophthalmoplegia; cerebellar syndromes, and acute or chronic myelopathy. In the PNS, symmetrical axonal sensorimotor polyneuropathy with a predominance of sensory symptoms or pure sensory neuropathy occur most frequently, but multiple cranial neuropathy, autonomic neuropathy, multiple mononeuropathies, polyradiculoneuropathy, and myositis are also reported.[1553, 4488]

Trigeminal sensory neuropathy and III and VIII cranial nerve involvement are uncommon. Intracerebral or subarachnoid hemorrhage is probably the most specific indicator of vasculitis, but ischemic lesions can also occur. Subacute or chronic aseptic meningitis or meningoencephalitis manifesting as dementia or encephalopathy may also rarely be seen.

Laboratory studies may show the presence of oligoclonal banding in the CSF. Abnormal visual-evoked potentials and findings of white matter lesions on MRI meeting the radiologic criteria for **multiple sclerosis** are well described. As both clinical and MRI findings may resemble those of multiple sclerosis (including the primary progressive form), screening for Sjögren syndrome in at least older female patients who are suspected of having multiple sclerosis may be warranted. Serum anti Ro/SS-A, anti-La/SS-B, and anti-Hu antibodies, polyclonal hyperglobulinemia, and positive tests for cryoglobulins may be detected.[3008]
A minority has antibodies to Ro (SSA).[1553]

Brief diagnostic criteria[4787] require positive Schirmer Test results, a positive result from the Rose Bengal dye test for keratoconjunctivitis, or abnormal minor salivary gland biopsy findings. Alternative criteria require the same but with the added demonstration of antinuclear factor or rheumatoid factor and objective evidence of diminished salivary flow in place of the salivary gland biopsy. A more recent and complex list of criteria follows.

Revised International Classification Criteria for Sjögren Syndrome[6555]

I. Ocular symptoms—A positive response to at least one of the following questions:

1. Have you had daily, persistent, troublesome dry eyes for more than 3 months?
2. Do you have a recurrent sensation of sand or gravel in the eyes?
3. Do you use tear substitutes more than 3 times a day?

II. Oral symptoms—A positive response to at least one of the following questions:

1. Have you had a daily feeling of dry mouth for more than 3 months?
2. Have you had recurrently or persistently swollen salivary glands as an adult?
3. Do you frequently drink liquids to aid in swallowing dry food?

III. Ocularsigns—objectiveevidenceofocular involvement defined as a positive result for at least one of the following two tests:

1. Schirmer's Test, performed without anesthesia (<<5 mm in 5 min)
2. Rose bengal score or other ocular dye score = 4 (according to van Bijsterveld's scoring system).

IV. Histopathology—In minor salivary glands (obtained through normal-appearing mucosa) focal lymphocytic sialoadenitis, evaluated by an expert histopathologist, with a focus score >1, defined as a number of lymphocytic foci (which are adjacent to normal-appearing mucous acini and contain more than 50 lymphocytes per 4 mm^2 of glandular tissue).

V. Salivary gland involvement—objective evidence of salivary gland involvement defined by a positive result for at least one of the following diagnostic tests:

1. Unstimulated whole salivary flow (≤1.5 ml in 15 min)
2. Parotid sialography showing the presence of diffuse sialectasiasis (punctate, caviatary, or destructive pattern) without evidence of obstruction in the major ducts.
3. Salivary scintigraphy showing delayed uptake, reduced concentration, and/or delayed excretion tracer.

VI. Autoantibodies—presence in the serum of the following autoantibodies—Antibodies to Ro (SSA) or La (SSB) antigens, or both.

Primary SS in patients without any potentially associated disease may be defined as follows:

a) The presence of any 4 of the 6 items is indicative of primary SS, as long as either item IV (histopathoogy) or VI (serology) is positive.
b) The presence of any 3 of the 4 objective criteria items (i.e., items III, IV, V, and VI).
c) The classification tree procedure represents a valid alternative method for classification, although it should be more properly used in clinical–epidemiological survey.

Exclusion criteria are past head and neck radiation treatment; hepatitis C infection; acquired immunodeficiency syndrome (AIDS); pre-existing lymphoma; sarcoidois; graft versus host disease, and use of anticholinergic drugs (since a time shorter than 4-fold the half life of the drug).

From Vitali C, Bombardieri S, Jonsson R, et al. Classification criteria for Sjogren's syndrome. *Ann.Rheumat.Dis.* 2002;61:554–8. Reproduced by kind permission of the BMJ Publishing Group Ltd. © 2002.

In *variant* forms, **polymyositis** and **dermatomyositis**[5311] occur in conjunction.

Sjögren, Henrik Samuel Conrad

(b. 1899) Swedish ophthalmologist, practicing in Stockholm. He described the association of filamentary keratitis with arthritis in 1933.

Sjögren–Larsson syndrome

(ichthyosis-Little disease; OMIM 270200) A recessively inherited leukodystrophy characterized by congenital ichthyosiform erythroderma (scaly hyperkeratosis), pigmentary retinopathy, dental enamel dysplasia, deficient scalp hair, spastic paraparesis, seizures, speech defect, and mental retardation.[5884] Impaired oxidation of long-chain fatty alcohols due to deficiency of the enzyme *FALDH* (fatty aldehyde dehydrogenase) carried on chromosome 17p11.2 may be the underlying mechanism.

Ichthyosis and neurological signs also occur together in **Rud** and in **Refsum syndromes**.

skeletal dysplasia-unusual facies-mental retardation

See **CAT syndrome**.

skeletal myoclonus

See **myorhythmia**.

skeleton–skin–brain syndrome

See **cerebellar syndromes** (congenital ataxias).

skew deviation

(Hertwig–Magendie syndrome) An acquired nonparetic ocular divergence in the vertical plane due to an imbalance of prenuclear inputs—a supranuclear lesion involving the brainstem tegmentum at any level between the medulla and the diencephalon. It is characterized by downward and inward rotation of one eye, accompanied by upward and outward rotation of the other, and by nystagmus.[5101]

The following criteria for the diagnosis have been suggested:[5920]

A. Sudden onset of vertical diplopia, usually in adults
B. Significant vertical deviation, comitant or noncomitant
C. No preceding strabismus
D. A laterally comitant deviation (e.g., no deviation in left gaze but vertical deviation in right gaze, essentially equal both up and right and down and right, and essentially the same in amount with either eye fixing in these positions)
E. Associated signs and symptoms
F. Clinical evidence of a brachium pontis lesion
G. Exclusion of III and IV cranial nerve disease, orbital fractures, etc.
H. Noncomitant skew deviation mimicking inferior or superior rectus or inferior oblique palsies or primary overaction of an oblique most commonly, but without other evidence of III or of IV cranial nerve disease

Reproduced by kind permission of the American Academy of Neurology and Lippincott Williams and Wilkins.

The condition was first recognized in laboratory animals by **Magendie** in 1824 and by Henry Hertwig 2 years later, but it was only reported in humans following the carnage of World War I. It is a sign of disease of the utricle (upward deviation of both eyes with different amplitudes); of the dorsal medulla (hypertropia of one eye); of the midbrain tegmentum (simultaneous hypertropia of one eye and hypotropia of the other, and inferred when pupillary or III cranial nerve abnormalities are also present); or of intrinsic brainstem or cerebellar disease (on the side of the lower eye).

A *variant* is *slowly alternating skew deviation*, in which one eye descends as the other ascends over 30–60 s, and which is a sign of a pretectal lesion.[1280]

skin roll test

Gentle pinching or rolling of the skin of the neck or head leads to a complaint of unusual pain in patients with migraine; in fibromyalgia the pain is increased in areas overlying the tender muscle trigger points. The problems with the method are the variability of the stimulus and the subjectivity of the estimate of pain felt, let alone the underlying pathogenesis.

skin wrinkling The ridged appearance of skin immersed for a period in warm water. This depends upon the capacity of keratin to bind water, which in turn requires the presence of salt. In the skin this is derived from sweat, so the phenomenon occurs only in the presence of an intact sympathetic system; its absence is suggested as a simple test of sympathetic function[795] and thus useful in the diagnosis of small fiber neuropathy.[6255]

skinache syndrome A syndrome of uncertain validity characterized by chronic pain of unknown etiology with numerous cutaneous trigger points and responsive to injection of local anesthetic.[435]

Skre syndrome See **hereditary spastic paraplegia**.

SKT test battery A scale designed to measure recent memory and attention in patients with cognitive impairment, containing 9 manually administered subtests, available in 5 alternate forms, and completed within 10–15 min. The test has been used in treatment trials that included patients with **Alzheimer disease**.[1910]

skull (Old Engl, skulle) The protective bony covering of the brain and organs of special sense, consisting of the cranium and the face.

skull noise Murmurs heard over the skull, as in patients with cervical or cranial vascular disease or intracranial arteriovenous communications, and in many normal children and others with anemia or with increased cerebral blood flow stemming from other causes. See also **cephalic bellows sound**.

sleep A heterogeneous and complicated physiological condition in which consciousness and activity are altered, occurring cyclically due to reductions in the activity of systems promoting wakefulness such as the ascending reticular activating system and the activation of other systems responsible for nonrapid eye movement sleep (median forebrain area, serotonergic median raphe nuclei) or for rapid eye movement sleep (gigantocellular tegmental field in the pons).

SLEEP The official journal of the Associated Professional Sleep Societies, a joint venture of the American Academy of Sleep Medicine (Web site: http://www.aasmnet.org/) and the Sleep Research Society (Web site: http://www.sleepresearchsociety.org/srs/index.php). Primary readers are scientists engaged in the study of sleep and its disorders and clinicians practicing sleep disorders medicine.

sleep apnea DIMS (disorders of initiating or maintaining sleep) syndrome Cessation of ventilation during sleep due to central causes (sometimes with obstructive causes as well), leading to complaints of insomnia as a result of multiple awakenings.[1574] This was the terminology of the original ASDA diagnostic classification of **sleep disorders**.[280]

sleep apnea disorder of excessive sleep (DOES) syndrome (sleep apnea, obstructive sleep apnea syndrome) A syndrome characterized by multiple obstructive or mixed apneas during sleep, loud snoring, and excessive daytime somnolence. Additional symptoms include **sleep drunkenness** and dulling of the sensorium; cardiac arrhythmias may occur and may cause death.[2627] This was the terminology used in the original ASDA diagnostic classification of **sleep disorders**.[280]

sleep apnea headache See **hypoxic headache**.

sleep apnea A condition in which repetitive nocturnal apneas result in recurrent hypoxemia and sleep disruption. The occurrence of at least 15 apneic or hypoapneic episodes per hour of sleep in association with symptoms, including snoring, restless nocturnal sleep with repeated awakenings, excessive daytime sleepiness, attacks of choking during the night, morning headaches, nocturia, and irritability, suggests the diagnosis of sleep apnea syndrome.[6763]

The cessation of ventilatory movements during sleep is due to a prolonged pause in the central brainstem upper airway motor neuron output at the end of expiration. Clinically, the condition presents most often with snoring, abnormal sleep behavior, excessive daytime sleepiness, intellectual deterioration, personality change, morning headache, and sleep disturbances. It occurs in association with a wide range of primary neurological diseases, most of which affect the brainstem or the brain in a diffuse manner.

Four types of sleep apnea have been defined (see Chart S–6), although all have the same neurological basis. The **Pickwickian syndrome** and **idiopathic hypoventilation** could also be classified as sleep apnea syndromes.

Chart S–6. The Four Types of Sleep Apnea

1. *Central sleep apnea syndrome* Respiratory movements cease so that there is no oronasal airflow. The disorder is characterized by a cessation or decrease of ventilatory effort during sleep, usually with associated oxygen desaturation. The following diagnostic criteria have been suggested:[1629]

   A. The patient has a complaint of either insomnia or excessive sleepiness. Occasionally, the patient may be unaware of clinical features observed by others
   B. Frequent episodes of shallow or absent breathing during sleep
   C. Associated features include at least one of the following:

      1. Gasps, grunts, or choking during sleep
      2. Frequent body movements
      3. Cyanosis during sleep

   D. Polysomnographic monitoring demonstrates:

      1. Central apneic pauses greater than 10 s (20 s in infancy) in duration, and one or more of the following:
      2. Frequent arousals from sleep associated with the apneas
      3. Bradytachycardia

4. Oxygen desaturation in association with the apneic episodes, with or without item 5 below.
5. A mean sleep latency test (MSLT) that demonstrates a mean sleep latency of less than 10 min

E. Other sleep disorders can be present, for example, periodic limb movement disorder, obstructive sleep apnea syndrome, or central alveolar hypoventilation syndrome

2. *Obstructive sleep apnea syndrome* A disorder characterized by repetitive episodes of upper airway obstruction that occur during sleep and are usually associated with a reduction in blood oxygen saturation. In this form, the diaphragm and chest wall move with variations in intrathoracic pressure, but there is no airflow at the nose or mouth. The problem is due to facial or palatal malformations, upper airway disease, or collapse of the muscular all of the pharynx.[3434] The following diagnostic criteria have been suggested:[1629]

A. The patient has a complaint of excessive sleepiness or insomnia Occasionally, the patient may be unaware of clinical features that are observed by others
B. Frequent episodes of obstructed breathing during sleep
C. Associated features include the following:

1. Loud snoring
2. Morning headaches
3. A dry mouth upon awakening
4. Chest retraction during sleep in young children

D. Polysomnographic monitoring demonstrates the following:

1. More than five obstructive apneic episodes, greater than 10 s in duration, per hour of sleep and one or more of the following:
2. Frequent arousals from sleep associated with the apneas
3. Bradytachycardia
4. Arterial oxygen desaturation in association with the apneic episodes; with or without:
5. An MSLT that demonstrates a mean sleep latency of less than 10 min

E. Can be associated with other medical disorders, for example, tonsillar enlargement
F. Other sleep disorders can be present, for example, periodic limb movement disorder or narcolepsy

3. *Mixed* Respiratory movements and airflow are absent early in the episode but are followed by unsuccessful attempts at breathing.
4. *Subobstructive* There is reduced airflow with increased respiratory effort.

Another *variant* is *infantile sleep apnea*, which is defined as the occurrence of central or obstructive apneas during sleep in infants.[248] The following diagnostic criteria have been suggested:[1629]

A. Clinical presentation includes one or more of the following:

1. An episode of cessation of breathing during sleep
2. An episode characterized by the following:

a. Color change (pallor or cyanosis)
b. Tone change (limpness, rarely stiffness)

3. Noisy breathing during sleep

B. Central or obstructive apneas occurring during sleep
C. Age of infant at presentation either

1. Less than 37 weeks postconceptional age, or
2. Greater than 37 weeks postconceptional age

D. Polysomnographic monitoring demonstrates one or more of the following:

1. Prolonged central apnea >20 s
2. Obstructive apnea >10 s
3. An apnea accompanied by cyanosis
4. An apnea accompanied by transient bradycardia (defined as a drop in heart rate to levels below 50 bpm, a heart rate below 60 bpm lasting more than 10 s or a drop below 60 bpm with a duration exceeding 30 s below baseline heart rate)
5. Arterial oxygen saturation less than 85% during sleep
6. Sustained hypoventilation (end tidal carbon dioxide partial pressure [$PETCO_2$] >45 mmHg) during sleep

E. An identifiable cause for the apnea was either

1. Found following a thorough diagnostic evaluation and is believed to be the cause of the apnea, or
2. Not found following a thorough diagnostic evaluation

From the ASDA Diagnostic Classification Steering Committee. The International Classification of Sleep Disorders Diagnostic and Coding Manual. *Rochester, MN. American Sleep Disorders Association, 1990. Reproduced by kind permission of the American Academy of Sleep Medicine.*

The recurrent headache associated with sleep apnea is a frequently occurring bilateral, pressing pain experienced on waking, lasting less than half an hour, without nausea, photophobia or phonophobia. It ceases after effective treatment of the sleep apnea.

Narcolepsy, cervical cordotomy, **Chiari malformation**, kyphoscoliosis, bulbar polio, and brainstem infarct or tumor are other causes of sleep-related apnea, and may be accompanied by disturbed sleep with abnormal movements, hypnagogic hallucinations, enuresis, and somnambulism.[2626]

sleep architecture The disposition of rapid eye movement and nonrapid eye movement sleep periods relative to one another.

sleep attacks Overpowering attacks of sleepiness, occurring typically as part of the **narcolepsy** syndrome.

sleep bruxism Bruxism (tooth-grinding or tooth-clenching) occurring during stage 2 nonrapid eye movement sleep, the contractions being forceful, rhythmic, of variable duration up to seconds and painful thereafter.

Faciomandibular myoclonus, a rare familial disorder, can mimic this.

sleep choking syndrome A syndrome of frequent abrupt awakenings during sleep with tachycardia, intense anxiety, and a sensation of impending death despite apparently normal ventilation during sleep. **Panic disorder, obstructive sleep apnea syndrome, sleep-related abnormal swallowing syndrome**, and **sleep terrors** may present in a similar way.[1629]

Chart S–7. The International Classification of Sleep Disorders—List of Syndromes

1. Dyssomnias

A. *Intrinsic sleep disorders*

Psychophysiologic insomnia
Sleep state misperception
Idiopathic insomnia
Narcolepsy
Recurrent hypersomnia
Idiopathic hypersomnia
Post-traumatic hypersomnia
Obstructive sleep apnea syndrome
Central sleep apnea syndrome
Central alveolar hypoventilation syndrome
Periodic limb movement disorder
Restless legs syndrome
Intrinsic sleep disorder not otherwise specified (NOS)

B. *Extrinsic sleep disorders*

Inadequate sleep hygiene
Environmental sleep disorder
Altitude insomnia
Adjustment sleep disorder
Insufficient sleep syndrome
Limit-setting sleep disorder
Sleep-onset association disorder
Food allergy insomnia
Nocturnal eating (drinking) syndrome
Hypnotic-dependent sleep disorder
Stimulant-dependent sleep disorder
Alcohol-dependent sleep disorder
Toxin-induced sleep disorder
Extrinsic sleep disorder NOS

C. *Circadian-rhythm sleep disorders*

Time zone change (jet lag) syndrome
Shift work sleep disorder
Irregular sleep–wake pattern
Delayed sleep-phase syndrome
Advanced sleep-phase syndrome
Non-24-h sleep-wake disorder
Circadian-rhythm sleep disorder NOS

2. Parasomnias

A. *Arousal disorders*

Confusional arousals
Sleepwalking
Sleep terrors

B. *Sleep–wake transition disorders*

Rhythmic movement disorder
Sleep starts
Sleep talking
Nocturnal leg cramps

C. *Parasomnias usually associated with REM Sleep*

Nightmares
Sleep paralysis
Impaired sleep-related penile erections
Sleep-related painful erections
REM sleep-related sinus arrest
REM sleep behavior disorder

D. *Other parasomnias*

Sleep bruxism
Sleep enuresis
Sleep-related abnormal swallowing syndrome
Nocturnal paroxysmal dystonia
Sudden unexplained nocturnal death syndrome
Primary snoring
Infant sleep apnea
Congenital central hypoventilation syndrome
Sudden infant death syndrome
Benign neonatal sleep myoclonus
Other parasomnia NOS

3. Sleep Disorders Associated with Mental, Neurologic, orOther Medical Disorders

A. *Associated with mental disorders*

Psychoses
Mood disorders
Anxiety disorders
Panic disorders
Alcoholism

B. *Associated with neurologic disorders*

Cerebral degenerative disorders
dementia
Parkinsonism
Fatal familial insomnia
Sleep-related epilepsy
Electrical status epilepticus of sleep
Sleep-related headaches

C. *Associated with other medical disorders*

Sleeping sickness
Nocturnal cardiac ischemia
Chronic obstructive pulmonary disease
Sleep-related asthma
Sleep-related gastroesophageal reflux
Peptic ulcer disease
Fibromyalgia

4. Proposed Sleep Disorders

Short sleeper
Long sleeper
Subwakefulness syndrome
Fragmentary myoclonus
Sleep hyperhidrosis
Menstrual-associated sleep disorder
Pregnancy-associated sleep disorder
Terrifying hypnagogic hallucinations
Sleep-related neurogenic tachypnea
Sleep-related laryngospasm
Sleep choking syndrome

From AASM Diagnostic Classification Steering Committee. The International Classification of Sleep Disorders Diagnostic and Coding Manual. *Rochester, MN. American Academy of Sleep Medicine 1991/2001. Reproduced by kind permission of the Academy.* See also http://www.sleepeducation.com/Disorders.aspx/.

sleep deprivation Unusual prevention of sleep, leading to decreased vigilance and creative efficiency, increase in microsleeps, improved affect, and a reduction in seizure thresholds. If sleep deprivation is prolonged, delirium may occur. Afterward, delta and later rapid eye movement sleep times increase.

sleep disorders A subspecialty within neurology, the problems subsumed including those in Chart S–7 as listed by Hauri[2795] and in the 2001 International Classification of Sleep Disorders.[1629]

sleep drunkenness (somnolentia) A **parasomnia** of adult life characterized by clouding of the sensorium with confusion and inappropriate impulsive behavior occurring during an abnormally prolonged period of transition between the states of being asleep (commonly in a deep nonrapid eye movement sleep stage) and being awake. Tiredness, impaired concentration, ataxia, headache, and drowsiness are other symptoms described.[5427] See also ASDA Diagnostic Classification,[1629] **sleep disorders**, and **confusional arousals**.

sleep efficiency The ratio of the total sleep time to the time designed for sleep by an individual.

sleep enuresis See **enuresis**.

sleep epilepsy Generalized or complex partial seizures occurring during any phase of sleep.

sleep fragmentation Repetitive interruption of sleep by arousals and awakenings.[280]

sleep hiccup The unusual occurrence of hiccups during sleep, recorded in a patient following severe head injury.[278]

sleep hyperhidrosis Excessive sweating during sleep, either idiopathic or due to conditions that can cause fever such as **tuberculosis, diabetes insipidus, hyperthyroidism, pheochromocytoma**, hypothalamic lesions, **epilepsy**, cerebral and brain stem **strokes, cerebral palsy, chronic paroxysmal hemicrania**, spinal cord infarction, head injury, and **familial dysautonomia**. Sleep hyperhidrosis can also occur in pregnancy, can be produced by the use of antipyretic medications, and may be seen in patients with **obstructive sleep apnea**.[1629]

sleep hypochondriasis See **subjective DIMS complaint without objective findings**.

sleep inertia The apparent paradoxical decrement in psychometric performance following a brief sleep, associated with the feeling of grogginess and nonrestoration on awakening. During this state, the EEG features of light nonrapid eye movement sleep are mingled with those of wakefulness.[883]

sleep latency The time between the subject's composing himself or herself for sleep and attaining it.

sleep maintenance insomnia The occurrence of frequent nocturnal arousals after initially falling asleep. This is usually due to incidental parasomnias or to anxiety.[280]

Sleep Medicine Home Page A Web site at http://www.users.cloud9.net/~thorpy/.

Sleep Medicine A comprehensive computerized textbook of sleep medicine listing sleep-related newsgroups and discussion groups; sources of patient information; an alphabetical listing of sleep disorders; resources regarding all aspects of sleep including its physiology, clinical sleep medicine, and sleep research; and business-related groups. Clinical practice parameters, professional associations, sleep-related foundations and associated organizations, professional journals and books, sleep research sites, and American federal and state information sources are also catalogued, as are sleep medications and neurotransmitters and contact information for sleep disorder centers worldwide. Web site: http://www. users.cloud9.net/~thorpy/.

Sleep Medicine A subspecialty journal published by Elsevier Science. Web site: http://www.elsevier.com/inca/publications/store/6/2/0/2/8/2/.

sleep mentation The imagery, thinking, and emotion experienced during sleep, most vividly in dreams and during the first entry into and last exit from nonrapid eye movement sleep.[280]

sleep myoclonus (periodic movements in sleep) Periodic, repetitive, brief, rhythmic myoclonic movements due to contraction of the tibialis anterior and more proximal muscles, occurring during any stage of nonrapid eye movement sleep in adults and afterward accompanied by features of the **restless limbs syndrome**.[1249] The condition was first reported by Symonds in 1953. See **periodic limb movement disorder**.

sleep onset The transition from the waking state to sleep, usually nonrapid eye movement stage 1, but, in infancy and in narcolepsy, into rapid eye movement sleep. (See ASDA diagnostic classification[280] and **sleep disorders**.)

sleep paralysis (catalepsy of awakening, daymares, waking cataplexy, postchalastic fits, nocturnal hemiplegia, Rosenthal syndrome) A dissociated rapid eye movement sleep inhibitory process, characterized by

Chart S–8. Diagnostic Criteria for Sleep Paralysis[1629]

A. A complaint of inability to move the trunk or limbs at sleep onset or upon awakening
B. Presence of a brief episode of partial or complete skeletal muscle paralysis
C. Episodes can be associated with hypnagogic hallucinations or dreamlike mentation
D. Polysomnographic monitoring demonstrates at least one of the following:
   1. Suppression of skeletal muscle tone
   2. A sleep-onset rapid eye movement period
   3. Dissociated rapid eye movement sleep
E. Not associated with other medical or psychiatric disorders, for example, hysteria or hypokalemic paralysis.

From AASM Diagnostic Classification Steering Committee. *The International Classification of Sleep Disorders Diagnostic and Coding Manual*. Rochester MN. American Academy of Sleep Medicine 1991/2001. Reproduced by kind permission of the Academy. See also http://www.sleepeducation.com/Disorders.aspx/.

periods of flaccid paralysis of all but the respiratory and extraocular muscles with areflexia, occurring for minutes during the waking stage immediately preceding or succeeding sleep and terminated by sleep or by sensory stimulation. The experience is frequently frightening. This may represent the tonelessness of normal rapid eye movement sleep occurring in the conscious state. **Cataplexy** is the equivalent in the waking state. The syndrome may occur in isolation or as a component of the **narcolepsy** syndrome, and may be familial. The diagnostic criteria in Chart S–8 have been suggested: [1629]

The condition was described by the American Dr. R. McNish in 1837, but Weir **Mitchell** in 1876 gave a more professional account.[4404] *Variants* include familial and sporadic or "isolated" cases in which an attack occurs in otherwise normal subjects and those linked with the **Pickwickian syndrome**. The first description may have been that told in the childrens' story of the *Sleeping Beauty*, who awoke from her slumber at the touch of the Prince's kiss. More mundane stimuli, however, are equally effective. See also **narcolepsy**.

sleep quality A term for the overall satisfaction with sleep by a person and assessed from sleep latency (in minutes); time awake after sleep onset, total sleep time, sleep efficiency (time asleep or time in bed) and latency to stage 2 and to rapid eye movement sleep in minutes.

sleep rebound The increase in the proportion of rapid eye movement sleep which occurs following a period of selective deprivation of that stage.

Sleep Research Society An American professional society composed of members with research interests in the realm of sleep. Address: One Westbrook Corporate Center, Suite 920, Westchester, IL 60154. Tel:708-492-0930. E-mail: JYore@aasmnet.org. Web site: http://www.sleepresearchsociety.org/contact/index.php/.

sleep reversal Wakefulness during darkness and sleep during the day; a phenomenon occurring in some demented patients and in the context of South African trypanosomiasis (**sleeping sickness**).

sleep spindles (sigma rhythm) Recurring bursts of increasing- and then decreasing-amplitude EEG activity at 11–16 Hz (but mostly at 12–14 Hz), lasting 0.5–2 s, signaling the onset of stage 2 nonrapid eye movement sleep. They are generally diffuse but of higher voltage over the central regions of the head. Their amplitude is variable but is mostly below 50 μV in adults. (Adapted from the 1974 report of the Committee on Terminology, IFCN. In: Chatrian GE, Bergamini L, Dondey M, et al. A glossary of terms most commonly used by clinical electroencephalographers. *EEG Clin Neurophysiol* 1974;**37**:538–48. Reproduced with kind permission from Elsevier Science.)

sleep stages Periods of sleep with individual distinguishing characteristics, as recorded with the measures used in **polysomnography**, in which stereotyped patterns of EEG, electro-oculographic, and EMG activity allow distinction between **nonrapid eye movement** (NREM) and **rapid eye movement** (REM) stages. Precise guidelines for scoring and naming these stages are available.[5223] **Nonrapid eye movement** stages are defined as shown in Chart S–9.

The first indication of the existence of different types of sleep was given by **von Economo**, who noted that drowsy postencephalitic patients had lesions in the posterior hypothalamus and mesencephalic tegmentum, while those who were insomniac had lesions in the forebrain. See also **REM sleep**.

sleep starts (hypnagogic jerks, hypnic jerks, predormital myoclonus, somnolescent starts) A sleep–wake transition parasomnia in the form of a partial arousal response, manifest as generalized, single, asymmetrical bodily jerks on falling asleep, unassociated with clinical or EEG abnormalities and of no pathological significance. They are occasionally accompanied by a perception of falling or a flash of dream prior to intense arousal, with return of alpha rhythms on the EEG.[4829] These brief, spontaneous, generalized, or localized nonperiodic myoclonic movements of the trunk and limbs occur mainly at the onset of the first periods of stages 3 and 4 of nonrapid eye movement sleep. They last less than a quarter of a second, mainly affect the legs, resemble the startle reaction of wakefulness,[1629] and occur in many normal people, usually during sleep onset. A positive family history is frequently found.

Diagnostic criteria have been suggested[1629] and are reproduced in Chart S–10.

In a *variant* form, the jerks are excessive and repeatedly interrupt sleep, without evidence of **hyperekplexia**.[882] See also **physiological hypnic myoclonus**.

sleep state misperception A dyssomnia in which there is a complaint of insomnia or excessive sleepiness without objective evidence of disturbance of sleep. Polysomnography reveals a normal sleep latency, and the multiple sleep latency test demonstrates a mean sleep latency of greater than 10 min.[1629]

sleep talking (somniloquy) The utterance of speech or sounds during any stage of sleep without simultaneous subjective detailed awareness of the event. Such talking during rapid eye movement

Chart S–9. Nonrapid Eye Movement Sleep Stages

Stage 1. A stage of sleep following directly upon wakefulness and characterized by the EEG appearance of low-voltage activity with alpha activity constituting less than 50%, with beta activity and vertex spikes, and with slow rolling eye movements. This usually comprises some 5% of total sleep time.

Stage 2. A stage of sleep characterized by the appearance of sleep spindles and K complexes on a low-voltage mixed-frequency background and with delta activity constituting up to 20% of the stage. This stage usually comprises some 50% of the total sleep time.

Stage 3. A stage of sleep characterized by the appearance of high-amplitude delta waves (>75 μV, <2 Hz) for between 20 and 50% of the time, which occurs in the first third of the sleep period.

Stage 4. A stage of sleep characterized by the appearance of high-amplitude delta waves (>75 μV, <2 Hz) for more than 50% of the time and comprising with NREM stage 3 and slow-wave or delta sleep.

Adapted from Rechtschaffen A, Kales A. A Manual of Standardized Terminology, Techniques and Scoring for Sleep Stages of Normal Subjects. Washington, DC: Dept. Heath, Education and Welfare, 1968.

Chart S–10. Diagnostic Criteria for Sleep Starts

A. A complaint of either difficulty initiating sleep or of an intense body movement at sleep onset
B. Sudden brief jerks at sleep onset, mainly affecting the legs or arms
C. Associated with at least one of the following:
  1. A subjective feeling of falling
  2. A sensory flash
  3. A hypnagogic dream
D. Polysomnographic monitoring during an episode demonstrates one or more of the following:
  1. Brief, high-amplitude muscle potentials during the transition from wakefulness to sleep
  2. Arousals from light sleep
  3. Tachycardia following an intense episode
E. Absence of any medical or psychiatric disorder that could produce the disorder, e.g., **hyperekplexia**.
F. Can occur in the presence of other sleep disorders producing insomnia.

From AASM Diagnostic Classification Steering Committee. The International Classification of Sleep Disorders Diagnostic and Coding Manual. *Rochester, M.N. American Academy of Sleep Medicine 1991/2001. Reproduced by kind permission of the Academy.* See also http://www.sleepeducation.com/Disorders.aspx/.

(REM) sleep may represent the vocal expression of dream experiences, but it also occurs during transient arousals from NREM sleep. It can be associated with psychiatric or medical disorders, febrile illness, and, for example, **sleepwalking, obstructive sleep apnea syndrome**, or **REM sleep behavior disorder**.

sleep terrors See **night terrors**.

sleep test A diagnostic procedure for **myasthenia gravis**, in which a temporary remission in ptosis and ocular muscle paresis is seen after resting for some 30 min in a quiet dark room, the differences being ascertained by photography.[6829]

sleeping sickness 1. (human African trypanosomiasis) Infection by the *Trypanosoma brucei gambiense* or *T. brucei rhodesiense* as a result of a bite of the tsetse fly. Neurological complications of the *West African* form include a chronic meningitis with focal gliosis. Clinically, this leads to neurological complications after a year of systemic symptoms, with evidence of progressive chronic encephalitis characterized particularly by tremor, ataxia, involuntary movements, and dementia.

In the *East African* form, a more acute illness occurs as a result of infection by *T. brucei rhodesiense*. Involvement of the nervous system occurs early with fever and evidence of diffuse encephalopathy, usually with associated cardiac involvement. The condition is usually fatal.[6858] 2. See **encephalitis lethargica**.

sleep-onset association disorder A condition of impaired sleep onset as a result of the absence of a certain object or set of circumstances—for example, a child cannot settle to sleep without a teddy bear. This is mainly a disorder of childhood and is eventually self-limiting.

sleep-onset insomnia (prolonged sleep latency) The occurrence of a delay in going to sleep of 30 min or more. This is usually due to psychological or environmental factors. See **delayed sleep phase syndrome**.

sleep-onset REM sleep period (SOREMP) The occurrence of rapid eye movement sleep without a preceding period of nonrapid eye movement sleep, as in infancy and with depressive illness and **narcolepsy**.[4904]

sleep-related abnormal swallowing syndrome A disorder in which inadequate swallowing of saliva results in aspiration, with coughing, choking, and frequent brief arousals or awakenings from sleep.[1629]

sleep-related asthma The occurrence of asthma attacks during sleep, usually as a sign of increasing severity of the condition. Patients awaken with dyspnea, wheezing, coughing, air hunger, or chest tightness, which are, however, amenable to the usual treatments. Upper GI reflux is a possible precipitant.[1629]

sleep-related bruxism See **bruxism**.

sleep-related enuresis (idiopathic enuresis) A disorder of partial arousal in which involuntary micturition occurs during the first period of nocturnal nonrapid eye movement stage 3 or 4 sleep in children more than 3 years old. See also the AASM International Classification of Sleep Disorders Diagnostic and Coding Manual.[1629]

sleep-related epilepsy The occurrence of seizures with particular frequency at night as opposed to seizures occurring by day. Any form of seizure can occur nocturnally, but benign focal epilepsy of childhood, seizures of "partial" origin, and **juvenile myoclonic epilepsy** are most likely to occur at night.[6039] Clinically, abrupt awakenings at night, unexplained urinary incontinence, unexplained bitten tongue, and abnormal movements witnessed during sleep are diagnostic clues.

sleep-related headaches The preferential occurrence of headaches during sleep. **Cluster headache, chronic paroxysmal hemicrania**, and **migraine** are leading examples. Raised intracranial pressure tends to lead to headaches on awakening. See also the AASM International Classification of Sleep Disorders Diagnostic and Coding Manual.[1629]

sleep-related headbanging See **jactatio capitis nocturna**.

sleep-related laryngospasm The occurrence of episodes of abrupt awakening from sleep with an intense sensation of inability to breathe, choking and stridor and tachycardia, intense anxiety, and a sense of impending death.[1629]

sleep-related myoclonus DIMS syndrome (nocturnal myoclonus) The occurrence of repetitive stereotyped attacks of leg myoclonus, starting during sleep but leading to multiple awakenings and complaints of insomnia, usually in adults. The movements occur every 20–120 s, last between 0.5 and 10 s, and occur in groups of

30 or more jerks.[3958] See also **hypnic jerks**, **myoclonus**, the ASDA Diagnostic Classification,[1629] **sleep disorders**, and **periodic limb movement disorder**.

sleep-related myoclonus DOES syndrome (nocturnal myoclonus) The occurrence of repetitive stereotyped attacks of leg myoclonus, starting during sleep but leading to multiple awakenings and complaints of excessive daytime sleepiness, usually in adults. The movements occur every 20–120 s, last between 0.5 and 10 s, and occur in groups of 30 or more jerks. The sleepiness is the sole feature differentiating this from the equivalent DIMS syndrome.[3958] See also **hypnic jerks**, **myoclonus**, the ASDA diagnostic classification,[1629] **sleep disorders**, and **periodic limb movement of sleep**.

sleep-related neurogenic tachypnea A sustained increase in respiratory rate during sleep from onset to arousal. It may cause excessive sleepiness or can be asymptomatic. The cause is not known, but the **central alveolar hypoventilation syndrome** is similar in presentation.[1629]

sleep-related painful erections The occurrence of prolonged, painful erections, subsiding over minutes and often recurring during the same night usually during rapid eye movement sleep periods, leading to arousal; without associated deficits in sexual functioning. Erections occurring during wakefulness are painless.[3302]

sleep-related upper GI reflux Recurrent awakenings from sleep with chest discomfort or burning substernal pain, a sour or bitter taste in the mouth, coughing or choking, and heartburn.[1629]

Sleep–Wake Disorders (Canada) A charitable organization providing support and information on this condition. Address: 5385 Yonge St., P. O. Box 45034, North York, ON M2N 5R7.

sleep–wake transition disorders Sleep disturbances which occur in the transition from wakefulness to sleep, in the transition from sleep to wakefulness, or occasionally in transitions from between different sleep stages. These include **rhythmic movement disorder**, **sleep starts**, **sleep talking**, and **nocturnal leg cramps**.

sleepwalking (somnambulism, semipurposeful automatisms) A sequence of complex behaviors during clouded consciousness which occur during the first nocturnal periods of nonrapid eye movement sleep stages 3 or 4, which are not thereafter recalled by the subject and which may end with confused awakening or with a return to normal sleep.[3275] Sitting up in bed, perseverated simple movements, and complex automatic activities such as walking, descending stairs, and opening doors may occur; attempts to restrain the subject usually lead to avoidance behavior.[5223] Such abnormal behavior is seen less in adults than in children, among whom it may be associated with **enuresis** and **night terrors**.[280]

Sleep deprivation and forced arousals during slow-wave sleep are inducers of this phenomenon.

The diagnostic criteria in Chart S–11 have been suggested by the AASM.[1629]

Chart S–11. Diagnostic Criteria for Sleepwalking

A. Ambulation that occurs in sleep
B. The onset typically occurs in prepubertal children
C. Associated features include the following:
   1. Difficulty in arousing the patient during an episode
   2. Amnesia following an episode
D. Episodes typically occur in the first third of the sleep episode
E. Polysomnographic monitoring demonstrates the onset of an episode during stage 3 or 4 sleep
F. Other medical and psychiatric disorders can be present but do not account for the symptom
G. The ambulation is not due to other sleep disorders, such as rapid eye movement sleep behavior disorder or **sleep terror**.

From AASM Diagnostic Classification Steering Committee. The International Classification of Sleep Disorders Diagnostic and Coding Manual. *Rochester, M.N. American Academy of Sleep Medicine 1991/2001. Reproduced by kind permission of the Academy.* See also http://www.sleepeducation.com/Disorders.aspx/.

slimmers' paralysis A neuropathy affecting the peroneal nerves in subjects on a weight-reducing diet. While the most likely reason would seem to be an unusual susceptibility of the nerve to the effects of compression when the knees are crossed, as a result of a reduction in the thickness of the subcutaneous tissues,[4122] a local cause has been considered unlikely by other authors.[5956]

slipping clutch gait See **isolated gait ignition failure**.

slit ventricle syndrome The occurrence of scattered pyramidal signs following the collapse of formerly enlarged ventricles, as a result of surgical shunting.[2599]

slit ventricles Abnormally narrow ventricles occurring in children with raised intracranial pressure whose shunts are blocked. The ventricles are not expanded probably because of the presence of subependymal gliosis, which has resulted from repeated distension of their walls in the past, stiffening them.[1881]

slow activity All EEG activity at a frequency lower than that of the alpha rhythm (8–13 Hz).

slow alpha variant rhythms EEG rhythms at 3.5–6 Hz (mostly at 4–5 Hz) recorded most prominently over the posterior regions of the head. They generally alternate with or are intermixed with alpha rhythms, to which they are often harmonically related. Their amplitude is variable but is frequently close to 50 μV and they are blocked or attenuated by attention, especially visual and mental effort.

Slow alpha variant rhythms should be distinguished from posterior slow waves which are characteristic of children and adolescents and are occasionally seen in young adults. (Adapted from the 1974 report of the Committee on Terminology, IFCN. In: Chatrian GE, Bergamini L, Dondey M, et al. A glossary of terms most commonly used by clinical electroencephalographers. *EEG Clin Neurophysiol* 1974;37:538–48. Reproduced with kind permission from Elsevier Science.)

slow channel syndrome (slow ion channel defect) A congenital, dominantly inherited myasthenic syndrome of selective weakness and fatigability in the face, neck, and arms, not responding to edrophonium or pyridostigmine, but with a decrementing response to repetitive nerve stimulation (which also causes a repetitive response to a single shock). It is also seen in infancy and childhood. It is due to abnormal gating of mutant acetylcholine receptors (AChRs) in the neuromuscular junction. The pathological hallmark is selective degeneration of the neuromuscular junction (*end-plate myopathy*). Caspase activation may lead to localized cellular degenerative processes without causing nuclear or cell death.[4488]

The characteristic laboratory features are prolonged decay phases of end-plate potentials and of minature end-plate potentials; repetitive compound motor action potentials; and degenerative changes of the postsynaptic membrane. The pathophysiology is considered to be a prolongation of the "open time" of the acetylcholine-induced ion channel, with a reduction in the safety factor due to decreased amplitudes of the normal miniature end-plate potentials.[1866, 1878] See also **myasthenia gravis**.

slow downward ocular bobbing See **dipping**.

slow eye movements See **pursuit eye movements** and **optokinetic nystagmus**.

slow fusional adaptive mechanism See **fusion**.

slow ion channel defect See **slow channel syndrome**.

slow motor neuron disease Those forms of **amyotrophic lateral sclerosis** in which patients survive for longer than 5 years.

slow saccades Reduction in the velocity of the saccadic movements of the eyes, due to focal or diffuse lesions in the pontine tegmentum. See *hypometric* **saccades**.

slow spike-and-wave activity See **generalized sharp-and-slow-wave discharges**.

slow stroke syndrome An ischemic stroke syndrome atypical because of its extended and gradual progression toward completion over weeks without the more usual stepwise deteriorations characteristic of multiple emboli.

slow syndrome The term of Plum[5051] for the somnolent, hypokinetic, apathetic state characterizing **thalamic dementia**.

slow upward ocular bobbing A variety of ocular bobbing seen in patients with pontine infarcts, in which the eye moves upward slowly, returning fast to the mid-position. See **ocular bobbing**.

slow wave An EEG waveform with a duration longer than that of alpha waves.

slowly alternating skew deviation A form of dysconjugate eye movement in which the findings resemble those of **skew deviation** but in which the cycles take 30–90 s. Mesodiencephalic lesions are responsible.[1280]

slowly progressive aphasia A syndrome in which the first symptom is typically an anomic, dysfluent dysphasia with phonemic paraphasic errors and relatively retained comprehension, resulting from initial involvement of the left perisylvian region. Eventually other cognitive losses appear, indicating the presence of a dementing illness (Pick, Alzheimer, spongiform, or other types).[4309, 4330]

slow-virus syndrome See **prion disease**.

slow-wave sleep The alternate of rapid eye movement sleep, in which a gradual reduction in the frequency and amplitude of the EEG rhythms occurs. Sleep spindles, vertex sharp waves, and kappa complexes also appear on this theta and delta background.

Sluder syndrome (sphenopalatine neuralgia, lower-half headache) Persistent pain felt intermittently in the face at the root of the nose and in the frontal region, temples, eye, occiput, mastoid, teeth, or hard palate, associated with homolateral reduction in the sense of taste, facial flushing, lachrymation, and salivation, and often following sphenoid or ethmoid sinusitis.

Its etiology is obscure; it may be a form of **cluster headache** but the (incomplete) descriptions given[5892] suggest that it is quite unlike any of the usual types of that disease, although later authors, in reviewing the condition, have incorporated features which Sluder did not describe. Sluder reported that this pain could be relieved by cocainization of the sphenopalatine ganglion.

Sluder, Greenfield (1865–1928) American laryngologist, who practiced in St. Louis. He believed that disease of the sphenopalatine ganglion was responsible for various facial and cranial pains.

Sly disease See **mucopolysaccharidoses**.

Small disease A recessively inherited syndrome of deafness, mental retardation, muscle atrophy with weakness and clumsiness, and vascular retinopathy.[5896] See also **Coats syndrome**.

small fiber sensory neuropathies Those neuropathies that selectively affect the small-diameter myelinated and unmyelinated fibers, leading to spontaneous neuropathic pains, hyperalgesias, paresthesias, loss of visceral pain, reduced thermal and pain sensitivity and autonomic function, or a combination of these, while proprioception and power are unaffected. Causes include **hereditary sensory neuropathy, diabetes, Fabry disease, amyloidosis, HIV** infection, **paraneoplastic** states, and certain toxins, but in many cases they remain idiopathic.

Routine nerve conduction studies may be normal and tests of intraepidermal nerve fiber analysis and quantitative sensory testing may be needed to confirm the diagnosis.[87]

See also **QSART, autonomic function tests, sympathetic skin response**.

small intensely fluorescent cells (SIF cells) Ganglion cells capable of releasing dopamine and epinephrine.

small sharp spikes (big or large sharp spikes, SSS, benign sporadic sleep spikes, **benign epileptiform transients of sleep**) Stereotyped unilateral, low-amplitude, brief, diphasic, single but repeated, transient needle-sharp spikes, recorded sporadically, mainly over temporal regions during nonrapid eye movement sleep stages 1 and 2 in normal adults and shifting between the two sides of the brain. These waveforms have no significance with regard to epilepsy.[3469, 6751]

smallpox (variola major) An acute infectious disease characterized by an abrupt onset of fever, rigors, backache, malaise, and prostration with headache, vomiting, delirium, and encephalopathy. An early erythematous rash gives way after a few days to a maculopapular rash on the face, hands, and forearms and axillae and upon oral mucous membranes, becoming vesicular and then pustular and eventually crusting. A 30% mortality rate is described in unvaccinated populations (3% in vaccinated populations).

Variola minor (alastrim, amaas) is a milder illness, with a 1% mortality in the unvaccinated population.

The disorder is noted here because of the potential for use of the organism in bioterrorism.[1204]

SMART See **stroke-like migraine attacks after radiation therapy**.

Smell Identification Test A multiple-choice "scratch and sniff" test using over three dozen odors. Although it also requires that the patient's language and memory be intact, it correlates well with other tests of olfactory thresholds.[1697]

smile–wink phenomenon The tendency for one eyelid to descend in patients with contralateral infarcts when they smile, if they smile.[3428]

smith's cramp A focal (occupational) dystonia. See **focal dystonia**.

Smith syndrome 1. (macular colobomas and dwarfism) A congenital dysmorphic syndrome characterized by short stature, macular pigmentation, colobomas of the retina, skeletal deformities, and pendular nystagmus.[5909] 2. (dwarfism, mental retardation, and dysmorphism) A congenital dysmorphic syndrome characterized by low birthweight, short stature, proportionate but prominent ears, strabismus, ptosis, seizures, dolichocephaly, and mental and developmental delay.[5909]

Smith–Lemli–Opitz syndrome A relatively common congenital, recessively inherited syndrome of dwarfism, microcephaly, holoproscencephaly, micrognathia, psychomotor retardation, ptosis, genital abnormalities, spasticity or hypotonia, seizures, and variable other musculoskeletal anomalies such as dwarfism[5910] due to a defect in cholesterol biosynthesis. In the brain, polymicrogyria, small brainstem and cerebellum, and absence of the corpus callosum are described. The genetic defect is at *DHCR7*. The authors are American pediatricians or geneticists.

Smith–Magenis syndrome An unusual syndrome caused by an interstitial deletion in the 17p11.2 region and characterized by facial dysmorphisms, brachydactylia, short stature, varying degrees of mental retardation, occasional neuropathy, and a specific behavioral phenotype that includes stereotypic movements, aggression phenomena, and sleep.[674]

SMON See **subacute myelo-optico-neuropathy**.

smooth endoplasmic reticulum A structural component of the axon, continuous distally from the perikaryon and responsible for the rapid transfer of large-molecular-weight proteins.

smooth pursuit system A reflex mechanism, not therefore under voluntary control, whereby the eyes track a mobile target so as to keep the image of that target on the fovea. The pathways responsible are not precisely known but must involve the frontal eye fields and the occipital cortex as well as subcortical connections. See also **fixation, saccades, optokinetic nystagmus**, and **pursuit eye movements**.

Sneddon syndrome A thrombotic vasculopathy leading to the rare association of idiopathic livedo reticularis and strokes, the latter being due to a noninflammatory arteriopathy affecting small- and medium-sized vessels. Seizures and dementia are also described as part of the syndrome. The condition appears in youth or adult life and is probably dominantly inherited. Complicated obstetrical histories, cardiac lesions, venous thromboses, thrombocytopenia, and disturbed sexual function in men are other features described.[5221, 5929]

In a *variant* form, a vascular dementing syndrome without livedo reticularis occurs in the presence of **antiphospholipid antibodies**. See also **Worster–Drought syndrome**.

sneeze center A cell cluster in the rostral dorsolateral pontomedullary area, damage to which may result in abortion of the normal sneezing phenomena.[2061]

sneeze reflex See **nasal reflex**.

sneeze syncope Fainting, produced by sneezing (or other methods of performing the Valsalva maneuver), and noted rarely as a complication of the **Chiari malformation**.[1279]

sneezing (ptarmus, sternutatio convulsiva) A compound reflex with various adequate afferent stimuli which induce involuntary spasmodic inspiration, followed by explosive expiration with initial brief nasopharyngeal closure and closure of the eyes. It is mediated by the V and VII cranial nerves and brainstem respiratory centers.

The Talmud describes sneezing as a pleasure sent from God, while Pope Gregory (AD 540–604) regarded it as a sign of impending plague and, following his lead, the benediction "God bless you" is commonly offered to a person who sneezes. Intractable sneezing is usually psychogenic but may have an epileptic or local basis.[1206] See also **ACHOO**.

Snellen, Hermann (1834–1908) Dutch ophthalmologist who in 1862 devised the first standard test types for assessing visual acuity. He also described the aural hyperemia that occurs with stimulation of the auriculotemporal nerve. See also **red ear syndrome.**

Sniffin' Sticks A proprietary test of olfactory functions assessing odor threshold, discrimination, and identification.

snoring (rhencospasm) (from Gr, snore + spasm) The occurrence of loud upper airway breathing sounds during sleep without episodes of apnea or hypoventilation, occurring mainly in males with large tonsils. Retrognathia, depression of the CNS, nasal congestion, and obesity also predispose to snoring. Although snoring is also a feature of forms of **sleep apnea**, the primary form is not associated with these conditions.[1629]

snout response Puckering or protrusion of the lower lip and depression of the corner of the mouth, elicited by a light tap below the nose or brief pressure above the upper lip. This is a developmental reflex (an augmentation of the **oral** reflex) which is present in cases of anterior cerebral artery occlusion, hepatic coma, toxic and traumatic states, and dementias[4939] and in subjects with diffuse cortical disease or bilateral corticobulbar tract lesions. See **buccal reflex**.

snouting See **buccal reflex**.

snow blindness See **photophthalmia**.

snowbanking Accumulation of the products of inflammation in the lower half of the anterior chamber of the eye as a result of gravity.

S-O syndrome See **sphenoidal fissure-optic canal syndrome**.

soap-bubble tumor A name suggested by the CT appearance of lymphoplasmacytoid lymphoma (cerebral immunocytoma).[6209]

sobbing spasms See **breathholding spells**, of which these attacks represent a *variant*, characterized by prolonged sobbing up to the point that the infant is performing a Valsalva maneuver.[2312]

Sobue disease See **monomelic amyotrophy.**

Social Ties checklist A 10-item scale that assesses the quantity and quality of social supports. Scores range from 0 to 10, higher scores indicating better social supports.

Sociedad Espanola de Neurologia A professional organization. Web site: http://www.sen.es/.

Sociedade Portuguesa de Neuroscienzias A professional organization. Web site: http://www.spn.org.pt/brain/brain01.asp.

Società Italiana di Neurologia A professional organization. Web site: http://www.neuro.it/modelli-organizzativi.php.

The following Italian organizations can also be accessed at this site: Società dei Neurologie, Neurochirurghie Neuroradiologi Ospedalieri; Società Italiana di Neurochirurgia; Società Italiana di Neurofisiologia Clinica; Società Italiana di Riabilitazione Neurologica.

Societa Italiana di Neuroradiologia Medica A professional organization. Web site: http://www.sirm.org/sirm/sezioni_studio/neuroradiologia.

Société Française de Neurologie A professional organization. Web site: http://www.sf-neuro.org/.

Society for Neuro-Oncology A professional organization. Web site: http://www.soc-neuro-onc.org/.

Society for Neuroscience A professional organization. Web site: www.sfn.org.

Society for Progressive Supranuclear Palsy Inc. An advocacy and mutual support group. Address: c/o David Saks 3737, Courtleigh Dr. Randallstown, MD 21133-4827.Tel: 410-655-1715; 1-800-457-4777. Web site: http://www.psp.org/.

Society for Progressive Supranuclear Palsy Inc. Johns Hopkins Outpatient Center, Suite 5065, 601 Caroline St., Baltimore, MD 21287. Web site: www.psp.org.

Society for Research into Hydrocephalus and Spina Bifida A charitable and research-oriented organization. Web site: http://www.srhsb. org/.

Society of British Neurological Surgeons A professional organization. Web siste: http://www.sbns.org.uk/.

Society of Neurological Surgeons A professional organization. Web site: http://www.societyns.org/society/search.aspx?MemberType=A.

Society of Neurosurgical Anesthesia and Critical Care A professional organization. Web site: http://www.snacc.org/.

socioeconomic scale An instrument designed to identify the socioeconomic needs of patients with **multiple sclerosis**, in which working ability; financial or economic status; residence; dependence; transportation; therapy services; psychosocial status; problem-solving capacity; and memory are each rated on a 6-point scale.[4296] See also **environmental status scale**.

SOD1 Copper or zinc superoxide dismutase, the gene for which appears remarkably likely to undergo mutations causing various phenotypic varieties of **amyotrophic lateral sclerosis**, etc.

sodium amytal test (Wada Test) The intracarotid injection of sodium amylobarbitone for the purpose of producing reversible inhibition of the functions of the ipsilateral hemisphere. The test was introduced by Dr. Jun Wada while at the Montreal Neurological Institute, in an attempt to determine the side where speech function is localized—important information in candidates for temporal lobectomy. See **Wada Test**.

Soederbergh pressure reflex Flexion of the second, third, and fourth fingers when the ulna is firmly stroked in a downward direction. When this is done over the radius, the thumb flexes. The phenomenon is seen in some cases of pyramidal and perhaps basal ganglion disease. Similar muscle contractions in response to pressure upon other bony prominences are also described.

Soemmerring, Samuel Thomas von (1755–1830) Prussian anatomist, professor of anatomy and surgery at a number of German universities, who in 1778 reclassified **Willis'** scheme of the cranial nerves into one recognizing 12 pairs, which is the system accepted today, albeit with some reluctance. He gave priority to **Vicq d'Azir** for discovering the substantia nigra but was an early describer of the difference between the gray and white matter of the cerebrum; he also described the macula lutea and the substantia gelatinosa and reported a case of achondroplasia.

soft exudates Organized edema fluid in the retina, the whitish clumps having ill-defined margins.

Chart S–12. Diagnostic Criteria for Somatization Disorder

A. There is a history of many physical complaints, beginning before age 30 years, that occur over a period of several years and result in treatment being sought or significant impairment in social, occupational, or other important areas of functioning.
B. Each of the following criteria must have been met, with individual symptoms occurring at any time during the course of the disturbance:

(1) *Four pain symptoms:* a history of pain related to at least four different sites or functions (e.g., head, abdomen, back, joints, extremities, chest, rectum, during menstruation, during sexual intercourse, or during urination)
(2) *Two gastrointestinal symptoms:* a history of at least two gastrointestinal symptoms other than pain (e.g., nausea, bloating, vomiting other than during pregnancy, diarrhea, or intolerance of several different foods)
(3) *One sexual symptom*: a history of at least one sexual or reproductive symptom other than pain (e.g., sexual indifference, erectile or ejaculatory dysfunction, irregular menses, excessive menstrual bleeding, vomiting throughout pregnancy)
(4) *One pseudo-neurological symptom:* a history of at least one symptom or deficit suggesting a neurological condition not limited to pain (conversion symptoms such as impaired coordination or balance, paralysis or localized weakness, difficulty swallowing or lump in throat, aphonia, urinary retention, hallucinations, loss of touch or pain sensation, double vision, blindness, deafness, seizures; dissociative symptoms such as amnesia; or loss of consciousness other than fainting)

C. Either (1) or (2): (1) After appropriate investigation, each of the symptoms in Criterion B cannot be fully explained by a known general medical condition or the direct effects of a substance (e.g., a drug of abuse or a medication)

(2) When there is a related general medical condition, the physical complaints or resulting social or occupational impairment are in excess of what would be expected from the history, physical examination, or laboratory findings

D. The symptoms are not intentionally feigned or produced (as in factitious disorder or malingering). (Author's comment: How a clinican determines that to be the case is not explained.)

Reproduced from American Psychiatric Association, Diagnostic and Statistical Manual of Mental Disorders, Fourth edition (DSM-IV TR). *Washington, DC: American Psychiatric Association, 2001 with paid permission.* The full *DSM–IV* criteria can be accessed at http://www.behavenet.com/capsules/disorders/dsm4TRclassification.htm/

soft neurological signs Clinical departures from the normal which because of their imprecision, inconstancy, or isolation are not adequate to convince the examiner of the presence of disease.

Sollier, Paul (1861–1938) French neurologist, for some years a pupil of **Charcot**, who encouraged him to work on the subject of memory. on which he did publish his observations. His work was known to Marcel Proust, his patient, and formed the basis for aspects of Prousts novel *A la récherche du temps perdu.*[764]

soma- (Gr, the body).

Somagyi sign Dilation of the pupils with full inspiration and constriction with full expiration. The feature is physiological but so small in degree that instrumentation may be needed to demonstrate it, which is why it is not a standard clinical method.

somatization disorder (conversion disorder, hysterical neurosis, dissociative or conversion disorder, Briquet syndrome) The expression of psychological conflicts as physical complaints, *or* "a tendency to experience and communicate somatic distress and symptoms unaccounted for by physical findings, to attribute them to physical illness and to seek medical help."[5371] The main features are multiple, recurrent, and frequently changing physical symptoms of at least 2 years' duration. Most patients have a long and complicated history of contact with both primary and specialist medical care services, during which many negative investigations or fruitless exploratory operations may have been carried out. Symptoms may be referred to any part or system of the body. The course of the disorder is chronic and fluctuating and is often associated with disruption of social, interpersonal, and family behavior. The diagnostic criteria proposed in the *DSM-IV TR* are given in Chart S–12.

In clinical practice, one sometimes hears a long list of somatic complaints which turn out to have no medical ("organic") basis but the patients' preoccupations persist despite appropriate medical evaluation and reassurance and they return with some variations to the initial complaint, focusing on the symptom itself and not on what it means. Their life seems to revolve around the symptom. Factors reinforcing or contributing to the condition include society itself (because such symptoms are socially approved and sometimes even rewarded) and a past background of disproportionate incidence of illness or injury while growing up.

One *variant* is *somatoform autonomic dysfunction* in which the patient presents cardiovascular, gastrointestinal, respiratory, and/or urogenital symptoms such as palpitations, sweating, flushing, tremor, and expression of fear and distress about the possibility of a physical disorder, and subjective complaints of a nonspecific or changing nature such as fleeting aches and pains, sensations of burning, heaviness, tightness, and feelings of being bloated or distended, which are referred by the patient to a specific organ or system. Terms used in this context include cardiac neurosis, Da Costa's syndrome, gastric neurosis, neurocirculatory asthenia, psychogenic forms of aerophagy, cough, diarrhea, dyspepsia, dysuria, flatulence, hiccough, hyperventilation, increased frequency of micturition, irritable bowel syndrome, and pylorospasm. Another is *persistent somatoform pain disorder*, in which the predominant complaint is of persistent, severe, and distressing pain, which cannot be explained fully by a physiological process or a physical disorder and which occurs in association with emotional conflict or psychosocial problems that can be considered to be the main causative influences. The result is usually a marked increase in support and attention, either personal or medical.

(Abstracted from the NIMH site: http://www.nimh.nih.gov/health/publications/adhd/symptoms.shtml/.)

somatoform disorder See **conversion disorder** and **hysteria**.

somatofugal axonal atrophy The process whereby altered synthesis of neurofilaments in the cell body of an axon leads to the delivery of axoplasm containing a low concentration of neurofilament protein to the distal part of the axon, which causes the axon to shrink.

somatognosia A distinct psychological function concerned with bodily orientation corresponding to body image or to the "body schema" of **Head** and **Holmes**. "A spatial quality in the awareness of various sensory impressions of the body" (Bonnier, 1905).[5059]

somatognosia The conscious awareness of the presence, disposition, and orientation of the parts of the body, forming a scheme or image of the body in the mind. This distinct body function is localized in the right hemisphere.

somatomotor seizures A form of simple partial seizure characterized by localized unilateral clonic movements affecting particularly the distal and the bulbar muscles.

In a *variant* form, the attacks begin with a brief period of tonic contraction and then become clonic.

somatosensory aura In the context of epilepsy, tingling, numbness, electric shock sensations, pain, a sense of movement, or a desire to move preceding the actual ictus.[16]

somatosensory blink response A blink response elicited by electrical stimulation of a peripheral nerve such as the median, recording from the inferior orbicularis oculi muscles. It represents a release phenomenon transmitted through the brainstem reticular activating system.

The criteria for the somatosensory blink response (SBR) elicited by electrical stimulation of the median nerve as suggested by Miwa et al.[4412] are as follows:

The latency to the onset of the EMG response of the orbicularis oculi muscle ranges from 35 to 60 ms

The EMG response is a bilateral response (at times, its appearance can be slightly more pronounced on the side ipsilateral to the stimulation)

The EMG response is a phasic response with a duration of less than 100 ms

If three consecutive electrical stimulations at intervals of at least 10 s fail to elicit any obvious EMG discharges, the SBR is considered negative

The amplitude of the obtained EMG response is at least threefold greater than the baseline activities of the orbicularis oculi muscles by inspection

somatosensory evoked potentials (SEPs) Electrical waveforms of biological origin elicited by electrical stimulation or physiological activation of peripheral sensory fibers, for example, of the median, common peroneal, or posterior tibial nerves.

The normal SEP is a complex waveform with several components which are specified by polarity and the average peak latency. The polarity and latency of individual components depend upon the following:

1. Subject variables, such as age and sex
2. Stimulus characteristics, such as intensity and rate of stimulation
3. Recording parameters, such as amplifier time constants, electrode placement, and electrode combinations

From the 2001 Report of the Nomenclature Committee of the American Academy of Neuromuscular and Electrodiagnostic Medicine.[19] Reproduced by kind permission of the AANEM.

See also **spinal evoked potential**.

somatosensory nystagmus See **arthrokinetic-induced nystagmus**.

somatosensory seizures Simple partial seizures in which paresthesias or abnormal somatognosis occurs, usually spreading through a geographical area of the body on one side.[4184]

somatosensory vertigo
1. A physiological illusion of bodily rotation which occurs when limbs are passively rotated about a vertical axis at the hips or shoulder joints. The phenomenon may be accompanied by **arthrokinetic-induced nystagmus**. 2. Vague sensorimotor symptoms occurring in patients with peripheral sensory neuropathy, especially when there is an abnormality in another afferent channel.[819] See **multisensory syndrome**.

somatostatin (growth hormone inhibitory factor) A neuropeptide transmitter substance found in the striatum and hypothalamopituitary axis. It inhibits the secretion of growth hormone but also depresses the secretion of insulin and glucagon. It is also found in the spinal cord, where it may act as a modulator of the pain pathway.

somatotopic localization The representation of particular regions of the body within specific areas of the CNS.

somesthesis The sensation of static position or movement of a part of the body.

somesthetic temporal discrimination The ability to perceive as separate two successive somesthetic stimuli applied to the same or to different places on the skin. The somatosensory pathways and parietal cortex, the supplementary motor area, and subcortical regions are all normally involved in such discrimination.[3635]

Sommer sector Ammon's horn, a part of the hippocampus, in which the pyramidal cells are unusually sensitive to oxygen deprivation. It was described by Wilhelm Sommer (1852–1900), a German physician.

Sommer syndrome A congenital dysmorphic syndrome of modern description, characterized by dysplasia of the iris, renal agenesis, hydrocephalus, wide cranial sutures, and mental and developmental delay.[381]

somnambulism See **sleepwalking**.

somniloquy See **sleeptalking**.

somnolence syndrome A reversible syndrome of lethargy, nausea, and headache with slowing of the EEG patterns, occurring in children treated with methotrexate and irradiation for leukemia. See also **necrotizing leukoencephalopathy**.[2188]

somnolence See **excessive daytime sleepiness** and **hypersomnia**.

somnolentia See **sleep drunkenness**.

somnolescent starts See **sleep starts**.

sonogenic reflex epilepsy See **musicogenic epilepsy**.

soporific (from Lat, deep sleep + making).

sorbinil An aldose reductase inhibitor, under scrutiny as a treatment for diabetic peripheral neuropathy.

sorbitol An alcohol sugar, the level of which is increased in the peripheral nerves of those with diabetes.

Sotos Syndrome Support Association A charitable organization in this field. E-mail: sssa@well.com. Web site: http://www.well.com/user/sssa/.

Sotos syndrome See **cerebral gigantism**.

Sottas, J. (1866–1953) French neurologist and naval historian. See **hereditary motor and sensory neuropathy**, type 3.

soul-deaf Totally destitute of hearing and of all reminiscence of sounds previously heard.

Souques disease (functional bent back) See **camptocormia**.

Souques signs 1. Elevation and extension of a paretic arm causes extension and spreading of all the fingers.[5960, 4449] See also **digiti quinti sign**. 2. (leg sign) When a Parkinsonian patient seated on a chair is suddenly tipped backward on the chair, the subject's legs do not extend because of the lack of associated movements.[2066] 3. See **Gordon sign**. 4. Abduction of all the fingers when the arm is outstretched, a sign of hemiparesis.[4449] See also **digiti quinti sign**.

Souques syndrome 1. See **palilalia**. 2. Congenital absence of the pectoral muscles, usually unilaterally.[5959] Hypotrophy of the corresponding arm may be associated.

Souques, Achille-Alexandre (1860–1944) French neuropsychiatrist who switched from the study of law to that of medicine at the Université de Paris. He worked under **Charcot**, eventually becoming *chef de clinique* under **Brissaud** and **Raymond** after Charcot's death. After some years spent elsewhere, he returned to the **Salpêtrière**, where he remained until his retirement in 1925.

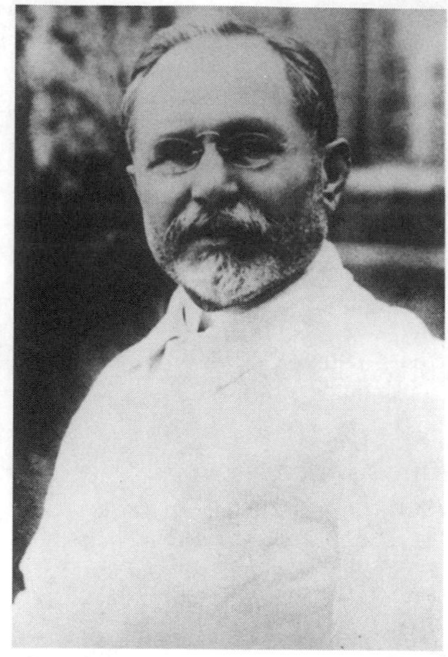

Figure S–5 Achille-Alexandre Souques

He described **palilalia**, the **inversion** of reflexes, and hypophyseal infantilism, but published principally on the topics of Parkinsonism, multiple sclerosis, epilepsy, **camptocormia**, and medical history.

South American trypanosomiasis (Chaga disease) A zoonosis caused by *Trypanosoma cruzi*, a protozoan organism with an animal reservoir in the southern United States and South America. In the chronic phase of the infection, parasympathetic degeneration occurs as a result of massive degeneration of autonomic ganglia, leading to digestive disturbances, motor neuropathy, and cardiac signs including sudden death. Clinically, an acute, mild febrile illness leads on to asymptomatic infection or cardiomyopathy, with or without systemic myositis.[6858] See also **sleeping sickness** (West African trypanosomiasis).

South Indian paraplegia See **Madras neuropathy**.

space motion sickness Vertigo experienced by astronauts during orbital flights following changes in environmental conditions and generated by active head movements. Episodes of dizziness, nausea, and a persistent feeling of movement occur during the switch from the earth's gravity to microgravity, as well as when astronauts come back to earth after a long period of weightlessness (*re-adaptation syndrome*). In each case, symptoms normally appear during the first hours in orbit or upon return to earth's gravity and may last hours to days.

The combined sensory inputs from the vestibular apparatus, eyes, and muscles allow our orientation on earth, but when the environment is altered such that information from the different receptors are conflicting, motion sickness may occur due to inequality of the weight of the otoliths or to an intravestibular mismatch between the otoliths and the semicircular canals.[819]

The condition is uncommon in general neurology practice.

space-occupying lesions A nonsense term signifying any solid or liquid intracranial lesion. It is difficult to think of anything affecting the brain that does not occupy some space, except perhaps for neurosis. See **mass lesions**, the preferred term.

Spanish toxic oil syndrome A clinical syndrome of myalgia, joint limitation, weight loss, cramps, progressive weakness and wasting, and sensory disturbances and changes in the skin due to a progressive mixed axonal neuropathy affecting both proximal and distal muscles. The condition was due to the ingestion of cooking oil adulterated with triorthocresyl phosphate and was described in Spain in 1981.[1367]

sparganosis Infection with the larvae of tapeworms belonging to the genus *Spirometra*, presenting usually as a solitary cyst in muscle containing the worm *Spirometra mansoni* or *Diphyllobothrium latum*. It results from the ingestion of uncooked fish or amphibians. Obstructive hydrocephalus, focal motor seizures, myelopathy, ptosis, and orbital cellulitis are described complications.[124] The condition is more common in the Orient and in Northern Canada.

sparing of fixation (macular sparing) Retention of the central 5° of the visual field in the presence of occipital lobe infarction.

This is considered to be due to the supplementary supply of blood through the middle cerebral artery to the occipital pole (which is the projection area for the macula), rather than to the bilateral representation of macular function.

spasm (Gr, muscular contraction) Involuntary reflex muscle contractions with accompanying electrical activity which is either normal or resembles that occurring in **tetany**. The cramps may be tonic or clonic and are usually painful. Prolonged muscle contraction and ischemia are the more common causes.

spasm faciale mediane See **cranial dystonias**.

spasm of conjugate gaze Conjugate deviation of the eyes when the patient attempts to close them against resistance. This is a sign of parietal lobe disease, the eyes deviating away from the side of the lesion. The sign would be of greater localizing value were it not often present with some lesions of the brainstem as well.[1219]

spasm of the near reflex Intermittent and painful attacks of convergence, accommodation, and miosis with failure of lateral movement of the globes. The condition resembles bilateral VI cranial nerve palsies except that there is miosis of the putative abducting eye on attempted lateral gaze.[1218] Normally the pupil dilates when abduction is attempted. See **convergence spasm**.

spasmodic crying See **emotionalism**.

spasmodic dysphonia (spastic dysphonia, inspiratory speech) A laryngeal dystonia leading to a form of speech which is constrained, harsh, and monotonous; enunciated *staccato* with variable but uncontrolled volume and accompanied by spillover movements of the face and bulbar muscles. Other descriptions note quiet, tremulous, hoarse, strangulated, or whispered speech, interrupted by irregular stoppages or catches. Whispering may, however, be relatively normal. The features of **Meige syndrome** or of other **dystonias** may coexist. The condition was first described by Traube in 1871.

Although all of the speech is uttered during expiration, the sound effect is unnatural and suggests the picturesque but incorrect alternative title given it. A good example will be given if the reader enunciates this entry during inspiration rather than expiration. No single pathology is suggested by such speech, which has parallels in certain other languages.[1326]

spasmodic laughter (Homeric laughter, sham mirth) Emotional expression in the absence of emotional experience, as occurs in some patients with brainstem or frontal lobe disease, intracranial hemorrhage, or **Lytico-Bodig**. Uncontrollable weeping without appropriate affect is a similar phenomenon.[4118]

spasmodic torticollis A common form of focal or segmental dystonia, characterized by involuntary tonic or intermittent spasms of the neck muscles, which typically lead to a deviation of the head from its normal position and which may be painful.

The condition was first described in detail by Jean **Cruchet** in 1907. Other dystonias and tremor are found in a proportion of patients and the condition may be a *forme fruste* of idiopathic torsion **dystonia**. Somehow, it has also been detected in fossil dinosaurs.[4100, 5372] Although assuredly there exists organic disease of the basal ganglia in this condition, which may also complicate cervical spinal lesions, the precise nature of this is not known. See also **cervical dystonia**, **antecollis**, and **retrocollis**.

spasmophilia 1. (latent **tetany**) An increased tendency to suffer tetanic attacks, as in patients with hypocalcemia.
2. (**hyperventilation syndrome**) A state characterized by hyperventilation and anxiety.

spasmus nictitans (nictitatio, blepharoclonus) Clonic spasms of the eyelids, seen in dystonias and in **hemifacial spasm**.

spasmus nutans (head nodding) The rare association of ocular oscillations at 2.4 Hz, head-nodding, tilt, and torticollis occurring in the first 2 years of life. It seldom lasts longer than 3 years, except in the unusual case in which it is due to a tumor in the region of the third ventricle. An accompanying pendular horizontal nystagmus is frequently bilateral but asymmetrical.[5965]

spastic ataxia of Charlevoix-Saguenay See **Charlevoix-Saguenay spastic ataxic syndrome**.

spastic diplegia See **Little disease**.

spastic dysphonia See **spasmodic dysphonia**.

spastic eyelids Uninhibited tonic lid elevation leading to the maintenance of eye opening in the unconscious state without blinking, associated with increased levator tone. It is thought to indicate the presence of a pontine lesion.[3353]

Spastic Paraplegia Foundation A charitable organization in this field promoting research and treatment of these conditions. Address: P.O. Box 1208, Forston, GA 31808. Tel: 888-572-7934. Web site: http://www.sp-foundation.org/. See also http://perso.wanadoo.fr/asl.spastic/, http://www.fsp-info.de and www.hspinfo.org.

spastic paraplegia The syndrome of pyramidal signs with a defined upper level corresponding to a spinal level, usually taken as below C8. The causes include **hereditary spastic paraparesis**, spinal tumors, transverse myelopathy, **multiple sclerosis**, and spinal trauma, as well as a range of less common conditions, but it may also occur after multiple cerebrovascular episodes, indicating that not all cases are of spinal origin.[6447]

spastic paraplegia, ataxia, mental retardation (SPAR) See **hereditary spastic paraparesis**.

spastic paraplegia, optic atrophy, and neuropathy A recessively inherited congenital neurodegenerative disorder characterized by amblyopia due to optic atrophy and with the onset of progressive spastic paraplegia in infancy and of progressive motor and sensory axonal neuropathy in late childhood or early adolescence. Dysarthria starts in the third decade and exacerbated acoustic startle response and progressive joint contractures and spine deformities follow. Motor handicap is severe and all patients are wheelchair-bound after 15 years. Linkage to 11q13 has been established.[3994]

spastic paretic facial contracture A chronic, persistent, unilateral facial contracture resulting from persistent **myokymia**, associated with facial weakness and due to intrinsic pontine disease.[5942] See also **Rasdolsky syndrome**.

spastic pelvic floor syndrome A disorder due to persistent contraction of normal pelvic floor muscles, causing a functional outlet obstruction during straining and resulting in severe constipation.[3591]

spastic pseudosclerosis See **Wilson disease**. The term has also been used for **Creutzfeldt–Jakob disease**.

spastic spinal paralysis (Erb spastic paraparesis) See **Erb–Charcot syndrome**.

spasticity of conjugate gaze The term of Cogan for ocular deviation contralateral to the side of a hemispheric (especially parietotemporal) lesion with attempted eye closure.[6123]

Spasticity Rating Scale A valid measure of disease severity in **hereditary spastic paraplegia**. It rates such items as walking distance without a pause, gait quality, maximum gait speed, climbing stairs and speed of doing so, arising from a chair, spasticity of hip adductors and knee extensors, weakness of hip abduction and of foot dorsiflexion, contractures of the legs, pain, and sphincter function.[5659]

spasticity "A motor disorder characterized by a velocity-dependent increase in tonic stretch reflexes (muscle tone) with exaggerated tendon jerks, resulting from hyperexcitability of the stretch reflex, as one component of the upper motor neuron syndrome."[3656, 3655] Loss of supraspinal control leads to excessive activity of motoneurons and lack of the normal reciprocal innervation, and thus to the firing off of agonists and antagonists at the same time, either spontaneously or as a response to stimulation. Hyperreflexia, clonus, and extensor spasms are associated.

This definition is but one among many; some others (in which the term denotes proprioceptive reflex release, generalized reflex release, the upper motor neuron syndrome, dystonic-rigid states, etc.) are reviewed by Landau.[3664]

spät apoplexy (Ger, late + Gr, stroke) Delayed intracerebral hemorrhage following cranial trauma, which may be minor.[2658] The mechanisms suggested for it include an acute rise in blood pressure, suddenly increased intracerebral blood flow after the relief of a focal obstruction, and reperfusion of ischemic regions.

spatial agnosia See **spatial neglect**.

spatial agraphia See **agraphia**.

spatial neglect (agnosia for the opposite half of space, spatial agnosia) A spontaneous orientation bias toward the right side, leading to neglect of objects or persons on the left. This leads to inattention to half of visual space—almost always the left half—occurring in patients with a right hemisphere lesion in the region of the parietooccipitotemporal junction which interferes with spatial analysis and visual perception of the left side. See also **extinction** and **neglect**.

spatial summation A phenomenon of synaptic transmission, whereby two inadequate impulses converging upon a synapse may together form an adequate stimulus for excitation or suppression at that site.

Spatz, H. (1888–1969) German neurologist, experimental neuropathologist, and neuroanatomist, who worked in **Kraepelin**'s clinic in Munich, whence came **Hallervorden** with the brain of a girl who had died with the syndrome until recently known by their names. Captured by the American forces after World War II, both were pressed into serving the Allied forces' medical services and were later installed in a laboratory in Vienna for the remainder of their professional careers.

special sensory ataxia Sensory ataxia caused by loss of muscle spindle (proprioceptive) afferent input to the cerebellum.

specificity theory of sensation The original concept of **von Frey** that four somatesthetic senses were mediated by four receptor types in the skin. This is now considered to be untenable, but the **pattern theory**, which in contradistinction stated that there were neither specific fibers nor receptors, has also been found wanting. A synthesis has been achieved by Melzack and Wall.[4302]

SPECT Acronym for Single Photon Emission Computed Tomography, a technique for measuring cerebral perfusion rate by using ^{99}Tc HMPAO or Iofetamine ^{123}I as the tracer agents, with computerized reconstruction of the isotopic emissions recorded by a rotating gamma camera.

spectacular shrinking deficit The dramatic improvement in the clinical appearance of a patient with cardiogenic brain embolism, occurring over the course of minutes to hours and considered to be due to rapid dissolution of the embolus within a large artery in the carotid system, with consequent re-establishment of adequate cerebral perfusion.[4429]

speech apraxia Selective impairment in ability to produce speech sounds.[3540]

speech audiometry The assessment of auditory perception using phonemically balanced word lists. Typically, patients with neural lesions exhibit a particular difficulty in hearing speech sounds, as opposed to pure tones.[745]

speech dyspraxia See **dysprosody**.

Speech Questionnaire A rating scale of communication impairment, completed during an interview of the relative(s) of a subject with aphasia, as that occurring after a stroke. The scale consists of 19 questions relating to expressive speech and comprehension, but ignores repetition and naming abilities.[3850]

speech 1. The enunciation of "words referring to one another in a particular manner" (Hughlings-**Jackson**) according to grammar, which allows a meaning to be derived over and above the sum of the meanings of the individual words uttered. 2. The expression and reception of ideas and feelings by way of verbal symbols such as words or other verbal tools. See also **propositional language** and **speech**.

spelling agraphia An agraphic syndrome characterized by a disturbance of letter choice, although the actual form of the written letters remains intact.[452]

spelling alexia Inability to read words and phrases with relative sparing of the ability to read individual letters.[5755]

Spens, Thomas (1769–1842) Edinburgh physician whose account of bradycardia with syncope antedated that of Stokes by over half a century.[5973]

spermatic neuralgia Severe unilateral paroxysms of pain radiating between the testis and the inguinal canal, with no known cause.[645]

sphenocavernous syndrome An inclusive term for the orbital apex, cavernous, and **superior orbital fissure syndromes**. The clinical features include involvement of the III, IV, VI, and first two divisions of the V cranial nerves, and sometimes of the optic and oculosympathetic nerves as well, with or without proptosis and pain.[2746]

sphenocephaly A malformation due to persisting patency of the anterior fontanelle and of the metopic suture, characterized by prominence of the bregma and by frontal bossing.[4]

sphenoid (Gr, like a wedge) Wedge-shaped. The sphenoid bone is so-named because it is placed as though "wedged" between its neighbors.

sphenoid sinus carcinoma Rare primary carcinomas, usually presenting in adult males who complain of severe deep-seated boring headaches and visual loss, and who show features of the **sphenocavernous syndrome**, diplopia due to isolated VI cranial nerve paresis, or visual obscurations due to optic nerve or chiasmal infiltration.[2746]

sphenoid sinus A rectangular midline structure within the sphenoid bone, bounded by the pituitary fossa above, the ethmoid sinus and nasal cavity in front, the nasopharynx and Eustachian tube below, the clivus and brainstem behind, and the superior orbital fissure, cavernous sinuses, and petrous temporal bone at the sides.

sphenoidal electrodes Long EEG recording wires which can be introduced through the mandibular notch to lie beneath the floor of the middle cranial fossa. They are used the better to record discharges emanating from the inferomedial aspect of the temporal lobe. The technique was originated by H.H. **Jasper**.

sphenoidal fissure syndrome (Tolosa–Hunt syndrome, orbital apex syndrome, Rollet syndrome, Rochon-Duvigneau syndrome, painful ophthalmoplegia) A syndrome of retroorbital pain, oculomotor palsies, and sometimes visual impairment, often with acute onset following trauma or a viral infection, but also commonly with a slower onset and then usually due to a neoplasm or to granulomatous inflammation.[5361] See **superior orbital fissure syndrome**.

sphenoidal fissure–optic canal syndrome (S-O Syndrome, orbital apex syndrome) Involvement of cranial nerves II, III, IV, VI, and the ophthalmic division of the V nerve; sympathetic fibers, and the ophthalmic artery and vein by an infiltrating malignancy in this region, such as a nasopharyngeal carcinoma. The **superior orbital fissure syndrome** is probably the same thing.

sphenopalatine neuralgia One of the 17 terms for **cluster headache** listed by Kudrow[3583]—suggesting, as does the term *periodic migrainous neuralgia*, that a firm neurogenic basis may be found for the condition. It may, but it has not yet been.

sphenopetrosal fissure syndrome See **superior orbital fissure syndrome**.

spheroid body myopathy A rare, dominantly inherited, benign myopathy (a desminopathy) characterized by the onset in youth of proximal weakness, pain and atrophy in the legs, and by the presence of filamentous spheroid bodies in type I fibers on muscle biopsy specimens. Serum CK levels are normal. See also **myofibrillar (desmin-storage) myopathy**; and for further data log on to http://www.neuro.wustl.edu/neuromuscular/maltbrain.html.

sphingolipidoses A group of lysosomal storage diseases characterized by the accumulation, variously, of gangliosides, sulfatides, cerebrosides, or sphingomyelin as a result of genetically determined enzymatic failure. They include **Fabry disease**, **Farber disease**, **Gaucher disease**, **GM_1 and GM_2 gangliosidoses**, **Krabbe disease**, the **mucosulfatidoses**, and **sphingomyelin storage disorders**, such as Niemann–Pick disease and the **sulfatidoses**.

sphingomyelin lipidosis See **sphingomyelin storage disorders**.

sphingomyelin storage disorders (sphingomyelin lipidoses) A group of uncommon, recessively transmitted lysosomal storage diseases affecting sphingomyelin metabolism and causing the deposition of sphingomyelin and cholesterol in the endothelial, mesenchymal, and parenchymal cells of all body organs. Six varieties are described. Types A, B, and F have detectable deficiency of sphingomyelinase and storage of sphingomyelin. In types C, D, and E, the sphingomyelinase activity is normal or only mildly reduced. The features of the different types of the disease are summarized in Chart S–13.

All are characterized by the presence of Niemann–Pick cells in the bone marrow and a greater or lesser deficiency of sphingomyelinase.

sphingomyelin A diaminophosphatide derived from sphingosine.

sphingomyelinase An enzyme responsible for breaking down sphingomyelin, absent in some **sphingomyelin storage disorders** such as **Niemann–Pick disease**.

sphingosine The base of the sphingolipids, so named by Johann Ludwig **Thudichum** (1829–1901), who left his native Germany when 25 years old and who eventually became director of chemistry at St. Thomas' Hospital, London. Because the substance remained insoluble in ether, and in commemoration of the many enigmas which it presented, he chose a name derived from that of the Sphinx, another enigma

Chart S–13. Summary of the Sphingomyelin Storage Disorders

I. *Type A. Classical infantile Niemann–Pick disease, acute neuropathic form* A familial condition marked by sphingomyelin storage in the viscera and nervous system, and clinically manifesting mental and motor deterioration beginning in the first year of life, with seizures, hypotonia and later hypertonia, gait disturbance, Mongoloid facies, emaciation, hepatosplenomegaly, and sometimes a cherry-red macular spot with visual failure.[4671]

This form is the most common. It occurs mainly in Jewish infants and is marked by the accumulation of foamy cells throughout the reticuloendothelial system, heart, spleen, and liver, and the deposition of sphingomyelin, gangliosides, and cholesterol in the CNS leading to demyelination, gliosis, and atrophy.

II. *Type B. Juvenile, non-neuropathic* or chronic *visceral form* A form in which there is visceral involvement only; neurological abnormalities have only been described in adults.[1725]

III. *Type C. Juvenile chronic neuropathic form* (downgaze paralysis–ataxia–foam cell syndrome; juvenile dystonic lipidosis; supranuclear vertical gaze palsy with sea-blue histiocytosis; neurovisceral storage disease with vertical supranuclear ophthalmoplegia) This was the phenotype originally described. This chronic form is recessively inherited and occurs in childhood with neurological involvement (vertical supranuclear ophthalmoplegia and disorders of other saccadic movements; variable mental and motor retardation; seizures; rigidity; ataxia, and dementia). The presence of foamy storage cells (sea-blue histiocytes) in the bone marrow, the occurrence of sphingomyelin storage in the spleen, and the presence of sphingomyelinase are also notable and most patients have a mutation of the *NPC1* gene at chromosome 18q11. Three phenotypes are described as follows:

1. An early-onset, rapidly progressive form with severe hepatic dysfunction and psychomotor delay in infancy, and with the later development of vertical gaze pareses, peripheral neuropathy, ataxia, spasticity, and dementia.[3677]
2. A delayed-onset form with a slower course, characterized by mild intellectual impairment in childhood, vertical gaze pareses, ataxia and variable dementia, seizures, and extrapyramidal defects. See **dystonic juvenile lipidosis**.
3. A late (adult-onset) slowly progressive form otherwise resembling the last.[2059] It may present as a schizophrenia-like psychosis, but dementia, ataxia, dysarthria, and gaze palsies later appear.[5660] This form is also known as type F.

IV. (*Type D; Nova Scotia variant*) A late-onset, slowly progressive form affecting only families of Acadian extraction from the south-west part of that Canadian Province. Clinical features are macular degeneration, hypotonia, gait disturbance, early jaundice, and sphingomyelin storage in the spleen. The hepatic involvement is more severe[1343] but otherwise the differences from type III are minimal.

V. *Type E. Chronic Niemann–Pick disease* with neurological involvement. In this form, dementia and peripheral sensorimotor neuropathy are the leading features. It resembles the infantile form in its onset and features but the juvenile form in its course, when it affects the nervous system at all.

VI. *Type F.* The adult form of type C.

Dr. L. Pick (1868–1944) was a German pathologist working in Berlin; he re-described Niemann's patients in fuller detail, and referred to the disease with both of their names attached.[5020]

(although that word comes from the Greek term for squeeze or strangle).[2185]

spiegelschrigt See **mirror writing**.

Spielmeyer, Walther (1879–1935) German neuropsychiatrist who graduated from Halle and trained in psychiatry and pathology. In 1905 he reported the variant of **neuronal ceroid lipofuscinosis** to which his name is attached and produced a book on cerebral histology during this period of his training. In 1912 he succeeded **Alzheimer** as professor at Munich at the invitation of **Kraepelin** and continued his work, which now included studies of the peripheral nervous system. He concluded his professional career as director of the Kaiser Wilhelm Institute, although in some danger of displacement on account of his antipathy to the Nazi régime.[2066]

Spielmeyer–Sjögren disease See **neuronal ceroid lipofuscinosis**.

Spielmeyer–Stock disease See **neuronal ceroid lipofuscinosis**.

Spielmeyer–Vogt disease See **neuronal ceroid lipofuscinosis**.

Spielmeyer–Vogt–Sjögren syndrome See **neuronal ceroid lipofuscinosis**.

spike 1. In cellular neurophysiology, a short-lived (usually 1–3 ms), all-or-none change in membrane potential that arises when a graded response passes a threshold. 2. The electrical record of a nerve impulse or similar event in muscle or elsewhere. 3. In clinical EEG recordings, a wave with a duration of less than 80 ms (usually 15–80 ms).[162] Its main component is generally negative relative to other areas and its amplitude is variable. EEG spikes should be differentiated from **sharp waves**, (transients having similar characteristics but longer durations) but this distinction is largely arbitrary and serves primarily descriptive purposes. In practical terms, spikes occupy 2 mm or less of paper width and sharp waves more than 2 mm in ink-written EEG records taken at 3 cm/s.

Such spikes are associated with clinical seizures states. They should be held in clear contradistinction to the brief unit spikes recorded from single cells with microelectrode techniques. (From the 1974 report of the Committee on Terminology, IFCN. In: Chatrian GE, Bergamini L, Dondey M, et al. A glossary of terms most commonly used by clinical electroencephalographers. *EEG Clin Neurophysiol* 1974;37:538–48. Reproduced with kind permission from Elsevier Science.)

spike-and-slow-wave complex An EEG pattern consisting of a spike regularly followed by a slow wave.

spike-wave stupor See **status epilepticus**, **twilight state**, and **absence status**.

Spillane syndrome See **neuralgic amyotrophy**.

Spiller syndrome (epidural ascending spinal paralysis) A syndrome resembling transverse myelitis, but resulting from thrombophlebitis of the meningeal veins in the presence of pachymeningitis, and leading to cord compression, pain in the back and chest, and the motor and sensory deficits of acute (ischemic) myelopathy.[5983] See **hypertrophic spinal meningitis**.

Spiller, William Gibson (1863–1940) American neurologist, pathologist, and psychiatrist who trained at the University of Pennsylvania and then in Europe with **Déjèrine**, **Gowers**, and **Edinger**. After his return to the United States, he became professor of neuropathology and later head of the department of neurology at the University of Pennsylvania and held senior academic appointments in that city until his retirement in 1932. He edited the *Journal of Nervous and Mental Diseases* from 1902–1913. His publications were mainly on the topics of brainstem vascular diseases, extraocular movements, facial pain and weakness, and on **Spiller syndrome**, which he described in 1911.

Spina Bifida or Hydrocephalus Association of Canada A charitable organization providing support and information on this condition. Web site: http://www.sbhac.ca/beta/index.php.

Spina Bifida Association of America A charitable association in this field. Web site: http://www.spinabifidaassociation. org/site/c.liKWL7P-LLrF/b.2642297/k.5F7C/Spina_Bifida_Association.htm.

spina bifida Nonfusion of the laminas of the spinal arches. When the fusion defect is yet more severe, **meningocele** or **meningomyelocele** results.

Spina bifida occulta is the term for nonfusion of the arches without any clinical manifestations unless a dermoid cyst or lipoma is also present, or if there is **diastematomyelia**. *Spina bifida manifesta* indicates the presence of some neurological or local evidence of disease.

The disorder was described and named by the Dutch physician Dr. Nicholas **Tulp** in his *Medical Observations* (1641), although he is better remembered as being the inspiration for Rembrandt's picture *The Anatomy Lesson of Dr. Tulp.*

spina (Lat, a thorn).

spinal adductor reflex See **spinoadductor reflex**.

spinal adhesive arachnoiditis See **spinal arachnoiditis**.

spinal and bulbar muscle atrophy See **bulbospinal neuronopathy**.

spinal angioma An arteriovenous malformation involving the spinal cord, where it causes a slowly progressive myelopathy due to local ischemia, the angioma acting as a shunt. See **subacute necrotizing myelitis**.

spinal arachnoid cyst See **arachnoid diverticula**.

spinal arachnoiditis (chronic spinal meningitis, adhesive spinal arachnoiditis, meningitis serosa circumscripta spinalis, spinal adhesive arachnoiditis) A rare condition of localized or generalized scarring of the leptomeninges. The condition usually follows meningeal infection, lumbar disk disease, spinal surgery, or repeated lumbar punctures performed for the administration of intrathecal drugs or for diagnostic purposes. Bilateral sciatic pain, clinical evidence of multilevel radiculopathy, and paraparesis are the more common presentations.[5771]

spinal arachnoiditis ossificans A rare form of arachnoiditis in which bone is deposited within the inflamed arachnoid membrane. Clinically, the condition may remain asymptomatic or may cause spinal cord or optic nerve compression.[6834]

spinal block Obstruction to the flow of CSF beside the spinal cord as a result of occlusion of the subarachnoid space by a lesion within the cord (*intramedullary* or *intrinsic*); outside the cord but within the dura mater (*intradural*); or outside the dura mater (*extradural*). See **Froin syndrome**.

spinal cholesterolosis A myelopathic syndrome resulting from heavy deposits of cholesterol within the spinal canal.[6469] See **Thiébaut syndrome**.

spinal cord gliomas Primary malignancies of the spinal cord, including pilocytic and diffuse fibrillary astrocytomas and ependymomas.[2863]

Spinal Cord Injury Hotline A charitable organization providing support and information on this condition. Address: 2201 Argonne Drive Baltimore, MD 21218. Tel: 410-554-5413; National Spinal Cord Injury Hotline at 1-800-962-9629. See also the MGH Neurosurgery Web site: http://neurosurgery.mgh.harvard.edu/Spine/lnkspine.htm.

spinal cord injury Traumatic or ischemic lesions of the spinal cord, proportionally more devastating at increasingly high levels, for which the search for remedies proceeds steadfastly but slowly. Web sites of relevance that summarize current knowledge and provide personal and research support include the following:

Canadian Spinal Research Organization An organization dedicated to the improvement of the physical quality of life for persons with a spinal cord injury through targeted scientific and medical research. Web site: http://www.csro.com/.

Center for Paralysis Research An organization that develops and clinically tests novel methods of treatment for spinal cord injury and the effects of paralysis. Web site: http://www.vet.purdue.edu/cpr/.

Christopher Reeve Paralysis Foundation A national nonprofit organization whose mission is to encourage and support research to find a cure for paralysis caused by spinal cord injury and related disorders, including the latest news and progress in research studies. Web site: http://www.christopherreeve.org/site/c.geIMLPOpGjF/b.899265/.

National Center for Medical Rehabilitation Research An organization that funds research in the rehabilitation of impairment, disability, and handicap; including that caused by spinal cord injury, brain injury, stroke, amputation, cerebral palsy, spina bifida, and other disabling conditions. Web site: http://www.nichd.nih. gov/about/org/ncmrr/.

Reeve-Irvine Spinal Cord Injury Research Center A center dedicated to spinal cord injury research and to finding a cure for spinal cord injury and neural degenerative disease. Web site: http://www.reeve.uci.edu/

Spinal Cord Injury: Hope through Research An informational booklet about efforts to develop better treatments. Web site: http://www.ninds.nih.gov/disorders/sci/detail_ sci.htmI.

Stem Cell Research in Spinal Cord Injury A site that summarizes current research in treating spinal cord injury and the new applications of stem cells in that field. Web site: http://www.namiscc.org/newsletters/December01/SCI-stem-cell-research.htm.

Spinal Cord Society A charitable organization in this field. Address: 19051 County Hwy. 1, Fergus Falls, MN 56537. Tel: 218-739-5252;218-739-5261. Web site: http://users.aol.com/scsweb/.

Spinal Cord The official journal of the International Spinal Cord Society. Web site: http://www.naturesj.com/sc/index.html.

spinal dural arteriovenous fistula The most common vascular anomaly affecting the spinal cord, causing slowly progressive myelopathy as a result of impaired venous drainage. See also **Foix–Alajouanine syndrome**.

spinal dysraphism Congenital defects in closure of the neural tube.

spinal epidermoid tumor A benign tumor resulting from the implantation of superficial tissue into the spinal canal during prior lumbar puncture. Local and radicular pain and radiculopathic signs are the usual clinical features.[2369]

spinal epidural abscess (pachymeningitis externa) Pyogenic infection in the epidural space as a result of hematogenous spread or direct local extension from an adjacent infection, such as vertebral osteomyelitis.[5226] It may also occur iatrogenically following lumbar puncture or epidural anesthesia. The usual clinical picture consists of the progression of back and radicular pain to weakness and paraparesis. The most common infecting organism is *Staphylococcus*.

spinal epidural hematoma Extravasation of venous blood into the epidural space, usually in low cervical or thoracolumbar areas and most often associated with local arteriovenous malformations or malignancy, or with coagulopathies in adults or birth injury in neonates. The clinical effect is usually acute myelopathy, which must be handled as an emergency if cord function is not to be lost permanently. MRI is the diagnostic procedure of choice.

Subacute or chronic presentations with evidence of cord compression may also occur.[3716]

spinal epidural lipomatosis An increase in the amount of epidural fat in lumbar or thoracic regions, occurring in Cushing disease, in patients treated with steroids for a prolonged period and occasionally without a known cause as a form of **lipoma**. Clinically, gradually progressive paraparesis, back pain, and radiculopathy are the usual syndromes resulting.[3294]

spinal evoked potential Electrical waveforms of biological origin recorded over the sacral, lumbar, thoracic, or cervical spine in response to electric stimulation or physiological activation of peripheral sensory fibers.[162] See **somatosensory-evoked potential**.

spinal monomelic amyotrophy See **monomelic amyotrophy**.

spinal muscular atrophy (SMA) A group of heterogeneous conditions with the common factor of damage to the anterior horn cells of the spinal cord and/or the bulbar nuclei, leading to denervation of muscles in variable distributions.

Those SMAs with a genetic basis are classified under the **hereditary motor neuropathies**. Acquired forms may have an acute onset (acute anterior **poliomyelitis**, Coxsackie, other enterovirus infections) or may be chronic (**amyotrophic lateral sclerosis**, anterior horn cell disease in the spinocerebellar degenerations, **Creutzfeldt–Jakob disease, Huntington disease, Parkinsonism**, Shy–Drager syndrome [**multiple system atrophy**], **Joseph disease**, and with remote neoplasms as a **paraneoplastic syndrome**).

spinal muscular atrophy and **optic atrophy with deafness** See **hereditary motor neuropathy** (*variants*).

Spinal Muscular Atrophy Foundation A charitable organization that provides information on spinal muscular atrophy and updates on research, treatment, and funding. Web site: http://www.smafoundation.org/.

Spinal Muscular Atrophy Information Page (SMA) A comprehensive account of clinical, diagnostic, and pathophysiologic material relating to spinal muscular atrophies. Web site: http://www.geneclinics.org/profiles/sma/index.html.

spinal muscular atrophy with calf hypertrophy See **hereditary motor neuropathy** (*variants*).

spinal muscular atrophy with deafness See **hereditary motor neuropathy** (*variants*).

spinal muscular atrophy with mental retardation See **hereditary motor neuropathy** (*variants*).

spinal muscular atrophy with microcephaly and mental retardation See **hereditary motor neuropathy**.

spinal muscular atrophy with myoclonus See **hereditary motor neuropathy** (*variants*).

spinal muscular atrophy with oculopharyngeal muscular atrophy See **hereditary motor neuropathy** (*variants*).

spinal muscular atrophy with ophthalmoplegia See **hereditary motor neuropathy** (*variants*).

spinal muscular atrophy with pallidonigral degeneration See **hereditary motor neuropathy** (*variants*).

spinal muscular atrophy with retinitis pigmentosa and hereditary spastic paraplegia See **hereditary motor neuropathy** (*variants*).

spinal muscular atrophy with retinitis pigmentosa See **hereditary motor neuropathy** (*variants*).

spinal muscular atrophy, Ryukyuan type See **hereditary motor neuropathy** (*variants*).

spinal myoclonus (focal myoclonus) Sudden, involuntary, near-rhythmic, focal muscle jerks of the arms or legs, usually at about 1 Hz, occurring during rest in the awake state and during sleep and anesthesia, without an accompanying EEG abnormality and not precipitated by sensory or motor stimuli. Their electrical origin is in the spinal cord at sites of ischemic damage, myelitis, degenerative or traumatic cord lesions, or tumors.[2987] See **segmental myoclonus**.

spinal nerve root That portion of the nerve fiber pathway which issues from the spinal cord and which is still within the extramedullary, intradural space.

spinal nerve That portion of the nerve fiber pathway issuing from the spinal cord which lies outside the intradural space.

spinal neuritis See **radiculitis**.

spinal schistosomiasis A myelopathy or radiculopathy resulting from granulomatous involvement of the spine and underlying dura mater, usually with *Schistosoma mansoni* or *haematobium*.[654]

spinal shock A condition lasting days or weeks during which the severely traumatized spinal cord conducts no impulses, consequent upon the sudden withdrawal of the normal tonic excitation playing down upon it from higher levels. The weakness, flaccidity, and areflexia may persist for months (Jackson, Bastian). The phenomenon was first remarked by Robert **Whytt**, but was so named by Marshall **Hall**.

spinal stenosis A syndrome of compression of the spinal nerve roots, usually at lumbar levels and as a result of soft tissue intrusion or disc prolapse into a congenitally narrow spinal canal with reduction in its caliber. Degenerative osteophyte formation, spondylosis or spondylolisthesis, and developmental abnormalities such as achondroplasia are other causes. Low back pain, poorly localized referred pain on exercise (**neurogenic claudication**), paresthesias, a flexed posture, weakness (foot drop or waddling gait), and areflexia in lumbar and sacral segments on exercise, relieved by rest, are the leading clinical features.

The *central* type often presents as drop attacks, back pain, and pain in the shins with prolonged standing or walking. At night, the patient may experience cold or rubbery legs, and neurological deficits may appear with exercise. In *lateral spinal stenosis*, the patient complains of radicular pain provoked by exercise, but the usual signs of root irritation are absent.

spinal subdural hematoma Extravasation of blood into the subdural space of the spine, usually as a result of birth injury in the newborn or of other trauma in older subjects. Clinically, radicular pain and local tenderness, often with evidence of myelopathy, are the major features.

spinal xanthomatosis A variant of **cerebrotendinous xanthomatosis** manifesting a slowly progressive, chronic myelopathy. MRI demonstrates white matter abnormalities in the lateral and dorsal columns of the spinal cord.[6536]

spindle coma The occurrence of physiological patterns of nonrapid eye movement sleep such as sleep spindles, vertex sharp waves, K complexes, and background theta and delta activity on the EEG following CNS trauma, metabolic, infectious or hypoxic problems.[3172] Spindle coma may represent a combination of true sleep and coma, the latter accounting for the failure of arousal that is attributed to impairment of the activating ascending reticular formation. The causative lesion is in the hypothalamic or upper mesencephalic regions. In post-traumatic cases, the prognosis for recovery may be good, but, in nontraumatic cases, it is significantly worse.[2742] The presence of spindles, vertex waves, and K complexes indicates relative integrity of the cerebral hemispheres.[1508]

spindle vertigo That state of fearfulness and "dizziness" reflecting a distortion of muscle sense and seen particularly in the aged in association with a loss of 1A afferent fiber (proprioceptive) activity or with age-related changes in the intramuscular nerve terminals.

spindle A group of rhythmic waves on the EEG, characterized by a progressively increasing then gradually decreasing amplitude. See also **sleep spindles**.

spindles Groups of encapsulated special muscle fibers within somatic muscles with the function of assessing the rate and force of stretch as a result of the contraction of surrounding muscle, thus modulating the strength of further muscle contraction. Two forms are described, according to their shape, as resembling either a *bag* or a *chain*.

spin-lattice relaxation time (T1, longitudinal relaxation time) The characteristic time constant for spins to achieve an equilibrium alignment within an applied magnetic field.[875, 6856]

spinoadductor reflex (Tschlenow reflex, spinal adductor reflex) Bilateral contraction of the adductors of the leg in response to the vibration set up by a tap over the spine. It is said to be present in normal subjects but increased in the setting of pyramidal disease. This is the corollary of the **scapulohumeral reflex** in the upper limb and has the same slight importance.

spinobulbar muscular atrophy See **bulbospinal neuronopathy** (Kennedy disease).

spinocerebellar ataxia and pupillary paralysis See **cerebellar ataxias** (*variants*).

spinocerebellar ataxia with dementia and plaquelike deposits See **Gerstmann–Straussler–Scheinker syndrome**.

spinocerebellar ataxias See **cerebellar ataxias**. A heterogeneous group of neurodegenerative disorders characterized by features of degeneration in the brainstem, cerebellum, and spinal cord.

spinocerebellar degeneration with motor system involvement See **cerebellar ataxias** (*variants*).

spinocerebellar degenerations A group of progressive diseases characterized clinically by disturbances in the coordination of movement, or ataxia, and pathologically by degeneration of those afferent and efferent neuronal systems upon which the smooth and efficient regulation of movement depends.[2565] See **cerebellar ataxias** (*variants*).

spino-olivocerebellar degeneration and ophthalmoplegia See **cerebellar ataxias** (*variants*).

spinopontine atrophy A dominantly inherited, progressive ataxic syndrome characterized by the onset in youth or young adult life of optic atrophy; dementia; cerebellar, pyramidal, and posterior column signs; and myoclonus.

It may be classified with the progressive late-onset **cerebellar ataxias** of unknown cause until the underlying biochemical defect is ascertained.[728] See also **Joseph disease**.

spinoscopy A method of assessing spinal movements using a high-resolution television camera which records the varying relative positions of markers placed on a subject's back during forward and lateral flexion, allowing the estimation of movement at the facet joints and at the intervertebral disk spaces. Despite the pretentious name, the operator does not look at (let alone into) the spine by this method.

spinothalamic system (anterolateral system) One of the two major somatosensory systems (the other is the posterior or **lemniscal**) comprising the ascending fiber pathways. It arises from the dorsal root cells concerned with the conduction of impulses subserving the sensations of pain, heat, and cold as well as sexual sensation, although the system also contains a number of lemniscal fibers. Its fibers terminate in the reticular activating system, in the intralaminar and centromedian thalamic nuclei, and in the ventrobasal thalamic complex. The system is characterized by wide receptive fields, lack of modality specificity, and slow adaptation. It was first described by **Edinger** but more fully by **Brown-Séquard**.

spin-spin relaxation time (T2, transverse relaxation time) The characteristic time constant for loss of phase coherence among spins oriented at an angle to the static magnetic field, due to interactions between the spins, with resulting decay of the transverse magnetization and MRI signal. Starting from a finite value, the transverse magnetization will decay so that it loses 63% of its initial value in a time (T2).[875, 6856]

spiral nerve bands of Fontana Zig-zag or spiraling lines most easily visible on the surface of nerves, using oblique lighting; the optical expression of the arrangement of nerve fibers in the nerve.[1192]

splenium The posterior third of the corpus callosum.

split brain The condition resulting from the severance of the neocortical commissures, leading to the inability to exchange information between the hemispheres and to the existence of two independent cognitive systems within the same brain. The right hemisphere, thus, appears to have some function in the processing of language.

The retention of abilities related to calculation, spatial orientation, and lexical decision making supports the view that the brainstem is implicated in the transfer of some cognitive processing.[5729]

split hand syndrome Preferential denervation of the thenar muscles and the first dorsal interosseus rather than the hypothenar muscles, recorded in some cases of **amyotrophic lateral sclerosis** or with distal ulnar lesions. The name was applied because of the involvement mainly of the muscles on the lateral side of the hand, such as the thenar muscles and the first dorsal interosseous.[6780] The underlying lesion may be at cortical or at spinal level.

split notochord syndrome See **diastematomyelia**.

spondyl (Gr, a vertebra).

spondylalgia Pain in the spine.

spondylitis (Gr, a vertebra + inflammation)

spondylolisthesis (Gr, a vertebra + a slippage) The name given by Killian in 1852 to the forward slippage of one vertebra upon the one below (usually L4 on L5, but in his case, L5 on S1), either due to a defect in the isthmus of the pars interarticularis (*true spondylolisthesis*) or to degeneration of the disk and facet joints (*degenerative spondylolisthesis*). **Lumbar spinal stenosis** is a possible result, but, in many cases, its occurrence causes no symptoms.[2222]

spondylolysis A defect in the pars interarticularis of the vertebra, and thus a cause of **spondylolisthesis**.

spondylopathy Any disease of the vertebra.

spondylosis A degenerative hypertrophy of the ligamentous, bony, and articular structures of the spinal column which occurs with aging. The unwanted effects of this may include compression of the emerging nerve roots and possibly of the spinal cord itself.

spongiform encephalopathies A group of slowly progressive, transmissible cerebral diseases affecting humans and animals, with the shared characteristics of cortical spongy change, neuronal loss, an accumulation of **prion** protein, and gliosis. They include **Creutzfeldt–Jakob disease**, **scrapie**, **kuru**, and **Gerstmann–Straussler–Scheinker syndrome**.[6790]

spongiform encephalopathy with white matter changes See **Creutzfeld–Jakob disease**, of which this is a *variant*.

spongioblast (Gr, a sponge + a germ) A cell of ectodermal origin which is the precursor of glial cells.

spongioblastoma polare (polar spongioblastoma) A malignant but relatively slowly growing cerebral tumor composed of primitive spongioblasts, occurring mainly in the cerebellum, brainstem, and optic chiasm.[3392] See also **primitive neuroectodermal tumors**.

spongy degeneration of infancy See **Canavan leukodystrophy**.

spongy degeneration The histological appearance of brain tissue which contains round, empty spaces separated by bands of more or less intact neural tissue. The agonal production of CO_2 from glycogen reservoirs just after the cessation of blood flow has been suggested as the cause.[1987] Such an appearance is also seen in many other metabolic, degenerative, and infectious conditions. See **Canavan leukodystrophy**.

spongy glioneuronal dystrophy A familial degenerative disorder of the nervous system of unknown cause, marked by spongy change in the thalamus, dentate nucleus, and cortex with sparing of white matter. It closely resembles **Alpers disease**. Clinical characteristics are the onset between the ages of 1 and 5 years of intellectual failure, seizures, myoclonus, involuntary movements, cerebellar signs, blindness, deafness, and eventual decerebration and death.[2989, 3191] See **glioneuronal dystrophies**.

spontaneous activity Electrical activity recorded from muscle or nerve at rest after insertion activity has subsided and when there is no voluntary contraction or external stimulus. Compare with **involuntary (EMG) activity**.

spontaneous corneomandibular reflex See **palpebromandibular synkinesia**.

spontaneous intracranial hypotension (idiopathic intracranial hypotension, low CSF-volume headache, hypoliquorrheic headache, aliquorrhea) A rare, postural headache syndrome occurring in the absence of a known dural tear but still almost invariably due to a CSF leak at a spinal level. Typically it presents with orthostatic headaches, pain or stiffness of the neck, nausea, emesis, horizontal diplopia, dizziness, change in hearing, visual blurring or visual field deficits, photophobia, interscapular pain, and occasionally face numbness or weakness or radicular upper-limb symptoms and often other features such as nausea, vomiting, vertigo, tinnitus, altered auditory acuity, photophobia, neck stiffness, diplopia due to VI cranial nerve palsy, and bradycardia. It can also present rarely with cognitive changes or with reversible coma.[1844, 774, 4433] The headache is relieved by recumbency.

The syndrome results from CSF hypovolemia due to a persistent leak of CSF through a meningeal defect, as after lumbar puncture (CSF opening pressure <60 mm H_2O in sitting position). The problem may rarely be complicated by subdural fluid collections.[5183, 1176] Diagnosis is best made by MRI, which typically shows dural enhancement, or by isotope cisternography. CSF pressures, by definition, are low. MRI shows diffuse pachymeningeal enhancement, often with imaging evidence of "sinking of the brain" with descent of the cerebellar tonsils and of the optic chiasm; less frequently subdural fluid collections, engorged cerebral venous sinuses, enlarged pituitary gland, or decreased size of the ventricles are shown. Radioisotope cisternography typically shows absence of activity over the cerebral convexities and early appearance of activity in the kidneys and urinary bladder; occasionally it reveals the site of the leak.[4433, 5968, 5566]

The headache is diffuse and/or dull and it worsens within 15 min after sitting or standing. Neck stiffness, tinnitus, hypacusis, photophobia, and nausea are common accompaniments.

spontaneous nystagmus Those forms of nystagmus that occur without provocation, as, for example, those elicited by **optokinetic** stimuli.

spontaneous periodic hypothermia A rare disturbance of thermoregulation leading to severe sweating and persistently low body temperatures, usually arising in patients with other evidence of hypothalamic damage. The condition has been considered to represent a form of diencephalic epilepsy.[2170]

spoon test Variable resistance is normally felt when a soup spoon is drawn across the skin, but the resistance is smooth and unopposed when the spoon crosses (anhidrotic) areas of sympathetic denervation.[6409]

sporadic degenerative visceral neuropathy Alteration in bowel function due to damage to the myenteric plexus of the colon in association with inflammatory conditions and paraneoplastic disorders.[6827]

sporadic juvenile amyotrophic lateral sclerosis See **amyotrophic lateral sclerosis** (*variants*).

sporadic myoclonic encephalopathy See **opsoclonus-myoclonus syndrome** and **Ohtahara syndrome**.

sporadic olivopontocerebellar degeneration See **cerebellar ataxias** (autosomal dominant, late-onset forms).[1545]

sporadic progressive thalamic atrophy The rare occurrence of isolated atrophy of any of the thalamic nuclei without a demonstrable neurological cause such as **Wernicke–Korsakoff syndrome**, **cerebellar ataxias**, or distant carcinoma. Abulia and dementia are the clinical accompaniments reported, but the very existence of the syndrome as an entity is unproved. See also **multiple-system atrophies**.

sporadic spongiform encephalopathies with myoclonus See **Creutzfeldt–Jakob disease**.

Spranger syndrome See **rhizomelic chondrodysplasia punctata**.

spread of comitance The reduction in the degree of primary and secondary deviation of the eyes in a patient with strabismus, as a function of time.

spreading depression of Leao Marked, enduring reduction in the electrical activity of the cortex (of rabbits) following an excitation wave produced by weak faradic or mechanical stimulation of the exposed cerebrum, associated with markedly increased blood flow in the surface arterioles and veins and followed by increased fast activity on the EEG.[3737]

Sprengel deformity A sporadic or dominantly inherited syndrome resulting from maldevelopment occurring during embryogenesis, wherein the scapulas fail to migrate to their usual position. This leads to scapular elevation, rotation, and winging. The condition was first described by Dr. O.G.K. Sprengel (1852–1915), a German surgeon.

springende pupille See **springing pupil**.

springing pupil (see-saw anisocoria, mydriasis à bascule, springende pupille)

A term variously employed, but generally taken to indicate the presence of periodic alternating dilation of the pupils of unknown cause (*type* 1), but often in a pupil affected by long-standing **Horner syndrome**. In *type* 2, unilateral iris paresis (as in **Adie syndrome**) leads to the appearance of unilateral pupillary dilation during accommodation and in bright light conditions. *Type* 3 is synonymous with **cyclic oculomotor spasm**.[2699]

springlike phenomenon See **rebound**.

sprouting The growth of new nerve fibers (neurites) in large numbers from the proximal end of a cut nerve in the process of repair.

sprung back The condition of rupture or stretching of the supra- and interspinous ligaments, usually at low lumbar levels, associated both with aging and with prolapse of intervertebral disks. Whether the problem is a cause or an effect has yet to be determined.[4647]

sprung pupil See **Riegel symptom**.

spurious diabetes See **diabetes insipidus**.

spurious hydrocephalus See **Hall syndrome**.

Spurling sign 1. Accentuation of the pain felt during **straight-leg raising** elicited by dorsiflexion of the ankle or the hallux, thus causing slight further traction on the sciatic nerve. This sign represents a combination of the signs of **Sicard** and of **Bragard**. 2. Pain in the shoulder or arm occurring with lateral flexion of the neck to that side, a sign of acute (or of severe chronic) cervical disk herniation.

Spurway syndrome See **Apert syndrome**.

Spurzheim, Johann Caspar (1776–1832) French physician and iconoblast. He forsook the study of theology for that of medicine in order to become a student of (and a highly partial proponent of the theories of) F.J. **Gall**, with whom he presented a major treatise on the anatomy of the brain to the *Institut de France* in 1808, and he produced between 1810 and 1819 a superb four-volume text on the anatomy and physiology of the nervous system and the brain, containing accounts of many new and definitive dissections. He lectured on **phrenology** on both sides of the Atlantic, but his enthusiastic and uncritical claims for that discipline (quite unlike the reserved and scholarly productions of **Gall** himself) could not be substantiated, and he thus accelerated the rejection of Gall's theories. Spurzheim withdrew from participation in the writing of Gall's major work after 4 years of labor due to disagreements between them.[5978]

sputtering positive potentials Small, irregular, positive potentials resembling nerve potentials, recorded on EMG in normal distal muscles. They are artifactual and have no clinical significance.[5021]

square window The angle between the hypothenar eminence and the plane of the forearm, made when the infant's wrist is passively flexed to the maximal extent, normally up against the forearm. Less acute angles suggest prematurity. The same maneuver can be applied at the ankle and scored according to the key provided in Dubowitz' test procedure.[1727]

square-wave jerks (square-wave oscillations, gegenrucke, hopping nystagmus, lightning eye movements, ocular myoclonus, saccadic intrusions, saccadic oscillations, zickzakbewegungen) Involuntary, 0.5–3° conjugate horizontal saccades occurring at 1–4 Hz, moving the eyes away from a point of fixation for 200 ms and followed after about 200 ms by a corrective saccadic return to the original fixation position, these cycles occurring at about 2 Hz.[1456] Thus they interrupt steady visual fixation upon a point and may also interrupt smooth pursuit movements.

The term is applied because of the rectangular waveform of the tracing of eye movements. They occur sometimes in normal subjects with the eyes closed, but more usually and obviously in patients with **progressive supranuclear palsy** or with cerebellar disease, whose eyes are open. See also **macro square-wave jerks**.[35]

square-wave oscillations See **square-wave jerks**.

square-wave pulses (kippdkviationen, kippnystagmus, pendular macro-oscillations, saccadic nystagmus, saccadic oscillations, saccadic intrusions) See **macro square-wave jerks**.

squat-jump myoglobinuria The occurrence of myoglobinuria following this provocative exercise as a result of excessive or unaccustomed use of the leg muscles.

squint syndrome of Braun See **Swan syndrome**.

squint (Old Engl, to escape or avoid) Lack of parallelism of the ocular axes so that the eyes look in different directions. See **strabismus**.

SREDA See **Subclinical Rhythmic Excitatory Discharges of Adults**. An orphan EEG phenomenon.

SSEP See **short-latency somatosensory evoked potential**.

S-shaped lid The appearance of the upper lid in patients with a neurofibroma in its outer part which droops as a result, while the inner half remains in its usual position.

SSS See **small sharp spikes**.

S-state Slow-wave sleep. See **nonrapid eye movement sleep**.

St Friedeswide English princess and abbess of a monastery in Oxford in the late seventh century. Most of those attempting to attack/ravish her were struck blind until she forgave them; parallels with **optic neuritis** have been drawn.

St. Anthony's dance Synonym for St. Vitus' dance (**chorea**).

St. Avertin's disease An antique name for epilepsy.

St. Avisius' disease An antique name for deafness.

St. Guy's dance Synonym for St. Vitus' dance (**chorea**).

St. Hubert disease See **rabies**.

St. Job's disease Syphilis.

St. John's dance See **dancing mania**.

St. John's evil An antique name for epilepsy.

St. Lazarus' disease Leprosy.

St. Louis encephalitis Direct infection of the brain by a flavivirus member of the togavirus group of arboviruses. The condition is mosquito-borne and occurs in all parts of South America, the United States, and south central Canada in particular. Clinically, the condition is most common in subjects over 50 years of age. The condition is usually asymptomatic, but fever and headaches as well as meningitis and encephalitic syndromes are recorded, the latter presenting with altered consciousness, tremors, dysarthria, and seizures.[841] See the CDC Web site: http://www.cdc.gov/ncidod/dvbid/sle/Sle_FactSheet.html.

St. Mathurin's disease An antique name for epilepsy, and also for insanity.

St. Modestus' dance Synonym for St. Vitus dance (**chorea**).

St. Paul (Saul of Tarsus) (c. AD 10–c. AD 48) Initially in the employ of the Jewish anti-Christian establishment, he was converted to Christianity during a journey to Damascus where (as described in Acts 9 and 22) he was suddenly blinded by a bright light, fell to the ground, and received the remonstrances of God. This episode has been interpreted as evidence of a complex "partial" seizure,[3679] especially as Paul wrote of a persistent "thorn in the flesh," and thus perhaps of a tendency to some such recurrent problems, but the conflicting evidence in the similar experiences of others in his party, the more usual occurrence of postictal blindness after generalized rather than after partial seizures and the retention of insight into his sightlessness have led to some scepticism regarding the epileptic basis of this extraordinary event.

St. Sement's disease Syphilis.

St. Valentine's disease An antique name for epilepsy.

St. Vitus' dance St. Vitus was a young Sicilian martyr, who died under the Roman Emperor Diocletian. He prayed that all who commemorated the day of his death should be protected against the **dancing mania**, a disease (probably a form of mass hysteria) which is no longer fashionable. In 1418, sufferers from this condition prayed successfully to the Saint for relief at his chapels in Zabern, near Strasbourg.

Although **Sydenham** described chorea in 1675, the association between dancing mania and chorea (St. Vitus' dance) has been maintained to some degree, but quite incorrectly since the two are completely different conditions. See **Sydenham chorea**.

stable stroke A form of stroke in which there is little change in the deficit over a specified period of time.[4678]

Staehli pigment line A crescent of brown pigment in the lower central quadrant of the cornea found in some elderly patients, in the region where the arcus senilis usually begins.

staircase phenomenon The progressive increase in the force of a muscle contraction in response to continued low rates of direct or indirect muscle stimulation.[162] This phenomenon may be produced by the increasingly efficient mobilization of acetylcholine quanta from the nerve terminals during muscular activity over a finite period.

stammering Abnormal speech in which the flow of words is interrupted by hesitations, during which the muscles of articulation function in the absence of laryngeal speech sounds. See also **stuttering**.

stamping gait The gait of a subject with **sensory ataxia**, which is markedly worse in dark places and on rough ground. The hips and knees are flexed to an unusual extent, and the regularity and precision with which they are brought down again to the ground are both impaired.

standard electrode placement The EEG electrode location(s) on the scalp determined by the **ten-twenty system**.

Stanford Sleepiness Scale A long and complicated instrument for assessing and rating sleepiness.[2930]

Stanford-Binet tests A test battery modifying and expanding upon the original intelligence scales developed in France by Alfred **Binet**.

Stanley syndrome (proctalgia fugax) (Gr, anus + pain + fleeting) A benign but uncomfortable condition of severe intermittent attacks of rectal pain, said to be common in elderly, myopic lexicophiles and caused by remaining in the sedentary position for long periods (Stanley J, cited by Jablonski[3113]).

stapedius myokymia Repetitive contractions of the stapedius muscle for reasons unknown, causing tinnitus.

stapedius reflex Bilateral reflex contraction of the stapedius muscles with sound stimulation of one ear, this contraction measurably altering the acoustical impedance of the middle ear.

stapedius reflexometry Measurement of the contractions of the stapedius muscle by means of an electroacoustic impedance bridge, the threshold and decay of the reflex allowing estimation of the degree or weakness and fatigability of the muscle, as in **myasthenia gravis**.

star walking Subjects with mild left vestibular disease who walk sets of three paces forward and three backward with the eyes closed will angle their course anticlockwise, and those with right-sided disease will veer clockwise (provided, of course, that they do not fall down in the meantime).[823] See also **stepping test**.

stare nystagmus See **look nystagmus**.

starfish hand Dystonic abduction and extension of the fingers, seen in some patients following contralateral hemispheric infarction, especially with lesions of the caudate, putamen, or thalamus.

Stargardt syndrome (familial juvenile macular degeneration) A recessively inherited syndrome of insidious deterioration of vision first detectable in infancy, leading eventually to total blindness. Bilateral macular pigmentation is the earliest sign, followed by the appearance of coalescing yellow retinal spots and pigmentary retinal degeneration of the outer layers of the retina.[6019]

Stargardt, K.B. (1875–1927) German ophthalmologist, who graduated from Kiel and trained further both there and at Strasbourg and Bonn. He succeeded **Bielschowsky** as professor and director of the eye clinic at Marburg.

Stark–Kaiser syndrome See **scapuloperoneal syndromes**.

startle disease See **startle epilepsy**.

startle disorder See **hyperekplexia**.

startle epilepsy (startle disease) An unusual form of reflex epilepsy in which the seizures consist of a startle response followed by a brief asymmetric tonic phase with falls and clonic jerks. They are precipitated by sudden, unexpected stimuli (usually a sudden sound and seldom in more than one sensory modality), and comprise an abrupt startle response followed by a phase of tonic posturing involving the paretic side, or by a generalized seizure.[4041] Autonomic manifestations, automatisms, laughter, and jerks may occur concurrently; atonic or myoclonic startle seizures are less common. The response to antiepileptic drugs is very poor.

Evidence of localized or diffuse **static encephalopathy** is usually present, such as developmental delay or hemiparesis occurring within the first 2 years of life and often pre- or perinatal. Brain imaging may show localized or diffuse lesions. The lateralized lesions usually involve sensorimotor and premotor cortex and white matter lesions on MRI. Dysplasias and **schizencephaly** have also been found. The condition may also complicate the **Lennox–Gastaut syndrome**, perinatal anoxic encephalopathy, **porencephaly, Down syndrome**, or other known cerebral disorders. It was first described by **Gowers**.[2530, 5496] See also **hyperekplexia, Coffin–Lowry syndrome**, and **hot water epilepsy**.

In a dominantly inherited *familial* form (**hyperekplexia**, congenital stiff-person syndrome, and hereditary stiff-baby syndrome), the responsible gene is located on chromosome 5q.

startle reflex Flexion of the arms in response to a sudden loud noise, normally present in babies up to 3 months of age.[896]

startle A basic alerting reaction seen in all mammals, consisting in humans of a stereotyped facial grimace, flexion of the head, trunk, elbows, and knees; and elevation of the shoulders in response to sudden stimuli, but diminishing somewhat with the repetition of such stimuli. The reflex is enhanced by tension, fatigue, and the expectation of the causal stimulus.[189, 744] Though a normal motor pattern, it may become excessive, in which case the disease is known as **hyperekplexia, jumping** or **startle epilepsy**, and it may be a precipitant of myoclonus or of other seizures.[187]

The disorders named **latah** in Malaysia, **myriatchit**, *ikota,* or *amurakh* in Siberia, and *ainu imu* elsewhere in Asia, *jauns* in Burmah, *bah-tsche* in Thailand, *mali mali* or *silok* in the Philippines, *panic* in Lapland, and the Bantu or southwest African disorder are also considered by some to represent the same condition.

startle-induced seizures A form of reflex epilepsy seen in some children with brain damage of any kind, comprising brief motor seizures characterized by sudden flexion of the neck, trunk, and limbs, elicited by visual, auditory, or proprioceptive stimuli and followed by tonic flexion of the arm and extension of the leg on the hemiparetic side. Consciousness is minimally affected. The EEG shows a muscle artifact corresponding to the seizure, followed by temporary suppression of activity. The attacks lessen with increasing age.[72]

startle-induced tics The occurrence of tics with this precipitant as part of **Tourette syndrome** of late onset.[6321]

start-stop-start phenomenon A pattern of electrographic activity in which the abnormal activity representing an electrographic seizure appears for a few seconds, disappears, and then recurs, usually from the same site.[691]

stasi-basophobia Immobility in the standing position due to a pathological fear of walking,[5984] usually in association with severe bilateral frontal cortical disease.

state dependent In the context of epilepsy, a manifestation occurring exclusively or primarily in the various stages of drowsiness, sleep, or arousal.[16]

static embryopathy A pathological state occurring during fetal life, caused by viral infections in utero and leading to developmental abnormalities of the brain which do not progress after birth. Cytomegalovirus, varicella, and rubella viruses are the best-known causative agents.

static encephalopathy (nonprogressive encephalopathy) A chronic, nonprogressive, genetic or developmental brain disorder resulting from lesions of the brain sustained before, during, or after birth. The clinical features are essentially those of **cerebral palsy**, mostly affecting intellectual functions and motor development. Basal ganglion calcification and dystonia are also common findings.

static perimetry (profile perimetry) That form of perimetry in which the contrast of a stimulus at given points in the visual field is gradually increased up to the threshold of perception. The technique is of particular value in the quantitative assessment of retinal sensitivity.[1840] See also **kinetic perimetry**.

The test is most accurately performed with the aid of a computerized program which monitors fixation and provides false-negative and false-positive scores, in which the target is of fixed size and is illuminated at different points programmed by the computer with variable and increasing intensity.

static positional nystagmus A form of nystagmus that persists during the maintenance of a particular position of the head, of no localizing value, though seen most often in the context of peripheral vestibular disease. **Positional alcohol nystagmus** is an example.

static reflex spasms See **saltatory spasm**.

static reflexes Those reflexes which employ the extensor muscles of the limbs in the maintenance of posture, their origin being in the mesencephalon. They are best expressed in decerebrate preparations and are lost in "spinal" animals (Sir Charles **Sherrington**).

static seizures See **myoclonic astatic seizures**.

static tremor See **cerebellar tremors**.

statin myopathy Skeletal muscle injury presenting as muscle pain, tenderness, weakness, cramping, and fatigue associated with the ingestion of statins. Creatine kinase levels may exceed the upper limit of normal by over 10x and myoglobulinuria may be associated with rhabdomyolysis.[2520, 6334] Statins can also exacerbate other acquired and genetic myopathies.

stationary night-blindness A familial syndrome, variably inherited and characterized by an inability to see at night as a result of absent secondary rod or cone adaptation. The fundi are normal. Day vision is unaffected in the dominantly inherited form, but it is abnormal in the recessively inherited and X-linked varieties (in part due to myopia).[1033]

statognosia The appreciation of the position of a limb in space.

statokinetic dissociation A difference in visual sensitivity for moving targets compared with that for stationary targets. In the presence of optic atrophy, dissociation is increasingly marked, the subject having a higher sensitivity for moving targets.[6691]

status dissociatus A severe form of **REM sleep behavior disorder** in which elements of rapid eye movement and of nonrapid eye movement sleep are mixed together, the sleep interrupted by dreaming, twitching, and vocalizations. Alcohol withdrawal, narcolepsy, and brainstem diseases have been associated.[5594]

status dysmyelinatus A congenital disorder of the lenticular nuclei characterized by loss of neurons and myelinated fibers, leading to athetosis in childhood and additional severe rigidity later. This may be the underlying mechanism of **juvenile paralysis agitans**.

The condition was described by the **Vogts** in 1919–1920, but the pathogenesis is still uncertain. See **double athetosis**.

status dystonicus (dystonic storm) A syndrome of unremitting, severe, generalized dystonic spasms occurring rarely in patients with primary or secondary dystonias, after intercurrent infection, and alteration in medications, or for no obvious reason. The complication is life-threatening due to the risks of respiratory or airway compromise, aspiration pneumonia, renal failure from secondary rhabdomyolysis, or exhaustion.

status epilepticus 1. Any seizure state lasting longer than half an hour; *or* a single epileptic seizure for more than 30 min in duration *or* a series of epileptic seizures during which function is not regained between ictal events after 30 min.[1265]

2. Recurrent seizures which occur without an intervening period of conscious awareness, reflecting a failure of the natural homeostatic seizure-suppressing mechanisms responsible for seizure termination.

3. An epileptic seizure that is sufficiently prolonged, or repeated at sufficiently brief intervals, so as to produce an unvarying and enduring epileptic condition.

Operationally, the simplest definition is "any seizure state which is not self-limiting." Generalized status may be convulsive (tonic/clonic/myoclonic) or nonconvulsive (absence). Partial status may comprise simple (somatomotor, aphasic) or complex partial seizures.[72] The various forms of status have been classified by Gastaut[2308] and these are summarized in Chart S–14. See also **serial seizures**.

status hemiparalyticus See **hemiparetic seizures.**

status marmoratus (Lat, state + marble) A pathological appearance of the basal ganglia in patients with hypoxic-ischemic cerebral injury (asphyxia neonatorum), characterized by irregular and excessive myelination of these structures,

Chart S–14. Classification of Status Epilepticus

Forms of generalized status epilepticus

Convulsive tonic-clonic and clonic status includes generalized tonic-clonic, clonic, absence, tonic and myoclonic forms, in which the seizure type is as indicated by the name. *Tonic status* is uncommon but very prolonged; it is usually seen in children with **Lennox–Gastaut syndrome**.

Myoclonic status is rare, and consists of the unremitting repetition of massive myoclonic jerks with retained consciousness, unless it is accompanied by generalized tonic-clonic or absence attacks. In all such cases there should be continuous seizure activity for 30 min or more and/or two or more seizures without recovery of consciousness between them.[1048]

Generalized nonconvulsive status epilepticus (**absence status**, petit mal status, minor epileptic status, spike-wave stupor, epilepsia minoris continua, epileptic twilight state) is characterized by some degree of clouding of mental processes, accompanied by bilateral spike-wave discharges on the EEG. Typical, atypical, and myoclonic forms are described. Diagnosis requires all of the following:[4125]

1. Depressed levels of consciousness (sometimes with coma), agitation, or disorientation
2. Absence of clinical convulsive activity
3. Continuous epileptiform discharges on the EEG.

Forms of focal status epilepticus

Focal (formerly *partial*) *convulsive status* is the persistence of convulsive activity within a restricted area on one side of the body. **Epilepsia partialis continua** of Kojevnikov, **aura continua,** limbic (psychomotor) status, **supplementary motor area status epilepticus,** and hemiconvulsive status epilepticus are examples. See also **subtle status epilepticus.**[1861]

Focal (formerly *partial*) *nonconvulsive status epilepticus* may present as recurrent, typical, complex, partial seizures without normalization of mental activity between seizures, or as prolonged continuous episodes of mental confusion and behavioral disturbance, with or without automatisms.[72]

Impending status epilepticus (early status epilepticus, early heralds of status) is defined as continuous or intermittent seizures lasting more than 5 min without full recovery of consciousness between seizures.[1129]

Supplementary motor area status epilepticus

Dyscognitive focal (limbic) status epilepticus (psychomotor status); medial temporal or neocortical forms

Hemiconvulsive status with hemiparesis

Adapted from Gastaut (1983)[2309] *and the ILAE classification at* http://www.ilae-epilepsy.org/Visitors/Centre/ctf/seizure_types.cfm/.

producing a marbled appearance. Clinically, this is associated with the later development of dystonia, chorea, spastic quadriparesis, and mental retardation. See **double athetosis** and **état marbré**.

status migrainosus A debilitating migraine attack lasting for more than 72 h. Diagnostic criteria have been defined as follows:

A. The present attack in a patient with **migraine without aura** is typical of previous attacks, except for its duration
B. Headache has both of the following features:
   1. Unremitting for > 72 h.
   2. Severe intensity
C. Not attributed to another disorder

From the International Classification of Headache Disorders (Headache Classification Committee of the International Headache Society. *Cephalalgia* 2004;**24**[Suppl 1]). Reproduced by kind permission of Dr. Jes Olesen, the International Headache Society, and Wiley-Blackwell Publications.

For practical purposes, this is a disabling headache of the migraine type, lasting for over 72 h, refractory to the usual analgesics and requiring hospitalization or repeated visits to the emergency room.

Steele–Richardson–Olszewski syndrome (heterogeneous system degeneration) A dementing illness with the added features of impairment of vertical gaze, especially downward; Parkinsonism; dystonic axial rigidity; and variable corticospinal and cerebellar signs. See **progressive supranuclear palsy**. The condition was described by these Canadian physicians in 1964.[6028]

steely hair disease See Menkes **syndrome**.

Steinbrocker disease (shoulder–hand syndrome) See **reflex sympathetic dystrophy**.

Steinert disease (Steinert–Batten–Curschmann disease) See **myotonic dystrophy**.

Steinert, Hans German physician who practiced in Leipzig and whose description of **myotonic dystrophy** was published in 1909.

Steinert–Batten–Curschmann disease See **myotonic dystrophy**.

Steinfeld syndrome (holoprosencephaly and limb defects) A congenital dysmorphic syndrome characterized also by optic atrophy, seizures, microcephaly, and holoprosencephaly or arhinencephaly with skeletal and visceral maldevelopments.[381]

Stellwag sign Infrequent and incomplete blinking, with retraction of the upper eyelid, resulting in a widening of the palpebral fissure, as seen in **dysthyroid ophthalmopathy** but also in **Parkinson disease**.

Stellwag, Karl (1823–1904) Austrian ophthalmologist.

Stengel syndrome The association of constructional apraxia, loss of spatial orientation, and all four features of **Gerstmann syndrome**.[6032]

stenosis (from Gr, to make narrow) The pathological narrowing of a hollow viscus or bony conduit.

Stephens syndrome A familial syndrome characterized by the combination of **chronic progressive external ophthalmoplegia**, cerebellar ataxia, and peripheral neuropathy resembling **hereditary motor and sensory neuropathy**, type 2.[6034]

stepless saccades See **saccadic pulses**.

steppage gait The gait of a subject with drop foot on one or both sides, who is aware that in order to prevent his feet catching on obstacles or irregularities on the ground, each foot must be lifted higher than is normal before being brought down again in front of him.

stepping-around nystagmus A non-vestibular form of ocular nystagmus occuring when a blindfolded subject actively walks for more than a minute at constant speed around a circular trajectory such as a slowly-rotating platform, thus not actually being displaced in space.

stepping response (walking reflex) When the held infant is lowered so that his or her feet touch the table, he or she makes stepping movements.[6898] The response normally appears after at least 34 weeks of gestation and disappears by 6 months of age.

stepping test The subject is asked to take 60 steps in place with the eyes closed and the arms held parallel to the ground. In the presence of unilateral vestibular disease, the subject tends to rotate more than 45° toward the affected side. With bilateral lesions, the tendency is to move forward or backward. See also **star walking**.

stereoanesthesia Lack of recognition of the shape or form of objects handled, due to lesions of the contralateral parietal lobe or ascending sensory pathways in the spinal cord.

stereognosis 1. Three-dimensional tactile feeling. 2. The ability to perceive objects in three dimensions or in a spatial relationship within a depth of field. In the visual form, this requires sight in each eye; in the tactile forms, this requires normal parietal lobe function. In each case the peripheral pathway is assumed to be functioning normally.

stereomorphometry Measurement of the distance between neuronal cell bodies in three dimensions.

stereopsis The ability to discriminate depth (i.e., three-dimensional perception) as a result of binocular vision, a function dependent upon normal activity in both cerebral hemispheres.

stereotactic (stereotaxic) depth electroencephalogram (SDEEG) A recording of the electrical activity of the brain by means of electrodes implanted within the brain substance according to stereotactic measurements. (From the 1974 report of the Committee on Terminology, IFCN. In: Chatrian GE, Bergamini L, Dondey M, et al. A glossary of terms most commonly used by clinical electroencephalographers. *EEG Clin Neurophysiol* 1974;**37**:538–48. Reproduced with kind permission from Elsevier Science.)

stereotypy An involuntary, patterned, repetitive, continuous, coordinated, purposeless or ritualistic movement, posture, or utterance (recurring utterances, verbal automatism, monophasia, formula speech). They may be simple, as exemplified by repetitive tongue protrusions or body-rocking movements, or complex, such as self-caressing, crossing and uncrossing of the legs, marching in place, and pacing.[6007] They differ from tics and mannerisms in that the latter are usually discontinuous steely attached hand. Such movements are a hallmark of **Rett syndrome**.

Sterling reflex The **Rossolimo reflex** applied to the fingers.[6037]

Sterling sign Adduction of the normal shoulder against resistance, accompanied by involuntary adduction of the opposite shoulder, indicating the presence of a pyramidal tract lesion affecting the latter side.

Sterling–Flatau progressive torsion spasm An alternating name for primary torsion **dystonia**.

sternal push test See **pull test**.

Sternberg-Cushing-Oppenheim syndrome See **Oppenheim disease**.

Sternberg-Oppenheim syndrome See **Oppenheim disease**.

Stern–Garcin syndrome A rapidly progressive dementing illness without focal cortical symptoms, first described by Dr. K. Stern in a 41-year-old patient admitted to the **National Hospital** under Dr. F.M.R. Walshe (and by Raymond Garcin in 1962) as "Severe dementia associated with bilateral symmetrical degeneration of the thalamus," although the temporal and parietal cortices were gliotic and showed neuronal loss. Garcin hinted that this may be the same condition as **Creutzfeld–Jakob disease**, but Stern rejected that possibility.[6042, 4258] See **familial myoclonic dementia**.

sternocleidomastoid test The demonstration of weakness of this muscle *on the same side* as a functional hemiparesis . Because this muscle is homolaterally innervated, with a left hemispheric lesion producing a right hemiparesis, it is the *left* sternomastoid that should be weak, so the strength of head turning to the *right* should be impaired. Weakness of head turning to the *left* in such a case would be considered evidence of **functional** weakness.[6074]

sternomastoid reflex Contraction of this muscle in response to a tap on its tendon at its insertion into the clavicle. The reflex is diminished in the presence of lesions of C3, 4 and augmented with pyramidal tract lesions above that level.

sternospinal reference A noncephalic reference achieved by interconnecting two electrodes, one placed over the right sternoclavicular junction and the other over the spine of the seventh cervical vertebra, the voltage between them being balanced by means of a potentiometer in order to reduce ECG artifact. (From the 1974 report of the Committee on Terminology, IFCN. In: Chatrian GE, Bergamini L, Dondey M, et al. A glossary of terms most commonly used by clinical electroencephalographers. *EEG Clin Neurophysiol* 1974;37:538–48. Reproduced with kind permission from Elsevier Science.)

sternotomy-related brachial plexopathy a lower trunk brachial plexopathy in which the ulnar sensory and motor amplitudes are the most affected responses. The predominant damage is in C8 distribution, suggesting that the focus of the lesion is localized at the level of the anterior primary rami of the cervical roots rather than in the lower trunk of the brachial plexus.[3805]

sternutation convulsiva See **sneezing**.

sternutatory reflex See **nasal reflex**.

steroid myopathy A syndrome of proximal muscle weakness and wasting preferentially affecting the legs. Type II fiber atrophy is the characteristic pattern on muscle biopsy. Serum creatine kinase activity is at the lower end of the normal range. A myopathic electromyogram and a raised 24-h urinary 3-methylhistidine/creatinine ratio on a creatine-free diet are also typical findings.[3412]

steroid-responsive myositis See **dropped head syndrome**.

steroid-responsive recurrent polyneuropathy See **chronic inflammatory demyelinating polyneuropathy**.

Stethoscope Loudness Imbalance Test A bedside test of stapedial muscle function. A strongly activated tuning fork placed close to the bell of a stethoscope worn by the subject with VII cranial nerve palsy affecting the nerve to stapedius leads to a louder sound on the side of stapedius paresis. Quieter vibrations are not so lateralized.[3967]

stethoscope neuropathy Compression of the greater auricular nerves by the metal arms of a stethoscope held in a resting position on the neck. Clinically, this presents with a sensation of increased warmth, numbness, burning, and paresthesias bilaterally along the posterior service of the auricle and lobule of the ears and over the retroauricular mastoid areas in the distribution of the nerves.[5225]

Stewart, J. Purves (1869–1949) English neurologist.

Stewart–Holmes syndrome See **Jackson cerebellar fits**.[6062]

Stewart–Morel–Morgagni syndrome A benign condition of increased thickness of the skull in the frontal regions, with which no neurological features are clearly associated. See **hyperostosis frontalis interna**.

Stickler syndrome (hereditary arthro-ophthalmopathy) A dominantly inherited congenital syndrome characterized by conductive and sensorineural deafness, cataract, detached retina, skeletal deformities including platyspondyly, and mental and developmental delay.[6064]

stick-man dystrophy A slowly progressive nonspecific myopathy with onset in early childhood, characterized by marked wasting of the limb muscles with retention of a surprising degree of power, and by contractures. See also **Emery–Dreifuss syndrome** and **congenital muscular dystrophy**.

stick-man syndrome See **congenital muscular dystrophy**.

stiff-baby syndrome (hereditary startle syndrome) A rare, dominantly inherited, congenital disease characterized by muscle stiffness, maximal at birth and tapering slowly during childhood.[3858] See **startle epilepsy**.

stiff-leg syndrome A syndrome of adults manifest as symmetric stiffness and spasms of the legs induced by voluntary movements and reflex stimuli. The nervous system is otherwise normal.[897]

stiff-limb syndrome A disorder of uncertain nature which resembles but also differs from the **stiff-person syndrome**, though also causing rigidity and spasm in the setting of continuous motor unit activity and with anti-GAD autoantibodies. Three subgroups have been defined:

1. Progressive encephalomyelitis with rigidity (PERM) is a rapidly progressive condition characterized by widespread rigidity which is lethal.
2. Stiff-person syndrome with rigidity and painful spasms of the lumbar paraspinal, abdominal, and occasionally proximal leg muscles associated with a lumbar hyperlordosis. The arms, lower legs, and cranial nerves are spared. Anti-GAD antibodies may be present. Neurophysiologically there is continuous motor unit activity. The condition responds to baclofen/ diazepam.
3. Truncal rigidity is uncommon and few patients in this group have anti-GAD antibodies. Neurophysiologically there is continuous motor unit activity in the affected limb and abnormally segmented EMG activity during spasms. The disease runs a protracted course and the response to baclofen or diazepam is suboptimal. Progression into typical **stiff-person syndrome** has been described, with added dementia, progressive ataxia, and the development of type 1 diabetes mellitus.

stiff-man syndrome. See **stiff-person syndrome**.

stiff-person syndrome (SPS) (Moersch-Woltman syndrome, stiff-man syndrome, progressive muscular rigidity) A rare, encephalomyelopathic syndrome with onset in adult life of persistent, progressive, painful rigidity of agonists and antagonists with powerful muscular spasms, of spinal origin, mainly affecting the axial and pelvic girdle muscles and inducing hyperlordosis. The face is spared. The spasms are triggered by stretching, emotion and sensory stimuli. The cause is considered to be diminution of activity in a spinal descending inhibitory pathway as a result of an autoimmune attack on glutamic acid decarboxylase, a precursor of GABA. Women are more affected than men, usually in the 30–50 year age group.

The Titanic spasms, which can be strong enough to break underlying bones, may be evoked by many exteroceptive stimuli and are at first intermittent but later become more or less continuous. They typically begin with an abrupt jerk followed by tonic activity that slowly subsides and are worsened by any attempt at active or passive movement or by noise, but diminish in sleep. In the classic stiff-person syndrome , muscle rigidity and superimposed episodic painful spasms begin insidiously over several months, affecting the lumbar and thoracic paraspinal and proximal legs muscles. In the trunk, the continuous muscle contractions produce a board-like appearance of the abdominal wall; co-contraction of abdominal and paraspinal muscles may lead to exaggeration of normal lumbar lordosis. Rarely the spasms last for days at a time (*status spasticus*). Associated oculomotor abnormalities include nystagmus, abduction weakness, impaired smooth pursuit, and saccade initiation. Paroxysmal autonomic dysfunction, seizures, arterial hypertension, rhabdomyolysis, and acute autonomic failure are associated complications.[1914]

High anti-GAD titers can be expected. EMG findings are of continuous action potentials indistinguishable from voluntary activity with superimposed brief bursts of 5–6 Hz rhythmic synchronous activity.

The spasms may be reduced by general anesthesia and by peripheral nerve block, as well as by high doses of diazepam, curare, baclofen, or sodium valproate.[4424] Associated disorders described include seizures, diabetes mellitus type 1, breast or lung cancer, thymoma, and other immune disorders such as thyroiditis, pernicious anemia, myasthenia gravis, and ovarian or adrenal failure. Sudden death may occur due to cardiac arrhythmias or restrictive respiratory arrest. For further analysis, access http://www.wustl.edu/neuromuscular.

The suggested diagnostic criteria[4558] include the presence of stiffness and rigidity in the axial muscles, progressing proximally and with superimposed muscle spasms, without involvement of the brainstem, upper or lower motor neuron systems, or the sphincters, sensation, or cognition. There should be an abnormal axial posture with lumbar lordosis and the EMG will show continuous motor unit activity in at least one axial muscle. A response to diazepam is another suggested criterion.

Separation into three categories has been suggested. In the first two the course is slow and the manifestations either distal (stiff-limb syndrome) or axial stiff trunk (man) syndrome. In the last the course is rapidly progressive to death within months (progressive encephalomyelitis with rigidity).[395]

Variants include the *jerking stiff-man syndrome*, a severe and rapidly progressive condition characterized by axial and lower-limb stiffness and rigidity followed by the appearance of spontaneous and stimulus-sensitive myoclonus and upper motor neuron signs, often accompanied by profuse sweating and other manifestations of dysautonomia. Nystagmus, ocular motor impairment, retinopathy, deafness, dysarthria, and dysphagia may be prominent. Death may occur between 6 weeks and 3 years from the onset of symptoms. Anti-GAD autoantibodies are usually detectable. The CSF shows a lymphocytic pleocytosis, elevated IgG, and oligoclonal bands, in which it is myoclonic jerks that are triggered by such stimulation; *congenital stiff-man syndrome;*[5528] *stiff-man syndrome with tremor;*[1661] and an association with thymoma and **myasthenia gravis**. See also **stiff-baby syndrome** and **startle epilepsy**.

In *SPS-plus syndromes* there is evidence of added encephalomyelitis or cerebellar deficits.

Arm, neck, and cranial nerve involvement occurs in paraneoplastic *variants*, such as occur with small cell lung cancer, breast cancer, thymoma, and Hodgkin lymphoma. When an arm is predominantly involved, a paraneoplastic stiff-limb syndrome should be suspected.[1914]

Focal lesions of the spinal cord can imitate this constellation of clinical features.[895]

See also the NIH Web site at http://www.ninds.nih.gov/disorders/stiffperson/stiffperson.htm.

stiff-skin-lipoma syndrome

A familial congenital syndrome characterized by generalized hirsutism, lipomas, conjunctivitis, scleroderma-like stiffness of the skin, digital flexion contractures, dental abnormalities, stomach ulcers, renal stones, arthropathy, strabismus, deafness, bulbar weakness, and loss of pain sensation.[1920]

stigmatic electrode The term of **Sherrington** for the **active**, or exploring, electrode.

Stiller disease (asthenia universalis congenita) An ill-defined entity comprising constitutional visceroptosis, neurasthenia, and vasomotor instability.

Stilling syndrome (ocular retraction syndrome) See **Duane syndrome**.

Stilling, Benedict (1810–1879) German anatomist and surgeon who described the solitary bundle and tract in the medulla in 1843 and who demonstrated the innervation of the walls of blood vessels. He published detailed accounts of the anatomy of the spinal cord, medulla, and pons—data which he acquired from his use of serial sections in three dimensions, using the microtome which he had introduced in 1824. Employing this technique, he described and differentiated almost all the cranial nerve nuclei recognized today. On the clinical side, he described various surgical procedures, but also wrote on psychosomatic symptoms, which he considered to be due to spinal cord irritation.

Stilling, Jakob (1842–1915) German ophthalmologist who graduated from Marburg and trained further in Paris, Berlin, and Vienna, returning to practice ophthalmology in Strasbourg for most of his career.

Stilling–Turk–Duane syndrome

A syndrome of complete or partial failure of abduction; a partial or complete adduction with retraction of the affected eye into the socket when it is adducted; an oblique movement of the eye up and in or down and in when it is adducted; and deficiency of convergence. See **Duane syndrome.** The account by Duane is complete, but was published 18 years after Stilling's original definition of the condition, which he acknowledged.

Stimmler syndrome (alaninuria–microcephaly–dwarfism–diabetes) A congenital dysmorphic syndrome characterized also by short stature, dental abnormalities, diabetes, aminoaciduria, ataxia, microcephaly, and mental and developmental delay.[381]

stimulant-dependent sleep disorder A disorder characterized by a reduction of sleepiness or suppression of sleep caused by central stimulants with resultant alterations in wakefulness following drug abstinence. Patients complain of insomnia or excessive sleepiness at times of the use of or withdrawal from a stimulant drug such as amphetamine and have reduced sleep efficiency and an increased number and duration of awakenings.[1629] Alcohol and toxins can produce a similar picture.

stimulating electrode A device used to deliver electric current. All electric stimulation requires two electrodes; the negative terminal is termed the *cathode* and the positive terminal is the *anode*. Electrical stimulation for nerve conduction studies generally requires application of the cathode to produce depolarization of the subjacent nerve. (Adapted from the 2001 Report of the Nomenclature Committee of the American Association of Electromyography and Electrodiagnosis.[19] Reproduced by kind permission of the AANEM.)

stimulation single fiber electromyography (stimulation SFEMG) Use of electrical stimulation instead of voluntary activation of motor units for analysis in single fiber electromyography, used in patients who are unable to produce a steady voluntary low-level muscle contraction. The stimulation can be delivered to intramuscular axons, nerve trunks, or muscle fibers. (From the 2001 Report of the Nomenclature Committee of the American Association of Electromyography and Electrodiagnosis.[19] Reproduced by kind permission of the AANEM.)

stimulation-produced analgesia

Lack of pain discrimination produced by stimulation of the ventrolateral periaqueductal gray matter of the midbrain.

stimulus (Lat, goad) Any external agent, state, or change that is capable of influencing the activity of a cell, tissue, or organism. In clinical nerve conduction studies, it usually refers to an electric current applied to a nerve. It may be described in absolute terms or with respect to the evoked potential of the nerve or muscle. In absolute terms, it is defined by a duration (ms), a waveform (square, exponential, linear, etc.), and a strength or intensity measured in voltage (V) or current (mA). With respect to the evoked potential, the stimulus may be graded as subthreshold, threshold, submaximal, maximal, or supramaximal.

A threshold stimulus is one just sufficient to produce a detectable response. Stimuli less than the threshold stimulus are termed *subthreshold*. The maximal stimulus is the stimulus intensity after which a further increase in intensity causes no increase in the amplitude of the evoked potential. Stimuli of intensity below this level but above threshold are *submaximal*. Stimuli of intensity greater than the maximal stimulus are termed *supramaximal*. Ordinarily, supramaximal stimuli are used for nerve conduction studies. By convention, an electric stimulus of approximately 20% greater voltage/current than required for the maximal stimulus is used for supramaximal stimulation. The frequency, number, and duration of a series of stimuli should be specified. (From the 2001 Report of the Nomenclature Committee of the American Association of Electromyography and Electrodiagnosis.[19] Reproduced by kind permission of the AANEM.)

stimulus-sensitive epilepsies

(reflex epilepsies) Seizures which are regularly and reproducibly evoked or facilitated by specific motor, sensory, or psychic stimuli. Visual stimuli are the most common of these. See also **photoconvulsive response**. More complex stimuli occasionally provoking seizures include music, hot water, eating, and thinking. Thus, *language-induced epilepsy* is that form in which seizures are induced by reading, writing, or speaking.[72]

stimulus-sensitive myoclonus

(reflex myoclonus) Myoclonus, often of the action or intention variety, which appears abruptly when a voluntary movement is initiated or during its performance. Such movements are often those requiring precision for their proper accomplishment.

stinger (burner) syndrome An upper trunk brachial plexopathy occurring secondary to traction when an athlete sustains a lateral flexion injury of the neck, leading to compression of the brachial plexus between the shoulder pad and the superior medial scapula when the pad is pushed into the area of Erb's point, where the brachial plexus is most superficial.[4090]

Stingle syndrome Loss of spatial orientation associated with the major features of **Gerstmann syndrome**.

Stocker sign The patient in typhoidal delirium fumbles with and tends to turn down or push away the bedclothes. In the presence of tuberculous meningitis, the patient is said to try to replace them.[5333]

Stock–Speilmeyer–Vogt disease See **neuronal ceroid lipofuscinosis**.

Stokes, William (1804–1878) Irish physician who practiced in Dublin. His description of syncopal attacks in association with a permanently slow pulse[6068] led to the attachment of his name to the syndrome, although **Spens** in Edinburgh had described the same thing 50 years before. See **Adams–Stokes–Morgagni syndrome**.

Stokes–Adams syndrome See **Adams–Stokes–Morgagni syndrome**.

stop See **voiceless bilabial**.

Storandt battery A screening instrument comprising a group of tests for intellectual impairment including some taken from other scales. The battery consists of two trailmaking tests—the Wechsler logical memory test and a test of mental control; but it is under revision.

Stormorken syndrome A dominantly inherited syndrome characterized by dyslexia, ichthyosis, short stature, migraine-like headache, photophobia, extreme miosis, impaired upward gaze, muscle fatigue, distal myopathic weakness, slow relaxation of muscle, absence of the spleen, thrombocytopathia, and red cell abnormalities.[6082]

strabismic amblyopia Visual failure in one eye due to an abnormality in neuronal maturation as a consequence of lack of use of the eye for fixation in early development. The usual reason for the neglect of the eye is muscular imbalance—a **strabismus**.

strabismus (from Gr, a squinting) Lack of parallelism of the ocular axes caused by the incoordinate action or developmental malposition of the extraocular muscles. The name was given by the Alexandrians to the geographer Strabo, who was so afflicted. See also **diplopia, ductions, phoria, tropia, vergence**, and **versions**.

Strachan syndrome (Strachan–Scott disease, Jamaican neuritis) A nutritional neuropathy resembling **pellagra**, manifest as the combination of amblyopia due to optic neuritis, painful areflexic sensorimotor neuropathy with sensory ataxia, hearing loss, and orogenital dermatitis. The syndrome was originally described in the residents of Jamaica[6086] in 1897 but occurs in malnourished people with low levels of riboflavin regardless of where they live. The epidemic neuropathy found in Cuba today may reflect the result of malnourishment occasioned by the economic embargo placed on that country. See also **Cuban optic neuropathy**.

Strachan, William Henry Williams (1857–1921) English physician, attached to the British West Indian garrison in Jamaica in the late nineteenth century.

Strachan–Scott disease See **Strachan syndrome**.

straight-leg raising A maneuver described by **Lasègue** in which the extended leg is passively flexed at the hip, thereby pulling on the sciatic nerve. Normally this is painless, but with meningeal irritation or root compression, pain is felt in the low back and in the back of the leg when the flexion reaches 60°, and spasm of the hip extensors occurs to prevent further flexion.[3729]

straight-thumb sign Inability to flex the terminal joint of the thumb when making a grasping movement. This is seen in the presence of anterior interosseous palsy and is due to weakness of the flexor pollicis longus.[1135] See also **Froment sign.**

Stransky nystagmus See **arthrokinetic-induced nystagmus**.

Stransky sign An alternative method of eliciting the **Babinski response**, whereby the little toe is pulled laterally and suddenly released. Its value is in its diminished tendency to cause withdrawal of the foot. See also **Allen reflex**.

Stransky syndrome A congenital dysmorphic syndrome characterized by short stature, aminoaciduria, renal tubular acidosis, osteoporosis, distal myopathy, and mental and developmental delay.[381]

strategic-infarct dementia Persistent cognitive impairment occurring as a result of a single left-sided cerebral infarct. This has been described following an acute syndrome of confusion, abulia, fluctuating alertness, inattention, memory disturbance, and psychomotor retardation, due to a small infarct in the lowest part of the genu of the internal capsule, causing thalamocortical disconnection.[6222]

strategy application disorder The inability to plan and execute complex tasks, requiring articulation of goals, specification of plans, self-monitoring, and the evaluation of outcomes. This disorder may reflect uni- or bilateral frontal lobe lesions.[5754]

strength testing See **functional muscle tests**.

strength-duration curve The graphic presentation of the relationship between the intensity (*Y* axis) and various durations (*X* axis) of the threshold electric stimulus of a nerve or muscle. The *rheobase* is the intensity of an electric current of infinite duration necessary to produce a minimal action potential. The *chronaxie* is the time required for an electric current twice the rheobase to elicit the first visible action potential. Measurement of the strength-duration curve is now more or less obsolete in electrodiagnostic medicine. (Adapted from the 2001 Report of the Nomenclature Committee of the American Association of Electromyography and Electrodiagnosis.[19] Reproduced by kind permission of the AANEM.)

strephosymbolia (Gr, turn + symbol) The occurrence of reversals of single letters such as "P" and "Q," or of words (e.g., *ten* and *net*), as seen in patients with **dyslexia**. *Spoonerisms* are similar errors in speech output, many of which (e.g. "Is it kisstomary to cuss the bride?") have been attributed to the Rev. Mr. William Spooner (1844–1930), Warden of New College, Oxford, often incorrectly.

stress 1. Any condition which poses a potential threat to the comfort or integrity of an organism or its constituents.
2. Accentuation of a spoken syllable.

stress convulsions Epileptic attacks in subjects without previous unprovoked seizures who have been exposed to stresses in the period immediately preceding the attack. Such stresses include lack of sleep, physical exhaustion, and emotional stress. The EEG is unhelpful in diagnosis or prognosis, and the incidence of epilepsy at followup is a little higher than the rate in normal subjects.[2209]

stress headache See **episodic tension-type headache**.

stretch reflex The reflex contraction of a muscle following sudden stretch, as by a tap on its tendon. The first physiological explanation was supplied by Sir Charles **Sherrington** in 1927. The principal sensory stimuli come to the cord via group I and group II afferents from muscle spindles. The earliest component is monosynaptic (the **muscle stretch reflex**), but there are also long-latency stretch reflexes. See also **T wave**.

stria (Lat, a furrow) A stripe or line, both elevated (ridges) and depressed lines (furrows) being so named.

stria terminalis A fiber pathway carrying impulses from the amygdala to the medial hypothalamic nuclei.

striatal degeneration A dominantly inherited, adult-onset, slowly progressive hypokinetic condition manifesting marked dysarthria and mild hypokinesia manifesting as gait disturbance without tremor and with no reduction in life expectancy, in which MRI scans demonstrate a distinctive lesion pattern restricted mainly to the putaminal and cordate nucleus. The disorder is mapped to chromosome 5q13.[3589]

striatal foot See **dystonic foot response**.

striatal hemiplegia An uncommon syndrome of athetosis proceeding to a fixed dystonic hemiplegia and resulting from lesions of the putamen and caudate nucleus.[1588]

striatal necrosis A syndrome with congenital or early childhood onset, characterized by cerebral atrophy with pyramidal and extrapyramidal signs (e.g., dystonia and choreoathetosis), seizures, apathy, depression, nystagmus, optic atrophy, and mental and developmental delay, and due to symmetrical degeneration of the caudate, putamen, and globus pallidus. It is mapped to chromosome 19q. A similar syndrome may complicate wasp-stings. See also **neurodegeneration with brain iron accumulation, infantile bilateral striatal necrosis, Wilson disease, Leigh disease**, and **cerebral palsy**.

striate cortex That area of cortex at the occipital pole forming the banks of the calcarine fissure in which the striae Gennarii are visible, and which receives input from the entire retina, relayed through the lateral geniculate bodies.

striate pseudobulbar palsy The state in which multiple lacunar infarcts lead to severe weakness of the bulbar muscles—in the opinion of **Wartenberg** it is sufficient to cause virtual anarthria.[645]

striatocapsular infarction A stroke syndrome in the territory of the lateral striate arteries, infarcting the head of the caudate and the anterior limb of the internal capsule and due to complete or partial occlusion of the proximal part of the middle cerebral artery. The usual clinical presentation is with arm weakness accompanied by such cortical signs as dysphasia, neglect, or dyspraxia.[1686]

striatocapsular infarcts Small infarcts of the caudate, the anterior limb of the internal capsule, or of the putamen, resulting from middle cerebral artery occlusion due to embolus, atheroma, arteritis, dissection, etc. and causing hemiparesis with hemiparesis (the arm weakness being greater than that of the face or leg) with neuropsychological dysfunction. Cortical signs may be minimal or absent. CT/MRI shows comma-shaped signals in the striatum.

striatonigral degeneration (striopallidonigral degeneration) A rare, sporadic, degenerative, akinetic-rigid syndrome of adult life, involving primarily the putamen and substantia nigra and leading to the clinical syndrome of Parkinsonism, with marked and progressive bradykinesia, rigidity, apathy, or depression, and urinary incontinence. Pyramidal and cerebellar signs are often detectable.[51, 6481] The clinical features suggested as most indicative of the diagnosis include the occurrence of unexplained falls, autonomic dysfunction, absence of rest tremor, and poor response to levadopa treatment.[1977] See also **multiple-system atrophies**.

In a *variant* form, the condition is dominantly inherited.[5411]

striatopallidal calcification (Fahr syndrome, idiopathic familial intracerebral arterial calcification, symmetrical cerebral calcification, dominant basal ganglion calcification, brain ferrocalcinosis) A rare heterogeneous group of conditions in which, bilaterally, the capillaries of the basal ganglia, dentate nucleus, and deeper cortical layers are affected by nonarteriosclerotic calcification of the vessels. The condition was first described in 1850; the later contribution of Fahr has been belittled and the eponym is no longer used.

Clinically, the condition may be asymptomatic or may be associated with any combination of dementia, seizures, evidence of raised intracranial pressure, and pyramidal, cerebellar, and extrapyramidal syndromes, including Parkinsonism, dystonia, or solitary tremor in young or middle adult life,[1953] coupled with evidence of parathyroid disturbance in the endocrine cases. Both dominantly and recessively inherited familial varieties, often with added ataxia and pigmentary retinal degeneration,[6092] are also delineated and have been reviewed by Baraitser.[379]

Idiopathic, pseudo-, and pseudo-pseudohypoparathyroidism are present in most sporadic cases, but the mineral deposition (not always calcium) may also be seen in various other neurological or metabolic diseases such as **Cockayne syndrome, Down syndrome, AIDS, NBIA, mitochondrial myopathy, Aicardi syndrome, Kearns–Sayre syndrome**, and **osteopetrosis**.[1843, 4516, 3938] A listing of *variant* forms is given in Chart S–15.

Chart S–15. Variants of Striopallidal Calcification

Basal ganglion calcification, mental retardation, and steatorrhea A recessively inherited syndrome characterized by these features.[1211]
Basal ganglion calcification with hypoparathyroidism A recessively inherited syndrome characterized by these features.[4501]
Familial basal ganglion calcification with neurological features A dominantly inherited syndrome of dense symmetrical calcification in the basal ganglia, with ataxia, spasticity, and mental deterioration and without evidence of pseudo- or pseudo-pseudohypoparathyroidism or evidence of infectious, toxic, or metabolic disease and with normal serum calcium and phosphate levels and a renal tubular response to parathyroid hormone.[2143, 4516]
Familial basal ganglion calcification with pseudo-hypoparathyroidism A dominantly inherited syndrome in which the endocrine features are accompanied by calcium deposition in the lenticular nuclei.[4662]
Familial calcifications of the brain, iron storage, and porphyria A condition in which calcifications are accompanied by deficient serum iron transport, hemochromatosis, and porphyria.[458]
Familial encephalopathy and basal ganglion calcification A recessively inherited congenital syndrome of microcephaly, seizures, spasticity, dystonia, abnormal eye movements, and lymphocytosis in the CSF.[77]
Idiopathic familial calcification of the basal ganglia A recessively inherited syndrome of dense basal ganglion, occipital lobe, and dentate nucleus calcification with (variously) Parkinsonism in middle life, dementia, spasticity, contractures, and athetosis, ataxia, or dystonia.[379]
Striatopallidal calcification with ataxia A rare variant also manifesting pigmentary retinopathy, described by Strobos, et al.[6092]

striatum The caudate, putamen, and globus pallidus; this group of structures being so called because of their striped appearance in fresh sections, as a result of the layers of fibers crossing the internal capsule to connect the caudate and putamen.

string sign An extended region of almost, but not quite, total occlusion of a major artery, seen on angiograms in patients with dissection of the carotid artery in the neck. The descriptor "rat tail" is also sometimes employed here.

striopallidodentate calcification The appearance of diffuse metallic signals from the basal ganglia. The causes include hypoparathyroidism and pseudohypoparathyroidism, familial striopallido-dentate calcification,[6092] and infantile or familial cases associated with microcephaly, pigmentary macular degeneration, and progeria. The appearances of iron deposition resemble those of calcium on CT scans.

In another *variant* syndrome, leukodystrophy and parenchymal brain cysts are associated.[3628]

Clinical features include seizures, EEG abnormalities, mental deterioration, signs of Parkinson disease, pyramidal signs, and endocrinological symptoms.[3938]
See also **mitochondrial myopathies**, **Urbach–Weithe disease**, and **lipomembranus polycystic osteodysplasia**.

striothalamic hand See **thalamic hand**.

Strohl, André (b. 1887) French physician who studied in Paris, where he was later elected professor of physical medicine. Most of his work was on the circulatory system, electrophysiology, and respiratory functions. He was, with **Guillain** and **Barré**, an author of the classic description of **acute inflammatory demyelinating polyneuropathy**.

stroke (cerebrovascular disease) A neurological deficit secondary to cerebral arterial or venous disease: A generic term for all neurovascular syndromes that occur due to infarction, hemorrhage, or subarachnoid hemorrhage.[4678]

Various classifications of stroke have been suggested;[2662, 4601] but the scheme of Prof. Vladimir Hachinski is reproduced in Chart S–16.

Chart S–16. Classification of Stroke

A. *Presumed stroke*

Presumed transient ischemic attack (TIA)
Other

B. *Anatomical classification*

By axial location:

Supratentorial	Lobar (specify)
Centrencephalic (specify)	Infratentorial
Cerebellar (specify)	Brainstem (specify)

By vascular territory:

Carotid (specify)	Vertebrobasilar (specify)

C. *Etiological classification*

By result:

Cerebral infarct (arterial, arteriolar [lacunar], venous)
Cerebral hemorrhage (intraparenchymal, subarachnoid)

By cause:

Ischemia (extracranial vascular disease, embolism, other)
Hemorrhage (hypertension, amyloid angiopathy, vascular malformation, other)

D. *Management classification:*

TIA and minor stroke
Major stroke
Deteriorating stroke
Stroke in the young
Stroke in the elderly

Web sites of relevance to stroke include the following:

http://www.ninds.nih.gov/disorders/tia/tia.htm Provides information on transient ischemic attack.

http://www.strokeassociation.org/presenter.jhtml?identifier=1200037 Offers data on prevention and recovery fact sheets for consumers and treatment guidelines for professionals from the American Stroke Association.

http://www.basp.ac.uk/ The Web site of the British Association of Stroke Physicians, a professional association whose objective is to advance stroke medicine within Great Britain.

http://www.strokeconsortium.ca/ The Web site of an academic alliance, the Canadian Stroke Consortium, pursuing anti-stroke therapies through research projects and clinical trials in Canada.

http://www.hemikids.org/ The Web site of the Children's Hemiplegia and Stroke Association, a nonprofit organization offering support for affected children and their families.

http://www.canadianstrokenetwork.ca/.

http://www.tandf.co.uk/journals/titles/13638491.html A Web site promoting scientific awareness, communication, and knowledge about recovery, development, and outcome.

http://www.world-stroke.org/ The Web site of the International Stroke Society, a professional association endeavoring to expand stroke-prevention efforts and improve stroke patients' care through research and education.

http://www.strokecenter.org/ A stroke resource for medical professionals and consumers at the Internet Stroke Center at Washington University in St. Louis, providing information about education and directories of clinical trials and stroke centers.

http://www.sirweb.org/patients/stroke/ An educational resource from the Society of Interventional Radiology, covering intra-arterial thrombolysis, aneurysm embolization, and carotid stenting.

http://www.stroke.org/ The Web site of the National Stroke Association, a nonprofit organization, providing services, including educational programs and community-based activities in prevention, treatment, and rehabilitation to stroke-affected families and the medical profession.

http://www.nemahealth.org/programs/nsc/ The Web site of the National Stroke Council, an organization established by the American National Emergency Medicine Association, to further research and education on the causes and effects of brain attack.

http://www.strokefoundation.com.au/ The Web site of the National Stroke Foundation, an organization dedicated to reducing the impact of stroke in Australia.

http://content.nejm.org/cgi/collection/stroke Provides access to *The New England Journal of Medicine: Stroke Collection* and lists literature covering topics such as antithrombotic therapy, cerebral thrombosis, and carotid stenosis from the archives of that journal.

http://www.ninds.nih.gov/disorders/stroke/stroke.htm The NINDS stroke information page, providing an introduction to stroke, with pointers to related fact sheets concerning symptoms, prevention, and rehabilitation.

http://www.pediatricstrokenetwork.com/ The Web source of the **Pediatric Stroke Network**, providing information and support to families dealing with this disease in infancy, childhood, or adolescence.

http://www.ninds.nih.gov/news_and_events/proceedings/stroke_proceedings/childneurology.htm Provides a review of current knowledge.

http://www.rcplondon.ac.uk/pubs/books/childstroke/index.asp A free online publication from the Royal College of Physicians of London, providing clinical guidelines for diagnosis, management, and rehabilitation for childhood stroke.

http://www.stroke.org.uk/media_centre/press_releases/children_and.html A fact sheet dealing with stroke in children and babies.

http://www.stroke.org.uk/ The Stroke Association, a charitable organization in the UK.

Stroke and Aphasia Quality-of-Life Scale 39 A scale measuring the quality of life of people with stroke causing aphasia.[2899]

Stroke Center A Web resource for information about stroke care and research. Web sites: www.strokecenter.org/ and www.neuro.wustl.edu/stroke/.

Stroke Data Bank A study initiated in 1978 by the National Institute of Neurological and Communicative Disorders **and Stroke** to amass information from a large number of patients as a data source for clinical research in stroke.[3602]

stroke delirium An acute confusional state following upon infarction of the lower division of the middle cerebral artery in the nondominant hemisphere.

Stroke Impact Scale-16 A stroke-specific, self-reported health status measure designed to assess multidimensional stroke outcomes, including strength, hand function, activities of daily living or instrumental activities of daily living (ADL/IADL), mobility, communication, emotion, memory and thinking, and participation 1–3 months after the event using items from the composite physical domain of the Stroke Impact Scale.[1751]

stroke scales Semiquantitative rating scales of the deficits resulting from stroke. Some of those most commonly employed are described more fully in this book. (See **Allen Scale, Barthel Index of Activities of Daily Living, Canadian Neurological Scale, European Stroke Scale, Frenchay Activities Index, Fugl–Meyer Assessment Scale,** Hemispheric Stroke Scale, **Mathew Stroke Scale, NIH Stroke Scale, Orgogozo Scale, Rankin Scale, Scandinavian Stroke Scale,** and **Toronto Stroke Scale.**) Van Gijn[6495] has reviewed 41 such scales in an assessment of outcome measures and de Haan has dissected five of them.[1497] See also **disability scales**. The Web site http://www.medal.org/visitor/www/active/ch17/ch17.aspx lists 35 such scales and over 20 more assessing stroke risk and prevention.

The National Institutes of Health Stroke Scale (NIHSS) correlates well with the simpler **Canadian Neurological Scale**, both quantifying neurological deficits. The **Barthel Index** is a functional scale and is widely acknowledged as of value in measuring activities of daily living (ADLs). The modified **Rankin Scale** (mRS) as well as the **Glasgow Outcome Scale** (GOS) are long-term measures of residual handicap and are generally used when the physical recovery seemed to have achieved a plateau.

Stroke A professional journal of the American Heart Association, publishing reports on clinical and basic investigation of any aspect of the cerebral circulation and its diseases. The journal does not follow the Vancouver style for references. Web site: http://intl-stroke.ahajournals.org.

Stroke-Adapted Sickness Impact Profile A condensation of the original 136-item Sickness Impact Profile, assessing quality of life in patients who have sustained a stroke.

stroke-in-evolution See **evolving stroke**.

stroke-like episodes and leukoencephalopathy A dominantly inherited syndrome characterized by the occurrence in mature adulthood of completed subcortical strokes or transient ischemic attacks, migraine-like headaches, and evidence from CT or MRI scanning of widespread white matter disease.[6362] See also **MELAS**.

stroke-like migraine attacks after radiation therapy (SMART) A syndrome which occurs as a long-delayed consequence of cerebral irradiation in patients with a previous history of **migraine with** or **migraine without aura**, without evidence of residual or recurrent neoplasm, who experience prolonged unilateral migrainous neurological symptoms such as confusion, visuospatial or hemisensory deficits, hemiparesis, aphasia, or seizures, any of these being accompanied by headaches. MRI shows transient, dramatic cortical gadolinium enhancement of the affected cerebral hemisphere. Ipsilateral slowing is seen on the EEG.[665]

Stroke-TIA.org An Internet site providing data on cerebrovascular diseases to health professionals. Web site: http://www.stroke-tia.org/stroke-tia/professional.html.

strongyloidiasis Infection with *angiostrongylus cantonensis*, a nematode usually acquired from tropical snails, with a tendency to invade all body tissues, including the brain and spinal cord. Clinical neurological signs of infection include headache, meningism, VI and VII cranial nerve palsies, and occasionally coma as a result of a chronic granulomatous encephalomyelitis, the response of the nervous system to the presence of the dead nematodes. The CSF shows an eosinophilic pleocytosis.

Stroop Word Color Test A test of perseverance and concentration, based on the fact that normal people read a word faster than they name an object or color associated with that word. In the test, subjects first read color words, then name the colors of dots, and finally name the color in which each of the 100 words is printed—but these colors do not match the word. Thus when the word *red* is printed in green ink, the correct response is "green."[6096] The test has been used extensively in the identification of simulated (malingering) syndromes. An online form of the test is available.

Strümpell disease 1. Acute polioencephalomyelitis; the cerebral form of poliomyelitis, with convulsions and hemiplegia added to the peripheral motor effects of the poliovirus.[6099] 2. See **Erb–Charcot syndrome**. 3. See **cerebral infantile paralysis**.

Strümpell hereditary spastic paraplegia (Strümpell–Lorrain syndrome) See **hereditary spastic paraplegia**.

Strümpell signs 1. Contraction of the tibialis anterior as an associated movement during hip flexion.[6102] See **tibialis phenomenon**. 2. Strong passive flexion of the forearm normally leads to pronation as well but this is increased in the presence of an upper motor neuron lesion. 3. Dorsiflexion of the hallux with leg paresis. (The preceeding three signs were noted in patients with pyramidal disease.) 4. (**radialis sign**) Inability to close the hand without dorsiflexion of the wrist, as seen in both spasticity and tetany. 5. An alternative method of producing the **Babinski response**, whereby the examiner firmly runs his finger and thumb down the spine of the tibia.

Strümpell, Ernst Adolf Gustav Gottfried von (1853–1925) German physician who studied philosophy, psychology, and the violin before turning to medicine, graduating from Leipzig in 1879 and later succeeding **Erb** as director of the medical clinic at Heidelberg. He was finally elected professor of medicine at Leipzig in 1910. Strümpell published extensively on the topics of **tabes dorsalis**, neuritis, muscular atrophy, **multiple sclerosis**, and traumatic disease and gave the first description of pure **hereditary spastic paraplegia** in 1880,[6098] completing this in 1886.[6100] He also published a classic study of polioencephalomyelitis and described spastic pseudosclerosis and (ankylosing) spondylitis deformans. The first of the 30 editions of his textbook of medicine was published in 1883, when he was 31.

Strümpell–Liechtenstern disease See **acute disseminated encephalomyelitis** and **acute hemorrhagic leukoencephalitis**.

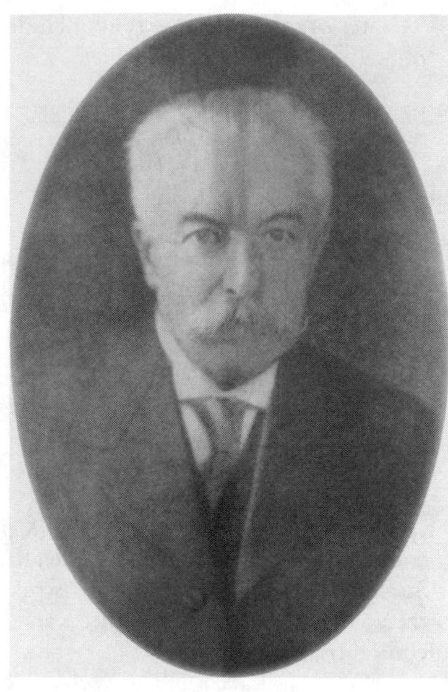

Figure S–6 Ernst Adolf Gustav Gottfried von Strümpell

Strümpell–Lorrain disease See **hereditary spastic paraplegia**.

Struthers ligament A band of aponeurotic tissue arising from the humerus and inserted into the medial epicondyle, occasionally compressing the median nerve and producing impairments resembling the **pronator teres syndrome** except for the absence of involvement of that muscle, innervation of which is achieved at a higher level. Sir John Struthers was an English physician and anatomist.

Stuart syndrome (Stuart–Bergstrom syndrome) A congenital dysmorphic syndrome characterized also by nerve deafness, papilledema, vascular abnormalities of the retina, callosal agenesis, and cutaneous pustules.[6105]

Stuart–Bergstrom syndrome See **Stuart syndrome**.

stuck-in-set perseveration Persistent and inappropriate repetition of a motor task; a sign of frontal lobe or mesolimbic disease.

stump dyskinesia The occurrence of motor sequelae such as chorea, dystonia, repetitive jerking spasms, and tremor in the stump after amputation, frequently associated with pain.[4084]

stump pain A sharp, jabbing pain felt locally at the site of amputation of a limb and worsened by local pressure. A neuroma of the cut nerve endings is held to be responsible.

stump pressure The intra-arterial pressure distal to the site of arterial occlusion.

stump spasm (convulsive movements of the stump, painful jumping amputation stumps, trépidation du moignon) Myoclonic or choreic movements of the remaining stump of an amputated limb, not always painful. The pathophysiology is unknown.[3593]

stunned brain Brain tissue within the **ischemic penumbra** surrounding a region of infarction, which is not now functioning but which may be expected to do so in time.

stupidity 1. The term of **Willis** for amentia or **dementia**; "A failure of the imagination, memory and judgement [in which] the eye of the intellect is . . . dulled."
2. Inability to share the insights of the observer.

stupor (Lat, insensibility) A state of reduced consciousness in which the subject retains the ability to make eye movements and limb motor and vocal (but not verbal) responses to vigorous stimulation; the range of awareness is markedly diminished but not lost, and there is little or no spontaneous activity. On the **Glasgow Coma Scale** the scores will be 3–5–3. The EEG will show diffuse slowing and caloric testing produces tonic deviation of the eyes. **Catatonia** looks very much the same but the EEG may be normal and caloric testing induces nystagmus.

Sturge, William Allen (1850–1919) English physician who trained at University College Hospital, London, and worked at the **National Hospital**, Queen Square, and in Paris with **Charcot**, returning to a staff position at the Royal Free Hospital. For the sake of his wife's health, he moved to Nice in France, practicing there for nearly 30 years, and only returning to England after his wife's death and his remarriage. His published output was small, papers on **amyotrophic lateral sclerosis** and on the disease bearing his name being those of lasting record.

In 1879, he presented a patient with a port-wine stain and focal motor seizures to a London medical society meeting, suggesting that the seizures were a result of an underlying lesion upon the brain, but he was not believed. Further delineation of the **Sturge–Weber syndrome** was provided by Parkes Weber in 1922.

Sturge–Weber Foundation
A support site for individuals and professionals dealing with Sturge–Weber syndrome, port-wine stains, and Klippel–Trenaunay syndrome.
Web site: http://www.sturge-weber.org/.

Sturge-Weber syndrome
(Sturge-Weber–Dimitri syndrome, Crouzon-Crostophy-Gaucher syndrome, neurocutaneous angiomatosis, Cushing–Bailey–Cobb auroral syndrome, cutaneocerebral angioma, encephalofacial or encephalotrigeminal angiomatosis, Parkes–Weber–Dimitri disease, Sturge–Kallischer–Weber disease, Schirmer–Sturge–Weber syndrome, Brushfield, Hebold, Krabbe, Lawford, Luschka, Milles, Jahnki or Wyatt syndrome, fourth phakomatosis; Weber himself called it Sturge–Kallischer disease) Venous angiomas of the meninges with overlying dermal angiomas (port-wine stain) in the trigeminal nerve distribution, frequently associated with atrophy of the underlying cortex, hemiparesis, and seizures, described by Sturge in 1879[6110] and by Weber in 1922. Choroidal angiomas may lead to glaucoma and visual loss.

Skull radiographs may show **tramline calcification** in the affected cortical layers; this calcium is also well seen on CT scans. The clinical features of note are the presence of a vascular nevus (port-wine stain) in the territory of the trigeminal nerve and of capillary and cavernous hemangiomas within the brain, the tendency to suffer recalcitrant seizures, glaucoma, macrocephaly, and mental or developmental delay. Jablonski[3113] lists 36 separate names for this condition, indicating either that many physicians have rushed into print without adequate familiarity with the literature or that the desire to coin Latin neologisms is an addiction of neurologists. The *variants* of the syndrome as classified by Francois[2175] are given in Chart S–17.

Other *variant forms* in which there is an association with **von Hippel–Lindau disease**, **neurofibromatosis**, or **tuberous sclerosis** are noted by Baraitser.[379]

Sturge-Weber Syndrome Center A clinical center dedicated to the treatment and study of the condition, based at Johns Hopkins University. Web site: http://sturgeweber.kennedykrieger.org/index.jsp.

Chart S–17. Classification of Sturge–Weber Syndrome

Complete, Three signs

Sturge–Weber (with glaucoma)
Jahnki (without glaucoma but with choroidal angioma)

Incomplete

A. *With ocular and cutaneous signs only*

Schirmer (with early glaucoma and buphthalmos)
Lawford (with late glaucoma, not buphthalmos)
Milles (with choroidal angioma)

B. *With two signs, one neurological*

Krabbe (with encephalotrigeminal angioma and bulbospinal symptoms)
Crouzon-Crostophy-Gaucher (with minor CNS signs only)
Cushing-Bailey-Cobb (with cutaneomedullary angiomatosis)
Arieti-Gray (with arterial aneurysms, multiple angiomatosis, mental deficiency, intracranial calcification, and seizures)
van Bogaert–Divry (with corticomeningeal telangiectatic angiomatosis) (infantile meningeal angiomatosis) A syndrome comprising seizures, spastic paraplegia, or quadriplegia, and associated with an increased incidence of meningioma or sarcoma in the brain.

Sturge-Weber–Dimitri syndrome See Sturge-Weber syndrome.

Stuttering Foundation of America A charitable organization providing support and information on this condition. Web site: http://www.stutteringhelp.org/.

stuttering Involuntary repetition, prolongation, or arrest of sounds in conversational speech. The precise etiology is unknown, but acquired forms may commence in association with traumatic or degenerative brain disease or aphasia and may be transient or persistent. They show no adaptation effect: Any syllable of any type of word may be affected, and there is no concurrent abnormal motor activity, but certain visuospatial and alternating motor tasks may be poorly performed by subjects suffering from acquired stuttering.

Aphasic stuttering may be etiologically linked; *stuttering with aphasia* is an emotional reaction to the lesion; and *dysarthric stuttering* occurs during recovery from expressive forms of dysphasia.[2847]

stylohyoid process syndrome See **Eagle syndrome**.

styloradial reflex See **brachioradialis reflex**.

Suarez–Kelly syndrome See **dropped head syndrome**.

sub- (Lat, under, beneath).

subacute (brainstem) encephalomyelitis A slowly progressive syndrome of distal more than proximal stiffness at its onset progressing to lower brainstem involvement manifest as nystagmus and ophthalmoplegia, deafness, blindness, and long-tract signs. The CSF contains inflammatory cells. The brainstem and cord pathology is that of inflammation and gliosis.

subacute AIDS encephalitis See **HIV-associated dementia complex**.

subacute angioendotheliopathy See **subacute diencephalic angioencephalopathy**.

subacute arteriosclerotic encephalopathy See **Binswanger disease**.

subacute cerebellar degeneration See **subacute cortical cerebellar degeneration**.

subacute cerebral degeneration See **Creutzfeldt–Jakob disease**.

subacute combined degeneration of the cord (Dana syndrome, posterolateral sclerosis, Putnam–Dana syndrome) Demyelination of the lateral columns and posterior columns of the spinal cord as a result of deficiency of vitamin B12. In the case of the posterior columns, the demyelination reflects primary damage to the large dorsal root ganglion cells, whose centripetal processes run therein.[5476] A pyramidal syndrome obscured by hyporeflexia, and diminution or loss of proprioception, discriminative touch and vibration are the classic findings; they are often accompanied by optic atrophy.[1438] Almost any degree of mental impairment, from mood change through drowsiness and intellectual dulling to confusion or paranoid states has also been recorded.

The condition was described by Lichtheim in 1887. The first clue as to the etiology was found by Minot, who observed improvement in a patient who ate *liverwurst* on a daily basis.

subacute cortical cerebellar degeneration (Lichtheim syndrome, subacute cerebellar degeneration) A rare **paraneoplastic syndrome** characterized by the acute or (more usually) subacute development of pancerebellar and brainstem dysfunction, sometimes with evidence of paraneoplastic **subacute motor neuronopathy** and dementia,[803] but usually without other motor or sensory signs. The syndrome is associated with small cell carcinomas of the lung, with ovarian carcinoma and with Hodgkin disease more commonly than with other malignancies. The major clinical features are progressive incoordination of gait and limb movements bilaterally, dysarthria, nystagmus, and oscillopsia.

Pathological examination reveals severe loss of the cerebellar Purkinje cells and perhaps lymphocytic infiltration of the meninges. A misdirected immune attack is considered the most likely etiology;[5098] high titers of anti-Hu and/or anti-Yo antibodies are typically detected.

subacute degeneration of the thalamus See **fatal familial insomnia**.

subacute degenerative polioencephalopathy of the presenium See **Creutzfeldt–Jakob disease**.

subacute demyelinating polyneuropathy See **chronic inflammatory demyelinating polyneuropathy**.

subacute diencephalic angioencephalopathy (subacute angioencephalopathy) A rare, fatal disease of unknown etiology causing confluent areas of necrosis and marked edema in the lower brainstem producing a syndrome of progressive impairment of intellect and memory, behavioral disturbances, abnormality in consciousness, apathy or depression, and myoclonus, associated with bilateral destructive lesions of the thalamus due to proliferative inflammatory lesions of the small blood vessels.[1530]

Neuropathology shows extensive fibromuscular thickening and luminal narrowing of venous meningeal vessels of the brainstem.[5208]

subacute encephalitis See also **HIV-associated cognitive/motor complex**.

subacute encephalomyelitis Acquired inflammatory disease of the brain due to direct viral invasion or postinfectious autoallergic responses, leading to a slowly progressive deterioration in functions. **Rabies, shingles, polymyoclonia, Reye syndrome**, and **acute cerebellar ataxia** are examples of such disorders.

subacute encephalomyelopathy See **Leigh disease**.

subacute familial thalamic atrophy A slowly progressive dementing disease, also characterized by sleep disturbances and associated with atrophy of the dorsomedial and anterior thalamic nuclei.[3257] See also **Stern-Garcin syndrome**.

subacute idiopathic demyelinating poly(radiculo)neuropathy A neuropathic syndrome which clinically and pathologically resembles mild **chronic inflammatory demyelinating polyneuropathy**, but which has a slowly progressive phase lasting 1–3 months;[3042] although "lumpers" would not accept this as an adequate differentiating feature.

subacute inclusion body encephalitis A form of encephalitis characterized by the presence of Type A intranuclear inclusion bodies in the CNS (Dawson, Greenfield). See **subacute sclerosing panencephalitis**.

subacute inflammatory demyelinating polyneuropathy A condition falling between **acute inflammatory polyneuropathy** and **chronic inflammatory demyelinating polyneuropathy** by virtue of the speed of its progression. Criteria for the former require less than 4 weeks of progression, and for the latter more than 2 months. This condition by definition, therefore, has a history of progression from 4 to 8 weeks. Its clinical features blend those of the acute and the chronic forms.[4765]

subacute motor neuronopathy A **paraneoplastic syndrome** occurring as a remote effect of Hodgkin disease or of other lymphomas and manifested as a subacute, painless, progressive lower motor neuron syndrome affecting the legs more than the arms, often asymmetrically. The symptoms may remit if the underlying cause is treated successfully.[5632, 6106]

subacute myelo-opticoneuropathy (SMON, acrodermatitis enteropathica) A central-distal axonopathy induced by the ingestion of clioquinol, in which axonal degeneration is found in the optic nerves, the distal corticospinal tracts, and the gracile columns at the cervicomedullary junction (the distal part of the central extension of the dorsal root ganglion cells).[6404, 6111] The pathophysiology appears to involve an abnormality in copper homeostasis. Clinical features of note when the disease was extant included painful distal hypesthesia and paresthesias, hyperreflexia, visual loss, ataxia, signs of autonomic neuropathy, seizures, and abdominal complaints. Also remarkable was the finding that the tongue and feces were stained green.[6366]

subacute myoclonic spinal neuronitis See **progressive encephalomyelitis with rigidity**.

subacute necrotizing encephalomyelopathy See **Leigh disease**.

subacute necrotizing myelitis A slowly progressive ischemic myelopathy, usually in the thoracic regions, due to an arteriovenous malformation or obliterative sclerosis of the small vessels of the cord in the affected areas causing cord necrosis, and leading to the usual motor, sensory, and autonomic signs of transverse myelitis extending upward from the legs. The initial spasticity is later replaced by flaccid paraparesis and the dissociated sensory alteration by complete loss of all modes.

The CSF protein level is increased but the cell counts remain low. Thrombophlebitis of the spinal thoracic and lumbosacral veins appears to be the most likely pathology.[2138] See **Foix–Alajouanine syndrome**.

subacute necrotizing myopathy A syndrome of muscular weakness with histological changes of muscle necrosis without inflammation. Whether this is a **paraneoplastic syndrome** or a *variant* of acute **polymyositis** is not yet determined.[6452]

subacute necrotizing polioencephalopathy A fatal, progressive disease of the cortex and brainstem of unknown cause, marked by disseminated areas of focal necrosis without inflammatory change.[5498]

subacute presenile polioencephalopathy See **Creutzfeldt–Jakob disease**.

subacute presenile spongy atrophy See **Creutzfeldt–Jakob disease**.

subacute reversible motor neuron disease See **amyotrophic lateral sclerosis**.

subacute sclerosing leukoencephalitis A slowly progressive form of encephalitis in which there is conspicuous gliosis of the white matter of the CNS.[6467] See **subacute sclerosing panencephalitis**.

subacute sclerosing panencephalitis (van Bogaert encephalitis, Dawson encephalitis, subacute inclusion body encephalitis, subacute sclerosing leukoencephalitis) A fatal, progressive encephalitis of children following exposure to the measles virus at an early age, the agent now acting as a slow virus. There is no evidence that immunization against measles is a cause. The clinical picture is initially that of a slight behavior disorder, but it is followed by mental deterioration and impairment of speech, leading on to generalized and partial seizures, myoclonus, ataxia, dementia, decerebration, and death.

Pathologically, there is both neuronal and white matter damage; eosinophilic inclusions are seen in neurons and oligodendroglia; and viral antigen is detectable in neurons in all parts of the brain except the cerebellum. The white matter lesions (perivascular edema, inflammation, and demyelination) are identical to those that are seen in progressive rubella encephalitis, subacute AIDS encephalomyelitis, tropical spinal paraparesis due to HTLV-1, and visna of Icelandic sheep; and deposits of immune complexes can be demonstrated in the walls of small cerebral blood vessels. The EEG appearance of paroxysmal slow-wave dysrhythmias (**burst–suppression**) is characteristic. A high titer of anti-measles antibodies is found in the CSF.[6467, 5093] Typical diagnostic criteria require clinical evidence of progressive subacute mental deterioration with, for example, myoclonus; periodic, stereotyped, high-voltage EEG discharges; raised gammaglobulin levels or oligoclonal bands in the CSF; a raised titer of anti-measles antibodies (>1:256) in the CSF; and brain biopsy evidence of panencephalitis.

subacute sensory neuropathy (primary sensory neuropathy, malignant sensory neuropathy, ganglioradiculitis, progressive sensory neuropathy, sensory neuronopathy) A debilitating **paraneoplastic syndrome** typically associated with small cell carcinoma of the lung most commonly among adult white female smokers, but also occurring in **Sjögren syndrome**, as a result of toxicity[3339] and Epstein-Barr virus infections.

Clinically, it is characterized by the subacute but progressive asymmetrical centripetal loss of all sensory modes, mainly in the limbs, with pain and dysesthesias but good motor power and with raised CSF protein levels. Sensory ataxia, pseudoathetosis, areflexia, and frequently other signs of neurological dysfunction such as limbic encephalitis, seizures, cerebellar, myelopathic or autonomic signs, a myasthenic syndrome, and inappropriate ADH secretion are also described. The pathological hallmark is inflammation and widespread degeneration of the dorsal root ganglia.[3003] The presence of anti-Hu antibodies staining neuronal nuclei is a marker for the small cell carcinoma.

The condition was first recognized by **Denny-Brown** in 1948.

subacute spongiform encephalopathy See **Creutzfeldt–Jakob disease**.

Subanaerobic Threshold Exercise Test A simple test identifying patients with abnormalities of muscle energy metabolism secondary to mitochondrial dysfunction, based on the venous lactate response to exercise at 90% of predicted work rate at the anaerobic threshold.[4594]

subarachnoid bolts Devices inserted through the skull in order to monitor intracranial pressure.

subarachnoid hemorrhage (meningeal apoplexy) The extravasation of blood into the subarachnoid space as a result of rupture of a berry aneurysm on an artery close to the circle of Willis, or as a result of bleeding from an arteriovenous malformation; less commonly other causes are responsible.

The first recorded incident was probably that described in 2 Kings 4:18, in which a boy became moribund after a sudden violent headache and was revived by the prophet Elisha, who apparently used mouth-to-mouth respiration. It was, however, Sir Charles **Symonds** who gave the most complete account of the findings in 1924–1925. Suggested criteria for the clinical diagnosis[4859] include the following:

1. The demonstration by CT scan of blood in the Sylvian fissure, the basal cisterns, the interhemispheric sulcus, or a ventricle, *or*
2. Any combination of

   Blood in the CSF (after a nontraumatic tap) or xanthochromia, *and* the presence of
   Severe headache at onset or on awakening after the ictus, *or*
   Depressed level of consciousness, *or*
   Clinical signs of meningeal irritation, *or*
   Retinal hemorrhages, *or*
   Focal neurological signs.

Subarachnoid Hemorrhage Grading Scale A scale designed to describe change in an individual patient at different times, to estimate prognosis and to standardize assessment and management in different groups of patients. It emphasizes level of consciousness (assessed with the **Glasgow Coma Scale**) and the presence or absence of hemiparesis or aphasia.[1709] (See Chart S–18). See also **Naidech Scale**.

Another simple grading scale recognizes five levels: (1) Headache only without neurological signs. (2) Minor extraocular signs only. (3) Significant neurological deficit (hemiparesis, etc.). (4) Significant disturbance in consciousness. (5) Moribund.

Yet other scoring systems addressing vasospasm and outcome, using CT scans and clinical assessments, are available at http://www.medal.org/visitor/www/active/ch17/ch17.aspx.

subclavian steal syndrome (brachial-basilar insufficiency) Symptoms of brainstem ischemia (vertebrobasilar insufficiency) occurring due to reversal of the flow of blood which has now ascended in one vertebral artery and down the other one, rather than continuing up the basilar artery. This occurs as a result of stenosis of the first part of the subclavian artery proximal to the takeoff of the vertebral, so that blood cannot ascend in that vessel. When that arm is exercised, its demand for blood increases; but as the demand cannot be met across the proximal stenosis, flow is diverted down the vertebral artery on that side to supply the arm, thus stealing from the basilar.[5262] The syndrome may only cause symptoms when flow in the carotid system is also reduced.

Symptoms include vertigo, limb paresis, binocular visual changes, paresthesias, ataxia, diplopia, syncope, and monocular visual changes, in that order of frequency.[2043]

Chart S–18. The Subarachnoid Hemorrhage Grading Scale

Grade	*Glasgow Score*	*Motor Deficit*
1	15	nil
2	14–13	nil
3	14–13	+
4	12–7	±
5	6–3	±

From Drake CG. Report of a World Federation of Neurosurgeons committee on a universal subarachnoid hemorrhage scale. J Neurosurg *1988;***68***:1985–86.*

subclinical rhythmic excitatory discharges of adults (SREDA; Pseudolarval electrographic seizure of the elderly) A rare EEG pattern resembling an epileptic discharge but without any known clinical association.[3469]

subclinical seizure A paroxysmal event without clinical, behavioral, or cognitive changes produced by an "epileptic" discharge on the EEG.

subcortical aphasia Forms of aphasia consequent upon circumscribed infarctions in the neostriatum and thalamus (territory supplied by the lenticulostriate branches of the middle cerebral artery) on the dominant side.

The characteristics of the resulting aphasic syndromes vary between cases, but, at least in those cases with thalamic infarctions, they may resemble those of the **transcortical aphasias**.[1432] See also **subcortical motor aphasia**.

subcortical arteriosclerotic encephalopathy See **Binswanger disease**.[320]

subcortical auditory aphasia See **pure word deafness**.

subcortical band heterotopia See **diffuse cortical dysplasia**.

subcortical dementia Dementia occurring in association with degenerative disorders involving the subcortical structures. The major clinical features include forgetfulness; marked slowing of thought processes; alterations of personality with inertia, apathy, and depression; occasional irritability or euphoria; inappropriate emotional display; and impaired ability to manipulate abstract knowledge (e.g., poor abstraction ability and calculation). Dysarthria and motor signs are also common.

These changes are thought to stem from a primary problem of excessive delay in the performance of intellectual tasks. **Parkinson disease, progressive supranuclear palsy, Huntington disease, progressive subcortical gliosis, NBIA, multisystem atrophy,** paramedian thalamic infarctions,[3325] and **normal-pressure hydrocephalus**[106] are representative disorders.

Clinically, the condition may be suspected when the dementia is accompanied by prominent motor disturbances, while typically "cortical" signs such as aphasias, apraxias, agnosias, and visual field deficits are less evident,[3022] and memory loss is relatively slight. Verbal and perceptual-motor abilities are also relatively well preserved if the subject is not pressed for time.[106]

Criticisms of this clinical differentiation have been reviewed, but its validity is as yet unproved.[6753]

subcortical dysequilibrium (tottering, astasia-abasia, thalamic astasia) A gait disorder characterized by prominent dysequilibrium with absent or ineffective postural responses. Sometimes the postural responses are inappropriate; for example, the patient may hyperextend the trunk and neck and fall backward. Other patients appear inattentive to their posture and unable to generate postural responses, although EMG recordings show that there are postural responses, but these are ineffective. Locomotion is primarily impaired because of the dysequilibrium. There is, thus, an inability to stand in the absence of muscle weakness or marked sensory loss, usually due to a unilateral vascular lesion.

The pattern is associated with lesions of the midbrain, thalamus, or basal ganglia, and associated signs include ocular palsies (vertical gaze palsies and pupillary abnormalities), dysarthria, and extrapyramidal signs. (Adapted from Nutt JG, et al.[4722] and Masdeu and Gorelick.[4135] Reproduced by kind permission of the American Academy of Neurology and Lippincott Williams and Wilkins.).

subcortical functions Those endowments which preferentially serve fundamental functions, such as arousal, motivation, and mood. Dysfunction is considered to lead to slowing of information processing, with disturbance of memory, cognition, mood, and behavior. The memory disturbance, however, is mainly a difficulty in spontaneous recall rather than in encoding or storing new material, so memory assisted by clues and cues is better than free recall.

subcortical gliosis (Neumann type dementia) An autosomal dominantly inherited condition presenting in the fifth or sixth decades with personality change and degeneration of social ability which later develop into profound dementia with mutism, dysphagia, and extrapyramidal signs as in **Pick disease**.

Pathologically, moderately severe atrophy with preferential involvement of the frontal and temporal lobes is seen but without the knife-edge pattern characteristic of Pick disease. There is fibrillary astrocytosis, particularly in the U fibers and in the subpial cortex and laminar spongiosis as in Pick and Alzheimer diseases, but not pancortical as in **Creutzfeldt–Jakob disease**. Neuronal inclusions and amyloid deposits are absent.

subcortical junctional infarcts Infarcts in the periventricular regions, resulting from distal middle cerebral artery occlusions(usually due to extracranial carotid artery disease) and causing hemipareses with hemisphere-specific neuropsychological dysfunction.

subcortical laminar heterotopia An X-linked or dominantly inherited neuronal migration disorder giving a "double cortex" appearance on MRI scans.[5030] See also **lissencephaly** and **pachygyria**.

subcortical motor aphasia An aphasic syndrome characterized by the acute onset of mutism, progressing to hypophonia with dysarthria and paraphasia, while comprehension, naming, and reading are variably affected or spared and repetition may be good, with progressive reduction in paraphasic errors. The likelihood of ultimate recovery is high. Hemiparetic and hemisensory deficits are usually present in the early stages at least. See **aphemia** and **subcortical aphasia**.

subcortical neglect Neglect produced by subcortical lesions. Compare with **neglect**.

subcortical reflex myoclonus See **reticular reflex myoclonus**.

subcortical sensory aphasia See **Lichtheim aphasia**.

subcortical vascular dementia A subtype of **vascular dementia**. Diagnostic criteria require radiologic evidence of subcortical cerebrovascular disease and a neuropsychological profile demonstrating greater impairment of executive functions relative to delayed recognition memory.[5118]

subcortical visual aphasia See **pure word blindness**.

subdural abscess See **subdural empyema**.

subdural effusion A collection of fluid beneath the cranial dura mater. The term is used to describe acute, subacute, or chronic subdural hemorrhage; subdural hygroma; and subdural empyema. The fluid contained is usually xanthochromic and may be hemorrhagic, but is usually sterile.

The effusion is commonly the result of birth or other head injuries, meningitis, or cranial surgery, but it usually stems from the organization of a subdural hematoma. Its clinical features include seizures, vomiting, irritability, and failure to thrive in infants who are found to have a bulging fontanel, hyperactive reflexes, and enlargement of the head, sometimes with evidence of the fluid-containing cyst shown by transillumination.

In adults, the clinical features are those of subdural hematoma.[4170]

subdural empyema (subdural abscess, cortical abscess, circumscript meningitis, internal purulent pachymeningitis) Pyogenic infection of the meninges in which the pus lies between the arachnoid and dural membranes. The condition was first recorded in 1886. It is usually a complication of chronic otitic or sinus infection with adjacent osteomyelitis and presents clinically with rapidly progressive local symptoms, headache, fever and meningism, alteration of consciousness, focal seizures, and neurological signs, depending on the site of the empyema.[3581]

subdural grid electrodes A line of electrodes placed on the cortex at open operation in an attempt to determine the precise origin of abnormal electrical discharges in epileptic patients. **Magnetometry** may in the future accomplish the same thing better and noninvasively.

subdural hematoma (subdural hemorrhage) A collection of blood or blood products beneath the dura of the skull or in the spinal cord, stemming from rupture of the bridging veins, usually due to trauma. Both *acute* and *chronic* forms exist. Clinically, these are signs of increased intracranial pressure, focal signs, and occasionally seizures due to compression of the underlying cortex.

The presence of hemiparetic signs on the side opposite the skull lesion was first noted in the Edwin Smith Papyrus, and appears again in Hippocratic writings, with a description of post-traumatic seizures. Ambrose Paré described the underlying pathology and most of the physical signs resulting, although LeDran was the first to comment on the **lucid interval** (which, however, is more common with **epidural hematoma**). Pupillary dilation as a result of compression of the III cranial nerve was drawn by Hans Wachtlin of Basle in 1527, but the sign was not recognized further until remarked by Richard **Bright** in 1827, again in a case of epidural hematoma. Jonathan **Hutchinson** gave a full account of the stages of pupillary dilation in 1867.[2119] An early record of the (successful) evacuation of a **subdural hematoma** was that of Dr. Thomas Kirkland (1792).

subdural hemorrhage See **subdural hematoma**.

subdural hygroma A collection of fluid in the subdural space, usually remotely following trauma and presenting with symptoms similar to those of chronic subdural hematoma.[4572]

subependymal cell plate See **germinal zone**.

subependymal giant cell astrocytoma See **astrocytoma**.

subependymal zone See **germinal zone**.

subependymoma An uncommon, slowly growing, malignant, primary neuroectodermal cerebral tumor, likely a variant of **ependymoma**, occurring mainly in males. It is usually located in the fourth ventricle, less often in periventricular regions of the brain and rarely in the spinal cord. It carries a fair prognosis if completely removed, and in some cases remains asymptomatic. Pathologically, the lobulated tumor is characterized by the presence of nests of fibrillary astrocytes with round nuclei containing chromatin, separated by areas filled with glial processes and by the presence of calcium and hyalinized, partly obliterated vessels within it.[5590] The underlying glial layer also proliferates.

subjective DIMS complaint without objective findings (pseudoinsomnia, sleep hypochondriasis) Complaints of insomnia (and of its usual associated symptoms) which cannot be verified by polysomnography. See ASDA diagnostic classification,[280] **sleep disorders**.

subjective tinnitus See **tinnitus**.

sublimis syndrome See **pseudo-carpal tunnel syndrome**.

submandibular, rectal, and ocular pain and flushing A dominantly inherited syndrome of infancy characterized by severe, brief attacks of pain in the eyes, rectum, and submandibular regions, with local skin flushing and bowel movement. The cause is not known.[2805]

submedullary syndrome See **Opalski syndrome**.

subnormal period A time interval that immediately follows the supernormal period of nerve which is characterized by reduced excitability compared to the resting state. Its duration is variable and is related to the refractory period. (From the 2001 Report of the Nomenclature Committee of the American Association of Electromyography and Electrodiagnosis.[19] Reproduced with kind permission from the AANEM.)

subpial cerebral siderosis The deposition of iron-containing pigment within the subpial layers of the CNS following previous bleeding into the subarachnoid space stemming from any cause.[4226]

substance P A vasoactive oligopeptide hormone found in the hypothalamus and elsewhere in the CNS, in the dorsal horn of the spinal cord, and in the gastrointestinal tract. It functions as a primary sensory neurotransmitter in the pain pathways and is capable of activating pain receptors. Its release is inhibited by morphine and endorphins.

substantia gelatinosa A curved band capping the posterior part of the dorsal horn of gray matter in the spinal cord, distinguished from the surrounding structures by its transparency and consistency. It receives the bulk of the C-fiber afferent projections in the cord as well as many small, myelinated afferent fibers.

Described first by the Italian anatomist **Rolando** in 1824, this is the only structure in the spinal cord extending continuously from the brainstem to the filum terminale. While its relevance in the transmission of impulses to do with pain is a keystone of the **gate theory**, other authors have concluded that its function is still unknown and have cast doubt upon its role as a functional entity.[1071]

substantia nigra (Lat, substance + black) A pigmented area in the mesencephalon dorsal to the crura cerebri, but ventral to the red nuclei.

subtentorial lesions Lesions within the posterior fossa, beneath the tentorium and above the foramen magnum. Their clinical effects are manifest through their effects on the brainstem, the cerebellum, and the passage of CSF.

subthalamic nuclear degeneration See **dentatorubropallidoluysian atrophy**.

subthalamic syndrome The clinical features following occlusion of the thalamoperforating arteries, comprising extension at the interphalangeal joints, most marked at the fifth finger and progressively less toward the thumb; slight flexion at the metacarpophalangeal joints; and choreoathetotic movements of the hand, with added tremor, ataxia, and choreoathetosis but minimal sensory disturbances.[645]

subtle seizures (fragmentary seizures) See **automatism** and **minimal seizures**.

subtle status epilepticus An end stage of prolonged generalized tonic–clonic status epilepticus characterized by focal or multifocal myoclonic movements, coma, and pseudoperiodic lateralized epileptiform discharges (PLEDs) superimposed upon a slow low-voltage EEG background. The myoclonic movements reflect severe brain damage caused by prolonged status epilepticus.[1861]

subwakefulness syndrome A rare form of hypersomnolence of unknown cause, characterized by excessive daytime sleepiness with repetitive nonrapid eye movement stage 1 or 2 sleep episodes but normal nocturnal sleep patterns.[280, 4523] See **idiopathic CNS hypersomnolence**.

succinate semi-aldehyde dehydrogenase deficiency A rare recessively inherited disorder of childhood with mental retardation, seizures, hypotonia, hyporeflexia, and nonprogressive ataxia. Marked language impairment and behavioral abnormalities including aggressiveness, anxiety, hallucinations, and self-injurious behaviors are also seen. MRI scans show symmetrically increased T2 signals in the globus pallidus. The condition is diagnosed by finding 4-hydroxybutyrate on urine organic acid analysis.[4953]

succinylcholine sensitivity A recessive condition with a locus on chromosome 3, in which exposure to succinylcholine as a muscle relaxant in anesthesia leads to prolonged muscle paralysis with apnea. Screening tests for the disorder use quantitative assays of plasma pseudocholinesterase, which are low.

succinylpurinemic autism An inherited syndrome due to deficiency of adenylsuccinase for which the responsible gene maps to chromosome 22.

succubus A female devil, thought in the Middle Ages to be seeking sexual intercourse with men during their sleep. See also **incubus**.

sucking reflex Stimulation of the lips by a finger introduced between them (or stimulation of the cheek); elicits sucking movements involving the lips, tongue, and jaw, and turning of the head toward the stimulus.

The reflex is normally present from 30 weeks' gestation, is lost by 4 months, and reappears only in the presence of diffuse bilateral cortical disease or bilateral corticobulbar lesions.[6898]

sudanophilic (orthochromatic) leukodystrophies A group of congenital dysmyelinating syndromes characterized by optic atrophy, seizures, nystagmus, spasticity, low densities in the periventricular white matter on T2 weighted MRI scans, and the accumulation of sudanophilic lipids in microglia and astrocytes.[5109] See **adrenoleukodystrophy**.

sudden bodily jerks on falling asleep See **periodic limb movement disorder**.

sudden infant death syndrome (SIDS) A syndrome of uncertain cause, one candidate being failure of the automatic control of respiration, leading to periodic apnea, alveolar hypoventilation, and death. Structural changes in the brainstem affecting the neural controlling mechanisms are present in a number of infants dying from this cause. **Ondine's curse** is a similar condition in adults. See also the *International Classification of Sleep Disorders Diagnostic and Coding Manual*[1629] and **sleep disorders**.

sudden unexpected death in epilepsy (SUDEP) Deaths occurring in subjects with epilepsy either directly as a result of seizures or without that explanation. Some of the latter may, however, be due to unwitnessed seizures, leading to severe bradycardia, and/or asystole, pulmonary edema, or respiratory arrest. Identified risk factors for SUDEP are the occurrence of frequent tonic-clonic seizures, youth, male gender, alcohol abuse, treatment with more than two anticonvulsants, nonadherence to therapy, and a full-scale IQ of less than 70.[6594]

sudden unexplained nocturnal death syndrome The occurrence of sudden death during sleep in young adults previously considered healthy. This is most commonly seen in subjects of Southeast Asian decent and appears to be based upon episodic ventricular fibrillation. Suggested diagnostic criteria[1629] are given in Chart S–19.

Sudeck atrophy See **reflex sympathetic dystrophy** and **causalgia**.

Chart S–19. Diagnostic Criteria for Sudden Unexplained Nocturnal Death Syndrome

A. Sudden cardiorespiratory arrest during sleep
B. Occurs in persons of Southeast Asian descent
C. Associated features include one or more of the following:

1. Male sex
2. Choking, gurgling, gasping, or labored breathing during the episode
3. The episode occurs during the habitual sleep period
4. A history of prior sleep terror episodes

E. Cardiac studies of survivors have demonstrated spontaneous ventricular fibrillation after initial resuscitation
F. No evidence of any medical or psychiatric disorder that could account for the features, e.g., ischemic heart disease
G. May be associated with **sleep terrors** but does not meet the criteria for other sleep disorders producing a risk of cardiopulmonary arrest, e.g., **obstructive sleep apnea syndrome** or rapid eye movement sleep–related sinus arrest

From AASM Diagnostic Classification Steering Committee. The International Classification of Sleep Disorders Diagnostic and Coding Manual. *Rochester, MN. American Academy of Sleep Medicine 1991/2001. Reproduced by kind permission of the Academy.* See also **sudden unexpected death in epilepsy** and http://www.sleepeducation.com/Disorders.aspx/.

Sudeck, Paul Hermann Martin (1866–1938) German surgeon, professor at Hamburg.

Sugiura sign Depigmentation within the corneal limbus, seen in patients with **uveomeningoencephalitic syndrome**.

sulfatide antibody-related neuropathy A rare, slowly progressive, painful axonal sensory neuropathy of later adult life with IgM binding to trisulfated heparin disaccharide and presenting with distal symmetrical sensory loss affecting all modalities except proprioception; areflexia; and mild weakness in the feet associated with serum IgM antibodies to trisulfated heparin disaccharide. Nerve conduction studies show axonal loss; SNAP amplitudes are reduced, and biopsy reveals a loss of unmyelinated axons and the presence of IgM deposited around the outside of the wall of medium- and larger-sized vessels.[4992]

sulfatide lipidosis See **metachromatic leukodystrophy**.

sulfatidoses Forms of sphingolipidosis characterized by the accumulation of sulfatides and, in some cases, steroid, heparan, or dermatan sulfate; they include the various forms of **metachromatic leukodystrophy** and **mucosulfatidosis**.

sulfite oxidase deficiency (sulfituria) A syndrome of severe neurological dysfunction with mental retardation, microcephaly, seizures, blindness, and extrapyramidal and pyramidal signs, also characterized by dislocation of the lenses and the excretion of inorganic sulfite, thiosulfite, and S-sulfocysteine.[889]

sulfituria See **sulfite oxidase deficiency**.

Suliman syndrome A congenital dysmorphic syndrome characterized by short stature, ptosis, skeletal and genital abnormalities, and mental and developmental delay. See also **Marden-Walker syndrome**, which is similar.

Sulzberger–Bloch disease See **incontinentia pigmenti**.

summation hyperpathia The awareness of excessive pain during stimulation of the same area in two modes. The lesion may be either in the thalamus or in the cerebral cortex.[4347]

Summerskill sign Widening of the palpebral fissure in patients with hepatic insufficiency.[6127]

Summitt syndrome A recessively inherited congenital syndrome characterized by craniosynostosis, syndactyly, obesity, strabismus and high-arched palate.[6128] See **craniosynostosis** and **acrocephalopolysyndactyly**.

SUNA syndrome (Short lasting Unilateral Neuralgiform headache attacks with cranial Autonomic symptoms). A *variant* of **SUNCT** (see below) based largely upon timing. Characteristics are brief orbital, supraorbital, or temporal head pains, migrating elsewhere in the cranium, the attack types including brief stabs or groups of stabs, and saw-tooth attacks lasting between 1 min and 3 h with a mean attack frequency of about 60/day. Conjunctival injection or tearing (not both) and nasal blockage, rhinorrhea, eyelid edema, facial sweating or flushing, and ear flushing accompany the pains. Agitation is common in the attacks.[1227] The following diagnostic criteria have been suggested by the IHS.[2819]

A. At least 20 attacks fulfilling criteria B–E
B. Attacks of unilateral orbital, supraorbital, or temporal stabbing pain lasting from 2 s to 10 min
C. Pain is accompanied by one of
    1. Conjunctival injection and/or tearing
    2. Nasal congestion and/or rhinorrhea
    3. Eyelid edema
D. Attacks occur with a frequency of one or more per day for more than half the time
E. Not attributed to another disorder

In *episodic SUNA*, attacks occur for 7 days to 1 year with pain-free intervals longer than 1 month, while in *chronic SUNA* at least two attack periods last 7 days to 1 year separated by remission periods of less than 1 month, if untreated. See also **red ear syndrome** and **SUNCT syndrome**.

From the International Classification of Headache Disorders (Headache Classification Committee of the International Headache Society. *Cephalalgia* 2004;**24**[Suppl 1]) and reproduced by kind permission of Dr. Jes Olesen, the International Headache Society, and Wiley-Blackwell Publications.

sunbath polyneuritis A subacute sensory polyneuropathy with photosensitivity usually resulting from treatment with phenothiazines or their derivatives with a good prognosis. VII nerve palsy may be associated.[5351]

SUNCT syndrome (Short-lasting Unilateral Neuralgiform Headache Attacks with Conjunctival Injection and Tearing) A distinctive, rare trigeminal-autonomic cephalalgia characterized by intermittent head pains (unilateral neuralgia-like paroxysms lasting 5–250 s [mean 50 s]) up to about 20 times daily accompanied by marked autonomic activation such as conjunctival injection, tearing, rhinorrhea, subclinical sweating, raised intraocular pressure, and bradycardia, the attacks being precipitated by stimulation of regions innervated by the V cranial nerve.[5881] They seldom occur at night.[2416]

Males are much more commonly affected. The frequency may also vary in bouts. A systematic study of attack frequency demonstrated a mean of 28 attacks per day, ranging from 6 to 77. Other less-prominent autonomic symptoms include sweating of the forehead or rhinorrhea.

Although usually a central disorder, cerebellopontine angle and pituitary lesions and brainstem arteriovenous malformations can cause the same syndrome. The following diagnostic criteria have been suggested:

A. At least 20 attacks fulfilling criteria B–E
B. Attacks of unilateral, orbital, supraorbital, or temporal, stabbing or pulsating pain lasting 5–240 s
C. Pain is accompanied by ipsilateral conjunctival injection and lacrimation
D. Attacks occur with a frequency from 3 to 200 per day
E. Not attributed to another disorder.

From the International Classification of Headache Disorders (Headache Classification Committee of the International Headache Society. *Cephalalgia* 2004;**24**[Suppl 1]). Reproduced by kind permission of Dr. Jes Olesen, the International Headache Society, and Wiley-Blackwell Publications.

A SUNCT Headache Information Page is found at http://www.ninds.nih.gov/disorders/sunct/sunct.htm.

sundown syndrome The onset or exacerbation of delirium during the evening or night, with reduction or disappearance of the delirium during the day. Reduced ability to maintain attention to external stimuli, disorganized thinking and speech, restlessness and agitation, perceptual disturbances such as illusions, and hallucinations and emotional disturbances are common features. The problem is common in the setting of dementing illnesses.[6556]

sunflower cataract The appearance of the cataract in **Wilson disease**.

sunflower syndrome (Gr, the sun + movement; thus an attraction toward strong light) Heliotropism followed by the performance of movements of the arm on the side to which the gaze is directed, perhaps to induce flickering of the solar image and leading to heterogeneous (photosensitive) epileptic attacks, which presumably either induce pleasurable sensations or blot out unpleasant ones—the subjects are amnesic for the events during the seizures.[174]

sunglasses sign The wearing of sunglasses by a patient complaining of ocular symptoms but with no obvious ophthalmologic reason to do so is highly suggestive of nonorganic visual loss.[514]

It is always a joy when scientific research confirms one's long-held but unsubstantiated opinions.

Sunnybrook Scale A scale for evaluating patients with spinal cord injury.[3678]

Motor	*Sensory*	*Grade*
Complete loss	Complete loss	1
Complete loss	Incomplete loss	2
Incomplete loss, useless	Complete loss	3
Incomplete loss, useless	Incomplete loss	4
Incomplete loss, useless	Normal	5
Incomplete loss, useful	Complete loss	6
Incomplete loss, useful	Incomplete loss	7
Incomplete loss, useful	Normal	8
Normal	Incomplete loss	9
Normal	Normal	10

(Useless = MRC scale 1–2; Useful = MRC scale 3–4)

sunrise (sunset) sign Depression of the eyeball with failure of upward gaze and retraction of the upper lid, such that only the upper rim of the cornea shows above the lower lid margin; seen in children with pressure on the mesencephalic tegmentum due to hydrocephalus.

super- (Lat, above).

superficial anal reflex A superficial reflex manifested by contraction of the anal sphincter in response to stroking or scratching the perianal skin. The reflex arc employed is at S4–5.

superficial radial nerve palsy Damage to the nerve, causing pain, numbness, and paresthesias in the space between the thumb and the index finger, most commonly as a result of **handcuff** or watch-strap pressure[6077] or within the syndrome of **multiple mononeuropathy**. See **cheiralgia paresthetica**.

superficial reflexes Reflex muscle contraction elicited by stimulating cutaneous receptors. Such reflexes are relatively long in latency and duration, are graded in proportion to the strength of the stimulus, and show both summation and exhaustion; in all of which characteristics they differ from the **muscle stretch reflexes**. See also **cutaneous reflexes**.

superficial siderosis of the central nervous system A disorder characterized by deposition of hemosiderin in the leptomeninges and the subpial tissue following repeated episodes of bleeding into the subarachnoid space from any cause; following the treatment of cerebellar tumors; or for unknown reasons.

Clinically, the disease causes any combination of myelopathy, sensorineural deafness, cerebellar ataxia, and dementia.[3039] Anterior horn cell disease has also been reported. The diagnosis is suggested by the T2-weighted MRI findings of hypointensities overlying the brainstem, cerebellar vermis, VIII nerve, spinal cord, and sometimes the cerebral cortex and in the basal cisterns as a result of the deposition of iron-containing compounds such as hemosiderin.[3512] Pathologically, there is discoloration of the leptomeninges and adjacent parenchyma especially of the superior vermis, crests of the cerebellar folia, basal frontal lobe, temporal cortex, brainstem, spinal cord, nerve roots, and cranial nerves I and VIII.

Antecedent events include subarachnoid hemorrhage, prior intradural surgery or trauma, root avulsions, epidural cysts, tumors, or vascular abnormalities. There is a sharp cutoff in the spinal roots and cranial nerves at the junction between the peripheral Schwann cell and central glial segments.[3596]

superior canal dehiscence syndrome A syndrome of vertigo, oscillopsia, and chronic dysequilibrium induced by sound (**Tullio phenomenon**) or by changes of middle ear (**Hennebert sign**) or intracranial pressure and showing vertical pendular nystagmus or oscillopsia and Valsalva-induced up-and-counterclockwise-beating jerk nystagmus. Hyperacusis to bone-conducted sounds and chronic dysequilibrium are also described features. The diagnosis is suggested by the presence of vertical–torsional eye movements evoked by sound or pressure stimuli (excitation with a Valsalva maneuver against pinched nostrils, tragal compression, loud sounds) or inhibition (Valsalva against a closed glottis or jugular venous compression) of the affected superior semicircular canal. Lowered thresholds for responses to vestibular-evoked myogenic potentials also assist.[355, 4394]

Provocative tests exciting the affected superior semicircular canal include using the Valsalva maneuver against pinched nostrils, tragal compression, or exposure to loud sounds. Inhibiting it may be possible using the Valsalva against a closed glottis or jugular venous compression.

Abnormal communication between the inner ear and the intracranial space is considered to explain the nystagmus, modulated by increased intracranial pressure. Dehiscence of bone overlying the superior semicircular canal on the affected side can be confirmed on CT scanning,[6323] but MRI is even better.

Dehiscence of the posterior canal causes a similar syndrome.

superior cerebellar peduncle syndrome See **cerebellar tremors**.

superior cerebellar peduncle tremor See **cerebellar tremors**.

superior Foville syndrome See **Raymond–Cestan syndrome**.

superior gluteal nerve entrapment syndrome A syndrome of aching gluteal pain and weakness of the gluteus medius muscle causing weakness of leg abduction and limping, and considered to be due to compression of the nerve by the piriformis muscle.[5199] See also **piriformis syndrome**.

superior laryngeal nerve syndrome

See **Avellis syndrome**.

superior laryngeal neuralgia

(Arnold syndrome, auriculotemporal neuralgia) A rare syndrome of severe lancinating paroxysmal pain in the side of the neck, extending up to the face as high as the zygoma, down to the upper portion of the thorax and medially perhaps as far as the mid-larynx, almost invariably unilateral and triggered by swallowing, yawning, coughing, or stretching the neck. The attack lasts from seconds to a minute or even more.[5922] The syndrome was first described fully by Avellis in 1900. The IHS criteria are as follows:

A. Pain paroxysms lasting for seconds or minutes in the throat, submandibular region and/or under the ear and fulfilling criteria B–D
B. Paroxysms are triggered by swallowing, straining the voice, or head turning
C. A trigger point is present on the lateral aspect of the throat overlying the hypothyroid membrane
D. The condition is relieved by local anesthetic block and cured by section of the superior laryngeal nerve
E. Not attributed to another disorder; other causes, in particular a structural lesion, have been ruled out by history, physical examination, and special investigations.

From the International Classification of Headache Disorders (Headache Classification Committee of the International Headache Society. *Cephalalgia* 2004; **24**[Suppl 1]). Reproduced by kind permission of Dr. Jes Olesen, the International Headache Society, and Wiley-Blackwell Publications.

superior oblique myokymia

A variant form of **saccadic intrusion**, characterized by a rapid, intermittent, small-amplitude, torsional, vertical jerk nystagmus in one eye, as a result of repetitive contraction of the superior oblique muscle. This leads to complaints of oscillopsia and often of oblique diplopia. The condition was first described by Duane in 1906. It is not really myokymia at all, but a chronic microtremor[5404] caused by any form of partial damage to the IV cranial nerve such as microvascular compression.[6935]

superior oblique tendon syndrome

(Brown syndrome) A restrictive ophthalmopathy in which fibrosis and shortening with tethering of the superior oblique tendon within its sheath causes failure of elevation of the adducted eye due to prevention of the normal upward and inward movement of the globe of the eye. It is caused by contraction of the inferior oblique muscle and gives the impression of paresis of that muscle. The condition is usually congenital, but has also been described as an acquired and intermittent problem.[2449, 3113]

superior orbital fissure syndrome

(intermittent painful ophthalmoplegia, superior orbital fissuritis, anterior cavernous sinus syndrome, Colio syndrome, Rollet syndrome, orbital apex syndrome, Tolosa–Hunt syndrome, sphenoidal fissure syndrome, cavernous sinus–lateral wall syndrome, cavernous sinus syndrome of Raeder, syndrome of Bonnet and Bonnet, sphenopetrosal fissure syndrome) A syndrome of episodic acute or subacute orbital pain associated with paralysis of one or more of the muscles supplied by the III, IV, or VI cranial nerves, which resolves spontaneously but may relapse and remit. It is considered to result from a nonspecific inflammatory process affecting the structures traversing the superior orbital fissure, including the three oculomotor nerves, the first division of the trigeminal nerve and the sympathetic and parasympathetic fibers destined for the eye. Involvement of the optic nerve has also been recorded.[5361] Trauma, neoplasm, and aneurysm affecting the superior orbital fissure may produce identical findings.[3480]

The symptoms include painful unilateral ophthalmoplegia, headache, ocular pain, and sensory loss on the upper face and scalp. The condition resembles **orbital pseudotumor syndrome** in its responsiveness to steroids and may represent the same pathology sited more posteriorly.

No conclusive diagnostic test exists,[2700, 6342] but the following diagnostic criteria are suggested by the Headache Classification Committee of the International Headache Society.[2820]

A. One or more episodes of unilateral orbital pain persisting for weeks if untreated
B. Paresis of one or more of the III, IV, and/or VI cranial nerves and/or demonstration of granuloma by MRI or biopsy
C. Paresis coincides with the onset of pain or follows it within 2 weeks
D. Pain and paresis resolve within 72 h when treated adequately with corticosteroids
E. Other causes have been excluded by appropriate investigations

From the International Classification of Headache Disorders (Headache Classification Committee of the International Headache Society. *Cephalalgia* 2004; **24**[Suppl 1]). Reproduced by kind permission of Dr. Jes Olesen, the International Headache Society, and Wiley-Blackwell Publications.

Hunt (an American neurosurgeon in Columbus, Ohio) proposed that the diagnostic criteria should include the presence of a **Horner syndrome**, involvement of the first division of the trigeminal nerve, spontaneous remission and recurrence, and the absence of features suggesting the presence of lesions outside the cavernous sinus; and he contributed six new cases. Collier gave an account of such features in 1921. Steroid responsiveness was suggested as another criterion in 1966. Other features reported include chemosis, proptosis, papilledema, and irregular constriction of the carotid syphon on angiography (**arterial stationary wave**). The causes vary; both vasculitis and nonspecific granulomas of the retro-orbital region have been described.[6342, 2414, 2734]

An identical condition is unusually common in Asia, where it is known as *polyneuritis cranialis*.[6583, 6228]

Other causes of painful ophthalmoplegia include tumors, vasculitis, basal meningitis, sarcoid, diabetes mellitus, and ophthalmoplegic "migraine."

superior thoracic aperture syndrome

See **thoracic outlet syndrome**.

supermarket neuropathy

Proper digital neuropathies causing numbness and tingling of the fingers, occasioned by the constricting effects of the handles of filled plastic shopping bags.[4817]

supernormal period

A time interval that immediately follows the refractory period which corresponds to a very brief period of partial depolarization. It is characterized by increased nerve excitability and is followed by the subnormal period.

(From the 2001 Report of the Nomenclature Committee of the American Academy of Neuromuscular disease and Electrodiagnostic Medicine.[19] Reproduced by kind permission of the AANEM.)

supernumerary first rib Usually a feminine disorder; a harmless condition until detected during the search for a cause of the complaints of dragging pain, discomfort, paresthesias, and minor vascular changes in an arm or hand; but when found, it is cast in the role of malefactor, for which nothing but radical extirpation will suffice. When symptoms persist thereafter, treatment of a **carpal tunnel syndrome** often provides relief.

superoxide dismutase A cell enzyme inactivating superoxide.

supination (from Lat, bent back, lying on the back) The posture of the body lying with the face up and the arms externally rotated and thus also facing up.

supinator channel syndrome See **posterior interosseous syndrome**.

supinator reflex See **brachioradialis reflex**.

supplementary motor area aphasia See **transcortical aphasia**.

supplementary motor area status epilepticus Frequently repeated seizures originating in the supplementary motor area, usually presenting as a type of focal status epilepticus but with preserved consciousness and individual tonic motor seizures occurring every few minutes or consisting of secondarily generalized seizures that evolve into repetitive asymmetrical tonic motor seizures with profound impairment of consciousness.[1861]

supplementary motor cortex An area situated on the mesial surface of the frontal lobe of the human brain, above the cingulate gyrus, and anterior to the primary motor areas of the foot and leg (part of Brodmann's area 6).[4980] It is considered to play an important role in the intentional process, whereby internal thought content sparks the elaboration of action.

Goldberg suggests that the area is crucial in the programming and fluent execution of extended action sequences. It was defined by Penfield and Welch[4980] on the basis of the motor responses obtained with electrical stimulation which differed from those produced by stimulating the primary motor cortex.[2439, 4979]

supplementary motor epilepsy An epileptic syndrome in which the seizure patterns are postural, focal, and tonic, with vocalization, speech arrest, and fencing postures. (From Dreifuss, F.E. et al. Commission for classification and terminology, ILAE. Proposal for Revised Classifications of Epilepsies and Epileptic syndromes. *Epilepsia* 1989;**30**:389–99. Reproduced by kind permission of Wiley-Blackwell Publications.)

The seizures begin abruptly and occur frequently, without warning. They consist of tonic posturing of one or more limbs and twisting truncal movements, with vocalization and speech arrest, ending with rhythmic or clonic movements of the extremities, such as the elevation of one arm (fencing posture). Awareness is preserved even though all four limbs may be affected. The seizures are highly resistant to current medical treatments.[4495]

This form of seizure was first described by **Penfield** and his colleagues. An increase in seizure frequency during rapid eye movement sleep is also described. The interictal EEG record is usually normal.

supplementary sensation Retention of pressure sensation in an area insensitive to pinprick after nerve injury.[2818]

supporting reactions The involuntary contractions of antigravity muscles which maintain the body upright.[4723]

supporting response If an infant is held vertically above a table and his feet allowed to come into contact with its surface, there will be simultaneous contraction of the leg flexors and extensors as if to provide standing support for the body. This is a normal reflex, persisting from birth. See also **stepping response**.

supra- (Lat, above).

supramarginal gyrus Area 40 of Brodmann, located at the junction of the frontal, parietal, and temporal lobes. Lesions in this region are associated with **Wernicke aphasia** and with the **Gerstmann syndrome**.

suprameatal triangle See **MacEwen triangle**.

supramodal 1. Attending to more than one single sensory channel. Thus the parietal lobe considers both visual and auditory representations in the analysis of information about spatial relationships. 2. Processes that are above the perceptual modalities, such as vision, hearing, and touch.

supranuclear gaze palsy See **progressive supranuclear palsy** and **sphingolipidoses**.

supranuclear upgaze paresis A form of dysconjugate eye movement in which there is limitation of elevation of one eye in all positions of horizontal gaze, due to a contralateral pretectal lesion.

supraorbital neuralgia An uncommon disorder characterized by pain in the region of the supraorbital notch and medial aspect of the forehead in the area supplied by the supraorbital nerve. The following diagnostic criteria have been defined:

A. Paroxysmal or constant pain in the region of the supraorbital notch and medial aspect of the forehead in the area supplied by the supraorbital nerve
B. Tenderness over the nerve in the supraorbital notch
C. Pain is abolished by local anesthetic blockade or ablation of the supraorbital nerve.

From the International Classification of Headache Disorders (Headache Classification Committee of the International Headache Society. *Cephalalgia* 2004;**24**[Suppl 1]). Reproduced by kind permission of Dr. Jes Olesen, the International Headache Society, and Wiley-Blackwell Publications.

Related conditions are *other terminal branch neuralgias* resulting from injury or entrapment of peripheral branches of the trigeminal nerve other than the nasociliary and supraorbital nerves. These may give rise to pain referred to the area innervated by the branch affected. Examples are neuralgias of the infraorbital, lingual, alveolar, and mental nerves. Their diagnostic criteria are as above. See also **nummular headache**.

supraorbital reflex See **orbicularis oculi reflex** and **glabellar tap**.

suprapatellar reflex Contraction of the quadriceps with extension of the knee in response to a tap on the top of the patella, with the knee flexed. This is just another way of obtaining the knee jerk and is best seen in patients with hyperactive muscle stretch reflexes due to a pyramidal lesion.

suprarubral syndrome A syndrome of intention tremor, ophthalmoparesis, and disturbed conjugate eye movements occurring as a result of **multiple sclerosis** or of a vascular lesion in the basilar artery territory, in subthalamic regions.[1153]

suprascapular neuropathy Wasting and weakness of the supra- and infraspinatus muscles as a result of entrapment of the nerve. This usually occurs at the upper trunk of the brachial plexus or at the suprascapular notch; less commonly it is more distal, at the spinoglenoid notch,[3530] in which case only the infraspinatus muscle is affected.

suprasellar cysts Benign tumor masses having the same site and origin as **craniopharyngiomas**, but lined with keratinizing squamous epithelium and thus also resembling epidermoid cysts elsewhere.[6]

supratentorial cavernous hemangioma See **cavernoma**.

sural neuropathy A syndrome of numbness on the lateral aspect of the foot as a result of damage to the sural nerve, due to compression or stretch at the popliteal fossa or in the calf, or due to direct local trauma.[3435]

surface electrode A conducting device for stimulating or recording when placed on the surface of the skin.

Surgical Neurology A neurosurgical journal published by Elsevier. Web site: http://www.elsevier.com/locate/surneu.

sursumduction See **ductions**.

Susac syndrome (arterial occlusive retinopathy and encephalopathy with retinocochleocerebral arteriolopathy; microangiopathy of the retina, brain, and cochlea) A rare microangiopathy of unknown etiology, occurring most often in young adult women. Its features may resemble **multiple sclerosis** with added hearing loss, usually remitting within 2 years.[6137] The encephalopathy is associated with branch retinal artery occlusion, headache, confusion, dementia, and behavioral changes. The disease is typically self-limited, with acute exacerbations followed by remission after a few years with some residual neurologic dysfunction.

In exacerbations, brain MRI shows enhancing supratentorial white matter lesions involving the corpus callosum, gray matter, posterior fossa, and leptomeninges. See also **RED-M syndrome**.

suspended sensory loss See **hanging sensory loss**.

sustension Sustained forward extension of the upper limbs against gravity, used to demonstrate drifts or abnormal movements or tremors. The term may also be applied to other sustained motor activities, such as vocal sustension (HJM).

Sutton, Thomas (1767–1835) English physician practicing in Kent, who wrote *Tracts on Delirium Tremens* (1813) which he so-named and in which he gave the first definitive description of the condition, although he noted the prior contributions of Thomas **Saunders.** His peculiar familiarity with the disease was, as he recognized, due to its frequency among those who, living on the Kentish coast, were able to procure alcohol smuggled in from France at knock-down prices.

swallow syncope A rare occurrence of syncope during or immediately after swallowing, and due to reflexly enhanced vagal tone and thus sinus bradycardia, during eating in patients with esophageal or cardiac abnormalities.[2606] See **deglutition syncope**.

Swan syndrome 1. (squint syndrome of Braun) A physiological method for the abolition of diplopia by turning the head 12°–18°. This allows light from the object viewed to fall on the physiological blind spot of the deviating eye, thus eliminating the false image.[6150] 2. The association of insufficiency of the inferior oblique muscle with proptosis, entropion, epicanthus, and hypotelorism.[6151]

sweat testing See **quantitative sudomotor axon reflex test** and **thermoregulatory sweat test**.

Swedenborg, Emanuel (1688–1772) Swedish scientist, (some have said psychotic) visionary, and philosopher whose accomplishments in neurology included the identification of the cortical motor areas and the localization of representation therein. He also ascribed motor functions to the basal ganglia and differentiated upper from lower motor neuron lesions.

Swediaur disease See **achillodynia**.

Swedish National Association for Disabled Children and Young People (RBU) A charitable organization and member society of the European Alliance of Muscular Dystrophy Societies.

swim-goggle headache A headache described as feeling like a tight band constricting the head, probably because of a tight band constricting the head, in this case the elastic strap of the goggles worn during swimming. See **external compression headache**.

swimmer's migraine Acute, benign, pulsating headache related to swimming; a form of **effort headache**.[3084]

swimming reflex When a baby is supported in water in the prone position, rhythmic movements of all extremities and the trunk are made.[6898]

swinging flashlight test A most sensitive clinical test for afferent lesions of the anterior visual pathway. A bright flashlight is directed into one eye and then swung rapidly across to the other one. When the normal eye is stimulated, both direct and consensual pupillary constriction occurs. When the light passes across from a normal eye to an eye with an afferent defect, the stimulus to constrict is less effective, and so both pupils dilate; but the examiner is looking at the illuminated one, which is said to dilate "paradoxically."[1355]

The phenomenon of dilatation of the pupil which is being examined in this circumstance is wrongly named for **Marcus Gunn**, the test having been described by Levatin.

Swiss Neuropathological Society A professional organization based at Institut. für Pathologie, Neuropathologie Abt., Kantonsspital, CH-5001 Aarau, Switzerland.

Swiss syndrome See **familial Cushing syndrome** and **Carney complex**.

switching-on, switching-off Fluctuations in the clinical state of Parkinsonian patients on long-term levadopa therapy in which the facilitation or inhibition of movements occurs at times of rising or falling levadopa levels, respectively.

Sybert syndrome A congenital dysmorphic syndrome characterized by skeletal and cutaneous abnormalities, short stature, optic atrophy, pigmentary retinopathy, microcephaly, and mental and developmental delay.[381]

Sydenham chorea (chorea minor, rheumatic chorea, infectious chorea, **St. Vitus' dance**, danse de St. Guy) Acute, benign, and self-limited chorea, incoordination of voluntary movement and muscle weakness occurring in the limbs, face, and trunk of children; carditis (which is much less benign) may also be found.[6169] The condition may complicate Group A β-hemolytic *Streptococcus* infection and is due to the formation of autoantibodies against the caudate nucleus and endothelium. Girls are more commonly affected. **Wilson**[6819] quoted the saying that a choreic child is punished thrice before her condition is recognized—once for general fidgetiness, once for breaking crockery, and once for making faces at her grandmother.

Sydenham cough Spasm of the respiratory muscles, as a hysterical manifestation. It was described by Thomas **Sydenham** in his *Epistolary Dissertation to Dr. Cole* in 1682 as follows: "When it falls on the lungs, the patient coughs continually, but without spitting; and although this cough may not shake the chest so much as the true convulsive sort, the fits are much more frequent, and the patient is less able to master them. Women with an excess of phlegm are most liable to this cough; which, otherwise, is very rare."

Sydenham, Thomas (1624–1689) Prominent English physician, born in Dorset. He attended the University of Oxford for a short spell, leaving to enter military service on the side of Parliament (as opposed to the Royalist cause), but returned, graduated, and succeeded in being elected to a Fellowship of All Souls College thanks to the expulsion of a Royalist member.

Before the restoration of legal government he had moved to France, later returning to London where he remained in practice for the rest of his life. He was known as the English Hippocrates, his reputation resting upon his first-hand accounts of diseases such as hysteria, gout, dysentery, scarlatina, smallpox, malaria, tuberculosis, and rheumatism; but he is best remembered today for his account of chorea minor (1686), now named for him.[7]

syllogomania The compulsion to hoard rubbish, usually a sign of a failing brain.

Sylvester disease A dominantly inherited syndrome of progressive deafness with optic atrophy, cerebellar ataxia, and muscle wasting, mainly of the shoulder girdle and hands, with onset in childhood.[6170]

Sylvian aqueduct syndrome (Kestenbaum syndrome, Koerber–Salus–Elschnig syndrome) The association of light-near dissociation, anisocoria, impaired conjugate upward gaze, convergence and retraction nystagmus, vertical nystagmus on up- or down-gaze, and extraocular palsies, occurring due to lesions of the rostral periaqueductal gray matter, usually tumors.[1851, 3513] Salus' first case had a *Cysticercus* cyst in the aqueduct and rostral fourth ventricle.[5517] See **Parinaud syndrome**.

The aqueduct itself was first described by Jacobus Sylvius (1478–1555), a French anatomist. See **dorsal midbrain syndrome**.

Sylvian aqueduct The pathway for CSF drainage from the third ventricle to the fourth.

Sylvian epilepsy See **benign childhood epilepsy with centrotemporal spikes**.

Sylvian fissure (lateral fissure) The first fissure to be described; it separates the frontal lobe before and above from the temporal and parietal lobes behind and below. It was named after Sylvius (who did not write anything about it until 1663) by Caspar Bartholin, a Danish anatomist, in 1641.

Sylvian spikes See **central-midtemporal spikes**.

Sylvius (François de la Böe, 1614–1672) A physician of French origin but born in Germany, training in medicine in Sedan, Leiden, and Basel. As professor of medicine in Leiden his most significant publications were on cerebral anatomy, even though most of the structures now named after him had been identified previously.[1670] He did, however, break new ground in proposing that the cerebral cortex, rather than the ventricles, was responsible for brain function.

Symbol-Digit Modalities Test A simple oral test assessing the speed of information processing, and not requiring the patient to make any nonverbal motor responses.[5899] See also **Wechsler Adult Intelligence Scale**.

symmetrical calcification of the basal ganglia with familial ataxia and pigmentary macular degeneration A syndrome of symmetrical basal gangliar calcifications usually recessively inherited. It is often associated with progressive ataxia, impairment of central vision due to macular degeneration, and onset in the fourth decade.[6092] See **striatopallidal calcification**.

symmetrical cerebral calcification See **striatopallidal calcification**.

symmetrical degeneration of the neostriatum See **infantile bilateral striatal necrosis**.

symmetrical proximal lower extremity motor neuropathy See **diabetic amyotrophy**. Such convoluted appellations emphasize the relevance of eponyms.

symmetry 1. The approximately equal amplitude, frequency, and form of EEG activities over homologous areas on opposite sides of the head. 2. The approximately equal distribution of potentials of unlike polarity on either side of a zero isopotential axis (see also **true phase reversal**). 3. The approximately equal distribution of EEG waves about the baseline. (Adapted from the 1974 report of the Committee on Terminology, IFCN. In: Chatrian GE, Bergamini L, Dondey M, et al. A glossary of terms most commonly used by clinical electroencephalographers. *EEG Clin Neurophysiol* 1974;37:538–48. Reproduced with kind permission from Elsevier Science.)

Symonds syndrome See **idiopathic intracranial hypertension**.

Symonds, Sir Charles Putnam (1890–1978) English neurologist who trained as a postgraduate at the **National Hospital**, Queen Square, and was subsequently appointed as the first physician for diseases of the nervous system at Guy's Hospital and later at the National Hospital as well. His clinical analyses of disease were outstanding, as typified by his correct diagnosis of a ruptured berry aneurysm in a patient of **Cushing**, made while Symonds was on a traveling Fellowship to the United States; this was the first occasion on which such a diagnosis had been made in life.

Many of his classic publications on head injury, cluster headache, multiple sclerosis, neuropathies, myelopathies, **idiopathic intracranial hypertension**,[6172] and other topics have been preserved in his *Studies in Neurology*.[6178] During World War II, he rose to the rank of Air Vice Marshal (in the first he had been wounded as a dispatch rider) and was later knighted. He retired in 1970.

sympathalgia See **reflex sympathetic dystrophy**.

sympathetic delirium See **delirium**.

sympathetic dyspraxia The appearance of dyspractic responses on the left side in a patient with a right hemiparesis. See **apraxia**.

sympathetic skin response The electrical potential resulting from electrodermal activity in sweat glands in response to both direct and reflex peripheral or sympathetic trunk stimulation of autonomic activity. Typically the response is obtained from one hand following stimulation of the contralateral median nerve. It is absent in patients with autonomic neuropathy as in patients with the **systemic inflammatory response syndrome**. See **psychogalvanic response**.

sympathetic system The division of the autonomic nervous system originating in the hypothalamus, its second-order neurons departing from the spinal cord through white rami exclusively at thoracic and upper lumbar levels and thence running to relay in ganglia of the sympathetic chain.

Galen had recognized the existence of the structure which **Willis** called the *intercostal nerves*. The current name was first applied by Winslow in 1732, when he thus described the nerves to the heart and gastrointestinal tract because they regulated the "sympathies" of the body using nervous energy.[3113] Their anatomy was well delineated by Dr. Benjamin Kent in his 1831 thesis presented to Edinburgh University. Gaskell in 1885 noted that the three outflows (bulbar, thoracolumbar, and sacral) are organized into two antagonistic systems and named them the *involuntary nervous system*. The term ***autonomic nervous system*** was the invention of Langley in 1889.

sympathotonic orthostatic hypotension A syndrome in which receptor insensitivity leads to orthostatic hypotension accompanied by tachycardia, without other evidence of central or peripheral nervous system disease.[5064]

symphysis pubis reflex Contraction of the lower abdominal muscles in response to a tap over the symphysis pubis. If the stimulus is applied more laterally, the hip adductors may also contract (*puboadductor reflex*).[1500]

symphysis sign See **Brudzinski signs**.

symptomatic diabetic neuropathy A stage of diabetic neuropathy in which any of the features listed in Chart S–20 appear, but not to the extent that they produce **disabling diabetic neuropathy**.

symptomatic epilepsy syndrome A syndrome in which epileptic seizures result from the presence of structural lesions of the brain.[1861]

symptomatic focal epilepsies (and *"probably symptomatic" focal epilepsies*) Focal (anatomical, topographical, or localization-related) epilepsies defined by seizures that emanate from an epileptogenic

Chart S–20. Features of Symptomatic Diabetic Neuropathy

Motor

1. Symptoms of muscle weakness in acts of daily living

Sensory

1. Absence of feeling: reported deficiency of tactile, thermal, or nocioceptive sensation encountered in acts of daily living
2. Sensory ataxia: reported unsteadiness in walking
3. Numbness or paresthesia ("dead," "asleep," "prickly asleep," "like hand gone asleep," "tightly bound feeling," etc.): judged by its distribution, persistence, and duration to be due to neuropathy and not due to physiological compression, as occurs in acts of daily living or entrapment syndromes
4. Neuropathic pain: burning, aching, excessive discomfort of feet or hands with use, and lancinating pain

Autonomic

Any of the following symptoms due to diabetes mellitus and not to medications, psychologic disturbance, intercurrent illness, disease of the organ, or previous injury or surgery: gastric atony; urinary retention; urinary incontinence; rectal incontinence; diarrhea; impotence in males <65 years of age; postural hypotension, light-headedness, or fainting (with postural decrease of systolic BP >30 mmHg)[1770]

Adapted from Dyck PJ. Detection, characterization and staging of polyneuropathy: assesed in diabetics. Muscle Nerve *1988;11:21–32.* Reproduced by kind permission of Lippincott Williams and Wilkins.

focus anywhere within the brain. These may be idiopathic, symptomatic, and cryptogenic (probably symptomatic). Ictal symptoms, particularly at onset, are determined by localization and not by etiology, but their anatomical origins are cannot always be assigned to specific loci.[4882]

These are not the same as idiopathic focal epilepsies because the prognosis and treatment of the latter differ significantly. Examples are **mesial temporal lobe epilepsy with hippocampal sclerosis** (hippocampal epilepsy); **lateral temporal lobe epilepsy;** and **frontal, parietal,** and **occipital lobe epilepsies.**

symptomatic generalized epilepsies and syndromes Epilepsies most often occurring in infancy and childhood and characterized by generalized seizures with clinical and EEG features different from those of idiopathic generalized epilepsies. There may be only one type, but more often there are several, including myoclonic jerks, tonic seizures, atonic seizures, and atypical absences. The EEG expression is bilateral but less rhythmic than that seen in idiopathic generalized epilepsies, and it is more or less asymmetrical.

The interictal EEG abnormalities differ from those of idiopathic generalized epilepsies, appearing as suppression bursts, hypsarrhythmia, slow spike-waves, or generalized fast rhythms. Focal abnormalities may be associated with any of the above. There are clinical, neuropsychological, and neuroradiologic signs of a usually diffuse, specific, or nonspecific encephalopathy. (Adapted from Dreifuss FE, et al. Commission for classification and terminology, ILAE. Proposal for revised classifications of epilepsies and epileptic syndromes. *Epilepsia* 1989;30:389–99. Reproduced by kind permission of the ILAE and Wiley-Blackwell Publications.)

symptomatic internal carotid artery The internal carotid artery supplying the territory of that eye or that side of the brain manifesting dysfunction due to ischemia.[2730]

The actual internal carotid artery might not, however, actually be the site of the causal pathology; for example, the middle cerebral artery is the site of the lesion in some cases.

symptomatic migraine Headaches which fulfill the International Headache Society diagnostic criteria but which are considered to arise as a result of the presence of such disorders as meningioma or hydrocephalus.

symptomatic myoclonus See **myoclonus.**

synalgies See **referred itch.**

synapse The term of Foster and Sherrington (1897) for their functional conception of the structure which forms the junction of two or more neurons. This represented the final seal of approval of the neuron theory, contradicting the idea that neurons are in substantial continuity. Sherrington had considered *syndesm*, but abandoned that name in favor of *synapse* (from Gr, a clasp), as advised by Verrall, a Greek scholar with whom he was acquainted.

synaptic dysgenesis The abnormal formation of synapses as a result of environmental insults or defective genetic control of neuronal proliferation and differentiation.[471]

synaptopathy An end-plate disorder in which the neuromuscular junctions are small and simplified, as in some forms of congenital **myasthenia.**

synaptosomes Specialized sites in the membranes of cells adapted for the reception of nerve transmission.

synchiria The sensation of bilateral stimulation following stimulation on one side only.

synchronized fibrillation See **complex repetitive discharge.**

synchronized sleep Nonrapid eye movement sleep, in which the EEG shows waveforms that are regular or sinusoidal in all areas.

synchrony The simultaneous occurrence of EEG waves over regions on the same or opposite sides of the head.

synchysis scintillans Showers of glistening particles composed of cholesterol, falling within the eye with ocular movement.

synclonus (Gr, together + great shaking) Continuous repetitive contractions of muscle groups.

syncopal migraine See **basilar migraine.**

syncope (Gr, a cutting short) A transient reduction in consciousness accompanied by visual and postural impairments due to global diminution in cerebral perfusion. The most common causes are excessive vagal tone leading to bradycardia (vasovagal, vasodepressor, or **reflex syncope**) and, in the elderly, orthostatic hypotension or cardiac dysrhythmias. Various specific types have been named according to their antecedent causes, such as **swallow, micturition, defecation, sneeze,** and **cough syncope** (each a form of **situational syncope**); also **cardiac** and **respiratory syncope** as well as the **carotid sinus syndrome.** See also **neurocardiogenic syncope, oculocardiac reflex.**

Reflex or *vasovagal syncope* is due to overactive cardiac reflexes and occurs mainly in healthy young people, triggered by attainment of the erect posture, by straining, or by emotionally significant stimuli. There is often a prodrome of nausea, dimmed vision, or malaise. The spells last less than a minute and the patient is pallid, sweaty, and cold on sinking to the floor, but recovers quickly without confusion or other sequelae.[5926] Differentiation from seizures may be difficult since multifocal and generalized myoclonus, incontinence, head injury, tonic body extension, automatisms, vocalizations, eye deviations, and visual and auditory hallucinations can occur in both conditions. With syncope, however, the predominant movement pattern (if there is any) consists of multifocal arrhythmic jerks in proximal and distal muscles, generalized myoclonus being frequently superimposed. Head turns, oral automatisms, and righting movements are also described. The eyes usually remain open and initial upward deviation is usual. Such motor elements have led to the use of the term *convulsive syncope*; it occurs in about 10% of syncopal episodes, especially those that are vasovagal in origin.[3773, 3774]

An ingenious system for differentiating seizure and syncope has been published using nine weighted criteria: tongue biting +2; déjà or jamais vu +1; emotional stress associated with loss of consciousness +1;

head turning during a spell +1; confusion after the spell +1; lightheaded spells −2; sweating before the spell −2; spell associated with prolonged sitting or standing −2. If the score is 1 or above, the likelihood is seizure, and if it is below 1, the likelihood is syncope with 94% sensitivity and specificity.[5779]

syndactylic craniovertebral anomalies A group of syndromes linked by the common characteristics of syndactyly and premature fusion of the cranial sutures. See **craniosynostosis**.

syndrome de spasmes en flexion See **flexor spasms**.

syndrome of approximate answers See **Ganser syndrome**.

syndrome of Bonnet and Bonnet See **superior orbital fissure syndrome**.

syndrome of caudal regression See **caudal regression syndrome**.

syndrome of Charles Bonnet (ophthalmopathic hallucinations) See **Bonnet syndrome**.

syndrome of inappropriate ADH secretion (SIADH, Schwartz syndrome) Excessive, nonphysiological secretion of antidiuretic hormone by the posterior pituitary, in the absence of the usual stimuli of hyperosmolality or hypervolemia, leading to dilutional hyponatremia as a result of impaired water excretion at a time that sodium excretion is normal.

Essential diagnostic features include hyponatremia, hypo-osmolality of the serum, inappropriately high urinary osmolality, normovolemia, and urinary sodium levels >20 mEq/l in the presence of normal acid–base and potassium balance and normal renal, adrenal, and thyroid function. Clinically it presents with fatigue, anorexia, headache, nausea, and vomiting, progressing, if untreated, to a confusional state, agitated delirium, convulsions, coma, and death.[5390] The condition may complicate many neurological diseases affecting both the central and peripheral nervous systems, or it may occur as a paraneoplastic syndrome or as a reaction to certain drugs.

syndrome of Jacobson's nerve and plexus See **tympanic neuropathy**.

syndrome of Mount and Reback See **familial paroxysmal dystonic choreoathetosis**.

syndrome of Rochon-du Vigneau See **orbital pseudotumor syndrome**.

syndrome of the basilar communicating artery of Percheron See **paramedian diencephalic syndrome**.

syndrome of the cerebral peduncle See **Weber syndrome**.

syndrome of the corpus striatum See **Vogt syndrome**.

syndrome of the decussation See **hemiplegia cruciata**.

syndrome of the interpeduncular space Bilateral III cranial nerve palsies with quadriparesis, due either to large central mesencephalic lesions or to others affecting the cerebral peduncles bilaterally.

syndrome of the mesencephalic artery See **top of the basilar syndrome**.

syndrome of the mesencephalic gray matter (aqueduct syndrome, Lyle syndrome) A periaqueductal lesion causing bilateral III cranial nerve palsy, bilateral mydriasis, somnolence, and vertical nystagmus or gaze palsy. Irritative phenomena may include miosis and convergence spasms. See **mesoencephalothalamic syndrome**.

syndrome of the neural crest See **neural crest** and **hereditary sensory and autonomic neuropathy**.

syndrome of the paramedian thalamic arteries Sudden alteration of consciousness followed by fluctuating hypersomnia and bilateral ophthalmoplegia due to asymmetric, paramedian thalamic and midbrain lesions as a result of emboli to the rostral basilar artery originating from a fibrillating heart.[638]

syndrome of the posterior commissure External ophthalmoplegia due to a central mesencephalic lesion; the association of a reduction in conjugate upward gaze movements with lid retraction (**Collier** sign), gaze disturbances including spasm and retraction nystagmus and frequently impaired saccades on downward gaze, downbeat nystagmus, light-near dissociation of the pupillary reactions and skew deviation of the eyes. The horizontal movements remain intact. See **Parinaud syndrome**.

syndrome of the posterior-inferior cerebellar artery See **lateral medullary syndrome**.

syndrome of the sea-blue histiocyte See **sea-blue histiocytosis**.

syndrome of the thalamoperforating pedicle of Foix and Hillemand See **paramedian diencephalic syndrome**.

syndrome paralytique unilateral global des nerfs craniens See **Garcin syndrome**.

syndrome (Gr, to run with, or together) "A group of symptoms constantly associated in a particular disease and together presenting a characteristic picture of that disease or condition."[5886]

In philosophical terms, a syndrome is a chain of physiological processes which when interrupted produces the same impairment of bodily functions, as opposed to it occurring as a result of specific disease factors. Thus a further definition might be: "a recurrent association of clinical signs for which a single pathogenesis or localization may be postulated."

Some syndromes are eponymic, some descriptive. The first use of the word was in Copland's translation of Galen.[1765]

synechiae Intraocular adhesion(s) classified as anterior (iridicorneal) and posterior (iridolenticular).

synergist A muscle which by its contraction assists the action of an **agonist** muscle, either by stabilizing the joint or by exerting a weaker action in the same direction as that of the agonist.

synergy (Gr, with + work) The term of **Babinski** for the ability to accomplish simultaneously all of those movements which together are required to execute a purposeful movement. Failure to do so results in **decomposition of movement.**

synesthesia (Gr, together + perception) A permanent, involuntary spillover of sensory impressions such that stimulation of one sensory channel leads to a perception in another one or more than one. From synesthetes, the statement, "I see what you're saying" could be taken literally. The condition is reported to have affected the composers Scriabin, Sibelius, and Rimsky-Korsakov, for some of whom certain keys evoked particular colors.[6646]

The condition was reported in 1690 in a studious blind man who perceived sound-induced colored visions, understanding scarlet to be the sound of a trumpet; and again by Thomas Woolhouse (an English ophthalmologist).[1399] Erasmus Darwin and Isaac Newton next experimented with its production, resulting in the *clavacin oculaire*, an instrument which produces sound and light simultaneously. Modern electronic versions are available.

Clinical examples of synesthesias include geometrically shaped tastes and colored smells, but the evocation of colors following the presentation of sounds is the most common form and is known as *chromesthesia*.[1399] In the idiopathic form, nonright-handers predominate; the condition is extant in childhood and may be an autosomal dominant trait with incomplete penetrance. It is more common in women and can probably be localized in the left hemisphere, since many synesthetes display elements of **Gerstmann syndrome** without other neurological abnormalities other than phenomenal memories, while mathematical and spatial navigational skills suffer. The phenomena are distinguished from imagery by the following five criteria:

1. The sensations are involuntary and insuppressible.
2. They are perceived as external and real.
3. They are discrete and few in number.
4. They are highly memorable.
5. They are accompanied by strong emotion.

Synesthesia can also occur during epileptic seizures involving the hippocampus, with hallucinogenic intoxication, brainstem lesions, and sometimes following concussion, in which case sudden noises or bright lights may actually cause pain.[1400]

syngnathia with fusion of the gums and jaws A congenital developmental anomaly in which fusion of the maxilla and mandible is accompanied by facial weakness, microcephaly, nystagmus, hemivertebrae, an atrial septal defect, and mental and developmental delay.[381]

synkinesis (Gr, together + movement) Involuntary movements made by muscles distant from those being activated voluntarily due to aberrant reinnervation and/or ephaptic transmission, as during recovery after facial neuropathy in some cases.

synkinetic blepharoclonus A benign, sporadic, or familial condition manifesting blepharoclonus with eye closure, vertical gaze, speech or postural changes, sometimes with other movement disorders such as tremor, myoclonus, or restless legs.[3140]

synophrys The condition of hair growth linking the eyebrows across the **glabella**; it is of no known pathological significance, although to the timid it appears mildly threatening.

synoptophore A device for testing the normal fusion of visual images when these are presented separately to the eyes.

syntactic alexia A failure to recognize relational words in the presence of preserved recognition of substantive words (written in this case), as occurs in **anterior alexia**. The inability to comprehend graphically presented sentences when their meaning depends on the syntax. Although the condition often occurs with **Broca aphasia**, the usual cause is considered to be a lesion in the dominant supramarginal gyrus.[5430]

syntactic aphasia The term of Sir Henry **Head** for that form of speech disturbance in which the internal balance of a word as an orderly rhythmic expression is disturbed, and jargon results. Articulation, speech rhythm, and grammaticism are severely affected.[2814] See **Wernicke aphasia**.

syntactic structure Descriptions of the structural relationships between words in a sentence—the representations of the grammatical pattern of sentence; for example, "The man is going to the store" consists of a noun phrase + auxilliary + verb *-ing* + preposition + noun phrase.[3949]

syntactic transformations Rules which serve to define the structures of different sentence types in a language and describe the relationships between words, the overall form of sentences and how simple sentences are changed from one type to another, such as questions, commands, passives, and embedded sentences.
For example, transformations of the sentence, "You are holding the boy up" might include "Are you holding the boy up?" (question); "Hold the boy up" (command); "The boy is being held up by you" (passive); and "I can see that you are holding the boy up" (embedded sentence).[3949]

syntax The ordering of words, their alteration, and the insertion among them of qualifying words in accordance with a set of grammatical rules peculiar for each language.

synucleinopathies A diverse group of neurodegenerative disorders that share the characteristic of aggregates of the protein α-synuclein in certain vulnerable populations of neurons and glia. The filaments produced are toxic and lead to degeneration in certain brain regions.[2264] Conditions comprising this group are listed below.[2262] It is also associated with the appearance of **REM sleep behavior disorder** in the setting of dementia or Parkinson disease.

Synuclein is a nonamyloid component structural protein normally found in synaptic terminals. It also accumulates within **Lewy bodies**. While important in the learning processes of singing birds, its accumulation is toxic to neurons in man. See also **tauopathies**.

Listing of Synucleinopathies

Synucleinopathies commonly associated with dementia

- **Parkinson disease** (the most common synucleinopathy)
- **Dementia with Lewy bodies**

Other synucleinopathies

- **Multiple system atrophy**
- **Pure autonomic failure**

syphilis (Gr, a hog + to love)
1. A wayward shepherd, a character in

Chart S–21. Classification of the Forms of Syphilis

1. **Syphilitic meningitis**
2. *Spinal syphilis*

 Meningomyelitis, leading to any syndrome of myelopathy
 Erb–Charcot syndrome (spinal syphilitic paralysis, a slowly progressive spastic paraparesis)[1902]
 Systematized spinal sclerosis, a pure pyramidal syndrome
 Systemic amyotrophy resembling **amyotrophic lateral sclerosis**

3. *Cerebral syphilis*

 General, a mild dementing or delirious syndrome
 Local (basal, convexity, intracerebral, midbrain), leading to cranial nerve palsies and hydrocephalus, focal signs, or a Parkinsonian syndrome.

4. *Cerebrospinal syphilis* (disseminated syphilitic sclerosis) Any form of cerebral and spinal syphilis in combination such as **tabes dorsalis, general paresis,** or **syphilitic optic atrophy**
5. Syphilitic neuroses
6. **Syphilitic optic atrophy**
7. **Syphilitic neuritis**, syphilitic osteitis

From Wilson SAK. Neurology. *London, Edwin Arnold, 1940.*
See also **congenital syphilis, gumma,** and **Erb–Charcot syndrome.**

Morbus Gallicorum, a book of poetry published by Girolamo Fracastoro in 1530. The book was described as a call to righteousness and piety as well as a medical text, since in it he described the transmission and manifestations of the disease at some length. The author dedicated the book to the College of Cardinals in Rome. 2. Infection by the spirochete **treponema pallidum**, classified by Kinnier **Wilson**[6819] as shown in Chart S–21. Eighty-two synonyms are listed by Whitwell (*Syphilis in Earlier Days*, HK Lewis, London, 1940); most attribute the disease to infection brought by visiting traders or conquerors in an attempt at self-exculpation. It was not brought to Europe by sailors returning with Columbus, but had been recorded by Pliny in ancient Rome.

syphilis serology (serological tests for syphilis) A set of tests used to confirm syphilitic infection and to measure the activity of the disease. *Nontreponemal* tests such as the **VDRL** detect nonspecific antibodies (reagins) which react with the lipoidal antigens of *Treponema pallidum* or others produced by interaction with the host.

Treponemal tests detect antibodies which are specific for the organism and which include the **FTA-Abs, TPI**, and the **TPHA**, or **MHA–TPA**. More recently, specific assays of treponemal immunoglobulin antibodies have become available.

syphilitic "osteitis" A manifestation of congenital **syphilis**, characterized by severe pain in the limb bones with disinclination of the child to move the limb as a result of syphilitic osteochondritis. The condition was described by **Parrot** in 1871.

syphilitic amyotrophy (syphilitic neuritis) A widespread lower motor neuron degeneration with onset in the small hand muscles and radial extensors, occurring in patients with the meningovascular form of tertiary syphilis.

The classic description indicated an absence of myelopathic signs, but the existence of such a syndrome is disputed today, as a lower motor neuron syndrome associated with syphilitic myelopathy (**Erb–Charcot syndrome**) does occur, which must be the same condition.

syphilitic meningitis Latent, acute, chronic patchy, or generalized inflammation of the spinal or cerebral membranes. See **meningovascular syphilis** and **syphilitic amyotrophy**.

syphilitic myelitis See **Erb–Charcot syndrome**.

syphilitic neuritis See **syphilitic amyotrophy**.

syphilitic optic atrophy A form of primary optic atrophy characteristically seen alone or in the setting of **tabes dorsalis** or **general paresis** as a manifestation of tertiary **syphilis**. It does not differ from other forms of primary optic atrophy except in its association with **Argyll Robertson pupils**.

syphilitic wristdrop Weakness of the radial extensors of the forearm occurring in the setting of **syphilitic amyotrophy**.[2822]

syringal hemorrhage Slow bleeding into hydrosyringomyelia, perhaps due to tearing of an intraspinal vein, described first by Gowers in 1904. It is a condition of extreme rarity.[4987]

syringobulbia A condition in which brainstem signs are detectable in patients with syringomyelia resulting from distortion of the hindbrain due to pressure differences acting downward upon it. Clefts may extend from the fourth ventricle into the substance of the medulla oblongata, or may occur as a result of upward impulsive fluid movements from the cavity in the cervical cord. Hydrocephalus is commonly associated.

In descending order of frequency, the most common clinical signs are headache, vertigo, dysphonia or dysarthria, facial paresthesias, dysphagia, diplopia, and palatal and lingual palsies.[4476]

syringomeningocele (Gr, a pipe + a membrane + a rupture) Protrusion of a cystic mass composed of the membrane and posterior wall of the dilated central canal of the spinal cord through a spinal defect (spina bifida).

syringomesencephalia A cystic cavity in the CNS extending through the brainstem into the mesencephalon, and possibly representing a diverticulum from the aqueduct. The condition is far less common than **syringomyelia** or **syringobulbia**.[5519]

syringomyelia (Gr, a pipe + the marrow) The formation of an elongated fluid-containing cavity running from the center of the spinal cord posterolaterally beside a posterior horn, expanding the cord. The abnormality occurs most often in the cervical or thoracic regions.

The term was first applied by **Chiari** in 1888. Clinically, signs of compromise of the spinothalamic and pyramidal tracts, and of the cord and the anterior horn cells at the levels of the cavity, are the usual features; the triad of dissociated sensory loss, distal arm weakness, and pyramidal signs in the legs is classic. **Gull** gave the first account of the clinical manifestations in 1862.[2634] See also **secondary syringomyelia** and **hydromyelia**.

A *variant* familial form is also reported.[4547] The Web site http://www.ninds.nih.gov/disorders/syringomyelia/syringomyelia.htm provides further information from the NIH.

syrinx (Gr, a pipe) The fluid-filled abnormal cavity in the spinal cord in the setting of **syringomyelia**. The name was applied by Ollivier d'Angers in 1824, but the condition had been recognized by Estienne in 1546.

system degenerations

1. Selective atrophy or demyelination of distinct anatomical fiber pathways in the CNS. These may be genetic (e.g., **Friedreich ataxia**) or acquired (e.g., **subacute combined degeneration of the cord, tabes dorsalis**). A more restricted definition is that of Oppenheimer,[4807] who lists autonomic nervous system failure (**idiopathic orthostatic hypotension**), olivopontocerebellar atrophy (**late-onset cerebellar ataxias**), **striatonigral degeneration**, and **dentatorubropallidoluysian atrophy**, to which Baraitser suggests the addition of **pure pallidal atrophy, pallidoluysian atrophy**, and **pallidostriatonigral degeneration**.

2. A heterogeneous group of neurological diseases characterized by cell loss and variable gliosis occurring in one or more neuronal groups (or "systems"). These disorders are characterized by the spontaneous dysfunction and death of certain systems within the nervous system. Almost all are inherited.

The syndromes resulting appear to be the functional result of various combinations of localizable lesions within the neuraxis including retinal degeneration, optic atrophy, mid-brain lesions with pupillary dysreflexia, or progressive external ophthalmoplegia; atrophy of the cerebellar nuclei, pons, or olives; degeneration of the cochleas, the posterior columns, the spinocerebellar or the pyramidal tracts, the anterior horn cells or roots, or the dorsal ganglion cells.[1208] See also **multiple system atrophies**.

system A whole compounded of several parts; a compounding of things assembled to create a complex functioning scheme.

systemic achromic nevus See **hypomelanosis of Ito**.

systemic angiomatosis See **Ullmann syndrome**.

systemic carnitine deficiency

A fatal disorder of lipid metabolism in which the effects of carnitine deficiency include recurrent attacks of metabolic encephalopathy (resembling that of **Reye syndrome**), hypoketotic hypoglycemia, cardiomyopathy, and a proximal lipid-storage myopathy with muscle weakness and failure to thrive. Carnitine levels in red cells, muscle, and liver are low, and those in the serum are variable.[3312, 5222] See **carnitine deficiency**.

systemic histiocytosis See **histiocytosis**.

systemic inflammatory response syndrome (SIRS)

A syndrome of multiple organ failure, frequently in the context of sepsis, seen in patients who have critical illnesses, and who are usually in intensive care unit. In this condition, cellular and humoral responses are activated to produce changes in the microcirculation of the whole body.[729] It is commonly associated with **septic encephalopathy** and **critical illness polyneuropathy** or myopathy and affects the central and peripheral nervous systems and also the autonomic system.

Typical features are two or more of the following:

1. Body temperature above 38° or below 36°C.
2. Heart rate above 90/min
3. Tachypnea above 20 breaths/min or hyperventilation with $PaCO_2 < 32$ torr
4. White cell count above 12,000 cells/mm^3 or less than 4000 cells/mm^3 or the presence of 10% or more immature neutrophils (bands)

Critical illness polyneuropathy and **critical illness myopathy** commonly occur in such patients.

systemic late infantile lipidosis

See **GM$_1$ gangliosidosis**.

systemic lupus erythematosus

A relapsing and remitting multisystem inflammatory disease of unknown cause, characterized by dermal, vascular, serosal, and neural manifestations.

The American Rheumatological Association has suggested that at least four of the following features must be present for the diagnosis to be made:[6199]

Malar skin rash; discoid photosensitivity; oral or nasal ulceration; nonerosive peripheral polyarthritis; pleurisy or pericarditis; renal disorder (with proteinuria or cellular casts); neuropsychiatric disorder; hematological disorder (hemolytic anemia, leukopenia, lymphopenia, thrombocytopenia); immunological disorder (LE cells, anti-DNA antibodies, anti-sM antibodies, false-positive test for syphilis); and antinuclear antibody.

The neurological signs most commonly reported reflect the effects of widespread vasculitis or of scattered demyelination and include cognitive dysfunction; seizures; focal strokelike syndromes; psychoses and affective disorders; diffuse encephalopathy; cranial neuropathy; retinal vasculitis; papilledema; brainstem disorders; chorea, Parkinsonism, or ataxia; headache; aseptic meningitis; transverse myelopathy; syndromes resembling almost any form of multiple sclerosis; and multiple mononeuropathy or polyneuropathy.[4385, 78] The occurrence of neuropsychiatric manifestations is closely linked to higher levels of anticardiolipin antibodies.

The American Rheumatological Association has provided case definitions for 19 of the neuropsychiatric lupus syndromes.[46]

systemic mastocytosis

A generalized disorder with headaches and autonomic features such as hypotension, flushing, and lacrimation as potential neurological complications.[3533]
See **mastocytosis**.

systemic necrotizing vasculitis See **polyarteritis nodosa**.

systemic sclerosis A multisystem disease that can involve several other organs besides the skin. Reports of neurological involvement have primarily referred to the peripheral nervous system; CNS involvement is rare, although transverse myelitis has been reported.

systemic sclerosis See **progressive systemic sclerosis**.

systemic vasculitic neuropathy A multiple mononeuropathy resulting from multifocal vasculitis causing occlusion of epineurial arterioles.[1773]

Szabo sign Diminished sensation in only one small cutaneous nerve territory at a time in patients with sciatic nerve lesions. The sign was described by a Hungarian physician whose other contributions are less well recorded.

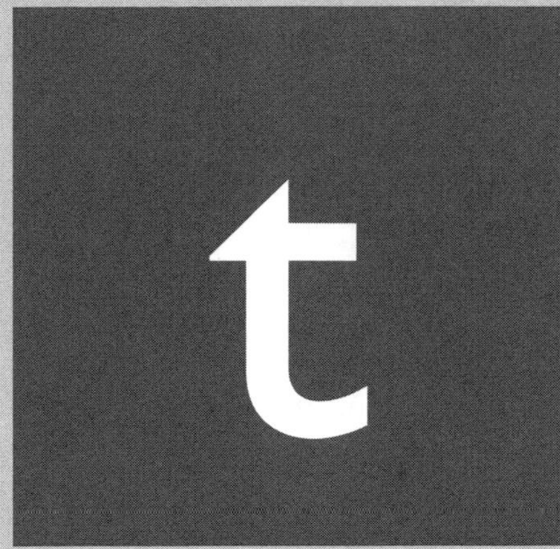

T wave A compound muscle action potential evoked from a muscle by rapid stretch of its tendon, as part of the muscle stretch reflex.[162]

T1 spin-lattice (longitudinal relaxation time) A term in MRI for the characteristic time constant for spins to achieve an equilibrium alignment, returning to their original position within the external magnetic field. In the case of water, this may be as long as 500 ms.

T1 weighting (inversion-recovery) An MRI image generated by a pulse sequence that does not allow the magnetization of the tissues of interest to attain their equilibrium values. Contrast in the image is determined by the differential T1 values of the tissues, with short T1 tissues, such as fat, appearing bright. The gray scale brightness is inversely proportional to T1. This sequence provides the greatest T1 weighting with a short T1 value. Using this technique, H^+ protons (as in water) show as lucencies.[875]

T2 spin-spin (transverse relaxation time) The characteristic time constant for the loss of phase coherence among proton spins, due to lack of homogeneity of the magnetic field. It is due to interactions between the spins, with resulting decay of the transverse magnetization and the MRI signal. This is much shorter than the T1 time constant, and is usually less than 100 ms.

T2-weighted image (spin-echo) An MRI image generated by a pulse sequence with a long repetition time and long echo time, so that only those tissues with a sufficiently long T2 value will still have any remaining transverse magnetization to contribute to the signal. Using this technique, H^+ protons (as in water) are bright.

When the TE value is extended beyond 100 ms, the image obtained is referred to as a *heavily T2-weighted image*. This gives improved demonstration of brain lesions such as tumor, and edema because of the longer T2 values relative to normal brain.[875]

tabes dorsalis (Lat, wasting + back) Wasting (of the dorsal columns), the most noticeable pathological abnormality in the most common form of tertiary neurosyphilis, much more commonly seen in men. It is characterized clinically by a triad of symptoms (lightning pains, ataxia, and urinary incontinence with dysuria) and a second triad of signs (Argyll Robertson pupils, areflexia, and loss of joint position sense), but also by acute (lightning) pains (**crises**),[1107] paresthesias, patchy sensory loss, deafness, impotence and rectal incontinence, and by optic atrophy, Charcot joints, painless perforating ulcers of the feet, ptosis, and oculomotor palsies. The CSF is usually abnormal.[5852]

Although **Romberg** had described the condition well in 1846, the term was first applied by **Remak**.[5263] That tabes is a form of syphilis was the (initially controversial) opinion (1876) of Jean Alfred Fournier (1832–1914), a French physician.

The major damage is incurred by the large dorsal root ganglion cells, the central processes of which run in the posterior columns; their atrophy led to the name given. **Duchenne** (1858) called it *locomotor ataxia*; his description[1735] was so complete that the condition was many years known as *Duchenne disease*.

Many signs once regarded as specific for tabes (**Frankel, Gowers, Pitres, Remak, Sarbo, Westphal**) are no longer considered to be so. The lightning pains and arthropathies were first recorded by **Charcot** and Bouchard in 1866[1107] and Delamarre described gastric crises in the same year. The arthropathy was described independently in 1869 by the English physician Thomas Clifford Allbutt (1836–1925).

tabetic ciliary neuralgia See **Pel crises**.

tache cérébrale Excessive dermal hyperemia along the track scratched by a finger, described by Trousseau in the setting of meningitis, but in fact not specific to that condition.

tachistoscope A device for the instantaneous presentation of visual images.

tachylalia Rapid speech.

tachyphemia See cluttered speech.

tachyphylaxis (Gr, fast + guard) Increasing tolerance to the pharmacological effect of a drug.

tacrolimus encephalopathy A form of posterior reversible **leukoencephalopathy** due to the ingestion of tacrolimus, an immunosuppressive agent and calcineurin inhibitor.

tactile (Lat, touching) Of or to do with the sense of touch.

tactile agnosia (agraphesthesia) Loss of the power of appreciating size, shape, and form in three dimensions, as well as consistency and texture,[2816] due to a lesion in the contralateral hemisphere which is usually post-Rolandic.

tactile aphasia The inability to name objects felt by one hand or foot, although they can be named when heard or seen, in the presence of normal spontaneous speech. This represents a **disconnection syndrome** in which somatesthetic impulses fail to cross to the opposite hemisphere because of a lesion in the anterior part of the corpus callosum.[2339, 2338]

tactile apraxia Impairment of hand movements for the use of and interaction with an object, in the presence of preserved intransitive movements.[3540] See **apraxia**.

tactile discrimination The ability to recognize unseen objects by touch. It is usually tested on the hands or fingers with a two-point discriminator or a pair of compasses, but figure-writing on the palms tests the same function. Loss of tactile discrimination in the absence of peripheral or spinal lesions suggests damage to the contralateral parietal lobe. See also **direction of scratch test**.

Tactile Form Recognition Test A test of visual perceptual function in which the subject touches an unseen cutout of a shape and must then select the matching figure from a group of visually presented drawings.[533]

tactile hallucinations (haptic hallucinations) Hallucinations of touch; an uncommon phenomenon in the settings of partial epilepsy or delirious states. See **haptic hallucinations**.

tactile perception of direction A specific sensory function of the dorsal columns, which appear to be alone in providing a centripetal pathway that transmits impulses concerning the direction of a moving cutaneous stimulus. Clinical findings suggest that the length of the scratch should be 2 cm[2729] although 2 mm can usually be discerned on the palms. See **direction of scratch test**.

tactile perseveration Continued perception of a tactile stimulus after its removal; a sign of right parietal lobe lesions.

tactile projection See **projection**.

tacts Comments made about external stimuli.[1336] See also **mands**.

tadpole pupil Intermittent spasm of one segment of the pupillodilator muscle, causing the pupil to assume a comma-shaped appearance. The pupil is often of the **springing** type. The condition is benign.[6302]

Takayasu disease See **aortic arch disease**.

talantropia See **pendular nystagmus**.

talipes equinovarus (Lat, to walk on the ankles) Clubfoot.

Talma, Sape (1847–1918) Dutch surgeon and physician who graduated from Utrecht and practiced in that city as professor of pathological anatomy or medicine.

Talma disease (myotonia acquisita) Myotonia occurring for the first time in adult life, without a positive family history.[6196]

Tamari-Goodman upper limb–cardiovascular syndrome A congenital dysmorphic syndrome characterized also by short stature, strabismus, kyphosis, atrial septal defect, pulmonary stenosis, winged scapulae, radioulnar synostosis, microcephaly, and mental and developmental delay.[381]

Tamminga Marfanoid syndrome with leukodystrophy A congenital dysmorphic syndrome, characterized also by tall stature; ocular, cardiac, and skeletal anomalies; hypotonia; cerebral atrophy; hydrocephalus; and mental and developmental delay.[381]

tandem gait test The subject is asked to take 10 steps along a straight line without walking aids or support and with the eyes open. The number of steps taken to the side is counted. The performance on the test correlates with a history of falls in patients with atypical Parkinsonism in whom more than one side-step is usually taken during the test, whereas patients with Parkinson disease usually have a normal stance width during gait, and do not tend to veer to the side.[32]

tandem Romberg test The subject stands with one foot directly in front of the other with the arms folded and the eyes closed. A normal subject can maintain this position for at least 5 s. Failure to do so indicates impairment of conscious proprioception.

Tang sign An alternative method for eliciting the **Babinski** response in which the lateral plantar and dorsal surfaces of the foot are stroked simultaneously.

tangent screen A piece of black material, upon which a grid is faintly marked and with a central point for uniocular gaze fixation. Hand-held stimuli are brought in from the periphery toward the center by the examiner, allowing charting of the central 25° of the visual field.

Tangier disease (analphalipoproteinemia, high-density lipoprotein deficiency) An inherited, clinically heterogeneous multisystem disease due to mutations at *ABCA1*, with two main forms:

1. A slowly progressive peripheral neuropathy, clinically resembling **syringomyelia** with dissociated sensory loss and facio-brachial weakness.
2. Prominent but relapsing–remitting small-fiber multiple mononeuropathies.[1885]

Both varieties are characterized by hepatosplenomegaly, diarrhea, tonsillar enlargement, cataracts, accelerated atherosclerosis, and low serum cholesterol and α-lipoprotein levels, but raised triglycerides.

The name comes from the small island in Chesapeake Bay (United States) where the disorder was first recognized by Fredrickson in 1961[2184, 5072] and not from the North African city.

tapetoretinal degeneration A form of retinal pigmentary degeneration, usually dominantly inherited but expressed more commonly in boys, who complain of impaired twilight vision (**nyctalopia**) which progresses in some cases to blindness.

Tapia, Antonio Garcia (1875–1950) Spanish otolaryngologist in Madrid, who in 1904 described the syndrome named for him, his patient being a matador who had suffered an occupational injury.

Tapia syndrome (ambiguohypoglossal paralysis) Unilateral damage to the IX, X, and XI cranial nerves in the brainstem, usually as a result of vascular disease, or due to lesions at the base of the skull or in the retroparotid space, such as infiltration by tumors.[6210] Paralysis of the pharynx, larynx, and tongue results but the trapezius and sternomastoid are spared.

Differentiation between the syndromes of **Avellis, Collet, Jackson, Schmidt, Tapia**, and **Vernet** is an exercise in grand roundmanship but is clinically irrelevant.[5631] However, some instances of Tapia syndrome (possibly including Tapia's original case) may be the result of dissection of the external carotid artery, thus signifying imminent endangerment of the internal carotid artery as well.[3235]

tapping test 1. A test of repetitive motor abilities using agonist and antagonistic muscles. The subject is required to tap the wrist, elbow, and shoulder and then the ankle, knee, and hip on each side with his finger, the number of taps completed at each site on each side in 30 s being counted. 2. The subject is asked to tap out rhythms, such as groups of double or triple taps, changing between them on command. Difficulty in executing the taps rhythmically suggests a lesion of (usually the left) prefrontal area.

tarantism See **dancing mania**.

Tarchanov phenomenon See **psychogalvanic reflex**.

Tardieu Scale An instrument assessing spasticity in children with cerebral palsy in which the supine patient's limb is moved passively at different velocities; V1: As slow as possible, slower than the natural drop of the limb segment under gravity; V2: Speed of limb segment falling under gravity; V3: As fast as possible, faster than the rate of the natural drop of the limb segment under gravity. It is scored as follows:

0. No resistance throughout the course of the passive movement
1. Slight resistance throughout the course of the passive movement, but with no clear catch at a precise angle
2. There is a clear catch at a precise angle, interrupting the passive movement and followed by release
3. Fatigable clonus (lasting <10 s) when maintaining the pressure and appearing at the precise angle
4. Unfatigable clonus (lasting >10 s) when maintaining the pressure and appearing at a precise angle
5. Joint is immovable.[6211]

The scale can be accessed at http://www.mdvu.org/library/ratingscales/spasticity/Tardieu_Scale.pdf/.

tardive akathisia (Lat, late + Gr, not sitting) A form of chronic **akathisia** that occurs at a late stage of neuroleptic therapy, coinciding with a reduction in the dose of the drug.[945]

tardive dyskinesia (cervicolinguomasticatory syndrome, Tarnow–Kulenkampff syndrome) An involuntary movement disorder (dystonic, choreic, or athetotic) complicating the prolonged ingestion of dopamine antagonists such as the butyrophenones, reserpine, or the phenothiazines.[2281] Research diagnostic criteria have been formulated[5639] and are given in Chart T–1.

Tardive Dyskinesia Rating Scale A 43-item scale scoring abnormal movements in five general body areas (face, neck and trunk, upper extremities, lower extremities, and entire body) with an attached list of definitions of the abnormal movements that can occur.[5859]

An abbreviated form of the scale has also been validated; its 16 items examine the periocular areas (blinking, eyelid tremor); lip movements; chewing; the **bonbon sign**; tongue protrusion and tongue tremor; **rabbit syndrome**; axial hyperkinesia; rocking movement; torsion movements; head and neck movements; movements of fingers and wrists, and of ankles and toes; stamping movements; repetitive thumb movements; and **akathisia**.

Tardive Dyskinesa/Tardive Dystonia National Association A charitable organization providing support and information on this condition. Address: Tardive Dyskinesia/Tardive Dystonia National Association. P.O. Box 45732, Seattle, WA 98145-0732. Tel: 206-522-3166.

tardive dystonia 1. Persistent late-onset dystonia occurring as a result of the ingestion of antipsychotic drugs at least within the previous 2 months, in the absence of a positive family history of dystonia and of evidence of any other known cause. Opisthotonos, retrocollis, torticollis, scoliosis, and isolated limb dystonias have been the movements described.[943, 6198] 2. The same, occurring after head injury.

tardive myoclonus Sudden brief, shocklike movements, occurring singly or repetitively, after a period of treatment with dopamine receptor blocking drugs.

tardive stereotypy A common form of **tardive dyskinesia** characterized by involuntary, patterned, repetitive, continuous, coordinated, purposeless, or ritualistic movements, postures, or utterances, occurring after prolonged treatment with dopamine receptor blocking agents.[6007] See also **stereotypy**.

tardive tremor An involuntary oscillatory movement disorder, the tremor

Chart T–1. Diagnostic Criteria for Tardive Dyskinesia

Prerequisites:

1. A history of at least 3 months total cumulative neuroleptic exposure, continuous or discontinuous. Patients who have failed to meet this criterion should receive the appropriate diagnosis with the qualification "less than 3 months' neuroleptic exposure."
2. The presence of at least moderate abnormal involuntary movements in one or more body areas or at least mild movements in two or more body areas (face, lips, jaw, tongue, upper extremities, lower extremities) because of the variability of the movements associated with tardive dyskinesia (TD). If the examination reveals movements that are only minimal or mild in only one body area, the examination should be repeated in 1 week to confirm their presence. Determination of the presence of these movements should be made using a standarized examination procedure and a rating scale such as the **Abnormal Involuntary Movement Scale** or the **Tardive Dyskinesia Rating Scale**.
3. Absence of other conditions that might produce abnormal involuntary movements.

Diagnosis of clinical types:

1. *Probable TD.* The patient needs all three of the above prerequisites.
2. *Masked TD.* The patient meets the criteria for probable TD but within the 2 weeks following an increase in dosage in the case of concurrent neuroleptics or reinstitution of neuroleptic treatment in the case of a neuroleptic-free patient (movements no longer meet the second prerequisite).
3. *Transient TD.* The patient meets the criteria for probable TD, but, on subsequent examination within 3 months, movements meeting the second prerequisite are no longer observed and neuroleptic treatment has not been reinstituted nor the dose increased.
4. *Withdrawal TD.* The patient does not meet the second prerequisite while receiving neuroleptics, but does so within 2 weeks following their discontinuation. If within 3 months of drug withdrawal, the movements meeting the second prerequisite are no longer observed, the diagnosis stands.
5. *Persistent TD.* The patient meets the criteria for probable TD and continues to do so over a 3-month period. The diagnosis may be qualified as "concurrent neuroleptic" if the patient has been receiving the neuroleptics continuously during the 3-month period; as "neuroleptic free" if the patient has received no neuroleptics during the 3-month period or has met the criteria for withdrawal TD, but the movements meeting the second prerequisite have persisted for at least 3 months with no neuroleptic administration; or as "unspecified" if the patient has received neuroleptics for part but not all of the three month period.
6. *Masked persistent TD.* The patient meets the criteria for persistent TD, but, within 3 weeks following an increase in dosage or reinstitution of neuroleptic treatment for movements, no longer meets the second prerequisite.

Adapted from Schooler NR, Kane JM.[5638] *© American Medical Association. Reproduced by kind permission.*

having a frequency range of 3–5 Hz, appearing at all times but especially during maintenance of a posture and induced by long-term neuroleptic treatment. Other tardive movement disorders (see previous entries) are also frequently present.[6008]

tardy ulnar palsy Ulnar nerve paresis developing slowly after trauma to that nerve at the elbow. See **cubital tunnel syndrome**.

target fibers Myofibrils, usually of type I, found in ATPase preparations, in which a densely stained ring of tissue is interposed between an inner core, which does not take up the stain, and a normally stained outer ring of tissue. The appearance is due to streaming of the Z-disk material and to alterations in the distribution of muscle enzymes.

The fibers represent a variant of the muscle cores seen in slowly progressive denervating diseases, in which there appear three concentric zones composed of a central mass, a light halo, and a surrounding region of normal myofibrils. They are most commonly seen in slowly progressive denervating diseases and after tenotomy.[1883]

Tarlov cyst A perineurial cyst compressing the sacral roots and capable of causing sciatic pain[6213] and rarely intracranial hypotension.

Tarnow–Kulenkampff syndrome (cervicolinguomasticatory syndrome) See **tardive dyskinesia**.

tarsal tunnel syndrome Compression of the posterior tibial nerve in the fibro-osseous compartment beneath the flexor retinaculum at the medial malleolus, leading to complaints of pain, weakness, and sensory loss in the distribution of one or all of the three branches (medial, lateral plantar, calcaneal) of that nerve.[1813] In the *anterior* form of the syndrome, there is pain and sensory loss in the distal parts of the dorsum of the foot. The *posterior* type presents with pain in the sole of the foot. Entrapment of the medial calcaneal branch leads to chronic pain in the heel. The electrodiagnostic features have been described.[1559]

tarsophalangeal response See **dorsal foot response**.

Tarui disease (phosphofructokinase deficiency) See **glycogen storage diseases**.

task-specific tremor Tremor of the limbs occurring during the performance of specific activities, such as writing (**primary writing tremor**). Other task-specific tremors include **bowlers' cramp** and the **yips** observed in golfers, while tremors occurring in musicians may be associated with the later appearance of signs of essential tremor or of **Parkinson disease**.[3265] See also **tremor**.

taste disorders Disorders in the dedifferentiation of sweet, salt, sour, bitter, or umami (savory). See **ageusia, dysgeusia**.

Tatasuki syndrome See POEMS.

tau (τ) protein A microtubule-associated protein capable of aggregating and accumulating within the microtubules, causing metabolic dysfunction, which is expressed pathologically as neurofibrillary tangles. Various dementia syndromes are associated with the many mutations of the gene that have been described. Tau protein is normally found in microtubules but can accumulate in different subcellular compartments of the neurons. In neurofibrillary tangles, tau accumulates in the cell body of the neuron as paired helical filaments. Neuropil threads occur when tau accumulates in the processes of the neurons, again as paired helical filaments. The corona of neuritic plaques is composed of tau protein in the axons surrounding their amyloid core. CSF tau levels are a marker for various brain diseases. See **tauopathies**.

tauopathies Conditions associated with the presence of mutated tau protein on 17q21; they include *dementia lacking distinctive histopathology* and *progressive subcortical gliosis* (**fronto-temporal dementia** linked to chromosome 17 with the dementia-predominant or the Parkinsonism-predominant phenotype); **Alzheimer** and **Pick** diseases, variant **Creutzfeldt–Jakob disease, corticobasal degeneration**, and **progressive supranuclear palsy**. Other conditions with defined tau pathology have been reviewed.[255, 1552] See also **synucleopathies**. Galpern and Lang[2262] have reviewed the tauopathies and provide this listing:

Tauopathy with possible Parkinsonism

- Alzheimer disease

Tauopathies with predominant Parkinsonism

- Corticobasal degeneration
- Progressive supranuclear palsy
- Frontotemporal dementia and Parkinsonism linked to chromosome 17 (FTPD-17)
- Parkinsonism–dementia complex of Guam
- Post encephalitic Parkinsonism
- Dementia pugilistica
- Pantothenate kinase-associated neurodegeneration

Other tauopathies

- Pick disease
- Down syndrome
- Argyrophilic grain disease
- Myotonic dystrophy
- Dementia with tangles with or without calcification
- Familial British dementia
- Familial Danish dementia
- Gerstmann–Straussler–Scheinker syndrome
- Niemann–Pick disease type C
- Subacute sclerosing panencephalitis

Neurodegeneration with brain iron accumulation, some forms of muscular dystrophy and **inclusion body myositis** are other conditions in which tau pathology is found.

A Yorkshire kindred has also been reported[4661] suffering from an aggressive early-onset recessively inherited tauopathy with respiratory failure and clinical features resembling **familial fatal parkinsonism with alveolar hypoventilation and depression**.

Tay, Warren (1843–1927) English ophthalmologist who trained at the London Hospital, where he was later appointed to the staff. He was also surgeon at Moorfields Eye Hospital and thus a colleague of Jonathan **Hutchinson**. In 1880 he described the ocular findings in the disease named in part for him, in the first volume of the transactions of the London Ophthalmological Society, of which he was a founding member.

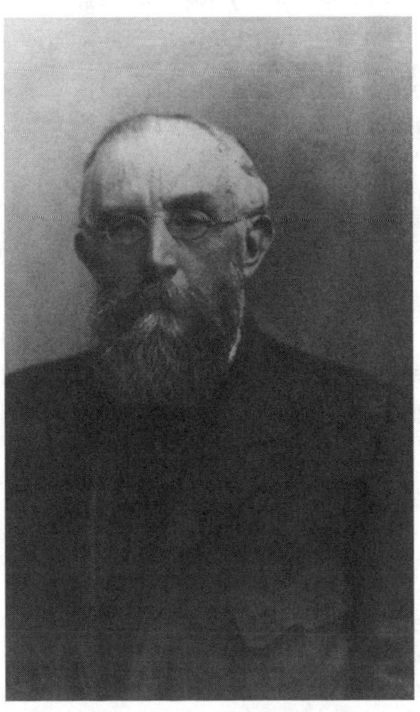

Figure T–1 Warren Tay

Tay sign The cherry-red foveal spot seen in certain **gangliosidoses**.[6229] The term *cherry-red spot*, however, originated with Herman Knapp, a New York ophthalmologist.

Tay syndrome (ichthyosiform erythroderma) A recessively inherited dysmorphic syndrome, characterized also by congenital ichthyosis, dermal atrophy, brittle hair, physical and mental retardation, hypogonadism, and frequently skin photosensitivity. Neurological complications are variable, but may include microcephaly, intracerebral calcifications, seizures, and pyramidal and cerebellar signs. The condition was originally reported from Singapore,[6227] but is not confined to the Orient.

Taybi syndrome A form of generalized skeletal dysplasia, manifesting also mental retardation, small stature, conductive deafness, thin frontal skull, hypotelorism, cleft palate, and limited extension of the elbows.[6230] See **oropalatodigital syndrome**.

Taybi–Rubinstein syndrome See **Rubinstein–Taybi syndrome**.

Tay–Sachs disease See **GM_2 gangliosidosis**.

tea-kettle calves The appearance of the calves in pseudohypertrophic muscular dystrophy (Sir William **Gowers**).

tea party epilepsy Seizures occurring as a result of hyponatremia induced by excessive water intake, as in primary polydipsia.[5054] The same syndrome has been observed in the residents of Labrador and Scandinavia as a result of the excessive consumption of low-sodium-containing, home-made beer. See **hyponatremic encephalopathy**.

tectocerebellar dysraphia with encephalocele A congenital dysmorphic syndrome, manifesting also ventricular septal defect, encephalocele, hydrocephalus, cerebellar lesions, and neuronal heterotopias.[381]

tectorial (Lat, Covering or roofing over) Covering like a roof.

tectorial membrane Part of the cochlea in which the cilia of the hair cells are embedded.

tectospinal tract (Lowenthal's tract [or bundle], predorsal bundle) An extrapyramidal motor pathway first identified by Wilhelm Lowenthal (1850–1894), a German physician.[4502]

tectum (Lat, a roof) A lid or roof.

tegmen (Lat, a covering) A covering or coating.

tegmental mesencephalic paralysis See **Benedikt syndrome.**

tegmental syndrome See **Benedikt syndrome.**

teichopsia (Gr, *teichos*, a wall + seeing) The experience of visual hallucinations as part of the migraine aura, in which blurred vision leads to bilateral homonymous paracentral scotomata which expand with a jagged edge, likened by Dr. Hubert Airy in 1870 to the plan of some northern European medieval castles (*'fortification spectra'*). The same design is used today in oceanic gravity-based oil extraction rigs, in order to withstand icebergs.

Tel-Hashomer camptodactyly A recessively inherited congenital dysmorphic syndrome characterized also by dwarfism, frontal bossing, telecanthus, high-arched palate, winged scapulae, abnormal palmar creases, camptodactyly, syndactyly, clubfoot, joint laxity, brachycephaly, absent muscles, and myopathic muscle atrophy.[2480]

The condition was described in Jewish children of Bedouin descent; the name is that of the hospital in Israel where it was identified.[3113]

tela choroidea (Lat, a web + Gr, membrane) The layer of pia mater inside the ventricles forming the choroid plexus.

telangiectasia (Gr, the end + a vessel + an extension) A congenital dilatation of capillaries and other small vessels.

telecanthus (Gr, far + corner of the eye) A congenital malformation consisting of an increase in the distance between the medial canthi, as commonly seen with **Waardenburg syndrome, meningoencephalocele,** or **blepharophimosis.**[4]

telegrammatism See **telegraphic speech.**

telegraphic speech (telegrammatism) That type of aphasic speech or writing in which propositions, articles, and conjunctions tend to be omitted, while nouns, verbs, and adjectives (which are usually more concrete in their nature) tend to be spared; thus, the type of speech which results after the sacrifice of the shorter terms, which are less heavily charged with reference, function, or meaning.[1330] Such agrammatical, nonfluent speech resembles the typical style used in telegrams, only the words with the highest substantive content being included and the filler words that form the grammatical mesh being omitted. The same form of speech is beloved of Hollywood dialogue experts when writing parts for simple people ("Me no want write more book"). See **agrammatism.**

telegraphist's cramp A focal (occupational) dystonia. See **occupational cramp.**

telencephalon (Gr, end + brain) The cerebrum.

telencephalosynapsis See **holoprosencephaly.**

teleopsia A visual distortion, in which objects appear to have receded into the distance. When unilateral, local retinal disease or chiasmal diseases are usually found, but when bilateral, temporal lobe lesions are the most common pathology.

teleorbitism See **hypertelorism.**

telephone epilepsy A form of **reflex epilepsy** induced by a complex auditory stimulus involving the lateral temporal areas.

telethoninopathy (LGMD2G) A rare autosomal recessive form of **limb girdle muscular dystrophy.**[3454]

television-induced seizures (television epilepsy) One of the commoner types of **photosensitive epilepsy,** seen in photosensitive adolescents who sit close o a TV screen or observe one that is flickering. Clinically, myoclonic jerks,generalized tonic-clonic seizures (GTCS), or absences occur (in that order of frequency). Focal seizures resembling the occipital seizures of idiopathic photosensitive occipital lobe epilepsy are also described. In most subjects no other epileptic syndrome is manifest. *Video game epilepsy* is a small-screen variant. See also **Jeavons syndrome.**

Telfer syndrome A dominantly inherited cochleovestibular atrophy characterized by variable depigmentation of the skin, white forelocks, mild deafness, mental retardation, and ataxia.[6248]

temperature sensation A misnomer, since, between the limits of a physiological range (21–38°C), the body registers not absolute temperature but the rate of loss or gain of heat.

temple (from Lat, temple) The anterior portion of the lateral side of the head. Hair in this region is the first to go gray and, as the Greeks considered time to be an isolated portion of eternity, and the temple a place where a blow might well be fatal, so the structures in this area are called *temporal*. The word has been in use in English for some 700 years.

temporal arteritis (cranial arteritis) See **giant cell arteritis.**[1050] The alternative term is preferred in recognition of the fact that involvement of the temporal arteries in this condition is the least serious complication of a disorder that can involve any or all branches of the carotid system.

temporal crescent The extreme temporal peripheral field, with only monocular representation, in the occipital lobe. They extend some 45° further laterally than the binocular field, which subtends about 120° horizontally. Nasal retinal and postgeniculate lesions lead to impairment of vision in this region, best identified with Goldman perimetry.

temporal dispersion Relative desynchronization of components of a compound muscle action potential due to different rates of conduction of each synchronously evoked component from the stimulation point to the recording electrode. It may be due to normal variability in individual axon conduction velocities, especially when assessed over a long nerve segment, or to disorders that affect myelination of nerve fibers. (Adapted from the 2001 Report of the Nomenclature Committee of the American Association of Electromyography and Electrodiagnosis.[19] Reproduced by kind permission of the AANEM).

temporal lobe epilepsy See **temporal lobe syndromes**.

Temporal Lobe Rating Scale A system for assessing localized atrophy on MRI scans.[2263]

temporal lobe syndromes (temporal lobe epilepsy) Seizure syndromes characterized by simple partial seizures, complex partial seizure, and secondarily generalized seizures, or any combination of these. Their onset is frequently in childhood or young adult life. The seizures occur in clusters at intervals or randomly; frequently there is a history of febrile seizures, a residue of which may be hippocampal sclerosis, but almost any local pathology may be responsible.

Memory deficits may occur. Features which, when present, strongly suggest the diagnosis include the following:

1. Simple focal seizures which are typically characterized by autonomic and/or psychic symptoms and certain sensory phenomena such as olfactory and auditory hallucinations or illusions. Most common are the often rising epigastric sensation (the **epigastric aura**) and **déjà vu** phenomena.
2. Focal seizures with altered consciousness which often (but not always) begin with motor arrest, typically succeeded by oroalimentary automatisms; other automatisms frequently follow. They typically last longer than 1 min. Recovery is gradual, often with postictal confusion and amnesia for the ictal events. *Amygdalohippocampal* and *lateral temporal* varieties are defined on the basis of EEG and surgical studies.[1264]

In interictal periods, the subject may have no psychiatric morbidity, but, in a few cases, a schizophrenia-like psychosis occurs[5890] and psychosis may also arise after temporal lobectomy.[4038] Facial asymmetries are described,[5264] but there are seldom other neurological signs peculiar to the more common temporal lobe lesions causing seizures.

On metabolic imaging (e.g., positron emission tomography), hypometabolism is frequently observed. Uni- or bilateral temporal lobe spikes are common on the interictal EEG. Posterior lateralized slow waves are typical of lateral temporal lobe epilepsy (TLE). In mesial TLE, many subjects have unilateral or bilateral anterior temporal spikes.

Electroencephalographic characteristics. The interictal scalp EEG may show the following:

1. No abnormality.
2. Slight or marked asymmetry of the background activity.
3. Temporal spikes, sharp waves, and/or slow waves, which are unilateral or bilateral, and usually synchronous but also asynchronous. These findings are not always confined to the temporal region.
4. In addition to scalp EEG findings, intracranial recordings may allow better definition of the intracranial distribution of the interictal abnormalities.

Various EEG patterns may accompany the initial clinical ictal symptomatology, including a unilateral or bilateral interruption of background activity and temporal or multilobar low-amplitude fast activity, rhythmic spikes, or rhythmic slow waves. The onset of the EEG disturbance may not correlate with the clinical onset, depending on the methodology used. Intracranial recordings may provide additional information regarding the chronological and spatial evolution of the discharges. (Reproduced by kind permission (but adapted) from Commission for Classification and Terminology, ILAE. Proposal for revised classifications of epilepsies and epileptic syndromes. *Epilepsia* 1989;**30**:389–99.) See also **amygdalohippocampal seizures**.

In *mesial temporal lobe epilepsy*, the characteristics have been defined by Engel (*Neurology* 1993;**43**:1613) and are reproduced by kind permission of the American Academy of Neurology and Lippincott Williams and Wilkins.

A. History

There is an increased incidence of preceding complicated febrile convulsions or a family history of epilepsy.

The onset is in the latter half of the first decade of life. Auras are common and occur in isolation.

Secondarily generalized seizures occur infrequently. Seizures often remit for several years until adolescence or early adulthood, but in time often become medically intractable. Interictal behavioral disturbances can occur (most commonly depression).

B. Clinical seizure

1. An aura is usually present; most common is the epigastric rising aura, often with other autonomic or psychic symptoms including emotion (e.g., fear). Olfactory or gustatory sensations lasting several seconds are also described.
2. The seizures often begin with alteration of consciousness (and subsequent amnesia), motor arrest, and staring; oroalimentary and other complex automatisms are also common. Posturing of one upper extremity may occur on the side opposite to the ictal discharge and last 1–2 min.
3. The postictal phase usually includes disorientation, recent memory deficit, amnesia for the event, and dysphasia if the seizure began in the language-dominant hemisphere; it lasts several minutes.

C. The neurologic examination is generally normal, although recent memory deficit may be detected.

D. EEG

This may be normal, in which case prolonged EEG monitoring, with sleep, is appropriate. Otherwise

1. Unilateral or bilateral independent anterior temporal spikes are recorded with their maximum amplitude in the basal electrodes.
2. There may be intermittent or continuous rhythmic slowing in one mesial temporal area.
3. Extracranial ictal activity appears only with complex partial symptoms, and usually consists of initial or delayed focal-onset pattern of 5–7/s rhythmic activity with its maximum amplitude in one basal temporal derivation.
4. Depth electrode studies show that the onset of the ictus is usually with high-amplitude rhythmic spikes or sharp waves. Low-voltage waves or suppression are less common.
5. Propagation to the contralateral side is slow (>5 s, and may be minutes) or may not occur at all.

E. Usual focal functional deficits

1. Temporal lobe hypometabolism is seen on interictal FDG-PET, often involving the ipsilateral thalamus and basal ganglia also.

2. Temporal lobe hypoperfusion is documented on interictal SPECT and there is a characteristic pattern of hypo- and hyperperfusion on ictal SPECT.
3. Material-specific memory disturbances are shown by neuropsychological testing, and contralateral intracarotid sodium amylobarbitone injection produces amnesia.
4. Mesial temporal lobe slowing and attenuation of normal rhythms can be seen with scalp/sphenoidal electrodes, but is shown better with depth electrodes. This is exacerbated by IV thiopental administration.

F. Structural Imaging MRI scans may show a reduction in size of the hippocampus and temporal lobe with enlargement of the temporal horn on one side.

G. Pathophysiology

1. Hippocampal sclerosis (>30% cell loss with specific patterns).
2. Sprouting of dentate granule cell mossy fibers.
3. Selective loss of certain hilar neurons (Somatostatin and NPY-containing cells).
4. Hamartomas and heterotopias may occur as "dual pathology."
5. Microdysgenesis common.
6. Seizures may originate in sclerotic hippocampi but much larger area appears to be included in the epileptogenic region.

H. Features that cast doubt on the diagnosis

1. A history of severe head trauma, encephalitis, or other specific causal events.
2. The occurrence of focal motor or specific sensory symptoms at seizure onset or postictally.
3. Interictal focal neurologic deficits.
4. Marked cognitive impairment on neuropsychological testing.
5. Bilaterally synchronous, generalized, or extratemporal focal EEG spikes.
6. Diffuse or extratemporal focal EEG slowing.
7. The presence of any cerebral lesion other than hippocampal sclerosis on MRI scans.

In *lateral temporal lobe epilepsy*, simple seizures occur, characterized by auditory hallucinations or illusions or dreamy states, visual misperceptions, or language disorders in the case of a focus in the hemisphere dominant for language. These may progress to complex focal (partial) seizures with alteration in consciousness if propagation to mesial temporal or extratemporal structures occurs. Motor ictal symptoms include clonic movements of facial muscles, grimacing, finger and hand automatisms, dystonic posturing of an upper extremity, leg automatisms, restlessness, and unformed vocalizations. Lack of an epigastric aura or fear and the occurrence of rotation of the whole body differentiate this condition from mesial TLE. The scalp EEG shows unilateral or bilateral midtemporal or posterior temporal spikes which are most prominent in the lateral derivations.[1264]

This form comprises a third of all temporal lobe epilepsies and about 10%–15% of all epilepsies. Any temporal lobe pathology may be responsible.[4882]

A *variant* autosomal dominantly inherited form is described with the onset in youth or young adult life of visual and auditory and a benign course. Mapping to chromosome 10q has been achieved.[5104]

temporal lobectomy Resection of the anterior 5–6 cm of a temporal lobe (back to the vein of Labbé) in the treatment of medically intractable seizures arising from this region. Other stereotactic or surgical approaches are also available.

temporolimbic epilepsy See **temporal lobe syndromes.**

temporomandibular dysfunction (Costen syndrome [?], oromandibular dysfunction, facial arthromyalgia, Schwartz syndrome, craniomandibnular disorder) A painful syndrome arising from dysfunction of the temporomandibular joint (TMJ), characterized by facial or jaw pains often radiating to the temple and neck, tenderness of the masticatory muscles, clicking arising from the TMJ, and restriction of jaw opening.[6946] The syndrome has been critically reviewed.[4614]

The ICHD[2820] suggests diagnostic criteria, including the demonstration of TMJ disorder by imaging; precipitation of pain by jaw movements, such as chewing of hard or tough food; a reduced range of or irregular jaw opening; crepitus from a TMJ during jaw movements; and tenderness of the joint capsule(s). The headache should resolve within 3 months and not recur after successful treatment of the TMJ disorder.

Temtamy syndrome A dominantly inherited congenital syndrome characterized by brachydactyly, affecting mainly the second and fifth digits of the hand and the lateral four toes.[3113] Obesity, hirsutism, blindness, scoliosis, platyspondyly, sclerosis of the skull, optic atrophy, pendular nystagmus, metaphyseal dysplasia, and skin atrophy have also been described in association.

tenalgia Pain arising from tendons of muscles overtaxed by protracted contraction. See **repetitive strain injury, overuse syndromes**.

tenascin An extracellular matrix glycoprotein expressed predominantly on glioma tissue in the CNS. Its assay may be useful in the evaluation and monitoring of the progress of brain tumors.[6919]

tendinous xanthomatosis See **cerebrotendinous xanthomatosis**.

tendon reflex (deep tendon reflex) See **muscle stretch reflexes**. That the percussion of a tendon should lead to reflex contraction of that muscle was not appreciated until 1875, when the German physicians **Erb** and **Westphal** each described the phenomenon. Despite the fact that Erb introduced this term, it remains a misnomer, as tendons have no part to play in the generation of the reflex, except for providing a convenient place to hit the patient. See also **deep tendon reflex**, an even worse misnomer.

TENDS See **transient episodes of neurological dysfunction**.

tennis elbow See **lateral epicondylitis**.

tensilon See **edrophonium**.

Tensilon Test The observation of a patient with suspected **myasthenia gravis**, who shows fatigability after exercise and who is then given an intravenous injection of edrophonium chloride (Tensilon®; an inhibitor of cholinesterase) in an attempt to reverse the fatigability temporarily.

A 2-mg dose is usually injected first; if there are no untoward effects within 2 min more is given, either as one 8-mg dose or as two doses (3 mg followed by 5 mg). Salivation, sweating, and fasciculations are common; hypotension and bradycardia are less common side effects. Cardiac arrhythmias and asthma are contraindications. Atropine should be available in the event of marked bradycardia. Cynics give a placebo dose of saline first.

Improvement in ocular signs is the easiest to assess clinically, though better accuracy is obtained with the **Lancaster red-green test**. Unfortunately, ptosis and oculomotor weakness do not respond to the Tensilon in all cases of **myasthenia gravis**.[5745, 1457]

tensilon tonography A test for **myasthenia gravis** in which increased ocular pressure occurs after the intravenous injection of Tensilon (edrophonium chloride) in myasthenic patients as a result of contraction of the extraocular muscles in response to the drug; no such increase is seen in normal subjects.[6876]

tension (-type) headache A class of headaches subdivided as follows in the International Classification of Headache Disorders.[2820] As a template, one definition will be reproduced here:

Infrequent episodic tension-type headache Infrequent episodes of headache lasting minutes to days. The pain is typically bilateral, pressing, or tightening in quality and of mild to moderate intensity, and it does not worsen with routine physical activity. There is no nausea but photophobia or phonophobia may be present. Diagnostic criteria have been defined:

A. At least 10 episodes occurring on <1 day per month on average (<12 days per year) and fulfilling criteria B–D
B. Headache lasting from 30 min to 7 days
C. Headache has at least two of the following characteristics:
  1. Bilateral location
  2. Pressing/tightening (nonpulsating) quality
  3. Mild or moderate intensity
  4. Not aggravated by routine physical activity such as walking or climbing stairs
D. Both of the following:
  1. No nausea or vomiting (anorexia may occur)
  2. No more than one of photophobia or phonophobia
E. Not attributed to another disorder

Adapted from the International Classification of Headache Disorders (Headache Classification Committee of the International Headache Society. *Cephalalgia* 2004;**24**[Suppl 1]) by kind permission of Dr. Jes Olesen, the International Headache Society and Wiley-Blackwell Publications.[2820]

Subcategories delineated are as follows:

Infrequent episodic tension-type headache associated with pericranial tenderness, which have the same diagnostic criteria but in which there is increased pericranial tenderness on manual palpation.
Infrequent episodic tension-type headache not associated with pericranial tenderness.
Frequent episodic tension-type headache, again with the same criteria except that the headaches occur on ≥1 but <15 days per month for at least 3 months (≥12 and <180 days per year).
Chronic tension-type headache, is a disorder evolving from episodic tension-type headache, with daily or very frequent episodes of headache lasting minutes to days. The pain is typically bilateral, pressing, or tightening in quality and of mild to moderate intensity, and it does not worsen with routine physical activity. There may be mild nausea, photophobia, or phonophobia. The ICHD criteria are the same as for *infrequent episodic tension-type headache* except that the headache has to occur on ≥15 days per month on average for >3 months (≥180 days per year).
Chronic tension-type headache associated with pericranial tenderness is yet a further, minor, subcategory, as is *chronic tension-type headache not associated with pericranial tenderness*.

If all but one of the major criteria for these entities are fulfilled, the word *probable* is added in the ICHD system. See also **new daily-persistent headache**.

tensor (from Lat, to stretch) A muscle which tightens or stretches a body part.

tensor fascia lata reflex Contraction of this muscle in response to a tap applied at its origin from the anterior superior iliac spine. The reflex informs about the state of the reflex arcs between L4 and S1.

tentorium (Lat, a tent, from Lat, to stretch) The tentorium cerebelli is indeed shaped similarly and forms a roof for the posterior fossa.

ten-twenty system A standardized system of scalp electrode placement recommended by the International Federation of Societies for Electroencephalography and Clinical Neurophysiology. According to this system, electrode placements are determined by measuring the head from external landmarks and taking 10 or 20% of each such measurement. (Adapted from the 1974 report of the Committee on Terminology, IFCN. In: Chatrian GE, Bergamini L, Dondey M, et al. A glossary of terms most commonly used by clinical electroencephalographers. *EEG Clin Neurophysiol* 1974;37:538–48. Reproduced by kind permission of Elsevier Science and the IFCN.)

tephromalacia The term of Marie for softening of the anterior part of the spinal cord in patients thought to have syphilitic arteritis.

teratoid tumor of head or neck See **dermoid cyst**.

teratoma A rare, slowly growing tumor containing a range of tissue components as a result of differentiation along various embryonic lines. They occur mainly in the region of the pineal, in the posterior fossa, or within mixed germ cell tumors.[6] The term *malignant teratoma* (teratocarcinoma) is used both for embryonal carcinomas and for regions of malignancy within an otherwise well-differentiated teratoma.

terminal innervation ratio (TIR) The ratio of the number of terminals at the distal ends of **neurites** to the number of motor end-plates innervated. The ratio is normally 1:1, but, in the process of regeneration following axonal section, there are temporarily excessive numbers of neurites; in chronic atrophic diseases, the few surviving axons each innervate an unusually large number of motor end-plates. Thus, only a small minority of healthy axons innervate more than one muscle fiber. The innervation ratio increases in the presence of motor neuropathies and in **myotonic dystrophy**.[1213]

The ratio is a histological measurement of axonal branching within muscles; the *absolute TIR* is the number of subterminal motor arborizations arising from a given number of motor axons, and the *functional TIR* is the number of muscle fibers innervated by these axons.

terminal latency The interval between the stimulation of a nerve distally and the muscle's response.

terminal latency index An electrographic measure of demyelination in peripheral nerves, calculated as follows:[157]

$$\mathrm{TLI} = \frac{\text{distal distance}}{(\text{proximal conduction velocity} \times \text{distal latency})}$$

terminal transverse with orofacial manifestation Inherited syndromes characterized by the presence of cranial nerve palsies associated with a variety of craniofacial and limb malformations. These include **Möbius syndrome, Duane syndrome**, and single VI and VII cranial nerve palsies.[4371]

terrifying hypnagogic hallucinations Intensely frightening hallucinatory phenomena that occur at sleep onset. They may occur alone or be associated with narcolepsy.[1629] See also **sleep terrors**.

Terson syndrome Intraocular hemorrhage (retinal, subhyaloid, or vitreous) following a sudden increase in intracranial pressure, as occurs with **subarachnoid hemorrhage** or trauma.[6257]

tertiary position The position of the eyes when they have deviated from the primary position to any position other than that obtaining with pure adduction, abduction, elevation, or depression.

Tesla, Nikola Yugoslavian physicist, who worked for much of his life in the United States, mainly in the area of magnetic fields. The units of magnetic field strength are named for him. To honor his scientific achievements he was offered the Nobel Prize, but he refused it.

Tesla The preferred unit of measurement of a magnetic field. One Tesla is equal to 10,000 gauss, where the Earth's magnetic field has a strength of about 1 gauss.

Test for Severe Impairment A validated measure sensitive to cognitive changes in severely demented patients with **Alzheimer disease.**[103]

test types Samples of print of different sizes, standardized such that the smallest print which can be read by a subject allows the assignment of a score that reflects his or her acuity relative to the acuity of the normal population.

tetanic contraction The contraction produced in a muscle through repetitive maximal direct or indirect stimulation at a sufficiently high frequency to produce a smooth summation of successive maximum twitches. The term may also be applied to maximum voluntary contractions in which the firing frequencies of most or all of the component motor units are sufficiently high that successive twitches of individual motor units fuse smoothly. Their combined tensions produce a steady, smooth, maximum contraction of the whole muscle. (From the 2001 Report of the Nomenclature Committee of the American Association of Electromyography and Electrodiagnosis.[19] Reproduced by kind permission of the AANEM.)

tetanic neuromyopathy syndrome Strong tetanic muscle contractions with encephalopathy and myoclonus occurring as part of the syndrome of uremic encephalopathy.[1935]

tetanoid chorea The term of Gowers for **athetosis**.

tetanus 1. Maximal and unphysiological tonic contraction of muscle fibers, as a result of repetitive stimulation of the muscle itself or of its nerve. This was first achieved by Volta in 1792, using electrical stimulation. 2. A disease caused by the exotoxin of *Clostridium tetani* which selectively blocks inhibitory interneuronal transmission in the brainstem and spinal cord. The condition was known in Egypt 3000 years ago and was well described by both Hippocrates and Aretaeus; the nature of the underlying disorder was elucidated by Rosenbeck in 1887.

Clinically, after an incubation period of up to 3 weeks following a breach of the skin or mucosa, the patient manifests muscle rigidity, hyperreflexia, and later strong, painful intermittent spasms in a localized or generalized distribution, involving the agonist and antagonist muscles and precipitated by any form of sensory stimulation initially, though later spontaneous. The spinal extensors and face are particularly affected, the former leading to stiffness of the neck and opisthotonos, and the latter to the *risus sardonicus*. (It should be noted here that facial involvement is *not* a feature of the **stiff-person syndrome.**) Rigidity of the chest and abdominal muscles and laryngeal spasm are other features of note. The muscle spasm and secondary myofibrillar damage may lead to myoglobinuria and renal failure.[1935] The condition itself[1969] and the electrophysiological manifestations of diseases associated with excessive motor unit activity have been reviewed.[293] *Variants* are as follows:

Chronic tetanus, a protracted form of tetanus occurring in partially immune subjects presenting with risus sardonicus, trismus, and stimulus-sensitive spasms of somatic muscles, and causing denervation with reinnervation of the affected muscles.[5321]

Neonatal tetanus, in which infants are infected through the umbilical cord, and present within 2 weeks of birth with failure to suck, restlessness, muscle stiffness, opisthotonos, fever, and seizures.

See also **trismus, local tetanus, cephalic tetanus**. A *hemiplegic* form is also described.

tetanus-like seizures See **diencephalic autonomic seizures**.

tetany Involuntary tonic muscle contraction as a result of excessive spontaneous repetitive activity in the motor nerve, as occurs with hypocalcemia or alkalosis causing a reduction in ionized calcium levels. Clinically, this is seen preferentially in distal muscles (*carpopedal spasm*), including those of the face (**Chvostek sign, Schultze sign**). Muscle twitching, cramps, and carpal and pedal spasms are manifestations of peripheral and central nervous system nerve irritability stemming from several causes. Tetany is the only neuromuscular complication of hypoparathyroidism, but hypocalcemia, the usual cause, may be asymptomatic until the nerve is made ischemic (see **Trousseau sign**) or until the patient hyperventilates (*latent tetany*).[3100]

In these conditions, repetitive discharges (double discharge, triple discharge, multiple discharge) occur frequently with voluntary activation of motor unit action potentials or appear as spontaneous activity, enhanced by systemic alkalosis or local ischemia. Tetany was first described by **Erb** in 1873 and by **Trousseau** in 1880,[6402] although Walter Harris (1647–1732) was the first to use calcium (in the treatment of infantile tetany) in 1689. George Kellie (1777–1846), a Scottish physician, first described the laryngospasm in this condition.[5619] Twelve eponymous signs are listed by Robertson and Robertson,[5333] all manifesting the excessive irritability of peripheral nerves to mechanical or electrical stimulation, but only the **Chvostek** and **Trousseau** signs are regarded as important today.

tethered cord syndrome (tethering, filum terminale syndrome) A midline embryological defect in which there is anchoring of the conus medullaris within the confines of the sacrum, usually by a lipomatous growth. The condition is considered to be a form of spinal **dysraphism**. The neurologic symptoms are caused by longitudinal traction on the conus medullaris, and usually present in infancy. The conus is deemed to be abnormally low if it begins at or below the L1–2 disc space.

Clinically, progressive neurological defects in the legs, scoliosis, enuresis, foot ulcers, and deformities appear, usually when the child attains the erect posture or during the rapid pubertal growth phase,[6905] but presentation may be delayed until adult life.[4131] In some cases, muscle hypertrophy is noted in the affected regions.[594] Other features include diffuse and diffuse leg or anorectal pain, bladder or bowel dysfunction, foot and spine deformities in children, leg weakness, and decreased sensation in the perineum and legs. Symptoms may be precipitated by a sudden stretching of the conus associated with any form of exertion or disc herniation. See also **diastematomyelia**.

tethering See **tethered cord syndrome**.

tetra-amelia with multiple malformations (Gr, four + no + limb) See **Zimmer syndrome**.

tetrahydrobiopterin Defects in the metabolism of this substance lead to raised levels of phenylalanine in infants, in whom myoclonic seizures, rigidity, and dystonia develop. See **phenylketonuria**.

tetraphasic action potential Action potential with three baseline crossings, producing four phases.

tetrodotoxin (puffer fish toxin) A potent inhibitor of the initiation and propagation of the action potentials of excitable cells, through its absolute inhibition of the passage of sodium ions across cell membranes.[3515, 3516] It occurs after the ingestion of improperly prepared puffer fish or salamanders. The clinical syndrome results from conduction block in the peripheral nerves and comprises facial paresthesias, numbness, peculiar sensory experiences, nausea, sweating, pallor, salivation, and hypotension, leading on to flaccid paralysis with areflexia and ventilatory failure. It is potentially lethal.[2484]

The condition is mainly seen in people who have ingested fish from the southeastern Asian seas. Puffer fish bred in captivity do not encounter (and so do not ingest) the toxic microorganism that causes this syndrome.

Texidor twinge (precordial catch syndrome) A recurrent, acute, brief, and self-limited pain localized to the anterior left chest wall, associated with the slouched position and relieved by standing erect or by taking a deep breath. The etiology is unknown, but unless the subjects agree to full cardiological investigation, the condition is harmless.[4361]

thalamencephalon (Gr, an inner chamber + the brain) Those parts of the brain around the third ventricle which are derived from the first primary vesicle.

thalamic amnesia An acute, persistent amnesic syndrome caused by bilateral paramedian thalamic infarction due to occlusion of a thalamosubthalamic artery supplying both medial thalami. Clinically, after a period of transient coma, the patient enters an apathetic and hypersomnolent state, accompanied by severe anterograde verbal and visual amnesia and bilateral vertical gaze palsies, evolving to a condition of **subcortical dementia**.[2607]

thalamic aphasia A fluent dysnomic aphasia, complicated by fluctuations of attention and of performance, resulting from thalamic hemorrhagic or ischemic strokes. This is not necessarily a causative association, however, as all patients studied more recently have had evidence of diminished cortical perfusion or the cortical effects have been interpreted in terms of the interruption of neural connections.

thalamic astasia See **subcortical dysequilibrium**.

thalamic ataxia Unilateral ataxia, coarse action tremor, hemisensory loss, and mild hemiparesis as a result of contralateral midthalamic or posterior thalamic infarction.[4054, 5944]

thalamic Creutzfeld–Jakob syndrome See **thalamic dementia**.

thalamic degeneration with multiple system atrophy See **thalamic dementia**.

thalamic dementia Global psychological defects in adult patients with paramedian diencephalic lesions. The syndrome is characterized clinically by optic atrophy, ophthalmoplegias, myoclonic seizures, dystonias, spasticity, and autonomic disturbances. Mental signs include impairment of attention and mental control with apathy, poor motivation, slowness in response, amnesia, and emotional lability.[713] Three types have been defined:

Selective thalamic degeneration includes familial or sporadic types, characterized by severe thalamic atrophy without pathology elsewhere. This may be the same condition as **fatal familial insomnia**.[5001]

Thalamic degeneration with multiple-system atrophy includes sporadic or familial cases in combination with with cerebellar ataxia or **hereditary motor neuropathy.**

Thalamic **Creutzfeld–Jakob syndrome** comprises those sporadic cases in which there is substantial gliosis or spongy change in the cerebral cortex as well as the thalamic pathology.[5001]

The condition may also occur as a **lacunar syndrome**.[2092, 2106] See also **Stern–Garcin syndrome, subcortical dementia**.

thalamic esotropia Sustained convergence of the eyes as a result of acute thalamic disease.[2459]

thalamic hand 1. Permanent sensory loss of part of the arm down into the hand, in association with a small thalamic infarction (pseudoradicular infarction). 2. (striothalamic hand) The flexed, pronated, and adducted posture of the hand and fingers in some patients with basal ganglion disorders.

thalamic infarcts Small infarcts resulting from in situ disease of small vessels or at the mouth of the parent artery or cardioembolism, producing a variety of syndromes with moderate motor and sensory signs, memory impairment, dysphasia (if the left thalamus is involved), and neglect (if the right is involved). Other clinical features include confusion, behavioral changes, eye movement disorders, and contralateral ataxia. Posterior choroidal artery infarcts may produce an isolated homonymous horizontal sectoranopia.

thalamic neglect A neglect syndrome resulting from a lesion of the medial thalamic nuclei which, like the mesencephalic reticular activating system, are involved with tonic arousal.[6672]

thalamic overreaction The occurrence of spontaneous pains and of **hyperpathia** following thalamic lesions.[645]

thalamic pain Unilateral facial pain and dysesthesia attributed to a lesion of the quintothalamic pathway or the thalamus, usually on the right side. The symptoms also involve the trunk and limbs on the same side. The pain and dysesthesias affect one half of the face and are associated with impaired sensation to pinprick, not explicable by a lesion of the trigeminal nerve. In addition, one or more of the following is present: a history of sudden onset suggesting a vascular lesion; a remitting and relapsing history of symptoms in the face or elsewhere suggesting **multiple sclerosis**; and the demonstration of a lesion in an appropriate site by CT or MRI. (Based on Classification of headache disorders, cranial neuralgias and facial pains; and diagnostic criteria for primary headache disorders. *Cephalalgia* 1988;8[Suppl]:1–96).

Allodynia, **hypoesthesia** and **hypalgesia**, **dysesthesia**, and motor and sensory signs are also commonly found, and symptoms more commonly affect half the body than the face alone. Déjèrine and Roussy described the pains as follows: "lively pains on the hemiparetic side which are persistent, paroxysmal, often intolerable and refractory to any analgesic therapy." See also **central pain**.

thalamic sensory loss More or less complete loss of all forms of sensation of the contralateral side of the face and body as a result of a lesion of the posterior thalamic nuclei.

thalamic syndrome (Déjèrine–Roussy syndrome, capsulothalamic syndrome) **Thalamic pain** following lesions of the ventroposterior thalamic nuclei (occlusion of thalamogeniculate branches of the posterior cerebral artery) or of the deep white matter of the parietal lobe. This usually succeeds a period of mild contralateral hemiparesis, hemiataxia and choreoathetosis, complete astereognosis, and persistent hemianesthesia, although superficial sensation may be more or less spared.

The severe, persistent, paroxysmal, and often intolerable pain is variously described with a wealth of verbal detail. Any outside stimulus appears capable of aggravating it. Therapy is seldom effective.[1543] The various thalamic infarct syndromes have been reviewed.[713]

Isolated anterior thalamic infarctions lead to acute, severe perseverative behavior in thinking, speech, and memory tasks with increased sensitivity to interference and **palipsychism**, anterograde memory impairments with impairment of delayed recall, and difficulty in programming motor sequences.[2350]

See also **paramedian thalamic artery syndrome**.

thalamic tremor Unilateral resting and postural 3-Hz tremor of the upper limb, occurring as a delayed manifestation of thalamic stroke.[4411]

thalamocapsular stroke See **sensorimotor stroke**.

thalamosubthalamic infarction syndrome See **paramedian diencephalic syndrome**.

thalamus (Gr, room or inner chamber) (optic thalamus) The name applied by Galen to the final major relay station in the ascending sensory pathways, reaffirmed as such by **Willis** in 1664.

thalassemia A heterogeneous group of hereditary disorders characterized by a decrease in the production of one or more globin chains and leading to multiple complications due to chronic anemia or transfusion related hemosiderosis.

thalassemic myopathy (Gr, sea + blood + muscle + disease) A myopathic syndrome occurring uncommonly in patients with (homozygous) thalassemia major and presenting with proximal weakness (mainly in the legs) and a myopathic EMG pattern.[3898]

thalassemic neuropathy A sensory neuropathy present in a majority of patients with thalassemia but not always symptomatic.[5567]

thallium poisoning A syndrome of peripheral neuropathy, ataxia, somnolence, seizures, and sometimes cranial nerve palsies, including optic neuritis, resulting from the ingestion of thallium-containing substances (usually pesticides). Ataxia and some degree of dementia may be permanent sequelae.[1061]

thanatophoric dwarfism (Gr, death + bringing) (nanism) A rare congenital asphyxiating syndrome of skeletal deformities resulting from complicated achondroplasia. The clinical features of note include dwarfism and platyspondyly, anal atresia, Kleeblattschädel (cloverleaf malformation of the skull), widened cranial sutures and fontanelles, and heterotopias with CNS dysplasias.[3549]

thanatophoric dysplasia A dominantly inherited lethal congenital syndrome of craniosynostosis and short-limbed dwarfism, mapped to chromosome 4p.

thanos syndrome A rare congenital dysmorphic syndrome said to be characterized by myopia, macrocephaly, craniosynostosis, thickened calvarium, sclerosis of the skull bones, epidermoid nevi, and mental and developmental delay. However, it has also been argued that the syndrome does not exist.

Thaysen syndrome See **proctalgia fugax, familial rectal pain**.

Theile syndrome A congenital dysmorphic syndrome characterized also by scoliosis, cryptorchidism, microcephaly, and mental and developmental delay.

thenar The flat part or hollow of the hand. The name was used by Homer, Hippocrates, and Galen for the small hand muscles, but the separation into thenar muscles (at the base of the thumb) and hypothenar muscles (on the ulnar side) was the invention of Riodan in 1649.[5886]

thenar hypoplasia A sporadic developmental anomaly characterized by the occurrence of hypoplastic thenar muscles on one or both sides. The differential diagnosis of this condition from **carpal tunnel syndrome** is not easy, especially because it may not lead to referral for medical care until adult life; but there are no sensory changes in this anomalous form.[1063]

therapeutic embolization The intra-arterial injection of foreign substances with the aim of obliterating a vascular lesion such as an arteriovenous malformation or an aneurysm fed by the appropriate artery. The precise indications for the procedure are still in the process of determination.[2169]

thermanesthesia Loss of temperature sensation.

thermesthesia Temperature sensation.

thermhypesthesia Partial loss of temperature sensation.

thermography A technique for the measurement of skin temperature using either a liquid-crystal device applied to the skin or infrared detection equipment. Its reliability in the diagnosis of radiculopathies and neuropathies is disputed. An American Academy of Neurology subcommittee concluded that it is of limited value in characterizing neurological dysfunctions.[164, 1005] Those who possess a machine, however, find its use profitable.

thermoregulatory sweat test A technique for assessing the integrity of the central and peripheral efferent sympathetic pathways. It consists of measuring the sweat distribution using an indicator powder while applying a controlled heat stimulus to raise body temperature sufficient to induce sweating.

In performing the test, the naked patient is heated by 1°C, and coated with starch powder and iodine; in the presence of moisture (sweat) the starch–iodine reaction causes a dark blue-gray color change. See **autonomic function tests**.

Thermotest A commercial device (Somedic Thermotest apparatus; Somedic AS, Stockholm, **Sweden**) useful in the assessment of small fiber neuropathies.

theta wave A waveform recorded on the EEG, with a duration of < 0.25 s and >0.125 s.

theta rhythm An EEG rhythm with a frequency of 4 to <8 Hz.

Thévenard disease (l'acropathie ulcéro-mutilante familiale) Neurogenic plantar ulceration, as may occur in **hereditary sensory and autonomic** and **alcoholic neuropathies, syringomyelia, tabes dorsalis**, the **cerebellar ataxias**, and low spinal cord lesions.[6269]

thiamine-dependent lactic acidemia A rare congenital or childhood syndrome characterized by mental retardation, episodic ataxia, choreoathetosis, hypotonia with areflexia, and chronic lactic acidosis. The condition is considered a manifestation of pyruvate decarboxylase deficiency.[1759] See also **Leigh disease**.

thiamine-dependent maple syrup urine disease (thiamine-responsive branched-chain ketoaciduria) A milder variant of **maple syrup urine disease** in which there is an error in the degradation of the branched-chain amino acids leucine, isoleucine, and valine and presenting with ketoacidosis and seizures in the neonatal period. The clinical disease resolves in those infants treated permanently with thiamine.[1759]

thiamine-dependent megaloblastic anemia, sensorineural deafness, and diabetes mellitus A rare syndrome of unknown cause characterized by the combination of these features.[2802]

thiamine-responsive branched-chain ketoaciduria See **thiamine-dependent maple syrup urine disease. thick-filament myopathy** See **acute quadriplegic myopathy**.

Thiebaut syndrome (spinal cholesterolosis) A syndrome of spastic paraparesis with hypercholesterolemia and large tendinous masses. It is probably a form of **cerebrotendinous xanthomatosis** but has so far been reported only without pathological verification.[6270]

Thiebaut–Refsum disease See **hereditary motor and sensory neuropathy** (type 4; Refsum disease).

thigmesthesia General tactile sensibility, the receptors for which are around the hair follicles and in Merkel's disks.

thinking epilepsy A rare form of **reflex epilepsy** induced by specific cognitive tasks, mainly occurring in patients with idiopathic generalized epilepsies. Focal epilepsies are exceptionally triggered by the action of mind.

third alexia See **alexia**.

third and fourth pharyngeal pouch syndrome See **DiGeorge syndrome**.

third circulation The CSF system, this term being suggested by **Cushing** in 1926.

third occipital headache A constant aching occipital or suboccipital head pain worsened by neck movement and resulting from irritation of the third occipital nerve (a branch of the C3 root) by pressure from osteophytes around the C2–3 zygapophyseal joints[701] and following "**whiplash**" injury.[3913]

thirty:fifteen ratio The ratio of the pulse rates at 30 compared with 15 beats after standing; a measure of parasympathetic autonomic function.[3085] Normally the ratio is 1.04 or more; 1.00 or less is definitely abnormal. See also **expiration:inspiration ratio, autonomic function tests**.

Thomas, André See **André-Thomas**.

Thomas atrophy See **olivopontocerebellar atrophies**.

Thomas disease (André-Thomas disease, pure cerebellar cortical atrophy) An ataxic syndrome best classified as an

olivopontocerebellar atrophy even though described separately[6272] from that on which André-Thomas and **Déjèrine** had published an account 5 years before.[1545]

Thomas reflex A rather different method of eliciting the **Babinski** plantar response, in which the examiner smartly rubs the sole of the patient's foot with the back of the knuckles two or three times. The particular indications for this technique are not defined. It is named for the late Prof. P.K. Thomas, a Welsh neurologist working in London, UK.

Thomsen, Asmus Julius Thomas (1815–1896) Danish physician and lyric poet, who suffered from **myotonia congenita** (Strümpell, 1881), the disorder subsequently named after him by **Westphal** (1883). His family history was strongly positive over five generations (not surprisingly in a condition with likely autosomal dominant inheritance), but he refrained from publishing his observations on "Ataxia Muscularis" or "Tonic Cramp" until 1876, when his son, who was also affected, was accused of feigning symptoms in order to avoid military service.[3226, 6305]

The production of muscle spasms by emotion led Thomsen to consider the condition a disease of the central rather than of the peripheral nervous system. Unknown to him, Ernst **Leyden** had published a good account of the same disorder 2 years before, and Wilhelm **Erb** wrote an exhaustively complete account of it 10 years later.

Thomsen disease Dominantly inherited myotonia with secondary hypertrophy of muscles and without loss of power, unlike **paramyotonia**. See **myotonia congenita**.

Thompson disease See **glycogen storage diseases**.

Thompson syndrome A congenital form of optic atrophy.

Thompson Test The patient kneeling with the foot hanging over the edge of a couch, the calf is pinched just below its widest point. Passive plantar flexion of the foot is the normal response, but this is absent in the presence of rupture of the Achilles' tendon.[2044]

thoracic inlet syndrome See **thoracic outlet syndrome**.

thoracic outlet An anatomical artifact, variously described as including the interscalene triangle, the costoclavicular passage, and the axillary passage, through which passes the neurovascular bundle composed of the brachial plexus and the subclavian artery and vein as they leave the chest to enter the arm.

thoracic outlet syndrome (Falconer–Weddell syndrome, scalenus anticus syndrome, costo-clavicular syndrome, hyperabduction syndrome, Naffziger syndrome, neurogenic or vascular thoracic outlet compression syndromes, thoracic inlet syndrome, superior thoracic aperture syndrome) A collection of disorders, linked by the common (but thin) thread of supposed compression of the brachial plexus and subclavian vessels along the costoclavicular passages by, for example, a cervical rib at C7, a fibrous band passing from the scalenus medius to the first rib, or the scalenus anterior muscle itself. *Neurogenic* and *vascular* (both arterial and venous) forms are described.[1369] The description by Falconer and Weddell[1956] of the "costo-clavicular compression syndrome" is among the most complete.

Clinically, combinations of aching pain in the forearm or shoulder, reproduced by traction on the arms; paresthesias in the medial part of the forearm; weakness and occasionally wasting of the hand; and coldness and color changes are the more common symptoms. Supraclavicular bruits and sensory or motor findings appropriate to compression of the lower fibers of the brachial plexus may be found, but the diagnosis is suggested by the symptoms rather than by the signs, of which there may be none.

The *neurogenic* form is characterized by pain and sensory disturbance in the ulnar side of the forearm and hand, made worse by use of the arm, combined with weakness and wasting of the intrinsic hand muscles (especially the abductor, flexor, and opponens of the thumb). The presence of a cervical rib assists in the diagnosis, but a long C7 transverse process and a fibrous band (visible only to surgeons) have also been incriminated at causal.[3734] Its electrophysiological signs are inconstant and disputed, though abnormal medial antebrachial cutaneous sensory studies are reported as being abnormal in all such cases.[3543] A recent dispassionate review was by le Forestier et al. (1998).[3734]

The *vascular* form presents with evidence of arterial insufficiency in the hand presumed to be as a result of subclavian artery or vein compression.

A host of names has been ascribed to the syndrome of arm pain and subjective sensory disturbance; some are given above. The syndrome represents a major source of controversy because the pathology can exist without any symptoms, the clinical features are not specific, the operation is attended by potential important complications, and there exists no definitive confirmatory test. Thus the condition perplexes neurologists, vexes electromyographers, and activates surgeons. Recent disputations have been published.[5375, 6777] In 40 years of EMG practice, this author has encountered two patients in whom both the clinical evidence was complete and the surgical intervention beneficial. See also **droopy shoulder syndrome**.

http://www.ninds.nih.gov/disorders/thoracic/thoracic.htm is the relevant NINDS site.

thoracic radiculopathy See **diabetic truncal neuropathy**.

thoracic-pelvic-phalangeal dystrophy See **Jeune syndrome, Langer–Gierdon syndrome**.

thoraco-abdominal neuropathy See **diabetic truncal neuropathy**.

Thorburn phenomenon Involuntary muscle contractions associated with mechanical or other insults to adjacent regions of the spinal cord; adoption of a position of abduction of the shoulders and flexion of the elbows as a result of bilateral C7 lesions. See **Bradborn sign**. As a regrettable example, the tragic shooting of President John Kennedy caused an immediate initial elevation of his shoulders and flexion of his arms (C5, 6 activation) when the bullet pierced the cord at C6.

thought Conscious mental content, whether in linguistic form or not.

three clap test The patient is asked to clap three times as quickly as possible after demonstration by the examiner. An abnormal result is for the patient to clap four or more times or to perseverate in clapping (*applause sign*) as is common in patients with **frontotemporal dementia** or **progressive supranuclear palsy**.[1724]

three-Hertz spike-and-slow waves A paroxysm of EEG activity consisting of a regular sequence of spike-and-slow-wave complexes which repeat at 3–3.5 Hz (measured during the first few seconds of the paroxysm). They are bilateral in their onset and termination, generalized, and usually of maximal amplitude over the frontal areas, and are approximately synchronous and symmetrical on the two sides of the head throughout the paroxysm. Their amplitude is variable but can reach values of 1000 μV. See also **atypical repetitive spike-and-slow waves.** (Adapted from the 1974 report of the Committee on Terminology, IFCN. In: Chatrian GE, Bergamini L, Dondey M, et al. A glossary of terms most commonly used by clinical electroencephalographers. *EEG Clin Neurophysiol* 1974;37:538–48. Reproduced by kind permission of Elsevier Science and the IFCN.)

Three Paper Test A test of reading comprehension using verbal instruction, introduced by Pierre **Marie**. The patient is given a piece of paper on which is written,"When you have finished reading this, tear the paper into three. Give one piece to me. Throw a second piece on the floor. Put the third piece in your pocket."

Three Words, Three Shapes Test A test of verbal and nonverbal memory wherein the subject copies three simple shapes, each labeled with an unrelated word, and then attempts to reproduce these without further stimulation after various intervals.[4332]

threshold In any context, the level at which a clear and abrupt transition occurs from one state to another. The term is generally used to refer to the voltage level at which an action potential is initiated in a single axon or muscle fiber or a group of axons or muscle fibers. (From the 2001 Report of the Nomenclature Committee of the American Association of Electromyography and Electrodiagnosis.[19] Reproduced by kind permission of the AANEM.)

Throckmorton sign Extension of the hallux when the metatarsophalangeal region is repeatedly struck just medial to the tendon of the extensor hallucis longus. This is a variant of the **Babinski reflex**, but of rather less utility. It was described by T.B. Throckmorton (b. 1885), an American neurologist.

thrombocythemia (primary thrombocythemia) A condition characterized by platelet counts greater than 400×10^9/l and an increase in the number of clustered mature megakaryocytes in bone marrow biopsy specimens, in the absence of any cause for reactive thrombocytosis. Neurological complications include transient ischemic attacks and other evidence of microvascular disease such as erythromelalgia, presenting with burning paresthesias and pains in the extremities, and painful acrocyanosis, but the peripheral pulses are normal.[4349]

thrombophlebitis, cerebral See **cerebral venous thrombosis**.

thrombosis Occlusion of a blood vessel as a result of coagulation of the blood contained therein, triggered either by hematological disease or by disease of the vessel wall. See **cavernous sinus thrombosis, cerebral thrombosis, cerebral venous thrombosis**.

thrombotic microangiopathy See **Moschcowitz disease**.

thrombotic thrombocytopenic purpura See **Moschcowitz disease**.

Thudichum, Johann Ludwig Wilhelm (1828–1901) German physician and neurochemist who emigrated to England and was appointed to the staff of St. Thomas' Hospital in London in 1853. He studied the normal chemical composition of the brain, isolating and naming the phosphatides, sphingomyelin, sulfatides, cerebrosides, and cholesterol, in many cases giving an account of their chemical composition. His overview of his research results[6310] laid the foundations of modern neurochemistry but his observations were not well received in his time. He also invented a nasal speculum and published on gastronomy.

thumb adductor response Adduction and flexion of the thumb in response to gentle stroking of the ulnar side of the palm; seen in patients with pyramidal tract lesions. The reflex was described by **Marie** and **Foix**.

thumb extensor and finger aplasia A recessively inherited syndrome with these features.

thumb reflex Tapping the tendon of the flexor pollicis longus above the pronator quadratus leads to flexion of the distal phalanx. This reflex is usually appreciated only in patients with pyramidal tract disease.

thumb sign Protusion of the thumbs over the ulnar aspect of the palm when the fist is clenched; a sign in **Marfan syndrome** resulting both from elongation of the phalanges and metacarpals and hypermotility of the joints. See also **arachnodactyly**.

thumb-chin reflex Contraction of the mentalis muscle when the underside of the patient's thumbnail is flicked up by the index finger nail of the examiner; a variation of the **palmomental reflex**, with the same significance.

thunderclap headaches Paroxysmal, excruciatingly severe, generalized headaches presenting with extreme abruptness. The pathophysiology is unknown but the condition is usually benign unless caused by subarachnoid hemorrhage, but in the benign forms, bolded below, there is no evidence of intracranial bleeding. Diagnostic criteria were suggested by Dodick (2002)[1677]

1. Very severe pain intensity.
2. Instantaneous to hyperacute onset of pain (<30 s).
3. Appropriate investigations exclude the presence of an underlying cause such as subarachnoid hemorrhage, cerebral venous sinus thrombosis, pituitary apoplexy, arterial dissection, spontaneous intracranial hypotension, and acute hypertensive crisis.

The ICHD-2 criteria for primary thunderclap headache are somewhat similar, requiring severe head pain with sudden onset, reaching maximum intensity in <1 min and lasting from 1 h to 10 days, not recurring regularly over subsequent weeks or months and not attributed to another disorder.

Dodick also pointed out that the attacks are spontaneous or may be precipitated by the Valsalva maneuver, sexual activity, or strenuous exercise, and that they may recur infrequently over 1–2 weeks. Their occurrence is also described in migraine (*crash migraine*). In all cases, full investigation (e.g., a CT head scan) is urgently required.

See also **reversible cerebral vasoconstriction syndrome, sentinel headache, and headache associated with sexual activity**, (coital cephalgia, benign sex headache) which, like cervical spinal disorders, may present with pain of a similar nature.[1490]

thunderstruck disease An antique colloquialism for apoplexy.

thymectomy Removal of the thymus gland, first performed by Alfred Blalock (b. 1899), an American surgeon, for the treatment of **myasthenia gravis.**

thymoma (Gr, thymus + cutting out) A tumor of the thymus gland, usually benign and frequently without any associated symptoms. The tumor is usually in the lateral lobes of the thymus, and is characterized by mixed epithelial or lymphothelial cell nests with many lymphocytes, rosettes, and some gland-like formations. A relationship with **myasthenia gravis** is, however, established.

thyrocerebrorenal syndrome A recessively inherited congenital dysmorphic syndrome, characterized by sensorineural deafness, goiter with hypothyroidism, platelet abnormalities, seizures, and cerebellar signs.[1397]

thyroid ophthalmopathy See **dysthyroid orbitopathy**.

thyroid storm See **thyrotoxic crises.**

thyrotoxic crises (thyroid storm, acute thyrotoxic encephalomyelopathy) An agitated delirious state with tremor and hyperkinesia, and later lethargy, obtundation, or coma. Pyramidal signs, aphasia, chorea, bulbar palsy, and respiratory insufficiency are also recorded. Other features include insomnia, fever, tachycardia, diarrhea and vomiting, atrial fibrillation, and cardiac failure. The disorder is precipitated by infection, trauma, and by hot summer weather, and may occur in hypothyroid subjects given too much thyroxine. The best early description was that of Waldenström in 1945; he also pointed out the difficulty in deciding whether the bulbar weakness was due to myopathy or to encephalopathy.

thyrotoxic myopathy A syndrome of symmetrical proximal muscle weakness and wasting, found almost universally in patients with hyperthyroidism.

thyrotoxic periodic paralysis (Kitamura syndrome) Recurrent attacks of flaccid paralysis of the limbs more than the trunk, lasting for between 2 and 72 h, in association with hypokalemia. The condition is described mainly in young Japanese, Chinese, and Thai males with hyperthyroidism.[2267, 4707]

thyrotropin releasing hormone A hypothalamic hypophysiotropic peptide hormone, one of the first to be identified. Like other brain peptides, it is localized within nerve terminals, is released as a result of depolarization, and acts as a supplementary neurotransmitter—in this case to cause the release of thyrotropin.

TIAs See **transient ischemic attacks.**

tibial muscular dystrophy (OMIM 600334) A late-onset, autosomal dominant distal myopathy with weakness and atrophy confined to the anterior compartment of the lower leg muscles, particularly the tibialis anterior and the long toe extensors. The first symptoms are of impaired ankle dorsiflexion occuring in young adult life, mild or moderate proximal lower limb weakness occuring later. Pathologically, the affected muscles show rimmed vacuoles and the usual myopathic features. The disease is mapped to chromosome 2q31 and is linked to **Markesbery–Griggs disease**, to dilated cardiomyopathy, and to **autosomal dominant myopathy with proximal weakness and early respiratory muscle involvement**.[6437]

tibial neuropathy Lesions of the main trunk of the nerve, usually in the thigh, as a result of compression, trauma, or ischemic disease and causing sural sensory and lower motor neurone lesions in the gastrocnemius, soleus, and plantar muscles. See **posterior tibial neuropathy**.

tibialis anterior reflex The contraction of the tibialis anterior in response to sudden stretch resulting from a tap on the dorsal aspect of the hallux. The reflex is not usually visible in the healthy subject, but can be recorded electromyographically.[6013] At the bedside, therefore, the clinician has to rely on the lateral hamstrings to provide a site for the assessment of the L5 reflex arc.[6013]

tibialis anterior hypertrophy A syndrome of localized painful hypertrophy of this muscle in association with persistent complex repetitive discharges within it, arising neurogenically.[4683]

tibialis phenomenon (Strümpell sign) Marked dorsiflexion at the ankle when the patient attempts to flex the thigh on the hip; a pathological associated movement seen in patients with pyramidal lesions.

tibialis posterior reflex The contraction of the tibialis posterior in response to sudden stretch resulting from a tap on its tendon above and behind the medial malleolus. The contraction is not usually visible in the healthy subject, but can be recorded electromyographically. The reflex informs about the state of the reflex arcs at L5 and S1.

tic A sudden, brief, stereotyped, more or less complex, repetitive, normally coordinated but inappropriate movement which can be suppressed for a period by an effort of will, but only at the expense of rising psychic tension (which in turn is only relieved by expression of the tic).[2443] In brief, these are irresistible, inapposite involuntary movements.

Motor (including vocal) and sensory tics are described; these may be either simple or complex, and represent either *transient* or *chronic tic disorders*. See also **coprolalia, palilalia**, and **echolalia**.[3159]

The international classification[6868] distinguishes elementary, complex, and generalized tics. Examples of the *elementary* forms are mimicking, blinking, sniffing, tooth-grinding, or swallowing, stuttering, neck, shrugging, trunk and leg, and vocal tics, the last including barking, shouting, grunting, and swearing. Any of these in combination are regarded as *complex tics*, while the *generalized tic* category includes those tics affecting a number of separate body areas, with or without vocal expression. All of these forms are met with in **Tourette syndrome**.[2443] A rating scale for the disorder has been devised.[2432]

tic convulsif See **trigeminal neuralgia**.

tic disorder Diseases of unknown origin (but with a genetic predisposition) in which tics are manifested as a major feature. Criteria for this diagnosis[3608] are listed in Chart T–2, but see also **Tourette syndrome**.

In a *variant* form, a familial tic disorder is accompanied by signs of Parkinson disease, motor neuron disease, and acanthocytosis.[5994] See also **neuroacanthocytosis**.

tic douloureux See **trigeminal neuralgia**.

tick-borne encephalitis An acute meningoencephalitis with or without myelitis due to a flavivirus transmitted by *Ixodes* spp. ticks from western Europe to the east coast of Japan. Morbidity is highest in adults, half of whom develop encephalitis. A third of patients have long-lasting sequelae, frequently with cognitive dysfunction and substantial impairment in quality of life. Serological diagnosis is available. There is no specific treatment for the disease; immunization is the main preventive measure.[3856]

tick paralysis A syndrome of neuromuscular blockade, capable of inducing a subacute generalized flaccid paralysis starting in the legs, with areflexia, respiratory and bulbar paralyses, and even death, usually occurring in children and due to envenomation by the ticks *Ixodes holocyclus* (in Australia) or *Dermacentor andersoni* or *variabilis* (in North America), which are most commonly hidden in the hair. Sensory functions are normal. The clinical features have been ascribed both to impairment of nerve conduction and of neurotransmission.[1134] The condition is more frequent in children who live in abundantly forested areas.

ticq A seventeenth-century French term denoting unsightly muscular activity.

Tietz syndrome See **dominant albinism and congenital deafness**.

Chart T–2. Research Diagnostic Criteria for Tic Disorders

A–1. Definite Tourette syndrome

1. Both multiple motor and one or more phonic tics have been present at some time during the illness, although not necessarily concurrently.
2. The tics occur many times a day (usually in bouts), nearly every day or intermittently throughout a period of more than a year.
3. The anatomical location, number, frequency, complexity, type and severity of the tics change over time.
4. Onset before age 21 years.
5. Involuntary movements and noises cannot be explained by other medical conditions.
6. Motor and/or phonic tics must be witnessed by a reliable examiner directly at some point in the illness, or be recorded by videotape or cinematography.

A–2. Tourette syndrome by history

1. Both multiple motor and one or more phonic tics have been present at some time during the illness, although not necessarily concurrently.
2. The tics occur many times a day (usually in bouts), nearly every day or intermittently throughout a period of more than a year.
3. The anatomical location, number, frequency, complexity, type and severity of the tics change over time.
4. Onset before age 21 years.
5. Involuntary movements and noises cannot be explained by other medical conditions.
6. Tics have not been witnessed by a reliable examiner, but tics were witnessed by a reliable family member or close friend, and the description of the tics as demonstrated is accepted by a reliable examiner.

B–1. Definite chronic multiple motor or phonic tic disorder

1. Either multiple motor or phonic tics, but not both, have been present at some time during the illness.
2. The tics occur many times a day (usually in bouts), nearly every day or intermittently throughout a period of more than a year.
3. The anatomical location, number, frequency, complexity, type, and severity of the tics change over time.
4. Onset before age 21 years.
5. Involuntary movements or noises cannot be explained by other medical conditions.
6. Motor and/or phonic tics must be witnessed by a reliable examiner directly at some point in the illness, or be recorded by videotape or cinematography.

B–2. Chronic multiple motor or phonic tic disorder by history

1. Either multiple motor or phonic tics, but not both, have been present at some time during the illness.
2. The tics occur many times a day, (usually in bouts), nearly every day or intermittently throughout a period of more than a year.
3. The anatomical location, number, frequency, complexity, type, and severity of the tics change over time.
4. Onset before age 21 years.
5. Involuntary movements or noises cannot be explained by other medical conditions.
6. Tics have not been witnessed by a reliable examiner, but were witnessed by a reliable family member or close friend, and the description of the tics as demonstrated is accepted by a reliable examiner.

continued

Chart T–2. (*continued*)

C. Chronic single motor or phonic tic disorder (by history)

1. Same as B–1 (and B–2), but with single motor or phonic tic.

D–1. Definite transient tic disorder

1. Single or multiple motor and/or phonic tics.
2. The tics occur many times a day (usually in bouts), nearly every day for at least 2 weeks, but for no longer than 12 consecutive months.
3. The anatomical location, number, frequency, complexity, type, and severity of the tics change over time.
4. No history of Tourette syndrome or chronic motor or phonic tic disorder.
5. Onset before age 21 years.
6. Motor and/or phonic tics must be witnessed by a reliable examiner directly at some point in the illness or be recorded by videotape or cinematography.

D–2. Transient tic disorder by history

1. Single or multiple motor and/or phonic tics.
2. The tics occur many times a day (usually in bouts), nearly every day for at least 2 weeks, but for no longer than 12 consecutive months.
3. No history of Tourette syndrome or chronic motor or phonic tic disorder.
4. Onset before age 21 years.
5. Tics have not been witnessed by a reliable examiner, but tics were witnessed by a reliable family member or close friend, and the description of the tics as demonstrated is accepted by a reliable examiner.

E–1. Definite nonspecific tic disorder

1. Tics that do not meet the criteria for a specific tic disorder. An example is a tic disorder with onset in adulthood.
2. Motor and/or phonic tics must be witnessed by a reliable examiner directly at some point in the illness or be recorded by videotape or cinematography.

E–2. Nonspecific tic disorder by history

1. Tics that do not meet the criteria for a specific tic disorder. An example is a tic disorder with onset in adulthood.
2. Tics have not been witnessed by a reliable examiner, but tics were witnessed by a reliable family member or close friend, and the description of the tics as demonstrated is accepted by a reliable examiner.

F. Definite tic disorder, diagnosis deferred

1. Meets all criteria for a tic disorder, but duration of illness has not yet extended to one year, so that a distinction between a chronic and transient tic disorder cannot be made.

G. Probable ***Tourette syndrome***

Type 1. Fulfills all criteria for definite Tourette syndrome (A–1) completely, except for criteria 3 and/or 4.
Type 2. Fulfills all criteria for definite Tourette syndrome (A–1) except for criterion 1. This type can be either a single motor tic with phonic tics or multiple motor tics with possible phonic tic(s).
Subjects can be assigned to more than one diagnostic category. For example, an individual with definite chronic motor tics, but possible phonic tics, may be classified as having a definite chronic motor tic disorder, probably Tourette syndrome.

Adapted from Kurlan R. Tourette's syndrome: current concepts. Neurology 1989;**39**:1625–30. *Reproduced by kind permission of the American Academy of Neurology and Lippincott Williams and Wilkins.*

Tietze syndrome A syndrome of acute chest wall pain, probably due, for example, to Coxsackie virus infection.

tigroid demyelination Mottled hypointensity of the white matter on MRI scans in a radiating pattern, caused by the sparing of perivascular myelin in the context of dysmyelinating disease such as **Pelizaeus–Merzbacher disease** or other **leukodystrophies**. See also **leopard skin appearance**.

tilt test (tilt-table test) The measurement of heart rate and blood pressure over sequential 30-s periods, recorded both with the subject supine and with upright tilt to 65° after an initial 15-min lying supine. The normal response is for both heart rate and diastolic blood pressure to increase, while systolic pressure declines. The test examines aspects of sympathetic autonomic function. See also **neurocardiogenic syncope** and **postural orthostatic tachycardia syndrome**.

tilted disks An ocular anomaly occurring when the optic nerve leaves the globe at an unusually oblique angle. Focal ectasia or hypoplasia of the inferonasal retina is the underlying defect. The syndrome is characterized by high myopia and angulation of the optic disks which now point nasally and/or inferiorly, and which may lead to incomplete field defects, usually bitemporally.[6933]

tilting reaction Large labyrinthine postural reactions affecting the whole body and excited by bodily instability, especially angular displacement of the supporting base relative to the horizontal plane. They are designed to maintain the center of gravity of the individual within the vertical projection of its base. Such reactions are impaired or lost in the settings of Parkinsonism and other diseases of the basal ganglia.[4119]

time agnosia The illusionary appreciation of the passage of time without impairment of orientation in other spheres and in an otherwise unclouded sensorium, occurring as a feature of a chronic organic psychosyndrome. It has no precise localization.[1480]

time constant, EEG channel (TC) The product of the values of the resistance (in megohms) and the capacitance (in microfarads) which make up the time constant control of an EEG channel. This product represents the time required for the pen to fall to 37% of the deflection initially produced when a D.C. voltage difference is applied to the input terminals of the amplifier and is expressed in seconds (s). For a simple R-C coupling network, the time constant is related to the percentage reduction in sensitivity of the channel at a given stated low frequency by the equation $TC = 1/2f$, where f is the frequency at which a 30% (3 Db) attenuation occurs at 0.5 Hz. Thus, either the time constant or the percentage attenuation at a given stated low frequency can be used to designate the same position of the low-frequency filter of the EEG channel. See also **low-frequency filter**. (Adapted from the 1974 report of the Committee on Terminology, IFCN. In: Chatrian GE, Bergamini L, Dondey M, et al. A glossary of terms most commonly used by clinical electroencephalographers. *EEG Clin Neurophysiol* 1974;**37**:538–48. Reproduced by kind permission of Elsevier Science and the IFCN.)

time dotting test A test of repetitive motor activity, in which the subject is required to place dots in small squares with the right and left hands separately, in each case for 30 s.

time zone change syndrome (jet lag) A condition characterized by difficulty in initiating or maintaining sleep, excessive sleepiness, decrements in subjective daytime alertness and performance, and somatic symptoms following rapid travel across multiple time zones.[1629]

timed functional testing Tests of the capacity of patients (with neuromuscular disease) to perform complex movements that reflect activities of everyday living (**functional tests**). The trials employed vary slightly for various diseases; thus, in **Duchenne dystrophy**, the ability to stand, climb 4 steps, and walk 30 ft (9 m) are examined; in **amyotrophic lateral sclerosis,** the ability to stand, climb 4 steps, walk 15–20 ft (4.5–6 m), speech rate, and pegboard tests are assessed; in **hereditary motor neuropathy,** the tests comprise the time taken to drink 120 ml of water, to stand, to climb 4 steps, and to walk 30 ft, and pegboard tests; while in **myotonic dystrophy,** standing, climbing 4 steps, walking 30 ft, and cutting out a 3-inch (7.5 cm) square are the activities examined.[4524]

timed manual performance test An instrument for assessing the performance of structured fine and gross manual motor tasks, based on observations of activities performed under timed conditions.[6800]

Tinel, Jules (1879–1952) French neurologist who trained in Rouen and Paris, becoming a student of **Landouzy** and **Déjèrine** during his further training. He became chef de clinique at the **Salpêtrière** but left to perform military service.

His description of the sign of regenerating nerve fibers appeared in his book on gunshot injuries to nerves, and arose from his experiences in World War I. Before World War II he had reduced active practice because of cardiac disease but, with all his family, played an active role in the Resistance, for which his son paid with his life.

Tinel sign Paresthesias felt in the distal distribution of a sensory nerve when it is percussed, indicating the presence of regenerating nerve fibers at the site percussed.[6327] A motor variant has been described[4452] in which tapping a motor nerve leads to twitching of distal muscles supplied by that nerve.

Hoffmann also described the sign in 1915, a few months before Tinel did, but from the opposing side at a time when it was not literature that was being exchanged.

tinnitus (Lat, ringing in the ears) (tinnitus aurium, subjective tinnitus) Hallucinatory sounds caused by disturbance of the cochlea or VIII cranial nerve (in 80% of cases) or occurring with disease in the CNS (in 20% of cases).[3741] In either case, the perception of sounds originating from inside the head. Such sounds may be constant or intermittent, steady or pulsatile, and may be described as humming, buzzing, whistling, or ringing.[3969] The causes are legion, but the pathophysiology is poorly defined, both neural and cochlear mechanisms being suggested. In most cases, some hearing loss is associated.

Objective tinnitus signifies the presence of such sounds appropriately heard by a patient with, for example, carotid artery stenosis, an arteriovenous communication such as a **glomus jugulare tumor** or **palatal myoclonus**.

tinnitus aurium See **tinnitus**.

tip-of-the-tongue phenomenon A form of anomia or word-finding difficulty in which the subject is keenly aware that the word sought is partially recalled and close to discovery, but still cannot be brought forth without facilitatory phonetic or semantic cues. The phenomenon occurs in normal subjects and in those with Parkinsonism.[1169] See also **word production anomia**.

tired arm syndrome See **Wartenberg cheiralgia paresthetica**.

Tissot, Simon-André (1728–1797) Swiss physician who trained in Geneva and Montpelier before entering practice in Lausanne, where his early fame rested on his success in combating an outbreak of the smallpox using Jennerian vaccination. In 1750 he published *Traité de l'onanisme*, a work strongly condemning masturbation; this was widely successful on account of its popular appeal and brought him a pension, membership of the Royal Society of London, and an international reputation, which would not quite have been justified by his other publications on psychiatric topics—although many of his ideas seem to have antedated those of Freud and he did give the first recorded descriptions of simple absence and of myoclonic seizures.

titinopathies Rare recessively inherited forms of limb girdle muscular dystrophy due to mutations of titin, a large peptide, which are the cause of **tibial muscular dystrophy**, **limb-girdle muscular dystrophy** (LGMD2J), and dilated cardiomyopathy.[3454]

titubation (from Lat, to stagger)
1. A rhythmic anteroposterior (to-and-fro) or side-to-side head or body tremor at about 2–5 Hz resulting from cerebellar lesions.
2. Restlessness, a staggering gait, and incoordination due to cerebellar disease (nineteenth century).

tobacco-alcohol amblyopia (nutritional optic neuropathy) Optic atrophy resulting from deficiency of B complex vitamins, initially confined to the papillomacular bundle, described first by Dr. Wordsworth, an English physician, in 1863. See **nutritional amblyopia**.

Tobey, George Loring (1881–1947) American otolaryngologist.

Tobey–Ayer Test Failure of the CSF pressure (measured at lumbar puncture) to rise during compression of one jugular vein, while pressure on the other one does cause a pressure increase. It suggests the presence of lateral sinus thrombosis on that side where compression does not change the CSF pressure. See also **Crowe Test**. The MRI is a much better guide, however.

Todd, Robert Bentley (1809–1860) Irish physician who trained in medicine in Dublin with **Graves** and at Oxford and was afterwards appointed professor of physiology and morbid anatomy and later dean of King's College, London, while continuing the practice of medicine. There he was a founder of the nursing school that trained Florence Nightingale.

He is remembered by neurologists for his (1854) description of postepileptic paralysis in a volume of clinical lectures in neurology, which was followed by two others on general medical topics. His full descriptions of the neurological symptoms, signs, and syndromes led to his depiction as "the greatest neurologist that Britain had produced until the time of Hughlings-**Jackson**" (Collier, cited by Spillane[5978]).

Todd paralysis (postepileptic paralysis, postconvulsive palsy, postictal hemisyndrome) A neurological deficit in a body part following a focal epileptic seizure, associated with focal or generalized slowing or absence of EEG activity and lasting for up to 36 h. The paralysis (or aphasia, or sensory deficit) is in many cases an aid to the localization of the underlying lesion and a confirmation of the focal rather than the generalized nature of the seizure.[6337]

Todd described both hemiparesis and hemianesthesia ("epileptic hemiplegia") as postepileptic manifestations in a book of lectures that he had given at Kings College Hospital over the previous 10 years (London, Churchill, 1854), but the phenomenon had already been described by J.C. Prichard in 1822. He pointed out that the paralysis may be bilateral but worse on one side, and that it may last from hours to days. In the few cases examined pathologically, focal or generalized brain disease was remarked.

It would be reasonable to regard the confusion and generalized weakness which follow generalized tonic-clonic (grand mal) seizures (postictal confusion) as having exactly the same mechanism, namely either active inhibition due to postictal hyperpolarization or else functional exhaustion of the overstimulated area due to local (or generalized) cortical anoxia.[4342]

toe reflex Forcible flexion of the hallux leads to tightening of all the leg muscles below the knee in normal people, but more so in patients with pyramidal tract lesions.

1. The *great toe phenomenon of Edelmann* consists of dorsiflexion of the hallux in response to passive flexion of the hip when the knee is extended. It is a minor sign of meningeal irritation.[1500]
2. The *little toe reflex of Puusepp* consists of slow adduction of the little toe when the outer border of the foot is stroked.[1500] Although a sign of extrapyramidal disease, it has no precise localizing value.

toe walking Tightness of the heel cords (Achilles' tendon), either as an isolated problem or as a manifestation of muscle contracture in severe dystrophies.[869]

toilet seat neuritis See **saturday night palsy**.

Token test A test for latent receptive dysphasia in patients with hemispheric lesions, the results yielded correlating strongly with the results of tests of auditory verbal comprehension.[1605] In the test, subjects are instructed verbally to touch or otherwise manipulate large and small, round and square counters of five different colors in response to commands of increasing complexity.[1517, 725]

Tollner syndrome A congenital dysmorphic syndrome characterized by atrioventricular septal defect, horseshoe kidneys, polydactyly, macrocephaly, and hydrocephalus.[6339]

Tolosa, Eduardo Spanish neurosurgeon in Barcelona who described the **superior orbital fissure syndrome** in 1954.[6342]

Tolosa–Hunt syndrome See **superior orbital fissure syndrome**.

toluene encephaloneuropathy See **glue sniffers' neuropathy**.

tomaculae Strings of sausage-shaped swellings in peripheral nerves, representing segmental expansion of the damaged myelin sheaths.

tomaculous neuropathy (from Lat, a sausage) A pathological feature in some neuropathies, consisting of sausage-shaped thickenings of the myelin sheaths of between 80 and 250 μM, affecting fibers of all sizes and usually accompanied by segmental demyelination with remyelination and early onion bulb formation. The clinical accompaniments include recurrent brachial plexus neuropathy, pressure-sensitive neuropathy, or sensorimotor polyneuropathy.[4969] In most cases there is a genetic basis.[5530] See **hereditary pressure-sensitive neuropathy**.

Tondeur syndrome See **sialuria**.

tone (tonus) 1. The resistance of muscles to passive stretch. 2. A defined frequency of vibration. 3. A manner of speech or other behavior.

tone decay A hearing test using pure tone audiometry in which continuous tones are repeatedly presented at threshold intensity. Patients with cochlear nerve lesions, but not those with lesions of the cochlea itself, perceive such tones as decreasing in loudness and eventually disappearing.

Tong sign An alternative method for eliciting the **Babinski** response, in which the lateral plantar surface is stroked while the knee is hyperextended.

tongue-blade (tongue-point) sounds See **linguals**.

tonic (from Gr, pitch or tension) 1. See **tone** (definition 1). 2. Continuously occurring or persistent.

tonic absences (retropulsive absences) Atypical absences accompanied by mild tonic contractions, especially in the neck muscles.

tonic arousal A state of alert arousal for which the mesencephalic RAS is responsible. Unilateral lesions of that structure produce contralateral neglect, while bilateral lesions cause coma.[6672]

tonic cerebellar fits 1. Acute attacks of vertigo, with clouding of consciousness seen in patients with cerebellar tumors, described by Sir Gordon **Holmes** in 1904. 2. Attacks of retraction of the head, arching of the back, flexion and supination of the elbows, and plantar flexion of the toes, occurring in association with tumors of the cerebellar vermis and likely to be a form of decorticate response.

tonic-clonic motor seizures Epileptic sequences consisting of a tonic followed by a clonic phase.[16] They may involve the brainstem, possibly the prefrontal cortex and basal ganglia. Ictal initiation of primarily bilateral events is predominantly disinhibitory, but other mechanisms are responsible for ictal evolution to the clonic phase, involving gradual periodic introduction of seizure-suppressing mechanisms. The mechanism of tonic seizures is probably not the same as of the tonic phase of GTCS. They are seen in **Lennox–Gastaut syndrome** and occasionally with **myoclonic astatic seizures**.[1861]

tonic convergence reaction of pupils See **Holmes–Adie syndrome**.

tonic foot response Persistent plantar flexion of the ankle as a result of diffuse cerebral disease. It interferes with walking, as the foot may remain "stuck" to the ground—the *magnetic foot*.

tonic innervation The term of **Wilson** and **Walshe**[6820] for a delay in the relaxation of a voluntary contraction, resulting in an inability to relax the grasp in the paretic arm of a patient affected by hemiparesis due to frontal lobe lesions affecting the premotor area (Area 6 of Brodmann).

Differentiation from **gegenhalten** and **perseveration** is difficult, but tonic innervation is often associated with motor apraxia and always with pyramidal signs. **Grasping** and **groping** reactions are often associated.

tonic inverse masticatory activity Paradoxical contraction of a muscle that normally closes the mouth only when the subject is trying to open it. This form of **dystonia** is seen with lesions in the cerebello-pontine angle. The condition thus resembles hemimasticatory dystonia caused by brainstem lesions.[3754]

tonic labyrinthine reflexes Extension of the neck of babies lying in the supine position, and flexion of the neck when lying in the prone position; also extension of the arms of the prone child aged more than 4 months when the chin is passively raised. Children of this age with cerebral palsy may respond to chin elevation with flexion of the arms or tonic extension of the arms and flexion of the legs.[3080]

tonic motor seizure A sustained increase in muscle contraction lasting between seconds and minutes.

tonic neck reflex 1. *Asymmetrical response*: extension of the arm on turning of the head to one side while the normal baby is lying quietly in the supine position. The arm may extend fully with further rotation of the neck. This reflex is normally lost by the third month but persists in children with spasticity. 2. *Symmetrical response*: extension of the arms with flexion or extension of the neck.[6898] Such postural changes induced by afferent stimuli from the neck muscles were first demonstrated by Magnus and de Kleijn in animals after total labyrinthine extirpation. See also **developmental reflexes**.

tonic palmar reflex Slow flexion and adduction of the thumb, flexion of the other fingers, and increased palmar concavity in response to linear tactile stimulation of the palm going from proximal to distal.[757]

tonic perseveration The term of Liepmann for the inability to relax any muscle group or groups owing to the presence of a central lesion. Wilson and Walshe[6820] substituted the term **tonic innervation**.

tonic plantar response Slow and persistent flexion and adduction of the toes and of the ankle in response to gentle stroking of the sole of the foot. This is a sign of extrapyramidal disease, but is otherwise not localizing.

tonic pupil See **Holmes–Adie syndrome**.

tonic seizures Epileptic seizures lasting 10–20 s and predominantly occurring during the night, almost exclusively during NREM sleep in children, and consisting of tonic contractions of various muscle groups without progression to any clonic phase but sometimes causing the child to fall to the ground as a result of leg flexion. Respiratory arrhythmias, tachycardia, mydriasis, flushing, salivation, and loss of consciousness, accompanied by slow-spike and slow-wave complexes on the EEG are other features. During the tonic seizure, the EMG shows muscle activity similar to that occurring during voluntary contraction.

This seizure pattern is seen most commonly in the **Lennox–Gastaut syndrome** among individuals who are intellectually impaired and who may manifest multiple other seizure types.[2315]

tonic status epilepticus A restricted form of seizure, most commonly seen in patients with symptomatic generalized epilepsy, but also in those with the idiopathic form. Characteristically, the supine patient's neck is flexed with the arms flexed at the elbow and slightly elevated. The tonic spasms are brief and can continue intermittently for hours—longer still in symptomatic generalized epilepsy.[1861] See also **status epilepticus**.

tonic tics See **tics**.

tonic torsion neurosis See **dystonia**.

tonic vibration reflex Tonic muscle contraction normally evoked by the effect of vibration on primary spindle endings. It is diminished on the side of a hemiparesis and lost below a spinal cord lesion.[941]

tonotopy Functional localization in the auditory cortex, wherein there is spatial representation of different tones.

tonsillar herniation Downward extrusion of the cerebellar tonsils into the foramen magnum, leading to compression of the caudal medulla. This typically results from expansion of a mass lesion in the posterior fossa. Reduction in conscious level, neck rigidity, skew deviation of the eyes, and vomiting are the associated clinical signs, preceding the appearance of irregular respirations, apnea, bradycardia, and death.

tonus See **muscle tone**.

Tooth, Howard Henry
(1856–1926) English neurologist who trained at Cambridge and St. Bartholomew's Hospital, where he was later appointed physician. He was also on the staff at the **National Hospital** and was active in army medicine during the Boer and First World wars.

He described **hereditary motor and sensory neuropathy** as *the peroneal type of progressive muscular atrophy* (London, 1886) and wrote importantly on the pathology of spinal cord degeneration and on cerebral tumors.

toothbrushing epilepsy An unusual form of **reflex epilepsy** provoked by the act (or the thought of the act) of toothbrushing. A medial temporal lobe origin is likely.

toothed trochlea phenomenon See **Negro sign**.

top of the basilar syndrome A stroke syndrome characterized by visual, oculomotor, and behavioral abnormalities, often without significant motor dysfunction, in which the lesions are confined to the territory of the distal branches of the posterior cerebral artery (or arteries). Rostral brainstem infarction produces oculomotor and pupillary signs identical to those in thalamic hemorrhage, sometimes with somnolence, vivid hallucinations, and dreamlike behavior. Temporal and occipital infarctions are often accompanied by hemianopia with distinctive characteristics such as fragments of the Balint syndrome, amnestic dysfunction, and agitated behavior. The cause is usually embolic.[1007] Two major forms are defined:

1. *Rostral brainstem infarction* (the syndrome of the mesencephalic artery) is characterized by disorders of vertical gaze, convergence spasm on attempted lateral gaze, convergence retraction nystagmus, pseudo-sixth, Collier sign, lightning-like oscillations of the eyes, skew deviation of the eyes, and corectopia with loss of the pupillary responses.
2. *Posterior cerebral artery territory hemispheric infarction* commonly leads to partial hemianopia with awareness of the deficit and complaints of surrounding scintillations, visual perseveration, and anomic aphasia, alexia without agraphia, or visual agnosia when the infarct is unilateral. With bilateral infarcts, asimultagnosia, apraxia of gaze, metamorphopsia, memory deficits, sensory loss, and agitated delirium are typical findings.[1007]

topesthesia (Gr, a place + sensation) Local sensibility to touch.

topognosis (locognosis) Localization of a point of contact on the body; a function identified by A.W. Volkmann in 1844.

topographic amnesia (topographical disorientation) A disorder of finding one's way about familiar environments and of learning to navigate new ones. The problem may represent the effect of a disorder of spatial memory coupled with a failure to recognize places and has been described in a patients with right temporal lobe disease.[4201]

topographical agnosia (body-image agnosia) 1. Failure of localization of a point of contact on the body. 2. Failure to identify the proper placing of cities, etc., on a map, inability to find defined places within a town, or to locate a specific room in a house. The disturbance in visuospatial memory is a form of visual agnosia and is associated with bilateral or right-sided posterior (occipitoparietal) lesions.

topography The distribution of the amplitudes of EEG activity at the surface of the head, in the cerebral cortex, or in the depths of the brain.

topographic disorientation See **topographic amnesia**.

TOPOSCOUT A "user-friendly" computer-based system designed to analyze the presenting clinical features in a case of cerebrovascular disease in order to identify the most likely stroke territory.[5995] See also **microstroke**.

torcular Herophili (Lat, wine-press, from the verb *to twist*) The confluence of the dural venous sinuses posteriorly.

Toriello–Carey syndrome A rare syndrome comprising agenesis of the corpus callosum, telecanthus, small palpebral fissures, Pierre Robin sequence, abnormal ears, nuchal laxity and cardiac defects, Hirschsprung disease, and moderate to severe developmental delay.[67]

Torkildsen shunt The operation of ventriculocisternostomy, performed as a palliative procedure for aqueductal stenosis. It was introduced by A. Torkildsen, a Norwegian neurosurgeon, in 1939.[6357]

tornado epilepsy (epilepsia rotatoria) A form of seizure disorder characterized by recurrent vertigo and falling; it is only differentiated from **benign paroxysmal vertigo of childhood** by the greater age of the patient and by the abnormality in the EEG, which usually suggests the presence of a lesion in a temporal lobe. The condition was first described (as *epilepsia rotatoria*) by Arnold Pick in 1903.[4668]

Tornwaldt disease The presence of a cyst formed by occlusion of the orifice of a nasopharyngeal bursa, leading to local abscess formation and nasopharyngeal stenosis and presenting clinically with occipital headache or glossopharyngeal neuralgia.[6043] Dr. Gustav Tornwaldt (1843–1910) was a German physician.

Toronto Stenosis index A method of determining the degree of narrowing of the internal carotid artery (ICA) from angiograms in which the diameter of the stenotic region is compared with the expected diameter of the ICA as assessed by its usual relationship (120%) to that of the common carotid artery.[672]

Toronto Western Spasmodic Torticollis Rating Scale (TWSTRS) A new instrument for rating this disorder. See the Web site: http://www.mdvu.org/library/ratingscales/dystonia/PadwChart.11.pdf/.

torosity (from Lat, muscular sheath) Muscular strength.

torpescence See **torpor**.

torpid (Lat, to be sluggish) Dull, stupid, or inactive.

torpor (torpescence) The state in which a part of the body or the whole organism becomes numbed, unreactive to external stimuli, and disinclined to move.

torsion dystonia See **dystonia**.

torsion dystonia with basal ganglion lucencies See **dystonia**.

torsion dystonia, X-linked A *variant* X-linked dystonic syndrome of childhood or early adult onset, manifesting also sensorineural deafness and mental and developmental delay. See **dystonia**.

torsion spasm Slow, forceful, twisting dystonic movements at the neck, shoulder, hip, and trunk, representing proximal dystonic movements.[6868]

torsional nystagmus (rotary nystagmus) That form of central vestibular nystagmus in which the movement of the globe is about the anteroposterior axis, increases after active rotation of the head and is suppressed by convergence. Such rotations of the eyes occur when they are close to the central position, are usually associated with lesions of the medulla and are often accompanied by an **ocular tilt reaction**.[5731] The upper pole of the iris usually beats (has its fast component) away from the damaged side. The disorder may be congenital in origin, but is also seen with thalamic, pontine, or lateral medullary lesions disrupting central vestibular connections.[4500, 4710] See also **rotatory nystagmus**.

torticollis (from Lat, twist + a neck) (wry-neck) A focal dystonia causing intermittent or persistent rotation of the neck, and frequently part of a generalized dystonic state. Cruchet gave the first modern description.[1362] In infancy, torticollis may occur in association with hematomas of the sternomastoid.[3840] Guillaume Dupuytren (1823) in France and W.W. Keen (1891) in America advised, respectively, section of the sternocleidomastoid muscle and of the spinal accessory nerve for its relief.[5617]

In a *variant* form, the torticollis is associated with sternomastoid myopathy and neuropathy of the spinal accessory nerve.[5550] See **spasmodic torticollis**.

torulosis *Cryptococcus neoformans* meningitis, often combined with granulomatous pulmonary, dermal, and mucosal lesions. See **cryptococcal meningitis**. The condition was described first in man by James L. Stoddard (b. 1899) and Elliott C. Cutler, both American pathologists.

total lipodystrophy An uncommon condition characterized by the complete loss of body fat, sometimes associated with diabetes mellitus, hepatomegaly, hyperpigmentation, hyperlipidemia, and renal disease. Peripheral neuropathy is an occasional complication.[6415]

Total Neuropathy score A composite measure of peripheral nerve function, scoring sensory and motor and autonomic symptoms, pinprick and vibration sensibility, motor power, muscle stretch reflexes, quantitative vibratory sensory testing, and the amplitude of sural and peroneal sensory nerve action potentials.[1287]

total sleep period The period of time from the onset of sleep to final awakening, and including the time spent in brief arousals.

total sleep time The total amount of time spent asleep during a sleep period, not including the time spent in arousals.

tottering gait See **subcortical dysequilibrium**.

touch epilepsy (tap seizures) A rare form of stimulus-sensitive seizure disorder in which myoclonic seizures are evoked by touch without clinical, radiologic, or EEG evidence of lateralized lesions in children who are usually developmentally normal and who have normal EEG background activity. It has also been reported in children with diffuse degenerative encephalopathies.[605]

touch sensation The faculty of awareness of the contact of an object with the skin. Though not obviously subdivisible, nevertheless the sensation is bipartite, consisting both of a crude awareness of a contact and a discriminative perception of the nature of the object. Impulses subserving the former are considered to be carried centrally in the spinothalamic tracts, and possibly even perceived at the thalamic level; those for the latter ascend in the posterior columns and relay in the thalamus, because they require the discriminatory functions of the parietal cortex.

Toulouse reflex See **buccal reflex**.

Tourette, George-Edmond-Albert-Brutus Gilles de la (1857–1904) A colorful and versatile French neuropsychiatrist who was born in Vienne and died in Lausanne. Described as a clever but unruly boy, he studied medicine in Poitiers and afterwards went to Paris, becoming a favorite pupil of **Charcot** at the **Salpêtrière**, but (like **Babinski**) he was never appointed to its faculty. He was prolific in his literary output in medicine (concentrating upon syphilis, hysteria, and neurasthenia), and also published on social and political reform, literature, forensic medicine, and aspects of medical history. In 1884, the year he joined Charcot, he described Jumping, Latah, and Myriatchit (considering all to be the same condition) and in the following year gave a complete description of the syndrome which bears his euphonious name, stimulated by his reading of George **Beard**'s account of jumping disease (**hyperekplexia**). The disease, however, had already been described by **Itard** in 1825.

In 1893, two tragedies occurred from which Tourette never fully recovered—his son died and he himself was shot by a paranoid female patient in his consulting room, but he returned to active practice and to historical and other writing until his death.[5704]

Tourette syndrome (maladie des tics compulsifs/impulsifs, compulsive tics, multiple tic syndrome, imubacco)

A dominantly inherited syndrome with incomplete penetrance, characterized by recurrent, involuntary, repetitive, rapid, purposeless motor movements of variable intensity affecting several muscle groups; similar involuntary utterances occur at some time during the duration of the disorder, which lasts for over a year. The tics can be suppressed voluntarily for a short time. They often occur daily, with variable location, severity, and complexity, and last a lifetime. The responsible gene maps to 18q22.1.

The first recorded sufferer was the French Prince of Condé, who had to stuff cloths into his mouth to stop himself barking at King Louis XIX. In 1825, Dr. Jean-Marie-Gaspard Itard reported (*Arch Gen Med* 8:403–7) the case of the Marquise de Dampierre, who had begun to tic at the age of seven and later uttered bizarre cries and meaningless phrases; her symptoms abated with milk-bath treatments in Switzerland, but worsened after her marriage, and henceforward included severe coprolalia, forcing her to become a recluse for the rest of her life. She died, still cursing, at the age of 85. **Trousseau** mentioned her case briefly in his *Clinique médicale* of 1867. More important people who may have suffered from this disorder include Dr. Samuel Johnson and W.A.Mozart.

Tourette gave a long, broad but incomplete description of the syndrome in 1885,[6360] while a 28-year-old student of **Charcot**, and the eponym was granted when C.L. **Dana** attributed it in the following year, even though Tourette had incorporated Itard's case into his paper. In the same year, Georges Guinon described five further cases, commenting on the abnormal mental state but not emphasizing the compulsive behavior. Ten years later, **Brissaud** described "chorea variabilis," which is now considered to be Tourette syndrome. In 1899, Tourette wrote a summary paper, accepting that mental symptoms were also characteristic of the disease. Despite Tourette's original title, **latah, myriachit** and **jumping** (the jumping Frenchmen of Maine) are different diseases. Tourette mentioned in his thesis (1885) that Itard (1825) and Trousseau had also noted this syndrome, but they did not explore it in depth. He described nine cases (five of them his own), all characterized by the combination of tics, jumps, and echo- and coprolalia.

Criteria for the diagnosis of Tourette syndrome include the following:[172]

A. Presence of multiple motor and/or vocal tics at some time during the course of the illness, not necessarily concurrently.
B. Tics occur many times a day (usually in bouts), nearly every day or intermittently throughout a period of more than 1 year.
C. The anatomical location, number, frequency, and severity of the tics change over time.
D. Onset before the age of 21 years.
E. Occurrence not exclusively during psychoactive substance intoxication or known CNS disease such as **Huntington disease** and postviral encephalitis.

Echolalia (Gr, echo + speech) (the repetition of words or phrases) is also common, but **coprolalia** (the uttering of obscenities) occurs in only a third of patients, though it captures the imagination of everybody. Associated obsessive-compulsive behavior, attention-deficit disorder, and sleep disturbances are other characteristics.[172] Tic disorders other than Tourette syndrome are distinguishable only by the absence of coprophenomena and of vocalizations. Whether they are regarded merely as partial expressions of a dominant condition depends on the attitude of the observer rather than upon evidence. See also **tic disorder**.

Tourette Syndrome Association A national, nonprofit organization dedicated to finding the cause and cure of Tourette syndrome. Web site: http://www.tsa-usa.org/. See also the National Institute of Neurological Disorders and Stroke: Tourette Syndrome Fact Sheet at http://.ninds.nih.gov/disorders/tourette/tourette.htm/, which includes definitions, possible causes, treatments, and information on current research.

Tourette Syndrome Diagnostic Confidence index A weighted diagnostic schedule rating coprolalia, echo phenomena, complex tics, temporal features, subjective experiences, tic severity and duration, and confirmatory features.[5331]

Tourette Syndrome Association of Australia A nonprofit organization of people with Tourette syndrome, their families, health and education professionals, and other interested people. It provides educational materials, telephone counseling, parent advocacy, a newsletter, and support groups. Web site: http://www.tourette.org.au/.

Tourette Syndrome Foundation of Canada A charitable organization providing support and information on this condition. Address: 238 Davenport Road, Box 343, Toronto, ON M5R 1J6 Canada. Tel: 416-351-7757; 1-800-361-3120. Web site: http://www.tourette.ca/.

Tourette syndrome global scale A scale attempting to give semiquantitative ratings of the various phenomena of Tourette syndrome such as simple and complex motor tics or rituals, simple or complex phonic tics, and aspects of social functioning such as behavior in the company of other people, motor restlessness, and difficulties in school or at work.[2747] A quality-of-life scale for this condition has also been developed. (Cavanna AE, et al. *Neurology* 2008;71:1410)

Tourette Syndrome "Plus" A Web site providine information and support in this disease area, at http://www.tourettesyndrome.net/.

Tournay sign (Gianelli sign) Dilation of the pupil of the abducting eye after about 5 s of extreme lateral deviation, seen in normal people and in those with **Horner syndrome.**[5333] The sign has no known diagnostic value. Dr. A. Tournay (b. 1878) was a French ophthalmologist who described the sign in 1917, 10 years after Gianelli did.

tourniquet paralysis (pneumatic tourniquet paralysis) Persisting conduction block at the upper and lower edges of an area of compression of peripheral nerves due to compressive ischemia, as occurs with the use of a tourniquet, which disrupts the myelin sheath of the nerves and causes conduction block.[730, 4435]

tourniquet test A test of pain tolerance and perception in which the subject is required to perform precisely graded manual exercise with occlusion of the circulation to the arm.[5911]

tower skull (turricephaly) Vertical enlargement of the skull as a result of premature fusion of the coronal and lambdoid sutures. See **Crouzon syndromes**.

toxic encephalopathy See **Dupré syndrome**.

toxic hydrocephalus (postinfectious encephalopathy, serous meningitis) Raised intracranial pressure following nasopharyngeal or otitic infections, occurring in children and adolescents. See **idiopathic intracranial hypertension, otitic hydrocephalus.**

toxic leukoencephalopathy White matter damage resulting from exposure to drugs, irradiation, chemicals, or environmental toxins and clinically causing variable degrees of cognitive deficit, impairment of consciousness, and reduction in movement. Pathological features progress from white matter edema through demyelination to axonal loss, particularly affecting white matter tracts devoted to higher cognitive functions.[2050] Inhalation of heroin vapor is a potent cause.

toxic oil syndrome (Spanish toxic oil syndrome) A syndrome of fever, pneumonitis, headache, myalgia, hepatitis, and eosinophilia, causing appreciable mortality in the acute stage and leading on to chronic sensorimotor peripheral neuropathy.

Adulteration of the olive oil used for cooking by aniline-treated rapeseed oil led to an epidemic of the disease in Spain in 1980.[6181] In other outbreaks in which cooking oil has been poisoned (for instance, in Jamaica and in Algeria), acrylamide or TOCP was the offending toxin.

toxic pseudomeningitis See **idiopathic intracranial hypertension**.

toxic psychosis An encephalopathy produced by metabolic disease or intoxication, presenting as a paranoid, delusional, or hallucinatory state in which the psychotic disturbance rather than inattention is the most salient feature. See **confusional state.**[4332]

toxic shock syndrome An acute illness induced by staphylococcal exotoxins, characterized by mucosal and skin lesions, upper respiratory symptoms, hypotension, nausea, vomiting and diarrhea, myalgia, and delirium proceeding in some cases to coma and death. Laboratory abnormalities include evidence of hepatic and renal damage, thrombocytopenia, and raised serum CK and myoglobin levels (in cases with muscle destruction).[1138]

toxic-nutritional amblyopia A form of optic neuropathy leading to subacute loss of the central fields, in some cases due to cyanide poisoning as a result of excessive tobacco exposure; in others due to the ingestion of alcohol or of other toxins.

toxin-induced sleep disorder A disorder characterized by either insomnia or excessive sleepiness produced by poisoning with heavy metals or organic toxins.[1629]

toxocariasis (visceral larva migrans) A systemic infection due to ingestion of the eggs of *Toxocara canis*, the developing larvae of which migrate extensively within the body. Encephalitis, myelitis, optic neuritis, and/or seizures are the usual clinical manifestations of neurological involvement, which is, however, uncommon. Some cases of **acute inflammatory demyelinating polyneuropathy** have been ascribed to this organism.[5016, 5949]

toxoplasmosis Infection with the protozoon *Toxoplasma gondii*. Acquired CNS toxoplasmosis was highly uncommon (except in immunosuppressed patients) before the AIDS epidemic, but syndromes of diffuse encephalopathy with or without seizures, of meningoencephalitis, or of progressively enlarging intracerebral mass lesions are now well-recognized neurological presentations.[5445, 6364, 1791] The usual systemic illness comprises an acute febrile illness with which lymphadenopathy and uveitis may be associated.

An association with **polymyositis** or **dermatomyositis** has been suggested but not proved. Congenital toxoplasmosis is an important cause of mental retardation with microcephaly and chorioretinopathy.[122]

TPHA, MHA-TP (*Treponema pallidum* hemagglutination test, microhemagglutination *treponema pallidum* test) Treponemal tests for syphilis which are more sensitive and more specific than the VDRL, and which, unlike that test, are persistently reactive following infection.[5852]

TPI (*Treponema pallidum* immobilization test) A specific diagnostic test for syphilis in which the motility of treponemes exposed to the patient's serum is recorded. Though sensitive, it is hard to perform and is not widely available.[5852]

trace alternant A discontinuous EEG pattern of nonrapid eye movement (quiet) sleep seen in preterm infants of 34 weeks conceptional age or older and which can persist for up to 3–4 weeks after birth in full-term infants. The pattern is characterized by bursts of predomintly slow waves (1–3 Hz, 50–100 μV) appearing approximately every 4–5s with intervening periods of low voltage activity (<50 μV, 4–7 Hz) (After Noachtar S, et al. A glossary of terms most commonly used by clinical electroencephalographers. *EEG Clin Neurophysiol* 1999;52[Suppl]:21–41. Reproduced by kind permission of the IFCN and Elsevier Science.)

trace continu Continuous EEG activity replacing a previously marked intermittent record during the evolution of the EEG in preterm infants. (After Noachtar S, et al. A glossary of terms most commonly used by clinical electroencephalographers. *EEG Clin Neurophysiol* 1999;52[Suppl]:21–41. Reproduced by kind permission of the IFCN and Elsevier Science.)

trace discontinu An EEG pattern of preterm infants below 34 weeks of conceptional age, characterized by mixed-frequency high-voltage bursts, separated by periods of very low background activity. (After Noachtar S, et al. A glossary of terms most commonly used by clinical electroencephalographers. *EEG Clin Neurophysiol* 1999;52[Suppl]:21–41. Reproduced by kind permission of the IFCN and Elsevier Science.)

tract (Lat, a pathway) An anatomically defined bundle of nerve fibers.

traction headache The headache of raised intracranial pressure, as a result of distortion of pain-sensitive structures inside the cranium.

traction response That flexion of the neck occurring when the infant lying supine is pulled gently and slowly up to the sitting position. Such flexion is usually seen by the end of the first month of life; by 3–5 months, the infant can pull against the examiner, flexing the arms at the elbow, and holding the neck and trunk in a straight line without any head lag.[6898, 3]

traction spurs Osteophytes projecting away from the disk space, as seen in the **segmental instability syndrome.**

tractotomy Surgical section of a specific fiber pathway in the spinal cord or medulla, usually for the relief of pain. High spinothalamic tractotomy was introduced by Achille Mario Dogliotti (1897–1966), an Italian neurosurgeon, for this purpose in 1938, the same year as Carl Sjoqvist (b. 1901) reported medullary trigeminal tractotomy.[4502]

trailmaking test A test of concentration, conceptual shifting, perceptual motor speed, and resistance to interference, wherein the subject first connects successive printed numbers with a pencil, and then connects 13 numbers/letters (e.g., 1-A-2-B-3-C and so on), thus continually alternating response strategies. As a result, it provides a sensitive indicator of the presence of **perseveration**. The trailmaking test is a part of the Halstead–Reitan Battery, and is sensitive to brain damage in either hemisphere. It is used mainly in the assessment of aging and dementia.[5259, 6639]

train nystagmus See **optokinetic nystagmus**.

train of stimuli A group of successive stimuli.

tramer reflex (contralateral abdominal proprioceptive reflex) Contraction of the abdominal muscles on the side opposite that on which a tap was made on the upper abdominal wall, described as a sign of basal ganglion disorders such as **Huntington disease**.[6368]

tramline calcification An X-ray appearance best seen in the occipital lobes in **Sturge–Weber** syndrome, consisting of a thin double line of calcification in two of the deeper cortical layers.

transcortical aphasias Those aphasias that are caused by large lesions of the cortex in the watershed areas, as occur after severe global reduction in cerebral perfusion, and which are characterized by preserved repetition with variably impaired comprehension and spontaneous output. They represent **disconnection syndromes**, the language areas now being out of touch with concepts and memories stored elsewhere in the brain. Three types are described, and are summarized in Chart T–3.

Chart T–3. The Transcortical Aphasias

Motor form: Spontaneous speech is nonfluent, effortful, and sparse with poor naming and a reduction in the drive to speak, but articulation, repetition, and comprehension are unaffected. The anomia is for category naming; object naming may be unimpaired. The causative lesion, anterior and superior to Broca's area, disconnects the frontal perisylvian speech zone from the supplementary motor area.[2186, 2905]

Sensory form: Speech is fluent and paraphasic, but comprehension and naming are impaired, as in Wernicke aphasia; repetition is retained. The lesion is usually at the border between the parietal and temporal lobes. While patients lose the meaning of words, they retain fluency and can carry on a conversation as articulation, phonology, and syntax remain intact. However, they do not comprehend well and have word finding difficulties.[2839, 3398]

Mixed form ("isolation of the speech area"): The findings resemble those of global aphasia, in that spontaneous speech is nonfluent or nonexistent, and comprehension, naming, reading, and writing are severely impaired and semantic paraphasias are evident. Repetition is, however, retained to the extent that the totality of the patient's speech echoes that of the examiner. The lesion is at the watershed areas between the middle and the anterior and the posterior cerebral arteries,[3408] and may be due to internal carotid occlusion with both pial and watershed infarcts.

Supplementary motor area aphasia is probably an identical condition.

transcortical aprosodia See **aprosodia**.

transcortical syndromes See **disconnection syndromes**.

transcranial Doppler sonography (TCD) The extension of the principles used in **continuous-wave Doppler sonography** of the carotid bifurcation to the basal cerebral arteries. A low-frequency pulsed Doppler sound wave is sent through the temporal bone, the orbit, and the foramen magnum, allowing determination of the direction and character of blood flow in the circle of Willis. Two- and three-dimensional representations of the velocity of blood flow in various vessels can be obtained by the newer machines, noninvasively.

TCD is used chiefly to detect cerebral vasospasm and to evaluate of the intracranial collateral pathways, but also to assess the degree of any intracranial vasoconstriction, to detect arteriovenous malformations, and to demonstrate absent blood flow in the case of suspected brain death.[1621, 4678]

transcranial electrical stimulation (TES) Stimulation of the cortex of the brain through the intact skull and scalp by means of a brief, very high voltage, electrical stimulus. Activation is more likely under the anode rather than the cathode. Because it is painful, this technique has largely been replaced by transcranial magnetic stimulation. (From the 2001 Report of the Nomenclature Committee of the American Association of Electromyography and Electrodiagnosis.[19] Reproduced by kind permission of the AANEM.)

transcranial magnetic stimulation Stimulation of the cerebral cortex by the creation of a brief intense magnetic field in the order of 1 to 2 Tesla generated by a bank of capacitors placed beside the cranium, which induces an electrical field in the subjacent tissues capable of depolarizing neurones and dendrites presynaptically. The procedure is thus able to provide measurements of **central conduction time** from the cortex to the spinal cord and to the muscles from which standard recordings of the compound muscle action potentials are made. (From the 2001 Report of the Nomenclature Committee of the American Association of Electromyography and Electrodiagnosis.[19] Reproduced by kind permission of the AANEM.)

The procedure is easily tolerated (each stimulus feels like a brisk blow to the head of a person wearing an army helmet) and apart from a possible risk of causing deafness, appears safe. Normative data for typical recording modes have been published.[1824]

transformed migraine A headache syndrome that represents an alteration in the patterm of previous migraine headaches, usually as a result of the too-frequent ingestion of agents that can cause medication-induced headache. The proposed diagnostic criteria are as follows,[5833] reproduced by kind permission of the American Academy of Neurology and Lippincott Williams and Wilkins.

A. Daily or almost-daily (>15 days/month) head pain for >1 month.
B. Average headache duration of >4 h/day (if untreated).
C. At least one of the following:
   1. History of episodic migraine meeting any IHS criteria 1.1–1.6.
   2. History of increasing headache frequency with decreasing severity of migrainous features over at least 3 months.
   3. Current headache meets IHS criteria for migraine 1.1–1.6 other than duration.
D. At least one of the following:
   1. There is no suggestion of one of the disorders listed in the ICHD, groups 5–11.
   2. Such disorder is suggested, but it is ruled out by appropriate investigations.
   3. Such disorder is present, but first migraine attacks do not occur in close temporal relation to the disorder.

transformational migraine

See **migraine with interparoxysmal headaches.**

transient and situational DIMS

A period of sleep disturbance related to a psychologically disturbing situation and lasting less than 3 weeks after this has ended, as defined in the ASDC Diagnostic Classification.[280] See also ASDA Diagnostic Classification,[1629] **sleep disorders**.

transient and situational DOES

The condition in which the normal sleep–wake pattern is disrupted as a result of a psychological disturbance related to life stress; the subject has trouble staying awake or is aware of an abnormal need to sleep, although the sleep architecture remains normal. The ASDC diagnostic classification[280] defined this state as occurring only for a maximum of 3 weeks after the initiating events. See also ASDA diagnostic classification,[1629] **sleep disorders**.

transient CNS deficits

A common, benign syndrome in young adults. The neurological deficits last less than 24 h. Losses of vision, power, balance, or coordination are those most commonly noted. Although the same definition may be used for **transient ischemic attacks**, in this context the term refers to episodes of neurological dysfunction unaccompanied by evidence of vasculopathy in young people who, over a median 5-year follow-up, exhibit no other evidence of neurological disease.[3814]

transient epileptic amnesia

An epileptic syndrome of older males, often with a history of heart disease, who have an average of three episodes per year comprising multiple brief (less than 1 h) episodes of pure amnesia, often preceded by an aura and occurring usually after a period of sleep. It may also cause brief episodes of transient anomia for people's names. Affected subjects frequently have a personal or past medical history of seizures and a history of past or current lesions of the brain in or near the mesial aspects of the temporal lobes. It is thought that the syndrome results from a disruption of antegrade and/or retrograde memory consolidation during sleep.[2349, 960]

Despite the lack of responsiveness, inappropriate speech and behavior, involuntary stereotyped movements, and reduction in ability to retain new information presented during the period of the event, some recollection of the episode may be possible afterwards. Bilateral mesial temporal lobe dysfunction is considered to be responsible and sleep EEGs may show bilateral temporal lobe discharges.[3300] See also **transient global amnesia**.

Diagnostic features have been suggested[2931] and are reproduced by kind permission of BMJ Publishing Group.

1. A history of recurrent episodes of transient amnesia.
2. Cognitive functions other than memory must be judged intact during a typical episode by a reliable witness.
3. Evidence of underlying partial epilepsy (reproducible epileptiform discharges on EEG; co-occurrence of other seizure types, if concurrent onset or close association with episodes of transient amnesia suggests a connection); and abolition or definite reduction in frequency of amnesic episodes with anticonvulsant therapy.

"Dr. Z," a patient of Hughlings **Jackson**, was so afflicted.

transient episodes of neurological dysfunction (TENDs)

This author's inclusive term for a symptom complex characterized by the occurrence of neurological deficits with a definable onset and termination and with periods of normality intervening. The term is proposed in order to recall the differential diagnosis of typical **transient ischemic attacks** which includes **migraine,** labyrinthine disorders, **papilledema,** cerebral tumor, epileptic seizures, **narcolepsy,** glaucoma, **multiple sclerosis, periodic paralyses,** nondystrophic **myotonias, episodic ataxias,** paroxysmal **dyskinesias, transient CNS deficits,** and long QT syndrome, all of which share the feature of being episodic and often brief in their occurrence. Almost another dozen similar conditions are entered below.

transneuronal degeneration

See **transsynaptic degeneration.**

transient global amnesia

An acquired syndrome of anterograde amnesia characterized by the sudden onset of inability to form new memories (and thus inability to recall newly presented information) and of uncertainty with regard to the current situation, leading to the futile repetitive questioning of companions. It occurs in elderly people and lasts minutes up to about 4 h, with a variable period of retrograde amnesia ensuing. There is no loss of consciousness, personal identity, nor insight, and the patient remains alert and may be able to perform complex activities. There are no physical signs.

Although once considered a manifestation of epilepsy, transient ischemia of the mesial temporal lobe structures is now considered the likely pathophysiology, perhaps as a manifestation of migraine or due to insufficiency of the jugular vein valves. The first description was that of Bender,[506] but 2 years later Fisher and Adams[2104] proposed the term now used. The following diagnostic criteria are modified from those of Caplan:[1009]

A. Attacks must be witnessed and reported by a capable observer present during the attack.
B. Anterograde amnesia occurs during the attack.
C. Consciousness is not clouded and there is no loss of personal identity; the cognitive impairment is limited to amnesia.
D. No focal neurological symptoms are present during the attack, nor are there significant neurological signs afterward.
E. No epileptic features occur.

F. The attack resolves within 24 h.
G. The patient does not have an active seizure disorder and has not suffered a recent head injury.

Adapted from Caplan LR. TGA criteria: what's in a name? *Neurology* 1986;36:1625. Reproduced by kind permission of the American Academy of Neurology and Lippincott Williams and Wilkins.)

A *variant* familial form has been reported.[1318, 4871]

Chart T–4. Diagnostic Criteria for Transient Ischemic Attacks

Time course: Symptoms develop within seconds, affecting several different parts of the body (e.g., face and arm) at the same time and resolve completely on clinical examination within 24 h., and usually within 1h. (Note: Any "march" of symptoms is more suggestive of migraine)
Symptoms of carotid TIA: Hemiparesis, aphasia, or transient monocular blindness.
Symptoms of vertebrobasilar TIA: Bilateral or alternating weakness or sensory symptoms. Sudden bilateral blindness in patients over 40 years of age.Vertigo, diplopia, dysphagia, ataxia, or drop attacks are accepted only if two or more of these occur together.
Symptoms of uncertain arterial territory: Hemianopia alone or dysarthria alone.
Symptoms explicitly not acceptable as TIA: Syncope, loss of consciousness or confusion, convulsion, incontinence of urine or of feces, dizziness, focal pain, focal symptoms associated with migraine headache, scintillating scotomata.

Based upon Dennis M, Bamford JM, Sandercock JM, Warlow CP. A comparison of risk factors and prognosis for transient ischemic attacks and minor ischemic strokes. Stroke *1989;20:1494–9.*
Comments: 1. While drop attacks are acceptable if occurring with other evidence of posterior circulation involvement, syncope is not, which may make for a difficult clinical decision.
2. By the older definition of TIA there should be no abnormality on imaging but that criterion has now been superseded by advances in technique.

transient headache with neurologic deficits and CSF lymphocytosis (HaNDL) A syndrome of unknown cause characterized by recurrent episodes of severe headache with temporary neurological deficits in various parts of the brain and increased CSF lymphocytes (and sometimes pressure). The patients are typically normal between attacks.[550]

transient idiopathic dystonia of infancy A form of segmental dystonia affecting infants in the first year of life, who present with an abnormal posture of one arm or on one side of the body while at rest. The problem disappears usually by the age of 18 months. The etiology is unknown.[6792]

transient ischemic attacks (from Lat, temporary + Gr, shortage + blood) Acute episodes of focal cerebral or ocular dysfunction lasting less than 24 h (actually usually 2–15 min) and caused by ischemia of the appropriate part of the cerebrum or retina and without neuroimaging evidence of acute infarction. Such ischemia may be either due to thromboembolism or to spasm of the arterial wall. Denny-Brown[1587] reviewed the phenomenology of such transient cerebrovascular episodes. The attacks can usually be localized to that portion of the brain supplied by one vascular system (left or right carotid or vertebrobasilar system).[4678] Diagnostic criteria (Chart T–4) have been suggested:[1581]

transient lone bilateral blindness The occurrence in youth or young adult life of transient bilateral blindness with abrupt onset over seconds, unaccompanied by any other features, lasting minutes and with a benign outcome. The cause is unkown but the condition is precipitated usually by exercise or postural change.[783]

transient monocular blindness (amaurosis fugax) Sudden temporary failure of sight; a term introduced by Posey in 1902, and now preferred to the alternative one named here.[2100] The usual cause is the presence of emboli from the carotid artery that have migrated to the retinal circulation, but glaucoma, migraine, and raised intracranial pressure are among the other causes.

transient movement disorders See **epilepsy, myoclonus, palatal essential tremor, jitteriness, shuddering attacks, transient idiopathic dystonia of infancy, spasmus nutans, benign paroxysmal torticollis of infancy, benign paroxysmal tonic upgaze, benign myoclonus of the newborn, benign myoclonus of infancy,** and **transient tic disorder.**[2024]

transient neonatal myasthenia See **neonatal myasthenia.**

transient tic disorder A condition with the same diagnostic criteria as **Tourette syndrome**, except that the tics have occurred for less than a year at the time of examination. It is a common event in school-aged children, and probably represents partial expression of the same condition, which is itself not uncommon.[3610]

transient tumor attacks The occurrence of episodes of nonepileptic, reversible cerebral dysfunction as a result of the presence of an intracranial tumor. The episodes include loss of vision, motor power, sensation, speech, or posture and last between minutes and 2 or 3 days. They allow no conclusion as to the nature or localization of the tumor, and their pathophysiology is also uncertain.[5419]

transient topographical amnesia A benign cognitive disorder of later adult life without sequelae or known cause, manifest as a temporary difficulty in finding ones way in a familiar place.[6085] See **topographic amnesia, transient global amnesia.**

transient visual obscurations Painless and fleeting reductions in vision of one or both eyes, classically in association with raised intracranial pressure but also occasionally due to other causes of elevated pressure in the optic nerve head.[5494]

transient wave Any isolated EEG wave or complex which can be distinguished from background activity.

transillumination test Applicable to the paranasal sinuses as well as to the head, the test compares the amount of light passing through the part examined to that transmitted in a normal subject. This subjective determination does not invalidate the test, so long as it has been performed and verified on numerous prior occasions. Increased transillumination of the skull suggests hydrocephalus. Decreased transillumination of the sinuses suggests local tumor or infection.

transitional diffuse sclerosis A leukoencephalopathy. The term is probably best regarded as a synonym for **adrenoleukodystrophy**.

transitional meningioma See **meningioma**.

transitional progressive multiple sclerosis An unusual presentation and course of **multiple sclerosis**.[2048]

transmantle pressure The difference between the ambient pressure in the subarachnoid space over the convexity and the intraventricular pressure. The difference is greatest with obstructive, and least with communicating, hydrocephalus.

transmissible dementias Prion diseases which involve an aberrant isoform of prion protein, present within the amyloid plaques of patients with such conditions and causing encephalopathy in animals and man. These include **scrapie** (in sheep and goats), **transmissible mink encephalopathy, chronic wasting disease** (in deer and elk), sporadic and familial **Creutzfeldt–Jakob disease, Gerstmann–Straussler syndrome, kuru**, and **bovine spongiform encephalopathy**.

transmissible mink encephalopathy A slow virus disease characterized by spongy changes and gliosis of the gray matter, occurring in mink and possibly analogous to **Creutzfeldt–Jakob disease** and **kuru** in man.

transmissible spongiform encephalopathies See **prion diseases**.

transplantation Neuromuscular complications in transplant recipients include **acute and chronic inflammatory demyelinating polyneuropathies** and toxic **myopathies**, related to the changes in immune modulation that occur after transplantation or to toxicity of immunosuppressant drugs. Myositis, **myasthenia gravis**, and multiple mononeuropathy result from a dysimmune systemic disorder such as posttransplant lymphoproliferative disorder, graft-versus-host disease, or hepatitis C virus or hepatitis B virus chronic infection. Compression or stretch of individual nerves or plexuses is common postoperatively.[1804]

transsynaptic degeneration (transneuronal degeneration) Secondary atrophy of neurons, whose cell bodies receive major excitatory influences from other neurons in the CNS, which themselves have atrophied as a result of disease. Thus, it is the result of a loss of afferent impulses. An example is the degeneration of some lower motor neurons in the spinal cord that occurs after a stroke in the contralateral hemisphere, and thus involves damage to the descending pyramidal tracts. The precise mechanism of the change is not known. See also **diaschisis**.

transtentorial herniation (clivus edge syndrome) See **uncal syndrome, Kernohan notch syndrome**.

transthyretin (prealbumin) An abnormal form of this substance polymerizes into amyloid fibrillary protein, deposited in the tissues of patients with **familial amyloid neuropathy**.

transverse bipolar montage See **coronal bipolar montage**.

transverse myelitis (idiopathic transverse myelitis) See **acute transverse myelitis**.

http://www.ninds.nih.gov/disorders/transversemyelitis/transversemyelitis.htm/ is an information site from the NIH.

transverse myelopathy An acute intrinsic ("intra-medullary") dysfunction of the spinal cord occurring bilaterally, affecting numerous segments and appearing without prior evidence of cord disease. Ropper and Poskanzer[5386] have summarized the causes as infectious, peri- or postinfectious or vaccinial, vascular, demyelinating, paraneoplastic, postirradiative, and secondary to vascular malformations.

transverse relaxation time See **T2 spin-spin**.

transverse temporal gyri See **Heschl gyri**.

trapezius (From Gr, a four-sided figure with no two sides parallel) A large superficial muscle of the upper back and neck.

trapezius aplasia A dominantly inherited syndrome mapped to 8q12.2, genetically close to hydrocephalus, **Duane syndrome**, and **Holt–Oram syndrome**.

trapezius hump A mound of the muscle which can be seen like the sunrise above the middle third of the clavicle in patients with girdle atrophy, both at rest and with arm elevation, when the trapezius contracts in an effort to fix the scapula.

trapshooter's cramp An occupational dystonia of the trigger finger occurring in competitive marksmen, the finger not obeying the willed command to squeeze the trigger at the appropriate time.[80] See **dystonias, yips, bowlers' cramp**.

Traquair, Harry Moss (b. 1876) Scottish ophthalmologist who refined and amplified the methodology and significance of charting the visual fields and introduced the concept of the "hill of vision," whereby not only the planar extent of the field but also its differing sensitivities on differing parts of the retina are charted.[6373]

Traquair scotoma (junctional scotoma) A central scotoma superimposed upon a bitemporal hemianopia due to compression of the optic chiasm.[6372]

Traub–Hering waves See C waves.

traumatic brain (injury) disease Brain injury following head trauma, usually as a result of abrupt deceleration. It may be diagnosed in the presence of the following:

A. Loss of consciousness of any duration following head injury.
B. Evidence of a neurological deficit following the trauma.
C. Evidence of focal brain damage revealed by clinical or laboratory methods.

The severity of brain injuries has been classified (Chart T–5).

Relevant Web sites include the following:

http://www.neuro.pmr.vcu.edu/ (National Resource Center for Traumatic Brain Injury) This provides information for professionals and people with brain injury.

http://www.ninds.nih.gov/disorders/tbi/tbi.htm (NINDS Traumatic Brain Injury Information) A fact sheet on definitions, treatment methods, prognosis, current research projects, and references.

http://www.nidcd.nih.gov/health/voice/tbrain.asp (Traumatic Brain Injury: Cognitive and Communication Disorders) A fact sheet discussing oblems, assessment, treatment, and research related to TBI.

http://www.tbidirectory.com/ (The Traumatic Brain Injury Directory) providing a list of brain injury programs, services, and resources in the USA.
http://www.mja.com.au/public/issues/178_06_170303/kha11095_fm.html/ (Rehabilitation After Traumatic Brain Injury) reviews the types of TBI and their treatment and prognosis (from the Medical Journal of Australia).

traumatic neuralgia See causalgia.

traumatic neuroma (amputation neuroma) A bulbous mass at the end of an injured peripheral nerve, largely composed of disorganized neurites and fibrous tissue.

Chart T–5. Classification of Traumatic Brain Disease

Mild brain injury: Following a transient loss of consciousness there is no focal neurological deficit and consciousness is regained rapidly. Posttraumatic amnesia (PTA) is less than 1 h.
Moderate brain injury: There is still impaired consciousness or disorientation 1 h after injury but the the patient can obey commands; or the patient is alert but shows evidence of a focal deficit. PTA is from 1–24 h.
Severe brain injury: The patient cannot follow commands after the injury and, if he can speak, words are used inappropriately. The best motor response is the ability to localize stimuli. PTA of 1–7 days is usual.
Very severe brain injury: The patient's eyes are closed soon after the injury, despite intense stimulation; words cannot be uttered, nor commands followed, and the best motor response is posturing. The threat to life is severe; if death does not occur, a **persistent vegetative state** may ensue. PTA is longer than 7 days, if it can be assessed.

See also **mild brain injury**.
In *severe traumatic brain injury* the combination of focal and diffuse brain lesions leads to a complex syndrome characterized by disorders of memory, attention, and executive function, slowed information processing and changes in personality and behavior, correlating poorly with the results of brain imaging studies.[2151]

traumatic spreading depression syndrome (postcontusion seizure syndrome, **juvenile** head trauma syndrome) Early convulsions following mild or trivial head injuries in infants and young children, or other transient neurological signs (headache, nausea, somnolence, vomiting, confusion, alteration in consciousness, aphasia, hemiparesis) occurring in the same context but following a lucid (asymptomatic) interval in children and adolescents, with complete recovery. The condition is considered by Ohtahara et al.[4777] to represent the clinical effects of the **spreading depression of Leao**.

Treacher Collins syndrome See **mandibulofacial dysostosis.**

Tredgold, Alfred Frank (1870–1952) English physician who trained at the London Hospital and devoted his life to the subject of mental retardation. His book *Mental Deficiency* (1908) was a landmark, consolidating knowledge to that time. In it, Tredgold gave the first account of *idiots savants*.

trefoil canal The fancied cloverleaf shape of the spinal canal in a congenital variant of the normal, or as a result of degenerative hypertrophy of the lumbar facets. In either case, the cross-sectional area of the canal is diminished, and symptoms of **spinal stenosis** may appear.[252]

Treft syndrome A dominantly inherited syndrome of childhood characterized by optic atrophy, visual failure, ophthalmoplegia with ptosis, and deafness.[5449]

trekker's shoulder See **upper brachial plexus palsy, rucksack palsy.**

tremblement affirmatif A vertical or nodding movement of the head, in which the amplitude of the oscillations increases rather than decreases with voluntary movement. It is seen in **essential tremor**, but also in some elderly people who have no other evidence of that condition.

tremblement negatif A horizontal shaking movement of the head, in which the amplitude of the oscillations increases rather than decreases with voluntary movement. It is seen in **essential tremor**, but also in some elderly people who have no other evidence of that condition.

tremor (Lat, to shake) Involuntary rhythmic and regular oscillations of a body part in any plane, due to the alternate or synchronous action of groups of muscles and their antagonists. Tremors may be regular or irregular in rate and amplitude. They are classified according to the state of motor activity of the body part when they occur: **rest tremor; postural tremor**; tremor during goal-directed activity (**intention** or action tremor) or at the completion of a complex and skilled activity. Using etiology as the basis for a classification, **cerebellar, dystonic, essential, flapping, functional, neuropathic, Parkinsonian, physiological, postural**, and **wing-beating** (hepatic) forms are defined.[6868]

A classification suggested by Jankovicz is adapted in Chart T–6 with some definitions after Bain.[340] See also Movement Disorder Society Consensus Statement.[1615] and the Website: http://www.wemove.org/.

Tremor Action Network A charitable organization. Web site: http://tremoraction.org/.

tremor and cognitive decline (FXTAS) See **cerebellar syndromes** (congenital ataxias).

tremor saturninus A fine, irregular, distal tremor of the fingers and lips, seen in the setting of lead and other heavy metal poisoning.

tremorgenic encephalopathy A syndrome of kinesigenic tremor and reversible dementia, thought to occur as a result of the inhalation of neurotoxins derived from the fungi within mouldy silage.[2490] Such toxins may be produced by *Aspergillus flavus*, *fumigatus*, and *clavatus*, and *Penicillium cyclopium* and *claviceps*; in animals, they are recognized as able to produce a syndrome of transient tremor and weakness. See also **woodtrimmers disease.**

trench foot (immersion foot) A syndrome of ulceration, maceration, and trophic changes in the skin of the legs and feet consequent upon prolonged immersion in cold water, as occurred in soldiers fighting from the trenches during World War I. The cold injury also damages both the arterial supply and the nerves in the legs, resulting in ischemia and distal sensorimotor neuropathy.

Chart T–6. A Classification of Tremors

A. Rest tremor (tremor occurring when the limb is supported against the effects of gravity and in which muscle contraction is voluntarily inhibited):

1. Parkinsonian tremor: **Parkinson disease**, other Parkinsonian disorders; **Parkinsonism-plus**
2. **Spasmus nutans**
3. **Hereditary chin quivering (tremor)**
4. Other: **midbrain (rubral) tremor, severe essential tremor,** and tremors in **Roussy–Lévy syndrome, Wilson disease, acquired hepatocerebral degeneration, myorhythmia, tardive tremor**

B. Action Tremor (tremor which occurs during any voluntary muscle activation)

1. Postural (tremor which occurs when a posture is maintained voluntarily)

A. **Physiologic tremor**

1. Normal physiologic tremor
2. **Accentuated physiologic tremor** (stress-induced, endocrine, drugs, toxins)

B. **Essential tremor**

1. Autosomal dominant
2. Sporadic
3. With **hereditary motor and sensory neuropathy** (See **Roussy–Lévy syndrome**)
4. With other movement disorders (e.g., dystonia, Parkinsonism, myoclonus)
5. With metabolic disorder (e.g., Vitamin E deficiency)

C. Action tremor of Parkinsonism
D. **Neuropathic tremor**
E. Cerebellar (hypotonic) postural tremor (**titubation**)
F. **Rubral tremor** (Holmes' tremor; midbrain tremor, thalamic tremor, myorhythmia)
G. **Dystonic tremor**

2. Kinetic (intention or action) (tremor occurring during the performance of a voluntary movement; *terminal tremor* is that form of kinetic tremor in which the amplitude of the tremor is increased at the end of the goal-directed movement)

A. **Cerebellar tremors**
B. Cerebellar outflow tremor with midbrain lesions (**rubral tremor**)

3. Other Tremors

A. **Psychogenic tremor.** Abnormal repetitive movements which do not fit the patterns described here, occurring in patients with suspected disorders of personality or of emotional control. With adequate follow-up, many turn out to have organic neurological disease
B. **Task-specific tremor**, in which the tremor occurs only during one or more particular highly-skilled activities, such as playing a musical instrument or writing (**primary handwriting tremor**), and in certain sports (see **bowlers cramp, yips**)
C. **Isometric tremor,** occurring when muscle activity is exerted at maximal force against an unyielding object, or against the antagonists of the muscle in question
D. **Orthostatic tremor**
E. Isometric tremor, present when muscles are contracting against an unyielding force
F. Palatal tremor See **patalal myoclonus** although it is actually a tremor

After Dr. Joseph Jankowicz' personal communication (2003), with many thanks.

Trendelenburg, Friedrich (1844–1924) German surgeon.

Trendelenburg gait A waddling gait, due to weakness in the pelvic girdle muscles.[6379]

Trendelenburg Test When the patient stands on one foot, the buttock of the unsupported foot usually rises, but falls in patient with weak gluteal muscles, as in radiculopathy, high sciatic neuropathy, and the **piriformis syndrome**.

Trendelenberg position Flexion of the hips and the knees by the supine patient with <20° head-down tilt. Although mainly of gynecological importance, the position is of value in the diagnosis of low CSF pressure syndromes, the adoption of this posture usually relieving the headache promptly.

Trends in Neurosciences (*Trends Neurosci*, TINS) A basic science neurological journal. Web site: http://www.trends.com/tins/default.htm/.

trepanning See **trephining**.

trephining (trepanning) The surgical opening of the skull. The original word was *trepan* (Gr, a gimlet); *trephine* was introduced by Woodall in 1628 as the name for an instrument which he had devised for this purpose. **Osler** stated that this operation is the oldest known surgical procedure, but it is likely to have been preceded by circumcision.

trepidant abasia (from Lat, fearful + Gr, not + going) See **isolated gait ignition failure.**

trépidation du Moignon See **stump spasm.**

triad syndrome See **prune belly syndrome.**

triangular bipolar montage A montage consisting of derivations from pairs of electrodes in a group of three electrodes arranged in a triangular pattern. (From the 1974 report of the Committee on Terminology, IFCN. In: Chatrian GE, Bergamini L, Dondey M, et al. A glossary of terms most commonly used by clinical electroencephalographers. *EEG Clin Neurophysiol* 1974;37:538–48. Reproduced by kind permission of Elsevier Science and the IFCN.)

triceps (from Lat, three + heads) 1. The major extensor muscle of the elbow (triceps brachii). 2. The gastrocnemius and soleus muscles (triceps surae).

triceps surae reflex The correct name for the Achilles reflex or **ankle jerk**, use of the term being a custom honored entirely in the breach rather than the observance, perhaps in part because there is no alternative to the name of **triceps reflex** in the arm. The reflex is best obtained by tapping the tendon of the muscle with the patient kneeling on a chair or, if supine, with the ankle in slight passive dorsiflexion, tapping the sole of the foot or the belly of the tibialis anterior muscle. (**Gowers' frontal tap**).

trichinosis Infection by the nematode *Trichinella spiralis* following the oral ingestion of inadequately cooked meat (especially pork and wild boar). Clinically, after prodromal diarrhea, symptoms of myopathy appear usually within a month, with diffuse myalgia, swelling and weakness, and with systemic fever; periorbital edema, a maculopapular rash; splinter hemorrhages; and evidence of encephalitis and/or of congestive cardiac failure and arrhythmias resulting from the larval encystment in muscles. Encephalitis is a rare complication. The CSF is normal but the blood shows marked eosinophilia and high CK levels. Muscle biopsy shows the encysted larvae in the early stages, and calcified cysts, which at this stage may be seen on plain X-rays. Antibody titers are positive after the first week or two. Despite this, the condition is usually subclinical.[1486]

tricho-onycho-oligophrenia See **Sabinas syndrome.**

trichopoliodystrophy (Gr, hair + gray + wrong + growth) See **Menkes disease.**

trichopsia Central blindness with scintillating scotomata, as in **migraine**.

trichotillomania (Gr, hair + pluck + madness) Compulsive pulling-out of the hair, leading to patchy baldness. The patients may also eat the hair pulled out. **Bulimia** is associated in some cases.[6162]

trickle angiography A technique for visualizing blood clots in the carotid bulb and internal carotid artery, introduced by Hugh in 1970.[3033]

trident tongue See **triple-furrowed tongue**.

trientine A chelating agent of value in the treatment of **Wilson disease**.

trifacial neuralgia See **trigeminal neuralgia.**

trigeminal autonomic cephalgias A group of headaches whose pathophysiology is based upon the trigeminal-autonomic reflex. They are characterized by pain in a unilateral trigeminal nerve distribution with marked cranial autonomic (mainly parasympathetic) features such as conjunctival and nasal congestion, tearing, rhinorrhea, pupillary changes, and sweating resulting from activation in the posterior hypothalamus.

Although generally considered "idiopathic" (and thus suggesting that there is no structural pathology responsible) tumors (especially including pituitary tumors) can cause an identical clinical picture, for which reason neuroimaging should always be considered in patients with syndromes such as **cluster headache, paroxysmal hemicrania,** SUNA, and SUNCT.[2416, 2412]

trigeminal autonomic reflex Increased facial blood flow and temperature resulting from stimulation of trigeminal afferents, the facial and greater superficial petrosal nerves carrying the efferent vasodilating responses. The reflex is employed in the generation of the **trigeminal autonomic cephalgias.**[6966, 2418]

trigeminal nerve (Lat, three + twins; thus triplets, appropriate since the nerve has three branches) The V cranial nerve, described by Fallopius.

trigeminal neuralgia (tic douloureux, trifacial neuralgia, facial chorea, Fothergill syndrome, tic convulsif) A syndrome of brief facial pains, considered to be one of the most severe afflicting humans. The pain is commonly evoked by trivial stimuli including washing, shaving, smoking, talking, and/or brushing the teeth (trigger factors) but frequently occurs spontaneously. Small areas in the nasolabial fold and/or chin may be particularly susceptible to the precipitation of pain (trigger areas). It occurs in patients older than 55 years, is unilateral, and is felt in the second or third divisions of the V cranial nerve; when any of these conditions is not met, *symptomatic trigeminal neuralgia* is diagnosed and a structural lesion along the path of the nerve is to be sought.

The condition was known to Galen and to Avicenna, and was described by **Fothergill**, first in 1776 and again (more fully) in his book 30 years later.[2158] However, Johannes Fehr and Elias Schmidt were probably describing the same condition in their 1671 eulogy of Dr. Johannes Bausch who had died while suffering from this condition.[5619]

Two forms (*idiopathic* and *symptomatic*) are described by the Headache Classification Committee of the International Headache Society[2820] and their definitions and diagnostic criteria are reproduced in Chart T–7.

Chart T–7. Definition and Diagnostic Criteria for Trigeminal Neuralgia

Classical (idiopathic) trigeminal neuralgia

A. Paroxysmal attacks of pain lasting from a fraction of a second to 2 min, affecting one or more divisions of the trigeminal nerve and fulfilling criteria B and C
B. Pain has at least one of the following characteristics:
   1. Intense, sharp, superficial, or stabbing
   2. Precipitated from trigger areas or by trigger factors
C. Attacks are stereotyped in the individual patient
D. There is no clinically evident neurological deficit
E. Not attributed to another disorder

Symptomatic trigeminal neuralgia is pain indistinguishable from classical trigeminal neuralgia but caused by a demonstrable structural lesion other than vascular compression. Diagnostic criteria are as follows:

A. Paroxysmal attacks of pain lasting from a fraction of a second to 2 min, with or without persistence of aching between paroxysms, affecting one or more divisions of the trigeminal nerve and fulfilling criteria B and C
B. Pain has at least one of the following characteristics:
   1. Intense, sharp, superficial, or stabbing
   2. Precipitated from trigger areas or by trigger factors
C. Attacks are stereotyped in the individual patient
D. A causative lesion, other than vascular compression, has been demonstrated by special investigations and/or posterior fossa exploration. Unlike the classic form, symptomatic trigeminal neuralgia demonstrates no refractory period after a paroxysm. Central lesions (as in **multiple sclerosis**) can cause a similar pain. See also **Hellsing syndrome.**

Adapted from the International Classification of Headache Disorders (Headache Classification Committee of the International Headache Society. Cephalalgia 2004;*24(Suppl 1)) by kind permission of Dr. Jes Olesen, the International Headache Society, and Wiley-Blackwell Publications.*

Trigeminal Neuralgia Association A nonprofit, voluntary organization founded in 1990, providing information and support to patients with trigemonal neuralgia and their families through informational mailings, a support network, and support groups. The association also endeavors to increase public and professional awareness of this disorder. Address: P.O. Box 785, Barnegat Light, NJ 08006. Tel: 609-361-1014. Web site: http://www.tna-support.org/.

trigeminal sensory neuropathy Usually a benign syndrome of slowly progressive sensory loss affecting one or more branches of the V cranial nerve, sometimes preceded by paresthesias and mild pain and accompanied by impairment of taste sensation but with the corneal reflex preserved.[5982] The clinical syndrome is the same in isolation as it is when accompanying various connective tissue diseases, particularly **progressive systemic sclerosis** and mixed connective tissue disease.

In a *variant* form with degeneration and amyloid deposition in the trigeminospinal system, nasal ulceration and myelopathy accompany the facial numbness.[5981]

trigeminobrachial reflex Flexion and supination of the forearm in response to stimulation of the contralateral side of the face, as seen in patients with bilateral corticobulbar tract disease.

trigemino-cardiac reflex (trigeminal depressor response) Sinus bradycardia occurring reflexly in response to stimulation of trigeminal nerve afferents.

trigeminocervical reflex 1. Rotation of the neck in the direction away from the side on which the face is stimulated; a sign of bilateral corticobulbar tract disease. 2. A short latency reflex that can normally be recorded from the sternocleidomastoid muscle after electrical stimulation of the supra- or infraorbital nerves. It may be absent with medullary lesions.[1626]

trigemino-encephalo-angiomatosis See **Sturge–Weber syndrome.**

trigeminofacial reflex The **blink reflex,** elicited by electrical stimulation of the supra- or infraorbital nerves. The reflex is employed clinically in the study of brainstem reflex circuits. See **orbicularis oculi reflex**.

trigemino-ocular synkinesis See **Gunn phenomenon**.

trigemino-orbicularis reflex See **palpebral reflex**.

trigeminopalpebral reflex See **palpebral reflex**.

trigeminosympathetic neuralgia See **trigeminal neuralgia, Bonnet syndrome**.

trigeminovascular system A network of intracranial and extracranial blood vessels innervated by the V cranial nerve. Stimulation through the nerve leads to vasodilatation.[4515]

trigemino-cerebrovascular system Those neurons with cell bodies in the trigeminal ganglion innervating the cerebral vessels and dura mater and supplying all of the sensory innervation of the cerebral vessels through the neurotransmitters, NKA and CGRP. The system is considered responsible for mediating the pain of **migraine** and of the **trigeminal autonomic cephalgias**.[2418]

trigger points (trigger zones) Focal areas of pain within specific muscles in any part of the body but most commonly in the neck and shoulder girdle regions. A firm nodule may be felt within the muscle, palpation of which increases the pain, but there is no known pathology and EMG study of the area reveals no abnormality.

trigonocephaly (Gr, triangle + head) An unusual cranial malformation characterized by synostosis of the midline frontal (metopic) suture, giving the forehead a triangular, pointed shape. Radiologically, the orbits are closer than normal with parallel inner walls. The malformation is sometimes associated with arhinencephaly and hypotelorism.[4] See also **Opitz–Frias syndrome**.

trihexose ceramide lipidosis See **Anderson–Fabry disease**.

trilaminar muscle fiber disease A rare congenital myopathy presenting with weakness at birth, manifested as poor sucking and swallowing as well as limb weakness, but abating with time.[6] Trichrome stains of muscle fibers reveal three concentric rings, the center zone (which contains no contractile elements) staining red, the (normal) middle zone staining green, and the outside (containing variously glycogen, mitochondria, and lipid) staining purple.[5314]

trilateral retinoblastoma The concurrence of **pinealoblastoma** and **retinoblastoma**.

TRIM32-related dystrophy (LGMD2H) A rare autosomal recessive form of **limb girdle muscular dystrophy**.[3454]

trinucleotide repeat disorders Conditions due to unstable mutations, in most of which there is an expansion of the CAG repeat in the coding sequence of a gene. See **cerebellar ataxias** (SCA types 1, 2, 3 and 7), **X-linked spinal-bulbar muscular atrophy, fragile X syndrome, FRAXE mental retardation, myotonic dystrophy, Huntington disease, dentatorubropallidodoluysian atrophy**.

triorthocresylphosphate An organophosphate with a strong anticholinesterase effect and with a delayed neurotoxic effect causing a motor neuropathy. See **toxic oil syndrome**.

triose phosphate isomerase deficiency An inborn error of metabolism (a corencephalopathy) in which the enzyme is deficient in muscle, skin fibroblasts, and blood cells. Clinically, denervation atrophy of muscles, pyramidal signs, tremor, and dystonia with hemolytic anemia develop in young children.[5065]

Trip Database An attempt to bring together all the evidence-based health care resources on the Internet, with a dedicated neurology section and e-mail updates. It provides a synthesis of reliable evidence about the effects of health care. Web site: www.tripdatabase.com.

triphasic action potential Action potential with two baseline crossings, producing three phases.

triphasic wave An EEG manifestation consisting of a waveform with an initial negative (upward), then a major downward deflection followed by a second upward deflection before return to baseline. Such waves are common in all metabolic encephalopathies, such as those due to hepatic or renal failure, in which they are said to have an earlier onset in frontal regions; and in **Alzheimer disease**, hyperthyroidism, and **Mollaret meningitis** as well as after strokes.[2146]

triple A syndrome See **Allgrove syndrome**.

triple discharge (triplet) Three motor unit action potentials of the same form and nearly the same amplitude occurring consistently in the same relationship to one another and generated by the same axon. The interval between the second and third action potentials often exceeds that between the first two, and both are usually in the range of 2 to 20 ms. See also **double discharge, multiple discharge**. (After the 2001 Report of the Nomenclature Committee of the American Association of Electromyography and Electrodiagnosis.[19] Reproduced by kind permission of the AANEM.)

triple E syndrome Bilateral posterior fracture-dislocations of the shoulders, as a result of sudden extreme extensor and internal rotator contractions of the shoulder girdle musculature. The more common causes of this are epilepsy, extreme trauma, and electrocution.[790]

triple response The formation of a weal, surrounded by a tâche and flare at the site of a linear scratch on the skin, due to local axon reflex activity, described by Lewis. The existence of such a response, representing in part the liberation of histamine and in part an axon reflex, indicates that the smallest cutaneous nerve fibers are intact.

triple-furrowed tongue (trident tongue) The presence of three longitudinal fissures in the tongue, said to be characteristic in **myasthenia gravis**.

triple symptom complex See **Behçet syndrome**.

triplet See **triple discharge**.

triplet repeat disease Any of several familial diseases resulting from expansion in length of a segment of repeated nucleotide triples within an affected gene (see table). Many (but not all) of the triplet repeat diseases arise from expansion of a repeated cytosine-adenine-guanine $(CAG)_n$ triple in an exon of the gene, which causes a corresponding increase in length of a polyglutamine $(Gln)_n$ segment of the affected protein. This expanded $(Gln)_n$ tract can produce a toxic gain of function, and the mutant protein often has a propensity to coalesce as intracellular inclusion bodies. The triplet repeat of the gene may be prone

Triplet Repeat Diseases*

Disease	*Gene locus*	*Affected protein*	*Number of triplet repeats*		*Mechanism/ Inheritance**
			Normal	*Diseased*	
I. Diseases caused by $(CAG)_n$ expansions					
Haw River syndrome (dentatorubropallidoluysianz atrophy, DRPLA)	12p13.31	Atrophin-1	6–35	49–88	$(Gln)_n$/AD Ant
Huntington disease	4p16.3	Huntingtin	6–35	36–121	$(Gln)_n$/AD Ant
Kennedy disease (spinobulbar muscular atrophy, SBMA)	Xq13–21	Androgen receptor	9–36	38–62	$(Gln)_n$[a]/SLR
Spinocerebellar ataxia type 1†	6p23	Ataxin-1	6–44	39–82	$(Gln)_n$[b]/AD Ant
Spinocerebellar ataxia type 2†	12q24.1	Ataxin-2	15–31	36–63	$(Gln)_n$/AD Ant
Machado–Joseph disease (spinocerebellar ataxia type 3†	14q32.1	Ataxin-3	12–40	55–84	$(Gln)_n$/AD Ant
Spinocerebellar ataxia type 6†	19p13	α_{1A}-voltage-dependent Ca^{2+} channel subunit	4–18	21–33	$(Gln)_n$/AD Ant ?
Spinocerebellar ataxia type 7†	13p12–13	Ataxin-7	4–35	37–306	$(Gln)_n$/AD
Spinocerebellar ataxia type 12†	5q31–33	PP2A-PR55β	7–28	66–78	5' UTR/SLR
Spinocerebellar ataxia type 17	6q27	TATA-binding protein	24–42	47–55	
II. Diseases caused by other trinucleotide expansions					
Fragile X syndrome (FRAXA)/CGG	Xq27.3	FMR-1	6–53	>230	5' UTR/SLR
Fragile XE syndrome (FRAXE)/GCC	Xq28	FMR-2	6–35	>200	5' UTR/SLR
Friedreich ataxia/GAA	9q13–21.1	Frataxin	7–34	>100	intron 1/AR
Myotonic dystrophy/CTG	19q13.3	Dystrophia myotonica protein kinase (DMPK)	5–37	>50	3' UTR/AD Ant
Oculopharyngeal muscular dystrophy/GCC	14q11	PABP2	6	8–13	$(Ala)_n$/AD
Spinocerebellar ataxia type 8/CTG (SCA8)	13q21	KLHL1	16–37	>110	3' UTR/AD

* *Modified from Tables 1 and 2 in Cummings CI and Zoghb iHY. Hum Molec Genet 2000;9:906–16, with thanks to Dr. Homer J. Moore.*
† *See cerebellar ataxia.*

to increase in length during replication so that each affected generation possesses a successively longer expansion. This results in genetic anticipation, wherein each generation expresses the phenotype of the disease at successively younger age. Note, however, that triplet repeat expansions can also occur within an intron, or within an altogether untranslated segment of the gene, and in these cases the resulting disease arises by some other mechanism. Expansions of runs involving other triplet combinations including thymine (T) also occur. (HJM)

triplopia The complaint that when one object is regarded, three are seen. The symptom is usually regarded as functional (especially when monocular) but sometimes is due to eye movement abnormalities such as **oscillopsia** or binocular diplopia.

trismus (Gr, grinding) Involuntary, painful spasm of the masseter muscles leading to an inability to open the mouth.

Classically, it is a sign of **tetanus**, but it also occurs with dystonic reactions to drugs, with local disease of the muscles or joints and in psychogenic disease.

trismus nascentium Neonatal **tetanus**.

trisomy 8 syndrome An uncommon congenital chromosomal disorder with marked phenotypic variation. Dysmorphic facies, skeletal deformities, clino- and camptodactyly, mental and motor delay, agenesis of the corpus callosum, and the presence of deep furrows on the palms and soles are characteristic and representative findings.[3] See **Warkany syndrome**.

trisomy 9p A relatively common syndrome of mental retardation, seizures, microcephaly, short stature, kyphosis, other dysmorphic features, and extra chromosomal material on the short arm of chromosome.[9, 6041]

trisomy 12p syndrome A congenital dysmorphic syndrome manifesting hypotonia, enlarged fontanelle, turricephaly, hypertelorism, severe mental retardation, and a seizure disorder resembling **progressive myoclonic epilepsy** accompanied by 4-Hz slow waves and polyspikes on the EEG.[2613]

trisomy 13 syndrome (Patau syndrome, chromosome 13 trisomy syndrome) An uncommon congenital chromosomal dysmorphic syndrome in which the extra chromosome is responsible for causing microcephaly, physical and mental retardation, feeding difficulties, breath-holding spells, atypical minor motor seizures with **hypsarrhythmia**, agenesis of the olfactory apparatus, optic atrophy, deafness, **holoprocencephaly**, microphthalmia, congenital cardiac and genital malformations, polydactyly, and multiple other skeletal anomalies. Numerous other associated anomalies, such as cleft lip or palate, capillary hemangiomas of the scalp, and genital anomalies, have been described in a minority of cases.[5908] A report of Bartholin (a Danish physician) in 1657 was probably of the same condition.[4925]

trisomy 18 syndrome An uncommon congenital chromosomal dysmorphic syndrome, characterized by low birth weight, cardiac and skeletal anomalies (e.g., micrognathia, long narrow head, flexed fingers, and pelvic and foot deformities), and hypoplasia of the cerebellum, anterior commissure, and corpus callosum. Mental retardation, seizures, and spasticity are common. Most affected infants die before they are 3 months old.[1812] See **Edwards syndrome**.

trisomy 21 syndrome See **Down syndrome**.

TRISS An acronym deviated from TRauma score and Injury Severity Score, noting also the age of the patient and whether the injury is blunt or penetrating, in order to provide a measure of the probability of survival. The *injury scale* is derived from the abbreviated injury scale booklet (AIS 1990) obtainable from the Northwestern Injury Research Centre, University of Manchester, Hope Hospital, Salford England, M6 8HD. The *trauma score* combines coded measurements of respiration, systolic blood pressure, and the **Glasgow Coma Scale** to provide a general assessment of physiological derangement.[6908]

tritanopia Dominantly inherited yellow-blue color blindness. In a *variant* rare, dominantly inherited syndrome, the tritanopia is associated with optic atrophy.[3565, 6879]

triton tumor A rare, high-grade malignant tumor of the peripheral nerve sheath showing rhabdomyosarcomatous degeneration, commonly in the context of **neurofibromatosis**.[878]

trochanter reflex The **adductor reflex** elicited by the vibration set up by a tap over the greater trochanter.

trochlear nerve (from Lat, a pulley) The IV cranial nerve, described by Alessandro Achillini (1463–1512), an Italian anatomist.

TROG Acronym for the Test for the Reception of Grammar, an instrument for assessing language comprehension in which the child is asked to select which of four pictures best fits the verbal cue given by the examiner.

Trolard, Paulin (1842–1910) Professor of anatomy in Algiers.

Trolard's vein The great annectent vein of the cerebral cortex, described by Trolard in his graduation thesis (University of Paris) in 1868.

trombone tongue Repetitive protrusion and replacement of the tongue, seen characteristically in **Huntington disease** and other choreic states, but also in tertiary syphilis.

Trömner reflex Flexion of the fingers in response to a tap on the volar surface of the tip of the patients second or third finger; a sign with the same significance as the **finger flexion reflex**, of which it is a *variant*.

Tromner–Hoffman reflex See **Hoffmann reflex**.

trophic 1. Causing movement. 2. Stimulating growth.

trophic influences Factors causing growth or differentiation of the targeted structures.

tropias Manifest deviation of the eyes (with misalignment of the visual axes), present when both eyes are viewing a target. See **heterotropia, phoria**.

tropical ataxic neuropathy See **Nigerian neuropathy**.

tropical neuropathy See **brucellosis, leprosy, Nigerian neuropathy, HIV, HTLV, cassava, ciguatoxin, scombroid**. Poisoning by *coyotillo* and *gloriosa suberba* may also cause acute neuropathies.[6280]

tropical nutritional ataxia See **Nigerian neuropathy**.

tropical pyomyositis See **pyomyositis**.

tropical spastic paraparesis (HTLV-1-associated myelopathy [HAM]) An insidiously progressive paraparesis occurring in the third to fifth decades as a result of cytotoxic T-cell-mediated demyelination following infection with HTLV-1. Clinically, the major features include "burning feet" and later spastic gait, spastic bladder, and impotence in men. Additional features include lumbar girdle pains, leg spasticity and hyper-reflexia, myoclonic jerks, and slowly progressing loss of vibration and common sensation in the feet with paresthesia in both the hands and the feet. The ankle reflexes are diminished at a later stage.[5365, 5364]

The disease is more prevalent in tropical, rain-forested countries such as India, Africa, the Seychelles, Jamaica, and Colombia, but has extended with the spread of the virus elsewhere in the world. The clinical features resemble those of pure spinal **multiple sclerosis**.[1365]

tropical sprue A malabsorption syndrome of unknown cause, seen particularly in India and Africa. Clinical features include steatorrhea with xylose malabsorption, and (later) progressive muscle weakness, sensory neuropathy, and features of both **tetany** and **subacute combined degeneration of the cord**.[6208]

tropomyosin A protein constituent of muscle with contractile properties, manifest when contacted by troponin.

Trotter, Wilfred Batten Lewis (1872–1939) English physician.

Trotter syndrome (sinus of Morgagni syndrome) Malignant infiltration of the lower cranial nerves unilaterally by a malignant tumor in the lateral pharyngeal recess, producing facial pain and numbness, palatal paresis, and weakness of the masticatory and facial muscles with conductive deafness due to infiltration of the eustachian tube.[6398] See also **pterygopalatine fossa syndrome**.

trouble du sens de l'éspace See **visuomotor ataxia**.

Trousseau, Armand (1801–1867) French physician who was trained in medicine and practiced in Paris. He introduced the procedure of tracheotomy; wrote two successful textbooks on medicine and therapeutics; and described what is now known as Hodgkin disease independently in 1864, hemochromatosis in 1859, his sign in tetany in 1861, and the occurrence of thrombophlebitis in association with a visceral carcinoma (in himself) shortly before his death.[2066]

Trousseau sign 1. A test for latent **tetany**; the appearance within 3 min of paresthesias, muscle tightening, and **carpopedal spasm** distal to a blood pressure cuff inflated to 20 mmHg above the systolic blood pressure in the arm. 2. The **tâche cerebrale**.

Troyer syndrome (hereditary spastic paraparesis with wasting and growth retardation) A recessively inherited syndrome of **hereditary spastic paraparesis** with onset in early childhood, complicated by **pseudobulbar palsy**, distal muscle wasting, choreoathetosis, and short stature, and detected in the Amish people of Ohio.[1355]

true Broca aphasia See **Broca aphasia**.

true myoclonic epilepsy See **centrencephalic myoclonic-astatic epilepsy**.

true phase reversal The occurrence of simultaneous pen deflections in opposite directions in two referential derivations using a suitable common reference electrode and displaying the same wave. This phenomenon is rarely observed in scalp EEGs, but when demonstrated beyond doubt in appropriate recording conditions, it indicates a 180° change in phase of an EEG wave between adjacent areas of the brain on either side of a zero isopotential axis. See also **instrumental phase reversal**. (Adapted from the 1974 report of the Committee on Terminology, IFCN. In: Chatrian GE, Bergamini L, Dondey M, et al. A glossary of terms most commonly used by clinical electroencephalographers. *EEG Clin Neurophysiol* 1974;37:538–48. Reproduced by kind permission of Elsevier Science and the IFCN.)

trunk control test See **motricity index**.

trunk extension test The subject extends the spine while standing. Pain felt in the back, radiating to the leg, indicates the presence of root compression at lower lumbar levels.

trunkal dystonia Rare, isolated, focal dystonias affecting the trunk alone, and causing trunk flexion, extension, scoliosis, or torsion, often increased by walking.[4101]

trunkal incurvation See **developmental reflexes, Galant reflex**.

trunkal mononeuropathy See **diabetic truncal neuropathy**.

trunk-thigh sign Flexion of the thigh with elevation of a paretic leg from the bed when the subject attempts to sit up from the supine position without using his arms for support. The normal response is for the legs to remain in contact with the bed during this movement.

trypanosomiasis (human African) See **sleeping sickness**.

trypanosomiasis (American) See **Chagas disease**.

tryptophan-eosinophilia-myalgia syndrome A form of **eosinophilic fasciitis** presenting as a scleroderma-like syndrome, and caused by the oral ingestion of tryptophan products. Whether the cause of the syndrome is the tryptophan or something in the excipient is not determined.

tryptophanuria A rare syndrome resulting from a block in the pathway of tryptophan metabolism. The clinical features resemble those of **Hartnup disease** and include cerebellar ataxia, dermal photosensitivity, small stature, and mental retardation.[1409]

tsara'ath See **leprosy**.

Tschlenow reflex See **spino-adductor reflex**.

tsiminakis syndrome Chorea.

tsutsugamshi fever An infectious disease manifesting rash, fever, meningoencephalitis, and a positive Weil–Felix reaction.

The disease is frequently complicated by peripheral neuropathy, seizures, and residual nerve deafness.[4685] See **scrub typhus**.

tuberculoid leprosy (maculoanesthetic leprosy) That form of the disease in which the body's immune response to the bacillus is relatively successful. Clinical manifestations include raised anesthetic maculopapules involving the face, buttocks, and limb extensor surfaces and a nodular hypertrophic multiple mononeuropathy.[5485] See **leprosy**.

tuberculoma (tuberculous granuloma) Encapsulated nodules of granulation tissue which range in size from millimeters to centimeters in diameter. They are composed of acid fast bacilli; necrotic caseous material; lymphoid, epitheliomatous, and plasma cells; histiocytes; and giant cells, and are surrounded by a zone of vascularity in the periphery.[6206] Tuberculomas result from the hematogenous spread of *Mycobacterium tuberculosis* to any part in the body. In the nervous system they are usualy intracerebral and supratentorial.

tuberculoma dolorosa The **glomus tumor**.

tuberculous alcoholic polyneuritis See **Lemierre–Boltanski–Justin–Besançon syndrome**.

tuberculous encephalopathy A rare syndrome of diffuse brain damage, apparently restricted to children and characterized by edema of the white matter with perivascular demyelination and sometimes hemorrhagic leukoencephalopathy. The condition is considered due to an allergic reaction to proteins released by the mycobacteria.[1466]

tuberculous granuloma See **tuberculoma**.

tuberculous meningitis A chronic basal meningitis characterized by the usual features of meningeal irritation, increased intracranial pressure, and involvement of the cranial nerves, usually with a protracted but accelerating course culminating in death if untreated. The infection of the meninges proceeds from the spillage of acid-fast bacilli from a small tuberculoma anywhere within the nervous system. The first description was that of Robert **Whytt**, published posthumously in 1768.

tuberous sclerosis (tuberose sclerosis, Bourneville disease, Bourneville–Brissaud disease, Bourneville–Pringle disease, Brushfield–Wyatt disease, Bourneville–Pellizzi disease, Sherlock epiloia, Pellizzi disseminated cortical dysplasia; OMIM 191090, 1911092).[5704] A complex syndrome inherited as an irregular autosomal dominant trait, and manifesting mental deficiency, multifocal seizures including infantille spasms, and **adenoma sebaceum**. Bourneville's early description made all the important clinical points.[770] The responsible genes map variously to 9q34.1–9q34.2, to 11q14–q23, or to 16p13.3.

Complications of the numerous calcifying subependymal tubers and of those scattered elsewhere in the brain include focal neurological signs and obstructive hydrocephalus. Elsewhere in the body, simian hands, short in-curved little fingers, accessory thumbs, deformities of the ears, rhabdomyoma of the heart, hypernephroma, spina bifida, dental enamel abnormalities, cardiac tumors, honeycomb lung, renal cysts, renal tumors, osteosclerosis, skeletal cysts, and thickened calvarium may also be found.[771, 2460, 1323] Bourneville gave the first report of the disease at the **Salpêtrière** in 1867 and published his observations in 1880, the same year as the condition was described by Hartgeden from Germany. Pringle described the skin signs in 1890.

In a *variant form*, tuberous sclerosis is associated with the **Klippel–Trenaunay–Weber syndrome** in childhood. The clinical features then include pseudogliomas of the retina, seizures, bony abnormalities, and mental and developmental delay. Diagnostic criteria for tuberous sclerosis complex have been proposed[5325] and can be found at http://www.tsalliance.org//pages.aspx?content=54/. They are summarized, without the explanatory notes on the Web site, in Chart T–8.

Chart T–8. Diagnostic Features of Tuberous Sclerosis

Major features	*Minor features*
Facial angiofibromas (best seen above the philtrum) or forehead plaque	Multiple, randomly distributed pits in dental enamel
Nontraumatic ungual or periungual fibroma	Hamartomatous rectal polyps
Three or more hypomelanotic patches (best seen with Woods light)	Multiple renal cysts
Shagreen patch (connective tissue nevus)	Bone cysts
Multiple retinal nodular hamartomas	Cerebral white matter radial migration lines
Cortical tubers	Gingival fibromas
Subependymal nodules	Nonrenal hamartoma
Subependymal giant cell astrocytoma	Retinal achromatic patch
Cardiac rhabdomyoma, single or multiple	"Confetti" skin lesions
Lymphangiomyomatosis	
Renal angiomyolipoma	

Definite Tuberous Sclerosis Complex (TSC): Two major or one major and two minor features
Probable TSC: One major and one minor feature
Possible TSC: Either one major or two or more minor features.

However, revised criteria (2004) require tuberous sclerosis complex-associated lesions of two or more organ systems or at least two dissimilar lesions of the same organ to be found in order to confirm the diagnosis. DNA testing complements the clinical diagnosis and allows more precise genetic counseling and perhaps prenatal diagnosis, but it carries a 15% false-negative rate, further complicated by germline mosaicism in about 2% of people with tuberous sclerosis complex.

From Roach ES. et al. J Child Neurol *1988;13:624–8 and* J Child Neurol *2004;19:643–9.*

Tuberous Sclerosis Alliance

A charitable organization providing support and information on this condition. Web site: http://www.tsalliance.org/. See also http://www.kumc.edu/gec/support/tuberous.html.

tubular aggregate myopathies

(myopathy with tubular aggregates) Rare, slowly progressive, dominantly or recessively inherited myopathies presenting in adult life. Clinical complaints include cramps, muscle stiffness, and myalgias which are brought on by exertion and relieved by prolonged rest, as well as proximal muscle weakness[2376] and fatigability without atrophy. Compact collections of tubules are seen on electron microscopy preparations in the subsarcolemmal regions of some of the muscle fibers of each type (especially type II), associated with some type II fiber atrophy.[4484, 4485, 5356] This pathological change may also be a feature of the **familial periodic paralyses**.[869]

In a *variant* form progressive muscular weakness occurs with contractures and skeletal deformity and with pupillary abnormalities. The tubular aggregates are found in both type I and type II muscle fibers.

tubular aggregates

Densely packed, subsarcolemmal, basophilic tubules with doubled walls, found in type IIb myofibrils, which stain red on trichrome staining.[4485] They derive from proliferations of the sarcoplasmic reticulum and are detectable in a variety of diseases, including a myasthenic syndrome, dominantly and recessively inherited myopathies (**tubular aggregate myopathies**), a syndrome of myalgias and cramps without other pathological change,[5405] familial and nonfamilial myopathies and hyperornithinemia, and after poisoning with diazepam or alcohol.[5356]

tubular constriction

See **gun-barrel constriction of the visual fields**.

tubulomembranous inclusion disease

A progressive myopathy of youth resembling limb-girdle dystrophy, with facial involvement, marked fatigability, and elevated serum CK levels, in which these inclusions are seen on electron microscopy preparations of muscle.[2233]

tucked-lid sign

Retraction of the upper eyelid, with scleral show. A finding in **Parinaud syndrome**. See **Collier sign**.

Tuck–McLeod syndrome

A sporadic disorder characterized by onset in childhood or middle adult life of a predominantly sensory peripheral polyneuropathy, cerebellar ataxia, and sensorineural hearing loss without distinguishing biochemical abnormalities.[6414]

Tufts Quantitative Neuromuscular examination

A 29-item protocol assessing the neuromuscular deficits at various levels of the neuraxis in **amyotrophic lateral sclerosis**. The items include the results of pulmonary function tests, tests of bulbar function, timed functional tests of hand activities, and measurements of isometric strength. To date, it has been used mainly in research studies (Chart T–9).[200]

tullidora

See **buckthorn neuropathy**.

Tullio phenomenon

Vertigo, nystagmus, and postural instability induced by high-intensity sound stimulation in patients who are congenitally deaf or who have labyrinthine fistulas. The effect is due to physical activation of the vestibular system by the sound vibrations.[819, 6673]

Tulp, Nicholaas

(Claes Pieteszoon, 1593–1674) Physician of Amsterdam who trained in Leyden. He gave the first full description of **spina bifida** in his *Observationes medicae* (1641),[7] but is better remembered because his anatomy lesson at the Amsterdam surgeon's guild was painted by Rembrandt in 1631.

Tumarkin otolithic crisis

See **otolithic catastrophe**.

tumor

(Lat, swelling) See **brain tumor** and specific entries.

tumor circoidius

See **arteriovenous malformation**.

Tunbridge–Paley syndrome

A recessively inherited syndrome of progressive deafness with pigmentary retinopathy, optic atrophy, and diabetes mellitus, commencing in the first decade of life.[6421]

tunnel vision

Symmetrical constriction of the visual fields as though the subject were looking down a hollow cylinder. The diameter of the field is identical, whether the target object is close or far away, unlike the physiological "funnel vision" in which the field's diameter increases with distance.

turban tumors

See **cylindromatosis**.

Turck, Ludwig

(1810–1868) Austrian anatomist and chief of a neurology service in Vienna, who showed in 1851 that degeneration in a nerve fiber corresponds to the direction in which it conducts impulses physiologically, degeneration in ascending tracts being above the lesion and in descending

Chart T–9. The Tufts Quantitative Neuromuscular Examination

Pulmonary function:

1. Forced vital capacity; best of two trials
2. Maximum voluntary ventilation

Oropharyngeal:

1. Time (seconds) to say "pa" 20 times
2. Time (seconds) to say "pata" 15 times

Timed motor activities:

1. Dialing 764–7172 on a spring-loaded dial phone
2. Number of pegs placed on the Purdue peg board in 30 s
3. Time (seconds) taken to walk 15 ft (4.5 m) with any aid or assistance as needed

Scores for *isometric arm and leg strength* (measured using an electronic strain gauge) are awarded on the basis of assessments of maximum voluntary contractions, which reliably quantitate motor unit losses

(Adapted from Andres PL, Hedlund W, Finison L, et al. Quantitative assessment in amyotrophic lateral sclerosis. Neurology *1986;36:937–41. Reproduced by kind permission of the American Academy of Neurology and Lippincott Williams and Wilkins.)*

tracts, below it.[4502] The *bundle of Turck* comprises the motor fibers that run from the parietotemporal cortex through the posterior limb of the internal capsule to the cerebral peduncle, and thence to the pons. Turck also described the anterior corticospinal tract in 1849 and demonstrated overlap of innervation in adjacent dermatomes.

Turcot syndrome (intestinal polyposis and glioma) A rare, genetically transmitted (dominant or recessive) syndrome, characterized by the co-occurrence of multiple colorectal tumors such as familial adenomatous polyposis, and cerebral glioblastoma or medulloblastoma.[2718]

turn The point of change in polarity of a waveform and the magnitude of the voltage change following the turning point. It is not necessary that the voltage change pass through the baseline. The minimal excursion required to constitute a change should be specified. (Adapted from the 2001 Report of the Nomenclature Committee of the American Association of Electromyography and Electrodiagnosis.[19] Reproduced by kind permission of the AANEM.)

turns analysis An automated method of analyzing EMG activity during isometric voluntary contraction whereby the number of positive and negative potential changes exceeding 100 µV is counted over a specific period. The method provides some data distinguishing primary myopathic from neurogenic muscle disease.[2273]

Turner, William (1832–1916) Professor of anatomy at the University of Edinburgh, noted for his description of the gyri, fissures, and lobes of the cerebral cortex in today's accepted form.

turns-amplitude analysis A computerized method of assessing the muscle recruitment patterns recorded by EMG. The parameters studied are the maximal number of turns to mean amplitude (peak ratio or PR); the mean amplitude; and the number of time intervals between turns at different degrees of voluntary contraction. The technique assists in the EMG diagnosis of myopathy.[6012]

turricephaly (Lat, tower + Gr, head) See **tower skull**.

turtle headache A condition described only in colder climates, characterized by the occurrence of dull, generalized matutinal headaches, presumed to be due to the hypercapnia resulting from sleeping with the head completely under the bedclothes.[2410]

tussive syncope (Lat, cough + Gr, faint) (Laryngeal vertigo) See **cough syncope**.

twilight state (absence status, état confusionnel simple, spike-wave stupor, fugue state) A syndrome characterized by prolonged confusion, diminished responsiveness, speech arrest, automatic behaviour, and subsequent amnesia as a result of petit mal or of subconvulsive complex partial seizure (psychomotor) status.

In the former, diffuse, irregular 1.5- to 4-Hz multispike-wave complexes are recorded, there is no complete loss of responsiveness, and the episode represents one single prolonged attack. In the latter, the episode is due to repetitive, discontinuous attacks; total unresponsiveness may ensue; and the EEG patterns are variable and include both fast and slow-wave discharges, rhythmic diffuse bilateral spikes, and anterior temporal sharp waves.[491] Twilight states may also occur as postictal manifestations.[1912]

twitch-convulsive syndrome A symptom of uremic encephalopathy in the setting of other metabolic disorders such as **delirium tremens**, diabetes, and **systemic lupus erythematosus**. Clouding of consciousness, seizures, and multifocal myoclonus occur, the latter in any area of the body in both the waking and sleeping states.

two-point discrimination The discrimination of two points of simultaneous contact on the skin or mucosa. On the fingertips, 2 mm of separation should be detectable in normal young people; on the back the separation may have to be 8 cm for discernment. The fingetip threshold rises (greater separation of the two points being needed) with advancing age.[6504]

TWUD index (Time Wasted in Unnecessary Discussion) The relationship between the frequency with which a condition is considered and its actual prevalence. Informal, introspective analysis suggests a TWUD index of 4800 for **normal-pressure hydrocephalus**, 320 for **Creutzfeldt–Jakob disease**, and 15 for **Bell palsy**. The occurrence of bedsores in demented patients has a negative score.{JF}

The lengthy discussion of differential diagnoses (i.e., describing many conditions that could possibly be considered, all but one of which are wrong) is rather similar.

tylosis-optic atrophy A rare syndrome of adult life consisting of thickening of the palms and soles and the later development of optic atrophy.[1658]

tympanic neuropathy (syndrome of Jacobson's nerve and plexus) Loss of secretion by the parotid gland as a result of damage to the nerve, usually as a result of cranial trauma.[3807]

tympanic plexus neuralgia See **glossopharyngeal neuralgia**.

type grouping The presence of unusually large numbers of fibers (50 or more) of the same histochemical type, arranged contiguously in groups within a microscopic preparation of muscle. The appearance is considered to indicate the collateral sprouting of motor axons in cases of chronic motor neuropathy.[3315] See **fiber type grouping**.

type/token ratio A measure of verbal diversification in which the number of times a particular word appears in a block of language is expressed as its ratio to the total number of words in the block. All the words in the block are counted (*Tokens*), but the count of the number of different words is the *Type*. In the shortest and simplest sentences, in old age and in dementia, the ratio is low (e.g., <0.5).[1338]

type 1 acrocephalosyndactyly See **Apert syndrome**.

type I fiber atrophy Selective atrophy of type I muscle fibers, found in numerous conditions such as nemaline myopathy, congenital fiber-type disproportion,[868] and myotonic dystrophy and also as a lone familial occurrence when it presents with congenital nonprogressive muscle wasting and weakness.[5557]

type I fiber hypotrophy with central nuclei An X-linked recessive disorder characterized by this microscopic appearance which is associated clinically with congenital severe diffuse weakness and hypotonia and enlargement of the tongue, the disease resembling **hereditary motor neuropathy**, type 1.[1888] Biopsy specimens show fiber hypertrophy or hypotrophy with central nuclei and the presence of cytoplasmic bodies.[381]

type I fiber predominance The appearance on muscle biopsy specimens when the number of histochemically type I fibers shown exceeds the normal for the muscle biopsied. For the vastus lateralis, for example, >55% would be abnormal.

The finding is present in cases of **congenital** and **Duchenne muscular dystrophies,** various **congenital myopathies, hypothyroid myopathy**, and **benign congenital hypotonia**, and also in some children with hypotonia without other evidence of neuromuscular disease.[3625]

type I myofibrils Slow-twitch muscle fibers containing substantial amounts of myoglobin and staining well for dehydrogenases. ATPase stains at pH 9.4 color these fibers poorly, but they stain dark at pH 4.35.

type II myofibrils Fast-twitch muscle fibers staining well for phosphorylase, glycogen, and α-glycerophosphate dehydrogenase. ATPase stains at pH 9.4 stain these fibers dark. At pH 4.35 they are unstained and at pH 4.63, two fiber subtypes (colorless IIa and intermediate IIb) can be differentiated.

type-specific atrophy Selective atrophy of type I or type II myofibrils. Type IIb atrophy is seen in the settings of cachectic wasting, or systemic malignancy or prolonged immobilization.

typhus A louse-borne *rickettsial* infection causing generalized vasculitis. Clinical features consist of fever, headache, vomiting, respiratory symptoms, conjunctival injection, and diarrhea, followed by the appearance of a purpuric rash.

The neurological complications are those of a meningoencephalitis causing delirium and stupor, and any of many possible focal deficits, occurring either during or following the acute illness.[2872]

typical absence attacks See **typical absence epilepsy**.

typical absence epilepsy (typical absence attacks) A term applied to a number of epileptic syndromes including frequent absence attacks occurring in isolation between the ages of 4 and 10 years (pyknolepsy); **typical absence epilepsy of adolescents,** sometimes with associated tonic-clonic seizures, etc.; **petit mal epilepsy; myoclonic absences** (clonic absences); and typical absence epilepsies with unusual EEG features. The latter include adversive absence, absences occurring with focal clinical features, absence with evidence of a brain lesion, and absences induced by visual stimuli.[72] The condition was first described by Poupart in 1705.

Simple typical absences are characterized by a sudden decrease in mental functioning of brief duration, usually 5–15 s, with abolition or diminution of awareness, responsiveness, and memory for the event when the subject returns from this period of unawareness and unresponsiveness. Hyperventilation and stimulation are strong precipitants.

In *complex typical absences*, the impairment of consciousness is associated with motor manifestations, including gaze deviation, head rotation, clonic jerks, or decreased muscle tone.

typical absence epilepsy of adolescence (primary generalized epilepsy of adolescence) A syndrome of repetitive absences clustering within the hour following awakening, in which the attacks are shorter and less frequent than the similar syndrome in younger children, and sometimes without complete loss of contact with the surroundings. Generalized tonic-clonic seizures also occur in some cases.[6844] See also **juvenile myoclonic epilepsy of Janz**.

tyramine infusion test A test of postganglionic sympathetic fiber integrity, wherein tyramine is infused intravenously at rates of 60–500 μg/min until there is an elevation of systolic blood pressure of 15 mmHg or more.

An exaggerated response (e.g., with 300 μg/min) suggests the presence of denervation hypersensitivity, and an impaired response, severe postganglionic damage.[374] The test is based on the fact that normally the tyramine is taken up by sympathetic vesicles and leads to the secretion of norepinephrine, and hence an increase in blood pressure.[374]

tyrosine hydroxylase The rate-limiting enzyme in catecholamine synthesis.

tyrosinemia I (OMIM 276700) A rare recessively inherited disorder of aminoacid metabolism due to a deficiency of the gene for fumarylacetoacetate hydrolase, leading to hepatic disease, neuropathy, and other neurological features resembling those of porphyria.[2587]

tyrosinemia II A diffuse encephalopathy presenting with cataracts, skin lesions, and mental delay.[4400] The responsible gene maps to 16q22.1–q22.3. See **Richner–Hanhart syndrome**.

tyrosinosis A recessively inherited dysmetabolic state seen in neonates, and due to impairment of hepatic tyrosine transaminase function. The condition is characterized by hepatic and renal impairment, vitamin D-resistant rickets, blepharospasm, and mental and motor delay in the survivors.[6947]

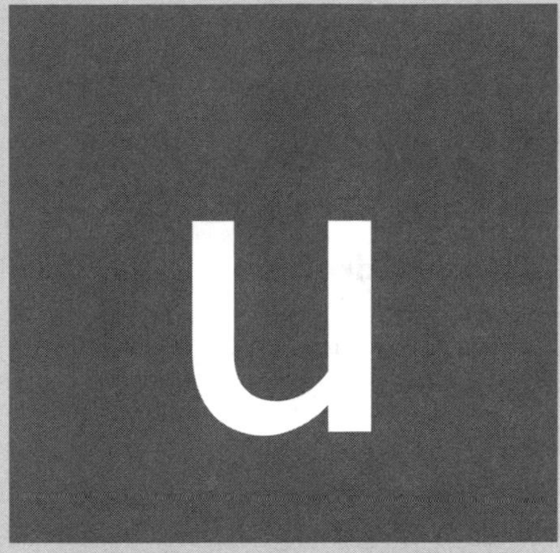

U fibers The longitudinal (*arcuate*, from Lat, bow-shaped) myelinated fibers of the cerebral cortex which course beneath the sulci. They are spared in **Binswanger disease**, in some leukodystrophies, and in **cerebral amyloid angiopathy**.

ubiquitin An abnormal protein component of neuronal inclusions in **Alzheimer, Parkinson,** and **Pick diseases**.

UBOs See **unidentified bright objects**.

Udorn encephalopathy A syndrome described in the population of Thailand which closely resembles **Reye syndrome**, but which is due to aflatoxin poisoning.[4790]

Uhthoff symptom (hot-bath sign) Deterioration of neural function in association with a rise in local body temperature.[6439] It is seen in patients with demyelinating disease as a result of the increased conduction block occurring at higher temperatures, and is usable as a sign of demyelination when nystagmus, motor power, or visual acuity are measured before and after heating a patient by as little as 1°C. While present in many patients with **multiple sclerosis**, the sign is not diagnostic of that condition. Dr. Wilhelm Uhthoff (1853–1927) was a German physician who described the phenomenon in 1889.

An *inverse Uhtoff sign* has been reported, in which vision *improves* with warming.[153]

ulcerative mutilating acropathy with abnormal CSF aminoacids A rare *variant* of **hereditary sensory and autonomic neuropathy**.

ulceromutilating acropathy See **hereditary sensory and autonomic neuropathy**.

ulceromutilating acropathy (mutilating acropathy) The trophic changes, including impaired circulation and loss of hair, nonhealing ulceration of the skin, and infection of soft tissues and bone, occurring usually in the distal parts of limbs as a result of peripheral sensory neuropathies impairing pain sensation and autonomic functions. See **hereditary sensory and autonomic neuropathy, familial amyloid neuropathy**.

Lesions of the conus medullaris and central cord may do the same. Compare with **Charcot joint** (in which the damage is usually more proximal).

ulegyria (mantle sclerosis, nodular cortical sclerosis) A localized destruction of the deepest parts of the cortical wall in the sulci with relative sparing of the cortex at the surface. The abnormality may be generalized or localized, but in either case is usually a result of perinatal hypoxia.

Ullmann Syndrome (systemic angiomatosis) A heterogeneous syndrome characterized by the presence of cavernous and telangiectatic angiomas in the brain with associated dural abnormalities. The condition is probably a form of **Osler–Rendu–Weber disease**.

Ullrich muscular dystrophy (*atonic-sclerotic type*) The second most common form of **congenital muscular dystrophy**; a slowly progressive form due to mutations of collagen type VI, subunits $\alpha 1$, $\alpha 2$, or $\alpha 3$. All are inherited as either recessive or dominant traits (the same gene as **Bethlem myopathy**). Typical features include presentation in the neonatal period with hypotonia, kyphosis of the spine, proximal joint contractures, torticollis, and hip dislocation. Historically there may have been reduced fetal movements.

Variable weakness mainly affecting the neck and distal musculature and early hyperlaxity of distal joints are notable in infancy. Sometimes distal arthrogryposis is present. Congenital contractures are more proximal than distal but the long finger flexors are much affected. Spinal rigidity, kyphoscoliosis, and torticollis are also common. Respiratory insufficiency is notable even in childhood, and death occurs before the end of the second decade. The skin shows follicular hyperkeratosis, keloids, atrophic scars, striae, and petechiae. The serum CK is normal or high and the EMG is myopathic. Muscle biopsy shows varied muscle fiber size with some very small fibers and increased endomysial connective tissue.[4992, 4555]

Ullrich syndrome A benign form of muscular dystrophy associated with hyperexcitability in the CNS. See **minimal change myopathy**.

Ullrich, Otto (1894–1957) German pediatrician who practiced in Essen, Berlin, and Rostock, and who described what is now known as *Turner syndrome* and *hypophosphatemic renal rickets* as well as the syndromes described in the adjacent entries.

Ullrich–Noonan syndrome See **Noonan syndrome**.

ulnar flexion maneuver Flexion of the elbow and flexion and ulnar deviation of the wrist increase paresthesias in the fourth and fifth digits in cases of ulnar nerve entrapment beneath the flexor carpi ulnaris.[2054]

ulnar nerve palsy (tardy ulnar palsy) Sensory deficits with weakness and wasting of the muscles supplied by the ulnar nerve, usually as a result of its compression in the cubital tunnel or distally, in **Guyon's canal**. The former is far more common (**cubital tunnel syndrome**); the interossei, adductor pollicis, and hypothenar muscles are affected, and there is reduced common sensation in the ulnar palm and the ulnar 1½ digits. The **Tinel sign** is frequently positive at the cubital tunnel.

Damage to the *deep palmar branch* of the nerve in **Guyon's canal** occurs in carpenters, cobblers, cyclists, and others who repeatedly compress the nerve there in the course of work or play. Weakness and wasting of the interossei and adductor pollicis without hypothenar muscle involvement and without sensory changes are the characteristic findings. The most useful electrodiagnostic test compares the latencies of the median and ulnar mixed nerve action potentials between the wrist and the elbow.[4324]

Isolated damage to the *dorsal sensory branch* of the nerve on the dorsum of the hand is a rarity, and almost always due to local trauma. See also **all-ulnar hand**.

Ulnar nerve palsies sometimes occur in the perioperative period, usually after 24 h have passed; it has been thought that this is a result of poor positioning of the outstretched arm during the surgery, but postoperative compression of the nerve as a result of sitting in a chair or bed with the elbows flexed is a much more likely cause.[6058]

ultimum moriens The superior portion of the trapezius muscle, which **Gowers** considered to be remarkable in that it does not atrophy in certain myopathic states although other muscles do.

ultraterminal sprouting The growth of neuronal shoots at the motor nerve terminal to innervate orphaned end-plates, seen when the release of acetylcholine from the terminal is blocked, as in **botulism**.

ultraviolet keratitis See **photophthalmia**.

umami The savory taste associated with cured meats, Parmesan cheese, and monosodium glutamate, additional to the usually recognized sweet, salt, sour, and bitter quartet.

uncal herniation (Lat, hook + rupture) (lateral transtentorial herniation) Downward displacement of the uncus and parahippocampal gyrus through the tentorial opening due to increased intracranial pressure, as may result from an expanding mass in the temporal lobe. One of the earliest and still surely the most perfect image of **uncal herniation** is that engraved by Robert Hooper and published in his *The Morbid Anatomy of the Human Brain* (London: Longman, 1826; Plate XIII) although the artist did not comment on the appearance which was only spotted later by Sir Geoffrey Jefferson, an English neurosurgeon.

uncal syndrome The clinical effect of herniation of the uncus downward through the tentorium cerebelli as a result of increased intracranial pressure, usually resulting from a temporal lobe mass on the same side. Lateral displacement of the brainstem may be as important as the downward shift, however.[5383] The herniating tissue compresses the brainstem at the level of the peduncles and distorts the III cranial nerve, leading to III nerve palsy, diminution in conscious level, Cheyne–Stokes respirations, and direct compression of the same and secondary compression of the opposite cerebral peduncle, leading to ipsi- and contralateral hemiparesis with a grave prognosis.[5053]

Compression of the posterior cerebral artery may lead to occipital infarction, the resultant homonymous hemianopia then representing a false localizing sign.

uncinate (Lat, hooked) To do with the uncus.

uncinate fits Complex focally-originating seizures in which olfactory hallucinations occur as part of the consciously appreciated manifestations of the seizure, and assumed to be due to electrical excitation of the uncus and olfactory cortex.[1426] The name was applied by Hughlings-**Jackson** in 1899: "There is at the onset of the paroxysm a crude sensation of smell or of taste or in which there are movements of chewing, smacking of the lips, and sometimes spitting, etc." Jackson was aware of the researches of **Ferrier** showing that the functions of smell and taste in animals are localized in the uncinate gyrus.

uncrossed diplopia That form of diplopia which results from **esotropia**, and in which the false image is displaced toward the side of the paretic eye. See also **crossed diplopia.**

Underwood, Michael (1737–1820) English physician, pediatrician, and obstetrician, who gave the first modern account of **poliomyelitis** in 1789.[4938]

undifferentiated jargon See **jargon**.

undulatory nystagmus See **pendular nystagmus**.

unformed hallucinations Visual hallucinations, the images not being recognizable as people or objects, or, in the case of auditory hallucinations, those in which the sound heard does not resemble that from any recognized source.

unidentified bright objects (UBOs) Areas of brightness on T2-weighted (long spin-echo) MRI scans indicating the presence in those areas of high concentrations of H^+ protons (i.e., water or glial cells); such areas may be multiple sclerosis plaques, infarcts, or other pathologies.

Unified Batten Disease Rating Scale An instrument quantifying the physical, behavioral, and functional aspects of **juvenile neuroceroid lipofuscinosis**. Visual acuity, fundoscopy, speech clarity, tongue protrusion, initiation and velocity of saccades, ocular pursuit, passive motion of the neck and of each limb, power in each limb, hand tapping on each side, maximal dystonia bilaterally, overall body bradykinesia, gait, tandem walking, retropulsion (pull-test), heel stomping bilaterally, motor tics, myoclonus, rest and action tremor, finger-to-nose dysmetria, and appendicular chorea are all assessed on a 0–4 scale.[4109]

Unified Dystonia Rating Scale An instrument for this purpose, accessible at the Web site: http://www.mdvu.org/library/ratingscales/dystonia/TWSTRS_09_29_02.pdf/.

Unified Form for Neurological Stroke Scales A combination scale constituting reconciliations of the neurological scale for middle cerebral artery infarction (MCANS) and the Scandinavian stroke scale (SNSS). It also allows the generation of scores on the **Canadian Stroke Scale**.[4810] (Chart U–1)

Unified Multiple System Atrophy Rating Scale A rating scale for **multiple system atrophy** including the following items:[6723]

I. Historical (speech, swallowing, handwriting, cutting food and handling utensils, dressing, hygiene, walking, falling [in the past month], orthostatic symptoms)
II. Motor examination (facial expression, speech, ocular motor dysfunction, tremor at rest, action tremor, increased tone, rapid alternating movements of hands, finger-tapping, leg agility, heel-shin test, arising from chair, posture, body sway, and gait)
III. Autonomic examination (urinary, sexual, and bowel functions; systolic and diastolic blood pressures, supine and standing for 2 min; heart rate supine and standing for 2 min; orthostatic symptoms)
IV. A 5-point global disability scale.

Chart U–1. Unified Form for Neurological Stroke Scale

Item	*SNSS*	*MCANS*
Consciousness:		
Normal/fully conscious	6	15
Somnolent/drowsiness	4	10
Reacts to verbal command	2	10
Stupor (reacts to pain only)	0	5
Coma	0	0
Speech/Verbal communication:		
Normal/no aphasia	10	10
Limited vocabulary or incoherent speech/difficult	6	5
More than yes/no but not longer sentences/difficult	3	5
Only yes/no or less/extremely difficult or impossible	0	0
Eye movements/Eyes and head shift:		
No gaze/palsy/none	4	10
Gaze palsy/gaze failure	2	5
Conjugate eye deviation/forced	0	0
Facial Palsy:		
None/dubious/slight paresis	2	5
Present/paralysis or marked paresis	0	0
Arm: Motor power/Raising:		
Raises with normal strength/normal	6	10
Raised with reduced strength/possible	5	10
Raises with flexion in elbow/incomplete	4	5
Can move but not against gravity/impossible	2	0
Paralysis	0	0
Hand: Motor power/Movements:		
Normal strength/normal	6	15
Reduced strength/skilled	4	10
Fingertips do not reach palm/useful	2	5
Paralysis/useless	0	0
Leg: Motor power/Raising:		
Normal strength	6	15
Raises with reduced strength/against resistance	5	10
Raises with flexion of knee/against gravity	4	5
Can move, but not against gravity/impossible	2	0
Paralysis	0	0
Foot Dorsiflexion:		
Against resistance/normal	—	10
Against gravity	—	5
Foot drop	—	0
Upper limb tone:		
Normal (even if brisk reflexes)	—	5
Overtly spastic or flaccid	—	0
Lower limb tone:		
Normal (even if brisk reflexes)	—	5
Overtly spastic or flaccid	—	0
Orientation:		
Correct for time, place, and person	6	—
Two of these	4	—
One of these	2	—
Completely disoriented	0	—

continued

Chart U–1. (*continued*)

Item	*SNSS*	*MCANS*
Gait:		
Walks at least 5 m without aids	12	—
Walks with aids	9	—
Walks with help of another person	+6	—
Sits without support	3	—
Bedridden/wheelchair	0	—
Total		

(From Orgogozo JM. A unified form for neurological scoring of hemispheric stroke with motor impairment. *Stroke* 1992;**23**:1678–9, with paid permission from Lippincott, Williams and Wilkins)

Unified Myoclonus Rating Scale An instrument for this purpose, accessible at the Web site: http://www.mdvu.org/library/ratingscales/myo/UMRS.pdf/.

Unified Rating Scale for Parkinsonism A popular and comprehensive scale for the determination of disability in Parkinson disease.[6044] The headers of a modified version from the Movement Disorder Society are presented in Chart U–2. See also http://www.wemove.org/.

uniform fiber-type myopathy A form of muscle disorder in which histochemical staining demonstrates that more than 99% of the muscle fibers belong to one histochemical type.[4762]

unihemispheric sleep The biological changes of sleep occurring in but one of the cerebral hemispheres; an attribute of dolphins. For a human to be "half-asleep," however, suggests the presence of stage 1 non–rapid eye movement sleep on both sides.

unilateral atonic seizures See **hemiparetic seizures**.

unilateral jaw and masticatory spasm A focal dystonic syndrome with onset in youth or early adult life, characterized by spasm and secondary hypertrophy of the masseters. See **oromandibular dystonia**.

unilateral juvenile muscular atrophy of upper limbs See **monomelic amyotrophy**.

unilateral lobar atrophy A form of unilateral frontotemporal atrophy causing slowly progressive aphasia without dementia, and associated with neuronal loss, gliosis, and spongiform change in the affected cortical region.[3455]

unilateral pursuit paresis The association of saccadic (rather than smooth) pursuit when the eyes follow toward the side of a hemispheric lesion, and contralateral homonymous hemianopia.[6311]

unilateral spatial agnosia Massive neglect of the left half of visual space, leading to loss of topographical orientation and caused by a lesion of the right parietal region.

Chart U–2. Revised MDS–Unified Rating Scale for Parkinsonism

Part I: Nonmotor Aspects of Experiences of Daily Living

Cognitive impairment
Hallucinations and psychosis
Depressed mood
Anxious mood
Apathy
Features of **dopamine dysregulation syndrome**
Sleep problems
Daytime sleepiness
Pain and other sensations
Urinary problems
Constipation problems
Lightheadedness on standing
Fatigue

Part II: Motor Experiences of Daily Living

Speech
Saliva and drooling
Chewing and swallowing
Eating tasks
Dressing
Hygiene
Handwriting
Doing hobbies and other activities
Turning in bed
Tremor impact on activities
Getting in and out of bed
Walking and balance
Freezing

Part III: Motor Examination

Speech
Facial expression
Rigidity
Finger tapping
Hand movements
Pronation–supination movements of hands
Toe tapping
Leg agility
Arising from chair
Gait
Freezing of gait
Postural stability
Posture
Global spontaneity of movement (body bradykinesia)
Postural tremor of hands
Kinetic tremor of hands
Rest tremor amplitude
Constancy of rest tremor

Part IV: Motor Complications

Dyskinesias: time spent with dyskinesias
Dyskinesias: functional impact of dyskinesias
Dyskinesias: painful *off* state dystonia
Motor fluctuations: time spent in the *off* state
Motor fluctuations: functional impact of fluctuations
Motor fluctuations: complexity of motor fluctuations
The patient's blood pressure, pulse, and weight are also to be recorded on the scoring form.

The Movement Disorder Society–Unified Rating Scale for Parkinsonism (UPDRS) retains the previous UPDRS structure of four parts with a total summed score, but the parts have been modified to provide a section that integrates nonmotor elements of Parkinson disease: All items have five response options with uniform anchors.[2431] The full scale is accessible at the Web site: http://www.movementdisorders.org/UserFiles/New%20UPDRS%207%203%2008%20final.pdf.

See also **Hoehn and Yahr Scale**,[2933] **Columbia Rating Scale**,[1942] **Parkinson Disease Impairment Index**, and **SCOPA**.

unimacular nystagmus See **latent nystagmus**.

unimodal apraxia Any form of apraxia that is specific to actions demonstrated in a single modality, e.g., visual but not auditory.[3540] See **apraxia**.

uniocular nystagmus Vertical oscillations of one eye in association with long-standing visual loss. The amplitude of the oscillations ranges from 3 to 50° and the frequency from 0.1 to 5 Hz, inversely correlated with the amplitudes.[5125]

unipolar See **referential derivation**.

unipolar needle electrode See **monopolar needle recording electrode**.

United Cerebral Palsy Association A charitable organization. Address: 1522 K Street NW Suite 1112, Washington, DC 20005. Tel: 202-842-1266; 202-842-3519. Web site: http://www.ucpa.org/.

United Cerebral Palsy Association A charitable organization in this field. Web site: http://www.ucpa.org/.

United Leukodystrophy Foundation A charitable association in this field. Web site: http://www.ulf.org/.

United Mitochondrial Disease Foundation A charitable organization promoting research and providing support to families of people with mitochondriopathies. Address: P.O. Box 1151, Monroeville, PA 15146-1151. Tel: 412-856-1297. Web site: http:/biochemgen.ucsd.edu/umdf/.

United Mitochondrial Disease Foundation An American charitable association promoting research and supporting families of people with mitochondriopathies. Web site: http://biochemgen.ucsd.edu/umdf.

United Parkinson Foundation An organization dedicated to funding research on Parkinson disease, publishing educational materials for patients and health care professionals, and providing support for patients with the disease. It is based at Saint Louis University, St. Louis, MO 63103-2097. Web site: http://www.pdf.org/AboutPDF/history.cfm/.

unloading reflex A biphasic response characterized by an initial reduction or absence of electrical potentials recorded on the EMG, followed by an abrupt increase in electrical activity, when a muscle is contracted against an external load and the load is then suddenly removed.[148]

unprovoked seizures of unknown etiology[1265] Cases of unprovoked seizures for which no clear antecedent etiology can be detected. One form comprises the *idiopathic epilepsies*, which are defined by the ILAE as certain partial or generalized epileptic syndromes with particular clinical characteristics and with specific EEG findings; the term should not be used to refer to epilepsy or seizures without obvious cause.

Unverricht, Heinrich (1853–1912) German physician, practicing in Jena, Austria. His graduating thesis, in which he asserted that all seizures required the presence of cortex, aroused great interest and within 6 years he had been appointed professor of medicine at Dorpat. He published his account of familial myoclonic epilepsy in 1891.

Unverricht–Lundborg–Lafora syndrome (Lafora body epilepsy, Unverricht–Lundborg disease, Baltic or Nordic myoclonus, myoclonic encephalopathy with progressive cranial nerve palsies, progressive familial myoclonic epilepsy, progressive myoclonic epilepsy type 1 [EPM1] OMIM 254800)[568, 6449] A recessively inherited **mitochondrial encephalomyelopathy** presenting between the ages of 6 and 16 years with tonic–clonic seizures; spontaneous, stimulus-sensitive and action myoclonus (**cortical myoclonus**); drop attacks, ataxia; rigidity; cerebellar signs; and, later, ataxia, incoordination, intentional tremor, dysarthria, and progressive mental deterioration. Repetitive morning myoclonus is common. The biochemical cause is unknown but one responsible gene maps to chromosome 21q22.3 (*EPM1*) and another to chromosome 12 (*EPM1B*). This is the commonest cause of **progressive myoclonic epilepsy**.[3280]

The Marseilles consensus group defined the condition as follows: "Myoclonus with epileptic seizures and progressive neurological decline, particularly ataxia and dementia." The syndrome was first reported by Unverricht in 1891 and appears to occur mainly in the populations of eastern Sweden and Finland, determining the name *Baltic*, but it has also been reported from distant shores. It is probably the same condition as many (but not all) cases of the **dyssynergia cerebellaris myoclonica** of **Ramsay Hunt**.[6221] Lundborg contributed by adding new cases, demonstrating autosomal recessive inheritance, and confirming that the disease is indeed progressive. **Lafora** contributed by identifying the presence of intracytoplasmic inclusions (**Lafora bodies**) within the nervous system.

Myoclonic encephalopathy with progressive cranial nerve palsies and a form with younger onset mapped to chromosome 12 (*EPM1B*)[570] are *variants*.

See also **progressive myoclonic ataxias, dentate-rubropallidoluysian atrophy**.

Unverricht–Wagner syndrome See **dermatomyositis**.

upbeat nystagmus A form of central vestibular jerk nystagmus in which the fast component is upward and which is present in the primary position but increases on upward gaze. Defective upward pursuit but intact vestibulo-ocular movements are characteristic accompaniments. Bilateral lesions of the ventral tegmental pathways at the pontomesencephalic junction or in the caudal brainstem close to the perihypoglossal nuclei and lesions of the anterior vermis are most commonly incriminated.[3362, 5181]

up-gaze palsy Failure of conjugate upward deviation of the eyes as a result of a pretectal lesion in which the posterior commissure is damaged. Other features of the **Parinaud syndrome** are usually present as well.

upper airway resistance syndrome Anatomical constriction of the airways at levels above the larynx, considered relevant in the genesis of some cases of **idiopathic hypersomnia**.[113]

upper brachial plexus palsy (Erb palsy, cadet palsy, Duchenne–Erb palsy, **rucksack palsy**, knapsack palsy, **pallbearers' palsy**) Weakness and atrophy of the muscles supplied by C5–6 through the upper trunk of the brachial plexus, leading to the posture of the arm described as the "porter's tip" position. It is commonly caused by violent falls on the shoulder, excessive traction on the head during delivery, or direct injury to the upper fibers of the brachial plexus.[1896]

Erb's name is popularly attached to this condition, although he attributed its delineation to **Duchenne**, whose adequate account had been provided 19 years before.[5729] Another, by William Smellie, a Scottish obstetrician, had been published in 1768.

upper motor neuron lesion

(pyramidal lesion, corticospinal tract lesion) A lesion of the descending motor pathways between the cortex and the brainstem or spinal cord, producing a relatively constant syndrome of postural disturbance, increased tone (spasticity), decreased power especially in the arm extensors and the leg flexors, hyperreflexia of the muscle stretch reflexes and loss of superficial reflexes, and an upgoing plantar (positive Babinski) response. Both the corticospinal and the corticoreticulospinal pathways are considered to be involved.

The alternative term *pyramidal lesion* is used synonymously, but could be considered inappropriate in those cases in which the lesion affects the corticopontine fibers, because obviously these do not go as far as the pyramids. Lesions of the extrapyramidal pathways are also upper motor neuron lesions, but the syndrome resulting is different and by convention such disturbances are not included under this heading. On electromyographic examination of weak muscles, there is slow motor unit action potential firing at maximal effort.

upper syndrome of the brainstem tegmentum Infarction of the nucleus of the IV cranial nerve, and perhaps of the III; with superior cerebellar peduncle and medial lemniscus involvement.

upside-down ptosis The elevation of the lower lid accompanying drooping of the upper lid in **Horner syndrome**.

upward transtentorial herniation Upward herniation of the cerebellum through the tentorial incisura, usually due to a cerebellar tumor, abscess, or hemorrhage, but lesions of the cerebellopontine angle, pons, or medulla may occasionally be responsible. Forward compression of the brainstem and downward herniation of the cerebellar tonsils precede the upward movement. Clinically, the patients are in coma with unreactive miotic pupils, loss of vertical doll's head movements, asymmetrical or absent caloric responses, and decerebrate posturing.[1380]

Urbach–Wiethe disease

(hyalinosis cutis et mucosae) A rare, recessively inherited lipid storage disorder, characterized by hoarse voice, waxy infiltration of the skin and mucous membranes, skin nodules over the upper body, photosensitivity, alopecia, short stature, ocular and dental abnormalities, intracranial calcifications, seizures, rage attacks, and memory disturbances (sometimes without other evidence of dementia).[4653] Although some of the children have little cognitive abnormality, they differ emotionally and in their judgment of all emotions in facial expressions from their peers.[5828] The manifestations reflect damage in the amygdaloid region, usually symmetrically.

A *variant* is an hereditary small vessel disease of the brain, its mutated gene distinct from *NOTCH3*, and a potential cause of lacunar infarcts with leukoaraiosis.[6535] See also **lipoid proteinosis**.

ureal diabetes See **diabetes insipidus**.

uremic encephalopathy Diffuse cerebral dysfunction occurring in the context of acute or chronic renal failure, but more severe in the former, and presenting with fatigue, impaired concentration, clumsiness leading to asterixis, myoclonus or generalized seizures, confusion, and eventual coma. In the chronic form, lability of mood, asthenia, inverted sleep rhythms, and impaired frontal lobe functions are the most common findings.

uremic myopathy A syndrome of proximal weakness and wasting with myopathic EMG findings, occurring in patients with chronic renal failure.[2131]

uremic polyneuropathy A distal, symmetrical axonal neuropathy often complicating end-stage kidney disease (glomerular filtration rates less than 12 ml/min), typically presenting with slowly progressive involvement of the legs more than the arms. The paresthesias, diminished muscle stretch reflexes, impaired vibration sense, and muscle wasting and weakness reflect large-fiber involvement. Autonomic features include postural hypotension, impaired sweating, diarrhea, constipation, and/or impotence. Chronic hyperkalemic depolarization is the most likely mechanism.[262, 3567]

urethral crisis Acute paroxysms of pain felt along the course of the urethra in patients with **tabes dorsalis**.

urethral reflex The fancied gripping of a catheter or sound passed into the penile lumen. The mechanism and purpose of this reflex are equally obscure.

urogenital triangle The anatomical space whose floor is the deep transverse perineal muscles and the external sphincter, forming the urogenital diaphragm. On each side are the bulbocavernosus (perineal nerve) and ischiocavernosus muscles, while the base is formed by the superior transverse perineal muscles.

useless hand (useless arm) Lack of control of the hand or arm as a result of rigidity, dystonia, apraxia, or akinesia with sensory deafferentation, despite the retention of normal power. It is described in **multiple sclerosis** affecting the posterior columns at cervical level and can also be a presenting feature in **corticobasal degeneration**. The condition was first described by Oppenheim in 1910.[1247, 4066]

Usher syndrome (Hallgren syndrome, recessive retinitis pigmentosa with congenital deafness) The recessively inherited combination of progressive visual loss resulting from retinitis pigmentosa (tapetoretinal degeneration), moderate to severe congenital sensorineural deafness, vestibular impairment, cerebellar atrophy, and mental retardation or other mental disorders.[3515, 6454]

Both *severe (type 1)* and *mild (type 2)* forms of the condition are described. Although vision is preserved until later life and there are no vestibular symptoms in the type 2 form, it is uncertain whether this is a single condition or more than one.[4229]

utilization behavior A disturbance in the response to external stimuli, which indicates an exaggerated and disinhibited dependency on the environment for behavioral clues, and which indicates the presence of damage to one or both frontal lobes, with loss of frontal inhibition of posterior perceptual and perceptuomotor processing.[3826] Paramedian thalamic infarcts have also been described as leading to this behavior. Such activity can be considered as an extension of bimanual grasping behavior (**magnetic apraxia**), in which the patient appears compelled to grasp and use any object presented visually or through touch; it is associated with uni- or bilateral lesions of the frontal lobe. See also **forced hyperphasia**.

utilization time See **latency of activation**.

utricle A part of the labyrinthine structures, with the saccule and semicircular canals. It contains specialized sensory epithelium from which the hair cell processes project into mucilaginous material within it, where they are stimulated by the movement of otoliths.

uveal tract The iris, ciliary body, and choroid in the eye.

uveitis Inflammation of the uvea; classified as *anterior* (inflammation of the iris and/or the ciliary body, i.e., iritis, cyclitis, iridocyclitis) and *posterior* (inflammation of the choroid, i.e., choroiditis).

uveomeningitic syndrome See **uveomeningoencephalitic syndrome**.

uveomeningoencephalitic syndrome (Vogt–Koyanagi–Harada syndrome) A rare multisystem inflammatory disorder comprising uveitis or sympathetic ophthalmia, dysacousis, alopecia, leukoderma, whitening of the eyelashes and eyebrows, and acute encephalitic and fluctuating meningitic signs.[6560]

The initial acute meningitic phase may be complicated by delirium, cranial nerve palsies and other pareses, and loss of sphincter control, and is accompanied by pleocytosis of the CSF. Acute bilateral uveitis with widely dilated pupils then supervenes and retinal detachment and acute glaucoma may ensue. Decreased visual acuity, macular edema, papillitis, and visual field defects are common findings. The remaining systemic features of the disease, listed above, appear during the convalescent phase. Abortive forms also occur.[5] **Sarcoidosis** is an important cause of the uveomeningitic syndrome (without the encephalitis); **Behçet disease, syphilis, Wegener granulomatosis**, and viral infections are others. Other uveomeningeal syndromes occur in acute or chronic infections and in **multiple sclerosis**, in **primary CNS lymphoma**, or as a **paraneoplastic syndrome** associated with breast carcinoma.

Vogt gave the first modern report in 1906, but the condition was described in part at least by Ali-ibn-Isa (940–1010), an Arabian physician.[4936] The clinical features and stages have been delineated[3091] and are given in Chart U–3.

uveoparotid fever A variety of sarcoidosis. See **Heerfordt syndrome**.

Chart U–3. Stages of Uveomeningoencephalitic Syndrome

I. Early acute stage (uveoauditomeningitis)

1. Bilateral uveitis

   Loss of visual acuity
   Cells in the anterior chamber
   Exudative retinal detachment
   Multifocal dye leakage from retinal pigment epithelium on angiography

2. Auditory disturbance

   Auditory disturbance
   Tinnitus, vertigo
   Nerve deafness

3. Meningitis

   Meningitis
   Headache, nausea
   CSF pleocytosis

II. Recovery stage (oculodermal depigmentation)

1. Ocular depigmentation

   Depigmentation of the iris
   Depigmentation of the ciliary body
   Sunset glow fundus
   Dalen–Fuchs nodules
   Multiple window defects of retinal pigment epithelium with angiography
   Perilimbal vitiligo (**Sugiura sign**)

2. Dermal depigmentation

   Poliosis in eyebrow and eyelash
   Alopecia
   Vitiligo of face, chest, hands, and back

Adapted from Inomata H, Kato M. Vogt-Koyanagi-Harada disease. In: Bruyn GW, Vinken PJ, eds. *Handbook of Clinical Neurology*, pp. 611–626. Reprinted with kind permission from Elsevier Science.

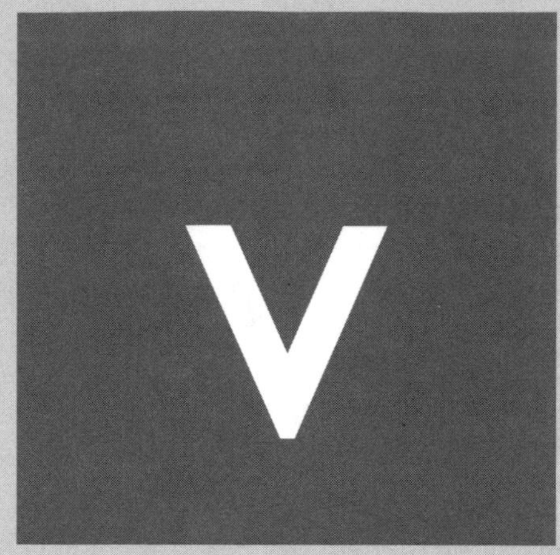

V pattern deviation A nonparalytic form of horizontal strabismus or **tropia** in which the visual axes are directed to closer objects (**esotropia**) as the subject looks down, or separate (**exotropia**) as the subject looks up. The phenomenon is described in patients with mesencephalic lesions. See also **A pattern deviation**.

V wave See **vertex sharp transient**.

vacor An organophosphate rodenticide capable of inducing neuropathy and neuromuscular junction disease.

vacuolar myelopathy
See **HIV-associated myelopathy**.

vacuolar myopathies Disorders of muscle in which the occurrence of widespread irregular vacuoles with a well-defined wall is the major or the only histological abnormality. Such myopathies include those due to **glycogen storage diseases, familial periodic paralysis**, steroid myopathy, and myopathies complicating collagen vascular diseases. A recessive X-linked form is also described, with juvenile onset, slow progression of proximal myopathic weakness. Pathologically there is vacuolation of muscle fibers without necrosis but with excessive autophagy. In a second form, cardiomyopathy and mental retardation are associated.[297] See also **hereditary inclusion body myopathy**, a form in which the quadriceps muscles are spared.

vacuoliting megalencephalitic leukoencephalopathy (OMIM 604004) A rare, recessively inherited leukodystrophy with infantile onset, characterized by diffuse swelling of the white matter, large subcortical cysts, and megalencephaly. The condition has been mapped to chromosome 22qtel.[6351]

vagal neuralgia A form of neuralgia resembling **glossopharyngeal neuralgia**, but in which the pain is felt in the throat and laryngeal regions.

vagal stimulation A technique whereby chronic stimulation of one vagus nerve by an implanted electrode is used to reduce the frequency of generalized and partial epileptic seizures. The precise mode of action of this intervention remains undetermined, but it appears to be effective for the treatment of uncontrolled seizures of focal origin, **Lennox–Gastaut syndrome**, and depression.

vagal syncope See **carotid sinus syncope**.

vaginismus Retentive spasm of the vagina, described by a certain Y. Davis. Davis was supposed at the time to be a real person but in fact the name was the pseudonym of Sir William **Osler** in mellow mood. The condition, fortunately, does not exist either.

vagoaccessory syndrome
See **Schmidt syndrome**.

vagus nerve (pneumogastric nerve)
A mixed nerve, supplying the entire cranial parasympathetic outflow as well as having somatic motor and sensory functions. It was described by Marinus in about 100 A.D. as the VI cranial nerve and was known to Galen, but was named by Domenico di Marchetti of Padua (1626–1688). The nerve's long course and wide distribution led to the derivation of the name from the Latin word *vagari* (a wanderer).

Vail neuralgia See **Vidian neuralgia, cluster headache**.

Vail vidian neuralgia See **cluster headache**.

valgus Having the calf of the leg bent outward. "Applied originally to a bow-legged man, the meaning {became} reversed and the term 'genu valgum' is now used for a knock-kneed person."[5886]

Valleix points 1. Local areas of tenderness along the course of peripheral nerves both proximal and distal to a site of compression, which persist between paroxysms of neuralgia.[6461] 2. Regions where nerves are accessible to palpation. As is known to exponents of oriental martial arts, such points are extremely sensitive to pressure, but, in cases of nerve irritation or neuralgia, even light pressure may be agonizing, which suggests the presence of such nerve pathology.

Valleix sign Tenderness of the sciatic nerve in the buttock or posterior thigh. The sign is said to be positive with root irritation, but muscle tenderness is easily confused with nerve pain at that site.

Valleix, François-Louis-Isidore (1807–1855) French physician who trained in Toulouse and Paris, but whose advancement in the Paris hospitals was disappointing, although he published over a hundred papers before his early death from diphtheria contracted from a patient. He described the points on nerves, now named for him, in his book *Traité des névralgies ou affections douloureuses des nerfs* (Paris, 1841).

Valsalva, Antonio Mario (1666–1723) Italian anatomist who trained in Bologna, where he was later professor of anatomy. In 1704 he described the increase in intrathoracic pressure as a means to express pus from the middle ear in otitis. Valsalva also observed that hemiparesis occurs on the side opposite to a hemispheric stroke.

Valsalva maneuver Forcible expiration against a closed glottis, as by exhaling hard against resistance, leading to an increase in intrathoracic pressure to about 30–40 mmHg, usually maintained for 10 s in the test situation. In the normal subject, this results in a substantial rise in intrathoracic pressure and a transient increase in blood pressure (*phase 1*); a reduction in venous return to the heart and in blood pressure with an increase in the pulse rate (*phase 2*); further increase in pulse rate and decrease in blood pressure occurring immediately after the pressure is released (*phase 3*); and a restitution of blood pressure after an initial overshoot, with a fall in pulse rate, following this (*phase 4*). Absence of any of these changes suggests disturbance in the parasympathetic system. See **autonomic function tests**.

Valsalva ratio A test of baroceptor afferent and both sympathetic and parasympathetic efferent functions. The maximum heart rate generated by the Valsalva maneuver is divided by the minimum heart rate occurring within 30 s of the maximum, measured by a continuously running EKG. The ratio of the longest R-R interval to the shortest should be 1.45 or more in healthy young people. The measurement is more accurate using invasive techniques.[4252] See also **thirty:fifteen ratio, autonomic function tests**.

Van Allen, Maurice (1918–1986) American neurologist, born in Iowa, where he received his early training in medicine, who before and again after wartime service trained in neurosurgery and neurology, although his practice was in the latter discipline. He became professor at the University of Iowa in 1965 and later chairman of the department. His greatest impact was as editor of the **Archives of Neurology** from 1976, but his introductory text on the neurological examination was also hugely successful. See also **familial amyloid neuropathy** (type III).

van Bogaert encephalitis See **subacute sclerosing panencephalitis**.

van Bogaert, Ludo (1897–1989) Belgian neurologist who trained in Brussels and who later studied in Paris under Pierre **Marie** and Marcel Labbé. His graduation thesis was on the mental changes that occur in **amyotrophic lateral sclerosis**. He practiced as a neurologist and neuropathologist in Belgium, developing a special interest in neurometabolic disorders, multiple sclerosis, and hypothalamic tumors, as well as the subjects suggested by the following entries. He contributed 753 publications to the literature and was the founder and president of **the World Federation of Neurology**.

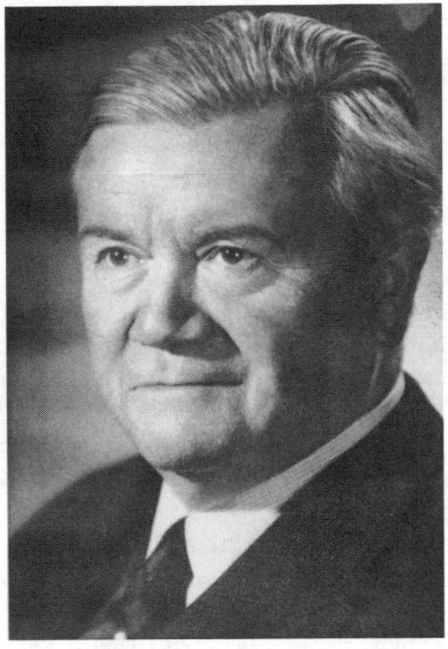

Figure V–1 Ludo Van Bogaert

van Bogaert syndrome (Divry–van Bogaert syndrome, corticomeningeal diffuse angiomatosis, Hozay–Van Bogaert syndrome) A recessively inherited or sporadic syndrome of mental retardation, seizures, spastic paraparesis, extrapyramidal disorders, hemianopia, marbled skin, and telangiectasia[6470] associated with diffuse, noncalcifying angiomatosis of the cortex and meninges and demyelination of the centrum semiovale,[2290] resembling the changes in **Binswanger disease**. Death usually occurs within 20 years of presentation.

van Bogaert–Bertrand disease The same condition as **Canavan disease**. See **glial degenerations, glioneuronal degenerations**.

van Bogaert–Divry syndrome See **Sturge–Weber syndrome, van Bogaert syndrome**.

van Bogaert–Nissen–Pfeiffer syndrome See **metachromatic leukodystrophy**.

van Bogaert–Scherer–Epstein syndrome See **cerebrotendinous xanthomatosis**.

van Buchem syndrome See **hyperostosis corticalis generalisata familiaris.**

van Deen, Isaac (1805–1869) Danish physician who graduated from the University of Leyden in Holland. An ingenious experimenter, he demonstrated that in frogs the posterior columns of the cord carry sensory impulses and the anterior columns motor impulses, conclusions which assisted **Brown-Séquard** in the elucidation of the basis of cord lesions. He was eventually appointed professor of physiology at Groningen.[3511]

van der Hoeve phakomatosis
1. (Ekbom–Lobstein syndrome)
A dominantly inherited cochleovestibular atrophy with onset between 10 and 30 years of age, and manifesting progressive conductive deafness, blue sclerae, and the other features of **osteogenesis imperfecta.**[6482] 2. Pediculate tumors on the optic nerve head associated variously with **Sturge–Weber disease, tuberous sclerosis, von Hippel–Lindau disease,** and **neurofibromatosis,** described by van der Hoeve (1878–1952), a Dutch ophthalmologist and professor at Leyden.[2934]

van der Hoeve syndrome See **Apert syndrome.**

van der Hoeve–Halbertsma–Waardenburg–Klein syndrome See **Waardenburg syndrome.**

van der Kolk's law The sensory fibers of a mixed nerve are distributed to parts that are moved by muscles supplied with motor fibers from the same nerve.

van Dyke–Hanson syndrome A rare syndrome of contractures with continuous muscle discharges, titubation, and episodic ataxia. See **hereditary myokymia with periodic (episodic) ataxia.**

vanillylmandelic acid The product of the metabolism of norepinephrine, used as a marker of norepinephrine production as it is a stable substance and is freely excreted in the urine.

vanishing white matter disease See **fatal infantile leukodystrophy.**

vapours A term commonplace in Victorian England for a state of reluctance to engage in any exertion on account of a sense of extreme fatigue; and also used for presyncope, usually with an emotional cause. In those days, such affections were considered evidence of the most exalted sensibility. Today, see **chronic fatigue syndrome.**

variant Creutzfeldt–Jakob disease (vCJD) See **Creutzfeldt–Jakob disease.** A Web site containing collected resources from the *British Medical Journal*, with links to scientific papers from other journals, is at http://www.bmj.com/cgi/collection/mad_cow/.

variant hereditary motor and sensory neuropathy The association of retinitis pigmentosa, ataxia, and peripheral neuropathy without any increase in the serum phytanic acid level. Sensorineural deafness and radiological evidence of cerebellar atrophy are occasional features. Sensory conduction is more affected than motor conduction. Biopsy specimens show a reduction of myelinated fibers without onion bulb formations.

The cases reported resemble Refsum disease (**hereditary motor and sensory neuropathy,** type 4) but have neither detectable biochemical abnormality nor peripheral nerve hypertrophy.[6414]

varicella-zoster myelitis A self-limiting motor paraparetic syndrome, sometimes with a relapsing–remitting course, with variable sensory and sphincter involvement, occurring after acute varicella or zoster infection and considered to be on the basis of a postinfectious myelitis. More severe and acute syndromes are also described.[2378]

variegate porphyria A dominantly inherited form of **porphyria** in which protoporphyrin is not converted into heme and coproporphyrin is continuously excreted in the stools. The disorder is commonest in South Africans (Afrikaaners).[5370, 1322] Neurological features complicate some acute attacks, and include the acute or subacute occurrence of proximal motor neuropathy affecting the arms more than the legs (often asymmetrically) and also the face and autonomic system, in the setting of other features of the disease, including skin photosensitivity, abdominal pain, vomiting, tachycardia, hypertension, and often seizures and delirium.

Variot–Pironneau senile dwarfism See **progeria.**

Varoli, Costanzo (1543–1575) Italian anatomist, who described the pons (in a book published posthumously in 1591) and also named the hippocampus.

varus Bent or grown inward, knock-kneed (Lat), but the meaning is now reversed and the term is used to describe bowleggedness.[5886] See also **valgus.**

vascular cognitive impairment (vascular dementia, multi-infarct dementia, progressive cognitive disturbance due to thromboembolic cerebrovascular disease) The vascular component of all dementias and the only treatable element of a disease that has a highly significant impact on the health of older adults at risk of both strokes and coronary artery disease. Other forms of cerebrovascular disease such as hypoperfusion, subdural hematoma, vasculitis, and subarachnoid hemorrhage are equally capable of leading on to cognitive impairment, and the same may be true for states of chronically impaired cardiac output.

Erkinjuntti et al.[1907] regard vascular dementia as that form in which there is a history of focal or acute signs and symptoms referable to disturbed cerebral circulation, and they suggest the following subcategories: *Vascular dementia of hemodynamic type* is that form of dementia evolving in connection with cardiac arrhythmias and systemic hypotension. *Probable vascular dementia* is that form clinically considered to be related to disturbances of the cerebral circulation without any clear temporal connection with the evolution of the dementia, and without evidence of multiple vascular lesions on the CT scan. This group includes patients with combined degenerative and vascular dementias. *Multi-infarct dementia* is that form which evolves in connection with acute neurological symptoms and signs and/or CT scan findings indicating multiple cortical or deep vascular lesions of the brain.

For dementia to result from vascular disease, it is estimated that at least 100 ml of brain tissue has to have been destroyed. A high **Hachinski ischemic score** may be helpful in predicting the presence of cerebral infarcts, but does not predict the pathology causing the dementia in any given case.[5589]

There are no clinical clues to the presence of vascular as opposed to other pathologies to be gleaned from the features of the dementia itself.

Two of at least five sets of criteria extant for the diagnosis (CERAD,[4396] APA-DSM,[172] Hachinski,[2663] Chui et al.,[1173] and the NINCDS-AIREN Workshop[5366]) are presented in Charts V–1 and V–2; the critique of Drachman[1706] should be imbibed prior to their ingestion.

A suggested data collection form has been published.[5345]

vascular dementia See vascular **cognitive impairment**.

vascular malformations

Collections of abnormal blood vessels of various sizes, most often found in the cerebral lobar white matter, and ranging in size from small capillary telangiectasias through **venous** and **cavernous angiomas** to **arteriovenous malformations**. They represent occasional causes of

Chart V–1. Criteria for the Diagnosis of Vascular (Dementia) Cognitive Impairment

Vascular dementia (VaD) is a complex disorder characterized by cognitive impairment resulting from ischemic or hemorrhagic stroke or from ischemic-hypoxic brain lesions.

The clinical criteria for the diagnosis of probable, possible, and definite VaD are summarized:

I. Criteria for the clinical diagnosis of *Probable VaD* include all of the following:

1. Dementia defined by cognitive decline from a previously higher level of functioning and manifested by impairment of memory and of two or more cognitive domains (orientation, attention, language, visuospatial functions, executive functions, motor control, and praxis), preferably established by clinical examination and documented by neuropsychological testing. Deficits should be severe enough to interfere with activities of daily living, not due to physical effects of stroke alone.

Exclusion criteria include cases with disturbance of consciousness, delirium, psychosis, severe aphasia, or major sensorimotor impairment precluding neuropsychological testing. Also excluded are systemic disorders or other brain diseases such as AD that in and of themselves could account for deficits in memory and cognition.

2. CVD defined by the presence of focal signs on neurological examination consistent with stroke, with or without a history of stroke, and evidence of relevant CVD by brain imaging (CT or MRI), including multiple large vessel infarcts or a single strategically placed infarct (angular gyrus, thalamus, forebrain, or posterior or anterior cerebral artery territories) as well as multiple basal ganglia and white matter lacunes or extensive periventricular white matter lesions or combinations thereof.
3. A relationship between the above two disturbances manifested by one or more of the following: (a) onset of dementia within 3 months following a recognized stroke; (b) abrupt deterioration in cognitive functions; or fluctuating, stepwise progression of cognitive deficits.

II. Clinical features consistent with the diagnosis of *Probable VaD* include the following:

1. Early presence of a gait disturbance (small step gait or marche à petits pas, or magnetic, apraxic-ataxic or parkinsonian gait);
2. History of unsteadiness and frequent, unprovoked falls;
3. Early urinary frequency, urgency, and other urinary symptoms not explained by urologic disease;
4. Pseudobulbar palsy; and
5. Personality and mood changes, abulia, depression, emotional incontinence, or other subcortical deficits including psychomotor retardation and abnormal executive function.

III. Features that make the diagnosis of VaD uncertain or unlikely include:

1. Early onset of memory deficit and progressive worsening of memory and other cognitive functions, such as language (transcortical sensory aphasia), motor skills (apraxia), and perception (agnosia), in the absence of corresponding focal lesions on brain imaging;
2. Absence of other focal neurological signs other than cognitive disturbance; and
3. Absence of cerebrovascular lesions on brain CT or MRI scans.

IV. Clinical diagnosis of *Possible VaD* may be made in the presence of dementia (Section I-1) with focal neurological signs in patients in whom brain imaging studies to confirm definite CVD are missing; or in the absence of clear temporal relationships between dementia and stroke; or in patients with subtle onset and variable course (plateau or improvement) of cognitive deficits and evidence of relevant CVD.

V. Criteria for the diagnosis of *Definite VaD* are as follows:

1. Clinical criteria for probable vascular dementia;
2. Histopathological evidence of CVD obtained from biopsy or autopsy;
3. Absence of neurofibrillary tangles and neuritic plaques exceeding those expected for age; and
4. Absence of other clinical or pathological disorder capable of producing dementia.

VI. Classification of vascular dementia for research purposes may be made on the basis of clinical, radiological, and neuropathologic features for subcategories or defined conditions such as cortical vascular dementia, subcortical vascular dementia, Binswanger dementia, and thalamic dementia.

The term *AD with CVD* should be reserved to classify patients fulfilling the clinical criteria for possible AD and who also present clinical or brain imaging evidence of relevant CVD. Traditionally, these patients have been included with VaD in epidemiological studies. The term *mixed dementia*, used hitherto, should be avoided.

AD, Alzheimer disease; CVD, cerebrovascular disease; VaD, vascular dementia. (Adapted from Román GC, Tatemichi TK, Erkinjuntti T, et al. Vascular dementia: diagnostic criteria for research studies. *Neurology* 1993;43:250–60. Reproduced by kind permission of the American Academy of Neurology and Lippincott Williams and Wilkins.)

Chart V–2. Diagnostic Criteria for Ischemic Vascular Cognitive Impairment

Probable ischemic vascular dementia

A. The criteria for the clinical diagnosis of probable IVD include all of the following:

1. Dementia;
2. Evidence of two or more ischemic strokes by history, neurological signs, and/or neuroimaging studies (CT or T_1-weighted MRI); or occurrence of a single stroke with a clearly documented temporal relationship to the onset of dementia;
3. Evidence of at least one infarct outside the cerebellum by CT or T_1-weighted MRI.

B. The diagnosis of probable IVD is supported by:

1. Evidence of multiple infarcts in brain regions known to affect cognition;
2. A history of multiple transient ischemic attacks;
3. History of vascular risk factors (e.g., hypertension, heart disease, diabetes mellitus);
4. Elevated Hachinski ischemia scale (original or modified version).

C. Clinical features that are thought to be associated with IVD, but await further research, include:

1. Relatively early appearance of gait disturbance and urinary incontinence;
2. Periventricular and deep white matter changes on T_2-weighted MRI that are excessive for age;
3. Focal changes in electrophysiological studies (e.g., EEG, evoked potentials) or physiological neuroimaging studies (e.g., SPECT, PET, NMR spectroscopy).

D. Other clinical features that do not constitute strong evidence either for or against a diagnosis of probable IVD include:

1. Periods of slowly progressive symptoms;
2. Illusions, psychosis, hallucinations, delusions;
3. Seizures.

E. Clinical features that cast doubt on a diagnosis of probable IVD include:

1. Transcortical sensory aphasia in the absence of corresponding focal lesions on neuroimaging studies;
2. Absence of central neurological symptoms/signs, other than cognitive disturbance.

Possible ischemic vascular dementia

A clinical diagnosis of possible IVD may be made when there is

1. Dementia; and one or more of the following:

2a. A history or evidence of a single stroke (but not multiple strokes) without a clearly documented temporal relationship to the onset of dementia, or

2b. Binswanger's syndrome (without multiple strokes) that includes all of the following:

- i. Early-onset urinary incontinence not explained by urological disease, or gait disturbance (e.g., Parkinsonian, magnetic, apraxia, or senile gait) not explained by peripheral cause;
- ii. Vascular risk factors; and
- iii. Extensive white matter changes on neuroimaging.

Definite ischemic vascular dementia

A diagnosis of definite IVD requires histopathological examination of the brain, as well as

1. Clinical evidence of dementia;
2. Pathological confirmation of multiple infarcts, some outside of the cerebellum.

If there is evidence of Alzheimer disease or some other pathological condition that is thought to have contributed to the dementia, a diagnosis of **mixed dementia** should be made. *{But see footnote to Chart V–1}*

IVD, ischemic vascular cognitive impairment. (Adapted from Chiu HC, Victoroff JI, Margolin D, et al. Criteria for the diagnosis of ischemic vascular dementia proposed by the State of California Alzheimer's disease diagnostic and treatment centers. *Neurology* 1992;**42**:473–80. Reproduced by kind permission of the American Academy of Neurology and Lippincott Williams and Wilkins.)

intraparenchymal or intraventricular hemorrhage in the CNS (especially in younger patients) but are often asymptomatic.

vascular thoracic outlet compression syndrome See **thoracic outlet syndrome**.

vasculitic neuropathy Painful mononeuropathies, multiple mononeuropathies, or polyneuropathies associated with systemic vasculitic diseases.[5582] A review of the many causes of the syndrome has been published.[5582] These have been classified by Scott.[5687] HIV infection and hepatitis are prominent causes.

Diagnostic criteria for clinically probable vasculitic neuropathy in patients lacking biopsy-proven necrotizing vasculitis have been suggested.[1257] and are reproduced below. Common to all is necrotizing arteritis of the epi- and perineurial vessel walls with nerve fiber loss, Wallerian degeneration, and electrodiagnostic evidence of regions of conduction block.

The diagnosis requires at least three of the first five criteria for nonsystemic vasculitic neuropathy; criterion 6 is also mandatory for systemic vasculitis.

1. Clinical presentation typical for a vasculitic neuropathy

   Asymmetric or multifocal, painful, sensorimotor neuropathy
   Acute/subacute relapsing, progressive, or relapsing progressive course
   No spontaneous remission

2. Elevated sedimentation rate or other laboratory evidence of a systemic inflammatory state
3. Electrodiagnostic evidence of an active, asymmetric, axonal, sensorimotor neuropathy
4. Suggestive neuromuscular pathology

   Vascular thickening or sclerosis, narrowing or obliteration of the vascular lumen, thrombosis, periadventitial capillary proliferation, hemosiderin deposits, nonrandom nerve fiber loss, or Wallerian-like degeneration

5. Clinical response to immunosuppressive therapy
6. Clinicopathologic evidence of a systemic/secondary etiology

   Concurrent condition known or suspected to predispose to vasculitis (connective tissue diseases, certain infections or drugs, malignancies/paraproteinemias, cryoglobulinemia)
   Simultaneous multiorgan, nonperipheral nerve involvement
   Biopsy-proven vasculitis in other tissues

(Reproduced by kind permission of the American Academy of Neurology and Lippincott Williams and Wilkins.)

A variant is *nonsystemic vasculitic neuropathy* which is a relatively benign vasculitis, most often presenting as multiple mononeuropathy without evidence of any underlying disease, nor of CNS or other site of vasculitis. See also **Churg–Strauss syndrome, diabetic amyotrophy, polyarteritis nodosa, rheumatoid arthritis, Sjögren syndrome, sytemic lupus erythematosus, and Wegener granulomatosis**.

vasculitis Inflammation and necrosis of the walls of blood vessels, as part of a multisystem disease that is drug related or isolated within the CNS. The various syndromes have been classified; the one in Chart V–3 is freely modified from Moore and Cupps.[4460]

See also **cryoglobulinemic neuropathy, diabetes mellitus, rheumatoid neuropathy, Sjogren syndrome, systemic lupus erythematosus**.

vasoactive intestinal peptide (VIP) A peptide hormone found in the gut and CNS of humans, with its highest concentrations in the cerebral cortex, where it acts as a modulator of vasodilation, as well as having a release function for growth hormone and prolactin and a neurotrophic action on neuronal survival.

vasoconstriction syncope See **Gowers syndromes**.

vasogenic cerebral edema An increase in the volume of the brain's extracellular space due to the accumulation of water, electrolytes, and protein within it, as a result of damage to the **blood–brain barrier**. This occurs most typically in the tissue surrounding cerebral tumors, infarcts, abscesses, and contusions.

vasopressin (antidiuretic hormone) A peptide with highest concentration in the supraoptic and paraventricular nuclei of the hypothalamus and in their nerve terminals in the posterior pituitary gland, with effects upon learning as well as on renal water excretion.

vasoregulation The process whereby blood vessels adapt to the metabolic needs of the tissues they supply. Carbon dioxide and oxygen tensions and pH are the most effective stimuli leading to alterations in the caliber of the cerebral arterioles.

vasovagal (vasodepressor) syncope A mechanism of fainting, typically precipitated by unpleasant physical or emotional stimuli (e.g., pain, fright, sight of blood), usually in the upright posture and often preceded by vagally mediated warning symptoms such as nausea, weakness, and yawning. Other features include apprehension, visual blurring, sweating, malaise, anxiety,

Chart V–3. Classification of the Vasculitides

1. *Systemic necrotizing vasculitis*:

   Classic **polyarteritis nodosa**
   Allergic angiitis and granulomatosis (**Churg–Strauss disease**)
   Wegener granulomatosis
   Overlap syndromes
   Cerebral vasculitis with ulcerative colitis
   Sjögren syndrome
   Sytemic lupus erythematosus

2. *Hypersensitivity vasculitis*:

   Henoch–Schönlein purpura
   Serum sickness
   Vasculitis associated with infections, connective tissue disease, or malignancy.
   Drug-induced vasculitis (amphetamines, heroin, cocaine).

3. *Giant cell arteritides*:

   Cranial arteritis
   Takayasu **aortic arch arteritis**

4. *Localized vasculitis*:

   Isolated peripheral nervous system vasculitis (nonsystemic neuropathy)
   Isolated angiitis of the nervous system
   Cutaneous polyarteritis
   Essential mixed cryoglobulinemia
   Lymphomatoid granulomatosis
   Behçet disease
   Proximal diabetic neuropathy
   Multiple mononeuropathy in **rheumatoid arthritis**

Adapted from Moore PM, Cupps TR. Neurological complications of vasculitis.[4460] Ann. Neurol. 1983; 14:155. Reprinted by permission of Wiley-Blackwell Publications.

pallor, and brief convulsive movements during the period of unconsciousness.

Neurally mediated, prolonged asystolic pauses, mainly due to sinus arrest, preceded for a few minutes by progressive bradycardia or progressive tachycardia–bradycardia appear to be the commonest cause.[4526, 6839] The mechanism was described in 1932 by Thomas Lewis (1881–1945), an English cardiologist.[5619]

A series of weighted diagnostic questions to determine whether syncope is vasovagal or due to another cause has been formulated.[5778]

The patient probably has vasovagal syncope if the point score is ≥–2. See also **encephalosyncope, reflex syncope**.

Question (with points given for "yes" answers)	
Is there a history of at least one of bifascicular block, asystole, supraventricular tachycardia, diabetes?	−5
At times have bystanders noted you to be blue during your faint?	−4
Did your syncope start when you were 35 years of age or older?	−3
Do you remember anything about being unconscious?	−2
Do you have lightheaded spells or faint with prolonged sitting or standing?	1
Do you sweat or feel warm before a faint?	2
Do you have lightheaded spells or faint with pain or in medical settings?	3

Vater, Abraham (1684–1751) German anatomist, the first to describe the encapsulated nerve endings now named for **Pacini**.

VDRL See **Venereal Disease Research Laboratory Test**.

Vegas neuropathy An ulnar neuropathy at the elbow, resulting from leaning the elbow on the edges of gaming tables for prolonged periods.[3170]

vegetative nervous system See **autonomic nervous system**.

vegetative state A state of altered consciousness occurring as a residuum from severe cortical damage in which wakefulness appears to be present because the eyes are open and a sleep–wake cycle is retained, but in which there is no evidence of conscious awareness, the patients neither speaking nor obeying commands given in any modality, nor showing evidence of emotional awareness. There is thus arousal without awareness. The **Glasgow Coma Scale** scores will be 4–4–2 or worse. The condition is most often seen after severe head injury or hypoxic-ischemic injury.

Suggested criteria require that there shall be no evidence of awareness of the self or of the environment and no volitional responses to external stimuli. Language will not be comprehended nor expressed. Cycles of eye closure and eye opening will simulate sleep and wakefulness. Hypothalamic and brainstem functions are sufficient to maintain respiration and circulation.[5218]

See also **persistent vegetative state**[5053] and **minimally conscious state**.

vein of Galen A large deep cerebral vein draining into the straight sinus. It is subject to massive dilation as a congenital anomaly (**aneurysm of the vein of Galen**) which may lead to compression of the midbrain, bleeding, seizures, macrocephaly with hydrocephalus, and, by virtue of the volume of blood shunted, heart failure in infants.[4455]

vein of Labbé See **Labbé's vein**.

vein of Trolard See **Trolard's vein**.

Venereal Disease Research Laboratory Test (VDRL)
A nontreponemal test for syphilis, detecting flocculation in reaction to nonspecific antibodies of, or in response to, *Treponema pallidum* infection of the host. Though widely used as a screening test, the result is negative in up to a quarter of the cases of tertiary syphilis and may be positive in collagen-vascular disease, after other infections or recent immune challenges, in leprosy and in old age.[5852] See also **TPI**.

Venezuelan equine encephalitis
Direct brain infection by an arthropod-borne alphavirus of the togavirus group, causing cycles of encephalitic disease throughout Central and South America and the southern United States. Clinically, adults exhibit an influenzal disease with marked myalgia, fevers, nausea and vomiting, headaches, conjunctivitis, and pharyngitis. A few children suffer severe neurological complications such as seizures, paralysis, and coma.[1820]

venoarteriolar reflex Arteriolar constriction in the skin and muscles of the legs reducing blood flow during limb dependency (when venous pressure is raised by 25 mmHg) as a result of a local sympathetic C-fiber reflex.[4525]

venous angiomas Rare tumor-like masses comprising dilated veins with slight or no arterial contribution. See **venous malformation**.

venous infarction Ischemic damage to tissues resulting from impairment of their venous drainage. This occurs most often in the retina and in the spinal cord, and as a result of thrombosis of the dural venous sinuses. See **central retinal vein thrombosis, Foix–Alajouanine syndrome, sinus thrombosis, cerebral venous thrombosis**.

venous lakes Benign demineralized areas of the skull seen on either side of the midline on plain X-ray and CT studies, and of no pathological import, unless they prompt invasive investigations.

venous malformation A congenital **vascular malformation** consisting of a mass of dilated venous channels, within or on the surface of the cerebrum. Bleeding may be clinically inapparent and lesions may be detected fortuitously, especially if they calcify. See **venous angiomas, arteriovenous malformation**.

venous sinus thrombosis
Occlusion of the superior sagittal or of the transverse sinus, usually as a result of infection or dehydration. See **sinus thrombosis**.

venous stasis retinopathy
A syndrome of unilateral, slowly progressive visual loss with a funduscopic picture of venous engorgement and dot-and-blot hemorrhages, with low central retinal artery pressure, resulting from central retinal vein occlusion and usually associated with severe carotid artery disease. Anterior segment ischemia may also be present.[3363]

ventral brainstem syndrome See **locked-in syndrome**.

ventral cerebellum See **inverse cerebellum**.

ventral pontine syndrome See **locked-in syndrome**.

ventral suspension A test of motor abilities used in determining **gestational age**, in which the infant is suspended in the prone position with the examiner's hand under the infant's chest (one hand in a small infant, two in a large infant). Normally, there will be obvious extension of the neck and lower spine with some flexion of the arms and legs.[1728] However, an infant with congenital 'hypotonia' and marked truncal weakness will also droop in flexion with this manoeuvre.

ventricle of Arantius See **cava septi pellucidi et vergae**.

ventricles (Lat, a small belly) A hollow part of an organ. The paired lateral and the third and the fourth ventricles were considered to be "cells" by the ancient Greeks, wherein resided mental functions. The ventricular contents were considered to be animal spirits that were pumped out through small tubes to the rest of the body. Hierophilus of Alexandria in 300 B.C. located the seat of the soul in the fourth ventricle. These concepts remained essentially unaltered until the sixteenth century.

ventricular empyema See **ventriculitis**.

ventricular germinal zone See **germinal zone**.

ventriculitis (ependymitis, pyocephalus, ventricular empyema) Inflammation of the cerebral ventricles which contain suppurative fluid, usually as a complication of **meningitis**.

ventriculography A procedure for outlining the internal proportions of the cerebral ventricles with X-radiography after the introduction of air or contrast medium at operation. The procedure was introduced by **Dandy** in 1913,[1439, 5619] after Dr. W.H. Luckett had published an account of intraventricular air following a compound skull fracture.

ventriculostium A communication between the cerebral ventricles and the subarachnoid space, occurring spontaneously.[3285]

VEP See **visual evoked potential**.

verb phrase The part of a sentence which contains the verb (the predicate) as well as all words, clauses, and sentences modifying the verb.[3949]

verbal adynamia See **dynamic aphasia**.

verbal alexia Inability to interpret the written word, although isolated letters can be identified. The phenomenon is seen in patients with dominant angular gyrus lesions.[1336]

verbal aphasia (motor aphasia) The term of Sir Henry **Head** for that form of speech disturbance (a defect in word formation) in which words are evoked with difficulty and tend to be abnormal in structure and the vocabulary restricted. See **Broca aphasia**.

verbal asomatognosia Distorted awareness of a body part, manifested by verbal denial of ownership of a limb, accompanied by hemispatial neglect. The lesion is considered to lie in the right supramarginal gyrus.[1988]

verbal auditory agnosia See **word deafness**.

verbal automatism Single or repetitive utterances consisting of words, phrases, or brief sentences. See **stereotypy**.

verbal dissociation, apraxia A condition in which patients cannot gesture normally to command while they can imitate and can use tools and objects. It is suggested that the conceptual system for action and action production are intact but cannot be accessed by verbal command.[2561]

verbal dysdecorum A syndrome resulting from focal damage to the medial, sagittal, and or dorsal convolutions of the right frontal lobe, in which patients voice bizarre and caustic descriptions of themselves, of everyday occurrences and of those about them, and fail to monitor the undesirable effects of this output and so to inhibit it.[521]

verbal paraphasia The substitution of incorrect words within sentences; a characteristic of dysphasic syndromes.

verbal perseveration Repetition of the same word or phrase. See **verbigeration**.

verbal standstill The interruption of flowing speech because the correct word fails to come to mind. When it is offered by another, it is immediately recognized as correct and speech continues. Paraphasic errors and substitutions do not occur. This occurs commonly in elderly people and in those of any age who are under stress or fatigued.[1338]

verbal sterotypy See **stereotypy**.

verbal–motor dissociation apraxia See **apraxia**.

Verbiest syndrome See **lumbar spinal stenosis**.

verbigeration The meaningless repetition by the patient of the same words or phrases over and over again, with appropriate gestural accompaniment; an example of verbal stereotypy.

Vereniging Spierziekten Nederland A member society of the European Alliance of Muscular Dystrophy Societies based at Lt-Gen. van Heutszlaan, 6 NL-743 JN Baarn, The Netherlands.

Vereniging Spierzielcten België A member society of the European Alliance of Muscular Dystrophy Societies. Address: c/o Weyneshoflei 1 B-820 Rymenam, Belgium.

Verga, Andrea (1811–1895) Italian anatomist and physician who first described the Cavum Vergae, a cavity within the septum pellucidum.

vergence (Lat, turn downward) (disjunctive eye movements) Simultaneous movements of the eyes, but in different directions. This is usually seen as an in-turning of the eyes (which thus lose the parallelism of their axes), in order to allow focused close vision. Refixation movements and visual tracking movements are of this type, and other forms are described.[2400]

Four components of vergence are described:

1. *Tonic vergence* determines the baseline alignment of the visual axis in darkness.
2. *Accommodator vergence* is an involuntary in-turning of the eyes induced by blurring of vision.
3. *Fusional vergence*, which is induced by retinal disparity.
4. *Proximal vergence* (nearness), which is induced by a sense of distance of the target and is based on a number of sensory cues.[6767]

See also **versions**.

Verger, Theodore-Paul-Henri (1873–1930) French neurologist who trained in Bordeaux, **Pitres** being one of his teachers. He was appointed in succession to the chairs of forensic and then internal Medicine. He wrote on proprioceptive sensation and the functions of the parietal lobe, experimental thalamic syndromes, neuralgias, encephalitis, syringomyelia, the traumatic neuroses, and medical ethics.

Verger–Déjèrine syndrome (Déjèrine syndrome, Déjèrine–Mouzon syndrome, Claude topoanesthesia) A syndrome of the parietal lobe in which discriminative tactile sensations and proprioception are lost, while sensations of pain, temperature, vibration, and crude light touch remain intact.[1542]

vermis (Lat, worm-like) The appearances of the folia of the cerebellar vermis bear a fanciful resemblance to the segmented body of a worm.

vermis syndrome (Bailey syndrome) Disturbance of equilibrium with nystagmus and some degree of limb ataxia as a result of a lesion of the vermis of the cerebellum. Depending on the cause, there may also be evidence of increased intracranial pressure.

Vernant syndrome (recurrent optic neuromyelitis with endocrinopathies) A syndrome described in young black women in the West Indies, comprising recurrent optic neuritis, cervical myelopathy with a syringomyelia-like syndrome, and amenorrhea with galactorrhea. The cause is not known[6532] but tuberculous neuropathy and hemorrhagic fevers may be associated.[5362] See **disseminated vasculomyelinopathy**.

Vernet syndrome (Vernet–Sargon syndrome, Collet–Sicard syndrome) Unilateral paralysis of cranial nerves IX, X, and XI, due to a lesion at the level of the jugular foramen in front of the anterior occipital condyles. The clinical consequences of this include loss of taste in the posterior third of the tongue; paresis of the vocal cords and palate with resulting dysarthria, dysphagia, and dysphonia; anesthesia of the soft palate and throat; and weakness of the trapezius and sternomastoid muscles.[6147, 6533] The pathology is usually a malignancy, aneurysm, or fracture. See also **jugular foramen syndrome**.

Vernet, Maurice (b. 1887) French neurologist, who described the preceding syndrome in his graduation thesis (University of Lyon) in 1916.

Vernet–Sargon syndrome See **Vernet syndrome**.

vernicomyelia The presence of the contents of the amniotic fluid sac in the spinal subarachnoid space, accompanied by a foreign-body giant cell reaction in the leptomeninges. The condition may complicate a lumbar meningomyelocele in infants.[3131]

Verocay nodule A mass of nuclei formed by polar cells seen within neurinomas, tightly opposed in palisades and forming a nodule within the tumor; the arrays of palisaded cells within **Schwannomas**.[6]

Verocet neurilemmoma See **Schwannoma**.

verruga peruana See **Oroya fever**.

versions Normal, conjugate deviations of the eyes in any direction, in parallel. *Fast versive eye movements* of this type include **saccades**, microsaccades, saccadic pursuit, the fast phase of jerk nystagmus, **saccadic intrusions, saccadic oscillations**, and the rapid eye movements of (paradoxical) **REM Sleep**.[2400] *Slow versive eye movements* include **pursuit eye movements, microdrift, glissades**, the slow phase of jerk nystagmus, and the movements of **pendular nystagmus**. Other forms are also recorded.[2400] See also **vergence**.

versive motor seizure A sustained, forced conjugate ocular, cephalic, and/or truncal rotation or lateral deviation from the midline.[16]

versive movements See **versive seizures**.

versive seizures (versive movements) A variety of simple seizures of focal origin involving conjugate deviation of the head and eyes, usually but not invariably away from the side of the hemispheric discharge.[72] They are evidence of a frontal lobe lesion in most cases, but disease of other cortical regions may occasionally be responsible.

Nonversive movements are smaller-amplitude, ill-sustained, and wandering eye movements in any direction, and although likely to be electrically driven, have no localizing significance.[6887] Compare with **Vulpian sign**.

vertebra prominens The (longest) spinous process, of C7; and thus that which is most easily palpated or seen in the low neck. The longest (the middle) finger also is innervated by C7.

vertebral artery hypoplasia A congenital reduction in the diameter of one vertebral artery to less than 2 or 3 mm, predisposing a subject to stroke in the posterior circulation.[4988]

vertebral artery stump syndrome The occurrence of posterior circulation strokes after occlusion of a vertebral artery when a thrombus formed at the distal end of a vertebral artery occlusion is carried into the cerebral circulation through cervical artery collaterals.[4023]

vertebral dysplasia-spinal dysraphism (Curry syndrome) A congenital dysmorphic syndrome characterized by dwarfism, short webbed neck, kyphosis, platyspondyly, spina bifida occulta, skeletal deformities of the thorax and sacrum, inguinal hernia, absent testes, and cutis gyrata of the scalp.[381]

vertebrobasilar dolichoectasia Elongation and tortuosity of the basilar artery, which may be benign or can cause cranial nerve or brainstem compression, obstructive hydrocephalus, vertebrobasilar ischemia, or intracranial bleeding.

vertebrobasilar Ds A mnemonic to assist the recall of common symptoms of hind-brain ischemia: dysphagia, dysarthria, diplopia, drop attacks, dysmetria, and dysesthesia.

vertebrobasilar insufficiency (Millikan–Siekert syndrome) Transient ischemic attacks in the territory of the posterior circulation, first recognized by Denny-Brown in 1951[1583, 1584] (who, however, argued against vasospasm but in favor of endarteritis as the cause of transient ischemic attacks [TIAs] in the anterior and posterior circulations) and by Millikan 2 years later.[4382] The symptoms may be precipitated by extrinsic compression of the vertebral artery, by spasm or dissection of its wall, by emboli within the lumen, or by diversion of blood (as in the **subclavian steal syndrome**). The clinical localization of the vascular lesion is frequently incorrect.

The diagnosis is suggested by the finding of any two of the following motor or sensory symptoms or both occurring bilaterally in one attack; ataxia of gait or clumsiness of both extremities; diplopia; dysphagia; and bilateral homonymous hemianopia.[299, 6744]

vertebrobasilar insufficiency nystagmus See **cervical nystagmus**.

vertebrobasilar migraine See **basilar migraine**.

vertex sharp transient (vertex sharp wave, V wave) A sharp potential, maximal at the vertex, usually negative in relation to other areas and occurring apparently spontaneously during sleep or in response to a sensory stimulus during sleep or wakefulness. It may be single or repetitive and its amplitude varies but rarely exceeds 250 μV. See also **K-complex**.

vertex sharp wave See **vertex sharp transient**.

vertical gaze paresis Inability to deviate the eyes voluntarily in the vertical plane as a result of a mesencephalic lesion involving the posterior commissure. See **dorsal midbrain syndrome**.

vertical nystagmus A form of central vestibular nystagmus resulting from an imbalance in central vestibulo-ocular reflex pathways, in which the deviations of the eyes are in the vertical plane. Upbeat nystagmus is likely due to pontine lesions resulting from damage to the ventral tegmental tract, originating in the superior vestibular nucleus, coursing through the ventral pons, and transmitting excitatory upward vestibular signals to the III nerve nucleus. In **internuclear ophthalmoplegia**, the medial longitudinal fasciculus is involved in the transmission of both upward and downward vestibular signals. The main focal lesions resulting in downbeat nystagmus affect the cerebellar flocculus and/or paraflocculus.[5022] If purely vertical, nystagmus is never of peripheral origin. See **upbeat nystagmus, downbeat nystagmus**.

vertical one-and-a-half syndrome 1. The combination of paralysis of up-gaze in both eyes and of down-gaze in one of them.[1555] 2. A supranuclear down-gaze paralysis with monocular paralysis of elevation.

In each case, the precise nature of the responsible brainstem lesion is unknown.

vertical retraction syndrome A rare syndrome characterized by limitation of elevation or depression of the globe of the eye, with retraction and narrowing of the palpebral fissure. The condition is likely to be a synkinesis due to aberrant reinnervation following injury to the III cranial nerve.[5]

vertical vestibulo-ocular reflex Ocular deviation resulting from vertical head movement or bilateral caloric stimulation. Bilateral cold stimulation induces downward deviation of the eyes and warm stimulation, upward deviation, the corrective fast component (taken as the direction of the nystagmus) naturally being in the opposite direction in each case.

vertige épileptique See **affective-psychic seizure**.

vertige larynge of Charcot See **cough syncope**.

vertige paralysant (kubisagari) The acute onset of vertigo and pareses of the elevators of the eyes and weakness of the neck and limbs, occurring in those who work in and around stables in Geneva and Japan. The cause of the condition is not known. See **Gerlier disease**.

vertiginous epilepsy Brief seizures which include a sensation of rotational or linear vertigo accompanied by versive movements of the head, eyes, and body. They are usually due to a focus in the temporal or parietal lobe.[377]

vertigo (Lat, dizziness) A hallucination of movement; the distortion of static gravitational orientation, or the erroneous perception of movement of the self or of the environment, frequently accompanied by nystagmus, ataxia, and nausea. Episodic or paroxysmal; sustained; and positional forms are differentiated.[6104] It represents a mismatch between the sense of motion provided by the vestibular apparatus and that provided by visual or proprioceptive inputs. Its presence may be **physiological** or pathological, the latter indicating dysfunction in the vestibular, visual, or somatosensory systems or (rarely) in the cortex of the superior temporal gyrus.

Central (brainstem) and *peripheral* (vestibular apparatus) forms exist, the difference at a clinical level being the absence of nausea in many cases of central vertigo, and the form of the accompanying nystagmus. See **benign positional vertigo, central nystagmus, peripheral nystagmus, migrainous vertigo**.

Vesalius, Antonio (1514–1564) Belgian anatomist. After study at the Universities of Louvain, Montpellier, and Paris, he worked in Venice and Madrid and was successively professor of anatomy at Padua, Bologna, and Pisa, and at one time was surgeon to the Emperor Charles V.

He introduced eponyms into anatomy, but is thus remembered himself only for a small bone and a foramen, although his monumental work *De humani corporis diffusa libri septum* (Basel, 1543) assured him a permanent monument as one of the greatest anatomists of all time. In the fourth and seventh books, he corrected Galen's error that the human has a rete mirabile and that the vapor rather than the fluid was the important part of the third (CSF) circulation, though he agreed with the flow pattern suggested.

He began to reject what is now called the *medieval cell doctrine* on the basis of his human dissections, which latter led him to be the first to describe internal hydrocephalus.

vesical crises (Lat, bladder + Gr, sudden change) Acute paroxysmal neuralgic pain in the bladder region experienced by patients with **tabes dorsalis**. The same may occur in the larynx and the abdomen. See also **gastric crises, rectal crises**.

vesical reflex Stimulation of the bladder mucosa through bladder distension leads to contraction of the detrusor muscle, relaxation of the internal sphincter, and voiding of the bladder contents. The reflex is mediated through reflex arcs at S2–4.

vesperal hallucinations (Lat, evening + wandering in mind) Hallucinations occurring at nightfall, as is typically the case with **peduncular hallucinations**. See also **sundown syndrome**.

vespers curse Pain in the low back and legs with features of the **restless limb syndrome,** waking the subject from sleep in the early morning. The mechanism is considered to be the combination of congestive cardiac failure and lumbar spinal stenosis, the increased right atrial filling pressure being transmitted to the epidural venous plexus and causing increased pressure in the constricted spinal canal.[3627]

Vestibular Disorders Association A charitable organization in this field providing services to patients and professionals. Address: P.O. Box 13305, Portland, OR 97213-0305. Tel: 800-837-8428. Web site: http://www.vestibular.org/index.php/.

vestibular epilepsy (vestibulogenic epilepsy) 1. A variety of sensory-evoked epilepsy precipitated by excessive provoked or spontaneous stimulation of the vestibular apparatus.[377] 2. Recurrent, transient postepileptic vertigo, possibly a variant of that form of epilepsy in which the seizures are provoked by excessive spontaneously arising discharges of the vestibular apparatus.[485]

vestibular migraine The occurrence of rotational or "to-and-fro" vertigo lasting minutes to hours in adults, often without currently accompanying headache.[1640]

vestibular neuronitis A form of recurrent unilateral labyrinthine dysfunction presenting as acute severe rotatory vertigo with postural imbalance, nausea, and vomiting lasting for about a week, without cochlear or other neurological symptoms.[1666, 6104] Reactivation of a latent HSV1 infection is suspected in some cases, but the unique identity of the syndrome is not universally agreed. See **acute peripheral vestibulopathy**.

vestibular nystagmus (electrical nystagmus) A form of acquired horizontal, horizontal-rotatory, or vertical direction-changing jerk nystagmus resulting from dysfunction of the central or peripheral vestibular system and commonly associated with the clinical complaint of vertigo.

Its amplitude is increased with gaze in the same direction as the fast phase, and, when due to peripheral end-organ disorder, the fast phase is away from the side of the lesion. When due to *peripheral lesions*, the nystagmus is unidirectional, the fast phase is away from the side of the lesion, a rotatory component is common, visual fixation tends to inhibit it, the nystagmus is not always reproducible with testing, and the vertigo is usually marked. By contrast, in the presence of *central lesions* the nystagmus is uni- or bidirectional, it is usually purely vertical or rotatory, fixation has no effect on the amplitude, and any accompanying vertigo is mild.[5]

Forms described include **apogeotropic**, alternating current, **Bechterew, caloric, after-caloric, compensatory**, compression, Faradic, Galvanic, **geotropic, head-shaking**, induced, **labyrinthine**, perverted, pneumatic, **positional**, positioning, **post-rotational**, pseudocaloric, **rotational, upbeat, downbeat**, and secondary phase nystagmus.

vestibular pseudoneuritis A vestibular syndrome due to central (brainstem) rather than peripheral lesions. The manifestations of the two sites of lesions are very similar except for the increased prevalence of **skew deviation** with central pathologies.

vestibular Schwannoma See **Schwannoma, neurofibromatosis**.

vestibular vertigo Vertigo due to disorders affecting the semicircular canals or the otoliths in the utricle and saccule. The first of these causes a spontaneous rotational vertigo of the self or the surroundings, associated with spontaneous nystagmus with the fast phase beating away from the side of the lesion; and with severe nausea, postural imbalance, and homolateral horizontal canal paresis on irrigation. The second produces more of a sensation of tilt or levitation, with postural imbalance, vibration oscillopsia, and moderate nausea, but without nystagmus, although there is diminution of ocular counter-rolling on head tilt.[819]

vestibular-evoked myogenic potentials A short-latency reflex mediated by the otoliths and recorded from the sternocleidomastoid muscle, usually in response to loud auditory clicks. The test evaluates otolith function[6715] and can demonstrate a return to normal function after plugging in **superior canal dehiscence**.

vestibule (Lat, a room within an entrance) A cavity leading on to another one, of larger size.

vestibulitis An acute acquired, presumably viral, infection of the vestibular apparatus, leading to acute vertigo, nystagmus, nausea and vomiting, and imbalance. See also **vestibular nystagmus, vestibular vertigo, vestibular neuronitis**.

vestibulocephalic response See **vestibulocerebral response**.

vestibulocerebral response (oculocephalic response, vestibulocephalic response, doll's head response) Ocular deviation, with or without nystagmus, occurring as a result of head movements causing labyrinthine stimulation.

vestibulocollic reflex (vestibular evoked myogenic potential) Short-latency myogenic responses evoked in the tonically contracted ipsilateral sternocleidomastoid muscle in response to auditory click-stimuli,[1244] in which case a cochlear component would appear likely as well. The reflex can also be obtained by tapping the head with a reflex hammer. The homolateral reflex is absent in cases of unilateral vestibular disease[3110] and in **Ménière disease, acoustic neuroma, vestibular neuritis, multiple sclerosis**, and **basilar-type migraine**. The reflex depends upon a rapidly conducting oligosynaptic brainstem pathway between the vestibular nuclei and motor neurons of the XI n nucleus.

vestibulogenic epilepsy A variety of sensory-evoked seizure, the stimulus here being of the peripheral labyrinth. See **vestibular epilepsy**.

vestibulo-ocular reflex (VOR) A short-latency reflex ensuring stability of the position of the eyes (and thus stable retinal imaging) during rapid changes in head position, through the execution of smooth, conjugate, restitutive, slow eye movements. The pathway runs from the semicircular canals to the superior vestibular nuclei in the brainstem and thence to the oculomotor nerve nuclei. The reflex and its mechanisms and disturbances are fully reviewed by Leigh and Zee.[3762] See **oculovestibular reflex**.

vestibulo-oculogyric reflex (labyrinthine reflex) Lateral deviation of the eyes, with or without nystagmus, away from the side of stimulation of one labyrinth, as in **caloric testing** using cold water. See **oculovestibular response**.

vestibulopathy Any affection of the vestibular apparatus. Acute vestibulopathy provokes the acute or subacute onset of vertigo, dizziness or imbalance, tinnitus, aural fullness, and hearing loss with or without ocular-motor, sensory, postural, or autonomic symptoms and signs, lasting from seconds to days. Its causes include acute peripheral disorders (benign paroxysmal positioning vertigo, vestibular neuritis, **Ménière disease, perilymph fistula** as with **superior canal dehiscence syndrome**, and vestibular paroxysmia); and acute central vestibular disorders such as vestibular **migraine**. Predisposing factors to the peripheral form include blowing the nose, lifting heavy goods, and landing in an airplane.[6103]

A dominantly inherited form of bilateral vestibulopathy has been linked to a mutation at 6q and two syndromes of dominantly inherited hearing loss (DFNA9 and DFNA11) are associated with bilateral vestibulopathy.[3194] Another dominantly inherited form is described in which episodic vertigo is succeeded by gait imbalance and oscillopsia in the presence of normal hearing.[363]

vestibulopupillary response Dilation of the pupil in response to labyrinthine stimulation.

Veterans Administration (VA) Seizure Frequency and Severity Scale A scale recording the frequency and severity of partial seizures based on the reports of the patient and observers.[1750]

Vialetto–van Laere syndrome (bulbar spinal muscular atrophy with deafness, bulbar palsy with deafness) A recessively inherited form of bulbar palsy seen in children and occurring in two forms:

1. Eighth nerve deafness and bulbar palsy accompanied by extraocular palsies and facial weakness; the condition is fatal within 18 months of onset.[6501]
2. A form that has similar clinical features, but its onset is in the second decade and the deafness and facial, bulbar, and truncal neurogenic weakness progress slowly enough to allow life until the fourth decade. **Madras neuropathy** may be identical. See also **progressive bulbar palsy**.

vibrameter A device that emits continuous sinusoidal vibrations at frequencies and intensities under the control of the operator. The subject is exposed to such varying stimuli in the bedside quantitation of large-diameter afferent fiber conduction or the assessment of posterior column function.

vibration oscillopsia Reduced visual acuity during walking due to damage to the otoliths in the utricle and saccule.[819]

vibration white finger See **hand-arm vibration syndrome**.

vibration-induced nystagmus Nystagmus induced by a vibrating tuning fork placed on the mastoid process, with the fast component away from the side of the vestibular lesion.

vibratory sensation (pallesthesia) (from Gr, shake + sensation) A sensory mode considered at the end of the nineteenth century to be a discrete modality, with receptors in the periosteum conveying the "shocks of locomotion." (The ability of the penis, cheek, breast, and skin of the abdominal wall to feel vibration was not considered.) The modality was first examined in the clinical context by Rumpf in 1889; it had not been noticed by Gowers in his textbook the previous year.

von Frey believed that vibration was mediated by pressure receptors, and Pacinian corpuscles are now regarded as the relevant end-organs. The central transmission pathway includes a route through the posterior columns and almost certainly others, perhaps even in the lateral columns and spinocerebellar tracts, which would support the suggestion that the pathway from the skin is the same as that for touch, but from deeper structures, it is the same as that for postural sensibility.

The sensation of vibration itself represents the temporal modulation of tactile sense, analogous to the relationship between flicker and vision. Loss of vibratory sense is due to the desynchronization of the afferent pattern of impulses in demyelinated peripheral nerves or in the central processes of the large dorsal root ganglion cells.[983] The tuning fork was invented by John Shore, an English musician, in 1711.

vibroacoustic disease A systemic disorder caused by exposure to large pressure amplitude and low-frequency noise and characterized by proliferation of the extracellular matrix of connective tissue. Clinical presentations include cognitive problems, balance disorders, and seizures.

Vicq d'Azir, Felix (1748–1794) French physician and comparative anatomist, physician to the French Queen Marie Antoinette, and secretary of the French Academy of Medicine. He gave a rudimentary account of the lobes of the cerebrum, his anterior, middle, and posterior lobes corresponding to the frontal, parietal, and occipital, but the temporal lobe was only differentiated by **Arnold** in 1838. He also described the insula well before Reil, the substantia nigra ("locus niger crurum cerebri") in 1786 and the mammillothalamic tract (bundle of Vicq d'Azir), although this observation was not published until 1805.[4895]

Victor, Maurice (1920–2001) Canadian neurologist who trained initially in Winnipeg and later in Utah and Boston. He accompanied Dr. Raymond Adams to the Massachusetts General Hospital in 1951 and moved to Cleveland in 1962. An outstanding teacher and clinician, he wrote on many neurological topics, especially on those related to alcohol abuse, but is most widely remembered for his joint authorship of a textbook on the *Principles of Neurology* (with Dr. Raymond Adams), to which he brought huge knowledge, perspicacity, and common sense in its descriptions of the basic and clinical aspects of the discipline.

video game-induced seizures Usually generalized and less often occipital seizures with or without photosensitivity, induced by playing games on a video monitor or hand-held liquid crystal display and due to pre-existing photosensitivity, pattern sensitivity, emotional and cognitive excitation, and/or proprioceptive stimulation. Fatigue, sleep deprivation, and prolonged playing are facilitating factors.[4882]

Vidian neuralgia (Vail neuralgia, **cluster headache**) A syndrome of facial pain resembling **Sluder syndrome**, the pain radiating as far back as the ear, mastoid, neck, and shoulder (as it may also in the latter condition; the distinction between the two is too fine for this author to perceive).[6457] The condition may represent another form of **cluster headache**. Vidus Vidius (1500–1569) was an Italian, physician to King Francis I of France and later professor of medicine at Pisa.

Viets test Manual compression of the jugular veins until the subject feels fullness in the head. Increased pain radiating from the back into the legs represents a positive result, suggesting irritation of the lumbosacral nerve roots. The **Naffziger test** is similar except that it employs a blood pressure cuff around the neck, inflated to 40 mmHg for 10 min, whereby the patient is made to suffer extreme discomfort in order to add a degree of spurious precision to an observation of minor importance.

Vieusseux, Gaspard Swiss physician who himself suffered a lateral medullary syndrome (**Vieusseux–Wallenberg syndrome**), his case being discussed and reported in 1810. He gave the first description of bacterial meningitis in 1806, in Geneva.

Vieusseux, Raymond (1641–1716) French physician, professor of anatomy at Montpellier. He described the inferior olives, the pyramids, the centrum ovale, and the semilunar ganglion.

Vieusseux–Wallenberg syndrome See **lateral medullary syndrome**.

vigilance The ability to sustain sensory attention. A state of the nervous system manifested at all levels and capable of either local or general depression; the high-grade physiological efficiency in those neural structures responsible for certain activities and allowing diverse and varying modes of response. Conscious processes would thus be the expressions of physiological vigilance.[2814]

Viliuisk encephalomyelitis A neurodegenerative disorder expressed as subacute meningoencephalitis progressing to a more prolonged pan-encephalitic syndrome with a fatal outcome in 1–10 years. Some patients survive to a steady state of global dementia and severe spasticity that may last over 20 years. Multiple micronecrotic foci surrounded by inflammatory infiltrates are observed throughout the cerebral cortex and other gray matter areas. An infectious etiology is strongly suspected, but the causative agent has not been identified but most patients show evidence for intrathecal IgG synthesis correlating with the clinical manifestations of the disease.[126]

Villaret, Maurice (1877–1946) French physician and physiologist with major interests outside medicine, who wrote on cirrhosis and the portal circulation and was expert in the therapeutic value of spas.[2066]

Villaret syndrome (retroparotid space syndrome, posterior retropharyngeal syndrome, posterior retroparotid syndrome) Unilateral paralysis of the muscles supplied by cranial nerves IX, X, XI, and XII, and sometimes cranial nerve VII, with **Horner syndrome**, as a result of compression of these nerves in the posterior retroparotid space, usually by a malignancy.[6550]

The difference between this and the **Collet–Sicard syndrome** is minimal. The cranial nerves affected in other syndromes resulting from disease of this area include the following:

- **Jackson syndrome** (complete unilateral X, XI, XII);
- **Mackenzie syndrome** (IX, X, XI, XII);
- **Collet–Sicard syndrome** (IX, X, XI, XII);
- **Avellis syndrome** (X);
- **Schmidt syndrome** (X, XI);
- **Tapia syndrome** (XI, XII);
- **Lannois and Jouty syndrome** (IX, X, XI, XII);
- **Vernet syndrome** (VII, IX, X, XI, XII with or without involvement of the cervical sympathetic pathway and hemiparesis).[6147]

Villar–Rose syndrome See **cephalic tetanus**.

Vincent sign The **Argyll Robertson pupil**.

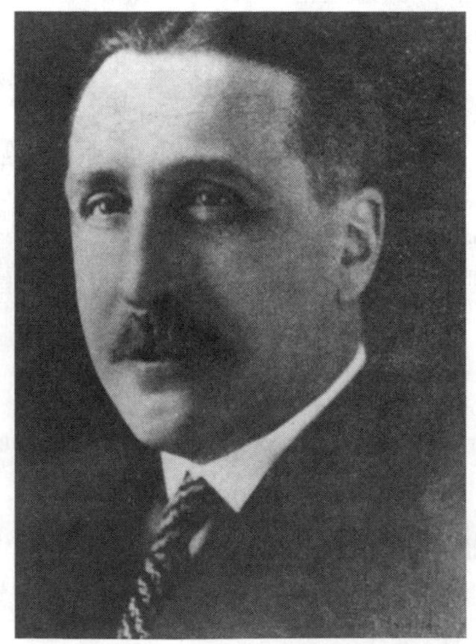

Figure V–2 Maurice Villaret

Vineland Adaptive Behavior Scale A set of scales measuring self-help skills such as communication, daily living skills, socialization, motor skills, and maladaptive behavior, based upon a questionnaire and a structured interview. The instrument is appropriate for cognitively impaired people at all ages from infancy to adult.[5966]

violaceous hue The light purple color of the skin of the eyelids in some patients with **dermatomyositis** or with the skin lesions of morphoea. The French word *mauve* would be equally appropriate, if less memorable.

violinists' cramps Focal (occupational) dystonias occurring either in the hand fingering the strings or in that holding the bow.

viral myoglobinuria The occurrence of rhabdomyolysis with spilling of myoglobin into the urine, as a result of viral (e.g., influenzal, Coxsackie) infections.

Virchow disease Acute congenital encephalitis. The nature of this condition is now uncertain.[6554]

Virchow, Rudolf Ludwig Karl (1821–1902) German pathologist who graduated from Berlin. After he reported that the cause of a typhus epidemic into which he had been sent to inquire was largely social and directly the fault of the government, he was dismissed from his posts in Berlin, but was appointed at once as professor of pathological anatomy at Würzburg and eventually was able to return to Berlin as professor in 1856.

The father of modern pathology, particularly cellular pathology, he founded *Virchow's Archives*, the prestigious journal of pathology, in 1847, and was a preeminent medical scientist, historian, and politician during his active career. He first identified the neuroglia in 1846, and also described thrombosis, infarction, vascular emboli, subdural hematomas, spina bifida occulta, and leontiasis ossea. The terms *agenesis*, *heterotopia*, *ochronosis*, and *leukocytosis* were initially his, and Virchow's name is also given to the following three items.

Virchow–Robin spaces (Virchow spaces) Extensions of the subpial spaces forming gaps around blood vessels in the brain. They are filled with interstitial fluid and house penetrating arteries and veins.[1961] They were described by Virchow 4 years after they had been identified by Charles-Philippe Robin (1821–1885), a French physician.

Larger spaces of this kind, more than 1.5 cm in diameter, are most commonly seen in the midbrain and are known as *giant perivascular spaces*. These have variously been thought able to cause headaches, dementia, syncope, seizures, visual changes, stroke, impaired memory and concentration, and imbalance on the basis of mere association and many diseases are alleged to be associated. MRI scans show that they are located along the path of a penetrating vessel, are isointense with CSF, contain no calcium, and are surrounded by normal appearing brain tissue.[1961]

Virchow–Seckel syndrome See **Seckel syndrome**.

virile reflex See **bulbocavernosus reflex**.

visceral epilepsy Epigastric auras consisting of indescribable feelings, pain (**Moores syndrome**), and cardiac, respiratory, or gastrointestinal symptoms as manifestations of "partial" epilepsies.[4537]

visceral larva migrans See **toxocariasis**.

visceral neuropathy See **familial visceral neuropathy**.

visceral pain Dull or cramping abdominal discomfort and pain, often associated with nausea and autonomic reactions. It may occur in the absence of any abdominal organ dysfunction, and represent a neuropathic type of pain. **Autonomic dysreflexia** may complicate patients with spinal cord lesions above the splanchnic outflow (sixth thoracic level).

visceromotor symptoms Lip-smacking, swallowing, or chewing movements, most commonly recognized as part of a seizure originating in the temporal lobe. See **temporal lobe syndromes**.

viscosity 1. Stickiness of thought processes, leading to a tendency to talk repetitively and circumstantially on a narrow range of topics. 2. Enhanced intrapersonal adhesiveness; a tendency to "cling" to certain other people. In each case, the trait is associated with temporal lobe epilepsy, especially with left-sided or bilateral foci.[5190]

vision (from Lat, the sense of seeing) The faculty of sight.

visual adaptation The disappearance from sight of a stationary visual target after the subject has gazed at it for a few seconds. The phenomenon is occasionally found with some cases of lesions of the optic radiations.[454]

visual agnosia A disorder of recognition confined to the realm of vision in which alert, intelligent, and nondysphasic patients with normal visual perception fail to comprehend the nature or meaning of nonverbal visual stimuli which formerly had been understood.

Two forms are recognized: In *visual apperceptive agnosia*, the subject cannot name, copy, or match an object, although the visual fields are full and acuity is unaffected. The lesion (usually ischemic) affects the calcarine cortex bilaterally, or its pathways.[758] In *visual associative agnosia* discrimination is retained but identification fails. Thus, the subject can recognize or draw an object named and presented among others, but cannot recognize objects visually without such cues.[5028] The lesion is likely to be in the anterior left temporal lobe.

visual agnosia or apraxia without dementia A progressive syndrome in which there is an impairment of visuoperceptive abilities in the absence of dementia or oral language disorders, starting in adult life and with slow progression. The relationship to other primary progressive dementias is not yet clarified.[1515] See also **agnosia**.

visual allesthesiae The transfer of visual images from one half-field to the other—thus a form of **palinopsia**.[3133]

Visual Analog Mood Scale A method of assessing mood levels whereby the subjects select a point along a visually presented scale corresponding to their assessment of their level of, for example, happiness–sadness.[2148]

Visual Analog Test A method for scoring the amount of pain felt, whereby subjects are required to mark on a line the place corresponding to the intensity of their pain, from *no pain* to *the worst pain I ever felt*.[732]

visual apperceptive agnosia See **visual agnosia**.

visual associative agnosia See **visual agnosia**.

visual aura The perception of flashing or flickering lights, spots, simple patterns, scotomata, or amaurosis, in epilepsy or in migraine.

Visual Aura Rating Scale A scale developed to differentiate migraine visual aura and non-aura features, assessing duration, speed of development, the presence of scotomata and zigzag lines, and unilateral/homonymous visual loss.

visual axis A line between the fovea and the point of fixation.

visual confusion A visual error consisting of the perception that two different objects are occupying the same position in space. See also **diplopia**.

visual disorientation (Holmes syndrome, Riddoch syndrome) Defective visuospatial orientation as a result of lesions in the region of the supramarginal and angular gyri; there is, thus, an inability to localize objects in the three planes of space, and especially to estimate absolute and relative distances. When occurring in a single homonymous half-field, it is due to a contralateral parietal lobe lesion.[5292] See **simultagnosia**.

visual dysesthesia The tendency for stimuli in one half-field to have an unpleasant quality, tending to elicit an exaggerated **startle** reaction; an uncommon manifestation in disease of the visual cortex.

visual evoked potential (visual evoked response) Electric waveforms of biologic origin recorded over the cerebrum and elicited in response to visual stimuli. They are classified by stimulus rate as *transient* or *steady state*, and they can be further divided by stimulus presentation mode. The normal transient VEP to checkerboard pattern reversal or shift has a major positive occipital peak at about 100 ms (P100), often preceded by a negative peak (N75). The precise range of normal values for the latency and amplitude of P100 depends on several factors: (1) subject variables, such as age, gender, and visual acuity, (2) stimulus characteristics, such as type of stimulator, full-field or half-field stimulation, check size, contrast, and luminescence, and (3) recording parameters, such as placement and combination of recording electrodes. (From the 2001 Report of the Nomenclature Committee of the American Association of Electromyography and Electrodiagnosis.[19] Reproduced by kind permission of the AANEM.)

visual evoked response See **visual evoked potential**.

visual field That portion of space in which objects are visible at the same moment during steady fixation of the gaze in one direction.[6374] See also **field of vision**.

visual grasp reflex The return of gaze to a target despite commands to look elsewhere. Reflex saccadic movements are made toward a transiently presented visual stimulus, while gaze is meant to be directed upon a different, fixed target.[2127]

visual hallucinations Perception of visual images in the absence of objective stimuli. See **ophthalmopathic hallucinations, hemianopic hallucinations, peduncular hallucinosis, hypnagogic hallucinations**. The subject has been reviewed in depth by Miller Fisher.[2101]

visual illusions of movement The appearance of movement or of displacement of the visual field with respect to an observer when no such movement has occurred.

Three forms are differentiated:

1. *Autokinetic illusions* are the apparent wanderings of a small light source in a dark environment.
2. *Oculogyral illusions* arise when the observer experiences the stimulus of angular acceleration, again best seen when the observer fixes a small light source in a dark place.
3. *Oculogravic illusions*, linked with the stimulus of linear acceleration, can be seen in any condition of illumination, and consist of illusions of tilt and of movement.

All three forms have been ascribed to small, involuntary, and physiological eye movements resulting from labyrinthine activity.[6756]

visual inversion Transient complete 180° inversion of the visual image resulting from ischemic, traumatic, or inflammatory pathology in the occipital lobes.[4284]

visual neglect A defective ability to attend to one or more components of the total visual environment as a result of lesions of one or other cerebral hemisphere, especially the right. Accompanying visual field defects are not always demonstrable. The area of neglect is more frequently central or bilateral than contralateral to the site of the cerebral lesion. It occurs with either left or right hemisphere damage but is more severe with the latter. It is also more common in the center of the page or bilaterally than unilaterally and so is probably a bilateral phenomenon. It may occur without a visual field defect.[104]

Visual Neglect Recovery Index A battery of tests modified from the **Behavioral Inattention Test** and used to evaluate visual and other forms of neglect following acute stroke, and to predict recovery.[6071]

visual object agnosia A failure of generic class recognition—even worse than the usual visual agnosia. See also **agnosia**.

visual orbicularis reflex (of Descartes) (palpebral reflex) See **orbicularis oculi reflex**.

visual paresthesias Disagreeable qualities of sensation coming from the affected side in patients with partial hemianopias.

visual paraneoplastic syndrome (photoreceptor degeneration, **cancer-associated retinopathy**, paraneoplastic retinopathy)A syndrome of night blindness, visual hallucinations, or other visual impairments in subjects with small cell carcinoma of the lung (or less often cervical, endometrial, or breast carcinomas, malignant melanomas, and other lung carcinomas) due to the production of antibodies directed against the antigens shared by the tumor and the retina and/or optic nerve.

visual perseveration (paliopsia) 1. Recurrence of visual perceptions after the stimulus-object has been removed. A variety of this affection (*illusory visual spread*) comprises an illusory extension of the visual perception over an area greater than that which the stimulus-object would be expected to excite; thus, a metamorphopsia in which objects appear elongated in one dimension only. The causative lesion is in the posterior part of the hemisphere, on either side.[1328] 2. A phenomenon characterized by the prolonged persistence of a visual image without late recurrences, in the presence of evidence of ictal activity but without any associated hemianopia.[1376] See also **palinopsia**.

visual reproduction test A test of visuospatial praxis in which the subject has to reproduce increasingly complex geometric figures after a 10-s study period, and then to copy the stimulus figures (to assess visuoperceptual dysfunction).[5474]

visual static agnosia Impaired recognition of statically presented stimuli, with relatively retained recognition of those that are moving.[759]

visual vertigo Vertiginous symptoms provoked by visual stimuli, usually evidence of a peripheral vestibular rather than a psychogenic disorder.[865]

visual vertigo 1. (optokinetic motion sickness) The physiological effect of a mismatch between the visual sensation of movement and the concomitant vestibular and somatosensory inputs which signal that movement is not occurring—as occurs when viewing chase scenes on a wide-angle cinema screen. 2. Vertigo induced by distorted visual input, as with incorrect refraction, strong plus-lenses after cataract surgery, or oculomotor paresis (ocular vertigo).

visual-constructive derangement See **visuospatial agnosia**.

visual-palpebral reflex See **palpebral reflex**.

visual-sensitive seizures Seizures provoked by visual stimuli or alteration of such stimuli. See **photosensitive epilepsies**. (Even though not the officially recommended term, the latter is the one best known and more etymologically correct).

visual–verbal test A test of abstraction ability wherein the subject is required to determine the common attributes of three of the four patterns printed on cards, there being two sets, each card with three patterns sharing such attributes.[2002]

visuomotor ataxia (disturbance in visual orientation, trouble du sens de l'éspace) A disorder of the visual control of motor activity despite intact motor, cerebellar, and somatosensory functions, and with normal praxis and visual perception. One or both half-fields and the contralateral or the homolateral hand may be affected; bilateral involvement indicates the presence of a callosal lesion; unilateral involvement, a lesion of the occipitofrontal pathways subserving the visual control of movement.[5373] See **optic ataxia**.

visuopatial agraphia See **agraphia**.

visuospatial ability The capacity to recognize the presence, position, and spatial relationships of objects seen, and to manipulate them appropriately in space.

visuospatial acalculia See **acalculia**.

visuospatial agnosia (planotopokinesia, apractagnosia for spatial orientation, visual-constructive derangement) A defect in the analysis of spatial relationships and in the execution of constructional tasks under visual control, particularly those demanding a fine appreciation of spatial structure such as drawing, copying, and the manipulation of patterns, caused by a lesion of the "minor" hemisphere parietal lobe,[5247] due in part to unilateral visual inattention.

visuospatial neglect A relative imperception of objects in one half of the visual field, most commonly occurring with right hemisphere lesions in the early stages after, for example, stroke, but later found with equal incidence after lesions of either hemisphere.

visuovestibulo-ocular response A combination of the **vestibulo-ocular response** and **optokinetic nystagmus**, providing the mechanism for the stability of the retinal image when not only the head but also the object of fixation is moving.

vitamin E deficiency A consequence of chronic malabsorption syndromes in which dysarthria, an ataxic syndrome with or without musculoskeletal changes (especially in children), an areflexic sensorimotor peripheral neuropathy, and extensor plantar responses have been described.[2759] Other manifestations may include cranial neuropathy with ophthalmoplegia and dysarthria; psychomotor impairment; posterior column dysfunction; myopathy; and pigmentary retinopathy. This deficiency has been held responsible for the neurological syndromes of children with severe chronic liver disease and of **hypo-** and **a-betalipoproteinemia**. The syndrome resembles **Friedreich ataxia**, but in that condition plasma α-tocopherol levels are normal and there is no response to vitamin E supplementation.

Isolated vitamin E deficiency is inherited as an autosomal recessive disease mapped to chromosome 8q13 and presents with cerebellar and peripheral neuropathic signs.[3120]

vitamin E deficiency myopathy A syndrome complicating chronic cholestasis, in which low serum vitamin E levels, absent reflexes, mild weakness, ataxia, and sensory loss in the arms and legs occur in association with the presence of multiple autofluorescent inclusions within skeletal muscle fibers, showing strong acid phosphatase reactivity.[4638]

vocal agnosia Difficulty in recognizing a known human voice due to bilateral temporal lobe damage.

vocal automatisms Single or repetitive utterances consisting of sounds such as grunts or shrieks, in the context of epilepsy.

vocal cord abductor paralysis A potential life-threatening complication of multiple system atrophy through its ability to cause nocturnal airway obstruction.[3105]

vocal spasmodic dystonia A primary focal dystonia affecting phonation, the speech having a "strangled" or tight quality.

Vogt syndrome 1. (Wilson–Vogt syndrome, congenital chorea, syndrome of the corpus striatum) A form of cerebral palsy with athetosis, chorea, and eventually dystonias, and usually with mental retardation, characterized by the abnormal presence of myelinated fibers in the corpus striatum (**état marbré**).[6561] The clinical syndrome results from destruction of the cells of the caudate nucleus and putamen, leading to spastic diplegia without pyramidal tract involvement, dysarthria, athetosis, rhythmic oscillations, and pseudobulbar palsy as a consequence of damage to all cell types in the neostriatum.[6561] See also **double athetosis**.

2. A form of **acrocephalosyndactyly** once regarded as type II, but so similar to type I (**Apert syndrome**) that the difference is illusory.

Vogt, A. (1879–1943) Swiss ophthalmologist, working in Zurich.

Vogt, Cécile (1875–1931) French neuroanatomist, who trained in Paris and worked for a year with **Marie** at the **Salpêtrière**, where she met Oskar **Vogt**, whom she later married. Her earlier interests were in myelination, but she and her husband later concentrated upon **cytoarctitectonic** and stimulation studies in primates, which led to the differentiation of 100 separate cortical areas—minutiae no longer accepted as meaningful. She also studied the basal ganglia and was the first to ascribe a specific disease state (double athetosis) to disease of the striatum and to apply the term **état marbré**.

Vogt, Heinrich (1875–1937) German psychiatrist who graduated from Heidelberg and became professor of psychiatry in Göttingen. He described the features of the juvenile form of **neuronal ceroid lipofuscinosis** (Spielmeyer–Vogt disease) before, but published after, Spielmeyer.[7]

Vogt, Oskar (1870–1959) Danish-German neuroanatomist and neuropathologist. He was born in Schleswig-Holstein and trained with **Binswanger** and **Forel**, **Marie**, and the **Déjèrines** in biological sciences and neurology. His goal was to found an institute where scientists of various disciplines could work together on problems of the nervous system, and he did so with the founding of the Neurologische Zentralstation in Berlin (1898), later incorporated into the University of Berlin and in 1931 becoming the Kaiser Wilhelm-Institut with over a hundred staff members and himself as director, funded in large part by the Rockefeller Foundation.

Political factors led to his removal in 1937 to a smaller institute in Neustadt, from which he was called up for military service as a private soldier at the age of 69. However, he proved intractable and was discharged to resume his cytological studies on the huge collection of brains collected in the Institut by **Bielschowsky, Brodmann, Foerster, Liepmann, Oppenheim**, and others, and preserved over the years.

Both Oskar and Cecile Vogt had as their goal the correlation of normal and abnormal behavior with brain morphology, and to this end they published their works on cytoarchitectonics from 1903, assisted by Brodmann, and on myeloarchitectonics in numerous animals as well as in humans. The Vogts also studied the variable susceptibility to disease manifested by different brain areas, noting that the vulnerability of each neuron system is determined by the distinctive physicochemical composition of its cells (pathoclisis).[5704, 2808]

Vogt–Koyanagi syndrome See **uveomeningoencephalitic syndrome**.

Vogt–Koyanagi–Harada syndrome See **uveomeningoencephalitic syndrome**.

Vohwinkel syndrome See **deafness, keratopachydermia, and digital constrictions**.

voice-induced epilepsy A form of **reflex epilepsy** in which the seizures are triggered by a certain quality of the voice heard.[2155]

voiceless bilabial (stop) A consonant made by occluding air flow completely at the lips, letting pressure build up, then releasing it in a sudden burst. The only voiceless bilabial stop in English is "P".[3949]

volitional activity Activity performed as a result of conscious decision.

volitional facial palsy Weakness of the lower quadrant of one side of the face for the performance of willed movements, as a result of damage to some of the corticobulbar fibers supplying the VII cranial nerve nucleus. Cf. **mimetic facial palsy**.

Volkmann ischemic contracture Muscle fibrosis and sensorimotor neuropathy with distal muscle atrophy resulting from prolonged compressive ischemia, as in the **compartment syndromes** and thus most commonly seen in forearm and pretibial muscles after vascular injury due, for example, to supracondylar fractures. Features of **Sudeck atrophy** are also commonly present.[6563]

Volkmann, Richard von (1830–1889) German surgeon who graduated in Berlin and later became professor of surgery in Halle.

Vollmer reflex Lordosis of the spine, flexion of the limbs, and a loud cry occurring when the spine of the infant held in ventral suspension is firmly stroked. This reflex is normally present for the first 3 months of life.[6898]

voltage The potential difference between two sites, expressed in volts (V) or millivolts (mV).

volume conduction The propagation of electrical currents from external sources within the body, but through extraneural tissues.[1748]

voluntary (from Lat, of free will) Under conscious control.

voluntary activity In electromyography, the electric activity recorded from a muscle during consciously controlled contraction. The effort made to contract the muscle may be specified relative to that of a corresponding normal muscle, e.g., minimal, moderate, or maximal. If the recording remains isoelectric during the attempted contraction and equipment malfunction has been excluded, it can be concluded that there is no voluntary activity. (From the 2001 Report of the Nomenclature Committee of the American Association of Electromyography and Electrodiagnosis.[19] Reproduced by kind permission of the AANEM.)

voluntary flutter See **psychogenic flutter**.

voluntary nystagmus A series of repetitive, conjugate eye movements (back-to-back saccades) which are consciously induced. They can seldom be sustained for more that 15 s at a time and usually occur horizontally at high frequency, often accompanied by facial grimacing. Rarely, the same can be seen in one eye only. The condition has also been reported to occur as a dominant characteristic, but in such cases the movements do not represent true nystagmus.[264, 3746] See also **psychogenic flutter**.

volvular epilepsy A form of complex partial seizure in which the patient walks around in small circles; a generalized tonic–clonic attack may or may not follow. The seizure focus is in the temporal or frontal region.[1684]

vomiting reflex Reverse peristalsis of the esophagus with vomiting in response to stimulation of the posterior pharyngeal wall or elsewhere in the upper part of the gastrointestinal tract. This is a normal response unless markedly disinhibited.

von Ammon syndrome See **Apert syndrome**.

von Angyal syndrome A variant of **Gerstmann syndrome**, characterized by right–left confusion, dysgraphia, and thumb-mouth agnosia.[6564]

von Bekesy, Georg (1899–1972) Hungarian otologist and physicist whose work (mainly at Harvard) clarified the functions of the cochlea for which he was awarded the Nobel prize for Physiology in 1961. He invented the patient-controlled audiometer that bears his name.

von Bekhterev reflex See **carpometacarpal reflex**.

von Bonsdorff technique A method of increasing the yield in the **Trousseau** test, whereby a blood pressure cuff on the arm is inflated to just below the diastolic pressure for 10 min, after which the patient hyperventilates for a minute. Tetany in the arm tested represents a positive result.

von Burdach, Karl Friedrich See **Burdach**.

von Economo encephalitis See **encephalitis lethargica**.

von Economo, Baron Konstantin (1876–1931) Austrian neurologist and neuropathologist. Born in Romania of wealthy Greek parents, he grew up in Trieste and studied engineering in Vienna before commencing medical studentship. After graduation he trained with Pierre **Marie** in Paris, but later returned to Vienna and eventually became professor of psychiatry and neurology in 1921. Having numerous other interests, however, he refused further promotion. He was passionately interested in aeronautics (and was the first Austrian to hold an international pilot's licence) and in ballooning.

He published on the topics of pontine tumors, the trigeminal nerve, sleep, **Wilson disease**, and cortical cytoarchitecture, his 1925 treatise clarifying much of the prevailing confusion about the extent of the different areas and their characteristics. As a result of a paper on accelerated dementia, von Economo narrowly escaped having his name attached to what is now known as **Creutzfeldt–Jakob disease**. His published account of **encephalitis lethargica** (May 10, 1917)[6567] immediately followed that of **Cruchet** of Bordeaux (April 27, 1917) and the latter began a squabble, loudly claiming that precedence which was then considered important; as delicately adjudicated by **van Bogaert**, he failed in his claim, because von Economo had defined the condition as a single disease entity, which Cruchet and his colleagues had not.[6473]

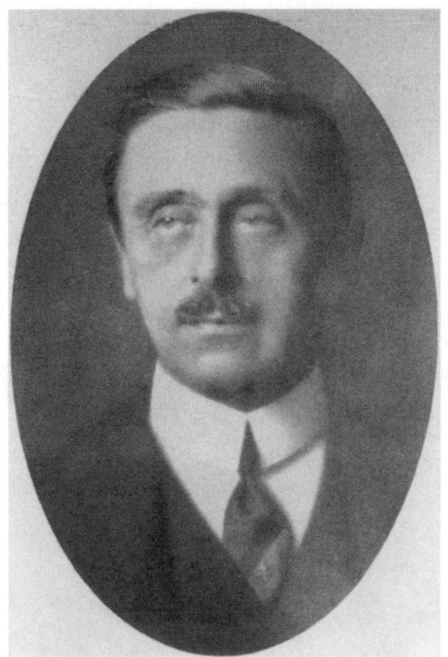

Figure V–3 Konstantin von Economo

von Frey hairs Bristles of varying thicknesses, mounted upon suitable holders, for the semi-quantitative examination of the sense of touch.

von Frey, Max Originator (1895) of the specificity theory of sensation, he considered that heat, cold, touch, and pain were the four specific modalities, each subserved by specific receptors and fibers. He believed that skin receptors are differentiated with respect to the lowest threshold to particular energy categories: Meissner corpuscles and hair cells for touch, Ruffini end-organs for warm, Krause end-bulbs for cold, and free nerve endings for pain. These opinions are no longer held.

von Gierke disease (glycogenosis type 1) A recessively inherited deficiency of glucose-6-phosphatase, leading to the deposition of glycogen in the liver and kidneys. Clinically, obesity, hepatomegaly, renal impairment, lactic acidosis, and failure to thrive are the most obvious features; seizures represent the only neurological problem.[6568] See **glycogen storage diseases**.

von Graefe cramp See **blepharospasm**.

von Graefe sign Lid lag—the failure of the upper lid to maintain its normal position relative to the globe during down-gaze, although the lid descends normally with eye closure. The sign is an inconstant feature of hyperthyroidism, and is also seen in facial nerve palsy (in which, however, there is ptosis of the brow) and in **myasthenia gravis**.[2540] See also **pseudo-Von Graefe sign**.

von Graefe syndrome See **chronic progressive external ophthalmoplegia, progressive external ophthalmoplegia**.

von Graefe, Friedrich Wilhelm Ernst Albrecht See Graefe.

von Graefe–Sjögren syndrome (Hallgren syndrome) A recessively inherited condition characterized by pigmentary retinal degeneration, deafness, and spinocerebellar ataxia, often with mental retardation.[6571]

von Gudden, Bernhard Aloys (1824–1886) See **Gudden**. He demonstrated the presence of both crossed and uncrossed fibers in the optic nerve and showed that secondary thalamic atrophy occurs after a lesion of the occipital cortex.

von Hippel, Eugen (1867–1939) German ophthalmologist who trained in Heidelberg, where he became assistant to **Leber**, working mainly on angiomatosis retinae. He later became Professor at Halle and then at Göttingen.

von Hippel did not report the autosomal dominant inheritance of the condition named for him, nor its intracranial complications, nor the occurrence of pancreatic cysts, pheochromocytomas, and renal and pancreatic tumors which may also be features of the disorder; such insights were the work of Arvid **Lindau** (1926).

von Hippel-Lindau disease (cerebro-retinal angiomatosis: OMIM 193300) A rare, dominantly inherited, multisystem tumor syndrome with variable expression, in which diffuse hemangiomatoses are found (in descending order of frequency) in the retinas, adrenal glands, cerebellum, spinal cord, and kidney.[2908] The gene is carried on the short arm of chromosome 3 at 3p25–p24.

Renal carcinoma, multiple visceral cysts, and pheochromocytoma are important and specific complications; cerebral tumors are detected by enhanced MRI in 70% of cases. Endolymphatic sac tumors, which can cause tinnitus or deafness, are also described.

The diagnosis is likely if a patient with a positive family history of von Hippel–Landau disease (VHL):

A. Has more than one retinal or cerebellar hemangioblastoma; or
B. Has an isolated lesion in association with a visceral manifestation of the disease such as renal cell carcinoma or pheochromocytoma, and, possibly, multiple pancreatic cysts; or
C. When there is only one manifestation in the presence of a positive family history.

In the absence of a family history of von Hippel–Lindau disease, the presence of two or more retinal or cerebellar hemangioblastomas, or one hemangioblastoma with one visceral tumor, is required for diagnosis.

The condition was first described in England by Collins in 1894, but it was von Hippel who 10 years later recognized that the lesions were **hemangioblastomas**,[3060] while Lindau reported the cerebellar features. The abnormal gene is found at 3p25, a site normally possessed of tumor-suppressant activity.

von Mickulicz disease Sarcoidosis affecting the parotid glands.

von Monakow See Monakow.

von Monakow bundle See **rubrospinal tract**.

von Monakow reflex See **lateral foot reflex**.

von Monakow syndrome See **anterior choroidal artery syndrome**.

von Recklinghausen disease See **neurofibromatosis**.

von Recklinghausen, Friedrich Daniel (1833–1910) See **Recklinghausen**.

von Soemmerring, Samuel Thomas See **Soemmerring**.

von Stein tests 1. Performance of the **Romberg test** while the patient stands on one leg or with one foot in front of the other. This adds sensitivity but subtracts specificity; in a positive test, it also requires the examiner to be very vigilant. 2. Tilt-table tests.

von Stockert phenomenon The prompt induction of sleep by certain visual stimuli in subjects who have recovered from an acute attack of **encephalitis lethargica**.

von Strümpell, E.A.G.G. See **Strümpell**, E.A.G.G.

von Willebrand's knee A looping-forward of crossing fibers in the optic chiasm, such that a lesion of the posterior part of the homolateral optic nerve also affects these fibers, causing a field defect in the opposite eye.

vorbeirenden (Ger, talking past [or beside] the point) Although this word is used to describe the characteristic feature of Ganser syndrome, Ganser never used it himself, preferring *verbeigehen*, translated as "to pass by," which actually gives a better feeling for the abnormal verbal output.

Vulpian sign (Prévost sign) The tendency of the eyes to turn toward the side of a cortical lesion and thus away from the paralyzed side, as after a hemispheric stroke. The integrity of the frontal eye fields appears necessary for normal deviations to occur in either direction, but the sign does occur with some more posterior lesions in the right hemisphere and, according to the original publications, with deep lesions as well.[2483]

Vulpian, Edmé-Felix-Alfred (1826–1887) French physician, a pupil of Flourens who assisted him to enter medical school in Paris. Vulpian later worked with **Charcot** at the **Salpêtrière**, where he later succeeded **Cruveilhier** as professor of pathological anatomy. A retiring man, he was somewhat overshadowed by Charcot, although considered an outstanding teacher. His research output included studies of peripheral nerve regeneration, the **scapuloperoneal syndrome**, the chromaffin system, the motor end-plate, and the pathological anatomy of the spinal cord.[2066]

Vurpas reflex See **buccal reflex**.

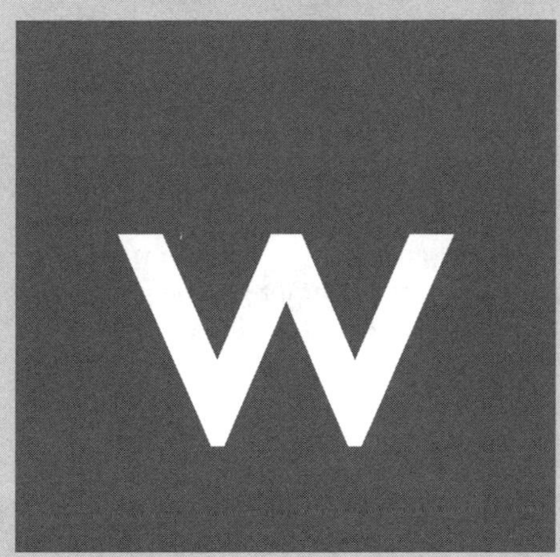

Waaler anomaly (hydrocephalus, costovertebral dysplasia with Sprengel deformity) A dominantly inherited congenital dysmorphic syndrome characterized by white forelock, deafness, and numerous musculoskeletal abnormalities affecting the face, ribs, spine, and limbs.

Waardenberg syndrome 1. (van der Hoeve–Halbertsma–Waardenburg–Klein syndrome) A relatively common dominantly inherited syndrome characterized by nerve deafness, heterochromia iridis, confluence of the eyebrows (**synophrys**), a white forelock, lateral displacement of the lacrimal canthi, abnormal skin pigmentation, and impaired vestibular responses.[6579, 6578]

In a *variant* form, *Mende syndrome*, the features of **Down syndrome** are also present.

2. A singularly rare form of **acrocephalosyndactyly** (variously *type* III or V), characterized by hypertelorism, facial dysmorphism, syndactyly of the hands, and abnormal genitalia.[6251] See also **Apert syndrome.**

Waardenburg, Petrus Johannes (1886–1979) A Dutch ophthalmic geneticist working in Utrecht.

Wada Test The intracarotid injection of sodium amylobarbitone, given in order to ascertain the lateralization of the speech centers in patients under consideration for excision of a temporal lobe for the management of intractable seizures.[3207]

By causing temporary (10 min) inactivity of the injected hemisphere, the functions of the other one can be assessed, although questions to do with its interpretation have been discussed.[4270] The technique was described in 1949 by Dr. Jun Wada of Vancouver, Canada, but it is likely that the use of functional MRI will make it obsolete in the foreseeable future.

Waddell signs Physical findings that suggest that the back pain complained of by a patient has its root in some behavioral disturbance. The signs are grouped into five classes:[6580]

1. Tenderness which is superficial (dermal) or nonanatomical. (See also **cellulalgia, skin roll test.**)
2. Simulation tests, which give the patient the impression that a test is being performed, when actually it is not. Back pain felt with downward compression on the head or rotation of the patient's shoulders and pelvis in the same plane are examples.
3. Distraction tests, such as the examination of straight-leg raising with the patient in the lying and then in the sitting position. In many cases found not to have structural pathology, the test is painless when the subject is seated.
4. Regional disturbances. "Giving way" of many muscle groups that cannot be explained on a localized neurological basis and sensory disturbances following a glove-and-stocking distribution (often terminating abruptly at the groin or shoulder) rather than in a dermatomal pattern are examples.
5. Behavioral and verbal overreaction to the manipulations of the examiner.

Such signs were shown to correlate with each other, but not with the presence of organic causes for back pain. (After Waddell G, McCulloch JA, Kummell E, et al. Nonorganic physical signs in low back pain. *Spine* 1980;5:117–25.)

Wadia–Swamy spinocerebellar degeneration A dominantly inherited cerebellar ataxic syndrome, characterized also by unusually slow saccades and ocular pursuit.[6586]

Wagener retinopathy See **Keith–Wagener Scale.**

Waggoner syndrome A recessively inherited syndrome characterized by mental retardation and agenesis of the cerebral white matter.[6589]

Wagner syndrome (Wagner–Unverricht syndrome, Wagner–Hepp disease, Potain dermatomyositis, Bergouignan edematous polymyositis) See **dermatomyositis.**

Wagner von Jauregg, Julius (1857–1940) German physician, awarded the Nobel prize in 1927 for his introduction of malarial treatment for **general paresis** in 1918, which he had actually first proposed 40 years before.

Wagner, Ernst Leberecht (1829–1888) German physician who described acute generalized polymyositis in 1863.[6591]

Wagner–Hepp disease See **Wagner syndrome.**

Wagner–Unverricht syndrome See **Wagner syndrome.**

WAGR syndrome A rare syndrome characterized by the association of Wilms tumor, Aniridia, Genital abnormality, and mental Retardation. The responsible gene maps to 11–p13.

Waida dystrophy See **benign X-linked muscular dystrophy.**

WAIS, WAIS-R Acronyms for the **Wechsler Adult Intelligence Scale** (Revised), the most used of all the comprehensive intelligence tests available.

wakefulness without awareness See **persistent vegetative state.**

wake-up stroke The first awareness of a neurological deficit when a patient wakes, usually indicating an ischemic infarct that had occurred during sleep.

wake-up test A procedure used most commonly in spinal surgery. During critical portions of an operation in which the spinal cord is at risk of injury, the level of general anesthesia is allowed to decrease to the point where the patient can respond to commands. The patient is then asked to move hands and feet, and a movement in response to commands indicates the spinal cord is intact. This procedure is used routinely in some centers. Somatosensory evoked potential monitoring is an alternative in surgical situations where the possibility of spinal cord injury exists. (Adapted from the 2001 Report of the Nomenclature Committee of the American Association of Electromyography and Electrodiagnosis.[19] Reproduced by kind permission of the AANEM.)

waking cataplexy See **sleep paralysis.**

waking epilepsy Generalized seizures occurring only during the waking hours.

Waldenström macroglobulinemia (hyperviscosity syndrome) A syndrome characterized by excessive IgM production and circulation following the uncontrolled proliferation of lymphocytes and plasma cells. It occurs either in isolation among elderly men (primary macroglobulinemia) or as a **paraneoplastic syndrome** associated with multiple myeloma and leukemia. Clinical characteristics include easy bruising and bleeding, anemia with systemic malaise and fatigue, chorioretinopathy with retinal hemorrhages, optic disk edema, focal cerebral deficits, sensorimotor peripheral neuropathy, hepatosplenomegaly, lymphadenopathy, and Raynaud syndrome.

Laboratory findings include anemia, raised ESR, abnormal protein immunoelectrophoresis, and hyperviscosity of the serum.[6596]

Waldenström syndrome See **acute thyrotoxic encephalomyelopathy.**

Waldeyer, Heinrich German physician who formulated the concept that the unit structure of the nervous system is the "neuron," which he so named in 1881.

Walker effect Induced fatigabilty of remote muscles (e.g., ptosis) after the forearm muscles have been exercised repeatedly with an inflated blood pressure cuff occluding the arm circulation, and then removed. Temporarily high lactic acid levels have been suggested as the cause.

Walker syndrome See **Marden–Walker syndrome.**

Walker, Mary Broadfoot (1888–1974) English physician who discovered the beneficial effect of physostigmine in **myasthenia gravis** in 1934. For some months she had been trying the effect of a number of different agents on a close friend with the disease[6600] but experimented with this one on a hospital patient after discussing the similarity of myasthenic symptoms to those of curare poisoning with Dr. D. **Denny-Brown,** who was then consultant to the London hospital in which she was a junior staff member.[3366]

She was also the first to describe hypokalemia in **familial periodic paralysis.**

Walker–Warburg syndrome (lissencephaly, encephalo-optic dysplasia; oculocerebral malformative syndrome; muscle–eye–brain disease; cerebro-ocular dysgenesis; cerebro-oculo-muscular syndrome; retinal dysplasia with hydrocephalus; hydrocephalus, agyria, retinal dysplasia, and encephalocele/HARD ± E syndrome, Fukuyama-type muscular dystrophy) A lethal recessive congenital α-dystroglycanopathy characterized by cobblestone **lissencephaly** (cortical agyria with a lack of cortical laminations; type 2 lissencephaly), congenital muscular dystrophy with contractures, cerebellar and pyramidal tract aplasia, callosal agenesis, aqueductal stenosis with severe hydrocephalus, ocular abnormalities such as buphthalmos, micro-ophthalmia, corneal opacities, and retinal dysplasia and detachment, hypoplasia; atrophy of the optic nerve and macula and colobomas also occur, all in the absence of such known causes as toxoplasmosis, cytomegalovirus, or other viral disease.[746, 6757, 4555]

Other manifestations include seizures, severe mental retardation, the **Dandy-Walker malformation,** and **encephalocele.** HARD ± E is the acronym for Hydrocephalus, Agyria and absent cortical laminar structure, Retinal Dysplasia ± Encephalocele,[6606] a condition that is usually lethal during the first year of life.

The condition has been mapped variously to 9q34 (*POMT1*); 14q24 (*POMT2*); and 9q31 (*fukutin*), as have some of the other conditions listed above.[6335] Diagnostic criteria have been suggested.[1671] **Muscle–eye–brain disease** is a similar but possibly less severe *variant*; both are genetically heterogeneous.

Other *variant* forms include those due to mutations in *POMT1*, associated with congenital muscle dystrophy, microcephaly, and mental retardation but without structural brain changes on MRI;[1404] and *o-mannosyltransferase 2 deficiency* (14q24.3, *POMT2*), a recessively inherited form which is clinically similar to the above.[4992]

walking reflex (stepping response) When a baby is supported upright over a table and its feet allowed to come into contact with the surface of the table, reciprocal flexion and extension of the legs is induced, simulating walking. The reflex normally disappears after the age of 6 weeks.

Wallenberg syndrome (Vieusseux–Wallenberg syndrome) See **lateral medullary syndrome.**[6608]

Wallenberg, Adolf (1862–1949) German neurologist who graduated from Heidelberg and worked in Danzig, where he was elected titular professor of neurology. Forbidden to publish by the Nazi régime, he left Germany for Oxford, moving to the United States in 1943. The syndrome named for him is his major legacy, but he also published important work on poliomyelitis, cerebellar vascular disease, and neuroanatomy.

Waller, Augustus Volney (1816–1870) English physician and physiologist who lived in France for much of his childhood, graduating from medical school in Paris. He practiced in London for a few years and continued his physiological research, studying nerve regeneration in the frog (1860) and pointing out that a divided nerve fiber will only survive when it retains its continuity with its cell body and that degeneration thus will only occur distal to the site of injury. He left England in 1851 to work with Budge in Berlin on pupillary innervation before going in turn to Paris, Birmingham, and finally Geneva, where he died.

Waller's Law "If a spinal nerve be divided, the peripheral parts degenerate completely. If the anterior root be divided, the peripheral fibres degenerate. If the posterior root be divided, the central fibres degenerate. If the ganglion on the posterior root be divided, both central and peripheral nerve fibres degenerate. Hence it is assumed that the trophic center for the fibres in the anterior root lie in the multipolar cells of the anterior grey cornu of the cord, and the trophic center for the fibres of the posterior root in the cells of the ganglion in this root."

No more succinct description has yet been provided.

Wallerian degeneration (axonal degeneration) Those changes occurring distal to the site of transection of a nerve fiber, and thus in that part of an axon separated from its perikaryon. They are characterized by fragmentation, dissolution, and removal of the myelin sheath and the subsequent departure of Schwann cells, and by the dissolution of the axis cylinder distally, as a result of failure of the energy processes required to maintain the exclusion of calcium ions from the interior of the cell. Similar changes also occur for a very short distance in a proximal direction, and the neuronal cell body swells and shows a degree of **chromatolysis.** These events were first observed in 1850 by Waller[6610] in the glossopharyngeal nerve of the frog.

wallet neuritis See **piriformis syndrome.**

wall-eyed bilateral internuclear ophthalmoplegia syndrome (WEBINO syndrome) Lateral deviation of both eyes (exotropia) and loss of the power of convergence, with bilateral internuclear ophthalmoplegia, as a result of bilateral midbrain lesions affecting the nuclei of both medial recti and both median longitudinal fasciculi.[6093]

Wallgren, Arvid Johan (1889–1973) Swedish physician who described aseptic meningitis.

Walsh, Frank Burton (1895–1978) Canadian neuro-ophthalmologist, born and trained in Manitoba, who was invalided out of the army after active service in World War I. He later trained in ophthalmology, from which he developed the specialty of neuro-ophthalmology at the Willmer Eye Institute, Baltimore, where he was in his later years professor emeritus. Described as an "optimath" (one who never ceases to learn), he provided the world with superb teaching in his subspecialty, epitomized by his classic book *Clinical Neuro-Ophthalmology*, which reached its third edition before his death; by his co-authored *Neuropathology of Vision*; and by over a hundred original clinical papers.

Walshe, Sir Francis (1886–1973) English neurologist, philosopher, writer, and critic, the outstanding intellectual of British neurology in his time. He trained in medicine at University College Hospital, where he was at one time house surgeon to Sir Victor **Horsley,** and with **Sherrington** at Oxford. He was later appointed to the staff of University College hospital and of the **National Hospital,** Queen Square. He was at various times in his career the editor of ***Brain***, and president of the Royal Society of Medicine and of the Association of British Neurologists, which he had helped to found. He was elected to fellowship of the Royal Society.

He was a devout admirer of Hughlings-**Jackson** and, like him, was a supremely capable clinical observer who deduced physiology in the wards rather than experimenting in the laboratory. His books, in particular his textbook of neurology and *Critical Studies in Neurology*, reflect his precise critical analyses of neurological mechanisms and phenomena.

A highly principled man, he accepted no government salary for his hospital work because he remained unreconciled with the concept of the British National Health Service. He was a towering figure in neurology; yet, it must be accounted as a regrettable loss to the advancement of learning that he was also a polemicist of mean repute whose emotional defense of his opinions did nothing to encourage the uncertain, while his barbed comments, commonly appearing in academic journals, provided brief entertainment for the reader but must have inhibited constructive discourse. Nevertheless, seven of his publications are referenced in this book.[6620, 6626, 6623, 6624, 6622, 6621, 6625]

waning discharge A repetitive discharge gradually decreasing in frequency or amplitude before it stops. cf. **myotonic discharge.**

Warburg syndrome See **Walker–Warburg syndrome, HARD + E syndrome.**

Ward–Romano syndrome Abnormal prolongation of the Q-T interval on the EKG, leading to cardiac arrhythmia and reduction of cerebral perfusion sufficient to cause **occasional seizures,** as in **Stokes-Adams attacks.**[5025]

warehouse worker's headache

Headache due to chronic, mild to moderate, and sublethal occupational carbon monoxide poisoning that occurs when internal combustion engines are run in an enclosed space with poor ventilation. Apart from the nonspecific headache, nausea, light-headedness or syncope, and rarely more protracted loss of consciousness are typical features.[10]

warfarin embryopathy

A congenital dysmorphic syndrome occurring in infants born to mothers treated with warfarin during pregnancy. The clinical features include microcephaly, blindness with optic atrophy, seizures, hypotonia, epiphyseal lesions, and mental and developmental delay.[1628]

Warkany syndrome (trisomy 8 syndrome) A congenital dysmorphic syndrome with great phenotypic variability, characterized by facial and skeletal anomalies and by any combination of mild physical and mental retardation, corneal opacities, nystagmus, callosal agenesis, aqueductal stenosis with hydrocephalus, seizures, and developing hypertonia.[1495]

warm-up effect The reduction in myotonic stiffness and weakness with exercise; a peripheral rather than a central phenomenon due to altered excitation and contractile performance.[1275] **Paradoxical myotonia** represents the opposite condition, the myotonia worsening with activity.

warning headache See **sentinel headache.**

Wartenberg cheiralgia paresthetica (nocturnal arm dysesthesias, tired arm syndrome) Pain, paresthesias, and numbness following intercurrent stretching or compression of peripheral nerves and described as a syndrome of the superficial radial nerves.[6657] **Handcuff neuropathy** is identical.[6001, 6654]

Wartenberg migrant sensory neuritis A self-limiting condition characterized by the occurrence of pain and numbness in the territory of sensory nerves which have suffered a stretching injury.[4180]

Wartenberg Pendulum Test

With the patient sitting with his legs hanging over the side of the bench, the examiner extends the knee and then drops it to swing freely under the action of gravity. The pattern of the swinging movements reflects the balance of suprasegmental motor influences (mainly affecting the quadriceps), and is decreased with spasticity. The test was originally introduced by Wartenberg to assess rigidity in patients with **Parkinson disease,**[6659] in whom a marked reduction in the maximum velocity of the first swing has been shown, while the reduction in spastic limbs is much less.[899, 898]

Wartenberg signs 1. Decreased arm swing on walking, in cases of pyramidal, cerebellar, or basal ganglion disease. 2. Active flexion of the terminal phalanges of the four fingers of a paretic hand about a firm object, or against resistance offered by the examiner's fingers similarly flexed, is followed by adduction, flexion, and opposition of the thumb (in a normal extremity the thumb remains in abduction and extension); this pathological associated movement is seen in pyramidal tract disease.[6656] 3. Intense pruritus of the nostrils and the tip of the nose felt by patients with cerebral tumor.[6652] 4. Abduction of the little finger in cases of ulnar nerve palsy[6653] (Wartenberg's oriental prayer sign). 5. Reduced vibration felt in the upper eyelid when the patient with facial palsy closes his eyes.[6651] 6. The "useless arm" as a sign of a parietal plaque in **multiple sclerosis.** 7. The **finger flexor reflex** (a pyramidal sign with excessive flexion of the fingers). 8. Diminished abduction of the thumb in cases of median nerve palsy. 9. The **corneomandibular reflex.**

Wartenberg syndrome 1. See **Parry–Romberg syndrome.** 2. Brachialgia statica paresthetica. See **carpal tunnel syndrome.**[6654]

Wartenberg wheel A small wheel upon a handle, set with radially projecting spikes, which is run over the surface of the skin in testing superficial pain sensation. Use of the instrument is ill-advised today due to its capacity for transmitting such diseases as AIDS and hepatitis.

Wartenberg winking-jaw phenomenon (corneomandibular reflex, pterygocorneal reflex, reverse Marcus Gunn phenomenon, inverse Marcus Gunn phenomenon) Involuntary deviation of the jaw to the opposite side when the cornea is stimulated; seen with supranuclear lesions of the V cranial nerve.[6658]

Wartenberg, Robert (1887–1956) Lithuanian-American neurologist who graduated *cum laude* from Rostock, worked with **Foerster,** and headed the neurology service at Freiburg before emigrating to the United States in 1935 (after his teaching permit had been withdrawn by the Nazi government). He was eventually made clinical professor at San Francisco where he built and led a strong teaching, research, and clinical service.

His publications were eclectic; initially, they were much influenced by the epidemic encephalitis raging in Europe, while later he became interested in the employment of new technologies for the examination of neurological disease, and in the clinical examination. In this area, his book *The Examination of Reflexes* was acclaimed as a perfect simplification of an hitherto complex subject. He was a superb clinical neurologist, and some of his clinical insights are indicated in the preceding entries.[5606, 5084] His facility with the English language was admirable, but his detailed editorial corrections of F.M.R. **Walshe**'s book *Diseases of the Nervous System* were not appreciated by its author.

Wassermann, August Paul von

(1866–1925) German bacteriologist, who worked mainly in Berlin. He described the Wassermann reaction for the diagnosis of syphilis, a modification of the Bordet–Gengou complement-fixation reaction in 1906.

wasting Atrophy of skin, bone, or muscle.

water babies A term applied to children suffering from pitressin-resistant **diabetes insipidus,** fancifully emulating the title of the classic children's book by Charles Kingsley.

water-deprivation headache

A suggested primary headache, the pain arising from the meninges with accompanying impaired concentration and irritability. The pain can be localized or generalized, is accentuated by head movement, and is relieved in most cases within 30 min by drinking water.[677]

Waterhouse, Rupert (1873–1958) English physician who in 1911 gave the definitive account of the syndrome bearing his name.[6666] Friedreichsen published 7 years later.

Waterhouse–Friedreichsen syndrome Adrenal hemorrhage leading to adrenal failure, complicating meningococcemia. The condition was actually first described by Dr. Arthur Voelcker (1861–1946), an English physician, in a brief report in 1894.The major clinical features are petechiae leading on to extensive purpura, hypotensive hypovolemic shock, and reducing consciousness up to coma.[6666]

watershed areas The boundary zones between the territories of the three major cerebral arteries (anterior/middle; middle/posterior) of the brain, representing the sites most likely to show evidence of infarction when cerebral perfusion is globally diminished, as occurs with impaired cardiac output and decreased perfusion pressure of the brain.

watershed infarcts (border-zone, borderline, distal field, extraterritorial, low-flow, or terminal zone infarcts) Cerebral infarcts of two types, each occurring at the point furthest from the systemic arterial supply: The *macro*-type occurs between the territories of supply of the major arteries (anterior, middle, and posterior cerebral). The *micro*-watershed infarct is sited between the columnar, penetrating arteries of the cortex. Both usually occur as a result of systemic hypotension with critical reduction in cerebral blood flow. In addition, "internal" watershed infarcts occur in the centrum semi-ovale between the arterial territories of the deep branches of the basal cerebral arteries and those of the superficial pia-arachnoid plexus and also between the territories of the major arteries supplying the cerebellum.[1085] See also **transcortical aphasia.**

Watson–Schwarz Test A chemical reaction of value in the diagnosis of acute intermittent porphyria.[6115]

wave A transient change in voltage represented as a line of differing directions over time.

wave-and-spike phantom See **phantom spike and wave.**

waveform The shape of a wave.

We Move (Worldwide Education and Awareness for Movement Disorders) A nonprofit organization providing education and awareness for movement disorders, including treatment information for patients and medical professionals. Web site: www.wemove.org/. See also WE MOVE's Movement Disorder Virtual University at the Web site: www.mdvu.org.

weakness A decrease in the force of muscular activity exerted in the performance of a resisted task, as judged by the patient or the examiner.

weakness of one leg with ease of falling A **lacunar syndrome** suspected to be due to a lesion of the brainstem, in which the hypertensive patient notes mild weakness of one leg, or of the arm and leg, with a marked tendency to fall toward that side.[2106, 2092]

wear and tear pigment See **lipofuscin.**

wearing-off effect See **end-of-dose deterioration.**

weaver mutant A murine mutation causing ataxia.

Weaver syndrome A dysmorphic syndrome, manifesting also accelerated skeletal maturation, flat occiput, hypertelorism, hoarse voice, camptodactyly and clinodactyly, congenital cardiac anomalies, hypertonia, and mental and developmental delay.[6680]

Weaver–Williams syndrome A congenital dysmorphic syndrome, characterized also by deafness, dental and skeletal malformations, microcephaly, and mental and developmental delay.[381]

Weber law (Weber–Fechner Law) The variation in the intensity of a stimulus that causes the least appreciable change in sensation maintains an approximately fixed ratio to the strength of the whole stimulus already acting. Thus, perception is proportional to stimulus strength. This designates the relationship between the magnitude of the stimulus and that of the response, the sensation being a logarithmic function of the stimulus as the sensation increases only arithmetically when the stimuli increase geometrically.[6609] The law was elaborated by E.H. Weber.

Weber syndrome (Weber–Gubler syndrome, Leyden paralysis, hemiplegia alternans superior peduncularis, syndrome of the cerebral peduncle) Unilateral III nerve palsy with contralateral hemiparesis, due to a lesion of the mesencephalon.[6684, 6685] The syndrome is named for H.D. Weber, who described it in 1863, although Gubler had already described it 4 years previously.

Weber Test A test of auditory function. A vibrating tuning fork placed in the scalp in the midline should be heard equally by each ear but will be heard more loudly in the ear affected by conduction (middle-ear) deafness. In the presence of nerve deafness, the sound will be localized to the normal ear. Thus, if the sound is heard more loudly in the right ear, then either there is conductive deafness on the right or nerve deafness on the left, and tests of acuity will be needed to determine which is the case. The test was described by E.H. Weber in 1834.

Weber, Ernst Heinrich (1795–1878) German anatomist and physiologist, born and educated in Wittenberg, where he graduated with a thesis on the sympathetic nerves.

Weber, Frederick Parkes (1863–1962) The son of Sir Hermann David **Weber,** he studied medicine at Cambridge and St. Bartholomew's Hospital, London, as well as in Paris, and Vienna and was a prolific writer (over 1200 papers published). Neurological publications included studies of amyotrophies and cerebral tumors, but he is best known for his description of *multiple hereditary developmental angiomata (telangiectases) of the skin and mucous membranes associated with recurring haemorrhages* **(Rendu–Osler–Weber hemangiomatosis)** (London: Lancet, 1907;**2**:160–2), **Weber–Christian disease,** *Weber disease* (localized epidermolysis bullosa), and the **Klippel–Trenaunay–Weber syndrome.**

Weber, Sir Herman David (1823–1918) German-English physician who was born in Germany and graduated in

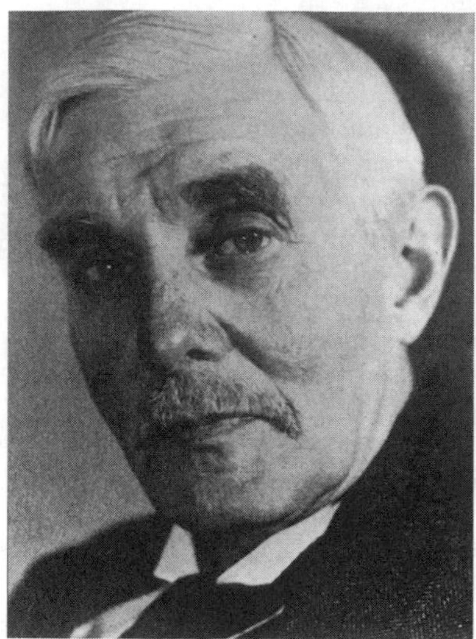

Figure W–1 Frederick Parkes Weber

medicine from Bonn. He became enamored of England and emigrated there, entering as a student at Guy's Hospital to re-qualify. Thereafter, he created a successful practice in London; his patients included five prime ministers.

His own clinical research output was also notable (e.g., the Weber **cerebral peduncle syndrome**), but it was his son, Frederick Parkes Weber (1863–1962), whose name is applied to **Osler–Rendu–Weber disease, Weber–Christian disease** (relapsing febrile nodular nonsuppurative panniculitis), **Sturge–Weber syndrome,** and **Weber disease** (localized epidermolysis bullosa).

Weber–Christian disease

(relapsing panniculitis) A syndrome of later adult life characterized by repetitive episodes of pain felt in fatty subcutaneous tissue nodules, mainly over the thighs and hips.[6683] Myopathy is an uncommon complication. The syndrome was named after H.D. Weber.

Weber–Gubler syndrome See **cerebral peduncle syndrome.**

WEBINO syndrome See **wall-eyed bilateral internuclear ophthalmoplegia syndrome.**

WebMD A source of medical (including neurological) information for physicians. Web site: http://www.webmd.com/.

Webster Rating Scale A rating scale designed to provide a semiquantitative assessment of the disabilities of patients with **Parkinson disease.** The items scored are *bradykinesia, rigidity, posture, arm-swing, gait, tremor, facial movement, seborrhea, speech, and self-care.* As with other scales, this one provides a template for the physical examination and arbitrarily selects common clinical features for scrutiny. See also **Hoehn and Yahr Scale, Columbia Rating Scale, Unified Rating Scale.**

Wechsler Adult Intelligence Scale (WAIS) A classic psychometric instrument in use for over 30 years, but requiring both training and experience to administer reliably. It is composed of six verbal and five (nonverbal) performance subtests, yielding verbal, performance, and composite (intelligence quotient) scores.

A relative retention of abilities on the verbal as opposed to the performance items is commonly used as an indicator of a decline in cognitive functioning. Scores on the information and vocabulary subtests are the best measures of original ability, or "that ubiquitous test factor which appears to be the statistical counterpart of learning capacity plus mental alertness, speed and efficiency." The scale has been revised (WAIS-R), mainly with respect to scoring.[6688]

The *Wechsler Intelligence Scale for Children* is an adapted form of this test battery.

Wechsler Memory Scale

A standardized measurement tool for the assessment of aspects of memory including information and orientation, mental control, visual pattern reproduction, and digit recall forwards and reversed.[6686] A revised version is now available.

weckblitz Noise-induced phosphenes, occurring in the hypnagogic state and commonly associated with disease of the eye or optic nerve.

wedge hemianopia A sectoral field loss caused by a lesion of the lateral geniculate body.

weekend migraine The occurrence of caffeine-withdrawal headaches on Saturdays in people who do not go to the office on weekends.

Wegener granulomatosis

A granulomatous vasculitis of the upper respiratory tract accompanied by glomerulonephritis, systemic necrotizing vasculitis of arteries and veins, with eventual necrotizing pulmonary vasculitis and glomerulonephritis.[1973] Neurological complications include cranial and painful peripheral (vasculitic) neuropathies, meningism with diffuse meningeal enhancement on MRI, diabetes insipidus, and focal or diffuse brain or cord lesions (stroke, seizures, cerebritis, meningitis); these occur in a quarter of all cases.[1704, 4680] Elevated cytoplasmic antineutrophil cytoplasmic antibody (cANCA) titers may be confirmatory, having a specificity of 98% and sensitivity of 96% for active disease and sensitivity of 65% for initial or inactive disease.

Dr. Friedreich Wegener (b. 1907) was a German pathologist.

Weichselbaum syndrome

Cerebrospinal (meningococcal) meningitis.

Weichselbaum, Anton

(1845–1920) German pathologist who discovered the *meningococcus* as the cause of cerebrospinal fever.

Weigel Test A modified color-sorting test, in which blocks are sorted according to any one of five principles which can be derived.[5269]

Weigert, Karl (1843–1905) German professor of pathology at Frankfort. Weigert's myelin stain (1882) was modified by Jakob Pal 6 years later and is known now as the *Weigert-Pal stain*, but his own modification of the Van Gieson/hematoxylin stain is still in use.

weightlifters migraine An acute exertional headache.[4940] See **benign exertional headache.**

Weil disease Infection by *Leptospira icterohaemorrhagica*, usually from rodents or other small mammals. The clinical manifestations include fever, severe headache with meningism, widespread petechiae later running into purpura, conjunctival hemorrhages, jaundice due to hepatic necrosis, myalgia, myoglobinuria, and encephalopathy with cranial nerve palsies and drowsiness, progressing (if untreated) to coma. Dr. M.P. Weil, (b. 1884) was a French physician.

Weil stain An iron-alum-hematoxylin method for staining myelin sheaths, now superseded by more effective methods.

Weil-Cornell LINCL Scale An instrument allowing quantitation of the deficits of children with late infantile **neuronal ceroid lipofuscinosis.** It rates feeding, gait, motor, disturbances (involuntary movements, myoclonus, and pyramidal signs), and language.[6866]

Weill–Marchesani syndrome (brachydactylyspheroplakia) A recessively inherited congenital dysmorphic syndrome, manifesting also short stature, broad skull, dental anomalies, brachydactyly, myopia, ectopia lentis, and sometimes glaucoma leading to blindness.[6693] The syndrome was further defined by Oswald Marchesani (1900–1952), an Austrian ophthalmologist working in Münster, in 1939.

Weill–Reys syndrome See **Adie pupil, Holmes–Adie syndrome.**

Weinstein Enhanced Sensory Test (WEST) A commercial method for testing sensation wherein calibrated forces are delivered to intact skin by means of five force-calibrated monofilaments.[6699]

Weir Mitchell room A hospital room occupied by a patient considered by Dr. Weir Mitchell to have factitious or hysterical paralysis, a condition that was briefly relieved by the emotional trauma she sustained when he set fire to her bedclothes.

In this context it should however be noted that when there was a fire in a London hospital ward occupied by patients with chronic postencephalitic Parkinsonism, they were the first out of the building, unassisted.

Weir Mitchell syndrome (erythromelalgia) The sudden onset of a vasomotor disorder causing pain, redness, and thickening of the terminal phalanges and nail beds in the hands and feet, and engorgement of the peripheral veins. The pain is worsened by heat and relieved by cold. The temperature sense may be diminished.

Weir Mitchell treatment Rest in isolation, exercise, good food, and massage as a treatment for hysteria.

Weir Mitchell, Silas (1829–1914) American physiologist, neurologist, and novelist. He was regarded by his father as "wanting in nearly all the qualities that go to make a success in Medicine," but was stimulated to investigate the nervous system by **Claude Bernard**, under whom he had studied in Paris for a year after graduation from Jefferson Medical College and before returning to Philadelphia.

He published extensively in pharmacology, toxicology, and physiology both before and after his experience as a contract surgeon to the Union forces in the American Civil War, collaborating at times with **Hammond**, but it was his experiences in what became a 400-bed neurological hospital under his direction that led to his greatest work, *Gunshot Wounds and Other Injuries of Nerves* (1864), later enlarged as *Injuries of Nerves and their Consequences* (1872),[4403] which became a standard text internationally. In this book, Weir Mitchell described ascending neuritis, pressure effects upon peripheral nerves, neural anatomy and physiology, trophic changes, the overlap of cutaneous sensation, referred sensation, and current forms of treatment with accounts of 66 patients. A final chapter described **causalgia** in complete detail. The 1864 edition also contains an excellent description of what we call **Horner syndrome.** Nearly 30 of the patients originally described therein were subsequently re-examined by his son Dr. John Mitchell (1857–1917), whose findings were published in his book *Remote Consequences of Injuries to Nerves* (1895).

After the war, Weir Mitchell practiced successfully as a neurologist and continued to publish extensively on the topics of muscle stretch reflexes (he described what amounts to the **Jendrassik maneuver**), ankle clonus, erythromelalgia, epilepsy, hysteria and malingering, the circle of Willis, the cerebellum, and numerous other subjects.

In the latter half of his life, he published nearly a score of historical novels as well as books of poetry, a biography of George Washington, and other medical and historical tracts, the total amounting to over 250 publications between 1852 and 1917. He was elected a Fellow of the Royal Society (London) on the recommendation of Sir William **Osler**, whose appointment as professor of clinical medicine in Philadelphia he had assisted. The two were close friends and Osler, in his obituary of Mitchell, quoted Dr. Samuel Johnson's remark about Richard Mead: "No man ever lived more in the sunshine of life,"[4232] while perhaps less charitably, **Cushing** remarked that he was vain, but had much to be vain about.

Weisenberg syndrome See **glossopharyngeal neuralgia.**

Weisenberg–Sicard–Robineau syndrome See **Collet–Sicard syndrome.**

Weiss sign Contraction of the facial muscles when they are tapped lightly, as occurs in tetany, neurasthenia, hyperthyroidism, and hysteria.[6706]

Weiss syndrome 1. A rare congenital syndrome characterized by congenital deafness, dwarfism, obesity, and hypogenitalism, sometimes with mental retardation, described by Dr. E. Weiss in 1932.[6704] 2. A dominantly inherited syndrome characterized by craniosynostosis, medially deviated halluces, and syndactyly.[6705]

Weiss, Soma (1898–1942) Hungarian-American physician and physiologist who emigrated to the United States in 1920 and trained in medicine at Cornell. After further work in Boston, he was appointed professor of the theory and practice of physick and physician-in-chief at the Peter Bent Brigham Hospital. Most of his publications were concerned with cardiovascular disease, including the elucidation of the mechanism of **carotid sinus syncope.**[6707]

Weiss–Charcot–Baker syndrome See **carotid sinus hypersensitivity.**[6707]

Welander distal myopathy A dominantly inherited distal myopathy with adult onset, mapped to 2p13.[71] It is complicated by mild disturbances of temperature sensation.[6711] See also **distal muscular dystrophy, inclusion body myositis.**

Welander–Kugelberg–Wohlfart syndrome See **hereditary motor neuropathy,** *type 3.*

Wellcome Department of Imaging Neuroscience A functional imaging center with downloadable software. Web site: www.fil.ion.ac.uk.

well-leg compartment syndrome A syndrome resulting from incorrect positioning of the leg, almost exclusively associated with maintenance of the lithotomy or hemilithotomy position for 2 h or more during surgery and due to direct external compression causing vascular insufficiency or hypoperfusion of the calf muscles, or a combination of the two. The common pathway may be hypo-oxygenation, leading to local ischemia, tissue edema, and a fulminant compartment syndrome.[2871]

Wepfer, Johann Jakob (1620–1695) A German physician who wrote the first major treatise on stroke in 1658, in which he showed that the rete mirabile does not exist in the human; described intra- and extracranial occlusion of the carotid artery, transient ischemic attacks, and reversible ischemic neurological deficits; and established that most cases of apoplexy were due to intracerebral hemorrhage or vascular occlusion. He anticipated Willis in his description of the arterial anatomy of the major cerebral arteries.

He seems to have been unaware of the decussation of the motor pathways as in cases of stroke; he usually looked for the pathology on the same side as the paralysis, an error corrected during his lifetime by Antonio Maria **Valsalva** (1666–1738).

Werdnig, Guido (1844–1919) Austrian neurologist who spent most of his professional life in Graz or Vienna, and who, independently of **Hoffmann**, published a series of papers between 1891–1900 on the clinical and pathological findings in infants suffering from the disease named for him.

Werdnig–Hoffmann disease See **hereditary motor neuropathy**, *type 1*.

Werner syndrome See **progeria.**[6728]

Werner, Otto German physician who, while still a medical student at Kiel, described the syndrome named for him in four siblings.

Wernicke aphasia (Bastian aphasia, dissociated aphasia, auditory receptive dysphasia, cortical receptive aphasia) A form of fluent aphasia containing verbal and phonemic **paraphasias,** in which comprehension, repetition, and naming are severely impaired and writing is poor, while grammar, articulation, prosody, and phrase length are often normal although the actual speech may be meaningless. The patient is not aware of this.[2905]

It was described by Wernicke in 1874[6729] (but also by Bastian in 1869), and occurs with large lesions of the posterior temporal, inferior parietal, and lateral posterior temporal lobes. It has also been described with a right hemisphere lesion (*dissociated aphasia*). The composer Ravel was ultimately so afflicted.

Wernicke cramp A rare form of local muscle cramp precipitated by movement, described by him in a lecture-demonstration in 1904.[6732]

Wernicke hemianopic pupil Loss of the pupillary reflex when a thin pencil of light is shone exclusively upon the "blind" side of the retina, indicating that the lesion is anterior to the point at which the pupillary fibers leave the optic tract for the superior colliculus, because, when the lesion is more posterior, these fibers are spared, and so pupillary constriction still occurs even when the "blind" retina is stimulated.[6731]

Wernicke, Karl (1848–1905) German neuropsychiatrist, born in Silesia and dying (after a bicycle accident) in Thuringia. He studied medicine at Breslau and, on graduating in 1870, worked there and in Vienna under Meynert. He was later assistant to **Westphal** in Berlin and, in 1885, was elected to the faculty in neurology and psychiatry in Berlin, then Breslau, and, shortly before his death, Halle.

He left neurology such major legacies as his description of the encephalopathy named for him, and the anatomy and phenomenology of dysphasia (1874); he conceived that sensory aphasia was due to damage to the left temporal lobe where auditory images were stored, motor dysphasia to lesions of Broca's area, conduction aphasia to the pathways between them, and total dysphasia to lesions of both areas. The encephalopathy (which he first described in his major textbook in 1881) was named for him and for **Korsakoff,** although it had been recognized previously by **Gayet** in 1875. He also described the major cerebral convolutions, predicted the occurrence of pseudobulbar palsy, demonstrated the existence of a brainstem center for lateral gaze, and helped to establish the concept of unilateral cerebral dominance.

Wernicke's area The posterior part of the dominant auditory association cortex together with the heteromodal cortex on the banks of the superior temporal sulcus, and part of the inferior parietal lobule. Damage to this region leads to **Wernicke aphasia.**

Wernicke–Korsakoff encephalopathy (Wernicke syndrome, polioencephalitis hemorrhagica superior, Meynert amentia, Gayet disease, Gayet–Wernicke syndrome) The association of nystagmus, ophthalmoplegia, cerebellar signs, neuropathy, and inability to record new information ("loss of recent memory") as a result of thiamine deficiency, with bilateral pinhead-sized hemorrhages in the mamillary bodies and in the periventricular and periaqueductal gray matter.

This classical syndrome was first described by a Swedish physician, Magnus Huss (1807–1890), who had spent the greater part of his career in the study of alcoholic diseases. **Strümpell** in 1883 and **Charcot** in the following year also called attention to the association of mental manifestations and polyneuropathy in alcoholism, while Charles Gayet described the pathology in 1875. Wernicke[6730] described three cases: the first a seamstress who had developed pyloric stenosis after swallowing sulfuric acid; and the other two alcoholics. He named the disease *acute superior hemorrhagic polioencephalitis*, considering it to be an infectious process in part because of the symmetrical capillary hemorrhages around the III and IV ventricles, periaqueductal gray matter, etc. **Meynert's** account of the amnesic syndrome was as accurate as **Korsakoff's** but was published a year later, in 1890. Korsakoff considered the pathology to be cortical and probably vascular.[3537,6541] The role of vitamin deficiency in the causation was only established following the studies of thiamine deficiency in pigeons conducted by Peters in 1936. Diagnostic criteria have been suggested[975] as follows:

Two of the following features are present:

Dietary deficiencies
Oculomotor abnormalities
Cerebellar dysfunction

Altered mental state or mild memory impairment

In a *variant* form, the condition is associated with paraneoplastic nutritional deficiency states.

Wernicke–Korsakoff syndrome

A site providing information including definition, symptoms, prevention, signs, tests, treatment, prognosis, and possible complications.

Wernicke–Mann paralysis A form of hemiparesis with remarkable variability in the severity of involvement of different muscle groups, or the inequality of weakness in different muscle groups in a paretic limb during recovery. The sign was described by these authors in 1889 and 1896, respectively.[5619] The peronei; knee flexors; extensors of the elbow, wrists, and fingers; and supinators are muscle groups in which functional recovery is the least, compared with their antagonists,[645] which leads to the typical posture of the patient with unilateral spastic hemiparesis.

West Haven–Yale Multidimensional Pain Inventory A series of 12 scales examining the impact of pain on people's lives, the responses of others to their communications about pain, and the extent to which they are able to participate in usual daily activities.[3394]

West Indian (Jamaican) amblyopia Optic atrophy occurring in subjects with **Jamaican neuropathy.**

West Indian spastic-ataxic syndrome The insidious onset of deafness, visual scotomas, optic atrophy, ataxia, and spasticity associated with HTLV-1 infection. Some patients have more spasticity, some more ataxia.[4453] See **tropical spastic paraparesis.**

West Nile encephalitis Direct infection of brain due to a flavivirus member of the togavirus group of arboviruses, endemic in Israel and Egypt, but also further east and west, mainly affecting elderly adults. It is now the most common cause of epidemic viral encephalitis in the United States. Clinical syndromes include asymptomatic infection, West Nile fever and West Nile neuroinvasive disease (WNND) (syndromes of meningitis, encephalitis, and acute flaccid paralysis resembling poliomyelitis). Initial symptoms include malaise, anorexia, nausea and vomiting, headache, myalgias, back pain and arthralgias, lymphadenopathy, and a maculopapular or morbilliform rash lasting for about a week. In a very small percentage of cases, a neurological syndrome follows comprising meningoencephalitis with ataxia, cranial nerve palsies, polyradiculitis, and a pure motor syndrome of acute flaccid paralysis resembling **poliomyelitis** or **acute inflammatory polyneuropathy,** sometimes asymmetrically. If the anterior horn cell damage is severe, disabilities may be permanent.[953] Rarely, Parkinsonism, tremors, or myoclonus may be seen.

Diagnosis depends predominantly on demonstration of West Nile virus (WNV)-specific IgM antibodies in cerebrospinal fluid. A profound lymphopenia and elevated serum lipase or ferritin levels are suggestive laboratory findings. Recovery from neurological sequelae of WNV infection including cognitive deficits and weakness may be prolonged and incomplete.[1484]

http://www.cdc.gov/ncidod/dvbid/westnile/ is a Web site from the US Centre for Disease Control addressing all aspects of this infection.

West syndrome (infantile spasms, massive infantile spasms, blitz-nick-salaam krämpfe) The most common epileptic encephalopathy of infancy and childhood with onset before the age of 1 year, characterized by brief muscle contractions resembling massive myoclonic attacks, sometimes with tonic or atonic components,[6735] and accompanied by a characteristic chaotic EEG appearance of high-voltage bursts of slow waves and spikes pattern known as **hypsarrhythmia.** Microphthalmia, colobomas of the optic nerve and retina with optic atrophy, pigmentary retinopathy, strabismus, nystagmus, dementia, microcephaly, and callosal abnormalities have also been recorded in affected children. The cause of the condition is not known.

Usually the syndrome consists of a characteristic triad: infantile spasms, arrest of psychomotor development, and EEG hypsarrhythmia, although any one element may be missing. The spasms may be flexor, extensor, lightning, or simple nodding, but most commonly they are mixed. The age of onset peaks between 4 and 7 months and is always before the end of the first year. Boys are more commonly affected. The prognosis is generally poor.[6833]

The syndrome may be divided between two groups. The *symptomatic* group, characterized by the previous existence of brain damage signs (psychomotor retardation, neurological signs, radiological signs, or other types of seizures) or by a known etiology (metabolic, dysgenetic, or infectious, or due to perinatally acquired disease or tumors such as tuberous sclerosis.[2462] A smaller, *cryptogenic* group is characterized by a lack of previous signs of brain damage and of known etiology. The prognosis appears to be partly based on early therapy with adrenocorticotrophic hormone or oral steroids. (Adapted from Commission for Classification and Terminology, ILAE. Proposal for Revised Classifications of Epilepsies and Epileptic syndromes. *Epilepsia* 1989;**30**:389–99.)

Variants are as follows:

Infantile spasms, hemimegalencephaly, and hemihypsarrhythmia, a congenital epileptic syndrome manifesting infantile spasms with hypsarrhythmia, polymicrogyria, megalencephaly, and heterotopias.

Infantile spasms, X-linked (OMIM 308350), an inherited form in which the onset of infantile spasms, myoclonic seizures, and mental and developmental deterioration is in the first few months of life.[1186]

Forms characterized by spasms and mental retardation without hypsarrhythmia but with paroxysmal EEG abnormalities; with spasms and hypsarrhythmia but without mental retardation; with hypsarrhythmia and mental retardation but without spasms; with mental retardation, hypsarrhythmia, and staring seizures (see **Lennox–Gastaut syndrome**) with onset before 3 months of age; and **Aicardi syndrome.** See also **salaam attacks.**

West, W.J. (1794–) English general practitioner working in Tunbridge Wells, whose son James was affected by repetitive flexion seizures (*salaam attacks* in the words of Sir Charles Clarke, whom he had consulted), pareses, and mental deterioration. He reported the syndrome in a letter to the *Lancet* in 1841.

Western Aphasia battery

A formal, validated scale for assessing language, in particular spontaneous speech, naming, repetition, comprehension of oral language, reading, and writing, but also apraxia and constructional and visuospatial tasks.[3401]

Western equine encephalitis

Direct infection of brain by an α-virus member of the togavirus group, a virus with a reservoir in birds and small rodents. The condition is seen mainly in the central and western United States and in Southern Canada. The major vector is a mosquito; despite the name, horses play no role in transmission.

Clinically, the encephalitis is relatively mild and subclinical infection is common. The usual course in adults is for the mild encephalitis to lead on to recovery within 10 days. The illness may be more serious in small children, among whom many exhibit seizures, pyramidal signs, or behavioral problems.[2063] See also the CDC Fact Sheet: Western Equine Encephalitis.

Westphal maneuver The use of kinesthetic clues in order to identify large print, by dint of sweeping movements of the eyes or of the head and neck, named for A.K.O. Westphal.

Westphal nucleus See **Edinger–Westphal nucleus**. Edinger's paper (1885) was 2 years earlier than that of C.F.O. Westphal.

Westphal reflex See **knee jerk.**

Westphal sign Abolition of the knee jerks in **tabes dorsalis,** named after C.F.O. Westphal. **Erb** described the same thing independently, but at the same time.

Westphal syndrome

1. Agoraphobia; the dread of open spaces, nicely described by Westphal in 1872, but also previously noted by the Dutch physician Pieter Forest (1522–1597) in 1592 and by many others subsequently (Wepfer in 1727, de Sauvages in 1768, Stoll in 1788, Herz in 1791, Bruck in 1832, Reynolds in 1855, Delasiauve in 1854, Perroud in 1863, and Kohler in 1867). This is thus a prime example of an eponymous attribution which is wholly unjustified, although one must credit Westphal with the generation of the term and with an accurate description.

The author defends the inclusion of this condition in a book that claims a neurological leaning on the grounds that patients complaining of dizziness or vertigo commonly present to neurologists and many are ultimately found to have agoraphobia.

2. See **familial periodic paralysis.**

Westphal, Alexander Karl Otto

(1863–1941) German physician, the son of Karl Westphal. He trained at Berlin and studied with **Erb** and others in psychiatry and neurology, eventually becoming professor of neurology at Bonn. He described pathologic sleep attacks as well as the phenomena now given his name.

Westphal, Carl Friedreich Otto

(1833–1890) German psychiatrist, neurologist, and anatomist who held the chair of psychiatry in Berlin, where his son became professor of neurology. He gave the first account of what is now known as **Wilson disease** (which he called pseudosclerosis) in 1883, and at the same time as **Erb** he described muscle stretch reflexes in any detail.

Westphal–Leyden syndrome See **acute cerebellar ataxia,** described by Leyden in 1890,[3824] 13 years after the shorter account of A.K.O. Westphal.

Westphal–Piltz phenomenon

(paradoxical pupil phenomenon) Contraction followed by dilation of the pupil after forceful eye closure, when the tension of the orbicularis muscle is increased,[6738] named after A.K.O. Westphal.

Westphal–Strümpell pseudosclerosis See **Wilson disease.** Westphal described most of the neurological features in 1883,[6740] and **Strümpell** did the same 15 years later (but still without remarking the hepatic cirrhosis, which observation was the particular contribution of S.A.K. **Wilson** in 1912).

wet beriberi Cardiac failure with edema as a result of thiamine deficiency.

wheelchair palsy A form of compression neuropathy of the radial nerve at the level of the elbow. See also **posterior interosseous syndrome.**

whiplash amnesia Transient loss of memory following extension-flexion injury of the cervical spine. The mechanism is unknown.[2093]

whiplash injury (cervical acceleration injury syndrome, whiplash-associated disorder) An acceleration/deceleration mechanism of energy transfer to the neck, described by Crowe in 1928 and more fully by Gay and Abbott in 1953. **Erichsen** however described "railway spine" in the nineteenth century and it is the same condition. It may result from rear-end or side-impact motor vehicle collisions but can also occur during diving or other mishaps. In humans, the injury is usually of the hyperextension-flexion type.[4951] The impact may result in bony or soft-tissue injuries (*whiplash injuries*) which in turn may lead to a variety of clinical manifestations (*whiplash-associated disorders*).[5996] The definition should exclude damage to the cervical disks, the nerve roots, or the spinal cord.[971, 4952]

The pathology is not known but cervical facet (zygo-apophyseal) joint strain has been incriminated as the source of the pain, without proof. The commoner symptoms include neck, head and thoracic pain, dizziness, tinnitus, blurred vision, psychological distress, impaired concentration and memory, and intolerance of alcohol.[5946] Such features are identical with those of **postconcussion syndrome.**

For unknown reasons, up to 20% of subjects fail to return to normal capacity within a year. This is most likely if there is reduced range of motion of the neck early on.[702, 3320] There is no good evidence that the persistence of symptoms is associated with a search for compensation, nor with psychogenic factors. Patients with whiplash-associated headache are not significantly different from those with other forms of posttraumatic headache or with whiplash-associated neck pain without headache, but they do have higher scores on somatization, obsessive-compulsive, depression, and hostility subscales and global severity, implying that patients with whiplash-associated headache suffer psychological distress, perhaps as a result of chronic pain. The presence of an underlying CNS disturbance may be suggested by the occurrence of circadian rhythm disorders in some patients.

Staging of whiplash-associated disorders was attempted by the Quebec Task force:[9]

WAD 1:Neck pain, stiffness, and tenderness
WAD 2: Added signs of point tenderness and reduced range of neck motion
WAD 3: The presence of neurologic signs with the above

WAD 4: The presence of fractures or dislocations.

One may speculate that the lack of such symptoms in people who participate in, for example, "demolition derbys" or professional sports with extreme body contact may be explained by a state of anticipatory readiness in such situations, such that a protective degree of muscle contraction is in place prior to each "hit," unlike the surprise impacts of motor vehicle collisions among the general public. A biopsychosocial explanation synthesizing physical and societal perceptive causes has been proposed.[2027]

Acute and chronic headache attributed to whiplash injury are new diagnostic entities in the International Classification of Headache Disorders, 2nd edition. However, there is some evidence that acute headaches after rear-end car collisions mainly represent episodes of a primary headache induced by the stress of the situation.[5649]

Freeman et al. (1999) have asserted that there is an epidemiologic or scientific basis for the following statements,[2190] greatly adapted here:

1. Acute whiplash injuries lead to chronic pain.
2. Chronic pain resulting from whiplash injuries is not usually psychogenic.
3. Whiplash injuries are likely to result in chronic pain in countries where there is no compensation for injury.
4. Rear-impact collisions that do not result in vehicle damage are still able to cause injury.
5. Whiplash trauma is not biomechanically comparable with common movements of daily living.
6. There is sufficient force generated at the temporomandibular joint (TMJ) during whiplash trauma to cause injury.
7. TMJ injuries are associated with whiplash trauma.
8. There is no direct correlation between the extent of vehicle damage and the probability of developing chronic pain after whiplash trauma.
9. Chronic pain following acute whiplash injury is not caused or worsened by treatment and diagnostic testing.
10. The risk of chronic neck pain among acutely injured whiplash victims is not the same as the prevalence of chronic neck pain in the general population.

A *variant* of the syndrome is the *whiplash-shaken infant syndrome*, a form of nonaccidental injury to infants presenting with a suspiciously uncertain history from the parents or guardians that is at odds with the physical findings; evidence of epileptic seizures; retinal hemorrhages; CT or MRI scan findings of intradural surface hemorrhages; and new or healing rib or limb bone fractures.[173, 971]

Whipple disease (intestinal lipodystrophy) A multisystem infective enteropathy with *Tropheryma whipplei*, actinomycetes involving many organ systems, most commonly presenting in elderly men as described by George Whipple in 1907. Typical clinical features include the insidious onset of seronegative migratory arthropathy accompanied by malabsorption, intermittent, low-grade fever with night sweats and lymphadenopathy, weight loss, episodic watery diarrhea, or steatorrhea with colicky abdominal pain, and sometimes a chronic nonproductive cough or chest pain. Hyperpigmentation of the skin occurs in one third of cases.

Features reflecting CNS involvement occur in up to 40% of patients and comprise progressive lethargy and hypersomnia, cognitive, behavioral, and personality changes, ocular and facial myoclonus, and increased intracranial pressure. Less commonly found are polydipsia, hyperphagia, ataxia, diplopia, ocular palsies, internuclear and supranuclear ophthalmoplegias typically limiting vertical gaze, and **oculomasticatory myorhythmia** (pendular vergence oscillations of 0.5–1 Hz combined with contraction of the jaw muscles). Though rare, this is pathognomonic when seen.[193]

Those with possible CNS Whipple disease should undergo small-bowel biopsy; this is likely to show diastase-resistant, PAS-positive, intracellular inclusions within macrophages in the lamina propria of the small bowel. In the CNS, the findings are cerebral atrophy and diffuse or focal, small chalky granulomas. The CSF shows pleocytosis and elevated protein levels. In the CNS, the unculturable PAS-positive, rod-shaped inclusions within macrophages (*Tropheryma whippelii*) are found in the temporal lobes; scattered cortical and subcortical lymphocytic infiltrates[2706,5928] and MRI lesions are also described. The condition usually responds to protracted antibiotic treatment.[3924]

Whipple triad Confusion, faintness, seizures, or coma in the fasting state; hypoglycemia; and recovery with administration of glucose,[6743] named after A.O. Whipple. However, most postprandial symptoms are not due to hypoglycemia.

Whipple, Allen Oldfather (b. 1881) American surgeon who practiced in New York.

Whipple, George Hoyt (b. 1878) American physician who worked at Johns Hopkins University.

whispering The utterance of language without vibration of the vocal cords.

whispering dysphonia (whispering dystonia) 1. A dominantly inherited syndrome characterized by the onset in childhood or adult life of facial spasms, bulbar palsies, torticollis, and an inability to converse normally in anything above a whisper, although affected subjects can yell under adequate emotional stress. Other dystonic symptoms often eventually supervene.[4903] See **hereditary whispering dysphonia.** 2. That form of dystonia in which the muscles of the larynx are involved, producing adduction of the vocal cords and whispered speech.

whispering dystonia See **whispering dysphonia.**

whispering stroke Strokes evident on brain imaging accompanied by only the mildest of symptoms or deficits. These clinically consistent symptoms fail to result in a diagnosis of stroke or transient ischemic attack either because the symptoms are insufficiently pronounced or persistent to raise concerns in the participant or they were not sufficiently defined to allow the diagnosis of stroke.

whistle-smile sign (Hanes sign) Failure of the patient to smile when asked by the examiner to whistle, suggested as a sign of **Parkinson disease.**[2725]

whistling-face syndrome (craniocarpotarsal dysplasia, Freeman–Sheldon syndrome) A dominantly inherited or sporadic congenital dysmorphism, characterized by microstomia, flat mid-face, high palate, talipes equinovarus, and ulnar deviation of the fingers. Strabismus, ptosis, and hypertelorism may also be present. It was described in 1938 by Freeman and

Sheldon,[2187] while the name used here was applied independently by Burian in 1963.

white breath-holding attacks See **reflex anoxic seizure.**

white centered retinal hemorrhages (Roth spots) Small retinal hemorrhages seen in sepsis such as bacterial endocarditis, and in subarachnoid hemorrhage, leukemia, myeloma, diabetes, and anemia. They were first described by Litten in 1880; the retinal lesions described by Roth are now thought to have been cytoid bodies.[6506]

white cerebellum sign A CT appearance in children with acute cerebral edema in which there is loss of the normal gray–white matter differentiation, obliteration of cortical sulci, and diffuse low density but sparing of the cerebellum and basal ganglia, which appear relatively hyperdense.

white muscles The light-colored striated muscles, best seen in animals or birds. Such muscles are composed mainly of type 2 myofibrils with fast-twitch capacity, and are seen particularly in the phasically contracting limb muscles of humans. Compare with **red muscles.**

white rami B fibers of the sympathetic efferent system, bearing nicotinic cholinergic synapses at the ganglia.

white-liver disease See **Reye syndrome.**

white-matter medullary infarcts Infarcts in the centrum semi-ovale or the external/extreme capsule due to emboli or small vessel disease. Clinically, hemiparesis of variable severity is the main feature.

Whole Brain Atlas An Internet site providing anatomical images of the CNS at www.med.harvard.edu/AANUB.

whonamedit.com A biographical dictionary of medical eponyms, also useful for finding bibliographical data.

Whytt disease Acute hydrocephalus resulting from tuberculous meningitis.

Whytt reflex Loss of the pupillary reaction to light due to damage to the superior corpora quadrigemina.[5704]

Whytt, Robert (1714–1766) Scottish physician, who became professor of the institutes of medicine at Edinburgh at the age of 33. He was elected a Fellow of the Royal Society and later president of the Royal College of Physicians of Edinburgh.[208]

Whytt demonstrated reflex activity in frogs and in 1751 was the first to describe the pupillary light reflex and its anatomy.[6764] He also wrote a full description of the clinical features of increased intracranial pressure, probably in patients with communicating hydrocephalus resulting from tuberculous meningitis, and described "dropsy of the brain" (cerebral edema), transient monocular blindness, and diphtheria.[6765] In 1764 he published the first textbook of neurology since that of Thomas **Willis.**[5886, 891]

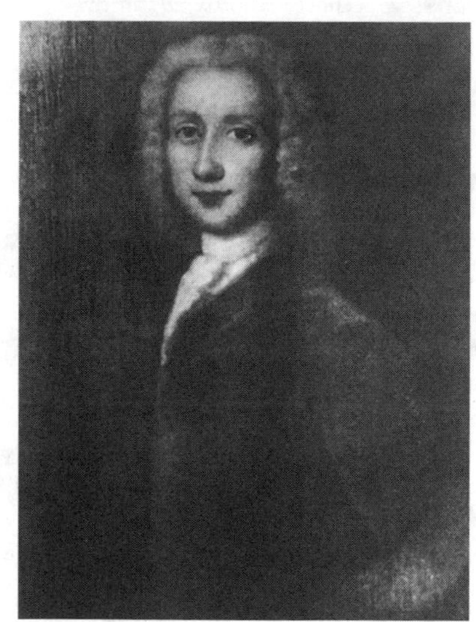

Figure W–2 Robert Whytt

wicket rhythm An EEG finding, consisting of a fragment of medium voltage mu-like rhythm at 6–11 Hz, occurring singly or in trains during wakefulness or sleep and recorded in temporal lobe regions. The phenomenon has no clinical significance.[3469]

wicket spikes Benign EEG phenomena comprising a brief run of μ-like rhythm, occurring asymmetrically in the temporal regions of adults in alert or drowsy states.[5243] They have no known clinical significance. See **mu rhythm.**

Wide Range Achievement Test A brief test of reading, spelling, and arithmetic, used as an objective assessment of academic progress.[3173]

Widowitz sign See **Cantelli sign.**

Wieacker syndrome (contractures, muscle atrophy, and ocular lesions syndrome) A congenital, X-linked recessive dysmorphic syndrome characterized also by abnormal pupils, strabismus, ptosis, dysarthria, clubfoot, muscle contractures, neural or myopathic weakness, scoliosis, and mental and developmental delay.[6768] See **Cogan syndrome** (definition 1).

Wildervanck syndrome (Franceschetti–Klein–Wildervanck syndrome, cervico-osteofacial syndrome, cervico-oculo-acoustic syndrome; OMIM 314600) A polygenic, autosomal dominant or X-linked disorder seen almost exclusively in females and characterized by congenital deaf-mutism, **Klippel-Feil syndrome, Duane retraction syndrome,** facial dysmorphism, and abnormal tethering of the hair.[1627]

Dysraphism, skeletal deformities, deafness, torticollis, spina bifida occulta, and psychomotor delay may also be associated.[6782]

Wilhelmsen–Lynch disease A dominantly inherited neurologic multisystem disease characterized by dementia, Parkinsonism, amyotrophy, and behavioral disinhibition.[3976]

Wilks, Sir Samuel (1824–1911) English physician to Guy's Hospital. He was a general physician who, like his colleague Richard **Bright,** was unusually interested in neurological problems. He published accounts of alcoholic paraplegia,[6787] of bulbar palsy, and of **myasthenia gravis,**[6788] as well as a major summation of neurological knowledge in his collected *Lectures on Diseases of the Nervous System* (London, 1878).

Williams Syndrome Association A charitable organization in this field. Address: P.O. Box 297, Clawson, MI 48017-0297. Tel: 248-541-3630.

E-mail: Tmonkaba@aol.com. Web site: http://www.williams-syndrome.org/.

Williams–Beuren syndrome

(elfin face syndrome, infantile hypercalcemia) A dominantly inherited contiguous gene syndrome (7q11.23, with the deletion of the genes *elastin*, *RFC2*, *LIM-kinase*, *GTF3 muscle transcription factor {MusTRD1}*, and *GTF2I*). The syndrome manifests short stature, idiopathic hypercalcemia, congenital heart disease such as supravalvular aortic stenosis or coarctation, pulmonary stenosis, and peripheral arterial stenoses; and craniosynostosis with microcephaly, blue irides with a stellate pattern, strabismus, and a constellation of facial dysmorphisms such as medial eyebrow flare, malar flattening, elongated philtrum, full lips, upturned nasal tip, and low nasal bridge resulting in the "pixie face." Dental anomalies, skeletal contractures and synostoses, and retardation of mental and somatic growth with relative preservation of affective skills are other characteristics.[6798, 4562] Neurological features include disproportionate skills in and attraction to music and language (despite hyperacusis with high-frequency hearing loss and phonophobia), squint, muscle hypertonia, and hyperreflexia.

It has been suggested that the folklore surrounding pixies, elves, and leprechauns and their musical talents may be based upon the features of this syndrome.[3776]

Willis headache A vascular headache following a stroke, possibly as a result of increased blood flow through the branches of the external carotid artery when the internal is occluded, or in the vessels at the base of the brain (which do have pain fiber innervation) in the presence of occlusion of one of the arteries contributing to the circle of Willis. It may also occur on the side opposite to that of the internal carotid artery occlusion, suggesting increased flow, presumably as a result of increased demand.

Willis, Thomas (1621–1675) English physician who took up arms in defense of King Charles I before entering upon the study of medicine. He later practiced in Oxford, at which university he obtained the Sedlian Chair of Natural Philosophy in 1660 as a result of family connections and patronage, then even more than now a common method. On moving to London in 1666, he obtained an appointment as physician to the family of the Duke of York (later King James II), in which eminent position he did not long remain on account of the forthrightness of his clinical diagnoses.

He was a founder of the Royal Society. Like **Sylvius,** he ascribed behavioral functions to the cortex rather than to the ventricles of the brain. His name is given to the arterial anastomotic circle at the base of the brain (**circle of Willis**), which he described in precise detail and with the first commentary on its physiological significance, along with a re-classification of the cranial nerves into nine pairs and a description of the sympathetic chain, in his "*Cerebri Anatome*" (1664), for which Sir Christopher Wren drew many of the plates, and which, with great political acumen, he dedicated to the Archbishop of Canterbury.

Willis described the XI cranial nerve, which was known by his name for some years thereafter, and the ciliary ganglion, thalamus, lentiform body, corpus striatum, and intercostal nerves. He also described meningococcal meningitis, **hysteria, general paresis, narcolepsy,** and a body of physiological observations in his *De Anima Brutorum* (*Two Discourses of the Soul of Brutes which is the Vital and Sensitive* (*soul*) *of Man*; London, 1672).[6804] Other observations concerned the intercostal and spinal nerves (1684) and the differentiation of diabetes insipidus and diabetes mellitus in 1674. He distinguished cerebral and meningeal inflammation and gave a good clinical description of **myasthenia gravis** in his book *De anima brutorum* (London, 1672) and *The London Practice of Physick* (London, 1685). In the words of Sherrington, "'Thomas Willis practically refounded the anatomy and physiology of the brain and nerves .... He collated bedside observation with anatomical fact. He, as had Fernel, a century before him, shifted the seat of the anima from the chambers of the brain to the actual substance of the brain itself.... Willis put the brain and the nervous system on their modern footing so far as that could be then done."[6975]

Willis described the epidemiology of (probably) meningococcal meningitis; carotid occlusion with headache (**Willis headache**); transient ischemic attacks ("the irradiation of the spirits is wont ... to be interrupted with little clouds, as it were, scattered here and there"); migraine; vertebral occlusion; Epilepsy (due to "an explosion of the animal spirits in the brain"); focal seizures; Parkinsonism; palilalia; torsion **dystonia;** referred pain; **internuclear ophthalmoplegia;** posttraumatic dementia; and traumatic quadriplegia.[2891, 3103, 6806]

Again like Sylvius, he denied that either the **rete mirabile** or the ventricles were the site of production of "animal spirits," although he did consider that these were secreted by the cortex. The word *neurology* was his invention; he derived this from the Greek name for a tendon, sinew, or bowstring and defined it as "the doctrine of the nerves."[3038]

Willis discounted the existence of Galen's channels from intracranial to extracranial regions and introduced the concept of CSF absorption into the veins as well as through the infundibulum; he suggested active CSF secretion by the choroid, but still accepted drainage through the nose until this was refuted by Richard Lower.[6174, 3037]

A fine, recent, critical biography is *Soul Made Flesh: The English Civil War and the Mapping of the Mind* (Zimmer C, 2004. London: Heinemann)

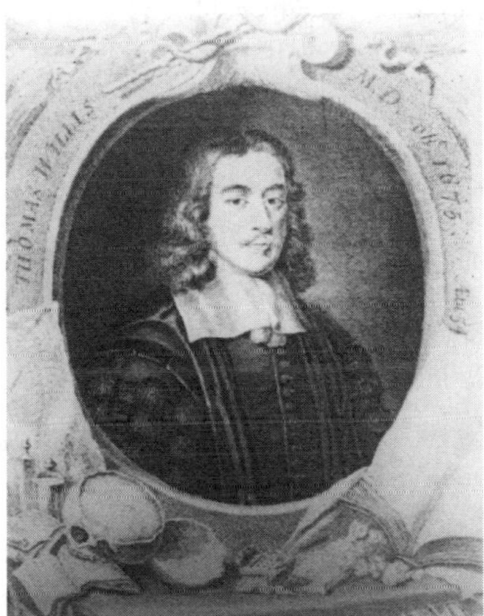

Figure W–3 Thomas Willis

Willvonseder syndrome

(dementia, vertical gaze palsy, copper dysmetabolism syndrome) A dysmorphic syndrome of abnormal copper metabolism presenting in childhood with speech defect, vertical gaze palsy, splenomegaly, platelet abnormalities, dementia, sleep disorders, and cerebellar ataxia.[6809]

Wilson disease (Westphal–Strümpell syndrome, Hall disease, cerebral pseudosclerosis, hepatolenticular degeneration, progressive lenticular degeneration, Gowers tetanoid chorea) A recessively inherited syndrome linked to markers on chromosome 13 (13q14.21, *atpase, Cu++ transporting β polypeptide; atp7b*), originally described in 1861 by Friedrich **Frerichs** (1819–1885), by **Westphal** (also in Germany) in 1883, and by **von Strümpell** in 1898, but only widely recognized after the independent report by Wilson in 1912, in which, however, the characteristic corneal changes were not described.[6818]

The essential features are due to the deposition of copper in the basal ganglia, corneas, liver, and kidneys, and comprise **Kayser–Fleischer rings,** evidence of hepatic cirrhosis and its complications, and progressive incoordination of fine movements, such as those required for handwriting and speech. Sunflower cataracts may also be seen. Dystonias, chorea, or athetosis, pyramidal and cerebellar signs, Parkinsonian features, dysarthria, mental deterioration, psychiatric syndromes, seizures, and flapping tremor of the arms and hands are the other major features. Low serum ceruloplasmin and bound serum copper levels, and high tissue and urine copper levels are diagnostic,[2827,1305] the urine copper levels rising after a dose of penicillamine. On T2-weighted MRI scans, a bilateral hyperintense stripe is classically seen in each putamen.

The disease has been subdivided into two types: In *pseudosclerosis*, dysarthria and the flapping wing-beating tremor are accompanied by cirrhosis, which is asymptomatic and progresses slowly. In the *juvenile* type, onset is also during childhood or adolescence, but hepatic involvement is obvious and the first neurological sign is usually dystonia, while the flapping tremor is rare.[1589]

Because the disease is eminently treatable if detected early (using agents to chelate and excrete copper), the index of suspicion should be high in young people manifesting any involuntary movement disorder whatsoever. An information sheet "Wilson's Disease" has been compiled by the National Institute of Neurological Disorders and Stroke. Vanderbilt Medical Center has also produced information on this and other conditions: http://www.vanderbiltchildrens.com/interior.php?mid=38&typeID=7.

Variant forms are reported:

> In an X-linked variety, the clinical findings (dementia, dysarthria, gait disturbance, tremor, vertical gaze paresis, hypersomnia, splenomegaly) are similar, but Kayser–Fleischer rings are absent, ceruloplasmin levels are normal, and the metabolic disorder is copper depletion due to abnormal membrane transport.[6809, 2421]

Involuntary movements such as dystonia, myoclonus, athetosis, dysarthria, and rapid orobuccal movements occur in the presence of slightly low urinary and serum copper levels.[6184]

See also **acquired (non-Wilsonian) hepatocerebral degeneration, Menkes syndrome, hepatic encephalopathy.**

Wilson sign See **pronator sign.**

Wilson, Samuel Alexander Kinnier (1874–1937) Irish-American neurologist, born in the United States, who trained at Edinburgh and in Europe with Pierre **Marie** and others before going to the **National Hospital** in 1904. He practiced there for the rest of his life, the first "pure" neurologist in the United Kingdom, holding successively more senior appointments despite unfriendly relationships with most of his contemporaries. He was also variously on the staff of the Westminster and King's College hospitals and was editor of the *British Journal of Neurology* before founding the ***Journal of Neurology (Neurosurgery) and Psychiatry***, the first issue of which appeared just after his death.

His fame was early achieved by his description in 1912 of the disease bearing his name, but rests also upon his superbly lucid textbook *Neurology* (edited by A.N. Bruce), published in 1940, which is filled with historical fact and a distillate of his clinical wisdom; and upon his other studies on the basal ganglia, the extrapyramidal system (so named by him), apraxia,[6817] and aphasia.

Wilson's Disease An information sheet compiled by the National Institute of Neurological Disorders and Stroke.

Wilson's Disease Association A charitable organization providing support and information on this condition. The Wilson's Disease Association Web site http://www.wilsonsdisease.org/ provides data on the copper content of various foods and much more.

Wilson's Disease Support Group UK An organization providing support, outreach, and information for people interested in Wilson's disease.

Wilson–Vogt syndrome See **Vogt syndrome.**

windmill nystagmus (alternating windmill nystagmus) A form of **periodic alternating nystagmus** seen in some patients with severe or total visual loss, and characterized by vertical and horizontal oscillations that are out of phase in the two eyes.[5533]

wind-up Increased dorsal horn neuronal responses with ongoing stimulation by Aλ and C afferent fibers, plateauing after about 20 stimuli. It is considered to be a factor in the prolongation of pain responses.[2411]

wing-beating tremor A proximal, wide-amplitude, regular tremor of the upper limbs due to lesions of the dentatorubral pathway; it is best elicited with the shoulders abducted and the elbows flexed, at which the elbows move up and down.

Winiwater–Buerger disease (Buerger disease) Thromboangiitis obliterans of the cerebral as well as of the peripheral vessels. It is an entity of doubtful validity; most cases are actually either due to atherosclerosis or due to other identified forms of angiitis.

wink reflex See **orbicularis oculi reflex.**

winking jaw See **Wartenberg winking-jaw phenomenon.**

Winkleman disease (Winkleman–Dercum disease) See **progressive pallidal atrophy, NBIA.**

Winkleman sign Described as a mild, permanent hyperextension of the great toe on the side affected by pyramidal tract disease, but more commonly evidence of disease of the basal ganglia.

Winkleman–Dercum disease See **Winkleman disease.**

Winter–Baraitser Dysmorphology Database (London Dysmorphology Database) A comprehensive, computerized, menu-driven database assisting in the recognition of over 4000 defined neurogenetic syndromes by means of a listing of selected features; allowing a search for a differential diagnosis of specific clinical features; reviewing the clinical manifestations of named disorders; and providing references to recent or seminal papers. The database was conceived and compiled by Dr. Michael Baraitser and Dr. Robin Winter, and is published by Oxford University Press, Walton St., Oxford, UK OX2 6DP. A dysmorphology photographic library of over 7500 images is also available. See also **London Neurogenetics Database.**

The database includes dysmorphic, multiple congenital anomaly and mental retardation syndromes, single gene disorders, sporadic conditions, and those caused by environmental agents.

wire electrodes Thin wires that are insulated except for the tips, which are bare, and which are inserted into a muscle through a needle for kinesiologic EMG studies, in which they are superior to surface electrodes because they are less affected by **cross talk** from adjacent muscles.

Wisconsin Card Sorting Test A test of ability to respond selectively to different aspects of a situation. In this case, the color, form, and number of designs printed on cards shown to the subject have to be matched by the subject, using response cards, on which are printed the same symbols in various colors and numbers. Subjects are told when they make a correct match and when they are wrong, and are expected to learn from these clues which cards to use to make the match in future; but the rules are changed after 10 successful matches, so that, successively, form, then color, and then number are the criteria for matching successfully.[2552]

The test is sensitive in detecting lesions of the dorsolateral regions of the frontal lobes.[2551]

WISC-R Acronym for the *Wechsler Intelligence Scale for Children-Revised*, a compound instrument for the assessment of intelligence with 12 verbal or performance subtests adapted from the **WAIS** for use in children over the age of 7 years. Verbal subtests examine information, similarities, arithmetic, vocabulary, comprehension, and digit span; performance tests are of picture arrangement and completion, block design, object assembly, coding, and maze drawing.[6687] Below this age, the Revised Wechsler Preschool and Primary Scale of Intelligence (**WPPSI-R**), which has a parallel structure, can be employed.[6689]

Wishart syndrome Multiple meningiomas or neurilemmomas of the VIII cranial nerves or of the spinal roots, or a glioma associated with neurofibromatosis. See **neurofibromatosis.**

Wishart, John (1782–1834) Scottish surgeon who graduated in medicine at Edinburgh, where he returned to practice after study in Europe, working with **Argyll Robertson.** He was at some time president of the Royal College of Surgeons at Edinburgh. His contributions were mainly in the areas of ophthalmia neonatorum, ophthalmic surgery, and methods of pupillary dilation.

withdrawal emergent dyskinesias A transient syndrome seen usually in children, characterized by the occurrence of chorea and ataxia with autonomic hyperreactivity when neuroleptic agents are suddenly withdrawn.[2282]

withdrawal headaches Those forms of headache consequent upon discontinuation of such substances as caffeine, opiods, and estrogens.

withdrawal reflex A painful stimulus to the sole of the foot will cause withdrawal of the stimulated limb and sometimes also of the unstimulated limb.[6898]

Wittmarck–Ekbom syndrome See **restless legs (limbs) syndrome.**

witzelsucht A German term for a state of unwonted and unwarranted cheerfulness, characterized by mild euphoria, jocularity, and an abnormal tendency to make rhyming or punning word associations. Frontal lobe disease (cortical atrophy, tumor) is usually responsible.

wobbler mouse A murine mutation, with some features resembling those of **amyotrophic lateral sclerosis.**

Wohlfarht–Kugelberg–Welander disease See **hereditary motor neuropathy,** *type 3*.

Wohwill–Andrade syndrome See **Andrade neuropathy.**

Wolff, Harold G. (1898–1963) American neurologist, born in New York and educated at Harvard, who worked mainly at Bellvue and became Anne Parrish Titzel Professor of Neurology at Cornell and director of the neurological service at the New York Hospital. His best-remembered studies were those dealing with aspects of headache, psychosomatic diseases, and pain, and for his studies with Stewart Wolf on Alexis St. Martin, whose stomach wall had been eventrated since a childhood accident; the secretions of the stomach and its vascularity were observed during the daily activities of St. Martin and the influences on them were reported in a series of classic studies. Wolff was editor of the ***Archives of Neurology*** from its inception to his death and an important figure in American neurological research and administration.

Wolfflin nodules Small regular and uniform spots found in the periphery of the iris in 10–25% of normal subjects, and, apart from their similarity with **Brushfield spots,** of no clinical significance.[6801]

Wolf–Hirschorn syndrome (4p.16.3 deletion; midline fusion defect syndrome) A chromosomal dysmorphic syndrome characterized by low birth weight, failure to thrive, asymmetrical microcephaly, micrognathia, abnormal ear structure, hypertelorism, and midline fusion defects such as cleft palate and defects in the scalp.[6781] Myoclonic and other seizures, strabismus, hypotonia, and insensitivity to pain are also reported.

Wolfing reflex (atz, mastication reflex: OMIM 194190) Sucking, chewing, and swallowing movements, representing an exaggerated **sucking reflex;** seen in subjects with severe diffuse cortical disease or with bilateral corticobulbar lesions.

Wolfram syndrome (DIDMOAD) A rare, recessively inherited syndrome presenting in youth with widespread cerebral atrophy, characterized by the presence of four cardinal signs: Diabetes Insipidus, Diabetes Mellitus, Optic Atrophy, and nerve Deafness. Numerous other neurological, endocrine, and urinary tract abnormalities are also found, but variably.[6852, 5184]

Wolman disease A lysosomal storage disease (an inborn error of metabolism) due to absence of acid lipase, presenting in infancy and characterized by hepatosplenomegaly, steatorrhea, anemia, and adrenal calcifications. There is a heavy deposition of cholesterol esters and triglycerides in many tissues.[6853, 6720]

Woltman sign Slowness of both the contraction and the relaxation of muscles in hypothyroid patients, best seen as the "hung-up" ankle jerk and occurring due both to mechanical factors and to slowness of contraction time, as in myotonia and pseudomyotonia.

Dr. H.W. Woltman (1889–1964) was an American physician.

Woods–Black–Norbury Syndrome An X-linked dominantly inherited immunoneurologic disorder (Xq26) presenting as neonatal hypotonia which is lethal in males. Females develop spastic paraparesis and have impaired night vision.[4992]

Woodcock–Johnson Scales of Independent Behavior A set of scales used in assessing children's abilities, based on data acquired by interviewing the parents and by assessing motor and communication skills, social interaction, and personal and community independence.[3]

Woodhouse Sakati syndrome A rare autosomal recessive neuroendocrine disorder characterized by the combination of alopecia, hypogonadism, diabetes mellitus, mental retardation, sensory neural deafness, and extrapyramidal features. Movement disorders mainly consist of dystonia and chorea of the limbs with onset in adolescence. The facial muscles are usually spared but dysarthria is common. Pyramidal features and peripheral abnormalities are inconsistent features. Most of the reported families are from the Middle Eastern countries although rare europoid cases have been described.[5628, 381]

Woods-Pendleton syndrome A familial condition manifesting dystonia, dysequilibrium and speech disturbance observed during a famine in China but not reported in the Western hemisphere since. (Osler, quoted by Durham.[1765])

woodtrimmer's disease A syndrome of transient tremor resulting from overexposure to the mycotoxins contained in sawdust. See **tremorgenic encephalopathy.**

Woon syndrome A congenital dysmorphic syndrome characterized also by spinal, skeletal and gastro-intestinal malformations, brachycephaly and craniosynostosis. See **craniosynostosis.**

word blindness 1. (developmental dyslexia) The term suggested by Rudolph Berlin (1833–1897), a German ophthalmologist, for the difficulties experienced by children in mastering the comprehension and production of written words. The degree of dyslexia is variable; it has been estimated that 10% of all children have some degree of congenital language difficulty. Errors in reading, spelling and writing occur in the presence of normal recognition of letters and understanding of the meaning of pictures, objects and diagrams. The condition is somewhat susceptible to steady and prolonged educational effort. See **alexia**. 2. **aphasia,** (here, an inability to understand the language value of written symbols), as suggested by Adolf Kussmaul (1822–1902), a German physician, in 1877.

word deafness (developmental receptive aphasia, verbal auditory agnosia, auditory imperception, central deafness) The inability to understand the accepted content and symbolic meaning of words heard; difficulty in the comprehension and discrimination of spoken language, while spontaneous speech, reading, writing and comprehension of nonlanguage sounds are relatively intact.

Repetition is also affected, but reading, writing and spontaneous speech are not. *Pure word deafness* is described, but appears to be a vanishing rarity. The condition was first described by Bastian in 1869 and attributed to disturbance of the auditory perceptive center in the first temporal convolution; Lichtheim applied the name in 1885. The condition is somewhat susceptible to steady and prolonged educational effort.[929]

Word List Generation Test A test of word fluency, perseverance and concentration (and indirectly of intelligence), wherein subjects generate as many words within a category as they can think of (e.g., words beginning with "D", items to be found in a supermarket, or names of animals or of plants) within a defined period of time, usually 1 min.[5998]

word list recall A standard, sensitive method of testing recent memory (new learning), as in the assessment of mild-to-moderate age-related cognitive dysfunction. Usually up to ten three-letter words (which may be nonsense words) are presented, and the number recalled after a delay, with or without distraction during this time, represents the subject's score.

word production anomia Difficulty in word-finding, which, however, is assisted by phonetic or semantic cues, and is seen in aphasics with dominant frontal lobe lesions.[523] See also **anomia.**

word rests See **stereotypy.**

word-form dyslexia An acquired form of dyslexia characterized by letter-by-letter reading, whole word reading being impossible. Reading is thus exceptionally slow. It is considered to be due to a lesion of the system whereby a visual word-form is obtained.[5755]

word-selection anomia See **anomia.**

work shift change The occurrence of excessive sleepiness and impaired work performance during a subject's conventional sleep-wake schedule, when daytime activities are re-scheduled to that period, as occasioned by shift work, and of insomnia with shortened and fragmented sleep during the new sleep period. (See also ASDA Diagnostic Classification,[1629] **sleep disorders.**)

working memory The process whereby information is temporarily stored and manipulated. This requires a number of inter-related systems including a central executive system controlling an articulatory loop (which is concerned with the storage of speech) and a third system that maintains and manipulates visuospatial material.[1667] Forgetting why one went into a room, or a telephone number just heard but not yet written down, are examples of temporary impairment of this faculty. The length of storage is usually seconds unless there is conscious rehearsal of the data.

The *structural capacity* of working memory refers to the number of distinct informational units that can be remembered at one time; while the *operational capacity* is the number of processing operations that can be performed while still preserving the products of earlier operations.[5516] See also **short-term memory.**

World Federation of Interventional and Therapeutic Neuroradiology A specialist professional organization. Website: www.wfitn.org.

World Federation of Neurologic Societies Grading System A system for grading subarachnoid hemorrhage. A scale with less inter-observer variability than others.[6242]

	Major Focal	
Glasgow Coma Score	*Motor Deficit*	*Grade*
15	absent	1
13–14	absent	2
13–14	present	3
7–12	present or absent	4
3–6	present or absent	5

World Federation of Neurology http://www.wfneurology.org/wfn/ An international organization for the advancement of research and education in neurology.

World Federation of Neurology Research Committee on Parkinsonism and Related Disorders An international research committee established by the **World Federation of Neurology** to promote and monitor research developments, and to foster communication among neuroscientists in this field. It sponsors occasional symposia on Parkinson disease. Web site: http://www.elsevier.com/inca/publications/store/3/0/5/4/1/.

World Federation of Neurosurgical Societies An organization including all national neurosurgical societies, based at: Academic Hospital, Radboud, P.O. Box 9101, NL-6500 HB Nijmegen, The Netherlands.

World Health Organization Handicap Scale Six scales, based on six "survival roles", each intended to classify the circumstances in which individuals find themselves as a result of disease. Each scale has 9 levels, 0 reflecting the best and 8 the worst functional state. Detailed descriptions are given in an accompanying manual. The concept of Handicap refers to discordance between the individual's performance or status and the expectations of the individual himself or of the particular group of which he is a member. The scales deal with *orientation, physical independence, mobility, occupation, social integration,* and *economic self-sufficiency,* using semantic gradations.[6870]

World Muscle Society An international, multidisciplinary, scientific society, dedicated to the advancement and dissemination of knowledge in the field of neuromuscular disorders. Web site: http://www.ior.it/wms/.

World of Multiple Sclerosis http://www.ifmss.org.uk/ A website maintained by the International Federation of MS Societies, providing information and advice particularly to people with multiple sclerosis.

Worldwide Education & Awareness for Movement Disorders (WE MOVE) A charitable organization in this field. Web site: http://www.wemove.org/.

Worm disease Bulbar **tetanus.** See also **cephalic tetanus.**

Worm, Ole (1588–1654) Danish anatomist.

Wormian bones Small areas of bone lying in the cranial sutures like islands in a river, described by Ole **Worm** and named for him by Thomas Bartholin, his nephew, in 1656.[5619]

Worster-Drought syndrome 1. (congenital suprabulbar palsy) A dominantly inherited congenital syndrome of weakness of the face, soft palate and tongue, sometimes complicated by seizures and mental retardation.[379] See **congenital suprabulbar paresis.** 2. (familial spastic paraparesis and dementia) A dominantly inherited spastic syndrome with onset in mature adult life, characterized by slowly progressive dysarthria, spastic paraparesis and dementia with widespread ischemic damage to the deep white matter and corpus callosum.[6873] See also **familial multiinfarct dementia, multiinfarct dementia.**

Worster-Drought-Allen syndrome (congenital auditory imperception, idiotic aphasia, atavistic speech, congenital pure word deafness) A congenital syndrome in which the child who has normal hearing is unable to comprehend spoken language but can lip read and can repeat sounds and words that he hears, but not a long series of them. Speech is absent or very defective and the comprehension of written language at least slightly impaired. Inability to appreciate musical sounds may also be found.[6872]

WPPSI-R Acronym for the Wechsler Preschool and Primary Scale of Intelligence (Revised), an instrument adapted from the **WISC-R** for use in children between 3 and 7 years of age. Subtests include information, arithmetic, vocabulary, similarities, geometric design, design recognition, animal pegs and sentences.[6689]

Wren, Sir Christopher (1632–1723) English scientist, anatomist, artist and architect. He was the illustrator for **Willis'** book *Cerebri Anatome.*

Wright manoeuvre Hyperabduction and elevation of the arms as a test for the vascular form of the **thoracic outlet syndrome.** Obliteration of the radial pulse is the end point sought but as this may also occur in normal subjects, the two sides have to be compared. See also **Adson Test.**

wrinkly skin syndrome A recessively inherited congenital disorder of connective tissue, characterized by short stature, skeletal malformations, premature aging, wrinkled skin, optic atrophy, pigmentary retinopathy, myopia, microcephaly, and mental and developmental delay.[2322]

Wrisberg, Heinrich (1739–1808) Professor of anatomy at Göttingen, where he was **Soemerring**'s assistant. The nerve of Wrisberg is the nervus intermedius, the sensory component of the VII nerve. Wrisberg also the first to identify the medial cutaneous nerve of the arm and he gave a good account of the phrenic, vagus and trigeminal nerves.

wrist drop A persistent posture of flexion of the wrist due to loss of power in the radial-innervated long extensor muscles of the forearm. The lesion is high, in the upper arm or in the brachial plexus, as the branch of the nerve to the extensor carpi radialis longus comes off above the elbow.

wrist extension reflex Contraction of the extensor muscles of the wrist when they are tapped, with the arm supported and the wrist hanging flexed; this represents a normal phenomenon when just visible and a sign of pyramidal tract disease when increased in amplitude.

wrist flexion reflex Contraction of the long flexor muscles of the wrist when they are tapped at the volar aspect of the wrist, with the arm supported in supination; this represents a normal phenomenon when just visible and a sign of pyramidal tract disease when increased in amplitude.

wrist sign See **Chaddock reflex.**

writers' cramp (scrivener's palsy, la crampe des écrivains, graphospasm, mogographia) A focal (occupational) task-specific dystonia usually manifest in adults who earn their living by writing, typing or otherwise communicating language mechanically, preventing the further performance of writing tasks because of clumsiness, cramp, aching, tremor, "freezing" or involuntary movement of the hand.[5174, 3271]

It was first described in detail by **Bell** in 1830, and although in fact a focal dystonia, it was long considered to be psychogenic in origin. It differs only in form and site from other occupational cramps, which have been listed as affecting people in at least 55 different activities.

In the *simple* form of writer's cramp, only writing is affected. In the *dystonic* form, the disorder spills over into other activities. Psychiatric morbidity is not increased among such patients.[5775] A (complex) rating scale to assess the benefit of local botulinus toxin injection into the forarm muscle has been published.[6837]

A *variant* is a familial form with onset in adult life.[381] See also **myoclonic writers' cramp.**

writing tremor A variant of **essential tremor** characterized by the adult onset of tremor at 5–6 Hz while writing, and occasionally complicated by other dystonias or by myoclonic seizures. See **primary writing tremor.**

wrong-way deviation 1. Deviation of the eyes *away from* the side of the lesion and *toward* the paretic side in patients with medial thalamic hemorrhage who have blood in the third ventricle.[2086] (The usual, though not invariable, finding with supratentorial lesions is that the eyes deviate toward the side of the cerebral lesion and away from the paretic limbs). 2. Acute hemiparesis should be accompanied by deviation of the protruded tongue to the paretic side; a minority of patients with hysterical hemiparesis protrude their tongue toward the normal side. Such wrong-way deviation, however, also occurs in **Jackson syndrome** in which a low medullary lesion damages the XII cranial nerve nucleus and the pyramidal tract which has not yet crossed.[3358]

wry head See **plagiocephaly.**

wry neck See **torticollis.**

Wyatt syndrome See **Sturge-Weber syndrome.**

Wyatt-Brushfield disease See **Sturge-Weber syndrome.**

Wyburn-Mason syndrome (Bonnet-Déchaume-Blanc syndrome, retino-cephalic angiomatosis, cerebroretinal arteriovenous aneurysms, multiple cerebra-retinal arteriovenous malformations) Tortuosity of the retinal vessels unilaterally, with cirsoid aneurysms or huge overgrowths of the vessels; arteriovenous angiomas of the optic nerve, thalamus and mesencephalon; and often trigeminal vascular nevi.

Clinically, the main presenting features are headache, facial palsy and hydrocephalus with oculomotor paresis, visual field deficits and hemangiomas of the optic disk, due to brainstem and subarachnoid hemorrhages.[739, 6886] See **Bonnet syndrome.**

Wynter, Walter Essex (1860–1945) A physician at the Middlesex Hospital, London, and sometime editor of the *British Medical Journal*. While on the junior staff of the Middlesex Hospital he made the first attempt at lumbar puncture, (reported by him in the *Lancet* on May 2, 1891). Each of his four patients had meningitis, and each one died.

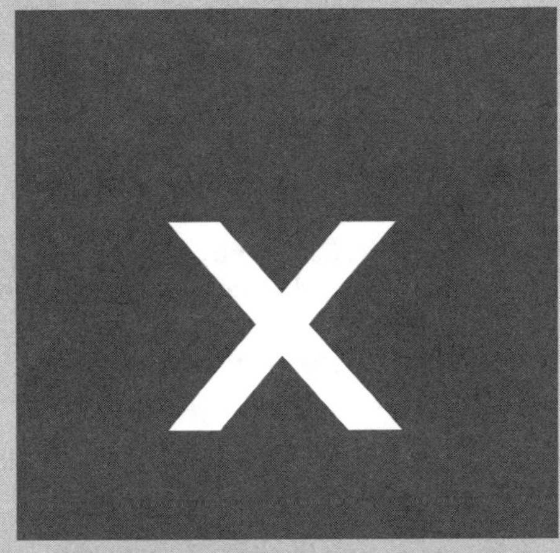

xanthinuric myopathy A syndrome due to xanthine oxidase deficiency, characterized by proximal weakness, wasting, and muscle discomfort, with electrical and biopsy evidence of myopathy. Electron microscopy study reveals intracellular aggregates of crystalline material within muscle fibers.[1083]

xanthochromia (from Gr, yellow + color) (of CSF) A yellow discoloration of the CSF, usually due to the presence of protein which has had time to absorb bilirubin from blood spilled into this foreign compartment. The protein level is commonly more than 300 mg/dl. When the protein level is very high but the cell count is low (**albumino-cytological dissociation**), spinal block, **acute inflammatory demyelinating polyneuropathy,** and eighth nerve Schwannomas are the commonest causes.

xanthoma 1. (fibroxanthoma, fibrohistiocytoma) A benign tumor of histiocytes containing uni- or multinucleated cells and giant cells and usually attached to the dura mater. 2. (xanthosarcoma, malignant fibrous histiocytoma) A rare malignant form of fibroxanthoma.

xanthomatosis 1. See **cerebrotendinous xanthomatosis.** 2. See **Hand–Schüller–Christian disease** (generalized xanthomatosis).

xanthomatous neuropathy A rare complication of biliary cirrhosis in which cholesterol esters are deposited within the peripheral nerves.[3952]

xanthopsia A condition in which all visual perceptions have a yellow tinge, as occurs in chronic digitalis, sulfonamide, and other drug poisoning, as well as in jaundice and in eclampsia.

xanthurenic aciduria An hereditary disorder due to deficiency of the enzyme kyureninase, manifesting mental retardation, which is responsive to treatment with pyridoxine.

X-disease See **Murray valley encephalitis.**

xenografts Grafts taken from one species and placed in another. Man-to-mouse is the most common example.

xeroderma pigmentosum (Gr, dry + skin pigment) (xerodermic idiocy) A rare, recessively inherited heterogeneous **neurocutaneous syndrome** due to failure of DNA repair and manifested by extreme cutaneous sensitivity to ultraviolet light, with telangiectasias, pigment changes, keratoses, and skin malignancies of all types.

The condition was first described by Hebra and Kaposi in 1872. de Sanctis and Cacchione noted its association with mental retardation, microcephaly, hypogonadism, and dwarfism 60 years later.[1610] See **de Sanctis–Cacchione syndrome.**

Since then, seizures, cerebellar ataxia, choreoathetosis, dysarthria, deafness, spasticity, peripheral neuropathy, glycogen storage myopathy, dementia, areflexia, abnormal EEG, and neuropathic EMG and muscle biopsy findings have been added as components of the syndrome.[4388, 6308]

xeroderma with talipes equinovarus and enamel defects A congenital dysmorphic syndrome, a *variant* of xeroderma pigmentosum, manifesting also skeletal malformations, abnormalities of the hair, teeth, nails, and skin and psychomotor retardation.[381]

xerodermic idiocy See **xeroderma pigmentosum.**

xerophthalmia An ocular disorder due to deficiency of vitamin A, and characterized by keratomalacia, night blindness, and Bitot spots.

xerostomia Dryness of the mouth.

XK-aproscencephaly A congenital dysmorphic syndrome characterized by cyclopia, cardiac and genital maldevelopment, microcephaly, and aproscencephaly or arhinencephaly.[381]

X-linked adrenoleukodystrophy See **adrenoleukodystrophy.**

X-linked bulbospinal neuronopathy (Kennedy syndrome, familial progressive bulbospinal muscular atrophy, bulbospinal neuronopathy) A rare, slowly progressive hereditary motor neuropathy with onset in young adult life, characterized by androgen insensitivity (gynecomastia, oligozoospermia, raised serum gonadotrophins), pelvic girdle and proximal limb weakness with postural tremor, prominent lingual and perioral fasciculations, hyporeflexia, and muscle cramps. Masseteric and facial weakness, dysphagia, and dysarthria appear later. EMG, sensory conduction, and biopsy studies show typical changes resulting from degeneration of the anterior horn cells and dorsal root ganglia.[3385, 2764, 2025] But sensory nerve action potentials are small or absent despite clinically normal sensation.[4323]

Variants are as follows:

- A form in which hexosaminidase A and B deficiencies exist, as in **Sandhoff disease.**[6290, 4788]
- A form resembling **hereditary spastic paraparesis.**[4085]
- *X-linked spinal muscular atrophy with bulbar involvement*, a syndrome of proximal limb, facial and bulbar weakness, and wasting with adult onset, associated with gynecomastia and raised CSF protein levels, differing from *Kennedy syndrome* mainly in its later age of onset.[5313]
- *A form with early onset and rapid progression.*

X-linked cerebellar ataxia An X-linked ataxic syndrome with onset in infancy. Pyramidal signs appear later and myoclonic seizures, ophthalmoplegia, sensorimotor peripheral neuropathy, lordosis, scoliosis, and pes cavus have been reported in association.[5988] See also **X-linked periodic ataxia, cerebellar ataxias.**

X-linked congenital muscle fiber hypotrophy with central nuclei[276] See **centronuclear myopathies.**

X-linked congenital neural deafness An X-linked disease manifesting congenital severe neural hearing loss but normal vestibular function.[1600]

X-linked dominant myopathy A proximal myopathic syndrome seen only in females, because it is lethal in hemizygous boys.[2870]

X-linked early-onset neural deafness An X-linked recessive syndrome of severe neural hearing loss with early onset.[4427]

X-linked external ophthalmoplegia and myopia A rare syndrome in males characterized by bilateral ptosis, weakness of the external ocular muscles, high myopia, ectopic pupils, hyporeflexia, and scoliosis.[5512] See also **familial static ophthalmoplegia.**

X-linked humeroperoneal muscular disease An inclusive term describing mild and slowly progressive muscular disorders so inherited, with onset in the first decade. The clinical features include mainly distal neurogenic and proximal myopathic EMG findings and cardiomyopathy.[6669] See **Emery–Dreifuss syndrome.**

X-linked hydrocephalus Familial **aqueductal stenosis** causing obstructive hydrocephalus, so inherited.[619]

X-linked leukodystrophies A large and ill-defined group of **peroxisomal diseases** in which cholesterol esters are deposited. These stain red with fat stains engendering the alternative term *sudanophilic leukodystrophy*. See **adrenoleukodystrophy, Pelizaeus–Merzbacher disease.**

X-linked lissencephaly and subcortical band heterotopias A genetically determined or sporadic condition presenting with mental retardation and epilepsy, mainly in females, and mapped to Xq22.3. See **also heterotopias, bilateral periventricular nodular heterotopia.**[1673]

A *variant* is *X-linked lissencephaly with abnormal genitalia*, a rare syndrome of postnatal growth retardation, microcephaly, hypotonia, impaired hypothalamic function, seizures, micropenis, and cryptorchidism in the presence of lissencephaly and agenesis of the corpus callosum, associated with mutations in the *ARX* gene.

X-linked mental retardation A nonspecific condition of intellectual impairment associated with congenital microcephaly and due to amputations in the protein kinase gene.[635] Syndromic and nonsyndromic varieties are differentiated on the presence or absence of dysmorphic and somatic features. The entire group of over 200 entities comprises various developmental disabilities; **fragile X syndrome** is the single most common form. Oligophrenin mutations have been described in over 10% of the remaining cases.[6951] See http://www.ggc.org/xlmr.htm.

One *variant* is mapped to Xq24 and is a syndrome with early onset characterized by low birth weight, delayed milestones, short stature, hyperextensible joints, kyphosis, obesity, small testes, fine finger tremor, distal leg weakness and wasting, impaired motor coordination, and mental retardation with behavioral disturbances.[3306] Another is *X-linked mental retardation with short stature, small testes, muscle wasting, and tremor*. See **cerebellar syndromes** (congenital ataxias).

X-linked mental retardation with fragile site See **fragile-X syndrome.**

X-linked microcephaly A congenital dysmorphic syndrome manifesting also microcephaly, sensorineural deafness, psychomotor retardation, seizures, and spasticity.[381]

Obesity is also present in a *variant* form.

X-linked moderate hearing loss A sex-linked disease manifesting the childhood onset of a slowly progressive, moderate neural hearing loss, but normal vestibular responses.[3880]

X-linked muscular dystrophy (Mabry muscular dystrophy) A pseudohypertrophic muscular dystrophy manifesting features similar to those of **Becker muscular dystrophy**, but with a later onset and slower course.[3983]

X-linked muscular dystrophy with humeropelvic distribution, contractures, and cardiomyopathy See **Emery–Dreifuss syndrome.**

X-linked myoclonic epilepsy with generalized spasticity and intellectual disability (XMESID) A rare X-linked recessive form of myoclonic epilepsy, presenting with spasticity and intellectual disability, while carrier women are hyperreflexic. It is associated with a missense mutation in *ARX* and is allelic with X-linked infantile spasms (ISSX; MIM 308350) in which polyalanine tract expansions represent the molecular defect.[5587] Mutations of *ARX* are associated with a wide range of phenotypes.

X-linked myopathies A group of muscle diseases sharing this pattern of inheritance. Such conditions include **bulbospinal neuronopathy, Duchenne muscular dystrophy, Becker muscle dystrophy**[472] and related forms,[3983] **Emery–Dreifuss syndrome,**[1854] **X-linked humeroperoneal muscular disease, X-linked dominant myopathy, dystrophin partial deficiency, Barth syndrome, X-linked myopathy with excessive autophagy,** and **McLeod syndrome**[6160] as well as other X-linked disorders separately listed under this letter.

X-linked myopathy with excessive autophagy A benign, slowly progressive X-linked recessive proximal myopathy with onset in childhood or youth mapped to Xq28 with mild and slowly progressive limb-gridle weakness, slight increase in serum CK levels, and a myopathic EMG. Neither cardiac nor intellectual involvement is present. Biopsy evidence shows a vacuolar myopathy.[3276, 4390] For further data, see http://www.neuro.wustl.edu/neuromuscular/maltbrain.html/.

X-linked periodic ataxia A form of pyruvate dehydrogenase deficiency characterized by symptoms and pathology resembling those of **Leigh disease,** with intermittent episodes of ataxia and dysarthria lasting days, with onset in childhood and abating during adolescence.[3883]

X-linked pigmentary abnormalities and congenital deafness A congenital, X-linked recessive disease characterized by severe neural deafness, large irregular spots of hypo- and hyperpigmentation, and impaired vestibular function.[3526]

X-linked recessive congenital muscle fiber hypotrophy with central nuclei A fatal congenital myopathy with the features suggested by the title.[276] In a *variant* form, there is an added axonal neuropathy without segmental demyelination.[1535]

X-linked recessive myotubular myopathy (XLMTM; MIM 310400) A rare congenital muscle disorder resulting from mutations in the *MTMl* gene, located in Xq28, and characterized by severe hypotonia and generalized muscle weakness at birth in affected males, most of whom die within the first year of life from respiratory failure. The characteristic muscle histopathology consists of small rounded muscle cells with centrally located nuclei resembling fetal myotubes, suggesting that the disorder results from a defect in the structural organization or in the normal development of the muscle fibers. Autosomal centronuclear myopathies (CNM) are disorders with similar histopathological findings, but the age of onset is later with a progressive clinical course.

X-linked recessive myotubular myopathy (XLMTM; OMIM 310400) A rare, frequently lethal congenital muscle disorder resulting from mutations in the *MTMl* gene located at Xq28, and characterized by severe hypotonia and generalized muscle weakness at birth in affected males, most of whom die within the first year of life from respiratory failure.[6508]

The characteristic muscle histopathology consists of small rounded muscle cells with centrally located nuclei resembling fetal myotubes, suggesting that the disorder results from a defect in the structural organization or in the normal development of the muscle fibers. Autosomal centronuclear myopathies (CNM) are disorders with similar histopathological findings, but the age of onset is later with a progressive clinical course. For further data, access http://www.neuro.wustl.edu/neuromuscular/maltbrain.html/.

However, neonatal asphyxia alone is not a symptom that may distinguish between an unfavorable and a more favorable prognosis. The latter prognosis applied to a milder form marked by development of spontaneous breathing, whereas such a development does not occur in the rapidly fatal form. Thus, an adult age (though not complete well-being) may be reached by patients with milder XLMTM.

X-linked recessive ophthalmoplegia and myopia Complete or partial ophthalmoplegia with ptosis, abnormal pupillary shape, myopia, choroido-retinal degeneration, and sometime hyporeflexia.[5512]

X-linked scapuloperoneal muscular dystrophy One of a heterogeneous group of diseases manifesting weakness and wasting of the proximal arm and distal leg muscles which may have a myopathic or a neurogenic etiology; in this case, an X-linked, childhood-onset muscular dystrophy manifesting joint contractures and pes cavus as well as the muscular involvement but without pseudohypertrophy. Type 2 fiber group atrophy is detectable on muscle biopsy specimens.[5888] Progression is slow, but a lethal cardiomyopathy may develop in adult life.[560] The condition is linked to deutan color blindness.[6281] See also **Emery–Dreifuss syndrome;** the differences between these disorders are minimal.

X-linked sideroblastic anemia with ataxia A very rare syndrome characterized by motor delay, ataxia with onset in early childhood, and dysarthria; these are almost nonprogressive until later adult life. The haematological features are ineffective erythropoiesis with marked iron loading of the red cell precursors.[2846]

X-linked spastic paraplegia A congenital syndrome manifesting optic atrophy, strabismus, dysarthria, joint contractures, pyramidal signs, and psychomotor retardation. The responsible gene maps to Xq12–q22. See also **hereditary**

spastic paraparesis and **hereditary motor neuropathy.**

X-linked spinal and bulbar muscular atrophy See X-linked bulbospinal neuronopathy.

X-linked spinal muscular atrophy See X-linked bulbospinal neuronopathy.

X-linked spinal muscular atrophy with bulbar involvement See X-linked bulbospinal neuronopathy.

X-linked spinobulbar muscular atrophy See X-linked bulbospinal neuronopathy.

X-linked torsion dystonia An X-linked dystonic syndrome of childhood or early adult onset, manifesting also sensorineural deafness and psychomotor retardation. See **dystonia.**

X-linked West syndrome A variant due to mutations in the *ARX* gene.

Xp21 myopathy See McLeod **syndrome.**

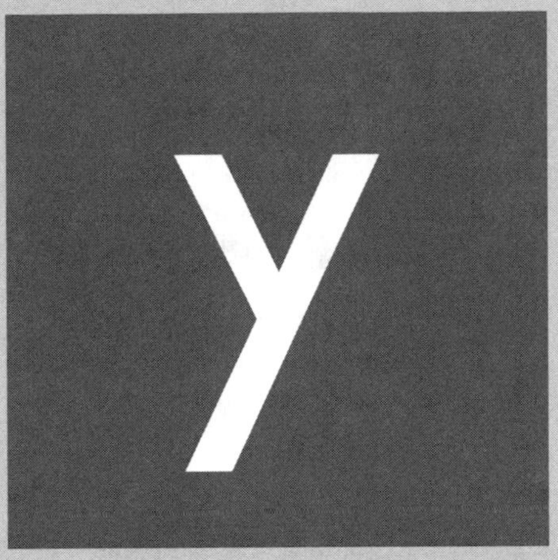

Yakolev, Paul Ivan (1894–1983) Russian-born neurologist and neuropathologist who trained at St. Petersburg, where at first he considered psychiatry as a career, but was dissuaded after listening to Pavlov's lectures. After graduating with high honors, he escaped from revolutionary Russia to Finland in 1919. After some time in England, he was later able to study in Paris with **Marie** and **Babinski and there** obtained his M.D. degree after which he went to America and was appointed to positions in neurology and neuropathology at the Boston City Hospital under Stanley **Cobb** and later at the Harvard Medical School. He improved upon the methods then available for sectioning brains and published widely on cerebral malformations, mainly in the context of epilepsy. He eventually became clinical professor of neuropathology; his large collection of neuropathological specimens is now located at the Armed Forces Institute of Pathology as it is regarded as a national resource.

Yakolev's most important publications were on the functional anatomy of the limbic system and of thalamocortical relationships, and on neuroanatomy.[3380]

Yale Children's inventory A child-rating instrument responsive to *DSM-III* terminology used to assess pediatric neurobehavioral disorders. The inventory rates attention, habituation, activity, impulsivity, tractability, academic performance, and fine motor skills. (Shaywitz SE et al. Pediatrics 1988;81:562–566)

yawning (chasma, oscedo) (Gr, open mouth, Lat, yawning) "A slow inspiration and depression of the lower jaw, followed by brief tonic spasm of the muscles of inspiration, of the depressors and elevators of the lower jaw, of some of the facial muscles and of the muscles of the neck so that the head is drawn backward" (Sir William **Gowers**). It can often be inhibited and frequently is associated with stretching.

Its occurrence is thought to be associated with an integrated discharge in a bulbospinal motor complex, which appears at a certain (depressed) level of excitability of the reticular activating system but the teleological benefit of this primitive movement pattern, a commonplace phenomenon halfway between a reflex and an expressive movement, is obscure. Pathologically, it is described in migraine, epilepsy, basal ganglion disorders, multiple sclerosis, and brain tumors. Most of the lesions, however, are infratentorial and a diencephalic yawning center has been hypothesized.

Year Book of Neurology and Neurosurgery An annual review book published by Elsevier. Web site: http://www.us.elsevierhealth.com/fcgi-bin/displaypage.pl?isbn=05135117/.

yellow-blue color blindness (tritanopia) A dominantly inherited syndrome of confusion between blue-green and yellow-pink shades, considered due to a deficiency in the blue pigment in the retinal cones.[6879]

Yim syndrome A congenital dysmorphic syndrome, manifesting also severe skeletal and ocular maldevelopments, macrocephaly, cerebral atrophy, and hydrocephalus.[381]

yips Involuntary movements occurring during the execution of skilled, focused, finely controlled motor behavior, as in the game of golf. The movements emerge particularly during putting; golfers have used such descriptive terms for them as *yips,* *twitch, staggers, waggles, jitters, jerks,* or "*them,*" suggesting that muscle spasms, myoclonus, cramps, or tremor may variously be responsible.[4212] Such eminent golfers as Sam Snead and Ben Hogan are reported to have been afflicted. The movements probably represent a form of focal dystonia resembling those of other sporting activities such as **bowlers' cramp.**

yoga footdrop A common peroneal palsy resulting from remaining in the customary cross-legged position for a prolonged period. See also **lotus footdrop.**

Yolken syndrome A congenital dysmorphic syndrome, manifesting also genital and skeletal maldevelopments, deafness, blindness, and microcephaly.[381]

Yom Kippur headache
A generalized nonthrobbing headache experienced in the middle of the day and associated with fasting. It is thought to reflect the effects of dehydration and is relieved by lying down.[4509]

Yoshimura reflex Yet another way of eliciting the plantar response, this time by stimulating the middle of the sole. Bekhterev, Guillain, Sicard, and others have also found that a noxious stimulus here is an effective way of eliciting the response. For neurologists who aspire to immortality, the bad news is that there is scarcely a square inch of the foot left for *de novo* stimulation, interpretation, and publication.

Young syndrome 1. A dominantly inherited distal form of **hereditary motor neuropathy** with onset in adolescence, affecting the arms before the legs and associated with laryngeal paresis.[6930]
2. (macrocephaly and callosal agenesis) A congenital dysmorphic syndrome manifesting also intestinal and cerebellar abnormalities, hydrocephalus, and mental and developmental delay.[381]

young-onset benign occipital lobe epilepsy A form of focal epilepsy with an onset in the first decade of occasional prolonged (<30 min) seizures with headache, vomiting, and tonic deviation of the eyes, sometimes progressing to tonic-clonic seizures. On the EEG, occipital discharges are associated with eye closure. After about three episodes the condition remits.[4039]

young-onset Parkinson disease
Arbitrarily defined as that form of otherwise typical **Parkinson disease** which produces symptoms between the ages of 21 and 39 inclusively and which is either sporadic or dominantly inherited. *Dominantly inherited early-onset Parkinsonism* is one *variant*.

Although similar to Parkinson disease in older patients, slower progression of symptoms, an onset with dystonia, a greater incidence of levadopa-related fluctuations, and the earlier appearance of dyskinesias, as with **juvenile Parkinsonian syndromes**, are distinguishing characteristics.[2434]

yo-yo-ing Rapid fluctuations in the clinical status of Parkinsonian patients on long-term levadopa therapy.[4105] See **on-off phenomenon, fluctuations.**

Yunis–Varon craniocleidal dysostosis plus A recessively inherited congenital dysmorphic syndrome, characterized also by severe skeletal maldevelopments, including brachydactyly and absence of the thumbs, dolichocephaly, scaphocephaly, and microcephaly with delayed closure of the fontanelles.[6941]

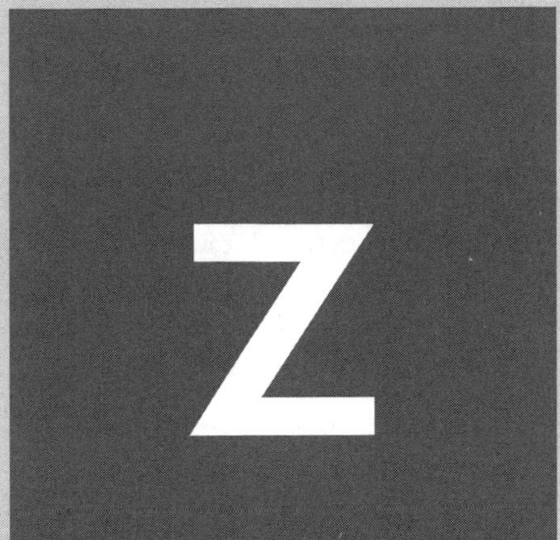

Zackai syndrome A congenital dysmorphic syndrome, manifesting also microcephaly, fusion of cervical vertebrae, and psychomotor retardation.[381] See also **Klippel–Feil syndrome.**

Zadik syndrome A congenital dysmorphic syndrome, manifesting also hypothyroidism; abnormalities of the teeth, skin, and skeleton; dermoid cysts; strabismus; and extra fontanelles in the skull.[381]

Zange–Kindler syndrome (cerebrospinal block syndrome, cisternal block syndrome) Arrest of CSF flow through the cisterna magna due to chronic meningitis or to mass lesions such as tumor and abscess, producing early signs of compromise of brainstem function and obstructive hydrocephalus.[6949]

Zappert syndrome (Zappert–Heller syndrome) See **acute cerebellar ataxia, cerebellar ataxias** (*variants*).

ZASPopathy A **congenital (distal) myopathy** with phenotypes of myofibrillar myopathy or Markesbery dominant distal myopathy caused by ZASP mutation A165V.[2580]

Zazzo Test A test of attention and of visuomotor abilities in which the subject is required within a 2-min period to mark every box with each of two particular designs on them; such boxes being randomly placed among a thousand boxes with 25 different designs printed on a chart placed before him or her.[6955]

zebra body myopathy An inherited nonprogressive myopathy reported in two sporadic cases[4992] and characterized by congenital onset, weak fetal movements, mild and nonprogressive proximal myopathic weakness, atrophy, hypotonia, areflexia, raised serum CK levels, and the presence of targets and nemaline rods in type 2 fibers in extraocular muscle biopsy specimens.[3648] Hypertonia and contractures are also described. The zebra bodies are thin actin filaments (Z-line material) arranged in parallel to the plasma membranes. See also **congenital myopathies with intracytoplasmic inclusions.**

Zeh syndrome The association of acalculia, dysgraphia, and noncomprehension of facial expression in pictures.[6961, 1335]

zeitgebers Indicators of the passage of time, required to synchronize the circadian rhythms. They include mealtimes, shifts, broadcasts, clocks, etc.

Zellweger, H.V. (1909–1990) Swiss geneticist, pediatrician, and neurologist who trained in Hamburg, Rome, and Berlin before graduating from Zurich in 1934. After residency training in Switzerland and a period spent with Dr. Albert Schweitzer in Africa, he moved to the United States as a Rockefeller Fellow, and, after further experience in Lebanon, returned to Iowa, where he later became professor of pediatrics. He founded one of the earliest neuromuscular clinics and was instrumental in founding regional genetic counselling services in his state. He was the author of *Chromosomes of Man* and of *Genetics in Neurology*, each in collaboration.

Zellweger spectrum The peroxisome biogenesis disorders including neonatal **adrenoleukodystrophy,** infantile **Refsum disease,** and **Zellweger syndrome.**

Zellweger syndrome

1. (cerebrohepatorenal syndrome). A rare, recessively inherited lethal multisystrem disorder caused by deficiency of multiple peroxisomes and, therefore, of the enzymes contained therein. It is characterized by dysgenesis of the cerebral cortex (micropolygyria, macrogyria, heterotopias), lissencephaly, callosal agenesis, cerebellar and olivary dysplasias, and white matter degeneration (sudanophilic leukodystrophy), as well as renal cortical cysts, hepatic periportal fibrosis, and bone pathology. Other clinical features include low birth weight, hypertelorism, abnormal ears, an open metopic suture, and generalized hypotonia.[4922, 1506, 427] MRI shows neocortical dysplasia, germinolytic cysts, and delayed myelination.

Three genotypes are recognized on the basis of peroxisomal disorder complementation groups.[4512] The chromosomal abnormality is at 7q11.23. Clinical manifestations in each include congenital facial dysmorphism, megalencephaly, multifocal seizures, cataract, optic atrophy, hepatomegaly, hypotonia, areflexia, and diminution of motor activity in infancy; death ensues within a few months.

The clinical and morphological features strongly resemble those of other **peroxisomal disorders.**[780]

2. The combination of **narcolepsy** and petit mal epilepsy.[6964]

In a *variant* form, survival is prolonged.[430]

Zeman–King syndrome

(anterior midline structure syndrome) The association of slowly progressive intellectual deterioration and affective lability, associated with a paroxysmal confusional state, gait ataxia, vertigo, weakness, nystagmus, pyramidal signs, and disturbances of sensation due to tumors of the septal region. The syndrome was first described by the American neurologists Wolfgang Zeman and Frederick King in 1958,[6968] who noted that an English physician, W.B. Ransom, had already described the same findings in a heterogeneous group of patients in 1895.

Zenker fluid

A fixative for pathological specimens, compounded by Friedrich Zenker (1825–1898), a German pathologist. The active ingredients are mercuric chloride and potassium dichromate.[5619]

Zenker paralysis

Peroneal nerve palsy.

zickzakbewegungen

See **square-wave jerks/oscillations.**

Ziehen, Georg Theodor

(1862–1924) German psychiatrist, professor at Jena, who described **dystonia** in the same year as **Oppenheim.**

Ziehen syndrome

(Ziehen–Oppenheim disease) See **dystonia.**

Zimmer syndrome

(tetra-amelia with multiple malformations) A congenital dysmorphic syndrome, manifesting also severe ocular and skeletal maldevelopments, hydrocephalus, and agenesis of the corpus callosum.[381]

Zimmerlin dystrophy

Hereditary muscular dystrophy with onset in the shoulder girdle.[6976] This probably a *variant* of the **scapuloperoneal syndrome**.

Zimmerlin, F.

(1858–1932) Swiss physician in Basel who gave an early account of *scapulohumeral muscular dystrophy*.

Zonana syndrome

A congenital dysmorphic syndrome, manifesting also hypotonia, nystagmus, and psychomotor retardation.[381]

zoster arteritis

(Gr, a girdle) Contralateral hemiparesis occurring some weeks after the onset of herpes zoster ophthalmicus. It is considered that the virus infects the appropriate artery (usually the middle cerebral) directly, spreading by way of the first division of the trigeminal nerve, and causing a necrotizing arteritis with occlusion, producing characteristic radiological findings.[4238]

Zung self-rating depression scale

A popular self-rating inventory that lists 20 attitudes (e.g., "I feel downhearted, blue and sad") which the patient scores (alone or with an interviewer) according to the frequency with which he experiences them. Eight items relate to physiological disturbances, the remainder to affect and to psychological and psychomotor changes.[6986] The test yields unusually high scores in subjects older than 65 years, and so is best not employed for individual screening nor for the evaluation of change in depressive symptoms in the elderly. See also **depression rating scales, Hamilton rating scale.**

Zunich syndrome

A congenital dysmorphic syndrome, manifesting also retinal colobomas, ichthyosis, seizures, and psychomotor delay.[381]

zygomatic reflex

Deviation of the mandible to the side on which the zygoma is tapped; a sign of bilateral corticobulbar tract lesions.

References

1. *The Lennox-Gastaut Syndrome.* Trevathan E. New York: Alan R. Liss, 1988.
2. *Disablement in the Community,* Patrick DL and Peach H (eds) Appendices 1,2. Oxford: Oxford University Press, 1989.
3. *Pediatric Neurology.* Swaiman KF (ed.) St. Louis: C.V. Mosby Company, 1989.
4. *Craniofacial Malformations.* Stricker M, van der Meulen J, Raphael B, and Mazzola R (eds) Edinburgh: Churchill, 1990.
5. *Neuro-Ophthalmology.* (Walsh and Hoyt) 5th edition. Philadelphia: Lippincott, 1990.
6. *Systemic Pathology Nervous System, Muscle and Eyes.* Weller RO (ed.) Edinburgh: Churchill Livingstone, 1990.
7. *The Founders of Child Neurology.* Ashwal S (ed.) San Francisco: Norman Publishing, 1990.
8. Proceedings of a consensus development conference on standardized measures in diabetic neuropathy. *Neurology* 1992;42:1823–39.
9. Scientific monograph of the Québec task force on whiplash associated disorders: Redefining whiplash and its management. *Spine* 1995;20:S1–S735.
10. *Ellenhorn's Medical Toxicology.* Ellenhorn, MJ. Philadelphia: Williams & Wilkins, 1997.
11. *Dictionary of Biological Psychology.* Winn P (ed.) London: Routledge, 2001.
12. Posterior reversible encephalopathy in infancy. (Arrovo HA et al.) *Rev Neurol (Paris)* 2003;37:506–10.
13. Relapsing focal myositis . . . Misu T et al. The localization detected by gallium citrate ga 67 scintigraphy. *Arch Neurol* 2005;62:1930–1.
14. Cerebellar ataxia with spasmodic cough: Coutinho P. et al. A new form of dominant ataxia. *Arch Neurol* 2006;63:553–5.
15. Alladi S, Xuereb J, Bak T, et al. Focal cortical presentations of Alzheimer's disease. *Brain* 2007;130:2636–45.
16. A proposed diagnostic schema for people with epileptic seizures and with epilepsy: Report of the ILAE task force on classification and terminology. *ILAE* 2008. (Electronic Citation)
17. Gene table of monogenic neuromuscular disorders (nuclear genome only). *Neuromuscular Disorders* 2008;18:101–29.
18. Jacobson DM. Relative pupil-sparing third nerve palsy: Etiology and clinical variables predictive of a mass. *Neurology* 2001;56:797–8.
19. AAEM subcommittee. Glossary of terms in electrodiagnostic medicine. *Muscle Nerve* 2001;(**Suppl.** 10):S5–S28.
20. AAN AIDS Task Force. Research criteria for diagnosis of chronic inflammatory demyelinating polyneuropathy (CIDP). *Neurology* 1991;41:617–8.
21. AAN quality standards subcommittee. *Practice Parameters: Carpal Tunnel Syndrome* 1993.
22. AAN therapeutic and technology assessment committee. The clinical usefulness of Botulinus Toxin A in treating neurologic disorders. *Neurology* 1990;40:1332–6.
23. AAN therapeutic and technology assessment committee. *Assessment: Posturography* 1993.
24. AAN therapeutic and technology assessment committee. Melodic intonation therapy. *Neurology* 1994;44:566–8.
25. Aase JM, Smith DW. Congenital anemia and triplalangeal thumbs: A new syndrome. *J Pediatr* 1969;74:417.
26. Abadi R. Mechanisms underlying nystagmus. *J Roy Soc Med* 2002;95: 231–5.
27. Abadie CA. *Traité des maladies des yeux.* Paris: O. Dain, 1887.
28. Abarbanel JM, Bashan N, Potashnik R et al. Adult muscle phosphorylase "b" kinase deficiency. *Neurology* 1986;36:560–2.
29. Abbie AA. The clinical significance of the anterior choroidal artery. *Brain* 1933;56:233–46.
30. Abboud FM. Neurocardiogenic syncope. *N Engl J Med* 1993;328:1117–20.
31. Abdo A, Coderre S, Bridges R. Leptomeningeal carcinomatosis secondary to gastroesophageal adenocarcinoma: A case report and review of the literature. *Can J Gastroenterol* 2002;16:807–11.

32. Abdo WF, Bor GF, Munneke M et al. 10 steps to identify atypical parkinsonism. *J Neurol Neurosurg Psychiatr* 2006;77:1369.
33. Abe K, Fujimura H, Tatsumi C et al. Eyelid "apraxia" in patients with motor neuron disease. *J Neurol Neurosurg Psychiatry* 1995;59:629–32.
34. Abel LA, Parker L, Daroff RB et al. End point nystagmus. *Invest Ophthalmol* 1978;17:539–44.
35. Abel LA, Traccis S, Dell'Osso LF. Square wave oscillation. The relation of saccadic intrusions and oscillations. *Neuroophthalmology* 1984;4:21.
36. Aberfeld DC. The hypertrophic degeneration of the olives. *Acta Neurol Scand* 1966;42:296–306.
37. Aberfeld DC, Hinterbuchner LP, Schneider M. Myotonia, dwarfism, diffuse bone disease and unusual ocular and facial abnormalities (A new syndrome). *Brain* 1965;88:313–22.
38. Aberfeld DC, Namba T. Progressive ophthalmoplegia in Kugelberg-Welander disease. *Arch Neurol* 1969;20:253–6.
39. Abid F, Hall R, Hudgson P et al. Möbius syndrome, peripheral neuropathy and hypogonadotrophic hypogonadism. *J Neurol Sci* 1978;35:309–15.
40. Abrahamson J, Bell L. Carotid-cavernous-fistula syndrome. *Am J Ophthalmol* 1955;39:521.
41. Absher JR, Benson DF. Disconnection syndromes. *Neurology* 1993;43:862–7.
42. Achaibar K, Moore S, Bain PG. Ciguatera poisoning. *Practical Neurol* 2007;7:316–22.
43. Achard J. *Rev Neurol* 1924;41:270–6.
44. Achenbach T, Edelbrock C. The child behavior profile II. Boys aged 12–16 and girls aged 6–11 and 12–16. *J Consult Clin Psychol* 1979;47:223.
45. Ackerknecht EH. The history of the discovery of the vegetative (autonomic) nervous system. *Med Hist* 1974;18:1–8.
46. ACR ad hoc committee on neuropsychiatric lupus nomenclature. The ACR nomenclature and case definitions for neuropsychiatric lupus syndromes. *Arth Rheum* 1999;42:599–608.
47. Adamolekun B. Epidemiological studies of the etiology of a seasonal ataxia in Nigerians. *Neurology* 1993;43:1419.
48. Adams CBT. Hemispherectomy – A modification. *J Neurol Neurosurg Psychiatry* 1983;46:61–9.
49. Adams D. Hereditary and acquired amyloid neuropathies. *J Neurol* 2001;248:647–57.
50. Adams RD. Cases of diseases of the heart, accompanied with pathological observations. *Dublin Hosp Rep* 1827;4:353–453.
51. Adams RD. Striatonigral degeneration. *J Neuropath Exp Neurol* 1964;24: 584–608.
52. Adams RD, Fisher CM, Hakim S et al. Symptomatic occult hydrocephalus with "normal" cerebrospinal fluid pressure: A treatable syndrome. *N Engl J Med* 1965;273:117–26.
53. Adams RJ, Meador KJ, Sethi KD et al. Graded neurological scale for use in acute hemispheric stroke protocols. *Stroke* 1987;18:665–9.
54. Addonizio G, Susman VL, Roth SD. Neuroleptic malignant syndrome: Review and analysis of 115 cases. *Biol Psychiatr* 1987;22:1004–20.
55. Adie WJ. Pseudo-Argyll Robertson pupils with absent tendon reflexes: A benign disorder simulating tabes dorsalis. *Brit Med J* 1931;1:928–30.
56. Adie WJ, Critchley M. Forced grasping and groping. *Brain* 1927;50:142–70.
57. Adler FH, Schie HC. The site of the disturbance in tonic pupils. *Trans Amer Ophth Soc* 1940;38:183–9.
58. Adolfsson R, Forsell A, Johansson G. Hereditary polycystic osteodysplasia with progressive dementia in Sweden. *Lancet* 1978;i:120.
59. Adornato BT, Carlini WG. Pushing palsy: A case of self-induced bilateral peroneal palsy induced during natural childbirth. *Neurology* 1992;42:936–7.
60. Adour KK. Mona Lisa syndrome: Solving the enigma of the Gioconda smile. *Ann Otol Rhinol Laryngol* 1989;98:196–9.
61. Adrian ED. General principles of nervous activity. *Brain* 1947;70:1–17.
62. Adrian ED, Forbes A. The all-or-nothing response of sensory nerve fibres. *J Physiol* 1922;56:301–30.
63. Adrilq A, Lopez MV. Paroxysmal aphasias. *Epilepsia* 1988;29:630–4.
64. Adson AW, Coffey JR. Cervical rib: A new method of anterior approach for relief of symptoms by division of the scalenus anticus. *Ann Surg* 1927;85:839–57.
65. Affi AK, Rebeiz JJ, Mire J et al. The myopathology of the prune belly syndrome. *J Neurol Sci* 1972;15:153–65.
66. Afifi AK. Idiopathic hyperCKemia revisited. *J Child Neurol* 1998;13:251–2.
67. Aftimos S, McGaughran J. Toriello-Carey syndrome: Case report with additional findings. *Am J Med Genet* 2001;98:273–6.
68. Agrup C, Gleeson M, Rudge P. The inner ear and the neurologist. *J Neurol Neurosurg Psychiatr* 2007;78:114–22.
69. Aguayo A, Nair CPV, Bray GM. Peripheral nerve abnormalities in Riley-Day syndrome. *Arch Neurol* 1971;24:105–16.
70. Aguilar L, et al. A new syndrome characterized by mental retardation, epilepsy, palpebral conjunctival telangiectasias and IgA deficiency. *Clin Genet* 1978;13:154–8.
71. Ahlberg G, Borg K, Edstrom L et al. Welander hereditary distal myopathy: A molecular genetic comparison to hereditary myopathies with inclusion bodies. *Neuromuscular Disorders* 1998;8:111–4.
72. Aicardi J. *Epilepsy in Children*. New York: Raven Press, 1986.
73. Aicardi J. Alternating hemiplegia of childhood. *Int Pediatr* 1987;2:115–9.
74. Aicardi J. *Diseases of the Nervous System in Infancy and Childhood*. London: MacKeith Press, 1992.
75. Aicardi J. The place of neuronal migration abnormalities in child neurology. *Can J Neurol Sci* 1994;21:185–93.
76. Aicardi J, Barbosa C, Andermann E et al. Ataxia-ocular motor apraxia: A syndrome mimicking ataxia-telangiectasia. *Ann Neurol* 1988;24:497–502.
77. Aicardi J, Goutieres F. A progressive familial encephalopathy in infancy with calcifications of the basal ganglia and chronic cerebrospinal fluid lymphocytosis. *Ann Neurol* 1984;15: 49–54.
78. Ainiala H, Loukkala J, Peltola J et al. The prevalence of neuropsychiatric syndromes in systemic lupus erythematosus. *Neurology* 2001;57:496–500.
79. Aird C, McIntosh RAC. Shakespeare's Richard III and the Ellis-van Creveld syndrome. *Practitioner (London)* 1978;220:656–62.
80. Ajax ET. Trapshooters cramp. *Arch Neurol* 1982;39:131.
81. Akesson HO. Cutis verticis gyrata and mental deficiency in Sweden. *Acta Med Scand* 1964;175:115–27.
82. Al-Deeb SM, Yaqub BA, Sharif HS et al. Neurobrucellosis. *Neurology* 1989;39:498–501.
83. Al-Din ASN, Anderson M, Bickerstaff ER et al. Brainstem encephalitis and the syndrome of Miller Fisher: A clinical study. *Brain* 1982;105:481–95.
84. Al-Hakim M, Katirji MB, Osorio I et al. Cerebral venous thrombosis in paroxysmal nocturnal hemaglobinuria. *Neurology* 1993;43:742–6.
85. Al-Lozi MT, Pestronk A, Yee WC et al. Rapidly evolving myopathy with myosin deficient muscle fibers. *Ann Neurol* 1994;35:273–9.
86. Al-Shahwan SA, Singh B, Riela A et al. Hemisomatic spasms in children. *Neurology* 1994;44:1332–3.
87. Al-Shekhlee A, Chelimsky T, Preston D. Small fibre neuropathies. *Neurologist* 2002;8:237–53.
88. Al-Shekhlee A, Hachwi RN, Preston DC. New criteria for early electrodiagnosis of

acute inflammatory demyelinating polyneuropathy. *Muscle Nerve* 2005;32:66–73.

89. Al-Yahyaee S, AlGazali LI, De Jonghe P et al. A novel locus for hereditary spastic paraplegia with thin corpus callosum and epilepsy. *Neurology* 2006;66:1230–4.
90. Alafuzoff I. The pathology of dementias: An overview. *Acta Neurol Scand* 1992; (**Suppl.** 139):8–15.
91. Alajouanine T. Quatre cas d'une affection congénitale caracterisée par un double pied bot, une double paralysie faciale et une double paralysie de la sixième paire. *Rev Neurol* 1930;2:501–11.
92. Alajouanine T. Baillarger, Jackson: The principle of Baillarger and Jackson in aphasia. *J Neurol Neurosurg Psychiatry* 1960;23:191–3.
93. Alajouanine T. Trouble with expressive language activities in aphasia, and their relationship with apraxias. *Rev Neurol* 1960;102:604–33.
94. Alajouanine T. Dostoiewski's epilepsy. *Brain* 1963;86:209–18.
95. Alam CN, Merskey H. Neuralgia: The history of a meaning. *Pain Res Manage* 1996;1:165–72.
96. Alayza Escardo F. Arnold's neuralgia. *JAMA* 1966;161:391
97. Alba A, Trainor FS, Ritter W et al. A clinical rating scale for Parkinson patients. *J Chronic Disease* 1968;21:507–22.
98. Alberca R, Montero C, Ibanez A et al. Progressive bulbar paralysis associated with neural deafness. *Arch Neurol* 1980;37:214–6.
99. Alberca R, Romero M, Chaparro J. Jerking stiff man syndrome. *J Neurol Neurosurg Psychiatry* 1982;45:1159–60.
100. Albers JW, Allan AA, Bastron JA et al. Limb myokymia. *Muscle Nerve* 1981;4:494–504.
101. Albers JW, Kelly JJ. Acquired inflammatory demyelinating polyneuropathies: Clinical and electrodiagnostic features. *Muscle Nerve* 1989;12:435–51.
102. Albers-Schonberg HE. *Fortschr Rontgensr* 1903;7:158–9.
103. Albert M, Cohen C. The test for severe impairment: An instrument for the assessment of patients with severe cognitive dysfunction. *J Am Geriatr Soc* 1992;40:449–53.
104. Albert ML. A simple test of visual neglect. *Neurology* 1973;23:658–64.
105. Albert ML. Henry Hécaen. MD: Neurologist – neuropsychologist 1912–1983. *Arch Neurol* 1984;41:458–9.
106. Albert ML, Feldman RG, Willis AL. The "subcortical dementia" of progressive supranuclear palsy. *J Neurol Neurosurg Psychiatry* 1974;37:121–30.
107. Albert ML, Reches A, Silverberg R. Associative visual agnosia without alexia. *Neurology* 1975;25:322–6.
108. Albert ML, Sparks RW, Helm NA. Melodic intonation therapy for aphasia. *Arch Neurol* 1973;29:130–1.
109. Albert MS, Butters N, Levin J. Temporal gradients in the retrograde amnesia of patients with alcoholic Korsakoff's disease. *Arch Neurol* 1979;36:211.
110. Albright F, Butler AM, Hampton AO et al. Syndrome characterized by osteitis fibrosa disseminata, areas of pigmentation and endocrine dysfunction, with precocious puberty in females. *N Engl J Med* 1937;216:727.
111. Albright F, et al. Pseudo-hypoparathyroidism – example of "Seabright bantam" syndrome. *Endocrinology* 1942;30:922–32.
112. Alcock NS. A note on the pathology of senile chorea (non-hereditary). *Brain* 1936;59:376–87.
113. Aldrich MS. Diagnostic aspects of narcolepsy. *Neurology* 1998;50:S2–S7.
114. Aldrich MS, Alessi AG, Beck RW, Gilman S. Cortical blindness: Etiology, diagnosis and prognosis. *Ann Neurol* 1987;21:149–58.
115. Aldrich MS, Beck RW, Albers JW. Familial recurrent Bell's palsy with ocular motor palsies. *Neurology* 1987;37:1369–71.
116. Aleck KA, Shapiro LJ. Genetic-metabolic considerations in the sick neonate. *Pediatr Clins N Am* 1978;25:431–51.
117. Aleksic S, Budzilovich GN, Chou A et al. Congenital ophthalmoplegia in Oculo-auriculo-vertebral dysplasia – hemifacial microsomia (Goldenhar-Gorlin syndrome). *Neurology* 1976;26:638–44.
118. Alexander MP. Mild traumatic brain injury. *Neurology* 1995;45:1253–60.
119. Alexander WS. Progressive fibrinoid degeneration of fibrillary astrocytes associated with mental retardation in a hydrocephalic infant. *Brain* 1949;72:373–81.
120. Alexopoulos GS, Abrams RC, Young RC et al. Cornell scale for depression in dementia. *Biol Psychiatr* 1988;23: 271–84.
121. Alfonso I, et al. Spinal cord involvement in encephalocutaneous lipomatosis. *Ped Neurol* 1986;2:380–4.
122. Alford CA, Stagno S, Reynolds DW. Congenital toxoplasmosis: Clinical, laboratory, and therapeutic considerations, with special reference to subclinical case. *Bull NY Acad Med* 1974;50:160–81.
123. Alhalabi M, Moore PM. Serial angiography in isolated angiitis of the nervous system. *Neurology* 1994;44: 1221–6.
124. Ali-Khan Z, Irving RT, Wignall N et al. Imported sparganosis in Canada. *Can Med Assn J* 1973;108:590–3.
125. Alison MR, Sarraf CE. Apoptosis: A gene-directed programme of cell death. *J Roy Coll Phys London* 1992;26(**no.1**):25.
126. Alison S, Greena JE, Sivtsevab TM et al. Viliuisk encephalomyelitis: Intrathecal synthesis of oligoclonal IgG. *J Neurol Sci* 2003;212:69–73.
127. Allan JD et al. A disease, probably hereditary, characterized by severe mental deficiency and a constant gross abnormality of aminoacid metabolism. *Lancet* 1958;1:182–7.
128. Allbutt TG. On the ophthalmoscopic signs of spinal disease. *Lancet* 1870;1:76.
129. Allen CMC. Clinical diagnosis of the acute stroke syndrome. *Quart J Med* 1983;52:515–23.
130. Allen CMC. Predicting the outcome of acute stroke. *J Neurol Neurosurg Psychiatry* 1984;47:457–80.
131. Allen IM. Speech defects apparently congenital in origin. *Brit J Child Dis* 1932;29:98.
132. Allen IV, Dermott E, Connally J et al. A study of a patient with the amyotrophic form of Creutzfeldt-Jakob disease. *Brain* 1971;94:715–24.
133. Allen RJ, Young W, Read S et al. "Galactosemic encephalopathy": The effect of early versus late neonatal detection and treatment on neurological outcome. *Ann Neurol* 1991;30:465.
134. Allen RP, Picchietti D, Hening WA et al. Restless legs syndrome: Diagnostic criteria, special considerations, and epidemiology. *Sleep Med* 2003;4:101–19.
135. Allen T, Carman H. Homonymous hemianoptic paracentral scotoma. *Arch Ophthal Berlin* 1938;20:846–9.
136. Allgrove J, Clayden GS, Grant DB et al. Familial glucocorticoid deficiency with achalasia of the cardia and deficient tear production. *Lancet* 1978;1:1284–6.
137. Allison RS. Perseveration as a sign of diffuse and focal brain damage. *Brit Med J* 1966;2:1027–32.
138. Allison RS, Millar J. Prevalence and familial incidence of disseminated sclerosis. *Ulster Med J* 1954;(**Suppl. 23**): 1–92.
139. Allman P. Crying and laughing after brain damage (letter). *J Neurol Neurosurg Psychiatry* 1990;53:1439–40.
140. Allsop JL, Martins L, Lebris H. Neurological manifestations of ciguatera. *Rev Neurol* 1986;142:590–7.
141. Al Otaibi SF, Blaser S, MacGregor DL. Neurological complications of kernicterus. *Can J Neurol Sci* 2005;32:311.

142. Alpers BJ. Diffuse progressive degeneration of the gray matter of the cerebrum. *Arch Neurol* 1931;25:469–505.

143. Alpers BJ, Grant FC. The clinical syndrome of corpus callosum. *J Nerv Ment Dis* 1931;121:205–14.

144. Alpers BJ, Yaskin BJ. The Bruns syndrome. *J Nerv Ment Dis* 1944;100:115–34.

145. Alpert JN. Failure of fixation suppression: A pathologic effect of vision on caloric nystagmus. *Neurology* 1974;24:891–6.

146. Alpert JN, Coats AC, Perusquia E. Saccadic nystagmus in cerebellar cortical atrophy. *Neurology* 1975;25:676–80.

147. Alport AC. Hereditary familial congenital hemorrhagic nephritis. *Brit Med J* 1927;1:504–6.

148. Alston W, Angel RW, Fink FS et al. Motor activity following the silent period in human muscle. *J Physiol* 1967;190:189.

149. Alstrom CH, Hallgren B, Nilsson LB et al. Retinal degeneration combined with obesity, diabetes mellitus and neurogenous deafness. *Acta Psychiatr Neurol* 1959;S.129.

150. Alter M. The digiti quinti sign of mild hemiparesis. *Neurology* 1973;23:503–5.

151. Alter M, Schaumann B. Hereditary amyotropic lateral sclerosis. A report of two families. *Europ Neurol* 1976;14: 250–65.

152. Altrocchi PH. Spontaneous oral-facial dyskinesia. *Arch Neurol* 1972;36:506.

153. Alvarez SL, Jacobs NA, Murray IJ. Visual changes mediated by beer in retrobulbar neuritis – an investigative report. *Br J Ophthalmol* 1986;70:141–6.

154. Alvord EC, Lofton S. Gliomas of optic nerve or chiasm. *J Neurosurg* 1988;68:85–98.

155. Alzheimer A. Uber eine eigenartige Erkrangkung der Hirnrinde. *All Z Psychiatr* 1907;64:146–8.

156. Amalric P. A new type of tapetoretinal degeneration in the course of deaf-mutism. *Bull Fr Soc Ophthal* 1960;73:196–212.

157. Amato AA, Barohn RJ. Hereditary neuropathy with liability to pressure palsies: Association with central nervous system demyelination. *Muscle Nerve* 1996;19:770–3.

158. Amato AA, Jackson CE, Ridings LW et al. Childhood-onset oculopharygodistal myopathy with chronic instestinal pseudo-obstruction. *Muscle Nerve* 1995;18:842–7.

159. Amato AA, Kagan-Hallet K, Jackson CE et al. The wide spectrum of myofibrillar myopathy suggests a multifactorial etiology and pathogenesis. *Neurology* 1998;51:1646–55.

160. Ambler MW, Trice J, Grauerholz J et al. Infantile osteopetrosis and neuronal storage disease. *Neurology* 1983;33:437–41.

161. Ameli NO. Avicenna and trigeminal neuralgia. *J Neurol Sci* 1965;2:105–7.

162. American Academy of Electrodiagnostic Medicine. AAEE glossary of terms in clinical electromyography. *Muscle Nerve* 1987;10S:G5–G23.

163. American Academy of Neurology. The Dolman-Delcato treatment of neurologically handicapped children. *Neurology* 1968;18:1214–6.

164. American Academy of Neurology. Assessment: Thermography in neurologic practice. *Neurology* 1990;40:523–5.

165. American Academy of Neurology. Assessment and management of patients in the persistent vegetative state. *Neurology* 1995;45:1015–8.

166. American Academy of Neurology AIDS task force. Nomenclature and case definitions for neurological manifestations of HIV type 1 infection. *Neurology* 1991;41:778–85.

167. American Academy of Neurology Quality Standards Committee. Practice parameters: Lumbar puncture. *Neurology* 1993;43:625–7.

168. American Academy of Neurology Therapeutics Subcommittee. Assessment: Positron emission tomography. *Neurology* 1991;41:163–7.

169. American Diabetes Association. Report and recommendations of the San Antonio conference on diabetic neuropathy. *Muscle Nerve* 1988;11:661–7.

170. American Neurological Association Committee on Ethical Affairs. Persistent vegetative state. *Ann Neurol* 1993;33:386–90.

171. American Psychiatric Association. *APA Diagnostic and Statistical Manual of Mental Disorders*. Washington, DC: APA, 1994.

172. American Psychiatric Association. *Diagnostic and Statistical Manual of Mental Disorders* (DSM-IV TR). Washington: American Psychiatric Association, 2000.

173. American Society of Pediatric Surgeons. Identifying the infant with nonaccidental central nervous system injury (the whiplash-shake syndrome). *Pediatr Neurosurg* 1993;19:170.

174. Ames FR, Saffer D. The sunflower syndrome. *J Neurol Sci* 1983;59:1–11.

175. Amico L, Caplan LR, Thomas C. Cerebrovascular complications of mucinous cancers. *Neurology* 1989;39:522–6.

176. Amiel-Tison C, Grenier A. Neurological assessment during the first year of life. New York, Oxford: Oxford University Press, 1986.

177. Aminoff MJ. Acanthocytosis and neurological disease. *Brain* 1972;95:749–60.

178. Aminoff MJ. Vascular anomalies in intracranial dura mater. *Brain* 1973;96:601–2.

179. Aminoff MJ, Dedo HH, Izdebski K. Clinical aspects of spasmodic dysphonia. *J Neurol Neurosurg Psychiatry* 1978;41:361–5.

180. Amir RE, van den Veyver IB, Wan M et al. Rett syndrome is caused by mutations in X-linked MECP2, encoding methyl-CpG-binding protein 2. *Nat Genet* 1999;23:185–8.

181. Amit R, Bashan N, Abarbanel JM et al. Fatal familial infantile glycogen storage disease: Multisystem phosphofructokinase deficiency. *Muscle Nerve* 1992;15:455–8.

182. Amit R, Glick B, Itzchak Y et al. Acute severe combined demyelination. *Childs Nerv Syst* 1992;8:354–6.

183. Amoiridis G. Median – ulnar nerve communications and anomalous innervation of the intrinsic hand muscles: An electrophysiological study. *Muscle Nerve* 1993;15:576–9.

184. Andermann E, Andermann F, Silver K et al. Benign familial nocturnal alternating hemiplegia of childhood. *Neurology* 1994;44:1812–4.

185. Andermann E et al. Agenesis of the corpus callosum with sensorimotor neuropathy. *Vth Int Conf Birth Defects* 1977; Amsterdam. Excerpta Medica

186. Andermann F. Nicolaus Friedreich and degenerative atrophy of the posterior columns of the spinal cord. *Can J Neurol Sci* 1976;3:275–7.

187. Andermann F, Andermann E. Excessive startle syndromes: Startle disease, jumping, and startle epilepsy. *Adv Neurol* 1986;43:321–38.

188. Andermann F, Andermann E, Carpenter S et al. Action myoclonus-renal failure: A new autosomal recessive syndrome in three families. *Adv Neurol* 1986;43:87–103.

189. Andermann F, Keene DL, Andermann A, Quesney LF. Startle disease or hyperekplexia. *Brain* 1980;103:985–97.

190. Andermann F, Olivier A, Melanson D et al. Epilepsy due to focal cortical dysplasia with macrogyria and the forme fruste of tuberous sclerosis: A study of 15 patients. In Wolf P, Dam M, Janz D et al., ed.s. *Advances in Epileptology*, pp 35–8. New York: Raven Press, 1987.

191. Andersen DH. Familial cirrhosis of the liver with storage of abnormal glycogen. *Lab Invest* 1956;5:11–20.

192. Anderson B, McCann SM. The effects of hypothalamic lesions on the water intake of the dog. *Acta Physiol Scand* 1956;35:312–20.

193. Anderson M. Neurology of Whipple's disease. *J Neurol Neurosurg Psychiatry* 2000;68:2–5.
194. Anderson W. A case of "Angiokeratoma". *Brit J Dermatol* 1898;10:113.
195. Andersson M, Alvarez-Cermeno J, Bernadi G et al. Cerebrospinal fluid in the diagnosis of multiple sclerosis: A consensus report. *J Neurol Neurosurg Psychiatry* 1994;57:897–902.
196. Andrade C. A peculiar form of peripheral neuropathy. *Brain* 1952;75:408–27.
197. Andrade C, Araki S, Block WD et al. Hereditary amyloidosis. *Arth Rheum* 1970;13:902–15.
198. Andrasik F, Blanchard EB, Arena JG et al. Psychological functioning in headache sufferers. *Psychosom Med* 1982;44:171–82.
199. Andre-Thomas. Atrophie lamellaire des cellules de Purkinje. *Rev Neurol* 1905;13:917–24.
200. Andres PL, Hedlund W, Finison L et al. Quantitative motor assessment in amyotrophic lateral sclerosis. *Neurology* 1986;36:937–41.
201. Andres PL, Skerry LM, Munsat TL. Measurement of strength in neuromuscular disease. In Munsat TL, ed. *Quantification of Neurologic Deficit*, pp 87–100. Boston: Butterworths, 1989.
202. Andrews PI, Massey J, Howard JF et al. Race, sex and puberty influence onset, severity and outcome in juvenile myasthenia gravis. *Neurology* 1994;44:1208–14.
203. Angel RW. Shortening reaction in patients with cerebellar ataxia. *Ann Neurol* 1982;11:2722–2728.
204. Angelman H. Puppet children. *Dev Med Child Neurol* 1965;7:681–8.
205. Angelucci A. Di una sindrome sconoscita negli infermi di cattaro primaverile. *Arch di ottal* 1897;4:270.
206. Anon. Eosinophilia-Myalgia syndrome and L-tryptophan containing products. *MMWR* 1989;38:785.
207. Anon. Obituary. *J Neurophysiol* 1942;5:1–17.
208. Anon. Richard Whytt (editorial). *JAMA* 1964;189:150–1.
209. Anthony JH, Procopis PG, Ouvrier RA. Benign acute childhood myositis. *Neurology* 1979;29:1068–71.
210. Antinori A, Arendt G, Becker JT et al. Updated research nosology for HIV-associated neurocognitive disorders. *Neurology* 2007;69:1789–99.
211. Anton G. Ueber den Ausdruck der Gemuthsbewegungen beim gesunden und kranken Menschen. *Psychiat Wschr* 1900;17:165–9.
212. Antonaci F, Bono G, Chimento P. Diagnosing cervicogenic headache. *J Headache Pain* 2006;7:145–8.
213. Antonaci F, Ghimmai S, Bono G, et al. Cervicogenic headache; evaluation of the original criteria. *Cephalalgia* 2001;21:583.
214. Antozzi C, Garavaglia B, Mora M et al. Late-onset riboflavine-responsive myopathy with combined multiple acyl coenzyme A dehydrogenase and respiratory chain deficiency. *Neurology* 1994;44:2153–8.
215. Anzil AP, Gessaga E. Late-life cavitating dystrophy of cortical and cerebellar white matter. *Europ Neurol* 1972;7:79–94.
216. Apert E. De l'acrocephalosyndactylie. *Bull Soc Med Hop Paris* 1906;23:1310–30.
217. Apgar V. A proposal for a new method of evaluation of the newborn infant. *Anesth Analg* 1953;32:260–7.
218. Appel V, et al. A rating scale for amyotrophic lateral sclerosis. *Arch Neurol* 1987;22:328–33.
219. Appelt J, et al. Tetraphokomelie mit Lippen – Kiefer – Gaumenspalte und Clitorishhypertrophie – ein Syndrom. *Padiatr Padol* 1966;2:119–24.
220. Appen RE, Wray SH, Cogan DG. Central retinal artery occlusions. *Am J Ophthalmol* 1975;79:374–81.
221. Appenzeller O, Amick L. Paralysis with paradoxic myotonia. *Trans Amer Neurol Assn* 1972;97:245–7.
222. Appenzeller O, Biehl JP. Mouthing in the elderly: A cerebellar sign. *J Neurol Sci* 1968;6:249–60.
223. Appenzeller O, Hanson JC. Parietal ataxia. *Arch Neurol* 1966;15:264–9.
224. Appenzeller O, Kornfeld M. Macrodactyly and localized hypertrophic neuropathy. *Neurology* 1974;24:767–71.
225. Appenzeller O, Parks RD, MacGee J. Peripheral neuropathy in chronic disease of the respiratory tract. *Amer J Med* 1968;44:873–80.
226. Appleton RE, Panayiotopoulos CP, Acomb BA et al. Eyelid myoclonia with typical absences: An epilepsy syndrome. *J Neurol Neurosurg Psychiatry* 1993;56:1312–6.
227. Apuzzo MLJ, Davey LM, Manuelidise EE. Pineal apoplexy associated with anticoagulant therapy. *J Neurosurg* 1976;45:223–6.
228. Aramideh M, Koelman JH, Speelman JD et al. Eyelid movement disorders and electromyography. *Lancet* 2001;357:805–6.
229. Aran FA. Récherches sur un maladie non encore décrite du système musculaire (atrophie musculaire progressive). *AGMP* 1850;24:172–214.
230. Arbisser A, et al. A syndrome manifested by brittle hair, with morphologic and biochemical abnormalities, developmental delay and normal stature. *Birth Defects Orig Artic Ser* 1976;12:219–28.
231. Arbogast SD, Khanna S, Koontz DW et al. Chronic apraxic neuropathy mimicking dorsal mid brain syndrome. *J Neurol Neurosurg Psychiatr* 2007;78:1276–7.
232. Arden JB, Barrada A, Kelsey JH. New clinical test of retinal function based on the standing potential of the eye. *Br J Ophthalmol* 1962;46:449–67.
233. Ardinger HH, Bell WE. Hypomelanosis of Ito. *Arch Neurol* 1986;43:848–50.
234. Arend R, Handzel L, Weiss B. Dysphatic stuttering. *Folia Phoniatrica* 1962;14:55–66.
235. Aretaeus. On epilepsy. In Adams F, trans., ed. *Extant Works*, London, 1856.
236. Arezzo JC, Schaumberg HH. The use of the Optacon as a screening device for detecting sensory loss in individuals exposed to neurotoxins. *J Occupat Med* 1980;22:461–4.
237. Argov Z, Eisenberg I, Grabov-Nardini G et al. Hereditary inclusion body myopathy. *Neurology* 2003;60:1519–23.
238. Argov Z, Navon R. Clinical and genetic variations in the syndrome of adult GM2 gangliosidosis resulting from hexosaminidase A deficiency. *Ann Neurol* 1984;16:14–20.
239. Argyll Robertson J. Four cases of spinal myosis. With remarks on the action of light on the pupil. *Edinburgh Med J* 1869;15:487–93.
240. Arias D, Passarge E, Engle MA et al. Human chromosomal deletion: Two patients with the 4p syndrome. *J Pediatr* 1970;76:82–8.
241. Arias-Carrion O, Olivares-Bunuelos T, Drucker-Colin R. Neurogenesis in the adult brain. *Rev Neurol* 2007;44:541–50.
242. Arieff AJ, Tigay EL, Kurtz JF. The Hoover sign. *Arch Neurol* 1961;5:673–8.
243. Arii J, Tanabe Y, Miyake M et al. Clinical and pathologic characteristics of non-typhoidal salmonella encephalopathy. *Neurology* 2002;58:1641–5.
244. Arjundas G. Experiences with neuromuscular disorders in South India. *Neurology (Bombay)* 1977;25:1–18.
245. Armendares S, Antillar F, del Castillo V et al. A newly recognized inherited syndrome of dwarfism, craniosynostosis, retinitis pigmentosa, and multiple congenital malformations. *J Pediatr* 1974;85:872–3.
246. Armon C. The alternating eye deviation sign. *Neurology* 1991;41:1845.
247. Armon C, Radtke RA, Friedman AH. Inhibitory simple partial (non-convulsive) status epilepticus after intracranial surgery. *J Neurol Neurosurg Psychiatry* 2000;69:18–24.
248. Armstrong D, Sachis P, Bryan C et al. Pathological features of persistent infantile sleep apnea with reference to the pathology

of sudden infant death syndrome. *Ann Neurol* 1982;12:169–74.

249. Arnason BGW. Inflammatory polyradiculoneuritis. In Dyck PJ, Thomas PK, Lambert EH, eds. *Peripheral Neuropathy*, pp 1110–48. Philadelphia: Saunders, 1975.
250. Arness MK, Brown JD, Dubey JP et al. An outbreak of acute eosinophilic myositis attributed to human sarcocystis parasitism. *Am J Trop Med Hyg* 1999;61:548–53.
251. Arnold J. Myelocyste, Transposition von Gewebskeinem und Sympodie. *Beitr Path Anat* 1894;16:1–28.
252. Arnoldi CC, Brodsky AE, Cauchoix J et al. Lumbar spinal stenosis and nerve root entrapment syndromes: Definition and classification. *Clin Orthop* 1976;115:4–5.
253. Arts WFM, Busch HFM, v de Brand HJ et al. Hereditary neuralgic amyotrophy. *J Neurol Sci* 1983;62:261–79.
254. Arts WFM, Loonen MCB, Sengers RCA et al. X-linked ataxia, weakness, deafness and loss of vision in early childhood with a fatal course. *Ann Neurol* 1993;33:535–9.
255. Arvanitakis Z, Wszolek ZK. Recent advances in the understanding of tau protein and movement disorders. *Current Opinion in Neurology* 2001;14:491–7.
256. Asberg MA, Montgomery SA, Perris C et al. A comprehensive psychopathological rating scale. *Acta Psychiatrica et Neurologica* 1978;271: S5–S27.
257. Asbury AK. Renaut bodies – A forgotten endoneurial structure? *J Neuropath Exp Neurol* 1973;324:334–43.
258. Asbury AK, Arnason BGW, Karp H et al. Criteria for the diagnosis of Guillain-Barré syndrome. *Ann Neurol* 1978;3:565–6.
259. Asbury AK, Cornblath DR. Assessment of current diagnostic criteria for Guillain-Barré syndrome. *Ann Neurol* 1990;27: S21–S24.
260. Asbury AK, Picard EH, Baringer JR. Sensory perineuritis. *Arch Neurol* 1972;26:302–12.
261. Asbury AK, Prensky AL. Graphogenic epilepsy. *Trans Amer Neurol Assn* 1963;88:193–4.
262. Asbury AK, Victor M, Adams RD. Uremic polyneuropathy. *Arch Neurol* 1963;8:413–28.
263. Asby A, Guerrini R, David P et al. Facial hemangioma and cerebral corticovascular dysplasia. *Neurology* 2003;60:1030–2.
264. Aschoff JC, Becker W, Rettelbach R. Voluntary nystagmus in five generations. *J Neurol Neurosurg Psychiatry* 1976;39:300–4.
265. Aserinsky E, Kleitman N. Regularly occurring periods of eye motility and concomitant phenomena during sleep. *Science* 1953;118:273–4.
266. Ashe J, Hain TC, Zee DS et al. Microsaccadic flutter. *Brain* 1991;114:461–72.
267. Asher R. Myxoedematous madness. *Brit Med J* 1949;ii:555–62.
268. Asher R. Munchausen's syndrome. *Lancet* 1951;1:339–41.
269. Asher SW, Berg BO. Progressive hemifacial atrophy: Report of three cases, including one observed over 43 years, and computed tomographic findings. *Arch Neurol* 1982;39:44–6.
270. Asherson N. Trotter's syndrome and associated lesions. *J Laryng Otol* 1951;65:349–66.
271. Ashizawa T, Butler IJ, Harati Y et al. A dominantly inherited syndrome with continuous motor neuron discharges. *Ann Neurol* 1983;13:285–90.
272. Ashizawa T, Rolak LA, Hines M. Spastic pure motor monoparesis. *Ann Neurol* 1986;20:638–41.
273. Ashwal S, Thrasher TV, Rice DR et al. A new form of sea-blue histiocytosis associated with progressive anterior horn cell and axonal degeneration. *Ann Neurol* 1984;16:184–92.
274. Ashworth B. Preliminary triaı of carisoprodol in multiple sclerosis. *Practitioner (London)* 1964;192:540–2.
275. Askanas V, Engel WK, Kwan HH et al. Autosomal dominant syndrome of lipid neuromyopathy with normal carnitine: Successful treatment with long chain fatty acid free diet. *Neurology* 1985;35:66–72.
276. Askanas V, Engel WK, Reddy NB et al. X-linked recessive congenital muscle fiber hypotrophy with central nuclei. *Arch Neurol* 1979;36:604–9.
277. Askenasy H, Wijsenbeek H, Hertzberger E. Retraction nystagmus and retraction of the eyelids due to arteriovenous aneurysm of the midbrain. *Arch Neurol Psychiatry* 1953;69:236.
278. Askenasy JJM. Sleep hiccup. *Sleep* 1988;11:187–94.
279. Assmann H, Bielenstein H, Hobs H et al. Beobachtungen und Untersuchungen bei der Haffkrankeit. *Dtsch Med Wschr* 1933;59:122–6.
280. Association of Sleep Disorder Centers. Diagnostic classification of sleep and arousal disorders. *Sleep* 1979;2:1–137.
281. Astrom K-E, Mancall EL, Richardson EPJ. Progressive multifocal leuko-encephalopathy: A hitherto unrecognized complication of chronic lymphatic leukaemia and Hodgkin's disease. *Brain* 1958;81:93–111.
282. Astrup J, Siesjo BK, Symon L. Thresholds in cerebral ischemia: The ischemic penumbra. *Stroke* 1981;12:723–5.
283. Atchison PR, Thompson PD, Frackowiak RS et al. The syndrome of gait ignition failure: A report of six cases. *Mov Disord* 1993;8:285–92.
284. Atkin A, Bender MB. Lightning eye movements (ocular myoclonus). *J Neurol Sci* 1964;1:2–12.
285. Atkin BM, Buist NRM, Utter MF et al. Pyruvate carboxylate deficiency and lactic acidosis in a child without Leigh's disease. *Pediat Res* 1979;13:109.
286. Atkin JF, Flaitz K, Patil S et al. An X-linked mental retardation syndrome. *Am J Med Genet* 1985;21: 697–705.
287. Atkins EJ, Biousse V, Newman NJ. The natural history of optic neuritis. *Rev Neurol Dis* 2006;3:45–56.
288. Atsuta N, Watanabe H, Ito M et al. Natural history of spinal and bulbar muscular atrophy (SBMA): A study of 223 Japanese patients. *Brain* 2006;129:1446–55.
289. Auberger G, Ratzlaff T, Lunkes A et al. A gene for autosomal dominant paroxysmal choreoathetosis/spasticity (CSE) maps to the vicinity of a potassium channel gene cluster on chromosome 1p. *Genomics* 1996;31:90–4.
290. Aubert H. *Physiologie der Netzhaut.* Breslau: Morgenstern, 1865.
291. Auer-Grumbach M, Strasser-Fuchs S, Wagner K et al. Roussy Levy syndrome is a phenotypic variant of Charcot-Marie-Tooth syndrome associated with a duplication on chromosome 17p11.2. *J Neurol Sci* 1998;154:72–5.
292. Auerbach SH. Central razzle: A central auditory pain syndrome? *Arch Neurol* 1981;38:671.
293. Auger RG. Diseases associated with excess motor unit activity. *Muscle Nerve* 1994;17:1250–63.
294. Auger RA, Daube JR, Gomez MR et al. Hereditary form of sustained muscle activity of peripheral nerve origin causing generalized myokymia and muscle stiffness. *Ann Neurol* 1984;15:13–21.
295. Aujesky, A. Ueber eine neue Infektionskrankheit bei Haustieren. *Zbl F Bakt* 1902; 32:535–57.
296. Aula P, Autio S, Raivio KO et al. "Salla disease": A new lysosomal storage disorder. *Arch Neurol* 1979;36:88–94.
297. Auranen M, Villanova M, Muntoni F et al. X-linked vacuolar myopathies: Two separate loci and refined genetic mapping. *Ann Neurol* 2000;47:666–9.
298. Auré K, Ogier de Baulny H, Laforêt P et al. Chronic progressive ophthalmoplegia with large-scale mtDNA rearrangement: Can we predict progression? *Brain* 2007;130:1516–24.

299. Ausman JI, Shrontz CE, Pearce JE et al. Vertebrobasilar insufficiency: A review. *Arch Neurol* 1985;42:803–8.
300. Austin EJ, Wilkus RJ, Longstreth WT. Etiology and Prognosis of alpha coma. *Neurology* 1988;38:773–7.
301. Austin J. Studies in metachromatic leukodystrophy. XII. Multiple sulfatase deficiency. *Arch Neurol* 1973;28:258–64.
302. Austin J, Armstrong D, Fouch S et al. Metachromatic leukodystrophy (MLD). *Arch Neurol* 1968;18:225–40.
303. Authier FJ, Cherin P, Creange A et al. Central nervous system disease in patients with macrophagic myofasciitis. *Brain* 2001;124:974–83.
304. Authier FJ, Kondo H, Ghnassia RT et al. Necrotizing myopathy with pipestem capillaries and minimal cellular infiltration: A case associated with cutaneous signs of dermatomyositis. *Neurology* 1996;46:1448–51.
305. Avellis G. Klinische Beitrage zur halbseitigen Kehlkopflamung. *Berl Klin Wochenschr* 1891;40:1–26.
306. Aver'ianov I, Il'ina NA, Nechkina NP et al. Ophthalmoplegia plus (multisystem mitochondrial cytopathy) in childhood. *Zh Nevropatol Psikiatr* 1983;83:1624–8.
307. Averback P. Primary cerebral venous thrombosis in young adults: The diverse manifestations of an underrecognized disease. *Ann Neurol* 1978;3:81–6.
308. Averbuch-Heller L, Zivotovsky AZ, Das VE et al. Investigations of the pathogenesis of acquired pendular nystagmus. *Brain* 1995;118:369–78.
309. Avoni P, Monari L, Carelli V et al. Congenital encephalomyopathy with Epilepsy, Chorioretinitis, Basal Ganglia Involvement and Muscle Minicores. *Ann Neurol* 2000;47:399.
310. Awang DVC. Feverfew. *Pharmaceutical Journal* 1987;239:487.
311. Axenfeld T. Cyclic oculomotor paralysis. *Klin Mbl Augenh* 1901;39:64–73.
312. Ay H, Buonanno FS, Price BH et al. Sensory alien hand syndrome: Case report and review of the literature. *J Neurol Neurosurg Psychiatry* 1998;65:366–9.
313. Azher SN, Jankovic J. Camptocormia. *Neurology* 2005;65:355–9.
314. Azouvi P, Bergigo C, Robel L et al. Slowly progressive apraxia: Two case studies. *J Neurol* 1993;240:347–50.
315. Azzarelli B, Roessmann U. Diffuse anoxic myelopathy. *Neurology* 1977;27:1049–52.
316. B'chir Hamzaoui S, Bouslama K, Abdallah M. Familial mediterranean fever. *Rev Neurol (Paris)* 2007;163:93–5.
317. Baar HS, Gabriel AM. Sex linked spastic paraplegia. *Am J Ment Defic* 1966;71:13–8.
318. Baastrup CI. On the spinous processes of the lumbar vertebra and the soft tissues between them, and on pathological changes in that region. *Acta Radiol* 1933;14:52–4.
319. Babel J. Association d'un diabete Juvenile Insulino-dépendant et d'atrophie optique. *Rev Med Suisse Rom* 1980;100:337–41.
320. Babikian V, Ropper AH. Binswanger's disease: A review. *Stroke* 1987;18:2–12.
321. Babinski J. Sur le réflexe cutane plantaire dans certains affections organique de système nerveux central. *C R Soc Biol* 1896;48:207–8.
322. Babinski J. Des troubles pupillaires dans les anévrismes de l'aorte. *Bull Soc Hop Paris* 1901;18:1121–4.
323. Babinski J. De l'équilibre volitionnel statique et de l'équilibre volitionnel cinétique. *Rev Neurol* 1902;10:470–4.
324. Babinski J. Hemispasme faciale periphérique. *Nouv Icon Salpet* 1905;18:418–23.
325. Babinski J. Contribution a l'étude des troubles mentaux dans l'hemiplégie organique cérébrale (anosognosie). *Rev Neurol* 1914;22:845–8.
326. Babinski J, Froment JC. *Bull Acad Med Paris* 1916;75:40–7.
327. Babinski J, Nageotte J. Hemiasynergie, lateropulsion et miosis bulbaire. *Nouv Icon Salpet* 1902;492.
328. Backonja M, Krause S. Neuropathic pain questionnaire – short form. *Clin J Pain* 2003;19:315–6.
329. Badhwar A, Berkovic SF, Dowling JP et al. Action myoclonus-renal failure syndrome: Characterization of a unique cerebro-renal disorder. *Brain* 2004;127:2173–82.
330. Bahill AT, Hsu FK, Stark L. Glissadic overshoots are due to pulse width errors. *Arch Neurol* 1978;35:138–42.
331. Bahill AT, Troost BT. Types of saccadic eye movements. *Neurology* 1979;29:1150–2.
332. Bailey P. Reflections aroused by an unusual tumor of the cerebellum. *J Mt Sinai Hosp* 1942;9:299–310.
333. Bailey P, Cushing HW. Medulloblastoma cerebelli: A common type of midcerebellar glioma in childhood. *Arch Neurol Psychiatry* 1925;14:192–225.
334. Bailey P, Cushing HW. *A Classification of the Tumors of the Glioma Group on a Histogenetic Basis with a Correlated Study of Prognosis.* Philadelphia: J.B. Lippincott, 1926.
335. Bailey RO, Dentinger MP, Tome ME et al. Benign muscular dystrophy with contractures. *Acta Neurol Scand* 1986;73:439–43.
336. Bailey RO, Markules DL, Hans MTS. Infantile facioscapulohumeral muscular dystrophy. *Acta Neurol Scand* 1986;74:51–8.
337. Baillarger J-G-F. General paralysis – a new symptom. *Gaz Hop Civ Milit* 1850;2:225.
338. Baillarger J-G-F. *Récherches sur l'anatomie, la physiologie et la pathologie du système nerveux.* Paris: Victor Masson, 1872.
339. Bain P, Brin M, Deuschl G et al. Criteria for the diagnosis of essential tremor. *Neurology* 2000;54:5–7.
340. Bain P. A combined clinical and neurophysiological approach to the study of patients with tremor. *J Neurol Neurosurg Psychiatry* 1993;69:839–44.
341. Bain P, Brin M, Deuschl G et al. Criteria for the diagnosis of essential tremor. *Neurology* 2000;54 **(Suppl. 4)**: S7.
342. Bajaj NPS, Waldman A, Orrel R et al. Familial adult onset of Krabbe disease resembling hereditary spastic paraplegia with normal neuroimaging. *J Neurol Neurosurg Psychiatry* 2002;72: 635–8.
343. Baker AB, Adams JM. Lipomatosis of the central nervous system. *Am J Cancer* 1938;34:214.
344. Baker GA, Smith DF, Dewey M et al. The development of a seizure severity scale as an outcome measure in epilepsy. *Epilepsy Research* 1991;8:245–51.
345. Baker RS, Ross PA, Baumann RJ. Neurologic complications of the epidermal nevus syndrome. *Arch Neurol* 1987;44:227–32.
346. Balasubramanian M, Ramamurthi B. An unusual location of Guinea worm infestation. *J Neurosurg* 1965;23:537.
347. Balduzzi O. A new reflex of the contralateral adductor muscles. *Rev Neurol* 1926;2:243–6.
348. Bale JF. Human cytomegalovirus infection and disorders of the nervous system. *Arch Neurol* 1984;41:310–20.
349. Balestrini MR, Cavaletti G, D'Angelo A, Tredici G. Infantile hereditary neuropathy with hypomyelination: Report of two siblings with different expressivity. *Neuropediatrics* 1991;22:65–70.
350. Balint R. Seelenlahmung des "Schauens", optische Ataxia, raumliche Storung der Aufmerskameit. *Mschr Psychiat Neurol* 1909;25:51–81.
351. Baller F. Radiusaplasie und Inzucht. *Z Menschl Vererb Konstit Lehre* 1950;29:782–790.
352. Ballet G. External ophthalmoplegia and bulbar palsy. *RMP* 1888;8:337, 355, 513–546.
353. Balo J. Encephalitis periaxalis concentrica. *Arch Neurol* 1928;19:242–64.
354. Baloh RB. Charles Skinner Hallpike and the beginnings of neurotology. *Neurology* 2000;54:2138–46.

355. Baloh RB. Superior semicircular canal dehiscence syndrome. *Neurology* 2004;62:684–5.
356. Baloh RB, Foster CA, Yue Q et al. Familial migraine with vertigo and essential tremor. *Neurology* 1996;46:458–60.
357. Baloh RB, Jacobson K, Honrubia V. Horizontal semicircular canal variant of benign positional vertigo. *Neurology* 1993;43:2542–9.
358. Baloh RB, Yue Q, Jacobson KM et al. Persistent direction-changing positional nystagmus. *Neurology* 1995;45:1297–301.
359. Baloh RW. Robert Bárány and the controversy surrounding his discovery of the caloric reaction. *Neurology* 2002;58:1094–9.
360. Baloh RW, DeRossett SE, Cloughesy TF et al. Novel brainstem syndrome associated with prostate carcinoma. *Neurology* 1993;43:2591–6.
361. Baloh RW, Furman JMR, Yee RD. Dorsal midbrain syndrome: Clinical and oculographic findings. *Neurology* 1985;35:54–60.
362. Baloh RW, Honrubia V, Jacobson K. Benign positional vertigo. *Neurology* 1987;37:371–8.
363. Baloh RW, Jacobson K, Fife T. Familial vestibulopathy. *Neurology* 1994;44:20–5.
364. Baloh RW, Konrad HR, Dirks D et al. Cerebellar-pontine angle tumors. *Arch Neurol* 1976;33:507–12.
365. Baloh RW, Sills AW, Kumley WE et al. Quantitative measurement of saccade amplitude, duration and velocity. *Neurology* 1975;25:1065–70.
366. Bamberger Hv. Saltatorischer Refelexkrampf, eine merkwurdige Form vom Spinal-Irritation. *Wien Med Wschr* 1859;49–67.
367. Bamford JM. Interobserver agreement for the assessment of handicap in stroke. *Stroke* 1989;20: 828.
368. Bamford JM, Sandercock P, Dennis M et al. Classification and natural history of clinically identifiable subtypes of cerebral infarction. *Lancet* 1991;337:1521–6.
369. Bancaud J. Kojewnikow's syndrome (epilepsia partialis continua) in children. In Roger J, Dravet C, Bureau M et al., eds. *Epileptic Syndromes*, pp 286–98. London: John Libbey, 1985.
370. Banfield GK, Crate ID, Griffiths CL. Long-term sequelae of Palmar-Plantar erythrodysaesthesia syndrome secondary to 5-fluouracil therapy. *J Roy Soc Med* 1995;88:365P–57P.
371. Banker BQ, Chester CS. Ischemic infarction of thigh muscle in the diabetic patient. *Neurology* 1973;23:667–77.
372. Banker BQ, Victor M, Adams RD. Arthrogryposis multiplex due to congenital muscular dystrophy. *Brain* 1957;80:319–34.
373. Banks G, Short P, Martinez AJ et al. The Alien hand syndrome. *Arch Neurol* 1989;46:456–9.
374. Bannister R, Davis B, Holly E et al. Defective cardiovascular reflexes and supersensitivity to sympathomimetic drugs in autonomic failure. *Brain* 1979;102:144–9.
375. Bannwarth A. Chronische lymphocytare Meningitis, entzundliche Polyneuritis und "Rheumatismus." *Arch Psychiat (Berlin)* 1941;113:284–376.
376. Baquis GD, Pessin MS, Scott RM. Limb shaking – a carotid TIA. *Stroke* 1985;16:444–8.
377. Barac B. Vertiginous epileptic attacks and so-called vestibulogenic seizures. *Epilepsia* 1968;9:137–44.
378. Baraitser M. The Orofaciodigital (OFD) syndromes. *J Med Genet* 1986;23:116–9.
379. Baraitser M. *The Genetics of Neurological Disorders*. Oxford: Oxford University Press, 1990.
380. Baraitser M, Burn J, Fixsen J. A female infant with features of Mohr and Majewsky syndromes: Variable expression, a genetic compound or a distinct entity. *J Med Genet* 1983;20:65–7.
381. Baraitser M, Tomiwa K, Wilson J et al. A database of genetically determined neurological conditions for clinicians. *J Neurol Neurosurg Psychiatry* 1989;52:106–7.
382. Baraitser M, Winter RM, Brett EM. Greig cephalopolysyndactyly: Report of 13 affected individuals in three families. *Clin Genet* 1983;24:257–65.
383. Barak Y, Lavie M, Achiron A. Screening for cognitive impairment in multiple sclerosis patients using the clock drawing test. *J Clin Neurosci* 2002;9: 629–32.
384. Barany R. Vestibularapparat und Centralnervensystem. *Med Klin Berlin* 1911;7:1818–21.
385. Barbeau A. Distribution of ataxia in Quebec. In Sobue I, ed. *Spino-cerebellar degeneration*, pp 120–2. Tokyo: Tokyo University Press, 1980.
386. Barber HS. Myalgic syndrome with constitutional effects; polymyalgia rheumatica. *Ann Rheumat Dis* 1957;16:230–7.
387. Barbieri F, Pellechia MT, Esposito E et al. Adult onset familial laryngeal abductor paralysis, cerebellar ataxia and pure motor neuropathy. *Neurology* 2001;56:1412–4.
388. Barbieri F, Santangelo R, Capperelli G et al. Autosomal recessive motor and sensory neuropathy with excessive myelin outfolding in two siblings. *Can J Neurol Sci* 1994;21:29–33.
389. Barcia-Goyanes JJ, Calvo W, Barcia-Salorio JL. A new method for exploration of the cerebral circulation. *Rev Esp Oto-neuro-oftal* 1953;241–6.
390. Bardet G. *Sur un syndrome d'obesity congenitale avec polydactylie et retinite pigmentaire.* Paris: Thèse, Université de Paris, 1920.
391. Bardosi A, DiMauro S, Servidei S et al. Myo-neuro-gastro-intesting-encephalopathy. *Muscle Nerve* 1986;9:177–81.
392. Bardwick PA, Zvaifler NJ, Gill GN, et al. Plasma cell dyscrasia with polyneuropathy, organomegaly, M protein and skin changes; the POEMS syndrome. *Medicine* 1980;59:311–22.
393. Barer N, Nouri F. Measurement of activities of daily living. *Clin Rehabil* 1990;3:179–87.
394. Barjon P, Labauger R, Cazaban R et al. Primary optic atrophy, hearing loss and juvenile diabetes mellitus. *Diabetes* 1964;11:231–7.
395. Barker RA, Revesz T, Thom M et al. Review of 23 patients affected by the stiff man syndrome: Clinical division into stiff trunk (man) syndrome, stiff limb syndrome and progressive encephalomyelitis with rigidity. *J Neurol Neurosurg Psychiatry* 1998;65:633–40.
396. Barkhaus PE, Morgan O. Jamaican neuropathy: An electrophysiological study. *Muscle Nerve* 1988;11:380–5.
397. Barkhof F, Rocca M, Francis G et al. Validation of diagnostic magnetic resonance imaging criteria for multiple sclerosis and response to interferon β1a. *Ann Neurol* 2003;53:718–24.
398. Barkovich AH, Jackson DE, Boyer RS. Band heterotopias: A newly recognized neuronal migration anomaly. *Radiology* 1989;171:455–8.
399. Barkovich AH, Kuzniecky R, Jackson GD et al. A developmental and genetic classification for malformations of cortical development. *Neurology* 2005;65:1873–87.
400. Barkovich AJ, Chuang SH. Unilateral megalencephaly. *Am J Neuroradiol* 1990;11:523–31.
401. Barkovich AJ, Kock TK, Carrol CL. The spectrum of lissencephaly: Report of 10 patients analyzed by magnetic resonance imaging. *Ann Neurol* 1991;30:139–46.
402. Barkovich AJ, Kuzniecky R. Gray matter heterotopia. *Neurology* 2000;55:1603–8.
403. Barkovich AJ, Kuzniecky R, Bollen AW et al. Focal transmantle dysplasia: A specific malformation of cortical development. *Neurology* 1997;49:1148–52.
404. Barkovich AJ, Kuzniecky R, Jackson GG et al. Classification system for

malformations of cortical development. *Neurology* 2001;57:2168–78.
405. Barkovich AJ, Millen KJ, Dobyns WB. A developmental classification of malformations of the brainstem. *Ann Neurol* 2007;62:625–39.
406. Barlow CF. *Headaches and Migraine in Childhood*. Philadelphia: Lippincott, 1984.
407. Barmada MA, Moosy J, Painter M. Pontosubicular necrosis and hyperoxemia. *Pediatrics* 1980;66:840.
408. Barnard RI, Scholz RO. Ophthalmoplegia and retinal degeneration. *Am J Ophthalmol* 1944;27:621–4.
409. Barnes D, Misra VP, Young EP et al. An adult onset hexosaminidase A deficiency syndrome with sensory neuropathy and internuclear ophthalmoplegia. *J Neurol Neurosurg Psychiatry* 1991;54:1112–3.
410. Barnes HD. Further South African cases of porphyrinuria. *South African J Clin Sci* 1951;2:117–69.
411. Barnes MP, Saunders M, Walls TJ. The syndrome of Karl Ludwig Kahlbaum. *J Neurol Neurosurg Psychiatry* 1986;49:991.
412. Barnett HJM, Wortzman G, Gladstone RM et al. Diversion and reversal of cerebral blood flow. *Neurology* 1970;20:1–14.
413. Barohn RJ, Kissel JT, Warmolts JR et al. Chronic inflammatory demyelinating polyradiculopathy: Clinical characteristics, course, and recommendations for diagnostic criteria. *Arch Neurol* 1989;46:878–84.
414. Barohn RJ, Miller RG, Griggs RC. Autosomal recessive distal dystrophy. *Neurology* 1991;41:1365–70.
415. Baron DN, Dent CE, Harris H, Hart EW, Jepson JB. Hereditary pellagra-like skin rash with temporary cerebellar ataxia, constant renal amino-aciduria and other bizarre biochemical features. *Lancet* 1956;2:421–8.
416. Baron JC, Bousser M-G, Comar D et al. "Crossed cerebellar diaschisis" in human supratentorial brain infarction. *Trans Amer Neurol Assn* 1980;105:459–61.
417. Baron JC, Busser M-G, Comar D et al. Crossed cerebellar diaschisis in human supratentorial infarction. *Ann Neurol* 1980;8:128.
418. Baron R, Levine JD, Fields HL. Causalgia and reflex sympathetic dystrophy: Does the sympathetic nervous system contribute to the generation of pain? *Muscle Nerve* 1999;22:678–95.
419. Barre JA. Chronic vertebral arthritis and medullar disturbances; chronic vertebral arthritis and tumor of the spinal cord. *Paris Med* 1925;2: 226.
420. Barre MJ. Sur un syndrome sympathique cervical posterieur et sa cause fréquent, l'arthrite cervicale. *Rev Neurol* 1926;1:1246–8.
421. Barrows HS. Neurological eponyms. *Arch Neurol* 1960;3:91–7.
422. Barry DT, Gooch J. Evoked acoustic signals as a measure of contractile properties of muscles. *Muscle Nerve* 1986;9:651a.
423. Barry MJ, VanSwearingen JM, Albright AL. Reliability and responsiveness of the Barry-Albright dystonia scale. *Devel Med Child Neurol* 1999;41:404–11.
424. Barsky RJ, Borus JF. Functional somatic syndromes. *Ann Int Med* 1999;130:910–21.
425. Bart RS, Pumphrey RE. Knuckle pads, leukonychia and deafness: A dominantly inherited syndrome. *N Engl J Med* 1967;276:202–7.
426. Barth PG, Blennow G, Lenard HG et al. The syndrome of autosomal recessive pontocerebellar hypoplasia, microcephaly and extrapyramidal dyskinesia (pontocerebellar hypoplasia type 2). *Neurology* 1995;45:311–7.
427. Barth PG, Gootjes J, Bode H et al. Late onset white matter disease in peroxisome biogenesis disorder. *Neurology* 2001;57:1949–55.
428. Barth PG, Hoffmann GF, Jaeken J et al. L-2-hydroxyglutaric acidemia: A novel inherited neurometabolic disease. *Ann Neurol* 1992;32:66–71.
429. Barth PG, Majoie CB, Caan MWA et al. Pontine tegmental cap dysplasia: A novel brain malformation with a defect in axonal guidance. *Brain* 2007;130:2258–66.
430. Barth PG, Majoie C, Gotjes J et al. Neuroimaging of peroxisome biogenesis disorders (Zellweger syndrome) with prolonged survival. *Neurology* 2004;62:444.
431. Bartt R. Listeria and atypical presentations of *Listeria* in the central nervous system. *Semin Neurol* 2000;20:361–73.
432. Bassen FA, Kornzweig AL. Malformation of the erythrocytes in a case of atypical retinitis pigmentosa. *Blood* 1950;5:381–7.
433. Bassetti C, Bogousslavsky J, Mattle H et al. Medial medullary stroke: Report of seven patients and review of the literature. *Neurology* 1997;48:882–90.
434. Bassetti C, Bogousslavsky J, Regli F. Sensory syndromes on parietal stroke. *Neurology* 1993;43:1942–9.
435. Bassoe CF. The skinache syndrome. *J Roy Soc Med* 1995;88:565–9.
436. Bassoe HH. Familial congenital muscular dystrophy with gonadal dysgenesis. *J Clin Endocrinology* 1956;16:1614–21.
437. Bassuk AG, McLone D, Bowman R et al. Autosomal dominant occipital cephalocele. *Neurology* 2004;62:1888.
438. Bastian AJ, Mink JW, Kaufman JA et al. Posterior vermal split syndrome. *Ann Neurol* 1998;44:601–10.
439. Bastian HC. On the various forms of loss of speech in cerebral disease. *Brit Med Chir Rev* 1869;43:209–36.
440. Bastian HC. On the symptomatology of total transverse lesions of the spinal cord, with special reference to the condition of the various reflexes. *Med Chir Trans* 1890;73:151–217.
441. Bateman DE, Saunders M. Cyclic oculomotor palsy: Description of a case and hypothesis of the mechanism. *J Neurol Neurosurg Psychiatry* 1983;46:451–3.
442. Batshaw ML. Inborn errors of urea synthesis. *Ann Neurol* 1994;35:133–41.
443. Battaglia A, Gurrieri F, Bertini E et al. The inv dup(15) syndrome. *Neurology* 1997;48:1081–6.
444. Batten FE. Cerebral degeneration with symmetrical changes in the maculae in two members of a family. *Trans Opthal Soc U K* 1903;23:386–90.
445. Batten FE. Acute poliomyelitis. *Brain* 1916;39:115–211.
446. Battistella PA et al. Carnitine deficiency induced during haemodialysis. *Lancet* 1978;i:939.
447. Baumann CR, Bassetti CL. Hypocretins (orexins) and sleep-wake disorders. *Lancet Neurology* 2005;4:673–82.
448. Baumann N, Turpin J-C. Adult-onset leukodystrophies. *J Neurol* 2000;247:751–9.
449. Baumgarten M, Becker R, Gauthier S. Validity and reliability of the dementia behavior disturbance scale. *J Am Geriatr Soc* 1990;38:221.
450. Baumgartner MR, Poll-The BT, Verhoeven NM et al. Clinical approach to genetic peroxisomal disorders: A series of 27 patients. *Ann Neurol* 1998;44:720–30.
451. Bautista J, Rafel E, Castilla JM et al. Hereditary distal myopathy with onset in early infancy. *J Neurol Sci* 1978;37:149–58.
452. Baxter DM, Warrington EK. Ideational agraphia: A single case study. *J Neurol Neurosurg Psychiatry* 1986;369:374.
453. Baxter DW, Olszewski J. Congenital universal insensitivity to pain. *Brain* 1983;83:381–93.
454. Bay E. Disturbances of visual perception and their examination. *Brain* 1953;76:515–50.
455. Bayle ALJ. *Récherches sur la maladie mentale: Thèse de Paris*. Paris: Université de Paris, 1822.
456. Beal MF, Fisher CM. Neoplastic angioendotheliosis. *J Neurol Sci* 1982;53:359–75.
457. Beal MF, Richardson EPJ. Primary lateral sclerosis: A case report. *Arch Neurol* 1981;38:630–3.
458. Beall SS, Patten BM, Janovik J. Familial calcification of the brain, iron storage and

porphyria: A new syndrome. *Ann Neurol* 1984;16:137.

459. Beard GM. Neurasthenia, or nervous exhaustion. *Boston Med Surg J* 1869;80:217–21.
460. Beard GM. Remarks on "jumpers" or "jumping frenchmen". *J Nerv Ment Dis* 1878;5:526.
461. Beard GM. *A Practical Treatise on Nervous Exhaustion (Neurasthenia)*. New York: W.Wood & Co., 1880.
462. Beatty RA. The piriformis muscle syndrome: A simple diagnostic maneuver. *Neurosurgery* 1994;34:512–4.
463. Beauchesne P, Pialat J, Duthel R et al. Aggressive treatment with complete remission in primary diffuse leptomeningeal gliomatosis – a case report. *J NeuroOncol* 1998;37:161–7.
464. Beauvieux J. Quelques aspects de syncinésies oculaires. *Concours Med* 1952;74:369–72.
465. Beauvois M-F, Derouesne J. Lexical or orthographic agraphia. *Brain* 1981;104:21–49.
466. Bech-Azeddine R, Hogh P, Juhler M et al. Idiopathic normal pressure hydrocephalus. *J Neurol Neurosurg Psychiatr* 2007;78:157–61.
467. Beck AT, Ward CH, Mendelson M et al. An inventory for measuring depression. *Arch Gen Psychiat* 1961;4:561–71.
468. Beck K. The syndrome of anterior spinal artery thrombosis. *Dtsch Z Nervenklinik* 1952;164–86.
469. Becker DP, Grossman RG, McLaurin RL et al. Head injuries – panel 3. *Arch Neurol* 1979;36:750–8.
470. Becker GD, Davis JL, Parell J. Pseudocaloric nystagmus. *Arch Neurol* 1978;35:93–4.
471. Becker LE. Synaptic dysgenesis. *Can J Neurol Sci* 1991;18:170–80.
472. Becker PE. Neue Ergebnisse der Genetik der Muskeldystrophien. *Acta Genet* 1957;7:303–10.
473. Beckham JC, Krug LM, Penzien DB et al. The relationship of ovarian steroids, headache activity and menstrual distress: A pilot study with female migraineurs. *Headache* 1992;32:292–7.
474. Beckman E. A celebrated case of cerebral injury. *Bull Med Hist* 1945;17:521–6.
475. Bedry R, Baudrimont I, Deffieux G et al. Wild-mushroom intoxication as a cause of rhabdomyolysis. *N Engl J Med* 2001 Sep 13;345(11):798–802.
476. Beede HE, Newcomb RW. Lower motor neurone paralysis in association with asthma. *Johns Hopkins Med J* 1980;147:186–7.
477. Beeson D, Newland C, Croxen R et al. Congenital myasthenic syndromes. Studies of the AChR and other candidate genes. *Ann N Y Acad Sci* 1998;841:181–3.
478. Beeson D, Palace J, Vincent A. Congenital myasthenic syndromes. *Curr Opin Neurol* 1997;10:402–7.
479. Beevor CE. The cerebral arterial supply. *Brain* 1907;30:403.
480. Begbie J. Remarks on rheumatism and chorea; their relation and treatment. *Month J Med Sci* 1847;7:740–54.
481. Beghi E, Kurland LT, Mulder DW et al. Brachial plexus neuropathy in the population of Rochester, Minnesota, 1970–1981. *Ann Neurol* 1985;18:320–3.
482. Behcet H. Uber rezidivierende, aphthose durch ein Virus verurasachte Geschwure am Mund, am Auge und an dem Genitalien. *Derm Wschr* 1937;105:1152–7.
483. Behr C. Die komplizierte, hereditar-familiare Optikusatrophie des Kindesalters. Ein bisher nicht beschreibener Symptomkomplex. *Klin Mbl Augenh* 1909;47:138–60.
484. Behr C. Die Heredodegeneration der Makula. *Klin Mbl Augenh* 1920;65:465–505.
485. Behrman S. Vestibular epilepsy. *Brain* 1955;78:471–86.
486. Behrman S. Pathology of papilledema. *Brain* 1966;89:1–14.
487. Beighton P et al. Osteoglophonic dwarfism. *Pediat Radiol* 1980;10:46–50.
488. Beighton PH, Hamersma H, Raad M. Oculodento-osseous dysplesia – variability of expression within a large family. *Clin Genet* 1979;16:169–77.
489. Bejsovec M, Kulenda Z, Ponca E. Familial intrauterine convulsions in pyridoxine dependency. *Arch Dis Child* 1967;42:201–7.
490. Bekhterev VM. Die Bedeutung der Sehhugel auf Grund von experimentalen und pathologische Daten. *Virchow's Arch Path Anat Physiol* 1887;110:102–54.
491. Belafsky MA, Rosman NP, Miller P et al. Prolonged epileptic twilight state. *Neurology* 1978;28:239–45.
492. Belal S, Cancel G, Stevanin G et al. Clinical and genetic analysis of a Tunisian family with autosomal dominant cerebellar ataxia type 1 linked to the SCA2 locus. *Neurology* 1994;44:1423–6.
493. Bell C. On the nerves; giving an account of some experiments on their structure and functions which lead to a new arrangement of the system. *Phil Trans Roy Soc Lond* 1821;111:398–424.
494. Bell C. On the motions of the eye, an illustration of the uses of the muscles and nerves of the orbit. *Phil Trans Roy Soc Lond* 1823;113:166–86.
495. Bell HS. Cruciate paralysis. *J Neurosurg* 1970;33:376–90.
496. Bell JA, Fielder AR, Viney S. Congenital double elevator palsy in identical twins. *J Clin Neuroophthalmol* 1990;10:38–40.
497. Bell R, Font RL. Granulomatous anterior uveitis caused by *Coccidioides immitis*. *Am J Ophthalmol* 1972;74:93–8.
498. Bell WE, Van Allen MW. Agenesis of the corpus callosum with associated facial abnormalities. *Neurology* 1959;9:694–8.
499. Bell SP, Frankel A, Brown EA. Cholesterol emboli syndrome – uncommon or unrecognized? *J Roy Soc Med* 1997;90:543–6.
500. Belman AL, Lantos G, Houroupian D et al. AIDS: Calcification of the basal ganglia in infants and children. *Neurology* 1986;36:1192.
501. Ben Hamida M, Belal S, Sirugo G et al. Friedreich's ataxia phenotype not linked to chromosome 9 and associated with selective autosomal recessive vitamin E deficiency in two inbred Tunisian families. *Neurology* 1993;43:2179–83.
502. Ben Hamida M, Fardeau M, Attia N. Severe childhood muscular dystrophy affecting both sexes and frequent in Tunisia. *Muscle Nerve* 1983;6:469.
503. Ben Yaou R, Bécane HM, Demay L et al. Autosomal dominant limb-girdle muscular dystrophy associated with conduction defects (LGMD1B): A description of 8 new families with the LMNA gene mutations. *Rev Neurol (Paris)* 2005;161:42–54.
504. Benbadis SR, Lancman ME, King LM et al. Preictal pseudosleep: A new finding in psychogenic seizures. *Neurology* 1996;47:63–7.
505. Bender L. *A Visual Motor Gestalt Test and Its Clinical Use*. New York: American Orthopsychiatric Association, 1938.
506. Bender MB. Syndrome of isolated episode of confusion with amnesia. *J Hillside Hosp* 1956;5:212–5.
507. Bender MB. Oscillopsia. *Arch Neurol* 1965;13:204–13.
508. Bender MB, Fink M, Green M. Patterns in perception on simultaneous test of face and hand. *Arch Neurol Psychiatry* 1951;66:355–62.
509. Bender MB, Stacy C, Cohen J. Agraphesthesia. *J Neurol Sci* 1982;53:531–55.
510. Bender MD. Polyopia and monocular diplopia of cerebral origin. *Arch Neurol Psychiatry* 1945;54:323.
511. Benedek L. Zwangsmassig Schreien in Anfallen als postencephalitische Hyperkinese. *Z Ges Neurol Psychiat* 1925;98:17–26.
512. Benedict RH, Munschauer F, Linn R et al. Screening for multiple sclerosis cognitive impairment using a

self-administered 15 item questionnaire. *Mult Scler* 2003;9:95–101.
513. Benedikt M. Tremblement avec paralysie croissée du moteur oculaire commun. *Bull Soc Med Hop Paris* 1889;3:547–8.
514. Bengtzen R, Woodward M, Lynn MJ et al. The "sunglasses" sign predicts nonorganic visual loss in neuro-ophthalmologic practice. *Neurology* 2008;70:218–21.
515. Benhaiem-Sigaux N, Gray F, Gherardi R et al. Expanding cerebellar lacunes due to dilatation of the perivascular space associated with Binswanger's subcortical arteriosclerotic encephalopathy. *Stroke* 1987;18:1087–92.
516. Bennett BM, Bong DM, Spargo BH. Neuropsychiatric problems in mixed connective tissue disease. *Amer J Med* 1978;65:955–62.
517. Bennett CL, Lawson VH, Brickness KL et al. Late-onset hereditary axonal neuropathies. *Neurology* 2008;71:14–20.
518. Bennett DA, Wilson RS, Gilley DW et al. Clinical diagnosis of Binswanger's disease. *J Neurol Neurosurg Psychiatry* 1990;53:961–5.
519. Bennett NM. Murray valley encephalitis, 1974: Clinical features. *Med J Aust* 1976;ii:446–50.
520. Benomar A, Le Guern E, Durr A et al. Autosomal Dominant Cerebellar Ataxia with Retinal Degeneration (ADCA Type II) is genetically different from ADCA Type I. *Ann Neurol* 1994;35: 439–44.
521. Benson DF. The aphasias and related disturbances. In Baker AB, Baker LH, eds. *Cli Neurol* pp 1–26. New York: Harper and Row, 1971.
522. Benson DF. The third alexia. *Arch Neurol* 1977;34:327–31.
523. Benson DF. Neurologic correlates of anomia. In Whitaker H, ed. *Studies in Neurolinguistics* pp 293–328. New York: Academic Press, 1979.
524. Benson DF, Davis JR, Synder BD. Posterior cortical atrophy. *Arch Neurol* 1988;45:789–93.
525. Benson DF, Djenderedjian A, Miller BL et al. Neural basis of confabulation. *Neurology* 1996;46:1239–43.
526. Benson DF, Geschwind N. The alexias. In Vinken PJ, Bruyn GW, eds. *Handbook of Neurology* pp 112–40. Amsterdam: North Holland Publishing Co., 1969.
527. Benson DF, Geschwind N. Aphasia and related disorders: A clinical approach. In Mesulam M-M, ed. *Principles of Behavioral Neurology* pp 193–238. Philadelphia: F.A. Davis Co., 1985.
528. Benstead TJ, Grant IA. Charcot-Marie-Tooth disease and related inherited peripheral neuropathies. *Can J Neurol Sci* 2001;28:199–214.
529. Bentley JF, Smith JR. Developmental posterior enteric remnants and spinal malformations: The split notochord syndrome. *Arch Dis Child* 1960;35:76–86.
530. Benton AL. Differential behavioral effects in frontal lobe disease. *Neuropsychologia* 1968;6:53–60.
531. Benton AL. *Revised Visual Retention Test: Clinical and Experimental Applications.* New York: Psychological Corporation, 1974.
532. Benton AL. Historical notes on hemispheric dominance. *Arch Neurol* 1977;34:127–9.
533. Benton AL, Hamsher KdS, Varney N et al. *Contributions to Neuropsychological Assessment*. New York: Oxford University Press, 1983.
534. Benton AL, Joynt RJ. Early descriptions of aphasia. *Arch Neurol* 1960;3:205–22.
535. Benton AL, Levin HS. An experimental study of "obscuration". *Neurology* 1972;22:1176–81.
536. Benton JW, Nellhaus G, Huttenlocher PR et al. The bobble-head doll syndrome: Report of a unique truncal tremor associated with third ventricular cyst and hydrocephalus in children. *Neurology* 1966;16:725–9.
537. Benzer A, Mitterschlifftbaler G, Marosi M et al. Prediction of non-survival after trauma: Innsbruck coma scale. *Lancet* 1991;338:977–8.
538. Beradinelli W. An undiagnosed endocrine metabolic syndrome. *J Clin Endocrinol* 1954;14:193.
539. Berant W, Berant N. Radioulnar synostosis and craniosynostosis syndromes. *Birth Defects Orig Artic Ser* 1992;11:137–89.
540. Berchtold MW, Brinkmeier H, Muntener M et al. Calcium ions in skeletal muscle: Its crucial role for muscle function, plasticity and disease. *Physiol Rev* 2000;80:1215–65.
541. Berciano J. Olivopontocerebellar atrophy. *J Neurol Sci* 1982;53:253–72.
542. Berciano J, Boesch S, Pérez-Ramos JM et al. Olivopontocerebellar atrophy: Toward a better nosological definition. *Mov Disord* 2006;21:1607–13.
543. Berciano J, Gallardo E, Dominguez-Perlez R et al. Autosomal dominant distal myopathy with a myotilin S55F mutation. *J Neurol Neurosurg Psychiatry* 2007;79:205–8.
544. Berenberg RA, Pellock JM, DiMauro S et al. Lumping or splitting? "Ophthalmoplegia plus" or Kearns-Sayre syndrome? *Ann Neurol* 1977;1:37–54.
545. Beresford OD, Graham AM. Chorea gravidarum. *J Obstet Gynecol Br Empire* 1950;57:616–25.
546. Berg AT, Panayiotopoulos CP. Diversity in epilepsy and a newly recognized benign childhood syndrome. *Neurology* 2000;55:1073–4.
547. Berg BO, Rosenberg S, Asbury AK. Giant axonal neuropathy. *Pediatrics* 1972;49:894–9.
548. Berg L. Clinical dementia rating (CDR). *Psychopharm Bull* 1988;24:637.
549. Berg L. Mild senile dementia of the Alzheimer type: Diagnostic criteria and natural history. *Mt Sinai J Med* 1988;55:87–96.
550. Berg MJ, Williams LS. The transient syndrome of headache with neurologic deficits and CSF lymphomatosis. *Neurology* 1995;45:1648–54.
551. Bergara C. Un nuevo signo de paralisis facial. *Rev Espec Asoc Med Argentina* 1929;4:556–60.
552. Berger E. Pupillary and other disturbances in tabes. *Arch Augenheilk* 1889;19:305–53.
553. Berger J. Uber das Elektrenkephalogramm des Menschen. *Arch Psychiat Nervenkr* 1929;87:527–70.
554. Berger J, Moser HW, Forss-Petter S. Leukodystrophies: Recent developments in genetics, molecular biology, pathogenesis and treatment. *Curr Opin Neurol* 2001;14:305–12.
555. Berger JR, Oral EA, Taylor SI. Familial lipodystrophy associated with neurodegeneration and congenital cataracts. *Neurology* 2002;58:43–7.
556. Berger JR, Weaver A, Greenlee JE et al. Neurologic consequences of autoimmune polyglandular syndrome type 1. *Neurology* 2008;70:2248–51.
557. Berger L, Luc, Richard. L'esthesioneuroepitheliome olfactif. *Bull Assoc Fr Etude Cancer* 1924;13:410–21.
558. Berger MS, Wilson CB. Epidermoid cysts of the posterior fossa. *J Neurosurg* 1985;62:214–9.
559. Bergia B, Sybers HD, Butler IJ. Familial lethal cardiomyopathy with mental retardation and scapulo-peroneal muscular dystrophy. *J Neurol Neurosurg Psychiatry* 1986;49:1423–6.
560. See 559.
561. Berginer VM, Salen G, Shefer S. Cerebrotendinous xanthomatosis. *Neurol Clin* 1989;7:55–74.
562. Bergner M, Bobbit RA, Carter J et al. The sickness impact profile. Development and final revision of a health status measure. *Medical Care* 1981;19:787–805.
563. Bergstedt M, Johansson S, Muller R. Hereditary spastic ataxia with central retinal degeneration and vestibular impairment. *Neurology* 1962;12:124–32.
564. Beri M, Klugman MR, Kohler JA et al. Anterior ischemic optic neuropathy: VII.

Incidence of bilaterality and various influencing factors. *Ophthalmology* 1987;94:1020–8.
565. Beric A. Central pain: "New" syndromes and their evaluation. *Muscle Nerve* 1994;16:1017–24.
566. Beric A, Light JK. Anorgasmia in anterior spinal cord syndrome. *J Neurol Neurosurg Psychiatry* 1993;56:548–51.
567. Berkovic S, Carpenter S, Andermann F et al. Kufs' disease: A critical reappraisal. *Brain* 1988;111:27–62.
568. Berkovic S et al. Progressive myoclonus epilepsies: Specific causes and diagnosis. *N Engl J Med* 1986;315:296–305.
569. Berkovic S, McIntosh AM, Howell RA et al. Familial temporal lobe epilepsy: A common disorder identified in twins. *Ann Neurol* 1996;40:227–35.
570. Berkovic SF, Mazarib A. A new clinical and molecular form of Unverricht-Lundborg disease localized by homozygosity mapping. *Brain* 2005;128:652–8.
571. Berkovic SF, Scheffer IE. Genetics of the epilepsies. *Curr Opin Neurol* 1999;12:177–82.
572. Berkowitz BW. Matutinal vertigo: Clinical characteristics and possible management. *Arch Neurol* 1985;42: 874–7.
573. Berlin C. Congenital generalized melanoleucoderma associated with hypodontia, hypotrichosis, stunted growth, and mental retardation occurring in two brothers and two sisters. *Dermatologica* 1961;123:227–43.
574. Berlin L. A peroneal muscle stretch reflex. *Neurology* 1971;21:1177–8.
575. Berlin R. *Eine Besondere Art Der Wortblindheit.* Wiesbaden: J.F. Bergmann, 1887.
576. Berlit P. Car toll neuropathy. *J Neurol Neurosurg Psychiatry* 1993;56:1329.
577. Berman B. Voluntary propulsion of the eyeballs. *Arch Int Med* 1966;117:648.
578. Berman ER, Livni N, Shapira E et al. Congenital corneal clouding with abnormal systemic storage bodies: A new variant of mucolipidosis. *J Pediatr* 1974;84:519–26.
579. Berman W, Haslam RHA, Konigsmark BW et al. A new familial syndrome with ataxia, hearing loss, and mental retardation. *Arch Neurol* 1973;29:258–61.
580. Bermils C, Tassin S, Brvela J-M et al. Idiopathic recurrent myoglobinuria and persistent weakness. *Neurology* 1983;33:1613–5.
581. Bernard C. Experience sur les fonctions de la portion cephalique du grand sympathique. *C R Soc Biol* 1854;5:77.
582. Bernard C. Des phenomenes oculo-pupillaires produits par la section du nerf sympathique cervical: Ils sont independents des phénomènes vasculaires caloriques de la tête. *C R Acad Sci (Paris)* 1862;55:381–8.
583. Bernhardt M. Ueber isoliert im Gebiete des N. cutaneous femoris externus vorkommende Parasthesien. *Neurol Centralbl* 1895;14:242–4.
584. Bernier FP, Boneh A, Dennett X et al. Diagnostic criteria for respiratory chain disorders in adults and children. *Neurology* 2002;59:1406–11.
585. Bernstein EF, Browse NL. The CHAT classification of stroke. *Ann Surg* 1989;209:242–8.
586. Berrios GE. Depressive pseudodementia or melancholic dementia: A 19th century view. *J Neurol Neurosurg Psychiatry* 1985;48:393–400.
587. Berry H. Examination of the central portion of the visual fields at the bedside. *Brit J Ophth* 1963;47:435–40.
588. Berry H, MacDonald EA, Mrazek AC. Accessory nerve palsy: A review of 23 cases. *Can J Neurol Sci* 1991;18:337–41.
589. Berry-Kravis E, Abrams L, Coffey SM et al. Fragile X-associated tremor/ataxia syndrome: Clinical features, genetics, and testing guidelines. *Mov Disord* 2008;22:2018–30.
590. Bertola L, Pedrocca A. Oste opatie nevralgiformi lombosciatalgiche a localizzazioni vertebrali e paravertebrali (Sindrome del Camera). *Minerva Orthop* 1953;4:215–8.
591. Bertolotti M. Les syndromes lombo-ischialgiques d'origine vertèbrale. *Rev Neurol* 1922;38:1112–25.
592. Bertoni JM, Schwartzman RJ, Van Horn G et al. Asterixis and encephalopathy following metrizamide myelography: Investigations into possible mechanisms and review of the literature. *Ann Neurol* 1981;9:366–70.
593. Bertoni JM, von Loh S, Allen RJ. The Aicardi syndrome: Report of 4 cases and review of the literature. *Ann Neurol* 1979;5:475–82.
594. Bertorini T, Woodhouse C, Horner L. Muscle hypertrophy secondary to the tethered cord syndrome. *Muscle Nerve* 1994;17:331–5.
595. Bertorini T, Yeh Y-Y, Trevisan C et al. Carnitine palmitoyl transferase deficiency: Myoglobinuria and respiratory failure. *Neurology* 1980;30:263–71.
596. Bertrand J. *Anatomico-Clinical Study of Ollivier's Disease*. Lyon, France: Université de Lyon, 1932.
597. Besana G, Comi G, del Maschio A et al. Electrophysiological and MRI evaluation of neurological involvement in Behcet's disease. *J Neurol Neurosurg Psychiatry* 1989;52:749–54.
598. Bessman SP, Baldwin R. Imidazole aminoaciduria in cerebromacular degeneration. *Science* 1962;135:789–91.
599. Bethlem J, Van Gool J, Hulsmann WC, Meijer AEFH. Familial non-progressive myopathy with muscle cramps after exertion. *Brain* 1966;89:569–88.
600. Bethlem J, Van Wijngaarden GK. The incidence of ringed fibres and sarcoplasmic masses in normal and diseased muscle. *J Neurol Neurosurg Psychiatry* 1963;26:326–32.
601. Bethlem J, Van Wijngaarden GK. Centronuclear myopathy with type 1 fiber atrophy and myotubes. *Arch Neurol* 1970;23:70–3.
602. Betz VA. Anatomischer Nachweis zweiter Gehirncentra. *Zbl Med Wiss* 1874;12:578–95.
603. Beversdorf BQ, Heilman K. Facilitatory paratonia and frontal lobe functioning. *Neurology* 1998;51:968–71.
604. Bhagat K, Vallance P. Nitric oxide 9 years on. *J Roy Soc Med* 1996;89:667–73.
605. Bhandari B, Gupta BM, Garg AR. Touch epilepsy. *Indian J Pediatr* 1973;40:111–3.
606. Bharucha NE, Morgan-Hughes JA. Chronic focal polymyositis in the adult. *J Neurol Neurosurg Psychiatry* 1981;44:419–25.
607. Bhatia KP. The paroxysmal dyskinesias. *J Neurol* 1999;246:149–55.
608. Bhatia KP, Bhatt MH, Marsden CD. The causalgia-dystonia syndrome. *Brain* 1993;116:843–51.
609. Bhatia KP, Brown P, Gregory R et al. Progressive myoclonic ataxia associated with coeliac disease. *Brain* 1995;118:1087–93.
610. Bhatia KP, Quinn NP, Marsden CD. Clinical features and natural history of axial predominant adult onset primary dystonia. *J Neurol Neurosurg Psychiatry* 1997;63:788–91.
611. Bhatia KP, Soland VL, Bhatt MH et al. Paroxysmal exercise-induced dystonia: Eight new sporadic cases and a review of the literature. *Mov Disord* 1997;12: 1007–12.
612. Bianchi E et al. A family with Saethre-Chotzen syndrome. *Am J Med Genet* 1985;22:649–58.
613. Bianchi L. La sindrome parietale. *Med Ital* 1911;9:187, 243–333.
614. Bianchine JW, Lewis RC. The MASA syndrome: A new heritable mental retardation syndrome. *Clin Genet* 1974;21:123–9.
615. Biary N, Cleeves L, Findley LJ et al. Post-traumatic tremor. *Neurology* 1989;39:103–6.
616. Bichat MFX. Nerfs de la vie organique. *Traite d'anatomie descriptive*, p 319. Paris: Masson, 1802.

617. Bicjnese AR, May W, Hickey WF et al. Early childhood hepatocerebral degeneration misdiagnosed as valproate toxicity. *Ann Neurol* 1992;32:767–75.
618. Bick RL, Baker WF. Anticardiolipin antibodies and thrombosis. *Hematol/Oncol Clin N Amer* 1992;6:1287–99.
619. Bickers DS, Adams RD. Hereditary stenosis of the aqueduct of Sylvius as a cause of congenital hydrocephalus. *Brain* 1949;72:246–62.
620. Bickerstaff ER. Basilar artery migraine. *Lancet* 1961;1:15–7.
621. Bickerstaff ER, Cloake PCP. Mesencephalitis and rhombencephalitis. *Brit Med J* 1951;2:77–81.
622. Bickford RG. Sensory precipitation of seizures. *J Mich State Med Soc* 1954;53:1018–20.
623. Bickford RG, Billinger TW, Fleming NI et al. The compressed spectral array (CSA): A pictorial EEG. *Proc San Diego Biomed Symp* 1972;11:365–70.
624. Bickford RG, Klass DW, Whelan JL et al. Reading epilepsy: Clinical and electrographic studies of a new syndrome. *Trans Amer Neurol Assn* 1956;81:100–2.
625. Bickford RG, Sem-Jacobsen CW, Whithe PT et al. Some observations on the mechanism of photic and photo-metrazol activation. *EEG Clin Neurophysiol* 1952;4:275–82.
626. Bickford RG, Whelan JL, Klass DW et al. Reading epilepsy: Clinical and EEG studies of a new syndrome. *Trans Amer Neurol Assn* 1956;**100**.
627. Bicknell JM, Holland JV. Neurologic manifestations of Cogan syndrome. *Neurology* 1978;28:278–81.
628. Bielschowsky A. Die innervation der Musculi recti interni als Seitenwender. *Ber Deut Ophth Ges* 1902;30:164–71.
629. Bielschowsky M. Uber spatinfantilefamiliare amautotische Idiotie mit Kleinhirnsymptomen. *Dtsch Z Nervenklinik* 1914;50:7–29.
630. Biemond A. Brachydactyly, nystagmus and cerebellar ataxia: A familial syndrome. *Ned Tschr Geneesk* 1934;78:1423.
631. Biemond A. Het syndroom van Laurence-Biedl en een aanverwant, niuew syndroom. *Ned Tschr Geneesk* 1934;78:1801–9.
632. Biemond A. La forme radiculo-cordonalle posterieure des dégénerescences spino-cerebelleuses. *Rev Neurol* 1954;91:3–21.
633. Bien CG, Granata T, Antozzi C et al. Pathogenesis, diagnosis and treatment of Rasmussen encephalitis a European consensus statement. *Brain* 2005;128:454–71.
634. Bienfait HME, Baas F, Koelman JHTM et al. Phenotype of Charcot-Marie-Tooth disease type 2. *Neurology* 2007;68:1658–67.
635. Bienvenu T, des Portes V, McDonell N et al. Missense mutation in PAK3, R67C, causes X-linked non-specific mental retardation. *Am J Med Genet* 2000;93:294–8.
636. Bignami A, MacCagnami F, Zappella M et al. Familial infantile spasms and hypsarrhythmia associated with leukodystrophy. *J Neurol Neurosurg Psychiatry* 1966;29:129–34.
637. Bill PLA, Cole G, Proctor NSF. Centronuclear myopathy. *J Neurol Neurosurg Psychiatry* 1979;42:548–56.
638. Biller J, Sand JJ, Corbett JJ et al. Syndrome of the paramedian thalamic arteries: Clinical and neuroimaging correlation. *Clinical Neuroophthalmology.* 1985;5:217–23.
639. Billiard M, Guilleminault C, Dement WC. A menstruation-linked periodic hypersomnia. *Neurology* 1975;25:436–43.
640. Bilous RW, Murty G, Parkinson DB et al. Brief report: Autosomal dominant familial hypoparathyroidism, sensorineural deafness and renal dyspslasia. *N Engl J Med* 1992;327:1069–74.
641. Binder JR, Lazar RM, Tatemichi TK et al. Left hemiparalexia. *Neurology* 1992;42:562–9.
642. Bindl L, Emons D, Haverkamp F et al. Das Megazystis – Mikrokolon – intestinale Hypoperistaltik – Syndrom: Eine Neuropathie? *Z Kinderchir* 1989;44:249–52.
643. Bing Zhou B, Westaway S, Levinson B et al. A novel pantothenate kinase gene (*PANK2*) is defective in Hallervorden-Spatz syndrome. *Nature Genetics* 2001;28:345–9.
644. Bing J, Neel AV. Two cases of hyperglobulinemia with affection of the central nervous system on a toxi-infectious basis (myelitis, polyradiculitis, spinal-fluid change). *Acta Med Scand* 1936;88:492–506.
645. Bing R. *Textbook of Nervous Diseases.* London: Kimpton, 1939.
646. Binnie CD, Macgillivray BB. Brain mapping – useful tool or dangerous toy? *J Neurol Neurosurg Psychiatry* 1992;55:527–9.
647. Binnie CD, Prior PF. Electroencephalography. *J Neurol Neurosurg Psychiatry* 1994;57:1308–19.
648. Binswanger OL. Die Abgrenzung der allgemeinen progressiven Paralyse. *Berl Klin Wochenschr* 1894;31:1103–5.
649. Biot C. Contribution to the study of Cheyne-Stokes breathing. *Lyon Med* 1876;23:517–28, 561–567.
650. Biousse V, Bousser M-G. The myth of carotidynia. *Neurology* 1994;44:993–5.
651. Biran I, Chatterjee A. Alien hand syndrome. *Arch Neurol* 2004;61:292–4.
652. Biran I, Cohen O, Diment J et al. Focal, steroid responsive myositis causing droppped head syndrome. *Muscle Nerve* 1999;22:769–71.
653. Birch-Machin MA, Taylor RW, Cochran B et al. Late-onset optic atrophy, ataxia and a myopathy associated with a mutation of a complex II gene. *Ann Neurol* 2000;48:330–5.
654. Bird AV. Schistosomiasis of the central nervous system. In Vinken PJ, Bruyn GW, eds. *Handbook of Clinical Neurology*, vol. 35, pp 231–41. Amsterdam: Elsevier/North Holland Biomedical Press, 1978.
655. Bird TA, Nicolaus A. Friedreich's description of peripheral facial nerve paralysis in 1798. *J Neurol Neurosurg Psychiatry* 1979;42:56–8.
656. Bird TD, Carlson CB, Hall JG. Familial essential (benign) chorea. *J Med Genet* 1976;13:357–62.
657. Bird TD, Koerker RM, Leaird BJ et al. Lipomembranous polycystic osteodysplasia (brain, bone and fat disease): A genetic cause of presenile dementia. *Neurology* 1983;33:81–6.
658. Birke RN. Congenital ptosis: A classification of 200 cases. *Arch Ophthalmol* 1949;41:188.
659. Birnbaum G. Chronisch-progressive Chorea mit Kleinhirnatrophie. *Arch Psychiat (Berlin)* 1941;114:160–82.
660. Bischoff A, Flerz U, Regli F et al. Fabry disease. *Fall Klin Wschr* 1968;46:666–71.
661. Bishop D. *Test for Reception of Grammar.* Manchester: Univ. Manchester, 1990.
662. Bisno AL, Stevens DL. Streptococcal infections of skin and soft tissues. *N Engl J Med* 1996;334:240–5.
663. Bjerrum JP. *Vejledning i anveldesen of ojespejlet.* Copenhagen: Priors, 1890.
664. Bjornstadt R. *Pili Torti and Sensory-neural Loss of Hearing.* Copenhagen: Scand. Dermatol. Assn., 1965.
665. Black DF, Bartleson JD, Bell MH et al. SMART: Stroke-like migraine attacks after radiation therapy. *Cephalalgia* 2006;26:1137–42.
666. Black DN, Booth F, Watters GV et al. Leukoencephalopathy among native Indian infants in northern Quebec and Manitoba. *Ann Neurol* 1988;24:490–6.
667. Black DN, Watters GV, Andermann E et al. Encephalitis among Cree children in Northern Quebec. *Ann Neurol* 1988;24:483–9.
668. Black DW. Pathological laughter. *J Nerv Ment Dis* 1982;170:67–71.
669. Black PM. Brain tumors. *N Engl J Med* 1991;324:1471–6.
670. Blackburn CRB, McLeod JG. CNS lesions in cystinuria. *Arch Neurol* 1977;34:638–9.

671. Blackmer J. Autonomic dysreflexia. *Can Med Assn J* 2003;**169**:931–5.
672. Bladin CF, Alexandrov AV, Murphy J et al. The Toronto stenosis index. *Can J Neurol Sci* 1994;21(**Suppl. 2**):S7.
673. Blanchet P. Unilateral lumbar polyradiculopathy with sympathetic features. *Presse Med* 1945;53:383–4.
674. Blanco-Barca O, Gallego-Blanco M, Ruiz-Ponte C et al. Smith-Magenis syndrome: A report of two new cases and an approximation to their characteristic behavioural phenotype. *Rev Neurol* 2004;**38**:1038–42.
675. Blass JP. Inborn errors of pyruvate metabolism. In Stanbury JB, Wyngaarden JB, Fredrickson DS et al., eds. *The Metabolic Basis of Inherited Disease*, pp 193–203. New York: McGraw-Hill, 1983.
676. Blau EB. Ectodermal dysplasia, osteosclerosis, atrial septal defect, malabsorption, neutropenia, growth and mental retardation: The Cote-Katsantoni syndrome? *Am J Med Genet* 1987;**26**:729–32.
677. Blau JN. Water-deprivation headache: A new headache with two variants. *Headache* 2004;**44**:79–83.
678. Blau JN. Ponytail headache: A pure extracranial headache. *Headache* 2004;**44**:411–3.
679. Bleecker ML, Ford DP, Celio MA et al. Impact of cognitive reserve on the relationship of lead exposure and neurobehavioral performance. *Neurology* 2007;**69**:470–6.
680. Bleicher RJ, Sherman HF, Latenser BA. Bilateral gluteal compartment syndrome. *J Trauma* 1997;**42**:118–22.
681. Blessed G, Tomlinson BE, Roth M. The association between quantitative measures of dementia and of senile change in the cerebral grey matter of elderly subjects. *Brit J Psychiatry* 1968;**114**:797.
682. Blethen SL, Weldon VV. Hypopituitarism and septo-optic dysplasia in first cousins. *Am J Med Genet* 1985;**21**:123–9.
683. Bloch B. Eigentumliche bisher nicht beschriebene Pigmentaffekton (Incontinentia pigmenti). *Schweiz Med Wschr* 1926;**56**:404–5.
684. Blocq P. Sur une affection caracterisée par de l'astasie et de l'abasie. *Arch Neurol (Paris)* 1888;**15**:24–51.
685. Bloor K. Gustatory sweating and other responses after cervico-thoracic sympathectomy. *Brain* 1969;**92**: 137–46.
686. Blume G, Pestronk A, Goodnough LT. Anti-MAG antibody-associated polyneuropathies. *Neurology* 1995;**45**:1577–80.
687. Blume RS, Wolff SM. The Chediak-Higashi syndrome: Studies in four patients and a review of the literature. *Medicine* 1972;**51**:247–80.
688. Blume WT. Clinical and electroencephalographic correlates of the multiple independent spike foci pattern in children. *Ann Neurol* 1978;**4**:541–7.
689. Blume WT. Hemispheric epilepsy. *Brain* 1996;**121**:1937–49.
690. Blume WT. Clinical and basic neurophysiology of generalized epilepsies. *Can J Neurol Sci* 2002;**29**:6–18.
691. Blume WT, Kaibara M. The "start-stop-start" phenomenon in subdural recordings of epileptic patients. *Neurology* 1991;41 **Suppl.**:261.
692. Blumenthal HJ. Great auricular neurlgia. *Headache* 1992;**32**:413–5.
693. Blumstein SE, Alexander MP, Ryalls JH et al. On the nature of the foreign accent syndrome: A case study. *Brain Lang* 1987;**31**:215–44.
694. Bobker DH, Deloughery TG. Natural killer cell leukemia presenting with a peripheral neuropathy. *Neurology* 1993;**43**:1853–4.
695. Bode M, Tikkakoski T, Tuisku S et al. Isolated neurosarcoidosis – MR findings and pathologic correlation. *Acta Radiol* 2001;**42**:563–7.
696. Bodian D. A new method for staining nerve fibers and nerve endings in mounted paraffin sections. *Anat Rec* 1936;**65**:89–97.
697. Bodner RA, Lynch TLL et al. Serotonin syndrome. *Neurology* 1995;**45**:219–23.
698. Boehme DH, Cottrel JC, Leonberg SC et al. A dominant form of neuronal ceroid lipofuscinosis. *Brain* 1971;**94**:745–60.
699. Boeri R, Passerini A. The megadolichobasilar anomaly. *J Neurol Sci* 1964;**1**:475–84.
700. Boeve BF, Lang A, Litvan I. Cortico-basal degeneration and its relationship to progressive supranuclear palsy and frontotemporal dementia. *Ann Neurol* 2003;**54**:S15–S23.
701. Bogduk N, Marsland A. On the concept of third occipital headache. *J Neurol Neurosurg Psychiatry* 1986;**49**:775–80.
702. Bogduk N, Teasell R. Whiplash. *Arch Neurol* 2000;**57**:590–1.
703. Boghen DR, Glaser JS. Ischaemic optic neuropathy: The clinical profile and natural history. *Brain* 1975;**98**:689–708.
704. Bogorad FA. A syndrome of crocodile tears. *Vrach Delo* 1928;**11**:1328–30.
705. Bogousslavsky J, Maeder P, Regli F, Meuli R. Pure midbrain infarction: Clinical syndromes, MRI, and etiologic patterns. *Neurology* 1994;**44**:2032–40.
706. Bogousslavsky J, Gaio J-M, Caplan LR et al. Encephalopathy, deafness and blindness in young women: A distinct retinocochleocerebral arteriolopathy? *J Neurol Neurosurg Psychiatry* 1989;**52**:43–6.
707. Bogousslavsky J, Kumral E, Regli F et al. Acute hemiconcern: A right anterior parietal syndrome. *J Neurol Neurosurg Psychiatry* 1995;**58**:428–32.
708. Bogousslavsky J, Maeder P, Regli F et al. Pure midbrain infarction. *Neurology* 1994;**44**:2032–40.
709. Bogousslavsky J, Martin R, Moulin T. Homolateral ataxia and crural paresis: A syndrome of anterior cerebral artery territory infarction. *J Neurol Neurosurg Psychiatry* 1992;**55**:1146–9.
710. Bogousslavsky J, Regli F. Response-to-next-patient-stimulation: A right hemisphere syndrome. *Neurology* 1988;**38**:1225–7.
711. Bogousslavsky J, Regli F. Capsular genu syndrome. *Neurology* 1990;**40**:1499–502.
712. Bogousslavsky J, Regli F. Centrum ovale infarcts: Subcortical infarction in the superficial territory of the middle cerebral artery. *Neurology* 1992;**42**: 1992–8.
713. Bogousslavsky J, Regli F, Uske A. Thalamic infarcts – clinical syndromes, etiology, and prognosis. *Neurology* 1988;**38**:837–47.
714. Bogousslavsky J, Regli F, Van Melle G et al. Migraine stroke. *Neurology* 1988;**38**:223–7.
715. Bogousslavsky J, Regli F, Zografos L et al. Optico-cerebral syndrome: Simultaneous hemodynamic infarction of optic nerve and brain. *Neurology* 1987;**37**:263–8.
716. Bogousslavsky J, Regli F, Zogratos L et al. Optico-cerebral syndrome. *Neurology* 1987;**37**:263–8.
717. Bohan A, Azizi F. Allan-Herndon-Dudley syndrome. *Arch Neurol* 2004;**61**:1470.
718. Bohan A, Peter JB. Polymyositis and dermatomyositis. *N Engl J Med* 1975;**292**:344–7.
719. Bohan A, Peter JB, Bowman RL et al. A computer assisted analysis of 153 patients with polymyositis and dermatomyositis. *Medicine* 1977;**56**:255–86.
720. Bohannon RW, Andrews AW. Interrater reliability of hand-held dynamometry. *Phys Ther* 1987;**67**:931–3.
721. Bohm E, Strang RR. Glossopharyngeal neuralgia. *Brain* 1962;**85**:371–88.
722. Boland RP. The Neurocristopathies. *Human Neurobiology* 1974;**5**:409–28.
723. Bolger G, Bojanic S, Sheahan N et al. Ocular microtremor (OMT): A new neurophysiological approach to multiple sclerosis. *J Neurol Neurosurg Psychiatry* 2000;**68**:639–42.

724. Boller F. Johann Baptist Schmidt: A pioneer in the history of aphasia. *Arch Neurol* 1977;34:306–7.
725. Boller F, Bignolo LA. Latent sensory aphasia in hemisphere-damaged patients: An experimental study with the Token test. *Brain* 1966;89:815–31.
726. Boller F, Cole M, Kim Y et al. Optic ataxia: Clinical-radiological correlations with the EMI scan. *J Neurol Neurosurg Psychiatry* 1975;38:954–8.
727. Boller F, Keefe NC, Zoccolotti P. Luigi Galvani, body electricity and the "galvanic skin response". *Neurology* 1989;39: 868–70.
728. Boller F, Segarra JM. Spino-pontine degeneration. *Europ Neurol* 1969;2: 356–73.
729. Bolton CF. Neuromuscular manifestations of critical illness. *Muscle Nerve* 2005;32:140–63.
730. Bolton CF, McFarlane RM. Human pneumatic tourniquet paralysis. *Neurology* 1978;28:787–93.
731. Bolton CF, Young GB, Zochodne DW. The neurological complications of sepsis. *Ann Neurol* 1993;33:94–100.
732. Bond MR, Pilowsky I. The subjective assessment of pain and its relationship to the administration of analgesics in patients with advanced cancer. *J Psychosom Res* 1966;10:203–7.
733. Bondin G, Barbizet J. D'association epilepsie-endocrinopathie. *Rev Neurol* 1954;91:330–47.
734. Bonhoeffer KL. Ein Beitrag zur Localisation der Choreatischen Bewegungen. *Mschr Psychiat Neurol* 1897;1:6–41.
735. Bonkalo A. Hypersomnia, a discussion of psychiatric implication based on three cases. *Brit J Psychiat* 1968;114:69–75.
736. Bonneau D, Toutain A, Laquerriere A et al. X-linked lissencephaly with absent corpus callosum and ambiguous genitalia (XLAG). *Ann Neurol* 2005;51:340–9.
737. Bonnet C. *Essai analytique sur les facultés de l'ame.* Copenhagen: Les frères C & A. Philibert. 1760.
738. Bonnet P. Les syndromes trigeminosympathiques. *Arch Ophth (Paris)* 1956;16:361–79.
739. Bonnet P, Dechaume J, Blanc E. L'aneurysme cirsoide de la rétine (aneurysme racemeux). Ses relations avec l'aneurysme cirsoide de la face et avec l'aneurysme cirsoide du cerveau. *J Med Lyon* 1937;18:163–78.
740. Bonnet P, Dechaume J, Blanc E. L'aneurisme cirsoide de la rétine (aneurisme racemeux). Ses rélations avec l'aneurisme cirsoide du cerveau. *Bull Fr Soc Ophthal* 1938;51:521–4.
741. Bonnette H, Roelofs R, Olson WH. Multicore disease: Report of a case with onset in middle age. *Neurology* 1974;24:1039–44.
742. Bonney G. The value of axon responses in determining the site of the lesion in traction injuries of the brachial plexus. *Brain* 1954;77:588–609.
743. Bonnier P. Un nouveau syndrome bulbaire. *Presse Med* 1903;11:174–7.
744. Booker HE, Forster FM, Klove H. Extinction factors in startle (acousticomotor) seizures. *Neurology* 1965;15:1095–103.
745. Boothroyd A. Developments in speech audiometry. *Sound* 1968;2:3.
746. Bordarier C, Aicardi J, Goutières F. Congenital hydrocephalus and eye abnormalities with severe developmental brain defects: Warburg's syndrome. *Ann Neurol* 1984;16:60–5.
747. Bordini C, Antonaci F, Stovner LJ et al. "Hemicrania Continua": A clinical review. *Headache* 1991;31:20–6.
748. Borenstein S, Desmedt J. Local cooling in myasthenia. *Arch Neurol* 1975;32:1152–157.
749. Boringa JB, Lazeron RH, Reuling IE et al. The brief repeatable battery of neuropsychological tests: Normative values allow application in multiple sclerosis clinical practice. *Multiple Sclerosis* 2001;7:263–7.
750. Borjeson M, Forssman H, Lehmann O. Zusammentreffen von idiotie, epilepsie, zwergwuchs, keimdrusen-unterfunktion, myxodem und morphologischen besonderheiten als ezessiv erbliches syndrom. *Int Cong Psych Entwickg Kind.* 1961.
751. Born JD. The Glasgow-Liége Scale. Prognostic value and evolution of motor response and brain stem reflexes after severe head injury. *Acta Neurochir* 1988;91:1–11.
752. Borrett D, Becker LE. Alexander's disease. A disease of astrocytes. *Brain* 1985;108:367–85.
753. Borries T. Otogene encephalitis. *Zschr Gesamte Neurol Psychiatr* 1921;70:93–101.
754. Bors E. Urological aspects of rehabilitation in spinal cord injuries. *JAMA* 1951;146:225–9.
755. Bosley TM, Oystreck DT, Robertson RL et al. Neurological features of congenital fibrosis of the extraocular muscles type 2 with mutations in PHOX2A. *Brain* 2006;129:2362–4.
756. Bosley TM, Salih MH, Jen JC et al. Neurologic features of horizontal gaze palsy and progressive scoliosis with mutations in ROBO3. *Neurology* 2005;64:1196–203.
757. Botez MI. The tonic palmar reflex. *Acta Neurol Psychiat Belg* 1957;57:551–61.
758. Botez MI. Two visual systems in clinical neurology: Readaptive role of the primitive system in visual agnostic patients. *Europ Neurol* 1975;13:101.
759. Botez MI, Serbanescu T, Vernea I. Visual static agnosia with special reference to literal agnosic alexia. *Neurology* 1964;14:1101–11.
760. Bots GTAM, Staal A. Amyotrophic lateral sclerosis-dementia complex, neuroaxonal dystrophy and Hallervorden Spatz disease. *Neurology* 1973;23:35–9.
761. Bottini G, Sterzi R, Vallar G. Directional hypokinesia in spatial neglect: A case study. *J Neurol Neurosurg Psychiatry* 1992;55:562–5.
762. Bouchard J-P, Barbeau A, Bouchard R, Bouchard RW. Autosomal recessive spastic ataxia of Charlevoix-Saguenay. *Can J Neurol Sci* 1978;5:61–9.
763. Bougneres PF, Saudubray JM, Marsac C et al. Fasting hypoglycemia resulting from hepatic carnitine palmitoyltransferase deficiency. *J Pediatr* 1981;98:742–6.
764. Bogousslavsky J. Memory after Charcot: Paul Sollier's visionary work. *J Neurol Neurosurg Psychiatr* 2007;1373–4.
765. Bouhouche A, Birouk N, Azzedine H et al. Autosomal recessive axonal Charcot-Marie-Tooth disease (ARCMT2): Phenotype-genotype correlations in 13 Moroccan families. *Brain* 2007;130:1062–75.
766. Bouillaud JB. Récherches cliniques propres a démontrer que la perte de la parôle correspond a la lésion des lobules anterieurs de cerveau. *AGMP* 1825;8:25.
767. Bouma PAD, Westendorp RGJ, van Dijk JG et al. The outcome of absence epilepsy: A meta-analysis. *Neurology* 1996;47:802–8.
768. Bour H, Tutin M, Pasquier P. The central nervous system and carbon monoxide poisoning. 1.Clinical data with reference to 20 fatal cases. *Progr Brain Res* 1967;24:1.
769. Bourne RB, Rorabeck CH. Compartment syndromes of the lower leg. *Clin Orthop Rel Res* 1988;40:97–104.
770. Bourneville DM. Contribution a l'étude de l'idiotie. *Arch Neurol (Paris)* 1880;1:69–91.
771. Bourneville DM, Brissaud E. Encephalite ou sclérose tubereuse des circonvolutions cérébrales. *Arch Neurol (Paris)* 1880;1:397–412.
772. Bourque CN, Anderson BA, del Campo CM et al. Sensorimotor perineuritis – an autoimmune disease? *Can J Neurol Sci* 1985;12:129–33.
773. Bousser M-G. Cerebral venous thrombosis: Diagnosis and management. *J Neurol* 2000;247:252–8.

774. Bousser M-G. Headache in spontaneous cerebrospinal fluid hypotension. *Rev Neurol (Paris)* 2005;161:700–2.
775. Bousser M-G. Patent foramen ovale and migraine. *Rev Neurol (Paris)* 2007;163:17–25.
776. Bousser M-G, Chiras J, Bories J et al. Cerebral venous thrombosis – a review of 38 cases. *Stroke* 1985;16:199–213.
777. Boustany RMN et al. Autosomal dominant familial spastic paraplegia. *Neurology* 1987;37:910.
778. Bouwsma G,Van Wijngaarden GIC. Spinal muscular atrophy with hypertrophy of the calves. *J Neurol Sci* 1980;44:275–9.
779. Bowen P, Conradi GJ. Syndrome of skeletal and genitourinary anomalies with unusual facies and failure to thrive in Hutterite sibs. *Birth Defects Orig Artic Ser* 1976;12:101–8.
780. Bowen P et al. A familial syndrome of multiple congenital defects. *Bull Johns Hopkins Hosp* 1964;114:402–14.
781. Bower BD, Jeavons PM. The "happy puppet" syndrome. *Arch Dis Child* 1967;42:298–302.
782. Bower JH, Hammack JE, McDonnell SK et al. The neurological complications of B-cell chronic lymphocytic leukemia. *Neurology* 1997;48:407–12.
783. Bower S, Dennis M, Warlow C et al. Long term prognosis of transient lone bilateral blindness in adolescents and young adults. *J Neurol Neurosurg Psychiatry* 1994;57:734–6.
784. Boyce WF, Gowland C, Rosenbaum PI et al. The gross motor performance measure: Validity and responsiveness of a measure of quality of movement. *Phys Ther* 1995;75:603–13.
785. Boyd Y, Buckle VJ. Cytogenetic heterogeneity of translocations associated with Duchenne muscular dystrophy. *Clin Genet* 1986;29:108–15.
786. Boylan KB, Ferriero DM, Greco CM et al. Congenital hypomyelination neuropathy with arthrogryposis multiplex. *Ann Neurol* 1992;31:337–40.
787. Boyle RS, Shakir RA, Weir AI, McInnes A. Inverted knee jerk: A neglected localising sign in spinal cord disease. *J Neurol Neurosurg Psychiatry* 1979;42:1005–7.
788. Braak H, Del Tredici K, Rüb Ueal. Staging of brain pathology related to sporadic Parkinson's disease. *Neurobiol Aging* 2003;24:197–210.
789. Braakhekke JP, Bruin MId, Stegeman DF et al. The second wind phenomenon in McArdle's disease. *Brain* 1986;109:1087–101.
790. Brackstone M, Patterson SD, Kertesz A. Triple E syndrome: Bilateral locked posterior fracture dislocation of the shoulders. *Neurology* 2001;56:1403–4.
791. Bradley WG, Chad DA, Verghese JP et al. Painful lumbosacral plexopathy with elevated erythrocyte sedimentation rate: A treatable inflammatory syndrome. *Ann Neurol* 1984;15:457–64.
792. Bradley WG, Fewings JD, Cumming WJK et al. Delayed myeloradiculopathy produced by spinal irradiation in the rat. *J Neurol Sci* 1977;31:51.
793. Bradley WG, Hudgson P, Gardner-Medwin D et al. The syndrome of myosclerosis. *J Neurol Neurosurg Psychiatry* 1973;36:651–60.
794. Bradley WG, Madrid R, Thrush DC. Recurrent brachial plexus neuropathy. *Brain* 1975;98:381–98.
795. Braham J, Sadeh M, Sarova-Pinhas I. Skin wrinkling on immersion of hands: A test of sympathetic function. *Arch Neurol* 1979;36:113–4.
796. Braheny, S. Hangman's vs Non-Hangman's Fracture. 1993. (Personal Communication)
797. Braille L. *Procéde pour écrire au moyen des points.* Paris, 1837.
798. Brain WR. On the rotated or "cerebellar" posture of the head. *Brain* 1926;49: 61–76.
799. Brain WR. Visual disorientation with special reference to lesions of the right cerebral hemisphere. *Brain* 1941;64:244–72.
800. Brain WR. The physiological basis of consciousness. *Brain* 1958;81:426–55.
801. Brain WR, Curran RD. The grasp-reflex of the foot. *Brain* 1932;55:347–56.
802. Brain WR, Northfield D, Wilkinson M. The neurological manifestations of cervical spondylosis. *Brain* 1952;75: 187–225.
803. Brain WR,Wilkinson M. Subacute cerebellar degeneration associated with neoplasms. *Brain* 1965;88:465–78.
804. Brais B. The third left frontal convolution plays no role in language: Pierre Marie and the Paris debate on aphasia (1906–1908). *Neurology* 1992;42:690.
805. Brait K, Fahn S, Schwarz GA. Sporadic and familial parkinsonism and motor neurone disease. *Neurology* 1973;23: 990–1002.
806. Bramwell B. *The Diseases of the Spinal Cord*. Edinburgh: Maclachlan and Stewart, 1882.
807. Brancatelli G, Lagalla R. Reversal sign after cardiopulmonary arrest. *J Neurol Neurosurg Psychiatry* 2000;68:525.
808. Branch LG, Meyers AR. Assessing physical function in the elderly. *Clin Geriatr Med* 1987;3:29–51.
809. Branconnier RJ. A computerized battery for behavioural assessment in Alzheimer's disease. In Poon LW, Crook T, Davis KL et al., eds. *Handbook for Clinical Memory Assessment in Older Adults*, pp 189–96. Washington, DC: American Psychological Association, 1986.
810. Brandel J-P, Delasnerie-Lauprêtre N, Laplanche J-P et al. Diagnosis of Creutzfeldt–Jakob disease. *Neurology* 2000;54:1095–9.
811. Brandt IK, Hsia YE, Clement DH et al. Proprionic acidemia (ketotic hyperglycinemia). *Pediatrics* 1974;53:391–5.
812. Brandt J. The Hopkins verbal learning test. Development of a new memory test with six equivalent forms. *Clin Psychol* 1991;5:125–42.
813. Brandt NJ. Symptoms and signs in organic acidurias. *J Inherit Metab Dis* 1984;(**Suppl.** 1):23–7.
814. Brandt NJ, Brandt S, Christensen E et al. Glutamic aciduria in progressive choreo-athetosis. *Clin Genet* 1978;13:77–80.
815. Brandt NJ, Terenius L, Jacobsen BB et al. Hyper-endorphin syndrome in a child with necrotizing encephalomyelopathy. *N Engl J Med* 1980;303:914–6.
816. Brandt S, Carlsen N, Glenting P et al. Encephalopathia myoclonica infantilis (Kinsbourne) and neuroblastoma in children. A report of three cases. *Dev Med Child Neurol* 1974;16:286–94.
817. Brandt T. Phobic postural vertigo. *Neurology* 1996;46:1515–9.
818. Brandt T, Bronstein AM. Cervical vertigo. *J Neurol Neurosurg Psychiatry* 2001;71:8–12.
819. Brandt T, Daroff RB. The multisensory physiological and pathological vertigo syndromes. *Ann Neurol* 1980;7:195–203.
820. Brashear A, DeLeon D, Bressman SB et al. Rapid-onset dystonia-parkinsonism in a second family. *Neurology* 1997;48: 1066–9.
821. Brashear A, Dobyns WB, de Carvalho Aguiar Ozelius P et al. The phenotypic spectrum of rapid-onset dystonia-parkinsonism (RDP) and mutations in the ATP1A3 gene. *Brain* 2007;130:828–35.
822. Bray PF, Bale JF, Anderson RE. Progressive neurological disease associated with chronic cytomegalovirus infection. *Ann Neurol* 1981;9:499–502.
823. Brazis PW, Masdeu JC, Biller J. *Localization in Clinical Neurology*. Boston: Little, Brown, 1990.
824. Brazis PW, Volger JB, Shaw KE. The "numb cheek – limp lower lid" syndrome. *Neurology* 1991;41:327–8.
825. Breathnach CS. Sir Gordon Holmes. *Med Hist* 1975;19:194–200.
826. Bregeat P, Juge P, Pouliquen Y et al. A propos d'une angiomatose orbito-thalamencéphalique. *Bull Fr Soc Ophthal* 1958;581–94.

827. Bremer FW. On the etiology of syringomyelia and the dysraphic state. *Dtsch Klin Nervenheilk* 1926;95:1–103.
828. Bremer FW. Cerveau isolé et physiologie du sommeil. *C R Soc Biol* 1935;118:1235–41.
829. Brenner RP, Atkinson R. Generalised paroxysmal fast activity: Electroencephalographic and clinical features. *Ann Neurol* 1982;11:386–90.
830. Bresolin N, Miranda A, Chang HW et al. Phosphoglycerate kinase deficiency myopathy. *Muscle Nerve* 1984;5:542–55.
831. Bressman S. Dystonia. *Curr Opin Neurol Neurosurg* 1998;11:363–72.
832. Bressman S, Fahn S. Essential myoclonus. *Adv Neurol* 1986;43:287–94.
833. Brett EM. On a particular mode of onset of epilepsy in childhood. *J Neurol Sci* 1967;4:315–38.
834. Brewerton DA, Sandifer PH, Sweetnam DR. Idiopathic pes cavus. *Br Med J* 1963;1:659–61.
835. Brey RL. Antiphospholipid antibodies and ischemic stroke. *Heart Dis Stroke* 1992;1:379–82.
836. Brice JEH. Congenital varicella resulting from infection during second trimester of pregnancy. *Arch Dis Child* 1976;51:474–6.
837. Brickner RM. Oscillopsia: A new symptom commonly occurring in multiple sclerosis. *Arch Neurol Psychiatry* 1936;36:586–9.
838. Bright R. Fatal epilepsy, from suppuration between the dura mater and arachnoid in consequence of blood having been effused in that situation. *Guy's Hosp Rep* 1836;1:36–40.
839. Brill AA. Piblokto or hysteria among Peary's Eskimos. *J Nerv Ment Dis* 1913;40:514–20.
840. Brinar VV, Poser C. Disseminated vasculomyelinopathy. *Clin Neurol Neurosurg* 2006;108:295–310.
841. Brinker KR, Paulson G, Monath TP et al. St.Louis encephalitis in Ohio, September 1975: Clinical and EEG studies in 16 cases. *Arch Int Med* 1979;139:561–6.
842. Brinkman C. Lesions in supplementary motor area interfere with a monkey's performance of a bimanual co-ordination task. *Neurosci Lett* 1981;27:267.
843. Brinkmann R, von Cramon D, Schultz H. The Munich coma scale (MCS). *J Neurol Neurosurg Psychiatry* 1976;39:788–93.
844. Briquet P. *Traité clinique et thérapeutique de l'hysteria*. Paris, 1859.
845. Brissaud E. La chorée variable des dégénerés. *Rev Neurol* 1896;4.
846. Brissaud E. L'infantilisme vrai. *Nouv Icon Salpet* 1907;20:1–17.
847. Brissaud E. La sinistrose. *Bull Med-chir Accid Trav* 1908;2:97–109.
848. Brissaud E, Lereboullet P. Deux cas d'hemicraniose. *Rev Neurol* 1903;11:37–40.
849. Brissaud E, Marie P. De la déviation faciale dans l'hémiplegie hysterique. *Progr Med (Paris)* 1887;15:84, 128–85, 131.
850. Brissaud E, Sicard JA. L'hemispasme facial alterne. *Presse Med* 1908;16:234–6.
851. Brissaud EA, Sicard J. Type spéciale de syndrome alterne. *Rev Neurol* 1908;16:86.
852. Brissaud EW. Spasmodic laughing and crying. *Rev Sci Paris* 1894;1:38–46.
853. Britton JW, Ghearing GR, Benarroch EE et al. The ictal bradycardia syndrome: Localization and lateralization. *Epilepsia* 2006;47:737–44.
854. Britton JW, Uitti RJ, Ahlskog JE et al. Hereditary late-onset chorea without significant dementia. *Neurology* 1995;45:443–7.
855. Broadbent DE, Cooper PF, FitzGerald P et al. The cognitive failures questionnaire and its correlates. *Brit J Clin Psychol* 1982;21:1–16.
856. Broadbent W. Hughlings Jackson as pioneer in nervous physiology and pathology. *Brain* 1903;26:305–66.
857. Broadbent WH. On ingravescent apoplexy. *Proc Roy Med Chir Soc* 1876;8:103–8.
858. Broca P-P. Remarques sur le siège de la faculté du language articulé, suivie d'une observation d'aphemie (perte de la parôle). *Bull Soc Anat Paris* 1861;36:330–57.
859. Broca P-P. Sur la siége de la faculté de language articule. *Bull Soc Anthrop Paris* 1865;6:398–407.
860. Brockmann K, Wang D, Korenke CG et al. Autosomal dominant Glut-1 deficiency syndrome and familial epilepsy. *Ann Neurol* 2001;50:476–85
861. Brodie B. *Local Nervous Affections*. London: Longman, 1837.
862. Brody IA. Muscle contracture induced by exercise: A syndrome attributed to decreased relaxation factor. *N Engl J Med* 1969;2821:187–92.
863. Brogna CG, Lee SI, Dreifuss FE. Pilomotor seizures: Magnetic resonance imaging and electroencephalographic localization of originating focus. *Arch Neurol* 1986;43:1085–6.
864. Bromberg MB. Comparison of electrodiagnostic criteria for primary demyelination in chronic polyneuropathy. *Muscle Nerve* 1991;14:968–76.
865. Bronstein AM. Visual vertigo syndrome: Clinical and posturography findings. *J Neurol Neurosurg Psychiatry* 1995;59:472–6.
866. Bronstein AM, Gresty MA, Mossman SS. Pendular pseudonystagmus arising as a combination of head tremor and vestibular failure. *Neurology* 1992;42:1527–31.
867. Bronstein AM, Hood JD. The cervico-ocular reflex in normal subjects and patients with absent vestibular function. *Brain Res* 1986;373:399–408.
868. Brooke MH. Congenital fiber type disproportion. In Kakulas BA, ed. *Proc 2nd Int Cong on Muscle Diseases, Perth, Australia, Part 2*, pp 147–59. Amsterdam: Excerpta Medica, 1973.
869. Brooke MH. *A Clinician's View of Neuromuscular Diseases*. Baltimore: Williams & Wilkins, 1986.
870. Brooke MH, Carroll JE, Davis JE et al. The prolonged exercise test. *Neurology* 1979;29:636–43.
871. Brooke MH, et al. Clinical investigation in Duchenne dystrophy:2. Determination of the "power" of therapeutic trials based on the natural history. *Muscle Nerve* 1983;6:91–103.
872. Brooke MH, King-Engel W. Histological biopsy with regard to fiber types. *Neurology* 1969;19:591–605.
873. Brooke MH, Miller R. Fatigue testing. *Muscle Nerve* 1990;S13.S35–S7.
874. Brooke MH, Neville HE. Reducing body myopathy. *Neurology* 1972;22:829–40.
875. Brookeman JR. MRI: Physical principles and glossary. *Va Med* 1986;113:343–6.
876. Brooks BR, Miller RG, Swash M et al. El Escorial revisited: Revised criteria for the diagnosis of ALS. *ALS, Other Motor Neuron Disord* 2000;1:293–299.
877. Brooks DJ. PET: Its clinical role in neurology. *J Neurol Neurosurg Psychiatry* 1991;54:1–5.
878. Brooks JSJ, Freeman M, Enterline HT. Malignant triton tumours. *Cancer* 1985;55:2543–9.
879. Brooks WS, Kwok JBJ, Kril JJ et al. Alzheimer's disease with spastic paraparesis and cotton wool plaques: Two pedigrees with PS-1 exon 9 deletions. *Brain* 2003;126:783–91.
880. Brossard J. *Clinical Study of an Hereditary Type of Progressive Muscular Atrophy Beginning in the Legs*. Paris: Université de Paris, 1886.
881. Broughton R, Tolentino M, Krelina M. Fragmentary pathological myoclonus in NREM sleep: A report of 38 cases. *EEG Clin Neurophysiol* 1985;61:123–33.
882. Broughton RJ. Pathological fragmentary myoclonus, intensified "hypnic jerks" and hypnagogic foot tremor: Three unusual sleep-related disorders. In Koella WP, Obal F, Schulz H et al., eds. *Sleep* 1986, pp 240–3. Stuttgart: Fischer Verlag, 1988.
883. Broughton RJ. Sleep attacks, naps, and sleepiness in medical disorders. In Dinges DF, Broughton RJ, eds. *Sleep and Alertness: Chronological, Behavioral, and Medical Aspects of Napping*, pp 267–98. New York: Raven Press, 1989.
884. Broughton RJ, Hasan J, Dunham W. Anterior slow alpha of drowsiness EEG

patterns do not represent the alpha rhythm. *Can J NeurolSci* 1994;21(**Suppl.** 2):S30.

885. Brousolle E, Tommasi M, Mauguiere F et al. Progressive anarthria with secondary parkinsonism: A clinicopathological case report. *J Neurol Neurosurg Psychiatry* 1992;55:577–80.

886. Brouwer OF, Padberg GW, Ruys CJM et al. Hearing loss in facioscapulohumeral muscular dystrophy. *Neurology* 1991;41:1878–81.

887. Brown CL, Symmers D. Acute serous encephalitis. A newly recognized disease of children. *Am J Dis Childh* 1925;29:174–81.

888. Brown GC, Shields JA, Patty BE et al. Congenital pits of the optic nerve head. *Arch Ophthalmol* 1979;97:1341–4.

889. Brown GK, Scholem RD, Croll HB et al. Sulfite oxidase deficiency: Clinical, neuroradiologic and biochemical features in two new patients. *Neurology* 1989;39:252–7.

890. Brown J, Lantos P, Stratton M et al. Familial progressive supranuclear palsy. *J Neurol Neurosurg Psychiatry* 1993;56: 473–6.

891. Brown JA, Braun MA, Namey TC. Pyriformis syndrome in a 10-year old boy. *Neurosurgery* 1988;23:117–9.

892. Brown JR. The early years of the American Academy of Neurology. *Neurology* 1974;24:1–9.

893. Brown JW, Podosin R. A syndrome of the neural crest. *Arch Neurol* 1966;15:294–301.

894. Brown M, Asbury AK. Diabetic neuropathy. *Ann Neurol* 1984;15:2–12.

895. Brown P, Marsden CD. The stiff man and stiff man plus syndromes. *J Neurol* 1999;246:648–52.

896. Brown P, Rothwell JC. New observations on the normal auditory startle reflex in man. *Brain* 1991;114:1891–902.

897. Brown P, Rothwell JC, Marsden CD. The stiff leg syndrome. *J Neurol Neurosurg Psychiatry* 1997;62:31–7.

898. Brown RA, Lawson DA, Leslie GC et al. Does the Wartenberg pendulum test differentiate quantitatively between spasticity and rigidity? A study in elderly stroke and Parkinsonian patients. *J Neurol Neurosurg Psychiatry* 1988;51:1178–86.

899. Brown RA, Lawson DA, Leslie GC, et al. Observations on the applicability of the Wartenberg pendulum test to healthy elderly subjects. *J Neurol Neurosurg Psychiatry* 1988;51:1171–7.

900. Brown RG, Jahanshahi M, Marsden CD. The execution of bimanual movements in patients with Parkinson's, Huntington's and cerebellar disease. *J Neurol Neurosurg Psychiatry* 1993;56:295–7.

901. Brown RJ, Trimble MR. Dissociative psychopathology, non–epileptic seizures and neurology. *J Neurol Neurosurg Psychiatry* 2000;69:285–91.

902. Brown WF,Yates SK. Percutaneous localization of conduction abnormalities in human entrapment neuropathies. *Can J Neurol Sci* 1982;9:391–400.

903. Brown-Séquard CE. De la transmission croisée des impressions sensitives par la moelle épinière. *CR Soc Biol* 1850;2:33–4.

904. Browne CD, Nolan BM, Faithfull DK. Occupational repetition strain injuries: Guidelines for diagnosis and management. *Med J Aust* 1984;140: 329–32.

905. Browne F, Bayer JF. Familial nephrosis associated with deafness and urinary tract anomalies in siblings. *J Pediatr* 1962;60:33.

906. Browne TR, Mirsky AF. Absence (petit mal) seizures. In Browne TR, Feldman RG, eds. *Epilepsy, Diagnosis and Management*, pp 61–74. Boston: Little, Brown, 1983.

907. Brownell AKW, Severson DL, Thompson CD. Cold-induced rhabdomyolysis in carnitine palmitoyl transferase deficiency. *Can J Neurol Sci* 1979;6:367–70.

908. Brudzinski J. Un signe nouveau sur les membres inferieurs dans les meningites chez les enfants. *Arch Med Enf Paris* 1909;12:745.

909. Brudzinski J. A new symptom of tuberculous meningitis and irritation in children. *Berl Klin Wochenschr* 1916;53:686–90.

910. Brugger P, Agosti R, Regard MN et al. Heautoscopy, epilepsy and suicide. *J Neurophysiol* 1994;57:838–9.

911. Brumback RA, Staton RD, Susaq ME. Exercise-induced pain, stiffness and tubular aggregation in skeletal muscle. *J Neurol Neurosurg Psychiatry* 1981;44: 250–4.

912. Brun A, Englund B, Mann DMA, Neary D et al. Consensus on Clinical and Neuropathological Criteria for FrontoTemporal Dementia. *J Neurol Neurosurg Psychiatry* 1994;57.

913. Bruni J, Bilbao JM, Pritzker KP et al. Myopathy associated with amyloid. *Can J Neurol Sci* 1977;4:77–9.

914. Bruno C, van Diggelen OP, Cassandrini D et al. Clinical and genetic heterogeneity of branching enzyme deficiency (glycogenesis type IV). *Neurology* 2004;63:1053–8.

915. Bruno MK, Lee H-Y, Auburger GWJ. Genotype-phenotype correlation of paroxysmal nonkinesigenic dyskinesia. *Neurology* 2007;68:1782–9.

916. Bruno MK, Hallett M, Gwinn-Hardy K et al. Clinical evaluation of idiopathic paroxysmal kinesigenic dyskinesia. *Neurology* 2004;63:2280–7.

917. Bruns L. Gait disorders in frontal lobe tumors. *Dtsch Med Wschr* 1892;18: 138–40.

918. Bruns L. Neuropathologische Demonstrationen. *Neurol Zbl* 1902;21:561–7.

919. Bruns L, Cramer A, Ziehen T. *Handbuch der Nervenkrankheiten im Kindesalter.* Berlin: S. Karger, 1912.

920. Brushfield T. Mongolism. *Brit J Dis Child* 1924;21:241–58.

921. Brushfield T, Wyatt W. Hemiplegia associated with extensive naevus and mental defect. *Brit J Child Dis* 1927;24:98–106.

922. Brust JCM. Music and Language. *Brain* 1980;103:367–92.

923. Brust JCM, Behrens MM. Release hallucinations as the major symptom of posterior cerebral artery occlusion. *Ann Neurol* 1977;2:432–6.

924. Brust JCM, List TA, Catalaro LW et al. Ocular myasthenia gravis mimicking progressive external ophthalmoplegia. *Neurology* 1974;24:755–60.

925. Bruyn GW, Staathof LJA, Raymakers GMJ. Mollaret's meningitis: Differential diagnosis and diagnostic pitfalls. *Neurology* 1962;12:745–53.

926. Bruyn GW, Vielvoye GJ, Went LJ. Hereditary spastic dystonia: A new mitochondrial encaphalopathy? *J Neurol Sci* 1991;103:195–202.

927. Bryceson ADM, Parry EHO, Perine PL et al. Louse-borne relapsing fever. A clinical and laboratory study of 62 cases and a reconsideration of the literature. *Quart J Med* 1970;39:129–70.

928. Buchem FSPv, Hadders HN, Ubbens R. An uncommon familial systemic disease of the skeleton: Hyperostosis corticalis generalisata familiaris. *Acta Radiol* 1955;44:109–20.

929. Buchman AS, Garron DC, Trost-Cardamone JE et al. Word deafness: One hundred years later. *J Neurol Neurosurg Psychiatry* 1986;49:4899–9.

930. Buckley DJ, Hall MS, Penney S. Shuddering attacks mimicking infantile spasms. *Can J.Neurol. Sci.* 1994;21 (**Suppl.** 2):S33–4.

931. Budd MA, Tanaka K, Holmes LB et al. Isovaleric acidemia. *N Engl J Med* 1967;277:321–7.

932. Budka H. Cerebral pathology in AIDS. *Curr Opin Neurol Neurosurg* 1992;5: 917–23.

933. Bugiani M, Al Shahwan S, Lamantea E et al. GJA12 mutations in children with recessive hypomyelinating

leukoencephalopathy. *Neurology* 2006;67:273–9.

934. Bull JWD, Nixon WLB, Pratt RTC. The radiological criteria and familial occurrence of primary basilar impression. *Brain* 1955;78:229–47.
935. Bullard DE. Diencephalic seizures: Responsiveness to bromocriptine and morphine. *Ann Neurol* 1987;21:609–11.
936. Bundey S. A genetic study of infantile and juvenile myasthenia gravis. *J Neurol Neurosurg Psychiatry* 1972;35:41–51.
937. Bundey S, Griffiths MI. Recurrent risks of families of children with symmetrical spasticity. *Dev Med Child Neurol* 1977;19:179–81.
938. Bundey S, Harrison MJG, Marsden CD. A genetic study of torsion dystonia. *J Med Genet* 1975;12:12–9.
939. Burde RM. Amaurosis fugax. *J Clin Neuroophthalmol* 1989;9:185–9.
940. Burger PC, Vogel FS, Green SB et al. Glioblastoma multiforme and anaplastic astrocytoma: Pathologic criteria and prognostic implications. *Cancer* 1985;56:1106–111.
941. Burke D, Andrews CJ, Lance JW. Tonic vibration reflex in spasticity, Parkinson's disease, and normal subjects. *J Neurol Neurosurg Psychiatry* 1972;35:477–86.
942. Burke RE, Brin MF, Fahn S et al. Analysis of the clinical course of non-Jewish, autosomal dominant torsion dystonia. *Mov Disord* 1986;1:163–78.
943. Burke RE, Fahn S, Jankovic J et al. Tardive dystonia: Late-onset and persistent dystonia caused by antipsychotic drugs. *Neurology* 1982;32:1335–46.
944. Burke RE, Fahn S, Marsden CD et al. Validity and reliability of a rating scale for the primary torsion dystonias. *Neurology* 1985;35:73–7.
945. Burke RE, Kang UJ, Fahn S. Tardive akathisia: Motor phenomena and treatment. *Neurology* 1987;37(**Suppl.** 1):124–5.
946. Burneo JG, Shatz R, Nikolaoa IH et al. Amusement park stroke. *Neurology* 2000;55:564–5.
947. Burnett C, Commons RR, Albright F et al. Hypercalcemia without hypercalciuria or hypophosphatemia, calcinosis and renal insufficiency: A syndrome following prolonged intake of milk and alkali. *N Engl J Med* 1949;240:787–94.
948. Burnham HH. Anterior ethmoidal nerve syndrome: Referred pain and headache from lateral nasal wall. *Arch Otolaryngol* 1949;50:640–6.
949. Burnier LR. A new hypophysial syndrome. *Ann Ophthalmol* 1912;21:263–73.
950. Burns FS. A case of generalised congenital erythroderma. *J Cutan Dis* 1915;32:255.
951. Burns RJ, Bretag AH, Blumbergs PC et al. Benign familial disease with muscle mounding and rippling. *J Neurol Neurosurg Psychiatry* 1994;57:344–7.
952. Burstein R, Cutrer M, Yarnitsky D. The development of cutaneous allodynia during a migraine attack: Clinical evidence for the sequential recruitment of spinal and supraspinal nociceptive neurons in migraine. *Brain* 2000 Aug;123(Pt 8):1703–1709.
953. Burton JM, Kern RZ, Halliday W et al. Neurological manifestations of west Nile virus infection. *Can J Neurol Sci* 2004;31:185–93.
954. Burton MJ, Brochwitz-Lewinski ML. Frey and the auriculotemporal syndrome. *J Roy Soc Med* 1991;84:619–20.
955. Burwell CS, Robin ED, Whaley RD, Bickemann AG. Extreme obesity associated with alveolar hypoventilation—a Pickwickian syndrome. *Amer J Med* 1956;21:811.
956. Buschke F. Selective reminding for analysis of memory and learning. *J Verb Learn Verb Behav* 1973;12:543–50.
957. Buschke H. Cued recall in amnesia. *J Clin Neuropsychol* 1984;6:433–40.
958. Buschke H, Kuslansky G, Katz M et al. Screening for dementia with the memory impairment screen. *Neurology* 1999;52:231–8.
959. Butinar D, Zidar J, Leonardis L et al. Hereditary auditory, vestibular, motor and sensory neuropathy in a Slovenian Roma (Gypsy). *Ann Neurol* 1999;46:36–44.
960. Butler CR, Graham KS, Hodges JR et al. The syndrome of transient epileptic amnesia. *Ann Neurol* 2007;61:587–98.
961. Butterworth B, Warrington EK. Two routes to repetition: Evidence from a case of "Deep Dysphasia". *Neurocase* 1995;1: 55–66.
962. Butterworth T, Strean LP. The ichthyosiform genodermatosis. *Postgrad Med J* 1965;37:175.
963. Buzzard T. On the simulation of hysteria by organic disease of the nervous system. *Brain* 1890;13:1–44.
964. Bynke O, Hillman J. Role of transsphenoidal operation in the management of pituitary adenomas with surasellar extension. *Arch Neurochir* 1989;100:50–5.
965. Byrne E, Thomas PK, Zilkha KJ. Familial extrapyramidal disease with polyneuropathy. *J Neurol Neurosurg Psychiatry* 1982;45:372–4.
966. Byrne E, White O, Cook M. Familial dystonic choreoathetosis with myokymia: A sleep responsive disorder. *J Neurol Neurosurg Psychiatry* 1991;54:1090–2.
967. Byrne EJ. Diffuse Lewy body disease: Clinical features in 15 cases. *J Neurol Neurosurg Psychiatry* 1989;52:709–17.
968. Bywaters EGL. The Cheshire cat syndrome. *Postgrad Med J* 1968;44:19–22.
969. Bywaters EGL, Beall D. Crush injuries with impairment of renal function. *Brit Med J* 1941;1:427–32.
970. Caccavale A, Mignemi L. Acute onset of a bilateral areflexical mydriasis in Miller-Fisher syndrome: A rare neuro-ophthalmologic disease. *J Neuroophthalmol* 2000;20:61–2.
971. Caffey J. The whiplash shaken infant syndrome. *Pediatrics* 1974;54:396–403.
972. See 971
973. Caffey J, Silverman WA. Infantile cortical hyperostosis. *Am J Roentgenol* 1945;54:1–16.
974. Cagnoli C, Mariotti C, Taroni F et al. SCA28, a novel form of autosomal dominant cerebellar ataxia on chromosome 18p11.22q11.2. *Brain* 2006;129:235–42.
975. Caine D, Halliday GM, Kril JJ et al. Operational criteria for the classification of chronic alcoholics: Identification of Wernicke's encephalopathy. *J Neurol Neurosurg Psychiatry* 1997;62:51–60.
976. Cairns H. Surgical aspects of meningitis. *Brit Med J* 1949;1:969–76.
977. Cairns H, Oldfield RC, Pennybacker JB, Whitteridge D. Akinetic mutism with an epidermoid cyst of the 3rd ventricle. *Brain* 1941;64:273–90.
978. Cairns NJ, Grossman M, Arnold SE et al. Clinical and neuropathologic variation in neuronal intermediate filament inclusion disease. *Neurology* 2004;63:1376–84.
979. Calabrese LH, Dodick DW, Schwedt TJ et al. Narrative review: Reversible cerebral vasoconstriction syndromes. *Ann Int Med* 2007;146:34–44.
980. Calabrese LO, Mallek JA. Primary angiitis of the central nervous system. Report of 8 new cases, review of the literature, and proposal for diagnostic criteria. *Medicine* 1988;67:20–39.
981. Calabresi PA, Silvestri G, DiMauro S et al. Ekbom's syndrome: Lipomas, ataxia, and neuropathy with MERRF. *Muscle Nerve* 1994;17:943–5.
982. Calleja J, Carpizo R, Berciano J. Orgasmic epilepsy. *Epilepsia* 1988;29:635–9.
983. Calne DB, Pallis CA. Vibratory sense: A critical review. *Brain* 1966;89:723–46.
984. Calne DB, Snow BJ, Lee C. Criteria for diagnosing Parkinson's disease. *Ann Neurol* 1992;32:S125–7.
985. Calvert RJ, Caplin G. The Houssay syndrome. *Brit Med J* 1957;2:71–4.
986. Cambier J, Dehen H. Imitation synkinesia and sensory control of movement. *Neurology* 1977;27:646–9.

987. Camfield PR, Metrakos K, Andermann F. Basilar migraine, seizures, and severe epileptiform EEG abnormalities. *Neurology* 1978;28:584–8.
988. Camins MB, Mount LA. Primary suprasellar atypical teratoma. *Brain* 1974;97:447.
989. Campbell AMG, Rosenberg LE, Snodgrass PJ et al. Orthinine transcarbamylase deficiency: A cause of lethal neonatal hyperammonemia in males. *N Engl J Med* 1973;288:1–6.
990. Campbell AMG, Williams CR, Barltrop D. Motor neurone disease and exposure to lead. *J Neurol Neurosurg Psychiatry* 1970;33:877–85.
991. Campbell WW. The numb cheek syndrome: A sign of infraorbital neuropathy. *Neurology* 1986;36:421–3.
992. Campbell WW. Ulnar neuropathy at the elbow. *Muscle Nerve* 2000;23:450–2.
993. Campbell WW, Buschbacher R, Pridgeon RM et al. Selective finger drop in cervical radiculopathy: The pseudopseudoulnar claw hand. *Muscle Nerve* 1995;18:108–10.
994. Camponovo F, Meier C. Neuropathy of vasculitic origin in a case of Garin-Boujadoux-Bannwarth syndrome with positive borrelia antibody response. *J Neurol* 1986;233:69–72.
995. Canadian Medical Association. Eating disorders: Anorexia nervosa and bulimia. Ottawa, Canada: Dept. of Communications and Government Relations, 1989.
996. Canavan M. Schilder's encephalitis periaxalis diffusa. Report of a case in a child aged sixteen and one-half months. *Arch Neurol* 1931;25:299–308.
997. Cancilla PA, Kalyanaraman K, Verity MA et al. Familial myopathy with probably lysis of myofibrils in type 1 fibre. *Neurol Minneap* 1971;21:579–85.
998. Canter GJ, De la Torre R, Mier M. A method for evaluating disability in Parkinson disease. *J Nerv Ment Dis* 1961;133:143–7.
999. Cantu JM et al. Autosomal recessive microcephaly associated with chorioretinopathy. *Hum Genet* 1977;36:243–7.
1000. Cantu RC. Second-impact syndrome. *Clin Sports Med* 1998;17:37–44.
1001. Cantwell RJ. Congenital sensorineural deafness associated with onycho-osteodystrophy and mental retardation. *Humangenetik* 1975;26:261–5.
1002. Capasso M, Caporale CM, Pomilio F et al. Acute motor conduction block neuropathy. *Neurology* 2003;61:617–22.
1003. Capetto JR, et al. A syndrome of arterial occlusive retinopathy and encephalopathy. *Am J Ophthalmol* 1984;98:189–202.
1004. Capgras J. L'illusion des "sosies" dans une délire systematisée chronique. *Ann Med Psychol* 1923;81:186.
1005. Capistrant TD, Gumnit RJ. Thermography and extracranial vascular disease. *Arch Neurol* 1970;22:499–503.
1006. Caplan LR. Ptosis. *J Neurol Neurosurg Psychiatry* 1974;37:1–7.
1007. Caplan LR. "Top of the Basilar" syndrome. *Neurology* 1980;30:72–9.
1008. Caplan LR. Bilateral distal vertebral artery occlusion. *Neurology* 1983;33:552–8.
1009. Caplan LR. TGA criteria: What's in a name? *Neurology* 1986;36:1625.
1010. Caplan LR. Intracranial branch atheromatous disease. *Neurology* 1989;39:1246–50.
1011. Caplan LR. Charles Foix – the first modern stroke neurolgist. *Stroke* 1990;21:348–56.
1012. Caplan LR. Binswanger's disease revisited. *Neurology* 1995;45:626–33.
1013. Caplan LR. Dilatative arteriopathy dolichoectasia: What is known and not known. *Ann Neurol* 2005;57:469–71.
1014. Caplan LR. Cardiac encephalopathy and congestive heart failure. *Neurology* 2006;66:99–101.
1015. Caplan LR, Gorelick PB. "Salt and pepper on the face" pain in acute brainstem ischemia. *Ann Neurol* 1983;13:344–7.
1016. Caress J, Walker F. The spectrum of ectopic motor nerve behavior: From fasciculations to neuromyotonia. *Neurology* 2002;8:41–6.
1017. Carfi J, Ma DM. Posterior interosseous syndrome revisited. *Muscle Nerve* 1985;8:499–502.
1018. Carleton A, Biggs R. Diffuse mesodermal pigmentation with cranial abnormality. *Brit J Dermatol* 1948;60:102.
1019. Carmel PW. Tumors of the third ventricle. *Acta Neurochir* 1985;75: 136–46.
1020. Carney JA, Bianco AJ JR, Sizemore GW et al. Multiple endocrine neoplasia with skeletal manifestations. *J Bone Joint Surg* 1981;63:405–10.
1021. Carney JA, Gordon H, Carpenter PC et al. The complex of myxomas, spotty pigmentation, and endocrine overactivity. *Medicine* 1985;64:270–83.
1022. Carney LR. The dimple sign in peroneal palsy. *Neurology* 1967;17:922.
1023. Carney RGJ. Incontinentia pigmenti. *Arch Derm* 1976;112:535–42.
1024. CarodArtal FJ, Vargas AP, Marinho PB et al. Tourettism, hemiballism and juvenile Parkinsonism: Expanding the clinical spectrum of the neurodegeneration associated to pantothenate kinase deficiency (Hallervorden Spatz syndrome). *Rev Neurol* 2004;38:327–31.
1025. Carol WL, Godfried EG, Prakken JR et al. v. Recklinghausensche Neurofibromatosis, Atrophodermia vermiculata und kongenitale Herzanomalie als Hauptkennizeichen eines familiar–hereditaren Syndroms. *Dermatologica* 1940;81:345–65.
1026. Carota A, Rossetti AO, Karapanayiotides T et al. Catastrophic reaction in acute stroke: A reflex behaviour in aphasic patients. *Neurology* 2001;57:1902–5.
1027. Carota A, Staub F, Bogousslavsky J. Emotions, behaviours and mood changes in stroke. *Current Opinion in Neurology* 2002;15:57–69.
1028. Carpay JA, Vermeulen J, Stropink J et al. Seizure severity in children with epilepsy; a parent-completed scale compared with clinical attacks. *Epilepsia* 1997;38: 346–52.
1029. Carpenter G. Two sisters showing malformation of the skull and other congenital abnormalities. *Rep Soc Study Dis Childr (London)* 1901;1:110–8.
1030. Carpenter S, Karpati G, Rothman S et al. The childhood type of dermatomyositis. *Neurology* 1976;26:952–62.
1031. Carpio A, Placencia M, Santillan F et al. A proposal for classification of neurocysticercosis. *Can J Neurol Sci* 1994;21:43–7.
1032. Carr JA, van der Walt P, Nakayama J et al. FAME 3. *Neurology* 2007;68:1382–9.
1033. Carr RE, Ripps H, Sequal IM et al. Visual function in congenital night-blindness. *Invest Ophthalmol* 1976;5:508.
1034. Carr-Locke DL, Nair HJ. Neurological presentation of psittacosis during a small outbreak in Leicestershire. *Brit Med J* 1976;ii:853–4.
1035. Carraro A. Congenital absence of the tibia and deafness in 4 siblings. *Chir di Org di Movimento* 1931;16:429–38.
1036. See 1035
1037. Carroll FD. Optic nerve complications of cataract extraction. *Trans Am Acad Ophthal Otolaryng* 1973;77:623.
1038. Carroll GJ, Willis K, Peter JB. Penicillamine-induced polymyositis or dermatomyositis. *J Rheumatol* 1987;14:995–9.
1039. Carroll JE, Brooke MH, DeVivo DC et al. Biochemical and physiologic consequences of carnitine palmityl transfersase deficiency. *Muscle Nerve* 1978;1:103–10.
1040. Carroll JE, Shumate JB, Brooke MH et al. Riboflavine-responsive lipid myopathy and carnitine deficiency. *Neurology* 1981;31:1557–9.
1041. Carroll RA, Bornstein SS, Hoffman SG. Rehabilitation networking: A solution for the future. In Granger CV, Gresham GE, eds. *Functional Assessment in Rehabilitation*

Medicine, pp 364–77. Baltimore: Williams and Wilkins, 1984.

1042. Carruthers A, Carruthers J, Wright P. Necrotizing fasciitis with polymyositis. *Brit Med J* 1975;3:355–6.

1043. Carskadon MA, Dement WC, Mitler MM et al. Guidelines for the multiple sleep latency test. *Sleep* 1986;9:519–24.

1044. Carson NA, Scally BG, Neill DW et al. Saccharopinuria: A new inborn error of lysine metabolism. *Nature* 1968;218:679.

1045. Carter RF et al. Primary amebic meningoencephalitis. *Rep Roy Soc Trop Med Hygiene* 1972;66:193.

1046. Carton H, Kayembe K, Kabeya et al. Epidemic spastic paraparesis in Bandundu (Zaire). *J Neurol Neurosurg Psychiatry* 1986;49:620–7.

1047. Casaer P. *Migraine and Other Headaches*. Pearl River, NJ: Parthenon, 1989.

1048. Cascino GD. Generalized convulsive status epilepticus. *Mayo Clin Proc* 1996;71:787–92.

1049. Caselli RJ, Boeve BF, Scheithauer BW et al. Nonvasculitic autoimmune inflammatory meningoencephalitis (NAIM): A reversible form of encephalopathy. *Neurology* 1999;53:1579–81.

1050. Caselli RJ, Hunder GG, Whisnant JP. Neurologic disease in biopsy-proven giant cell (temporal) arteritis. *Neurology* 1988;38:352–8.

1051. Caselli RJ, Jack CR. Asymmetric cortical degenerative syndromes: A proposed clinical classification. *Arch Neurol* 1992;49:770–80.

1052. Caselli RJ, Jack CR, Peterson RC et al. Assymetric cortical degenerative syndromes: Clinical and radiologic correlations. *Neurology* 1992;42:1462–8.

1053. Caselli RJ, Windebank AJ, Peterson RC et al. Rapidly progressive aphasic dementia and motor neuron disease (MND): Six new cases of a distinctive clinical syndrome. *Neurology* 1991;41 **Suppl.**:176.

1054. Cassidy SB. Prader-Willi syndrome: Characteristics, management, and etiology. *Ala J Med Sci* 1987;24:169–75.

1055. Cassim F. Myoclonic dystonia. *Rev Neurol (Paris)* 2003;159:1–892.

1056. Castelnovo G, Levade T, Riise Stensland HM et al. Adult leukoencephalopathy caused by alpha-mannosidosis deficiency. *Rev Neurol (Paris)* 2007;163:359–61.

1057. Castillo M, Davis PC, Takei Y et al. Intracranial ganglioglioma: MR, CT, and clinical findings in 18 patients. *AJR* 1990;154:607–12.

1058. Castillo P, Woodruff B, Caselli R. Steroid-responsive encephalopathy associated with autoimmune thyroiditis. *Arch Neurol* 2006;63:197–202.

1059. Cavanagh JB. Peripheral nerve changes in orthocresyl phosphate poisoning in the rat. *J Path Bact* 1964;87:365–83.

1060. Cavanagh JB. The "dying-back" process: A common denominator in many naturally occurring and toxic neuropathies. *Arch Pathol Lab Med* 1979;103:659–64.

1061. Cavanagh JB et al. The effects of thallium salts, with particular reference to the nervous system changes. *Quart J Med* 1974;43:293.

1062. Cavanagh NPC, Eames RA, Galvin RJ et al. Hereditary sensory neuropathy with spastic paraplegia. *Brain* 1979;102:79–94.

1063. Cavanagh NPC, Yates DAH, Sutcliffe J. Thenar hypoplasia with associated radiologic abnormalities. *Muscle Nerve* 1979;2:431–6.

1064. Cedarbaum JM, Stambler N, Malta E et al. The ALSFRS -R: A revised rating scale that incorporates assessments of respiratory function. *J Neurol Sci* 1999;169:13–21.

1065. Cederbaum SD et al. Argininosuccinic aciduria. *Am J Ment Defic* 1973;77: 395–404.

1066. Celani MG, Righetti E, Migliacci R et al. Comparability and validity of two clinical scores in the early differential diagnosis of acute stroke. *Brit Med J* 1994;308:1674–6.

1067. Celesia GC. Disorders of membrane channels or channelopathies. *Clin Neurophysiol* 2001;112:2–18.

1068. Celesia GC, Andermann F, Wiglesworth FW, Robb JP. Monomelic myopathy. *Arch Neurol* 1967;17:69–77.

1069 Cerebral Embolism Task Force. Cardiogenic brain embolism. *Arch Neurol* 1986;43:71–84.

1070. Cereda C, Ghika J, Maeder P et al. Strokes restricted to the insular cortex. *Neurology* 2002;59:1950–5.

1071. Cervero F, Iggo A. The substantia gelatinosa of the spinal cord. *Brain* 1980;103:717–72.

1072. Cestan EJM, Chenais J. Du miosis dans certains lesions bulbaires en foyer (hemiplegie du type Avellis associés au syndrome oculaire sympathique). *Gaz Hop Paris* 1903;76:1229–33.

1073. Ceuterick-de Groote C, Lehtokari VL, de Jonghe P et al. Cap disease caused by heterozygous deletion of the beta-tropomyosin gene TPM2. *Neuromuscul Disord* 2007;17:433–42.

1074. Chabriat H, Levy C, Taillia H et al. Patterns of MRI lesions in CADASIL. *Neurology* 1998;51:452–7.

1075. Chad DA, Lacomis D. Critically ill patients with newly acquired weakness: The clinico-pathological spectrum. *Ann Neurol* 1994;35:257–9.

1076. Chaddock CG. A preliminary communication concerning a new diagnostic nervous sign. *Interstate Med* 1911;18:742–6.

1077. Chadwick D, Clear DB, Eldridge P et al. Golf ball epilepsy. *J Neurol Neurosurg Psychiatry* 2000;68:251–2.

1078. Chahin N, Engel AG. Correlation of muscle biopsy, clinical course and outcome in PM, and sporadic IBM. *Neurology* 2008;70:418–24.

1079. Chahin N, Klein C, Mandrekar J et al. Natural history of spinal-bulbar muscular atrophy. *Neurology* 2008;70:1967–71.

1080. Chalela JA, Kasner SE. The fogging effect. *Neurology* 2000;55:315.

1081. Chalk CH, Mills KR, Jacobs JM et al. Familial multiple symmetric lipomatosis with peripheral neuropathy. *Neurology* 1990;40:1246–50.

1082. Chalk CH, Windebank AJ, Kimmel DW et al. The distinctive clinical features of paraneoplastic sensory neuropathy. *Can J Neurol Sci* 1992;19:346–51.

1083. Chalmers RA, Johnson M, Pallis CA et al. Xanthenuria with myopathy. *Quart J Med* 1969;38:493–512.

1084. Chalmers RM, Bird AC, Harding AE. Autosomal dominant optic atrophy with asymptomatic peripheral neuropathy. *J Neurol Neurosurg Psychiatry* 1996;60: 195–6.

1085. Chambers BR, Bladin CF. Internal watershed infarction. In Donnan GA, Norrving B, Bamford JM, eds. *Lacunar and Other Subcortical Infarctions*, pp 139–48. Oxford: Oxford University Press, 1995.

1086. Chan CC, Egbert PR, Herrick MK et al. Oculocerebral malformations: A Reappraisal of Walker's "Lissencephaly". *Arch Neurol* 1980;37:104–8.

1087. Chan D, Rossor M. ". . . but who is that on the other side of you?" Extracampine hallucinations revisited. *Lancet* 2002;360:2064–6.

1088. Chan DKY, Hung WT, Wong A et al. Validating a screening questionnaire for parkinsonism in Australia. *J Neurol Neurosurg Psychiatry* 2000;69:117–20.

1089. Chanarin et al. Chanarin-Miranda syndrome: Lipid storage myopathy and congenital ichthyosis. *Brit Med J* 1975;1:203.

1090. Chancellor MB, Lavelle J, Ozawa H et al. Ice water test in the urodynamic evaluation of spinal cord injured patients. *Tech Urol* 1998;4:87–91.

1091. Chandler D, Angelicheva D, Heather L et al. Hereditary motor and sensory neuropathy-Lom (HMSNL): Refined genetic mapping in Romani (Gypsy) families from several European countries. *Neuromuscular Disorders* 2000;10:584–91.

1092. Chandler KE, Del Rio A, Rakshi K et al. Leucodysplasia, microcephaly, cerebral malformation (LMC): A novel recessive disorder linked to 2p16. *Brain* 2006;129:272–277.
1093. Chang BS, Piao X, Giannini C et al. Bilateral generalized polymicrogyria (BGP). *Neurology* 2004;62:1722–1728.
1094. Chang CM, Yu CW, Fong KY et al. N-hexane neuropathy in offset printers. *J Neurol Neurosurg Psychiatry* 1993;56: 538–42.
1095. Chapman SB, Rosenberg RN, Weiner MF et al. Autosomal dominant progressive syndrome of motor-speech loss without dementia. *Neurology* 1997;49:1298–306.
1096. Chapple CC. A duosyndrome of the laryngeal nerve. *J Dis Child* 1956;91: 14–8.
1097. Charcot J-M. Histologie de la sclèrose en plaques. *Gaz Hop Paris* 1868;41:554, 555, 557–558.
1098. Charcot J-M. Sur quelques arthropathies qui paraissent dépendre d'une lésion du cerveau ou de la moelle épinière. *Arch Physiol (Paris)* 1868;1:161–78.
1099. Charcot J-M. *Leçons sur les maladies du système nerveux faites at la Salpêtrière.* Paris: Delahnye, 1872.
1100. Charcot J-M. Séance du 13 mai. *C R Soc Biol* 1873;**serie 5e iii, 1871**:32–8.
1101. Charcot J-M. Des amyotrophies spinales chroniques. *Progr Med (Paris)* 1874;2:573–4.
1102. Charcot J-M. On chorea in old people. *Med Times Gaz* 1878;1:245–6.
1103. Charcot J-M. Diagnostic des formes frustes de la sclèrose en plaques. *Progr Med (Paris)* 1879;7:97–9.
1104. Charcot J-M. Du vertige larynge. *Progr Med (Paris)* 1879;7:317–9.
1105. Charcot J-M. Un cas de suppression brusque et isolée de la vision mentale des objects (formes et couleurs). *Progr Med (Paris)* 1883;11:568.
1106. Charcot J-M. *Clinical Lectures on Diseases of the Nervous System.* London: The New Sydenham Society, 1889.
1107. Charcot J-M, Bouchard A. Douleurs fulgurantes de l'ataxie sans incoordination des mouvements; sclérose commençante des cordons posterièures de la moêle épinière. *Gaz Med (Paris)* 1866;21:122–4.
1108. Charcot J-M, Joffroy A. Deux cas d'atrophie musculaire progressive avec lesions de la substance grise et des faisceaux anterolateraux de la moelle épinière. *Arch Physiol Norm Pathol (Paris)* 1869;2:354–67.
1109. Charcot J-M, Marie P. Sur une forme particulière d'atrophie musculaire progressive, souvent familiale, débutant par les pieds et les jambes et attéignant plus tard les mains. *RMP* 1886;6:97–138.
1110. Charleston AJ, Andserson NE, Willoughby EW. Idiopathic steroid responsive chronic lymphocytic meningitis – clinical features and long-term outcome in 17 patients. *Aust NZ J Med* 1998;28:784–9.
1111. Charlin C. Le syndrome du nerf nasal. *Ann d'ocul* 1931;168:86.
1112. Charnas LR, Luciano CA, Dalakas M et al. Distal vacuolar myopathy in nephropathic cystinosis. *Ann Neurol* 1994;35:181–8.
1113. Charnas LR, Marini JC. Communicating hydrocephalus, basilar invagination and other features in osteogenesis imperfecta. *Neurology* 1993;43:2603–8.
1114. Charous DI, Saxe BI. The Landry Guillain Barré syndrome: Report of an unusual case. *N Engl J Med* 1962;267:1334–8.
1115. Chaslin P. Note sur l'anatomie pathologique de l'epilepsie dite essentielle. La sclerose nevroglique. *C R Soc Biol* 1889;1:169–71.
1116. Chassaignac P. De la paralysie douloureuse des jeunes enfants. *AGMP* 1856;1: 653–69.
1117. Chatrian GE, Bergamini L, Dondey M et al. A glossary of terms most commonly used by clinical electroencephalographers. *EEG Clin Neurophysiol* 1974;37:538–48.
1118. Chatrian GE, Shaw C-M, Leffman H. The significance of periodic, lateralized epileptiform discharges in EEG: An electrographic, clinical, and pathologic study. *EEG Clin Neurophysiol* 1964;17:177–93.
1119. Chaudhuri A, Behan PO. The clinical spectrum, diagnosis, pathogenesis and treatment of Hashimoto's encephalopathy (Recurrent acute disseminated encephalomyelitis). *Curr Med Chem* 2003;10:1645–53.
1120. Chaudhuri KR, Healy DG, Schapira AHV. Non–motor symptoms of Parkinson's disease: Diagnosis and management. *Lancet Neurology* 2006;5:235–245.
1121. Chaudhuri KR, Pal S, DiMarco A et al. The Parkinson's disease sleep scale. *J Neurol Neurosurg Psychiatr* 2002;73: 629–35.
1122. Chavanay J-A, Brunhes J. Syndromes cephalgiques et psychoneurotiques avec calcification de la faux du cerveau. *Rev Neurol* 1938;69:113–31.
1123. Chavanay J-A, Taptas JN, Haggenmuiller D. Les faux syndromes alternes d'origine hemispherique; l'hemiplegia cruciata par lesions corticales bilaterales. *Presse Med* 1952;60:1126–8.
1124. Chee K-Y, Sachdev P. A controlled study of sensory tics in Gilles de la Tourette syndrome and obsessive-compulsive using a structured interview. *J Neurol Neurosurg Psychiatry* 1997;62:188–92.
1125. Chelluri L, Jastremski MS. Bilateral optic atrophy after cardiac arrest in a patient with acute respiratory failure on positive pressure ventilation. *Rescuscitation* 1998;16:45–8.
1126. Chen C-L, Shen C-C, Wang J et al. Central neurocytoma. *Clin Neurol Neurosurg* 2008;110:129–36.
1127. Chen D-W, Cimino PJ, Ranum LPW et al. The clinical and genetic spectrum of spinocerebellar ataxia 14. *Neurology* 2005;64:1258–60.
1128. Chen HC, Marcharani U. Hashimoto's encephalopathy. *South Med J* 2000;93:504–6.
1129. Chen JWY, Wasterlain CG. Status epilepticus: Pathophysiology and management in adults. *Lancet Neurology* 2006;5:246–56.
1130. Chen R, Collins S, Remtulla H et al. Phrenic nerve conduction study in normal subjects. *Muscle Nerve* 1995;18: 330–5.
1131. Chen R, Sahjpaul R, Del Maestro RF et al. Initial enlargement of the opposite pupil as a false localizing sign in intraparenchymal frontal hemorrhages. *J Neurol Neurosurg Psychiatry* 1994;57:1126–8.
1132. Chen Y-Y, Lirng J-F, Fuh JL et al. Primary cough headache is associated with posterior fossa crowdedness: A morphometric MRI study. *Cephalalgia* 2004;24:694–9.
1133. Cherington M. Botulism: Clinical and therapeutic observations. *Rocky Mt Med J* 1972;69:55–8.
1134. Cherington M. Botulism: Ten year experience. *Arch Neurol* 1974;30:432–7.
1135. Cherington M. Anterior interosseous nerve syndrome straight thumb sign. *Neurology* 1977;27:800–1.
1136. Cherington M. Neurologic manifestations of lightning strikes. *Neurology* 2003;60:182–5.
1137. Cherington M, Yarnell P, Hallmark D. MRI in lightning encephalopathy. *Neurology* 1993;43:1437–8.
1138. Chesney PJ, Davis JP, Purdy WK et al. Clinical manifestations of toxic shock syndrome. *JAMA* 1981;246:741–8.
1139. Chester EM, Agamanolis DP, Banker BQ et al. Hypertensive encephalopathy: A clinicopathologic study of 20 cases. *Neurology* 1978;28:928–39.
1140. Cheung C, Ezzat S, Smyth H, Asa S. The spectrum and significance of primary hypophysitis. *J Clin Endocrinol Metab* 2001;86:1048–53.
1141. Cheyne J. *The English malady, or a Treatise of Nervous Diseases of All Kinds, as Spleen and Vapours, Lowness of Hypochondriacal Distempers Etc.* London: Powell, 1773.

1142. Cheyne J. A case of apoplexy in which the fleshy part of the heart was converted into fat. *Dublin Hosp Rep* 1818;2:216–23.

1143. Chia L-G, Chu F-L. A clinical and genetic study of patients with PCB poisoning. *J Neurol Neurosurg Psychiatry* 1985;**48**: 894–901.

1144. Chiappa KH, Gladstone KJ, Young RR. Brain stem auditory evoked responses: Studies of waveform variations in 50 normal human subjects. *Arch Neurol* 1979;**36**:81–7.

1145. Chiappa KH, Ropper AH. Evoked potentials in clinical medicine. *N Engl J Med* 1982;**306**:1140–50;–1205–1211.

1146. Chiari H. Concerning changes in the cerebellum due to hydrocephalus of the cerebrum. *Dtsch Med Wschr* 1891;**17**:1172–5.

1147. Chiba S, Saitoh M, Hatanaka Y et al. Autosomal dominant muscle cramp syndrome in a Japanese family. *J Neurol Neurosurg Psychiatry* 1999;**67**:116–9.

1148. Childs B, Nyhan WR, Borden M et al. Idiopathic hyperglycinemia and hyperglycinuria. *Pediatrics* 1961;**27**: 522–38.

1149. Chin RL, Sander HW, Brannagan TH et al. Celiac neuropathy. *Neurology* 2003;**60**:1581–5.

1150. Chinnery PF, Crompton D, Birchall D et al. Clinical features and natural history of neuroferritinopathy caused by the *FTL1* 460InsA mutation. *Brain* 2007;**130**:110–9.

1151. Chinnery PF, Johnson MA, Walls TJ et al. A novel autosomal dominant distal myopathy with early respiratory failure: Clinico-pathologic characteristics and exclusion of linkage to candidate genetic loci. *Ann Neurol* 2001;**49**:443–52.

1152. Chinnery PF, Schon EA. Mitochondria. *J Neurol Neurosurg Psychiatr* 2003;**74**: 1188–99.

1153. Chiray P, Foix C, Nicolesco I. Hemi-tremblement du type de la sclérose en plaques par lesion rubro-thalamo-sous-thalamique. *Ann Med* 1923;**14**:173–91.

1154. Chitanondh H, Rosen L. Fatal eosinophilic encephalomyelitis caused by the nematode Gnathostoma sphingerum. *Am J Trop Med* 1967;**16**:638.

1155. Cho H, Skowera A, Cleare A, Wessely S. Chronic fatigue syndrome: An update focusing on phenomenology and pathophysiology. *Curr Opin Psychiatry* 2006;**19**:67–73.

1156. Chodzko W. On a new symptom of organic CNS lesions. *Rev Neurol* 1936;**65**:131–4.

1157. Choi KD, Shin HY, Kim JS et al. Rotational vertebral artery syndrome. *Neurology* 2005;**65**:1287–90.

1158. Chokroverty S, Bruetman ME, Berger V et al. Progressive dialytic encephalopathy. *J Neurol Neurosurg Psychiatry* 1976;**39**:411–9.

1159. Chokroverty S, Khedekar R, Derby B et al. Pathology of olivopontocerebellar atrophy with glutamate dehydrogenase deficiency. *Neurology* 1984;**34**:1451–5.

1160. Chokroverty S, Reyes MG, Rubino FA et al. Hemiplegic amyotrophy: Muscle and motor point biopsy study. *Arch Neurol* 1976;**33**:104–10.

1161. Chokroverty S, Walters A, Zimmerman T et al. Propriospinal myoclonus. *Neurology* 1992;**42**:1591–5.

1162. Chollet P, Rigal J-P, Pignide L. Une complication méconnue de l'hyperthyroidie: La neuropathie péripherique. *Presse Med* 1971;**79**:145.

1163. Cholod EJ, Haust MD, Hudson AJ et al. Myopathy in primary familial hyperparathyroidism. *Amer J Med* 1970;**48**:700–7.

1164. Chou SM. Myxovirus-like structures in a case of human chronic polymyositis. *Science* 1967;**158**:1453.

1165. Chouinard G, Ross-Chouinard A, Annable L et al. The extrapyramidal symptom rating scale. *Can J Neurol Sci* 1980;**7**:233.

1166. Chow CW, Frerman FE, Goodman SI et al. Striatal degeneration in glutaric acidemia Type 2. *Acta Neuropathologica* 1989;**77**:554–6.

1167. Chretien JH, Fermaglich J, Garagusi VF. Ciguatera poisoning: Presentation as a neurologic disorder. *Arch Neurol* 1981;**38**:783.

1168. Christian JC, Bixsler D, Blythe SC et al. Familial telecanthus with associated abnormalities. *Birth Defects Orig Artic Ser* 1969;**5**:82.

1169. Christian JC et al. X-linked skeletal dyspslasia with mental retardation. *Clin Genet* 1977;**11**:128–36.

1170. Christian JC et al. The adducted thumbs syndrome: An autosomal recessive disease with arthrogryposis, dysmyelination, craniostenosis, and cleft palate. *Clin Genet* 1971;**2**:95–103.

1171. Christodoulou K, Zamba E, Tsingis M et al. A novel form of distal hereditary motor neuropathy maps to chromosome 9p21.1-p12. *Ann Neurol* 2000;**48**: 877–84.

1172. Chroni E, Panayiotopoulos CP. F tacheodispersion. *J Neurol Neurosurg Psychiatry* 1993;**56**:1103–8.

1173. Chui HC, Victoroff JI, Margolin D et al. Criteria for the diagnosis of ischemic vascular dementia. *World Neurology* 1992;**7**:12–3.

1174. Chung MH, Sum J, Morrell MJ et al. Intracerebral involvement in Scleroderma en Coup de Sabre: Report of a case with neuropathologic findings. *Ann Neurol* 1995;**37**:679–81.

1175. Chung S, Gerber P, Kirlin KA. Ictal eye closure is a reliable indicator for psychogenic nonepileptic seizures. *Neurology* 2007;**69**:963.

1176. Chung SJ, Kim JS, Lee MC. Syndrome of cerebral spinal fluid hypovolemia. *Neurology* 2000;**55**:1321–7.

1177. Chusid J, DeGutierrez-Mahoney CG. Syndrome of bilateral vestibular paralysis. *J Nerv Ment Dis* 1946;**103**:172–80.

1178. Chutkow JG. Posterior femoral cutaneous neuralgia. *Muscle Nerve* 1988;**11**:1146–8.

1179. Chutkow JG, Heffner RRjr, Kramer AA, Edwards JA. Adult-onset autosomal dominant limb-girdle muscular dystrophy. *Ann Neurol* 1986;**20**:240–8.

1180. Chvostek F. Beitrag zur Tetanie. *Wein Med Presse* 1876;**17**:1201–3.

1181. Ciardo F, Costantino S, Curatolo P. Neurological aspects of adenylosuccinate lysase deficiency. *J Child Neurol* 2001;**16**:301–8.

1182. Cilicchia CF, Gol A, Ericksen EE. Diffuse central nervous system involvement in papulosis atrophica maligna. *Neurology* 1962;**12**:503–9.

1183. Cincotta M, Borgheresi A, Liotta P et al. Reorganization of the motor cortex in a patient with congenital hemiparesis and mirror movements. *Neurology* 2000;**55**:129–31.

1184. Citak KA, Dickoff DJ, Simpson DM. Progressive sensory radiculopathy responsive to corticosteroid therapy. *Muscle Nerve* 1993;**16**:679–80.

1185. Cittadini EM, Matharu MS, Goadsby PJ. Paroxysmal hemicrania. A prospective clinical study of 31 cases. *Brain* 2008;**131**:1142–56.

1186. Claes S, Devrient K, Lagae L et al. The X-linked infantile spasms syndrome. *Ann Neurol* 1997;**42**:360–4.

1187. Clancy RR, Kurtz MB, Baker D et al. Neurologic manifestations of the organoid nevus syndrome. *Arch Neurol* 1985;**42**:236–40.

1188. Clara R, Lowenthal A. Familial and congenital lysine-cystinuria with benign myopathy and dwarfism. *J Neurol Sci* 1966;**3**:433–4.

1189. Clark JR, d'Agostino AN, Wilson J et al. Autosomal dominant myofibrillar inclusion body myopathy. *Neurol Minneap* 1978;**28**:399.

1190. Clarke CRA, Harrison MJG. Neurological manifestations of Paget's disease. *J Neurol Sci* 1978;**38**:171–8.

1191. Clarke E. Apoplexy in the Hippocratic writings. *Bull Hist Med* 1963;**37**:301–14.

1192. Clarke E, Bearn JG. The spiral nerve bands of fontana. *Brain* 1972;**95**:1–20.

1193. Clarke E, Dewhurst K. *An Illustrated History of Brain Function*. Oxford: Sandford Publications, 1972.
1194. Clarke TH, Saunders BS, Feldman B. Pyridoxine-dependent seizures requiring high doses of pyridoxine for control. *Am J Dis Childh* 1979;133:963.
1195. Clarren SK, Alvord EC, Sumi SM et al. Brain malformations related to prenatal exposure to alcohol. *J Pediatr* 1978;92:64.
1196. Classen J. Focal hand dystonia – a disorder of neuroplasticity? *Brain* 2003;126:2571–2.
1197. Claude H. Syndrome pédonculaire de la région du noyau rouge. *Rev Neurol* 1912;23:311–3.
1198. Claude H, Lhermitte JJ. Le syndrome infundibulaire dans les tumeurs de l'encéphale. *Presse Med* 1918.
1199. Clay SA, Ramseyer JC, Fishman LS et al. Acute infantile motor unit disorder. *Arch Neurol* 1977;34:226–43.
1200. Cleckley H. *The Mask of Sanity*. St. Louis: Mosby, 1964.
1201. Cleland JB, Campbell AW. The Australian epidemics of an acute polio-encephalomyelitis (X disease). *Rep Dir-Gen Publ Hlth New S Wales*. 1917;150–280.
1202. Clemens PR, Yamamoto M, Engel AG. Adult phosphorylase b kinase deficiency. *Ann Neurol* 1990;28:529–38.
1203. Clements SD, Peters JE. Minimal brain dysfunctions in school-age child. *Arch Gen Psychiat* 1962;6:185–97.
1204. Cleri D, Villota F, Porwancher R. Smallpox, bioterrorism, and the neurologist. *Arch Neurol* 2003;60:489–94.
1205. Clouston HC. An hereditary ectodermal dystrophy. *Can Med Assn J* 1929;21:18–31.
1206. Co S. Intractable sneezing: Case report and literature review. *Arch Neurol* 1979;36:111–2.
1207. Cobb S. Haemangioma of the spinal cord associated with skin naevi of the same metamere. *Ann Surg* 1915;62:641–9.
1208. Cobb S, Bereday M. Familial system diseases of the neuraxis. *Trans Amer Neurol Assn* 1953;78:12–4.
1209. Cobben JM, de Visser M, Scheffer H et al. Confirmation of clinical diagnosis in requests for prenatal prediction of SMA type 1. *J Neurol Neurosurg Psychiatry* 1993;56:319–21.
1210. Cockayne EA. Dwarfism with retinal atrophy and deafness. *Arch Dis Child* 1936;11:1–8.
1211. Cockel R, Hill EE, Rushton DI et al. Familial steatorrhea with calfcification of the basal ganglia and mental retardation. *Quart J Med* 1973;42:771–83.
1212. Coers C, Telerman-Toppet N, Durdu J. Neurogenic benign fasciculations, pseudomyotonia, and pseudotetany: A disease in search of a name. *Arch Neurol* 1981;38:282–7.
1213. Coers C, Telerman-Toppet N, Gerard J-M. Terminal innervation ratio in neuromuscular disease: Methods and controls. *Arch Neurol* 1973;29:210–4.
1214. Coffin GS. A syndrome of retarded development with characteristic appearance. *Am J Dis Childh* 1968;115:698–702.
1215. Cogan DG. Syndrome of nonsyphilitic interstitial keratitis and vestibuloauditory symptoms. *Arch Ophthalmol* 1945;33:144–9.
1216. Cogan DG. A type of congenital motor apraxia presenting jerky head movements. *Am J Ophthalmol* 1953;36:433–41.
1217. Cogan DG. Ocular dysmetria, flutter-like oscillations of the eyes and opsoclonus. *Arch Ophthalmol* 1954;51:318–35.
1218. Cogan DG. *Neurology of the Ocular Muscles*. Springfield: Charles C Thomas, 1956.
1219. Cogan DG. Hemianopia and associated symptoms due to Parieto-temporal lesions. *Am J Ophthalmol* 1960;50: 1056–66.
1220. Cogan DG. Myasthenia gravis. A review of the disease and a description of lid twitch as a characteristic sign. *Arch Ophthalmol* 1965;74:217–21.
1221. Cogan DG. Opsoclonus, body tremulousness and benign encephalitis. *Arch Ophthalmol* 1968;79:545–51.
1222. Cogan DG, Adams RD. Type of paralysis of conjugate gaze (ocular motor apraxia). *Arch Ophthalmol* 1953;50:434–42.
1223. Cogan DG, Chu FC, Reingold DB. Ocular signs of cerebellar disease. *Arch Ophthalmol* 1982;100:755.
1224. Cogan DG, Freese CG. Spasm of the near reflex. *Arch Ophthalmol* 1955;54:752–9.
1225. Coggins CH, Lillington GA, Gray CP. Micturition syncope. *Arch Int Med* 1964;113:14–8.
1226. Cognard C, Gobin YP et al. Cerebral dural arteriovenous fistulas: Clinical and angiographic correlation with a revised classification of venous drainage. *Radiology* 1995;194:671–80.
1227. Cohen AS, Matharu MS, Goadsby PJ. Short-lasting unilateral neuralgiform headache attacks with conjunctival injection and tearing (SUNCT) or cranial autonomic features (SUNA)-a prospective clinical study of SUNCT and SUNA. *Brain* 2006;129:2746–60.
1228. Cohen D. Magnetoencephalography: Evidence of magnetic fields produced by alpha rhythm currents. *Science* 1968;161:784–6.
1229. Cohen L, Benoit N, Van Eeeckhout P et al. Pure progressive aphemia. *J Neurol Neurosurg Psychiatry* 1993;56:923–4.
1230. Cohen LG, Hallett M. Hand cramps. *Neurology* 1988;38:1005–12.
1231. Cohen M, Campbell R, Yaghmai F. Neuropathological abnormalities in developmental dysphasia. *Ann Neurol* 1989;25:567–70.
1232. Cohen M, Lanska D, Roessmann U et al. Amyloidoma of the CNS. *Neurology* 1992;42:2019–23.
1233. Cohen MM et al. Syndrome with cephalocele. *Teratology* 1982;25:161–72.
1234. Cohen MM JR. Craniosynostosis and syndromes with craniosynostosis: Incidence, genetics, penetrance, variability, and new syndrome updating. *Birth Defects Orig Artic Ser* 1979;15:13–63.
1235. Cohen MM JR. *The Child with Multiple Birth Defects*. New York: Raven Press, 1982.
1236. Cohen MM JR, Gorlin RJ. Prader-Willi syndrome. *Am J Dis Childh* 1969;117:213–8.
1237. Cohen MM JR, et al. A new syndrome with hypotonia, obesity, mental deficiency and facial, oral, ocular and limb anomalies. *J Pediatr* 1973;83:280–4.
1238. Cohen HA, Nussinovitch M, Ashkenazi A et al. Benign abducens nerve palsy of childhood. *Ped Neurol* 1993;9:394–5.
1239. Cohen HA, Nussinovitch M, Ashkenazi A et al. Benign paroxysmal torticollis in infancy. *Ped Neurol* 1993;9:488–90.
1240. Cohn R. Phantom vision. *Arch Neurol* 1971;25:468–71.
1241. Cohn R. Eyeball movements in homonymous hemianopia following simultaneous bitemporal object presentation. *Neurology* 1972;22:12–4.
1242. Cohn R, Neumann MA, Wood DH. Prosopagnosia: A clinical study. *Ann Neurol* 1977;1:177–82.
1243. Colby MY, Kearns TP. Radiation therapy of pituitary adenomas with associated visual impairment. *Proc Staff Meet Mayo Clin* 1962;37:15.
1244. Colebatch JG, Halmagyi GM, Skuse NF. Myogenic potentials generated by a click-evoked vestibulocollic reflex. *J Neurol Neurosurg Psychiatry* 1994;57: 190–7.
1245. Coleman AE, Norman DJ. OKT3 encephalopathy. *Ann Neurol* 1990;28:837–8.
1246. Coleman DI, Gambetti P, DiMauro S. Muscle in Lafora disease. *Arch Neurol* 1974;31:396–406.
1247. Coleman RJ, Russon L, Blanshard K et al. Useless hand of Oppenheim-magnetic resonance imaging findings. *Postgrad Med J* 1993;69:149–50.
1248. Coleman RM. *Periodic Nocturnal Myoclonus in Disorders of Sleep and Wakefulness*. Ann Arbor, Michigan: Yeshiva University Microfilms, 1979.

1249. Coleman RM, Pollak CP, Weitzman ED. Periodic movements in sleep (nocturnal myoclonus): Relation to sleep disorders. *Ann Neurol* 1980;8:416–21.

1250. Collen FM. Rivermead Mobility Index. *Int Disabil Stud* 1991;13:50–4.

1251. Collet FJ. Sur un nouveau syndrome paralytique pharyngo–larynge par blessure de guerre (hemiplégie glosso–laryngo–scapulo–pharyngée). *Lyon Med* 1915;124:121–9.

1252. Collie A, Maruff P, Darby DG et al. The effects of practice on the cognitive test performance of neurologically normal individuals assessed at brief test-retest intervals. *J Int Neuropsychol Soc* 2003;9:419–428.

1253. Collier J. Epilepsy. In Bett WR, ed. *A Short History of Some Common Diseases*, pp 119–36. Oxford: Oxford University Press, 1934.

1254. Collier M. Ophthalmological findings in Kartagener syndrome. *Bull Fr Soc Ophthal* 1961;74:429–47.

1255. Collinge J. Molecular neurology of prion disease. *J Neurol Neurosurg Psychiatry* 2005;76:906–19.

1256. Collins ET. Case with symmetrical congenital notches in the outer parts of each lower lid and defective development of the malar bones. *Trans Ophthal Soc UK* 1900;20:190.

1257. Collins MP, Mendell JR, Periquet MI et al. Superficial peroneal nerve/peroneus brevis muscle biopsy in vasculitic neuropathy. *Neurology* 2000;55:636–43.

1258. Collins SJ, Ahlskog JE, Parisi J et al. Progressive supranuclear palsy: Neuropathologically based diagnostic clinical criteria. *J Neurol Neurosurg Psychiatry* 1995;58:167–73.

1259. Coltheart M, Patterson K, Marshall JC. *Deep Dyslexia*. London: Routledge and Kegan Paul, 1980.

1260. Combs JT, Grunt JA, Brandt IK. New syndrome of neonatal hypoglycemia, association with visceromegaly, macroglossia, microcephaly and abnormal umbilicus. *N Engl J Med* 1966;275: 236–43.

1261. Comi G, Fortunato F, Lucchiari S et al. Beta-enolase deficiency, a new metabolic myopathy of distal glycolysis. *Ann Neurol* 2001;50:202–7.

1262. Comi G, Testa D, Cornelio F et al. Potassium depletion myopathy. *Muscle Nerve* 1985;8:17–21.

1263. Comings DE, Amromin GD. Autosomal dominant insensitivity to pain with hyperplastic myelinopathy. *Neurology* 1974;24:838–48.

1264. Commission for Classification and Terminology I. Proposal for revised classification of epilepsies and epileptic syndromes. *Epilepsia* 1989;30:389–99.

1265. Commission of Epidemiology and Prognosis I. Guidelines for epidemiological studies in epilepsy. *Epilepsia* 1993;34:592–6.

1266. Confavreux C, Compston DAS, Hommes OR et al. EDMUS, a European database for multiple sclerosis. *J Neurol Neurosurg Psychiatry* 1992;55:671–6.

1267. Conics BW, Hollander MB, Berlin CI. Familial neural hearing loss and atopic dermatitis. *JAMA* 1968;204:953.

1268. Conn HO et al. Comparison of lactulose and neomycin in the treatment of chronic portal-systemic encephalopathy. *Gastroenterology* 1977;72:573–83.

1269. Connett MC, Lansche JM. Fibromuscular hyperplasia of the internal carotid artery. *Ann Surg* 1969;162:59–62.

1270. Connolly AM, Dodson WE, Prensky AL et al. Course and outcome of acute cerebellar ataxia. *Ann Neurol* 1994;35:673–9.

1271. Conradi E. Hypoplastic fetal chondrodystrophia. *Jb Kinderheilk* 1914;80:86–7.

1272. Consensus Panel. Report and recommendations of the San Antonio conference on diabetic neuropathy. *Diabetes* 1988;37:1000–4.

1273. Cook AW, Nathan PW, Smith MC. Sensory consequences of commissural myelotomy. *Brain* 1984;107:547–68.

1274. Cooke SF, Bliss TV. Plasticity in the human central nervous system. *Brain* 2006;129:1659–73.

1275. Cooper RG, Stokes MJ, Edwards RHT. Physiological characteristics of the "warm-up" effect of activity in patients with myotonic dystrophy. *J Neurol Neurosurg Psychiatry* 1988;51:1134–41.

1276. Coplan J. *The Early Language Milestone Scale.* Austin, Texas: PRO-ED Inc., 1987.

1277. Coppack SW, Watkins PJ. The natural history of diabetic femoral neuropathy. *Quart J Med* 1991;79:307–13.

1278. Coppeto JR, Lessell S. A familial syndrome of dystonia, blepharospasm, and pigmentary retinopathy. *Neurology* 1990;40:1359–63.

1279. Corbett JJ, Butler AB, Kaufman B. "Sneeze syncope," basilar invagination and Arnold-Chiari type I malformation. *J Neurol Neurosurg Psychiatry* 1976;39: 381–4.

1280. Corbett JJ, Schatz NJ, Shults WT et al. Slowly alternating skew deviation. *Ann Neurol* 1981;10:540–6.

1281. Corbin D, Martyr T, Graham AC. Migraine coma. *J Neurol Neurosurg Psychiatry* 1991;54:744.

1282. Corbin D, Williams A, Johnson AP. Dystonia complicated by respiratory obstruction. *J Neurol Neurosurg Psychiatry* 1987;50:1707.

1283. Cordonnier C, Al-Shahi Salman R, Wardlaw JM. Spontaneous brain microbleeds: Systematic review, subgroup analyses and standards for study design and reporting. *Brain* 2007;130:1988–2003.

1284. Cori GT. Biochemical aspects of glycogen deposition disease. *Bibl Pediat Basel* 1958;66:344–58.

1285. Corkin S. Acquisition of motor skill after bilateral medial temporal lobe excision. *Neuropsychologia* 1968;6:255–65.

1286. Cormand B, Pihko H, Bayés M et al. Clinical and genetic distinction between Walker-Warburg syndrome and muscle-eye-brain disease. *Neurology* 2001;56:1059–69.

1287. Cornblath DR, Chaudhry V, Carter K et al. Total neuropathy score. *Neurology* 1999;53:1660–4.

1288. Cornblath DR. Radiculopathy in AIDS. *Ann Neurol* 1987;21:32.

1289. Corry IS, Cosgrove APDCM. Botulinum toxin A as an alternative to serial casting in the conservative management of equinus in cerebral palsy. *Dev Med Child Neurol* 1995;37:20–1.

1290. Corsellis JAN, Goldberg GJ, Norton AR. "Limbic encephalitis" and its association with carcinoma. *Brain* 1968;91:481–96.

1291. Cortez MA, McKerlie C, Snead OC. A model of atypical absence seizures. *Neurology* 2001;56:341–9.

1292. Cossa PM, Berard-Badier M, Camuzard S et al. Familial polyradiculopathy syndrome. *Rev Neurol* 1957;97:450–65.

1293. Costeff H, Elpeleg O, Apter N et al. 3-Methylglutaconic aciduria in "optic atrophy plus". *Ann Neurol* 1993;33: 103–4.

1294. Costen JB. A syndrome of ear and sinus symptoms dependent upon disturbed function of the temporo-mandibular joint. *Annals of Otology and Rhinology* 1934;43: 1–15.

1295. Coté R, Battista RN, Wolfson C et al. The Canadian Neurological Scale: Validation and reliability assessment. *Neurology* 1989;39:638–43.

1296. Cotugno D. *A Treatise of the Nervous Sciatia or Nervous Hip Gout*. London: Wilkie, 1775.

1297. Coulon A, Lafitte F, Hoang-Xuan K et al. Radiographic findings in 37 cases of primary CNS lymphoma in immunocompetent patients. *Eur Radiol* 2002;12:329–40.

1298. Coulter DL, Allen RJ. Benign neonatal sleep myoclonus. *Arch Neurol* 1982;39:191–2.

1299. Coulter DL, Beals TF, Allan IJ. Neurotrichosis: Hair abnormalities associated with neurological disease. *Devel Med Child Neurol* 1982;24:634.

1300. Courtois A. Unilateral reflex flexion of the leg with flexion of the neck in cases of coma due to focal cerebral lesions. *Ann Med Psychol* 1931;89:506–11.
1301. Courville CB. *Birth and Brain Damage.* Pasadena,TX: M.F.Courville, 1971.
1302. Coutinho A, Andrade C. Autosomal dominant system degeneration in Portuguese families of the Azores Islands. *Neurology* 1978;28:703–9.
1303. Coutinho P, Barros J, Zemmouri R et al. Clinical heterogeneity of autosomal recessive spastic paraplegias: Analysis of 106 patients in 46 families. *Arch Neurol* 1999;56:943–9.
1304. Coutinho P, Cruz VT, Tuna A et al. Cerebellar ataxia with spasmodic cough a new form of dominant ataxia. *Arch Neurol* 2006;63:553–5.
1305. Cox DW. Factors influencing ceruloplasmin levels in normal individuals. *J Lab Clin Med* 1966;68: 893–904.
1306. Cox JM. *Low Back Pain: Mechanism, Diagnosis and Treatment*. BValtimore: Williams and Wilking, 1985.
1307. Cox TA. Pupillary escape. *Neurology* 1992;42:1271–3.
1308. Cox TM. Hereditary fructose intolerance. *Quart J Med* 1988;68:585–94.
1309. Coyle PK, Wolinsky JS. Characterization of immune complexes in progressive rubella panencephalitis. *Ann Neurol* 1981;9:557–62.
1310. Cram RH. A sign of sciatic nerve pressure. *J Bone Jt Surg* 1905;35B:192.
1311. Cramer JA, French J. Quantitative assessment of seizure severity for clinical trials: A review of approaches to seizure components. *Epilepsia* 2001;42:119–29.
1312. Crandall BF. A familial syndrome of deafness, alopecia and hypogonadism. *J Pediatr* 1973;82:461–5.
1313. Cravens G, Kline DG. Posterior interosseous nerve palsies. *Neurosurgery* 1990;27:397–402.
1314. Cravioto H, Feigin I. Noninfectious granulomatous angiitis with a predilection for the nervous system. *Neurology* 1959;9:599–609.
1315. Crawford JR, Santi MR, Vezina G et al. CNS germ cell tumor (CNSGCT) of childhood. *Neurology* 2007;68:1668–73.
1316. Cremer PD, Halmagyi GM, Goadsby PJ. Secondary cluster headache responsive to sumatriptan. *Journal of Neurology, Neurosurgery and Psychiatry* 1995;59: 633–634.
1317. Cremers FPM, Molloy CM, van der Pol DJR et al. An autosomal homologue of the choroideremia gene colocalizes with the Usher syndrome type II locus on the distal part of chromosome 1q. *Hum Mol Genet* 1992;1:71–5.
1318. Creston RN, Godwin-Austen RB. Transient global amnesia in four brothers. *J Neurol Neurosurg Psychiatry* 1982;45:375–7.
1319. Creutzfeldt HG. On a peculiar type of disease of the central nervous system: A preliminary communication. *Z Ges Neurol Psychiat* 1920;57:1–18.
1320. Crevits L. Brachial radial pruritus - a peculiar neuropathic disorder. *Clin Neurol Neurosurg* 2006;108:803–5.
1321. Crevits L, Vander Ecken H. Ocular lateropulsion in Wallenburg's syndrome. *Acta Neurol Scand* 1982;65:219.
1322. Crimlisk H. The little imitator-porphyria: A neuropsychiatric disorder. *J Neurol Neurosurg Psychiatry* 1997;62:319–28.
1323. Crino PB, Henske EP. New developments in the neurobiology of the tuberous sclerosis complex. *Neurology* 1999;53:1384–90.
1324. Critchley M. The anterior cerebral artery and its syndromes. *Brain* 1930;53:120–65.
1325. Critchley M. Musicogenic epilepsy. *Brain* 1937;60:13–27.
1326. Critchley M. Spastic dysphonia ("inspiratory speech"). *Brain* 1939;62:96–103.
1327. Critchley M. *The Language of Gesture*. London: Edward Arnold, 1939.
1328. Critchley M. Types of visual perseveration: Paliopsia and illusory visual spread. *Brain* 1951;74:267–99.
1329. Critchley M. The *Parietal Lobes*. London: Arnold, 1953.
1330. Critchley M. *Aphasiology and Other Disorders of Speech*. London, Edwin Arnold. 1957.
1331. Critchley M. Head's contribution to Aphasia. *Brain* 1961;84:551–60.
1332. Critchley M. Periodic hypersomnia and megaphagia in adolescent males. *Brain* 1962;85:627–56.
1333. Critchley M. Acquired anomalies of colour perception of central origin. *Brain* 1965;88:711–24.
1334. Critchley M. Neurology's debt to F.J. Gall. *Brit Med J* 1965;2:775–81.
1335. Critchley M. The enigma of Gerstmann's syndrome. *Brain* 1966;89:183–98.
1336. Critchley M. *Aphasiology and Other Aspects of Language*. London: Edward Arnold, 1970.
1337. Critchley M. *Aphasiology and Other Disorders of Speech*. London: Arnold, 1980.
1338. Critchley M. And all the daughters of musick shall be brought low: Language function in the elderly. *Arch Neurol* 1984;41:1135–9.
1339. Critchley M, Earl CJC. Tuberose sclerosis and allied conditions. *Brain* 1932;55:311–46.
1340. Critchley M, Henson RA. *Music and the Brain - Studies in the Neurology of Music.* London: Heinemann, 1977.
1341. Crock HV. Isolated lumbar disk resorption as a cause of nerve root canal stenosis. *Clin Orthop* 1976;115:109–15.
1342. Crock HV. Internal disk disruption: A challenge to disc prolapse fifty years on. *Spine* 1986;11:650–3.
1343. Crocker AC, Farber S. Niemann-Pick disease: A review of 18 patients. *Medicine* 1958;37:1–95.
1344. Croft PB, Urich H, Wilkinson M. Peripheral neuropathy of sensorimotor type associated with malignant disease. *Brain* 1967;90:31.
1345. Croft PB, Wilkinson M. The course and prognosis in some types of carcinomatous neuromyopathy. *Brain* 1969;92:1.
1346. Croisile B, Astier JL, Beaumont C. Standardization of the 5-word test in a group of 191 normal subjects aged 50 to 90 years. *Rev Neurol (Paris)* 2007;163:323–33.
1347. Crome L et al. Congenital cataracts, renal tubular necrosis and encephalopathy in two sisters. *Arch Dis Child* 1963;38:505–15.
1348. Crome L, Hanefeld F, Patrick D et al. Late onset globoid cell leukodystrophy. *Brain* 1973;96:841–8.
1349. Crome L, Williams C. The problem of familial multilocular encephalomalacia. *Acta Pediatr Scand* 1960;49:175.
1350. Crook TH, Bartus RT, Ferris SH et al. Age-associated memory impairment: Proposed diagnostic criteria and measures of clinical change: Report of a National Institute of Mental Health work group. *Dev Neuropsychol* 1986;2:261–76.
1351. Crook TH, Ferris SH, McCarthy M. The misplaced objects task: A brief test for memory dysfunction in the aged. *J Am Geriatr Soc* 1979;7:284–7.
1352. Crook TH, Larrabee GJ. Age-associated memory impairment: Diagnostic criteria and treatment strategies. *Psychopharm Bull* 1988;2:509–14.
1353. Crosby L, Parsons LC. Clinical neurological assessment tool. *Heart Lung* 1989;18:121–9.
1354. Cross HE, McKusick VA. The mast syndrome. *Arch Neurol* 1967;16:1–13.
1355. Cross HE, McKusick VA. The Troyer syndrome: A recessive form of spastic paraplegia with distal muscle wasting. *Arch Neurol* 1967;16:473–85.
1356. Cross HE, McKusick VA, Breen W. A new oculocerebral syndrome with hypopigmentation. *J Pediatr* 1967;70:398–406.
1357. Crouzon E. De l'acrocephalosyndactylie. *Bull Soc Med Hop Paris* 1906;23:1310–30.

1358. Crouzon O. Dysostose cranio–faciale hereditaire. *Bull Soc Med Hop Paris* 1912;33:545–55.
1359. Crouzon O, Justin-Besancon L-E. Post-traumatic parkinsonism. *Presse Med* 1929;37:1325–7.
1360. Crow RS. Peripheral neuritis in myelomatosis. *Brit Med J* 1956;2:802–4.
1361. Croxen R, Newland C, Betty M et al. Novel functional ε-subunit polypeptide generated by a single nucleotide deletion in acetylcholine receptor deficiency congenital myasthenic syndrome. *Ann Neurol* 1999;46:639–47.
1362. Cruchet JR. *Traité des torticollis spasmodiques*. Paris: Masson, 1907.
1363. Cruchet JR, Moutier J, Calmettes R. Quarante cas d'encephalomyelite subaîgue. *Bull Soc Med Hop Paris* 1917;41:814–6.
1364. Crue BL. *Medulloblastoma*. Springfield Illinois: Charles C. Thomas, 1958.
1365. Cruickshank JK, Rudge P, Dalgleish AG et al. Tropical spastic paraparesis and human T-cell lymphotropic virus Type 1 in the United Kingdom. *Brain* 1989;112:1057.
1366. Cruveilhier J. *Anatomie pathologique du corps humain.* Paris: Baillière, 1829.
1367. Cruz Martinez A, Conde MCP, Ferrer MT et al. Neuromuscular disorders in a new toxic syndrome. *Muscle Nerve* 1984;7:12–22.
1368. Cuba Neuropathy Field Investigation Team. Epidemic optic neuropathy in Cuba – clinical characterization and risk factors. *N Engl J Med* 1995;333:1176–82.
1369. Cuetter AC, Bartoszek DM. The thoracic outlet syndrome: Controversies, overdiagnosis, overtreatment and recommendations for management. *Muscle Nerve* 1989;12:410–9.
1370. Cullen B, O'Neill B, Evans JJ et al. A review of screening tests for cognitive impairment. *J Neurol Neurosurg Psychiatry* 2007;78:790–9.
1371. Cumming WJK. Lipid myopathy. *J Neurol Sci* 1984;64:73–7.
1372. Cumming WJK, Weiser R, Teoh R et al. Localized nodular myositis: A clinical and pathological variant of polymyositis. *Quart J Med* 1977;46:531–46.
1373. Cummings J, Benson DF, LoVerne S. Reversible dementias. *JAMA* 1980;243:2434–9.
1374. Cummings JL, Gittinger JW Jr. Central dazzle: A thalamic syndrome? *Arch Neurol* 1981;38:372–4.
1375. Cummings JL, Mega M, Gray K et al. The neuropsychiatric inventory. *Neurology* 1994;44:2308–14.
1376. Cummings JL, Syndulko K, Goldberg Z et al. Palinopsia reconsidered. *Neurology* 1982;32:444–7.
1377. Cummings JL, Uwming WJK, Weiser TR et al. *Quart J Med* 1977;46:531–46.
1378. Cummings JN, Kremer M. Clinical effects of hypoglycemia. *Biochemical Aspects of Neurological Disorders*, pp 159–68. Philadelphia: Lippincott, 1965.
1379. Cummins D. Arenaviral haemorrhagic fevers. *Blood Rev* 1991;5:129–37.
1380. Cuneo RA, Caronna JJ, Pitts L et al. Upward transtentorial herniation: Seven cases and a literature review. *Arch Neurol* 1979;36:618–23.
1381. Cunliffe WJ, Hudgson P, Fulthorpe JJ et al. A calcitonin–secreting medullary thyroid carcinoma associated with mucosal neuromas, marfanoid features, myopathy and pigmentation. *Amer J Med* 1970;48:120–6.
1382. Curless RG, Flynn JT, Olsen KR et al. Leber congenital amaurosis in siblings with diffuse demyelination. *Ped Neurol* 1991;7:223–5.
1383. Curran T, Grewal K, Frecker M. Dystonia, acanthocytosis, basal ganglia "calcification" and eye abnormalities (DACE syndrome). 1993. (Personal Communication)
1384. Currie S, Noronha M, Harriman DGF. Minicore disease. *Excerpta Medica Int. Congr. Ser* 1974;334:12.
1385. Currie S, Roberts AH, Urich H. The nosological position of concentric lacunar leucoencephalopathy. *J Neurol Neurosurg Psychiatry* 1970;33:131–7.
1386. Currier RD, Giles CL, DeJong RN. Some comments on Wallenberg's lateral medullary syndrome. *Neurology* 1961;11:778–91.
1387. Curschmann H. Ueber die diagnostische Bedeutung des Babinskischen Phaenomens im praeuraemischen Zustand. *Munch Med Wschr* 1911;39:2054–7.
1388. Curtius F. Kongenitaler partieller Riesenwuchsmit endocrinen Storungen. *Arch Klin Med* 1925;147:310–9.
1389. Cushing HW. Concerning a definite regulatory system mechanism of the vasomotor center which controls blood pressure during cerebral compression. *John Hopkins Hosp Bull* 1901;12:290–2.
1390. Cushing HW. *Tumors of the Nervus Acousticus and the Syndrome of the Cerebellopontine Angle*. Philadelphia: Saunders, 1917.
1391. Cushing HW. The meningiomas (dural endotheliomas): Their source and favoured seats of origin. *Brain* 1922;5:282–316.
1392. Cushing HW. The chiasmal syndrome of primary optic atrophy with bitemporal field defects in adults with a normal sella turcica. *Arch Ophthalmol* 1930;3:505–51.
1393. Cushing HW. The basophil adenomas of the pituitary body and their clinical manifestations (pituitary basophilism). *Bull Johns Hopkins Hosp* 1932;50:137–95.
1394. Cushing HW, Walker CB. Distortions of the visual fields in cases of brain tumour. *Brain* 1915;37:341–400.
1395. Cushman J, Floccare D. Flicker illness: An under-recognized but preventable complication of helicopter transport. *Prehosp Emerg Care* 2007;11:85–8.
1396. Cusimano MD, Bilbao JM, Cohen SM. Hypertrophic brachial plexus neuritis: A pathological study of two cases. *Ann Neurol* 1988;24:615–22.
1397. Cutler EA et al. A familial thyrocerebral-renal syndrome. *Birth Defects Orig Artic Ser* 1978;14:265–74.
1398. Cutler RWP,Spertell RB. Cerebrospinal fluid: A selective review. *Ann Neurol* 1982;11:1–10.
1399. Cytowic RE. *Synesthesia: A Union of the Senses*. New York: Springer–Verlag, 1988.
1400. Cytowic RE. Synesthesia: Phenomenology and neuropsychology: A review of current knowledge. *Psyche* 1995;2:723–93.
1401. D'Addario R, Greenberg J, O'Neill JE et al. Pneumocephalus: An unusual cause. *J Neurol Neurosurg Psychiatry* 1974;37:271–4.
1402. D'Agostino MD, Bastos A, Pisas C et al. Posterior quadrantic dysplasia or hemi-hemimegalencephaly. *Neurology* 2004;62:2214–20.
1403. D'Alessio JG, Rosenblum M. The Bezold-Jarisch reflex. *Anesth Analg* 1996;83:201–2.
1404. D'Amico A, Tessa A, Bruno C et al. Expanding the clinical spectrum of POMT1 phenotype. *Neurology* 2006;66:1564–7.
1405. D'Amico D, Rigamonti A, Spina L et al. Migraine, celiac disease and cerebral calcifications. *Headache* 2005;45:1263–6.
1406. D'Avanzo R, Scuotto A, Natale M et al. Transient "cerebellar" mutism in lesions of the mesencephalic-cerebellar region. *Acta Neurologica* 1993;15:289–96.
1407. D'Costa DF, Abbott RJ, Pye IF et al. The apomorphine test in Parkinsonian syndromes. *J Neurol Neurosurg Psychiatry* 1991;54:870–2.
1408. Daentl DL, Berg BO, Layzer RB et al. A new familial arthrogryposis without weakness. *Neurology* 1974;24:55–60.
1409. Dal Canto MC, Rapin I, Suzuki K. Neuronal storage disease with chorea and curvilinear bodies. *Neurology* 1974;24:1026.
1410. Dalakas M. Progress in inflammatory myopathies: Good but not good enough. *J Neurol Neurosurg Psychiatry* 2001;70:569–73.
1411. Dalakas MC. Chronic idiopathic ataxic neuropathy. *Ann Neurol* 1986;19:545–54.
1412. Dalakas MC, Elder G, Hallett M et al. A long-term follow-up study of patients

with post-poliomyelitis neuromuscular symptoms. *N Engl J Med* 1986;314: 959–63.

1413. Dalakas MC et al. Late post-polio muscular atrophy. *Rev Inf Dis* 1984;6 (**Suppl.** 2):S562.

1414. Dalakas MC, Hallett M. Post-polio muscular atrophy. In Plum F, ed. *Advances in Contemporary Neurology*, pp 61–83. Philadelphia: F.A. Davis, 1988.

1415. Dalal PM. The aortic arch syndrome. In Spillane JD, ed. *Tropical Neurology*, pp 92–8. London: Oxford, 1973.

1416. Dalby MA. Epilepsy and 3 per second spike wave rhythms. A clinical, EEG and prognostic analysis of 346 patients. *Acta Neurol Scand* 1969;40 **Suppl.**:1–183.

1417. Dale RC, Church AJ, Surtees RAH et al. Encephalitis lethargica syndrome:20 new cases and evidence of basal ganglia autoimmunity. *Brain* 2004;127:21–33.

1418. Daley ML, Swank RL, Ellison CM. Flicker fusion thresholds in multiple sclerosis: A functional measure of neurological damage. *Arch Neurol* 1979;36:292–5.

1419. Dalla Bernardina B, Bureau M, Dravet C et al. Epilepsie benigne de l'enfant avec crises a semeiologie affective. *Rev Electroencephalogr Neurophysiol Clin* 1980;10:8–18.

1420. Dalmau J, Graus F, Villarejo A et al. Clinical analysis of anti-Ma2-associated encephalitis. *Brain* 2004;127:1831–44.

1421. Dalmau J, Posner JB. Neurologic paraneoplastic antibodies (anti-Yo; anti-Hu; anti-Ri). *Neurology* 1994;44:2241–6.

1422. Dalmau JO, Posner JB. Paraneoplastic syndromes. *Arch Neurol* 1999;56:405–8.

1423. Dalton J. Extraordinary facts relating to the vision of colours with observations. *Mem Lit and Phil Soc (Manchester)* 1798;5:28–45.

1424. Dalton K, Dalton MJT. Characteristics of pyridoxine overdose neuropathy syndrome. *Acta Neurol Scand* 1987;76: 8–11.

1425. Daltroy LH, Fossel AH et al. The POSNA pediatric musculoskeletal functional health questionnaire: Report on reliability, validity, and sensitivity to change. *J Pediatr Orthop* 1988;18:561–71.

1426. Daly DD. Uncinate fits. *Neurology* 1958;8:250–60.

1427. Daly RF, Forster FM. Inheritance of reading epilepsy. *Neurol Minneap* 1975;25:1051–4.

1428. Damas-Mora J, Skelton-Robinson, Jenner FA. The Charles Bonnet syndrome in perspective. *Psychol Med* 1982;12:251–61.

1429. Damasio AR. Autism. *Arch Neurol* 1984;41:481.

1430. Damasio AR. Disorders of complex visual processing: Agnosias, achromatopsia, Balint's syndrome, and related difficulties of orientation and construction. In Mesulam M-M, (ed). *Principles of Behavioral Neurology*, pp 259–89. Philadelphia: F.A. Davis Co., 1985.

1431. Damasio AR. Aphasia. *N Engl J Med* 1992;326:531–9.

1432. Damasio AR, Damasio H, Rizzo M et al. Aphasia with non-hemorrhagic lesions in the basal ganglia and internal capsule. *Arch Neurol* 1982;39:15–20.

1433. Damasio AR, Damasio H, Van Hoesen GW. Prosopagnosia: Anatomic basis and behavioral mechanisms. *Neurology* 1982;32:331–41.

1434. Damasio AR, Galaburda AM. Norman geschwind. *Arch Neurol* 1985;42:500–4.

1435. Damasio H, Damasio AR. The anatomical basis of conduction aphasia. *Brain* 1980;103:337–50.

1436. Dan D, Grubb BP, Mouhaffel AH et al. Use of serotonin re-uptake inhibitors as primary therapy for carotid sinus hypersensitivity. *Clinical Electrophysiology* 1997;20:1633–5.

1437. Dana CL. Hereditary tremor, a hitherto undescribed form of motor neurosis. *Amer J Med Sci* 1887;94:386–93.

1438. Dana CL. The degenerative diseases of the spinal cord with the description of a new type. *J Nerv Ment Dis* 1891;18:205–16.

1439. Dandy WE. Ventriculography following the injection of air into the cerebral ventricles. *Ann Surg* 1918;68:5–11.

1440. Dandy WE. Rontgenography of the brain after the injection of air into the spinal canal. *Ann Surg* 1919;70:397–403.

1441. Dandy WE. The diagnosis and treatment of hydrocephalus due to occlusion of the foramina of Luschka and Magendie. *Surg Gyn Obst* 1921;32:112–24.

1442. Danek A, Rubio JP, Rampoldi L et al. McLeod neuroacanthocytosis: Genotype and phenotype. *Ann Neurol* 2001;50:755–64.

1443. Danielssen DC, Boeck CW. *Om spedalskheden.* Christiana: Grondahl, 1847.

1444. Danon MJ, Carpenter S, Manaligod R et al. Fatal infantile glycogen storage disease. *Neurology* 1981;31:1302–7.

1445. Danon MJ, Oh SJ, DiMauro S et al. Lysosomal glycogen storage diseases with normal acid maltase. *Neurology* 1981;31:51–7.

1446. Danpure J, Angelini C, Vergani L. Enzymic diagnosis of primary hyperoxaluria, type 1 by measurement of hepatic alanine: Glyoxalate aminotransferase activity. *Lancet* 1987;1:289–91.

1447. Danta G. Familial carpal tunnel syndrome with onset in childhood. *J Neurol Neurosurg Psychiatry* 1975;38:350–5.

1448. Danta G, Hilton RC, Lynch PG. Chronic progressive external ophthalmoplegia. *Brain* 1975;98:473–92.

1449. Danzl DF, Pozos RS. Accidental hypothermia. *N Engl J Med* 1994;331:1756–60.

1450. Daras M, Koppel BS, Atos-Radzien E. Cocaine-induced choreoathetoid movements (crack dancing). *Neurology* 1994;44:751–2.

1451. Darby DY, Domman GA, Saling MA. Primary interventricular hemorrhage. *Neurology* 1988;38:68–75.

1452. Darin N, Kyllerman M, Wahlstrom J et al. Autosomal dominant myopathy with congenital joint contractures, ophthalmoplegia and rimmed vacuoles. *Ann Neurol* 1998;44:242–8.

1453. Darley FL, Aronson AE, Brown JR. Differential diagnostic pattern of dysarthria. *J Speech Hear Res* 1969;12:246–9.

1454. Darley FL, Aronson AE, Brown JR. *Audioseminars in Speech Pathology – Motor Speech Disorders*. Philadelphia: Saunders, 1975.

1455. Darnell RB, Arbit E. Reversible diencephalic dysfunction. *Neurology* 1993;43:579–82.

1456. Daroff R. Ocular oscillations. *Ann Otol Rhinol* 1977;86:1–6.

1457. Daroff RB. The office tensilon test for ocular myasthenia gravis. *Arch Neurol* 1986;43:843–4.

1458. Daroff RB, Deller JJ, Kastl AJ et al. Cerebral malaria. *JAMA* 1967;202:679–82.

1459. Daroff RB, Hoyt WF. Supranuclear disorders of ocular motor control systems in man. In Bach-y-Rita P, Collins CC, Hyde JE, eds. *The Control of Eye Movements*, pp 191–5. New York: Academic Press, 1971.

1460. Daroff RB, Hoyt WF, Sanders MD et al. Gaze-evoked eyelid and ocular nystagmus inhibited by the near reflex. *J Neurol Neurosurg Psychiatry* 1968;31:362–7.

1461. See 1462.

1462. Darsee JR, Miklozek L, Heynsfield S et al. Mitral valve prolapse and ophthalmoplegia. *Ann Int Med* 1980;92:735–41.

1463. Darvesh S, Leach L, Black SE et al. The behavioural neurology assessment. *Can J Neurol Sci* 2005;32:167–77.

1464. Darwish H, Sarnat HB, Archer C et al. Congenital cervical spinal muscular atrophy. *Muscle Nerve* 1981;4:106–10.

1465. Dastur DK, Manghani DK, Osuntokun BO et al. Neuromuscular and related changes in malnutrition. *J Neurol Sci* 1982;55:207–30.

1466. Dastur DK, Udani PM. The pathology and pathogenesis of tuberculous encephalopathy. *Acta Neuropathol* 1992;6:311–26.

1467. Dau PC. Plasmapheresis: Therapeutic or experimental procedure? *Arch Neurol* 1984;41:647–53.
1468. Daube JR. Rucksack paralysis. *JAMA* 1969;208:2447–52.
1469. Daube JR, Peters HA. Hereditary essential myoclonus. *Arch Neurol* 1966;15:587–94.
1470. Dauer WT, Burke RE, Greene P et al. Current concepts on the clinical features, aetiology and management of idiopathic cervical dystonia. *Brain* 1996;121:547–60.
1471. Daum RS, Scriver CR, Mamer OA et al. An inherited disorder of isoleucine catabolism causing accumulation of alpha methylacetoacetate and alpha-methyl-beta-hydroxybutyrate, and intermittent acidosis. *Pediat Res* 1973;7:149.
1472. Daum RS, Lamm PH, Mamer OA et al. A "new" disorder of isoleucine catabolism. *Lancet* 1971;2:1289–90.
1473. Daumas-Duport C. Histological grading of gliomas. *Curr Opin Neurol Neurosurg* 1992;5:924–31.
1474. Daumas-Duport C, Scheithauer B, O'Fallon J et al. Grading of astrocytomas: A simple and reproducible method. *Cancer* 1988;62:2152–65.
1475. David AS, Jeste DV, Folstein MF et al. Voluntary movement dysfunction in Huntington's disease and Tardive dyskinesia. *Acta Neurol Scand* 1987;75:130–9.
1476. David DJ, Proudman TW. Cephaloceles: Classification, pathology and management. *World J Surg* 1989;13: 349–57.
1477. David NJ. Optokinetic nystagmus. *J Clin Neuro-Ophthalmol* 1989;9:258–66.
1478. David TJ. Nature and etiology of the Poland anomaly. *N Engl J Med* 1972;287:487–9.
1479. Davidenkow S. Scapuloperoneal amyotrophy. *Arch Neurol Psychiatry* 1939;41:694–701.
1480. Davidson G. Time agnosia. *J Nerv Ment Dis* 1941;94:336–43.
1481. Davidson S. Cryptococcal spinal arachnoiditis. *J Neurol Neurosurg Psychiatry* 1968;31:76.
1482. Davion S, Johnson N, Weintraub S et al. Clinicopathologic correlation in PGRN mutations. *Neurology* 2007;69:1113–21.
1483. Davis FA, Bergen D, Schauf C et al. Movement phosphenes in optic neuritis: A new clinical sign. *Neurology* 1967;26:1100–4.
1484. Davis LE, DeBiasi R, Goade DE et al. West Nile virus neuroinvasive disease. *Ann Neurol* 2006;60:286–300.
1485. Davis LE, Greenlee JE. Pneumococcal meningitis: Antibiotics essential but insufficient. *Brain* 2003;126:1013–4.
1486. Davis MJ, Cilo M, Plaitakis A et al. Trichinosis: Severe myopathic involvement with recovery. *Neurology* 1976;26:37–40.
1487. Davis RL, Holohan PD, Shrimptom AE et al. Familial encephalopathy with neuroserpin inclusion bodies. *Am J Path* 1999;155:1901–13.
1488. Dawson G. Glycosphingolipid levels in an unusual neurovisceral storage disease: Lactosylceramidosis. *J Lipid Res* 1972;13:207–19.
1489. Dax M. Lesions de la moitié gauche de l'encéphale coincident avec l'oublie des signes de la pensée. *Gaz Hebd Med Chir* 1865;2:259.
1490. Day JW, Raskin NH. Thunderclap headache: Symptom of unruptured cerebral aneurysm. *Lancet* 1986;ii:1247–8.
1491. Dayan AD, Williams R. Demyelinating peripheral neuropathy in liver disease. *Lancet* 1967;2:133–4.
1492. de Barsy AM, Moens E, Dierckx L. Dwarfism, oligophrenia and degeneration of the elastic tissue in skin and cornea: A new syndrome? *Helv Pediat Acta* 1968;23:305–13.
1493. de Falco FA, Striano P, de FalcoA et al. Benign adult familial myoclonic epilepsy. *Neurology* 2003;60:1381–5.
1494. De Gasperi R, Gama Sosa MA, Battinisti S et al. Late onset GM2 gangliosidosis. *Neurology* 1996;47:547–52.
1495. de Grouchy J, Turleau C, Leonard C. Etude en fluorescence d'une trisomy C mosaique, probablement 8:46, XY-47, XY:8+. *Ann Genet* 1971;14:69.
1496. de Haan R, Aaronson N, Limburg M et al. Measuring quality of life in stroke. *Stroke* 1993;24:320–7.
1497. de Haan RJ. *Clinimotrics in Stroke*. Univ. Amsterdam. 1994. (Thesis)
1498. De Jong JGY. Over families met hereditaires disposities tpt het optreden van neuritiden gecorreleerd met migraine. *Psychiat Neurol (Belg)* 1947;50:60–76.
1499. De Jong JGY, Sloof JL, van der Erden AAJJ. A family with paramyotonia congenita, with the report of an autopsy. *Acta Neurol Scand* 1973;49:480–94.
1500. de Jong RN. *The Neurological Examination*. Hagerstown, MD.: Harper and Row, 1979.
1501. De Kruijk JR, Leffers P, Menheere PP et al. Prediction of post-traumatic complaints after mild traumatic brain injury: Early symptoms and biochemical markers. *J Neurol Neurosurg Psychiatry* 2002;73:727–32.
1502. de la Monte SM, Horowitz SA, Larocque AA et al. Keyhole aqueduct syndrome. *Arch Neurol* 1986;43:926–9.
1503. de Lange C. Sur un type nouveau de dégenération (typus amstelodamnus). *Arch Med Enf Paris* 1933;36:713–9.
1504. de Lange C. Congenital hypertrophy of the muscles, extrapyramidal motor disturbances and mental deficiency. A clinical entity. *Am J Dis Childh* 1934;48:243–68.
1505. de Lange FP, Kalkman JS, Bleijenberg G et al. Neural correlates of the chronic fatigue syndrome-an fMRI study. *Brain* 2004;127:1948–57.
1506. De Leon GA, Grover WD, Huff DS et al. Globoid cells, glial nodules and peculiar fibrillary changes in the cerebro-hepato-renal syndrome of Zellweger. *Ann Neurol* 1977;2:473–84.
1507. De Lisi L. Su di un fenomeno motorio costante del sonno normale: Le mioclonie ipniche fisiolische. *Riv Pat Nerv Ment* 1932;39:481–96.
1508. de Melo A, Krauss GL, Niedermeyer E. Spindle coma: Observations and thoughts. *Clin Electroenceph* 1990;21:151–61.
1509. de Morsier G. Pathologie du diencephale. Le syndrome psychologique et le syndrome sensori-moteur. *Schweiz Arch Neur* 1944;54:161–226.
1510. de Morsier G. Median cranioencephalic dysraphias and olfactogenital dysplasia. *World Neurol* 1962;3:485–506.
1511. de Morsier G. Contribution a l'étude clinique des alterations de la formation reticulée: Le syndrome sensori-moteur et psychologique. *J Neurol Sci* 1966;4:15–49.
1512. de Morsier G. Amyotrophic lateral sclerosis with Pick disease. *Rev Neurol* 1967;116:373.
1513. De Myer W. Megalencephaly: Types, clinical syndromes and management. *Ped Neurol* 1986;2:321–7.
1514. De Paepe A, Devereux RB, Dietz HC et al. Revised diagnostic criteria for the Marfan syndrome. *Am J Med Genet* 1996;62:417–426.
1515. De Renzi E. Slowly progressive visual agnosia or apraxia without dementia. *Cortex* 1986;22:171–80.
1516. De Renzi E, Faglione P. Normative data and screening power of a shortened version of the token test. *Cortex* 1978;14:41–9.
1517. De Renzi E, Vignolo LA. The token test: A sensitive test to detect receptive disturbances in aphasics. *Brain* 1962;85:665–78.
1518. De Sanctis C, Cacchione A. L'idiozia xerodermica. *Riv Sper Freniatr* 1932;56:269.
1519. de Silva RN. A diagnostic sign in migraine? *J Roy Soc Med* 2001;94:286–7.
1520. De Simone R. Hypnic headache: An update. *J Neurol Sci* 2006;27.
1521. de Visser M, Scholte HR, Schutgens RS et al. Riboflavine responsive hereditary storage myopathy and glutaric aciduria Type II of early adult onset. *Neurology* 1986;36:367–72.

1522. De Wytt CN, Dickson PL, Holt GW. Cryptococcal meningitis. *J Neurol Sci* 1982;53:283–92.

1523. de Yebenes JG, Vacquez A, Rabarro J et al. Hereditary branchial myoclonus with spastic paraparesis and cerebellar ataxia. *Neurology* 1988;38:569–72.

1524. Deady JP, Morrell AJ, Sutton GA. Recognising aponeurotic ptosis. *J Neurol Neurosurg Psychiatry* 1989;52:996–8.

1525. Dearborn G. A case of congenital general pure analgesia. *J Nerv Ment Dis* 1932;75:612–5.

1526. DeBassio WA, Kemper TL, Knoefel JE. Coffin-Siris syndrome: Neuropathological findings. *Arch Neurol* 1985;42:350–3.

1527. Debré R, Semelaigne G. Hypertrophie musculaire generalisée du petit enfant. *Bull Soc Pediat Paris* 1934;32:699–706.

1528. Dechambre A. Memoire sur la curabilité du ramollissement cérébral. *Gaz Med (Paris)* 1838;6:305–14.

1529. DeCroix JP, Graveleau PH, Masson M et al. Infarction in the territory of the anterior choroidal artery: A clinical and computerized tomographic study of 16 cases. *Brain* 1986;109:1071–85.

1530. deGirolami U, Haas ML, Richardson EP JR. Subacute diencephalic angioencephalopathy – a clinico-pathologic case study. *J Neurol Sci* 1974;22:197–210.

1531. Degos R, Delort J, Tricot R. Dermatite papulo-squameuse atrophiante. *Bull Soc France Derm Syph* 1942;49:148–281.

1532. Degoul F, Pou-Serradell A, Lloreta J et al. Myo-leukoencephalopathy in twins: Study of 3243 myopathy, encephalopathy, lactic acidosis and strokelike episodes of mitochondrial mutation. *Ann Neurol* 1994;35:365–70.

1533. DeGrouchy J, Royer P, Salmon CH et al. Deletion partielle des bras longs du chromosome 18. *Path et Biol* 1964;12:5–79.

1534. Dehan M, Quilleron D, Navelet Y et al. Les convulsions du cinquieme jour de vie: Un nouveau syndrome? *Arch Fr Ped* 1977;34:730–42.

1535. Dehkharghani F, Sarnat H, Brewster M et al. Congenital muscle fiber type disproportion in Krabbe's leukodystrophy. *Arch Neurol* 1981;38:585–7.

1536. Dejean MC. Le syndrome du plancher de l'orbite. *Bull Fr Soc Ophthal* 1935;48: 473–85.

1537. Déjèrine JJ. Sur un cas de paraplégie par névrites périphèriques, chez un ataxique morphiomane. *C R Soc Biol* 1887;4:137–43.

1538. Déjèrine JJ. Sur un cas de cécité verbal avec agraphie, suivie d'autopsie. *C R Soc Biol* 1891;3:197–201.

1539. Déjèrine JJ. *Diseases of the Spinal Cord.* Paris: Baillière, 1909.

1540. Déjèrine JJ. *Sémiologie des affections du système nerveux.* Paris: Masson, 1914.

1541. Déjèrine JJ, Déjerine-Klumpke H. *Anatomie des centres nerveux.* Paris: J. Rueff, 1901.

1542. Déjèrine JJ, Mouzon J. Two cases of a sensory cortical syndrome. *Rev Neurol* 1914;28:388–92.

1543. Déjèrine JJ, Roussy G. Le syndrome thalamique. *Rev Neurol* 1906;14:521–32.

1544. Déjèrine JJ, Sottas J. Sur la névrite interstitielle hypertrophique et progressive de l'enfant. *C R Soc Biol* 1890;2:43–53.

1545. Déjèrine JJ, Thomas A. L'atrophie olivo-ponto-cerebelleuse. *Nouv Icon Salpet* 1900;13:330–70.

1546. DeJong JGY, Sloof JL, van der Erden AAJJ. A family with paramyotonia congenita with the report of an autopsy. *Acta Neurol Scand* 1973;49:480–94.

1547. DeJong R. *The Neurological Examination.* N.Y.: Harper & Row, 1967.

1548. Dejoun HH. *Experimental Catatonia.* Baltimore: Williams and Wilkins, 1945.

1549. Dekaban AS. Anencephaly in human embryos. *J Neuropath Exp Neurol* 1963;22:533.

1550. Del Brutto OH, Rajshekhar V, White AC et al. Proposed diagnostic criteria for neurocysticercosis. *Neurology* 2001;57:177–83.

1551. Del Brutto OH, Wadia NH, Dumas M et al. Proposal of diagnostic criteria for human cysticercosis and neurocysticercosis. *J Neurol Sci* 1996;142:1–6.

1552. Delacourte A, Buée L. Tau pathology: A marker of neurodegenerative disorders. *Curr Opin Neurol* 2000;13:371–6.

1553. Delalande S, de Seze J, Fauchais A et al. Neurologic manifestations in primary Sjögren syndrome: A study of 82 patients. *Medicine (Baltimore)* 2004;83:280–91.

1554. Delaney P. Neurologic manifestations of sarcoidosis. *Ann Int Med* 1977;87: 336–45.

1555. Deleu D, Buisseret T, Ebinger G. Vertical one and a half syndrome. *Arch Neurol* 1989;46:1361–3.

1556. Delgado-Escueta AV. Epileptogenic paroxysms: Modern approaches and clinical correlations. *Neurology* 1979;29:1014–22.

1557. Delgado-Escueta AV, Greenberg D. Classification of the epilepsies for genetic studies. *Ann Neurol* 1984;16: (Suppl. 1) 11.

1558. Delis DC, Kramer JH, Kaplan E et al. *The California Verbal Learning Test.* New York: Psychological Corporation, 1987.

1559. DeLisa JA, Saeed MA. The tarsal tunnel syndrome. *Muscle Nerve* 1983;6:664–70.

1560. Delitto A. Isokinetic dynamometry. *Muscle Nerve* 1990;S53–S57.

1561. Dell'Osso LF. Nystagmus, saccadic intrusions/oscillations and oscillopsia. In Lessell S, van Dalen JTW, eds. *Current Neuro-Ophthalmology*, pp 153–91. St.Louis: Mosby-Year Book, 1991.

1562. Dell'Osso LF, Schmidt D, Daroff RB. Latent, manifest latent and congenital nystagmus. *Arch Ophthalmol* 1979;97:1877–85.

1563. Dell'Osso LF, Troost BT, Daroff RB. Macro square wave jerks. *Neurology* 1975;25:975–9.

1564. Dell'Osso LF, Weissman BM, Leigh RJ et al. Hereditary congenital nystagmus and gaze-holding failure. *Neurology* 1993;43:1741–9.

1565. Delleman JW, Oorthuys JWE. Orbital cysts in addition to congenital cerebral and focal dermal malformations: A new entity? *Clin Genet* 1984;25:470–2.

1566. DeLong GR, Bean SC, Brown FR. Acquired reversible autistic syndrome in acute encephalopathic illness in children. *Arch Neurol* 1981;38:191–4.

1567. Delwaide PJ, Pepin JL, Maertens de Noordhout A. The audiospinal reaction in Parkinsonian patients reflects functional changes in reticular nuclei. *Ann Neurol* 1993;33:63–9.

1568. DeMarco P, Tassinari CA. Extreme somatosensory evoked potential (ESEP): An EEG sign forecasting the possible occurrence of seizures in children. *Epilepsia* 1981;22:569–75.

1569. DeMatteo C, Law M, Russell D et al. *QUEST Quality of Upper Extremity Skills Test Manual.* Hamilton, ON, Canada: Neurodevelopmental Research Unit, McMaster University, 1992.

1570. Demeurisse G, Demol O, Robaye E. Motor evaluation in vascular hemiplegia. *Europ Neurol* 1980;19:382–9.

1571. DeMeyer W, Zeman W, Palmer CG. The face predicts the brain: Diagnostic significance of median facial anomalies for holoprosencephaly. *Pediatrics* 1964;34:256–63.

1572. Demir E, Bomont P, Erdem S et al. Giant axonal neuropathy: Clinical and genetic study in 6 cases. *J Neurol Neurosurg Psychiatry* 2004;76:825–32.

1573. Demirkiran M, Jankovic J. Paroxysmal dyskinesias: Clinical features and classification. *Ann Neurol* 1995;38:571–9.

1574. Dempsey JA, Skatrud JB. A sleep induced apneic threshold and its consequences. *Am Rev Respir Dis* 1986;133:1163–70.

1575. DeMyer W. Megalencephaly: Types, clinical syndromes, and management. *Ped Neurol* 1986;2:321.

1576. Deng H, Weidong Le, Jankovic J. Genetics of essential tremor. *Brain* 2007;139:1456–64.

1577. Dengler R, Wohlfarth K, Zierz S et al. Muscle fatigue, lactate and pyruvate in mitochondrial myopathy with progressive external ophthalmoplegia. *Muscle Nerve* 1996;19:456–62.
1578. Denier C, Ducros A, Vahedi K et al. High prevalence of CACNA1A truncations and broader clinical spectrum in episodic ataxia type 2. *Neurology* 1999;52:1816–21.
1579. Denmark A. An example of symptoms resembling tic doulereux produced by a wound in the radial nerve. *Med Chir Trans* 1813;3:48–52.
1580. Dennie C. Partial paralysis of the lower extremities in children accompanied by backward mental development. *Amer J Syph* 1929;13:157–63.
1581. Dennis M, Bamford JM, Sandercock P, Warlow CP. A comparison of risk factors and prognosis for transient ischemic attacks and minor ischemic strokes. *Stroke* 1989;20:1494–9.
1582. Dennis M, Warlow C. Migraine aura without headache; transient ischemic attack or not? *J Neurol Neurosurg Psychiatry* 1992;55:437–40.
1583. Denny-Brown D. The treatment of recurrent cerebrovascular symptoms and the question of "Vasospasm". *Med Clin N Amer* 1951;35:1457–74.
1584. Denny-Brown D. Basilar artery syndromes. *Bull NE Md Center* 1953;15:53–60.
1585. Denny-Brown D. Primary sensory neuropathy with muscular changes by carcinoma. *J Neurol* 1948;11:73–87.
1586. Denny-Brown D. Hereditary sensory radicular neuropathy. *J Neurol Neurosurg Psychiatry* 1951;14:237–52.
1587. Denny-Brown D. Recurrent cerebrovascular episodes. *Arch Neurol* 1960;2:194–210.
1588. Denny-Brown D. *The Basal Ganglia*. Oxford: Oxford University Press, 1962.
1589. Denny-Brown D. Hepato-lenticular degeneration (Wilson's disease). Two different components. *N Engl J Med* 1964;270:1149.
1590. Denny-Brown D. The release of deep pain by nerve injury. *Brain* 1965;88:725–38.
1591. Denny-Brown D. Clinical symptomatology of diseases of the basal ganglia. In Vinken PJ, Bruyn GW, eds. *Handbook of Clinical Neurology*, pp 133–72. Amsterdam: North Holland, 1975.
1592. Denny–Brown D. Spasm of visual fixation. In Rose FC, ed. *Physiological Aspects of Clinical Neurology*, p 68. Oxford: Blackwell, 1977.
1593. Denny-Brown D, Banker BQ. Amorphosynthesis from left parietal lesions. *Arch Neurol Psychiatry* 1954;71:302–13.
1594. Denny-Brown D, Chambers RA. Pseudo-thalamic syndrome. *Res Publ Assn Nerv Ment Dis* 1958;36:35.
1595. Denny-Brown D, Foley JM. Myokymia and benign fasciculations of muscular cramps. *Trans Am Acad Physicians* 1948;61:88–96.
1596. Denny-Brown D, Rose AS, Sahs AL. *Centennial Anniversary Volume, American Neurological Association*. New York: Springer Publishing Co., 1975.
1597. Deonna TW. *Neuropediatrics* 1986;17: 81–5.
1598. Deonna TW. Paroxysmal disorders which may be migraine or may be confused with it. In Hockaday JM, ed. *Migraine in Childhood*, pp 75–87. London: Butterworths, 1988.
1599. Der Meche FGA v, Gijn J v. Hypotonia: An erroneous clinical concept? *Brain* 1986;109:1169–78.
1600. Deraemaeker R. Sex-linked congenital deafness. *Acta Genet* 1958;8:228–31.
1601. Dercum FX. A subcutaneous connective tissue dystrophy of the arms and neck, associated with symptoms resembling myxedema. *University Med Mag* 1888;1:140–50.
1602. Dercum FX. Three cases of an hitherto unclassified affection resembling in its grosser aspects obesity, but associated with special nervous symptoms, adiposis dolorosa. *Amer J Med Sci* 1892;104:521 35.
1603. DeRenzi E, Ferrari C. The reporter's test: A sensitive test to detect expressive disturbances in aphasics. *Cortex* 1978;14:279–93.
1604. DeRenzi E, Gentilini M, Bazolli C. Eyelid movement disorders and motor impersistence on acute hemisphere disease. *Neurology* 1986;36:414.
1605. DeRenzi E, Vignolo LA. The token test: A sensitive test to detect disturbances in aphasics. *Brain* 1962;85:665.
1606. Derkay CS, Bramhall TC. Epstein-Barr viral infectious mononucleosis. *Otolaryngol Head Neck Surg* 1995;113:334–7.
1607. Derogatis LR, Spencer PM. *The Brief Symptom Inventory (BSI) - Administration, Scoring and Procedures Manual*. Baltimore: Clinical Psychometric Research, 1982.
1608. Derry CP, Duncan JS, Berkovic SF. Paroxysmal motor disorders of sleep: The clinical spectrum and differentiation from epilepsy. *Epilepsia* 2007;47:1775–91.
1609. Desai BT, Porter RJ, Penry JK. Psychogenic seizures: A study of 42 attacks in six patients, with intensive monitoring. *Arch Neurol* 1982;39:202–9.
1610. DeSanctis C, Cacchione A. L'idiozia xerodermica. *Riv Sperimentale di Freniatria e Medicina Legale delle Alienazione* 1932;56:269–92.
1611. Desforges JF. Medical problems associated with underwater diving. *N Engl J Med* 1992;326:30–5.
1612. Desmeules J, Cedraschi C, Rapiti E et al. Neurophysiologic evidence for a central sensitization in patients with fibromyalgia. *Arthritis Rheum* 2003;48:1420–9.
1613. Desmond NM, Wilson GS, Melnick JL et al. Congenital rubella encephalitis. *J Pediatr* 1967;71:311.
1614. Destee A, Cassim F, Defebvre L et al. Hereditary chin trembling or hereditary chin myoclonus? *J Neurol Neurosurg Psychiatry* 1997;63:804–7.
1615. Deuschl G, Bain P, Brin M. Consensus statement of the movement disorder society on tremor. *Mov Disord* 1998;13: 2–23.
1616. Devereaux MW, Kleane JR, Davis RL. Automatic respiratory failure associated with infarction of the medulla. *Arch Neurol* 1973;29:46–52.
1617. Devic ME. Myélite aîgue dorso-lombaire avec névrite optique. Autopsie. *Cong Fr Med Lyon* 1894;1:434–9.
1618. Devonport H, Oworu O, Mahla A et al. Purtshcher's like retinopathy as the presenting feature of acute alcoholic pancreatitis. *Eye* 2005;20:255–7.
1619. Devos D, Vuillame I, De BA et al. New syndromic form of benign hereditary chorea is associated with a deletion of TITF-1 and PAX-9 contiguous genes. *Mov Disord* 2006;21:2237–40.
1620. Dewey RB, Maraganore DM. Isolated eyelid-opening apraxia. *Neurology* 1994;44:1752–4.
1621. DeWitt LD, Wechsler L. Transcranial doppler. *Stroke* 1988;19:915–21.
1622. Di Chiro G, Reames PM, Matthews WB. RISA-ventriculography and RISA-cisternography. *Neurology* 1964;14: 185–91.
1623. Di Costanzo A, Tedeschi G, Di Salle F et al. Pineal cysts: An incidental MRI finding? *J Neurol Neurosurg Psychiatry* 1993;56:207–8.
1624. Di Donato D, Garavaglieri B, Striociuglio P et al. Multisystem triglyceride storage disease is due to a specific defect in the degradation of endocellularly synthesized triglycerides. *Neurology* 1988;38:1107–10.
1625. Di Donato S, Gellera C, Peluchetti D et al. Normalization of short-chain acylcoenzyme A dehydrogenase. *Arch Neurol* 1989;25:479–84.
1626. Di Lazzaro V, Restuccia D, Nardone R et al. Preliminary observations on a new trigeminal reflex. *Neurology* 1996;46: 479–85.
1627. Di Maio L, Marcelli V, Vitale V et al. Cervico-oculo-acoustic syndrome in a

male with consanguineous parents. *Can J Neurol Sci* 2006;33:237–9.
1628. Di Saia PJ. Pregnancy and delivery of a patient with Starr-Edwards mitral valve prosthesis. *Obstet Gynec* 1966;28:469–71.
1629. Diagnostic Classification Steering Committee. *ICSD - International Classification of Sleep Disorders, Revised: Diagnostic and Coding Manual American Academy of Sleep Medicine*. Rochester, MN: American Sleep Disorders Association, 2001.
1630. Diamond S, Markham CH. Evaluating the evaluations: Or how to weigh the scales of parkinsonian disability. *Neurology* 1983;33:1098–9.
1631. Diaz-Arrastia R, Younger DS, Hair L et al. Neurolymphomatosis. *Neurology* 1992;42:1136–41.
1632. Dick AP, Massey EW. Neurological presentations of decompression sickness and air embolism in sport divers. *Neurology* 1985;35:667–71.
1633. Dick AP, Stevenson CJ. Hereditary spastic paraplegia. Report of a family with associated extrapyramidal signs. *Lancet* 1953;i:921–3.
1634. Dick JPR, Cantello R, Buruma O et al. The Bereitschaftspotential, L-DOPA and Parkinson's disease. *EEG Clin Neurophysiol* 1987;66:263–74.
1635. Dickson D, Bergeron C, Chin S et al. Office of rare diseases neuropathologic criteria for corticobasal degeneration. *J Neuropathol Exp Neurol* 2002;61:935–46.
1636. Dide M. Persisting amnesia, pure speech loss and atopagnosia with bilateral lingual lobe lesions. *Rev Neurol* 1902;10:676–80.
1637. Dide M. Les désorientations temporo-spatiale et la préponderance de l'hemisphere droit dans les agnoso-akinesies proprioceptives. *Encephale* 1938;33:276–94.
1638. Dieterich M, Brandt T. Wallenberg's syndrome. *Ann Neurol* 1992;31:399–408.
1639. Dieterich M, Brandt T. Ocular torsion and tilt of subjective visual vertical are sensitive brainstem signs. *Ann Neurol* 1993;33:292–9.
1640. Dieterich M, Brandt T. Episodic vertigo related to migraine (90 cases): Vestibular migraine? *J Neurol* 1999;246:883–92.
1641. DiGeorge AM. A new concept of the cellular basis of immunity. *J Pediatr* 1965;67:907–8.
1642. Diliberti JH et al. The fetal valproate syndrome. *Am J Med Genet* 1984;19: 473–81.
1643. Dilli E, Dodick DW. Extracephalic cluster (cluster sine headache). *Neurology* 2008;70:1362–3.
1644. Dillmann U, Heide G, Dietz B et al. Hereditary motor and sensory neuropathy with spastic paraplegia and optic atrophy: Report on a family. *J Neurol* 1997;244:562–5.
1645. DiMauro S, Bonilla E, Zeviani M et al. Mitochondrial myopathies. *Ann Neurol* 1985;17:521–38.
1646. DiMauro S, Bresolin N. Newly recognized defects in distal glycolysis. In Engel WK, Banker BQ, eds. *Myology*, pp 1619–51. New York: McGraw-Hill, 1986.
1647. DiMauro S, Dalakas MC, Miranda AF. Phosphoglycerate kinase deficiency, another cause of recurrent myoglobinuria. *Ann Neurol* 1983;13:11–9.
1648. DiMauro S, DiMauro PMM. Muscle carnitine palmityltransferase deficiency and myoglobinuria. *Science* 1973;182:929–31.
1649. DiMauro S et al. Metabolic myopathies. *Am J Med Genet* 1986;25:635–51.
1650. DiMauro S, Hartlege PL. Fatal infantile form of muscle phosphorylase deficiency. *Neurology* 1978;28:1124–9.
1651. DiMauro S, Hartwig GB, Hays A et al. Debrancher deficiency: Neuromuscular disorder in 5 adults. *Ann Neurol* 1979;5:422–36.
1652. DiMauro S, Hirano M. Mitochondrial encephalomyopathies: An update. *Neuromuscular Disorders* 2005;15:276–86.
1653. DiMauro S, Mendell JR, Sahenk Z et al. Fatal infantile mitochondrial myopathy and renal dysfunction due to cytochrome *c* oxidase deficiency. *Neurology* 1980;30:795–804.
1654. DiMauro S, Miranda AF, Hays AF et al. Myoadenylate deaminase deficiency. *J Neurol Sci* 1980;47:191–202.
1655. DiMauro S, Miranda AF, Olarte M et al. Muscle phosphoglycerate mutase deficiency. *Neurology* 1982;32:584–91.
1656. DiMauro S, Schotland DL, Bonilla E et al. Progressive ophthalmoplegia, glycogen storage and abnormal mitochondria. *Arch Neurol* 1973;29:170–9.
1657. DiMauro S, Trevisan C, Hays A. Disorders of lipid metabolism in muscle. *Muscle Nerve* 1980;3:369–88.
1658. Dimsdale H. Hereditary optic atrophy in family with keratodermia palmaris et plantaris (tylosis). *Proc Roy Soc Med* 1949;42:796.
1659. Dinarello CA et al. New concepts on the pathogenesis of fever. *Rev Infect Dis* 1988;10:1.
1660. Dincer P, Leturcq F, Richard I et al. A biochemical, clinical and genetic study of autosomal recessive limb girdle muscular dystrophies in Turkey. *Ann Neurol* 1997;42:222–9.
1661. Diniz MA, Cunha L, Goncalves F et al. Two cases of stiff man syndrome with tremor. *J Neurol* 1986;142:918–20.
1662. Dinsdale HB. Hypertensive encephalopathy. *Stroke* 1982;13,No.5:717–9.
1663. DiNubile MJ. Septic thrombosis of the cavernous sinuses – neurological review. *Arch Neurol* 1988;45:567–74.
1664. Direkze M, Fernando BL. Transient anterior horn cell dysfunction in diphenylhydantoin therapy. *Europ Neurol* 1977;15:131.
1665. Disertori B, Ducati A, Piazza M et al. Brainstem auditory evoked potentials in a case of "Manto syndrome" or spasmodic torticollis with thoracic outlet syndrome. *Ital J Neurol Sci* 1982;3:359–363.
1666. Dix MR. Modern tests of vestibular function, with special reference to their value in clinical practice. *Brit Med J* 1969;270:317.
1667. Dobbs AR, Rule BG. Adult age differences in working memory. *Psychol Aging* 1989;4:500–503.
1668. Dobkin BH, Verity MA. Spinal muscular atrophy with bulbar palsy. *Neurology* 1976;26:754.
1669. Dobkin BH, Verity MA. Familial neuromuscular disease with Type I fiber hypoplasia, tubular aggregates, cardiomyopathy and myasthenic features. *Neurology* 1978;28:1135–40.
1670. Dobson J. *Anatomical Eponyms*. London: Bailliere, Tindall & Cox, 1946.
1671. Dobyn WB, Pagon RA, Armstrong D et al. Diagnostic criteria for Walker-Warburg syndrome. *Am J Med Genet* 1989;32:195–210.
1672. Dobyns WB. The neurogenetics of lissencephaly. *Neurol Clin* 1989;7:89–105.
1673. Dobyns WB, Andermann E, Andermann F et al. X-linked malformations of neuronal migration. *Neurology* 1996;47:331–9.
1674. Dobyns WB et al. Familial cavernous malformations of the central nervous system and retina. *Ann Neurol* 1987;21:578–83.
1675. Dobyns WB, Ozelius LJ, Kramer PL et al. Rapid-onset dystonia-Parkinsonism. *Neurology* 1993;43:2596–602.
1676. Dobyns WB, Stratton RF, Greenberg F. Syndromes with lissencephaly. I: Miller-Dieker and Norman-Roberts syndromes with isolated lissencephaly. *Am J Med Genet* 1984;18:509–26.
1677. Dodick DW. Thunderclap headache. *J Neurol Neurosurg Psychiatry* 2002;72:6–11.
1678. Dodwell DG, Jampol LM et al. Optic nerve involvement associated with multiple evanescent white-dot syndrome. *Ophthalmology* 1990;97:862–8.
1679. Domazetovska A, Ilkovski B, Kumar V et al. Intranuclear rod myopathy:

Molecular pathogenesis and mechanisms of weakness. *Ann Neurol* 2007;62: 597–608.

1680. Donadio V, Montagna P, Nolano M et al. Generalized anhidrosis: Different lesion sites demonstrated by microneurography and skin biopsy. *J Neurol Neurosurg Psychiatr* 2005;76:588–91.

1681. Donaghy M. Classification and clinical features of motor neurone diseases and motor neuropathies in adults. *J Neurol* 1999;246:331–3.

1682. Donaghy M, Hakin RN, Bamford JM et al. Hereditary sensory neuropathy with neurotrophic keratitis. *Brain* 1987;110:563–83.

1683. Donaire A, Carreno M, Gómez B et al. Cortical laminar necrosis related to prolonged focal status epilepticus. *J Neurol Neurosurg Psychiatry* 2006;77:104–6.

1684. Donaldson IM. Volvular epilepsy: A distinctive and underreported seizure type. *Arch Neurol* 1986;43:260–2.

1685. Donat JR, Auger R. Familial periodic ataxia. *Arch Neurol* 1979;36:568–9.

1686. Donnan GA, Bladin PF, Berkovic S et al. The stroke syndrome of striatocapsular infarction. *Brain* 1991;114:51–70.

1687. Donnan GA, O'Malley HM, Quang L et al. The capsular warning syndrome. *Neurology* 1993;43:957–62.

1688. Donofrio PD. Monomelic amyotrophy. *Muscle Nerve* 1994;17:1129–34.

1689. Donohue WL. Dysendocrinism. *J Pediatr* 1948;32:739–48.

1690. Dooley JM, Gordon K, Camfield P. The Rushes. *Clin Ped* 1990;29:536–8.

1691. Dooley JM, Hayde. Benign febrile myoclonus in childhood. *Can J Neurol Sci* 2004;31:504–5.

1692. Doose H, Baier WK. Epilepsy with primarily generalized myoclonic-astatic seizures. *Eur J Pediatr* 1987;146:550–4.

1693. Doose H, Gerken H, Leonhardt R et al. Centrencephalic myoclonic-astatic petit mal. *Neuropediatrics* 1970;2:59–78.

1694. Dorfman LJ, Forno LS. Paraneoplastic encephalomyelitis. *Acta Neurol Scand* 1972;48:556–74.

1695. Dorfman LJ, Pedley TA, Tharp BR et al. Juvenile neuroaxonal dystrophy: Clinical, electrophysiological and neuropathological features. *Ann Neurol* 1978;3:419–28.

1696. Doshi R, Fowler T. Proximal myopathy due to carcinomatous metastasis in muscle. *J Neurol Neurosurg Psychiatry* 1983;46:358–60.

1697. Doty RL, Sharman P, Dann M. Development of the University of Pennsylvania smell identification test. *Physiol Behav* 1984;32:489–502.

1698. Douglas AC, MacLeod JG, Matthews JD. Symptomatic sarcoidosis of skeletal muscle. *J Neurol Neurosurg Psychiatry* 1973;36:1034–40.

1699. Douglas EF, White PT. Abdominal epilepsy: A reappraisal. *J Pediatr* 1951;78:59–67.

1700. Douglas VI. Attentional and cognitive problems. In Rutter M, ed. *Developmental Neuropsychiatry*, pp 280–329. New York: The Guilford Press, 1983.

1701. Down JL. Marriages of consanguinity in relation to degeneration of race. *London Hosp Clin Lect Rep* 1866;3:224–36.

1702. Doyle JB. Neurologic complications of serum sickness. *American Journal of Medical Science* 1933;185:484–92.

1703. Drachman D, Banker BQ. Arthrogryposis multiplex congenita. *Arch Neurol* 1961;5:89–105.

1704. Drachman DA. Neurological complications of Wegener's granulomatosis. *Arch Neurol* 1963;8:145–55.

1705. Drachman DA. Ophthalmoplegia plus: The neurodegenerative disorders associated with progressive external ophthalmoplegia. *Arch Neurol* 1968;18:654–74.

1706. Drachman DA. New criteria for the diagnosis of vascular dementia: Do we know enough yet? *Neurology* 1993;43:243–5.

1707. Drachman DA, Hart CW. Approach to the dizzy patient. *Neurology* 1972;22:323–34.

1708. Drachman DA, Richardson EP JR. Aqueductal narrowing, congenital and acquired. *Arch Neurol* 1961;5:552–9.

1709. Drake CG. Report of a World Federation of Neurosurgeons committee on a universal subarachnoid hemorrhage scale. *J Neurosurg* 1988;68:1985–6.

1710. Drake ME, Jackson RL, Miller CA. Paroxysmal choreoathetosis after head injury. *J Neurol Neurosurg Psychiatry* 1986;49:837–8.

1711. Dravet C. Les epilepsies graves de l'enfant. *Vie Med* 1978;8:543–8.

1712. Dreifuss FE. Discussion of absence and photosensitive epilepsy. In Roger J, Dravet C, Bureau M et al., eds. *Epileptic Syndromes in Infancy, Childhood and Adolescence*, pp 237–41. London: John Libbey, 1985.

1713. Dreifuss FE. The epilepsies: Clinical implications of the international classification. *Epilepsia* 1990;31:S3–S10.

1714. Drislane FW. Evidence against permanent neurological damage from nonconvulsive status epilepticus. *J Clin Neurophysiol* 1999;16:323–31.

1715. Druckman R, Chao D, Alvord EC. A case of atonic cerebral diplegia with lissencephaly. *Neurology* 1959;9:806–14.

1716. Drummond KN et al. The blue diaper syndrome: Familial hypocalcemia with nephrocalcinosis and indicanuria. *Am J Med* 1964;37:928–48.

1717. Drummond PD, Lance JW. Site of autonomic deficit in harlequin syndrome: Local autonomic failure affecting the arm and the face. *Ann Neurol* 1993;34:814–6.

1718. Druschky K-F. Hereditary putaminal necrosis. In Vinken PJ, Bruyn GW, Klawans HL, eds. *Extrapyramidal Disorders. Handbook of Clinical Neurology*, vol.5, pp 493–8. Amsterdam: Elsevier Science Publishers, 1986.

1719. Du Pasquier R, Vingerhoets F, Safran AB et al. Periodic downbeat nystagmus. *Neurology* 1998;51:1478–80.

1720. du Petit P. A memoir showing that the intercostal nerves supply branches to the eyes. *Mem Acad Sci Paris* 1727;1:1–19.

1721. Duane A. Congenital deficiency of abduction, associated with impairment of adduction, retraction movements, contraction of the palpebral fissure and oblique movements of the eye. *Arch Ophthalmol* 1905;34:133–59.

1722. Dubini A. Primi cenni sulla corea elettrica. *Ann Univ Med (Milano)* 1846;117:5–50.

1723. Dubois B, Slachevsky A, Litvan I, et al. The FAB. *Neurology* 2000;55:1621–6.

1724. Dubois B, Slachevsky A, Pillon B et al. Applause sign helps to discriminate PSP from FTD and PD. *Neurology* 2005;64:2132–3.

1725. Dubois G, Mussini J-M, Auclair M et al. Adult sphingomyelinase deficiency. *Neurology* 1990;40:132–6.

1726. Dubourg O, Barhoumi C, Azzedine H et al. Clinical, electrophysiological and genetic study of a family with autosomal dominant hereditary sensory neuropathy and predominant weakness. *Muscle Nerve* 2000;23:1508–14.

1727. Dubowitz L, Dubowitz V. *The Neurological Assessment of the Preterm and Full-Term Newborn Infant*. Heinemann: Clinics in Developmental Medicine, 1981.

1728. Dubowitz LMS, Dubowitz V, Goldberg C. Scoring system for neurologic criteria. *J Pediatr* 1970;77:1.

1729. Dubowitz V. Familial low birthweight dwarfism with an unusual facies and a skin eruption. *J Med Genet* 1965;2:12–7.

1730. Dubowitz V. Pseudo-muscular dystrophy. In Research committee of the muscular dystrophy group of Great Britain, ed. *Research in Muscular Dystrophy. Proceedings of the Third Symposium. Research Committee of the Muscular Dystrophy Group of Great Britain*, pp 57–73. London: Pitman Medical, 1965.

1731. Dubowitz V. Rigid spine syndrome: A muscle syndrome in search of a name. *Proc Roy Soc Med* 1973;66:219.

1732. Dubowitz V. What is muscular dystrophy? *J Roy Coll Phycns* 2000;34:464–8.
1733. Dubowitz V, Brooke MH. *Muscle Biopsy: A Modern Approach.* London: Saunders, 1973.
1734. Dubrovsky T, Curless R, Scott G et al. Cerebral aneurysmal arteriopathy in childhood AIDS. *Neurology* 1998;51: 560–565.
1735. Duchenne de Boulogne GBA. De l'ataxie locomotrice progressive; récherches sur une maladie caracterisée spécialement par les troubles généraux de la coordination des mouvements. *AGMP* 1858;12: 641–52.
1736. Duchenne de Boulogne GBA. Paralysie musculaire progressive de la langue, du voile, du palais et des lèvres, affection non encore décrite comme éspéce morbide distincte. *AGMP* 1860;16:283–96.
1737. Duchenne de Boulogne GBA. Récherches sur la paralysie musculaire pseudohypertrophique ou paralysie myo-sclerosique. *AGMP* 1868;11:5–25.
1738. Duchenne de Boulogne GBA. De l'electrisation localisée et de son application a la pathologie et a la thérapeutique. Paris: J.B. Baillière, 1872.
1739. Duchowny M, Jayakar P, Resnick T et al. Posterior temporal epilepsy: Electroclinical features. *Ann Neurol* 1994;35:427–31.
1740. Ducros A, Boukobza M, Porcher R et al. The clinical and radiological spectrum of reversible cerebral vasoconstriction syndrome. A prospective series of 67 patients. *Brain* 2007;130:3091–101.
1741. Duddung BA, Gorlin RJ. The oto-palato-digital syndrome. *Am J Dis Childh* 1967;113:214–21.
1742. Duffy CJ. The legacy of association cortex. *Neurology* 1984;34:192–7.
1743. Duffy CJ. Implicit memory. *Neurology* 1997;49:1200–2.
1744. Duffy FH, Burchfiel JL, Lombroso CT. Brain electrical activity mapping (BEAM): A method for extending the clinical utility of EEG and evoked potential data. *Ann Neurol* 1979;5: 309–21.
1745. Duffy PE, Sassin JF, Summers DS et al. Rhombencephalitis due to Listeria monocytogenes. *Neurology* 1964;14: 1067–72.
1746. Duhamel B. From the mermaid to anal imperforation: The syndrome of caudal regression. *Arch Dis Child* 1961;36: 152–5.
1747. Dulcan MK. Attention deficit disorder: Evaluation and treatment. *Ped Ann* 1985;14: 5:383–400.
1748. Dumitru D, DeLisa JA. AAEM minimonograph #10: Volume conduction. *Muscle Nerve* 1991;14:605–24.
1749. Duncan JS. Idiopathic generalized epilepsies with typical absences. *J Neurol* 1997;244:403–11.
1750. Duncan JS, Sander JWA. The Chalfont seizure severity scale. *J Neurol Neurosurg Psychiatry* 1991;54:873–6.
1751. Duncan PW, Lai SM, Bode RK et al. Stroke impact scale-16. *Neurology* 2003;60:291–6.
1752. Dunn HG. Ataxia-telangiectasia. *Dev Med Child Neurol* 1973;15:324.
1753. Dunn LM. *Expanded Manual for the Peabody Picture Vocabulary Test.* Minneapolis: American Guidance Service, 1970.
1754. Dunne JW, Summers QA, Stewart Wynne EG. Non-convulsive status epilepticus: A prospective study in an adult population. *Quart J Med* 1987;62:117–26.
1755. Duplay ES. De la peri–arthrite scapulo–humerale et des raideurs de l'épaule qui en sont la consequence. *AGMP* 1872;20:513–42.
1756. Dupre E. Le meningisme. *Cong Fr Med Lyon* 1894;1:411–23.
1757. Dupre N, Howard HC, Mathieu J et al. Hereditary motor and sensory neuropathy with agenesis of the corpus callosum. *Ann Neurol* 2003;54:9–18.
1758. Duquette A, Tetreault M, Thiffault I et al. A new form of congenital muscular dystrophy with joint hyperlaxity maps to 3p23–21. *Brain* 2006;129:2077–84.
1759. Duran M, Wadman SK. Thiamine responsive inborn errors of metabolism. *J Inherit Metab Dis* 1985;8 **(Suppl. 1)**:70.
1760. Durand N, Favre J. Lymphogranulomatose inguinale subaïgue d'origine génitale probable peut-être vénérienne. *Bull Soc Med Hop Paris* 1913;35:274–88.
1761. Durand P, Borrone C, Della Cella G. A new mucopolysaccharide lipid storage disease? *Lancet* 1966;ii:1313–4.
1762. Durand P, Zunin C. Associazione de agenesia del setto pellucido, cranio lacunare, spina bifida ed altri segni malformativi. *Minerv Pediatr* 1955;7:1249–56.
1763. Duret H. Récherches anatomiques sur la circulation de l'encèphale. *Arch Physiol Norm Pathol (Paris)* 1874;1:60, 316–664, 919.
1764. Duret H. *Etudes experimentales et cliniques sur les traumatismes cerebraux.* Paris: V.Adrien Delahaye, 1878.
1765. Durham RH. *Encyclopedia of Medical Syndromes.* New York: Paul Hoeber, 1960.
1766. Durr A, Brice A, Serdaru M et al. The phenotype of "pure" autosomal dominant spastic paraplegia. *Neurology* 1994;44:1274–7.
1767. Duvoisin RC, Golbe LI, Lepore FE. Progressive supranuclear palsy. *Can J Neurol Sci* 1987;14:547–54.
1768. Dwork AJ, Balmaceda C, Fazzini OD et al. Dominantly inherited, early-onset parkinsonism: Neuropathology of a new form. *Neurology* 1993;43:69–74.
1769. Dyck PJ. Inherited neuronal degeneration and atrophy affecting peripheral motor, sensory, and autonomic neurons. In Dyck PJ, Thomas PK, Lambert EH, eds. *Peripheral Neuropathy*, pp 825–67. Philadelphia: W.B. Saunders, 1975.
1770. Dyck PJ. Detection, characterization and staging of polyneuropathy: Assessed in diabetics. *Muscle Nerve* 1988;11:21–32.
1771. Deleted: see 1770
1772. Dyck PJ. Hypoxic neuropathy: Does hypoxia play a role in diabetic neuropathy? *Neurology* 1989;39:111–8.
1773. Dyck PJ, Benstead TJ, Conn DL et al. Nonsystemic vasculitic neuropathy. *Brain* 1987;110:843–54.
1774. Dyck PJ, Carney JA, Sizemore GW et al. Multiple endocrine neoplasia, type 2b: Phenotype recognition; neurological features and their pathological basis. *Ann Neurol* 1979;6:302–14.
1775. Dyck PJ, Conn DL, Okazaki H. Necrotizing angiopathic neuropathy. *Mayo Clin Proc* 1972;47:461–75.
1776. Dyck PJ, Curtis DJ, Buskek W et al. Description of Minnesota thermal disks and normal values of cutaneous thermal discrimination in man. *Neurology* 1974;24:325–30.
1777. Dyck PJ, Karnes J, O'Brien PC et al. Neuropathy symptom profile in health, motor neurone disease, diabetic neuropathy and amyloidosis. *Neurology* 1986;36:1300–8.
1778. Dyck PJ, Kratz KM, Lehman KA et al. The Rochester diabetic neuropathy study. *Neurology* 1991;41:799–807.
1779. Dyck PJ, Lambert EH. Lower motor and primary sensory neuron diseases with peroneal muscular atrophy. I. Neurologic, genetic and electrophysiological findings in hereditary polyneuropathies. *Arch Neurol* 1968;80:603–18.
1780. Dyck PJ, Lambert EH. Polyneuropathy associated with hypothyroidism. *J Neuropath Exp Neurol* 1970;29:631–58.
1781. Dyck PJ, Litchy WJ, Minnerath S et al. Hereditary motor and sensory neuropathy with diaphragm and vocal cord paresis. *Ann Neurol* 1994;35:608–15.
1782. Dyck PJ, Norell JE, Dyck PJ JR. Non–diabetic lumbosacral radiculoplexus neuropathy: Natural history, outcome and comparison with the diabetic variety. *Brain* 2001;124:1197–207.
1783. Dyck PJ, Sherman WR, Hallcher LM et al. Human diabetic endoneurial sorbitol, fructose and myo-inositol related to sural nerve morphometry. *Ann Neurol* 1980;8:590–6.

1784. Dyck PJ, Yao JK, Knickerbocker DE et al. Multisystem neuronal degeneration, hepatosplenomegaly and adrenocortical deficiency associated with reduced tissue arachidonic acid. *Neurology* 1981;31:925–34.

1785. Dyel J. Differentiation between optic neuritis in Bright's disease from that due to Cerebral Tumor. *Sem Med* 1901;21:247.

1786. Dyggve HV, Melchior JC, Clausen J et al. Morquio-Ulrich's disease. An inborn error of metabolism. *Arch Dis Child* 1962;37:525–34.

1787. Dyke CG, Davidoff LM, Masson CB. Cerebral hemiatrophy with homolateral hypertrophy of the skull and sinuses. *Surg Gyn Obstet* 1933;57:588–600.

1788. Dyken P, Kolar O. Dancing eyes, dancing feet: Infantile polymyoclonia. *Brain* 1968;91:305–20.

1789. Dyken P, Krawiecki N. Neurodegenerative diseases of infancy and childhood. *Ann Neurol* 1983;13:351–64.

1790. Dyken PR, Miller M. *Facial Features of Neurologic Disease.* St.Louis: Mosby, 1980.

1791. Dyken PR, Morales V, John-Sanchez F et al. Chronic toxoplasmosis of the central nervous system: Another neurological "degenerative" disease. *Proc Child Neurol Soc* 1976;5:27.

1792. Dzierzynsky W. Dystrophia periostalic hyperplastica familiaris. *Zbl Ges Neurol Psychiat* 1913;20:547.

1793. Eadie MJ. Olivpontocerebellar degeneration (Menzel type). In Vincken PJ, Bruyn GW, eds. *Handbook of Clinical Neurology*, pp 433–49. Amsterdam: North Holland, 1975.

1794. Eagle WW. Facial pain from an elongated styloid process. *Arch Otolaryngol* 1948;47:630–40.

1795. Eagleton WP. *Cavernous Sinus Thrombosis.* New York: Macmillan, 1926.

1796. Eales H. Cases of retinal hemorrhage, associated with epistaxis and constipation. *Birmingh Med Rev* 1880;9:262–73.

1797. Eames P. Hysteria following brain injury. *J Neurol Neurosurg Psychiatry* 1992;55:1046–53.

1798. Earl CJC, Fullerton PM, Wakefield GS et al. Hereditary neuropathy with liability to pressure palsies. *Quart J Med* 1964;33:481–98.

1799. Eastman JR, Bixler D. Facio-cardio-renal syndrome. *Clin Genet* 1977;11:424–30.

1800. Ebers GC. Optic neuritis and multiple sclerosis. *Arch Neurol* 1985;42:702–4.

1801. Ebke M, Dichgans M, Bergmann M et al. CADASIL: Skin biopsy allows diagnosis in early stages. *Acta Neurol Scand* 1997;95:351–7.

1802. Ebrahim S, Nouri F, Barer D. Measuring disability after stroke. *J Epidem Comm Health* 1985;39:86–9.

1803. Eccles JC, Gibson WC. *Sherrington: His Life and Thought*. Berlin: Springer, 1979.

1804. Echaniz-Laguna A. Neuromuscular complications in transplant recipients. *Rev Neurol (Paris)* 2007;163:275–85.

1805. Edelman RR, Warach S. Magnetic resonance imaging. *N Engl J Med* 1993;328:708, 785–16, 791.

1806. Edelson RN, Levy DE. Transient benign pupillary dilatation in young adults. *Arch Neurol* 1974;31:12–4.

1807. Edmeads J. The cervical spine and headache. *Neurology* 1988;38:1874–8.

1808. Edmeads J. Headache of cervical origin. *Rev Prat* 1990;40:399–402.

1809. Edstrom L, Thornell LE, Eriksson A. A new type of hereditary distal myopathy with characteristic sarcoplasmic bodies and intermediate (skeletin) filaments. *J Neurol Sci* 1980;47:171–90.

1810. Edwards JA, Sethi PK, Scoma AJ et al. A new familial syndrome characterized by pigmentary retinopathy, hypogonadism, mental retardation, nerve deafness, and glucose intolerance. *Amer J Med* 1976;60:23–32.

1811. Edwards JH. Sign of the Cheshire cat. *Lancet* 1987;2:581.

1812. Edwards JH, Harnden DG, Cameron AH et al. A new trisomic syndrome. *Lancet* 1960;1:787–90.

1813. Edwards WG, Lincoln CR, Bassett FH et al. The tarsal tunnel syndrome, diagnosis and treatment. *JAMA* 1969;207:716–20.

1814. Efron R. An extension of the Pulfrich effect. *Brain* 1963;86:295–300.

1815. Egas Moniz AC. L'encephalographie arterielle, son importance dans la localisation des tumeurs cerébrales. *Rev Neurol* 1927;2:72–90.

1816. Egas Moniz AC. Essai d'un traitement chirurgical de certaines psychoses. *Bull Acad Med Paris* 1936;115:385–92.

1817. Eggenberger E. Eight-and-a-half syndrome: One-and-a-half syndrome plus cranial nerve VII palsy. *J Neuroophthalmol* 1998;18:114–6.

1818. Ehle A, Co S, Jones MG. Clinical correlates of midline spikes: An analysis of 21 patients. *Arch Neurol* 1981;38:355–7.

1819. Ehlers E. Cutis Laxa. *Derm Z* 1901;8:173.

1820. Ehrenkranz NJ, Ventura AK. Venezuelan equine encephalitis virus infection in man. *Ann Rev Med* 1974;25:9–14.

1821. Ehrenpeis P. *Hirschsprung's Disease.* Chicago: Year Book Medical, 1970.

1822. Ehret H. Ueber eine functionelle Lahrmungsform der Peronealmuskeln traumatischen Ursprunges. *Arch Unfallh (Stuttgart)* 1898;2:32–56.

1823. Eidelberg D, Sotrel A, Vogel H et al. Progressive polyradiculopathy in acquired immune deficiency syndrome. *Neurology* 1986;36:912–6.

1824. Eisen A, Shtybel W. Clinical experience with transcranial magnetic stimulation. *Muscle Nerve* 1990;13:995–1011.

1825. Eisendrath SJ, Rand DC, Feldman MC. Factitious disorders in the legal setting. In Feldman MC, Eisendrath SJ, eds. *The Spectrum of Factitious Disorders*, pp 65–82. American Psychiatric Press, 1996.

1826. Eisenson J. *Examination for Aphasia.* New York: Psychological Corporation, 1954.

1827. Eisler T, Wilson JH. Muscle fibre-type disproportion: Report of a family with symptomatic and asymptomatic members. *Arch Neurol* 1978;35:823–6.

1828. Ekbom KA. Asthenia crurum paresthetica ("Irritable Legs"). A new syndrome consisting of weakness, sensation of cold and nocturnal paresthesia in the legs, responding to a certain extent to treatment in general. *Acta Med Scand* 1944;118:197–209.

1829. Ekbom KA. Restless legs. A clinical study of a hitherto overlooked disease in the legs characterized by peculiar paresthesia (anxietas tibiarum), pain and weakness and occurring in two main forms, asthenia crurum paraesthetica and asthenia crurum dolorosa. A short review of paraesthesias in general. *Acta Med Scand* 1945;(**Suppl.** 158):1–123.

1830. Ekbom KA. Hereditary ataxia, photomyoclonus, skeletal deformities and lipoma. *Acta Neurol Scand* 1975;51:393–404.

1831. Ekbom KA, Hed R, Kirstein L et al. Muscular affections in chronic alcoholism. *Arch Neurol* 1964;10:449–58.

1832. Ekbom KA, Jernelius B, Kugelberg E. Perioral reflexes. *Neurology* 1952;2:103–11.

1833. El Masry WS, Biyani A. Incidence, management and outcome of post-traumatic syringomyelia. *J Neurol Neurosurg Psychiatry* 1996;60:141–6.

1834. Elble RJ. Diagnostic criteria for essential tremor and differential diagnosis. *Neurology* 2000;54(**Suppl.** 4):S2–S6.

1835. Eldjarn L, Jellum E, Stokke O. Betahydroxyvaleric aciduria and betamethyl crotanyl glycinuria: A new inborn error of metabolism. *Lancet* 1970;2:54–5.

1836. Eldridge R, Anayiotos CP, Schlesinger S et al. Hereditary adult-onset leukodystrophy simulating chronic progressive multiple sclerosis. *N Engl J Med* 1984;311:948–53.

1837. Elia M, Musumeci SA, Ferri R et al. Familial cortical tremor, epilepsy and mental retardation: A distinct clinical entity? *Arch Neurol* 1998;55:1569–73.

1838. Elkon D, Hightower SI, Lim ML et al. Esthesioneuroblastoma. *Cancer* 1979;44:1087–94.

1839. Ellenberg M. Diabetic neuropathic cachexia. *Diabetes* 1974;23:418–23.

1840. Ellenberger C. Modern perimetry in neuro-ophthalmic diagnosis. *Arch Neurol* 1974;30:193–201.

1841. Ellenberger C, Messner KH. Papillophlebitis: Benign retinopathy resembling papilledema or papillitis. *Ann Neurol* 1978;3:438–44.

1842. Eller KM, Kuller JA. Fetal porencephaly: A review of etiology, diagnosis and prognosis. *Obstet Gynecol Surv* 1995;50:684–7.

1843. Ellie E, Julien J, Ferrer X. Familial idiopathic striopallidodentate calcifications. *Neurology* 1989;39:381–5.

1844. Ellis K, Speed J, Balbierz JM. Post-craniectomy intracranial hypotension: Potential impact on rehabilitation. *Brain Inj* 1998;12:895–9.

1845. Ellis RWB, van Crefeld S. A syndrome characterized by ectodermal dysplasia, polydactyly, chondrodysplasia and congenital morbus cordis. *Arch Dis Child* 1940;15:65.

1846. Ellis SJ, Small M. Denial of illness in stroke. *Stroke* 1993;24:757–9.

1847. Ellison PH, Farina MA. Progressive central nervous system deterioration: A complication of advanced chronic lung disease and prematurity. *Ann Neurol* 1980;8:43–6.

1848. Ellner JJ. Chronic meningitis. In Mandell GL, Douglas RG, Bennett JE, eds. *Principles and Practice of Infectious Diseases*, pp 573–9. New York: Wiley, 1985.

1849. Elsahy NI, Waters WR. The brachio-skeleto-genital syndrome. *Plast Reconstr Surg* 1971;48:542–50.

1850. Elsberg CA. Experiences in spinal surgery. Observations upon 60 laminectomies in spinal disease. *Surg Gyn Obstet* 1931;16:117.

1851. Elschnig A. Nystagmus retractorius, ein cerebrales Herdsymptom. *Med Klin Berlin* 1913;1:8–11.

1852. Elston JS. A new variant of blepharospasm. *J Neurol Neurosurg Psychiatry* 1992;55:369–71.

1853. Elston JS, Casgranje F, Lees AJ. The relationship between eye-winking tics, frequent eye-blinking and blepharospasm. *J Neurol Neurosurg Psychiatry* 1989;52:477–80.

1854. Emery AEH, Dreifuss FE. Unusual type of benign X-linked muscular dystrophy. *J Neurol Neurosurg Psychiatry* 1966;29:338–42.

1855. Emre M, Aarsland D, Brown R et al. Clinical diagnostic criteria for dementia associated with parkinson's disease. *Mov Disord* 2007;22.

1856. Emslie-Smith AM, Engel AG. Necrotizing myopathy with pipestem capillaries, microvascular deposition of the complement membrane attack complex (MAC), and minimal cellular infiltration. *Neurology* 1991;41:936–9.

1857. Enderby PM, Wade DTeal, Hewer RL. Frenchay Aphasia Screening Test (FAST). *Int Rehabil Med* 1986;8:166–70.

1858. Endicott J, Spitzer RL. A diagnostic interview for affective disorders and schizophrenia. *Arch Gen Psychiat* 1978;35:837–44.

1859. Enevoldson TP, Sanders MD, Harding AE. Autosomal dominant cerebellar ataxia with pigmentary macular dystrophy: A clinical and genetic study of eight families. *Brain* 1994;117:445–60.

1860. Eng L, Vanderhaegen J, Bignami A et al. An acidic protein isolated from fibrous astrocytes. *Brain Res* 1971;28:351–4.

1861. Engel JJ. ILAE classification of epilepsy syndromes. *Epilepsy Res* 2006;70:5–10.

1862. Engel AG. Light on limb-girdle myasthenia. *Brain* 2006;129:1938–9.

1863. Engel AG, Ohno K, Sine SM. Congenital myasthenic syndromes: Progress over the past decade. *Muscle Nerve* 2003;27:4–25.

1864. Engel AG. Late onset rod myopathy (a new syndrome?). Light and electron microscopic observations in two cases. *Mayo Clin Proc* 1966;41:713–41.

1865. Engel AG. Acid maltase deficiency in adults: Studies in four cases of a syndrome which may mimic muscular dystrophy or other myopathies. *Brain* 1970;93:599–616.

1866. Engel AG. Myasthenia gravis and myasthenic syndromes. *Ann Neurol* 1984;16:519–34.

1867. Engel AG. Congenital myasthenic syndromes. *Neurol Clin* 1994;12:401–37.

1868. Engel AG, Angelini C. Carnitine deficiency of human skeletal muscle with associated lipid storage myopathy: A new syndrome. *Science* 1973;173:899–902.

1869. Engel AG, Angelini C, Gomez MR. Fingerprint body myopathy: A newly recognized congenital muscle disease. *Mayo Clin Proc* 1972;47:377–88.

1870. Engel AG, Banker BQ. *Myology*. 1986.

1871. Engel AG, Gomez MR. Congenital myopathy associated with multifocal degeneration of muscle fibers. *Trans Amer Neurol Assn* 1966;91:222–3.

1872. Deleted; see 1871.

1873. Engel AG, Gomez MR, Groover RJ. Multicore disease. *Mayo Clin Proc* 1971;46:666–81.

1874. Deleted; see 1873

1875. Engel AG, Gomez MR, Seybold ME et al. The spectrum and diagnosis of acid maltase deficiency. *Neurology* 1973;23:95–106.

1876. Engel AG, Lambert EH, Gomez MR. A new myasthenic syndrome with endplate acetylcholinesterase deficiency, small nerve terminals, and reduced acetylcholine release. *Ann Neurol* 1977;1:315–30.

1877. Engel AG, Lambert EH, Gomez MR. A new myasthenic syndrome with end–plate acetylcholinesterase deficiency, small nerve terminals, and reduced acetylcholine release. *Ann N Y Acad Sci* 1981;377:614–39.

1878. Engel AG, Lambert EH, Gomez MR. A newly recognised congenital myasthenic syndrome attributed to a prolonged open time of the actylcholine-induced ion channel. *Ann Neurol* 1982;11:553–69.

1879. Engel AG, Uchitel OD, Walls TJ. Newly recognized congenital myasthenic syndrome associated with high conductance and fast closure of the acetylcholine channel. *Ann Neurol* 1993;34:38–47.

1880. Engel J JR, Rapin I, Giblin DR. Electrophysiological studies in two patients with cherry-red spot-myoclonus syndrome. *Epilepsia* 1977;18:73–87.

1881. Engel M, Carmel PW, Chutorian AM. Increased intraventricular pressure without ventriculomegaly in children with shunts: "Normal volume" hydrocephalus. *Neurosurgery* 1979;5:549–52.

1882. Engel W, Askanas V. Inclusion body myositis. *Neurology* 2006;66:S20–S29.

1883. Engel WK. Muscle target fibers: A newly recognized sign of denervation. *Nature* 1961;191:389–90.

1884. Engel WK. Brief, small, abundant motor-unit action potentials. *Neurology* 1975;25:173–6.

1885. Engel WK, Dorman JD, Levy RI et al. Neuropathy in Tangier disease: A-lipoprotein deficiency manifesting as familial recurrent neuropathy and intestinal lipid storage. *Arch Neurol* 1967;17:1–9.

1886. Engel WK et al. A recently-recognized congenital myopathy associated with multifocal degeneration of muscle fibers. *Mayo Clin Proc* 1971;46:666–81.

1887. Engel WK, Eyerman EL, Williams HE. Late onset type of skeletal muscle phosphorylase deficiency. A new familial variety with completely and partially affected subjects. *N Engl J Med* 1963;268:135–7.

1888. Engel WK, Gold GN, Karpati G. Type I fiber hypotrophy and central nuclei. *Arch Neurol* 1968;18:435–44.

1889. Engel WK, Hawley RJ. Focal lesions of muscle in peripheral vascular disease. *J Neurol* 1977;215:161–8.

1890. Engel WK, Kurland LT, Klatzo I. An inherited disease similar to amyotrophic lateral sclerosis with a pattern of posterior column involvement. *Brain* 1959;82:203–20.

1891. England AC, Denny-Brown D. Severe sensory changes and trophic disorder, in peroneal muscular atrophy (Charcot-Marie-Tooth type). *Arch Neurol Psychiatry* 1952;67:1–22.

1892. Enzinger FM, Dulcey F. Proliferative myositis. Report of 33 cases. *Cancer* 1967;20:2213–23.

1893. Epley JM. Particle repositioning for benign paroxysmal positional vertigo. *Otolaryngol Clin North Am* 1996;29: 323–31.

1894. Epstein CJ, Martin GM, Schultz AL, Motulsky AG. Werner's syndrome: A review of it's symptomatology, natural history, pathologic features, genetics and relationship to the natural aging process. *Medicine* 1966;45:177–221.

1895. Epstein SH. History of the Boston Society of psychiatry and neurology. *Arch Neurol* 1985;42:391–2.

1896. Erb WH. Uber eine eigentumliche Lokalisation von Lahmung im Plexus brachialis. *VHMVH* 1874;2:130–7.

1897. Erb WH. Ueber einen wenig bekannten spinalen Symptomencomplex. *Berl Klin Wochenschr* 1875;12:357–9.

1898. Erb WH. Ueber die spastische Spinalparalyse (Tabes dorsalis spasmodique). *Arch Path Anat Berlin* 1877;70:241–67.

1899. Erb WH. Casuistik der bulbaren Lahmungen. *Arch Psychiat (Berlin)* 1879;9:325–50.

1900. Erb WH. Ueber einen eigenthumlichen bulbaren Symptomenkomplex. *Arch Psychiat Nervenkr* 1879;9:172–3.

1901. Erb WH. Ueber die "juvenile Form" der progressiven Muskelatrophie, ihre Beziehungen zur sogenannten Pseudohypertrophie der Muskeln. *Arch Klin Med* 1884;34:467–519.

1902. Erb WH. Ueber syphilitische Spinalparalyse. *Neurol Zbl* 1892;11: 161–8.

1903. Erba G, Browne TR. Atypical absence, myoclonic, atonic, and tonic seizures and the "Lennox-Gastaut syndrome". In Browne TR, Feldman RG, eds. *Epilepsy, Diagnosis And Management*, pp 75–94. Boston: Little, Brown, 1983.

1904. Erdheim J. On complications of acromegaly. *Virchow's Arch Path Anat Physiol* 1931;281:197–296.

1905. Erickson TC. Neurogenic hyperthermia. *Brain* 1998;172:1039.

1906. Erikson A. Hereditary syndrome consisting of recurrent attacks resembling brachial plexus neuritis, special features and cleft palate. *Acta Pediatr Scand* 1974;63:885–8.

1907. Erkinjuntti T, Haltia M, Palo J et al. Accuracy of the clinical diagnosis of vascular dementia. *J Neurol Neurosurg Psychiatry* 1988;51:1037–44.

1908. Eronen M et al. A digito-reno-cerebral syndrome. *Am J Med Genet* 1985;22:281–5.

1909. Ertekin C, Reel F. Bulbocavernosus reflex in normal men and in patients with neurogenic bladder and/or impotence. *J Neurol Sci* 1976;28:1–15.

1910. Erzigkeit H. The SKT – a short cognitive performance test as an instrument for the assessment of clinical efficacy of cognition enhancers. In Berenger M, Reisberg B, eds. *Diagnosis and Treatment of Senile Dementia*, p 164. Berlin: Springer-Verlag, 1989.

1911. Escobar V et al. Multiple pterygium syndrome. *Am J Dis Child* 1978;132: 609–11.

1912. Escueta AV, Boxley J, Stubbs N et al. Prolonged twilight state and automatisms: A case report. *Neurology* 1974;24:331–9.

1913. Eslinger PJ, Dennis K, Moore P et al. Metacognitive deficits in frontotemporal dementia. *J Neurol Neurosurg Psychiatr* 2005;76:1630–5.

1914. Espay AJ, Chen R. Rigidity and spasms from autoimmune encephalomyelopathies: Stiff-person syndrome. *Muscle Nerve* 2006;34:677–90.

1915. Espildora-Luque C. Sindrome oftalmico-silviano (ceguera monocular y hemiplejia alternas). *Arch Oft Hisp Amer* 1934;34:616–21.

1916. Espinosa PS, Berger JR. Acute central cord syndrome with bodybuilder sign. *Clin Neurol Neurosurg* 2007;109:354–6.

1917. Esquirol JE-D. *Des maladies mentales considerees sous les rapports medical, hygenique et modico-legal*. Paris: Baillière, 1838.

1918. Estanol BV, Marin OSM. Mechanism of the inverted supinator reflex: A clinical and neurophysiological study. *J Neurol Neurosurg Psychiatry* 1976;39:905–8.

1919. Esteban-García A. Blepharospasm and blepharocolysis. Different sides of the same coin. *Rev Neurol* 2005;40:298–302.

1920. Esterly NB, McKusick VA. Stiff skin syndrome. *Pediatrics* 1971;47:360–9.

1921. Ethelberg S. Symptomatic "Cataplexy" or chalastic fits in cortical lesion of the frontal lobe. *Brain* 1950;73:499–512.

1922. Etiemble J, Picort Ceal, Simeon J. Inherited erythrocyte PFK deficiency. *Hum Genet* 1980;55:383–90.

1923. Eulenberg A. Uber eine familiare durch 6 Generationen verfolgbare Form kongenitaler Paramyotonie. *Zbl Neur* 1886;5:265.

1924. Eunson LH, Rea R, Zuberi SM et al. Clinical, expression and genetic studies of mutations in the potassium channel gene KCNA1 reveal new phenotypic variability. *Ann Neurol* 2000;48:647–56.

1925. European Malignant Hyperpyrexia Group. A protocol for the investigation of malignant hyperpyrexia (MH) susceptibility. *Br J Anaesth* 1984;56:1267–9.

1926. Evans BK, Donley DK. Pseudohypoparathyroidism, Parkinsonism syndrome, with no basal ganglia calcification. *J Neurol Neurosurg Psychiatry* 1988;51:709–13.

1927. Evans BM, Milen M. Potassium losing nephritis presenting as a case of periodic paralysis. *Brit Med J* 1954;2:1067.

1928. Evans DGR, Mason S, Huson SM et al. Spinal and cutaneous schwannomatosis is a variant form of type 2 neurofibromatosis: A clinical and molecular study. *J Neurol Neurosurg Psychiatry* 1997;62:361–6.

1929. Evans J. Rocking at night. *J Child Psychol Psychiatr* 1961;2:71–85.

1930. Evans PR. Referred itch (Mitempfidungen). *Brit Med J* 1976;2:839–41.

1931. Evans RW. The postconcussion syndrome and the sequelae of mild head injury. *Neurol Clin* 1992;10:815–47.

1932. Eve FR. Pterygoid-levator synkinesis. *J Clin Neuro-Ophthalmol* 1987;7:61–2.

1933. Everett HC. Sneezing in response to light. *Neurology* 1964;14:483–90.

1934. Ewenczyk C, Leroux A, Roubergue A et al. Recessive hereditary methaemoglobinaemia, type II: Delineation of the clinical spectrum. *Brain* 2008;131:760–1.

1935. Ewer RW, Bissonnette RP, Brakel FJ et al. Tetanic neuromyopathy and renal failure. *JAMA* 1965;192:1117–20.

1936. Ewing DJ, Campbell IW, Murray A et al. Immediate heart rate response to standing: Simple test for autonomic neuropathy in diabetes. *Brit Med J* 1978;1:145–7.

1937. Ewing DJ, Irving IB, Kerr F et al. Cardiovascular responses to sustained handgrip in normal subjects and in subjects with diabetes mellitus: A test of autonomic function. *Clin Sci Mol Med* 1974;46:295–306.

1938. Eymard B, Hauw JJ. Mitochondrial encephalomyelopathies. *Curr Opin Neurol Neurosurg* 1992;5:909–16.

1939. Eymard B, Ioos C, Barois A et al. Congenital myasthenic syndromes due to mutations in the rapsyn gene. *Rev Neurol (Paris)* 2004;160: S78–S84.

1940. Eymard B, Romero N, Leturcq F et al. Primary adhalinopathy: (Alpha-sarcoglycanopathy). *Neurology* 1997;48:1227–34.

1941. Eysenck HJ, Eysenck SGB. *Handbook of the Eysenck Personality Inventory.* London: University of London Press, 1964.

1942. Fabbrini G, Juncos J, Mourdian MM et al. Levadopa pharmacokinetic mechanisms and motor fluctuations in Parkinson disease. *Ann Neurol* 1987;21:370–6.

1943. Fabian TC, Hoots AV, Stanford DS et al. Fat embolism syndrome. *Crit Care Med* 1990;18:42–6.

1944. Fabrizi GM, Cavallaro T, Angiari C. Charcot-Marie-Tooth disease type 2E, a disorder of the cytoskeleton. *Brain* 2007;130:368–80.

1945. Fabry J. Ein Beitrag zur Kenntnis der Purpura haemorrhagica nodularis (Purpura papulosa haemorrhagica Hebrae). *Arch Derm Syph* 1898;43: 187–200.

1946. Factor S, Podskalny G, Molho E. Psychogenic movement disorders: Frequency, clinical profile, and characteristics. *J Neurol Neurosurg Psychiatry* 1995;59:406–12.

1947. Fahn S. Rating scales for blepharospasm. *Adv Ophthalmic Reconstr Surg* 1985;4: 97–101.

1948. Fahn S. Generalized dystonia: Concept and treatment. *Clin Neuropharmacol* 1986;9 (**Suppl.2**):S37–S48.

1949. Fahn, S. *AAN Course Manual, 1989*. 1989. (Unpublished Work)

1950. Fahn S. Clinical variants of idiopathic torsion dystonia. *J Neurol Neurosurg Psychiatry* 1989;(**Suppl. June**):96–100.

1951. Fahn S, Marsden CD, Calne DB. Classification and investigation of dystonias. In Marsden CD, Fahn S, eds. *Movement Disorders* 2, pp 332–58. Butterworth, 1987.

1952. Fahn S,Williams D. Psychogenic dystonia. *Adv Neurol* 1998;50:431–55.

1953. Fahr T. Idiopathische Verkalkung der Hirngefasse. *Zbl Allg Path* 1930;50: 129–33.

1954. Falconer MA. Mesial temporal (Ammon's horn) sclerosis as a common cause of epilepsy. *Lancet* 1974;2:767–70.

1955. Falconer MA, Taylor DC. Surgical treatment of drug-resistant epilepsy due to mesial temporal lobe sclerosis. *Arch Neurol* 1968;19:353–61.

1956. Falconer MA,Weddell G. Costoclavicular compression of the subclavian artery and vein. Relation to the scalenus anticus syndrome. *Lancet* 1943;2:539–43.

1957. Fallon MD, Teitelbaum SL. Hypophosphatasia: Clinicopathologic comparison of the infantile, childhood and adult forms. *Medicine* 1984;63:12–24.

1958. Falls HF. Sex-linked ocular albinism displaying typical fundus changes in female heterozygotes. *Am J Ophthalmol* 1951;34:41.

1959. Fanconi G. Familial infantile pernicious anemia. *Jahrb Kinderh* 1927;117:257–80.

1960. Fanconi G, Turler U. Kongenitale Kleinhirnatrophie Mit Supranuclearen Storungen der Motilitat der Augenmuskeln. *Helv Pediat Acta* 1951;6:475–83.

1961. Fanous R, Midia M. Perivascular spaces: Normal and giant. *Can J Neurol Sci* 2007;34:5–10.

1962. Fantini ML, Ferini-Strambi L, Montplaisir J. Idiopathic REM sleep behavior disorder. *Neurology* 2005;64:780–6.

1963. Fara M et al. Dysmorphic Oto-Facio-Cervical abnormalities. *Acta Chir Orthop Traum Cech* 1967;34:511–20.

1964. Farber S. A lipid metabolic disorder - disseminated lipogranulomatosis - a syndrome with similarity to, and important differences from Nieman-Pick and Hand-Schuller-Christian disease. *Am J Dis Childh* 1952;84:499–500.

1965. Farbu E, Gilhus NE, Barnes MP et al. EFNS guideline on diagnosis and management of post-polio syndrome. Report of an EFNS task force. *Eur J Neurol* 2006;13:795–81.

1966. Fardeau M. Some orthodox and non-orthodox considerations on congenital myopathies. In Ellinson RJ, Murray NMF, Halliday AM, eds. *The London Symposia* (EEG) (**Suppl.** 39), pp 85–90. Elsevier Science Publishers, 1987.

1967. Fardin P, Negrin P, Sparta S et al. Posterior interosseous nerve neuropathy: Clinical and electromyographic aspects. *EMG Clin Neurophysiol* 1992;32:229–34.

1968. Farlow MR, DeMyer W, Dlouhy S et al. X-linked recessive inheritance of ataxia and adult onset dementia. *Neurology* 1987;37:602–7.

1969. Farrar JJ, Yen LM, Cook T et al. Tetanus. *J Neurol Neurosurg Psychiatry* 2000;69: 292–301.

1970. Farrell DF, Starr A. Delayed neurologic sequelae of electrical injuries. *Neurology* 1968;18:601–6.

1971. Fasler JJ, Rose FC. West Indian amblyopia. *Postgrad Med J* 1980;56:494.

1972. Fauci AS, Haynes BF, Katz P. The spectrum of vasculitis: Clinical, pathologic, immunologic, and therapeutic considerations. *Ann Int Med* 1978;89:660–76.

1973. Fauci AS,Wolff SM. Wegener's granulomatosis: Studies in eighteen patients and a review of the literature. *Medicine* 1973;52:535–61.

1974. Faull K, Bolton P, Halpern B et al. Patient with defect in leucine metabolism. *N Engl J Med* 1976;294:1013.

1975. Fauquembergue M, Tilikete C, Perret-Liaudet A et al. Heidenhain's variant of Creutzfeldt-Jakob's disease. *Rev Neurol* 2005;161:578–81.

1976. Fazio M. Eredetarieta della paralisi bulbare progressiva. *Rif Med* 1892;8:327.

1977. Fearnley JM, Lees AJ. Striatonigral degeneration. *Brain* 1990;113, **No.6**:1823–42.

1978. Feasby TE, Burton SR, Hahn AF. Obstetrical lumbosacral plexus injury. *Muscle Nerve* 1992;15:937–40.

1979. Feasby TE, Gilbert JJ, Brown WF et al. An acute axonal form of Guillain-Barré polyneuropathy. *Brain* 1986;109:1115–26.

1980. Feddersen B, Klopstock T. The puppy sign. *J Neurol Neurosurg Psychiatry* 2007;78:1055.

1981. Feder HM, Gerber MA. Saxophone headaches. *N Engl J Med* 1991;325:1888.

1982. Federico A, Cecio A, Apponi Battini G et al. Macular cherry-red spot and myoclonus syndrome: Juvenile form of sialidosis. *J Neurol Sci* 1980;48:157–69.

1983. Federico A, Guazzi G, Gruschelli C et al. Glycopeptidosis: A new inherited disorder of glycoconjugate metabolism affecting the central nervous system. *J Inhetited Metab Dis* 1981;4:141–2.

1984. Feeney DM, Baron JC. Diaschisis. *Stroke* 1986;17:817–30.

1985. Feeney DM, Walker AE. The prediction of posttraumatic epilepsy: A mathematical approach. *Arch Neurol* 1979;36:8–12.

1986. Feibel JH, Campa JF. Thyrotoxic neuropathy (Basedow's paraplegia). *J Neurol Neurosurg Psychiatry* 1976;39: 491–7.

1987. Feigin I, Pena CE, Budzilovich GN. The infantile spongy degenerations. *Neurology* 1968;18:153–66.

1988. Feinberg TE, Haber LD, Leeds NE. Verbal asomatognosia. *Neurology* 1990;40: 1391–4.

1989. Feinberg TE, Shapiro AK, Shapiro E. Paroxysmal myoclonic dystonia with vocalisations: New entity or variant of preexisting syndromes? *J Neurol Neurosurg Psychiatry* 1986;49:52–7.

1990. Feindel W. Herbert Henri Jasper (1906–1999): An appreciation. *Can J Neurol Sci* 1999;26:224–9.

1991. Feit H, Glasberg M, Ireton C et al. Peripheral neuropathy and starvation after gastric partitioning for morbid obesity. *Ann Int Med* 1982;96:453–5.

1992. Feit H, Silbergleit A, Schneider LB et al. Vocal cord and pharyngeal weakness with autosomal dominant distal myopathy: Clinical description and gene localization to 5q31. *Am J Hum Genet* 1998;63:1732–42.

1993. Feldman AB, Haley SM, Coryell J. Concurrent and construct validity of the pediatric evaluation of disability inventory. *Phys Ther* 1990;70:602–10.

1994. Feldman EL, Stevens MJ et al. A practical two-step quantitative clinical and electrophysiological assessment for the diagnosis and staging of diabetic neuropathy. *Diabetes Care* 1994;17:1281–9.

1995. Feldman EL, Russell JW, Sullivan KA et al. New insights into the pathogenesis of diabetic neuropathy. *Current Opinion in Neurology* 1999;12:553–63.

1996. Feldman EL, Stevens MJ. Clinical testing in diabetic peripheral neuropathy. *Can J Neurol Sci* 1994;21:S3–S7.

1997. Feldman GL, Weaver DD, Lovrein EW. The fetal trimethadione syndrome. *Am J Dis Childh* 1977;131:1389–92.

1998. Feldman H, Kertesz A. Diagnosis, classification and natural history of degenerative dementias. *Can J Neurol Sci* 2001;28:S17–S27.

1999. Feldman H, Schulzer M, Wang S et al. The functional rating scale in Alzheimer's disease assessment: A longitudinal study. In Iqbal K, Mortimer JA, Winblad B et al., eds. *Research Advances in Alzheimer's Disease and Related Disorders*, pp 235–41. John Wiley and Sons Ltd., 1995.

2000. Feldman M, Todman L, Bender MB. Flight of colours in lesions of the visual system. *J Neurol Neurosurg Psychiatry* 1974;37:1265–72.

2001. Feldman MD. The syndrome of anticholinergic intoxication. *Am Fam Physcn* 1986;34:113–6.

2002. Feldman MJ, Drasgow J. *The Visual-Verbal Test.* Los Angeles: Western Psychological Services, 1959.

2003. Felice K, Meredith C, Bonz N et al. Autosomal dominant distal myopathy not linked to the known distal myopathy loci. *Neuromuscular Disorders* 1999;9:59–65.

2004. Felice KJ, North WA, Moore SA et al. FSH dystrophy 4q35 deletion in patients presenting with facial-sparing scapular myopathy. *Neurology* 2000;54:1927–31.

2005. Felice KJ, Schwarta RC, Brown CA et al. Autosomal dominant Emery-Dreifuss dystrophy due to mutations in rod domain of the lamin A/C gene. *Neurology* 2000;55:275–80.

2006. Felice KJ, Whitaker CH, Grunnet ML. Benign calf amyotrophy. *Arch Neurol* 2003;60:1415–20.

2007. Fenichel GM. Clinical syndromes of myasthenia in infancy and childhood: A review. *Arch Neurol* 1978;35:97–103.

2008. Fenichel GM. Congenital muscular dystrophies. *Neurol Clin* 1988;6:519–28.

2009. Fenichel GM, Emery ES, Hunt P. Neurogenic atrophy simulating facioscapulohumeral dystrophy. *Arch Neurol* 1967;17:257–60.

2010. Fenichel GM, Olson WH, Kilroy AW. Hereditary dystonia associated with unique features in skeletal muscle. *Adv Neurol* 1971;25:552–9.

2011. Fenichel GM, Sul YC, Kilroy AW et al. An autosomal dominant dystrophy with humero-pelvic distribution and cardiomyopathy. *Neurology* 1982;32:1399–401.

2012. Féré C. Note sur les modifications de la resistance electrique sous l'influence des excitations sensorielles et des emotions. *CR Soc Biol* 1888;217.

2013. Féré MC. Le fou rire prodromique. *Rev Neurol* 1903;11:353.

2014. Ferell MR, Smallberg G, Lesis LD et al. A benign motor neuron disorder: Delayed cramps and fasciculations after poliomyelitis or myelitis. *Ann Neurol* 1982;11:423–7.

2015. Ferguson F, Critchley M. A clinical study of an heredo-familial disease resembling disseminated sclerosis. *Brain* 1929;52:203–25.

2016. Ferguson IT, Mahon M, Cinnings WJK. An adult case of Andersen's disease - Type IV glycogenosis. *J Neurol Sci* 1983;60:337–51.

2017. Feringa ER, Weatherbee L. Hypertrophic granulomatous cranial pachymenigitis causing progressive blindness in a chronic dialysis patient. *J Neurol Neurosurg Psychiatry* 1975;38:1170–6.

2018. Ferm D. Behavioral activities in demented geriatric patients. *Gerontol Clin (Basel)* 1974;16:185–94.

2019. Fernandes CM, Daya MR. A roller coaster headache: Case report. *J Trauma* 1994;37:1007–10.

2020. Fernandez C, Maues de Paula A, Figarella-Branger D et al. Diagnostic evaluation of clinically normal subjects with chronic hyperCKemia. *Neurology* 2006;66:1585–7.

2021. Fernandez HH, Friedman JH. Punding on L-dopa. *Mov Disord* 1999;14:836–8.

2022. Fernandez M, Raskind W, Matsushita M et al. Hereditary benign chorea. *Neurology* 2001;57:106–10.

2023. Fernandez M, Raskind W, Wolff J et al. Familial dyskinesia and facial myokymia (FDFM): A novel movement disorder. *Ann Neurol* 2001;49:486–92.

2024. Fernandez-Alvarez E. Transient movement disorders in children. *J Neurol* 1998;245:1–5.

2025. Ferrante MA, Wilbourn AJ. The characteristic electrodiagnostic features of Kennedy's disease. *Muscle Nerve* 1997;20:323–9.

2026. Ferrari G, Taddei L, Vivenza C et al. Paraparesis in hereditary multiple exostoses. *Neurology* 1979;29:973–7.

2027. Ferrari R, Schrader H. The late whiplash syndrome: A biopsychological approach. *J Neurol Neurosurg Psychiatry* 2001;70:722–6.

2028. Ferreiro A, Estournet B, Chateau D et al. Multi-minicore disease - searching for boundaries: Phenotype analysis of 38 cases. *Ann Neurol* 2000;48:745–57.

2029. Ferreiro A, Monnier N, Romero NB et al. A recessive form of central core disease, transiently presenting as multi-minicore disease, is associated with a homozygous mutation in the ryanodine receptor type I gene. *Ann Neurol* 2002;51:750–9.

2030. Ferrer I, Santpere G, van Leeuwen FW. Argyrophilic grain disease. *Brain* 2008;131:1416–32.

2031. Ferrier D. Experimental researches in cerebral physiology and pathology. *The West Riding Lunatic Asylum Medical Reports* 1873;3:30.

2032. Ferriman D. *Acrocephaly and Acrocephalosyndactyly.* London: Oxford U.P., 1941.

2033. Ferris SH, Crook TH, Clarke E et al. Facial recognition of memory deficits in normal aging and senile dementia. *J Gerontol* 1988;35:707–14.

2034. Ferris SH, Flicker C, Reisberg B. NYU computerized test battery for assessing cognition in aging and dementia. *Psychopharm Bull* 1988;24:699.

2035. Ferro JM, Kertesz A, Black SE. Subcortical neglect: Quantitation, anatomy, and recovery. *Neurology* 1987;37:1487.

2036. Fertleman CR, Ferrie CD, Aicardi J et al. Paroxysmal extreme pain disorder (previously familial rectal pain syndrome). *Neurology* 2007;69:586–95.

2037. Fetell MR, Smallberg G, Lewis L et al. A benign motor neurone disorder: Delayed cramps and fasciculations after poliomyelitis or myelitis. *Ann Neurol* 1982;11:423–7.

2038. Feuerstein RC, Mims LC. Linear nevus sebaceous with convulsions and mental retardation. *Am J Dis Childh* 1962;104:675–9.

2039. Feyrter F. Uber eine eigenartige Geschwulstform des Nervengewebes im menschlichen Verdauungsschlauch. *Virchow Arch* 1935;295:480–501.

2040. Fidueira F. Cephaloplegic syndrome in children. *Arch Med Enf Paris* 1919;22:113–25.

2041. Fidzianska A, Badurska B, Ryniewicz B et al. "Cap disease": New congenital myopathy. *Neurology* 1981;31:1113–20.

2042. Field CE. Albers-Schonberg disease. A typical case. *Proc Roy Soc Med* 1939;32:3220–4.

2043. Fields WS, Lemak NA. Joint study of extracranial arterial occlusion: VII. subclavian steal: A review of 168 cases. *JAMA* 1972;222:1139–43.

2044. Fiero RA, Groth M, Hurewitz A et al. Chronic hemoptysis: An unusual manifestation of fungal sinusitis. *South Med J* 1995;88:782–5.

2045. Fife T, Iverson DJ, Lempert T et al. Therapies for paroxysmal positional vertigo (an evidence-based review). *Neurology* 2008;70:2067–74.

2046. Fife TD, Baloh RB. Disequilibrium of unknown cause in older people. *Ann Neurol* 1993;34:694–702.

2047. Filipek PA, Accardo PJ, Ashwal S et al. Practice parameter: Screening and diagnosis of autism. *Neurology* 2000;55:468–79.

2048. Filippi M, Campi A, Martinelli V et al. Transitional progressive multiple sclerosis: MRI and MTI findings. *Acta Neurol Scand* 1995;92:178–82.

2049. Filla A, De Michele G, Cocozza S et al. Early onset autosomal dominant dementia with ataxia, extrapyramidal features and epilepsy. *Neurology* 2002;58:922–8.

2050. Filley CM, Kleinschmidt-DeMasters BK. Toxic leukoencephalopathy. *N Engl J Med* 2001;345:425–32.

2051. Findlay JM, Hao C, Emery D. Non-atherosclerotic fusiform cerebral aneurysms. *Can J Neurol Sci* 2002;29:41–8.

2052. Findley LJ, Gresty MA. Tremor. In Harrison MJG, ed. *Contemporary Neurology*, London: Butterworths, 1983.

2053. Findley LJ, Koller WC. Essential tremor: A review. *Neurology* 1987;37:1194–7.

2054. Fine EJ and Wongjirad C. The Ulnar Flexion Maneuver. 1985. (Unpublished Work)

2055. Fine JD, Arndt KA. The TORCH syndrome: A clinical review. *J Am Acad Derm* 1985;12:697–706.

2056. Finisterer J, Milvay E. Lactate stress testing in 155 patients with mitochondriopathy. *Can J Neurol Sci* 2002;29:49–53.

2057. Fink JK. The hereditary spastic paraplegias. *Arch Neurol* 2003;60:1045–9.

2058. Fink JK. Hereditary spastic paraplegia spastin phenotype and function. *Arch Neurol* 2004;61:830–3.

2059. Fink JK, Filling-Katz MR, Sokol J et al. Clinical spectrum of Niemann-Pick disease. *Neurology* 1989;39:1040–9.

2060. Fink JK, Heiman-Paterson T. Hereditary spastic paraplegias: Advances in genetic research. *Neurology* 1996;46:1507–14.

2061. Fink JN, Localization of the "sneeze center". *Neurology* 2001;56:138.

2062. Fink M, Green MA, Bender MB. The face-hand test as a diagnostic sign of organic mental syndrome. *Neurology* 1952;2:46–58.

2063. Finley KH. Post-encephalitic manifestations in viral encephalitis. In Field WS, Blattner RL, eds. *Viral encephalitis*, pp 69–94. Springfield: C.C. Thomas, 1958.

2064. Fins JJ, Master MG, Gerber LM. The minimally conscious state a diagnosis in search of an epidemiology. *Arch Neurol* 2007;64:1400–5.

2065. Finsterer J. Mitochondriopathies. *Europ J Neurol* 2004;11:163–86.

2066. Firkin BG, Whitworth JA. *Dictionary of Medical Eponyms*. Lancashire U.K., New Jersey, U.S.A.: The Parthenon Publishing Group, 1987.

2067. Firth D. *The Case of Augustus D'Este*. Cambridge: Cambridge University Press, 1970.

2068. Fischer D, Herasse M, Bitoun M et al. Characterization of the muscle involvement in dynamin 2-related centronuclear myopathy. *Brain* 2006;129:1463–9.

2069. Fischer H. A familial syndrome. *Derm Zschr (Berlin)* 1921;32–33:114–42.

2070. Fischer MH, Gerritsen T, Opitz JM. Aminoadipic aciduria: A non-deleterious inborn metabolic defect. *Humangenetik* 1974;24:265–70.

2071. Fischer P-A, Enzensberger W. Neurological complications in AIDS. *J Neurol* 1987;234:269–79.

2072. Fischer-Perroudon C, Mouret J, Jouvet M. Four months without sleep (agrypnia) in a case of "choree fibrillaire de Morvan" – improvement after 5HTP. In Chase MH, Stern WC, Walter PL, eds. *Sleep Research*, p 148. Los Angeles: BIS, UCLA, 1973.

2073. Fischer-Perroudon C, Mouret J, Jouvet M. Sur un cas d'agrypnie (4 mois sans sommeil) au cours d'une maladie de Morvan. Effet favorable du 5–hydroxytryptophane. *EEG Clin Neurophysiol* 1974;36:1–18.

2074. Fischer-Williams M, Bosanquet FD, Daniel PM. Carcinomatosis of the Meninges. *Brain* 1955;78:42–58.

2075. Fisher A, Gresty MA, Chambers B, Rudge P. Primary position upbeating nystagmus. *Brain* 1983;106:949–64.

2076. Fisher CM. Lacunes: Small deep cerebral infarctions. *Neurology* 1954;15:774–84.

2077. Fisher CM. An unusual variant of acute idiopathic polyneuritis (syndrome of ophthalmoplegia, ataxia and areflexia). *N Engl J Med* 1956;255:57–65.

2078. Fisher CM. Left hemiplegia and motor impersistence. *J Nerv Ment Dis* 1956;123:201–18.

2079. Fisher CM. A simple test of cordination in the fingers. *Neurology* 1960;10:745–6.

2080. Fisher CM. An improved test of motor coordination in the lower limbs. *Neurology* 1961;11:335–6.

2081. Fisher CM. Concerning recurrent transient cerebral ischemic attacks. *Can Med Assn J* 1962;86:1091–9.

2082. Fisher CM. Ocular bobbing. *Arch Neurol* 1964;11:543–6.

2083. Fisher CM. Pure sensory stroke involving face, arm and leg. *Neurology* 1965;15:76–80.

2084. Fisher CM. Concussion amnesia. *Neurology* 1966;16:826–30.

2085. Fisher CM. A lacunar stroke. *Neurology* 1967;17:614–7.

2086. Fisher CM. Some neuro-ophthalmological observations. *J Neurol Neurosurg Psychiatry* 1967;30:383–92.

2087. Fisher CM. Nonsense speech – amphigory. *Trans Amer Neurol Assn* 1970;95:238–40.

2088. Fisher CM. Pure spastic paralysis of corticospinal origin. *Can J Neurol Sci* 1977;4:251–8.

2089. Fisher CM. Transient paralytic attacks of obscure nature:The question of non-convulsive seizure paralysis. *Can J Neurol Sci* 1978;5:267–73.

2090. Fisher CM. Oval pupils. *Arch Neurol* 1980;37:502–3.

2091. Fisher CM. Disorientation for place. *Arch Neurol* 1982;39:33–6.

2092. Fisher CM. Lacunar strokes and infarcts: A review. *Neurology* 1982;32:871–6.

2093. Fisher CM. Whiplash amnesia. *Neurology* 1982;32:667–8.

2094. Fisher CM. Cataclysmic migraine. *Can J Neurol Sci* 1986;13:1–5.

2095. Fisher CM. Late-life migraine accompaniments – further experience. *Stroke* 1986;17:1033–42.

2096. Fisher CM. The posterior cerebral artery syndrome. *Can J Neurol Sci* 1986;13:232–9.

2097. Fisher CM. Neurologic fragments. I. Clinical observations in demented patients. *Neurology* 1988;38:1868–73.

2098. Fisher CM. The "herald hemiparesis" of basilar artery occlusion. *Arch Neurol* 1988;45:1301–3.

2099. Fisher CM. Neurologic fragments. II. *Neurology* 1989;39:127–32.

2100. Fisher CM. Transient monocular blindness versus amaurosis fugax. *Neurology* 1989;39:1622–4.

2101. Fisher CM. Visual hallucinations on eye closure associated with atropine toxicity. A neurological analysis and comparison with other visual hallucinations. *Can J Neurol Sci* 1991;18:18–27.

2102. Fisher CM. Brain herniation: A revision of classical concepts. *Can J Neurol Sci* 1995;22:83–91.

2103. Fisher CM. Alien hand phenomena: A review with the addition of six personal cases. *Can J Neurol Sci* 2000;27:192–203.

2104. Fisher CM, Adams RD. Transient global amnesia. *Acta Neurol Scand* 1964;40:1–83.

2105. Fisher CM, Cole M. Homolateral ataxia and crural paresis: A vascular syndrome. *J Neurol Neurosurg Psychiatry* 1965;28: 48–55.

2106. Fisher CM, Curry HB. Pure motor hemiplegia of vascular origin. *Arch Neurol* 1965;13:30–44.

2107. Fisher GR. Binswanger's encephalopathy: A review. *Arch Neurol* 1999.
2108. Fisher M, Mateer JE, Ullrich I et al. Pyramidal tract deficits and polyneuropathy in hyperparathyroidism. *Amer J Med* 1985;78:1041–4.
2109. Fisher M, Sargent J, Drachman D. Familial inverted choreoathetosis. *Neurology* 1979;29:1627–31.
2110. Fisher O. Zur Frage der anatomischen Grundlage der athetose double und der posthemiplegischen Bewegungsstorung uberhaupt. *Z Ges Neurol Psychiat* 1911;7:463.
2111. Fishman LM, Zybert PA. Electrophysiological evidence of pyriformis syndrome. *Arch Phys Med Rehab* 1992;73:359–64.
2112. Fishman LS, Samson JH, Sperling D. Primary alveolar hypoventilation syndrome (Ondine's curse). *Am J Dis Childh* 1965;110:155–61.
2113. Fishman L, Anderson C, Rosner B. BOTOX and physical therapy in the treatment of piriformis syndrome. *Am J Phys Med Rehabil* 2002;81:936–42.
2114. Fishman MA et al. Lacunar skull deformity and intelligence. *J Pediatr* 1977;59:296.
2115. Fishman RA. *Cerebrospinal Fluid in Diseases of the Nervous System.* Philadelphia: Saunders, 1980.
2116. Fisk JD, Pontefract A, Ritvo PG et al. The impact of fatigue on patients with multiple sclerosis. *Can J Neurol Sci* 1994;21:9–14.
2117. Fitch N, Karpati G, Pinsky L. Congenital blepharophimosis, joint contractures and muscular hypotonia. *Neurology* 1971;21:1215–20.
2118. Fitzsimmons JS et al. Four brothers with mental retardation, spastic paraplegia and palmoplantar hyperkeratosis. *Clin Genet* 1983;23:329–35.
2119. Flamm ES. The dilated pupil and head trauma. *Med Hist* 1972;16:194–8.
2120. Flamm ES. The neurology of Jean Cruveilhier. *Med Hist* 1973;17:343–55.
2121. Flanagan DE, Ibrahim AE, Ellison DW et al. Inflammatory hypophysitis: The spectrum of disease. *Acta Neurochir (Wien)* 2002;144:47–56.
2122. Flanagan D, Ibrahim A, Ellison D et al. Inflammatory hypophysitis – the spectrum of disease. *Acta Neurochir (Wien)* 2002;1444:47–56.
2123. Flanigan KM, Kerr L, Bromberg MB et al. Congenital muscular dystrophy with rigid spine syndrome: A clinical, pathological, radiological, and genetic study. *Ann Neurol* 2000;47:152–61.
2124. Flatau E. Atlas des menschlichen Gehirns und des Faserverlaufes. Berlin: Karger, 1894.
2125. Flatau E. On an epidemic of disseminated inflammation of the nervous system. *Encephale* 1929;25:619–60.
2126. Fletcher WA, Imes RK, Goodman D et al. Acute idiopathic blind spot enlargement. A big blind spot syndrome without disc edema. *Arch Ophthalmol* 1988;106:44–9.
2127. Fletcher WA, Sharpe JA. Saccadic eye movement dysfunction in Alzheimer's disease. *Ann Neurol* 1986;20:464.
2128. Fleury P, Hageman G. A dominantly-inherited lower motor neurone disorder presenting at birth with associated arthrogryposis. *J Neurol Neurosurg Psychiatry* 1985;48:1037–48.
2129. Flink EB, McCollister R, Prasad AS et al. Evidences for clinical magnesium deficiency. *Ann Int Med* 1957;47:956–68.
2130. Flourens MJP. *Récherches experimentales sur les proprietés et les fonctions du système nerveux dans les animaux vertèbres.* Paris: J.B. Baillière, 1842.
2131. Floyd P, Ayyar DR, Barwick DD. Myopathy in chronic renal failure. *Quart J Med* 1974;43:509–23.
2132. Flusser H, Kormann SH, Sato K et al. Mild glycine encephalopathy (NKH) in a large kindred due to a silent exonic GLDC splice mutation. *Neurology* 2005;64: 1426–30.
2133. Flynn P, Aird RB. A neuroectodermal syndrome of dominant inheritance. *J Neurol Sci* 1965;2:161–82.
2134. Foerster O. Der atonisch-astatische Typus der infantilen Cerebrallahmung. *Arch F Klin Med* 1909;48:216–44.
2135. Foerster O. The dermatomes in man. *Brain* 1933;56:1–39.
2136. Foix C. Syndrome de la paroi externe du sinus caverneux. *Rev Neurol* 1922;38: 827–32.
2137. Foix C. Le syndromes de la region thalamique. *Presse Med* 1925;33:113–7.
2138. Foix C, Alajouanine T. Myélite necrotique subaigue (myélite contrale angiohypertrophique à evolution progressive). *Rev Neurol* 1926;2:1–42.
2139. Foix C, Chavanay J-A, Marie J. Diplegie facio-linguo-masticatrice d'origine cortico-sous-corticale sans paralysie des membres. *Rev Neurol* 1926;33:214–9.
2140. Foix C, Chavany H, Hillemand P et al. Obliteration de l'artère choroidienne anterieure. Ramollissment de son territoire cerebral. Hemiplegie, hemianesthesie, hemianopsie. *Bull Fr Soc Ophthal* 1925;221–3.
2141. Foldes FF, Klonymus DH, Maisel W et al. A new curare test for diagnosis of myasthenia gravis. *JAMA* 1968;203: 183–8.
2142. Foley J. The athetoid syndrome: A review of a personal series. *J Neurol Neurosurg Psychiatry* 1983;46:289–98.
2143. Foley JM. Calcification of the corpus striatum and dentate nuclei occurring in a family. *J Neurol Neurosurg Psychiatry* 1951;14:253–61.
2144. Foley JM. Benign forms of intracranial hypertension – "toxic" and "otitic" hydrocephalus. *Brain* 1955;78:1–41.
2145. Foley JM. Derek Ernest Denny-Brown, 1901–1981. *Ann Neurol* 1982;11:413–9.
2146. Foley JM, Watson CW, Adams RD. Significance of the electroencephalographic changes in hepatic coma. *Trans Amer Neurol Assn* 1950;75:161–4.
2147. Folstein MF, Folstein SE, McHugh PR. Mini-mental state. A practical method for grading the cognitive state of patients for the clinician. *J Psychiatr Res* 1975;12:189–98.
2148. Folstein MF, Luria R. Reliability, validity, and clinical application of the visual analogue mood scale. *Psychol Med* 1973;3:479.
2149. Folstein SE, Leigh RJ, Parhad IM, Folstein MF. The diagnosis of Huntington's disease. *Neurology* 1986;36:1279–83.
2150. Fons-Estupina MC, Poo P, Colomer J et al. Moebius sequence: Clinico-radiological findings. *Rev Neurol* 2007;44:583–8.
2151. Fontaine A, Azouvi P, Remy P et al. Functional anatomy of neuropsychological deficit after severe traumatic brain injury. *Neurology* 1999;53:1963–8.
2152. Ford CV. A type of disability neurosis: The Humpty-Dumpty syndrome. *Intl J Psychiat Med* 1978;8:285–93.
2153. Ford FR, Wilkins L. Congenital universal insensitiveness to pain: A clinical report of three cases in children, with discussion of the literature. *Bull Johns Hopkins Hosp* 1938;62:448–66.
2154. Forsius H, Eriksson AW. A new X-linked syndrome *Klinische Monatsblatter Augenheilkunde* 1964;144:447.
2155. Forster FM, Hansotia P, Cleeland CS et al. A case of voice induced epilepsy treated by conditioning. *Neurology* 1969;19:325–31.
2156. Forsythe WI. Congenital hereditary vertical nystagmus. *J Neurol Neurosurg Psychiatry* 1955;18:196–8.
2157. Fothergill J. Of a painful affection of the face. *Med Obs & Inq* 1773;5:129.
2158. Fothergill J. *A Concise and Systematic Account of a Painful Affection of the Nerves of the Face, commonly called Tic Douloureux.* London: C. Dilly, 1794.
2159. Fotopoulos A. Spinal muscular atrophy with Huntington disease. *Psychiat Neurol Med Psychol (Leipzig)* 1966;18:129.
2160. Fountain RB. Familial bone abnormalities, deaf mutism, mental retardation and skin granuloma. *Proc Roy Soc Med* 1974;67:878–9.
2161. Fourcade G, Bengler C, Campello CH et al. Bickerstaff's syndrome presenting

with coma, tetraplegia and blindness. *Rev Neurol* 2007;163:231–4.

2162. Fourman P. Hereditary deafness in a family with ear pits. *Brit Med J* 1955;2:13542–1356.

2163. Fourney DR, Tong KA, Macoulay RJB et al. Spinal angiolipoma. *Can J Neurol Sci* 2001;28:82–8.

2164. Foville A. Note sur un paralysie peu connu dans certains muscles de l'oeil et sa liason avec quelques points de l'anatomie et la physiologie de la protuberance annulaire. *Bull Soc Anat Paris* 1858;30:393–414.

2165. Fowler EPA. A method for the early detection of otoslerosis; a study of sounds well above threshold. *Arch Otolaryngol* 1936;24:731.

2166. Fowler HL. Machado-Joseph-Azorean disease: A ten year study. *Arch Neurol* 1984;41:921–5.

2167. Fowler M, Dow R, White TA et al. Congenital hydrocephalus – hydrancephaly in five siblings with autopsy studies: A new disease. *Dev Med Child Neurol* 1972;14:173–88.

2168. Fowler WM, Layzer RB, Taylor RG et al. The Schwartz-Jampel syndrome. *J Neurol Sci* 1974;22:127–46.

2169. Fox AJ, Vinuela F. Neurological deficit from an inoperable arteriovenous malformation: An indication for therapeutic embolization? *Arch Neurol* 1986;43:510–1.

2170. Fox RH, Wilkins DC, Bell JA et al. Spontaneous periodic hypothermia: Diencephalic epilepsy. *Brit Med J* 1973;2:693–5.

2171. Francalcini P, Eymard-Pierre E, Dionisi-Vici C et al. Fatal infantile leukodystrophy: A severe variant of CACH/VWM syndrome, allelic to chromosome 3q27. *Neurology* 2001;57:265–70.

2172. Francis DA, Bronstein AM, Rudge P et al. The site of brainstem lesions causing semicircular canal paresis: An MRI study. *J Neurol Neurosurg Psychiatry* 1992;55:446–9.

2173. Francis DA, Heron JR. Ocular flutter in suspected multiple sclerosis: A presenting paroxysmal manifestation. *Postgrad Med J* 1985;61:333–4.

2174. Franco-Paredes C, Martin K. Extranodal Rosai–Dorfman disease involving the meninges. *South Med J* 2002;95: 111–2.

2175. Francois J. Oculo-cutaneous angiomatosis of Lawford. *Acta Neurol Psychiat Belg* 1951;8:503–20.

2176. Francois J. The phakomatoses: Introduction. In Vincken PJ, Bruyn GW, eds. *Handbook of Clinical Neurology*, pp 1–18. Amsterdam: North Holland Publishing Co., 1972.

2177. Frank JW, Kuschner BJ, France TD. Paradoxical pupillary phenomena: A review of patients with pupillary constriction to darkness. *Arch Ophthalmol* 1988;106:1564.

2178. Frankel HL, Hancock DO, Hyslop G et al. The value of postural reduction in the initial management of closed injuries of the spine with paraplegia and tetraplegia. *Paraplegia* 1969;7:179–92.

2179. Frankenburg WK, Dodds J, Archer P et al. Denver II. *Denver Developmental Materials* 1990.

2180. Frankl-Hochwart J. Uber Diagnose der Zirbeldrusentumoren. *Dtsch Z Nervenklinik* 1909;37:455–65.

2181. Fraser CL. Hepatic encephalopathy. *N Engl J Med* 1985;313, No.14:865–73.

2182. Fraser FC, Lytwyn A. Spectrum of abnormalities in the Meckel syndrome. *Am J Med Genet* 1981;9:67–73.

2183. Fraser JL, Olney RK. The relative diagnostic sensitivity of different F-wave parameters in various polyneuropathies. *Muscle Nerve* 1992;15:912–8.

2184. Fredrickson DS, Altrocchi PH, Avioli LV et al. Tangier disease. *Ann Int Med* 1961;55:1016–31.

2185. Freedman BJ. *Just a Word, Doctor*. Oxford: Oxford University Press, 1987.

2186. Freedman M, Alexander MP, Naeser MA. Anatomic basis of transcortical motor aphasia. *Neurology* 1984;34:409–17.

2187. Freeman EA, Sheldon JH. Cranio-carpo-tarsal dystrophy. An undescribed congenital formation. *Arch Dis Child* 1938;13:277–83.

2188. Freeman JE et al. Somnolence after prophylactic cranial irradiation in children with acute lymphoblastic leukaemia. *Brit Med J* 1973;4:523–5.

2189. Freeman JM, Finkelstein JD, Mudd SH et al. Homocystinuria presenting as reversible "schizophrenia": A new defect in methionine metabolism with reduced methylene-tetrahydrofolate reductase activity. *Pediat Res* 1972;6:423.

2190. Freeman MD, Croft A, Rossignol AM et al. A review and methodologic critique of the literature refuting whiplash syndrome. *Spine* 1999;24:86–96.

2191. Freeman RW, Bleecker ML, Comstock GW et al. Validation of self-administered questionnaire for study of peripheral neuropathy. *Am J Epidem* 1985;121: 291–300.

2192. Freeman T, Gathercole CE. Perseveration: The clinical symptoms in chronic schizophrenia and organic dementia. *Brit J Psychiat* 1966;112:27–32.

2193. Freeman W, Watts JW. *Psychosurgery*. Springfield: CC Thomas, 1950.

2194. Freeman W, Watts JW. Prefrontal lobotomy in agitated depression. Report of a case. *Med Ann Distr Columbia* 1936;5:326–8.

2195. Frei KP, Patronas N, Crutchfield KE et al. Mucolipidosis type IV. *Neurology* 1998;51:565–9.

2196. Freiberg AH. Sciatic pain and its relief by operations on muscle and fascia. *Arch Surg* 1937;34:337–49.

2197. Freke J. A case of extraordinary exostoses on the back of a boy. *Phil Trans Roy Soc Lond* 1740;41:369–70.

2198. Frey E. Hereditary quivering of the chin. *Deut Z Nervenheilk* 1930;115:9–26.

2199. Frey L. Le syndrome du nerf auriculo-temporal. *Rev Neurol* 1923;2:97–104.

2200. Fridenberg SM, Hermann RC. The breathing hand: Obstetric brachial plexopathy reinnervation from thoracic roots? *J Neurol Neurosurg Psychiatry* 2004;75:158–60.

2201. Friedburg D. Pseudoneuritis und Drusenpapille beim Alport-Syndrom. *KMA*. 1968;152:379.

2202. Friede RL. *Developmental Neuropathology*. Vienna: Springer-Verlag, 1975.

2203. Friedman DI, Jacobson DM. Diagnostic criteria for idiopathic intracranial hypertension. *Neurology* 2002;59:1492–5.

2204. Friedmann M. *On the Pathology and Anatomy of Widespread Chronic Encephalitis.* [in German] Vienna: C. Fromme, 1883.

2205. Friedmann M. *Ueber die nicht epileptischen absenscen oder Kurzen Narkoleptischen anfalle. Dtsch Z Nervenklinik* 1906;30:462–92.

2206. Friedreich N. Uber degenerative Atrophie der spinalen Hiterstrange. *Arch Path Anat Berlin* 1863;26:391–419.

2207. Friedreich N. Ueber congenitale halbseitige Kopfhypertrophie. *Virchow's Arch Path Anat Physiol* 1863;28:474–81.

2208. Friedreich N. Paramyoclonus multiplex. *Arch Path Anat Berlin* 1881;86:421–30.

2209. Friis ML, Lund M. Stress convulsions. *Ann Neurol* 1994;31:155–9.

2210. Frijns CJM, Van Deutekom J, Frants RR et al. Dominant congenital benign spinal muscular atrophy. *Muscle Nerve* 1994;17:192–7.

2211. Frisen L. Quadruple sectoranopia and sectorial optic atrophy: A syndrome of the distal anterior choroidal artery. *J Neurol Neurosurg Psychiatry* 1979;42:590–4.

2212. Frisoni GB. Structural imaging in the clinical diagnosis of Alzheimer's disease: Problems and tools. *J Neurol Neurosurg Psychiatry* 2001;70:711–8.

2213. Frith JA, McLeod JG, Nicholson GA et al. Peroneal muscular atrophy with pyramidal tract features (hereditary motor and sensory neuropathy type V). *J Neurol Neurosurg Psychiatry* 1994;57:1343–6.

2214. Fritsch GT, Hitzig E. Ueber die elektrische Erregbarkeit des

Grosshirns. *Arch Anat Physiol u wiss Med* 1870;300–32.

2215. Frohlich A. Ein fall von tumor der hypophysis cerebri ohne akromegalie. *Wien Klin Rdsch* 1901;15:883–906.

2216. Froin G. Inflammations meningées avec reactions chronique, fibrineuse et cytologique du liquide cephalo-rachidien. *Gaz Hop Paris* 1903;76:1005–6.

2217. Froment JC. La préhension dans les paralysies du nerf cubital et le signe du pouce. *Presse Med* 1915;23:409.

2218. Froment JC, Gardene H. La rigidité et la rue dentée Parkinsoniene s'effacent au repos. *Rev Neurol* 1926;1:52–3.

2219. Fromm GH, Graff-Radford SB, Terrence CF et al. Pre-trigeminal neuralgia. *Neurology* 1990;40:1493–5.

2220. Fry JH. Overuse syndrome in musicians – 100 years ago: An historical review. *Med J Aust* 1986;145:620–5.

2221. Frydman M et al. Oculo-palato-cerebral dwarfism: A new syndrome. *Clin Genet* 1985;27:414–9.

2222. Frymoyer JW. Back pain and sciatica. *N Engl J Med* 1988;318:291–300.

2223. Frymoyer JW, Selby DK. Segmental instability: Rationale for treatment. *Spine* 1985;10:280–6.

2224. Fryns JP et al. A new lethal syndrome with cloudy corneae, diaphragmatic defects and distal limb deformities. *Human Genetics* 1979;50:65–70.

2225. Fugl-Meyer AR, Jaasko L, Leyman I et al. The post-stroke hemiplegic patient: 1. A method for evaluation of physical performance. *Scand J Rehab Med* 1975;7:13–31.

2226. Fujii T, Okuno T, Ito M et al. Non-Menkes-type copper deficiency with regression, lactic acidosis, and granulocytopenia. *Neurology* 1991;41:1263–6.

2227. Fujita T, Kanno T, Kobayashi S. *The Paraneuron*. Tokyo and London: Springer, 1988.

2228. Fukatsu R, Yamadori A, Fujii T. Impaired recall and preserved encoding in prominent amnesic syndrome: A case of basal forebrain amnesia. *Neurology* 1998;50:541.

2229. Fukazawa T, Sasaki H, Kikuchi S et al. Dominantly inherited leukodystrophy showing cerebellar deficits and spastic paraparesis: A new entity? *J Neurol* 1997;244:446–9.

2230. Fukuda K, Straus S, Hickie J et al. The chronic fatigue syndrome; a comprehensive approach to its definition and study. *Ann Int Med* 1994;121:953–9.

2231. Fukuda K, Tanaka T, Hyodo S et al. Hyperphenylalaninaemia due to impaired dihydrobiopterin biosynthesis: Leukocyte function and effect of tetrahydrobiopterin therapy. *J Inherit Metab Dis* 1985;8:49–52.

2232. Fukuhara N. Myoclonus epilepsy and mitochondrial myopathy. In Scarloto G, Cerri C, eds. *Mitochondrial Pathology in Muscle Diseases,* pp 89–110. Padova: Piccin, 1983.

2233. Fukuhara N, Kumamoto T, Hirahara H, Tsubaki T. A new myopathy with tubulomembranous inclusions. *J Neurol Sci* 1981;50:95–107.

2234. Fukunaga H, Osame M, Igata A. A case of nemaline myopathy with ophthalmoplegia and mitochondrial abnormalities. *J Neurol Sci* 1980;46: 169–77.

2235. Fukutate T, Kita K, Sakakibara R et al. Late onset hereditary ataxia with global thermoanalgesia and absence of fungiform papillae on the tongue in a Japanese family. *Brain* 1996;119:1011–21.

2236. Fukuyama Y, Audo T, Yokota J. Acute fulminant myoglobinuria polymyositis with picornavirus-like crystals. *J Neurol Neurosurg Psychiatry* 1977;40:775–81.

2237. Fukuyama Y, Osaw M, Suzuki H. Congenital muscular dystrophy of the Fukuyama type – clinical, genetic, and pathological considerations. *Brain Dev* 1981;3:1–29.

2238. Fuld PA, Katzman R, Davies P et al. Intrusions as a sign of Alzheimer dementia: Chemical and pathological verification. *Ann Neurol* 1982;11:155–9.

2239. Fuller GN, Marshall A, Flint J et al. Migraine madness: Recurrent psychosis after migraine. *J Neurol Neurosurg Psychiatry* 1993;56:416–8.

2240. Fullerton PM, Gilliatt RW. Axon reflexes in human motor nerve fibres. *J Neurol Neurosurg Psychiatry* 1965;28:1–11.

2241. Funakoshi M, Goto K, Arahata K. Epilepsy and mental retardation in a subset of early onset 4q35-facioscapulohumeral muscular dystrophy. *Neurology* 1998;50:1791–4.

2242. Furman JM, Balaban CD, Jacob RG et al. Migraine anxiety-related dizziness (MARD). *J Neurol Neurosurg Psychiatr* 2005;76:1–8.

2243. Furman JMR, Crumrine PK, Reinmuth O. Epileptic nystagmus. *Ann Neurol* 1990;27:686–8.

2244. Furman JMR et al. Infantile cerebellar atrophy. *Ann Neurol* 1985;17:399–402.

2245. Furman JMR, Jacob RG. Psychiatric dizziness. *Neurology* 1997;48:1161–6.

2246. Furst W, Ostrum HW. Platybasia, Klippel-Feil syndrome and Sprengel's deformity. *Am J Roentgen* 1942;47: 588–90.

2247. Furukawa T. Numb chin syndrome in the elderly. *J Neurol Neurosurg Psychiatry* 1990;53:173.

2248. Furukawa T, Akagami N, Maruyama S. Chronic neurogenic quadriceps amyotrophy. *Ann Neurol* 1977;2:528–30.

2249. Furukawa T, Takogi A, Nakao K et al. Hereditary muscular atrophy with ataxia, retinitis pigmentosa and diabetes mellitus. *Neurology* 1968;18:942–7.

2250. Furukawa T, Toyokura V. Congenital hypotonic-sclerotic muscular dystrophy. *J Med Genet* 1977;14:426–9.

2251. Furukawa T, Toyokura Y. Alternating Horner's syndrome. *Arch Neurol* 1974;30:311–4.

2252. Fuzukawa T, Sasaki H, Kikuchi S et al. Dominantly inherited leukodystrophy showing cerebellar deficits and spastic paraparesis: A new entity? *J Neurol* 1997;244:446–9.

2253. Gafni J, Fischel B, Reit R et al. Amyloidotic polyneuropathy in a Jewish family. *Quart J Med* 1985;55:33–43.

2254. Gagliardi ART et al. GAPO syndrome: Report of three affected brothers. *Am J Med Genet* 1984;19:217–23.

2255. Gaillard JM. Electrophysiological semeiology of sleep. *Experientia* 1980;36:3–7.

2256. Gainer JV JR, Chou SM, Chadduck WM. Familial cerebral sarcomas. *Arch Neurol* 1975;32:665–8.

2257. Gajusdek DC, Zigas V. Degenerative disease of the central nervous system in New Guinea. The endemic occurrence of "Kuru" in the native population. *N Engl J Med* 1957;257:974–8.

2258. Galer BS. Neuropathic pain of peripheral origin. *Neurology* 1995;45:S17–S25.

2259. Galer BS, Jensen MP. Development and preliminary validation of a pain measure specific to neuropathic pain. *Neurology* 1997;48:332–8.

2260. Gallai V, Hockaday JM, Hughes JT et al. Ponto-bulbar syndrome with deafness (Brown-Vialetto-Van Laere Syndrome). *J Neurol Sci* 1981;50:259–75.

2261. Gallop TR. Fronto-facio-nasal-dysostosis: A new autosomal recessive syndrome. *Am J Med Genet* 1981;10:409–12.

2262. Galpern WR, Lang AE. Interface between tauopathies and synucleinopathies. *Ann Neurol* 2006;59:449–58.

2263. Galton CJ, Gomez-Anson B, Antoun N et al. Temporal lobe rating scale; application to Alzheimer's disease and frontal lobe dementia. *J Neurol Neurosurg Psychiatry* 2001;70:165–73.

2264. Galvin JE, Lee VM-Y, Trojanowski JQ. Synucleinopathies. *Arch Neurol* 2001;58:186–90.

2265. Galvin JE, Roe CM, Powlishta KK et al. The AD8. *Neurology* 2005;65:559–64.

2266. Gambardella A, Andermann F, Shorvon S et al. Limited chronic focal encephalitis. *Neurology* 2008;70:374–7.

2267. Gamstorp I. Adynamia episodica hereditaria. *Acta Pediatr Scand* 1956;(**Suppl 108**):1–126.
2268. Gamstorp I, Wohlfart G. Myokymia, hyperhydrosis, impaired muscle relaxation. *Acta Psychiatr Scand* 1959;**34**:181.
2269. Gancher ST, Nutt JG. Autosomal dominant episodic ataxia: A heterogenous syndrome. *Mov Disord* 1986;**1**:239–53.
2270. Gandevia SC, McCloskey DI. Sensations of Heaviness. *Brain* 1977;**100**:345–54.
2271. Ganser SJA. Ueber einen eigenartigen hysterischen Dammerzustund. *Arch Psychiat (Berlin)* 1898;**30**:633–40.
2272. Garcia Albea E. The ecstatic epilepsy of Teresa of Jesus. *Rev Neurol* 2003;**37**: 879–87.
2273. Garcia HA, Milner-Brown HS, Fisher MA. "Turns" analysis in the physiological evaluation of neuromuscular disorders. *J Neurol Neurosurg Psychiatry* 1980;**43**:1091–7.
2274. Garcin R, Raverdy Ph, Delthil S et al. Sur une affection heredo-familiale associant cataracte, atrophis optique, signes extra pyramidaux et certains stigmates de la maladie de Friedreich. *Rev Neurol* 1961;**101**:373–9.
2275. Gardner RC. Confirmed case and diagnosis of Pseudocarpal tunnel (sublimis) syndrome. *N Engl J Med* 1970;**282**:858.
2276. Gardner WJ. Cross Talk – The paradoxical transmission of a nerve impulse. *Arch Neurol* 1966;**14**:149–56.
2277. Gardner WJ, Frazier CH. Bilateral acoustic neurofibromas. *Arch Neurol Psychiatry* 1930;**23**:266–302.
2278. Gardner-Medwin D, Johnston HM. Severe muscular dystrophy in girls. *J Neurol Sci* 1984;**64**:79–87.
2279. Gardner-Thorpe C, Pearn J. The Cotard syndrome. Report of two patients: With a review of the extended spectrum of "délire des négations". *Eur J Neurol* 2004;**11**: 563–6.
2280. Gardner-Thorpe C. Muscle weakness due to sarcoid myopathy. *Neurology* 1972;**22**:917–28.
2281. Gardos G, Cole JO, Salomon M et al. Clinical forms of severe tardive dyskinesia. *Am J Psychiatry* 1987;**144**:895–902.
2282. Gardos G, Simmelgaard H. Tardive dyskinesia during and following treatment. *Psychopharmacol Berlin* 1978;**59**:105–12.
2283. Gareis FJ, Mason JD. X-linked mental retardation associated with bilateral clasp-thumb anomaly. *Am J Med Genet* 1984;**17**:333–8.
2284. Garfield J. Brain abscesses and focal suppurative infections. In Vinken PJ, Bruyn GW, eds. *Handbook of Clinical Neurology*, vol. 33, Pt1. Amsterdam: North Holland Publishing Co., 1978.
2285. Garfinkel PE. The validity of the distinction between bulimia with and without anorexia nervosa. *Am J Psychiatry* 1985;**143**:581–7.
2286. Garg BP. Colpocephaly: An error of morphogenesis? *Arch Neurol* 1982;**39**:243–6.
2287. Garies FJ, Johnson J. Inanition in infants associated with diencephalic neoplasms. *J Dis Child* 1965;**109**:349.
2288. Garland HG. Central nervous deficiency syndrome. *Proc Roy Soc Med* 1946;**39**: 178–80.
2289. Garland HG, Astley CE. Hereditary spastic paraplegia with amyotrophy and pes cavus. *J Neurol Neurosurg Psychiatry* 1950;**13**:130–3.
2290. Garland HG, Taverner D. Diabetic myelopathy. *Brit Med J* 1953;**1**:1405–8.
2291. Garlepp MJ, Dawkins RL, Christiansen FT. Penicillamine-induced myasthenia. *Brit Med J* 1983;**286**:338–40.
2292. Garlepp MJ, Mastaglia FL. Inclusion body myositis. *J Neurol Neurosurg Psychiatry* 1996;**60**:251–5.
2293. Garthe E, States J, Mango N. Abbreviated injury scale unification: The case for a unified injury system for global use. *J Trauma* 1999;**47**:309–23.
2294. Garvey MA, Giedd J, Swedo SE. PANDAS: The search for environmental triggers of pediatric neuropsychiatric disorders. Lessons from rheumatic fever. *J Child Neurol* 1998;**13**:413–23.
2295. Gascon GG, Barlow CF. Juvenile migraine presenting as an acute confusional state. *Pediatrics* 1970;**45**: 628–35.
2296. Gascon GG, Gilles FH. Limbic dementia. *J Neurol Neurosurg Psychiatry* 1973;**36**:421–30.
2297. Gascon GG, Lombroso CT. Epileptic (gelastic) laughter. *Epilepsia* 1971;**12**: 63–76.
2298. Gass A, Barker GJ, Kidd D et al. Correlation of magnetisation transfer ratio with clinical disability in multiple sclerosis. *Ann. Neurol.* 1994. 36 (1) 997–1003.
2299. Gass JD. The syndrome of keratoconjunctivitis, superficial monoliaisis, idiopathic hypoparathyroidism and Addison's disease. *Am J Ophthalmol* 1962;**54**: 660–74.
2300. Gass JD. Cavernous hemangioma of the retina: A neuro-oculo-cutaneous syndrome. *Am J Ophthalmol* 1971;**71**:799.
2301. Gass JMD. Acute posterior multifocal placoid pigment epithiliopathy. *Arch Ophthalmol* 1968;**80**:177–85.
2302. Gassell MM. False localising signs. *Arch Neurol* 1961;**4**:526–54.
2303. Gassell MM, Williams D. Visual function in patients with homonymous hemianopia. Part III. *Brain* 1963;**86**:229–60.
2304. Gastaut H. Le syndrome "hemiconvulsion-hemiplegie-epilepsie". *Rev Neurol* 1957;**97**:37–52.
2305. Gastaut H. *Dictionary of Epilepsies. Part I: Definitions*. Geneva: World Health Organization, 1973.
2306. Gastaut H. Fyodor Dostoevsky's involuntary contribution to the symptomatology and prognosis of epilepsy. *Epilepsia* 1978;**19**:186–190.
2307. Gastaut H. A new type of epilepsy: Benign partial epilepsy of childhood with occipital spike-waves. *Clin Electroenceph* 1982;**13**:13–22.
2308. Gastaut H. Classification of status epilepticus. In Delgado-Escueta AV, Wasterlain DG, Traimen DM et al., eds.*Advances in Neurology,* vol.34; *Status Epilepticus*, p 75. New York: Raven Press, 1983.
2309. Gastaut H. Classification of status epilepticus. *Adv Neurol* 1983;**34**:75.
2310. Gastaut H. Benign epilepsy of childhood with occipital paroxysms. In Roger J, Dravet C, Bureau M et al., eds. *Epileptic Syndromes in Infancy, Childhood and Adolescence*, pp 159–70. London: John Libbey, 1985.
2311. Gastaut H, Broughton RJ. Paroxysmal psychological events and certain phases of sleep. *Percept Mot Skills* 1963;**17**:362.
2312. Gastaut H, Broughton RJ. *Epileptic Seizures*. Springfield, Illinois: C.C. Thomas, 1972.
2313. Gastaut H, Gastaut Y. Syncopes et convulsions. A propos de la nature syncopal de certains spasmes du sanglot et de certains convulsions essentielles, hyperthermiques et a froid. *Rev Neurol* 1957;**96**:158–63.
2314. Gastaut H, Naquet R. Etude electroencéphalographiquede l'insuffisance circulatoire cérebral (ICC). Symposium International sur la Circulation Cérebrale 1966;163–191. (Abstract)
2315. Gastaut H, Roger J, Ouahchi S et al. An electro-clinical study of generalized epileptic seizures of tonic expression. *Epilepsia* 1963;**4**:15–44.
2316. Gates AI, McGintie WH. *Gates-McGintie Reading Exercises.* New York: Teachers College Press, 1965.
2317. Gatfield PD, Taller E, Hinton GG et al. Hyperpipecolatemia. A new metabolic disorder associated with neuropathy and hepatomegaly: A case study. *Can Med Assn J* 1968;**99**:1215–33.
2318. Gaucher PCE. *De l'epithelioma primitif de la rate: Hypertrophie idiopathique de la rate sans leucémie.* Paris: Univ. Paris, 1882.

2319. Gaull GE, Bender AN, Vulovic D et al. Methioninemia and myopathy: A new disorder. *Ann Neurol* 1980;9:423–32.
2320. Gautier-Smith PC. Neurological complications of Glandular fever (Infectious mononucleosis). *Brain* 1965;88:323–34.
2321. Gaymard B, Lafitte C, Gelot A et al. Plus-minus lid syndrome. *J Neurol Neurosurg Psychiatry* 1992;55:846–8.
2322. Gazit E et al. The wrinkly skin syndrome: A new heritable disorder of connective tissue. *Clin Genet* 1973;4:186–92.
2323. Geiger LR, Mancall EL, Penn AS et al. Familial neuralgic amyotrophy: Report of three families with review of the literature. *Brain* 1974;97:87–102.
2324. Gelinas I, Gauthier L, McIntyre M et al. Development of a functional measure for persons with Alzheimer's disease: The disability assessment for dementia. *Am J Occup Ther* 1999;53:471–81.
2325. Gelineau JBE. De la narcolepsie. *Gaz Hop Paris* 1880;53:626–8.
2326. Gellis SS, Feingold M. Spondylothoracic dysplasia (costo-vertebral dysplasia, Jarcho-Levin syndrome). *Am J Dis Childh* 1976;130:513–4.
2327. Gelwan MJ, Seidman M, Kupersmith MJ. Pseudo-pseudo Foster Kennedy syndrome. *J Clin Neuro-Ophthalmol* 1985;5:209–12.
2328. Geminginani F. Spinocerebellar ataxia with localized amyotrophy of the hands, sensorineural deafness and spastic paraparesis in 2 brothers. *J Neurogenet* 1986;3:125–33.
2329. Gent M, Blakeley J, Easton JD et al. Canadian-American ticlopidine study: Thrombo-embolic stroke. *Stroke* 1988;19:1203–10.
2330. Gerhardt C. Encephalitis: Stimmbandlahmung ohne Stimmveranderung. *Berlin: Arch F Path Anat,* Berl., 1863.
2331. Gerle B. Dynamite encephalosis. *Acta Psychiatrica et Neurologica* 1946;21:319.
2332. Gerlier EF. Une epidemie de vértige paralysant. *Rev Med Suisse Rom* 1887;7: 5–29.
2333. Gershanik OS, Nygaard TG. Parkinson's disease beginning before age 40. *Adv Neurol* 1990;53:251–8.
2334. Gerstmann J. Fingeragnosie und isolierte Agraphie – ein neues syndrom. *Zschr Gesamte Neurol Psychiatr* 1927;108:152–77.
2335. Gerstmann J, Straussler E, Scheinker IM. Uber eine eigenartige hereditar-familiare erkrankung des zentralnervensystems zugleich ein beitrag zur frage des vorzeitigen lokalen alterns. *Z Neurol* 1936;154:736–62.
2336. Gertz MA, Kyle RA. Myopathy in primary systemic amyloidosis. *J Neurol Neurosurg Psychiatry* 1999;60:655–60.
2337. Geschwind DH, Perlman S, Figueroa K et al. Spinocerebellar ataxia type 6. *Neurology* 1997;49:1247–51.
2338. Geschwind N. Disconnexion syndromes in animals and man. *Brain* 1965;88: 237–94.
2339. See 2338.
2340. Geschwind N. Derek Ernest Denny-Brown. *J Neurol Sci* 1982;53:137–9.
2341. Geschwind N,Galaburda AM. Cerebral lateralization: Biological mechanisms, associations, and pathology:1.A hypothesis and a program for research. *Arch Neurol* 1985;42:428, 521, 63–459, 552, 65.
2342. Geschwind N, Sherwin I. Language-induced epilepsy. *Arch Neurol* 1967;16:25–31.
2343. Geyelin HR, Penfield W. Cerebral calcification and epilepsy. *Arch Neurol Psychiatry* 1929;21:1020–43.
2344. Geyer JD, Payne TA, Drury I. The value of pelvic thrusting in the diagnosis of seizures and pseudoseizures. *Neurology* 2000;54:227–9.
2345. Gfeller JD, Chibnall JT, Duckro JN. Postconcussion symptoms and cognitive functioning in posttraumatic headache patients. *Headache* 1994;34:503–7.
2346. Ghadimi H, Bimington VI, Pecora F. Hyperlysinemia associated with retardation. *N Engl J Med* 1965;273: 723–9.
2347. Gherardi R, Chretien F, Delfau-Larue M-H et al. Neuropathy in diffuse infiltrative lymphocytosis syndrome. *Neurology* 1998;50:1041–4.
2348. Ghezzi A, Zaffaroni M. Neurological manifestations of gastrointestinal disorders with particular reference to the differential diagnosis of multiple sclerosis. *Neurol Sci* 2001;22:S117–S122.
2349. Ghika-Schmid F, Nater B. Anomia for people's names, a restricted form of transient epileptic amnesia. *Eur J Neurol* 2003;10:651–4.
2350. Ghika-Schmid F, Bogousslavsky J. The acute behavioral syndrome of anterior thalamic infarction: A prospective study of 12 cases. *Ann Neurol* 2000;48:220–7.
2351. Ghosh D, Mohanty GPS. Ictal deafness – a report of three cases. *Seizure* 2001;10: 130–3.
2352. See 2353.
2353. Giacino JT, Ashwal S, Chinnery PF et al. The minimally conscious state. *Neurology* 2002;58:349–53.
2354. Giacino JT, Kezmarsky MA, DeLuca J et al. Monitoring rate of recovery to predict outcome in minimally-responsive patients. *Arch Phys Med Rehab* 1991;72:897–901.
2355. Gibb WRG. Neuropathology in movement disorders. *J Neurol Neurosurg Psychiatry* 1989;**Suppl.**:55–67.
2356. Gibb WRG, Esiri MM, Lees AJ. Clinical and pathological features of diffuse cortical Lewy Body disease (Lewy Body dementia). *Brain* 1987;110:1131–53.
2357. Gibb WRG, Lees A. The relevance of the Lewy body in the genesis of idiopathic Parkinson's disease. *J Neurol Neurosurg Psychiatr* 1998;51:745–52.
2358. Gibb WRG, Lees AJ. The clinical phenomenon of akathisia. *J Neurol Neurosurg Psychiatry* 1986;49:861–6.
2359. Gibb WRG, Luthert PJ, Janota I, Lantos PL. Cortical Lewy body dementia: Clinical features and classification. *J Neurol Neurosurg Psychiatry* 1989;52:185–92.
2360. Gibb WRG, Mountjoy CQ, Mann DMA, Lees AJ. A pathological study of the association between Lewy body disease and Alzheimer's disease. *J Neurol Neurosurg Psychiatry* 1989;52:701–8.
2361. Gibb WRG, Narabayashi H, Yokochi M et al. New pathologic observations in juvenile onset parkinsonism with dystonia. *Neurology* 1991;41:820–2.
2362. Gibberd FB, Gavrilescu K. A familial neuropathy associated with a paraprotein in serum, CSF and urine. *Neurology* 1966;16:130–44.
2363. Gibbon NO. Nomenclature of neurogenic bladder. *Urology* 1976;8:423–31.
2364. Gibbons A. The Chinese paralytic syndrome. *Science* 1991;253:26.
2365. Gibbons CH. Delayed orthostatic hypotension. *Neurology* 2006;67:28–32.
2366. Gibbons CH, Illigens BMW, Centi J et al. QDIRT. *Neurology* 2008;70:2299–304.
2367. Gibbs FA, Davis H, Lennox WG. The electroencephalagram in epilepsy and in conditions of impaired consciousness. *Arch Neurol Psychiatry* 1935;34:1133.
2368. Gibbs RC, Frank SB. Keratoma hereditaria mutilans (Vohwinkel syndrome). *Arch Derm* 1966;94:619.
2369. Gibson T, Noris W. Skin fragments removed by injection needles. *Lancet* 1958;2:983.
2370. Gieron MA, Korthais JK, Koussett BG. Facioscapulohumeral dystrophy with cochlear hearing loss and tortuosity of the retinal veins. *Am J Med Genet* 1985;22:143–7.
2371. Giladi N, Turezkite T, Harel D. Myelopathy as a complication of diabetes mellitus. *Israeli Journal of Medical Sciences* 1991;27:316–9.
2372. Gilbert GJ. Ménière's syndrome and cluster headache. Recurrent paroxysmal focal vasodilatation. *JAMA* 1965;191:691–4.

2373. Gilbert GJ. Lightning-induced robotic speech. *Neurology* 1994;44:991.

2374. Gilbert GJ, McEntee WJ, Glaser GH. Familial myoclonus and ataxia: Pathophysiologic implications. *Neurology* 1963;13:365.

2375. Gilbert JG, Levee RF. Patterns of declining memory. *J Gerontol* 1971;26:70.

2376. Gilchrist JM, Ambler MW, Agatiello P. Steroid-responsive tubular aggregate myopathy. *Muscle Nerve* 1991;14:233–6.

2377. Gilchrist JM, Leschner RT. Humeroperoneal myopathy. *Arch Neurol* 1986;43:734–5.

2378. Gilden DH, Beinlich BR, Rubinstein EM et al. Varicella-zoster virus myelitis. *Neurology* 1994;44:1818–23.

2379. Gilden DH, Dueland AN, Cohrs R et al. Preherpetic neuralgia. *Neurology* 1991;41:1215–8.

2380. Gillepsy T3, Gillespy T JR, Revak C. Progressive senile scoliosis: Seven cases of increasing spinal curves in elderly patients. *Skeletal Radiol* 1985;13:280–6.

2381. Gilles FH, Averil DR, Kerr CS. Neonatal endotoxin encephalopathy. *Ann Neurol* 1977;2:49–56.

2382. Gillespie FD. Aniridia, cerebellar ataxia and oligophrenia in siblings. *Arch Ophthalmol* 1965;73:338–41.

2383. Gilliam F, Steinhoff BJ, Bitterman HJ et al. Adult myoclonic epilepsy: A distinct syndrome of idiopathic generalized epilepsy. *Neurology* 2000;55:1030–3.

2384. Gilliam F,Wyllie E. Ictal amaurosis: MRI, EEG and clinical features. *Neurology* 1995;45:1619–21.

2385. Gilman S, Horenstein S. Familial amyotrophic dystonic paraplegia. *Brain* 1964;87:51–66.

2386. Gilman S, Little R, Johanns J et al. Evolution of sporadic olivopontocerebellar atrophy into multiple system atrophy. *Neurology* 2000;55:527–32.

2387. Gilman S, Low P, Quinn NP. Consensus statement on the diagnosis of multiple system atrophy. *J Neurol Sci* 1999;163: 94–8.

2388. Gilman S, Low PA, Quinn NP et al. Consensus statement on the diagnosis of multiple system atrophy. *J Aut Nerv Syst* 1998;74:189–92.

2389. Ginsberg L, DiFerrante DT, Caskey CT et al. Glucosamine-6-SO_4 sulfatase deficiency: A new mucopolysaccharidosis. *Clin Res* 1977;25:471a.

2390. Ginsberg L, Malik O, Kenton AR et al. Coexistent hereditary and inflammatory neuropathy. *Brain* 2004;127:193–202.

2391. Giraud P, Thobois S, Hermier M et al. Intravenous hypertrophic Paccioni granulations: Differentiation from venous dural thrombosis. *J Neurol Neurosurg Psychiatry* 2001;70:700–1.

2392. Gironi M, Lamperti C, Nemni R et al. Late onset cerebellar ataxia with hypogonadism and muscle coenzyme Q10, deficiency. *Neurology* 2004;62: 818–20.

2393. Giroud M, Creisson E, Fayolle H et al. Homolateral ataxia and crural paresis: A crossed cerebral-cerebellar diaschisis. *Journal of Neurology, Neurosurgery and Psychiatry* 1994;57:221–2.

2394. Giroux JM, Barbeau A. Erythrokeratodemia with ataxia. *Arch Derm* 1972;106:183–8.

2395. Gisselin S, Kyle RA, Dyck PJ. Neuropathy associated with monoclonal gammopathy of undetermined significance. *Ann Neurol* 1991;30:54–61.

2396. Gittinger JW JR. Functional hemianopsia: A historical perspective. *Surv Ophthalmol* 1988;32:427–32.

2397. Gitzelmann R. Deficiency of erythrocyte galactokinase in a patient with galactose diabetes. *Lancet* 1965;2:670.

2398. Giurgea CE. The nootropic concept - twenty years on. *Proc Third Congress, International Psychogeriatric Association,* 1987 #369. (Abstract)

2399. Gladstone RM. Development and significance of heterochromia iridis. *Arch Neurol* 1969;21:184–92.

2400. Glaser JS. *Clinical Neuroophthalmology*. Philadelphia, PA.: Lippincott, 1990.

2401. Glaser JS, Savino PJ, Sumers KD et al. The photostress recovery test in the clinical assessment of visual function. *Am J Ophthalmol* 1977;83:255–60.

2402. Glasgow BJ, Brown HH, Hannah JB et al. Ocular pathologic findings in neonatal adrenoleukodystrophy. *Ophthalmology* 1987;94:1054–60.

2403. Glass GA, Ahlskog JE, Matsumoto J. Orthostatic myoclonus. *Neurology* 2007;68:1826–30.

2404. Glass J, Hochberb FH, Miller DC. Intravascular lymphomatosis: A systemic disease with neurologic manifestations. *Cancer* 1993;71:3156–64.

2405. Glass JD, Levey AI, Rothstein JD. The Dysarthria-Clumsy hand syndrome: A distinct entity related to pontine infarction. *Arch Neurol* 1990;27:487–94.

2406. Glass-Marmor L, Paperna T, Ben-Yosef Y, Miller A. Chronotherapy using corticosteroids for multiple sclerosis relapses. *J Neurol Neurosurg Psychiatry* 2007;78:886–8.

2407. Glew RH, Basu A, Prence EM, Remaley AT. Lysosomal storage diseases. *Lab Invest* 1985;53:250–69.

2408. Glick B, Shapira Y, Stein A et al. Congenital fiber type disproportion. *Ann Neurol* 1984;16:405–6.

2409. Gloor P. Consciousness. *Epilepsia* 1986;27 **(Suppl. 2)**:S14–S26.

2410. Goadsby P. Turtle headaches. *Neurology* 2003;60:905–9.

2411. Goadsby P. Migraine, allodynia, sensitization and all of that. *Europ Neurol* 2005;53:10–6.

2412. Goadsby P. Trigeminal autonomic cephalalgias. *J Neurol Neurosurg Psychiatr* 2005;76:301–5.

2413. Goadsby PJ. Paratrigeminal paralysis of the oculopupillary sympathetic system. *J Neurol Neurosurg Psychiatry* 2002;72:297–9.

2414. Goadsby PJ, Lance JW. Clinicopathological correlation in a case of painful ophthalmoplegia: Tolosa-Hunt syndrome. *J Neurol Neurosurg Psychiatry* 1989;52:1290–3.

2415. Goadsby PJ, Lipton RB. A review of paroxysmal hemicranias, SUNCT syndrome and other short-lasting headaches with autonomic features. *Brain* 1997;120:–193.

2416. Goadsby PJ, Lipton RB. A review of paroxysmal hemicranias, SUNCT syndrome and other short-lasting headaches with autonomic features, including new cases. *Brain* 1999;120:193–209.

2417. Goadsby PJ, Schoenen J, Ferrari MD et al. Towards a definition of intractable headache for use in clinical practice and trials. *Cephalalgia* 2008;26:1168–70.

2418. Goadsby P. *Acta Neurol Psychiat Belg* 2001;101:10–9.

2419. Godtfredsen E. Ophthalmological and neurological symptoms in malignant naso-pharyngeal tumors. *Acta Path Microbiol Scand* 1944;**(Suppl. 55)**: 120–85.

2420. Godtfredsen E. Ophthalmoneurological symptoms in malignant naso-pharyngeal tumors. *Brit J Ophth* 1947;31:78–100.

2421. Godwin-Austen RB, Robinson A, Evans K, Lascelles PT. An unusual neurological disorder of copper metabolism clinically resembling Wilson's disease but biochemically a distinct entity. *J Neurol Sci* 1978;39:85–98.

2422. Goebel HH. Desmin-related neuromuscular disorders. *Muscle Nerve* 1995;18:1306–20.

2423. Goebel HH. Congenital myopathies. *Seminars in Pediatric Neurology* 1996;3:152–61.

2424. Goebel HH. Congenital myopathies at their molecular dawning. *Muscle & Nerve* 2003;27:527–48.

2425. Goebel HH et al. Subacute necrotizing encephalomyelopathy (Leigh's disease). *Muscle Nerve* 1986;9:1657.

2426. Goebel HH, Heipertz R, Scholz W et al. Juvenile Huntington's chorea: Clinical ultrastructural and biochemical studies. *Neurol Minneap* 1978;28:23–31.

2427. Goebel HH, Lenard HG, Langenbeck U et al. A form of congenital muscular dystrophy. *Brain Dev* 1980;2:387–400.
2428. Goebel HH, Muller J, DeMyer W. Myopathy associated with Marfan syndrome. *Neurology* 1973;23:1257–68.
2429. Goeminne F. A new, probably X-linked syndrome; congenital muscular torticollis, multiple keloids, cryptorchidism and renal dysplasia. *Acta Genet (Roma)* 1968;17:439.
2430. Goetz CG. *Charcot the Clinician*. New York: Raven Press, 1987.
2431. Goetz CG, Fahn S, Martinez-Martin P et al. Movement Disorder Society-sponsored revision of the Unified Parkinson's Disease Rating Scale (MDS-UPDRS): Process, format, and clinimetric testing plan. *Mov Disord* 2007;22:41–7.
2432. Goetz CG, Tanner CM, Wilson RS et al. Tourette rating scale. *Neurology* 1987;37:1542–4.
2433. Golabi M, Rosen L. A new X-linked mental retardation-overgrowth syndrome. *Am J Med Genet* 1984;17:345–58.
2434. Golbe LI. Young-onset Parkinson's disease: A clinical review. *Neurology* 1991;41:168–73.
2435. Golbe LI, Lazzarini AM, Schwarz KO et al. Autosomal dominant parkinsonism with benign course and typical Lewy-body pathology. *Neurology* 1993;43:2222–7.
2436 Golbe LI, Ohman-Strickland PA. A clinical rating scale for progressive supranuclear palsy. *Brain* 2007;130:1552–65.
2437. Gold K, Rabins PV. Isolated visual hallucinations and the Charles Bonnet syndrome. *Compr Psychiatr* 1989;30:90–8.
2438. Gold M, Shuren J, Heilman KM. Proximal intentional neglect: A case study. *J Neurol Neurosurg Psychiatry* 1994;57:1395–400.
2439. Goldberg G. Supplementary motor area structure and function: Review and hypotheses. *Behav Brain Sci* 1985;8: 567–615.
2440. Goldberg MF, Cotlier E, Fichenscher LG et al. Macular cherry-red spot, corneal clouding and B-galactosidase deficiency. *Arch Int Med* 1971;128:387–98.
2441. Golden JA. Holoprosencephaly: A defect in brain patterning. *J Neuropath Exp Neurol* 1998;57:991–9.
2442. Golden CJ. A standardized version of Luria's neuropsychological tests. In Filskov S, Boll TJ, eds. *Handbook of Clinical Neuropsychology*, New York: Wiley-Interscience, 1981.
2443. Golden GM. Tics and Tourettes: A continuum of symptoms. *Ann Neurol* 1978;4:145–8.
2444. Golden GS. Stroke Syndromes in childhood. *Neurol Clin* 1985;3:59–75.
2445. Goldenhar M. Associations malformatives de l'oeil et de l'oreille, en particulier le syndrome dermoide epibulbaire-appendices auriculaires-fistula auris congenita et ses relations avec la dysostose mandibulo-faciale. *J Genet Hum* 1952;1:243–83.
2446. Goldfarb LG, Vicart P, Goebel HH et al. Desmin myopathy. *Brain* 2004;127:723–34.
2447. Goldfield M, Sussman O. The 1959 outbreak of eastern encephalitis in New Jersey. 1. Introduction and description of outbreak. *Am J Epidem* 1968;87:1–10.
2448. Goldfischer SL, Collins J, Rapin I et al. Pseudo-Zellweger syndrome: Deficiencies in several peroxisomal oxidative activities. *J Pediatr* 1986;108:25–32.
2449. Goldhammer Y, Lawton Smith J. Acquired intermittent Brown's syndrome. *Neurology* 1974;24:666–8.
2450. Goldhammer Y, Smith JL. Optic nerve anomalies in basal encephalocele. *Arch Ophthalmol* 1975;93:115–8.
2451. Goldie WD, Holtzman D, Suzuki K. Chronic hexosaminidase A and B deficiency. *Ann Neurol* 1977;2:156–8.
2452. Goldman RL. Gliomyosarcoma of the cerebrum. *Am J Clin Path* 1969;52:741–4.
2453. Goldstein K. Acute cerebellitis. *Munch Med Wschr* 1915;92:1439–42.
2454. Goldstein K. Account of the symptoms and lesions of the cerebellum. *Arch Psychiat Nervenkr* 1916;56:466–521.
2455. Goldstein K. *Language and Language Disturbances*. New York: Grune and Stratton, 1948.
2456. Goldstein LB, Bertels C, Davis JN. Interrater reliability of the NIH stroke scale. *Arch Neurol* 1989;46:660–2.
2457. Gollin ES. Developmental studies of visual recognition of incomplete objects. *Percept Mot Skills* 1960;11:289.
2458. Goltz RW. Focal dermal hypoplasia. *Arch Derm* 1962;86:708–17.
2459. Gomez CR, Gomez SM, Selhorst JB. Acute thalamic esotropia. *Neurology* 1988;38:1759.
2460. Gomez MR. *Tuberous Sclerosis*. New York: Raven Press, 1979.
2461. Gomez MR, Clermont V, Bernstein J. Progressive bulbar paralysis in childhood. *Arch Neurol* 1962;6:317–23.
2462. Gomez MR, Klass DW. Epilepsies of infancy and childhood. *Ann Neurol* 1983;13:113–24.
2463. Gomez-Aranda F, Canadillas F, Marti-Masso JF et al. Pseudomigraine with temporary neurological symptoms and lymphocytic pleocytosis. *A Report of 50 cases. 120* 1997;7:1113.
2464. Gommans IMP, Davis M, Saar K et al. A locus on chromosome 15q for a dominantly inherited nemaline myopathy with core-like lesions. *Brain* 2003;126:1545–51.
2465. Gomori AJ, Partnow AJ, Houroupian DS et al. Ataxic form of Creutzfeldt-Jakob disease. *Arch Neurol* 1973;29:318–23.
2466. Gonce M, Delwaide PJ. Exteroceptive reflex myoclonus: Clinical and electrophysiological study. *J Neurol Neurosurg Psychiatry* 1986;49:1195–8.
2467. Gondim FA, Thomas FP, Oliveira GR et al. Fou rire prodromique and history of pathological laughter in the XIXth and XXth centuries. *Rev Neurol (Paris)* 2004;160:277–83.
2468. Gondim FAA, Brannagan THI, Sander HT et al. Peripheral neuropathy in patients with inflammatory bowel disease. *Brain* 2007;128:867–79.
2469. Gonzalez J, Lacomis D, Kramer DJ. Mushroom myopathy. *Muscle Nerve* 1996;19:790–2.
2470. Gooddy W. On the nature of pain. *Brain* 1957;80:118–31.
2471. Gooddy W, Reinhold M. The function of the cerebral cortex. *Brain* 1954;77:416–26.
2472. Goodenough DJ, Fariello RG, Annis BL et al. Familial and acquired paroxysmal dyskinesias. A proposed classification with delineation of clinical features. *Arch Neurol* 1978;35:827–31.
2473. Goodglass H, Berko J. Agrammatism and inflectional morphology in English. *J Speech Hear Res* 1960;3:257–67.
2474. Goodglass H, Kaplan E. *The Assessment of Aphasia and Related Disorders*. Philadelphia: Lea & Febiger, 1972.
2475. Goodglass H, Kaplan E. *The Assessment of Aphasia and Related Disorders*. Philadelphia: Lea & Febiger, 1983.
2476. Goodin DS, Squires KC, Henderson BH et al. Age-related variations in evoked potentials to auditory stimuli in normal human subjects. *EEG Clin Neurophysiol* 1978;44:447–58.
2477. Goodkin DE, Hertsgaard D, Seminary J. Upper extremity function in multiple sclerosis: Improving assessment sensitivity with box and block and nine-hole peg tests. *Arch Phys Med Rehab* 1988;69:850–4.
2478. Goodman BW. Temporal arteritis. *AmerJ Med* 1979;77:839–52.
2479. Goodman G, Ripps H, Siegal IM. Cone dysfunction syndromes. *Arch Ophthalmol* 1963;70:214.
2480. Goodman RM et al. Camptodactyly: Occurrence in two new genetic syndromes and its relationship to other syndromes. *J Med Genet* 1972;9:203–12.
2481. Goodman RM, Lockareff S, Gwinup G. Hereditary congenital deafness with onychodystrophy. *Arch Otolaryngol* 1969;90:474.

2482. Goodman SI, Mace JW, Pollak S. Serum gamma-glutamyl transpeptidase deficiency. *Lancet* 1971;1:234.

2483. Goodwin JA, Kansu T. Vulpian's sign: Conjugate eye deviation in acute cerebral hemisphere lesions. *Neurology* 1986;**36**:711–2.

2484. Goonetilleke A, Harris JB. Envenomation and consumption of poisonous seafood. *J Neurol Neurosurg Psychiatry* 2003;**73**: 103–9.

2485. Gopalan C. The "burning feet" syndrome. *Indian Med Gaz* 1946;**81**:22–6.

2486. Gordon A. A new reflex: Paradoxic flexor reflex. Its diagnostic value. *Amer Med* 1904;8:971.

2487. Gordon A. Paradoxical flexor reflexes and their relationship with the knee jerk and the Babinski response. *Rev Neurol* 1904;**21**:1083.

2488. Gordon AM, Capute AJ, Konigsmark BW. Progressive quadriparesis, mental retardation, retinitis pigmentosa and hearing loss – report of 2 sibs. *Johns Hopkins Med J* 1976;**138**:142–5.

2489. Gordon AM, Capute AJ, Konigsmark BW. Progressive quadriparesis, mental retardation, retinitis pigmentosa and hearing loss – report of 2 sibs. *John Hopkins Hosp Bull* 1976;138:142–5.

2490. Gordon KE, Masotti RE, Waddell WR. Tremorgenic encephalopathy: A role of mycotoxins in the production of CNS disease in humans? *Can J Neurol Sci* 1993;**20**:237–9.

2491. Gordon NS, Marsden HB, Noronha MJ. Neuronal ceroid lipofuscinosis (Batten's disease). *Arch Dis Child* 1972;**47**:285–91.

2492. Gordon PH, Cheng B, Katz IB et al. The natural history of primary lateral sclerosis. *Neurology* 2006;**66**:647–53.

2493. Gorelick PB, Rosenberg M, Pagano RJ. Enhanced ptosis in myasthenia gravis. *Arch Neurol* 1981;**38**:531.

2494. Gorelick PB, Sullivan M, Lansky L. Cerebral auscultation. *Neurology* 1987;**37**:1523–4.

2495. Gorelick PB, Zych D. Corning, James Leonard and the early history of spinal puncture. *Neurology* 1987;**37**:672–4.

2496. Goren H, Steinberg MC, Farbourg GH. Familial oculoleptomeningeal amyloidosis. *Brain* 1980;**103**:473–8.

2497. Gorham DR. A proverbs test for clinical and experimental use. *Psychol Rep* 1956;1:1.

2498. Gorlin RJ. Some facial syndromes. *Birth Defects Orig Artic Ser* 1969;5:65–76.

2499. Gorlin RJ, Chaudhry AP, Moss ML. Craniofacial dysostosis, patent ductus arteriosus, hypertrichosis hypoplasia of labia majora, dental and eye anomalies, a new syndrome? *J Pediatr* 1960;**56**: 778–85.

2500. Gorlin RJ, Cohen MM JR. Frontometaphyseal dysplasia: A new syndrome. *Am J Dis Childh* 1969;**118**:487–94.

2501. Gorlin RJ et al. Genetic craniotubular bone dysplasias and hyperostoses: A critical analysis. *Birth Defects Orig Artic Ser* 1969;5:79–95.

2502. Gorlin RJ et al. Multiple lentigines syndrome, complex comprising multiple lentigines, electrocardiographic conduction abnormalities, ocular hypertelorism, pulmonary stenosis, abnormalities of genitalia, retardation of growth, sensorineural deafness, and autosomal dominant hereditary pattern. *Am J Dis Childh* 1969;117:652–62.

2503. Gorlin RJ, Jue R, Jacobsen K et al. Oculoauriculovertebral dysplasia. *J Pediatr* 1963;63:991–9.

2504. Gorlin RJ, Pindborg JJ, Cohen MM JR. *Syndromes of the Head and Neck*. New York: McGraw-Hill Book Co., 1976.

2505. Gorlin RJ, Psaume J. Orodigitofacial dysostosis – a new syndrome. *J Pediatr* 1962;61:250.

2506. Gorlin RJ, Sedano H, Anderson VE. The syndrome of palmaro-plantar hyperkeratosis and premature periodontal destruction of the teeth, a clinical and genetic analysis of the Papillon-Lefevre syndrome. *J Pediatr* 1964;**65**:895–908.

2507. Gorlin RJ, Sedano HO. Multiple nevoid basal cell carcinoma syndrome. In Vincken PJ, Bruyn GW, eds. *Handbook of Clinical Neurology*, pp 455–73. Amsterdam: North Holland Publishing, 1972.

2508. Gorlin RJ, Vickers RA, Kelln E et al. The multiple basal cell Nevi syndrome. *Cancer* 1965;18:89.

2509. Gormley JB. Treatment of postspinal headache. *Anesthesiology* 1960;**21**:565–6.

2510. Gormley RK. Low back pain with special reference to the articular facets with presentation of an operative procedure. *Coll Papers Mayo Clinic* 1933;25:813–23.

2511. Gorospe JR, Singhal BS, Kainu T et al. Indian Agarwal megalencephalic leukodystrophy with cysts is caused by a common *MLC1* mutation. *Neurology* 2004;62:878–82.

2512. Gorson KC, Hermann DN, Thiagarajan R et al. Non-length dependent small fiber neuropathy/ganglionopathy. *J Neurol Neurosurg Psychiatr* 2008;79:163–9.

2513. Gorson KC, Ropper AH, Adelmann LS et al. Chronic motor axonal neuropathy: Pathological evidence of inflammatory polyradiculoneuropathy. *Muscle Nerve* 1999;22:266–270.

2514. Gospe SM, Lazaro RP, Lava NS et al. Familial X-linked myalgia and cramps. *Neurology* 1989;**39**:1277–80.

2515. Gospe S JR, Lazaro RP, Lava NS et al. Familial X-linked myalgia and cramps: A nonprogressive myopathy associated with a deletion in the dystrophin gene. *Neurology* 1989;**39**:1277–80.

2516. Gotham JE, Wein H, Meyer JS. Clinical studies of neuropathy due to macroglobulinemia (Waldenstrom's syndrome). *Can Med Assn J* 1963;89:806.

2517. Goto I, Kanazawa Y, Kobagashi T et al. Oculopharyngeal myopathy with distal and cardiomyopathy. *J Neurol Neurosurg Psychiatry* 1977;**40**:600–7.

2518. Goto I, Nakai H, Tabira T et al. Juvenile neurogenic muscular atrophy with lysosomal deficiencies: A new variant or a variant of mucopolysaccharidosis? *J Neurol* 1983;**229**:45–54.

2519. Gotschall C. The functional capacity index, second revision: Morbidity in the first year post injury. *Int J Inj Contr Saf Promot* 2005;12:254–6.

2520. Gotto AJ, Sanford I. Risks and benefits of continued aggressive statin therapy. *Clin Cardiol* 2003;**26**:11–2.

2521. Gottschaldt K. Uber den Einfluss, Der Erfahrung auf Die Wahrnehmung Von Figuren. *Psychol Forsch* 1928;8:18–317.

2522. Gouider R, LeGuern E, Emile J et al. Hereditary neuralgic amyotrophy and hereditary neuropathy with liability to pressure palsies. *Neurology* 1994;**44**: 2250–2.

2523. Gouider-Khouja N, Ben Youssef-Turki I. Type I glutaric aciduria: An unrecognized cause of progressive dystonia. *Rev Neurol (Paris)* 2006;162:858–61.

2524. Gourie-Devi M, Suresh TG, Shankar SK. Monomelic amyotrophy. *Arch Neurol* 1984;**41**:388–94.

2525. Goutieres F, Aicardi J, Farakas E. Anterior horn cell disease associated with pontocerebellar hypoplasia in infants. *J Neurol Neurosurg Psychiatry* 1977;**40**: 370–8.

2526. Goutieres F, Bogicevic D, Aicardi J. A predominantly cervical form of spinal muscular atrophy. *J Neurol Neurosurg Psychiatry* 1991;**54**:223–5.

2527. Gouw LG, Digre KB, Harris CP et al. Autosomal dominant cerebellar ataxia with retinal degeneration. *Neurology* 1994;44:1441–7.

2528. Gowers WG. *The Border-Land of Epilepsy*. London: Churchill, 1907.

2529. Gowers WR. On saltatoric spasm. *Lancet* 1877;2:42– 45 and152–155.

2530. Gowers WR. *Epilepsy and other Chronic Convulsive Diseases*. London: J&A Churchill, 1881.

2531. Gowers WR. *A Manual of Diseases of the Nervous System*. Philadelphia: Blakiston, 1888.

2532. Gowers WR. Myopathy of a distal form. *Brit Med J* 1902;2:89–92.

2533. Gowers WR. Vasovagal attacks. *Lancet* 1907;1:1551.
2534. Gowland C, Stratford P, Ward M et al. Measuring physical impairment and disability with the Chedoke-McMaster stroke assessment. *Stroke* 1993;24:58–63.
2535. Goyal RK, Hirano I. The enteric nervous system. *N Engl J Med* 1996;334:1106–15.
2536. Goyer RA, Reynolds J, Burke J et al. Hereditary renal disease with neurosensory hearing loss, prolinuria and ichthyosis. *American Journal of Medical Science* 1968;256:166–79.
2537. Graaf AS et al. An early-onset recessive cerebellar disorder with distal amyotrophy and, in two patients, gross myoclonia: A probable ataxia telangiectasia variant. *Clin Neurol Neurosurg* 1995;97:1–7.
2538. Grabow JD, Chou SM. Thyrotropic hormone deficiency with polyneuropathy. *Arch Neurol* 1968;19:284–91.
2539. Gradenigo G. Sulla leptomeningite circonscritta e sulla paralisi dell'abducente di origine attica. *Gior Acad Med Torino* 1904;4:59–84.
2540. Graefe Av. Ueber Basedow'sche Krankheit. *Dtsch Klinik* 1864;16:158–9.
2541. Graf CJ. Spontaneous carotid-cavernous fistula. *Arch Neurol* 1965;13:662–72.
2542. Graff-Radford NR. A recessively-inherited ataxia with episodes of dystonia. *J Neurol Neurosurg Psychiatry* 1986;49:591–4.
2543. Graff-Radford NR, Tranel D, Van Hoesen GW et al. Diencephalic amnesia. *Brain* 1990;113:1–25.
2544. Graham FK, Kendall BS. Memory for designs test: Revised general manual. *Percept Mot Skills* 1960;11:147–88.
2545. Graham J, Greenwood R, Lecky B. Cortical deafness: A case report and review of the literature. *J Neurol Sci* 1980;48:35–49.
2546. Graham K, Paterson K Hodges JR. Progressive pure anomia: Insufficient activation of phonology by meaning. *Neurocase* 1995;1:25–38.
2547. Graham RC, Hughes R. A modified peripheral neuropathy scale: The overall neuropathy limitations scale. *J Neurol Neurosurg Psychiatr* 2006;77:973–6.
2548. Grand MG, Kaine J, Fulling K et al. Cerebroretinal vasculopathy: A new hereditary syndrome. *Ophthalmology* 1988;95:649–59.
2549. Grandas F, Elston J, Quinn NP. Blepharospasm: A review of 264 patients. *J Neurol Neurosurg Psychiatry* 1988;51:767–72.
2550. Grant AC, Hunter S, Partin WC. A case of acutre monocytic Ehrlicosis with prominent neurologic signs. *Neurology* 1997;48:1619–23.
2551. Grant DA, Berg EA. A behavioural analysis of degree of reinforcement and ease of shifting to new responses in a Weigl-type card sorting problem. *J Exper Psychol* 1948;38:404–11.
2552. Grant DA, Berg EA. *The Wisconsin Card Sort Test Random Layout: Directions for Administration and Scoring.* Madison,Wisconsin: Wells Printing Co. Inc., 1980.
2553. Graus F, Delattre J-Y, Antoine JC et al. Recommended diagnostic criteria for paraneoplastic neurological syndromes. *J Neurol Neurosurg Psychiatr* 2004;75:1135–40.
2554. Graus F et al. Neuronal antinuclear antibody in sensory neuropathy from lung cancer. *Neurology* 1985;35:538–43.
2555. Gray F, Eisenbaum JF, Gherardi R et al. Luyso-Pallido-Nigral atrophy and amyotrophic lateral sclerosis. *Acta Neuropathologica* 1985;66:78–82.
2556. Gray F, Louarn F, Gherardi R et al. Adult form of Leigh's disease: A clinicopathological study with CT scan examination. *J Neurol Neurosurg Psychiatry* 1984;47:1211–5.
2557. Green AJE, Thompson EJ, Stewart GE et al. Use of 14-3-3 and other brain-specific proteins in CSF in the diagnosis of variant Creutzfeldt-Jakob disease. *J Neurol Neurosurg Psychiatry* 2001;70:744–8.
2558. Green JB. Pilomotor seizures. *Neurology* 1984;34:837–9.
2559. Green JS, Parfrey PS, Harnett JD et al. The cardinal manifestations of Bardet-Biedl syndrome, a form of Laurence-Moon-Biedl syndrome. *N Engl J Med* 1989;321:1002–10.
2560. Greenberg R. Dream interruption insomnia. *J Nerv Ment Dis* 1967;144:18–21.
2561. Greene JDW. Apraxia, agnosias and higher visual function abnormalities. *Practical Neurol* 2005;76:v25–234.
2562. Greenfield ADM, Sheperd JT, Whelen RF. The part played by the nervous system in the response to cold of the circulation through the finger tip. *Clin Sci* 1951;10:347–60.
2563. Greenfield JG. A form of progressive cerebral sclerosis in infants associated with primary degeneration of the interfascicular glia. *J Neurol Psychopath* 1933;13:289–302.
2564. Greenfield JG. Encephalitis and encephalomyelitis in England and Wales during the last decade. *Brain* 1950;73:141–66.
2565. Greenfield JG. *The Spinocerebellar Degenerations*. Oxford: Oxford University Press, 1954.
2566. Greenfield JG, Matthews WB. Post-encephalitic parkinsonism with amyotrophy. *J Neurol Neurosurg Psychiatry* 1954;17:50–6.
2567. Greenfield JG, Turner JWA. Acute and subacute necrotic myelitis. *Brain* 1939;62:227–52.
2568. Greenhalgh J, Ford H, Long AF et al. The MS symptom and impact diary: Psychometric evaluation of a new instrument to measure the day-to-day impact of multiple sclerosis. *J Neurol Neurosurg Psychiatry* 2004;75:577–82.
2569. Greenhouse AH, Bicknell JM, Pesch RN et al. Myotonia, myokymia, hyperhidrosis and wasting of muscle. *Neurology* 1967;17:263–8.
2570. Greenwood RS, Nelson JS. Atypical neuronal ceroid lipofuscinosis. *Neurology* 1978;28:710–7.
2571. Greer HD, Massey EW. Neurologic injury from undersea diving. *Neurol Clin* 1992;10:1031–45.
2572. Gregg N. Congenital cataract following German measles in the mother. *Trans Ophthal Soc Aust* 1941;3:35.
2573. Greig DM. Hypertelorism, a hitherto undifferentiated congenital cranio-facial deformity. *Edinburgh Medical Journal* 1924;31:560–93.
2574. Gresty MA, Ell JJ, Findley LJ. Acquired pendular nystagmus: Its characteristics, localizing value and pathophysiology. *J Neurol Neurosurg Psychiatry* 1982;45:431.
2575. Gribaa M, Salih M, Anheim C. A new form of childhood onset, autosomal recessive spinocerebellar ataxia and epilepsy is localized at 16q21-q23. *Brain* 2007;130:1921–8.
2576. Gribbin B, Pickering TG, Sleight P et al. Effect of age and high blood pressure on baroreflex sensitivity in man. *Circ Resp* 1971;29:424–31.
2577. Griesinger W. Ueber Muskelhypertrophie. *Arch Heilk* 1865;6:1–13.
2578. Griffin JW, Goren E, Schaumberg HH et al. Adrenomyeloneuropathy: A probable variant of adrenoleukodystrophy. *Neurology* 1977;27:1107–13.
2579. Griffiths RA, Mortimer TF, Oppenheimer DR, Spalding JMK. Congophilic angiopathy of the brain: A clinical and pathological report on two siblings. *J Neurol Neurosurg Psychiatry* 1982;45:396–408.
2580. Griggs R, Vihola P, Hackman P et al. Zaspopathy in a large classic late-onset distal myopathy family. *Brain* 2007;130:1477–84.
2581. Griggs RC, Askanas V, DiMauro S et al. Inclusion body myositis and myopathies. *Ann Neurol* 1995;38:705–15.
2582. Griggs RC, Moxley RT, Lafrance RA et al. Hereditary paroxysmal ataxia: Response to acetazolamide. *Neurology* 1978;28:1259–64.
2583. Grimes DA. Tremor. *Can J Neurol Sci* 2003;30:S59–S63.

2584. Grisold W, Drlicek M. Paraneoplastic neuropathy. *Current Opinion in Neurology* 1999;12:617–25.

2585. Groenblad E. Angioid streaks – pseudoxanthoma elasticum. *Acta Ophth Kopenhagen* 1929;7:329.

2586. Grohmann K, Varon R, Stolz P et al. Infantile spinal muscular atrophy with respiratory distress type I. *Ann Neurol* 2003;54:719–24.

2587. Grompe M, St. Louis M, Demers SI et al. A single mutation of the fumarylacetoacetate hydrolase gene in French Canadians with hereditary tyrosinemia type 1. *N Engl J Med* 1994;331:353–7.

2588. Gronwall DMA. Paced auditory serial-addition task: A measure of recovery from concussion. *Percept Mot Skills* 1977;44:367–73.

2589. Grosberg BM, Solomon S, Friedman DI et al. Retinal migraine reappraised. *Cephalalgia* 2005;**26**:1275–86.

2590. Gross DW, Rajput AH, Yeung M. Distal hereditary upper limb muscular atrophy. *J Neurol Neurosurg Psychiatry* 1998;64: 217–20.

2591. Gross KB, Skrivanek JA, Carlson KC et al. Familial amyotrophic chorea with acanthocytosis: New clinical and laboratory investigations. *Arch Neurol* 1985;42:753–6.

2592. Gross MLP et al. Rejection encephalopathy. An acute neurological syndrome complicating renal transplantations. *J Neurol Sci* 1982;56: 23–34.

2593. Gross S, Fioravanti A, Biasi G et al. Linear scleroderma associated with progressive brain atrophy. *Brain Dev* 2003;**25**:57–61.

2594. Grove AS. Evaluation of exophthalmos. *N Engl J Med* 1975;**292**:1005.

2595. Grubb BP. Neurocardiogenic syncope. *N Engl J Med* 2008;**352**:1004–10.

2596. Grubb BP, Kosinski DJ, Boehm K et al. The postural orthostatic tachycardia syndrome: A neurocardiogenic variant identified during head-up tilt table testing. *Pacing Clin Electrophysiol* 1997;**20**:2205–12.

2597. Grubb B, Kosinski DJ, Boehm K, Kip K. The postural orthostatic tachycardia syndrome: A neurocardiogenic variant identified during head-up tilt table testing. *Pacing Clin Electrophysiol* 1997;**20**:2205–12.

2598. Gruber GB. Gruber syndrome. *Beitr Path Anat* 1934;93:459.

2599. Gruber R et al. Experiments with anti-siphon device in shunt therapy of pediatric hydrocephalus. *J Neurosurg* 1984;61: 156–62.

2600. Grunnett ML. Gomori's trichrome stain: Its use with myelin sheaths. *Arch Neurol* 1978;35:692.

2601. Grunnett ML, Bale JF. Brain abnormalities in infants with Potter syndrome (oligohydramnios tetrad). *Neurology* 1981;31:1571–4.

2602. Guarino JR. Auscultatory percussion of the head. *Brit Med J* 1982;**284**:1075–7.

2603. Guarnaschelli J. "Fallen fontanelle" (caida de mollera): A variant of the battered child syndrome. *JAMA* 1972;**222**:1545–6.

2604. Guazzi GC, D'Amore I, van Hoef F et al. Type III chronic GM1 gangliosidosis presenting as infantile choreo-athetosis and dementia without epilepsy in three sisters. *Neurology* 1988;**38**:1124–7.

2605. Guberman A. Clinical significance of the corneomandibular reflex. *Arch Neurol* 1982;39:578–80.

2606. Guberman A, Catching J. Swallow syncope. *Can J Neurol Sci* 1986;13:267–9.

2607. Gubermann A, Stuss D. The syndrome of bilateral paramedian infarction. *Neurology* 1983;33:540–6.

2608. Gubler AM. De l'hemiplégie alterne envisagee comme signe de lesion de la protuberance annulaire et comme preuve de la decussation des nerfs faciaux. *Gaz Hebd Med Chir* 1856;3:749–et.seq.

2609. Gudden BAL. Experimentaluntersuchungen uber das peripherische und central Nernensystem. *Arch Psychiat(Berlin)* 1870;2:693–723.

2610. Guerin JR. *Récherches sur les déformités congenitales chex les monstres.* Paris:48 v de Vauvigard. 1880.

2611. Guerreiro MM, Andermann E, Guerrini R et al. Familial perisylvian polymicrogyria: A new familial syndrome of cortical maldevelopment. *Ann Neurol* 2000;48:39–48.

2612. Guerrini R, Barkovich AJ, Sztriha L et al. Bilateral frontal polymicrogyria. *Neurology* 2000;54:909–13.

2613. Guerrini R, Bureau M, Mattei M-G et al. Trisomy 12p syndrome: A chromosomal disorder associated with generalized 3 Hz spike and wave discharges. *Epilepsia* 1990;31:557–66.

2614. Guerrini R, Dobyns WB. Bilateral periventricular nodular heterotopia with mental retardation and frontonasal malformation. *Neurology* 1998;51: 499–503.

2615. Guerrini R, Dravet C, Genton P et al. Epileptic negative myoclonus. *Neurology* 1993;43:1078–83.

2616. Guerrini R, Moro F, Kato M et al. Expansion of the first PolyA tract of ARX causes infantile spasms and status dystonicus. *Neurology* 2007;69: 427–33.

2617. Guggenheim MA, McCabe ERB, Rogi M et al. Glycerol kinase deficiency with neuromusculoskeletal and adrenal abnormalities. *Ann Neurol* 1980;7:441–9.

2618. Guignon G. L'oedème bleu des hysteriques. *Progr Med (Paris)* 1890;12:259–64.

2619. Guillain G. On a clinical form of syphilis affecting the neuraxis and lying between tabes, GPI and myelitis. *C R Soc Biol* 1905;63:49–51.

2620. Guillain G, Alajouanine R, Garcin R. Le syndrome paralytique unilateral global des nerfs craniens. *Bull Soc Hop Paris* 1926;50:456–60.

2621. Guillain G, Barre J, Strohl A. Sur un syndrome de radiculo–névrite avec hyperalbuminose du liquide cerebro–rachidien sans réaction cellulaire. Remarques sur les caractères cliniques et graphiques des réflexes tendineux. *Bull Soc Med Hop Paris* 1916;40:1462–70.

2622. Guillain G, Bertrand I, Lerebouillet J. Myoclonies arythmiques unilaterale des membres par lesion de noyau dentele du cervelet. *Rev Neurol* 1934;2:73–8.

2623. Guillain G, Mollaret P. Deux cas de myoclonies synchrones et rhythmées velo-pharyngo-laryngo-oculo-diaphragmatiques. *Rev Neurol* 1931;2:545–66.

2624. Guillamo J-S, Doz F, Delattre J-Y. Brain stem gliomas. *Current Opinion in Neurology* 2001;14:711–5.

2625. Guilleminault C. Narcolepsy 1985. *Sleep* 1986;9:99–291.

2626. Guilleminault C, Billiard M, Montplaisir J, Dement WC. Altered states of consciousness in disorders of daytime sleepiness. *J Neurol Sci* 1975;26: 377–93.

2627. Guilleminault C, Dement WC. 235 cases of excessive daytime sleepiness. *J Neurol Sci* 1977;31:13–27.

2628. Guilleminault C, Eldridge FL, Phillips JR et al. Two occult cases of insomnia and their therapeutic problems. *Arch Gen Psychiat* 1976;33:1241–5.

2629. Guilleminault C, Phillips R, Dement WC. A syndrome of hypersomnia with automatic behaviour. *EEG Clin Neurophysiol* 1975;38:403.

2630. Guilleminault C, Stoohs R, Quera-Salva M-A. Sleep-related obstructive and nonobstructive apneas and neurologic disorders. *Neurology* 1992;42 **(Suppl. 6)**:53–60.

2631. Guiloff RJ. Evidence for linkage of Type I hereditary motor and sensory neuropathy to the duffy locus on chromosome 1. *Ann Hum Genet* 1982;46:25–7.

2632. Guinter RH, Hernreid LS, Kaplan AM. Infantile neurogenic muscular atrophy with prolonged survival. *J Pediatr* 1977;90:95–7.

2633. Gulick EE. Model confirmation of the MS-related symptom checklist. *Nurs Res* 1989;38:147–53.

2634. Gull WW. Case of progressive atrophy of the muscles of the hands: Enlargement of the ventricle of the cord in the cervical region, with atrophy of the gray matter. *Guy's Hosp Rep* 1862;**8**:244–50.
2635. Gull WW. On a cretinoid state supervening in adult life in women. *Trans Clin Soc London* 1874;7:180–5.
2636. Gullstrand A. Om Braunlinier vid Astigmatism. *Nord Ophth Tidsskr Kjobenh* 1890;3:1–18.
2637. Gultekin SH, Rosenfeld MR, Voltz R et al. Paraneoplastic limbic encephalitis: Neurological symptoms, immunological findings and tumour association in 50 patients. *Brain* 2000;**123**:1481–94.
2638. Gumpert J, Hansotia P, Upton ARM. Gelastic epilepsy. *J Neurol Neurosurg Psychiatry* 1970;**33**:479–83.
2639. Gunderson CH, Lehmann CR, Sidell FR et al. Nerve agents: A review. *Neurology* 1992;**42**:946–50.
2640. Gunn RM. Congenital ptosis with peculiar associated movements of the affected lid. *Trans Ophthal Soc UK* 1883;3:283–7.
2641. Gur AY, Lampl Y, Gross B et al. A new scale for assessing patients with vertebrobasilar stroke – the Israel vertebrobasilar stroke scale. *Clin Neurol Neurosurg* 2007;**109**:317–22.
2642. Gurdjian ES. History of occlusive cerebrovascular disease. 1 from Wepfer to Moniz. *Arch Neurol* 1979;**36**:340–3.
2643. Gurel L, Linn MW, Linn BB. Physical and mental impairment-of-function in the aged the pamie scale. *J Gerontol* 1972;**27**:83–90.
2644. Gurland B, Golden RR, Teresi JA et al. The SHORT-CARE: An efficient instrument for the assessment of depression, dementia and disability. *J Gerontol* 1984;**39**:166–9.
2645. Gurland B, Kuriansky J, Sharpe L et al. The comprehensive assessment and referral evaluation (CARE). Rationale, development and reliability. *Int J Aging Hum Devel* 1977;**8**1:9–42.
2646. Gurney GE. Chronic bilateral benign hypertrophy of masseter muscles. *Amer J Surg* 1947;**73**:137–9.
2647. Gustafson L. Clinical classification of dementia conditions. *Acta Neurol Scand* 1992;(**Suppl. 139**):16–20.
2648. Gutmann L. Management of the quinizarine sweat test. *Postgrad Med J* 1947;**23**:332–6.
2649. Gutmann L. Facial and limb myokymia. *Muscle Nerve* 1991;**14**:1043–9.
2650. Gutmann L, Libell D, Gutmann L. When is myokymia neuromyotonia? *Muscle Nerve* 2001;**24**:151–3.
2651. Gutschalk A, Harting I, Cantz M et al. Adult α mannosidosis. *Neurology* 2004;**63**:1744–6.
2652. Guze BH, Baxter LR. Neuroleptic malignant syndrome. *N Engl J Med* 1985;**313**:163–6.
2653. Guzzetta F, Ferriere G, Lyon G. Congenital hypomyelination polyneuropathy. *Brain* 1982;**105**:395–416.
2654. Gwinn-Hardy K, Chen JY, Liu H-C et al. Spinocerebellar ataxia type 2 with parkinsonism in ethnic Chinese. *Neurology* 2000;**55**:800–5.
2655. Haan J, Roos RAC, Algra PR et al. Hereditary cerebral hemorrhage with amyloidosis – Dutch type. *Brain* 1990;**113**:1251–67.
2656. Haar F, Dyken P. Hereditary nonprogressive athetotic hemiplegia: A new syndrome. *Neurology* 1977;**27**:849–54.
2657. Haas DC. Chronic post-traumatic headaches classified and compared with natural headaches. *Cephalalgia* 1996;**16**:486–93.
2658. Haas DC, Lourie H. Delayed deterioration of consciousness after trivial head injury in childhood. *Brit Med J* 1984;**289**:1625.
2659. Haas RH, Robinson A, Evans K et al. An X-linked disease of the nervous system with disordered copper metabolism and features differing from Menkes disease. *Neurology* 1981;**31**:852–9.
2660. Habel A. Typus Edinburgensis? *Pediatrics* 1974;**53**:425–30.
2661. Haberland C, Perou J. Encephalocraniocutaneous lipomatosis. *Arch Neurol* 1970;**22**:144.
2662. Hachinski VC. Classification of stroke for clinical trials. *Stroke* 1990;21 (**Suppl II**):27–29.
2663. Hachinski VC, Iloff L, Zilkha K et al. Multi-infarct dementia. *Arch Neurol* 1975;**32**:632–7.
2664. Hachinski VC, Lassen N et al. Multi-infarct dementia. *Lancet* 1974;**2**:207–9.
2665. Hachinski VC, Potter P, Merskey H. Leuko-araiosis. *Arch Neurol* 1987;**44**: 21–3.
2666. Hackett PH, Rennie D. Acute mountain sickness. *Sem Resp Med* 1983;**5**:132–9.
2667. Hackett PH, Yarnell PR, Hill R. High altitude cerebral edema evaluated with magnetic resonance imaging: Clinical correlation and pathophysiology. *JAMA* 1998;**280**:1920–5.
2668. Haddock DRW, Ebrahim GJ, Kappur BB. Ataxic neurological syndrome found in Tanganyika. *Brit Med J* 1962;**2**: 1442–3.
2669. Hademenos GJ, Alberts MJ, Awad I et al. Advances in the genetics of cerebrovascular disease and stroke. *Neurology* 2001;**56**:997–1008.
2670. Hadjivassiliou M, Boscolo S, Davies-Jones DAB et al. The humoral response in the pathogenesis of gluten ataxia. *J Neurol Neurosurg Psychiatr* 2002;72:563.
2671. Hadjivassiliou M, Grunewald RA, Kandler RH et al. Neuropathy associated with gluten sensitivity. *J Neurol Neurosurg Psychiatry* 2006;**77**:1262–6.
2672. Hadjivassiliou M, Chattopadhyay AK, Grünewald RA et al. Myopathy associated with gluten sensitivity. *Muscle & Nerve* 2007;**35**:443–50.
2673. Haenel H. Ein neues Tabessymptom. *Neurol Zbl* 1909;**28**:1199.
2674. Haerer AF, Currier RD. Mirror movements. *Neurology* 1966;**16**:737–60.
2675. Haerer AF, Currier RD, Jackson JF. Hereditary nonprogressive chorea of early onset. *N Engl J Med* 1967;**276**:1220–4.
2676. Hagberg B, Aicardi J, Dias K, Ramos O. A progressive syndrome of autism, dementia ataxia and loss of purposeful hand use in girls: Rett's syndrome: Report of 35 cases. *Ann Neurol* 1983;**14**:471–9.
2677. Hagberg B, Sanner G, Steen G. The dyseqilibrium syndrome in cerebral palsy. *Acta Pediatr Scand* 1972;61 (**Suppl 226**):1–63.
2678. Hageman G, Ippel PF, te Nijenhuis FCAM. Autosomal dominant congenital Horner's syndrome in a Dutch family. *J Neurol Neurosurg Psychiatry* 1992;**55**: 28–30.
2679. Hageman G, Ramaekers V, Hilhorst BGJ et al. Congenital cervical spinal muscular atrophy: A non-familial, non-progressive condition of the upper limbs. *J Neurol Neurosurg Psychiatry* 1993;**56**:365–8.
2680. Hagemans MLC, Van Doorn PA, Winkel LPF et al et al. Clinical manifestation and natural course of late-onset Pompe's disease in 54 Dutch patients. *Brain* 2005;**128**:671–7.
2681. Hagerman RJ, Hagerman PJ. Fragile X-associated tremor/ataxia syndrome an aging face of the fragile X gene. *Arch Neurol* 2008;**65**:19–25.
2682. Haig AJ, Talley C, Grobler LJ et al. Paraspinal mapping: Quantified needle electromyography in lumbar radiculopathy. *Muscle Nerve* 1993;**16**: 477–84.
2683. Hainfellner JA, Schmidbauer M, Schmutzhard E et al. Devic's neuromyelitis optica and Schilder's myelinoclastic diffuse sclerosis. *J Neurol Neurosurg Psychiatry* 1992;**55**: 1194–6.
2684. Hajdu N, Kauntze R. Cranio-skeletal dysplasia. *Brit J Radiol* 1948;**21**:42–8.
2685. Haley EC JR, Brashear HR, Barth JT et al. Deep cerebral venous thrombosis. *Arch Neurol* 1989;**46**:337–40.
2686. Hall AJ. Encephalitis lethargica. *Lancet* 1923;**1**:731.
2687. Hall BD. Choanal atresia and associated multiple anomalies. *J Pediatr* 1979;**95**:395–8.

2688. Hall BM, Walsh JC, Horvath JS et al. Peripheral neuropathy complicating primary hyperoxaluria. *J Neurol Sci* 1976;29:343–9.
2689. Hall JAS. Diphtheritic pseudodotabes. *West Ind Med J* 1963;12:47.
2690. Hall JG, Pellester PD et al. Congenital hypothalamic hamartoblastoma, hypopituitarism, imperforate anus and post-axial polydactyly – a new syndrome? *Am J Med Genet* 1980;7:47–74.
2691. Hall JG, Reed SD, Scott CI et al. 3 distinct types of X-linked arthrogryposis seen in 6 families. *Clin Genet* 1982;21: 81–97.
2692. Hall M. On the reflex function of the medulla oblongata and medulla spinalis. *Phil Trans Roy Soc Lond* 1833;123:635–59.
2693. Hallermann W. Bird-like face and congenital cataract. *Klin Mbl Augenh* 1948;113:315–8.
2694. Hallervorden J, Spatz H. Einartige Erkrankung im extrapyramidalen System mit besonderer Beiteiligung im des Globus pallidus uind der Substantia nigra: Ein Beitrag zu den beziehungen zwischen diesen beiden Zentren. *ZN* 1922;79: 254–302.
2695. Hallett M. Myoclonus: Relation to epilepsy. *Epilepsia* 1985;26(**Suppl** 1):S67–S77.
2696. Hallett M. The pathophysiology of myoclonus. *Trends Neurosci* 1987;10: 69–73.
2697. Hallett M. NINDS Myotatic reflex scale. *Neurology* 1993;43:2923.
2698. Hallett M, Chadwick D, Marsden CD. Ballistic movement overflow myoclonus: A form of essential myoclonus. *Brain* 1977;100:299–312.
2699. Hallett M, Cogan DG. Episodic unilateral mydriasis in otherwise normal patients. *Arch Ophthalmol* 1970;84:130–6.
2700. Hallpike JF. Superior orbital fissure syndrome. *J Neurol Neurosurg Psychiatry* 1973;36:486–90.
2701. Halmagyi GM, Curthoys IS, Gresty MA et al. Hemi see-saw nystagmus due to unilateral diencephalic lesion. *Ann Neurol* 1987;(**Suppl.** 22):147.
2702. Halmagyi GM, Gresty MA, Gibson WPR. Ocular tilt reaction with peripheral vestibular lesion. *Ann Neurol* 1979;6:80–3.
2703. Halmagyi GM, Gresty MA, Leech J. Reversed optokinetic nystagmus (OKN): Mechanism and clinical significance. *Ann Neurol* 1980;7:429–35.
2704. Halmagyi GM, Rudge P, Gresty MA et al. Downbeating nystagmus: A review of 62 cases. *Arch Neurol* 1983;40:777–84.
2705. Halmagyi MB, Evans WA, Hallinan JM. Failure of downward gaze: The site and nature of the lesion. *Arch Neurol* 1978;35:22–6.
2706. Halperin JJ, Landis DMD, Kleinman GM. Whipple disease of the nervous system. *Neurology* 1982;32:612–7.
2707. Halperin JJ, Logigian EL, Finkel MF et al. Practice parameters for the diagnosis of patients with nervous system Lyme borreliosis (Lyme disease). *Neurology* 1996;46:619–27.
2708. Halpern L, Bental E. Epileptic cephalea. *Neurology* 1958;8:615–20.
2709. Halstead LS, Rossi CD. Post-polio syndrome: Clinical experience with 132 consecutive outpatients. In Halstead LS WD, ed. *Research and Clinical Aspects of the Late Effects of Poliomyelitis. Birth Defects Original Article Series*, pp 13–27. 1987.
2710. Halstead WC. *Brain and Intelligence.* Chicago: Univ. Chicago Press, 1947.
2711. Halstead WC, Wepman JM. The Halstead-Wepman aphasia screening test. *J Speech Hear Dis* 1959;14:9–15.
2712. Haltia M, Somer H, Palo J et al. Neuronal intranuclear inclusion disease in identical twins. *Ann Neurol* 1984;15:316–21.
2713. Haltia T, Palo J, Haltia M et al. Juvenile metachromatic leukodystrophy. *Arch Neurol* 1980;37:42–6.
2714. Hamida MB, Fardeau M, Attia N. Severe childhood muscular dystrophy affecting both sexes and frequent in Tunisia. *Muscle Nerve* 1983;6:469–72.
2715. Hamida MB, Hentati F, Hamida CB. Hereditary motor system diseases (chronic juvenile amyotrophic lateral sclerosis). *Brain* 1990;113:347–63.
2716. Hamilton M. A rating scale for depression. *J Neurol Neurosurg Psychiatry* 1960;23:56–62.
2717. Hamilton M. Development of a rating scale for primary depressive illness. *Br J Soc Clin Psychol* 1967;6:278–96.
2718. Hamilton SR, Liu B, Parsons RE et al. The molecular basis of Turcot's syndrome. *N Engl J Med* 1995;332:839–47.
2719. Hammans SR. The inherited ataxias and the new genetics. *J Neurol, Neurosurg Psychiatr* 1996;61; 327–32.
2720. Hammond WA. Athetosis. *Med Times Gaz* 1871;2:747–8.
2721. Hanaway J, Lee SI, Netsky MG. Pachygyria: Relation of findings to modern embryologic concepts. *Neurology* 1968;18:791–9.
2722. Hancock N, Poon M, Taylor B et al. Hereditary diffuse leukoencephalopathy with spheroids. *J Neurol Neurosurg Psychiatr* 2003;74:1345–7.
2723. Hand A. Polyuria and tuberculosis. *Arch Pediat* 1893;10:673–5.
2724. Handforth A, Nag S, Sharp D et al. Paraneoplastic subacute necrotic myelopathy. *Can J Neurol Sci* 1983;10:204–7.
2725. Hane FM. The whistle-smile reflex in the parkinsonian syndrome. *JAMA* 1989;121:1152.
2726. Hanemann CO. Magic but treatable? Tumours due to loss of Merlin. *Brain* 2008;131:606–15.
2727. Hanigan WC, Winer SJ. Saxophone headache. *N Engl J Med* 1991;325: 1888–9.
2728. Hankey GJ. Isolated angiitis/angiopathy of the central nervous system. *Cerebrovascular Diseases* 1991;1:2–15.
2729. Hankey GJ, Edis RH. The utility of testing tactile perception of direction of scratch as a sensitive clinical sign of posterior column dysfunction in spinal cord disorders. *J Neurol Neurosurg Psychiatry* 1989;52:395–8.
2730. Hankey GJ, Warlow CP. Symptomatic carotid ischaemic events: Safest and most cost effective way of selecting patients for angiography, before carotid endarterectomy. *Brit Med J* 1990;300:1485–90.
2731. Hansen GH. Indberetning til det Norske medicinske Selskab i Christiania om en med understottelseof selskabet foretagen rise for at anstille undersogelser angaende spedalskhedens arsager, tildels udforte sammen med forstander Hartwig. *Norsk* 1874;4**Suppl**:1–88.
2732. Hansen L, Salmon D, Galasko D et al. The Lewy Body variant of Alzheimer's disease. *Neurology* 1990;40:1–8.
2733. Hansen LA, Galasko D. Lewy body disease. *Curr Opin Neurol Neurosurg* 1992;5:889–94.
2734. Hansen SL, Borelli-Moller L, Strange P et al. Ophthalmoplegic migraine: Diagnostic criteria, incidence of hospitalization and possible etiology. *Acta Neurol Scand* 1990;81:54–60.
2735. Hanson PA, Chodos R. Hemiparetic seizures. *Neurology* 1978;28:920–3.
2736. Hanson PA, Farber RE, Armstrong RA. Distal muscle wasting, nephritis and deafness. *Neurology* 1970;20:427–34.
2737. Hanson PA, Mastrianni AF, Post L. Neonatal ophthalmoplegia with microfibers: A reversible myopathy? *Neurology* 1977;27:974–80.
2738. Hanson PA, Mincy JE. Adolescent familial cramps. *Neurology* 1975;25: 454–8.
2739. Hanson PA, Rowland LP. Möbius' syndrome with facioscapulohumeral muscular dystrophy. *Arch Neurol* 1971;24:31–9.
2740. Hanson PA, Urizar RE. Myopathy in Reye's syndrome. *Ann Neurol* 1977;1:431.
2741. Hanson PA, Urizar RE. Ultrastructural lesions of muscle and immunofluorescent deposits in vessels in Reye's syndrome. *Arch Neurol* 1977;1:431–7.

2742. Hansotia P. Spindle coma. *Neurology* 1981;31:83–7.
2743. Hantson L, De Weerdt W et al. The European stroke scale. *Stroke* 1994;25:2215–9.
2744. Harada E. A clinical study of non-suppurative choroiditis. Acute diffuse choroiditis. *Acta Soc Ophth Japan* 1926;30:356.
2745. Haravuori H, Makela-Bengs P, Udd B et al. Assignment of the tibial muscular dystrophy locus to chromosome 2q31. *Am J Hum Genet* 1998;62: 620–6.
2746. Harbison JW, Lessell S, Selhorst JB. Neuro-ophthalmology of sphenoid sinus carcinoma. *Brain* 1984;107:855–70.
2747. Harcherik DF, Leckman JF, Detleor J et al. A new instrument for clinical studies of Tourette's syndrome. *J Amer Acad Child Psychiatr* 1984;23:153–60.
2748. Hardesty WH, Roberts B, Toole JF et al. Studies of carotid blood flow in man. *N Engl J Med* 1960;263:944–6.
2749. Hardie RJ, Lees AJ, Stern GM. On-off fluctuations in Parkinson's disease: A clinical and neuropharmacological study. *Brain* 1984;107:487–506.
2750. Hardie RJ, Pullon HWH, Harding AE et al. Neuroacanthocytosis. *Brain* 1991;114:13–49.
2751. Harding AE. "Idiopathic" late-onset cerebellar ataxia: A clinical and genetic study of 36 families. *J Neurol Sci* 1981;50:259–71.
2752. Harding AE. Friedreich's ataxia: A clinical and genetic study of 90 families with an analysis of early diagnostic criteria and intrafamilial clustering of clinical features. *Brain* 1981;104:589–620.
2753. Harding AE. The clinical features and classification of the late onset autosomal dominant cerebellar ataxias. *Brain* 1982;105:1–28.
2754. Harding AE. *The Spinocerebellar Degenerations and Related Disorders*. Edinburgh: Livingstone, 1983.
2755. Harding AE. Clinical features and classification of inherited ataxias. In Harding AE, Deufel T, eds. *Advances in Neurology*, pp 1–14. New York: Raven Press, 1993.
2756. Harding AE. From the syndrome of Charcot, Marie and Tooth to disorders of peripheral myelin proteins. *Brain* 1995;118:809–18.
2757. Harding AE, Bradbury PG, Murray NMF. Chronic asymmetrical spinal muscular atrophy. *J Neurol Sci* 1983;59:69–83.
2758. Harding AE, Diengdoh JV, Lees AJ. Autosomal recessive late onset multisystem disorder with cerebellar cortical atrophy at necropsy. *J Neurol Neurosurg Psychiatry* 1984;47:853–6.
2759. Harding AE, Muller DPR, Thomas PK et al. Spinocerebellar degeneration secondary to chronic intestinal malabsorption: A vitamin E deficiency syndrome. *Ann Neurol* 1982;12:419–24.
2760. Harding AE, Sweeney MG, Miller DH et al. Occurrence of multiple sclerosis-like illness in women who have a Leber's hereditary optic neuropathy mitochondrial DNA mutation. *Brain* 1992;115:979–89.
2761. Harding AE, Thomas PK. Hereditary distal spinal muscular atrophy. *J Neurol Sci* 1980;45:337–48.
2762. Harding AE, Thomas PK. The clinical features of hereditary motor and sensory neuropathy types I and II. *Brain* 1980;103:259–80.
2763. Harding AE, Thomas PK. Progressive muscular atrophy with pyramidal features. *J Neurol Neurosurg Psychiatry* 1984;47:168–72.
2764. Harding AE, Thomas PK, Baraitser M et al. X-linked recessive bulbospinal neuronopathy: A report of 10 cases. *J Neurol Neurosurg Psychiatry* 1982;45:1012–9.
2765. Harding BN. Familial olivopontocerebellar atrophy with neonatal onset: A recesssively inherited syndrome with systemic and biochemical abnormalities. *J Neurol Neurosurg Psychiatry* 1988;51:385–90.
2766. Hardison J. Are the jumping Frenchmen of Maine goosey? *JAMA* 1980;70:244.
2767. Hare ES. Tumour involving certain nerves. *Lond Med Gaz* 1838;1:16–8.
2768. Harik SI, Ghandour MH, Farah FS, Affi AK. Postganglionic cholinergic dysautonomia. *Ann Neurol* 1977;1:393–6.
2769. Harkin LA, McMahon JM, Iona X et al. The spectrum of SCN1A-related infantile epileptic encephalopathies. *Brain* 2007;130:843–52.
2770. Harley RD, Rodriguez MM, Crawford JS. Congenital fibrosis of the extraocular muscles. *Trans Amer Ophth Soc* 1978;76:197.
2771. Harlow JW. Passage of an iron rod through the head. *Boston Med Surg J* 1848;20:381.
2772. Harmon DC. Case discussion. *N Engl J Med* 1994;331:1079–84.
2773. Harms E, Bahr M, Klock F. The HELPP syndrome - a severe complication of pre-eclampsia. *Z Geburtshilfe Perinatol* 1991;195:187–92.
2774. Harnett JD, Green JS, Cramer BC et al. The spectrum of renal disease in Laurence-Moon-Biedel syndrome. *N Engl J Med* 1988;319:615–8.
2775. Harper A. *Myotonic Dystrophy*. London: Saunders, 1088.
2776. Harper CM. Hemifacial spasm: Preoperative diagnosis and intraoperative management. Muscle Nerve 1991;14:213–8.
2777. Harriman DGF. The histochemistry of reactive masticatory muscle hypertrophy. Muscle Nerve 1996;19:1447–56.
2778. Harriman DGF et al. Ekbom syndrome "restless legs". Brain 1970;93:393.
2779. Harriman DGF, Sumner DW, Ellis FR. Malignant hyperpyrexia myopathy. *Quart J Med* 1973;42:639–64.
2780. Harris H, Penrose LS, Thomas DHH. Cystathioninuria. *Am J Hum Genet* 1959;23:442.
2781. Harris W. *Neuritis and Neuralgia*. London: Oxford University Press, 1926.
2782. Harrison MJG. Muscle wasting after prolonged hypoglycemic coma: Case report with electrophysiological data. *J Neurol Neurosurg Psychiatry* 1976;39:465–70.
2783. Hart MN, Earle KM. Primitive neuroectodermal tumors of the brain in children. *Cancer* 1973;32:890–7.
2784. Hart MN, Malamud N, Ellis WG. The Dandy-Walker syndrome. *Neurology* 1972;22:771–80.
2785. Hart RG, Gardner DP, Howieson J. Acoustic tumors: Atypical features and recent diagnostic tests. *Neurology* 1983;33:211–21.
2786. Hart RG, Kanter MC. Acute autonomic neuropathy: Two cases and a clinical review. *Arch Int Med* 1990;150:2373–6.
2787. Hart ZH, Sahashi K, Lambert EH et al. A congenital familial myasthenic syndrome caused by a presynaptic defect of transmitter resynthesis or mobilization. *Neurology* 1979;29:556–7.
2788. Hartmann E, Baekeland F, Zwilling GR. Psychological differences between long and short sleepers. *Arch Gen Psychiat* 1972;26:463–8.
2789. Hartmann F. Beitrage zur Apraxielehre. *Mschr Psychiat Neurol* 1907;21:97–118.
2790. Harvey CC, Haworth JC, Lorber J. A new heredofamilial neurological syndrome. *Arch Dis Child* 1955;30:338–44.
2791. Harvey DG, Torack RM, Rosenbaum HE. Amyotrophic lateral sclerosis with ophthalmoplegia. *Arch Neurol* 1979;36:615–7.
2792. Harwood RH, Gompertz P, Ebrahim S. Handicap one year after stroke: Validity of a new scale. *J Neurol Neurosurg Psychiatry* 1994;57:825–9.
2793. Hathaway SR, McKinley JC. *The Minnesota Multiphasic Personality Inventory Manual*. New York: Psychological Corporation, 1951.
2794. Hauptmann A. Luminal bei Epilepsie. *Munch Med Wschr* 1912;59:1907–9.

2795. Hauri P. *The Sleep Disorders*. Kalamazoo: Upjohn (Scope), 1982.
2796. Hauri P, Fischer J. Persistent psychophysiological (learned) insomnia. *Sleep* 1986;9:38–53.
2797. Hauser SL, Dawson DM, Lehrich JR et al. Intensive immunosuppression in progressive multiple sclerosis. *N Engl J Med* 1983;308:173–80.
2798. Hauw J-J, Daniel SE, Dickson D et al. Preliminary NINDS neuropathologic criteria for Steele-Richardson-Olszewski syndrome (progressive supranuclear palsy). *Neurology* 1994;44:2015–9.
2799. Hauw J-J, De Baecque C, Hausser-Hauw C et al. Chromatolysis in alchoholic encephalopathies. Pellagra-like changes in 22 cases. Brain 1988;111:843–57.
2800. Haven H. Neurocirculatory scalenus anticus syndrome in presence of developmental anomaly of first rib. *Yale J Biol Med* 1939;11:443–8.
2801. Hawkes CH, Thorpe JW. Acute polyneuropathy due to lightning injury. *J Neurol Neurosurg Psychiatry* 1992;55: 388–90.
2802. Haworth C, Evans DIK, Mitra J et al. Thiamine responsive anemia: Study of two further cases. *Br J Haematol* 1982;50:549.
2803. Haxton HA. Gustatory sweating. Brain 1948;71:16–25.
2804. Hayashi Y, Nagashima K, Urano Y et al. Spinocerebellar degeneration with prominent involvement of the motor neurone system. *Acta Neuropathologica* 1986;70:82–5.
2805. Hayden R, Grossman M. Rectal, ocular, and submaxillary pain: A familial autonomic disorder related to proctalgia fugax. Report of a family. *Am J Dis Childh* 1959;97:479–82.
2806. Hayes DJ, Lecky BRF, Landon DN et al. A new mitochondrial myopathy. Brain 1984;107:1165–77.
2807. Hayes DJ, Taylor DJ, Bore PJ et al. An unusual metabolic myopathy – a malate-aspartate shuttle defect. *J Neurol Sci* 1987;82:27–39.
2808. Haymaker W. Oskar and Cecile Vogt. *Arch Neurol* 1961;4:675–84.
2809. Hayman M, Harvey AS, Hopkins IJ. Paroxysmal tonic upgaze: A reappraisal of outcome. *Ann Neurol* 1998;43: 514–20.
2810. Head H. On disturbances of sensation with especial reference to the pain of visceral disease. Brain 1893;16:1–133.
2811. Head H. Hughlings Jackson on aphasia and kindred disorders of speech. Brain 1915;38:1–42.
2812. Head H. Sensation and the cerebral cortex. Brain 1918;41:57–253.
2813. Head H. Some principles of neurology. *Brain* 1918;41:344–54.
2814. Head H. *Aphasia and Kindred Disorders of Speech*. Cambridge: Cambridge, 1926.
2815. Head H, Campbell AW. The pathology of herpes zoster and its bearing on sensory localisation. Brain 1900;23:353–523.
2816. Head H, Holmes G. Sensory disturbances from cerebral lesions. Brain 1911;34:102–254.
2817. Head H, Riddoch G. The automatic bladder, excessive sweating and some other reflex conditions in gross injuries of the spinal cord. Brain 1917;40:188–263.
2818. Head H, Sherren J. The consequences of injury to the peripheral nerves in man. Brain 1905;28:118–338.
2819. Headache Classification Committee of the IHS. International classification of headache disorders. *Cephalalgia* 2004;24(**Suppl.** 1):1.
2820. Headache Classification Subcommittee of the International Headache Society. The International classification of headache disorders. *Cephalalgia* 2004;24:16–151.
2821. Healton EB, Brust JCM, Kerr DL et al. Presumably autosomal dominant motor system degeneration in a presumably non-Portuguese family. *Neurology* 1980;30:1084–9.
2822. Heathfield KWG, Turner JWA. Syphilitic wrist-drop. *Lancet* 1951;2: 566–9.
2823. Hebb DO. Intelligence, brain function and the theory of mind. Brain 1959;82:260–75.
2824. Heberden W. Of the night-blindness or nyctalopia. *Med Trans Coll Phys Lond* 1768;1:60–3.
2825. Hecaen H, Angelergues R, Houillier S. Les varietes cliniques des acalculies au cours des lesions retrorolandiques: Approche statistique du problème. *Rev Neurol* 1961;105:85–103.
2826. Hecaen H, Penfield W, Bertrand C et al. The syndrome of apractognosia due to lesions of the minor cerebral hemisphere. *A M A Arch Neurol Psychiat* 1956;75: 400–34.
2827. Heckman J, Saffer D. Abnormal copper metabolism: Another "non-Wilson's" case. *Neurology* 1988;38:1493–5.
2828. See 2827.
2829. Hed R, Lundmark C, Fahlgren H et al. Muscular affections in chronic alcoholism. *Acta Med Scand* 1962;171: 585–99.
2830. Hedera P, Blair MA, Andermann E et al. Familial mesial temporal lobe epilepsy maps to chromosome 4q13.2–q21.3. *Neurology* 2007;68:2107–12
2831. Hedley-Whyte T. Case records of the MGH: Case 30:1992. *N Engl J Med* 1992;327:265–7.
2832. Heerfordt CF. Uber eine "Febris uveo–parotidea subchronica", and der Glandula parotis und der Uvea des Auges lokalisiert und haufig mit Paresen cerebrospinaler Nerven komplizert. *Graefe's Arch Ophth* 1909;70:254–73.
2833. Heffner HE. Ferrier and the study of auditory cortex. *Arch Neurol* 1987;44:218–21.
2834. Heffner RR JR. Myopathy of embolic type in patients with carcinoma. *Neurology* 1971;21:841–6.
2835. Heffner RR JR, Barron SA. Polymyositis beginning as a focal process. *Arch Neurol* 1981;38:439–42.
2836. Heggie P et al. Cerebro-ocular dysplasia-muscular dystrophy syndrome. *Arch Ophthalmol* 1987;105:520–4.
2837. Heidenhain A. Klinische und anatomische Untersuchungen uber eine eigenartige organische Erkrankung des Zentralnervensystems im Praesenium. *Zschr Gesamte Neurol Psychiatr* 1929;118:49–114.
2838. Heilman KM. Orthostatic tremor. *Arch Neurol* 1984;41:880–1.
2839. Heilman KM, Rothi L, McFarling DA et al. Transcortical sensory apahasia with relatively spared spontaneous speech and naming. *Arch Neurol* 1981;38:236–9.
2840. Heilman KM, Scholes R, Watson RT. Auditory affective agnosia: Disturbed comprehension of affective speech. *J Neurol Neurosurg Psychiatry* 1975;38:69–72.
2841. Heilman KM,Valenstein E. Mechanisms underlying hemispatial neglect. *Ann Neurol* 1979;5:166–70.
2842. Heilman KM, Watson R, Valenstein E. Neglect and related disorders. In Heilman K, Valenstein E, eds. *Clinical Neuropsychology*, pp 243–93. New York: Oxford Univ. press, 1985.
2843. Heimburger RF, Reitan RM. Easily administered written test for lateralizing brain lesions. *J Neurosurg* 1961;18:301–12.
2844. Heine J. Beobachtungenuber Lahrmungstande der untern Extremitaten undd eren Behandlung. Stuttgart: Kohler, 1840.
2845. Heller T. Ueber Dementia infantilis. *Ztschr f Kinderforsch* 1930;37:661–7.
2846. Hellier KD, Hatchwell E, Duncombe AS et al. X-linked sideroblastic anaemia with ataxia: Another mitochondrial disease? *J Neurol Neurosurg Psychiatry* 2001;70:65–9.
2847. Helm NA, Butler RB, Benson DF. Acquired stuttering. *Neurology* 1978;28:1159–65.
2848. Helm-Estabrooks N, Fitzpatrick PM, Barresi B. Visual action therapy for global aphasia. *J Speech Hear Dis* 1982;47:385–9.

2849. Helmchen C, Glasauer S, Buttner U. Pathological torsional eye deviation during voluntary saccades: A violation of Listing's law. *J Neurol Neurosurg Psychiatry* 1997;62:253–60.

2850. Helmes E, Csapo KG, Short JA. Standardization and validation of the Multidimensional Observation Scale for Elderly Subjects (MOSES). *J Gerontol* 1987;42:395–405.

2851. Helmholtz HLFv. Beschreibung eines Augen-Spiegels zur Untersuchung der Netzhaut im lebenden Auge. Berlin: A. Forstner, 1851.

2852. Helweg-Larsen HF, Ludvigsen K. Congenital familial anhidrosis and neurolabyrinthitis. *Acta Derm Vener Stockh* 1946;26:489–505.

2853. Hemphill J et al. The ICH score. *Stroke* 2001;32:891–7.

2854. Henderson VW. Speech fluency in crossed aphasia. Brain 1983;106:837–57.

2855. Henderson VW. Jules Déjèrine and the third alexia. *Arch Neurol* 1984;41:430–2.

2856. Henderson VW. Paul Broca's less heralded contributions to aphasia research: Historical perspective and contemporary relevance. *Arch Neurol* 1986;43:609–12.

2857. Henderson WR, Smyth GE. Phantom limbs. *J Neurol Neurosurg Psychiatry* 1948;11:88.

2858. Henkind P, Siegel IM, Carr RE. Mesodermal dysgenesis of the anterior segment; Rieger's anolamy. *Arch Ophthalmol* 1965;73:810.

2859. Henley FA. Pelvic colectomy for obstinate constipation. *Proc Roy Soc Med* 1967;60:806–7.

2860. Hennebert C. Reactions vestibularies dans les labyrinthes heredo-syphilitiques. *Arch Internat Laryngol (Paris)* 1909;28:93–6.

2861. Hennebert C. Vestibular reaction auf die pneumonitische. *Ohr Rhinolaryngol* 1909;8:532.

2862. Henneke M, Preuss N, Engelbrecht V et al. Cystic leukoencephalopathy without megalencephaly. *Neurology* 2005;64:1411–6.

2863. Henson JW. Spinal cord gliomas. *Current Opinion in Neurology* 2001;14:679–82.

2864. Henson RA. Henry Head's work on sensation. Brain 1961;84:535–50.

2865. Henson RA. Henry Head: His influence on the development of ideas on sensation. *Brit Med Bull* 1977;33:91–6.

2866. Henson RA. The editors of brain. *Practitioner (London)* 1978;221:639–44.

2867. Henson RA, Hoffman HL, Urich H. Encephalomyelitis with carcinoma. Brain 1965;88:449–64.

2868. Henson RA, Russell DS, Wilkinson M. Carcinomatous neuropathy and myopathy: A clinical and pathological study. Brain 1954;77:82–121.

2869. Henson RA, Urich H. *Cancer and the Nervous System: The Neurological Manifestations Of Systemic Malignant Disease.* Oxford: Blackwell Scientific, 1982.

2870. Henson TE, Muller J, DeMyer WE. Hereditary myopathy limited to females. *Arch Neurol* 1967;17:238–47.

2871. Heppenstall B, Tan V. Well-leg compartment syndrome. *Lancet* 1999;354:970–1.

2872. Herman E. Neurological syndromes in typhus fever. *J Nerv Ment Dis* 1949;109:25–36.

2873. Hernandez A et al. Cortical blindness, growth and psychomotor retardation and postaxial polydactyly. *Clin Genet* 1985;28:251–4.

2874. Herrick JB. Peculiar elongated and sickle-shaped red corpuscles in a case of severe anemia. *Arch Int Med* 1910;6:517.

2875. Herrmann DN, Griffin JW. Intermediate filaments. *Neurology* 2002;58:1143.

2876. Herrmann C, Anguilar M, Sacks O. Hereditary photomyoclonus associated with diabetes mellitus, deafness, nephropathy and cerebral dysfunction. *Neurology* 1964;14:213–21.

2877. Herrmann J et al. A familial dysmorphogenetic syndrome of limb deformities, characteristic facial appearance and associated anomalies: The "pseudothalidomide" or SC-syndrome. *Birth Defects Orig Artic Ser* 1969;5:81–9.

2878. Herrmann J, Opitz JM. An unusual form of acrocephalosyndactyly. *Birth Defects Orig Artic Ser* 1969;5:39–42.

2879. Hers HG. Etudes enzymatiques sur fragments hepatiques: Application a la classification des glycogenoses. *RIH* 1959;9:35–55.

2880. Hersch EL. Development and application of the extended scale for dementia. *J Am Geriatr Soc* 1979;26:348.

2881. Hershey AD, Powers SW, Vockell A-LB et al. PedMIDAS. *Neurology* 2001;57:2034–9.

2882. Herskovitz S, Lipton RB, Lantos G. Neuro-Behcet's disease. *Neurology* 1988;38:1714–20.

2883. Herskovitz S, Loh F, Berger AR et al. Erythromelalgia: Association with hereditary sensory neuropathy and response to amitryptline. *Neurology* 1993;43:621–2.

2884. Hertzman PA, Blevins WL, Mayer J et al. Association of the eosinophilia – myalgia syndrome with the ingestion of tryptophan. *N Engl J Med* 1990;322: 869–73.

2885. Herva R, Leisti J, Kerkinen P et al. A lethal autosomal recessive syndrome of multiple congenital contractures. *Am J Med Genet* 1985;20:431–439, 431.

2886. Herxheimer A. Gustatory sweating and piloerection. *Brit Med J* 1958;1:688–9.

2887. Hess DC. Stroke associated with antiphospholipid antibodies. *Stroke* 1992;23 **(Suppl. 1)**:23–8.

2888. Hewer E, Danek A, Schoser BG et al. McLeod myopathy revisited: More neurogenic and less benign. Brain 2007;130:3285–96.

2889. Heymans A, Nelck G, Oorthuys JWE et al. Rhizomelic chondrodysplasia punctata. *N Engl J Med* 1985;313:187–8.

2890. Hicks EP. Hereditary perforating ulcer of the foot. *Lancet* 1922;1:319–21.

2891. Hierons R. Willis' Contribution to clinical medicine and neurology. *J Neurol Sci* 1967;4:1–13.

2892. Hietaharju A, Jaaskelainen S, Kalimo H. Peripheral neuromuscular manifestations in systemic sclerosis (scleroderma). Muscle Nerve 1993;16:1204–12.

2893. Higashi K et al. Cerebral paragonimiasis. *J Neurosurg* 1971;34:515.

2894. Higgins JJ, Kaneski CR, Bernadini I. Pyridoxine-responsive hyper-β-alaninemia associated with Cohen's syndrome. *Neurology* 1994;44:1728–32.

2895. Higgins JJ, Morton DH, Patronas N et al. An autosomal recessive disorder with posterior column ataxia and retinitis pigmentosa. *Neurology* 1997;49:1717–20.

2896. Higgins JJ, Patterson M, Papadopoulos NM et al. Hypoprebetalipoproteinemia, acanthocytosis, retinitis pigmentosa and pallidal degeneration (HARP syndrome). *Neurology* 1991;41 **(Suppl. 1)**:243.

2897. Higgins JJ, Rosen DR, Loveless JM et al. A gene for nonsyndromic mental retardation maps to chromosome 3p25-pter. *Neurology* 2000;55:335–40.

2898. Highet WB. Grading of motor and sensory recovery in nerve injuries. In Seddon HJ, ed. *Peripheral Nerve Injuries*, London: HMSO, 1954.

2899. Hilari K, Owen S, Farell S. Proxy and self report agreement on the stroke and aphasia quality-of-life scale 39. *J Neurol Neurosurg Psychiatry* 2007;78:1072–5.

2900. Hilden T, Svendsen TL. Electrolyte disturbance in beer drinkers. *Lancet* 1975;2:245–7.

2901. Hilger JA. Carotid pain. *Laryn* 1949;59:829–38.

2902. Hillbom M, Muuronen A, Holm L et al. The clinical versus radiological diagnosis of alcoholic cerebellar degeneration. *J Neurol Sci* 1986;73:45–53.

2903. Hillemand P. Charles Foix and his life-work. *Clio Medicale* 1976;11:269–87.

2904. Hilliquin P, Menkes CJ, Laoussadi S et al. Camptocormia in the elderly. A new entity with paravertebral muscle involvement?. *Rev Rheum Mal Osteoarth* 1992;59:169–75.

2905. Hillis AE. Aphasia. *Neurology* 2007;69:200–13.
2906. Hilz MJ, Dutsch M. Quantitative studies of autonomic function. *Muscle & Nerve* 2006;33:6–20.
2907. Hinchey J, Chaves C, Appignani B et al. A reversible posterior leukoencephalopathy syndrome. *N Engl J Med* 1996;334:494–500.
2908. Hippel Ev. Vorstellung eines Patienten mit einem sehr ungewohnlichen Aderhautleiden. In Bericht u.d.24 Versammlung, ed. *Ophthl Ges* p 269. 1895.
2909. Hippocrates. The sacred disease. In Jones WHS, Withington ET, eds. *Works*, pp 127–83. London: 1990.
2910. Hirano A, Kurland LT, Krooth RS et al. Parkinsonism-dementia complex, endemic disease on island of Guam. I. Clinical features. Brain 1961;84:642–61.
2911. Hirano A, Kurland LT, Sayre GP. Familial amyotrophic lateral sclerosis. *Arch Neurol* 1967;16:232–43.
2912. Hirano M, Angelini C, Montagna P et al. Amyotrophic lateral sclerosis with ragged-red fibers. *Arch Neurol* 2008;65:403–6.
2913. Hirano M, Ott BR, Raps EC et al. Acute quadriplegic myopathy: A complication of treatment with steroids, non-depolarizing blocking agents, or both. *Neurology* 1992;42:2082–7.
2914. Hirano M, Ricci E, Koenigsburger MR. MELAS: An original case and clinical criteria for diagnosis. *Neuromuscular Disorders* 1992;2:125–35.
2915. Hirayama K, Tomonaga M, Kitano K et al. Focal cervical poliopathy causing juvenile muscular atrophy of the distal upper extremity. *J Neurol Neurosurg Psychiatry* 1987;50:285–90.
2916. Hirayama K, Toyakura Y, Tsubaki T. Juvenile muscular atrophy of unilateral upper extremity: A new clinical entity. *Psychiat Neurol (Jap)* 1959;6140:2190–7.
2917. Hirayama T, Takemitsu Y. Isolated paralysis of the descending branch of the posterior interosseous nerve. *J Bone Jt Surg* 1988;70–A:1402–3.
2918. Hirsch AE, Ommaya AK, Mahone RH. Tolerance of subhuman primate brain to cerebral concussion. In Gurdijan ES, Lange WA, Patrick LM et al., eds. *Impact Injury and Crash Protection*, pp 352–71. Springfield, IL: C.C. Thomas, 1970.
2919. Hirschowitz BI, Groll A, Ceballos R. Hereditary nerve deafness in three sisters with absent gastric motility, small bowel diverticulitis and ulceration and progressive sensory neuropathy. *Birth Defects Orig Artic Ser* 1972;8(2): 27–41.
2920. Hisanaga K, Hosokawa M, Sato N et al. "Neuro–Sweet disease". *Arch Neurol* 1999;56:1010–3.
2921. Hitchings RA, Corbett AA, Winklemam J et al. Hemorrhages with optic nerve drusen. *Arch Neurol* 1976;33:675–7.
2922. Hjorth RJ, Willison RG. The electromyogram in facial myokymia and hemifacial spasm. *J Neurol Sci* 1973;20:117–26.
2923. Ho K-L, Meyer KR. The medial medullary syndrome. *Arch Neurol* 1981;38:385–7.
2924. Ho SS, Berkovic SF, Newton MR et al. Parietal lobe epilepsy. *Neurology* 1994;44:2277–84.
2925. Hobart J, Lamping D, Fitzpatrick R et al. The multiple sclerosis impact scale (MSIS 29): A new patient-based outcome measure. Brain 2001;1124:962–73.
2926. Hobart JC, Thompson AJ. The five item Barthel index. *J Neurol Neurosurg Psychiatry* 2001;71:225–30.
2927. Hobson DE. Clinical manifestations of Parkinson's disease and parkinsonism. *Can J Neurol Sci* 2003;30:S2–S9.
2928. Hochsinger C. Concerning tetany in children. *Verh Ges Kinderheilk* 1900;16:107–15.
2929. Hockaday JM, Whitty CWM. Patterns of referred pain in the normal subject. Brain 1967;90:481–96.
2930. Hoddes E, Zarcone V, Smythe H et al. Quantification of sleepiness: A new approach. *Psychophysiology* 1973;10: 431–6.
2931. Hodges JR, Bonface S. Transient epileptic amnesia: A description of the clinical and neuropsychological features in 10 cases and a review of the literature. *J Neurol Neurosurg Psychiatry* 1998;64:435–43.
2932. Hodges JR, Rhys Davies R, Xuereb JH et al. Clinicopathological correlates in frontotemporal dementia. *Ann Neurol* 2004;56:399–406.
2933. Hoehn MH,Yahr MD. Parkinsonism: Onset, progression and mortality. *Neurology* 1967;17:427–42.
2934. Hoeve Jvd. Signs in tuberose sclerosis. *Graefe's Arch Ophth* 1921;105:880–98.
2935. Hoffmann EP et al. Characterization of dystrophin in muscle biopsy specimens from patients with Duchenne's or Becker's muscular dystrophy. *N Engl J Med* 1988;318:1363–8.
2936. Hoffmann EP et al. Hoffmann syndrome (adults). *Dtsch Z Nervenheilk* 1897;9:278.
2937. Hoffmann EP et al. Amyotrophic lateral sclerosis due to HIV. *N Engl J Med* 1985;313:324.
2938. Hoffmann J. Ueber chronische spinale Muskelatrophie im Kindesalter, auf familiarer Basis. *Dtsch Z Nervenklinik* 1891;1:95–120.
2939. Hoffmann J. Weiterer Beitrag zur lehre von der Tetanie. *Dtsch Z Nervenklinik* 1897;9:278–80.
2940. Hoffmann PM, Stuart WH, Earle KM et al. Hereditary late-onset cerebellar degeneration. *Neurology* 1971;21:771–7.
2941. Hogan EL, Krigman MR. Herpes myelitis. *Arch Neurol* 1973;29:309–13.
2942. Hogan PJ, Greenberg MK, McCarty GE. Neurological complications of lymphomatoid granulomatosis. *Neurology* 1981;31:619–20.
2943. Hognestad S. Hereditary nerve deafness associated with diabetes. *Acta Otolaryngol* 1967;64:219.
2944. Hogrel J-Y, Laforêt P, Yaou RB et al. A non-ischemic forearm exercise test for the screening of patients with exercise intolerance. *Neurology* 2001;56:1733–8.
2945. Hohol MJ, Orav EJ, Weiner HL. Disease steps in multiple sclerosis: A longitudinal study comparing disease steps and EDSS to evaluate disease progression. *Multiple Sclerosis* 1999;5:349–54.
2946. Hoke A, Rewcastle NB, Zochodne DW. Acute quadriplegic myopathy unrelated to steroids or paralyzing agents: Quantitative EMG studies. *Can J Neurol Sci* 1999;26:325–9.
2947. Holbrook J, Bennett JB. Brachial plexus injury associated with chest restraint seatbelt: Case report. *J Trauma* 1990;30:1413–4.
2948. Holbrook M, Skilbeck CE. An activities index for use with stroke patients. *Age and Ageing* 1983;12:166–70.
2949. Holden JD. The Russell-Silver's dwarf. *Dev Med Child Neurol* 1967;9:457–9.
2950. Holden KR, Dekaban AS. Neurological involvement in nevus unis lateralis and nevus linearis sebaceus. *Neurology* 1972;22:879–87.
2951. Hollander H, Levy JA. Neurologic abnormalities and recovery of human immunodeficiency virus from cerebrospinal fluid. *Ann Int Med* 1987;106:692–5.
2952. Hollenhorst RW. The neuro-ophthalmology of strokes. In Smith JL, ed. *Neuro–Ophthalmology*, p 109. St. Louis: Mosby CV, 1965.
2953. Hollenhorst RW, Svien HJ, Benoit CF. Unilateral blindness occurring during anesthesia for neurosurgical operations. *Arch Ophthalmol* 1954;52:819.
2954. Holmagyi GM, Curthoys IS. A clinical sign of (inner ear) canal paresis. *Arch Neurol* 1988;45:737–9.
2955. Holman CB. Radiologic manifestations of glioma of the optic nerve and chiasm. *Am J Radiol* 1959;82:462.
2956. Holmes G. A form of familial degeneration of the cerebellum. *Brain* 1907;30:466–89.

2957. Holmes G. The symptoms of acute cerebellar injuries due to gunshot injuries. *Brain* 1917;**40**:461–535.
2958. Holmes G. Disturbances of visual orientation. *Brit J Ophth* 1918;2:449–68.
2959. Holmes G. Spasm of fixation. *Tr Ophth Soc U Kingdom* 1930;50:253–62.
2960. Holmes G. Partial iridoplegia associated with symptoms of other disease of the nervous system. *Trans Ophthal Soc UK.* 1931;51:209–24.
2961. Holmes G. The cerebral integration of the ocular movements. *Brit Med J* 1938;2:107–12.
2962. Holmes G. The cerebellum of man. *Brain* 1939;**62**:1–30.
2963. Holmes G. *The National Hospital, Queen Square 1860–1948*. London: Livingstone, 1954.
2964. Holmes G. *Selected Papers of Gordon Holmes*. Oxford: Oxford University Press, 1979.
2965. Holmes G, Lister WT. Disturbances of vision from cerebral lesions. *Brain* 1916;**39**:35–73.
2966. Holmes G, Russman J. Shuddering Attacks. *Am J Dis Childh* 1986;**140**:72–3.
2967. Holmes GL, Logan WJ. A syndrome of infantile CNS degeneration. *American Journal of Diseases of Children* 1980;134:262–6.
2968. Holmes GL, McKeever M, Adamson M. Absence seizures in children: Clinical and electroencephalographic features. *Ann Neurol* 1987;21:268–73.
2969. Holmes GP, Kaplan JE, Gantz NM et al. Chronic fatigue syndrome: A working case definition. *Ann Int Med* 1988;**108**:387–9.
2970. Holtermuller K, Wiedemann HR. Kleeblattschadel-Syndrome. *Med Wschr* 1960;14:439–46.
2971. Homeida J et al. Dapsone motor neuropathy. *Brit Med J* 1980;**281**:1180.
2972. Homen EA. Eine eigenthumliche Familienkrankheit, unter der Form einer progressiven Dementia, mit besonderem anatomischen Befund. *Neurol Zbl* 1890;9:514–8.
2973. Hood JD, Kayan A, Leech J. Rebound nystagmus. *Brain* 1973;**96**:507–26.
2974. Hood JD, Korres S. Vestibular suppression in peripheral and central vestibular disorders. *Brain* 1979;102:785–804.
2975. Hooft C, DeLacey P, Herpol J et al. Familial hypolipidemia and retarded development without steatorrhea. *Helv Pediat Acta* 1962;17:1.
2976. Hoogendijk JE, Amato AA, Lecky B. Trial design in adult idiopathic inflammatory myopathies with the exception of inclusion body myositis. *Neuromuscul Disord* 2004;**14**: 337–45.
2977. Hooper HE. *The Hooper Visual Organization Test Manual.* Los Angeles: Western Psychological Services, 1958.
2978. Hooshmand H, Martinez AJ, Rosenblum WI. Arthrogryposis multiplex congenita. *Arch Neurol* 1971;24:561–72.
2979. Hootnick D, Holmes LB. Familial polysyndactyly and craniofacial anomalies. *Clin Genet* 1972;3:128–34.
2980. Hoover CF. A new sign for the detection of malingering and functional paresis of the lower extremities. *JAMA* 1908;51:746.
2981. Hope T, Fairburn CG. The present behavioral examination (PBE): The development of an interview to measure current behavioral abnormalities. *Psychol Med* 1992;22:223–30.
2982. Hopf H. Topodiagnostic value of brainstem reflexes. Muscle Nerve 1994;17:475–84.
2983. Hopf HC. Peripheral neuropathy in Acrodermatitis chronica atrophicans. *J Neurol Neurosurg Psychiatry* 1975;38:452–8.
2984. Hopf HC, Ehhrich J, Hundemer H. The pterygoid reflex in man and its clinical application. Muscle Nerve 1992;15:1278–83.
2985. Hopkins A, Rudge P. Hyperpathia in the cervical cord syndrome. *J Neurol Neurosurg Psychiatry* 1973;36:637–42.
2986. Hopkins AP, Harvey PKP. Chronic benign lymphocytic meningitis. *J Neurol Sci* 1973;18:443–53.
2987. Hopkins AP, Michael WF. Spinal myoclonus. *J Neurol Neurosurg Psychiatry* 1974;37:1112–5.
2988. Hopkins IJ. A new syndrome: Poliomyelitis-like illness associated with acute asthma. *Aust Paediatr J* 1974;10:273–6.
2989. Hopkins IJ, Turner B. Spongy glio-neural dystrophy: A degenerative disease of the nervous system. *J Neurol Neurosurg Psychiatry* 1973;36:50–6.
2990. Hopper KD et al. Poland-Möbius syndrome. *South Med J* 1985;78:523–7.
2991. Hormes JT, Filley CM, Rosenberg NL. Neurological sequelae of chronic solvent vapor abuse. *Neurology* 1986;36:698–702.
2992. Horn JL. Psychometric studies of aging and intelligence. In Gershon S, Raskin A, eds. *Aging*, pp 19–43. New York: Raven Press, 1975.
2993. Horner F. Uber ein form von Ptosis. *Klin Mbl Augenh* 1869;7:193–8.
2994. Horner J, Massey EW. Dynamic spelling alexia. *J Neurol Neurosurg Psychiatry* 1986;49:455–7.
2995. Horoupian DS. Hereditary sensory neuropathy with deafness. *Neurology* 1989;39:244–8.
2996. Horowitz SH, Schmalbruch H. Autosomal dominant distal myopathy with desmin storage: A clinicopathologic and electrophysiologic study of a large kinship. Muscle Nerve 1994;17:151–60.
2997. Horsley VAH. *The Structure and Functions of the* Brain *and Spinal Cord.* London: Charles Griffin and Co., 1892.
2998. Horsley VAH. The Linacre lecture on the function of the so-called motor area of the brain. *Brit Med J* 1909;2:125–32.
2999. Horsley VAH, Clarke RH. The structure and functions of the cerebellum examined by a new method. *Brain* 1908;31:45–124.
3000. Horten BC, Rubinstein LJ. Primary cerebral neuroblastoma: A clinicopathological study of 35 cases. *Brain* 1976;99:735–56.
3001. Horton BT, Magath TB, Brown GE. Arteritis of the temporal vessels. A previously undescribed form. *Arch Int Med* 1934;53:400–9.
3002. Horton JC Hoyt WF. Occipital visual field defects respecting the horizontal meridian: A hallmark of extrastriate cortical lesions. 1990. (Unpublished Work)
3003. Horwich MS, Cho L, Poro RS, Posner JB. Subacute sensory neuropathy: A remote effect of carcinoma. *Ann Neurol* 1977;2: 7–19.
3004. Hosking G. Special forms: Variants of migraine in childhood. In Hockaday JM, ed. *Migraine in Childhood*, pp 35–53. London: Butterworths, 1988.
3005. Hoskins TA, Squires JE. Developmental assessment: A test for gross motor and reflex development. *Phys Ther* 1973;2:117–26.
3006. Houlden H, King R, Blake J et al. Clinical, pathological and genetic characterization of hereditary sensory and autonomic neuropathy type 1 (HSAN I). *Brain* 2006;129:411–25.
3007. House JR, Gwathmey FW, Fidler MO. A dynamic approach to the thumb-in-palm deformity in cerebral palsy. *J Bone Joint Surg* 2008;**63A**:216–25.
3008. How A, Dent PB, Liao SK et al. Antineuronal antibodies in neuropsychiatric systemic lupus erythematosus. *Arth Rheum* 1985;28:789–95.
3009. Howard D, Patterson K. *Pyramids and Palm Trees*. Bury St. Edmunds: Thames Valley Test Co., 1992.
3010. Howard RS, Greenwood R, Gawler J et al. A familial disorder associated with palatal myoclonus, other brainstem signs, tetraparesis, ataxia and Rosenthal fiber formation. *J Neurol Neurosurg Psychiatry* 1993;56:977–81.
3011. Howe JR, Miller CA. Midbrain deafness following head injury. *Neurology* 1975;25:286–9.

3012. Howell JT, Monto RW. Syndrome of anemia, dysphagia, and glossitis (Plummer-Vinson syndrome). *N Engl J Med* 1953;**249**:1009–12.
3013. Howell SJL, Owen L, Chadwick DW. Pseudostatus epilepticus. *Quart J Med* 1989; 515–8.
3014. Howlett WP, Brubaker GR, Mlingi N et al. Konzo, an epidemic upper motor neurone disease studied in Tanzania. *Brain* 1990;**113**:223–35.
3015. Howship J. *Practical Remarks on the Discrimination and Appearance of Surgical Disease.* London: Churchill, 1840.
3016. Hsia YE et al. Genetics of the Meckel Syndrome (dysencephalia splanchnocystica). *Pediatrics* 1971;**48**:237–47.
3017. Huang C-C, Chu N-S, Chen T-J et al. Acute hemorrhagic leucoencephalitis with a prolonged clinical course. *J Neurol Neurosurg Psychiatry* 1988;**51**:870–4.
3018. Huang C-C, Chu N-S, Lu C-S et al. Long-term progression in chronic manganism. *Neurology* 1998;**50**:698–700.
3019. Huang C, Broe G. Isolated facial palsy: A new lacunar syndrome. *J Neurol Neurosurg Psychiatry* 1984;**47**:84–6.
3020. Hubble JP, Busenbark KL, Koller WC. Essential tremor. *Clin Neuropharmacol* 1989;**12**:453–82.
3021. Huber A. Electrophysiology of the retraction syndromes. *Br J Ophthalmol* 1974;**58**:293.
3022. Huber SJ, Paulson GW. The concept of subcortical dementia. *Am J Psychiatry* 1985;**142**:1312–7.
3023. Huchard H. Character and mental state of hysterics. *Arch Neurol* 1882;**3**:187–211.
3024. Hudgins RJ, Edwards MSB, Ousterhouk DK et al. Pediatric neurosurgical implications of the amniotic band syndrome. *Pediatr Neurosci* 1986;**12**:232–9.
3025. Hudgson P. Subacute or chronic proximal metabolic myopathies. *Brit Med J* 1984;**1**:585.
3026. Hudgson P, Peter JB. Classification (of polymyositis). *Clin Rheum Dis* 1984;**10**:3–8.
3027. Hudson AJ. Amyotrophic lateral sclerosis and its association with Dementia, Parkinsonism and other neurological disorders. *Brain* 1981;**104**:217–47.
3028. Hudson AJ, Brown WF, Gilbert JJ. The muscular pain-fasciculation syndrome. *Neurology* 1978;**28**:1105–9.
3029. Hudson AJ, Grace GM. Misidentification syndromes related to face specific area in the fusiform gyrus. *J Neurol Neurosurg Psychiatry* 2000;**69**:645–8.
3030. Hudson AJ, Kiernan JA, Munoz D et al. Clinicopathological features of primary lateral sclerosis are different from amyotrophic lateral sclerosis. *Brain Res Bull* 1993;**30**:359–64.
3031. Hudson G, Amati-Bonneau P, Blakely EL et al. Mutation of OPA1 causes dominant optic atrophy with external ophthalmoplegia, ataxia, deafness and multiple mitochondrial DNA deletions: A novel disorder of mtDNA maintenance. *Brain* 2008;**131**:329–37.
3032. Hug G, Bove KE, Soukup S. Lethal neonatal multiorgan deficiency of carnitine palmitoyltransferase II. *N Engl J Med* 1991;**325**:1862–4.
3033. Hugh AE. Trickle Arteriography. *Brit Med J* 1970;**2**:574–6.
3034. Hughes A, Daniel SE, Lees AJ. Improved accuracy of the clinical diagnosis of Lewy body Parkinson's disease. *Neurology* 2001;**57**:1497–9.
3035. Hughes CA, Byrne PC, Webb S et al. SPG15, a new locus for autosomal recessive complicated HSP on chromosome 14q. *Neurology* 2001;**56**:1230–3.
3036. Hughes CP, Berg L, Danziger WL et al. A new clinical scale for the staging of dementia. *Br J Psychiatry* 1982;**140**:566–72.
3037. Hughes JT. *Thomas Willis: His Life and Work.* London: Royal Society of Medicine, 1991.
3038. Hughes JT. *Thomas Willis 1621–1675. His Life and Work.* London: RSM Services, 1992.
3039. Hughes JT, Oppenheimer DR. Superficial siderosis of the central nervous system. A report on nine cases with autopsy. *Acta Neuropathol* 1969;**13**:556–74.
3040. Hughes RAC, Bensa S, Willison H et al. Randomized controlled trial of intravenous immunoglobulin versus oral prednisolone in chronic inflammatory demyelinating polyneuropathy. *Ann Neurol* 2001;**50**:195–201.
3041. Hughes RAC, Newsom-Davis J, Perkin GD et al. Controlled trial of prednisolone in acute polyneuropathy. *Lancet* 1978;**2**:750–3.
3042. Hughes RAC, Sanders E, Hall S et al. Subacute idiopathic demyelinating polyradiculoneuropathy. *Arch Neurol* 1992;**49**:612–6.
3043. Hughes R, Umapathi T, Gray I et al. A controlled investigation of the cause of chronic idiopathic axonal polyneuropathy. *Brain* 2004;**127**:1723–30.
3044. Humphreys P, Whiting S, Pham B. Hemiparetic cerebral palsy: Clinical pattern and imaging in prediction of outcome. *Can J Neurol Sci* 2000;**27**:210–9.
3045. Hund E. Neurological complications of sepsis: Critical illness polyneuropathy and myopathy. *J Neurol* 2001;**248**: 929–34.
3046. Hunt AD. Pyridoxine dependency: Report of a case of intractable convulsions in an infant, controlled by pyridoxine. *Pediatrics* 1954;**13**:140–5.
3047. Hunt JR. On herpetic inflammation of the geniculate ganglion. A new syndrome and its complications. *J Nerv Ment Dis* 1907;**34**:73–96.
3048. Hunt JR. Dyssynergia cerebellaris progressiva – a chronic progressive form of cerebellar tremor. *Brain* 1914;**37**:247–68.
3049. Hunt JR. Progressive atrophy of the globus pallidus (primary atrophy of the pallidal system). *Brain* 1917;**40**:58–148.
3050. Hunt JR. Dyssynergia cerebellaris myoclonica – primary atrophy of the dentate system; a contribution to the pathology and symptomatology of the cerebellum. *Brain* 1921;**44**:490–538.
3051. Hunt JR. On the occurrence of static seizures in epilepsy. *J Nerv Ment Dis* 1922;**56**:351–6.
3052. Hunt WE, Hess RM. Surgical risks as related to time of intervention in the repair of intracranial aneurysms. *J Neurosurg* 1968;**28**:14–20.
3053. Hunter AG et al. Absence of cerebellar granular layer, mental retardation, tapetoretinal degeneration, and progressive glomerulopathy: An autosomal recessive ocular-renal-cerebellar syndrome. *Am J Med Genet* 1982;**11**:383–95.
3054. Hunter AGW, McAlpine PJ, Rudd NL et al. A "new" syndrome of mental retardation with characteristic facies and brachyphalangy. *J Med Genet* 1977;**14**:430–7.
3055. Hunter C. A rare disease in two brothers. *Proc Roy Soc Med* 1917;**10**:104–16.
3056. Huntington G. On Chorea. *Med Surg Report.* 1872;**26**:317–21.
3057. Huott AD, Madison DS, Niedermeyer E. Occipital lobe epilepsy. *Europ Neurol* 1974;**11**:325–39.
3058. Hurler G. Uber einen Typ multipler Abartungen vorwiegend am Skelettsystem. *Zschr Kinderh* 1919;**24**:220–34.
3059. Hurst EW. Acute haemorrhagic leucoencephalitis; previously undefined entity. *Med J Aust* 1941;**2**:1–6.
3060. Huson SM, Harper PS, Hourihan MD et al. Cerebellar haemangioblastoma and von Hippel-Lindau disease. *Brain* 1986;**109**:1297–310.
3061. Hutchinson J. On the different forms of inflammation of the eye consequent on inherited syphilis. *Ophth Hosp Rep* 1858;**1**:191, 226–303, 244.
3062. Hutchinson J. Report on the effect of infantile syphilis in marring the development of teeth. *TPSL* 1858;**9**: 449–55.

3063. Hutchinson J. Case of congenital absence of hair with atrophic condition of the skin and its appendages. *Lancet* 1886;1:923.

3064. Hutchinson R. Suprarenal sarcoma in children with metastasis in the skull. *Quart J Med* 1907;1:33.

3065. Huttenlocher PR, Gilles FH. Infantile neuroaxonal dystrophy. *Neurology* 1967;**17**:1174–84.

3066. Hwang YM, Lee MC, Suh DC et al. Coxiella (Q-fever)-associated myelopathy. *Neurology* 1993;**43**:338–42.

3067. Hyland K, Surtees RAH, Rodeck C et al. Aromatic L-amino acid decarboxylase deficiency: Clinical features, diagnosis, and treatment of a new inborn error of neurotransmitter amine synthesis. *Neurology* 1992;42:1980–8.

3068. Hymas N, Lees A, Bolton D et al. The neurology of obsessional slowness. *Brain* 1991;114:2203–33.

3069. IASP Taxonomy Committee. Classification of chronic pain. *Pain* 1986;**27**:S1–S226.

3070. Igarashi O, Iguchi H, Ogura N et al. Cheiro-oral-pedal syndrome due to brainstem hemorrhage. *Clin Neurol Neurosurg* 2006;**108**:507–10.

3071. Iglesias S, Chapon F, Baron J-C. Familial occipital calcifications, hemorrhagic strokes, leukoencephalopathy, dementia and external carotoid dysplasia. *Neurology* 2000;**55**:1661–7.

3072. Iizuka R et al. Dentato-rubro-pallido-luysian atrophy. *J Neurol Neurosurg Psychiatry* 1984;**47**:1288–98.

3073. Iizuka T, Sakai F, Ide T et al. Anti-NMDA receptor encephalitis in Japan. *Neurology* 2008;**70**:504–11.

3074. Ikeda A, Kakigi R, Funai N et al. Cortical tremor: A variant of cortical reflex myoclonus. *Neurology* 1990;**40**:1561–5.

3075. Ikeda K, Iwasaki Y, Kinoshita M. Amyotrophic lateral sclerosis associated with isolated adrenocorticotrophic hormone deficiency. *Muscle Nerve* 1995;**18**:111–3.

3076. Ikeda S, Yakazi M, Takei Y et al. Type II (adult onset) citrullinemia: Clinical pictures and the therapeutic effect of liver transplantation. *J Neurol Neurosurg Psychiatry* 2001;**71**:663–70.

3077. Ikida S, Kondo K, Oguchi K et al. Adult fucosidosis. *Neurology* 1984;**334**:451–6.

3078. Iliceto G, Thompson PD, Day BL et al. Diaphragmatic flutter, the moving umbilicus syndrome and "belly-dancers' dyskinesia". *Mov Disord* 1990;**5**:15–22.

3079. Illa I, Serrano-Munuera C, Gallardo E et al. Distal anterior compartment myopathy: A dysferlin mutation causing a new muscular dystrophy phenotype. *Ann Neurol* 2001;**49**:130–4.

3080. Illingworth RS. *The Development of the Infant and the Young Child: Normal and Abnormal.* Edinburgh etc.: Churchill Livingstone, 1987.

3081. Illis LS. Central pain. *Brit Med J* 1990;**300**:1284–6.

3082. Ince B, Petty GW, Brown JR et al. Dolichoectasia of the intracranial arteries in patients with first ischemic stroke. *Neurology* 1998;**50**:1694–8.

3083. Ince PG, Duffey P, Cochrane HR et al. Relapsing ischemic encephaloenteropathy and cryoglobulinemia. *Neurology* 2000;**55**:1579–81.

3084. Indo T, Takahashi A. Swimmer's migraine. *Headache* 1990;**30**:485–7.

3085. Ingall TJ, McLeod JG, Tamura N. Autonomic function and unmyelinated fibres in chronic inflammatory demyelinating polyradiculoneuropathy. *Muscle Nerve* 1990;**13**:70–6.

3086. Inghilleri M, Bernadelli A, Cioni B et al. The conduction velocity of the corticospinal tract in man. In Rossini PM, Marsden CD eds. *Non-Invasive Stimulation of Brain and Spinal Cord*, pp 123–30. New York: Liss, 1988.

3087. Ingle VN, Talwalker YB, Neil JV. Bilateral congenital anophthalmos. *J Pediatr* 1966;**33**:149.

3088. Ingram TTS. *Paediatric Aspects of Cerebral Palsy*. Edinburgh: Livingstone, 1964.

3089. Ingram TTS, Naughton JA. Paediatric and psychological aspects of cerebral palsy associated with hydrocephalus. *Dev Med Child Neurol* 1962;**4**:287–92.

3090. Ingvar DH, Nyman GE. Epilepsia arithmetices. *Neurology* 1962;**12**:282–7.

3091. Inomata H, Kato M. Vogt-Koyanagi-Harada disease. In Bruyn GW, Vinken PJ, eds. *Handbook of Clinical Neurology*, pp 611–26. Amsterdam: Elsevier, 1989.

3092. Inouye SK, van Dyck CH, Alessi CA et al. Clarifying confusion: The confusion assessment method. *Ann Int Med* 1990;**113(12)**:941–8.

3093. International Continence Society Standardisation Committee. Fourth report on the standardisation of terminology of lower urinary tract dysfunction. *Brit J Urol* 1981;**53**:333.

3094. International Federation of Multiple Sclerosis Societies. Minimal record of disability for multiple sclerosis. *Acta Neurol Scand* 1984;**S101**:15–217.

3095. Ionasescu VV, Burns TL, Searby C et al. X-linked dominant Charcot-Marie-Tooth neuropathy with 15 cases in a family genetic linkage study. *Muscle Nerve* 1988;**11**:1154–6.

3096. Iqbal A, Alter M, Lee SH. Pseudoxanthoma elasticum: A review of neurological complications. *Ann Neurol* 1978;**4**:18–20.

3097. Iragui VJ. The Charcot-Bouchard controversy. *Arch Neurol* 1986;**43**:290–5.

3098. Isaacs B, Kennie AT. The set test as an aid to the detection of dementia in old people. *Br J Psychiatry* 1973;**123**:467–70.

3099. Isaacs H. A syndrome of continuous muscle fibre activity. *J Neurol Neurosurg Psychiatry* 1961;**24**:319–25.

3100. Isgren WP. Normocalcemic tetany. A problem of erethism. *Neurology* 1976;**26**:825–34.

3101. Ishihara S. Tests for colour-blindness. Tokyo: Kanehawa Shuppan Co. Ltd. 1917.

3102. Ishiyama A, Ishiyama G, Lopez I et al. Temporal bone histopathology in dominantly inherited audiovestibular syndrome. *Neurology* 2004;**63**:1859–62.

3103. Isler H. Thomas Willis' two chapters on headache of 1672: A first attempt to apply the 'new science' to this topic. *Headache* 1986;**26**:95–8.

3104. Ismael SS, Ameranco G, Bayle B et al. Postpartum lumbosacral plexopathy limited to autonomic and perineal manifestations: Clinical and electrophyiological study of 19 patients. *J Neurol Neurosurg Psychiatry* 2000;**68**:771–3.

3105. Isozaki E, Naito A, Horiguchi S et al. Early diagnosis and stage classification of vocal cord abductor paralysis in patients with multiple system atrophy. *J Neurol Neurosurg Psychiatry* 1996;**60**:399–402.

3106. Israels S, Haworth JC, Dunn HG et al. Lactic acidosis in childhood. *Adv Pediatr* 1976;**22**:267–303.

3107. Itigaki S, McGeer PL, Akiyama H et al. A case of adult onset dementia with argyrophilic grains. *Ann Neurol* 1989;**26**:685–9.

3108. Ito M. Nevus fusco-ceruleus acromio-deltoideus. *Tohoku J Exp Med* 1954;**60**:10.

3109. Ives EJ, Houston CS. Autosomal recessive microcephaly and micromelia in Cree Indians. *Am J Med Genet* 1980;**7**:351–60.

3110. Iwasaki S, McGarvie LA, Halmagyi GM et al. Head taps evoke a crossed vestibulo-ocular reflex. *Neurology* 2007;**68**:1227–96.

3111. Iwashita H, Ohnishi A, Asada M et al. Polyneuropathy, skin hyperpigmentation, edema and hypertrichosis in localised osteosclerotic myeloma. *Neurology* 1977;**27**:675–81.

3112. Jablecki CK. Lateral antebrachial cutaneous neuropathy in a windsurfer. *Muscle Nerve* 1999;**22**:944–5.

3113. Jablonski S. *Illustrated Dictionary of Eponymic Syndromes and Diseases and their Synonyms.* Philadelphia: W.B.Saunders, 1969.

3114. Jablonski S. *Jablonski's Dictionary of Syndromes and Eponymic Diseases.* Malabar, Fla.: Krieger, 1991.

3115. Jabre JF. Surface recording of the H-reflex of the flexor carpi radialis. *Muscle Nerve* 1981;**4**:435–8.

3116. Jabre JF. Concentric macro electromyography. *Muscle Nerve* 1991;14:820–5.
3117. Jabre JF, Bryan RW. Bent-knee pulling in the diagnosis of upper lumbar root lesions. *Arch Neurol* 1982;39:669–70.
3118. Jackson AC. Acute viral infections. *Current Opinion in Neurology* 1995;8: 170–4.
3119. Jackson AC, Gilbert JJ, Young GB, Bolton CF. The encephalopathy of sepsis. *Can J Neurol Sci* 1985;12:303–7.
3120. Jackson CE, Amato AA, Barohn RJ. Isolated Vitamin E deficiency. *Muscle Nerve* 1996;19:1161–5.
3121. Jackson CE, Barohn RJ. Improvement of the exercise test in thyrotoxic periodic paralysis. *Muscle Nerve* 1992;15:1069–71.
3122. Jackson CE, Barohn RJ, Gronseth G et al. Inclusion body myositis functional rating scale: A reliable and valid measure of disease severity. *Muscle Nerve* 2008;37:473–6.
3123. Jackson CE, et al. "Brittle" hair with short stature, intellectual impairment with decreased fertility: An autosomal recessive syndrome in an Amish kindred. *Pediatrics* 1974;54:201–7.
3124. Jackson JH. Unilateral epileptiform seizures, attended by temporary defect of sight. *Med Times Gaz* 1863;1:588.
3125. Jackson JH. Case of paralysis of the tongue from haemorrhage in the medulla oblongata. *Lancet* 1872;2:770–3.
3126. Jackson JH. Contribution to the comparative study of convulsions. *Brain* 1886;9:1–23.
3127. Jackson JH. On a particular variety of epilepsy. *Brain* 1889;11:179–207.
3128. Jackson JH. Case of tumor of the middle lobe of the cerebellum: Cerebellar paralysis with rigidity (cerebellar attitude), occasional tetanus-like seizures. *Brain* 1906;29:425–40.
3129. Jackson MJ, Schaefer JA, Johnson MA et al. Presentation and clinical investigation of mitochondrial respiratory chain disease. *Brain* 1995;118:339–57.
3130. Jackson R. The facet syndrome. Myth or reality? *Clin Orthop* 1992;279:110–21.
3131. Jacobs EB, Landing BH, Thomas W. Vernicomyelia. Its bearing on theories of genesis of the Arnold-Chiari complex. *Am J Path* 1961;39:345–53.
3132. Jacobs JW, Bernhard MR, Delgado A et al. Screening for organic mental syndromes in the medically ill. *Ann Int Med* 1977;86:40–6.
3133. Jacobs L. Visual allesthesia. *Neurology* 1980;30:1059–63.
3134. Jacobs L, Grossman MD. Three primitive reflexes in normal adults. *Neurology* 1980;30:184–8.
3135. Jacobsen P. Ptosis, oligomimia and motor dysphasia in mental retardation. *Lancet* 1966;1:1379.
3136. Jacobson GP, Ramadan NR, Aggarwal SK et al. The Henry Ford Hospital headache disability inventory. *Neurology* 1994;44:837–42.
3137. Jacobson PL, Farmer TW. The hypernormal CT scan in dementia. *Neurology* 1979;29:1522–7.
3138. Jacobson RI. Classification of craniosynostosis. *Neurol Clin* 1985;3:117.
3139. Jacod M. Sur la propagation intracranienne des sarcomes de la trompe d'Eustache, syndrome du carrefour petro–sphenoidal, paralysie des 2, 3, 4, 5, et 6 paires craniennes. *Rev Neurol* 1921;37:33–8.
3140. Jacome DE. Synkinetic blepharoclonus. *J Neuroophthalmol* 2000;20:276–84.
3141. Jacome DE. Dracula's teeth syndrome. *Headache* 2001;41:892–4.
3142. Jacome DE, FitzGerald R. Monocular ictal nystagmus. *Arch Neurol* 1982;39:653–6.
3143. Jacome DE, Risko M. Pseudocataplexy: Gelastic-atonic seizures. *Neurology* 1984;34:1381–3.
3144. Jacquemont S, Hagerman RJ, Leehey M et al. Fragile X pre-mutation tremor/ ataxia syndrome. *Am J Hum Genet* 2003;72:869–78.
3145. Jadassohn J, Lewandowsky K. Pachyonychia congenita. In Neisser A, Jacobi E, eds. *Ikonographia Dermatologica*, pp 29–31. Berlin: Urban & Schwarzenberg, 1906.
3146. Jaeken J, Carchon H. Congenital disorders of glycosylation; the rapidly growing tip of the iceberg. *Current Opinion in Neurology* 2001;14:811–5.
3147. Jafari H, Couratier P, Camu W. Motor neuron disease after electrical injury. *J Neurol Neurosurg Psychiatry* 2001;71: 265–7.
3148. Jaffe HL. Osteoid osteoma. Benign osteoblastic tumor composed of osteoid (atypical bone). *Arch Surg* 1935;31: 709–28.
3149. Jahanshahi M, Hunter M, Philips C. The headache scale: An examination of its reliability and validity. *Headache* 1986;26:76–82.
3150. Jakob AM. Ueber eigenartige Erkrankungen der Zentralnervensystems mit bemerkenswertem anatomischem Befunde. *Z Ges Neurol Psychiat* 1921;64:147–228.
3151. Jamal JA, Hansen S, Apertopoulos Feal. The "Gulf War syndrome". Is there evidence of dysfunction of the nervous system? *J Neurol Neurosurg Psychiatry* 1996;60:449–51.
3152. James DG, Sharma OP. Neurologic complications of sarcoidosis. *Proc Roy Soc Med* 1967;60:1169–70.
3153. James PB. Dysbarism: The medical problems from high and low atmospheric pressures. *J Roy Coll Phycns* 1993;27:367–74.
3154. James W. *Textbook of Psychology*. London: Macmillan, 1892.
3155. Jamieson PW, Katorji MB. Idiopathic generalized myokymia. *Muscle Nerve* 1994;17:42–51.
3156. Jampel RS et al. Ophthalmoplegia and retinal degeneration associated with spinocerebellar ataxia. *Arch Ophthalmol* 1961;6:247–59.
3157. Jankovic J. Neuroacanthocytosis syndrome. *Neurology* 1985;35:1679.
3158. Jankovic J. Post-traumatic movement disorders. *Neurology* 1994;44:2006–14.
3159. Jankovic J, Fahn S. The phenomenology of tics. *Mov Disord* 1986;1:17–26.
3160. Jankovic J, Ford J. Blepharospasm and oro-facial-cervical dystonia: Clinical and pharmacological findings in 100 patients. *Ann Neurol* 1983;13:407–11.
3161. Jankovic J, Kirkpatric JB, Blomquist KA. Late-onset Hallervorden-Spatz disease presenting as familial parkinsonism. *Neurology* 1985;35:227–34.
3162. Jankovic J, Leder S, Warner D et al. Cervical dystonia: Clinical findings and associated movement disorders. *Neurology* 1991;41:1088–91.
3163. Jankovic J, Rivera VM. Hereditary myoclonus and progressive distal muscular atrophy. *Ann Neurol* 1979;6:227–31.
3164. Jannetta PJ. Hemifacial spasm. In Samii M, Jannetta PJ, eds. *The Cranial Nerves*, pp 484–93. Berlin: Springer-Verlag, 1981.
3165. Jannetta PJ, Moller MB, Moller AR. Disabling positional vertigo. *N Engl J Med* 1984;310:1700–5.
3166. Jansen CM, Cao H, Kaplan P et al. Sanfilippo Syndrome Type D. *Arch Neurol* 2007;64:1629–34.
3167. Janz D. Epilepsy with impulsive petit mal (juvenile myoclonic epilepsy). *Acta Neurol Scand* 1985;72:339–59.
3168. Jaretzki A III, Barohn RJ, Ernstoff RM et al. Myasthenia gravis: Recommendations for clinical research standards. Task force of the medical scientific advisory board of the Myasthenia Gravis Foundation of America. *Neurology* 2000;55:16–23.
3169. Jaretzki A III, Barohn RJ, Ernstoff RM et al. Myasthenia gravis: Recommendations for clinical research standards. *Ann Thoracic Surg* 2000;70:327–34.
3170. Jarrell HR. Vegas neuropathy. *N Engl J Med* 1981;319:1487.
3171. Jarry J, Rioux MF, Bolduc V. A novel autosomal recessive limb-girdle muscular dystrophy with quadriceps atrophy maps to 11p13-p12. *Brain* 2007;130.

3172. Jasper HH, Van Buren J. Interrelationships between cortex and subcortical structures: Clinical electroencephalographic studies. *EEG Clin Neurophysiol* 1953;4:168–202.

3173. Jastakj S. *The Wide Range Achievement Test.* Wilmington, Delaware: Guidance Associates, 1965.

3174. Jayam AV, Hass WK, Carr RE, Kumar AJ. Saturday night retinopathy. *J Neurol Sci* 1974;22:413–8.

3175. Jeannet P-Y, Bassez G, Eymard B et al. Clinical and histologic findings in autosomal centronuclear myopathy. *Neurology* 2004;62:1484–90.

3176. Jeannet PY, Mittaz L, Dunand M et al. Autosomal dominant nemaline myopathy: A new phenotype unlinked to previously known genetic loci. *Neuromuscular Disorders* 2007;17:6–12.

3177. Jeavons PM. Nosological problems of myoclonic epilepsies in childhood and adolescence. *Dev Med Child Neurol* 1977;19:3–8.

3178. Jeavons PM, Harding GFA. Television epilepsy. *Lancet* 1970;2:926–7.

3179. Jefferson G. Compression of the chiasma, optic nerves and optic tracts by intracranial aneurysms. *Brain* 1937;60:444–97.

3180. Jefferson G. On the saccular aneurysms of the internal carotid artery in the cavernous sinus. *Brit J Surg* 1938;26:267–302.

3181. Jefferson G. Memories of Hugh Cairns. *J Neurol Neurosurg Psychiatry* 1959;22: 155–66.

3182. Jeffreys R. Clinical and surgical aspects of posterior fossa haemangioblastomata. *J Neurol Neurosurg Psychiatry* 1975;38: 105–11.

3183. Jelic V, Kivipelto M, Winblad B. Clinical trials in mild cognitive impairment: Lessons for the future. *J Neurol Neurosurg Psychiatry* 2006;77:429–38.

3184. Jelliffe S. Nervous and mental disturbances of influenza. *NY Med J* 1918;108:725–8.

3185. Jelliffe SE. Sigmund Freud as a neurologist. *J Nerv Ment Dis* 1937;85:696–711.

3186. Jellinek EH. The orbital pseudotumour syndrome and its differentiation from endocrine exophthalmos. *Brain* 1969;92:35–58.

3187. Jellinek EH, Kelly RE. Cerebellar syndrome in myxoedema. *Lancet* 1960;2:225–7.

3188. Jellinger K. Progressive pallidal atrophy. *J Neurol Sci* 1968;6:19–44.

3189. Jellinger K, Neumayer E. Progressive vascular myelopathy. *Acta Neurol Psychiat Belg* 1962;62:944.

3190. Jellinger K, Seitelberger F. Protracted Post-traumatic encephalopathy: Pathology, pathogenesis and clinical implications. *J Neurol Sci* 1970;10:51–94.

3191. Jellinger K, Seitelberger F. Spongy glioneural dystrophy in infancy and childhood. *Acta Neuropathol* 1970;16:125–40.

3192. Jen J, Cohen AH, Yue Q et al. Hereditary endotheliopathy with retinopathy, nephropathy and stroke (HERNS). *Neurology* 1997;49:1322–30.

3193. Jen J, Coulin CJ, Bosley TM et al. Familial horizontal gaze palsy with progressive scoliosis maps to chromosome 11 to 23–25. *Neurology* 2002;59:432–5.

3194. Jen JC, Wang H, Lee H et al. Suggestive linkage to chromosomes 6q. in families with bilateral vestibulopathy. *Neurology* 2004;63:2376–9.

3195. Jendrassik E. Beitrage zur Lehre von den Sehnenreflexen. *Arch Klin Med* 1883;33:177–99.

3196. Jenis EH, Lindquist RR, Lister RC. New congenital myopathy with crystalline intranuclear inclusions. *Arch Neurol* 1969;20:281–7.

3197. Jenkins JE. The Mozart effect. *J Roy Soc Med* 2001;94:170–2.

3198. Jenkyn LR, Walsh DB, Culver RG, Reeves AG. Clinical signs in diffuse cerebral dysfunction. *J Neurol Neurosurg Psychiatry* 1977;40:956–66.

3199. Jenkyn LR, Walsh DB, Walsh BT et al. The nuchocephalic reflex. *J Neurol Neurosurg Psychiatry* 1975;38:561–6.

3200. Jennekens FGI, Busch HFM, van Hemel NM. Inflammatory myopathy in scapulo-ilio-peroneal atrophy with cardiomyopathy. *Brain* 1975;98:709–22.

3201. Jennekens FGI, Veldman H, Vroegindeweij-Claessens LJHM et al. Congenital oculo-bulbar palsy. *J Neurol Neurosurg Psychiatry* 1992;55:404–6.

3202. Jennekens FGI, Wokke JHJ. Proximal weakness of the extremities as main feature of amyloid myopathy. *J Neurol Neurosurg Psychiatry* 1987;50:1353–8.

3203. Jennett B. Post-traumatic epilepsy. *Arch Neurol* 1974;30:396–8.

3204. Jennett B. *Epilepsy After Non-Missile Head Injuries*. London: Heinemann, 1975.

3205. Jennett B, Bond M. Assessment of outcome after severe brain damage. *Lancet* 1975;1:480.

3206. Jennett B, Teasedale G, Braakman R et al. Prognosis in series of patients with severe head injury. *Neurosurgery* 1979;4: 283–300.

3207. Jennum P, Friberg L, Fuglsang-Frederiksen A et al. Speech localization using repetitive transcranial magnetic stimulation. *Neurology* 1994;44: 269–73.

3208. Jensen PK. Nerve deafness, optic nerve atrophy, and dementia: A new X-linked recessive syndrome? *Am J Med Genet* 1981;9:55–60.

3209. Jequier M, Deonna TW. A propos des dégenérescences neurosensorielles. *Schweiz Arch Neurol Psychiatry* 1973;112:219–27.

3210. Jerritsen T, Waisman HA. Hypersarcosinemia. *N Engl J Med* 1966;275:66.

3211. Jerusalem F, Angelini C, Engel AG et al. Mitochondria-lipid-glycogen (MLG) disease of muscle. *Arch Neurol* 1973;29:162–9.

3212. Jerusalem F, Engel AG, Gomez MR. Sarcotubular myopathy. *Neurology* 1973;23:897–906.

3213. Jerusalem F, Ludin H, Bischoff A, Hartmann G. Cytoplasmic body neuromyopathy presenting as respiratory failure and weight loss. *J Neurol Sci* 1979;441:1–9.

3214. Jerusalem F, Spiess H, Baumgartner G. Lipid storage myopathy with normal carnitine levels. *J Neurol Sci* 1975;24: 273–82.

3215. Jervell A, Lange-Nielson F. Congenital deaf-mutism, functional heart disease with prolongation of the Q-T interval, and sudden death. *Am Heart J* 1957;54:59–68.

3216. Jervis GA. Early familial cerebellar degeneration (report of three cases in one family). *J Nerv Ment Dis* 1950;111: 398–407.

3217. Jestico JV, Urry PA, Efphimiou J. An hereditary sensory and autonomic neuropathy transmitted as an X-linked recessive trait. *J Neurol Neurosurg Psychiatry* 1985;48:1259–64.

3218. Jett DA. Neurological aspects of chemical terrorism. *Ann Neurol* 2007;61:9–13.

3219. Jeune M et al. Syndrome familial associant ataxie, surdité et oligophrenic sclérose myocardique d'evolution fatale chez l'un des enfants. *Pediatrie* 1963;18:984–7.

3220. Jewsbury ECO. Insensitivity to pain. *Brain* 1951;74:336–53.

3221. Jia J, Pollock M. Cold nerve injury is enhanced by intermittent cooling. *Muscle Nerve* 1999;22:1644–52.

3222. Jinnah HA, Visser JE, Harris JC et al. Delineation of the motor disorder of Lesch-Nyhan disease. *Brain* 2007;129:1201–17.

3223. Jobsis GJ, Boers JM, Barth PG et al. Bethlem myopathy: A slowly progressive congenital muscular dystrophy with contractures. *Brain* 1999;122:649–55.

3224. Joffroy A. Nature et traitement du goitre exophthalmique. *Progr Med (Paris)* 1893;18:477–80.

3225. Jog MS, Lang AE. Chronic acquired hepatocerebral degeneration: Case reports and new insights. *Mov Disord* 1995;10:714–22.

3226. Johnson J. Thomsen and myotonia congenita. *Med Hist* 1968;**12**:190–4.
3227. Johnson KP, Lepow ML, Johnson RT. California encephalitis. 1. Clinical and epidemiological studies. *Neurology* 1968;**18**:250–4.
3228. Johnson LC, Karpan W. Autonomic correlates of the spontaneous K-complex. *Psychophysiology* 1968;**4**:444–52.
3229. Johnson LM, Randall MJ, Reddihough DS et al. Development of a clinical assessment of quality of movement for unilateral upper-limb function. *Dev Med Child Neurol* 1994;**36**:965–73.
3230. Johnson LV. Adherence syndrome: Pseudoparalysis of lateral or superior rectus muscles. *Arch Ophthal Berlin* 1950;**44**:870–8.
3231. Johnson PC, Rolak LA, Hamilton RH et al. Paraneoplastic vasculitis of nerve: A remote effect of cancer. *Ann Neurol* 1979;**5**:437–44.
3232. Johnson RJ, Bonfiglio M. Lipofibromatous hamartoma of the median nerve. *J Bone Joint Surg* 1969;**51A**:984.
3233. Johnson RT. The pathogenesis of acute viral encephalitis and post-infectious encephalomyelitis. *J Infect Dis* 1987;**155**:359–64.
3234. Johnson RV, Kaplan SR, Blailock ZR. Cerebral venous thrombosis in paroxysmal nocturnal hemoglobinuria. *Neurology* 1970;**20**:681–6.
3235. Johnson TM, Moore HJ. Cranial nerve X and XII paralysis (Tapia's Syndrome) after an interscalene brachial plexus block for a left shoulder Mumford procedure. *Anesthesiology* 1999;**90**:311–2.
3236. Johnson WG. The clinical spectrum of hexoaminidase deficiency diseases. *Neurology* 1981;**31**:1453–6.
3237. Johnson WG, Chutorian AM, Miranda A. A new juvenile hexosaminidase deficiency disease presenting as cerebellar ataxia. *Neurology* 1977;**27**:1012–8.
3238. Johnson WG, Wigger HJ, Karp HR et al. Juvenile spinal muscular atrophy: A new hexosaminidase deficiency phenotype. *Ann Neurol* 1982;**11**:11–6.
3239. Johnston AW, Mckay E. X linked muscular dystrophy with contractures. *J Med Genet* 1986;**23**:591–5.
3240. Johnston JC, Rosenbaum DM, Picone CM et al. Apraxia of eyelid opening secondary to right hemisphere infarction. *Ann Neurol* 1989;**25**:622.
3241. Johnston W, Karpati G, Carpenter S. Late-onset mitochondrial myopathy. *Ann Neurol* 1995;**37**:16–23.
3242. Joliffe N et al. Nicotinic acid deficiency encephalopathy. *JAMA* 1940;**114**:307–12.
3243. Jolly F. Pseudoparalysis myasthenica. *Neurol Zbl* 1895;**14**:34–6.
3244. Jones HR. EMG evaluation of the floppy infant: Differential diagnosis and technical aspects. *Muscle Nerve* 1990;**13**:338–47.
3245. Joplin RJ. The proper digital nerve, vitallium stem arthroplasty and some thoughts about foot surgery in general. *Clin Orthop* 1971;**76**:199–212.
3246. Jordan A, Kelsall AR. Observations on a case of idiopathic hypoparathyroidism. *Arch Internal Medicine* 1951;**87**:242–58.
3247. Jordan BD. Neurologic aspects of boxing. *Arch Neurol* 1987;**44**:453–9.
3248. Jorgenson RJ. Ectodermal dysplasia with hypotrichosis, hypohydrosis, defective teeth, and unusual dermatoglyphics (Basan syndrome?). *B.D.* 1974;**10(4)**:323–5.
3249. Joseph R et al. Maladie familiale associant des convulsions a debut tres précoce, une hyperalbuminorachie et une hyperaminoaciduruie. *Arch Fr Ped* 1958;**15**:374–87.
3250. Josephs KA, Holton JL, Rossor MN. Neurofilament inclusion body disease: A new proteinopathy? *Brain* 2003;**126**:2291–303.
3251. Joubert M, Eisenring JJ, Robb JP, Andermann F. Familial agenesis of the cerebellar vermis. *Neurology* 1969;**19**:813–25.
3252. Joutel A, Tournier-Lasserve E, Bousser MG et al. Hemiplegic migraine. *Presse Med* 1995;**24**:411–4.
3253. Juba A. Contribution to the pathology of ballism. *Psychiatr Neurol (Belg)* 1957;**134**:81–96.
3254. Juberg RC, Hayward JR. A new familial syndrome of oral, cranial, and digital anomalies. *J Pediatr* 1969;**74**:755–62.
3255. Juberg RC, Hellman CD. A new familial form of convulsive disorder and mental retardation, limited to females. *J Pediatr* 1971;**79**:726–32.
3256. Juguilon A, Chad DA, Bradley WG et al. Familial granulovacuolar lobular myopathy with electrical myotonia. *J Neurol Sci* 1983;**62**:261–79.
3257. Julien J, Vital C, Deleplanque B et al. Subacute familial thalamic atrophy with memory disorders and complete insomnia. *Rev Neurol* 1990;**146**:173–8.
3258. Julien J, Vital C, Vallant J et al. Inclusion body myositis. *J Neurol Sci* 1982;**55**:15–24.
3259. Juncos JL, Beal MF. Idiopathic cranial polyneuropathy. *Brain* 1987;**110**:197–211.
3260. Juneja I, Yovic A. Hepatic decerebration. *Neurology* 1972;**22**:537–9.
3261. Jung HH, Hergersberg M, Kneifel S et al. McLeod syndrome: A novel mutation, predominant psychiatric manifestations and distinct striatal imaging findings. *Ann Neurol* 2001;**49**:384–92.
3262. Jungbluth H, Zhou H, Hartley L et al. Minicore myopathy with ophthalmoplegia caused by mutations in the ryanodine receptor type I gene. *Neurology* 2005;**65**:1930–5.
3263. Jusic A, Dogan S, Stojanovic V. Hereditary persistent distal cramps. *J Neurol Neurosurg Psychiatry* 1972;**35**:379–84.
3264. Juvonen V, Hietala M, Paivarinta M et al. Clinical and genetic findings in Finnish ataxia patients with the spinocerebellar ataxia 8 repeat expansion. *Ann Neurol* 2000;**48**:354–61.
3265. Kachi T, Rothwell JC, Cowan JM et al. Writing tremor: Its relation to benign essential tremor. *J Neurol Neurosurg Psychiatry* 1985;**48**:545–50.
3266. Kachi T, Sobue G, Yamamoto M et al. Sensory conduction study in chronic sensory ataxic neuropathy. *J Neurol Neurosurg Psychiatry* 1994;**57**:941–4.
3267. Kaeser HE. Scapuloperoneal muscular atrophy. *Brain* 1965;**88**:407–18.
3268. Kahn A, Mozin MJ, Rebuffat E et al. Difficulty in initiating and maintaining sleep associated with cow's milk allergy in infants. *Sleep* 1987;**10**:116–21.
3269. Kahn E. A neurologic syndrome in infants recovering from malnutrition. *Arch Dis Child* 1954;**29**:256–61.
3270. Kahn RL, Goldfarb AI, Pollack M, Peck A. Brief objective measures for the determination of mental status in the aged. *Am J Psychiatry* 1960;**117**:326–8.
3271. Kaji R. Facts and fancies on Writer's cramp. *Muscle Nerve* 2000;**23**:1313–5.
3272. Kakigi R, Shibasaki H. Generator mechanism of giant somatosensory potentials in cortical reflex myoclonus. *Brain* 1987;**110**:1359–73.
3273. Kakzanis KF. Ideomotor prosodic apraxia. *J Neurol Neurosurg Psychiatry* 2000;694–5.
3274. Kalbe E, Kessler J, Calabresi PA et al. DemTect: A new, sensitive cognitive screening test to support the diagnosis of minimal cognitive impairment and early dementia. *J Geriatr Psychiatry* 2004;**19**:136–43.
3275. Kales A, Jacobson A, Paulson MJ et al. Somnambulism. *Arch Gen Psychiatry* 1966;**14**:586–94.
3276. Kalimo H, Savontaus M-L, Lang H et al. X-linked myopathy with excessive autophagy: A new hereditary muscle disease. *Ann Neurol* 1988;**23**:258–65.
3277. Kalkers NF, de Groot V, Lazeron RHC et al. MS functional composite. *Neurology* 2000;**54**:1233–9.
3278. Kallmann FJ et al. The genetic aspects of primary eunuchoidism. *Am J Ment Defic* 1943;**48**:203–36.
3279. Kalpakian B, Choy AE, Sparkes RS et al. Duane syndrome associated with features

of the cat-eye syndrome and mosaicism for a supernumerary chromosome probably derived from number 22. *J Pediatr Ophthalmol Strabismus* 1988;25:293–7.

3280. Kälviäinen R, Khyuppenen J, Koskenkorva P et al. Clinical picture of EPM1-Unverricht-Lundborg disease. *Epilepsia* 2008;49:549–56.

3281. Kamaki M, Kawamura M, Moriya H et al. Crossed homonymous hemianopia and crossed left hemispatial neglect in a case of Marchiafava-Bignami disease. *J Neurol Neurosurg Psychiatry* 1993;56:1027–32.

3282. Kamm C, Healy DG, Quinn NP et al. The fragile X tremor ataxia syndrome in the differential diagnosis of multiple system atrophy: Data from the EMSA Study Group. *Brain* 2005;128:1855–60.

3283. Kane RE. Neurologic deficits following epidural and spinal anesthesia. *Anesth Analg* 1981;60:150–61.

3284. Kanemoto K, Watanabe Y, Tsuji T et al. Rub epilepsy: A somatosensory evoked reflex epilepsy induced by prolonged cutaneous stimulation. *J Neurol Neurosurg Psychiatry* 2001;70:541–3.

3285. Kanjilal GC. Spontaneous cerebral ventriculostium: Two cases. *J Neurol Neurosurg Psychiatry* 1972;35:676–81.

3286. Kankirawatana P, Leonard H, Ellaway C et al. Early progressive encephalopathy in boys and MEPC2 mutations. *Neurology* 2006;67:164–6.

3287. Kanner L. Autistic disturbances of affective contact. *Nerv Child* 1943;2:217.

3288. Kanno T, Sudo K, Takeuchi I et al. Hereditary deficiency of lactate dehydrogenase M subunit. *Clin Chem Acta* 1980;108:267–76.

3289. Kanouchi T, Yokota T, Kamata T et al. Central pathway of photic reflex myoclonus. *J Neurol Neurosurg Psychiatry* 1997;62:414–7.

3289a. Kannoth S, Thomas SV, Nair S, Sarma PS. Proposed diagnostic criteria for intracranial infectious aneurysms. *J Neurol Neurosurg Psychiatry* 2008;79:943–6.

3290. Kantarjian AD. A syndrome clinically resembling amyotrophic lateral sclerosis following mercurialism. *Neurology* 1961;11:639–44.

3291. Kantola IM, Tarssanen LT. Diagnosis of familial hypokalemic periodic paralysis: Role of the potassium exercise test. *Neurology* 1992;42:2158–61.

3292. Kaplan E, Goodglass H, Weintraub S. *The Boston Naming Test.* Philadelphia: Lea & Febiger, 1983.

3293. Kaplan H. Collateral circulation of the brain. *Neurology* 1961;11:S9–S15.

3294. Kaplan KG, Barasch E, Hirschfeld A et al. Spinal epidural lipomatosis. *Neurology* 1989;39:1031–4.

3295. Kaplan P. X linked recessive inheritance of agenesis of the corpus callosum. *J Med Genet* 1983;20:122–4.

3296. Kaplan P, Genoud D, Ho TW et al. Etiology, neurologic correlations and prognosis in alpha coma. *Aust NZ J Med* 1979;9:448–50.

3297. Kaplan RE, Lacey DJ. Benign familial neonatal and infantile seizures. *Am J Med Genet* 1983;16:595–9.

3298. Kapur NP, Abbott AL, Willison RG. The neuropsychological profile associated with variant Creutzfeldt-Jakob disease. *Brain* 2003;126:2693–702.

3299. Kapur N. The coin-in-the-hand test. *J Neurol Neurosurg Psychiatry* 1993;56:385–6.

3300. Kapur N. Transient epileptic amnesia – a clinical update and a reformulation. *J Neurol Neurosurg Psychiatry* 1993;56:1184–90.

3301. Kar NC, Pearson CM, Verity MA. Muscle fructose 1,6 diphosphate deficiency associated with an atypical central core disease. *J Neurol Sci* 1980;48:243–56.

3302. Karacan I. Painful nocturnal penile erections. *JAMA* 1971;215:1831.

3303. Karadimas CL, Greenstein P, Sue CM et al. Recurrent myoglobinuria due to a missense mutation in the COX 1 gene of mitochondrial DNA. *Neurology* 2000;55:644–9.

3304. Karapanayiotides T, Piechowski-Jozwiak B, Michel P. Hyperechogenic rim sign in internal carotid artery thrombus. *Arch Neurol* 2004;61:773–4.

3305. Karch SB, Urich H. Medulloepithelioma: Definition of an entity. *J Neuropath Exp Neurol* 1972;31:27–53.

3306. Karnath H-O, Johanssen L, Broetz D et al. Posterior thalamic hemorrhage induces pusher syndrome. *Neurology* 2005;64:1014–9.

3307. Karnath H-O, Ferber S, Dichgans J. The origin of contraversive pushing. *Neurology* 2000;55:1298–304.

3308. Karnofsky DA, Burchenal JH, Armistead GC et al. Triethylenemelamine in the treatment of malignant disease. *Arch Int Med* 1951;87:477–516.

3309. Karp BI, Hallett M. Extracorporeal "phantom" tics in Tourette's syndrome. *Neurology* 1996;46:38–40.

3310. Karpati G, Carpenter S. Idiopathic inflammatory myopathies. *Curr Opin Neurol Neurosurg* 1988;1: 806–14.

3311. Karpati G, Carpenter S, Eisen A et al. Multiple peripheral nerve entrapments. *Arch Neurol* 1974;31:418–22.

3312. Karpati G, Carpenter S, Engel AG et al. The syndrome of systemic carnitine deficiency. *Neurology* 1975;25: 16–24.

3313. Karpati G, Carpenter S, Larbrisseau A, Lafontaine R. The Kearns-Shy syndrome. *J Neurol Sci* 1973;19:133–51.

3314. Karpati G, Carpenter S, Wolfe LS et al. Juvenile dystonic lipidosis: An unusual form of neurovisceral storage disease. *Neurology* 1977;27:32–42.

3315. Karpati G, Engel WK. "Type grouping" in skeletal muscles after experimental reinnervation. *Neurology* 1968;18:447–55.

3316. Karpati G et al. Myopathy caused by a deficiency of calcium-ATP in sarcoplasmic reticulum. *Ann Neurol* 1986;20:33–49.

3317. Karsch J. Erbliche Augenmissbildung in Verbindung mit Spalyhand und -Fuss. *Zschr Augenheilk* 1936;89:274–9.

3318. Karson CN. Spontaneous eye-blink rates and dopaminergic systems. *Brain* 1983;106:643–53.

3319. Kasarskis EJ, Winslow M. When did Lou Gehrig's personal illness begin? *Neurology* 1989;39:1243–5.

3320. Kasch H, Bach FW, Jensen TS. Handicap after acute whiplash injury. *Neurology* 2001;56:1637–43.

3321. Kase CS. Case records of the M.G.H. (cerebral amyloid angiopathy). *N Engl J Med* 1988;318:623–31.

3322. Kasim S, Moo LR, Zschocke J et al. Phenylketonuria presenting in adulthood as progressive spastic paraparesis with dementia. *J Neurol Neurosurg Psychiatry* 2001;71:795–7.

3323. Kasman M, Bernstein L, Schulman S. Chronic polyradiculoneuropathy of infancy. *Neurology* 1976;26:565–73.

3324. Katz DA, Naseem A, Horoupian DS et al. Familial multisystem atrophy with possible thalamic dementia. *Neurology* 1984;34:1213–7.

3325. Katz DI, Alexander MP, Mandell AM. Dementia following strokes in the mesencephalon and diencephalon. *Arch Neurol* 1987;44:1127–33.

3326. Katz J, Wolfe GI, Burns DK et al. Isolated neck extensor myopathy: A common cause of dropped head syndrome. *Neurology* 1996;46:917–21.

3327. Katz JD, Ropper AH. Progressive necrotic myelopathy. *Arch Neurol* 2000;57:355–61. (Abstract)

3328. Katz JS, Rando TA, Barohn RJ. Late-onset distal muscular dystrophy affecting the posterior calves. *Muscle Nerve* 2003;28:443–8.

3329. Katz JS, Barohn RJ, Kojan S et al. Axonal multifocal motor neuropathy, without conduction block or other features of demyelination. *Neurology* 2002;58: 615–20.

3330. Katz JS, Saperstein DS, Gronseth G et al. Distal acquired demyelinating symmetric neuropathy. *Neurology* 2000;54:615–20.

3331. Katz JS, Wolfe GI, Anderss PB et al. Brachial amyotrophic diplegia – a slowly progressive motor neurone disorder. *Neurology* 1999;53:1071–6.

3332. Katz MM, Lyerly SB. Methods of measuring adjustment and social behaviour in the community 1. *Psychol Rep* 1963;13:503–35.

3333. Katz S. Assessing self-maintenance: Activities of daily living, mobility and instrumental activities of daily living. *J Am Geriatr Soc* 1983;31:721.

3334. Katz S, Ford AB, Moskowitz RW et al. Studies of illness in the aged: The index of ADL – a standardized measure of biological and psychosocial function. *JAMA* 1963;185:914–9.

3335. Katzin RC. Arm rolling test. *Neurology* 1995;45:203.

3336. Katzman R. Alzheimer's disease. *N Engl J Med* 1986;314:964–73.

3337. Kaufman B. The "Empty Sella Turcica": A manifestation of the intrasellar subarachnoid space. *Radiology* 1968;90:931–41.

3338. Kaufman DK, Kimmel DW, Parisi J et al. A familial syndrome with cutaneous malignant melanoma and cerebral astrocytoma. *Neurology* 1993;43:1728–31.

3339. Kaufman MD, Hopkins LC, Hurwitz BJ. Progressive sensory neuropathy in patients without carcinoma. *Ann Neurol* 1981;9:237–42.

3340. Kaufman RL, et al. An oculocerebral facial syndrome. *Birth Defects* 1971;7(1):135–8.

3341. Kaufman S, et al. Phenylketonuria due to a deficiency of dihydropteridine reductase. *N Engl J Med* 1975;293:785.

3342. Kaufman S et al. Hyperphenylalaninemia due to a deficiency of biopterin. *N Engl J Med* 1978;299:673.

3343. Kaufmann WE, Galaburda AM. Cerebrocortical microdysgenesis in neurologically normal subjects: A histopathologic study. *Neurology* 1989;39:238–44.

3344. Kavanaugh GJ, Svien HJ, Holman CB et al. "Pseudoclaudication" syndrome produced by compression of the cauda equina. *JAMA* 1968;206:2477–81.

3345. Kavèiè DB, Vodusek OB. A historical perspective on cerebral palsy as a concept and a diagnosis. *Eur J Neurol* 2005;12:582–7.

3346. Kawamura M, Hirayama K, Shinohara Y et al. Alloesthesia. *Brain* 1987;110: 225–36.

3347. Kawanami T, Kato T, Daimon M et al. Hereditary ceruloplasmin deficiency: Clinicopathological study of a patient. *J Neurol Neurosurg Psychiatry* 1996;61: 506–9.

3348. Kayden NJ, Reagan TJ, Mize CE et al. Diffuse cerebral sclerosis erroneously reported as Refsum's disease. *Arch Neurol* 1973;28:304–7.

3349. Kaye JA. Diagnostic challenges in dementia. *Neurology* 1998;51(**Suppl.** 1):S45–S52.

3350. Kaye K, Grigsby J, Robbins LJ et al. Prediction of independent functioning and behavior problems in geriatric patients. *J Am Geriatr Soc* 1990;38:1304–10.

3351. Kayser B. Ueber einen Fall von angeborener grunlicher Verfarbung der Cornea. *Klin Mbl Augenh* 1902;40:22–5.

3352. Kazemi-Esfarjani P, Skomorowska E, Jensen TS et al. A nonischemic forearm exercise test for McArdle disease. *Ann Neurol* 2002;52:153–9.

3353. Keane JR. Spastic eyelids: Failure of levator inhibition in unconscious states. *Arch Neurol* 1975;32:695–8.

3354. Keane JR. Gaze-evoked blepharoclonus. *Ann Neurol* 1978;3:243–5.

3355. Keane JR. Neuro-ophthalmologic signs and symptoms of hysteria. *Neurology* 1982;32:757–62.

3356. Keane JR. Galloping tongue: Post-traumatic, episodic, rhythmic movements. *Neurology* 1984;34:251–2.

3357. Keane JR. Pretectal pseudobobbing: Five patients with "V"-pattern convergence nystagmus. *Arch Neurol* 1985;42:592–4.

3358. Keane JR. Wrong-way deviation of the tongue with hysterical hemiparesis. *Neurology* 1986;36:1406–7.

3359. Keane JR. Lid opening apraxia in Wilson's disease. *J Clin Neuro-Ophthalmol* 1988;8:31.

3360. Keane JR. Neurectasy. *Neurology* 1990;40:829–31.

3361. Keane JR. The pretectal syndrome:206 patients. *Neurology* 1990;40:684–90.

3362. Keane JR, Itabashi HH. Upbeat nystagmus: Clinicopathologic study of two patients. *Neurology* 1987;37:491.

3363. Kearns TP. Differential diagnosis of central retinal vein obstruction. *Ophthalmology* 1983;90:475–80.

3364. Kearns TP, Sayre GP. Retinitis pigmentosa, external ophthalmoplegia and complete heart block. *Arch Ophthal Berlin* 1958;60:280–9.

3365. Keay AJ, Lewis IC. The Bonnevie-Ullrich syndrome. *Arch Dis Child* 1954;29:424.

3366. Keesey JC. Contemporary opinions about Mary Walker. *Neurology* 1998;51:1433–9.

3367. Keime-Guibert F, Napolitano M, Delattre J-Y. Neurological complications of radiotherapy and chemotherapy. *J Neurol* 1998;245:695–708.

3368. Keipert JA et al. A new syndrome of broad terminal phalanges and facial abnormalities. *Aust Paediatr J* 1973;9:10–3.

3369. Keith RA, Granger CV, Hamilton BB, Sherwin FS. The functional independence measure: A new tool for rehabilitation. In Eisenberg MG, Grzesiak RC eds. *Advances in Clinical Rehabilitation*, New York: Springer, 1987.

3370. Keller M, Hiltbrunner B, Dill C et al. Reversible neuropsychological deficits after mild traumatic brain injury. *J Neurol Neurosurg Psychiatry* 2000;68:761–4.

3371. Kelley RI et al. Neonatal adrenoleukodystrophy: New cases, biochemical studies and differentiation from Zellweger and related peroxisomal polydystrophy syndromes. *Am J Med Genet* 1986;23:869–901.

3372. Kelley RI, Moser HW. Hyperpipecolic acidemia in neonatal adrenoleukodystrophy. *Am J Med Genet* 1984;19:791–5.

3373. Kelly EC. *Encyclopedia of Medical Sources*. Baltimore: Williams and Wilkins, 1948.

3374. Kelly JJ. Peripheral neuropathies associated with monoclonal proteins: A clinical review. *Muscle Nerve* 1985;8:138–50.

3375. Kelly JP, Rosenberg JH. Diagnosis and management of concussion in sports. *Neurology* 1997;48:575–80.

3376. Kelly R. Colloid cysts of the third ventricle. *Brain* 1951;74:23–65.

3377. Kelly RI, Data NS, Dobyns WB et al. Neonatal adrenoleukodystrophy. *Am J Med Genet* 1986;23:869.

3378. Kelly RI et al. The association of the DiGeorge anomaly with partial monosomy of chromosome 22. *J Pediatr* 1982;101:197.

3379. Kelly TE. Teratogenicity of anticonvulsant drugs. *Am J Med Genet* 1984;19:413–34.

3380. Kemper T. Paul Ivan Yakovlev:1894 – 1983. *Arch Neurol* 1984;41:536–40.

3381. Kendall FP, McCreary EK, Provance PG. *Muscles: Testing and Function*. Baltimore: Williams and Wilkins, 1993.

3382. Kennard C, Swash M. Acute viral encephalitis. *Brain* 1981;104:129–48.

3383. Kennaway NG, Buist NRM. Metabolic studies in a patient with hepatic cytosol tyrosine aminotransferase deficiency. *Pediatr Res* 1971;5:287.

3384. Kennedy F. Retrobulbar neuritis as an exact diagnostic sign of certain tumors and abscesses in the frontal lobes. *Am J Med* 1911;142:355–68.

3385. Kennedy WR, Alter M, Sung JH. Progressive proximal spinal and bulbar muscular atrophy of late onset. A sex-linked recessive trait. *Neurology* 1968;18:671–80.

3386. Kennedy WR, Sakuta M, Sutherland D et al. Quantitation of the sweating defect in diabetes mellitus. *Ann Neurol* 1984;15:482–8.

3387. Kenney C, Diamond A, Mejia N. Psychogenic tremor. *J Neurol Sci* 2007;263:94–9.

3388. Kerber KA, Jen JC, Lee H. A new episodic ataxia syndrome with linkage to chromosome 19q13. *Arch Neurol* 2007;64:749–52.

3389. Kerkhoff G. Neurovisual rehabilitation: Recent developments and future directions. *J Neurol Neurosurg Psychiatry* 2000;68:691–706.

3390. Kern WH. Proliferative Myositis: A pseudosarcomatous reaction to injury. *Arch Path* 1960;69:209–16.

3391. Kernig VM. Ein Krankheitssymptom der acuten Meningitis. *St Petersb Med Wschr* 1882;7:398.

3392. Kernohan JW, Sayre GP. *Atlas of Tumor Pathology: Tumors of the CNS.* Washington, DC: Armed Forces Institute of Pathology, 1993.

3393. Kernohan JW, Woltman HW. Incisura of the crus due to contralateral brain tumour. *Arch Neurol Psychiatry* 1929;21:274–87.

3394. Kerns RD, Turk DC, Rudy TE. The West Haven-Yale multidimensional pain inventory. *Pain* 1985;23:345–56.

3395. Kerr A, Derbes VJ. The syndrome of cough syncope. *Ann Int Med* 1953;39:1240–53.

3396. Kerr GW, Parke TR. Scombroid poisoning – a pseudoallergic syndrome. *J Roy Soc Med* 1998;91:83–4.

3397. Kerrigan JF, Aleck KA, Tarby TJ et al. Fumaric aciduria: Clinical and imaging features. *Ann Neurol* 2000;47:583–8.

3398. Kertesz A. Frontotemporal dementia-Pick's disease. *Can J Neurol Sci* 2006;33:141–8.

3399. Kertesz A, Munoz D. Relationship between frontotemporal dementia and corticobasal degeneration/progressive supranuclear palsy. *Dement Geriatr Cogn Disord* 2004;17:282–6.

3400. Kertesz A. Paroxysmal kinesigenic choreoathetosis. *Neurology* 1967;17:680–90.

3401. Kertesz A. *The Western Aphasia Battery.* New York: Grune and Stratton, 1982.

3402. Kertesz A, Benson F. Neologistic jargon – a clinicopathological study. *Cortex* 1970;6:362–86.

3403. Kertesz A, Davidson W, Fox H. Frontal behavioral inventory: Diagnostic criteria for frontal lobe dementia. *Can J Neurol Sci* 1997;24:29–36.

3404. Kertesz A, Hudson L, MacKenzie IRA et al. The pathology and nosology of primary progressive aphasia. *Neurology* 1994;44:2065–72.

3405. Kertesz A, Martinez-Lage P, Davidson W et al. The corticobasal degeneration syndrome overlaps progressive aphasia and frontotemporal dementia. *Neurology* 2000;55:1368–75.

3406. Kertesz A, Nicholson I, Cancelliere A et al. Motor impersistence: A right-hemisphere syndrome. *Neurology* 1985;35:662–6.

3407. Kertesz A, Poole E. The aphasia quotient: The taxonomic approach to measurement of aphasic disability. *Can J Neurol Sci* 1974;1:7–16.

3408. Kertesz A, Sheppard A, MacKenzie R. Localization in transcortical sensory aphasia. *Arch Neurol* 1982;39:475–8.

3409. Keshavan MS. The ear wigglers: Tics of the ear in ten patients. *Am J Psychiatry* 1988;145:1462–3.

3410. Keutel J et al. Eine wahrscheinlich autosomal recessive vererbte Skeletmissbildung mit Humeroradialsynostose. *Humangenetik* 1970;9:43–53.

3411. Keynes G. The history of myasthenia gravis. *Med Hist* 1961;5:313–25.

3412. Khaleeli AA, Levy RD, Edwards RH et al. The neuromuscular features of acromegaly: A clinical and pathological study. *J Neurol Neurosurg Psychiatry* 1984;47:1009–115.

3413. Khalifeh RR, Zellweger H. Hereditary sensory neuropathy with spinal cord disease. *Neurol Minneap* 1963;13: 405–11.

3414. Khan SF, Ashalatha R, Syam K. Periodic EEG pattern in neuro-dengue – a novel observation. *Eur J Neurol* 2005;12: 1009–14.

3415. Khurana RK, Watabiki S, Hebel JR et al. Cold face test in the assessment of trigeminal-brainstem-vagal function in humans. *Ann Neurol* 1980;7:144–9.

3416. Khurana VG, Perez-Terzic CM, Petersen R et al. Singing paraplegia: A distinictive manifestation of a spinal dural arteriovenous malformation. *Neurology* 2002;58:279–81.

3417. Kibler RF, Rose FC. Peripheral neuropathy in the collagen diseases. *BMJ* 1960;1:1781–4.

3418. Kidd D, Burton B, Plant GT et al. Chronic relapsing inflammatory optic neuropathy (CRION). *Brain* 2003;126:276–84.

3419. Kidd D, Steuer A, Denman AM et al. Neurological complications in Behcet's syndrome. *Brain* 1999;122:2183–94.

3420. Kidd D, Wilson PL, Unwin B. Paroxysmal intracranial hypertension. *Eur J Neurol* 2005;12:1002–5.

3421. Kidd M. An electron microscopical study of a case of atypical cerebral lipidosis. *Acta Neuropathol* 1967;9:70.

3422. Kienbock R. Kritik der sogenannten "traumatischen Syringomyelie". *Jb Psychiat* 1902;21:50–210.

3423. Kilaru S, Bergqvist AGC. Myoclonic astatic epilepsy: The Children's Hospital of Philadelphia experience. *Epilepsia* 2005;46(Suppl. 8):153 Abs No.2. 185.

3424. Kilgare S, Laker GW. Hallervorden-Spatz syndrome and brain iron metabolism. *Arch Neurol Psychiatry* 1946;56:401.

3425. Kiloh LG, Nevin S. Progressive dystrophy of external ocular muscles (ocular myopathy). *Brain* 1951;74:115–43.

3426. Kiloh LG, Nevin S. Isolated neuritis of the anterior interosseous nerve. *BM J* 1952;1:850–1.

3427. Kim JH, Shucart WA, Haimovici H. Symptomatic arachnoid diverticula. *Arch Neurol* 1974;31:35–7.

3428. Kim JS. Smile-wink phenomenon. *J Neurol* 2001;248:389–93.

3429. Kim JY, Lee KW, Roh JK et al. A clinical study of benign focal amyotrophy. *J Korean Med Sci* 1994;9:145–54.

3430. Kim Y, Pakiam AS-I, Lang AE. Historical and clinical features of psychogenic tremor: A review of 70 cases. *Can J Neurol Sci* 1999;2:190–5.

3431. Kim JS, Lopez I, DiPatre DL et al. Internal auditory artery infarction. *Neurology* 1999;52:40–4.

3432. Kimber E, Tajsharghy H, Kroksmark A-K et al. A mutation in the fast skeletal muscle troponin I gene causes myopathy and distal arthrogryposis. *Neurology* 2006;67:597–601.

3433. Kimber J, McLean BN, Prevett M, Hammans SR. Allgrove or 4 "A" syndrome: An autosomal recessive syndrome causing multisystem neurological disease. *J Neurol Neurosurg Psychiatry* 2003;74:654–7.

3434. Kimoff RJ, Cosio MG, McGregor M. Clinical features and treatment of obstructive sleep apnea. *Can Med Assn J* 1991;144:689–95.

3435. Kimura J. *Electrodiagnosis in Diseases of Nerve and Muscle.* Philadelphia: F.A. Davis, 1983.

3436. Kindler P. Morning glory syndrome: Unusual congenital disk abnormality. *Am J Ophthalmol* 1970;69:376.

3437. Kindstrand E, Nilsson BY, Hovmark A et al. Peripheral neuropathy in acrodermatitis chronica atrophicans – a late Borrelia manifestation. *Acta Neurol Scand* 1997;95:338–45.

3438. King JO, Denborough MA. Anesthetic induced malignant hyperexia in children. *J Pediatr* 1973;83:37–40.

3439. King N, Crawford S, Wenden FJ et al. The Rivermead post concussion symptoms questionnaire: A measure of symptoms commonly experienced after head injury and its reliability. *J Neurol* 1995;242:587–92.

3440. Kingston W, Moxley RT, Griggs RC et al. Flier syndrome: Muscle cramps, acanthocytosis nigricans, acral hypertrophy and insulin resistance. *Ann Neurol* 1982;12:79.

3441. Kinney H, Burger PC, Vogel FSY. Subacute diencephalic angioencephalopathy: Report of an additional case. *J Neurol Sci* 1980;45: 73–81.

3442. Kinney HC, Filiano JJ, Brazy JE et al. Congenital apnea with medullary and olivary hypoplasia. *Clin Neuropathol* 1989;8:163–73.

3443. Kinsbourne M. Myoclonic encephalopathy of infants. *J Neurol Neurosurg Psychiatry* 1962;25:271–6.

3444. Kinsbourne M. Hiatus hernia with contortions of the neck. *Lancet* 1964;1:1058–61.

3445. Kinsbourne M. The cerebral basis of lateral asymmetries in attention. *Acta Psychol* 1970;33:193–201.

3446. Kinsbourne M, Warrington EK. A study of finger agnosia. *Brain* 1962;85:47–66.

3447. Kinsella SM, Tuckey JP. Perioperative bradycardia and asystole: Relationship to vasovagal syncope and the Bezold-Jarisch reflex. *Br J Anaesth* 2001;86:859–68.

3448. Kinton L et al. Partial epilepsy with pericentral spikes. *Ann Neurol* 2002;51:740–9.

3449. Kipps CM, Hodges JR. Cognitive assessment for clinicians. *J Neurol Neurosurg Psychiatry* 2005;76:i22–i30.

3450. Kirby DM, Crawford M, Cleary MA et al. Respiratory chain complex 1deficiency: An underdiagnosed energy generation disorder. *Neurology* 1999;52:1255–64.

3451. Kirk A Boyle CAJ. Radial neglect is caused by vertical neglect of an internal representation. *Can J Neurol Sci* 1994;21(**Suppl.** 2):S51. (Abstract)

3452. Kirk A, Heilman KM. Auricular myoclonus. *Can J Neurol Sci* 1991;18:503–4.

3453. Kirkham TH. The ocular symptomatology of pituitary tumours. *Proc Roy Soc Med* 1972;65:517–8.

3454. Kirschner J, Bönnemann CG. The congenital and limb-girdle muscular dystrophies. *Arch Neurol* 2004;61: 189–99.

3455. Kirshner HS, Tanridag O, Thurman L et al. Progressive aphasia without dementia: Two cases with focal spongiform degeneration. *Ann Neurol* 1987;22:527–32.

3456. Kisch B. Horners syndrome: An American discovery. *Bull Med Hist* 1951;25:284–8.

3457. Kish SJ, Dixon LM, Burnham WM et al. Brain neurotransmitters in glycine encephalopathy. *Ann Neurol* 1988;24:458–61.

3458. Kissel P, Arnould G, Andre JM. Incidence des accidents vasculaires cerebraux au cours des conjonctivo dysplasies héréditaires. *J Genet Hum* 1972;29: 151–67.

3459. Kistler JP, Lott IT, Kolodny EH et al. Mannosidosis: New clinical presentation, enzyme studies, and carbohydrate analysis. *Arch Neurol* 1977;34:45–51.

3460. Kitagawa M, Fukushima J, Tashiro K. Relationship between antisaccades and the clinical symptoms in Parkinson's disease. *Neurology* 1994;44:2285–9.

3461. Kitamoto T, Amano N, Terao Y et al. A new inherited prion disease (PrP-P105L mutation) showing spastic paraparesis. *Ann Neurol* 1993;34:808–13.

3462. Kite WC. Seizures associated with the Catlin mark. *Neurology* 1961;11:345–8.

3463. Kitka DG, Breuer A, Wilbourn AJ. Thoracic root pain in diabetes. *Ann Neurol* 1982;11:80–3.

3464. Kiuru S, Seppalainen A-M. Neuropathy in familial amyloidosis, Finnish type (FAF): Electrophysiological studies. *Muscle Nerve* 1994;17:299–304.

3465. Kivlin JD, Sanborn GE, Myers GG. The cherry-red spot in Tay-Sachs and other storage diseases. *Ann Neurol* 1985;17:356–60.

3466. Kiwaki T, Umehara F, Takashima H et al. Hereditary motor and sensory neuropathy with myelin folding and juvenile onset glaucoma. *Neurology* 2000;55:392–7.

3467. Kjellin K. Familial spastic paraplegia with amyotrophy, oligophrenia and central retinal degeneration. *Arch Neurol* 1959;1:133–40.

3468. Kjer P. Infantile optic atrophy with dominant mode of inheritance. *Acta Ophthalmol* 1959;(**Suppl.** 54):1.

3469. Klass DW, Westmoreland BF. Nonepileptogenic epileptiform electroencephalographic activity. *Ann Neurol* 1985;18:627–35.

3470. Klatzky RL. *Human Memory*. San Francisco: W.H. Freeman and Co., 1980.

3471. Klawans HL. Hemiparkinsonism as a late complication of hemiatrophy: A new syndrome. *Neurology* 1981;31:625–8.

3472. Klebe S, Hamid Azzedine H, Durr A et al. Autosomal recessive spastic paraplegia (SPG30) with mild ataxia and sensory neuropathy maps to chromosome 2q37.3. *Brain* 2006;122:1456–62.

3473. Klein C. Myoclonus and myoclonus-dystonia. In Pulst SM ed. *Genetics of Movement Disorders*, pp 451–71. New York: Academic press, 2003.

3474. Klein D. *Archiv Julius Klaus-Stift* 1947;22:336.

3475. Klein O, Pierre-Kahn A et al. Dandy-Walker malformation: Prenatal diagnosis and prognosis. *Childs Nerv Syst* 2003;19:484–9.

3476. Klein R, Hadow JE, DeLuca C. Familial congenital disorder resembling Stiff–Man syndrome. *Am J Dis Child* 1972;124: 730–1.

3477. Kleine BU, Stegeman DF, Schelhaas HJ. Firing patterns of fasciculations in ALS. *Neurology* 2008;70:353–9.

3478. Kleine W. Periodische Schlafsucht. *Mschr Psychiat* 1925;57:285–320.

3479. Kleist K. Gegenhalten (Motorischer Negativsmus) Zwangsgreifen und Thalamus Opticus. *Monatsschr Psychiatr Neurol* 1927;65:317.

3480. Kline LB, Hoyt WF. The Tolosa-Hunt syndrome. *J Neurol Neurosurg Psychiatry* 2001;71:577–82.

3481. Klingele TC, Burde RM, Rappazzo JA et al. Paraneoplastic retinopathy. *J Clin Neuro-Ophthalmol* 1984;4:239–45.

3482. Klingman WO, Hodges RG. Acute ataxia of unknown origin in children. *J Pediatr* 1944;24:536–43.

3483. Klintworth GK. The neurological manifestations of osteopetrosis. *Neurology* 1963;13:512–9.

3484. Klippel M. Concerning spontaneous thumb flexion in hemiplegic contractures. *Rev Neurol* 1909;17:506–7.

3485. Klippel M, Feil A. Un cas d'absence des vertèbres cervicales avec cage thoracic remontant jusqu'a la base du crâne (cage thoracique cervicale). *Nouv Icon Salpet* 1912;25:223–50.

3486. Klippel M, Felstein E. L'hypertrophie cranienne simple familiale. *Nouv Icon Salpet* 1913;26:445–51.

3487. Klippel M, Trenaunay P. Du noevus variqueux osteo-hypertrophique. *AGMP* 1900;3:641–72.

3488. Klockgether T, Ludkte R, Kramer B et al. The natural history of degenerative ataxia: A retrospective study in 466 patients. *Brain* 1998;121:589–600.

3489. Kloepfer HW. *Proc 10th Int Conf Genet Montreal* 1958;2:146. Toronto, Univ. Toronto Press.

3490. Kluin KJ, Foster NL, Berent S et al. Perceptual analysis of speech disorders in progressive supranuclear palsy. *Neurology* 1993;43:563–6.

3491. Kluver H, Bucy PC. "Psychic blindness" and other symptoms following bilateral temporal lobectomy in rhesus monkeys. *Am J Physiol* 1937;119:352–3.

3492. Kmiec T, Jurkiewicz E, Jozwiak S et al. Usefulness of brain MRI in diagnosis of NBIA in PKAN and non–PKAN patients. *Neuropediatrics* 2006;37.

3493. Knapp HJ. On the formation of dark angioid streaks as an unusual metamorphosis of retinal hemorrhage. *Arch Ophthalmol* 1892;21:289–92.

3494. Knapp PC. Astasia-abasia, with the report of a case of paroxysmal trepidant abasia, associated with paralysis agitans. *J Nerv Ment Dis* 1891;17:673–703.

3495. Knaus WA, Draper EA, Wagner DP et al. APACHE II: A severity of disease classification system. *Crit Care Med* 1985;13:818–29.

3496. Knaus WA et al. Trauma severity classification. *Crit Care Med* 1985;13:818–29.

3497. Knight MA, McKinlay Gardner J, Bahlo M et al. Dominantly inherited ataxia and dysphonia with dentate calcification: Spinocerebellar ataxia type 20. *Brain* 2004;127:1172–81.

3498. Knight RSG, Anslow P, Theaker JM. Neoplastic angioendotheliosis: A case of subacute dementia with unusual cerebral CT appearances and a review of the literature. *J Neurol Neurosurg Psychiatry* 1987;50:1022–8.

3499. Knopman DS, Knapp MJ, Gracon SI et al. The Clinician Interview-Based Impression (CIBI). *Neurology* 1994;44: 2315–21.

3500. Knopman DS, Mastri AR, Frey WH et al. Dementia lacking distinctive histological features. *Neurology* 1990;40:251–6.

3501. Knopman DS, Sung JH, Davis D. Progressive familial leukodystrophy of late onset. Neurology 1996;46:429–34.

3502. Knox DL. Ischemic ocular inflammation. Am J Ophthalmol 1965;60:995–1001.

3503. Knox DL, Clark DB, Schuster FF. Benign VI nerve palsies in children. Pediatrics 1967;40:560–4.

3504. Kny E. Concerning paramyoclonus multiplex (Friedreich). *Arch Psychiatr Nervenkr* 1888;19:577–90.

3505. Kobari M, Nogawa S, Sugimoto Y et al. Familial idiopathic brain calcification with autosomal dominant inheritance. Neurology 1997;48: 645–9.

3506. Kobayashi JS, Clarke M, Sullivan T. Familial congenital corneal anesthesia. *Can J Neurol Sci* 1993;(**Suppl.** 2):S37.

3507. Kobayashi O, Hayashi Y, Arahata K et al. Congenital muscular dystrophy. Neurology 1996;46:815–8.

3508. Kobori JA, Herrick MK, Urich H. Arhinencephaly. *Brain* 1987;110: 237–60.

3509. Kocher T. Zur Verhuntung des Cretinismus und cretinoider Zustande nach neuen Forschungen. *Dtsch Z Nervenklinik* 1892;34:556–626.

3510. Koebbe CJ, Sherman JD, Warnick RE. Distant wounded glioma syndrome: Report of two cases. *Neurosurgery* 2001;48:940–3.

3511. Koehler PJ, Endtz LJ. Between Magendie and Brown–Séquard: Isaac van Deen's spinal hemisections. *Neurology* 1989;39:446–8.

3512. Koeppen AH, Dickson AC, Chu RC et al. The pathogenesis of superficial siderosis of the central nervous system. Ann Neurol 1993;34:646–53.

3513. Koerber HL. Ueber drei Falle von Retraktionsbewegung des Bulbus. *Ophth Klin* 1903;7:65–7.

3514. Kohlschutter A, Chappuis D, Meier C et al. Familial epilepsy and yellow teeth – a disease of the CNS associated with enamel hypoplasia. *Helv Pediat Acta* 1974;29:283–94.

3515. Koizumi J, Ofuku K, Sakuma K et al. CNS changes in Usher's syndrome with mental disorder: CT, MRS, and PET findings. *J Neurol Neurosurg Psychiatry* 1988;51:987–90.

3516. Koizumi K, Levine DG, Brooks CM. Effect of tetrodotoxin (puffer fish toxin) on the central nervous system. *Neurology* 1967;17:395–404.

3517. Kolker S, Koeller DM, Okun JG et al. Pathomechanisms of neurodegeneration in Glutaryl-CoA cyst dehydrogenase deficiency. *Arch Neurol* 2004;55:7–12.

3518. Koller WC. Adult onset foot dystonia. *Neurology* 1984;34:703.

3519. Koller WC. How accurately can Parkinson's disease be diagnosed? *Neurology* 1992;42**Suppl.**:6–16.

3520. Kolmel HW. Complex visual hallucinations in the hemianopic field. *J Neurol Neurosurg Psychiatry* 1985;48: 29–38.

3521. Kolodny EH. Agenesis of the corpus callosum: A marker for inherited metabolic disease? *Neurology* 1989;39:847–8.

3522. Kolodny EH, Cable WJL. Inborn errors of metabolism. Ann Neurol 1982;11: 221–32.

3523. Koman LA, Smith BP, Shilt JS. Cerebral palsy. *Lancet* 2004;363:1619–31.

3524. Komar J, Varga B. Syndrome of the rectus abdominis muscle. *J Neurol* 1975;210:121–5.

3525. Kondo K, Tsubaki T, Sakamoto F. The Ryukyuan muscular atrophy. J Neurol Sci 1970;11:359–82.

3526. Konigsmark BW. Hereditary deafness in man. *N Engl J Med* 1969;281: 713–20.

3527. Konigsmark BW, Weiner LP. The olivopontocerebellar atrophies: A review. *Medicine* 1970;49:227–41.

3528. Kono N, et al. Amyotrophy with acute haemorrhagic conjunctivitis. *J Infect Dis* 1974;129:590.

3529. Konrad PN et al. Gamma glutamyl cysteine deficiency. *N Engl J Med* 1972;286:557.

3530. Kopell HP, Thompson WAL. *Peripheral Entrapment Neuropathies*. Malabar: Robert Krieger Publ Co, 1976.

3531. Kopell HP, Thompson WAL, Postel AH. Entrapment neuropathy of the ilioinguinal nerve. *N Engl J Med* 1962;266:16.

3532. Korein J, Codder DR, Mowrey FH. The clinical syndrome of paroxysmal paralytic myoglobinuria. *Neurology* 1959;9: 767–85.

3533. Korenblat P, Wedner H, Whyte M et al. Systemic Mastocytosis. *Arch Int Med* 1984;144:2249–53.

3534. Korf B, Waldman JK, Levy HL et al. Bilateral lucency of the globus pallidus complicating methylmalonic acidemia. *Ann Neurol* 1986;20:364–6.

3535. Kori SH. Interventional neurology. *Neurology* 1993;43:2395–9.

3536. Kors EE, Terwindt GM, Vermeulen FLMG et al. Delayed cerebral edema and fatal coma after minor head trauma: Role of the CACNA1A calcium channel subunit gene and relationship with familial hemiplegic migraine. *Ann Neurol* 2001;49:753–60.

3537. Korsakov SS. Ob alkogol'nom paraliche. *Vest Psikhiat* 1887;4.

3538. Korten JJ, Notermans SLH, Frenken CWGM et al. Familial essential myoclonus. *Brain* 1974;97:131–8.

3539. Kosaka K. Diffuse neurofibrillary tangles with calcification: A new presenile dementia. *J Neurol Neurosurg Psychiatry* 1994;57:594–6.

3540. Koski L, Lacoboni MN, Mazziotta JC. Deconstructing stroke: Understanding disorders of intentional movement after stroke. *Curr Opin Neurol Neurosurg* 2002;15:363–71.

3541. Koskinen T, Sainio K, Rapola J et al. Sensory neuropathy in infantile onset spinocerebellar ataxia (IOSCA). *Muscle Nerve* 1994;17:509–15.

3542. Kost GJ, Verity MA. A new variant of late-onset myophopsphorylase deficiency. *Muscle Nerve* 1980;3:195–201.

3543. Kothari MJ, Macintosh K, Heistand M et al. Medial antebrachial cutaneous sensory studies in the evaluation of neurogenic thoracic outlet syndrome. *Muscle Nerve* 1998;21:647–9.

3544. Koussa S, Roukoz H, Rizk T et al. Megalencephalic leukoencephalopathy with subcortical cysts: A study of a Lebanese family and a review of the literature. *Rev Neurol (Paris)* 2005;161:183–91.

3545. Kousseff BG. Sacral meningocele with conotruncal heart defects: A possible autosomal recessive trait. *Pediatrics* 1984;74:395–8.

3546. Koutras A. Myositis with Kawasaki's disease. *Am J Dis Child* 1982;136:78–9.

3547. Kovanen J, Somer Heal, Schroeder P. Acute myopathy associated with gasoline sniffing. *Neurology* 1983;33:629.

3548. Kozhevnikov AY. Osobyi: vid kortikalnoi epilepsii. *Med Obozr* 1894;42:97–118.

3549. Kozlowski K, Maroteaux P, Spranger J. La dysostose spondylometaphysaire. *Presse Med* 1967;75:2769–74.

3550. Krabbe KH. A new familial infantile form of diffuse brain sclerosis. *Brain* 1916;39:74–114.

3551. Krabbe KH. Congenital generalised muscular atrophies. *Acta Psychiatr Scand* 1958;33:94.

3552. Kral VA. Senescent forgetfulness: Benign and malignant. *Can Med Assn J* 1962;86:257–60.

3553. Kramer JH, Reed BR, Mungas D et al. Executive dysfunction in subcortical ischaemic vascular disease. *J Neurol Neurosurg Psychiatry* 2002;72:217–20.

3554. Kramer RE, Luders H, Goldstick LP et al. Ictus emeticus: An electroclinical analysis. *Neurology* 1988;38:1048–52.

3555. Krams M, Quinton R, Mayston MJ et al. Mirror movements in X-linked Kallmann's syndrome. II A PET study. *Brain* 1997;120(7):217–229.

3556. Krane RJ, Siroky MB. *Clinical Neuro-Urology*. Boston: Little, Brown, 1979.

3557. Krarup C, Stewart JD, Sumner AJ et al. A syndrome of asymmetric limb weakness with motor conduction block. *Neurology* 1990;40:118–27.

3558. Krarup-Hansen A, Helweg-Larsen S, Schmalbruch H et al. Neuronal involvement in cisplatin neuropathy: Prospective clinical and neurophysiological studies. *Brain* 2007;130:1076–68.

3559. Kratz R, Brooke MH. *Distal Myopathy*. Amsterdam: North-Holland, 1979.

3560. Krause AC. Congenital encephalo-ophthalmic dysplasia. *Arch Ophthal Berlin* 1946;36:387–444.

3561. Krayenbuhl H, Siebermann R. Small vascular malformations as a cause of primary intracerebral hemorrhage. *J Neurosurg* 1965;22:7–20.

3562. Kretschmer E. Das apallische Syndrom. *Zschr Ges Neur* 1940;169:576–9.

3563. Kriegstein AR. The pathogenesis of epilepsy: Relevance to therapy. *Curr Opin Neurol Neurosurg* 1988;1:200–5.

3564. Krill AE, Kline BA. Retinal syndrome. *Arch Ophthalmol* 1965;74:496.

3565. Krill AE, Smith VC, Pokorny J. Further studies supporting the identity of congenital tritanopia and hereditary dominant optic atrophy. *Invest Ophthalmol* 1971;10:457–65.

3566. Krishaber M. *Gaz Hebd Med Chir* 1872.

3567. Krishnan AV, Kiernan MC. Uremic neuropathy: Clinical features and new pathophysiological insights. *Muscle Nerve* 2007;35:273–90.

3568. Kritschevsky M, Squire LR. Permanent global amnesia with unknown etiology. *Neurology* 1993;43:326–32.

3569. Krugliak L, Gadofi N, Behan AJ. Neuropathic form of arthrygryposis multiplex congenita. *J Neurol Sci* 1978;37:179–85.

3570. Kruiansky J, Gurland B. The performance test of activities of daily living. *Int J Aging Hum Dev* 1976;7:343–52.

3571. Kruit MC, Launer LJ, Ferrari MD et al. Infarcts in the posterior circulation territory in migraine. The population-based MRI CAMERA study. *Brain* 2005;128:2068–77.

3572. Krumholz A. Nonepileptic seizures: Diagnosis and management. *Neurology* 1999;53:S76–S83.

3573. Krumholz A, Bergey GK, Nathanson N. John Hughlings Jackson's observations on "lower level" or "pontobulbar" fits and their relevance to current concepts of seizures and myoclonus. *Neurology* 1994;44:1527–30.

3574. Krupp LB, Banwell B, Tenembaum S. Consensus definitions proposed for pediatric multiple sclerosis and related disorders. *Neurology* 2007;68:S7–S12.

3575. Krupp LB, Pollina DA. Mechanisms and management of fatigue in progressive neurological disorders. *Curr Opin Neurol* 1996;9:456–60.

3576. Krupp LBLNG, Muir-Nash J et al. The fatigue severity scale. Application to patients with multiple sclerosis and systemic lupus erythematosus. *Arch Neurol* 1989;46:1121–3.

3577. Krupp LJ, Elkins LE. Fatigue and declines in cognitive functioning in multiple sclerosis. *Neurology* 2000;55:934–9.

3578. Ksiasek SM, Repka MX, Maguire A et al. Divisional oculomotor nerve paresis caused by intrinsic brainstem disease. *Ann Neurol* 1989;26:714–8.

3579. KU A, Kern H, Lachman E et al. Sciatic nerve impingement from piriformis hematoma due to prolonged labor. *Muscle Nerve* 1995;789–90.

3580. Kuban KCK, Leviton A. Cerebral palsy. *N Engl J Med* 1994;330:188–95.

3581. Kubik CS, Adams RD. Subdural empyema. *Brain* 1943;66:18–42.

3582. Kudo T. Spontaneous occlusion of the circle of Willis. *Neurology* 1968;18:485–96.

3583. Kudrow L. *Cluster Headache: Diagnosis and Management*. New York: Oxford, 1980.

3584. Kudrow L, Esperanca P, Vijayan N. Episodic paroxysmal hemicrania? *Cephalalgia* 1987;7:197–201.

3585. Kufs A. Uber heredopofamiliare angiomatose des gehirns und der Retina, ihre Beziehungen zueinader und Angiomatose der Hant. *Zbl Ges Neurol Psychiat* 1928;112:651–86.

3586. Kufs H. Uber eine Spatform der amaurotischen Idiotie und ihre heredofamiliaren Grundlagen. *Zschr Gesamte Neurol Psychiatr* 1925;95:169–88.

3587. Kugelberg E. Facial reflexes. *Brain* 1952;75:385–96.

3588. Kugelberg E, Welander L. Heredofamilial juvenile muscular atrophy simulating muscular dystrophy. *Arch Neurol Psychiatry* 1956;75:500–9.

3589. Kuhlenbaumer G, Ludemann A, Schirmacher A et al. Autosomal dominant striatal degeneration. *Neurology* 2004;62:2203–8.

3590. Kuhlenbäumer G, Stögbauer F, Young P et al. Hereditary recurrent focal neuropathies: Clinical and molecular features. *Neurology* 2000;54(3):546–51.

3591. Kuijpers HC, Bleijenberg G. The spastic pelvic floor syndrome: A cause of constipation. *Dis Colon Rectum* 1985;28:669–72.

3592. Kulenkampff C. Ein eigentumliches Syndrom im oralen Bereich bei Megaphenapplikation. *Nervenarzt* 1956;27:178–80.

3593. Kulisevsky J, Marti-Fabregas J, Grau JM. Spasms of amputation stumps. *J Neurol Neurosurg Psychiatry* 1992;55:626–7.

3594. Kumandas S, Akcakus M, Coskun A. Joubert syndrome: Review and report of seven new cases. *Eur J Neurol* 2004;11:505–10.

3595. Kumar AJ, Kohler W, Kruse B et al. MR findings in adult-onset adrenoleukodystrophy. *Am J Neuroradiol* 1995;16:1227–37.

3596. Kumar N. Superficial siderosis. *Arch Neurol* 2007;64:491–6.

3597. Kumar N, Gross JB JR, Ahlskog JE. Myelopathy due to copper deficiency. *Neurology* 2004;61:273–4.

3598. Kumral E, Gulluolgu H, Dramali B. Thalamic chronotaraxis: Isolated time disorientation. *J Neurol Neurosurg Psychiatry* 2007;78:880–2

3599. Kun LE. Postirradiation myelopathy in children. *Ann Neurol* 1979;5:106.

3600. Kuncl RW, Wiggins WW. Toxic myopathies. *Neurol Clin* 1988;6:593–619.

3601. Kunishio K, Yamamoto Y, Sunami N. Histologic investigation of a case of meningoangiomatosis not associated with von Recklinghausen's disease. *Surg Neurol* 1987;27:575–9.

3602. Kunitz SC, Gross CR, Heyman A et al. The pilot stroke data bank: Definition, design, and data. *Stroke* 1984;15:740–6.

3603. Kuntzer T, Van Melle G, Regli F. Clinical and prognostic features in unilateral femoral neuropathies. *Muscle Nerve* 1997;20:205–11.

3604. Kupersmith MJ, Martin V, Heller G et al. Idiopathic hypertrophic pachymeningitis. *Neurology* 2004;62:686–94.

3605. See 3604.

3606. Kuriansky JB, Gurland BJ, Fleiss JL et al. The assessment of self-care capacity in geriatric psychiatric patients by objective and subjective methods. *J Clin Psychol* 1990;32:95–102.

3607. Kurihara T, Landau WM, Torack RM. Progressive supranuclear palsy with action myoclonus, seizures. *Neurology* 1974;24:219–23.

3608. Kurlan R. Tourette's syndrome; Current concepts. *Neurology* 1989;39:1625–30.

3609. Kurlan R. Tourette's syndrome and PANDAs. *Neurology* 1998;50:1530–4.

3610. Kurlan R, Behr J, Medved L et al. Transient tic disorder and the spectrum of Tourette's syndrome. *Arch Neurol* 1989;45:1200–1.

3611. Kurlan R, Behr J, Shoulson I. Hereditary myoclonus and chorea: The spectrum of hereditary nonprogressive hyperkinetic movement disorders. *Mov Disord* 1987;2:301–6.

3612. Kurtzke JF. Rating neurological impairment in multiple sclerosis: An expanded disability status scale (EDSS). *Neurology* 1983;33:1444–52.

3613. Kurtzke JF. Neuroepidemiology. *Ann Neurol* 1984;16:265–77.

3614. Kurtzke JF. Optic neuritis or multiple sclerosis. *Arch Neurol* 1985;42:704–10.

3615. Kushner MJ, Parrish M, Burke A et al. Nystagmus in motor neuron disease. *Ann Neurol* 1984;16:71–7.

3616. Kussmaul A. Die Storungen der Sprache. Versuch einer Pathologie der Sprache. In von Ziemssen HW ed. *Handbuch der speciellen Pathologie und Therapie*, pp 211–2. Leipzig: FCW Vogel, 1881.

3617. Kuter I. Systemic mastocytosis. *N Engl J Med* 1992;326:472–81.

3618. Kuzniecky R, Andermann F, Guerrini R et al. The epileptic spectrum in the congenital bilateral perisylvian syndrome. *Neurology* 1994;44:379–85.

3619. Kuzniecky R, Andermann F, Tampieri D et al. Bilateral cerebral macrogyria: Epilepsy, pseudobulbar palsy, and mental retardation – a recognisable neuronal migration disorder. *Ann Neurol* 1989;25:547–54.

3620. Kuzniecky R, Berkovic S, Andermann F et al. Focal cortical myoclonus and rolandic cortical dysplasia: Clarification by magnetic resonance imaging. *Ann Neurol* 1988;23:317–25.

3621. Kuzuhara S, Kanakawa I, Sasaki H et al. Gerstmann-Straussler-Scheinker's disease. *Ann Neurol* 1983;14:216–25.

3622. Kwok RHM. Chinese restaurant syndrome. *N Engl J Med* 1968;278:1122.

3623. Kwon SE, Heilman K. Ipsilateral neglect in a patient following a unilateral frontal lesion. *Neurology* 1991;41: 2001–4.

3624. Kyle RA, Bayrd ED. Benign monoclonal gammopathy (monoclonal gammopathy of undetermined significance). *The Monoclonal Gammopathies*, pp 284–368. Springfield, IL: CC Thomas, 1976.

3625. Kyriakides T, Silberstein JM, Jongpiputvanich S et al. The clinical significance of Type 1 fiber predominance. *Muscle Nerve* 1993;16:418–23.

3626. La Spada AR, Paulson HL, Fishbeck KH. Trinucleotide repeat expansion in neurological disease. *Ann Neurol* 1994;36:814–22.

3627. LaBan MM, Viola SL, Femminineo AF et al. Restless legs syndrome associated with diminished cardiopulmonary compliance and lumbar spinal stenosis – a motor concomitant of Vespers curse. *Arch Phys Med Rehab* 1990;71:384–8.

3628. Labrune P, Lacroix C, Goutieres F et al. Extensive brain calcifications, leukodystrophy and formation of parenchymal cysts. *Neurology* 1996;46:1297–301.

3629. Lacerte D, Gagné F, Copty M. Intracranial chondroma. Report of cases and review of the literature. *Can J Neurol Sci* 1996;23:132–7.

3630. Lach B, Russell NA, Benoit B, Atack D. Cellular blue nevus (melanocytoma) of the spinal meninges. *Neurosurgery* 1988;22:773–80.

3631. Lachaud S, Soriani MH, Delmont E et al. Mills' syndrome: A rare clinical entity. *Rev Neurol (Paris)* 2007;163:335–40.

3632. Lacheretz M, Walbum CH, Tourgis R. L'acrocephalosynankie. A propos d'une observation avec synostoses multiples. *Pediatrie* 1974;29:169–77.

3633. Lacomis D, Smith TW, Chad DA. Acute myopathy and neuropathy in status asthmaticus: Case report and literature review. *Muscle Nerve* 1993;16:84–90.

3634. Lacomis D, Zochodne DW, Bird SJ. Critical illness myopathy. *Muscle Nerve* 2000;23:1785–8.

3635. Lacruz F, Artieda J, Pastor MA et al. The anatomical basis of somaesthetic temporal discrimination in humans. *J Neurol Neurosurg Psychiatry* 1991;54:1077–81.

3636. Lacson AG, Seshia SS, Sarnat HB et al. Autosomal recessive, fatal infantile hypertrophic muscular dystrophy among Canadian natives. *Can J Neurol Sci* 1994;21:203–212.

3637. Ladame P. Friedreich's disease. *Brain* 1890;13:467–537.

3638. Lader MH, Montagu JD. The psychogalvanic reflex: A pharmacological study of the peripheral mechanism. *J Neurol Neurosurg Psychiatry* 1962;25:126–33.

3639. Lado C, Eirís-Puñal J, Blanco-Barca O et al. Hypomelanosis of Ito. A possibly under-diagnosed heterogeneous neurocutaneous syndrome. *Rev Neurol* 2004;38:223–8.

3640. Laff R, Mesad S, Devinsky O. Epileptic kinetopsia. *Neurology* 2003;61:1262–4.

3641. Lafora GR. Beitrag zur Histopathologie der Myoklonischen Epilepsie. *Z Ges Neurol Psychiat* 1911;6:1–14.

3642. Lagier R, Cox JN. Pseudomalignant myositis ossificans. *Human Pathology* 1975;6:653–65.

3643. Lagueny A. Cramp-fasciculation syndrome. *Rev Neurol (Paris)* 2005;161:1260–6.

3644. Lagueny A, Bouillot S, Vital C et al. POEMS syndrome (or Crow–Fukase syndrome). *Rev Neurol (Paris)* 2004;160:285–95.

3645. Lagueny P et al. Amyotrophy after radiotherapy. *Rev Neurol* 1985;141:222.

3646. Laing NG, Laing BA, Meredith C et al. Autosomal dominant distal myopathy: Linkage to chromosome 14. *Am J Hum Genet* 1995;56:422–7.

3647. Lairy GC, Harrison A, Leger EM. Foyers EEG bioccipitaux asynchrones de pointes chez l'enfant mal voyant et aveugle d'age scolaire. *Rev Neurol* 1964;111:351–3.

3648. Lake BD, Wilson J. Zebra body myopathy. *J Neurol Sci* 1975;24:437–46.

3649. Lamantea E, Tiranti V, Bordoni A et al. Mutations of mitochondrial DNA polymerase ýA are a frequent cause of autosomal dominant or recessive progressive external ophthalmoplegia. *Ann Neurol* 2002;52:211–9.

3650. Lambert CD,Young JRB. Hypertrophy of the branchial muscles. *J Neurol Neurosurg Psychiatry* 1976;39:810–6.

3651. Lambert EH, Eaton LM, Rooke ED. Myasthenia associated with small-cell carcinoma of the bronchus. *Am J Physiol* 1956;187:612–3.

3652. Lamey P-J, Lamb AB. Prospective study of aetiological factors in burning mouth syndrome. *BMJ* 1988;296:1243–6.

3653. Lamont PJ, Udd B, Mastaglia F et al. Lang early-onset distal myopathy. *J Neurol Neurosurg Psychiatr* 2006;77:208–15.

3654. Lance JW. Familial paroxysmal dystonic choreoathetosis and its differentiation from related syndromes. *Ann Neurol* 1977;2:285–93.

3655. Lance JW. Spasticity. In Feldman RG, Young RR, Koella WP eds. *Spasticity: Disordered Motor Control*, Chicago: Year Book Medical Publishers, 1980.

3656. Lance JW. Symposium synopsis. In Feldman RG, Young RR, Koella WP eds. *Spasticity: Disordered Motor Control*, pp 485–94. Chicago: Year Book Medical Publishers, 1980.

3657. Lance JW. Solved and unsolved headache problems. *Headache* 1991;31:439–45.

3658. Lance JW. The red ear syndrome. *Neurology* 1996;47:617–20.
3659. Lance JW. Transient sensations of impending loss of consciousness; the "blip" syndrome. *J Neurol Neurosurg Psychiatry* 1996;60:437–8.
3660. Lance JW, Adams RD. The syndrome of intention or action myoclonus as a sequel to hypoxic encephalopathy. *Brain* 1963;86:111–36.
3661. Lance JW, Anthony M. Neck-tongue syndrome on sudden turning of the head. *J Neurol Neurosurg Psychiatry* 1980;43: 97–101.
3662. Lance JW, Burke D, Pollard J. Hyperexcitability of motor and sensory neurons in neuromyotonia. *Ann Neurol* 1979;5:523–32.
3663. Lance JW, Drummond PD, Gandevia SC, Morris JGL. Harlequin syndrome: The sudden onset of unilateral flushing and sweating. *J Neurol Neurosurg Psychiatry* 1988;51:635–42.
3664. Landau WM. Spasticity: The fable of a neurological demon and the emperor's new therapy. *Arch Neurol* 1974;31:217–9.
3665. Landau WM. Au clair de lacune. *Neurology* 1989;39:725–30.
3666. Landau WM. Reflex dementia: Disinhibited primitive thinking. *Neurology* 1989;39:133–7.
3667. Landau WM, Kleffner FR. Syndrome of acquired aphasia with convulsive disorder in children. *Neurology* 1957;7:523–30.
3668. Landau WM, Torack RM, Guggenheim MA. Congenital retardation and later evolution to a seizure disorder, orofacial dysplasia and amyotrophy. *Neurology* 1976;26:869–73.
3669. Lander CM, Eadie MJ, Tyrer JH. Hereditary motor peripheral neuropathy predominantly affecting the arms. *J Neurol Sci* 1976;28:389–94.
3670. Landi G, Motto C, Cella E et al. Pathogenetic and prognostic features of lacunar transient ischemic attack syndromes. *J Neurol Neurosurg Psychiatry* 1993;56:1265–70.
3671. Landing BH, Shirkley HS. A syndrome of recurrent infection and infiltration of viscera by pigmented lipid histiocytes. *Pediatrics* 1957;20:431–8.
3672. Landis DMD, Rosenberg RN, Landis C. Olivopontocerebellar degeneration. *Arch Neurol* 1974;31:295–307.
3673. Landouzy L. De la sciatique et de l'atrophie musculaire qui peut la compliquer. *Arch Gen Med Paris* 1875;1:303–25.
3674. Landouzy L. De la déviation conjugée des yeux et de la rotation de la tête par excitation ou paralysie des 6e et 11e paires. *Bull Soc Anat Paris* 1879;54: 293–352.
3675. Landouzy L. De la myopathie atrophique progressive; myopathie sans neuropathie, débutant d'ordinaire dans l'enfance par la face. *Rev Med Paris* 1885;5:81–117.
3676. Landouzy L. Camptodactylie. *Presse Med* 1906;251–3.
3677. Landrieu P, Said G. Niemann-Pick disease. *Acta Neuropathol* 1984;63:66–71.
3678. Landry O. Note sur la paralysie ascendante aigue. *GHMP* 1859;6:472–4.
3679. Landsborough D. St. Paul and temporal lobe epilepsy. *J Neurol Neurosurg Psychiatry* 1987;50:659–64.
3680. Landy S, Rice K, Lobo B. Central sensitization and cutaneous allodynia in migraine. *CNS Drugs* 2004;18:337–42.
3681. Lane RJM. Cardiogenic dementia. *Lancet* 1977;i:27–8.
3682. Lane RJM, Mastaglia FL. Malignant hyperpyrexia. *Lancet* 1978;2:562.
3683. Lang AE. Psychogenic dystonia: A review of 18 cases. *Can J Neurol Sci* 1995;22:136–43.
3684. Lang AE, Consky E, Sandor P. Signing tics. *Ann Neurol* 1993;33:212–5.
3685. Lang AH, Hirvasniemi A, Siivola J et al. Neurophysiological findings in the Northern epilepsy syndrome. *Acta Neurol Scand* 1997;95:1–8.
3686. Lang H, Wurzburg U. Creatine kinase, an enzyme of many forms. *Clin Chem* 1982;28:1439–47.
3687. Lange C. Die Ausflockung Kolloidalen Goldesdurch zebrospinalflussgeit bei Luetischen Affektionen des Zentralnervensystems. *Z Chemotherap* 1912;1:44–78.
3688. Langley JN. The autonomic nervous system. *Brain* 1903;26:1–26.
3689. Langley JN, Sherrington CS. *J Physiol* 1891;12:278.
3690. Langston JW, Dorfman LJ, Forno LS. Encephalomyeloneuritis in the absence of cancer. *Neurology* 1975;25:633–7.
3691. Lanska D. Anthrax meningoencephalitis. *Neurology* 2002;59:327–34.
3692. Lanska D, Remler BF. Benign paroxysmal positioning vertigo. Neurology 1997;48:1167–77.
3693. Lanska DJ. The history of reflex hammers. Neurology 1989;39:1542–9.
3694. Lanska DJ, Currier RD, Cohen M et al. Familial progressive subcortical gliosis. *Neurology* 1994;44:1633–43.
3695. Lanska DJ, Goetz C. Romberg's sign. *Neurology* 2000;55:1201–6.
3696. Lanthier S, Lortie A, Michaud J et al. Isolated angiitis of the CNS in children. *Neurology* 2001;56:837–42.
3697. Lantos PL, Papp MI. Cellular pathology of multiple system atrophy: A review. *J Neurol Neurosurg Psychiatry* 1994;47:129–33.
3698. Lapresle J, Annabi A. OPCA with velopharyngolaryngeal paralysis. *J Neuropath Exp Neurol* 1979;38:401–6.
3699. Larbrisseau A, Vanasse M, Brochu P et al. The Andermann syndrome: Agenesis of the corpus callosum associated with mental retardation and progressive sensorimotor neuropathy. *Can J Neurol Sci* 1984;11:257–61.
3700. Larner AJ. False localizing signs. *J Neurol Neurosurg Psychiatry* 2008;74:415–8.
3701. Larrabee GJ, Crook TH. A computerized everyday memory battery for assessing treatment effects. *Psychopharm Bull* 1988;24:695–7.
3702. Larrabee GJ, Pathy MSJ, Bayer A et al. Memory clinics: State of the art and future prospects. In Bergener M, Finkel SI eds. *Clinical and Scientific Psychogeriatrics*, pp 83–97. Berlin: Springer-Verlag, 1988.
3703. Larsen R, Ashwal S, Peckham N. Incontinentia pigmenti and anterior horn cell degeneration. *Neurology* 1987;37:446–50.
3704. Larsen R, Ashwall S, Peckham N. Incontinentia pigmenti. *Neurology* 1987;37:446–50.
3705. Larsen R et al. Infantile spinal muscular atrophy in incontinentia pigmenti. *Neurology* 1987;37:446.
3706. Lascelles RG, Baker IA, Thomas PK. Hereditary polyneuropathy of Roussy-Levy type with associated cardiomyopathy. *Guy's Hosp Rep* 1970;119:253–62.
3707. Lasègue E-C. Considerations sur la sciatique. *AGMP* 1852;28:129–50.
3708. Lasègue E-C. De l'anesthesie et de l'ataxie hysteriques. *AGMP* 1864;3:385–402.
3709. Lasègue E-C. Des hysteriques peripheriques. *AGMP* 1878;1:641–56.
3710. Lashley KS. *Brain Mechanisms and Intelligence: A Quantitative Study of Injuries to the Brain*. Chicago: University of Chicago Press, 1929.
3711. Lassen NA. The luxury-perfusion syndrome and its possible relation to acute metabolic acidosis localised with the brain. *Lancet* 1966;2:1113–5.
3712. Latham AD, Munro TA. Familial myoclonus epilepsy associated with deaf mutism in a family showing other psychobiological abnormalities. *Ann Eugen* 1937;8:166–75.
3713. Latov S et al. Peripheral Neuropathy and anti-MAG antibodies. *CRC Crit Rev Clin Neurobiol* 1988;3:301–31.
3714. Laurence JZ, Moon RC. Four cases of "retinitis pigmentosa", occurring in the same family, and accompanied by general imperfections of development. *Ophth Rev London* 1866;2:32–41.
3715. Lauritzen M. Cortical spreading depression as a putative migraine mechanism. *TINS* 1987 Jan;8–13.
3716. Laursen J, Fode K, Dahlerup B. Spinal epidural hematomas. *Clin Neurol Neurosurg* 1987;89:247–53.

3717. Laux W. In Memoriam - Hans-Gerhard Creutzfeldt. *Med Klin Berlin* 1965;60:553–4.
3718. Lavade T, Graber D, Flurin V et al. Human Beta-mannosidase deficiency associated with peripheral neuropathy. *Ann Neurol* 1994;35:116–9.
3719. Law EM, Masterson JG. Partial deletion of chromosome 18. *Lancet* 1966;2:1137.
3720. Lawford JB. Naevus of left side of face, nevus of choroid, subretinal hemorrhage and detached retina in left eye. *Trans Ophthal SocUK* 1885;5:136–9.
3721. Lawton MP, Brody EM. Assessment of elder people: Self-maintaining and instrumental activities of daily living. *Gerontologist* 1969;9:179–86.
3722. Lawton MP, Moss M, Fulcomer M et al. A research and service oriented multilevel assessment instrument. *J Gerontol* 1982;37:91–9.
3723. Laxova R et al. A further example of lethal autosomal recessive condition in sibs. *J Ment Defic Res* 1972;16:139–43.
3724. Layzer RB. *Neuromuscular Manifestations of Systemic Disease*. Philadelphia: F.A. Davis, 1985.
3725. Layzer RB. The origin of muscle fasciculations and cramps. *Muscle Nerve* 1994;17:1243–9.
3726. Layzer RB, Rowland LP, Ranney HM. Muscle phosphofructokinase deficiency. *Arch Neurol* 1967;17:512–23.
3727. Layzer RB, Shearn MA, Satya-Murti S. Eosinophilic polymyositis. *Ann Neurol* 1977;1:65–71.
3728. Lazare A. Conversion symptoms. *N Engl J Med* 1981;305:745–8.
3729. Lazarevic LK. Ischias postica Cotunnii. *Allg Wien Med Ztg* 1884;29:425.
3730. Lazawow PB, Moser HW. Disorders of peroxisomal biogenesis. In Scriver CR ed. *The Metabolic Basis of Inherited Disease*, New York: McGraw-Hill, 1989.
3731. Le Ber I, Moreira M-C, Rivaud-Péchoux C. Cerebellar ataxia with oculomotor apraxia type 1: Clinical and genetic studies. *Brain* 2003;126:2761–72.
3732. Le Ber IE, Clot F, Vercueil L et al. Predominant dystonia with marked cerebellar atrophy. Neurology 2006;67:1773.
3733. Le Douarin NM. Embryonic chimeras: A tool for studying the development of the nervous and immune systems. *Proc Roy Soc Med* 1988;235:1–17.
3734. Le Forestier N, Moulonguet A, Maisonobe T et al. True neurogenic thoracic outlet syndrome: Electrophysiological diagnosis in six cases. *Muscle Nerve* 1998;21:1129–34.
3735. Le Fort D, Safran AB, Picard F et al. Elicited repetitive daily blindness. Neurology 2004;63:348–50.
3736. Le Roux K, Streichenberger N, Vial C. Granulomatous myositis: A clinical study of thirteen cases. *Muscle Nerve* 2007;35(**Suppl.** 2):171–7.
3737. Leao AAP. Spreading depression of activity in the cerebral cortex. *J Physiol* 1944;7:358–90.
3738. Leber T. Beitrage zur Kenntniss der Atrophischen Veranderungen des Sehnerven nebst Bemerkungen uber die normale Structur des Nerven. *Arch Ophthal Berlin* 1868;14:164–76.
3739. Leber T. Uber hereditare und kongenital–angelegte Sehnervenleiden. *Arch Ophthal Berlin* 1871;17:249–91.
3740. Lebrun C, Bensa C, Debouverie M et al. Unexpected multiple sclerosis. *J Neurol Neurosurg Psychiatry* 2008;79:195–8.
3741. Lechtenberg R, Shulman A. The neurologic implications of tinnitus. *Arch Neurol* 1984;41:718–21.
3742. Lecube A, Francisco G, Ortega A. Lymphocytic hypophysitis successfully treated with azathioprine: First case report. *J Neurol Neurosurg Psychiatry* 2003;74:1581–3.
3743. Lederman RJ, Calabrese LH. Overuse syndromes in instrumentalists. Med Probl Perform Art 1986;1:7–11.
3744. Lee BI, Lesser RP, Pippinger CE et al. Familial paroxysmal hypnogenic dystonia. Neurology 1985;35:1357–60.
3745. Lee EK, Maselli RA, Ellis WG et al. Morvan's fibrillary chorea: A paraneoplastic manifestation of thymoma. *J Neurol Neurosurg Psychiatry* 1998;65:857–62.
3746. Lee J, Gresty M. A case of "voluntary nystagmus" and head tremor. *J Neurol Neurosurg Psychiatry* 1993;56:1321–2.
3747. Lee JA, Madrid RE, Sperle K. Spastic paraplegia type 2 associated with axonal neuropathy and apparent *PLP1* position effect. *Ann Neurol* 2006;59:398–403.
3748. Lee K, Lee Y, Kim S et al. Occipital lobe epilepsy: Clinical characteristics, surgical outcome, and role of diagnostic modalities. *Epilepsia* 2007;46:688–95.
3749. Lee VH, Wijdicks EFM, Manno EM et al. Clinical spectrum of reversible posterior leukoencephalopathy syndrome. *Arch Neurol* 2008;65:205–10.
3750. Lee YS, Yip WCL. A fatal congenital myopathy with severe Type 1 fibre atrophy, central nuclei and multicores. *J Neurol Sci* 1981;50:227–90.
3751. Leech J, Gresty MA, Hess K et al. Gaze failure, drifting eye movements, and centripetal nystagmus in cerebellar diseases. *Br J Ophthalmol* 1977;61:774–81.
3752. Lees AJ. Familial static ophthalmoplegia. *J Neurol Neurosurg Psychiatry* 1960;23:46.
3753. Lees AJ. *Tics and Related Disorders*. Edinburgh: Churchill Livingstone, 1985.
3754. Lees A. Odd and unusual movement disorders. *J Neurol Neurosurg Psychiatry* 2002;72:17–21.
3755. Leeuwenhoek Av. *Selected Works*. London: Nicol, 1798.
3756. Lehmann-Horn F, Rüdel R. Hereditary nondystrophic myotonias and periodic paralyses. *Curr Opin Neurol* 1995;8:402–10.
3757. Leichtenstern OML. Concerning epidemic meningitis. *Dtsch Med Wschr* 1885;11:537–40.
3758. Leigh D. Subacute necrotizing encephalomyelopathy in an infant. *J Neurol Neurosurg Psychiatry* 1951;14:216–21.
3759. Leigh RJ, Foley JM, Remler BF et al. Oculogyric crises: A syndrome of thought disorder and ocular deviation. *Ann Neurol* 1987;22:13–7.
3760. Leigh RJ, Robinson DA, Zee DS. A hypothetical explanation for periodic alternating nystagmus: Instability in the optokinetic-vestibular system. *Ann N Y Acad Sci* 1981;374:619.
3761. Leigh RJ, Tusa RJ. Disturbance of smooth pursuit caused by infarction of occipito-parietal cortex. *Ann Neurol* 1985;17:185.
3762. Leigh RJ, Zee DS. *The Neurology of Eye Movements*. Philadelphia: F.A. Davis, 1991.
3763. Leiguarda R, Starkstein S, Nogues M et al. Paroxysmal alien hand syndrome. *J Neurol Neurosurg Psychiatry* 1993;56:788–92.
3764. Leiguarda RC, Marsden CD. Limb apraxias. *Brain* 2000;123:860–79.
3765. Leis AA, Ross MA, Summers AK. Psychogenic seizures: Ictal characteristics and diagnostic pitfalls. *Neurology* 1992;42:95–9.
3766. Leisti J et al. The floating harbor syndrome. *Birth Defects* 1975;11:305.
3767. Lejeune J, LaFourcade J, Berger R et al. Three cases of deletion of the short arm of chromosome 5. *CR Acad Sci (Paris)* 1963;257:3098.
3768. Lejonne P, Lhermitte JJ. Olivo-Rubro-Cerebellar Atrophy. *Nouv Icon Salpet* 1909;2:605–19.
3769. Leli DA, Furlow TW, Falgout JE. Benign familial chorea. *J Neurol Neurosurg Psychiatry* 1984;47:471–4.
3770. LeMarquand HS, Hausmann W, Hemsted EH. Myxoedema as a cause of death: Report of two cases. *BMJ* 1953;1:704–6.
3771. Lemierre A-A, Boltanski E, Justin-Besancon L-E. Les polynevrites alcoolo-tuberculeuses. *Bull Acad Med Paris* 1931;105:676–8.
3772. Lemieux G, Neemeh JA. Charcot-Marie-Tooth disease and nephritis. *Can Med Assn J* 1967;97:1193–8.
3773. Lempert T. Syncope. Phenomenology and differentiation from epileptic seizures. *Nervenarzt* 1997;68:620.

3774. Lempert T, Bauer MS, Schmidt D. Syncope: A videometric analysis of 56 episodes of transient cerebral hypoxia. *Ann Neurol* 1994;**36**:233–7.

3775. Lendon CL, Lynch.T, Norton J et al. Hereditary dysphasic disinhibition dementia. *Neurology* 1998;**50**:1546–55.

3776. Lenhoff HM, Wang PP, Greenberg F et al. Williams syndrome and the brain. *Sci Am* 1997;277:63–73.

3777. Lennox WG. *Epilepsy and Related Disorders.* Boston: Little, Brown, 1960.

3778. Lenoble E, Aubineau E. Une variété nouvelle de myoclonie congénitale pouvant être héréditaire et familiale a nystagmus constant. *Rev Med Paris* 1906;**26**:471–515.

3779. Lenz W. Recessiv-geschlechtsgebundene Mikrophthalmie mit multiplen Missbildungen. *Z Kinderheilkd* 1955;77:384–90.

3780. Leonard JV, Schapira AHV. Mitochondrial respiratory chain disorders. *Lancet* 2000;**355**:299–304;–389–393.

3781. Leonhard K. Agraphia and constructional apraxia. *Arch Psychiatr Z Neurol* 1952;**188**:504–10.

3782. Lepore F. Bilateral cerebral ptosis. *Neurology* 1987;**37**:1043–6.

3783. Lerche H, Weber YG, Baier H et al. Generalized epilepsy with febrile seizures plus. *Neurology* 2001;**57**:1191–8.

3784. Leri A. A reflex phenomenon in the arm. *Rev Neurol* 1913;**25**:277.

3785. Leriche R. Resection of the aorto-iliac bifurcation and bilateral sympathectomy for distal aortic arteritis. *Presse Med* 1940;**48**:601–4.

3786. Lerman P, Kivity S. Benign focal epilepsy of childhood: A follow-up study of 100 recovered patients. *Arch Neurol* 1975;**32**:261–4.

3787. Lerman P, Kivity S. The benign focal epilepsies of childhood. In Pedley TA, Meldrum BS eds. *Recent Advances in Epilepsy* - 3, pp 137–56. Edinburgh: Churchill Livingstone, 1986.

3788. Lermoyez M. La vertige qui fait entendre (angiospasme labyrinthique). *Presse Med* 1919;**27**:1–3.

3789. Leroy MR. Syndrome of lilliputian hallucinations. *J Nerv Ment Dis* 1922;**56**:325–33.

3790. Lesca G, Eymard-Pierre E, Santorelli FM et al. Infantile and ascending hereditary spastic paralysis. *Neurology* 2003;**60**:674–82.

3791. Lesch M, Nyhan WL. A familial disorder of uric acid metabolism and central nervous system function. *Am J Med* 1964;**36**:561–70.

3792. Lescher FG. The nervous complications of infective hepatitis. *BMJ* 1944;1:554.

3793. Lessell S. Supranuclear paralysis of monocular elevation. *Neurology* 1975;**25**:1134–43.

3794. Lessell S, Lessell IM, Rizzo IJF. Ocular neuromyotonia after radiation therapy. *Am J Ophthalmol* 1986;**102**:766–70.

3795. Lessell S, Wolf PA, Benson MD et al. Scalloped pupils in familial amyloidosis. *N Engl J Med* 1975;**293**:914–5.

3796. Leuzzi V, De Negri AM, Gallucci M et al. Bilateral striatal necrosis, dystonia and optic atrophy in two siblings. *J Neurol Neurosurg Psychiatry* 1992;**55**:16–9.

3797. Leuzzi V, Rinna A, Gallucci M et al. Ataxia, deafness, leukodystrophy: Inherited disorder of the white matter in three related patients. *Neurology* 2000;**54**:2325–8.

3798. Levenson JL. Neuroleptic malignant syndrome. *Am J Psychiatry* 1985;**142**:1137–45.

3799. Levic ZM, Stefanovic BS, Nikolic MZ et al. Progressive nuclear ophthalmoplegia associated with mental deficiency, lingua scrotalis, and other neurologic and ophthalmologic signs in a family. *Neurology* 1975;**25**:68–71.

3800. Levin M, Ward TN. Ophthalmoplegic migraine. *Curr Pain Headache Rep* 2004;**8**:306–9.

3801. Levin AB. A simple test of cardiac function based upon the heart rate changes during the Vansalva maneuver. *Am J Cardiol* 1966;**18**:90–9.

3802. Levin BE. The clinical significance of spontaneous pulsations of the retinal vein. *Arch Neurol* 1978;**35**:37–40.

3803. Levin HS, High WM, Goethe AE et al. The neurobehavioral rating scale. *J Neurol Neurosurg Psychiatry* 1987;**50**:183–93.

3804. Levin HS, O'Donnell VM, Grossman RG. The Galveston orientation and aphasia test. *J Nerv Ment Dis* 1979;**167**:675–84.

3805. Levin KH, Wilbourn AJ, Maggiano HJ. Cervical rib and median sternotomy-related brachial plexopathies: A reassessment. *Neurology* 1998;**50**:1407–13.

3806. Levin LS et al. A heritable syndrome of craniosynostosis, short, thin hair, dental abnormalities, and short limbs: Cranioectodermal dysplasia. *J Pediatr* 1977;**90**:55–61.

3807. Levin SL. The syndrome of isolated disturbance of the tympanic nerve. *Arch Neurol* 1983;**40**:106–8.

3808. Levine DN, Lee JM, Fisher CM. The visual variant of Alzheimer's disease. *Neurology* 1993;43:305–13.

3809. Levine IM, Estes JW, Looney JM. Hereditary neurological disease with acanthocytosis. *Arch Neurol* 1968;**19**:403–9.

3810. Levine SR, Welch KMA. Cerebrovascular ischemia associated with lupus anticoagulant. *Stroke* 1987;**18**:257–63.

3811. Levine SR, Welch KMA. Antiphospholipid antibodies. *Ann Neurol* 1989;**26**:386–9.

3812. Levine T, Pestronk A. Inflammatory myopathy with cytochrome oxidase negative muscle fibers: Methotrexate treatment. *Muscle Nerve* 1998;**21**:1724–8.

3813. Leviton A, Gilles FH. An epidemiologic study of perinatal telencephalic leucoencephalopathy in an autopsy population. *J Neurol Sci* 1973;**18**:53–66.

3814. Levy DE. Transient CNS deficits. *Neurology* 1988;**38**:831–6.

3815. Levy IS, Wright JE, Lloyd GAS. Orbital and Retro-orbital Pseudo-tumors. *Mod Prob Ophthalmol* 1975;**14**:364–7.

3816. Levy ML, Cummings JL, Fairbanks LA et al. Apathy is not depression. *J Neuropsychiatr Clin Neurosci* 1998;**10**:314–9.

3817. Lewis AJ, Besant DF. Muscular dystrophy in infancy. *J Pediatr* 1962;**60**:376–84.

3818. Lewis DW, Tucker SH. Central nervous system involvement in cat scratch disease. *Pediatrics* 1986;**77**:714–21.

3819. Lewis JM, Kline LB. Periodic alternating nystagmus with periodic alternating skew deviation. *J Clin Neuro-Ophthalmol* 1983;**3**:115.

3820. Lewis P. Familial orthostatic hypotension. *Brain* 1964;**87**:719–28.

3821. Lewis RA, Sumner AJ, Brown MJ. Multifocal demyelinating neuropathy with conduction block. *Neurology* 1982;**32**:958–64.

3822. Lewy FH. Zur pathologischen Anatomie der Paralysis agitans. *Dtsch Z Nervenklinik* 1913;**50**:50.

3823. Leyden E. *Klinik der Ruchenmarks-Krantheiten*. Berlin:1876;2.

3824. Leyden E. Ueber acute Ataxie. *Zschr Klin Med* 1890;**18**:576–87.

3825. Lezak MD. *Neuropsychological Assessment*. New York: Oxford University Press, 1995.

3826. Lhermitte F. "Utilization behaviour" and its relation to lesions of the frontal lobes. *Brain* 1983;**106**:237–55.

3827. Lhermitte F, Pillon B, Serdaru M. Human autonomy and the frontal lobes. *Ann Neurol* 1986;**19**:326–34–335–343.

3828. Lhermitte JJ. Les maladies du sommeil et des narcolepsies. *J de Neurologie* 1910;**15**:1–17.

3829. Lhermitte JJ. L'encéphalite léthargique; anatomie et physiologie pathologiques. *Arch Ophthal Berlin* 1921;**38**.

3830. Lhermitte JJ, Cornil L, Quesnel. Le syndrome de la degeneration pyramido–pallidale progressive. *Rev Neurol* 1920;**27**:262–9.

3831. Lhermitte JJ, Delthil, Garnier. Syndrome contralateral du noyau rouge avec hallucinations visuelles et auditives. *Rev Neurol* 1938;**70**:623–8.

3832. Lhermitte JJ, Levy G. L'hallucinose pédonculaire. *Rev Neurol* 1931;55:312–8.

3833. Lhermitte JJ, McAlpine D. A clinical and pathological resume of combined disease of the pyramidal and extrapyramidal systems with special reference to a new syndrome. *Brain* 1926;49:157–81.

3834. Lhermitte JJ, Nicholas M. Les douleurs à type de décharge electrique consecutives a la flexion cephalique dans la sclèrose en plaques. Un cas de forme sensitive de la sclèrose multiple. *Rev Neurol* 1924;2:56–62.

3835. Liao Y, Fuh J, Lirng J et al. Bathing headache: A variant of idiopathic thunderclap headache. *Cephalalgia* 2003;23:854–9.

3836. Libman LJ, Matthews JH. "Oblongata" crises in tabes dorsalis. *J Neurol Neurosurg Psychiatry* 1976;39:1240–1.

3837. Lichtenstein H, Knorr A. Uber einige Falle von forschreitender Schwerhorig–keit bei hereditarer Ataxie. *Dtsch Z Nervenklinik* 1930;114:1–28.

3838. Lichtheim L. Ueber Aphasie. *Arch Klin Med* 1885;36:204–68.

3839. Liddell EGT, Sherrington CS. Reflexes in response to stretch (myotatic reflexes). *Proc Roy Soc Med* 1924;B96:212–42.

3840. Lidge RT, Bechtol RC, Lambert CM. Congenital muscular torticollis: Etiology and pathology. *J Bone Jt Surg* 1957;39A:1165–82.

3841. Lidsky TI, Schneider JS. Lead neurotoxicity in children: Basic mechanisms and clinical correlates. *Brain* 2003;126:5–19.

3842. Liebow AS, Carrington CRB, Friedman RJ. Lymphomatoid granulomatosis. *Human Pathology* 1972;3:457–538.

3843. Lien J, Nyhan WL, Barshop BA et al. Fatal initial adult–onset presentation of urea cycle defect. *Arch Neurol* 2007;64:1777–9.

3844. Liepert J, Kotterba S, Tegenthoff M et al. Central fatigue assessed by transcranial stimulation. *Muscle Nerve* 1996;19: 1429–34.

3845. Liepmann HK. Das Krankheitsbild der Apraxie (motorischen Asymbolie) auf Grund eines Falles von einseitiger Apraxie. *Mschr Psychiat Neurol* 1900;8:15, 102, 182–44, 132, 197.

3846. Lilly R, Cummings JL, Benson DF et al. The human Kluver–Bucy syndrome. *Neurology* 1983;33:1141–5.

3847. Lim J, Yagnik P, Schraeder P et al. Ictal catatonia as a manifestation of nonconvulsive status epilepticus. *J Neurol Neurosurg Psychiatry* 1986;49:833–6.

3848. Lin JT-Y, Ziegler DK, Lai C-W, Bayer W. Convulsive syncope in blood donors. *Ann Neurol* 1982;11:525–8.

3849. Lincoln N, Leadbitter D. Assessment of motor function in stroke patients. *Physiotherapy* 1979;65:48–51.

3850. Lincoln NB. The speech questionnaire: An assessment of functional language ability. *Int Rehabil Med* 1982;4:114–7.

3851. Lincoln NB, Edmans JA. A re-validation of the Rivermead ADL scale for elderly patients with stroke. *Age Ageing* 1990;19:9–24.

3852. Lind J. *A Treatise of the Scurvy in three parts, containing an inquiry into the nature, causes and cure of that disease, together with a critical and chronological view of what has been published on the subject.* Edinburgh: A Kincaid and A Donaldson, 1753.

3853. Lindenov H. *The Aetiology of Deaf-Mutism with Special Reference to Heredity.* Copenhagen: Munksgard, 1945.

3854. Lindenstrom E, Boysen G, Waage Christiansen L et al. Reliability of Scandinavian neurological stroke scale. *Cerebrovasc Dis* 1991;1:103–7.

3855. Lindgren K-A, Manninen H, Rytkonen H. Thoracic outlet syndrome – a functional disturbance of the thoracic upper aperture? *Muscle Nerve* 1995;18:526–30.

3856. Lindquist L, Vapalahti O. Tick-borne encephalitis. *Lancet* 2008;371:1861–71.

3857. Lindsberg J, Hallenbeck JM, Feuerstein G. Platelet-activating factor in stroke and brain injury. *Ann Neurol* 1991;30: 117–29.

3858. Lingam S, Read S, Hart EW. Hereditary stiff-baby syndrome. *Am J Dis Childh* 1981;135:909–11.

3859. Lingjaerde O, Bratlid T, Hansen T. Insomnia during the dark period in northern Norway: An explorative controlled trial with light treatment. *Acta Psychiatr Neurol* 1985;71:506–12.

3860. Linn MW, Linn BS. The rapid disability rating scale 2. *J Am Geriatr Soc* 1982;30:378–82.

3861. Linnankivi T, Valanne L, Paetau A et al. Cerebroretinal microangiopathy with calcifications and cysts. *Neurology* 2006;67:1437–43.

3862. Lippa CF, Zhukareva V, Kararai T et al. Frontotemporal dementia with novel tau pathology and a Glu342Val *tau* mutation. *Ann Neurol* 2000;48:850–8.

3863. Lisak RP, Lebeau J, Tucker SH. Hyperkalemic periodic paralysis and cardiac arrhythmia. *Neurology* 1972;22:810–5.

3864. Lishman WA. Cerebral disorder in alcoholism. *Brain* 1981;104:1–20.

3865. Lishman WA. What is neuropsychiatry? *J Neurol Neurosurg Psychiatry* 1992;55: 983–5.

3866. Lishman WA, Russell WR. The brachial neuropathies. *Lancet* 1961;2:941–7.

3867. Lison M, Kombrut B, Feinstein A et al. Progressive spastic paraparesis, vitiligo, premature graying and distinct facial appearance: A new genetic syndrome in three sibs. *Am J Med Genet* 1981;9:361–7.

3868. Lissauer H. Ein Fall von Seelenblindheit nebst einem Beitrag zur Theorie derselban. *Arch Psychiatr Nervenkr* 1890;21:222–70.

3869. List CF. Neurologic syndromes accompanying developmental anomalies of occipital bone, atlas, and axis. *Arch Neurol Psychiatry* 1941;45:577–616.

3870. List CF. Interhemispheric subdural suppuration. *J Neurosurg* 1950;7:313–24.

3871. Lister GD, Belso LB, Clivert HE. The radial tunnel syndrome. *J Hand Surg* 1979;4:52.

3872. Little BW, Brown PW, Rodgers-Johnson P et al. Familial myoclonic dementia masquerading as Creutzfeldt-Jakob disease. *Ann Neurol* 1986;20:231–6.

3873. Little BW, Park DP. Oculopharyngeal muscular dystrophy. *J Neurol Sci* 1982;53:145–58.

3874. Little JR, Opitz JM. The G syndrome. *Am J Dis Childh* 1971;121:505–7.

3875. Little WJ. Course of lectures on the deformities of the human frame. Lecture IX. *Lancet* 1843;1:350–4.

3876. Little WJ. On the influence of abnormal parturition, difficult labours, premature birth, and asphyxia neonatorum, on the mental and physical condition of the child especially in relation to deformities. *Trans Obstet Soc London* 1861;3:293–344.

3877. Litvan I, Agid Y, Calne DB et al. Clinical research criteria for the diagnosis of progressive supranuclear palsy (Steele-Richardson-Olszewski syndrome). *Neurology* 1996;47:1–9.

3878. Litvan I, Agid Y, Goetz C et al. Accuracy of the clinical diagnosis of corticobasal degeneration. *Neurology* 1997;48: 119–25.

3879. Litvan I, Mangone CA, Werden W et al. Reliability of the NINDS myotatic reflex scale. *Neurology* 1996;47:969–72.

3880. Livan M. Contributo alla conoscenza della sordita ereditarie. *Arch Ital Otol* 1961;72:331–9.

3881. Livingston S, Torres I. Photic epilepsy: Report of an unusual case and review of the literature. *Clin Ped* 1964;3:304–7.

3882. Livingston WK. Back disabilities due to strain of multifidus muscle; cases treated by novocain injection. *Western J Surg* 1941;49:259–65.

3883. Livingstone IR, Gardner-Medwin D, Watkins PJ. Familial intermittent ataxia with possible X-linked recessive inheritance. *J Neurol Sci* 1984;64: 89–97.

3884. Livingstone MG, Livingstone HM. The Glasgow assessment schedule: Clinical and research assessment of head injury outcome. *Int Rehabil Med* 1985;7:145–9.

3885. Lloyd AR, Hales JP, Gandevia SC. Muscle strength, endurance and recovery in the post-infection fatigue syndrome. *J Neurol Neurosurg Psychiatry* 1988;51:1316–22.
3886. Lloyd KG, Hornykiewicz O, Davidson L et al. Biochemical evidence of dysfunction of brain transmitters in the Lesch-Nyhan syndrome. *N Engl J Med* 1981;305: 1106–11.
3887. Lloyd ME, Spector TD, Howard R. Osteoporosis in neurological disorders. *J Neurol Neurosurg Psychiatry* 2000;68: 543–9.
3888. Lobstein J. *De l'appairaissment des os*. Paris: Traite de l'anatomie pathologique, 1833.
3889. Lockwood AH. Medical problems of musicians. *N Engl J Med* 1989;320:221–7.
3890. Locock C. In discussion of Sieveking EH. Analysis of 52 cases of epilepsy observed by the author. *Lancet* 1857;1:527–8.
3891. Lodder J, Baard WC. Paraballism caused by bilateral hemorrhagic infarction in basal ganglia. *Neurology* 1981;31:484–6.
3892. Loeb C, Gandolfo C, Mancardi GL et al. The Lacunar syndromes: A review with personal contribution. In Meyer JS, Lechner H, Eichorn O, eds. *Cerebrovascular Disease: Research and Clinical Management*, pp 107–56. Amsterdam: Elsevier, 1986.
3893. Loeffen J, Elpeleg O, Smeitink J et al. Mutations in the complex 1 NDUFS2 gene of patients with cardiomyopathy and encephalomyopathy. *Ann Neurol* 2001;49:195–201.
3894. Loewen SC, Anderson BA. Reliability of the modified motor assessment scale and the Barthel index. *Phys Ther* 1988;68:1077–81.
3895. Loewenfeld IE, Thompson HS. Oculomotor paresis with cyclic spasms. *Surv Ophthalmol* 1975;20:81.
3896. Logan JL, Harveyson KB, Wisdom GB et al. Hereditary caeruloplasmin deficiency, dementia and diabetes mellitus. *Quart J Med* 1994;87:663–70.
3897. Logigian EL, Kolodny EH, Griffith JF et al. Myoclonus epilepsy in two brothers. *Brain* 1986;109:411–29.
3898. Logothetis J, Constantoulakis M, Economidou J et al. Thalassemia major (homozygous beta-thalassemia). *Neurology* 1972;22:294–304.
3899. Logsdail SJ,Toone BK. Post-ictal psychosis: A clinical and phenomenological description. *Br J Psychiatry* 1988;152:246–52.
3900. Loiseau H, Marchal C, Vital A et al. Occurrence of polyglucosan bodies in temporal lobe epilepsy. *J Neurol Neurosurg Psychiatry* 1992;55:1092–3.
3901. Loiseau J, Loiseau P, Duclo B et al. A survey of epileptic disorders in southwest France: Seizures in elderly patients. *Ann Neurol* 1990;27:231–8.
3902. Loiseau P, Guyot M, Loiseau H et al. Eating seizures. *Epilepsia* 1986;27:161–3.
3903. Lomas DA. Molecular mousetraps, alpha, antitrypsin deficiency and the serpinopathies. *Clin Med* 2005;5:249–57.
3904. Lombroso CT. Sylvian seizures and midtemporal spike foci in children. *Arch Neurol* 1967;17:52–9.
3905. Lombroso CT, Fejerman N. Benign polymyoclonus of early infancy. *Ann Neurol* 1977;1:138–43.
3906. Lombroso CT, Lerman P. Breathholding spells (cyanotic and pallid infantile syncope). *Pediatrics* 1967;39:563–81.
3907. Lomen-Hoerth C, Anderson T, Miller B. The overlap of amyotrophic lateral sclerosis and frontotemporal dementia. *Neurology* 2002;59:1077–9.
3908. Long RR, Sargent JC, Pappas AM et al. Pitcher's arm: An electrodiagnostic enigma. *Muscle Nerve* 1996;19:1276–81.
3909. Loonen MCB, Busch HFM, Koster JF et al. A family with different forms of acid maltase deficiency glycogenosis Type II. *Neurology* 1981;31:1209–16.
3910. Lopez JR, Adornato BT, Hoyt WF. Entomopia: A remarkable case of cerebral polyopia. *Neurology* 1993;43:2145–6.
3911. Lopez PF, Lawton Smith J. Leber's optic atrophy. *J Clin Neuro-Ophthalmol* 1986;6:144–52.
3912. Lopez-Hernandez A. Craniosynostosis, ataxia, trigeminal anaesthesia and parietal alopecia with pons-vermis fusion anomaly (atresia of the fourth ventricle). Report of two cases. *Neuropediatrics* 1982;13:99–102.
3913. Lord SM, Barnsley L, Walis BJ et al. Third occipital nerve headache: A prevalence study. *J Neurol Neurosurg Psychiatry* 1994;57:1187–90.
3914. Lorentzen SE. Drusen of the optic disk, an irregularly dominant hereditary affection. *Acta Ophthalmol* 1961;39:626–43.
3915. Loseth S, Torbergsen T, Brautaset N et al. A new non-dystrophic painful myotonia with dominant inheritance. *J Neurol Neurosurg Psychiatr* 2001;71:419. (Abstract)
3916. Lossos A, Baala L, Soffer D et al. A novel autosomal recessive myopathy with external ophthalmoplegia linked to chromosome 17p13.1-p12. *Brain* 2005;128:42–51.
3917. Lossos A, Barash V, Soffer D et al. Hereditary branching enzyme dysfunction in adult polyglucosan body disease: A possible metabolic cause in two patients. *Ann Neurol* 1991;30:655–62.
3918. Lossos A, Cooperman H, Soffer D et al. Hereditary leukoencephalopathy and palmoplantar keratoderma. *Neurology* 1995;45:331–7.
3919. Lossos A, Dobson-Stone C, Monaco AP et al. Early clinical heterogeneity in choreoacanthocytosis. *Arch Neurol* 2005;62:611–4.
3920. Lotz BP, Stubgen J-P. The rigid spine syndrome: A vacuolar variant. *Muscle Nerve* 1993;16:530–6.
3921. Louis ED, Lynch T, Ford B et al. Delayed onset cerebellar syndrome. *Arch Neurol* 1996;53:450–4.
3921a. Lou M, Safdar A, Mehdiratta M et al. The HAT score. Neurology 2008;71:1417–23
3922. Louis-Bar D. Sur un syndrome progressif comprénant des telangiectasies capillaires cutanées et conjontivales symmetriques, a disposition naevoide et des troubles cerebelleux. *Confin Neurol* 1941;4:32–42.
3923. Louis-Bar D, Legros J. Les hypertrophies partielles avec angiome (syndrome de Klippel-Trenaunay) et leurs rapports avec les phacomatoses. *Confin Neurol* 1946;7–8:245.
3924. Louis ED, Lynch T, Kaufmann Peal. Diagnostic guidelines in central nervous system Whipple's disease. *Ann Neurol* 1996;40:561–8.
3925. Love S, Duchen LW. Familial cerebellar ataxia with cerebrovascular amyloid. *J Neurol Neurosurg Psychiatry* 1982;45:271–3.
3926. Lovell HW. Familial progressive bulbar paralysis. *Arch Neurol Psychiatry* 1932;28:394–8.
3927. Low PA, Burke WJ, McLeod JG. Congenital sensory neuropathy with selective loss of small myelinated nerve fibers. *Ann Neurol* 1978;3:179–82.
3928. Low PA, Dyck PJ, Lambert EH et al. Acute panautonomic neuropathy. *Ann Neurol* 1983;13:412.
3929. Low PA, et al. The sympathetic nervous system in diabetic neuropathy. *Brain* 1975;98:341–56.
3930. Low PA, Fealey RD, Sheps SG et al. Chronic idiopathic anhidrosis. *Ann Neurol* 1985;18:344–8.
3931. Low VA. *Muscle Nerve* 2006;34:57–61.
3932. Lowden JA, O'Brien JS. Sialidosis: A review of human neuramindase deficiency. *Am J Hum Genet* 1979;31:1–18.
3933. Lowe CU, Terrey M, MacLachlan EA. Organic aciduria, decreased renal ammonia production, hydrophthalmos, and mental retardation. A clinical entity. *Am J Dis Childh* 1952;83:164–84.
3934. Lowe J, Spillantini MG. Non-Alzheimer degenerative dementias. *Brain Pathol* 1998;8:295–7.
3935. Lowenberg K, Hill TS. Diffuse sclerosis with preserved myelin islands. *Arch Neurol Psychiatry* 1933;29:1232–45.
3936. Lowenstein O, Levine AS. Pupillographic studies. *Arch Ophthal Berlin* 1944;31:74–94.
3937. Lowenthal A. On a congenital and familial form of generalized muscle sclerosis with blepharoptosis. *Acta Neurol Psychiatr Belg* 1952;52:141–55.

3938. Lowenthal A. Striopallidodentate calcifications. In Vinken PJ, Bruyn GW, Klawans HL eds. *Extrapyramidal Disorders. Handbook of Clinical Neurology*, vol.5, pp 417–36. Amsterdam: Elsevier Science Publishers, 1986.

3939. Lowry RB. Congenital absence of the fibula and craniosynostosis in sibs. *J Med Genet* 1972;9:227–9.

3940. Lowry RB, Wood BJ. Syndrome of epiphyseal dysplasia, short stature, microcephaly and nystagmus. *Clin Genet* 1975;8:269–74.

3941. Lubbers WJ, Brunt ERP, Scheffer H et al. Hereditary myokymia and paroxysmal ataxia linked to chromosome 12 is responsive to acetazolamide. *J Neurol Neurosurg Psychiatry* 1995;59:400–5.

3942. Lubin B. *Depression Adjectives Checklist (Manual)*. San Diego: Educational and Industrial Testing Service, 1967.

3943. Lubkin V. The inverse Marcus Gunn phenomenon: An electromyographic contribution. *Arch Neurol* 1978;35:249.

3944. Lublin FD, Tsairis P, Streletz LJ et al. Myokymia and impaired muscular relaxation with continuous motor unit activity. *J Neurol Neurosurg Psychiatry* 1979;42:557–62.

3945. Lubs M-LE, Bauer MS, Formas ME et al. Lisch nodules in neurofibromatosis type 1. *N Engl J Med* 1991;324:1264–5.

3946. Luccelli F, De Renzi E. Primary dyscalculia after a medial frontal lesion of the left hemisphere. *J Neurol Neurosurg Psychiatry* 1993;56:304–7.

3947. Lucchelli F, De Renzi E, Perani D et al. Primary amnesia of insidious onset with subseqent stabilisation. *J Neurol Neurosurg Psychiatry* 1994;57:1366–70.

3948. Luders H, Lesser RP, Dinner DS et al. The second sensory area in humans: Evoked potential and electrical stimulation studies. *Ann Neurol* 1985;17:177–84.

3949. Ludlow CL. Children's language disorders: Recent research advances. *Ann Neurol* 1980;7:497–507.

3950. Ludolph AC, Hugon J, Dwivedi MP et al. Studies on the aetiology and pathogenesis of motor neuron diseases. I. Lathyrism: Clinical findings in established cases. *Brain* 1987;110:149–66.

3951. Ludwig CL, Smith MT, Godfrey AD et al. A clinicopathological study of 323 patients with oligodendrogliomas. *Ann Neurol* 1986;19:15–21.

3952. Ludwig J, Dyck PJ, LaRusso NF. Xanthomatous neuropathy of liver. *Human Pathology* 1982;137:1049–51.

3953. Luft R et al. A case of severe hypermetabolism of nonthyroid origin with a defect in the maintenance of mitochondrial respiratory control: A correlated clinical, biochemical, and morphological study. *J Clin Invest* 1962;41:1776–804.

3954. Lugaresi, Cirignotta F. Hypnogenic paroxysmal dystonia: Epileptic seizure or a new syndrome? *Sleep* 1981;4:129–38.

3955. Lugaresi E. *Abnormal Movements Occurring During Sleep (AAN Course Handout)*, 1989.

3956. Lugaresi E, Cirignotta F, Montagna P. Occipital lobe epilepsy with scotosensitive seizures: The role of central vision. *Epilepsia* 1984;25:115–20.

3957. Lugaresi E, Cirignotta F, Montagna P. Nocturnal paroxysmal dystonia. *J Neurol Neurosurg Psychiatry* 1986;49:375–80.

3958. Lugaresi E, Coccagna G, Gambi D et al. Symond's nocturnal myoclonus. *EEG Clin Neurophysiol* 1967;23:289.

3959. Lugaresi E, Pazzaglia P, Roger J. Evolution and prognosis of petit mal. In Harris P, Mawdsley C eds. *Epilepsy: Proceedings of the Hans Berger Centenary*, pp 151–3. Edinburgh: Churchill Livingstone, 1974.

3960. Lundberg A. Myalgia cruris epidemica. *Acta Pediatr Scand* 1957;46:18.

3961. Lundberg N. Continuous recording and control of ventricular fluid pressure in neurosurgical practice. *Acta Psychiatr Neurol* 1960;36:1–193.

3962. Lundberg PO. Hereditary polyneuropathy, oligophrenia, premature menopause and acromicria. *Eur Neurol* 1971;5:84–98.

3963. Lundberg PO, Westerberg CE. A hereditary neurological disease with facial spasm. *J Neurol Sci* 1968;8:85–100.

3964. Lundberg PO, Wranne I, Brun A. A family with optic atrophy and neurological symptoms. *Acta Neurol Scand* 1967;43:87–105.

3965. Luria AR. *Human Brain and Psychological Processes.* New York: Harper & Row, 1966.

3966. Luria AR. *The Mind of a Mnemonist*. New York: Basic Books, 1968.

3967. Luscher E. Function of the stapedius muscle. *Z Hals-Nasen-Ohrenheilkd* 1929;105:23.

3968. Luscher TF, Lie JT, Stanson AW et al. Arterial fibromuscular dysplasia. *Mayo Clin Proc* 1987;62:931–52.

3969. Luxon LM. Disorders of hearing. In Asbury AK, McKhann GM, McDonald WI eds. *Diseases of the Nervous System*, pp 544–60. Philadelphia: Saunders, 1987.

3970. Lyell A. Delusions of parasitosis. *Br J Dermatol* 1983;108:489.

3971. Lying-Tunell U. Quantitative methods of estimating CSF flow. *Radiol Clin N Amer* 1974;12:503–11.

3972. Lyle DJ. The ocular syndrome of cataract and papilledema in the manifest form of parathyroid deficiency. *Am J Ophthalmol* 1948;31:580.

3973. Lynch DR, Chance PF. Inherited peripheral neuropathies. *The Neurologist* 1997;3:277–92.

3974. Lynch PG, Bansal DV. Granulomatous polymyositis. *J Neurol Sci* 1973;18:1–9.

3975. Lynch SA, Hall K, Precious S et al. Two further cases of Sener syndrome. *J Med Genet* 2000;37:466–70.

3976. Lynch T, Sano M, Marder KS et al. Clinical characteristics of a family with chromosome 17-linked disinhibition-dementia-parkinsonism-amyotrophy complex. *Neurology* 1994;44:1878–84.

3977. Lyon G, Arita F, Le Galloudec E et al. A disorder of axonal development, necrotizing myopathy, cardiomyopathy and cataracts: A new familial disease. *Ann Neurol* 1990;27:193–9.

3978. Lyon G, Ponsot G, Lebon P. Acute measles encephalitis of the delayed type. *Ann Neurol* 1977;2:322–7.

3979. Lyon LW. Neurological manifestations of cat-scratch disease. Report of a case and review of the literature. *Arch Neurol* 1971;25:23–7.

3980. Lyons JB. *The Citizen Surgeon: A Biography of Sir Victor Horsley.* London: Dawnay, 1966.

3981. Lyons JB. Sir Victor Horsley. *Med Hist* 1967;11:361–73.

3982. Lyu R-K, Chen S-T. Acute multiple cranial neuropathy: A variant of Guillain–Barré syndrome? *Muscle Nerve* 2004;30:433–6.

3983. Mabry CC, Roeckel IE, Munich RL et al. X-linked pseudohypertrophic muscular dystrophy with a late onset and slow progression. *N Engl J Med* 1965;273:1062–70.

3984. Macalpine I, Hunter R. A clinical reassessment of the insanity of King George III and some of its historical implications. *Bull Inst Hist Res* 1967;40:166–85.

3985. Maccario M et al. A sibship with neuroaxonal dystrophy and renal tubular acidosis. *Ann Neurol* 1983;13:608–15.

3986. Maccario M, Lustman LI. Paroxysmal nocturnal dystonia presenting as excessive daytime somnolence. *Arch Neurol* 1990;47:291–4.

3987. MacCollin M, Chiocca EA, et al. Diagnostic criteria for schwannomatosis. *Neurology* 2005;64:1838–45.

3988. MacCollin M, De Vivo DC, Moser AB et al. Ataxia and peripheral neuropathy: A benign variant of peroxisome dysgenesis. *Ann Neurol* 1990;28:833–6.

3989. MacCollin M, Woodfin W, Kronn D et al. Schwannomatosis: A clinical and pathologic study. *Neurology* 1996;46:1072–9.

3990. Macdermot KD, Walker RWH. Autosomal recessive hereditary motor and sensory neuropathy with mental retardation, optic atrophy and pyramidal signs. *J Neurol Neurosurg Psychiatry* 1987;50:1342–7.

3991. Macdonald RL, Deck JHN. Immunohistochemistry of ecchordosis physaliphora and chordoma. *Can J Neurol Sci* 1990;17:420–423.

3992. Mace CJ, Trimble MR. "Hysteria","functional", or "psychogenic"? A survey of British neurologists' preferences. *J Roy Soc Med* 1991;84: 471–5.

3993. Mace JW, Sponaugle HD, Mitsunaga RY et al. Congenital hereditary non-progressive external ophthalmoplegia. *Am J Dis Childh* 1971;122:261–3.

3994. Macedo-Souza LI, Kok F, Santos S. Spastic paraplegia, optic atrophy, and neuropathy is linked to chromosome 11q13. *Ann Neurol* 2005;57:730–7.

3995. McEwen W. A Consideration of the means we possess for distinguishing between coma arising from alcoholic intoxication and that produced by apoplexy, fracture of the base of the skull, and other causes. *Glasgow Med J* 1879;2:1.

3996. McEwen W. Pyogenic infective diseases of the brain and spinal cord. Glasgow: J.Maclehose & Sons, 1893.

3997. MacFarlin DE, Strober W, Waldmann TA. Ataxia telangiectasia. *Medicine* 1972;51:281–314.

3998. Mack WJ, Freed DM, Williams BW. Boston naming test: Shortened version for use in Alzheimer's disease. *J Gerontol* 1992;47:154–8.

3999. Mackay MT, Kornberg AJ, Shield LK et al. Benign acute childhood myositis: Laboratory and clinical features. *Neurology* 1999;53:2127–31.

4000. Mackay RP. Congenital demyelinating encephalopathy. *Arch Neurol Psychiatry* 1940;43:111–8.

4001. MacKeith RC. The placing response and primary walking. *Guy's Hosp Gaz* 1965;79:394.

4002. Mackenzie I. The clinical presentation of the cerebral angioma. *Brain* 1953;76:184–214.

4003. Mackenzie S. Two cases of associated paralysis of the tongue, soft palate and vocal chord on the same side. *Trans Clin Soc London* 1886;19:317–9.

4004. Mackin GA, Bird SJ, Adams CA et al. EMG indicators of critical illness myopathy following prolonged neuromuscular blockade and high dose corticosteroids. *Muscle Nerve* 1994;17:168. (Abstract)

4005. Maclaren NK, Max SR, Cornblath M et al. GM3 gangliosidosis: A novel human sphingolipodystrophy. *Pediatrics* 1976;57:106–11.

4006. MacLean JB, Sassin JF. Paroxysmal vertical ocular dyskinesia. *Arch Neurol* 1973;29:117–9.

4007. Macleod AD. Shell shock, Gordon Holmes and the great war. *J Roy Soc Med* 2004;37:86–9.

4008. MacLeod PM, Wood S, Jan JE et al. Progressive cerebellar ataxia, spasticity, psychomotor retardation and hexosaminidase deficiency in a 10-year old child: Juvenile Sandhoff disease. *Neurology* 1977;27:571–3.

4009. MacPherson RI. Craniodiaphyseal dysplasia, a disease or group of diseases? *J Can Assoc Radiol* 1974;25:22.

4010. Madonick MJ, Gilbert S, Stern WZ. Partial agenesis of septum pellucidum with cave of septum pellucidum. *Arch Neurol* 1964;11:324–9.

4011. Madrid R, Bradley WG. The pathology of neuropathies with focal thickenings of the myelin sheath (tomaculous neuropathy). *J Neurol Sci* 1975;25:415–48.

4012. Maeda K, Horiguchi S, Hosokawa M. History of the studies on occupational cervicobrachial disorder in Japan and remaining problems. *J Human Ergol* 1982;11:17–29.

4013. Magee KR, DeJong RN. Hereditary distal myopathy with onset in infancy. *Arch Neurol* 1965;13:387–90.

4014. Magee R. Genitofemoral causalgia. *Can Med Assn J* 1942;46:326–9.

4015. Magendie F. Memoire sur un liquide qui se trouve dans le crâne et le canal vertebral de l'homme et des animaux mammiferes. *J Physiol Exp* 1825;5:27.

4016. Maguadda A, Bernardino BD, de Marco P et al. Bilateral occipital calcification, epilepsy and celiac disease: Clinical and neuroimaging features of a new syndrome. *J Neurol Neurosurg Psychiatry* 1993;56:885–9.

4017. Magy L, Birouk N, Vallat JM et al. Hereditary thermosensitive neuropathy. *Neurology* 1997;48:1684–90.

4018. Mahjneh I, Udd B, Haravuori H et al. A distinct phenotype of distal myopathy in a large Finnish family. *J Neurol* 2000;3:247.

4019. Mahloudji M, Livingston KE. Familial and congenital simple anhidrosis. *Am J Dis Childh* 1967;134:77.

4020. Mahloudji M, Pikielny RT. Paramyoclonus multiplex. *Trans Am Neurol Assn* 1966;91:289–90.

4021. Mahloudji M, Pikielny RT. Hereditary essential myoclonus. *Brain* 1967;90: 669–74.

4022. Mahloudji M, Teasdall RD, Adamkiewicz JJ et al. The genetic amyloidoses: With particular reference to hereditary neuropathic amyloidosis, type II (Indiana Rukavina type). *Medicine* 1969;48:1–37.

4023. Mahmoud M, Raymond J, Mahmoud M et al. Vertebral artery stump syndrome. *J Neurol Neurosurg Psychiatry* 2008;79: 91–3.

4024. Mahoney FI, Barthel DW. Functional evaluation: The Barthel index. *Md State Med J* 1965;14:61–5.

4025. Mahowald MW, Ettinger MG. Things that go bump in the night: The parasomnias revisited. *J Clin Neurophysiol* 1990;7:119–43.

4026. Mahowald MW, Schenck CH. REM sleep behavior disorder. In Kryger MH, Roth T, Dement WC eds. *Principles and Practice of Sleep Medicine*, Philadelphia: W.B. Saunders Co., 1989.

4027. Mahowald MW, Schenck CH. Dissociated states of wakefulness and sleep. *Neurology* 1992;42:44–52.

4028. Mai FM, Merskey H. Briquet's concept of hysteria: An historical perspective. *Can J Psychiatry* 1981;26:57–63.

4029. Maigne R. Douleur d'origine vertébrale et traitment par manipulation. Paris: Expansion Scientifique, 1977.

4030. Mailander JC. Hereditary gustatory sweating. *J AmMed Assoc* 1967;202: 203–4.

4031. Mainzer F, Saldino RM, Ozonoff MB et al. Familial nephropathy associated with retinitis pigmentosa, cerebellar ataxia and skeletal abnormalities. *Am J Med* 1970;49:556–62.

4032. Maitland CG, Abiko S, Hoyt WF et al. Chiasmal apoplexy: Report of four cases. *J Neurosurg* 1982;56:118–22.

4033. Maitland C. Perilymphatic fistula. *Curr Neurol Neurosci Rep* 2001;1:486–91.

4034. Majewski F et al. Polysyndactyly . . . An original syndrome?. *Zschr Kinderh* 1971;111:118–38.

4035. Makin GJV, Brown WF, Ebers GC. C7 radiculopathy: Importance of scapular winging in clinical diagnosis. *J Neurol Neurosurg Psychiatry* 1986;49:640–4.

4036. Malm J, Kristensen B, Karlsson T et al. The predictive value of cerebrospinal fluid dynamic tests in patients with the idiopathic hydrocephalus syndrome. *Arch Neurol* 1995;52:783–9.

4037. Mancall EL, Patel AN, Hirschorn AM. Hypertrophic branchial myopathy. *Neurology* 1974;24:1166–70.

4038. Manchanda R, Miller H, McLachlan RS. Post-ictal psychosis after right temporal lobectomy. *J Neurol Neurosurg Psychiatry* 1993;56:277–9.

4039. Manford M. Assessment and investigation of possible epileptic seizures. *J Neurol Neurosurg Psychiatry* 2001;70:113–8.

4040. Manford M, Andermann F. Complex visual hallucinations: Clinical and neurobiological insights. *Brain* 1992;121:1819–40.

4041. Manford MRA, Fish DR, Shorvon SD. Startle provoked epileptic seizures: Features in 19 patients. *J Neurol Neurosurg Psychiatry* 1996;61:151–6.
4042. Mann L. Concerning some physical signs after brain contusion. *Dtsch Med Wschr* 1931;57:2072–5.
4043. Mann MD, MacFarlane CM, Verburg CJ et al. The bromide partition test and CSF adenosine deaminase activity in the diagnosis of tuberculosis meningitis in children. *S Afr Med J* 1982;62:431–3.
4044. Mann SC, Caroff SN, Blein HR et al. Lethal catatonia. *Am J Psychiatry* 1986;143:1374–81.
4045. Manni JJ, Scaf JJ, Huygen PLM et al. Hyperostosis cranialis interna: A new hereditary syndrome with cranial nerve entrapment. *N Engl J Med* 1990;322:450.
4046. Manor-Esperrilat M, Gothe B, Adams N et al. Familial sleep apnea plus syndrome. *Neurology* 1988;38:190–3.
4047. Manschot S, van Passel L, Buskens E et al. Mayo and NINDS scales for assessment of tendon reflexes: Between observer agreement and implications for communication. *J Neurol Neurosurg Psychiatry* 1998;64:253–5.
4048. Mansour AH, Shoch D, Logani S. Optic disk size in ischemic optic neuropathy. *Am J Ophthalmol* 1988;106:587–9.
4049. Manta P, Kalfakis N, Bassilopoulos D et al. An unusual case of lower motor neuron disease. *J Neurol* 1983;230:141–2.
4050. Manta P, Kalfakis N, Vassipoulos D et al. Neuropathy of vasculitic origin in a case of Garin-Boujadoux-Bannwarth syndrome with a positive Borrelia antibody response. *J Neurol* 1986;233:69–72.
4051. Manto M, Goldman S, Bodur H. Cerebellar syndrome associated with Hashimoto's encephalopathy. *Rev Neurol* 1996;152:202–4.
4052. Manzur AY, Keyes RD, Bennett M et al. Progressive axial muscle rigidity during infancy: A new entity. *Can J Neurol Sci* 1994;21(**Suppl. 2**):S34. (Abstract)
4053. Mao C-C, Coull BM, Golper AC et al. Anterior operculum syndrome. *Neurology* 1989;39:1169–72.
4054. Maraist TA, Soloman DH, Barohn RJ et al. Thalamic ataxia. *Neurology* 1991;41 (**Suppl. 1**):125.
4055. Maramattom BV, Wijdicks EF. Arrow sign in MCA trifurcation aneurysm. *Neurology* 2004;63.
4056. Marburg O. Die sogenannte "akute multiple Sklerose". *Jhrb Psychiatr Neurol* 1906;27:211–312.
4057. Marchall C. Some clinical correlates of the wave and spike phantom. *EEG Clin Neurophysiol* 1955;77:63343.
4058. Marchiafava E, Bignami A. Sopra un alterazione del corpo calloso osservata da sogetti alcolisti. *Riv Pat Nerv delle Alienazione* 1903;8:544–9.
4059. Marden PM, Walker WA. A new generalized connective tissue syndrome. *Am J Dis Childh* 1966;112:225–8.
4060. Marelli FL. Lichtheim syndrome: Neurologic study. *Revista Argentina de Neurol y Psquiat; Rosario* 1942;7:143.
4061. Mareska M, Gutmann L. Lambert-Eaton myasthenic syndrome. *Semin Neurol* 2004;24:149–53.
4062. Marfan ABJ. A case of congenital deformation of all four limbs. *Bull Soc Med Hop Paris* 1896;13:220.
4063. Margo CE, Levy MH, Beck RW. Bilateral idiopathic inflammation of the optic nerve sheaths. *Ophthalmology* 1989;96:200–6.
4064. Margolis E. A new hereditary syndrome – sex-linked deaf mutism associated with total albinism. *Acta Genet* 1962;12:12.
4065. Margolis RL, O'Hearn E, Rosenblatt A et al. A disorder similar to Huntington's disease is associated with a novel CAG repeat expansion. Ann Neurol 2001;50:373–80.
4066. Mahapatra RK, Edwards MJ, Schott JM et al. Cortico-basal degeneration. *Lancet Neurol* 2004;3:736–42.
4067. Maricich SM, Neul JL, Lotze TE et al. Neurologic complications associated with influenza A in children during the 2003–2004 influenza season in Houston, Texas. *Pediatrics* 2004;114: e626–e633.
4068. Maridort P. Un nouveau signe d'alcoolisme. *Med Mod* 1900;11:397.
4069. Marie J, See G. Hydrocephalie aigue benigne du nourrisson apres ingestion d'une dose massive et unique de vitamine A et D. *Arch Fr Ped* 1951,8:563–5.
4070. Marie P. Sur l'heredo-ataxie cerebelleuse. *Sem Med* 1893;13:444–7.
4071. Marie P. Existe-t-il une atrophie musculaire progressive Aran-Duchenne? *Rev Neurol* 1897;5:686.
4072. Marie P. Revision de la question de l'aphasie; la troisième circonvolution frontale gauche ne joue aucun rôle special dans la fonction du language. *Sem Med* 1906;26:241.
4073. Marie P, Foix C. Symmetrical and centrilobar intracerebral sclerosis. *Rev Neurol* 1914;27:1–16.
4074. Marie P, Meige ET, Patrikios H. Paralysie radiale disociée simulant une griffe cubitale. *Rev Neurol* 1917;24:123–4.
4075. Mariën P, Verhoeven J, Engelborghs S et al. A role for the cerebellum in motor speech planning: Evidence from foreign accent syndrome. *Clin Neurol Neurosurg* 2006;108:518–522.
4076. Marin Amat M. Contribucion al esudio de la curabilidad de las paralisis oculares de origen traumatico – substitucion funcional del VII par el V par craneal. *Arch Oft Hisp Amer* 1918;18:70–99.
4077. Marin R, Dillingham TR, Chang CM et al. Extensor digitorum brevis reflex in normals and patients with radiculopathies. *Muscle Nerve* 1995;18:52–9.
4078. Marin-Padilla M. Cephalic axial skeletal-neural dysraphic disorders: Embryology and pathology. *Can J Neurol Sci* 1991;18:153–69.
4079. Marin-Padilla M, Parisi J, Armstrong D et al. Shaken infant syndrome: Developmental neuropathology, progressive cortical dysplasia and epilepsy. *Acta Neuropathol (Berl)* 2002;103:321–32.
4080. Marinacci AA, von Hagen KO. Misleading all median hand. *Arch Neurol* 1965;12:80–3.
4081. Marinesco G. *Succulent Hand and Muscle Atrophy in Syringomyelia.* Paris: Université de Paris, 1897.
4082. Marinesco G, Draganesco S, Vasili U. Nouvelle maladie familiale caracterisèe par une cataracte congenitale et un arrêt du developpement somato-neuro-psychique. *Encephale* 1931;26:97–109.
4083. Marini C, King MA, Archer JS et al. Idiopathic generalized epilepsy of adult onset: Clinical syndromes and genetics. *J Neurol Neurosurg Psychiatr* 2003;74: 192–6.
4084. Marion MH, Gledhill RF. Spasms of amputation stumps: A report of two cases. *Mov Disord* 1989;4:354–8.
4085. Maris T, Androulidakis EJ, Tzagournissakis M et al. X-linked adrenolcukodystrophy presenting a neurologically pure familial spastic paraparesis. *Neurology* 1994;45: 1101–4.
4086. Markand ON, Daly DD. Juvenile type of slowly progressive bulbar palsy: Report of a case. *Neurology* 1971;21:753–8.
4087. Markesbery WR, Griggs RC, Herr B. Distal myopathy: Electron microscopic and histochemical studies. *Neurology* 1977;27:727–35.
4088. Markesbery WR, Griggs RC, Leach RP et al. Late onset hereditary distal myopathy. *Neurology* 1974;23: 127–34.
4089. Markesbery WR, Schmitt FA, Kryscio RJ et al. Neuropathologic substrate of mild cognitive impairment. *Arch Neurol* 2006;63:38–46.
4090. Markey K, Di Benedetto M, Curl W. Upper trunk brachial plexopathy. The stinger syndrome. *Am J Sports Med* 1993;21:650–5.
4091. Markson EW, Levitz G. A Guttman scale to assess memory loss among the elderly. *Gerontologist* 1973;13:337–40.

4092. Markson L, Jarman P, Bril V. Response to therapy in demyelinating motor neuropathy. *Muscle Nerve* 1998;21: 1769–71.

4093. Maroon JC. Burning hands in football spinal cord injuries. *JAMA* 1977;**238**:2049–51.

4094. Maroteaux P. Le syndrome camptomyelique. *Presse Med* 1971;79:1157–62.

4095. Maroteaux P, Lamy M. Pyknodysostosis. *Presse Med* 1962;70:999.

4096. Maroteaux P, Lamy M. Hurler's disease, Morquio's disease, and related mucopolysaccharidoses. *J Pediatr* 1965;67:312–23.

4097. Marquez S, Turley JJ, Peters WJ. Neuropathy in burn patients. *Brain* 1993;116:471–83.

4098. Mars H, Lewis LA, Robertson AL et al. Familial hypo-β-lipoproteinemia. *Am J Med* 1969;46:886–900.

4099. Marsden CD. Blepharospasm-oromandibular dystonia syndrome (Brueghel's syndrome): A variant of adult-onset torsion dystonia? *J Neurol Neurosurg Psychiatry* 1976;39:1204–9.

4100. Marsden CD. The problem of adult-onset idiopathic torsion dystonia and other isolated dyskinesias in adult life. In Eldridge R, Fahn S eds. *Advances in Neurology: Dystonia*, pp 259–76. New York: Raven Press, 1976.

4101. Marsden CD. The Focal dystonias. *Clin Neuropharmacol* 1986;9(**Suppl.** 2):S49–S60.

4102. Marsden CD, Harrison MJG. Idiopathic torsion dystonia (dystonia musculorum deformans). *Brain* 1974;97:793–810.

4103. Marsden CD, Obeso JA, Rothwell JC. Benign essential tremor is not a single entity. In Yahr MD ed. *Current Concepts in Parkinson's Disease*, pp 31–6. Amsterdam: Excerpta Medica, 1983.

4104. Marsden CD, Obeso JA, Zarranz JJ et al. The anatomical basis of symptomatic hemidystonia. *Brain* 1985;108:463–83.

4105. Marsden CD, Parkes JD. "On-off" effects in patients with Parkinson's disease on chronic levodopa therapy. *Lancet* 1976;1:292–6.

4106. Marsden CD, Reynolds EH, Parsons V. Myopathy associated with anticonvulsant osteomalacia. *B MJ* 1973;4:526–7.

4107. Marseille Consensus group. Classification of progressive myoclonus epilepsies and related disorders. *Ann Neurol* 1990;28:113–6.

4108. Marshall JC, Halligan PW, Fink GR et al. The functional anatomy of a hysterical paralysis. *Cognition* 1997;64:B1–B8.

4109. Marshall FJ, de Blieck EA, Mink JW et al. A clinical rating scale for Batten disease. *Neurology* 2005;65:275–9.

4110. Marshall J. Observations of reflex changes in the lower limbs in spastic paraplegia in man. *Brain* 1954;77:290–304.

4111. Marshall J. Dominant saddle nose, cataract and hearing loss. *Am J Ophthalmol* 1958;45:143–56.

4112. Marshall JC, Newcombe F. Patterns of paralexia - a psycholinguistic approach. *J Psychol Res* 1973;2:175–99.

4113. Marshall LF, Marshall LB, Klauber MR et al. The diagnosis of head injury requires a classification based on computed axial tomography. *J Neurotrauma* 1992;9 (**Suppl.** 1): S287–S292.

4114. Marshall LF, Marshall SB, Klauber MR et al. A new classification of head injury based on computerized tomography. *J Neurosurg* 1991;75:S14–S20.

4115. Martensson B. Dominant hereditary nerve deafness. *Acta Oto-Rhino-Laryngol (Belg)* 1960;52:270–4.

4116. Martin J-J, Brucher J-M, Evrard P et al. On an autosomal dominant form of retino-cerebellar degeneration: An autopsy study of four patients in a Belgian family. *Neurology* 1991;41 (**Suppl.**):424.

4117. Martin J, Swash M. Myopathy with absence of muscle glycogen and neutral lipid in the neuroleptic malignant syndrome. *J Neurol* 1987;235:120–1.

4118. Martin JP. Fits of laughter (sham mirth) in organic cerebral disease. *Brain* 1950;73:453–64.

4119. Martin JP. Tilting reactions and disorders of the basal ganglia. *Brain* 1965;88: 855–74.

4120. Martin NA. A proposed grading system for arteriovenous malformations. *J Neurosurg* 1986;65:476–83.

4121. Martinelli P, Fabbri R, Gabellini AS. Familial hypertrophy of the masseter muscles. *J Neurol* 1987;234:251–3.

4122. Martinez AC. Slimmer's paralysis: Electrophysiological evidence of compressive lesion. *Eur Neurol* 1987;26:189.

4123. Martinez BA, Lake BD. Childhood nemaline myopathy – a review of clinical presentation in relation to prognosis. *Dev Med Child Neurol* 1987;29:815–20.

4124. Martínez-Juárez IE, Alonso ME, Medina MT et al. Juvenile myoclonic epilepsy subsyndromes: Family studies and long-term follow-up. *Brain* 2007;129:1269–80.

4125. Martinez-Rodriguez JE, Barriga FJ. Nonconvulsive status epilepticus associated with cephalosporins in patients with renal failure. *Am J Med* 2001;111:115–9.

4126. Martinsson T, Darin N, Kyllerman M et al. Dominant hereditary inclusion-body myopathy gene (IBM3) maps to chromosome region 17p13.1. *Am J Hum Genet* 1999;64:1420–6.

4127. Martsolf JT, Cracco JB, Carpenter GG et al. Pfeiffer syndrome: An unusual type of acrocephalosyndactyly with broad thumbs and great toes. *Am J Dis Childh* 1971;121:257–62.

4128. Martsolf JT et al. Severe mental retardation, cataracts, short stature and primary hypogonadism in two brothers. *Am J Med Genet* 1978;1:291–9.

4129. Martuza RL, Eldridge R. Neurofibromatosis 2. *N Engl J Med* 1988;318:684–8.

4130. Martyn CN, Ewing DJ. Pupil cycle time: A simple way of measuring an autonomic reflex. *J Neurol Neurosurg Psychiatry* 1986;49:771–4.

4131. Marushima A, Matsumura A et al. Adult tethered cord syndrome presenting with refractory diarrhoea. *J Neurol Neurosurg Psychiatry* 2003;74:1596–7.

4132. Marxmiller J, Trenkle I, Ashwal S. Rud syndrome revisited. *Dev Med Child Neurol* 1985;27:335–43.

4133. Mas JL, Dilouya A, de Recondo J. A familial disorder with subcortical ischemic strokes, dementia and leukoencephalopathy. *Neurology* 1992;42:1015–9.

4134. Masdeu JC et al. Pseudo-abducens palsy with midbrain lesions. *Trans Am Neurol Assn* 1981;105:184.

4135. Masdeu JC, Gorelick PB. Thalamic astasia: Inability to stand after unilateral thalamic lesions. *Ann Neurol* 1988;23:596–603.

4136. Masdeu JC, Quinto C, Olivera C et al. Open-ring imaging sign. *Neurology* 2000;54:1427–33.

4137. Masdeu JC, Ross ER. Medullary satiety. *Neurology* 1988;38:1643–5.

4138. Maselli RA, Kong DZ, Bowe CM et al. Presynaptic congenital myasthenic syndrome due to quantal release deficiency. *Neurology* 2001;57:279–89.

4139. Maselli RA, Rosenberg RS, Spire J-P. Episodic nocturnal wanderings in non-epileptic young patients. *Sleep* 1988;11:156–61.

4140. Maset AL, Marmarou A, Ward JD et al. Pressure-volume index in head injury. *J Neurosurg* 1987;67:832–40.

4141. Masjuan J, Alvarez-Cermeno JC, Garcia-Barragan N et al. Clinically isolated syndromes. *Neurology* 2006;66:576–8.

4142. Mass A. Retinopathy, encephalopathy and deafness. *Neurology* 1988;38 (**Suppl.** 1):215.

4143. Massey EW. Familial occurrence of meralgia paresthetica. *Arch Neurol* 1978;35:182.

4144. Massey EW. Effort headache in runners. *Headache* 1982;22:99–100.

4145. Massey EW, Blannon WL, Friedman AJ, Pleet AB. Cylindroma (adenoid cyctic

carcinoma) causing unilateral cranial neuropathy. *South Med J* 1979;72:1003–5.
4146. Massey EW, Brannon WL, Moreland M. Nevus of Ota and intracranial arteriovenous malformation. *Neurology* 1979;29:1625–7.
4147. Massey EW, Massey J. Elongated styloid process (Eagle's syndrome) causing hemicrania. *Headache* 1979;19:339.
4148. Massey EW, McHenry LC JR. Hysteroepilepsy in the nineteenth century: Charcot and Gowers. *Neurology* 1986;36:65–7.
4149. Massey EW, Moore J, Schold SC. Mental neuropathy from systemic cancer. *Neurology* 1981;31:1277–81.
4150. Massey EW, Schoenberg B. Foster Kennedy syndrome. *Arch Neurol* 1984;41:658–9.
4151. Massion-Verniory L, Dumont E, Potvin AM. Rétinite pigmentaire familiale compliquée d'une amyotrophie neurale. *Rev Neurol* 1946;78:561–71.
4152. Masson C, Henin D, Hauw JJ et al. Cranial pachymeningitis of unknown origin. *Neurology* 1993;43:1329–34.
4153. Mastaglia FL, Ojeda V. Inflammatory myopathies. *Ann Neurol* 1985;17:215–27–317–323.
4154. Mastaglia FL, Garlepp MJ, Phillips BA et al. Inflammatory myopathies: Clinical, diagnostic and therapeutic aspects. *Muscle Nerve* 2003;27:407–25.
4155. Mastaglia FL, Barwick DD, Hall R. Myopathy in acromegaly. *Lancet* 1970;2:907–9.
4156. Mastaglia FL, Laing NG. Distal myopathies: Clinical and molecular diagnosis and classification. *J Neurol Neurosurg Psychiatry* 1999;67:703–9.
4157. See 4153.
4158. Mastaglia FL, Walton JN. Inflammatory myopathies. In Mastaglia FL, Walton JN eds. *Skeletal Muscle Pathology*, pp 360–92. Edinburgh: Churchill Livingstone, 1991.
4159. Masters CL, Harris JO, Gajusdek DC et al. Creutzfeldt-Jakob disease: Patterns of worldwide occurrence and the significance of familial and sporadic clustering. *Ann Neurol* 1979;5:177–88.
4160. Masucci EF, Kurtzke JF, Saini N. Myorhythmia: A widespread movement disorder. *Brain* 1984;107:53–79.
4161. Masuzugawa S, Kuzuhara S, Natita Y et al. Autosomal dominant hyaline body myopathy presenting as scapuloperoneal syndrome. *Neurology* 1997;48:253–7.
4162. Mata M, Dorovini-Zis K, Wilson M et al. New form of familial Parkinson-dementia syndrome. *Neurology* 1983;33:1439–43.
4163. Mathers SE, Kempster PA, Swash M, Lees AJ. Constipation and paradoxical puborectalis contraction in anismus and Parkinson's disease: A dystonic phenomenon? *J Neurol Neurosurg Psychiatry* 1988;51:1503–7.
4164. Mathew NT, Meyer JS, Rivera VM et al. Double blind evaluation of glycerol treatment in acute cerebral infarction. *Lancet* 1972;2:1327–9.
4165. Mathew NT, Tietgen NE, Lucker C et al. Serotonin syndrome complicating migraine pharmacotherapy. *Cephalalgia* 1996;16:323–7.
4166. Mathews KD, Moore SA. Limb-girdle muscular dystrophy. *Curr Neurol Neurosci Rep* 2003;3:78–85.
4167. Mathiesen B, Reumert T. Blue jeans syndrome. *Ugersk Laeger* 1981;143:1333.
4168. Mathuranath PS, Nestor PJ, Berrios GE et al. A brief cognitive test battery to differentiate Alzheimer's disease and frontotemporal dementia. *Neurology* 2000;55:1613–20.
4169. Matison R, Mayeux R, Rosen J et al. "Tip-of-the-tongue" phenomenon in Parkinson's disease. *Neurology* 1982;32:567–70.
4170. Matson DD. *Neurosurgery of Infancy and Childhood*. Springfield, IL: CC Thomas, 1969.
4171. Matsumoto J, Fuhr P, Nigro M et al. Physiological abnormalities in hereditary hyperekplexia. *Ann Neurol* 1992;32: 41–50.
4172. Matsumoto K, Natori Y, Hirokawa E et al. Hypertrophic pachymeningitis as a result of a retropharyngeal inflammatory pseudotumor: Case report. *Neurosurgery* 2002;51:1061–4.
4173. Matsumoto S. Cheiro-oral syndrome with bilateral involvement: A study of pontine lesions by high-resolution MRI. *J Neurol Neurosurg Psychiatry* 1989;52:792–4.
4174. Matsunaga M, Inokudi T, Ohnishi A et al. Oculopharyngeal involvement in familial neurogenic muscular atrophy. *J Neurol Neurosurg Psychiatry* 1973;36:104–11.
4175. Matsuo F, Ajax ET. Palatal myoclonus and denervation supersensitivity in the central nervous system. *Ann Neurol* 1979;5:72–8.
4176. Matthews BJ, Crutchfield MB. Painful nocturnal penile erections associated with rapid eye movement sleep. *Sleep* 1987;10:184–7.
4177. Matthews PM, Jezzard P. Functional magnetic resonance imaging. *J Neurol Neurosurg Psychiatry* 2004;75:6–12.
4178. Matthews WB. Sarcoidosis of the nervous system. *J Neurol Neurosurg Psychiatry* 1965;28:23.
4179. Matthews WB. Footballer's migraine. *BMJ* 1972;2:326–7.
4180. Matthews WB, Esiri MM. The migrant sensory neuritis of Wartenberg. *J Neurol Neurosurg Psychiatry* 1983;46:1–4.
4181. Matthews WB, Howell DA, Stevens DL. Progressive myoclonus epilepsy without Lafora bodies. *J Neurol Neurosurg Psychiatry* 1969;32:116–22.
4182. Matthews WB, Rundle AT. Familial cerebellar ataxia and hypogonadism. *Brain* 1964;87:463–8.
4183. Mattis S. Mental status examination for organic mental syndrome in the elderly patient. In Bellak L, Karasu TB eds. *Geriatric psychiatry: A Handbook For Psychiatrists and Primary Care Physicians*, pp 77–121. New York: Grune & Stratton, 1976.
4184. Mauguiere F, Courjon J. Somatosensory epilepsy: A review of 127 cases. *Brain* 1978;101:307–32.
4185. Maumenee AE. Congenital hereditary corneal dystrophy. *Am J Ophthalmol* 1960;50:1114–24.
4186. Maxwell RE. Surgical control of chronic migrainous neuralgia by ganglio-rhizolysis. *J Neurosurg* 1982;57:459–66.
4187. May DL, White DL. Familial myoclonus, cerebellar ataxia and deafness: Specific genetically-determined disease. *Arch Neurol* 1968;19:331–8.
4188. Mayer C, Ostheimer S. *Arch Psychiatr Nervenkr* 1918;59:462–83.
4189. Mayer EA, Schuffler MD, Rotter JI et al. Familial visceral neuropathy with autosomal dominant transmission. *Gastroenterology* 1986;91:1528–35.
4190. Mayer-Gross W. Some observations on apraxia. *Proc Roy Soc Med* 1935;28:1203–12.
4191. Mayeux R, Alexander MP, Benson DF et al. Poriomania. *Neurology* 1979;29:1616–9.
4192. Maynard R, Garrel S. Les crises de nouveau- né: Intêret de la polygraphie. *Rev Electroencephalogr Neurophysiol Clin* 1983;13:219–23.
4193. Maytum CK. Tetany caused by functional dyspnea with hyperventilation: Report of a case. *Proc Staff Meet Mayo Clin* 1933;8:282–4.
4194. Mazars G. Criteria for identifying cingulate epilepsies. *Epilepsia* 1970;11:41–7.
4195. Mbakop A et al. Lethal multiple pterygium syndrome: Report of a new case with hydranencephaly. *Am J Med Genet* 1986;25:575–9.
4196. McAllister VL, Kendle BL, Bull JW. Symptomatic vertebral hemangiomas. *Brain* 1975;98:71.
4197. McAlpine D, Araki S. Minamata disease: An unusual neurological disorder caused by contaminated fish. *Lancet* 1958;2:629–31.
4198. McArdle B. Myopathy due to a defect in muscle glycogen breakdown. *Clinical Science (London)* 1951;10:13–35.
4199. McArthur J, Harrison MJG. HIV-associated dementia. In Appel SH ed.

Current Neurology, pp 231–74. St. Louis: Mosby, 1994.
4200. McArthur JB. Neurologic manifestations of AIDS. *Medicine* 1987;66:407–37.
4201. McCarthy RA, Evans JJ, Hodges JR. Topographic amnesia: Spatial memory disorder, perceptual dysfunction, or category specific semantic memory impairment? *J Neurol Neurosurg Psychiatry* 1996;60:318–25.
4202. McCarthy RA,Warrington EK. The double dissociation of short-term memory for lists and sentences. Evidence from aphasia. *Brain* 1987;110:1545–63.
4203. McCauley SR, Levin HS, Vanier M et al. The neurobehavioural rating scale revised: Sensitivity and validity in closed head injury assessment. *J Neurol Neurosurg Psychiatry* 2001;71:643–51.
4204. McComas AJ. Motor unit estimation: Anxieties and achievements. *Muscle Nerve* 1995;18:369–79.
4205. McCombe PA, Pollard JD, McLeod JG. Chronic inflammatory demyelinating polyradiculoneuropathy: A clinical and electrophysiological study of 92 cases. *Brain* 1987;110:1617–30.
4206. McCormick GF, Zee C-S, Heiden J. Cysticercosis cerebri: Review of 127 cases. *Arch Neurol* 1982;39:534–9.
4207. McCormick K et al. Partial pyruvate decarboxylase deficiency with profound lactic acidosis and hyperammonemia: Response to dichloroacetate acid benzoate. *Am Med Genet* 1985;22:291–9.
4208. McCormick WF, Lemmi H. Familial degeneration of the pallidonigral system. *Neurology* 1965;15:141–53.
4209. McCrory PR, Berkovic S. Concussion. *Neurology* 2001;57:2283–9.
4210. McCrory PR, Berkovic SF. Second impact syndrome. *Neurology* 1998;50:677–83.
4211. McCune DJ, Bruch H. Osteodystrophia fibrosa. *Am J Dis Childh* 1937;54:806–12.
4212. McDaniel KD, Cummings JL, Shain S. The "yips": A focal dystonia of golfers. *Neurology* 1989;39:192–5.
4213. McDermott CJ, Burness CE, Kirby J et al. Clinical features of hereditary spastic paraplegia due to spastin mutation. *Neurology* 2006;67:45–51.
4214. McDermott CJ, White K, Bushby K et al. Hereditary spastic paraparesis: A review of new developments. *J Neurol Neurosurg Psychiatry* 2000;69:150–69.
4215. McDonald JW, Bautista RE, Gutmann DH. Pseudocervical cord syndromes. *Arch Neurol* 1996;53.
4216. McDonald WI, Compston DAS, Edan G et al. Recommended diagnostic criteria for multiple sclerosis: Guidelines from the international panel on the diagnosis of multiple sclerosis. *Ann Neurol* 2001;50:121–7.
4217. McDonald WI, Halliday AM. Diagnosis and classification of multiple sclerosis. *Br Med Bull* 1977;33:4–9.
4218. McDowell F, Lee JE, Swift T et al. Treatment of Parkinson's syndrome with Levadopa. *Ann Int Med* 1970;72:29–35.
4219. McEntee WJ, Biber MP, Perl DP et al. Diencephalic amnesia: A reappraisal. *J Neurol Neurosurg Psychiatry* 1976;39: 436–41.
4220. McEntee WJ, Crook TH. Age-associated memory impairment. *Neurology* 1990;40, No.3(Part1):526–30.
4221. McEntee WJ, Mancall EL. Neuromyositis: A reappraisal. *Neurology* 1965;15:69–75.
4222. McFarland HR, Wood WG, Drowns BV et al. Papulosis atrophicans maligna (Kohlmeier-Degos disease): A disseminated occlusive vasculopathy. *Ann Neurol* 1978;3:388–92.
4223. McFarland RA. Air travel across time zones. *Am Sci* 1975;63:23–30.
4224. McFarlin DE, Strober W, Barlow M et al. The immunological deficiency state in ataxia-telangiectasia. *Res Publ Assn nerv ment Dis* 1972;49:275–92.
4225. McFarling DA, Susac JO. Hoquet diabolique: Intractable hiccups as a manifestation of multiple sclerosis. *Neurology* 1979;29:797–801.
4226. McGee DA, Van Patter HJ, Marotta J et al. Subpial cerebral siderosis. *Neurology* 1962;12:108–13.
4227. McGeer EG, McGeer PL. The Dystonias. *Can J Neurol Sci* 1988;15:447–85.
4228. McGeoch KL, Gilmour WH, Taylor W. Sensorineural objective tests in the assessment of hand-arm vibration syndrome. *Occup Envir Med* 1994;51: 57–61.
4229. McGovern FH. Association of nerve deafness and retinitis pigmentosa. *Acta Otolaryngol* 1942;36:827–36.
4230. McGuire SA, Fischbeck KH. Autosomal recessive Duchenne-like muscular dystrophy: Molecular and histochemical results. *Muscle Nerve* 1991;14:1209–12.
4231. McHenry LC. Rheoencephalography. *Neurology* 1965;15:507–17.
4232. McHenry LC JR. Introduction. In Weir Mitchell S, ed. *Injuries to Nerves*, New York: Dover (Reprint), 1965.
4233. McHenry LC JR. *Garrison's History of Neurology*. Springfield, Il: CC Thomas, 1969.
4234. McHugh HE, Souden KA, Levitt MN. Facial paralysis and muscle agenesis in the newborn. *Arch Otolaryngol* 1969;89:131.
4235. McJunkin JE, de los Reyes EC, Irazuzta JE et al. La Crosse encephalitis in children. *N Engl J Med* 2001;344:801–7.
4236. McKay C, Casey JE, Wertheimer J et al. Reliability and validity of the RBANS in a traumatic brain injured sample. *Arch Clin Neuropsychol* 2007;22:91–8.
4237. McKenna P, Warrington EK. Testing for nominal dysphasia. *J Neurol Neurosurg Psychiatry* 1980;43:781–8.
4238. McKenzie RA, Forbes GS, Karnes WE. Angiographic findings in herpes zoster arteritis. *Ann Neurol* 1981;10:458–64.
4239. McKeon A, Pittock S, Glass G et al. Isolated generalized polymyoclonus. *Arch Neurol* 2007;64:1322.
4240. McKeon A, Pittock SJ, Glass GA. Whole-body tremulousness: Isolated generalized polymyoclonus. *Arch Neurol* 2007;64:1318–22.
4241. McKhann A et al. Clinical and electrophysiological aspects of acute paralytic diseases of children and young adults in northern China. *Lancet* 1991;338:593–7.
4242. McKhann GM, Cornblath DR, Griffin JW et al. Acute motor axonal neuropathy: A frequent cause of acute flaccid paralysis in China. *Ann Neurol* 1993;33:333–42.
4242a. McKeon A, Frye MS, Delanty N. The alcohol withdrawal syndrome. *JNNP* 2008;79:854–62.
4243. McKusick VA. Dwarfism in the Amish:1. The Ellis-van Creveld Syndrome. *Bull Johns Hopkins Hosp* 1964;115:306–36.
4244. McKusick VA. *Mendelian Inheritance in Man*. Baltimore: Johns Hopkins University Press, 1983.
4245. McKusick VA et al. Chorioretinopathy with hereditary microcephaly. *Arch Ophthalmol* 1966;75:597–600.
4246. McLachan RS, Girvin JP, Blume WT et al. Rasmussen's chronic encephalitis in adults. *Arch Neurol* 1993;50:269–74.
4247. McLaurin RL. Parietal cephaloceles. *Neurology* 1964;14:764–72.
4248. McLean B, Allen J, Ferdinandusse S et al. A new defect of peroxisomal function involving pristanic acid: A case report. *J Neurol Neurosurg Psychiatry* 2002;72: 396–9.
4249. McLeod JG, Baker WdC et al. Centronuclear myopathy with autosomal dominant inheritance. *J Neurol Sci* 1972;15:375–87.
4250. McLeod JG, Low PA, Morgan JA. Charcot–Marie–Tooth disease with Leber optic atrophy. *Neurology* 1978;28:179–84.
4251. McLeod JG, Tuck RR. Disorders of the autonomic nervous system, Part 1. Pathophysiology and clinical features. *Ann Neurol* 1987;21:419–30.
4252. McLeod JG, Tuck RR. Disorders of the autonomic nervous system, Part 2. *Ann Neurol* 1987;21:519–29.
4253. McLeod JG, Tuck RR, Pollard JD et al. Chronic polyneuropathy of unknown cause. *J Neurol Neurosurg Psychiatry* 1984;47:530–5.

4254. McLeod JG, Walsh JC. Peripheral neuropathy associated with lymphomas and other reticuloses. In Dyck PJ, Thomas PK, Lambert EH, Bunge R eds. *Peripheral Neuropathy*, pp 2192–203. Philadelphia: Saunders, 1984.

4255. McManis PG, Lambert EH, Daube JR. The exercise test in periodic paralysis. *Muscle Nerve* 1986;9:704–10.

4256. McManis PG, Sharborough FW. Orthostatic tremor: Clinical and electrophysiological characteristics. *Muscle Nerve* 1993;16:1254–60.

4257. McMaster KR, Powers JM, Hennigar GR et al. Nervous system involvement in Type IV glycogenosis. *Arch Pathol Lab Med* 1979;103:105.

4258. McMenemey WH et al. Two examples of presenile dementia (Pick's disease and Stern-Garcin syndrome) with a history of trauma. *Arch Psychiatr Nervenkr* 1965;207:128–40.

4259. McMillan DE. A brief history of the neurobehavioral toxicity of manganese. *Neurotoxicology* 1999;20:499–507.

4260. McMurray WC, Rathbun JC, Mohyuddin F et al. Citrullinuria. *Pediatrics* 1963;32:347–57.

4261. McNair D, Lorr M, Droppleman LF. *Profile of Mood States, Bipolar Form.* San Diego: Educational and Industrial Testing Service, 1971.

4262. McNamara JO. Kindling: An animal model of complex partial epilepsy. *Ann Neurol* 1984;16(**Suppl.**):S72–S76.

4263. McNamara JO, Curran JR, Hideo H et al. Congenital ichthyosis with spastic paraplegia of adult onset. *Arch Neurol* 1975;32:699–701.

4264. McNaughton S. *Communicating with Blissymbolics.* Don Mills, ON, Canada: Blissymbolics Communication International, 1985.

4265. McQuarrie I. Idiopathic spontaneously occurring hypoglycemia in infants. *Am J Dis Childh* 1954;87:399–428.

4266. McQuillen MP. Familial limb-girdle myasthenia. *Brain* 1966;89:121–32.

4267. McQuillen MP, Cantor H, O'Rourke JR. Myasthenic syndrome associated with antibiotics. *Arch Neurol* 1968;18:402–15.

4268. Mead S, James-Galton M, Revesz T et al. Familial British dementia with amyloid angiopathy. Early clinical, neuro-psychological and imaging findings. *Brain* 2000;123:975–99.

4269. Mead S, Proukakis C, Wood N et al. A large family with hereditary spastic paraparesis due to a frame shift mutation of the spastin (SPG4) gene. *J Neurol Neurosurg Psychiatry* 2001;71: 788–91.

4270. Meador KJ, Loring DW. The Wada test. *Neurology* 1999;52:1535–6.

4271. Meador KJ, Watson RT, Bowers D et al. Hypometria with hemispatial and limb motor neglect. *Brain* 1986;109: 293–305.

4272. Meadow R. Fictitious epilepsy. *Lancet* 1984;2:25–8.

4273. Meadow SR. Who's to blame – mothers, Munchausen or medicine? *J Roy Coll Physicians* 1994;28:332–7.

4274. Meadows JC. Dysphagia in unilateral cerebral lesions. *J Neurol Neurosurg Psychiatry* 1973;36:853–60.

4275. Meadows JC. Observations of a case of monocular diplopia of cerebral origin. *J Neurol Sci* 1973;18:249.

4276. Meadows JC, Marsden CD, Harriman DGF. Chronic spinal muscular atrophy in adults, Part I (The Kugelberg-Welander syndrome). *J Neurol Sci* 1969;9:527–50.

4277. Medina JL, Diamond S. Cluster headache variant: Spectrum of a new headache syndrome. *Arch Neurol* 1981;38:705–9.

4278. Medlock MD, Cruse RS, Winek SJ et al. A 10-year experience with postpump chorea. *Ann Neurol* 1993;34:820–6.

4279. Medori R, Fritscher HJ, leBlanc A et al. Fatal familial insomnia: A prion disease with a mutation at Codon 178 of the prion protein gene. *Neurology* 1992;32:444–9.

4280. Meenakashisundaram E, Jagganathan K, Ramamurthi B. Clinical pattern of motor neuron disease in younger age groups. *Neurology (Bombay)* 1970;8(**Suppl.** 1):–104.

4281. Mega MS, Masterman DL, Benson DF et al. Dementia with Lewy bodies. *Neurology* 1996;47:1403–9.

4282. Mehegan CC, Driefuss MB. Hyperlexia. *Neurology* 1092;22:1105–11.

4283. Mehler M. The rostral basilar artery syndrome. *Neurology* 1989;39:9–16.

4284. Mehler MF. Complete visual inversion in vertebrobasilar ischemic disease. *J Neurol Neurosurg Psychiatry* 1988;51:1235–41.

4285. Mehler MF. The clinical spectrum of ocular bobbing and ocular dipping. *J Neurol Neurosurg Psychiatry* 1988;51: 725–7.

4286. Mei Liu H, Loew JM, Hunt CE. Congenital central hypoventilation syndrome: A pathologic study of the neuromuscular system. *Neurology* 1978;28:1013–9.

4287. Meier C et al. Spinal muscular atrophy with phenylketonuria. *Dev Med Child Neurol* 1975;17:625.

4288. Meier C, Vodlony W, Gatsch M et al. Nemaline myopathy appearing in adults as cardiomyopathy. *Arch Neurol* 1984;41:443–5.

4289. Meierkord H, Shorvon S. Variations on a theme – singing as an epileptic automatism. *J Neurol Neurosurg Psychiatry* 1991;54:1114–6.

4290. Meige H. Les convulsions de la face, une forme clinique de convulsion faciale, bilaterale et mediane. *Rev Neurol* 1910;20:437–43.

4291. Meissner I, Sapir S, Kokmen E et al. The paramedian diencephalic syndrome: A dynamic phenomenon. *Stroke* 1987;18:380–5.

4292. Melberg A, Oldfors A, Bloomstrom-Lundqvist C et al. Autosomal dominant myofibrillar myopathy with arrhythmogenic right ventricular cardiomyopathy linked to chromosome 10q. *Ann Neurol* 1999;46:684–92.

4293. Meleney F. Hemolytic streptococcal gangrene. *Arch Surg* 1924;9:317–64.

4294. Melins RB, Balfour HH, Turino GM, Winters RW. Failure of automatic control of ventilation – (Ondine's curse). *Medicine* 1973;49:487.

4295. Melkersson E. Ett fall av recidiverande facialispares i samband med angioneurotiskt odem. *Hygiea* 1928;90:737–41.

4296. Mellarup E, Fog T, Raun N et al. The socio-economic scale. *Acta Neurol Scand* 1981;S87:130–8.

4297. Mellon CD, Carter JE, Owen DB. Ollier's disease and Maffuci's syndrome: Distinct entities or a continuum? *J Neurol* 1988;235:376–8.

4298. Melo TP, Bogousslavsky J. Hemiataxia-hypesthesia: A thalamic stroke. *J Neurol Neurosurg Psychiatry* 1992;55:581–4.

4299. Melotte G. Idiopathic paralysis of the facial nerve. *Arch Neurol* 1981;38:349–53.

4300. Melzack R, Coderre T, Katz J, Vaccarino A. Central neuroplasticity and pathological pain.*Ann N Y Acad Sci* 2001;933:157–74.

4301. Melzack R. The McGill pain questionnaire: Major properties and scoring methods. *Pain* 1975;1:277–99.

4302. Melzack R, Wall PD. On the nature of cutaneous sensory mechanisms. *Brain* 1962;85:331–56.

4303. Melzack R, Wall PD. Pain mechanisms: A new theory. *Science* 1965;150:971–9.

4304. Mendaz MF, Selwood A, Mastri AR et al. Pick's disease versus Alzheimer's disease. *Neurology* 1993;43:289–92.

4305. Mendel K. Ein Reflex ein Fussrucken. *Neurol Zbl* 1904;23:197–8.

4306. Mendell JR, Florence J. Manual muscle testing. *Muscle Nerve* 1990;13(S):S16–S20.

4307. Mendell JR, Kilkin S, Kissel JT et al. Evidence for central nervous system demyelination in chronic inflammatory demyelinating polyneuropathy. *Neurology* 1987;37:1291–4.

4308. Mendez MF, Cherrier MM, Perryman KM. Epileptic forced thinking from left frontal lesions. *Neurology* 1996;47:79–83.

4309. Mendez MF, Zander BA. Dementia presenting with aphasia: Clinical characteristics. *J Neurol Neurosurg Psychiatry* 1991;54:542–5.

4310. Menge T, Hemmer B, Nessler S. Acute disseminated encephalomyelitis: An update. *Arch Neurol* 2005;62:1673–80.

4311. Mengel MC, Konigsmark BW, Berlin CI. Recessive early onset neural deafness. *Acta Otolaryngol* 1967;64:313–26.

4312. Ménière P. Sur une forme particulière de surdité grave dependant d'une lesion de l'oreille interne. *Gaz Med (Paris)* 1861;16:21.

4313. Menkes JH. *Textbook of Child Neurology*. Philadelphia: Lea and Febiger, 1985.

4314. Menkes JH, Alter M, Stiegleder GK et al. A sex-linked recessive disorder with retardation of growth, peculiar hair, and focal cerebral and cerebellar degeneration. *Pediatrics* 1962;29:764–79.

4315. Menkes JH, Hurst PL, Craig JM. A new syndrome: Progressive familial infantile cerebral dysfunction associated with an unusual urinary substance. *Pediatrics* 1954;14:462–7.

4316. Menkes JH, Philippart M, Clark DB. Hereditary partial agenesis of corpus callosum. *Arch Neurol* 1964;11:198–208.

4317. Menzel P. Beitrag zur Kenntniss der hereditaren Ataxie und Kleinhirnatrophie. *Arch Psychiatr (Berlin)* 1891;22:160–90.

4318. Meola G, Sansone V, Radice S et al. A family with an unusual myotonic and myopathic phenotype and no CTG expansion (proximal myotonic myopathy syndrome): A challenge for future molecular studies. *Neuromuscul Disord* 1996;6:143–50.

4319. Mercimek-Mahmutoglu S, Stoeckler-Ipsiroglu S, Adami A et al. GAMT deficiency. *Neurology* 2006;67:480–4.

4320. Meredith J, Grantham E. Cervical spine trauma associated with injury to the head and shoulder girdle. *Am J Surg* 1940;49:203.

4321. Meretoja J. Familial systemic paramyloidosis. *Ann Clin Res* 1969;1:314–24.

4322. Meretoja J, Teppo L. Histopathological findings of familial amyloidosis with cranial neuropathy as principal manifestation. *Acta Path Microbiol Scand* 1971;79:432–40.

4323. Meriggioli M, Rowin J, Sanders D. Distinguishing clinical and electrodiagnostic features of X-linked bulbospinal neuronopathy. *Muscle Nerve* 1999;22:1693–7.

4324. Merlevede K, Theys P, van Hees J. Diagnosis of ulnar neuropathy: A new approach. *Muscle Nerve* 2000;23:478–81.

4325. Merritt HH, Putnam TJ. Sodium diphenylhydantoinate in the treatment of convulsive disorders. *JAMA* 1938;111:1068.

4326. Merskey H, Bogduk N. *Descriptions of Chronic Pain Syndromes, and Definitions of Pain Terms*. Seattle,WA: IASP Press, 1994.

4326a. Merlini L, Martoni E, Grumati P et al. Autosomal recessive myosclerosis myopathy is a collagen VI disorder. *Neurology* 2008;71:1245–53

4327. Mertens H-G, Zschocke S. Neuromyotonie. *Klin Wschnschr* 1965;43:917–25.

4328. Merwarth HR. Hemiplegia of cortical or venous origin (occlusion of Rolandic veins). *Brooklyn Hosp J* 1940;2:193–212.

4329. Mestre D, Blin O, Serratrice GT. Contrast sensitivity is increased in a case of nonparkinsonian freezing gait. *Neurology* 1992;42:189–94.

4330. Mesulam M-M. Slowly progressive aphasia without generalised dementia. *Ann Neurol* 1982;11:592–8.

4331. Mesulam M-M. Norman Geschwind, 1926–1984. *Ann Neurol* 1985;18:98–100.

4332. Mesulam M-M. *Principles of Behavioral Neurology*. Philadelphia: F.A. Davis Co., 1985.

4333. Mesulam M-M. Frontal cortex and behavior. *Ann Neurol* 1986;19:320–5.

4334. Mesulam M-M. Primary progressive aphasia. *Ann Neurol* 2001;49:425–32.

4335. Metcalfe RA, Macdermott N, Chalmers RJG. Restless red legs. *J Neurol Neurosurg Psychiatry* 1986;49:820–3.

4336. Mettinger KL, Ericson K. Fibromuscular dyspasia and the brain: Observations on angiographic, clinical, and genetic characteristics. *Stroke* 1982;13:46–58.

4337. Meulen EFJ, Schmand CJ et al. The seven minute screen. *J Neurol Neurosurg Psychiatry* 2004;75:700–5.

4338. Meyer A. Karl Friedrich Burdach and his place in the history of neuroanatomy. *J Neurol Neurosurg Psychiatry* 1970;33:553–61.

4339. Meyer A. The frontal lobe syndrome, the aphasias and related conditions (a contribution to the history of cortical localization). *Brain* 1974;97:565–600.

4340. Meyer A, Leigh D, Bagg CF. Heidenhain's disease. *J Neurol Neurosurg Psychiatry* 1954;17:129–31.

4341. Meyer B-U, Irlbacker K, Meierkord H. Analysis of stimuli triggering attacks of paroxysmal dystonia induced by exertion. *J Neurol Neurosurg Psychiatry* 2001;70:247–51.

4342. Meyer JS, Portnoy HD. Post-epileptic paralysis: A clinical and experimental study. *Brain* 1959;82:162–85.

4343. Meyer MA. Neurologic complications of anthrax. *Arch Neurol* 2003;60:483–8.

4344. Meyer-Betz F. Beobachtungen an einem eigenartigen mit Muskellahmungen verbundenem Fall von Hamoglobinurie. *Arch Klin Med* 1910;101:85–127.

4345. Meyers R. The extrapyramidal system. *Neurology* 1953;3:627–55.

4346. Meyrier A, Fardeau M, Richet G. Acute asymmertical neuritis associated with rapid ultrafiltration dialysis. *BMJ* 1972;2:252–4.

4347. Michel D, Laurent B, Convers P et al. Cortical pain: Clinical, electrophysiological and mapping study in 12 cases. *Rev Neurol* 1990;146:405–14.

4348. Michel P-J. Linea fusca. A study of 13 cases. *Ann Dermatol Syphil* 1958;85:509–21.

4349. Michiels JJ, Koudstaal PJ, Mulder AH et al. Transient neurologic and ocular manifestations in primary thrombocythemia. *Neurology* 1993;43:1107–10.

4350. Mickeviciene D, Schrader H, Nestvold K et al. A controlled historical cohort study on the post-concussion syndrome. *Eur J Neurol* 2002;9:581–7.

4351. Mickey MR, Ellison GW, Myers LW et al. An illness severity score for multiple sclerosis. *Neurology* 1984;34:1343–7.

4352. Middleton PJ, Alexander RM, Szymanski MT. Severe myositis during recovery from influenza. *Lancet* 1970;2:533–5.

4353. Midroni G, Dyck PJ. Chronic inflammatory demyelinating polyradiculoneuropathy. *Neurology* 1996;46:1206–12.

4354. Mietens C, Weber H. A syndrome characterized by corneal opacity, nystagmus, flexion contracture of the elbows, growth failure and mental retardation. *J Pediatr* 1966;69:624.

4355. Mikati MA, Maguire H, Barlow CF et al. A syndrome of autosomal dominant alternating hemiplegia: Clinical presentation mimicking intractable epilepsy; chromosomal studies; and physiologic investigations. *Neurology* 1992;42:2251–7.

4356. Miles JH et al. Macrocephaly with hamatomas: Bannayan-Zonana syndrome. *Am J Med Genet* 1984;19:225–34.

4357. Milhorat AT. Studies in disease of muscle. XIV Progressive muscular atrophy of peroneal type associated with atrophy of the optic nerves: Report on a family. *Arch Neurol Psychiatry* 1943;50:279–87.

4358. Milhorat TH. *Pediatric Neurosurgery*. Philadelphia: F.A. Davis, 1978.

4359. Millard A. Extrait du Rapport. *Bull Soc Anat Paris* 1855;30:206.

4360. Miller A, Nathanson N. Rabies: Recent advances in pathogenesis and control. *Ann Neurol* 1977;2:511–9.

4361. Miller A, Texidor T. Precordial catch. *JAMA* 1955;**159**:1364–5.

4362. Miller BL, Ikonte C, Ponton M et al. A study of the Lund-Manchester research criteria for fronto-tempoal dementias. *Neurology* 1997;**48**:937–42.

4363. Miller D, Barkhof F, Montalban X et al. Clinically isolated syndromes suggestive of multiple sclerosis, part one: Natural history, pathogenesis, diagnosis and prognosis. *Lancet Neurol* 2005;4:281–8.

4364. Miller DH, Leary SM. Primary progressive multiple sclerosis. *Lancet Neurol* 2007;6:903–11.

4365. Miller GM, Sears JC, Guggenheim MA et al. Schizencephaly: A clinical and CT study. *Neurology* 1984;**34**:997–1001.

4366. Miller JD. Intracranial pressure monitoring. *Arch Neurol* 1985;**42**:1191–3.

4367. Miller JQ. Lissencephaly in two siblings. *Neurology* 1963;**13**:841–50.

4368. Miller JQ, Price TR. The nervous system in Rocky Mountain spotted fever. *Neurology* 1972;**22**:561–6.

4369. Miller LA, McLachan RS, Bouwer S et al. Amygdalar sclerosis: Preoperative indicators and outcome after temporal lobectomy. *J Neurol Neurosurg Psychiatry* 1994;**57**:1099–105.

4370. Miller ME, Kido D, Horner F. Cavum vergae. *Arch Neurol* 1986;**43**:821.

4371. Miller MT, Ray V, Owens P et al. Mobius and Mobius-like syndromes (TTV-OFM, OMLH). *J Pediatr Ophthalmol Strabismus* 1989;**26**:176–88.

4372. Miller RG, Layzer RB, Mellenthen MA et al. Emery-Dreifuss muscular dystrophy with autosomal dominant transmission. *Neurology* 1985;**35**:1230–3.

4373. Miller RG, Nielsen SL, Sumner AJ. Hereditary sensory neuropathy and tonic pupils. *Neurology* 1976;**26**:931–5.

4374. Miller RM, Sparkes RS. Segmental neurofibromatosis. *Arch Dermatol* 1977;**113**:837–8.

4375. Miller SD, Thompson HS. Edge-light pupil cycle time. *Br J Ophthalmol* 1978;72:495–500.

4376. Miller SP, Latal B et al. Clinical signs predict 30-month neurodevelopmental outcome after neonatal encephalopathy. *Am J Obstet Gynecol* 2004;**190**:93–9.

4377. Miller TA, Mogyoros I, Burke D. Homonymous and heteronymous monosynaptic reflexes in biceps brachii. *Muscle Nerve* 1995;**18**:585–92.

4378. Miller TM. Differential diagnosis of myotonic disorders. *Muscle Nerve* 2008;37:293–9.

4379. Miller TM, Layzer RB. Muscle cramps. *Muscle Nerve* 2005;**32**:431–42.

4380. Miller TN. Differential diagnosis of myotonic disorders. *Muscle Nerve* 2008;37:293–9.

4381. Miller VT, Rothrock JF, Pearce LA et al. Ischemic stroke in patients with atrial fibrillation. *Neurology* 1993;**43**:332–36.

4382. Millikan CH, Siekert RG. Studies in cerebrovascular disease. 1.The syndrome of intermittent insufficiency of the basilar arterial system. *Proc Mayo Clin* 1955;**30**:61–8.

4383. Millns JL, Dicken CH. Hereditary acrolabial telangiectasia. A report of familial blue lips, nails and nipples. *Arch Dermatol Chicago* 1979;**115**:474–8.

4384. Mills CK. Unilateral ascending paralysis and unilateral descending paralysis. Their clinical varieties and their pathological causes. *JAMA* 1906;**47**:1638–45.

4385. Mills JA. Systemic lupus erythematosus. *N Engl J Med* 1994;**330**:1871–9.

4386. Mills KR, Murray NMF. Corticospinal tract conduction time in multiple sclerosis. *Ann Neurol* 1985;**18**:601–5.

4387. Milner B. Interhemispheric differences in the localization of psychological processes in man. *Br Med Bull* 1971;**27**:272.

4388. Mimaki T, Itoh N, Abe J et al. Neurological manifestations in xeroderma pigmentosum. *Ann Neurol* 1986;**20**:70–5.

4389. Min J-H, Jang J-S, Lee SH. Clinical significance of redundant nerve roots of the chorda equina in lumbar spinal stenosis. *Clin Neurol Neurosurg* 2008;**110**:14–8.

4390. Minassian BA, Aiyar R, Alic S et al. Narrowing in on the causative defect of an intriguing X-linked myopathy with excessive autophagy. *Neurology* 2002;**59**:596–601.

4391. Minauf E, Jellinger K. Amyotrophy in sporadic Pick disease. *Arch Psychiatr Nervenkr* 1969;**212**:279.

4392. Minchin R. Primary lateral sclerosis of South India: Lathyrism without lathyrus. *BMJ* 1940;**1**:253–5.

4393. Minor L. Central hematomyelia. *Arch Psychiatr Nervenkr* 1892;24:693–729.

4394. Minor LB, Solomon D, Zinreich JS et al. Sound and/or pressure induced vertigo due to bone dehiscence of the superior semicircular canal. *Arch Otolaryngol* 1998;**124**:249–58.

4395. Minshew N, Williams D. The new neurobiology of autism. *Arch Neurol* 2007;64:945–50.

4396. Mirra SS, Heyman A, McKeel D et al. The consortium to establish a registry of Alzheimer's disease II. *Neurology* 1991;**41**:479–86.

4397. Misiewick JJ, Waller SL, Anthony PP et al. Achalasia of the cardia. *Quart J Med* 1969;**38**:17.

4398. Mitchell et al. Buckhorn neuropathy. *Neuropath Exp Neurol* 1978;4:85.

4399. Mitchell DM, Olcszak SA. Remission from a syndrome indistinguishable from motor neurone disease after resection of a bronchial carcinoma. *BMJ* 1979;**2**:176–7.

4400. Mitchell G, Larochelle J, Lambert M et al. Neurologic crises in hereditary tyrosinemia. *N Engl J Med* 1990;**322**:432.

4401. Mitchell RG. The Landau reaction. *Dev Med Child Neurol* 1962;4:65.

4402. Mitchell SW. Phantom limbs. *Lippincott's Magazine* 1871;8:563–9.

4403. Mitchell SW. *Injuries of Nerves and their Consequences.* Philadelphia: J.B. Lippincott & Co., 1872.

4404. Mitchell SW. On some of the disorders of sleep. *Virginia Med Monthly* 1876(Feb);2:769–81.

4405. Mitler MM, Gujavarty KS, Browman CP. Maintenance of wakefulness test: A polysomnographic test for evaluating treatment in patients with excessive somnolence. *EEG Clin Neurophysiol* 1982;**53**:658–61.

4406. Mitros FA, Schuffler MD, Teja K et al. Pathologic features of familial visceral myopathy. *Hum Pathol* 1982;**13**:825–33.

4407. Mitsumoto H, Adelmann LS, Liu HC. A case of congenital Werdnig Hoffman disease with glial bundles in spinal roots. *Ann Neurol* 1982;**11**:214–6.

4408. Mitsumoto H, Estes ML, Wilbourn AJ et al. Perineurial cell hypertrophic mononeuropathy manifesting as carpal tunnel syndrome. *Muscle Nerve* 1992;**15**:1364–8.

4409. Mitsumoto H, Sliman RH, Schafer IA et al. Motor neurone disease and adult hexosaminidase – a deficiency in two families; Evidence for multisystem degeneration. *Arch Neurol* 1985;**17**: 378–85.

4410. Mitsumoto H, Wilbourn AJ, Subramony SH. Generalized myokymia and gold therapy. *Arch Neurol* 1982;**39**:449–50.

4411. Miwa H, Hatori K, Kondo T et al. Thalamic tremor. *Neurology* 1996;**46**:75–9.

4412. Miwa H, Yamaji Y, Abe H et al. Evaluation of the somatosensory evoked blink response in patients with neurological disorders. *J Neurol Neurosurg Psychiatry* 1996;**60**:539–43.

4413. Miyajima H, Nishimura Y, Mizoguchi K et al. Familial apoceruloplasmin deficiency associated with blepharospasm and retinal degeneration. *Neurology* 1987;**37**:761–7.

4414. Miyasaki JM, Sa DS, Galvez-Jiminez N et al. Psychogenic movement disorders. *Can J Neurol Sci* 2003;**30**:S94–S100.

4415. Miyoshi K, Kawai H, Masaru I et al. Autosomal recessive distal muscular dystrophy as a new type of progressive muscular dystrophy. *Brain* 1986;**109**:31–54.

4416. Miyoshi K, Matsuoka T, Mizushima S. Familial holotopistic striatal necrosis. *Acta Neuropathol* 1969;**13**:240–9.

4417. Mizuguchi M, Mikkaichi K, Noma S et al. Acute necrotizing encephalopathy of childhood: A new syndrome presenting with multifocal symmetric brain lesions. *J Neurol Neurosurg Psychiatry* 1995;58: 555–61.

4418. Mizuno Y, Hattori N, Mori H et al. Parkin and Parkinson's disease. *Curr Opin Neurol* 2001;14:477–82.

4419. Mizusawa H, Tagaki A, Sugita H et al. Mounding phenomenon: An experimental study *in vitro*. *Neurology* 1983;33:90–3.

4420. Möbius PJ. Ueber priodisch wiederkehrende Oculomotoriuslahmung. *Berl Klin Wochenschr* 1884;21:604–8.

4421. Möbius PJ. Ueber angeborene doppelseitige Abducens-facialis Lahmung. *Munch Med Wschr* 1888;35:108–11.

4422. Modarres H, Samuel M, Schon F. Isolated finger flexion: A novel form of focal neuromyotonia. *J Neurol Neurosurg Psychiatry* 2000;69: 110–3.

4423. Moerman P, Fryns JP, Godderis P et al. Multiple ankyloses, facial anomalies, and pulmonary hypoplasia associated with severe antenatal spinal muscular atrophy. *J Pediatr* 1983;103:238–41.

4424. Moersch FP, Woltman HW. Progressive fluctuating muscular rigidity and spasm ("stiff man syndrome"): Report of a case and some observations in 13 other cases. *Mayo Clin Proc* 1956;31:421–7.

4425. Moessinger AC. Fetal akinesia deformation sequence: An animal model. *Pediatrics* 1983;72:857–63.

4426. Mohnot D, Snead OC, Benton JW. Burn encephalopathy in children. *Ann Neurol* 1982;12:42–7.

4427. Mohr J, Magerpy K. Sex-linked deafness of a possibly new type. *Acta Genet* 1960;10:54–62.

4428. Mohr JP. Distal field infarction. *Neurology* 1969;12:279.

4429. Mohr JP, Barnett HJM. Classification of ischemic strokes. In Barnett HJM, Stein BM, Mohr JP, Yatsu FM eds. *Stroke: Pathophysiology, Diagnosis, and Management,* vol.1, pp 281–91. New York: Churchill Livingstone, 1986.

4430. Mohr JP et al. Right hemianopia with memory and color deficits in circumscribed left posterior cerebral artery territory infarction. *Neurology* 1971;21:1104–6.

4431. Mohr JP, Pessin MS, Finkelstein S et al. Broca's aphasia: Pathological and clinical. *Neurology* 1978;28:311–24.

4432. Mohr OL. An hereditary sublethal syndrome in man. *Avhandinger ugitt av det Norske Videnskaps*, Oslo: Norsk Videnskaps, 1941.

4433. Mokri B. Spontaneous intracranial hypotension. *Curr Neurol Neurosci Rep* 2001;1:109–17.

4434. Mokri B. Raeder's paratrigeminal syndrome: Original concept and subsequent deviations. *Arch Neurol* 1982;39:395–9.

4435. Moldaver J. Tourniquet paralysis syndrome. *Arch Surg* 1954;68:136–44.

4436. Molinari GF. Lobar hemorrhages. *Stroke* 1993;24:523–526.

4437. Moll JWB, Antoine JC, Brashear HR et al. Guidelines on the detection of paraneoplastic anti-neuronal-specific antibodies. *Neurology* 1995;45:1937–41.

4438. Moll JWB, Henzen-Logmans SC, Splinter TAW et al. Diagnostic value of anti-neuronal antibodies for paraneoplastic disorders of the nervous system. *J Neurol Neurosurg Psychiatry* 1990;53:940–3.

4439. Mollaret P. La méningite endothélio-leucocytaire multirecurrente benigne. Syndrome nouveau ou maladie nouvelle? (Documents cliniques). *Rev Neurol* 1944;76:57–76.

4440. Mollica F, Pavone L. Hyperprolinemia: A disease which does not need treatment. *Acta Pediatr Scand* 1976;65:206.

4441. Mom AM, Polak M, Fabitero JL et al. Psoriatic myopathy. *Dermatologia* 1970;140:214–8.

4442. Monakow K von. *Gehornpathologie.* Vienna: Holder, 1905.

4443. Monakow K von. Biologisches und Morphogenetisches uber die Mikrocephalia vera. *Schweiz Arch Neurol Psychiatr* 1926;18:3–39.

4444. Monbrun A, Benisty A. Symptoms in war-injured eyes. *Rev Neurol* 1916;23:906–11.

4445. Monday K, Jankovic J. Psychogenic myoclonus. *Neurology* 1993;43:349–52.

4446. Mongini T, Bosone I et al. Alpha-sarcoglycan deficiency featuring exercise intolerance and myoglobinuria. *Neuropediatrics* 2002;33:109–11.

4447. Monnens L, Heymans H. Peroxisomal disorders: Clinical characterization. *J Inherit Metab Dis* 1987;10 **(Suppl.)**:23–32.

4448. Monrad-Krohn GH. Dysprosody or altered melody of language. *Brain* 1947;70:405–15.

4449. Monrad-Krohn GH. *The Clinical Examination of the Nervous System*. New York: Paul B. Hoeber, 1955.

4450. Montagna P, Provini F, Plazzi G et al. Bilateral paramedian thalamic syndrome. *J Neurol Neurosurg Psychiatry* 2002;73:772–4.

4451. Montagna P. Nocturnal paroxysmal dystonia and nocturnal wandering. *Neurology* 1992;42:61–7.

4452. Montagna P. Motor Tinel sign: A new localizing sign in entrapment neuropathy. *Muscle Nerve* 1994;17:1493–4.

4453. Montgomery RD, Cruickshank EK, Robertson WB et al. Clinical and pathological observations on Jamaican neuropathy: A report on 206 cases. *Brain* 1964;87:425–62.

4454. Montgomery SA, Asberg MA. A new depression scale designed to be sensitive to change. *Br J Psychiatry* 1979;134:382–9.

4455. Montoya G, Dohn DF, Mercer RD. Arteriovenous malformation of the vein of Galen as a cause of heart failure and hydrocephalus in infants. *Neurology* 1971;21:1054–8.

4456. Montplaisir J, Godbout R. Restless legs syndrome and periodic movements during sleep. In Kryger MH, Roth T, Dement WC eds. *Principles and Practice of Sleep Medicine*, pp 402–9. Philadelphia: W.B. Saunders,Co., 1989.

4457. Monytigiani A, Cencetti S, Bandinelli G et al. The "harlequin sign". Case description and review of the literature. *Ann Ital Med Int* 1998;13:173–5.

4458. Moo LR, Slotnick SD, Tesoro MA et al. Interlocking finger test: A bedside screen for parietal lobe dysfunction. *J Neurol Neurosurg Psychiatry* 2003;74:530–2.

4459. Moore MT. Paroxysmal abdominal pain. *JAMA* 1944;124:561–3.

4460. Moore PM, Cupps TR. Neurological complications of vasculitis. *Ann Neurol* 1983;14:155.

4461. Moore RF. Physiology and pathology of the pupil reactions. *Trans Ophthal Soc UK* 1924;44:38–43.

4462. Moore RF. Subjective "lightning streaks". *Br J Ophthalmol* 1947;31:46.

4463. Moosa A, Dubowitz V. Peripheral neuropathy in Cockayne's syndrome. *Arch Dis Child* 1970;45:674–7.

4464. Mora M, Lambert EH, Engel AG. Synaptic vesicle abnormality in familial infantile myasthenia. *Neurology* 1987;37:206–14.

4465. See 4464.

4466. Moran LJ, Mefferd RB. Repetitive psychometric measures. *Psychol Rep* 1959;5:269–75.

4467. Moran NF, Fish DR, Kitchen N et al. Supratentorial cavernous hemangiomas and epilepsy: A review of the literature and case series. *J Neurol Neurosurg Psychiatry* 1999;66:561–8.

4468. Morariu MA, Taranu J. Clinico-genetic consideration of basilar impression. *StudiiCerc Neurol* 1968;13:441.

4469. Morava E, van der Heuvel I, Hol F et al. Mitochondrial disease criteria. *Neurology* 2006;67:1823–6.

4470. Morel F. Hyperostosis frontalis interna, its clinical signs and associated symptoms. *Schweiz Med Wschr* 1937;67:1235–7.

4471. Morel F. A special anatomo-clinical form of chronic alcoholism: Alcoholic laminated cortical sclerosis. *Rev Neurol* 1939;71:280–8.
4472. Morel F, Wildi E. Disseminated nodular dysgenesis of the frontal cortex. *Rev Neurol* 1952;87:251–70.
4473. Moretti G, Manzoni GC, Carrarra MD et al. "Benign recurrent vertigo" and its connection with migraine. *Headache* 1980;20:344–6.
4474. Moretti G, Manzoni GC, Mainini P et al. Empty sella headache. *Headache* 1981;21:211–7.
4475. Morgagni GB. *De sedibus et causis morborum peranatomen indagatis libri quinque.* Venetiis: Remondiniana, 1769.
4476. Morgan D, Williams B. Syringobulbia: A surgical appraisal. *J Neurol Neurosurg Psychiatry* 1992;55:1132–41.
4477. Morgan JP, Penovich P. Jamaica ginger paralysis: Forty-seven year follow-up. *Arch Neurol* 1978;35:530–2.
4478. Morgan WC. The probably systemic nature of Mikulicz's syndrome and its relation to Sjogren's syndrome. *N Engl J Med* 1954;251:5.
4479. Morgan-Hughes JA. Mitochondrial and lipid storage myopathies. In Engel AG, Banker BQ eds. *Myology*, pp 1709–43. New York, NY: McGraw Hill, 1993.
4480. Morgan Hughes JA, Darvenica P, Kahn SM et al. A mitochondrial myopathy characterized by a deficiency in reducible cytochrome *B*. *Brain* 1977;11:617–40.
4481. Morgan-Hughes JA, Darveniza P, Landon DN et al. A mitochondrial myopathy with a deficiency of respiratory chain NADH-Co-Q reductase activity. *J Neurol Sci* 1979;43:27–46.
4482. Morgan-Hughes JA, Hayes DJ, Clark JB et al. Mitochondrial encephalomyelopathies. *Brain* 1982;105:553–82.
4483. Morgan-Hughes JA, Hayes DJ, Cooper M et al. Mitochondrial myopathies: Deficiencies localised to complex I and complex III of the mitochondrial respiratory chain. *Biochem Soc Trans* 1985;13:648–50.
4484. Morgan-Hughes JA, Lecky BRF, Murray NMF et al. Alterations in the number and affinity of junctional acetylcholine receptors in a myopathy with tubular aggregates. *Brain* 1981;104:279–95.
4485. Morgan-Hughes JA, Mair WGP, Lascelles PT. A disorder of skeletal muscle associated with tubular aggregates. *Brain* 1970;93:873–80.
4486. Morgenlander JC, Goldstein RB. Recurrent transient ischemic attacks and stroke associated with an internal carotid argery web. *Stroke* 1991;22:94–8.
4487. Mori E, Yamadori A. Rejection behaviour: A human homologue of the abnormal behaviour of Denny-Brown and Chambers' monkey with bilateral parietal ablation. *J Neurol Neurosurg Psychiatry* 1989;52:1260–6.
4488. Mori K, Iijima M, Koike H et al. The wide spectrum of clinical manifestations in Sjögren's syndrome-associated neuropathy. *Brain* 2005;128:2518–34.
4489. Morin C, Dubé J, Robinson BH et al. Stroke-like episodes in autosomal: Recessive cytochrome oxidase deficiency. *Ann Neurol* 1999;45:389–92.
4490. Morin P, Lechevalier B, Bianco C. Atophie cérébelleuse et lesions pallido-luyso-nigriques avec corps de Lewy. *Rev Neurol* 1980;136:381–90.
4491. Morita H, Ikeda S, Yamamoto K et al. Hereditary ceruloplasmin deficiency with hemosiderosis: A clinicopathological study of a Japanese family. *Ann Neurol* 1995;37:646–56.
4492. Morley JS, Miles JB, Wells JC et al. Paradoxical pain. *Lancet* 1992;340:1045.
4493. Morquio L. Sur une forme de dystrophie osseuse familiale. *Bull Soc Pediat Paris* 1929;27:145.
4494. Morquio L. Sur une forme de dystrophie osseuse familiale. *Arch Med Enf Paris* 1929;32:129–40.
4495. Morris HH, Dinner DS, Luders H et al. Supplementary motor seizures: Clinical and electroencephalographic findings. *Neurology* 1988;38:1075–82.
4496. Morris HH, Peters BH. Pronator syndrome: Clinical and electrophysiological features of seven cases. *J Neurol Neurosurg Psychiatry* 1976;39:461–4.
4497. Morris JC, Cole M, Banker BQ et al. Hereditary dysphasic dementia and the Pick Alzheimer spectrum. *Ann Neurol* 1984;16:455–66.
4498. Morris JC, Heyman A, Mohs RC et al. The consortium to establish a registry for Alzheimer's disease (CERAD). Part 1. Clinical and neuropsychological assessment of Alzheimer's disease. *Neurology* 1989;39:1159–65.
4499. Morris JC, Mohs RC, Rogers H et al. CERAD clinical and psychological assessment of Alzheimer's disease. *Psychopharm Bull* 1988;24:641–51.
4500. Morrow MJ, Sharpe JA. Torsional nystagmus in the lateral medullary syndrome. *Ann Neurol* 1988;24:390–8.
4501. Morse WI, Cochrane WA, Landrigan PL. Familial hypoparathyroidism with pernicious anemia, steatorrhea and adrenocortical insufficiency. *N Engl J Med* 1961;264:1021–6.
4502. Morton LT. *A Medical Bibliography.* London: Andre Deutsch, 1970.
4503. Morton TG. A peculiar and painful affection of the fourth metatarsalphalangeal articulation. *Am J Med Sci* 1876;71:37–45.
4504. Moruzzi G, Magoun HW. Brain stem reticular formation and activation of EEG. *EEG Clin Neurophysiol* 1949;1:455–73.
4505. Morvan AM. De la parésie analgésique à panaris des extrémites supérieures ou paréso-analgésie des extrémites supérieures. *Gaz Hebd Med* 1883;20:580,590,–583,594.
4506. Morvan AM. De la chorée fibrillaire. *Gaz Hebd Med* 1890;27:173–176, 186–189.
4507. Mosberg WH. The Klippel-Feil syndrome: Etiology and treatment of neurologic signs. *J Nerv Ment Dis* 1953;117:479–91.
4508. Moschcowitz E. An acute febrile pleiochromic anemia with hyaline thrombosis of the terminal arterioles and capillaries. An undescribed disease. *Arch Int Med* 1925;36:89–93.
4509. Mosek A, Korcyzn AD. Yom Kippur headache. *Neurology* 1995;45:1953–5.
4510. Moseley I. *Magnetic Resonance Imaging in Diseases of the Nervous System*. Oxford: Blackwell, 1988.
4511. Moseley JL, Molinari JF, Walker AE. Respirator brain: Report of a survey and review of current concepts. *Arch Pathol Lab Med* 1976;100:61–4.
4512. Moser HW. The peroxisome: Nervous system role of a previously underrated organelle. *Neurology* 1988;38:1617–27.
4513. Moser HW, Moser AB, Kawamura N et al. Adrenoleukodystrophy: Elevated C_{26} fatty acid in cultured skin fibroblasts. *Ann Neurol* 1980;7:542–9.
4514. Moser HW, Naidu S, Kumar AJ et al. The adrenoleukodystrophies. *CRC Crit Rev Clin Neurobiol* 1987;3:29–88.
4515. Moskowitz MA, Henrikson BM, Beyerl BD. Headache. In Rose C ed. *Handbook of Clinical Neurology*, pp 107–16. Amsterdam: Elsevier, 1986.
4516. Moskowitz MA, Winickoff RN, Heinz ER. Familial calcification of the basal ganglions. *N Engl J Med* 1971;285:72–7.
4517. Moss M, Albert M, Butters N et al. Differential patterns of memory loss in patients with Alzheimer's disease, Huntington's disease and alcoholic Korsakoff's syndrome. *Arch Neurol* 1986;43:239–46.
4518. Moss-Morris R, Petrie KJ, Large RG et al. Neuropsychological deficits in chronic fatigue syndrome: Artifact or reality? *J Neurol Neurosurg Psychiatry* 1996;60: 474–7.
4519. Mossuto-Agatiello L. Caudal paramedian midbrain syndrome. *Neurology* 2006;66:1668–71.

4520. Motta J, Guilleminault C. Cardiac dysfunction during sleep. *Ann Clin Res* 1985;17:190–8.

4521. Mount LA, Reback S. Familial paroxysmal choreoathetosis. Preliminary report on a hitherto undescribed clinical syndrome. *Arch Neurol* 1940;44:841–7.

4522. Mouradian MM. Recent advances in the genetics and pathogenesis of Parkinson disease. *Neurology* 2002;58: 179–85.

4523. Mouret JB, Renaud P, Quenin D et al. Monoamines et regulation de la vigilance. In Girard P, Couteaux R eds. *Les Mediateurs Chimiques*, p 139. Paris: Masson, 1972.

4524. Moxley RT. Functional testing. *Muscle Nerve* 1990;13(S):S26–S29.

4525. Moy S, Opfer-Gehrking TL, Proper CJ. The venoarteriolar reflex in diabetic and other neuropathies. *Neurology* 1989;39:1490–2.

4526. Moya A, Brignole M, Menozzi C et al. Mechanism of syncope in patients with isolated syncope and in patients with tilt-positive syncope. *Circulation* 2001;104:1261–7.

4527. Moynahan EJ. Familial congenital alopecia, epilepsy, mental retardation with unusual electroencephalograms. *Proc Roy Soc Med* 1962;551:411–2.

4528. Mozaffar T, Pestronk A. Myopathy with anti-Jo-1 antibodies: Pathology in perimysium and neighbouring muscle fibres. *J Neurol Neurosurg Psychiatry* 2000;68:472–8.

4529. Mozes M, Ramon Y, Jahr J. The anterior tibial syndrome. *J Bone Joint Surg* 1962;44-A:730–5.

4530. Mrak RE, Griebel M, Brodsky MC. Broad A band disease: A new benign congenital myopathy. *Muscle Nerve* 1996;19:587–94.

4531. Mrak RE, Lange B, Brodsky MC. Broad A bands of striated muscle in Leber's congenital amaurosis: A new congenital myopathy? *Neurology* 1993;43:838–41.

4532. Mrissa N, Belal S, Ben Hamida M et al. Linkage to chromosome 13q11-12 of an autosomal recessive cerebellar ataxia in a Tunisian family. *Neurology* 2000;54:1408–14.

4533. Msall ME, DiGaudio K, Rogers BT et al. The functional independence measure for children. *Clin Pediatr* 1994;33:421–43.

4534. Mubarak SJ, Hargens SR. *Compartment Syndromes and Volkmann's Contracture.* Philadelphia: W.B. Saunders, 1981.

4535. Muckle TJ, Wells M. Urticaria, deafness, and amyloidosis: A new heredo-familial syndrome. *Quart J Med* 1962;31:235–48.

4536. Mulder DW, Baskan JA, Lambert EH. Hyperinsulin neuronopathy. *Neurology* 1956;6:627–35.

4537. Mulder DW, Daly DD, Bailey AA. Visceral epilepsy. *Arch Int Med* 1954;91:481–93.

4538. Mulder DW, Kurland LT, Offord KP et al. Familial adult motor neuron disease. *Neurology* 1986;36:511–7.

4539. Mulder DW, Rosenbaum RA, Layton DD JR. Late progression of poliomyelitis or forme fruste amyotrophic lateral sclerosis? *Mayo Clin Proc* 1972;47:756–61.

4540. Mulleners WM, Verhagen WI, Bartels RH. Cerebral salt wasting syndrome. *J Neurol Neurosurg Psychiatry* 1996;60: 234–5.

4541. Muller E. Ueber einige weniger bekannte Verlaufdformen der Multiplen Sklerose. *Neurol Zbl* 1905;24:593–601.

4542. Muller J, Wissel J et al. Craniocervical dystonia questionnaire (CDQ 24). *J Neurol Neurosurg Psychiatry* 2004;75:749–53.

4543. Muller J, Zeman W. Dégenérescence systematisée optico-cochleo-dentelée. *Acta Neuropathol* 1965;5:26–39.

4544. Müller JS, Herczegfalvi A, Vilchez JJ et al. Phenotypical spectrum of DOK7 mutations in congenital myasthenic syndromes. *Brain* 2007;130:1497–506.

4545. Muller M, Hubbard SL, Provias J et al. Malignant rhabdoid tumour of the pineal region. *Can J Neurol Sci* 1994;21:277.

4546. Multi-Society Task Force on PVS. Medical aspects of the persistent vegetative state. *N Engl J Med* 1994;330:1499–508.

4547. Mulvey BE, Reilly LA. Familial syringomyelia and status dysraphicus. *Ann Int Med* 1942;16:966.

4548. Munchau A, Valente EM, Shahidi GA et al. A new family with paroxysmal exercise induced dystonia and migraine: A clinical and genetic study. *J Neurol Neurosurg Psychiatry* 2000;68:609–14.

4549. Munchmeyer E. Ueber Myositis ossificans progressiva. *Z Rat Med* 1869;34:9–41.

4550. Munhoz RP, Li J-Y, Kurtinecz M et al. Evaluation of the pull test technique in assessing postural instability in Parkinson's disease. *Neurology* 2004;62:125–7.

4551. Munoz-Garcia D, Ludwin SK. Adult-onset neuronal intranuclear hyaline inclusion disease. *Neurology* 1986;36: 785–90.

4552. Munoz-Malaga A, Bautista J, Salazar JA et al. Lipomatosis, proximal myopathy and the mitochondrial 8344 mutation. A lipid storage myopathy? *Muscle Nerve* 2000;23:538–42.

4553. Munsat TL. A standardized forearm ischemic exercise test. *Neurology* 1970;20:1171–8.

4554. Muntoni F, Sewry CA. Central core disease: New findings in an old disease. *Brain* 2003;126:2339–40.

4555. Muntonia F, Voitb T. The congenital muscular dystrophies in 2004: A century of exciting progress. *Neuromuscul Disord* 2004;14:635–49.

4556. Murachi S, Nogami H, Oki T et al. The trichorhinophalangeal syndrome with exostoses: Four additional patients without mental retardation and a review of the literature. *Am J Med Genet* 1984;19:111.

4557. Muratov W. Pathogenesis of post-apoplectic chorea. *Mschr Psychiat Neurol* 1899;5:180–92.

4558. Murinson BB. Stiff person syndrome. *Neurologist* 2004;10:131–7.

4559. Murphy SF, Drachman DB. The oculopharyngeal syndrome. *JAMA* 1968;203:1003–8.

4560. Murray TJ. Congenital sensory neuropathy. *Brain* 1973;96:387–94.

4561. Murri A. Degeneratione cerebellare da intossicazione endogena. *Riv Crit Clin Med* 1900;1:593–609.

4562. Myers AR, Willis PW. Clinical spectrum of supravalvular aortic stenosis. *Arch Int Med* 1966;118:553–61.

4563. Myerson A. Contralateral periosteal reflexes of the arm. *J Nerv Ment Dis* 1914;41:162–4.

4564. Myhrman G. The secondary wave: A forgotten muscular phenomenon. *Acta Med Scand* 1939;98:542–60.

4565. Nabbout R, Baulac SDI et al. New locus for febrile seizures with absence epilepsy on 3p and a possible modifier gene on 18p. *Neurology* 2007;68: 1374–1381.

4566. Nachemson A. Lumbar spine instability: A critical update and symposium summary. *Spine* 1985;10:290–1.

4567. Nadeau A, Therrien C, Karpati G et al. Danon disease due to a novel splice mutation in the *LAMP2* gene. *Muscle Nerve* 2008;37:338–42.

4568. Nadeau SE, Trobe JD. Pupil sparing in oculomotor palsy: A brief review. *Ann Neurol* 1983;13:143–8.

4569. Nadkarni N, Lisak RP. Guillain–Barré syndrome with bilateral optic neuritis and central white matter disease. *Neurology* 1993;43:842–3.

4570. Nadler HL, Egan TJ. Deficiency of lysosomal acid phosphatase. *N Engl J Med* 1970;282:303–7.

4571. Nadol JB JR, Burgess B. Cochleosaccular degeneration of the inner ear and progressive cataracts inherited as an autosomal dominant trait. *Laryn* 1982;92:1028–37.

4572. Naffziger HC. Subdural fluid accumulation following head injury. *JAMA* 1924;82:1751–2.

4573. Naffziger HC. The scalenus syndrome. *Surg Gyn Obst* 1937;64:119–20.

4574. Nagae-Poetscher LM, Bibat G, Phillipart M et al. Leukoencephalopathy, cerebral calcifications and cysts. *Neurology* 2004;62:1206–9.
4575. Nagamitsu S, Matsuura T, Khajavi M et al. A "dystrophic" variant of autosomal recessive myotonia congenita caused by novel mutations in the CLCN1 gene. *Neurology* 2000;55:1697–703.
4576. Nahas SA, Duquette A, Roddier K et al. Ataxia-oculomotor apraxia 17. *Neuromuscul Disord* 2007;17:968–9.
4577. Naidech AM, Janjua N et al. Predictors and impact of aneurysmal rebleeding after subarachnoid hemorrhage. *Arch Neurol* 2005;62:410–6.
4578. Naidu S, Hoefler G, Watkins PA et al. Neonatal seizures and retardation in a girl with biochemical features of X-linked adrenoleukodystrophy: A possible new disease entity. *Neurology* 1988;38:1100–7.
4579. Najim al-Din AS, Wriekat A, Mubaidin A et al. Pallido-pyramidal degeneration, supranuclear gaze paresis and dementia: Kufor-Rakeb syndrome. *Acta Neurol Scand* 1994;89:347–52.
4580. Nakada T, Knight RT, Mani RL. Intermittent venous claudication of the upper extremity: The pectoralis minor syndrome. *Ann Neurol* 1982;11:433–4.
4581. Nakada T, Kwee IL. Oculopalatal myoclonus. *Brain* 1986;109:431–41.
4582. Nakada T, Kwee IL. See-saw nystagmus – role of visuovestibular interaction in its pathogenesis. *J Clin Neuro-Ophthalmol* 1988;8:171.
4583. Nakajima M, Hirayama K. Midcervical central cord syndrome: Numb and clumsy hands due to midline cervical disc protrusion at the C3-4 intervertebral level. *J Neurol Neurosurg Psychiatry* 1995;58:607–13.
4584. Nakano KK, Dawson DM, Spence A. Machado disease. *Neurology* 1972;22: 49–55.
4585. Nakano T, Ikeda S, Condo K et al. Adult GM 1 – gangliosidosis. *Arch Neurol* 1985;35:875–80.
4586. Namba T, Brown SB, Grob D. Neonatal myasthenia gravis. *Pediatrics* 1970;45:488–504.
4587. Namba T, Brunner NG, Brown SB. Familial myasthenia gravis: Report of 27 patients in 12 families and review of 164 patients in 73 families. *Arch Neurol* 1971;25:49–60.
4588. Namba T, Brunner NG, Grob N. Idiopathic giant cell polymyositis: Report of a case and review of the syndrome. *Arch Neurol* 1974;31:27–30.
4589. Nance WE et al. X-linked mixed deafness with congenital fixation of the stapedial footplate and perilymphatic gusher. *Birth Defects* 1971;7(4):64–9.
4590. Narabayashi H, Imai H, Yokochi M et al. Cases of pure akinesia without rigidity and tremor and with no effect by L-Dopa therapy. In Birkmayer W, Horniekiewicz O eds. *Advances in Parkinsonism*, pp 335–42. Basel: Roche, 1976.
4591. Narayan SB, Rakheja D, Tan L et al. CLN3P, the Batten's disease protein, is a novel palmitoyl-protein Δ-9 Desaturase. *Ann Neurol* 2006;60:570–7.
4592. Nardocci N, Orzi G, Arzaghi C et al. Myoclonus-dystonia syndrome: Clinical presentation, disease course, and genetic features in 11 families. *Mov Disord* 2008;23:28–34.
4593. Nardocci N, Zorzi G, Farina L et al. Infantile neuroaxonal dystrophy. *Neurology* 1999;52:1472–8.
4594. Nashef L, Lane RJM. Screening for mitochondrial cytopathies: The sub-anaerobic threshold exercise test (SATET). *J Neurol Neurosurg Psychiatry* 1989;52:1090–4.
4595. Nashold BS, Ostdahl RH, Bullitt E et al. Dorsal root entry zone lesions: A new neurosurgical therapy for deafferentation pain. In Bonica JJ ed. *Advances in Pain Research and Therapy*, pp 739–50. New York: Raven Press, 1983.
4596. Nasreddine JS et al. The Montreal cognitive assessment: A brief screening tool for mild cognitive impairment. *J Am Geriatr Soc* 2005;53:695–9.
4597. Nathan PW, Smith MC. The rubrospinal and central tegmental tracts in man. *Brain* 1982;105:223–69.
4598. Nathan PW, Smith MC, Cook AW. Sensory effects in man of lesions of the posterior columns and of some other afferent pathways. *Brain* 1986;109:1003–41.
4599. Nathanson M. Lou Gehrig. *Neurology* 1986;36:1349.
4600. National Institute of Neurological and Communicative Diseases and Stroke. Diagnostic criteria for Alzheimer disease. *Neurology* 1988;38:360–5.
4601. National Institute of Neurological Disorders and Stroke. Classification of cerebrovascular diseases III. *Stroke* 1990;21:637–76.
4602. Nausieda PA, Weiner WJ, Klawans HL. Dystonic foot response of Parkinsonism. *Arch Neurol* 1980;37:132–6.
4603. Navon R, Khosravi R, Korczyn Teal. A new mutation in the HEXA gene associated with a spinal muscular atrophy phenotype. *Neurology* 1995;45:539–43.
4604. Neary D, Snowden JS, Gustafson L et al. Frontotemporal lobar degeneration. *Neurology* 1998;5157:1546–54.
4605. Neary D, Snowden JS, Mann DMA. Frontotemporal dementia. *Lancet Neurology* 2005;4:771–80.
4606. Neary D, Snowden JS, Northen B, Goulden P. Dementia of frontal lobe type. *J Neurol Neurosurg Psychiatry* 1988;51:353–61.
4607. Needles W. Pseudotabes pituitaria. *J Nerv Ment Dis* 1934;80:651–7.
4608. Neelon FA, Goree JA, Lebovitz HE. The primary empty sella: Clinical and radiographic characteristics and endocrine function. *Medicine* 1973;52:73–92.
4609. Negro C. *Clinical and Pathological Study of the Nervous System*. Torino: Lattes, 1912.
4610. Neill CA, Dingwall MM. A syndrome resembling progeria. *Arch Dis Child* 1950;25:213–21.
4611. Neilson DE, Feiler HS, Wilhelmsen KC. Autosomal dominant acute necrotizing encephalopathy maps to 2q12.1-2q13. *Ann Neurol* 2004;55:291–4.
4612. See 4611.
4613. Nellhaus G. Composite international and inter-racial graphs. *Pediatrics* 1968;41:106.
4614. Nelson DA, Landau WM. Jaws: Diversities of gnathological history and temporomandibular joint enterprise. *J Neurol Neurosurg Psychiatry* 1999;67:141–7.
4615. Nelson DH, Meakin JW, Dealy JB et al. ACTH-producing tumour of the pituitary gland. *N Engl J Med* 1958;259: 161–4.
4616. Nelson HE. Wisconsin card sorting test. *Cortex* 1976;12:313–24.
4617. Nelson HE. *The National Adult Reading Test Manual*. 1. 1982. Windsor, NFER Nelson. (Pamphlet)
4618. Nelson I, Hanna MG, Alsamjari N et al. A new mitochondrial DNA mutation associated with progressive dementia and chorea: A clinical, pathological and genetic study. *Ann Neurol* 1995;37: 400–3.
4619. Nelson JR. The minimal ice water caloric test. *Neurology* 1970;20:577–85.
4620. Nelson JS, Prensky AL. Sporadic juvenile amyotrophic lateral sclerosis. *Arch Neurol* 1972;27:300–6.
4621. Nelson KB, Ellenberg JH. The asymptomatic newborn and risk of cerebral palsy. *Am J Dis Childh* 1987;141:1333.
4622. Nelson K, Mattingly M, Lee S, Schmitt F. Does the arousal system contribute to near death experience? *Neurology* 2006;66:1003–9.
4623. Nelson M, Lessell S, Sadun AA. Optic nerve hypoplasia and maternal diabetes mellitus. *Arch Neurol* 1986;43:20–5.

4624. Nelson MM, Thompson AJ. The acrocallosal syndrome. *Am J Med Genet* 1982;12:195–9.
4625. Nemni R, Bottacci E, Fazio R et al. Polyneuropathy in hypothyroidism. *J Neurol Neurosurg Psychiatry* 1987;50:1454–60.
4626. Nemni R, Galassi G, Cohen M et al. Symmetrical sarcoid polyneuropathy. *Neurology* 1981;31:1217–23.
4627. Neng T, Yi C, Xiu-Bao Z et al. Acute infectious torticollis. *Neurology* 1983;33:1344–6.
4628. Neri V. On a new sign of organic hemiplegia. *Nouv Icon Salpet* 1910;23:88–9.
4629. Neu RL, Kajii T, Gardner LI et al. A lethal syndrome of microcephaly with multiple genetic anomalies in three siblings. *Pediatrics* 1971;47:610–2.
4630. Neubauer BA, Stefanova I, Hubner CA et al. A new type of leukoencephalopathy with metaphyseal chondrodysplasia maps to Xq25-q27. *Neurology* 2006;67: 587–91.
4631. Neufeld MY, Blumen SC, Nisipeanu P et al. Lingual seizures. *Epilepsia* 1988;29:20–33.
4632. Neuhauser H, Lempert T. Vertigo and dizziness related to migraine: A diagnostic challenge. *Cephalalgia* 2004;24:83–91.
4633. Neuhauser H, Leopold M, von Brevern M et al. The interrelations of migraine, vertigo and migrainous vertigo. *Neurology* 2001;56:436–41.
4634. Neumann MA, Cohn R. Progressive subcortical gliosis - a rare form of presenile dementia. *Brain* 1967;90:405–17.
4635. Neuzelius C. Spontaneous cerebrospinal fluid otorrhea due to congenital malformation. *Acta Otolaryngol* 1951;39:314.
4636. Neville BGR, Boyd SG. Selective epileptic gait disorder. *J Neurol Neurosurg Psychiatry* 1995;58:371–3.
4637. Neville HE, Baumbach LL, Ringel SP et al. Familial inclusion body myositis. *Neurology* 1992;42:897–902.
4638. Neville HE, Ringel SP, Guggenheim MA et al. Ultrastructure and histochemical abnormalities of skeletal muscle in patients with chronic vitamin E deficiency. *Neurology* 1983;33:483–8.
4639. Nevin S. Gliomatosis cerebri. *Brain* 1938;61:170–91.
4640. Nevin S, Jones DP. Rapidly progressive cerebral degeneration (subacute vascular encephalopathy) with mental disorder, focal disturbances, and myoclonic epilepsy. *J Neurol Neurosurg Psychiatry* 1954;17:148–59.
4641. Nevin S, McMenemey WH, Behrman S, Jones DP. Subacute spongiform encephalopathy. *Brain* 1960;83:519–63.
4642. New GB, Eric JB. Dermoid cysts of head and neck. *Surg Gyn Obst* 1937;65:48.
4643. Newman LC, Lipton RB, Russell M et al. Hemicrania continua: Attacks may alternate sides. *Headache* 1992;32:237–8.
4644. Newman LC, Lipton RB, Solomon S. Hemicrania continua. *Neurology* 1994;44:2111–4.
4645. Newman NJ, Lessell S, Winterkorn MS. Optic chiasmal neuritis. *Neurology* 1991;41:1203–10.
4646. Newman NM, Tornambe PE, Corbett JJ. Ophthalmoscopy of the retinal nerve fiber layer: Use in detection of neurologic disease. *Arch Neurol* 1982;39:226–33.
4647. Newman PH. Sprung back. *J Bone Joint Surg* 1952;34B:30–7.
4648. Newmark J, Hochsinger C. Isolated painless manual incoordination in 57 musicians. *J Neurol Neurosurg Psychiatry* 1987;50(3):291–295.
4649. Newsom-Davis J. Lambert–Eaton myasthenic syndrome. *Rev Neurol (Paris)* 204;160:177–80.
4650. Newsom-Davis J. Diseases of the nervous system. In Campbell EJM, Agostoni E, Newsom Davis J eds. *The Respiratory Muscles*, pp 314–27. London: Lloyd-Luke, 1970.
4651. Newton CRJC, Hien TT, White N. Cerebral malaria. *J Neurol Neurosurg Psychiatry* 2000;69:433–41.
4652. Newton CRJC, Warrell DJ. Neurological manifestations of falciparum malaria. *Ann Neurol* 1998;43:695–702.
4653. Newton FH, Rosenberg RN, Lampert PW et al. Neurologic involvement in Urbach–Wiethe's disease (lipoid proteinosis). *Neurology* 1971;21:1205–13.
4654. Newton RW. Intracranial pressure and its monitoring in childhood: A review. *J Roy Soc Med* 1987;80:566–70.
4655. Neyman J. Statistics – servant of all sciences. *Science* 1955;122:401.
4656. Nezelof C, Dupont F, Jankers F et al. A lethal familial syndrome associating arthrogryposis multiplex congenita, renal dysfunction and a cholestatic and pigmentary liver disease. *J Pediatr* 1979;94:258–90.
4657. Ng H-Y, Lin S-H, Hsu C-Y et al. Hypokalemic paralysis due to Gitelman syndrome. *Neurology* 2006;67:1080–2.
4658. Nguyen DK, Botez MI. Diaschisis and neurobehavior. *Can J Neurol Sci* 1998;25:5–12.
4659. Nguyen K, Philip N, Suchet L et al. Progressive spastic paraplegia as a presentation of oculodentodigital syndrome. *Rev Neurol (Paris)* 2004;160:83–5.
4660. Nicholas G, Maisonobe T, Le Forestier N et al. Proposed revised electrophysiological criteria for chronic inflammatory demyelinating polyradiculoneuropathy. *Muscle Nerve* 2002;25:26–30.
4661. Nicholl DJ, Greenstone MA, Clarke CE et al. An English kindred with a novel recessive tauopathy and respiratory failure. *Ann Neurol* 2003;54:682–6.
4662. Nichols FL, Holdsworth DE, Reinfrank RF. Familial hypocalcemia latent tetany and calcification of the basal ganglia: Report of a kindred. *Am J Med* 1961;30:518–28.
4663. Nickel SN, Frame B, Bebin J et al. Myxedema neuropathy and myopathy. *Neurology* 1961;11:125–37.
4664. Nicolao P, Xiang F, Gunnarsson LG et al. Autosomal dominant myopathy with proximal weakness and early respiratory muscle involvement maps to chromosome 2q. *Am J Hum Genet* 1999;64:788–92.
4665. Nielsen JE, Johnsen B, Koefoed P et al. Hereditary spastic paraplegia with cerebellar ataxia: A complex phenotype associated with a new *SPG4* gene mutation. *Eur J Neurol* 2004;11:817–24.
4666. See 4665.
4667. Nielsen JM. *Agnosia, Apraxia, and Aphasia.* New York: Hoeber, 1946.
4668. Nielsen JM. Tornado epilepsy simulating Ménière's syndrome. *Neurology* 1959;9:794–6.
4669. Nielsen VK, Friis ML, Johnsen T. Electromyographic distinction between paramyotonia congenita and myotonia congenita: Effect of cold. *Neurology* 1982;32:827–32.
4670. Nielson JM. A subacute generalized neuromuscular exhaustion syndrome. *JAMA* 1940;126:801–6.
4671. Niemann A. Ein unbekanntes Krankheitsbild. *Jahrb Kinderh* 1914;29: 1–10.
4672. Nighoghossian N, Derex L, Loire R et al. Giant Lambl excrescences. *Arch Neurol* 1997;54:41–4.
4673. Nihira K, Foster R, Shellhaas M et al. *AAMD Adaptive Behavior Scale, 1974 Revision*. Washington, DC: AAMD, 1975.
4674. Niikawa N, Fukushima Y, Taniguchin M et al. Chromosome abnormalities involving 11p13 and low erythrocyte catalase activity. *Hum Genet* 1982;60:373–5.
4675. Nikawa N et al. Kabuki make-up syndrome. *J Pediatr* 1981;99:565–9.
4676. Nikolao P, Xiang F, Gunnarsson LG et al. Autosomal dominant myopathy with proximal weakness and early respiratory muscle involvement maps to chromosome 2 q. *Am J Hum Genet* 1999;64:788–92.
4677. Nikoskelainen EK, Marttila RJ, Huoponen K et al. Leber's "plus": Neurological abnormalities in patients with Leber's hereditary optic neuropathy.

J Neurol Neurosurg Psychiatry 1995;59:160–4.
4678. NINCDS Ad Hoc Committee. Classification of cerebrovascular disease. *Stroke* 1990;21:637–76.
4679. Nishimura RN, Barranger JA. Neurological complications of Gaucher's disease, type 3. *Arch Neurol* 1980;37: 92–3.
4680. Nishino H, Rubino FA, DeRemee RA et al. Neurological involvement in Wegener's granulomatosis: An analysis of 324 consecutive patients at the Mayo Clinic. *Ann Neurol* 1993;33:4–9.
4681. Nishio Y, Kazui H, Hashimoto M et al. Actions anchored by concepts: Defective action comprehension in the semantic dementia. *J Neurol Neurosurg Psychiatry* 2006;77:1313–7.
4682. Nissen JJ, Jones PA, Signorini DF et al. Glasgow head injury prediction program: An independent assessment. *J Neurol Neurosurg Psychiatry* 1999;67:796–9.
4683. Nix WA, Butler IJ, Roontga S et al. Persistent unilateral tibialis anterior muscle hypertrophy with complex repetitive discharges and myalgia. *Neurology* 1992;42:602–6.
4684. Noachtar S, Holthausen H, Luders HO. Epileptic negative myoclonus. *Neurology* 1997;49:1534–7.
4685. Noad KB, Haymaker W. The neurological features of Tsutsugamushi fever, with special reference to deafness. *Brain* 1953;76:113–31.
4686. Nobile-Orakio E, Baldini L, Barbieri S. Treatment of patients with neuropathy and anti-MAG IgM M-proteins. *Ann Neurol* 1988;24:93–7.
4687. Nobunga M, Yoskioka K, Yasuda M et al. Clinical studies of polymyalgia rheumatica. A proposal of diagnostic criteria. *Japan J Med* 1989;28:452–6.
4688. Nogen AG. Congenital muscular disease and abnormal findings on computerized tomography. *Dev Med Child Neurol* 1980;22:658–63.
4689. Nolano M, Provitera V, Perretti A et al. Ross syndrome: A rare or a misknown disorder of thermoregulation? A skin innervation study on 12 subjects. *Brain* 2006;129:2119–31.
4690. See 4689.
4691. Nomizu S, Person DA, Saito C et al. A unique case of reducing body myopathy. *Muscle Nerve* 1992;15:463–6.
4692. Nonaka I. Distal myopathies. *Curr Opin Neurol* 1999;12:493–9.
4693. Nonaka I, Sunohara N, Satoyoshi E et al. Autosomal recessive distal muscular dystrophy: A comparative study with distal myopathy with rimmed vacuole formation. *Ann Neurol* 1985;17:51–9.
4694. Noonan JA. Hypertelorism with Turner phenotype. *Am J Dis Childh* 1968;116:373–80.
4695. Nordborg C, Conradi N, Sourander P et al. A new type of non-progressive sensory neuropathy in children with atypical dysautonomia. *Acta Neuropathol* 1981;55:135–41.
4696. Nordlund A, Rolstad S, Hellestrom P et al. The Goteborg MCI study: Mild cognitive impairment is a heterogeneous condition. *J Neurol Neurosurg Psychiatry* 2005;76:1485–90.
4697. Norenberg MD, Leslie KO, Robertson AS. Association between rise in serum sodium and central pontine myelinolysis. *Ann Neurol* 1982;11:128–35.
4698. Norman MG, Roberts M et al. Lissencephaly. *Can J Neurol Sci* 1976;3:39–46.
4699. Norman RM, Tingey AH. Syndrome of microencephaly, strio-cerebellar calcification and leukodystrophy. *J Neurol Neurosurg Psychiatry* 1966;29:157–63.
4700. Norman RM, Urich H. Cerebellar hypoplasia associated with systemic degeneration early in life. *J Neurol Neurosurg Psychiatry* 1958;159:166.
4701 Norman RM, Wood N. A congenital form of amaurotic familial idiocy. *J Neurol Neurosurg Psychiatry* 1941;4:175–90.
4702. Norre ME, Stevens A. Cervical vertigo. *Acta Oto-Rhino-Laryngol (Belg)* 1987;41:436.
4703. Norregaard J, Bulow PM, Danneskiold-Samsoe B. Muscle strength, voluntary activation, twitch properties and endurance in patients with fibromyalgia. *J Neurol Neurosurg Psychiatry* 1994;57:1106–11.
4704. Norrie G. Causes of blindness in children. *Acta Ophthalmol* (Copenhagen) 1927;5:363–4.
4705. Norris FH. Amyotrophic lateral sclerosis score. *Neurology* 1974;24:721–8.
4706. Norris FH, Panner BJ. Hypothyroid myopathy. *Arch Neurol* 1966;14:574–89.
4707. Norris FH, Panner BJ, Stormont JM. Thyrotoxic periodic paralysis: Metabolic and ultrastructural studies. *Arch Neurol* 1968;19:88–98.
4708. Norton JV, Zager E, Grady JF. Erythromelalgia: Diagnosis and classification. *J Foot Ankle Surg* 1999;38:238–41.
4709. Norwood F, de Visser M, Eymard B et al. EFNS guideline on diagnosis and management of limb girdle muscular dystrophies. *Eur J Neurol* 2007;14: 1305–12.
4710. Noseworthy JH, Ebers GC, Leigh RJ et al. Torsional nystagmus: Quantitative features and possible pathogenesis. *Neurology* 1988;38:992–4.
4711. Noseworthy JH, Heffernan LP, Ross JB. Acne fulminans with inflammatory myopathy. *Ann Neurol* 1980;8:67–9.
4712. Notermans NC, Fransses H, Eurelings M et al. Diagnostic criteria for demyelinating polyneuropathy associated with monoclonal gammopathy. *Muscle Nerve* 2000;23:73–9.
4713. Noth J, Dietz V, Mauritz K-H. Cyclist's palsy. *J Neurol Sci* 1980;47:111–6.
4714. Nothnagel CWH. On vasomotor neuroses. *Arch Klin Med* 1867;2:173–91.
4715. Nothnagel H. *Topische Diagnostik der Gehirnkrankheiten.* Berlin: Hischwalden, 1879.
4716. Nouri FM, Lincoln NB. An extended activities of daily living scale for stroke patients. *Clin Rehabil* 1987;1:301–5.
4717. Noviaka I, Sunohara N, Isiki S et al. Familial distal myopathy with rimmed vacuoles and lamellar (myeloid) body formation. *J Neurol Neurosurg Psychiatry* 1981;51:141–55.
4718. Novotny HR, Alvis DL. A method of photographing fluorescence in circulating blood of the human eye. *Am J Ophthalmol* 1960;50:176.
4719. Nowak DA, Widenka DC. Neurosarcoidosis: A review of its intracranial manifestations. *J Neurol* 2001;248:363–72.
4720. Nudleman K, Andermann E, Andermann F et al. The hemi 3 syndrome. *Brain* 1984;107:533–46.
4721. Nukada H, McMorran PD, Shimizu J. Acute inflammatory demyelination in reperfusion nerve injury. *Ann Neurol* 2000;47:71–9.
4722. Nurr JG, Marsden CD, Thompson PD. Human walking and high-level gait disorders, particularly in the elderly. *Neurology* 1993;43:268–279.
4723. See 4722
4724. Nygaard TG, Marsden CD, Duvoisin RC. Dopa-responsive dystonia. *Adv Neurol* 1988;50:377–84.
4725. Nygaard TG, Raymond D, Chen C et al. Localization of a gene for myoclonus-dystonia to chromosome 7q21-q31. *Ann Neurol* 1999;46:794–8.
4726. O'Brien JG et al. Juvenile GM1 gangliosidosis: Clinical, pathological, chemical and enzymatic studies. *Clin Genet* 1972;3:411–34.
4727. O'Brien JS. The gangliosidoses. In Stanbury JS, Wyngaarden JB, Frederickson DS et al., eds. *The Metabolic Basis of Inherited Disease*, p 952. New York: McGraw-Hill, 1983.
4728. O'Brien MD, Upton ARM. Anterior interosseous nerve syndrome. *J Neurol Neurosurg Psychiatry* 1972;35:531–6.
4729. O'Brien TJ, Cascino GD, So EL et al. Incidence and clinical consequences of the

purple glove syndrome in patients receiving intravenous phenytoin. *Neurology* 1998;51:1034–9.

4730. O'Connell JEA, Du Boulay EPGH. Binasal hemianopia. *J Neurol Neurosurg Psychiatry* 1973;36:697–709.

4731. O'Connell JEA, Turner JWA. Basilar impression of the skull. *Brain* 1950;73:405–25.

4732. O'Donnell PP, Leschner RT, Campbell WW. Hypertrophia musculorum vera in familial ataxia. *Arch Neurol* 1986;43: 146–7.

4733. O'Duffy JD, Goldstein NP. Neurologic involvement in seven patients with Behcet's disease. *Am J Med* 1976;61: 170–8.

4734. O'Halloran HS, Berger JR Lee WB et al. Acute multifocal placoid pigment epitheliopathy and central nervous system involvement: Nine new cases and a review of the literature. *Ophthalmology* 2001;108(5):861–8.

4735. O'Hearn E, Holmes SE, Cavert PC et al. SCA-12: Tremor with associated cerebellar and cortical atrophy is associated with a CAG repeat expansion. *Neurology* 2001;56:299–303.

4736. O'Leary CP, Willison H. Autoimmune ataxic neuropathies (sensory ganglionopathies). *Curr Opin Neurol* 1997;10:366–70.

4737. O'Neill B, Butler AB, Young E et al. Adult onset GM2 gangliosidosis. *Neurol Minneap* 1978;28:117–1123.

4738. O'Neill BP, Aronson AE, Pearson BW et al. Superior laryngeal neuralgia: Carotidynia or just another pain in the neck? *Headache* 1982;22:6–9.

4739. O'Neill BP, Illig JJ. Primary central nervous system lymphoma. *Mayo Clin Proc* 1989;64:1005–20.

4740. O'Sullivan DJ, McLeod JG. Spinal muscular atrophy, sporadic, confined to hands. *J Neurol Neurosurg Psychiatry* 1978;41:653–8.

4741. Obal A. Nutritional amblyopia. *Am J Ophthalmol* 1951;34:857–65.

4742. Oberklaid F, Danks DM, Mayne V et al. Asphyxiating thoracic dysplasia. *Arch Dis Child* 1977;52:758–65.

4743. Oberman HA. Chemodectomas (nonchromaffin paraganglioma) of head and neck. *Cancer* 1968;21:838–51.

4744. Obersteiner H. On allochiria: A peculiar sensory disorder. *Brain* 1881;4:153–63.

4745. Obeso JA, Rothwell JC, Lang AE et al. Myoclonic dystonia. *Neurology* 1983;33:825–30.

4746. Ochipa C, Rothi LJG, Heilman KM. Conduction apraxia. *J Neurol Neurosurg Psychiatry* 1994;57:1241–4.

4747. Ochoa JL. Positive sensory symptoms in neuropathy: Mechanisms and aspects of treatment. In Asbury AK, Thomas PK eds. *Peripheral Nerve Disorders* 2, pp 44–58. Oxford: Butterworth-Heinemann, 1995.

4748. Ochoa JL, Yarnitsky D. Mechanical hyperalgesias in neuropathic pain patients: Dynamic and static subtypes. *Ann Neurol* 1993;33:465–72.

4749. Ochs S. The early history of nerve regeneration, beginning with Cruickshank's observations in 1776. *Med Hist* 1977;21:261–74.

4750. Ochsner A, Gage M, DeBakey M. Scalenus anticus (Naffziger) syndrome. *Am J Surg* 1935;28:669.

4751. Odaka M, Yuki N, Hirata K. Anti-GQ1b antibody syndrome: Clinical and immunological range. *J Neurol Neurosurg Psychiatry* 2001;70:50–5.

4752. Odaka M, Yuki N, Yamada M et al. Bickerstaff's brainstem encephalitis: Clinical features of 62 cases and a subgroup associated with Guillain–Barré syndrome. *Brain* 2003;126:2279–90.

4753. Oerlemans WG, de Visser M. Dropped head syndrome and bent spine syndrome: Two separate clinical entities or different manifestations of axial myopathy? *J Neurol Neurosurg Psychiatry* 1998;65:258–9.

4754. Offen ML, Davidoff RA, Troost BT et al. Dacrystic epilepsy. *J Neurol Neurosurg Psychiatry* 1976;39:829–34.

4755. Offenbacher H, Fazekas F, Schmidt R et al. Assessment of MRI criteria for a diagnosis of MS. *Neurology* 1993;43: 905–9.

4756. Oguni H, Olivier A, Andermann F et al. Anterior callosotomy in the treatment of medically intractable epilepsies: A study of 43 patients with a mean follow-up of 39 months. *Ann Neurol* 1991;30:357–364.

4757. Ogunyemi AO, Dreifuss FE. Syndromes of epilepsy in childhood and adolescence. *J Child Neurol* 1988;35:214–24.

4758. Ogunyemi AO, Murphy D. The pinky finger in neurological diagnosis. *Can J Neurol Sci* 1999;(**Suppl. 2**):S44. (Abstract)

4759. Oh SJ, Birmingham AL, Danon MJ et al. Mitochondrial myelo-myopathy (3-M syndrome). *Neurology* 1991;41 (**Suppl. 1**): 178.

4760. Oh SJ, Claussen GC, Kim DS. Motor and sensory demyelinating mononeuropathy multiplex (multifocal motor and sensory demyelinating neuropathy): A separate entity or a variant of chronic inflammatory demyelinating polyneuropathy? *J Periph Nerv Syst* 1997;2:362–9.

4761. Oh SJ, Claussen GC, Ryan H et al. Multifocal sensory demyelinating neuropathy: A heretofore unrecognized entity. *Ann Neurol* 2000;48(3):468. (Abstract)

4762. Oh SJ, Darron MJ. Nonprogressive congenital neuromuscular disease with uniform Type 1 fiber. *Arch Neurol* 1983;40:147–50.

4763. Oh SJ, Dwyer DS, Bradley RJ. Overlap myasthenia gravis and Eaton-Lambert syndrome. *Neurology* 1987;37:1411–4.

4764. Oh SJ, Joy JL, Kuruoglu R. "Chronic sensory demyelinating neuropathy": Chronic inflammatory demyelinating polyneuropathy presenting as a pure sensory neuropathy. *J Neurol Neurosurg Psychiatry* 1992;55:677–80.

4765. Oh SJ, Kurokawa K, de Almeida DF et al. Subacute inflammatory demyelinating polyneuropathy. *Neurology* 2003;61:1507–12.

4766. Oh SJ, Kuruoglu R. Chronic limb-girdle myasthenia gravis. *Neurology* 1992;42:1153–6.

4767. Oh SJ, Kwon KH, Hah JS et al. Lateral plantar neuropathy. *Muscle Nerve* 1999;22:1234–8.

4768. Oh SJ, LaGanke C, Claussen GC. Sensory Guillain–Barré syndrome. *Neurology* 2001;56:82–6.

4769. Oh SJ, Lee KW. Medial plantar neuropathy. *Neurology* 1987;37:1408–10.

4770. Oh SJ, Myers GJ, Wilson ER et al. A benign form of reducing body myopathy. *Muscle Nerve* 1983;6:278–82.

4771. Ohara S, Kondo K, Morita H et al. Progressive supranuclear palsy-like syndrome in two siblings of a consanguineous marriage. *Neurology* 1992;42:1009–14.

4772. Ohkawa S, Yamasaki H, Tabuchi M et al. Eyebrow lifting test. *J Neurol Neurosurg Psychiatry* 1997;63:256–7.

4773. Ohlsson L. Congenital renal disease, deafness, and myopia in one family. *Acta Med Scand* 1963;174:77–84.

4774. Ohnishi A, Matsuo H. X-linked motor and sensory neuropathy with pyramidal signs and cerebral white matter lesions. *Muscle Nerve* 2003;28:623–5.

4775. Ohno K, Engel AG, Brengman JM et al. The spectrum of mutations causing end-plate acetylcholinesterase deficiency. *Ann Neurol* 2000;47:162–70.

4776. Ohta M, Ellefson RD, Lambert EH et al. Hereditary sensory neuropathy Type II. *Arch Neurol* 1973;29:23–37.

4777. Ohtahara S, Ishida T, Oka E et al. On the age-dependent epileptic syndromes: The early infantile encephalopathy with suppression burst. *Brain Dev* 1976;8:270–88.

4778. Ohtahara S, Yamatogi Y, Ohtsuka Y et al. Prognosis of West syndrome with special reference to Lennox syndrome: A developmental study. In Wada J, Penry JK eds. *Advances in Epileptology: The Xth Epilepsy International Symposium*, pp 149–54. New York: Raven Press, 1980.

4779. Oka Y, Fukui K, Shoda D et al. Cerebral cysticercosis manifesting as hydrocephalus – case report. *Neurol Med Chir (Tokyo)* 1996;36:654–8.

4780. Okajima T, Yamamura S, Hamada K et al. Chronic autonomic and sensory neuropathy. *Neurology* 1983;33:1061–4.

4781. Okihiro MM et al. Duane syndrome and congenital upper limb anomalies. *Arch Neurol* 1977;34:174–9.

4782. Oldfors A. Hereditary myosin myopathies. *Neuromuscul Disord* 2007;17:355–67.

4783. Olesen J, Bousser M-G, Diener H-C. New appendix criteria open for a broader concept of chronic migraine. *Cephalalgia* 2006;26:742–6.

4784. See 4783

4785. Olivé M, Goldfarb LG, Shatunov A et al. Myotilinopathy: Refining the clinical and myopathological phenotype. *Brain* 2005;128:2315–26.

4786. Olivé M, Goldfarb LG, Moreno D et al. Desmin-related myopathy: Clinical, electrophysiological, radiological, neuropathological and genetic studies. *J Neurol Sci* 2004;219:125–37.

4787. Olney RK. Neuropathies in connective tissue disease. *Muscle Nerve* 1992;15: 531–42.

4788. Olney RK, Aminoff MJ, So YT. Clinical and electrodiagnostic features of X-linked recessive bulbospinal neuronopathy. *Neurology* 1991;41:823–7.

4789. Olney RK, Lewis RA et al. Consensus criteria for the diagnosis of multifocal motor neuropathy. *Muscle Nerve* 2003;27:117–21.

4790. Olson LC, Bourgeois CH, Cotton RB et al. Encephalopathy and fatty degeneration of the viscera in northeastern Thailand: Clinical syndrome and epidemiology. *Pediatrics* 1971;47:707.

4791. Olson WH, Bardin CW, Walsh GC et al. Möebius syndrome. *Neurology* 1970;20:1002–8.

4792. Omae T, Tsuchiya T, Yamaguchi T. Cheiro-oral syndrome due to lesions in the corona radiata. *Stroke* 1992;23:599–601.

4793. Omenn GS. Familial reticuloendotheliosis with eosinophilia. *N Engl J Med* 1965;273:427–32.

4794. Ommaya AK et al. Nontraumatic cerebrospinal fluid rhinorrhea. *J Neurol Neurosurg Psychiatry* 1968;31:214–25.

4795. Onanoff M. Du réflexe "bulbo-caverneux". *Paris Soc Biol* 1890;2:215–7.

4796. Oonk JGW, Van der Helm HJ, Martin JJ. Spinocerebellar degeneration: Hexosaminidase A and B deficiency in two adult sisters. *Neurology* 1979;29: 380–3.

4797. Opalski A. Nowy zespol podopuszkowy. Zespol czesciowy tetnicy kregowo-rezeniowej tylnej. *Pol Tyg Lek* 1946;1:397–402.

4798. Opitz JM, Frias JL, Gutenberger JE et al. The G syndrome of multiple congenital anomalies. The clinical delineation of birth defects: II Malformation syndromes. *b.d.* 1969;V:95–101.

4799. Opitz JM, Johnson RC, McCreadie SR et al. The C syndrome of multiple congenital anomalies. *b.d.* 1969;5:161–6.

4800. Opitz JM, Kaveggia EG. The FG syndrome. An X-linked recessive syndrome of multiple congenital anomalies and mental retardation. *S Kindrheilk* 1974;117:1–18.

4801. Oppenheim G. Multiple system atrophy. *J Neurol Neurosurg Psychiatry* 1989;28:34.

4802. Oppenheim H. Ueber allgemeine und localisierte Atonie der Muskulatur(Myatonie) im fruhen Kindersalter. Vorlaufige Mitteilung. *Mschr Psychiat* 1900;8:232–3.

4803. Oppenheim H. Zur Pathologie der Hautreflexe an den unteren Extremitaten. *Mschr Psychiat Neurol* 1902;12:421–3.

4804. Oppenheim H. Ueber eine eigenartige Krampfkrankheit des kindlichen und jugendlichen Alters (Dysbasia lordotica progressiva, Dystonia musculorum deformans). *Zbl Nervenheit* 1911;30:1090–109.

4805. Oppenheim H, Vogt C. Wesen und Localisation der Kongennitalen und infantilen Pseudobulbarparalyse. *J F Psychol U Neurol* 1911;18:293–308.

4806. Oppenheimer DR. A benign "tumour" of the cerebellum. *J Neurol Neurosurg Psychiatry* 1955;18:199–213.

4807. Oppenheimer DR. Diseases of the basal ganglia, cerebellum and motor neurons. In Blackwood W, Corsellis JAN eds. *Greenfield's Neuropathology*, p 615. London: Arnold, 1976.

4808. Optiz JM, Johnsons RC, McCreadie SR et al. The syndrome of multiple congenital anomalies. *b.d.* 1969;5:161–6.

4809. Orgogozo JM. Evaluation of treatments in ischemic-stroke patients. In Amery WK, Bousser MG, Rose FC eds. *Clinical Trial Methodology in Stroke*, pp 35–53. London: Balliere Tindall, 1989.

4810. Orgogozo JM. A unified form for neurological scoring of hemispheric stroke with motor impairment. *Stroke* 1992;23:1678–9.

4811. Orgogozo JM, Bougousslavsky J. Lacunar syndromes. In Toole JF ed. *Handbook of Clinical Neurology*, Amsterdam: North Holland, 1989.

4812. Orlacchio A, Kawarai T, Gaudiello F et al. New locus for hereditary spastic paraplegia maps to chromosome 1p31. 1-1p21.1. *Ann Neurol* 2005;58: 423–9.

4813. Orlacchio A, Patrono C, Gaudiello F et al. Silver syndrome variant of hereditary spastic paraplegia. *Neurology* 2008;70:1959–66.

4814. Ormandy L. Scapulocostal syndrome. *VA Med Q* 1994;121:105–8.

4815. Orrell RW, Marsden CD. The neck-tongue syndrome. *J Neurol Neurosurg Psychiatry* 1994;57:348–52.

4816. Orschansky J. Tabes dorsalis und das Kniewinkelphanomen. *Neurol Centralbl* 1906;25:401–5.

4817. Ortiz-Arduan A, Martin-Lionch N. Supermarket neuropathy. *Muscle Nerve* 1991;14:785.

4818. Ortner N. Recurrenslahmung bei Mitralstenose. *Wien Klin Wschr* 1897;10:753–5.

4819. Orzechowski K, Walichiewicz T. Operated cyst of the cerebellum. *Lwowski Tygodnik Lekarski* 1913;8:219–27.

4820. Oschmann P, Dorndorf W, Hornig C et al. Stages and syndromes of neuroborreliosis. *J Neurol* 1998;245: 262–72.

4821. Osher RH, Griggs RC. Orbicularis fatigue: The "peek" sign of myasthenia gravis. *Arch Ophthalmol* 1979;97:677.

4822. Osher RH, Shields JA, Schatz MJ. Axial myopia: A neglected case of proptosis. *Arch Neurol* 1978;35:237–41.

4823. Ostberg O. Study of interindividual differences in circadian fatigue patterns of shift workers. *Br J Ind Med* 1973;30: 341–51.

4824. Oster G. Phosphenes. *Sci Am* 1970;222:82.

4825. Oster J. Growing pain: A symptom and its significance. *Dan Med Bull* 1972;19:72–9.

4826. Ostergaard E, Hansen FJ, Sorensen N et al. Mitochondrial encephalomyopathy with elevated methylmalonic acid is caused by SUCLA2 mutations. *Brain* 2007;130:853–61.

4827. Osuntokun BO. An ataxic neuropathy in Nigeria: A clinical, biochemical and electrophysiological study. *Brain* 1968;91:215–48.

4828. Osuntokun BO, Odeku EL, Luzzato L. Congenital pain asymbolia and auditory imperception. *J Neurol Neurosurg Psychiatry* 1968;31:291–6.

4829. Oswald I. Sudden bodily jerks on falling asleep. *Brain* 1959;82:92–102.

4830. Otsubo H, Chitoku S, Ochi A et al. Malignant rolandic-sylvian epilepsy in children. *Neurology* 2001;57:590–6.

4831. Ott BR, Saver JL. Unilateral amnesic stroke. *Stroke* 1993;24:1033–42.

4832. Ouachi K, Arita M, Kayden H et al. Ataxia with isolated vitamin E deficiency is caused by mutations in alpha-tocopherol transfer protein. *Nat Genet* 1995;9:141–5.

4833. Ouvrier R, Geevasingha N, Ryan MM. Autosomal-recessive and X-linked forms of hereditary motor and sensory neuropathy in childhood. *Muscle Nerve* 2007;**36**:131–43.
4834. Ouvrier RA. Progressive dystonia with marked diurnal fluctuation. *Ann Neurol* 1978;**4**:412–7.
4835. Ouvrier RA et al. HMSN III, autosomal recessive inheritance. *Brain* 1987;**110**:121.
4836. Ouzonellis T. Some notes on quail myopathy. *J Am Med Assn* 1970;**211**: 1186–7.
4837. Overall JE, Gorham DR. Introduction – the brief psychiatric rating scale. *Psychopharm Bull* 1988;**24**:97–9.
4838. Overell J, Willison H. Chronic inflammatory demyelinating polyradiculoneuropathy. *Practical Neurol* 2006;**6**:102–10.
4839. Overell J, Willison HJ. Recent developments in Miller Fisher syndrome and related disorders. *Curr Opin Neurol* 2005;**18**:562–6.
4840. Owen CA, Woody PR, Mubarak SJ et al. Gluteal compartment syndromes. A report of three cases and management utilising the wick catheter. *Clin Orthop* 1978;**132**:57–60.
4841. Owen G, Mulley GP. The palmomental reflex: A useful clinical sign? *J Neurol Neurosurg Psychiatry* 2002;**73**:113–5.
4842. Oxbury JM, Oxbury SM, Humphrey NK. Varieties of colour anomia. *Brain* 1969;**92**:847–60.
4843. Oxbury JM, Whitty CWM. The syndrome of isolated epileptic status. *J Neurol Neurosurg Psychiatry* 1971;**34**: 182–4.
4844. Ozawa E, Noguchi S, Mizuno Y et al. From dystrophinopathy to sarcoglycanopathy: Evolution of a concept of muscular dystrophy. *Muscle Nerve* 1998;**21**:421–38.
4845. Ozawa K, Saida K, Saida T et al. Familial neuropathy with dementia, retinitis pigmentosa and dysautonomia. *Neurology* 1985;**35**:1184–7.
4846. Pace JB, Nagle D. Piriformis syndrome. *West J Med* 1976;**124**:435–9.
4847. Pachner AR, Delaney E. The polymerase chain reaction in the diagnosis of Lyme neuroborreliosis. *Ann Neurol* 1993;**34**:544–50.
4848. Pacia SV, Devinsky O, Lucioano DJ et al. The prolonged QT syndrome presenting as epilepsy. *Neurology* 1994;**44**:1408–10.
4849. Packman S, Sweetman L, Baker H et al. The neonatal form of biotin-responsive multiple carboxylase deficiency. *J Pediatr* 1981;**99**:418–20.
4850. Padberg GW, Schot JDL, Vielvoye GJ et al. Lhermitte–Duclos disease and Cowden disease: A single phakomatosis. *Ann Neurol* 1991;**29**:517–23.
4851. Page IH. A syndrome simulating diencephalic stimulation occurring in patients with essential hypertension. *Am J Med Sci* 1935;**190**:9–14.
4852. Page NGR, Bolger JP, Sanders MD. Auditory evoked phosphenes in optic nerve disease. *J Neurol Neurosurg Psychiatry* 1982;**45**:7–12.
4853. Pageot N, Vial C, Chazot G et al. Progressive chorea and amyotrophy without acanthocytes: A new case of Fotopoulos syndrome? *J Neurol* 2000;**247**:392–4.
4854. Pagon RA. Retinitis pigmentosa. *Surv Ophthalmol* 1988;**33**:137–77.
4855. Paige DG, Clayton P, Bowron A et al. Richner–Hanhart syndrome. *J Roy Soc Med* 1992;**85**:759–60.
4856. Paine RS. Evaluation of familial biochemically determined mental retardation in children, with special reference to aminoaciduria. *N Engl J Med* 1960;**262**:658–65.
4857. Paine RS, Efron ML. Atypical variants of "ataxia-telangiectasia syndrome". *Dev Med Child Neurol* 1963;**5**:14–23.
4858. Pakalnis A, Drake ME, John K et al. Forced normalization: Acute psychosis after seizure control in seven patients. *Arch Neurol* 1987;**44**:289–92.
4859. Pakarinen S. Incidence, etiology, and prognosis of primary subarachnoid hemorrhage. *Acta Neurol Scand* 1967;43 **(Suppl. 29)**.
4860. Pakiam AS-I, Parry GJ. Multifocal motor neuropathy without overt conduction block. *Muscle Nerve* 1998;**21**:243–5.
4861. Palace J, Lashley D, Newsom-Davis J et al. Clinical features of the DOK7 neuromuscular junction synaptopathy. *Brain* 2007;**130**:1507–15.
4862. Palace J, Wiles CM, Newsom-Davis J. 3,4-Diaminopyridine in the treatment of congenital (hereditary) myasthenia. *J Neurol Neurosurg Psychiatry* 1991;**54**:1069–72.
4863. Paladini D, Dellantonio R, Cinti A et al. Axillary neuropathy in volleyball players: Report of two cases and literature review. *J Neurol Neurosurg Psychiatry* 1996;**60**: 345–7.
4864. Palau F, De Michele G, Vilchez JJ et al. Early onset ataxia with cardiomyopathy and retained tendon reflexes maps to the Friedreich's ataxia locus on chromosome 9q. *Ann Neurol* 1995;**37**:359–62.
4865. Palisano RI, Hanna SE, Rosenbaum PL et al. Validation of a model of gross motor function for children with cerebral palsy. *Phys Ther* 2000;**80**:974–85.
4866. Palix C, Coignet J. A case of congenital neuropathy with absence of myelin in the peripheral nervous system. *Pediatrie* 1978;**33**:201–7.
4867. Pallis CA, Scott JT. Peripheral neuropathy in rheumatoid arthritis. *BMJ* 1965;**1**:1141–7.
4868. Pallister PD et al. The W syndrome. Studies of malformation syndromes of man XXVIII. *Birth Defects* 1974;**10(7)**:51–60.
4869. Pallister PD et al. The Pallister mosaic syndrome. *Birth Defects* 1977;**13(13B)**:103–10.
4870. Palma-da Cunha-Matta A, Soares-Moreno SA, Cardoso-de Almeida A et al. Neurological complications arising from dengue virus infection. *Rev Neurol* 2004;**39**:233–7.
4871. Palmer EP. Transient global amnesia and the amnestic syndromes. *Med Clin North Am* 1986;**70**:1361–74.
4872. Palmer JJ. Radiation myelopathy. *Brain* 1972;**95**:109–22.
4873. Palmini A, Andermann F, Aicardi J et al. Diffuse cortical dysplasia, or the "double cortex" syndrome. *Neurology* 1991;**41**:1656–62.
4874. Palmucci L, Mongini T, Doriguzzi C et al. Familial autosomal recessive rigid spine syndrome with neurogenic facio-scapulo-peroneal muscle atrophy. *J Neurol Neurosurg Psychiatry* 1991;**54**:42–5.
4875. Paloneva J, Autti T, Raininko R et al. CNS manifestations of Nasu-Hakola disease. *Neurology* 2001;**56**:1552–8.
4876. Palthe PMvW. A peculiar reflex phenomenon. *Brain* 1925;**48**:476–91.
4877. Pampiglione G, Maia M. Syndrome of rapid irregular movements of eyes and limbs in childhood. *BMJ* 1972;**1**:469–73.
4878. Pan C-L, Yuki N, Koga M et al. Acute sensory ataxic neuropathy associated with monospecific anti-GD1b IgG antibody. *Neurology* 2001;**57**:1316–8.
4879. Panayiotopoulos CP. Benign childhood epilepsy with occipital paroxysms: A 15-year prospective study. *Ann Neurol* 1989;**26**:51–6.
4880. Panayiotopoulos CP. Benign childhood partial epilepsies: Benign childhood seizure susceptibility syndromes. *J Neurol Neurosurg Psychiatry* 1993;**56**: 2–5.
4881. Panayiotopoulos CP. Early-onset benign childhood occipital seizure susceptibility syndrome: A syndrome to recognize. *Epilepsia* 1999;**40**:621–30.
4882. Panayiotopoulos CP. *A clinical guide to epileptic syndromes and their treatment.* London: Springer-Verlag, 2007.
4883. Panayiotopoulos CP, Chroni E. F waves in clinical neurophysiology: A review, methodological issues and overall value in peripheral neuropathies. *EEG Clin Neurophysiol* 1996;**101**:365–74.

4884. Pancoast HK. Superior pulmonary sulcus tumor. Tumor characterized by pain, Horner's syndrome, destruction of bone and atrophy of hand muscles. *JAMA* 1932;99:1391–6.

4885. Pansini S. On a cerebellar syndrome with dysarthria in acute malaria. *Rif Med* 1901;4:458–62.

4886. Pant SS, Benton JW, Dodge PR. Unilateral pupillary dilatation during and immediately following seizures. *Neurology* 1966;16:837–40.

4887. Paparella MM. The cause (multifactorial inheritance) and pathogenesis (endolymphatic malabsorption) of Meniere's disease and its symptoms. *Acta Otolaryngol* 1985;99:445–51.

4888. Paparella MM, Elfiky FM. Mondini's deafness. *Arch Otolaryngol* 1972;95: 134–40.

4889. Papez JW. A proposed mechanism of emotion. *Arch Neurol Psychiatry* 1937;38:725–43.

4890. Paping RHL, Annyas AA, Mouji JJA. Nasopharyngeal torticollis (Grisel's syndrome). *Ned Tschr Geneesk* 1985;129:1787–90.

4891. Paradiso G, Micheli F, Taratuto AL et al. Familial bulbospinal neuronopathy with optic atrophy: A distinct entity. *J Neurol Neurosurg Psychiatry* 1996;61:196–9.

4892. Pareja JA, Cuadrado ML, Fernández-de-las-Peñas C et al. Epicrania fugax: An ultrabrief paroxysmal epicranial pain. *Cephalalgia* 2004;28:257–63.

4893. Pareja JA, Vincent M, Antonaci F et al. Hemicrania continua: Diagnostic criteria and nosologic status. *Cephalalgia* 2001;21:874–7.

4894. Pareja J, Caminero A, Serra J et al. Nummular headache: A coin-shaped cephalgia. *Neurology* 2002;58:1678–9.

4895. Parent A. Felix Vicq d'Azir. *Can J Neurol Sci* 2007;34:30–7.

4896. Parent A, Parent M, Leroux-Hugon V. Jules Bernard Luys. *Can J Neurol Sci* 2002;29:282–8.

4897. Pareyson D. Charcot–Marie–Tooth disease and related neuropathies: Molecular basis for distinction and diagnosis. *Muscle Nerve* 1999;22: 1498–509.

4898. Parinaud H. Paralysie des mouvements associés des yeux. *Arch Neurol (Paris)* 1883;5:145–72.

4899. Parinaud H. Paralysie de la convergence. *Ann Ocul Paris* 1886;95:205–6.

4900. Parisi JE, Collins GH, Kim C et al. Prenatal symmetric thalamic degeneration with flexion spasticity at birth. *Ann Neurol* 1983;13:94.

4901. Parjiale JR, Hudgins TH, Fishman LM. The piriformis syndrome. *Am J Orthop* 1996;25:819–23.

4902. Park TA, Del Toro DR. Isolated inferior calcaneal neuropathy. *Muscle Nerve* 1996;19:106–8.

4903. Parker N. Hereditary whispering dysphonia. *J Neurol Neurosurg Psychiatry* 1985;48:218–24.

4904. Parkes JD. *Sleep and its Disorders.* London: W.B. Saunders Co., 1985.

4905. Parkinson D. Concussion. *Mayo Clin Proc* 1977;52:492–6.

4906. Parkinson J. *An Essay on the Shaking Palsy.* London: Whittingham and Rowland, 1817.

4907. Parks AG. Anorectal incontinence. *Proc Roy Soc Med* 1975;68:681–90.

4908. Parmar C, Blackburn C. Madelung's disease: An uncommon disorder of unknown aetiology? *Br J Oral Maxillofac Surg* 1996;34:467–70.

4909. Parmelee AH. Critical evaluation of the Moro reflex. *Pediatrics* 1964;33:773.

4910. Parr J, Terry TM, Larner J. Symptomatic hypoglycemia, visceral fatty acid metamorphosis and aglycogenosis in an infant lacking glycogen synthetase and phosphorylase. *Pediatrics* 1965;35:770.

4911. Parrott JMJ. Sur une pseudo-paralysie causée par une alteration du système osseux chez les nouveau-nés atteints de syphilis hereditaire. *Arch Physiol (Paris)* 1871;4:319–33.

4912. Parrott JMJ. Lesions of the skull as a result of congenital syphilis. *Progr Med (Paris)* 1879;7:268–9.

4913. Parrott JMJ. On a pupillary phenomenon observed in certain pathological states in infancy. *Rev Med Paris* 1882;2:809–24.

4914. Parry CH. *Collections from the Unpublished Medical Writings.* London: Underwood, 1825.

4915. Parry GJ. Are multifocal motor neuropathy and Lewis-Sumner syndrome distinct nosologic entities? *Muscle Nerve* 1999;22:557–9.

4916. Parsonage MJ, Turner JWA. Neuralgic amyotrophy: The shoulder girdle syndrome. *Lancet* 1948;1:973–8.

4917. Parton A, Malhotra P, Husain M. Hemispatial neglect. *J Neurol Neurosurg Psychiatr* 2004;75:13–21.

4918. Parziale JR, Hudgins TH, Fishman LM. The piriformis syndrome. *Am J Orthop* 1996;25:819–23.

4919. Pascucci RC. Head trauma in the child. *Intensive Care Med* 1988;14:185–95.

4920. Pascuzzi RM, Gratianne R, Azzarelli B et al. Schwartz–Jampel syndrome with dominant inheritance. *Muscle Nerve* 1990;13:1152–63.

4921. Pashayan HA. A family with blepharo-naso-facial malformations. *Am J Dis Childh* 1973;125:389–93.

4922. Passarge E, McAdams AJ. Cerebro-hepato-renal syndrome: A newly recognized hereditary disorder of multiple congenital defects, including sudanophilic leukodystrophy, cirrhosis of the liver, and polycystic kidneys. *J Pediatr* 1967;71:691–702.

4923. Passouant P. Historical note. Doctor Gelineau (1828–1906): Narcolepsy centennial. *Sleep* 1981;4:241–6.

4924. Passwell JL, Ziplowski D, Nelson A et al. A syndrome characterized by congenital ichthyosis, erythroderma, mental retardation, dwarfism and generalized aminoaciduria. *J Pediatr* 1973;82:466–71.

4925. Patau K, Smith DW, Therman E et al. Multiple congenital anomaly caused by an extra autosome. *Lancet* 1960;1:790–3.

4926. Patel AN, Razzak ZA, Dastur DK. Disuse atrophy of human skeletal muscles. *Arch Neurol* 1969;20:413–21.

4927. Patel H, Berry K, McLeod P et al. Cytoplasmic body myopathy. *J Neurol Sci* 1983;60:281–92.

4928. Paterson D, Carmichael EA. Form of familial cerebral degeneration chiefly affecting the lenticular nucleus. *Brain* 1924;47:207–31.

4929. Paterson D, Greenfield JG. Erythroedema polyneuritis (the so-called Pink disease). *Quart J Med* 1923;65:6–18.

4930. Paton JY, Swaminathan S, Sargent CW et al. Hypoxic and hypercapneic ventilatory responses in awake children with congenital central hypoventilation syndrome. *Am Rev Respir Dis* 1989;140:368–72.

4931. Patry G, Lyagoubi S, Tassinari CA. Subclinical "electrical status epilepticus" induced by sleep in children. *Arch Neurol* 1971;24:242–52.

4932. Patten BM, Pages M. Severe neurological disease associated with hyperparathyroidism. *Ann Neurol* 1984;15:453–6.

4933. Patterson JH. Presentation of a patient with leprechaunism. *b.d.* 1969;5(4): 117–21.

4934. Patterson JR, Grabois M. Locked-in syndrome: A review of 139 cases. *Stroke* 1986;17:758–64.

4935. Pattie AH, Gileard CJ. A brief psychogeriatric assessment schedule. *Br J Psychiatry* 1975;127:289–93.

4936. Pattison EM. Uveomeningoencephalitic syndrome (Vogt–Koyanagi–Harada). *Arch Neurol* 1965;12:197–205.

4937. Paty DW, Blume WT, Brown WF et al. Chronic progressive myelopathy: Investigation with CSF electrophoresis, evoked potentials, and CT scan. *Ann Neurol* 1979;6:419–24.

4938. Paul JR. *A History of Poliomyelitis.* New Haven: Yale U.P., 1971.

4939. Paulson G, Gottlieb G. Developmental reflexes: The reappearance of foetal and neonatal reflexes in aged patients. *Brain* 1968;91:37–52.

4940. Paulson GW. Weightlifter's headache. *Headache* 1983;23:193–4.

4941. Pavlakis SG, Phillips PC, DiMauro S et al. Mitochondrial myopathy, encephalopathy, lactic acidosis, and strokelike episodes: A distinctive clinical syndrome. *Ann Neurol* 1984;16:481–8.

4942. Pavlov I. *Conditioned Reflexes*. Oxford: Oxford University Press, 1927.

4943. Pavone L, Curatolo P, Rizzo R et al. Epidermal nevus syndrome: A neurologic variant with hemimegalencephaly, gyral malformation, mental retardation, seizures, and facial hemihypertrophy. *Neurology* 1991;41:266–71.

4944. Pavone P, Parano E, Polizzi A et al. Colobomatous microphthalmia, microcephaly with cerebellar hypoplasia: A new clincal syndrome. *Ann Neurol* 2000;48(3):530. (Abstract)

4945. Payan C, Hodgkinson I, Berard C et al. A motor function measure scale for neuromuscular diseases. Construction and validation study. *Neuromuscul Disord* 2005;15:463–70.

4946. Payne EE, Spillane JD. The cervical spine: An anatomico-pathological study of 70 specimens (using a special technique) with particular reference to the problem of cervical spondylosis. *Brain* 1957;80:571–96.

4947. Pearce JMS. Needle-in-the-eye syndrome. *World Medicine* 1979;14:77–8.

4948. Pearce JMS. Historical aspects of migraine. *J Neurol Neurosurg Psychiatry* 1986;49:1097–103.

4949. Pearce JMS. Aspects of the history of Parkinson's disease. *J Neurol Neurosurg Psychiatry* 1989;52**Suppl.**:6–10.

4950. Pearce JMS. Clinical features of the exploding head syndrome. *J Neurol Neurosurg Psychiatry* 1989;52:907–10.

4951. Pearce JMS. Whiplash injury: A reappraisal. *J Neurol Neurosurg Psychiatry* 1989;52:1329–31.

4952. Pearce JMS. Polemics of chronic whiplash injury. *Neurology* 1994;44:1993–7.

4953. Pearl PL, Gibson KM, Acosta MT et al. Clinical spectrum of succinic semialdehyde dehydrogenase deficiency. *Neurology* 2003;60:1413–7.

4954. Pearlman AL, Birch J, Meadows JC. Cerebral color blindness: An acquired defect in hue discrimination. *Ann Neurol* 1979;5:253–61.

4955. Pearn JH. Neurology of ciguatera. *J Neurol Neurosurg Psychiatry* 2001;70:4–8.

4956. Pearn JH, Gardner-Medwin D, Wilson J. A clinical study of chronic childhood spinal muscular atrophy. *J Neurol Sci* 1978;38:23–37.

4957. Pearn JH, Gardner-Thorpe C. Jules Cotard. *Neurology* 2002;58:1400–3.

4958. Pearn JH, Hudgson P, Walton JN. A clinical and genetic study of spinal muscular atrophy of adult onset. *Brain* 1978;101:591–606.

4959. Pearson CM. The periodic paralyses: Differential features and pathological observations in permanent myopathic weakness. *Brain* 1963;87:341.

4960. Pebenito R, Feretti C, Chaudary RR et al. Idiopathic torsion dystonia associated with lesions of the basal ganglia. *Clin Pediatr* 1984;23:232.

4961. Pederson E. Epidemic vertigo: Clinical picture, epidemiology and relation to encephalitis. *Brain* 1959;82:566–80.

4962. Pedley TA, Guilleminault C. Episodic nocturnal wanderings responsive to anticonvulsant drug therapy. *Ann Neurol* 1977;2:30–5.

4963. Pedraza S, Gamez J, Rovira A et al. MRI findings in Möbius syndrome: Correlation with clinical features. *Neurology* 2000;55:1058–60.

4964. Peiris JB, Senviratne KN, Wickremasinghe HR et al. Nonfamilial juvenile distal spinal muscular atrophy of upper extremity. *J Neurol Neurosurg Psychiatry* 1989;52:314–9.

4965. Pelayo R, Barasch E, Kang H et al. Progressively intractable seizures, focal alopecia and hemimegalencephaly. *Neurology* 1994;44:969–71.

4966. Peled R, Lavie P. Paroxysmal awakenings from sleep associated with excessive daytime somnolence: A form of nocturnal epilepsy. *Neurology* 1986;36:95–8.

4967. Pelizaeus F. Ueber eine eigentumliche Form spastischer Lahmung mit Cerebralerscheinungen auf hereditarer Grundlage (multiple Sklerose). *Arch Psychiatr (Berlin)* 1885;16:698–710.

4968. Pellechia MT, Scala R, Filla A et al. Idiopathic cerebellar ataxia associated with celiac disease: Lack of distinctive neurological features. *J Neurol Neurosurg Psychiatry* 1999;66:32–5.

4969. Pellissier JF, Pouget J, de Victor B et al. Tomaculous neuropathy. Histopathologic study and electro-clinical correlations in 10 cases. *Rev Neurol* 1987;143:263–78.

4970. Pelmear PL, Taylor W. Hand-arm vibration syndrome. *J Fam Pract* 1994;38:180–5.

4971. Pelz DM, Fox AJ, Vinuela F. Digital subtraction angiography: Current clinical applications. *Stroke* 1985;16:528–36.

4972. Pena CE, Miller F, Budzilovich GN. Arthrogryposis multiplex congenita. *Neurology* 1968;18:926–30.

4973. Pena SDJ, Shokeir MHK. Syndrome of campodactyly, multiple ankyloses, facial anomalies, and pulmonary hypoplasia: A lethal condition. *J Pediatr* 1974;85: 373–5.

4974. Pendred V. Deaf-mutism and goitre. *Lancet* 1896;2:532.

4975. Penfield W. Diencephalic autonomic epilepsy. *Arch Neurol Psychiatry* 1929;22:358–74.

4976. Penfield W. Engrams in the human brain. *Proc Roy Soc Med* 1968;61:831–40.

4977. Penfield W, Perot P. The brain's record of auditory and visual experience. *Brain* 1963;86:595–696.

4978. Penfield W, Ward A. Calcifying epileptogenic lesions. *Arch Neurol Psychiatry* 1948;60:20–36.

4979. Penfield W, Welch K. The supplementary motor area in the cerebral cortex of man. *Trans Am Neurol Assn* 1949;74:179–269.

4980. Penfield W, Welch K. The supplementary motor area of cerebral cortex. *Arch Neurol Psychiatry* 1951;66:289–317.

4981. Penisson-Besnier I, Dumez C, Chateau D et al. Autosomal dominant late adult onset distal leg myopathy. *Neuromuscul Disord* 1998;8:459–66.

4982. Percy ME, Thompson MW. Creatine kinase – no phospho-, please!". *Muscle Nerve* 1981;4:271–3.

4983. Peress NS, DiMauro S, Roxburgh VA. Adult polysaccharidosis: Clinicopathological, ultrastructural, and biochemical features. *Arch Neurol* 1979;36:840–5.

4984. Perheentupa J et al. Mulibrey nanism, an autosomal recessive syndrome with pericardial constriction. *Lancet* 1973;2:351–5.

4985. Perheentupa J, Visakorpi JK. Protein intolerance with deficient transport of basic amino acids. *Lancet* 1965;2:813.

4986. Peripheral Neuropathy Association. Quantitative sensory testing. *Neurology* 1993;43:1050–2.

4987. Perot P, Feindel W, Lloyd-Smith D. Hematomyelia as a complication of syringomyelia: Gowers' syringal haemorrhage. Case report. *J Neurosurg* 1966;25:447–51.

4988. Perren F, Poglia D, Landis T, Sztajzel R. Vertebral artery hypoplasia. *Neurology* 2007;68:65–7.

4989. Perret G. The epidemiology and clinical course of arteriovenous malformations. In Pia HW, Gleave JRW, Grote E et al. eds. *Cerebral Angiomas: Advances in Diagnosis and Therapy*, pp 21–6. New York: Springer Publishing Co., 1975.

4990. Perry TL, Bratty PJA, Hansen S et al. Hereditary mental depression and Parkinsonism with taurine deficiency. *Arch Neurol* 1975;32:108–13.

4991. Perry TL, Hansen S, Tischler B et al. Carnosinemia: A new metabolic disorder associated with neurologic disease and mental defect. *N Engl J Med* 1967;277:1219–27.

4992. Pestronk A. *Neuromuscular Home Page.* Washington University, St. Louis, 2008. (Electronic Citation)
4993. Pestronk A et al. Polyneuropathy syndromes associated with serum antibodies to sulfatide and myelin associated glycoprotein. *Neurology* 1991;41:357–62.
4994. Pestronk A, Kos K, Lopate G et al. Brachio-cervical inflammatory myopathies: Clinical, immune, and myopathologic features. *Arthritis Rheum* 2006;54:1687–96.
4995. Pestronk A, Lopate G, Kornberg AJ et al. Distal lower motor neuron syndrome with high-titer serum IgM anti GM1 antibodies. *Neurology* 1994;44:2027–31.
4996. Petajan JH. Antigravity posture for analysis of motor unit recruitment: The 45 degree test. *Muscle Nerve* 1990;13:355–9.
4997. Petajan JH, Danforth RC, D'Allesio D et al. Progressive sudomotor denervation and Adie's syndrome. *Neurology* 1965;15:172.
4998. Petajan JH, Momberger GL, Aase J et al. Arthrogryposis syndrome (Kuskokwim disease) in the Eskimo. *JAMA* 1969;209:1481.
4999. Peters JP, Welt LG, Sims EA et al. A salt wasting syndrome associated with cerebral disease. *Trans Am Acad Physicians* 1950;53:57–64.
5000. Petersen RC, Smith GE et al. Apolipoprotein E status as a predictor of the development of Alzheimer's disease in memory-impaired individuals. *JAMA* 1995;273:1274–8.
5001. Petersen RB, Tabaton M, Berg L et al. Analysis of the prion protein gene in thalamic dementia. *Neurology* 1992;42:1859–63.
5002. Petersen RB, Tabaton M, Chen SG et al. Familial progressive subcortical gliosis. *Neurology* 1995;45:1062–7.
5003. Peterson LR, Peterson MJ. Short-term retention of individual verbal items. *J Exp Psychol* 1959;58:193–8.
5004. Petito CK, Navia BA, Cho BD et al. Vacuolar myelopathy pathologically resembling subacute combined degeneration in patients with the acquired immunodeficiency syndrome. *N Engl J Med* 1985;312:874–9.
5005. Peto V, Jenkinson V, Fitzpatrick R et al. The development and validation of a short measure of functioning and well-being for individuals with Parkinson's disease. *Qual Life Res* 1995;4:241–8.
5006. Pettigrew LC, Jankovic J. Hemidystonia: A report of 22 patients and a review of the literature. *J Neurol Neurosurg Psychiatry* 1985;48:650–7.
5007. Petty RKH, Harding AE, Morgan-Hughes JA. The clinical features of mitochondrial myopathy. *Brain* 1986;109:915–38.
5008. Petzold A, Thom M, Powell M et al. Relapsing intracranial Rosai–Dorfman disease. *J Neurol Neurosurg Psychiatry* 2001;71:538–41.
5009. Pfeiffer E. A short portable mental status questionnaire for the assessment of organic brain deficit in elderly patients. *J Am Geriatr Soc* 1975;23:433–41.
5010. Phalen GS, Kendrick JI. Compression of the median nerve in the carpal tunnel. *JAMA* 1957;614:524–30.
5011. Phelps CD et al. The diagnosis and prognosis of atypical carotid-cavernous fistula (red-eyed shunt syndrome). *Am J Ophthalmol* 1982;93:423–36.
5012. Phillips B. Diagnostic criteria for periodic limb movement disorder. *Neurology* 2004;62:S9–S16.
5013. Phillips CI, Griffiths DL. Macular coloboma and skeletal abnormality. *Br J Ophth* 1969;53:346–9.
5014. Phillips CJ, Smith B, Broadhurst A. The draw-a-man test: A study in scoring methods, validity and norms with English children at 5 and 11 years. *Clinics in Developmental Medicine*, 1973.
5015. Phillips DG. The shoulder girdle disc. *J Neurol Neurosurg Psychiatry* 1976;39: 817–20.
5016. Phillips JA, McLean WT, Huntley CC. Co-existing Guillain–Barré and visceral larva migrans syndromes. *Pediatrics* 1969;44:142–3.
5017. Phillips LHI. Familial long thoracic nerve palsy: A manifestation of brachial plexus neuropathy. *Neurology* 1986;36:1251–3.
5018. Piccolo F, Roberds SL, Jeanpierre M et al. Primary adhalinopathy. A common cause of autosomal recessive muscular dystrophy of variable severity. *Nat Genet* 1995;10:243–5.
5019. Pick A. Clinical studies III. On reduplicative paramnesia. *Brain* 1903;26:260–7.
5020. Pick L. *Gaucher's Disease.* Berlin: Springer, 1926.
5021. Pickett JB, Schmidley JW. Sputtering positive potentials in the EMG. *Neurology* 1980;30:215–8.
5022. Pierrot-Deseilligny C, Milea C. Vertical nystagmus: Clinical facts and hypotheses. *Brain* 2005;128:1237–46.
5023. Pietrantoni L. Neuralgic and anesthetic zones in the face and mouth as early signs of malignancies of the paranasal cavities. *Arch Ital Otol* 1948;59: 105–28.
5024. Pietz J. Neurological aspects of adult phenylketonuria. *Curr Opin Neurol* 1998;11:679–88.
5025. Pignata C, Farina V, Andria G et al. Prolonged Q-T interval syndrome presenting as idiopathic epilepsy. *Neuropediatrics* 1983;14:235–6.
5026. Pihko H, Lehtinen I, Tikkanen H et al. Progressive unilateral hypertrophic myopathy: A case study. *Muscle Nerve* 1993;16:63–8.
5027. Pilley SF, Thompson HS. Pupillary dilatation lag in Horner's syndrome. *Br J Ophthalmol* 1975;59:731–5.
5028. Pillon B, Signoret JL, Lhermitte F. Associative visual agnosia: Role of the left hemisphere in visual perception. *Rev Neurol* 1981;137:831.
5029. Piltz J. Concerning a pupillary reflex. *Neurol Zbl* 1899;18:14–7.
5030. Pinard J-M, Motte J, Chiron C et al. Subcortical laminar heterotopia and lissencephaly in two families: A single X-linked dominant gene. *J Neurol Neurosurg Psychiatry* 1994;57:914–20.
5031. Pinckers A. Patterned dystrophies of the retinal pigment epithelium. *Ophthal Paed Gen* 1988;9:77–114.
5032. Pinckers AJL. Leber's congenital amaurosis as conceived by Leber. *Ophthalmologia* 1979;179:48–51.
5033. Pincus JH, Chutorian AM. Familial benign chorea with intention tremor: A clinical entity. *J Pediatr* 1967;70:724.
5034. Pineda M et al. Family agenesis of the corpus callosum with hypothermia and apnoeic spells. *Neuropediatrics* 1984;15:63–7.
5035. Pinel P. *Traité medico-philosophique sur l'alienation mentale ou la manie.* Paris: Richard, Caille, & Ravier, 1801.
5036. Pinsky L, Finlayson MH, Libman I et al. Familial amyotrophic lateral sclerosis with dementia. *Clin Genet* 1975;7:186–91.
5037. Pirini MG, Mascalchi M, Salvi F et al. Primary diffuse meningeal melanomatosis: Radiologic-pathologic correlation. *Am J Neuroradiol* 2003;24:115–8.
5038. Pitt DB, Rogers JG, Danks DM. Mental retardation, unusual face and intrauterine growth retardation. A new recessive syndrome? *Am J Med Genet* 1984;19: 307–13.
5039. Pitt M, Houlden H, Jacobs J et al. Severe infantile neuropathy with diaphragmatic weakness and its relationship to SMARD1. *Brain* 2003;126:2682–92.
5040. Pitt P, Hamilton EBD. Myositis ossificans progressiva. *J Roy Soc Med* 1984;77:68–70.
5041. Pittock SJ, Rabinstein AA, Edwards BS, Wijdicks EF. OKT3 neurotoxicity presenting as akinetic mutism. *Transplantation* 2003;75:1058–60.
5042. Pittock SJ, Joyce C, O'Keane V et al. Rapid-onset dystonia-parkinsonism. *Neurology* 2000;55:991–5.
5043. Pittock SJ, Lucchinetti CF, Arisi JE et al. Amphiphysin autoimmunity:

Paraneoplastic accompaniments. *Ann Neurol* 2005;58:96–107.

5044. Plant GT. The fortification spectra of migraine. *BMJ* 1986;293:1613–6.

5045. Planté-Bordeneuve V. The diagnosis and management of familial amyloid polyneuropathy. *Rev Neurol (Paris)* 2006;162:1138–46.

5046. Plaster NM, Uyama E, Uchino M et al. Genetic localization of the familial adult myoclonic epilepsy (FAME) gene to chromosome 8q24. *Neurology* 1999;53:1180–3.

5047. Platt BS, Burgess RC. Beriberi. *Fed Proc* 1958;17:3–56.

5048. Pleet AB, Massey EW. Notalgia paresthetica. *Neurology* 1978;28:1310–1.

5049. Pleet AB, Massey EW. Palmaris brevis sign in neuropathy of the deep palmar branch of the ulnar nerve. *Ann Neurol* 1978;3:469.

5050. Plum F. Mechanisms of "central" hyperventilation. *Ann Neurol* 1982;11:636–7.

5051. Plum F. Other disorders of consciousness. *Curr Opin Neurol Neurosurg* 1989;2:236–9.

5052. Plum F, Brown HW, Snoep E. Neurologic significance of posthyperventilation apnea. *JAMA* 1962;181:1050–5.

5053. Plum F, Posner JB. *The Diagnosis of Stupor and Coma.* Philadelphia: Davis, 1987.

5054. Plum F, Van Uitert R. Nonendocrine diseases and disorders of the hypothalamus. In Reichlin S, Baldessarini RJ, Martin JB eds. *The Hypothalamus*, pp 415–73. New York: Raven, 1978.

5055. Plutchik R, Conte H, Lieberman M et al. Reliability and validity of a scale for assessing the functioning of geriatric patients. *J Am Geriatr Soc* 1971;19:614–23.

5056. Poch GF, Sica EP, Taratuto A et al. Hypertrophia musculorum vera. Study of a family. *J Neurol Sci* 1971;12:53–61.

5057. Podoll K, Robinson D. Illusory splitting as visual aura symptom in migraine. *Cephalalgia* 2000;20:228–32.

5058. Podreka I, Suess E, Goldenberg G et al. Initial experience with technetium-99m HM-PAO and SPECT. *J Nucl Med* 1987;28:1657–66.

5059. Poeck K, Orgass B. The concept of the body schema. A critical review with some experimental results. *Cortex* 1971;7:254–77.

5060. Poels PJE, Wevers RA et al. Exertional rhabdomyolysis in a patient with calcium adenosine triphosphatase deficiency. *J Neurol Neurosurg Psychiatry* 1993;56:823–6.

5061. Poewe W, Willeit H, Surgon E. The rigid spine syndrome. *J Neurol Neurosurg Psychiatry* 1985;48:887–9.

5062. Pohowalla JN, Kaul KK, Bhandari NR, Singh SD. Infantile "meningoencephalitic syndrome". *Indian J Pediatr* 1960;27:49.

5063. Poland A. Deficiency of the pectoral muscles. *Guy's Hosp Rep* 1841;6:191–3.

5064. Polinsky J. Sympathotonic orthostatic hypotension. *Neurology* 1981;31:1–7.

5065. Poll-The B, Aicardi J, Girot R et al. Neurological findings in triosephosphate isomerase deficiency. *Ann Neurol* 1985;17:439–43.

5066. Pollack L, Klein C, Rabey J-M. The distance shortening phenomenon or the lazy arm sign as a subtle pyramidal sign. *Arch Neurol* 1997;54:935.

5067. Pollard WE, Bobbitt RA, Bergner M. The sickness impact profile: Reliability of a health status measure. *Med Care* 1976;14:146–55.

5068. Pollen RH. Cat-scratch encephalitis. *Neurology* 1968;18:1031–3.

5069. Pollitt RJ, Jenna FA, Mersky H. Aspartylglycosaminuria: An inborn error of metabolism associated with mental defect. *Lancet* 1968;2:253.

5070. Pollock M, Kies B. Benign hereditary cerebellar ataxia and extensive thermoanalgesia. *Brain* 1990;113:857–65.

5071. See 5070.

5072. Pollock M, Nukada H, Frith RW et al. Peripheral neuropathy in Tangier disease. *Brain* 1983;106:911–28.

5073. Polman CH, Reingold SC, Edan G et al. Diagnostic criteria for multiple sclerosis: 2005 revisions to the "McDonald criteria". *Ann Neurol* 2005;58:846.

5074. Polo A, Manganotti P, Zanette G et al. Polyneuritis cranialis: Clinical and electrophysiological findings. *J Neurol Neurosurg Psychiatry* 1992;55:398–400.

5075. Pomeranz HD, Lessell S. Palinopsia and palinopia in the absence of drugs or cerebral disease. *Neurology* 2000;54:855–9.

5076. Pompe JC. Over idiopatische hypertophie van het hart. *Ned Tschr Geneesk* 1932;76:304–5.

5077. Poppe M, Gree L, Bourke J et al. The phenotype of limb-girdle muscular dystrophy type 2I. *Neurology* 2003;60:1246–51.

5078. Poppelreuter W. *Die psychischen Schadigungen durch Kopfschuss im Kriege* 1914–16. Leipzig: Verlag von Leopold Voss, 1917.

5079. Poppi M, Giuliani G, Gambari PI et al. A hazard of craniotomy in the sitting position: The posterior compartment syndrome of the thigh. *J Neurosurg* 1989;71:618–9.

5080. Porch BE. *Porch Index of Communicative Ability.* Palo Alto: Consulting Psychologists Press, 1967.

5081. Porot A. Hemorragie limitée du pedoncle cerebelleux superieur droit: Hemisyndrome cerebelleux direct. *Lyon Med* 1906;106:1137–41.

5082. Portenoy RK. Mechanisms of clinical pain. In Portenoy RK ed. *Neurologic Clinics*, vol.7. *Pain: Mechanisms and Syndromes*, p 205. Philadelphia: W.B. Saunders, 1989.

5083. Portenoy RK, Duma C, Foley KM. Acute herpetic and postherpetic neuralgia: Clinical review and current management. *Ann Neurol* 1986;20:651–64.

5084. Porter L, Wartenberg R. The man. *J Nerv Ment Dis* 1952;116:469–74.

5085. Porter WB. Diaphragmatic flutter with symptoms of angina pectoris. *JAMA* 1936;106:992–4.

5086. Porteus SD. *Porteus Maze Test*. Palo Alto: Pacific Books, 1933.

5087. Portmann M, Aran JM. Electrocochleography. *Laryngoscope* 1971;81:899.

5088. Posas HN JR, Rivner MH. Deep peroneal sensory neuropathy. *Muscle Nerve* 1992;**June**:745.

5089. Poser CM. Myelinoclastic and diffuse sclerosis. In Vincken PJ, Bruyn GW eds. *Handbook of Clinical Neurology*, p 469. Amsterdam: North Holland, 1970.

5090. Poser CM. Diseases of the myelin sheath. In Baker AB, Baker LH eds. *Clin Neurol*, pp 80–104. Hagerstown, MD.: Harper & Row, 1978.

5091. Poser CM. Dysmyelination revisited. *Arch Neurol* 1978;35:401–8.

5092. Poser CM. Criteria for the diagnosis of the Guillain–Barré syndrome: A critique. *J Neurol Sci* 1981;52:191–9.

5093. Poser CM. Notes on the pathogenesis of subacute sclerosing panencephalitis. *J Neurol Sci* 1990;95:219–24.

5094. Poser CM, Paty DW, Scheinberg L et al. New diagnostic criteria for multiple sclerosis: Guidelines for research protocols. *Ann Neurol* 1983;13:227–31.

5095. Poser CM, Paty DW, Scheinberg L et al. *The Diagnosis of Multiple Sclerosis*. New York: Thieme-Stratton, 1984.

5096. Poser CM, van Bogaert L. Natural history and evolution of the concept of Schilder's diffuse sclerosis. *Acta Psychiatr Neurol* 1956;31:285–331.

5097. Poskanzer DC, Kerr DNS. A third type of periodic paralysis with normokalemia and a favourable response to sodium chloride. *Amer J Med* 1961;31:328–42.

5098. Posner JB. Paraneoplastic cerebellar degeneration. *Can J Neurol Sci* 1993;20:S117–S122.

5099. Pott P. *Remarks on that kind of palsy of the lower limbs which is frequently found to accompany a curvature of the spine and is supposed to be caused by it, together with its method of cure*. London: Johnson, 1779.

5100. Potzl O. Word- and color-blindness. *Zbl Neur* 1919;52:241.

5101. Potzl O, Sittig O. Klinische Befunde mit Hertwig-Magendiescher Augeneinstellung. *Z Ges Neurol Psychiat* 1925;95:701.
5102. Pouget J, Philip N, Faugere G et al. Andersen syndrome: A particular form of paralysis with cardiac dysrhythmia. *Rev Neurol* 2004;160:S38–S42.
5103. Power H, Sedgwick LW. *Lexicon of Medicine and the Allied Sciences.* London: The New Sydenham Society, 1882.
5104. Poza JJ, Saenz A, Martinez-Gil A et al. Autosomal dominant lateral temporal lobe epilepsy: Clinical and genetic study of a large Basque pedigree linked to chromosome 10q. *Ann Neurol* 1999;45:182–8.
5105. Pradat P-F, Bruneteau G, de Aguilar JL et al. Muscle Nogo-A expression is a prognostic marker in lower motor neuron syndromes. *Ann Neurol* 2007;62:15–20.
5106. Pradhan S. Calf-head sign in Miyoshi myopathy. *Arch Neurol* 2006;63:1414–7.
5107. Pranzatelli MR, Huang Y, Tate E et al. Cerebrospinal fluid 5-hydroxyindoleacetic acid and homovanillic acid in the pediatric opsoclonus-myoclonus syndrome. *Ann Neurol* 1995;37:189–97.
5108. Prasad AN, Kaye EM, Alroy J. Electron microscopic examination of skin biopsy as a cost effective tool in the diagnosis of lysosomal storage diseases. *J Child Neurol* 1996;11:301–8.
5109. Prasad AN, Prasad C, Stafstrom C. Recent advances in the genetics of epilepsy: Insights from human and animal studies. *Epilepsia* 1999;40:1329–52.
5110. Pratt RK, Fairbank JC, Virr A. The reliability of the shuttle walking test, the Swiss spinal stenosis Questionnaire, the Oxford spinal stenosis score, and the Oswestry disability index in the assessment of patients with lumbar spinal stenosis. *Spine* 2002;27:84–91.
5111. Prechtl HF, Stemmer CJ. The choreiform syndrome in children. *Dev Med Child Neurol* 1962;4:119.
5112. Prendes JL, Rosenberg SJ. Rip van Winkle syndrome: Confusion and irresistible somnolence after stroke. *South Med J* 1986;179:1162–4.
5113. Preobrashenski PA. Syphilitic paraplegia with dissociated disturbance of sensation. *Zh Nevropatol Psikiatr* 1904;4:388.
5114. Preston DC, Kelly JJ. "Pseudospasticity" in Guillain–Barré syndrome. *Neurology* 1991;41:131–4.
5115. Preston NW. Toxicity of pertussis vaccine. *BMJ* 1982;284:1817–8.
5116. Prévost J-L. *On Conjugate Deviation of the Eyes and Rotation of the Head in Some Cases of Hemiplegia*. Paris: Thèse de Paris, 1868.
5117. Price BH, Mesulam M-M. Behavioral manifestations of central pontine myelinolysis. *Arch Neurol* 1987;44:671–3.
5118. Price CC, Jefferson AL, Merino JG et al. Subcortical vascular dementia. *Neurology* 2005;65:376–82.
5119. Price RW, Brew BJ. The AIDS-dementia complex. *J Infect Dis* 1988;158:1079–83.
5120. Price TR, Netsky MG. Myxedema and ataxia. *Neurology* 1966;16:957–62.
5121. Prichard JW, Brass LM. New anatomical and functional imaging methods. *Ann Neurol* 1992;32:395–400.
5122. Prineas JW, Hall R, Barwick DD et al. Myopathy associated with pigmentation following adrenalectomy for Cushing disease. *Quart J Med* 1968;37:63–77.
5123. Pringle CE, Belden J, Veitch JE et al. Multifocal motor neuropathy presenting as ophthalmoplegia. *Muscle Nerve* 1997;20:347–51.
5124. Pringle CE, Hudson AJ, Munoz KC et al. Primary lateral sclerosis. *Brain* 1992;115:495–520.
5125. Pritchard C, Flynn JT, Smith JL. Waveform characteristics of vertical oscillations in long standing visual loss. *J Pediatr Ophthalmol Strabismus* 1988;25:233–6.
5126. Probst A et al. Sensory ganglioneuropathy in infantile muscular atrophy. *Neuropediatrics* 1981;12:215–31.
5127. Prusiner S. Prions and neurodegenerative diseases. *N Engl J Med* 1987;317: 1571–80.
5128. Prusiner S. Prion diseases of humans and animals. *J Roy Coll Physicians* 1993;28: 1–30.
5129. Prusiner SB. Neurodegenerative disease and prions. *N Engl J Med* 2001;344: 1516–25.
5130. Prynn WL, Kates DE, Pollack CV. Gluteal compartment syndrome. *Ann Emerg Med* 1994;24:1180–3.
5131. Pryse-Phillips WEM. Bowlers cramp. *Med J Aust* 1967;1:61–2.
5132. Pryse-Phillips WEM. An olfactory reference syndrome. *Acta Psychiatr Scand* 1971;47:484–509.
5133. Pryse-Phillips WEM. Validation of a diagnostic sign in carpal tunnel syndrome. *J Neurol Neurosurg Psychiatry* 1984;47:870–2.
5134. Pryse-Phillips WEM, Johnson GJ, Larsen B. Incomplete manifestations of myotonic dystrophy in a large kinship in Labrador. *Ann Neurol* 1982;8:582–91.
5135. Przelomski MM, O'Rourke E, Grady GF et al. Eastern equine encephalitis in Massachusetts. *Neurology* 1988;38: 736–9.
5136. Psychopharmacology Research Branch N. ECDEU Assessment Manual for Psychopharmacology. Revised DEW Publication No. ADM 76–338. Rockville, MD: DHEW, 1976.
5137. Ptácek LJ, Fu Y-H. Channels and disease. *Arch Neurol* 2004;61:1665–8.
5138. Ptacek LJ, Johnson KJ, Griggs RC. Genetics and physiology of the myotonia muscle disorders. *N Engl J Med* 1993;328:482–9.
5139. Puce A, Kalnins RM, Berkovic S et al. Limbic P3 potentials, seizure localization and surgical pathology in temporal lobe epilepsy. *Ann Neurol* 1989;26:377–85.
5140. Pullicino PM, Jacobs L. Palpebromandibular synkinesia. *Ann Neurol* 1991;30:318. (Abstract)
5141. Pullicino PM, Jacobs L, McCall WD et al. Spontaneous palpebromandibular synkinesia: A localizing clinical sign. *Ann Neurol* 1994;35:222–8.
5142. Purdy A, Hahn AF, Barnett HJM et al. Familial fatal parkinsonism with alveolar hypoventilation and mental depression. *Ann Neurol* 1979;6:523–31.
5143. Purves-Stewart JPM. Paralysis agitans, with an account of a new symptom. *Lancet* 1898;2:1258–60.
5144. Putnam JJ. A series of cases of paraesthesia, mainly of the hands, of periodical recurrence, and possibly of vaso-motor origin. *Arch Med (New York)* 1880;4:147–62.
5145. Putnam JJ. A group of cases of system sclerosis of the spinal cord, associated with diffuse collateral degeneration: Occurring in enfeebled persons past middle life, and especially in women; studied with particular reference to etiology. *J Nerv Ment Dis* 1891;16:69.
5146. Putnam T. The progressive confusional syndrome following injuries to cervical portion of the spinal cord. *Science* 1937;86:542–3.
5147. Pyeritz RE, Conant J. *The Marfan Syndrome.* 1. 1984. New York, National Marfan Foundation. (Pamphlet)
5148. Pyeritz RE, McKusick VA. The Marfan syndrome: Diagnosis and management. *N Engl J Med* 1979;300:772–7.
5149. Pyle E. Case of unusual bone development. *J Bone Joint Surg* 1931;13:874–80.
5150. Quality Standards Committee of the American Academy of Neurology. The management of concussions in sports. *Neurology* 1997;48:581–5.
5151. Quarles RH, Weiss MD. Autoantibodies associated with peripheral neuropathy. *Muscle Nerve* 1999;22:800–22.
5152. Quay HC, Peterson DR. *Interim Manual for the Revised Behavior Problem Checklist*. Coral Gables: University Miami, 1983.
5153. Queckenstedt H. Diagnosis of compression of the spinal cord. *Dtsch Z Nervenklinik* 1916;55:325–33.

5154. Queckenstedt H. Changes in spinal fluid in peripheral neuritis. *Dtsch Z Nervenklinik* 1917;57:316–29.

5155. Quincke H. Die lumbarpunction des hydrocephalus. *Klin Wschnschr* 1981;28:929–33.

5156. Quinn J, Stiel I, McDermott D et al. Derivation of the San Francisco syncope rule to predict patients with short-term serious outcomes. *Ann Emerg Med* 2004;43:224–32.

5157. Quinn NP. Multiple system atrophy – the nature of the beast. *J Neurol Neurosurg Psychiatry* 1989;(**Suppl.**):78–89.

5158. Quinn NP. Classification of fluctuations in patients with Parkinson's disease. *Neurology* 1998;51(**Suppl.** 2):S25–S29.

5159. Quinn NP, Rothwell JC, Thompson PD, Marsden CD. Hereditary myoclonic dystonia. In Fahn S et al. eds. *Advances in Neurology*, pp 391–6. New York: Raven Press, 1988.

5160. Quinn NP, Wenning G, Marsden CD. The Shy–Drager syndrome. *Arch Neurol* 1995;52.:656–7.

5161. Qureshi AI, Choudhry MA, Akbar MS et al. Plasma exchange versus intravenous immunoglobulin treatment in myasthenic crisis. *Neurology* 1999;52:629–32.

5162. Qureshi HI, Tuhrim S, Broderick JP et al. Spontaneous intracerebral hemorrhage. *N Engl J Med* 2001;344:1450–60.

5163. Rabin BA, Griffin JW, Crain BJ et al. *Autosomal Dominant Juvenile Amyotrophic Lateral Sclerosis. 122* 1999;8:1550.

5164. Rademaker GGJ. On the lengthening and shortening reactions and their occurrence in man. *Brain* 1947;70: 109–26.

5165. Radloff LS. The CES-D scale. *Appl Psychol Meas* 1977;1:385–401.

5166. Raeder JG. Paratrigeminal paralysis of oculo-pupillary sympathetic. *Brain* 1924;47:149–58.

5167. Rafya MF, Halliday W, Bril V. Hyaline body myopathy: Adulthood manifestations. *Can J Neurol Sci* 2005;32:253–6.

5168. Ragge NK, Hoyt WF. Midbrain myasthenia: Fatigable ptosis, 'lid twitch' sign, and ophthalmoparesis from a dorsal midbrain glioma. *Neurology* 1992;42:917–9.

5169. Rail D, Scholtz C, Swash M. Post-encephalitic Parkinsonism: Current experience. *J Neurol Neurosurg Psychiatry* 1981;44:670–6.

5170. Raimondi AJ, Hirschauer J. Head injury in the infant and toddler: Coma scoring and outcome scale. *Child's Brain* 1984;11:12–35.

5171. Raitta C, Perheentupa J. Congenital ophthalmoplegia plus. *Neuroophthalmology* 1985;5:27–31.

5172. Ramachandran VS, Altschuler EL, Hillyer S. Mirror agnosia. *Proc Roy Soc London* 1997;264:645–7.

5173. Ramat S, Zee DS, Minor L et al. Translational vestibulo-ocular reflex evoked by a "head heave" stimulus. *Ann NY Acad Sci* 2001;942:95–113.

5174. Ramazzini M. Diseases of scribes and notaries. *Privately Printed* 1713.

5175. Ramirez F, Arana IR. The hypothalamic crossroads syndrome. *An Fac Med Montev* 1952;37:109.

5176. Ramon Y Cajal S. *Manual de anatomia patologica general.* Madrid: N. Moya, 1909.

5177. Ramon Y Cajal S. *Recollections of My Life.* London: MIT Press, 1989.

5178. Ramos Arroyo MA, Weaver DD, Beals RK. Congenital contractural arachnodactyly. *Clin Genet* 1985;27:570–81.

5179. Rana PVS, Wadia RS. The Marin-Amat syndrome: An unusual facial synkinesia. *J Neurol Neurosurg Psychiatry* 1985;48:939–41.

5180. Ranalli PJ, Sharpe JA. Contrapulsion of saccades and ipsilateral ataxia: A unilateral disorder of the rostral cerebellum. *Ann Neurol* 1986;20:311.

5181. Ranalli PJ, Sharpe JA. Upbeat nystagmus and the ventral tegmental pathway of the upward vestibulo-ocular reflex. *Neurology* 1988;38:1329–30.

5182. Rand RW, Crowdall PH. Central spinal cord syndrome in hyperextension injuries of the cervical spine. *J Bone Joint Surg* 1962;44:1415.

5183. Rando TA, Fishman RA. Spontaneous intracranial hypotension: Report of two cases and review of the literature. *Neurology* 1992;42:481–7.

5184. Rando TA, Horton JC, Layzer RB. Wolfram syndrome. *Neurology* 1992;42:1220–4.

5185. Rangel-Guerra R, Martinez HR, Saenz C. Mucormycosis: Report of 11 cases. *Arch Neurol* 1985;42:578–81.

5186. Rankin J. Cerebrovascular accidents in patients over the age of 60: II. Prognosis. *Scot Med J* 1957;2:200–15.

5187. Rankine JJ. Adult traumatic brachial plexus injury. *Clin Radiol* 2004;59:767–74.

5188. Rantamaki M, Krahe R, Paetau A et al. Adult-onset autosmal recessive ataxia with thalamic lesions in a Finnish family. *Neurology* 2001;57:1043–9.

5189. Rao KC, Kanipp HC, Waggoner EJ. CT findings in cerebral sinus and venous thrombosis. *Radiology* 1981;140: 391–75.

5190. Rao SM, Devinsky O, Grafman J et al. Viscosity and social cohesion in temporal lobe epilepsy. *J Neurol Neurosurg Psychiatry* 1992;55:149–52.

5191. Rao SM, Leo GJ, Bernardin L et al. Cognitive dysfunction in multiple sclerosis 1. Frequency, patterns and prediction. *Neurology* 1991;41:685–91.

5192. Rapcsak SZ, Polster MR, Glisky ML et al. False recognition of unfamiliar faces following right hemisphere damage: Neuropsychological and anatomical observations. *Cortex* 1996;32:593–611.

5193. Rapin I, Goldfischer S, Katzman R et al. The cherry-red spot – myoclonus syndrome. *Ann Neurol* 1978;3:234–42.

5194. Rapin I, Susuki K, Valsamis MP. Adult (chronic) Gm2-gangliosidosis – atypical spinocerebellar degeneration in a Jewish sibship. *Arch Neurol* 1976;33:120–30.

5195. Rapoport AM. Analgesic rebound headache. *Headache* 1988;28:662–5.

5196. Rappaport M, Hall KM, Hopkins K et al. Disability rating scale for severe head trauma: Coma to community. *Arch Phys Med Rehab* 1982;63:118–23.

5197. Rapscak S, Cimino CR, Heilman KM. Altitudinal neglect. *Neurology* 1988;38:277–81.

5198. Rasdolsky I. Dorsal-Pontins Tumorsyndrom. *Zschr Gesamte Neurol Psychiatr* 1935;152:530–7.

5199. Rask MR. Superior gluteal nerve entrapment syndrome. *Muscle Nerve* 1980;3:304–7.

5200. Raskin A. *Validation of a Battery of Tests to Assess Psychopathology in the Elderly.* London: John Levi, 1985.

5201. Raskin A, Crook TH. Mood scales – elderly. *Psychopharm Bull* 1988;24: 727–32.

5202. Raskin NH. Hypnic headache. *Headache* 1988;28:534–6.

5203. Raskin NH. The cough headache syndrome: Treatment. *Neurology* 1995;45:1784.

5204. Raskin NH, Schwartz RK. Icepick like-pain. *Neurology* 1980;30:203–5.

5205. Raskind RH. Problems at the reading distance. *Am Orthop J* 1976;26:53.

5206. Rasmussen A, Matsuura T, Ruano L et al. Clinical and genetic analysis of four Mexican families with spinocerebellar ataxia type 10. *Ann Neurol* 2001;50: 234–9.

5207. Rasmussen T, Olszewski J, Lloyd-Smith D. Focal seizures due to chronic localised encephalitis. *Neurology* 1958;8:435–45.

5208. Rauschka H, Retzl J, Baumhackl U et al. Subacute brainstem angioencephalopathy: A case report and review of the literature. *J Neurol Sci* 2003;208:101–4.

5209. Raven JC. *Guide to Using the Standard Progressive Matrices.* New York: The Psychological Corporation, 1956.

5210. See 5209.

5211. Ravits J. Autonomic system testing. *Muscle Nerve* 1997;20:919–37.

5212. Ravits J, Hallett M, Baker M et al. Primary writing tremor and myoclonic writer's cramp. *Neurology* 1985;35: 1387–91.
5213. Raychaudhuri R, Batjer HH, Awad IA. Intracranial cavernous angioma: A practical review of clinical and biological aspects. *Surg Neurol* 2005;63:319–28.
5214. Raymond AA, Fish DR, Stevens JM et al. Subependymal heterotopia: A distinct neuronal migration disorder associated with epilepsy. *J Neurol Neurosurg Psychiatry* 1994;57:1195–202.
5215. Raymond F, Cestan R. Trois observations de paralysie des mouvements associès des globes oculaires. *Rev Neurol* 1901;9:70–7.
5216. Raymond GV. Peroxisomal disorders. *Curr Opin Neurol* 2001;14:783–7.
5217. Raynaud M. *De l'asphyxie locale et de la gangrène symmetrique des extremities.* Paris: Rignoux, 1862.
5218. RCP working group. The permanent vegetative state. *J Roy Coll Physicians* 1996;30:119–21.
5219. Reagan TJ, Thomas JE, Colby MYj. Chronic progressive radiation myelopathy. *JAMA* 1968;203:106–10.
5220. Rebeiz JJ, Kolodny EH, Richardson EPj. Corticodentatonigral degeneration with neuronal achromasia. *Arch Neurol* 1968;18:20–33.
5221. Rebollo M, Val JF, Garijo F et al. Livedo reticularis and cerebrovascular lesions (Sneddon's Syndrome). *Brain* 1983;106:965–79.
5222. Rebouche J, Engel AG. Systemic carnitine deficiency. *Neurology* 1981;31:813–8.
5223. Rechtschaffen A, Kales A. *A Manual of Standardized Terminology, Techniques and Scoring for Sleep Stages of Human Subjects.* Washington, DC: Dept. Health, Education and Welfare, 1968.
5224. Recklinghausen FD. *Uber die multiplen Fibrome der Haut und ihre Beziehungen zu den Neuromen*. Berlin: Festschr. R. Viirchow, 1882.
5225. Reddy AN. The stethoscope neuropathy. *Ann Int Med* 1987;106:913. (Letter ed.)
5226. Redekop GJ, Del Maestro RF. Diagnosis and management of spinal epidural abscess. *Can J Neurol Sci* 1992;19:180–7.
5227. Reding MJ, Orto L, Willensky P et al. The dexamethasone suppression test: An indicator of depression in stroke but not a predictor of rehabilitation outcome. *Arch Neurol* 1985;42:209–12.
5228. Redlich FC, Dorsey JF. Denial of blindness by patients with cerebral disease. *Arch Neurol Psychiatry* 1945;53:407.
5229. Reed DM, Kurland LT. Muscle fasciculations in a healthy population. *Arch Neurol* 1963;9:363–7.
5230. Reed LA, Grabowski TJSML et al. Autosomal dominant dementia with widespread neurofibrillary tangles. *Ann Neurol* 1997;42:564–72.
5231. Reed WB, Stone VM, Boder E et al. Hereditary syndrome with auditory and dermatological manifestations. *Arch Derm* 1967;95:456–61.
5232. Rees JH. Paraneoplastic syndromes. *J Neurol Neurosurg Psychiatr* 2007;75:ii. 43–ii.50.
5233. Rees JR et al. Lentiginosis and left atrial myxoma. *Br Heart J* 1973;35:874–6.
5234. Refetoff S, DeWind LT, DeGroot LJ. Familial syndrome combining deaf-mutism, stipple deficiencies, goitre and abnormally high PBI: Possible target organ refractory to thyroid hormone. *J Clin Endocrinology* 1967;27:279.
5235. Refsum S. Heredoataxia hemeralopica polyneuritiformis et tidligere ikke beskrevet familiaert syndrome? En forelobig moddelelse. *Nord Med* 1945;28:2682–5.
5236. Regard M, Landis T. Gourmand syndrome. *Neurology* 1997;48:1185–90.
5237. Regueiro AM, Segurado OG, Mata P et al. Acquired selective signature dysgraphia. *Ann Neurol* 1992;31:115.
5238. Reich SG. Psychogenic movement disorders. *Semin Neurol* 2006;26:289–96.
5239. Reichert FL. Tympanic plexus neuralgia. True tic douloureux of the ear or so-called geniculate ganglion neuralgia: Cure effected by intracranial section of the glossopharyngeal nerve. *JAMA* 1933;100:1744–6.
5240. Reichmann H, Goebel HH, Schneider C et al. Familial mixed congenital myopathy with rigid spine phenotype. *Muscle Nerve* 1997;20:411–6.
5241. Reid E. The hereditary spastic paraplegias. *J Neurol* 1999;246:995–1003.
5242. Reid RL, Quigley ME, Yen SSC. Pituitary apoplexy: A review. *Arch Neurol* 1985;42:712–9.
5243. Reiher J, Lebel M. Wicket spikes: Clinical correlates of a previously undescribed EEG pattern. *Can J Neurol Sci* 1977;4:39–47.
5244. Reik L, Steere AC, Bartenhagen NH, Shope RE, Malawista SE. Neurologic abnormalities of Lyme disease. *Medicine* 1979;58:281–94.
5245. Reilly M. Sorting out the inherited neuropathies. *Practical Neurol* 2007;7: 93–105.
5246. Reinfeld H, Louis S. Unilateral asterixis. *NY State J Med* 1983;83:206–8.
5247. Reinhold M. A case of auditory agnosia. *Brain* 1950;73:203–23.
5248. Reis DJ. The palmo-mental reflex. A fragment of a general nocioceptive skin reflex: A physiological study in normal man. *Arch Neurol* 1961;4:486–98.
5249. Reis J, Eber A-M, Warter J-M et al. Alternating nystagmus and infectious mononucleosis. *Neuroophthalmology* 1989;9:289–92.
5250. Reisberg B. Functional assessment staging (FAST). *Psychopharm Bull* 1988;24:653.
5251. Reisberg B, Borenstein J, Franssen E et al. BEHAVE-AD: A clinical rating scale for assessment of pharmacologically remediable behavioral symptomatology in Alzheimer's disease. In Altman HJ ed. *Alzheimer's disease: Problems, prospects and perspectives*, p 1. New York: Plenum Press, 1987.
5252. Reisberg B, Ferris SH. The Brief Cognitive Rating Scale (BCRS). *Psychopharm Bull* 1988;24:629.
5253. Reisberg B, Ferris SH, De Leon MJ et al. The global deterioration scale in assessment of primary degenerative dementia. *Am J Psychiatry* 1982;139:1136–9.
5254. Reisberg B, Ferris SH, De Leon MJ et al. The global deterioration scale (GDS). *Psychopharm Bull* 1988;24:661.
5255. Reisberg B, London E, Ferris SH et al. The Brief Cognitive Rating Scale: Language, motoric and mood concomitants in primary degenerative dementia. *Psychopharm Bull* 1983;19:702–8.
5256. Reisecker F, Lebelhuber F, Lexner R et al. A sporadic form of hereditary neuropathy with liability to pressure palsies. *Neurology* 1994;44:753–5.
5257. Reisman LE, Kashara S, Chung C-Y et al. Antimongolism. *Lancet* 1966;1:394.
5258. Reisner SH et al. Cutis laxa associated with severe intrauterine growth retardation and congenital dislocation of the hip. *Acta Pediatr Scand* 1971;60:357.
5259. Reitan RM. Validity of the trail-making test as an indication of organic brain damage. *Percept Mot Skills* 1958;8:271.
5260. Reitan RM, Davison LA. *Clinical Neuropsychology: Current Status and Applications.* Tucson: Neuropsychology Press, 1985.
5261. Reitan RM, Wolfson D. *The Halstead-Reitan Neuropsychological Test Battery: Theory and Clinical Interpretation.* Tucson: Neuropsychology Press, 1985.
5262. Reivich M, Holling HE, Roberts B et al. Reversal of blood flow through the vertebral artery and its effect on cerebral circulation. *N Engl J Med* 1961;265:878–85.
5263. Remak E. Zur Pathogenese der Bleilahmungen. *Arch Psychiatr (Berlin)* 1878;6:1–56.
5264. Remillard GM, Andermann F, Rhi-Sausi A et al. Facial asymmetry in patients with temporal lobe epilepsy. *Neurology* 1977;27:109–14.
5265. Remillard GM, Ethier R, Andermann F. Temporal lobe epilepsy and perinatal

occlusion of the posterior cerebral artery. A syndrome analogous to infantile hemiplegia and a demonstrable etiology in some patients with temporal lobe epilepsy. *Neurology* 1974;24:1001–9.

5266. Renehan AG, Booth C, Potten CS. What is apoptosis and why is it important? *BMJ* 2001;322:1536–8.

5267. Renfrew S, Melville ID. The somatic sense of space (choraesthesia) and its threshold. *Brain* 1960;83:93–112.

5268. Rennert OM, Greer M. Hereditary fructosemia. *Neurology* 1970;20:421–5.

5269. Rensi E, Faglione P, Savoiardo M. The influence of aphasia and of the hemisphere side of the cerebral lesion on abstract thinking. *Cortex* 1966;2:399–420.

5270. Requena I, Arias M, Lopez-Ibor L et al. Cavernomas of the central nervous system: Clinical and neuroimaging manifestations in 47 patients. *J Neurol Neurosurg Psychiatry* 1991;54:590–4.

5271. Requena I, Indakoextea B, Lema C et al. Coma associated with migraine. *Rev Neurol* 1999;29:1048–51.

5272. Reszel PA, Janes JM, Spittell JA. Ischemic necrosis of the peroneal musculature: A lateral compartment syndrome: Report of a case. *Proc Staff Meet Mayo Clin* 1963;38:130–6.

5273. Rett Syndrome Diagnostic Criteria Working Group. Diagnostic criteria for Rett Syndrome. *Ann Neurol* 1988;23:425–8.

5274. Retzlaff JA, Kearns TP, Howard FM et al. Lancaster red-green testing in evaluation of edrophonium effect in myasthenia gravis. *Am J Ophthalmol* 1969;67:13–21.

5275. Reuber M, Pukrop R, Bauer J et al. Outcome in psychogenic nonepileptic seizures:1 to 10-years, follow-up in 164 patients. *Ann Neurol* 2003;53:305–11.

5276. Revilliod JLA. Left hemiplegia in a left-hander from embolism of the brachiocephalic trunk: Orbicularis sign. *Rev Med Suisse Rom* 1889;9:595–606.

5277. Rey A. L'examen psychological en cas d'encephalopathie traumatique. *Arch Psychiol Norm Pathol (Paris)* 1941;28: 286–340.

5278. Rey A. L'examen clinique en psychologie. Paris: Presses Universitaires de France, 1964.

5279. Reye RD, Morgan G, Baral J. Encephalopathy and fatty degeneration of the viscera. *Lancet* 1963;2:749–52.

5280. Reyes MG, Noronha P, Thomas V et al. Myositis of chronic graft-versus-host disease. *Neurology* 1983;33:1222–4.

5281. Reynolds DW, Stagno S, Stubbs G et al. Inapparent congenital cytomegalovirus infection with elevated cord IgM levels: Causal relation with auditory and mental deficiency. *N Engl J Med* 1974;290: 291–6.

5282. Rhys Davies R, Hodges JR, Kril JJ et al. The pathological basis of semantic dementia. *Brain* 2005;128:1984–95.

5283. Richards BW, Rundle AT. A familial hormonal disorder associated with mental deficiency, deaf mutism and ataxia. *J Ment Defic* 1959;3:33–55.

5284. Richardson JK, Forman GM, Riley B. An electrophysiological exploration of the double crush hypothesis. *Muscle Nerve* 1999;22:71–7.

5285. Richieri-Costa A et al. Adult proximal spinal muscular atrophy. *Am J Med Genet* 1981;9:119–23.

5286. Richman DP, Agius MA. Acquired myasthenia gravis: Immunopathology. *Neurol Clin* 1994;12:273–4.

5287. Ricker K, Kock MC, Lehmann-Horn F et al. Proximal myotonic myopathy. *Arch Neurol* 1995;52:25–31.

5288. Ricker K, Lehmann-Horn F, Moxley RT. Myotonia fluctuans. *Arch Neurol* 1990;47:268–72.

5289. Ricker K, Mertens H-G. Okulare neuromyotonie. *Klin Mbl Augenh* 1970;156:837.

5290. Ricker K, Moxley RT, Rohkamm R. Rippling muscle disease. *Arch Neurol* 1989;46:405–8.

5291. Riddoch G. The reflex functions of the completely divided spinal cord in man, compared with those associated with less severe lesions. *Brain* 1917;40: 264–402.

5292. Riddoch G. Visual disorientation in homonymous half-fields. *Brain* 1935;58:376–82.

5293. Riddoch G. Phantom limbs and body shape. *Brain* 1941;64:197–222.

5294. Ridley A, Kennard C, Scholtz CL et al. Omnipause neurons in two cases of opsoclonus associated with oat cell carcinoma of the lung. *Brain* 1987;110:1699.

5295. Rieder H. Die "Steintrager-Lahmung." Eine Form der combinirten Armnerven-oder Brachialplexus-Lahmung. *Munch Med Wschr* 1893;40:121–3.

5296. Riegel W. On alternating mydriasis. *Dtsch Z Nervenklinik* 1900;17:169–70.

5297. Rieger H. Beitrage zur Kenntnis seltener Missbildungen der Iris. *Arch Ophthal Berlin* 1935;133:602.

5298. Riese W. The early history of aphasia. *Bull Med Hist* 1947;21:322–34.

5299. Riese W. The sources of Hughlings Jackson's view on Aphasia. *Brain* 1965;88:811–22.

5300. Riggs JE, Klingberg WG, Flink EB et al. Cardioskeletal mitochondrial myopathy associated with chronic magnesium deficiency. *Neurology* 1992;42:128–30.

5301. Riggs JE, Schochet SS, Fakadi AV et al. Mitochondrial encephalomyopathy with decreased succinate cytochrome reductase activity. *Neurology* 1984;34:48–53.

5302. Riggs JE, Schochet SS, Gutmann L et al. Lysosomal glycogen storage disease with acid maltase deficiency. *Neurology* 1983;33:873–7.

5303. Riley CM, Day RL, Greeley DM et al. Central autonomic dysfunction with defective lacrymation: Report of 5 cases. *Pediatrics* 1949;3:468–78.

5304. Riley CM, Schwachman H. Unusual osseous disease with neurologic changes. *Am J Dis Child* 1990;150–4.

5305. Riley DE, Lang AE. Non-Parkinson akinetic-rigid syndromes. *Curr Opin Neurol* 1996;9:321–6.

5306. Riley HD, Smith WR. Macrocephaly, pseudopapilledema, and multiple hemangiomata. *Pediatrics* 1960;26:293–300.

5307. Rimel RW, Giodani B, Barth JT et al. Disability caused by minor head injury. *Neurosurgery* 1981;9:221–8.

5308. Riminton DS, Chambers ST, Parkin PJ et al. Inclusion body myositis presenting solely as dysphagia. *Neurology* 1993;43:1241–3.

5309. Ringel SP, Bailey OT. Rathke's cleft cyst. *J Neurol Neurosurg Psychiatry* 1972;35:693–7.

5310. Ringel SP, Claman HN. Amyloid-associated muscle pseudohypertrophy. *Arch Neurol* 1982;39:413–7.

5311. Ringel SP, Forstot JZ, Tau EM et al. Sjogren's syndrome with polymyositis or dermatomyositis. *Arch Neurol* 1982;39:157–68.

5312. Ringel SP, Kenny CE, Neville HE et al. Spectrum of inclusion body myositis. *Arch Neurol* 1987;44:1154–7.

5313. Ringel SP, Lava NS, Treihaft MM et al. Late onset X-linked recessive spinal and bulbar muscular atrophy. *Muscle Nerve* 1978;1:297–307.

5314. Ringel SP, Neville HE, Duster MC et al. A new congenital neuromuscular disease with trilaminar muscle fibers. *Neurology* 1978;28:282–9.

5315. Ringertz N. Grading of gliomas. *Acta Path Microbiol Scand* 1950;27:51–64.

5316. Ringrose RE et al. Hemihypertrophy. *Pediatrics* 1965;36:434–48.

5317. Riordan-Eva P, Sanders MD, Govan GG et al. The clinical features of Leber's hereditary optic neuropathy defined by the presence of a pathogenic mitochondrial mutation. *Brain* 1995;118:319–37.

5318. Rippon GA, Scarmeas N, Gordon PH. An observational study of cognitive impairment in amyotrophic lateral sclerosis. *Arch Neurol* 2006;63:345–52.

5319. Ripps H, Noble KG, Greenstein VC et al. Progressive cone dystrophy. *Ophthalmology* 1987;94:1401.

5320. Riser M, Geraud J, Ducoudray J et al. Dolicho-carotide interne avec syndrome vertigineux. *Rev Neurol* 1951;**85**:145–7.
5321. Risk WS, Bosch EP, Kimura J et al. Chronic tetanus: Clinical report and histochemistry of muscle. *Muscle Nerve* 1981;**4**:363–6.
5322. Ritvo PG, Fischer JS, Miller F et al. *Multiple Sclerosis Quality of Life Inventory: A Users Manual*. New York: National Multiple Sclerosis Society, 1997.
5323. Rivers WH, Head H. A human experiment in nerve division. *Brain* 1908;**31**:323–450.
5324. Rizzo M, Hurtig R, Damasio AR. The role of scanpaths in facial recognition and learning. *Ann Neurol* 1987;**22**:41–5.
5325. Roach ES, Gomez MR, Northrup MH. Tuberous sclerosis complex consensus conference: Revised clinical diagnostic criteria. *J Child Neurol* 1998;**13**:624–8.
5326. Roaf R. Lateral flexion injuries of the cervical spine. *J Bone Joint Surg* 1963;**45**:36–8.
5327. Robb JP. A footnote to medical history: David Alexander Shirres on spinal cord regeneration. *Can J Neurol Sci* 1991;**18**:361–2.
5328. Roberts TA, Jenkyn LR, Reeves AG. On the notion of doll's eyes. *Arch Neurol* 1984;**41**:1242–3.
5329. Robertson A. On an interesting series of eye-symptoms in a case of spinal disease, with remarks on the action of Belladonna on the iris, etc. *Edinburgh Medical Journal* 1868;**14**:696–708.
5330. Robertson D, Hollister AS, Biaggioni I et al. The diagnosis and treatment of baroreflex failure. *N Engl J Med* 1993;**329**:1449–55.
5331. Robertson MM, Banerjee S, Kurlan R et al. The Tourette syndrome diagnostic confidence index. *Neurology* 1999;**53**:2108–12.
5332. Robertson WC, Fariello RG. Eating epilepsy associated with a deep forebrain glioma. *Ann Neurol* 1979;**6**:271–3.
5333. Robertson WE, Robertson HF. *Diagnostic Signs, Reflexes and Syndromes*. Philadelphia: F.A. Davis, 1947.
5334. Robin P. La glossoptose: Son diagnostic, ses conséquences, son traitement. *J Med (Paris)* 1923;**43**:235–7.
5335. Robins LN, Helzer JE, Croughan J et al. NIMH diagnostic interview schedule. *Arch Gen Psychiatry* 1981;**38**:381–9.
5336. Robinson B, Johnson R, Abernethy D et al. Familial distal dysautonomia. *J Neurol Neurosurg Psychiatry* 1989;**52**:1281–5.
5337. Robinson D. Pyriformis syndrome in relation to sciatic pain. *Am J Surg* 1947;**73**:355–8.
5338. Robinson DA, Zee DS, Hain TC et al. Alexander's law: Its behavior and origin in the human vestibulo-ocular reflex. *Ann Neurol* 1984;**16**:714–22.
5339. Robinson G, Blair J, Cipolotti L. Dynamic aphasia: An inability to select between competing verbal responses? *Brain* 1998;**121**:77–89.
5340. Robinson GC, Miller JR, Bensimon JR. Familial ectodermal dysplasia with sensorineural deafness and other anomalies. *Pediatrics* 1962;**30**:797.
5341. Robinson LK et al. Carpenter syndrome: Natural history and clinical spectrum. *Am J Med Genet* 1985;**20**:461–9.
5342. Robinson RO, Thornett CEE. Benign hereditary chorea response to steroids. *Dev Med Child Neurol* 1985;**27**:814–6.
5343. Robitaille Y, Carpenter S, Karpati G et al. A distinct form of adult polyglucosan body disease with massive involvement of central and peripheral neuronal processes and astrocytes. A report of four cases and a review of the occurrence of polyglucosan bodies in other conditions such as Lafora's disease and normal ageing. *Brain* 1980;**103**:315–36.
5344. Rochon-Duvigneau A. Some cases of paralysis of all the orbital nerves. *Arch Ophthal Berlin* 1896;**16**:746–60.
5345. Rockwood K, Parhad I, Hachinski V et al. Diagnosis of vascular dementia. *Can J Neurol Sci* 1994;**21**:358–64.
5346. Rode G, Michel C, Rosetti Y et al. Left size distortion (hyperschematia) after right brain damage. *Neurology* 2006;**67**:1801–8.
5347. Rodiet A, Cans F. Differentiation of toxic and general paralytic cerebral diseases. *Ann Med Psychol* 1906;**4**:408–20.
5348. Rodolico C, Toscano A, Autunno M et al. Limb-girdle myasthenia: Clinical, electrophysiological and morphological features in familial and autoimmune cases. *Neuromuscul Disord* 2002;**12**:964–9.
5349. Rodríguez-Gómez FJ, López-Domínguez JM, Borrero-Martín JJ. Cystinosis: An infrequent cause of distal myopathy. *Rev Neurol* 2005;**40**:156–8.
5350. Rodriquez B, Rodriquez BR, Oreggia A. A new type of peduncular syndrome. *Am J Ophthalmol* 1946;**29**:511.
5351. Roelcke U, Hornstein C, Hund E et al. "Sunbath polyneuritis": Subacute axonal polyneuropathy in perazine-treated patients after intense sun exposure. *Muscle Nerve* 1996;**19**:438–41.
5352. Roessmann U, Schwartz JF. Familial striatal degeneration. *Arch Neurol* 1973;**29**:314–7.
5353. Roger J, Dravet C, Bureau M et al. Epileptic syndromes in infancy, childhood and adolescence. London & Paris: John Libby Eurotext, 1985.
5354. Roger J, Genton P, Bureau M et al. Dyssynergia cerebellaris myoclonica (Ramsay Hunt's syndrome) associated with epilepsy: A study of 32 cases. *Neuropediatrics* 1987;**18**:117.
5355. Rogers L. The posterior fossa compression syndrome. *BMJ* 1933;**2**:100–1.
5356. Rohkamm R, Boxler K, Ricker K et al. A dominantly inherited myopathy with excessive tubular aggregates. *Neurology* 1983;**33**:331–6.
5357. Rolak LA. The flight of colors test in multiple sclerosis. *Arch Neurol* 1985;**42**:759–60.
5358. Roland PE. Lack of appreciation of compressibility. *J Neurol Sci* 1973;**20**: 51–61.
5359. Roles NC, Maudsley RH. Radial tunnel syndrome: Resistant tennis elbow as nerve entrapment. *J Bone Joint Surg* 1972;**54**:499–508.
5360. Rolfs A, Koeppen AH, Bauer I et al. Clinical features and neuropathology of autosomal dominant spinocerebellar ataxia. *Ann Neurol* 2003;**54**:367–75.
5361. Rollet J, Colrat. Syndrome de l'apex orbitaire (ophthalmoplègie sensorio-sensitivo-motrice d'origine traumatique). *Bull Soc Ophth Lyon* 1926;**16**:13–4.
5362. Roman G. Epidemic neuropathy in Cuba: A public health problem related to the Cuban Democracy Act of the United States. *Neuroepidemiology* 1998;**17**:111–5.
5363. Roman G, Fisher M, Perl DP et al. Neurological manifestations of hereditary hemorrhagic telangiectasia (Rendu–Osler–Weber disease): Report of 2 cases and review of the literature. *Ann Neurol* 1978;**4**:130–44.
5364. Roman GC, Roman LN, Spencer PS et al. Tropical spastic paraparesis - a neuroepidemiological study in Colombia. *Ann Neurol* 1985;**17**:361–5.
5365. Roman GC, Spencer PS, Schoenberg BS. Tropical myeloneuropathies. *Neurology* 1985;**35**:1158–70.
5366. Roman GC, Tatemichi TK, Erkinjuntti T et al. Vascular dementia: Diagnostic criteria for research studies. *Neurology* 1993;**43**:250–60.
5367. Romberg MH. *Klinische Ergebnisse*. Berlin: A. Forstner, 1846.
5368. Romberg MH. Hyperesthesia of the nerves of muscular sense. In Sieveking EH ed. *Manual of the Nervous Diseases of Man*, London: New Sydenham Society, 1853.
5369. See 5368.
5370. Romeo G. Enzymatic defects of hereditary porphyrias: An explanation of dominance at a molecular level. *Hum Genet* 1977;**39**:261–76.
5371. Ron MA. Somatisation in neurological practice. *J Neurol Neurosurg Psychiatry* 1994;**57**:1161–4.
5372. Rondot P, Marchand MP, Dellatolas G. Spasmodic torticollis – review of 220

patients. *Can J Neurol Sci* 1991;18: 143–51.

5373. Rondot P, Recondo Jd, Dumas JLR. Visuomotor ataxia. *Brain* 1977;100: 355–76.

5374. Ronen GM, Rosales TO, Connolly M et al. Seizure characteristics in chromosome 20 benign familial neonatal convulsions. *Neurology* 1993;43:1355–60.

5375. Roos DB. Thoracic outlet syndrome. *Muscle Nerve* 1999;22:126–9.

5376. Roos RAC, van Dijk JC. Reflex epilepsy induced by immersion in hot water: Case report and review of the literature. *Europ Neurol* 1992.

5377. Ropper AH. Case records of the Massachusetts General Hospital #35 – 1981. *N Engl J Med* 1981;305:507–14.

5378. Ropper AH. Ocular dipping in anoxic coma. *Arch Neurol* 1981;38:297–9.

5379. Ropper AH. Self-grasping: A focal neurological sign. *Ann Neurol* 1982;12:575–7.

5380. Ropper AH. Unusual spontaneous movements in brain-dead patients. *Neurology* 1984;1089:1092.

5381. Ropper AH. In favor of intracranial pressure monitoring and aggressive therapy in neurologic practice. *Arch Neurol* 1985;42:1194–5.

5382. Ropper AH. Seronegative, non-neoplastic acute cerebellar degeneration. *Neurology* 1993;43:1602–5.

5383. Ropper AH. Syndrome of transtentorial herniation: Is vertical displacement necessary? *J Neurol Neurosurg Psychiatry* 1993;56:932–5.

5384. Ropper AH, Davis KR. Lobar cerebral hemorrhages: Acute clinical syndromes in 26 cases. *Ann Neurol* 1980;8:141–7.

5385. Ropper AH, Gorson KC. Concussion. *N Engl J Med* 2007;356:166–72.

5386. Ropper AH, Poskanzer DC. The prognosis of acute and subacute transverse myelopathy based on early signs and symptoms. *Ann Neurol* 1978;4:51–9.

5387. Ropper AH, Wijdicks EFM, Truax BT. *Guillain–Barré Syndrome.* Philadelphia: F.A. Davis, 1991.

5388. Ros R, Gómez P, Garre MH et al. Genetic linkage of autosomal dominant progressive supranuclear palsy to 1q31.1. *Ann Neurol* 2005;57:634–41.

5389. Roscher A, Hofler S, Hofler G et al. Neonatal adrenoleukodystrophy (ALD) and cerebral-hepato-renal syndrome (CHRS): Genetic complementation analysis of impaired peroxisomal plasmalogen biosynthesis. 24th International Symposium, Society for the Study of Inborn Errors in Metabolism. 1986. Boston, MA.

5390. Rose BD. Hypoosmolal states – hyponatremia. *Clinical Physiology of Acid-Base and Electrolyte Disorders*, pp 651–94. McGraw-Hill, 1989.

5391. Rose E. Uber den Starrkrampf. *Pitha-Billroths Handbuch* 1870. 1–118.

5392. Rosemberg S. Neuropathology of San Paulo south coast epidemic encephalitis. *J Neurol Sci* 1980;45:1–12.

5393. Rosen HJ, Allison SC, Ogar JM et al. Behavioral features in semantic dementia vs other forms of progressive aphasias. *Neurology* 2006;67:1752–6.

5394. Rosen S. Tic douloureux of the chorda tympani. *Arch Neurol Psychiatry* 1953;69:275–8.

5395. Rosen SM et al. Hemodialysis disequilibrium. *Brit Med J* 1964;2:672–5.

5396. Rosen WG, Mohs RC, Davis KL. A new rating scale for Alzheimer's disease. *Am J Psychiatry* 1984;14:1356–64.

5397. Rosen WG, Terry RD, Fuld PA et al. Pathological verification of ischemic score in differentiation of dementias. *Ann Neurol* 1980;7:486–8.

5398. Rosenbach O. Ein Beitrag zur sympt cerebraler Hemiplegien. *Arch Psychiatr (Berlin)* 1876;6:845.

5399. Rosenbaum DH, Siegel M, Barr WB et al. Epileptic aphasia. *Neurology* 1986;36:822–5.

5400. Rosenberg AL, Bergstrom L, Troost BT et al. Hyperuricemia and neurological deficits. *N Engl J Med* 1970;282:992–7.

5401. Rosenberg LE, Durant JL, Elsas LJ. Familial iminoglycinuria: An inborn error of renal tubular transport. *N Engl J Med* 1968;278:1407–13.

5402. Rosenberg ML. Congenital trigeminal anesthesia. *Brain* 1984;107:1073–82.

5403. Rosenberg ML, Clark JB. Familial trembling of the chin. *Neurology* 1987;37(**Suppl.** 1):190.

5404. Rosenberg ML, Glaser JS. Superior oblique myokymia. *Ann Neurol* 1983;13:667–9.

5405. Rosenberg NL, Neville HE, Ringel SP. Tubular aggregates: Their association with neuromuscular diseases, including the syndrome of myalgias/cramps. *Arch Neurol* 1985;42:973–6.

5406. Rosenberg R, Fowler HL. Spinal muscular atrophy with Joseph disease. *Neurology* 1981;31:1124.

5407. Rosenberg R, Greenberg J. Linear scleroderma as a cause for hemiatrophy. *Ann Neurol* 1979;5:307.

5408. Rosenberg RN, Chutorian AM. Familial opticoacoustic nerve degeneration and polyneuropathy. *Neurology* 1967;17: 827–32.

5409. Rosenberg RN, Green JB, White CL et al. Dominantly inherited dementia and Parkinsonism, with non-Alzheimer amyloid plaques. *Ann Neurol* 1989;25:152–8.

5410. Rosenberg RN, Grossman A. Hereditary ataxia. In Johnson WG ed. *Neurologic Clinics*, pp 25–36. Philadelphia: W.B. Saunders, 1989.

5411. Rosenberg RN, Nyhan WL, Bay C et al. Autosomal dominant striatonigral degeneration. *Neurology* 1976;26:703–14.

5412. Rosenberg S, Lancellotti CLP, Anta F et al. Progressive bulbar paralysis of childhood (Fazio–Londe disease) with deafness. *Eur Neurol* 1982;21:84–9.

5413. Rosenblatt B, Kaplan P. A distinctive facies in neurofibromatosis. *Am J Human Genet* 1983;35(6):115A.

5414. Rosenthal R, Hall JA, Archer D et al. *The PONS Test Manual.* New York: Irvington Publishers, 1979.

5415. Rosow I, Breslau N. A Guttman scale for the aged. *J Gerontol* 1966;21:556–9.

5416. Ross AT. Progressive selective sudomotor denervation: A case with coexisting Adie's syndrome. *Neurology* 1959;8:809–17.

5417. Ross BG, Fradet G, Nedzelski JM. Development of a sensitive clinical facial grading system. *Otolaryngol Head Neck Surg* 1996;114:380–6.

5418. Ross ED. The aprosodias: Functional-anatomic organization of the affective components of language in the right hemisphere. *Arch Neurol* 1981;38:561–9.

5419. Ross RT. Transient tumor attacks. *Arch Neurol* 1983;40:633–6.

5420. Rossi F, Triggs WJ, Gooch J et al. Bilateral medial pectoral neuropathy in a weight lifter. *Muscle Nerve* 1999;22: 1597–9.

5421. Rossi G, Macchi G, Porro M et al. Fatal familial insomnia. *Neurology* 1998;50:688–92.

5422. Rossi PW, Kleiferts S, Reding MJ. Fresnel prisms improve visual perception in stroke patients with homonymous hemianopia or unilateral visual neglect. *Neurology* 1990;40:1597–9.

5423. Rossolimo GI. De la myotonie atrophique: Contribution a la théorie des myopathies. *Nouv Icon Salpet* 1902;15:63–77.

5424. Rosvold HE, Mirsky AF, Sarason I et al. A continuous performance test of brain damage. *J Clin Consult Psychol* 1956;20:343.

5425. Rot WK. *Meralgia Paresthetica.* Berlin: Karger, 1895.

5426. Roth B, Bruhova S, Berkova L. Familial sleep paralysis. *Arch Suisse Neurol Neurochir Psychiat* 1968;102:321–30.

5427. Roth B, Nevsimalova S, Rechtschaffen A. Hypersomnia with "sleep drunkenness". *Arch Gen Psychiatry* 1972;26:456–62.

5428. Roth CJ, Williams HE. The muscular variant of Pompe's disease. *J Pediatr* 1967;71:567–73.

5429. Roth M, Tym E, Mountjoy MQ. CAMDEX: A standardised instrument for the diagnosis of mental disorder in the elderly with special reference to the early detection of dementia. *Br J Psychiatry* 1986;149:698–709.

5430. Rothi LJ, McFarling DA, Heilman KM. Conduction aphasia, syntactic alexia, and the anatomy of syntactic comprehension. *Arch Neurol* 1982;39:272–5.

5431. Rothi LJG, Mack L, Heilman KM. Pantomime agnosia. *J Neurol Neurosurg Psychiatry* 1986;49:451–4.

5432. Rothman S. Physiology of itching. *Physiol Rev* 1941;21:357–81.

5433. Rothstein TL, Alvord EC. Posterior internuclear ophthalmoplegia. *Arch Neurol* 1971;24:191–202.

5434. Rothwell JC, Traub MM, Marsden CD. Primary writing tremor. *J Neurol Neurosurg Psychiatry* 1979;42:1106–14.

5435. Rothwell P. Investigation of sensory or motor symptoms: Frequency of neurological pathology depends on side of symptoms. *J Neurol Neurosurg Psychiatry* 1994;57:1401–2.

5436. Rotthauwe HW, Kowalewski S, Mumenthaler M. Congenital muscle dystrophy. *Zschr Kinderh* 1969;106:131–62.

5437. Roulet E, Deonna T, Despland PA. Prolonged intermittent drooling and oromotor dyspraxia in benign childhood epilepsy with centrotemporal spikes. *Epilepsia* 1989;30:564–8.

5438. Roussy G, Cornil L. Névrite hypertrophique progressive non-familial de l'adulte. *Ann Med* 1919;6:296–305.

5439. Roussy G, Levy G. Sept cas d'une maladie particulaire: Troubles de la marche, pieds bots et areflèxie tendineuse generaliseé, avec accessoirement, legère maladresse des mains. *Rev Neurol* 1926;1:427–50.

5440. Roussy G, Lhermitte JJ. *Les blessures de la moelle et de la queue de cheval.* Paris: Masson, 1918.

5441. Rowin J, Lewis SL. Copper deficiency myeloneuropathy and pancytopenia secondary to overuse of zinc supplementation. *J Neurol Neurosurg Psychiatry* 2005;76:750–1.

5442. Rowland LP. Myoglobinuria. *Can J Neurol Sci* 1984;11:1–6.

5443. Rowland LP. Cramps, spasms and muscle stiffness. *Rev Neurol* 1985;141:261–73.

5444. Rowland LP, Fetel M, Olarte A et al. Emery–Dreifuss muscular dystrophy. *Ann Neurol* 1979;5:111–7.

5445. Rowland LP, Greer M. Toxoplasmosis. *Neurology* 1961;11:367.

5446. Rowland LP, Penn AS. Myoglobinuria. *Med Clin N Amer* 1972;56:1233–4.

5447. Rowland LP, Shneider NA. Amyotrophic lateral sclerosis. *N Engl J Med* 2001;344:1688–99.

5448. Roxburgh RHSR, Seaman SR, Masterman T et al. Multiple sclerosis severity score. *Neurology* 2005;64:1144–51.

5449. Roy FH. *Ocular Syndromes and Systemic Diseases*. Philadelphia: W.B. Saunders, 1989.

5450. Roy PR, Emanual R, Ismail SA et al. Hereditary prolongation of the Q-T interval: Genetic observations. *Am J Cardiol* 1976;37:237–43.

5451. Royall DR, Cabello M, Polk M. Executive dyscontrol: An important factor affecting the level of care received by elderly retirees. *J Am Geriatr Soc* 1988;46: 1519–24.

5452. Royall DR, Chiodo LK, Polk M. Correlates of disability among elderly retirees with "sub-clinical" cognitive impairment. *J Gerontol* 2000;55A:M541–M546.

5453. Royall DR, Cordes JA, Polk M. CLOX: An executive drawing task. *J Neurol Neurosurg Psychiatry* 1999;64:588–94.

5454. Royall DR, Mahurin RK, Gray KF. Bedside assessment of executive cognitive impairment: The executive interview. *J Am Geriatr Soc* 1992;40:1221–6.

5455. Rozear MP, Pericak-Vance S, Pericaz-Vance MA et al. Hereditary motor and sensory neuropathy, X-linked. *Neurology* 1987;37:1460–5.

5456. Rubens O, Logina I, Kravale I et al. Peripheral neuropathy in chronic occupational inorganic lead exposure: A clinical and electrophysiological study. *J Neurol Neurosurg Psychiatry* 2001;71:200–4.

5457. Rubenstein JH, Taybi H. Broad thumbs and toes and facial abnormalities. *Am J Dis Childh* 1963;105:588.

5458. Rubin SA, Sylves P, Vogel M et al. Borna disease virus-induced hippocampal dentate gyrus damage is associated with spatial learning and memory deficits. *Brain Res Bull* 1998;48:23–30.

5459. Rubin SE, Wagner RS. Ocular torticollis. *Surv Ophthalmol* 1986;30:366.

5460. Rubinstein AE, Weinapel SF. Acute hypokalemic myopathy of alcoholism. *Arch Neurol* 1977;34:553–5.

5461. Rubio-Golalbo ME, Smeitink JA, Ruitenbeek W et al. Spinal muscular atrophy-like picture, cardiomyopathy, and cytochrome *c* oxidase deficiency. *Neurology* 1999;52:383–6.

5462. Ruchoux MM, Maurage CA. CADASIL. Cerebral autosomal dominant arteriopathy with subcortical infarcts and leukoencephalopathy. *J Neuropath Exp Neurol* 1997;56:947–64.

5463. Rud E. Et tilfaelde af infantilisme med tetani, epilepsi, polyneuritis, ichthyosis og anaemi of pernicios type. *Hospitalstidende* 1927;70:525–38.

5464. Rudick RA, Cutter G, Baier M et al. Use of the multiple sclerosis functional composite to predict disability in relapsing MS. *Neurology* 2001;56:1324–30.

5465. Ruggieri M, Tigano G, Mazzone D et al. Involvement of the white matter in hypomelanosis of Ito. *Neurology* 1996;46:485–92.

5466. Ruiz-Sandoval JL, Gutierrez-Aceves GA et al. Linear scleroderma en coup de sabre: Neurological symptoms, images and review. *Rev Neurol* 2005;41:534–7.

5467. Rukavina JG, Block WD, Jackson CF et al. Amyloidosis Type II. *Medicine (Baltimore)* 1956;35:239–334.

5468. Rush PJ, Inman R, Bernstein M et al. Isolated vasculitis of the central nervous system in a patient with celiac disease. *Am J Med* 1986;81:1092–4.

5469. Rushton AR, Genel G. Hereditary ectodermal dysplasia, olivopontocerebellar degeneration, short stature and hypogonadism. *J Med Genet* 1981;18:335–9.

5470. Rushworth G. Observations on blink reflexes. *J Neurol Neurosurg Psychiatry* 1962;25:93–108.

5471. Russell AA. A diencephalic syndrome of emaciation in infancy and childhood. *Arch Dis Child* 1951;26:274.

5472. Russell DJ, Avery LM et al. Improved scaling of the gross motor function measure for children with cerebral palsy: Evidence of reliability and validity. *Phys Ther* 2000;80:873–85.

5473. Russell DS, Marshall AHE, Smith FB. Microgliomatosis. *Brain* 1948;71:1–15.

5474. Russell EW. A multiple scoring method for the assessment of complex memory functions. *J Consult Clin Psychol* 1975;43:800–9.

5475. Russell GFM. Bulimia nervosa: An ominous variant of anorexia nervosa. *Psychol Med* 1979;9:429–48.

5476. Russell JSR, Batten FE, Collier J. Subacute combined degeneration of the spinal cord. *Brain* 1900;23:39–110.

5477. Russo LS, Aron A, Anderson PJ. Alexander's disease: A report and reappraisal. *Neurology* 1976;26:607–14.

5478. Russomano S, Herbison GJ, Baliga A et al. Riche–Cannieu anastomosis with partial transection of the median nerve. *Muscle Nerve* 1995;18:120–2.

5479. Ruvalcaba RHA, Reichert A, Smith DW. A new familial syndrome with osseous dysplasia and mental deficiency. *J Pediatr* 1971;79:450–5.

5480. Ryan AJ, Stephens RE. *Dance Medicine. A Comprehensive Guide.* Chicago: Pluribus Press, 1987.

5481. Ryan L, Warden DL. Post concussion syndrome. *Int Rev Psychiatry* 2003;15:310–6.

5482. Ryan MM, Schnell C, Strickland CD et al. Nemaline myopathy: A clinical study of 143 cases. *Ann Neurol* 2001;**50**:312–20.
5483. Rylander G. Psychoses and the punding and choreiform syndromes in addiction to central stimulant drugs. *Psychiatr Neurol Neurochir (Amst)* 1972;**75**:203–12.
5484. Ryvlin P, Rheims S, Risse G. Nocturnal frontal lobe epilepsy. *Epilepsia* 2006;**47**:83–6.
5485. Sabin TD, Swift TR. Leprosy. In Dyck PJ, Thomas PK, Lambert EH eds. *Peripheral Neuropathy*, p 1198. Philadelphia: Saunders, 1975.
5486. Sabra AF, Hallett M. Action tremor with alternating activity in antagonist muscles. *Neurology* 1984;**34**:151–6.
5487. Sachdev PS, Smith JS, Angus-Lepan H et al. Pseudodementia twelve years on. *J Neurol Neurosurg Psychiatry* 1990;**53**:254–9.
5488. Sachev P, Loneragan C. Low dose apomorphine challenge in tardive akathisia. *Neurology* 1993;**43**:544–7.
5489. Sachs B. On arrested cerebral development, with special reference to its cortical pathology. *J Nerv Ment Dis* 1887;**14**:541–53.
5490. Sachs GM, Raynor EM, Schefner JM. The all ulnar motor hand without forearm anastomosis. *Muscle Nerve* 1995;**19**:309–13.
5491. Sadeghian H. Mount Fuji sign in tension pneumocephalus. *Arch Neurol* 2000;**57**:1366.
5492. Sadeh M, Blatt I, Goldhammer Y. Single fiber EMG in a congenital myasthenic syndrome associated with facial malformations. *Muscle Nerve* 1993;**16**:177–80.
5493. Sadler RM, Rahey S. Prescience as an Aura of temporal lobe epilepsy. *Epilepsia* 2004;**45**:982–4.
5494. Sadun AA, Currie JN, Lessell S. Transient visual obscurations with elevated optic discs. *Ann Neurol* 1984;**16**:489–94.
5495. Saenger A. On a form of myotonic pupil. *Neurol Centralbl* 1902;**21**:1137–8.
5496. Saenz-Lope E, Herranz FJ, Masdeu JC. Startle epilepsy: A clinical study. *Ann Neurol* 1984;**16**:78–81.
5497. Saethre H. Ein Beitrag zum Turmschadelproblem (Pathogenese, Erblichkeit und Symptomatolgie). *Dtsch Z Nervenheilk* 1931;**117**:533–55.
5498. Safdari H, Richardson EPj. Subacute necrotizing polioencephalopathy. *Arch Neurol* 1979;**36**:638–42.
5499. Sagin K. Le réfléxe de la malleole éxterne et le phénomène de Piotrowski. *Rev Neurol* (Paris) 1927;**1**:319–25.
5500. Sahgal V, Sahgal S. A new congenital myopathy: A morphological, cytochemical and histochemical study. *Acta Neuropathol* 1977;**37**:255.
5501. Said G. Chronic inflammatory demyelinating polyneuropathy. *Neuromuscular Dis* 2006;**16**:293–303.
5502. Said G. A clinicopathological study of acrodystrophic neuropathies. *Muscle Nerve* 1980;**3**:491–501.
5503. Said G, Goulon-Goeau C, Lacroix C et al. Nerve biopsy findings in different patterns of proximal diabetic neuropathy. *Ann Neurol* 1994;**35**:559–69.
5504. Saiz A, Arpa J, Sagasta A et al. Autoantibodies to glutamic acid decarboxylase in three patients with cerebellar ataxia, late onset insulin dependent diabetes mellitus and polyendocrine abnormality. *Neurology* 1997;**49**:1026–30.
5505. Saka E, Saygi S, Ciger A et al. Circling seizures. *Seizure* 1996;**5**:299–302.
5506. Sakakibara R, Hirano S, Asahina S et al. Primary Sjôgren's syndrome presenting with generalized autonomic failure. *Europ J Neurol* 2004;**11**:635–8.
5507. Sakati N et al. A new syndrome with acrocephalopolysyndactyly, cardiac disease, and distinctive defects of the ear, skin, and lower limbs. *J Pediatr* 1971;**79**:104–9.
5508. Sakuraba H, Suzuki Y, Akagi M et al. Beta galactosidase - neuraminidase deficiency (galactosialidosis): Clinical, pathological, and enzymatic studies in a postmortem case. *Ann Neurol* 1983;**13**:497–503.
5509. Salanova V, Andermann F, Rasmussen T et al. Parietal lobe epilepsy. *Brain* 1995;**118**:607–27.
5510. Salbert BA, Pellock JM, Wolf B. Characterization of seizures associated with biotinidase deficiency. *Neurology* 1993;**43**:1351–5.
5511. Saldino RM, Mainzer F. Cone-shaped epiphyses in siblings with hereditary renal disease and retinitis pigmentosa. *Radiology* 1971;**98**:39–45.
5512. Salleras A, Ortiz J, Zarate JC. Recessive sex-linked inheritance of external ophthalmoplegia and myopia coincident with other dysplasias. *Brit J Ophth* 1950;**34**:662.
5513. Salman MS, Ackerley C, Senger C et al. New insights into the pathogenesis of molybdenum cofactor deficiency. *Can J Neurol Sci* 2002;**29**:91–6.
5514. Salomons GS, vanDooren SJM, Darmin P et al. A novel X-linked mental retardation syndrome: Creatine transporter deficiency. *Neurology* 2004;**62**:A22.
5515. Salonen R, Herva R, Norio R. The hydrolethalus syndrome: Delineation of a "new", lethal malformation syndrome based on 28 patients. *Clin Genet* 1981;**19**:321–30.
5516. Salthouse TA, Mitchell DRD. Structural and operational capacities in integrative spatial ability. *Psychology and Aging* 1989;**4**:18–25.
5517. Salus R. Acquired retraction movements of the globe. *Archiv Fur Augenheilkunde* 1910;**68**:61–76.
5518. Samii A, Pal PK, Schulzer M et al. Post-traumatic cervical dystonia: A distinct entity? *Can J Neurol Sci* 2000;**27**:55–9.
5519. Samples JR, Howard FM, Okazaki H. Syringomesencephalia: Report of a case. *Arch Neurol* 1983;**40**:757–9.
5520. Samuel M, Torun N, Tuite PJ et al. Progressive ataxia and palatal tremor (PAPT): Clinical and MRI assessment with review of palatal tremors. *Brain* 2004;**127**:1268.
5521. Samuels OB, Duffy CJ, Griggs RC. Cacacusis: Frightening echoes in neurologic disease. *Neurology* 1996;**46Suppl.**A293–A294. (Abstract)
5522. San Antonio V, Sachs P, Monier A. Aicardi-Goutières syndrome: An oft unrecognised familial early-onset encephalopathy. *Rev Neurol (Paris)* 2005;**161**:445–50.
5523. San Pedro EC, Mountz JM, Ojha B et al. Anterior cingulate gyrus epilepsy: The role of SPECT in seizure localization. *Epilepsia* 2000;**41**:594–600.
5524. Sanborn GE, Magargal L. Neuro-ophthalmology enters the nineties. Hialeah: Dutton, 1988.
5525. Sanchez-Carpintero R, McLellan A, Parmeggiani R et al. Pallister-Killian syndrome: An unusual cause of epileptic spasms. *Dev Med Child Neurol* 2005;**47**:776–9.
5526. Sander HW, Latov N. Research criteria for defining patients with CIDP. *Neurology* 2003;**60**:S8–S15.
5527. Sander HW, Tavoulareas GP, Quinto CM et al. The exercise test distinguishes myotonic myopathy from myotonic dystrophy. *Muscle Nerve* 1997;**20**:2325–237.
5528. Sander JE, Layzer RB, Goldsobel AB. Congenital stiffman syndrome. *Ann Neurol* 1980;**8**:195–7.
5529. Sander JE, Sharp FR. Lumbosacral plexus neuritis. *Neurology* 1981;**31**:470–3.
5530. Sander S, Ouvrier RA, McLeod JG et al. Clinical syndromes associated with tomacula or myelin swellings in sural nerve biopsies. *J Neurol Neurosurg Psychiatry* 2000;**68**:483–8.
5531. Sanders DB. Myotonia congenita with painful muscle contractions. *Arch Neurol* 1976;**33**:580–2.
5532. Sanders DB, Stalberg E. Single-fiber electromyography. *Muscle Nerve* 1996;**19**:1069–83.
5533. Sanders MD. Alternating windmill nystagmus. In Smith JL, Glaser JS eds. *Neuro-Ophthalmology*, pp 133–6. St. Louis: Mosby, 1973.

5534. Sanders MD. Retinal arteritis, retinal vasculitis and autoimmune retinal vasculitis. *Eye* 1987;1:441.
5535. Sanders MD, Hoyt WF, Daroff RB. Lid nystagmus evoked by ocular convergence: An ocular electromyographic study. *J Neurol Neurosurg Psychiatry* 1968;31:368–71.
5536. Sandhoff K, Andreae U, Jatkewitz H. Deficient hexosaminidase activity in an exceptional case of Tay-Sachs disease with additional storage of kidney globoside in visceral organs. *Life Sci* 1968;7:283–8.
5537. Sandhoff K, Harzer K, Wassle W et al. Enzyme alteration and lipid storage in three variants of Tay-Sachs disease. *J Neurochem* 1971;18:2469.
5538. Sandok BA, Houser OW, Baker HL et al. Fibromuscular dysplasia: Neurologic disorders associated with disease involving the great muscles in the neck. *Arch Neurol* 1971;24:462–6.
5539. Sandson J, Albert ML. Varieties of perseveration. *Neuropsychologia* 1984;22:715–32.
5540. Sandvig K. Pseudoglaucoma of autosomal dominant inheritance. *Acta Ophth Kopenhagen* 1961;39:33.
5541. Sanfilippo SJ et al. Mental retardation associated with mucopolysacchariduria (heparitin sulfate type). *J Pediatr* 1963;63:832–8.
5542. Sano Y, Date H, Igarashi S et al. Aprataxin, the causative protein for EAOH is a nuclear protein with a potential role as a DNA repair protein. *Ann Neurol* 2004;55:241–9.
5543. Santavuori P, Haltia M, Rapola J, Raitta C. Infantile type of so-called neuronal ceroid-lipofuscinosis. *J Neurol Sci* 1973;18:257–67.
5544. Santavuori P, Leisti J, Kruus J et al. Muscle, eye and brain disease: A new syndrome. *Doc Ophthalmol* 1978;17: 393–6.
5545. Saper JR. The mixed headache syndrome: A new perspective. *Headache* 1982;22:284–6.
5546. Saper JR. Daily chronic headache. *Neurol. Clin.* 1990;8(4):891–901.
5547. Saper JR, Holt JF. Cranial metaphyseal dysplasia: A cause of recurrent bilateral facial palsy. *Arch Neurol* 1974;31:204–7.
5548. Saperstein DS, Amato AA, Wolfe GI et al. Multifocal acquired demyelinating sensory and motor neuropathy: The Lewis-Sumner syndrome. *Muscle Nerve* 1999;22:560–6.
5549. Saperstein DS, Katz JS, Barohn RJ. Clinical spectrum of chronic acquired demyelinating polyneuropathies. *Muscle Nerve* 2001;24:311–24.
5550. Sarnat H, Morrissey RT. Idiopathic torticollis, sternocleidomastoid myopathy and accessory neuropathy. *Muscle Nerve* 1981;4:374.
5551. Sarnat HB, Case ME, Graviss R. Sacral agenesis. *Neurology* 1976;26:1124–9.
5552. Sasanuma S, Monoi H. The syndrome of Gogi (word-meaning) aphasia. *Neurology* 1975;25:627–32.
5553. Sass JO, Olbrich H, Mohr V et al. Neurological findings in aminoacyclase 1 deficiency. *Neurology* 2007;68:2151–3.
5554. Satoh A, Tsuijihata M, Yokimura T. Myasthenia gravis associated with the Satayoshi syndrome. *Neurology* 1983;33:1209–11.
5555. Satoh T, Harada Y. Electrophysiological study on tooth-grinding during sleep. *EEG Clin Neurophysiol* 1973;35:267–75.
5556. Satoyoshi E. A syndrome of progressive muscle spasm, alopecia and diarrhea. *Neurology* 1978;28:458–71.
5557. Satoyoshi E, Kinoshita M. Oculopharyngodistal myopathy: Report of four families. *Arch Neurol* 1977;34: 89–92.
5558. Satoyoshi E, Kowa H. A myopathy due to glycolytic abnormality. *Arch Neurol* 1967;17:248–55.
5559. Satoyoshi E, Yamada K. Recurrent muscle pains of central origin. *Arch Neurol* 1967;16:254–64.
5560. Satran R. Déjèrine-Sottas disease revisited. *Arch Neurol* 1980;37:67–8.
5561. Satya-Murti S, Navada S, Eames F. Central nervous system involvement in blue-rubber-bleb-nevus syndrome. *Arch Neurol* 1986;43:1184–6.
5562. Saunders JB, Aasland OG, Babor TF et al. Development of the alcohol use disorders identification test (AUDIT) A WHO collaborative project on detection of persons with harmful alcoholic consumption. *Addiction* 1993;88: 791–803.
5563. Saunders-Pullman R, Shriberg J, Heiman G et al. Myoclonus dystonia. *Neurology* 2002;58:242–5.
5564. Saunders-Pullman R, Soto-Valencia J, Costan-Toth C et al. A new screening tool for cervical dystonia. *Neurology* 2005;64:2046–9.
5565. Savage DCL, Forbes M, Pearce GW. Idiopathic rhabdomyolysis. *Arch Dis Child* 1971;46:594–607.
5566. Savoiardo M, Minati L, Farina L et al. Spontaneous intracranial hypotension with deep brain swelling. *Brain* 207;130:1884–93.
5567. Sawaya RA, Zahed L, Taher A. Peripheral neuropathy in thalassaemia. *Ann Saudi Med* 2006;26:358–63.
5568. Sawayama T, Kurihara T, Araki S. Non-invasive cardiovascular findings in familial amyloid polyneuropathy. *Br Heart J* 1978;40:1288–92.
5569. Sawyer RN, Hanna JP, Ruff RL et al. Asymmetry of forearm rolling as a sign of unilateral cerebral dysfunction. *Neurology* 1993;43:1596–8.
5570. Saxton J, Swihart AA. Neuropsychological assessment of the severely impaired elderly patient. *Clin Geriatr Med* 1989;5:531–43.
5571. Say B, Meyer J. Familial trigonocephaly associated with short stature and development delay. *Am J Dis Child* 1981;135:711–2.
5572. Scaglione C, Salvi F, Riguzzi P et al. Symptomatic unruptured capillary telangiectasia of the brain stem: Report of three cases and a review of the literature. *J Neurol Neurosurg Psychiatry* 2001;71: 390–3.
5573. Scarfone H, McComas AJ, Pape K et al. Denervation and reinnervation in Congenital Brachial Palsy. *Muscle Nerve* 1999;22:600–7.
5574. Scarrfge R. *J Nerv Ment Dis* 1947;106:605–7.
5575. Scelsa S, Yakubov B, Salzman SH. Dyspnea-fasciculation syndrome: Early respiratory failure in ALS with minimal motor signs. *Amyotroph Lateral Scler Other Motor Neuron Disord* 2002;3:239–43.
5576. Schady W, Meara RJ. Hereditary progressive chorea without dementia. *J Neurol Neurosurg Psychiatry* 1988;51: 295–7.
5577. Schady W, Smith CML. Sensory neuropathy in hereditary spastic paraplegia. *J Neurol Neurosurg Psychiatry* 1994;57:693–8.
5578. Schaefer M. On an antagonistic reflex. *Neurol Zbl* 1899;18:1016–8.
5579. Schaible HG. Peripheral and central mechanisms of pain generation. *Handb Exp Pharmacol* 2007;177:3–28.
5580. Schapira AHV. Inborn and induced defects of mitochondria. *Arch Neurol* 1998;55:1293–6.
5581. Scharli AF, Meier-Ruge W. Localized and disseminated forms of neuronal intestinal dysplasia mimicking Hirschsprung's disease. *J Pediatr Surg* 1981;16:164–70.
5582. Schaublin GA, Michet CJ JR, Dyck PJB et al. An update on the classification and treatment of vasculitic neuropathy. *Lancet Neurology* 2005;4:853–65.
5583. Schaul N, Luders H, Sachdev KK. Generalized bilaterally synchronous bursts of slow waves in the EEG. *Arch Neurol* 1981;38:690–2.
5584. Scheffer IE, Lones L, Pozzebon M et al. Autosomal dominant rolandic epilepsy and speech dyspraxia: A new syndrome with anticipation. *Ann Neurol* 1995;38:633–42.
5585. Scheffer IE, Phillips HA, Mulley J et al. Autosomal dominant partial epilepsy with

variable foci is not allelic with autosomal dominant frontal lobe epilepsy. *Epilepsia* 1995;36(**Suppl.** 3):S28. (Abstract)
5586. Scheffer IE, Phillips HA, O'Brien CE et al. Familial partial epilepsy with variable foci. *Ann Neurol* 1998;44:890–9.
5587. Scheffer IE, Wallace RH, Phillips FL et al. X-linked myoclonic epilepsy with spasticity and intellectual disability. *Neurology* 2002;59:348–56.
5588. Scheie HG et al. A new recognized forme fruste of Hurler's disease (gargoylism). *Am J Ophthalmol* 1962;53:753–69.
5589. Scheinberg P. Dementia due to vascular disease - A multifactorial disorder. *Stroke* 1988;19:1291–9.
5590. Scheinker IM. Subependymoma: A newly-recognized tumor of subependymal origin. *J Neurosurg* 1945;2:232–40.
5591. Schelhaas HJ, Ippel PF, Beemer FA et al. Similarities and differences in the phenotype, genotype and pathogenesis of different spinocerebellar ataxias. *Europ J Neurol* 2000;7:309–314.
5592. Schellack J, Fulenwider JT, Olson RA et al. The carotid sinus syndrome: A frequently overlooked cause of syncope in the elderly. *J Vasc Surg* 1986;4:376–83.
5593. Schenck CH, Bundle SR, Mahowald MW. Human REM sleep chronic behaviour disorders; A new category of parasomnia. *Sleep Res* 1985;14:208.
5594. Schenck CH, Mahowald MW. REM sleep parasomnias. *NC* 1996;14:697–718.
5595. Schenck CH, Milner DM, Hurwitz TD et al. Dissociative disorders presenting as somnabulism: Polysomnographic, video and clinical documentation (8 cases). *Dissociation* 1989;2:194–204.
5596. Schenkenberg T, Bradford DC, Ajax ET. Line bisection and unilateral visual neglect in patients with neurological impairment. *Neurology* 1980;30:509–17.
5597. Schenone A, Mancardi GL. Molecular basis of inherited neuropathies. *Current Opinion in Neurology* 1999;12:603–16.
5598. Schiff HB, Alexander MP, Naeser MA et al. Aphemia: Clinical-anatomical correlations. *Arch Neurol* 1983;40:720–7.
5599. Schiffmann R, Moller JR, Trapp BD et al. Childhood ataxia with diffuse central nervous system hypomyelination. *Ann Neurol* 1994;35:331–40.
5600. Schiffmann R, Moller JR, Trapp BD et al. CACH syndrome - vanishing white matter. Childhood ataxia with central nervous system hypomyelination. *Ann Neurol* 1994;35:331–40.
5601. Schilder P. Zur Kenntnis der sogenannten diffusen Sklerose (uber Encephalitis periaxialis diffusa). *ZN* 1912;10:1–60.
5602. Schilder P. *Psych Anal Rev* 1931;18:1.
5603. Schiller F. The reflex hammer. *Med Hist* 1967;11:75–85.
5604. Schiller F. Coenesthesis. *Bull Hist Med* 1984;58:496–515.
5605. Schiller F. The inveterate paradox of dreaming. *Arch Neurol* 1985;42:903–6.
5606. Schiller F. Wartenberg R.; The neurologist. *J Nerv Ment Dis* 1952;116:480–7.
5607. Schimke RN et al. A new X-linked syndrome comprising progressive basal ganglion dysfunction, mental and growth retardation, external ophthalmoplegia, postnatal microcephaly and deafness. *Am J Med Genet* 1984;17:323–32.
5608. Schindler RJ, Feinberg TE, Flanagan NG et al. Two syndromes of the alien hand. *Neurology* 1991;41 (**Suppl.** 1):187.
5609. Schinzel A. Post-axial polydactyly, hallux duplication, absence of the corpus callosum, macrocephaly and severe mental retardation: A new syndrome. *Helv Pediat Acta* 1979;34:141–6.
5610. Schinzel A, Hayashi K, Schmid W. Further delineation of the clinical picture of trisomy for the distal segment of chromosome 13. *Human Genetics* 1976;32:1–12.
5611. Schlitt M, Dempsey PJ, Robinson RK, Cervical butterfly-block vertebra. A case report. *Clin Imaging* 1989;13:167–70.
5612. Schmahmann JD, Sherman JC. The cerebellar cognitive affective syndrome. *Brain* 1996;121:561–79.
5613. Schmand B, Lindeboom J, Schagen S et al. Cognitive complaints after whiplash injury: The impact of malingering. *J Neurol Neurosurg Psychiatry* 1998;64:339–43.
5614. Schmid RH, Luedtke H, Wilhelm BJ et al. Pupil campimetry in patients with visual field loss. *Eur J Neurol* 2005;12:602–8.
5615. Schmidley JW, Levinsohn MW, Maratto V. Infantile X-linked ataxia and deafness. *Neurology* 1987;37:1344–9.
5616. Schmidt. Ocular myasthenia. In Daroff RB, Neetens A, eds. *Neurological Organization of Extraocular Movement*, New York, NY.: Kugler Publicns, 1989.
5617. Schmidt A. Doppelseitige Accessormslahmung bei Syringomyelie. *Dtsch Med Wschr* 1892;18:606–8.
5618. Schmidt D, Dell'Osso LF, Abel LA et al. Myasthenia gravis: Dynamic changes in saccadic wavefor, gain and velocity. *Exp Neurol* 1980;68:365.
5619. Schmidt JE. *Medical Discoveries.* Springfield: Charles C. Thomas, 1959.
5620. Schmidt S, Hertfelder H-J, von Speigel T et al. Lethal capillary leak syndrome after a single administration of interferon beta-1b. *Neurology* 1999;53:220–3.
5621. Schmitt HP, Bersch W, Feustel HP. Acute abdominal rhabdomyolysis after body building exercise. *Muscle Nerve* 1983;6:228–32.
5622. Schmitt HP, Emser W, Heimes C. Familial occurrence of amyotrophic lateral sclerosis, parkinsonism, and dementia. *Ann Neurol* 1984;16:642–8.
5623. Schmitz-Hubsch T, Tezenas du Montcel S, Baliko L et al. Scale for the assessment and rating of ataxia. *Neurology* 2006;66:1717–20.
5624. Schneider H. On an epidemic of serous meningitis. *Wien Klin Wschr* 1831;44:350–2.
5625. Schneider JW, Gurucharti LM, Gutierrez AL et al. Health-related quailty of life and functional outcome measures for children with cerebral palsy. *Dev Med Child Neurol* 2001;43:601–8.
5626. Schneider RC, Cherry G, Pantek H. The syndrome of acute central cervical spinal cord injury. *J Neurosurg* 1954;11:546–77.
5627. Schneider SA, Aggarwal A, Bhatt MH. Severe tongue protrusion dystonia. *Neurology* 2006;67:940–3.
5628. Schneider SA, Bhatia KP. Dystonia in the Woodhouse Sakati syndrome: A new family and literature review. *Mov Disord* 2008;23:592–6.
5629. Schneider SA, Edwards MJ, Grill SE et al. Adult-onset primary lower limb dystonia. *Mov Disord* 2006;21:767–71.
5630. Schnider A, Benson DF, Rosner LJ. Callosal disconnection in multiple sclerosis. *Neurology* 1993;43:1243–5.
5631. Schoenberg B, Massey EW. Tapia's syndrome. *Arch Neurol* 1979;36:257–60.
5632. Schold SC, Cho E-S, Somasundaram M et al. Subacute motor neuropathy: A remote effect of lymphoma. *Ann Neurol* 1979;5:271–87.
5633. Scholte HR, Jennekens FGI, Bonvy JJBJ. Carnitine palmitoyl transferase II deficiency with normal carnitine palmitoyl transferase I in skeletal muscle and leucocytes. *J Neurol Sci* 1979;40: 39–51.
5634. Scholtz CL, Swash M. Cerebellar degeneration in dominantly inherited spastic paraplegia. *J Neurol Neurosurg Psychiatry* 1985;48:145–9.
5635. Schon F, Blau JN. Post-epileptic headache and migraine. *J Neurol Neurosurg Psychiatry* 1987;50:1148–52.
5636. Schon F, Martin RJ, Prevett M et al. CADASIL coma: An undiagnosed acute encephalopathy. *J Neurol Neurosurg Psychiatry* 2003;74:249–52.
5637. Schondorf R, Low PA. Idiopathic postural orthostatic tachycardia syndrome: An attenuated form of acute pandyautonomia? *Neurology* 1993;43:132–7.
5638. Schooler NR, Kane JM. Research diagnoses for tardive dyskinesia. *Arch Gen Psychiatry* 1982; –486.
5639. See 5638.

5640. Schott GD. Distant referral of cutaneous sensation. *Exp Neurol* 1973;1:451–6.
5641. Schott GD. Some neurological observations on Leonardo da Vinci's handwriting. *J Neurol Sci* 1979;42:321–9.
5642. Schott GD. A chronic and painless form of idiopathic brachial plexus neuropathy. *J Neurol Neurosurg Psychiatry* 1983;46: 555–7.
5643. Schott GD. Mechanisms of causalgia and related clinical conditions: The role of the central and of the sympathetic nervous systems. *Brain* 1986;109:717–38.
5644. Schott GD. Reflex sympathetic dystrophy. *J Neurol Neurosurg Psychiatry* 2001;71:291–5.
5645. Schott GD. Mirror writing: Neurological reflections on an unusual phenomenon. *J Neurol Neurosurg Psychiatr* 2007;78: 5–13.
5646. Schott GD,Wills MR. Myopathy in hypophosphatemic osteomalacia presenting in adult life. *J Neurol Neurosurg Psychiatry* 1975;38:297–304.
5647. Schott GD, Wyke MA. Obligatory bimanual associated movements. *J Neurol Sci* 1977;33:301–12.
5648. Schott J. A neurological MRI menagerie. *Practical Neurol* 2007;7:186–90.
5649. Schrader J, Stovner L, Obelieniene D. Examination of the diagnostic validity of 'headache attributed to whiplash injury': A controlled, prospective study. *Eur J Neurology* 2006;13:1226–32.
5650. Schrag A, Selai C, Jahanshahi M et al. The EG-5D - a generic quality of life measure - is a useful instrument to measure quality of life in patients with Parkinson's disease. *J Neurol Neurosurg Psychiatry* 2000;68:67–73
5651. Schrag A, Trimble M, Quinn N et al. The syndrome of fixed dystonia: An evaluation of 103 patients. *Brain* 2005;127:2360–72.
5652. Schreiber MM, McGregor JG. Pseudolymphoma syndrome. A sensitivity to anticonvulsant drugs. *Arch Derm* 1968;97:297–300.
5653. Schroder JM, Kramer KG, Hopf HC. Granular nuclear inclusion body disease. *Muscle Nerve* 1985;8:52–9.
5654. Schroeder AH. Diagnostico del quiste hidatico cerbral y su tratamiento. *Anales del Instituto de Neurologia (Montevideo)* 1941;3:11–38.
5655. Schroeder AH, Medoc J. Vertebral hydatidosis. *J Nerv Ment Dis* 1952;116:1025–45.
5656. Schubert R, Cracco JB. Familial rectal pain; A type of reflex epilepsy? *Ann Neurol* 1992;32:824–6.
5657. Schuell H. *Differential Diagnosis of Aphasia with the Minnesota Test.* Minneapolis: Univ. Minnesota Press, 1965.
5658. Schuffler M, Pagon RA, Schwartz R et al. Visceral myopathy of the gastrointestinal and genitourinary tracts in infants. *Gastroenterology* 1988;94:892–8.
5659. Schule R, Holand-Letz T, Klimpe S et al. The spastic paraplegia rating scale. *Neurology* 2006;67:430–4.
5660. Schulman LM, David NJ, Weiner WJ. Psychosis as the initial manifestation of adult-onset Niemann-Pick disease. *Neurology* 1995;45:1739–43.
5661. Schulz U, O'Leary CP. Spinal AVM, epidermal nevus and rhabdomyosarcoma: A rare neurocutaneous syndrome? *Neurology* 2001;56:395–7.
5662. Schulz V, Ward D, Moulin DE. Segmental hyperhidrosis as a manifestation of spinal and paraspinal disease. *Can J Neurol Sci* 1998;25:325–7.
5663. Schumacher GA, Beebe G, Kibler RF et al. Problems of experimental trials of therapy in multiple sclerosis: Report by the panel on the evaluation of experimental trials of therapy in multiple sclerosis. *Ann N Y Acad Sci* 1965;122:552–68.
5664. Schuman JS, Lieberman KV, Friedman AH et al. Senior-Loken syndrome (familial renal-retinal dystrophy) and Coat's disease. *Am J Ophthalmol* 1985;100:822–5.
5665. Schurch B, Wichmann W, Rossier AB. Post-traumatic syringomyelia (cystic myelopathy): A prospective study of 449 patients with spinal cord injury. *J Neurol Neurosurg Psychiatry* 1996;60:61–7.
5666. Schurr PH. The Cairns Tradition. *J Neurol Neurosurg Psychiatry* 1990;53:188–93.
5667. Schuster H-P, Dick W. Scoresysteme in der Notfallmedizine? *Anaesthesist* 1994;43:30–5.
5668. Schut JW, Haymaker W. Hereditary ataxia: A pathologic study of five cases of common ancestry. *J Neuropath Clin Neurol* 1951;1:183–213.
5669. Schwalbe MW. *Eine eigentumliche tonische Krampfform mit hysterischen Symptomen.* Berlin: Inaug. Diss., 1907.
5670. Schwankhaus JD, Parisi J, Gulledge WR et al. Hereditary adult-onset Alexander's disease with palatal myoclonus, spastic paraparesis and cerebellar ataxia. *Neurology* 1995;45:2266–71.
5671. Schwartz AS, Marchok PL, Flynn RE. A sensitive test for tactile extinction: Results in patients with parietal and frontal lobe disease. *J Neurol Neurosurg Psychiatry* 1977;402:228–33.
5672. Schwartz CE, Vollmer T, Lee H et al. Reliability and validity of two self-report measures of impairment and disability for MS. *Neurology* 1999;52:63–70.
5673. Schwartz E. Craniometaphyseal dysplasia. *Am J Roentgenol* 1960;84:461–6.
5674. Schwartz GE. Geriatric evaluation by relatives rating instrument. *Psychol Rep* 1983;53:479–88.
5675. Schwartz HG, O'Leary J. Section of the spinothalamic tract in the medulla with observations on the pathway for pain. *Surgery* 1941;9:183–93.
5676. Schwartz JT, Brumback RJ, Lakatos M. Acute compartment syndrome of the thigh. *Am J Med Genet* 1999;85:147–56.
5677. Schwartz MA, Selhorst JB, Ochs AL et al. Oculomasticatory myorhythmia: A unique movement disorder occurring in whipple's disease. *Ann Neurol* 1986;20:677–83.
5678. Schwartz ML, Rowed DW, Schwartz DL. Sunnybrook cord injury scales for assessing neurologic injury and neurological recovery. In Tator CH, ed. *Early Management of Acute Spinal Cord Injury*, pp 7–24. New York: Raven Press, 1982.
5679. Schwartz MS, Swash M. Scapulo-peroneal atrophy with sensory involvement: Davidenkow's syndrome. *J Neurol Neurosurg Psychiatry* 1975;38:1063–7.
5680. Schwartz O, Jampel R. Congenital blepharophimosis associated with an unique generalized myopathy. *Arch Ophthalmol* 1962;68:52–7.
5681. Schwartz RA, Tedesco AS, Stern LZ et al. Myopathy associated with sclerodermal facial hemiatrophy. *Arch Neurol* 1981;38:592–4.
5682. Schwartz S, Mohr A, Knauth M et al. Acute disseminated encephalomyelitis. *Neurology* 2001;56:1313–8.
5683. Schwartzman RJ, McLellan TL. Reflex sympathetic dystrophy: A review. *Arch Neurol* 1987;44:555–61.
5684. Scolding NJ, Joseph F, Kirby PA. Aß-related angiitis: Primary angiitis of the central nervous system associated with cerebral amyloid angiopathy. *Brain* 2005;128:500–15.
5685. Scoppetta C, Vaccario ML, Casali C et al. Distal muscle dystrophy with autosomal recessive inheritance. *Muscle Nerve* 1984;7:478–81.
5686. Scott CR, Bryant JI, Graham CB. A new craniodigital syndrome with mental retardation. *Journal of Pediatrics* 1971;78:658–63.
5687. Scott DGI. Classification and treatment of systemic vasculitis. *Br J Rheumatol* 1988;27:251.
5688. Scott K, Kothari M. Hereditary Neuropathies. *Semin Neurol* 2005;25: 174–84.
5689. Scott O, Macartney FJ, Deverall PB. Sick sinus syndrome in children. *Arch Dis Child* 1976;51:100–5.
5690. Scott OM, Goddard C, Dubowitz V. Quantitation of muscle function in

children: A prospective study in Duchenne muscular dystrophy. *Muscle Nerve* 1982;5:291–301.

5691. Scott RM, Brody JA. Benign early-onset Parkinsons disease: A syndrome distinct from classic post-encephalitis Parkinson disease. *Neurology* 1970;20:400.

5692. Scott TF. Neurosarcoidosis. *Neurology* 1993;43:8–12.

5693. Scott TF, Yager JG, Gross JA. Handcuff neuropathy revisited. *Muscle Nerve* 1989;12:219–20.

5694. Scottish Motor Neurone Disease Research Group. The Scottish motor neurone disease register. *J Neurol Neurosurg Psychiatry* 1992;55:536–41.

5695. Scribanu N, Kennedy C. Familial syndrome with dystonia, nerve deafness and possible intellectual impairment. *Adv Neurol* 1976;14:235–43.

5696. Scrimgeour EM, Mastaglia FL. Oculopharyngeal and distal myopathy. A case study from Papua New Guinea. *Am J Med Genet* 1984;17:763–71.

5697. Scriver CR, Levy HL. Histidinemia 1. *J Inherit Metab Dis* 1983;6:51.

5698. Scriver CR, Pueschel S, Davis E. Hyperbetaalaninemia associated with beta aminoaciduria and gamma aminoacidurea. *N Engl J Med* 1966;174:636.

5699. Seah ABH, Azran MS, Newman NJ. Cat-scratch encephalopathy. *Arch Neurol* 2004;61:145–7.

5700. Seashore CE, Lewis D, Saetveit DL. Seashore Measures of Musical Talents. New York: The Psychological Corporation, 1960.

5701. Sebire G, DeVistor D, Hualt G et al. Coma associated with intense bursts of abnormal movements and long-lasting cognitive disturbances: An acute encephalopathy of obscure origin. *J Pediat* 1992;121:845–51.

5702. Sébire G, Tabarki B, Saunders DE et al. Cerebral venous sinus thrombosis in children: Risk factors, presentation, diagnosis and outcome. *Brain* 2005;128:477–89.

5703. Seckel HPG. *Bird-headed Dwarfs: Studies in Developmental Anthropology Including Human Proportions.* Springfield: Thomas, 1960.

5704. Seckersen ALG. *Neuroscience Biographies.* 1989. (Unpublished Work)

5705. Seddon HJ. Three types of nerve injury. *Brain* 1943;66:237–88.

5706. Seeligmuller O. Ueber spastiche spinale Paralysen bei Kindern. *Amtl Ber Deutsch Naturf U Aertze* 1877;50:299.

5707. Seeligmuller O. On syphilitic neuralgia. *Dtsch Med Wschr* 1883;9:624–5.

5708. Seemenova E et al. Familial microcephaly with normal intelligence, immunodeficiency and risk for lymphoreticular malignancies: A new autosomal recessive syndrome. *Am J Med Genet* 1985;20:639–48.

5709. Segawa M, Hosaka A, Miyagawa F et al. Hereditary progressive dystonia with marked diurnal fluctuation. *Adv Neurol* 1976;14:215–33.

5710. Seifert T, Enzinger C, Ropele S et al. Relapsing acute transverse myelitis: A specific entity. *Europ J Neurology* 2005;12:681–4.

5711. Seitelberger E. Pelizaeus-Merzbacher disease. In Vincken PJ, Bruyn GW eds. *Handbook of Clinical Neurology*, pp 150–202. Amsterdam. North Holland Publishing Co., 1990.

5712. Seitelberger F. Eine unbekannte Form von infantiler lipoidspeicher Krankheit des Gehirns. *Proc 1st Internat Cong Neuropath (Turin)* 1952;3:323–33.

5713. Seitelberger F, Simma A. On the pigment variant of amaurotic idiocy. In Aronson SM, Volk BM eds. *Cerebral Sphingolipidoses*, pp 29–47. New York: Academic Press, 1962.

5714. Seitz RJ et al. Congenital Leigh's disease: Panencephalomyelopathy and peripheral neuropathy. *Acta Neuropathol* 1984;64:167–71.

5715. Selcen D, Ohno K, Engel AG. Myofibrillar myopathy: Clinical, morphological and genetic studies in 63 patients. *Brain* 2004;127:439–51.

5716. Selcen D, Stilling G, Engel AG. The earliest pathological alterations in dysferlinopathy. *Neurology* 2001;56:1472–81.

5717. Selhorst JB, Hoyt WF, Feinsod M et al. Midbrain Corectopia. *Arch Neurol* 1976;33:193–5.

5718. Selhorst JB, Stark L, Ochs A et al. Disorders of cerebellar oculomotor control: II. Macrosaccadic oscillation. *Brain* 1976;99:509–22.

5719. Selye H. The general adaptation syndrome and the diseases of adaptation. *J Clin Endocrinology* 1946;6:117–230.

5720. Selye H. The physiology and pathology of exposure to stress: A treatise based on the concepts of the general-adaptation syndrome and the diseases of adaptation. Montreal: Acta, 1950.

5721. Selye H, Gabbiani G, Tuchweber B. Neurotropic calcergy. *Neurology* 1964;14:1084–90.

5722. Semon F. On the proclivity of the abductor fibers of the recurrent laryngeal nerve to become affected sooner than the adductor fibers, or even exclusively, in cases of undoubted central or peripheral injury or disease of the roots or trunks of the pneumogastric, spinal accessory, or recurrent nerves. *Arch Laryngol* 1881;2:197–222.

5723. Semont A, Freyss G, Vitte E. Curing the BPPV with a liberatory maneuver. *Adv Otorhinolaryngol* 1988;42:290–3.

5724. Sen Gupta PC, Sanyal NN, Bhattacharya B et al. Avitaminosis in Kala-Azar: Preliminary observations. *Indian Med Gaz* 1952;87:444.

5725. Sencer W. Neurological manifestations of the malabsorption syndrome. *J Mt Sinai Hosp* 1957;24:331.

5726. Senelick RC. Ping-Pong alternating gaze deviation. *Neurology* 1976;26:532–5.

5727. Seneviratne U, Gunasekera S. Acute small fibre sensory neuropathy: Another variant of Guillain-Barré syndrome? *J Neurol Neurosurg Psychiatr* 2002;72:540–2.

5728. Serdaru M, Chiras J, Cujas M et al. Isolated benign vasculitis or migrainous vasospasm? *J Neurol Neurosurg Psychiatry* 1984;47:73–6.

5729. Sergent J. A new look at the human split brain. *Brain* 1987;110:1375–92.

5730. Sergott RC. Neuro-ophthalmic evaluation of the red orbit syndrome. *NC* 1983;1:897–908.

5731. Serra A, Leigh RJ. Diagnostic value of nystagmus: Spontaneous and induced ocular oscillations. *J Neurol Neurosurg Psychiatr* 2002;73:615–8.

5732. Serra S, Millgren SI, Bergsholm R et al. Amyotrophic choreo-acanthocytosis. *Acta Neurol Scand* 1986;66:78–82.

5733. Serratrice GT, Azulay J-P, Serratrice J et al. Palmaris brevis spasm syndrome. *J Neurol Neurosurg Psychiatry* 1999;59:182–4.

5734. Serratrice GT, Pellissier JF, Cros D et al. Relapsing eosinophilic perimyositis. *J Rheumatol* 1980;7:199–205.

5735. Serratrice GT, Pouget J, Pellissier JF. Bent spine syndrome. *J Neurol Neurosurg Psychiatry* 1996;60:51–4.

5736. Serratrice GT, Toga M, Pellissier JF. Chronic spinal muscular atrophy and pallidonigral degeneration: Report of a case. *Neurology* 1983;33:306–10.

5737. Serratrice J, Gastaut JL, Dubois D. Peripheral neurogenic atrophy in Marinesco-Garland syndrome. *Rev Neurol* 1973;128:432–41.

5738. Servidei S, Capon F, Spinazzola M et al. A distinctive autosomal dominant vacuolar neuromyopathy linked to 19p13. *Neurology* 1999;53:830–7.

5739. Servidei S, Zeviani M, Manfredi G et al. Dominantly inherited mitochondrial myopathy with multiple deletions of mitochondrial DNA: Clinical, morphologic, and biochemical studies. *Neurology* 1991;41:1053–9.

5740. Seshia SS, McLachlan RS. Aura continua. *Epilepsia* 2005;46:454–5.

5741. Sethi KD, Rivner MH, Swift TR. Ice pack test for myasthenia gravis. *Neurology* 1987;37:1383–5.

5742. Sethi PK, Rao TS. Gelastic, quiritanian and cursive epilepsy. *J Neurol Neurosurg Psychiatry* 1976;39:823–8.
5743. Severinghaus JW, Mitchell RA. Ondine's curse - failure of respiratory center automaticity while awake. *Clin Res* 1962;10:122.
5744. Sevilla T, Cuesta A, Chumillas MJ et al. Clinical, electrophysiological and morphological findings of Charcot–Marie–Tooth neuropathy with vocal cord palsy and mutations in the GDAP1 gene. *Brain* 2003;126:2023–33.
5745. Seybold ME. The office Tensilon test for ocular myasthenia gravis. *Arch Neurol* 1986;43:842–3.
5746. Seyffarth H. The reaction to passive straining of joints (Bending reflex) in patients with frontal lobe lesions. *Brain* 1953;76:457–72.
5747. Seyffarth H, Denny-Brown D. The grasp reflex and the instinctive grasp reaction. *Brain* 1948;71:109–83.
5748. Sghirlanzoni A, Pareyson D, Lauria G. Sensory neuron diseases. *Lancet Neurology* 2005;4:349–61.
5749. Shabtai F, Halbrecht I. Bloom's syndrome, missing Y, hypogonadism and cancer. *Clin Genet* 1980;18:93.
5750. Shader RI, Harmantz JS, Salzman C. A new scale for assessment in geriatric populations: Sandoz clinical assessment-geriatric. *J Am Geriatr Soc* 1974;22:107–13.
5751. Shaikh AG, Miura K, Optican LM et al. A new familial disease of saccadic oscillations and limb tremor provides clues to mechanisms of common tremor disorders. *Brain* 2007;130:3020–31.
5752. Shakir RA, Al-Din ASN, Araj GF et al. Clinical categories of neurobrucellosis. *Brain* 1987;110:213–23.
5753. Shallice T. Phonological agraphia and the lexical route in writing. *Brain* 1981;104:413–29.
5754. Shallice T, Burgess PW. Deficits in strategy application following frontal lobe damage in man. *Brain* 1991;114:727–41.
5755. Shallice T, Warrington EK. Word form dyslexia. *Brain* 1980;103:99–112.
5756. Shamay-Tsoory SG, Tibi-Elhanany Y, Aharon-Peretz J. The green-eyed monster and malicious joy: The neuroanatomical bases of envy and gloating (schadenfreude). *Brain* 2007;130:1663–78.
5757. Shane et al. Hypoparathyroidism with myopathy. *Neurology* 1980;30:192.
5758. Shapiro AK, Shapiro ES, Young JG. *Gilles de la Tourette Syndrome*. New York: Raven Press, 1988.
5759. Shapiro K, Shulman K. Facial nevi associated with anomalous venous return and hydrocephalus. *J Neurosurg* 1976;45:20–5.
5760. Shapiro LJ et al. Metachromatic leukodystrophy without arylsulfatase A deficiency. *Pediat Res* 1979;13:1179–81.
5761. Shapiro WR, Williams GH, Plum F. Spontaneous recurrent hypothermia accompanying agenesis of the corpus callosum. *Brain* 1969;92:423–36.
5762. Sharief MK, Hentges R, Ciardi M. Intrathecal immune response in patients with post-polio syndrome. *N Engl J Med* 1991;325:749–55.
5763. Sharief MK, Priddin J, Delamont RS et al. Neurophysiologic analysis of neuromuscular symptoms in UK Gulf War veterans. *Neurology* 2002;59:1518–25.
5764. Sharp FR, Rando TA, Greenberg SA et al. Pseudochoreoathetosis. Movements associated with loss of proprioception. *Arch Neurology* 1994;51:1103–1109.
5765. Sharpe JA, Hoyt WF, Rosenberg ML. Convergence-evoked nystagmus. *Neurology* 1990;40:161–2.
5766. Sharpe JA, Lo AW. Voluntary and visual control of the vestibulo-ocular reflex after cerebral hemidecortication. *Ann Neurol* 1981;10:164–72.
5767. Sharpe JA, Rosenberg MA, Hoyt WF et al. Paralytic pontine exotropia. *Neurology* 1974;24:1076–81.
5768. Sharpe JA, Silversides JL, Blair RDG. Familial paralysis of horizontal gaze. *Neurology* 1975;25:1035–40.
5769. Shaw C-M, Alvord EC. Cava septi pellucidi et vergae: Their normal and pathological states. *Brain* 1969;92:213–24.
5770. Shaw EB et al. Aminopterin-induced fetal malformation. *Am J Dis Childh* 1968;115:477.
5771. Shaw MDM, Russell JA, Grossart KW. The changing pattern of spinal arachnoiditis. *J Neurol Neurosurg Psychiatry* 1978;41:97–107.
5772. Shaw MW, Falls HF, Neil JV. Congenital aniridia. *Am J Hum Genet* 1960;12:389.
5772a. Shaw PJ, Walls TJ, Newman PK et al. Hashimoto's encephalopathy: A steroid responsive disorder associated with high anti-thyroid antibody titers - report of 5 cases. Neurology 1991;41:228–233.
5773. Sheaff HM. Hereditary myokymia. *Arch Neurol Psychiatry* 1952;68:236–47.
5774. Sheehan HL. Atypical hypopituitarism. *Proc Roy Soc Med* 1961;54:43–8.
5775. Sheehy MP, Marsden CD. Writer's cramp - a focal dystonia. *Brain* 1982;105:461–80.
5776. Sheen VL, Wheless JW, Bodell A et al. Periventricular heterotropia associated with chromosome 5p anomalies. *Neurology* 2003;60:1033–6.
5777. Sheldon JH. On the natural history of falls in old age. *Brit Med J* 1960;2:1685–90.
5778. Sheldon R, Rose S, Connolly S et al. Diagnostic criteria for vasovagal syncope based on a quantitative history. *Eur Heart J* 2006;27:344–50.
5779. Sheldon R, Rose S, Ritchie D et al. *J Am Coll Cardiol* 2002;46:142–8.
5780. Shelley ED, Shelley WB. The fish odor syndrome. *JAMA* 1984;251:253–6.
5781. Shelley WB, Livingood CS. Familial multiple nevi flammei. *Arch Derm Syph* 1949;59:343–5.
5782. Shelton P, Knopman DS. Isolated gait apraxia with bilateral posterior subcortical lesions. *Neurology* 1986;36 **Suppl**:164.
5783. Sher JH, Rimalovski AB, Athanassiades TJ et al. Familial centronuclear myopathy: A clinical and pathological study. *Neurol Minneap* 1967;17:727–42.
5784. Sheridan MD. *The Developmental Progress of Infants and Young Children, 2*. London, UK: Ministry of Health, 1968. (Pamphlet)
5785. Sherman L, Goldberg M, Larson FC. The Achilles reflex: A diagnostic test of thyroid function. *Lancet* 1963;1:243–5.
5786. Sherrington CS. Decerebrate rigidity, and reflex coordination of movements. *J Physiol* 1898;22:319–32.
5787. Sherrington CS. *The Integrative Action of the Nervous System.* New Haven: Yale University Press, 1906.
5788. Sherrington CS. On plastic tonus and proprioceptive reflexes. *Quart J Exp Physiol* 1909;2:109–56.
5789. Sherrington CS. *The Brain and its Mechanisms.* Cambridge: Cambridge University Press, 1933.
5790. Sherrington CS. *Selected Writings of Sir Charles Sherrington.* Oxford: Oxford University Press, 1979.
5791. Shetan AH, Lawton Smith J, O'Connor P et al. The phantom optic nerve. *J Clin Neuro-Ophthalmol* 1985;5:209–12.
5792. Shevell M. Racial hygiene, active euthanasia, and Julius Hallervorden. *Neurology* 1992;42:2214–9.
5793. Shevell M. Familial acephalgic migraines. *Neurology* 1997;48:776–7.
5794. Shevell M, Rosenblatt B, Silver K et al. Congenital inflammatory myopathy. *Neurology* 1990;40:1111–4.
5795. Shibasaki H. Electrophysiologic studies of myoclonus. *Muscle Nerve* 1988;11:899–907.
5796. See 5795
5797. Shibasaki H. et al. Pigmentary degeneration of the retina in heredodegenerative neurological disease. *Acta Neurol Scand* 1979;59:331–42.
5798. Shibasaki H, Hallett M. Electrophysiological studies of myoclonus. *Muscle Nerve* 2005;31:157–74.
5799. Shibasaki H, Yamashita Y, Neshige R et al. Pathogenesis of somatosensory

evoked potentials in progressive myoclonic epilepsy. *Brain* 1985;**108**: 225–40.

5800. Shibasaki Y et al. Linkage of autosomal recessive familial spastic paraplegia with mental impairment and thin corpus callosum to chromosome 15q13-15. *Ann Neurol* 2000;**48**:108–12.

5801. Shields CL, Eagle RC JR. Pseudo-Schnabel's cavernous degeneration of the optic nerve secondary to intraocular silicone oil. *Arch Ophthalmol* 1989;**107**:714–7.

5802. Shih VE, Efron ML, Moser HW. Hyperornithinemia, hyperammonemia and homocitrullinuria: A new disorder of amino acid metabolism associated with myoclonic seizures and mental retardation. *Am J Dis Childh* 1969;**117**:83.

5803. Shilkin KB, Chen BTM, Khoo OT. Rhabdomyolysis caused by hornet venom. *Brit Med J* 1972;**1**:156.

5804. Shill H, Gerber P. Evaluation of clinical diagnostic criteria for psychogenic movement disorders. *Mov Disord* 2008;**21**:1163–8.

5805. Shin RK, Galetta SL, Ting TY et al. Ross syndrome plus. *Neurology* 2000;**55**:1841–6.

5806. Shinar D, Cross CR, Price TR et al. Screening for depression in stroke patients: The reliability and validity of the center for epidemiologic studies depression scale. *Stroke* 1986;**17**:241–5.

5807. Shipley WC. *Institute of Living Scale.* Los Angeles: Western Psychological Services, 1946.

5808. Shore JW, McCord CD. Anatomical changes in involutional blepharoptosis. *Am J Ophthalmol* 1984;**98**:21.

5809. Short DW. Tardy median palsy following injury. *Glasgow Medical Journal* 1951;**32**:315. (Abstract)

5810. Shorvon HJ. The depersonalisation syndrome. *Proc Roy Soc Med* 1946;**39**:779–92.

5811. Shorvon S. What is nonconvulsive status epilepticus, and what are its subtypes? *Epilepsia* 2007;**48**:35–8.

5812. Shuaib A, Becker WJ. Variants of Guillain-Barré syndrome: Miller Fisher syndrome, facial diplegia and multiple cranial nerve palsies. *Can J Neurol Sci* 1987;**14**:611–6.

5813. Shuaib A, Paasuke RT, Brownell AKW. Central core disease. *Medicine* 1987;**66**:389–96.

5814. Shulman DI, Martinez CR, Bercu BB et al. Hypothalamic-pituitary dysfunction in primary empty sella syndrome in childhood. *J Pediatr* 1986;**108**:540.

5815. Shulman LE. Diffuse fasciitis with eosinophilia: A new syndrome. *Arth Rheum* 1977;**20S**:S205–S215.

5816. Shuman RM, Leech RW, Scott CR. The neuropathology of the nonketotic and ketotic hyperglycinemias: Three cases. *Neurology* 1978;**28**:139–46.

5817. Shuman RM, Selednik LJ. Periventricular leukomalacia: A one-year autopsy study. *Arch Neurol* 1980;**37**:231–5.

5818. Shuren J, Geldmacher D, Heilman KM. Nonoptic aphasia. *Neurology* 1993;**43**:1900–7.

5819. Shy GM, Drager GA. A neurological syndrome associated with orthostatic hypotension. *Arch Neurol* 1960;**2**:511–27.

5820. Shy GM, Engel WK, Somers JE et al. Nemaline myopathy, a new congenital myopathy. *Brain* 1963;**86**:793–810.

5821. Shy GM et al. A generalized disorder of nervous system, skeletal muscle and heart resembling Refsum's syndrome and Hurler's syndrome. *Am J Med* 1967;**42**:163.

5822. Shy GM, Gonatas NK, Perez M. Two childhood myopathies with abnormal mitochondria: I. megaconial myopathy. II. pleoconial myopathy. *Brain* 1966;**89**:133–58.

5823. Shy GM, Magee KR. A new congenital non-progressive myopathy. *Brain* 1956;**79**:610–21.

5824. Shy ME, Blake J, Krajewski K et al. Reliability and validity of the CMT neuropathy score as a measure of disability. *Neurology* 2005;**64**:1209–14.

5825. Shy ME, Rowland LP, Smith T et al. Motor neurone disease and plasma cell dyscrasia. *Neurology* 1986;**36**:1429–32.

5826. Siao Tick Chong P, Tian D et al. Facial onset sensory and motor neuronopathy (FOSMN syndrome): A novel syndrome in neurology. *Brain* 2006;**129**:3384–90.

5827. Siddall PJ, McClelland J. Non-painful sensory phenomena after spinal cord injury. *J Neurol Neurosurg Psychiatry* 1999;**66**:617–22.

5828. Siebert M, Markowitsch HJ, Bartel P. Amygdala, affect and cognition: Evidence from 10 patients with Urbach-Wiethe disease. *Brain* 2003;**126**:2627–37.

5829. Siemen HW. Siemen syndrome. *Arch Derm Syph* 1926;**152**:372–80.

5830. Siintola E, Partanen S, Strömme P et al. Cathepsin D deficiency underlies congenital human neuronal ceroid-lipofuscinosis. *Brain* 2006;**129**:1438–45.

5831. Silber E, Sonnenberg P, Collier DJ et al. Clinical features of headache at altitude. *Neurology* 2003;**60**:1167–71.

5832. Silberstein SD. Tension-type headaches. *Headache* 1994;**34**:S2–S7.

5833. Silberstein SD, Lipton RB, Sliwinski M et al. Classification of daily and near-daily headaches. *Neurology* 1996;**47**:871–5.

5834. Silburn PA, Nicholson GA, Teh BT et al. Charcot–Marie–Tooth disease and Noonan syndrome with giant proximal nerve hypertrophy. *Neurology* 1998;**50**:1067–73.

5835. Silver JR. Familial spastic paraplegia with amyotrophy of the hands. *Ann Hum Genet* 1966;**30**:69–73.

5836. Silver MM, Gilbert JJ, Stewart S et al. Morphologic and morphometric analysis of muscle in X-linked myotubular myopathy. *Human Pathology* 1986;**17**:1167–78.

5837. Silverdale MA, Schneider SA, Bhatia KP et al. The spectrum of orolingual tremor: A proposed classification system. *Mov Disord* 2008;**23**:159–65.

5838. Silverman FN et al. Cerebro-costo-mandibular syndrome. *J Pediatr* 1980;**97**:406–16.

5839. Silverman IE, Liu GT, Volpe NJ et al. The crossed paralyses. *Arch Neurol* 1994;**52**:635–8.

5840. Silverstein A, Siltzbach LE. Muscle involvement in Sarcoidosis. *Arch Neurol* 1969;**21**:235–41.

5841. Silvis SE, Paragas PD. Paresthesias, weakness, seizures and hypophosphatemia in patients receiving hyperalimentation. *Gastroenterology* 1972;**62**:513–20.

5842. Sima AAF, Caplan M, D'Amato CJ et al. Fulminant multiple system atrophy in a young adult presenting as motor neurone disease. *Neurology* 1993;**43**: 2031–5.

5843. Simell O et al. Lysinuria protein intolerance. *Am J Med* 1975;**59**:229.

5844. Simmonds NJ, Hoffbrand BI. Contracturing granulomatous myositis: A separate entity. *J Neurol Neurosurg Psychiatry* 1990;**53**:998–1000.

5845. Simmons Z, Felgoise FH, Bremer BA et al. The ALSSQOL. *Neurology* 2006;**67**:1659–64.

5846. Simon A, Kremer HPH, Wevers RA et al. Mevalonate kinase deficiency. *Neurology* 2004;**62**:994–7.

5847. Simon DB, Ringel SP, Sufit RL. Clinical spectrum of fascial inflammation. *Muscle Nerve* 1982;**5**:525–37.

5848. Simon DK, Nishino S, Scammell TE. Mistaken diagnosis of psychogenic gait disorder in a man with status cataplecticus (Limp Man Syndrome). *Mov Disord* 2004;**19**:838–40.

5849. Simon F, Slatt BK. Light-induced nystagmus. *Can J Ophthalmol* 1971;**6**:128–32.

5850. Simon LT, Horoupian DS, Dorfman LJ et al. Polyneuropathy, ophthalmoplegia, leukoencephalopathy, and intestinal pseudo-obstruction: POLIP syndrome. *Ann Neurol* 1990;**28**:349–60.

5851. Simon LT, Ricuarte GA, Forno LS. Chronic idiopathic ataxic neuropathy. *Acta Neuropathologica* 1989;**79**:104–7.

5852. Simon RP. Neurosyphilis. *Arch Neurol* 1985;42:606–13.
5853. Simone DA, Alreja M, LaMotte RH. Psychophysical studies of the itch sensation and itchy skin ("allokinesis") produced by intracutaneous injection of histamine. *Somatosens Motor Res* 1991;8:271–9.
5854. Simons RC. Resolution of the latah paradox. *J Nerv Ment Dis* 1980;168: 195–206.
5855. Simpson CA. Practical use of the ring finger in sensory conduction for the early carpal Tunnel syndrome. *Can J Neurol Sci* 1978;5:353.
5856. Simpson DM. Pseudoneurogenic thoracic outlet syndrome. *Muscle Nerve* 1994;17:242–4.
5857. Simpson DM, Bender AN, Farraye J et al. Human immunodeficiency virus wasting syndrome may represent a treatable myopathy. *Neurology* 1990;40:535–8.
5858. Simpson DM, Olney RK. Peripheral neuropathies associated with human immunodeficiency virus infection. In Dyck PJ ed. *Neurological Clinics: Peripheral Neuropathy*, pp 685–711. Philadelphia: Saunders, 1992.
5859. Simpson GM, Lee JH, Zoubokb L. A rating scale of Tardive dyskinesia. *Psychopharmacol Berlin* 1979;64:171–9.
5860. Sinclair DC. Cutaneous sensation and the doctrine of Specific Energy. *Brain* 1955;78:584–614.
5861. Singer HS, Naidu S. Rett syndrome. *Neurology* 2001;56:582–5.
5862. Singer MA, Statland JM, Wolfe GI et al. Primary lateral sclerosis. *Muscle & Nerve* 2007;35:291–302.
5863. Singh A, Jolly SS, Bansal BC. Skeletal flourosis and its neurological complications. *Lancet* 1961;1:197.
5864. Singh B, Jamil A, Al-Shahwah SA et al. Choroido-cerebral calcification syndrome with retardation. *Neurology* 1993;43:2387–9.
5865. Singh H, Sham R. Heredofamilial ataxia with muscle fasciculations. *Brit J Cln Pract* 1964;18:91–2.
5866. Singh N, Grewal MS, Austin JH. Familial anosmia. *Arch Neurol* 1970;22:40–4.
5867. Singh N, Sachdev KK, Susheela AK. Juvenile muscular atrophy localized to arms. *Arch Neurol* 1980;37:297–9.
5868. Singh R, Scheffer IE, Crossland K et al. Generalized epilepsy with febrile seizures plus: A common childhood-onset genetic epilepsy syndrome. *Ann Neurol* 1999;45:75–81.
5869. Singleton EB et al. Peripheral dysostosis. *Am J Roentgenol* 1960;84:499–505.
5870. Sinha D, Zemlan FP, Nelson S et al. A new scale for assessing behavioral agitation in dementia. *Psychiatry Res* 1992;41:73–88.
5871. Sinniah D, Lin HP, Loh TG. Inhibitory epilepsy. *Aust NZ J Med* 1979;9:448–50.
5872. Sinnreich M, Klein CJ, Daube JR et al. Chronic immune sensory polyradiculopathy. *Neurology* 2004;63:1662–9.
5873. Sipe JC, Knobler RL, Braheny SL et al. A neurological rating scale for use in multiple sclerosis. *Neurology* 1984;34:1368–72.
5874. Sipila I, Simell O, Rapola J et al. Gyrate atrophy of the choroid and retina with hyperornithinemia: Tubular aggregates and Type 2 fiber atrophy in muscle. *Neurology* 1979;29:996–1005.
5875. Siqueira EB, Murray KJ. Calcified aneurysm of the vein of Galen. *Neurochirurgia* 1972;15:106–12.
5876. Siva A. Vasculitis of the nervous system. *J Neurol* 2001;248:451–68.
5877. Sjaastad O, Apfelbaum R, Caskey W et al. Chronic paroxysmal hemicrania: The clinical manifestations. *Uppsala J Med Psy* 1980;31:27–35.
5878. Sjaastad O, Berstad J, Gjesdahl P et al. Homocarnosinosis. *Acta Neurol Scand* 1976;53:275–90.
5879. Sjaastad O, deSouza CD, Fragoso YD et al. Cluster headache: On the significance of so-called minibouts. *Cephalalgia* 1988;8:285–91.
5880. Sjaastad O, Fredriksen TA, Pfaffenrath V. Cervicogenic headache: Diagnostic criteria. *Headache* 1990;30:725–6.
5881. Sjaastad O, Saunte C, Salveson R et al. Shortlasting, unilateral neuralgiform headache attacks with conjunctival injection, tearing, sweating, and rhinorrhea. *Cephalalgia* 1989;9:147–56.
5882. Sjaastad O, Spierings ELH. Hemicrania continua: Another headache absolutely responsive to indomethacin. *Cephalalgia* 1984;4:65–70.
5883. Sjögren HSC. Zur Kenntnis der Keratoconjunctivitis sicca (Keratitis filiformis bei hypofunktion der Tranendrusen). *Acta Ophth Kopenhagen* 1933;2:151.
5884. Sjögren T, Larsson T. Oligophrenia in combination with congenital ichthyosis and spastic disorders. A clinical and genetic study. *Acta Psychiatrica et Neurologica* 1957;(Suppl.113):1–112.
5885. Skelton AK, Fried RA. Headphone neuralgia. *N Engl J Med* 1995;333: 1786–7.
5886. Skinner HA. *The Origin of Medical Terms*. Baltimore: Williams and Wilkins, 1949.
5887. Skipper JJ, Barnes GR. Eye movements induced by linear acceleration are modified by visualisation of imaginary targets. *Acta Otolaryngol* 1989;S.468:289–93.
5888. Skre H. Unusual type of neural muscular atrophy with a possible X-linked inheritance pattern. *Acta Neurol Scand* 1978;58:249–60.
5889. Slater E. Diagnosis of hysteria. *Brit Med J* 1965;1:1395–9.
5890. Slater E, Beard AW, Glitheroe E. The schizophrenia-like psychosis of epilepsy. *Br J Psychiatry* 1963;109:95–150.
5891. Slavotinek A, Tifft C. Fraser syndrome and cryptophthalmos: Review of the diagnostic criteria and evidence for phenotypic modules in complex malformation syndromes. *J Med Genet* 2002;39:623–33.
5892. Sluder G. The role of the sphenopalatine (or Meckel's) ganglion in nasal headaches. *NY Med J* 1908;87:989–90.
5893. Sly WS, Lang R, Avioli J et al. Recessive osteopetrosis: New clinical phenotype. *Am J Hum Genet* 1972;24:34A.
5894. Sly WS, Quinton BA, McAlister WH et al. Beta glucuronidase deficiency. *J Pediatr* 1973;82:249–57.
5895. Smaje JC, McLellan DL. Depth sense aesthesiometry: An advance in the clinical assessment of sensation of the hands. *J Neurol Neurosurg Psychiatry* 1981;44:950–6.
5896. Small RG. Coats' disease and muscular dystrophy. *Trans Am Acad Ophthal Otolaryng* 1968;72:225–31.
5897. Smit LS, Roofthooft D, van Ruissen F et al. Congenital hypomyelinating neuropathy, a long term follow-up study in an affected family. *Neuromuscular Disorders* 2008;18:59–62.
5898. Smith JL. Whence pseudotumor cerebri? *J Clin Neuro-Ophthalmol* 1985;5:55–6.
5899. Smith A. *Symbol Digit Modalities Test Manual*. Los Angeles: Western Psychological Services, 1973.
5900. Smith AB. Unilateral hereditary deafness. *Lancet* 1939;2:1172–3.
5901. Smith AG, Urbanits S, Blaivas M et al. Clinical and pathologic features of focal myositis. *Muscle Nerve* 2000;23:1569–75.
5902. Smith AJ, Strang LB. An inborn error of metabolism with the urinary excretion of alpha-hydroxy-butyric acid and phenylpyruvic acid. *Arch Dis Child* 1958;33:109–13.
5903. Smith BE. Inflammatory sensory polyganglionopathies. In Dyck PJ ed. *Neurological Clinics: Peripheral Neuropathy*, pp 735–59. Philadelphia: Saunders, 1992.
5904. Smith CG, Linell EA. Microgyria: A case report. *Neurology* 1959;9:689–93.
5905. Smith DB, Sidman R, Hencke J. A reliable method for localizing both depth and superficially generated EEG potentials. *Neurology* 1983;33(Suppl. 2):70.
5906. Smith DC, Mitchell DA, Peterson GW et al. Medial brachial fascial compartment syndrome: Anatomic basis of neuropathy after transaxillary arteriopathy. *Radiology* 1989;173:149–54.

5907. Smith DP. Diagnostic criteria in dominantly inherited juvenile optic atrophy. *Am J Optom* 1972;49:183.

5908. Smith DW. The 18 trisomy and 13 trisomy syndromes. *B.D.* 1969;5:67–71.

5909. Smith DW. *Recognizable Patterns of Human Malformations.* Philadelphia: Saunders, 1976.

5910. Smith DW, Lemli L, Opitz JM. Newly recognized syndrome of multiple congenital anomalies. *J Pediatr* 1964;64:210–7.

5911. Smith GM, Egbert LD, Markowitz RA et al. An experimental pain method sensitive to morphine in man: The submaximal effort tourniquet technique. *J Pharm Exper Ther* 1966;154:324–32.

5912. Smith I, Clayton BE, Wolff OH. New variant of phenylketonuria with progressive neurological illness unresponsive to phenylalanine restriction. *Lancet* 1975;i:1108.

5913. Smith IS, Kahn SN, Lacey BW et al. Chronic demyelinating polyneuropathy associated with benign IgM paraproteinemia. *Brain* 1983;106:169.

5914. Smith JR. Accessory enteric formations: A classification and nomenclature. *Arch Dis Child* 1960;35:87.

5915. Smith J, Zellweger H, Affi AK. Muscular form of glycogenosis Type II (Pompe). *Neurology* 1967;17:537–49.

5916. Smith JK, Gonda VE, Malamud N. Unusual form of cerebellar ataxia. Combined dentato rubral and pallido-Luysian degeneration. *Neurology* 1958;8:205–9.

5917. Smith JL. Whence pseudotumor cerebri? *J Clin Neuro-Ophthalmol* 1985;5:55–6.

5918. Smith JL, Cogan DG. Internuclear ophthalmoplegia - a review of 58 cases. *Arch Ophthalmol* 1959;61:687.

5919. Smith JL, David NJ. Internuclear ophthalmoplegia: Two new clinical signs. *Neurology* 1964;14:307.

5920. Smith JL, David NJ, Klintworth GK. Skew deviation. *Neurology* 1964;14:96–105.

5921. Smith JL, Flynn JT, Spiro JT. Monocular vertical oscillations of amblyopia. *J Clin Neuro-Ophthalmol* 1982;2:85–91.

5922. Smith LA, Moersch HJ, Love JG. Superior laryngeal neuralgia. *Proc Staff Meet Mayo Clin* 1941;16:164–7.

5923. Smith ME, Katz DA, Harris JO et al. Systemic histiocytosis presenting as multiple sclerosis. *Ann Neurol* 1993;33:549–54.

5924. Smith MT, Huntington HW. Inverse cerebellum and occipital encephalocele: A dorsal fusion defect. *Neurology* 1977;27:246–51.

5925. Smith NJ, Espir ML, Matthews WB. Familial myoclonus epilepsy with ataxia and added features of Friedreich's ataxia and peroneal muscular atrophy. *Brain* 1978;101:461–72.

5926. Smith P. If it's not epilepsy. . . *J Neurol Neurosurg Psychiatry* 2001;70:ii9–ii14.

5927. Smith R, Stern G. Myopathy osteomalacia and hyperparathyroidism. *Brain* 1967;90:593–602.

5928. Smith WT, French JM, Gottsman M et al. Cerebral complications of Whipple's disease. *Brain* 1965;88:137–50.

5929. Sneddon IB. Cerebrovascular lesions and livedo reticularis. *Brit J Dermatol* 1965;77:180–5.

5930. Sneddon W, Mellor CS, Martin JR. Hypertryptophanemia in two mentally subnormal siblings. *N Engl J Med* 1982;307:1405.

5931. Snider WD, Simpson DM, Nielsen S et al. Neurological complications of acquired immunodeficiency syndrome. *Ann Neurol* 1983;14:403–18.

5932. Snorrasson E. Cranial deformation in the reign of Akhnaton. *Bull Med Hist* 1946;20:601–10.

5933. Snowden JS, Mann DMA, Neary D. Distinct neuropsychological characteristics in Creutzfeldt-Jakob disease. *J Neurol Neurosurg Psychiatry* 2002;73:613–4.

5934. Snyder TM, Little BW, Roman-Campos G et al. Successful treatment of familial idiopathic lipid storage myopathy with L-carnitine and a modified lipid diet. *Neurology* 1982;32:1106–15.

5935. Snyderman SE. Clinical aspects of disorders of the urea cycle. *Pediatrics* 1981;68:284–9.

5936. Snyderman SE et al. Argininemia. *J Pediatr* 1975;90:563.

5937. So YT, Olney RK. Acute lumbosacral polyradiculopathy in acquired immunodeficiency syndrome: Experience in 23 patients. *Ann Neurol* 1994;35:53–8.

5938. Sobrido MJ, Fernández JM, Fontoira E et al. Autosomal dominant congenital fibre type disproportion: A clinicopathological and imaging study of a large family. *Brain* 2005;128:1716–27.

5939. Sobue I, Saito N, Lida M et al. Juvenile type of distal and segmental muscular atrophy of upper extremities. *Ann Neurol* 1978;3:429–32.

5940. Sockeel P, Dujardin K, Devos D et al. The Lille apathy rating scale (LARS), a new instrument for detecting and quantifying apathy: Validation in Parkinson's disease. *J Neurol Neurosurg Psychiatry* 2006;77:579–84.

5941. Soffer D, Grotsky HW, Rapin I et al. Cockayne syndrome: Unusual neuropathological findings and review of the literature. *Ann Neurol* 1979;6:340–8.

5942. Sogg RL, Hoyt WF, Boldrey E. Spastic paretic facial contracture. *Neurology* 1963;13:607–12.

5943. Solders G, Andersson T, Borin Y et al. Electroneurography index: A standardized neurophysiological method to assess peripheral nerve function in patients with polyneuropathy. *Muscle Nerve* 1993;16:941–6.

5944. Solomon DH, Barohn RJ, Bazan C et al. The thalamic ataxia syndrome. *Neurology* 1994;44:810–4.

5945. Solomon GE, Hilal SK, Gold AP, Carter S. Natural history of acute hemiplegia in childhood. *Brain* 1970;93:107–20.

5946. Solomon S. Chronic post traumatic neck and head pain. Headache 2005;45:53–67.

5947. Solomon S, Karfunkel P, Gugliemo KM. Migraine-cluster headache syndrome. *Headache* 1985;25:236–9.

5948. Solomon T, Dung NM, Kneen R et al. Japanese encephalitis. *J Neurol Neurosurg Psychiatry* 2000;68:405–15.

5949. Sommer C, Ringelstein EB, Biniek R et al. Adult Toxocara canis encephalitis. *J Neurol Neurosurg Psychiatry* 1994;57:229–31.

5950. Sommerville RB, Noble JM, Vonsattel JP et al. Eosinophilic vasculitis in an isolated central nervous system distribution. *J Neurol Neurosurg Psychiatr* 2007;78:85–8.

5951. Sone J, Hishikawa N, Koike H et al. Neuronal intranuclear, hyaline inclusion disease, showing motor-sensory and autonomic neuropathy. *Neurology* 2005;65:1538–43.

5952. Sonninen V, Savontaus M-L. Hereditary multi-infarct dementia. *Europ Neurol* 1987;27:209–15.

5953. Sonoo M. Abductor sign: A reliable new sign to detect unilateral non-organic paresis of the lower limb. *J Neurol Neurosurg Psychiatry* 2004;75:121–5.

5954. Sorenson EJ, Sima AAF, Blaivas M et al. Clinical features of perineuritis. *Muscle Nerve* 1997;20:1153–7.

5955. Soros P, Vo O, Husstedt I-W et al. Phantom eye syndrome. *Neurology* 2003;60:1542–3.

5956. Sotaniemi KA. Slimmer's paralysis—peroneal neuropathy during weight reduction. *J Neurol Neurosurg Psychiatry* 1984;47:564–6.

5957. Sotgiu S, Pugliatti M, Rosati G et al. Neurological disorders associated with *Mycoplasma pneumoniae* infection. *Europ J Neurol* 2003;10:165–8.

5958. Sotos JF, Dodge PR, Muirhead D et al. Cerebral giantism in childhood, a report of two cases and a review of the literature. *N Engl J Med* 1964;271:109–16.

5959. Souques AA. Congenital absence of the pectoralis major and minor muscles. *Nouv Icon Salpet* 1902;15:131–7.

5960. Souques AA. On the interosseous or digital phenomenon in organic hemiplegia. *Bull Soc Med Hop Paris* 1907;24:677–8.
5961. Souques AA. Palilalie. *Rev Neurol* 1908;16:340–2.
5962. Souques AA. Rapport sur les syndromes parkinsoniens. *Rev Neurol* 1921;28:534–73.
5963. Souques M, Rosanoff-Saloff M. Camptocormia: Incurvation of the trunk following trauma of the back and lumbar region: Morphological considerations. *Rev Neurol* 1914;28:937–9.
5964. Soylu A, Kasap B, Mehmet T et al. Febrile myalgia syndrome in familial Mediterranean fever. *J Clin Rheumatol* 2006;12:93–6.
5965. Spaide RF, Klara PM, Restuccia RD. Spasmus nutans as a presenting sign of arachnoid cyst. *Pediatr Neurosci* 1986;12:311–4.
5966. Sparrow SS, Cicchetti DV. Diagnostic uses of the Vineland adaptive behavior scales. *J Pediatr Psychol* 1985;10:215–25.
5967. Spector GJ, Druck NS, Gado M. Neurologic manifestations of glomus tumours in the head and neck. *Arch Neurol* 1976;33:270–4.
5968. Spelle L, Boulin A, Tainturier C et al. Neuroimaging features of spontaneous intracranial hypotension. *Neuroradiology* 2001;43:622–7.
5969. Spencer PS. Guam ALS/parkinsonism-dementia: A long latency neurotoxic disorder caused by "slow toxin(s)" in food? *Can J Neurol Sci* 1987;14:347–57.
5970. Spencer PS, Nunen PB, Hugar J et al. Guam amyotrophic lateral sclerosis-Parkinsonism-Dementia linked to a plant excitant neurotoxin. *Science* 1987;237:517–22.
5971. Spencer SE, Walker FO, Moore SA. Chorea-amyotrophy with chronic hemolytic anemia. *Neurology* 1987;37:645–9.
5972. Spengos K, Tsivgoulis G, Toulas P et al. Spinal cord stroke in a ballet dancer. *J Neurol Sci* 2006;244:159–61.
5973. Spens T. History of a case in which there took place a remarkable slowness of the pulse. *Med Commentaries, Edinburgh* 1793;7:458–65.
5974. Spetzler RF, Martin NH. A proposed grading system of arteriovenous malformations. *J Neurosurg* 1986;65: 476–83.
5975. Spiegel EA, Wycic HT, Orchinik C et al. Thalamic chronotaraxis. *Am J Psychiatry* 1956;113:97–105.
5976. Spilker B, Molinek FRj, Johnston KA et al. Quality of life bibliography and indexes. *Med Care* 1990;28:DS1–DS77.
5977. Spillane JD. Familial pes cavus and absent ankle jerks. *Brain* 1940;63:275–90.
5978. Spillane JD. *The Doctrine of the Nerves*. Oxford: Oxford Medical Publications, 1981.
5979. Spillane JD, Nathan PW, Kelly RE, Marsden CD. Painful legs and moving toes. *Brain* 1971;94:541–56.
5980. Spillane JD, Pallis CA, Jones AM. Developmental abnormalities in the region of the foramen magnum. *Brain* 1957;80:11–48.
5981. Spillane JD, Urich H. Trigeminal neuropathy with nasal ulceration: Report of two cases and one necropsy. *J Neurol Neurosurg Psychiatry* 1976;39:105–13.
5982. Spillane JD, Wells CEC. Isolated trigeminal neuropathy: A report of 16 cases. *Brain* 1959;82:391–416.
5983. Spiller WG. Epidural ascending spinal paralysis. *Rev Neur Psychiat* 1911;9: 494–8.
5984. Spiller WG. Akinesia algera. *Arch Neurol Psychiatry* 1933;30:842–84.
5985. Spiller WG, Martin E. The treatment of persistent pain of organic origin in the lower part of the body by division of the anterolateral column of the spinal cord. *JAMA* 1912;58:1489–90.
5986. Spina-Franca A, Mattosinho-Franca LC. Chagas disease and the nervous system. In Spillane JD ed. *Tropical Neurology*, pp 397–407. London: Oxford, 1973.
5987. Spinella GM, Sheridan PH. Research initiatives on Machado-Joseph disease: National Institute of Neurological Disorders and stroke workshop summary. *Neurology* 1992;42:2048–51.
5988. Spira PJ, McLeod JG, Evans WE. A spinocerebellar degeneration with X-linked inheritance. *Brain* 1979;102: 27–41.
5989. Spire J-P, Maselli RA. Episodic nocturnal wandering: Further evidence of an epileptic disorder. *Neurology* 1983;33,(Suppl. 2):215.
5990. Spiro A. Minipolymyoclonus: A neglected sign in childhood spinal muscular atrophy. *Neurology* 1970;20:1124–6.
5991. Spiro AJ, Fogelson MH, Goldberg AC. Microcephaly and mental subnormality in chronic progressive spinal muscular atrophy of childhood. *Dev Med Child Neurol* 1967;9:594–601.
5992. Spiro AJ, Shy GM, Gonatas NK. Myotubular myopathy. *Arch Neurol* 1966;14:1–14.
5993. Spiro JJ, Folgelson MH, Goldberg AB. Microcephaly and mental subnormality in chronic progressive spinal muscular dystrophy of childhood. *Devel Med Child Neurol* 1987;9:594–601.
5994. Spitz MC, Jankovic J, Killian JM et al. Familial Tic disorder, Parkinson disease, motor neurone disease and acanthocytosis. *Neurology* 1985;35:366–70.
5995. Spitzer K, Thie A, Caplan LR, Kunze K. The TOPOSCOUT expert system for stroke diagnosis. *Stroke* 1989;20:1195–201.
5996. Spitzer WO, Skovron MI, Salmi LR et al. Scientific monograph of the Quebec task force on Whiplash-associated disorders. *Spine* 1995;20Suppl.:1S–73S.
5997. Spoor TC, Hartel WC. Orbital myositis. *J Clin Neuro-Ophthalmol* 1983;3:67–74.
5998. Spreen O, Benton AL. Neurosensory Center Comprehensive Examination for Aphasia. Victoria, B.C., Canada: Neuropsychological laboratory, Dept.Psych.Univ.of Victoria, 1969.
5999. Spreen O, Benton AL. Neurosensory Center Comprehensive Examination for Aphasia. Victoria: Univ. Victoria, 1977.
6000. Sprenger JW et al. Cerebrodigital syndrome: A newly recognized formal genesis syndrome in three patients. *Am J Med Genet* 1985;13:24.
6001. Sprofkin BE. Cheiralgia paresthetica – Wartenberg's disease. *Neurology* 1954;4:857–62.
6002. Spruance SL, Bailey A. Colorado tick fever. A review of 115 laboratory confirmed cases. *Arch Int Med* 1973;131:288–93.
6003. Spuler S, Kalbhenn T, Zabozszeza J et al. Muscle and nerve pathology in Dunnigan familial partial lipodystrophy. *Neurology* 2007;68:677–83.
6004. Squire LR. Remote memory as affected by aging. *Neuropsychologia* 1974;12:429–35.
6005. Srinivasan R, Rhodes J. The median-ulnar anastomosis (Martin-Gruber) in normal and congenitally abnormal fetuses. *Arch Neurol* 1981;38:418–9.
6006. Staal A, Went LW. Juvenile amyotrophic lateral sclerosis-dementia complex in a Dutch family. *Neurol Minneap* 1968;18:800–6.
6007. Stacy M, Cardodo F, Jankovic J. Tardive stereotypy and other movement disorders in tardive dyskinesias. *Neurology* 1993;43:937–41.
6008. Stacy M, Jankovic J. Tardive tremor. *Mov Disord* 1992;7:53–7.
6009. Stahl SM, Layzer RB, Aminoff MJ et al. Continuous cataplexy in a patient with a midbrain tumor: The Limp Man syndrome. *Neurology* 1980;30:1115–8.
6010. Stalberg E. Macro EMG. *Muscle Nerve* 1983;6:619–30.
6011. Stalberg E, Bischoff C, Falck B. Outliers, a way to detect abnormality in quantitative EMG. *Muscle Nerve* 1994;17:392–9.
6012. Stalberg E, Chu J, Bril V et al. Automatic analysis of the EMG interference pattern. *EEG Clin Neurophysiol* 1983;56: 672–81.
6013. Stam J. The tibialis anterior reflex in healthy subjects and in L5 radicular

compression. *J Neurol Neurosurg Psychiatry* 1988;51:397–402.

6014. Stamey W, Jankovic J. The other Babinski sign in hemifacial spasm. *Neurology* 2007;69:402–3.

6015. Stanley CH. New genetic defects in mitochondrial fatty acid oxidation and carnitine deficiency. *Adv Pediatr* 1987;34:59.

6016. Stanton-Hicks M, Janig W, Hassenbrusch S et al. Reflex sympathetic dystrophy: Changing concepts and taxonomy. *Pain* 1995;63:127–33.

6017. Stanzac DE, White DE, White JG et al. Comprehensive level of consciousness scale. *J Neurosurg* 1984;60:955–60.

6018. Stapleton SR, Harkness W, Wilking PR et al. Gliomyosarcoma: An immunohostochemical analysis. *J Neurol Neurosurg Psychiatry* 1992;55:728–30.

6019. Stargardt KB. On progressive familial macular degeneration. *Graefe's Arch Ophth* 1909;71:534–51.

6020. Stark P. Etude clinique et genetique d'une famille atteinte d'atrophie musculaire progressive neuronale (amyotrophie de Charcot–Marie). *J Genet Hum* 1958;7: 1–32.

6021. Starkstein S, Federoff JP, Price TR et al. Catastrophic reaction after cerebrovascular lesions: Frequency, correlates and validation of a scale. *J Psychiatr Clin Neurosci* 1993;5:189–94.

6022. Starmark J-E, Stalhammar D, Holmgren E. The reaction level scale (RLS85): Manual and guidelines. *Acta Neurochir* 1988;91:12–20.

6023. Starr A, Picton TW, Siininger Y et al. Auditory neuropathy. *Brain* 1996;119:741–53.

6024. Staunton T, Andermann F, Melanson D et al. Focal macrogyria: A recognizable developmental disorder presenting with intractable focal seizures. *Ann Neurol* 1983;14:152A.

6025. Staunton TG. A left-sided hemisensory phenomenon more common in women. *Canadian Journal of Neurological Sciences* 1994;21(**Suppl.** 2): S.38. (Abstract)

6025a. Starkstein S, Leentjens AFG. The nosological position of apathy in clinical practice. *J Neurol Neurosurg Psychiatry* 2008;79:1088–92

6026. Staunton TG. Traumatic pudendal neuropathy and the dimple sign. *Can J Neurol Sci* 1994;21(**Suppl.** 2): S.63. (Abstract)

6027. Steegman AT, Roberts DJ. The syndrome of the anterior choroidal artery. *JAMA* 1935;104:1695–7.

6028. Steele JC, Richardson JC, Olszewski J. Progressive supranuclear palsy. A heterogeneous degeneration involving the brain stem, basal ganglia and cerebellum with vertical gaze and pseudobulbar palsy, nuchal dystonia and dementia. *Arch Neurol* 1964;10:333–59.

6029. Steere AC. Lyme disease. *N Engl J Med* 1989;321:586–96.

6030. Stein BM, Wolpert SM. Arteriovenous malformations of the brain. 1.Current concepts and treatment. *Arch Neurol* 1980;37:1–5.

6031. Steinman GS, Rorke LB, Brown MJ. Infantile neuronal degeneration masquerading as Werdnig-Hoffmann disease. *Ann Neurol* 1980;8:317–24.

6032. Stengel E. Loss of spatial orientation, constructional apraxia and Gerstmann's syndrome. *J Ment Sci* 1944;90:753.

6033. Stephens FE. Hereditary nerve deafness. *Am J Hum Genet* 1949;1:37–51.

6034. Stephens J, Hoover ML, Denst J. On familial ataxia, neural amyotrophy and their association with progressive external ophthalmoplegia. *Brain* 1958;81:556–66.

6035. Stephens RE. The biomechanical aspects of injuries in elite ballet dancers. *La récherche en danse*, pp 226–8. Paris: University of Paris, Sorbonne, 1986.

6036. Stephenson J. Two types of febrile seizure: Anoxic (syncopal) and epileptic mechanisms differentiated by oculocardiac reflex. *Brit Med J* 1978;2:726–8.

6037. Sterling W. A finger phenomenon like that of Rossolimo or Babinski. *Rev Neurol* 1926;2:82–8.

6038. Sterman AB, Schaumberg HH, Asbury AK. The acute sensory neuronopathy syndrome: A distinct clinical entity. *Ann Neurol* 1980;7:354–8.

6039. Sterman MB, McGinty DJ, Harper PM et al. Developmental comparison of sleep EEG power spectral patterns in infants at high and at low risk for sudden death. *EEG Clin Neurophysiol* 1982;53:166–81.

6040. Stern BJ, Krumholz A, Johns C et al. Sarcoidosis and its neurological manifestations. *Arch Neurol* 1985;42:909–17.

6041. Stern JM. The epilepsy of trisomy 9p. *Neurology* 1996;47:821–4.

6042. Stern K. Severe dementia associated with bilateral, symmetrical degeneration of the thalamus. *Brain* 1939;62:157–70.

6043. Stern LZ, Hall SW. Tornwaldt's disease. *Neurology* 1972;22:1182–5.

6044. Stern MB. The clinical characteristics of Parkinson's disease and Parkinsonian syndromes: Diagnosis and assessment. In Stern MB, Hurtig HM, eds. *The Comprehensive Management of Parkinson's Disease*, pp 33–41. New York: PMA Publishing Corp., 1988.

6045. Sternbach H. The serotonin syndrome. *Am J Psychiatry* 1991;148:705–13.

6046. Sternbach H. The serotonin syndrome. *Neurology* 1998;51:276–9.

6047. Sternberg D. High-speed scanning in human memory. *Science* 1966;153:652.

6048. Stevanin G, Azzedine H, Denora P et al. Mutations in SPG11 are frequent in autosomal recessive spastic paraplegia with thin corpus callosum, cognitive decline and lower motor neuron degeneration. *Brain* 2008;131:772–84.

6049. Stevanin G, Bouslam N, Thobois S et al. Spinocerebellar ataxia with sensory neuropathy (SCA25) maps to chromosome 2p. *Ann Neurol* 2004;55:97–104.

6050. Stevanin G, Durr A, David G et al. Clinical and molecular features of spinocerebellar ataxia type 6. *Neurology* 1997;49:1243–6.

6051. Stevanin G, Paternotte C, Coutinho P et al. A new locus for autosomal recessive spastic paraplegia on chromosome 14q12-q21. *Neurology* 2007;68:1837–40.

6052. Stevens DL, Matthews WB. Cryptogenic drop attacks: An affliction of women. *Brit Med J* 1973;1:439–42.

6053. Stevens H. Jumping Frenchmen of Maine. *Arch Neurol* 1965;12:311–4.

6054. Stevenson VL, Hardie RJ. Acanthocytosis and neurological disorders. *J Neurol* 2001;248:87–94.

6055. Stewart BM. The hypertrophic neuropathy of acromegaly. *Arch Neurol* 1966;14:107–10.

6056. Stewart JD. Diabetic truncal neuropathy: Topography of the sensory deficit. *Ann Neurol* 1989;25:233–8.

6057. Stewart JD, Low PA, Fealey RD. Distal small fiber neuropathy: Results of tests of sweating and autonomic cardiovascular reflexes. *Muscle Nerve* 1992;15:661–2.

6058. Stewart JD, Shantz SH. Peri-operative ulnar neuropathies. *Can J Neurol Sci* 2003;30:15–19.

6059. Stewart JM, Bergstrom L. Familial hand abnormality and sensorineural deafness. *J Pediatr* 1971;78:102–10.

6060. Stewart PM, Hensley WJ. Acute polymyopathy. *Brit Med J* 1981;283:1578.

6061. Stewart RM, Turnell G, Ehle A. Familial spastic paraplegia, peroneal neuropathy and crural hypopigmentation: A new neurocutaneous syndrome. *Neurology* 1981;31:754–7.

6062. Stewart TG, Holmes G. Symptomatology of cerebellar tumours: A study of forty cases. *Brain* 1904;27:522–91.

6063. Stibler H, Blennow G, Kristiannsson B et al. Carbohydrate-deficient glycoprotein syndrome: Clinical expression in adults with a new metabolic disease. *J Neurol Neurosurg Psychiatry* 1994;57:552–6.

6064. Stickler GB et al. Hereditary progressive arthro-ophthalmopathy. *Mayo Clin Proc* 1965;40:433–55.

6065. Stickroot FL, Schaeffer RL, Bergo HL. Myasthenia gravis occurring in an infant of a myasthenic mother. *JAMA* 1942;120:1207–9.

6066. Stocks P. Facial spasm inherited through four generations. *Biometrika* 1923;14:311–5.

6067. Stogbauer F, Young P, Kuhlenbaumer G et al. Autosomal dominant burning feet syndrome. *J Neurol Neurosurg Psychiatry* 1999;67:78–81.

6068. Stokes W. Observations on some cases of permanently slow pulse. *Quart J Med Sci (Dublin)* 1846;2:73–85.

6069. Stokke O et al. Beta-methyl-crotonol-CoA-carboxylase deficiency: New metabolic error in lysine degradation. *Pediatrics* 1972;49:726.

6070. Stoll BA, Andrews JT. Radiation-induced peripheral neuropathy. *Brit Med J* 1966;1:834–6.

6071. Stone BW, Wilson B, Wroot A et al. The assessment of visuospatial neglect after acute stroke. *J Neurol Neurosurg Psychiatry* 1991;54:345–50.

6072. Stone J, Franks AJ, Guthrie JA et al. Scleroderma "en coup de sabre": Pathological evidence of intracerebral inflammation. *J Neurol Neurosurg Psychiatry* 2001;70:382–5.

6073. Stone J, Zeman A, Sharpe M. Functional weakness and sensory disturbance. *J Neurol Neurosurg Psychiatry* 2002;73:241–5.

6074. See 6073

6075. Stone JL, Goodrich JT. The craniopagus malformation: Classification and implications for surgical separation. *Brain* 2006;129:1084–95.

6076. Stone SP, Halligan PW, Wilson B et al. Performance of age-matched controls on a battery of visuo-spatial neglect tests. *J Neurol Neurosurg Psychiatry* 1991;54: 341–4.

6077. Stopford J. Neuritis produced by a wristlet watch. *Lancet* 1922;1:993.

6078. Storch E. On an atypical form of progressive paralysis. *Mschr Psychiat Neurol* 1901;9:401–34.

6079. Stores G. Dramatic parasomnias. *J Roy Soc Med* 2001;94:173–6.

6080. Storey E, Gardner RJM, Knigyht MA et al. A new autososmal dominant pure cerebellar ataxia. *Neurology* 2001;57:1913–5.

6081. Storey JE, Rowlane JTJ, Conforti DA et al. The Rowland universal dementia assessment scale. *Int Psychogeriatr* 2004;16:13–31.

6082. Stormorken H, Sjaastad O, Langslet A et al. A new syndrome: Thrombocytopathia, muscle fatigue, asplenia, miosis, migraine, dyslexia and ichthyosis. *Clin Genet* 1985;28: 367–74.

6083. Stothers HH. Prosper Ménière. *Annals of Otology and Rhinology* 1961;70:319–37.

6084. Stowens D. Neuroblastoma and related tumors. *Arch Pathol* 1957;63:451–9.

6085. Stracciari A, Lorusso S, Pazzaglia P. Transient topographical amnesia. *J Neurol Neurosurg Psychiatry* 1994;57:1423–5.

6086. Strachan H. On a form of multiple neuritis prevalent in the West Indies. *Practitioner (London)* 1897;59:477–84.

6087. Strauss L, Churg J, Zak FG. Cutaneous lesions of allergic granulomatosis: A histiopathologic study. *J Invest Dermat* 1951;17:349–59.

6088. Straussberg R, Basel-Vanagaite L, Kivity S et al. An autosomal recessive cerebellar ataxia syndrome with upward gaze palsy, neuropathy and seizures. *Neurology* 2005;64:142–4.

6089. Straussberg R, Shorer Z, Weitz R et al. Familial infantile bilateral striatal necrosis. *Neurology* 2002;59:983–9.

6090. Streib EW. AAEE minimonograph #27: Differential diagnosis of myotonic syndromes. *Muscle Nerve* 1987;10:603–15.

6091. Streib EW, Sun SF, Yarkowski T. Transient paresis in myotonic syndromes: A simplified electrophysiological approach. *Muscle Nerve* 1982;5:719–23.

6092. Strobos RRJ, Torre Edl, Martin JF. Symmetrical calcification of the basal ganglia with familial ataxia and pigmentary macular degeneration. *Brain* 1957;80:313–8.

6093. Strominger MB, Mincy EJ, Strominger NL. Bilateral internuclear movements ophthalmoplegia with absence of convergent eye movements - clinicopathologic correlation. *J Clin Neuro Ophthalmol* 1986;6:57.

6094. Strong E, Davila J. The cluneal nerve syndrome. *Indust Med* 1957;26:417–29.

6095. Strong MJ. The evidence for ALS as a multisystems disorder of limited phenotypic expression. *Can J Neurol Sci* 2001;28:283–98.

6096. Stroop JR. Studies of interference in serial verbal reactions. *J Exp Psychol* 1935;18:643.

6097. Strother CM, Sackett JF, Crummy AB et al. Clinical applications of computerized fluoroscopy: The extracranial carotid arteries. *Radiology* 1980;136:781–3.

6098. Strumpell EAGG von. Beitrage zur Pathologie des Ruckenmarks. *Arch Psychiatr (Berlin)* 1880;10: 676–717.

6099. Strumpell EAGG von. On acute encephalitis in children. *Jb Kinderheilk* 1885;22:173–8.

6100. Strumpell EAGG von. Uber eine bestimmte Form der primaren kombinierten Systemerkrankungen des Ruckenmarks. *Arch Psychiatr (Berlin)* 1886;17:217–38.

6101. Strumpell EAGG von. Ueber primare acute Encephalitis. *Arch Klin Med* 1890;47:53–74.

6102. Strumpell EAGG von. On the tibialis phenomenon and muscle synergies in spastic pareses. *Dtsch Z Nervenklinik* 1901;20:436–44.

6103. Strupp M, Arbusow V. Acute vestibulopathy. *Curr Opin Neurol* 2001;14:11–20.

6104. See 6103

6105. Stuart JM, Bergstrom L. Familial hand abnormality and sensorineural deafness. *J Pediatr* 1971;78:102–10.

6106. Stübgen J-P. Neuromuscular disorders in systemic malignancy and its treatment. *Muscle Nerve* 1995;18:636–48.

6107. Stubgen J-P. Limb girdle muscular dystrophy: Description of a phenotype. *Muscle Nerve* 1994;17:1449–55.

6108. Stubgen J-P. Neuromuscular disorders in systemic malignancy and its treatment. *Muscle Nerve* 1995;18:636–48.

6109. Stunkard AJ, Grace WJ, Wolfe HG. The night eating syndrome. *Amer J Med* 1955;7:78–86.

6110. Sturge WA. A case of partial epilepsy apparently due to a lesion of one of the vasomotor centers of the brain. *Clin Soc Tr* 1879;12:162.

6111. Sturtevant FM. Zinc deficiency, acrodermatitis enteropathica, optic atrophy, subacute myelo-optic neuropathy and 5, 7-dihalo-8-quinolinols. *Pediatrics* 1980;65:610–3.

6112. Sturznegger M, Newell DW, Douville CM et al. Transcranial and Doppler findings in adolescent stretch syncope. *J Neurol Neurosurg Psychiatry* 1995;58: 367–70.

6113. Suarez GA, Kelly JJ. The Dropped head syndrome. *Neurology* 1992;42:1625–7.

6114. Suarez GA, Opfer-Gehrking TL, Offord KP et al. The autonomic symptom profile. *Neurology* 1999;53:523–8.

6115. Suarez JI, Cohen ML, Larkin J et al. Acute intermittent porphyria: Clinicopathologic correlation. *Neurology* 1997;48:1678–83.

6116. Subramony SH, Filla A. Autosomal dominant spicocerebellar ataxias ad infinitum? *Neurology* 2001;56: 287–9.

6117. Sudeck P. Ueber die acute entzundliche Knochenatrophie. *Arch Klin Chir Berlin* 1900;62:147–56.

6118. Sugar HS. The cryptophthalmos—syndactyly syndrome. *Am J Ophthalmol* 1968;66:897–9.

6119. Sugarman GI, Katakia M, Menkes JH. See-Saw winking in a familial oro-facio-digital syndrome. *Clin Genet* 1971;2: 248–54.

6120. Sugiura K, Muraoka K, Chishiki T et al. The Edinburgh-2 coma scale: A new scale for assessing impaired consciousness. *Neurosurgery* 1983;12:411–5.

6121. Sugiura Y, Aoki T, Sugiyama Y et al. Temperature-sensitive sodium channelopathy with heat-induced myotonia and cold-induced paralysis. *Neurology* 2000;54:2179–81.

6122. Suhr JA, Gunstad J. Postconcussive symptom report: The relative influence of head injury and depression. *J Clin Exp Neuropsychol* 2002;24:981–93.

6123. Sullivan HC, Kaminski HJ, Maas EF et al. Lateral deviation of the eyes on forced lid closure in patients with cerebral lesions. *Arch Neurol* 1991;48:310–1.

6124. Sullivan JJL, Edgley K, Dehoux E. A survey of multiple sclerosis, Part 1: Perceived cognitive problems and compensatory strategy use. *Canadian Journal of Rehabilitation* 1990;4:99–105.

6125. Sumi SM, Bird TD, Nochlin D et al. Familial presenile dementia with psychosis associated with cortical neurofibrillary tangles and degeneration of the amygdala. *Neurology* 1992;42: 120–7.

6126. Summerskill WHJ. Aguecheek's disease. *Lancet* 1955;2:288.

6127. Summerskill WHJ, Molnar GD. Eye signs in hepatic cirrhosis. *N Engl J Med* 1962;266:1244.

6128. Summitt RL. Recessive acrocephalosyndactyly with normal intelligence. *B.D.* 1969;5:35–8.

6129. Sunderland A, Tinson D, Bradley L et al. Arm function after stroke. *J Neurol Neurosurg Psychiatry* 1989;52:1267–72.

6130. Sunderland S. A classification of peripheral nerve injuries producing loss of function. *Brain* 1951;74:491–516.

6131. Sunderland T, Hill JL, Lawlor BA et al. NIMH dementia mood assessment scale (DMAS). *Psychopharm Bull* 1988;24:747.

6132. Sunderland T, Hill JL, Mellow AM, Lawlor BA. Clock drawing in Alzheimer's disease: A novel measure of dementia severity. *J Am Geriatr Soc* 1989;37:725–9.

6133. Sung JH, Ramirez-Lassepas M, Mastro AR et al. An unusual degenerative disorder of neurons associated with a novel intranuclear hyaline inclusion (Neuronal intranuclear hyaline inclusion disease). *J Neuropath Exp Neurol* 1980;39:107–30.

6134. Sunohara N, Mano Y, Ando K et al. Idiopathic dystonia-parkinsonism with marked diurnal fluctuation of symptoms. *Ann Neurol* 1985;17:39–45.

6135. Suomalainen A, Majander A, Wallin M et al. Autosomal dominant progressive external ophthalmoplegia with multiple deletions of mtDNA. *Neurology* 1997;48:1244–1253.

6136. Surtees R. Inherited ion channel disorders. *Eur J Pediatr* 2000;159:S199–S203.

6137. Susac JO. Susac's syndrome. *Neurology* 1994;44:591–3.

6138. Susuki J, Kodama N. Moyamoya disease: A review. *Stroke* 1983;14:104–8.

6139. Susuki K, Atsumi M, Koga M et al. Acute facial diplegia and hyperreflexia. *Neurology* 2004;62:825–7.

6140. Sutherland JM. Familial spastic paraplegia: Its relationship to mental and cardiac abnormalities. *Lancet* 1957;**ii**: 169–70.

6141. Sutherland JM, Tyrer JH, Eadie MJ. Atrophie spino- cérebelleuse familiale avec mydriase fixé. *Rev Neurol* 1963;108:439–42.

6142. Sutherling WW, Hershman LM, Miller JQ et al. Seizures induced by playing music. *Neurology* 1980;30:1001–4.

6143. Sutton GG, Mayer RF. Focal reflex myoclonus. *J Neurol Neurosurg Psychiatry* 1974;37:207–17.

6144. Sutton JR. Mountain sickness. *Neurol Clin* 1992;10:1015–30.

6145. Sutton T. *Tracts on Delirium Tremens, on Peritonitis, and on Some Other Internal Inflammatory Infections, and on the Gout.* London: Underwood, 1813.

6146. Suzuki J, Takaku A. Cerebrovascular moyamoya disease. *Arch Neurol* 1969;20:277–99.

6147. Svien HJ. Jugular foramen syndrome and allied syndromes. *Neurology* 1963;13:796–809.

6148. Swaiman K. Hallervorden-Spatz syndrome and brain iron metabolism. *Arch Neurol* 1991;48:1285–93.

6149. Swaiman KF, Garg BP, Lockman LA. Sea-blue histiocyte and posterior column dysfunction: A familial disorder. *Neurol Minneap* 1975;25:1084–7.

6150. Swan KC. A squint syndrome. *Arch Ophthal Berlin* 1947;37:149–54.

6151. Swan KC. Syndrome of congenital epiblepharon and inferior oblique insufficiency. *Am J Ophthalmol* 1955;39:130–6.

6152. Swanson AG. Congenital insensitivity to pain with anhidrosis. *Arch Neurol* 1963;8:299–306.

6153. Swartz MN. The chronic fatigue syndrome—one entity or many? *N Engl J Med* 1988;319:1726–7.

6154. Swash M. Acute fatal carcinomatous neuromyopathy. *Arch Neurol* 1974;30:324–6.

6155. Swash M. John Hughlings-Jackson: A sesquicentennial tribute. *J Neurol Neurosurg Psychiatry* 1986;49: 981–5.

6156. Swash M, Fox KP, Davidson AR. Carcinoid myopathy. *Arch Neurol* 1975;32:572–4.

6157. Swash M, Heathfield W. Quadriceps myopathy. A variant of the limb girdle dystrophy syndrome. *J Neurol Neurosurg Psychiatry* 1983;46:355–7.

6158. Swash M, Schwartz MS. Familial multicore disease with focal loss of cross striations and ophthalmoplegia. *J Neurol Sci* 1981;52:1–10.

6159. Swash M, Schwartz MS. *Neuromuscular Diseases.* London: Springer-Verlag, 1988.

6160. Swash M, Schwartz MS, Carter ND et al. Benign X-linked myopathy with acanthocytes (McLeod Syndrome). *Brain* 1983;106:717–33.

6161. Swash M, van der Noorts S, Craig JW. Late onset proximal myopathy with diabetes mellitus in 4 sisters. *Neurology* 1970;20:694–9.

6162. Swedo SE, Leonard HL, Rapoport JL et al. A double-blind comparison of clomipramine and desipramine in the treatment of trichotillomania (hair-pulling). *N Engl J Med* 1989;321: 497–501.

6163. Swedo S, Leonard H, Garvey M et al. Pediatric autoimmune neuropsychiatric disorders associated with streptococcal infections: Clinical description of the first 50 cases. *Am J Psychiatr* 1998;155: 264–71.

6164. Sweeney CJ, Gilden DH. Ramsay Hunt syndrome. *J Neurol Neurosurg Psychiatry* 2001;71:149–54.

6165. Sweet RA, Nimgaonkar VL, Devlin B et al. Increased familial risk of the psychotic phenotype of Alzheimer disease. *Neurology* 2002;58:907–11.

6166. Swift TR, Leschner RT, Gross JA. Arm-diaphragm synkinesis: Electrodiagnostic studies of aberrant regeneration of phrenic motor neurons. *Neurology* 1980;30:339–44.

6167. Swift TR, Nichols FT. The droopy shoulder syndrome. *Neurology* 1984;34:212–5.

6168. Swisher H. Semantic Pragmatic syndrome. *Neuropsychologica* 1972;10:137.

6169. Sydenham T. *Schedula monitoria de novae febris ingressu.* London: Kettleby, 1636.

6170. Sylvester PE. Some unusual findings in a patient with Friedreich's ataxia. *Arch Dis Child* 1958;33:217–21.

6171. Symmans WA, Beresford CH, Bruton D et al. Cyclic eosinophilic myositis and hyperimmunoglobuinemia E. *Ann Int Med* 1986;104:26–32.

6172. Symonds CP. Otitic hydrocephalus. *Brain* 1931;54:55.

6173. Symonds CP. Nocturnal myoclonus. *J Neurol Neurosurg Psychiatry* 1953;16: 166–71.

6174. Symonds CP. Thomas Willis. *Brit Med J* 1955;1:119–23.

6175. Symonds CP. A particular variety of headache. *Brain* 1956;79:217–32.

6176. Symonds CP. Cough headache. *Brain* 1956;79:557–68.
6177. Symonds CP. Excitation and inhibition in epilepsy. *Brain* 1959;82:133–46.
6178. Symonds CP. *Studies in Neurology.* London: Oxford Univ. Press, 1970.
6179. Synek VM. Prognostically important EEG coma patterns in diffuse anoxic and traumatic encephalopathies in adults. *Journal of Clinical Neurophysiology* 1988;5:161–74.
6180. Taaka K, Kean EA, Johnson B. Jamaican vomiting sickness: Biochemical investigation of two cases. *N Engl J Med* 1976;295:461–7.
6181. Tabuenca JM. Toxic-allergic syndrome caused by ingestion of rapeseed oil denatured with aniline. *Lancet* 1981;2:567.
6182. Tada K, Wada Y, Arakawa T. Hypervalinemia. *Am J Dis Childh* 1967;113:64.
6183. Taeusch HW, Sniderman S. Neonatal resuscitation. In Taeusch HW, Christiansen RO, Buescher ES eds. *Pediatric and Neonatal Tests and Procedures*, pp 1–3. Philadelphia: W.B. Saunders Co., 1996.
6184. Tagawa A, Ono S, Shibata M et al. A new neurological entity manifesting as involuntary movements and dysarthria with possible abnormal copper metabolism. *J Neurol Neurosurg Psychiatry* 2001;71:780–3.
6185. Tahmoush AJ, Alopnso RJ, Tarmoush GP. Cramp-fasciculation syndrome: A treatable hyperexcitable peripheral nerve disorder. *Neurology* 1991;41:1021–4.
6186. Tahmoush AJ, Alpers DH, Feigin RD et al. Hartnup disease. *Arch Neurol* 1976;33:797–807.
6187. Takahashi H, Nakamura H, Okada E. Hereditary amyotrophic lateral sclerosis, histochemical and electron microscopic study of hyaline inclusions in motor neurones. *Arch Neurol* 1972;27:292–9.
6188. Takahashi H, Ohama E, Naito H et al. Hereditary dentatorubral-pallidoluysian atrophy. *Neurology* 1988;38:1065–70.
6189. Takahata N, Ito K, Yoshimura Y et al. Familial chorea and myoclonus epilepsy. *Neurol Minneap* 1978;28:913–9.
6190. Takamori M, Gutmann L, Crosby TW et al. Myasthenic syndrome with hypothyroidism. *Arch Neurol* 1972;26:326–35.
6191. Takayasu MA. A case with peculiar changes in the central retinal vessels. *Amer J Med* 1962;32:379–(abstract).
6192. Takeuchi H, Hattori N, Misu K et al. Chronic sensory ataxic neuropathy. *Neurology* 2000;54:1008.
6193. Takeuchi Y, Yoshikawa M, Tsujino T et al. A case of aceruloplasminemia: Abnormal serum cereuplasmin protein without ferroxidase activity. *J Neurol Neurosurg Psychiatry* 2002;72:543–5.
6194. Talks SJ, Elston JS. Oculopalatal myoclonus: Eye movement studies. *Eye* 1997;11:19–24.
6195. Tallaksen CME, Dürr A, Brice A. Recent advances in hereditary spastic paraplegia. *Current Opinion in Neurology* 2001;14: 457–63.
6196. Talma S. On acquired myotonia. *Dtsch Z Nervenklinik* 1892;2:210–6.
6197. Talwar D, Smith SA. CAMFAK syndrome: A demyelinating disease similar to Cockayne's syndrome. *Am J Med Genet* 1989;34:194–8.
6198. Tan E-K, Jankovic J. Tardive and idiopathic oromandiblar dystonia: A clinical comparison. *J Neurol Neurosurg Psychiatry* 2000;68:186–90.
6199. Tan EM, Cohen AS, Fines JF et al. The 1982 revised criteria for the diagnosis of systemic lupus erythematosus. *Arth Rheum* 1982;25:1271–7.
6200. Tan N, Urich H. Postictal cerebral hemiatrophy: With a contribution to the problem of crossed cerebellar atrophy. *Acta Neuropathologica* 1984;62:332–9.
6201. Tanaka K, Shimazu S, Oya N et al. Muscular form of glycogenosis type II (Pompe's disease). *Pediatrics* 1979;63:124.
6202. Tanaka Y, Albert ML, Hara H et al. Forced hyperphasia and environmental dependency syndrome. *J Neurol Neurosurg Psychiatry* 2000;68:224–6.
6203. Tandan R, Bradley WG. Amyotrophic lateral sclerosis: Part 1. Clinical features, pathology, and ethical issues in management. *Ann Neurol* 1985;18: 271–80.
6204. Tandan R, Taylor R, Adesina A et al. Benign autosomal dominant syndrome of neuronal Charcot–Marie–Tooth disease, ptosis, parkinsonism and dementia. *Neurology* 1990;40:773–9.
6205. Tandon PN, Bajpai BC. The infantile tremor syndrome. In Spillane JD ed. *Tropical Neurology*, pp 114–9. London: Oxford, 1973.
6206. Tandon PN, Pathak SN. Tuberculosis of the CNS. In Spillane JD ed. *Tropical Neurology*, pp 37–62. London: Oxford, 1973.
6207. Tani T, Yamamoto H, Kimura J. Cervical spondylotic myelopathy in elderly people: A high incidence of conduction block at C3-4 or C4-5. *J Neurol Neurosurg Psychiatry* 1999;66:456–64.
6208. Taori GM, Iyer GV. Neurological complications in tropical Sprue. In Spillane JD ed. *Tropical Neurology*, pp 73–7. London: Oxford, 1973.
6209. Taphoorn MJB, Tulleken CAF, Jansen GH et al. A "soap-bubble" tumour in the brain: Isolated cerebral immunocytoma. *J Neurol Neurosurg Psychiatry* 1998;65:217.
6210. Tapia Garcia A. Un caso de paralisis del lado derecho de la laringe y de la lengua, con paralisis del esterno-cleido-mastoidea y trapecio del mismo lado; accompanado de hemiplejia total temporal del lado izquierdo del cuerpo. *Siglo Med Madrid* 1905;52:211–3.
6211. Tardieu G, Shentoub S, Delarue R. A la récherche d'une technique de mésure de la spasticité. *Neurologue* 1954;91:143–4.
6212. Tariot PN, Mack JL, Patterson MB et al. The behavioral rating scale for dementia. *Am J Psychiatry* 1995;152:1349–57.
6213. Tarlov IM. Cysts (perineurial) of the sacral roots. Another cause (removable) of sciatic pain. *JAMA* 1948;138:740–4.
6214. Tarui S et al. Typical form of glycogenosis type 7 (Tarui's disease) due to phosphofructokinase deficiency, lack of M subunit. *Biochem Biophys Res Comm* 1965;19:571.
6215. Tarui S, Kono N, Kuwajima M et al. Type VII Glycogenoses. *Monogr Hum Genet* 1978;9:42–7.
6216. Tashiro K. Reversed Chaddock method: A new method to elicit the upgoing great toe. *J Neurol Neurosurg Psychiatry* 1986;49:1321.
6217. Tashiro K, Kikuchi S, Itoyama Y et al. Nationwide survey of juvenile muscular atrophy of distal upper extremity (Hirayama disease) in Japan. *Amyotrophic Lateral Sclerosis* 2006;7:38–45.
6218. Tassinari CA et al. Dyssynergia cerebellaris myoclonica (Ramsay Hunt syndrome): A condition unrelated to mitochondrial encephalomyopathies. *J Neurol Neurosurg Psychiatry* 1989;52: 262–5.
6219. See 6218.
6220. Tassinari CA, Bureau M. Epilepsy with myoclonic absences. In Roger J, Bureau M eds. *Epileptic Syndromes in Infancy, Childhood and Adolescence*, London: Eurotext Ltd., 1985.
6221. Tassinari CA, Michelucci R, Genton P et al. Dyssynergia cerebellaris myoclonica (Ramsay Hunt syndrome): A condition unrelated to mitochondrial encephalomyopathies. *J Neurol Neurosurg Psychiatry* 1989;52:262–5.
6222. Tatemichi TK, Desmond DW, Prohovnik I et al. Confusion and memory loss from capsular genu infarction. *Neurology* 1992;42:1966–79.
6223. Tattevin P, Jauréguiberry S, Gangneux JP. Cerebral aspergillosis. *Rev Neurol (Paris)* 2004;160:597–606.
6224. Tatum WO, Coker SB, Ghobrial M, Abd-Allah S. The open opercular sign: Diagnosis and significance. *Ann Neurol* 1989;25:196–9.

6225. Tawil R, Figlwwicz DA, Griggs RC et al. Facioscapulohumeral dystrophy: A distinct regional myopathy with a novel molecular pathogenesis. *Ann Neurol* 1998;43:279–82.
6226. Tawil R, Ptacek LJ, Pavlakis SG et al. Andersen's syndrome: Potassium sensitive periodic paralysis, ventricular ectopy, and dysmorphic features. *Ann Neurol* 1994;35:326–30.
6227. Tay CH. Ichthyosiform erythroderma, hair shaft abnormalities and mental and growth retardation. *Arch Derm* 1971;104:4–13.
6228. Tay CH, Tan YT, Cheah JS et al. Ocular palsies of obscure origin in South East Asia. *J Neurol Neurosurg Psychiatry* 1974;37:739–44.
6229. Tay W. Symmetrical changes in the region of the yellow spot in each eye of an infant. *Trans Ophthal Soc UK* 1880;1: 55–7.
6230. Taybi H. Generalized skeletal dysplasia with multiple anomalies. *Am J Roentgenol* 1962;88:450.
6231. Taylor D, Falconer M, Bruton C et al. Focal dysplasia of the cerebral cortex in epilepsy. *J Neurol Neurosurg Psychiatry* 1971;34:369–87.
6232. Taylor D, Lewis S. Delirium. *J Neurol Neurosurg Psychiatry* 1993;56:742–51.
6233. Taylor DA, Carroll JE, Smith ME et al. Facioscapulohumeral dystrophy associated with hearing loss and Coat's syndrome. *Ann Neurol* 1982;12:395–8.
6234. Taylor DC. One hundred years of epilepsy surgery: Sir Victor Horsley's contribution. *J Neurol Neurosurg Psychiatry* 1986;49:485–8.
6235. Taylor DC, Marsh SM. Hughlings Jackson's Dr. Z. The paradigm of temporal lobe epilepsy. *J Neurol Neurosurg Psychiatry* 1980;43:758–67.
6236. Taylor HA, Thomas GH, Miller CS et al. Mucolipidosis III (pseudo-Hurler polydystrophy). Cytological and ultrastructural observations in cultural fibroblast cells. *Clin Genet* 1973;4: 388–97.
6237. Taylor I, Scheffer IE, Berkovic SF. Occipital epilepsies: Identification of specific and newly recognized syndromes. *Brain* 2004;124:753–69.
6238. Taylor J. The ophthalmological observations of Hughlings Jackson and their bearing on nervous and other diseases. *Brain* 1915;38:391–417.
6239. Taylor KL, Sandberg E, Baum KF. Medial medullary syndrome and meningovascular syphilis. *Neurology* 1994;44:2231–5.
6240. Taylor RA. Heredofamilial mononeuritis multiplex with brachial predilection. *Brain* 1960;83:113–37.
6241. Taylor W. The hand-arm vibration syndrome. *J Roy Soc Med* 1993;86:101–4.
6242. Teasdale GM, Drake CG et al. A universal subarachnoid hemorrhage scale: Report of a committee of the World Federation of neurosurgical societies. *J Neurol Neurosurg Psychiatry* 1988;51:1457.
6243. Teasedale G, Jennett B. Assessment of coma and impaired consciousness: A practical scale. *Lancet* 1974;2:81–4.
6244. Tein I, De Vivo DC, Hale DE et al. Short-chain L-3-hydroxyacyl-CoA dehydrogenase deficiency in muscle: A new cause for recurrent myoglobinuria and encephalopathy. *Ann Neurol* 1991;30:415–9.
6245. Teitelbaum JS, Eliasziw M, Garner M. Tests of motor function in patients suspected of having mild unilateral cerebral lesions. *Can J Neurol Sci* 2002;29:337–44.
6246. Teitelbaum JS, Zatorre RJ, Carpenter S et al. Neurologic sequelae of domoic acid intoxication due to the ingestion of contaminated mussels. *N Engl J Med* 1990;322:1781–7.
6247. Telerman-Toppet N, Khoubesserian P, Bacq M et al. Unclassified familial myopathy resembling Steinert disease, without myotonia. *Muscle Nerve* 1984;7:439–41.
6248. Telfer MA et al. Dominant piebald trait (white forelock and leucoderma) with neurological impairment. *Am J Hum Genet* 1971;23:383–9.
6249. Temkin O. Gall and the phrenological movement. *Bull Med Hist* 1947;21:275–321.
6250. Temtamy SA. Hand malformations. *J Pediatr* 1974;85:345–9.
6251. Temtamy SA, McKusick VA. Synopsis of hand malformations with particular emphasis on genetic factors. *B.D.* 1969;V:125–84.
6252. Tenconi R et al. Chorio-retinal dysplasia, microcephaly, and mental retardation. An autosomal dominant syndrome. *Clin Genet* 1981;20:347–51.
6253. Tenembaum S, Chitnis T, Ness J et al. Acute disseminated encephalomyelitis. *Neurology* 2007;68:S23–S36.
6254. Teng EL, Chui HC. The modified mini-mental state (3MS) examination. *J Clin Psychiatr* 1987;48:314–8.
6255. Teoh HL, Chow A, Wilder-Smith EP. Skin wrinkling for diagnosing small fibre neuropathy: Comparison with epidermal nerve density and sympathetic skin response. *J Neurol Neurosurg Psychiatry* 2008;79:835–7.
6256. Terrence CF, Rao GR, Pepper JA. Neurogenic pulmonary edema in unexpected, unexplained death of epileptic patients. *Ann Neurol* 1980;9:458–64.
6257. Terson A. An unusual ophthalmoscopic sign. *Annales Oculist* 1912;147:410–7.
6258. Terwindt GM, Hann J, Ophoff RA et al. Clinical and genetic analysis of a large Dutch family with autosomal dominant vascular retinopathy, migraine and Raynaud's phenomenon. *Brain* 1998;121:303–16.
6259. Tessitore E, Tessitore A. Tolosa-Hunt syndrome preceded by facial palsy. *Headache* 2000;40:393–6.
6260. Tetreault M, Duquette A, Thiffault I. A new form of congenital muscular dystrophy with joint hyperlaxity maps to 3p23-21. *Brain* 2006;129:2077–84.
6261. Thauvin-Robinet C, Roze E, Couvreur G et al. The adolescent and adult form of cobalamin C disease: Clinical and molecular spectrum. *Neurology* 2008;70:725–8.
6262. The Multi-Society Task Force on PVS. Medical aspects of the persistent vegetative state (2). *N Engl J Med* 1994;330:1572–9.
6263. The Quality Standards Subcommittee of the American Academy of Neurology. Practice parameters for determining brain death in adults (summary statement). *Neurology* 1995;45:1012–4.
6264. The Transverse Myelitis Consortium working group. Proposed diagnostic criteria and nosology of acute transverse myelitis. *Neurology* 2002;59:499–505.
6265. Théaudin M, Saint-Maurice JP, Chapot R et al. Diagnosis and treatment of dural carotid-cavernous fistulas. *J Neurol Neurosurg Psychiatry* 2007;78:174–9.
6266. Theodorakis GN, Markianos M, Livanis EG et al. Central serotonergic responsiveness in neurocardiogenic syncope: A clomipramine test challenge. *Circulation* 1998;98:2724–30.
6267. Theodore WH, Porter RJ, Penryk JK. Complex partial seizures: Clinical characteristics and differential diagnosis. *Neurology* 1983;33:1115–21.
6268. Theunissen EJJM, Huygen PLM, Verhagen WIM. Familial vestibulocerebellar dysfunction: A new syndrome? *J Neurol Sci* 1989;89:149–55.
6269. Thévenard A. L'acropathie ulcéro-mutilante familiale. *Rev Neurol* 1942;74:193–212.
6270. Thiebaut F. Spastic paraplegia and tendinous xanthomata with csf cholesterinosis. *Rev Neurol* 1942;74:313–5.
6271. Thiffault I, Rioux MF, Tetreault M et al. A new autosomal recessive spastic ataxia associated with frequent white matter changes maps to 2q33-34. *Brain* 2006;129:2332–40.
6272. Thomas A. Atrophie lamellaire des cellules de Purkinje. *Rev Neurol* 1905;13:917–24.

6273. Thomas HL. *Hunterian Oration.* London: Royal College of Surgeons, 1827.
6274. Thomas JE, Howard FM. Herpes Zoster. *Neurology* 1972;22:459–66.
6275. Thomas JE, Klass DW. 6 Hz spike and wave pattern. *EEG Clin Neurophysiol* 1968;23:591.
6276. Thomas JE, Schirger A. Idiopathic orthostatic hypotension. *Arch Neurol* 1970;22:289–93.
6277. Thomas JE, Schirger A, Fealey RD et al. Orthostatic hypotension. *Mayo Clin Proc* 1981;56:117–25.
6278. Thomas M, Jankovic J, Suteerawattananon M. Clinical gait and balance scale (GABS): Validation and utilization. *J Neurol Sci* 2004;217:89–99.
6279. Thomas P, Beaumanoir A, Genton P et al. "De novo" absence status of late onset: Report of 11 cases. *Neurology* 1992;42:104–10.
6280. Thomas PK. *Tropical Neuropathies.* 1997;244:482.
6281. Thomas PK, Calne DB, Elliott CF. X-linked scapulo-peroneal syndrome. *J Neurol Neurosurg Psychiatry* 1972;35:208–15.
6282. Thomas PK, Claus D, Jaspert A et al. Focal upper limb demyelinating neuropathy. *Brain* 1996;119:765–74.
6283. Thomas PK, Claus D, King RHM. Autosomal recessive type II hereditary motor and sensory neuropathy with acrodystrophy. *J Neurol* 1999;246:107–12.
6284. Thomas PK, Kalaydjieva L, Youl B et al. Hereditary motor and sensory neuropathy-Russe. *Ann Neurol* 2001;50:452–7.
6285. Thomas PK, Ormerod IEC. Hereditary neuralgic amyotrophy associated with a relapsing multifocal sensory neuropathy. *J Neurol Neurosurg Psychiatry* 1993;56: 107–9.
6286. Thomas PK, Schaumberg HH, Spencer PS et al. Central-distal axonopathy syndromes: Newly recognized models of naturally occurring human degenerative disease. *Ann Neurol* 1984;15:313–5.
6287. Thomas PK, Walker JG. Xanthomatous neuropathy in primary biliary cirrhosis. *Brain* 1965;88:1079.
6288. Thomas PK, Walker RWH, Rudge P et al. Chronic demyelinating peripheral neuropathy associated with multifocal central nervous system demyelination. *Brain* 1987;110:53–76.
6289. Thomas PK, Workman JM, Thage O. Behr's syndrome. A family exhibiting pseudodominant inheritance. *J Neurol Sci* 1984;64:137–48.
6290. Thomas PK, Young E, King RHM. Sandhoff disease mimicking adult-onset bulbospinal neuronopathy. *J Neurol Neurosurg Psychiatry* 1989;52:1103–6.
6291. Thomas PS, Carson NAJ. Homocystinuria: The evolution of skeletal changes in relation to treatment. *Ann Radiol* 1978;21:95–104.
6292. Thomas SV. Neurological aspects of eclampsia. *J Neurol Sci* 1998;155:37–43.
6293. Thomasen E. *Myotonia, Thomsen's Disease, (Myotonia Congenita?), Paramyotonia and Dystrophia Myotonica.* Danmark: Universitetforlaget i Aarhus, 1992.
6294. Thomashevsky AJ, Horwitz SJ, Feingold MH. Acute autonomic neuropathy. *Neurology* 1972;22:251–5.
6295. Thomke F, Hopf HC. Pontine lesions mimicking acute peripheral vestibulopathy. *J Neurol Neurosurg Psychiatry* 1999;66:340–9.
6296. Thompson AJ, Kermode AG, Wicks D et al. Major differences in the dynamics of primary and secondary multiple sclerosis. *Ann Neurol* 1991;29:53–62.
6297. Thompson AJ, Montalban X, Barkhof F et al. Diagnostic criteria for primary progressive multiple sclerosis: A position paper. *Ann Neurol* 2000;47:831–5.
6298. Thompson BM, Corbett JJ, Kline LB et al. Pseudo-Horner's syndrome. *Arch Neurol* 1982;39:108–11.
6299. Thompson CE. Infantile myositis. *Dev Med Child Neurol* 1982;24:307–13.
6300. Thompson HC. Associated movements in hemiplegia: Their origin and physiological significance. *Brain* 1903;26:514–23.
6301. Thompson HS. Binasal field loss. In Thompson HS ed. *Neuro-Ophthalmology*, pp 82–5. Baltimore: Williams and Wilkins, 1979.
6302. Thompson HS, Zackon DH, Czarnecki JSC. Tadpole-shaped pupils caused by segmental spasm of the iris dilator muscle. *Am J Ophthalmol* 1983;96:467.
6303. Thompson P, Obeso JA, Delgado G et al. Focal dystonia of the jaw and the differential diagnosis of unilateral jaw and masticatory spasm. *J Neurol Neurosurg Psychiatry* 1986;49:651–6.
6304. Thompson PN, Carroll WM. Hemimasticatory spasm - a peripheral paroxysmal cranial neuropathy? *J Neurol Neurosurg Psychiatry* 1983;46:274–6.
6305. Thomsen J. Tonische Krampfe in willkurlich beweg lichen Muskeln in Folge von ererbter psychischer Disposition (Ataxia muscularis?). *Arch Psychiatr (Berlin)* 1875;6:706–18.
6306. Thomson MS. Poikiloderma congenitale. *Brit J Dermatol* 1936;48:221–34.
6307. Thrush DC. Congenital insensitivity to pain. *Brain* 1973;96:369–86.
6308. Thrush DC, Holt H, Bradley WG et al. Neurological manifestations of xeroderma pigmentosum in two siblings. *J Neurol Sci* 1974;22:91–104.
6309. Thrush DC, Morris CJ, Salmon MV. Paramyotonia congenita: A clinical, histochemical and pathological study. *Brain* 1972;95:537–52.
6310. Thudichum JLW. *A Treatise on the Chemical Constitution of the Brain.* London: Bailliere,Tindall and Cox, 1884.
6311. Thurston SE, Leigh RJ, Crawford T et al. Two distinct deficits of visual tracking caused by unilateral lesions of cerebral cortex in humans. *Ann Neurol* 1988;23:266–73.
6312. Thuy LF et al. Multiple carboxylase deficiency due to deficiency of biotinidase. *J Neurogenet* 1986;3:357–63.
6313. Thyagarajan D, Bressman S, Bruno C et al. A novel mitochondrial 12SrRNA point mutation in Parkinsonism, deafness and neuropathy. *Ann Neurol* 2000;48:730–6.
6314. Thyagarajan D, Shanske S, Vazquez-Memiji M et al. A novel mitochondrial ATPase 6 point mutation in familial bilateral striatal necrosis. *Ann Neurol* 1995;38:468–72.
6315. Tibbetts RW. Spasmodic torticollis. *J Psychosom Res* 1971;15:461–9.
6316. Tibbles JAR, Cohen MM jr. The proteus syndrome: The elephant man diagnosed. *Brit Med J* 1986;293:683.
6317. Tiberin P, Beller AJ. Observations on so-called brain stones or cerebral calculi. *Neurology* 1963;13:464–76.
6318. Tien R, Arieff AI, Kucharczyk W et al. Hyponatremic encephalopathy: Is central pontine myelinolysis a component? *Amer J Med* 1992;92:513–22.
6319. Tietz W. A syndrome of dominant deaf-mutism associated with albinism showing dominant autosomal inheritance. *Am J Hum Genet* 1963;15:259–64.
6320. Tijssen CC, van Gisbergen JAM, Schulte BPM. Conjugate eye deviation: Side, site, and size of hemispheric lesion. *Neurology* 1991;41:846–50.
6321. Tijssen MAJ, Brown P, Morris HR et al. Late-onset startle induced tics. *J Neurol Neurosurg Psychiatry* 1999;67:782–4.
6322. Tiliket C, Ventre-Dominey J, Vighetto A et al. Room tilt illusion. *Arch Neurol* 1996;53:1259–64.
6323. Tilikete C, Krolak-Salmon P, Truy E, Vighetto A. Pulse-synchronous eye oscillations revealing bone superior canal dehiscence. *Ann Neurol* 2004;56: 556–60.
6324. Tilikete C, Vial C, Niederlaender M et al. Idiopathic ocular neuromyotonia: A neurovascular compression syndrome? *J Neurol Neurosurg Psychiatry* 2000;69: 642–4.
6325. Tim RW, Sanders DB. Repetitive nerve stimulation studies in the Lambert-Eaton myasthenic syndrome. *Muscle Nerve* 1994;17:995–1001.

6326. Tindall RSA et al. Preliminary results of a trial of cyclosporine in Myasthenia Gravis. *N Engl J Med* 1987;316: 719–24.

6327. Tinel J. *Les blessures des nerfs.* Paris: Masson, 1916.

6328. Tinetti ME, Williams TF, Mayewski R. Fall risk index for elderly patients based on number of chronic disabilities. *Am J Med* 1986;80:429–34.

6329. Ting J. Hyperosmolar diabetic non-ketotic coma, hyperkalaemia and an unusual near death experience. *Europ J Emerg Med* 2001;8:57–63.

6330. Tintore M, Rovira A, Rio J et al. Baseline MRI predicts future attacks and disability in clinically isolated syndromes. *Neurology* 2006;67:968–72.

6331. Tinuper P, Montagna P, Cortelli P et al. Idiopathic recurring stupor: A case with possible involvement of the gamma-aminobutyric acid. *Ann Neurol* 1992;31:503–6.

6332. Tinuper P, Montagna P, Plazzi G et al. Idiopathic recurring stupor. *Neurology* 1994;44:621–5.

6333. Tipton RE, Gorlin RJ. Growth retardation, alopecia, pseudo-anodontia, and optic atrophy - The GAPO syndrome: Report of a patient and review of the literature. *Am J Med Genet* 1984;19: 209–16.

6334. Tiwari A, Bansal V, Chugh A et al. Statins and myotoxicity: A therapeutic limitation. *Expert Opin Drug Saf* 2006;5:651–66.

6335. Toda T, Yoshioka M, Nakahori Y et al. Genetic identity of Fukayama-type congenital muscular dystrophy and Walker-Warburg syndrome. *Ann Neurol* 1995;37:99–101.

6336. Todd J. The syndrome of Alice in Wonderland. *Can Med Assn J* 1955;73:701–4.

6337. Todd RB. *Clinical Lectures on Paralysis, Certain Diseases of the Brain.* London: Churchill, 1856.

6338. Tokumaru A, Obata T, Kohyama S et al. Intracranial meningeal involvement in Churg-Strauss syndrome. *Am J Neuroradiol* 2002;23:221–4.

6339. Tollner U et al. Hepta-octatarso-dactyly combined with multiple malformations. *Eur J Pediatr* 1981;136:207–10.

6340. Tolone S. La sindroma Alterna Parabulbar Laterale. *J Nerv Ment Dis* 1952;116: 1017–22.

6341. Tolosa E, Wenning G, Poewe W. The diagnosis of Parkinson's disease. *Lancet Neurology* 2006;5:75–86.

6342. Tolosa ES. Periarteritic lesions of the cavernous syphon with clinical features of a carotid infraclinoid syndrome. *J Neurol Neurosurg Psychiatry* 1954;17:300–2.

6343. Tolosa ES. Clinical features of Meige's disease (idiopathic orofacial dystonia). *Arch Neurol* 1981;38:147–51.

6344. Toma S, Shiozawa Z. Amyotrophic cervical myelopathy in adolescence. *J Neurol Neurosurg Psychiatry* 1995;58: 56–64.

6345. Tomasulo RA. Aberrant conduction in human nerve: Ephaptic transmission? *Neurology* 1982;32:712–9.

6346. Tomelleri G, Palmucci L, Tonin P et al. SERCA1 and calsequestrin storage myopathy: A new surplus protein myopathy. *Brain* 2006;129:2085–92.

6347. See 6346

6348. Tomsak RL et al. Bilateral central scotomas. In Smith JL ed. *Neuro-ophthalmology Focus*, New York: Manor, 1982.

6349. Tondeur M, Ubert J, Vamos E et al. Infantile form of sialic acid storage disorder. *Eur J Pediatr* 1982;139:142–7.

6350. Toole JF, Weeks FD. Stimulation of the carotid sinus in man. *Amer J Med* 1959;27:952.

6351. Topcu M, Gartioux C, Ribierre P et al. Vacuoliting megalencephalic leukoencephalopathy with subcortical cysts, mapped to chromosome 22qtel. *Am J Hum Genet* 2000;66:733–9.

6352. Topcu M, Saatei I, Topucuoglu A et al. Megalencephaly and leukodystrophy with mild clinical course. *Brain Dev* 1998;20:142–53.

6353. Torack RM. Historical aspects of normal and abnormal brain fluids. 1. Cerebrospinal fluid. *Arch Neurol* 1982;39:197–201.

6354. Torack RM. Historical aspects of normal and abnormal brain fluids. 2. Hydrocehalus. *Arch Neurol* 1982;39: 276–9.

6355. Torack RM. Historical aspects of normal and abnormal brain fluids. 3. Cerebral edema. *Arch Neurol* 1982;39:355–7.

6356. Torack RM, Morris JC. Mesolimbocortical dementia: A clinicopathologic case study of a putative disorder. *Arch Neurol* 1986;43:1074–8.

6357. Torkildsen A. A new palliative operation in cases of inoperable occlusion of the Sylvian aqueduct. *Acta Chiurg Scand* 1939;82:117–24.

6358. Tosi L, Rigoli G, Beltramello A. Fibrocartilaginous embolism of the spinal cord: A clinical and pathological reconsideration. *J Neurol Neurosurg Psychiatry* 1996;60:55–60.

6359. Tosun F, Gerek M, Ozkaptan Y. Nasal surgery for contact point headaches. *Headache* 2000;40:237–40.

6360. Tourette Gdl. Étude sur une affection nerveuse caracterisée par l'incordination motrice accompagné d'echolalie et de coprolalie. *Arch Neurol (Paris)* 1885;9:19–153.

6361. Tournev I, Kalydjieva L, Youl B et al. Congenital cataracts-facial dysmorphism-neuropathy syndrome, a novel complex genetic disease in Balkan gypsies: Clinical and electrophysiological observations. *Ann Neurol* 1999;45:742–50.

6362. Tournier-Lasserve E, Iba-Zizen M-T, Romero N et al. Autosomal dominant syndrome with strokelike episodes and leukoencephalopathy. *Stroke* 1991;22:1297–302.

6363. Towfighi J, Gonatas NK, Pleasure D et al. Glue sniffer's neuropathy. *Neurology* 1976;26:238–43.

6364. Townsend JJ, Wolinsky JS, Baringer JR et al. Acquired toxoplasmosis: A neglected cause of treatable nervous system disease. *Arch Neurol* 1975;32:335–43.

6365. Toyka KV. Ptosis in myasthenia gravis: Extended fatigue and recovery bedside test. *Neurology* 2006;67:1524.

6366. Toyokura Y, Takasu T. Clinical features of SMON. *Jap J Med Sci Biol* 1975;28:87–99.

6367. Tozlavanu V, Forget R, Iancu A et al. Prolonged orbicularis oculi activity: A major factor in apraxia of lid opening. *Neurology* 2001;57:1013–8.

6368. Tramer T. *Schweiz Arch Neurol Psychiatr* 1945;55:306–16.

6369. Tranchant C, Auclair M, Mohr M et al. A new peroxisomal disease with impaired phytanic and pipecolic acid oxidation. *Neurology* 1993;43:2044–8.

6370. Tranebjaerg L, Schwartz C, Eriksen H et al. A new X-linked recessive deafness syndrome with blindness, dystonias, fractures and mental deficiency is linked to Xq 22. *J Med Genet* 1995;32: 257–63.

6371. Tranier S, Durey A, Chevallier B et al. Value of somatosensory evoked potentials in saphenous entrapement neuropathy. *J Neurol Neurosurg Psychiatry* 1992;55: 461–5.

6372. Traquair HM. Bitemporal hemiopia: The later stages and the special features of the scotoma. With an examination of current theories of the mechanism of production of the field defects. *Br J Ophth* 1917;1:216, 239,281– 294.

6373. Traquair HM. *Clinical Perimetry.* Edinburgh: Henry Kimpton, 1927.

6374. Traquair HM. *An Introduction to Clinical Perimetry*. London: Henry Kimptom, 1957.

6375. Travers RF. Limbic epilepsy. *J RSM* 1991;84:454–6.

6376. Treft RL et al. Dominant optic atrophy, deafness, ptosis, ophthalmoplegia, dystaxy and myopathy. *Ophthalmology* 1984;91:908–15.

6377. Trelles JO. Aspectes neurologiques de la verruga Peruvienne. *Rev Neurol* 1955;93:357–68.
6378. Tremlett H, Paty DW, Devonshire V. The natural history of primary progressive MS in British Columbia, Canada. *Neurology* 2005;65:1919–23.
6379. Trendelenburg F. Ueber den Gang bei angeborener Huftgelenksluxation. *Dtsch Med Wschr* 1895;21:21–4.
6380. Trenel J. Quelques observations sur le délire aîgu. *Presse Med* 1930;2:257–68.
6381. Trenkwalder C, Paulus W, Walters AS. The restless legs syndrome. *Lancet Neurol* 2005;4:465–75.
6382. Trethowan WH, Enoch M. *Some Uncommon Psychiatric Syndromes.* Bristol: John Wright, 1970.
6383. Trevathan E et al. Diagnostic criteria for Rett Syndrome. *Ann Neurol* 1988;23: 425–8.
6384. Triarhou LC, Cerro M. Freud's contribution to neuroanatomy. *Arch Neurol* 1985;42:282–7.
6385. Triggs WJ, Beric A, Butler IJ et al. A congenital myasthenic syndrome refractory to acetylcholinesterase inhibitors. *Muscle Nerve* 1992;15:267–72.
6386. Triggs WJ, Owens J, Gilmore RL et al. Central conduction abnromalities after electrical injury. *Muscle Nerve* 1994;17:1068–70.
6387. Triggs WJ, Roe CR, Read WJ et al. Neuropsychiatric manifestations of defect in mitochondrial beta oxidation response to riboflavin. *J Neurol Neurosurg Psychiatry* 1992;55:209–11.
6388. Trimble MR. Behavior and personality disturbances. In Bradley WG, Daroff RB et al., eds. *Neurology in Clinical Practice.* London: Butterworth-Heinemann, 2000.
6389. Tristani-Firouzi M, Jensen J, Donaldson M et al. Functional and clinical characterization of *KCNJ2* mutations associated with LQT7 (Andersen syndrome). *J Clin Invest* 2002;110: 381–8.
6390. Tritschler HJ, Andreeta F, Moraes CT et al. Mitochondrial myopathy of childhood onset associated with depletion of mitochondrial DNA. *Neurology* 1992;42:209–17.
6391. Trobe JD, Acosta PC, Krischer JP et al. Confrontation field techniques in the detection of anterior visual pathway lesions. *Ann Neurol* 1981;10:28–34.
6392. Trockel U et al. Multiple exercise-related mononeuropathy with abdominal colic. *J Neurol Sci* 1983;60:431–42.
6393. Trojan D, Cashman N. Post-poliomyelitis syndrome. *Muscle Nerve* 2005;31:6–19.
6394. Trommer BL, Homer D, Mikhael MA. Cerebral vasospasm and eclampsia. *Stroke* 1988;19:326–9.
6395. Troost BT, Newton TH. Occipital lobe arteriovenous malformations. *Arch Ophthalmol* 1975;93:250.
6396. Troost BT, Troost EG. Functional paralysis of horizontal gaze. *Neurology* 1979;29:82.
6397. Trosch RM, Hasbani M, Brass LM. "Bottoms up" dissection. *N Engl J Med* 1989;320:1564–5.
6398. Trotter W. On certain clinically obscure malignant tumours of the naso-pharyngeal wall. *Brit Med J* 1911;2:1057–9.
6399. Trotter W. Chronic subdural haematoma. *Am J Dis Childh* 1930;39:980.
6400. Trouillas P, Brudon F, Froment JC et al. Cerebellar imitation synkineses. *Rev Neurol* 1990;146:107–15.
6401. Trouillas P, Takayanagi T, Hallett M et al. International cooperative ataxia rating scale for pharmacological assessment of the cerebellar syndrome. *J Neurol Sci* 1997;145:205–11.
6402. Trousseau A. *Clinique medicale de l'Hotel Dieu de Paris.* Paris: J.B. Baillière, 1861.
6403. Trowell HC, Davies JNP, Dean RFA. *Kwashiorkor.* London: Edwin Arnold, 1954.
6404. Trubaki T, Tiyokura Y, Tsukagoshi H. *Japan J Med* 1965;4:181.
6405. Truswell AS. Osteopetrosis with syndactyly: A morphological variant of Albers-Schonberg's disease. *J Bone Jt Surg* 1958;40:208–18.
6406. Trzepacz PT, Mittal D, Torres R et al. Validation of the delirium rating scale revised-98. *J Neuropsychiatry Clin Neurosci* 2001;13:229–42.
6407. Tsai SY. Eponym and identity. *Arch Gen Psychiatry* 1968;19:104–9.
6408. Tsao CY, Mendell JR. The childhood muscular dystrophies: Making order out of chaos. *Semin Neurol* 1999;19:9–23.
6409. Tsementzis SA, Hitchcock ER. The spoon test: A simple bedside test for assessing sudomotor autonomic failure. *J Neurol Neurosurg Psychiatry* 1985;48:378–80.
6410. Tsujino S, Kanazawa N, Ohashi T et al. Three novel mutations in the ORNT1 gene of Japanese patients with the HHH syndrome. *Ann Neurol* 2000;47:625–31.
6411. Tsujino T, Tonin P, Shanske S et al. A splice junction mutation in a new myopathic variant of phosphoglycerate kinase deficiency (PGK North Carolina). *Ann Neurol* 1994;35:349–53.
6412. Tsukagoshi H. Spinal muscular atrophy, X-linked, juvenile, proximal. *Neurology* 1970;20:1188.
6413. Tsunoda I, Awano H, Kayama H et al. Idiopathic AA amyloidosis manifested by autonomic neuropathy, vestibulocochleopathy and lattice corneal dystrophy. *J Neurol Neurosurg Psychiatry* 1994;57:635–7.
6414. Tuck RR, McLeod JG. Retinitis pigmentosa, ataxia, and peripheral neuropathy. *J Neurol Neurosurg Psychiatry* 1983;46:206–13.
6415. Tuck RR, McLeod JG, Basten A. Total Lipodystrophy. A report of a case with peripheral neuropathy and glomerulonephritis. *Aust NZ J Med* 1983;13:65–9.
6416. Tucker T. Central nervous system AIDS. *J Neurol Sci* 1989;89:119–33.
6417. Tucker T, Layzer RB, Miller RG et al. Subacute reversible motor neuron disease. *Neurology* 1991;41:1541–4.
6418. Tuckett RP. Neurophysiology and neuroanatomy of pruritis. In Bernhard JD, ed. *Itch*, pp 1–22. New York, NY: McGraw-Hill, 1994.
6419. Tukahashi K, Ohama E, Nerito H et al. Hereditary dentato-rubral-pallido-luysian atrophy. *Neurology* 1988;38:1065–70.
6420. Tumarkin A. The otolithic catastrophe. *Brit Med J* 1936;2:175.
6421. Tunbridge RE, Paley RG. Primary optic atrophy in diabetes mellitus. *Diabetes* 1956;5:295–6.
6422. Tunkel AR, Kaye D. Infective endocarditis. *Neurol Clin* 1993;11: 419–40.
6423. Turnbull GK, Hoare C, Ritvo PG et al. *The Assessment of Bowel and Bladder Dysfunction in Clinic-Attending MS Patients.* 1995. Halifax, NS, Canada: Dept. Medicine Research Symposium, Dalhousie University.
6424. Turner JWA. The relationship between amyotonia congenita and congenital myopathy. *Brain* 1940;63:163–77.
6425. Turner JWA. On amytonia congenita. *Brain* 1949;72:25–34.
6426. Tyler HR. Abnormalities of perception with defective eye movements. *Cortex* 1968;4:154–70.
6427. Tyler HR,Tyler KL. Charles Edouard Brown-Sequard. *Neurology* 1984;34:1231–6.
6428. Tyrrell P, Rossor M. The association of gegenhalten in the upper limb with dyspraxia. *J Neurol Neurosurg Psychiatry* 1988;51:995–7.
6429. Tyrrell PJ. Hypertonia of opposition. *J Neurol Neurosurg Psychiatry* 1988;51: 995–7.
6430. Tyrrell PJ, Feher MD, Rossor MN. Sciatic nerve damage due to toilet seat entrapment: Another Saturday night palsy. *J Neurol Neurosurg Psychiatry* 1989;52:1113–4.
6431. Tyson J, Ellis D, Fairbrother U et al. Hereditary demyelinating neuropathy of infancy: A genetically complex syndrome. *Brain* 199;120:47–63.
6432. Uchihara T, Tsukagoshi H. Jolt accentuation of headache: The most

sensitive sign of CSF pleocytosis. *Headache* 1991;31:167–71.

6433. Uchitel O, Engel AG, Walls TJ et al. Congenital myasthenic syndromes: II. Syndrome attributed to abnormal interaction of acetylcholine with its receptor. *Muscle Nerve* 1993;16: 1293–301.

6434. Udd B, Griggs RC. Distal myopathies. *Current Opinion in Neurology* 2001;14: 561–6.

6435. Udd B, Krahe R, Walgren-Petersson C et al. Proximal myotonic dystrophy–a family with autosomal dominant muscular dystrophy, cataracts, hearing loss and hypogonadism: Heterogeneity of proximal myotonic syndromes? *Neuromuscular Disorders* 1997;7:217–28.

6436. Udd B, Partanen J, Haloinen P et al. Tibial muscular dystrophy: Late adult-onset distal myopathy in 66 Finnish patients. *Arch Neurol* 1993;50:604–8.

6437. Udd B, Vihola A, Sarparanta J et al. Titinopathies and extensional of the M-line mutation phenotype beyond distal myopathy and LGMD2J. *Neurology* 2005;64:636–42.

6438. Ugawa Y, Inoue K, Takamura T et al. Accumulation of glycogen in Sural nerve axons in Adult-onset Type III Glycogenosis. *Ann Neurol* 1986;19: 294–7.

6439. Uhthoff W. Untersuchungen uber die bei der multiplen Herdsklerose vorkommenden Augenstorungen. *Arch Psychiatr Nervenkr* 1889;21:303–410.

6440. Ullrich O. Kongenitale, atonisch-sklerotische Muskel Dystrophie. *Z Ges Neurol Psychiat* 1930;126:171–201.

6441. Ulrich S. The natural history of myoclonic astatic epilepsy (Doose syndrome) and Lennox-Gastaut syndrome. *Epilepsia* 2006;47:53–6.

6442. Umapathi T, Chaudhry V, Cornblath D et al. Head drop and camptocormia *J Neurol Neurosurg Psychiatry* 2002; 72:1–7.

6443. See 6442

6444. Umehara F, Matsumuro K, Kurono Y et al. Neurologic manifestations of Kanzaki disease. *Neurology* 2004;62:1604–6.

6445. Uncini A, Sabatelli M, Mignogna T et al. Chronic progressive steroid responsive axonal polyneuropathy: A CIDP variant or a primary axonal disorder? *Muscle and Nerve* 1996;19:365–71.

6446. Uncini A, Servidei S, Silvestri G et al. Ophthalmoplegia, demyelinating neuropathy, leukoencephalopathy, myopathy and gastrointestinal dysfunction with multiple deletions of mitochondrial DNA. *Muscle Nerve* 1994;17:667–74.

6447. Ungar-Sargon JY, Lovelace RE, Brust JCM. Spastic Paraplegia-Paraparesis. *J Neurol Sci* 1980;46:1–12.

6448. Unverricht H. Dermatomyositis acuta. *Dtsch Med Wschr* 1891;17:41–4.

6449. Unverricht H. *Die Myoclonie*. Leipzig: Franz Deuticke, 1891.

6450. Upshaw BY, Montgomery H. Hereditary anhidrotic ectodermal dysplasia. *Arch Derm* 1949;60:1170.

6451. Upton ARM, McComas AJ. The double crush in nerve entrapment syndromes. *Lancet* 1973;2:359–62.

6452. Urich H, Wilkinson M. Necrosis of muscle with carcinoma: Myositis or myopathy? *J Neurol Neurosurg Psychiatry* 1970;33:398–407.

6453. Ursell MR, Marras CL, Farb R et al. Recurrent intracranial hemorrhage due to postpartum cerebral angiopathy: Implications for management. *Stroke* 1998;29:1995–8.

6454. Usher CH. On the inheritance of retinitis pigmentosa, with notes of cases. *Roy Lond Ophthalmol Hosp Rep* 1914;19:130–236.

6455. Uswatte G, Taub E, Morris D et al. The Motor Activity Log- 28. *Neurology* 2006;67:1189–94.

6456. Vahedi K, Massin P, Guichard J-P et al. Hereditary infantile hemiparesis, retinal arteriolar tortuosity and leukoencephalopathy. *Neurology* 2003;60:57–63.

6457. Vail HH. Vidian neuralgia. *Ann Otolarynol* 1932;41:837.

6458. Vajsar J, Becker LE, Freedom RM et al. Familial desminopathy: Myopathy with accumulation of desmin-type intermediate filaments. *J Neurol Neurosurg Psychiatry* 1993;56:644–8.

6459. Valdmanis PN, Brunet D, St.Onge J et al. A founder haplotype for autosomal dominant sensory ataxia in Eastern Canada. *Neurology* 2006;67: 2239–42.

6460. Valdmanis PN, Dupré N, Rouleau G. A locus for primary lateral sclerosis on chromosome 4ptel-4p16.1. *Arch Neurol* 2008;65:383–6.

6461. Valleix FLI. *Traite des nevralgies ou affections douloureuses des nerfs*. Paris: J.B. Bailliere, 1841.

6462. Van Acker R. Rett syndrome: A review of current knowledge. *Autism Devel Dis* 1991;21:381–406.

6463. Van Allen MW, Blodi FC. Neurologic aspects of the Möbius syndrome. *Neurology* 1960;10:249–59.

6464. Van Allen MW et al. Amyloidosis type III. *Neurology* 1969;19:10.

6465. Van Allen MW, Frohlich JA, Davis JR. Inherited predisposition to generalized amyloidosis: Clinical and pathological study of a family with neuropathy, nephropathy and peptic ulcer. *Neurol Minneap* 1969;19:10–25.

6466. van Bogaert L. Tendinous areflexia without pupillary changes. *J Neurol Psychiatr* 1939;29:193–202.

6467. van Bogaert L. Une leuco-encèphalite sclerosante subaîgue. *J Neurol* 1945;8:101–20.

6468. van Bogaert L. La mélanose neurocutanée diffuse heredofamiliale. *Bull Acad Roy Med Belg 6th Series* 1948;13:397.

6469. van Bogaert L. Spinal cholesterolosis. *Brain* 1965;88:687–96.

6470. van Bogaert L, Divry P. Sur une maladie familiale caracterisée par une angiomatose diffuse cortico-meningée et une demyelinisation de la substance blanche du centre ovale. *Bruxelles Med* 1945;25:1090–1.

6471. van Bogaert L, Moreau M. Combination of Charcot–Marie–Tooth neuropathy and Friedreich ataxia. *Encéphale* 1939;1: 312–20.

6472. van Bogaert L, Scherer HJ, Epstein E. *Une forme cérebrale de la cholesterinose generalisée.* Paris: Masson, 1937.

6473. van Bogaert L, Theorides J. *Constantin Von Economo - The Man and the Scientist*. Vienna: Verlag, 1979.

6474. van Buchem FSP, Hadders HN, Ubbens R. An uncommon, familial systemic disease of the skeleton. *Acta Radiol* 1955;44:109–20.

6475. van de Warrenberg BPC, Giunti P, Schneider S et al. The syndrome of (predominantly cervical) dystonia and cerebellar ataxia. *J Neurol Neurosurg Psychiatry* 2006;774–5.

6476. Van den Berg-Vos RM, Visser J, Franssen H et al. Sporadic lower motor neuron disease with adult onset: Classification of subtypes. *Brain* 2003;126: 1036–47.

6477. Van den Berg-Vos RM, Franssen H, Wokke JHJ et al. Multifocal motor neuropathy: Diagnostic criteria that predict the response to immunoglobulin treatment. *Ann Neurol* 2000;48:919–26.

6478. Van den Berg-Vos RM, Van den Berg LH, Franssen H et al. Multifocal inflammatory demyelinating neuropathy. *Neurology* 2000;54:26–32.

6479. van den Bergh PYK, Thonnard J-L, Duprez T et al. Chronic demyelinating hypertrophic brachial plexus neuropathy. *Muscle Nerve* 2000;23:283–8.

6480. Van den Burg W, Saan RJ, Deelman BG. *15-Woordetest. Provisional Manual*. Groningen: University Hospital, 1985.

6481. Van der Eecken H, Adams RD, van Bogaert L. Striato-pallidal degeneration. An hitherto undescribed lesion in paralysis agitans. *J Neuropath Exp Neurol* 1960;19:159–61.

6482. van der Hoeve J, Kleyn A. *Ned Tschr Geneesk* 1917;1:1003.
6483. van der Knapp MS, Barth PG, Gabreels FJ et al. A new leukoencephalopathy with vanishing white matter. *Neurology* 1997;48:845–55.
6484. van der Knapp MS, Kamphorst W, Barth PG et al. Phenotypic variation in leukoencephalopathy with vanishing white matter. *Neurology* 1998;51:540–7.
6485. van der Knapp MS, Ramesh V, Schiffmann R et al. Alexander disease. *Neurology* 2006;66:494–8.
6486. van der Knapp MS, van der Voorn P, Barkhof F et al. A new leukodystrophy with brainstem and spinal cord involvement and high lactate. *Ann Neurol* 2003;53:252–8.
6487. van der Ploeg RJO, Oosterhuis HJGH. The "make\break test" as a diagnostic tool in functional weakness. *J Neurol Neurosurg Psychiatry* 1991;54:248–51.
6488. Van der Viel HL, Van Gijn J. Horner's syndrome. *J Neurol Sci* 1982;56:293–8.
6489. Van der Zee SPM et al. Citrullinaemia with a rapidly fatal neonatal outcome. *Arch Dis Child* 1971;48:847.
6490. van Dijk JG, Pondaag W, Malessy MJA. Obstetric lesions of the brachial plexus. *Muscle Nerve* 2001;24:1451–61.
6490a. van der Knapp MS, Arts WFM, Garbern JY et al. Cerebellar leukoencephalopathy. *Neurology.* 2008;71:1361–7.
6491. van Dongen HR, Catsman-Berrevoets CE, van Mourik M. The syndrome of 'cerebellar' mutism and subsequent dysarthria. *Neurology* 1994;44:2040–6.
6492. Van Dyke DH, Griggs RC, Murphy MJ, Goldstein MN. Hereditary myokymia and periodic ataxia. *J Neurol Sci* 1975;25: 109–18.
6493. van Erven PMM, Cillessen JPM, Eekhoff EMW et al. Leigh syndrome, a mitochondrial encephalo(myo)pathy. *Clin Neurol Neurosurg* 1987;89:217–30.
6494. van Geel BM, Assies J, Wanders RJA, Barth PG. X linked adrenoleukodystrophy: Clinical presentation, diagnosis and therapy. *J Neurol Neurosurg Psychiatry* 1997;63: 4–14.
6495. Van Gijn J. Measurement of outcome in stroke prevention trials. *Cerebrovascular Diseases* 1992;2(**Suppl.** 1):23–34.
6496. Van Gijn J. The Babinski sign: The first hundred years. *J Neurol* 1996;243: 675–83.
6497. Van Gijn J. Cerebral venous thrombosis: Pathogenesis, presentation and prognosis. *J Roy Soc Med* 2000;93:230–3.
6498. Van Goethem G et al. OLG mutations in neurodegenerative disorders with ataxia but no muscle involvement. *Neurology* 2004;63:1251–7.
6499. Van Hove JL, Kishnani PS, Demaerel P et al. Acute hydrocephalus in nonketotic hyperglycemia. *Neurology* 2000;54: 754–6.
6500. van Huffelen AC. A tribute to Martinus Rulandus. *Arch Neurol* 1989;46:445–7.
6501. Van Laere JE. Paralysie bulbo-pontine chronique progressive famiiale avec surdité: Un cas de syndrome de Klippel-Trenaunay dans la même fratrie. *Rev Neurol* 1966;115:289–95.
6502. van Mook WNKA, Rennenberg RJNW, Schurink GW et al. Cerebral hyperperfusion syndrome. *Lancet Neurology* 2005;4:877–87.
6503. Van Munster ETL, Joosten EMG et al. The rigid spine syndrome. *J Neurol Neurosurg Psychiatry* 1986;49:1292–7.
6504. van Nes SI, Faber CG, Hamers RMTP et al. Revising two-point discrimination assessment in normal aging and in patients with polyneuropathies. *J Neurol Neurosurg Psychiatr* 2008;79:832–4.
6505. Van Praagh R. Diagnosis of kernicterus in the neonatal period. *Pediatrics* 1961;28:870–6.
6506. Van Uitert RL, Solomon GE. White-centered retinal hemorrhages: A sign of intracranial hemorrhage. *Neurology* 1979;29:236–9.
6507. van Vugt P, Paquier PF, Kees L et al. Increased writing activity in neurological conditions: A review and clinical study. *J Neurol Neurosurg Psychiatry* 1996;61: 510–4.
6508. Van Wijngaarden GK, Fleury P, Bethlem J et al. Familial "myotubular" myopathy. *Neurology* 1969;19:901–8.
6509. van Zomeren AH, ten Duis H-J, Minderhoud JM et al. Lightning stroke and neuropsychological impairment: Cases and questions. *J Neurol Neurosurg Psychiatry* 1998;64:763–9.
6510. Vance JM. The many faces of Charcot–Marie–Tooth disease. *Arch Neurol* 2000;57:638–40.
6511. Vandertop W,Bosma NJ. The piriformis syndrome. *J Bone Joint Surg* 1991; 73–A:1095–7.
6512. Vanhatalo S, Riikonen R. Markedly elevated nitrate/nitrite levels in the cerebrospinal fluid of children with progressive encephalopathy with edema (PEHO syndrome). *Epilepsia* 2000;41:705–8.
6513. VanLandingham KE, Heinz ER, Cavazos JE et al. Magnetic resonance imaging evidence of hippocampal injury after prolonged focal febrile convulsions. *Ann Neurol* 1998;43:413–26.
6514. Vanneste JAL. Three decades of normal pressure hydrocephalus: Are we wiser now? *J Neurol Neurosurg Psychiatry* 1994;57:1021–5.
6515. Vargas-Diaz J, Garófalo-Gómez N, Rodríguez U et al. Mondini dysplasia: Recurrent bacterial meningitis in adolescence. *Rev Neurol* 2004;39:935–9.
6516. Varma JS, Smith AN, McInnes A. Electrophysiological observations on the human pudendal - anal reflex. *J Neurol Neurosurg Psychiatry* 1986;49:1411–6.
6517. Varni JW, Seid M, Kurtin PS. PedsQL 4.0: Reliability and validity of the pediatric quality of life inventory version 4.0 generic core scales in healthy and patient populations. *Med Care* 2001;39:800–12.
6518. Vassilescu C, Alexianu M, Dan A. Neuronal type of Charcot–Marie–Tooth disease with a syndrome of continuous motor unit activity. *J Neurol Sci* 1984;63:11–25.
6519. Vazquez V, Sotelo J. The course of seizures after treatment for cerebral cysticercosis. *N Engl J Med* 1992;327:696–701.
6520. Veit C, Ware J. The structure of psychological distress and well-being in general populations. *Journal of Consulting and Clinical Psychology* 1983;51:730–732.
6521. Velamoor V, Norman R, Caroff S et al. Progression of symptoms in neuroleptic malignant syndrome. *J Nerv Ment Dis* 1994;182:168–73.
6522. Venance SL, Cannon SC, Fialho D et al. The primary periodic paralyses: Diagnosis, pathogenesis and treatment. *Brain* 2006;129:8–17.
6523. See 6522.
6524. Ventruto V, Di Garolamo R, Festa B et al. Family study of inherited syndrome with multiple congenital deformities: Symphalangism, carpal and tarsal fusion, brachydactyly, craniosynostosis, strabismus, hip osteochondritis. *J Med Genet* 1976;13:394–8.
6525. Verbiest H. Primaire stenose van het lumbale wervelkanal bij volwassenen, een nieur ziektebeeld. *Ned Tschr Geneesk* 1950;94:2415–33.
6526. Verdugo R, Ochoa JL. Quantitative somatosensory thermotest: A new method for functional evaluation of small calibre afferent channels. *Brain* 1992;115: 893–913.
6527. Verhagen WI, Horstink MWIM, Notermans SLH. Painful arm and moving fingers. *J Neurol Neurosurg Psychiatr* 1985;48:384–5.
6528. See 6527
6529. Verity MA, Roitberg B, Kepes JJ. Mesolimbocortical dementia: Clinico-pathological studies on two cases. *J Neurol Neurosurg Psychiatry* 1990;53:492–5.
6530. Verma A, Bradley WG. High dose IVIg therapy in chronic progressive lumbosacral plexopathy. *Neurology* 1994;44:248–50.

6531. Verma P, Oger J. Treatment of acquired autoimmune Myasthenia Gravis. *Can J Neurol Sci* 1992;19:360–75.
6532. Vernant JC, Cabre P, Smadja D et al. Recurrent optic neuromyelitis with endocrinopathies. *Neurology* 1997;48: 58–64.
6533. Vernet M. *Les paralysies laryngées associés*. Lyon: Univ. de Lyon (Thesis), 1916.
6534. Vernino S, Sandroni P, Singer W, Low PA. Autonomic ganglia. *Neurology* 2008;70:1926–32.
6535. Verreault S, Joutel A, Riantet F et al. A novel hereditary small vessel disease of the brain. *Ann Neurol* 2006;59:353–7.
6536. Verrips A et al. Spinal xanthomatosis: A variant of cerebrotendinous xanthomatosis. *Brain* 1999;122:1589–95.
6537. Verzijl HTFM, Padberg GG, Zwarts MJ. The spectrum of Möbius syndrome: An electrophysiological study. *Brain* 2005;128:1728–36.
6538. Verzijl H, vann der Zwaag BL, Lammens M et al. The neuropathology of hereditary congenital facial palsy vs Möbius syndrome. *Neurology* 2005;64:649–53.
6539. Vetrugno R, Provini F, Plazzi G et al. Catathrenia (nocturnal groaning): A new type of parasomnia. *Neurology* 2001;56:681–3.
6540. Viala K, Renié L, Maisonobe T et al. Follow-up study and response to treatment in 23 patients with Lewis-Sumner syndrome. *Brain* 2004;127:2010–7.
6541. Victor M. The Wernicke-Korsakoff syndrome. *Handb Clin Neurol* 1989;28:243–70.
6542. Victor M. Alcholic dementia. *Can J Neurol Sci* 1994;21:88–99.
6543. Vidailhet M. Paroxysmal dyskinesias as a paradigm of paroxysmal movement disorders. *Current Opinion in Neurology* 2000;13:457–62.
6544. Vigevano F. Benign familial infantile seizures. Brain Dev 2005;27(3):172–177.
6545. Vignaendra V, Wilkus RJ, Copass MK, Chatrian GE. Electroencephalographic rhythms of alpha frequency in comatose patients after cardiac arrest. *Neurology* 1974;24:582–8.
6546. Vigouroux C, Capeau J. A-type lamin-linked lipodystrophies. *Novartis Found Symp* 2005;264:166–77.
6547. Vijayan N, Dreyfus PM. Posttraumatic dysautonomic cephalalgia: Clinical observations and treatment. *Arch Neurol* 1975;32:649–52.
6548. Vijayan N, Watson C. Site of injury headache. *Headache* 1989;29:502–6.
6549. Villanova M, Louboutin JP, Chateau D et al. X-linked vacuolated myopathy: Complement membrane attack complex on surface membrane of injured muscle fibers. *Ann Neurol* 1995;37: 637–45.
6550. Villaret M. Le syndrome nerveux de l'éspace retroparotidien posterieur. *Rev Neurol* 1916;23:188–90.
6551. Vincent FM. Benign masturbatory cephalalgia. *Arch Neurol* 1982;39:673.
6552. Vincent KA, Carr AJ, Walburn J et al. Construction and a validation of a quality of life questionnaire for neuromuscular disease. *Neurology* 2007;68:1051–7.
6553. Vinchon M, Blond S, Lejeune JP et al. Association of Lhermitte-Duclos and Cowden disease: Report of a new case and review of the literature. *J Neurol Neurosurg Psychiatry* 1994;57:699–704.
6554. Virchow RLK. On the pathologic anatomy of children. *Virchow's Arch Path Anat Physiol* 1867;38:129–38.
6555. Vitali C, Bombardieri S, Jonsson R et al. Classification criteria for Sjögren's syndrome. *Ann Rheumat Dis* 2002;61:554–8.
6556. Vitiello MV, Bliwise DL, Prinz PN. Sleep in Alzheimer's disease and the sundown syndrome. *Neurology* 1992;42(**Suppl.** 6):83–94.
6557. Vodusek OB. Pudendal and Bulbo-Cavernosus reflexes in women. *EEG Clin Neurophysiol* 1990;77:134–6.
6558. Vogel CM, Albin R, Albers JW. Lotus footdrop: Sciatic neuropathy in the thigh. *Neurology* 1991;41:605–6.
6559. Vogel P, Gabriel M, Goebel HH, Dyck PJ. Hereditary motor sensory neuropathy type II with neurofilament accumulation. *Ann Neurol* 1985;17:455–61.
6560. Vogt A. Fruhzeitiges Ergrauen der Zilien ud Bemerkungen uber den sogenanten plotzlichen Eintritt dieser Veranderung. *Klin Mbl Augenh* 1906;44:228–42.
6561. Vogt C, Vogt O. Zur Lehre der Erkrankungen des striaten Systems. *J Psychol Neur (Leipzig)* 1920;25: 627–846.
6562. Vogt H. Uber familiare amaurotische Idiotie und verwandte Krarankheitsbilder. *Mschr Psychiat* 1905;18:161–171,310–357.
6563. Volkmann Rv. Die ischamischen Muskellahmungen und Kontrakturen. *Zbl f Chir* 1881;8:801–3.
6564. von Angyal L. Thumb-Mouth agnosia: A special form of Gerstmann syndrome. *Confin Neurol* 1940;3:245–52.
6565. von Brevern M, Zeise D, Neuhauser H et al. Acute migrainous vertigo: Clinical and oculographic findings. *Brain* 2005;128:365–74.
6566. von Brevern M, Radyke M, Lezius F et al. Epidemiology of benign paroxysmal positional vertigo: A population based study. *J Neurol Neurosurg Psychiatry* 2007;78:710–5.
6567. Von Economo K. Encephalitis lethargica. *Wien Klin Wschr* 1917;30:581–5.
6568. Von Gierke E. Hepato-nephromegalia glycogenica. *Beitr Path Anat* 1929;82:497–513.
6569. von Giesen H-J, Neuen-Jacob E, Dorries K et al. Diagnostic criteria and clinical procedures in HIV-1 associated progressive multifocal leukoencephalopathy. *Arendt G Med Clin (Batrc)* 1999;113:210–4.
6570. von Giesen H-J, Stoll G, Koch MA et al. Mixed axonal-demyelinating polyneuropathy as predominant manifestation of myotonic dystrophy. *Muscle Nerve* 1004;17:701–3.
6571. Von Graefe AF. Exceptionelles Verhalten des Gessichtsfeldes bei Pigmentatartung der Netzhaut. *Arch Ophthal Berlin* 1848;4:250.
6572. Von Graefe AF. Demonstration in der Berliner Medizinischen Gesellschaft. *Berl Klin Wochenschr* 1868;5:127.
6573. Von Graefe AF. Verhandlungen artzlicher Gessellschaften. *Berl Klin Wochenschr* 1868;5:125–7.
6574. Voon V, Hassan K, Zurowski M et al. Prevalence of repetitive and reward-seeking behaviors in Parkinson disease. *Neurology* 2006;67:1254–7.
6575. Vowles G, Scholtz CL. Diffuse axonal injury in early infancy. *J Clin Pathol* 1987;40:185–9.
6576. Vuardens P, Bogousslavsky J. Face-arm-trunk-leg sensory loss limited to the contralateral side in lateral medullary infarction: A new variant. *J Neurol Neurosurg Psychiatry* 1998;65:255–7.
6577. Vuillaume I, Devos D, Schraen-Maschke S et al. A new locus for spinocerebellar ataxia (SCA21) maps to Chromosome 7p21.3-p15.1. *Ann Neurol* 2002;52: 666–70.
6578. Waardenburg A. Das mensch. auge u.seine Erblagen. Haag: M Nijhoff. 1932.
6579. Waardenburg PJ. A new syndrome combining developmental anomalies of the eyelids, eyebrows and nose root with pigmentary defects of the iris and head hair and with congenital deafness. *Am J Hum Genet* 1951;3:195–253.
6580. Waddell G, McCulloch JA, Kummell E et al. Nonorganic physical signs in low back pain. *Spine* 1980;5:117–25.
6581. Wade DT. *Measurement in Neurological Rehabilitation.* Oxford: Oxford Medical, 1992.
6582. Wadia NH. Atlantoaxial dislocation. *Neurology (Bombay)* 1960;8:81.
6583. Wadia NH. An introduction to neurology in India. In Spillane JD ed. *Tropical Neurology*, pp 25–36. London: Oxford, 1973.
6584. Wadia NH. Congenital atlanto-axial dislocation and its manifestations due to

spinal cord compression. In Spillane JD ed. *Tropical Neurology*, pp 99–107. London: Oxford, 1973.

6585. Wadia NH, Ivari PF, Katrak SM. Amyotrophy with acute hemorrhagic conjunctivitis. *Lancet* 1972;2:970–1.

6586. Wadia NH, Swami RK. A new form of heredofamilial spinocerebellar degeneration with slow eye movements (nine families). *Brain* 1971;94:359–74.

6587. Wadia RS, Wadgaonkar SU, Amin RB et al. An unusual family of benign "X" linked muscular dystrophy with cardiac involvement. *J Med Genet* 1976;13:352–6.

6588. Wadsworth TG. Tennis elbow. *Brit Med J* 1987;294:621–4.

6589. Waggoner RW et al. Agenesis of white matter with idiocy. *Am J Ment Defic* 1942;47:20–4.

6590. Wagner von Jauregg J. Ueber die Einwirkung der Malaria auf die progressive Paralyse. *Psychiat Neurol (Belg)* 1918;20:132–134, 251–255.

6591. Wagner EL. Fall einer seltenen Muskelkrankheit. *Arch Heilk* 1863;4:282–3.

6592. Wakai S, Ikehata M, Nihira H et al. Obtundation status (Dravet) caused by complex partial status epilepticus in a patient with severe myoclonic epilepsy in infancy. *Epilepsia* 1996;37:1020–2.

6593. Wakamiya M, Matsuura T, Liu Y et al. The role of ataxin 10 in the pathogenesis of spinocerebellar ataxia type 10. *Neurology* 2006;67:607–13.

6594. Walczak TS, Leppik IE, D'Amelio M et al. Incidence and risk factors in sudden unexpected death in epilepsy. *Neurology* 2001;56:519–25.

6595. Waldenstrom J. Acute thyrotoxic encephalo- or myopathy, its cause and treatment. *Acta Med Scand* 1945;121:251–94.

6596. Waldenstrom J. Two interesting syndromes with hyperglobulinemia. purpura, hyperglobinuria and macroglobulinemia. *Schweiz Med Wschr* 1948;78:927–8.

6597. Waldvogel D, Mattle HP, Sturzenegger M et al. Pulsatile tinnitus: A review of 84 patients. *J Neurol* 1998;245:137–42.

6598. Walk D, Kang S-S, Horwitz A. Intermittent encephalopathy, reversible nerve conduction slowing, and MRI evidence of cerebral white matter disease in methylene tetrahydrofolate reductase deficiency. *Neurology* 1994;44:344–7.

6599. Walker FO. Voice fatigue in myasthenia gravis: The sinking pitch sign. *Neurology* 1997;48:1135–6.

6600. Walker MB. Treatment of myasthenia gravis with physostigmine. *Lancet* 1934;1:1200–1.

6601. Walker R, Rasmussen A, Rudnicki D et al. Huntington's disease-like 2 can present as chorea-acanthocytosis. *Neurology* 2003;61:1002–4.

6602. Walker RH, Jung HH, Dobson-Stone C et al. Neurologic phenotypes associated with acanthocytosis. *Neurology* 2007;68:92–8.

6603. Walker RW. Idiopathic intracranial hypertension: Any light on the mechanism of the raised pressure? *J Neurol Neurosurg Psychiatry* 2001;71:1–7.

6604. Wall M, Rosenberg M, Richardson D. Gaze-evoked tinnitus. *Neurology* 1987;37:1034–6.

6605. Wall M, Wray SH. The one-and-a-half syndrome. A unilateral disorder of the pontine tegmentum: A study of 20 cases and review of the literature. *Neurology* 1983;33:971–80.

6606. Wall PD, Noordenbos W. Sensory functions which remain in man after complete transection of dorsal columns. *Brain* 1977;100:641–53.

6607. Wallace MR, Dwulet FE, Conneally M et al. Biochemical and molecular genetic characteristics of a new variant prealbumin associated with hereditary amyloidosis. *J Clin Invest* 1986;78:6–12.

6608. Wallenberg A. Acute bulbaraffection (Embolie der Arteria cerebelli posterior inferior sinistra?). *Arch Psychiatr (Berlin)* 1895;27:504–40.

6609. Waller AD. Points relating to the Weber-Fechner law. *Brain* 1895;18:200–16.

6610. Waller AV. Experiments on the section of the glossopharyngeal and hypoglossal nerves of the frog, and observations of the alterations produced thereby in the structure of their primitive fibers. *Phil Trans Roy Soc Lond* 1850;423–9.

6611. Wallgren-Pattersson C, Laing NG. *Report of the 70th ENMC International Workshop: Nemaline Myopathy.* 2000;10(4–5): 299–306.

6612. Wallgren-Pattersson C, Lehtokari VLL, Kalimo H et al. Distal myopathy caused by homozygous missense mutations in the nebulin gene. *Brain* 2007;130:1476.

6613. Walser M. Urea cycle disorders and other hereditary hyperammonemic syndromes. In Stanbury JB, Wyngaarden JB, Fredrickson DS et al., eds. *The Metabolic Basis of Inherited Disease*, pp 402–38. New York: McGraw-Hill, 1983.

6614. Walsh EG. Clonus: Beats provoked by the application of a rhythmic force. *J Neurol Neurosurg Psychiatry* 1976;39: 266–74.

6615. Walsh FB. Third nerve regeneration. *Br J Ophthalmol* 1957;41:577–98.

6616. Walsh FB, Gass JD. Concerning the optic nerve. *Am J Ophthalmol* 1960;50: 1031–47.

6617. Walsh FB, Hoyt WF. *Clinical Neuro-Ophthalmology.* Baltimore: Williams & Wilkins Co., 1969.

6618. Walsh FB, King AB. Ocular signs of intracranial saccular aneurysms. *Arch Ophthal Berlin* 1942;12 **Suppl.**:1–33.

6619. Walsh JC. Neuromyotonia: An unusual presentation of intrathoracic malignancy. *J Neurol Neurosurg Psychiatry* 1976;39:1086–91.

6620. Walshe F. Diagnosis of hysteria. *Brit Med J* 1965;2:1451–4.

6621. Walshe FMR. The physiological significance of the reflex phenomena in spastic paralysis of the lower limbs. *Brain* 1915;37:269–336.

6622. Walshe FMR. On certain tonic or postural reflexes in hemiplegia. *Brain* 1923;46: 1–37.

6623. Walshe FMR. On the "syndrome of the premotor cortex"(Fulton) and the definition of the terms "premotor" and "motor": With a consideration of Jackson's views on the cortical representation of movements. *Brain* 1935;58:49–80.

6624. Walshe FMR. On the role of the pyramidal system in willed movements. *Brain* 1947;70:329–54.

6625. Walshe FMR. Contributions of John Hughlings Jackson to neurology: A brief introductions to his teachings. *Arch Neurol* 1961;5:119–31.

6626. Walshe FMR, Robertson EG. Observations upon the form and nature of the "grasping" movements and "tonic innervation" seen in certain cases of lesion of the frontal lobe. *Brain* 1933;56:40–70.

6627. Walter MC, Reilich P, Huebner A et al. Scapuloperoneal syndrome type Kaeser and a wide phenotypic spectrum of adult-onset, dominant myopathies are associated with the desmin mutation R350P. *Brain* 2007;130:1485–96.

6628. Walter WG. Epilepsy. In Hill JDN, Parr G eds. *Electroencephalography*, p 246. New York: Macmillan, 1950.

6629. Walter WG, Cooper R, Aldridge VJ. Contingent negative variation: An electrical sign of sensori-motor association and expectancy in the human brain. *Nature* 1964;203:380–4.

6630. Walters AS. Toward a better definition of restless legs syndrome. *Mov Disord* 1995;10:634–42.

6631. Walton JN. Amyotonia congenita. A follow-up study. *Lancet* 1956;1:1023–8.

6632. Walton JN. The limp child. *J Neurol Neurosurg Psychiatry* 1957;20:144–54.

6633. Walton W. *Dictionary of Psychiatry.* Oxford: Blackwell, 1993.

6634. Waltz G, Harik SI, Kaufman B. Adult metachromatic leukodystrophy. *Arch Neurol* 1987;44:225–7.

6635. Wan CL, Lin TK, Lu CH et al. Mah-Jong-induced epilepsy: A special reflex epilepsy in Chinese society. *Seizure* 2005;**14**:19–22.
6636. Wanamaker WM. Firearm recoil palsy. *Arch Neurol* 1974;**31**:208–9.
6637. Wang S, Yang S, Chen CC et al. Darier's disease associated with bipolar affective disorder: A case report. *Kaohsiung J Med Sci* 2002;**18**:622–6.
6638. Wang Z, Low PA, Jordan J et al. Autoimmune autonomic ganglionopathy. *Neurology* 2007;**68**:1917–21.
6639. War Department. *Army Individual Test Battery.* Washington, D.C.: Adjutant General's Office, 1944.
6640. Wardlaw JM, Dennis MS, Lindlay RI et al. The validity of a simple clinical classification of acute ischaemic stroke. *J Neurol* 1996;**243**:274–9.
6641. Ware JC. Evaluation of impotence - Monitoring periodic penile erections during sleep. *Psychiatr Clin N Amer* 1987;**10**:675–86.
6642. Warier RP et al. Opsomyoclonus and neuroblastoma. *Clin Ped* 1985;**24**:32.
6643. Warmolts JR, Mendell JR. Neurotonia: Impulse-induced repetitive discharges in motor nerves in peripheral neuropathy. *Ann Neurol* 1980;**7**:245–50.
6644. Warner TT, Jarman P. The molecular genetics of the dystonias. *J Neurol Neurosurg Psychiatry* 1998;**64**:427–9.
6645. Warrell DA, Godfrey S, Olsen EJG. Giant cell arteritis with peripheral neuropathy. *Lancet* 1968;**1**:1010–3.
6646. Warren JD. Variations on the musical brain. *J Roy Soc Med* 1999;**92**:571–5.
6647. Warrington EK. *Warrington Recognition Memory Test.* Windsor, UK.: NFER-Nelson, 1984.
6648. Warrington EK, Langdon D. Spelling dyslexia: A deficit of the visual word-form. *J Neurol Neurosurg Psychiatry* 1994;**57**:211–6.
6649. Warrington K, Shallice T. Category specific semantic impairments. *Brain* 1984;**107**:829–54.
6650. Warshawsky I, Rudick RA, Staugaitis SM et al. Primary progressive multiple sclerosis as a phenotype of a *PLP1* gene mutation. *Ann Neurol* 2005;**58**: 470–3.
6651. Wartenberg R. A sign of facial palsy. *Dtsch Z Nervenklinik* 1930;**116**:144–5.
6652. Wartenberg R. Nasal pruritis with cerebral tumours. *Klin Wschnschr* 1932;**11**:461.
6653. Wartenberg R. A sign of ulnar palsy. *JAMA* 1939;**112**:1688.
6654. Wartenberg R. Brachialgia statica paresthetica (nocturnal arm dysesthesias). *J Nerv Ment Dis* 1944;**99**:877–87.
6655. Wartenberg R. Progressive facial hemiatrophy. *Arch Neurol Psychiatry* 1945;**54**:75–96.
6656. Wartenberg R. *The Examination of Reflexes: A Simplification.* Chicago: The Year Book Publishers, 1945.
6657. Wartenberg R. Multiple sensory neuritis: A clinical entity. *Trans Amer Neurol Assn* 1946;**71**:101–4.
6658. Wartenberg R. Winking-jaw phenomenon. *Arch Neurol Psychiatry* 1948;**59**:734–53.
6659. Wartenberg R. Pendulousness of the legs as a diagnostic test. *Neurology* 1951;**1**: 18–24.
6660. Wartenberg R. Digitalia paresthetica and gonyalgia paresthetica. *Neurology* 1954;**4**:106–15.
6661. Wartenberg R. On neurologic terminology, eponyms and the Lasègue sign. *Neurology* 1956;**6**:853–8.
6662. Warwick R. The so-called nucleus of convergence. *Brain* 1955;**78**:92–114.
6663. Wasserstrom WR, Glass JP, Posner JB. Diagnosis and treatment of leptomeningeal metastases from solid tumors: Experience with 90 patients. *Cancer* 1982;**49**:759–72.
6664. Watanabe I et al. Early lesion of Pelizaeus-Merzbacher's disease: Electron microscope and biochemical study. *J Neuropath Exp Neurol* 1973;**32**:313–33.
6665. Watanabe T, Katamaya Y. Evaluation by magnetic resonance imaging of the entrapped temporal horn syndrome. *J Neurol Neurosurg Psychiatry* 1999;**66**:113.
6666. Waterhouse R. A case of suprarenal apoplexy. *Lancet* 1911;**1**:577–8.
6667. Waters CH, Miller CA. Autosomal dominant Lewy body Parkinsonism in a four-generation family. *Ann Neurol* 1994;**35**:59–64.
6668. Waters CH, Takahashi H, Wilhelmsen KC et al. Phenotypic expression of X-linked dystonia-parkinsonism (lubag) in two women. *Neurology* 1993;**43**: 1555–8.
6669. Waters DD, Nutter DO, Hopkins LC et al. Cardiac features of an unusual X-linked humeroperoneal neuromuscular disease. *N Engl J Med* 1975;**293**:1017–22.
6670. Watson CPN. Postherpetic neuralgia. In Portenoy RK ed. *Neurologic Clinics,* vol.7, *Pain: Mechanisms and Syndromes*, p 231. Philadelphia: W.B. Saunders, 1989.
6671. Watson RT, Heilman KM. Callosal apraxia. *Brain* 1983;**106**:391–403.
6672. Watson RT, Valenstein E, Heilman KM. Thalamic neglect: Possible role of the medial thalamus and nucleus reticularis in behavior. *Arch Neurol* 1981;**38**:501–6.
6673. Watson SR, Halmagyi GM, Colebatch JG. Vestibular hypersensitivity to sound (Tullio phenomenon): Structural and functional assessment. *Neurology* 2000;**54**:722–8.
6674. Watters GV, Fitch N. Familial laryngeal abductor paralysis and psychomotor retardation. *Clin Genet* 1973;**4**:429–33.
6675. Waxman SG. The flexion-adduction sign in neuralgic amyotrophy. *Neurology* 1979;**29**:1301–4.
6676. Waxman SG, Dib-Hajj SD. Erythromelalgia: A hereditary pain syndrome enters the molecular era. *Ann Neurol* 2005;**57**:785–8.
6677. Waxman SG, Geschwind N. Hypergraphia in temporal lobe epilepsy. *Neurology* 1974;**24**:629–36.
6678. Waziri M et al. Abnormality of chromosome 11 in patients with features of Beckwith-Wiedermann syndrome. *J Pediatr* 1983;**102**:873.
6679. Weatherby E, Wiley NH. Left sided weakness, unequal blood pressure in the two arms and left optic atrophy: A new syndrome? *J Nerv Ment Dis* 1940;**92**: 151–6.
6680. Weaver DD, Graham B, Thomas IT et al. A new overgrowth syndrome with accelerated skeletal maturation, unusual facies and camptodactly. *J Pediatr* 1974;**84**:547–52.
6681. Webb S, Coleman D, Byrne P et al. Autosomal dominant hereditary spastic paraparesis with cognitive loss linked to chromosome 2p. *Brain* 1998;**121**:601–9.
6682. Webb WB, Agnew HW. Sleep and waking in a time-free environment. *Aerosp Med* 1974;**45**:617–22.
6683. Weber FP. A case of relapsing, non-suppurative nodular panniculitis, showing phagocytosis of subcutaneous fat-cells by macrophages. *Brit J Dermatol* 1925;**37**:301–11.
6684. Weber H. A contribution to the pathology of the crura cerebri. *Med Chir Trans* 1863;**46**:121–39.
6685. See 6684
6686. Wechsler D. A standardised memory scale for clinical use. *J of Psychology* 1954;**19**:87–95.
6687. Wechsler D. *The Wechsler Intelligence Scale for Children (Revised).* New York: Psychological Corp., 1976.
6688. Wechsler D. *The Wechsler Adult Intelligence Scale (Revised).* New York: Psychological Corp., 1986.
6689. Wechsler D. *The Wechsler Primary and Preschool Scale of Intelligence (Revised).* New York: Psychological Corp., 1990.
6690. Wedderburn C, Wear H, Brown J et al. The utility of the Cambridge behavioural inventory in neurodegenerative disease. *J Neurol Neurosurg Psychiatr* 2008;**79**: 500–3.
6691. Wedemeyer L, Johnson CA, Keltner JL. Statokinetic dissociation in optic nerve

disease. In Heijl A ed. *Proceedings of the Eighth International Visual Field Symposium*, pp 9–14. Amsterdam: Kugler, 1989.

6692. Weglinski MR, Wedel DJ. Malignant hyperthermia testing in patients with persistently increased serum creatine kinase levels. *Anesthesiology and Analgesia* 1997;84:1038–41.

6693. Weill G. Ectopia of the crystalline lens and general malformations. *Annales Oculist* 1932;169:21–44.

6694. Weiner LP, Konigsmark BW, Stoll J et al. Hereditary olivopontocerebellar atrophy with retinal degeneration. *Arch Neurol* 1967;16:364–76.

6695. Weiner WJ, Koller WC, Perlik S et al. Drug holiday and management of Parkinson disease. *Neurology* 1980;30:1257–61.

6696. Weiner WJ, Nora LM, Glantz RH. Elderly inpatients: Postural reflex impairment. *Neurology* 1984;34:945–7.

6697. Weinshenker BG, Bass B et al. The natural history of multiple sclerosis: A geographically based study. 2. Predictive value of the early clinical course. *Brain* 1989;112:1419–28.

6698. Weinstein EA, Kahn RL, Malitz S, Rozanski J. Delusional reduplication of parts of the body. *Brain* 1954;77:45–60.

6699. Weinstein S. Fifty years of somatosensory research: From the Semmes-Weinstein monofilaments to the Weinstein enhanced sensory test. *J Hand Therapy* 1993;6: 11–22.

6700. Weisberg LA. The syndrome of increased intracranial pressure without localizing signs: A reappraisal. *Neurology* 1975;25:85–8.

6701. Weisberg LA. Lacunar infarcts: Clinical and computed tomography correlations. *Arch Neurol* 1982;39:37–40.

6702. Weiser HG. The phenomenology of limbic seizures. In Weiser HG, Speckmann EJ, Engel J eds. *The Epileptic Focus*, pp 113–36. London: John Libbey, 1987.

6703. Weiskrantz L. *Blindsight: A Case Study and Implications.* Oxford: Oxford University Press, 1986.

6704. Weiss E. Cerebral adiposity with nerve deafness, mental deficiency and genital dystrophy: A variant of the Lawrence-Biedl syndrome. *American Journal of Medical Science* 1932;183:268–72.

6705. Weiss L. Syndromes II. In Smith DW ed. *Birth Defects*, pp 309–10. Amsterdam: Excerpta Medica, 1974.

6706. Weiss N. Zur Messung der Intensitat galvanischer Strome in der Elektrotherapie. *Zbl Ges Therap* 1883;1: 9–14.

6707. Weiss S, Baker JB. The carotid sinus in health and disease: Its role in the causation of fainting and convulsions. *Medicine* 1933;12:297–354.

6708. Weisscher N, Post B, de Haan RJ et al. The AMC . . . disability score in patients with newly diagnosed Parkinson disease. *Neurology* 2007;69:2155–61.

6709. Weissleder R et al. Limb girdle type muscular dystrophy associated with Wolff-Parkinson-White syndrome. *J Neurol Neurosurg Psychiatry* 1987;50: 500–1.

6710. Weitzman ED, Czeisler CA, Coleman RM et al. Delayed sleep phase syndrome: A chronobiological disorder with sleep-onset insomnia. *Arch Gen Psychiatry* 1985;38:737–46.

6711. Welander L. Myopathia distalis tarda heredetaria. *Acta Med Scand* 1951;14 S265:1–124.

6712. Welch JP, Alterman K. The syndrome of caudal dysplasia: A review. *Pediatr Pathol* 1984;2:313.

6713. Weleber RG, Beals RK. Hajdu-Cheney syndrome: Report of two cases and review of the literature. *J Pediatr* 1976;88:243–9.

6714. Weleber RG, Tongue AC, Kennaway NG et al. Ophthalmic manifestations of infantile phytanic acid storage disease. *Arch Ophthalmol* 1984;102:1317–21.

6715. Welgampola MS, Colebatch JG. Characteristics and clinical applications of vestibular evoked myogenic potentials. *Neurology* 2005;64:1682–8.

6716. Wellner VP et al. Glutathione synthetase deficiency: An inborn error of metabolism. *Proc Nat Acad Sci* 1974;71:2505.

6717. Wells CR, Jankovic J. Familial spastic paraparesis and deafness: A new X-linked neurodegenerative disorder. *Arch Neurol* 1986;43:943–6.

6718. Wells GAH, Scott AC, Johnson CT et al. A novel progressive spongiform encephalopathy in cattle. *Vet Rec* 1987;121:134–40.

6719. Wendel U, Rudiger HW, Pryzrembel H et al. Alpha-ketoadipic aciduria: Degradation studies with fibroblasts. *Clin Chem Acta* 1975;58:271.

6720. Wenger DA, Coppola S, Liu S-L. Insights into the diagnosis and treatment of lysosomal storage diseases. *Arch Neurol* 2003;60:322–8.

6721. Wennberg R. Electroclinical analysis of postictal noserubbing. *Can J Neurol Sci* 2000;27:131–6.

6722. Wenning G, Ben-Schlomo Y, Hughes A et al. What clinical features are most useful to distinguish definite multiple system atrophy from Parkinson's disease? *J Neurol Neurosurg Psychiatry* 2000;68:434–40.

6723. Wenning GK, Tison F, Seppi K et al. Development and validation of the Unified Multiple System Atrophy Rating Scale (UMSARS). *Mov Disord* 2004;19:1391–402.

6724. Werdnig G. Zwei fruhinfantile hereditare Falle von progressiver Muskelatrophie unter dem Bilde der Dystrophie, aber auf neurotischer Grundlage. *Arch Psychiatr (Berlin)* 1891;22:437–80.

6725. Werhahn KJ, Brown P, Thompson PD et al. The clinical features and prognosis of chronic posthypoxic myoclonus. *Mov Disord* 1997;12:216–20.

6726. Wermer P. Genetic aspects of adenomatosis of endocrine glands. *Am J Med* 1954;16:363–71.

6727. Werner C-O. Lateral elbow pain and posterior interosseous nerve entrapment. *Acta Orthop Scand* 1979;**(Suppl.** 174):1.

6728. Werner CWO. Ueber Katarackt in Verbindung mit Sclerodermie. *Diss Kiel* 1904.

6729. Wernicke K. Der aphasische Symptomenkomplex. Eine psychologische Studie auf anatomischer Basis. Breslau: M. Cohn, 1874.

6730. Wernicke K. Die acute hamorrhagische der Polioencephalitis superior (in) Lehrbuch der Gehirenkrankheiten. Kassel: Fischer, 1881.

6731. Wernicke K. Ueber hemiopische Pupillenreaction. *Fort d Med* 1883;1: 49–53.

6732. Wernicke K. A note on Cramp-Neurosis. *Berl Klin Wochenschr* 1904;43:1121–4.

6733. Wertham FL. A new sign of cerebellar diseases. *J Nerv Ment Dis* 1929;69: 4986–493.

6734. Wertsch JJ, Sanger JR, Marloub HS. Pseudo anterior interosseous nerve syndrome. *Muscle Nerve* 1985;8:68–70.

6735. West WJ. On a peculiar form of infantile convulsions. *Lancet* 1840;1:724–5.

6736. Wester K, Hugdahl K. Arachnoid cysts of the left temporal fossa: Impaired preoperative cognition and postoperative improvement. *J Neurol Neurosurg Psychiatry* 1995;59:293–8.

6737. Westheimer G, Blair SM. The ocular tilt reaction - a brainstem oculomotor routine. *Invest Ophthalmol* 1975;14:833–9.

6738. Westphal A. Ueber ein bischer nicht beschriebene Pupillenphanomen. *Neurol Centralbl* 1899;18:161–4.

6739. Westphal CFO. Die Agoraphobie, eine neuropathische Erscheinung. *Arch Psychiatr Nervenkr* 1871;3:138–61.

6740. Westphal CFO. Ueber eine dem Bilde der cerebrospinalen grauen Degeneration ahnliche Erkrankung des centralen Nervensystems ahne anatomischen Befund, nebst einigen Bemerkungen uber paradoxe Contraction. *Arch Psychiatr Nervenkr* 1883;14:87–134.

6741. Wexler N. Huntington's disease. *Curr Opin Neurol Neurosurg* 1988;1:319–23.
6742. Wheaton LA, Hallett M. Ideomotor apraxia: A review. *J Neurol Sci* 2007;**260**:1–10.
6743. Whipple AO. Criteria for diagnosis of islet cell adenoma. Surgery of the pancreas. *N Engl J Med* 1942;**226**:513–26.
6744. Whisnant JP, Cartlidge NEF, Elvebach LR. Carotid and vertebral-basilar transient ischemic attacks: Effects of anticoagulants, hypertension, and cardiac disorders on survival and stroke occurrence - a population study. *Ann Neurol* 1978;3:107–15.
6745. White AA, McBride ME, Wiltse LL et al. The management of patients with back pain and idiopathic vertebral sclerosis. *Spine* 1986;11:607–16.
6746. White AM. What happened? alcohol, memory blackouts, and the brain. *Health. Alcohol Research and Health* 2003;**27**:186–96.
6747. White BD, Firth JL. Anterior spinal hernia: An increasingly recognised cause of thoracic cord dysfunction. *J Neurol Neurosurg Psychiatry* 1994;**57**:1433–5.
6748. White BV. *Stanley Cobb: A Builder of the Modern Neurosciences.* Charlottesville,VA: University Press of Virginia, 1984.
6749. White HH, Rowland LP, Araki S et al. Homocystinuria. *Arch Neurol* 1965;**13**:455–70.
6750. White JC. A case of keratosis (ichthyoses) follicularis. *J Cutan Dis* 1889;**7**:201–9.
6751. White JC, Langston JW, Pedley TA. Benign epileptiform transients of sleep. *Neurology* 1977;**27**:1061–8.
6752. White JC, Sweet WH. *Pain and the Neurosurgeon.* Springfield, IL: C.C. Thomas, 1989.
6753. Whitehouse PJ. The concept of subcortical dementia: Another look. *Ann Neurol* 1986;**19**:1–6.
6754. Whiteley AM, Hauw J-J, Escourolle R. A pathological survey of 41 cases of acute intrinsic spinal cord disease. *J Neurol Sci* 1979;**42**:229–42.
6755. Whiteley AM, Swash M, Urich H. Progressive encephalomyelitis with rigidity: Its relation to "subacute myoclonic spinal neuronitis" and to the "stiff man syndrome". *Brain* 1976;**99**:27–42.
6756. Whiteside TCD, Graybiel A, Niven JI. Visual illusions of movement. *Brain* 1965;**88**:193–210.
6757. Whitley CB et al. Warburg syndrome: Lethal neurodysplasia with autosomal recessive inheritance. *J Pediatr* 1983;**102**:547–51.
6758. Whitley RJ, Nahmias AJ, Visintine AM et al. The natural history of herpes simplex virus infection of mother and newborn. *Pediatrics* 1980;**66**:489–94.
6759. Whitman BW, Packer RJ. The photic sneeze reflex. *Neurology* 1993;**43**:868–71.
6760. Whitty CWM. On the so-called "laryngeal epilepsy". *Brain* 1943;**66**: 43–54.
6761. Whitwell JL, Weigand SD, Shiung MM et al. Focal atrophy in dementia with Lewy bodies on MRI: A distinct pattern from Alzheimer's disease. *Brain* 2007;**130**:708–19.
6762. WHO Study Group. Assessment of fracture risk and its application to screening for post-menopausal osteoporosis. *WHO Tech Rep Ser* 1994;**843**:1–129.
6763. Whyte KF, Alan MB, Jeffery AA et al. Clinical features of the sleep apnoea, hypopnoea syndrome. *Quart J Med* 1989;**72**:659–66.
6764. Whytt R. *An Essay on the Vital and Other Involuntary Motions of Animals.* Edinburgh: Hamilton, Balfour, and Neill, 1751.
6765. Whytt R. Observations on the Dropsy in the Brain. Edinburgh: J. Balfour, 1768.
6766. Wichman A, Frankl M, Kelly TE. Autosomal recessive congenital cerebellar hypoplasia. *Clin Genet* 1985;**27**:373–82.
6767. Wick B, Bedell HE. Magnitude and velocity of proximal vergence. *Invest Ophthamol Vis Sci* 1989;**30**:755–60.
6768. Wieacker P, Wolff G et al. A new X-linked syndrome with muscle atrophy, congenital contractures and oculomotor apraxia. *Am J Med Genet* 1985;**20**: 597–606.
6769. Wiebers DO, Swanson JW, Cascino TL et al. Bilateral loss of vision in bright light. *Stroke* 1989;**20**:554–8.
6770. Wiese JA, Gentry LR, Menezes AH. Bobble head doll syndrome: Review of the pathology and CSF dynamics. *Ped Neurol* 1985;**1**:361.
6771. Wigboldus JM, Bruyn GW. Hallervorden-Spatz disease. In Vinken PJ, Bruyn GW eds. *System Disorders and Atrophies, Part I. Handbook of Clinical Neurology,* vol.21, pp 604–31. Oxford: North Holland Publishing Co., 1975.
6772. Wijdicks EFM, Bamler WR et al. Validation of a new coma scale: The FOUR score. *Ann Neurol* 2005;**58**: 585–93.
6773. Wijdicks EF, Bamlet WR, Maramattom BV et al. Validation of a new coma scale: The FOUR score. *Ann Neurol* 2005;**58**:585–93.
6774. Wijemanne S, Jankovic J. Hemiparkinsonism-hemiatrophy syndrome. *Neurology* 2007;**69**:1585–94.
6775. Wik B, Hillestad L. Deglutition syncope. *Brit Med J* 1975;**2**:747.
6776. Wilbourn AJ. Clinical neurophysiology in the diagnosis of amyotrophic lateral sclerosis. *J Neurol Sci* 1998;**160(Suppl. 1)**: S25–S29.
6777. Wilbourn AJ. Thoracic outlet syndrome is overdiagnosed. *Muscle Nerve* 1999;**22**(1):130–5.
6778. Wilbourn AJ, Aminoff MJ. The electrodiagnostic examination in patients with radiculopathies. *Muscle Nerve* 1998;**21**:1612–31.
6779. Wilbourn AJ, Furlan AJ, Hulley W et al. Ischemic monomelic neuropathy. *Neurology* 1983;**33**:447–51.
6780. Wilbourn AJ, Sweeney PJ. Dissociated wasting of medial and lateral hand muscles with motor neurone disease. *Can J Neurol Sci* 1994;**21**:S9.
6781. Wilcox LM JR, Bercovith K, Howard RO. Ophthalmic features of chromosome deletion 4p- (Wolf-Hirschorn syndrome). *Am J Ophthalmol* 1978;**86**:834.
6782. Wildervanck LS. Een cervico-oculo-acusticus syndroom. *Ned Tschr Geneesk* 1960;**104**:2600–5.
6783. Wiles CM, Karni Y. The measurement of strength in patients with peripheral neuromuscular disorders. *J Neurol Neurosurg Psychiatry* 1983;**46**:1006–13.
6784. Wilhelmsen KC, Weeks DE, Nygaard TG et al. Genetic mapping of "Lubag" (X-linked dystonia-Parkinsonism) in a Filipino kindred to the pericentromeric region of the X chromosome. *Ann Neurol* 1991;**29**:124–31.
6785. Wilkins DE, Hallett M, Erba G. Primary generalised epileptic myoclonus: A frequent manifestation of minipolymyoclonus of central origin. *J Neurol Neurosurg Psychiatry* 1985;**48**:506–16.
6786. Wilkinson IMS, Anderson JR, Holmes AE. Oligodendroglioma: An analysis of 42 cases. *J Neurol Neurosurg Psychiatry* 1987;**50**:304–12.
6787. Wilks S. Drunkard's or alcoholic paraplegia. *Med Times Gaz* 1868;**2**:470.
6788. Wilks S. On cerebritis, hysteria, and bulbar paralysis, as illustrative of arrest of function of the cerebro-spinal centres. *Guy's Hosp Rep* 1877;**22**:7–55.
6789. Will AD, Sale EJ, Price S et al. Quantitative measurement of the "milkmaid" sign in Huntington's disease. *Ann Neurol* 1991;**30**:320.
6790. Will RG. The spongiform encephalopathies. *J Neurol Neurosurg Psychiatry* 1991;**54**:761–3.
6791. Will RG. Prion related disorders. *J Roy Coll Physicians* 1999;**33**:311–5.
6792. Willemse J. Benign idiopathic dystonia with onset in the first year of life. *Dev Med Child Neurol* 1986;**28**:355–60.
6793. Williams AO, Osuntokun BO. Peripheral neuropathy in tropical (Nutritional) ataxia in Nigeria. *Arch Neurol* 1969;**21**:475–92.
6794. Williams D, de Silva R, Paviour D et al. Characteristics of two distinct clinical phenotypes in pathologically proven progressive supranuclear palsy:

Richardson's syndrome and PSP-parkinsonism. *Brain* 2005;128:1235–6.

6795. Williams DR. Psychogenic palatal tremor. *Mov Disord* 2004;19:333–5.

6796. Williams DR, Hadeed A, Najim al-Din AS et al. Kufor Rakeb disease: Autosomal recessive, levodopa-responsive parkinsonism with pyramidal degeneration, supranuclear gaze palsy, and dementia. *Mov Disord* 2005;20:1264–71.

6797. Williams DR, Reardon K, Roberts L et al. A new dominant distal myopathy affecting posterior leg and anterior upper limb muscles. *Neurology* 2005;64: 1245–54.

6798. Williams J, Barrett-Boyes B, Lowe J et al. Supravalvular aortic stenosis. *Circulation* 1961;24:1311–8.

6799. Williams JC et al. Progressive neurologic deterioration and renal failure due to storage of glutamyl ribose-5-phosphate. *N Engl J Med* 1984;311:152.

6800. Williams ME, Hadler NM, Earp JA. Manual ability as a marker of dependency in geriatric women. *J Chronic Disease* 1982;35:115–22.

6801. Williams RDB. Brushfield spots and Wolfflin nodules in the iris: An appraisal in handicapped children. *Dev Med Child Neurol* 1981;23:646–50.

6802. Williamson PD, Boon PA, Thadani VM et al. Parietal lobe epilepsy: Diagnostic considerations and results of surgery. *Ann Neurol* 1992;31:193–201.

6803. Williamson PD, Spencer DD, Spencer SS et al. Complex partial seizures of frontal lobe origin. *Ann Neurol* 1985;18:497–504.

6804. Willis T. *De anima brutorum.* Oxonii, R.: Davis, 1672.

6805. Willis T. *The London Practice of Physick.* London: T. Basset, 1685.

6806. Willis T. *Willis' Oxford Lectures.* Oxford: Sandford Press, 1980.

6807. Willison HJ. Antiglycolipid antibodies in peripheral neuropathy: Fact or fiction? *J Neurol Neurosurg Psychiatry* 1994;57:1303–6.

6808. Willoughby EW, Eason R. The crossed upgoing toe sign: A clinical study. *Ann Neurol* 1983;14:480–2.

6809. Willvonseder R, Goldstein NP, McCall JT et al. A hereditary disorder with dementia, spastic dysarthria, vertical eye movement paresis, gait disturbance, splenomegaly and abnormal copper metabolism. *Neurology* 1973;23:1039–49.

6810. Wilson B, Cockburn J, Baddeley AD. *The Rivermead Behavioural Memory Test.* Reading, UK.: Thames Valley Test Co., 1985.

6811. Wilson BA, Alderman N, Burgess P et al. *Behavioural Assessment of the Dysexecutive Syndrome (BADS).* Bury St. Edmunds, Thames Valley Test Co., 1996. (Pamphlet)

6812. See 6811.

6813. Wilson BA, Cockburn J, Halligan P. *Behavioural Inattention Test.* Titchfield, Hants, UK: Thames Valley Test Company, 1987.

6814. Wilson JX, Young. Sepsis-associated encephalopathy. *Can J Neurol Sci* 2005;30:98–105.

6815. Wilson MG, Towner JW, Forsman I et al. Syndromes associated with deletion of the long arm of chromosome 18. *Am J Med Genet* 1979;3:155–74.

6816. Wilson MS, Wherrett BA, Mahdy MS. Powassan virus meningoencephalitis. *Can Med Assn J* 1979;121:320–2.

6817. Wilson SAK. A contribution to the study of apraxia. *Brain* 1908;31:164.

6818. Wilson SAK. Progressive lenticular degeneration: A familial nervous disease associated with cirrhosis of the liver. *Brain* 1912;34:295–509.

6819. Wilson SAK. *Neurology.* London: Edward Arnold & Co., 1940.

6820. Wilson SAK, Walsh FMR. The phenomenon of tonic innervation and its relation to motor apraxia. *Brain* 1914;37:199–246.

6821. Wilson WA, Gharave AE, Koike T et al. International consensus statement on preliminary classification criteria for definite antiphospholipid syndrome. *Arth Rheum* 1999;42:1309–11.

6822. Winawer MR, Ottman R, Hauser WA et al. Autosomal dominant partial epilepsy with auditory features: Defiining the phenotype. *Neurology* 2000;54: 2173–6.

6823. Winer JB. Bickerstaff's encephalitis and the Miller Fisher syndrome. *J Neurol Neurosurg Psychiatry* 2001;71:433–5.

6824. Wing JK, Cooper E, Sartorius N. *Measurements and Classification of Psychiatric Symptoms.* Cambridge: Cambridge University Press, 1974.

6825. Wingerchuk DMHWFOPC et al. The clinical course of neuromyelitis optica. *Neurology* 2008;53:1107–14.

6826. Winkelman NW. Progressive pallidal degeneration: A new clinicopathologic syndrome. *Arch Neurol Psychiatry* 1932;27:1–21.

6827. Winter HS. Case records of the Massachusetts General Hospital. *N Engl J Med* 1991;325:1865–73.

6828. Winter JH, Neville JB, Henderson AF et al. Life-threatening respiratory failure due to a previously undescribed myopathy. *Quart J Med* 1986;61:1171.

6829. Winterkorn JMS, Odel JG, Behrens MM. Sleep test for myasthenia gravis. *International Neuro-Ophthalmology Symposium VIIIth Symposium.* 1990. (Abstract)

6830. Winterthun S et al. Autosomal recessive mitochondrial ataxic syndrome due to mitochondrial polymerase gamma mutations. *Neurology.* 2005 Apr 12;64(7):1204–8.

6831. See 6830.

6832. Wintzen AR, Plomb JJ, Molenaar PC et al. Acquired slow-channel syndrome: A form of myasthenia gravis with prolonged open time of the acetylcholine receptor channel. *Ann Neurol* 1998;44:657–64.

6833. Wirrell E, Farrell K, Whiting S. The epileptic encephalopathies of infancy and childhood. *Can J Neurol Sci* 2005;32: 409–18.

6834. Wise BL, Smith M. Spinal arachnoiditis ossificans. *Arch Neurol* 1965;13:391–4.

6835. Wisniewski KE, French JH, Fernando S et al. Fragile X syndrome: Associated neurological abnormalities and developmental disabilities. *Ann Neurol* 1985;18:665–9.

6836. Wisniewski KE, Zhong N, Phillipart M. Pheno/genotypic correlations of neuronal ceroid lipofuscinosis. *Neurology* 2001;57:576–81.

6837. Wissel J, Kabus C, Klepsch S et al. Botulinum toxin in writer's cramp: Objective response evaluation in 31 patients. *J Neurol Neurosurg Psychiatry* 1996;61:172–5.

6838. Witt TN, Danek A, Hein MUeal. McLeod syndrome: A distinct form of neuroacanthocytosis. *J Neurol* 1992;239:302–6.

6839. Landau W, Nelson D. Clinical neuromythology XV. Feinting science: Neurocardiogenic syncope and collateral vasovagal confusion. *Neurology* 1996;46:609–18.

6840. Wohlfart G. Zwei Falle von Dystrophia musculorum progressiva mit fibrillaren Zuckungen und atypischen Muskelbefund. *Dtsch Z Nervenklinik* 1942;153:189–204.

6841. Wohrle JC, Spengos K, Steinke W et al. Alcohol-related acute axonal polyneuropathy: A differential diagnosis of Guillain-Barré syndrome. *Arch Neurol* 1998;55:1329–34.

6842. Wolf A, Morton BF. Ganglion cell tumours of the central nervous system. *NY Neurol Inst Bull* 1937;6:453–88.

6843. Wolf NL, Harting I, Bolthauser E et al. Leukoencephalopathy with ataxia, hypodontia and hypomyelination. *Neurology* 2005;64:1461–4.

6844. Wolf P. Juvenile absence epilepsy. In Roger J, Dravet C, Bureau M et al., eds.

Epileptic Syndromes in Infancy, Childhood and Adolescence, pp 242–6. London: John Libbey, 1985.

6845. Wolf P, Goosses R. Relation of photosensitivity to epileptic syndromes. *J Neurol Neurosurg Psychiatry* 1986;49:1386–91.

6846. Wolfe F, Smythe HA, Yunus MB et al. Fibromyalgia; The American College of Rheumatology 1990 criteria for the classification of fibromyalgia: Report of the multicenter criteria committee. *Arthritis Rheum* 1990;33:160–72.

6847. See 6846.

6848. Wolfe GI, Baker NS, Amato AA et al. Chronic cryptogenic sensory polyneuropathy: Clinical and laboratory characteristics. *Arch Neurol* 1999;56:540–7.

6849. Wolfe GI, Bank WJ. Pseudokyphosis in motor neuron disease corrected by the 'Pocket sign'. *Muscle and Nerve,* 1994:113. (Abstract)

6850. Wolff B, Grier RE, Lukvoy JRS et al. Biotinidase deficiency: A novel vitamin recycling defect. *J Inherit Metab Dis* 1985;8 (**Suppl.** 1):53–8.

6851. Wolff M, Cassé-Perrot C, Dravet C. Severe myoclonic epilepsy of infants (Dravet Syndrome): Natural history and neuropsychological findings. *Epilepsia* 2006;47:45–8.

6852. Wolfram DJ. Diabetes mellitus and simple optic atrophy among siblings: Report of four cases. *Proc Staff Meet Mayo Clin* 1938;13:715–8.

6853. Wolman M et al. Primary familial xanthomatosis with involvement and calcification of the adrenals. *Pediatrics* 1961;28:742–57.

6854. Wolpe J. *Psychotherapy by Reciprocal Inhibition.* Stanford, Ca.: Stanford Univ. Press, 1958.

6855. Wong KW et al. Ocular involvement associated with Chronic Epstein-Barr virus Disease. *Arch Ophthalmol* 1987;105:788–92.

6856. Wong W, Tsuruda J, Kortman K et al. Practical MRI. Rockville, Aspen Publishers, 1987.

6857. Wood DH. Cerebrovascular complications of sickle cell anemia. *Stroke* 1977;9:73–5.

6858. Wood M, Anderson M. *Neurological Infections.* London: W.B. Saunders Co., 1988.

6859. Wood N. Genes and Parkinsonism. *J Neurol Neurosurg Psychiatry* 1997;62:305–9.

6860. Woodman R, Shin K, Pineo G. Primary non-Hodgkin's lymphoma of the brain: A review. *Medicine* 1985;64:425–30.

6861. Woods BT, Schaumberg HH. Nigro-spino-dentatal degeneration with nuclear ophthalmoplegia. *J Neurol Sci* 1972;17:149–66.

6862. Woody RC et al. Ophthalmoplegic migraine in infancy. *Clin Ped* 1986;25:82–4.

6863. Woolf CM, Dolowitz DA, Aldous HE. Congenital deafness associated with piebaldness. *Arch Otolaryngol* 1965;82:244–50.

6864. Woolley JD, Gorno-Tempini M-L, Seeley WW et al. Binge eating is associated with right orbitofrontal-insular-striatal atrophy in frontotemporal dementia. *Neurology* 2007;69:1424–33.

6865. Wooten GF, Lopes MBS, Harris WO et al. Pallidoluysian atrophy. *Neurology* 1993;43:1764–8.

6866. Worgall S, Kekatpure MV, Heier L et al. Neurological deterioration in late infantile neuronal ceroid lipofuscinosis. *Neurology* 2007;629:521–35.

6867. World Federation of Neurology ad hoc committee. Criteria for diagnosis of amyotrophic lateral sclerosis. *World Neurol* 1990;5:12.

6868. World Federation of Neurology ad hoc Committee. Classification of extrapyramidal disorders. *J Neurol Sci* 1981;51:311–27.

6869. World Federation of Neurology Classification Subcommittee. Classification of neuromuscular diseases. *J Neurol Sci* 1988;86:333–60.

6870. World Health Organisation. *International Classification of Impairments, Disabilities and Handicaps.* Geneva: WHO, 1980.

6871. World Health Organization. T*he ICD-10 Classification of Mental and Behavioral Disorders.* Geneva: WHO, 1992.

6872. Worster-Drought C, Allen IM. Congenital auditory imperception (congenital word deafness) and its relation to idioglossia and other speech defects. *J Neurol Psychopath* 1930;10:193–235.

6873. Worster-Drought C, Greenfield JC, McMenemey WH. A form of familial presenile dementia with spastic paralysis. *Brain* 1940;63:237–54.

6874. Worth HM, Wollin DG. Hyperostosis corticalis generalisata congenita. *J Can Assoc Radiol* 1966;17:67–74.

6875. Wray SH. Extracranial internal carotid disease. In Bernstein EF ed. *Amaurosis Fugax*, New York: Springer-Verlag, 1987.

6876. Wray SH, Pavan-Langston D. A reevaluation of edrophomium chloride (Tensilon) tonography in the diagnosis of myasthenia gravis. *Neurology* 1971;21:586–93.

6877. Wright J, Morley DC. Encephalitis tremens. *Lancet* 1958;1:871–3.

6878. Wright RA, Hermann RC, Parisi JE. Neurological manifestations of Erdheim-Chester disease. *J Neurol Neurosurg Psychiatry* 1999;66:72–5.

6879. Wright WD. Characteristics of tritanopia. *J Optic Amer* 1952;42:509.

6880. Wszolek ZK, Baba Y, Mackenzie IR et al. Autosomal dominant dystonia-plus with cerebral calcifications. *Neurology* 2008;67:620–5.

6881. Wszolek ZK, Pfeiffer RF, Bhatt MH et al. Rapidly progressive autosomal dominant Parkinsonism and dementia with pallido-ponto-nigral degeneration. *Ann Neurol* 1992;32:312–20.

6882. Wu LJC, Jankovic J. Runner's dystonia. *J Neurol Sci* 2006;251:73–6.

6883. Wulff EA, Simpson DM. Neuromuscular complications of the human immunodeficiency virus type 1 infection. *Semin Neurol* 1999;19:157–64.

6884. Wulfften Palthe PMv. Leiodystonia, an endocrine-autonomic neurosis of the tropics. *Brain* 1933;56:479–90.

6885. Wyatt HV. Injection paralysis. *Bull Hist Med* 1981;55:543–57.

6886. Wyburn-Mason R. Arterio-venous aneurysm of midbrain and retina, facial naevi and mental changes. *Brain* 1943;66:163–203.

6887. Wyllie E, Luders H, Morris HH et al. The lateralizing significance of versive head and eye movements during epileptic seizures. *Neurology* 1986;36:606.

6888. Wynter E. Four cases of tubercular meningitis in which paracentesis of the theca vertebralis was performed for the relief of fluid pressure. *Lancet* 1891;981–2.

6889. Xiang F, Nicolao P, Chapon F et al. A second locus for autosomal dominant myopathy with proximal muscle weakness and early respiratory muscle involvement: A likely chromosomal locus on 2q21. *Neuromuscular Disorders* 1999;9:308–12.

6890. Yabe I, Kikuchi S, Higashi T et al. A Japanese case of steroid responsive myopathy with deficient chondroitin sulphate. *J Neurol Neurosurg Psychiatry* 2002;73:89–90.

6891. Yaffe MG, Kaback M, Goldberg M et al. An amyotrophic lateral sclerosis-like syndrome with hexosaminidase-A deficiency: A new type of Gm2-gangliosidosis. *Neurology* 1979;29:611.

6892. Yagishita S, Itoh Y, Nakano T et al. Pleomorphic intra-neuronal polyglucosan bodies mainly restricted to the pallidum. *Acta Neuropathologica* 1983;62:159–63.

6893. Yahr MD. A physician for all seasons. *Arch Neurol* 1978;35:185–8.

6894. Yamada M, Ohno S, Okayasu I et al. Chronic manganese poisoning. *Acta Neuropathol* 1986;71:273–8.

6895. Yamada S, Ogawa T, Nishimiya J. Masticator myopathy. *Muscle & Nerve* 2003;28:123–7.

6896. Yamadori A, Mori E, Tabuchi M et al. Hypergraphia: A right hemisphere syndrome. *J Neurol Neurosurg Psychiatry* 1986;**49**:1160–4.
6897. Yandell RW. Epidemic Convulsions. *Brain* 1881;4:339–50.
6898. Yang DC. Neurologic status of newborn infants on first and third days of life. *Neurology* 1962;**12**:72–7.
6899. Yanguela J, Sanchez -del-Rio M, Bueno A et al. Primary trochlear headache. *Neurology* 2004;**62**:1134–40.
6900. Yap CB, Mayo C, Barron K. "Ocular bobbing" in palatal myoclonus. *Arch Neurol* 1968;**18**:304–10.
6901. Yap PM. The latah reaction. Its pathodynamics and nosological position. *J Ment Sci* 1952;**98**:515–64.
6902. Yaqub BA, Al-Deeb SM, Daif AK et al. Bickerstaff brainstem encephalitis: A grave non-demyelinating disease with benign prognosis. *J Neurol Sci* 1990;**96**:29–40.
6903. Yarnell PR, Lynch S. The 'ding': Amnestic states in football trauma. *Neurology* 1973;**23**:196–7.
6904. Yasargil GM, Von Ammon K, Von Diem Ling A et al. Central neurocytoma: Histopathological variants and therapeutic approaches. *J Neurosurg* 1992;**76**:32–7.
6905. Yashon D, Beatty RA. Tethering of the conus medullaris within the sacrum. *J Neurol Neurosurg Psychiatry* 1966;**29**: 244–50.
6906. Yassa R. The Pisa syndrome: A report of two cases. *Br J Psychiatry* 1984;**146**:93–5.
6907. Yasuda M, Takamatsu J, D'Souza I et al. A novel mutation at Position +12 in the intron following exon 10 of the tau gene in Familial Frontotemporal Dementia (FTD-Kumamoto). *Ann Neurol* 2000;**47**:422–9.
6908. Yates DW. Scoring systems for trauma. *Brit Med J* 1990;**301**:1090–4.
6909. Yatsu FM, Fields WS. Asymptomatic carotid bruits: Stenosis or ulceration, a conservative approach. *Arch Neurol* 1985;**42**:383–5.
6910. Yee RD, Wong EK, Baloh RW et al. A study of congenital nystagmus: Waveforms. *Neurology* 1976;**26**:326–33.
6911. Yee WC, Hahn AF, Gilbert JJ. Adult onset scapuloperoneal myopathy: Diagnostic value of nerve morphometry and multiple muscle biopsies. *J Neurol Neurosurg Psychiatry* 1988;**51**:808–13.
6912. Yeoman W. The relation of arthritis of the sacro-iliac joint to sciatica. *Lancet* 1928;**2**:1119–22.
6913. Yesavage JA, Brink TL. Development and validation of a geriatric depression screening scale: A preliminary report. *J Psychiatr Res* 1983;**17**:41.
6914. Yiannikas C, McLeod JG, Pollard JD et al. Peripheral neuropathy associated with mitochondrial myopathies. *Ann Neurol* 1986;**20**:249–57.
6915. Yilmaz N, Unal O, Kiymaz N et al. Intracranial lipomas - a clinical study. *Clin Neurol Neurosurg* 2006;**108**:363–8
6916. Yilmaz U, Yang CC, Berger RE. Dartos reflex: A sympathetically mediated scrotal reflex. *Muscle Nerve* 2006;**33**:363–8.
6917. Yip, P-K. Bilateral ptosis, ataxia and areflexia - a variant of Fisher's syndrome. *J Neurol, Neurosurg Psychiatr* 1991;**54**:1121. (Abstract)
6918. Yokochi M et al. Juvenile Parkinsonism - some clinical, pharmacological and neuropathological aspects. *Adv Neurol* 1984;**40**:407–13.
6919. Yoshida J, Wakabayashi T, Okamoto S et al. Tenascin in cerebrospinal fluid is a useful biomarker for the diagnosis of brain tumour. *J Neurol Neurosurg Psychiatry* 1994;**57**:1212–5.
6920. Yoshiyama A, Tokuymaru Y, Hattori T et al. The pseudo polyneuropathy type sensory disturbances in cervical spondylotic myelopathy. *Rinsho Shinkeigaku* 1995;**35**:141–6.
6921. Yoss RE, Corbin KB, MacCarty CS et al. Significance of symptoms and signs in localization of involved roots in cervical disk protrusion. *Neurology* 1957;**7**:673–83.
6922. Yoss RE, Daly DD. Criteria for the diagnosis of the narcoleptic syndrome. *Mayo Clin Proc* 1957;**33**:320–8.
6923. Young AW, Robertson IH, Hellawell DJ et al. Cotard delusion after brain injury. *Psychol Med* 1992;**22**:799–804.
6924. Young GB. Status epilepticus and brain damage: Pathology and pathophysiology. *Adv Neurol* 2006;**97**:217–20.
6925. Young GB, Barr HWK, Blume WT. Painful epileptic seizures involving the second sensory area. *Ann Neurol* 1986;**19**:412.
6926. Young GB, Kark RM. Richard Bright, pioneer epileptologist. *Neurology* 1988;**38**:661–2.
6927. Young GB, McLachan RS, Kreeft JH et al. An EEG Classification for Coma. *Can J Neurol Sci* 1994;**21**(**Suppl.** 2):S.37. (Abstract)
6928. Young GB, McLachan RS, Kreeft JH et al. An electroencephalographic classification for coma. *Can J Neurol Sci* 1997;**24**:320–5.
6929. Young GF, Leon-Barth CA, Green J. Familial hemiplegic migraine, retinal degeneration, deafness and nystagmus. *Arch Neurol* 1970;**23**:201–9.
6930. Young ID, Harper PS. Hereditary distal spinal muscular atrophy with vocal cord paralysis. *J Neurol Neurosurg Psychiatry* 1980;**43**:413–8.
6931. Young RR. Asterixis: One type of negative myoclonus. In Fahn S ed. *Advances in Neurology: Myoclonus*, pp 123–53. New York: Raven Press, 1985.
6932. Young RR, Asbury AK, Corbett JL et al. Pure pan-dysautonomia with recovery: Description and discussion of diagnostic criteria. *Brain* 1975;**98**:613–36.
6933. Young SE et al. The tilted disk syndrome. *Am J Ophthalmol* 1976;**82**:16–23.
6934. Young WB, Gangal KS, Aponte RJ et al. Migraine with unilateral. Motor symptoms: A case-control study. *J Neurol Neurosurg Psychiatr* 2007;**78**:600–4.
6935. Yousry I, DietrichM, Naidich TP et al. Superior oblique myokymia: Magnetic resonance imaging support for the neurovascular compression hypothesis. *Ann Neurol* 2002;**51**:361–8.
6936. Yu G-Y, Howell MJ, Roller MJ et al. Spinocerebellar ataxia type 26 maps to chromosome 19p13.3 adjacent to *SCA6*. *Ann Neurol* 2005;**57**:349–54.
6937. Yuen EC, Olney RK, So YT. Sciatic neuropathy. *Neurology* 1994;**44**:1669–74.
6938. Yuill GM, Lynch PG. Congenital non-progressive peripheral neuropathy with arthrogryposis multiplex. *J Neurol Neurosurg Psychiatry* 1974;**37**:316–23.
6939. Yukawa Y, Kate F. Isolated spinal cord sarcoidosis mimicking an intramedullary tumor. *Spinal Disorders* 1999;**12**:530–3.
6940. Yung WA, Horten BC, Shapiro WR. Meningeal gliomatosis: A review of 12 cases. *Ann Neurol* 1980;**8**:605–8.
6941. Yunis E, Varon H. A new genetic syndrome. *Am J Dis Childh* 1980;**134**:649–53.
6942. Yunus MB. Diagnosis, etiology and management of fibromyalgia syndrome: An update. *Compr Ther* 1988;**14**:8–20.
6943. Zadikoff C, Lang AE. Apraxia in movement disorders. *Brain* 2005;**128**:1480–97.
6944. Zajicek J, Scolding N, Foster O et al. Central nervous system sarcoidosis: Diagnosis and management. *Quart J Med* 1999;**92**:103–17.
6945. Zaki MS, Abdel-Aleem A, Abdel-Salaam G et al. The molar tooth sign. *Neurology* 2008;**70**:556–65.
6946. Zakrzewska J. Facial pain: Neurological and non-neurological. *J Neurol Neurosurg Psychiatry* 2002;**72**:1127–32.
6947. Zaleski W, Hill A. Tyrosinosis: A new variant. *Can Med Assn J* 1973;**108**:477–84.
6948. Zalin A, Darby V, Vaughan S et al. Primary neuropathic amyloidosis in three brothers. *Brit Med J* 1974;**1**:65–6.
6949. Zange J. On subarachnoid blockage in the region of the cerebromedullary cistern (Cistern Block). *Munch Med Wschr* 1926;**173**:1150–2.
6950. Zanna C, Ghelli A, Porcelli A. OPA1 mutations associated with dominant optic

atrophy impair oxidative phosphorylation and mitochondrial fusion. *Brain* 2008;131:362–7.

6951. Zanni G, Saillour Y, Nagara M et al. Oligophrenin 1 mutations frequently cause X-linked mental retardation with cerebellar hypoplasia. *Neurology* 2005;65:1364–9.

6952. Zappert J. Dementia infantilis (Heller). *Mschr Kinderh* 1921;389–97.

6953. Zaslavskii ES. Scapulo-costal syndrome. *Ortop Travmatol Protez* 1972;33:78–80.

6954. Zatz M, de Paula F, Starling A et al. The 10 autosomal recessive limb-girdle muscular dystrophies. *Neuromuscul Disord* 2003;13:532–44.

6955. Zazzo R. *Manuel pour l'examen psychologique de l'enfant.* Neuchatel: Delachaux, Niestle, 1969.

6956. Zee DS. Adaptive control of eye movements: Clinical implications. *Can J Neurol Sci* 1994;21:177–84.

6957. Zee DS, Chu FC, Leigh RJ et al. Blink-saccade synkinesis. *Neurology* 1983;33:1233–6.

6958. Zee DS, Robinson DA. A hypothetical explanation of saccadic oscillations. *Ann Neurol* 1979;5:405.

6959. Zee DS, Yee RD, Cogan DG. Ocular motor abnormalities in hereditary cerebellar ataxia. *Brain* 1976;99:207–34.

6960. Zee DS, Yee RD, Singer HS. Congenital ocular motor apraxia. *Brain* 1977;100:581–99.

6961. Zeh W. Storung des ausdrucksenkennens beim Gerstmannschen Syndrom. *Arch Psychiatr Nervenkr* 1950;185:193–210.

6962. Zehender W, Ackermann E, Manz K. Eine Missbildung mit hautuberzogenen Augen order Kryptophthalmus. *Klinische Monatsblatter Augenheilkunde* 1872;10:225–34.

6963. Zeki S. Cerebral akinetopsia. *Brain* 1991;114:811–24.

6964. Zellweger H. Narcolepsy and epilepsy: Case of narcolepsy with spike and waves in the EEG. *Helv Pediat Acta* 1956;11: 269–74.

6965. Zellweger H, Bell WE. Congenital muscular hypertrophy. *Neurology* 1959;9:160–6.

6966. Zellweger H, Simpson J, McCormick WF et al. Spinal muscular atrophy with autosomal dominant inheritance. *Neurology* 1972;22:957–63.

6967. Zeman A, McLean B, Keir G et al. The significance of serum oligoclonal bands in neurological diseases. *J Neurol Neurosurg Psychiatry* 1993;56:32–5.

6968. Zeman W, King FA. Tumours of the septum pellucidum and adjacent structures with abnormal affective behavior: An anterior midline structure syndrome. *J Nerv Ment Dis* 1958;127:490–502.

6969. Zentner J, Wolf HK, Ostertun B et al. Gangliogliomas: Clinical, radiological and histopathological findings in 51 patients. *J Neurol Neurosurg Psychiatry* 1994;57:1502–i.

6970. Zeviani M, Servidei S, Gellera C et al. An autosomal dominant disorder with multiple deletions of mitochondrial DNA starting at the D-loop region. *Nature* 1989;339:309–11.

6971. Ziegler DK. Familial acephalgic migraine. *Neurology* 1995;45:2293–4.

6972. Ziegler DW, Schimke RN, Kepes JJ et al. Late onset ataxia, rigidity and neuropathy. *Arch Neurol* 1972;27:52–66.

6973. Zifkin B, Andermann E, Andermann F et al. An autosomal dominant syndrome of hemiplegic migraine, nystagmus, and tremor. *Ann Neurol* 1980;8:329–32.

6974. Zihl J, Von Cramon D. The Contribution of the 'Second Visual System' to directed visual attention in man. *Brain* 1979;102:835–56.

6975. Zimmer C. *Soul Made Flesh: The English Civil War and the Mapping of the Mind.* London:2004.

6976. Zimmerlin F. On hereditary progressive muscular atrophy. *Zschr Klin Med* 1884;7:15–35.

6977. Zimprich F, Djamshidian A, Hainfellner J et al. An autosomal dominant early adult onset distal muscular dystrophy. *Muscle Nerve* 2000;23:1876–9.

6978. Zinn AB, Kerr DS, Hoppel CL. Fumarase deficiency: A new cause of mitochondrial encephalopathy. *N Engl J Med.* 1986;315:469–75.

6979. Zivin JA. Lateral cervical puncture: An alternative to lumbar puncture. *Neurology* 1978;28:616–8.

6980. Zivkovic SA, Lacomis D, Clemens PR. Chronic eosinophilic perimyositis with persistent myalgias. *Muscle Nerve* 2002;25:461–5.

6981. Zochodne DW, Bolton CF, Wells GA et al. Critical illness polyneuropathy. *Brain* 1987;110:819–42.

6982. Zochodne DW, Ramsay DA, Saly V et al. Acute necrotizing myopathy of intensive care: Electrophysiological features. *Muscle Nerve* 1994;17:285–92.

6983. Zorly T. Kofferath's syndrome. *Forum Medicum (Istanbul)* 1955;1:255–7.

6984. Zuckerman E, Peres MF, Kaup AO et al. Chronic paroxysmal hemicrania-tic syndrome. *Neurology* 2000;54: 1524–6.

6985. Zuckerman M, Lubin B. *Multiple Affect Adjective Checklist (Manual).* San Diego: Educational and Industrial Testing Service, 1965.

6986. Zung WAK. A self-rating depression scale. *Arch Gen Psychiatry* 1965;12: 63–70.

6987. Zuniga G, Ropper AH, Frank J. Sarcoid peripheral neuropathy. *Neurology* 1991;41:1558–61.